A to Z DRUG FACTS

6th Edition

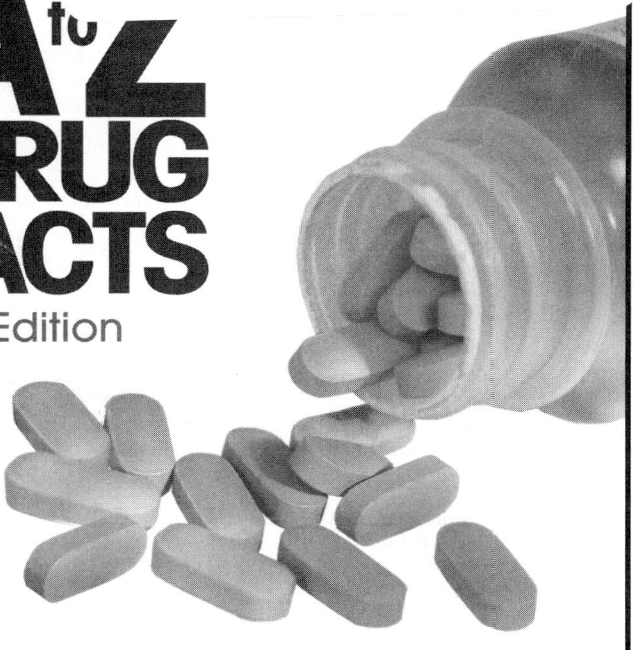

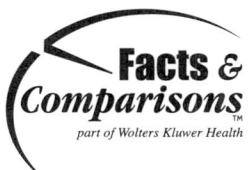

Facts & Comparisons™
part of Wolters Kluwer Health

A to Z Drug Facts™

© Wolters Kluwer Health, Inc., 2005

All rights reserved. No part of this publication may be reproduced or transmitted in any form or by any means, electronic or mechanical, including photocopy, recording, stored in a data base or any information storage or retrieval system or put into a computer, without prior permission in writing from Wolters Kluwer Health, Inc., the publisher.

Manuscript indexed by Coughlin Indexing Services, Inc., Annapolis, Maryland.

ISBN 1-57439-219-0

Printed in the United States of America

The information contained in this publication is intended to supplement the knowledge of health care professionals regarding drug information. This information is advisory only and is not intended to replace sound clinical judgment or individualized patient care in the delivery of health care services. Wolters Kluwer Health, Inc. disclaims all warranties, whether express or implied, including any warranty as to the quality, accuracy or suitability of this information for any particular purpose.

The information contained in *A to Z Drug Facts* is available for licensing as source data. For more information on data licensing, please call 1-800-223-0554.

Facts and Comparisons
part of Wolters Kluwer Health
77 Westport Plaza, Suite 450
St. Louis, Missouri 63146-3125
www.drugfacts.com
Phone: 314/216-2100 • 800/223-0554
Fax: 314/878-5563

A to Z Drug Facts Editorial Review Panel

Editor	**David S. Tatro, PharmD**
	Drug Information Analyst
	San Carlos, California
Assistant Editor	**Lawrence R. Borgsdorf, PharmD, FCSHP**
	Ambulatory Care Pharmacist
	Kaiser Permanente
	Bakersfield, California

Facts and Comparisons Staff

Vice President and Publisher	Cathy H. Reilly
Senior Managing Editor	Renée M. Wickersham
Managing Editor	Jill A. O'Dell
Senior Editor	Sara L. Schwein
Associate Editors	Sarah W. Lenzini
	Sharon M. McCarron
Senior Quality Control Editor	Susan H. Sunderman
Senior Composition Specialist	Beverly A. Donnell
Senior SGML Specialist	Linda M. Jones
Purchasing Specialist	Heather L. Broad
Clinical Director	Renée Rivard, PharmD
Clinical Manager	Cathy A. Meives, PharmD
Clinical Editors	Lori A. Buss, PharmD
	Shanti Divvela, PharmD
	Kim S. Dufner, PharmD
	Paul B. Johnson, RPh
	Andrea L. Raftery, RPh
	Paula S. Welker, RPh
Vice President, Strategic Development	David Zirkle
Director, Referential Product Manager	Teri Hines Burnham
Cover Design	Mark L. Wickersham

Facts and Comparisons™ Editorial Advisory Panel

Lawrence R. Borgsdorf, PharmD, FCSHP
Pharmacist Specialist-Ambulatory Care
Kaiser Permanente
Bakersfield, California

Dennis J. Cada, PharmD, FASHP, FASCP
Executive Editor
The Formulary
Editor in Chief
Hospital Pharmacy
Laguna Niguel, California

Michael Cirigliano, MD, FACP
Associate Professor of Medicine
University of Pennsylvania
School of Medicine
Philadelphia, Pennsylvania

Timothy R. Covington, PharmD, MS
Executive Director
Managed Care Institute
Bruno Professor of Pharmacy
McWhorter School of Pharmacy
Samford University
Birmingham, Alabama

Joyce A. Generali, RPh, MS, FASHP
Director, Drug Information Center
Clinical Professor
University of Kansas Medical Center
Department of Pharmacy
Drug Information Service
Kansas City, Kansas

Daniel A. Hussar, PhD
Remington Professor of Pharmacy
Philadelphia College of Pharmacy
University of the Sciences in Philadelphia
Philadelphia, Pennsylvania

James R. Selevan, BSEE, MD
Founder and Member of the Board of Directors
Monarch Healthcare
Vice President of Pharmacy Relations
Syntiro Healthcare Services, Inc.
Laguna Beach, California

Richard W. Sloan, MD, RPh
Chairman
Department of Family Practice
York Hospital
Clinical Associate Professor
Pennsylvania State University
York, Pennsylvania

Burgunda V. Sweet, PharmD
Director, Drug Information and Investigational Drug Services
Clinical Associate Professor of Pharmacy
University of Michigan Health System and College of Pharmacy
Ann Arbor, Michigan

David S. Tatro, PharmD
Drug Information Analyst
San Carlos, California

Thomas L. Whitsett, MD
Professor of Medicine and Pharmacology
Director of Vascular Medicine Program
University of Oklahoma Health Sciences Center
Oklahoma City, Oklahoma

Table of Contents

Introduction	vi
Standard Abbreviations	ix
Drug Monographs A to Z	1
Combination Drugs	1913
Orphan Drugs	1919
AIDS Drugs in Development	1963
FDA Pregnancy Categories	1968
General Management of Acute Overdosage	1969
Management of Acute Hypersensitivity Reactions	1971
Calculations	1972
International System of Units	1974
Normal Laboratory Values	1976
Drug Names That Look and Sound Alike	1981
Oral Dosage Forms That Should Not Be Crushed or Chewed	1995
Childhood Immunization Schedule	2004
Index	2009

Introduction

A to Z Drug Facts was developed with the health care provider in mind. It is designed to provide vital drug information in a format that is easy to understand and readily accessible. *A to Z Drug Facts* contains many full drug monographs, plus abbreviated monographs for combination drugs, orphan drugs, and AIDS drugs in development. Each monograph covers pharmacology considerations and patient care considerations.

Monographs are organized alphabetically by generic drug name. Consistent sections are used to create a visual roadmap to help navigate the information. The standard format used throughout the book makes the information clear and easy to find. The following outlines what is in each category.

Monograph Organization

Pharmacology considerations: The top half of each monograph contains detailed drug information. The following sections are included:

Drug Name: Generic drug name and common synonyms are listed in each monograph header. A slash between drug names indicates a combination product.

Class: Facts and Comparisons'® drug classification is used. A slash separates two equal therapeutic classes (eg, Cardiovascular/Antineoplastic).

Phonetic Pronunciation: A guide is provided for generic drug names. Pronunciations for commonly used terms, such as acid, have not been given. The pronunciations are based on the USAN Council officially designated pronunciations. The syllable in capital letters receives the emphasis.

Trade Name: US trade names are listed for each drug along with doseform and strength. If none are available, the statement *available as generic only* appears. Common Canadian trade names are provided whenever possible following the list of US names. A maple leaf appears at the beginning of the Canadian list. If a trade name is available in the US and Canada, it appears under the US list only.

Action: A brief, simple description of the drug's action, including pharmacology, pharmacokinetics, and pharmacodynamics, is provided.

Indications: All approved indications are included. For some antibiotics, a general statement regarding susceptible microorganisms is listed instead of listing the entire microbial spectrum, which could be quite lengthy. Common unlabeled uses and orphan drug uses are included when appropriate.

Contraindications: All known contraindications are included. Hypersensitivity to a given drug is always a contraindication and, therefore, this fact is assumed and has not been repeated for every monograph. *Standard Considerations* appears when there are no specific contraindications other than hypersensitivity.

Route/Dosage: Route of administration and the pertinent dosages are provided. Standard abbreviations are used when possible (see Standard Abbreviations, page ix). Route and dosage are organized by age group, route, and specific condition when appropriate.

Interactions: Potential drug interactions are listed alphabetically followed by any incompatibilities. *None well documented* appears when there is no specific information.

Lab Test Interferences: Potential lab test interferences are listed alphabetically. *None well documented* appears when there is no specific information.

Adverse Reactions: Common (at least 1% incidence), life-threatening, and postmarketing reactions are included. Adverse reactions are classified according to abbreviated body system (see Standard Abbreviations, page ix).

Warning Box: A brief description of the drug's warning box information is provided.

Precautions: Information regarding pregnancy (including FDA category), lactation, children, elderly, and special risk patients is included. For pregnancy Category X drugs, any applicable information regarding birth control use also is included.

Overdosage: Information not available for all drugs. Specific signs and symptoms that might signal an overdose are included when appropriate.

Patient Care Considerations: The bottom half of each monograph contains information specific to nursing care. The following sections are included:

Administration/Storage: Information includes timing of administration, methods of administration, whether or not to crush, chew, or swallow certain dose forms, reconstitution/dilution specifics, general storage guidelines, safe handling, and disposal. Storage temperature ranges are given and generally are as follows:

Controlled Room Temperature	=	20° to 25°C (68° to 77°F)
Refrigeration	=	2° to 8°C (36° to 46°F)
Freezing	=	−20° to 10°C (−4° to 14°F)

Assessment/Interventions: Information includes actions to take before/during/after drug administration, assessing for allergy, history, preconditions, dietary and social habits.

Patient/Family Education: Information to share with patient or family is listed, including how/when to take medication, side effects to watch for, actions to take to counteract/minimize side effects, cautions on hazardous activities, and general safety precautions.

The following information is not stated because it is assumed that, for every drug, the health care provider will take these patient education actions:
1. Discuss name, action, and side effects of drug.
2. Instruct patient to take medication exactly as prescribed. Tell patient not to adjust dosage, skip dose, or discontinue medication without notifying the prescriber.
3. Advise patient that if a dose is missed, contact prescriber.
4. Instruct patient to complete full course of medication as prescribed unless otherwise directed by prescriber.
5. Instruct patient to keep medication out of reach of children.
6. Give patient written information if appropriate.

Combination Drugs

Combination drugs not included in the general monograph section are summarized in table format. Generic name, trade name, strength, and average adult dose are listed.

Orphan Drugs

Drug or biological products for the diagnosis, treatment, or prevention of rare diseases or conditions. A rare disease is one that affects less than 200,000 people in the US or one that affects more than 200,000 people but for which there is no reasonable expectation that the cost of developing the drug and making it available will be recovered from sales of that drug in the US.

AIDS Drugs in Development

Investigational agents specific to AIDS that are in any phase of clinical trials, usually Phase II or later.

Appendices

The appendices include a variety of reference material designed to offer a quick guide to often needed information. They include the FDA Pregnancy Categories, General Management of Acute Overdosage, Management of Hypersensitivity Reactions, Calculations, International System of Units, and Normal Laboratory Values.

Using the Index

The index includes generic and trade drug names (including Canadian trade names) followed by the number of their monograph page. Trade drug names appear in italics and Canadian trade names are indicated with a [C].

Standard Abbreviations

ABGs	arterial blood gases	EMIT	enzyme-multiplied immunoassay test
AIDS	acquired immunodeficiency syndrome	ENDO	endocrine
ALT	alanine aminotransferase	°F	degrees Fahrenheit
APTT	activated partial thromboplastin time	FDA	Food and Drug Administration
ARDS	adult respiratory distress syndrome	G-6-PD	glucose-6-phosphate dehydrogenase
AST	aspartate aminotransferase	GABA	gamma-aminobutyric acid
AUC	area under the curve	GI	gastrointestinal
AV	atrioventricular	gtt	drops
bid	twice daily	GU	genitourinary
bpm	beats per minute	Hct	hematocrit
BP	blood pressure	HDL	high-density lipoprotein
BSA	body surface area	HEMA	hematologic
BUN	blood urea nitrogen	HEMA/LYMPH	hematologic-lymphatic
°C	degrees Celsius	HEPA	hepatic
Cal	calorie (kilocalorie)	Hgb	hemoglobin
CBC	complete blood count	HIV	human immunodeficiency virus
Cc	cubic centimeter		
Ccr	creatinine clearance	hr	hour
CDC	Centers for Disease Control and Prevention	HYPERSENS	hypersensitivity reactions
		I&O	intake and output
		IM	intramuscular
CHF	congestive heart failure	IND	investigational new drug
Cl	clearance	IOP	intraocular pressure
C_{max}	maximum serum concentration	IU	international units
		IV	intravenous
C_{min}	minimum serum concentration	kg	kilogram
		L	liter
CN	cranial nerve	LABTESTABS	laboratory test abnormalities
CNS	central nervous system		
COPD	chronic obstructive pulmonary disease	lb	pound
		LDH	lactate dehydrogenase
CPK	creatine phosphokinase	LDL	low-density lipoprotein
CSF	cerebrospinal fluid	LFT	liver function test
CT	computed tomography	LOC	level of consciousness
cu	cubic	LOCAL	location reactions
CV	cardiovascular	LYMPH	lymphatic
CVP	central venous pressure	m	meter
D5W	5% Dextrose in Water	m^2	square meter
D10W	10% Dextrose in Water	MAO	monoamine oxidase
DERM	dermatologic	max	maximum
DIC	disseminated intravascular coagulation	mcg	microgram
		mEq	milliequivalent
dL	deciliter (100 mL)	META	metabolic
DNA	deoxyribonucleic acid	mg	milligram
DSM	Diagnostic and Statistical Manual of Mental Disorders	MI	myocardial infarction
		min	minute
		mL	milliliter
ECG	electrocardiogram	mm	millimeter
EDTA	ethylenediamine tetraacetic acid	mm^3	cubic millimeter
		mm Hg	millimeters of mercury
EEG	electroencephalogram	M/N	metabolic/nutritional
EENT	eye, ear, nose, throat	mo	month
ELECDIST	electrolyte disturbance	mOsm	milliosmole
ELISA	enzyme-linked immunosorbent assay	MRI	magnetic resonance imaging

A TO Z DRUG FACTS

MUSC	musculoskeletal
ng	nanogram
NK	natural killer (cells)
npo	nothing by mouth
NSAID	nonsteroidal anti-inflammatory drug
OPHTH	ophthalmic
OTC	over-the-counter (nonprescription)
oz	ounce
PABA	para-aminobenzoic acid
PAC	premature atrial contraction
pH	negative log of hydrogen ion concentration
PMS	premenstrual syndrome
pCO_2	carbon dioxide pressure (tension)
pO_2	oxygen pressure (tension)
PO	by mouth
ppm	parts per million
prn	as needed
PR	per rectum
pt	pint
PT	prothrombin time
PTT	partial thromboplastin time
PULM	pulmonary
PVC	premature ventricular contraction
q	every
qd	every day
q hr	every hour
qid	four times daily
qod	every other day
q 2 hr	every 2 hours
qt	quart
RBC	red blood cell count
RDA	Recommended Dietary Allowance
RDS	respiratory distress syndrome
RENAL	renal
RNA	ribonucleic acid
SC	subcutaneous
sec	second
SIADH	syndrome of inappropriate secretion of antidiuretic hormone
SL	sublingual
SLE	systemic lupus erythematosus
SPF	sun protection factor
SPEC	SENSES special senses
STD	sexually transmitted disease
SYST	systemic
$t\frac{1}{2}$	elimination/terminal half-life
Tbsp	tablespoon
tid	three times daily
T_{max}	time to reach maximum concentration
TPN	total parenteral nutrition
TSH	thyroid-stimulating hormone
tsp	teaspoon
U	unit
ULN	upper limits of normal
UTI	urinary tract infection
Vd	volume of distribution
VHDL	very high density lipoprotein
VLDL	very low density lipoprotein
WBC	white blood cell count
WHO	World Health Organization
wk	week
yr	year

Monographs

Abacavir Sulfate

(ab-ah-KAV-ear)

Class Antiretroviral/Nucleoside reverse transcriptase inhibitor

How Supplied
Ziagen Tablets 300 mg, Oral solution 20 mg/mL

Action

PHARMACOLOGY: Converted by cellular enzymes to carbovir triphosphate, which inhibits HIV-1 reverse transcriptase and interferes with DNA synthesis.

PHARMACOKINETICS/DYNAMICS:

Absorption: Rapidly and extensively absorbed. Bioavailability is 83% (tablets). C_{max} is approximately 3 mcg/mL and AUC_{0-12} is approximately 6.02 mcg•hr/mL.

Distribution: Vd after IV administration is approximately 0.86 L/kg. Plasma protein binding is approximately 50%.

Metabolism: Metabolized to inactivate metabolites by alcohol dehydrogenase and glucuronyl transferase.

Excretion: Urine is 1.2% as abacavir, 81% as inactive metabolites; feces is 16% of dose. The t½ is approximately 1.54 hr and Cl is approximately 0.8 L/hr/kg (after IV administration).

Special Populations:
Hepatic Function Impairment – Mild hepatic impairment (Child-Pugh score 5 to 6) AUC increased 89% and t½ increased 58%.

Indications Treatment of HIV-1 in combination with other antiretroviral agents.

Contraindications Moderate or severe hepatic impairment; hypersensitivity to any component of the product.

Route/Dosage

ADULTS: **PO** 300 mg bid in combination with other antiretroviral agents.

ADOLESCENTS AND CHILDREN 3 MO TO UP TO 16 YR: **PO** 8 mg/kg bid (max dose, 300 mg bid) in combination with other antiretroviral agents.

Hepatic Impairment – **PO** 200 mg bid in patients with mild hepatic impairment (Child-Pugh score 5 to 6).

PATIENT CARE CONSIDERATIONS

Administration/Storage

- Do not administer to patient with moderate to severe hepatic impairment.
- Administer prescribed dose bid without regard to meals.
- Administer with food if GI upset occurs.
- Store tablets and solution at controlled room temperature (68° to 77°F). Solution may be refrigerated but do not freeze.

Interactions
Ethanol: Increases exposure to abacavir by decreasing the elimination and prolonging the t½.
Methadone: Plasma levels of methadone may be decreased in some patients, reducing the therapeutic effect.

Lab Test Interferences None well documented.

Adverse Reactions
CNS: Insomnia; sleep disorders; headache.
DERM: Skin rashes; Stevens-Johnson syndrome, toxic epidermal necrolysis, erythema multiforme (postmarketing).
GI: Nausea; vomiting; diarrhea; loss of appetite; anorexia; pancreatitis.
METAB: Elevated blood glucose; elevated triglycerides; redistribution/accumulation of body fat (postmarketing).
OTHER: Hypersensitivity reactions (eg, fever, rash, fatigue, GI symptoms, malaise, lethargy, myalgia, arthralgia, edema, shortness of breath, paresthesia, hypotension, death); fever.

> WARNING:
>
> *Fatal hypersensitivity reactions:* Associated with therapy. Drug should not be restarted after suspected reaction.
>
> Lactic acidosis and hepatomegaly reported with steatosis (including fatal cases) reported with the use of nucleoside analogues alone or in combination with other antiretrovirals.

Precautions
Pregnancy: Category C.
Lactation: Undetermined; however, HIV-infected mothers should not breastfeed infants.
Children: Safety and efficacy not established in children under 3 mo.
Elderly: Select dose with caution, reflecting greater frequency of decreased hepatic, renal, or cardiac function and comorbidity.
Fat redistribution: Redistribution/accumulation of body fat have been observed (eg, buffalo hump, peripheral/facial wasting, central obesity).

Solution:

- Measure prescribed dose using dosing spoon or dosing syringe.

Assessment/Interventions

- Obtain patient history, including drug history and any known allergies. Note hepatic impairment and history of previous hypersensitivity reaction to abacavir.

- Ensure that medication is used in combination with other antiretroviral agents.
- Ensure that patient has received the *Medication Guide* and Warning Card before therapy is started.
- Ensure that reduced dose is administered to patient with mild hepatic impairment.
- Monitor patient for signs and symptoms of hypersensitivity reaction to abacavir. Discontinue use and notify health care provider immediately if skin rash or 1 or more symptoms from at least 2 of the following groups are noted: fever; nausea, vomiting, diarrhea, abdominal pain; fatigue, muscle aches, malaise; sore throat, shortness of breath, cough. If hypersensitivity reaction is documented, ensure that reaction is reported to Abacavir Hypersensitivity Register as noted in the package insert.
- Monitor patient for signs of lactic acidosis. If patient develops profound weakness or tiredness, unexpected stomach discomfort, feeling cold, dizzy or lightheaded, or slow or irregular heartbeat, withhold drug and contact health care provider.
- Monitor patient for evidence of CNS, GI, and general body side effects. Inform health care provider if noted and significant.

Patient/Family Education
- Explain name, dose, action, and potential side effects of drug.
- Advise patient to review *Medication Guide* before starting therapy and with each refill of the medication.
- Advise patient to review, and carry with them at all times, the Warning Card summarizing the symptoms of abacavir hypersensitivity reaction.
- Instruct patient to take exactly as prescribed and not to change the dose or discontinue therapy unless advised by health care provider.
- Advise patient to take drug bid without regard to meals but to take with food if GI upset occurs.
- Advise patient, family, or caregiver to measure prescribed dose of solution using dosing spoon or dosing syringe.
- Instruct patient that if a dose is missed, to take as soon as remembered, take the next dose at the usual scheduled time.
- Instruct patient to continue to take other HIV medications as prescribed by health care provider.
- Instruct patient to discontinue use and notify health care provider immediately if skin rash or 1 or more symptoms from at least 2 of the following groups are noted: fever; nausea, vomiting, diarrhea, abdominal pain; fatigue, muscle aches, malaise; sore throat, shortness of breath, cough.
- Instruct patient to report the following symptoms immediately to health care provider: profound weakness or tiredness; feeling cold, dizzy, or lightheaded; slow or irregular heartbeat; pain or tingling in the hands or feet; muscle or joint pain.
- Inform patient that drug does not completely eliminate HIV virus and, therefore, does not reduce risk of transmitting HIV. Appropriate precautions must still be followed.
- Advise patient that drug is not a cure for HIV infection. Illnesses associated with HIV infection, including opportunistic infections, may continue to be acquired, and patients should remain under a physician's care.
- Inform patient that redistribution or accumulation of body fat may occur.
- Instruct patient not to take any prescription or OTC medications or dietary supplements unless advised by health care provider.
- Caution breastfeeding mother to discontinue nursing while receiving medication because of potential for adverse effects from the medication in nursing infant as well as transmission of HIV virus.
- Advise women to notify health care provider if pregnant, planning to become pregnant, or breastfeeding.
- Remind patient that examinations and laboratory tests will be required to monitor therapy and to keep appointments.

Abacavir Sulfate/ Lamivudine/Zidovudine

(ab-ah-KAV-ear SULL-fate/la-MIH-view-deen/zie-DOE-view-DEEN)

Class Antiretroviral combination

How Supplied
Trizivir Tablets 300 mg abacavir sulfate/150 mg lamivudine/300 mg zidovudine

Action
PHARMACOLOGY: Inhibits replication of HIV by incorporation into HIV DNA and producing incomplete, nonfunctional DNA.

PHARMACOKINETICS/DYNAMICS:
Absorption: Rapidly and extensively absorbed. Bioavailability is 83% (tablets). C_{max} is about 3 mcg/mL. AUC_{0-12} is about 6.02 mcg•hr/mL.
Distribution: Vd after IV administration is about

0.86 L/kg. Plasma protein binding is about 50%.

Metabolism: Metabolized to inactive metabolites by alcohol dehydrogenase and glucuronyl transferase.

Excretion: Urine is 1.2% as abacavir; 81% as inactive metabolites. Feces is 16% of dose. $T_{1/2}$ is about 1.54 hr. Cl is about 0.8 L/hr/kg (after IV administration).

Indications Use alone and in combination with other antiretroviral agents for the treatment of HIV-1 infection.

Contraindications Abacavir has been associated with fatal hypersensitivity reactions and should not be restarted following a hypersensitivity reaction to abacavir; hypersensitivity to any component of the product.

Route/Dosage

ADULTS AND ADOLESCENTS (40 KG OR GREATER): **PO** 1 tablet bid.

Interactions

Doxorubicin, ribavirin, stavudine: Antagonistic relationship has been demonstrated between these agents and zidovudine.

Ganciclovir, interferon-alpha, other bone marrow suppressive or cytotoxic agents: May increase the hematologic toxicity of zidovudine.

Trimethoprim/sulfamethoxazole: Serum concentrations of lamivudine may be elevated, increasing the pharmacologic and adverse effects.

Zalcitabine: Lamivudine and zalcitabine may inhibit the intracellular phosphorylation of each other.

Lab Test Interferences None well documented.

Adverse Reactions

CV: Cardiomyopathy.

CNS: Loss of appetite; anorexia; insomnia; sleep disorders; headache; malaise; fatigue; neuropathy; dizziness; depression; paresthesia; peripheral neuropathy; seizures.

DERM: Skin rash; alopecia; Stevens-Johnson syndrome; toxic epidermal necrolysis; erythema multiforme.

EENT: Nasal signs and symptoms.

GI: Nausea; vomiting; diarrhea; pancreatitis; abdominal pain; dyspepsia; stomatitis; oral mucosal pigmentation.

GU: Gynecomastia.

HEMA: Neutropenia; anemia; thrombocytopenia; aplastic anemia; lymphadenopathy; pure red cell aplasia; splenomegaly.

HEPA: Increased ALT, AST, and bilirubin; hepatic steatosis; posttreatment exacerbation of hepatitis.

METAB: Redistribution of body fat; hyperglycemia.

RESP: Cough; abnormal breath sounds; wheezing.

OTHER: Hypersensitivity; fever; chills; musculoskeletal pain; myalgia; arthralgia; vasculitis; weakness; muscle weakness; CPK elevation; rhabdomyolysis.

Precautions

Pregnancy: Category C.

Lactation: HIV-infected mothers should not breastfeed their infants.

Zidovudine – Excreted in breast milk.

Abacavir and lamivudine – Undetermined.

Children: Safety and efficacy not established in children weighing less than 40 kg.

Elderly: Select dose with caution, reflecting greater frequency of decreased hepatic, renal, or cardiac function and comorbidity.

Hypersensitivity: Fatal hypersensitivity reactions have been associated with abacavir use and have occurred within hours after reintroduction of abacavir in patients who have no identified history or unrecognized symptoms of hypersensitivity. If hypersensitivity cannot be ruled out, do not restart therapy.

Renal function impairment: Because this is a fixed-dose tablet, do not use for patients requiring dosage adjustments (eg, Ccr less than 50 mL/min or patients experiencing dose-limiting adverse effects).

Bone marrow suppression: Use with caution in patients who have bone marrow compromise evidenced by granulocyte count less than 1000 cells/mm^3 or hemoglobin less than 9.5 g/dL.

Lactic acidosis/Severe hepatomegaly: Steatosis have been reported.

Overdosage: Signs and Symptoms

Nausea, vomiting, headache, dizziness, drowsiness, lethargy, confusion.

PATIENT CARE CONSIDERATIONS

Administration/Storage

- Administer twice daily without regard to meals.
- Administer with food if GI upset occurs.
- Store tablets at controlled room temperature (59° to 86° F).

Assessment/Interventions

- Obtain patient history, including drug history and any known allergies. Note patient's weight and history of renal impairment (Ccr less than 50 mL/min) or liver impairment.
- Ensure that patient is not receiving abacavir, lamivudine, or zidovudine in other dose forms.

- Do not administer to patient weighing less than 90 lbs.
- Ensure that CBC is obtained prior to starting and periodically during therapy.
- Monitor patient for signs of lactic acidosis. If patient develops profound weakness or tiredness, unexpected stomach discomfort, feeling cold, dizzy, or lightheaded, or slow or irregular heartbeat, withhold drug and contact health care provider.
- Monitor patient for signs/symptoms of allergic reaction to abacavir. Discontinue use and notify health care provider immediately if skin rash or 1 or more symptoms from at least 2 of the following groups are noted: fever; nausea, vomiting, diarrhea, abdominal pain; fatigue, muscle aches, malaise; sore throat; shortness of breath; cough. If hypersensitivity reaction is documented then ensure that reaction is reported to Abacavir Hypersensitivity Register as noted in the package insert.
- Assess for evidence of peripheral neuropathy (eg, numbness, tingling, burning or pain in hands or feet) or evidence of opportunistic infections. Notify health care provider if these occur.
- Monitor patient for evidence of CNS, GI, musculoskeletal, and general body side effects. If noted and significant, inform health care provider.

Patient/Family Education
- Explain name, dose, action, and potential side effects of drug.
- Advise patient to review Medication Guide before starting therapy and with each refill of the medication.
- Advise patient to take drug twice daily without regard to meals but to take with food if GI upset occurs.
- Instruct patient that if a dose is missed to take as soon as remembered then take the next dose at the usual scheduled time.
- Instruct patient to continue taking other HIV medications as prescribed by health care provider.
- Instruct patient to discontinue use and notify health care provider immediately if skin rash or 1 or more symptoms from at least 2 of the following groups are noted: fever; nausea, vomiting, diarrhea, abdominal pain; fatigue, muscle aches, malaise; sore throat; shortness of breath; cough.
- Instruct patient to report the following symptoms immediately to health care provider: profound weakness or tiredness; feeling cold, dizzy or lightheaded; slow or irregular heartbeat; pain or tingling in the hands or feet; muscle or joint pain.
- Advise patient to carry Warning Card at all times.
- Inform patient that drug does not completely eliminate HIV virus and therefore does not reduce risk of transmitting HIV. Appropriate precautions must still be followed.
- Advise patient that drug is not a cure for HIV infection and that he/she may continue to acquire illnesses associated with HIV infection, including opportunistic infections and to remain under a health care provider's care.
- Instruct patient to not take any prescription or OTC medications or dietary supplements unless advised to do so by their health care provider.
- Instruct women to notify health care provider if pregnant, planning to become pregnant, or breastfeeding.
- Remind patient that examinations and laboratory tests will be required to monitor therapy and to keep appointments.

Abarelix

(ab-ah-RELL-ix)
Class Antineoplastic
How Supplied
Plenaxis Injectable Suspension 113 mg
Action
PHARMACOLOGY: Directly suppresses luteinizing hormone and follicle stimulating hormone secretion, thereby reducing the secretion of testosterone by the testes.

PHARMACOKINETICS/DYNAMICS:
Absorption: Slowly absorbed following IM injection, reaching a peak concentration of 43.4 ng/mL approximately 3 days after injection.
Distribution: Vd is about 4040 L. AUC is about 500 ng•day/mL; 96% to 99% is protein bound.
Metabolism: Major metabolites are formed via hydrolysis of peptide bonds.
Excretion: Approximately 13% unchanged in the urine. The $t_{½}$ is about 13.2 days.

Indications Palliative treatment of advanced symptomatic prostate cancer in men in whom luteinizing hormone-releasing hormone agonist therapy is not appropriate and who refuse surgical castration, and have 1 or more of the following: risk of neurological compromise caused by metastases; ureteral or bladder outlet obstruction caused by local encroachment or metastatic disease; or severe bone pain from skeletal metastases persisting on narcotic analgesia.

Contraindications Women; pediatric

patients; pregnancy; hypersensitivity to any component of the product.

Route/Dosage
ADULTS: **IM** 100 mg to buttock on days 1, 15, 29 (week 4) and q 4 wk thereafter.

Interactions
Class IA (eg, quinidine, procainamide), class III (eg, amiodarone, sotalol) antiarrhythmic agents: Because the QT interval may be prolonged by abarelix, benefits of use should outweigh risk of potential QT prolongation.

Lab Test Interferences None well documented.

Adverse Reactions
CNS: Sleep disturbances (44%); dizziness, headache (12%); fatigue (10%).
GI: Constipation (15%); diarrhea (11%); nausea (10%).
GU: Breast enlargement (30%); breast pain/nipple tenderness (20%); dysuria, micturition frequency, urinary retention, UTI (10%).
LABTESTABS: Increased serum triglycerides (10%); increased ALT (8%); increased AST (3%).
RESP: Upper respiratory tract infection (12%).
OTHER: Hot flushes (79%); pain (31%); back pain (17%); peripheral edema (15%); immediate-onset systemic allergic reactions.

> **WARNING:**
> Immediate-onset systemic allergic reactions, some resulting in hypotension and syncope, can occur. May only be prescribed by physicians who have enrolled in the *Plenaxis* PLUS program.

Precautions
Pregnancy: Category X.
Lactation: Undetermined.
Children: Safety and efficacy not established.
Effectiveness: A decrease in overall effectiveness with increased duration of treatment may occur, especially in patients weighing more than 225 pounds.
Prolongation of QT interval: May occur.

PATIENT CARE CONSIDERATIONS

Administration/Storage
- For IM administration only. Not for intradermal, SC, or IV administration
- Reconstitute powder following manufacturer's guidelines.
- Do not administer if particulate matter, cloudiness, or discoloration noted.
- Administer solution by IM injection into buttock within 1 hr of reconstitution.
- Discard any unused solution. Do not save for future use.
- Dose is usually administered on days 1, 15, and 29 (wk 4) and then q 4 wk thereafter.
- Store vials at controlled room temperature (59° to 86°F).

Assessment/Interventions
- Obtain patient history, including drug history and any known allergies. Note congenital QT prolongation or concurrent use of class IA (eg, quinidine) or class III (eg, amiodarone) antiarrhythmic medications.
- Ensure that risks and benefits of treatment with abarelix have been reviewed with the patient and that the patient has signed the *Patient Information* signature page before starting therapy. Place original signed form in patient's medical record and provide copy of *Patient Information* leaflet with signed page to patient.
- Ensure that medication is not administered to women or pediatric patients.
- Monitor for treatment failure by ensuring that serum total testosterone concentration is measured just prior to administration of medication on day 29 of therapy and q 8 wk thereafter for duration of treatment.
- Ensure that liver enzymes and prostate-specific antigen are evaluated before starting therapy and periodically during treatment.
- Monitor patient for immediate-onset allergic reaction (hives, itching, hypotension, syncope) for at least 30 min following each injection. Immediately inform health care provider if noted and be prepared to treat appropriately.
- Periodically assess and document response to treatment. Inform health care provider if any of the symptoms of advanced prostate cancer (eg, bone pain, neurological compromise, urinary symptoms) are not improving or are worsening.
- Assess patient for CNS, GI, GU, and general body side effects. Inform health care provider if noted and significant.
- Ensure that serious adverse events (eg, immediate-onset allergic reaction) are reported to the manufacturer or to the FDA's MedWatch program.

Patient/Family Education
- Explain name, dose, action, and potential side effects of drug.
- Advise patient that medication is not a cure for prostate cancer but is being used to provide relief of symptoms caused by the prostate cancer.
- Review dosing schedule with patient (injec-

tions on days 1, 15, and 29 then q 4 wk thereafter).
- Advise patient that medication will be prepared and administered by a health care professional in a medical setting.
- Advise patient that allergic reactions can occur following the injection and to remain in the medical setting for at least 30 min following each injection so that a reaction can be treated if it occurs.
- Advise patient that hot flushes and sleep disturbances are the most common side effects and to inform health care provider if they occur and are intolerable or if any other side effect becomes bothersome.
- Advise patient that drug may cause dizziness and to use caution while driving or performing other tasks requiring mental alertness until tolerance is determined.
- Instruct patient to not take any prescription or OTC medications or dietary supplements unless advised by health care provider.
- Advise patient that follow-up visits and lab tests will be required to monitor therapy and to keep appointments.

Abciximab

(ab-SICK-sih-mab)
Class Antiplatelet
How Supplied
ReoPro Injection 2 mg/mL
Action
PHARMACOLOGY: Binds to glycoprotein IIb/IIIa receptors on surface of platelets, thereby preventing platelet aggregation.
PHARMACOKINETICS/DYNAMICS:
Distribution: Rapidly binds to glycoprotein IIb/IIIa receptors.
Excretion: Initial t½ is less than 10 min. Second phase $t_{1/2}$ is about 30 min.
Duration: Platelet function generally recovers over 48 hr.
Indications Adjunct to percutaneous coronary intervention (PCI) to prevent ischemic complications in patients at high risk of abrupt closure of the treated vessel. Intended for use with aspirin and heparin.
Contraindications Active internal bleeding; recent (6 wk) GI/GU bleeding, major surgery, or trauma; history of CVA in the past 2 yr of CVA with significant residual neurological deficit; use of oral anticoagulants within 7 days unless prothrombin time is less than 1.2 times control; thrombocytopenia; severe uncontrolled hypertension; vasculitis; intracranial neoplasm, aneurysm, or arteriovenous malformation; or the recent or current use of IV dextran.

Route/Dosage
ADULTS: IV 0.25 mg/kg bolus 10 to 60 min before PCI followed by continuous infusion of 0.125 mcg/kg/min (to a max of 10 mcg/min) for 12 hr.
Interactions None well documented.
Lab Test Interferences None well documented.
Adverse Reactions
CV: Hypotension; bradycardia; atrial fibrillation; pulmonary edema; AV block; supraventricular tachycardia.
CNS: Hypesthesia; headache; confusion; dizziness.
EENT: Abnormal vision.
GI: Nausea, vomiting.
HEMA: Bleeding; thrombocytopenia; anemia; leukocytosis.
RESP: Pleural effusion; pneumonia.
OTHER: Pain; peripheral edema.
Precautions
Pregnancy: Category C.
Lactation: Undetermined.
Children: Safety and efficacy not established.
Readministration: Abciximab may cause antibody development. Readministration may be associated with allergic reactions.
Bleeding: Because risk of bleeding is increased, use cautiously, if at all, with thrombolytics, oral anticoagulants, NSAIDs, dipyridamole, and ticlopidine. Institute bleeding precautions.
Thrombocytopenia: Monitor platelet counts.

PATIENT CARE CONSIDERATIONS
Administration/Storage
- Use only NS or D5W for IV infusion. Add no other medication for the infusion.
- Do not use drug if vial contains visibly opaque particles.
- Withdraw medication through a 0.2 or 2.2 micron filter.
- Administer drug through a separate IV line with filter.
- Store vials at 2° to 8°C (36° to 46°F). Do not freeze. Do not shake. Discard any unused portion.

Assessment/Interventions
- Obtain patient history.
- If symptoms of sensitivity occur any time during therapy, discontinue drug and initiate symptomatic and supportive therapy. Have epinephrine, dopamine, theophylline, antihis-

tamines, and corticosteroids available.
- If serious bleeding occurs that is not controlled with pressure, stop infusion of abciximab and heparin.
- Avoid noncompressible sites when obtaining IV access.
- Discontinue heparin at least 4 hr prior to removal of arterial sheath. Following removal, apply pressure for at least 30 min, then apply a pressure dressing.
- Maintain the patient on bedrest for 6 to 8 hr.
- Frequently check insertion site and distal pulses while sheath is in place and 6 hr after removal. Measure any hematoma and monitor for enlargement.
- Avoid other invasive procedures during therapy.
- Prior to administration, check platelet count, PTT, and APTT. Monitor during and after treatment.

Patient/Family Education
- Advise patient to report any bleeding or bruising to health care provider immediately.

Acamprosate Calcium

(a-kam-PROE-sate KAL-see-uhm)
Class Antialcoholic agent

How Supplied
Campral Tablets, delayed-release 333 mg acamprosate calcium (equiv. to 300 mg acamprosate)

Action
PHARMACOLOGY: Chronic alcohol exposure may alter normal balance between neuronal and excitation and inhibition. In vitro and in vivo animal data suggest acamprosate interacts with glutamate and GABA neurotransmitter systems, restoring this balance.

PHARMACOKINETICS/DYNAMICS:
Absorption: Bioavailability about 11%. Steady state reached within 5 days. Steady-state concentrations average 350 ng/mL and occur 3 to 8 hr postdose. C_{max} and AUC approximately 42% and 23%, respectively.

Distribution: Vd estimated to be 72 to 109 L (1 L/kg). Protein binding is negligible.

Metabolism: Does not undergo metabolism.

Excretion: Terminal t½ ranges from about 20 to 33 hr. Major route of excretion is via kidneys.

Special Populations:
Renal impairment – C_{max} in patients with moderate or severe renal impairment were 2- and 4-fold higher, respectively. Elimination t½ were 1.8- and 2.6-fold longer, respectively.

Indications Maintenance of abstinence from alcohol in patients with alcohol dependence who are abstinent at treatment initiation.

Contraindications Severe renal impairment (Ccr 30 mL/min or less); hypersensitivity to any component of product.

Route/Dosage
ADULTS: PO Two 333 mg tablets tid.

Renal Impairment
ADULTS: PO Start with 333 mg tid in patients with moderate renal impairment (Ccr 30 to 50 mL/min). Do not administer to patients with severe renal impairment (Ccr 30 mL/min or less).

Interactions
Antidepressants: Weight gain and loss reported more frequently compared with either agent alone.
Naltrexone: Acamprosate levels may be increased; however, no dosage adjustment is recommended.

Lab Test Interferences None well documented.

Adverse Reactions
CV: Palpitation, syncope (at least 1%).
CNS: Insomnia (7%); asthenia, anxiety (6%); depression (5%); dizziness (3%); dry mouth, paresthesia (2%); headache, somnolence, decreased libido, amnesia, abnormal thinking, tremor, vasodilatation, hypertension (at least 1%).
DERM: Pruritus (4%); sweating (2%); rash (at least 1%).
EENT: Pharyngitis, abnormal vision, taste perversion (at least 1%).
GI: Diarrhea (16%); nausea (4%); anorexia, flatulence (3%); vomiting, dyspepsia, constipation, increased appetite (at least 1%).
GU: Impotence (at least 1%); acute kidney failure (postmarketing).
M/N: Peripheral edema, weight gain (at least 1%).
MUSC: Back pain, myalgia, arthralgia (at least 1%).
RESP: Rhinitis, increased cough, dyspnea, bronchitis (at least 1%).
OTHER: Accidental injury, pain (3%); abdominal pain, infection, flu syndrome, chest pain, chills, suicide attempt (at least 1%).

Precautions
Pregnancy: Category C
Lactation: Undetermined.
Children: Safety and efficacy not established.
Elderly: Because elderly are more likely to have decreased renal function, select dose with care and monitor renal function.
Renal function impairment: Reduce dose in patients with moderate renal impairment. Do

not administer to patients with severe renal impairment.
Suicide: While infrequent, suicide is more common than in patients receiving placebo.
Withdrawal: Alcohol withdrawal symptoms are not eliminated or diminished by acamprosate administration.

Overdosage: Signs and Symptoms
Diarrhea.

PATIENT CARE CONSIDERATIONS

Administration/Storage
- Do not administer to patient with severe renal impairment (Ccr 30 mL/min or less).
- Do not administer to patient who has not undergone detoxification or has not achieved alcohol abstinence.
- Administer prescribed dose without regard to meals but administer with food if GI upset occurs or if administration with food increases compliance.
- Store tablets at controlled room temperature (59° to 86°F).

Assessment/Interventions
- Obtain patient history, including drug history and any known allergies. Note renal impairment.
- Ensure that patient is participating in a comprehensive management program that includes psychosocial support.
- Ensure that reduced dose (333 mg tid) is used in patient with moderate renal impairment (Ccr 30 to 50 mL/min).
- Monitor patient for depression or suicidal tendencies often associated with alcohol dependence. Immediately inform health care provider if depression or suicidal behaviors or thoughts are noted.
- Monitor patient for GI, CNS, PSYCH, and general body side effects. Report to health care provider if noted and significant.

Patient/Family Education
- Explain name, dose, action, and potential side effects of drug.
- Ensure patient understands that acamprosate only helps maintain abstinence from alcohol and will not work if alcohol is still being ingested when therapy is started.
- Advise patient that medication will be most effective when taken exactly as prescribed and combined with participation in a comprehensive treatment program that includes counseling and support.
- Advise patient to take without regard to meals but to take with food if stomach upset occurs or if taking with food helps patient remember to take each dose.
- Advise patient to continue acamprosate therapy as directed, even in the event of a relapse. Instruct patient to discuss any renewed drinking with health care provider.
- Instruct family members and/or caregiver to monitor patient for development of symptoms of depression or suicidality often associated with alcohol dependence and to immediately inform health care provider if any symptoms of depression or suicidal behaviors or thoughts are noted.
- Advise patient that drug may impair judgment, thinking, or motor skills and to use caution while driving or performing other tasks requiring mental alertness and coordination until tolerance is determined.
- Advise women to inform health care provider if pregnant, planning to become pregnant, or breastfeeding.
- Instruct patient not to take any prescription or OTC drugs, herbal preparations, or dietary supplements unless advised by health care provider.
- Advise patient that follow-up visits and lab tests may be necessary to monitor therapy and to keep appointments.

Acarbose

(A-car-bose)

Class Antidiabetic

How Supplied
Precose Tablets 25 mg, Tablets 50 mg, Tablets 100 mg

Action
PHARMACOLOGY: Inhibits intestinal enzymes that digest carbohydrate, thereby reducing carbohydrate digestion after meals. This lowers postprandial glucose elevation in diabetics.

PHARMACOKINETICS/DYNAMICS:
Absorption: Less than 2% is absorbed as active drug. T_{max} is approximately 1 hr.

Metabolism: Metabolized within the GI tract by intestinal bacteria and digestive enzymes. At least 13 metabolites have been separated from urine specimens, with 1 being active.

Excretion: Less than 2% is recovered in the urine as active. The plasma elimination t½ is approximately 2 hr. Drug accumulation does not

occur with tid oral dosing.
Special Populations:
Renal Function Impairment – In those with Ccr less than 25 mL/min per 1.73 m^2, the C_{max} was approximately 5 times higher, and the AUC was 6 times larger. Treatment with acarbose is not recommended.
Elderly – AUC and C_{max} are approximately 1.5 times higher in the elderly, although not statistically significant.

Indications Patients with non-insulin-dependent diabetes mellitus who have failed dietary therapy. May be used alone or in combination with sulfonylureas, insulin, or metformin.

Contraindications Diabetic ketoacidosis; cirrhosis; inflammatory bowel disease; colonic ulceration; intestinal disorders of digestion or absorption; partial or predisposition to intestinal obstruction; conditions that may deteriorate as a result of increased intestinal gas production.

Route/Dosage
ADULTS: **PO** 25 mg tid with the start of each meal. To minimize GI side effects, some patients may benefit from more gradual dose titration. This may be achieved by initiating treatment at 25 mg daily and increasing the frequency to achieve 25 mg tid. Increase by 25 mg/dose at 4- to 8-wk intervals, according to response, up to a max based on blood glucose response (max, 150/day if no more than 60 kg, 300 mg/day if above 60 kg).

Interactions
Drugs that produce hyperglycemia (eg, corticosteroids, diuretics, thyroid preparations), phenothiazines, estrogens, oral contraceptives, phenytoin, nicotinic acid, sympathomimetics, calcium channel-blocking drugs, isoniazid: May lead to loss of glucose control.
Intestinal adsorbents (eg, charcoal); digestive enzymes: May lower the efficacy of acarbose.

Lab Test Interferences None well documented.

Adverse Reactions
GI: Flatulence (74%); diarrhea (31%); abdominal pain (19%).

HEPA: Elevated serum transaminases rarely associated with jaundice.
OTHER: Hypersensitivity skin reactions such as rash, edema (rare); decreased hematocrit; low serum calcium; low plasma vitamin B_6 levels.

Precautions
Pregnancy: Category B. Insulin is recommended to maintain blood glucose levels during pregnancy.
Lactation: Undetermined.
Children: Safety and efficacy not established.
Renal function impairment: Acarbose plasma concentrations may increase relative to the degree of renal dysfunction.
Elevated serum transaminase levels: In long-term studies (up to 12 mo, and including acarbose doses up to 300 mg tid), treatment-emergent elevations of serum transaminases (AST and/or ALT) above the upper limit of normal (ULN), greater than 1.8 times the ULN, and greater than 3 times the ULN occurred in acarbose-treated patients. Although these differences between treatments were statistically significant, these elevations were asymptomatic, reversible, more common in women, and, in general, were not associated with other evidence of liver dysfunction. Serum transaminase elevations appeared to be dose related. In studies including acarbose doses up to the max approved dose of 100 mg tid, treatment-emergent elevations of AST and/or ALT at any level of severity were similar between acarbose-treated patients and placebo-treated patients.
Hypoglycemia: Acarbose does not produce hypoglycemia; however, hypoglycemia may develop if used together with sulfonylureas or insulin.
Loss of blood glucose control: Certain medical conditions (eg, surgery, fever, infection, trauma) and drugs (eg, diuretics, corticosteroids, oral contraceptives) affect glucose control. In these situations, it may be necessary to adjust dose of acarbose and other antidiabetic drugs.

Overdosage: Signs and Symptoms
Increased flatulence, diarrhea, abdominal discomfort.

PATIENT CARE CONSIDERATIONS
Administration/Storage
- May be used alone or in combination with insulin, sulfonylureas, or metformin.
- Administer prescribed dose at the start (with the first bite) of each main meal.
- Store tablets at controlled room temperature (less than 77°F). Protect from moisture.

Assessment/Interventions
- Obtain patient history, including drug history and any known allergies. Note renal impairment, cirrhosis, inflammatory bowel disease, colonic ulceration, partial intestinal obstruction or predisposition to intestinal obstruction, chronic intestinal disease associated with disorders of digestion or absorption, or diabetic ketoacidosis.
- Ensure that dose does not exceed 50 mg tid in patient who weighs less than 60 kg (132 pounds).
- Ensure that medication is not used in patient with significant renal impairment (eg, serum creatinine greater than 2 mg/dL).

- Ensure that serum transaminase levels are evaluated before starting therapy, every 3 mo for the first year of therapy, and then periodically thereafter. Inform health care provider if elevated transaminase levels are noted and be prepared to reduce the dose or discontinue therapy.
- Check blood sugars frequently and observe for signs of hypoglycemia. Inform health care provider if blood sugar readings are outside target range or if hypoglycemic events are noted. Be prepared to treat hypoglycemic reactions with IV or oral glucose instead of cane sugar (table sugar) because absorption of cane sugar is inhibited by acarbose.
- Assess patient for GI and general body side effects. Inform health care provider if noted and significant.

Patient/Family Education
- Explain name, dose, action, and potential side effects of drug.
- Educate patient regarding type 2 diabetes and its management, including target ranges for blood sugar control. Instruct patient that medication is not a substitute for diet and exercise and to continue to follow prescribed regimens.
- Educate patient or caregiver regarding potential long-term complications of diabetes and need for regular general physical and eye examinations.
- Advise patient to read *Patient Information* leaflet before starting therapy and with each refill.
- Advise patient to take prescribed dose at the start (ie, with the first bite) of each main meal.
- Advise patient that medication will be started at a low dose and then gradually increased as tolerated until max benefit is obtained.
- Advise patient to take as prescribed and not to stop taking or change the dose unless advised by health care provider.
- Advise patient to continue to take other medications for diabetes as prescribed by health care provider.
- Advise patient that GI side effects (eg, gas, diarrhea, stomach discomfort) are common when therapy is started or the dose is increased, but that they should become less intense or frequent with continued therapy. Advise patient to inform health care provider if GI side effects persist or become intolerable.
- Ensure that patient understands how to use home glucose monitor and has a plan for monitoring and recording blood sugar measurements (eg, log). Advise patient to take log to each visit with health care provider.
- Educate patient regarding value of periodic hemoglobin A1c testing to confirm level of glucose control.
- Advise patient to discuss with health care provider a plan for managing each of the following situations: medication dosing during intercurrent conditions (eg, vomiting, infection, trauma, stress, sick days); accidental administration of too little or too much medication; missed dose; inadequate food intake or a skipped meal; travel across time zones; change in physical activity.
- Advise patient to carry medical identification of diabetes (eg, *Medi-Alert*).
- Review symptoms of hypoglycemia and hyperglycemia and action plans to undertake in the event either occur. Caution patient to use only readily available sources of glucose (dextrose) for treatment of hypoglycemic reactions and to avoid using table sugar (cane sugar) because acarbose prevents cane sugar from being absorbed.
- Instruct patient to notify health care provider if experiencing hypoglycemic episodes or if measured blood sugars are outside target range.
- Advise women to notify health care provider if pregnant, planning to become pregnant, or breastfeeding.
- Instruct patient not to take prescription or OTC drugs, dietary supplements, or herbal preparations without consulting health care provider.
- Advise patient that follow-up visits and lab tests will be necessary to monitor therapy and to keep appointments.

Acebutolol Hydrochloride

(ass-cee-BYOO-toe-lahl HIGH-droe-KLOR-ide)

Class Beta-adrenergic blocker

How Supplied
Sectral Capsules 200 mg, Capsules 400 mg
✤ *Apo-Acebutolol* ◆ *Gen-Acebutolol* ◆ *Gen-Acebutolol Type S* ◆ *Monitan* ◆ *Novo-Acebutolol* ◆ *Nu-Acebutolol* ◆ *Rhotral*

Action
PHARMACOLOGY: Blocks beta-receptors, primarily affecting heart (slows rate), vascular musculature (decreases BP), and lungs (reduces function).

PHARMACOKINETICS/DYNAMICS:
Absorption: Well absorbed. T_{max} is 2.5 hr (acebutolol) and 3.5 hr (diacetolol). Bioavailability is about 40%. Food may decrease the rate of absorption and C_{max} slightly.

Distribution: About 26% protein bound. Hydrophilic (minimally excreted into CSF). Crosses placenta and is excreted in breast milk.

Metabolism: Extensive first-pass hepatic biotransformation. Major metabolite is diacetolol (active; equipotent to acebutolol).

Excretion: $T_{1/2}$ is about 3 to 4 hr (acebutolol) and 8 to 13 hr (diacetolol). About 30% to 40% eliminated by kidneys, 50% to 60% eliminated by nonrenal mechanisms (ie, bile, feces). Dialyzable.

Onset: 1.5 hr.

Peak: 3 to 8 hr.

Special Populations:
Renal Function Impairment – Decreased elimination of diacetolol resulting in a 2- to 3-fold increase in its $t_{1/2}$. Administer with caution.
Elderly – Bioavailability increased about 2-fold.

Indications Management of hypertension and premature ventricular contractions.

Contraindications Hypersensitivity to beta-blockers; persistently severe bradycardia; greater than first-degree heart block; CHF, unless secondary to tachyarrhythmia treatable with beta-blockers; overt cardiac failure; sinus bradycardia; cardiogenic shock.

Route/Dosage

Hypertension
ADULTS: **PO** 400 mg qd initially in single or divided doses; usual response range is 200 to 1200 mg/day.
ELDERLY: May require lower maintenance doses. Do not exceed 800 mg qd.

Ventricular Arrhythmia
ADULTS: **PO** 400 mg (200 mg bid); may be titrated up to 1200 mg qd.

Interactions
Clonidine: May enhance or reverse acebutolol's antihypertensive effect; potentially life-threatening situations may occur, especially on withdrawal.
NSAIDs: Some agents may impair antihypertensive effect.
Prazosin: May cause increase in orthostatic hypotension.
Verapamil: Effects of both drugs may be increased.

Lab Test Interferences Antinuclear antibodies may develop; usually reversible on discontinuation. Acebutolol may interfere with glucose or insulin tolerance tests. May cause changes in serum lipids.

Adverse Reactions
CV: Hypotension; bradycardia; CHF; cold extremities; heart block.
CNS: Insomnia; fatigue; dizziness; depression; lethargy; drowsiness; forgetfulness.
DERM: Rash; hives; fever; alopecia.
EENT: Dry eyes; blurred vision; tinnitus; slurred speech; sore throat.
GI: Nausea; vomiting; diarrhea; dry mouth.
GU: Impotence; painful, difficult or frequent urination.
HEMA: Agranulocytosis; thrombocytopenia purpura.
RESP: Bronchospasm; dyspnea; wheezing.
OTHER: Weight changes; facial swelling; muscle weakness.

Precautions
Pregnancy: Category B.
Lactation: Excreted in breast milk.
Children: Safety and efficacy not established.
Renal function impairment: Reduction in daily dose is advised.
Hepatic function impairment: Reduction in daily dose is advised.
Abrupt withdrawal: Abrupt withdrawal is associated with adverse effects; gradually decrease dose over 1 to 2 wk.
Anaphylaxis: Serious reactions may occur; aggressive therapy may be required.
CHF: Administer cautiously in patients taking digitalis and diuretics for CHF.
Diabetes: Acebutolol may mask signs of hypoglycemia (eg, tachycardia, BP changes). May potentiate insulin-induced hypoglycemia.
Nonallergic bronchospasm (eg, chronic bronchitis, emphysema): In general, do not give beta blockers to patients with bronchospastic disease.
Peripheral vascular disease: Acebutolol may precipitate or aggravate symptoms of arterial insufficiency.
Thyrotoxicosis: Acebutolol may mask clinical signs of developing or continuing hyperthyroidism (eg, tachycardia). Abrupt withdrawal may exacerbate symptoms of hyperthyroidism, including thyroid storm.

PATIENT CARE CONSIDERATIONS

Administration/Storage
- Before giving initial dose, take patient's pulse. If pulse is less than 60 bpm, do not administer medication; notify health care provider.
- During initial phase of therapy, continue taking patient's pulse before administering each dose. After initial phase, take pulse before first dose of day and measure BP twice weekly.
- Store at room temperature.

Assessment/Interventions
- Obtain patient history, including drug history and any known allergies.

- Monitor serum lipid levels and thyroid function.
- Assess for signs of CHF (eg, shortness of breath, edema, decreased output) or respiratory involvement (eg, dyspnea, cough); if present, withhold drug and notify health care provider.

Patient/Family Education
- Teach patient to take pulse every day and record. If less than 60 bpm, tell not to take medication and to notify health care provider.
- Instruct diabetic patients to monitor blood sugar level q 6 hr. Drug may mask symptoms of hypoglycemia.
- Caution patient not to stop taking drug suddenly because doing so may exacerbate angina and increase possibility of MI.
- Explain that drug may cause dizziness. Advise patient to avoid sudden position changes to prevent orthostatic hypotension.
- Advise patient that drug may cause drowsiness and to use caution while driving or performing other tasks requiring mental alertness.
- Instruct patient not to take any otc medications without consulting health care provider.

Acetaminophen (N-Acetyl-p-Aminophenol; APAP)

(ass-cet-ah-MEE-noe-fen)

Class Analgesic/Antipyretic

How Supplied
Acephen Suppositories 120 mg, Suppositories 325 mg, Suppositories 650 mg ◆ Aceta Tablets 325 mg, Tablets 500 mg, Elixir 120 mg/5 mL ◆ Acetaminophen Unisents Suppositories 120 mg, Suppositories 325 mg, Suppositories 650 mg ◆ Apacet Tablets, chewable 80 mg, Solution 100 mg/mL ◆ Aspirin Free Anacin Maximum Strength Tablets 500 mg, Caplets 500 mg, Gelcaps 500 mg ◆ Aspirin Free Pain Relief Tablets 325 mg, Tablets 500 mg, Caplets 500 mg ◆ Children's Dynafed Jr. Tablets, chewable 80 mg ◆ Children's Feverall Suppositories 120 mg, Tablets, chewable 120 mg, Capsules, sprinkle 80 mg ◆ Children's Genapap Tablets, chewable 80 mg, Elixir 160 mg/5 mL ◆ Children's Halenol Liquid 160 mg/5 mL ◆ Children's Mapap Tablets, chewable 80 mg, Elixir 160 mg/5 mL ◆ Children's Panadol Tablets, chewable 80 mg, Liquid 160 mg/5 mL ◆ Children's Silapap Elixir 80 mg/2.5 mL ◆ Children's Tylenol Tablets, chewable 80 mg, Elixir 160 mg/5 mL ◆ Children's Tylenol Soft Chews Tablets, chewable 80 mg ◆ Dapacin Capsules 325 mg ◆ Extra Strength Dynafed E.X. Tablets 500 mg ◆ Feverall, Junior Strength Suppositories 325 mg, Capsules, sprinkle 160 mg ◆ Feverall, Infants Suppositories 80 mg ◆ Genapap Tablets 325 mg ◆ Genapap, Infants' Drops Solution 100 mg/mL ◆ Genapap Extra Strength Tablets 500 mg, Caplets 500 mg ◆ Genebs Tablets 325 mg ◆ Genebs Extra Strength Tablets 500 mg, Caplets 500 mg ◆ Infants' Pain Reliever Drops 80 mg/0.8 mL ◆ Infants' Silapap Solution 100 mg/mL ◆ Liquiprin Drops for Children Solution 80 mg/1.66 mL ◆ Mapap Extra Strength Tablets 500 mg ◆ Mapap Infant Drops Solution 100 mg/mL ◆ Mapap Regular Strength Tablets 325 mg ◆ Maranox Tablets 325 mg ◆ Meda Cap Capsules 500 mg ◆ Meda Tab Tablets 325 mg ◆ Neopap Suppositories 125 mg ◆ Oraphen-PD Elixir 120 mg/5 mL ◆ Panadol Tablets 500 mg, Caplets 500 mg ◆ Panadol, Infants' Drops Solution 100 mg/mL ◆ Redutemp Tablets 500 mg ◆ Ridenol Elixir 80 mg/5 mL ◆ Tapanol Extra Strength Tablets 500 mg, Caplets 500 mg, Gelcaps 500 mg ◆ Tapanol Regular Strength Tablets 325 mg ◆ Tempra Tablets 160 mg ◆ Tempra 1 Solution 100 mg/mL ◆ Tempra 2 Syrup Liquid 160 mg/5 mL ◆ Tempra 3 Tablets, chewable 80 mg ◆ Tylenol Arthritis Tablets, extended-release 650 mg ◆ Tylenol Caplets Tablets 325 mg ◆ Tylenol Extended Relief Caplets 650 mg ◆ Tylenol Extra Strength Tablets 500 mg, Gelcaps 500 mg, Liquid 500 mg/15 mL ◆ Tylenol Infants' Drops Solution 100 mg/mL ◆ Tylenol Junior Strength Tablets 160 mg ◆ Tylenol Regular Strength Tablets 325 mg ◆ Uni-Ace Solution 100 mg/mL ❀ Abenol ◆ Apo-Acetaminophen ◆ Atasol ◆ Pediatrix

Action

PHARMACOLOGY: Inhibits prostaglandins in CNS but lacks anti-inflammatory effects in periphery; reduces fever through direct action on hypothalamic heat-regulating center.

PHARMACOKINETICS/DYNAMICS:

Absorption: Rapid and complete from the GI tract. T_{max} is 0.5 to 2 hr; 4 hr after overdosage.

Distribution: Distributed throughout most body fluids. Binding to plasma proteins is variable.

Metabolism: Primarily metabolized by hepatic conjugation (94%), and about 4% is metabolized by CYP450 oxidase to toxic metabolite.

Excretion: $T_{1/2}$ is about 2 hr. 90% to 100% is recovered in the urine within the first day, primarily as inactive metabolites. 2% is excreted as unchanged drug.

Special Populations:
Neonates and cirrhotic patients – Half-life is slightly prolonged.

Indications Relief of mild to moderate pain; treatment of fever. **Unlabeled use(s):** Pain and fever prophylaxis after vaccination.

Contraindications Standard considerations.

Route/Dosage
ORAL
ADULTS: **PO** 325 to 650 mg prn q 4 to 6 hr or 1 g 3 to 4 times/day. Do not exceed 4 g/day.
CHILDREN: **PO** 10 to 15 mg/kg dose prn q 4 to 6 hr; do not exceed 5 doses/24 hr.

SUPPOSITORIES
ADULTS: **PR** 650 mg q 4 to 6 hr; do not exceed 6 suppositories/24 hr.
CHILDREN 3 TO 6 YR: **PR** 120 mg q 4 to 6 hr; do not exceed 720 mg/24 hr.
CHILDREN 6 TO 12 YR: **PR** 325 mg q 4 to 6 hr; do not exceed 2.6 g/24 hr.

Interactions
Ethanol: Chronic excessive use may increase risk of hepatotoxicity.
Hydantoins, sulfinpyrazone: May decrease therapeutic effect of APAP; concomitant long-term use may increase risk of hepatotoxicity.

Lab Test Interferences With *Chemstrip bG, Dextrostix, Visidex II* home blood glucose measurement systems, drug may cause more than 20% decrease in mean glucose.

Adverse Reactions
HEMA: Hemolytic anemia; neutropenia; leukopenia; pancytopenia; thrombocytopenia.
HEPA: Jaundice.
OTHER: Hypoglycemia; allergic skin eruptions or fever.

Precautions
Pregnancy: Category B.
Lactation: Excreted in breast milk.
Hepatic function impairment: Chronic alcoholics should not exceed 2 g/day.
Persistent pain or fever: May indicate serious illness. Consult health care provider.

Overdosage: Signs and Symptoms
Nausea, vomiting, abdominal pain, diarrhea, anorexia, malaise, diaphoresis, confusion, low BP, cardiac arrhythmias, jaundice, acute renal failure, liver failure.

PATIENT CARE CONSIDERATIONS
Administration/Storage
- Administer with water 30 min before or 2 hr after meals.
- Store tablets and capsules at room temperature in tightly closed container. Refrigerate suppositories. Refrigeration of elixir improves palatability.

Assessment/Interventions
- Obtain patient history, including drug history and any known allergies.
- Assess for pain and fever before and 1 to 2 hr after administration.
- Assess serum glucose and liver enzyme levels before long-term therapy.

Patient/Family Education
- Instruct family to consult health care provider for use in children less than 3 yr and, not to continue taking drug more than 5 days unless advised by health care provider.
- Instruct adult patients not to continue taking drug more than 10 days for pain or 3 days for fever.
- Instruct patient/family to contact health care provider if pain or fever (above 103°F) persists for more than 3 days.
- Advise diabetic patients to use sugar-free form of drug.

Acetaminophen with Codeine Phosphate

(ass-cet-ah-MEE-noe-fen with KOE-deen FOSS-fate)

Class Narcotic analgesic combination

How Supplied
Tylenol w/Codeine Elixir 12 mg codeine phosphate/120 mg acetaminophen ♦ *Capital w/Codeine* Suspension 12 mg codeine phosphate/120 mg acetaminophen ♦ *Tylenol w/Codeine No. 2* Tablets 15 mg codeine phosphate/300 mg acetaminophen ♦ *Aceta w/Codeine* Tablets 30 mg codeine phosphate/300 mg acetaminophen ♦ *Tylenol w/Codeine No. 3* Tablets 30 mg codeine phosphate/300 mg acetaminophen ♦ *Phenaphen w/Codeine No. 3* Capsules 30 mg codeine phosphate/325 mg acetaminophen ♦ *Tylenol w/Codeine No. 4* Tablets 60 mg codeine phosphate/300 mg acetaminophen ♦ *Phenaphen w/Codeine No. 4* Capsules 60 mg codeine phosphate/325 mg acetaminophen
※ *Triatec-30* ♦ *Tylenol Elixir with Codeine* ♦ *Tylenol with Codeine No. 4*

Action
PHARMACOLOGY: Inhibits synthesis of prostaglandins; binds to opiate receptors in CNS and peripherally blocks pain impulse generation; produces antipyresis by direct action on hypothalamic heat-regulating center; causes cough suppression by direct central action in medulla; may produce generalized CNS depression; does not have significant anti-inflammatory or antiplatelet effects.

Indications Relief of mild to moderate pain; analgesic-antipyretic therapy in presence of aspirin allergy, hemostatic disturbances, bleeding diatheses, upper GI disease and gouty arthritis.

Contraindications Hypersensitivity to codeine phosphate or similar compounds.

Route/Dosage
Tylenol No. 2 equals 15 mg codeine, 300 mg acetaminophen. *Tylenol No. 3* equals 30 mg codeine, 300 mg acetaminophen. *Tylenol No. 4* equals 60 mg codeine, 300 mg acetaminophen.
Max adult dose:
Codeine equals 360 mg/day; acetaminophen equals 4 g/day.

Tablets
ADULTS: **PO** Usually 1 to 2 tablets q 4 hr (varies according to product).
CHILDREN UNDER 12 YR: **PO** 0.5 to 1 mg codeine/kg/dose q 4 to 6 hr; 10 to 15 mg acetaminophen/kg/dose q 4 hr to max 2.6 g/24 hr.

Elixir
CHILDREN OLDER THAN 12 YR: **PO** 15 mL q 4 hr prn.
CHILDREN 7 TO 12 YR: **PO** 10 mL tid to qid prn.
CHILDREN 3 TO 6 YR: **PO** 5 mL tid to qid prn.

Interactions
Carbamazepine, hydantoins, sulfinpyrazone: May result in increased risk of hepatotoxicity.
Cimetidine: Effects of codeine may be enhanced, increasing toxicity.
CNS depressants (eg, barbiturates, ethyl alcohol, other narcotics): May result in additive CNS depressant effects and toxicity.
Tricyclic antidepressants, phenothiazines: May cause additive CNS depressant effects and toxicity.

Lab Test Interferences With *Chemstrip bG*, *Dextrostix*, and *Visidex II* home blood glucose systems, drug may cause false decrease in mean glucose values. False-positive results may occur in urinary 5-hydroxy-indoleacetic acid test.

Adverse Reactions
CV: Flushing.
CNS: Lightheadedness; dizziness; sedation; euphoria; insomnia; disorientation; incoordination.
DERM: Pruritus.
GI: Nausea; vomiting; dry mouth; constipation; abdominal pain.
RESP: Dyspnea; respiratory depression; decreased cough reflex.
OTHER: Histamine release.

Precautions
Pregnancy: Category C.
Lactation: Excreted in breast milk.
Hepatic function impairment: Acetaminophen intake must be limited to 2 g/day or less.
Sulfite sensitivity: Caution is needed with sulfite sensitive patients; some commercial preparations contain sodium bisulfite.

Overdosage: Signs and Symptoms
Blood dyscrasias, respiratory depression, hepatic damage (may occur up to several days after overdose).

PATIENT CARE CONSIDERATIONS
Administration/Storage
- Give with food or milk if GI distress occurs.
- Store in airtight, light-resistant container at room temperature.

Assessment/Interventions
- Obtain patient history, including drug history and any known allergies. Note pulmonary or hepatic disease, alcoholism, head injury, Addison disease, hypothyroidism, or previous addiction to narcotic drugs.
- Assess baseline level of pain before administration.
- Take vital signs before administration. Withhold dose if respiratory rate is less than 12 breaths/min (less than 20 in children) and notify health care provider.
- Consider related factors that may lower pain threshold (eg, anxiety, fear, boredom, environmental stressors).
- Assess cough for productiveness and effectiveness; auscultate for rales.
- Administer scheduled dose before pain becomes severe.
- Use the following adjunctive pain relief measures: massage, emotional support, diversion.
- If visual acuity is decreased by pupil constriction, keep room well lit during waking hours.
- Assess therapeutic effectiveness 1 hr after administration of dose based on patient's report of relief. Do not rely on objective signs.
- Reassess respiratory rate, depth, and rhythm after each dose. Notify health care provider if rate is less than 10 breaths/min or breathing is shallow.
- Assess for dizziness, sedation, euphoria, or confusion.
- Monitor for urinary retention or constipation.
- Monitor the following special-risk patients carefully: elderly, debilitated, those with increased intracranial pressure, pulmonary disease or conditions involving hypoxia or hypercapnia, history of drug dependence.
- Record degree and duration of pain relief. Notify health care provider if therapy is ineffective.
- Record any adverse or unusual reactions.
- If drowsiness or sedation occurs, institute safety precautions.
- Provide diet high in fiber; increase fluids to 2

to 3 L unless contraindicated.
- If constipation occurs, notify health care provider.
- Encourage patient to void q 3 to 4 hr.

Patient/Family Education
- Caution patient that drug dependency or tolerance may result from long-term use.
- Instruct patient not to discontinue medication abruptly after long-term regular use.
- Caution patient to avoid intake of alcohol and other CNS depressants without consulting health care provider.
- Advise patient that drug may cause drowsiness, and to use caution while driving or performing other tasks requiring mental alertness.
- Instruct patient to notify health care provider if the following signs/symptoms occur: persistence or recurrence of pain before next scheduled dose; difficulty breathing; blurred vision; increased drowsiness; severe nausea; vomiting; urinary retention; or yellowing of skin, sclera, or gums.
- Warn patient that orthostatic hypotension may occur; instruct patient to change positions slowly and to sit or lie down if symptoms occur.
- Explain that diaphoresis is a common side effect and does not indicate a problem.
- Warn patient that constipation may occur. Advise patient to increase dietary fiber and fluids unless contraindicated.
- Caution patient against taking *otc* medications that contain acetaminophen.

Acetazolamide

(uh-seet-uh-ZOLE-uh-mide)

Class Anticonvulsant/Carbonic anhydrase inhibitor

How Supplied
Acetazolamide Tablets 250 mg, Powder for injection, lyophilized 500 mg ◆ *Diamox Sequels* Capsules, sustained-release 500 mg
🍁 *APO-Acetazolamide*

Action
PHARMACOLOGY: Inhibits carbonic anhydrase enzyme, reducing rate of aqueous humor formation and thus lowering IOP; produces diuretic effect; retards neuronal conduction in brain.

PHARMACOKINETICS/DYNAMICS:
Absorption: Sustained release (SR) T_{max} is 3 to 6 hr. Immediate release (IR) T_{max} is 1 to 4 hr.
Onset: SR is 2 hr; IR is 1 to 1.5 hr; IV is 2 min.
Peak: SR is 3 to 6 hr; IR is 1 to 4 hr; IV is 15 min.
Duration: SR is 18 to 24 hr; IR is 8 to 12 hr; IV is 4 to 5 hr.

Indications Prevention or lessening of symptoms associated with acute mountain sickness (tablet only); adjunctive treatment of chronic simple (open-angle) glaucoma and secondary glaucoma; preoperative treatment of acute congestive (closed-angle) glaucoma; adjunctive treatment of 1) edema caused by CHF or drug-induced edema and 2) centrencephalic epilepsies (eg, petit mal, generalized seizures).

Contraindications Hypersensitivity to other sulfonamides; depressed sodium and/or potassium serum levels; marked kidney and liver disease or dysfunction; suprarenal gland failure; hyperchloremic acidosis; adrenocortical insufficiency; severe pulmonary obstruction with increased risk of acidosis; cirrhosis; long-term use in chronic noncongestive angle-closure glaucoma. Sustained release dosage form is not recommended for use as anticonvulsant or for treatment of edema caused by CHF or drug-induced edema.

Route/Dosage
Acute Mountain Sickness
ADULTS: **PO** 500 to 1,000 mg per day in divided doses.

Chronic Simple (Open-Angle) Glaucoma
ADULTS: **PO** 250 mg to 1 g per day, usually in divided doses for amounts above 250 mg.

Diuresis in CHF
ADULTS: **PO/IV** Initially 250 to 375 mg (5 mg/kg) every morning; then give on alternate days or for 2 days alternating with 1 day of rest.

Drug-Induced Edema
ADULTS: **PO/IV** 250 to 375 mg daily for 1 to 2 days, alternating with a day of rest.

Epilepsy
ADULTS: **PO/IV** 8 to 30 mg/kg per day in divided doses; optimum range 375 to 1,000 mg/day. When drug is given in combination with other anticonvulsants, initial dosage is 250 mg daily.

Secondary Glaucoma/Preoperative Treatment of Closed-Angle Glaucoma
ADULTS (SHORT-TERM CARE): **PO** 250 mg q 4 hr or 250 mg bid.
ACUTE CARE: **PO** Initially 500 mg; then 125 to 250 mg q 4 hr. IV therapy may be used for rapid relief of increased IOP. Direct IV administration is preferred because IM route is painful.

Interactions

Diflunisal: May cause significant decrease in IOP.
Primidone: Primidone concentrations may be altered.
Quinidine: Quinidine serum levels may be increased.
Salicylates: May cause acetazolamide accumulation and toxicity, including CNS depression and metabolic acidosis.

Lab Test Interferences
False-positive urinary protein results may occur because of alkalinization of urine.

Adverse Reactions

CNS: Drowsiness; confusion; sensory disturbances, including paresthesia and loss of appetite; convulsions.
DERM: Skin rash; urticaria.
EENT: Transient myopia; hearing disturbances; sore throat; tinnitus.
GI: Nausea; vomiting; diarrhea; melena; taste alterations.
GU: Polyuria; hematuria; glycosuria.
HEMA: Blood dyscrasias, including agranulocytosis and aplastic anemia; unusual bleeding or bruising.
HEPA: Hepatic insufficiency; fulminant hepatic necrosis.
METAB: Metabolic acidosis; electrolyte imbalance.
OTHER: Flaccid paralysis; fever; flank or loin pain; severe adverse reactions associated with sulfonamides, including Stevens-Johnson syndrome and toxic epidermal necrolysis; photosensitivity.

Precautions

Pregnancy: Category C.
Lactation: Undetermined.
Children: Safety and efficacy not established.
Dose increases: Increasing dose does not augment diuresis but may increase drowsiness and paresthesias.
Pulmonary conditions: Use in pulmonary obstruction and emphysema may aggravate or precipitate acidosis.

Overdosage: Signs and Symptoms
Electrolyte imbalance, acidosis, CNS effects.

PATIENT CARE CONSIDERATIONS

Administration/Storage

- Dose is individualized depending on condition being treated.
- May be used alone or in combination with other antiepileptic drugs (AEDs).
- Is used as an adjunct to usual therapy when treating glaucoma.
- Store sustained-release capsules at controlled room temperature (68° to 77°F). Store tablets and powder for injection at ambient room temperature (59° to 86°F). Store reconstituted injectable solution in refrigerator (36° to 46°F) for up to 3 days or use within 12 hr of reconstitution if stored at room temperature (59° to 86°F).

Tablets and Sustained-Release Capsules:

- Administer prescribed dose with a full glass of water.
- Administer without regard to meals but administer with food if GI upset occurs.
- Administer sustained-release capsules whole. Caution patient not to crush or chew capsule.

Powder for Injection:

- Direct IV administration is preferred because IM administration is painful due to alkaline pH of reconstituted solution. Not for intradermal, subcutaneous, or intra-arterial administration.
- Reconstitute following manufacturer's guidelines using at least 5 mL of sterile water for injection.
- Do not administer if particulate matter, cloudiness, or discoloration noted
- Discard any unused solution.

Assessment/Interventions

- Obtain patient history, including drug history and any known allergies. Note renal or hepatic impairment, hypokalemia, hyponatremia, hyperchloremic acidosis, adrenocortical insufficiency, angle-closure glaucoma, high dose aspirin therapy, COPD, or allergy to sulfonamide antibiotics or chemically related drugs (eg, sulfonylureas, thiazide and loop diuretics).
- Ensure that for patient being treated for glaucoma that IOPs are measured and documented in the patient's record before starting therapy and periodically during therapy.
- Ensure that CBC with differential and platelet count, urinalysis, and serum electrolytes are evaluated before therapy is started and periodically thereafter during prolonged therapy.
- Monitor patient for signs of allergic reaction. Discontinue therapy and immediately notify health care provider if noted. Be prepared to treat appropriately.
- Implement seizure precautions for patient being treated for epilepsy. Provide a quiet, nonstimulating environment.
- Monitor patient for GI, CNS, DERM, and general body side effects. Report to health care provider if noted and significant.
- Withhold drug and notify health care provider immediately if any of the following

symptoms occur: sore throat, fever, pallor, purpura, hematuria, unusual bleeding or bruising.

Patient/Family Education
- Explain name, dose, action, and potential side effects of drug.
- Advise patient or caregiver that injection will be prepared and administered by a health care provider in a health care setting.
- Advise patient with glaucoma to continue to use other glaucoma medications prescribed by health care provider unless advised otherwise.
- Advise patient with epilepsy to continue to use other AEDs prescribed by health care provider unless advised otherwise.
- Review dosing schedule with patient.
- Advise patient to take each dose with a full (8 oz) glass of water without regard to meals. Advise patient to take with food if stomach upset occurs.
- Advise patient using sustained-release capsules to swallow whole. Caution patient not to crush or chew capsule.
- Advise patient urine production may increase following the first few doses of the medication and that this is normal and of no concern. Advise patient to inform health care provider if excessive urine production occurs.
- Advise patient to drink fluids liberally (eg, eight 8 oz glasses of water daily) while taking this medication.
- Advise patient using medication for preventing symptoms of high altitude sickness that if rapid ascent produces symptoms of high altitude sickness, rapid descent is necessary.
- Advise patient to discontinue therapy and contact health care provider immediately if any of the following occur: rash, hives, itching, sore throat, unexplained fever, pallor, purple spots under the skin, unusual bleeding or bruising, blood in urine, tingling or tremors in hands or feet, ringing in ears or hearing changes, flank or loin pain.
- Advise patient to avoid unnecessary exposure to sunlight or tanning lamps and to use sunscreen and wear protective clothing to avoid photosensitivity reactions.
- Advise patient that drug may cause drowsiness and to use caution while driving or performing other tasks requiring mental alertness until tolerance is determined.
- Advise women to notify health care provider if pregnant, planning to become pregnant, or breastfeeding.
- Instruct patient to not take any prescription or OTC medications, dietary supplements, or herbal preparations unless advised by health care provider.
- Advise patient that follow-up examinations and lab tests will be required to monitor therapy and to keep appointments.

Acetohexamide

(uh-seet-toe-HEX-uh-mide)

Class Antidiabetic/Sulfonylurea

How Supplied
Dymelor Tablets 250 mg, Tablets 500 mg

Action
PHARMACOLOGY: Decreases blood glucose by stimulating release of insulin from pancreas.

PHARMACOKINETICS/DYNAMICS:
Absorption: Rapidly absorbed.
Metabolism: Active metabolite is hydroxyhexamide.
Excretion: Plasma $t_{1/2}$ is 1.3 hr (acetohexamide) and 6 hr (hydroxyhexomide). More than 80% is excreted in 24 hr, mostly as metabolites.
Peak: 3 hr.
Duration: 12 to 24 hr.
Special Populations:
Renal Function Impairment – May have elevated blood levels of acetohexamide.
Hepatic Function Impairment – May have elevated blood levels of acetohexamide.

Indications Adjunctive therapy, used with dietary modification, in patients with noninsulin-dependent diabetes mellitus (type II) for lowering blood glucose level.

Contraindications Hypersensitivity to sulfonylureas; diabetes complicated by ketoacidosis; sole therapy of insulin-dependent (type I) diabetes mellitus; diabetes complicated by pregnancy.

Route/Dosage
ADULTS: PO 250 mg to 1.5 g/day. In patients receiving 1 g/day or less, condition can be controlled with once-daily dosage; 1.5 g/day is given bid (max, 1.5 g/day).

Interactions
Androgens, chloramphenicol, clofibrate, fenfluramine, H_2 antagonists, MAOIs, phenylbutazone, probenecid, salicylates, sulfonamides: Hypoglycemic effect may be increased.
Diazoxide, rifampin, thiazide diuretics: Hypoglycemic effect of acetohexamide may be decreased.

Lab Test Interferences Elevated liver function. Mild to moderate elevations in BUN and creatinine.

Adverse Reactions

CV: Possible increased risk of cardiovascular mortality as compared with treatment with diet alone.
CNS: Dizziness; vertigo.
DERM: Allergic skin reactions; eczema; pruritus; erythema; urticaria; morbilliform or maculopapular eruptions, lichenoid reactions; photosensitivity.
EENT: Tinnitus.
GI: Nausea; epigastric fullness; heartburn; cholestatic jaundice (rare, discontinue drug if this occurs).
GU: Mild diuresis.
HEMA: Leukopenia; thrombocytopenia; aplastic anemia; agranulocytosis; hemolytic anemia; pancytopenia.
HEPA: Hepatic porphyria.
METAB: Hypoglycemia.
OTHER: Disulfiram-like reaction; weakness; paresthesia, fatigue; malaise.

Precautions

Pregnancy: Category C. Insulin is recommended to maintain blood glucose levels during pregnancy. Prolonged severe neonatal hypoglycemia can occur if sulfonylureas are administered at time of delivery.
Lactation: Undetermined.
Children: Safety and efficacy not established.
Elderly: Particularly susceptible to hypoglycemic effects of drug.
Renal function impairment: Cautious use is necessary.
Hepatic function impairment: Cautious use is necessary.
Disulfiram-like syndrome: Alcohol may cause facial flushing and breathlessness.
Hypoglycemia: May be difficult to recognize in elderly patients or in patients receiving beta-blockers.
Loss of blood glucose control: Stress (eg, fever, surgery) or secondary drug failure may precipitate loss of blood glucose control.

Overdosage: Signs and Symptoms

Hypoglycemia, mild hypoglycemia without loss of consciousness and no neurologic findings, severe hypoglycemic reactions.

PATIENT CARE CONSIDERATIONS

Administration/Storage

- Administer at same time each day, with food if desired.
- Do not give more than 1.5 g/day.
- For amounts over 1 g, administer in divided doses before morning and evening meals.
- Store tablets in tightly closed container at room temperature.

Assessment/Interventions

- Obtain patient history, including drug history and any known allergies.
- Assess condition of patient's feet, and routinely perform foot care.
- Note baseline liver function, BUN, and creatinine. Monitor for elevated levels.
- Assess current blood glucose levels. Observe patient for signs of hyperglycemia (eg, frequent urination, thirst, weakness, weight loss, ketoacidosis) and hypoglycemia (eg, tingling of lips and tongue, nausea, diminished cerebral function [eg, lethargy, confusion], tachycardia, sweating, convulsions, coma). Have oral glucose or carbohydrates and IV glucose available.
- Monitor liver and renal function regularly.
- Monitor effectiveness of diabetes control through individualized treatment plan, including diet, daily blood glucose levels, medication, and exercise.

Patient/Family Education

- Advise patient that drug may be taken with food if nausea occurs.
- Review symptoms of hypoglycemia and hyperglycemia.
- Emphasize importance of wearing *Medi-Alert* bracelet at all times.
- Instruct patient to call health care provider if any of the following symptoms occur: nausea, vomiting, heartburn, diarrhea, fever, sore throat, rash, itching, weakness, unusual bruising, bleeding.
- Caution patient about the following possible effects of alcohol intake: flushing, weakness, dizziness, tingling sensation, headache.
- Caution patient to avoid exposure to sunlight, and to use sunscreen or wear protective clothing to avoid photosensitivity reaction.
- Advise patient not to take any OTC medications without consulting health care provider.

Acetylcysteine (N-Acetylcysteine)

(ASS-cee-till-SIS-teen)

Class Respiratory inhalant/Mucolytic

How Supplied
Acetadote Injection 20% (200 mg/mL) ♦
Mucomyst Solution 10% (as sodium), Solution 20% (as sodium)
 *Parvolex*

Action

PHARMACOLOGY: Decreases thickness of mucous secretions in lung.

PHARMACOKINETICS/DYNAMICS:

Absorption:
Oral – C_{max} is 0.35 to 4 mg/L; T_{max} is 1 to 2 hr.

Distribution:
IV – Vd is 0.47 L/kg, and 83% protein bound.
Oral – About 50% protein bound. Vd is 0.33 to 0.47 L/kg.

Metabolism:
Inhalation – Undergoes rapid deacetylation to yield cysteine or oxidation to yield diacetylcysteine.

Excretion:
IV – The t½ is 5.6 hr. The mean Cl is 0.11 L/hr/kg, renally about 30% of total Cl.
Oral – The t½ is 6.25 hr. About 70% is excreted by nonrenal mechanisms.

Special Populations:
Hepatic Function Impairment – For severe liver impairment, primary and/or secondary biliary cirrhosis, t½ increased 80%, Cl decreased 30%.
Children – The t½ is increased to 11 hr.

Indications Reduction of viscosity of bronchopulmonary mucous secretions in patients with chronic or acute lung diseases, pulmonary complications associated with cystic fibrosis, surgery, anesthesia, or atelectasis caused by mucous obstruction; diagnostic bronchial studies; tracheostomy care, posttraumatic chest conditions (oral solution); prevention or lessening of liver damage after potentially toxic quantity of acetaminophen (oral or IV). **Unlabeled use(s):** Ophthalmic preparation for dry eyes; enema for bowel obstruction.

Contraindications Standard considerations.

Route/Dosage

ADULTS: **Nebulization (face mask, mouthpiece, tracheostomy)** 1 to 10 mL (usually 3 to 5 mL) of 20% solution or 2 to 20 mL (usually 6 to 10 mL) of 10% solution q 2 to 6 hr (usually tid or qid); (nebulization tent) large volumes (up to 300 mL) during treatment period. **Instillation:** 1 to 2 mL of 10% to 20% solution as often as q 1 hr.

Diagnostic Bronchograms
2 to 3 administrations of 1 to 2 mL of 20% solution or 2 to 4 mL of 10% solution by nebulization or tracheal instillation before procedure.

Acetaminophen Overdose
After appropriate overdose procedures (eg, lavage, induction of emesis), **PO** 140 mg/kg as oral loading dose (diluted with diet soft drink). Then 70 mg/kg orally 4 hr after loading dose and repeated at 4-hr intervals for total of 17 doses, unless acetaminophen assay indicates otherwise. **IV** On admission, draw a serum blood sample at least 4 hr after ingestion to determine the acetaminophen level, which will serve as a basis for determining the need for acetylcysteine treatment. If patient presents 4 hr postingestion, determine acetylcysteine serum sample immediately. Administer acetylcysteine within 8 hr from acetaminophen ingestion for max protection against hepatic injury. If time of ingestion is unknown, or acetaminophen level is not available, administer acetylcysteine immediately if 24 hr or less has elapsed from the time of the reported overdose ingestion of acetaminophen, regardless of quantity reported to have been ingested. Critical ingestion-treatment interval for max protection against severe hepatic injury is 0 to 8 hr. Efficacy diminishes progressively after 8 hr and treatment initiated 15 hr postingestion of acetaminophen yields limited efficacy. However, it does not appear to worsen the condition and should not be withheld.
Loading dose – 150 mg/kg in 200 mL of 5% dextrose; infuse over 15 min.
Maintenance dose – 50 mg/kg in 500 mL of 5% dextrose; infuse over 4 hr followed by 100 mg/kg in 1,000 mL of 5% dextrose infused over 16 hr.

Interactions None well documented.
INCOMPATIBILITIES: Do not mix with tetracycline, chlortetracycline, oxytetracycline, erythromycin lactobionate, amphotericin B, ampicillin sodium, iodized oil, chymotrypsin, trypsin, or hydrogen peroxide.

Lab Test Interferences None well documented.

Adverse Reactions
CV: Tachycardia, hypotension, hypertension, chest tightness (oral); tachycardia, chest tightness (greater than 1%; IV).
CNS: Drowsiness (oral).
DERM: Rash, pruritus, angioedema (oral); pruritus, rash, flushing (greater than 1%; IV).
EENT: Rhinorrhea (oral); ear pain, pharyngitis, throat tightness (greater than 1%; IV).
GI: Nausea, vomiting, stomatitis (oral); nausea, vomiting (greater than 1%; IV).
HYPERSEN: Anaphylactoid reactions (greater than 1%; IV).
RESP: Bronchospasm, bronchial irritation

(oral); rhinorrhea, rhonchi (greater than 1%; IV).
OTHER: Fever, clamminess (oral).

Precautions
Pregnancy: Category B.
Lactation: Undetermined.
Anaphylactoid reaction: Serious anaphylactoid reactions, including death, have been reported with IV administration.
Antidotal use: If allergic reaction, encephalopathy, or severe, persistent vomiting occurs, discontinuation of drug may be necessary.
Asthmatic bronchospasm: Use with caution. If bronchospasm progresses, medication must be discontinued immediately.
Bronchial secretions: Increased secretion volume may occur. When cough is inadequate, open airway may need to be maintained by mechanical suction.
Cutaneous reactions: Acute flushing and erythema may occur with IV use.

PATIENT CARE CONSIDERATIONS
Administration/Storage
Mucolytic:
- For inhalation or direct instillation into bronchial tree. Not for parenteral administration.
- The 10% solution may be used undiluted.
- The 20% solution may be diluted to a lesser concentration using sodium chloride for injection or inhalation, or sterile water for injection or inhalation.
- Because compatibility with other medications may vary between manufacturers of acetylcysteine, refer to individual manufacturer's guidelines before combining with other medications or solvents. If an admixture is prepared, administer as soon as possible after preparation. Do not store admixtures for future use.
- When using nebulizer, administer prescribed dose q 2 to 6 hr by mouthpiece, facemask, or tracheostomy, as ordered by health care provider.
- Do not use nebulization equipment that contains iron, copper, or rubber because of potential for corrosion. Use glass, plastic, aluminum, anodized aluminum, chromed metal, tantalum, sterling silver, or stainless steel equipment. Silver may become tarnished after exposure to acetylcysteine, but this is not harmful to the patient and does not reduce the effectiveness of the medication.
- Clean nebulizing equipment immediately after use to prevent clogging of small orifices or corrosion of metal parts.
- To prevent concentration of medication during prolonged nebulization add sterile water for injection to canister when three fourths of initial volume of acetylcysteine has been administered. The amount of sterile water for injection added should be approximately equal to the volume of solution remaining.
- When using nebulization tent or croupette, use enough volume of acetylcysteine to maintain a heavy mist in the tent or croupette for the prescribed length of therapy (eg, overnight).
- When administering directly into bronchial tree, prescribed dose may be used q 1 to 4 hr.
- Store unopened vials at controlled room temperature (59° to 86°F). Once opened, store any unused solution in refrigerator (36° to 46°F). Discard any unused solution after 96 hr.

Oral Solution for Acetaminophen Overdose:
- Administer initial dose as soon as possible within 24 hr of ingestion. Max protection is obtained if acetylcysteine is administered within 8 hr of ingestion.
- To reduce propensity of oral acetylcysteine to cause or aggravate vomiting, dilute 10% and 20% solution with diet cola or other diet soft drink to provide an oral solution with a final concentration of 5%. Administer diluted solution within 1 hr of preparation.
- Repeat any oral dose if patient vomits within 1 hr of administration.
- May dilute with water and administer via duodenal intubation if patient is unable to retain the orally administered acetylcysteine.
- Store unopened vials at controlled room temperature (59° to 86°F). Once opened, store any unused solution in refrigerator (36° to 46°F). Discard any unused solution after 96 hr.

Injection for Acetaminophen Overdose:
- For IV infusion only. Not for IV bolus, intradermal, subcutaneous, IM, or intra-arterial administration.
- Administer initial dose as soon as possible within 24 hr of ingestion. Max protection is obtained if acetylcysteine is administered within 8 hr of ingestion.
- Dilute injection concentrate with 5% dextrose for loading dose and maintenance doses following manufacturer's guidelines.
- Do not mix with other IV medications or dilute with any IV solution other than 5% dextrose.
- Do not administer injection if particulate matter, cloudiness, or discoloration noted.
- Discard any remaining injection concentrate from single dose vial. Do not save for future

use or use if vial has been previously opened.
- Store unopened vials at controlled room temperature (68° to 77°F). Diluted solution is stable for up to 24 hr at controlled room temperature.

Assessment/Interventions

- Obtain patient history, including drug history and any known allergies. Note history of asthma, bronchospasm, or previous anaphylactoid reaction to acetylcysteine.

Mucolytic:

- Assess airway patency, baseline lung sounds, and effectiveness of cough.
- Assess response to treatment. If increased volume of liquified secretions is noted and cough is inadequate to clear, maintain airway by mechanical suction.
- Assess patient for development of airway obstruction. If rapid onset of bronchospasm occurs, discontinue therapy and notify health care provider immediately. Be prepared to treat with a nebulized, short-acting bronchodilator.
- Monitor patient for GI, RESP, and general body side effects. Inform health care provider if noted and significant.

Acetaminophen Overdose:

- Ensure that appropriate emergency treatment of the ingestion (eg, gastric emptying) has been completed before administering oral acetylcysteine. If activated charcoal has been administered, ensure that gastric lavage to remove it has been performed before administering oral acetylcysteine.
- Ensure that blood for baseline acetaminophen plasma level, liver enzymes, bilirubin, prothrombin time, electrolytes, blood sugar, BUN, and creatinine has been drawn before initiating therapy and then daily for duration of therapy.
- Ensure that supportive treatment of acetaminophen overdose (eg, maintain fluid and electrolyte balance, treatment of hypoglycemia, vitamin K, or fresh frozen plasma for coagulopathy) is provided.
- Monitor patient for signs and symptoms of anaphylactic or serious allergic reactions. Be prepared to treat appropriately. Discontinue acetylcysteine unless it is deemed necessary and the allergic reaction can be controlled with appropriate treatment.
- Frequently assess patient for encephalopathy caused by hepatic failure. If encephalopathy develops, be prepared to discontinue acetylcysteine to avoid further administration of nitrogenous substances.
- Ensure that appropriate follow-up counseling is provided for patient who deliberately ingested acetaminophen.

Patient/Family Education

- Explain name, dose, action, and potential side effects of drug.

Mucolytic:

- Instruct patient or caregiver not to change the dose or stop taking unless advised by health care provider.
- Advise patient or caregiver that medication has a disagreeable odor (rotten eggs) but that this should become unnoticeable after continued use.
- Advise patient or caregiver that treatment is expected to increase volume of respiratory secretions and that effective coughing will be required to clear the secretions. Advise patient or caregiver to immediately notify health care provider if respiratory secretions cannot be adequately removed by coughing.
- Advise patient or caregiver that administration using face mask may leave a sticky residue on the face that can be easily removed by washing with water.
- Advise patient that medication may turn a light purple color after opening bottle. Advise patient that this is normal and does not alter the safety or effectiveness of the medication.
- Caution patient or caregiver to dilute the nebulizer solution with sterile water for injection to prevent the solution from becoming concentrated and plugging the nebulizer.
- Caution patient or caregiver not to add other medications or solutions to nebulizer canister unless advised by health care provider.
- Advise patient or caregiver to notify health care provider if any of the following occur: rash or other signs or allergic reaction, new or worsening wheezing, chest tightness or difficulty breathing, persistent nausea or vomiting, coughing up blood, fever, or other signs of respiratory infection.
- Advise women to notify health care provider if pregnant, planning to become pregnant, or breastfeeding.
- Instruct patient not to take any prescription or OTC medications, dietary supplements, or herbal preparations unless advised by health care provider.
- Advise patient that follow-up visits will be required to monitor therapy and to keep appointments.

Acetaminophen Overdose:

- Advise patient, family, or caregiver that medication will be prepared and administered by a health care professional in a hospital setting.

Acitretin

(ASS-ih-TREH-tin)

Class Retinoid

How Supplied
Soriatane Capsules 10 mg, Capsules 25 mg

Action

PHARMACOLOGY: Unknown.

PHARMACOKINETICS/DYNAMICS:

Absorption: Absorption is linear and proportional with increasing doses; approximately 72% is absorbed following a 50 mg dose. C_{max} (mean 416 ng/mL) is achieved in 2 to 5 hr.

Distribution: Plasma protein binding is 99.9%, primarily to albumin.

Metabolism: Undergoes extensive metabolism to cis-acitretin.

Excretion: Excreted in the feces (34% to 54%) and urine (16% to 53%). Terminal t½ of acitretin is 49 hr; t½ of cis-acitretin is 63 hr.

Special Populations:
Elderly – Higher plasma concentrations are seen; however, no changes occur in the t½.
Renal failure – Plasma concentrations are lower in end-stage renal failure. Acitretin is not removed by dialysis.

Indications Treatment of severe psoriasis.

Contraindications Pregnancy; severe liver or kidney function impairment; chronic abnormal elevation in blood lipid values; concurrent use of methotrexate or tetracyclines; hypersensitivity to other retinoids or any component of the product.

Route/Dosage

ADULTS: **PO** Start with 25 to 50 mg/day given as a single dose with the main meal. Maintenance doses of 25 to 50 mg/day may be given dependent upon the patient's response to initial treatment.

Relapse

ADULTS: **PO** Relapses may be treated as outlined for initial treatment.

Phototherapy

ADULTS: **PO** When used with phototherapy, the phototherapy dose should be decreased by the prescriber based upon the patient's individual response.

Interactions

Ethanol: Concurrent use of alcohol and acitretin may lead to the formation of etretinate, which increases the duration of teratogenic potential in women.

Glyburide: The glucose-lowering effect of glyburide may be potentiated.

Methotrexate: Because the risk of hepatitis may be increased, concurrent use is contraindicated.

Phenytoin: Protein binding of phenytoin may be reduced.

Progestin "minipill": Acitretin may interfere with the contraceptive effect.

Tetracyclines: Because acitretin and tetracyclines can cause increased intracranial pressure, concurrent use is contraindicated.

Vitamin A, oral retinoids: Because the risk of hypervitaminosis A is increased, concurrent use is contraindicated.

Lab Test Interferences None well documented.

Adverse Reactions

CV: Acute MI, thromboembolism, stroke (postmarketing).
CNS: Rigors (10% to 25%); headache, pain, depression, insomnia, somnolence (1% to 10%); myopathy with peripheral neuropathy, aggressive feelings and/or suicidal thoughts (postmarketing).
DERM: Alopecia, skin peeling (60% to 75%); dry skin, nail disorder, pruritus (25% to 50%); erythematous rash, hyperesthesia, paresthesia, paronychia, skin atrophy, sticky skin (10% to 25%); abnormal skin odor, abnormal hair texture, bullous eruption, cold/clammy skin, dermatitis, increased sweating, psoriasiform rash, purpura, pyogenic granuloma, rash, seborrhea, skin fissures, skin ulceration, sunburn, infection (1% to 10%); skin thinning, skin fragility and scaling (postmarketing).

EENT: Rhinitis (25% to 50%); dry eyes (23%); xerophthalmia, epistaxis (10% to 25%); eye irritation (9%); brow and lash loss (5%); Bell palsy, blepharitis, crusting of eye lids, blurred vision, conjunctivitis, corneal epithelial abnormality, cortical cataract, decreased night vision/night blindness, diplopia, itchy eyes or eyelids, nuclear cataract, pannus, papilledema, photophobia, posterior subcapsular cataract, recurrent sties, subepithelial corneal lesions (less than 5%); eye pain, sinusitis, earache, taste perversion, tinnitus (1% to 10%).
ELECDIST: Increased phosphorus, potassium, sodium, magnesium, decreased magnesium (10% to 25%); increased calcium, chloride, decreased calcium, chloride, phosphorus, potassium, sodium (1% to 10%).
GI: Cheilitis (greater than 75%); dry mouth (10% to 25%); abdominal pain, diarrhea, nausea, tongue disorder, stomatitis, ulcerative stomatitis (1% to 10%).
GU: White blood cells in urine (25% to 50%); acetonuria, hematuria, red blood cells in urine (10% to 25%); glycosuria, proteinuria (1% to 10%); vulvo-vaginitis from *Candida albicans* (postmarketing).
HEMA: Increased reticulocytes (25% to 50%); decreased hematocrit, hemoglobin, WBC (10% to 25%); increased haptoglobin, neutrophils, WBC (10% to 25%); increased bands, basophils, eosinophils, hematocrit, hemoglobin, lymphocytes, monocytes, platelets, red blood cells, decreased haptoglobin, lymphocytes, neutrophils, reticulocytes, platelets, RBC (1% to 10%).
HEPA: Increased cholesterol, LDH, AST, ALT, decreased HDL (25% to 50%); increased alkaline phosphatase, direct bilirubin, gamma-glutamyl transpeptidase (10% to 25%); increased globulin, total bilirubin, total protein, serum albumin, decreased serum albumin (1% to 10%).
MUSC: Arthralgia, spinal hyperostosis (10% to 25%); arthritis, arthrosis, back pain, hypertonia, myalgia, osteodynia, peripheral joint hyperostosis (1% to 10%).
RENAL: Increased uric acid (10% to 25%); increased BUN, creatinine (1% to 10%).
OTHER: Increased triglycerides (50% to 75%); increased CPK, fasting blood glucose (25% to 50%); decreased fasting blood sugar, high occult blood (10 to 25%); anorexia, edema, fatigue, hot flashes, increased appetite, gingival bleeding, gingivitis, increased salivation, thirst, infection, decreased and increased iron, flushing (1% to 10%).

> **WARNING:**
> Acitretin must not be used by women who are pregnant or intend to become pregnant during therapy or at any time for at least 3 yr following discontinuation of therapy. Acitretin must not be used by women who may not use reliable contraception while undergoing treatment or for at least 3 yr following discontinuation of treatment. Women must sign a Patient Agreement/Information Consent Form that contains warnings about the risk of potential birth defects. An acitretin medication guide must be given to patients each time acitretin is dispensed, as required by law. If pregnancy occurs during therapy or at any time for at least 3 yr after stopping therapy, the prescriber and patient should discuss the possible effects on the pregnancy.
>
> *Hepatotoxicity:* Hepatotoxicity, hepatitis, and hepatitis related deaths may occur.

Precautions
Pregnancy: Category X.
Lactation: Excreted in breast milk.
Children: Safety and efficacy not established.
Photosensitivity: May occur; avoid excessive use of sunlamps, exposure to sunlight, and ultraviolet light.
Blood donation: Patients should not donate blood during and for at least 3 yr following completion of acitretin therapy.
Hyperostosis: Examine patient for possible ossification abnormalities.
Lipid effects and CV risk: Elevation in triglycerides and cholesterol may occur; decreased HDL may occur. CV risk status may be increased.
Pancreatitis: Pancreatitis (including fatal fulminant pancreatitis) with or without elevated triglyceride levels may occur.
Pseudotumor cerebri: May occur.
Psychiatric disorder: Depression and other psychiatric symptoms such as aggressive feeling or thought of self-harm may occur.
Vision: Night vision and tolerance to contact lenses may be decreased.

Overdosage: Signs and Symptoms
Identical to acute hypervitaminosis A (headache, vertigo).

PATIENT CARE CONSIDERATIONS
Administration/Storage
- Administer prescribed dose qd with the main meal.
- Store capsules at controlled room temperature (59° to 77°F). Protect from light. Avoid exposure to high temperatures and humidity after bottle is opened.

Assessment/Interventions
- Obtain patient history, including drug history and any known allergies. Note renal impairment, hepatic impairment, pregnancy, breastfeeding, hyperlipidemia, CV disease, depression or history of depression, history of taking etretinate, and concurrent use of methotrexate, tetracyclines, phenytoin, vitamin A supplements, St. John's wort, etretinate, or phototherapy.
- Ensure that blood lipids are evaluated before starting therapy and q 1 to 2 wk thereafter until the lipid response to acitretin is determined.
- Ensure that liver enzymes are determined before starting therapy and q 1 to 2 wk until stable and then periodically thereafter as clinically indicated.
- Ensure that Patient Agreement/Informed Consent for Female Patients has been reviewed with and signed by female patient.
- Ensure that sexually active women have 2 negative pregnancy tests before starting therapy.
- Ensure that sexually active women who are not clearly postmenopausal or have undergone a hysterectomy are using 2 reliable forms of contraception beginning 1 mo before starting therapy, during therapy, and understand the need to continue effective contraception for 3 yr following cessation of therapy.
- Ensure that women of childbearing potential do not consume alcohol or products containing alcohol during and for 2 mo following cessation of therapy.
- Monitor blood sugar levels frequently in diabetic patients receiving acitretin. Inform health care provider if significant changes are noted.
- Monitor patients for signs and symptoms of pseudotumor cerebri (headache, nausea, vomiting, visual changes). Inform health care provider if noted.
- Monitor patient for psychiatric side effects. Notify health care provider immediately if depression or other psychiatric symptoms are noted.
- Monitor patient for GI, CNS, DERM, musculoskeletal, and general body side effects. Inform health care provider if noted and significant.

Patient/Family Education
- Advise patient to review *Medication Guide* before starting therapy and with each refill.
- Explain name, dose, action, and potential side effects of drug.
- Advise patient that dose may be adjusted based on tolerance and effectiveness.
- Instruct patient to take prescribed dose qd with main meal. Advise patient that food increases absorption and beneficial effects.
- Advise patient that if a dose is missed to skip the missed dose and resume the normal schedule. Caution patient not to double the dose to try to catch up.
- Advise patient that psoriasis may worsen during the initial treatment period but that gradual improvement should follow and max benefit may not be noted for 2 to 3 mo. Advise patient to notify health care provider if symptoms do not improve as expected or continue to worsen.
- Caution women of childbearing potential not to consume alcohol or products containing alcohol during and for 2 mo following cessation of therapy.
- Instruct sexually active women who are not clearly menopausal or have undergone a hysterectomy to use 2 reliable forms of contraception beginning 1 mo before starting therapy, during therapy, and for 3 yr following cessation of therapy. Caution patient that micro-dosed progestin "minipills" are not recommended during therapy with acitretin.
- Advise women of childbearing potential to notify health care provider immediately if pregnant, miss a period, or have sex without using 2 effective forms of birth control either while taking acitretin or for 3 yr following cessation of therapy.
- Caution both men and women not to donate blood during and for at least 3 yr following cessation of therapy because women of childbearing potential must not receive blood from patients being treated with acitretin.
- Advise patient, family, or caregiver to inform health care provider of the following: persistent severe headache; persistent nausea and/or vomiting; yellowing of the skin or eyes; dark urine; persistent appetite loss; frequent urination; great thirst or unexplained hunger; sudden vision changes; severe skin or mucus membrane dryness; depression or other mental symptoms; shortness of breath; dizziness; chest pain; sudden weakness; trouble speaking; swelling of a leg.

- Advise patient that medication can cause chapped lips, peeling of the fingertips, palms, and soles, itching or scaly skin, runny or dry nose, or nosebleeds and to inform health care provider if any of these occur and are bothersome. Advise patient that health care provider or pharmacist can recommend a lotion or cream to help treat drying or chapping.
- Advise patient that drug may cause decreased night vision and to avoid driving at night if any sudden vision problems occur.
- Advise diabetic patient to monitor blood sugars more frequently when medication is started or after a dose adjustment and to inform health care provider if significant changes in blood sugar are noted.
- Caution patient that medication can increase sensitivity to UV light and to avoid use of sun lamps and unnecessary exposure to sunlight while undergoing treatment.
- Advise patient wearing contact lenses that decreased tolerance to lenses may be experienced during treatment and after therapy has been stopped.
- Instruct patient not to take any prescription or OTC medications or dietary supplements unless advised by health care provider. Caution patient against taking vitamin A supplements in excess of recommended daily allowances.
- Advise patient that follow-up examinations and lab tests will be required to monitor therapy and to keep appointments.

Acrivastine/ Pseudoephedrine Hydrochloride

(ACK-rih-VASS-teen/SUE-doe-eh-FED-rin HIGH-droe-KLOR-ide)

Class Antihistamine/Decongestant

How Supplied
Semprex-D Capsules 8 mg acrivastine/60 mg pseudoephedrine

Action
PHARMACOLOGY: Acrivastine: Competitively blocks histamine at H_2 receptor sites; pseudoephedrine: causes vasoconstriction and subsequent shrinkage of nasal mucous membranes by alpha-adrenergic stimulation, promoting nasal drainage.

Indications
Relief of symptoms associated with seasonal allergic rhinitis.

Contraindications
Hypersensitivity to any ingredient of product; known sensitivity to other alkylamine antihistamines (eg, triprolidine); patients with severe hypertension or coronary artery disease; MAO inhibitor therapy or within 14 days of stopping MAO inhibitor therapy.

Route/Dosage
ADULTS AND CHILDREN (12 YR OR OLDER): PO 1 capsule (8 mg acrivastine/60 mg pseudoephedrine) q 4 to 6 hr (up to qid).

Interactions
Acrivastine:
Alcohol; other CNS depressants – Additional decrease in alertness and impairment of CNS performance may occur.

Pseudoephedrine:
Antihypertensive agents that interfere with sympathetic activity (eg, mecamylamine, methyldopa, reserpine, veratrum alkaloids) – Antihypertensive effects of these agents may be reduced.
Digitalis – Increased ectopic pacemaker activity may occur.
MAO inhibitors – Contraindicated in patients taking MAO inhibitors and for 14 days after stopping use of an MAO inhibitor.

Lab Test Interferences May diminish or prevent positive reactions to skin tests.

Adverse Reactions
CV: Palpitations, tachycardia, pressor activity, cardiac arrhythmias, cardiovascular collapse (pseudoephedrine).
CNS: Somnolence; headache; dizziness; nervousness; insomnia.
EENT: Pharyngitis; increased cough.
GI: Nausea; dyspepsia.
GU: Dysmenorrhea.
OTHER: Asthenia; hypersensitivity (anaphylaxis, angioedema, bronchospasm, erythema multiforme).

Precautions
Pregnancy: Category B.
Lactation: Acrivastine: Undetermined; pseudoephedrine: excreted in breast milk.
Children: Safety and efficacy not established in children less than 12 yr.
Elderly: More likely to cause dizziness, sedation, bladder-neck obstruction, and hypertension.
Renal function impairment: Use is not recommended.
Special risk patients: Use with caution in patients with hypertension, diabetes mellitus, ischemic heart disease, increased intraocular pressure, hyperthyroidism, psoriatic hypertrophy, stenosing peptic ulcer, or pyloroduodenal obstruction.

Overdosage: Signs and Symptoms
Convulsions, CNS stimulation or depression, cardiovascular collapse with hypotension, fear, anxiety, tenseness, restlessness, tremor, weakness, pallor, respiratory difficulty, dysuria, insomnia, hallucinations, convulsions, arrhythmia.

PATIENT CARE CONSIDERATIONS
Administration/Storage
- Give q 4 to 6 hr, up to qid, with a full glass of water.
- Store capsules at controlled room temperature (59° to 86°F). Protect from light and moisture.

Assessment/Interventions
- Obtain patient history, including drug history and any known allergies. Note history of renal impairment, narrow angle glaucoma, urinary retention, severe hypertension or coronary artery disease, concurrent use of or within 2 wk of stopping MAO-inhibitor therapy, or allergy to alkylamine antihistamines (eg, triprolidine) or sympathomimetic amines.
- Assess for allergy symptoms (eg, rhinitis, nasal congestion, sneezing, itching, watery eyes) before and periodically throughout therapy.
- Monitor pulse and BP periodically during therapy.
- Monitor patient for nervousness, dizziness, and insomnia. If noted, hold therapy and notify health care provider.

Patient/Family Education
- Explain name, dose, action, and potential side effects of drug.
- Advise patient to take q 4 to 6 hr, up to qid, with a full glass of water.
- Advise patient to take last dose late in the afternoon or early in the evening to reduce chance of drug causing sleepiness.
- Advise patient that if allergy symptoms are not controlled not to increase the dose of medication but to inform a health care provider.
- Caution patient that drug may cause drowsiness and to use caution while driving or performing other tasks requiring mental alertness until tolerance is determined.
- Advise patient to avoid alcohol and other CNS depressants because of the risk of excessive sedation.
- Caution patient not to take any OTC antihistamines or decongestants while taking this medication unless advised by a health care provider.
- If patient is to have allergy skin testing, advise to not take the medication for at least 2 days before the skin testing.
- Advise women to notify health care provider if pregnant, planning to become pregnant, or breastfeeding.
- Instruct patient to stop taking drug and immediately report any of these symptoms to health care provider: nervousness, dizziness, sleeplessness.
- Caution patient to not take any prescription or OTC medications or dietary supplements unless advised by health care provider.

Acyclovir

(A-SIKE-low-vihr)

Class Anti-infective/Antiviral

How Supplied
Acyclovir Injection 50 mg/mL (as sodium), Powder for injection 500 mg/vial (as sodium), Powder for injection 1,000 mg/vial (as sodium) ♦ *Zovirax* Tablets 400 mg, Tablets 800 mg, Capsules 200 mg, Suspension 200 mg per 5 mL, Powder for injection, lyophilized 500 mg/vial (as sodium), Powder for injection, lyophilized 1,000 mg/vial (as sodium), Ointment 5%, Cream 5%
🍁 *Apo-Acyclovir* ♦ *Gen-Acyclovir* ♦ *Nu-Acyclovir*

Action
PHARMACOLOGY: Inhibits viral DNA replication by interfering with viral DNA polymerase.

PHARMACOKINETICS/DYNAMICS:

Absorption:
Oral – Bioavailability is 10% to 20%. C_{max} is 0.83 to 1.61 mcg/mL (200 to 800 mg at steady state).
IV – C_{max} is 9.8 mcg/mL (5 mg/kg dose), 22.9 mcg/mL (10 mg/kg).
Topical – Systemic absorption is minimal.

Distribution: 9% to 33% protein bound.
IV – CSF concentrations are about 50% of plasma values.

Excretion: The $t_{½}$ is 2.5 to 3.3 hr. Cl and $t_{½}$ are dependent on renal function.
IV – 62% to 91% is excreted unchanged in the urine. Cl is 5.1 mL/min/kg.

Special Populations:
Renal Function Impairment – Total body Cl and

t½ are dependent on renal function. Dosage adjustment recommended.
Elderly – Increased plasma concentrations. Dosage adjustment may be required.

Indications
Parenteral: Treatment of initial or recurrent mucosal and cutaneous herpes simplex viruses (HSV) and varicella zoster (shingles) infections in immunocompromised patients; treatment of herpes simplex encephalitis; treatment of severe initial clinical episodes of genital herpes; treatment of neonatal herpes infections.
Oral: Treatment of initial and recurrent episodes of genital herpes in certain patients; acute treatment of shingles and chickenpox.
Topical: Treatment of initial episodes of herpes genitalis and nonlife-threatening mucotaneous HSV infections in immunocompromised patients (ointment); recurrent herpes labialis (cold sores) (cream). **Unlabeled use(s):** Treatment of cytomegalovirus and HSV infection after bone marrow or renal transplant; treatment of infectious mononucleosis, varicella pneumonia, chickenpox, and other HSV infections.

Contraindications Hypersensitivity to acyclovir or valacyclovir.

Route/Dosage
PARENTERAL
For IV infusion only; rapid or bolus IV must be avoided.
Herpes Simplex Infections in Immunocompromised Patients
ADULTS AND ADOLESCENTS 12 YR OF AGE AND OLDER: **IV** 5 mg/kg infused at a constant rate over 1 hr q 8 hr for 7 days.
CHILDREN YOUNGER THAN 12 YR OF AGE: **IV** 10 mg/kg infused at a constant rate over 1 hr q 8 hr for 7 days.

Severe Initial Genital Herpes
ADULTS AND ADOLESCENTS 12 YR OF AGE AND OLDER: **IV** 5 mg/kg at a constant rate over 1 hr q 8 hr for 5 days.

Varicella Zoster Infections in Immunocompromised Patients
ADULTS AND ADOLESCENTS 12 YR OF AGE AND OLDER: **IV** 10 mg/kg infused at a constant rate over 1 hr q 8 hr for 7 days.
CHILDREN YOUNGER THAN 12 YR OF AGE: **IV** 20 mg/kg infused at a constant rate over 1 hr q 8 hr for 7 days.

Herpes Simplex Encephalitis
ADULTS AND ADOLESCENTS 12 YR OF AGE AND OLDER: **IV** 10 mg/kg infused at a constant rate over 1 hr q 8 hr for 10 days.
CHILDREN 3 MO TO 12 YR OF AGE: **IV** 20 mg/kg infused at a constant rate over 1 hr q 8 hr for 10 days.

Neonatal Herpes Infections (CDC Recommendations)
IV Disseminated and CNS disease: 20 mg/kg q 8 hr for 21 days. Mucocutaneous disease: 20 mg q 8 hr for 14 days.

ORAL
Chickenpox
ADULTS AND CHILDREN (GREATER THAN 40 KG): **PO** 800 mg qid for 5 days.
CHILDREN 2 YR OF AGE AND OLDER (40 KG OR LESS): **PO** 20 mg/kg qid for 5 days.

Herpes Zoster
ADULTS: **PO** 800 mg q 4 hr 5 times/day for 7 to 10 days.

Initial Genital Herpes
ADULTS: **PO** 200 mg q 4 hr 5 times/day for 10 days.

Suppressive Therapy for Recurrent Genital Herpes
ADULTS: **PO** 400 mg bid for up to 12 mo.

Intermittent Therapy for Recurrent Genital Herpes
ADULTS: **PO** 200 mg q 4 hr 5 times/day for 5 days at earliest sign or symptom of recurrence.

TOPICAL
Initial Genital Herpes and Herpes Simplex Infections in Immunocompromised Patients
ADULTS: **Ointment** Apply sufficient quantity to cover all lesions q 3 hr, 6 times/day, for 7 days.

Recurrent Herpes Labialis (Cold Sores)
ADULTS AND CHILDREN 12 YR OF AGE AND OLDER: **Cream** Apply to lesion 5 times/day for 4 days.

Interactions
Probenecid: IV acyclovir plasma levels may be increased, and the duration of action prolonged, while the urinary excretion and renal Cl may be reduced.
Zidovudine: Increased propensity for lethargy.
INCOMPATIBILITIES: Precipitation may occur with bacteriostatic water. Do not add acyclovir to biologic or colloidal fluids.

Lab Test Interferences None well documented.

Adverse Reactions
CV: Phlebitis at injection site (9%); hypotension (postmarketing).
CNS: Headache, agitation, coma, confusion, delirium, dizziness hallucinations, obtundation, psychosis, seizure, somnolence (postmarketing).
DERM: Itching, rash, hives (2%); alopecia, erythema multiforme, photosensitive rash, pruritus, rash, Stevens-Johnson syndrome, toxic epidermal necrolysis, urticaria (postmarketing).
EENT: Visual abnormalities.

GI: Nausea, vomiting (7%); diarrhea, GI distress, abdominal pain (postmarketing).
GU: Transient elevations of serum creatinine or BUN (5% to 10%); renal failure, elevated blood urea nitrogen, elevated creatinine.
HEMA: Anemia, neutropenia, thrombocytopenia, thrombocytosis, leukocytosis, neutrophilia (less than 1%); leukopenia (postmarketing).
HEMA/LYMPH: Disseminated intravascular coagulation, hemolysis, lymphadenopathy (postmarketing).
HEPA: Elevated transaminases (1% to 2%); hepatitis, jaundice (postmarketing).
MUSC: Myalgia (postmarketing).
OTHER: Anaphylaxis, fever, pain, peripheral edema (postmarketing).

Precautions
Pregnancy: Category B.
Lactation: Excreted in breast milk.
Children:
Oral – Safety and efficacy in children under 2 yr of age not established.
Topical – Safety and efficacy not established in pediatric patients.
Elderly: Use with caution because of the greater frequency of decreased hepatic, renal, or cardiac function, and concomitant diseases or other drug therapy.

Renal function impairment: Dosage adjustment may be needed. With parenteral use, acyclovir may precipitate as crystals in renal tubules.
Chickenpox: Chickenpox in otherwise healthy children is usually a self-limiting disease of mild to moderate severity; however, adolescents and adults tend to have more severe disease.
Cutaneous use: Care must be taken to avoid getting drug in eyes.
Encephalopathic changes: Patients with underlying neurologic abnormalities or severe hypoxia may have increased risk of neurotoxic effects.
Genital herpes: Sexual intercourse must be avoided when lesions are present. Use of acyclovir does not prevent transmission.
Herpes zoster infection: There are no data on treatment started more than 72 hr after the onset of the rash.
Thrombotic thrombocytopenic purpura/hemolytic uremic syndrome: May occur and has resulted in death in immunocompromised patients.

Overdosage: Signs and Symptoms
Increased BUN and serum creatinine, renal failure, convulsions, lethargy, acyclovir precipitation, renal tubules, agitation, coma.

PATIENT CARE CONSIDERATIONS

Administration/Storage
- Route of administration, dose, dosing frequency, and duration of therapy are variable, depending on condition being treated.

Oral:
- Capsules, tablets, and suspension are interchangeable on a mg to mg basis.
- Administer prescribed dose without regard to meals. Administer with food if GI upset occurs.
- Shake suspension well before measuring dose. Measure and administer prescribed dose using dosing syringe, dosing dropper, or medicine cup.
- Store tablets, capsules, and suspension at controlled room temperature (59° to 77°F). Protect from moisture.

Topical:
- For cutaneous use only. Not for use in the nose, mouth, or eyes.
- Use finger cot or rubber glove when applying ointment to prevent spread of infection.
- When using ointment, apply a sufficient quantity to adequately cover all lesions. Apply ointment q 3 hr (6 times/day) for 7 days. A ½ inch of ribbon of ointment covers about 4 square inches.
- When using cream, apply 5 times/day for 4 days.

- Store ointment at controlled room temperature (59° to 77°F). Store cream at controlled room temperature (59° to 86°F).

Injection:
- For IV infusion only. Not for oral, topical, ophthalmic, intradermal, subcutaneous, IM, intra-arterial, or IV bolus administration.
- Reconstitute powder for injection, following manufacturer's guidelines, with sterile water for injection to produce a solution containing 50 mg/mL.
- Further dilute prescribed dose in any appropriate IV solution at a volume selected for administration over 1 hr.
- Infuse prescribed dose over a period of at least 1 hr to reduce risk of renal tubular damage.
- Do not administer if particulate matter, cloudiness, or discoloration noted.
- Discard any unused solution. Do not save for future use.
- Store powder for injection at controlled room temperature (59° to 77°F). Use reconstituted solution within 12 hr. Refrigeration of reconstituted solution may result in formation of a precipitate that will redissolve at room temperature. Use diluted solution within 24 hr.

Assessment/Interventions
- Obtain patient history, including drug history

and any known allergies. Note impaired renal function, dehydration, electrolyte abnormalities, hypoxia, hypersensitivity to valacyclovir, or concurrent therapy with potentially nephrotoxic medications.
- Following manufacturer's guidelines, ensure that reduced dose and/or prolonged dosing interval is used in patient with renal impairment.
- Ensure that patient receiving IV acyclovir is well hydrated during therapy and that max dose of 20 mg/kg q 8 hr is not exceeded.
- For herpes zoster (shingles), assess for history of present illness and time of rash onset. Treatment should be started no later than 72 hr after onset of rash.
- For genital herpes, assess for history of present illness and time of onset of symptoms. Treatment should be started no later than 6 hr after onset of symptoms of recurrent episode.
- For chickenpox (varicella), assess for history of present illness and time of rash onset. Treatment should be started no later than 24 hr after onset of rash.
- For recurrent genital herpes, assess history of frequency of recurrence.
- Frequently assess patient for response to treatment. Notify health care provider if condition does not appear to be improving or is worsening.
- Ensure that therapy is periodically reviewed to determine if it needs to be continued without change or if a dose change (eg, increase, decrease, discontinuation) is indicated.
- Monitor patient for GI, CNS, general body side effects, and injection site reactions. Report to health care provider if noted and significant.

Patient/Family Education

- Explain name, dose, action, and potential side effects of drug.

Injection:
- Advise patient, family, or caregiver that medication will be prepared and administered by a health care provider in a health care setting.
- Advise patient, family, or caregiver to report injection site pain or redness.

Topical:
- Advise patient not to cover the cold sore with a bandage or dressing.
- Advise patient that the cream dose form is not to be used for genital herpes.
- Advise patient or caregiver using ointment to use finger cot or rubber glove when applying to prevent spread of infection and to wash hands with soap and water after applying ointment.

- Advise patient or caregiver to apply enough ointment to adequately cover all lesions q 3 hr (6 times/day) for 7 days. Advise patient or caregiver that a ½ inch ribbon of ointment should cover about 4 square inches.
- Advise patient or caregiver using cream to apply to lesions 5 times/day for 4 days and to wash hands with soap and water after each application.
- Advise patient or caregiver to notify health care provider if lesions do not appear to be improving, are getting worse, or if application site reactions (eg, burning, stinging, redness, itching) develop.

Tablets, capsules, or suspension:
- Review dose and appropriate dosing schedule depending on condition being treated (shingles, chickenpox, recurrent genital herpes). Instruct patient to take medication exactly as prescribed and not to stop taking or change the dose unless advised by health care provider.
- Advise patient that medication can be taken without regard to meals but to take with food if stomach upset occurs.
- Advise patient or caregiver using suspension to shake it well before measuring dose and to measure and administer prescribed dose using a dosing syringe, dosing dropper, or medicine cup.
- Remind patient using medication for recurrent episodes of genital herpes to initiate therapy at the first sign or symptom or recurrence and that medication may not be effective if started more than 6 hr after onset of signs or symptoms of recurrence.
- Advise patient with genital herpes that this drug is not a cure for genital herpes and does not prevent transmission of virus. Instruct patient to avoid sexual intercourse when lesions and/or symptoms are present to avoid infecting partner.
- Advise patient to contact health care provider if medication does not seem to be controlling lesions and/or symptoms or if intolerable side effects develop.
- Advise women to notify health care provider if pregnant, planning to become pregnant, or breastfeeding.
- Instruct patient not to take any prescription or OTC medications, dietary supplements, or herbal preparations unless advised by health care provider.
- Advise patient that follow-up visits may be necessary to monitor therapy and to keep appointments.

Adalimumab

(ah-dah-LIM-you-mab)

Class Immunologic agent

How Supplied
Humira Injection 40 mg/0.8 mL

Action

PHARMACOLOGY: Blocks interaction of human tumor necrosis factor (TNF)-alpha with receptors and modulates biological responses induced or regulated by TNF.

PHARMACOKINETICS/DYNAMICS:

Absorption: C_{max} is approximately 4.7 mcg/mL following a single 40 mg SC injection. T_{max} is approximately 131 hr. The average absolute bioavailability is 64%.

Distribution: Vd_{ss} is 4.7 to 6 L.

Excretion: Mean terminal t½ is approximately 14 days. Systemic Cl is approximately 12 mL/hr.

Indications Reduce signs and symptoms and inhibit progression of structural damage in patients with moderate to severe active rheumatoid arthritis who have had an inadequate response to 1 or more disease-modifying antirheumatic drugs.

Contraindications Standard considerations.

Route/Dosage

ADULTS: **SC** 40 mg every other wk. Patients not receiving methotrexate concurrently may benefit from 40 mg every wk.

Interactions

Immunosuppressive therapy: May increase risk of serious infection.
Live vaccines: Do not give concurrently.
Methotrexate: Reduces apparent Cl of adalimumab; however, adjustments in the dose of either drug do not appear necessary.

Lab Test Interferences None well documented.

Adverse Reactions

CV: Hypertension (at least 5%); arrhythmia, atrial fibrillation, CV disorder, chest pain, CHF, coronary artery disorder, heart arrest, hypertensive encephalopathy, MI, palpitation, pericardial effusion, pericarditis, syncope, tachycardia, vascular disorder (less than 5%).
CNS: Headache (at least 5%); confusion, multiple sclerosis, paresthesia, subdural hematoma, tremor (less than 5%).
DERM: Injection site reactions including erythema, itching, hemorrhage, pain, swelling (approximately 20%); rash (at least 5%); cellulitis, erysipelas, herpes zoster (less than 5%).
EENT: Sinusitis (at least 5%); esophagitis, cataract (less than 5%).
GI: Nausea, abdominal pain (at least 5%); cholecystitis, cholelithiasis, gastroenteritis, GI disorder and hemorrhage, vomiting (less than 5%).
GU: UTI, hematuria (at least 5%); cystitis, kidney calculus, menstrual disorder, pyelonephritis (less than 5%).
HEMA: Agranulocytosis, granulocytopenia, leukopenia, lymphoma-like reaction, pancytopenia, polycythemia (less than 5%).
HEPA: Hepatic necrosis (less than 5%).
METAB: Hypercholesterolemia, hyperlipidemia, increased alkaline phosphatase (at least 5%); dehydration, abnormal healing, ketosis, paraproteinemia, peripheral edema (less than 5%).
MUSC: Arthritis, bone disorder, bone fracture, bone necrosis, joint disorder, muscle cramps, myasthenia, pyogenic arthritis, synovitis, tendon disorder.
RESP: Upper respiratory tract infection, sinusitis, flu syndrome (at least 5%); asthma, bronchospasm, dyspnea, lung disorder, decreased lung function, pleural effusion, pneumonia (less than 5%).
OTHER: Accidental injury, back pain (at least 5%); fever, infection, pain in extremity, pelvic pain, sepsis, thorax pain, reactivated tuberculosis, lupus erythematosus syndrome, parathyroid disorder, adenoma, carcinoma (including breast, GI, skin, urogenital), lymphoma, malignancies, melanoma; leg thrombosis (less than 5%); serious infection (0.04%).

> **WARNING:**
> Tuberculosis, frequently disseminated or extrapulmonary, has been observed in patients receiving adalimumab. Evaluate patients for latent tuberculosis infection with a tuberculin skin test. Initiate treatment of latent tuberculosis infection prior to therapy.

Precautions

Pregnancy: Category B.
Lactation: Undetermined.
Children: Safety and efficacy not established.
Elderly: Use with caution, reflecting greater frequency of infections and malignancies.
Immunization: Do not administer live vaccines while on therapy.
Immunogenicity: May result in formation of autoantibodies and, rarely, in the development of a lupus-like syndrome.
Immunosuppression: May affect host defenses against infection and malignancies.
Infection: Serious, fatal infections and sepsis have occurred. Do not initiate treatment in patients with active infections, including chronic or local infections. Rare cases of tuberculosis have been observed.
Malignancy: Lymphomas have occurred.

Neurologic events: Rare cases of exacerbation of clinical symptoms and/or radiographic evidence of demyelinating disease have occurred.

PATIENT CARE CONSIDERATIONS

Administration/Storage
- For SC administration only. Not for intradermal, IM, or IV administration.
- Dose is usually administered every other wk.
- Do not administer if particulate matter, cloudiness, or discoloration noted.
- Rotate injection sites (thigh, abdomen, upper arm). Give new injections at least 1 inch from old site and never into areas where the skin is tender, bruised, red, or hard.
- Do not rub injection site after injection has been completed.
- Methotrexate, glucocorticoids, salicylates, NSAIDs, or other DMARDs (disease-modifying antirheumatic drugs) may be continued during treatment with adalimumab.
- Discard any unused solution. Do not save unused solution for later administration.
- Store syringes in refrigerator (36° to 46°F). Do not freeze. Store in original carton until time of administration. Protect from light.

Assessment/Interventions
- Obtain patient history, including drug history and any known allergies. Note history of the following: latex sensitivity; recurrent infections; conditions predisposing to infections; prior residence in areas where tuberculosis or histoplasmosis are endemic; preexisting or recent-onset demyelinating disorders; concurrent use of immunosuppressant therapy.
- Ensure that patient does not have an active chronic or localized infection prior to starting therapy.
- Ensure that patient is evaluated for presence of latent tuberculosis using a tuberculin skin test prior to starting therapy. If latent infection is identified ensure that patient is started on appropriate prophylaxis before adalimumab therapy is started.
- Monitor patient for signs and symptoms of infection and immediately report to health care provider if noted.
- Discontinue use if patient experiences a serious infection during therapy.
- Monitor patient for signs and symptoms of anaphylactic or serious allergic reactions. Be prepared to discontinue therapy and treat appropriately.
- Monitor patient for CNS, GI, CV, respiratory, musculoskeletal, and general body side effects, and injection-site reactions. Report to health care provider if noted and significant.
- Do not administer live virus vaccines while patient is on adalimumab therapy.

Patient/Family Education
- Explain name, dose, action, and potential side effects of drug.
- Advise patient or caregiver to review *Patient Information* insert before starting therapy and with each refill.
- If administered at home, ensure that patient or caregiver understands how to store, prepare, and administer the dose, and how to dispose of used equipment and supplies. The first injection should be performed under the supervision of a qualified health professional.
- Advise patient that if a dose is missed, to inject the missed dose as soon as remembered and inject the next dose at the regularly scheduled time.
- Instruct patient to continue taking other arthritis medications prescribed by the health care provider.
- Advise patient that injection site reactions are common and that placing a towel soaked in cold water on the reaction site should decrease reaction symptoms.
- Advise patient to report any of the following to health care provider: intolerable injection-site reactions, fever or other signs of infection, sore throat, persistent cough, wasting or weight loss, low grade fever, numbness or tingling, vision problems, leg weakness, dizziness, persistent chest pain, unexplained shortness of breath, new or worsening joint pain, or rash on cheeks or arms that is sensitive to the sun.
- Advise women to notify health care provider if pregnant, planning to become pregnant, or breastfeeding.
- Instruct patient not to take any prescription or OTC medications or dietary supplements unless advised by health care provider.
- Remind patient that office visits and laboratory tests will be required to monitor therapy and to keep appointments.

Adapalene

(ADE-ah-PALE-een)
Class Retinoid
How Supplied
Differin Cream 0.1%, Gel 0.1%, Solution 0.1%
Action
PHARMACOLOGY: May normalize the differentiation of follicular epithelial cells, resulting in decreased microcomedone formation.
Indications Topical treatment of acne vulgaris.
Contraindications Standard considerations.
Route/Dosage
ADULTS AND CHILDREN (12 YR AND OLDER):
Topical Apply a thin film once daily to affected areas after washing in the evening before bedtime.
Interactions
Potentially irritating topical products (eg, medicated or abrasive soaps and cleansers, soaps and cosmetics that have strong drying effect, products with high concentrations of alcohol, spices or limes), products containing sulfur, resorcinol, or salicylic acid: Because of increased risk of local irritation, use with caution.
Lab Test Interferences None well documented.
Adverse Reactions
DERM: Erythema; scaling; dryness; pruritus, skin discomfort, burning, stinging, and irritation; sunburn; acne flares.
Precautions
Pregnancy: Category C.
Lactation: Undetermined.
Children: Safety and efficacy not established in children less than 12 yr.
Photosensitivity: Photosensitivity may occur. Patients should minimize exposure to sunlight, including sunlamps, and use sunscreens and protective clothing over treated areas.
External use: Avoid contact with eyes, lips, angles of the nose, other mucous membranes, and open wounds.
Irritation: May cause local irritation. May need to use less often or discontinue use.
Overdosage: Signs and Symptoms
Redness, peeling, discomfort.

PATIENT CARE CONSIDERATIONS
Administration/Storage
- For topical use only. Not for ophthalmic, oral, or intravaginal use.
- Avoid contact with eyes, lips, angles of the nose, and mucus membranes.
- Cleanse area with a mild or soapless cleanser before applying medicated cream.
- Cream, gel, or solution are usually applied to affected areas once daily at nighttime.
- Apply a thin film of cream, gel, or solution to cover the affected area(s).
- Store at controlled room temperature (68° to 77°F). Keep tube tightly capped. Keep bottle tightly capped and stored upright. Protect from freezing.

Solution:
- Apply directly to affected area(s) using supplied applicator. Replace cap after each use.

Pledgets:
- Do not use if seal is broken. Remove pledget from foil pouch just before using. Discard pledget after single use. Do not reuse pledget.

Assessment/Interventions
- Obtain patient history, including drug history and any known allergies.
- Assess the skin and identify areas where medication is to be applied and areas that are sunburned, have cuts, eczema, or abrasions; avoid these areas.
- Assess and document skin condition before initial application and periodically throughout treatment.
- Monitor for side effects, including redness, scaling, dryness, or persistent itching or burning. Inform health care provider if noted and significant.

Patient/Family Education
- Explain name, dose, action, and potential side effects of drug.
- Advise patient that medication is applied topically to skin lesions once daily at nighttime.
- Teach patient the following proper technique for applying medication: wash hands; cleanse area with mild or soapless cleanser first then apply a thin film of cream, gel, or solution to cover skin areas with acne lesions; wash hands after applying medication.
- Inform patient that a mild sensation of warmth or slight stinging may be felt shortly after application and that this is expected and should be of no concern.
- Warn patient that applying medication more often than prescribed or in excessive quantities will not produce more rapid improvement or better results but will result in greater side effects such as redness, scaling, and discomfort.
- Warn patient to avoid contact with the eyes,

lips, angles of the nose, and mucous membranes.
- Advise patient to not apply to skin areas where there are cuts, abrasions, or eczema, or to sunburned skin.
- Advise patient that moisturizers may be used but to avoid those containing alpha hydroxy or glycolic acids.
- Advise patient that acne may appear to worsen during the first few weeks of therapy but to continue to use the cream. Improvement may not be seen for at least 2 wk but may take up to 8 wk.
- Advise patient that local redness, drying, scaling, burning, or itching may occur during the first 2 to 4 wk of treatment and usually will lessen with continued use of medication. However, if these symptoms are bothersome or do not go away, the frequency of application may need to be reduced or the medication discontinued completely.
- Advise patient that if severe dermal reactions occur to stop using the medication and contact the health care provider.
- Advise patient to talk to the health care provider before using any other topical agents (eg, medicated soaps, astringents, cosmetics, or other acne products) on treated skin.
- Advise patient to not use wax epilation on treated skin because of risk of skin erosions.
- Warn patient to avoid unnecessary exposure to sun and sun lamps while using this medication. Advise patient to use sunscreens and protective clothing over treated areas when exposure cannot be avoided.
- Caution patient that while using the medication, exposure to extreme weather conditions (eg, wind or cold air) may be irritating to the treated areas.
- Advise women to contact health care provider if pregnant, planning to become pregnant, or breastfeeding.
- Warn patient not to take any prescription or OTC drugs or dietary supplements without consulting the health care provider.
- Advise patient that follow-up visits to examine the skin lesions may be necessary and to keep appointments.

Adefovir Dipivoxil

(Ah-DEF-fah-vihr die-pihv-VOX-ill)
Class Antiviral Agent
How Supplied
Hepsera Tablets 10 mg
Action
PHARMACOLOGY: Inhibits HBV DNA polymerase (reverse transcriptase) by competing with the natural substrate deoxyadenosine triphosphate and by causing DNA chain termination after its incorporation into viral DNA.
PHARMACOKINETICS/DYNAMICS:
Absorption: Bioavailability of adefovir is approximately 59%. C_{max} is approximately 18.4 ng/mL and T_{max} is approximately 1.75 hr.
Distribution: Up to 4% is protein bound. Vd is approximately 352 to 392 mL/kg (IV doses at steady state).
Metabolism: Adefovir dipivoxil (prodrug) is rapidly converted to adefovir (active).
Excretion: The t½ is approximately 7.48 hr; 45% of dose is recovered as adefovir in the urine over 24 hr.
Special Populations:
Renal Function Impairment – The C_{max}, AUC, and t½ increased in those with moderate or severe renal impairment or with end-stage renal disease. Dosing interval modification is recommended.
Indications Treatment of chronic hepatitis B in adults with evidence of active viral replication and evidence of persistent elevations in serum aminotransferases (ALT or AST) or histologically active disease.
Contraindications Standard considerations.
Route/Dosage
ADULTS: PO 10 mg qd.
Renal Impairment
ADULTS: PO For Ccr 50 mL/min or less, administer 10 mg q 24 hr; for Ccr 20 to 49 mL/min, administer 10 mg q 48 hr; for Ccr 10 to 19 mL/min, administer 10 mg q 72 hr; hemodialysis patients, administer 10 mg q 7 days following dialysis.
Interactions
Ibuprofen, drugs that reduce renal function: May increase plasma concentrations of adefovir.
Lab Test Interferences None well documented.
Adverse Reactions Treatment-related adverse events reported in pre- and postliver transplantation patients include the following:
CNS: Headache.
DERM: Pruritus; rash.
EENT: Pharyngitis.
GI: Nausea; vomiting; diarrhea; flatulence.
GU: Increases in creatinine; renal failure; renal insufficiency.
HEPA: Hepatic failure; increases in ALT and AST; abnormal liver function.
RESP: Increased cough; sinusitis.
OTHER: Asthenia; abdominal pain; fever.

> **WARNING:**
>
> *Hepatitis:* Acute exacerbations have occurred in patients who have discontinued anti-hepatitis B therapy, including therapy with adefovir.
>
> Nephrotoxicity related to chronic administration in patients at risk or those with underlying renal dysfunction. Close monitoring required. Dosage adjustment may be necessary.
>
> HIV resistance may occur in unrecognized or untreated HIV infection.
>
> Lactic acidosis and hepatomegaly reported with steatosis (including fatal cases) reported with the use of nucleoside analogues alone or in combination with other antiretrovirals.

Precautions
Pregnancy: Category C.
Lactation: Undetermined.
Children: Safety and efficacy not established.
Elderly: Select dose with caution, reflecting greater frequency of decreased hepatic, renal, or cardiac function and comorbidity.

Overdosage: Signs and Symptoms
GI side effects.

PATIENT CARE CONSIDERATIONS
Administration/Storage
- Administer with or without food. Administer with food if GI upset occurs.
- Give prescribed dose once daily to patient with normal renal function.
- Follow manufacturer's guidelines for dosing intervals in patients with renal impairment.
- Store tablets at controlled room temperature (59° to 86°F).

Assessment/Interventions
- Obtain patient history, including drug history and any known allergies. Note renal impairment, HIV infection, and concurrent use of potentially nephrotoxic medications (eg, NSAIDs).
- Ensure that HIV testing is done prior to starting therapy in patients whose HIV status is unknown.
- Monitor renal function and liver enzymes periodically during therapy. Be prepared to adjust dosing interval should evidence of renal impairment be noted.
- Monitor patient for evidence of lactic acidosis (eg, extreme fatigue, unexplained muscle pain, dyspnea, dizziness, lightheadedness, abdominal pain with nausea and vomiting, chills, tachycardia, irregular heartbeat) and hepatitis (eg, jaundice, right upper quadrant pain, dark urine, light stools). If noted, discontinue therapy and notify health care provider immediately.
- Monitor patient for evidence of CNS, GI, and general body side effects. If noted and significant, inform health care provider.

Patient/Family Education
- Advise patient to review the Patient Information pamphlet carefully before starting therapy and to read and check for new information each time the medication is refilled.
- Explain name, dose, action, and potential side effects of therapy.
- Review dosing schedule with patient.
- Advise patient that tablets can be taken without regard to food but can be taken with food if GI upset occurs.
- Advise patient that if a dose is missed to take it as soon as remembered on that day. Caution patient to not take more than 1 dose of adefovir dipivoxil in a day nor to take 2 doses at the same time.
- Caution patient to not change the dose or stop taking unless advised to do so by their health care provider. Stopping therapy may result in severe exacerbation of the hepatitis.
- Advise patient to get an HIV test before starting therapy and any time after that when there is a chance of exposure to HIV.
- Advise patient that medication will not cure hepatitis B infection nor any other viral infection (eg, HIV) and to continue to take other antiviral medications as prescribed.
- Advise patient that this therapy will not prevent transmission of hepatitis B to others nor is it know if it can prevent cirrhosis, liver failure, or liver cancer that may develop as a result of hepatitis B infection.
- Advise patient to immediately report any of the following to their health care provider: difficulty breathing, unusual muscle pain, generalized body discomfort, unexplained drowsiness, dizziness, lightheadedness, fast or irregular heart beat, stomach pain with nausea and vomiting, cold feeling, especially in arms and legs, yellowing of the skin or eyes, appetite

loss, bowel movements turn light in color, or urine turns very dark in color.
- Instruct women to notify health care provider if planning on becoming pregnant or breastfeeding.
- Instruct patient to not take any prescription or OTC medications or dietary supplements unless advised by health care provider.
- Advise patient that laboratory tests and follow-up visits will be required to monitor therapy and to keep appointments.

Adenosine

(ah-DEN-oh-seen)

Class Antiarrhythmic

How Supplied
Adenocard Injection 3 mg/mL ♦ Adenoscan Injection 3 mg/mL

Action
PHARMACOLOGY: Slows conduction through atrioventricular (AV) node; can interrupt reentry pathways through AV node and restore normal sinus rhythm.

PHARMACOKINETICS/DYNAMICS:
Distribution: Rapidly cleared from circulation via cellular uptake, primarily by erythrocytes and vascular endothelial cells.
Metabolism: Rapidly metabolized intracellularly to adenosine monophosphate or inosine. Inosine is ultimately degraded to uric acid.
Excretion: Extracellular adenosine has a $t_{1/2}$ of less than 10 sec in whole blood.

Indications Conversion to sinus rhythm of paroxysmal supraventricular tachycardia (PSVT), including that associated with Wolff-Parkinson-White syndrome. **Unlabeled use(s):** Noninvasive assessment of patients with suspected coronary artery disease in conjunction with thallium tomography. Used with BCNU for treatment of brain tumors.

Contraindications Second- or third-degree AV block or sick sinus syndrome (except in patients with functioning artificial pacemaker); atrial flutter; atrial fibrillation; ventricular tachycardia.

Route/Dosage
INITIAL DOSE (ADULTS): **IV** 6 mg as rapid IV bolus (over 1 to 2 sec).
REPEAT ADMINISTRATION (ADULTS): If first dose does not eliminate PSVT within 1 to 2 min, give 12 mg as rapid IV bolus; 12 mg dose may be repeated a second time if necessary. Doses over 12 mg are not recommended.

Interactions
Caffeine, theophylline: Antagonize effects of adenosine; larger doses of adenosine may be needed.
Carbamazepine: May produce higher degrees of heart block.
Dipyridamole: Potentiates effects of adenosine; smaller doses may be adequate.

Lab Test Interferences None well documented.

Adverse Reactions
CV: Facial flushing; headache; chest pain; hypotension.
CNS: Lightheadedness, dizziness, tingling in arms; numbness.
GI: Nausea.
RESP: Dyspnea; shortness of breath; chest pressure.

Precautions
Pregnancy: Category C.
Lactation: Undetermined.
Arrhythmias: At time of conversion to normal sinus rhythm, new arrhythmias may appear on ECG; these are usually self-limiting.
Asthma: Adenosine may cause bronchoconstriction.
Heart block: Drug may produce short-lasting heart block. Patients in whom high-level heart block (eg, third-degree) develops after one dose should not receive repeat doses.

PATIENT CARE CONSIDERATIONS

Administration/Storage
- Administer by rapid IV bolus only.
- Administer either directly into vein or, if given into IV line, in most proximal IV line and follow with rapid saline solution flush.
- Do not administer if solution is cloudy or if sediment is present.
- Discard unused portion.
- Store at room temperature.
- Do not refrigerate because crystallization may occur. If crystallization has occurred, dissolve crystals by warming to room temperature.

Assessment/Interventions
- Obtain patient history, including drug history and any known allergies or asthma.
- Monitor BP and cardiac rhythm during and after administration.
- Monitor for transient asystole, which may develop during administration.

Patient/Family Education
* Inform patient to report the following symptoms to health care provider: facial flushing, headache, shortness of breath, chest pressure, lightheadedness, dizziness, tingling in arms, numbness or nausea.

Agalsidase Beta

(aye-GAL-sih-dace BAY-tah)

Class Enzyme replacement therapy

How Supplied
Fabrazyme Powder for injection, lyophilized 37 mg (5 mg/mL when reconstituted)

Action
PHARMACOLOGY: Provides exogenous source of α-galactosidase A.

PHARMACOKINETICS/DYNAMICS:
Excretion: Terminal t½ ranges from 45 to 102 min.

Indications Treatment of Fabry disease.

Contraindications Standard considerations.

Route/Dosage
ADULTS: **IV** 1 mg/kg infused every 2 wk.

Interactions None well documented.
INCOMPATIBILITIES: Do not infuse in the same IV line with other products.

Lab Test Interferences None well documented.

Adverse Reactions
CV: Stroke; bradycardia; cardiac arrhythmia; cardiac arrest; decreased cardiac output; cardiomegaly (10%); hypertension (10%); hypotension (14%); dependent edema (21%).
CNS: Ataxia; vertigo; dizziness (14%); headache (45%); paresthesia (14%); anxiety (28%); depression.
EENT: Hypoacousia; laryngitis; pharyngitis.
GI: Dyspepsia (10%); nausea (28%).
GU: Nephrotic syndrome; testicular pain (7%).
RESP: Bronchitis (10%); bronchospasm (7%); rhinitis (38%); sinusitis (7%).
OTHER: Infusion reactions (eg, tachycardia, hypertension, throat tightness, chest pain/tightness, dyspnea, fever (48%), chills/rigors, abdominal pain, pruritus, urticaria, nausea, vomiting, lip or ear edema, rash); pain (21%); chest pain (17%); pallor (14%); rigors (52%); sensations of temperature change (17%); arthrosis (10%); skeletal pain (21%).

Precautions
Pregnancy: Category B.
Lactation: Undetermined.
Children: Safety and efficacy not established.
Elderly: Undetermined.
Antibodies: Most patients develop IgG antibodies and some develop IgE antibodies to treatment. Consider testing for IgE if a suspected allergic reaction develops.
Cardiac Function: Patients with Fabry disease may have compromised cardiac function, that may predispose them to higher risk of severe complications from infusion reactions. Monitor cardiac function closely in patients with compromised cardiac function.
Infusion Reactions: Infusion-related hypersensitivity reactions may occur. Some reactions may be severe. Reactions may include fever, rigors, chest tightness, and hypertension. Prior to infusion, patients should receive antipyretics. If an infusion reaction occurs, decreasing the infusion rate, temporarily stopping the infusion, and/or administration of additional antipyretics, antihistamines, and/or steroids may ameliorate the symptoms.

PATIENT CARE CONSIDERATIONS

Administration/Storage
* For IV administration only. Not for intradermal, IM, or SC administration.
* Administer prescribed dose by IV infusion q 2 wk.
* Follow manufacturer's instructions for reconstitution of powder and final dilution for infusion solution.
* Do not shake or agitate vials during reconstitution or dilution. Do not use filter needles during preparation of infusion.
* Inspect solution visually before administration. Do not administer if solution is cloudy, discolored, or contains particulate matter.
* Discard any unused product. Vials are for single-use only. Do not save medication for future use.
* Initial IV infusion rate should be no more than 15 mg/hr. After patient tolerance to the infusion has been established, each subsequent infusion may be increased in increments of 3 to 5 mg/hr.
* Infusion may be filtered through in-line low protein-binding 0.2 μm filter during administration.
* Do not administer in same IV line with other products.
* Store vials in refrigerator (36° to 46°F). Do not freeze. Use reconstituted and diluted solutions immediately. If immediate use is not possible, the reconstituted and diluted solutions may be stored for up to 24 hr in refrigerator (36° to 46°F).

Assessment/Interventions

- Obtain patient history, including drug history and any known allergies. Note compromised cardiac function.
- Ensure that an antipyretic (eg, acetaminophen) and an antihistamine (eg, diphenhydramine) are administered at least 60 min prior to infusion to decrease or prevent infusion-associated reactions.
- Monitor patient for development of infusion reaction (fever, chills or rigors, throat tightness, chest pain or tightness, rash, pruritus, hives, myalgia, dyspnea, abdominal pain, headache, hypotension, or hypertension). If infusion reaction develops, be prepared to decrease the infusion rate, temporarily stop the infusion, and/or administer additional antipyretics, antihistamines, and/or corticosteroids.
- Closely monitor patient with compromised cardiac function during therapy.
- Consider testing for IgE or skin test reactivity specific to agalsidase beta in patient who experienced allergic reaction during treatment.
- Assess patient for CNS, CV, GI, respiratory, psychiatric, and general body side effects. Inform health care provider if noted and significant.

Patient/Family Education

- Explain name, action, dosing regimen, and potential side effects of drug.
- Advise patient, family, or caregiver that medication will be prepared and administered by a health care provider in a health care setting.
- Advise patient, family, or caregiver that an antipyretic (eg, acetaminophen) and an antihistamine (eg, diphenhydramine) will be administered before each treatment to prevent or reduce severity of infusion reactions.
- Advise patient, family, or caregiver to report any signs or symptoms of infusion-reaction (eg, fever, chills or rigors, throat tightness, chest pain or tightness, rash, itching, hives, muscle aches, difficulty breathing, stomach pain, or headache).
- Advise women to notify health care provider if pregnant, planning to become pregnant, or breastfeeding.
- Instruct patient not to take any prescription or OTC medications or dietary supplements unless advised by health care provider.
- Encourage patient to enroll and participate in the Fabry Registry as noted in the manufacturer's product information.
- Advise patient, family, or caregiver that follow-up visits and lab tests will be required to monitor response to therapy and to keep appointments.

Albumin Human (Normal Serum Albumin)

(al-BYOO-MIN human)

Class Plasma protein fraction

How Supplied

Albuminar-5 Injection 5% ♦ *Albuminar-25* Injection 25% ♦ *Albunex* Injection 5% ♦ *Albutein* 5% Injection 5% ♦ *Albutein* 25% Injection 25% ♦ *Buminate* 5% Injection 5% ♦ *Buminate* 25% Injection 25% ♦ *Human Albumin Grifols* Injection 25% ♦ *Plasbumin-5* Injection 5% ♦ *Plasbumin-25* Injection 25%

Action

PHARMACOLOGY: Maintains plasma colloid osmotic pressure and serves as carrier of intermediate metabolites in transport and exchange of tissue products.

Indications Symptomatic relief and supportive treatment in management of shock, burns, hypoprothrombinemia, adult respiratory distress syndrome, cardiopulmonary bypass, acute liver failure, acute nephrosis, sequestration of protein-rich fluids, erythrocyte resuspension, hypotension or shock during renal dialysis, hyperbilirubinemia and erythroblastosis fetalis.

Contraindications Severe anemia; cardiac failure; renal insufficiency; presence of normal or increased intravascular volume; chronic nephrosis; hypoprothrombinemic states associated with chronic cirrhosis; malabsorption; protein-losing enteropathies, pancreatic insufficiency; undernutrition.

Route/Dosage

Burns

Initial treatment usually consists of large amounts of crystalloid infusions (eg, normal saline, Lactated Ringer's) with lesser amounts of 5% albumin to maintain adequate plasma volume. After first 24 hr, ratio of albumin and crystalloid should maintain plasma albumin level of about 2.5 g ± 0.5 g/100 mL or total plasma protein level about 5.2 g/100 mL. This is best achieved with albumin 25% solution.

NORMAL SERUM ALBUMIN, 5%

Shock

Give as rapidly as necessary to improve patient's condition and restore normal blood volume. ADULTS: **IV** Initial dose is 500 mL of 5% albumin given as rapidly as tolerated. If response in 30 min is inadequate, give additional 500 mL. In patients with slightly low or normal blood volume, rate is 2 to 4 mL/min.

CHILDREN: **IV** Rate of administration is 25% to 50% adult rate.
NEWBORNS AND INFANTS: **IV** 10 to 20 mL/kg 5% albumin based on clinical response, BP, and assessment of anemia.

Hypoproteinemia
To replace protein loss, 5% albumin may be given.

ALBUMIN HUMAN, 25%
Shock
ADULTS AND CHILDREN: **IV** Initial dose is determined by patient's condition and response to treatment. Therapy is guided by degree of venous or pulmonary congestion or Hct measurements.

Hypoproteinemia
ADULTS: **IV** 50 to 75 g/day at rate not exceeding 2 mL/min.
CHILDREN: **IV** 25 g/day at rate not exceeding 2 mL/min.

Acute Nephrosis
ADULTS: **IV** 100 mL 25% albumin in combination with loop diuretic repeated daily for 7 to 10 days.

Renal Dialysis
ADULTS: **IV** Approximately 100 mL 25% albumin.

Hyperbilirubinemia and Erythroblastosis Fetalis
NEWBORNS AND INFANTS: **IV** 1 g/kg 1 to 2 hr before transfusion.

Interactions None well documented.

Lab Test Interferences None well documented.

Adverse Reactions
CV: Hypotension after rapid infusion (above 10 mL/min) or intra-arterial administration to patients undergoing cardiopulmonary bypass; rapid administration may cause vascular overload, dyspnea or pulmonary edema.
OTHER: Allergic or pyogenic reactions (characterized by fever and chills).

Precautions
Pregnancy: Category C.
Lactation: Undetermined.
Renal function impairment: Caution is needed because of added protein load.
Hepatic function impairment: Caution is needed because of added protein load.
Special risk patients: Circulatory overload may develop in patients with CHF, renal insufficiency or stabilized chronic anemia.
Blood coadministration: Relative anemia can be avoided by supplementing or replacing large quantities of albumin with whole blood.

PATIENT CARE CONSIDERATIONS
Administration/Storage
- Administer by IV infusion only, using accompanying administration set and large-gauge needle or catheter.
- Give medication as supplied; do not dilute.
- Administer slowly to prevent too-rapid expansion of blood volume. The exception may be administered rapidly if there is severe loss of plasma volume.
- Do not administer if solution is cloudy or sediment is present.
- Store at room temperature. Do not freeze.

Assessment/Interventions
- Obtain patient history, including drug history and any known allergies. Note severe anemia, hepatic, or renal impairment.
- Assess baseline Hct before infusion.
- Take pulse and BP before and during infusion.
- Monitor liver and kidney function, Hct, electrolytes, plasma albumin, and total serum protein before and during therapy.
- Assess for signs of fluid overload before and during infusion.
- If venous or pulmonary congestion worsens or if hypotension occurs, slow or discontinue infusion and notify health care provider.
- Monitor I&O.
- Monitor for dehydration. Patient may require additional fluids.
- If patient has sustained injury or has had surgery, observe for new bleeding points as BP increases.
- Monitor for allergic or pyogenic reactions characterized by fever and chills. If these symptoms occur, discontinue treatment and notify health care provider.
- Do not infuse if intravascular volume is normal or increased or if patient has potential for fluid volume overload.

Patient/Family Education
- Explain rationale for infusion of drug and need for frequent monitoring.
- Instruct patient to report the following symptoms to health care provider: fever, chills, headache, back pain.

Albuterol

(al-BYOO-ter-ahl)
Class Bronchodilator/Sympathomimetic
How Supplied
Airet Solution for inhalation 0.083% (as sulfate) ♦ *Proventil* Tablets 2 mg (as sulfate), Tablets 4 mg (as sulfate), Syrup 2 mg (as sulfate) per 5 mL, Aerosol Each actuation delivers 90 mcg albuterol, Solution for inhalation 0.083% (as sulfate), Solution for inhalation 0.5% (as sulfate) ♦ *Proventil HFA* Aerosol Each actuation delivers 90 mcg albuterol (as sulfate) ♦ *Ventolin* Tablets 2 mg (as sulfate), Tablets 4 mg (as sulfate), Syrup 2 mg (as sulfate) per 5 mL, Solution for inhalation 0.5% (as sulfate) ♦ *Ventolin Nebules* Solution for inhalation 0.083% (as sulfate) ♦ *Ventolin Rotacaps* Capsules for inhalation 200 mcg microfine (as sulfate)
✽ *Airomir* ♦ *Alti-Salbutamol Sulfate* ♦ *Apo-Salvent* ♦ *Gen-Salbutamol Respirator Solution* ♦ *Gen-Salbutamol Sterinebs P.F.* ♦ *Novo-Salmol* ♦ *Nu-Salbutamol Solution* ♦ *PMS-Salbutamol Respirator Solution* ♦ *ratio-Salbutamol* ♦ *Rho-Salbutamol* ♦ *Rhoxal-salbutamol* ♦ *Ventodisk Disk* ♦ *Ventolin Diskus* ♦ *Ventolin Oral Liquid*

Action
PHARMACOLOGY: Produces bronchodilation by relaxing bronchial smooth muscle through beta-2 receptor stimulation.
PHARMACOKINETICS/DYNAMICS:
Absorption:
Tablets – Rapidly absorbed; T_{max} is 2 hr; C_{max} is about 18 ng/mL.
Inhalation – Less than 20% absorbed; T_{max} is 0.5 hr; C_{max} is 2.1 ng/mL.
Excretion: $T_{1/2}$ is 5 to 6 hr. 76% recovered in urine over 3 days with 60% as metabolites; 4% excreted in feces.
Onset:
Oral – Within 30 min.
Inhalation – Within 5 min.
Duration:
Oral – 4 to 8 hr.
Inhalation – 3 to 6 hr.

Indications Prevention and treatment of reversible bronchospasm associated with asthma and other obstructive pulmonary diseases.
Unlabeled use(s): Adjunctive treatment of hyperkalemia in patients undergoing dialysis.
Contraindications Cardiac tachyarrhythmias.

Route/Dosage
INHALATION AEROSOL
ADULTS AND CHILDREN AT LEAST 4 YR (AT LEAST 12 YR FOR *PROVENTIL*): 1 to 2 inhalations q 4 to 6 hr.
PREVENTION OF EXERCISE-INDUCED BRONCHOSPASM: 2 inhalations 15 min before exercise.

INHALATION SOLUTION
ADULTS AND CHILDREN AT LEAST 2 YR: 2.5 mg/dose 3 to 4 times/day by nebulization.
CHILDREN 2 TO 12 YR (*ACCUNEB*): 1.25 mg or 0.63 mg 3 to 4 times/day by nebulization.

ORAL
ADULTS AND CHILDREN AT LEAST 12 YR: PO 2 to 4 mg/dose 3 to 4 times/day. Do not exceed 32 mg/day.
CHILDREN 6 TO 12 YR: PO 2 mg/dose 3 to 4 times/day. Do not exceed 24 mg/day.
CHILDREN 2 TO 6 YR: PO 0.1 to 0.2 mg/kg/dose 3 times/day. Do not exceed 12 mg/day.
ADULTS AND CHILDREN ABOVE 12 YR, EXTENDED-RELEASE (*PROVENTIL REPETABS*): PO 4 to 8 mg q 12 hr. May be cautiously increased stepwise to a max of 16 mg bid (max, 32 mg/day).
CHILDREN 6 TO 12 YR, EXTENDED-RELEASE (*PROVENTIL REPETABS*): PO 4 q 12 hr. May be cautiously increased stepwise to a max of 12 mg bid.

SYRUP
ADULTS AND CHILDREN ABOVE 12 YR: 2 or 4 mg (1 to 2 tsp) 3 or 4 times/day. Doses of above 4 mg 4 times/day may be appropriate when patient fails to respond.
CHILDREN 6 TO 12 YR: 2 mg (1 tsp) 3 or 4 times/day. Doses of 2 mg 4 times/day may be cautiously increased. Do not exceed 24 mg/day in divided doses.
CHILDREN 2 TO 6 YR: Initiate at 0.1 mg/kg 3 times/day. Dose may be increased 2 mg 3 times/day. Do not exceed 2 mg 3 times/day. Dose may be increased to 0.2 mg/kg 3 times/day, but not to exceed 4 mg 3 times/day.
ELDERLY AND THOSE SENSITIVE TO BETA-ADRENERGIC STIMULATION: Restrict initial dose to 2 mg (1 tsp) 3 or 4 times/day. Individualize dosage thereafter.

Interactions
Beta-blockers: Severe bronchospasms may be produced in asthmatic patients taking albuterol.

Digoxin: Albuterol may decrease serum digoxin levels.
Diuretics: ECG changes and hypokalemia associated with these diuretics may worsen with albuterol coadministration.

Lab Test Interferences None well documented.

Adverse Reactions
CV: Palpitations; tachycardia; elevated BP; chest tightness; angina.
CNS: Tremor; dizziness; hyperactivity; nervousness; headache; insomnia; weakness; drowsiness; restlessness.
EENT: Dry mouth; throat irritation.
GI: Nausea; vomiting; heartburn; diarrhea.
GU: Urinary retention.
RESP: Cough; bronchospasm; wheezing; dyspnea.
OTHER: Flushing; sweating; anorexia; unusual sensory changes.

Precautions
Pregnancy: Category C.
Lactation: Unknown.
Children: Albuterol aerosol and inhalation powder in children below 4 yr and albuterol solution for inhalation in children below 2 yr not established.
Labor and delivery: May inhibit uterine contractions.
Cardiovascular effects: Toxic symptoms may occur in patients with cardiovascular disorders.
CNS effects: CNS stimulation may occur; use cautiously in patients with history of seizures or hyperthyroidism.
Diabetes: Dosage adjustment of insulin or oral hypoglycemic agent may be required.
Excessive use: Paradoxical bronchospasm and cardiac arrest have been associated with excessive inhalant use.
Hypokalemia: Decreases in potassium levels have occurred.
Tolerance: If previously effective dose fails to provide relief, therapy may need to be reassessed.

Overdosage: Signs and Symptoms
Tremor, palpitations, tachycardia, elevated BP, seizures.

PATIENT CARE CONSIDERATIONS

Administration/Storage
- Do not crush or chew tablets.
- Administer oral preparations with meals to minimize GI upset.
- Use before other inhalation therapy and before postural drainage.
- Allow 1 to 2 min between metered-dose inhalations and 5 min before administering other inhalant medications. Permit patient to rinse mouth after each completed inhalation dose.
- Store at room temperature. Refrigeration of syrup improves palatability.

Assessment/Interventions
- Obtain patient history, including drug history and any known allergies.
- Check pulse, BP, respiration, and lung sounds before and after administration.
- Review baseline and any follow-up ECG. If patient takes digoxin, check baseline and any follow-up serum digoxin levels.
- If patient is diabetic, check baseline and follow-up blood sugar levels.
- If bronchospasm occurs, withhold drug and report to health care provider.
- During pregnancy, monitor fetal heart rate and report tachycardia (more than 140 bpm).

Patient/Family Education
- Tell patient not to chew or crush capsules.
- Teach patient correct method for using metered-dose inhaler. Have patient demonstrate proper technique, including timing between inhalations.
- Instruct patient in home monitoring of pulse and BP.
- Advise patient to maintain fluid intake of 2000 mL/day and to rinse mouth after each complete dose.
- Instruct patient not to use OTC inhalers without consulting health care provider.
- Instruct patient to contact health care provider if symptoms are not relieved by normal dose.
- Tell patient to report adverse reactions or side effects.

Alclometasone Dipropionate

(al-kloe-MEH-tah-zone die-PRO-pee-oh-nate)

Class Corticosteroid/Topical

How Supplied
Aclovate Cream 0.05%, Ointment 0.05%

Action
PHARMACOLOGY: Topical glucocorticoid with anti-inflammatory, antipruritic, and vasoconstrictive properties. Thought to act by inducing phospholipase A_2 inhibitory proteins, thus controlling biosynthesis of potent mediators of inflammation.

Indications Relief of inflammatory and pruritic manifestations of corticosteroid-responsive dermatoses.

Contraindications Standard considerations.

Route/Dosage
ADULTS AND CHILDREN AT LEAST 1 YR OF AGE: **Topical** Apply thin film to affected area bid to tid.

Interactions None well documented.

Lab Test Interferences None well documented.

Adverse Reactions
DERM: Itching, burning, erythema, dryness, irritation, papular rashes (2%).

Precautions
Pregnancy: Category C.
Lactation: Undetermined.
Children: May be used with caution in pediatric patients at least 1 yr of age, although the safety and efficacy of drug use for more than 3 wk not established. Children may absorb proportionally larger amounts of topical corticosteroids and, therefore, be more susceptible to systemic toxicity. Use is not recommended in children under 1 yr of age. Pediatric patients are at higher risk than adults of hypothalamic-pituitary-adrenal (HPA) axis suppression and Cushing syndrome when they are treated with topical corticosteroids. Do not use to treat diaper rash.
Systemic: Systemic absorption may produce HPA axis suppression and systemic side effects, particularly when used over 20% of body surface area.

PATIENT CARE CONSIDERATIONS
Administration/Storage
- For topical use only. Not for ophthalmic, oral, or intravaginal use.
- Apply cream or ointment sparingly but in sufficient quantity to cover affected areas; rub in gently until medication disappears.
- Apply cream or ointment 1 to 3 times daily as prescribed.
- Avoid contact with the eyes.
- Store cream and ointment in refrigerator (36° to 46°F) or at ambient room temperature (below 86°F). Keep tube tightly capped.

Assessment/Interventions
- Obtain patient history, including drug history and any known allergies.
- Ensure that appropriate antifungal or antibacterial therapy is used in patient who has a concomitant skin infection.
- Assess and document skin condition before initial application and periodically throughout treatment. Inform health care provider if condition does not improve, worsens, or if application site reactions develop.
- Ensure that patient applying medication to a large surface area, or to areas under occlusion, is periodically evaluated for evidence of HPA axis suppression (eg, adrenocorticotropic hormone stimulation, morning plasma cortisol, urinary free cortisol tests).

Patient/Family Education
- Explain name, action, and potential side effects of drug.
- Teach patient or caregiver proper technique for applying cream or ointment: Wash hands; apply sufficient cream or ointment to cover affected areas sparingly and gently massage into skin; wash hands after applying cream or ointment.
- Advise patient to apply cream or ointment to affected areas 1 to 3 times a day as directed by health care provider.
- Advise patient that if a dose is missed, to apply it as soon as remembered and then continue on the regular schedule. If it is almost time for the next application, instruct patient to skip the dose and continue on the regular schedule. Caution patient not to apply double doses.
- Caution patient not to apply to face, underarms, or groin area unless directed by health care provider.
- Caution patient not to bandage, cover, or wrap treated skin areas or use cosmetics or other skin products over treated areas unless advised by health care provider.
- Caution patient to avoid contact with eyes. Advise patient that if cream does come into contact with the eyes, to wash eyes with large amounts of cool water and contact health care provider if eye irritation occurs.
- Caution parents of pediatric patients not to use alclometasone cream or ointment to treat diaper rash.
- Advise patient that symptoms should begin to improve fairly soon after starting treatment and to notify health care provider if condition does not improve, worsens, or if application site reactions (eg, burning, stinging, redness, itching) develop.
- Advise patient that therapy is usually discontinued when control has been achieved.
- Advise women to notify health care provider if pregnant, planning to become pregnant, or breastfeeding.
- Warn patient not to take any prescription or OTC drugs, dietary supplements, or herbal

preparations without consulting health care provider.
* Advise patient that follow-up visits to monitor response to treatment may be required and to keep appointments.

Aldesleukin

(al-dess-LOO-kin)

Class Biologic response modifier

How Supplied
Proleukin Preservative-free lyophilized powder for reconstitution 22 million IU (1.3 mg) vials (18 million IU [1.1 mg] per mL when reconstituted)

Action
PHARMACOLOGY: Enhancement of lymphocyte mitogenesis and stimulation of long-term growth of human IL-2 dependent cell lines. Enhancement of lymphocyte cytotoxicity. Induction of killer cell (lymphokine-activated [LAK] and natural [NK]) activity. Induction of interferon-gamma release.

PHARMACOKINETICS/DYNAMICS:
Distribution: Rapidly distributed into extravascular space; about 30% detectable in plasma. Distribution t½ is 13 min.

Excretion: Elimination t½ is 85 min. Eliminated by kidneys with little or no bioactive protein excreted in urine. Cl is 268 mL/min.

Indications Metastatic renal cell carcinoma, metastatic melanoma.

Contraindications Hypersensitivity to interleukin-2 or any component of the formulation; abnormal thallium stress test or pulmonary function tests; organ allografts; retreatment in patients experiencing CLS toxicities during initial therapy.

Route/Dosage
Metastatic Renal Cell Carcinoma, Metastatic Melanoma
ADULTS: IV 600,000 IU/kg q 8 hr by a 15 min IV infusion for 14 doses. Repeat regimen after 9 days recovery for a total of 28 doses/course. Evaluate tumor response 4 wk after therapy. If tumor shrinkage is evident and further treatment is not contraindicated, another course of aldesleukin may be given using the same regimen. Allow at least 7 wk between treatment courses (from date of hospital discharge). If toxicity occurs, hold or interrupt doses rather than decrease them. If hepatic failure occurs, discontinue further treatment for that course. Further courses may be given at least 7 wk after resolution of hepatic failure or hospital discharge, whichever is most recent.

Required Dosage Modification Because of Adverse Effects
CV – Permanently discontinue therapy if sustained ventricular tachycardia (at least 5 beats), uncontrolled or unresponsive arrhythmias, recurrent chest pain with ECG changes, documented angina, MI, or pericardial tamponade occur. Delay subsequent doses if atrial fibrillation, supraventricular tachycardia, or bradycardia, which requires therapy, recurs or persists. If systolic BP under 90 mm Hg with increasing pressor requirements occurs. If ECG changes consistent with MI, myocarditis, or ischemia with or without chest pain, or suspected cardiac ischemia occur. Continue with subsequent doses if asymptomatic with full recovery to normal sinus rhythm, or if MI is ruled out, there is a low suspicion of angina, systolic BP is at least 90 mm Hg and stable, and patient asymptomatic, or if no ventricular hypokinesia is present.
CNS – Permanently discontinue therapy if coma or toxic psychoses lasting more than 48 hr or if repetitive or refractory seizures occur. Delay subsequent doses if mental status changes occur (eg, moderate confusion, agitation). Continue with subsequent doses if complete resolution of mental status changes occurs.
DERM – Delay subsequent doses if bullous dermatitis or if marked worsening of preexisting skin condition occur. Continue with subsequent doses if complete resolution of bullous dermatitis occurs.
GI – Permanently discontinue therapy if bowel ischemia, perforation, or bleeding requiring surgery occur. Delay subsequent doses if stool guaiac is more than 3 to 4+, repeatedly. Continue with subsequent doses if negative stool guaiac occurs.
HEPA – Delay subsequent doses if signs of hepatic failure (eg, encephalopathy, increased ascites, liver pain, hypoglycemia) occur. Continue with subsequent doses if resolution of hepatic failure occurs.
RENAL – Permanently discontinue therapy if dysfunction requiring dialysis for more than 72 hr occurs. Delay subsequent doses if serum creatinine above 4.5 mg/dL or serum creatinine of above 4 mg/dL with severe volume overload, acidosis, or hyperkalemia. Persistent oliguria or urine output less than 10 mL/hr for 16 to 24 hr with increasing serum creatinine. Continue with subsequent doses if serum creatinine is below 4 mg/dL with stable fluid and electrolytes, or if urine output is above 10 mL/hr with normalization or decrease (over 1.5 mg/dL) in creatinine.
RESP – Permanently discontinue therapy if intubation is required for more than 72 hr. Delay subsequent doses if oxygen saturation is

below 90%. Continue with subsequent doses if oxygen saturation above 90%.
SYST – Delay subsequent doses if sepsis syndrome occurs. Continue with subsequent doses if resolution of sepsis syndrome occurs, patient is clinically stable, or if infection is under treatment.

Interactions
Beta-blockers and other antihypertensives: May exacerbate aldesleukin-induced hypotension.
Cardiotoxic drugs (eg, doxorubicin): May exacerbate aldesleukin cardiotoxicity.
CNS depressants (eg, narcotics, analgesics, alcohol, antiemetics, benzodiazepines, sedatives, tranquilizers): May exacerbate aldesleukin CNS adverse effects.
Corticosteroids: May reduce the antineoplastic effect of aldesleukin.
Hepatotoxic drugs (eg, methotrexate, asparaginase): May exacerbate aldesleukin hepatotoxicity.
Myelotoxic drugs (eg, cytotoxic chemotherapy): May exacerbate aldesleukin myelotoxicity.
Nephrotoxic drugs (eg, aminoglycosides, NSAIDs): May exacerbate aldesleukin nephrotoxicity.
Protease inhibitors (eg, indinavir): Protease inhibitor levels may be elevated, increasing risk of toxicity.

Lab Test Interferences None well documented.

Adverse Reactions
CV: Hypotension (71%); tachycardia (23%); supraventricular tachycardia (12%); CV disorder (eg, asymptomatic ECG changes, CHF, BP fluctuations [11%]); arrhythmia (10%); MI, ventricular tachycardia; heart arrest (1%); myocarditis, pericarditis, transient ischemic attacks, atrial arrhythmia, second-degree AV block, bradycardia, coronary artery disorders, endocarditis, myocardial ischemia, pericardial effusion, syncope, thrombosis, ventricular extrasystoles, stroke, peripheral gangrene, phlebitis (less than 1%); cardiomyopathy, cerebral hemorrhage, fatal endocarditis, hypertension (postmarketing).
CNS: Confusion (34%); somnolence (22%); anxiety (12%); dizziness (11%); coma (2%); psychosis, stupor (1%); cerebral edema, meningitis, agitation, convulsion, delirium, grand mal convulsion, hyperthermia, neuropathy, paranoid reaction, shock somnolence, malignant hyperthermia, severe depression leading to suicide (less than 1%); cerebral lesions, encephalopathy, extrapyramidal syndrome, insomnia, neuralgia, neuropathy (demyelination), neuritis (postmarketing).
DERM: Rash (42%); pruritus (24%); exfoliative dermatitis (18%); cellulitis, injection-site necrosis, urticaria (postmarketing).
EENT: Mydriasis, papillary disorder (less than 1%).
GI: Diarrhea (67%); vomiting (50%); nausea (35%); stomatitis (22%); anorexia (20%); abdominal pain (11%); enlarged abdomen (10%); bowel necrosis, duodenal ulceration, tracheo-esophageal fistula, bloody diarrhea, GI hemorrhage, hematemesis, intestinal perforation, nausea, stomatitis, vomiting. pancreatitis (less than 1%); cholecystitis, colitis, gastritis, intestinal obstruction (postmarketing).
GU: Oliguria (63%); anuria (5%); acute kidney failure (1%); abnormal kidney function, acute tubular necrosis, increased BUN, kidney failure, hyperuricemia (less than 1%).
HEPA: Increased AST (23%); abnormal LFTs, liver failure (less than 1%); hepatitis, hepatosplenomegaly (postmarketing).
HEMA/LYMPH: Thrombocytopenia (37%); anemia (29%); leukopenia (16%); coagulation disorders (including, intravascular coagulopathy [1%]); leukocytosis, hemorrhage (less than 1%); neutropenia (postmarketing).
LABTESTABS: Increased nonprotein nitrogen (less than 1%).
M/N: Bilirubinemia (40%); increased creatinine (33%); peripheral edema (28%); weight gain (16%); edema (15%); acidosis, hypomagnesemia, (12%); hypocalcemia (11%); increased alkaline phosphatase (10%).
MUSC: Myopathy, myositis, rhabdomyolysis (postmarketing).
RENAL: Renal failure (less than 1%).
RESP: Dyspnea (43%); lung disorder (including, pulmonary congestion, rales, rhonchi [24%]); respiratory disorder (including, ARDS, chest x-ray infiltrates, unspecified pulmonary changes, increased cough (11%); rhinitis (10%); apnea (1%); pulmonary edema, pulmonary emboli, asthma, hemoptysis, hyperventilation, hypoventilation. hypoxia, pneumothorax, respiratory acidosis, respiratory arrest, respiratory failure (less than 1%); pneumonia (bacterial, fungal, viral [postmarketing]).
OTHER: Chills (52%); fever (29%); malaise (27%); asthenia (23%); infection (13%); pain

(12%); sepsis (1%); anaphylaxis, hyperthyroidism, retroperitoneal hemorrhage (postmarketing).

> **WARNING:**
> Therapy with aldesleukin for injection should be restricted to patients with normal cardiac and pulmonary functions.
>
> Aldesleukin should be administered in a hospital setting under the supervision of a qualified physician experienced in the use of anticancer agents. An intensive care facility and specialists skilled in cardiopulmonary or intensive care medicine must be available.
>
> Aldesleukin administration has been associated with CLS. CLS results in hypotension and reduced organ perfusion which may be severe and can result in death. CLS may be associated with cardiac arrhythmias (supraventricular and ventricular), angina, MI, respiratory insufficiency requiring intubation, GI bleeding or infarction, renal insufficiency, edema, and mental status changes.
>
> Aldesleukin treatment is associated with impaired neutrophil function (reduced chemotaxis) and with an increased risk of disseminated infection, including sepsis and bacterial endocarditis. Treat preexisting infections prior to initiation of therapy.
>
> Aldesleukin administration should be withheld in patients developing moderate to severe lethargy or somnolence; continued administration may result in coma.

Precautions

Pregnancy: Category C.
Lactation: Undetermined. Because of the potential for serious adverse reactions in nursing infants, decide whether to discontinue nursing or to discontinue the drug, taking into account the importance of the drug to the mother.
Children: Safety and efficacy not established.
Hypersensitivity: Reactions have been reported in patients receiving combination regimens containing sequential high-dose aldesleukin and antineoplastic agents.

PATIENT CARE CONSIDERATIONS

Administration/Storage

♦ For IV infusion only. Not for IV bolus, intradermal, SC, IM, or intra-arterial administration.

♦ Follow institutional procedures for handling,

Renal function impairment: Impairment of renal function occurs during treatment.
Hepatic function impairment: Impairment of hepatic function occurs during treatment.
Fertility impairment: It is recommended that this drug not be administered to fertile people of either sex not practicing effective contraception.
Allograft rejection: Enhancement of cellular immune function may increase the risk of allograft rejection in transplant patients.
Autoimmune diseases: Aldesleukin may exacerbate autoimmune disease.
CLS: Begins immediately after initiation of treatment and results from extravasation of plasma proteins and fluid into the extravascular space and loss of vascular tone. Watch for a drop in mean arterial BP within 2 to 12 hr after the start of treatment and reduced organ perfusion, which may be severe and result in death.
CNS effects: New neurologic signs, symptoms, and anatomic lesions have been reported in patients without evidence of CNS metastases.
CNS metastases: May exacerbate disease symptoms in patients with clinically unrecognized or untreated CNS metastases.
Iodinated contrast media: Acute, atypical adverse reactions (eg, fever, chills, nausea, vomiting, pruritus, rash, diarrhea, hypotension, edema) have been reported in patients administered iodine contrast media subsequent to IL-2 treatment.
Mental status changes: Mental status changes including irritability, confusion, or depression may occur and may be indicators of bacteremia or early bacterial sepsis.
Retreatment: Contraindicated in patients who experienced the following toxicities while receiving an earlier course of therapy: sustained ventricular tachycardia (at least 5 beats); cardiac rhythm disturbances uncontrolled or unresponsive; recurrent chest pain with ECG changes, consistent with angina or MI; intubation required more than 72 hr; pericardial tamponade, renal dysfunction requiring dialysis more than 72 hr; coma or toxic psychosis lasting more than 48 hr; repetitive or difficult to control seizures; bowel ischemia/perforation; GI bleeding requiring surgery.
Thyroid function impairment: Impairment has occurred following treatment.

Overdosage: Signs and Symptoms
Dose-related side effects.

administration, and disposal of anticancer drugs.

♦ Reconstitute powder for injection with 1.2 mL sterile water for injection following manufacturer's guidelines. Swirl to mix; do

not shake vial. Dilute prescribed amount of reconstituted solution with appropriate volume of 5% dextrose injection following manufacturer's guidelines.
- Do not reconstitute or dilute with bacteriostatic water for injection or 0.9% sodium chloride injection or mix with any other medications.
- Do not administer if particulate matter or cloudiness is noted. A slight yellow coloration is normal and of no concern.
- Administer premedications (eg, NSAIDs, meperidine, H_2 antagonists) as ordered before beginning infusion and for 12 hr after the final aldesleukin dose.
- Administer prescribed dose by IV infusion over 15 min. Do not use in-line filters.
- Dose is usually repeated q 8 hr for 14 doses unless toxicity or severe side effects develop.
- For single-use only. Discard unused portions of vial. Do not save any unused portions for future use.
- Store unopened vials, reconstituted and diluted solutions in refrigerator (36° to 46°F). Do not freeze. Administer within 48 hr of reconstitution. Bring refrigerated solution to room temperature prior to infusion. Discard solution if not used within 48 hr.

Assessment/Interventions

- Obtain patient history, including drug history and any known allergies. Note renal or hepatic impairment, history of cardiac or respiratory disease, abnormal thallium stress test or pulmonary function tests, organ allograft, history of CLS with previous treatment, autoimmune disease, inflammatory disorder, seizure disorder, concurrent treatment with nephrotoxic, or hepatotoxic, myelotoxic, or cardiotoxic medications.
- Do not administer to patient with abnormal thallium stress test or pulmonary function test, or organ allograft.
- If considering retreatment, review patient history for any previous toxicity to aldesleukin that would contraindicate further treatment: sustained ventricular tachycardia; uncontrolled cardiac arrhythmias; chest pain with ECG changes consistent with angina or MI; intubation for greater than 72 hr; cardiac tamponade; renal dysfunction requiring dialysis for greater than 72 hr; coma or toxic psychosis lasting more than 48 hr; repetitive or difficult to control seizures; bowel ischemia or perforation; GI bleeding requiring surgery.
- Do not administer to patient with serum creatinine greater than 1.5 mg/dL.
- Review guidelines for discontinuing, or holding and restarting, aldesleukin therapy because of CV, CNS, DERM, GI, PULM, renal, hepatic, or systemic complications, before starting therapy.
- Ensure that preexisting bacterial infections have been treated before initiating therapy.
- Ensure that CNS metastases have been treated prior to initiating therapy and patient has a negative CT scan.
- Ensure that use of prophylactic antibiotics have been considered for patient with indwelling central line(s).
- Ensure that pulmonary function tests, arterial blood gasses and stress thallium study are performed, and the results documented before initiating therapy.
- Ensure that CBC with differential and platelet count, serum electrolytes, renal function, liver enzymes, and chest x-ray are evaluated before starting therapy and then daily during drug administration.
- Assess vital signs, weight, and fluid intake and output daily during treatment. If patient develops a decreased systolic BP (below 90 mm Hg), conduct constant cardiac rhythm monitoring and take vital signs hourly.
- Monitor pulmonary function (clinical examination, pulse oximetry, vital signs) on regular basis during therapy. Further assess patient with dyspnea or clinical signs of respiratory impairment (eg, tachypnea, rales) with arterial blood gas determinations.
- Monitor cardiac function (clinical examination, vital signs) daily during therapy. Further assess patient with new signs or symptoms of cardiac dysfunction (eg, chest pain, irregular rhythm) with an ECG and cardiac enzyme evaluation. Hold aldesleukin therapy and perform a repeat thallium studies if there is evidence of cardiac ischemia or CHF.
- Monitor patient for signs and symptoms of CLS (eg, hypotension, tachycardia, edema). Inform health care provider immediately and be prepared to treat appropriately with close monitoring (eg, BP, pulse, weight, urine output), IV fluids (eg, colloids, crystalloids), and vasopressors (eg, dopamine). Discontinue aldesleukin therapy if evidence of failure to maintain organ perfusion (eg, altered mental status, reduced urine output, cardiac arrhythmias, or systolic BP less than 90 mm Hg) develop.
- Monitor patient for signs and symptoms of CNS toxicity (eg, change in mental status, speech difficulties, hallucinations, agitation, cortical blindness, limb or gait ataxia, obtundation, coma). Immediately notify health care provider and be prepared to discontinue therapy.

- Monitor patient for signs and symptoms of anaphylactic or serious allergic reactions. Be prepared to treat appropriately.
- Ensure that women of childbearing potential are not pregnant or attempting to become pregnant.
- Assess patient for GI, DERM, HEMA, and general body side effects. Report to health care provider if noted and significant.

Patient/Family Education
- Explain name, action, and potential side effects of drug.
- Advise patient, family, or caregiver that medication will be prepared and administered by health care provider in a health care setting.
- Review dosing schedule with patient, family, or caregiver.
- Advise patient, family, or caregiver to immediately report any of the following to health care provider: fever, mental status changes, hallucinations, agitation, speech difficulties, vision changes, incoordination, swelling, difficulty breathing, shortness of breath or unexplained rapid breathing, chest pain, pounding in chest, changes in heart rhythm.
- Caution women of childbearing potential to avoid becoming pregnant during therapy.
- Advise women of childbearing potential to notify health care provider if pregnant, planning to become pregnant, or breastfeeding.
- Instruct patient not to take any prescription or OTC medications or dietary supplements unless advised by health care provider.
- Advise patient, family, or caregiver that frequent follow-up visits and laboratory tests will be required after discharge to monitor therapy and to keep appointments.

Alefacept

(ah-LEE-fah-sept)

Class Anti-Psoriatic/Immunosuppressant

How Supplied
Amevive Powder for injection, lyophilized 7.5 mg, Powder for injection, lyophilized 15 mg

Action
PHARMACOLOGY: Interferes with lymphocyte activation.

PHARMACOKINETICS/DYNAMICS:
Absorption: Bioavailability of alefacept after IM injection is 63%.

Distribution: The mean Vd of alefacept is 94 mL/kg after IV injection.

Excretion: The mean elimination t½ and Cl are approximately 270 hr and 0.25 mL/kg, respectively, following IV injection.

Indications Treatment of adult patients with moderate to severe chronic plaque psoriasis who are candidates for systemic therapy orphototherapy.

Contraindications Standard considerations.

Route/Dosage
Should only be used under the guidance and supervision of a health care professional.
Adults:
IV/IM 7.5 mg once weekly as an **IV** bolus or 15 mg once weekly as an **IM** injection for 12 weekly injections. After a minimum of a 12-wk interval since the initial treatment, retreatment, with an additional 12-wk course may be initiated provided the CD4+ T-lymphocyte counts are within the normal range.

Interactions None well documented.

INCOMPATIBILITIES: Do not add other medications to solutions containing alefacept and do not reconstitute with other diluents.

Lab Test Interferences None well documented.

Adverse Reactions
CV: Coronary artery disorder; MI.
CNS: Dizziness; nausea.
DERM: Pruritus.
RESP: Pharyngitis; increased cough.
OTHER: Hypersensitivity reactions (eg, urticaria, angioedema, anaphylactic reactions); malignancies; serious infections; lymphopenia; myalgia; chills; injection site reactions (eg, pain, inflammation, bleeding, edema, nonspecific reaction, mass, skin hypersensitivity); accidental injury.

Precautions
Pregnancy: Category B.
Lactation: Undetermined.
Children: Safety and efficacy not established.
Elderly: Use with caution because the incidence of infection and certain malignancies is higher.
Immunosuppressive system: Because of the risk of excessive immunosuppression, do not use with other immunosuppressive agents or phototherapy.
Lymphopenia: Because alefacept induces dose-dependent reductions in circulating CD4+ and CD8+ T-lymphocyte counts, do not initiate therapy in patients with a CD4+ T-lymphocyte count below normal.
Malignancies: May increase the risk of malignancies.
Serious infections: Because alefacept is an immunosuppressive agent, it may increase the risk of

infection and reactivate latent, chronic infections.

PATIENT CARE CONSIDERATIONS
Administration/Storage
- For IV or IM administration only. Not for SC or intradermal administration.
- Dose is administered once weekly.
- Reconstitute powder for injection following manufacturer's instructions.
- Do not shake or vigorously agitate vial during reconstitution.
- Do not filter solution during preparation or administration.
- Do not administer if particulate matter, cloudiness, or discoloration noted.
- Do not add other medications to solution.
- Rotate IM injection sites (thigh, abdomen, upper arm). Give new injections at least 1 inch from old site and never into areas where the skin is tender, bruised, red, or hard.
- Administer IV dose over no more than 5 sec using 3 mL normal saline for pre- and postadministration flush.
- Discard any unused solution. Do not save unused solution for later administration.
- Store dose tray with lyophilized powder at controlled room temperature (59° to 86°F). Store in original carton until time of use. Protect from light.
- Use reconstituted product immediately or within 4 hr if stored in refrigerator (36° to 46°F). Discard if not used within 4 hr of reconstitution.

Assessment/Interventions
- Obtain patient history, including drug history and any known allergies. Note history of chronic infections, recurrent infections, conditions predisposing to infections, or concurrent immunosuppressive therapy or phototherapy.
- Ensure that patient does not have an active chronic or localized infection prior to starting therapy.
- Ensure that CD4+ T-lymphocyte counts are determined prior to starting therapy and weekly throughout entire 12 wk course of therapy.
- Withhold therapy if CD4+ T-lymphocyte count is below 250 cells/mcL.
- Discontinue therapy if CD4+ T-lymphocyte counts are below 250 cells/mcL for 1 mo.
- Monitor patient for signs and symptoms of infection and immediately report to health care provider if noted.
- Monitor patient for signs and symptoms of anaphylactic or serious allergic reactions. Be prepared to treat appropriately.
- Monitor patient for CNS, GI, respiratory, and general body side effects, and injection site reactions. Report to health care provider if noted and significant.
- Do not administer live virus vaccines while patient is on alefacept therapy.

Patient/Family Education
- Explain name, dose, action, and potential side effects of drug.
- Advise patient that medication will be prepared and administered by a health care professional in a medical setting.
- Advise patient to report any of the following symptoms to health care provider: intolerable injection site reactions, fever or other signs of infection, sore throat.
- Instruct women to notify health care provider if pregnant or planning to become pregnant during and for 8 wk following discontinuation of therapy.
- Instruct women to notify health care provider if considering breastfeeding while taking this medication.
- Instruct patient to not take any prescription or OTC medications or dietary supplements unless advised to do so by health care provider.
- Remind patient that office visits and laboratory tests will be required to monitor therapy and to keep appointments.

Overdosage: Signs and Symptoms
Chills, headache, arthralgia, sinusitis.

Alemtuzumab
(ah-lem-TOO-ze-mab)
Class Monoclonal antibody
How Supplied
Campath Sterile, preservative-free solution for injection 30 mg/3 mL in a single-use ampule
Action
PHARMACOLOGY: Alemtuzumab is a recombinant DNA-derived humanized monoclonal antibody. Alemtuzumab binds to CD52, a nonmodulating antigen that is present on the surface of essentially all B- and T- lymphocytes, a majority of monocytes, macrophages, and NK cells, and a subpopulation of granulocytes. The proposed mechanism of action is antibody-dependent lysis of leukemic cells following cell surface binding. The maximum serum concen-

tration and the AUC has shown relative dose proportionality.

Pharmacokinetics/Dynamics:
Absorption: Time to reach steady-state is about 6 wk.
Excretion: $T_{1/2}$ is about 12 days.

Indications Refractory B-cell chronic lymphocytic leukemia. **Unlabeled use(s):** Rheumatoid arthritis, multiple sclerosis.

Contraindications Patients who are allergic to alemtuzumab, in patients with active systemic infections, and in patients with underlying immunodeficiency.

Route/Dosage
Refractory B-cell Chronic Lymphocytic Leukemia
ADULTS (INITIAL DOSE): **IV** 3 mg/dose daily until tolerated. Increase to 10 mg/dose IV daily until tolerated, then switch to maintenance regimen. Most patients start the maintenance regimen within 3 to 7 days of initiating therapy.
ADULTS (MAINTENANCE): **IV** 30 mg/dose, given 3 times weekly for 4 to 12 wk. Give doses on alternate days, with 1 day between doses (such as Mondays, Wednesdays, and Fridays). Gradually increase to the recommended maintenance dose when initiating therapy or when therapy is interrupted for at least 7 days. To reduce the risk of pancytopenia, avoid giving single doses that are more than 30 mg or cumulative doses more than 90 mg/week.

Dosage Adjustment
ADULTS: **IV** Discontinue alemtuzumab if any serious toxicity occurs, including severe infection, profound hematologic toxicity, or other serious adverse effects. Resume treatment after the event resolves, using the following dosage adjustment information. Treatment may resume with 3 mg once daily or 3 times weekly on alternate days, at the health care provider's discretion. Similarly, the regimen may be escalated to 10 mg once daily or 3 times weekly on alternate days. No specific guidelines are available for making this determination. Permanently discontinue therapy if autoimmune anemia or thrombocytopenia is evident.

Dosage Adjustment for Hematologic Toxicity (Patients with Normal Baseline Values, ANC less than 250, or Platelet Count 25,000 or less)
ADULTS (FIRST OCCURRENCE): **IV** Delay therapy until ANC at least 500 and platelet count at least 50,000. If therapy is delayed less than 7 days, resume therapy at same dose. If delayed at least 7 days, resume therapy at 3 mg, increasing to 10 and 30 mg as tolerated. *Second occurrence:* Delay therapy until ANC at least 500 and platelet count at least 50,000. If therapy is delayed less than 7 days, resume therapy at 10 mg. If delayed at least 7 days, resume therapy at 3 mg and increase to 10 mg (maximum) as tolerated. *Third occurrence:* Permanently discontinue therapy.

Dosage Adjustment for Hematologic Toxicity (Patient with Baseline ANC 500 or less or Baseline Platelet Count 25,000 or less)
ADULTS (ANC OR PLATELET COUNT DECREASE AT LEAST 50%): **IV** Delay therapy until ANC and platelet count return to baseline. If therapy is delayed less than 7 days, resume therapy at same dose. If delayed at least 7 days, resume therapy at 3 mg, increasing to 10 and 30 mg as tolerated.

Interactions None well documented.

Lab Test Interferences An immune response to alemtuzumab may interfere with subsequent diagnostic serum tests that utilize antibodies.

Adverse Reactions
CV: Hypotension; peripheral edema; hypertension; supraventricular tachycardia.
CNS: Fatigue; headache; dysesthesias; asthenia; dizziness; insomnia.
DERM: Rash; urticaria; pruritus; increased sweating.
GI: Moderate to low potential for nausea and vomiting; diarrhea; anorexia; mucositis;, abdominal pain; and dyspepsia common.
HEMA: Myelosuppression (80% to 85%); fatal pancytopenia; marrow hypoplasia; autoimmune anemia; autoimmune thrombocytopenia.
MUSC: Skeletal pain; myalgias; back pain; chest pain.
RESP: Dyspnea; cough; bronchitis or pneumonitis; pneumonia; pharyngitis.
OTHER: Rigors; fever; pain. Infections in 43% of patients despite antimicrobial prophylaxis; fatal infections (18% of patients receiving prophylaxis).
Infusion reactions – Rigors and fever in more than 80% of patients during the infusion or within 45 to 60 minutes afterward. Nausea; vomiting; rash; urticaria; dyspnea; hypotension; and chills also may occur.

> **WARNING:**
> Alemtuzumab has been associated with infusion-related events including hypotension, rigors, fever, shortness of breath, bronchospasm, chills, or rash. In order to ameliorate or avoid infusion-related events, premedicate patients with an oral antihistamine and acetaminophen prior to dosing and monitor closely. In addition, initiate alemtuzumab at a low dose with gradual escalation to the effective dose. Careful monitoring of blood pressure and hypotensive symptoms is recommended, especially in patients with ischemic heart disease and in patients on antihypertensive medications. If therapy is interrupted for at least 7 days, reinstitute alemtuzumab with gradual dose escalation.
>
> Serious, potentially fatal (rare) pancytopenia, marrow hypoplasia, autoimmune idiopathic thrombocytopenia, and autoimmune hemolytic anemia have occurred.
>
> Serious sometimes fatal opportunistic infections (bacterial, viral, fungal, and protozoan) reported.

Precautions

Pregnancy: Category C.
Lactation: Undetermined. Discontinue breastfeeding during treatment and for at least 3 mo following the last dose of alemtuzumab.
Children: Safety and efficacy in children not established.
Hypersensitivity: Discontinue further therapy if the patient experiences anaphylaxis. Patients who are hypersensitive to alemtuzumab may react to other monoclonal antibodies.
Cardiovascular: Use additional caution in patients with ischemic heart disease or patients receiving antihypertensive medications.
Immunization: Because of their immunosuppression, do not immunize patients who have recently received alemtuzumab with live viral vaccines.
Immunogenicity: Four (1.9%) of 211 patients evaluated for development of an immune response were found to have antibodies to alemtuzumab.
Immunosuppression: Alemtuzumab may cause profound immunosuppression and increased risk of infection during treatment and for up to 12 mo afterward. Immune response to vaccines may be decreased and vaccine efficacy reduced. However, risk of infection caused by live attenuated vaccines may increase.
Lymphopenia: Patients with profound lymphopenia are at risk for graft-vs-host disease when nonirradiated blood products are given. Administration of irradiated blood products is recommended.

PATIENT CARE CONSIDERATIONS

Administration/Storage

- Refrigerate; do not freeze. Protect from direct sunlight.
- Discard ampule if solution has been frozen.
- Avoid shaking the ampule before use.
- Withdraw appropriate dose from ampule, then filter with a sterile 5 micron filter prior to dilution.
- Visually inspect solution and discard if particulates or discoloration are present.
- Dilute in 100 mL 0.9% Sodium Chloride or 5% Dextrose. Mix the solution by gently inverting the bag.
- Diluted solutions are preservative-free and should be used within 24 hr to reduce the risk of microbial contamination. The manufacturer recommends use within 8 hr.
- Store diluted solutions at room temperature or in the refrigerator. Protect from light.
- Administer by IV infusion. Do not administer as an IV push or bolus.
- Infuse over 2 hr. Observe patients for infusion-related symptoms (eg, rigors, fever).

Pretreatment regimen:
- Give acetaminophen 650 mg (oral or rectal) and diphenhydramine 50 mg (oral or IV) 30 min before administering alemtuzumab. In patients who experience severe infusion reactions, hydrocortisone sodium succinate 200 mg IV may be added to the pretreatment regimen prior to subsequent doses. Give premedication before the first dose, before dose escalation, and as needed.

Antimicrobial prophylaxis:
- Give prophylactic antimicrobials to reduce the risk of serious infections, starting on the first day of alemtuzumab therapy. Continue prophylaxis for 2 mo after the last alemtuzumab dose or until the $CD4^+$ count is at least 200 cells/mcL, whichever is later. Although the manufacturer recommends the following regimen, other agents with similar spectrums of activity may be used. Co-trimoxazole 800/160 (eg, *Bactrim DS*, *Septra DS*) orally twice daily, 3 times per week, plus famciclovir *Famvir*) 250 mg orally twice daily.

Assessment/Interventions
Infusion reactions:
- If the patient experiences a reaction, the infusion may be continued at the same rate at the health care provider's discretion. Temporarily interrupt the infusion or decrease the rate for severe reactions, including hypotension, hypertension, shortness of breath, or rash. Symptoms may be treated with hydrocortisone (eg, *Solu-Cortef*) 200 mg IV, diphenhydramine (eg, *Benadryl*), acetaminophen (eg, *Tylenol*), bronchodilators, oxygen, or IV fluids. Monitor the patient until symptoms resolve completely. Patients who react to alemtuzumab infusions may receive additional doses. Hydrocortisone or an equivalent corticosteroid may be added to the pretreatment regimen at the practitioner's discretion.
- Monitor vital signs (eg, heart rate, blood pressure, respiratory rate, temperature) q 15 to 30 min during the infusion and for 4 hr afterward.
- Hyperuricemia may occur caused by rapid cell lysis; monitor serum uric acid. Minimize effects of hyperuricemia with hydration, urinary alkalinization, and allopurinol.
- Monitor CBC, differential, and platelet count at baseline and once weekly during therapy. Patients may need red blood cell transfusions or erythropoietin therapy to maintain adequate counts. After treatment, monitor $CD4^+$ count until it is at least 200 cells/mcL.
- Avoid immunization with live attenuated vaccines during this period, including BCG, measles, mumps, rubella, Ty21a typhoid, varicella, yellow fever, and others.
- Use alemtuzumab cautiously in patients who are allergic to neomycin or to hamsters, especially Chinese Hamster Ovary cell proteins.

Patient/Family Education
- Women of childbearing age and men of reproductive potential should use effective contraceptive methods during treatment and for at least 6 mo after alemtuzumab therapy.

Alendronate Sodium

(al-LEN-droe-nate SO-dee-uhm)
Class Hormone/Bisphosphonates
How Supplied
Fosamax Tablets 5 mg, Tablets 10 mg, Tablets 40 mg

Action
PHARMACOLOGY: Inhibits bone resorption and increases bone density.
PHARMACOKINETICS/DYNAMICS:
Absorption: Oral bioavailability is 0.64% (women) and 0.59% (men). Food decreases bioavailability significantly.

Distribution: Distributes to soft tissues, then rapidly to bone. Vd is at least 28 L (exclusive of bone); about 78% protein bound.

Metabolism: Not metabolized.

Excretion: About 50% excreted in urine. $T_{1/2}$ is more than 10 years.

Special Populations:
Renal Function Impairment – Elimination may be reduced. No dosage adjustment is necessary in those with mild to moderate renal insufficiency. Alendronate is not recommended in those with severe renal insufficiency (Ccr less than 35 mL/min).

Indications Treatment of osteoporosis in postmenopausal women; prevention of osteoporosis in postmenopausal women at risk of developing osteoporosis; treatment of osteoporosis in men; treatment of glucocorticoid-induced osteoporosis in men and women; treatment of Paget disease of the bone.

Contraindications Hypocalcemia.
Route/Dosage
Osteoporosis (Postmenopausal Women)
ADULTS (TREATMENT): PO 70 mg once weekly or 10 mg once daily.
ADULTS (PREVENTION): PO 35 mg once weekly or 5 mg once daily.

Osteoporosis (Men)
ADULTS: PO 10 mg once daily.

Glucocorticoid-Induced Osteoporosis
ADULTS: PO 5 mg once daily. For postmenopausal women not receiving estrogen, 10 mg once daily.

Paget Disease
ADULTS: PO 40 mg once daily for 6 mo. Retreatment may be considered for patients who relapse after a 6-mo observation period.

Interactions
Aspirin: Risk of upper GI adverse effects is increased by concomitant use of aspirin and alendronate doses over 10 mg/day.
Calcium supplements, antacids: Decreased alendronate absorption.
Food: Absorption of alendronate is decreased by food.
Liquids: Beverages other than water decrease absorption.
Ranitidine: Increased alendronate absorption; clinical importance unknown.

Lab Test Interferences None well documented.

Adverse Reactions
CNS: Headache.
GI: Abdominal pain; constipation; diarrhea; flatulence; esophageal ulcer; dysphagia.

OTHER: Musculoskeletal pain.
Precautions
Pregnancy: Category C.
Lactation: Undetermined.
Children: Safety and efficacy not established.
Renal function impairment: Not recommended for patients with Ccr below 35 mL/min.
Absorption: Food, beverages other than water, and medication inhibit absorption. Must be taken first thing in the morning with a full glass of water at least 30 min before any food, beverages, or medications. Must remain sitting or standing for 30 min after taking.
Concomitant estrogen replacement therapy: Not recommended.
GI Disorders: Not recommended for patients with upper GI problems.
Hypocalcemia: Correct before starting alendronate.
Nutrition: Maintain adequate calcium and vitamin D intake during alendronate therapy.

Overdosage: Signs and Symptoms
Hypocalcemia, hypophosphatemia, upper GI adverse effects.

PATIENT CARE CONSIDERATIONS
Administration/Storage
- Divide dose if GI upset occurs.
- Avoid high calcium food, vitamins with mineral supplements, and antacids high in metals within 2 hr of dosing.
- Take 30 min before first meal, medication, or drink of the day. Take with 6 to 8 oz of plain water only.
- Store at room temperature in well-closed container.

Assessment/Interventions
- Obtain patient history.
- Assess for hypersensitivity reaction.
- Assess for severe renal insufficiency prior to administration.

Patient/Family Education
- Instruct patient to take medication with plain water 30 min before the first food or drink of the day.
- Take medication with a full glass of water. Patient should not lie down for 30 min following administration.
- Instruct patient not to suck or chew on tablet; swallow whole.
- Have patient take supplemental calcium (1500 mg) and vitamin D (400 IU PO daily) if dietary intake is not adequate.
- Encourage patient to perform weight-bearing exercises and modify behaviors that promote osteoporosis (ie, avoid alcohol and cigarette smoking).
- Have patient read package insert before starting therapy.

Alfentanil Hydrochloride
(al-FEN-tuh-NILL HIGH-droe-KLOR-ide)

Class Narcotic agonist analgesic

How Supplied
Alfenta Injection 500 mcg (as HCL)/mL

Action
PHARMACOLOGY: Binds opioid receptors in CNS.

PHARMACOKINETICS/DYNAMICS:
Distribution: Vd is 0.4 to 1 L/kg. Protein binding is about 92%. Sequential distribution $t_{1/2}$ is 1 and 14 min.
Metabolism: Metabolized in the liver.
Excretion: Terminal $t_{1/2}$ is 90 to 111 min. Plasma clearance is about 5 mL/kg/min. One percent is excreted as unchanged drug; urinary excretion is the major route for metabolites.
Special Populations:
Hepatic Function Impairment – Reduced plasma clearance and extended terminal elimination may develop.
Elderly – Reduced plasma clearance and extended terminal elimination may develop.

Indications Induction of analgesia and anesthesia in specific situations, monitored anesthesia care (MAC).

Contraindications Hypersensitivity to narcotics; diarrhea caused by poisoning until toxic agent is identified; acute bronchial asthma; upper airway obstruction.

Route/Dosage
Obese Patients
Calculate dosage on basis of lean body weight.

Spontaneously Breathing/Assisted Ventilation
ADULTS (INITIAL DOSE): IV 8 to 20 mcg/kg.
ADULTS (MAINTENANCE DOSE): IV 0.5 to 1 mcg/kg/min.

Incremental Injection
ADULTS (INITIAL DOSE): IV 20 to 50 mcg/kg.
ADULTS (MAINTENANCE DOSE): IV 5 to 15 mcg/kg q 5 to 20 min.

Anesthetic Induction
ADULTS (INITIAL DOSE): IV 130 to 245 mcg/kg.
ADULTS (MAINTENANCE DOSE): IV 0.5 to 1.5 mcg/kg/min (or use general anesthetic).

Continuous Infusion
ADULTS (INITIAL DOSE): **IV** 50 to 75 mcg/kg.
ADULTS (MAINTENANCE DOSE): **IV** 0.5 to 3 mcg/kg/min.

MAC
ADULTS (INITIAL DOSE): **IV** 3 to 8 mcg/kg; total dose, 3 to 40 mcg/kg.
ADULTS (MAINTENANCE DOSE): **IV** 3 to 5 mcg/kg q 5 to 20 min to 1 mcg/kg/min.

Interactions
Cimetidine: Reduces alfentanil clearance.
CNS depressants: May increase CNS and cardiovascular effects of alfentanil.
Diazepam: May produce cardiovascular depression when given with high doses of alfentanil.
Erythromycin: May increase levels of alfentanil, causing prolonged or delayed respiratory depression.
Protease inhibitors: May increase CNS and respiratory depression.

Lab Test Interferences Amylase or lipase concentration test results may be unreliable for 24 hr after administration of alfentanil.

Adverse Reactions
CV: Hypotension; hypertension; tachycardia; bradycardia; asystole hypercarbia; arrhythmia.
CNS: Sedation; dizziness.
EENT: Blurred vision.
GI: Nausea; vomiting.
RESP: Respiratory depression; bronchospasm; apnea.
OTHER: Muscular rigidity.

Precautions
Pregnancy: Category C.
Lactation: Undetermined.
Children: Hypotension has occurred in newborns receiving alfentanil. Not recommended for children under 12 yr.
Elderly: Decreased dosage may be necessary.
Labor and delivery: Narcotics cross placenta and can affect newborn.
Cardiac effects: Drug may cause bradycardia and hypotension; may aggravate arrhythmias.
CNS depression: Patient may be sensitive to depressive effects of alfentanil.
Head injury: Alfentanil may increase intracranial pressure.
Respiratory effects: Alfentanil may decrease respiratory drive and cause apnea.
Seizures: Alfentanil may cause or aggravate seizure disorder.
Skeletal muscle rigidity: Alfentanil may cause skeletal muscle rigidity, particularly of the truncal muscle.

Overdosage: Signs and Symptoms
Respiratory depression, CNS depression, circulatory collapse (usually after rapid IV administration).

PATIENT CARE CONSIDERATIONS
Administration/Storage
- Drug is to be administered only by those qualified to give IV anesthetics.
- For accurate administration of small volumes, use tuberculin syringe or equivalent.
- Slow IV administration (90 sec to 3 min) reduces incidence of adverse reactions.
- Infusion should be discontinued 10 to 15 min before surgery is complete.

Assessment/Interventions
- Obtain patient history, including drug history and any known allergies.
- Monitor vital signs frequently during and after administration.
- Monitor serum amylase or lipase concentrations for elevations.
- Assist patient with ambulation.

Patient/Family Education
- Instruct preoperative patient about possible side effects.
- Advise postoperative patient to rise from bed slowly and to call for assistance in ambulation.
- Instruct patient to avoid intake of alcoholic beverages or other CNS depressants for 24 hr after outpatient surgery.

Alfuzosin Hydrochloride

(al-FEW-zoe-sin HIGH-droe-KLOR-ide)

Class Alpha$_1$-adrenergic blocker

How Supplied
Uroxatral Tablets, extended release 10 mg

Action
PHARMACOLOGY: Selective blockade for alpha$_1$-adrenergic receptors in the lower urinary tract, which cause smooth muscle in the bladder neck and prostate to relax, resulting in improved urine flow and a reduction in symptoms of benign prostatic hyperplasia (BPH).

PHARMACOKINETICS/DYNAMICS:
Absorption: Bioavailability is about 49%. Time to reach C_{max} is about 8 hr. The C_{max} and AUC are about 13.6 ng/mL and 194 ng•hr/mL, respectively.

Distribution: Following IV administration, the Vd is about 3.2 L/kg. Protein binding is 82% to 90%.

Metabolism: Extensive hepatic metabolism

with only 11% excreted unchanged in the urine. The major isozyme responsible for metabolism is CYP3A4.

Excretion: After 7 days, 69% is recovered in the feces and 24% in the urine.

Renal impairment: The mean C_{max} and AUC values were increased about 50% in patients with mild, moderate, or severe renal impairment.

Hepatic insufficiency: In patients with moderate or severe hepatic insufficiency, plasma concentrations of alfuzosin were increased 3- to 4-fold.

Indications Treatment of signs and symptoms of benign prostatic hyperplasia.

Contraindications Patients with moderate or severe hepatic insufficiency; coadministration with potent CYP3A4 inhibitors (eg, itraconazole, ketoconazole, ritonavir); hypersensitivity to any component of the product.

Route/Dosage
ADULTS: **PO** 10 mg/day, immediately after the same meal each day.

Interactions
Atenolol: Plasma levels may be elevated by alfuzosin, increasing the pharmacologic and adverse effects.

Cimetidine: Alfuzosin levels may be elevated, increasing the pharmacologic and adverse effects.

Moderate CYP3A4 inhibitors (eg, diltiazem): Alfuzosin plasma levels may be elevated, increasing the pharmacologic and adverse effects.

Potent CYP3A4 inhibitors (eg, itraconazole, ketoconazole, ritonavir): Because plasma concentrations of alfuzosin may be increased more than 2-fold, coadministration of these agents is contraindicated.

Lab Test Interferences None well documented.

Adverse Reactions
CV: Orthostatic hypotension (7%); tachycardia (postmarketing).
CNS: Dizziness (6%); headache, fatigue (3%).
DERM: Rash (postmarketing).
EENT: Sinusitis, pharyngitis (1% to 2%).
GI: Abdominal pain, dyspepsia, constipation, nausea (1% to 2%).
GU: Impotence (1% to 2%); priapism (postmarketing).
RESP: Upper respiratory tract infection (3%); bronchitis (1% to 2%).
OTHER: Pain (1% to 2%); chest pain (postmarketing).

Precautions
Pregnancy: Category B.
Lactation: Use not indicated.
Children: Safety and efficacy not established.
Alpha-blockers: Do not use in combination with other alpha-blockers.
Coronary insufficiency: Discontinue if symptoms of angina pectoris appear or worsen.
Hepatic insufficiency: Do not administer to patients with moderate or severe hepatic insufficiency.
Hypotension: Postural hypotension with or without symptoms may occur within a few hr following administration of alfuzosin.
Prostate carcinoma: Rule out presence of carcinoma of the prostate before starting alfuzosin.
QT prolongation: Use with caution and monitor patients with a known history of QT prolongation or patients taking medication known to prolong the QT interval.
Renal insufficiency: Use with caution.

Overdosage: Signs and Symptoms
Hypotension.

PATIENT CARE CONSIDERATIONS

Administration/Storage
- Not indicated for use in women.
- Do not cut, chew, or crush tablet. Instruct patient to swallow tablet whole.
- Give qd immediately following the same meal each day.
- Store at controlled room temperature (59° to 86°F). Protect from light and moisture.

Assessment/Interventions
- Obtain patient history, including drug history and any known allergies. Note renal or hepatic impairment, history of symptomatic hypotension, QT prolongation, hypotensive response to other medications, or concomitant use of antihypertensives, potent CYP3A4 inhibitors (eg, ketoconazole) or medication known to prolong QT interval (eg, quinidine).
- Do not administer to patient with moderate to severe hepatic impairment.
- Monitor BP and pulse after each dose.
- Assess changes in urinary symptoms such as frequency, hesitancy, weak stream, volume, dribbling, and nocturia.
- Monitor patient for GI, CNS, CV, and general body side effects. Report to health care provider if noted and significant.
- Monitor patient for orthostatic hypotension. Notify health care provider if symptomatic orthostatic hypotension or new onset or worsening of angina pectoris is noted.
- Implement safety precautions for patients who experience dizziness.

Patient/Family Education
- Explain name, dose, action, and potential side effects of drug.
- Advise patient to take prescribed dose qd, immediately after the same meal each day.
- Advise patient not to cut, crush, or chew tablet and to swallow the tablet whole with a full glass of water.
- Caution patient to avoid sudden position changes to prevent orthostatic hypotension.
- Caution patient that drug may cause dizziness or fainting and to use caution while driving or performing other tasks requiring mental alertness until tolerance is determined.
- Advise patient to contact health care provider if urinary symptoms do not improve or worsen while taking this medication.
- Instruct patient to report the following symptoms to health care provider: dizziness, fainting, chest pain, prolonged or painful erection, or bothersome side effects.
- Caution patient not to take any prescription or OTC drugs or dietary supplements unless advised by health care provider.
- Advise patient that follow-up visits may be necessary to monitor therapy and to keep appointments.

Alitretinoin

(al-ih-TRET-ih-no-in)

Class Retinoid

How Supplied
Panretin Gel 0.1%

Action
PHARMACOLOGY: Binds to and activates all known intracellular retinoid receptor substrates. Once activated, these receptors function as transcription factors that regulate the expression of genes that control the process of cellular differentiation and proliferation of both normal and neoplastic cells.

PHARMACOKINETICS/DYNAMICS:

Absorption: Indirect evidence indicates that absorption is not extensive. Plasma levels are similar to circulating, naturally occurring 9-cis-retinoic acid levels.

Indications Topical treatment of cutaneous lesions of AIDS-related Kaposi sarcoma (KS).

Contraindications Hypersensitivity to retinoids or any component of the product.

Route/Dosage
ADULTS: **Topical** Start with bid application to KS lesions. Application can be gradually increased to tid or qid or reduced according to individual lesion tolerance or application site toxicity. If severe irritation occurs, application of drug can be temporarily stopped for a few days until symptoms subside. Apply a sufficient amount of gel to cover the lesion with a generous coating. Allow to dry for 3 to 5 min before covering with clothing. A response to KS lesions may be seen as soon as 2 wk; however, some patients have required over 14 wk.

Interactions
N,N-diethyl-m-toluamide (DEET): Avoid concurrent use of products containing DEET (a common component of insect repellents).

Lab Test Interferences None well documented.

Adverse Reactions
DERM: Rash (77%); pain (34%); pruritus (11%); exfoliative dermatitis (9%); edema, skin disorder (including excoriation, cracking, scab, crusting, drainage, eschar, fissure, oozing [8%]); paresthesia (3%).

Precautions
Pregnancy: Category D. Could cause fetal harm if absorption were to occur in pregnant women.
Lactation: Undetermined.
Children: Safety and efficacy not established.
Photosensitivity: May occur with this class of agent; avoid excessive sunlight and ultraviolet light.

PATIENT CARE CONSIDERATIONS
Administration/Storage
- For topical use only. Not for ophthalmic, oral, or intravaginal use.
- Apply gel bid to qid as prescribed.
- Do not apply gel on or near mucosal surfaces or on healthy skin surrounding lesion(s).
- Apply sufficient gel to cover the lesion(s) with a generous coating. Allow gel to dry for 3 to 5 min before covering with clothing.
- Do not allow patient to shower, bathe, or swim for at least 3 hr following application of gel.
- Do not cover with occlusive dressings.
- Store gel at controlled room temperature (59° to 86°F). Keep tube tightly capped.

Assessment/Interventions
- Obtain patient history, including drug history and any known allergies. Note pregnancy, breastfeeding, or systemic anti-KS treatment.
- Do not use gel on patient who requires systemic anti-KS therapy (eg, more than 10 new KS lesions in prior month, symptomatic pulmonary KS, symptomatic visceral involvement).

- Do not apply other topical products unless advised by health care provider. Assess the skin and identify areas where medication is to be applied and areas that should be avoided (eg, healthy skin).
- Assess and document skin condition before initial application and periodically throughout treatment. Inform health care provider if condition does not improve, worsens, or if application site reactions are bothersome.

Patient/Family Education
- Explain name, action, and potential side effects of drug.
- Advise patient that gel will not work immediately but to expect a slow improvement over several wk.
- Advise patient to apply gel to skin lesion(s) bid to qid as directed by health care provider.
- Caution patient not to apply gel on or near mucosal surfaces (eg, eyes, nostrils, mouth, lips, vagina, tip of penis, rectum, anus) or on healthy skin surrounding lesion(s).
- Caution patient that gel contains alcohol and is flammable and to keep away from open flame.
- Teach patient or caregiver proper technique for applying gel: wash hands; apply sufficient gel to generously coat lesion(s); wash hands after applying gel; allow gel to dry for 3 to 5 min before covering with clothing.
- Caution patient not to scratch or cover treated areas with bandages, dressings, or wraps and not to swim, bathe, or shower for at least 3 hr after application.
- Advise patient not to stop treatment after lesion(s) have improved and that daily application of gel will be required to maintain the improvement.
- Advise patient that application site reactions occur commonly and to notify health care provider if swelling, blistering, oozing, drainage, pain, or intense redness or itching occurs.
- Advise patient that medication does not prevent the appearance of new KS lesions or increased growth of KS lesions not being treated, nor does the medication treat lung or intestinal KS.
- Instruct patient to avoid use of other topical products on treated lesion(s) except for mineral oil, which may be used 2 hr before or after alitretinoin applications to help prevent excessive dryness and itching.
- Advise patient that if gel comes in contact with the eyes to wash eyes with large amounts of cool water and to contact health care provider if eye irritation persists.
- Advise patient to talk to health care provider before using any other topical agents (eg, medicated soaps, astringents, cosmetics) on treated skin.
- Caution patient that medication can increase sensitivity to UV light and to avoid use of sun lamps and unnecessary exposure to sunlight while undergoing treatment.
- Caution patient not to use insect repellants containing DEET while using alitretinoin. Advise patient that toxicity from DEET may occur if applied together.
- Advise women to inform health care provider if pregnant, planning to become pregnant, or breastfeeding.
- Warn patient not to take any prescription or OTC drugs or dietary supplements without consulting health care provider.
- Advise patient that follow-up visits to monitor KS disease will be necessary and to keep appointments.

Allopurinol

(AL-oh-PURE-ee-nahl)
Class Analgesic/Gout/Cytoprotective
How Supplied
Aloprim Powder for injection, lyophilized 500 mg
- *Zyloprim* Tablets 100 mg, Tablets 300 mg
- 🍁 *Apo-Allopurinol* • *Novo-Purol*

Action
PHARMACOLOGY: Inhibits xanthine oxidase, the enzyme responsible for conversion of hypoxanthine to xanthine and then to uric acid.
PHARMACOKINETICS/DYNAMICS:
Absorption: About 90% absorbed from GI tract. T_{max} is 1.5 hr (allopurinol) and 4.5 hr (oxipurinol). C_{max} is 3 mcg/mL (allopurinol 300 mg) and 6.5 mcg/mL (oxipurinol).
Metabolism: Rapidly oxidized to oxipurinol.
Excretion: About 20% is excreted in the feces. Allopurinol is essentially cleared by glomerular filtration, whereas oxipurinol is reabsorbed in the kidney tubules. $T_{1/2}$, plasma is about 1 to 2 hr (allopurinol) and about 15 hr (oxipurinol).
Onset: Uric acid decreases in about 2 to 3 days.
Peak: May require a week or more of treatment.
Duration: Xanthine oxidase inhibition is maintained over 24 hr; however, uric acid levels may not return to pretreatment levels until 7 to 10 days following cessation of therapy.

Indications
Tablets: Treatment of primary or secondary gout,

hyperuricemia resulting from chemotherapy for malignancies, recurrent calcium oxalate renal calculi.

Tablets and injections: Management of patients with leukemia, lymphoma, and solid tumor malignancies when concurrently receiving cancer therapy that causes elevations of serum and urinary uric acid levels. Use injection in patients who cannot tolerate oral therapy. **Unlabeled use(s):** Prevention of fluorouracil-induced stomatitis and fluorouracil-induced granulocyte suppression.

Contraindications Standard considerations.

Route/Dosage

Control of Gout/Hyperuricemia
ADULTS: **PO** 100 to 800 mg/day. For amounts over 300 mg, give divided doses.

Secondary Hyperuricemia Associated with Malignancies
CHILDREN 6 TO 10 YR: **PO** 300 mg/day.
CHILDREN UNDER 6 YR: **PO** 150 mg/day.

Prevention of Uric Acid Nephropathy in Vigorous Chemotherapy of Neoplastic Disease
ADULTS: **PO** 600 to 800 mg/day for 2 to 3 days.

Reduction of Risk of Acute Gouty Attacks
ADULTS (INITIAL DOSE): **PO** 100 mg/day, increased by 100 mg at weekly intervals until adequate response is achieved or max recommended dose (800 mg/day) is reached.

Leukemia, Lymphoma, Solid Tumor Malignancies
ADULTS: **IV** 200 to 400 mg/m^2/day (max 600 mg/day).
CHILDREN: **IV** Starting dose 200 mg/m^2/day.

Interactions

Aluminum salts, uricosuric agents: May lessen effectiveness of allopurinol.
Ampicillin: May increase incidence of ampicillin-induced skin rash.
Cyclophosphamide: May enhance bone marrow suppression.
Theophyllines: Theophylline clearance may be decreased, leading to toxicity.
Thiopurines (eg, azathioprine, mercaptopurine): Toxicity of these drugs may be increased.
Drugs that are physically incompatible in solution with allopurinol sodium for injection are the following: amikacin; amphotericin B; carmustine; cefotaxime; chlorpromazine; cimetidine; clindamycin; cytarabine; dacarbazine; daunorubicin; diphenhydramine; doxorubicin; doxycycline; droperidol; floxuridine; gentamicin; haloperidol; hydroxyzine; idarubicin; imipenem plus cilastatin; mechlorethamine; meperidine; metoclopramide; methylprednisolone sodium succinate; minocycline; nalbuphine; netilmicin; ondansetron; prochlorperazine edisylate; promethazine; sodium bicarbonate; streptozocin; tobramycin; vinorelbine tartrate.

Lab Test Interferences None well documented.

Adverse Reactions

CNS: Drowsiness; generalized seizure (injectable); headache; neuritis; paresthesias; peripheral neuropathy.
DERM: Allergic vasculitis; alopecia; ecchymosis; skin rash. Allergic reactions may be severe and sometimes fatal.
EENT: Epistaxis; myopathy; taste disturbance.
GI: Abdominal pain; diarrhea; dyspepsia; gastritis; granulomatous changes; nausea; vomiting.
GU: Renal failure; uremia.
HEMA: Bone marrow depression; eosinophilia; leukocytosis; leukopenia; thrombocytopenia.
HEPA: Cholestatic jaundice; elevated liver enzymes; hepatic necrosis; hepatitis; reversible hepatomegaly. Acute gouty attacks; arthralgia; fever; myopathy; necrotizing angiitis.

Precautions

Pregnancy: Category C.
Lactation: Excreted in breast milk.
Children: Allopurinol is rarely indicated for use in children, except for hyperuricemia resulting from malignancy or with certain rare inborn errors of purine metabolism.
Hypersensitivity: Discontinue drug at first appearance of skin rash or other signs of allergic reaction. Rash may be followed by more severe hypersensitivity reactions and, rarely, death.
Renal function impairment: Reduced dose is given in patients with this condition. Drug may exacerbate renal failure in certain patients.
Acute gouty attacks: May occur during initial stages of therapy.
Bone marrow depression: Reported in patients given allopurinol.

PATIENT CARE CONSIDERATIONS

Administration/Storage

- Administer immediately after meals. For patients who have difficulty swallowing, crush tablets and mix with food.
- Store tablets in tightly closed container in cool location.
- Store unreconstituted powder at room temperature.
- Store reconstituted solution at 20° to 25°C; do not refrigerate or dilute product.

Assessment/Interventions

- Obtain patient history, including drug history and any known allergies.
- Assess for renal toxicity and failure.
- Increase fluid intake to 2000 to 3000 mL/day

(unless contraindicated) to prevent calculi formation.
- Obtain baseline CBC. Monitor frequently.
- For treatment of gout, obtain baseline uric acid level. Monitor q 1 to 2 wk for dosage adjustment, then monitor every few months.
- Monitor liver and kidney function, including BUN, serum creatinine, and Ccr, especially during early therapy.
- Monitor for decrease in joint swelling and pain.
- If urine output is decreased, dosage may need to be decreased. Consult health care provider.

Patient/Family Education
- Encourage patient to focus on weight loss or control.
- Tell patient to avoid purine-rich foods (eg, organ meats).
- Caution patient to avoid excessive intake of alcohol.
- Explain that gouty attacks may not end for 2 to 6 wk after beginning therapy.
- Instruct patient to stop taking medication and notify health care provider if rash or flu-like symptoms develop.
- Advise patient that drug may cause drowsiness, and to use caution while driving or performing other tasks requiring mental alertness.
- Instruct patient not to take otc medications without consulting health care provider.

Almotriptan Malate

(al-moe-TRIP-tan MAL-ate)
Class Analgesic/Migraine

How Supplied
Axert Tablets 6.25 mg, Tablets 12.5 mg

Action
PHARMACOLOGY: Selective agonist for vascular serotonin (5-HT) receptor subtype, causing vasoconstriction of cranial arteries.

PHARMACOKINETICS/DYNAMICS:
Absorption: Well absorbed. T_{max} is 1 to 3 hr. C_{max} is 49.5 to 64 mcg/L.
Distribution: Bioavailability is about 70%. About 35% is protein bound. Vd is about 180 to 200 L.
Metabolism: Metabolized to inactive metabolites by MAO-mediated oxidation (about 27%), CYP450 (3A4 and 2D6)-mediated oxidation (about 12%), and flavin mono-oxygenase (minor).
Excretion: The t½ is 3 to 4 hr. About 75% is excreted by the kidneys (about 40% as unchanged drug). About 13% is excreted in feces.
Special Populations:
Renal Function Impairment – Cl is decreased about 65% in those with Ccr 10 to 30 mL per min and decreased about 40% in those with Ccr 31 to 71 mL per min. C_{max} increased about 80%.

Indications Acute treatment of migraine with or without aura.

Contraindications Ischemic heart disease (eg, angina pectoris, history of MI, documented silent ischemia); symptoms or findings consistent with ischemic heart disease, coronary artery vasospasm (including Prinzmetal variant angina); significant underlying CV disease; uncontrolled hypertension; within 24 hr of treatment with another 5-HT$_1$ agonist, or an ergotamine-containing or ergot-type medication; hemiplegic or basilar migraine; hypersensitivity to any component of the product.

Route/Dosage
ADULTS: PO 6.25 to 12.5 mg, if headache returns, may repeat dose after 2 hr (max, 2 doses per 24 hr).

Hepatic or Renal Impairment
ADULTS: PO 6.25 mg initially (max, 12.5 mg per 24 hr).

Interactions
Ergot-containing drugs (eg, methysergide): May cause prolonged vasospastic reactions; therefore, contraindicated within 24 hr of almotriptan administration.
Other 5-HT$_{1B/1D}$ agonists (eg, sumatriptan): Contraindicated within 24 hr of each other.
Potent CYP3A4 inhibitors (eg, erythromycin, itraconazole ketoconazole, ritonavir): Almotriptan plasma levels may be elevated, increasing the risk of side effects.
Selective serotonin reuptake inhibitors (eg, fluoxetine): Weakness, hyperpyrexia, and incoordination have been reported.

Lab Test Interferences None well documented.

Adverse Reactions
CV: Coronary artery vasospasm; transient myocardial ischemia; MI; ventricular tachycardia and fibrillation.
CNS: Somnolence; headache; paresthesia; dizziness (at least 1%).
EENT: Dry mouth (at least 1%).
GI: Nausea (2%).

Precautions
Pregnancy: Category C.
Lactation: Undetermined.
Children: Safety and efficacy not determined.

Elderly: Safety and efficacy in patients above 65 yr of age not established.
Renal function impairment: Cl is reduced; use with caution.
Hepatic function impairment: Cl is reduced; use with caution.
Cardiac events/Vasoconstriction: Serious coronary events, though rare, can occur after administration of 5-HT$_1$ agonists. Administer first dose in the health care provider's office or similarly staffed and equipped facility to patients with risk factors predictive of coronary artery disease (CAD). Coronary artery vasospasm, acute MI, life-threatening cardiac rhythm disturbances, and death have been reported.
Cerebrovascular events: Cerebral hemorrhage, subarachnoid hemorrhage, stroke, and other cerebrovascular events have been reported with 5-HT$_1$ agonists.
Hypertensive crisis: Elevations in systemic BP, including hypertensive crisis, have been reported.

Overdosage: Signs and Symptoms
Hypertension, serious CV symptoms.

PATIENT CARE CONSIDERATIONS

Administration/Storage

- Administer prescribed dose at onset of migraine symptoms.
- Administer without regard to meals.
- Do not administer within 24 hr of treatment with another 5-HT$_1$ agonist or ergot-containing drug.
- If headache recurs after initial relief, a second dose may be administered provided there is an interval of at least 2 hr between doses.
- If first dose is ineffective, do not administer a second dose unless prescribed by health care provider.
- Do not administer more than 2 doses per 24-hr period.
- Store tablets at ambient room temperature (59° to 86°F).

Assessment/Interventions

- Obtain patient history, including drug history and any known allergies. Note history of ischemic or vasospastic CAD, uncontrolled hypertension, hemiplegic or basilar migraine.
- Note recent (within 24 hr) use of other 5-HT$_1$ agonists or ergotamine-containing or ergot-type drugs.
- Note recent (within 72 hr) use of ketoconazole and any other potent CYP3A4 inhibitor.
- Assess pain location, intensity, duration, and associated symptoms of migraine attack and response to treatment.
- Provide quiet, calm environment. Decrease stimuli, noise, and light.
- Ensure that patients with potential for CAD, including postmenopausal women, men over 40 yr of age, patients with risk factors for CAD (eg, hypertension, hypercholesterolemia, obesity, diabetes, smokers, family history), undergo a CV evaluation before initiating therapy.
- Administer first dose in physician's office or other adequately staffed medical facility to patient with potential for CAD whose CV evaluation provided clinical evidence that patient is reasonably free of coronary artery and ischemic myocardial disease or other significant underlying CV disease. Consider obtaining an ECG during the interval immediately following administration of the first dose of medication to patient with potential for CAD.
- Monitor patient for signs of allergic reaction. Discontinue therapy and immediately notify health care provider if noted. Be prepared to treat appropriately.
- Ensure that patient who is a long-term user of triptans, such as almotriptan, undergoes periodic CV evaluation.
- Monitor patient for CNS, CV, GI, and general body side effects. Report to health care provider if noted and significant.

Patient/Family Education

- Explain name, dose, action, and potential side effects of drug.
- Advise patient to read the *Patient Information* leaflet before starting therapy and again with each refill.
- Explain that drug is to be used only during migraine and does not prevent or reduce the number of attacks. Emphasize that drug is used only to treat actual migraine attack.
- Advise patient that drug is to be taken as soon as symptoms of migraine appear. Second dose may be taken if symptoms return, but no sooner than 2 hr following the first dose. For a given attack, if there is no response to the first tablet, do not take a second tablet without first consulting health care provider. Do not take more than 2 tablets in any 24-hr period.
- Advise patient that safety of treating more than 4 headaches in a 30-day period has not been established and to inform health care provider if headaches are occurring more frequently.
- Advise patient that if tightness, pain, pressure, or heaviness in chest or throat occurs

when using almotriptan, to notify the health care provider before using the drug again. If chest pain is severe or does not go away, tell patient to notify health care provider immediately.
• Advise patient to notify health care provider if feeling tingling, heat, heaviness, or pressure after treatment.
• Advise patient that drug may cause drowsiness or dizziness and to use caution while driving or performing other activities requiring mental alertness.
• Advise patient to avoid unnecessary exposure to sunlight or tanning lamps and to use sunscreen and wear protective clothing to avoid photosensitivity reactions.
• Instruct patient that if migraine prophylactic medications are prescribed, to continue to take daily as directed.
• Advise patient not currently taking a migraine prophylactic drug to discuss the use of such drugs with health care provider.
• Advise women to notify health care provider if pregnant, planning to become pregnant, or breastfeeding.
• Warn patient not to take any prescription or OTC drugs, dietary supplements, or herbal preparations without consulting health care provider.
• Advise patient that follow-up visits may be necessary to monitor therapy and to keep appointments.

Alosetron

(al-OH-seh-trahn)
Class 5HT$_3$ receptor antagonist
How Supplied
Lotronex Tablets 1.124 mg (equivalent to 1 mg alosetron base)
Action
PHARMACOLOGY: Selective serotonin (5HT$_3$) receptor antagonist that inhibits serotonin receptors in the GI tract.

PHARMACOKINETICS/DYNAMICS:
Absorption: Rapidly absorbed. T_{max} is 1 hr; C_{max} is about 5 ng/mL (males) and about 9 ng/mL (females). Bioavailability is about 50% to 60%. Food decreases absorption about 25% and increases T_{max} 15 min.
Distribution: Vd is about 65 to 95 L; 82% protein bound.
Metabolism: Extensively metabolized by CYP2C9 (30%), CYP3A4 (18%), CYP1A2 (10%), and non-CYP mediated phase I metabolic conversion (11%).
Excretion: T½ is about 1.5 hr. Plasma clearance is about 600 mL/min. Renal clearance is about 94 mL/min. About 73% is excreted in the urine, 24% in the feces (1% as unchanged drug), and 7% of dose is recovered as unchanged drug.
Special Populations:
Elderly – Plasma concentrations are about 40% increased.
Gender – Plasma concentrations are 30% to 50% lower and less variable in men.

Indications Treatment of irritable bowel syndrome (IBS) in women whose predominant bowel syndrome is diarrhea. **Unlabeled use(s):** Treatment of IBS in men; carcinoid diarrhea.

Contraindications History of chronic or severe constipation or sequelae from constipation; history of intestinal obstruction, stricture, toxic megacolon, GI perforation, or adhesions; history of ischemic colitis; current or history of Crohn disease or ulcerative colitis; active diverticulitis. Do not initiate therapy in patients with constipation (fewer than 3 bowel movements a week, hard or lumpy stools, or straining during a bowel movement).

Route/Dosage
ADULTS: **PO** 1 mg/day initially. If after 4 wk the 1 mg/day dose is well tolerated but does not adequately control IBS symptoms, the dose can be increased to 1 mg bid.

Interactions None well documented.

Lab Test Interferences None well documented.

Adverse Reactions
CV: Hypertension.
CNS: Sleep disorders; depressive disorders.
GI: Constipation; nausea; GI discomfort and pain; abdominal discomfort and pain; GI gaseous symptoms; viral GI infections; dyspeptic symptoms; abdominal distention; hemorrhoids.
RESP: Allergic rhinitis; throat and tonsil discomfort and pain; bacterial ear, nose, and throat infections.

> **WARNING:**
> *Gastrointestinal:* Serious adverse events, some fatal have been reported with use, including ischemic colitis and serious complications of constipation have resulted in hospitalization, blood transfusions, surgery, and death.
> *Restricted prescribing program:* Only for women with severe diarrhea predominant irritable bowel syndrome refractory to conventional therapy.
> Patient signed patient-physician agreement.
> Discontinue immediately upon signs of constipation or symptoms ischemic colitis.

Precautions
Pregnancy: Category B.
Lactation: Undetermined.
Children: Safety and efficacy not established.
Elderly: May be at greater risk of constipation.
Hepatic function impairment: Increased exposure to alosetron is likely to occur in patients with hepatic insufficiency; use with caution.

PATIENT CARE CONSIDERATIONS

Administration/Storage
- Do not administer if patient is constipated.
- Administer without regard to meals.
- Initial dose is 1 mg once daily for 4 wk.
- Store at controlled room temperature (59° to 86°F).

Assessment/Interventions
- Obtain patient history, including drug history and any known allergies. Note history of liver disease, kidney disease, and concurrent use of medications that decrease GI motility.
- Review patient's health history for any condition that could contraindicate therapy with alosetron: chronic or severe constipation; complications from constipation; intestinal obstruction, stricture, toxic megacolon, GI perforation, or adhesions; ischemic colitis, impaired intestinal circulation, thrombophlebitis, or hypercoagulable state; or Crohn disease or ulcerative colitis.
- Ensure that patient has read, understands, and has signed the "Patient-Physician Agreement" before starting therapy.
- Assess IBS symptoms prior to starting therapy and periodically during therapy.
- Assess patient for GI side effects. Discontinue use and contact health care provider immediately if any of the following are noted: constipation, rectal bleeding, bloody diarrhea, or new or worsening stomach pain.

Patient/Family Education
- Explain name, dose, action, and potential side effects of drug.
- Instruct patient to read the "Medication Guide" before starting therapy and with each refill.
- Advise patient that medication is started at 1 tablet once daily for 4 wk and then may be increased by health care provider to 1 tablet bid if needed for improved symptom control and if no side effects have been noted.
- Advise patient to take prescribed dose without regard to meals.
- Instruct patient to not change the dose or stop taking unless advised by health care provider.
- Instruct patient that if a dose is missed, to skip that dose and wait until the next time scheduled to take the prescribed dose. Caution patient to never take 2 doses to try to catch up.
- Instruct patient to stop using and contact health care provider immediately if any of the following symptoms occur: constipation, rectal bleeding, bloody diarrhea, new or worsening stomach pain.
- Instruct patient to discontinue use and contact health care provider after 4 wk of therapy if IBS symptoms not controlled.
- Warn patient that if medication has caused constipation and has been stopped, to not restart medication unless advised by health care provider.
- Advise women to notify health care provider if pregnant, planning to become pregnant, or breastfeeding.
- Instruct patient to not take any prescription or OTC medications or dietary supplements unless advised by health care provider.
- Advise patient that follow-up visits will be required to monitor therapy and to keep appointments.

Alpha₁-Proteinase Inhibitor (Human) [α₁-PI]

(AL-fah WON PRO-teen-ace)

Class Respiratory enzyme

How Supplied
Aralast Powder for Injection (lyophilized) 400 mg (greater than or equal to 16 mg /mL α_1-PI when reconstituted), Powder for Injection (lyophilized) 800 mg (greater than or equal to 16 mg/mL α_1-PI when reconstituted) ◆ *Prolastin* Powder for Injection (lyophilized) 500 mg (greater than or equal to 20 mg/mL α_1-PI when reconstituted), Powder for Injection (lyophilized) 1000 mg (greater than or equal to 20 mg/mL α_1-PI when reconstituted) ◆ *Zemaira* Powder for injection, lyophilized 1000 mg

Action
PHARMACOLOGY: Inhibits serine proteases (eg, neutrophil elastase), which are capable of degrading protein components of the alveolar walls and which are chronically present in the lung.

PHARMACOKINETICS/DYNAMICS:
Metabolism: Metabolic t½ 5.9 days.

Indications Chronic augmentation therapy in patients with congenital deficiency of α_1-PI with clinically evident emphysema.

Contraindications Individuals with selective IgA deficiencies (IgA level less than 15 mg/dL) who have known antibodies against IgA. *Zemaira:* History of anaphylaxis or severe systemic response to α_1-PI products.

Route/Dosage
ADULTS: **IV** 60 mg/kg infusion once weekly. Administer at a rate not exceeding 0.08 mL/kg/min.

PATIENT CARE CONSIDERATIONS
Administration/Storage
- For IV administration only. Do not administer intradermal, IM, or SC.
- Administer prescribed dose by IV infusion once weekly.
- Follow manufacturer's instructions for reconstitution of powder with supplied diluent and final dilution for infusion solution.
- Do not shake or agitate vials during reconstitution or dilution.
- Inspect solution visually before administration. Do not administer if solution is cloudy, discolored, or contains more than a few small particles.
- Discard any unused product. Vials are for single-use only. Do not save medication for future use.

Interactions None well documented.
INCOMPATIBILITIES: Do not mix with other agents or diluting solutions.

Lab Test Interferences None well documented.

Adverse Reactions
CV: *Prolastin:* Hypotension, tachycardia (postmarketing).
CNS: *Zemaira:* Headache (3%); dizziness (1%).
DERM: *Prolastin:* Rash (postmarketing); *Zemaira:* Pruritus (1%).
EENT: *Zemaira:* Sinusitis (2%); *Aralast:* Pharyngitis (2%).
HEPA: *Aralast:* ALT or AST elevations (11%).
MUSC: *Zemaira:* Asthenia (1%).
PULM: COPD.
RESP: *Aralast:* Upper and lower respiratory tract infections (96%); *Prolastin:* dyspnea (postmarketing); *Zemaira:* upper respiratory tract infection (2%).
OTHER: *Prolastin:* Fever (1%); flu-like symptoms, allergic-like reactions, chills (postmarketing); *Zemaira:* Injection site pain, paresthesia (1%).

Precautions
Pregnancy: Category C.
Lactation: Undetermined.
Children: Safety and efficacy not established.
Anaphylaxis: Immediately discontinue the infusion if severe anaphylactoid or anaphylactic reactions occur.
Circulatory overload: Use with caution in patients at risk of circulatory overload.
Infection: Because α_1-PI is derived from pooled human plasma, there is a risk of transmitting infectious agents (eg, viruses) and, theoretically, Creutzfeldt-Jakob disease.

- Infuse prescribed dose over period of 30 min or so. Do not exceed IV infusion rate of 0.8 mL/kg/min.
- Infuse *Zemaira* reconstituted solution through supplied in-line filter.
- Do not administer in same IV line with other products.
- Store vials in refrigerator (36° to 46°F). Do not freeze. Vials may be removed from refrigerator and stored at controlled room temperature (not to exceed 77°F). *Aralast* must be used within 1 mo once removed from refrigeration. Use solution within 3 hr of reconstitution. Do not refrigerate solution after reconstitution.

Assessment/Interventions
- Obtain patient history, including drug history

and any known allergies. Note selective IgA deficiency with known antibody against IgA, heart failure, or other conditions in which circulatory overload would be problematic, and allergic reaction to previous α_1-protease inhibitor therapy.
- Ensure that lung disease is associated with congenital deficiency of α_1-proteinase inhibitor deficiency and not another cause.
- Ensure that patient receiving *Prolastin* is immunized against hepatitis B before beginning therapy.
- Monitor vital signs and carefully observe patient throughout the infusion.
- Monitor patient for signs and symptoms of anaphylactic or serious allergic reaction. Be prepared to discontinue infusion and treat appropriately if reaction occurs.
- Monitor patient for development of infusion reaction. If infusion reaction develops, decrease the infusion rate or temporarily stop the infusion until symptoms subside. Resume infusion at rate tolerated by patient.
- Assess patient for CNS, CV, respiratory, and general body side effects. Inform health care provider if noted and significant.
- Notify manufacturer if patient develops any infection (eg, hepatitis C) thought to be transmitted by the medication.

Patient/Family Education
- Explain name, action, dosing regimen, and potential side effects of drug.
- Advise patient, family, or caregiver that medication will be prepared and administered by a health care provider in a health care setting.
- Advise patient, family, or caregiver to report any signs or symptoms of hypersensitivity reaction (eg, hives, rash, chest tightness, wheezing, difficulty breathing, faintness).
- Advise patient, family, or caregiver to report the following symptom complex to health care provider: fever, drowsiness, chills, and runny nose followed 2 wk later by rash and joint pain.
- Advise women to notify health care provider if pregnant, planning to become pregnant, or breastfeeding.
- Instruct patient not to take any prescription or OTC medications or dietary supplements unless advised by health care provider.
- Advise patient, family, or caregiver that follow-up visits will be required to monitor response to therapy and to keep appointments.

Alprazolam

(al-PRAY-zoe-lam)

Class Antianxiety/Benzodiazepine

How Supplied
Alprazolam Intensol Oral solution 1 mg/mL ♦ *Xanax* Tablets 0.25 mg, Tablets 0.5 mg, Tablets 1 mg, Tablets 2 mg ♦ *Xanax XR* Tablets, extended-release 0.5 mg, Tablets, extended-release 1 mg, Tablets, extended-release 2 mg, Tablets, extended-release 3 mg
✤ Apo-Alpraz ♦ Apo-Alpraz TS ♦ Gen-Alprazolam ♦ Novo-Alprazol ♦ Nu-Alpraz ♦ ratio-Alprazolam ♦ Xanax TS

Action
PHARMACOLOGY: Potentiates action of GABA, an inhibitory neurotransmitter, resulting in increased neuronal inhibition and CNS depression, especially in limbic system and reticular formation.

PHARMACOKINETICS/DYNAMICS:
Absorption: Readily absorbed; T_{max} is 1 to 2 hr; C_{max} is 8 to 37 ng/mL (0.5 to 3 mg doses).
Distribution: 80% protein bound. Crosses the placenta and is excreted in breast milk.
Metabolism: Metabolized in the liver to alpha-hydroxy-alprazolam (activity is approximately 50% that of alprazolam) and a benzophenone derivative (inactive).
Excretion: The t½ may be increased to approximately 16.3 hr. Excreted in the urine.
Special Populations:
Hepatic Function Impairment – The t½ may be increased to approximately 19.7 hr in those with alcoholic liver disease.
Elderly – The t½ may be increased to approximately 16.3 hr.
Obese – T½ may be increased to approximately 21.8 hr.

Indications
Treatment of panic disorders with or without agoraphobia (*Xanax* and *Xanax XR*); management of anxiety disorders or for short-term relief of symptoms of anxiety, including anxiety associated with depression (immediate-release tablets and oral solution). **Unlabeled use(s):** Treatment of irritable bowel syndrome, depression, PMS, agoraphobia with social phobia.

Contraindications
Hypersensitivity to other benzodiazepines; psychoses; acute narrow-angle

glaucoma; patients receiving itraconazole or ketoconazole.

Route/Dosage
Anxiety Disorder (Immediate-Release Tablets and Oral Solution)
ADULTS: **PO** Immediate-release tablets: 0.25 to 0.5 mg tid (max, 4 mg/day in divided doses). Extended-release tablets: Start with 0.5 mg qd and gradually increase if needed.

Elderly/Debilitated Patients
ADULTS: **PO** 0.25 mg bid to tid; may increase dose gradually.

Panic Disorder
INITIAL DOSE: **PO** Immediate-release tablets: 0.5 mg tid; if needed, increase by max 1 mg/day q 3 to 4 day. May require more than 4 mg/day. Extended-release tablets: start with 0.5 to 1 mg qd (suggested daily dose ranges between 3 and 6 mg).

Interactions
Alcohol and other CNS depressants: Produce additive CNS depressant effects.
Cimetidine, oral contraceptives, disulfiram: May increase effects of alprazolam, producing excessive sedation and impaired psychomotor function.
Digoxin: Serum digoxin concentrations may increase.
Diltiazem, fluvoxamine, grapefruit juice, isoniazid, macrolide antibiotics (eg, erythromycin), nefazodone, non-nucleoside reverse transcriptase inhibitors (eg, delavirdine, efavirenz), protease inhibitors (eg, indinavir): May increase alprazolam plasma concentrations.
Itraconazole, ketoconazole: Concurrent use with alprazolam is contraindicated.
Omeprazole: May increase serum levels of alprazolam and enhance alprazolam's effects.
Rifamycins: May decrease alprazolam plasma concentrations.
Theophyllines: May antagonize sedative effects of alprazolam.

Lab Test Interferences
None well documented.

Adverse Reactions
CV: Tachycardia (15%); hypotension (5%); palpitation (at least 1%).
CNS: Drowsiness (77%); fatigue/tiredness (49%); sedation (45%); irritability, memory impairment (33%); cognitive disorder (29%); somnolence (23%); light-headedness (21%); decreased libido (14%); depression (12%); dysarthria (11%); confusional state (10%); abnormal coordination (9%); ataxia, mental impairment (7%); disturbed attention, impaired balance, disinhibition (3%); disorientation, paresthesia, dyskinesia, talkativeness, derealization, abnormal dreams, lethargy (2%); anxiety, hypoesthesia, hypersomnia, fear, warm feeling (1%); malaise, weakness, headache, dizziness, tremor, irritability, insomnia, nervousness, increased libido, restlessness, agitation, depersonalization, nightmare (at least 1%).
DERM: Rash (11%); increased sweating (at least 1%); Stevens-Johnson syndrome (postmarketing).
EENT: Nasal congestion (17%); allergic rhinitis (1%); vertigo, blurred vision (at least 1%).
GI: Constipation (26%); nausea/vomiting (22%); diarrhea (21%); abdominal distress (18%); dry mouth (15%); increased salivation (6%); dyspepsia, abdominal pain (at least 1%).
GU: Micturition difficulties (12%); menstrual disorders (10%); dysmenorrhea (4%); sexual dysfunction, premenstrual syndrome, incontinence (2%); gynecomastia (postmarketing).
HEPA: Increased liver enzymes, hepatitis, hepatic failure (postmarketing).
M/N: Increased appetite (33%); decreased appetite (28%); weight gain (27%); weight loss (23%); edema (5%); anorexia (2%).
MUSC: Rigidity (4%); arthralgia, myalgia (2%); limb pain (1%); back pain, muscle cramps, muscle twitching (at least 1%).
RESP: Upper respiratory tract infection (4%); dyspnea (2%); hyperventilation (at least 1%).
OTHER: Chest pain (at least 1%); hyperprolactinemia (postmarketing).

Precautions
Pregnancy: Category D.
Lactation: Excreted in breast milk.
Children: Safety and efficacy in children under 18 yr not established.
Elderly: Use smallest effective dose to preclude development of ataxia or overdosage.
Renal function impairment: Caution is needed to avoid accumulation of drug.
Hepatic function impairment: Caution is needed to avoid accumulation of drug.
Dependence: Prolonged use can lead to physical and psychological dependence. Withdrawal syndrome has occurred within 4 to 6 wk of treatment, especially if abruptly discontinued. Cautious use and tapering of dosage are necessary.
Psychiatric disorders: Not intended for patients with primary depressive disorder, psychoses, or disorders in which anxiety is not prominent.
Seizures: May occur during abrupt drug discontinuation or dose reduction.
Suicide: Use with caution in patients with suicidal tendencies; do not allow access to large quantities of drug.

Overdosage: Signs and Symptoms
Somnolence, confusion, impaired coordination, diminished reflexes, coma, death.

PATIENT CARE CONSIDERATIONS
Administration/Storage
- Immediate-release and extended-release tablets are interchangeable on a daily mg-to-mg basis.
- Administer prescribed dose without regard to meals but administer with food if GI upset occurs.
- Immediate-release tablets may be administered sublingually to patient who has difficulty swallowing tablets.
- Administer extended-release tablets qd, preferably in the morning. Have patient swallow whole. Do not crush, chew, divide, or break tablet.

Oral Solution:
- Use calibrated dropper to measure prescribed dose.
- Add prescribed dose to a liquid (eg, juice, water, soda) or semisolid food (eg, applesauce, pudding), stir for a few seconds then immediately administer entire amount of mixture. Do not prepare and store doses for future use.
- Increase dose no more often than q 3 to 4 days.
- Store immediate-release tablets below 77°F. Store extended-release tablets and oral solution at controlled room temperature (59° to 86°F).

Assessment/Interventions
- Obtain patient history, including drug history and any known allergies. Note hepatic or renal impairment, pulmonary disease, acute narrow-angle glaucoma, depression, suicidal tendency, seizure disorder, history of drug abuse or sensitivity to other benzodiazepines, or concurrent use of other psychotropic medications, CNS depressants, or strong CYP3A inhibitors (eg, ketoconazole, erythromycin) or inducers (eg, carbamazepine).
- Ensure that reduced dose and slower dose escalation is used in elderly patient or patient with advanced liver disease or debilitating disease.
- Ensure that women of childbearing potential are not pregnant when therapy is initiated.
- Ensure that CBC with differential, urinalysis, and blood chemistries are evaluated periodically in patient on prolonged therapy.
- Frequently assess patient for response to treatment. Notify health care provider if condition does not appear to be improving or is worsening.
- Ensure that therapy is periodically reviewed to determine if it needs to be continued without change or if a dose change (eg, increase, decrease, discontinuation) is indicated.
- If treatment is to be discontinued, or the dose reduced, gradually taper the dose (eg, no more than 0.5 mg q 3 days). Monitor patient for withdrawal symptoms (eg, increased anxiety, tremor, muscle or abdominal cramps, sweating). If significant withdrawal symptoms develop, reinstitute previous dosing schedule and attempt a less rapid tapering regimen after patient has stabilized.
- Monitor patient for CNS, GI, psychiatric, and general body side effects. Report to health care provider if noted and significant. Implement safety precautions if excessive drowsiness or dizziness occurs.

Patient/Family Education
- Explain name, dose, action, and potential side effects of drug.
- Advise patient or caregiver to read the *Patient Information* leaflet before starting therapy and with each refill.
- Advise patient that medication is usually started at a low dose and then gradually increased until max benefit is obtained.
- Caution patient that medication may be habit forming and to take as prescribed and not to stop taking or change the dose unless advised by health care provider.
- Advise patient to take each dose without regard to meals but to take with food if stomach upset occurs.
- Advise patient using extended-release tablets to take prescribed dose qd, preferably in the morning. Caution patient to swallow tablets whole and not to crush, chew, divide, or break the tablet.
- Advise patient or caregiver using oral solution to measure prescribed dose using calibrated dropper and then add solution to a liquid (eg, juice, water, soda) or semisolid food (eg, applesauce, pudding), stir for a few seconds then immediately take (give) the entire mixture. Caution patient or caregiver not to prepare mixtures ahead of time and store.
- Advise patient that if a dose is missed to skip that dose and take the next dose at the regularly scheduled time. Caution patient to never take 2 doses at the same time.
- Advise patient that if medication needs to be discontinued it will be slowly withdrawn over a period of 2 wk or more unless safety concerns (eg, rash) require a more rapid withdrawal.
- Instruct patient to avoid alcoholic beverages and other depressants while taking this medication.
- Advise patient with anxiety to take as needed and to seek alternative methods for control-

ling or preventing anxiety (eg, stress reduction, counseling).
- Instruct patient to contact health care provider if symptoms do not appear to be getting better, are getting worse, or if bothersome side effects (eg, drowsiness, memory impairment) occur.
- Advise patient that drug may cause drowsiness or impair judgment, thinking, or reflexes and to use caution while driving or performing other tasks requiring mental alertness until tolerance is determined.
- Advise women to notify health care provider if pregnant, planning to become pregnant, or breastfeeding.
- Warn patient not to take any prescription or OTC drugs or dietary supplements without consulting health care provider.
- Advise patient that follow-up visits may be necessary to monitor therapy and to keep appointments.

Alprostadil (PGE$_1$; Prostaglandin E$_1$)

(al-PRAHST-uh-dill)

Class Prostaglandin/Patent ductus arteriosus/ Agent for impotence

How Supplied
Caverject Powder for injection, lyophilized 6.15 mcg (5 mcg/mL), Powder for injection, lyophilized 11.9 mcg (10 mcg/mL), Powder for injection, lyophilized 23.2 mcg (20 mcg/mL) ♦ *Edex* Powder for injection, lyophilized 6.225 mcg (5 mcg/mL), Powder for injection, lyophilized 12.45 mcg (10 mcg/mL), Powder for injection, lyophilized 24.9 mcg (20 mcg/mL) ♦ *Muse* Pellet 125 mcg, Pellet 250 mcg, Pellet 500 mcg, Pellet 1000 mcg ♦ *Prostin VR Pediatric* Injection 500 mcg/mL (in 1 mL dehydrated alcohol)

Action
PHARMACOLOGY: Relaxes smooth muscle of ductus arteriosus. Produces vasodilation, inhibits platelet aggregation and stimulates intestinal and uterine smooth muscle. Induces erection by relaxation of trabecular smooth muscle and by dilation of cavernosal arteries.

PHARMACOKINETICS/DYNAMICS:
Absorption:
Urethral suppository – About 80% absorbed within 10 min.
Distribution: About 81% bound to albumin and about 55% bound to alpha-globulin IV-4.
Metabolism: About 80% metabolized in one pass through the lungs.
Urethral suppository – Also rapidly metabolized locally by enzymatic oxidation.
Excretion: Metabolites excreted by kidneys; about 90% of IV dose excreted in urine within 24 hr and remainder is excreted in feces. $T_{1/2}$ is 0.5 to 10 min.
Special Populations:
Pulmonary disease – May have reduced capacity to clear the drug.

Indications Palliative therapy to maintain patency of ductus arteriosus temporarily, until surgery can be performed, in newborns who have congenital heart defects (eg, pulmonary stenosis, tricuspid atresia) and who depend on patent ductus for survival. Treatment of erectile dysfunction caused by neurogenic, vasculogenic, psychogenic, or mixed etiology. Intracavernosal alprostadil (*Caverject* only) may be useful adjunct to other diagnostic tests in the diagnosis of erectile dysfunction.

Contraindications Standard considerations. *Caverject*: Conditions that might predispose patients to priapism (eg, sickle cell anemia or trait, multiple myeloma leukemia); patients with anatomical deformation of the penis (eg, angulation, cavernosal fibrosis, Peyronie disease); patients with penile implants; use in women, children or newborns; use in men for whom sexual activity is inadvisable or contraindicated.

Route/Dosage
Ductus Arteriosus
NEWBORNS: **IV** 0.01 to 0.4 mcg/kg/min. Drug is infused for shortest time and at lowest effective dose.

Impotence (Erectile Dysfunction of Vasculogenic, Psychogenic, or Mixed Etiology)
Intracavernosal Initiate dose titration at 2.5 mcg. If there is a partial response, the dose may be increased by 2.5 mcg to a dose of 5 mcg and then in increments of 5 to 10 mcg, depending on erectile response, until the dose that produces an erection suitable for intercourse and not exceeding a duration of 1 hr is reached. If there is no response to the initial 2.5 mcg dose, the second dose may be increased to 7.5 mcg, followed by increments of 5 to 10 mcg. If there is no response, then the next higher dose may be given within 1 hr. If there is a response, then there should be a 1-day interval before the next dose is given.

Erectile Dysfunction of Pure Neurogenic Etiology (Spinal Cord Injury)
Initiate dosage titration at 1.25 mcg. The dose may be increased by 1.25 mcg to a dose of

2.5 mcg, followed by an increment of 2.5 mcg to a dose of 5 mcg, and then in 5 mcg increments until the dose that produces an erection suitable for intercourse and not exceeding a duration of 1 hr is reached. If there is no response, then the next higher dose may be given within 1 hr. If there is a response, then there should be at least 1-day interval before the next dose is given.

Maintenance therapy – The first injections of alprostadil must be done at the health care provider's office by medically trained personnel. Self-injection therapy by the patient can be started only after the patient is properly instructed and well-trained in the self-injection technique. The health care provider should make a careful assessment of the patient's skills and competence with the procedure.

Intraurethral Administer as needed to achieve an erection. The onset of injection is 5 to 10 min after administration. Duration of effect is approximately 30 to 60 min. Titrate dose under the supervision of health care provider.

CAVERJECT
Adjunct to Diagnosis of Erectile Dysfunction
ADULTS: **Intracavernosal** Monitor patients for occurrence of an erection after an intracavernosal injection of alprostadil. Extensions of this testing are the use of alprostadil as an adjunct to laboratory investigations (eg, duplex or Doppler imaging) to allow visualization and assessment of penile vasculature. For these tests, use a single dose of alprostadil that induces a rigid erection.

Interactions
Anticoagulants (eg, heparin, warfarin): After intracavernosal injection, risk of bleeding may be increased.

Lab Test Interferences
None well documented.

Adverse Reactions
CV: Flushing; bradycardia; hypotension; tachycardia; cardiac arrest; edema. Other rare, but serious, cardiovascular effects include CHF; hyperemia; second-degree heart block; shock; spasm of right ventricle infundibulum; supraventricular tachycardia; ventricular fibrillation.
CNS: Fever; seizures; cerebral bleeding.
GI: Diarrhea.
GU: Urethral pain; urethral burning; urethral bleeding/spotting; testicular pain (*Muse* only).
HEMA: DIC; bleeding.
RESP: Apnea.
OTHER: Cortical proliferation of long bones; sepsis; penile pain; prolonged erection; penile fibrosis; injection site hematoma; penis disorder; injection site ecchymosis (*Caverject* only); back pain; pain; pelvic pain; accidental injury (*Muse* only).

> **WARNING:**
> Apnea is experienced by about 10% to 12% of neonates with congenital heart defects treated with *Prostin VR Pediatric* solution. Apnea is most often seen in neonates weighing less than 2 kg at birth and usually appears during the first hr of drug infusion. Monitor respiratory status throughout treatment.

Precautions
Pregnancy: Category C.
Hemostatic effects: Use cautiously in newborns with bleeding tendencies because alprostadil inhibits platelet aggregation.
Respiratory status: Apnea has occurred in some newborns treated with alprostadil.
Priapism (erection lasting more than 6 hr): Prolonged erection has been known to occur following intracavernosal administration of vasoactive substances, including alprostadil. To minimize the chances of priapism, titrate slowing to the lowest effective dose. If priapism is not treated immediately, penile tissue damage and permanent loss of potency may result.
Penile fibrosis: Discontinue treatment in patients who develop penile angulation, cavernosal fibrosis, or Peyronie disease.

Overdosage: Signs and Symptoms
Apnea, bradycardia, pyrexia, hypotension, flushing.

PATIENT CARE CONSIDERATIONS
Administration/Storage
Prostin VR Pediatric:
- Drug is to be given only by trained personnel in PICU via continuous IV infusion into large vein or through umbilical artery catheter.
- Dilute medication with normal saline or D5W only.
- Use volumetric IV pump to regulate delivery.
- Monitor infant closely during administration.
- Discard preparation after 24 hr and mix new solution.

Caverject:
- Bacteriostatic water for injection or sterile water, both preserved with benzyl alcohol 0.945% w/v, must be used as the diluent for reconstitution.
- After reconstitution, immediately use the solution and do not store or freeze.
- Do not shake the contents of the reconstituted vial.
- Discard vials with precipitates or discoloration.

- The intracavernosal injection must be done under sterile conditions. The site of injection is usually along the dorsolateral aspect of the proximal third of the penis. Avoid visible veins. The side of the penis that is injected and the site of injection must be alternated; the injection site must be cleansed with an alcohol swab.

Muse:
- The max frequency of use is 2 systems or less per 24-hr period.
- Store unopened foil pouches in a refrigerator at 2° to 8°C (36° to 46°F). It may be kept at room temperature (below 30°C; 86°F).

Assessment/Interventions
- Obtain patient history, including drug history and any known allergies.
- Assess infant's cardiac status before administration.
- Do not administer if infant is in respiratory distress.
- Obtain baseline CBC, ABGs, PT, PTT, and pulmonary function tests.
- Monitor arterial pressure intermittently. If pressure decreases significantly, notify health care provider immediately. Infusion rate will need to be decreased.
- Monitor respiratory status throughout treatment. Have ventilatory equipment at bedside.
- Monitor BP during administration.
- Notify health care provider and decrease or stop infusion if infant develops: increased respiratory distress; bleeding, bruising or hematoma formation; sudden changes in cardiac status (eg, decreased BP, bradycardia, cardiac arrest, cyanosis). Decrease or stop infusion until health care provider gives new orders.

Caverject:
- Exercise careful follow-up of the patient while in the self-injection program. This is especially true for the initial self-injections, since adjustments in the dose of alprostadil may be needed. While on self-injection treatment, it is recommended that the patient visit the prescribing health care provider's office q 3 mo. At that time, assess the efficacy and safety of the therapy and adjust the dosage.

Patient/Family Education
Prostin VR Pediatric:
- Explain to parents about infant's congenital heart disease and purpose and expected outcome of treatment.
- Keep parents/family informed of course of treatment; alert them to usual side effects (eg, flushing of skin).
- Promote parent-infant bonding by encouraging parental involvement in infant's care.
- Encourage parents to express their emotions. Show compassion and understanding, and help them to cope.

Caverject:
- Thoroughly instruct and train patient in the self-injection technique before beginning intracavernosal treatment at home. Establish the desired dose in the health care provider's office.
- Inform patient that the established dose should not be changed without consulting the health care provider.
- The patient may expect an erection to occur within 5 to 20 min. A standard treatment goal is to produce an erection lasting no longer than 1 hr.
- Instruct patient that alprostadil generally should be used 3 times/wk or less, with at least 24 hr between each use.
- Instruct patient to seek immediate medical attention if an erection persists for more than 6 hr.
- Patient should report any penile pain that was not previously present or that increased in intensity, as well as the occurrence of nodules or hard tissue in the penis to health care provider as soon as possible.
- Advise patient that the use of intracavernosal alprostadil offers no protection from the transmission of STDs. Counsel individuals who use alprostadil about the protective measures necessary to guard against the spread of STDs, including HIV.
- The injection can induce a small amount of bleeding at the site of injection. In patients infected with blood-borne diseases, this could increase the risk of transmission of blood-borne diseases between partners.

Intraurethral:
- Instruct patient on proper technique for administering alprostadil prior to self-administration.

Muse:
- Instruct patient on the proper technique for administering alprostadil prior to self-administration.
- The max frequency of use is 2 systems or less per 24-hr period.

Alteplase, Recombinant

(AL-tuh-PLACE)

Class Tissue plasminogen activator

How Supplied
Activase Powder for injection, lyophilized 50 mg (29 million IU), Powder for injection, lyophilized 100 mg (58 million IU) ♦ *Cathflo Activase* Powder for injection, lyophilized 2 mg
🍁 *Activase rt-PA*

Action
PHARMACOLOGY: Aids in dissolution of blood clots.

PHARMACOKINETICS/DYNAMICS:
Absorption: C_{max} is 3 to 4 mg/L.
Distribution: Vd is 2.8 to 4.6 L and doubles at steady state.
Excretion: Initial t½ is less than 5 min. Plasma Cl is 380 to 570 mL/min; total body Cl is 34.3 to 38.4 L/hr. More than 80% is cleared from plasma within 10 min.

Indications Lysis of thrombi in management of acute MI or acute massive pulmonary embolism, management of acute ischemic stroke (*Activase* only). Restoration of function to central venous access device as assessed by the ability to withdraw blood (*Cathflo Activase* only).

Contraindications Active internal bleeding; history of cerebrovascular accident; intracranial hemorrhage; recent (within 3 mo) intracranial or intraspinal surgery or trauma; recent previous stroke; seizure at the onset of stroke; intracranial neoplasm; arteriovenous malformation or aneurysm; bleeding diathesis; severe uncontrolled hypertension; evidence of intracranial hemorrhage on pretreatment evaluation; suspicion of subarachnoid hemorrhage; uncontrolled hypertension at time of treatment; current use of oral anticoagulants; prothrombin time longer than 15 sec, administration of heparin within 48 hr preceding stroke onset with an elevated activated partial thromboplastin time at presentation; platelet count below 100,000/mm³.

Route/Dosage
Acute Ischemic Stroke
ADULTS: **IV** The recommended dose is 0.9 mg/kg (max, 90 mg) infused over 60 min with 10% of the total dose administered as an initial IV bolus over 1 min. The safety and efficacy of this regimen with coadministration of heparin and aspirin during the first 24 hr after symptom onset has not been investigated. Doses 0.9 mg/kg may be associated with an increased incidence of ICH. Do not use doses more than 0.9 mg/kg (max, 90 mg).

Acute MI
Administer as soon as possible after the onset of symptoms. Do not use a dose of 150 mg because it has been associated with an increase in intracranial bleeding.
Accelerated infusion – The recommended dose is based upon patient weight; do not exceed 100 mg. For patients weighing more than 67 kg, the recommended dose administered is 100 mg as a 15 mg IV bolus, followed by 50 mg infused over the next 30 min and then 35 mg infused over the next 60 min. For patients weighing 67 kg or less, the recommended dose is administered as a 15 mg IV bolus, followed by 0.75 mg/kg infused over the next 30 min not to exceed 50 mg and then 0.5 mg/kg over the next 60 min not to exceed 35 mg. (The safety and efficacy of this accelerated infusion of alteplase regimen has only been investigated with coadministration of heparin and aspirin).
3-hr infusion – 100 mg given as 60 mg (34.8 million IU) in the first hour (with 6 to 10 mg given as a bolus over the first 1 to 2 min), 20 mg (11.6 million IU) over the second hour and 20 mg (11.6 million IU) over the third hour. For smaller patients (less than 65 kg), use a dose of 1.25 mg/kg given over 3 hr as described above.
Coadministration – Although the use of anticoagulants during and following alteplase has been shown to be of equivocal benefit, heparin has been given concomitantly for at least 24 hr in more than 90% of patients. Aspirin or dipyridamole has been given during or following heparin treatment.

Pulmonary Embolism
ADULTS: **IV** 100 mg administered over 2 hr. Initiate or reinstate heparin therapy near the end of or immediately following the alteplase infusion when the partial thromboplastin time or thrombin time returns to twice normal or less.

Restoration of Function to Central Venous Catheter (*Cathflo Activase* only)
ADULTS: **IV** Instill into dysfunctional catheter at a concentration of 1 mg/mL. For patients weighing 30 kg or more, use 2 mg/2 mL; for patients weighing 10 kg or more to less than 30 kg, use 110% of the internal lumen volume of the catheter (max, 2 mg/2 mL). If catheter function is not restored in 120 min after 1 dose, a second dose may be instilled.

Interactions
Anticoagulants (eg, warfarin, heparin), aspirin, drugs affecting platelet function (eg, abciximab, dipyridamole), vitamin K antagonists: May increase the risk of bleeding.

Nitroglycerin: May reduce alteplase concentrations, decreasing the thrombolytic effect.
INCOMPATIBILITIES: Do not add other medications to infusion solution.

Lab Test Interferences Results of tests for coagulation or fibrinolytic activity may be unreliable because of degradation of fibrinogen in blood.

Adverse Reactions
CV: All strokes (2%); arrhythmia; AV block; cardiogenic shock; heart failure; cardiac arrest; recurrent ischemia; myocardial reinfarction; myocardial rupture; electromechanical dissociation; pericardial effusion; pericarditis; mitral regurgitation; cardiac tamponade; thromboembolism; pulmonary edema; hypotension; pulmonary re-embolization.
Cathflo Activase – Venous thrombosis; major hemorrhage; intracranial hemorrhage; pulmonary emboli; upper extremity deep vein thrombosis.
CNS: Cerebral edema; cerebral herniation; seizure.
DERM: Ecchymosis (1%); injection-site hemorrhage.
GI: Bleeding (5%); nausea; vomiting.
GU: Bleeding (4%).
HYPERSEN: Allergic-type reactions (eg, anaphylactoid reactions, laryngeal edema, orolingual angioedema, rash, urticaria).
OTHER: Fever; pleural effusion.
Cathflo Activase – Sepsis; death.

PATIENT CARE CONSIDERATIONS
Administration/Storage
- Administer only by IV infusion or into central venous access device. Not for intradermal, SC, IM, or intra-arterial administration.
- Initiate treatment for stroke only within 3 hr after onset of symptoms and after exclusion of intracranial hemorrhage.
- Do not use 50 mg vial if vacuum is not present.
- Reconstitute lyophilized powder following manufacturer's recommendations using sterile water for injection. Do not reconstitute with bacteriostatic water for injection.
- Reconstituted solution may be further diluted immediately before injection for treatment of acute MI or pulmonary embolus with an equal volume of 0.9% sodium chloride injection or 5% dextrose injection.
- Mix by gentle swirling or gentle inversion. Avoid excessive agitation during reconstitution.
- Use reconstituted solution immediately or within 8 hr if stored properly.
- Do not add any other medications to infusion solution.

Precautions
Pregnancy: Category C.
Lactation: Undetermined.
Children: Safety and efficacy not established (*Activase*); safety and efficacy in children under 2 yr or who weigh less than 10 kg have not been established (*Cathflo Activase*).
Hypersensitivity: There is no experience with readministration of alteplase.
Acute ischemic stroke: Risk of alteplase therapy to treat acute ischemic stroke may be increased by severe neurological deficit at presentation and major early infarct on a CT scan and should be weighed against the benefit.
Acute MI: In patients who are at low risk of death from cardiac causes and who have high BP at time of presentation, risk of stroke may offset survival benefit produced by thrombolytic therapy.
Bleeding: Most frequent and serious adverse effect.
Cholesterol embolism: May occur rarely in patients treated with thrombolytic agents.
Infection: Use with caution in presence of known or suspected infection in a catheter because use may release a localized infection into the systemic circulation.
Pulmonary embolism: Alteplase does not constitute treatment of underlying deep vein thrombosis; therefore, consider the risk of re-embolism caused by lysis of underlying deep vein thrombi.

- Do not administer if particulate matter or discoloration noted. A pale yellow color is normal and is of no concern.
- Discard any unused solution.
- Store unopened vials in refrigerator (36° to 46°F). Fifty and 100 mg vials may also be stored at controlled room temperature (less than 86°F). Protect from excessive exposure to light. Reconstituted solution may be stored for up to 8 hr in refrigerator (36° to 46°F) or at controlled room temperature (less than 86°F)

Restoration of function to central venous catheter:
- Assess catheter function 30 min after instilling alteplase solution. If catheter function has been restored, aspirate 4 to 5 mL of blood to remove alteplase and residual clot. Gently irrigate catheter with 0.9% sodium chloride for injection. If catheter is nonfunctional, reassess catheter function 120 min after instilling alteplase. If catheter function has been restored, aspirate 4 to 5 mL of blood to remove alteplase and residual clot. Gently irrigate catheter with 0.9% sodium chloride for injection. If catheter is still nonfunctional,

a second dose of alteplase may be instilled and the process repeated.

Assessment/Interventions

- Obtain patient history, including drug history and any known allergies.

Management of acute MI, pulmonary embolism, or acute ischemic stroke:

- Review patient's health history for any of the following conditions that would contraindicate alteplase use in acute MI or pulmonary embolism: active internal bleeding; history of cerebrovascular accident; recent intracranial or intraspinal surgery or trauma; intracranial neoplasm, arteriovenous malformation, or aneurysm; severe uncontrolled hypertension; known bleeding diatheses; hypersensitivity to alteplase.
- Review patient's health history for any of the following conditions that would contraindicate alteplase use in acute ischemic stroke: evidence or history of intracranial hemorrhage; suspicion of subarachnoid hemorrhage; recent (within 3 mo) intracranial or intraspinal surgery, serious head trauma, or previous stroke; uncontrolled hypertension at time of treatment; seizure at onset of stroke; active internal bleeding; intracranial neoplasm, arteriovenous malformation, or aneurysm; known bleeding diatheses; hypersensitivity to alteplase.
- Review patient's health history for any of the following conditions that could increase the risk of bleeding complications: severe neurological deficit (eg, National Institutes of Health Stroke Scale [NIHSS] greater than 22) at time of presentation; major early infarct signs on CT scan (eg, midline shift, substantial edema, mass effect); recent trauma, major surgery, GI bleeding, obstetrical delivery, organ biopsy, previous puncture of noncompressible vessel, or GI or GU bleeding; hypertension; likelihood of left heart thrombus; subacute bacterial endocarditis; acute pericarditis; hemostatic defects including those caused by liver or kidney disease; pregnancy; diabetic hemorrhagic retinopathy or other hemorrhagic ophthalmic conditions; septic thrombophlebitis or occluded AV cannula at seriously infected site; cerebrovascular disease; age greater than 75 yr; concurrent use of oral anticoagulants.
- Review patient's medication record for use of drugs that present special risks when used in conjunction with alteplase (other thrombolytic agents, anticoagulants, or antiplatelet agents).
- Do not administer alteplase if patient is on warfarin and INR is greater than 1.7 or PT is greater than 15 sec; if heparin had been administered within 48 hr preceding stroke onset and aPTT was elevated at time of presentation.
- Ensure that CBC with differential is evaluated before therapy is started. Do not administer alteplase if platelet count is less than 100,000/mm^3.
- Monitor patient for signs of internal and superficial bleeding throughout therapy, paying particular attention to recent puncture and cutdown sites. If bleeding develops (epistaxis, hematuria, hematemesis, bloody or black, tarry stools) notify health care provider immediately. Should uncontrollable bleeding occur, discontinue alteplase therapy and concurrent heparin. Be prepared to administer protamine to reverse heparin effects.
- Monitor BP during administration. If hypertension or hypotension develops, notify health care provider immediately. Be prepared to treat appropriately.
- Monitor patient for signs of anaphylaxis or severe allergic reaction. Discontinue therapy and immediately notify health care provider if noted. Be prepared to treat appropriately.
- Avoid IM injections, noncompressible arterial punctures, internal jugular and subclavian venous punctures, and nonessential handling of patient during treatment. Perform venipunctures carefully and as infrequently as possible during therapy.
- If arterial puncture is necessary, ensure that upper extremity vessel is used. Following puncture, apply pressure for at least 30 min. Apply pressure dressing and check puncture site frequently.

Patient/Family Education

- Explain name, action, and potential side effects of drug.
- Advise patient, family, or caregiver that medication will be prepared and administered by a health care professional in a medical setting.
- Instruct patient, family, or caregiver to report any unusual symptoms or feelings, signs of bleeding, or allergic reaction immediately.
- Caution patient to avoid getting out of bed without assistance during treatment.

Altretamine

(ahl-TRETT-uh-meen)

Class Alkylating agent/Ethylenimines/Methylmelamines

How Supplied
Hexalen Gelatin capsules 50 mg

Action
PHARMACOLOGY: The precise mechanism by which altretamine exerts its cytotoxic effect is unknown. Synthetic monohydroxymethylmelamines and products of altretamine metabolism in vitro and in vivo can form covalent adducts with tissue macromolecules including DNA, but the relevance of these reactions to antitumor activity is unknown.

PHARMACOKINETICS/DYNAMICS:
Absorption: Well absorbed; T_{max} of 0.5 to 3 hr; C_{max} is 0.2 to 20.8 mg/L.
Distribution: Does bind to plasma proteins.
Metabolism: Metabolism occurs in the liver with rapid and extensive demethylation to 2 metabolites.
Excretion: $T_{1/2}$ of the beta-phase is 4.7 to 10.2 hr. 90% is excreted in the urine at 72 hr. Less than 1% of unmetabolized altretamine is excreted at 24 hr.

Indications Palliative therapy of refractory ovarian cancer.

Contraindications Hypersensitivity to altretamine; pre-existing severe bone marrow depression or severe neurologic toxicity. Careful monitoring of neurologic function in these patients is essential.

Route/Dosage
Refractory Ovarian Cancer
ADULTS: PO 260 mg/m^2/day for 14 or 21 days in a 28-day cycle, given in 4 divided doses (round dose to the nearest 50 mg) after meals and at bedtime (usual dose, 400 mg/day). Discontinue therapy for at least 14 days and resume at 200 mg/m^2/day in any of the following situations: treatment-resistant GI adverse effects; WBC less than 2000/mm^3; granulocyte count less than 1000/mm^3; platelet count less than 75,000/mm^3; progressive neurotoxicity. Discontinue permanently if neurologic symptoms persist after dose reduction.

PATIENT CARE CONSIDERATIONS
Administration/Storage
- Administer prescribed number of capsules 4 times a day, after meals and at bedtime.
- Dose is administered daily for either 14 or 21 days in a 28-day cycle.
- Follow procedures for proper handling and disposal of anticancer drugs. Wear gloves and avoid skin exposure and inhalation of fumes.

Interactions
Cimetidine: May increase altretamine's half-life and toxicity.
Cytochrome P450 enzymes: Altretamine elimination may be altered by agents that inhibit or induce cytochrome P450 enzymes.
Tricyclic antidepressants or monoamine oxidase inhibitors: Coadministration of altretamine with these drugs may cause orthostatic hypotension.

Lab Test Interferences None well documented.

Adverse Reactions
CNS: Reversible peripheral neuropathy; ataxia; depression; vertigo; agitation; confusion; hallucinations.
DERM: Rash; pruritus.
GI: Moderate potential for nausea and vomiting.
HEMA: Bone marrow suppression; nadir at 3 to 4 wk with intermittent therapy (for 14 to 21 days in a cycle) and at 6 to 8 wk with continuous administration.

> **WARNING:**
> *Neurotoxicity:* Altretamine causes mild to moderate neurotoxicity. Peripheral neuropathy and CNS symptoms (eg, mood disorders, disorders of consciousness, ataxia, dizziness, vertigo) have occurred. These are more likely to occur in patients receiving continuous high-dose daily altretamine. Neurologic toxicity appears to be reversible when therapy is discontinued.
> Perform neurologic exams regularly during therapy.
> *Hematologic:* Altretamine causes mild to moderate dose-related myelosuppression.
> Perform peripheral blood counts at baseline; prior to each course, at least monthly and when clinically indicated.

Precautions
Pregnancy: Category D.
Lactation: Undetermined.
Children: Safety and efficacy not established.
Carcinogenesis: Drugs with similar mechanisms of actions are carcinogenic.
Nausea and vomiting: With continuous high-dose daily altretamine, nausea and vomiting of gradual onset occur frequently.

- Store capsules at controlled room temperature in a tightly closed container.

Assessment/Interventions
- Obtain patient history, including drug history and any known allergies. Note history of bone marrow depression and neurologic toxicity.
- Ensure that CBC and differential are determined at baseline, prior to each course, and as indicated during therapy.
- Ensure that a neurologic examination is performed at baseline, prior to each course, and as indicated during therapy.
- Temporarily discontinue therapy (for 14 days or longer) and then restart with lower dose if any of the following occurs: GI intolerance; WBC less than 2000/mm^3; granulocyte count less than 1000/mm^3; platelet count less than 75,000/mm^3; or progressive neurotoxicity.
- Implement infection control measures if WBC drops; implement bleeding precautions if platelet count drops.

Patient/Family Education
- Explain name, dose, action, and potential side effects of drug.
- Review dosing schedule with patient (ie, 14 or 21 consecutive days in a 28-day cycle).
- Advise patient to take prescribed dose 4 times a day, after meals, and at bedtime.
- Advise patient that if a dose is missed, take it as soon as possible, but if close to the next dose, do not double the dose to catch up and take the next dose as scheduled.
- Advise patient to immediately report any of the following to their health care provider: fever, chills or other signs of infection; sore throat; persistent nausea, vomiting or appetite loss; unusual bruising or bleeding, skin rash; abnormal skin sensations; mood changes; feeling of a whirling motion; incoordination.
- Advise patient that drug may cause dizziness and to use caution while driving or performing other tasks requiring mental alertness.
- Instruct women of child bearing potential to notify health care provider if pregnant, planning to become pregnant, or breastfeeding.
- Instruct patient to not take any prescription or OTC medications or dietary supplements unless advised to do so by their health care provider.
- Advise patient that follow-up examinations and lab tests will be required to monitor therapy and to keep appointments.

Amantadine Hydrochloride

(uh-MAN-tuh-deen HIGH-droe-KLOR-ide)

Class Antiparkinson/Antiviral

How Supplied
Symmetrel Tablets 100 mg, Syrup 50 mg/5 mL ◆ *Amantadine hydrochloride* Capsules 100 mg
✽ *Endantadine* ◆ *Gen-Amantadine* ◆ *Symmetrel*

Action
PHARMACOLOGY: Exact mechanism is unknown; thought to facilitate dopamine release from intact dopaminergic terminals, increasing dopamine concentration at dopaminergic terminals. Exhibits antiviral activity against influenza A virus by inhibiting entry of virus into host cell.

PHARMACOKINETICS/DYNAMICS:
Absorption: Well absorbed. C_{max} is about 0.22 mcg/mL and T_{max} is about 3.3 hr.

Distribution: Vd is 3 to 8 L/kg and about 67% protein bound.

Metabolism: 8 metabolites were identified.

Excretion: Primarily excreted unchanged in the urine. Cl is about 0.28 L/hr/kg. The t½ is about 17 hr. Excretion increases when urine is acidic.

Special Populations:
Renal Function Impairment – Elimination t½ increased 2- to 3-fold or greater when Ccr is less than 40 mL/min/1.73 m^2.

Elderly – Cl reduced and plasma t½ and concentrations are increased.

Indications Symptomatic treatment of several forms of Parkinson disease or syndrome and drug-induced extrapyramidal reactions; prevention and treatment of influenza A viral respiratory illness, especially in high-risk patients.

Contraindications Standard considerations.

Route/Dosage
Parkinson Disease
ADULTS: PO 100 mg bid when used as single agent.
Initial dose: PO 100 mg/day if patient is debilitated or receiving high doses of other antiparkinson drugs. If necessary, dose may be titrated to max of 400 mg/day.

Drug-Induced Extrapyramidal Reactions
ADULTS: PO 100 mg bid; up to 300 mg/day may be given in divided doses.

Influenza A Viral Infection (Symptomatic Treatment)
ADULTS: PO 200 mg/day as single dose or 100 mg bid. If CNS effects develop on a once-daily dosage, split dosage schedule may reduce complaints.
ELDERLY OVER 65 YR: PO 100 mg qd.
CHILDREN 9 TO 12 YR: PO 100 mg bid.
CHILDREN 1 TO 9 YR: PO 4.4 to 8.8 mg/kg/day; not to exceed 150 mg/day.

Renal Impairment
ADULTS: **PO** Ccr 30 to 50 mL/min: Administer 200 mg first day followed by 100 mg/day thereafter; Ccr 15 to 29 mL/min: Administer 200 mg first day followed by 100 mg on alternate days; Ccr less than 15 mL/min and hemodialysis patients: Administer 200 mg q 7 days.

Influenza A Viral Infection (Prophylaxis)
Same dosages as for symptomatic treatment. However, start in anticipation of contact or as soon as possible after exposure. Continue drug administration for at least 10 days after known exposure. When influenza A virus vaccine is unavailable or contraindicated, administer amantadine for up to 90 days. In conjunction with the vaccine, administer amantadine for 2 to 3 wk after vaccination.

Interactions
Anticholinergic agents, quinidine, quinine, triamterene, thiazide diuretics, trimethoprim-sulfamethoxazole: May increase the effects of amantadine.
CNS stimulants: The effects of the CNS stimulant may be increased by amantadine.

Lab Test Interferences None well documented.

Adverse Reactions
CV: Orthostatic hypotension (1% to 5%); cardiac arrest, arrhythmias (including malignant arrhythmias), hypotension, tachycardia (postmarketing).
CNS: Dizziness, lightheadedness, insomnia (5% to 10%); depression, anxiety, irritability, hallucinations, confusion, headache, somnolence, nervousness, abnormal dreams, agitation (1% to 5%); coma, stupor, delusions, aggressive behavior, paranoid reaction, manic reaction, involuntary muscle contractions, abnormal gait, paresthesia, EEG changes, tremor, (postmarketing).
DERM: Pruritus, diaphoresis (postmarketing).
EENT: Dry nose (1% to 5%); keratitis, mydriasis (postmarketing).
GI: Nausea (5% to 10%); dry mouth, constipation, diarrhea (1% to 5%); dysphagia (postmarketing).
HEMA: Leukocytosis (postmarketing).
LABTESTABS: Elevated CPK, BUN, serum creatinine, alkaline phosphatase, LDH, bilirubin, glucose tolerance test, AST, ALT.

RESP: Acute respiratory failure, pulmonary edema, tachypnea (postmarketing).
OTHER: Ataxia, livedo reticularis, peripheral edema, fatigue (1% to 5%); allergic reactions (including anaphylactic reactions, edema, and fever), neuroleptic malignant syndrome (postmarketing).

Precautions
Pregnancy: Category C.
Lactation: Excreted in breast milk.
Children: Safety and efficacy in newborns and infants under 1 yr not established.
Elderly: Decreased dosage is necessary.
Renal function impairment: Reduced dose is required in renal impairment.
Hepatic function impairment: Use with caution.
Special risk patients: Use with caution in patients with a history of recurrent eczematoid rash, psychosis, or severe psychoneurosis not controlled by chemotherapeutic agents.
CHF: CHF has developed in patients taking amantadine.
Glaucoma: Because amantadine has anticholinergic effects and may cause mydriasis, do not give to patients with untreated angle-closure glaucoma.
Neuroleptic malignant syndrome: Neuroleptic malignant syndrome may occur in association with dose reduction or withdrawal of amantadine therapy.
Seizures: Reduced dose is necessary in patients with prior seizure disorders, including epilepsy.
Suicide: Successful suicide and suicide attempts have been reported in patients with and without a history of psychiatric illness.

Overdosage: Signs and Symptoms
Death, cardiac, respiratory, renal, or CNS toxicity, cardiac dysfunction (including arrhythmia, tachycardia, and hypertension), pulmonary edema, respiratory distress (including adult respiratory distress syndrome), renal dysfunction (including increased BUN, decreased Ccr and renal insufficiency), CNS effects (including insomnia, anxiety, agitation, aggressive behavior, hypertonia, hyperkinesias, ataxia, gait abnormality, tremor, confusion, disorientation, depersonalization, fear, delirium, hallucinations, psychotic reactions, lethargy, somnolence, and coma), seizures, hyperthermia.

PATIENT CARE CONSIDERATIONS

Administration/Storage
- Administer qd or bid as prescribed without regard to meals.
- Administer with food if GI upset occurs.
- Avoid administering dose late in evening to reduce risk of causing insomnia.
- Store tablets, capsules, and syrup at controlled room temperature (59° to 86°F).

Assessment/Interventions
- Obtain patient history, including drug history and any known allergies. Note renal or hepatic impairment, untreated angle-closure glau-

coma, heart failure, orthostatic hypotension, or peripheral edema. Note history of substance abuse, psychiatric disorder, seizures, or recurrent eczematoid rash.
- If CNS side effects occur with once-daily dosing, consider dividing the dose into 2 portions and giving bid.
- Administer reduced dose, per manufacturer's guidelines, to patient 65 yr or older or to patient with renal impairment (Ccr less than 50 mL/min).
- Monitor patient for GI, CNS, and general body side effects. Inform health care provider if noted and significant. Notify health care provider immediately if any of the following are noted: psychotic or abnormal behavior, seizure activity, orthostatic hypotension.

Patient/Family Education
- Explain name, dose, action, and potential side effects of drug.
- Advise patient to take dose qd or bid as prescribed and not to stop taking or change the dose unless advised by health care provider.
- Advise patient to take without regard to meals but to take with food if GI upset occurs.
- Caution patient taking amantadine for Parkinson disease that rapid discontinuation of the medication can worsen Parkinson symptoms and cause other severe neurological changes (eg, agitation, delusions, hallucinations). Advise patient that if medication needs to be discontinued, it should be done by slowly reducing the dose.
- Caution patient to avoid alcohol and other CNS depressants (eg, sedatives) while using this medication.
- Caution patient that drug may cause blurred vision and impaired mental alertness and to use caution driving or performing other tasks requiring mental alertness until tolerance is determined.
- Advise patient to take frequent sips of water, suck on ice chips or sugarless hard candy, or chew sugarless gum if dry mouth occurs.
- Advise patient to arise slowly from a lying or sitting position to reduce the chances of dizziness occurring.
- Advise women to notify health care provider if pregnant, planning to become pregnant, or breastfeeding.
- Advise patient to report any of the following to health care provider: mood changes or changes in thinking or behavior, dizziness or lightheadedness when arising from a sitting or lying position, swelling of the arms or legs, difficulty urinating, shortness of breath.
- Caution patient not to take any prescription or OTC medications or dietary supplements unless advised by health care provider.

Amifostine

(am-ih-FOSS-teen)
Class Selective tissue chemoprotectant and radioprotectant

How Supplied
Ethyol Powder for injection, lyophilized 500 mg (anhydrous basis)

Action
PHARMACOLOGY: Organic thiophosphate cytoprotective agent that can reduce the toxicity of cisplatin. It binds to and thereby detoxifies, reactive metabolites of cisplatin. It scavenges reactive oxygen species generated by exposure to cisplatin radiation.

PHARMACOKINETICS/DYNAMICS:
Distribution: Distribution t½ is less than 1 min.
Metabolism: Amifostine is a prodrug that is dephosphorylated by alkaline phosphatase in tissues to the active free thiol metabolite. A disulfide metabolite is then subsequently produced.
Excretion: Rapidly cleared from plasma; elimination t½ is about 8 min. Renal excretion is 0.69% to 2.64% (parent compound and metabolites).

Indications Prevent or reduce renal damage in patients receiving repeated cisplatin doses for advanced ovarian or non-small cell lung cancer; reduce incidence of moderate to severe xerostomia in patients undergoing radiation of the parotid gland for head and neck cancer.
Unlabeled use(s): Prevent or reduce cisplatin-induced neurotoxicity and cyclophosphamide-induced granulocytopenia; prevent or reduce toxicity of radiation therapy to other areas; reduce toxicity of paclitaxel.

Contraindications Sensitivity to aminothiol compounds.

Route/Dosage
Reduction of Cumulative Renal Toxicity with Chemotherapy
ADULTS: **IV** Amifostine 910 mg/m^2 once daily as a 15 min IV infusion, 30 min before chemotherapy.

Reduction of Moderate to Severe Xerostomia from Radiation of the Head and Neck
ADULTS: **IV** Amifostine 200 mg/m^2 once daily as a 3 min IV infusion, 15 to 30 min prior to standard fraction radiation therapy (1.8 to 2 Gy).

Interactions
Antihypertensives: Coadministration of drugs

with similar pharmacologic effects may potentiate hypotension or cause additive side effects, including toxicity.

Lab Test Interferences None well documented.

Adverse Reactions

CV: Hypotension (all grades 61%); hypotension (associated with apnea, dyspnea, hypoxia, tachycardia, bradycardia, extrasystoles, chest pain, MI, respiratory and cardiac arrest); arrhythmias (including atrial fibrillation/flutter and supraventricular tachycardia); cardiac arrest; transient hypertension; exacerbation of preexisting hypertension; syncope.
CNS: Dizziness; somnolence; seizures.
DERM: Erythema multiforme; exfoliative dermatitis; Stevens-Johnson syndrome; toxic epidermal necrolysis.
GI: Nausea and vomiting (all grades 96%).
METAB: Hypocalcemia.
RENAL: Renal failure.
RESP: Sneezing; hiccoughs.
OTHER: Flushing; feeling of warmth; chills, feeling of coldness; fever; allergic reactions (including hypotension, fever, chills, rigors, dyspnea, hypoxia, chest tightness, cutaneous eruption, urticaria, laryngeal edema); anaphylactoid reactions.

Precautions

Pregnancy: Category C.
Lactation: Undetermined.
Children: Safety and efficacy not established.
Elderly: Safety and efficacy not established.
Hypersensitivity: Allergic manifestations including anaphylaxis and severe cutaneous reactions have occurred rarely.
Special risk patients: Avoid use in patients with hypersensitivity to amifostine and/or aminothiol compounds. Use cautiously in patients with cerebrovascular or CV disease or hypocalcemia.
Effectiveness of the cytotoxic regimen: Do not use in patients receiving chemotherapy for malignancies in which chemotherapy can produce a significant survival benefit or cure.
Effectiveness of radiotherapy: Do not administer in patients receiving definitive radiotherapy.
Hypotension: Do not give to patients who are hypotensive or dehydrated.

Overdosage: Signs and Symptoms

Anxiety, reversible urinary retention, hypotension.

PATIENT CARE CONSIDERATIONS

Administration/Storage

- For IV administration only. Not for intradermal, subcutaneous, IM, or intra-arterial administration.
- Reconstitute powder with 9.7 mL of 0.9% NaCl for a final amifostine concentration of 50 mg/mL.
- Prior to infusion further dilute amifostine in 0.9% NaCl to a final concentration of 5 to 40 mg/mL.
- Do not mix with other IV medications or IV fluids.
- To reduce nephrotoxicity with chemotherapy, administer as a 15 min infusion, starting 30 min prior to chemotherapy.
- To reduce xerostomia from radiation therapy, administer as a 3 min infusion, starting 15 to 30 min before radiation treatment.
- Do not administer if cloudiness or particulate matter is noted.
- Store vials at controlled room temperature (68° to 77°F). Reconstituted and diluted solutions are stable for up to 5 hr at controlled room temperature or for up to 24 hr if refrigerated (36° to 46°F).

Assessment/Interventions

- Obtain patient history, including drug history and any known allergies. Note if patient is hypotensive, dehydrated, or taking antihypertensive medications. Note history of preexisting CV or cerebrovascular conditions.
- Ensure that patient is well hydrated prior to infusion.
- Ensure that patient remains supine while receiving the infusion and for at least several minutes after completion of the infusion.
- Monitor BP q 5 min during the 15 min infusion and thereafter as clinically indicated. Follow manufacturer's guidelines for interrupting and restarting amifostine if a decrease in systolic BP is noted. Stop the infusion for significant decreases in systolic BP. If systolic BP returns to normal and the patient is asymptomatic within 5 min, restart the infusion and continue to monitor BP. If systolic BP remains low, do not administer remainder of dose but administer reduced dose for subsequent cycles.
- Monitor BP before and immediately after the 3 min infusion and thereafter as clinically indicated.
- If symptomatic hypotension develops, discontinue the infusion, place the patient in the Trendelenburg position, and administer normal saline via a separate IV line.
- Ensure that appropriate antiemetic medication is administered prior to and in conjunction with amifostine.
- Monitor fluid balance when highly emetogenic chemotherapy is being used.

- Ensure that serum calcium is monitored in patients at risk of hypocalcemia (eg, nephritic syndrome). Administer calcium supplements if necessary.
- Monitor patient for signs of allergic reaction during and shortly after infusion. Be prepared to respond if a serious reaction occurs.

Patient/Family Education
- Explain name, dose, action, and potential side effects of drug.
- Advise patient that medication will be prepared and administered by health care provider in a health care setting just before chemotherapy or radiation therapy.
- Advise patient to remain supine for 15 min after completion of infusion and to use caution when standing up.
- Instruct patient to inform health care provider if noting any of the following during the administration of drug: anxiety, sweating, rapid heart beat, shortness of breath or difficulty breathing, swelling of the throat, rash, itching.
- Instruct patient not to take any prescription or OTC medications, dietary supplements, or herbal preparations unless advised by health care provider.
- Advise women to notify health care provider if pregnant, planning to become pregnant, or breastfeeding.
- Advise patient that follow-up visits and laboratory tests will be required to monitor therapy and to keep appointments.

Amikacin Sulfate

(am-ih-KAE-sin SULL-fate)

Class Antibiotic/Aminoglycoside

How Supplied
Amikin Injection 250 mg/mL, Pediatric injection 50 mg/mL

Action
PHARMACOLOGY: Inhibits production of bacterial protein, causing bacterial cell death.

PHARMACOKINETICS/DYNAMICS:
Absorption:
IM – Rapidly absorbed. C_{max} is 12 to 21 mcg/mL (250 to 500 mg doses). T_{max} is 1 hr.
IV – Single doses (500 mg over 30 min) produced C_{max} 38 mcg/mL.

Distribution: Vd is 24 L and protein binding is 0% to 11%. Crosses the placenta.

Excretion:
IM – 98.2% is excreted in the urine as unchanged drug within 24 hr.
IV – 94% is excreted in the urine within 24 hr. $T_{1/2}$ is about 2 hr. Serum Cl is 100 mL/min; renal Cl is 94 mL/min.

Special Populations:
Renal Function Impairment – Rate of excretion is decreased and $t_{1/2}$ is prolonged. Dosage adjustment may be needed.

Indications Treatment of infections caused by susceptible strains of microorganisms, especially gram-negative bacteria.

Contraindications Generally not indicated for long-term therapy because of ototoxicity and nephrotoxicity.

Route/Dosage
ADULTS, CHILDREN, AND INFANTS: **IV/IM** 15 mg/kg (ideal body weight)/day in 2 or 3 divided doses. Treatment in heavier patients should not exceed 1.5 g/day.
Uncomplicated utis: **IV/IM** 250 mg bid.
NEWBORNS: **IV/IM** Loading dose of 10 mg/kg is recommended followed by 7.5 mg/kg q 12 hr. Lower doses may be needed in first 2 wk of life.

Interactions
Drugs with nephrotoxic potential (eg, cephalosporins, enflurane, methoxyflurane, vancomycin): May increase risk of nephrotoxicity.
Loop diuretics (eg, furosemide): May increase risk of auditory toxicity.
Neuromuscular blocking agents (eg, tubocurarine): Amikacin may enhance effects of these agents.
INCOMPATIBILITIES: Do not mix with betalactam antibiotics (eg, carbenicillin, ticarcillin).

Lab Test Interferences None well documented.

Adverse Reactions
EENT: Hearing loss; deafness; loss of balance.
GU: Oliguria; proteinuria; increased serum creatinine; urinary casts; red and white blood cells in urine; azotemia.
OTHER: Decreased serum magnesium.

> **WARNING:**
> *Neurotoxicity:* Manifests as both auditory and vestibular ototoxicity, and primarily occurs in patients with pre-existing renal damage or with prolonged therapy. Partial or total irreversible deafness may continue to develop after drug is stopped. Other features of neurotoxicity include paresthesias, twitching, and seizures.
> *Nephrotoxicity:* Usually reversible.
> Teratogenic in pregnancy.
> Renal and eighth nerve function closely monitored in patients with suspected renal dysfunction. Monitor peak and trough concentrations.
> Dosage adjustments required in renal impairment.

> Neuromuscular blockade and respiratory paralysis have been reported following use of aminoglycosides. The possibility of these phenomena should be considered if aminoglycosides are administered by any route, especially in patients receiving anesthetics; neuromuscular blocking agents or in patients receiving massive transfusions of citrate-anticoagulated blood.

Precautions
Pregnancy: Category D.
Lactation: Undetermined.
Children: Cautious use is necessary in premature infants and newborns because of renal immaturity.
Renal function impairment: Dosage adjustment is needed in patients with this condition.

PATIENT CARE CONSIDERATIONS

Administration/Storage
- Dilute with normal saline or D5W according to instructions.
- Administer by IV or IM route only.
- Use volumetric IV pump to regulate delivery.
- Avoid overrapid administration, which may result in respiratory depression and arrest; give over 30 to 60 min.
- Do not mix with or administer within 1 hr of other IV medications because of potential for incompatibility or inactivation.
- Discard diluted solution after 24 hr.
- When giving by IM route, use deep, slow injection; rotate sites to prevent tissue irritation or breakdown.

Assessment/Interventions
- Obtain patient history, including drug history and any known allergies. Note hypersensitivity to aminoglycosides.
- Assess renal and auditory function before administration and monitor periodically during therapy to detect nephrotoxicity or ototoxicity.
- Send blood for culture and sensitivity before beginning therapy.
- Monitor patient for signs and symptoms of yeast infections during therapy.
- Monitor I&O during therapy; maintain good hydration.
- Assess patient for signs of infection to determine effectiveness of therapy.
- Notify health care provider and stop infusion if patient has signs of oliguria or shows signs of renal failure (eg, edema, shortness of breath, pruritus), ototoxicity or anaphylactic reaction.

Patient/Family Education
- Encourage patient to increase fluid intake to 2000 to 3000 mL/day, unless contraindicated.
- Warn patient that diarrhea and abdominal bloating are common side effects of antibiotics.
- Inform patient that improvement should be seen in 3 to 5 days.
- Instruct patient to report the following signs to health care provider: Hypersensitivity, tinnitus, vertigo, hearing loss.
- Teach patient to look for signs of renal failure and to notify health care provider immediately if these signs occur.

Amiloride Hydrochloride
(uh-MILL-oh-ride HIGH-droe-KLOR-ide)

Class Potassium-sparing diuretic

How Supplied
Midamor Tablets 5 mg

Action
PHARMACOLOGY: Interferes with sodium reabsorption at distal tubule, resulting in increased excretion of water and sodium and decreased excretion of potassium.

PHARMACOKINETICS/DYNAMICS:
Absorption: 15% to 25% is absorbed; t_{max} is 3 to 4 hr.

Distribution: About 23% is protein bound.
Metabolism: Not metabolized.

Excretion: $T_{1/2}$ is 6 to 9 hr. About 50% is excreted unchanged in the urine; about 40% in the feces.
Onset: Within 2 hr.
Peak: 6 to 10 hr.
Duration: 24 hr.

Indications Treatment of CHF or hypertension (in combination with thiazide or loop diuretics) and diuretic-induced hypokalemia.
Unlabeled use(s): Reduction of lithium-induced polyuria; slowed reduction of pulmonary function in patients with cystic fibrosis (aerosol form).

Contraindications Serum potassium more than 5.5 mEq/L; potassium supplementation; impaired renal function: spironolactone or triamterene therapy.

Route/Dosage
ADULT: **PO** 5 to 10 mg/day.

Lithium-Induced Polyuria
PO 10 to 20 mg/day.

Cystic Fibrosis
Dissolve in 0.3% saline and deliver by nebulizer.

Interactions
Angiotensin-converting enzyme inhibitors: May result in severely elevated serum potassium levels.
Potassium preparations: May severely increase serum potassium levels, possibly resulting in cardiac arrhythmias or cardiac arrest. Do not administer to patients taking potassium preparations.

Lab Test Interferences None well documented.

PATIENT CARE CONSIDERATIONS
Administration/Storage
- Administer medication with food, preferably in the morning.
- Store in tightly closed container in cool location.

Assessment/Interventions
- Obtain patient history, including drug history and any known allergies. Note BP and renal disease or history of potassium supplement use.
- Monitor potassium, BUN, and creatinine levels.
- If sudden elevation in serum potassium level (more than 5.5 mEq/L) occurs, withhold dose and notify health care provider.
- Monitor fluid and electrolyte balance during therapy (eg, I&O, daily weight, edema).
- If drug is given in combination with another antihypertensive, monitor BP throughout administration.
- If hypokalemia is suspected, obtain periodic ECG during therapy.
- If ECG changes occur (eg, peaked T waves, abnormal S or P waves), withhold dose and notify health care provider.
- Monitor for signs of hyperkalemia (eg, fatigue, muscle weakness, cardiac irregularities).
- Monitor for signs of hyponatremia.
- Monitor renal function.

Patient/Family Education
- Explain that dietary considerations are very important while taking this medication. Advise patient to avoid the following: Eating excessive amounts of potassium-rich foods (bananas, citrus fruits, raisins, nuts), using salt substitutes, taking medications high in potassium and eating foods high in sodium (tomatoes, pickled foods, canned foods, luncheon meats).
- Teach patient to monitor BP daily.
- Instruct patient to take medication as directed, even if feeling well.

Adverse Reactions
CV: Angina pectoris; orthostatic hypotension; arrhythmia.
CNS: Headache; dizziness; encephalopathy; paresthesia; tremors; vertigo; nervousness; mental confusion; insomnia; decreased libido; depression.
DERM: Skin rash; itching; pruritus.
EENT: Visual disturbances; tinnitus; nasal congestion.
GI: Nausea; anorexia; diarrhea; vomiting; abdominal pain; gas pain; appetite changes; constipation; GI bleeding; abdominal fullness; thirst; dry mouth; heartburn; flatulence.
GU: Impotence; polyuria; dysuria; urinary frequency.
HEMA: Aplastic anemia; neutropenia.
HEPA: Jaundice.
METAB: Increased serum potassium levels.
RESP: Cough; dyspnea.
OTHER: Musculoskeletal (eg, weakness; fatigue; muscle cramps; joint/back/chest pain; neck or shoulder ache).

Precautions
Pregnancy: Category B.
Lactation: Undetermined.
Children: Safety and efficacy not established.
Renal function impairment: Use cautiously in patients with this condition.
Hepatic function impairment: With severe liver disease, hepatic encephalopathy (eg, tremors, confusion, coma, jaundice) may occur.
Diabetes mellitus: Hyperkalemia may occur.
Electrolyte imbalances and BUN increase: Hyperkalemia, hyponatremia, hypochloremia, and increases in BUN may occur.

- Encourage patient to avoid sudden changes in position to prevent orthostatic hypotension.
- Advise patient that drug may cause dizziness and blurred vision, and to use caution while driving or performing other tasks requiring mental alertness.
- Inform patient that this medication causes increased urine output.
- Teach patient signs and symptoms of hyperkalemia and hyponatremia.
- Caution patient to notify health care provider or dentist about taking this medication and notify health care provider of cramps or chronic fatigue and weakness, which are serious side effects.

Amiloride Hydrochloride/ Hydrochlorothiazide (HCTZ)

(Uh-MILL-oh-ride HIGH-droe-KLOR-ide/ high-droe-klor-oh-THIGH-uh-zide)

Class Potassium-sparing diuretic/Thiazide diuretic

How Supplied
Moduretic Tablets 5 mg amiloride/50 mg HCTZ
✥ Apo-Amilzide ♦ Moduret ♦ Novamilor ♦ Nu-Amilzide

Action
PHARMACOLOGY:
Amiloride: Interferes with sodium reabsorption at distal tubule, resulting in increased water and sodium excretion and decreased potassium excretion.
HCTZ: Increases chloride, sodium, and water excretion by interfering with transport of sodium ions across renal tubular epithelium.

Indications Treatment of hypertension or congestive heart failure in patients who develop hypokalemia when thiazide or other kaliuretic diuretics are used alone, or in patients in whom maintenance of normal serum potassium levels is clinically important (eg, digitalized patients); alone or as adjunctive treatment with other antihypertensive agents.

Contraindications Hyperkalemia (serum potassium levels greater than 5.5 mEq/L); concurrently with other potassium-sparing diuretics (eg, spironolactone), potassium supplements (including potassium-rich diet) except in severe or refractory cases of hypokalemia; impaired renal function; sensitivity to any components of product.

Route/Dosage
ADULTS: **PO** 1 to 2 tablets (5 mg amiloride/ 50 mg hydrochlorothiazide) daily with meals.

Interactions
Amiloride:
ACE inhibitors (eg, captopril) – May result in severely elevated potassium levels.
Potassium preparations – May severely increase serum potassium levels, possibly resulting in cardiac arrhythmias or cardiac arrest. Do not coadminister.

Hydrochlorothiazide:
Bile acid sequestrants – May reduce thiazide absorption; give thiazide at least 2 hr before sequestrant.
Diazoxide – May cause hyperglycemia.
Digitalis glycosides – Diuretic-induced hypokalemia and hypomagnesemia may lead to digitalis-induced arrhythmias.
Lithium – Renal excretion of lithium may be reduced.
Loop diuretics (eg, furosemide) – Synergistic effects may occur, resulting in profound diuresis and serious electrolyte abnormalities.
Sulfonylureas (eg, chlorpropamide) – Hypoglycemic effect of sulfonylurea may be decreased, necessitating an increase in sulfonylurea dosage.

Lab Test Interferences Hydrochlorothiazide may decrease serum protein-bound iodine levels without signs of thyroid disturbances. May cause diagnostic interference of serum electrolyte levels, blood and urine glucose levels, serum bilirubin levels, and serum uric acid levels.

Adverse Reactions
CV: Arrhythmia, tachycardia, palpitations (amiloride).
CNS: Headache, fatigue, tiredness, weakness, dizziness, encephalopathy, tremors, decreased libido (amiloride); restlessness (hydrochlorothiazide).
DERM: Mild skin rash, pruritus, alopecia (amiloride); urticaria, purpura (hydrochlorothiazide).
EENT: Increased ocular pressure, tinnitus (amiloride); transient blurred vision, xanthopsia (hydrochlorothiazide).
GI: Nausea, anorexia, GI and abdominal pain, flatulence, activation of peptic ulcer, dyspepsia, heartburn, dry mouth (amiloride); pancreatitis, cramping, GI irritation, sialadenitis (hydrochlorothiazide).
GU: Bladder spasm, polyuria, urinary frequency (amiloride); interstitial nephritis (hydrochlorothiazide).
HEMA: Aplastic anemia, neutropenia (amiloride); agranulocytosis, leukopenia, hemolytic anemia, thrombocytopenia (hydrochlorothiazide).
HEPA: Jaundice.
METAB: Hyperkalemia, hyperglycemia, glucos-

uria, hyperuricemia (hydrochlorothiazide).
RESP: Shortness of breath, cough (amiloride); respiratory distress, including pneumonitis and pulmonary edema (hydrochlorothiazide).
OTHER: Leg pain, painful extremities, neck/shoulder ache, fatigue, itching (amiloride); anaphylactic reactions, necrotizing angiitis, photosensitivity, fever (hydrochlorothiazide).

Precautions
Pregnancy: Category B.
Lactation: Amiloride: undetermined; hydrochlorothiazide: excreted in breast milk.
Children: Safety and efficacy not established.
Hyperkalemia: Hyperkalemia may occur. The risk of hyperkalemia may be increased in patients with renal impairment or diabetes mellitus. If possible, avoid use in patients with renal impairment or diabetes mellitus.

Overdosage: Signs and Symptoms
Dehydration, electrolyte imbalance (eg, hyperkalemia), electrolyte depletion (hypokalemia, hypochloremia, hyponatremia).

PATIENT CARE CONSIDERATIONS
Administration/Storage
- Give once daily in the morning with food.
- Administer alone or in combination with other antihypertensives.
- Store tablets at controlled room temperature (59° to 86°F). Protect from moisture, freezing, and excessive heat.

Assessment/Interventions
- Obtain patient history, including drug history and any known allergies. Note history of diabetes, lupus erythematosis, hyperkalemia, anuria, kidney disease, concurrent use of potassium-conserving medications, or potassium-containing salt substitute, or allergy to sulfonamides.
- Ensure that serum electrolytes, BUN, and creatinine are monitored periodically.
- Monitor and record BP and pulse. Should hypotension result, hold medication and notify health care provider.
- Take safety precautions if orthostatic hypotension occurs.
- Monitor blood sugar in diabetic patient when drug is started or dose is changed. Report significant changes to health care provider.
- Monitor patient for GI, CV, and general body side effects. Inform health care provider if paresthesia, weakness, fatigue, bradycardia, or other significant effects are noted.

Patient/Family Education
- Explain name, dose, action, and potential side effects of drug.
- Advise patient to take prescribed dose once daily in the morning with food.
- Inform patient that drug controls, but does not cure, hypertension and to continue taking medication as prescribed even when BP is not elevated.
- Caution patient not to change the dose or stop taking unless advised by health care provider.
- Instruct patient to continue taking other BP medications as prescribed by health care provider.
- Instruct patient in BP and pulse measurement skills.
- Advise patient to monitor and record BP and pulse at home and to inform health care provider should abnormal measurements be noted. Also, advise patient to take record of BP and pulse to each follow-up visit.
- Instruct patient to lie or sit down if experiencing dizziness or lightheadedness when standing.
- Caution patient that inadequate fluid intake, excessive perspiration, diarrhea, or vomiting can lead to excessive fall in BP, resulting in lightheadedness or fainting.
- Instruct diabetic patient to monitor blood glucose more frequently when drug is started or dose is changed and to inform health care provider of significant changes in readings.
- Caution patient to avoid unnecessary exposure to UV light (sunlight, tanning booths) and to use sunscreen and wear protective clothing when exposed to UV light to avoid photosensitivity reaction.
- Emphasize to hypertensive patient importance of other modalities on BP: weight control, regular exercise, smoking cessation, and moderate intake of alcohol and salt.
- Advise women to notify health care provider if pregnant, planning to become pregnant, or breastfeeding.
- Instruct patient to stop taking drug and immediately report any of these symptoms to health care provider: abnormal skin sensations, muscle weakness, or slow pulse.
- Caution patient to not take any prescription or OTC medications, salt substitutes, or dietary supplements unless advised by health care provider.
- Advise patient that follow-up visits and lab tests may be required to monitor therapy and to keep appointments.

Aminocaproic Acid

(uh-mee-no-kuh-PRO-ik acid)

Class Hemostatic

How Supplied
Amicar Injection 250 mg/mL, Tablets 500 mg, Syrup 250 mg/mL

Action
PHARMACOLOGY: Inhibits fibrinolysis to stop bleeding.

PHARMACOKINETICS/DYNAMICS:
Absorption:
Oral – Zero order process; absorption rate of 5.2 g/hr. C_{max} is about 164 mcg/mL; T_{max} is about 1.2 hr.

Distribution:
Oral – Vd is about 23.1 L.
IV – Vd is about 30 L.

Metabolism: Metabolite is adipic acid.

Excretion: Renally eliminated. 65% is recovered in the urine as unchanged drug and 11% as the metabolite adipic acid. Renal clearance is 116 mL/min and total body clearance is 169 mL/min. $T_{1/2}$ is about 2 hr.

Duration: 3 hr for single IV dose.

Indications Treatment of excessive bleeding from systemic hyperfibrinolysis and urinary fibrinolysis. **Unlabeled use(s):** Prevention of recurrence of subarachnoid hemorrhage; management of amegakaryocytic thrombocytopenia; abortion; or prevention of attacks of hereditary angioneurotic edema.

Contraindications Active intravascular clotting; DIC; administration to newborns.

Route/Dosage
ADULTS: **IV/PO** 4 to 5 g in first hour; then 1 to 1.25 g/hr for 8 hr or until bleeding is controlled.

Dosage over 30 g/24 hr is not recommended.

Interactions
Oral contraceptives or estrogens: May lead to increase in clotting factors, producing state of hypercoagulation.

Lab Test Interferences
Serum potassium levels: Serum potassium level may be elevated, especially in impaired renal function.

Adverse Reactions
CV: Bradycardia; hypotension; peripheral ischemia; thrombosis.
CNS: Dizziness; headache; delirium; hallucinations; confusion; intracranial hypertension; stroke; syncope.
DERM: Rash; pruritus.
EENT: Tinnitus; decreased vision; watery eyes.
GI: Nausea; diarrhea; abdominal pain; vomiting.
GU: Increased BUN; renal failure.
HEMA: Agranulocytosis; coagulation disorder; leukopenia; thrombocytoperia.
RESP: Dyspnea; nasal congestion; pulmonary embolism.
OTHER: Injection site reaction; pain and necrosis; myalgia; myositis; myopathy (characterized by muscle weakness, fatigue, elevated creatinine phosphokinase, rhabdomyolysis associated with myoglobinuria and renal failure); edema; allergic and anaphylactic reactions; anaphylaxis; malaise.

Precautions
Pregnancy: Category C.
Lactation: Undetermined.
Children: Safety and efficacy not established.
Upper urinary tract bleeding: Not used in treatment of hematuria of upper UT origin unless possible benefits outweigh risks.

Overdosage: Signs and Symptoms
Hypotension, severe acute renal failure.

PATIENT CARE CONSIDERATIONS

Administration/Storage
IV infusion:
- Dilute as 1 g/50 mL diluent. Compatible diluents include Sterile Water for Injection, normal saline, D5W, and Ringer's solution.
- Use infusion pump for IV administration. Closely monitor rate of infusion because this drug is not intended for rapid IV injection or in undiluted form.
- Infuse dose over 30 min to 1 hr.

Oral administration:
- Give with full glass of water.
- Encourage fluid intake between doses.
- Store in tightly closed container at room temperature.

Assessment/Interventions
- Obtain patient history, including drug history and any known allergies.
- Determine baseline BP and pulse before starting IV infusion.
- Assess patient's respiratory and neurologic status.
- Note presence of menstrual bleeding.
- Monitor serum potassium levels, clotting factors, and platelet counts.
- Monitor vital signs, especially BP and pulse, and respiratory and neurologic status throughout therapy.
- Monitor I&O. Note any increase or decrease in urinary output.

- Observe for signs of internal bleeding (eg, petechiae, gingival oozing, hematuria, epistaxis, ecchymosis).
- Have vitamin K or protamine sulfate available for emergency use.

Patient/Family Education
- Caution patient to avoid sudden position changes to prevent orthostatic hypotension.
- Advise patient to use soft toothbrush or sponge for dental care.
- Instruct patient to report the following symptoms to health care provider: gingival bleeding, epistaxis, hematuria, skin changes (eg, ecchymosis, petechiae), difficulty in urination, reddish-brown urine, chest or leg pain, or difficulty breathing.

Aminoglutethimide

(ah-MEE-no-glue-TETH-ih-mide)
Class Adrenal cortex suppressant

How Supplied
Cytadren Tablets 250 mg

Action
PHARMACOLOGY: Aminoglutethimide inhibits the enzymatic conversion of cholesterol to Δ^5-pregnenolone, thereby reducing the synthesis of adrenal glucocorticoids, mineralocorticoids, estrogens, and androgens.

PHARMACOKINETICS/DYNAMICS:
Absorption: Rapidly and completely absorbed. C_{max} is about 5.9 mcg/mL; T_{max} is about 1.5 hr.
Distribution: Minimally bound to proteins.
Excretion: $T_{1/2}$ is about 12.5 hr. 34.54% is excreted in urine as unchanged drug.

Indications Suppression of adrenal function in patients with Cushing syndrome. **Unlabeled use(s):** Suppression of adrenal function in advanced breast carcinoma or metastatic prostate carcinoma.

Contraindications Standard considerations.

Route/Dosage
Cushing Syndrome
ADULTS: PO 250 mg q 6 hr. Titrate to adrenal response in increments of 250 mg/day q 1 to 2 wk. Max daily dose is 2000 mg.

Dosage Adjustment
ADULTS: PO Dosage reduction may be required for a Ccr less than 10 mL/min; specific guidelines are not established. Discontinue therapy if patient develops severe rash or rash that lasts more than 5 to 8 days. Therapy may be continued at a lower dose after resolution of mild to moderate skin rashes.

Interactions
CNS depressants: Concurrent use with CNS depressants (eg, narcotics, analgesics, alcohol, antiemetics, benzodiazepines, sedatives, tranquilizers) may potentiate CNS effects.
Dexamethasone, digitoxin, medroxyprogesterone, tamoxifen, theophylline, warfarin: Aminoglutethimide increases oxidative metabolism of these drugs. Higher doses of these agents may be required to achieve therapeutic response during concomitant therapy.

Lab Test Interferences None well documented.

Adverse Reactions
CV: Orthostatic or persistent hypotension; tachycardia.
CNS: Headache; dizziness; drowsiness; lethargy.
DERM: Morbilliform rash; pruritus.
ENDO: Adrenocortical insufficiency; hypothyroidism; masculinization and hirsutism in females.
GI: Low potential for nausea and vomiting; elevated LFTs; cholestatic jaundice.
GU: Aminoglutethimide crosses the placenta and has caused pseudohermaphroditism in female infants whose mothers took this agent and anticonvulsants during pregnancy.
MUSC: Myalgia.

Precautions
Pregnancy: Category D.
Lactation: Undetermined.
Children: Safety and efficacy not established.
Cortical hypofunction: May cause adrenal cortical hypofunction, especially under conditions of stress.
Hypotension: Aminoglutethimide may suppress aldosterone production by the adrenal cortex and may cause orthostatic or persistent hypotension. Monitor BP.

Overdosage: Signs and Symptoms
Ataxia, somnolence, lethargy, dizziness, fatigue, coma, hyperventilation, respiratory depression, nausea and vomiting, loss of sodium and water, hyponatremia, hypochloremia, hyperkalemia, hypoglycemia, hypovolemic shock caused by dehydration, hypotension.

PATIENT CARE CONSIDERATIONS
Administration/Storage
* Administer PO.
* Store at room temperature. Protect from light.

Assessment/Interventions
* Adrenal function usually returns to normal within 36 to 72 hr of discontinuing aminoglutethimide, although recovery may be slower after prolonged therapy.
* Monitor plasma cortisol to assess response to therapy for suppression of adrenal function.
* Thyroid function may decrease during therapy. Monitor at baseline and throughout therapy. Some patients may require thyroid supplements.
* Monitor LFTs at baseline and throughout therapy.
* Monitor periodically for any electrolyte or hematologic changes.
* Patients may require replacement of mineralocorticoids with fludrocortisone.
* Patients may require replacement of glucocorticoids. Hydrocortisone 20 to 30 mg PO every morning replaces endogenous secretion. Discontinuation of aminoglutethimide and additional steroids may be required in situations that cause stress, such as shock, trauma, or infections.

Patient/Family Education
* May produce drowsiness or dizziness; use caution while driving or performing other tasks requiring alertness, coordination, or physical dexterity.
* May cause rash, fainting, weakness, or headache; notify health care provider if pronounced.
* Nausea and loss of appetite may occur during the first 2 wk of therapy; notify health care provider if these persist or become pronounced.

Aminophylline (Theophylline Ethylenediamine)
(am-in-AHF-ih-lin)

Class Bronchodilator/Xanthine derivative

How Supplied
Phyllocontin Tablets, controlled-release (12 hr) 225 mg (equiv. to 178 mg theophylline) ♦ *Truphylline* Suppositories 250 mg (equiv. to 197.5 mg theophylline), Suppositories 500 mg (equiv. to 395 mg theophylline)
🍁 *Phyllocontin* ♦ *Phyllocontin-350*

Action
PHARMACOLOGY: Relaxes bronchial smooth muscle and pulmonary blood vessels; stimulates central respiratory drive; increases diaphragmatic contractility.

PHARMACOKINETICS/DYNAMICS:

Absorption: (Note: Information for the pharmacokinetics/dynamics section was taken from theophylline because aminophylline is a mixture of theophylline and base.) Rapidly and completely absorbed in solution or immediate-release. C_{max} is 10 mcg/mL (5 to 15 mcg/mL). T_{max} is 1 to 2 hr. Food and antacid does not cause any clinically significant changes; therapeutic range (10 to 20 mcg/mL).

Distribution: 40% protein bound (primarily albumin). Unbound theophylline distributes throughout the body water, but distributes poorly into body fat. Vd is 0.45 L/kg (0.3 to 0.7 L/kg) based on idea body weight. Freely passes across the placenta into breast milk and into CSF.

Metabolism: Does not undergo any measurable first-pass elimination. About 90% of dose is metabolized in the liver in adults and children over 1 yr. Caffeine and 3–methytxanthine are the only theophylline metabolites with pharmacological activity.

Excretion: In neonates, about 50% of theophylline dose is excreted unchanged in the urine (ie, excretion is by the kidneys) 10% of theophylline dose is excreted unchanged in the urine in children 0 to 3 mo.

Special Populations:
Renal Function Impairment – No dosage adjustment required in adults and children over 3 mo. Neonates with reduced renal function, dose reduction and frequent monitoring of serum concentrations are required.
Special risk patients – Pharmacokinetics vary widely among similar patients and cannot be predicted by age, sex, body weight or other demographic parameters. However, a prolonged $t_{1/2}$ may occur in CHF, liver dysfunction, alcoholism, and respiratory infection patients.

Indications Prevention or treatment of reversible bronchospasm associated with asthma or COPD. **Unlabeled use(s):** Treatment of apnea and bradycardia of prematurity.

Contraindications Hypersensitivity to xanthines (eg, caffeine, theobromine) or ethylenediamine; peptic ulcer; seizure disorders not treated with medication. Aminophylline suppositories are contraindicated in presence of irritation or infection of rectum or lower colon.

Route/Dosage
Dosage is calculated on basis of lean body weight.

ORAL/RECTAL
Dose is determined by percentage of theophylline content in aminophylline salt. Aminophylline is 79% theophylline.

Loading Dose
ADULTS AND CHILDREN: **PO/PR** 5 mg/kg.

Maintenance Dose
HEALTHY NONSMOKERS: **PO/PR** 3 mg/kg q 8 hr.
ELDERLY AND PATIENTS WITH COR PULMONALE: 2 mg/kg q 8 hr.
CHF PATIENTS: 1 to 2 mg/kg q 12 hr.
CHILDREN 9 TO 16 YR AND YOUNG ADULT SMOKERS: 3 mg/kg q 6 hr.
CHILDREN 1 TO 9 YR: 4 mg/kg q 6 hr.

PARENTERAL
Loading Dose
ADULTS AND CHILDREN NOT RECEIVING THEOPHYLLINE: **IV** 6 mg/kg.
ADULTS AND CHILDREN RECEIVING THEOPHYLLINE: **IV** 0.6 to 3.1 mg/kg.

Maintenance Dose
HEALTHY NONSMOKERS: **IV** 0.5 to 0.7 mg/kg/hr.
ELDERLY AND PATIENTS WITH COR PULMONALE: **IV** 0.3 to 0.6 mg/kg/hr.
CHF PATIENTS: **IV** 0.1 to 0.5 mg/kg/hr.
CHILDREN 9 TO 16 YR AND YOUNG ADULT SMOKERS: **IV** 0.8 to 1 mg/kg/hr.
CHILDREN 1 TO 9 YR: **IV** 1 to 1.2 mg/kg/hr.
NEWBORNS TO INFANTS UNDER 6 MO: Not recommended. Weigh benefits against risks.
INFANTS 26 TO 52 WK: Divide into q 6 hr dosing.
INFANTS UNDER 26 WK: Divide into q 8 hr dosing.
INFANTS 6 TO 52 WK: 24 hr dosage (mg).
PREMATURE INFANTS OLDER THAN 4 DAYS POSTNATAL: **IV** 1.5 mg/kg q 12 hr.
PREMATURE INFANTS LESS THAN 24 DAYS POSTNATAL: **IV** 1 mg/kg q 12 hr.

Interactions
Allopurinol, nonselective beta blockers, calcium channel blockers, cimetidine, oral contraceptives, corticosteroids, disulfiram, ephedrine, influenza virus vaccine, interferon, macrolide antibiotics, mexiletine, quinolone antibiotics, thyroid hormones: May increase aminophylline levels.
Aminoglutethimide, barbiturates, hydantoins, ketoconazole, rifampin, smoking (tobacco and marijuana), sulfinpyrazone, sympathomimetics: May decrease aminophylline levels.
Benzodiazepines, propofol: Aminophylline may antagonize sedative effects.
Beta-agonists: Effects of both drugs may be antagonized.
Carbamazepine, isoniazid, loop diuretics: May increase or decrease aminophylline levels.
Food: Sustained-released medications are taken on empty stomach to avoid rapid drug release. Low-protein, high-carbohydrate diet may increase aminophylline levels. Charcoal-broiled foods or high-protein, low-carbohydrate diet may decrease aminophylline levels.
Halothane: May cause catecholamine-induced arrhythmias.
Ketamine: May result in seizures.
Lithium: Aminophylline may reduce lithium levels.
Nondepolarizing muscle relaxants: May antagonize neuromuscular blockade.
INCOMPATIBILITIES: Do not mix with anileridine hydrochloride, ascorbic acid, chlorpromazine, codeine phosphate, dimenhydrinate, dobutamine hydroxide, epinephrine, erythromycin gluceptate, hydralazine, insulin, levorphanol tartrate, meperidine, methadone, methicillin, morphine sulfate, norepinephrine bitartrate, oxytetracycline, penicillin G potassium, phenobarbital, phenytoin, prochlorperazine, promazine, promethazine, tetracycline, vancomycin, verapamil, vitamin B complex with vitamin C.

Lab Test Interferences
None well documented.

Adverse Reactions
CV: Palpitations; tachycardia; hypotension; arrhythmias.
CNS: Irritability; headache; insomnia; muscle twitching; seizures.
GI: Nausea; vomiting; anorexia; diarrhea; gastroesophageal reflux; epigastric pain.
GU: Proteinuria; diuresis.
RESP: Tachypnea; respiratory arrest.
OTHER: Fever; flushing; hyperglycemia; inappropriate antidiuretic hormone secretion; sensitivity reactions (exfoliative dermatitis and urticaria).

Precautions
Pregnancy: Category C.
Lactation: Excreted in breast milk.
Children: Safety and efficacy not established in children under 1 yr.
Cardiac effects: Aminophylline may cause or worsen preexisting arrhythmias.
GI effects: Aminophylline may cause or worsen preexisting ulcers or gastroesophageal reflux.
Status asthmaticus: In this medical emergency parenteral medication and close monitoring in

intensive care unit are recommended.
Toxicity: Patients with liver impairment or cardiac failure and those more than 55 yr are at greatest risk.

PATIENT CARE CONSIDERATIONS
Administration/Storage
* Store at room temperature.

Tablets and liquid:
* Give on empty stomach (30 min to 1 hr before meals or 2 hr after meals).
* Do not crush or chew extended-release forms; capsules may be opened and contents mixed with soft food. Scored tablets can be cut in half and then swallowed.

IV infusion:
* Do not administer if solution is discolored or if crystals are present.
* Rapid infusion may cause cardiac arrest.
* Give undiluted drug at rate of 25 mg/min.
* Dilute in Dextrose or saline solutions or Lactated Ringer's. Administer diluted drug at rate of 25 mg/min (max). Once mixed, solution must be refrigerated and used within 24 hr.
* Use of infusion pump is recommended for precise administration.
* Do not mix aminophylline solution in syringe with other drugs. Separate IV infusion is recommended because of IV incompatibilities.

Suppositories:
* Do not use rectal route when irritation or infection is present.
* May have special storage requirements.

IM injection:
* IM route is usually not used because this method produces intense prolonged pain.

Assessment/Interventions
* Obtain patient history, including drug history and any known allergies. Note sensitivity to xanthines (eg, caffeine, chocolate), peptic ulcer, seizure disorders, liver disease and current medication regimen.
* Take vital signs before and after administration.
* Note baseline ECG.
* Assess lung sounds.
* Measure and record I&O.
* Position patient with head of bed elevated or place in position of comfort to reduce dyspnea.
* Encourage fluid intake to liquefy bronchial secretions.
* Reduce patient's intake of cola, coffee, and chocolate and use of cigarettes.
* Report carbohydrate or protein restrictions in patient's diet because theophylline dosage may need to be adjusted.
* Monitor vital signs and cardiac status. If significant tachycardia or ventricular arrhythmias occur, withhold drug and report to health care provider.
* In patients receiving theophylline products, monitor serum theophylline levels for toxicity. If levels are above therapeutic range (10 to 20 mcg/mL), report to health care provider.
* In patients receiving erythromycin, beta-blockers (eg, atenolol, metoprolol, nadolol, propanolol), cimetidine, or allopurinol, monitor for toxicity.
* In patients receiving phenobarbital, rifampin, carbamazepine, or lithium, monitor effectiveness of aminophylline; dosage may not be sufficient.

Patient/Family Education
* Advise patient not to smoke. If patient changes smoking habits or stops smoking, dosage adjustment may be necessary.
* Instruct patient to report the following symptoms to health care provider: unusual worsening of symptoms, nausea, vomiting, excessive nervousness, insomnia, irregular heartbeat.
* For patients taking theophylline, emphasize that serum theophylline levels should be tested q 6 to 12 mo.
* Advise elderly patients to take safety precautions (eg, rise slowly, use handrails, request assistance in ambulation) if dizziness occurs.
* Instruct patient to avoid foods or beverages containing caffeine and to limit intake of charcoal-broiled foods.
* Advise patient not to take OTC cough, cold, or breathing medications without consulting health care provider.

Aminosalicylate Sodium (Para-Aminosalicylate Sodium; PAS)

(uh-MEE-no-suh-LIS-ih-late SO-dee-uhm)
Class Anti-infective/Antitubercular

How Supplied
Paser Granules, delayed-release 4 g

Action
PHARMACOLOGY: Competitively antagonizes metabolism of para-aminobenzoic acid, resulting in bacteriostatic activity against *Mycobacterium tuberculosis*.

PHARMACOKINETICS/DYNAMICS:
Absorption: T_{max} is about 6 hr; C_{max} is about 20 mcg/mL.

Distribution: About 50% to 60% is protein bound.

Excretion: 80% is excreted in the urine with at least 50% excreted in acetylated form. The $t_{1/2}$ of free aminosalicylic acid is 26.4 min.

Special Populations:
Renal Function Impairment – Drug and its acetyl metabolite may accumulate.

Indications Treatment of tuberculosis (in combination with other antituberculous drugs) caused by susceptible strains of tubercle bacilli.

Contraindications Severe hypersensitivity to aminosalicylate sodium and its congeners.

Route/Dosage
ADULTS AND CHILDREN: **PO** 150 mg/kg (max, 12 g/day).

Interactions
Digoxin: May reduce oral absorption and serum levels of digoxin.
Rifampin: May decrease absorption of rifampin.
Vitamin B_{12}: May decrease GI absorption of oral vitamin B_{12}.

PATIENT CARE CONSIDERATIONS
Administration/Storage
- Administer with food or meals. Product may cause GI upset.
- Sprinkle granules on acidic food or drink.
- Do not leave medication in extreme heat or direct sunlight. Moisture, extreme heat, or direct sunlight may reduce effectiveness of product.
- Do not use products that are brown or purple in color.

Assessment/Interventions
- Obtain patient history, including drug history and any known allergies.
- Review results of renal and hepatic function tests, and assess patient for undesirable side effects and adverse reactions. Notify health care provider of any unfavorable response.
- Check patient record for notation of prescription for parenteral administration of vitamin B_{12} when aminosalicylate sodium will be given for more than a few weeks or if patient is malnourished.
- Do not discontinue without consulting health care provider.

Lab Test Interferences None well documented.

Adverse Reactions
GI: Nausea; vomiting; diarrhea; abdominal pain.
METAB: Goiter with or without myxedema.
OTHER: Hypersensitivity (eg, fever, skin eruptions, infectious mononucleosis-like syndrome, leukopenia, agranulocytosis, thrombocytopenia, hemolytic anemia, jaundice, hepatitis, encephalopathy, Loffler syndrome, vasculitis).

Precautions
Pregnancy: Category C.
Lactation: Excreted in breast milk.
Hypersensitivity: Stop medication if hypersensitivity symptoms develop. Restart cautiously.
Renal function impairment: Use with caution.
Hepatic function impairment: Use with caution.
CHF: Use with caution because of high sodium content (55 mg of sodium per 500 mg tablet).
Crystalluria: Maintain urine at neutral or alkaline pH to avoid crystalluria.
Gastric ulcer: Use with caution.

- Monitor urine pH and report any change toward acidity or crystal formation.
- If patient is taking digoxin, monitor for signs of reduced serum levels of digoxin and notify health care provider of any associated signs, symptoms, or lab data.

Patient/Family Education
- Instruct patient to take medication with meals or immediately after meals to minimize GI symptoms, and to maintain adequate fluid intake.
- Explain to patient taking digoxin that dose may be increased while taking aminosalicylate sodium.
- Instruct patient to report the following symptoms to health care provider: fever, sore throat, unusual bleeding or bruising, rash.
- Teach patient importance of maintaining urine at neutral or alkaline pH and demonstrate method for testing urine pH.
- Instruct patient not to take OTC medications or dietary supplements without consulting health care provider.

Amiodarone

(A-MEE-oh-duh-rone)
Class Antiarrhythmic

How Supplied
Cordarone Tablets 200 mg, Injection 50 mg/mL
- *Pacerone* Tablets 200 mg, Tablets 400 mg

🍁 *Gen-Amiodarone* ♦ *Novo-Amiodarone* ♦ *ratio-Amiodarone* ♦ *Rhoxal-amiodarone*

Action
PHARMACOLOGY: Prolongs action potential duration and refractory period in myocardial cells; acts as noncompetitive inhibitor of alpha- and beta-adrenergic receptors.

Pharmacokinetics/Dynamics:

Absorption:
Oral – Bioavailability is 35% to 65%; t_{max} is 3 to 7 hr. Concentrations of 1 to 2.5 mg/L are effective with acceptable toxicity. Food increases rate and extent of absorption.

Distribution:
Oral – Vd is about 60 L/kg.
Oral/IV – Crosses the placenta; excreted in breast milk. More than 96% protein bound.
IV – Rapidly distributed; serum concentrations decline to 10% of peak values within 30 to 45 min after the end of the infusion. Vd is 40 to 84 L/kg (amiodarone) and 68 to 168 L/kg (N-desethyl amiodarone [DEA]).

Metabolism: Metabolized by CYP3A4 to DEA (active).

Excretion: Eliminated primarily by hepatic excretion into bile; some enterohepatic recirculation may occur; negligible renal excretion. Biphasic elimination with initial 50% reduction in plasma levels after 2.5 to 10 days; terminal $t_{1/2}$ is 26 to 107 days (mean, about 53 days) (oral) and 20 to 47 days (IV). Not dialyzable.

Onset: 2 to 3 days but more commonly 1 to 3 wk.

Special Populations:
Elderly – Clearance is lower and $t_{1/2}$ is increased. Monitor closely.
Severe left ventricular dysfunction: – $T_{1/2}$ of DEA is prolonged. Monitor closely.

Indications

Oral: Treatment of life-threatening, recurrent ventricular arrhythmias (ie, ventricular fibrillation and hemodynamically unstable ventricular tachycardia) that do not respond to other antiarrhythmic agents. Use only in patients with the indicated life-threatening arrhythmias because its use is accompanied by substantial toxicity.
Parenteral: Initiation of treatment and prophylaxis of frequently recurring ventricular fibrillation and hemodynamically unstable ventricular tachycardia in patients refractory to other therapy; treatment of ventricular tachycardia and fibrillation when oral amiodarone is indicated but patient is unable to take oral medication. **Unlabeled use(s):** Conversion of atrial fibrillation and maintenance of sinus rhythm; treatment of supraventricular tachycardia; IV amiodarone has been used to treat AV nodal reentry tachycardia.

Contraindications

Oral: Severe sinus-node dysfunction, causing marked sinus bradycardia; second- or third-degree atrioventricular (AV) block; when bradycardia produces syncope, unless used with pacemaker; hypersensitivity to the drug.
Parenteral: Marked sinus bradycardia; second- and third-degree atrioventricular block unless functioning pacemaker is available; cardiogenic shock.

Route/Dosage

Life-Threatening Recurrent Ventricular Arrhythmias
Loading dose – **PO** 800 to 1600 mg/day for 1 to 3 wk. Reduce doses of other antiarrhythmic agents gradually. When adequate arrhythmia control is achieved, reduce dose to 600 to 800 mg/day for 1 mo.
Usual maintenance dose – **PO** 400 mg/day.
ADULTS: **IV** Recommended starting dose is approximately 1000 mg over the first 24 hr administered as follows: rapid administration of 150 mg over first 10 min (15 mg/min), followed by 360 mg over next 6 hr (1 mg/min), then 540 mg over remaining 18 hr (0.5 mg/min). After first 24 hr, continue maintenance infusion rate of 0.5 mg/min (720 mg/24 hr).

Paroxysmal Atrial Fibrillation, PSVT, Symptomatic Atrial Flutter
ADULTS: **PO** 600 to 800 mg/day for 7 to 10 days, then 200 to 400 mg/day.

Arrhythmias in Patients with CHF
ADULTS: **PO** 200 mg/day.

IV to Oral Transition
ADULTS: Clinical monitoring is recommended when changing from IV to oral therapy. **PO** 800 to 1600 mg amiodarone if duration of IV infusion less than 1 wk; 600 to 800 mg amiodarone if duration of IV infusion 1 to 3 wk; 400 mg amiodarone if duration of IV infusion more than 3 wk.

Interactions

Anticoagulants: Effect of anticoagulant may be increased. Use of product may require 30% to 50% decrease in anticoagulant dose.
Beta-blockers: Increased risk of hypotension and bradycardia as well as increased effect of beta blockers eliminated by hepatic metabolism.
Calcium channel blockers: Increased risk of atrioventricular block with verapamil or diltiazem as well as hypotension with other calcium blockers.
Cisapride, disopyramide, fluoroquinolones (eg, gatifloxacin, moxifloxacin, sparfloxacin): Possible prolongation of the QT interval, increasing the risk of life-threatening cardiac arrhythmias (including torsades de pointes).
Cholestyramine, rifamycins (eg, rifampin): Amiodarone plasma levels may be reduced, decreasing the pharmacologic effect.
Cimetidine, ritonavir: Amiodarone plasma levels may be elevated, increasing the risk of side effects.
Cyclosporine: Elevated plasma concentrations of cyclosporine resulting in elevated creatinine.

Dextromethorphan: Increased dextromethorphan plasma levels.
Digoxin: Serum digoxin levels may be increased.
Fentanyl: Increased risk of hypotension and bradycardia and decreased cardiac output.
Flecainide: Serum levels of flecainide may be increased.
Hydantoins (eg, phenytoin): Serum concentrations of hydantoins may be increased with potential for symptoms of hydantoin toxicity; also, amiodarone levels may be decreased.
Methotrexate, theophylline: Amiodarone may elevate plasma levels of these agents, increasing the risk of toxicity.
Procainamide: Serum levels of procainamide may be increased.
Quinidine: Serum quinidine levels may increase, creating potential for fatal cardiac arrhythmias.

Lab Test Interferences May alter results of thyroid and LFTs.

Adverse Reactions

CV: Exacerbation of arrhythmias, CHF, bradycardia, sinoatrial node dysfunction, heart block, sinus arrest, flushing (oral); hypotension, asystole/cardiac arrest, cardiogenic shock, ventricular tachycardia, atrioventricular block (parenteral).
CNS: Fatigue; malaise; tremor/abnormal involuntary movements; lack of coordination; abnormal gait/ataxia; dizziness; paresthesias; decreased libido; insomnia; headache; sleep disturbances; abnormal sense of smell.
DERM: Photosensitivity, solar dermatitis, blue discoloration of skin (oral); Stevens-Johnson syndrome (parenteral).
EENT: Visual disturbances; visual impairment; blindness; reversible asymptomatic corneal microdeposits; photophobia; abnormal taste.
GI: Nausea, vomiting, constipation, anorexia, abdominal pain, abnormal salivation (oral); diarrhea (parenteral).
HEMA: Coagulation abnormalities (oral); thrombocytopenia (parenteral).
HEPA: Nonspecific hepatic disorders.
RESP: Pulmonary inflammation or fibrosis, progressive dyspnea, pulmonary toxicosis and death (oral); lung edema, respiratory disorder (parenteral).
OTHER: Edema, hyperthyroidism or hypothyroidism (oral); fever (parenteral).

> **WARNING:**
> Only indication for amiodarone is life-threatening arrhythmias.
>
> Potentially pulmonary fatal toxicities include hypersensitivity pneumonitis or interstitial/alveolar pneumonitis. Rates as high as 10% to 17% in series of patients with ventricular arrhythmias given doses approximating 400 mg daily. Fatality rate approximates 10%.
>
> Liver injury may occur and has been fatal in a few cases.
>
> Proarrhythmic effects, significant heart block, or sinus bradycardia has occurred. Patients must be hospitalized during loading dose administration.

Precautions

Pregnancy: Category D.
Lactation: Excreted in breast milk.
Children: Safety and efficacy not established.
Adult respiratory distress syndrome (ARDS): ARDS has been reported.
Benzyl alcohol: Benzyl alcohol, contained in some of these products as a preservative, has been associated with fatal "gasping syndrome" in children.
Ophthalmic effects: Optic neuropathy or neuritis, resulting in visual impairment may occur.

PATIENT CARE CONSIDERATIONS

Administration/Storage

- Only use amiodarone in patients with the indicated life-threatening arrhythmias because its use is accompanied by substantial toxicity.
- Administer with meals.
- Store at room temperature and protect from light.

Assessment/Interventions

- Obtain patient history, including drug history and any known allergies.
- Review baseline clotting factor studies and serum levels of digoxin, flecainide, quinidine, procainamide, and theophylline, as available, and continue to monitor these parameters during treatment.
- Review thyroid and LFT results, and note any changes after initiation of therapy.
- Consult chest x-ray, and review findings from any pulmonary function tests performed prior to and after initiation of therapy.
- Repeat history and physical examination q 3 to 6 mo, and consult chest radiographs as available.
- Assess for changes in pulmonary status, and notify health care provider of any trends that could be associated with pulmonary toxicity (eg, dyspnea, fatigue, cough, pleuritic pain). Document and report any fever to health care provider.
- Assess for symptoms of hyperthyroidism or hypothyroidism.
- Assess baseline pulse and BP and monitor during treatment. Report symptomatic bradycardia (eg, fatigue, lightheadedness, syncope).

- Assess for CNS side effects (eg, muscle weakness) and report to health care provider.
- Monitor cardiac rhythm continuously during initiation of treatment and regularly during maintenance therapy. Notify health care provider of exacerbation of presenting arrhythmia, bradycardia, heart block, or sinus arrest.
- Cases of optic neuropathy or optic neuritis, usually resulting in visual impairment (in some cases permanent blindness), have occurred in patients treated with amiodarone. If symptoms of visual impairment appear, prompt ophthalmic examination is recommended. Appearance of optic neuropathy or neuritis calls for re-evaluation of therapy.

Patient/Family Education
- Instruct patient to report any cough or shortness of breath.
- Show patient how to take pulse. Explain that heart rates less than 60 bpm should be reported to health care provider.
- Advise patient that regular ophthalmic examination is recommended during administration of amiodarone. Prompt evaluation is required if visual impairment occurs.
- Caution patient to avoid exposure to sunlight, and to use sunscreen and wear protective clothing to avoid photosensitivity reaction. Sun-exposed skin may appear blue-gray. Also, explain that discomfort of photophobia may be decreased by wearing sunglasses.
- Explain that eating small, frequent meals or dividing daily dose and taking 2 or 3 doses with meals may help if patient experiences GI upset.
- Instruct patient to report the following symptoms to health care provider: halos around lights; any vision problems; GI distress; loss of appetite; tremors; twitches; fatigue; unsteady walking; dizziness; numbness and tingling in hands or feet; insomnia; headache; slowing of heartbeat; irregular heart rhythm; difficulty breathing; coughing; sensitivity to sunlight, including blue-gray patches on skin; dermatitis; bruising; hair loss; flushing; abnormal sense of taste or smell; fluid retention; loss of sex drive.

Amitriptyline Hydrochloride

(am-ee-TRIP-tih-leen HIGH-droe-KLOR-ide)

Class Tricyclic antidepressant

How Supplied
Amitriptyline Tablets 10 mg, Tablets 25 mg, Tablets 50 mg, Tablets 75 mg, Tablets 100 mg, Tablets 150 mg ◆ *Elavil* Injection 10 mg/mL
✤ *APO-Amitriptyline*

Action
PHARMACOLOGY: Inhibits presynaptic reuptake of norepinephrine and serotonin in CNS.

PHARMACOKINETICS/DYNAMICS:
Absorption: Rapidly absorbed.

Metabolism: Metabolized in the liver by N-demethylation and bridge hydroxylation. Nortriptyline is an intermediate active metabolite.

Excretion: 50% to 66% excreted in the urine within 24 hr. Excreted as glucuronide or sulfate conjugate of metabolites. A small amount of unchanged drug excreted in the urine. $T_{1/2}$ is 31 to 46 hr.

Special Populations:
Elderly – May have increased plasma levels. Dosage adjustment may be necessary.

Indications Relief of depression. Endogenous depression is more likely to be alleviated than are other depressive states. **Unlabeled use(s):** Management of chronic pain associated with migraine, tension headache, phantom limb pain, tic douloureux, diabetic neuropathy, peripheral neuropathy, cancer or arthritis; treatment of panic and eating disorders.

Contraindications Hypersensitivity to any tricyclic antidepressant; use during acute recovery phase of MI; concomitant use with MAOIs, except under close medical supervision; may block the antihypertensive action of guanethidine or similarly active compounds.

Route/Dosage
ADULTS: Titrate dosage over 2 wk to 1 mo. Give maintenance dose 6 mo to 1 yr. Do not interrupt therapy abruptly; reduce over 2 wk period.
OUTPATIENTS: **PO** 75 to 150 mg/day in divided doses; give in evening or at bedtime because of sedative effects.
HOSPITALIZED PATIENTS: **PO** 100 to 300 mg/day.
ADOLESCENTS AND ELDERLY: **PO** 10 mg tid and 20 mg at bedtime.
MAINTENANCE: **PO** 40 to 100 mg/day.

PARENTERAL FORM
PO Do not use IV route.
IM 20 to 30 mg qid. Change to oral dosing as soon as possible.

Interactions
Barbiturates, charcoal: May cause decreased

blood levels of amitriptyline.
Cimetidine, fluoxetine: May cause increased blood levels of amitriptyline.
Clonidine: Use with product may result in hypertensive crisis.
CNS depressants: Depressant effects may be additive.
MAOIs: May cause hyperpyretic crises, severe convulsions, and death when given with amitriptyline.

Lab Test Interferences None well documented.

Adverse Reactions
CV: Orthostatic hypotension; hypertension; tachycardia; palpitations; arrhythmias; ECG changes.
CNS: Confusion; hallucinations; disturbed concentration; decreased memory; delusions; nervousness; restlessness; agitation; panic; insomnia; nightmares; mania; exacerbation of psychosis; drowsiness; dizziness; weakness; emotional lability; numbness; tremors; extrapyramidal symptoms (eg, pseudoparkinsonism, movement disorders, akathisia); seizures.
DERM: Rash; pruritus; photosensitivity reaction; dry skin; acne; itching.
EENT: Conjunctivitis; blurred vision; increased IOP; mydriasis; tinnitus; nasal congestion; peculiar taste in mouth.
GI: Nausea; vomiting; anorexia; GI distress; diarrhea; flatulence; dry mouth; constipation.
GU: Impotence; sexual dysfunction; menstrual irregularities; dysmenorrhea; nocturia; urinary frequency; UTI; vaginitis; cystitis; urinary retention and hesitancy.
HEMA: Bone marrow depression, including agranulocytosis; eosinophilia; purpura; thrombocytopenia; leukopenia.
HEPA: Jaundice.
METAB: Elevation or depression of blood sugar levels.
RESP: Pharyngitis; rhinitis; sinusitis; cough.
OTHER: Breast enlargement.

Precautions
Pregnancy: Category D.
Lactation: Excreted in breast milk.
Children: Not recommended for children less than 12 yr.
Special risk patients: Caution is needed with history of seizures; urinary retention; urethral or ureteral spasm; angle-closure glaucoma or increased IOP; cardiovascular disorders; hyperthyroidism and patients receiving thyroid medication; hepatic or renal impairment; schizophrenia; paranoia.
Changing from MAOI to amitriptyline: Waiting period of 7 to 10 days is necessary to prevent hypertensive crisis.
Serotonin syndrome: Some TCAs inhibit neuronal reuptake of serotonin and can increase synaptic serotonin levels.

Overdosage: Signs and Symptoms
Confusion, agitation, hallucinations, seizures, status epilepticus, clonus, choreoathetosis, hyperactive reflexes, positive Babinski's sign, coma, cardiac arrhythmias, renal failure, flushing, dry mouth, dilated pupils, hyperpyrexia.

PATIENT CARE CONSIDERATIONS

Administration/Storage
- Use IM route only if patient is unable to take oral form.
- Give drug with or immediately after food or fluid and in late afternoon or at bedtime because of sedative effect. Tablets may be crushed.
- Store at room temperature and protect from light.

Assessment/Interventions
- Obtain patient history, including drug history and any known allergies.
- Take vital signs and monitor during initial therapy.
- Assess patient's mental status, affect, energy level, sleeping, and eating habits, and suicidal tendencies.
- Record I&O, noting bowel elimination pattern.
- Encourage high intake of fiber and fluid, and offer laxatives or stool softeners as necessary.
- Restrict amount of medication available to patient. Check patient's mouth after administration to detect possible hoarding of medication or noncompliance with therapy.
- Provide frequent oral hygiene.
- Assist patient in rising slowly. Supervise ambulation and institute measures to prevent falling.
- Monitor ECG, WBC with differential, serum glucose level, and cardiac, renal, and hepatic function regularly.
- Perform baseline and periodic leukocyte and differential counts and liver function studies.
- Document patient's mental status and vital signs every shift until response to therapy is evaluated.
- Monitor closely for oversedation, especially if patient is taking antihistamines, narcotic analgesics, or sedatives/hypnotics.
- If systolic BP increases or decreases 10 to 20 mm Hg from baseline or if pulse rate or rhythm shows significant change, withhold drug and notify health care provider.

Patient/Family Education
- Caution patient not to stop taking medication abruptly without consulting health care provider.
- Warn patient of the risk of seizure.
- Reinforce importance of follow-up visits to health care provider for monitoring drug's effectiveness and side effects.
- Explain that drug effects may not be evident for 4 to 6 wk but that side effects are usually noted early.
- Patient should complete the full course of therapy.
- Tell patient that side effects are reduced if drug is taken at bedtime.
- Advise patient that weight gain often results from increased appetite caused by drug.
- Inform patient that urine may turn blue-green.
- Emphasize the need for regular dental care because oral dryness can increase risk for dental caries.
- Instruct patient to report the following symptoms to health care provider: blurred vision, sore throat, fever, increased heart rate, impaired coordination, difficult urination, excessive sedation, or seizures.
- Instruct patient to take sips of water frequently, suck on ice chips or sugarless hard candy, or chew sugarless gum if dry mouth occurs.
- Caution patient to avoid sudden position changes to prevent orthostatic hypotension.
- Instruct patient to avoid intake of alcohol beverages or other CNS depressants.
- Advise patient that drug may cause drowsiness, and to use caution while driving or performing other tasks requiring mental alertness.
- Caution patient to avoid exposure to sunlight, and to use sunscreen or wear protective clothing to avoid photosensitivity reaction.
- Instruct patient not to take OTC medications without consulting health care provider.

Amlodipine

(am-LOW-dih-PEEN)

Class Calcium channel blocker

How Supplied
Norvasc Tablets 2.5 mg, Tablets 5 mg, Tablets 10 mg

Action
PHARMACOLOGY: Inhibits movement of calcium ions across cell membrane in systemic and coronary vascular smooth muscle.

PHARMACOKINETICS/DYNAMICS:
Absorption: T_{max} is 6 to 12 hr.
Distribution: Bioavailability is 64% to 90%. About 93% is protein bound.
Metabolism: About 90% is converted to inactive metabolites in the liver.
Excretion: 10% of the parent compound and 60% of the metabolites are excreted in the urine. Elimination is biphasic. $T_{1/2}$ is about 30 to 50 hr.

Duration: 24 hr.

Special Populations:
Hepatic Function Impairment – Clearance is decreased and AUC may increase about 40% to 60%. May require lower initial dose.
Elderly – Clearance is decreased and AUC may increase about 40% to 60%. May require lower initial dose.
Moderate to severe heart failure – Clearance is decreased and AUC may increase about 40% to 60%. May require lower initial dose.

Indications Hypertension; chronic stable angina; vasospastic (Prinzmetal or variant) angina.

Contraindications Sick sinus syndrome; second- or third-degree atricventricular (AV) block, except with a functioning pacemaker.

Route/Dosage
ADULTS: PO 5 to 10 mg qd.
ELDERLY: PO Initially 2.5 mg qd.

Hepatic Impairment
PO Initially 2.5 mg qd.

Interactions
Beta-blockers: May cause increased adverse cardiac effects as a result of myocardial depression.
Fentanyl: Severe hypotension or increased fluid volume requirements have occurred with similar drug.

Lab Test Interferences None well documented.

Adverse Reactions
CV: Palpitations; peripheral edema; syncope; tachycardia; bradycardia; arrhythmias; ventricular asystoles.
CNS: Headache; dizziness; lightheadedness; fatigue; lethargy; somnolence.
DERM: Dermatitis; rash; pruritus; urticaria.
GI: Nausea; abdominal discomfort; cramps; dyspepsia.
RESP: Shortness of breath; dyspnea; wheezing.
OTHER: Flushing; sexual difficulties; muscle cramps, pain or inflammation.

Precautions
Pregnancy: Category C.
Lactation: Undetermined.
Children: Safety and efficacy not established.

Hepatic function impairment: Cautious use is required.
CHF: Cautious use is required with this condition.

PATIENT CARE CONSIDERATIONS

Administration/Storage
- Administer medication in morning.
- If patient has difficulty swallowing, crush tablets.
- Store in tightly closed container in cool location.

Assessment/Interventions
- Obtain patient history, including drug history and any known allergies. Note any diabetes, liver disease, cardiac disease or sensitivity to calcium channel blockers.
- Monitor BP and pulse before administration.
- Review baseline ECG.
- Assess for signs of withdrawal syndrome. Abrupt withdrawal may cause increased frequency and duration of angina. Gradual tapering of dose is necessary.
- Assess patient for signs of CHF during therapy.
- If chest pain occurs, assess for location, intensity, duration, and radiation. Nitroglycerin preparations may be administered in conjunction with this medication.
- If drug is used with other calcium channel blockers or beta-blockers, observe for intensification of side effects.
- Withhold medication and notify health care provider if any of the following signs and symptoms occur: Sudden severe dyspnea; edema of hands and feet; changes in ECG (widened QRS, prolonged QT segments); pulse falls below 50 bpm.
- If the patient experiences chest pain not relieved by medication, continue medication and notify health care provider.

Overdosage: Signs and Symptoms
Nausea, weakness, dizziness, drowsiness, confusion, slurred speech, hypotension, bradycardia, second- or third-degree AV block.

Patient/Family Education
- Teach patient how to monitor pulse before taking medication. Tell patient not to take medication if pulse if less than 50 bpm and to call health care provider.
- Explain to patient how to monitor BP daily.
- Instruct patient not to stop taking this medication suddenly because doing so can cause chest pain and MI.
- Teach patient importance of good oral hygiene and frequent visits to dentist while taking medication.
- Inform patient that frequent follow-up appointments with health care provider are important to adjust medication dosage.
- Caution patient to avoid sudden position changes to prevent orthostatic hypotension.
- Instruct patient to avoid intake of alcoholic beverages or other CNS depressants.
- Advise patient that drug may cause drowsiness, and to use caution while driving or performing other tasks requiring mental alertness.
- Instruct patient not to take *otc* medications without consulting health care provider.

Amlodipine Besylate/ Atorvastatin Calcium

(am-LOW-duh-PEEN BEH-sih-LATE/ah-TORE-vah-STAT-in KAL-see-uhm)

Class Calcium channel blocker/Antihyperlipidemic/HMG-CoA reductase inhibitor

How Supplied
Caduet Tablets 5 mg amlodipine per 10 mg atorvastatin, Tablets 5 mg amlodipine per 20 mg atorvastatin, Tablets 5 mg amlodipine per 40 mg atorvastatin, Tablets 5 mg amlodipine per 80 mg atorvastatin, Tablets 10 mg amlodipine per 10 mg atorvastatin, Tablets 10 mg amlodipine per 20 mg atorvastatin, Tablets 10 mg amlodipine per 40 mg atorvastatin, Tablets 10 mg amlodipine per 80 mg atorvastatin

Action
PHARMACOLOGY:
Amlodipine: Inhibits movement of calcium ions across cell membrane in systemic and coronary vascular smooth muscle.
Atorvastatin: Increases rate at which body removes cholesterol from blood and reduces production of cholesterol in body by inhibiting enzyme that catalyzes early rate-limiting step in cholesterol synthesis; increases HDL; reduces LDL, VLDL, and triglycerides (TG).

Indications
Amlodipine: Treatment of hypertension; chronic stable angina; confirmed or suspected vasospastic angina (Prinzmetal or Variant angina).
Atorvastatin: As an adjunct to diet to reduce elevated total cholesterol (C), LDL-C, apo B, and TG levels in patients with primary hyper-

cholesterolemia and mixed dyslipidemia; adjunct to diet for treatment of elevated serum TG levels (Fredrickson Type IV); treatment of primary dysbetalipoproteinemia (Fredrickson Type III); reduce total-C and LDL-C in patients with homozygous familial hypercholesterolemia, and apo B levels in boys and postmenarchal girls, 10 to 17 yr of age, with heterozygous familial hypercholesterolemia if after an adequate trial of diet therapy the following are present: LDL-C remains at 190 mg/dL or higher; LDL-C remains at 160 mg/dL or higher and there is positive family history of premature cardiovascular disease (CVD) or 2 or more CVD risk factors are present in pediatric patients.

Contraindications Active liver disease; unexplained persistent elevations of serum transaminases; pregnancy; nursing mothers hypersensitivity to any component of the product.

Route/Dosage
Dosage must be individualized based on effectiveness and tolerance for each individual component in the treatment of hypertension/angina and hyperlipidemia. Amlodipine/Atorvastatin may be substituted for its individually titrated components. Patients may be given the equivalent dose of amlodipine/atorvastatin or a dose of amlodipine/atorvastatin with increased amounts of amlodipine, atorvastatin, or both for additional antianginal effects, BP lowering, or lipid-lowering effect. As initial therapy for one indication and continuation of treatment of the other, select the recommended starting dose of amlodipine/atorvastatin based on the continuation of the component being used and the recommended starting dose of the added monotherapy. The max dose of amlodipine component is 10 mg once daily; the max dose of atorvastatin component is 80 mg daily.

Interactions
Antacids, colestipol: Atorvastatin plasma concentrations may be decreased.
Digoxin, oral contraceptives (eg, ethinyl estradiol, norethindrone): Plasma concentrations of these agents may be elevated by atorvastatin, increasing the risk of side effects.
Erythromycin: Atorvastatin plasma concentrations may be increased, increasing the pharmacologic and adverse effects.

Lab Test Interferences None well documented.

Adverse Reactions
CV:
Amlodipine – Palpitation (5%); vasodilation, syncope, migraine, postural hypotension, phlebitis, arrhythmia, angina pectoris, hypertension (less than 2%).

CNS:
Amlodipine – Fatigue (5%); dizziness (3%); somnolence (2%).
Atorvastatin – Headache (17%); asthenia (4%); insomnia, dizziness (more than 2%); paresthesia, somnolence, amnesia, abnormal dreams, decreased libido, emotional lability, incoordination, peripheral neuropathy, torticollis, facial paralysis, hyperkinesia, depression, hypesthesia, hypertonia (less than 2%).
DERM:
Atorvastatin – Rash (4%); photosensitivity, pruritus, contact dermatitis, alopecia, dry skin, sweating, acne, urticaria, eczema, seborrhea, skin ulcer (less than 2%); bullous rash including erythema multiforme, Stevens-Johnson syndrome, and toxic epidermal necrolysis (postmarketing).
EENT:
Amlodipine – Rhinitis (less than 2%).
Atorvastatin – Amblyopia, tinnitus, dry eyes, refraction disorder, eye hemorrhage, deafness, glaucoma, parosmia, taste loss, taste perversion (less than 2%).
GI:
Amlodipine – Nausea (3%); abdominal pain (2%).
Atorvastatin – Abdominal pain, diarrhea, dyspepsia (4%); constipation, flatulence (3%); nausea (more than 2%); gastroenteritis, colitis, vomiting, gastritis, dry mouth, rectal hemorrhage, esophagitis, eructation, glossitis, mouth ulceration, anorexia, increased appetite, stomatitis, biliary pain, cheilitis, duodenal ulcer, dysphagia, enteritis, melena, gum hemorrhage, stomach ulcer, tenesmus, ulcerative stomatitis, pancreatitis, (less than 2%).
GU:
Amlodipine – Gynecomastia (postmarketing).
Atorvastatin – UTI (more than 2%); urinary frequency, cystitis, hematuria, impotence, dysuria, kidney calculus, nocturia, epididymitis, fibrocystic breast, vaginal hemorrhage, albuminuria, breast enlargement, metrorrhagia, nephritis, urinary incontinence, urinary retention, urinary urgency, abnormal ejaculation, uterine hemorrhage (less than 2%).
HEMA/LYMPH:
Atorvastatin – Ecchymosis, anemia, lymphadenopathy, thrombocytopenia petechiae (less than 2%).
HEPA:
Amlodipine – Jaundice, hepatic enzyme elevations (postmarketing).
Atorvastatin – Abnormal LFTs, hepatitis, cholestatic jaundice (less than 2%).
HYPERSEN:
Atorvastatin – Anaphylaxis (postmarketing).
M/N:
Atorvastatin – Peripheral edema (more than

2%); hyperglycemia, increased creatine phosphokinase, gout, weight gain, hypoglycemia (less than 2%).
MUSC:
Atorvastatin – Arthralgia (5%); back pain (4%); myalgia (3%); arthritis (more than 2%); leg cramps, bursitis, tenosynovitis, myasthenia, tendinous contracture, myositis (less than 2%); rhabdomyolysis (postmarketing).
RESP:
Atorvastatin – Sinusitis (6%); pharyngitis (3%); bronchitis (more than 2%); pneumonia, dyspnea, asthma, epistaxis (less than 2%).
OTHER:
Amlodipine – Edema (15%); flushing (5%).
Atorvastatin – Infection (10%); accidental injury (4%); flu syndrome, allergic reaction (3%); chest pain (at least 2%); face edema, fever, malaise (less than 2%); angioneurotic edema (postmarketing).

Precautions
Pregnancy: Category X.
Lactation: Undetermined (see contraindications).

Children:
Amlodipine – Safety and efficacy not established for treating hypertension in patients under 6 yr of age.
Atorvastatin – Safety and efficacy not established for pre-pubertal patients or patients younger than 10 yr of age.
Angina/MI: Rarely, patients have developed increased frequency, duration and severity of angina, or acute MI on starting or increasing the dose of calcium channel blocker therapy.
CHF: Use amlodipine with caution.
Liver dysfunction: HMG-CoA reductase inhibitors have been associated with biochemical abnormalities of liver function.
Skeletal muscle: Rare cases of rhabdomyolysis with acute renal failure secondary to myoglobinuria have been reported.

Overdosage: Signs and Symptoms
Might be expected to cause excessive peripheral vasodilation with marked hypotension and possible reflex tachycardia.

PATIENT CARE CONSIDERATIONS

Administration/Storage
- Administer alone or in combination with other lipid-lowering therapy (eg, bile acid sequestrant) or with other cardiovascular medications for the treatment of hypertension and angina.
- Administer prescribed dose once daily without regard to meals. Administer with food if GI upset occurs.
- Store tablets at controlled room temperature (59° to 86°F).

Assessment/Interventions
- Obtain patient history, including drug history and any known allergies. Note active liver disease, hepatic insufficiency, unexplained elevations of serum transaminases, alcohol consumption, aortic stenosis, heart failure, and concurrent therapy with medications known to increase the risk of myopathy (eg, cyclosporine, gemfibrozil).
- Ensure secondary causes of hypercholesterolemia (eg, poorly controlled diabetes, hypothyroidism) are excluded before starting therapy.
- Ensure patient is on a cholesterol-lowering diet before starting therapy and that diet is continued during treatment.
- Ensure women of child-bearing potential are not pregnant when therapy is initiated and use effective contraception during treatment.
- Ensure therapy is temporarily withheld in patient with an acute, serious condition suggestive of myopathy or predisposing to the development of renal failure secondary to rhabdomyolysis (eg, sepsis, hypotension).
- Monitor and record BP and pulse frequently during treatment. Should hypotension and/or bradycardia develop, hold medication and notify health care provider.
- Implement safety precautions if orthostatic hypotension occurs.
- Ensure serum cholesterol and triglycerides are measured before therapy is started and within 2 to 4 wk of starting therapy or changing the atorvastatin dose, and then periodically thereafter.
- Ensure LFTs (transaminases) are determined before and 12 wk following initiation of therapy, or after increase in dose of atorvastatin, and periodically thereafter (eg, q 6 mo).
- If elevated serum transaminase levels develop during treatment, repeat levels more frequently. If transaminase levels rise to 3 times upper limit of normal and persist, notify health care provider. Be prepared to reduce dose or discontinue therapy if ordered.
- If muscle pain, tenderness, and/or weakness develop during therapy, determine CPK levels. Notify health care provider if CPK levels are markedly increased or if muscle symptoms continue or worsen, or are accompanied by malaise or fever.
- Assess patient for CV, GI, CNS, MUSC, and general body side effects. Inform health care provider if noted and significant.

Patient/Family Education
- Explain name, dose, action, and potential side effects of drug.
- Advise patient to take once daily as prescribed, without regard to meals, but to take with food if stomach upset occurs.
- Advise patient to try to take each dose at about the same time each day.
- Inform patient that drug helps control, but not does cure, high BP, angina, or cholesterol abnormality, and to continue taking drug as prescribed to maintain beneficial effects.
- Advise patient that dose of medication may be adjusted periodically to obtain max benefit.
- Caution patient not to change the dose or stop taking unless advised by health care provider.
- Advise patient that if a dose is missed, to take as soon as remembered. If several hours have passed, advise patient to skip that dose and take the next dose at the regularly scheduled time. Caution patient to never take more than 1 dose of medicine a day.
- Instruct patient to continue taking other BP, angina, or cholesterol medications as prescribed by health care provider.
- Instruct patient being treated for angina to notify health care provider if frequency or severity of chest pain, or need for sublingual nitroglycerin appears to be increasing.
- Emphasize to patient importance of the following other modalities on cholesterol and BP control: dietary changes (reduced saturated fat intake, increased soluble fiber intake, moderate intake of salt and alcohol); weight control; regular exercise; smoking cessation.
- Instruct patient in BP and pulse measurement skills.
- Advise patient to monitor and record BP and pulse at home and to inform health care provider if abnormal measurements are noted. Also advise patient to take record of BP and pulse to each follow-up visit.
- Instruct patient to lie or sit down if experiencing dizziness or lightheadedness when standing.
- Advise patient to notify health care provider of any of the following: unexplained muscle pain, tenderness, and/or weakness; frequent episodes of dizziness when arising; slow heart beat; persistent fatigue; or any other unusual or unexplained symptom or sign.
- Advise women of childbearing potential to use effective contraception during treatment.
- Advise women of childbearing potential to notify health care provider if pregnant, planning to become pregnant, or breastfeeding.
- Caution patient not to take any prescription or OTC medications, herbal preparations, or dietary supplements unless advised by health care provider.
- Advise patient that follow-up visits and lab tests will be required to monitor therapy and to keep appointments.

Amlodipine/Benazepril Hydrochloride

(am-LOW-dih-PEEN/BEN-AZE-uh-pril HIGH-droe-CLOR-ide)

Class Calcium channel blocker/Antihypertensive/ACE inhibitor

How Supplied
Lotrel Capsule 2.5 mg amlodipine/10 mg benazepril, Capsule 5 mg amlodipine/10 mg benazepril, Capsule 5 mg amlodipine/20 mg benazepril, Capsule 10 mg amlodipine/20 mg benazepril

Action
PHARMACOLOGY: Amlodipine: Inhibits movement of calcium ions across cell membrane in systemic and coronary vascular smooth muscle; benazepril: competitively inhibits angiotensin I-converting enzyme, resulting in the prevention of angiotensin I conversion to angiotensin II, a potent vasoconstrictor that stimulates aldosterone secretion. This action results in a decrease in sodium and fluid retention, increase in diuresis, and a decrease in blood pressure.

Indications Treatment of hypertension.

Contraindications Hypersensitivity to amlodipine, benazepril, or any other ACE inhibitor.

Route/Dosage
ADULTS: PO 1 capsule (2.5 to 10 mg amlodipine/10 to 20 mg benazepril)/day.

Interactions
Diuretics: Increased risk of excessive reduction of blood pressure after initiation of amlodipine/benazepril therapy.
Potassium supplements, potassium-sparing diuretics (eg, spironolactone): Increased risk of hyperkalemia.
Lithium: Plasma levels of lithium may be elevated, increasing the risk of toxicity.

Lab Test Interferences None well documented.

Adverse Reactions
CV: Palpitations.
CNS: Headache; dizziness; somnolence; fatigue; insomnia; nervousness; anxiety; tremor; decreased libido.
DERM: Rash; skin nodule; dermatitis; Stevens-Johnson syndrome.

EENT: Esophagitis.
GI: Dry mouth; nausea; abdominal pain; constipation; diarrhea; dyspepsia.
GU: Impotence; polyuria.
HEMA: Hemolytic anemia; thrombocytopenia.
HEPA: Jaundice; hepatic enzyme elevations consistent with cholestasis.
METAB: Hypokalemia.
RESP: Cough; pharyngitis.
OTHER: Edema; flushing; hot flashes; angioedema; asthenia; back pain; musculoskeletal pain; cramps; muscle cramps.

Precautions

Pregnancy: Category D (second and third trimester); Category C (first trimester). ACE inhibitors (eg, benazepril) can cause injury or death to fetus if used during second or third trimester. When pregnancy is detected, discontinue as soon as possible.
Lactation: Amlodipine: Undetermined; benazepril: excreted in breast milk.
Children: Safety and efficacy not established.
Renal function impairment: Use with caution.
Angioedema: Has been reported and may be fatal.
Hypotension: Has been reported, especially in patients who are volume or salt depleted (eg, those undergoing dialysis, dietary salt restriction, or prolonged diuretic therapy, or who are experiencing diarrhea or vomiting); use with caution.
Neutropenia/agranulocytosis: Has occurred with ACE inhibitors.

PATIENT CARE CONSIDERATIONS

Administration/Storage

- Give once daily, with or without food.
- Administer alone or in combination with other antihypertensives.
- Store capsules at controlled room temperature (59° to 86°F). Protect from moisture and light.

Assessment/Interventions

- Obtain patient history, including drug history and any known allergies. Note history of congestive heart failure, diabetes, anuria, lupus erythematosus, kidney or liver disease, and concomitant use of potassium-sparing diuretics, potassium supplements, or potassium-containing salt substitutes.
- Do not administer to pregnant women as fetal and neonatal morbidity and death can occur.
- Administer with caution and reduced dosage in patients with possible depletion of intravascular volume or history of hepatic impairment.
- Ensure that serum electrolytes and renal function are monitored periodically.
- Monitor and record BP and pulse. Should hypotension result, hold medication and notify health care provider.
- Take safety precautions if orthostatic hypotension occurs.
- Monitor for signs of hypersensitivity including angioedema involving swelling of the face, lips, eyelids, and tongue. Discontinue medication and notify health care provider immediately if noted. Be prepared to treat appropriately.

Patient/Family Education

- Explain name, dose, action, and potential side effects of drug.
- Advise patient to take once daily as prescribed, without regard to meals.
- Advise patient to try to take each dose at about the same time each day.
- Inform patient that drug controls, but does not cure, hypertension and to continue taking drug as prescribed even when BP is not elevated.
- Caution patient not to change the dose or stop taking unless advised by health care provider.
- Instruct patient to continue taking other BP medications as prescribed by health care provider.
- Instruct patient in BP and pulse measurement skills.
- Advise patient to monitor and record BP and pulse at home and to inform health care provider should abnormal measurements be noted. Also advise patient to take record of BP and pulse to each follow-up visit.
- Instruct patient to lie or sit down if experiencing dizziness or lightheadedness when standing.
- Caution patient that inadequate fluid intake, excessive perspiration, diarrhea, or vomiting can lead to excessive fall in BP resulting in lightheadedness or fainting.
- Emphasize to hypertensive patient importance of other modalities on BP: weight control, regular exercise, smoking cessation, and moderate intake of alcohol and salt.
- Advise women to contact health care provider if pregnant, planning to become pregnant, or breastfeeding.
- Instruct patient to stop taking drug and immediately report any of these symptoms to health care provider: fainting, swelling of the face, lips, eyelids, or tongue.
- Instruct patient to inform health care pro-

vider if a persistent cough or swelling of the ankles or feet develop while taking this medication.
- Caution patient to not take any prescription or OTC medications, salt substitutes, or dietary supplements unless advised by health care provider.
- Advise patient that follow-up visits and lab tests may be required to monitor therapy and to keep appointments.

Amobarbital Sodium

(am-oh-BAR-bih-tahl SO-dee-uhm)
Class Sedative/Hypnotic/Barbiturate

How Supplied
Amytal Sodium Powder for injection 500 mg
❀ Amytal

Action
PHARMACOLOGY: Depresses sensory cortex; decreases motor activity; alters cerebellar function and produces drowsiness, sedation and hypnosis.

PHARMACOKINETICS/DYNAMICS:
Distribution: Rapidly distributed to all tissues and fluids, with high concentrations in brain, liver, and kidneys. Bound to plasma and tissue proteins.
Metabolism: Metabolized by hepatic microsomal enzyme system.
Excretion: Plasma $t_{1/2}$ is about 25 hr. Metabolites excreted in urine and to a lesser extent in the feces. Negligible amount eliminated unchanged in urine.
Onset: 0.75 to 1 hr.
Duration: 6 to 8 hr.

Indications
Relief of anxiety; short-term therapy for insomnia; induction of preanesthetic sedation.

Contraindications
Hypersensitivity to barbiturates; history of addiction to sedative-hypnotic drugs; history of porphyria; severe liver impairment; respiratory disease with dyspnea; patients with nephritis.

Route/Dosage
Insomnia
ADULTS: **PO/IM/IV** 65 to 200 mg at bedtime.

Sedation
ADULTS: **PO/IM/IV** 30 to 50 mg bid or tid.
CHILDREN: **PO/IM** 2 to 6 mg/kg/dose.

Interactions
Alcohol, CNS depressants: Depressant effects of these drugs may be enhanced.
Anticoagulants, beta-blockers, calcium-channel blockers (eg, verapamil), theophyllines: Activity of these drugs may be reduced.
Anticonvulsants: Serum concentrations of carbamazepine, valproic acid and succinimides may be reduced. Valproic acid may increase barbiturate serum levels.
Corticosteroids: Effectiveness may be reduced.
Estrogens, estrogen-containing oral contraceptives: Effectiveness may be reduced.

Lab Test Interferences
Decreased serum bilirubin; false-positive phentolamine test results.

Adverse Reactions
CV: Bradycardia; hypotension; syncope.
CNS: Drowsiness; agitation; confusion; headache; hyperkinesia; ataxia; CNS depression; paradoxical excitement; nightmares; psychiatric disturbances; hallucinations; insomnia; dizziness.
GI: Nausea; vomiting; constipation.
HEMA: Blood dyscrasias (agranulocytosis, thrombocytopenia).
HEPA: Liver damage.
RESP: Hypoventilation; apnea; laryngospasm; bronchospasm.
OTHER: Hypersensitivity reactions (eg, angioedema, rashes, exfoliative dermatitis); fever; injection site reactions (eg, local pain, thrombophlebitis).

Precautions
Pregnancy: Category D.
Lactation: Excreted in breast milk.
Children: Safety and efficacy not established in children less than 6 yr.
Elderly: Reduce dosage.
Renal function impairment: Use with caution; reduce dosage.
Hepatic function impairment: Use with caution; reduce dosage.
Drug dependence: Tolerance or psychologic and physical dependence may occur with continued use.

Overdosage: Signs and Symptoms
Respiratory depression, CNS depression progressing to Cheyne-Stokes respiration, oliguria, tachycardia, hypotension, hypothermia, coma, shock, cessation of electrical activity in brain (extreme overdose).

PATIENT CARE CONSIDERATIONS
Administration/Storage
- May be given in oral, IM (deep), or IV form. Do not administer SC.
- Reconstitute solution with Sterile Water for Injection, rotating vial to mix. Do not shake vial. Solution should clear within 5 min.
- Do not dilute with Lactated Ringer's solution.
- Do not administer if solution is discolored or

if precipitate is present.
- After reconstitution, inject solution within 30 min.
- Do not exceed IV infusion rate of 1 mL/min or 100 mg/min. Over-rapid administration may result in respiratory depression, apnea, and hypertension.
- To avoid tissue irritation, do no inject more than 5 mL IM into any one site.
- Store at room temperature. Do not freeze.

Assessment/Interventions
- Obtain patient history, including drug history and any known allergies.
- Ensure that serum bilirubin level has been determined before beginning long-term therapy, especially in patients with hepatic disease.
- Monitor vital signs before and during IV infusion.
- Assess sleep patterns and mental status before beginning therapy and monitor periodically during therapy.
- Observe IV site during and after infusion. Extravasation or inadvertent intra-arterial injection may cause tissue necrosis, arterial spasm, thrombosis, or gangrene.
- Monitor children and elderly patients for adverse reactions, including marked excitement, confusion, restlessness, or depression.
- If hypersensitivity reaction develops, withhold dose and notify health care provider.
- When administering by IV infusion, keep resuscitation equipment at bedside.
- If signs of extravasation or phlebitis appear at injection site, discontinue IV infusion and notify health care provider.
- Implement safety measures to prevent falls, especially with elderly patients.
- Restrict amount of drug available to patient during early therapy.

Patient/Family Education
- Advise patient not to increase dosage or stop therapy without advice of health care provider.
- Instruct patient to avoid alcohol, nicotine, and caffeine products.
- Advise patient that drug may cause drowsiness, and to use caution while driving or performing other tasks requiring mental alertness.
- Inform patient to report the following symptoms to health care provider: excessive sleepiness, fatigue, nausea, vomiting.

Amobarbital/Secobarbital

(am-oh-BAR-bih-tahl/see-koe-BAR-bih-tahl)
Class Sedative/Hypnotic/Barbiturate

How Supplied
Tuinal 100 mg Pulvules Capsules 50 mg amobarbital sodium/50 mg secobarbital sodium ♦
Tuinal 200 mg Pulvules Capsules 100 mg amobarbital sodium/100 mg secobarbital sodium

Action
PHARMACOLOGY: Depresses sensory cortex, decreases motor activity, alters cerebellar function and produces drowsiness, sedation and hypnosis.

Indications Treatment of short-term insomnia; induction of preanesthetic sedation.

Contraindications Hypersensitivity to barbiturates; history of addiction to sedative-hypnotic drugs; history of porphyria; severe liver impairment; respiratory disease with dyspnea; nephrosis.

Route/Dosage
ADULTS: **PO** 1 capsule (50 mg/ 50 mg or 100 mg/100 mg) at bedtime or 1 hr before surgery.

Interactions
Alcohol, CNS depressants: Depressant effects of these drugs may be enhanced.
Anticoagulants, beta-blockers, calcium channel blockers (eg, Verapamil), theophyllines: Activity of these drugs may be reduced.
Anticonvulsants: Serum concentrations of carbamazepine, valproic acid and succinimides may be reduced. Valproic acid may increase barbiturate serum levels.
Corticosteroids: Effectiveness may be reduced.
Estrogens, estrogen-containing oral contraceptives : Effectiveness may be reduced.

Lab Test Interferences Decreased serum bilirubin; false-positive phentolamine test results.

Adverse Reactions
CV: Bradycardia; hypotension; syncope.
CNS: Drowsiness; agitation; confusion; headache; hyperkinesia; ataxia; CNS depression; paradoxical excitement; nightmares; psychiatric disturbances; hallucinations; insomnia; dizziness.
GI: Nausea; vomiting; constipation.
HEMA: Blood dyscrasias (agranulocytosis, thrombocytopenia).
HEPA: Liver damage.
RESP: Hypoventilation; apnea; laryngospasm; bronchospasm.
OTHER: Hypersensitivity reactions (eg, angioedema, rashes, exfoliative dermatitis); fever; injection site reactions (eg, local pain, thrombophlebitis).

Precautions
Pregnancy: Category D.
Lactation: Excreted in breast milk.
Children: Safety and efficacy not established.
Elderly: Reduce dosage.

Renal function impairment: Use with caution; reduce dosage.
Hepatic function impairment: Use with caution; reduce dosage.
Drug dependence: Tolerance or psychologic and physical dependence may occur with continued use.

PATIENT CARE CONSIDERATIONS
Administration/Storage
- Administer at bedtime or 1 to 2 hr prior to procedure.
- May be crushed and given mixed with food or fluid.
- Store at room temperature in tightly closed container.

Assessment/Interventions
- Obtain patient history, including drug history and any allergies. Note history of drug abuse.
- Assess patient's sleep patterns and mental status before beginning therapy and monitor periodically during long-term therapy.
- Assess vital signs prior to initial dose.
- Ensure that hepatic function tests have been performed and hematology test results and serum folate and vitamin D levels have been determined before beginning long-term therapy.
- Darken room, provide quiet environment and offer caffeine-free warm beverage to promote sleep at bedtime.
- If signs of respiratory depression or overdosage develop, withhold dose and notify health care provider.
- Report unexpected responses (particularly in elderly) such as marked excitement, confusion, restlessness, or depression.
- Implement safety measures to prevent falls, especially in elderly patients.

Patient/Family Education
- Instruct patient to avoid intake of alcohol or other CNS depressants (eg, sedatives or tranquilizers).
- Caution patient to avoid nicotine and caffeine.
- Advise patient that drug may cause drowsiness, and to avoid driving or performing other activities requiring mental alertness or coordination.
- Instruct patient to keep medication in daily-dose system or in locked cabinet to avoid accidental overdosage.
- Teach patient appropriate exercise and stress-reduction techniques to promote rest.

Overdosage: Signs and Symptoms
Respiratory depression, CNS depression progressing to Cheyne-Stokes respiration, oliguria, tachycardia, hypotension, hypothermia, coma, shock, cessation of electrical activity in brain (extreme overdose).

Amoxapine
(am-OX-uh-peen)
Class Tricyclic antidepressant

How Supplied
Asendin Tablets 25 mg, Tablets 50 mg, Tablets 100 mg, Tablets 150 mg

Action
PHARMACOLOGY: Inhibits reuptake of norepinephrine and serotonin in CNS.

PHARMACOKINETICS/DYNAMICS:
Absorption: Rapidly absorbed; t_{max} is about 90 min.
Distribution: About 90% protein bound.
Metabolism: Extensively metabolized. Major metabolite is 8-hydroxyamoxapine.
Excretion: $T_{1/2}$ is 8 hr. Biologic $t_{1/2}$ of 8-hydroxyamoxapine is 30 hr. Metabolites excreted in urine in conjugated form as glucuronides.

Indications Relief of symptoms of depression.
Unlabeled use(s): Management of chronic pain associated with migraine, chronic tension headache, diabetic neuropathy, phantom limb pain, tic douloureux, cancer pain, peripheral neuropathy, postherpetic neuralgia, and arthritic pain.

Contraindications Hypersensitivity to tricyclic antidepressants; not recommended for use during acute recovery phase of MI. Do not use drug concomitantly with MAOIs except under close medical supervision.

Route/Dosage
ADULTS: **PO** Initial dose: 200 to 300 mg/day; may be given in single daily dose at bedtime once effective dosage is established. Divided doses are given for amounts more than 300 mg/day. Hospitalized patients refractory to antidepressant therapy and with no history of seizures may be cautiously titrated to 600 mg/day in divided doses.
MAINTENANCE: Single daily dose of 300 mg or less at bedtime.
ELDERLY: **PO** Initially 25 mg bid or tid. If well tolerated, may be increased to 50 mg bid or tid. Some patients may need up to 300 mg/day.

Interactions
Barbiturates, charcoal: May decrease amoxapine blood levels.
Cimetidine, fluoxetine: May increase amoxapine blood levels.
Clonidine: May result in hypertensive crisis.
CNS depressants: Depressant effects may be additive.
MAOIs: May cause serious and possibly fatal hypertensive crisis.

Lab Test Interferences
None well documented.

Adverse Reactions
CV: Orthostatic hypotension; hypertension; tachycardia; palpitations; arrhythmias; ECG changes.
CNS: Confusion; hallucinations; delusions; nervousness; restlessness; disturbed concentration; decreased memory; agitation; panic; insomnia; nightmares; mania; exacerbation of psychosis; drowsiness; dizziness; weakness; emotional liability; seizures.
DERM: Rash; pruritus; photosensitivity reaction; dry skin; acne; itching.
EENT: Conjunctivitis; blurred vision; increased intraocular pressure; mydriasis; tinnitus; nasal congestion; peculiar taste in mouth.
GI: Nausea; vomiting; anorexia; GI distress; diarrhea; flatulence; dry mouth; constipation.
GU: Impotence; sexual dysfunction; nocturia; urinary frequency, retention or hesitancy; urinary tract infection; vaginitis; cystitis.
HEMA: Bone marrow depression including agranulocytosis; eosinophilia; purpura; thrombocytopenia; leukopenia.
HEPA: Hepatitis; jaundice.
METAB: Elevation or depression of blood glucose levels.
RESP: Pharyngitis; rhinitis; sinusitis; cough.
OTHER: Numbness; tremors; menstrual irregularities, dysmenorrhea; breast enlargement in men and women; extrapyramidal symptoms (pseudoparkinsonism, movement disorders, akathisia); tardive dyskinesia. Effects can generally be minimized by starting with low doses and increasing gradually.

Precautions
Pregnancy: Category C.
Lactation: Excreted in breast milk.
Children: Not recommended in children less than 16 yr.
Special risk patients: Use with caution in patients with history of seizures, urinary retention, urethral or ureteral spasm, angle-closure glaucoma or increased intraocular pressure, cardiovascular disorders, hyperthyroid patients or those patients receiving thyroid medication, hepatic or renal impairment, schizophrenia, or paranoia.
Neuroleptic malignant syndrome (NMS): Potentially fatal condition that has been reported with amoxapine. Signs and symptoms include hyperpyrexia, muscle rigidity, altered mental status, irregular pulse, irregular BP, tachycardia, and diaphoresis. Notify health care provider. Discontinue amoxapine and nonessential drugs.
Patients switching from MAOI to amoxapine: Wait 7 to 10 days to prevent hypertensive crisis.

PATIENT CARE CONSIDERATIONS

Administration/Storage
- Administer by oral route only.
- Administer with or immediately after meals to reduce GI irritation.
- May be crushed and given mixed with food or fluid.
- Dosage is titrated during first week(s). Once effective dosage is determined, may be given as single bedtime dose.
- Store at room temperature in tightly closed container.

Assessment/Interventions
- Obtain patient history, including drug history and any allergies. Note glaucoma, preexisting cardiovascular disease, history of prostatic hypertrophy, and seizures.
- Restrict amount of drug available to patient during early therapy.
- Implement suicide precautions.
- Assist patient to ambulate and change positions to prevent orthostatic hypotension.
- Offer frequent liquids or oral hygiene.
- Assess mental status, affect, and suicidal tendencies.
- Obtain baseline BP and monitor daily.
- Ensure that baseline hepatic, renal, and pancreatic function tests have been performed before therapy and monitor results during long-term therapy.
- Review baseline ECG and monitor CBC and differential counts during long-term therapy.
- Monitor for sedation and initial antidepressant effect during first 4 to 7 days of therapy.
- Monitor I&O and evaluate bowel elimination.
- In diabetic patient, monitor blood glucose levels periodically during therapy.
- Perform baseline and periodic leukocyte and differential counts and liver function studies.

Patient/Family Education
- Explain that full effectiveness of drug may not occur for up to 2 to 3 wk after initiation of drug therapy and that dosage will be tapered slowly before stopping.

- Advise patient that changes in smoking habits can alter drug effectiveness.
- Instruct patient to monitor food intake; weight gain can occur because of increased appetite and craving for sweets.
- Emphasize importance of regular dental care because oral dryness can increase risk for dental caries.
- Instruct patient to report the following symptoms to health care provider: Persistent dry mouth, constipation, urinary retention, fever, sore throat, or muscle rigidity.
- Instruct patient to take sips of water frequently, suck on ice chips or sugarless hard candy, or chew sugarless gum if dry mouth occurs. Suggest patient increase fluids and fiber in diet to alleviate constipation.
- Instruct patient to avoid intake of alcohol or other CNS depressants.
- Caution patient to avoid exposure to sunlight, and to use sunscreen or wear protective clothing to avoid photosensitivity reaction.
- Instruct patient not to take OTC medications without consulting health care provider.

Amoxicillin

(uh-MOX-ih-sil-in)

Class Antibiotic/Penicillin

How Supplied
Amoxil Tablets, chewable 200 mg (as trihydrate), Tablets, chewable 400 mg (as trihydrate), Tablets 500 mg (as trihydrate), Tablets 875 mg (as trihydrate), Capsules 250 mg (as trihydrate), Capsules 500 mg (as trihydrate), Powder for oral suspension 125 mg/5 mL (as trihydrate) when reconstituted, Powder for oral suspension 200 mg/5 mL (as trihydrate) when reconstituted, Powder for oral suspension 250 mg/5 mL (as trihydrate) when reconstituted, Powder for oral suspension 400 mg/5 mL (as trihydrate) when reconstituted ♦ *Amoxil Pediatric Drops* Powder for oral suspension 50 mg/mL (as trihydrate) when reconstituted ♦ *Trimox* Tablets, chewable 125 mg (as trihydrate), Tablets, chewable 250 mg (as trihydrate), Capsules 250 mg (as trihydrate), Capsules 500 mg (as trihydrate), Powder for oral suspension 125 mg/5 mL (as trihydrate) when reconstituted, Powder for oral suspension 250 mg/5 mL (as trihydrate) when reconstituted
❀ APO-Amoxi ♦ Gen-Amoxicillin ♦ Lin-Amox ♦ Novamoxin ♦ Nu-Amoxi

Action
PHARMACOLOGY: Inhibits bacterial cell wall mucopeptide synthesis.

PHARMACOKINETICS/DYNAMICS:
Absorption: Rapidly absorbed. T_{max} is 1 to 2 hr; C_{max} is 3.5 mcg/mL (250 mg dose), 5 mcg/mL (500 mg dose), and approximately 13.8 mcg/mL (875 mg dose).

Distribution: Diffuses into most body tissues and fluids; penetration in CNS is poor unless meninges are inflamed. Approximately 20% protein bound.

Excretion: $T_{½}$ is 61.3 min; approximately 60% excreted in the urine within 6 to 8 hr as unchanged drug.

Indications Treatment of ear, nose, throat, GU, skin and skin structure lower respiratory tract, and acute uncomplicated gonorrhea infections caused by susceptible strains of specific organisms.

Contraindications Hypersensitivity to penicillins, cephalosporins, or imipenem. Not used to treat severe pneumonia, empyema, bacteremia, pericarditis, meningitis, and purulent or septic arthritis during acute stage.

Route/Dosage
Ear, Nose, Throat, Skin And Skin Structure, GU Tract Infections
ADULTS AND CHILDREN WEIGHING AT LEAST 40 KG:
Mild to moderate infections: **PO** 500 mg q 12 hr or 250 mg q 8 hr.
Severe infections: **PO** 875 mg q 12 hr or 500 mg q 8 hr.
CHILDREN (OLDER THAN 3 MO AND WEIGHING LESS THAN 40 KG):
Mild to moderate infections: **PO** 25 mg/kg/day in divided doses q 12 hr or 20 mg/kg/day in divided doses q 8 hr.
Severe infections: **PO** 45 mg/kg/day in divided doses q 12 hr or 40 mg/kg/day in divided doses q 8 hr.

Lower Respiratory Tract Infections
ADULTS AND CHILDREN WEIGHING AT LEAST 40 KG: **PO** 875 mg q 12 hr or 500 mg q 8 hr.
CHILDREN (OLDER THAN 3 MO AND WEIGHING LESS THAN 40 KG): **PC** 45 mg/kg/day in divided doses q 12 hr or 40 mg/kg/day in divided doses q 8 hr.

Acute, Uncomplicated Gonorrhea
ADULTS: **PO** 3 g as a single dose.
PREPUBERTAL CHILDREN (2 YR AND OLDER): **PO** 50 mg/kg amoxicillin combined with 25 mg/kg probenecid as a single dose.

Interactions
Contraceptives, oral: May reduce efficacy of oral contraceptives.
Tetracyclines: May impair bactericidal effects of amoxicillin.

Lab Test Interferences May cause false-positive urine glucose test results with *Benedict's Solution*, *Fehling's Solution*, or *Clinitest* tablets (enzyme-based tests, eg, *Clinistix*, *Tes-Tape*, are recommended); false-positive direct *Coombs'* test result in certain patient groups; false-positive protein reactions with sulfosalicylic acid and boiling test, acetic acid test, biuret reaction and nitric acid test (bromphenol blue test, *Multi-Stix*, is recommended).

Adverse Reactions
CNS: Dizziness; fatigue; insomnia; reversible hyperactivity.
DERM: Urticaria; maculopapular to exfoliative dermatitis; vesicular eruptions; erythema multiforme; skin rashes.
EENT: Itchy eyes; glossitis; stomatitis; sore or dry mouth or tongue; black "hairy" tongue; abnormal taste sensation; laryngospasm; laryngeal edema.
GI: Gastritis; anorexia; nausea; vomiting; abdominal pain or cramps; epigastric distress; diarrhea or bloody diarrhea; rectal bleeding; flatulence; enterocolitis; pseudomembranous colitis.
GU: Interstitial nephritis (eg, oliguria, proteinuria, hematuria, hyaline casts, pyuria); nephropathy; vaginitis.
HEMA: Anemia; hemolytic anemia; thrombocytopenia; thrombocytopenic purpura; eosinophilia; leukopenia; granulocytopenia; neutropenia; bone marrow depression; agranulocytosis; reduced hemoglobin or hematocrit; prolonged bleeding and prothrombin time; increased or decreased lymphocyte count; increased monocytes, basophils, platelets.
HEPA: Transient hepatitis; cholestatic jaundice.
METAB: Elevated serum alkaline phosphatase and hypernatremia; reduced serum potassium, albumin, total proteins, and uric acid.
OTHER: Hyperthermia.

Precautions
Pregnancy: Category B.
Lactation: Excreted in breast milk.
Hypersensitivity: Reactions range from mild to life threatening. Use cautiously in cephalosporin-sensitive patients because of possible cross-allergenicity.
Superinfection: May result in overgrowth of nonsusceptible bacterial or fungal organisms.
Streptococcal infections: Minimum 10 days required for effective treatment.

Overdosage: Signs and Symptoms
Hyperexcitability, convulsions.

PATIENT CARE CONSIDERATIONS

Administration/Storage
- Use liquid preparations for patients with swallowing difficulties. Shake liquid preparations well before using.
- Time doses for equal distribution throughout day to achieve optimal blood levels.
- Be certain chewable tablets are crushed or chewed before swallowing. Supply water after each dose.
- Refrigerate liquid preparations as indicated after reconstitution. Discard after 14 days. Use tight lid to avoid evaporation of moisture.

Assessment/Interventions
- Obtain patient history, including drug history and any known allergies.
- Review results of culture and sensitivity testing as available.
- Monitor patient closely for several hours after administering first dose even when there is no history of allergy. Notify health care provider of any signs of potential hypersensitivity or anaphylactic reaction.
- Monitor renal and GI function. Notify health care provider of severe GI distress.

Patient/Family Education
- Instruct patient to time doses evenly over a 24-hr period.
- Inform patient that the medication works best on empty stomach but may be taken with food if there is GI upset.
- Instruct patient to increase fluid intake to 2000 to 3000 mL/day unless contraindicated.
- Advise patient to discard oral liquid preparations that are more than 14 days old.
- If therapy is changed because of allergic reaction, explain significance of penicillin allergy and inform patient of potential sensitivity to cephalosporins.
- Instruct patient to report the following symptoms to health care provider: rash, difficulty breathing.

Amoxicillin/Clavulanate Potassium

(uh-MOX-ih-sil-in/CLAV-you-lah-nate poe-TASS-ee-uhm)

Class Aminopenicillin

How Supplied
Augmentin Tablets 250 mg amoxicillin/125 mg clavulanic acid, Tablets 500 mg amoxicillin/125 mg clavulanic acid, Tablets 875 mg amoxicillin/125 mg clavulanic acid, Chewable tablets 125 mg amoxicillin/31.25 mg clavulanic acid, Chewable tablets 200 mg amoxicillin/28.5 mg clavulanic acid, Chewable tablets 250 mg amoxicillin/62.5 mg clavulanic acid, Chewable tablets 400 mg amoxicillin/57 mg clavulanic acid, Powder for oral suspension 125 mg amoxicillin/31.25 mg clavulanic acid/5 mL, Powder for oral suspension 200 mg amoxicillin/28.5 mg clavulanic acid/5 mL, Powder for oral suspension 250 mg amoxicillin/62.5 mg clavulanic acid/5 mL, Powder for oral suspension 400 mg amoxicillin/57 mg clavulanic acid/5 mL ♦ *Augmentin ES-600* Powder for oral suspension 600 mg amoxicillin (as trihydrate) and 42.9 mg clavulanic acid/5 mL (as the potassium salt). ♦ *Augmentin XR* Tablets 1000 mg amoxicillin/62.5 mg clavulanic acid

✤ *Apo-Amoxi-Clav* ♦ *Clavulin* ♦ *ratio-Amoxi Clav*

Action
PHARMACOLOGY: Amoxicillin inhibits bacterial cell wall mucopeptide synthesis. Clavulanic acid inactivates a wide range of beta-lactam enzymes found in bacteria resistant to penicillins and cephalosporins.

Indications Treatment of infections caused by susceptible strains of microorganisms.

Contraindications History of amoxicillin/clavulanate-associated cholestatic jaundice or liver disease. *Augmentin XR*: Severe renal impairment (Ccr less than 30 mL/min); hemodialysis patients.

Route/Dosage
AUGMENTIN
Strength listed below is based on amoxicillin content.
ADULTS AND CHILDREN OVER 12 YR: **PO** One 500 mg tablet q 12 hr or one 250 mg tablet q 8 hr (500 and 250 mg tablets contain the same amount of clavulanate; thus two 250 mg tablets are not equivalent to one 500 mg tablet).

Severe Infections
PO 500 mg q 8 hr; 875 mg q 12 hr.
CHILDREN UNDER 3 MO: **PO** Elimination impaired in children under 3 mo. 30 mg/kg/day divided q 12 hr.

CHILDREN OVER 3 YR: **PO** For otitis media, sinusitis, lower respiratory tract infections, severe infections, 45 mg/kg/day if given q 12 hr; 40 mg/kg/day if given q 8 hr.
Less Severe Infections for Children: **PO** 25 mg/kg/day if given q 12 hr; 20 mg/kg/day if given q 8 hr.

AUGMENTIN XR
The recommended starting dose is 4000 mg/25 mg/day.
Acute Bacterial Sinusitis: **PC** 2 tablets q 12 hr for 10 days.
Community-acquired Pneumonia: **PO** 2 tablets q 12 hr for 7 to 10 days.

AUGMENTIN ES-600
Augmentin ES-600 (5 mL) does not contain the same amount of clavulanic acid as any of the other *Augmentin* suspensions (5 mL). Therefore, *Augmentin ES-600* and *Augmentin* are not interchangeable. The dose listed below is based on the amoxicillin component.
CHILDREN 3 MO AND OLDER: **PO** 90 mg/kg/day divided q 12 hr for 10 days.

Interactions
Allopurinol: May increase incidence of rash.
Contraceptives, oral: May reduce effectiveness of oral contraceptives.
Probenecid: May increase and prolong blood levels of amoxicillin.
Tetracyclines: May reduce antibacterial effectiveness of amoxicillin.

Lab Test Interferences May cause false-positive urine glucose test results with *Benedict* solution, *Fehling* solution, or *Clinitest* tablets (enzyme-based tests [eg, *Clinistix*, *Tes-Tape*] are recommended); false-positive direct *Coombs'* test result in certain patient groups; false-positive protein reactions with sulfosalicylic acid and boiling test, acetic acid test, biuret reaction, and nitric acid test (*Bromphenol Blue Test*, *Multi-Stix* is recommended).

Adverse Reactions
CNS: Dizziness; fatigue; insomnia; reversible hyperactivity.
DERM: Erythema multiforme; maculopapular to exfoliative dermatitis; skin rashes; vesicular eruptions; urticaria.
EENT: Abnormal taste sensation; black hairy tongue; glossitis; itchy eyes, laryngeal edema; laryngospasm; sore or dry mouth or tongue; stomatitis.
GI: Abdominal pain or cramps; anorexia; diarrhea or bloody diarrhea; enterocolitis; epigastric distress; flatulence; gastritis; nausea; pseudomembranous colitis; rectal bleeding; vomiting.
GU: Interstitial nephritis (eg, oliguria, proteinuria, hematuria, hyaline casts, pyuria); nephropathy; vaginitis.

HEMA: Agranulocytosis; anemia; increased basophils; bone marrow depression; eosinophilia; granulocytopenia; hemolytic anemia; increased monocytes; increased or decreased lymphocyte count; leukopenia; neutropenia; increased platelets; prolonged bleeding and prothrombin time; reduced hemoglobin or hematocrit; thrombocytopenia; thrombocytopenic purpura.
HEPA: Cholestatic jaundice; transient hepatitis.
METAB: Reduced albumin; elevated serum alkaline phosphatase and hypernatremia; reduced serum potassium; reduced total proteins and uric acid.
OTHER: Hyperthermia; superinfection.

Precautions
Pregnancy: Category B.
Lactation: Secreted into breast milk.
Children: Safety and efficacy of *Augmentin ES-600* in children weighing 40 kg or more not established.
Renal function impairment: Dose reduction or q 12 hr recommended with severe impairment.
Hepatic function impairment: Use with caution. *Adults:* Safety and efficacy of *Augmentin ES-600* not established.
Mononucleosis patients: Increased risk of skin rash. Use not recommended.
Phenylalanine: Contains phenylalanine in 200 and 400 mg chewable tablets, 200 mg/5 mL and 400 mg/5 mL only.

PATIENT CARE CONSIDERATIONS
Administration/Storage
- Do not administer suspension or chewable tablets to patients with phenylketonuria.
- The 250 mg chewable tablet and 250 mg tablets are not interchangeable and should not be substituted for each other.
- Administer each dose at the start of a meal or snack to minimize GI intolerance.
- Shake suspension well before measuring dose.
- Use a medicine dropper or dosing spoon to administer suspension to children.
- Use suspension for adults with swallowing problems.
- Chewable tablets can be swallowed whole or crushed or chewed before swallowing. Supply water after each dose.
- Store suspension in refrigerator. Discard any unused suspension after 10 days. Store tablets at controlled room temperature (59° to 77°F).

Assessment/Interventions
- Obtain patient history, including drug history and any known allergies. Note current liver dysfunction, and history of phenylketonuria, drug-induced jaundice or liver dysfunction, or history of penicillin allergy.
- Review results of culture and sensitivity testing as available.
- Monitor patient for signs of anaphylaxis or severe allergic reaction. Discontinue therapy and immediately notify health care provider if noted. Be prepared to treat appropriately.
- Monitor patient for GI side effects. Report to health care provider if noted and significant.

Patient/Family Education
- Explain name, dose, action, and potential side effects of drug.
- Review dosing schedule with patient, family, or caregiver: q 8 hr or 12 hr, depending on strength of product prescribed.
- Instruct patient to take each dose at the start of a meal or snack to minimize GI side effects.
- Remind patient, family, or caregiver to complete entire course of therapy, even if symptoms of infection have disappeared.
- Instruct patient, family, or caregiver administering suspension to keep suspension refrigerated, shake well before each use, use dosing spoon or medicine dropper when administering to child, and to discard any unused suspension at end of treatment period.
- Advise patient, family, or caregiver to notify health care provider if severe diarrhea, diarrhea lasting 2 to 3 days, or diarrhea containing blood or puss occurs.
- Advise patient, family, or caregiver to report signs of superinfection to health care provider: black furry tongue, white patches in mouth, foul-smelling stools, vaginal itching or discharge.
- Advise patient, family, or caregiver to discontinue therapy and contact health care provider immediately if skin rash, hives, itching, or shortness of breath occurs.
- Instruct patient not to take any prescription or OTC medications or dietary supplements unless advised by health care provider.
- Advise patient, family, or caregiver that follow-up examinations and lab tests may be required to monitor therapy and to keep appointments.

Amoxicillin/Lansoprazole/ Clarithromycin

(uh-MOX-ih-sil-in/lan-SO-pruh-zole/kluh-RITH-row-MY-sin)

Class H. Pylori Agent/Gastrointestinal/ Antibiotic

How Supplied
Prevpac Capsules and tablets Two 30 mg lansoprazole capsules, four 500 mg amoxicillin capsules, two 500 mg clarithromycin tablets
❀ Hp-PAC

Action
PHARMACOLOGY:
Lansoprazole: Suppresses gastric acid secretion by blocking acid (proton) pump within gastric parietal cells.
Amoxicillin: Inhibits bacterial cell wall mucopeptide synthesis.
Clarithromycin: Inhibits microbial protein synthesis.

Indications Eradication of H. pylori to reduce risk of duodenal ulcer recurrence.

Contraindications Coadministration with cisapride or pimozide, known hypersensitivity to any component of formulation (ie, lansoprazole, any macrolide antibiotic, any penicillin).

Route/Dosage
ADULTS: PO 30 mg lansoprazole/1 g amoxicillin/500 mg clarithromycin given together bid (morning and evening) for 14 days. Not recommended in patients with Ccr less than 30 mL/min.

Interactions
Anticoagulants, oral: Coadministration may potentiate the effects of the oral anticoagulants. Carefully monitor prothrombin times while patients are receiving clarithromycin and oral anticoagulants simultaneously.
Carbamazepine: Coadministration of single doses of clarithromycin and carbamazepine has been shown to result in increased carbamazepine concentrations. Blood level monitoring of carbamazepine may be considered.
Cytochrome P-450 metabolized drugs: Concurrent use of clarithromycin and drugs metabolized by the cytochrome P-450 system may be associated with elevations in serum levels of these other drugs: cyclosporine, tacrolimus, hexobarbital, phenytoin, alfentanil, disopyramide, bromocriptine, valproate, pimozide, and rifabutin. Closely monitor serum concentrations of drugs metabolized by the cytochrome P-450 system in patients concurrently receiving these drugs.
Digoxin: Coadministration may potentiate the effects of digoxin. Some patients have shown clinical signs consistent with digoxin toxicity, including potentially fatal arrhythmias. Carefully monitor serum digoxin levels while patients are receiving digoxin and clarithromycin simultaneously.
Ergotamine or dihydroergotamine: Concurrent use of clarithromycin and ergotamine or dihydroergotamine has been associated in some patients with acute ergot toxicity characterized by severe peripheral vasospasm and dysthesia.
HMG-CoA reductase inhibitors (eg, lovastatin, simvistatin): Clarithromycin has been reported to increase concentrations of HMG-CoA reductase inhibitors. Rhabdomyolysis has been reported.
Sucralfate: When coadministered, the absorption of lasoprazole was delayed and bioavailability was reduced 17%. Take lansoprazole 30 min prior to sucralfate.
Theophylline: Plasma theophylline levels may be increased which may necessitate additional titration of theophylline when lansoprazole is started or stopped.
Triazolam: Clarithromycin has been reported to decrease the clearance of triazolam and may increase the CNS effects (eg, somnolence, confusion) on concomitant use.

Lab Test Interferences
Amoxicillin: May cause false-positive urine glucose test results with *Benedict's Solution*, *Fehling's Solution*, or *Clinitest* tablets (enzyme-based tests, eg, *Clinistix*, *TesTape*, are recommended); false-positive direct *Coombs* test result in certain patient groups; false-positive protein reactions, acetic acid test, biuret reaction, and nitric acid test (bromphenol blue test *Multi-Stix*, is recommended).The following changes in laboratory parameters were reported as adverse events: abnormal liver function tests, AG ratio, RBC, bilirubinemia, eosinophilia, or hyperlipemia; increased SGOT (AST), SGPT (ALT), creatinine, alkaline phosphatase, globulins, GGTP, gluconcorticoids, LDH, or gastrin levels; increased, or decreased electrolytes, cholesterol; increased, decreased, or abnormal WBC or platelets. Additional isolated laboratory abnormalities were reported.

Adverse Reactions
CNS: Headache; confusion; dizziness.
DERM: Skin reactions.
EENT: Taste perversion; glossitis.
GI: Diarrhea; abdominal pain; dark stools; dry mouth; rectal itching; nausea; oral moniliasis; stomatitis; tongue discoloration; tongue disorder; vomiting.
GU: Vaginitis; vaginal moniliasis.
RESP: Respiratory disorders.
OTHER: Thirst; myalgia.

Precautions
Pregnancy: Category C.
Lactation: Amoxicillin is excreted in breast milk in very small amounts.
Children: Safety and efficacy not established.
Elderly: Because these patients may suffer from asymptomatic renal or hepatic dysfunction, administer with caution.
Hypersensitivity: Serious and occasionally fatal hypersensitivity (anaphylactoid) reactions may occur; because cross-allergenicity may occur with cephalosporins, use with caution in patients allergic to either class of antibiotic.
Renal function impairment: Use with caution and adjust dosage in patients with severe renal impairment with or without impaired coexisting hepatic impairment. Dosage adjustment is not necessary in patients with impaired hepatic function and normal renal function.
Hepatic function impairment: Use with caution and adjust dosage in patients with severe renal impairment with or without impaired coexisting hepatic impairment. Dosage adjustment is not necessary in patients with impaired hepatic function and normal renal function.
Superinfection: Prolonged use may result in bacterial and fungal overgrowth.
Pseudomembranous colitis: Consider possibility in patients in whom diarrhea develops.

PATIENT CARE CONSIDERATIONS
Administration/Storage
- Each packet contains 2 doses (8 pills).
- Each dose consists of 4 pills (1 pink and black capsule; 2 maroon and light pink capsules; 1 yellow tablet).
- Administer all 4 pills bid before meals.
- Do not open capsules or chew or crush tablet. Instruct patient to swallow each pill whole.
- Store at controlled room temperature. Protect from light and moisture.

Assessment/Interventions
- Obtain patient history, including drug history and any known allergies. Note history of renal or hepatic impairment.
- Review patient's other medications for potentially serious interactions.
- Ensure that woman of child bearing potential is not pregnant before starting therapy.
- Monitor patient for signs of allergic reaction.
- Monitor patient for headache, taste perversion, and GI side effects.

Patient/Family Education
- Explain name, dose, action, and potential side effects of drug.
- Inform patient that each dose consists of 4 pills and should be taken bid before meals.
- Advise patient not to open capsules or crush or chew tablet and to swallow whole.
- Advise patient that the entire course of therapy (10 or 14 days) must be completed to ensure maximal benefit and to complete full course of therapy even if symptoms have resolved.
- Inform patient that headache, abnormal taste, and GI symptoms are most common side effects. Inform health care provider if any symptoms occur and are intolerable.
- Advise patient to notify health care provider if severe diarrhea or diarrhea lasting 2 to 3 days develops during or shortly after completing therapy.
- Advise patient to discontinue therapy and contact health care provider immediately if skin rash, hives, itching, or shortness of breath occurs.
- Instruct women to notify physician if they become pregnant, plan on becoming pregnant, or are breastfeeding.
- Instruct patient to not take any prescription or OTC medications or dietary supplements unless advised by a health care provider.

Amphetamine (Racemic Amphetamine Sulfate)

(am-FET-uh-meen)
Class CNS stimulant/Amphetamine
How Supplied
Adderall Tablets 5 mg (1.25 mg dextroamphetamine sulfate, 1.25 mg dextroamphetamine saccharate, 1.25 mg amphetamine aspartate, 1.25 mg amphetamine sulfate), Tablets 7.5 mg (1.875 mg dextroamphetamine sulfate, 1.875 mg dextroamphetamine saccharate, 1.875 mg amphetamine aspartate, 1.875 mg amphetamine sulfate), Tablets 10 mg (2.5 mg dextroamphetamine sulfate, 2.5 mg dextroamphetamine saccharate, 2.5 mg amphetamine aspartate, 2.5 mg amphetamine sulfate), Tablets 12.5 mg (3.125 mg dextroamphetamine sulfate, 3.125 mg dextroamphetamine saccharate, 3.125 mg amphetamine aspartate, 3.125 mg amphetamine sulfate), Tablets 15 mg (3.75 mg dextroamphetamine sulfate, 3.75 mg dextroamphetamine saccharate, 3.75 mg amphetamine aspartate, 3.75 mg amphetamine sulfate), Tablets 20 mg (5 mg dextroamphetamine sulfate, 5 mg dextroamphetamine saccharate, 5 mg amphetamine aspartate, 5 mg amphetamine sulfate), Tablets 30 mg (7.5 mg dextroamphetamine sulfate, 7.5 mg dextroamphetamine saccharate, 7.5 mg

amphetamine aspartate, 7.5 mg amphetamine sulfate) ♦ *Adderall XR* Capsules 5 mg (1.25 mg dextroamphetamine saccharate, 1.25 mg amphetamine aspartate monohydrate, 1.25 mg dextroamphetamine sulfate, 1.25 mg amphetamine sulfate), Capsules 10 mg (2.5 mg dextroamphetamine saccharate, 2.5 mg amphetamine asparatate monohydrate, 2.5 mg dextroamphetamine sulfate, 2.5 mg amphetamine sulfate), Capsules 15 mg (3.75 mg dextroamphetamine saccharate, 3.75 mg amphetamine aspartate monohydrate, 3.75 mg dextroamphetamine sulfate, 3.75 mg amphetamine sulfate), Capsules 20 mg (5 mg dextroamphetamine saccharate, 5 mg amphetamine aspartate monohydrate, 5 mg dextroamphetamine sulfate, 5 mg amphetamine sulfate), Capsules 25 mg (6.25 mg dextroamphetamine saccharate, 6.25 mg amphetamine aspartate monohydrate, 6.25 mg dextroamphetamine sulfate, 6.25 mg amphetamine sulfate), Capsules 30 mg (7.5 mg dextroamphetamine saccharate, 7.5 mg amphetamine aspartate monohydrate, 7.5 mg dextroamphetamine sulfate, 7.5 mg amphetamine sulfate)

Action

PHARMACOLOGY: Activates noradrenergic neurons, causing CNS and respiratory stimulation; stimulates satiety center in brain, causing appetite suppression.

PHARMACOKINETICS/DYNAMICS:

Absorption: T_{max} is approximately 3 hr (immediate release) and approximately 7 hr (extended release). Food prolongs the T_{max} by 2.5 hr for the extended-release formulation.

Distribution: Excreted in breast milk.

Excretion: $T_{1/2}$ is 10 hr (d-amphetamine) and 13 hr (l-amphetamine).

Special Populations:
Children – The rate of elimination is faster in children, and the $t_{1/2}$ is decreased.

Indications Narcolepsy; attention deficit disorder with hyperactivity; short-term (ie, few weeks) exogenous obesity adjunct used only when alternative therapy has been ineffective.

Contraindications Advanced arteriosclerosis; symptomatic cardiovascular disease; moderate to severe hypertension; hyperthyroidism; hypersensitivity to sympathomimetic amines; glaucoma; agitated states; history of drug abuse. Do not use concomitantly with or within 14 days of MAOI use.

Route/Dosage

Narcolepsy
ADULTS AND CHILDREN OVER 12 YR: **PO** 10 mg/day; may be increased weekly by 10 mg to max 60 mg/day in divided doses.
CHILDREN 6 TO 12 YR: **PO** 5 mg/day; may be increased weekly by 5 mg to max 60 mg/day in divided doses.

Attention Deficit Disorder
CHILDREN 6 YR OR MORE: **PO** 5 mg/day; may be increased weekly by 5 mg to max 40 mg/day in divided doses. Usual range: 0.1 to 0.5 mg/kg/dose q AM.
CHILDREN 3 TO 5 YR: **PO** 2.5 mg/day; may be increased weekly by 2.5 mg. Usual range: 0.1 to 0.5 mg/kg/dose in morning.

Exogenous Obesity
ADULTS AND CHILDREN OVER 12 YR: **PO** 5 to 10 mg 30 to 60 min before meals, up to 30 mg/day.

Interactions
Guanethidine: Effectiveness may be decreased.
MAOIs, furazolidone: May cause hypertensive crisis and intracranial hemorrhage.
Tricyclic antidepressants: May decrease amphetamine effect.
Urinary acidifiers (ammonium chloride, ascorbic acid): May decrease amphetamine effect.
Urinary alkalinizers (acetazolamide, sodium bicarbonate): May increase amphetamine effect.

Lab Test Interferences
Plasma and urine steroid levels may be altered.

Adverse Reactions
CV: Palpitations; tachycardia; hypertension; arrythmias.
CNS: Hyperactivity; dizziness; restlessness; tremors; insomnia; euphoria; headache.
DERM: Urticaria.
EENT: Dry mouth; unpleasant taste.
GI: Diarrhea; constipation; anorexia.
GU: Impotence.

> **WARNING:**
> *High abuse/diversion potential:* Drug dependence may develop with chronic use. Avoid prolonged periods of use.
> Prescribe/dispense sparingly due to high diversion potential.

Precautions
Pregnancy: Category C.
Lactation: Excreted in breast milk.
Children: Should not be used as anorectic agent in children less than 12 yr. Not recommended for attention deficit disorder in children less than 3 yr.
Tolerance: May occur; do not exceed recommended dose.

Overdosage: Signs and Symptoms
Restlessness, tremor, hyperreflexia, confusion, hallucinations, panic, fatigue, depression, convulsions, coma, arrhythmias, hypertension, hypotension, circulatory collapse, nausea, vomiting, diarrhea, abdominal cramps.

PATIENT CARE CONSIDERATIONS

Administration/Storage
- Administer drug as supplied; do not crush or have patient chew sustained-release or long-acting tablets.
- Administer in AM or at least 6 hr before bedtime to avoid insomnia.
- Store at room temperature.

Assessment/Interventions
- Obtain patient history, including drug history and any allergies (particularly aspirin). Note cardiovascular disease, hypertension, history of drug abuse.
- Obtain BP initially and monitor periodically during therapy.
- Ensure that serum thyroxine (T_4), plasma corticosteroid and urinary steroid levels have been obtained before beginning therapy.
- Review ECG for arrhythmias before beginning therapy.
- Assess mental status. Depressed patients are more likely to misuse drug to induce euphoria and mood elevation.
- Implement safety precautions to prevent falls.
- If hypertensive crisis occurs, administer phentolamine.
- Monitor patient drug use pattern closely. Physical and psychologic dependency can occur quickly with these agents.
- Observe for the following early signs of overdosage: restlessness, irritability, fever, hyperpnea, confusion.
- Closely monitor growth rate of children during therapy. Effect of drug on growth rate is unknown.
- Observe for dizziness and dry mucous membranes.

Patient/Family Education
- Caution patient to take medication exactly as ordered and not to increase dosage unless advised by health care provider.
- Advise patient to avoid caffeine, which increases drug effect.
- Instruct patient to report the following symptoms to health care provider: insomnia, skin discolorations, GI disturbances.
- Instruct patient to take sips of water frequently, suck on ice chips or sugarless hard candy, or chew sugarless gum if dry mouth occurs.
- Advise patient that drug may cause drowsiness, and to use caution while driving or performing tasks requiring mental alertness.

Amphotericin B

(am-foe-TER-ih-sin B)

Class Anti-infective/Antifungal

How Supplied

Amphotericin B Desoxycholate
Fungizone Oral suspension 100 mg/mL

Amphotericin B Lipid-Based
Abelcet Suspension for injection 100 mg/20 mL (as lipid complex) ♦ AmBisome Powder for injection 50 mg (as liposomal) ♦ Amphotec Powder for injection 50 mg (as cholesteryl), Powder for injection 100 mg (as cholesteryl)

Amphotericin B Cholesteryl
Amphotec Powder for injection 50 mg (as cholesteryl), Powder for injection 100 mg (as cholesteryl)

Action
PHARMACOLOGY: Alters fungal cell membrane permeability.

PHARMACOKINETICS/DYNAMICS:

Absorption:
Deoxycholate – C_{max} is approximately 0.5 to 2 mcg/mL.
Lipid based – C_{max} is approximately 1.7 mcg/mL (Abelcet) and approximately 7.3 to 83 mcg/mL (Ambisome; 1 to 5 mg/kg/day).
Cholesteryl – C_{max} is approximately 2.6 to 2.9 mcg/mL (Amphotec).

Distribution:
Deoxycholate – More than 90% protein bound.
Lipid based – Vd is approximately 131 L/kg (Abelcet) and 0.1 to 0.44 L/kg (Ambisome; 1 to 5 mg/kg/day).
Cholesteryl – Vd is approximately 3.8 to 4.1 L/kg; distribution $t_{1/2}$ is approximately 3.5 min (Amphotec).

Metabolism: Not known.

Excretion:
Deoxycholate – Elimination $t_{1/2}$ is approximately 15 days, plasma $t_{1/2}$ is approximately 24 hr; excreted very slowly by the kidneys with 2% to 5% of a dose excreted in the active form.
Lipid based – $T_{1/2}$ is approximately 173.4 hr (Abelcet), approximately 7 to 10 hr (Ambisome; measured within 24 hr dosing interval), and approximately 100 to 153 hr (Ambisome; measured up to 49 days after dosing). Clearance is approximately 436 mL/hr/kg (Abelcet) and 11 to 51 mL/hr/kg (Ambisome).
Cholesteryl – $T_{1/2}$ is approximately 27.5 to 28.2 hr, clearance is approximately 0.105 to 0.112 L/hr/kg (Amphotec).

Indications
Treatment of progressive, potentially fatal infections caused by certain fungal species.
Amphotericin B desoxycholate: Treatment of

American mucocutaneous leishmaniasis.
Amphotericin B lipid-based: Treatment of invasive fungal infections in patients refractory to conventional amphotericin B desoxycholate or when renal impairment or unacceptable toxicity precludes use of the desoxycholate formulation (lipid complex); treatment of infections caused by *Aspergillus, Candida,* or *Cryptococcus* species (liposomal); empirical treatment of febrile, neutropenic patients with presumed fungal infections (liposomal); treatment of visceral leishmaniasis (liposomal).
Amphotericin B cholesteryl: Treatment of invasive aspergillosis.
Amphotericin B (topical): Treatment of cutaneous and mucocutaneous mycotic infections caused by *Candida* sp. **Unlabeled use(s):** Prophylaxis of fungal infections in patients with bone marrow transplantation; treatment of primary amoebic meningoencephalitis caused by *Naegleria fowleri;* subconjunctival or intravitreal treatment of ocular aspergillosis; bladder irrigation for candidal cystitis; chemoprophylaxis of aspergillosis; intrathecal treatment of severe meningitis unresponsive to IV therapy; intraarticular or IM treatment of coccidioidal arthritis.

Contraindications Standard considerations.

Route/Dosage

AMPHOTERICIN B DESOXYCHOLATE
ADULTS: IV Test dose of 0.05 mg/mL infused slowly over 20 to 30 min. Record patient's temperature, pulse, respiration, and BP q 30 min for 2 to 4 hr.

Systemic Fungal Infections
ADULTS: IV Initial recommended dose is 0.25 to 0.3 mg/kg/day infused slowly over 2 to 6 hr. Dose is increased gradually up to 0.5 to 0.7 mg/kg/day and up to 1.5 mg/kg/day for some mycoses (max daily dose, 1.5 mg/kg). Daily dose varies with type of infection, ranging from 0.5 to 1.5 mg/kg/day for 4 to 12 wk. However, aspergillosis regimen is 1 to 1.5 mg/kg/day up to a total treatment dose of 3.6 g; rhinocerebral phycomycosis regimen is 0.25 to 1.5 mg/kg/day to a total treatment dose of 3 to 4 g; sporotrichosis regimen is 0.5 mg/kg/day up to a total treatment dose of 2.5 g.

Leishmaniasis
ADULTS: IV 0.5 mg/kg/day on alternate days for 14 doses.

AMPHOTERICIN B LIPOSOMAL
Empirical Fungal Infection
ADULTS: IV 3 mg/kg/day.

Systemic Fungal Infection
ADULTS: IV 3 to 5 mg/kg/day as a 1 to 2 mg/mL dilution.

CHILDREN: IV 3 to 5 mg/kg/day as a 0.2 to 0.5 mg/mL dilution.

Leishmaniasis
ADULTS: IV 3 mg/kg/day on days 1 through 5, and days 14 and 21 to immunocompetent patients; administer 4 mg/kg/day on days 1 through 5, and days 10, 17, 24, 31, and 38 to immunosuppressed patients.

AMPHOTERICIN B LIPID COMPLEX
Systemic Fungal Infection
ADULTS: IV 5 mg/kg/day as a 1 mg/mL dilution; patients with cardiovascular disease dilute to 2 mg/mL.
CHILDREN: IV 5 mg/kg/day as a 2 mg/mL dilution.

AMPHOTERICIN B CHOLESTERYL
Systemic Fungal Infection
ADULTS: IV Test dose advisable (eg, 10 mL containing 1.6 to 8.3 mg infused over 15 to 30 min); recommended treatment dose is 3 to 4 mg/kg/day.

AMPHOTERICIN B
Topical 2 to 4 times/day for 1 to 4 wk.

Interactions
Corticosteroids: Increased potential for hypokalemia.
Cyclosporine: May increase nephrotoxic effects.
Nephrotoxic agents (eg, aminoglycosides): Possible synergistic nephrotoxicity.
INCOMPATIBILITIES: Do not mix with other IV medications.

Lab Test Interferences None well documented.

Adverse Reactions
CV: Arrhythmias; ventricular fibrillation; cardiac arrest; hypotension; chest pain; hypertension; tachycardia.
CNS: Headache; convulsions; peripheral neuropathy; anxiety; confusion.
DERM: Topical preparations may cause local irritation (eg, erythema, pruritus, burning sensation) or dryness; pruritus; rash; sweating.
EENT: Hearing loss.
GI: Anorexia; nausea; vomiting; dyspepsia; diarrhea; cramping; epigastric pain; hemorrhagic gastroenteritis.
GU: Hypokalemia; azotemia; hyposthenuria; nephrocalcinosis; renal tubular acidosis; anuria; oliguria; permanent renal damage; kidney failure; hematuria.
HEMA: Normochromic, normocytic anemia; thrombocytopenia; leukopenia; agranulocytosis; eosinophilia; leukocytosis.
METAB: Increased ALT and AST; bilirubinemia.
RESP: Respiratory failure; dyspnea; respiratory

disorder; increased cough; epistaxis; hypoxia; lung disorder; pleural effusion; rhinitis.
OTHER: Fever (sometimes with shaking chills); malaise; generalized pain, including muscle and joint pain; venous pain at injection site with phlebitis and thrombophlebitis; weight loss; anaphylactoid reactions; sepsis.

> **WARNING:**
> Do not use to treat noninvasive forms of fungal diseases (eg, oral thrush, vaginal candidiasis and esophageal candidiasis) in patients with normal neutrophil counts.
>
> Exercise caution to prevent inadvertent overdose.

Precautions
Pregnancy: Category B.
Lactation: Undetermined.

Children:
Amphotericin B desoxycholate – Safety and efficacy not established.
Amphotericin B, lipid-based (ie, cholesteryl, lipid complex, liposomal) – Safety and efficacy in children less than 1 mo not established.
Nephrotoxicity: Drug is toxic and should be used with caution under close supervision. Renal damage is most important toxic effect. Despite its dangerous side effects, amphotericin B frequently is the only effective treatment for potentially fatal fungal diseases.
Topical use: Avoid contact with eyes.
Pulmonary reactions: Acute dyspnea, hypoxemia, and interstitial infiltrates can occur in neutropenic patients receiving amphotericin B and leukocyte transfusions.

Overdosage: Signs and Symptoms
Cardiorespiratory arrest.

PATIENT CARE CONSIDERATIONS

Administration/Storage
Amphotericin B deoxycholate:
- Administer IV infusion only in acute care setting under close supervision. Test dose is usually given before administering first therapeutic dose.
- Follow manufacturer's instructions for reconstitution and administration. Use Sterile Water for Injection without a bacteriostatic agent. Do not reconstitute with saline. Preservatives, bacteriostatic agents, and saline may cause precipitation.
- Use solutions prepared for IV infusion promptly after reconstitution.
- Use aseptic technique while handling medication.
- Wear gloves while applying topical ointments.
- Use volumetric IV pump to regulate delivery over the recommended 6-hr period. Shorter infusion times have also been used.
- Use IV filter (at least 1 micron) during administration.
- Agitate hanging solution to mix q 30 to 60 min.
- Do not mix with other IV medications.
- Do not administer if solution is discolored or if precipitate is present.
- Medication is stable for 24 hr at room temperature or 7 days if kept refrigerated.
- Store in dark area. Protect from light during administration.
- Do not exceed a total daily dose of 1.5 mg/kg.

Liposomal amphotericin B:
- Administer IV at a rate of 2.5 mg/kg/hr. If the infusion time exceeds 2 hr, mix the contents by shaking the infusion bag q 2 hr.
- Follow manufacturer's instructions for reconstitution and administration. Use 5% Dextrose Injection for reconstitution. Do not reconstitute with other drugs or electrolytes as compatibility of liposomal amphotericin B has not been established. Flush an existing IV line with 5% Dextrose Injection before infusion of liposomal amphotericin B, or use a separate infusion line.
- Shake the vial gently until there is no yellow sediment at the bottom.
- Do not use an in-line filter less than 5 microns.
- Do not freeze. Retain in the carton until time of use.
- May be stored for 15 hr if refrigerated or 6 hr at room temperature.
- Discard any unused material.

Amphotericin B cholesteryl:
- Administer diluted in 5% Dextrose for Injection by IV infusion rate of 1 mg/kg/hr.
- Test dose is usually given before administering first therapeutic dose.
- Follow manufacturer's instructions for reconstitution and administration. Reconstitute by using Sterile Water for Injection. Do not reconstitute with saline or dextrose solutions or admix with saline or electrolytes.
- Do not filter or use an in-line filter.
- Do not mix with other IV medications.
- Use within 24 hr after reconstitution.
- Store unopened vials at room temperature.

- Refrigerate after reconstitution.

Assessment/Interventions
- Obtain patient history, including drug history and any allergies.
- Ensure that fungal culture (blood or urine, as appropriate) of organism has been obtained before beginning therapy.
- Monitor pulse and BP q 15 min during test dose.
- Monitor IV injection site closely during administration for signs of infiltration.
- Monitor laboratory values, including LFTs, CBC, renal function tests, and magnesium levels during therapy.
- Monitor I&O during therapy.
- Monitor temperature 4 hr after administration; may be elevated.
- Assess for symptoms of hypokalemia, especially disorientation and weakness.
- If the patient experiences infusion-related symptoms (eg, chills, fever, hypotension, joint pain), NSAID, corticosteroid, or other antipyretic may be given before administering drug. Administration of heparin, rapid infusion, removal of needle after infusion, rotation of infusion sites, and administration through large central vein or distal vein may lessen incidence of thrombophlebitis.
- If severe side effects or signs of anaphylactic reaction occur, stop infusion and notify health care provider.

Patient/Family Education
- Explain need for prolonged therapy and for close monitoring during course of therapy.
- Encourage patient to increase fluid intake to 2000 to 3000 mL/day, if allowed.
- Inform patient to report any discomfort at injection site immediately.
- Instruct patient to report symptoms of chills, malaise, or fever.
- Warn patient that contact with topical preparation can cause discoloration of fabrics. However, this is easily removed by washing with soap and water or applying common stain removers.

Amphotericin B Cholesteryl Sulfate Complex

(am-foe-TER-ih-sin B)

Class Anti-infective/Antifungal

How Supplied
Amphotec Powder for injection 50 mg (as cholesteryl), Powder for injection 100 mg (as cholesteryl)

Action
PHARMACOLOGY: Alters fungal cell membrane permeability.

Indications Treatment of invasive aspergillosis when renal impairment or unacceptable toxicity precludes use of amphotericin B deoxycholate and where prior amphotericin B deoxycholate therapy has failed.

Contraindications Hypersensitivity to amphotericin B, unless condition requiring treatment is life-threatening and amenable only to amphotericin B.

Route/Dosage
ADULTS AND CHILDREN:
Test dose: **IV** Infusion of small amount of final preparation (eg, 10 mL containing 1.6 to 8.3 mg) over 15 to 30 min and observe the patient carefully for 30 min.
Initial dose: **IV** 3 to 4 mg/kg as required at a rate of 1 mg/kg/hr. Dose may be increased to 6 mg/kg if no improvement or there is evidence of progression of the fungal infection.

Interactions
Antineoplastic agents: Enhanced potential for nephrotoxicity, bronchospasm and hypotension.
Corticosteroids: Increased potential for hypokalemia.
Cyclosporine, tacrolimus: May increase nephrotoxic effects.
Flucytosine: Increased flucytosine toxicity.
Nephrotoxic agents (eg, aminoglycosides): Possible synergistic nephrotoxicity.
INCOMPATIBILITIES: Do not mix with other medications.

Lab Test Interferences None well documented.

Adverse Reactions
CV: Hypotension; tachycardia; hypertension; arrhythmia; edema.
CNS: Headache; confusion; depression; abnormal thinking.
DERM: Sweating; rash; pruritus.
EENT: Eye hemorrhage.
GI: Nausea, vomiting; abdominal pain.
GU: Increased creatinine; hematuria; kidney failure.
HEMA: Thrombocytopenia.
HEPA: Abnormal LFTs; bilirubinemia.
METAB: Hypokalemia; hypomagnesemia; hypocalcemia; hyperglycemia.
RESP: Dyspnea; hypoxia; epistaxis, increased cough; hemoptysis; hyperventilation; apnea.

OTHER: Chills; fever; pain; anaphylactoid reactions.

Precautions
Pregnancy: Category B.
Lactation: Undetermined.
Nephrotoxicity: Drug is toxic; use with caution under close supervision; however, amphotericin B frequently is the only effective treatment for potentially fatal fungal diseases.

Overdosage: Signs and Symptoms
Cardiorespiratory arrest.

PATIENT CARE CONSIDERATIONS
Administration/Storage
- Reconstitute using only Sterile Water for Injection. Further dilution can be made with 5% Dextrose in water. Do not admix with saline or electrolytes or fluids containing preservatives.
- Do not mix with any other drug. Administer through separate IV line or flush existing line with 5% dextrose in water.
- Give test dose before full IV dose.
- Administer full dose at 1 mg/kg/hr.
- Administer IV form only to patients who are hospitalized or in an outpatient medical facility under close supervision.
- Do not administer solutions that have precipitates or foreign matter.
- Unopened vials can be stored at room temperature (59° to 86°F) until reconstituted.
- Wear gloves during reconstitution and administration.
- Reconstituted solutions can be stored under refrigeration (36° to 46°F) and used within 24 hr. Discard any unused solution.

Assessment/Interventions
- Monitor patient closely during test administration for fever, chills, headache, nausea or vomiting.
- Obtain patient history, including drug history and any allergies.
- Ensure that fungal culture (blood or urine, as appropriate) of organism has been obtained before beginning therapy.
- Monitor pulse and BP q 15 min during test dose.
- Monitor IV injection site closely during administration for signs of infiltration.
- Monitor laboratory values, including LFTs, CBC, renal function tests, potassium, and magnesium levels.
- Monitor I&O during therapy.
- Monitor temperature 4 hr after administration; may be elevated.
- If patient experiences infusion-related symptoms (eg, chills, fever, hypotension, nausea), antihistamines and corticosteroids may be given before the infusion. Reducing the rate of infusion also may be helpful.

Patient/Family Education
- Explain need for prolonged therapy and for close monitoring during course of therapy.
- Encourage patient to increase fluid intake to 2000 to 3000 mL/day if allowed.
- Inform patient to report any discomfort at injection site immediately.
- Instruct patient to report symptoms of chills, malaise, or fever.

Ampicillin

(am-pih-SILL-in)

Class Antibiotic/Penicillin

How Supplied
Principen Capsules 250 mg (as trihydrate), Capsules 500 mg (as trihydrate), Powder for oral suspension 125 mg/5 mL (as trihydrate) when reconstituted, Powder for oral suspension 250 mg/5 mL (as trihydrate) when reconstituted
♦ *Ampicillin Sodium* Powder for injection 250 mg, Powder for injection 500 mg, Powder for injection 1 g, Powder for injection 2 g
✤ *APO-Ampi* ♦ *Novo Ampicillin* ♦ *Nu-Ampi*

Action
PHARMACOLOGY: Inhibits bacterial cell wall mucopeptide synthesis.

PHARMACOKINETICS/DYNAMICS:
Absorption: Well absorbed from GI tract. C_{max} is approximately 3 mcg/mL (500 mg capsules) and 3.4 mcg/mL (500 mg oral suspension). Food affects absorption; take on empty stomach.

Distribution: Diffuses readily into most body tissues and fluids; penetrates into the CSF and brain only when meninges are inflamed. Approximately 20% protein bound; excreted in breast milk.

Excretion: Excreted largely unchanged in the urine.

Special Populations:
Renal Function Impairment – $T_{1/2}$ may be prolonged. Dosing interval adjustments may be necessary.

Indications Treatment of respiratory, GI, and GU tract and soft tissue infections, bacterial meningitis and enterococcal endocarditis, septicemia and gonococcal infections caused by susceptible microorganisms. **Unlabeled use(s):**

AMPICILLIN

Prophylaxis in Cesarean section in certain high risk patients.

Contraindications Hypersensitivity to penicillins, cephalosporins or imipenem. Oral form not used to treat severe pneumonia, empyema, bacteremia, pericarditis, meningitis, and purulent or septic arthritis during acute stage.

Route/Dosage

Enterococcal Endocarditis
ADULTS: IV 12 g/day either continuously or in equally divided doses q 4 hr plus mg/kg IM or IV gentamicin q 8 hr for 4 to 6 wk.

Respiratory Tract and Soft Tissue Infections
ADULTS AND CHILDREN (AT LEAST 40 KG): IV/IM 250 to 500 mg q 6 hr.
CHILDREN (LESS THAN 40 KG): IV/IM 25 to 50 mg/kg/day in equally divided doses q 6 to 8 hr.
ADULTS AND CHILDREN (MORE THAN 20 KG): PO 250 mg q 6 hr.
CHILDREN (20 KG OR LESS): PO 50 mg/kg/day in equally divided dose q 6 to 8 hr.

Bacterial Meningitis
ADULTS AND CHILDREN: Initial treatment is usually IV followed by IM 150 to 200 mg/kg/day in equally divided doses q 3 to 4 hr.

Septicemia
ADULTS AND CHILDREN: IV 150 to 200 mg/kg/day for at least 3 days followed by IM q 3 to 4 hr.

GI and GU Infections (Other Than N. gonorrhea)
ADULTS AND CHILDREN (MORE THAN 20 KG): PO 500 mg q 6 hr; use larger doses for severe or chronic infections, if needed.
CHILDREN (20 KG OR LESS): PO 100 mg/kg/day in equally divided doses q 6 hr.

GI and GU infections (N. gonorrhea)
ADULTS: PO 3.5 g administered simultaneously with 1 g probenecid.
ADULTS AND CHILDREN (AT LEAST 40 KG): IV/IM 500 mg q 6 hr.
CHILDREN (LESS THAN 40 KG): IV/IM 50 mg/kg/day in equally divided doses q 6 to 8 hr.

Urethritis caused by N. gonorrhea
ADULT MALES: IV/IM Two 500 mg doses at an interval of 8 to 12 hr. Dose may be repeated if necessary. In complicated gonorrheal urethritis, intensive therapy is recommended.

Interactions
Allopurinol: Increases potential for ampicillin-induced skin rash.
Atenolol: Antihypertensive and antianginal effects may be impaired.
Contraceptives, oral: May reduce efficacy of oral contraceptives.
Tetracyclines: May impair bactericidal effects of ampicillin.
INCOMPATIBILITIES: Do not mix with aminoglycosides (eg, gentamicin).

Lab Test Interferences May cause false-positive urine glucose test results with *Benedict's Solution, Fehling's Solution,* or *Clinitest* tablets (enzyme-based tests, eg, *Clinistix, Tes-tape,* are recommended); false-positive direct *Coombs'* test result in certain patient groups; false-positive protein reactions with sulfosalicylic acid and boiling test, acetic acid test, biuret reaction and nitric acid test (the bromphenol blue test, *Multistix,* is recommended).

Adverse Reactions
CV: Thrombophlebitis at injection site.
CNS: Dizziness; fatigue; insomnia; reversible hyperactivity; neurotoxicity (eg, lethargy, neuromuscular irritability, hallucinations, convulsions, seizures).
DERM: Urticaria; maculopapular to exfoliative dermatitis; vesicular eruptions; erythema multiforme; skin rashes.
EENT: Itchy eyes; laryngospasm; laryngeal edema.
GI: Diarrhea; pseudomembranous colitis.
GU: Interstitial nephritis (eg, oliguria, proteinuria, hematuria, hyaline casts, pyuria); nephropathy; increased BUN and creatinine; vaginitis.
HEMA: Decreased Hgb, Hct, RBC, WBC, neutrophils, lymphocytes, platelets; increased lymphocytes, monocytes, basophils, eosinophils, and platelets.
METAB: Elevated serum alkaline phosphatase, glutamic oxaloacetic transaminase, ALT, AST, and LDH; reduced serum albumin and total proteins.
OTHER: Pain at injection site; hyperthermia.

Precautions
Pregnancy: Category B.
Lactation: Excreted in breast milk.
Hypersensitivity: Reactions range from mild to life threatening. Use cautiously in cephalosporin-sensitive patients because of possible cross-allergenicity.
Renal function impairment: Use cautiously with altered dosing interval.
Superinfection: May result in overgrowth of nonsusceptible bacterial or fungal organisms.

Overdosage: Signs and Symptoms
Hyperexcitability, convulsive seizures.

PATIENT CARE CONSIDERATIONS

Administration/Storage
- Use liquid preparations for patients with swallowing difficulties. Follow manufacturer's instructions for reconstitution, and handle liquids carefully to prevent contact dermatitis.
- Time doses at equal intervals to achieve optimal blood levels.
- To achieve max benefit, administer 1 hr before or 2 hr after a meal.
- Monitor renal function.
- Shake liquid preparations well before using.
- Administer IM and IV solutions within 1 hr of reconstitution.
- Allow foaming to subside before administering IV preparations. Do not administer if discolored or cloudy. Use volumetric IV pump to regulate delivery over 10- to 15-min period. Do not mix with other IV medications.
- Be sure certain chewable tablets are crushed or chewed before swallowing. Supply water following dose.
- Refrigerate liquid preparations after reconstitution, and discard after 14 days. Discard after 7 days if not refrigerated.
- Store tablets and capsules in dry, tightly closed container.

Assessment/Interventions
- Obtain patient history, including drug history and any known allergies.
- Review results of culture and sensitivity testing, as available.
- Monitor patient's condition closely for several hours after administering the first dose even when there is no history of allergy. Notify health care provider of any signs or symptoms of hypersensitivity or anaphylactic reaction.
- Monitor renal and GI function during therapy, and notify health care provider of severe GI distress.
- Evaluate skin daily for presence of classic ampicillin rash, usually maculopapular, pruritic, and generalized.
- Monitor for bleeding in patients receiving anticoagulant therapy.

Patient/Family Education
- Instruct patient to time the doses evenly over a 24-hr period.
- Inform patient that medication works best on an empty stomach, but may be taken with food if there is GI upset.
- Tell patient to increase fluid intake to 2000 to 3000 mL/day, unless contraindicated.
- Advise patient to refrigerate oral liquid preparations, and to discard unrefrigerated preparations that are more than 7 days old.
- Inform patient to notify health care provider immediately if rash develops or if having difficulty breathing.
- Warn diabetic patient that product may cause false-positive glucose urine test results, and identify alternative tests.
- If therapy is changed because of allergic reaction, explain the significance of penicillin allergy and inform of potential sensitivity to cephalosporins.

Ampicillin Sodium/Sulbactam Sodium

(am-pih-SILL-in SO-dee-uhm/sull-BAK-tam SO-dee-uhm)

Class Antibiotic/Penicillin

How Supplied
Unasyn Powder for injection 1.5 g (1 g ampicillin sodium/0.5 g sulbactam sodium), Powder for injection 3 g (2 g ampicillin sodium/1 g sulbactam sodium), Powder for injection 10 g (10 g ampicillin sodium/5 g sulbactam sodium)

Action
PHARMACOLOGY: Ampicillin inhibits bacterial cell wall mucopeptide synthesis. Sulbactam inhibits plasmid-medicated beta-lactamase enzymes commonly found in microorganisms resistant to ampicillin.

Indications Treatment of infections of skin and skin structure, intra-abdominal and gynecologic infections caused by susceptible microorganisms, and mixed infections caused by ampicillin-susceptible organisms and beta-lactamase–producing organisms.

Contraindications Hypersensitivity to penicillins, cephalosporins, or imipenem.

Route/Dosage
ADULTS: **IV/IM** 1.5 to 3 g q 6 hr, not to exceed 4 g/day sulbactam (1.5 g of product contains 0.5 g sulbactam).
CHILDREN AT LEAST 1 YR (LESS THAN 40 KG): **IV** 300 mg/kg/day (200 mg ampicillin/100 mg sulbactam) in divided doses q 6 hr.
CHILDREN AT LEAST 40 KG: **IV** Dose according to adult recommended doses; do not exceed total sulbactam dose of 4 g/day.

Interactions
Allopurinol: Increases potential for ampicillin-induced skin rash.
Contraceptives, oral: May reduce efficacy of oral contraceptives.
Tetracyclines: May impair bactericidal effects of

ampicillin/sulbactam.
INCOMPATIBILITIES: Do not mix with aminoglycosides (eg, gentamicin).

Lab Test Interferences May cause false-positive urine glucose test results with *Benedict's Solution, Fehling's Solution,* or *Clinitest* tablets (enzyme-based tests, eg, *Clinistix, Tes-tape,* are recommended); false-positive direct *Coombs'* test result in certain patient groups; false-positive protein reactions with sulfosalicylic acid and boiling test, acetic acid test, biuret reaction and nitric acid test (the bromphenol blue test, *Multistix,* is recommended).

Adverse Reactions
CV: Thrombophlebitis at injection site.
CNS: Dizziness; fatigue; insomnia; reversible hyperactivity.
DERM: Urticaria; maculopapular to exfoliative dermatitis; vesicular eruptions; erythema multiforme; skin rashes.
EENT: Itchy eyes; laryngospasm; laryngeal edema.
GI: Diarrhea; pseudomembranous colitis.
GU: Interstitial nephritis (eg, oliguria, proteinuria, hematuria, hyaline casts, pyuria); nephropathy; increased BUN and creatinine; vaginitis.
HEMA: Decreased Hgb, Hct, RBC, WBC, neutrophils, lymphocytes, platelets; increased lymphocytes, monocytes, basophils, eosinophils and platelets.
METAB: Elevated serum alkaline phosphatase, glutamic oxaloacetic transaminase, ALT, AST, and LDH; reduced serum albumin and total proteins.
OTHER: Pain at injection site; hyperthermia.

Precautions
Pregnancy: Category B.
Lactation: Excreted in breast milk.
Children: Safety and efficacy not established.
Hypersensitivity: Reactions range from mild to life-threatening. Use cautiously in cephalosporin-sensitive patients because of possible cross-allergenicity.
Renal function impairment: Use cautiously with altered dosing interval.
Superinfection: May result in overgrowth of nonsusceptible bacterial or fungal organisms.

Overdosage: Signs and Symptoms
Hyperexcitability, convulsive seizures.

PATIENT CARE CONSIDERATIONS

Administration/Storage
* Do not mix in same IV solution with aminoglycosides.
* Administer IM and IV solutions within 1 hr of reconstitution.
* Allow foaming to subside before administering IV preparations. Do not administer if discolored or cloudy. Use volumetric IV pump to regulate delivery over 10- to 15-min period.
* Do not infuse with other IV medications.
* Do not administer other antibiotics within 1 hr.
* Do not routinely exceed 14 days of IV therapy in children. Safety and efficacy of IM administration have not been established.
* Monitor renal function.
* Rotate IM injection sites.
* Keep refrigerated after reconstitution. Medication is stable for 2 hr at room temperature, 72 hr if refrigerated.

Assessment/Interventions
* Obtain patient history, including drug history and any known allergies.
* Review results of culture and sensitivity testing as available.
* Monitor I&O during therapy.
* Monitor patient's condition closely for several hours after administration even if there is no history of known penicillin allergy. Notify health care provider of any signs and symptoms of hypersensitivity or anaphylactic reaction.

Patient/Family Education
* Explain rationale for hospitalization during course of therapy.
* Inform patient of potential side effects, and encourage a report of any problems.
* Encourage patient to increase fluid intake to 2000 to 3000 mL/day, unless contraindicated.
* Inform diabetic patients that this medication may cause false-positive glucose urine test results, and identify types that will be more reliable.
* If therapy is changed because of allergic reaction, explain significance of penicillin allergy, and inform of potential sensitivity to cephalosporins.

Amprenavir

(am-PREN-ah-veer)

Class Antiretroviral/Protease inhibitor

How Supplied
Agenerase Capsules 50 mg, Capsules 150 mg, Oral solution 15 mg/mL

Action
PHARMACOLOGY: Inhibits HIV protease, the enzyme required to form functional proteins in HIV-infected patients.

PHARMACOKINETICS/DYNAMICS:
Absorption: Rapidly absorbed. T_{max} is 1 to 2 hr. C_{max} is approximately 7.66 mcg/mL. AUC_{0-12} is approximately 17.7 mcg•hr/mL. Oral solution is 14% less bioavailable than the capsules. Food high in fat decreased C_{max} and AUC, and increased T_{max}. Do not take with high-fat meals.

Distribution: Vd is approximately 430 L; approximately 90% protein bound (primarily alpha-1-acid glycoprotein).

Metabolism: Metabolized in the liver by CYP3A4.

Excretion: Less than 3% excreted unchanged by the kidney; approximately 14% of dose excreted in urine and approximately 75% excreted in the feces (more than 90% as metabolites). The $t_{1/2}$ is 7.1 to 10.6 hr.

Special Populations:
Renal Function Impairment – Oral solution contraindicated because of propylene glycol excipient.
Hepatic Function Impairment – Moderate cirrhosis increased AUC; severe cirrhosis increased AUC and C_{max}. Dosage reduction required for capsules. Oral solution is contraindicated in those with hepatic failure.
Children – Oral solution contraindicated because of propylene glycol excipient.

Indications
Treatment of HIV-1 infections in combination with other antiretroviral agents.

Contraindications
Concomitant therapies with cisapride, dihydroergotamine, ergotamine, ergonovine, methylergonovine, or pimozide; midazolam and triazolam; drugs that are highly dependent on CYP3A4 for clearance and for which elevated plasma levels are associated with serious or life-threatening events; when administered in combination with ritonavir, flecainide, and propafenone are contraindicated; hypersensitivity to any component of the product; because of the propylene glycol content, the oral solution is contraindicated in infants and children under 4 yr, pregnant women, patients with renal or hepatic failure, and patients treated with disulfiram or metronidazole.

Route/Dosage
ADULTS AND CHILDREN 13 TO 16 YR: **PO (capsules)** 1200 mg bid in combination with other antiretroviral agents.
ADULTS AND CHILDREN 13 TO 16 YR WITH WEIGHT 50 KG OR MORE: **PO** 1400 mg bid.
CHILDREN 4 TO 12 YR OR 13 TO 16 YR WITH WEIGHT LESS THAN 50 KG: **PO (capsules)** 20 mg/kg bid or 15 mg/kg tid (max, 2400 mg/day) in combination with other antiretroviral agents.
CHILDREN 4 TO 12 YR OR 13 TO 16 YR WITH WEIGHT LESS THAN 50 KG: **PO (oral solution)** 22.5 mg/kg (1.5 mL/kg) bid or 17 mg/kg (1.1 mL/kg) tid (max, 2800 mg) in combination with other antiretroviral agents.

Interactions
Abacavir, aldesleukin, azole antifungal agents (eg, itraconazole), cimetidine, clarithromycin, delavirdine, dexamethasone, didanosine, erythromycin, ethanol, indinavir, itraconazole, ritonavir, zidovudine: May increase amprenavir plasma levels.

Alprazolam, clorazepate, diazepam, flurazepam, midazolam, triazolam: Amprenavir may increase blood levels of these drugs, which may produce extreme sedation and respiratory depression.

Amiodarone, bepridil, cisapride, ergot derivatives, lidocaine (systemic), quinidine, rifabutin, sildenafil, tricyclic antidepressants: Amprenavir may elevate blood levels of these drugs, which may increase the risk of arrhythmias, hematologic abnormalities, seizures, or other potential serious adverse effects.

Amlodipine, atorvastatin, cerivastatin, carbamazepine, clozapine, cylcosporine, dapsone, diltiazem, erythromycin, felodipine, fentanyl, isradipine, itraconazole, ketoconazole, loratadine, lovastatin, nicardipine, nifedipine, nimodipine, oral contraceptives, pimozide, pravastatin, sildenafil, simvastatin, tacrolimus, tricyclic antidepressants (eg, amitriptyline), verapamil, zidovudine: May have their plasma concentrations increased, which could increase activity or toxicity.

Antacids, carbamazepine, efavirenz, methadone, oral contraceptives, phenobarbital, phenytoin, rifabutin, rifampin, St. John's wort: May decrease plasma levels of amprenavir, which may reduce antiviral activity.

Cisapride, dihydroergotamine, disulfiram, ergotamine, ergonovine, methylergonovine, midazolam, pimozide, triazolam: Use with amprenavir is contraindicated.

Ritonavir: Plasma levels may be decreased by amprenavir.

Warfarin: Risk of bleeding may be increased.

Lab Test Interferences None well documented.

Adverse Reactions
CNS: Depression; paresthesia.
DERM: Rash; pruritus; Stevens-Johnson syndrome.
GI: Nausea; vomiting; diarrhea; abdominal pain; taste disorders.
HEMA: Acute hemolytic anemia.
METAB: Hyperglycemia; hypertriglyceridemia; hypercholesterolemia.

> **WARNING:**
> *Oral solution:*
> *Propylene glycol excipient:* Risk of toxicity from large amount of excipient contraindicates use in children less than 4 yr and in certain other populations and used with caution in others. Only use when capsules or other protease inhibitors are not therapeutic options.

Precautions
Pregnancy: Category C.
Lactation: HIV-infected mothers should not breastfeed their infants.
Children: Safety and efficacy not established in children less than 4 yr.
Elderly: Select dose with caution, reflecting greater frequency of decreased hepatic, renal, or cardiac function and comorbidity.
Hepatic function impairment: Use with caution; decreased amprenavir clearance may occur.

PATIENT CARE CONSIDERATIONS
Administration/Storage
- Store at room temperature (25°C; 77°F).
- Do not interchange capsules and oral solution on a mg per mg basis as amprenavir capsules and oral solution are not directly interchangeable.
- Avoid a high-fat meal, as it will decrease absorption.
- Do not take supplemental vitamin E because amprenavir capsules and solution contain large amounts of vitamin E.

Assessment/Interventions
- Obtain patient history, including drug history and any known allergies.
- Monitor for signs of hypersensitivity (eg, fever, rash, fatigue, nausea, vomiting, diarrhea, abdominal pain, malaise, lethargy, myalgia, arthralgia, edema, shortness of breath, paresthesia).
- Discontinue use of medicine immediately if signs of hypersensitivity are present, and notify health care provider.
- Assess contraindications as amprenavir is metabolized by cytochrome P450 CYP3A4 enzyme system and serious and life-threatening drug/drug interactions can potentially occur.
- Monitor for adverse reactions including signs of Steven-Johnson syndrome, new-onset diabetes, and increased bleeding in patients with hemophilia.
- Monitor for elevation of LFTs, increased creatine, phosphokinase or creatinine, elevated triglycerides or cholesterol, and hyperglycemia.
- Monitor for blood glucose and triglyceride elevation, which may require adjustment in therapy for some patients (eg, patients with diabetes).
- Administer with caution to patients with hepatic impairment. Dosage may need to be adjusted.

Patient/Family Education
- Advise patient to take medication exactly as prescribed.
- Advise patient that if a dose is missed by more than 4 hr, wait and take the next dose at the regularly scheduled time; however, if the dose is missed by less than 4 hr, take the missed dose immediately.
- Inform patient that amprenavir is not a cure for HIV infection and that he/she may continue to develop opportunistic infections and

other complications associated with HIV disease.
- Tell patients that there are currently no data demonstrating that therapy with amprenavir can reduce the risk of transmitting HIV to others through sexual contact.
- The long-term effects of amprenavir are unknown at this time.
- Advise patient to inform primary health care provider of any sulfa allergy. The potential for cross-sensitivity between drugs in the sulfonamides and amprenavir is unknown.
- To avoid drug/drug interactions, advise patient to report to the health care provider if planning to use any other prescription or nonprescription medication.
- Instruct patients taking antacids or didanosine to take amprenavir at least 1 hr before or after the antacid or didanosine use.
- Advise patient receiving sildenafil that there may be an increased risk of sildenafil-associated adverse events including hypotension, visual changes, and priapism. Patient should promptly report any of these symptoms.
- Instruct patient receiving hormonal contraceptive to use alternate contraceptive measures during therapy with amprenavir.
- Instruct patient to avoid high-fat meals.
- Inform patient that redistribution or accumulation of body fat may occur while receiving protease inhibitors. The cause and long-term health effects of these conditions are unknown at this time.
- Advise women to contact health care provider if pregnant, planning to become pregnant, or breastfeeding.
- Advise mothers not to breastfeed because of the risk of transmitting HIV.
- Advise adult and pediatric patients not to take supplemental vitamin E.

Amyl Nitrite

(A-mill NYE-trite)

Class Antianginal

How Supplied
Amyl Nitrite Aspirols Inhalant 0.3 mL ♦ *Amyl Nitrite Vaporole* Inhalant 0.3 mL

Action
PHARMACOLOGY: Relaxes smooth muscle of venous and arterial vasculature.

PHARMACOKINETICS/DYNAMICS:
Excretion: Approximately 33% excreted in the urine.
Onset: 0.5 min
Duration: 3 to 5 min.

Indications Relief of angina pectoris.

Contraindications Hypersensitivity to nitrates; pregnancy; severe anemia; closed-angle glaucoma; orthostatic hypotension; head trauma; cerebral hemorrhage.

Route/Dosage
ADULT: **Inhalation** 0.3 mL prn. 1 to 6 inhalations from 1 capsule are usually sufficient. May be repeated in 3 to 5 min.

Interactions
Alcohol: Severe hypotension and cardiovascular collapse may occur.
Aspirin: Increased nitrate concentration and actions may occur.
Calcium channel blockers: Symptomatic orthostatic hypotension may occur.
Heparin: Effects of heparin may be decreased.

Lab Test Interferences May cause false report of reduced serum cholesterol with Zlatkis-Zak color reaction.

Adverse Reactions
CV: Tachycardia; palpitations; hypotension; syncope; arrhythmias; edema.
CNS: Headache; apprehension; weakness; vertigo; dizziness; agitation; insomnia.
DERM: Cutaneous vasodilation with flushing.
EENT: Blurred vision.
GI: Nausea; vomiting; diarrhea; dyspepsia.
GU: Dysuria; impotence.
HEMA: Methemoglobinemia; hemolytic anemia.
RESP: Bronchitis; pneumonia.
OTHER: Arthralgia; perspiration; pallor; cold sweat.

Precautions
Pregnancy: Category X.
Lactation: Contraindicated.
Children: Safety and efficacy not established.
Angina: May aggravate angina caused by hypertrophic cardiomyopathy.
Drug abuse: May be abused for sexual stimulation or for effects of lightheadedness, dizziness, and euphoria.
Glaucoma: May increase intraocular pressure.
Orthostatic hypotension: May occur even with small doses; alcohol accentuates this reaction.
Withdrawal: Dose is gradually reduced to prevent withdrawal reaction.

Overdosage: Signs and Symptoms
Severe headache, severe hypotension, flushing, tachycardia, vertigo, confusion, syncope, nausea, slow breathing or dyspnea, cyanosis, metabolic acidosis, convulsions, coma, death.

PATIENT CARE CONSIDERATIONS
Administration/Storage
- Help patient into sitting or reclining position.
- Crush capsule, wave under patient's nose and instruct to breathe deeply; 1 to 6 inhalations are usually sufficient. May repeat in 3 to 5 min.
- Keep capsules in original container and keep container tightly closed.

Assessment/Interventions
- Obtain patient history, including drug history and any known allergies.
- Assess current status of cardiac, renal and hepatic function.
- Assess vital signs, especially BP and pulse. Also assess for signs of tolerance to or abuse of the product.
- Evaluate relief of symptoms and monitor for any adverse effects such as GI symptoms, headache, tachycardia, postural hypotension, skin flushing, rash, or possible arrhythmia.
- Note any changes in serum cholesterol levels.

Patient/Family Education
- Caution patient that this medication must not be taken during pregnancy or when pregnancy is possible. Advise patient to use reliable form of birth control while taking this drug.
- Advise use of acetaminophen for relief of headache.
- Show patient how to crush capsule. Remind patient not to remove cloth-like covering.
- Show patient how to keep record of usage, including frequency, dosage, and level of pain relief.
- Explain potential for abuse.
- Instruct patient to report these symptoms to health care provider: blurred vision, dry mouth or persistent headache occurs or symptoms are not relieved.
- Caution patient to avoid sudden position changes to prevent orthostatic hypotension.
- Instruct patient to avoid intake of alcoholic beverages or other CNS depressants and aspirin.

Anagrelide

(an-AGG-reh-lide)

Class Antiplatelet agent

How Supplied
Agrylin Capsules 0.5 mg, Capsules 1 mg

Action
PHARMACOLOGY: Mechanism is under investigation. Studies support a hypothesis of dose-related reduction in platelet production resulting from a decrease in megakaryocyte hypermaturation.

PHARMACOKINETICS/DYNAMICS:
Absorption: Food reduced AUC 13.8% and the C_{max} approximately 45% and increased the T_{max} 2 hr.
Metabolism: Extensively metabolized.
Excretion: More than 70% of dose recovered in urine with less than 1% recovered as anagrelide. Plasma t½ is 1.3 hr (fasting state) and 1.8 hr (fed state).

Indications Thrombocythemia caused by myeloproliferative disorders; to reduce elevated platelet count and risk of thrombotic events; to relieve associated symptoms, including thrombohemorrhagic events.

Contraindications Standard considerations.

Route/Dosage
Thrombocythemia
ADULTS (INITIAL DOSE): **PO** 0.5 mg qid or 1 mg bid for at least 7 days. Titrate to minimum effective dose required to maintain platelet count less than 600,000 cells/mcL, or within normal range. Avoid dosage increases more than 0.5 mg/day in any 1-wk period. The max recommended dose is 10 mg/day or 2.5 mg/dose.

Interactions
Sucralfate: May reduce the oral absorption of anagrelide.

Lab Test Interferences None well documented.

Adverse Reactions
CV: Palpitations (26%); chest pain, tachycardia (8%); arrhythmia, hemorrhage, CV disease, angina pectoris, heart failure, postural hypotension, vasodilation, hypertension, syncope, thrombosis (1% to less than 5%).
CNS: Headache (44%); asthenia (23%); dizziness (15%); paresthesia (6%); depression, somnolence, confusion, insomnia, nervousness, amnesia, migraine (1% to less than 5%).
DERM: Rash (including urticaria [8%]); pruritus (6%); skin disease, alopecia (1% to less than 5%).
EENT: Pharyngitis (7%); rhinitis, epistaxis, amblyopia, abnormal vision, tinnitus, visual field abnormality, diplopia (1% to less than 5%).
GI: Diarrhea (26%); nausea (17%); abdominal pain (16%); flatulence; vomiting (10%); anorexia (8%); dyspepsia (5%); GI distress or hemorrhage, constipation, gastritis, melena, aphthous stomatitis, eructation (1% to less than 5%).
GU: Dysuria, hematuria (1% to less than 5%).

HEMA/LYMPH: Anemia, thrombocytopenia, ecchymosis, lymphadenopathy (1% to less than 5%).
LABTESTABS: Elevated liver enzymes (1% to less than 5%).
M/N: Edema (21%); peripheral edema (9%); dehydration (1% to less than 5%).
MUSC: Back pain (6%); arthralgia, myalgia, leg cramps (1% to less than 5%).
RESP: Dyspnea (12%); cough (6%); respiratory disease, sinusitis, pneumonia, bronchitis, asthma (1% to less than 5%).
OTHER: Pain (15%); fever (9%); malaise (6%); flu-like symptoms, chills, photosensitivity (1% to less than 5%).

Precautions
Pregnancy: Category C.
Lactation: Undetermined.
Children: The safety and efficacy of anagrelide in patients younger than 16 yr of age not established.
Renal function impairment: Patients with renal insufficiency (creatinine at least 2 mg/dL) receive anagrelide when the potential benefits of therapy outweigh the potential risks. Monitor patients closely for signs of renal toxicity.
Hepatic function impairment: Patients with evidence of hepatic dysfunction (bilirubin, AST, or measures of liver function more than 1.5 times the upper limits of normal) receive anagrelide when the potential benefits of therapy outweigh the potential risks. Monitor patients closely for signs of hepatic toxicity.
CV: Use with caution in known or suspected heart disease because anagrelide may have positive inotropic effects. Monitor ECG and systolic ejection fraction at baseline and periodically during treatment.
Thrombocytopenia: Thrombocytopenia, which promptly recovers upon discontinuation, may occur.

Overdosage: Signs and Symptoms
Thrombocytopenia, which can potentially cause bleeding, cardiac and CNS toxicity.

PATIENT CARE CONSIDERATIONS
Administration/Storage
* Administer prescribed dose without regard to meals. Administer with food if GI upset occurs.
* Do not increase dose by more than 0.5 mg in any 1 wk.
* Do not administer more than 10 mg/day or 2.5 mg in a single dose.
* Store at controlled room temperature (59° to 77°F).

Assessment/Interventions
* Obtain patient history, including drug history and any known allergies. Note renal impairment, liver disease, or suspected or known heart disease.
* Ensure women of childbearing potential are not pregnant when therapy is started and that effective contraception is being used during therapy.
* Ensure a CV exam is performed before therapy is started.
* Ensure patient with renal insufficiency (serum creatinine of 2 mg/dL or greater) is closely monitored for signs of renal toxicity during therapy.
* Ensure patient with hepatic dysfunction (eg, elevated bilirubin or liver enzymes) is closely monitored for signs of hepatic toxicity during therapy.
* Ensure platelet counts are determined q 2 days for the first week of therapy and then at least weekly thereafter until the maintenance dose is reached.
* Be prepared to reduce the dose or discontinue therapy if thrombocytopenia (platelet count less than 100,000/mcL) develops.
* Ensure blood counts (WBC and hemoglobin), renal function (serum creatinine, BUN), and liver function (liver enzymes) are evaluated frequently while the platelet count is being lowered (usually first 2 wk of therapy).
* Monitor patient for GI, CNS, CV, MUSC, and general body side effects. Report to health care provider if noted and significant. Immediately report bleeding or unusual bruising, unexplained shortness of breath, difficulty breathing, palpitations, rapid or irregular heartbeat, or swelling of the feet or ankles.

Patient/Family Education
* Explain name, dose, action, and potential side effects of drug.
* Advise patient that dose of medication may be adjusted to obtain max benefit.
* Advise patient that each dose may be taken without regard to meals but to take with food if stomach upset occurs.
* Advise patient that if a dose is missed to skip that dose and take the next dose at the regularly scheduled time.
* Instruct patient not to change the dose or stop taking unless advised by health care provider.
* Instruct patient to immediately contact health care provider of the following: bleeding or unusual bruising, unexplained shortness of breath, difficulty breathing, palpitations,

rapid or irregular heartbeat, swelling of the feet or ankles.
- Advise patient to notify health care provider if persistent diarrhea, nausea, stomach pain, frequent vomiting, intolerable headache, or other unexplained feelings or symptoms occur.
- Advise patient that medication may cause photosensitivity (sensitivity to sunlight) and to avoid unnecessary exposure to sunlight or tanning lamps, and to use sunscreens and wear protective clothing until tolerance is determined.
- Advise women of childbearing potential that medication can harm a developing fetus and to use effective contraception during therapy.
- Advise women to notify health care provider if pregnant, planning to become pregnant, or breastfeeding.
- Caution patient not to take any prescription or OTC medications, herbal preparations, or dietary supplements unless advised by health care provider.
- Advise patient that follow-up visits and laboratory tests will be required to monitor therapy and to keep appointments.

Anakinra

(an-a-KIN-ra)
Class Immunomodulator
How Supplied
Kineret Solution 100 mg per 0.67 mL
Action
PHARMACOLOGY: Blocks the biologic activity of interleukin-1 (IL-1) by competitively inhibiting IL-1 binding to interleukin-1 type I receptor, which is expressed in a wide variety of organs and tissues.
PHARMACOKINETICS/DYNAMICS:
Absorption: Bioavailability is 95%; T_{max} is 3 to 7 hr.
Excretion: The t½ is 4 to 6 hr.
Special Populations:
Renal Function Impairment – Mean plasma Cl decreased 70% to 75% in those with Ccr less than 30 mL/min.
Indications Reduction in signs and symptoms and slowing the progression of structural damage in moderately to severely active rheumatoid arthritis in patients who have failed at least 1 disease-modifying antirheumatic drug.
Contraindications Hypersensitivity to *Escherichia coli*-derived proteins, anakinra, or any component of product.
Route/Dosage
ADULTS: **Subcutaneous** 100 mg/day.
Renal Function Impairment
Subcutaneous 100 mg every other day for severe renal impairment (Ccr less than 30 mL/min).

Interactions None well documented.
Lab Test Interferences None well documented.
Adverse Reactions
CNS: Headache (12%).
EENT: Sinusitis (7%).
GI: Nausea (8%); diarrhea (7%); abdominal pain (5%).
HEMA: Neutropenia.
LOCAL: Injection site reaction (71%).
RESP: Upper respiratory tract infection (14%).
OTHER: Worsening of rheumatoid arthritis (19%); arthralgia, flu-like symptoms (6%); hypersensitivity, serious infections (eg, cellulitis, pneumonia, bone and joint 3%]).
Precautions
Pregnancy: Category B.
Lactation: Undetermined.
Children: Safety and efficacy not established.
Elderly: Use with caution because of higher rate of infection in this population.
Renal function impairment: Because anakinra is substantially excreted by the kidneys, risk of toxicity is increased in patients with impaired renal function.
Hematologic: Decreased neutrophil count may occur.
Infection: Serious infections may occur.
Vaccinations: Do not give live vaccines concomitantly.

PATIENT CARE CONSIDERATIONS

Administration/Storage
- Medication is provided in prefilled syringes only.
- Dose is administered daily.
- Administer via subcutaneous route only at about the same time daily.
- Rotate injection sites (eg, thigh, abdomen, upper arm). Give new injection at least 1 inch from old site and never into areas where the skin is tender, bruised, red, or hard.
- Do not use prefilled syringe if particulate matter, cloudiness, or discoloration is noted.
- Disease-modifying antirheumatic drugs (except etanercept), glucocorticoids, salicylates, NSAIDs, and analgesics may be continued during treatment with anakinra.
- Discard any unused portion. Do not save unused solution for later administration.

- Store prefilled syringes in refrigerator (36° to 46°F). Do not freeze or shake. Protect from light.

Assessment/Interventions

- Obtain patient history, including drug history and any known allergies. Note any findings suggestive of active infection. Note history of allergy to *E. coli*-derived proteins, renal impairment, immunosuppression, or recurrent infections.
- Document baseline disease state activity (eg, number of tender or swollen joints, pain, disability). Reassess periodically to document response to therapy.
- Ensure that dosage reduction (ie, dose given every other day instead of daily) is considered in patient with severe renal insufficiency (Ccr less than 30 mL/min).
- Ensure that neutrophil count is assessed prior to starting therapy, then monthly for 3 mo, and thereafter quarterly for a period of up to 1 yr.
- Monitor patient for signs and symptoms of infection (eg, persistent fever, sore throat, cellulitis). Immediately report to health care provider if noted. Be prepared to discontinue therapy if a serious infection develops or is suspected.
- Monitor patient for signs and symptoms of anaphylactic or serious allergic reactions. Be prepared to treat appropriately.
- Monitor patient for CNS, GI, general body side effects, and injection site reactions. Report to health care provider if noted and significant.
- Do not administer live virus vaccines to patient receiving anakinra.

Patient/Family Education

- Explain name, dose, action, and potential side effects of drug.
- If patient or caregiver is administering at home, provide the *Information for Patients and Caregivers* insert. Ensure that the patient or caregiver understands how to store, prepare, and administer the dose, and how to dispose of used equipment and supplies. Perform the first injection under the supervision of a qualified health professional.
- Advise patient to administer daily at about the same time.
- Caution patient to discard any unused portions and not to save unused drug for later administration.
- Advise patient to continue other arthritis medications as recommended by health care provider.
- Advise patient or caregiver that beneficial effects develop slowly and may take up to 12 wk to occur.
- Advise patient to immediately report any of the following to health care provider: fever or other signs of infection, sore throat, unusual bruising or bleeding, rash, hives, sudden shortness of breath.
- Advise patient to report intolerable injection site reactions or unusual symptoms to health care provider.
- Advise women to notify health care provider if pregnant, planning to become pregnant, or breastfeeding.
- Instruct patient not to take any prescription or OTC medications, herbal preparations, or dietary supplements unless advised by health care provider.
- Remind patient that office visits and laboratory tests will be required to monitor therapy and to keep appointments.

Anastrozole

(an-ASS-troe-zole)

Class Nonsteroidal aromatase inhibitor

How Supplied
Arimidex Tablets for oral use 1 mg

Action
PHARMACOLOGY: A selective nonsteroidal aromatase inhibitor. It lowers serum estradiol concentrations.

PHARMACOKINETICS/DYNAMICS:
Distribution: 40% protein bound.
Metabolism: Metabolized in the liver (N-dealkylation, hydroxylation, and glucuronidation).
Excretion: $T_{\frac{1}{2}}$ is approximately 50 hr; approximately 10% is excreted in the urine as unchanged drug within 72 hr and approximately 60% is excreted in the urine as metabolites.

Special Populations:
Renal Function Impairment – Renal clearance decreased proportionally with Ccr and was approximately 50% lower in those with severe renal impairment (Ccr less than 30 mL/min/ 1.73 m^2); however, this did not influence total body clearance.
Hepatic Function Impairment – Oral clearance was approximately 30% lower in those with stable hepatic cirrhosis but plasma concentrations were within normal range.

Indications Advanced breast cancer in postmenopausal women with progression following tamoxifen therapy; first-line treatment of postmenopausal women with hormone receptor positive or hormone receptor unknown locally advanced or metastatic breast cancer.

Contraindications None well documented.

Route/Dosage
Breast Cancer
ADULTS: **PO** 1 mg qd.

Interactions No significant drug interactions have been noted. May reduce blood estradiol levels. This may affect the efficacy of oral contraceptives.

Lab Test Interferences Elevations of GGT levels have been observed among patients with liver metastases.

Adverse Reactions
CV: Hypertension; thrombophlebitis; edema; vasodilation; chest pain.
CNS: Asthenia; headache; paresthesias; somnolence; confusion; insomnia; anxiety; dizziness; depression; hypertonia; lethargy; paresthesia.
DERM: Alopecia; pruritus; rash; sweating.
GI: Low to moderate potential for nausea and vomiting; diarrhea; constipation; anorexia; increased LFTs (GGT, AST, ALT); GI disturbances; abdominal pain; dry mouth.
GU: UTIs; vaginal dryness; menstrual bleeding; sexual inactivity; atrophy of the female reproductive organs; pregnancy loss; pelvic pain.
RESP: Dyspnea; sinusitis; bronchitis; cough increased; pharyngitis.
OTHER: Myalgia; arthralgia; breast pain; hot flashes; pain; back pain; peripheral edema; bone pain; flu-syndrome; tumor flare; weight gain; leukorrhea; edema.

Precautions
Pregnancy: Category D.
Lactation: Exercise caution when administering to a breastfeeding woman.
Children: Safety and efficacy not established.
Estrogen receptor negative: Patients who did not respond to tamoxifen rarely respond to anastrozole.

PATIENT CARE CONSIDERATIONS

Administration/Storage
* Administer prescribed dose qd without regard to meals. Administer with food if GI upset occurs.
* Store tablets at controlled room temperature.

Assessment/Interventions
* Obtain patient history, including drug history and any known allergies.
* Ensure that patient of childbearing potential has negative pregnancy test before starting therapy.
* Monitor patient for CV, GI, CNS, RESP, and general body side effects. Report to health care provider if noted and significant.
* Notify health care provider of pain, swelling, redness or warmth in calves; sudden severe headache; visual disturbances; or weakness or numbness of arms or legs.

Patient/Family Education
* Explain name, dose, action, and potential side effects of drug.
* Advise patient to take 1 tablet qd.
* Advise patient that medication can be taken without regard to meals, but to take with food if GI upset occurs.
* Advise patient that if a dose is missed, take it as soon as possible, but if close to the next dose, do not double the dose to catch up, and take the next dose as scheduled.
* Instruct patient to immediately report any of the following to the health care provider: pain in groin or calves; sharp chest pain or sudden shortness of breath; sudden severe headache; dizziness or fainting; vision or speech problems; weakness or numbness of arms or legs.
* Advise patient that drug may cause dizziness and to use caution while driving or performing other tasks requiring mental alertness.
* Instruct women of child bearing potential to notify health care provider if pregnant, planning to become pregnant, or breastfeeding.
* Instruct patient not to take any prescription or OTC medications or dietary supplements unless advised to do so by their health care provider.
* Advise patient that follow-up examinations and lab tests will be required to monitor therapy and to keep appointments.

Anistreplase

(uh-NISS-truh-place)

Class Thrombolytic enzyme

How Supplied
Eminase Powder for injection, lyophilized 30 units (potency is expressed in units of anistreplase by using a reference standard that is specific for anistreplase and is not comparable with units used for other fibrinolytics)

Action
PHARMACOLOGY: Aids in dissolution of blood clots.

PHARMACOKINETICS/DYNAMICS:
Metabolism: Deacylation of anistreplase forms

lys-plasminogen-streptokinase activator complex (active).

Excretion: $T_{1/2}$ of fibrolytic activity is approximately 94 min.

Indications Lysis of obstructing coronary thrombi for management of acute MI.

Contraindications Hypersensitivity to streptokinase; active internal bleeding; history of cerebrovascular accident; recent (within 2 mo) intracranial or intraspinal surgery or trauma; intracranial neoplasm; arteriovenous malformation or aneurysm; known bleeding diathesis; uncontrolled hypertension.

Route/Dosage
ADULTS: IV 30 U over 2 to 5 min into IV line or vein.

Interactions
Anticoagulants (eg, heparin, warfarin) and antiplatelet agents (eg, aspirin, dipyridamole): May increase risk of bleeding.
INCOMPATIBILITIES: Do not add to any infusion fluids. Do not add other medications to vial or syringe containing anistreplase.

Lab Test Interferences Can cause decreases in plasminogen and fibrinogen levels and increases in thrombin time, activated partial thromboplastin time and prothrombin time, making results of coagulation tests unreliable.

Adverse Reactions
CV: Arrhythmia and conduction disorders; hypotension.
HEMA: Bleeding at puncture site, nonpuncture-site hematoma; hematuria; hemoptysis; GI hemorrhage; intracranial bleeding; mouth and gum hemorrhage; epistaxis; ocular hemorrhage; nonspecific hemorrhage.

Precautions
Pregnancy: Category C.
Lactation: Undetermined.
Children: Safety and efficacy not established.
Hypersensitivity: Rarely anaphylactic and anaphylactoid reactions (with bronchospasm or angioedema) may occur.
Readministration: Because of formation of antistreptokinase antibody, anistreplase may not be effective if administered more than 5 day to 6 mo after prior anistreplase or streptokinase therapy or after streptococcal infection.

PATIENT CARE CONSIDERATIONS

Administration/Storage
- Reconstitute powder with 5 mL of Sterile Water for Injection. Do not shake vial during reconstitution; try to minimize foaming. Do not further dilute reconstituted anistreplase.
- Administer 30 U of anistreplase by IV injection over 2 to 5 min.
- Store lyophilized anistreplase under refrigeration.
- Discard any reconstituted anistreplase not administered within 30 min of reconstitution.

Assessment/Interventions
- Obtain patient history, including drug history and any known allergies.
- Identify factors that may contribute to bleeding risk, including baseline coagulation, and fibrinolytic activity test results.
- Determine if and when previous fibrinolytic therapy was administered.
- Have epinephrine and emergency treatment provisions available during administration of anistreplase.
- Avoid nonessential handling of patient during anistreplase therapy.
- If arterial puncture is necessary after administration of anistreplase, it is preferable to use upper extremity vessel that is accessible to manual compression. Apply pressure dressing; check puncture site frequently for evidence of bleeding. Control minor bleeding with manual pressure.
- Remember that allergic-type reactions may occur in milder forms up to 1 to 2 wk after therapy.
- Evaluate data from cardiac monitoring, and report any arrhythmias.
- Monitor diligently for signs or symptoms of internal or surface bleeding. Remember that lab values for coagulation tests and measurements of fibrinolytic activity after anistreplase therapy may be unreliable.
- Monitor vital signs, especially BP and pulse, because severe hypotension may occur.

Patient/Family Education
- Explain to patient the need for bedrest and minimal handling of patient.
- Instruct patient to report the following symptoms to health care provider: bruising, bleeding, hypersensitivity reactions (eg, urticaria, flushing, itching, rashes).
- Caution patient to avoid sudden position changes to prevent orthostatic hypotension.

Anti-thymocyte Globulin (Rabbit)

(an-tee-THIGH-moe-site GLAH-byoo-lin)
Class Leporine (rabbit) polyclonal antibody

How Supplied
Thymoglobulin Powder for injection 25 mg vials

Action
PHARMACOLOGY: Mechanism of action is not fully understood. Possible mechanisms include the following: T-cell Cl from the circulation and modulation of T-cell activation, homing, and cytotoxic activities.

PHARMACOKINETICS/DYNAMICS:
Excretion: The t½ is 2 to 3 days.

Indications Treatment of acute allograft rejection in renal transplantation.

Contraindications Acute viral illness; hypersensitivity to leporine proteins; previous hypersensitivity to anti-thymocyte globulin.

Route/Dosage
Acute Renal Graft Rejection
ADULTS: **IV** 1.5 mg/kg/day for 7 to 14 days using a high-flow vein. Infuse over a minimum of 6 hr for first infusion and over at least 4 hr for subsequent doses.

Dosage Adjustment
ADULTS: **IV** Reduce 50% if the WBC is between 2,000 and 3,000 cells/mm³ or if the platelet count is between 50,000 and 75,000 cells/mm³. Consider stopping treatment if the WBC falls below 2,000 cells/mm³ or platelets below 50,000 cell/mm³.

Interactions
Immunosuppressants (antineoplastic agents, corticosteroids, cyclosporines) Risk of infection may increase.

Lab Test Interferences May interfere with rabbit antibody-based immunoassays and with cross-match or panel-reactive antibody cytotoxicity assays.

Adverse Reactions
CV: Hypertension (37%); tachycardia (27%).
CNS: Headache (40%); asthenia (27%); malaise (13%); dizziness (9%).
GI: Abdominal pain (38%); diarrhea, nausea (37%).
HEMA/LYMPH: Leukopenia (57%); thrombocytopenia (37%).
HYPERSEN: Anaphylaxis.
LABTESTABS: Hyperkalemia (27%).
RESP: Dyspnea (28%).
OTHER: Fever (63%); chills (57%); pain (46%); infection (37%); peripheral edema (34%).

Precautions
Pregnancy: Category C.
Lactation: Undetermined.
Children: Safety and efficacy not established.
Hypersensitivity: Anaphylaxis may occur.
Antibodies: Human anti-rabbit antibodies develop in 68% of patients.
Extravasation: Local irritation or phlebitis may occur. Refer to your institution specific protocol.

Overdosage: Signs and Symptoms
Leukopenia, thrombocytopenia.

PATIENT CARE CONSIDERATIONS

Administration/Storage

- For administration by IV infusion only. Not for intradermal, subcutaneous, IM, IV bolus, or intra-arterial administration.
- Premedicate with corticosteroids, acetaminophen, and/or antihistamine 1 hr before infusion of anti-thymocyte globulin as ordered.
- Allow vials to reach room temperature before reconstitution.
- Reconstitute each vial of powder for injection using 5 mL of supplied diluent (sterile water for injection) following manufacturer's guidelines. Do not shake vial during reconstitution. Gently rotate vial until powder is completely dissolved. Resulting solution provides 5 mg/mL of anti-thymocyte globulin.
- Transfer contents of appropriate number of reconstituted vials into bag of saline or dextrose infusion solution (recommended volume of 50 mL infusion solution per vial of anti-thymocyte globulin). Mix solution by gently inverting infusion bag once or twice.
- Do not administer if solution is discolored, cloudy, turbid, or if particulate matter is noted.
- Administer prescribed dose through a 0.22 micron filter into a high-flow vein.
- To reduce infusion-related adverse effects (eg, fever, chills) infuse first dose over no less than 6 hr and subsequent doses over no less than 4 hr. Infusion rate may be further slowed if infusion-related reactions occur.
- Store unopened vials in refrigerator (36° to 46°F). Protect from light and freezing. Use reconstituted vials within 4 hr. Diluted infusion solution must be used immediately. Discard any unused solution. Do not save unused solution for future use.

Assessment/Interventions

- Obtain patient history, including drug history and any known allergies. Note acute viral

illness, or history of allergy or anaphylaxis to rabbit proteins.
- Ensure lymphocyte count (total lymphocyte and/or T-cell subsets) is monitored during treatment to assess degree of T-cell depletion.
- Ensure CBC and differential are determined at baseline and periodically during course of therapy. Reduce anti-thymocyte dose by one-half if WBC is between 2,000 and 3,000 cells/mm^3, or if platelet count is between 50,000 and 75,000 cells /mm^3. Be prepared to discontinue treatment if WBC falls below 2,000 cells/mm^3, or if platelet count falls below 50,000 cells /mm^3.
- Implement infection control measures if WBC drops; implement bleeding precautions if platelet count drops.
- Ensure resuscitation equipment is readily available during infusion of anti-thymocyte immune globulin.
- Monitor patient for signs of anaphylaxis or severe allergic reaction. Discontinue therapy and immediately notify health care provider if noted. Be prepared to treat appropriately.
- Ensure that potential value of antiviral, antibacterial, antiprotozoal, and/or antifungal prophylaxis has been evaluated.
- Monitor patient for CV, GI, CNS, RESP, general body side effects, and infusion site reactions. Inform health care provider if noted and significant.

Patient/Family Education
- Explain name, actions, and potential side effects of the treatment regimen. Review the treatment regimen including dosing schedule, duration of treatment, and monitoring that will be required.
- Advise patient, family, or caregiver that medication will be prepared and administered by health care provider in a health care setting.
- Advise patient, family, or caregiver that medication will be used in combination with other agents to achieve max benefit possible.
- Advise patient, family, or caregiver to immediately report any of the following to health care provider: rash; itching; hives; difficulty breathing; fever, chills, or other signs of infection; bleeding or unusual bruising; pain, redness, or swelling at injection site.
- Advise patient, family, or caregiver that after discharge frequent follow-up visits and laboratory tests will be required to monitor therapy and to keep appointments.

Antipyrine/Benzocaine/Glycerin Dehydrated

(ann-tee-PIE-reen/BEN-zoe-caine/GLIH-suh-rin)

Class Otic

How Supplied
Auralgan Liquid 14 mg benzocaine/54 mg antipyrine/mL

Action
PHARMACOLOGY: Decongestant/Analgesic

Indications Treatment of acute otitis media of various etiologies; removal of cerumen.

Contraindications Perforated tympanic membrane; hypersensitivity to any of the components or related substances.

PATIENT CARE CONSIDERATIONS
Administration/Storage
- For otic use only. Not for oral, nasal, or ocular use.
- Instill prescribed number of drops into external ear canal as directed using supplied dropper, then insert cotton pledget moistened with solution.
- Do not touch ear with dropper.
- Do not rinse dropper after use.
- Store at controlled room temperature (59° to 86°F). Protect from light and heat.

Route/Dosage
Acute Otitis Media
ADULTS AND CHILDREN: **OTIC** Instill solution to run along the wall of the ear canal until filled, then insert cotton pledget moistened with the otic solution into meatus. Repeat every 1 to 2 hr until pain and congestion is relieved.

Removal of Cerumen
ADULTS AND CHILDREN: **OTIC** Instill solution 3 times/day for 2 or 3 days.

Interactions None well documented.

Lab Test Interferences None well documented.

Precautions
Pregnancy: Category C.
Lactation: Undetermined.

Assessment/Interventions
- Obtain patient history, including drug history and any known allergies. Note presence of perforated tympanic membrane.
- Monitor patient for relief of symptoms.
- Monitor patient for sensitization or irritation and report to health care provider if noted.

Patient/Family Education
- Explain name, dose, action, and potential side effects of medication.

- Remind patient, family, or caregiver that medication is for use in the ear only.
- Teach patient proper technique for instilling ear drops: wash hands; do not allow dropper to touch ear. Tilt head to side or lie on side; instill prescribed number of drops; moisten cotton pledget and insert into ear canal; replace dropper.
- Advise patient, family, or caregiver to only use supplied dropper and to not rinse dropper after use.
- Advise patient, family, or caregiver to notify health care provider if symptoms do not improve or if irritation, inflammation, or itching of ear canal is noted.
- Advise patient, family, or caregiver that follow-up examinations may be required to monitor therapy and to keep appointments.

Apraclonidine

(app-rah-KLOE-nih-deen)

Class Sympathomimetic

How Supplied
Iopidine Solution 0.5%, Solution 1%
🍁 *Iopidine 0.5%* ♦ *Iopidine 1%*

Action
PHARMACOLOGY: Relatively selective ophthalmic alpha-adrenergic agonist, used to reduce intraocular pressure (IOP) and has minimal effect on cardiovascular parameters.

Indications
1% solution: Control or prevent postsurgical elevations in IOP that occur in patients after argon laser trabeculoplasty or iridotomy.
0.5% solution: Short-term adjunctive therapy in patients on maximally tolerated medical therapy who require additional IOP reduction.

Contraindications Hypersensitivity to any component of this medication or to clonidine; concurrent monoamine oxidase inhibitor therapy.

Route/Dosage

0.5% SOLUTION

Ophthalmic Instill 1 to 2 drops in affected eye(s) 3 times daily. Apraclondine 0.5% will be used with other ocular glaucoma therapies, use approximately 5 min interval between instillation of each medication to prevent washout of previous dose.

1% SOLUTION

Ophthalmic Instill 1 drop in scheduled operative eye 1 hr before initiating anterior segment laser surgery. Instill second drop into same eye immediately upon completion of surgery.

Interactions Drugs that may interact include cardiovascular agents and MAOIs. May potentiate effects on pulse and blood pressure.

Lab Test Interferences None well documented.

Adverse Reactions
CNS: Decreased libido; depression; dizziness; dream disturbance; headache; insomnia; irritability; nervousness; somnolence.
CV: Arrhythmia; Asthenia; bradycardia; palpitations; orthostatic episode; peripheral edema.
EENT: Abnormal vision; blanching; blurred vision; burning; conjunctivitis; discharge; discomfort; dry eye; edema; hyperemia; lid edema; lid margin crusting; mydriasis; pruritus; photophobia; tearing.
GI: Abdominal pain; constipation; diarrhea; dry mouth; nausea.
RESP: Asthma; dry nose; dyspnea; pharyngitis; sinusitis.
OTHER: Abnormal coordination; body heat sensation; chest pain; contact dermatitis; fatigue; shortness of breath; taste perversion.

Precautions
Pregnancy: Category C.
Lactation: Consider discontinuing nursing for the day when apraclonidine is used.
Children: Safety and efficacy not established.
Cardiovascular: Use 0.5% with caution in patients with severe cardiovascular disease of hypertension. Use 1% with caution in patients with recent MI, cerebral vascular disease, coronary insufficiency, chronic renal failure, and Reynaud disease.
Depression: Infrequently associated with depression.
IOP reduction: Monitor patients for exaggerated reduction.

Aprepitant

(ap-REH-pih-tant)

Class Antiemetic

How Supplied
Emend Capsules 80 mg, Capsules 125 mg

Action
PHARMACOLOGY: Selective high-affinity antagonist of human substance P/neurokinin 1 receptors.

PHARMACOKINETICS/DYNAMICS:
Absorption: The bioavailability is approximately 60% to 65%. Following doses of 125 mg

on day 1 and 80 mg on days 2 and 3, the mean C_{max} occurs at approximately 4 hr and reaches about 1.5 mcg/mL.

Distribution: Plasma protein binding is greater than 95%. The mean Vd_{ss} is approximately 70 L. Aprepitant crosses the blood-brain barrier.

Metabolism: Data indicate aprepitant is extensively metabolized by CYP3A4 and to a lesser degree by CYP1A2.

Excretion: Following IV administration of a single 100 mg dose, 57% was excreted in the urine and 45% in the feces.

Indications In combination with other antiemetic agents for the prevention of acute and delayed nausea and vomiting associated with initial and repeat courses of highly emetogenic cancer chemotherapy, including high-dose cisplatin.

Contraindications Coadministration of pimozide or cisapride, hypersensitivity to any component of the product.

Route/Dosage

ADULTS: **PO** 125 mg 1 hr prior to chemotherapy treatment on day 1 and 80 mg/day in the morning on days 2 and 3.

Interactions

CYP3A4 inhibitors (eg, clarithromycin, diltiazem, itraconazole, ketoconazole, nefazodone, nelfinavir, ritonavir, troleandomycin): Plasma concentrations of aprepitant may be elevated, increasing the risk of side effects.

CYP3A4 inducers (eg, carbamazepine, phenytoin, rifampin): Plasma concentrations of aprepitant may be reduced, decreasing the therapeutic effect.

Paroxetine: Paroxetine and aprepitant AUC and C_{max} may be decreased by approximately 25% and 20%, respectively.

CYP2C9 substrates (eg, phenytoin, tolbutamide, warfarin): Plasma concentrations of these agents may be reduced. In patients receiving warfarin, monitor the INR in the 2-wk period (especially at 7 to 10 days) after starting aprepitant therapy.

CYP3A4 substrates (eg, alprazolam, cisapride, dexamethasone, docetaxel, etoposide, ifosfamide, imatinib, irinotecan, ketoconazole, methylprednisolone; midazolam, paclitaxel, pimozide, vinblastine, vincristine, vinorelbine): Plasma concentrations of these agents may be increased. Cisapride and pimozide are contraindicated with coadministration of aprepitant. The dose of dexamethasone should be reduced approximately 50%, the IV and oral dose of methylprednisolone should be reduced by 25% and 50%, respectively, when given with aprepitant.

Oral contraceptives: Because the efficacy of oral contraceptives may be reduced, patients may need an alternative or additional, nonhormonal, contraceptive.

Lab Test Interferences None well documented.

Adverse Reactions

CV: Bradycardia; deep venous thrombosis; MI pulmonary embolism; tachycardia.
CNS: Dizziness; headache; insomnia; depression; peripheral neuropathy.
EENT: Tinnitus.
GI: Abdominal pain; anorexia; constipation; diarrhea; epigastric discomfort; gastritis; heartburn nausea; vomiting; hiccups; perforating duodenal ulcer.
GU: Increased BUN, proteinuria; renal insufficiency.
HEMA: Neutropenia; thrombocytopenia.
HEPA: Increased ALT and AST.
METAB: Dehydration.
OTHER: Asthenia; fatigue; fever; mucous membrane disorder.

Precautions

Pregnancy: Category B.
Lactation: Undetermined.
Children: Safety and efficacy not established.
Chronic therapy: Long-term continuous use for prevention of nausea or vomiting is not recommended.

Overdosage: Signs and Symptoms
Drowsiness, headache.

PATIENT CARE CONSIDERATIONS

Administration/Storage

- Administer in combination with a corticosteriod and 5-HT$_3$ antagonist.
- May administer without regard to meals.
- Administer prescribed dose 1 hr before chemotherapy treatment and then once daily in the morning on the following 2 days.
- Store capsules at controlled room temperature (59° to 86°F). Do not remove desiccant from bottle.

Assessment/Interventions

- Obtain patient history, including drug history and any known allergies. Note history of severe hepatic insufficiency, prior use and effectiveness of antiemetic therapy.
- Note concurrent use of medications metabolized by CYP3A4.
- Monitor patient for antiemetic efficacy. Notify health care provider if nausea or vomiting are not prevented.
- Ensure that patient taking warfarin has INR determined more frequently during the 2-wk period following each use of aprepitant.
- Ensure that women taking oral contraceptives

are instructed to use alternative or back-up contraceptive methods while using aprepitant.
* Monitor patient for CNS, GI, and general body side effects. Inform health care provider if noted and significant.

Patient/Family Education
* Explain name, dose, action, and potential side effects of drug.
* Advise patient, family, or caregiver to read the "Patient Package Insert" before starting therapy and with each refill.
* Advise patient, family, or caregiver that medication is designed to prevent nausea and vomiting caused by chemotherapy. It is not to be used to try to treat nausea or vomiting once it has started.
* Review dosing schedule with patient, including concomitant use of other antiemetics. Caution patient that first dose of aprepitant must be taken 1 hr before chemotherapy administration to provide greatest protection against nausea and vomiting.
* Advise patient that medication regimen will greatly reduce likelihood of nausea or vomiting but these are still possible.
* Instruct patient to inform health care provider if medication regimen does not prevent nausea or vomiting.
* Advise patient to report any of the following symptoms to health care provider: intolerable headache; persistent or intolerable constipation, diarrhea, or nausea; persistent weakness or general body discomfort.
* Advise patient receiving warfarin therapy that clotting status will need to be closely monitored for 2 wk following use of aprepitant.
* Advise women taking oral contraceptives to use alternative or back-up contraceptive methods while using aprepitant.
* Advise women to notify health care provider if pregnant, planning to become pregnant, or breastfeeding.
* Instruct patient not to take any prescription or OTC medications or dietary supplements unless advised by health care provider.
* Advise patient, family, or caregiver that follow-up visits and lab tests will be required to monitor therapy and to keep appointments.

Argatroban

(ahr-GAT-troe-ban)

Class Anticoagulants/Thrombin inhibitor

How Supplied
Argatroban Injection 100 mg/mL

Action
PHARMACOLOGY: Binds reversibly to thrombin active site, exerting its anticoagulant effects by inhibiting thrombin-catalyzed or induced reactions, including activation of coagulation factors V, VIII, and XIII, protein C, and platelet aggregation.

PHARMACOKINETICS/DYNAMICS:
Distribution: Distributes mainly in the extracellular fluid. Vd is 174 mL/kg. Approximately 54% is protein bound (20% to albumin and 34% to alpha-1-glycoprotein).

Metabolism: Hydroxylation and aromatization in the liver. CYP3A4/5 plays a minor role.

Excretion: Cl is approximately 5.1 mL/kg/min; t½ is 39 to 51 min. Approximately 65% is excreted in the feces (through biliary secretion) and approximately 22% is excreted in the urine. At least 14% is recovered in the feces as unchanged drug and 16% in urine.

Onset: Immediate.

Peak: 1 to 3 hr (steady state).

Special Populations:
Hepatic Function Impairment – Cl is reduced and t½ is increased. Dosage adjustment is recommended.

Indications As an anticoagulant for prophylaxis and treatment of thrombosis in heparin-induced thrombocytopenia (HIT); as an anticoagulant in patients with or at risk for heparin-induced thrombocytopenia undergoing percutaneous coronary intervention (PCI).

Contraindications Overt major bleeding; hypersensitivity to this product or any component of this product.

Route/Dosage
Coadministration of Warfarin
ADULTS (RECEIVING ARGATROBAN UP TO 2 MCG/KG/MIN): Measure international normalized ratio (INR) daily during coadministration of argatroban and warfarin. In general, doses of argatroban up to 2 mcg/kg/min can be discontinued when the INR is greater than 4. Repeat INR 4 to 6 hr after stopping argatroban and, if the INR is below desired therapeutic range, resume argatroban infusion and repeat the procedure daily until desired therapeutic range on warfarin alone is achieved.
ADULTS (RECEIVING ARGATROBAN AT DOSES GREATER THAN 2 MCG/KG/MIN): Temporarily reduce dose of argatroban to 2 mcg/kg/min and repeat the INR on argatroban and warfarin 4 to 6 hr after reducing the argatroban dose; follow the process described above for administering warfarin and argatroban at doses up to 2 mcg/kg/min.

Hepatic Function Impairment
ADULTS: **IV** In patients with moderate hepatic function impairment, initial dose is 0.5 mcg/kg/min; monitor aPTT closely and adjust dose as clinically indicated.

HIT or Heparin-Induced Thrombocytopenia and Thrombosis Syndrome (HITTS)
ADULTS: **IV** Initial dose is 2 mcg/kg/min as a continuous infusion; after initial dose, the dose can be adjusted as clinically indicated (not exceeding 10 mcg/kg/min), until steady-state activated partial thromboplastin time (aPTT) is 1.5 to 3 times the initial baseline value (not to exceed 100 sec).

PCI in HIT or HITTS
ADULTS: **IV** Initial dose is 25 mcg/kg/min and bolus of 350 mcg/kg via large bore IV line administered over 3 to 5 min. Check activated clotting time (ACT) 5 to 10 min after bolus is completed. Proceed if ACT is greater than 300 sec. If ACT is less than 300 sec, administer an additional IV bolus dose of 150 mcg/kg, increase the infusion dose to 30 mcg/kg/min, and check the ACT 5 to 10 min later. If ACT is greater than 450 sec, decrease the infusion rate to 15 mcg/kg/min and check ACT 5 to 10 min later. Once ACT is between 300 and 450 sec, continue infusion dose for the duration of the procedure. In case of dissection, impending abrupt closure, thrombus formation during the procedure, or inability to achieve or maintain an ACT over 300 sec, additional bolus doses of 150 mcg/kg may be administered and the infusion dose increased to 40 mcg/kg/min. Check the ACT after each additional bolus or change in rate of infusion.

Interactions
Anticoagulants, antiplatelet agents, thrombolytics: May increase risk of bleeding.
Heparin: Allow sufficient time for effects of heparin on aPTT to decrease before starting argatroban therapy.

Lab Test Interferences
None well documented.

Adverse Reactions
CV: Hypotension (11%); cardiac arrest (6%); ventricular tachycardia, bradycardia (5%); MI (4%); atrial fibrillation (3%); cerebrovascular disorder, coronary thrombosis, myocardial ischemia, coronary occlusion, angina pectoris (2%); aortic stenosis, arterial thrombosis, cerebrovascular disorder, vascular disorder (1%).
CNS: Headache (5%).
DERM: Allergic skin reactions (including rash, bullous eruption; 1% to less than 10%).
GI: Minor hemorrhagic GI bleeding (14%); nausea (7%); diarrhea, vomiting (6%); abdominal pain (3%); major hemorrhagic GI bleeding (2%); gastroesophageal reflux disease (1%).
GU: Minor GU hemorrhage and hematuria (12%); UTI (5%); abnormal renal function (3%); major GU hemorrhage and hematuria (1%).
HEMA: Minor decrease in hemoglobin and hematuria (12%); sepsis (6%); overall bleeding (hemorrhagic [5%]); retroperitoneal hemorrhage, major decrease in hemoglobin and hematocrit (1%).
PULM: Hemoptysis, pneumonia (3%); lung edema (1%).
RESP: Allergic airway reactions (including coughing and dyspnea [10% or more]); dyspnea (8%); coughing (3%).
OTHER: Chest pain (15%); back pain (8%); minor hemorrhagic event/groin, pain (5%); infection, fever (4%); minor hemorrhagic event/brachial (2%); general allergic reactions (1% to less than 10%).

Precautions
Pregnancy: Category B.
Lactation: Undetermined.
Children: Safety and efficacy not established.
Hepatic function impairment: Use with caution.
Hemorrhage: Because hemorrhage can occur at any site in patients receiving argatroban, use with extreme caution in disease states or circumstances in which there is an increased danger of hemorrhage (eg, major surgery, severe hypertension, spinal anesthesia).

Overdosage: Signs and Symptoms
Excessive anticoagulation.

PATIENT CARE CONSIDERATIONS

Administration/Storage
- For IV administration only. Not for intradermal, subcutaneous, IM, or intra-arterial administration.
- Follow manufacturer's guidelines for diluting concentrated solution in 0.9% sodium chloride injection, 5% dextrose injection, or lactated Ringer's injection before infusing.
- Do not mix with other injections or infusions.
- Do not administer if particulate matter or discoloration noted.
- Store vials at controlled room temperature (59° to 86°F). Diluted solution can be kept at room temperature for up to 24 hr or in refrigerator (36° to 46°F) for up to 48 hr. Do not freeze or expose to direct sunlight.

Assessment/Interventions
- Obtain patient history, including drug history and any known allergies. Note the following: liver disease; severe hypertension; recent lum-

bar puncture or spinal anesthesia; major surgery, surgery involving the eye, brain, or spinal cord; GI lesions; hematologic conditions associated with increased bleeding tendencies; concurrent use of antiplatelet agents, thrombolytics, or anticoagulants.
* Review patient's health history for any condition that could contraindicate argatroban (active major bleeding or hypersensitivity to argatroban or any of its components).
* Ensure all parenteral anticoagulants have been discontinued before administering argatroban.
* Administer reduced dose to patient with moderate hepatic impairment or if transaminases are 3 or more times the upper limit of normal.
* Ensure baseline hematocrit or hemoglobin and platelet count are obtained and evaluated prior to starting therapy.
* Ensure aPTT is obtained prior to starting therapy for HIT or HITTS and again 2 hr after initiation of therapy. Adjust infusion rate to maintain aPTT between 1.5 to 3 times the initial baseline value (not to exceed 100 sec).
* Ensure an activated clotting time (ACT) is obtained prior to starting therapy, 5 to 10 min after the bolus dose or change in infusion rate, and at end of procedure in patients undergoing PCI. Repeat ACTs every 20 to 30 min during a prolonged procedure. Use bolus doses and infusion rate changes, following manufacturer's dosing chart, to maintain ACT between 300 and 450 seconds.
* Determine ACT prior to removal of arterial sheath. Do not remove sheath until ACT is less than 160 sec.
* When initiating warfarin therapy in patient who has been receiving argatroban at a dose up to 2 mcg/kg/min, ensure warfarin therapy is started without a loading dose and that therapy overlaps 4 to 5 days. Discontinue argatroban when the INR is greater than 4 on combined therapy. Repeat INR 4 to 6 hr after argatroban has been discontinued. If INR is below desired range, restart argatroban and repeat procedure daily until desired therapeutic range on warfarin alone is reached.
* When coadministering warfarin and argatroban in a patient who has been receiving argatroban at a dose greater than 2 mcg/kg/min, ensure argatroban dose is reduced to 2 mcg/kg/min for 4 to 6 hr before determining INR, then follow steps above.
* Monitor patient for GI, CV, and general body side effects. Report to health care provider if noted and significant.
* Monitor patient for signs of bleeding, especially at vascular access sites, throughout therapy. If excessive or unusual bruising develops, or if bleeding develops (eg, epistaxis, hematuria, hematemesis, bloody or black, tarry stools) or is suspected (eg, unexplained fall in hematocrit or BP, or any other unexplained symptom develops), notify health care provider immediately.

Patient/Family Education
* Explain name, action, and potential side effects of drug.
* Advise patient, family, or caregiver that medication will be prepared and administered by a health care professional in a hospital setting.
* Instruct patient, family, or caregiver to report any of the following immediately: bleeding or unusual bruising, coughing, difficulty breathing, skin rash or reaction.

Aripiprazole

(A-rih-PIP-ray-zole)
Class Antipsychotic agent
How Supplied
Abilify Tablets 5 mg, Tablets 10 mg, Tablets 15 mg, Tablets 20 mg, Tablets 30 mg
Action
PHARMACOLOGY: Partial agonist at dopamine D_2 and serotonin 5-HT_{1A} receptors, and antagonist at serotonin 5-HT_{2A} receptor.
PHARMACOKINETICS/DYNAMICS:
Absorption: Well absorbed; steady state is attained within 14 days. T_{max} is 3 to 5 hr and bioavailability is 87%.
Distribution: More than 99% is protein bound, primarily to albumin. Vd is 404 L or 4.9 L/kg.
Metabolism: Hepatic metabolism (dehydrogenation, hydroxylation, N-dealkylation) involves CYP2D6 and CYP3A4. Major metabolite is dehydro-aripiprazole (active).
Excretion: Approximately 25% excreted in urine (less than 1% unchanged) and 55% in feces (approximately 18% as unchanged drug). The elimination $t_{½}$ is 75 hr (aripiprazole) and 94 hr (dehydro-aripiprazole).

Special Populations:
Renal Function Impairment – In severe renal impairment (Ccr less than 30 mL/min), C_{max} increased 36% (parent drug) and 53% (metabolite), but AUC was 15% lower for aripiprazole and 7% higher for metabolite. No dosage adjustment needed.

Hepatic Function Impairment – AUC increased 31% in mild hepatic impairment, increased 8% in moderate impairment, and decreased 20% in severe impairment. No dosage adjustment required.
Elderly – Cl was 20% lower. No dosage adjustment required.
Gender – C_{max} and AUC are 30% to 40% higher in women than in men. No dosage adjustment required.

Indications Treatment of schizophrenia.

Contraindications Standard considerations.

Route/Dosage

Usual Dose
ADULTS: **PO** Start with 10 or 15 mg/day on a daily schedule. The effective dose range is 10 to 30 mg/day. Do not increase dosage before 2 wk.

Concurrent Use of CYP3A4 (eg, ketoconazole) or CYP2D6 Inhibitors (eg, fluoxetine, quinidine)
ADULTS: **PO** Reduce the usual dose of aripiprazole 50%. Increase the dose when the CYP3A4 or CYP2D6 inhibitor is discontinued.

Concurrent Use of CYP3A4 Inducers (eg, carbamazepine)
ADULTS: **PO** Double the usual dose of aripiprazole (to 20 to 30 mg). Base additional increases on clinical evaluation. Decrease the dose (to 10 to 15 mg) when the CYP3A4 inducer is discontinued.

Maintenance
No evidence is available from controlled trials. Periodically reassess patients to determine need for maintenance treatment.

Interactions

Alcohol: Avoid while taking aripiprazole.
CYP2D6 inducers (eg, carbamazepine): May reduce aripiprazole plasma levels, decreasing the therapeutic effect.
CYP2D6 inhibitors (eg, fluoxetine, paroxetine, quinidine), CYP3A4 inhibitors (eg, ketoconazole): May elevate aripiprazole plasma levels, increasing the adverse effects.

Lab Test Interferences None well documented.

Adverse Reactions

CV: Hypertension, tachycardia, hypotension, bradycardia (at least 1%).
CNS: Headache (32%); anxiety (25%); insomnia (24%); lightheadedness, somnolence (11%); akathisia (10%); tremor (3%); depression, nervousness, increased salivation, hostility, suicidal thought, manic reaction, abnormal gait, confusion, cogwheel rigidity (at least 1%).
DERM: Rash (6%); dry skin, pruritus, sweating, skin ulcer (at least 1%).
EENT: Rhinitis (4%); blurred vision (3%); conjunctivitis, ear pain (at least 1%).
GI: Nausea (14%); vomiting (12%); constipation (10%); anorexia (at least 1%).
GU: Urinary incontinence (at least 1%).
HEMA: Ecchymosis, anemia (at least 1%).
METAB: Weight gain (7%); weight loss, increased creatine phosphokinase (at least 1%).
RESP: Coughing (3%); dyspnea, pneumonia (at least 1%).
OTHER: Asthenia (7%); fever (2%); flu-like symptoms, peripheral edema, chest pain, neck pain, neck rigidity, muscle cramp (at least 1%).

Precautions

Pregnancy: Category C.
Lactation: Undetermined.
Children: Safety and efficacy not established.
Aspiration pneumonia: Antipsychotics have been associated with esophageal dysmotility and aspiration; use with caution in patients at risk for aspiration pneumonia.
Cognitive and motor skills: Cognitive and motor skills may be impaired; caution patients about operating hazardous machinery or driving until they are reasonably certain that therapy does not affect them adversely.
Hyperglycemia and diabetes mellitus: Hyperglycemia, in some cases extreme and associated with ketoacidosis or hyperosmolar coma or death, may occur. Monitor patients with established diagnosis of diabetes mellitus regularly for worsening of glucose control.
Neuroleptic malignant syndrome (NMS): NMS has occurred with antipsychotics and is potentially fatal. Signs and symptoms are hyperpyrexia, muscle rigidity, altered mental status, irregular pulse, irregular BP, tachycardia, and diaphoresis.
Orthostatic hypotension: Orthostatic hypotension may occur.
Psychosis associated with Alzheimer disease or dementia: Use with caution.
Seizures: Seizures may occur; use with caution in patients with a history of seizures or with conditions that potentially lower the seizure threshold.
Suicide: Closely supervise high-risk patients; do not give excessive quantities.
Tardive dyskinesia: A potentially irreversible syndrome of involuntary body and facial movements may occur.
Temperature regulation: Antipsychotics can disrupt the body's ability to reduce core temperature.

Overdosage: Signs and Symptoms
Somnolence, vomiting.

PATIENT CARE CONSIDERATIONS
Administration/Storage
- Administer prescribed dose daily without regard to meals.
- Administer with food if GI upset occurs.
- Store at controlled room temperature (59° to 86°F).

Assessment/Interventions
- Obtain patient history, including drug history and any known allergies. Note renal disease, liver disease, recent MI, CV disease, heart failure, cerebrovascular disease, cardiac arrhythmias, previous episode of NMS, seizures or conditions that predispose to seizures (eg, Alzheimer disease), or condition that would predispose to hypotension (eg, dehydration, hypovolemia, treatment with antihypertensive medications).
- Note concurrent use of CYP2D6 inhibitor, CYP3A4 inhibitor or inducer, or antihypertensive therapy.
- Ensure that dosage adjustment is considered when aripiprazole is used concomitantly with potential CYP3A4 inhibitor or inducer or with potential CYP2D6 inhibitor.
- Monitor cardiac patient during initiation of drug for orthostatic hypotension; notify health care provider if noted.
- Take safety precautions if orthostatic hypotension occurs.
- Monitor blood sugar in diabetic patient when drug is started or dose is changed. Report significant changes to health care provider.
- Ensure that fasting blood glucose is evaluated before starting therapy and periodically thereafter during therapy in patient with risk factors for diabetes mellitus (eg, obesity, family history of diabetes).
- Inform health care provider immediately if hyperpyrexia, muscle rigidity, altered mental status, irregular pulse and BP, tachycardia, and diaphoresis develop.
- Notify health care provider if any of the following develop: hypotension, tachycardia, excessive drowsiness, symptoms of hyperglycemia (polyuria, polydipsia, polyphagia), nausea, vomiting, constipation, indigestion.
- Assess baseline neurologic status; during treatment observe for involuntary body and facial movements, drowsiness, agitation, anxiety, aggressive reaction, or seizure activity.
- Frequently assess patient for response to treatment. Notify health care provider if condition does not appear to be improving or is worsening.
- Ensure that therapy is periodically reviewed to determine if it needs to be continued without change or if a dose change (eg, increase, decrease, discontinuation) is indicated.
- Monitor patient for suicidal tendencies often associated with schizophrenia.
- Assess medication compliance.
- Monitor patient for CNS, GI, CV, PSYCH, and general body side effects. Inform health care provider if noted and significant.

Patient/Family Education
- Explain name, dose, action, and potential side effects of drug.
- Instruct patient to take prescribed dose daily without regard to meals but to take with food if GI upset occurs.
- Instruct patient not to stop taking aripiprazole when feeling better.
- Advise patient to take frequent sips of water, suck on ice chips or sugarless hard candy, or chew sugarless gum if dry mouth occurs.
- Instruct diabetic patient to monitor blood glucose more frequently when drug is started or dose is changed and to inform health care provider of significant changes in readings.
- Tell patient to immediately report high fever, muscle rigidity, altered mental status, irregular pulse, sweating, racing thoughts, mood swings, irritability, unquenchable thirst, frequent urination, seizures, or rash to health care provider.
- Advise patient to avoid strenuous activity during periods of high temperature or humidity.
- Instruct patient to avoid alcoholic beverages while taking aripiprazole.
- Instruct patient to get up slowly from lying or sitting position and to avoid sudden position changes to prevent postural hypotension. Advise patient to report dizziness with position changes to health care provider. Caution patient that hot tubs or hot showers or baths may make dizziness worse.
- Advise patient taking antihypertensives to monitor BP at regular intervals.
- Advise patient that drug may impair judgment, thinking, or motor skills or cause drowsiness and to use caution while driving or performing other tasks requiring mental alertness.
- Advise women to notify health care provider if pregnant, planning to become pregnant, or breastfeeding.
- Advise patient to notify health care provider of the following symptoms: excessive drowsiness, increased agitation or anxiety, involuntary body or facial movements, rapid pulse, nausea, vomiting, constipation.
- Instruct patient not to take any prescription

or OTC medications, dietary supplements, or herbal preparations unless advised by health care provider.

- Advise patient that follow-up visits will be required to monitor therapy and to keep appointments.

Arsenic Trioxide

(AHR-sen-ik tri-OX-ide)

Class Antineoplastic

How Supplied
Trisenox Solution for injection 1 mg/mL in 10 mL ampules

Action
PHARMACOLOGY: Arsenic trioxide causes morphological changes and DNA fragmentation characteristic of apoptosis in NB4 human promyelocytic leukemia cells in vitro. Arsenic trioxide also causes damage or degradation of the fusion protein PML/RAR alpha.

PHARMACOKINETICS/DYNAMICS:

Metabolism: Pentavalent arsenic is reduced to trivalent arsenic by arsenate reductase. Trivalent arsenic is methylated to monomethyl arsenic, which is then converted to dimethyl arsenic by methyltransferase. Methylation reactions are done in the liver.

Excretion: Excreted in the urine as methylated metabolite.

Indications
Adult/Pediatric: Refractory or relapsed acute promyelocytic leukemia (APL). Safety and efficacy in children less than 5 yr not established.

Contraindications
Standard considerations.

Route/Dosage
Refractory or Relapsed Acute Promyelocytic Leukemia
INDUCTION (ADULT/PEDIATRIC): **IV** 0.15 mg/kg/day until bone marrow remission, do not exceed 60 doses.

CONSOLIDATION (ADULT/PEDIATRIC): **IV** 0.15 mg/kg/day for 25 doses over a period of up to 5 wk. Begin 3 to 6 wk following induction.

Interactions
Insulin, sulfonylureas (eg, glipizide, glyburide, tolbutamide, chlorpropamide), glucagon, or diazoxide: May increase and decrease blood glucose levels, necessitating dosage adjustment of these drugs.

Medications that prolong the QT interval (eg, thioridazine, antiarrhythmics) or that cause electrolyte abnormalities (eg, amphotericin B, diuretics): Risk of arrhythmias may increase when arsenic trioxide is given concomitantly with these medications.

Lab Test Interferences None well documented.

Adverse Reactions
CV: Tachycardia (55%); QTc interval greater than 500 msec (38%); palpitations; other ECG abnormalities; torsades de pointes; edema (40%); chest pain; hypotension; flushing; hypertension.
CNS: Fatigue; fever; headache (approximately 60%); insomnia; rigors; paresthesia; anxiety; dizziness; depression; tremor; weakness; convulsion; somnolence.
DERM: Dermatitis; pruritus; ecchymosis; dry skin; nonspecific erythema; increased sweating; pallor; facial edema; night sweats; petechiae; hyperpigmentation; nonspecific skin lesions; urticaria; local exfoliation; eyelid edema; injection site pain; erythema; edema (10% to 20%).
GI: Moderate potential for nausea and vomiting; abdominal pain (58%); diarrhea; constipation; decreased appetite; elevated ALT and AST; abdominal discomfort.
GU: Vaginal hemorrhage (21%); breakthrough bleeding (13%); fetal harm possible; bone marrow chromosome defects in pregnant mice and neural tube defects in pregnant hamsters.
HEMA: Leukocytosis (50%); thrombocytopenia; anemia; neutropenia (nadir 14 to 21 days); hemorrhage; disseminated intravascular coagulation; lymphadenopathy.
HYPERSEN: Rash (up to 5%).
METAB: Hypokalemia, hypomagnesemia, hyperglycemia (up to 15% to 50%); hyperkalemia; weight gain; hypocalcemia; hypoglycemia.
MUSC: Arthralgia; myalgia; bone pain; nonspecific back, neck, and limb pain.
RENAL: Renal dysfunction (up to 10%).
RESP: Cough; dyspnea; sore throat; epistaxis; hypoxia; pleural effusion; post nasal drip; wheezing; changes in breath sounds; hemoptysis; tachypnea.
SPEC SENSE: Eye irritation, blurred vision, dry eyes, earache, tinnitus, painful red eyes (up to 10%).
OTHER: Retinoic-acid acute promyelocytic leukemia (RA-APL) syndrome during induction in up to 31% characterized by fever, dyspnea, weight gain, radiographic pulmonary infiltrates, pleural or pericardial effusions. Mean time to diagnosis was 17 days after initiating treatment (range, 7 to 24 days).

> **WARNING:**
>
> *Cardiac arrhythmias:* The risk of torsades de pointes depends on the extent of QT interval prolongation. Use with caution in patients with a history of torsades de pointes, preexisting QT interval prolongation, or CHF, and in patients taking medications known to prolong the QT interval or cause electrolyte abnormalities.
>
> *RA-APL syndrome:* RA-APL syndrome has occurred in 31% of patients treated with arsenic trioxide. If suspected (eg, unexplained fever, dyspnea, abnormal chest exam), administer dexamethasone 10 mg IV q 12 hr for at least 3 days until symptoms resolve.
>
> Perform baseline 12 lead ECG with serum electrolytes and creatinine levels.
>
> Pre-existing electrolyte abnormalities should be corrected prior to therapy. Electrolyte profiles monitored at least twice weekly and more frequently for unstable patients during the induction phase and at least weekly during the consolidation phase.
>
> ECG obtained weekly and more frequently for unstable patients during induction and consolidation phases.
>
> Discontinue drugs known to prolong QT interval.

Precautions

Pregnancy: Category D.

Lactation: Arsenic is excreted in human milk. Decide whether to discontinue nursing or discontinue the drug, taking into account the importance of the drug to the mother.

Children: Safety and efficacy in pediatric patients less than 5 yr not studied.

Adjustment in renal insufficiency: Dosage reduction may be necessary in patients with impaired renal function; however, specific recommendations are not available. Use additional caution in these patients.

Extravasation risk: Arsenic trioxide is an irritant; mild injection site reactions have been reported (13%). Local irritation or phlebitis may occur. Refer to your institution specific protocol.

Hyperleukocytosis: Common (50%) during arsenic trioxide therapy. Patients with higher baseline WBC (3900 cells/mm^3 vs 1200 cells/mm^3) may be at greater risk for developing hyperleukocytosis.

Overdosage: Signs and Symptoms

Convulsions, muscle weakness, confusion.

PATIENT CARE CONSIDERATIONS

Administration/Storage

- Store at room temperature. Do not freeze.
- Withdraw the desired dose from the ampule, using aseptic technique.
- Use a filter needle and dilute with 100 to 250 mL 5% Dextrose or 0.9% Sodium Chloride prior to administration.
- Diluted solutions are stable for 24 hr at room temperature or 48 hr if refrigerated.
- Discard the undiluted solution within 24 hr of opening.
- Administer by IV infusion. May be given via a peripheral venous catheter.
- IV infusion over 1 to 2 hr. Increase the infusion time to 4 hr if acute vasomotor reactions occur, such as dizziness, hypotension, tachycardia, or flushing.

Assessment/Interventions

- Obtain a 12-lead ECG at baseline and at least weekly during therapy. Monitor serum electrolytes (eg, potassium, magnesium, calcium), and serum creatinine at baseline at least twice weekly during induction and at least once weekly during consolidation. Before starting therapy, correct any electrolyte abnormalities, and if possible, discontinue drugs known to prolong the QT interval.
- Maintain serum potassium concentrations greater than 4 mEq/dL and serum magnesium concentrations greater than 1.8 mg/dL during therapy.
- Evaluate patients with a QT interval greater than 500 msec and immediately correct any risk factors.
- Discontinue therapy temporarily in patients who experience syncope or irregular heartbeat. Hospitalize and monitor these patients.
- Therapy may be restarted when the QT interval is less than 460 msec, syncope or irregular heartbeat has resolved, and electrolyte abnormalities are corrected.

Patient/Family Education

- Explain name, dose, action, and potential side effects of drug.
- Review dosing schedule with patient (ie, Induction Regimen and Consolidation Regimen).
- Advise patient that medication will be prepared and administered by health care provider in a health care setting.
- Instruct patient to immediately inform health

care provider if fever, weight gain, difficulty breathing, or shortness of breath occur.
- Instruct patient to not take any prescription or OTC medications or dietary supplements unless advised to do so by health care provider.
- Instruct women of childbearing potential to notify health care provider if pregnant, planning to become pregnant, or breastfeeding.
- Advise patient that follow-up visits and laboratory tests will be required to monitor therapy and to keep appointments.

Ascorbic Acid (Vitamin C)

(ASS-kor-bik acid)

Class Vitamin

How Supplied
Cecon Solution 100 mg/mL ◆ *Cevi-Bid* Tablets 500 mg ◆ *Chewable Vitamin C* Tablets, chewable 250 mg vitamin C as sodium ascorbate and ascorbic acid, Tablets, chewable 500 mg vitamin C as sodium ascorbate and ascorbic acid ◆ *Dull C Powder* 1060 mg/tsp ◆ *Fruit C 500* Tablets, chewable 500 mg vitamin C as calcium ascorbate and ascorbic acid ◆ *Fruit C 100* Tablets, chewable 100 mg vitamin C as calcium ascorbate and ascorbic acid ◆ *Fruit C 200* Tablets, chewable 200 mg vitamin C as calcium ascorbate and ascorbic acid ◆ *N'ice Vitamin C Drops* Lozenges 60 mg ◆ *Sunkist Vitamin C* Tablets, chewable 60 mg vitamin C as sodium ascorbate and ascorbic acid, Tablets, chewable 250 mg vitamin C as sodium ascorbate and ascorbic acid, Tablets, chewable 500 mg vitamin C as sodium ascorbate and ascorbic acid ◆ *Vicks Vitamin C Drops* Lozenges 25 mg vitamin C as sodium ascorbate and ascorbic acid ◆ *Vita-C* Crystals 1000 mg/tsp
✤ *Proflavanol* ◆ *Revitalose-C-1000* ◆ *Timedose Vitamin C*

Action

PHARMACOLOGY: Essential vitamin believed important for synthesis of cellular components, catecholamines, steroids, and carnitine.

PHARMACOKINETICS/DYNAMICS:

Absorption: Absorbed almost completely from distal small intestine.

Distribution: Distributed throughout water-soluble compartments. Adrenal cortex, leukocytes, platelets, and pituitary gland contain high concentrations.

Excretion: Excreted in the urine.

Indications Prevention and treatment of scurvy. **Unlabeled use(s):** Treatment of idiopathic methemoglobinemia; combination therapy with methenamine to increase acidity of urine. Although not proven scientifically, prevention of common colds and treatment of cancer, asthma, atherosclerosis, burns, and other wounds. Topical vitamin C may photoprotect against UVR because of its antioxidant and anti-inflammatory properties.

Contraindications Standard considerations.

Route/Dosage
ADULTS: **PO** Recommended daily allowance 60 mg; average protective dose 70 to 150 mg/day.

Nicotine use
ADULTS: The RDA for smokers is 100 mg/day because of an increased utilization of vitamin C.

High Dose Therapy
ADULTS: Taper vitamin C prior to discontinuing supplementation.

Scurvy
ADULTS: **IV/IM/SC** 75 to 150 mg/day; up to 6 g/day has been administered without toxicity.

Enhanced Wound Healing
ADULTS: **PO** 300 to 500 mg/day for 7 to 10 days has been given.

PARENTERAL
ADULTS: Used in acute deficiency or when oral absorption is uncertain. Avoid rapid IV administration.

Interactions None well documented.

Lab Test Interferences
Amine-dependent tests for occult blood in stool: May cause false-negative results.
Urine glucose determinations: May cause false-negative determinations.

Adverse Reactions
CNS: Faintness or dizziness may occur with rapid IV administration.
GI: Diarrhea; nausea; vomiting.
GU: Excessive doses over long period of time may cause precipitation of cystine, oxalate or urate crystals in kidney.
OTHER: Injection site irritation may occur with IM or SC administration.

Precautions
Pregnancy: Category A. (Category C in doses above the RDA).
Lactation: Excreted in breast milk.
Tartrazine sensitivity: Some products contain tartrazine, which can precipitate breathing difficulties in sensitive individuals.

Sulfite sensitivity: Some products contain sulfites, which may precipitate a reaction in sensitive individuals.
Excessive doses: Diabetics, patients prone to renal calculi, patients on sodium restricted diets, and those taking anticoagulants should not take excessive doses (more than 5 g/day) over extended periods of time.

PATIENT CARE CONSIDERATIONS
Administration/Storage
- Check expiration date on container for oral tablets; product is relatively unstable after exposure to air and light.
- Cover IV bag to protect from light if being administered IV.
- Refrigerate when possible, although storage at room temperature is acceptable.
- Discard IV solution after 24 hr.

Assessment/Interventions
- Obtain patient history, including drug history and any known allergies.
- Evaluate patient for signs of vitamin C deficiency before and during therapy.
- Monitor pH of urine if patient is being treated for renal stones.
- If patient experiences dizziness or syncope, stop administration and notify health care provider.
- Rotate injection or infusion sites to reduce irritation.

Patient/Family Education
- Explain that taking product with foods high in iron will enhance absorption of iron.
- Explain to any patient scheduled for glucose studies that product should not be taken for at least 48 to 72 hr before test.
- Inform patient that abruptly stopping high-dose therapy may lead to loosening of teeth and bleeding gums.

Asparaginase
(ass-PAR-uh-jin-aze)

Class Enzyme

How Supplied
Elspar Powder for injection, lyophilized 10,000 international units
✤ *Kidrolase*

Action
PHARMACOLOGY: Asparaginase contains the enzyme L-asparagine amidohydrolase. In a significant number of patients with acute leukemia, the malignant cells depend on exogenous asparagine for survival. Administration of asparaginase hydrolyzes serum asparagine to nonfunctional aspartic acid and ammonia, depriving tumor cells of a required amino acid. Tumor cell proliferation is blocked.

PHARMACOKINETICS/DYNAMICS:
Absorption:
IM – T_{max} is 14 to 24 hr.

Distribution: Vd is approximately 70% to 80% of the estimated plasma volume.

Excretion: Trace amounts found in urine.
IV – $T_{1/2}$ is 8 to 30 hr.
IM – $T_{1/2}$ is 39 to 49 hr.

Indications
Adult: Combination therapy for acute lymphocytic leukemia. Do not use as the sole induction agent unless combination therapy is deemed inappropriate.
Pediatric: Acute lymphocytic leukemia. Do not use as the sole induction agent unless combination therapy is deemed inappropriate.

Contraindications
Anaphylactic reactions to asparaginase; pancreatitis or a history of pancreatitis.

Route/Dosage
Acute Lymphocytic Leukemia
PEDIATRIC: **IV** Give over 30 min through the side arm of an already running infusion of Sodium Chloride Injection or 5% Dextrose Injection. The drug has little tendency to cause phlebitis when given IV.

PEDIATRIC: **IM** Limit the volume at a single injection site to 2 mL. For a volume greater than 2 mL, use 2 injection sites.

Acute Lymphocytic Leukemia Induction Regimens
PEDIATRIC: One of the following combination regimens is recommended for acute lymphocytic leukemia in children.

Acute Lymphocytic Leukemia Induction Regimen I
PEDIATRIC:
Prednisone: 40 mg/m^2/day PO in 3 divided doses for 15 days, followed by tapering the dosage as follows: 20 mg/m^2 for 2 days, 10 mg/m^2 for 2 days, 5 mg/m^2 for 2 days, 2.5 mg/m^2 for 2 days, and then discontinue.
Vincristine sulfate: 2 mg/m^2 IV once weekly on days 1, 8, and 15. The maximum single dose should not exceed 2 mg.
Asparaginase: 1000 IU/kg/day IV for 10 successive days beginning on day 22. When remission is obtained, institute appropriate maintenance therapy. Do not use asparaginase as part of a maintenance regimen. Asparaginase has been used in other combination regimens. Administering the drug IV concurrently with or immediately before a course of vincristine and prednisone may be associated with increased toxicity.

Acute Lymphocytic Leukemia Induction Regimen II
PEDIATRIC:

Prednisone: 40 mg/m^2/day PO in 3 divided doses for 28 days (the total daily dose to the nearest 2.5 mg), then gradual discontinuation over 14 days.

Vincristine sulfate: 1.5 mg/m^2 IV weekly for 4 doses, on days 1, 8, 15, and 22. The maximum single dose should not exceed 2 mg.

Asparaginase: 6000 IU/m^2 IM on days 4, 7, 10, 13, 16, 19, 22, 25, and 28. When remission is obtained, institute appropriate maintenance therapy. Do not use asparaginase as part of a maintenance regimen

Acute Lymphocytic Leukemia Single Agent Induction Therapy
ADULT/PEDIATRIC: **IV** Use asparaginase as the sole induction agent only when a combined regimen is inappropriate because of toxicity or other specific patient-related factors, or in cases refractory to other therapy. Administer 200 IU/kg/day IV for 28 days. Complete remissions are of short duration, 1 to 3 mo.

Interactions
Methotrexate: Asparaginase may diminish or abolish methotrexate's effect on malignant cells. Do not use methotrexate with, or following asparaginase, while asparagine levels are below normal. Asparaginase may augment corticosteroid-induced hyperglycemia.
Vincristine and prednisone: IV administration may be associated with increased toxicity.

Lab Test Interferences May interfere with the interpretation of thyroid function tests by producing a rapid and marked reduction in serum concentrations of thyroxine-binding globulin within 2 days after the first dose.

Adverse Reactions
CNS: Depression; confusion; hallucinations; headache; Parkinson-like syndrome.
DERM: Rashes.
ENDO: Hyperglycemia.
GI: Moderate potential for nausea, vomiting. Pancreatitis, sometimes fulminant, and acute hemorrhagic pancreatitis have occurred, both may be fatal; fatty changes in the liver; elevation of LFTs.
HEMA: Hypofibrinogenemia; decreased synthesis of clotting factors and antithrombin III.
HYPERSEN: Acute anaphylactoid reactions are common; discontinuation of therapy and administration of fluids, corticosteroids, antihistamines, or pressors may be required.
RENAL: Azotemia, usually prerenal; transient proteinuria.
OTHER: Chills; fever; weight loss (usually mild); fatal hyperthermia; hypoglycemia.

> **WARNING:**
>
> *Anaphylaxis:* Be prepared to treat anaphylaxis at each administration.
> Intradermal skin test should be performed prior to initial administration of this drug and repeated when at least 1 wk separates doses.

Precautions
Pregnancy: Category C.
Lactation: Discontinue nursing or discontinue the drug.
Children: Toxicity is reported to be greater in adults than in children.
Acute lymphocytic leukemia dosage adjustments: Patients who have received a course of therapy, if treated again, have an increased risk of hypersensitivity reactions. Therefore, repeat treatment only when the benefit of such therapy is weighed against the increased risk.
Hematologic: Bone marrow depression, leukopenia, thrombosis, and clotting factors depressed; increase in blood ammonia during the conversion of asparagine to aspartic acid by the enzyme.

PATIENT CARE CONSIDERATIONS
Administration/Storage
- Be prepared to treat anaphylaxis at each administration.
- Store at 2° to 8°C (36° to 46°F). Store reconstituted solution at 2° to 8°C (36° to 46°F); discard after 8 hr or sooner if cloudy.
- Administer by IV bolus injection, IV infusion, or IM injection.
- Desensitization regimen is recommended for patients with positive skin test and for retreatment.

IM:
- Reconstitute by adding 2 mL Sodium Chloride Injection to the 10,000 unit vial. Use the resulting solution within 8 hr and only if clear.

IV:
- Reconstitute the 10,000 unit vial with 5 mL Sterile Water for Injection or with Sodium Chloride Injection. This solution may be used for direct IV administration within 8 hr following reconstitution. For administration by infusion, dilute solutions with Sodium Chloride Injection or 5% Dextrose Injection. Infuse within 8 hr and only if clear.
- Filtration through a 5 micron filter during administration will remove the particles with no loss of potency.

Assessment/Interventions
- The manufacturer recommends that a test dose (approximately 2 IU) be given before the first dose and any time when more than 1 wk has elapsed between doses.
- Perform an intradermal skin test prior to initial administration and when it is given after a wk or more has elapsed between doses.
- Administer the drug only after successful desensitization.
- Anaphylactic reactions require the immediate use of epinephrine, oxygen, and IV steroids.
- Monitor leukocyte counts and serum uric acid. Take appropriate preventive measures. Monitor peripheral blood count and bone marrow frequently.
- Obtain frequent serum amylase to detect early evidence of pancreatitis. If pancreatitis occurs, discontinue therapy.
- Monitor blood sugar.

Patient/Family Education
- Explain name, dose, action, and potential side effects of drug.
- Advise patient, family, or caregiver that medication will be prepared and administered by health care provider in a health care setting.
- Advise patient, family, or caregiver that medication will be used in combination with other agents to achieve maximum benefit possible.
- Review dosing schedule with patient, family, or caregiver.
- Advise patient, family, or caregiver that skin tests may be used prior to administration of medication.
- Advise patient, family, or caregiver to carefully follow instructions for supplemental therapies designed to protect the kidneys from excessive uric acid (eg, increased fluid intake, allopurinol, urinary alkalinizing agents).
- Advise patient, family, or caregiver to immediately report any of the following to health care provider: rash; hives; difficulty breathing; fever, chills, or other signs of infection; sore throat.
- Advise patient, family, or caregiver to report any of the following to health care provider: persistent nausea, vomiting, or appetite loss; persistent stomach pain; unusual bruising or bleeding.
- Instruct diabetic patient to monitor blood glucose more frequently when drug is started or dose is changed and to inform health care provider of significant changes in readings.
- Instruct patient not to take any prescription or OTC medications or dietary supplements unless advised to do so by health care provider.
- Instruct women of childbearing potential to notify health care provide if pregnant, planning to become pregnant, or breastfeeding.
- Advise patient that frequent follow-up visits and laboratory tests will be required to monitor therapy and to keep appointments.

Aspirin (Acetylsalicylic Acid; ASA)

(ASS-pihr-in)
Class Analgesic/Salicylate
How Supplied
Arthritis Foundation Pain Reliever Tablets 500 mg ◆ *Aspergum* Gum tablets 227.5 mg ◆ *Bayer Children's Aspirin* Tablets, chewable 81 mg ◆ *Bayer Low Adult Strength* Tablets, delayed-release 81 mg ◆ *Easprin* Tablets, enteric-coated 975 mg ◆ *Ecotrin* Tablets, enteric-coated 325 mg ◆ *Ecotrin Adult Low Strength* Tablets, enteric-coated 81 mg ◆ *Ecotrin Maximum Strength* Tablets, enteric-coated 500 mg ◆ *Empirin* Tablets 325 mg ◆ *Extended Release Bayer 8-Hour* Tablets, extended-release 650 mg ◆ *Extra Strength Bayer Enteric 500 Aspirin* Tablets, enteric-coated 500 mg ◆ *Genprin* Tablets 325 mg ◆ *Genuine Bayer* Tablets 325 mg ◆ *½ Halfprin* Tablets, enteric-coated 165 mg ◆ *Halfprin 81* Tablets, enteric-coated 81 mg ◆ *Heartline* Tablets, enteric-coated 81 mg ◆ *Maximum Bayer* Tablets 500 mg ◆ *Norwich Extra-Strength* Tablets 500 mg ◆ *Regular Strength Bayer Enteric Coated Caplets* Tablets, enteric-coated 325 mg ◆ *St. Joseph Adult Chewable Aspirin* Tablets, chewable 81 mg ◆ *ZORprin* Tablets, controlled-release 800 mg

🍁 *Alka-Seltzer Flavoured* ◆ *Asaphen* ◆ *Asaphen E.C.* ◆ *Entrophen* ◆ *MSD Enteric Coated ASA* ◆ *Novasen*

Action
PHARMACOLOGY: Inhibits prostaglandin synthesis, resulting in analgesia, anti-inflammatory activity and platelet aggregation inhibition; reduces fever by acting on the brain's heat-regulating center to promote vasodilation and sweating.

PHARMACOKINETICS/DYNAMICS:
Absorption: Rapidly and completely absorbed. T_{max} is 1 to 2 hr (salicylic acid).
Distribution: Widely distributed to all tissues and fluids including CNS, breast milk, and fetal tissues. Approximately 90% of salicylate is protein bound at concentrations of less than 100 mcg/mL and approximately 75% is bound at concentrations of more than 400 mcg/mL.

Metabolism: Rapidly hydrolyzed to salicylic acid (active). Salicylic acid is conjugated in the liver to the metabolites.

Excretion: Salicylic acid plasma $t_{1/2}$ is approximately 6 hr but may exceed 20 hr in higher doses. $T_{1/2}$ is approximately 15 to 20 min for aspirin. Elimination follows zero order kinetics. Renal elimination of unchanged drug depends on urine pH. A pH of more than 6.5 increases renal clearance of free salicylate from less than 5% to more than 80%.

Indications Treatment of mild to moderate pain; fever; various inflammatory conditions; reduction of risk of death or MI in patients with previous infarction or unstable angina pectoris or recurrent transient ischemia attacks or stroke in men who have had transient brain ischemia caused by platelet emboli. **Unlabeled use(s):** Prevention of cataract formation; prevention of toxemia of pregnancy; improvement of inadequate uteroplacental blood flow in pregnancy.

Contraindications Hypersensitivity to salicylates or NSAIDs; hemophilia, bleeding ulcers, or hemorrhagic states.

Route/Dosage
Analgesic/Antipyretic
ADULTS: **PO** 325 to 650 mg q 4 hr prn; 500 mg q 3 hr prn; 1000 mg q 6 hr prn.
CHILDREN (2 TO 12 YR): **PO** 10 to 15 mg/kg/dose q 4 hr prn (up to 80 mg/kg/day).

Arthritis and Other Rheumatic Conditions
ADULTS: **PO** 3.2 to 6 g/day in divided doses.

Juvenile Rheumatoid Arthritis
CHILDREN: **PO** 60 to 110 mg/kg/day in divided doses q 6 to 8 hr.

Acute Rheumatic Fever
ADULTS: **PO** 5 to 8 g/day, initially, for up to 2 wk. Subsequent doses are based on patient response.
CHILDREN: **PO** 75 to 100 mg/kg/day.

Transient Ischemic Attacks in Men
ADULTS: **PO** 1300 mg/day in 2 to 4 doses.

MI Prophylaxis
ADULTS: **PO** 160 to 325 mg/day.

Kawasaki Disease
CHILDREN: **PO** 80 to 180 mg/kg/day during acute febrile period; 10 mg/kg/day after fever resolves.

Interactions
Alcohol: May increase risk of GI ulceration and prolong bleeding time.
Antacids, urinary alkalinizers, and corticosteroids: May decrease aspirin levels.
Anticoagulants, oral and heparin: May increase risk of bleeding.
Carbonic anhydrase inhibitors (eg, acetohexamide), methotrexate, valproic acid: May increase levels of these drugs.
Probenecid, sulfinpyrazone: May decrease uricosuric effect.
Sulfonylureas, insulin: Aspirin (more than 2 g/day) may potentiate glucose lowering.

Lab Test Interferences May increase levels of serum uric acid, cause false-positive readings of urine glucose by copper reduction method (*Clinitest*) and false-negative readings by glucose oxidase method (*Clinistix*); may interfere with urine tests of 5-hydroxyindoleacetic acid, ketone, phenolsulfonphthalein, vanillylmandelic acid.

Adverse Reactions
EENT: Dizziness; tinnitus.
GI: Nausea; dyspepsia; heartburn; bleeding.
HEMA: Increased bleeding times; anemia; decreased iron concentration.
OTHER: Hypersensitivity reactions may include urticaria, hives, rashes, angioedema and anaphylactic shock.

Precautions
Pregnancy: Category D.
Lactation: Excreted in breast milk.
Children: Reye syndrome has been associated with aspirin administration to children (including teenagers) with acute febrile illness. Do not use without consulting health care provider.
Hypersensitivity: Reaction may include bronchospasm and generalized urticaria or angioedema; patients with asthma or nasal polyps have greatest risk.
Renal function impairment: May decrease renal function or aggravate kidney diseases.
Hepatic function impairment: May cause hepatotoxicity in patients with impaired liver function.
GI disorders: Can cause gastric irritation and bleeding.
Surgical patients: Aspirin may increase risk of postoperative bleeding. If possible, avoid use 1 wk before surgery.

Overdosage: Signs and Symptoms
Nausea, vomiting, tinnitus, dizziness, respiratory alkalosis, metabolic acidosis, hemorrhage, convulsions.

PATIENT CARE CONSIDERATIONS
Administration/Storage
♦ Administer after meals, with food or antacid to minimize gastric irritation.
♦ Do not crush or have patient chew enteric-coated or timed-release caplets.
♦ Store oral forms at room temperature in tightly closed container. Store suppositories in a cool location or refrigerate. Do not freeze.

Assessment/Interventions
- Obtain patient history, including drug history and any known allergies, particularly to tartrazine (yellow dye #5). Note asthma, hay fever, and nasal polyps.
- Ensure that bleeding time and prothrombin time have been evaluated before beginning large dose long-term therapy.
- Monitor hemoglobin or guaiac (hemoccult) stool periodically during therapy.
- Monitor during long-term therapy for tinnitus, GI disturbances, bleeding from gums, black tarry stools, or prolonged fever lasting more than 3 days.
- If signs of bleeding, black tarry stools, or tinnitus occur, withhold medication and notify health care provider.
- Observe for rash, urticaria, dyspnea, or anaphylactic reaction. If these occur, notify health care provider immediately.

Patient/Family Education
- Instruct patient to take drug with food or after meals and with full glass of water. Explain that antacids should be avoided within 1 to 2 hr after ingestion of enteric-coated tablets.
- Tell patient to discard any aspirin that has a vinegar-like odor.
- Instruct patient to report ringing in ears or unusual bleeding, bruising, or persistent GI pain.
- Advise patient on long-term therapy to inform health care provider or dentist before seeking surgery or dental care.
- Tell patient on sodium-restricted diet to limit use of effervescent or buffered aspirin preparations.
- Caution parents to avoid giving aspirin to children or teenagers with flu-like symptoms or chickenpox without first consulting health care provider.
- Instruct patient to avoid intake of alcoholic beverages or other CNS depressants.

Atazanavir Sulfate

(At-ah-zah-NAH-veer SULL-fate)
Class Antiviral

How Supplied
Reyataz Capsules 100 mg, Capsules 150 mg, Capsules 200 mg

Action
PHARMACOLOGY: Inhibits human immunodeficiency virus (HIV) protease, the enzyme required to form functional proteins in HIV-infected cells.

PHARMACOKINETICS/DYNAMICS:
Absorption: Rapidly absorbed with a T_{max} of approximately 2.5 hr. Mean C_{max} is 3152 ng/mL. Mean AUC is 22,262 ng•hr/mL. Mean t½ is 6.5 hr. Mean C_{min} is 273 ng/mL.

Distribution: Serum protein binding is 86%. Distributes into the cerebrospinal fluid.

Metabolism: Extensively metabolized. The major pathways are mono-oxygenation and dioxygenation. Minor pathways of metabolism are glucuronidation, N-dealkylation, hydrolysis, and oxygenation with dehydrogenation. In vitro studies using human liver microsomes suggest that atazanavir is metabolized by CYP3A.

Excretion: Elimination is 79% in the feces (20% unchanged) and 13% in the urine (7% unchanged). Mean elimination t½ is 7 hr at steady-state.

Special Populations:
Hepatic Function Impairment – Increased concentrations are expected in patients with moderate to severe impairment of hepatic function.

Indications In combination with other antiretroviral agents for the treatment of HIV-1 infection.

Contraindications Drugs (eg, cisapride, ergot derivative, midazolam, pimozide, triazolam) that are highly dependent on CYP3A for Cl and for which elevated plasma levels are associated with serious and/or life-threatening events; hypersensitivity to any component of the product.

Route/Dosage
When coadministered with efavirenz, it is recommended that atazanavir 300 mg and ritonavir 100 mg be given with efavirenz 600 mg (all as a single dose with food). Atazanavir without ritonavir should not be coadministered with efavirenz.

ADULTS: PO 400 mg qd with food.

Hepatic Impairment
ADULTS: PO Use with caution in patients with mild to moderate hepatic insufficiency. Consider a dose reduction to 300 mg qd in patients with moderate hepatic insufficiency. Do not use in patients with severe hepatic impairment.

Interactions
Antacids and buffered medications (eg, didanosine buffered preparation), efavirenz, H_2-receptor antagonists, proton pump inhibitors (eg, omeprazole), rifampin, St. John's wort: May reduce atazanavir plasma levels, decreasing the therapeutic effect. Coadministration of proton pump inhibitors, rifampin, or St. John's wort with

atazanavir is not recommended. Atazanavir without ritonavir should not be coadministered with efavirenz.

Antiarrhythmic agents (eg, amiodarone, quinidine, systemic lidocaine), calcium channel blockers (eg, bepridil, felodipine, nicardipine, verapamil), HMG-CoA reductase inhibitors (ie, atorvastatin, lovastatin, simvastatin), immunosuppressive agents (ie, cyclosporine, sirolimus, tacrolimus), irinotecan, oral contraceptives (eg, ethinyl estradiol and norethindrone), phenytoin, rifabutin, sildenafil, tricyclic antidepressants, warfarin: Atazanavir may increase plasma levels of these agents, increasing the risk of toxicity and, in some instances, life-threatening reactions. Coadministration of bepridil is not recommended. Up to a 75% reduction in the rifabutin dose is recommended. A 50% reduction in the dose of diltiazem should be considered and titrate the dose of other calcium channel blockers. Sildenafil should be used with caution and at a reduced dose of 25 mg q 48 hr and monitor for adverse reactions.

Clarithromycin: Plasma levels of clarithromycin may be elevated by atazanavir, which may result in QTc prolongation. A 50% reduction in clarithromycin dose should be considered. In addition, levels of the active metabolite (14-OH clarithromycin) may be reduced. Use alternative therapy for indications other than *Mycobacterium avium* complex.

Cisapride, ergot derivatives (eg, ergotamine), midazolam, pimozide, triazolam: Coadministration with atazanavir is contraindicated because of serious or life-threatening adverse effects.

H_2-receptor antagonists (eg, cimetidine): Atazanavir plasma levels may be reduced, decreasing the therapeutic effect and increasing the development of resistance.

Indinavir: Coadministration is not recommended because of the increased risk of indirect hyperbilirubinemia.

Lab Test Interferences None well documented.

Adverse Reactions
CV: Cardiac arrest; heart block; hypertension; myocarditis; palpitation; syncope; vasodilation.
CNS: Headache (14%); depression (4%); dizziness, insomnia (3%); peripheral neurologic symptoms (1%); abnormal dreams; abnormal gait; agitation; amnesia; anxiety; confusion; convulsion; decreased libido; emotional lability; hallucination; hostility; hyperkinesia; hypesthesia; increased reflexes; nervousness; psychosis; sleep disorder; somnolence; suicide attempt; twitch.
DERM: Alopecia; cellulitis; dermatophytosis; dry skin; eczema; nail disorder; pruritus; seborrhea; urticaria; vesiculobullous rash.
EENT: Otitis; taste perversion; tinnitus.
GI: Nausea (16%); vomiting, abdominal pain, diarrhea (6%); acholia; anorexia; aphthous stomatitis; colitis; constipation; dental pain; dyspepsia; enlarged abdomen; esophageal ulcer; esophagitis; flatulence; gastritis; gastroenteritis; GI disorder; hepatitis; hepatomegaly; hepatosplenomegaly; increased appetite; liver damage; liver fatty deposit; mouth ulcer; pancreatitis; peptic ulcer.
GU: Abnormal urine; amenorrhea; crystalluria; decreased male fertility; gynecomastia; hematuria; impotence; kidney calculus; kidney failure; kidney pain; menstrual disorder; oliguria; pelvic pain; polyuria; proteinuria; urinary frequency; UTI.
HEMA: Abnormal neutrophils (7%) and hemoglobin (5%).
HEPA: Abnormal total bilirubin (35%); jaundice/scleral icterus (7%); abnormal ALT (4%) and AST (2%).
METAB: Buffalo hump; dehydration; diabetes mellitus; dyslipidemia; gout; lactic acidosis; lipohypertrophy; obesity; weight decrease and gain.
RESP: Increased cough; dyspnea; hiccough; hypoxia.
OTHER: Rash (9%); fever (4%); increased cough, pain (3%); back pain, fatigue (2%); lipodystrophy (1%); bone pain; extremity pain; muscle atrophy; myalgia; myasthenia; myopathy; allergic reactions; angioedema; asthenia; burning sensation; chest pain; dysplasia; ecchymosis; edema; facial atrophy; generalized edema; heat sensitivity; infection; malaise; pallor; peripheral edema; photosensitivity; purpura; substernal chest pain; sweating.

Precautions
Pregnancy: Category B.
Lactation: Undetermined. HIV-infected mothers should not breastfeed their infants.
Children: Safety and efficacy not established in children under 3 mo because of risk of kernicterus.
Elderly: Use with caution because of the greater frequency of decreased hepatic, renal, or cardiac function, and concomitant diseases or other drug therapy.
Hepatic function impairment: Use with caution (see Route/Dosage).
Diabetes mellitus/hyperglycemia: New-onset diabetes mellitus, exacerbation of preexisting diabetes mellitus, and hyperglycemia have been reported during postmarketing surveillance in HIV-infected patients treated with protease inhibitor therapy.
Fat redistribution: Redistribution and accumulation of body fat, including central obesity,

dorsocervical fat enlargement (buffalo hump), peripheral wasting, facial wasting, breast enlargement and "cushingoid appearance" have occurred in patients receiving antiretroviral therapy.
Hemophilia: Increased bleeding, including spontaneous skin hematomas and hemarthrosis in patients with hemophilia type A and B, has occurred in patients treated with protease inhibitors.
Hyperbilirubinemia: Asymptomatic elevations in indirect bilirubin occur in most patients.
Lactic acidosis: Lactic acidosis syndrome, sometimes fatal, and symptomatic hyperlactemia has occurred in patients receiving atazanavir in combination with nucleoside analogs. Female gender and obesity are known risk factors.
PR interval prolongation: Concentration- and dose-dependent prolongation of the PR interval in the ECG has been reported.
Resistance/Cross-resistance: Various degrees of cross-resistance between protease inhibitors have been observed.

Overdosage: Signs and Symptoms
Bifascicular block and PR interval prolongation, jaundice, hyperbilirubinemia.

PATIENT CARE CONSIDERATIONS
Administration/Storage
- Administer prescribed dose qd.
- Administer each dose with food to increase absorption.
- Store capsules at controlled room temperature (59° to 86°F). Keep tightly capped and protect from moisture.

Assessment/Interventions
- Obtain patient history, including drug history and any known allergies. Note liver impairment, hemophilia, diabetes, concurrent infection with hepatitis B or C, concurrent use of medications metabolized by CYP3A (eg, midazolam), concurrent use of medications that induce CYP3A (eg, rifampin), and concurrent use of medications that prolong the PR interval (eg, digoxin).
- Ensure that medication is used in combination with other antiretroviral agents.
- Ensure that reduced dose is administered to patient with moderate hepatic insufficiency.
- Ensure that liver enzymes are determined before starting therapy and periodically during therapy in patient with history of hepatitis B or C infection.
- Monitor patient for signs of lactic acidosis. If patient develops profound weakness or tiredness, unexpected stomach discomfort, feeling cold, dizzy, or lightheaded, or slow or irregular heartbeat, withhold drug and contact physician.
- Assess patient for GI, CNS, musculoskeletal, and general body side effects. Inform health care provider if noted and significant.

Patient/Family Education
- Advise patient to read the "Patient Information" leaflet before starting therapy and with each refill.
- Explain name, dose, action, and potential side effects of drug.
- Warn patient that this drug is not to be used by itself but is combined with other antiviral agents and to not change the dose or stop taking any of the antiviral agents unless advised by health care provider.
- Advise patient that redistribution or accumulation of body fat may occur.
- Advise patient to take prescribed dose qd and to swallow capsules whole. Caution patient not to open capsules.
- Advise patient to take each dose with food or snack to increase absorption and effectiveness.
- Advise patient that if a dose is missed to take the dose as soon as possible and then return to the normal schedule. However, if it is within 6 hr of the next dose, skip the dose and take the next dose at the regular time. If a dose is skipped, caution patient to not double the dose to catch up but to continue with the normal schedule.
- Instruct patient taking antacids or *Videx* tablets to take atazanavir 2 hr before or 1 hr after these medicines.
- Instruct patient to report these symptoms immediately to health care provider: dizziness; lightheadedness; palpitations (pounding in the chest); yellowing of the skin or eyes; persistent nausea or vomiting; profound weakness or tiredness; unexpected stomach discomfort; or trouble breathing.
- Inform patient that drug does not completely eliminate HIV virus and, therefore, does not reduce risk of transmitting HIV to others. Appropriate precautions must still be followed.
- Advise patient that drug is not a cure for HIV infection and that illnesses associated with HIV infection, including opportunistic infections, may continue to be acquired. The patient should remain under a physician's care.
- Instruct patient not to take any prescription or OTC medications or dietary supplements unless advised by health care provider.
- Instruct diabetic patient to monitor blood glucose more frequently when drug is started or dose is changed and to inform health care provider of significant changes in readings.

- Caution patient to avoid unnecessary exposure to UV light (sunlight, tanning booths) and to use sunscreen and wear protective clothing when exposed to UV light to avoid photosensitivity reaction.
- Advise women to notify health care provider if pregnant, planning to become pregnant, or breastfeeding. Caution HIV-infected mother that breastfeeding her baby could cause HIV infection in the baby.
- Remind patient that examinations and laboratory tests will be required to monitor therapy and to keep appointments.

Atenolol

(ah-TEN-oh-lahl)

Class Beta-adrenergic blocker

How Supplied
Tenormin Tablets 25 mg, Tablets 50 mg, Tablets 100 mg, Injection 5 mg/10 mL
✤ *APO-Atenol* ♦ *Gen-Atenolol* ♦ *Med-Atenolol* ♦ *Novo-Atenol* ♦ *Nu-Atenol* ♦ *PMS-Atenolol* ♦ *ratio-Atenolol* ♦ *Rhoxal-atenolol*

Action
PHARMACOLOGY: Blocks beta receptors, primarily affecting heart (slows rate), vascular system (decreases BP) and, to lesser extent, lungs (reduces function).

PHARMACOKINETICS/DYNAMICS:
Absorption:
Oral – Rapid and consistent but incomplete; approximately 50% is absorbed from the GI tract. T_{max} is 2 to 4 hr.
IV – T_{max} is reached within 5 min.

Distribution: 6% to 16% bound to plasma proteins.

Metabolism: Little or no metabolism by the liver.

Excretion:
Oral – Approximately 50% is excreted unchanged in the feces. Approximately 50% is excreted in the urine within 24 hr. $T_{1/2}$ is approximately 6 to 7 hr.
IV – More than 85% is excreted in the urine within 24 hr.

Onset: 1 hr (oral).

Peak: 2 to 4 hr (oral); 5 min (IV).

Duration: 24 hr (oral). For both oral and IV administration, duration of action is dose related.

Special Populations:
Renal Function Impairment – Elimination is closely related to glomerular filtration rate. Significant accumulation occurs when Ccr falls below 35 mL/min/1.73 m^2.

Indications Treatment of hypertension (used alone or in combination with other drugs), angina pectoris resulting from coronary atherosclerosis, acute MI. **Unlabeled use(s):** Migraine prophylaxis, alcohol withdrawal syndrome, ventricular arrhythmias, supraventricular arrhythmias or tachycardias, esophageal varices rebleeding, anxiety.

Contraindications Hypersensitivity to beta-blockers; sinus bradycardia; greater than first-degree heart block; CHF unless secondary to tachyarrhythmia treatable with beta-blockers; overt cardiac failure; cardiogenic shock.

Route/Dosage
Hypertension
ADULTS: **PO** 50 to 100 mg/day.

Angina Pectoris
PO May require up to 200 mg/day.

Acute MI
ADULTS: **IV** 5 mg over 5 min; second IV follow with 5 mg dose 10 min later.
ADULTS: **PO** 50 to 100 mg/day.

Interactions
Aluminum salts, ampicillin, calcium salts: Plasma levels and pharmacologic effects may be decreased.
Clonidine: May add to or reverse antihypertensive effects; potentially life-threatening situations may occur, especially on withdrawal.
Diltiazem: Pharmacologic effects of atenolol may be increased; symptomatic bradycardia may occur.
Nifedipine, verapamil: Effects of both drugs may be increased.
NSAIDs: Some agents may impair antihypertensive effect.
Prazosin: May increase orthostatic hypotension.
Quinidine: Pharmacologic effects of atenolol may be increased.

Lab Test Interferences None well documented.

Adverse Reactions
CV: Hypotension; bradycardia; CHF; cold

extremities; second- or third-degree heart block.
CNS: Insomnia; fatigue; dizziness; depression; lethargy; drowsiness; forgetfulness; slurred speech.
DERM: Rash; hives; fever; alopecia.
EENT: Dry eyes; blurred vision; tinnitus; dry mouth; sore throat.
GI: Nausea; vomiting; diarrhea.
GU: Impotence; painful, difficult or frequent urination.
HEMA: Agranulocytosis; thrombocytopenic purpura.
HEPA: Elevated liver enzymes and bilirubin.
RESP: Bronchospasm; dyspnea; wheezing.
OTHER: Weight changes; facial swelling; muscle weakness; hyperglycemia; hypoglycemia; antinuclear antibodies; hyperlipidemia.

> **WARNING:**
>
> *Abrupt withdrawal:* In patients with angina pectoris or CAD, may cause exacerbation of angina, occurrence of MI and ventricular arrhythmias. Monitor patients closely. Because CAD is common and unrecognized it may be prudent not to discontinue beta-blocker therapy abruptly in patients treated only for hypertension.

PATIENT CARE CONSIDERATIONS

Administration/Storage
- May be administered with or without food.
- If patient has difficulty swallowing, tablet may be crushed and mixed with fluid.
- Store in a tightly-closed container in a cool location.

Assessment/Interventions
- Obtain patient history, including drug history and any allergies. Note diabetes, respiratory, liver, or cardiac disease, or sensitivity to other beta-blockers.
- Review baseline ECG.
- Assess BP and pulse before administration. If pulse is less than 60 bpm, withhold medication and notify health care provider.
- Monitor I&O and daily weight during therapy for signs of fluid retention.
- If sudden severe dyspnea or edema of hands and feet develops, withhold medication and notify health care provider.
- If chest pain occurs, assess for location, intensity, duration, and radiation. Nitroglycerin preparations may be administered in conjunction with this medication if ordered.
- If patient experiences chest pain not relieved by medication, continue medication and notify health care provider.

Precautions
Pregnancy: Category D.
Lactation: Excreted in breast milk.
Children: Safety not established.
Elderly: Dosage reduction may be necessary.
Renal function impairment: Reduce dose.
Hepatic function impairment: Reduce dose.
Anaphylaxis: Deaths have occurred; aggressive therapy may be required.
CHF: Administer cautiously in patients with CHF controlled by digitalis and diuretics.
Diabetes mellitus: May mask symptoms of hypoglycemia (eg, tachycardia, BP changes).
Nonallergic bronchospastic diseases (eg, chronic bronchitis, emphysema): In general, do not give beta-blockers to patients with bronchospastic diseases.
Peripheral vascular disease: May precipitate or aggravate symptoms of arterial insufficiency.
Thyrotoxicosis: May mask clinical signs (eg, tachycardia) of developing or continuing hyperthyroidism. Abrupt withdrawal may exacerbate symptoms of hyperthyroidism, including thyroid storm.

Overdosage: Signs and Symptoms
Bradycardia, hypotension, CHF, cardiogenic shock, hypertension, cardiac arrhythmias, seizures, respiratory depression, coma, pulmonary edema, bronchospasm, hypoglycemia.

- If there are changes in the ECG (eg, long PR interval, low- or high-grade heart blocks, ventricular ectopic beats), withhold dose and notify health care provider.

Patient/Family Education
- Explain that full effectiveness of drug may not occur for up to 1 to 2 wk after initiation of therapy, and that dosage will be tapered slowly before stopping. Warn that sudden discontinuation can cause chest pain or heart attack.
- Teach patient how to take pulse and instruct patient to check before taking drug. Warn patient not to take drug if pulse is less than 60 bpm, and to call health care provider.
- When medication is being used for treatment of hypertension, teach patient how to take daily BP.
- Advise patient that medication may cause increased sensitivity to cold.
- Inform diabetic patients to monitor blood glucose level carefully. It may be necessary to alter insulin dose while taking drug.
- Inform patient that frequent follow-up appointments with health care provider are important to adjust medication dosage.
- Instruct patient to report the following symp-

toms to health care provider: difficulty breathing; swelling of feet, legs, and hands; irregular heart beat; altered mood; depression.
• Caution patient to avoid sudden position changes to prevent orthostatic hypotension.
• Advise patient that drug may cause drowsiness, and to use caution while driving or performing other tasks requiring mental alertness.
• Caution patient not to take OTC medications without consulting health care provider.

Atenolol/Chlorthalidone

(ah-TEN-oh-lahl/klor-THAL-ih-dohn)

Class Antihypertensive

How Supplied
Tenoretic-50 Tablets 50 mg atenolol/25 mg chlorthalidone ♦ *Tenoretic-100* Tablets 100 mg atenolol/25 mg chlorthalidone

Action
PHARMACOLOGY: Atenolol is beta-adrenergic blocking agent that slows heart rate, reduces cardiac output and lowers BP. Chlorthalidone is diuretic agent that reduces body water by increasing urine output.

Indications Treatment of hypertension.

Contraindications Hypersensitivity to sulfonamide-derived drugs, sinus bradycardia, heart block greater than first degree, cardiogenic shock, overt cardiac failure, anuria. Not for initial therapy of hypertension.

Route/Dosage
ADULTS: **PO** 50 mg atenolol/25 mg chlorthalidone or 100 mg atenolol/ 25 mg chlorthalidone once daily.

Interactions
Clonidine: Beta blockers may exacerbate rebound hypertension associated with clonidine withdrawal. Atenolol/chlorthalidone should be tapered and withdrawn several days before gradual withdrawal of clonidine.
Digitalis glycosides: Diuretic-induced hypokalemia may potentiate digitalis toxicity.
Lithium: May increase therapeutic and toxic effects of lithium; avoid concomitant use.
Nondepolarizing muscle relaxants: May increase effects of these agents.
Norepinephrine: May decrease arterial responsiveness to norepinephrine.
Other antihypertensive agents: May increase antihypertensive effects.
Sulfonylureas: May decrease hypoglycemic effects.

Lab Test Interferences May increase serum protein-bound iodine levels without signs of thyroid disturbances.

Adverse Reactions
CV: Bradycardia; orthostatic hypotension; cold extremities; leg pain; CHF; slow atrioventricular (AV) conduction; intensification of AV block.
CNS: Fatigue; dizziness; vertigo; lightheadedness; lethargy; drowsiness; depression; dreaming.
DERM: Rash.
GI: Diarrhea; nausea.
GU: Peyronie disease; impotence; diminished libido.
HEMA: Thrombocytopenia; agranulocytosis.
HEPA: Elevated liver enzymes; jaundice; pancreatitis.
METAB: Hyperuricemia; hyponatremia; hypochloremic alkalosis; hypokalemia.
RESP: Bronchospasm; wheezing; dyspnea.
OTHER: Development of lupus syndrome with antinuclear antibodies.

Precautions
Pregnancy: Category D.
Lactation: Atenolol is excreted in breast milk and may produce clinically significant effects in infants.
Children: Safety and efficacy not established.
Elderly: Dose may need to be reduced.
Renal function impairment: Use with caution in patients with renal or hepatic disease; dose may need to be reduced.
Hepatic function impairment: Use with caution in patients with renal or hepatic disease; dose may need to be reduced.
Anaphylaxis: Deaths have occurred with anaphylactic reactions to beta-blockers; aggressive therapy may be required.
Cardiac failure: Use with caution in patients with history of heart failure.
Diabetes mellitus: May mask symptoms of hypoglycemia (eg, tachycardia, BP changes). May potentiate insulin-induced hypoglycemia.
Hypertension: Fixed-dose combinations of drugs are not intended for initial therapy of hypertension but are used for convenience once patient has been stabilized.
Nonallergic bronchospastic diseases (eg, chronic bronchitis, emphysema): In general, do not give beta-blockers to patients with bronchospastic diseases.
Peripheral vascular disease: May precipitate or aggravate symptoms of arterial insufficiency.
Thyrotoxicosis: May mask clinical signs (eg, tachycardia), of developing or continuing hyperthyroidism. Abrupt withdrawal may exacerbate symptoms of hyperthyroidism, including thyroid storm.

PATIENT CARE CONSIDERATIONS

Administration/Storage
- Give in morning with food or milk.
- If patient has difficulty swallowing, tablet may be crushed and mixed with fluid.
- Store at room temperature in tightly closed, light-resistant container.

Assessment/Interventions
- Obtain patient history, including drug history and any known allergies. Note asthma, diabetes and respiratory, liver or cardiac disease.
- Ensure that baseline Ccr levels have been obtained in patients with impaired renal function and monitor periodically during therapy, along with serum electrolytes.
- Assess BP and apical pulse before administering. If systolic BP is less than 90 mm Hg or pulse is less than 60 bpm, withhold drug and notify health care provider.
- Monitor I&O and daily weight during therapy for signs of fluid retention.
- Monitor for fluid overload (eg, jugular venous distension, dyspnea, rales, peripheral edema). Notify health care provider if these signs occur.
- Withhold medication and notify health care provider if the following symptoms occur: hypotension; bradycardia or dyspnea; difficulty breathing on exertion or lying down; night cough; edema of hands and feet.

Patient/Family Education
- Explain that dosage will be tapered slowly before stopping. Warn that sudden discontinuation may cause adverse effects (eg, exacerbation of angina, precipitation of MI).
- Teach patient proper technique for taking pulse and BP, and instruct to check before taking medication.
- Advise patient not to take medication in evening to avoid prolonged diuretic effects.
- Instruct diabetic patient to monitor blood glucose level carefully.
- Counsel patient that impotence or decrease in libido are common side effects, and advise patient to contact health care provider if either symptom occurs.
- Caution patient to avoid sudden position changes to prevent orthostatic hypotension.
- Advise patient that drug may cause drowsiness, and to use caution while driving or performing other tasks requiring mental alertness until individual effects can be determined.
- Instruct patient not to take *otc* medications without consulting health care provider.

Atomoxetine

(AT-oh-MOX-ah-teen)

Class Psychotherapeutic

How Supplied
Strattera Capsules 10 mg (as base), Capsules 18 mg (as base), Capsules 25 mg (as base), Capsules 40 mg (as base), Capsules 60 mg (as base)

Action
PHARMACOLOGY: Selective inhibition of the presynaptic norepinephrine transporter is suspected.

PHARMACOKINETICS/DYNAMICS:

Absorption: C_{max} is approximately 1 to 2 hr.

Distribution: Vd is 0.85 L/kg (IV dose) and 98% is protein bound, primarily to albumin.

Metabolism: Primarily metabolized by CYP2D6; CYP2C19 and other CYP450 enzymes are involved to a lesser extent. Major metabolite is 4Ohydroxyatomoxetine, which is equipotent to atomoxetine, but circulates at much lower concentrations.

Excretion: Cl is approximately 0.35 L/hr/kg and t½ is 5.2 hr for extensive metabolizers. Cl is approximately 0.3 L/hr/kg and t½ is 21.6 hr for poor metabolizers. More than 80% is excreted in urine and less than 17% in feces (as metabolite). Less than 3% is excreted as unchanged atomoxetine.

Special Populations:
Hepatic Function Impairment – AUC is increased in extensive metabolizers with moderate or severe hepatic insufficiency. Dosage adjustment is required.

Indications Treatment of attention-deficit/hyperactivity disorder (ADHD).

Contraindications Narrow angle glaucoma; MAO inhibitors or within 2 weeks after discontinuing an MAO inhibitor; hypersensitivity to any component of the product.

Route/Dosage
ADULTS AND CHILDREN (OVER 70 KG): PO Start with 40 mg/day and increase the dose after a minimum of 3 days to a target total daily dose of approximately 80 mg. After 2 to 4 additional wk, the dose may be increased to a max of 100 mg/day in patients who have not achieved an optimal response. In children over 70 kg receiving a strong CYP2D6 inhibitor (eg, fluoxetine), increase the 40 mg/day dose to the target dose of 80 mg/day if symptoms fail to improve after 4 wk and the initial dose is well-tolerated.
CHILDREN (UP TO 70 KG): PO Start with 0.5 mg/kg/day and increase the dose after a minimum of 3 days to a target total dose of

approximately 1.2 mg/kg/day (max, 1.4 mg/kg or 100 mg/day, whichever is less). In children up to 70 kg receiving a strong CYP2D6 inhibitor (eg, fluoxetine), increase the 0.5 mg/kg/day dose to the target dose of 1.2 mg/kg/day if symptoms fail to improve after 4 wk and the initial dose is well-tolerated.

Impaired hepatic function: PO Moderate hepatic function impairment (Child-Pugh Class B), reduce initial and target doses to 50% of the normal dose; severe hepatic function impairment (Child-Pugh Class C), reduce initial and target doses to 25% of normal.

Interactions

Albuterol: Use with caution, the cardiovascular effects of albuterol may be potentiated.
CYP2D6 inhibitors (eg, fluoxetine, quinidine): The area under the plasma concentration-time curve and peak plasma level of atomoxetine may be increased.
MAO inhibitors (eg, isocarboxazid): Coadministration is contraindicated.
Pressor agents: Possible increased effects of BP.

Lab Test Interferences None well documented.

Adverse Reactions

CV: Increased BP; sinus tachycardia; chest pain; palpitations; hot flushes; flushing; tachycardia.
CNS: Aggression; irritability; somnolence; fatigue; dizziness; mood swings; headache; crying; fatigue; insomnia; sedation; depression; decreased libido; abnormal dreams; paresthesia; sleep disorder; sinus headache; lethargy.
DERM: Dermatitis; pruritus; increased sweating.
EENT: Ear infection; mydriasis; sore throat; nasal congestion; nasopharyngitis; sinusitis.
GI: Vomiting; dyspepsia; nausea; abdominal pain; decreased appetite; constipation; dry mouth; diarrhea; anorexia; viral gastroenteritis; flatulence.
GU: Impaired sexual function; urinary retention and hesitancy; difficulty in micturition; dysmenorrhea; erectile disturbances; ejaculation failure or disorder; impotence; menstrual disorder; prostatitis; delayed menses; irregular menstruation; abnormal orgasm.
METAB: Weight decrease.
RESP: Cough; rhinorrhea; sinus congestion; upper respiratory tract infection.
OTHER: Allergic hypersensitivity (eg, angioneurotic edema, urticaria, rash); influenza; early morning awakening; tearfulness; arthralgia; tremor; myalgia; pyrexia; rigors; peripheral coldness.

Precautions

Pregnancy: Category C.
Lactation: Undetermined.
Children: Safety and efficacy not established in children less than 6 yr.
Cardiac effects: Use with caution in patients with hypertension, tachycardia, or cardiovascular or cerebrovascular disease because BP and heart rate may be increased.
Growth: Monitor growth during treatment, mean weight and growth changes have been reported to be less than occurs with placebo administration.

PATIENT CARE CONSIDERATIONS

Administration/Storage

- Discontinue MAO inhibitors at least 14 days before initiating therapy.
- Administer prescribed dose without regard to meals. Administer with food if GI upset occurs.
- Medication can be administered as a single daily dose or as evenly divided doses in the morning and late afternoon or early evening.
- Dosage increases should occur no more often than q 3 days.
- Store at controlled room temperature (59° to 86°F).

Assessment/Interventions

- Obtain patient history, including drug history and any known allergies. Note history of liver disease, hypertension, CV, or cerebrovascular disease, or narrow angle glaucoma.
- Note concurrent or recent MAO inhibitor therapy or concurrent use of potent inhibitors of CYP2D6 (eg, fluoxetine).
- Ensure that reduced dose is used in patient with liver impairment.
- With parental permission, consult with school personnel regarding drug effectiveness.
- Discontinue drug periodically to assess behavior and determine need for continued therapy.
- Assess ADHD symptoms before and periodically throughout therapy.
- Monitor height and weight in children.
- Measure pulse and BP before starting therapy, following dose increases, and periodically during therapy.
- Promote total treatment program (eg, psychological, educational, social) when treating attention-deficit disorder with hyperactivity.
- Monitor patient for CNS, CV, GI, GU, and general body side effects. Report to health care provider if noted and significant.

Patient/Family Education

- Explain name, dose, action, and potential side effects of drug.
- Advise patient, family, or caregiver that medi-

cation is started at a low dose and gradually increased as needed and tolerated.
- Advise patient, family, or caregiver that medication should be taken as prescribed and to not stop taking or change the dose unless advised to do so by health care provider.
- Advise patient, family, or caregiver that if a dose is missed that it should be taken as soon as remembered but to never take more than the prescribed total daily dose.
- Advise patient, family, or caregiver that this drug is part of a total treatment program that should also include psychological, educational, and social interventions.
- Advise parents to inform school or day care personnel about drug use and administration.
- Advise patient that drug may cause dizziness or other nervous system disorders and to use caution while driving or performing other tasks requiring mental alertness until tolerance is determined.
- Advise women to inform health care provider if pregnant, planning to become pregnant, or breastfeeding.
- Warn patient, family, or caregiver not to take any prescription or OTC drugs or dietary supplements without consulting health care provider.
- Advise patient, family, or caregiver that follow-up visits may be necessary to monitor therapy and to keep appointments.

Atorvastatin Calcium

(ah-TORE-vah-STAT-in)

Class Antihyperlipidemic/HMG-CoA reductase inhibitor

How Supplied
Lipitor Tablets 10 mg, Tablets 20 mg, Tablets 40 mg, Tablets 80 mg

Action
PHARMACOLOGY: Increases rate at which body removes cholesterol from blood and reduces production of cholesterol by inhibiting enzyme that catalyzes early rate-limiting step in cholesterol synthesis; increases HDL; reduces LDL, VLDL, and triglycerides.

PHARMACOKINETICS/DYNAMICS:

Absorption: Rapidly absorbed; T_{max} is 1 to 2 hr. Bioavailability is approximately 14%; low bioavailability is because of presystemic Cl in GI mucosa or hepatic first-pass metabolism. Food decreases rate and extent of absorption approximately 25% and 9%, respectively, but does not alter efficacy.

Distribution: Vd is approximately 381 L. At least 98% is protein bound.

Metabolism: Undergoes hepatic and extrahepatic metabolism, including first-pass metabolism and CYP3A4. Extensively metabolized to active metabolites, which produce approximately 70% of circulating inhibitory activity of HMG-CoA reductase.

Excretion: Atorvastatin and metabolites eliminated primarily in bile. Less than 2% of dose is recovered in the urine. Plasma t½ is approximately 14 hr.

Duration: The t½ of HMG-CoA reductase inhibitor is 20 to 30 hr.

Special Populations:
Hepatic Function Impairment – Plasma levels are markedly increased in patients with chronic alcoholic liver disease.

Indications
Elevated serum triglyceride: As an adjunct to diet for the treatment of patients with elevated serum triglyceride levels (Fredrickson type IV).
Heterozygous familial hypercholesterolemia in pediatric patients: Adjunct to diet to reduce total and LDL cholesterol and apolipoprotein B levels in boys and postmenarchal girls 10 to 17 yr if, after an adequate trial of diet therapy, and LDL remains 160 mg/dL or higher and there is a positive family history of premature CV disease or 2 or more other CV risk factors present.
Homozygous familial hypercholesterolemia: To reduce total cholesterol and LDL cholesterol in patients with homozygous familial hypercholesterolemia as an adjunct to other lipid-lowering treatments or if such treatments are unavailable.
Hypercholesterolemia: Adjunct to diet to reduce elevated total cholesterol, LDL cholesterol, apolipoprotein B, and triglyceride levels and to increase HDL cholesterol.
Type III familial hyperlipoproteinemia: To treat patients with primary dysbetalipoproteinemia (Fredrickson type III) who do not respond adequately to diet.

Contraindications Active liver disease or unexplained persistent elevation of serum transaminases; pregnancy; lactation; hypersensitivity to any component of the product.

Route/Dosage
ADULTS: **PO** 10 to 80 mg/day.

Heterozygous Familial Hypercholesterolemia
CHILDREN (10 TO 17 YR): PO Start with 10 mg/day (max, 20 mg/day).

Interactions
Antacids: Coadministration may decrease atorvastatin levels.

Azole antifungal agents (eg, itraconazole), cyclosporine, macrolide antibiotics (eg, erythromycin), gemfibrozil, grapefruit juice, niacin, protease inhibitors (eg, ritonavir), verapamil: Severe myopathy or rhabdomyolysis may occur.
Contraceptives, oral: Coadministration increases AUC for norethindrone and ethinyl estradiol.
Digoxin: Elevated digoxin levels may occur.

Lab Test Interferences None well documented.

Adverse Reactions
CNS: Headache (17%); insomnia, dizziness (at least 2%).
DERM: Rash (4%).
EENT: Sinusitis (6%); pharyngitis (3%); rhinitis (at least 2%).
GI: Diarrhea (4%); constipation (3%); nausea (at least 2%).
GU: UTI (at least 2%).
METAB: Peripheral edema (at least 2%).
MUSC: Myalgia (6%); arthralgia (5%); arthritis (at least 2%).
RESP: Bronchitis (at least 2%).
OTHER: Back pain, asthenia, abdominal pain (4%); flu-like symptoms (3%); chest pain (at least 2%); anaphylaxis, angioneurotic edema, bullous rashes (including erythema multiforme, Stevens-Johnson syndrome, toxic epidermal necrolysis), rhabdomyolysis (postmarketing).

Precautions
Pregnancy: Category X.
Lactation: Contraindicated in nursing women.
Children: Safety and efficacy not established, except in children 10 to 17 yr with heterozygous familial hypercholesterolemia.
LFTs: Ensure that LFTs (transaminases) are determined before and 12 wk following initiation of therapy, or after increase in dose, and periodically thereafter (eg, q 6 mo).
Liver disease: Use with caution in patients who consume substantial quantities of alcohol or have a history of liver disease.
Skeletal muscle effects: Rhabdomyolysis with renal dysfunction secondary to myoglobinuria has occurred in this class of drugs. Consider myopathy in any patient with diffuse myalgias, muscle tenderness or weakness, or marked elevation of CPK.

PATIENT CARE CONSIDERATIONS

Administration/Storage

- Administer alone or in combination with other lipid-lowering therapy.
- Give prescribed dose qd without regard to meals, preferably in the evening.
- Administer with food if GI upset occurs.
- Avoid administering with grapefruit juice.
- Store tablets at controlled room temperature (68° to 77°F).

Assessment/Interventions

- Obtain patient history, including drug history and any known allergies. Note active liver disease, hepatic insufficiency, unexplained elevations of serum transaminases, alcohol consumption, and concurrent therapy with medications known to increase the risk of myopathy (eg, cyclosporine, gemfibrozil).
- Ensure that secondary causes of hypercholesterolemia (eg, poorly controlled diabetes, hypothyroidism) are excluded before starting therapy.
- Ensure that patient is on a cholesterol-lowering diet before starting therapy and that diet is continued during treatment.
- Ensure that therapy is temporarily withheld in patient with an acute, serious condition suggestive of myopathy or predisposing to the development of renal failure secondary to rhabdomyolysis (eg, sepsis, hypotension).
- Ensure that serum cholesterol and triglycerides are measured before therapy is started and within 2 to 4 wk of starting therapy or changing the atorvastatin dose and then periodically thereafter.
- Ensure that LFTs (transaminases) are determined before and 12 wk following initiation of therapy, or after increase in dose, and periodically thereafter (eg, q 6 mo).
- If elevated serum transaminase levels develop during treatment, repeat levels more frequently. If transaminase levels rise to 3 times upper limit of normal and persist, notify health care provider. Be prepared to reduce dose or discontinue therapy if ordered.
- If muscle tenderness and/or weakness develop during therapy, determine CPK levels. Notify health care provider if CPK levels are markedly increased or if muscle symptoms continue or worsen.
- Assess patient for GI, CNS, MUSC, and general body side effects. If noted and significant inform health care provider.

Patient/Family Education

- Explain name, dose, action, and potential side effects of drug.
- Advise patient to take qd as prescribed, without regard to meals but to take with food if stomach upset occurs.
- Advise patient to take the drug with a liquid other than grapefruit juice.
- Advise patient to try to take each dose at about the same time each day, preferably in the evening.
- Inform patient that drug helps control, but

does not cure, cholesterol abnormality and to continue taking drug as prescribed if cholesterol levels are lowered.
* Caution patient not to change the dose or stop taking unless advised by health care provider.
* Advise patient that if a dose is missed to take as soon as remembered but to never take more than 1 dose of medicine a day.
* Instruct patient to continue taking other cholesterol-lowering medications as prescribed by health care provider.
* Emphasize to patient importance of the following other modalities on cholesterol control: dietary changes (reduced saturated fat intake, increase soluble fiber intake); weight control, regular exercise, and smoking cessation.
* Advise women of childbearing potential to use effective contraception during treatment with atorvastatin.
* Advise women to notify health care provider if they are pregnant, planning to become pregnant, or breastfeeding.
* Caution patient not to take any prescription or OTC medications or dietary supplements unless advised by health care provider.
* Instruct patient to notify health care provider if experiencing any unexplained muscle pain, tenderness, and/or weakness, or any other unusual feelings.
* Advise patient that follow-up visits and lab tests will be required to monitor therapy and to keep appointments.

Atovaquone

(uh-TOE-vuh-KWONE)
Class Anti-infective/Antiprotozoal

How Supplied
Mepron Suspension 750 mg/5 mL

Action
PHARMACOLOGY: Inhibits mitochondrial electron transport in metabolic enzymes of microorganisms. This may cause inhibition of nucleic acid and adenosine triphosphate synthesis.

PHARMACOKINETICS/DYNAMICS:
Absorption: Bioavailability is approximately 47%. Food increases absorption approximately 2-fold. AUC is approximately 280 hr•mcg/mL (fed) and approximately 169 hr•mcg/mL (fasting). C_{max} is approximately 15.1 mcg/mL (fed) and 8.8 mcg/mL (fasting).

Distribution: Highly lipophilic. May undergo enterohepatic recycling. Vd is 0.6 L/kg. 99.9% protein bound.

Excretion: $T_{1/2}$ is 67 to 77.6 hr. More than 94% is excreted unchanged in the feces; less than 0.6% is excreted in the urine.

Indications
Treatment of mild to moderate *Pneumocystis carinii* pneumonia (PCP) in patients who are intolerant of trimethoprim-sulfamethoxazole and acute oral treatment of mild to moderate PCP in patients who are intolerant to trimethoprim-sulfamethoxazole (TMP-SMZ).

Contraindications
Standard considerations.

Route/Dosage
Prevention of PCP
ADULTS AND CHILDREN 13 TO 16 YR: **PO** 1500 mg once daily with a meal.

Treatment of Mild to Moderate PCP
ADULTS AND CHILDREN 13 TO 16 YR: **PO** 750 mg administered with food twice daily for 21 days (total daily dose, 1500 mg).

Interactions
Food: Food, particularly fats, increases absorption 3-fold.
Highly protein-bound drugs: Atovaquone is highly protein bound; interactions may occur because of competition for binding sites.
Rifamycins: Decreases steady-state plasma concentrations of atovaquone and increases steady-state plasma concentrations of rifampin.

Lab Test Interferences
None well documented.

Adverse Reactions
CNS: Headache; insomnia; dizziness; anxiety.
DERM: Rash; pruritus.
EENT: Sinusitis; rhinitis; altered taste.
GI: Nausea; diarrhea; vomiting; abdominal pain; constipation; oral monilia; anorexia; dyspepsia.
GU: Elevated creatinine; elevated BUN.
HEMA: Anemia; neutropenia.
HEPA: Elevated liver enzymes.
RESP: Cough increased.
OTHER: Fever; sweating; weakness; decreased sodium concentration; elevated amylase; allergic reaction; rhinitis; asthenia; infection; dyspnea.

Precautions
Pregnancy: Category C.
Lactation: Undetermined.
Children: Safety and efficacy not established.
Elderly: Atovaquone has not been systematically evaluated in patients older than 65 yr.
Hepatic function impairment: Use caution and closely monitor administration.
Severe PCP: Treatment of severe episodes of PCP has not been evaluated. Efficacy in patients not responding to trimethoprim-sulfamethoxazole has not been established. Atovaquone has not been evaluated for prophylaxis of PCP.

PATIENT CARE CONSIDERATIONS

Administration/Storage
- Most effective if administered with food, particularly proteins and fats.
- Do not freeze.

Assessment/Interventions
- Obtain patient history, including drug history and any known allergies, particularly to antifungal medications. Note existing GI disorders, because these may limit absorption of orally-administered drug.
- Monitor patient closely for several hours after administering the first dose, even if there is no history of allergy.
- Monitor renal and GI function during therapy.
- Observe for signs of superinfection during therapy (eg, yeast infections, black "hairy" tongue, itching in groin area).
- Monitor for effectiveness during therapy (eg, decreased temperature, decreased lung congestion).
- If signs and symptoms of hypersensitivity occur (eg, rash, shortness of breath), withhold medication and notify health care provider.
- If no improvement in infection occurs within 5 days, notify health care provider.
- If severe GI side effects occur, notify health care provider.

Patient/Family Education
- Inform patient that medication is most effective when taken with food (particularly fatty foods), and to notify health care provider if unable to eat.
- Inform patient that slight rash may develop while taking medication.
- Teach patient to recognize signs of oral fungal infections.

Atovaquone/Proguanil Hydrochloride

(uh-TOE-vuh-KWONE/pro-GWAHN-ill HIGH-droe-KLOR-ide)

Class Anti-infective/Antimalarial

How Supplied
Malarone Tablets 250 mg atovaquone and 100 mg proguanil hydrochloride ◆ *Malarone Pediatric* Tablets 62.5 mg atovaquone and 25 mg proguanil hydrochloride

Action
PHARMACOLOGY: Atovaquone inhibits mitochondrial electron transport in metabolic enzymes of parasites, causing inhibition of nucleic acid and adenosine triphosphate synthesis.

Proguanil exerts its effect by means of the metabolite cycloguanil, which inhibits dihydrofolate reductase in the malarial parasite, disrupting deoxythymidylate synthesis.

Indications Prophylaxis of *P. falciparum* malaria; treatment of acute, uncomplicated *P. falciparum* malaria.

Contraindications Prophylaxis of *P. falciparum* in patients with severe renal impairment (Ccr less than 30 mL/min); hypersensitivity to any component of the product.

Route/Dosage
Malaria Prevention
ADULTS: **PO** 250 mg atovaquone/100 mg proguanil daily, starting 1 or 2 days before entering a malaria-endemic area, and continuing during the stay and for 7 days after return.
CHILDREN: **PO** Based on body weight. 11 to 20 kg: 62.5 mg atovaquone/25 mg proguanil daily; 21 to 30 kg: 125 mg atovaquone/50 mg proguanil daily; 31 to 40 kg: 187.5 mg atovaquone/75 mg proguanil; more than 40 kg: 250 mg atovaquone/100 mg proguanil. Start prophylaxis 1 or 2 days before entering a malaria-endemic area and continue during the stay and for 7 days after return.

Treatment of Acute Malaria
ADULTS: **PO** 1 g atovaquone/400 mg proguanil as a single daily dose for 3 consecutive days.
CHILDREN: **PO** Based on body weight. 5 to 8 kg: 125 mg atovaquone/50 mg proguanil daily for 3 consecutive days; 9 to 10 kg: 187.5 mg atovaquone/75 mg proguanil daily for 3 consecutive days; 11 to 20 kg: 250 mg atovaquone/100 mg proguanil daily for 3 consecutive days; 21 to 30 kg: 500 mg atovaquone/200 mg proguanil daily for 3 consecutive days; 31 to 40 kg: 750 mg atovaquone/300 mg proguanil daily for 3 consecutive days; more than 40 kg: 1 g atovaquone/400 mg proguanil daily for 3 consecutive days.

Interactions
Metoclopramide: May reduce the bioavailability of atovaquone, decreasing the therapeutic effect.
Rifamycins (eg, rifampin, rifabutin): Because atovaquone concentrations may be reduced, coadministration is not recommended.
Tetracycline: May reduce plasma concentrations of atovaquone, decreasing the therapeutic effect.

Lab Test Interferences None well documented.

Adverse Reactions

CNS: Headache, anorexia, dizziness (5% or more); abnormal dreams, insomnia (1% or more).
DERM: Pruritus (1% or more); photosensitivity, urticaria, erythema multiforme, Stevens-Johnson syndrome (postmarketing).
EENT: Visual difficulties (2%).
GI: Abdominal pain, nausea, vomiting, diarrhea, oral ulcers (5% or more).
RESP: Cough (5% or more).
OTHER: Asthenia (5% or more).

Precautions

Pregnancy: Category C.
Lactation: Undetermined.
Children: Safety and efficacy not established for the treatment of malaria in children weighing less than 5 kg or for the prophylaxis of malaria in children weighing less than 11 kg.
Elderly: Use with caution because of the greater frequency of decreased hepatic, renal, or cardiac function, and concomitant diseases or other drug therapy.

PATIENT CARE CONSIDERATIONS

Administration/Storage

- Take the daily dose at the same time each day with food or milk. Repeat dose if vomiting occurs within 1 hr.
- Use pediatric tablets in children weighing less than 88 pounds (40 kg).
- Tablets may be crushed and mixed with condensed milk for children who have difficulty swallowing them.

Malaria Treatment:

- Administer prescribed dose qd for 3 consecutive days.

Malaria Prophylaxis:

- Do not administer to patient with Ccr less than 30 mL/min.
- Prescribed dose is taken qd beginning 1 or 2 days before entering a malaria-endemic area, while in the malaria-endemic area, and for 7 days following return.
- Store tablets at controlled room temperature (59° to 86°F).

Assessment/Interventions

- Obtain patient history, including drug history and any known allergies. Note renal or hepatic impairment.
- Monitor patient for vomiting or diarrhea. Consider using antiemetic therapy in patient who has frequent or persistent vomiting. If patient has severe or persistent vomiting or diarrhea, evaluate patient for need of alternative therapy.
- Monitor patient for GI, CNS, MUSC, and general body side effects. Inform health care provider if noted and significant.

Renal function impairment: Atovaquone/proguanil is contraindicated in patients with severe renal impairment (Ccr less than 30 mL/min).
Hepatic function impairment: Studies have not been conducted in patients with severe hepatic impairment; however, no dosage adjustments are needed in patients with mild to moderate hepatic impairment.
Diarrhea/Vomiting: Absorption of atovaquone may be reduced.
Recrudescent: In the event of recrudescent P. falciparum infections after treatment or failure of chemoprophylaxis with atovaquone/proguanil, patients should be treated with a different blood schizonticide.
Severe malaria: Because atovaquone/proguanil has not been evaluated for treatment of cerebral malaria or other severe manifestations of complicated malaria, patients with these conditions are not candidates for oral therapy.

Overdosage: Signs and Symptoms

Epigastric discomfort, vomiting.

Patient/Family Education

- Explain name, dose, action, and potential side effects of drug.
- Advise patient to take tablets qd, at about the same time each day with food or milk.
- Instruct patient to repeat dose if vomiting occurs within 1 hr of taking a dose.
- Advise patient that if a dose is missed, to take the dose as soon as remembered then return to the normal dosing schedule. Advise patient that if it is nearing time for the next dose or if a dose is skipped, not to double the next dose.
- Instruct patient taking medication for prophylaxis that medication should be taken qd, beginning 1 to 2 days prior to arrival in malaria-infected area, while in the malaria-infected area, and for 7 days after leaving the malaria-infected area.
- Advise patient that protective clothing, insect repellants, and bednets are important components of malaria prophylaxis.
- Advise patient to notify health care provider if severe or persistent vomiting or diarrhea develop, other bothersome side effects occur, or therapy is prematurely discontinued for any reason.
- Advise women to notify health care provider if pregnant, planning to become pregnant, or breastfeeding.
- Advise women taking folate supplements that the folate supplements can be continued while taking this medication.
- Instruct patient not to take any prescription

or OTC medications or dietary supplements unless advised by health care provider.
- Advise patient that if a febrile illness develops during or after return from a malaria-endemic area, to seek health care and inform health care provider of possible exposure to malaria.

Atropine

(AT-troe-peen)

Class Anticholinergic/Antispasmodic

How Supplied

Atropine-1 Solution 1% ♦ *Atropine Care* Solution 1% ♦ *Isopto Atropine* Solution 0.5%, Solution 1% ♦ *Sal-Tropine* Tablets 0.4 mg
❀ *Atropine* ♦ *Atropine Injection* ♦ *Atropine Ointment* ♦ *Minims Atropine*

Action

PHARMACOLOGY: Inhibits action of acetylcholine or other cholinergic stimuli at postganglionic cholinergic receptors, including smooth muscles, secretory glands and CNS sites.

PHARMACOKINETICS/DYNAMICS:

Absorption: Rapidly absorbed after oral administration.

Distribution: Readily crosses blood-brain barrier.

Excretion: $T_{1/2}$ is 2.5 hr. 94% of dose is eliminated through urine in 24 hr.

Indications Administration prior to anesthesia to reduce or prevent secretions of respiratory tract; to control rhinorrhea; treatment of parkinsonism; restoration of cardiac rate and arterial pressure in some situations; treatment of peptic ulcers; management of hypersecretion, irritation or inflammation of stomach, intestines or pancreas; treatment of diarrhea; relief of infant colic; management of spasms of bile tract; treatment of hypertonicity of small intestine or uterus; management of hypermotility of colon; prevention of spasm of pylorus, biliary tree, ureters, and bronchi; treatment of frequent urination and bed-wetting; therapy for certain bradycardias and heart blocks; treatment of closed head injury with acetylcholine release; reduction of laughing and crying associated with brain lesions; treatment of alcohol withdrawal symptoms; relief of motion sickness. Antidote for cardiovascular collapse in certain overdoses or poisonings. Short-term treatment and prevention of bronchospasm associated with chronic bronchial asthma, bronchitis and COPD.
Ophthalmic preparation: Production of cycloplegia and mydriasis.

Contraindications Hypersensitivity to anticholinergics; narrow-angle glaucoma; adhesions between iris and lens; prostatic hypertrophy; obstructive uropathy; myocardial ischemia; unstable cardiac status caused by hemorrhage; tachycardia; myasthenia gravis; pyloric or intestinal obstruction; asthma; hyperthyroidism; renal disease; hepatic disease; toxic megacolon; intestinal atony or paralytic ileus.

Route/Dosage

ADULTS: 0.4 to 0.6 mg q 4 to 6 hr.
CHILDREN: **PO** Use lowest effective dose beginning at 0.01 mg/kg q 4 to 6 hr not to exceed 0.4 mg q 4 to 6 hr.

Surgery

ADULTS: **SC/IM/IV** 0.4 to 0.6 mg q 4 to 6 hr.
CHILDREN: **SC/IM/IV** 0.01 mg/kg to max of 0.4 mg q 4 to 6 hr.
INFANTS LESS THAN 5 KG: **SC/IM/IV** 0.04 mg/kg.
INFANTS OVER 5 KG: **SC/IM/IV** 0.03 mg/kg.

Bradyarrhythmias

ADULTS: **SC/IM/IV** 0.4 to 2 mg q 1 to 2 hr prn.
CHILDREN: **SC/IV/IM** 0.01 to 0.03 mg/kg, q 1 to 2 hr prn.

Antidote (Insecticide Poisoning)

ADULTS: **Parenteral** At least 2 to 3 mg, repeated until signs of poisoning subside or signs of intoxication appear.
CHILDREN: 0.02 to 0.05 mg/kg/dose q 10 to 20 min until signs of atropic effect are observed, then q 1 to 4 hr for at least 24 hr.

OPHTHALMIC

Uveitis

ADULT: 1 to 2 drops 0.5% to 1% solution qid or ointment tid.
CHILDREN: 1 to 2 drops 0.5% solution tid.

Refraction

ADULTS: 1 to 2 drops of 1% solution 1 hr before refraction examination.
CHILDREN: 1 to 2 drops 0.5% solution bid 1 to 3 days before refraction examination.

Interactions

Haloperidol: Worsened schizophrenic symptoms; decreased serum haloperidol concentrations.
Phenothiazines: Decreased antipsychotic effects and increased anticholinergic effects may occur.
Other anticholinergic agents: Additive anticholinergic effects.

Lab Test Interferences None well documented.

Adverse Reactions

CV: Palpitations; bradycardia; tachycardia; orthostatic hypotension.
CNS: Headache; nervousness; drowsiness; weakness; dizziness; confusion; insomnia; fever; excitability; restlessness; tremor.

DERM: Allergic reactions; urticaria; rash; flushing.
EENT: Nasal congestion; altered taste.
GI: Xerostomia; nausea; vomiting; dysphagia; heartburn; constipation; bloated feeling; paralytic ileus.
GU: Urinary hesitancy and retention; impotence.
RESP: Bronchospasm.
OTHER: Suppression of lactation; decreased sweating.

Precautions
Pregnancy: Category C.
Lactation: If possible, do not use.
Children: Use cautiously in infants.
Special risk patients: Use cautiously in elderly patients and in patients with Down syndrome, brain damage or spastic paralysis.
Anticholinergic psychosis: Has occurred in sensitive patients.

Diarrhea: May be an early symptom of incomplete intestinal obstruction.
Gastric ulcer: May delay gastric emptying time and complicate therapy.
Glaucoma: Determine intraocular IOP and depth of angle of anterior chamber before and during ophthalmic use to avoid glaucoma attacks.
Heat prostration: May occur at high ambient temperature.

Overdosage: Signs and Symptoms
Dry mouth, thirst, vomiting, nausea, abdominal distention, CNS stimulation, delirium, drowsiness, restlessness, stupor, fever, seizures, hallucinations, convulsions, coma, circulatory failure, tachycardia, weak pulse, hypertension, hypotension, respiratory depression, palpitations, urinary urgency, blurred vision, dilated pupils, photophobia, rash, dry and hot skin.

PATIENT CARE CONSIDERATIONS

Administration/Storage
Oral:
* Administer 30 min before meals and at bedtime for GI disorders.
* Store in airtight, light-resistant container at room temperature.

IM/SC:
* Draw solution carefully into syringe. Accidental eye exposure results in blurred vision.
* Administer 30 to 60 min before surgery if used for preanesthesia.
* Give after patient has voided.

IV:
* Do not add to IV solutions.

Ophthalmic:
* Compress inner canthus gently for 1 to 3 min after installation.
* Wash hands after administration to avoid accidental eye exposure.

Assessment/Interventions
* Obtain patient history, including drug history and any known allergies.
* Identify baseline signs and symptoms, and monitor patient according to indications for use: increased heart rate when used for bradycardia (notify health care provider of paradoxical bradycardia); decreased secretions for preanesthesia; decreased GI motility or decreased abdominal pain in GI disorders; pupil dilation in eye disorders; decreased tremor, rigidity and drooling in Parkinson disease.
* Monitor elderly patient for agitation or drowsiness.
* Monitor vital signs. Remember that pulse rate is particularly sensitive to atropine.
* Assess for urinary retention, particularly in elderly men and in those with pre-existing prostatic hypertrophy and other obstructive/retentive disorders.
* Dim room lighting to comfort level or provide sunglasses if necessary.
* Keep room cool and provide adequate hydration to prevent hyperpyrexia.
* Institute safety precautions if visual or CNS disturbances occur.
* Provide frequent oral hygiene, skin care, and lubricating eye drops if dry mouth/skin/eyes occur.
* Notify health care provider immediately if eye pain, diarrhea, or significant tachycardia or bradycardia occurs.

Patient/Family Education
* Warn patient that temporary mild stinging and blurred vision may occur with ophthalmic preparations.
* Instruct patient to withhold ophthalmic preparations if eye pain, redness, or rapid, irregular pulse occurs and to notify health care provider immediately.
* Instruct patient in and observe return demonstration of patient's technique for installation of ophthalmic preparations.
* Instruct patient to take oral dose 30 min before meals and at bedtime.
* Caution patient to avoid hazardous activities until vision clears.
* Advise patients that eyes may be more sensitive to light and to wear sunglasses, as needed.

- Tell patients to increase dietary fiber and fluids, unless contraindicated, to reduce constipation.
- Explain importance of frequent oral hygiene and regular dental care when mouth is dry. Explain that chewing sugarless gum or sucking on ice chips or hard candy may relieve dry mouth.
- Caution patient to avoid vigorous exercise in warm environment and to avoid hot baths or saunas.
- Advise men that if impotence occurs, it may be a result of drug therapy and to notify health care provider.
- Tell patient to notify health care provider immediately if the following symptoms occur: rapid, irregular pulse; headaches; hot, dry skin; difficulty swallowing; urinary retention; constipation; difficulty breathing; loss of coordination; restlessness; tremors; disorientation; hallucinations.
- If patient is taking drug for symptoms of Parkinson disease, warn patient that drug should not be discontinued abruptly, because withdrawal-like symptoms may occur.

Atropine Sulfate/Scopolamine Hydrobromide/Hyoscyamine Sulfate/Phenobarbital

(AT-troe-peen SULL-fate/skoe-POLE-uh-meen HIGH-droe-BROE-mide/high-oh-SIGH-uh-meen SULL-fate/fee-no-BAR-bih-tahl)

Class Anticholinergic/Antispasmodic

How Supplied
Barbidonna Tablets 0.025 mg atropine sulfate/0.0074 mg scopolamine HBr/0.1286 mg hyoscyamine sulfate/16 mg phenobarbital ♦ *Barbidonna No. 2* Tablets 0.025 mg atropine sulfate/0.0074 mg scopolamine HBr/0.1286 mg hyoscyamine sulfate/32 mg phenobarbital ♦ *Donnatal* Capsules 0.0194 mg atropine sulfate/0.0065 mg scopolamine HBr/0.1037 mg hyoscyamine HBr or sulfate/16.2 mg phenobarbital, Tablets 0.0194 mg atropine sulfate/0.0065 mg scopolamine HBr/0.1037 mg hyoscyamine HBr or sulfate/16.2 mg phenobarbital ♦ *Hyosophen* Tablets 0.0194 mg atropine sulfate/0.0065 mg scopolamine HBr/0.1037 mg hyoscyamine HBr or sulfate/16.2 mg phenobarbital ♦ *Spasmolin* Tablets 0.0194 mg atropine sulfate/0.0065 mg scopolamine HBr/0.1037 mg hyoscyamine HBr or sulfate/16.2 mg phenobarbital

Action
PHARMACOLOGY: Promotes peripheral anticholinergic/antispasmodic action (decreases GI motility); provides mild sedation.

Indications Possibly effective for treatment of irritable bowel syndrome and acute enterocolitis. Also may be useful as adjunctive therapy for duodenal ulcer.

Contraindications Glaucoma; obstructive uropathy; obstructive disease of the gastrointestinal tract; paralytic ileus; intestinal atony in elderly or debilitated patient; severe ulcerative colitis; toxic megacolon complicating ulcerative colitis; hepatic or renal disease; tachycardia; myocardial ischemia; unstable cardiovascular status in acute hemorrhage; myasthenia gravis; acute intermittent porphyrinuria.

Route/Dosage
ADULTS: **PO** 1 to 2 tablets or capsules tid to qid; 1 extended-release tablet q 12 hr; 5 to 10 mL elixir tid to qid according to condition and severity of symptoms.
CHILDREN: **PO** 0.5 to 5.0 mL elixir: q 4 hr to q 6 hr, according to body weight.

Interactions
Anticoagulants: Anticoagulant effects may be decreased.
Anticholinergic agents: Additive anticholinergic effects.
Haloperidol: Worsened schizophrenic symptoms; decreased haloperidol concentrations.
Phenothiazines: Decreased antipsychotic effects and increased anticholinergic effects may occur.

Lab Test Interferences None well documented.

Adverse Reactions
CV: Palpitations; bradycardia; tachycardia; flushing.
CNS: Headache; nervousness; drowsiness; weakness; dizziness; confusion; insomnia; fever (especially in children); mental confusion or excitement (especially in the elderly, even with small doses); CNS stimulation (restlessness, tremor), psychosis.
DERM: Urticaria and other dermal manifestations of allergic reaction.
EENT: Blurred vision; mydriasis; photophobia; cycloplegia; increased IOP; dilated pupils; nasal congestion; altered taste perception.
GI: Xerostomia; nausea; vomiting; dysphagia; heartburn; constipation; bloated feeling; paralytic ileus.
GU: Urinary hesitancy and retention; impotence.
OTHER: Severe allergic reactions, including anaphylaxis; suppression of lactation; decreased sweating.

Precautions
Pregnancy: Category C.
Lactation: If possible, do not use.
Elderly: May react with agitation, drowsiness and other untoward manifestations even with small doses.
Special risk patients: Used with caution in patients with neuropathy, hepatic or renal disease, hyperthyroidism, coronary artery disease, CHF, arrhythmias, hypertension or tachycardia. May complicate gastric ulcer treatment.
Diarrhea: May be symptom of incomplete intestinal obstruction, especially in patients with ileostomy or colostomy and, therefore, may serve as contraindication.
Heat prostration: Can occur in presence of high ambient temperature because of interference with normal sweating.
Potentially hazardous tasks: May produce drowsiness, dizziness or blurred vision.
Addiction potential: May be habit forming; when possible, not given to addiction-prone individual.

Overdosage: Signs and Symptoms
Dry mouth, thirst, vomiting, nausea, abdominal distention, CNS stimulation, delirium, drowsiness, restlessness, stupor, fever, seizures, hallucinations, convulsions, coma, "flat" EEG, circulatory failure, tachycardia, weak pulse, hypertension, hypotension, respiratory depression, palpitations, arrhythmias, urinary urgency, blurred vision, dilated pupils, photophobia, rash, dry and hot skin.

PATIENT CARE CONSIDERATIONS

Administration/Storage
- Available for oral use only.
- Store in a cool, dry place.

Assessment/Interventions
- Obtain patient history, including drug history and any known allergies.
- Monitor vital signs and LOC. Note any signs of hyperactivity or sedation.
- Monitor I&O and bowel sounds. Notify health care provider of abdominal distention.
- In patient with chronic lung disease, monitor lung sounds and effectiveness of cough.

Patient/Family Education
- Caution patient to have adequate oral intake.
- Advise patient to include fiber in diet to prevent constipation.
- Caution patient to limit exposure to high ambient temperatures.
- Advise patient that dilated pupils may be experienced.
- Warn patient that product may cause excitability or sedation. Remind patient not to drive or operate heavy machinery if sedation occurs.
- Advise patient to notify health care provider if confusion, disorientation, ataxia, nausea, vomiting, diarrhea, abdominal distention, or elevated body temperature occurs. With ophthalmic preparations, also tell the patient to notify the doctor if eye pain is experienced.

Auranofin

(or-RAIN-oh-fin)

Class Analgesic/Antirheumatic/Gold compound

How Supplied
Ridaura Capsules 3 mg

Action
PHARMACOLOGY: Gold compounds relieve symptoms of arthritis but do not cure this disease; decrease rheumatoid factor concentrations and immunoglobulins.

PHARMACOKINETICS/DYNAMICS:
Absorption: Because of rapid metabolism, intact auranofin has never been detected in the blood. Approximately 25% of the gold in auranofin is absorbed. Steady state gold concentrations of approximately 0.68 mcg/mL are achieved in approximately 3 mo.
Distribution: Approximately 40% of auranofin gold is associated with red cells, and 60% is associated with serum proteins.
Metabolism: Rapidly metabolized.
Excretion: Mean terminal plasma $t_{1/2}$ of auranofin gold at steady state is 26 days. Approximately 60% of absorbed gold of single auranofin dose is excreted in urine; remainder is excreted in the feces.

Indications Relief of symptoms of active adult rheumatoid arthritis poorly controlled with other therapies. **Unlabeled use(s):** Treatment of pemphigus and psoriatic arthritis.

Contraindications Standard considerations.

Route/Dosage
ADULTS: **PO** 6 mg/day or 3 mg bid. If no response by 6 mo, dose may be increased to 3 mg tid. Parenteral route may be used when control cannot be achieved by oral form.
CHILDREN: Auranofin is not recommended for children; safety and efficacy have not been established. If prescribed, however, the following doses have been recommended. 0.1 mg/kg/day (initial dose); 0.15 mg/kg/day (maintenance dose); 0.2 mg/kg/day (max dose).

Interactions None well documented.
Lab Test Interferences None well documented.
Adverse Reactions Reactions can occur months after therapy is discontinued.
CNS: Confusion; hallucinations; seizures.
DERM: Dermatitis; pruritus; grey-blue pigmentation on sun-exposed skin; exfoliative dermatitis; angioedema.
EENT: Mucositis that may be preceded by metallic taste; conjunctivitis; corneal gold deposition; metallic taste; inflammation of the upper respiratory tract; pharyngitis.
GI: Diarrhea; abdominal pain; anorexia; dyspepsia; flatulence; GI bleeding; enterocolitis; gastritis; colitis; tracheitis.
GU: Nephrotic syndrome and glomerulitis with proteinuria and hematuria.
HEMA: Anemia; thrombocytopenia; leukopenia; aplastic anemia.
HEPA: Elevated liver enzymes; jaundice; hepatitis.
RESP: Interstitial pneumonitis; pulmonary fibrosis.
OTHER: Vaginitis; glossitis.

Precautions
Pregnancy: Category C.
Lactation: Excreted in breast milk.
Children: Safety and efficacy not established.
Elderly: Tolerance decreases with age.
Special risk patients: Use with caution in patients with diabetes mellitus, CHF, history of blood dyscrasias, allergy or hypersensitivity to other gold products, skin rash, previous kidney or liver disease, marked hypertension, compromised circulation or inflammatory bowel disease.

Overdosage: Signs and Symptoms
Renal damage (eg, hematuria, proteinuria), hematologic reactions (eg, thrombocytopenia), nausea, vomiting, diarrhea, fever, skin disorders.

PATIENT CARE CONSIDERATIONS
Administration/Storage
- Administer with food or fluid.
- Protect product from light and moisture.

Assessment/Interventions
- Obtain patient history, including drug history and any known allergies.
- Observe patient for early symptoms of toxicity such as a metallic taste in the mouth, pruritus or rash.
- Review laboratory values for indications of gold toxicity such as decreased hemoglobin, less than 4000 WBC/mm^3, platelets less than 100,000 to 150,000/cu mm, proteinuria, and elevated liver enzymes.
- If given parenterally, stay with patient for 15 min after injection and monitor for the following signs of adverse reaction: anaphylactic shock; syncope; bradycardia; thickening of tongue; dysphagia; dyspnea; and angioneurotic edema. Notify health care provider of any problems.
- Observe for diarrhea and loose stools, a common adverse reaction that usually can be managed by a reduction in dosage.

Patient/Family Education
- Instruct patient to immediately report any adverse effects of therapy including dermatitis and pruritus, weakness, fatigue, hematuria, sore mouth, indigestion, diarrhea, metallic taste in mouth, or unusual bruising.
- Caution patient to minimize exposure to the sun and other sources of ultraviolet light. Explain the need to wear sunscreen and protective clothing outdoors.
- Advise patient to keep appointments with health care providers for continued assessment and monitoring of renal, hepatic and hematologic functions.
- Review oral hygiene, including use of soft toothbrush, daily flossing and avoidance of strong, commercial mouthwashes. If mild stomatitis develops, an isotonic NaCl and sodium bicarbonate solution can be used.
- Alert women to the potential risks of using gold therapy during pregnancy.

Azacitidine

(AZE-ah-SIGH-tih-deen)
Class DNA demethylating agent
How Supplied
Vidaza Powder for injection, lyophilized 100 mg
Action
PHARMACOLOGY: Believed to cause hypomethylation of DNA and direct cytotoxicity on abnormal hematopoietic cells in bone marrow.

PHARMACOKINETICS/DYNAMICS:
Absorption: Rapidly absorbed after subcutaneous administration; C_{max} 750 ng/mL in 0.5 hr. Subcutaneous bioavailability 89% compared with IV administration.

Distribution: Mean Vd is 76 L.

Excretion: Mean apparent subcutaneous Cl is 167 L/hr and mean t½ is 41 min. After subcutaneous administration, mean urinary excretion 50%. Mean elimination t½ 4 hr.

Indications Treatment of myelodysplastic syndrome subtypes: refractory anemia or refractory anemia with ringed sideroblasts (if accompanied by neutropenia or thrombocytopenia or requiring transfusions), refractory anemia with excess blasts, refractory anemia with excess blasts in transformation, and chronic myelomonocytic leukemia.

Contraindications Advanced malignant hepatic tumors; hypersensitivity to mannitol or azacitidine.

Route/Dosage
ADULTS: **Subcutaneous** Recommended starting dose is 75 mg/m^2 daily for 7 days, q 4 wk. Premedicate patient for nausea and vomiting. Increase dose to 100 mg/m^2 if no beneficial effect seen after 2 treatment cycles and if no toxicity other than nausea and vomiting occur. Recommended that patients be treated for a minimum of 4 cycles. Treatment may be continued as long as patient continues to benefit.

Dosage Adjustments Based on Hematologic Laboratory Values
ADULTS: **Subcutaneous** For patients with WBC at least 3×10^9/L, ANC at least 1.5×10^9/L and platelets at least 75×10^9/L at the start of treatment, adjust dose based on nadir counts for any given cycle as follows:
- ANC less than 0.5×10^9/L, platelets less than 25×10^9/L administer 50% of dose in next course.
- ANC 0.5 to 1.5×10^9/L, platelets 25 to 50×10^9/L administer 67% of dose in next course.
- ANC greater than 1.5×10^9/L, platelets greater than 50×10^9/L administer 100% of dose in next course.
- For patients with WBC less than 3×10^9/L, ANC less than 1.5×10^9/L, or platelets less than 75×10^9/L at the start of treatment, base dose adjustments on nadir counts and bone marrow biopsy cellularity at time of nadir as follows, unless there is clear improvement in differentiation (percentage of mature granulocytes is higher and ANC is higher than at onset of course) at time of next cycle, in which case continue the dose of the current treatment.
- WBC or platelet nadir percent decrease in counts from baseline is 50% to 75% and bone marrow biopsy cellularity at time of nadir is 30% to 60%, give 100% of dose in next course.
- WBC or platelet nadir percent decrease in counts from baseline is 50% to 75% and bone marrow biopsy cellularity at time of nadir is 15% to 30%, give 50% of dose in next course.
- WBC or platelet nadir percent decrease in counts from baseline is 50% to 75% and bone marrow biopsy cellularity at time of nadir is less than 15%, give 33% of dose in next course.
- WBC or platelet nadir percent decrease in counts from baseline is greater than 75% and bone marrow biopsy cellularity at time of nadir is 30% to 60%, give 75% of dose in next course.
- WBC or platelet nadir percent decrease in counts from baseline is greater than 75% and bone marrow biopsy cellularity at time of nadir is 15% to 30% give 50% of dose in next course.
- WBC or platelet nadir percent decrease in counts from baseline is greater than 75% and bone marrow biopsy cellularity at time of nadir is less than 15% give 33% of dose in next course.
- If a nadir as defined above has occurred, give the next course of treatment 28 days after the start of the preceding course provided that both WBC and platelet counts are greater than 25% above the nadir and rising. If a greater than 25% increase above nadir is not seen by day 28, reassess counts q 7 days. If a 25% increase is not seen by day 42, treat the patient with 50% of the scheduled dose.

Dosage Adjustments Based on Renal Function and Serum Electrolytes
ADULTS: **Subcutaneous** If unexplained reductions in serum bicarbonate levels to less than 20 mEq/L occur, reduce dosage 50% on next course. If unexplained elevations of BUN or serum creatinine occur, delay the next cycle until values return to normal or baseline and reduce dose 50% on next treatment course.

Interactions None well documented.

Lab Test Interferences None well documented.

Adverse Reactions
CV: Cardiac murmur (10%); tachycardia (9%); hypotension (7%); atrial fibrillation, cardiac failure, CHF, cardio-pulmonary arrest, congestive cardiomyopathy, orthostatic hypotension (less than 5%).
CNS: Fatigue (36%); headache (22%); dizziness (19%); anxiety, aggravated fatigue, decreased appetite (13%); depression (12%); insomnia (11%); syncope (6%); hypoesthesia (5%); convulsions, intracranial hemorrhage, confusion (less than 5%).
DERM: Petechiae (24%); erythema (17%); pallor (16%); skin lesion (15%); rash (14%); pruritus (12%); increased sweating (11%); night sweats (9%); urticaria (6%); skin nodule, dry skin (5%); pyoderma gangrenosum, pruritic rash,

skin induration (less than 5%).
EENT: Pharyngitis (20%); epistaxis (16%); nasopharyngitis (15%); rhinorrhea (10%); nasal congestion (6%).
GI: Nausea (71%); vomiting (54%); diarrhea (36%); constipation (34%); anorexia (21%); abdominal pain (16%); abdominal tenderness (12%); upper abdominal pain (11%); gingival bleeding (10%); oral mucosal petechiae, stomatitis (8%); hemorrhoids, dyspepsia (7%); abdominal distention, loose stools (6%); mouth hemorrhage, dysphagia, tongue ulceration (5%); diverticulitis, GI hemorrhage, melena, perirectal abscess (less than 5%).
GU: Dysuria, UTI (8%); hematuria, loin pain, renal failure (less than 5%).
HEPA: Cholecystitis (less than 5%).
HEMA/LYMPH: Anemia (70%); thrombocytopenia (66%); leukopenia (48%); neutropenia (32%); febrile neutropenia (16%); lymphadenopathy (10%); hematoma (9%); aggravated anemia, postprocedural hemorrhage (6%); agranulocytosis, bone marrow depression, splenomegaly (less than 5%).
HYPERSEN: Anaphylactic shock, hypersensitivity (less than 5%).
LABTESTABS: Hypokalemia (13%).
LOCAL: Injection site erythema (35%); ecchymosis (31%); injection site pain (23%); injection site bruising or reaction (14%); injection site pruritus (7%); injection site granuloma, injection site pigmentation changes, injection site swelling (5%); catheter site hemorrhage (less than 5%).
M/N: Peripheral edema (19%); decreased weight (16%); pitting edema (15%); peripheral swelling (7%); dehydration (less than 5%).
MUSC: Arthralgia (22%); myalgia (16%); muscle cramps (6%); aggravated bone pain, muscle weakness, neck pain (less than 5%).
RESP: Cough (30%); dyspnea (29%); exertional dyspnea (14%); upper respiratory tract infection (13%); productive cough, crackles in lung, pneumonia (11%); wheezing, rales (9%); decreased breath sounds, rales (8%); pleural effusion, rhonchi (6%); exacerbated dyspnea, atelectasis, sinusitis (5%); hemoptysis, lung infiltration, pneumonitis, respiratory distress (less than 5%).
OTHER: Pyrexia (52%); weakness (29%); rigors (26%); limb pain (20%); back pain, contusion (19%); chest pain (16%); pain, malaise (11%); herpes simplex (9%); cellulitis, lethargy (8%); transfusion reaction (7%); chest wall pain; postprocedural pain (5%); general physical health deterioration, systemic inflammatory response syndrome, limb abscess, bacterial infection, blastomycosis, Klebsiella sepsis, streptococcal pharyngitis, Klebsiella pneumonia, sepsis, staphylococcal bacteremia, staphylococcal infection, toxoplasmosis, leukemia cutis, cholecystectomy (less than 5%).

Precautions
Pregnancy: Category D.
Lactation: Undetermined.
Children: Safety and efficacy not established.
Elderly: Because elderly patients are more likely to have decreased renal function, it may be useful to monitor renal function.
Hematologic: Neutropenia and thrombocytopenia may occur; monitor CBC.
Hepatic impairment: Use with caution.
Renal abnormalities: Elevated serum creatinine, renal failure, and death may occur.
Renal impairment: Monitor for toxicity because azacitidine and its metabolites are primarily excreted by the kidneys.
Use in men: Advise men to use effective contraception during treatment.

Overdosage: Signs and Symptoms
Bone marrow suppression, diarrhea, nausea, vomiting.

PATIENT CARE CONSIDERATIONS
Administration/Storage
- For subcutaneous administration only. Not for intradermal, IM, IV, or intra-arterial administration.
- Follow institutional procedures for handling, administration, and disposal of anticancer drugs. Wear appropriate protective equipment when preparing and administering medication.
- Reconstitute powder with 4 mL sterile water for injection. Inject diluent slowly into vial then invert vial 2 to 3 times and gently rotate until a uniform suspension is obtained. Resulting suspension contains 25 mg/mL of azacitidine.
- Draw contents into syringe. Divide doses greater than 4 mL equally into 2 syringes.
- Immediately prior to administration resuspend the contents by inverting syringe 2 to 3 times and gently rolling the syringe between the palms for 30 sec.
- Rotate sites for each injection (eg, thigh, abdomen, upper arm). Give new injections at least 1 inch from an old site and never into

areas where the site is tender, bruised, red, or hard.
- Avoid contact with skin and mucus membranes. If accidental skin contact occurs, wash thoroughly with soap and water. If mucus membrane contact occurs, flush thoroughly with water. If eye contact occurs, flush eyes using standard irrigation techniques.
- Discard unused portions of vial. Do not save any unused portions for future use.
- Premedicate patient with antiemetics as ordered by health care provider.
- Store unopened vials at controlled room temperature (59° to 86°F). If not used immediately, reconstituted suspension may be held for up to 1 hr at room temperature (77°F) but must be administered within 1 hr of reconstitution. The reconstituted suspension may be refrigerated immediately and held in refrigerator (36° to 46°F) for up to 8 hr. After removal from refrigerator, the suspension may be allowed to equilibrate to room temperature for up to 30 min.

Assessment/Interventions
- Obtain patient history, including drug history and any known allergies. Note renal or hepatic impairment, advanced malignant hepatic tumor, or hypersensitivity to mannitol.
- Ensure that CBC with differential and platelet count is evaluated prior to starting therapy and, at a minimum, before each cycle. After first cycle, reduce or delay dose for subsequent cycles based on nadir counts and hematologic response, following manufacturer's guidelines.
- Implement infection control measures if WBC drops; implement bleeding precautions if platelet count drops.
- Ensure that renal function is evaluated prior to starting therapy and before each cycle. If unexplained elevations in BUN or creatinine occur, delay next cycle until values return to normal or baseline, and reduce the dose 50% on the next treatment course.
- Ensure that women of childbearing potential are not pregnant before starting therapy and use effective contraception during treatment.
- Ensure that men use effective contraception during therapy.
- Monitor patient for signs and symptoms of anaphylactic or serious allergic reactions. Be prepared to treat appropriately.
- Assess patient for GI, CNS, CV, DERM, RESP, general body side effects, and injection site reactions. Report to health care provider if noted and significant.

Patient/Family Education
- Explain name, action, and potential side effects of drug.
- Advise patient that medication will be prepared and administered by health care providers in a health care setting.
- Review dosing schedule with patient.
- Advise patient to immediately report any of the following to health care provider: rash; hives; difficulty breathing fever, chills, or other signs of infection; unusual bleeding or bruising; pain, redness, or swelling at injection site.
- Advise patient to report any of the following to health care provider: persistent nausea, vomiting or appetite loss; persistent or worsening general body weakness.
- Caution men to use effective contraception during therapy.
- Caution women of childbearing potential to avoid becoming pregnant during therapy.
- Advise women to notify health care provider if pregnant, planning to become pregnant, or breastfeeding.
- Instruct patient not to take any prescription or OTC medications, herbal preparations, or dietary supplements unless advised by health care provider.
- Advise patient that follow-up visits and laboratory tests will be required to monitor therapy and to keep appointments.

Azathioprine

(AZE-uh-THIGH-oh-preen)

Class Immunosuppressive

How Supplied
Azasan Tablets 25 mg, Tablets 50 mg, Tablets 75 mg, Tablets 100 mg ◆ *Imuran* Tablets 50 mg, Injection 100 mg (as sodium)/vial
✤ *Apo-Azathioprine* ◆ *Gen-Azathioprine* ◆ *ratio-Azathioprine*

Action

PHARMACOLOGY: Suppresses cell-mediated hypersensitivities; alters antibody production and may reduce inflammation.

PHARMACOKINETICS/DYNAMICS:
Absorption: Well absorbed after oral administration.
Distribution: Azathioprine and mercaptopurine are approximately 30% bound to serum proteins.

Metabolism: Extensively metabolized. Azathioprine is cleaved to mercaptopurine (active). Both compounds are oxidized or methylated in erythrocytes or liver. Converted to inactive 6-thiouric acid by xanthine oxidase.

Excretion: Azathioprine and mercaptopurine are rapidly eliminated from blood. No azathioprine or mercaptopurine is detectable in urine after 8 hr. Partially dialyzable.

Indications Adjunct for prevention of rejection in renal homotransplantation; treatment in adults for severe, active, erosive rheumatoid arthritis not responsive to conventional management. **Unlabeled use(s):** Treatment of chronic ulcerative colitis, Crohn disease, myasthenia gravis and Behcet syndrome.

Contraindications Pregnancy in patients with rheumatoid arthritis.

Route/Dosage
Renal Transplantation
ADULTS AND CHILDREN: **IV/PO** Initiate with 3 to 5 mg/kg/day as single daily dose. Maintenance levels are 1 to 3 mg/kg/day.

Rheumatoid Arthritis
ADULTS: **PO** Initial dose is 1 mg/kg given as single dose or twice daily. Dose is increased by 0.5 mg/kg/day at 6 to 8 wk, then q 4 wk if there are no serious toxicities and if initial response is unsatisfactory. Max dose is 2.5 mg/kg/day. **IV** Reserved for patients unable to tolerate oral medications.

Interactions
Allopurinol: Decreases metabolism of azathioprine. Dose of azathioprine is reduced to approximately one-third to one-fourth usual dose when used concomitantly.

Nondepolarizing muscle relaxants (eg, tubocurarine, pancuronium): Azathioprine may resist or reverse neuromuscular blockade.

Lab Test Interferences None well documented.

Adverse Reactions
DERM: Rash.
GI: Nausea; vomiting.
HEMA: Leukopenia; thrombocytopenia; macrocytic anemia; bleeding; selective erythrocyte aplasia.

OTHER: Serious infections; neoplasias.

> **WARNING:**
> Chronic immunosuppression with this agent may increase risk of neoplasia.
> Experienced physician should be very familiar with mutagenic potential and hematological profile.

Precautions
Pregnancy: Category D.
Lactation: Excreted in breast milk.
Children: Safety and efficacy not established.
Carcinogenesis: Chronic immunosuppression with azathioprine increases risk of neoplasia. Patients with rheumatoid arthritis previously treated with alkylating agents (eg, cyclophosphamide, chlorambucil, melphalan) may have prohibitive risk of neoplasia.
Mutagenesis: Chronic immunosuppression with azathioprine increases risk of neoplasia. Patients with rheumatoid arthritis previously treated with alkylating agents (eg, cyclophosphamide, chlorambucil, melphalan) may have prohibitive risk of neoplasia.
Superinfection: Serious fungal, viral, bacterial and protozoal infections may develop in patients on long-term immunosuppression.
GI toxicity: Hypersensitivity reaction with severe nausea and vomiting may occur. Frequency of gastric disturbances can be reduced by giving in divided doses or after meals.
Hematologic effects: Severe hematologic toxicities (leukopenia and/or thrombocytopenia) may occur; monitor complete blood counts weekly during the first month, twice monthly for the second and third months, then monthly. Perform more frequently if dosage alterations or other therapy changes are necessary.
Hepatoxicity: Occurs primarily in allograft recipients. Rare but life-threatening hepatic veno-occlusive disease has occurred in transplant patients; monitor LFTs.

Overdosage: Signs and Symptoms
Bone marrow hypoplasia, bleeding, infection, death.

PATIENT CARE CONSIDERATIONS
Administration/Storage
- Do not vigorously shake solution when reconstituting IV preparations.
- Divide daily dosage to reduce GI upset.
- Administer with food or immediately after meals.
- Store in a tightly closed container in a cool location.
- Discard reconstituted IV preparations after 24 hr. Follow any procedures required for proper disposal of immunosuppressant/antimetabolite.

Assessment/Interventions
- Obtain patient history, including drug history and any known allergies.
- Review baseline CBC, renal studies, and liver studies.
- Assess for signs of infection before administration.
- Monitor I&O and daily weight during therapy.
- Monitor patient for signs of superinfection during therapy.
- Notify health care provider if patient displays sudden, severe dyspnea, bleeding from the gums or mucous membranes, or blood in urine or stools.

Patient/Family Education
- Instruct patient that if once-daily dose is forgotten to skip the dose, but if 2 daily doses are missed to call the health care provider. Next dose may be doubled.
- Explain importance of precautions regarding contact with individuals who have active infections and individuals who have recently received oral polio vaccine.
- Identify signs of transplant rejection (eg, localized redness, tenderness and swelling in the area of the transplant, decreased transplant organ function), and remind patient that this or similar medication will be required indefinitely to prevent transplant rejection.
- Explain that frequent follow-up appointments with a health care provider are important to adjust medication dosage.
- Instruct patient to report the following symptoms to health care provider: unusual bleeding, decreased urine output, abdominal pain.
- Caution patient not to take otc medications without consulting health care provider.

Azelaic Acid

(aze-eh-LAY-ik AH-sid)

Class Topical Anti-infective

How Supplied
Azelex Cream 20% ♦ Finacea Gel 15%

Action
PHARMACOLOGY: Mechanism of action is unknown; however, inhibition of microbial cellular protein synthesis may be involved.

PHARMACOKINETICS/DYNAMICS:
Absorption:
Cream – Approximately 4% of topically applied dose is systemically absorbed.

Distribution:
Cream – Approximately 3% to 5% penetrates into the stratum corneum and up to 10% into the epidermis and dermis.
Gel – Mean plasma concentration in rosacea patients ranges from 42 to 63.1 ng/mL after at least 8 wk of treatment.

Excretion:
Cream – Primarily unchanged in the urine. The t½ after topical application is approximately 12 hr.
Gel – Primarily unchanged in the urine.

Indications Topical treatment of mild to moderate inflammatory acne vulgaris (cream); topical treatment of papules and pustules of mild to moderate rosacea.

Contraindications Standard considerations.

Route/Dosage
ADULTS AND CHILDREN 12 YR AND OLDER: Topical After washing and patting dry, gently but thoroughly massage a thin film of cream or gel into the affected areas bid, in the morning and evening. In the majority of patients with inflammatory lesions, improvement of the condition occurs within 4 wk.

Interactions None well documented.

Lab Test Interferences None well documented.

Adverse Reactions
DERM: Vitiligo depigmentation; small depigmented spots; hypertrichosis; reddening (signs of keratosis pilaris); exacerbation of recurrent herpes labialis (rare).
Cream – Pruritus, burning, stinging, tingling (1% to 5%); erythema, dryness, rash, peeling, irritation, dermatitis, contact dermatitis (less than 1%).
Gel – Burning, stinging, tingling (20%); pruritus (7%); scaling, dry skin, xerosis (6%); erythema, irritation (2%); contact dermatitis, acne, seborrhea (1%).
RESP: Worsening of asthma.
OTHER:
Cream – Edema (1%); allergic reactions.

Precautions
Pregnancy: Category B.
Lactation: Undetermined.
Children: Safety and efficacy not established in children under 12 yr.
Sensitivity/Irritation: Discontinue if sensitivity or severe irritation develops.

PATIENT CARE CONSIDERATIONS

Administration/Storage

- For topical use only. Not for ophthalmic, oral, or intravaginal use.
- Avoid contact with eyes, eyelids, lips, and mucus membranes.
- Cream or gel is usually applied to affected area(s) bid, morning and evening.
- For treatment of acne, thoroughly wash and pat area(s) to be treated dry, then apply a thin film of cream to cover skin areas with acne lesions. Gently massage cream or gel into skin.
- For treatment of rosacea cleanse affected area(s) with mild soap or soapless cleansing solution then gently pat dry; apply a thin film of gel to affected area(s) and gently massage into the skin.
- Store cream or gel at controlled room temperature (59° to 86°F). Keep tube tightly capped and protect from freezing.

Assessment/Interventions

- Obtain patient history, including drug history and any known allergies.
- Assess the skin and identify areas where medication is to be applied and areas that should be avoided (severely irritated or sunburned skin).
- Assess and document skin condition before initial application and periodically throughout treatment.
- Monitor for side effects, including redness, scaling, dryness, or persistent itching or burning. Inform health care provider if noted and significant.

Patient/Family Education

- Explain name, action, and potential side effects of drug.
- Advise patient that medication is applied topically to skin lesions bid, morning and evening.
- Teach patient with acne proper technique for applying cream: wash hands; thoroughly wash and pat area(s) to be treated dry, then apply a thin film of cream to cover skin areas with acne lesions. Gently massage cream into skin. Wash hands after applying medication.
- Advise patient with acne that improvement may not be seen for at least 4 wk and to continue using the medication.
- Teach patient with rosacea proper technique for applying gel: wash hands; cleanse affected area(s) with mild soap or soapless cleansing solution then gently pat dry; apply a thin film of gel to affected area(s) and gently massage into the skin. Wash hands after applying medication.
- Instruct patient using gel to avoid concurrent use of topical alcoholic cleansers, tinctures and astringents, abrasives and peeling agents, as well as any food or beverage that might cause redness, flushing, or blushing (eg, spicy food, alcoholic beverages, hot drinks such as coffee or tea).
- Caution patient not to cover treated areas with bandages or dressings.
- Warn patient that applying medication more often than prescribed or in excessive quantities will not produce more rapid improvement or better results but will result in greater side effects such as redness, scaling, and discomfort.
- Advise patient that if an application is missed, not to try to make it up but to return to normal application schedule as soon as possible.
- Warn patient to avoid contact with the eyes, eyelids, lips, and mucous membranes.
- Advise patient that if cream or gel comes in contact with the eyes to wash eyes with large amounts of cool water and to contact health care provider if eye irritation persists.
- Advise patient with dark complexion to report any change in skin color to health care provider.
- Advise patient that local stinging, burning, itching, and tingling are the most common side effects and to notify health care provider if bothersome.
- Advise patient that if severe skin reactions occur to stop using the medication and contact health care provider.
- Advise patient to talk to health care provider before using any other topical agents (eg, medicated soaps, astringents, cosmetics, other acne products) on treated skin.
- Advise women to notify health care provider if pregnant, planning to become pregnant, or breastfeeding.
- Warn patient not to take any prescription or OTC drugs or dietary supplements without consulting health care provider.
- Advise patient that follow-up visits to examine the skin lesions may be necessary and to keep appointments.

Azelastine Hydrochloride

(ah-ZELL-ass-teen HIGH-dore-KLOR-ide)

Class Antihistamine

How Supplied
Astelin Nasal spray 137 mcg/spray ♦ *Optivar* Ophthalmic solution 0.05%

Action
PHARMACOLOGY: Competitively antagonizes histamine at H_1 receptor sites.

PHARMACOKINETICS/DYNAMICS:
Absorption: Bioavailability of nasal spray is approximately 40% and C_{max} is 2 to 3 hr. Absorption following ocular administration is relatively low, reaching a level of 0.02 to 0.25 ng/mL after 56 days of treatment.

Distribution: Vd is 14.5 L/kg. Approximately 88% (azelastine) and 97% (desmethylazelastine) are protein bound.

Metabolism: Oxidatively metabolized to desmethylazelastine (active) by CYP450 system.

Excretion: The t½ is 22 hr for azelastine and 54 hr for desmethylazelastine. Plasma Cl is 0.5 L/hr/kg. Approximately 75% was excreted in the feces, with less than 10% as unchanged azelastine.

Special Populations:
Renal Function Impairment – Based on oral doses, AUC and C_{max} increased 70% to 75% in those with Ccr less than 50 mL/min.

Indications Treatment of symptoms of seasonal allergic rhinitis, such as rhinorrhea, sneezing, and nasal pruritus; treatment of symptoms of vasomotor rhinitis, such as rhinorrhea, nasal congestion, and postnasal drip (nasal inhalation); treatment of itching of eye associated with allergic conjunctivitis (ophthalmic).

Contraindications Standard considerations.

Route/Dosage
Seasonal Allergic Rhinitis
ADULTS AND CHILDREN (12 YR AND OVER): Nasal Inhalation 2 sprays per nostril bid.
CHILDREN (5 TO 11 YR): **Nasal Inhalation** 1 spray per nostril bid.

Vasomotor Rhinitis
ADULTS AND CHILDREN (12 YR AND OVER): Nasal Inhalation 2 sprays per nostril bid.
ADULTS AND CHILDREN (3 YR AND OVER): Ophthalmic Instill 1 drop into each affected eye bid.

Interactions
Alcohol, other CNS depressants: Effects may be enhanced by azelastine.
Cimetidine: May increase azelastine plasma levels, increasing the risk of side effects.

Lab Test Interferences May interfere with diagnostic test results for skin tests using allergen extracts.

Adverse Reactions
CV: Flushing, hypertension, tachycardia (less than 2%).
CNS: Headache (15%); somnolence (12%); fatigue, dizziness (2%); hyperkinesias, hypoesthesia, vertigo, anxiety, depersonalization, depression, nervousness, sleep disturbances, abnormal thinking (less than 2%); confusion (postmarketing).
Ophthalmic – Headache (15%); fatigue (1% to 10%).
DERM: Contact dermatitis, eczema, hair and follicle infection, furunculosis (less than 2%); application site irritation, pruritus, rash (postmarketing).
Ophthalmic – Pruritus (1% to 10%).
EENT: Rhinitis (6%); conjunctivitis (5%); nasal burning, pharyngitis (4%); paroxysmal sneezing, sinusitis, epistaxis (3%); glossitis, burning throat, laryngitis, eye abnormality, eye pain, watery eyes (less than 2%); nasal congestion, parosmia, abnormal vision, xerophthalmia (postmarketing).
Ophthalmic – Transient eye burning/stinging (30%); conjunctivitis, eye pain, temporary blurring, rhinitis, pharyngitis (1% to 10%).
GI: Bitter taste (20%); dry mouth, nausea (3%); constipation, gastroenteritis, ulcerative stomatitis, vomiting, aphthous stomatitis, loss of taste, abdominal pain (less than 2%); diarrhea (postmarketing).
Ophthalmic – Bitter taste (10%).
GU: Albuminuria, amenorrhea, breast pain, hematuria, increased urinary frequency (less than 2%); urinary retention (postmarketing).
HEPA: Increased ALT (less than 2%).
METAB: Weight increase (2%); increased appetite (less than 2%).
RESP: Cough (11%); asthma (5%); bronchospasm (less than 2%); dyspnea (postmarketing).
Ophthalmic – Asthma, dyspnea (1% to 10%).
OTHER: Dysesthesia (8%); myalgia, cold symptoms, temporomandibular dislocation, allergic reaction, back pain, herpes simplex, viral infection, pain in extremities, malaise (less than 2%); anaphylactoid reaction, chest pain, facial edema, involuntary muscle contractions, paresthesia, tolerance (postmarketing).
Ophthalmic – Influenza-like symptoms (1% to 10%).

Precautions
Pregnancy: Category C.
Lactation: Undetermined.
Children: Safety and efficacy not established in seasonal allergic rhinitis in children younger

than 5 yr (nasal inhalation). Safety and efficacy not established in children younger than 3 yr (ophthalmic).

Elderly: Select dose with caution, reflecting greater frequency of decreased hepatic, renal, or cardiac function and comorbidity.

Overdosage: Signs and Symptoms
Somnolence.

PATIENT CARE CONSIDERATIONS

Administration/Storage
Nasal Spray:
- For intranasal administration only. Avoid spraying into the eyes.
- Prime spray pump with 4 sprays before first use and with 2 sprays if unit has not been used for 3 or more days.
- Have patient administer prescribed number of sprays bid.
- Have patient instill into nostril with head upright. Have patient sniff for a few minutes after instillation.
- Do not allow tip of container to touch nasal passage.
- Do not use container on more than 1 patient.
- Store nasal spray at controlled room temperature (68° to 77°F). Keep in upright position. Keep tightly closed and protect from freezing.

Ophthalmic Solution:
- For topical ophthalmic use only. Not for injection or oral use.
- Instill 1 drop into affected eyes bid.
- Do not allow tip of container to touch any surface, the eyelids, or surrounding areas.
- If using other topical ophthalmic drugs, separate each medication by at least 10 min.
- Store ophthalmic solution in refrigerator (36° to 46°F) or at controlled room temperature (47° to 77°F). Keep in upright position. Keep tightly closed and protect from freezing.

Assessment/Interventions
- Obtain patient history, including drug history and any known allergies.

Nasal Spray:
- Assess for allergy symptoms (eg, rhinitis, nasal congestion, sneezing, nasal itching) before and periodically throughout therapy. Notify health care provider if symptoms are not controlled with medication.
- Monitor patient for dizziness and excessive drowsiness. If noted, hold therapy and notify health care provider.
- Monitor patient for CNS, GI, and general body side effects. Inform health care provider if noted and significant.

Ophthalmic Solution:
- Assess ophthalmic symptoms (eg, itching) before and periodically throughout therapy. Notify health care provider if symptoms are not controlled with medication.
- Monitor patient for ocular (eg, burning, stinging) and systemic reactions (eg, headaches). Inform health care provider if noted and significant.

Patient/Family Education
- Advise patient to read patient instruction sheet that accompanies each spray bottle of azelastine.
- Explain name, dose, action, and potential side effects of drug.
- Advise women to notify health care provider if pregnant, planning to become pregnant, or breastfeeding.
- Caution patient not to take any prescription or OTC medications or dietary supplements unless advised by health care provider.

Nasal Spray:
- Instruct patient to prime spray unit as directed in patient instruction sheet before first use and after storage for 3 or more days.
- Ensure that patient understands how to properly administer spray.
- Advise patient that if allergy symptoms are not controlled not to increase the dose of medication or frequency of use but to inform health care provider. Inform patient that larger or more frequent dosing does not increase effectiveness and may cause drowsiness or other unwanted effects.
- Advise patient that medication may cause drowsiness or dizziness and not to drive or perform other activities requiring mental alertness until tolerance is determined.
- Caution patient that alcohol and other CNS depressants (eg, sedatives) will have additional sedative effects if taken with azelastine.
- Caution patient not to take any OTC antihistamines while taking this medication unless advised by health care provider.
- Advise patient to take sips of water, suck on ice chips or sugarless hard candy, or chew sugarless gum if dry mouth occurs.
- Advise patient that bitter taste is a frequent side effect and to notify health care provider if this occurs and is bothersome.
- Instruct patient to stop taking drug and immediately report dizziness or excessive drowsiness to health care provider.

Ophthalmic Solution:
- Advise patient that usual dose is 1 drop instilled into the affected eyes bid.
- Teach patient proper technique for instilling eye drops: wash hands; do not allow dropper

tip to touch eye. Tilt head back, look up; pull lower eyelid down; instill prescribed number of drops. Close eye for 1 to 2 min and apply gentle pressure to bridge of nose for 3 to 5 min. Do not rub eye.
* Advise patient that if more than 1 topical ophthalmic drug is being used, to administer the drugs at least 10 min apart.
* Advise patient who wears contact lenses not to wear lenses if eyes are red.
* Advise patient who wears contact lenses, and whose eyes are not red, to remove lenses before instilling this medicine and to wait at least 10 min after instilling eye drop before inserting lenses.
* Inform patient that temporary burning or stinging of the eye, headaches, and bitter taste are the most common side effects and to contact health care provider if they occur and are bothersome.

Azithromycin

(UHZ-ith-row-MY-sin)
Class Antibiotic/Macrolide
How Supplied
Zithromax Tablets 250 mg (as dihydrate), Tablets 500 mg (as dihydrate), Tablets 600 mg (as dihydrate), Powder for injection, lyophilized 500 mg, Powder for oral suspension 100 mg/5 mL, Powder for oral suspension 200 mg/5 mL, Powder for oral suspension 1 g/packet (as dihydrate)
♣ *Z-Pak*

Action
PHARMACOLOGY: Interferes with microbial protein synthesis.

PHARMACOKINETICS/DYNAMICS:
Absorption:
Oral – Rapidly absorbed.
IV – C_{max} is approximately 3.63 mcg/mL; C_{min} is approximately 0.2 mcg/mL (at 24 hr), AUC_{24} is approximately 9.6 mcg•hr/mL.

Distribution: Widely distributed into body (ie, skin, lung, sputum, cervix, tonsils) but distributes poorly in the CSF. Higher concentrations in tissues than in plasma or serum. Vd is 31.1 L/kg (oral) and 33.3 L/kg (IV). Protein binding is 7% to 50% (concentration dependent).

Excretion: $T_{½}$ is approximately 68 hr. Plasma clearance is 630 mL/min (oral) and 10.18 mL/min/kg (IV). Excreted primarily in the bile, predominantly as unchanged drug. Approximately 6% is excreted in urine as unchanged drug (oral); approximately 11% is excreted in the urine after first dose and 14% after fifth dose (IV).

Indications
Adults: Treatment of infections of the respiratory tract, chronic obstructive pulmonary disease (COPD), community-acquired pneumonia, *Mycobacterium avium* complex, pelvic inflammatory disease, skin and skin structure, and sexually-transmitted diseases caused by susceptible organisms.
Children: Treatment of acute otitis media caused by susceptible organisms; community-acquired pneumonia, treatment of pharyngitis/tonsillitis caused by *Streptococcus pyogenes* in patients who cannot use first-line therapy.

Contraindications Hypersensitivity to azithromycin, erythromycin, or to any macrolide antibiotic.

Route/Dosage
Acute Otitis Media
CHILDREN 6 MO AND OLDER: PO 30 mg/kg given as a single dose or 10 mg/kg once daily for 3 days or 10 mg/kg as a single dose on the first day (not to exceed 500 mg/day) followed by 5 mg/kg on days 2 through 5 (not to exceed 250 mg/day).

Bacterial Infections
ADULTS: PO 500 mg as single dose on first day, then 250 mg/day on days 2 through 5.

Community-Acquired Pneumonia
ADULTS AND CHILDREN 16 YR AND OLDER: PO 500 mg as a single dose on the first day followed by 250 mg once daily on days 2 through 5.
ADULTS: IV 500 mg as a single daily dose for greater than or equal to 2 days. Follow IV therapy by the oral route at a single daily dose of 500 mg to complete 7- to 10-day course of therapy.
CHILDREN 6 MO AND OLDER: PO 10 mg/kg as a single dose on the first day (not to exceed 500 mg/day), followed by 5 mg/kg on days 2 through 5 (not to exceed 250 mg/day).

Gonorrhea
ADULTS: PO Single 2 g dose.

Mild to Moderate COPD
ADULTS AND CHILDREN 16 YR AND OLDER: PO 500 mg/day for 3 days or 500 mg as a single dose on the first day followed by 250 mg once daily on days 2 through 5.

Mycobacterium Avium Complex
ADULTS: PO Prevention: 1.2 g taken weekly. Treatment: 600 mg/day in combination with ethambutol (15 mg/kg).

Pelvic Inflammatory Disease
ADULTS: IV 500 mg as a single daily dose for 1 to 2 days. Follow IV therapy by the oral route at a single daily dose of 250 mg to complete a 7-day course of therapy.

Pharyngitis/Tonsillitis
ADULTS AND CHILDREN 16 YR AND OLDER: **PO** 500 mg as a single dose on the first day followed by 250 mg once daily on days 2 through 5.
CHILDREN AT LEAST 2 YR: **PO** 12 mg/kg/day for 5 days, not to exceed 500 mg/day.

***Genital Ulcer Disease caused by** H. ducreyi* (chancroid), Nongonococcal Urethritis/ Cervicitis caused by *C. trachomatis*
ADULTS: **PO** Single 1 g dose.

Uncomplicated Skin and Skin Structure Infections
ADULTS AND CHILDREN 16 YR AND OLDER: **PO** 500 mg as a single dose on the first day followed by 250 mg once daily for 4 days.

Interactions
HMG-CoA reductase inhibitors (eg, lovastatin): Increased risk of myopathy and rhabdomyolysis.
Tacrolimus: Increased tacrolimus plasma levels with increased risk of toxicity.
Warfarin: The anticoagulant effect may be increased, increasing the risk of hemorrhage.

Lab Test Interferences None well documented.

PATIENT CARE CONSIDERATIONS
Administration/Storage
Oral suspension/Tablets:
- Administer 1 hr before or 2 hr after meal.
- Tablets can be taken without regard to meals.
- Time doses evenly throughout day for optimal blood levels.
- Do not give antacids for greater than 2 hr after administration of product.
- Do not crush capsules.
- Give patient 6 to 8 oz of water or noncitrus juice with oral medication.
- Store reconstituted oral suspension at room temperature and use within 10 days. Discard after full dosing is completed.
- Store in tightly closed container at room temperature.

Injection:
- The infusate concentration and rate of infusion for azithromycin for injection should be either 1 mg/mL over 3 hr or 2 mg/mL over 1 hr. Do not administer as a bolus or IM injection.

Assessment/Interventions
- Obtain patient history, including drug history and any known allergies.

Adverse Reactions
CV: Palpitations; chest pain.
CNS: Dizziness; headache; vertigo; somnolence; fatigue.
DERM: Rash; photosensitivity.
GI: Diarrhea; nausea; vomiting; abdominal pain; dyspepsia; flatulence; melena.
GU: Vaginitis; monilia; nephritis.
HEPA: Cholestatic jaundice.
OTHER: Angioedema; anaphylaxis.

Precautions
Pregnancy: Category B.
Lactation: Undetermined.
Renal function impairment: Use cautiously.
Hepatic function impairment: Use cautiously.
Cardiac effects: Serious cardiovascular events have occurred with other macrolide antibiotics, especially when given concomitantly with certain antihistamines (eg, terfenadine).
Gonorrhea/Syphilis: Ineffective for treatment of these infections.
Pneumonia: Only effective for mild community-acquired pneumonia.
Pseudomembranous colitis: May be factor in patients who develop diarrhea.

- Review C&S report as available.
- Monitor renal, liver, and GI function during therapy. Notify health care provider of any GI side effects.
- Observe for signs of superinfection during therapy (eg, yeast infections, black hairy tongue, itching in groin area).
- Monitor for bleeding in patients receiving concomitant oral anticoagulant therapy.
- Notify health care provider if signs and symptoms of anaphylaxis occur.

Patient/Family Education
- Instruct patient to time doses for even distribution over a 24-hr period.
- Inform patient that the medication works best on empty stomach, but may be taken with food if there is GI upset.
- Instruct patient to take medication with full glass of water or noncitrus juice.
- Encourage patient to increase fluid intake to 2000 to 3000 mL/day, if not contraindicated.
- Instruct patient to notify health care provider if rash develops or difficult breathing occurs.
- Explain that antacids should be avoided while this medication is being taken.

Aztreonam

(AZZ-TREE-oh-nam)

Class Antibiotic/Monobactam

How Supplied
Azactam Powder for injection (lyophilized cake) 500 mg (with approximately 780 mg L-arginine per gram aztreonam), Powder for injection (lyophilized cake) 1 g (with approximately 780 mg L-arginine per gram aztreonam), Powder for injection (lyophilized cake) 2 g (with approximately 780 mg L-arginine per gram aztreonam)

Action
PHARMACOLOGY: Inhibits bacterial cell wall synthesis.

PHARMACOKINETICS/DYNAMICS:
Absorption:
IV – C_{max} is 54 mcg/mL (500 mg dose), 90 mcg/mL (1 g dose); and 204 mcg/mL (2 g dose) immediately after administration.
IM – T_{max} is approximately 1 hr; produces comparable serum concentrations to IV doses.

Distribution: Vd is approximately 12.6 L; approximately 56% protein bound. Widely distributed to fluids and tissues, including CSF (inflamed meninges) and breast milk; crosses placenta.

Excretion: $T_{1/2}$ is approximately 1.7 hr; serum clearance is 91 mL/min; renal clearance 56 mL/min; 60% to 70% is recovered in the urine by 8 hr; approximately 12% recovered in the feces.

Special Populations:
Renal Function Impairment – Serum $t_{1/2}$ may be prolonged.
Hepatic Function Impairment – Serum $t_{1/2}$ may be prolonged.
Elderly – Serum $t_{1/2}$ may be prolonged.

Indications
Treatment of infections of urinary tract, lower respiratory tract, skin and skin structure, intra-abdominal infections, gynecologic infections, surgical infections, and septicemia caused by susceptible microorganisms.

Unlabeled use(s): Treatment of acute, uncomplicated gonorrhea in patients with penicillin-resistant gonococci.

Contraindications
Standard considerations.

Route/Dosage
Urinary Tract Infection
ADULTS: IM/IV 500 mg or 1 g q 8 to 12 hr.

Systemic Infections
ADULTS: IM/IV 1 to 2 g q 6 to 12 hr.
CHILDREN: IM/IV 30 to 50 mg/kg q 4 to 8 hr.

Acute Uncomplicated Gonorrhea:
IM 1 g. Max recommended dosage is 8 g/day.

Interactions
Beta-lactamase-inducing antibiotics (eg, cefoxitin, imipenem): May antagonize activity of aztreonam and should not be used concurrently.
INCOMPATIBILITIES: Nafcillin sodium, cephradine, metronidazole: Incompatible in admixture.

Lab Test Interferences
Children: 15% to 20% of patients had elevations of AST and ALT more than 3 times the upper limit of normal.

Adverse Reactions
DERM: Rash.
CNS: Seizures.
GI: Diarrhea; nausea; vomiting; pseudomembranous colitis.
RESP: Dyspnea.
OTHER: Phlebitis/thrombophlebitis after IV administration; pain/swelling at IM injection site; fever.

Precautions
Pregnancy: Category B.
Lactation: Excreted in breast milk.
Children: Safety and efficacy for use in pediatric patients under 9 mo has not been established.
Hypersensitivity: Reactions range from mild to life-threatening. Administer cautiously to penicillin-or cephalosporin-sensitive patients because of possible cross-reactivity.
Renal function impairment: Reduced dose required.
Superinfection: May result in overgrowth of nonsusceptible bacterial or fungal organisms.

PATIENT CARE CONSIDERATIONS

Administration/Storage
- Follow manufacturer's instructions for reconstitution.
- Shake reconstituted solutions vigorously immediately after mixing. Reconstituted solutions stable at room temperature for 48 hr; stable under refrigeration for 7 days. Discard unused solutions.
- Avoid coadministering with other IV medications.
- Administer by deep IM injection in large muscle masses because of localized tissue irritation.
- Constitute the contents of aztreonam for injection 15 or 30 mL capacity vial with at least 3 mL of an appropriate diluent per gram of aztreonam.
- If the contents of a 15 to 30 mL capacity vial are to be transferred to an appropriate infusion solution, each gram of aztreonam should be initially constituted with at least 3 mL Sterile Water for Injection.

Assessment/Interventions
- Obtain patient history, including drug history and any known allergies.
- Review culture and sensitivity of organism as available.
- Monitor patient closely for several hours after initial dose even without a history of allergy.
- Closely monitor renal and GI function during therapy.
- In patients with hepatic impairment, monitor for signs of hepatitis and jaundice.
- Observe for signs of superinfection during therapy (eg, yeast infections, black hairy tongue, itching in groin area).
- Monitor IV site continuously during administration.
- Notify health care provider if signs and symptoms of hypersensitivity occur (eg, rash, shortness of breath), and stop medication.
- Notify health care provider if severe GI side effects occur.
- Call health care provider and stop infusion if infusion site becomes red, streaked, warm, or painful.
- Notify health care provider of any signs of unusual bleeding.

Patient/Family Education
- Encourage patient to increase fluid intake to 2000 to 3000 mL/day, if allowed.
- Inform patient to notify health care provider if rash or difficulty breathing is experienced.
- If therapy is discontinued because of allergic reaction, explain significance of penicillin allergy and of potential problems with cephalosporins.
- Caution patient against skipping doses or stopping treatment early, which could result in recurrence of symptoms and potential resistance of the organism to this product.

Bacitracin Zinc/Neomycin/Polymyxin B Sulfates/Hydrocortisone

(Bass-ih-TRAY-sin zingk/NEE-oh-MY-sin/pal-ee-MIX-in BEE SULL-fates/HIGH-droe-CORE-tih-sone)

Class Antibiotic/Corticosteroid

How Supplied
Cortisporin Ointment 400 U/g bacitracin zinc, 0.5% neomycin, 10,000 U/g polymyxin B sulfate, 1% hydrocortisone

Action
PHARMACOLOGY:
Neomycin: Inhibits protein synthesis by binding to ribosomal RNA, causing bacterial genetic code misreading.
Polymyxin B: Interacts with phospholipid components of bacterial cell membrane, increasing cell wall permeability.
Bacitracin: Interferes with bacterial cell wall synthesis by inhibiting regeneration of phospholipid receptors involved with paptidoglycan synthesis.
Hydrocortisone: Suppresses inflammatory response.

Indications
Treatment of corticosteroid-responsive dermatoses with secondary infection.

Contraindications
Use in the eyes or external ear canal (if the eardrum is perforated); tuberculosis; fungal or viral (eg, varicella zoster) lesions of the skin; hypersensitivity to any of components of product.

Route/Dosage
Topical Apply thin film to affected area bid to qid, not to exceed 7 days.

Interactions
None well documented.

Lab Test Interferences
None well documented.

Adverse Reactions
DERM: Skin sensitization; burning, itching, dryness, folliculitis, hypertrichosis, acneiform eruption, hypopigmentation, perioral dermatitis, allergic contact dermatitis, maceration of the skin, secondary infection, skin atrophy, striae, miliaria.
EENT: Ototoxicity.
GU: Nephrotoxicity.
OTHER: Allergic sensitivity.

Precautions
Pregnancy: Category C.
Lactation: Hydrocortisone is excreted in breast milk following oral administration.
Children: Safety and efficacy in pediatric patients not established.
Superinfection: Prolonged use may result in bacterial or fungal overgrowth of nonsusceptible microorganisms.
Adrenal suppression: Signs and symptoms of exogenous hyperadrenocorticism can occur with use of topical corticosteroids, especially if occlusive dressings are used.
Bacterial resistance: Bacterial resistance to components of the product may develop.

PATIENT CARE CONSIDERATIONS

Administration/Storage
- For topical use only. Not for ophthalmic or otic use, if eardrum is perforated.
- Apply a thin film to affected area(s) bid to qid as ordered. Use gloves or applicator as applicable.
- Store at controlled room temperature (59° to 86°F). Keep tube tightly closed.

Assessment/Interventions
- Obtain patient history, including drug history and any known allergies. Note history of viral, fungal, or mycobacterial skin infections.
- Review results of culture and sensitivity testing as available.
- Limit use to 7 days.
- Monitor patient's response to therapy.
- Notify health care provider if skin inflammation, irritation, or sensitization are noted or if symptoms do not improve or worsen.

Patient/Family Education
- Explain name, dose, action, and potential side effects of medication.
- Review prescribed dosing schedule with patient or caregiver.
- Remind patient or caregiver that ointment is not to be used in the eye or ear, if the eardrum is perforated.
- Teach patient or caregiver proper technique for applying ointment: Wash hands; apply thin film to affected area(s) using fingers or applicator. Wash hands after applying ointment.
- Advise patient or caregiver to contact health care provider if local redness or swelling develops or if skin lesions do not improve or worsen.
- Remind patient or caregiver that follow-up examinations may be necessary while using this medication and to keep appointments.

Bacitracin Zinc/Polymyxin B Sulfate

(Bass-ih-TRAY-sin zingk/pal-ee-MIX-in BEE SULL-fate)

Class Antibiotic

How Supplied
Polysporin Ophthalmic ointment 500 U/g bacitracin zinc and 10,000 U/g polymyxin B sulfate
♦ *AK-Poly-Bac* Ophthalmic ointment 500 U/g bacitracin zinc and 10,000 U/g polymyxin B sulfate
❋ *Optimyxin Ointment*

Action

PHARMACOLOGY:

Polymyxin B: Interacts with phospholipid components of bacterial cell membrane, increasing cell wall permeability.
Bacitracin: Interferes with bacterial cell wall synthesis by inhibiting regeneration of phospholipid receptors involved with peptidoglycan synthesis.

Indications Treatment of superficial ocular infections, involving the conjunctiva and/or cornea, caused by susceptible organisms.

Contraindications Standard considerations.

Route/Dosage
Ophthalmic Apply q 3 or 4 hr for 7 to 10 days, depending on severity of infection.

Interactions None well documented.

Lab Test Interferences None well documented.

Adverse Reactions
OTHER: Itching; swelling; eye redness; eye irritation; allergic reaction.

Precautions
Pregnancy:
Bacitracin – Category C.
Polymyxin B – Category B.
Lactation: Undetermined.
Superinfection: Prolonged use may result in bacterial or fungal overgrowth of nonsusceptible microorganisms.
Corneal healing: Corneal healing may be retarded.

PATIENT CARE CONSIDERATIONS

Administration/Storage
- For ophthalmic use only. Not for use on the skin.
- Instill prescribed amount of ointment q 3 to 4 hr as ordered.
- Do not allow tip of tube to touch eye, eyelid, fingers, or any other surface.
- Do not use if bottom ridge of cap is exposed.
- If using other topical ophthalmic medications, instill drops first, wait at least 5 min, and instill ointment last.
- Store at controlled room temperature (59° to 86°F). Keep tightly closed.

Assessment/Interventions
- Obtain patient history, including drug history and any known allergies.
- Monitor patient's response to therapy.
- Notify health care provider if eye or eyelid inflammation is noted or if symptoms do not improve or worsen.

Patient/Family Education
- Explain name, dose, action, and potential side effects of drug.
- Review prescribed dosing schedule with patient, family, or caregiver.
- Remind patient, family, or caregiver that ointment is for use in the eye only.
- Teach patient, family, or caregiver proper technique for instilling ointment: wash hands; do not allow tip of tube to touch eye, eyelid, fingers, or any other surface. Tilt head back, look up; pull lower eyelid down to form pocket; place prescribed amount of ointment in the pocket. Look downward before closing eye. Do not rub eye.
- Advise patient, family, or caregiver that if more than 1 topical ophthalmic drug is being used, instill eye drops first, wait at least 5 min, and then instill ointment last.
- Inform patient that temporary blurred vision and stinging of the eye are the most common side effects and to contact a health care provider if side effects occur and are bothersome.
- Advise patient to contact an eye doctor if eye or eyelid inflammation is noted or if eye symptoms do not improve or worsen.
- Advise patient that the entire course of therapy must be completed to ensure maximal benefit and to complete full course of therapy even if symptoms have resolved.
- Instruct patient not to wear contact lenses during treatment.
- Remind patient, family, or caregiver that follow-up eye examinations may be necessary while using this medication and to keep appointments.

Baclofen

(BACK-low-fen)

Class Skeletal muscle relaxant/Centrally acting

How Supplied

Lioresal Tablets 10 mg, Tablets 20 mg, Intrathecal 0.05 mg/mL (50 mcg/mL), Intrathecal 10 mg/20 mL (500 mcg/mL), Intrathecal 10 mg/5 mL (2000 mcg/mL)

✤ *APO-Baclofen* ♦ *Gen-Baclofen* ♦ *Med-Baclofen* ♦ *Nu-Baclo* ♦ *PMS-Baclofen* ♦ *ratio-Baclofen*

Action

PHARMACOLOGY: May inhibit transmission of reflexes at spinal level, possibly by action (hyperpolarization) at primary afferent fiber terminals resulting in relief of muscle spasticity; has CNS depressant properties.

PHARMACOKINETICS/DYNAMICS:

Absorption: Rapidly and extensively absorbed.

Excretion: Primarily by the kidney in unchanged form.

Indications

Oral: Treatment of reversible spasticity resulting from multiple sclerosis. May be of some value in patients with spinal cord injuries and other spinal cord diseases.

Intrathecal: Treatment of severe spasticity of spinal cord origin in patients who are unresponsive to or cannot tolerate oral baclofen therapy. Used intrathecally in single bolus test doses; chronic use requires implantable pump.

Unlabeled use(s):

Oral – Therapy for trigeminal neuralgia (tic douloureux); tardive dyskinesia.

Intrathecal – Cerebral palsy spasticity in children.

Contraindications
Treatment of spasms from rheumatic disorders, stroke, cerebral palsy and Parkinson disease; use of intrathecal form via IV, IM, SC, or epidural routes.

Route/Dosage

ADULTS:

Initial dose: **PO** 5 mg tid; may be increased by 5 mg/dose q 3 days prn to max 80 mg/day (20 mg qid). **Intrathecal** Refer to manufacturer's manual for implantable pump.

Screening

ADULTS: 1 mL of 50 mcg/mL dilution is administered into the intrathecal space by barbotage over 1 min and patient is observed for 4 to 8 hr; may be repeated 24 hr later with 75 mcg/1.5 mL and 48 hr later with 100 mcg/2 mL. Do not give implantable pump to patients not responding to 100 mcg bolus.

CHILDREN: The starting screening dose for pediatric patients is the same as in adult patients (eg, 50 mcg). However, for very small patients, a screening dose of 25 mcg may be tried first.

Postimplant Dose Titration Period

To determine the initial total daily dose of baclofen following implant, double the screening dose that gave a positive effect and administer over a 24-hr period.

Spasticity of Spinal Cord Origin

ADULTS: **Intrathecal** After the first 24 hr, increase the daily dosage slowly in 10% to 30% increments and only once q 24 hr, until desired effect is achieved.

Spasticity of Cerebral Origin

ADULTS: **Intrathecal** After the first 24 hr, increase the daily dose slowly 5% to 15% once q 24 hr, until desired clinical effect is achieved.

CHILDREN: After the first 24 hr, increase the daily dose slowly 5% to 15% only once q 24 hr, until the desired effect is achieved.

Maintenance Therapy for Spasticity of Spinal Cord Origins

Very often the maintenance dose needs to be adjusted during the first few months of therapy while patients adjust to changes in life-style because of the alleviation of spasticity.

ADULTS: **Intrathecal** During periodic refills of the pump, the daily dose may be increased 10% to 40%, but no more than 40%, to maintain adequate symptom control. Maintenance dose for long-term continuous infusion has ranged from 12 to 2003 mcg/day, with most patients adequately maintained on 300 to 800 mcg/day.

Maintenance Therapy for Spasticity of Cerebral Origin

Very often the maintenance dose needs to be adjusted during the first few months of therapy while patients adjust to changes in life-style because of the alleviation of spasticity.

ADULTS: **Intrathecal** During the periodic refills of the pump, the daily dose may be increased 5% to 20%, but no more than 20%. Ranges from 22 to 1400 mcg/day, with most patients adequately maintained on 90 to 703 mcg/day.

CHILDREN LESS THAN 12 YR: Average daily dose 274 mcg/day. Requires individual titration. Use the lowest dose with an optimal response.

CHILDREN AT LEAST 12 YR: Same as adult. Determination of the optimal dose requires individual titration. Use the lowest dose with an optimal response.

Interactions

CNS depressants: May cause increased sedative effects.

Morphine (epidural): May cause hypotension and dyspnea.

Lab Test Interferences May cause false

elevation of AST, alkaline phosphatase, or blood glucose.

Adverse Reactions
CV: Hypotension; palpitations; chest pain.
CNS: Drowsiness; weakness in lower extremities; dizziness; seizures; headache; numbness; euphoria; depression; confusion; lethargy; insomnia; hallucinations; paresthesia; asthenia; anxiety; agitation.
DERM: Pruritus; rash.
EENT: Tinnitus; blurred vision; taste disorder; nasal congestion.
GI: Nausea; vomiting; dry mouth; constipation; diarrhea; abdominal pain; anorexia.
GU: Urinary frequency; enuresis; dysuria; impotence.
RESP: Dyspnea; pneumonia; hypoventilation.
OTHER: Hypotonia; slurred speech; muscle pain; ankle edema; excessive perspiration; weight gain; back pain.

> **WARNING:**
>
> Intrathecal: Abrupt discontinuation has resulted in high fever, altered mental status, exaggerated rebound spasticity, and muscle rigidity that in rare cases advances to rhabdomyolysis, multiple organ system failure and death.
>
> Give special attention to patients at apparent risk (eg, spinal cord injuries at T-6 or above, communication difficulties, history of withdrawal symptoms from oral or intrathecal baclofen.

Precautions
Pregnancy: Category C.
Lactation: Excreted in breast milk.
Children: Safety of oral baclofen in children less than 12 yr and of intrathecal baclofen in children less than 4 yr has not been established.
Renal function impairment: Administer with caution. Dosage reduction may be necessary.
Intrathecal use: Only specially trained personnel should administer baclofen intrathecally because of potentially life-threatening CNS depression, cardiovascular collapse, or respiratory failure.
Epilepsy and psychotic disorders: Use with caution because of potential exacerbations.
Fatalities: Fatalities occurred in premarketing trials of intrathecal baclofen; baclofen's role in these deaths is unknown.
Infection: Patients should be infection-free before screening trial with baclofen intrathecal.
Stroke: Baclofen has not significantly benefited patients with stroke; these patients also have poor drug tolerance.

Overdosage: Signs and Symptoms
Vomiting, muscular hypotonia, muscle twitching, drowsiness, accommodation disorders, coma, respiratory depression, seizures (oral); drowsiness, lightheadedness, dizziness, somnolence, respiratory depression, seizures (intrathecal).

PATIENT CARE CONSIDERATIONS

Administration/Storage
Oral:
- Administer with milk or food to avoid GI upset.
- Dilute intrathecal medication per manufacturer's instructions.

Intrathecal:
- If there is not a substantive clinical response to increases in the daily dose, check for proper pump function and catheter patency.
- The daily maintenance dose may be reduced 10% to 20% if patients experience side effects.
- Have resuscitation equipment available during trial drug period if intrathecal administration is considered. Patient must have positive response to trial of intrathecal medication before use of implantable pump.
- Store at room temperature in tightly closed container.

Assessment/Interventions
- Obtain patient history, including drug history and any known allergies. Note any signs of infection.
- Assess muscle spasticity and monitor throughout course of therapy.
- Monitor renal function prior to administration.

Patient/Family Education
- Instruct patient to take drug exactly as prescribed. If dose is missed it should be taken within 1 hr. Warn patient not to double up on doses.
- Explain that full effectiveness of drug may not occur until several weeks after initiation of drug therapy.
- Warn patient not to discontinue medication abruptly. Explain that hallucinations or seizures may occur.
- Instruct patient to avoid intake of alcoholic beverages or other CNS depressants.
- Teach patient to avoid sudden position changes to prevent orthostatic hypotension.

- Caution diabetic patient that false elevation of blood glucose may occur. Instruct patient to monitor blood glucose carefully.
- Instruct patient to report the following symptoms to health care provider: dizziness, nausea, hypotension, urinary frequency, retention, painful urination, headache, seizures, weakness.
- Advise patient that drug may cause drowsiness, and to use caution while driving or performing other tasks requiring mental alertness.

Balsalazide Disodium

(bal-SAL-a-zide die-SO-dee-uhm)
Class Intestinal anti-inflammatory
How Supplied
Colazal Capsule 750 mg
Action
PHARMACOLOGY: Reduces inflammation of colon by preventing local production of substances involved in inflammatory process such as arachidonic acid.

PHARMACOKINETICS/DYNAMICS:
Absorption: Very low systemic absorption. T_{max} is approximately 1 to 2 hr.
Distribution: At least 99% protein bound.
Metabolism: In the colon, bacterial azoreductases cleave the balsalazide compound to release 5-aminosalicylic acid (5-ASA) (active) and 4-aminobenzoyl-beta-alanine.
Excretion:
Urine – Less than 1% as parent compound, 5-ASA, or 4-aminobenzoyl-beta-alanine; up to 25% as N-acetylated metabolites.
Feces – 65% as 5-ASA, 4-aminobenzoyl-beta-alanine and N-acetylated metabolites; less than 1% as parent compound.
Special Populations:
Ulcerative colitis – May have increased AUC.
Indications Treatment of mildly to moderately active ulcerative colitis.
Contraindications Hypersensitivity to salicylates or any of the components of balsalazide capsules or balsalazide metabolites.
Route/Dosage
ADULTS: PO 2.25 g (ie, three 750 mg capsules) tid (ie, 6.75 g/day) for 8 wk; some patients may require up to 12 wk of treatment.
Interactions None well documented.
Lab Test Interferences None well documented.
Adverse Reactions
CNS: Headache; insomnia; dizziness.
EENT: Rhinitis; pharyngitis; coughing; sinusitis.
GI: Abdominal pain; nausea; vomiting; rectal bleeding; flatulence; dyspepsia; anorexia; frequent stools; dry mouth; cramps; constipation.
GU: Urinary tract disorder.
HEPA: Hepatotoxicity; jaundice; cholestatic jaundice; cirrhosis; hepatocellular damage.
RESP: Respiratory disorder; infection.
OTHER: Arthralgia; fatigue; fever; pain; back pain; myalgia; flu-like symptoms.
Precautions
Pregnancy: Category B.
Lactation: Undetermined.
Children: Safety and efficacy not established.
Colitis exacerbation: Some patients may develop symptoms of colitis.

PATIENT CARE CONSIDERATIONS

Administration/Storage
- Do not chew or crush. Instruct patient to swallow capsule whole.
- Give tid with a full glass of water.
- Store at controlled room temperature.

Assessment/Interventions
- Obtain patient history, including drug history and any known allergies. Note history of pyloric stenosis.
- Monitor patient for GI, CNS, and musculoskeletal side effects and report to health care provider if noted and significant.
- Assess patient's colitis symptoms including the following: rectal bleeding, stool frequency and character, abdominal pain, and overall functional status.
- Store at controlled room temperature.

Patient/Family Education
- Explain name, dose, action, and potential side effects of drug.
- Advise patient to not crush or chew medication and to swallow the capsule whole with a full glass of water.
- Advise patient that usual course of therapy is 8 to 12 wk.
- Advise patient to report worsening of colitis symptoms to health care provider.
- Advise patients to inform the health care provider if experiencing side effects such as headache, stomach pain, nausea, or diarrhea.
- Advise patients that follow-up visits and examinations may be required to monitor therapy; remind patients to keep appointments.

Basiliximab

(bah-sih-LICK-sih-mab)

Class Immunosuppressive

How Supplied
Simulect Powder for injection 20 mg

Action

PHARMACOLOGY: Blocks the interleukin-2 receptor α-chain, which is a critical pathway in allograft rejection.

PHARMACOKINETICS/DYNAMICS:
Absorption: C_{max} is about 7.1 mg/L (20 mg IV over 30 min).
Distribution: Vd is about 8.6 L.
Excretion: The t½ is about 7.2 days. Cl is about 41 mL/hr.
Special Populations:
Children – Distribution volume and Cl are reduced by about 50% compared with adult renal transplant patients.

Indications Prophylaxis of acute organ rejection in patients receiving renal transplantation when used as part of an immunosuppressive regimen that includes cyclosporine and corticosteroids.

Contraindications Standard considerations.

Route/Dosage

ADULTS: IV 20 mg within 2 hr prior to transplantation surgery, followed by 20 mg 4 days after transplantation. Withhold second dose if complications such as severe hypersensitivity reactions to basiliximab or graft rejection occur.

CHILDREN/ADOLESCENTS (UNDER 35 KG): IV 10 mg within 2 hr prior to transplantation surgery, followed by 10 mg 4 days after transplantation. Withhold second dose if complications such as severe hypersensitivity reactions to basiliximab or graft rejection occur.

CHILDREN/ADOLESCENTS (35 KG OR MORE): IV 20 mg within 2 hr prior to transplantation surgery, followed by 20 mg 4 days after transplantation. Withhold second dose if complications such as severe hypersensitivity reactions to basiliximab or graft rejection occur.

Interactions None well documented.
INCOMPATIBILITIES: No data available; do not add or infuse other drugs simultaneously through the same IV line.

Lab Test Interferences None well documented.

Adverse Reactions

CV: Hypertension; hypotension; angina pectoris; cardiac failure; abnormal heart sounds; arrhythmia; atrial fibrillation; tachycardia; vascular disorder.
CNS: Headache; tremor; dizziness; insomnia; hypoesthesia; neuropathy; paresthesia; agitation; anxiety; depression; fatigue; malaise.
DERM: Acne; surgical wound complications; cyst; herpes simplex; herpes zoster; hypertrichosis; pruritus; rash; skin ulceration.
GI: Constipation; nausea; diarrhea; abdominal pain; vomiting; dyspepsia; moniliasis; enlarged abdomen; flatulence; gastroenteritis; GI hemorrhage; gum hyperplasia; melena; esophagitis; ulcerative stomatitis.
GU: Dysuria; urinary tract infection; increased nonprotein nitrogen; impotence; genital edema; albuminuria; bladder disorder; hematuria; frequent micturition; oliguria; abnormal renal function; renal tubular necrosis; ureteral disorder; urinary retention.
HEMA: Anemia; hemorrhage; purpura; thrombocytopenia; thrombosis; polycythemia.
M/N: Hyperkalemia; hypokalemia; hyperglycemia; hypoglycemia; hyperuricemia; hypomagnesemia; hypophosphatemia; hypocalcemia; hypercholesterolemia; hyperlipidemia; hyperproteinemia; weight gain; acidosis; dehydration; diabetes mellitus; fluid overload.
RESP: Dyspnea; upper respiratory tract infection; coughing; rhinitis; pharyngitis; bronchitis; bronchospasm; abnormal chest sounds; pneumonia; pulmonary disorder; pulmonary edema.
SPEC SENSE: Cataracts; conjunctivitis; abnormal vision; sinusitis.
OTHER: Pain; chest pain; leg pain; back pain; asthenia; arthralgia; arthropathy; bone fracture; cramps; hernia; myalgia; hematoma; edema; peripheral edema; facial edema.

> **WARNING:**
> Should be administered under qualified medical supervision experienced in immunosuppression therapy and management of organ transplantation.
> Should be administered in equipped facility with supportive resources.

Precautions

Pregnancy: Category B.
Lactation: Undetermined.
Children: Safety and efficacy not established.
Elderly: Safety and efficacy not established.
Hypersensitivity: Although not reported, can occur following administration of proteins.
Opportunistic infections/lymphoproliferative disorders: Risk of developing these complications may be increased.

PATIENT CARE CONSIDERATIONS
Administration/Storage
* Store lyophilized basilixmab under refrigerated conditions at 2° to 8°C (36° to 46°F). The reconstituted solution can be refrigerated for 24 hr or at room temperature for 4 hr. Discard reconstituted solution if not used in 24 hr. Use the reconstituted solution immediately and dilute as directed.
* Inspect the bag for particulate matter or solution discoloration; do not use if present.
* Administer with care to assure sterility, as the solution contains no antimicrobial preservatives.
* Do not administer or add other drugs to the same bag or infuse simultaneously through the same IV line.
* Do not shake solution; invert bag gently to avoid foaming.
* Administer diluted solution through central or peripheral IV only over 20 to 30 min using sterile technique.

Assessment/Interventions
* Obtain patient history, including drug history and any known allergies.
* Monitor for signs of hypersensitivity. Have medications for the treatment of severe hypersensitivity available for immediate use.
* Discontinue infusion immediately if signs of hypersensitivity are present; keep IV line open, follow institution emergency protocol, and notify health care provider
* Monitor for adverse reactions.
* Maintain sterility and monitor infusion site, IV rate, and patient during infusion.

Patient/Family Education
* Instruct patient or family to monitor for signs and symptoms of adverse events and report immediately to primary health care provider.
* Instruct family or patient to monitor for signs and symptoms of infections and transplant rejection including fever, pain, and urinary tract infections. Report these symptoms immediately to primary care provider.
* Advise women to notify health care provider immediately if pregnant, planning to become pregnant, or planning to breastfeed.
* Instruct women of childbearing potential to use effective contraception before beginning therapy, during therapy, and for 2 mo after the completion of therapy.
* Nursing mothers should discontinue nursing prior to using the drug.
* Stress the importance of regular exams and laboratory work.
* Encourage patient to comply with the treatment regimen.

BCG Live
(BCG LIVE)

Class Biologic response modifier

How Supplied
TICE BCG Powder for suspension, lyophilized 1 to 8×10^8 CFU ♦ TheraCys Powder for suspension, lyophilized $10.5 \pm 8.7 \times 10^8$ CFU

Action
PHARMACOLOGY: BCG is a lyophilized preparation of an attenuated, live culture preparation of the Bacille Calmette-Guérin (BCG) strain of Mycobacterium bovis used in carcinoma in-situ of the urinary bladder and as prophylaxis of primary or recurrent stage Ta or T1 papillary tumors following transurethral resection (TUR).

Indications Intravesical use for the treatment of primary and relapsed carcinoma in-situ of the urinary bladder. Prevention of tuberculosis (TB) in the following: people not previously infected with Mycobacterium tuberculosis, infants and children with negative tuberculin skin test who are at high risk of intimate and prolonged exposure to persistently untreated or ineffectively treated patients with infectious pulmonary tuberculosis, health care workers in settings where a high percentage of TB patients are infected with M. tuberculosis strains resistant to both isoniazid and rifampin (BCG vaccine [TICE strain, lyophilized injection]). **Unlabeled use(s):** Local control of accessible tumor.

Contraindications Stage TaG1 papillary tumors unless judged to be at high risk of tumor recurrence; immunosuppressed patients with congenital or acquired immune deficiencies; cancer therapy; immunosuppressive therapy; vaccine for the prevention of cancer; as treatment of papillary tumors occurring alone; as an immunizing agent for the prevention of tuberculosis; positive Mantoux test; prevention of papillary tumors after TUR or for the treatment of papillary tumors occurring alone; active tuberculosis; papillary tumors of stages higher than T1; concurrent infections.

Route/Dosage
Carcinoma In-Situ of the Urinary Bladder
ADULTS (THERACYS): **Intravesical** Do not inject SC or IV. Each dose is administered intravesically via catheter once a wk for 6 wk followed by maintenance therapy consisting of 1 dose given at 3, 6, 12, 18, and 24 mo after initial treatment.
ADULTS (TICE BCG): **Intravesical** Do not inject SC or IV. Each dose is administered

intravesically via catheter once a wk for 6 wk. This schedule may be repeated once if tumor remission is not achieved and if deemed clinically necessary; thereafter, administer 1 dose at approximately monthly intervals for at least 6 to 12 mo.

TB Prevention for Individuals Negative to Recent Skin Test with 5 Tuberculin Units

ADULTS: **Percutaneous** 0.2 to 0.3 mL of vaccine on cleansed surface of the skin and spread over 1- by 2-inch area administered utilizing a sterile multiple-puncture devise. An additional 1 to 2 gtt of BCG vaccine may be added to ensure a very wet vaccination site. Repeat vaccination for individuals who remain tuberculin negative to 5TU of tuberculin after 2 to 3 mo.
CHILDREN UNDER 1 MO: **Percutaneous** Reduce the dose of vaccine by 50% by using 2 mL of sterile water when reconstituting.

Interactions

Antimicrobial therapy: Antimicrobial therapy for other infections may interfere with the effectiveness of TICE BCG therapy.
Bone marrow depressants/immunosuppressants/ radiation: Bone marrow depressants, immunosuppressants, or radiation may impair response to BCG.

Lab Test Interferences
May result in tuberculin skin reactivity.

Adverse Reactions

CNS: Malaise; fatigue.
GI: Nausea; vomiting; anorexia.
GU: Blood in urine; urinary frequency and urgency; painful urination; UTI; urinary incontinence.
HEMA: Anemia.
HYPERSEN: Tuberculin sensitivity; fever; chills; myalgia.
RESP: Cough.
OTHER: Joint pain.

> **WARNING:**
> *Fever:* Do not use in the presence of fever. If fever is caused by infection, withhold therapy until patient is afebrile and off all therapy.

Precautions

Pregnancy: Category C.
Lactation: Because of the potential for serious adverse reactions in nursing infants, discontinue nursing or discontinue the drug, taking into account the importance of the drug to the mother.
Children: Safety and efficacy not established.
Hypersensitivity: Systemic side effects (eg, malaise, fever, chills) of 1 or 2 days' duration may represent hypersensitivity reactions and can be treated with antihistamines.
BCG infection: Fever of 103°F or more, or acute localized inflammation persisting longer than 2 or 3 days suggest active infections and evaluation for serious infectious complications should be considered.
Immune deficiency syndromes: Administer with caution to individuals at high risk for HIV infection. Do not vaccinate children with a family history of immune deficiency disease.
Infection of aneurysms and prosthetic devices: BCG infection of aneurysms and prosthetic devices (eg, arterial grafts, cardiac devices, artificial joints) have been reported following intravesical administration of BCG. The risk is considered to be very small.
Management of BCG complications: The acute, localized irritative toxicities of BCG may be accompanied by systemic manifestations consistent with flu-like syndrome.
Rubber latex: The vial stopper for Thera-Cys contains natural rubber latex that may cause allergic reactions.
UTI: Do not use in the presence of a UTI because administration may result in the risk of disseminated BCG infection or in an increased severity of bladder irritation.

Overdosage: Signs and Symptoms
Overdosage occurs if more than 1 amp/vial is given per instillation.

PATIENT CARE CONSIDERATIONS

Administration/Storage

- The suspension is instilled into the bladder slowly by gravity flow, via the catheter. Do not force the flow.
- Reconstitute and dilute immediately prior to use. If there is a delay between reconstitution and administration, it must not exceed 2 hr.
- Keep BCG and any accompanying diluent refrigerated between 2° and 8°C (35° and 46°F). Use immediately after reconstitution and discard after 2 hr. Do not expose the freeze-dried or reconstituted BCG to sunlight, direct or indirect. Keep exposure to artificial light to a minimum. Do not use any reconstituted product that exhibits flocculation or clumping that cannot be dispersed with gentle shaking. Do not use after expiration date printed on label.
- After usage, immediately place all equipment and materials used for instillation of the prod-

uct into the bladder (eg, syringes, catheters, and containers that may have come into contact with BCG) into plastic bags labeled "Infectious Waste" and dispose of accordingly as biohazardous waste.

Assessment/Interventions
* Do not administer as an immunizing agent to prevent tuberculosis.
* Handle as biohazardous. Use aseptic technique.

Allergic reactions:
* Assess the possibility of allergic reactions. Do not attempt administration in individuals with severe immune deficiency disease.

Infection, systemic:
* Closely monitor for signs and symptoms of systemic infection.

TUR:
* Do not give intravesical BCG any sooner than 1 to 2 wk following TUR, biopsy, traumatic catherization, or gross hematuria.

Urinary tract status:
* Careful monitoring of urinary status is required.

Patient/Family Education
* Check with health care provider as soon as possible if there is an increase in existing symptoms, if symptoms persist even after receiving a number of treatments, or if any of the following symptoms develop: blood in urine, fever, chills, cough, skin rash, frequent urge to urinate, increased frequency of urination, increased tiredness/fatigue, joint pain, flu-like symptoms, painful urination.
* Notify health care provider immediately if a cough develops.
* Void in a seated position to avoid splashing of urine.
* Disinfect urine voided for 6 hr after instillation with an equal volume of 5% sodium hypochlorite solution (undiluted household bleach); allow to disinfect for 15 min before flushing.
* Increase fluid intake to flush the bladder in the hours following BCG treatment. Patients may experience burning with the first void after treatment.

Beclomethasone Dipropionate

(BEK-low-METH-uh-zone die-PRO-pee-oh-NATE)

Class Corticosteroid

How Supplied
QVAR Aerosol 40 mcg/actuation, Aerosol 80 mcg/actuation

🍁 Apo-Beclomethasone ♦ Gen-Beclo Aq. ♦ Nu-Beclomethasone ♦ Rivanase AQ

Action
PHARMACOLOGY: Has potent anti-inflammatory effect on respiratory tract and in nasal passages.

PHARMACOKINETICS/DYNAMICS:

Absorption: Rapidly absorbed.
Oral inhalation – Systemic bioavailability from lungs is about 20%.

Distribution: 87% protein bound.

Metabolism: Metabolized to beclomethasone 17-monopropionate (active) and free beclomethasone (very weak activity).

Excretion: Primarily excreted in feces. Less than 10% excreted in urine. The t½ is 2.8 hr for beclomethasone 17-monopropionate.

Onset:
Oral inhalation – Within 24 hr.
Nasal spray – Within 3 days, up to 2 wk.
Oral inhalation – 1 to 2 wk or longer.

Indications
Oral inhalation: QVAR: Maintenance prophylactic treatment of asthma in patients 5 yr and older; asthma patients requiring systemic corticosteroid administration in which adding an inhaled corticosteroid may reduce or eliminate need for systemic corticosteroids.

Contraindications
Oral inhalation: Primary treatment of status asthmaticus or acute episodes of asthma; systemic fungal infections; positive sputum cultures of *Candida albicans* or *Aspergillus niger*.

Route/Dosage
Bronchial Asthma
ADULTS AND CHILDREN (12 YR AND OLDER): PO QVAR: If previous therapy consisted of bronchodilators alone, start with 40 or 80 mcg bid (max dose, 320 mcg bid); if previous therapy consisted of inhaled corticosteroids, start with 40 to 160 mcg bid (max dose, 320 mcg bid).
CHILDREN (5 TO 11 YR): **Aerosol actuation** QVAR: If previous therapy consisted of bronchodilators alone or inhaled corticosteroids, start with 40 mcg bid (max dose, 80 mcg bid).

Interactions None well documented.

Lab Test Interferences None well documented.

Adverse Reactions
CNS: Headache; lightheadedness; agitation; depression; mental disturbances.
QVAR – Headache (at least 3%).
EENT: Nasal bleeding; sneezing; throat and nasal irritation, burning, or stinging; hoarseness

or dysphonia; nasal, laryngeal, or pharyngeal fungal infection.
QVAR – Pharyngitis, rhinitis, sinusitis (at least 3%).
GI: Dry mouth; dyspepsia; nausea; vomiting.
QVAR – Nausea (at least 3%).
GU:
QVAR – Dysmenorrhea (1% to 3%).
METAB: Suppression of hypothalamic-pituitary-adrenal (HPA) function.
RESP: Coughing; wheezing; pulmonary infiltrates.
QVAR – Upper respiratory tract infections (at least 3%); coughing (1% to 3%).
OTHER: Hypersensitivity reaction with rash, urticaria, angioedema, and bronchospasm; facial and tongue edema; pruritus; wheezing; dyspnea; acneiform lesions; atrophy; bruising; localized *Candida* or *Aspergillus* infections; cushingoid features; growth velocity reduction in children; weight gain.
QVAR – Increased asthma symptoms, oral symptoms (inhalation route), pain, back pain, dysphonia (at least 3%).

Precautions
Pregnancy: Category C.
Lactation: Undetermined. Because other corticosteroids are excreted in human milk, use caution.
Children: Safety and efficacy in children under 5 yr not established. Oral corticosteroids may suppress growth in children and adolescents, particularly with higher doses over extended periods.
Hypersensitivity: Immediate and delayed hypersensitivity reactions have occurred.
Acute asthma: Not indicated for relief of bronchospasm.
Fungal infections: Antifungal treatment or discontinuance of corticosteroid therapy may be necessary.
Immunology: Patients receiving immunosuppressant agents are more susceptible to infections than healthy adults. If a patient is exposed to measles or chickenpox, appropriate prophylaxis and treatment may be indicated.
Systemic effects: Use cautiously in patients taking daily or alternate-day prednisone; may increase likelihood of hypothalamic-pituitary axis suppression. Exceeding recommended dose may cause systemic effects.
Transfer: Use extreme caution when transferring patient from systemic corticosteroid to less systemically available inhaled corticosteroid because death caused by adrenal insufficiency has occurred in asthmatic patients.

PATIENT CARE CONSIDERATIONS
Administration/Storage
- May be administered alone or in combination with systemic corticosteroids.
- For oral inhalation only. Avoid spraying into the nose or eyes.
- If patient is also receiving bronchodilators by inhalation, administer bronchodilator 5 min before beclomethasone to enhance penetration of latter drug into bronchial tree.
- Aerosol does not need to be shaken before use.
- Test aerosol by spraying 2 times into the air before using the first time and/or when the inhaler has not been used for more than 10 days.
- Have patient place inhaler in mouth and close lips around mouthpiece, keeping tongue below mouthpiece. Tilt patient's head back slightly. Instruct patient to take a slow, deep breath while inhaler is being activated and to hold breath for 5 to 10 sec and then breathe out slowly. A spacing device (eg, *Aerochamber*) may be used to enhance delivery of medication. Have patient rinse mouth after inhalations are complete.
- If more than 1 spray/dose is ordered, administer each spray individually, waiting a few seconds between sprays.
- Store at controlled room temperature (59° to 86°F) on the concave end of the canister with the plastic actuator on top. For optimal results, canister should be at room temperature when used. Do not use actuator with any other inhalation drug product.
- Do not puncture canister or use near heat or open flame or discard into fire or incinerator.

Assessment/Interventions
- Obtain patient history, including drug history and any known allergies.
- If change is made from systemic (oral) corticosteroids to inhaled or intranasal corticosteroids, observe patient carefully for signs of adrenal insufficiency (nausea, fatigue, dizziness, hypotension, depression, or abdominal, joint, or muscle pain). Notify health care provider if these signs occur. Deaths caused by adrenal insufficiency have occurred during and after converting to aerosol corticosteroids.
- Assess patient's symptoms before initiating therapy and periodically during treatment. Notify health care provider if symptoms do not improve or worsen.

- Notify health care provider if oral, nasal, or pharyngeal irritation occurs or if symptoms worsen.

Patient/Family Education
- Explain name, dose, action, and potential side effects of drug.
- Advise patient to read the *Patient's Instructions* before starting therapy and again with each refill.
- Warn patient that drug is an asthma controller and is not to be used to treat an acute asthma attack. Patient must use rescue medication (bronchodilator) to obtain rapid relief of asthma symptoms.
- Instruct patient to carry Medi-Alert card if experiencing acute, severe asthma attacks requiring rapid systemic treatment.
- Advise patient to continue taking other medications for asthma as prescribed by health care provider.
- Review proper administration technique. Have patient demonstrate technique.
- Advise patient to rinse mouth with water after inhalations are complete. Instruct patient to spit rinse water out and not to swallow it.
- Advise patient to report the following symptoms to health care provider: sore throat or mouth, cough, dry mouth, rash, facial swelling, worsening asthma symptoms (increasing need for bronchodilator).
- Advise patient that dose may be changed periodically depending on how well symptoms are controlled.
- Instruct patient not to exceed prescribed dose.
- Explain that effects of drug are not immediate. Benefit requires daily use as instructed and usually occurs after 1 to 2 days, but full relief may take 1 to 2 wk.
- Instruct patient not to stop the medication once symptoms have been controlled. Continued daily use is necessary to control symptoms.
- Advise patient not to increase dose on own and to inform health care provider if symptoms do not improve or worsen.
- If patient is being converted from oral corticosteroids to inhaled corticosteroids, review signs and symptoms of adrenal insufficiency, which may occur days or weeks after conversion is complete. Advise patient to carry Medi-Alert card indicating that supplemental systemic corticosteroids during periods of stress or a severe asthma attack may be needed.
- Advise patient to discard the aerosol canister when the labeled number of doses have been used.
- Advise patient to avoid exposure to chickenpox and measles and to seek medical advice immediately if exposed.
- Advise women to notify health care provider if pregnant, planning to become pregnant, or breastfeeding.
- Caution patient not to take any prescription or OTC medications or dietary supplements unless advised by health care provider.
- Advise patient that follow-up visits may be required to monitor therapy and to keep appointments.

Belladonna/Opium

(Bell-ah-DON-ah/OH-pee-uhm)
Class Narcotic analgesic/Antispasmodic

How Supplied
B & O Suprettes No. 15A Suppositories 16.2 mg powdered belladonna, 30 mg powdered opium ♦
B & O Suprettes No. 16A Suppositories 16.2 mg powdered belladonna, 60 mg powdered opium

Action
PHARMACOLOGY: Contains more than a score of alkaloids, including morphine, narcotine, papaverine, and codeine, which act to relax smooth muscle, relieve pain, and cause sedation by depressant effect on cerebral cortex, hypothalamus, and medullary centers.

Indications Relief of moderate to severe pain associated with ureteral spasm not responsive to nonnarcotic analgesics and to space intervals between injections of opiates.

Contraindications Patients with glaucoma, severe hepatic, or renal disease; bronchial asthma; narcotic idiosyncrasies; respiratory depression; convulsive disorders; acute alcoholism; delirium tremens, premature labor; history of hypersensitivity to any component of product.

Route/Dosage
ADULTS: **Rectal** 1 or 2 suppositories/day (max, 4 doses/day).

Interactions None well documented.

Lab Test Interferences None well documented.

Adverse Reactions
CV: Rapid pulse.
CNS: Drowsiness, dizziness.
DERM: Pruritus, urticaria.
EENT: Blurred vision.
GI: Drug mouth; constipation, nausea, vomiting.

GU: Urinary retention.
OTHER: Photophobia.

Precautions

Pregnancy: Category C.
Lactation: Undetermined.
Children: Not recommended for use in children.
Special risk patients: Use with caution in patients with known idiosyncrasy to atropine or atropine-like compounds, cardiac disease, incipient glaucoma, prostatic hypertrophy, increased intracranial pressure, toxic psychosis, myxedema, and elderly or debilitated patients.
Drug dependence: Has abuse potential and may cause true addiction.

Overdosage: Signs and Symptoms

Respiratory depression, pinpoint pupils, coma, hot, dry, flushed skin, dry mouth, and hyperpyrexia.

PATIENT CARE CONSIDERATIONS

Administration/Storage

- Do not remove suppository from foil pack until immediately prior to insertion.
- Moisten gloved finger and suppository with water before inserting.
- Insert suppository qd to qid, or as ordered, as needed.
- Store suppositories in foil wrapping at controlled room temperature (59° to 86°F). Do not refrigerate.

Assessment/Interventions

- Obtain patient history, including drug history and any known allergies. Note history of asthma, COPD, seizures, pregnancy, hypothyroidism, enlarged prostate, narrow angle glaucoma, urinary retention, coronary artery disease, or kidney or liver impairment.
- Assess symptoms of ureteral spasm before and periodically throughout therapy.
- Assess patient for CNS, GI, GU, and general body side effects. Inform health care provider if noted and significant.

Patient/Family Education

- Explain name, dose, action, and potential side effects of drug.
- Advise patient or caregiver to insert suppository qd to qid, or as directed by health care provider, as needed for symptoms of ureteral spasm.
- Teach patient or caregiver proper technique for inserting suppository: Use gloves; remove suppository from foil wrap just before insertion; moisten gloved finger and suppository with water; insert suppository rectally with patient lying on side with legs flexed; remove and discard gloves; wash hands.
- Advise patient that if a dose is missed to take as soon as remembered unless it is nearing time for the next dose. Caution patient to not double the dose to catch up.
- Instruct patient to discontinue use and report any intolerable side effects to health care provider.
- Advise patient that if symptoms are not controlled not to increase the dose of medication but to inform health care provider.
- Advise women to notify health care provider if pregnant, planning to become pregnant, or breastfeeding.
- Caution patient to not take any prescription or OTC medications, or dietary supplements unless advised by health care provider.

Belladonna (levorotatory alkaloids)/Phenobarbital/ Ergotamine Tartrate

(Bell-ah-DON-ah/Fee-no-BAR-bih-tahl/ehr-GOT-ah-mean TAR-trate)

Class GI Anticholinergic/Antispasmodic

How Supplied

Bellamine Tablets 0.2 mg levorotatory alkaloids of belladonna/40 mg phenobarbital/0.6 mg ergotamine

Action

PHARMACOLOGY: Inhibition of the sympathetic and parasympathetic nervous system by ergotamine and belladonna, respectively, reinforced by the synergistic activity of phenobarbital in dampening the cortical centers.

Indications Management of disorders characterized by nervous tension and exaggerated autonomic response; menopausal disorders with hot flushes, sweats, restlessness, and insomnia; cardiovascular disorders with palpitation, tachycardia, chest oppression, and vasomotor disturbances; GI disorders with hypermotility, hypersecretion, "nervous stomach," diarrhea, constipation; interval treatment of recurrent, throbbing headache.

Contraindications Peripheral vascular disease; coronary heart disease; hypertension; impaired hepatic or renal function; sepsis; pregnancy; nursing mothers; glaucoma; coadministration of ergotamine and dopamine; history of manifest or latent porphyria; patients with history of restlessness and/or excitement with phenobarbital use; hypersensitivity to any component of the product.

Route/Dosage
ADULTS: PO 1 tablet in morning and evening.

Interactions
Beta-adrenergic blocking agents: Excessive vasoconstriction may occur.
CNS depressants (eg, alcohol, narcotic analgesics, phenothiazines, tricyclic antidepressants): Depressant action may be potentiated.
Doxycycline, estrogen, griseofulvin, quinidine: Pharmacologic effects of these agents may be decreased.
Hydantoins (eg, phenytoin): Effects of hydantoins may be increased or decreased.
Oral anticoagulants (eg, warfarin): Anticoagulant activity as measured by prothrombin time may be decreased.
Valproic acid: Pharmacologic effects of phenobarbital may be increased.

Lab Test Interferences
None well documented.

PATIENT CARE CONSIDERATIONS
Administration/Storage
- Administer 1 tablet bid, morning and evening, without regard to meals.
- Administer with food if GI upset occurs.
- Do not administer within 24 hr of treatment with another 5-HT$_1$ agonist or other ergot-containing or ergot-type drug (eg, methysergide).
- Store at controlled room temperature (59° to 86°F).

Assessment/Interventions
- Obtain patient history, including drug history and any known allergies. Note history of peripheral vascular disease, ischemic or vasospastic coronary artery disease, hypertension, hepatic or renal impairment, glaucoma, porphyria, asthma, prostatic enlargement, pregnancy, or childbearing potential.
- Note recent (within 24 hr) use of 5-HT$_1$ agonists or other ergotamine-containing or ergot-type drugs (eg, methysergide).
- Ensure that a woman of childbearing potential is not pregnant before administering medication.
- Assess symptoms before starting therapy and periodically during treatment.
- Obtain baseline vital signs, with special attention to pulse and BP.
- Monitor patient for CNS, CV, GI, musculoskeletal, and general body side effects. Report to health care provider if noted and significant.

Adverse Reactions
CV: Palpitations; tachycardia.
CNS: Drowsiness.
EENT: Blurred vision.
GI: Dry mouth; decreased GI motility.
GU: Urinary retention.
OTHER: Tingling and other paresthesias of the extremities; decreased sweating; flushing.

Precautions
Pregnancy: Category X.
Lactation: Ergot alkaloids excreted in breast milk.
Children: Safety and efficacy not established.
Special risk patients: Use with caution in patients with bronchial asthma or obstructive uropathy.
Drug dependence: Because of presence of phenobarbital, has abuse potential and may cause true addiction.

Overdosage: Signs and Symptoms
Symptoms may be attributable to any 1 or more of the 3 active ingredients; which toxic symptoms might predominate in an individual would be impossible to predict.

- Discontinue therapy and notify health care provider immediately if any of the following symptoms occur: numbness, tingling, coldness, or paleness in the fingers or toes; muscle pain in arms or legs; weakness in the legs; chest pain, tightness, or pressure; changes in heart rate; sudden worsening of headache; swelling; or itching.

Patient/Family Education
- Explain name, dose, action, and potential side effects of drug.
- Advise patient to take 1 tablet bid (morning and evening) without regard to meals but to take with food if GI upset occurs.
- Caution patient not to take more than 16 tablets in 1 wk because of the risk of toxic effects developing.
- Instruct patient to avoid alcoholic beverages and other depressants while taking this medication.
- Advise patient that drug may impair judgment, thinking, or motor skills or cause drowsiness and to use caution while driving or performing other tasks requiring mental alertness until tolerance is determined.
- Advise patient to stop taking the drug and notify health care provider if any of the following symptoms occur: numbness, tingling, coldness, or paleness in the fingers or toes; muscle pain in arms or legs; weakness in the legs; chest pain, tightness, or pressure; changes in heart rate; sudden worsening of

- headache; swelling; or itching.
- Advise women to contact health care provider if pregnant, planning to become pregnant, or breastfeeding.
- Warn patient not to take any prescription or OTC drugs or dietary supplements without consulting health care provider.
- Advise patient that follow-up visits may be necessary to monitor therapy and to keep appointments.

Benazepril Hydrochloride

(BEN-AZE-uh-prill HIGH-droe-KLOR-ide)
Class Antihypertensive/ACE inhibitor

How Supplied
Lotensin Tablets 5 mg, Tablets 10 mg, Tablets 20 mg, Tablets 40 mg

Action
PHARMACOLOGY: Competitively inhibits angiotensin I-converting enzyme, resulting in the prevention of angiotensin I conversion to angiotensin II, a potent vasoconstrictor that stimulates aldosterone secretion. Results in decrease in sodium and fluid retention, decrease in BP, and increase in diuresis.

PHARMACOKINETICS/DYNAMICS:

Absorption: T_{max} is 0.5 to 1 hr (benazepril), 1 to 2 hr (benazeprilat) in fasting state, and 2 to 4 hr (benazeprilat) in nonfasting state. Up to 37% absorbed.

Distribution: Protein binding is about 96.7% (benazepril) and about 95.3% (benazeprilat).

Metabolism: Converted to benazeprilat (active) by cleavage of ester group (primarily in liver). Also metabolized to glucuronide conjugates.

Excretion:
Urine – Benazepril (trace amounts), benazeprilat (about 20%), benazepril glucuronide (4%), benazeprilat glucuronide (8%).
Nonrenal (eg, biliary) – About 11% to 12% (benazeprilat).

Onset: Within 1 hr.

Peak: 2 to 4 hr.

Duration: 24 hr.

Special Populations:
Renal Function Impairment – In those with Ccr up to 30 mL/min, peak benzaprilat levels and initial t½ increase and time to steady state may be delayed.

Indications
Treatment of hypertension.

Contraindications
Hypersensitivity to ACE inhibitors.

Route/Dosage
ADULTS:
Initial dose: **PO** 10 mg qd for patients not receiving a diuretic. In patients taking diuretics that cannot be discontinued, give initial dose of 5 mg.
Maintenance: **PO** 20 to 40 mg/day as single dose or in 2 divided doses; doses up to 80 mg have been used.
Renal function impairment – Initial dose is 5 mg qd for patients with Ccr less than 30 mL/min. Dosage may be titrated upward until BP is controlled or to a total max daily dose of 40 mg.

Interactions
Antacids: May decrease bioavailability of benazepril; separate administration by 1 to 2 hr.
Diuretics: May cause symptomatic hypotension after initial dose of benazepril.
Lithium: May increase lithium levels and symptoms of lithium toxicity.
Potassium preparations, potassium-sparing diuretics: May increase serum potassium levels.
Salicylates (eg, aspirin): May reduce effects of benazepril, especially in low-renin or volume-dependent hypertensive patients.

Lab Test Interferences None well documented.

Adverse Reactions
CV: Hypotension.
CNS: Headache (6%); dizziness (4%); fatigue (3%); somnolence, postural dizziness (2%).
GI: Nausea (1%).
HEMA/LYMPH: Neutropenia; agranulocytosis.
LABTESTABS: Increased serum creatinine (2%).
RESP: Chronic dry cough (1%).
OTHER: Anaphylactoid reactions; angioedema.

> **WARNING:**
> *Pregnancy:* Use in second and third trimesters may cause injury and death to fetus.

Precautions
Pregnancy: Category D (second and third trimester); Category C (first trimester). When pregnancy is detected, discontinue ACE inhibitors as soon as possible.
Lactation: Excreted in breast milk; avoid use in nursing mothers if possible.
Children: Safety and efficacy not established.
Renal function impairment: Reduce dosage.
Angioedema: Use with extreme caution in patients with hereditary angioedema. Angioedema associated with laryngeal edema may be fatal.
Hepatic failure: Rarely, ACE inhibitors have been associated with a syndrome that starts with cholestatic jaundice and progresses to fulminant

hepatic necrosis and sometimes death.
Hypotension/first-dose effect: Significant decreases in BP may occur after first dose, especially in severely salt- or volume-depleted patients (eg, those undergoing dialysis or vigorous diuretic therapy) or those with heart failure. Risk is minimized by discontinuing use of diuretics, increasing salt intake about 1 wk before initiating benazepril, or decreasing benazepril dose.
Neutropenia/agranulocytosis: Has occurred with other ACE inhibitors.

Overdosage: Signs and Symptoms
Hypotension.

PATIENT CARE CONSIDERATIONS
Administration/Storage
- Administer alone or in combination with other antihypertensives.
- Give qd or bid as prescribed, without regard to meals. Administer with food if GI upset occurs.
- Do not administer to pregnant women during second and third trimesters as fetal and neonatal morbidity and death can occur.
- Store tablets at controlled room temperature (59° to 89°F). Protect from moisture.

Assessment/Interventions
- Obtain patient history, including drug history and any known allergies. Note renal or hepatic impairment, conditions predisposing to volume depletion (eg, prolonged diuretic therapy), diabetes, heart failure, anuria, hereditary or idiopathic angioedema, lupus erythematosus, left ventricular outflow obstruction, allergy to any other ACE inhibitor, and concurrent use of potassium-containing salt substitutes, potassium supplements, or potassium-sparing diuretics.
- Ensure that reduced dose is administered to patient with severe renal impairment (Ccr less than 30 mL/min).
- Ensure that volume and/or salt depletion have been corrected before initiating therapy.
- Ensure that serum electrolytes and renal function are monitored periodically.
- Ensure that CBC with differential are evaluated prior to starting therapy, at 2 wk intervals for 3 mo, and periodically thereafter in patient with renal impairment.
- Monitor and record BP and pulse. Should symptomatic hypotension occur, hold medication and notify health care provider.
- Take safety precautions if orthostatic hypotension occurs.
- Monitor for signs of hypersensitivity including angioedema involving swelling of the face, lips, eyelids, and tongue. Discontinue medication and notify health care provider immediately if noted. Be prepared to treat appropriately.
- Assess patient for GI, CNS, and general body side effects. Inform health care provider if noted and significant.

Patient/Family Education
- Explain name, dose, action, and potential side effects of drug.
- Advise patient to take qd or bid as prescribed, without regard to meals, but to take with food if stomach upset occurs.
- Advise patient to try to take each dose at about the same time each day.
- Inform patient that drug controls, but does not cure, hypertension and to continue taking drug as prescribed even when BP is not elevated.
- Caution patient not to change the dose or stop taking unless advised by health care provider.
- Instruct patient to continue taking other BP medications as prescribed by health care provider.
- Instruct patient in BP and pulse measurement skills.
- Advise patient to monitor and record BP and pulse at home and to inform health care provider if abnormal measurements are noted. Also advise patient to take record of BP and pulse to each follow-up visit.
- Caution patient to avoid sudden position changes to prevent orthostatic hypotension.
- Instruct patient to lie or sit down if experiencing dizziness or lightheadedness when standing.
- Emphasize importance of other modalities on BP control: weight control, regular exercise, smoking cessation, moderate intake of alcohol and salt.
- Advise patient to promptly report any indication of infection (eg, sore throat, fever), which could be a sign of neutropenia.
- Caution patient that inadequate fluid intake, excessive perspiration, diarrhea, or vomiting can lead to excessive fall in BP resulting in lightheadedness or fainting.
- Advise patient that medication may cause dizziness or lightheadedness and to use caution while driving or performing other tasks requiring mental alertness until tolerance is determined.
- Caution patient to avoid unnecessary exposure to UV light (sunlight, tanning booths)

and to use sunscreen and wear protective clothing when exposed to UV light to avoid photosensitivity reaction.
* Instruct women to inform health care provider if pregnant, planning to become pregnant, or breastfeeding.
* Instruct patient to stop taking drug and immediately report any of the following symptoms to health care provider: sore throat, fever, swelling of the hands or feet, irregular heartbeat, chest pains, fainting, swelling of the face, lips, eyelids, or tongue, difficulty breathing.
* Instruct patient to inform health care provider if a persistent cough develops while taking this medication.
* Caution patient not to take any prescription or OTC medications, potassium-containing salt substitutes, potassium supplements, or dietary supplements unless advised by health care provider.
* Advise patient that follow-up visits and lab tests will be required to monitor therapy and to keep appointments.

Benazepril Hydrochloride/ Hydrochlorothiazide

(BEN-AZE-uh-pril HIGH-droe-CLOR-ide/ high-droe-klor-oh-THIGH-uh-zide)
Class Antihypertensive

How Supplied
Lotensin HCT Tablets 20 mg benazepril, 25 mg hydrochlorothiazide, Tablets 20 mg benazepril, 12.5 mg hydrochlorothiazide, Tablets 10 mg benazepril, 12.5 mg hydrochlorothiazide

Action
PHARMACOLOGY:
Benazepril: Competitively inhibits angiotensin I-converting enzyme, resulting in the prevention of angiotensin I conversion to angiotensin II, a potent vasoconstrictor that stimulates aldosterone secretion. This action results in a decrease in sodium and fluid retention, increase in diuresis and a decrease in BP.
Hydrochlorothiazide: Increases chloride, sodium, and water excretion by interfering with transport of sodium ions across renal tubular epithelium.

Indications
Treatment of hypertension. This fixed combination drug is not intended for the initial therapy of hypertension.

Contraindications
Anuric patients; patients hypersensitive to benazepril or any other ACE inhibitor; hydrochlorothiazide or other sulfonamide derivative.

Route/Dosage
ADULTS: **PO** Combination therapy with qd doses of 5 to 20 mg benazepril and 6.25 to 25 mg of hydrochlorothiazide.

Interactions
Cholestyramine, colestipol: May impair the absorption of hydrochlorothiazide.
Insulin: In diabetic patients, requirements of insulin may be increased, decreased, or unchanged.
Lithium: Plasma levels of lithium may be elevated, increasing the risk of toxicity.
Potassium supplements, potassium-sparing diuretics (eg, spironolactone): Increased risk of hyperkalemia.
Tubocurarine: Effects may be increased.
Lab Test Interferences Hydrochlorothiazide may decrease serum protein-bound iodine levels without signs of thyroid disturbances.

Adverse Reactions
CV: Postural dizziness; hypotension; palpitations; syncope; tachycardia; peripheral vascular disorder; orthostatic hypotension.
CNS: Dizziness; headache; fatigue; somnolence; insomnia; nervousness; vertigo; lightheadedness; weakness; restlessness.
DERM: Rash; sweating; photosensitivity; purpura; urticarial rash; Stevens-Johnson syndrome.
EENT: Tinnitus; rhinitis; sinusitis; transient blurred vision; xanthopsia.
GI: Nausea; vomiting; diarrhea; dyspepsia; anorexia; constipation; dry mouth; paresthesia; taste perversion; pancreatitis; sialadenitis; cramping; gastric irritation.
GU: Impotence; urinary frequency; decreased libido.
HEMA: Aplastic anemia; agranulocytosis; leukopenia; thrombocytopenia.
HEPA: Intrahepatic cholestatic jaundice.
METAB: Gout; hyperglycemia; glucosuria.
RESP: Cough; upper respiratory infection; respiratory distress (including pneumonitis, pulmonary edema).
OTHER: Hypertonia; angioedema (including edema of lips and face); flushing; arthralgia; myalgia; asthenia; pain (including chest and abdominal); back pain; flu-like syndrome; muscle spasm; necrotizing angiitis.

Precautions
Pregnancy: Category D (second and third trimester); Category C (first trimester). ACE inhibitors (eg, benazepril) can cause injury or death to fetus if used during second or third trimester. When pregnancy is detected, discontinue as soon as possible.
Lactation: Excreted in breast milk.

Children: Safety and efficacy not established.
Renal function impairment: Use with caution.
Hepatic function impairment: Use with caution.
Angioedema: Use with extreme caution in patients with hereditary angioedema. Angioedema associated with laryngeal edema may be fatal.
Hypotension: Decreases in BP may occur, especially in salt- or volume-depleted patients as a result of dialysis, prolonged diuretic therapy, dietary salt restriction, diarrhea, or vomiting. Volume and salt depletion should be corrected before initiating therapy with benazepril/hydrochlorothiazide.
Neutropenia/agranulocytosis: Has occurred with other ACE inhibitors.

Overdosage: Signs and Symptoms
Dehydration, electrolyte disturbances, hypotension.

PATIENT CARE CONSIDERATIONS
Administration/Storage
- Give qd in the morning, with or without food.
- Administer alone or in combination with other antihypertensives.
- Do not administer to pregnant women as fetal and neonatal morbidity and death can occur.
- Store tablets at controlled room temperature (less than 86°F). Keep container tightly closed. Protect from moisture and light.

Assessment/Interventions
- Obtain patient history, including drug history and any known allergies. Note history of diabetes, anuria, lupus erythematosus, kidney or liver disease, or allergy to any other ACE inhibitor or sulfonamide-derived medications. Note concurrent use of potassium-containing salt substitutes, potassium supplements, or potassium-sparing diuretics.
- Ensure that serum electrolytes and renal function are monitored periodically.
- Ensure that volume and/or salt depletion have been corrected before initiating therapy.
- Monitor and record BP and pulse. Should hypotension result, hold medication and notify health care provider.
- Take safety precautions if orthostatic hypotension occurs.
- Monitor blood sugar in diabetic patient when drug is started or dose is changed. Report significant changes to health care provider.
- Monitor for signs of hypersensitivity including angioedema involving swelling of the face, lips, eyelids, and tongue. Discontinue medication and notify health care provider immediately if noted. Be prepared to treat appropriately.

Patient/Family Education
- Explain name, dose, action, and potential side effects of drug.
- Advise patient to take prescribed dose qd, without regard to meals.
- Advise patient to try to take each dose at about the same time each day.
- Inform patient that drug controls, but not does cure, hypertension and to continue taking drug as prescribed even when BP is not elevated.
- Caution patient not to change the dose or stop taking unless advised to do so by health care provider.
- Instruct patient to continue taking other BP medications as prescribed by health care provider.
- Instruct patient in BP and pulse measurement skills.
- Advise patient to monitor and record BP and pulse at home and to inform health care provider should abnormal measurements be noted. Also advise patient to take record of BP and pulse to each follow-up visit.
- Caution patient to avoid sudden position changes to prevent orthostatic hypotension.
- Instruct patient to lie or sit down if experiencing dizziness or lightheadedness when standing.
- Caution patient that inadequate fluid intake, excessive perspiration, diarrhea, or vomiting can lead to excessive fall in BP resulting in lightheadedness or fainting.
- Instruct diabetic patient to monitor blood glucose more frequently when drug is started or dose is changed and to inform health care provider of significant changes in readings.
- Caution patient to avoid unnecessary exposure to UV light (eg, sunlight, tanning booths) and to use sunscreen and wear protective clothing when exposed to UV light to avoid photosensitivity reaction.
- Emphasize to hypertensive patient importance of other modalities on BP: Weight control, regular exercise, smoking cessation, moderate intake of alcohol and salt
- Advise women to notify health care provider if pregnant, planning to become pregnant, or breastfeeding.

- Instruct patient to stop taking drug and immediately report any of the following symptoms to health care provider: fainting, swelling of the face, lips, eyelids, or tongue, difficulty breathing.
- Instruct patient to inform health care provider if a persistent cough develops while taking this medication.
- Caution patient to not take any prescription or OTC medications, potassium-containing salt substitutes, potassium supplements, or dietary supplements unless advised by health care provider.
- Advise patient that follow-up visits and lab tests may be required to monitor therapy and to keep appointments.

Bendroflumethiazide

(BEN-droe-flew-meth-EYE-ah-zide)
Class Thiazide diuretic
How Supplied
Naturetin Tablets 5 mg
Action
PHARMACOLOGY: Enhances excretion of sodium, chloride, and water by interfering with transport of sodium ions across renal tubular epithelium.

PHARMACOKINETICS/DYNAMICS:
Excretion: Eliminated rapidly by the kidney.
Onset: Approximately 2 hr.
Peak: Approximately 4 hr.
Duration: About 6 to 12 hr.

Indications Adjunctive therapy for edema associated with CHF, hepatic cirrhosis, and corticosteroid and estrogen therapy; treatment of edema associated with various forms of renal dysfunction (eg, nephrotic syndrome, acute glomerulonephritis, chronic renal failure); management of hypertension.

Contraindications Anuria, hypersensitivity to other sulfonamide-derived drugs.

Route/Dosage
Diuretic
ADULTS: PO Usual dose is 5 mg qd, preferably in the morning. Therapy may be initiated at 20 mg qd or in 2 divided doses. A single daily dose of 2.5 to 5 mg should be sufficient for maintenance. Alternatively, intermittent therapy (qod or 3 to 5 days/wk) may be administered.

Antihypertensive
ADULTS: PO Start with 5 to 20 mg/day. Maintenance dosage may range from 2.5 to 15 mg/day. Lower maintenance doses may be sufficient when used in combination with other antihypertensive agents.

Interactions
Alcohol, barbiturates, narcotics: May potentiate orthostatic hypotension.
Anticoagulants (eg, warfarin): May decrease anticoagulant effects. May need to adjust dose of anticoagulant.
Antigout medications: May require dosage adjustments caused by increase in uric acid levels.
Amphotericin B, corticosteroid, corticotropin: May intensify electrolyte imbalance, especially hypokalemia.
Bile acid sequestrants: May reduce bendroflumethiazide absorption; give thiazide at least 1 hr before or 4 to 6 hr after bile acid sequestrant.
Calcium salts: May decrease calcium excretion.
Diazoxide: May cause hyperglycemia, hyperuricemia, and antihypertensive effects.
Digitalis glycosides: Diuretic-induced hypokalemia and hypomagnesemia may precipitate digitalis-induced arrhythmias.
Ganglionic or peripheral adrenergic blocking agents: Bendroflumethiazide may potentiate effects. May need to adjust the dose.
Lithium: May decrease renal excretion of lithium.
Loop diuretics: Synergistic effects may result in profound diuresis and serious electrolyte abnormalities.
MAO inhibitors: May enhance hypotensive effects.
NSAIDs: May reduce effects of bendroflumethiazide.
Nondepolarizing muscle relaxants: May potentiate effects of these agents.
Pressor amines (eg, norepinephrine), anesthetic, and preanesthetic agents: Reduce dosage and discontinue bendroflumethiazide 1 wk prior to surgery.
Sulfonylureas, insulin: May decrease hypoglycemic effect of sulfonylureas. Because bendroflumethiazide may elevate blood glucose levels, dosage of sulfonylureas or insulin may need to be increased.

Lab Test Interferences May produce false-negative results with phentolamine and tyramine tests; may interfere with the phenolsulfonphthalein test due to decreased excretion; may cause diagnostic interference of serum electrolyte levels, blood and urine glucose levels, and a decrease in serum protein-bound iodine levels without signs of thyroid disturbance.

Adverse Reactions
CV: Hypotension.
CNS: Restlessness (not uncommon); dizziness, vertigo, paresthesia, headache (occasionally).
DERM: Purpura, exfoliative dermatitis, pruritus, ecchymosis, urticaria, necrotizing angitis (vasculitis, cutaneous vasculitis) (occasionally); photosensitivity; rash.

EENT: Xanthopsia, transient blurred vision (occasionally).
GI: Nausea, vomiting, cramping, anorexia (not uncommon); diarrhea, constipation, gastric irritation, abdominal bloating, sialoadenitis (occasionally); pancreatitis.
HEMA: Leukopenia; agranulocytosis; thrombocytopenia; hemolytic anemia; aplastic anemia.
HEPA: Jaundice (intrahepatic cholestatic); hepatitis (occasionally).
METAB: Hyperglycemia, glucosuria, metabolic acidosis, hyperuricemia (occasionally).
MUSC: Muscle spasm, weakness (not uncommon)
RENAL: Allergic glomerulonephritis (occasionally).
RESP: Respiratory distress (including pneumonitis [occasionally]).
OTHER: Fever (occasionally).

Precautions
Pregnancy: Category C.
Lactation: Excreted in breast milk.
Children: Safety and efficacy not established.
Hypersensitivity: May occur in patients with or without history of allergy or bronchial asthma; cross-sensitivity with sulfonamides also may occur.
Renal function impairment: Drug may precipitate azotemia; use drug with caution.
Hepatic function impairment: Minor alterations of fluid and electrolyte balance may precipitate hepatic coma; use with caution.
Lupus erythematosus: Exacerbation or activation may occur.
Postsympathectomy patients: Antihypertensive effects may be enhanced.
Diabetes mellitus: May become manifest.
Electrolytes: Increased urinary excretion of sodium, potassium, and magnesium may occur; decreased urinary excretion of calcium may occur.
Hyperuricemia: May occur or frank gout may be precipitated.

Overdosage: Signs and Symptoms
Temporary elevation of BUN, GI irritation, lethargy progressing to coma with minimal depression of respiration and CV function and without significant serum electrolyte changes or dehydration.

PATIENT CARE CONSIDERATIONS
Administration/Storage
* Administer qd in the morning without regard to meals. Administer with food if GI upset occurs.
* Administer alone or in combination with other antihypertensives.
* Store tablets at controlled room temperature (59° to 86°F). Protect from excessive heat.

Assessment/Interventions
* Obtain patient history, including drug history and any known allergies. Note liver or kidney disease, diabetes, lupus erythematosus, anuria, or allergy to sulfonamides.
* Ensure that serum electrolytes, BUN, creatinine, and uric acid are monitored periodically.
* Monitor and record BP and pulse. Should hypotension result, hold medication and notify health care provider.
* Take safety precautions if orthostatic hypotension occurs.
* Monitor blood sugar in diabetic patient when drug is started or dose is changed. Report significant changes to health care provider.
* Monitor patient for GI, CV, CNS, and general body side effects. Inform health care provider if paresthesia, weakness, fatigue, confusion, hypotension, tachycardia, or other significant effects are noted.

Patient/Family Education
* Explain name, dose, action, and potential side effects of drug.
* Advise patient to take prescribed dose qd in the morning without regard to meals but to take with food if stomach upset occurs.
* Advise patient that medication will initially increase urination but that this should go away after a few weeks of treatment.
* Advise patient that if a dose is missed to skip that dose and take the next dose at the regularly scheduled time. Caution patient not to double the dose to catch up.
* Inform patient that drug controls but does not cure hypertension and to continue taking medication as prescribed even when BP is not elevated.
* Caution patient not to change the dose or stop taking unless advised by health care provider.
* Instruct patient to continue taking other BP medications as prescribed by health care provider.
* Instruct patient in BP and pulse measurement skills.
* Advise patient to monitor and record BP and pulse at home and to inform health care provider if abnormal measurements are noted. Also advise patient to take record of BP and pulse to each follow-up visit.
* Instruct patient to lie or sit down if experiencing dizziness or lightheadedness when standing.
* Caution patient that inadequate fluid intake,

excessive perspiration, diarrhea, or vomiting can lead to excessive fall in BP, resulting in lightheadedness or fainting.
- Instruct diabetic patient to monitor blood glucose more frequently when drug is started or dose is changed and to inform health care provider of significant changes in readings.
- Caution patient to avoid unnecessary exposure to UV light (sunlight, tanning booths) and to use sunscreen and wear protective clothing when exposed to UV light until tolerance is determined.
- Emphasize to hypertensive patient importance of the following modalities on BP: weight control, regular exercise, smoking cessation, moderate intake of alcohol and salt.
- Advise women to notify health care provider if pregnant, planning to become pregnant, or breastfeeding.
- Instruct patient to inform health care provider if any of the following occur: muscle pain, weakness, or cramps; persistent nausea or vomiting; excessive thirst; unexplained tiredness; drowsiness; increased heart rate; unexplained joint pain; abnormal skin sensations.
- Caution patient to not take any prescription or OTC medications or dietary supplements unless advised by health care provider.
- Advise patient that follow-up visits and lab tests may be required to monitor therapy and to keep appointments.

Benzonatate

(ben-ZOE-nah-tate)
Class Nonnarcotic/Antitussive
How Supplied
Tessalon Capsules 100 mg, Capsules 200 mg
Action
PHARMACOLOGY: Reduces cough reflex by anesthetizing stretch receptors in respiratory passages.

PHARMACOKINETICS/DYNAMICS:
Onset: 15 to 20 min.
Duration: 3 to 8 hr.
Indications Symptomatic relief of cough.
Contraindications Standard considerations.
Route/Dosage
ADULTS AND CHILDREN AT LEAST 10 YR: PO 100 to 200 mg tid as required, up to 600 mg/day.
Interactions None well documented.

PATIENT CARE CONSIDERATIONS
Administration/Storage
- Swallow without chewing.

Lab Test Interferences None well documented.
Adverse Reactions
CNS: Sedation; headache; mental confusion; visual hallucinations.
DERM: Pruritus; skin eruptions.
GI: Constipation; nausea; GI upset.
HYPERSEN: Hypersensitivity reactions including bronchospasm, laryngospasm, cardiovascular collapse, possibly related to chewing the capsule.
OTHER: Nasal congestion; eye irritation; feeling cold; chest numbness.
Precautions
Pregnancy: Category C.
Lactation: Undetermined.
Children: Safety in children younger than 10 yr is not established.
Overdosage: Signs and Symptoms
CNS stimulation, restlessness, tremors, convulsions, profound CNS depression.

Benzoyl Peroxide

(BEN-zoyl per-OX-ide)
Class Topical Anti-infective
How Supplied
Benzac Liquid 2.5%, Liquid 5%, Liquid 10%, Gel 2.5%, Gel 5%, Gel 10% ◆ *Triaz* Liquid 3%, Liquid 6%, Liquid 9%, Gel 3%, Gel 6%, Gel 9%, Gel 10% ◆ *Triaz Cleanser* Lotion 3%, Lotion 6%, Lotion 10% ◆ *Brevoxyl* Liquid 4%, Liquid 8%, Lotion 4%, Lotion 8%, Gel 4%, Gel 8% ◆ *PanOxyl* Bar 5%, Bar 10%, Gel 2.5%, Gel 5%, Gel 10% ◆ *Desquam* Bar 10%, Gel 5%, Gel 10% ◆ *Neutrogena* Cleanser/Mask 3.5% ◆ *Oxy* Liquid 10% ◆ *Clearasil* Cream 10% ◆ *Clinac* Gel 7% ◆ *Benzagel* Gel 10%
✤ *Acetoxyl* 2.5% and 5% ◆ *Acetoxyl* 10% ◆ *Oxyderm* 5% ◆ *Oxyderm* 10% ◆ *Oxyderm* 20% ◆ *Panoxyl Aquagel* 2.5% and 5% ◆ *Panoxyl Aquagel* 10% and 20% ◆ *Panoxyl* 5% ◆ *Panoxyl 5% Wash* ◆ *Panoxyl* 10% ◆ *Panoxyl* 15% ◆ *Panoxyl* 20% ◆ *Solugel 4* ◆ *Solugel 8*

Action
PHARMACOLOGY: Release of active or free-radical oxygen capable of oxidizing bacterial proteins is suspected.

PHARMACOKINETICS/DYNAMICS:
Absorption: Absorbed by the skin, where it is metabolized to benzoic acid and excreted as benzoate in the urine.

Indications Treatment of mild to moderate acne vulgaris and as an adjunct to antibiotics, retinoic acid, and sulfur or salicylic acid-containing products in treating more severe cases of acne.

Contraindications Standard considerations.

Route/Dosage
ADULTS AND CHILDREN 12 YR AND OLDER:
Topical Cleansers Wash qd or bid. Wet skin areas to be treated prior to administration, rinse thoroughly, and pat dry. Control amount of drying or peeling by modifying dose frequency or concentration. Adjust frequency of use to obtain the desired clinical response. Visible improvement will normally occur by wk 3 with max lesion reduction approximately by wk 8 to 12.
Other dose forms After cleaning skin, smooth small amount over affected area qd or bid. Reduce dose frequency or concentration if bothersome dryness or peeling occurs. If excessive stinging or burning occurs after any single application, remove with mild soap and water, resuming use the next day.

Interactions
Tretinoin: Concurrent use may cause severe skin irritation.

Lab Test Interferences None well documented.

PATIENT CARE CONSIDERATIONS
Administration/Storage
- For topical use only. Not for ophthalmic, oral, or intravaginal use.
- Avoid contact with eyes, eyelids, lips, and mucus membranes.
- Cream, gel, or lotion is usually applied to affected area(s) qd or bid. Thoroughly wash and pat area(s) to be treated dry, then apply a thin film of cream, gel, or lotion to cover skin areas with acne lesions.
- Cleanser is usually used qd or bid. Wet skin area(s) to be treated prior to use of cleanser.
- Store at controlled room temperature (59° to 86°F).

Assessment/Interventions
- Obtain patient history, including drug history and any known allergies.
- Assess the skin and identify areas where medication is to be applied and areas that should be avoided (severely irritated or sun-burned skin).
- Assess and document skin condition before initial application and periodically throughout treatment.
- Monitor for side effects, including redness, scaling, dryness, or persistent itching or burning. Inform health care provider if noted and significant.

Adverse Reactions
DERM: Excessive drying, manifested by marked peeling, erythema, possible edema, and allergic contact sensitization/dermatitis.

Precautions
Pregnancy: Category C.
Lactation: Undetermined.
Children: Safety and efficacy not established in children under 12 yr.
Bleaching: Benzoyl peroxide is an oxidizing agent and may bleach hair and colored fabric.
Cross-sensitization: Cross-sensitization may occur with benzoic acid derivatives (eg, cinnamon, certain topical anesthetics).
External use only: Avoid contact with eyes, eyelids, lips, mucous membranes, and highly inflamed or damaged skin. Rinse with water if accidental contact occurs.
Irritation: If severe irritation develops, consult health care provider, discontinue use, and institute appropriate therapy. After reaction clears, treatment may often be resumed with less frequent application.
Sun exposure: Avoid unnecessary exposure to sun when using this product.

Overdosage: Signs and Symptoms
Excessive scaling, erythema, edema.

- If bothersome dryness or peeling occurs, consider reducing the frequency of application and/or the concentration of the medication.

Patient/Family Education
- Explain name, action, and potential side effects of drug.
- Advise patient that medication is applied topically to skin lesions qd or bid.
- Teach patient with acne proper technique for applying cream, gel, or lotion: wash hands; thoroughly wash and pat dry area(s) to be treated then apply a thin film of cream, gel, or lotion to cover skin areas with acne lesions. Wash hands after applying medication.
- Caution patient to avoid contact of medication with hair or colored fabrics because bleaching may occur.
- Instruct patient to avoid concurrent use of topical alcoholic cleansers, tinctures, astringents, abrasives, and peeling agents unless advised by health care provider.
- Caution patient not to cover treated areas with bandages or dressings.
- Warn patient that applying medication more often than prescribed or in excessive quantities will not produce more rapid improvement or better results but will result in greater side

effects such as redness, scaling, and discomfort.
- Advise patient if an application is missed, not to try to make it up but to return to normal application schedule as soon as possible.
- Warn patient to avoid contact with the eyes, eyelids, lips, and mucous membranes.
- Advise patient if cream or gel comes in contact with the eyes to wash eyes with large amounts of cool water and to contact health care provider if eye irritation persists.
- Advise patient that local stinging, burning, tingling, dryness, and redness are the most common side effects and to notify health care provider if they become bothersome.
- Advise patient if severe skin reactions occur to stop using the medication and contact health care provider.
- Warn patient to avoid unnecessary exposure to sun and sun lamps while using this medication. Advise patient to use sunscreens and protective clothing over treated areas when exposure cannot be avoided.
- Advise patient to talk to health care provider before using any other topical agents (eg, medicated soaps, astringents, cosmetics, or other acne products) on treated skin.
- Advise women to notify health care provider if pregnant, planning to become pregnant, or breastfeeding.
- Warn patient not to take any prescription or OTC drugs or dietary supplements without consulting health care provider.
- Advise patient that follow-up visits to examine the skin lesions may be necessary and to keep appointments.

Benzphetamine Hydrochloride

(benz-FET-uh-meen HIGH-droe-KLOR-ide)
Class CNS stimulant/Anorexiant
How Supplied
Didrex Tablets 25 mg, Tablets 50 mg
Action
PHARMACOLOGY: Stimulates satiety center in brain, causing appetite suppression.
Indications Short-term (few weeks) adjunct to diet plan to reduce weight.
Contraindications Hypersensitivity to sympathomimetic amines; pregnancy; advanced arteriosclerosis; symptomatic cardiovascular disease; moderate to severe hypertension; hyperthyroidism; glaucoma; agitated states; history of drug abuse; during or within 14 days of MAO inhibitor use; coadministration with other CNS stimulants.
Route/Dosage
ADULTS: **PO** 25 to 50 mg 1 to 3 times/day.
Interactions
Guanethidine: May decrease hypotensive effect.
MAO inhibitors, furazolidone: May cause hypertensive crisis and intracranial hemorrhage.
Selective serotonin reuptake inhibitors (eg, fluoxetine): Sympathomimetic effects of benzphetamine may be increased; increased risk of "serotonin syndrome."
Lab Test Interferences None well documented.

Adverse Reactions
CV: Palpitations; tachycardia; arrhythmias; hypertension; hypotension; chest pain.
CNS: Hypersensitivity; dizziness; insomnia; euphoria; tremor; headache; restlessness; overstimulation; nervousness; anxiety; agitation.
DERM: Urticaria; rash; erythema; hair loss.
EENT: Mydriasis; blurred vision; unpleasant taste.
GI: Dry mouth; nausea; diarrhea; constipation; stomach pain.
GU: Dysuria; urinary frequency; impotence; menstrual disturbances.
HEMA: Bone marrow depression; agranulocytosis; leukopenia.
OTHER: Excessive sweating; flushing; myalgia; gynecomastia.
Precautions
Pregnancy: Category X.
Lactation: Undetermined.
Children: Not recommended for children under 12 yr.
Tartrazine sensitivity: Some products contain tartrazine, which may cause allergic-type reactions in susceptible individuals.
Drug dependency: High potential for dependence and abuse; tolerance may occur.
Overdosage: Signs and Symptoms
Restlessness, tremor, rapid respirations, tachypnea, dizziness, confusion, mood changes, panic states, dysrhythmias, palpitations, and hypertension or hypotension.

PATIENT CARE CONSIDERATIONS
Administration/Storage
- Administer midmorning or midafternoon. Anorexiant effects occur within 1 to 2 hr and last up to 4 hr.
- Administer last dose several hours before bedtime.
- Store at room temperature in tightly closed, light-resistant container.

Assessment/Interventions
- Obtain patient history, including drug history and any known allergies. Note cardiovascular disease, hypertension, glaucoma, and history of drug or alcohol abuse.
- Monitor renal function.
- Take vital signs and auscultate heart and lungs before administration.
- Assess mental status. Depressed patients are more likely to misuse drug to induce euphoria and mood elevation.
- If hypertension, dysrhythmias, marked agitation, restlessness, depression, or other adverse effects occur, withhold medication and notify health care provider.
- For best results, administer medication concurrently with a program to improve eating habits, increase motivation, and improve self-image.

Patient/Family Education
- Caution patient that this medication must not be taken during pregnancy or when pregnancy is possible. Advise patient to use reliable form of birth control while taking this drug.
- Remind patient to take medication on empty stomach (1 hr before meal or 2 hr after meal).
- Instruct patient to avoid taking medication within 6 hr of bedtime because it may cause insomnia.
- Explain that anorexiant effects are temporary and tolerance to medication and dependence can occur.
- Instruct patient to notify health care provider immediately if the following symptoms occur: chest pain, palpitations, nervousness, or dizziness.
- Warn patient not to drive or perform tasks that require mental alertness if dizziness or blurred vision occurs. Notify health care provider of these disturbances.
- Tell patient to report excessive dryness of mouth, constipation, or prolonged insomnia because dosage may need to be adjusted.
- Inform patient that weight reduction requires strict adherence to dietary restrictions.

Benztropine Mesylate
(BENZ-troe-peen MEH-sih-LATE)

Class Antiparkinson/Anticholinergic

How Supplied
Cogentin Tablets 0.5 mg, Tablets 1 mg, Tablets 2 mg, Injection 1 mg/mL
✤ *Apo-Benztropine* ◆ *Benztropine Omega*

Action
PHARMACOLOGY: Thought to act by competitively antagonizing acetylcholine receptors in corpus striatum to restore neuromuscular balance.

Indications Treatment of all forms of parkinsonism; control of extrapyramidal disorders (except tardive dyskinesia) caused by neuroleptic drugs.

Contraindications Angle-closure glaucoma; myasthenia gravis; pyloric or duodenal obstruction; stenosing peptic ulcer; prostatic hypertrophy or bladder neck obstructions; megacolon; tardive dyskinesia; children under 3 yr.

Route/Dosage
Parkinsonism
ADULTS: PO 1 to 2 mg/day; range, 0.5 to 6 mg. Individualize dosage.

Idiopathic Parkinsonism
ADULTS: PO Initially 0.5 to 1 mg at bedtime; 4 to 6 mg/day may be required.

Postencephalitic Parkinsonism
ADULTS: PO 2 mg/day in 1 or more doses; some patients may require initial dose of 0.5 mg.

Drug-Induced Extrapyramidal Disorders
ADULTS: 1 to 4 mg qd or bid.

Acute Dystonic Reactions
ADULTS: PO/IM/IV Initial dose is IM/IV 1 to 2 mg; then PO 1 to 2 mg bid.

Interactions
Amantadine: May increase anticholinergic effects.
Digoxin: May increase digoxin serum levels, especially with slow-dissolution oral digoxin tablets.
Haloperidol: May worsen schizophrenic symptoms; may decrease haloperidol serum levels; tardive dyskinesia may develop.
Phenothiazines: May decrease action of phenothiazines. May increase incidence of anticholinergic effects.

Lab Test Interferences None well documented.

Adverse Reactions
CV: Tachycardia; bradycardia.
CNS: Toxic psychosis including confusion, disorientation, memory impairment, visual hallucinations; exacerbation of pre-existing psychosis; nervousness; depression; finger numbness.
DERM: Skin rash.
EENT: Blurred vision; dilated pupils; narrow-angle glaucoma.
GI: Paralytic ileus; constipation; nausea; vomiting; dry mouth.
GU: Urinary retention; dysuria.

OTHER: Heat stroke; hyperthermia; fever; weakness; inability to move particular muscle groups.

Precautions

Pregnancy: Category C.
Lactation: Undetermined.
Children: Safety and efficacy not established
Elderly: Patients above 60 yr may have increased side effects; dosage reduction and observation may be needed.
Special risk patients: Use with caution in patients with glaucoma, prostatic hypertrophy, epilepsy, cardiac arrhythmias, hypertension, hypotension, tendency toward urinary retention, liver or kidney disorders, obstructive disease of GI or GU tract, tachycardia or those who are taking other drugs with anticholinergic activity.
Heat illness: Fatal hyperthermia has occurred. Use with caution during hot weather.
Ophthalmic: Narrow-angle glaucoma may occur.
Tardive dyskinesia: May aggravate tardive dyskinesia.

Overdosage: Signs and Symptoms

Circulatory collapse, cardiac arrest, respiratory depression, CNS depression or stimulation, shock, coma, stupor, seizures, convulsions, ataxia, anxiety, incoherence, hyperactivity, foul-smelling breath, decreased bowel sounds, dilated and sluggish pupils.

PATIENT CARE CONSIDERATIONS

Administration/Storage

- When given PO, administer with food to prevent GI irritation.
- If patient has difficulty swallowing, tablet may be crushed.
- May be given IM or IV in acute dystonic reaction. However, because onset and efficacy are equivalent for IM and IV route, IV administration is usually unnecessary.
- Store in a dry place in tightly closed, light-resistant container.

Assessment/Interventions

- Obtain patient history, including drug history and any allergies. Note glaucoma, urinary retention, prostatic hypertrophy, or constipation.
- Monitor vital signs and I&O for anticholinergic side effects (eg, hypotension, urinary retention).
- Monitor patient for reduction of rigidity and decrease in tremors during therapy.
- Monitor frequency of bowel movements. Patient may need stool softener.

Patient/Family Education

- Explain that full effectiveness of drug may not occur for 2 to 3 days after initiation of drug therapy. Explain that doses will be tapered gradually before stopping.
- Advise patient that increasing fluid intake will help decrease dry mouth and constipation.
- Instruct patient to take sips of water frequently, suck on ice chips or sugarless hard candy, or chew sugarless gum if dry mouth occurs.
- Warn patient to pay particular attention to dental hygiene because of problems associated with decreased salivation.
- Tell patient that stool softeners may be used if constipation occurs.
- Warn patient to drink plenty of fluids and take precautions against hyperthermia in hot weather.
- Tell patient that vision may be blurry during the first 2 to 3 wk of treatment.
- Advise patient that wearing sunglasses outdoors will help to minimize photophobia.
- Instruct patient that drug may cause drowsiness and to use caution while driving or performing other tasks requiring mental alertness.
- Advise patient to avoid intake of alcoholic beverages or other CNS depressants.
- Instruct patient to obtain periodic eye examinations during long-term treatment to monitor for glaucoma.

Bepridil

(BEH-prih-dill)

Class Calcium channel blocker

How Supplied

Vascor Tablets 200 mg, Tablets 300 mg

Action

PHARMACOLOGY: Dilates peripheral arterioles and reduces total peripheral resistance.

PHARMACOKINETICS/DYNAMICS:

Absorption: Rapidly absorbed. T_{max} is approximately 2 to 3 hr.

Distribution: Greater than 99% protein bound. Crosses placenta.

Metabolism: Metabolized in the liver.

Excretion: Over 10 days, about 70% is excreted

in urine and 22% in feces as metabolites. Elimination is biphasic with distribution t½ of about 2 hr. Elimination t½ is about 42 hr (after multiple dosing) and t½ is less than 24 hr (during dosing interval).

Special Populations:
Elderly – C_{max} is increased 3-fold and t½ increased greater than 2-fold.
Angina pectoris – Clearance is decreased and plasma concentrations are increased.

Indications Treatment of chronic stable angina in patients who fail to respond optimally to, or who are intolerant of, other antianginal agents.

Contraindications History of serious ventricular arrhythmias; sick sinus syndrome; second- or third-degree block; uncompensated cardiac insufficiency; hypotension (less than 90 mm Hg systolic); congenital QT interval prolongation; concurrent drugs that prolong the QT interval; hypersensitivity to bepridil.

Route/Dosage
ADULTS: **PO** Start with 200 mg once daily, then, after 10 days, dosage may be adjusted upward depending on the response (max, 400 mg/day).

Interactions
Antiarrhythmic agents (eg, quinidine, procainamide), cardiac glycosides, cisapride, tricyclic antidepressants (eg, thioridazine), sparfloxacin, ritonavir: May increase the risk of serious adverse effects or life-threatening cardiac arrhythmias (including torsades de pointes).

Lab Test Interferences None well documented.

Adverse Reactions
CV: Palpitations; sinus tachycardia; sinus bradycardia; hypertension; vasodilation; edema; ventricular premature contractions; ventricular tachycardia; prolonged QT interval.
CNS: Insomnia; dizziness; tremor; hand tremor; nervousness; drowsiness; fainting; vertigo; akathisia; insomnia; depression; anxiousness; adverse behavior.
DERM: Rash; sweating; skin irritation.
EENT: Tinnitus; rhinitis; pharyngitis; blurred vision; taste change.
GI: Nausea; dyspepsia; GI distress; dry mouth; anorexia; diarrhea; constipation; flatulence; gastritis; increased appetite.
GU: Loss of libido; impotence.
HEPA: Abnormal LFTs; increased ALT.
RESP: Dyspnea; cough.
OTHER: Asthenia; flu-like syndrome; fever; pain; myalgic asthenia; superinfection; arthritis.

Precautions
Pregnancy: Category C.
Lactation: Excreted in breast milk.
Children: Safety and efficacy not established.
Elderly: Select dose with caution, reflecting greater frequency of decreased hepatic, renal, or cardiac function and comorbidity.
Renal function impairment: Risk of toxicity is increased.
QT interval: The QT and QTc interval are prolonged in a dose-related fashion, which may cause serious ventricular arrhythmias (including torsades de pointes).
Hematologic: Agranulocytosis has been associated with bepridil use.
Pulmonary infiltration: Noninfective, noncardiogenic pulmonary interstitial infiltrates, including cases of pulmonary fibrosis, have been associated with bepridil use.

Overdosage: Signs and Symptoms
Hypotension, high-degree AV block, ventricular tachycardia.

PATIENT CARE CONSIDERATIONS

Administration/Storage
- Administer prescribed dose once daily, with or without food. Administer with food if GI upset occurs.
- Store tablets at controlled room temperature (59° to 77°F). Protect from light.

Assessment/Interventions
- Obtain patient history, including drug history and any known allergies. Note history of the following: allergy to bepridil, serious ventricular arrhythmias, sick sinus syndrome, second- or third-degree AV block, hypotension (less than 90 mm Hg systolic), uncompensated CHF, congenital QT interval prolongation, concomitant use of other drugs that prolong the QT interval, severe liver or kidney dysfunction.
- Ensure that serum potassium and ECGs are monitored periodically.
- Monitor patient for GI, CNS, and general body side effects. Inform health care provider if noted and significant.
- Implement safety precautions if patient experiences dizziness.

Patient/Family Education
- Explain name, dose, action, and potential side effects of drug.
- Advise patient to take once daily as prescribed, without regard to meals.
- Advise patient to take with food if GI upset occurs.
- Advise patient to try to take each dose at about the same time each day.
- Inform patient that drug helps control, but not does cure angina, and to continue taking

drug as prescribed even when angina symptoms are not present and to keep sublingual nitroglycerin available for use if needed.
- Instruct patient to continue to take other antianginal medications (eg, beta blockers and daily nitrates) as prescribed by health care provider.
- Caution patient not to change the dose or stop taking unless advised by health care provider.
- Instruct patient to immediately report fainting or loss of consciousness, palpitations, or dizziness to health care provider.
- Instruct patient to notify health care provider if angina symptoms worsen or begin to occur more frequently or if their use of sublingual nitroglycerin suddenly increases.
- Instruct patient to continue taking potassium supplements or potassium-sparing diuretics as prescribed by health care provider.
- Instruct women to notify health care provider if pregnant, planning on becoming pregnant, or breastfeeding.
- Caution patient to not take any prescription or OTC medications or dietary supplements unless advised by health care provider.
- Advise patient that follow-up visits and lab tests, including ECGs and serum potassium levels, will be required to monitor therapy and to be sure and keep appointments.

Beractant

(ber-ACT-ant)
Class Lung surfactant

How Supplied
Survanta Suspension 25 mg phospholipids per mL suspended in 0.9% sodium chloride solution. With 0.5 to 1.75 mg triglycerides, 1.4 to 3.5 mg free fatty acids, and less than 1 mg protein per mL.

Action
PHARMACOLOGY: Replaces deficient endogenous pulmonary surfactant and restores surface activity of lung.

Indications Prevention and treatment ("rescue") of neonatal respiratory distress syndrome (RDS) in premature infants.

Contraindications Standard considerations.

Route/Dosage
NEWBORNS AND INFANTS: **Intratracheal**

Prevention: 25 mg/kg/instillation for 4 instillations (total dose of 100 mg/kg is administered in 4 quarter doses); dose is started within 15 min of birth.

Rescue: 25 mg/kg/instillation for 4 instillations (total dose 100 mg/kg). May be repeated for continued or progressive RDS.

Interactions None well documented.

Lab Test Interferences None well documented.

Adverse Reactions
CNS: Intracranial hemorrhage.

Precautions Administer drug only by trained personnel in a closely supervised setting.
Nosocomial sepsis: Occurred in controlled clinical trials.

Overdosage: Signs and Symptoms
Acute airway obstruction (based on animal studies).

PATIENT CARE CONSIDERATIONS

Administration/Storage
- Warm medication by allowing it to stand at room temperature for 20 min or in hand for 8 min. Do not use artificial warming methods.
- If settling has occurred, swirl gently; do not shake.
- If preventive dose is planned, begin preparation before infant's birth.
- Before administering, assure proper placement and patency of endotracheal (ET) tube. If suctioning is required, allow patient to stabilize before administering.
- Instill through small (5 Fr) catheter inserted into ET tube with tip above carina. Do not instill into main stem bronchus. Attach catheter to syringe. Fill with medication and discard any excess through catheter to ensure that total dose to be given remains in syringe. After each quarter dose, remove catheter and mechanically ventilate patient for 30 sec. Continue procedure until total dose is achieved. Administer each quarter dose with infant in different position.
- Store unopened vials under refrigeration and protect from light.
- Warmed unopened vials (under 8 hr) can be returned to refrigerator for future use. Drug should not be warmed and refrigerated more than once. Discard any open vials.

Assessment/Interventions
- If possible, review mother's patient history.
- Take baseline vital signs and monitor during and after medication administration.
- Avoid suctioning patient for 1 hr after administration unless airway is obstructed.
- Have emergency equipment available for cardiac or respiratory complications.

- Monitor lung sounds for any changes (eg, rales or moist sounds).
- Observe for signs of nosocomial infection/sepsis.
- Continually monitor oxygen and carbon dioxide measurements. If oxygen saturation decreases or bradycardia develops, discontinue administration until patient is stabilized.

Patient/Family Education
- Advise family of infant's condition and offer frequent updates.
- Encourage active family participation in care whenever possible.
- Provide emotional support; offer hospital services and support groups.

Betamethasone

(BAY-tuh-METH-uh-zone)

Class Adrenal cortical steroid/Glucocorticoid

How Supplied
Celestone Tablets 0.6 mg, Syrup 0.6 mg/5 mL

Betamethasone Sodium Phosphate
Celestone Phosphate Injection 4 mg betamethasone sodium phosphate (equivalent to 3 mg betamethasone alcohol) per mL solution
✤ *Betnesol*

Betamethasone Sodium Phosphate and Betamethasone Acetate
Celestone Soluspan Injection 3 mg betamethasone acetate and 3 mg betamethasone sodium phosphate per mL suspension

Betamethasone Valerate
Beta-Val Cream 0.1%, Lotion 0.1% ◆ *Valisone* Ointment 0.1%, Lotion 0.1%, Cream 0.1%
✤ *Valisone Scalp Lotion* ◆ *Luxiq* Foam 1.2 mg/g
Betacort ◆ *Celestoderm-V* ◆ *Celestoderm-V/2* ◆ *Prevex B*

Betamethasone Dipropionate
Diprosone Ointment 0.05%, Cream 0.05%, Lotion 0.05%, Aerosol 0.1% ◆ *Maxivate* Ointment 0.05%, Cream 0.05% ◆ *Teladar* Cream 0.05%
✤ *Betaprolene* ◆ *Diprolene Glycol* ◆ *Taro-Sone* ◆ *Topilene* ◆ *ratio-Topilene* ◆ *ratio-Topisone*

Augmented Betamethasone Dipropionate
Diprolene Ointment 0.05%, Gel 0.05%, Lotion 0.05% ◆ *Diprolene AF* Cream 0.05%

Action

PHARMACOLOGY: Synthetic, long-acting glucocorticoid that depresses formation, release, and activity of endogenous mediators of inflammation, including prostaglandins, kinins, histamine, liposomal enzymes, and complement system. Also modifies body's immune response.

PHARMACOKINETICS/DYNAMICS:
Excretion: The t½ is at least 300 min.

Indications Systemic treatment of primary or secondary adrenal cortex insufficiency, rheumatic disorders, collagen diseases, dermatologic diseases, allergic states, allergic and inflammatory ophthalmic processes, respiratory diseases, hematologic disorders, neoplastic diseases, edematous states (resulting from nephrotic syndrome), GI diseases, multiple sclerosis, tuberculous meningitis and trichinosis with neurologic or myocardial involvement.
Topical: Relief of inflammatory and pruritic manifestations of corticosteroid-responsive dermatoses.

Contraindications Systemic fungal infections; IM use in idiopathic thrombocytopenic purpura; administration of live virus vaccines when patient is receiving immunosuppressive doses.
Topical: Do not use as monotherapy in primary bacterial infections. Do not use on face, groin, or axilla or for ophthalmic treatments.

Route/Dosage

BETAMETHASONE
PO 0.6 to 7.2 mg/day.

BETAMETHASONE SODIUM PHOSPHATE
IV/IM or into joint or soft tissue up to 9 mg/day.

BETAMETHASONE SODIUM PHOSPHATE AND BETAMETHASONE ACETATE
Intrabursal, **intra-articular**, **intradermal**, or **intralesional** 0.5 to 9 mg/day, depending on site of administration or condition being treated.

BETAMETHASONE DIPROPIONATE, BETAMETHASONE VALERATE
Topical Apply sparingly to affected areas 2 to 4 times/day.

Interactions

Anticholinesterases: May antagonize anticholinesterase effects in myasthenia gravis.
Anticoagulants, oral: May alter anticoagulant dose requirements.
Barbiturates: May decrease pharmacologic effect of betamethasone.
Hydantoins: May increase clearance and decrease therapeutic efficacy of betamethasone. Nondepolarizing muscle relaxants (eg, tubocurarine). May potentiate or counteract neuromuscular blocking action.
Rifampin: May increase clearance and decrease therapeutic efficacy of betamethasone.
Salicylates: May reduce serum levels and efficacy of salicylates.

Troleandomycin: May increase effects of betamethasone.

Lab Test Interferences Increased urine glucose and serum cholesterol; decreased serum levels of potassium, T_3, and T_4; decreased uptake of I^{131}; false-negative nitrobluetetrazolium test.

Adverse Reactions

CV: Thromboembolism or fat embolism; thrombophlebitis; necrotizing angiitis; cardiac arrhythmias or ECG changes; syncopal episodes; hypertension; myocardial rupture; CHF.
CNS: Convulsions; increased intracranial pressure with papilledema (pseudotumor cerebri); vertigo; headache; neuritis/paresthesias; psychosis; fatigue; insomnia.
DERM: Impaired wound healing; thin, fragile skin; petechiae and ecchymoses; erythema; lupus erythematosus-like lesions; suppression of skin test reactions; SC fat atrophy; purpura; striae; hirsutism; acneiform eruptions; allergic dermatitis; urticaria; angioneurotic edema; perineal irritation; hyperpigmentation; hypopigmentation. Topical application may cause burning; itching; irritation; erythema; dryness; folliculitis; hypertrichosis; pruritus; perioral dermatitis; allergic contact dermatitis; numbness of fingers; stinging and cracking/tightening of skin; maceration of skin; secondary infections; skin atrophy; striae; miliaria; telangiectasia.
EENT: Posterior subcapsular cataracts; increased IOP, glaucoma; exophthalmos.
GI: Pancreatitis; abdominal distension; ulcerative esophagitis; nausea; vomiting; increased appetite and weight gain; peptic ulcer with perforation and hemorrhage; small and large bowel perforation.
GU: Increased or decreased motility and number of spermatozoa.
HEMA: Leukocytosis.
METAB: Sodium and fluid retention; hypokalemia; hypokalemic alkalosis; metabolic alkalosis; hypocalcemia; HPA axis suppression; endocrine abnormalities (eg, menstrual irregularities; cushingoid state; growth suppression in children secondary to adrenocortical and pituitary unresponsiveness; increased sweating; decreased carbohydrate tolerance; hyperglycemia; glycosuria; increased insulin or sulfonylurea requirements in diabetics; manifestations of latent diabetes mellitus; negative nitrogen balance caused by protein catabolism; hirsutism).
OTHER: Musculoskeletal (eg, weakness; myopathy; tendon rupture; osteoporosis; aseptic necrosis of femoral and humeral heads; spontaneous fractures, including vertebral compression fractures and pathologic fracture of long bones); hypersensitivity, including anaphylactic reactions; aggravation or masking of infections; malaise. Topical use may produce same adverse reactions seen with systemic use.

Precautions

Pregnancy: Safety not established (systemic). Category C (topical).
Lactation: Excreted in breast milk.
Children: Growth and development of infants and children on prolonged therapy must be monitored, even with topical treatment.
Elderly: May require lower doses. Consider benefits relative to risks.
Hypersensitivity: Anaphylactoid reactions have occurred rarely.
Adrenal suppression: Prolonged therapy may lead to HPA suppression.
Cardiovascular: Use with caution in patients with recent MI.
Fluid and electrolyte balance: Can cause elevated BP, salt and water retention, and increased potassium and calcium excretion. Dietary salt restriction and potassium supplementation may be necessary.
Hepatitis: May be harmful in chronic active hepatitis positive for hepatitis B surface antigen.
Infections: May mask signs of infection. May decrease host-defense mechanisms.
Ocular effects: Use cautiously in ocular herpes simplex because of possible corneal perforation.
Peptic ulcer: May contribute to peptic ulceration, especially in large doses.
Stress: Increased dosage of rapidly acting corticosteroid may be needed before, during, and after stressful situations.
Sulfites: Some products contain sulfites, which may cause allergic-type reactions in susceptible individuals.
Withdrawal: Abrupt discontinuation may result in adrenal insufficiency. Use is discontinued gradually, while supplementation is increased during times of stress.

Overdosage: Signs and Symptoms

Fever, myalgia, arthralgia, malaise, anorexia, nausea, skin desquamation, orthostatic hypotension, dizziness, fainting, dyspnea, hypoglycemia (acute overdosage); cushingoid changes, moonface, central obesity, striae, hirsutism, acne, ecchymoses, hypertension, osteoporosis, myopathy, sexual dysfunction, diabetes, hyperlipidemia, peptic ulcer, infarction, electrolyte and fluid imbalance (chronic overdosage).

PATIENT CARE CONSIDERATIONS

Administration/Storage

- Administer before 9 am for minimal suppression of adrenal cortex activity.
- Give with meals or snacks.
- For large doses, administer antacids between meals.

Assessment/Interventions
- Obtain patient history, including drug history and any known allergies.
- Review baseline lab results before therapy, including liver and renal function studies.
- Monitor BP, body weight, 2-hr postprandial blood glucose (at regular intervals), and electrolytes. Note potassium and calcium levels and any radiographic findings.
- Assess for signs of infection before initiation of therapy because product may mask signs of infection and exacerbate systemic fungal infections.
- Report to health care provider any weight increase, edema, elevated BP or low potassium, GI bleeding, nausea, or vomiting.

Patient/Family Education
- Tell patient to take with meals or snacks to avoid nausea.
- Explain that medication should be taken before 9 am for best results.
- When multiple doses are to be taken, show patient how to space them evenly throughout day.
- If patient has diabetes, discuss importance of closely monitoring blood glucose for possible increase in insulin dosage.
- If patient is receiving long-term therapy, tell patient to carry identification containing notification of steroid therapy.
- Tell patient not to stop taking medication suddenly.
- Instruct patient to report the following symptoms to health care provider: unusual weight gain or weight loss; swelling of lower extremities; muscle weakness; black tarry stools; vomiting blood; puffing face; prolonged sore throat, fever, or cold; anorexia; nausea; vomiting; diarrhea; weakness; dizziness.

Topical:
- Demonstrate proper technique for cleaning affected area before applying medication and for applying sparingly as a thin film.
- Tell patient to avoid contact with eyes and to avoid tight-fitting clothing on treated area.
- Explain that alcohol-containing preparations should not be applied to area because of drying/irritation.
- Caution patient to discontinue medication and notify health care provider if affected area worsens or develops irritation, redness, burning, swelling, or stinging.

Betamethasone/Clotrimazole
(BAY-tuh-METH-uh-zone/kloe-TRIM-uh-zole)

Class Topical/Corticosteroid/Antifungal

How Supplied
Lotrisone Cream 0.05% betamethasone (as dipropionate)/1% clotrimazole

Action
PHARMACOLOGY: Clotrimazole increases cell membrane permeability in susceptible fungi. Betamethasone has anti-inflammatory, antipruritic, and vasoconstrictive actions.

Indications Topical treatment of tinea pedis, tinea cruris, and tinea corporis caused by *Trichophyton rubrum*, *T. mentagrophytes*, *Epidermophyton floccosum*, *Microsporum canis*.

Contraindications Hypersensitivity to other corticosteroids or imidazoles.

Route/Dosage
Topical 1 application bid (2 wk for tinea cruris and tinea corporis; 4 wk for tinea pedis).

PATIENT CARE CONSIDERATIONS
Administration/Storage
- Wear gloves. Apply medication sparingly and rub in lightly. Notify health care provider if signs of hypersensitivity or irritation are noted.
- Avoid contact with eyes, mouth, and nose.

Interactions None well documented.

Lab Test Interferences None well documented.

Adverse Reactions
CNS: Paresthesias.
DERM: Maculopapular rash; erythema; stinging; blistering; peeling; pruritus; urticaria; burning; itching; dryness; acne; decreased pigmentation; striae; skin atrophy.
OTHER: Edema; secondary infection; adrenal suppression with long-term use over large areas of skin.

Precautions
Pregnancy: Category C.
Lactation: Undetermined.
Children: Safety and efficacy not established.
Adrenal suppression: Patients who receive large doses over large surface areas may experience HPA axis suppression.
Ophthalmic use: Do not use for eye infections.

- Do not cover treated area with dressings or use tight-fitting diapers, plastic pants, or underwear over treated area.
- Store cream at room temperature.

Assessment/Interventions
- Obtain patient history, including drug history and any known allergies.
- Monitor treated sites for irritation or signs of secondary infection, and report any adverse reactions to health care provider.

Patient/Family Education
- Remind patient that medication is for external application only and to avoid contact with eyes, nose, and mouth.
- Demonstrate application technique, cautioning patient to apply sparingly and to rub in lightly.
- Tell patient to notify health care provider if there is no improvement after 1 wk for tinea cruris or tinea corporis or after 2 wk for tinea pedis.
- Caution patient against using dressings, tight-fitting diapers, or plastic pants over treated area.
- Tell patients with tinea corporis (ringworm) to wash clothes separately from those of other family.
- Remind patient to wash hands before and after each application of product.
- Advise patient to complete prescribed treatment, even if infection clears, to prevent relapse.
- Instruct patient to report the following symptoms to health care provider: burning, itching, rash, swelling, redness or blistering in treated area.

Betaxolol Hydrochloride

(BAY-TAX-oh-lahl HIGH-droe-KLOR-ide)

Class Beta-adrenergic blocker

How Supplied
Betoptic Solution 5.6 mg (equivalent to 5 mg base) per mL (0.5%) ♦ *Betoptic S* Suspension 2.8 mg (equivalent to 2.5 mg base) per mL (0.25%) ♦ *Kerlone* Tablets 10 mg, Tablets 20 mg

Action
PHARMACOLOGY: Blocks beta receptors, primarily affecting cardiovascular system (decreases heart rate, cardiac contractility, and BP) and lungs (promotes bronchospasm). Ophthalmic use reduces IOP, probably by reducing aqueous production.

PHARMACOKINETICS/DYNAMICS:
Absorption:
Oral – Bioavailability is about 89%, C_{max} is about 21.6% ng/mL (10 mg dose), and T_{max} is about 3 hr.

Distribution:
Oral – Approximately 50% protein bound.

Metabolism:
Oral – Metabolized in liver to inactive metabolites.

Excretion:
Oral – The $t_{½}$ is 14 to 22 hr. More than 80% is recovered in urine as betaxolol and metabolites; about 15% excreted as unchanged drug.

Onset:
Oral – 24 hr.
Ophthalmic – Within 30 min.

Peak:
Oral – 7 to 14 days.
Ophthalmic – 2 hr.

Duration:
Ophthalmic – 12 hr.

Special Populations:
Renal Function Impairment – In moderate to severe impairment, Cl is decreased significantly. In those undergoing dialysis, the $t_{½}$ and AUC are approximately doubled. Dosage adjustment required for those with severe renal impairment and those undergoing dialysis.
Hepatic Function Impairment – The $t_{½}$ may be prolonged but Cl is unchanged. Dosage adjustments not needed.
Elderly – Elimination may be decreased. Dosage adjustment required.

Indications Hypertension.
Ophthalmic preparation: Lowering IOP; ocular hypertension; chronic open-angle glaucoma.

Contraindications Hypersensitivity to beta-blockers; sinus bradycardia; greater than first-degree heart block; CHF unless secondary to tachyarrhythmia treatable with beta-blockers; overt cardiac failure; cardiogenic shock.

Route/Dosage
Hypertension
ADULTS: **PO** 10 to 20 mg/day.
ELDERLY: **PO** Reduce initial dose to 5 mg/day.

Glaucoma
ADULTS: **Ophthalmic** 1 to 2 drops bid in affected eye(s). Consider concomitant therapy if IOP is not at satisfactory level.

Interactions
Clonidine: May enhance or reverse antihypertensive effect; potentially life-threatening situations may occur, especially on withdrawal.
NSAIDs: Some agents may impair antihypertensive effect.
Prazosin: May increase postural hypotension.

Verapamil: May increase effects of both drugs.

Lab Test Interferences None well documented.

Adverse Reactions

CV: Hypotension; bradycardia; CHF; cold extremities; second- or third-degree heart block; arrhythmias; syncope.
CNS: Insomnia; fatigue; dizziness; depression; lethargy; drowsiness; forgetfulness; headache.
DERM: Rash; hives; alopecia.
EENT: Dry eyes; blurred vision; tinnitus; slurred speech; dry mouth; sore throat. Ophthalmic use may cause eye discomfort or stinging; tearing; keratitis; blepharoptosis; visual disturbances; diplopia; ptosis.
GI: Nausea; vomiting; diarrhea; constipation.
GU: Impotence; painful, difficult, or frequent urination.
HEMA: Agranulocytosis; thrombocytopenic purpura.
HEPA: Elevated LFTs.
METAB: Acidosis; diabetes; hypercholesterolemia; hyperlipidemia; increased LDH; hypokalemia.
RESP: Bronchospasm; dyspnea; wheezing.
OTHER: Weight changes; fever; facial swelling; muscle weakness. Ophthalmic betaxolol may produce the same adverse drug reactions seen with systemic use; antinuclear antibodies may develop.

Precautions

Pregnancy: Category C.
Lactation: Excreted in breast milk.
Children: Safety and efficacy not established.
Elderly: Dosage reduction may be necessary.
Renal function impairment: Use with caution.
Hepatic function impairment: Use with caution.
Anaphylaxis: Deaths have occurred with anaphylactic reactions to beta-blockers; aggressive therapy may be required.
Angle-closure glaucoma: To effectively reduce elevated IOP in angle-closure glaucoma, use with miotic agent.
Cessation of therapy: Gradually withdraw over about 2 wk. Carefully observe patients and allow minimal physical activity.
CHF: Cautiously administer in patients whose CHF is controlled by digitalis and diuretics.
Diabetes mellitus: May mask symptoms of hypoglycemia (eg, tachycardia, BP changes). May potentiate insulin-induced hypoglycemia.
Nonallergic bronchospastic disease (eg, chronic bronchitis, emphysema): In general, beta-blockers are not given to patients with bronchospastic diseases.
Peripheral vascular disease: May precipitate or aggravate symptoms of arterial insufficiency.
Systemic absorption: Ophthalmic betaxolol may produce same adverse reactions seen with systemic use because of absorption.
Thyrotoxicosis: May mask clinical signs (eg, tachycardia) of developing or continuing hyperthyroidism. Abrupt withdrawal may exacerbate symptoms of hyperthyroidism, including thyroid storm.

Overdosage: Signs and Symptoms

Bradycardia, CHF, hypotension, bronchospasm, hypoglycemia.

PATIENT CARE CONSIDERATIONS

Administration/Storage

Ophthalmic:
- For ophthalmic solution, pull out lower eyelid to make pocket, administer drop without touching eye, release lower lid, close eye, and apply gentle pressure on inner canthus to avoid systemic absorption.
- Store ophthalmic form at room temperature. Do not freeze.

Oral:
- Store oral form in cool location.

Assessment/Interventions

- Obtain patient history, including drug history and any known allergies. Note CHF, diabetes mellitus, or hyperthyroidism.
- Ensure that baseline serum lipid and glucose levels have been obtained before initiating treatment with systemic medication.
- Monitor BP and pulse frequently when starting oral medication or when dosage is changed.
- In diabetic patient, monitor blood glucose and diabetic medication closely.
- Carefully monitor patients with CHF or chronic obstructive pulmonary disease who are taking oral form of medication.

Patient/Family Education

- Explain that full effectiveness of drug may not occur for up to 1 to 2 wk after initiation of therapy and that dosage will be tapered slowly before stopping to prevent adverse effects (eg, hypotension, tachycardia, anxiety, angina, MI).
- Teach patient how to monitor pulse before taking oral medication, and advise to contact health care provider if pulse remains < 50 bpm.
- Inform diabetic patient to monitor blood glucose level closely.
- Advise patient that ophthalmic solution may cause initial burning or stinging when first instilled in eye.
- Instruct patient to inform health care provider of any scheduled surgery or dental work;

dosage may need to be gradually tapered (and ophthalmic solution discontinued) before surgery or treatment.
- Explain that measurements of IOP will need to be performed on a regular basis to assess the therapeutic effect of the ophthalmic medication.
- Instruct patient to report the following symptoms to health care provider: dizziness, decreased pulse, shortness of breath, confusion, rash, or any unusual bleeding.
- Instruct patient not to take *otc* medications (including diet aids, cold or nasal preparations [alpha-adrenergic stimulants]) without consulting health care provider.
- Advise patient that drug may cause drowsiness, and to use caution while driving or performing other tasks requiring mental alertness.

Bethanechol Chloride

(beth-AN-ih-kole KLOR-ide)

Class Urinary tract product/Cholinergic stimulant

How Supplied
Urecholine Tablets 5 mg, Tablets 10 mg, Tablets 25 mg, Tablets 50 mg, Injection 5 mg/mL ♦ *Duvoid* Tablets 10 mg, Tablets 25 mg, Tablets 50 mg ♦ *Myotonachol* Tablets 10 mg, Tablets 25 mg
♣ *PMS-Bethanechol*

Action
PHARMACOLOGY: Stimulates parasympathetic nervous system, increasing tone to muscles of urinary bladder, stimulates gastric motility and tone and may restore rhythmic peristalsis.

PHARMACOKINETICS/DYNAMICS:
Distribution: Does not cross blood-brain barrier.
Onset:
Oral – 30 min.
SC – 5 to 15 min.
Peak:
Oral – 60 to 90 min.
Duration:
Oral – 1 hr, up to 6 hr for larger doses.
SC – 2 hr.

Indications
Treatment of acute postoperative and postpartum nonobstructive urinary retention and neurogenic atony of the urinary bladder with retention. **Unlabeled use(s):** Diagnosis and treatment of reflux esophagitis.

Contraindications
Hyperthyroidism; peptic ulcer; latent or active asthma; pronounced bradycardia; AV conduction defects; vasomotor instability; coronary artery disease; epilepsy; parkinsonism; coronary occlusion; hypotension; hypertension; bladder neck obstruction; spastic GI disturbances; acute inflammatory lesions of the GI tract; peritonitis; marked vagotonia. Not used when strength or integrity of GI or bladder wall is in question or in presence of mechanical obstruction, when increased muscular activity of GI tract or urinary tract may prove harmful (eg, after recent urinary bladder surgery, GI resection and anastomosis, possible GI obstruction).

Route/Dosage
ADULTS: **PO** 10 to 50 mg tid to qid on empty stomach.
SC 2.5 to 5 mg at 15 to 30 min intervals for max of 4 doses; then minimum effective dose may be repeated tid to qid prn.

Interactions
Cholinergic agents: Possible toxicity because of additive effects.
Ganglionic blocking compounds: Severe hypotension, usually preceded by severe abdominal symptoms.
Quinidine or procainamide: Antagonism of anticholinergic effects of bethanechol.

Lab Test Interferences
None well documented.

Adverse Reactions
CV: Fall in BP with reflex tachycardia; vasomotor response.
CNS: Headache.
DERM: Flushing with feeling of warmth; sensation of heat about face; sweating.
EENT: Lacrimation; miosis.
GI: Abdominal cramps or discomfort; colicky pain; nausea; belching; diarrhea; rumbling and gurgling of stomach; salivation.
GU: Urinary urgency.
RESP: Bronchial constriction; asthmatic attacks.
OTHER: Malaise.

Precautions
Pregnancy: Category C.
Lactation: Undetermined.
Children: Safety and efficacy not established.
Tartrazine sensitivity: Some products contain tartrazine, which may cause allergic-type reactions (eg, bronchial asthma) in susceptible individuals.
Reflux infection: May occur if bethanechol administration fails to relax urinary sphincter and urine is forced back into renal pelvis.

Overdosage: Signs and Symptoms
Abdominal discomfort, salivation, flushing of skin, sweating, nausea, vomiting, low BP, shock, cardiac arrest.

PATIENT CARE CONSIDERATIONS
Administration/Storage
- Give oral form on empty stomach.
- Use only SC route for parenteral administration. Violent symptoms of cholinergic overstimulation (eg, hypotension, circulatory collapse, cardiac arrest) may occur with IM or IV administration.
- Do not administer with quinidine or procainamide.

Assessment/Interventions
- Obtain patient history, including drug history and any known allergies.
- Note any history of GI or urinary tract surgery or obstructions.
- Establish baseline BP and pulse and monitor BP, pulse, and voiding patterns. Notify health care provider if urinary retention persists.
- Report symptoms of asthma or bronchial constriction.

Patient/Family Education
- Caution patient about potential side effects such as increased salivation, sweating, flushing, or stomach discomfort.
- Instruct patient to take medication on empty stomach.
- Show patient how to monitor I&O, and to report abdominal distention or urinary retention to health care provider.
- Instruct patient to report the following symptoms to health care provider: abdominal pain or discomfort, diarrhea, visual disturbances, dizziness, any other disturbing response to medication.

Bevacizumab

(beh-vuh-SIZ-uh-mab)http://www.fda.gov/medwatch/SAFETY/2004/safety04.htm#avastin

Class Monoclonal antibody/Antineoplastic

How Supplied
Avastin IV 4 mL, IV 16 mL

Action
PHARMACOLOGY: Binds to vascular endothelial growth factor, interfering with endothelial cell proliferation.

PHARMACOKINETICS/DYNAMICS:

Absorption: Time to reach steady state is predicted to be 100 days.

Excretion: Estimated t½ is approximately 20 days.

Indications In combination with IV 5-fluorouracil (5-FU)-based chemotherapy as first-line treatment of metastatic carcinoma of the colon or rectum.

Contraindications Standard considerations.

Route/Dosage
ADULTS: **IV** Recommended dose is 5 mg/kg once q 14 days until disease progression is detected.

Interactions None well documented.

Lab Test Interferences None well documented.

Adverse Reactions
CV: Hypertension (34%); hypotension (15%); deep vein thrombosis (9%); intra-abdominal thrombosis; syncope (3%); CHF.
CNS: Headache, dizziness (26%); confusion (6%); abnormal gait (5%).
DERM: Alopecia (32%); dry skin (20%); exfoliative dermatitis (19%); skin discoloration (16%); nail disorder (8%); skin ulcer (6%).
EENT: Epistaxis (35%); taste disorder (21%); excess lacrimation (18%).
GI: Abdominal pain (61%); vomiting (52%); anorexia (43%); constipation (40%); diarrhea (34%); stomatitis (32%); GI hemorrhage, dyspepsia (24%); flatulence (19%); dry mouth (7%); colitis (6%); minor gum bleeding, GI perforation (2%); intestinal obstruction; intestinal necrosis; mesenteric venous occlusion; anastomotic ulceration.
GU: Proteinuria (36%); urinary frequency/urgency (6%); vaginal hemorrhage (4%); ureteral stricture; nephrotic syndrome.
HEMA/LYMPH: Leukopenia (37%); neutropenia (21%); thrombocytopenia (5%); pancytopenia.
METAB: Weight loss, hypokalemia (16%); bilirubinemia (6%); hyponatremia.
MUSC: Myalgia (15%).
RESP: Upper respiratory tract infection (47%); dyspnea (26%); voice alteration (9%); hemoptysis.
OTHER: Asthenia (74%); pain (62%).

> **WARNING:**
> GI perforation and wound dehiscence, in some instances fatal, may occur. GI perforation, sometimes associated with intra-abdominal abscess, may occur throughout treatment. Serious, and in some instances fatal, hemoptysis may occur in patients with non-small cell lung cancer.

Precautions
Pregnancy: Category C.
Lactation: Undetermined.

Children: Safety and efficacy not established.
Hypersensitivity: Use with caution.
CHF: Risk of developing CHF may be increased compared with administration of other chemotherapy alone.
Hypertension: May occur. Permanently discontinue bevacizumab in patients with hypertensive crisis.
Immunogenicity: As with other proteins, immunogenicity may occur.
Nephrotic syndrome: Nephrotic syndrome may occur, in which case discontinue bevacizumab.
Proteinuria: Risk of developing proteinuria may be increased compared with administration of 5-FU alone.
Surgery: Do not initiate therapy for at least 28 days following major surgery.

PATIENT CARE CONSIDERATIONS

Administration/Storage

- For IV infusion only. Not for intradermal, subcutaneous, IM, or IV push or bolus administration.
- Dose is usually administered once q 14 days.
- Dilute prescribed dose in 100 mL of 0.9% sodium chloride injection.
- Administer diluted solution immediately after reconstitution; if necessary, store for up to 8 hr under refrigeration (36° to 46°F).
- Do not administer if particulate matter or discoloration noted.
- Do not administer or mix bevacizumab with dextrose solutions.
- Administer first dose via IV infusion over 90 min following chemotherapy. If first infusion is well tolerated, the second infusion may be administered over 60 min. If the 60-min infusion is well tolerated, subsequent infusions may be administered over 30 min.
- Discard any unused solution. Do not save for future administration.
- Store glass vials in refrigerator in original carton until time of use. Protect from light and freezing. Do not shake vials.

Assessment/Interventions

- Obtain patient history, including drug history and any known allergies. Note hypertension, proteinuria, CV disease, or recent surgery or hemoptysis.
- Ensure that bevacizumab is administered in combination with an IV 5-FU-based chemotherapy regimen.
- Ensure that women of child-bearing potential are using effective contraception during treatment and for at least 3 mo following discontinuation of therapy.
- Ensure that therapy is not started until at least 28 days following major surgery and complete healing of the surgical incision has occurred.
- Monitor patient for signs and symptoms of GI perforation (eg, abdominal pain in association with constipation and/or vomiting) or wound dehiscence. Notify health care provider immediately and be prepared to treat appropriately. Ensure that bevacizumab is permanently discontinued.
- Monitor BP regularly during treatment. Inform health care provider if hypertensive readings are noted. Ensure that therapy is temporarily suspended in patient who develops severe hypertension, which is not controlled by medical management. Permanently discontinue in patient who develops hypertensive crisis.
- Ensure that patient is monitored for development or worsening of proteinuria using serial urinalyses.
- Monitor patient for signs and symptoms of anaphylactic or serious allergic reaction. Discontinue therapy and immediately notify health care provider. Be prepared to treat appropriately.
- Monitor patient for CNS, GI, RESP, and general body side effects and injection site reactions. Report to health care provider if noted and significant.

Patient/Family Education

- Explain name, action, and potential side effects of drug, and administration schedule.
- Advise family or caregiver that medication will be prepared and administered by a health care professional in a health care setting.
- Advise patient or caregiver that medication will be administered in combination with other chemotherapy medications.
- Advise family or caregiver to report any of the following to health care provider: injection site reaction; rash, itching, or hives; swelling of the face, lips, eyes, or tongue; stomach pain in association with constipation and/or vomiting; coughing up blood; wheezing, shortness of breath, or difficulty breathing; any other unusual or unexplained feelings or symptoms.
- Advise women of child-bearing potential to use effective contraception during and for at least 3 mo following treatment.
- Advise women to notify health care provider if pregnant, planning to become pregnant, or breastfeeding.

* Instruct patient not to take any prescription or OTC medications, dietary supplements, or herbal preparations unless advised by health care provider.
* Advise family or caregiver that follow-up office visits will be required to administer and monitor therapy and to keep appointments.

Bexarotene

(bex-AIR-oh-teen)
Class Retinoids

How Supplied
Targretin Gelatin capsules for oral use 75 mg

Action
PHARMACOLOGY: Bexarotene selectively binds and activates retinoid X receptor subtypes (RXRα, RXRβ, RXRY). Once activated, these receptors function as transcription factors that regulate the expression of genes that control cellular differentiation and proliferation. Inhibits the growth in vitro of some tumor cell lines of hematopoietic and squamous cell origin and induces tumor regression in vivo in some animal models.

PHARMACOKINETICS/DYNAMICS:
Absorption:
Oral – T_{max} is about 2 hr. High-fat meal increased AUC 35% and C_{max} 48%.
Topical – Plasma concentrations generally are less than 5 ng/mL and do not exceed 55 ng/mL.

Distribution: Greater than 99% protein bound.

Metabolism: CYP3A4 may be responsible for the oxidative metabolites (active).

Excretion: The t½ is about 7 hr. Less than 1% is excreted in urine. Eliminated primarily through hepatobiliary system.

Indications Refractory cutaneous T-cell lymphoma (CTCL).

Contraindications Pregnancy; hypersensitivity to bexarotene or other product components.

Route/Dosage
Refractory CTCL
ADULTS: PO
Initial dose: 300 mg/m²/day as a single daily dose. An initial dose of 150 to 225 mg also has been used.
Maintenance dose: Increase dose to 400 mg/m²/day if no tumor response after 8 wk. A target maintenance dose of 450 to 525 mg also has been used. Continue therapy as response is favorable. See manufacturer product information for specific body surface area dosing.
ADULTS: **Topical** Apply topical gel to cutaneous lesions qod initially. Increase application at weekly intervals (eg, qd, bid, tid) up to target dose of qid as tolerated. Onset of response ranges from 4 to 56 wk. Continue therapy as long as response is favorable. Consider reducing frequency or discontinuing application if severe skin irritation occurs. Resume therapy after several days.

Dosage Adjustment (Oral Therapy)
ADULTS: PO Adverse reactions requiring dosage adjustment include AST, ALT, or bilirubin greater than 3 times the ULN, leukopenia or neutropenia, or hypertriglyceridemia unresponsive to therapy. Reduce dose to 200 mg/m²/day. If reaction does not resolve, decrease to 100 mg/m²/day or temporarily discontinue. Bexarotene is metabolized extensively by hepatic cytochrome P450 3A4 isoenzymes. Dosage adjustment in hepatic insufficiency is warranted; however, there are not specific guidelines.

Interactions
Antidiabetic agents (eg, insulin sulfonylureas, insulin-sensitizers): May enhance antidiabetic agents, resulting in hypoglycemia.
Contraceptives, oral: Potentially can induce metabolic enzymes and thereby theoretically reduce plasma concentrations of hormonal contraceptives. It is strongly recommended that 2 reliable forms of contraception be used concurrently, 1 of which should be nonhormonal.
CYP450 inducers (eg, rifampin, phenytoin, phenobarbital, primidone): May reduce plasma bexarotene concentrations.
CYP450 inhibitors (eg, ketoconazole, itraconazole, erythromycin, grapefruit juice): May increase plasma bexarotene concentrations.
DEET: For topical use, the absorption of DEET increases when used concomitantly with bexarotene gel, resulting in increased toxicity of DEET.
Gemfibrozil: Resulted in substantial increases in plasma concentrations of bexarotene.
Tamoxifen: Coadministration of bexarotene capsules and tamoxifen resulted in a modest decrease in plasma tamoxifen concentrations, possibly through an induction of cytochrome P450 3A4.
Vitamin A: Bexarotene is a member of the retinoids. Limit vitamin A supplements to avoid potential additive toxic effects (up to 15,000 IU/day).

Lab Test Interferences CA125 assay values in patients with ovarian cancer may be increased by bexarotene therapy.

Adverse Reactions
CV: Peripheral edema (oral).
CNS: Headache, asthenia (oral).
DERM: Photosensitivity; rash, dry skin, exfoliative dermatitis, alopecia (oral); pruritus, pain, skin disorder (topical).

ENDO: Hypothyroidism (oral).
GI: Nausea, vomiting, diarrhea, anorexia, hyperbilirubinemia, elevated LFTs (oral).
GU: Fetal malformation; developmental abnormality; developmental mortality.
HEMA: Leukopenia, anemia (oral).
M/N: Hyperlipidemia, hypercholesteremia (oral). Infection, flu-like symptom, fever, chills (oral).

> **WARNING:**
> Contraindication in pregnancy. Teratogenicity has been reported when administered orally to pregnant rats.

Precautions

Pregnancy: Category X.
Lactation: Undetermined. Because of the potential for serious adverse reactions in nursing infants from bexarotene, decide whether to discontinue nursing or to discontinue the drug, taking into account the importance of the drug to the mother.
Children: Safety and efficacy not established.
Hepatic function impairment: There is in vitro evidence of extensive hepatic contribution to bexarotene elimination.
Fertility impairment: Caused testicular degeneration when oral doses of 1.5 mg/kg/day were given to dogs for 91 days.
Photosensitivity: Retinoids as a class have been associated with photosensitivity.
Cataracts: Posterior subcapsular cataracts were observed in preclinical toxicity studies in rats and dogs administered bexarotene daily for 6 mo.

Diabetes mellitus: Use caution when administering in patients using insulin, agents enhancing insulin secretion (eg, sulfonlyureas), or insulin-sensitizers. Bexarotene could enhance the action of these agents, resulting in hypoglycemia.
Leukopenia: A total of 18% of patients with CTCL receiving an initial dose of 300 mg/m^2/day of bexarotene had reversible leukopenia in the range of 1000 to less than 3000 WBC/mm^3.
Lipid abnormalities: Induces major lipid abnormalities in most patients that must be monitored and treated during long-term therapy. Triglyceride levels greater than 2.5 times the ULN and cholesterol elevations greater than 300 mg/dL occurred in about 60% and 75% of patients with CTCL who received an initial dose of 300 mg/m^2/day, respectively. Decreases in HDL also were seen.
LFT abnormalities: Elevations in LFTs have been observed in 5% (AST), 2% (ALT) for those patients receiving initial doses.
Pancreatitis: Acute pancreatitis has been reported in 4 patients with CTCL and in 6 patients with non-CTCL cancers treated with bexarotene.
Thyroid abnormalities: Bexarotene induces biochemical evidence of clinical hypothyroidism in about 50% of all patients treated, causing a reversible reduction in thyroid hormone (total thyroxine [total T_4]) and TSH levels.
Vitamin A supplementation: Advise patients to limit vitamin A intake to up to 15,000 IU/day to avoid potential additive toxic effects.

PATIENT CARE CONSIDERATIONS

Administration/Storage

- Store at 2° to 25°C (36° to 77°F). Avoid exposing to high temperatures and humidity after the bottle is opened. Protect from light
- In women of childbearing potential, initiate therapy on the second or third day of a normal menstrual period.
- Disease severity, location of lesions, and number of lesions are the primary factors to consider when choosing between the available dosage forms. The capsules may be preferred in patients with more systemic involvement.

Topical:

- Gently apply gel to lesions without rubbing. Spread gel in an even, generous layer. Allow gel to dry for 5 to 10 min before covering with loose clothing. Do not cover with occlusive dressings. Keep treated lesions dry for 3 hr after applying gel.
- To minimize irritation and redness of healthy skin, apply bexarotene gel only to CTCL lesions. Avoid applying gel to surrounding healthy skin.
- Wipe hands and fingers with a disposable tissue immediately after applying bexarotene gel. Wash hands thoroughly with soap and water. Although systemic absorption of bexarotene is minimal with topical use, gloves may be worn at the health care provider's discretion.
- Avoid contact with eyes, mucous membranes, and unaffected skin.
- Give with food. There are no data about administration on an empty stomach.

Assessment/Interventions

- Monitor WBC prior to initiating and during therapy.
- Bexarotene is contraindicated in pregnancy. Perform a pregnancy test 1 wk before initiating bexarotene therapy in women. In all women of childbearing age, initiate 2 methods

of contraception 1 mo before starting bexarotene therapy, during therapy, and for 1 mo after bexarotene discontinuation. Repeat pregnancy test monthly and reinforce contraceptive counseling; dispense up to a 1 mo supply to facilitate these efforts. For men with partners of childbearing potential, recommend condom use during therapy and for 1 mo after discontinuation.

Oral:

- Monitor fasting lipid panels at baseline, weekly for 2 to 4 wk, and q 8 wk during therapy. Reduce triglyceride concentrations to less than 400 mg/dL before starting bexarotene. Lipid-lowering medications, such as the statins, may be helpful; do not use gemfibrozil.
- Maintain triglyceride concentrations less than 400 mg/dL to reduce risk of pancreatitis. Avoid bexarotene use in patients with risk factors for pancreatitis, including prior pancreatitis, uncontrolled hyperlipidemia, excessive alcohol consumption, biliary tract disease, and uncontrolled diabetes mellitus.
- Monitor LFTs (eg, bilirubin, AST, ALT) at baseline and 1, 2, and 4 wk after starting bexarotene. If results are stable, monitor q 8 wk throughout treatment.
- Monitor thyroid function (eg, total thyroxine and TSH) at baseline and periodically throughout treatment. Because hypothyroidism is centrally mediated, monthly monitoring of free thyroxine may be preferred. Consider supplementation with thyroid hormones if hypothyroidism occurs.
- In patients with ovarian cancer, bexarotene may increase measured CA125 concentrations.

Topical:

- Systemic absorption of bexarotene is minimal. However, plasma bexarotene concentrations increase with the fraction of body surface area treated and with the amount of gel applied.

Patient/Family Education

- Advise women of childbearing potential to avoid becoming pregnant when taking bexarotene. Effective contraception must be used for 1 mo prior to the initiation of therapy, during therapy, and for at least 41 mo following discontinuation of therapy; it is recommended that 2 reliable forms of contraception be used simultaneously unless abstinence is the chosen method.
- Advise patients to limit vitamin A supplements to avoid potential additive effects.
- Advise patients to minimize exposure to sunlight and artificial UV light.
- Instruct patients to avoid using insect repellents that contain DEET.

Bicalutamide

(BYE-kah-LOO-tah-mide)

Class Antiandrogen/Antineoplastic hormone

How Supplied
Casodex Tablets for oral use 50 mg.

Action

PHARMACOLOGY: Bicalutamide inhibits the action of androgens.

PHARMACOKINETICS/DYNAMICS:

Absorption: Well absorbed. T_{max} is 31.3 hr (active isomer). C_{max} is 0.77 mcg/mL (active isomer).

Distribution: 96% protein bound.

Metabolism: Undergoes stereospecific metabolism. The S-isomer (inactive) is metabolized by glucuronidation. The R-isomer (active) undergoes glucuronidation but is predominantly oxidized to an inactive metabolite.

Excretion: Eliminated in urine and feces; t½ is 5.8 days (active isomer).

Special Populations:
Hepatic Function Impairment – The t½ of the R-isomer is increased about 76% in patients with severe liver disease. No dosage adjustment is necessary.

Indications Advanced prostate cancer in combination with a luteinizing hormone releasing hormone (LHRH) analog. Safety and efficacy not established.

Contraindications Standard considerations.

Route/Dosage

Advanced Prostate Cancer

ADULTS: PO 50 mg (1 tablet) once daily at the same time of day with or without food.

Interactions

Warfarin: Prothrombin time may increase when bicalutamide is initiated in patients stabilized on chronic warfarin therapy.

Lab Test Interferences Elevated AST, ALT, bilirubin, BUN, and creatinine, and decreased hemoglobin and white cell count.

Adverse Reactions

CV: Angina pectoris; CHF; hypertension.
CNS: Myasthenia; anxiety; depression; confusion; somnolence; nervousness; loss of libido; neuropathy.
DERM: Dry skin; pruritus; alopecia.
ENDO: Hot flashes; gynecomastia; breast pain; diabetes mellitus.
GI: Anorexia; dyspepsia; rectal hemorrhage; melena; increased liver function enzymes.

GU: Impotence; nocturia; hematuria; reduced sperm count.
MUSC: Arthritis; myalgia; leg cramps; hypertonia.
RESP: Increased cough; pharyngitis; bronchitis; pneumonia; rhinitis; lung disorder.

Precautions
Pregnancy: Category X.
Lactation: Bicalutamide is not indicated for use in women.
Children: Safety and efficacy not established.
Hepatic function impairment: Use bicalutamide with caution in patients with moderate to severe hepatic impairment.
Gynecomastia/Breast pain: Reported in patients treated for prostate cancer.
Hepatotoxicity: Generally occurred within the first 3 to 4 mo of treatment.
Women: Do not use in women.

PATIENT CARE CONSIDERATIONS
Administration/Storage
- Store tablets at controlled room temperature.
- Initiate therapy simultaneously with the LHRH analog. Bicalutamide may be taken without regard to meals.

Assessment/Interventions
- Measure serum transaminase levels prior to starting treatment at regular intervals for the first 4 mo of treatment, and periodically thereafter. If clinical symptoms or signs suggestive of liver dysfunction occur (eg, nausea, vomiting, abdominal pain, fatigue, anorexia, "flu-like" symptoms, dark urine, jaundice, right upper quadrant tenderness), measure the serum transaminases immediately, in particular the serum ALT. If at any time a patient has jaundice, or their ALT rises above 2 times the ULN, immediately discontinue bicalutamide, with close follow-up of liver function.
- Regular assessments of serum prostate specific antigen (PSA) may be helpful in monitoring the patient's response.
- Monitor LFTs at baseline and at 3-mo intervals during therapy.

Patient/Family Education
- Notify health care provider if any of the following symptoms occur: nausea, vomiting, abdominal pain, fatigue, anorexia, "flu-like" symptoms, dark urine, jaundice, right upper quadrant tenderness.
- Bicalutamide and the LHRH analog will be initiated at the same time. Do not interrupt or stop taking these medications without consulting health care provider.

Bimatoprost
(bye-MAT-oh-proste)
Class Ophthalmic prostaglandin agonists

How Supplied
Lumigan Solution 0.03%

Action
PHARMACOLOGY: May lower IOP by increasing outflow of aqueous humor through the trabecular meshwork and uveoscleral routes.

Indications
Reduction of IOP in patients with open-angle glaucoma or ocular hypertension who are intolerant of other IOP-lowering agents or insufficiently responsive to other IOP-lowering medications.

Contraindications
Standard considerations.

Route/Dosage
ADULTS: **Ophthalmic** Instill 1 drop in affected eye(s) in evening.

Interactions
None well documented.

Lab Test Interferences
None well documented.

Adverse Reactions
CNS: Headache.
DERM: Hirsutism.
EENT: Conjunctival hyperemia; eyelash growth; ocular pruritus; ocular dryness; visual disturbances; ocular burning; foreign body sensation; eye pain; pigmentation of the periocular skin; blepharitis; cataract; superficial punctate dermatitis; eyelid erythema; ocular irritation; eyelash darkening; eye discharge; tearing; photophobia; allergic conjunctivitis; asthenopia; increase in iris pigmentation; conjunctival edema.
HEPA: Abnormal LFTs.
RESP: Upper respiratory infections.
OTHER: Cold; asthenia.

Precautions
Pregnancy: Category C.
Lactation: Undetermined.
Children: Safety and efficacy not established.
Active intraocular inflammation: Use with caution in patients with iritis/uveitis.
Bacterial keratitis: Bacterial keratitis has been reported with multiple-dose containers as a result of patient contamination.
Contact lenses: Remove contact lenses prior to and do not wear for 15 min following administration.
Macular edema: Use with caution in aphakic patients, pseudophakic patients with a risk of torn posterior lens capsule, or in patients with risk factors for macular edema.

Pigmentation changes: Permanent changes to pigmented tissue may occur, most frequently involving pigmentation of the iris and eyelid and increased pigmentation and growth of eyelashes. Gradual change in eye color (ie, increased amount of brown pigmentation in the iris) may occur.

PATIENT CARE CONSIDERATIONS
Administration/Storage
- If using other topical ophthalmic drugs, separate each medication by at least 5 min.
- Store at controlled room temperature. Keep container tightly closed.

Assessment/Interventions
- Obtain patient history, including drug history and any known allergies.
- Ensure that IOP has been measured and documented in the patient's record.

Patient/Family Education
- Explain name, dose, action, and potential side effects of drug.
- Warn patient not to instill more often than once a day in the evening. More frequent use may decrease efficacy of the medication.
- Teach patient proper technique for instilling eye drops. Wash hands; do not allow dropper to touch eye. Tilt head back, look up; pull lower eyelid down; instill drop. Close eye for 1 to 2 min and apply gentle pressure to bridge of nose. Do not rub eye.
- Advise patients who wear contact lenses to remove lenses before instilling medicine and to wait at least 15 min after instilling eye drop before inserting their lenses.
- Advise patient that if more than 1 topical ophthalmic drug is used, administer the drugs at least 5 min apart.
- Inform patient that medication may cause a gradual increase in brown pigment in the pupil, which may slowly change eye color.
- Inform patient that medication may cause eyelid skin darkening and increases in length, thickness, color, and number of eyelashes.
- Advise patient to contact the eye doctor if eye or eyelid inflammation is noted, or if eye is injured, or if eye surgery is planned.
- Remind patient that eye examinations and measurement of IOP are necessary while using this medication; advise patient to keep appointments.

Biperiden

(by-PURR-ih-den)

Class Antiparkinson/Anticholinergic

How Supplied
Akineton Tablets 2 mg (as hydrochloride), Injection 5 mg/mL (as lactate)

Action
PHARMACOLOGY: Biperiden is a weak peripheral anticholinergic agent and possesses nicotinolytic activity.

PHARMACOKINETICS/DYNAMICS:
Absorption: 29% bioavailable; C_{max} is 4 to 5 mcg/L; T_{max} is 1 to 1.5 hr.
Excretion: The t½ is 18.4 to 24.3 hr.

Indications Treatment of all forms of parkinsonism; control of extrapyramidal disorders secondary to neuroleptic drug therapy.

Contraindications Narrow angle glaucoma; bowel obstruction; megacolon.

Route/Dosage
Parkinsonism
ADULTS: PO 2 mg tid to qid to max 16 mg/day. Dosage must be individualized.

Drug-Induced Extrapyramidal Disorders
ADULTS: PO 2 mg qd to tid. IM/IV 2 mg repeated q 30 min until symptoms resolve, but not more than 4 consecutive doses (or 8 mg) per day.

Interactions
Amantadine: May increase anticholinergic side effects.
Digoxin: May increase digoxin serum levels, especially with slow-dissolution oral digoxin tablets.
Haloperidol: May worsen schizophrenic symptoms; may decrease haloperidol serum levels; tardive dyskinesia may develop. May decrease action of phenothiazines. May increase incidence of anticholinergic side effects.

Lab Test Interferences None well documented.

Adverse Reactions
CV: Mild transient orthostatic hypotension; bradycardia; tachycardia.
EENT: Blurred vision; narrow-angle glaucoma; pupillary dilation.
CNS: Drowsiness; euphoria; disorientation; agitation; memory loss; disturbed behavior.
DERM: Skin rash.
GI: Dry mouth; constipation; GI irritation.
GU: Urinary retention.
OTHER: Hyperthermia; heat stroke.

Precautions
Pregnancy: Category C.
Lactation: Undetermined.
Children: Safety and efficacy not established.
Elderly: Patients over 60 yr may have increased side effects; dosage reduction and observation may be needed.
Special risk patients: Use with caution in patients with glaucoma, prostatic hypertrophy, epilepsy, cardiac arrhythmias, hypertension, hypotension, tendency toward urinary retention, liver or kidney disorders, obstructive disease of GI or GU tract, tachycardia or those who are taking other drugs with anticholinergic activity.
Heat illness: Fatal hyperthermia has occurred. Use with caution during hot weather.

PATIENT CARE CONSIDERATIONS
Administration/Storage
- When given PO, administer with or after meals to prevent GI irritation.
- If patient has difficulty swallowing, tablet may be crushed.
- May be given IM or IV in acute dystonic reactions. When given IV, have patient remain recumbent during administration and for 15 min afterward.
- Store in dry place in tightly closed light-resistant container.

Assessment/Interventions
- Obtain patient history, including drug history and any known allergies. Note glaucoma, urinary retention, prostatic hypertrophy, or constipation.
- Monitor vital signs and I&O routinely for anticholinergic side effects (hypotension and urinary retention).
- Monitor patient for reduction of rigidity and decrease in tremors during therapy.
- Monitor frequency and consistency of bowel movement. Patient may need stool softeners or laxatives.

Patient/Family Education
- Explain that doses will be tapered gradually before stopping to avoid withdrawal reaction.
- Advise patient that increasing fluid intake will help decrease dry mouth and constipation.

Ophthalmic: Narrow-angle glaucoma may occur.

Overdosage: Signs and Symptoms
Characterized by adverse reactions. Also: Circulatory collapse, cardiac arrest, respiratory depression or arrest, CNS depression preceded or followed by stimulation, intensification of mental symptoms or toxic psychosis in mentally ill patients treated with neuroleptic drugs (eg, phenothiazines), shock, coma, stupor, seizures, convulsions, ataxia, anxiety, incoherence, hyperactivity, combativeness, anhidrosis, hyperpyrexia, fever, hot/dry/flushed skin, dry mucous membranes, dysphagia, foul-smelling breath, decreased bowel sounds, dilated and sluggish pupils.

- Instruct patient to pay particular attention to dental hygiene because of problems associated with decreased salivation (eg, increased risk of caries).
- Tell patient that stool softeners may be used if constipation occurs. Small doses of milk of magnesia may be helpful.
- Warn patient to drink plenty of fluids and take precautions against hyperthermia in hot weather.
- Instruct patient to obtain periodic eye exams during long-term treatment to monitor for glaucoma.
- Advise patient that wearing sunglasses outdoors will help to minimize photophobia.
- Tell patient that vision may be blurry during first 2 to 3 wk of treatment.
- Instruct patient to take sips of water frequently, suck on ice chips or sugarless hard candy or chew sugarless gum if dry mouth occurs.
- Caution patient to avoid sudden position changes to prevent orthostatic hypotension.
- Instruct patient to avoid intake of alcoholic beverages or other CNS depressants.
- Advise patient that drug may cause drowsiness, and to use caution while driving or performing other tasks requiring mental alertness.

Bisacodyl

(BISS-uh-koe-dill)

Class Laxative

How Supplied
Dulcolax Tablets, enteric-coated 5 mg, Suppositories 10 mg ♦ *Fleet Laxative* Tablets, enteric-coated 5 mg, Suppositories 10 mg ♦ *Modane* Tablets, enteric-coated 5 mg ♦ *Women's Gentle Laxative* Tablets, enteric-coated 5 mg ♦ *Bisac-Evac* Tablets, enteric-coated 5 mg, Suppositories 10 mg ♦ *Caroid* Tablets, enteric-coated 5 mg ♦ *Correctol* Tablets, enteric-coated 5 mg ♦ *Feen-a-mint* Tablets, enteric-coated 5 mg ♦ *Reliable Gentle Laxative* Tablets, enteric-coated and delayed-release 5 mg, Suppositories 10 mg ♦ *Bisacodyl Uniserts* Suppositories 10 mg
🍁 *APO-Bisacodyl* ♦ *ratio-Bisacodyl*

Action
PHARMACOLOGY: Acts as cathartic stimulant.
PHARMACOKINETICS/DYNAMICS:
Onset:
Tablets – 6 to 10 hr.
Suppositories – 15 to 60 min.

Indications Short-term treatment of constipation; evacuation of colon for rectal and bowel evaluations; preparation for delivery or surgery.

Contraindications Nausea, vomiting, or other symptoms of appendicitis; acute surgical abdomen; fecal impaction; intestinal obstruction; undiagnosed abdominal pain; ulcerative lesions of colon; rectal fissures; ulcerative hemorrhoids.

Route/Dosage
Oral
ADULTS: **PO** 10 to 15 mg.
PREPARATION OF LOWER GI TRACT: Up to 30 mg.
CHILDREN OVER 6 YR: **PO** 5 to 10 mg (0.3 mg/kg).

Suppository
ADULTS: **PR** 10 mg.
CHILDREN OVER 2 YR: **PR** 10 mg.
CHILDREN UNDER 2 YR: **PR** 5 mg.

Interactions
Milk or antacids: May cause enteric coating of tablets to dissolve, resulting in gastric lining irritation or gastric indigestion.

Lab Test Interferences None well documented.

Adverse Reactions
CV: Palpitations.
CNS: Dizziness, fainting.
GI: Excessive bowel activity (griping, diarrhea, nausea, vomiting); perianal irritation; bloating; flatulence; abdominal cramping; proctitis and inflammation.
OTHER: Sweating, weakness. Suppositories may cause proctitis and inflammation with long-term use.

Precautions
Pregnancy: Category B.
Lactation: Undetermined.
Children: Tablet form not recommended for children under 6 yr.
Drug dependency: Long-term use may lead to laxative dependency. Long-term abuse results in cathartic colon (poorly functioning colon).
Rectal bleeding or failure to produce bowel movement: May indicate serious condition that may require further medical attention.

PATIENT CARE CONSIDERATIONS
Administration/Storage
- Administer tablet at bedtime or before breakfast.
- Do not administer within 1 hr of patient ingesting antacids, milk, or cimetidine.
- Have patient take tablets whole with full glass of water. Tablets should not be crushed or chewed.
- Insert suppository at time bowel movement is desired or 1 to 2 hr before scheduled procedure. Onset of action is 6 to 10 hr for tablets and 15 to 60 min for suppositories.
- Moisten suppository with lukewarm water, insert high into rectum and instruct patient to retain suppository in rectum for as long as possible until urge to defecate is felt.
- Store tablets and suppositories in tightly closed containers in cool location.

Assessment/Interventions
- Obtain patient history, including drug history and any known allergies.
- Assess living and dietary habits, including bulk or fiber intake, exercise, fluid intake, and use of laxatives.
- Assess for presence of bowel sounds and usual pattern of bowel function.
- Assess for abdominal distention, excessive bowel activity, abdominal cramping, weakness, fluid and electrolyte imbalance, and perianal irritation.
- Monitor color, consistency, and amount of stool produced.
- Notify health care provider of unrelieved constipation, rectal bleeding, and signs and symptoms of electrolyte imbalance (eg, muscle cramps or pain, weakness, dizziness).

Patient/Family Education
- Inform patient not to take bisacodyl when constipation is accompanied by abdominal pain, fever, nausea or vomiting.
- Advise patient to use laxative only for short-term therapy; do not use > 1 wk.
- Caution patient that prolonged, frequent, or excessive use of drug may result in dependence and/or electrolyte imbalance.
- Encourage patient to incorporate high-fiber foods in diet, increase fluid intake ($\geq$ 6 to 8 glasses daily) and increase or maintain exercise level.
- Instruct patient to report the following symptoms to health care provider: unrelieved constipation, rectal bleeding, muscle cramps, pain, weakness, dizziness.

Bismuth Subsalicylate

(BISS-muth sub-suh-LIS-ih-late)

Class Antidiarrheal

How Supplied
Bismatrol Tablets, chewable 262 mg ♦ *Bismatrol Extra Strength* Liquid 524 mg/15 mL ♦ *Pepto-Bismol Maximum Strength* Liquid 524 mg/15 mL ♦ *Pepto-Bismol* Liquid 262 mg/15 mL, Tablets, chewable 262 mg, Caplets 262 mg ♦ *Pink Bismuth* Liquid 130 mg/15 mL, Liquid 262 mg/15 mL
✤ Pink Bismuth

Action
PHARMACOLOGY: Produces antisecretory and antimicrobial effects; may have anti-inflammatory effect.

PHARMACOKINETICS/DYNAMICS:
Absorption: In the GI tract, bismuth subsalicylate undergoes chemical dissociation to yield bismuth and salicylate. Bismuth absorption is negligible, and plasma levels of the salicylate are similar to levels achieved after a comparable dose of aspirin.
Metabolism: Chemical dissociation in the GI tract.
Excretion: Greater than 90% of salicylate is recovered in urine.

Indications
Treatment of indigestion without causing constipation, nausea, abdominal cramps; control of diarrhea, including traveler's diarrhea.
Unlabeled use(s): Treatment of recurrent ulcers, chronic infantile diarrhea, gastroenteritis associated with Norwalk virus; prevention of traveler's diarrhea.

Contraindications
Viral illness such as chickenpox or influenza in patients under 18 yr.

Route/Dosage
ADULTS: **PO** 2 tablets (262 mg each) or 30 mL suspension q 30 to 60 min prn (max, 8 doses/day).
CHILDREN 9 TO 12 YR: **PO** 1 tablet or 15 mL suspension q 30 to 60 min prn (max, 8 doses/day).
CHILDREN 6 TO 9 YR: **PO** ⅔ tablet or 10 mL suspension q 30 to 60 min prn (max, 8 doses/day).
CHILDREN 3 TO 6 YR: **PO** ⅓ tablet or 5 mL suspension q 30 to 60 min prn (max, 8 doses/day).
CHILDREN UNDER 3 YR: Consult health care provider.

Interactions
Aspirin or other salicylates: May cause salicylate toxicity.
Corticosteroids: May decrease effectiveness.
Insulin: Drug may increase glucose-lowering effect of insulin.
Methotrexate: Drug may increase effects and toxicity of methotrexate.
Spironolactone: Drug may interfere with diuretic effect.
Sulfinpyrazone: Drug may interfere with uricosuric effect.
Tetracyclines: Bismuth subsalicylate may reduce GI absorption of tetracyclines and diminish their effectiveness.
Valproic acid: Drug may increase free fraction of valproic acid, leading to toxicity.

Lab Test Interferences
Radiologic examination: Bismuth subsalicylate is radiopaque and may interfere with radiologic examination of GI tract.

Adverse Reactions
EENT: Tinnitus; discoloration of tongue.
GI: Discoloration of stools; impaction.

Precautions
Pregnancy: Category C.
Lactation: Excreted in breast milk.
Children: May cause impaction.
Debilitated patients: May cause impaction.

Overdosage: Signs and Symptoms
Ringing in ears, respiratory alkalosis, nausea, vomiting, hypokalemia, neurologic abnormalities (eg, disorientation, seizures), dehydration, hyperthermia, unusual bleeding or bruising.

PATIENT CARE CONSIDERATIONS

Administration/Storage
- Tablets may be crushed, chewed, or allowed to dissolve in mouth. Do not allow patient to swallow whole.
- Before administering, shake suspension well.
- Store at room temperature.
- Protect from light.

Assessment/Interventions
- Obtain patient history, including drug history and any known allergies.
- Assess patient for risk of Reye syndrome.
- Determine if patient is taking OTC medications for colds, fever, and pain; many contain salicylates, which may produce additive toxicity.
- Observe for discoloration of stool produced by drug (may mask GI bleeding).
- Discontinue use when symptoms subside.

Patient/Family Education
- Counsel patient to maintain adequate fluid intake (2 to 3 L/day) to prevent dehydration.
- Instruct patient to notify health care provider if diarrhea is accompanied by high fever or continues > 2 days or if abdominal pain occurs.
- Advise patient not to use medication if concurrent viral illness is present.
- Instruct patient to consult health care provider before taking drug if concurrently taking other salicylates, anticoagulants or medications for diabetes or gout.
- Instruct patient to inform health care provider regarding bismuth subsalicylate administration before any scheduled radiologic studies or stool examinations.
- Inform patient of possibility of salicylate toxicity and associated symptoms, and instruct patient to notify health care provider if these symptoms occur.
- Explain that stools may become black or gray and tongue may darken.

Bismuth Subsalicylate/Metronidazole/Tetracycline

(BISS-muth/meh-troe-NIH-dah-zole/teh-trah-SIGH-kleen)

Class H. pylori agents

How Supplied
Helidac Carton containing blister cards that, in total, contain: 112 bismuth subsalicylate chewable tablets, 262.4 mg; 56 metronidazole tablets, 250 mg; 56 tetracycline hydrochloride capsules, 500 mg

Action
PHARMACOLOGY: Each of the ingredients is individually active in vitro against most strains of H. pylori. The relative contribution of systemic versus local antimicrobial activity for H. pylori eradication is not established.

Indications Eradication of H. pylori for treatment of patients with H. pylori infection and duodenal ulcer disease. Used in combination with an H_2 antagonist.

Contraindications Pregnant or nursing women; children; renal or hepatic impairment; hypersensitivity to aspirin, salicylates, bismuth subsalicylate, metronidazole or other nitroimidazole derivatives, or any of the tetracyclines.

Route/Dosage
ADULTS: **PO** 2 bismuth subsalicylate tablets (chewed), 1 metronidazole tablet, and 1 tetracycline capsule taken together every 4 hr at meals and at bedtime with 8 oz of water.

Interactions
Alcohol: Avoid during metronidazole use and for at least 24 hr after.
Aluminum, calcium, and magnesium containing antacids: May decrease absorption of tetracycline.
Anticoagulants: Possible increased anticoagulant effect and risk of bleeding.
Antidiabetic agents: Possible increased antidiabetic effect.
Bactericidal antibiotics: Tetracycline may reduce effectiveness.
Cimetidine: May reduce clearance of metronidazole.
Contraceptives, Oral: Tetracycline may reduce effectiveness.
Dairy products: May decrease absorption of tetracycline.
Disulfiram: Metronidazole has been reported to cause psychosis.
Iron, Zinc, or Sodium Bicarbonate: May decrease absorption of tetracycline.
Lithium: Metronidazole may increase lithium blood levels.
Methoxyflurane: Tetracycline has caused fatal renal toxicity.
Phenobarbital: May increase elimination of metronidazole.
Phenytoin: May increase elimination of metronidazole. May reduce elimination of tetracycline.

Lab Test Interferences
X-ray procedures: Bismuth absorbs x-rays and may interfere with GI diagnostic procedures.
Metronidazole: May interfere with AST, ALT, LDH, TG, and nevu Kinase glucose

Adverse Reactions
CNS: Asthenia; anal discomfort; dizziness; headache; insomnia; pain; paresthesia.
GI: Abdominal pain; nausea; anorexia; constipation; diarrhea; discolored tongue; duodenal ulcer; dyspepsia; flatulence; GI hemorrhage; melena; metallic taste; stool abnormality; taste perversion, vomiting.
RESP: Sinusitis; upper respiratory infection.

Precautions
Pregnancy: Category D. Contraindicated during pregnancy.
Lactation: Secreted into breast milk.
Children: Safety and effectiveness not established. Contraindicated in children.
Elderly: May have pre-existing liver or renal disease. Use with caution.
Renal function impairment: Tetracycline may lead to azotemia, hyperphosphatemia, and acidosis.

Special risk patients:
Ultraviolet exposure – Tetracycline may increase susceptibility to sunburn.

CNS disease – Increased risk of seizures and peripheral neuropathy. Increased susceptibility to yeast infections.

Bisoprolol Fumarate/Hydrochlorothiazide

(bih-SO-pro-lahl FEW-mah-rate/high-droe-klor-oh-THIGH-uh-zide)

Class Antihypertensive

How Supplied
Ziac Tablets 6.25 mg hydrochlorothiazide/2.5 mg bisoprolol fumarate, Tablets 6.25 mg hydrochlorothiazide/5 mg bisoprolol fumarate, Tablets 6.25 mg hydrochlorothiazide/10 mg bisoprolol fumarate

Action
PHARMACOLOGY: Blocks beta receptors, primarily affecting cardiovascular system and lungs (bisoprolol); inhibits reabsorption of sodium and chloride in ascending loop of Henle and early distal tubules (hydrochlorothiazide).

Indications Management of hypertension.

Contraindications Cardiogenic shock; overt cardiac failure; second or third degree AV block; marked sinus bradycardia; anuria; hypersensitivity to either component of product or other sulfonamide derivatives.

Route/Dosage
ADULTS: **PO** Start with 2.5 mg bisoprolol/6.25 mg hydrochlorothiazide daily, increasing the dose in 14-day intervals until optimal response is obtained (max recommended dose 20 mg bisoprolol/12.5 mg hydrochlorothiazide).

Interactions
Bisoprolol:
Antiarrhythmic agents (eg, disopyramide), diphenylalkylamine calcium antagonists (eg, verapamil), benzothiazepine calcium antagonists (eg, diltiazem) – Use with caution.
Antihypertensives – Actions of other antihypertensive agents may be potentiated.
Beta-blockers – Do not combine with other beta-blockers.
Catecholamine-depleting agents (eg, guanethidine, reserpine) – Sympathetic action may be considerably reduced.
Clonidine – If discontinuing clonidine after coadministration with bisoprolol/hydrochlorothiazide, discontinue bisoprolol/hydrochlorothiazide several days before withdrawal of clonidine.
Hydrochlorothiazide:
Alcohol, barbiturates, narcotics – Increased risk of orthostatic hypotension.
Antidiabetic agents – Dose adjustments in antidiabetic agent may be needed.
Antihypertensives – Actions of other antihypertensive agents may be potentiated.
Cholestyramine, colestipol resins – Absorption of hydrochlorothiazide may be impaired.
Adrenocorticotropic hormone, corticosteroids – Increased risk of electrolyte depletion (eg, hypokalemia).
Pressor amines (eg, norepinephrine) – Decreased response to pressor amine.
Nondepolarizing skeletal muscle relaxants (eg, tubocurarine) – Responsiveness to muscle relaxant may be increased.
Lithium – Plasma levels of lithium may be elevated, increasing the risk of toxicity.
NSAIDs – The antihypertensive, diuretic, and natriuretic effect of hydrochlorothiazide may be reduced.

Lab Test Interferences Serum levels of protein-bound iodine may be decreased without signs of thyroid dysfunction.

Adverse Reactions
CV: Bradycardia; arrhythmia; peripheral ischemia; chest pain; palpitations and rhythm disturbances; cold extremities, claudication, hypotension; orthostatic hypotension, chest pain, CHF (bisoprolol); orthostatic hypotension (hydrochlorothiazide).
CNS: Fatigue; dizziness; headache; insomnia; somnolence; loss of libido; impotence; unsteadiness, vertigo, syncope, paresthesia, hyperesthesia, sleep disturbances, vivid dreams, depression, anxiety, restlessness, decreased concentration, catatonia, hallucinations, time and place disorientation, emotional lability, clouded sensorium (bisoprolol); vertigo, paresthesia, restlessness (hydrochlorothiazide).
DERM: Cutaneous vasculitis; rash, acne, eczema, psoriasis, skin irritation, pruritus, purpura, flushing, sweating, alopecia, dermatitis (bisoprolol); photosensitivity (hydrochlorothiazide).
GI: Diarrhea; constipation; nausea; dyspepsia; gastric, epigastric, and abdominal pain, peptic ulcer, gastritis, vomiting, dry mouth, taste abnormalities, mesenteric arterial thrombosis, ischemic colitis (bisoprolol); anorexia, gastric irritation, cramping, pancreatitis, sialadenitis, dry mouth (hydrochlorothiazide).
GU: Cystitis, renal colic, polyuria (bisoprolol); sexual dysfunction, renal failure, renal dysfunction, interstitial nephritis (hydrochlorothiazide).
HEMA: Agranulocytosis, thrombocytopenia; leukopenia, aplastic anemia, hemolytic anemia

(hydrochlorothiazide).
HEPA: Jaundice, cholecystitis (hydrochlorothiazide).
EENT: Rhinitis; pharyngitis, sinusitis, visual disturbances, ocular pain and pressure, abnormal lacrimation, tinnitus, decreased hearing, earache (bisoprolol); transient blurred vision, xanthopsia (hydrochlorothiazide).
METAB: Gout; increased serum triglycerides; small decrease in HDL cholesterol; weight gain (bisoprolol); hyperglycemia, glucosuria, edema, hyperuricemia, hypokalemia, hyperlipidemia, hypercalcemia (hydrochlorothiazide).
RESP: Bronchospasm; cough; upper respiratory infection; asthma, bronchitis, dyspnea (bisoprolol).
OTHER: Asthenia; peripheral edema; muscle cramps; myalgia; arthralgia, muscle and joint pain, back and neck pain, twitching, tremor, malaise, allergy (fever, aching, sore throat, laryngospasm, respiratory distress) (bisoprolol); weakness, muscle spasm, hypersensitivity (purpura, photosensitivity, rash, urticaria, necrotizing angitis [vasculitis and cutaneous vasculitis], fever, respiratory distress [including pneumonitis and pulmonary edema], anaphylactic reaction) (hydrochlorothiazide).

Precautions
Pregnancy: Category C.
Lactation:
Bisoprolol – Undetermined.
Hydrochlorothiazide – Excreted in breast milk.
Children: Safety and efficacy not established.
Renal function impairment: Dosage adjustment or discontinuation may be necessary; azotemia may be precipitated.
Hepatic function impairment: Use with caution.
Cardiac failure: Use with caution if therapy cannot be avoided.
Abrupt cessation of therapy: Exacerbations of angina pectoris and MI or ventricular arrhythmias may occur in patients with coronary artery disease following abrupt cessation of therapy.
Peripheral vascular disease: Precipitation or exacerbation of symptoms of arterial insufficiency in patients with peripheral vascular disease may occur.
Bronchospastic disease: Use with caution if therapy cannot be avoided.
Diabetes and hypoglycemia: May mask symptoms of hypoglycemia.
Thyrotoxicosis: May mask clinical signs of hyperthyroidism (eg, tachycardia).

Overdosage: Signs and Symptoms
Bradycardia, hypotension, lethargy, delirium, coma, convulsions, respiratory arrest, CHF, bronchospasm, hypoglycemia, acute loss of fluid and electrolytes (eg, hypokalemia, hyponatremia, hypochloremia), tachycardia, shock, weakness, confusion, dizziness, calf cramps, paresthesia, fatigue, impaired consciousness, nausea, vomiting, thirst, polyuria, oliguria, anuria, alkalosis, increased BUN.

PATIENT CARE CONSIDERATIONS

Administration/Storage
* Give once daily in the morning with or without food.
* Administer alone or in combination with other antihypertensives.
* Store tablets at controlled room temperature. Keep container tightly closed.

Assessment/Interventions
* Obtain patient history, including drug history and any known allergies. Note history of diabetes, lung disease, anuria, CHF, AV block, sinus bradycardia, renal or liver dysfunction, or gout.
* Ensure that serum electrolytes are monitored periodically.
* Monitor and record BP and apical pulse before each dose. If systolic BP is less than 90 mm Hg or pulse is less than 60 bpm, withhold drug and notify health care provider.
* Take safety precautions if orthostatic hypotension occurs.
* Monitor blood sugar in diabetic patient when drug is started or dose is changed. Report significant changes to health care provider.
* Withhold drug and notify health care provider if the following symptoms occur: hypotension, bradycardia, difficulty breathing, edema of hands or feet.

Patient/Family Education
* Explain name, dose, action, and potential side effects of drug.
* Advise patient to take medication every day as prescribed, without regard to meals.
* Advise patient to try to take each dose at the same time each day.
* Inform patient that drug controls, but does not cure, hypertension and to continue taking drug as prescribed even when BP is not elevated.
* Caution patient not to change the dose or stop taking unless advised to do so by health care provider.
* Instruct patient to not interrupt therapy or discontinue drug abruptly.
* Instruct patient to continue taking other BP medications as prescribed by health care provider.
* Instruct patient in blood pressure and pulse measurement skills.
* Advise patient to monitor and record BP and

- pulse at home. Patient should inform health care provider if abnormal measurements are noted. Also advise patient to take record of BP and pulse to each follow-up visit.
- Instruct patient to lie or sit down if experiencing dizziness or lightheadedness when standing.
- Caution patient that inadequate fluid intake, excessive perspiration, diarrhea, or vomiting can lead to excessive fall in BP, resulting in lightheadedness or fainting.
- Instruct diabetic patient to monitor blood glucose more frequently when drug is started or dose is changed. Patient should inform health care provider of significant changes in readings.
- Caution patient to avoid unnecessary exposure to UV light (sunlight, tanning booths) and to use sunscreen and wear protective clothing when exposed to UV light to avoid photosensitivity reaction.
- Advise patient that impotence or decreased libido are possible side effects and to notify health provider if either occur.
- Emphasize to hypertensive patient importance of other modalities on BP (eg, weight control, regular exercise, smoking cessation, moderate intake of alcohol and salt).
- Instruct patient to notify health care provider if becoming pregnant, planning on becoming pregnant, or breastfeeding.
- Instruct patient to report any of these symptoms to health care provider: difficulty breathing, slow heart rate, or swelling of ankles or feet.
- Advise patient that drug may cause drowsiness or dizziness and to use caution while driving or performing other tasks requiring mental alertness until tolerance is determined.
- Caution patient to not take any prescription or *otc* medications or dietary supplements unless advised by health care provider.
- Advise patient that follow-up visits and lab tests may be required and to keep appointments.

Bitolterol Mesylate

(by-TOLE-ter-ole MEH-sih-LATE)

Class Bronchodilator/Sympathomimetic

How Supplied
Tornalate Aerosol 0.8% (delivers 0.37 mg/actuation), Solution for inhalation 0.2%

Action
PHARMACOLOGY: Relaxes bronchial smooth muscle through beta-2 receptor stimulation.

PHARMACOKINETICS/DYNAMICS:
Metabolism: Bitolterol, a prodrug, is hydrolyzed by esterases in tissues and blood to active moiety colterol.
Excretion: Primarily excreted in the urine as metabolites.
Onset: 2 to 3 min.
Duration: At least 6 hr.

Indications Prevention and treatment of reversible bronchospasm associated with asthma or other obstructive pulmonary diseases.

Contraindications Standard considerations.

Route/Dosage
Acute Bronchospasm
ADULTS AND CHILDREN OVER 12 YR: **Oral inhalation** 2 inhalations at interval of 1 to 3 min, followed by third inhalation if necessary.

Prevention of Bronchospasm
ADULTS AND CHILDREN OVER 12 YR: **Oral inhalation** 2 inhalations q 8 hr, not to exceed 3 inhalations q 6 hr or 2 inhalations q 4 hr.

SOLUTION FOR INHALATION
Administer during a 10- to 15-min period.
Continuous flow nebulization – 1.5 to 3.5 mg (0.75 to 1.75 mL volume) 3 to 4 times/day with an interval of at least 4 hr between treatments. Max daily dose, 14 mg.
Intermittent flow nebulization – 0.5 to 1.5 mg (0.25 to 0.75 mL volume) 3 to 4 times/day with an interval of at least 4 hr between treatments. Max daily dose, 8 mg.

Interactions None well documented.

Lab Test Interferences May cause decreased potassium level.

Adverse Reactions
CV: Palpitations; tachycardia; irregular pulse; hypertension; angina.
CNS: Tremor; lightheadedness; dizziness; nervousness; headache; tiredness.
EENT: Throat and mouth irritation.
GI: Nausea; vomiting.
RESP: Cough; increased chest discomfort; dyspnea; bronchospasm.

Precautions
Pregnancy: Category C.
Lactation: Undetermined.
Children: Safety and efficacy in children under 12 yr not established.
Elderly: Lower doses may be required.
Labor and delivery: May inhibit uterine contractions and delay preterm labor.
Cardiovascular disorders: Toxic symptoms may occur.
CNS effects: Drug may cause CNS stimulation;

use cautiously in patients with history of seizures or hyperthyroidism.
Diabetes mellitus: Dosage adjustment of insulin or oral hypoglycemic agent may be required.
Excessive use: Paradoxical bronchospasm and cardiac arrest have been associated with excessive inhalant use.
Tolerance: May occur.
Combined therapy: Do not use 2 or more beta-adrenergic aerosol bronchodilators simultaneously because of the potential of additive effects. Do not use as a substitute for oral or inhaled corticosteroids.

Overdosage: Signs and Symptoms
Exaggerated side effects, such as tremors, tachycardia, seizures, hypokalemia, anginal pain, and hypertension.

PATIENT CARE CONSIDERATIONS
Administration/Storage
- To administer, instruct patient to tilt head back and put inhaler mouthpiece between lips or 2 inches from open mouth. Tell patient to inhale slowly, press down on canister, hold breath at least 10 sec or as long as comfortable, remove mouthpiece, then exhale slowly.
- Use spacing device (eg, *Aero-changer*) to enhance drug delivery.
- Administer pressurized inhalation during second half of inspiration to achieve better distribution of medication because airways are opened wider at this time. If second inhalation is necessary, wait at least 1 full min between inhalations.
- Store metered-dose inhaler in pressurized container at room temperature; do not freeze. Keep away from extreme heat. Do not store or use near open flame or discard in incinerator.
- For nebulizer use, find a location where patient can sit comfortably for 10 to 15 min. Do not mix different types of medications without permission from doctor or pharmacist. Have patient take slow, deep breaths and, if possible, hold breath 10 sec before slowly exhaling. Continue until medication chamber is empty.

Assessment/Interventions
- Obtain patient history, including drug history and any known allergies.
- Review baseline ECG for cardiac dysrhythmias associated with tachycardia.
- Take heart rate before administration of drug. If tachycardia, cardiac arrhythmia, or chest pain is present, hold medication and notify health care provider immediately.
- Have epinephrine 1:1000 available for immediate or delayed hypersensitivity reaction.
- Obtain baseline blood values and monitor during therapy. Notify health care provider of abnormal results.

Patient/Family Education
- Ask patient to demonstrate correct use of inhaler. It may be necessary to repeat instructions and demonstrations more than once. Consider use of spacing device.
- Explain that tolerance may occur with prolonged use, but temporary cessation of drug usually restores its original effectiveness. Instruct patient to notify health care provider if medication is ineffective.
- Warn patient to avoid excessive use, which can lead to side effects or loss of effectiveness.
- Instruct patient to rinse mouth with water or commercial mouthwash after use to remove residue and reduce irritation.
- Tell patient to store inhaler at room temperature, away from excessive heat or cold.
- Warn patient receiving concurrent corticosteroid therapy not to stop or reduce medication without consulting health care provider, even if patient feels better.
- Instruct patient to wash inhaler daily with warm water and to dry thoroughly.
- Caution patient to avoid getting aerosol spray in eyes.
- Instruct patient to report the following symptoms to health care provider: palpitations, chest pain, muscle tremors, dizziness, increased nervousness, headache, flushing, breathing problems, difficult urination.
- Instruct patient not to take *otc* medications without consulting health care provider.

Bivalirudin
(bye-VAL-ih-ruh-din)
Class Anticoagulants
How Supplied
Angiomax Powder for injection, lyophilized 250 mg

Action
PHARMACOLOGY: Inhibits thrombin by reversibly binding to the catalytic site and the anion-binding exosite of circulating and clot-bound thrombin. Inhibits clot-bound and free circulating thrombin, reducing the amount of active thrombin present for clot formation and extension.

PHARMACOKINETICS/DYNAMICS:

Absorption: Steady-state concentration is about 12.3 mcg/mL.

Distribution: Not bound to plasma proteins (other than thrombin).

Excretion: Cleared from plasma by renal mechanisms and proteolytic cleavage, elimination related to glomerular filtration rate. The $t_{½}$ is 25 min. Cl is 3.4 mL/min/kg.

Duration: Coagulation times return to baseline about 1 hr following end of administration.

Special Populations:
Renal Function Impairment – Cl is reduced about 20% in moderate to severe renal impairment and about 80% in dialysis-dependent patients.

Indications Anticoagulant in combination with aspirin in patients with unstable angina undergoing percutaneous transluminal coronary angioplasty (PTCA).

Contraindications Active major bleeding.

Route/Dosage

ADULTS: **IV** Bolus of 1 mg/kg followed by a 4-hr IV infusion at a rate of 2.5 mg/kg/hr. After the 4-hr infusion, an additional IV infusion of 0.2 mg/kg/hr for up to 20 hr may be given if needed. Bivalirudin is intended for concurrent use with aspirin (300 to 325 mg/day). Initiate treatment prior to PTCA.

Interactions

Heparin, thrombolytics, warfarin: The risk of major bleeding may be increased.

INCOMPATIBILITIES: Do not mix with other medications.

Lab Test Interferences None well documented.

Adverse Reactions

CV: Hypotension (12%); hypertension (6%); bradycardia (5%); major intracranial bleeding, syncope, vascular anomaly, ventricular fibrillation (less than 1%).
CNS: Headache (12%); insomnia (7%); anxiety (6%); nervousness (5%); cerebral ischemia, confusion, facial paralysis (less than 1%).
GI: Nausea (15%); vomiting (6%); abdominal pain, dyspepsia (5%).
GU: Urinary retention (4%); kidney failure, oliguria (less than 1%).
HEMA: Major hemorrhage (4%); sepsis (less than 1%).
PULM: Lung edema (less than 1%).
OTHER: Back pain (42%); pain (15%); injections site pain (8%); pelvic pain (6%); fever (5%); major retroperitoneal hemorrhage, infections (less than 1%).

Precautions

Pregnancy: Category B.
Lactation: Undetermined.
Children: Safety and efficacy not established.

PATIENT CARE CONSIDERATIONS

Administration/Storage

- For IV administration only. Not for intradermal, IM, or SC administration.
- Reconstitute vial with 5 mL sterile water for injection. Gently swirl until powder is dissolved.
- For initial infusion, each reconstituted vial should be further diluted in 50 mL of 5% dextrose in water or 0.9% sodium chloride for injection.
- For second or low-rate infusion, each reconstituted vial should be further diluted in 500 mL of 5% dextrose in water or 0.9% sodium chloride for injection.
- Administer bolus dose first and then adjust infusion rate to provide infusion over 4 hr using Dosing Table supplied with medication.
- A second (low-dose) infusion for up to 20 hr may follow the first infusion using Dosing Table suppled with medication.
- Do not mix with other IV medications.
- Do not administer if particulate matter or discoloration is noted.
- Store unopened vials at controlled room temperature (59° to 86°F). Reconstituted solution may be stored for up to 24 hr in refrigerator (36° to 46°F). Diluted solution may be stored for up to 24 hr at controlled room temperature (59° to 86°F). Protect reconstituted solutions from freezing.

Assessment/Interventions

- Obtain patient history, including drug history and any known allergies. Note active bleeding or concurrent use of anticoagulants, thrombolytics, or antiplatelet agents.
- Ensure that patient is also receiving aspirin therapy.
- Ensure that medication is administered just prior to PTCA.
- Avoid IM injections of other medications. Venipuncture sites may require pressure to prevent bleeding and hematoma formation.
- Monitor patient for signs of bleeding throughout therapy. If bleeding develops (epistaxis, hematuria, hematemesis, bloody or black, tarry stools) or is suspected (unexplained fall in hematocrit or BP), notify health care provider immediately.
- Monitor patient for unusual bleeding or bruising, especially at vascular access sites, and report to health care provider if noted.
- Monitor patient for CV, GI, and general body

side effects. Inform health care provider if noted and significant.

Patient/Family Education
* Explain name, action, and potential side effects of drug.
* Advise patient that medication will be prepared and administered by health care provider before PTCA is attempted and for several hr after the procedure.
* Instruct patient to inform health care provider if noting any of the following during the administration of drug: bleeding, back pain, pain, nausea, headache, pain at the injection site.

Bleomycin Sulfate

(BLEE-oh-MY-sin SULL-fate)

Class Antitumor antibiotic

How Supplied
Blenoxane Sterile powder for Injection 15 unit vial (15 units = 15 mg), Sterile powder for Injection 30 unit vial (30 units = 30 mg)

Action
PHARMACOLOGY: Bleomycin sulfate is a mixture of cytotoxic glycopeptide antibiotics. It inhibits DNA synthesis. When administered intrapleurally, bleomycin acts as a sclerosing agent.

PHARMACOKINETICS/DYNAMICS:
Distribution: High concentrations are found in the skin and lungs; low concentrations are found in bone marrow.

Excretion: The t½ is about 115 min; 60% to 70% is excreted in urine as active bleomycin.

Special Populations:
Renal Function Impairment – In those with Ccr less than 35 mL/min, the t½ increases.

Indications Lymphomas (Hodgkin and non-Hodgkin); testicular carcinoma (eg, embryonal cell, choriocarcinoma, teratocarcinoma); sclerosis of malignant pleural effusions (eg, treatment, prevention); treatment of squamous cell carcinomas (eg, head, neck). **Unlabeled use(s):** Mycosis fungoides, osteosarcoma, AIDS-related Kaposi sarcoma.

Contraindications Standard considerations.

Route/Dosage
Test Dose
ADULTS: **IV** , **IM** , or **subcutaneous** Because of the possibility of anaphylactoid reaction, treat lymphoma patents with 2 units or less for the first 2 doses. If no acute reaction occurs, follow the regular dosage schedule.

Hodgkin Disease
ADULTS: **IV** , **IM** , **subcutaneous** 10 to 20 units/m² 1 or 2 times/wk. After a 50% regression of tumor size, a maintenance dose of 1 unit/day or 5 units/wk can be given IV or IM. Response is usually seen within 2 wk. To minimize the risk of pulmonary toxicity, the max cumulative dose should not exceed 400 units. When bleomycin is used in combination with other antineoplastic agents, pulmonary toxicities may occur at lower doses.

Pleural Effusions
ADULTS: **Thoracostomy tube** 60 units diluted with 50 to 100 mL 0.9% sodium chloride is instilled into chest via a thoracotomy tube following drainage of excess pleural fluid and confirmation of complete lung expansion. The amount of drainage from the chest tube should be as minimal as possible prior to installation of bleomycin. The thoracotomy tube is then clamped. The patient is moved from the supine to the left and right lateral positions several times during the next 4 hr. The clamp is then removed and suction re-established. It is generally accepted that chest tube drainage should be below 100 mL in a 24-hr period prior to sclerosis. However, bleomycin instillation may be appropriate when drainage is between 100 and 300 mL under clinical conditions that necessitate sclerosis therapy.

Squamous Cell Carcinoma, non-Hodgkin Lymphoma, Testicular Carcinoma
ADULTS: **IV** , **IM** , **subcutaneous** 10 to 20 units/m² 1 or 2 times/wk. Response is usually seen within 3 wk. Squamous cell cancers respond more slowly, sometimes requiring 3 wk for improvement and testicular tumors is noticed within 2 weeks.

Interactions
Digoxin and phenytoin: Bleomycin may decrease serum concentrations of digoxin and phenytoin.

Lab Test Interferences None well documented.

Adverse Reactions
CV: Hypotension; cerebral arteritis, cerebrovascular accidents, MI, thrombotic microangiopathy, Raynaud phenomenon (with combination chemotherapy).
CNS: Malaise (postmarketing).
DERM: Alopecia, erythema, hyperkeratosis, hyperpigmentaion, nail changes, pruritus, rash, skin tenderness, stomatitis, striae, vesiculation (approximately 50%); scleroderma-like skin changes (postmarketing).
GI: Vomiting; anorexia.
LOCAL: Pain; pain at tumor site; phlebitis.
M/N: Weight loss (common).
PULM: Pneumonitis, pulmonary fibrosis, dyspnea, rales.

OTHER: Idiosyncratic reaction including chills, fever, hypotension, mental confusion, and wheezing (about 1% of lymphoma patients); chills; fever; acute chest pain.

> **WARNING:**
> Pneumonitis; life-threatening pulmonary fibrosis. Pulmonary toxicities occur in 10% of treated patients. In about 1%, the drug-induced nonspecific pneumonitis progresses to pulmonary fibrosis and death. Risk factors include the following: increased age, radiation to the lungs, oxygen therapy during or after bleomycin, recent cisplatin therapy, declining renal function. Toxicity may occur at cumulative doses more than 400 mg when risk factors are present, and it has occurred in young patients.
>
> The earliest symptom associated with bleomycin pulmonary toxicity is dyspnea. The earliest sign is rales.
>
> *Idiosyncratic reaction:* A severe idiosyncratic reaction consisting of hypotension, mental confusion, fever, chills, and wheezing has occurred in about 1% of lymphoma patients. These reactions may be immediate or delayed for several hours and usually occur after the first or second dose; careful monitoring is essential. Treatment is symptomatic including volume expansion, pressor agents, and antihistamines.

Precautions

Pregnancy: Category D.
Lactation: Undetermined. It is recommended that breastfeeding be discontinued by women receiving therapy.
Children: Safety and efficacy not established.
Elderly: Pulmonary toxicity was more common in patients older than 70 years of age.
Renal function impairment: Patients with a Ccr of less than 35 mL/min should receive a reduced dose of bleomycin. Guidelines for dosage reduction are empiric. Renal toxicity has occurred infrequently. This toxicity may occur at any time.
Hepatic function impairment: Hepatic toxicity has occurred infrequently. This toxicity may occur at any time.
Death: Death has been rarely reported in association with bleomycin pleurodesis in very seriously ill patients.
Extravasation: Local irritation or phlebitis may occur. Refer to your institution specific protocol.
Skin toxicity: Skin toxicity, a relatively late manifestation, appears to be related to the cumulative dose. It usually develops in the second and third week of treatment after administration of 150 to 200 units of the drug.

PATIENT CARE CONSIDERATIONS

Administration/Storage

- May be used alone or in combination with other chemotherapeutic agents.
- For subcutaneous, IM, IV, or intrapleural administration only. Not for intradermal, intra-arterial, or oral administration.
- Diligently follow institutional and NIH procedures for handling, administration, and disposal of anticancer drugs. Wear appropriate protective equipment when preparing and administering bleomycin. Avoid exposure by direct contact of the skin, mucous membranes, and eyes.
- If accidental skin or mucus membrane contact occurs, wash thoroughly with soap and water. If accidental eye contact occurs, immediately institute standard irrigation techniques.
- Do not reconstitute or dilute bleomycin with 5% dextrose in water or any other dextrose-containing diluent. Loss of bleomycin potency will occur.
- For subcutaneous or IM administration, reconstitute powder for injection with sterile water for injection, 0.9% sodium chloride for injection, or bacteriostatic water for injection. Reconstitute 15 unit vial with 1 to 5 mL of diluent; reconstitute 30 unit vial with 2 to 10 mL of diluent.
- For IV administration, reconstitute powder for injection with 0.9% sodium chloride for injection. Reconstitute 15 unit vial with 5 mL of diluent; reconstitute 30 unit vial with 10 mL of diluent. Infuse prescribed dose slowly over 10 min.
- For intrapleural administration, dissolve 60 units of bleomycin in 50 to 100 mL 0.9% sodium chloride for Injection. Clamp thoracostomy tube after instilling bleomycin. Move patient from supine to left and right lateral positions several times over next 4 hr, then remove clamp and reestablish suction.
- Do not administer if particulate matter or cloudiness is noted.
- Store powder for injection in refrigerator (36° to 46°F). Bleomycin is stable for 24 hr at

room temperature when reconstituted with 0.9% sodium chloride Injection. Discard any unused solution. Do not save any unused solution for future use.

Assessment/Interventions

- Obtain patient history, including drug history and any known allergies. Note renal impairment, compromised pulmonary function, or impending surgical intervention.
- Ensure women of childbearing potential are not pregnant before starting therapy and use effective contraception during treatment.
- Document total cumulative dose. Because of the risk of pulmonary toxicity, ensure that dosing beyond 400 units is only attempted after careful evaluation of the patient and clinical situation.
- Because of the risk of anaphylactoid-like reactions (ie, hypotension, mental confusion, fever, chills, and wheezing) in lymphoma patient, ensure that lymphoma patient receives no more than 2 units of bleomycin for the first 2 doses. Frequently monitor patient during and after therapy. Be prepared to treat reactions symptomatically. Regular dosing schedule can be followed if no acute reactions occur after either dose.
- Monitor renal function before starting therapy and periodically thereafter during treatment in elderly patient or patient with impaired renal function. Ensure that bleomycin therapy is reevaluated if evidence of deterioration in renal function noted.
- Ensure chest x-rays are obtained and evaluated every 1 to 2 wk during therapy to monitor for onset of pulmonary toxicity. If changes are noted ensure that therapy is discontinued until it is determined if changes are drug related.
- Ensure diffusion capacity for carbon monoxide (DLco) is determined before starting therapy and then monthly during treatment. Ensure that therapy is discontinued if DLco falls below 30% to 35% of pretreatment value.
- Monitor patient for signs of allergic reaction. Discontinue therapy and immediately notify health care provider if noted. Be prepared to treat appropriately.
- Monitor patient for RESP, GI, DERM, and general body side effects, and injection site reactions. Report to health care provider if noted and significant. Immediately report dyspnea or rales to health care provider.
- If patient is to undergo surgical intervention, ensure that surgical team (including anesthesiologist) is aware of treatment with bleomycin and that $FI\ O_2$ should be maintained, if possible, at concentrations no greater than 25%. Fluid replacement should consist of colloids rather than crystalloids to reduce the risk of lung damage.

Patient/Family Education

- Explain name, action, and potential side effects of the treatment regimen. Review the treatment regimen including dosing schedule, duration of treatment, and monitoring that will be required.
- Advise patient, family, or caregiver that medication will be prepared and administered by health care professionals in a health care setting.
- Advise patient, family, or caregiver that medication may be used in combination with other agents to achieve max benefit possible.
- Advise patient, family, or caregiver that medication may cause hair loss but that this is reversible when therapy is stopped.
- Advise patient, family, or caregiver to immediately report any of the following to health care provider: rash; hives; difficulty breathing or unexplained shortness of breath; chest pain; fever, chills, or other signs of infection; sores in mouth; pain, redness, or swelling at injection site.
- Advise patient, family, or caregiver to report any of the following to health care provider: persistent nausea, vomiting, or appetite loss; persistent or worsening general body weakness; skin changes; nail changes.
- Instruct patient not to take any prescription or OTC medications, herbal preparations, or dietary supplements unless advised by health care provider.
- Caution women of childbearing potential to avoid becoming pregnant during therapy.
- Advise women to notify health care provider if pregnant, planning to become pregnant, or breastfeeding.
- Advise patient that frequent follow-up visits, laboratory tests, x-rays, and breathing tests will be required to monitor therapy, and to keep appointments.

Bortezomib

(bore-TEZZ-oh-mib)

Class Proteasome inhibitor

How Supplied
Velcade Powder for Injection, lyophilized 3.5 mg

Action
PHARMACOLOGY: Inhibits 26S proteasome, disrupting normal homeostatic mechanisms and leading to cell death.

PHARMACOKINETICS/DYNAMICS:
Absorption: C_{max} 509 ng/mL following IV administration of 1.3 mg/m^2.
Distribution: 83% bound to plasma protein.
Metabolism: In vitro studies indicate metabolism is primarily oxidative via CYP 1A2, 2C9, 2C19, 2D6, and 3A4.
Excretion: Elimination t½ 9 to 15 hr at doses ranging from 1.45 to 2 mg/m^2.

Indications Treatment of multiple myeloma in patients who received at least 2 prior therapies and demonstrated disease progression on the last therapy.

Contraindications Hypersensitivity to boron, mannitol, or any component of the product.

Route/Dosage
ADULTS: IV 1.3 mg/m^2/dose administered as a bolus twice/wk for 2 wk (days 1, 4, 8, and 11) followed by a 10-day rest period (days 12 to 21), which constitutes a 3-wk treatment cycle. At least 72 hr should elapse between consecutive doses.

Reinstitution of Therapy
ADULTS: IV Withhold therapy at the onset of any Grade 3 nonhematological or Grade 4 hematological toxicities, excluding neuropathy discussed in the dose modification section (see below). Once symptoms of toxicity have resolved, reinitiate therapy at a 25% dose reduction (eg, 1.3 mg/m^2/dose reduced to 1 mg/m^2/dose).

Dose Modification
ADULTS: IV There is no dose modification for Grade 1 peripheral neuropathy (paresthesias and/or loss of reflexes) without pain or loss of function. For Grade 1 peripheral neuropathy with pain or Grade 2 (interfering with function but not with activities of daily living), reduce dose to 1 mg/m^2. For Grade 2 peripheral neuropathy with pain or Grade 3 (interfering with activities of daily living), withhold therapy until toxicity resolves, then reinitiate therapy with a reduced dose of 0.7 mg/m^2 and change treatment schedule to once weekly. Discontinue therapy for Grade 4 (permanent sensory loss that interferes with function).

Interactions
Oral hypoglycemic agents (eg, glipizide): Because hypoglycemia and hyperglycemia are reported, adjustment of antidiabetic dosages may be necessary.

Lab Test Interferences None well documented.

Adverse Reactions
CV: Hypotension (12%); aggravated atrial fibrillation; atrial flutter; cardiac amyloidosis; cardiac arrest; congestive cardiac failure; myocardial ischemia; MI; pericardial effusion; pulmonary edema; ventricular tachycardia; cerebrovascular accident; deep venous thrombosis; peripheral embolism.
CNS: Headache (28%); insomnia (27%); dizziness (21%); anxiety (14%); ataxia; coma; dizziness; dysarthria; dysautanomia; cranial palsy; grand mal convulsion; hemorrhagic stroke; motor dysfunction; spinal cord compression; transient ischemic attack; agitation; confusion; psychotic disorder; suicidal ideation.
65% – Fatigue; malaise; weakness.
DERM: Rash (21%); pruritus (11%).
EENT: Blurred vision (11%).
GI: Nausea (64%); diarrhea (51%); decreased appetite/anorexia, constipation (43%); vomiting (36%); dyspepsia, abdominal pain, dysgeusia (13%); ascites; dysphagia; fecal impaction; hemorrhagic gastritis; GI hemorrhage; hematemesis; paralytic ileus; large intestinal obstruction; paralytic intestinal obstruction; small intestinal obstruction; large intestinal perforation; stomatitis; melena; acute pancreatitis.
GU: Renal calculus; bilateral hydronephrosis; bladder spasm; hematuria; urinary incontinence; urinary retention; acute and chronic renal failure; proliferative glomerular nephritis.
HEMA: Thrombocytopenia (43%); anemia (32%); neutropenia (24%).
HEPA: Hyperbilirubinemia; portal vein thrombosis.
METAB: Dehydration (18%); hypocalcemia; hyperuricemia; hypokalemia; hyponatremia; tumor lysis syndrome.
RESP: Dyspnea (22%); upper respiratory tract infection (18%); cough (17%); pneumonia (10%); acute respiratory distress syndrome; atelectasis; exacerbated chronic obstructive airways disease; exertional dyspnea; epistaxis; hemoptysis; hypoxia; lung infiltration; pleural effusion; pneumonitis; respiratory distress; respiratory failure; pulmonary embolism.
OTHER: Asthenic conditions (65%); peripheral neuropathy (including peripheral sensory neuropathy and peripheral neuropathy [37%]); pyrexia (36%); edema (25%); paresthesia and dysesthesia (23%); dyspnea (22%); rigors (12%); herpes zoster (11%); anaphylactic reaction; drug

hypersensitivity; immune complex mediated hypersensitivity; bacteremia; skeletal fracture; subdural hematoma; disseminated intra-vascular coagulation.
26% – Arthralgia; pain in limb.
14% – Bone pain; myalgia; back pain; muscle cramps.

Precautions
Pregnancy: Category D.
Lactation: Undetermined.
Children: Safety and efficacy not established.
Hepatic function impairment: Use with caution.
GI: Nausea, diarrhea, constipation, and vomiting, sometimes requiring use of antiemetics and antidiarrheals may occur.
Hypotension: Because orthostatic/postural hypotension can occur, use with caution in treating patients with a history of syncope, patients receiving medications known to be associated with hypotension, and patients who are dehydrated.
Peripheral neuropathy: Peripheral neuropathy that is predominantly sensory may occur, although mixed sensori-motor neuropathy also has been reported.
Thrombocytopenia: May occur throughout therapy but is most common in cycles 1 and 2.

PATIENT CARE CONSIDERATIONS
Administration/Storage
* For IV administration only. Do not administer intradermal, IM, or SC.
* Administer prescribed dose by IV bolus twice/wk for 2 wk (days 1, 4, 8, and 11) followed by a 10-day rest period (days 12 to 21).
* Separate consecutive doses of medication by at least 72 hr.
* Follow manufacturer's instructions for reconstituting powder. Use caution during handling and preparation. Use gloves and other protective clothing to prevent skin contact.
* Inspect solution visually before administration. Do not administer if solution is cloudy, discolored, or contains particulate matter.
* Discard any unused product. Vials are for single-use only. Do not save medication for future use.
* Store unopened vials at controlled room temperature (59° to 86°F) in original package to protect from light. Reconstituted solution may be stored at controlled room temperature for up to 8 hr. Reconstituted solution may be stored for up to 3 hr in syringe prior to administration, however the total storage time for reconstituted solution must not exceed 8 hr when exposed to indoor lighting.

Assessment/Interventions
* Obtain patient history, including drug history and any known allergies. Note hepatic or renal impairment, dehydration, symptoms/signs of existing peripheral neuropathy, coadministration of medications known to cause hypotension or peripheral neuropathy, or history of syncope.
* Ensure that CBC including platelet count is frequently monitored throughout treatment.
* Ensure that women of childbearing potential are using effective contraception during therapy.
* Monitor patient for symptoms of peripheral neuropathy (eg, burning sensation, hyperesthesia, paresthesia, discomfort, neuropathic pain). Notify health care provider if detected and be prepared to change the dose and dosing schedule of bortezomib according to manufacturer's recommendations.
* Monitor BP, especially in patients concurrently receiving medications known to lower BP. Be prepared to adjust dose of antihypertensive medication(s) if hypotension occurs.
* Frequently monitor blood sugar in diabetic patient. Report significant changes to health care provider.
* Assess patient for injection site reactions, GI, CNS, CV, and general body side effects. Inform health care provider if noted and significant. Be prepared to administer antiemetics if vomiting is significant or antidiarrheals if diarrhea is significant.

Patient/Family Education
* Explain name, action, dosing regimen, and potential side effects of drug.
* Ensure that patient, family, or caregiver understands that medication is administered in "treatment cycles."
* Advise patient, family, or caregiver that medication will be prepared and administered by a health care provider in a health care setting.
* Advise patient that drug may cause fatigue, dizziness, fainting, and/or vision changes, and to use caution while driving or performing other tasks requiring mental alertness until tolerance is determined.
* Advise women to notify health care provider if pregnant, planning to become pregnant, or breastfeeding.
* Instruct breastfeeding women to discontinue breastfeeding while undergoing treatment.
* Advise patient to notify health care provider if any of the following occur: dizziness, lightheadedness, fainting, abnormal skin sensations, nerve pain, persistent vomiting or diarrhea, fever or other symptoms of infection.

- Instruct diabetic patient to monitor blood glucose more frequently during therapy and to inform health care provider of significant changes in readings.
- Instruct patient not to take any prescription or OTC medications or dietary supplements unless advised by health care provider.
- Advise patient, family, or caregiver that follow-up visits and lab tests will be required to monitor response to therapy, and to keep appointments.

Bosentan

(boe-SEN-tan)

Class Vasodilator/Endothelin receptor antagonist

How Supplied
Tracleer Tablets 62.5 mg, Tablets 125 mg

Action
PHARMACOLOGY: Antagonizes endothelin (ET) receptor by binding to ET_A and ET_B receptors in the endothelium and vascular smooth muscle.

PHARMACOKINETICS/DYNAMICS:
Absorption: T_{max} is 3 to 5 hr.

Distribution: Vd is about 18 L. Bosentan is more than 98% protein bound (mainly albumin).

Metabolism:
Liver – There are 3 metabolites, one of which contributes 10% to 20% of bosentan's effects. Bosentan induces CYP2C9, CYP3A4, and possibly CYP2C19; it may induce its own metabolism.

Excretion: The t½ is about 5 hr. Bosentan is eliminated by biliary excretion; less than 3% is recovered in urine. Cl is 8 L/hr.

Special Populations:
Renal Function Impairment – In those with severe renal impairment (Ccr 15 to 30 mL/min), concentrations of the 3 metabolites may increase 2-fold, although not clinically significant.

Hepatic Function Impairment – Exposure to bosentan would be significantly increased; avoid use in those with moderate or severe liver impairment or elevated aminotransferases more than 3 times the ULN.

Severe chronic heart failure – Exposure to bosentan may be increased 30% to 40%. Similar effects are expected in those with pulmonary arterial hypertension.

Indications
Treatment of pulmonary arterial hypertension in patients with WHO Class III and IV symptoms, to improve exercise ability and decrease the rate of clinical worsening.

Contraindications
Pregnancy; coadministration of cyclosporine or glyburide; hypersensitivity to bosentan or any component of the product.

Route/Dosage
ADULTS AND CHILDREN OVER 12 YR:
Initial dose: **PO** 62.5 mg bid for 4 wk; then increase to maintenance dose of 125 mg bid. If bosentan therapy is reintroduced, it should be at the starting dose.

PATIENTS UNDER 40 KG BUT OVER 12 YR:
Initial and maintenance dose: **PO** 62.5 mg bid. If bosentan therapy is reintroduced, it should be at the starting dose.

Interactions
Cyclosporine: Bosentan trough concentrations may be increased, while cyclosporine plasma levels may be decreased; coadministration is contraindicated.

Glyburide: Plasma concentrations of both glyburide and bosentan may be decreased; coadministration is contraindicated.

Ketoconazole: Plasma concentrations of bosentan may be increased.

Hormonal contraceptives (ie, oral, injectable, implantable), HMG-CoA reductase inhibitors (eg, simvastatin), warfarin: Plasma concentrations of these agents may be decreased.

Lab Test Interferences
None well documented.

Adverse Reactions
CV: Hypertension; palpitations; edema.
CNS: Headache; fatigue.
DERM: Pruritus.
EENT: Nasopharyngitis.
GI: Dyspepsia.
HEPA: Abnormal hepatic function.
OTHER: Flushing.

> **WARNING:**
>
> *Hepatotoxicity:* At least 3–fold increase in ALT or AST occurs in approximately 11% of patients and requires close monitoring.
>
> *Teratogenicity:* Use is contraindicated in pregnancy.

Precautions
Pregnancy: Category X. Pregnancy must be excluded before starting bosentan.
Lactation: Undetermined.
Children: Safety and efficacy not established.
Elderly: Select dose with caution, reflecting greater frequency of decreased hepatic, renal, or cardiac function and comorbidity.

Hepatic function impairment: In general, because monitoring liver injury may be more difficult in patients with hepatic impairment, avoid bosentan in patients with elevated aminotransferases (greater than 3 times the ULN). *Hepatotoxicity:* At least a 3-fold elevation of liver ALT and AST may occur in 11% of patients, which may indicate serious liver injury. *Hematologic:* Dose-related decreases in hemoglobin and hematocrit may occur.

Overdosage: Signs and Symptoms
Headache, nausea, vomiting, decreased blood pressure, increased heart rate.

PATIENT CARE CONSIDERATIONS

Administration/Storage
- This medication is available only through the *Tracleer* Access Program.
- Give prescribed dose bid, in the morning and evening, with or without food.
- Starting dose is 62.5 mg bid for 4 wk and then increased to 125 mg bid for maintenance.
- If bosentan is stopped and then restarted, restart with the lower starting dose and monitor liver enzymes after 3 days.
- Do not administer to pregnant women as major birth defects can occur.
- Administer reduced dose or interrupt treatment (per dosing guidelines) in patients with elevated liver enzymes.
- Administer reduced dose to patient with body weight less 40 kg but who are over 12 yr.
- If drug is to be discontinued, reduce dose to 62.5 mg bid for 3 to 7 days if possible.
- Store tablets at controlled room temperature (59° to 86°F).

Assessment/Interventions
- Obtain patient history, including drug history and any known allergies. Note history of liver disease.
- Ensure that liver enzymes are measured before starting therapy and monthly during treatment. Notify health care provider if any elevations are noted.
- Ensure that pregnancy has been excluded before starting bosentan in a woman of childbearing potential. Ensure that reliable contraceptive measures are being used during treatment. If patient is using hormonal contraception (eg, oral, injectable, implantable), ensure that another nonhormonal contraceptive is used. Ensure that monthly pregnancy tests are obtained after starting therapy.
- Ensure that hemoglobin is measured after 1 and 3 mo of therapy and then q 3 mo for duration of treatment.
- Document baseline disease state activity (eg, exercise capacity, walking distance). Reassess periodically to document response to therapy.
- Monitor for signs of liver injury (eg, nausea, vomiting, fever, abdominal pain, jaundice, unusual lethargy or fatigue). Discontinue medication and notify health care provider immediately if noted.

Patient/Family Education
- Advise patient to read the Medication Guide before beginning therapy.
- Explain name, dose, action, and potential side effects of drug.
- Advise patient to take morning and evening as prescribed, without regard to meals.
- Advise patient that monthly liver enzyme tests and pregnancy tests (in female patient of childbearing potential) will be required to use this medication safely.
- Inform patient that drug controls, but does not cure pulmonary hypertension, and to continue taking drug as prescribed.
- Caution patient not to change the dose or stop taking the drug unless advised to do so by health care provider.
- Caution patient that if drug is stopped for any period of time and then restarted, the lower initial dose should be used again.
- Instruct female patient of childbearing potential that reliable contraceptive measures must be used during treatment. Advise patient using hormonal contraception (eg, oral, injectable, implantable) that another nonhormonal contraceptive needs to be used.
- Instruct female patient to notify health care provider immediately if pregnancy is suspected (eg, delay in menses, have any other reason to suspect pregnancy), planning on becoming pregnant, or are breastfeeding.
- Instruct patient to stop taking drug and immediately report any of these symptoms to health care provider: nausea, vomiting, fever, abdominal pain, jaundice, unusual lethargy, fatigue.
- Caution patient to not take any prescription or OTC medications, or dietary supplements unless advised to do so by health care provider.
- Advise patient that follow-up visits and lab tests will be required to monitor therapy, and to keep appointments.

Botulinum Toxin Type A

(BOT-yoo-lin-um)

Class Botulinum toxins/Ophthalmic surgical adjunct

How Supplied
Botox Powder for injection 100 units vacuum-dried *Clostridium botulinum* toxin type A neurotoxin complex ♦ *Botox Cosmetic* Powder for injection 100 units vacuum-dried *Clostridium botulinum* toxin type A neurotoxin complex

Action
PHARMACOLOGY: Blocks neuromuscular conduction by binding to receptors on motor nerve terminals, entering the nerve terminals, and inhibiting the release of acetylcholine.

Indications Treatment of cervical dystonia in adults to decrease severity of abnormal head position and neck pain associated with cervical dystonia; treatment of strabismus and blepharospasm associated with dystonia, including benign essential blepharospasm or VII nerve disorder; for temporary improvement in appearance of moderate to severe glabellar lines associated with corrugator or procerus muscle activity in patients 65 yr of age or younger. **Unlabeled use(s):** Treatment of hemifacial spasms, spasmodic torticollis, oromandibular dystonia, spasmodic dysphonia, and other dystonias.

Contraindications Infection at the proposed injection site(s).

Route/Dosage
Blepharospasm
ADULTS AND CHILDREN AT LEAST 12 YR OF AGE: Initially, inject 1.25 to 2.5 units (0.05 to 0.1 mL volume at each site) into the medial and lateral pretarsal orbicularis oculi of the upper lid and into the lateral pretarsal orbicularis oculi of the lower lid.

Cervical Dystonia
ADULTS AND CHILDREN AT LEAST 16 YR OF AGE: In patients with known history of tolerance, tailor dosing in initial and sequential treatments to the individual patient based on patient's head and neck position, localized pain, muscle hypertrophy, patient response, and adverse event history. In patients without prior use, use lower dose than in patients with known history of tolerance, adjusting subsequent doses based on individual response.

Glabellar Lines (Botox Cosmetic only)
ADULTS (65 YR OF AGE OR YOUNGER): **IM** Total treatment dose is 20 units in 0.5 mL at intervals no more frequent than q 3 mo (duration of activity of botulinum toxin type A is approximately 3 to 4 mo).

Strabismus
ADULTS AND CHILDREN AT LEAST 12 YR OF AGE: Inject between 0.05 to 0.15 mL per muscle into extraocular muscles utilizing electrical activity recorded from tip of injection needle as guide to placement within target muscle.

Interactions
Aminoglycosides, drugs interfering with neuromuscular transmission: The effects of botulinum toxin may be potentiated.

Lab Test Interferences None well documented.

Adverse Reactions
CV: Arrhythmia; MI.
Botox cosmetic – Hypertension.
CNS: Headache; dizziness; drowsiness.
Botox cosmetic – Paresthesia, anxiety, twitch; decreased hearing, ear noise, blurred vision, retinal vein occlusion, glaucoma, vertigo with nystagmus (postmarketing).
DERM: Skin rash (including urticaria, psoriasiform eruption); erythema multiforme.
Botox cosmetic – Pruritus; skin tightness; localized numbness (postmarketing).
EENT: Dysphagia; rhinitis; oral dryness; diplopia; spatial disorientation, vertical deviation, or past-pointing (strabismus); superficial punctate keratitis; reduced blinking; eye dryness (blepharospasm).
Botox cosmetic – Sinusitis; pharyngitis; laryngitis.
GI: Nausea.
Botox cosmetic – Dyspepsia; tooth disorder.
GU:
Botox cosmetic – UTI.
HEMA:
Botox cosmetic – Ecchymosis.
HEPA:
Botox cosmetic – Abnormal liver function.
RESP: Cough; upper respiratory tract infection; dyspnea.
Botox cosmetic – Bronchitis; dyspnea.
OTHER: Flu syndrome; back pain; hypertonia; soreness at injection site; asthenia; speech disorder; fever; stiffness; numbness; ptosis; bruising; allergic reaction.
Botox cosmetic – Face pain; edema at injection site; muscle weakness; anaphylaxis, myasthenia gravis (postmarketing).

Precautions
Pregnancy: Category C.
Lactation: Undetermined.
Children: Botox Cosmetic is not recommended for use in children.
Blepharospasm and strabismus – Safety and efficacy in children younger than 12 yr of age not established.
Cervical dystonia – Safety and efficacy in children younger than 16 yr of age not established.

Elderly: Use with caution, reflecting greater frequency of decreased hepatic, renal, or cardiac function and comorbidity.
Albumin: Because this product contains albumin, a derivative of human blood, it carries a remote risk of viral disease transmission.
Dysphagia: Risk may be increased in patients requiring injections into the levator scapulae and in patients with smaller neck muscle mass and in patients requiring bilateral injections into sternocleidomastoid muscle.

Neuropathic disorders: Use with caution in patients with neuropathic diseases because of increased risk of systemic effects including severe dysphagia and respiratory compromise.
Strabismus: Botulinum toxin type A is ineffective in chronic paralytic strabismus, except to reduce antagonist contracture in conjunction with surgical repair.

Overdosage: Signs and Symptoms
Systemic weakness, muscle paralysis.

PATIENT CARE CONSIDERATIONS
Administration/Storage
- For IM administration only. Not for intradermal, subcutaneous, IV, or intra-arterial administration.
- Follow manufacturer's recommendations for dosing and frequency of administration.
- Reconstitute powder for injection following manufacturer's guidelines for dilution using sterile, non-preserved saline injection. Record date and time of reconstitution on vial.
- Discard vial if vacuum does not pull diluent into vial.
- Do not reconstitute with other diluents than sterile, non-preserved saline, or add other medications to vial.
- Do not administer if particulate matter, cloudiness, or discoloration noted.
- Use a new, sterile needle and syringe to enter vial on each occasion for removal of medication.
- Discard any unused solution that is not used within 4 hr of reconstitution.
- Follow institutional or organizational procedures for discarding medical waste and disposing unused solution, vials, and equipment used with the drug administration.
- Store unopened vials in refrigerator (36° to 46°F). Reconstituted solution may be stored for up to 4 hr if refrigerated. Do not freeze reconstituted solution.

Assessment/Interventions
- Obtain patient history, including drug history and any known allergies. Note infection or inflammation at proposed injection site, peripheral neuropathic motor disease (eg, amyotrophic lateral sclerosis), neuromuscular junctional disorders (eg, myasthenia gravis), weakness or atrophy of target muscles, or concurrent use of aminoglycosides or other agents known to interfere with neuromuscular transmission.
- Monitor patient for signs and symptoms of anaphylactic or serious allergic reaction. If noted, discontinue therapy immediately and be prepared to treat appropriately (eg, epinephrine).
- Ensure that precautions (eg, protective drops, ointment, patching) to prevent epithelial defect and corneal ulceration are implemented in patient treated for blepharospasm who experiences reduced blinking following treatment.
- Monitor patient for injection site reactions (eg, pain, tenderness, bruising), muscle weakness, CNS, DERM, GI, RESP, and general body side effects. Inform health care provider if noted and significant. Immediately notify health care provider if swallowing, speech, or breathing disorders develop.

Patient/Family Education
- Explain name, action, and potential side effects of drug.
- Advise patient or caregiver that medication will be prepared and administered by a health care provider in a health care setting.
- Advise patient being treated for cervical dystonia that improvement should be noted within the first 2 wk following treatment, and max improvement should be noted in about 6 wk. Advise patient that beneficial effects may last 3 mo before retreatment is needed.
- Advise patient being treated for blepharospasm that improvement should be noted within the first 3 days following treatment, and max improvement should be noted in about 1 to 2 wk. Advise patient that beneficial effects may last 3 mo before retreatment is needed.
- Advise patient being treated for stabismus that improvement should be noted within the first 2 days following treatment, and max improvement should be noted within the first week. Advise patient that beneficial effects may last 2 to 6 wk before the effects begin to wear off.
- Advise patient being treated for glabellar lines that improvement should be noted within the first 2 days following treatment, and max improvement should be noted within the first week. Advise patient that beneficial effects may last for 3 to 4 mo.
- Advise patient or caregiver to immediately

- seek medical assistance if swallowing, speech, or breathing problems develop.
- Advise patient to report intolerable injection site reactions or unusual symptoms to health care provider.
- Advise women to notify health care provider if pregnant, planning to become pregnant, or breastfeeding.
- Instruct patient not to take any prescription or OTC medications, dietary supplements, or herbal preparations unless advised by health care provider.
- Remind patient that office visits will be required to monitor therapy and to keep appointments.

Botulinum Toxin Type B

(BOT-yoo-lin-um)

Class Botulinum toxins

How Supplied
Myobloc Solution, injectable 5,000 units/mL

Action
PHARMACOLOGY: Interferes with neurotransmitter release by cleaving synaptic vesicle-associated membrane protein.

Indications Reduction of severity of abnormal head position and neck pain in adult patients with cervical dystonia.

Contraindications Standard considerations.

Route/Dosage
ADULTS: In patients with known history of tolerance, 2,500 to 5,000 units divided among affected muscles. In patients without a history of tolerating botulinum toxin, administer a lower initial dose than in patients with known history of tolerance, adjusting subsequent doses based on individual response.

Interactions
Aminoglycosides, drugs interfering with neuromuscular transmission: The effects of botulinum toxin may be potentiated.
Different botulinum serotypes: The effect of adding different botulinum neurotoxin serotypes at the same time or within less than 4 mo of each other is unknown. However, neuromuscular paralysis may be potentiated by coadministration or overlapping administration of different botulinum toxin serotypes.

Lab Test Interferences None well documented.

Adverse Reactions
CV: Migraine, vasodilation (at least 2%).
CNS: Headache (11%); dizziness (6%); anxiety, tremor, hyperesthesia, somnolence, confusion, vertigo (at least 2%).
DERM: Pruritus (at least 2%).
EENT: Amblyopia, otitis media, abnormal vision, taste perversion, tinnitus (at least 2%).
GI: Dry mouth (34%); dysphagia (25%); dyspepsia (10%); nausea (8%); vomiting, glossitis, stomatitis, tooth disorder (at least 2%).
GU: UTI, cystitis, vaginal moniliasis (at least 2%).
HEMA/LYMPH: Ecchymosis (at least 2%).
LOCAL: Injection site pain (15%).
M/N: Peripheral edema, edema, hypercholesterolemia (at least 2%).
MUSC: Arthralgia (7%); myasthenia (6%); arthritis, joint disorder (at least 2%).
RESP: Increased cough (7%); dyspnea, lung disorder, pneumonia (at least 2%).
OTHER: Neck pain related to cervical dystonia (17%); infection (15%); pain (13%); flu syndrome, torticollis (8%); back pain (7%); asthenia (6%); accidental injury (5%); allergic reaction, fever, chest pain, chills, hernia, malaise, abscess, cyst, neoplasm, viral infections (at least 2%).

Precautions
Pregnancy: Category C.
Lactation: Undetermined.
Children: Safety and efficacy not established.
Elderly: Safety and efficacy not established in patients 75 yr of age or older.
Albumin: Because this product contains albumin, a derivative of human blood, it carries a remote risk of viral disease transmission.
Dysphagia: Dysphagia is a commonly reported adverse effect of treatment with all botulinum toxins in cervical dystonia patients and may be severe enough in some cases to warrant insertion of a gastric feeding tube.
Neuropathic disorders: Use with caution in patients with neuropathic diseases because of increased risk of systemic effects, including severe dysphagia and respiratory compromise.

Overdosage: Signs and Symptoms
Systemic weakness, muscle paralysis.

PATIENT CARE CONSIDERATIONS
Administration/Storage
- For IM administration only. Not for intradermal, subcutaneous, IV, or intra-arterial administration.
- Follow manufacturer's recommendations for dosing and frequency of administration.
- May be diluted with sterile normal saline. Discard any unused solution that is not used within 4 hr of dilution.
- Do not add other medications to vial.

- Do not administer if particulate matter, cloudiness, or discoloration noted.
- Use a new, sterile needle and syringe to enter vial on each occasion for removal of medication.
- Follow institutional or organizational procedures for discarding medical waste when disposing unused solution, vials, and equipment used with the drug administration.
- Store unopened vials in refrigerator (36° to 46°F). Do not freeze. Do not shake vials.

Assessment/Interventions
- Obtain patient history, including drug history and any known allergies. Note infection or inflammation at proposed injection site, peripheral neuropathic motor disease (eg, amyotrophic lateral sclerosis), neuromuscular junctional disorders (eg, myasthenia gravis), weakness or atrophy of target muscles, or concurrent use of aminoglycosides or other agents known to interfere with neuromuscular transmission.
- Monitor patient for signs and symptoms of anaphylactic or serious allergic reaction. If noted, discontinue therapy immediately and be prepared to treat appropriately (eg, epinephrine).
- Monitor patient for injection site reactions (eg, pain, tenderness, bruising), CNS, GI, and general body side effects. Inform health care provider if noted and significant. Immediately notify health care provider if swallowing, speech, or breathing disorders develop.

Patient/Family Education
- Explain name, action, and potential side effects of drug.
- Advise patient or caregiver that medication will be prepared and administered by a health care provider in a health care setting.
- Advise patient being treated for cervical dystonia that improvement should be noted within the first 2 wk following treatment, and max improvement should be noted at about 6 wk following treatment. Advise patient that beneficial effects may last 3 to 4 mo before retreatment is needed.
- Advise patient or caregiver to immediately seek medical assistance if swallowing, speech, or breathing problems develop.
- Advise patient to report intolerable injection site reactions or unusual symptoms to health care provider.
- Advise women to notify health care provider if pregnant, planning to become pregnant, or breastfeeding.
- Instruct patient not to take any prescription or OTC medications, dietary supplements, or herbal preparations unless advised by health care provider.
- Remind patient that office visits will be required to monitor therapy and to keep appointments.

Botulism Immune Globulin Intravenous (BIG-IV)

(BOT-yoo-lizm ih-MYOON GLAH-byoo-lin intravenous)

Class Immune serum

How Supplied
BabyBIG Powder for injection, lyophilized 100 ± 20 mg (50 mg/mL when reconstituted)

Action
PHARMACOLOGY: Botulism immune globulin contains IgG antibodies representative of the immunized donors who contribute to the plasma pool of the derived product.
PHARMACOKINETICS/DYNAMICS:
Excretion: The t½ is approximately 28 days in infants.

Indications Treatment of patients younger than 1 yr of age with infant botulism caused by toxin type A or B.

Contraindications Prior history of severe reaction to other human immunoglobulin preparations; individuals with selective immunoglobulin A deficiency may develop antibodies to immunoglobulin A, resulting in anaphylactic reactions to subsequent administration of blood products containing immunoglobulin A.

Route/Dosage
CHILDREN YOUNGER THAN 1 YR: **IV** 50 mg/kg (1 mL/kg) as a single infusion as soon as clinical diagnosis of infant botulism is made.

Interactions
Live virus vaccines: May interfere with immune response to live virus vaccines (eg, polio, mumps, rubella); therefore, vaccination with live virus vaccines should be deferred until about 5 mo after administration of BIG-IV.

Lab Test Interferences None well documented.

Adverse Reactions
CV: Increased BP (75%); decreased BP (16%); cardiac murmur (15%); tachycardia (7%).
CNS: Irritability (41%); agitation (10%).
DERM: Contact dermatitis (24%); erythematous rash (22%).
EENT: Dysphagia (65%); nasal congestion (18%); otitis media (11%).
ELECDIST: Hyponatremia (6%).
GI: Loose stools (25%); vomiting (20%); oral

candidiasis (8%); nausea (less than 5%).
HEMA: Decreased hemoglobin (9%); anemia (5%).
METAB: Dehydration (10%); acidosis (5%).
RESP: Atelectasis (39%); rhonchi (34%); stridor (9%); lower respiratory tract infection (8%); dyspnea (6%); tachypnea (5%).
OTHER: Pallor (28%); edema (18%); pyrexia, decreased oxygen saturation (17%); decreased body temperature (16%); cough (13%); rales (13%); abdominal distension (11%); decreased breath sounds (10%); injection-site reactions (including erythema), peripheral coldness (7%); chills, muscle cramps, back pain, fever, wheezing (less than 5%).

Precautions
Pregnancy: Undetermined.
Lactation: Undetermined.
Children: Safety and efficacy not established in children (or adults) 1 yr of age or older.
Associated risks: Patients may be at increased risk of contracting or experiencing blood-borne viruses, anaphylaxis, angioneurotic edema, renal dysfunction, acute renal failure, osmotic nephrosis, and death.

Overdosage: Signs and Symptoms
Volume overload.

PATIENT CARE CONSIDERATIONS

Administration/Storage
- For IV infusion only. Not for intradermal, SC, IM, or intra-arterial administration.
- Reconstitute powder for injection following manufacturer's guidelines using the diluent provided with medication. Allow at least 30 min to reconstitute powder for injection.
- Do not shake the vial during reconstitution, reconstitute with diluents other than those supplied, or add other medications to vial.
- Do not administer if particulate matter, cloudiness, or discoloration noted.
- Begin infusion within 2 hr of reconstitution and conclude infusion within 4 hr of reconstitution.
- Infuse intravenously using low-volume tubing with disposable filter (18 mcm) and constant infusion pump following manufacturer's recommendations regarding rate of administration.
- Infuse using separate IV line. If separate IV line is not available, "piggyback" into preexisting line containing sodium chloride injection or dextrose in water (with or without sodium chloride) solutions.
- Discard any unused solution or reconstituted solution that is not used within 4 hr of reconstitution.
- Store unopened vials in refrigerator (36° to 46°F).

Assessment/Interventions
- Obtain patient history, including drug history and any known allergies. Note renal insufficiency or conditions predisposing to renal insufficiency (eg, diabetes mellitus, volume depletion, paraproteinemia, sepsis, concurrent use of nephrotoxic drugs), selective immunoglobulin A deficiency, or prior history of severe reaction to other human immunoglobulin preparations.
- Ensure that renal function is assessed prior to initial infusion.
- Ensure that medication is administered to patient with renal insufficiency, or condition predisposing to renal insufficiency, at minimum concentration available and at minimum rate of administration.
- Ensure that renal function and urine output are periodically assessed in patient judged to have potential risk for developing acute renal failure.
- Observe patient and monitor vital signs continuously during administration. If minor side effects develop, immediately slow the rate of infusion or temporarily interrupt the infusion. If hypotension develops, discontinue infusion immediately and be prepared to treat appropriately.
- Monitor patient for signs and symptoms of anaphylactic or serious allergic reaction. If noted, discontinue infusion immediately and be prepared to treat appropriately (eg, epinephrine).
- Monitor patient for signs and symptoms of aseptic meningitis (severe headache, nuchal rigidity, drowsiness, fever, photophobia, painful eye movements, nausea and vomiting) for 48 hr following infusion. Inform health care provider immediately if noted.
- Defer administration of live virus vaccines for at least 5 mo following treatment.

Patient/Family Education
- Explain name, action, and potential side effects of drug.
- Advise family or caregiver that medication will be prepared and administered by a health care provider in a hospital setting.

Bretylium Tosylate

(breh-TILL-ee-uhm TAH-sill-ate)

Class Antiarrhythmic

How Supplied
Bretylium Tosylate in 5% Dextrose Injection 2 mg/mL (500 mg/vial), Injection 4 mg/mL (1000 mg/vial) ♦ *Bretylium Tosylate* Injection 50 mg/mL

Action
PHARMACOLOGY: Causes a chemical sympathectomy-like state by inhibiting norepinephrine release and depressing adrenergic nerve terminal excitability; produces a positive inotropic effect on the myocardium.

PHARMACOKINETICS/DYNAMICS:
Metabolism: No metabolites identified.
Excretion: Eliminated intact by the kidneys; t½ is about 7.8 hr.
Onset: Rapid, usually within minutes.
Special Populations:
Renal Function Impairment – The t½ is increased.

Indications Prophylaxis and treatment of ventricular fibrillation; treatment of life-threatening ventricular arrhythmia that has failed to respond to first-line antiarrhythmic agents. **Unlabeled use(s):** Second-line therapy (following lidocaine) for the treatment of ventricular arrhythmia during advanced cardiac life support in CPR.

Contraindications Standard considerations.

Route/Dosage
Life-Threatening Ventricular Arrhythmias
ADULTS:
Initial dose: **IV** 5 to 10 mg/kg (undiluted) by rapid IV injection; if arrhythmia persists, adjust dosage as necessary.
Maintenance (for continuous suppression): **IV** Infuse diluted solution at 1 to 2 mg/min. Alternately, infuse diluted solution at 5 to 10 mg/kg over more than 8 min q 6 hr.
CHILDREN: **IV** 5 mg/kg/dose followed by 10 mg/kg at 10 to 30 min intervals (max total dose, 30 mg/kg).
Maintenance: 5 to 10 mg/kg/dose q 6 hr.

Other Ventricular Arrhythmias
ADULTS: **IV** 5 to 10 mg/kg (diluted) over 8 min; if arrhythmia persists, give subsequent doses q 1 to 2 hr.
Maintenance: Administer same dose q 6 hr or infuse 1 to 2 mg/min. **IM** 5 to 10 mg/kg (undiluted); if arrhythmia persists, give subsequent doses at 1 to 2 hr intervals. Maintain same dosage q 6 to 8 hr.
CHILDREN: 5 to 10 mg/kg/dose q 6 hr.

Interactions
Antihypertensives: May cause severe hypotension.
Catecholamines: Enhance pressor effects of catecholamines.
Digoxin: May aggravate arrhythmias caused by digitalis toxicity.

Lab Test Interferences None well documented.

Adverse Reactions
CV: Orthostatic hypotension; bradycardia; increased premature ventricular contractions and other arrhythmias; transient hypertension; angina; sensation of substernal pressure.
CNS: Dizziness; lightheadedness; syncope; vertigo.
GI: Nausea and vomiting after rapid IV injection.

Precautions
Pregnancy: Category C.
Lactation: Undetermined.
Children: Safety and efficacy not established.
Renal function impairment: Increase dosage interval.
Fixed cardiac output: Because severe hypotension may occur, avoid use in patients with fixed cardiac output (eg, severe aortic stenosis, pulmonary hypertension). Orthostatic hypotension is common (50%); keep patient supine until tolerance develops or medication is withdrawn.

Overdosage: Signs and Symptoms
Hypertension followed by refractory hypotension.

PATIENT CARE CONSIDERATIONS

Administration/Storage
- Use for short-term therapy only.
- For maintenance administration, dilute each dose in at least 50 mL of 5% Dextrose in Water or 0.9% Sodium Chloride for Injection. Larger amounts can be diluted in any amount of solution (1 g in 250 mL = 4 mg/mL; 1 g in 500 mL = 2 mg/mL; 1 g in 1000 mL = 1 mg/mL).
- Use slow injection (over 10 min) to prevent nausea and vomiting.
- Rotate IM injection sites frequently to prevent atrophy and necrosis of muscle tissue. Do not give more than 5 mL in any one site.
- Store at room temperature. Protect from freezing.

Assessment/Interventions
- Obtain patient history, including drug history and any known allergies.

- Anticipate nausea and vomiting to occur after rapid IV administration.
- Monitor patient's vital signs frequently, including cardiac rhythm. Transient increase in arrhythmias and hypertension may occur within 1 hr after initial administration. Especially note slow or irregular pulse or significant hypotension. If BP is less than 75 mm Hg, notify health care provider.
- Monitor I&O if nausea or vomiting develops or if patient has renal impairment or demonstrates decreased cardiac output.
- Take safety precautions if dizziness, lightheadedness, vertigo, or syncope occurs.
- Keep bed in low position and supervise ambulation.
- Keep the patient in supine position until tolerance to orthostatic hypotension develops.
- If systolic BP is less than 75 mm Hg, notify health care provider.
- Observe for increased anginal pain.

Patient/Family Education
- Instruct patient to make position changes slowly and to request assistance with ambulation.
- Advise men to sit on toilet while urinating.

Brimonidine Tartrate

Class Antiglaucoma/Alpha-2 adrenergic agonist

How Supplied
Alphagan P Solution 0.15%
♣ *ratio-Brimonidine*

Action
PHARMACOLOGY: Reduces aqueous humor production and increases uveoscleral outflow.

Indications Lowers IOP in open-angle glaucoma or ocular hypertension.

Contraindications Coadministration of MAO inhibitors.

Route/Dosage
ADULTS AND CHILDREN 2 YR AND OLDER: **Ophthalmic** Instill 1 drop into affected eye(s) tid (approximately 8 hr apart).

Interactions
Antihypertensives, beta blockers, cardiac glycosides: Brimonidine may reduce pulse and BP; use with caution.
CNS depressants (eg, alcohol, anesthetics, barbiturates, opiates, sedative): Additive or potentiating CNS depressant effect.
MAO inhibitors: Concurrent use contraindicated.
Tricyclic antidepressants: May decrease the effect of brimonidine by altering the metabolism and uptake of circulating amines.

Lab Test Interferences None well documented.

Adverse Reactions
CV: Hypertension; palpitations.
CNS: Headache; fatigue; drowsiness; dizziness; depression; anxiety; syncope.
EENT: Dry mouth; ocular hyperemia, burning, and stinging; blurred vision; foreign body sensation; conjunctival follicles; ocular allergy; ocular pruritus; corneal staining and erosion; photophobia; eyelid erythema and edema; ocular aching and pain; ocular dryness; tearing; conjunctival edema; blepharitis; ocular irritation; conjunctival blanching; abnormal vision; lid crusting; conjunctival hemorrhage; abnormal taste; conjunctival discharge; nasal dryness.
GI: GI symptoms.
RESP: Upper respiratory tract symptoms.
OTHER: Asthenia; muscle pain.

Precautions
Pregnancy: Category B.
Lactation: Undetermined.
Children: Safety and efficacy not established in children under 2 yr.
Renal function impairment: Use with caution.
Hepatic function impairment: Use with caution.
Soft contact lenses: Wait at least 15 min after instilling brimonidine before inserting contact lenses.

PATIENT CARE CONSIDERATIONS

Administration/Storage
- Discontinue MAO inhibitors at least 14 days before initiating therapy.
- Instill 1 drop in the affected eye(s) tid, approximately 8 hr apart.
- If using other topical ophthalmic drugs, separate each medication by at least 5 min.
- Store at controlled room temperature. Keep container tightly closed.

Assessment/Interventions
- Obtain patient history, including drug history and any known allergies. Note current or recent (within 14 days) use of MAO inhibitor.
- Ensure that IOPs have been measured and documented in the patient's record.

♦ Monitor patient for side effects and report to health care provider if noted and significant.

Patient/Family Education
♦ Explain name, dose, action, and potential side effects of drug.
♦ Advise patient that usual dose is 1 drop in the affected eye(s) tid, approximately 8 hr apart.
♦ Teach patient the following proper technique for instilling eye drops: wash hands; do not allow dropper to touch eye. Tilt head back, look up; pull lower eyelid down; instill prescribed number of drops.
♦ Close eye for 1 to 2 min and apply gentle pressure to bridge of nose. Do not rub eye.
♦ Advise patients who wear contact lenses to remove lenses before instilling this medicine and to wait at least 15 min after instilling eye drop before inserting lenses.
♦ Advise patient that if more than 1 topical ophthalmic drug is being used, administer the drugs at least 5 min apart.
♦ Advise patient that drug may cause drowsiness or fatigue and to use caution while driving or performing other activities requiring mental alertness.
♦ Advise patient to contact eye care physician if eye or eyelid inflammation, irritation, or itching is noted.
♦ Remind patient that eye examinations and measurement of IOP will be necessary while using this medication and make sure to keep appointments.

Brinzolamide

(brin-ZOE-lah-mide)

Class Carbonic anhydrase inhibitor

How Supplied
Azopt Ophthalmic suspension 1%

Action
PHARMACOLOGY: Inhibition of carbonic anhydrase in the ciliary processes of the eye decreases aqueous humor secretion, resulting in a reduction in IOP.

PHARMACOKINETICS/DYNAMICS:
Absorption: Following ocular administration, absorbed into the systemic circulation.

Distribution: Distributes extensively into RBCs. Protein binding is about 60%.

Metabolism: Metabolite is N-desethylbrinzolamide.

Excretion: Eliminated predominantly unchanged in the urine. Metabolites also found in the urine.

Indications Treatment of elevated IOP in patients with ocular hypertension or open-angle glaucoma.

Contraindications Standard considerations.

PATIENT CARE CONSIDERATIONS
Administration/Storage
♦ Shake dropper bottle well before instilling eye drops.
♦ Instill 1 gtt into affected eye(s) tid.
♦ If using other topical ophthalmic drugs, separate each medication by at least 10 min.
♦ Store below 86°F. Keep dropper bottle tightly closed.

Route/Dosage
ADULTS: **Ophthalmic** 1 gtt in affected eye(s) tid.

Interactions None well documented.

Lab Test Interferences None well documented.

Adverse Reactions
CNS: Headache (1% to 5%).
DERM: Dermatitis (1% to 5%).
EENT: Blurred vision (5% to 10%); blepharitis, dry eye, foreign body sensation, hyperemia, ocular discharge, ocular discomfort, ocular keratitis, ocular pain, ocular pruritus, rhinitis (1% to 5%).
GI: Bitter, sour, or unusual taste (5% to 10%).

Precautions
Pregnancy: Category C.
Lactation: Undetermined.
Children: Safety and efficacy not established.
Renal function impairment: Use not recommended.
Hepatic function impairment: Use with caution.
Sulfonamides: Brinzolamide is a sulfonamide and adverse reactions attributable to sulfonamides may occur (eg, Stevens-Johnson syndrome, toxic epidermal necrolysis, aplastic anemia, death).

Overdosage: Signs and Symptoms
Electrolyte imbalance, acidotic state, possible nervous system effects.

Assessment/Interventions
♦ Obtain patient history, including drug history and any known allergies. Note renal or hepatic impairment, sulfonamide sensitivity, or concurrent use of dorzolamide.
♦ Ensure that IOP has been measured and documented in the patient's record before starting therapy and periodically thereafter.

- Monitor patient for ocular and systemic reactions. Inform health care provider immediately if noted.

Patient/Family Education
- Explain name, dose, action, and potential side effects of drug.
- Advise patient that usual dose is 1 gtt instilled into the affected eye(s) tid.
- Teach patient proper technique for instilling eye drops: wash hands; shake well; do not allow dropper tip to touch eye. Tilt head back, look up; pull lower eyelid down; instill prescribed number of drops. Close eye for 1 to 2 min and apply gentle pressure to bridge of nose for 3 to 5 min. Do not rub eye.
- Advise patient that if more than 1 topical ophthalmic drug is being used, administer the drugs at least 10 min apart.
- Advise patients who wear contact lenses to remove lenses before instilling this medicine and to wait at least 15 min after instilling eye drops before reinserting lenses.
- Inform patient that blurred vision and taste abnormalities (bitter, sour, or unusual taste) are the most common side effects and to contact health care provider if they occur and are bothersome.
- Advise patient that medication may cause temporary blurring of vision and to use caution driving or performing other tasks requiring good vision until tolerance is determined.
- Advise patient to discontinue therapy and immediately notify health care provider if serious or unusual reactions occur in the eye (eg, eye or eyelid inflammation) or if experiencing any signs or symptoms of an allergic reaction (eg, rash, hives, itching).
- Advise patient to contact the eye doctor if eye injury occurs or eye surgery is forthcoming.
- Advise women to notify health care provider if pregnant, planning to become pregnant, or breastfeeding.
- Instruct patient not to take any prescription or OTC medications or dietary supplements unless advised by health care provider.
- Remind patient that eye examinations and measurement of IOP will be necessary while using this medication and to keep appointments.

Bromocriptine Mesylate

(BROE-moe-KRIP-teen MEH-sih-LATE)

Class Antiparkinson

How Supplied
Parlodel Tablets 2.5 mg (as mesylate), Capsules 5 mg (as mesylate)

Apo-Bromocriptine ♦ Parlodel ♦ PMS-Bromocriptine

Action
PHARMACOLOGY: Stimulates dopamine receptors in the corpus striatum, relieving parkinsonian symptoms. Inhibits prolactin, which is responsible for lactation, and lowers elevated blood levels of growth hormone in acromegaly.

PHARMACOKINETICS/DYNAMICS:
Absorption: 28% of oral dose absorbed.
Distribution: 90% to 96% bound to serum albumin.
Metabolism: Completely metabolized.
Excretion: Major elimination route is via the bile; 2.5% to 5% is excreted in urine and 84.6% is excreted in feces in 120 hr.

Indications Treatment of hyperprolactinemia-associated disorders (eg, amenorrhea with or without galactorrhea, infertility, hypogonadism) in patients with prolactin-secreting adenomas; therapy for female infertility associated with hyperprolactinemia; treatment of acromegaly; therapy for Parkinson disease (idiopathic or postencephalitic). **Unlabeled use(s):** Treatment of hyperprolactinemia associated with pituitary adenomas; therapy for neuroleptic malignant syndrome; treatment of cocaine addiction.

Contraindications Sensitivity to ergot alkaloids; severe ischemic heart disease or peripheral vascular disease; pregnancy.

Route/Dosage
Hyperprolactinemia-Associated Disorders
Initial dose – PO 1.25 to 2.5 mg/day; 2.5 mg may be added as tolerated q 3 to 7 days until optimum response. (Dosage range, 2.5 to 15 mg/day).

Acromegaly
Initial dose – PO 1.25 to 2.5 mg for 3 days at bedtime; may be increased by 1.25 to 2.5 mg as tolerated q 3 to 7 days until optimum response occurs. Dosage range, 20 to 30 mg/day, not to exceed 100 mg/day.

Parkinson Disease
Initial dose – PO 1.25 mg bid titrated individually. Dosage range, 10 to 40 mg/day, not to exceed 100 mg/day.

Interactions
Dopamine antagonists (eg, phenothiazines, butyrophenones, metoclopramide): May reduce bromocriptine efficacy.
Erythromycin: May increase bromocriptine serum levels.

Lab Test Interferences None well documented.

Adverse Reactions

CV: Hypotension (including orthostatic); syncope; hypertension; stroke; digital vasospasm.
CNS: Headache; dizziness; fatigue; lightheadedness; fainting; drowsiness; psychosis; seizures; abnormal involuntary movements; hallucinations; confusion; ataxia; insomnia; depression; vertigo; "on-off" phenomenon.
EENT: Visual disturbances, nasal congestion.
GI: Nausea; vomiting; abdominal cramps; constipation; diarrhea; anorexia; indigestion/dyspepsia; GI bleeding.
RESP: Shortness of breath; pulmonary infiltrates; pleural effusion; pleural thickening.
OTHER: Exacerbation of Raynaud syndrome; asthenia.

Precautions

Pregnancy: Pregnancy category undetermined.
Lactation: Contraindicated in nursing women.
Children: Safety and efficacy in children under 15 yr not established.
Acromegaly: Cold-sensitive digital vasospasms and severe GI bleeding from peptic ulcers have been reported in patients with acromegaly; institute appropriate treatment. Possible tumor expansion has occurred; monitor patient's condition and discontinue treatment if necessary.
Parkinson disease: Safe use longer than 2 yr has not been established. Periodic evaluation of hepatic, hematopoietic, cardiac, and renal functions is necessary.
Pituitary tumors: Evaluate pituitary before treatment to determine if tumor is present.
Symptomatic hypotension: Do not administer to postpartum patients until BP normalizes. Use caution in patients with pre-eclampsia and in those who have received other drugs that may alter BP.

PATIENT CARE CONSIDERATIONS

Administration/Storage

- Give with milk or meals to reduce gastric distress. Initial dose is usually given at bedtime because of adverse CNS reactions (eg, dizziness, fainting).
- Tablet may be crushed if patient has difficulty swallowing.
- If dose must be delayed for more than 4 hr, omit dose. Do not give double dose.
- Response to bromocriptine varies with individuals. Titrate dose to balance risks/benefits.
- Store at room temperature in tightly-closed container.

Assessment/Interventions

- Obtain patient history, including drug history and any known allergies.
- Monitor BP prior to and during drug therapy. Severe hypotension may occur. Have patient remain supine for several hours after initial dose.
- Observe for lessening of symptoms of Parkinson disease (eg, rigidity, akinesia, tremors, pill rolling, shuffling gait, mask facies) prior to and during drug therapy.
- Assess breasts for decrease in engorgement.
- Assess for exacerbation of Raynaud syndrome (eg, muscle cramps in hands or feet, cold feet).
- Ensure safety and assess for risk of falls if dizziness occurs.

Patient/Family Education

- Tell patient not to skip doses or take double doses.
- Caution patient not to discontinue drug suddenly, and to avoid rapid recurrence of original symptoms. Explain that dosage will be tapered slowly before stopping use of drug.
- Advise women of childbearing age to use nonhormonal methods of birth control during therapy.
- Instruct patient to inform health care provider immediately if pregnancy is suspected.
- When used for infertility, instruct patient to obtain daily basal body temperatures to determine when ovulation occurs.
- Advise patients who are taking drug to suppress lactation that breast engorgement may occur as therapy is discontinued.
- Inform patient that side effects are common, especially during initial phase of therapy.
- Instruct patient to notify health care provider if increasing dyspnea or nasal congestion occurs.
- Caution patient to avoid sudden position changes to prevent orthostatic hypotension.
- Advise patient to avoid intake of alcoholic beverages.
- Advise patient that drug may cause drowsiness, and to use caution while driving or performing other tasks requiring mental alertness.

Brompheniramine Maleate/Pseudoephedrine Hydrochloride

(brom-fen-AIR-uh-meen MAL-ee-ate/SUE-doe-eh-FED-rin HIGH-droe-KLOR-ide)

Class Antihistamine/Decongestant

How Supplied
Lodrane Liquid 4 mg brompheniramine/60 mg pseudoephedrine ♦ Lodrane 12 D Tablets 6 mg brompheniramine/45 mg pseudoephedrine ♦ Lodrane LD Capsules 6 mg brompheniramine/60 mg pseudoephedrine

Action
PHARMACOLOGY:
Brompheniramine: Competitively antagonizes histamine at H_1 receptor sites.
Pseudoephedrine: Causes vasoconstriction and subsequent shrinkage of nasal mucous membranes by alpha-adrenergic stimulation, which promotes nasal drainage.

Indications
Temporary relief of symptoms associated with seasonal and perennial allergic rhinitis and vasomotor rhinitis, including nasal congestion.

Contraindications
Hypersensitivity to any ingredients of product; nursing mothers, severe hypertension; severe coronary artery disease; narrow-angle glaucoma; urinary retention; peptic ulcer, asthma attack; MAO inhibitor therapy or for 2 wk after stopping MAO inhibitor therapy.

Route/Dosage
ADULTS AND CHILDREN OVER 12 YR: **PO** *Lodrane* extended-release tablet 1 or 2 tablets q 12 hr. *Lodrane* liquid: 1 tsp (5 mL) q 4 to 6 hr (max, 4 doses/24 hr).
CHILDREN 6 TO 12 YR: **PO** *Lodrane* extended-release tablet: 1 tablet q 12 hr. *Lodrane* liquid: ½ tsp (2.5 mL) q 4 to 6 hr (max, 4 doses/24 hr).
CHILDREN 2 TO 6 YR: **PO** *Lodrane* liquid: ¼ tsp (1.25 mL) q 4 to 6 hr (max, 4 doses/24 hr).
CHILDREN LESS THAN 2 YR: **PO** *Lodrane* liquid: as recommended by health care provider.

Interactions
Alcohol, barbiturates (eg, phenobarbital), tricyclic depressants (eg, amitriptyline), other CNS depressants: Effects may be enhanced by brompheniramine.
Antacids: Rate of pseudoephedrine absorption may be increased.
Antidepressants, antihypertensives: Do not use in patients receiving antidepressants or antihypertensive agents or within 14 days of stopping such treatment.
Digitalis: Increased ectopic pacemaker activity can occur with pseudoephedrine.
MAO inhibitors (eg, isocarboxazid): Do not use in patients receiving MAO inhibitor therapy or within 14 days of stopping such treatment. May prolong and intensify the effects of brompheniramine and increase the effects of pseudoephedrine.
Mecamylamine, methyldopa, reserpine, veratrum alkaloids: Antihypertensive effects may be reduced by pseudoephedrine.
Tricyclic antidepressants (eg, amitriptyline): May prolong or intensify the anticholinergic effects of brompheniramine.

Lab Test Interferences May interfere with diagnostic test results for skin tests using allergen extracts.

Adverse Reactions
CV: Palpitation; tachycardia; angina; elevated BP; circulatory collapse.
CNS: Drowsiness; confusion; restlessness; anorexia; dizziness; headache; insomnia; anxiety; tension; weakness; stimulation.
DERM: Rash; sweating.
GI: Nausea; vomiting; gastric distress; abdominal cramps.
GU: Dysuria.
OTHER: Vertigo; mydriasis.

Precautions
Pregnancy: Category C.
Lactation: Undetermined.
Children: Lodrane extended-release tablets: Safety and efficacy in children less than 6 yr not established. *Lodrane* liquid: Safety and efficacy in children less than 2 yr not established.
Elderly: More likely to cause dizziness, sedation, hyperexcitability, anticholinergic side effects (eg, urinary retention), confusion, hallucinations, seizures, CNS depression, and hypotension in the elderly.
Special risk patients: Use with caution in patients with hypertension, heart disease, asthma, hyperthyroidism, increased intraocular pressure, diabetes mellitus, prostatic hypertrophy, bronchial asthma.
Abuse: Pseudoephedrine is a CNS stimulant and has been abused.

Overdosage: Signs and Symptoms
Brompheniramine: Hallucination, convulsions and death, dizziness, sedation, hypotension
Pseudoephedrine: Cardiac arrhythmias, cerebral hemorrhage, pulmonary edema, palpitations, tremor, dizziness, vomiting, fear, labored breathing, headache, dryness of mouth, pallor, weakness, panic, anxiety, confusion, hallucination, delirium

PATIENT CARE CONSIDERATIONS
Administration/Storage
- Give sustained release tablet q 12 hr as needed, with a full glass of water.
- Give prescribed dose of liquid q 4 to 6 hr as needed, up to qid.
- Give with food or milk if GI upset occurs.
- Use dosing spoon or syringe for pediatric doses of liquid.
- Do not cut, chew, or crush tablet. Swallow whole.
- Store tablets and liquid at controlled room temperature (59° to 86°F). Protect tablets from light and moisture. Keep liquid tightly closed.

Assessment/Interventions
- Obtain patient history, including drug history and any known allergies. Note history of peptic ulcer disease, diabetes, hypertension, hyperthyroidism, enlarged prostate, asthma, narrow angle glaucoma, urinary retention, severe hypertension or coronary artery disease, concurrent use of or within 2 wk of stopping MAO-inhibitor therapy, or allergy to alkylamine antihistamines (eg, triprolidine) or sympathomimetic amines.
- Assess for allergy symptoms (eg, rhinitis, nasal congestion, sneezing, itching, watery eyes) before and periodically throughout therapy.
- Monitor pulse and BP periodically during therapy.
- Monitor patient for nervousness, dizziness, and insomnia. If noted hold therapy and notify health care provider.

Patient/Family Education
- Explain name, dose, action, and potential side effects of drug.
- Advise patient to take tablet dose q 12 hr as needed with a full glass of water. Liquid dose is taken q 4 to 6 hr as needed, up to qid.
- Advise caregiver to use dosing spoon or syringe when giving liquid dose to children.
- Advise patient to take with food or milk if GI upset occurs.
- Caution patient to not cut, chew, or crush tablet and to swallow whole.
- Advise patient to take last dose late in the afternoon or early evening to reduce chance of drug causing sleeplessness.
- Advise patient that if a dose is missed to take as soon as remembered unless it is nearing time for the next dose. Caution patient to not double the dose to catch up.
- Advise patient that if allergy symptoms are not controlled not to increase the dose of medication but to inform their health care provider.
- Caution patient that drug may cause drowsiness and to use caution while driving or performing other tasks requiring mental alertness until tolerance is determined.
- Advise patient to avoid alcohol and other CNS depressants due to risk of excessive sedation.
- Caution patient not to take any OTC antihistamines or decongestants while taking this medication unless advised to do so by their health care provider.
- If patient is to have allergy skin testing, advise to not take the medication for at least 6 days before the skin testing.
- Advise patient to notify health care provider if pregnant, planning to become pregnant, or breastfeeding.
- Instruct patient to stop taking drug and immediately report any of these symptoms to health care provider: nervousness, dizziness, or sleeplessness.
- Caution patient to not take any prescription or OTC medications, or dietary supplements unless advised by health care provider.

Brompheniramine Maleate/ Pseudoephedrine Hydrochloride/ Dextromethorphan HBr

(brom-fen-AIR-uh-meen MAL-ee-ate/SUE-doe-eh-FED-rin HIGH-droe-KLOR-ide/DEX-troe-meth-OR-fan HIGH-droe-BROE-mide)

Class Antihistamine/Decongestant/Antitussive

How Supplied
Rondec-DM Liquid 4 mg brompheniramine, 45 mg pseudoephedrine, 15 mg dextromethorphan

Action
PHARMACOLOGY:
Brompheniramine: Competitively antagonizes histamine at H_1 receptor sites.
Pseudoephedrine: Causes vasoconstriction and subsequent shrinkage of nasal mucous membranes by alpha-adrenergic stimulation, which promotes nasal drainage.
Dextromethorphan: Suppresses cough by central action on cough center in medulla.

Indications Relief of cough and upper respiratory tract symptoms (including nasal congestion) associated with allergy or common cold.

Contraindications Hypersensitivity or idiosyncratic reaction to any ingredients of product; severe hypertension; severe coronary artery disease; narrow-angle glaucoma; urinary retention; peptic ulcer; asthma attack; MAO inhibitor therapy or for 2 wk after stopping MAO inhibitor therapy.

Route/Dosage
ADULTS AND CHILDREN (6 YR AND OLDER): PO 1 tsp (5 mL) qid.
CHILDREN (2 TO 6 YR): PO ½ tsp (2.5 mL) qid.

Interactions
Alcohol, barbiturates (eg, phenobarbital), tricyclic antidepressants (eg, amitriptyline), other CNS depressants: Effects may be enhanced by brompheniramine.
MAO inhibitors (eg, isocarboxazid): May prolong and intensify the effects of brompheniramine and increase the effects of pseudoephedrine. Dextromethorphan is contraindicated with MAO inhibitors.
Mecamylamine, methyldopa, reserpine, veratrum alkaloids: Antihypertensive effects may be reduced by pseudoephedrine.
Narcotic antitussives (eg, codeine): May increase the cough suppressant effects of dextromethorphan.

Lab Test Interferences May interfere with diagnostic test results for skin tests using allergen extracts.

Adverse Reactions
CV:
Pseudoephedrine – Cardiac arrhythmia; increased heart rate; increased BP.
CNS:
Brompheniramine – Sedation; dizziness; headache; nervousness; excitability in children (rare).
Pseudoephedrine – Convulsions; CNS stimulation; hallucinations; tremors; nervousness; insomnia.
Dextromethorphan – Drowsiness; dizziness.
EENT:
Brompheniramine – Diplopia.
GI:
Brompheniramine – Vomiting; diarrhea; dry mouth; nausea; anorexia; heartburn.
Dextromethorphan – GI disturbance.
GU:
Brompheniramine – Polyuria; dysuria; urinary retention in patients with prostatic hypertrophy.
Pseudoephedrine – Dysuria.
RESP:
Pseudoephedrine – Respiratory difficulties.
OTHER:
Brompheniramine – Weakness.
Pseudoephedrine – Pallor.

Precautions
Pregnancy: Category C.
Lactation: Undetermined.
Children: Safety and efficacy in children less than 2 yr not established.
Elderly: Patients 60 yr and older are more likely to exhibit adverse effects.
Special risk patients: Use with caution in patients with hypertension, heart disease, asthma, hyperthyroidism, increased IOP, diabetes mellitus, prostatic hypertrophy.

Overdosage: Signs and Symptoms
Brompheniramine: Young children's predominant symptoms include: excitation, hallucination, ataxia, incoordination, tremors, flushed face, fever, convulsions, fixed and dilated pupils, coma, death; adults' common symptoms include: fever, flushing, excitation, convulsions, postictal depression preceded by drowsiness and coma, respiratory depression
Pseudoephedrine: Restlessness, dizziness, tremor, hyperactive reflexes, talkativeness, irritability, insomnia, cardiovascular and renal effects (eg, difficulty in micturition), headache, flushing, palpitation, cardiac arrhythmia, hypertension with subsequent hypotension and circulatory collapse, dry mouth, metallic taste, anorexia, nausea, vomiting, diarrhea, abdominal cramps
Dextromethorphan: Respiratory depression

PATIENT CARE CONSIDERATIONS
Administration/Storage
- Give prescribed dose q 4 to 6 hr prn, up to qid.
- Give with food if GI upset occurs.
- Store syrup at controlled room temperature (46° to 86°F). Keep tightly closed. Avoid exposure to heat.

Assessment/Interventions
- Obtain patient history, including drug history and any known allergies. Note history of peptic ulcer disease, diabetes, hypertension, hyperthyroidism, enlarged prostate, asthma, narrow-angle glaucoma, urinary retention, severe hypertension or coronary artery disease, concurrent use of or within 2 wk of stopping MAO inhibitor therapy, or allergy to alkylamine antihistamines (eg, triprolidine) or sympathomimetic amines.
- Assess for allergy symptoms (eg, cough, rhinitis, nasal congestion, sneezing, itching, watery eyes) before and periodically throughout therapy.

- Monitor pulse and BP periodically during therapy.
- Monitor patient for nervousness, dizziness, and insomnia. If noted, hold therapy and notify health care provider.

Patient/Family Education
- Explain name, dose, action, and potential side effects of drug.
- Advise patient to take dose q 4 to 6 hr prn, up to qid, as prescribed.
- Advise patient to take with food if GI upset occurs.
- Advise patient to take last dose late in the afternoon or early evening to reduce chance of drug causing sleeplessness.
- Advise patient that if a dose is missed, to take as soon as remembered unless it is nearing time for the next dose. Caution patient not to double the dose to catch up.
- Advise patient that if allergy symptoms are not controlled, not to increase the dose of medication but to inform health care provider.
- Caution patient that drug may cause drowsiness and to use caution while driving or performing other tasks requiring mental alertness until tolerance is determined.
- Advise patient to avoid alcohol and other CNS depressants because of risk of excessive sedation.
- Caution patient not to take any OTC antihistamines or decongestants while taking this medication unless advised by health care provider.
- If patient is to have allergy skin testing, advise not to take the medication for at least 6 days before the skin testing.
- Advise women to notify health care provider if pregnant, planning to become pregnant, or breastfeeding.
- Instruct patient to stop taking drug and immediately report any of the following symptoms to health care provider: nervousness, dizziness, sleeplessness.
- Caution patient not to take any prescription or OTC medications or dietary supplements unless advised by health care provider.

Brompheniramine Tannate

(brome-fen-AIR-uh-mee TAN-nate)

Class Antihistamine

How Supplied
Brovex Tablets, chewable 12 mg, Oral suspension 12 mg/5 mL

Action
PHARMACOLOGY: Competitively antagonizes histamine at H_1 receptor sites.
PHARMACOKINETICS/DYNAMICS:
Absorption: Well absorbed. T_{max} is 2 to 5 hr.
Excretion: The t½ is 25 hr. Renally eliminated.
Onset: Within 60 min.
Peak: 3 to 9 hr.
Duration: 4 to 8 hr.

Indications Relief of sneezing, itchy, watery eyes, itchy nose or throat, and runny nose because of hay fever (allergic rhinitis) or other respiratory allergies.

Contraindications Newborn or premature infants; nursing mothers; lower respiratory conditions, including asthma; MAO inhibitor therapy or for 2 wk after stopping MAO inhibitor therapy; allergy to any component of product.

Route/Dosage
BROVEX SUSPENSION
ADULTS AND CHILDREN 12 YR AND OLDER: PO 5 to 10 mL (1 to 2 tsp [max, 4 tsp/24 hr]).
CHILDREN 6 TO UNDER 12 YR: PO 5 mL (1 tsp [max, 2 tsp/24 hr]).
CHILDREN 2 TO UNDER 6 YR: PO 2.5 mL (½ tsp [max, 1 tsp/24 hr]).
CHILDREN 12 MO TO 2 YR: PO 1.25 mL (¼ tsp [max, ½ tsp/24 hr]).
BROVEX TABLETS
ADULTS AND CHILDREN 12 YR AND OLDER: PO 1 or 2 tablets (max, 4 tablets/24 hr).
CHILDREN 6 TO UNDER 12 YR: PO ½ to 1 tablet (max, 2 tablets/24 hr).
CHILDREN 2 TO UNDER 6 YR: PO ½ tablet (max, 1 tablet/24 hr).

Interactions
Alcohol, barbiturates (eg, phenobarbital), tricyclic antidepressants (eg, amitriptyline), other CNS depressants: Effects may be enhanced by brompheniramine.
MAO inhibitors: Do not use in patients receiving MAO inhibitor therapy or within 14 days of stopping such treatment.
Tricyclic antidepressants (eg, amitriptyline): May prolong or intensify the anticholinergic effects of brompheniramine.

Lab Test Interferences May interfere with diagnostic test results for skin tests using allergen extracts.

Adverse Reactions
CV: Hypotension; palpitations; tachycardia; extrasystoles.
CNS: Drowsiness; headache; sedation; sleepiness; dizziness; disturbed coordination; fatigue;

confusion; restlessness; excitation; nervousness; tremor; irritability; insomnia; euphoria; paresthesia; vertigo; hysteria; neuritis; convulsions.
DERM: Urticaria; drug rash.
EENT: Blurred vision; diplopia; tinnitus; acute labyrinthitis; nasal stuffiness.
GI: Dry mouth, nose, and throat; epigastric distress; anorexia; nausea; vomiting; diarrhea; constipation.
GU: Urinary frequency; difficult urination; urinary retention; early menses.
HEMA: Hemolytic anemia; hypoplastic anemia; thrombocytopenia; agranulocytosis.
RESP: Thickening of bronchial secretions; tightness of chest and wheezing.
OTHER: Anaphylactic shock; photosensitivity; excessive perspiration; chills.

Precautions
Pregnancy: Category B.
Lactation: Undetermined.
Elderly: More likely to cause dizziness, sedation, and hypotension in the elderly.
Special risk patients: Use with caution in patients with hypertension, heart disease, asthma, hyperthyroidism, increased IOP, diabetes mellitus, prostatic hypertrophy, bronchial asthma.

Overdosage: Signs and Symptoms
CNS depression and stimulation, dry mouth, fixed and dilated pupils, flushing, GI symptoms.

PATIENT CARE CONSIDERATIONS
Administration/Storage
- Give prescribed dose q 12 hr without regard to meals. Give with food if GI upset occurs.
- Shake suspension well before measuring dose.
- Provide small amount of water or juice after administering chewable tablet.
- Store tablets and suspension at controlled room temperature (68° to 77°F).

Assessment/Interventions
- Obtain patient history, including drug history and any known allergies. Note history of narrow angle glaucoma, stenosing peptic ulcer, pyloric obstruction, prostatic hypertrophy, bladder neck obstruction, hyperthyroidism, asthma, hypertension, cardiovascular disease, and concurrent or recent use of MAO inhibitors or oral anticoagulants.
- Assess for allergy symptoms (eg, rhinitis, nasal congestion, sneezing, itchy, watery eyes) before and periodically throughout therapy.
- Monitor patient for dizziness and excessive drowsiness. If noted, hold medication and notify health care provider.
- Monitor patient for CNS, CV, GI, RESP, and general body side effects. Inform health care provider if noted and significant.

Patient/Family Education
- Explain name, dose, action, and potential side effects of drug.
- Advise patient to take q 12 hr as prescribed without regard to meals, but to take with food if GI upset occurs.
- Advise patient that if allergy symptoms are not controlled not to increase the dose of medication or frequency of use but to inform health care provider. Inform patient that larger or more frequent dosing does not increase effectiveness and may cause drowsiness.
- Advise patient that medication may cause drowsiness or dizziness and to not drive or perform other activities requiring mental alertness until tolerance is determined.
- Caution patient that alcohol and other CNS depressants (eg, sedatives) will have additional sedative effects if taken with brompheniramine.
- Caution patient not to take any OTC antihistamines while taking this medication unless advised by health care provider.
- Advise patient to take sips of water, suck on ice chips or sugarless hard candy, or chew sugarless gum if dry mouth occurs.
- Caution patient that medication may cause sensitivity to sunlight and to avoid excessive exposure to the sun or UV light (eg, tanning booths) and to use protective clothing and sunscreens until tolerance is determined.
- If patient is to have allergy skin testing, advise to not take the medication for at least 7 days before the skin testing.
- Advise female patient to notify health care provider if pregnant, planning on becoming pregnant, or are breastfeeding.
- Instruct patient to stop taking drug and immediately report any of these symptoms to health care provider: dizziness or excessive drowsiness.
- Caution patient to not take any prescription or OTC medications or dietary supplements unless advised to do so by health care provider.

Budesonide

(byoo-DESS-oh-nide)

Class Corticosteroid

How Supplied
Entocort EC Capsules 3 mg budesonide (micronized) ♦ *Pulmicort Turbuhaler* Powder 200 mcg (each actuation delivers approximately 160 mcg)/metered dose ♦ *Pulmicort Respules* Inhalation suspension 0.25 mg per 2 mL, Inhalation suspension 0.5 mg per 2 mL ♦ *Rhinocort Aqua* Nasal spray 32 mcg budesonide/spray
❦ *Gen-Budesonide AQ* ♦ *Entocort Capsules* ♦ *Entocort Enema* ♦ *Pulmicort Nebuamp* ♦ *Rhinocort Turbuhaler*

Action
PHARMACOLOGY: Exhibits wide range of inhibitory activities against multiple cell types and mediators involved in allergic-mediated inflammation.

PHARMACOKINETICS/DYNAMICS:
Absorption:
Oral – 9% systemic availability.
Oral inhalation – 34% systemically available from lungs. T_{max} is within 30 min.
Intranasal – About 34% reaches systemic circulation. T_{max} is about 0.7 hr.

Distribution: Vd is 2 to 3 L/kg (or 200 L). Budesonide is 85% to 90% protein bound.

Metabolism:
Liver – Rapidly metabolized; CYP3A4 is involved in the formation of 2 metabolites (less than 1% of budesonide activity).

Excretion: The t½ is 2 to 3 hr. Budesonide is excreted in the urine (about 60%) and feces as metabolites; no unchanged drug is detected in the urine.

Special Populations:
Children – Plasma concentrations are approximately twice those of adults.

Indications
Intranasal: Management of seasonal and perennial allergic rhinitis symptoms in adults and children (*Rhinocort Aqua*).
Oral inhalation: For the maintenance treatment of asthma as prophylactic therapy in adults and children and for patients requiring oral corticosteroid therapy for asthma (inhaler).
Inhalation suspension: Maintenance treatment of asthma and prophylactic therapy in children 12 mo to 8 yr of age.
Oral capsule: Crohn disease.

Contraindications Untreated localized infections involving the nasal mucosa; relief of acute bronchospasm; primary treatment of status asthmaticus or other acute episodes of asthma when intensive measures are required; hypersensitivity to the drug or drug compound of the product. Not recommended for treatment of nonallergic rhinitis because of lack of data.

Route/Dosage
NASAL SPRAY
ADULT AND CHILDREN AT LEAST 12 YR OF AGE: **Spray** Start with 64 mcg/day administered as 1 spray in each nostril daily.
Maintenance: **Spray** Titrate to minimum effective dose (max, 256 mcg/day administered as 4 sprays in each nostril daily).
ADULT AND CHILDREN 6 TO UNDER 12 YR OF AGE: **Spray** Start with 64 mcg/day administered as 1 spray in each nostril daily.
Maintenance: **Spray** Titrate to minimum effective dose (max, 128 mcg/day administered as 2 sprays in each nostril daily).

AEROSOL, TURBUHALER
ADULTS: **Oral inhaler** 200 to 400 mcg bid (max, 800 mcg bid).
CHILDREN AT LEAST 6 YR OF AGE: **Oral inhaler** 200 mcg bid (max, 400 mcg bid).

RESPULES
CHILDREN 12 MO TO 8 YR OF AGE: **Inhalation suspension** Administer by inhaled route via jet nebulizer connected to air compressor.
CHILDREN RECEIVING BRONCHODILATORS ALONE: 0.5 mg/day administered daily or bid in divided doses (max, 0.5 mg/day).
CHILDREN RECEIVING INHALED CORTICOSTEROIDS: 0.5 mg/day administered daily or bid in divided doses (max, 1 mg/day).
CHILDREN RECEIVING ORAL CORTICOSTEROIDS: 1 mg/day administered as 0.5 mg bid or 1 mg daily (max, 1 mg/day).

ORAL CAPSULES
ADULTS: **PO** 9 mg daily in the morning for up to 8 wk (Crohn disease); can be tapered to 6 mg daily for 2 wk prior to complete cessation.

Interactions
Grapefruit juice, CYP3A4 inhibitors (eg, ketoconazole, ritonavir): May increase budesonide plasma levels, increasing the pharmacologic and adverse effects.

Lab Test Interferences None well documented.

Adverse Reactions
CV: Hypertension, palpitations, tachycardia (oral).
CNS: Headache, dizziness, fatigue, hyperkinesis, paresthesia, tremor, agitation, increased appetite, confusion, insomnia, nervousness, sleep disorder, somnolence (oral).
DERM: Acne, alopecia, dermatitis, eczema, skin

disorder, increased sweating (oral).
EENT: Nasal irritation/bleeding; burning; stinging; sneezing; pharyngitis; glossitis, ear infection, vertigo, eye abnormality, abnormal vision (oral).
GI: Dry mouth; indigestion; nausea, dyspepsia, abdominal pain, flatulence, vomiting, anus disorder, aggravated Crohn disease, enteritis, epigastric pain, GI fistula, hemorrhoids, intestinal obstruction, tongue edema, tooth disorder (oral).
GU: Intermenstrual bleeding, menstrual disorder, dysuria, micturition frequency, nocturia, hematuria, pyuria (oral).
HEMA: Leukocytosis, anemia, increased erythrocyte sedimentation rate (oral).
HYPERSEN: Immediate or delayed reactions including urticaria; angioedema; rash; bronchospasm; face and tongue edema; pruritus; wheezing; dyspnea.
METAB: Hypokalemia, weight increase (oral).
RESP: Increased cough; respiratory tract infection, bronchitis, dyspnea (oral).
OTHER: Symptoms of hypercorticism, back pain, pain, asthenia, increased C-reactive protein, chest pain, dependent edema, face edema, flu-like symptoms, malaise, aggravated arthritis, cramps, myalgia, moniliasis, flushing (oral).

Precautions

Pregnancy: Category B (inhalation). Category C (oral, intranasal).
Lactation: Undetermined. Use caution because other corticosteroids are excreted in human milk.
Children: Not recommended for children under 6 yr of age (intranasal, oral inhaler), or under 12 mo of age (respules); safety and efficacy not established in children for *Entocort EC*.
Corticosteroids may suppress growth in children and adolescents, particularly with higher doses over extended periods.
Elderly: Select dose with caution, reflecting greater frequency of decreased hepatic, renal, or cardiac function and comorbidity.
Hypersensitivity: Immediate hypersensitivity reactions have occurred.
Special risk patients: Use with caution in patients with tuberculosis infection, hypertension, diabetes mellitus, osteoporosis, peptic ulcer, glaucoma or cataracts, with a family history of diabetes or glaucoma, or with any condition in which glucocorticoids may have unwanted effects. Use inhaled corticosteroids with caution in patients with active or quiescent tuberculosis infection, untreated systemic fungal, bacterial, parasitic, or viral infections, or ocular herpes simplex.
Allergy: Transfer of patients from systemic steroids therapy to inhalation therapy may unmask allergic conditions previously suppressed by systemic steroid therapy (eg, rhinitis).
Bronchospasm: With inhaled asthma medications, bronchospasm may occur with an immediate increase in wheezing following dosing, which may require immediate treatment with a fast-acting inhaled bronchodilator.
Fungal infections: Antifungal treatment or discontinuation of corticosteroid therapy may be necessary.
Immunology: Patients receiving immunosuppressant agents are more susceptible to infections than healthy adults. If a patient is exposed to measles or chickenpox, appropriate prophylaxis and treatment may be indicated.
Pulmicort Turbuhaler: Transfer from oral corticosteroids to inhaled corticosteroids has resulted in death caused by adrenal insufficiency related to a lower systemic availability. A number of months are required for recovery of hypothalamic-pituitary adrenal (HPA) axis suppression. Patients maintained on 20 mg or more prednisone daily may be at higher risk. During periods of stress or severe asthma attack, instruct patients who have been withdrawn from systemic corticosteroids to resume oral steroids immediately.
Systemic effects: Use cautiously in patients taking daily or alternate-day steroid therapy; may increase likelihood of HPA suppression. Exceeding recommended dose may cause systemic effects.
Wound healing: Because of inhibitory effect of corticosteroids on wound healing, patients experiencing recent nasal septal ulcers, nasal surgery, or nasal trauma should not use nasal corticosteroids until healing has occurred.

Overdosage: Signs and Symptoms
Hypercorticoidism, adrenal suppression.

PATIENT CARE CONSIDERATIONS

Administration/Storage
PO:
- Administer prescribed dose daily in the morning. Administer without regard to meals but administer with food if GI upset occurs.
- Have patient swallow capsules whole. Do not crush, chew, or break capsules.
- Store capsules at ambient room temperature (59° to 86°F).

Oral Inhalation powder:
- May be administered alone or in combination with systemic corticosteroids.
- If patient is also receiving bronchodilators by inhalation, administer bronchodilator 5 min before budesonide to enhance penetration of latter drug into bronchial tree.
- Hold delivery canister in upright position (mouthpiece on top) during priming and

loading. Prime the unit before the first use by turning the brown grip fully to the right, then fully to the left until it clicks. Repeat a second time.
- Have patient exhale fully. Load inhaler by holding upright and turning brown grip fully to right, then fully to left until it clicks. Do not shake inhaler. While keeping inhaler in an upright or horizontal position, have patient place mouthpiece between lips and inhale forcefully and deeply. Have patient hold breath for 10 sec and breathe out slowly. Allow at least 1 min between inhalations. Have patient rinse mouth with water or mouthwash after each use.
- Do not use with a spacer device (eg, Aerochamber). Do not bite or chew mouthpiece, exhale into the inhalation device, wash or attempt to take the inhalation device apart. Replace cover securely after each use.
- Store inhalation device at controlled room temperature (68° to 77°F). Keep tightly capped and protect from moisture. Discard when red mark appears at bottom of indicator window.

Inhalation Suspension:
- Administer only via jet nebulizer. Not for injection or oral use or administration by ultrasonic nebulizer.
- Medication requires no dilution before administration and is added directly into the nebulizer reservoir. Gently shake vial using circular motion before adding to nebulizer reservoir.
- Once vial has been opened, administer promptly or discard.
- Discard any unused solution.
- Do not mix with other nebulized medications unless ordered by health care provider.
- Store unused vials in upright position in protective foil pouch at controlled room temperature (68° to 77°F). Protect from light. Do not refrigerate or freeze. After opening foil pouch, return unused vials to pouch to protect from light. Unused vials must be used within 14 days after pouch has been opened.

Nasal Inhalation:
- For intranasal use only. Avoid spraying into the nose or mouth.
- Shake gently before each use.
- Actuate the pump 8 times to prime before first use. If pump has not been used for 2 consecutive days, reprime the pump with 1 spray. If pump has not been used for more than 14 days, rinse the applicator and reprime the pump with 2 sprays.
- Clear nasal passages of secretions prior to use. If patient is congested, use topical, short-acting decongestant just before administration to ensure adequate penetration of spray. Saline nasal lavage may help remove secretions.
- Place nasal adapter into 1 nostril, gently close other nostril with finger. While inhaling from nostril, activate canister. Repeat process on other side.
- Do not blow nose immediately after administration.
- If 2 sprays per dose are ordered, administer 1 spray in each nostril, wait a few seconds, and administer second spray into each nostril.
- Store nasal spray at controlled room temperature (68° to 77°F). Protect from freezing. Discard bottle when labeled number of sprays have been used, even if bottle is not completely empty.

Assessment/Interventions

- Obtain patient history, including drug history and any known allergies. Note hepatic impairment, diabetes, osteoporosis, glaucoma, cataracts, peptic ulcer disease, untreated fungal, bacterial or systemic viral infection, active or quiescent tuberculosis, ocular herpes simplex, recent nasal surgery, trauma or septal ulcers (intranasal only), or concurrent use of CYP3A4 inhibitors (eg, ketoconazole).

Oral:
- If patient is being changed from a corticosteroid with high systemic effects (eg, prednisone) to budesonide, ensure that dose of systemic steroid is reduced cautiously. Observe patient carefully for signs of adrenal insufficiency (eg, nausea, fatigue, dizziness, hypotension, depression, abdominal, joint, or muscle pain). Notify health care provider if these signs occur.
- Document baseline disease state activity. Reassess periodically to document response to therapy.
- Ensure that therapy is periodically reviewed to determine if therapy needs to be continued without change or if a dose change (eg, increase, decrease, discontinuation) is indicated.
- Monitor blood sugar in diabetic patient when drug is started or dose is changed. Report significant changes to health care provider.
- Ensure that fasting blood glucose is evaluated before starting therapy and periodically thereafter during therapy in patient with risk factors for diabetes mellitus (eg, obesity, family history of diabetes).
- If treatment is to be discontinued after long-term use, ensure that dose is gradually tapered to prevent adrenal insufficiency from occurring. If symptoms of adrenal insufficiency occur, reinstitute previous dosing schedule

and attempt a less rapid tapering regimen after patient has stabilized.
- Monitor patient for GI, CNS, DERM, and general body side effects. Notify health care provider if noted and significant.

Oral Inhalation/Intranasal:

- If change is made from systemic (oral) to inhaled or intranasal corticosteroids, observe patient carefully for signs of adrenal insufficiency (eg, nausea, fatigue, dizziness, hypotension, depression, abdominal, joint, or muscle pain). Notify health care provider if these signs occur. Deaths caused by adrenal insufficiency have occurred during and after converting to aerosol corticosteroids.
- Assess patient's symptoms before initiating therapy and periodically during treatment. Notify health care provider if symptoms do not improve or worsen.
- Plot growth pattern in children on prolonged therapy with systemic product. Inform health care provider if abnormalities noted.
- Notify health care provider if oral, nasal, or pharyngeal irritation occurs or if symptoms worsen.

Patient/Family Education

- Explain name, dose, action, and potential side effects of drug.
- Advise patient to read the *Patient Information* leaflet before starting therapy and again with each refill.
- Advise patient to continue taking other medications for same condition as prescribed by health care provider.
- Advise patient that dose may be changed periodically, depending on how well symptoms are controlled.
- Explain that effects of drug are not immediate. Benefit requires daily use as instructed and usually begins to occur within 1 or 2 days, but full benefit may take 1 to 2 wk, depending on the condition being treated and the dose and route of administration of medication being used.
- Caution patient not to decrease the dose or stop taking unless advised by health care provider.
- Caution patient not to increase dose but to inform health care provider if symptoms do not seem to be improving or are worsening.
- If patient is being converted from oral to inhaled or intranasal corticosteroids, review signs and symptoms of adrenal insufficiency, which may occur days or weeks after conversion is complete. Advise patient to carry *Medi-Alert* card indicating possible need of supplemental systemic corticosteroids during periods of stress or a severe asthma attack.
- Instruct diabetic patient to monitor blood glucose more frequently when drug is started or dose is changed and to inform health care provider of significant changes in readings.
- Advise patient to immediately notify health care provider if any of the following occur: swelling of feet or ankles, muscle weakness, black tarry stools, vomiting of blood, fever, sore throat, or other signs of infection.
- Advise patient to avoid exposure to chickenpox and measles and to seek medical advice immediately if exposed.
- Advise women to notify health care provider if pregnant, planning to become pregnant, or breastfeeding.
- Caution patient to not take any prescription or OTC medications, dietary supplements, or herbal preparations unless advised by health care provider.
- Advise patient that follow-up visits may be required to monitor therapy and to keep appointments.

Oral Inhalation Powder:

- Review proper administration technique. Have patient demonstrate technique to ensure effective use of the delivery system.
- Warn patient that drug is an asthma controller and is not to be used to treat an acute asthma attack. Rescue medication (bronchodilator) must be used to obtain rapid relief of asthma symptoms.
- Instruct patient not to stop the medication once symptoms have been controlled. Continued daily use is necessary to control symptoms.
- Advise patient to discard the inhaler when red mark appears at bottom of indicator window.
- Instruct patient to carry *Medi-Alert* card if he or she experiences acute severe asthma attacks requiring rapid systemic treatment.
- Advise patient to report the following symptoms to health care provider: sore throat or mouth, cough, dry mouth, rash, facial swelling, worsening asthma symptoms (increasing need for bronchodilator).

Inhalation Suspension:

- Ensure caregiver can prepare, use, and clean the nebulizer without difficulty.
- Instruct caregiver not to mix with other nebulizer medications unless advised by health care provider.
- Instruct caregiver to use nebulizer solution immediately after opening. If solution is not used immediately, advise patient or caregiver to discard the solution.
- Advise caregiver to discard any unused nebulizer solution.

- Advise caregiver to rinse child's mouth and wash face after each treatment.

Nasal Inhalation:
- Review proper administration technique. Have patient demonstrate technique to ensure effective use of the nasal spray.
- Instruct patient not to stop the medication once symptoms have been controlled. Continued daily use is necessary to control symptoms.
- Instruct patient to use with caution if sores develop or injuries occur in nasal passages. Drug may prevent or slow proper healing.
- Advise patient to report the following symptoms to health care provider: sneezing, nasal irritation, nosebleed.
- Advise patient to discard bottle when labeled number of sprays have been used even if bottle is not completely empty.

Oral:
- Advise patient to take prescribed dose daily in the morning.
- Advise patient that medication can be taken without regard to meals but to take with food if stomach upset occurs.
- Advise patient to swallow capsules whole and not to chew, crush, or break the capsule.
- Caution patient to avoid consumption of grapefruit juice for duration of therapy.
- Advise patient to carry *Medi-Alert* card indicating use of corticosteroids, the condition(s) being treated, and possible need of supplemental systemic corticosteroids during periods of stress.
- Caution patient not to suddenly stop taking this medication after more than 1 mo of use. Advise patient that if medication needs to be discontinued after prolonged therapy (eg, greater than 1 mo), it will be slowly withdrawn to prevent adrenal insufficiency.
- Review signs and symptoms of adrenal insufficiency (eg, nausea, fatigue, dizziness, hypotension, depression, abdominal, joint, or muscle pain). Instruct patient to immediately seek medical care if symptoms suggestive of adrenal insufficiency develop.

Bumetanide

(BYOO-MET-uh-nide)

Class Loop diuretic

How Supplied
Bumex Tablets 0.5 mg, Tablets 1 mg, Tablets 2 mg, Injection 0.25 mg/mL
✤ *Burinex*

Action
PHARMACOLOGY: Inhibits reabsorption of sodium and chloride in proximal tubules and loop of Henle.

PHARMACOKINETICS/DYNAMICS:
Distribution: Bumetanide is 72% to 96% protein bound.
Metabolism: Oxidation of the N-butyl side chain.
Excretion: The t½ is 60 to 90 min; 81% is excreted in urine, 45% as unchanged drug, and 2% in bile.

Onset:
Oral – 30 to 60 min.
IV – Within minutes.

Peak:
Oral – 1 to 2 hr.
IV – 15 to 30 min.

Duration:
Oral – 4 to 6 hr.

Special Populations:
Renal Function Impairment – The t½ is prolonged.
Children – Elimination is considerably slower in neonates.

Indications Treatment of edema associated with CHF, hepatic cirrhosis and renal disease.
Unlabeled use(s): Relief of adult nocturia.

Contraindications Hypersensitivity to other loop diuretics or to sulfonylureas; anuria; hepatic coma or states of severe electrolyte depletion until condition is improved or corrected.

Route/Dosage
ADULTS: PO 0.5 to 2 mg/day as single dose. If inadequate response, give second or third dose at 4 to 5 hr intervals up to max 10 mg/day.
IM/IV 0.5 to 1 mg/day over 1 to 2 min. May repeat at 2- to 3-hr intervals, up to max 10 mg/day. Reserve parenteral route for situations in which GI absorption is impaired or when oral administration is not practical; replace with oral therapy as soon as possible.

Interactions
Aminoglycosides: Increased auditory toxicity.
Cisplatin: Additive ototoxicity.
Digitalis glycosides: Electrolyte disturbances may predispose to digitalis-induced arrhythmias.
Lithium: Increased plasma lithium levels and toxicity.
NSAIDs: Decreased effects of bumetanide.
Salicylates: Impaired diuretic response in patients with cirrhosis and ascites.
Thiazide diuretics: Synergistic effects that may result in profound diuresis and serious electrolyte abnormalities.

Lab Test Interferences None well documented.

Adverse Reactions
CV: Hypotension; ECG changes; chest pain.

CNS: Asterixis; encephalopathy with pre-existing liver disease; vertigo; headache; dizziness.
DERM: Hives; pruritus; itching; nipple tenderness; rash; photosensitivity.
EENT: Impaired hearing; ear discomfort; tinnitus; deafness.
GI: Upset stomach; dry mouth; nausea; vomiting; diarrhea; pain.
GU: Premature ejaculation; difficulty maintaining erection; renal failure.
HEMA: Thrombocytopenia; deviations in Hgb, Hct, prothrombin time and WBC, platelets, and differential counts.
METAB: Glucosuria and proteinuria; hyperuricemia; gout; hypochloremia; hypokalemia; azotemia; hyponatremia; increased serum creatinine; hyperglycemia; variations in phosphorus, CO_2 content, bicarbonate, and calcium; increases in LDL, total cholesterol, and triglycerides; decreases in HDL cholesterol.
RESP: Hyperventilation.
OTHER: Musculoskeletal weakness; arthritic pain; pain; muscle cramps; fatigue; dehydration; sweating.

> **WARNING:**
> Excessive amounts may cause profound diuresis and water/electrolyte depletion. Careful medical supervision required with dosage adjustment and schedule to individual patient need.

Precautions
Pregnancy: Category C.
Lactation: Undetermined.
Children: Safety and efficacy not established in children under 18 yr.
Renal function impairment: In severe chronic renal insufficiency, patients may benefit from continuous infusion (12 mg over 12 hr), rather than from intermittent bolus therapy. Monitor renal function and discontinue drug if renal function decreases further.
Dehydration: Excessive diuresis may cause dehydration and decreased blood volume with circulatory collapse and possible vascular thrombosis and embolism, especially in elderly patients.
Hepatic cirrhosis and ascites: Sudden alterations of electrolyte balance may precipitate hepatic encephalopathy and coma.
Ototoxicity: Associated with rapid injection, very large doses or concurrent use of other ototoxic drugs.
Systemic lupus erythematosus: May be exacerbated or activated.

Overdosage: Signs and Symptoms
Profound water loss, volume and electrolyte depletion (characterized by weakness, dizziness, mental confusion, anorexia, lethargy, vomiting, cramps), dehydration, reduction in blood volume, circulatory collapse with possible thrombosis and embolism.

PATIENT CARE CONSIDERATIONS
Administration/Storage
- Give with food or milk to reduce GI upset.
- Administer by parenteral route only in patients with impaired GI absorption or when oral route is not practical.
- Drug is most effective when given on alternate days or for 3 to 4 days with rest intervals of 1 to 2 days.
- If given by IV infusion, use solution within 24 hr of preparation.
- Store at room temperature in tightly closed container.

Assessment/Interventions
- Obtain patient history, including drug history and any known allergies. Note systemic lupus erythematosus or renal impairment.
- Ensure that baseline electrolytes have been obtained prior to administration. Do not administer to electrolyte-depleted patients.
- Check that baseline creatine, BUN, calcium, uric acid, and CBC have been obtained before beginning therapy and monitor throughout therapy.
- Monitor BP and pulse rate frequently.
- Monitor I&O and daily weight during therapy.
- Observe for ototoxicity, especially in patients receiving drug via IV infusion and in those taking other ototoxic drugs.
- Ensure that patient maintains adequate hydration to prevent dehydration.
- Have epinephrine 1:1000 available if hypersensitivity reaction occurs.
- If tinnitus, hearing impairment, or fullness in ears is reported, notify health care provider.

Patient/Family Education
- Instruct patient to take as single dose early in day. Drug can be taken with food or milk to reduce GI upset.
- Advise patient to drink adequate fluids to prevent dehydration unless fluid restrictions apply.
- Caution patient to get out of bed slowly on arising, and to avoid sudden position changes to prevent orthostatic hypotension.
- If patient is not taking a potassium supplement, advise patient to increase potassium-rich foods in daily diet.

- Instruct patient to report the following symptoms to health care provider: signs of bleeding, weakness, cramps, nausea or dizziness.
- Caution patient to avoid exposure to sunlight, and to use sunscreen or wear protective clothing to avoid photosensitivity reaction.
- Advise diabetic patients to monitor blood glucose carefully because drug may cause loss of glycemic control.

Buprenorphine Hydrochloride

BYOO-preh-NAHR-feen HIGH-droe-KLOR-ide

Class Narcotic agonist-antagonist analgesic

How Supplied
Buprenex Injection 0.324 mg (equiv. to 0.3 mg buprenorphine)/mL *Subutex* Tablets, sublingual 2 mg, Tablets, sublingual 8 mg

Action
PHARMACOLOGY: Analgesic effect caused by binding to opiate receptors in the CNS. Antagonist effects decrease abuse potential.

PHARMACOKINETICS/DYNAMICS:
Absorption: C_{max} is approximately 5.47 ng/mL (16 mg SL dose). AUC is approximately 32.63 hr•ng/mL (16 mg SL dose).
Distribution: Approximately 96% protein bound.
Metabolism: Undergoes CYP3A4-mediated N-dealkylation to norbuprenorphine (active) and glucuronidation.
Excretion: 30% is excreted in the urine and 69% in the feces. The t½ is 37 hr.
Onset: 15 min (IM).
Peak: 1 hr (IM).
Duration: At least 6 hr (IM).

Indications
Tablet: Treatment of opioid dependence.
Injection: Relief of moderate to severe pain.

Contraindications Standard considerations.

Route/Dosage
TABLETS

ADULTS: SL (Use limited to health care providers who meet certain qualifications and have notified the Health and Human Services of their intent to prescribe.) 12 to 16 mg/day.

INJECTION

ADULTS AND CHILDREN (13 YR AND OLDER): IM/IV 0.3 mg deep IM or slow IV (over at least 2 min) at up to 6 hr intervals, as needed. May repeat once (up to 0.3 mg) 30 to 60 min after initial dosage, if required.

Interactions
Barbiturate anesthetics: May have additive effects with buprenorphine, increasing the respiratory and CNS effects.
Benzodiazepines (eg, diazepam): Coma and death have been associated with misuse of buprenorphine and benzodiazepines.
CNS depressants (eg, alcohol, phenothiazines, sedative-hypnotics): Increased CNS depression may occur.
CYP3A4 inducers (eg, carbamazepine, phenytoin, rifampin): May reduce buprenorphine plasma levels, decreasing the efficacy.
CYP3A4 inhibitors (eg, erythromycin, ketoconazole, ritonavir): May elevate buprenorphine plasma levels, increasing the risk of side effects.

Lab Test Interferences None well documented.

Adverse Reactions
CV: Hypotension; hypertension; tachycardia; bradycardia.
CNS: Sedation; dizziness/vertigo; headache; confusion; dreaming; psychosis; euphoria; weakness/fatigue; malaise; hallucinations; depersonalization; coma; tremor; dysphoria; agitation; convulsions; lack of muscle coordination; insomnia.
DERM: Sweating; pruritus; injections site reaction; rash; pallor; urticaria.
EENT: Miosis.
GI: Nausea; vomiting; constipation; dry mouth; dyspepsia; flatulence; loss of appetite; diarrhea; abdominal pain.
HEPA: Hepatitis and hepatitis with jaundice.
RESP: Hypoventilation.
OTHER: Chronic and acute hypersensitivity; infection.

Precautions
Pregnancy: Category C.
Lactation: Excreted in breast milk.
Children: Safety and efficacy not established in children under 13 yr.
Special risk patients: Use with caution in elderly or debilitated patients; use with caution in patients with impaired hepatic, renal or pulmonary function, myxedema or hypothyroidism, adrenal cortical insufficiency (eg, Addison disease), CNS depression or coma, toxic psychoses, prostatic hypertrophy or urethral stricture, acute alcoholism, delirium tremens or kyphoscoliosis, biliary tract dysfunction.
Abdominal conditions: May obscure diagnosis or clinical course of patients with acute abdominal conditions.
Dependency: Buprenorphine has abuse potential. Psychological and physical dependence as well as tolerance may occur.
Head injury or increased intracranial pressure: Use with caution; drug can increase CSF pressure.

Narcotic dependent patients: Use in physically dependent individuals may result in withdrawal effects.

PATIENT CARE CONSIDERATIONS

Administration/Storage

Sublingual tablets:
- For sublingual use only. Do not chew, crush, or swallow tablets.
- Buprenorphine and buprenorphine/naloxone tablets are interchangeable.
- Do not initiate therapy until objective signs of opioid withdrawal are evident.
- Administer prescribed dose once daily.
- Place tablets under the tongue until they are dissolved. Swallowing tablets reduces effectiveness.
- For dose requiring more than 2 tablets, place all tablets under the tongue and allow to dissolve. If patient cannot fit more than 2 tablets under the tongue at one time, then place 2 tablets under the tongue at a time.
- Store tablets at controlled room temperature (59° to 86°F).

Injection:
- For deep IM or slow IV (over at least 2 min) administration only. Not for intradermal, SC, or intra-arterial administration.
- Prescribed dose may be given at up to q 6 hr, as needed for pain relief. May repeat dose once, if required for pain relief, 30 to 60 min after first dose.
- Administer reduced dose to high-risk patient (eg, elderly, debilitated, impaired respiratory function) or in patient receiving other CNS depressants (eg, postoperative).
- Store injection at controlled room temperature (59° to 86°F). Avoid freezing or exposure to excessive heat (over 104°F). Protect from prolonged exposure to light.

Assessment/Interventions

- Obtain patient history, including drug history and any known allergies. Note presence of hepatic or renal impairment, compromised respiratory function (eg, COPD), biliary tract dysfunction, acute abdominal condition, hypothyroidism, adrenal cortical insufficiency (Addison disease), CNS depression, toxic psychosis, prostatic hypertrophy or urethral stricture, acute alcoholism, delerium tremens, kyphoscoliosis, intracranial lesion, or history of recent head injury.
- Ensure that liver enzymes and hepatic function are evaluated prior to starting therapy and periodically during treatment.
- Document type of opioid dependence (eg, long-, short-acting), time since last opioid use, and degree of opioid dependence prior to starting sublingual tablets.
- Monitor patient for respiratory depression. If noted, re-establish adequate ventilation with mechanical assistance and notify health care provider immediately. Naloxone may not be effective in reversing respiratory depression caused by this drug.
- Monitor patient for narcotic withdrawal symptoms, CNS, GI, and general body side effects. Report to health care provider if noted and significant.

Patient/Family Education

- Explain name, dose, action, and potential side effects of drug.

Injection:
- Advise patient, family, or caregiver that medication is used to control pain and will be prepared and administered by a health care provider in a medical setting.

Sublingual tablets:
- Advise patient to take prescribed dose once daily by placing tablet under the tongue until dissolved. For dose requiring more than 2 tablets, advise patient to place all tablets under the tongue and allow to dissolve. If patient cannot fit more than 2 tablets under the tongue at one time, then advise patient to place 2 tablets under the tongue at a time and repeat until entire dose has been taken.
- Caution patient that swallowing tablets reduces effectiveness.
- Advise patient to not change the dose or stop taking unless advised by the health care provider.
- Caution patient to avoid alcoholic beverages and other CNS depressants (eg, narcotics, benzodiazepines) while taking this drug. Combined use may result in a serious overdose and possibly death.
- Advise patient to inform family members that, in the event of an emergency, the treating emergency personnel should be informed that the patient is physically dependent on narcotics and is being treated with buprenorphine.
- Advise patient that drug may impair mental or physical abilities required for the performance of potentially hazardous tasks and to use caution while driving or performing other tasks requiring mental alertness until tolerance is determined.
- Caution patient to avoid sudden position changes to prevent orthostatic hypotension.

Overdosage: Signs and Symptoms

Respiratory depression, pinpoint pupils, sedation, hypotension, death.

- Instruct patient to lie or sit down if they experience dizziness or lightheadedness when standing.
- Advise patient to contact health care provider if experiencing the following side effects: headache, insomnia, nausea, vomiting, or abdominal pain.
- Instruct patient not to take prescription or OTC drugs or dietary supplements without consulting health care provider.
- Advise women to notify health care provider if pregnant, planning to become pregnant, or breastfeeding.
- Advise patient that follow-up visits may be required to monitor therapy and to keep appointments.

Buprenorphine Hydrochloride/Naloxone Hydrochloride

BYOO-preh-NAHR-feen HIGH-droe-KLOR-ide/NAL-ox-ohn HIGH-droe-KLOR-ide

Class Narcotic agonist-antagonist analgesic

How Supplied
Suboxone Tablets, sublingual 2 mg buprenorphine base per 0.5 naloxone, Tablets, sublingual 8 mg buprenorphine base per 2 mg naloxone

Action

PHARMACOLOGY:

Buprenorphine: Analgesic effect caused by binding to opiate receptors in the CNS, while antagonist effects decrease abuse potential.
Naloxone: Possibly antagonizes opioid effects by competing for the same receptor sites.

Indications Treatment of opioid dependence.

Contraindications Standard consideration.

Route/Dosage

ADULTS AND CHILDREN (16 YR AND OLDER): SL Single daily dose in the range of 12 to 16 mg of buprenorphine. The dose should be adjusted in increments or decrements of 2 or 4 mg to a level that holds the patient in treatment and suppresses opioid withdrawal effects. This is likely to range between 4 and 24 mg/day.

Interactions

Barbiturate anesthetics: May have additive effects with buprenorphine, increasing the respiratory and CNS effects.
Benzodiazepines (eg, diazepam): Coma and death have been associated with misuse of buprenorphine and benzodiazepines.
CNS depressants (eg, alcohol, phenothiazines, sedative-hypnotics): Increased CNS depression may occur.
CYP3A4 inducers (eg, carbamazepine, phenytoin, rifampin): May reduce buprenorphine plasma levels, decreasing the efficacy.
CYP3A4 inhibitors (eg, erythromycin, ketoconazole, ritonavir): May elevate buprenorphine plasma levels, increasing the risk of side effects.

Lab Test Interferences None well documented.

Adverse Reactions

CV: Vasodilation.
CNS: Headache; insomnia; anxiety; depression; dizziness; nervousness; somnolence.
DERM: Sweating.
EENT: Rhinitis; pharyngitis; runny eyes.
GI: Abdominal pain; constipation; diarrhea; nausea; vomiting; dyspepsia.
RESP: Increased cough.
OTHER: Pain; back pain; withdrawal symptoms; abscess; asthenia; chills; fever; flu syndrome; infection; accidental injury.

Precautions

Pregnancy: Category C.
Lactation: Buprenorphine is excreted in breast milk.
Children: Safety and efficacy not established in children below the age of 16 yr.
Special risk patients: Use with caution in elderly or debilitated patients; use with caution in patients with impaired hepatic, renal, or pulmonary function (eg, chronic obstructive pulmonary disease), myxedema or hypothyroidism, adrenal cortical insufficiency (eg, Addison disease), CNS depression or coma, toxic psychoses, prostatic hypertrophy or urethral stricture, acute alcoholism, delirium tremens or kyphoscoliosis, or biliary tract dysfunction.
Dependency: Buprenorphine has abuse potential. Psychological and physical dependence as well as tolerance may occur.
Head injury or increased IOP: Use with caution; drug can increase CSF pressure.
Withdrawal: Marked and intense withdrawal symptoms are likely to occur if misused parenterally by individuals dependent on opioid agonists; sublingual use may cause opioid withdrawal symptoms if administered before the agonist effects of the opioid have subsided.

Overdosage: Signs and Symptoms
Pinpoint pupils, sedation, hypotension, respiratory depression, death.

PATIENT CARE CONSIDERATIONS

Administration/Storage
- For sublingual administration only. Do not chew, crush, or swallow tablets.
- Buprenorphine and buprenorphine/naloxone tablets are interchangeable.
- Do not initiate therapy until objective signs

of opioid withdrawal are evident.
- Administer prescribed dose once daily.
- Place tablets under the tongue until they are dissolved. Swallowing tablets reduces effectiveness.
- For dose requiring more than 2 tablets, place all tablets under the tongue and allow to dissolve. If patient cannot fit more than 2 tablets under the tongue at one time, then place 2 tablets under the tongue at a time.
- Store tablets at controlled room temperature (59° to 86°F).

Assessment/Interventions
- Obtain patient history, including drug history and any known allergies. Note presence of hepatic or renal impairment, compromised respiratory function (eg, COPD), biliary tract dysfunction, acute abdominal condition, hypothyroidism, adrenal cortical insufficiency (Addison disease), CNS depression, toxic psychosis, prostatic hypertrophy or urethral stricture, acute alcoholism, delerium tremens, kyphoscoliosis, intracranial lesion, or history of recent head injury.
- Document type of opioid dependence (eg, long-, short-acting), time since last opioid use, and degree of opioid dependence prior to starting therapy.
- Ensure that liver enzymes and hepatic function are evaluated prior to starting therapy and periodically during treatment.
- Monitor patient for respiratory depression. If noted, re-establish adequate ventilation with mechanical assistance and notify health care provider immediately. Naloxone may not be effective in reversing respiratory depression caused by this drug.
- Monitor patient for narcotic withdrawal symptoms, CNS, GI, and general body side effects. Report to health care provider if noted and significant.

Patient/Family Education
- Explain name, dose, action, and potential side effects of drug.
- Advise patient to take prescribed dose once daily by placing tablet under the tongue until dissolved. For dose requiring more than 2 tablets, advise patient to place all tablets under the tongue and allow to dissolve. If patient cannot fit more than 2 tablets under the tongue at 1 time, then advise patient to place 2 tablets under the tongue at a time and repeat until entire dose has been taken.
- Caution patient that swallowing tablets reduces effectiveness.
- Advise patient to not change the dose or stop taking unless advised by the health care provider.
- Caution patient to avoid alcoholic beverages and other CNS depressants (eg, narcotics, benzodiazepines) while taking this drug. Combined use may result in a serious toxicity and possibly death.
- Advise patient to inform family members that, in the event of an emergency, the treating emergency personnel should be informed that the patient is physically dependent on narcotics and is being treated with buprenorphine.
- Advise patient that drug may impair mental or physical abilities required for the performance of potentially hazardous tasks and to use caution while driving or performing other tasks requiring mental alertness until tolerance is determined.
- Caution patient to avoid sudden position changes to prevent orthostatic hypotension.
- Instruct patient to lie or sit down if experiencing dizziness or lightheadedness when standing.
- Advise patient to contact their health care provider if experiencing the following side effects: headache, insomnia, nausea, vomiting, abdominal pain.
- Instruct patient not to take prescription or OTC drugs or dietary supplements without consulting with their health care provider.
- Advise women to notify health care provider if pregnant, planning to become pregnant, or breastfeeding.
- Advise patient that follow-up visits may be required to monitor therapy and to keep appointments.

Bupropion Hydrochloride

(byoo-PRO-pee-ahn HIGH-droe-KLOR-ide)http://www.fda.gov/medwatch/SAFETY/2004/safety04.htm#antidepressants

Class Antidepressant/Smoking deterrent

How Supplied
Wellbutrin Tablets 75 mg, Tablets 100 mg ♦ *Wellbutrin SR* Tablets, sustained-release 100 mg, Tablets, sustained-release 150 mg, Tablets, sustained-release 200 mg ♦ *Wellbutrin XL* Tablets, extended-release 150 mg, Tablets, extended-release 300 mg ♦ *Zyban* Tablets, sustained-release 150 mg

Action
PHARMACOLOGY: Exact mechanism of antidepressant activity or as a smoking deterrent unknown; does not inhibit MAO.

Pharmacokinetics/Dynamics:
Absorption:
Immediate release (IR) – T_{max} within 2 hr.
Sustained release (SR) – T_{max} is 3 hr; C_{max} is 91 to 143 ng/mL.
Extended release (XL) – T_{max} is approximately 5 hr.
Hydroxybupropion – T_{max} is 6 hr; C_{max} is about 10 times that of bupropion.
Distribution: Bupropion is 84% protein bound. Vd is 1950 L.
Metabolism: Extensively metabolized by hydroxylation or oxidation in the liver. CYP2B6 is involved in formation of hydroxybupropion (comparable in potency to bupropion). The other 2 main metabolites are threohydrobupropion and erythrohydrobupropion, which are 10% to 50% as potent as bupropion.
Excretion: 87% is excreted in urine, 10% in feces, and 0.5% as unchanged drug; t½ is about 21 hr (bupropion), about 20 hr (hydroxybupropion), about 37 hr (threohydrobupropion), and about 33 hr (erythrohydrobupropion).

Special Populations:
Renal Function Impairment – Elimination of the major metabolite may be reduced. Dose adjustment may be needed.
Hepatic Function Impairment – Elimination of the major metabolite may be reduced. Dose adjustment may be needed.

Indications Treatment of depression; aid to smoking cessation treatment.

Contraindications Seizure disorder; current or prior diagnosis of bulimia or anorexia nervosa; concurrent treatment with or within 14 days of discontinuation of MAO inhibitors; concurrent treatment with multiple bupropion products (eg, coadministration of *Zyban* for smoking cessation and *Wellbutrin* for depression); abrupt discontinuation of alcohol or sedatives. Hypersensitivity to buproprion or any other component of the product.

Route/Dosage
Antidepressant
ADULTS: **PO** 100 mg bid initially; may increase to 100 mg tid after 3 days (max daily dose, 450 mg; max single dose, 150 mg).
Sustained/extended-release: 150 mg/day initially; may increase to 150 mg bid or qd (*Wellbutrin XL*) as early as day 4 (max daily dose, 400 mg or 450 mg [*Wellbutrin XL*]; max single dose, 200 mg).

Hepatic Function Impairment (Severe Hepatic Cirrhosis)
ADULTS: **PO** Do not exceed 75 mg qd.
Sustained/extended-release: Do not exceed 100 mg qd or 150 mg qod.
Mild to moderate cirrhosis: Use with caution; consider reduced dose and/or frequency.

Renal Function Impairment
ADULTS: **PO** Use with caution; consider reduced dose and frequency.

Smoking Deterrent
ADULTS: **PO**
Initial dose: 150 mg for first 3 days, increasing to 150 mg bid. Do not give doses greater than 300 mg/day. Initiate treatment while patient is still smoking. Patient should set target date to quit smoking within the first 2 wk of treatment; continue treatment for 7 to 12 wk.
Maintenance: Clinical data not available regarding long-term treatment (more than 12 wk) for smoking cessation. Whether to continue treatment must be determined for individual patients.
Combination treatment: Combination treatment with bupropion and nicotine transdermal system may be prescribed for smoking cessation.

Interactions
Alcohol: Adverse neuropsychiatric events or reduced alcohol tolerance may occur.
Amantadine, levodopa: Incidence of bupropion side effects may be increased.
Antidepressants, antipsychotics, systemic steroids, theophylline: May lower seizure threshold.
Carbamazepine: May decrease bupropion serum concentrations.
MAO inhibitors, selegiline: May increase risk of acute bupropion toxicity. Discontinue MAO inhibitors at least 14 days before starting bupropion.
Ritonavir: Plasma levels of bupropion may be elevated, increasing the risk of toxicity.
Tricyclic antidepressants (TCAs): TCA plasma concentrations may be elevated.

Lab Test Interferences None well documented.

Adverse Reactions
CV: Tachycardia (11%); palpitation (6%); cardiac arrhythmia (5%); flushing, migraine, hypertension (4%); hot flashes, hypotension (3%).
CNS: Headache (26%); insomnia (16%); dizziness (11%); agitation (9%); confusion (8%); anxiety, tremor, hostility (6%); nervousness (5%); impaired sleep quality, sensory disturbances (4%); somnolence, irritability, decreased memory, decreased libido (3%); paresthesia, CNS stimulation (2%).
DERM: Sweating (6%); rash (5%); pruritus (4%); urticaria (2%).
EENT: Pharyngitis (11%); tinnitus (6%); auditory disturbance (5%); amblyopia (3%).
GI: Dry mouth (24%); nausea (18%); constipation (10%); diarrhea (7%); anorexia (5%);

increased appetite, taste perversion (4%); dyspepsia, gustatory disturbance (3%); dysphagia (2%); vomiting.
GU: Urinary frequency, menstrual complaints (5%); urinary urgency, vaginal hemorrhage (2%); UTI (1%).
MUSC: Myalgia (6%); arthralgia (4%); arthritis, twitch, akathisia (2%).
RESP: Sinusitis (3%); increased cough (2%).
OTHER: Infection, abdominal pain (9%); asthenia, chest pain (4%); fever (2%).

Precautions
Pregnancy: Category B.
Lactation: Bupropion and its metabolites are secreted in breast milk.
Children: Safety and efficacy not established.
Elderly: Use with caution.
Renal function impairment: Use with caution; reduce frequency of dosing as needed.
Hepatic function impairment: Use with caution; reduce dose and frequency of bupropion as needed.
Allergic reaction: Anaphylactoid reactions characterized by symptoms such as pruritus, urticaria, angioedema, and dyspnea requiring medical treatment have been reported.

Cardiac effects: Hypertension requiring treatment may occur in patients receiving bupropion alone and in combination with nicotine replacement therapy.
CNS symptoms: Symptoms of restlessness, agitation, anxiety, and insomnia of sufficient magnitude to require treatment or discontinuation of therapy may occur.
Heart disease: Use with caution in patients with history of MI or unstable heart disease.
Psychosis or mania: May precipitate mania in bipolar patients or activate latent psychosis in other patients.
Seizures: May occur; dose-related risk. Use with caution in patients with history of head trauma or CNS tumor; in patients taking other drugs known to increase risk of seizures; in cases of excessive use of alcohol, addiction to opiates, cocaine, or other stimulants; anoretics; and diabetic patients treated with oral hypoglycemics or insulin.
Suicide: Patients at risk should not receive excessive quantities of drug.

Overdosage: Signs and Symptoms
Seizures, hallucinations, loss of consciousness, tachycardia, cardiac arrest.

PATIENT CARE CONSIDERATIONS
Administration/Storage
- Immediate-release tablets, sustained-release tablets, and extended-release tablets can be interchanged on a total mg-to-mg daily dose.
- Do not administer with, or within 14 days of MAO inhibitor.
- Increase dose gradually to reduce risk of seizures.
- Administer prescribed dose without regard to meals. Administer with food if GI upset occurs.
- Avoid bedtime doses to minimize insomnia.

Immediate-release tablets:
- Do not exceed dose increase of 100 mg/day in a 3-day period.
- Do not exceed 150 mg as a single dose or total daily dose of 450 mg.
- Separate doses by at least 6 hr.
- Store immediate-release tablets at controlled room temperature (59° to 77°F) out of direct sunlight.

Sustained-release tablets:
- Administer prescribed dose bid.
- Have patient swallow tablets whole. Do not crush, chew, or divide.
- Separate doses by at least 8 hr.
- Do not exceed single dose of 200 mg or total daily dose of 400 mg.
- Store sustained-release tablets at controlled room temperature (68° to 77°F) out of direct sunlight.

Extended-release tablets:
- Administer prescribed dose qd.
- Have patient swallow tablets whole. Do not crush, chew, or divide.
- Separate doses by at least 24 hr.
- Do not exceed total daily dose of 450 mg.
- Store extended-release tablets at controlled room temperature (59° to 86°F) out of direct sunlight.

Assessment/Interventions
- Obtain patient history, including drug history and any known allergies. Note hepatic or renal impairment, seizures, condition predisposing to seizures (eg, CNS tumor), current or prior diagnosis of bulimia or anorexia nervosa, recent MI or unstable heart disease, diabetes treated with insulin or oral hypoglycemic medications, addiction to narcotics, cocaine, or stimulants, concurrent use of OTC stimulants or appetite suppressants, concurrent or recent (eg, within 14 days) use of MAO inhibitor, concurrent use of other bupropion products (eg, *Zyban*), concurrent use of medications that can lower seizure threshold (eg, theophyllines), or concurrent abrupt discontinuation of alcohol or other sedatives (eg, benzodiazepines).

- Ensure that patient is not receiving any other bupropion-containing medication.
- Ensure that lower starting dose and slower dose escalation are used in patient with hepatic and/or renal impairment.
- Assess patient for insomnia. Inform health care provider if noted and problematic. Be prepared to reduce dose of bupropion or administer intermediate to long-acting sedative hypnotic if ordered.
- Monitor patient for evidence of psychiatric changes (eg, delusions, hallucinations, psychotic episodes, concentration disturbance, confusion, paranoia, personality change). Inform health care provider if noted and be prepared to reduce dose or discontinue therapy.
- Monitor BP in patient receiving bupropion and nicotine replacement therapy. Notify health care provider if BP becomes elevated.
- Monitor patient for signs and symptoms of anaphylactic or serious allergic reaction. Notify health care provider immediately and be prepared to treat appropriately.
- Assess baseline neurologic status and during treatment observe for delusions, hallucinations, personality change, agitation, paranoia, psychotic behavior, or seizure activity. Discontinue therapy and inform health care provider immediately if noted.
- Monitor patient for suicidal tendencies often associated with depression.
- Frequently assess patient for response to treatment. Notify health care provider if symptoms of depression do not appear to be improving or is worsening.
- Ensure that therapy is periodically reviewed to determine if therapy needs to be continued without change or if a dose change (eg, increase, decrease, discontinuation) is indicated.
- Monitor patient for CNS, GI, CV, MUSC, GU, and general body side effects. Report to health care provider if noted and significant.
- Assess medication compliance.

Smoking deterrent:

- Ensure that medication is started while patient is still smoking because it takes about 1 wk of therapy before bupropion reaches max stable blood levels.
- Ensure that patient sets a target quit date within the first 2 wk of treatment.

Patient/Family Education

- Explain name, dose, action, and potential side effects of drug.
- Advise patient to read *Patient Information* leaflet before starting therapy and with each refill.
- Advise patient that this medication contains the same active ingredients as the smoking cessation aid *Zyban*. Caution patient not to use these in combination or with any other medication containing bupropion.
- Advise patient that dose will be started low and then slowly increased as tolerated until max benefit is obtained.
- Explain to patient that medication has an unusual odor.
- Advise patient using bupropion as a smoking deterrent that counseling and support during cessation, and for a period of time afterwards, are an important part of therapy and increase the chances of successfully stopping smoking.
- Advise patient to take prescribed dose without regard to meals but to take with food if stomach upset occurs.
- Advise patient to avoid taking medication at bedtime to minimize problems with sleeping.
- Advise patient taking immediate-release tablets to take in equally divided doses, tid or qid, with at least 6 hr between doses to minimize risk of seizures.
- Advise patient taking sustained-release tablets in doses greater than 150 mg/day to take in 2 divided doses with at least 8 hr between doses to minimize risk of seizures
- Advise patient taking extended-release tablets to take prescribed dose qd with at least 24 hr between doses to minimize risk of seizures. Explain to patient that the medication in the extended-release tablet is contained in a plastic shell that slowly releases the medication over 24 hr and then is expelled in the stool.
- Caution patient taking sustained-release or extended-release tablets to swallow tablets whole and not to chew, divide, or crush the tablets.
- Caution patient that if a dose is missed not to take an extra dose to catch up because the risk of having a seizure increases. Advise patient that if a dose is missed to skip that dose and take the next dose at the regularly scheduled time.
- Advise patient that max improvement of depression symptoms may take 4 wk or longer to be noted and not to change the dose or stop taking unless advised by health care provider.
- Instruct patient not to stop taking the medication when feeling better.
- Instruct patient to contact health care provider if symptoms do not appear to be getting better, are getting worse, or if bothersome side effects (eg, agitation, concentration difficulties, headache, insomnia, excessive sedation,

excessive sweating, appetite loss, dry mouth) occur.
- Advise patient to take frequent sips of water, suck on ice chips or sugarless hard candy, or chew sugarless gum if dry mouth occurs.
- Instruct patient to stop taking the medication and immediately report seizures, delusions, hallucinations, confusion, change in personality, paranoid thoughts, rash, hives, difficulty breathing, or swelling of the lips, face, or throat to health care provider.
- Advise patient that medication may increase sensitivity to sunlight. Caution patient to avoid unnecessary exposure to UV light (sunlight, tanning booths) and to use sunscreen and wear protective clothing when exposed to UV light until tolerance is determined.
- Instruct patient to minimize or avoid consumption of alcoholic beverages while taking medication.
- Advise patient that drug may impair judgment, thinking, or motor skills or cause drowsiness or dizziness and to use caution while driving or performing other tasks requiring mental alertness until tolerance is determined.
- Advise women to notify health care provider if pregnant, planning to become pregnant, or breastfeeding.
- Instruct patient not to take any prescription or OTC medications or dietary supplements unless advised by health care provider.
- Advise patient that follow-up visits will be required to monitor therapy and to keep appointments.

Buspirone Hydrochloride

(byoo-SPY-rone HIGH-droe-KLOR-ide)

Class Antianxiety

How Supplied
BuSpar Tablets 5 mg (4.6 mg as base), Tablets 10 mg (9.1 mg as base), Tablets 15 mg (13.7 mg as base), Tablets 30 mg (27.4 mg as base)
✣ Apo-Buspirone ♦ Gen-Buspirone ♦ Lin-Buspirone ♦ Novo-Buspirone ♦ Nu-Buspirone ♦ PMS-Buspirone ♦ ratio-Buspirone

Action
PHARMACOLOGY: Mechanism unknown; does not exert anticonvulsant or muscle relaxant effects.

PHARMACOKINETICS/DYNAMICS:
Absorption: Rapidly absorbed. C_{max} is 1 to 6 mg/mL. T_{max} is 40 to 90 min.

Distribution: About 86% bound to plasma proteins.

Metabolism: Extensive first-pass metabolism. Primarily metabolized by oxidation (which is mediated by CYP3A4) to active metabolite.

Excretion: Within 24 hr, 29% to 63% excreted in urine, primarily as metabolites; 18% to 38% is excreted in feces. The $t_{½}$ is about 2 to 3 hr.

Special Populations:
Renal Function Impairment – AUC increased 4-fold.
Hepatic Function Impairment – AUC increased 13-fold.

Indications Treatment of anxiety disorders; short-term relief of anxiety symptoms.
Unlabeled use(s): Reduction of symptoms of PMS.

Contraindications Standard considerations.

Route/Dosage
ADULTS:
Initial dose: **PO** 7.5 mg bid; may increase by 5 mg/day q 2 to 3 days prn (max, 60 mg/day in divided doses).

Interactions
Diazepam: Dizziness, headache, and nausea can occur.
Fluoxetine: Buspirone effects may be decreased. Paradoxical worsening of OCD may occur.
Haloperidol: Buspirone may increase haloperidol plasma levels.
Inducers of CYP3A4 (eg, carbamazepine, dexamethasone, phenobarbital, phenytoin, rifampin): May reduce buspirone plasma levels, decreasing the therapeutic effect.
Inhibitors of CYP3A4 (eg, diltiazem, erythromycin, grapefruit juice, itraconazole, ketoconazole, nefazodone, ritonavir, verapamil): May elevate buspirone plasma levels, increasing the pharmacologic and adverse effects.
MAO inhibitors (eg, isocarboxazid): Risk of elevated BP may be increased.
Nefazodone: If used with buspirone, a low dose (eg, 2.5 mg/day) is recommended.
Trazodone: ALT may be elevated.

Lab Test Interferences None well documented.

Adverse Reactions
CV: Chest pain (at least 1%); tachycardia/palpitations (1%).
CNS: Dizziness (12%); drowsiness (10%); headache (6%); nervousness (5%); lightheadedness (3%); excitement, numbness, anger/hostility, confusion, weakness (2%); paresthesia, incoordination, tremor (1%); dream disturbances (at least 1%); cogwheel rigidity, dizziness, dystonic reactions, ataxia, extrapyramidal effects,

dyskinesias (acute and tardive), emotional lability, serotonin syndrome, difficulty in recall (postmarketing).
DERM: Skin rash, sweating/clamminess (1%); ecchymosis (postmarketing).
EENT: Blurred vision (2%); tinnitus, sore throat, nasal congestion (at least 1%); visual changes (postmarketing).
GI: Nausea (8%); diarrhea (2%).
GU: Urinary retention (postmarketing).
MUSC: Aches/pains (1%).
OTHER: Allergic reactions (including urticaria), angioedema (postmarketing).

Precautions
Pregnancy: Category B.
Lactation: Undetermined. Nursing should be avoided.
Children: The safety and efficacy of buspirone were evaluated in 2 placebo-controlled, 6-wk trials involving a total of 559 pediatric patients (ranging from 6 to 17 yr of age) with generalized anxiety disorder (GAD). Doses studied were 7.5 to 30 mg bid (15 to 60 mg/day). There were no significant differences between buspirone and placebo with regard to the symptoms of GAD following doses recommended for the treatment of GAD in adults. Pharmacokinetic studies have shown that, for identical doses, plasma exposure to buspirone and its active metabolite, 1-PP, are equal to or higher in pediatric patients than adults. No unexpected safety findings were associated with buspirone in these trials. There are no long-term safety or efficacy data in this population.
Renal function impairment: Administration of buspirone not recommended.
Hepatic function impairment: Administration of buspirone not recommended.

Overdosage: Signs and Symptoms
Nausea, vomiting, dizziness, drowsiness, miosis, gastric distress.

PATIENT CARE CONSIDERATIONS
Administration/Storage
- Do not administer with or within 14 days of MAO inhibitor administration.
- Administer prescribed dose in a consistent manner with respect to meals; either always with or without food.
- Increase dose no more often than q 2 to 3 days. Do not exceed 60 mg/day.
- Store tablets below 86°F.

Assessment/Interventions
- Obtain patient history, including drug history and any known allergies. Note hepatic or renal impairment, depression, suicidal tendency, history of drug abuse, concurrent or recent (eg, within 14 days) use of MAO inhibitor, or concurrent use of strong CYP3A inhibitors (eg, ketoconazole, erythromycin) or inducers (eg, carbamazepine).
- Frequently assess patient for response to treatment. Notify health care provider if condition does not appear to be improving or is worsening.
- Ensure that therapy is periodically reviewed to determine if it needs to be continued without change or if a dose change (eg, increase, decrease, discontinuation) is indicated.
- Monitor patient for CNS, GI, and general body side effects. Report to health care provider if noted and significant. Implement safety precautions if excessive drowsiness or dizziness occurs.

Patient/Family Education
- Explain name, dose, action, and potential side effects of drug.
- Advise patient or caregiver to read the *Patient Information* leaflet before starting therapy and with each refill.
- Advise patient that medication is usually started at a low dose and then gradually increased until max benefit is obtained.
- Advise patient that medication must be taken daily as prescribed in order to obtain max benefit and not to use on a prn basis.
- Advise patient to take each dose consistently either with or without food.
- Caution patient to avoid grapefruit and grapefruit juice while taking this medication.
- Caution patient to take as prescribed and not to stop taking or change the dose unless advised by health care provider.
- Advise patient that if a dose is missed to skip that dose and take the next dose at the regularly scheduled time. Caution patient to never take 2 doses at the same time.
- Instruct patient to avoid alcoholic beverages and other depressants while taking this medication.
- Instruct patient to contact health care provider if symptoms do not appear to be getting better, are getting worse, or if bothersome side effects (eg, drowsiness, dizziness) occur.
- Advise patient that drug may cause drowsiness or dizziness and to use caution while driving or performing other tasks requiring mental alertness until tolerance is determined.
- Advise women to notify health care provider if pregnant, planning to become pregnant, or breastfeeding.
- Caution patient not to take any prescription or OTC drugs or dietary supplements without

- Advise patient that follow-up visits may be necessary to monitor therapy and to keep appointments.

Busulfan

(byoo-SULL-fan)
Class Alkylating agent/Alkyl sulfonates

How Supplied
Myleran Tablets 2 mg, Solution for injection 6 mg/mL

Action
PHARMACOLOGY: Busulfan's predominant effect is against cells of the granulocytic series. Although a polyfunctional alkylating agent, it appears to interact with cellular thiol groups. The drug is cell cycle-phase nonspecific, however, alkylation of the DNA is felt to be an important biological mechanism for its cytotoxic effect.

PHARMACOKINETICS/DYNAMICS:
Absorption:
IV – C_{max} is about 1222 ng/mL.
Oral – Well absorbed.

Distribution: Concentrations in CSF are approximately equivalent to those in plasma. Busulfan is approximately 32.4% protein bound, primarily to albumin.

Metabolism: Metabolized predominantly by conjugation with glutathione. This conjugate is further oxidized in the liver.

Excretion: About 30% excreted in urine over 48 hr; negligible amounts are excreted in the feces; t½ is 2.5 hr.
IV – Cl is about 2.52 mL/min/kg.

Indications
Palliative treatment of chronic myelogenous leukemia (CML) (oral); allogeneic bone marrow transplantation for CML (IV).
Pediatric: Palliative treatment of CML (oral).
Unlabeled use(s): Severe thrombocytosis, polycythemia vera, myelofibrosis; bone marrow transplantation (oral).

Contraindications
Tablets: Do not use unless a diagnosis of CML has been adequately established. Contraindicated in patients whose disease has demonstrated prior resistance to the drug without a diagnosis of CML. Busulfan is of no value in chronic lymphocytic leukemia, acute leukemia, or in the "blastic crisis" of CML.
Injection: Hypersensitivity to any of its components.

Route/Dosage
Remission Induction of CML
ADULTS: PO 4 to 8 mg/day (60 mcg/kg or 1.8 mg/m²/day). When the total leukocyte count is less than 15,000/mm³, withhold drug. During remission, treatment is resumed when a monthly WBC reaches 50,000/mm³.
PEDIATRIC: PO 60 to 120 mcg/kg or 1.8 to 4.6 mg/m² once daily. When total leukocyte count is less than 15,000/mm³, withhold drug. During remission, treatment is resumed when a monthly WBC reaches 50,000/mm³.

Bone Marrow Ablation
ADULTS: PO 1 mg/kg q 6 hr for 16 doses (for a total dose of 16 mg/kg over 4 days) in combination with other agents. An alternate regimen is busulfan 0.4375 to 0.5 mg/kg q 6 hr for 16 doses (total dose of 7 to 8 mg/kg, respectively, over 4 days) alone or in combination with other chemotherapy agents.
ADULTS: IV 0.8 mg/kg q 6 hr for 16 doses (for a total dose of 12.8 mg/kg over 4 days). Base dose on ideal body weight or actual body weight, whichever is lower. For obese patients, base dosage on adjusted body weight.

Dosage Adjustment
PEDIATRIC: PO Reduce dose 50% for WBC between 30,000 to 40,000/mm³. Discontinue therapy if WBC count falls to 20,000/mm³ or less.

Interactions
Acetaminophen: May decrease busulfan clearance.
Itraconazole: Decreases busulfan clearance 25%, increasing serum levels and effects.
Phenytoin: Increases busulfan clearance at least 15%, reducing serum levels and effects.
Thioguanine: Long-term, concomitant use has resulted in hepatotoxicity and esophageal varices.

Lab Test Interferences
None well documented.

Adverse Reactions
CV: Tachycardia, thrombotic events, hypertension, generalized edema, chest pain, vasodilatation (IV).
CNS: Confusion; seizures; insomnia, anxiety, headache, asthenia, dizziness, depression (IV).
DERM: Hyperpigmentation, urticaria, alopecia; rash, pruritus (IV).
ENDO: Clinical syndrome similar to adrenal insufficiency.
GI: Nausea; vomiting; diarrhea; transient LFT elevations; hepatic veno-occlusive disease after bone marrow transplantation; stomatitis, anorexia, abdominal pain, hyperbilirubinemia, dyspepsia, constipation, dry mouth, jaundice (IV).
GU: Amenorrhea; ovarian failure; sterility; azo-

ospermia; testicular atrophy.
HEMA: Pancytopenia; delayed bone marrow suppression.
METAB: Hypomagnesemia, hypokalemia, hyperglycemia, hypocalcemia (IV).
RENAL: Uric acid nephropathy; renal stones; acute renal failure.
RESP: Interstitial pulmonary fibrosis; rhinitis, cough, epistaxis, dyspnea (IV).
SPEC SENSE: Cataracts.
OTHER: Acute leukemia and malignant tumors; cellular dysplasia; fever, chills (IV).

> **WARNING:**
> Bone marrow suppression.
> Leukemogenesis.
> Use with extreme caution in patients with prior radiation or chemotherapy.
> Perform hematological testing weekly during therapy.
> *Hematopoietic toxicity:* Most frequent and serious side effect is bone marrow failure, resulting in severe pancytopenia. Recovery from busulfan-induced pancytopenia may take from 1 mo to 2 yr. The most consistent dose-related toxicity is bone marrow suppression. This may be manifested by neutropenia, anemia, leukopenia, thrombocytopenia, or any combination of these. Busulfan-induced bone marrow suppression may be prolonged. The WBC may continue to drop for 2 to 3 wk after therapy is discontinued and may take up to 2 mo to recover.

Precautions
Pregnancy: Category D.
Lactation: Undetermined.
Children: Safety and efficacy not established.
Hepatic function impairment: High doses may be associated with an increased risk of developing hepatic veno-occlusive disease (VOD).
Carcinogenesis: Malignant tumors have occurred in patients on busulfan therapy; this drug may be a human carcinogen.
Adrenal insufficiency: A clinical syndrome closely resembling adrenal insufficiency and characterized by weakness, severe fatigue, anorexia, weight loss, nausea, vomiting, and melanoderma has developed after prolonged therapy.
Cardiovascular: Cardiac tamponade, which was often fatal, has been reported in a small number of pediatric patients with thalassemia (2% in 1 series) who received high doses of busulfan and cyclophosphamide as the preparatory regimen for bone marrow transplantation and hematopoietic progenitor cell transplantation. Abdominal pain and vomiting preceded the tamponade in most patients.
Cellular dysplasia: Busulfan may cause cellular dysplasia in many organs in addition to the lung. Giant hyperchromatic nuclei have been reported in the lymph nodes, pancreas, thyroid, adrenal glands, bone marrow, and liver.
Hyperuricemia and hyperuricosuria: May occur in patients with chronic myelogenous leukemia. Minimize adverse effects by increased hydration, urine alkalization, and the prophylactic administration of allopurinol.
Pulmonary effects: A rare but important complication of busulfan therapy is the development of bronchopulmonary dysplasia with pulmonary fibrosis. Symptoms have occurred within 8 mo to 10 yr after initiation of therapy. Clinically, patients report the insidious onset of cough, dyspnea, and low-grade fever. Pulmonary function studies reveal diminished diffusion capacity and decreased pulmonary compliance.
Seizures: Seizures have been reported in patients receiving high oral doses of busulfan. Risk of seizures may be reduced by prophylactic administration of phenytoin. Some clinicians administer a loading dose of phenytoin 15 to 18 mg/kg orally prior to starting busulfan followed by a maintenance dose of phenytoin 300 mg/day orally until 24 hr after administering the final busulfan dose. Maintenance doses ranging from 4 to 8 mg/kg/day orally have also been given, titrated to achieve therapeutic phenytoin serum levels (10 to 20 mcg/mL).

Overdosage: Signs and Symptoms
Bone marrow hypoplasia/aplasia, pancytopenia (tablets).

PATIENT CARE CONSIDERATIONS
Administration/Storage
- Store oral tablets at room temperature.
- Refrigerate solution for injection in unopened ampules.
- Withdraw dose from the ampule, using the provided 5 micron filter needle. Remove the filter needle and use a new needle to add busulfan to the diluent.
- Dilute solution for injection with 5% Dextrose or 0.9% Sodium Chloride, for a final busulfan concentration of about 0.5 mg/mL. Add the busulfan to the diluent; do not add the diluent to busulfan.
- To determine the approximate volume of diluent required, multiply the volume of busulfan injection by 10.
- Diluted busulfan solutions are stable for up to 8 hr at room temperature and for up to 12 hr

under refrigeration.
- Administer by oral, IV infusion
- Follow safe handling procedures and disposal of chemotherapy drugs. Wear gloves and avoid skin contact and inhalation of fumes.

IV:
- Infuse over 2 hr. Vigorous hydration reduces the risk of renal toxicity

Assessment/Interventions
- Monitor patients for signs of local or systemic infection or bleeding. Frequently evaluate their hematologic status.
- Periodic measurement of serum transaminases, alkaline phosphatase, and bilirubin is indicated for early detection of hepatotoxicity.
- It is recommended that evaluation of the hemoglobin or hematocrit, total WBC, CBC, including differential count and quantitative platelet count, be obtained weekly (daily for injection) while the patient is on busulfan therapy, and until engraftment has been demonstrated.
- Evaluate serum transaminase, alkaline phosphatase, and bilirubin daily through transplant day 28 to detect hepatotoxicity, which may herald the onset of hepatic VOD.
- Risk of seizures may be reduced by prophylactic administration of phenytoin. Some clinicians administer a loading dose of phenytoin 15 to 18 mg/kg orally prior to starting busulfan followed by a maintenance dose of phenytoin 300 mg/day orally until 24 hr after administering the final busulfan dose. Maintenance doses ranging from 4 to 8 mg/kg/day orally also have been given, titrated to achieve therapeutic phenytoin serum levels (10 to 20 mcg/mL).

PO:
- Some clinicians place patients on a clear-liquid diet to decrease the risk of vomiting. In addition, they may prescribe additional doses of busulfan if tablets are visible in emesis. A full replacement dose may be given if vomiting occurs within 30 min of a dose and pill fragments are visible in the vomitus. If vomiting occurs more than 30 min after a dose, the replacement dose may be estimated based on the number of visible pill fragments; patients typically receive 50% of the usual dose.

Patient/Family Education
- Inform patients beginning therapy with busulfan of the importance of having periodic blood counts.
- Notify health care provider if unusual bleeding or bruising; fever; persistent cough; congestion; shortness of breath; flank, stomach or joint pain; abrupt weakness; unusual fatigue; anorexia; or weight loss occurs.
- Tell patients that diffuse pulmonary fibrosis is an infrequent but serious and potentially life-threatening complication of long-term busulfan therapy.
- Inform patients that some toxicities to busulfan include infertility, amenorrhea, skin hyperpigmentation, drug hypersensitivity, dryness of the mucous membranes.
- Medication may cause darkening of skin, diarrhea, dizziness, fatigue, appetite loss, mental confusion, nausea, vomiting, and melanoderma that could be associated with a syndrome resembling adrenal insufficiency; notify health care provider if these become pronounced.
- Take medication at the same time each day.
- Extra fluid intake may be recommended.
- Contraceptive measures are recommended during therapy.
- If nausea or vomiting occurs, take the drug on an empty stomach.
- Explain the increased risk of a second malignancy to the patient.
- Instruct patients to promptly report the development of fever, sore throat, signs of local infection, bleeding from any site or symptoms suggestive of anemia.

Butabarbital Sodium

(byoo-tah-BAR-bih-tahl SO-dee-uhm)

Class Sedative and hypnotic/Barbiturate

How Supplied
Butisol Sodium Tablets 30 mg, Tablets 50 mg, Tablets 100 mg, Elixir 30 mg/5 mL

Action
PHARMACOLOGY: Depresses sensory cortex, decreases motor activity, alters cerebellar function and produces drowsiness, sedation, and hypnosis.

PHARMACOKINETICS/DYNAMICS:
Absorption: Rapidly absorbed.

Distribution: Rapidly distributed to all tissues and fluids with high concentrations in the brain, liver, and kidney. Bound to plasma and tissue proteins.

Metabolism: Primarily metabolized by the hepatic microsomal enzyme system.

Excretion: Most metabolic products excreted in the urine, with negligible amounts of unchanged drug excreted. Average plasma $t_½$ is 100 hr.

Indications Short-term use (2 wk) as a sedative or hypnotic.

Contraindications Hypersensitivity to barbiturates; history of manifest or latent porphyria.

Route/Dosage
Hypnotic
ADULTS: **PO** 50 to 100 mg at bedtime.

Sedative
ADULTS: **PO** Daytime sedative: 15 to 30 mg, tid or qid. Preoperative sedative: 50 to 100 mg, 60 to 90 min before surgery.
CHILDREN: **PO** Preoperative sedative: 2 to 6 mg/kg (max, 100 mg).

Interactions
Alcohol, CNS depressants: CNS depressant effects may be enhanced.
Anticoagulants (eg, warfarin), beta-blockers (eg, metoprolol), corticosteroids, doxycycline, felodipine, griseofulvin, methadone, metronidazole, nifedipine, quinidine, theophyllines, verapamil: Activity of these drugs may be reduced by butabarbital.
Anticonvulsants: Serum levels of carbamazepine, valproic acid, and succinimides may be reduced. Valproic acid may increase butabarbital levels.
Estrogens, estrogen-containing oral contraceptives: May reduce contraceptive effectiveness.
MAO inhibitors: The effects of butabarbital may be prolonged.
Methoxyflurane: Risk of renal toxicity may be increased.
Phenytoin: May increase butabarbital levels while phenytoin levels may increase or decrease.

Lab Test Interferences Decreased serum bilirubin; false-positive phentolamine test results; decreased response to metyrapone.

Adverse Reactions
CV: Bradycardia, hypotension, syncope (less than 1%).
CNS: Somnolence (1% to 3%); agitation, confusion, hyperkinesia, ataxia, CNS depression, nightmares, nervousness, psychiatric disturbance, hallucinations, insomnia, anxiety, dizziness, abnormal thinking, headache (less then 1%).
GI: Nausea, vomiting, constipation (less than 1%).
HEPA: Liver damage (less than 1%).
RESP: Hypoventilation, apnea (less than 1%).
OTHER: Hypersensitivity (angioedema, skin rashes, exfoliative dermatitis), fever (less than 1%).

Precautions
Pregnancy: Category D.
Lactation: Excreted in breast milk.
Children: May respond with excitement rather than depression.
Elderly: Use with caution because of the greater frequency of decreased hepatic, renal, or cardiac function, and concomitant diseases or other drug therapy.
Renal function impairment: Use with caution and in reduced dosage.
Hepatic function impairment: Use with caution and in reduced dosage.
Special risk patients: Use with caution in patients with a history of drug abuse, who are mentally depressed, or who have suicidal tendencies.
Acute or chronic pain: Because paradoxical excitement may be induced, use with caution.
Dependence: May be habit forming; tolerance or psychological and physical dependence may occur with continued use.

Overdosage: Signs and Symptoms
Unsteady gait, slurred speech, sustained nystagmus, CNS and respiratory depression, Cheyne-Stokes respiration, areflexia, constriction of pupils, oliguria, tachycardia, hypotension, lowered body temperature, coma, shock syndrome, pneumonia, pulmonary edema, cardiac arrhythmia, CHF, renal failure, death.

Butalbital/Acetaminophen/Caffeine

(BYOO-TAL-bih-tuhl/uh-seet-uh-MIN-oh-fen/kaff-EEN)

Class Nonnarcotic analgesic

How Supplied
Esgic Capsules 325 mg acetaminophen/40 mg caffeine/50 mg butalbital, Tablets 325 mg acetaminophen/40 mg caffeine/50 mg butalbital ◆ *Esgic-Plus* Tablets 500 mg acetaminophen/40 mg caffeine/50 mg butalbital, Capsules 500 mg acetaminophen/40 mg caffeine/50 mg butalbital ◆ *Fioricet* Tablets 325 mg acetaminophen/40 mg caffeine/50 mg butalbital ◆ *Margesic* Capsules 325 mg acetaminophen/40 mg caffeine/50 mg butalbital ◆ *Medigesic* Capsules 325 mg acetaminophen/40 mg caffeine/50 mg butalbital ◆ *Repan* Tablets 325 mg acetaminophen/40 mg caffeine/50 mg butalbital ◆ *Triad* Capsules 325 mg acetaminophen/40 mg caffeine/50 mg butalbital

Action
PHARMACOLOGY: Butalbital has generalized depressant effect on CNS and, in very high doses, has peripheral effects. Acetaminophen has analgesic and antipyretic effects; its analgesic effects may be mediated through inhibition of prostaglandin synthetase enzyme complex. Caffeine is thought to produce constriction of cerebral blood vessels.

Indications Relief of symptom complex of tension (or muscle contraction) headache.

Contraindications Hypersensitivity to acetaminophen, caffeine, or barbiturates; porphyria.

Route/Dosage
ADULTS: **PO** 1 to 2 tablets or capsules q 4 hr; max, 6 tablets or capsules/day.

Interactions
Beta-blockers (eg, propranolol), corticosteroids, doxycycline, estrogens (including oral contraceptives), felodipine, griseofulvin, nifedipine, phenylbutazone, quinidine, theophylline, warfarin: Effects of these drugs may be decreased.
Carbamazepine, sulfinpyrazone: May increase risk of hepatotoxicity.
MAO inhibitors: May increase CNS effects.
Other CNS depressants (ethanol, narcotics, general anesthetics, tranquilizers, sedative-hypnotics): Increased drowsiness, dizziness and other CNS depressive effects may occur.
Tricyclic antidepressants: Antidepressant effect may decrease.

Lab Test Interferences With *Chemstrip bG* and *Dextrostix* home blood glucose systems, may cause false decrease in mean glucose values; may give false-positive urinary 5-hydroxyindoleacetic acid test result.

Adverse Reactions
CNS: Drowsiness; dizziness; lightheadedness; confusion.
DERM: Rash.
GI: Nausea; vomiting; flatulence.

Precautions
Pregnancy: Category C.
Lactation: Undetermined.
Children: Safety and efficacy in children under 12 yr not established.
Drug dependency: Prolonged use may produce drug tolerance and dependency (psychologic and physical).

Overdosage: Signs and Symptoms
Blood dyscrasias, respiratory depression, hepatic damage, drowsiness, confusion, coma, hypotension, tachycardia, hypovolemic shock, nausea, vomiting, insomnia, restlessness, tremor.

PATIENT CARE CONSIDERATIONS

Administration/Storage
- Give with food or water.
- Store in airtight, light-resistant container at room temperature.

Assessment/Interventions
- Obtain patient history, including drug history and any known allergies.
- Assess pain before administration to establish baseline.
- Assess vital signs before administration.
- Assess related factors that may precipitate or worsen pain such as anxiety, fear, or stress.
- Administer scheduled dose before pain is severe.
- Utilize adjunct pain relief measures, such as massage, positioning, and maintaining quiet environment to enhance effectiveness.
- Assess therapeutic effectiveness 1 hr after dose based on patient report of relief. Do not rely on objective signs.
- Reassess vital signs.
- Assess for dizziness, sedation, or euphoria.
- Record degree and duration of pain relief. Notify health care provider if product is ineffective.
- Institute safety precautions if drowsiness or sedation occurs.

Patient/Family Education
- Caution patient that dependency/tolerance may result from regular long-term use.
- Tell patient to take drug with full glass of water.
- Instruct patient not to discontinue drug abruptly after long-term regular use.
- Caution patient to avoid intake of alcoholic beverages and other CNS depressants without health care provider approval.
- Advise patient to avoid any hazardous activity (driving or smoking) if dizziness, drowsiness or a decrease in mental acuity occurs.
- Warn patient that orthostatic hypotension may occur. Instruct patient to change positions slowly and to sit or lie down if symptoms occur.
- Instruct patient not to take OTC or other medications unless directed by health care provider.
- Inform patient to report the following symptoms to health care provider: persistent or recurrent pain before next scheduled dose, difficulty breathing, increased drowsiness, vomiting or yellowing of skin or gums.

Butalbital/Acetaminophen/ Caffeine/Codeine Phosphate

(BYOO-TAL-bih-tuhl/uh-seet-uh-MIN-oh-fen/kaff-EEN/KOE-deen FOSS-fate)

Class Narcotic analgesic

How Supplied
Fioricet with Codeine Capsules 30 mg codeine phosphate/325 mg acetaminophen/40 mg caffeine/50 mg butalbital

Action
PHARMACOLOGY: Butalbital has generalized depressant effect on CNS and, in very high doses, has peripheral effects. Acetaminophen has analgesic and antipyretic effects; its analgesic effects may be mediated through inhibition of prostaglandin synthetase enzyme complex. Caffeine is thought to produce constriction of cerebral blood vessels. Codeine binds to opiate receptors in the CNS, causing inhibition of ascending pain pathways and altering perception of and response to pain.

Indications Relief of symptom complex of tension (or muscle contraction) headache.

Contraindications Hypersensitivity to acetaminophen, caffeine, opiates, or barbiturates; porphyria.

Route/Dosage
ADULTS AND CHILDREN 12 YR AND OVER: **PO** 1 to 2 tablets or capsules q 4 hr; max, 6 tablets or capsules/day.

Interactions
Beta-blockers (eg, propranolol), corticosteroids, doxycycline, estrogens (including oral contraceptives), felodipine, griseofulvin, nifedipine, phenylbutazone, quinidine, theophylline, warfarin: Effects of these drugs may be decreased.
Carbamazepine, sulfinpyrazone: May increase risk of hepatotoxicity.
MAO inhibitors: May increase CNS effects.
Other CNS depressants (eg, ethanol, narcotics, general anesthetics, tranquilizers, sedative-hypnotics): Increased drowsiness, dizziness and other CNS depressive effects may occur.
Tricyclic antidepressants: Antidepressant effects may decrease.

Lab Test Interferences With *Chemstrip bG* and *Dextrostix* home blood glucose systems, may cause false decrease in mean glucose values; may increase serum amylase; may give false-positive urinary 5-hydroxyindoleacetic acid test results.

Adverse Reactions
CV: Tachycardia.
CNS: Drowsiness; dizziness; lightheadedness; confusion; intoxicated feeling.
DERM: Rash.
GI: Nausea; vomiting; flatulence; constipation.
RESP: Shortness of breath.

Precautions
Pregnancy: Category C.
Lactation: Undetermined.
Children: Safety and efficacy in children under 12 yr not established.
Labor and delivery: Delivery may be prolonged and newborn may experience respiratory depression or withdrawal.
Drug dependency: Prolonged use may produce drug tolerance and dependency (psychologic and physical).
Head injury: Respiratory depressant effects may be enhanced and CSF pressure may be increased.

Overdosage: Signs and Symptoms
Blood dyscrasias, respiratory depression, hepatic damage, drowsiness, confusion, coma, hypotension, hypovolemic shock, nausea, tremor, vomiting, tachycardia, insomnia, restlessness.

PATIENT CARE CONSIDERATIONS

Administration/Storage
- Give with food or water.
- Store in airtight, light-resistant container at room temperature.

Assessment/Interventions
- Obtain patient history, including drug history and any known allergies.
- Assess pain prior to administration to establish baseline.
- Assess related factors that may precipitate or worsen pain such as anxiety, fear, or stress.
- Take vital signs prior to administration. Withhold dose if respiratory rate less than 12 bpm (less than 20 bpm in children) and notify health care provider.
- Assess cough for productiveness and effectiveness. Auscultate for rales.
- Administer scheduled dose before pain is severe.
- Utilize adjunct pain relief measures (eg, massage, positioning, maintaining quiet environment and emotional support) to enhance effectiveness.
- Assess therapeutic effectiveness 1 hr after dose based on patient report of relief. Do not rely on objective signs.
- Record degree and duration of pain relief. Notify health care provider if product is ineffective.
- Reassess vital signs; notify health care provider if there is significant change.
- Assess for dizziness, sedation, or euphoria.

- Assess for urinary retention or constipation.
- Institute safety precautions if drowsiness or sedation occurs.
- Provide high-fiber diet with 2 to 3 L of fluids unless contraindicated.
- If constipation occurs, arrange for a stool softener or bulk laxative.
- Encourage patient to void q 3 to 4 hr.

Patient/Family Education
- Caution patient that dependency/tolerance may result from long-term use.
- Remind patient to take medication with full glass of water.
- Instruct patient not to discontinue drug abruptly after long-term regular use.
- Caution patient to avoid intake of alcoholic beverages and other CNS depressants without health care provider approval.
- Caution patient to avoid any hazardous activity (eg, driving, operating heavy machinery) if dizziness, drowsiness or a decrease in mental acuity occurs.
- Warn patient that orthostatic hypotension may occur. Instruct patient to change positions slowly and to sit or lie down if symptoms occur.
- Instruct patient not to take otc or other medications without consulting health care provider.
- Warn patient that constipation could occur. Advise patient to increase dietary fiber and fluids unless contraindicated.
- Instruct patient to report these symptoms to health care provider: persistent or recurrent pain occurs before next scheduled dose, difficulty breathing, blurred vision, increased drowsiness, vomiting, constipation, urinary retention, yellowing of skin or gums.

Butalbital/Aspirin/Caffeine

(BYOO-TAL-bih-tuhl/ASS-pihr-in/kaff-EEN)

Class Nonnarcotic analgesic combination

How Supplied
Fiorinal Capsules 325 mg aspirin/40 mg caffeine/50 mg butalbital ◆ *Fiortal* Capsules 325 mg aspirin/40 mg caffeine/50 mg butalbital ◆ *Butalbital Compound* Capsules 325 mg aspirin/40 mg caffeine/50 mg butalbital, Tablets 325 mg aspirin/40 mg caffeine/50 mg butalbital

Action
PHARMACOLOGY: Butalbital has generalized depressant effect on CNS and, in very high doses, has peripheral effects. Aspirin has analgesic, antipyretic, anti-inflammatory, and antirheumatic effects; its analgesic and anti-inflammatory effects may be mediated through inhibition of prostaglandin synthetase enzyme complex. Aspirin also irreversibly inhibits platelet aggregation. Caffeine is thought to produce constriction of cerebral blood vessels.

Indications Relief of symptom complex of tension (or muscle contraction) headache.

Contraindications Hypersensitivity to salicylates, aspirin, caffeine, or barbiturates; porphyria; bleeding disorders; syndrome of nasal polyps, angioedema, and bronchospastic reactivity to aspirin or other NSAIDs; peptic ulcer.

Route/Dosage
ADULTS AND CHILDREN 12 YR AND OVER: PO 1 to 2 tablets or capsules q 4 hr; max, 6 tablets or capsules/day.

Interactions
Beta-blockers (eg, propranolol), doxycycline, estrogens (including oral contraceptives), felodipine, griseofulvin, nifedipine, phenylbutazone, quinidine, theophylline: Effects of these drugs may be increased.
Corticosteroids: May enhance renal clearance of aspirin; sudden discontinuation of corticosteroids may result in symptoms of salicylism; effects of corticosteroids may be decreased.
Insulin, oral antidiabetic agents: Hypoglycemic effects may be increased.
MAO inhibitors: May increase CNS effects.
Methotrexate, 6-mercaptopurine: Bone marrow toxicity may occur.
NSAIDs: Increased GI ulceration or bleeding may occur.
Other CNS depressants (ethanol, narcotics, general anesthetics, tranquilizers, sedative-hypnotics): Increased drowsiness, dizziness and other CNS depressive effects may occur.
Sulfinpyrazone, probenecid: Uricosuric effects may be decreased.
Tricyclic antidepressants: Antidepressant levels/effect may decrease.
Warfarin: Anticoagulant effects may be increased or decreased.

Lab Test Interferences
Blood tests: Serum amylase; fasting blood glucose; cholesterol; protein; serum hepatic aminotransferase (ALT); uric acid; prothrombin time.
Urine tests: Glucose, 5-hydroxyindoleacetic acid; Gerhardt ketone, vanillylmandelic acid; uric acid; diacetic acid; spectrophotometric detection of barbiturates.

Adverse Reactions

CV: Tachycardia.
CNS: Drowsiness; dizziness; lightheadedness; confusion; mental depression; unusual excitement; nervousness.
DERM: Rash.
GI: Nausea; vomiting; flatulence; heartburn; abdominal pains; constipation.

Precautions

Pregnancy: Category C.
Lactation: Undetermined.
Children: Safety and efficacy in children under 12 yr not established.
Renal function impairment: Use with caution because of decreased elimination.
Hepatic function impairment: Use with caution because of decreased elimination.
Drug dependency: Prolonged use may produce drug dependency (psychologic and physical) and tolerance.
Peptic ulcer, coagulation abnormalities and preoperative states: Use with extreme caution because of increased bleeding time.
Reye syndrome: May occur in children because of aspirin component; do not use for chickenpox or flu symptoms.

Overdosage: Signs and Symptoms

Hyperthermia, tachycardia, respiratory depression, bleeding, drowsiness, confusion, coma, hypotension, hypovolemic shock, nausea, vomiting, tremor, tinnitus, fluid and electrolyte abnormalities, insomnia, restlessness.

PATIENT CARE CONSIDERATIONS

Administration/Storage

- Give with food or water.
- Discard if strong vinegar-like odor is present.
- Store in airtight, light-resistant container at room temperature.

Assessment/Interventions

- Obtain patient history, including drug history and any known allergies.
- Assess pain prior to administration to establish baseline.
- Take vital signs prior to administration.
- Assess related factors that may precipitate or worsen pain such as anxiety, fear, or stress.
- Administer scheduled dose before pain is severe.
- Record degree and duration of pain relief. Notify health care provider if product is ineffective.
- Assess therapeutic effectiveness 1 hr after dose based on patient report of relief. Do not rely on objective signs.
- Reassess vital signs.
- Assess for dizziness, sedation, or euphoria.
- Institute safety precautions if drowsiness or sedation occurs.
- Use adjunct pain relief measures (eg, massage, positioning, maintaining quiet environment and emotional support) to enhance effectiveness.

Patient/Family Education

- Caution patient that dependency/tolerance may result from long-term use.
- Tell patient to take with food or full glass of water.
- Instruct patient not to discontinue abruptly after long-term regular use.
- Caution patient to avoid intake of alcoholic beverages and other CNS depressants without health care provider approval.
- Warn patient to avoid any hazardous activity (eg, driving, smoking) if dizziness, drowsiness, or decrease in mental acuity occurs.
- Instruct patient to avoid sudden position changes to avoid orthostatic hypotension.
- Advise patient to notify health care provider if any surgical procedures are required. Discontinue aspirin therapy 5 days prior to surgery to reduce potential for bleeding problems.
- Instruct patient not to take *otc* medications without consulting health care provider.
- Advise patient to report these symptoms to health care provider: persistent or recurrent pain before next scheduled dose, difficulty breathing, buzzing in ears, increased drowsiness, vomiting, abdominal pain, tarry stools, unusual bruising or bleeding.

Butalbital/Aspirin/Caffeine/Codeine Phosphate

(BYOO-TAL-bih-tuhl/ASS-pihr-in/Kaff-EEN/KOE-deen FOSS-fate)

Class Narcotic analgesic combination

How Supplied

Fiorinal with Codeine Capsules 30 mg codeine phosphate/325 mg aspirin/40 mg caffeine/50 mg butalbital

Action

PHARMACOLOGY: Butalbital has generalized depressant effect on CNS and, in very high doses, has peripheral effects. Aspirin has analgesic, antipyretic, anti-inflammatory, and antirheumatic effects; its analgesic and anti-inflammatory effects may be mediated through inhibition of prostaglandin synthetase enzyme complex. Aspirin also irreversibly inhibits platelet aggregation. Caffeine is thought to produce constriction of cerebral blood vessels. Codeine binds to opiate receptors in CNS, causing inhibition of ascending pain pathways and altering perception of and response to pain.

Indications Relief of symptom complex of tension (or muscle contraction) headache.

Contraindications Hypersensitivity to salicylates, aspirin, caffeine, opiates, or barbiturates; porphyria; bleeding disorders; syndrome of nasal polyps, angioedema, and bronchospastic reactivity to aspirin or other NSAIDs; peptic ulcer.

Route/Dosage

ADULTS AND CHILDREN 12 YR AND OVER: **PO** 1 to 2 tablets or capsules q 4 hr; max, 6 tablets or capsules/day.

Interactions

Beta-blockers (eg, propranolol), doxycycline, estrogens (including oral contraceptives), felodipine, griseofulvin, nifedipine, phenylbutazone, quinidine, theophylline: Effects of these drugs may be decreased.
Corticosteroids: May enhance renal clearance of aspirin; sudden discontinuation of corticosteroids may result in symptoms of salicylism; effects of corticosteroid may be decreased.
Insulin, oral antidiabetic agents: Hypoglycemic effects may be increased.
MAO inhibitors: May increase CNS effects.
Methotrexate, 6-mercaptopurine: Bone marrow toxicity may occur.
NSAIDs: Increased GI ulceration may occur.
Other CNS depressants (ethanol, narcotics, general anesthetics, tranquilizers, sedative-hypnotics): Increased drowsiness, dizziness and other CNS depressive effects may occur.
Probenecid, sulfinpyrazone: Uricosuric effects may be decreased.
Tricyclic antidepressants: Antidepressant effects may decrease.
Warfarin: Anticoagulant effects may be increased or decreased.

Lab Test Interferences

Blood tests: Serum amylase; fasting blood glucose; cholesterol; protein; serum hepatic aminotransferase (ALT); uric acid; prothrombin time.
Urine tests: Glucose; 5-hydroxyindoleacetic acid; Gerhardt ketone, vanillylmandelic acid; uric acid; diacetic acid; spectrophotometric detection of barbiturates. Codeine component may increase serum amylase or lipase levels.

Adverse Reactions

CV: Tachycardia.
CNS: Drowsiness; dizziness; lightheadedness; confusion; mental depression; unusual excitement; nervousness.
DERM: Rash; pruritus.
GI: Nausea; vomiting; flatulence; heartburn; abdominal pain; constipation.

Precautions

Pregnancy: Category C.
Lactation: Undetermined.
Children: Safety and efficacy in children under 12 yr not established.
Renal function impairment: Use caution because of decreased elimination.
Hepatic function impairment: Use caution because of decreased elimination.
Drug dependency: Prolonged use may produce drug tolerance and dependency (psychologic and physical).
Head injury: Respiratory depressant effects may be enhanced and CSF pressure may be increased.
Peptic ulcer, coagulation abnormalities, and preoperative states: Use extreme caution because of increased bleeding time.
Reye syndrome: May occur in children because of aspirin component; do not use for chickenpox or flu symptoms.

Overdosage: Signs and Symptoms

Hyperthermia, tachycardia, respiratory depression, bleeding, drowsiness, confusion, coma, hypotension, hypovolemic shock, nausea, vomiting, tremor, fluid and electrolyte abnormalities, insomnia, restlessness.

PATIENT CARE CONSIDERATIONS

Administration/Storage

- Give with food or water.
- Discard if strong vinegar-like odor is present.
- Store in airtight, light-resistant container at room temperature.

Assessment/Interventions

- Obtain patient history, including drug history and any known allergies.
- Assess pain before administration to establish baseline.
- Assess vital signs before administration. Withhold dose if respiratory rate under 12 bpm (under 20 bpm in children) and notify health care provider.
- Assess related factors that may precipitate or worsen pain such as anxiety, fear, or stress.
- Assess cough for productiveness and effectiveness. Auscultate for rales.
- Administer scheduled dose before pain is severe.
- Assess therapeutic effectiveness 1 hr after dose based on patient report of relief. Do not rely on objective signs.

- Record degree and duration of pain relief. Notify health care provider if product is ineffective.
- Reassess vital signs. Notify health care provider of any significant change.
- Assess for dizziness, sedation, or euphoria. Institute safety precautions as needed.
- Assess for urinary retention or constipation.
- Use adjunct pain relief measures (eg, massage, positioning, maintaining quiet environment and emotional support) to enhance effectiveness.
- Provide high-fiber diet with 2 to 3 L of fluid unless contraindicated.
- If constipation occurs, arrange for a stool softener or bulk laxative.
- Encourage patient to void q 3 to 4 hr.

Patient/Family Education
- Caution patient that dependency/tolerance may result from long-term use.
- Tell patient to take with food or full glass of water.
- Instruct patient not to discontinue abruptly after long-term regular use.
- Caution patient to avoid intake of alcoholic beverages and other CNS depressants.
- Warn patient to avoid any hazardous activity (eg, driving, operating heavy machinery) if dizziness, drowsiness or a decrease in mental acuity occurs.
- Instruct patient to avoid sudden position changes to prevent orthostatic hypotension.
- Tell patient to notify health care provider if any surgical procedures are required. Aspirin therapy should be discontinued 5 days before surgery to reduce potential for bleeding problems.
- Instruct patient not to take OTC medications without consulting health care provider.
- Advise patient to report the following symptoms to health care provider: persistent or recurring pain before next scheduled dose, difficulty breathing, blurred vision, buzzing in ears, increased drowsiness, vomiting, abdominal pain, tarry stools, unusual bruising or bleeding.

Butenafine Hydrochloride

(byoo-TEN-ah-feen HIGH-droe-KLOR-ide)

Class Antifungal agent

How Supplied
Lotrimin Ultra Cream 1% ♦ *Mentax* Cream 1%

Action
PHARMACOLOGY: Appears to inhibit biosynthesis of the ergosterol component of fungal cell membranes.

Indications Interdigital tinea pedis (athlete's foot); tinea corporis (ringworm); tinea cruris (jock itch); tinea (pityriasis) versicolor caused by susceptible organisms.

Contraindications Standard considerations.

Route/Dosage
Tinea Pedis
ADULTS AND CHILDREN 12 YR AND OLDER:

Topical Apply to affected and surrounding area(s) bid for 7 days or qd for 4 wk.

Tinea Corporis, Tinea Cruris, and Tinea (Pityriasis) Versicolor
ADULTS AND CHILDREN 12 YR AND OLDER:
Topical Apply qd for 2 wk.

Interactions None well documented.

Lab Test Interferences None well documented.

Adverse Reactions
DERM: Worsening of condition, burning, stinging, itching (1%).

Precautions
Pregnancy: Category B.
Lactation: Undetermined.
Children: Safety and efficacy in children under 12 yr not established.

PATIENT CARE CONSIDERATIONS

Administration/Storage
- For external use only. Not for use on mucous membranes.
- For topical use only. Not for ophthalmic, oral, or intravaginal use.
- Avoid contact with eyes, eyelids, lips, and mucus membranes.
- Cream is applied to affected area(s) qd or bid as prescribed.
- Apply enough cream to cover affected area(s) and the immediately surrounding skin and gently massage cream into skin.
- Thoroughly dry area(s) to be treated if cream is applied after bathing.
- Store at controlled room temperature or in refrigerator (41° to 86°F). Keep tube tightly capped.

Assessment/Interventions
- Obtain patient history, including drug history and any known allergies.
- Assess the skin and identify areas where medication is to be applied.
- Assess and document skin condition before initial application and periodically throughout treatment. Notify health care provider if condition does not improve by end of

treatment period, or sooner, if the condition is getting worse (eg, blistering, oozing, swelling).
- Monitor for side effects at application site (eg, burning, stinging, itching, redness). Inform health care provider if noted and significant.

Patient/Family Education
- Explain name, action, and potential side effects of drug.
- Advise patient that medication is applied topically to skin lesions qd or bid.
- Teach patient proper technique for applying cream: wash hands; ensure that area to be treated is dry; apply a thin film of cream to cover affected area(s) and immediately surrounding skin areas; gently massage into skin; wash hands after applying medication.
- Advise patient that improvement may take several days to weeks to occur and to continue applying the medication for the entire treatment time recommended by health care provider.
- Instruct patient to notify health care provider if improvement is not noted after the end of the treatment period, or sooner if the condition worsens.
- Caution patient not to cover treated areas with bandages or dressings unless advised by health care provider.
- Advise patient that if an application is missed to not try to make it up but to return to the normal application schedule as soon as possible.
- Warn patient to avoid contact with the eyes, eyelids, lips, and mucous membranes.
- Advise patient that if cream comes in contact with the eyes to wash eyes with large amounts of cool water and to contact health care provider if eye irritation persists.
- Advise patient that local stinging, burning, itching, and redness are the most common side effects and to notify health care provider if they become bothersome.
- Advise patient to stop using the medication and contact health care provider if severe skin reactions occur (eg, blistering, swelling, oozing).
- Advise women to notify health care provider if pregnant, planning to become pregnant, or breastfeeding.
- Warn patient not to take any prescription or OTC drugs or dietary supplements without consulting health care provider.
- Advise patient that follow-up visits to examine the skin lesions may be necessary and to keep appointments.

Butoconazole Nitrate

(BYOO-toe-KOE-nuh-zole NYE-trate)

Class Topical/Antifungal

How Supplied
Femstat 3 Vaginal cream 2%

Action
PHARMACOLOGY: Increases cell membrane permeability in susceptible fungi.

Indications Local treatment of vulvovaginal candidiasis (moniliasis).

Contraindications Hypersensitivity to imidazoles.

Route/Dosage
Nonpregnant Women
Intravaginal 1 applicator (about 5 g) at bedtime for 3 days; may continue up to 6 days if needed.

PATIENT CARE CONSIDERATIONS
Administration/Storage
- Open applicator immediately before administration to prevent contamination.
- Use care not to contaminate applicator during use.
- With patient in supine position, (at bedtime or while in bed) insert medication high in vagina.

Pregnant Women
Intravaginal Use only during second or third trimester, 1 applicator (about 5 g) at bedtime for 6 days.

Interactions None well documented.

Lab Test Interferences None well documented.

Adverse Reactions
GU: Vulvar/vaginal burning; urinary frequency.

Precautions
Pregnancy: Category C.
Lactation: Undetermined.
Children: Safety and efficacy not established.
Intractable candidiasis: May be symptom of unrecognized diabetes or reinfection; evaluate patient carefully.
Irritation or sensitization: If this occurs, discontinue use.

- Complete full course of therapy even during menstrual period.
- Store at room temperature. Avoid heat above 40°C (104°F). Do not freeze.

Assessment/Interventions
- Obtain patient history, including drug history and any known allergies.

- Observe for vulvar or vaginal burning or urinary frequency. Notify health care provider of any signs of tissue changes at site of application.
- If patient has diabetes, monitor blood sugar and provide necessary interventions to control condition.

Patient/Family Education
- Teach patient correct application technique.
- Instruct patient to use sanitary napkin to prevent staining clothing.
- Caution patient to refrain from sexual intercourse or advise partner to use condom to prevent reinfection.
- Explain importance of informing sexual partner of possible infection and of seeking appropriate medical treatment.
- Caution patient against using tampons during treatment.
- Tell patient to notify health care provider if any of the following symptoms occur after initiation of therapy: headache; body aches; local irritation, burning or rash; vaginal swelling or discharge; sensitivity to light.

Butorphanol Tartrate

(byoo-TORE-fan-ahl TAR-trate)

Class Narcotic agonist-antagonist analgesic

How Supplied
Stadol Injection 1 mg/mL (1 mg of tartrate salt is equal to 0.68 mg base), Injection 2 mg/mL (1 mg of tartrate salt is equal to 0.68 mg base)
❧ *Apo-Butorphanol*

Action
PHARMACOLOGY: Potent analgesic that stimulates and inhibits opiate receptors in CNS. Antagonist effects decrease (but do not eliminate) abuse potential and may cause withdrawal symptoms in patients with opiate dependence.

PHARMACOKINETICS/DYNAMICS:
Absorption:
IM – T_{max} is 20 to 40 min.
Distribution: Butorphanol is about 80% protein bound. Vd is 305 to 901 L. Butorphanol crosses the blood-brain barrier and placenta; it is excreted into human milk.
Metabolism: Metabolized in liver to hydroxybutorphanol and norbutorphanol.
Excretion: 70% to 80% is excreted in urine (5% as unchanged drug); 15% is excreted in feces. The t½ is 2.1 to 8.8 hr (IV). Cl is 52 to 154 L/hr.
Onset:
IV – A few min.
IM – 10 to 15 min.
Peak:
IV/IM – 30 to 60 min.
Duration:
IV/IM – 3 to 4 hr.
Special Populations:
Renal Function Impairment – For those with Ccr less than 30 mL/min, the t½ is approximately doubled and the total body clearance is approximately ½.
Hepatic Function Impairment – The t½ may be tripled and total body clearance is approximately ½.
Elderly – The t½ is increased by 25%.

Indications Management of pain, including postoperative and migraine; preoperative or preanesthetic medication (to supplement balanced anesthesia); relief of pain during labor.

Contraindications Standard considerations.

Route/Dosage
Pain
ADULTS: **IV** 0.5 to 2 mg q 3 to 4 hr prn. **IM** 1 to 4 mg q 3 to 4 hr prn. Single doses should not exceed 4 mg.
ELDERLY: **IV/IM** ½ normal dose at twice normal interval. Titrate subsequent doses to response.
Nasal Initial dose is 1 mg. Wait 90 to 120 min before giving second 1 mg dose.

Preoperative/Preanesthetic
ADULTS:
Usual dose: **IM** 2 mg 60 to 90 min before surgery.

Labor
ADULTS: **IV/IM** 1 to 2 mg in early labor at term; repeat after 4 hr.

Kidney or Liver Impairment
ADULTS: **IM/IV** Increase dosing interval to q 6 to 8 hr initially. Titrate subsequent doses to response.

Interactions
Barbiturate anesthetics: Increased CNS and respiratory depression.
CNS depressants (eg, tranquilizers, sedatives, alcohol): Additive CNS depression.

Lab Test Interferences None well documented.

Adverse Reactions
CV: Vasodilation; palpitations.
CNS: Sedation; floating sensation; dizziness; confusion; headache; lethargy; insomnia.
DERM: Sweating; clammy skin.
GI: Nausea; vomiting; anorexia; constipation; dry mouth.
RESP: Respiratory depression.

Precautions
Pregnancy: Category C.

Lactation: Excreted in breast milk.
Children: Not recommended for children under 18 yr.
Elderly: More sensitive to effects; reduce dose.
Cardiovascular disease: Drug increases cardiac workload. Severe hypertension has occurred.
Drug dependency: Although potential for physical dependence is low, abuse may occur. Tolerance and psychological and physical dependence may occur with long-term use. Use in patients physically dependent on opiate agonists may precipitate withdrawal symptoms.
Head injury or increased intracranial pressure: Use with caution; drug can increase CSF pressure.

Overdosage: Signs and Symptoms
Hyperventilation, cardiovascular insufficiency, coma.

PATIENT CARE CONSIDERATIONS

Administration/Storage
- When giving by IM route, use deep, slow injection.
- When giving by direct IV infusion, drug may be given undiluted. Administer over 3 to 5 min.
- Store at room temperature, away from light.

Assessment/Interventions
- Obtain patient history, including drug history and any known allergies. Note history of drug abuse; neurologic, cardiovascular, renal, or liver disease.
- Take vital signs and auscultate heart and lungs before administration. Do not administer if respiratory rate is under 12 breaths/min.
- Institute fall precautions and assist with ambulation after administration.
- Monitor BP frequently to check for widening pulse pressure. If hypertension develops, withhold medication and call health care provider.
- Shallow respirations (under 10 breaths/min) may indicate impending respiratory arrest and need for respiratory assistance or stimulation.
- If drug is used during labor, observe fetal heart rate for signs of distress and newborn for signs of respiratory depression.

Patient/Family Education
- Demonstrate proper use of nasal spray for patients receiving drug via this route.
- Advise elderly patients to take safety precautions (eg, rise slowly, use handrails, request assistance with ambulation) if dizziness occurs.
- Explain that physical dependency can result from extended use.
- Instruct patient to avoid intake of alcoholic beverages or other CNS depressants.
- Advise patient that drug may cause drowsiness, and to use caution while driving or performing other tasks requiring mental alertness.
- Instruct patient not to take *otc* medications without consulting health care provider.

Caffeine

(KAF-een)

Class CNS stimulant

How Supplied
Caffedrine Tablets 200 mg ◆ *Maximum Strength NoDoz* Tablets 200 mg ◆ *Stay Awake* Tablets 200 mg ◆ *Vivarin* Tablets 200 mg ◆ *Keep Alert* Tablets 200 mg ◆ *357 HR Magnum* Tablets 200 mg ◆ *Overtime* Tablets 200 mg ◆ *20–20* Tablets 200 mg ◆ *Valentine* Tablets 200 mg ◆ *Keep Going* Tablets 200 mg ◆ *.44 Magnum* Capsules 200 mg ◆ *Molie* Capsules 200 mg ◆ *Fastlene* Capsules 200 mg ◆ *Enerjets* Lozenges 75 mg ◆ *Cafcit* Oral solution 20 mg/mL (caffeine citrate; 2 mg caffeine citrate is equivalent to 1 mg caffeine base), Injection 20 mg/mL (caffeine citrate; 2 mg caffeine citrate is equivalent to 1 mg caffeine base)

Action
PHARMACOLOGY: Increases calcium permeability in sarcoplasmic reticulum, inhibiting phosphodiesterase-promoting accumulation of cyclic AMP.

PHARMACOKINETICS/DYNAMICS:
Absorption: 99% absorbed orally. C_{max} is 5 to 25 mcg/mL; T_{max} is 15 to 120 min.
Distribution: Rapidly distributed throughout tissues; crosses the blood-brain barrier and placenta; excreted in breast milk. 17% to 36% protein bound. Vd is 0.64 kg.
Metabolism: Rapidly metabolized in the liver to 1-methyluric acid, 1-methylxanthine, and 7-methylxanthine; CYP1A2 is involved in the biotransformation.
Excretion: The $t_{½}$ is 3 to 5 hr. Approximately 1% is excreted in the urine as unchanged drug.
Special Populations:
Pregnancy, smoking, and cirrhosis – The $t_{½}$ is increased.

Indications
Fatigue and drowsiness; analgesia; apnea of prematurity; respiratory depression.

Contraindications
Caffeine and sodium benzoate solution in pediatrics.

Route/Dosage
Fatigue/Drowsiness
ADULTS AND CHILDREN (OVER 12 YR): **PO** 100 to 200 mg q 3 to 4 hr as needed.

Apnea of Prematurity
PRETERM INFANTS:
Loading dose (caffeine citrate): **IV** 20 mg/kg (1 mL/kg) over 30 min once.
Maintenance dose (caffeine citrate): **IV** (over 10 min) or PO 5 mg/kg (0.25 mL/kg) q 24 hr.

Interactions
Aspirin, clozapine, theophylline: Plasma levels of these agents may be elevated by caffeine, increasing their pharmacologic and adverse effect.
Cimetidine, disulfiram, fluoroquinolones, mexiletine, oral contraceptives: May increase caffeine levels, enhancing the effects.
Lithium: Plasma levels may be reduced by caffeine, decreasing the pharmacologic effect.
Phenytoin, smoking: May decrease caffeine levels.

Lab Test Interferences
False-positive elevations in serum urate measured by Bittner method; may increase urine levels of vanillymandelic acid, catecholamines, and 5-hydroxyindoleacetic acid, resulting in false-positive diagnosis of pheochromocytoma and neuroblastoma.

Adverse Reactions
CV: Tachycardia; extrasystoles; palpitations; other cardiac arrhythmias.
CNS: Insomnia; restlessness excitement; nervousness; tinnitus; scintillating scotoma; muscular tremor; headache; lightheadedness.
DERM: Urticaria; rash, dry skin, skin breakdown (caffeine citrate).
EENT: Retinopathy of prematurity (caffeine citrate).
GI: Vomiting; nausea; diarrhea; stomach pain; necrotizing enterocolitis, gastritis, GI hemorrhage (caffeine citrate).
GU: Diuresis; kidney failure (caffeine citrate).
HEMA: Disseminated intravascular coagulation (caffeine citrate).
METAB: Hyperglycemia; acidosis (caffeine citrate).
RESP: Dyspnea, lung edema (caffeine citrate).
OTHER: Hypersensitivity (eg, dermatitis, rhinitis, bronchial asthma); feeding intolerance, sepsis, accidental injury, hemorrhage, cerebral hemorrhage (caffeine citrate).

Precautions
Pregnancy: Category C.
Lactation: Excreted in breast milk.
Children: Caffeine and sodium benzoate injection is contraindicated in children.
Necrotizing enterocolitis: Other methylxanthines have been associated with development of necrotizing enterocolitis.
Depression: Too-vigorous treatment with parenteral caffeine can worsen depression.

GI effects: Caffeine may aggravate diarrhea in patients with irritable colon or exacerbate duodenal ulcers.
Seizure disorder: Seizures have been reported with caffeine overdose; use caffeine citrate with caution in infants with seizure disorders.
Cardiovascular disease: Caffeine can increase heart rate, left ventricular output, and stroke volume; use caffeine citrate with caution in infants with cardiovascular disease.
Metabolic effects: Caffeine stimulates glycogenolysis and lipolysis, which increases free fatty acids and produces hyperglycemia.
Bone mineral density: Caffeine is associated with decreased bone density.
Withdrawal: Symptoms may occur within 12 hr after cessation of chronic caffeine ingestion and persist up to 7 days.

Overdosage: Signs and Symptoms
Vomiting, myoclonus, agitation, myocardial irritability, cardiac arrhythmia, seizures, hematemesis, opisthotonus, decerebrate posturing, generalized muscular hypertonicity, rhabdomyolysis with renal failure, pulmonary edema, hyperglycemia; hypokalemia, leukocytosis, ketosis, metabolic acidosis, death.

PATIENT CARE CONSIDERATIONS
Administration/Storage
- Do not administer caffeine and sodium benzoate to neonates.
- Use syringe to carefully measure each oral dose of caffeine citrate oral solution.
- Do not administer tablets, capsules, or lozenges late in the day to avoid insomnia.
- Store capsules, tablets, lozenges, and oral solution at controlled room temperature (59° to 86°F). Keep oral solution tightly capped.
- Citrated caffeine parenteral solution may be stored for up to 24 hr at room temperature following dilution.

Assessment/Interventions
- Obtain patient history, including drug history and any known allergies. Note concurrent use of caffeine-containing beverages, foods, dietary supplements, or OTC products.
- Ensure that caffeine serum levels have been determined in neonates who have been treated with theophylline before starting caffeine citrate therapy for apnea.
- Monitor neonates for apnea events and notify health care provider if noted.
- Monitor patient for CNS, CV, GI, and general body side effects. Report to health care provider if noted and significant.

Patient/Family Education
- Explain name, dose, action, and potential side effects of drug.
- Caution patient to not exceed recommended dose.
- Inform patient that caffeine is not a substitute for normal sleep.
- Advise pregnant women to limit intake of caffeine and caffeine-containing beverages to a minimum.
- Warn patient that withdrawal symptoms may occur within 12 to 24 hr following cessation of chronic caffeine ingestion. Symptoms consist of headache, fatigue, depression, anxiety or insomnia and may last for up to 7 days.
- Advise patient to discontinue use if increased or abnormal heart rate, palpitations, dizziness, agitation, nervousness, or insomnia occur.
- Caution patient not to take any prescription or OTC drugs or dietary supplements without consulting their health care provider.

Caffeine citrate:
- Instruct parents or caregiver in proper measurement of dose.
- Caution parents or caregiver that if baby continues to have apnea events to contact the baby's health care provider and to not increase the dose of caffeine citrate unless advised to do so by health care provider.
- Advise parents or caregivers to contact the baby's health care provider if the baby seems lethargic or develops abdominal distention, vomiting, or bloody stools.

Calcipotriene
(kal-sih-POE-try-een)

Class Antipsoriatic/Synthetic vitamin D_3

How Supplied
Dovonex Ointment 0.005%, Cream 0.005%, Scalp solution 0.005%

Action
PHARMACOLOGY: Calcipotriene is a synthetic vitamin D_3 analog. In a manner similar to vitamin D, calcipotriene regulates skin cell production and development, thereby modifying the abnormal growth and production of keratinocytes, responsible for the scaly red patches characteristic of psoriasis.

Indications
Ointment and cream: Treatment of plaque psoriasis.
Scalp solution: Topical treatment of chronic, moderately severe psoriasis of the scalp.

Contraindications
Standard considerations; patients with acute psoriatic eruptions; patients with hypercalcemia or vitamin D toxicity.

Route/Dosage
OINTMENT
ADULTS: **Topical** Apply a thin layer to the affected skin once or twice daily; rub in gently and completely.

CREAM
ADULTS: **Topical** Apply a thin layer to the affected skin twice daily; rub in gently and completely.

SCALP SOLUTION
ADULTS: **Topical** Comb the hair to remove scaly debris and, after suitably parting, apply twice daily only to the lesions and rub in gently and completely, taking care to prevent the solution from spreading onto the forehead.

Interactions None well documented.

PATIENT CARE CONSIDERATIONS
Administration/Storage
- For topical use only.
- Avoid contact with the face and eyes.
- Cream is usually applied to affected skin areas bid.
- Apply a thin film of cream to affected area(s) and rub in gently and completely.
- Solution is usually applied to affected scalp areas bid.
- Comb hair to remove scaly debris, then part the hair and apply solution to lesions, rubbing in gently and completely.
- Do not allow solution to spread to the forehead.
- Store at controlled room temperature.
- Protect from freezing.
- Protect solution from sunlight.

Assessment/Interventions
- Obtain patient history, including drug history and any known allergies.
- Note history of hypercalcemia or evidence of vitamin D toxicity.
- Assess the skin and identify areas where medication is to be applied.
- Monitor for side effects, including irritation, dermatitis, rash, or itching.

Lab Test Interferences None well documented.

Adverse Reactions
DERM: Erythema, dry skin, peeling, rash, dermatitis, worsening of psoriasis, transient burning, stinging, tingling.

Precautions
Pregnancy: Category C.
Lactation: Undetermined.
Children: Safety and efficacy not established.
Elderly: May experience higher incidence of adverse effects.
Route: For topical dermatological use only; avoid contact with eyes and uninvolved skin. Scalp solution is flammable, keep away from open flame. Wash hands after every use. Monitor serum calcium.

Patient/Family Education
- Explain name, dose, action, and potential side effects of drug.
- Advise patient that medication is applied topically to skin lesions bid.
- Teach patient proper technique for applying cream: Wash hands; apply thin film of cream to affected area(s), rubbing in gently and completely. Wash hands after applying cream.
- Teach patient proper technique for applying solution to scalp: Wash hands; comb hair to remove scaly debris, then part the hair and apply solution to lesions, rubbing in gently and completely; do not allow solution to spread to the forehead. Wash hands after applying solution.
- Warn patient that scalp solution is flammable; keep away from open flame.
- Advise patient that improvement may not be seen for 2 wk or longer and may take up to 8 wk.
- Advise patient to stop using the product and contact the health care provider if skin irritation develops.
- Advise patient that follow-up visits to examine the skin lesions may be necessary and to keep appointments.

Calcitonin-Salmon

(kal-sih-TOE-nin–salmon)
Class Hormone

How Supplied
Calcimar Injection 200 IU/mL ♦ *Miacalcin* Injection 200 IU/mL, Nasal Spray 200 IU/activation (0.09 mL/dose) ♦ *Osteocalcin* Injection 200 IU/mL ♦ *Salmonine* Injection 200 IU/mL
✤ *Caltine* ♦ *Miacalcin* NS

Action
PHARMACOLOGY: Decreases rate of bone turnover, presumably by regulating bone metabolism (blocking bone resorption). In conjunction with parathyroid hormone, endogenous calcitonin regulates serum calcium.

PHARMACOKINETICS/DYNAMICS:

Absorption:
Injection – T_{max} is 16 to 25 min.
Nasal – Rapidly absorbed. T_{max} is 31 to 39 min. Bioavailability is approximately 3%.

Distribution: Calcitonin does not cross the placenta.

Metabolism: Rapidly metabolized to inactive fragments, primarily by the kidneys, but also in the blood and peripheral tissues.

Excretion: A small amount is excreted in the urine. The t½ is 43 min.

Duration: 5 to 8 days (after chronic dosing).

Indications Treatment of moderate to severe Paget disease, postmenopausal osteoporosis, hypercalcemia. Nasal spray for treatment of symptomatic Paget disease.

Contraindications Standard considerations.

Route/Dosage

Paget Disease
ADULTS:
Initial dose: **SC/IM** 100 IU/day.
Maintenance dose: **SC/IM** 50 IU/day or qod is usually sufficient.

Postmenopausal Osteoporosis
ADULTS: **SC/IM** 100 IU/day with supplemental calcium and adequate vitamin D intake. **Intranasal** 200 IU/day, alternating nostrils.

Hypercalcemia
ADULTS:
Starting dose: **SC/IM** 4 IU/kg q 12 hr. Titrate gradually on basis of response to maximum dose of 8 IU/kg q 6 hr.

Interactions None well documented.

Lab Test Interferences None well documented.

Adverse Reactions

DERM: Injection site inflammation; flushing of face or hands; pruritus of ear lobes; edema of feet; skin rashes.
EENT: Eye pain; salty taste.
GI: Nausea with or without vomiting (decreases with continued administration); anorexia; diarrhea; epigastric discomfort; abdominal pain.
GU: Nocturia.
OTHER: Feverish sensation.

Precautions

Pregnancy: Category C.
Lactation: Undetermined.
Children: Safety and efficacy not established.
Allergy: Systemic allergic reactions, including anaphylaxis, may occur.
Antibody formation: Circulating antibodies to calcitonin-salmon may occur after 2 to 18 mo of treatment. Treatment may or may not remain effective.
Hypocalcemic tetany: May occur with calcitonin, although no cases have been reported.
Osteogenic sarcoma: Known to increase in Paget disease.

Overdosage: Signs and Symptoms
Nausea, vomiting.

PATIENT CARE CONSIDERATIONS

Administration/Storage

- Administer by SC or IM injection. For doses greater than 2 mL, use IM site.
- Rotate injection sites to prevent skin irritation.
- Give medication at bedtime to reduce nausea and flushing.
- Keep medication under refrigeration.

Assessment/Interventions

- Obtain patient history, including drug history and any known allergies. Inquire about possible allergy to fish protein.
- Consider intradermal testing before first full therapeutic dose is given, to determine hypersensitivity.
- Have epinephrine (1:1000), antihistamines, and resuscitation equipment available in case anaphylaxis occurs.
- Use padded siderails and keep bed in low position if twitching or paresthesia occurs.
- Institute safety precautions to prevent falls.
- During early therapy have parenteral calcium available in case hypocalcemia occurs.
- Monitor serum calcium levels weekly during initial therapy.
- Periodically monitor BUN, serum creatinine, alkaline phosphatase, urinary hydroxyproline excretion (q 24 hr), parathyroid hormone levels, and electrolytes.
- Observe for signs of anaphylaxis, especially early in treatment. Notify health care provider immediately if any of these signs occur.
- Assess patient for signs of hypocalcemia: tachycardia, paresthesia, muscle cramps, laryngospasm, twitching, colic, Chvostek or Trousseau sign. Notify health care provider if any of these signs occur.

Patient/Family Education

- Teach patient aseptic injection technique.
- Instruct patient to rotate injection sites.
- Explain comfort measures to be used for injection sites.
- Emphasize importance of maintaining adequate intake of vitamin D.
- Explain that nausea is a common side effect, usually occurring 30 min after injection, and will lessen during course of therapy.

- Tell patient that other side effects include anorexia, vomiting, diarrhea, and flushing of face, ears, hands, and feet.
- If patient is taking medication for osteoporosis, explain need for maintaining proper levels of total calcium (1.5 g/day) and vitamin D.
- Remind patient that follow-up office visits and lab tests are necessary.
- Caution patient to follow low-calcium diet if ordered and to avoid high-calcium foods such as bok choy, broccoli, canned salmon/sardines, clams, cream soups, milk and dairy products, blackstrap molasses, oysters, spinach, tofu.
- Instruct patient not to take otc medications without consulting health care provider.

Calcitriol

(Kal-si-TRYE-ole)

Class Fat-soluble vitamin

How Supplied
Calcijex Injection 1 mcg/mL ♦ *Rocaltrol* Capsules 0.25 mcg, Capsules 0.5 mcg, Oral solution 1 mcg/mL ♦ *Calcitriol Injection* Injection 2 mcg/mL

Action
PHARMACOLOGY: Supply of vitamin D depends mainly on exposure to ultraviolet rays of the sun for conversion of 7-dehydrocholesterol in the skin to vitamin D_3 (cholecalciferol). Vitamin D_3 is activated in the liver and kidney before fully active as a regulator of calcium and phosphorus metabolism at target tissues.

PHARMACOKINETICS/DYNAMICS:
Absorption:
Oral – Rapidly absorbed from the intestine. T_{max} is 3 to 6 hr.

Distribution: Approximately 99.9% protein bound. Excreted in breast milk in low levels.

Metabolism: The first pathway involves 24-hydroxylase to produce calcitroic acid; the second pathway involves hydroxylation and cyclization. Calcitrol also undergoes enterohepatic recycling.

Excretion: The t½ is about 5 to 8 hr. About 27% is excreted in the feces and 7% in the urine within 24 hr.

Special Populations:
Renal Function Impairment – The t½ is increased by at least 2-fold.
Children – The t½ is prolonged.

Indications
Dialysis (Oral, IV): Hypocalcemia and resultant metabolic bone disease in patients on chronic renal dialysis.
Predialysis (Oral): Secondary hyperparathyroidism and resultant metabolic bone disease in patients with moderate to severe chronic renal failure (Ccr 15 to 55 mL/min) not yet on dialysis.
Hypoparathyroidism (Oral): Hypocalcemia in patients with postsurgical hypoparathyroidism, idiopathic hypoparathyroidism, and pseudohypoparathyroidism. **Unlabeled use(s):** Decreased severity of psoriatic lesions with an initial oral dose of 0.25 mcg bid and topically 0.1 to 0.5 mcg/g petrolatum.

Contraindications Hypercalcemia or patients with vitamin D toxicity; hypersensitivity to any component of this product.

Route/Dosage
Dialysis
PO 0.25 mcg/day. Unsatisfactory response, increase dose by 0.25 mcg/day at 4- to 8-wk intervals. Obtain serum calcium levels at least twice weekly during this titration. Normal or only slightly reduced calcium levels may respond to doses of 0.25 mcg every other day.
IV 0.02 mcg/kg (1 to 2 mcg) 3 times/wk, every other day. May increase 0.5 to 1 mcg, q 2 to 4 wk. During this titration, obtain serum calcium levels twice weekly.

Hypoparathyroidism
PO Initial dose is 0.25 mcg/day in the morning. Unsatisfactory response, increase dose at 2- to 4-wk intervals. During this titration, obtain serum calcium levels 2 times/wk.
ADULTS AND CHILDREN (6 YR OF AGE AND OVER): PO 0.5 to 2 mcg daily.
CHILDREN (1 TO 5 YR OF AGE): PO Have usually been given 0.25 to 0.75 mcg daily. Discontinue if hypercalcemia or serum calcium times phosphate product (Ca × P) totals more than 70.

Predialysis
PO Initial dose is 0.25 mcg/day in adults and pediatric patients over 3 yr of age. Dosage may be increased up to 0.5 mcg/day. In patients under 3 yr of age, dosage is 10 to 15 ng/kg/day.

Interactions
Calcium supplements: Avoid uncontrolled intake of additional calcium-containing preparations.
Cholestyramine: May reduce intestinal absorption of fat soluble vitamins.
Ketoconazole: May reduce endogenous calcitriol concentrations.
Magnesium: Magnesium-containing products may cause hypermagnesemia and should be avoided during calcitriol administration to patients on chronic renal dialysis.
Phenytoin/Phenobarbital: Inhibits endogenous synthesis of calcitriol, therefore may require higher doses if given simultaneously.

Phosphate-binding agents: Because phosphate transport in the intestine, kidneys, and bones may be affected, the dosage of phosphate-binding agents must be adjusted based on serum phosphate concentration.
Thiazides: Known to induce hypercalcemia by the reduction of calcium excretion.
Vitamin D: To avoid possible additive effects and hypercalcemia, withhold pharmacologic doses of vitamin D and its derivatives.

Lab Test Interferences None well documented.

Adverse Reactions See overdosage section.

Precautions
Pregnancy: Category C.
Lactation: May be excreted in breast milk.
Children: Safety and efficacy not established in dialysis patients.

Elderly: Dose selection should be cautious, starting at the low end of the dosage range.

Overdosage: Signs and Symptoms
Adverse effects are associated with excessive intake. The early stage of toxicity includes the following: weakness, headache, somnolence, nausea, vomiting, dry mouth, constipation, muscle pain, bone pain, metallic taste. The late stage symptoms of toxicity include the following: cardiac arrhythmias, hypertension, pruritus, conjunctivitis (calcific), anorexia, weight loss, pancreatitis, polyuria, polydipsia, nocturia, elevated BUN, nephrocalcinosis, hypercholesterolemia, elevated AST/ALT, albuminia, decreased libido, hyperthermia, photophobia, rhinorrhea, ectopic calcification, overt psychosis, dystrophy, sensory disturbances, dehydration, apathy, arrested growth, UTI.

PATIENT CARE CONSIDERATIONS
Administration/Storage
Oral:
- Administer prescribed dose without regard to meals, but administer with food if GI upset occurs.
- Administer dose in the morning to patient with hypoparathyroidism.
- Administer prescribed dose of oral solution using disposable graduated oral dispensers supplied with medication.
- Store capsules and oral solution at controlled room temperature (59° to 86°F). Protect from light.

Injection:
- For IV bolus injection only. Not for intradermal, subcutaneous, IM, or intra-arterial administration.
- Do not administer if particulate matter, cloudiness, or discoloration noted.
- Administer prescribed dose 3 times weekly.
- Discard any unused solution. Do not save for future use.
- Store injection at controlled room temperature (59° to 86°F).

Assessment/Interventions
- Obtain patient history, including drug history and any known allergies. Note hypercalcemia, vitamin D toxicity, concurrent use of vitamin D-containing products, concurrent use of digitalis products, or concurrent use of magnesium-containing products (dialysis patient only).
- Ensure that patient undergoing dialysis is using a nonaluminum phosphate binder and is on a low phosphate diet.
- Ensure that patient is receiving an adequate daily intake of calcium. Consider adding a calcium supplement if dietary calcium intake is less than 600 mg/day.
- Ensure that serum calcium is evaluated before starting therapy, twice weekly during dosage adjustment, and then periodically thereafter, and that blood samples are taken without a tourniquet. If hypercalcemia is noted or if the serum calcium times phosphate product (Ca × P) is greater than 70, immediately discontinue therapy and notify health care provider.
- Ensure that serum calcium and phosphorous are evaluated daily during periods of hypercalcemia.
- Ensure that serum calcium, phosphorous, magnesium, and alkaline phosphatase are determined periodically in patient on dialysis.
- Ensure that serum calcium, phosphorous, alkaline phosphatase, creatinine, and intact parathyroid hormone (iPTH) are determined before starting therapy in predialysis patient. Thereafter, serum calcium, phosphorous, alkaline phosphatase, and creatinine should be determined monthly for 6 mo and then periodically thereafter. The iPTH should be determined q 3 to 4 mo.
- Ensure that serum calcium, phosphorous, and 24-hr urinary calcium are determined periodically in hypoparathyroid patient.
- Frequently assess patient for signs and symptoms of hypercalcemia (eg, weakness, headache, drowsiness, nausea, vomiting, bone pain, metallic taste, appetite loss, weight loss, polyuria, polydipsia, nocturia, photophobia, mental status change). Immediately inform health care provider if noted.

Patient/Family Education
- Explain name, dose, action, and potential side effects of drug.
- Instruct patient to carefully follow the diet

and calcium supplementation instructions supplied by health care provider.
- Advise patient to take prescribed dose without regard to meals but to take with food if GI upset occurs.
- Advise patient or caregiver using oral solution to use disposable graduated oral dispensers supplied with medication.
- Instruct dialysis patient to avoid using any magnesium-containing products (eg, antacids).
- Educate patient regarding signs and symptoms of hypercalcemia. Instruct patient to immediately inform health care provider if they occur.
- Advise women to notify health care provider if pregnant, planning to become pregnant, or breastfeeding.
- Caution patient not to take any prescription or OTC medications, dietary supplements, or herbal preparations unless advised by health care provider.
- Advise patient that follow-up examinations and lab tests may be required to monitor therapy and to keep appointments.

Calfactant

(Kal-FACK-tant)
Class Lung surfactant

How Supplied
Infasurf Suspension, intrathecal 35 mg phospholipids/mL suspended in 0.9% sodium chloride solution and 0.65 mg proteins. With 26 mg phosphatidylcholine, of which 16 mg is disaturated phosphatidylcholine. Also includes 0.26 mg of SP-B.

Action
PHARMACOLOGY: Extract of natural surfactant from calf lungs that restores lung surfactant in premature infants with lung surfactant deficiency causing respiratory distress syndrome (RDS).

Indications RDS in premature infants under 29 wk of gestational age at high risk for RDS and for the treatment rescue of premature infants under 72 hr of age who develop RDS and require endotracheal intubation.

Contraindications None well documented.

Route/Dosage
NEWBORN INFANTS: **Intratracheal** 3 mL/kg body weight at birth. Dose may be repeated q 12 hr for total of 3 doses.

Interactions None well documented.

Lab Test Interferences None well documented.

PATIENT CARE CONSIDERATIONS

Administration/Storage
- Refrigerate (36° to 46°F) and protect from light.
- Discard any unused drug after opening.
- Unopened, unused vials that have been warmed to room temperature can be returned to refrigerator within 24 hr for future use. Avoid repeated warming.
- For intratracheal administration only. Administer through an endotracheal tube. Draw dose into a syringe from the single-use vial using a 20-gauge or larger needle; avoid

Adverse Reactions
CV: Bradycardia.
RESP: Cyanosis; airway obstruction.
OTHER: Reflux of surfactant into endotracheal tube; requirement for manual ventilation; reintubation.

Precautions
Monitoring: Calfactant can rapidly improve oxygenation and lung compliance; monitor patients carefully so that oxygen therapy and ventilatory support can be modified in response to changes in respiratory status.
Administration: Administer calfactant intratracheally through an endotracheal tube and only in an acute care unit organized, staffed, equipped, and experienced with intubation, ventilation management, and general care of newborns with, or at risk for, RDS.
Dosing precautions: If any of the following situations occur while administering calfactant, interrupt administration and stabilize the infant's condition before resuming administration: bradycardia; reflux of calfactant into endotracheal tube; airway obstruction; cyanosis; hypoventilation; dislodgment of endotracheal tube.

Overdosage: Signs and Symptoms
Overloading of the lungs with isotonic solution.

excessive shaking and foaming.
- Administer only in an acute care setting under clinicians experienced with ventilator management, intubation, and acute and general care of high-risk infants in respiratory distress.
- Do not shake, dilute, or sonicate. If settling has occurred, swirl or roll gently.
- Calfactant is not to be reconstituted.
- Visible flecks in the suspension and foaming at the surface are normal and warming before administration is not necessary.

- Before administration, ensure proper placement and patency of endotracheal tube. If suctioning is required, be sure patient is adequately oxygenated and stabilized before administering.
- Administer calfactant via the intratracheal route through a side-port adapter into the endotracheal tube. Two qualified medical professionals experienced in the care of high-risk infants should facilitate the dosing: one to instill the calfactant and the other to monitor the patient and assist in positioning. After each aliquot is instilled, position the infant on the right or left side to facilitate distribution.
- Cafactant also can be administered through a 5 French feeding catheter inserted into the endotracheal tube with the tip above the carina. Do not instill into the main stem bronchus. Attach the catheter to syringe. Fill with medication and discard any excess through catheter to ensure the total dose to be given remains in syringe. Instill the total dose in 4 equal aliquots with the catheter removed between each of the instillations and mechanical ventilation resumed for 30 sec to 2 min. Administer each of the aliquots in 1 of 4 different positions (eg, prone, supine, right, left lateral) to facilitate even distribution of the surfactant. Continue the procedure until the total dose is achieved.
- Repeat doses can be administered as early as 6 hr after the previous dose for a total of 4 doses or less if the infant is still intubated and required at least 30% inspired oxygen to maintain acceptable PaO_2 values.

Assessment/Interventions
- Take baseline vital signs and monitor during and after medication administration.
- During administration of calfactant liquid suspension into the airway, monitor the infant for bradycardia, reflux of calfactant into the endotracheal tube, airway obstruction, cyanosis, dislodgment of the endotracheal tube, or hypoventilation. If any of these events occur, interrupt administration and stabilize the infant's condition using appropriate interventions before resuming administration.
- Monitor lung sounds carefully for any changes (eg, moist rales).
- Continually monitor oxygen and carbon dioxide levels. If oxygen saturation decreases or bradycardia develops, discontinue administration until the infant is stabilized.
- Be prepared for possible endotracheal suctioning or re-intubation if signs of airway obstruction are present during administration.
- Monitor respiratory and oxygen status closely following administration and adjust oxygen therapy and ventilator pressures appropriately.
- Avoid suctioning patient for 1 hr after administration unless airway obstruction is present.
- Assess for signs and symptoms of common complications of prematurity and RDS not necessarily related to calfactant therapy (eg, apnea, patent ductus arteriosus, intracranial hemorrhage, sepsis, pulmonary air leaks, pulmonary interstitial emphysema, pulmonary hemorrhage, necrotizing enterocolitis) and institute appropriate action.

Patient/Family Education
- Provide family with drug information pamphlet.
- Offer frequent updates to the parents and other family members on the infant's condition.
- Encourage whole family participation in the infant's care whenever possible.
- Provide emotional support.
- Make appropriate referrals to hospital services and support groups.

Candesartan Cilexetil

(kan-deh-SAHR-tan sigh-LEX-eh-till)

Class Antihypertensive/Angiotensin II antagonist

How Supplied
Atacand Tablets 4 mg, Tablets 8 mg, Tablets 16 mg, Tablets 32 mg

Action
PHARMACOLOGY: Antagonizes the angiotensin II effect (vasoconstriction and aldosterone secretion) by blocking the angiotensin II receptor (AT_1 receptor) in vascular smooth muscle and the adrenal gland, producing decreased BP.

PHARMACOKINETICS/DYNAMICS:

Absorption: Bioavailability is about 15%. T_{max} is 3 to 4 hr.

Distribution: Vd is 0.13 L/kg. More than 99% protein bound.

Metabolism: Candesartan cilexetil is bioactivated by ester hydrolysis during absorption from the GI tract to candesartan. Candesartan undergoes minor hepatic metabolism by O-deethylation to an inactive metabolite.

Excretion: The $t_{½}$ is about 9 hr. Plasma Cl is 0.37 mL/min/kg. Renal Cl is 0.19 mL/min/kg.

About 26% is excreted unchanged in urine. Not dialyzable.

Special Populations:
Renal Function Impairment – In hypertensive patients, serum concentrations are elevated. In patients with Ccr less than 30 mL/min/1.73 m^2, the AUC and C_{max} are approximately doubled.
Hepatic Function Impairment – The AUC and C_{max} increased 30% and 56% in mild impairment and 145% and 73% in moderate impairment, respectively.
Elderly – C_{max} is about 50% higher; AUC is about 80% higher.

Indications Treatment of hypertension.

Contraindications Standard considerations.

Route/Dosage
ADULTS: PO *Initial dose:* 16 mg/day; consider lower dose if volume-depleted. Total daily doses range from 8 to 32 mg in 1 or 2 doses.

Interactions
Lithium: Plasma concentrations may be increased by candesartan, resulting in an increase in the pharmacologic and adverse effects of lithium.

Lab Test Interferences None well documented.

Adverse Reactions
CNS: Headache; dizziness; fatigue.
EENT: Rhinitis; sinusitis; pharyngitis.
GI: Nausea; abdominal pain; diarrhea; vomiting.
RESP: Upper respiratory tract infection; bronchitis; cough.
OTHER: Back pain; chest pain; edema; arthralgia; albuminuria.

> **WARNING:**
> *Pregnancy:* Use in second and third trimesters may cause injury and death to fetus.

Precautions
Pregnancy: Category D (second and third trimester); Category C (first trimester). Can cause injury or death to fetus if used during second or third trimester.
Lactation: Undetermined.
Children: Safety and efficacy not established.
Renal function impairment: Use caution in treating patients whose renal function may depend on the activity of the renin-angiotensin-aldosterone system (eg, patients with severe CHF).
Hepatic function impairment: Consider using a lower starting dose in patients with moderate hepatic impairment.
Hypotension/Volume-depleted patients: Symptomatic hypotension may occur after initiation of candesartan in patients who are intravascularly volume depleted (eg, those treated with diuretics). Correct these conditions prior to administration of candesartan or use a lower starting dose.
Black patients: Candesartan may not be as effective in black patients.

Overdosage: Signs and Symptoms
Hypotension, tachycardia.

PATIENT CARE CONSIDERATIONS

Administration/Storage
- Administer without regard to food.
- Check BP before administration.
- Anticipate a synergistic or additive effect with concomitant use of thiazides and other antihypertensive medications.
- Do not administer if patient is pregnant, breastfeeding, or otherwise contraindicated.
- Store at controlled room temperature (59° to 86°F) in a tightly closed container. Protect from moisture.

Assessment/Interventions
- Obtain complete drug history, including any known allergies.
- Closely monitor infants exposed to candesartan in utero for hypotension, oliguria, and hyperkalemia. Supportive measures for renal perfusion and BP stabilization may be necessary. Exchange transfusions and dialysis may be required.
- Monitor BP and pulse. Should hypotension, tachycardia, or bradycardia result, withhold the medication and notify health care provider.
- Monitor for symptomatic hypotension especially in salt- or volume-depleted patients such as those on diuretics. Correct condition prior to treatment or monitored under close medical supervision. If hypotension occurs, place the patient in the supine position and have an IV infusion of normal saline available.
- Institute fall precautions in unstable patients.
- Closely monitor patients with severe CHF or progressive azotemia and (rarely) symptoms of acute renal failure.
- Monitor patients with impaired renal function for decreased urinary output and for adverse reactions.
- Assess patient for signs of hyperkalemia, especially if they are using a potassium-sparing diuretic.
- Review available laboratory tests for the following abnormal findings: creatine and BUN,

hemoglobin, hematocrit, WBCs, platelets, LFTs.
- Monitor for signs of hypersensitivity, which includes angioedema, involving swelling of the face, lips, and tongue. Where there is involvement of the tongue, glottis, or larynx likely to cause airway obstruction, promptly administer emergency therapy, which could include epinephrine.

Patient/Family Education
- Provide patient information pamphlet.
- Instruct patient to take the medication as prescribed at the same time each day.
- Inform patient that candesartan can control but does not cure hypertension.
- Caution patient to take the dose exactly as prescribed and not to stop taking the medication even if feeling better.
- Instruct patient not to decrease or increase the dosage without talking with health care provider.
- Inform patient of the following possible adverse effects: dry cough, renal function impairment, fetal injury.
- Advise women to notify health care provider if pregnant, planning to become pregnant, or breastfeeding.
- Instruct the patient in BP and pulse measurement skills. Caution patient to call health care provider should abnormal readings occur.
- Instruct patient that other methods of fall prevention, including rising slowly and sitting on the side of the bed before standing, especially early in therapy.
- Instruct patient of other medications, especially hypertensive medications, can have additive or synergistic effects. Have patient inform health care provider of all medication, including OTC drugs, presently being taking.
- Inform patient of the importance of adjunct therapies such as dietary planning, a regular exercise program, weight reduction, a low sodium diet, smoking cessation program, alcohol reduction, and stress management.
- Instruct patient to monitor renal, hepatic, and hematologic symptoms including urinary output and any discomfort during urination, weakness, fatigue, dizziness, lightheadedness, and jaundice. Patient should inform primary caregiver if symptoms occur.
- Warn patient that inadequate fluid intake, excessive perspiration, diarrhea, or vomiting, resulting in reduced fluid volume, may lead to an excessive fall in BP, lightheadedness, and possible fainting.
- Tell patient not to use potassium supplement or salt substitutes containing potassium to prevent possible hyperkalemia.
- Instruct patient to report any indications of an infection such as a sore throat, which could indicate neutropenia.
- Caution patient to inform health care provider or dentist of drug therapy prior to surgery or treatment.

Candesartan Cilexetil/ Hydrochlorothiazide

(kan-deh-SAHR-tan sigh-LEX-eh-till/high-droe-klor-oh-THIGH-uh-zide)

Class Antihypertensive/Angiotensin II antagonist/Thiazide diuretic

How Supplied
Atacand HCT Tablets 16 mg candesartan, 12.5 mg hydrochlorothiazide, Tablets 32 mg candesartan, 12.5 mg hydrochlorothiazide
✤ Atacand Plus

Action
PHARMACOLOGY:
Candesartan: Antagonizes the effect of angiotensin II (vasoconstriction and aldosterone secretion) by blocking the angiotensin II receptor (AT_1 receptor) in vascular smooth muscle and the adrenal gland, producing decreased BP.
Hydrochlorothiazide (HCTZ): Increases chloride, sodium, and water excretion by interfering with transport of sodium ions across renal tubular epithelium.

Indications Treatment of hypertension.

Contraindications Any component of product; patients with anuria or hypersensitivity to sulfonamide-derived drugs.

Route/Dosage
ADULTS: **PO** *Atacand HCT* may be substituted for previously titrated individual components. The daily dose range for *Atacand HCT* tablets is candesartan 16 mg combined with HCTZ 12.5 mg to candesartan 32 mg combined with HCTZ 25 mg.

Interactions
Candesartan:
Alcohol, barbiturates, narcotics – Increased risk of orthostatic hypotension.
Antidiabetic agents (oral and insulin agents) – Dosage adjustment of antidiabetic agent may be necessary.
Corticosteroids, ACTH – Increased electrolyte depletion, increasing risk of hypokalemia.
Non-steroidal anti-inflammatory agents – The diuretic, natriuretic, and hypertensive effects of loop, potassium-sparing, and thiazide diuretics may be reduced.
Pressor amines (eg, norepinephrine) – Decreased responsiveness of the pressor amine.

Skeletal muscle relaxants, nondepolarizing (eg, tubocurarine) – Increased responsiveness of the muscle relaxant.
HCTZ:
Bile acid sequestrants – May reduce HCTZ absorption; give HCTZ at least 2 hr before sequestrant.
Diazoxide – May cause hyperglycemia.
Digitalis glycosides – Diuretic-induced hypokalemia and hypomagnesemia may lead to digitalis-induced arrhythmias.
Lithium – Because renal excretion of lithium may be reduced, avoid use if possible.
Loop diuretics (eg, furosemide) – Synergistic effects may occur, resulting in profound diuresis and serious electrolyte abnormalities.
Sulfonylureas (eg, chlorpropamide) – Hypoglycemic effect of sulfonylurea may be decreased, necessitating an increase in sulfonylurea dosage.

Lab Test Interferences HCTZ may decrease serum protein-bound iodine levels without signs of thyroid disturbances; may cause diagnostic interference of serum electrolyte levels, blood and urine glucose levels, serum bilirubin levels, and serum uric acid levels.

Adverse Reactions
CV:
Candesartan – Tachycardia; palpitation; extrasystoles; bradycardia; abnormal ECG.
HCTZ – Hypotension (including orthostatic hypotension).
CNS:
Candesartan – Dizziness; vertigo; paresthesia; hypesthesia; depression; insomnia; anxiety; somnolence.
HCTZ – Restlessness; headache.
DERM:
Candesartan – Eczema; increased sweating; pruritus; dermatitis; rash; urticaria.
HCTZ – Erythema multiforme (including Stevens-Johnson syndrome); exfoliative dermatitis (including toxic epidermal necrolysis); alopecia.
EENT:
Candesartan – Sinusitis; pharyngitis; rhinitis; conjunctivitis; tinnitus.
HCTZ – Transient blurred vision; xanthopsia.
GI:
Candesartan – Nausea; abdominal pain; diarrhea; dyspepsia; gastritis; gastroenteritis; vomiting.
HCTZ – Pancreatitis; sialadenitis; cramping; constipation; gastric irritation; anorexia.
GU:
Candesartan – UTI; hematuria; cystitis; albuminuria.
HCTZ – Renal failure; renal dysfunction; interstitial nephritis; impotence.
HEMA:
Candesartan – Epistaxis; neutropenia; leukopenia; agranulocytosis.
HCTZ – Aplastic anemia; hemolytic anemia; thrombocytopenia.
HEPA:
Candesartan – Abnormal hepatic function; increased transaminase levels.
METAB:
Candesartan – Hyperuricemia; hyperglycemia; hypokalemia; increased BUN; increased creatine phosphokinase; hypertriglyceridemia.
HCTZ – Electrolyte imbalance; glycosuria.
RESP:
Candesartan – Upper respiratory tract infection; influenza-like symptoms; bronchitis; cough; dyspnea.
HCTZ – Respiratory distress (including pneumonitis and pulmonary edema).
OTHER:
Candesartan – Back pain; fatigue; pain; chest pain; peripheral edema; asthenia; arthralgia; myalgia; arthrosis; arthritis; leg cramps; sciatica; infection; viral infection.
HCTZ – Fever; weakness; anaphylactic reactions; necrotizing angiitis; photosensitivity; muscle spasm; purpura.

Precautions
Pregnancy: Category D (second and third trimester); Category C (first trimester). Can cause injury and death to fetus if used during second or third trimester.
Lactation: Candesartan: Undetermined; HCTZ: excreted in breast milk.
Children: Safety and efficacy in children less than 18 yr not established.
Renal function impairment: Use with caution.
Hepatic function impairment: Use with caution.
Diabetics: May require adjustments of insulin or oral hypoglycemic agents; hyperglycemia may occur.
Hyperuricemia: May occur, or acute gout may be precipitated.
Hypotension/Volume-depleted patients: Symptomatic hypotension may occur after initiation of therapy in patients who are intravascularly volume depleted. Correct these conditions prior to administration.
Systemic lupus erythematosus: May be activated or exacerbated.

Overdosage: Signs and Symptoms
Candesartan: Hypotension, dizziness, tachycardia, bradycardia.
HCTZ: Electrolyte depletion (eg, hypokalemia, hypochloremia, hyponatremia), dehydration.

PATIENT CARE CONSIDERATIONS

Administration/Storage

- Give qd in the morning, with or without food.
- Administer alone or in combination with other antihypertensives.
- Do not administer to pregnant women as fetal and neonatal morbidity and death can occur.
- Administer with caution and reduced dosage in patients with possible depletion of intravascular volume.
- Store tablets at controlled room temperature (59° to 86°F). Keep container tightly closed.

Assessment/Interventions

- Obtain patient history, including drug history and any known allergies. Note history of diabetes, anuria, lupus erythematosus, kidney or liver disease, or allergy to sulfonamide-derived drugs.
- Ensure that serum electrolytes are monitored periodically.
- Monitor and record BP and pulse. Should hypotension result, hold medication and notify health care provider.
- Take safety precautions if orthostatic hypotension occurs.
- Monitor blood sugar in diabetic patient when drug is started or dose is changed. Report significant changes to health care provider.
- Monitor for signs of hypersensitivity, including angioedema involving swelling of the face, lips, eyelids, and tongue. Discontinue medication and notify health care provider immediately if noted.

Patient/Family Education

- Explain name, dose, action, and potential side effects of drug.
- Advise patient to take qd as prescribed, without regard to meals.
- Advise patient to try to take each dose at about the same time qd.
- Inform patient that drug controls, but does not cure, hypertension and to continue taking drug as prescribed even when BP is not elevated.
- Caution patient not to change the dose or stop taking unless advised by health care provider.
- Instruct patient to continue taking other BP medications as prescribed by health care provider.
- Instruct patient in BP and pulse measurement skills.
- Advise patient to monitor and record BP and pulse at home and to inform health care provider if abnormal measurements are noted. Also advise patient to take record of BP and pulse to each follow-up visit.
- Caution patient to avoid sudden position changes to prevent orthostatic hypotension.
- Instruct patient to lie or sit down if experiencing dizziness or lightheadedness when standing.
- Caution patient that inadequate fluid intake, excessive perspiration, diarrhea, or vomiting can lead to excessive fall in BP resulting in lightheadedness or fainting.
- Instruct diabetic patient to monitor blood glucose more frequently when drug is started or dose is changed and to inform health care provider of significant changes in readings.
- Caution patient to avoid unnecessary exposure to UV light (sunlight, tanning booths), use sunscreen, and wear protective clothing when exposed to UV light to avoid photosensitivity reaction.
- Emphasize to hypertensive patient importance of other modalities on BP: weight control, regular exercise, smoking cessation, and moderate intake of alcohol and salt.
- Advise women to notify health care provider if pregnant, planning to become pregnant, or breastfeeding.
- Instruct patient to stop taking drug and immediately report any of the following symptoms to health care provider: fainting, swelling of the face, lips, eyelids, or tongue.
- Caution patient to not take any prescription or OTC medications, potassium salt substitutes, or potassium dietary supplements unless advised by health care provider.
- Advise patient that follow-up visits and lab tests may be required to monitor therapy and to keep appointments.

Capecitabine

(cap-eh-SITE-ah-bean)
Class Pyrimidine/Antimetabolite

How Supplied
Xeloda Tablets 150 mg, Tablets 500 mg

Action
PHARMACOLOGY: Capecitabine is an oral systemic prodrug that is enzymatically converted to 5-fluorouracil (5-FU). Healthy and tumor cells metabolize 5-FU to 5-fluoro-2-deoxyuridine monophosphate (FdUMP) and 5-fluorouridine triphosphate (FUTP). These metabolites cause cell injury by 2 different mechanisms. First, they inhibit the formation of thymidine triphosphate, which is essential for the synthesis of DNA. Second, nuclear transcriptional enzymes can mistakenly incorporate FUTP during the synthesis of RNA. This metabolic error can interfere with RNA processing and protein synthesis.

PHARMACOKINETICS/DYNAMICS:
Absorption: T_{max} is approximately 1.5 hr for capecitabine and 2 hr for 5-FU. Food decreased C_{max} 60% and AUC 35% for capecitabine and decreased C_{max} 4.3% and AUC 21% for 5-FU. Food delayed T_{max} 1.5 hr.

Distribution: Less than 60% protein bound (about 35% bound to albumin).

Metabolism: Enzymatically metabolized to 5-FU (active) in tissues; also metabolized to inactive metabolites in the liver.

Excretion: The t½ is about 0.75 hr (for capecitabine and 5-FU). About 95.5% is excreted in urine (57% of the dose as inactive metabolite and 3% of the dose as unchanged drug); 2.6% is excreted in feces.

Special Populations:
Renal Function Impairment – In moderate to severe renal impairment, there is increased exposure to inactive metabolites and a 25% increase in exposure to capecitabine.
Hepatic Function Impairment – Capecitabine AUC and C_{max} increased 60%; 5-FU was not affected.

Indications Treatment of resistant metastatic breast cancer alone or in combination with docetaxel; colorectal cancer.

Contraindications Hypersensitivity to 5-FU; severe renal impairment (Ccr below 30 mL/min); dihydropyrimidine dehydrogenase deficiency.

Route/Dosage
ADULTS: PO 2500 mg/m²/day in 2 divided doses, about 12 hr apart, for 2 wk. After a 1-wk rest period, this 3-wk cycle is repeated. Round to the nearest dose that gives a whole tablet size, rather than cutting tablets in half. Dosing adjustments are needed for toxicities. Once the capecitabine dose is reduced, it should not be increased. Please see manufacturer's recommendations.

Interactions
Antacids: May increase capecitabine levels.
Cimetidine or metronidazole: May increase serum concentrations of fluorouracil and potentially increase toxicity
Fluorouracil: Drug interactions have been reported with fluorouracil, the principal active metabolite of capecitabine.
Leucovorin: May enhance GI toxicity of fluorouracil.
Levamisole: Risk of hepatotoxicity may be increased by coadministration with fluorouracil.
Phenytoin: Levels may be elevated by capecitabine, increasing the risk of side effects.
Warfarin: May alter warfarin's effects

Lab Test Interferences None well documented.

Adverse Reactions
CV: Venous thrombosis (8%).
CNS: Paresthesia (21%); peripheral sensory neuropathy, headache (10%); dizziness (8%); insomnia (7%); taste disturbances (6%); mood alteration, depression (5%).
DERM: Hand-and-foot syndrome (54%); dermatitis (27%); skin discoloration, nail disorder (7%); alopecia (6%).
EENT: Eye irritation (15%); pharyngeal disorder, abnormal vision (5%); sore throat (2%); laryngitis (1%).
GI: Diarrhea (55%); nausea (43%); abdominal pain (35%); vomiting (27%); decreased appetite (26%); stomatitis (25%); constipation (14%); GI motility disorder, oral discomfort (10%); upper GI inflammatory disorders, dyspepsia (8%); GI hemorrhage, ileus (6%).
HEMA: Lymphopenia (94%); anemia (80%); thrombocytopenia (24%); neutropenia (26%); idiopathic thrombocytopenia purpura (1%).
HEPA: Hyperbilirubinemia (48%); hepatic failure (postmarketing).
METAB: Dehydration (7%).
RESP: Dyspnea (14%); cough (7%); epistaxis (3%).
OTHER: Fatigue/weakness (42%); pyrexia (18%); edema (15%); pain (12%); back pain (10%); myalgia (9%); arthralgia (8%); chest pain, pain in limb (6%); viral infections (5%).

> **WARNING:**
>
> *Warfarin:* Interaction with oral coumarin derivative anticoagulants. Altered coagulation parameters, bleeding, and death have been reported with combination. Increases in INR have occurred several days up to several months after initiating capecitabine, and in some cases, within 1 mo after stopping the capecitabine. Risk factors include 60 yr of age and older cancer. INRs or prothrombin time monitoring required with great frequency and appropriate adjustment of anticoagulant dose.

Precautions

Pregnancy: Category D.
Lactation: Undetermined.
Children: Safety and efficacy not established.
Elderly: Patients 80 yr and over may experience a greater incidence of grade 3 or 4 adverse events.
Renal function impairment: Patients with moderate renal impairment at baseline require dosage modification. Carefully monitor patients with mild or moderate renal impairment for adverse effects.

Hepatic function impairment: Carefully monitor patients with mild to moderate hepatic dysfunction caused by liver metastases.
Cardiac effects: Cardiotoxicity has been associated with fluorinated pyrimidine therapy.
Diarrhea: Capecitabine can induce diarrhea, sometimes severe. If grade 2, 3, or 4 diarrhea occurs, immediately interrupt administration until the diarrhea resolves or decreases in intensity to grade 1. Following grade 3 or 4 diarrhea, decrease subsequent doses of capecitabine.
Dihydropyrimidine dehydrogenase deficiency (DDD): Rarely, unexpected, potentially fatal toxicity (eg, diarrhea, neutropenia, neurotoxicity) cannot be excluded in patients with inadequate DDD activity.
Hand-and-foot syndrome: If grade 2 or 3 hand-and-foot syndrome occurs, interrupt administration of capecitabine until the event resolves or decreases in intensity to grade 1. Following grade 3 hand-and-foot syndrome, decrease subsequent doses of capecitabine.
Hyperbilirubinemia: If grade 2 to 4 elevations in bilirubin occur, immediately interrupt administration until the hyperbilirubinemia resolves or decreases in intensity to grade 1.

Overdosage: Signs and Symptoms

Nausea, vomiting, diarrhea, GI irritation and bleeding, bone marrow depression.

PATIENT CARE CONSIDERATIONS

Administration/Storage

- Do not administer to patient with Ccr less than 30 mL/min.
- May be administered alone or in combination with other chemotherapy medications.
- Administer prescribed dose bid, morning and evening. Administer each dose with water within 30 min after a meal.
- Medication is administered in 3-wk cycles, 2 wk of bid therapy, then 1 wk rest period.
- Store tablets at controlled room temperature (59° to 86°F).

Assessment/Interventions

- Obtain patient history, including drug history and any known allergies. Note renal or hepatic impairment, coronary artery disease, dihydropyrimidine deficiency, or concurrent use of oral anticoagulant (eg, warfarin), phenytoin, or folic acid.
- Administer reduced dose to patient with renal impairment (Ccr 30 to 50 mL/min).
- Ensure that dose is reduced or therapy interrupted per manufacturer's recommendations in patient who develops toxicity.
- Ensure that women of childbearing potential use effective contraception before initiating therapy and for duration of treatment.

- Monitor patient for development of hand-and-foot syndrome (eg, redness, swelling, numbness, discomfort of the hands and feet), stomatitis, nausea, and vomiting. Inform health care provider if noted.
- Monitor patient for development of diarrhea. Consider use of antidiarrheal therapy (eg, loperamide) and be prepared to administer fluid and electrolyte replacement if severe.
- Monitor patient for CNS, GI, respiratory, dermatologic, and general body side effects. Report to health care provider if noted and significant.

Patient/Family Education

- Advise patient or caregiver to review patient package insert before starting therapy and with each refill.
- Explain name, action, and potential side effects of drug.
- Review the following cyclic dosing schedule with patient or caregiver: bid for 2 wk, rest for 1 wk, then repeat cycle.
- Advise patient to take prescribed dose in the morning and evening with a glass of water within 30 min after a meal.
- Advise patient or caregiver that if a dose is missed not to take the missed dose and do

not double the next dose. Take the next dose at the regularly scheduled time.
- If patient is using a combination of different tablet strengths, ensure that patient or caregiver can correctly identify the correct dose.
- Advise patient that medication may be used in combination with other chemotherapy agents to achieve max benefit possible.
- Advise patient to discontinue therapy and notify health care provider if any of the following occur: diarrhea with 4 to 6 stools/day or diarrhea at night; nausea or sores in the mouth that interfere with eating; vomit 2 to 5 times within 24 hr; redness, swelling, and pain of the hands or feet.
- Advise patient or caregiver that OTC antidiarrheals (eg, loperamide) can be used to treat mild diarrhea.
- Advise patient to report fever, chills, or other signs of an infection to health care provider immediately.
- Caution women of childbearing potential to avoid becoming pregnant while being treated.
- Advise women to notify health care provider if pregnant, planning to become pregnant, or breastfeeding.
- Instruct patient not to take any prescription or OTC medications or dietary supplements unless advised by health care provider.
- Advise patient that frequent follow-up visits and laboratory tests will be required to monitor therapy and to keep appointments.

Capreomycin

(CAP-ree-oh-MY-sin)

Class Anti-infective/Antitubercular

How Supplied
Capastat Sulfate Powder for injection 1 g (as sulfate)/vial

Action
PHARMACOLOGY: Interferes with protein synthesis.

PHARMACOKINETICS/DYNAMICS:
Absorption: The T_{max} is 1 to 2 hr following IM administration.
Excretion: Approximately 52% of capreomycin is excreted unchanged in the urine within 12 hr.

Indications Treatment of tuberculosis concomitantly with other antituberculous agents.

Contraindications Standard considerations.

Route/Dosage
ADULTS: **IV/IM** 1 g/day (max, 20 mg/kg/day) for 60 to 120 days, followed by 1 g **IV** or **IM** 2 or 3 times weekly.

Interactions
Aminoglycosides (eg, streptomycin): May increase the risk of respiratory paralysis and renal dysfunction.
Nondepolarizing neuromuscular blocking agents (eg, tubocurarine): Neuromuscular blockade may be enhanced.

Lab Test Interferences None well documented.

Adverse Reactions
EENT: Ototoxicity; hearing loss.
GU: Nephrotoxicity.
HEMA: Leukocytosis; leukopenia; eosinophilia; thrombocytopenia.
HEPA: Decreased bromosulfophthalein excretion; abnormal liver function tests.
OTHER: Hypersensitivity (including febrile reactions, urticaria, maculopapular rash); pain; induration and excessive bleeding at injection site; sterile abscesses.

Precautions
Pregnancy: Category C.
Lactation: Undetermined.
Children: Safety and efficacy not established.
Renal function impairment: Dosage reduction is necessary.
Special risk patients: Use with great caution in patients with preexisting renal insufficiency or auditory impairment.
Hypokalemia: May occur during therapy.
Nephrotoxicity: Renal injury with tubular necrosis, elevation of BUN or serum creatinine, and abnormal urinary sediment may occur.
Ototoxicity: May occur; perform audiometric measurements and assess vestibular function prior to therapy and at regular intervals during treatment.

PATIENT CARE CONSIDERATIONS

Administration/Storage
- For IM or IV administration only. Do not administer intradermal or SC.
- Reconstitute following manufacturer's instructions.
- Inspect reconstituted solution visually before administration. Do not administer if solution is cloudy, discolored, or contains particulate matter. Reconstituted solution may acquire a pale straw color and darken with time, but this is not associated with loss of potency.
- For IM administration, give reconstituted capreomycin by deep IM injection into large muscle mass.
- For IV infusion, dilute reconstituted capreomycin in 100 mL of 0.9% Sodium Chloride

injection and infuse prescribed dose over 60 min.
- Do not add other medications to IV container.
- Store powder for injection at controlled room temperature (59° to 86°F). Reconstituted solution may be stored for up to 24 hr in refrigerator (36° to 46°F).

Assessment/Interventions
- Obtain patient history, including drug history and any known allergies. Note history of auditory, renal, or hepatic impairment, or coadministration of medications with ototoxic or nephrotoxic potential.
- Administer reduced dose to patients with known or suspected renal impairment following manufacturer's guidelines.
- Assess mycobacterial studies and susceptibility tests before and periodically throughout therapy to detect possible resistance.
- Ensure that at least one other antituberculosis agent is being used concurrently.
- Ensure that audiometric measurements and assessment of serum potassium, liver function, and vestibular function are performed prior to starting therapy and periodically during therapy.
- Ensure that renal function is evaluated prior to starting therapy and weekly during therapy.
- Assess patient for auditory and vestibular dysfunction. Notify health care provider immediately if noted.
- Assess IM injection sites for pain, bleeding, induration, or evidence of abscess formation. Inform health care provider if noted and significant.

Patient/Family Education
- Explain name, dose, action, and potential side effects of drug.
- Advise patient that medication will be prepared and administered by a health care provider in a health care setting.
- Review dosing schedule and prescribed length of therapy with patient. Emphasize to patient that treatment will be lengthy.
- Instruct patient to report the following symptoms to health care provider: ringing in the ears, vertigo (feeling of whirling motion), dizziness, hearing loss, itching, rash, pain, lumps, bleeding at injection site.
- Instruct women to notify health care provider if pregnant, planning to become pregnant, or breastfeeding.
- Instruct patient to not take any prescription or OTC medications or dietary supplements unless advised to do so by health care provider.
- Advise patient that follow-up visits and lab tests will be required to monitor therapy and to keep appointments.

Capsaicin

(kap-SAY-uh-sin)

Class Topical/Analgesic

How Supplied
Capsin Lotion 0.025%, Lotion 0.075% ♦ *Capzasin•P* Cream 0.025% ♦ *Dolorac* Cream 0.25% in emollient base ♦ *No Pain-HP* Roll-On 0.075% ♦ *Pain Doctor* Cream 0.025% ♦ *Pain-X* Gel 0.05% ♦ *R-Gel* Gel 0.025% ♦ *Zostrix* Cream 0.025% in emollient base ♦ *Zostrix-HP* Cream 0.075% in emollient base
✤ *Antiphlogistine Rub A-535 Capsaicin* ♦ *Capsaicin HP*

Action
PHARMACOLOGY: May deplete and prevent reaccumulation of substance P, principal transmitter of pain impulses, from periphery to CNS.

Indications Temporary relief of pain from rheumatoid arthritis and osteoarthritis; relief of neuralgias (eg, pain after shingles, diabetic neuropathy). **Unlabeled use(s):** Temporary relief of pain of psoriasis, vitiligo, intractable pruritus, postmastectomy and postamputation neuroma (phantom limb syndrome), vulvar vestibulitis, apocrine chromidrosis, reflex sympathetic dystrophy.

Contraindications Standard considerations.

Route/Dosage
ADULTS AND CHILDREN 2 YR AND OVER: Apply to affected area 3 to 4 times/day or less. Wash hands immediately after application.

Interactions None well documented.

Lab Test Interferences None well documented.

Adverse Reactions
DERM: Burning; stinging; erythema.
RESP: Cough; respiratory irritation.

Precautions
Pregnancy: Safety undetermined.
Lactation: Undetermined. Capsaicin is for external use only.

PATIENT CARE CONSIDERATIONS

Administration/Storage
- Wear gloves during application and avoid contact with eyes and broken or irritated skin.
- If bandage is needed, apply loosely to application area.
- Store at room temperature.

Assessment/Interventions
- Obtain patient history, including drug history and any known allergies.
- Note that transient burning may occur during initial course of therapy but will decrease in a few days. Burning is more common when medication is applied more than 3 times/day.
- Assess location and intensity of pain periodically throughout therapy.

Patient/Family Education
- Remind patient that this medication is for external use only.
- Teach patient correct method of application: wear gloves, avoid contact with eyes and broken or irritated skin, wash hands immediately after application.
- Caution patient to use care when handling contact lenses after application.
- Advise patient to keep bandage placed loosely over application area.
- Emphasize that following prescribed regimen reduces transient burning associated with infrequent administration. Remind patient not to apply medication more than 3 times/day.
- Instruct patient to discontinue treatment and notify health care provider if pain persists 14 to 28 days or returns a few days after initiation of therapy, or if signs of infection occur.
- Counsel patient to notify health care provider if persistent cough accompanies therapy.

Captopril

(KAP-toe-prill)

Class Antihypertensive/ACE inhibitor

How Supplied
Capoten Tablets 12.5 mg, Tablets 25 mg, Tablets 50 mg, Tablets 100 mg
🍁 *APO-Capto* ♦ *Gen-Captopril* ♦ *Novo-Captoril* ♦ *Nu-Capto* ♦ *PMS-Captopril* ♦ *ratio-Captopril*

Action
PHARMACOLOGY: Competitively inhibits angiotensin I-converting enzyme, preventing conversion of angiotensin I to angiotensin II, a potent vasoconstrictor that also stimulates aldosterone secretion. Results in decreased BP, potassium retention, and reduced sodium reabsorption.

PHARMACOKINETICS/DYNAMICS:
Absorption: T_{max} is about 1 hr. Food reduces absorption 30% to 40%.
Distribution: About 25% to 30% protein bound.
Excretion: More than 90% of a dose is eliminated in the urine; 40% to 50% is unchanged drug. The t½ is less than 3 hr.
Peak: 60 to 90 min.
Special Populations:
Renal Function Impairment – Excretion is reduced. Dosage reduction may be needed.

Indications Treatment of hypertension, CHF, left ventricular dysfunction after MI, diabetic nephropathy. **Unlabeled use(s):** Treatment of hypertensive crisis, neonatal and childhood hypertension, rheumatoid arthritis, diagnosis of anatomic renal artery stenosis and primary aldosteronism, treatment of hypertension related to scleroderma renal crisis and Takayasu disease, idiopathic edema, Bartter and Raynaud syndromes, asymptomatic left ventricular dysfunction after MI.

Contraindications Hypersensitivity to ACE inhibitors.

Route/Dosage

Diabetic Nephropathy
ADULTS: PO 25 mg tid.

Heart Failure
ADULTS:
Initial dose: PO 6.25 to 12.5 mg tid; then titrate to usual daily dosage within next several days. Generally to be used in conjunction with a diuretic and digitalis.

Hypertension
ADULTS:
Initial dose: PO 25 mg bid to tid; gradually increase q 1 to 2 wk if satisfactory effect is not achieved. Usual dose: 25 to 150 mg bid to tid. Usual dose does not exceed 50 mg tid. Max daily dose is 450 mg.

Left Ventricular Dysfunction after MI
ADULTS: PO 6.25 mg 3 days after MI; then 12.5 mg tid and 25 mg tid for next several days. Target dose: 50 mg tid over next several weeks.

Interactions
Food: Reduces bioavailability of captopril.
Indomethacin, salicylates (eg, aspirin): Hypotensive effects may be reduced, especially in low-renin or volume-dependent hypertensive patients.
Lithium: Increased lithium levels and symptoms

of lithium toxicity may occur.
Potassium preparations, potassium-sparing diuretics: May increase serum potassium levels.

Lab Test Interferences False-positive urine acetone test may occur.

Adverse Reactions
CV: Chest pain; palpitations; tachycardia; orthostatic hypotension.
CNS: Headache; sleep disturbances; paresthesias; dizziness; fatigue; malaise; ataxia; confusion; depression; nervousness.
DERM: Rash; pruritus; alopecia.
EENT: Rhinitis; cough.
GI: Nausea; abdominal pain; vomiting; gastric irritation; aphthous ulcers; peptic ulcer; jaundice; cholestasis; diarrhea; dysgeusia; anorexia; constipation; dry mouth.
GU: Oliguria; proteinuria.
HEPA: Elevated liver enzymes and serum bilirubin.
HEMA: Neutropenia; agranulocytosis; thrombocytopenia; pancytopenia.
METAB: Hyperkalemia; hyponatremia; elevated uric acid and blood glucose.
RESP: Chronic dry cough; dyspnea; eosinophilic pneumonitis.
OTHER: Gynecomastia; myasthenia.

> **WARNING:**
> *Pregnancy:* Use in second and third trimesters may cause injury and death to fetus.

Precautions
Pregnancy: Category D (second and third trimester); Category C (first trimester). ACE inhibitors can cause injury or death to fetus if used during second or third trimester. When pregnancy is detected, discontinue ACE inhibitors as soon as possible.
Lactation: Excreted in breast milk.
Children: Safety and efficacy not established.
Renal function impairment: Because captopril is excreted primarily by the kidneys, patients with impaired renal function may require smaller or less frequent doses.
Angioedema: Use with extreme caution in patients with hereditary angioedema.
Hepatic failure: Rarely, ACE inhibitors have been associated with a syndrome that starts with cholestatic jaundice and progresses to fulminant hepatic necrosis and sometimes death.
Hypotension/first-dose effect: Significant decreases in BP may occur after first dose, especially in patients with severe salt or volume depletion or those with CHF.
Neutropenia and agranulocytosis: Risk appears greater with renal dysfunction, CHF.
Proteinuria: May occur, especially in patients with prior renal disease or those receiving high doses of drug (more than 150 mg/day); generally resolves within 6 mo.

Overdosage: Signs and Symptoms
Hypotension.

PATIENT CARE CONSIDERATIONS

Administration/Storage
- Administer alone or in combination with other antihypertensives.
- Give prescribed dose 1 hr before or 2 hr after meals.
- Do not administer to pregnant women during second and third trimesters as fetal and neonatal morbidity and death can occur.
- Store tablets at controlled room temperature (59° to 89°F). Protect from moisture.

Assessment/Interventions
- Obtain patient history, including drug history and any known allergies. Note renal or hepatic impairment, conditions predisposing to volume depletion (eg, prolonged diuretic therapy), diabetes, heart failure, anuria, hereditary or idiopathic angioedema, lupus erythematosus, left ventricular outflow obstruction, allergy to any other ACE inhibitor, and concurrent use of potassium-containing salt substitutes, potassium supplements, or potassium-sparing diuretics.
- Ensure that small initial dose and gradual escalation of dose are used in patient with heart failure or moderate to severe renal impairment (Ccr less than 50 mL/min).
- Ensure that volume and/or salt depletion have been corrected before initiating therapy.
- Ensure that serum electrolytes and renal function are monitored periodically.
- Ensure that CBC with differential are evaluated prior to starting therapy, at 2 wk intervals for 3 mo, and periodically thereafter in patient with renal impairment.
- Monitor and record BP and pulse. If symptomatic hypotension occurs, hold medication and notify health care provider.
- Take safety precautions if orthostatic hypotension occurs.
- Assess heart failure patient for evidence of worsening failure (eg, daily weights, evaluation of peripheral edema, shortness of breath). Inform health care provider if rapid weight gain (eg, 2 pounds in 1 day or 5 pounds in 1 wk) is noted or if patient is experiencing worsening edema or other symptoms of heart

failure (eg, worsening shortness of breath).
- Monitor for signs of hypersensitivity including angioedema involving swelling of the face, lips, eyelids, and tongue. Discontinue medication and notify health care provider immediately if noted. Be prepared to treat appropriately.
- Assess patient for GI, CNS, and general body side effects. Inform health care provider if noted and significant.

Patient/Family Education
- Explain name, dose, action, and potential side effects of drug.
- Advise patient to take prescribed dose 1 hr before or 2 hr after meals because food can reduce absorption and benefits of medication.
- Advise patient to try to take each dose at about the same time each day.
- Inform hypertensive patient that drug controls, but does not cure, hypertension and to continue taking drug as prescribed even when BP is not elevated.
- Caution patient not to change the dose or stop taking unless advised by health care provider.
- Instruct patient to continue taking other medications for the condition as prescribed by health care provider.
- Instruct patient in BP and pulse measurement skills.
- Advise patient to monitor and record BP and pulse at home and to inform health care provider if abnormal measurements are noted. Also advise patient to take record of BP and pulse to each follow-up visit.
- Caution patient to avoid sudden position changes to prevent orthostatic hypotension.
- Instruct patient to lie or sit down if experiencing dizziness or lightheadedness when standing.
- Emphasize to hypertensive patient the importance of other modalities on BP control: weight control, regular exercise, smoking cessation, and moderate intake of alcohol and salt.
- Emphasize to heart failure patient the importance of other modalities that can help control heart failure symptoms: weight control, progressive exercise program, smoking cessation, and moderate intake of alcohol and salt.
- Advise heart failure patient to weigh daily, keep a record of daily weights, and notify health care provider if rapid weight gain (eg, 5 pounds in 1 wk) is noted or if edema or shortness of breath worsen.
- Caution patient that inadequate fluid intake, excessive perspiration, diarrhea, or vomiting can lead to excessive fall in BP resulting in lightheadedness or fainting.
- Advise patient that medication may cause dizziness or lightheadedness and to use caution while driving or performing other tasks requiring mental alertness until tolerance is determined.
- Caution patient to avoid unnecessary exposure to UV light (sunlight, tanning booths) and to use sunscreen and wear protective clothing when exposed to UV light to avoid photosensitivity reaction.
- Instruct women to inform health care provider if pregnant, planning to become pregnant, or breastfeeding.
- Instruct patient to stop taking drug and immediately report any of the following symptoms to health care provider: sore throat, fever, irregular heartbeat, chest pains, fainting, signs or symptoms of angioedema (eg, swelling of the hands, feet, face, lips, eyelids, or tongue, hoarseness, difficulty swallowing or breathing).
- Instruct patient to inform health care provider if a persistent cough or changes in taste develop while taking this medication.
- Caution patient not to take any prescription or OTC medications, potassium-containing salt substitutes, potassium supplements, or dietary supplements unless advised by health care provider.
- Advise patient that follow-up visits and lab tests will be required to monitor therapy and to keep appointments.

Captopril/ Hydrochlorothiazide

(KAP-toe-prill/high-droe-klor-oh-THIGH-uh-zide)

Class Antihypertensive/Thiazide diuretic

How Supplied
Capozide 50/25 Tablets 50 mg captopril and 25 mg hydrochlorothiazide ◆ *Capozide* 25/25 Tablets 25 mg captopril and 25 mg hydrochlorothiazide ◆ *Capozide* 50/15 Tablets 50 mg captopril and 15 mg hydrochlorothiazide ◆ *Capozide* 25/15 Tablets 25 mg captopril and 15 mg hydrochlorothiazide

Action
PHARMACOLOGY:
Captopril: Competitively inhibits angiotensin I-converting enzyme, resulting in the prevention of angiotensin I conversion to angiotensin II, a potent vasoconstrictor that also stimulates aldosterone secretion. This action results in a decrease in sodium and fluid retention, increase in diuresis, and a decrease in BP.

Hydrochlorothiazide (HCTZ): Increases chloride, sodium, and water excretion by interfering with transport of sodium ions across renal tubular epithelium.

Indications Treatment of hypertension.

Contraindications Anuric patients; patients hypersensitive to captopril or any other ACE inhibitor, HCTZ, or other sulfonamide derivative.

Route/Dosage

ADULTS: PO *Capozide* may be substituted for previously titrated individual components. Alternatively, therapy may be started with a single *Capozide* tablet (25 mg captopril combined with 15 mg HCTZ) qd. For patients not responding sufficiently, the dose may be titrated upward, usually at 6-wk intervals. Maximum daily dose should not exceed 150 mg of captopril or 50 mg of HCTZ.

Interactions

Alcohol, barbiturates (eg, phenobarbital), narcotics: Orthostatic hypotension may be potentiated.
Anticoagulants (eg, warfarin): Anticoagulant effect may be decreased.
Antidiabetic agents (eg, insulin, sulfonylureas): Dosage adjustment may be necessary because of possible HCTZ-induced elevation in blood glucose levels.
Antigout agents (eg, probenecid): Dosage adjustment may be necessary because of possible HCTZ-induced elevation in blood uric acid levels.
Cardiac glycosides (eg, digoxin): Possible digitalis toxicity associated with hypokalemia.
Cholestyramine, colestipol: May impair the absorption of HCTZ.
Food: Reduces bioavailability of captopril.
Lithium: Plasma levels of lithium may be elevated, increasing the risk of toxicity.
NSAIDs: May reduce the natriuretic and antihypertensive effect of HCTZ.
Potassium supplements, potassium-sparing diuretics (eg, spironolactone): Increased risk of hyperkalemia.
Nondepolarizing muscle relaxants (eg, tubocurarine): Effects may be increased.

Lab Test Interferences

Captopril: May cause false-positive urine acetone test.
HCTZ: May cause diagnostic interference of bentiromide test; may decrease serum protein-bound iodine levels without signs of thyroid disturbances; may cause diagnostic interference of serum electrolyte levels, blood and urine glucose levels, serum bilirubin levels, and serum uric acid levels.

Adverse Reactions

CV:
Captopril – Hypotension; tachycardia; chest pain; palpitations; angina pectoris; MI; Raynaud syndrome; CHF; cardiac arrest; cerebrovascular accident; rhythm disturbances; orthostatic hypotension; syncope.
HCTZ – Orthostatic hypotension; necrotizing angiitis.
CNS:
Captopril – Ataxia; confusion; depression; nervousness; somnolence.
HCTZ – Dizziness; vertigo; paresthesia; headache; xanthopsia; restlessness.
DERM:
Captopril – Rash; pruritus; pemphigoid-like lesion; photosensitivity; bullous pemphigus; erythema multiforme (including Stevens-Johnson syndrome); exfoliative dermatitis.
HCTZ – Purpura; photosensitivity; rash; urticaria.
EENT:
Captopril – Glossitis; blurred vision.
HCTZ – Transient blurred vision.
GI:
Captopril – Dysgeusia; pancreatitis; dyspepsia.
HCTZ – Anorexia; gastric irritation; nausea; vomiting; cramping; diarrhea; constipation; jaundice (intrahepatic cholestatic jaundice); pancreatitis; sialadenitis.
GU:
Captopril – Proteinuria; gynecomastia; impotence.
HCTZ – Glycosuria.
HEMA:
Captopril – Neutropenia; agranulocytosis; anemia; thrombocytopenia; pancytopenia; eosinophilia; aplastic anemia; hemolytic anemia.
HCTZ – Leukopenia; agranulocytosis; thrombocytopenia; aplastic anemia; hemolytic anemia.
HEPA:
Captopril – Jaundice; hepatitis, including necrosis and cholestasis.
METAB:
Captopril – Hyponatremia; hyperkalemia.
HCTZ – Hyperglycemia; hyperuricemia; hypokalemia; hyponatremia.
RESP:
Captopril – Bronchospasm; eosinophilic pneumonitis; rhinitis; persistent dry cough.
HCTZ – Respiratory distress, including pneumonitis.
OTHER:
Captopril – Fever; arthralgia; angioedema; anaphylactoid reactions; asthenia; myalgia; myasthenia; syndrome including fever, myalgia, arthralgia, interstitial nephritis, vasculitis, rash or other dermatologic symptoms, eosinophilia, and

elevated erythrocyte sedimentation rate.
HCTZ – Muscle spasm; weakness; fever; anaphylactic reactions.

Precautions

Pregnancy: Category D (second and third trimester); Category C (first trimester). ACE inhibitors (eg, captopril) can cause injury or death to fetus if used during second or third trimester. When pregnancy is detected, discontinue as soon as possible.
Lactation: Excreted in breast milk.
Children: Safety and efficacy not established.
Renal function impairment: Use with caution.
Hepatic function impairment: Use with caution.
Angioedema: Use with extreme caution in patients with hereditary angioedema. Angioedema associated with laryngeal edema may be fatal.
Hypotension: Decreases in BP may occur, especially in salt- or volume-depleted patients as a result of dialysis, prolonged diuretic therapy, dietary salt restriction, diarrhea, or vomiting. Volume and salt depletion should be corrected before initiating therapy with benazepril/HCTZ.
Neutropenia/agranulocytosis: Has occurred with other ACE inhibitors.

Overdosage: Signs and Symptoms

Dehydration, electrolyte disturbances, hypotension, CNS depression, lethargy, coma.

PATIENT CARE CONSIDERATIONS

Administration/Storage

- Give prescribed dose qd in the morning or, if ordered bid, give in morning and late afternoon.
- Give each dose 1 hr before meals.
- Administer alone or in combination with other antihypertensives.
- Do not administer to pregnant women as fetal and neonatal morbidity and death can occur.
- Administer with caution and reduced dosage in patients with possible depletion of intravascular volume.
- Store tablets at controlled room temperature (59° to 86°F). Keep container tightly closed and protect from moisture.

Assessment/Interventions

- Obtain patient history, including drug history and any known allergies. Note history of diabetes, anuria, lupus erythematosus, kidney or liver disease, or allergy to sulfonamide-derived drugs.
- Ensure that serum electrolytes are monitored periodically.
- Ensure that WBC with differential is determined prior to starting treatment, q 2 wk for 3 mo, and periodically thereafter in hypertensive patients with impaired renal function.
- Monitor and record BP and pulse. Should hypotension result, hold medication and notify health care provider.
- Take safety precautions if orthostatic hypotension occurs.
- Monitor blood sugar in diabetic patient when drug is started or dose is changed. Report significant changes to health care provider.
- Monitor for signs of hypersensitivity, including angioedema involving swelling of the face, lips, eyelids, and tongue. Discontinue medication and notify health care provider immediately if noted.

Patient/Family Education

- Explain name, dose, action, and potential side effects of drug.
- Advise patient to take every day as prescribed. Advise patient that if more than 1 daily dose is prescribed to take the second dose late in the afternoon to avoid excessive urination at night.
- Instruct patient to take each dose at least 1 hr before meals.
- Advise patient to try to take each dose at about the same time each day if possible.
- Inform patient that drug controls, but does not cure, hypertension and to continue taking drug as prescribed even when BP is not elevated.
- Caution patient not to change the dose or stop taking unless advised by health care provider.
- Instruct patient to continue taking other BP medications as prescribed by health care provider.
- Instruct patient in BP and pulse measurement skills.
- Advise patient to monitor and record BP and pulse at home and to inform health care provider if abnormal measurements are noted. Also advise patient to take record of BP and pulse to each follow-up visit.
- Caution patient to avoid sudden position changes to prevent orthostatic hypotension.
- Instruct patient to lie or sit down if experiencing dizziness or lightheadedness when standing.
- Caution patient that inadequate fluid intake, excessive perspiration, diarrhea, or vomiting can lead to excessive fall in BP, resulting in lightheadedness or fainting.
- Instruct diabetic patient to monitor blood

glucose more frequently when drug is started or dose is changed and to inform health care provider of significant changes in readings.
- Caution patient to avoid unnecessary exposure to UV light (eg, sunlight, tanning booths), use sunscreen, and wear protective clothing when exposed to UV light to avoid photosensitivity reaction.
- Emphasize to hypertensive patient importance of other modalities on BP: weight control, regular exercise, smoking cessation, and moderate intake of alcohol and salt.
- Advise women to notify health care provider if pregnant, planning to become pregnant, or breastfeeding.
- Instruct patient to stop taking drug and immediately report any of the following symptoms to health care provider: persistent cough; fainting; swelling of the face, lips, eyelids or tongue; sore throat; fever or other signs of infection; yellowing of skin or eyes; persistent nausea or vomiting; swelling of the feet or ankles.
- Caution patient to not take any prescription or OTC medications, salt substitutes, or dietary supplements unless advised by health care provider.
- Advise patient that follow-up visits and lab tests may be required to monitor therapy and to keep appointments.

Carbamazepine

(KAR-bam-AZE-uh-peen)

Class Anticonvulsant

How Supplied
Carbatrol Capsules, extended-release 100 mg, Capsules, extended-release 200 mg, Capsules, extended-release 300 mg ♦ *Epitol* Tablets 200 mg ♦ *Tegretol* Tablets, chewable 100 mg, Tablets 200 mg, Suspension 100 mg per 5 mL ♦ *Tegretol XR* Tablets, extended-release 100 mg, Tablets, extended-release 200 mg, Tablets, extended-release 400 mg

♣ *APO-Carbamazepine* ♦ *Gen-Carbamazepine CR* ♦ *Novo-Carbamaz* ♦ *Nu-Carbamazepine* ♦ *PMS-Carbamazepine CR* ♦ *Taro-Carbamazepine*

Action

PHARMACOLOGY: Mechanism appears to act by reducing polysynaptic responses and blocks posttetanic potentiation.

PHARMACOKINETICS/DYNAMICS:

Absorption: Therapeutic levels are 4 to 12 mcg/mL.
Suspension – T_{max} is about 1.5 hr.
Tablets – T_{max} is 4 to 5 hr.
Extended-Release – T_{max} is 3 to 12 hr.

Distribution: 76% protein bound. Rapidly crosses the placenta.

Metabolism: Induces its own metabolism; metabolized in the liver by CYP3A4 to the active metabolite carbamazepine-10,11-epoxide (shown to be equipotent to carbamazepine).

Excretion: Initial t½ is 25 to 65 hr, decreasing to 12 to 17 hr on repeated doses. 72% is excreted in urine (3% as unchanged drug) and 28% in feces.

Special Populations:
Children – More rapidly metabolized to carbamazepine-10,11-epoxide.

Indications Treatment of epilepsy (eg, partial seizures with complex symptoms, generalized tonic-clonic seizures [grand mal], mixed seizure patterns, other partial or generalized seizures) in patients refractory to or intolerant of other agents. Treatment of pain associated with trigeminal neuralgia. **Unlabeled use(s):** Treatment of certain psychiatric disorders; management of alcohol withdrawal; relief of restless legs syndrome; treatment of postherpetic neuralgia.

Contraindications Hypersensitivity to tricyclic antidepressants or carbamazepine; history of bone marrow depression; concomitant use of MAO inhibitors. Discontinue MAO inhibitors at least 14 days before administration of carbamazepine.

Route/Dosage
Epilepsy
ADULTS AND CHILDREN OVER 12 YR OF AGE:
Initial dose: PO 200 mg bid (tablets) or 100 mg qid (suspension). Increase weekly by up to 200 mg per day in 2 divided doses for extended-release or 3 to 4 divided doses for other formulations to reach minimum effective dose (max, 1,000 mg per day in children 12 to 15 yr of age; 1,200 mg per day in children above 15 yr of age; 1,600 mg per day in adults).
Maintenance: 800 to 1,200 mg per day.
ADULTS AND CHILDREN OVER 12 YR OF AGE (EXTENDED-RELEASE):
Initial dose: PO 200 mg bid.
CHILDREN 6 TO 12 YR OF AGE:
Initial dose: PO 100 mg bid (tablets) or 50 mg qid (suspension). Increase weekly by 100 mg per day in 3 to 4 divided doses (extended-release formulations use a bid regimen) to reach minimum effective dose (max, 1,000 mg per day).
Maintenance: 400 to 800 mg per day in 3 to 4 divided doses.
CHILDREN 6 YR OF AGE AND YOUNGER:
Initial dose: PO 10 to 20 mg/kg per day in 2 or 3 divided doses (tablet) or 10 to 20 mg/kg per day in 4 divided doses (suspension). Increase weekly to achieve optimal clinical response

when administered in 3 or 4 divided daily doses (max, 35 mg/kg per day).
Maintenance: Less than 35 mg/kg per day.

Trigeminal Neuralgia
ADULTS:
Initial dose: **PO** 100 mg bid (tablets) or 50 mg qid (suspension). May increase by up to 200 mg per day in 3 to 4 divided doses (tablets: 100 mg increments q 12 hr; suspension: 50 mg qid) prn (max, 1,200 mg per day).
Maintenance: Usually 400 to 800 mg per day. Use minimum effective dose or discontinue drug once q 3 mo.
ADULTS (EXTENDED-RELEASE):
Initial dose: **PO** 100 mg bid (tablets) or 200 mg once daily (capsules).

Interactions
Acetaminophen, benzodiazepines (eg, midazolam), bupropion, clozapine, cyclosporine, olanzapine, succinimides (eg, ethosuximide), tiagabine, topiramate, ziprasidone: Levels may be reduced by carbamazepine.
Anticoagulants: May decrease anticoagulant effects.
Azole antifungal agents, diltiazem, verapamil, danazol, propoxyphene, macrolide antibiotics (except azithromycin): May increase carbamazepine levels and may result in toxicity.
Barbiturates: May result in decreased carbamazepine serum concentrations, possibly leading to decreased effectiveness.
Charcoal, activated: May reduce absorption of carbamazepine.
Cimetidine: May result in carbamazepine toxicity.
Contraceptives, oral: Causes breakthrough bleeding and reduces effectiveness of contraceptives.
Doxycycline hyclate: May decrease doxycycline hyclate levels.
Felbamate: May decrease concentrations of felbamate or carbamazepine.
Felodipine: May decrease effects of felodipine.
Haloperidol: May decrease effects of haloperidol.
Hydantoins (eg, phenytoin): May decrease carbamazepine levels; may alter hydantoin levels.
Isoniazid: May result in toxicity of isoniazid, carbamazepine, or both.
Lamotrigine: Lamotrigine levels may be decreased, while levels of the active metabolite of carbamazepine may be increased.
Lithium: May cause adverse CNS effects regardless of drug levels.
MAO inhibitors, voriconazole: Coadministration with carbamazepine is contraindicated.
Nondepolarizing muscle relaxants: May make these agents less effective.
Primidone: Decreased carbamazepine levels. Primidone's active metabolite (phenobarbital) may be increased.
Protease inhibitors (eg, indinavir): Carbamazepine levels may be elevated, while protease inhibitor levels may be decreased, resulting in antiretroviral treatment failure.
Selective serotonin reuptake inhibitors (eg, fluoxetine, fluvoxamine): Increased carbamazepine levels with possible toxicity.
Theophylline: May reduce effects of theophylline and carbamazepine. Theophylline levels may be increased or decreased.
Tricyclic antidepressants: May increase carbamazepine levels; may decrease tricyclic antidepressant levels.
Valproic acid: May decrease valproic acid levels; may alter carbamazepine levels.

Lab Test Interferences
None well documented.

Adverse Reactions
CV: AV block; CHF; hypertension; hypotension; syncope; edema; thrombophlebitis; aggravation of coronary artery disease; arrhythmias.
CNS: Dizziness; drowsiness; unsteadiness; confusion; headache; hyperacusis; fatigue; speech disturbances; abnormal involuntary movements; peripheral neuritis and paresthesias; depression with agitation; talkativeness; behavior changes (children); paralysis.
DERM: Pruritic and erythematous rashes; exfoliative dermatitis; erythema multiforme and nodosum; purpura; aggravation of disseminated lupus erythematosus; toxic epidermal necrolysis; urticaria; photosensitivity; pigment changes; alopecia; diaphoresis; Stevens-Johnson syndrome.
EENT: Blurred vision; visual hallucinations; diplopia; nystagmus; punctate cortical lens opacities; conjunctivitis; tinnitus; dryness and irritation of the mouth and throat.
GI: Nausea; vomiting; gastric distress; abdominal pain; diarrhea; constipation; anorexia.
GU: Urinary frequency or retention; oliguria with hypertension; renal failure; azotemia; impotence; albuminuria; glycosuria; elevated BUN; urinary microscopic deposits.
HEMA: Aplastic anemia; leukopenia; agranulocytosis; eosinophilia; leukocytosis; thrombocytopenia; pancytopenia; bone marrow depression.
HEPA: Abnormal LFTs; jaundice; hepatitis.
METAB: Hyponatremia; hypothyroidism.
RESP: Pulmonary hypersensitivity (eg, fever, dyspnea, pneumonitis, pneumonia).
OTHER: Aching joints and muscles; leg cramps; adenopathy; lymphadenopathy; fever; chills; syndrome of inappropriate antidiuretic hormone secretion.

> **WARNING:**
>
> *Aplastic anemia and agranulocytosis:* Has been reported with use. The risk is 5 to 8 times greater than in the general population.
>   Obtain complete pretreatment hematological testing as a baseline. If in the course of treatment a patient exhibits low or decreased WBC or platelet counts, monitor the patient closely.

Precautions
Pregnancy: Category D.
Lactation: Excreted in breast milk.

PATIENT CARE CONSIDERATIONS
Administration/Storage
- May be used alone or in combination with other antiepileptic drugs (AEDs) for treatment of seizures or with analgesics for treatment of trigeminal neuralgia.
- Do not administer with or within 14 days of MAO inhibitor.
- Store tablets, extended-release tablets, extended-release capsules, and suspension at ambient room temperature (59° to 86°F). Protect from moisture.

Tablets:
- Administer prescribed dose with food.

Extended-Release Tablets:
- When converting from tablets to extended-release tablets, administer same number of mg per day divided into 2 daily doses.
- Inspect tablet for chips or cracks. Do not administer damaged tablets.
- Administer prescribed dose with food. Advise patient to swallow tablet whole and not crush or chew the tablet.

Extended-Release Capsules:
- Administer without regard to meals. Administer with food if GI upset occurs.
- Advise patient to swallow whole and not crush or chew the capsule.
- Capsules may be opened and beads sprinkled over food (eg, tsp of applesauce or similar food product) and swallowed, without chewing, immediately. Caution patient not to chew the beads.

Suspension:
- When converting from tablets to suspension, administer same number of mg per day in smaller, more frequent doses (eg, bid tablets to tid suspension).
- Shake suspension well before measuring dose. Measure dose using dosing cup, spoon, or syringe.
- Do not administer carbamazepine suspension simultaneously with other liquid medications or diluents.

Children: Management of epilepsy in children is derived from clinical investigations in adults.
Special risk patients: Use with caution in patients with prior adverse hematologic reactions to any drug; cardiac, hepatic, or renal disease; and mixed seizure disorders, including absence seizures.

Overdosage: Signs and Symptoms
Irregular breathing, respiratory depression, tachycardia, hypotension, hypertension, shock, coma, LOC, convulsions, muscle twitching, tremor, ataxia, drowsiness, dizziness, nystagmus, nausea, vomiting, anuria, urinary retention, abnormal EEG.

Assessment/Interventions
- Obtain patient history, including drug history and any known allergies. Note renal or hepatic impairment, CV disease, atypical absence seizures, history of bone marrow depression, history of hematologic reaction to other medications, increased IOP, sensitivity to tricyclic compounds (eg, amitriptyline, oxcarbazepine), phenobarbital, or hydantoins, concurrent use of CYP3A4 inhibitors or inducers, or current or recent (within 14 days) use of an MAO inhibitor.
- Ensure that carbamazepine blood levels are evaluated if seizures are not controlled or worsen, if there are questions regarding patient compliance, or if toxic symptoms develop in patient on more than one AED.
- Ensure that CBC with differential and platelet count is evaluated before initiating therapy and periodically thereafter during prolonged therapy. Inform health care provider if decreased WBC and/or platelets are noted. Be prepared to discontinue therapy in patient who develops evidence of significant bone marrow depression.
- Implement infection control measures if neutrophil count drops; implement bleeding precautions if platelet count drops.
- Ensure that transaminases are evaluated before starting therapy and periodically thereafter during prolonged therapy. Immediately notify health care provider if transaminases become elevated or if patient develops jaundice or other signs or symptoms of hepatic dysfunction.
- Ensure that baseline and periodic eye examinations (eg, slit lamp, funduscopy, tonometry) and urinalysis and BUN are performed.
- Ensure that serum sodium is evaluated periodically during prolonged therapy, especially

in patient receiving other medications known to decrease serum sodium (eg, medications for syndrome of inappropriate antidiuretic hormone secretion).
- Evaluate serum sodium if symptoms possibly indicating hyponatremia develop (eg, nausea, malaise, headache, lethargy, confusion, obtundation, or increase in seizure frequency or severity).
- Closely observe patient and monitor plasma levels of other coadministered antiepileptic drugs when adding, or increasing or decreasing the dose of carbamazepine.
- Ensure that therapy is periodically reviewed to determine if therapy needs to be continued without change or if a dose change (eg, increase, decrease, discontinuation) is indicated.
- Avoid sudden discontinuation of therapy if possible. Attempt to gradually reduce dose over a period of several weeks if decision to discontinue medication is made.
- Monitor patient for GI, CNS, PSYCH, GU, OPHTH, MUSC, and general body side effects. Report to health care provider if noted and significant.
- Implement safety precautions for patients who experience dizziness or ataxia.

Suspension:
- Ensure that lower initial doses and slower dose escalation are used when treating with suspension because a given dose of suspension will produce higher blood levels than the same dose given as a tablet.

Patient/Family Education
- Explain name, dose, action, and potential side effects of drug.
- Advise patient to read the *Patient Information* leaflet before starting therapy and with each refill.
- Instruct patient to continue to take other antiepileptic medications as prescribed by health care provider.
- Instruct patient to take exactly as prescribed and not to change the dose or discontinue unless advised by health care provider.
- Advise patient using suspension or tablets to take each dose with food.
- Advise patient that dose is gradually increased as tolerated until max benefit has been obtained.
- Caution patient to avoid grapefruit products while taking carbamazepine because of the risk of toxicity.
- Advise patient that if a dose is missed to take it as soon as remembered. If several hours have passed, or it is nearing the time for the next scheduled dose, advise the patient to skip that dose and take the next dose at the regularly scheduled time. Caution patient to never double the dose to catch up.
- Advise patient that if medication needs to be discontinued it will be slowly withdrawn over a period of several weeks unless safety concerns (eg, rash) require a more rapid withdrawal.
- Caution patient being treated for trigeminal neuralgia that carbamazepine is not a simple analgesic (pain reliever) and not to use for treatment of trivial aches or pains.
- Advise patient to avoid alcoholic beverages and other depressants while taking this medication.
- Instruct patient or caregiver to immediately notify health care provider if any of the following occur: unusual bleeding or bruising, fever, sore throat, rash, ulcers in mouth, swollen glands, small purple spots under the skin, persistent nausea or headache, confusion, appetite loss, yellowing of eyes or skin.
- Instruct patient to contact health care provider if difficulty with concentration, speech or language problems, excessive drowsiness or fatigue, or coordination problems develop.
- Instruct patient with seizures to inform health care provider if seizures get worse, if new types of seizures develop, or if bothersome side effects occur.
- Caution patient that drug may cause drowsiness and dizziness and to use caution while driving or performing other tasks requiring mental alertness until tolerance is determined.
- Advise patient to avoid unnecessary exposure to sunlight or tanning lamps and to use sunscreen and wear protective clothing to avoid photosensitivity reactions
- Advise women using combination oral contraceptive to use additional nonhormonal form of contraception because carbamazepine causes a reduction in effectiveness of combination oral contraceptives.
- Advise women to notify health care provider if pregnant, planning to become pregnant, or breastfeeding.
- Advise patient not to take any prescription or OTC medications, dietary supplements, or herbal preparations unless advised by health care provider.
- Advise patient that laboratory tests and follow-up visits will be required to monitor therapy and to keep appointments.

Suspension:
- Advise patient or caregiver to shake suspension well before measuring dose and to mea-

sure prescribed dose using dosing cup, spoon, or syringe.
- Caution patient or caregiver not to administer carbamazepine suspension simultaneously with other liquid medications or diluents.

Extended-Release Tablets:
- Instruct patient using extended-release tablet to inspect each tablet for chips or cracks in the outer coating and not to take if a tablet is damaged.
- Advise patient that the extended-release coating is not absorbed and may be seen in the stool. Advise patient not to be concerned because this is normal and does not reduce the effectiveness of the medication because the medication inside the tablet has already been released and absorbed into the body.

Extended-Release Capsules:
- Advise patient to take prescribed dose without regard to meals but to take with food if stomach upset occurs. Caution patient to swallow capsule whole and not to crush or chew the capsule.
- Advise patient that capsules may be opened and the beads sprinkled over food (eg, teaspoon of applesauce or similar food product) and swallowed, without chewing, immediately. Caution patient not to chew the beads.

Carbenicillin Indanyl Sodium

(car-BEN-ih-SILL-in IN-duh-nil SO-dee-uhm)

Class Antibiotic/Penicillin

How Supplied
Geocillin Tablets 382 mg carbenicillin (118 mL indanyl sodium ester)

Action
PHARMACOLOGY: Inhibits mucopeptide synthesis in bacterial cell wall.

PHARMACOKINETICS/DYNAMICS:
Absorption: Rapidly absorbed. T_{max} is 1 hr. C_{max} is about 6.5 mcg/mL.

Distribution: 50% protein bound.

Metabolism: Rapidly converted to carbenicillin by hydrolysis of the ester linkage.

Excretion: About 30% is excreted in the urine unchanged within 12 hr.

Indications Treatment of acute and chronic infections of the upper and lower urinary tract, prostatitis, and asymptomatic bacteriuria caused by susceptible microorganisms.

Contraindications Hypersensitivity to penicillins, cephalosporins, or imipenem. Do not treat severe pneumonia, empyema, bacteremia, pericarditis, meningitis, and purulent or septic arthritis with oral carbenicillin during acute stage.

Route/Dosage
ADULTS: PO 382 to 764 mg qid.

Interactions
Contraceptives, oral: May reduce efficacy of oral contraceptives. Use nonhormonal form of contraception during carbenicillin therapy.
Tetracyclines: May impair bactericidal effects of carbenicillin.

Lab Test Interferences Antiglobulin (*Coombs'*) test: Drug may cause false-positive results. Urine glucose test: Drug may cause false-positive results with copper sulfate tests (*Benedict's* test, *Fehling's* test or *Clinitest* tablets); enzyme-based tests (eg, *Clinistix*, *Tes-tape*) are not affected. Urine protein determinations: May cause false-positive reactions with sulfosalicylic acid and boiling test, acetic acid test, biuret reaction and nitric acid test; bromphenol blue test (*Multi-Stix*) is not affected.

Adverse Reactions
CNS: Dizziness; fatigue; insomnia; reversible hyperactivity.
DERM: Urticaria; vesicular eruptions; erythema multiforme; skin rash.
EENT: Itchy eyes; furry tongue; black "hairy" tongue; abnormal taste sensation; laryngeal edema; laryngospasm.
GI: Gastritis; nausea; vomiting; abdominal pain or cramps; diarrhea or bloody diarrhea; flatulence; pseudomembranous colitis.
GU: Interstitial nephritis (eg, oliguria, proteinuria, hematuria, hyaline casts, pyuria); nephropathy; increased BUN and creatinine.
HEMA: Anemia; hemolytic anemia; thrombocytopenia; thrombocytopenic purpura; eosinophilia; leukopenia; granulocytopenia; neutropenia; bone marrow depression; agranulocytosis; reduced hemoglobin or hematocrit; prolonged bleeding and prothrombin time; increased or decreased lymphocyte count; increased monocytes, basophils, platelets.
HEPA: Transient hepatitis and cholestatic jaundice.
METAB: Elevated serum alkaline phosphatase and hypernatremia; reduced serum potassium, albumin, total proteins and uric acid.
OTHER: Hypersensitivity reactions (eg, urticaria, angioneurotic edema, laryngospasm, bronchospasm, hypotension, vascular collapse, death, maculopapular to exfoliative dermatitis, vesicular eruptions, erythema multiforme, serum sickness, laryngeal edema, skin rash, prostration); vaginitis; hyperthermia; fever.

Precautions
Pregnancy: Category B.
Lactation: Excreted in breast milk.
Children: Safety and efficacy in infants and children under 12 yr not established.

PATIENT CARE CONSIDERATIONS
Administration/Storage
- Administer on empty stomach 1 hr before meals or 2 hr after meals. Give with full glass of water.

Assessment/Interventions
- Obtain patient history, including drug history and any known allergies, especially to drugs in penicillin family or related drugs (eg, cephalosporins).
- Obtain specimens for culture and sensitivity before beginning therapy.
- Keep epinephrine, antihistamine, and resuscitation equipment close by in event of anaphylactic reaction.
- Monitor renal function throughout therapy.
- If rash, itching, hives, shortness of breath, wheezing, or other signs of allergic reaction and anaphylaxis occur, withhold drug and notify health care provider.
- If dizziness, black tongue, sore throat, nausea, diarrhea, vomiting, fever, swollen joints, or any unusual bruising occurs, withhold drug and notify health care provider.

Patient/Family Education
- If allergy to carbenicillin is demonstrated, inform patient that this allergy extends to all penicillins, cephalosporins and imipenem.
- Advise patient to take medication with full glass of water, not with food, fruit juice or carbonated beverages because doing so may inactivate drug.
- Caution patient to stop taking drug and notify health care provider if difficulty breathing, rash or other allergic response occurs.
- Advise patient to take medication at even intervals if possible.
- Instruct patient to report these symptoms to health care provider: decreased urinary output, nausea, vomiting, unpleasant aftertaste and smell, dry mouth, "furry" tongue, unexplained bruising or nosebleeds, foul-smelling diarrhea/stool or vaginal discharge.

Renal function impairment: Use drug cautiously; dosage adjustment may be required.
Cystic fibrosis: Associated with higher incidence of side effects with drug (eg, rash, fever).

Carbidopa
(CAR-bih-doe-puh)
Class Antiparkinson
How Supplied
Lodosyn Tablets 25 mg

Action
PHARMACOLOGY: Inhibits peripheral decarboxylation of levodopa, making more levodopa available for transport to brain.

Indications Has no effect as single agent. For use with levodopa in treatment of idiopathic Parkinson disease, postencephalitic parkinsonism and symptomatic parkinsonism associated with carbon monoxide or manganese poisoning.

Unlabeled use(s): Reduction of breakdown of L-5-hydroxytryptophan for treatment of postanoxic intention myoclonus.

Contraindications Hypersensitivity to carbidopa or levodopa.

Route/Dosage
ADULTS: **PO** in 1:10 ratio to levodopa (eg, 10 mg carbidopa/100 mg levodopa) tid to qid. With regimen of 1 mg carbidopa/100 mg levodopa, additional 12.5 to 25 mg carbidopa may be administered qd or qod with first dose if needed. With regimen of 25 mg carbidopa/250 mg levodopa, 12.5 to 25 mg carbidopa may be added by ½ to 1 tablet qd or qod to max of 8 tablets/day (2 tablets qid) for optimal therapeutic response (max, 200 mg/day).
Initiating combination therapy: Do not give carbidopa and levodopa together until at least 8 hr after last dose of levodopa was taken alone. Lower levodopa dose to 20% to 25% of previous daily dose and administer both drugs at same time.

Interactions None well documented (see *Levodopa*).

Lab Test Interferences May cause false-positive test result for urinary ketones when test tape is used to determine ketonuria. False-negative test results may occur with glucose-oxidase methods of testing for urinary glucose.

Adverse Reactions Only adverse reactions seen with carbidopa have been associated with combined use of carbidopa and levodopa.

Precautions
Pregnancy: Undetermined.
Lactation: Undetermined. Do not administer to nursing mothers.
Children: Safety and efficacy not established for children under 18 yr.
Elderly: May require lower doses of carbidopa/levodopa.
Dyskinesias: Dyskinesias caused by levodopa may occur sooner or at lower doses of levodopa

when levodopa and carbidopa are given concomitantly than when levodopa is administered alone.
Neuroleptic malignant-like syndrome: Muscular rigidity, fever, mental changes and increased serum CPK may occur when dose of levodopa is reduced abruptly or discontinued.

Overdosage: Signs and Symptoms
Blepharospasm.

PATIENT CARE CONSIDERATIONS
Administration/Storage
- Do not administer carbidopa and levodopa together until at least 8 hr after last dose of levodopa was taken alone.
- Administer carbidopa at same time as levodopa.
- Administer with food to reduce GI upset.
- Instruct patient not to crush or chew sustained-release tablets.
- Store in light-resistant container at room temperature.

Assessment/Interventions
- Obtain patient history, including drug history and any known allergies.
- Monitor vital signs during period of dose adjustment.
- Monitor glucose closely in diabetic patients. Report any abnormal results to health care provider.
- If patient experiences any CNS effects (eg, uncontrollable movements of the face, eyelids, mouth, tongue, neck, arms, hands or legs; mood or mental changes) notify health care provider.

Patient/Family Education
- Remind patient to take medication with food to prevent GI upset.
- Advise patient that onset of effect of first morning dose may be delayed by up to 1 hr.
- Inform patient it may take several wk to few mo to experience benefit from this drug.
- Caution patient that this drug may interfere with results of urine tests for glucose/ketones.
- Advise patient that harmless darkening of urine and sweat may occur.
- Caution patient to avoid sudden position changes to prevent orthostatic hypotension.
- Advise patient that this drug may cause drowsiness and to use caution while driving or performing tasks requiring mental alertness.
- Instruct patient not to take *otc* medications without consulting health care provider.

Carbidopa/Levodopa/ Entacapone

(CAR-bih-doe-puh/LEE-voe-DOE-puh/en-TACK-ah-pone)

Class Antiparkinson

How Supplied
Stalevo 50 Tablets 12.5 mg carbidopa, 50 mg levodopa, 200 mg entacapone ◆ *Stalevo 100* Tablets 25 mg carbidopa, 100 mg levodopa, 200 mg entacapone ◆ *Stalevo 150* Tablets 37.5 mg carbidopa, 150 mg levodopa, 200 mg entacapone

Action
PHARMACOLOGY:
Carbidopa: Inhibits peripheral decarboxylation of levodopa, making more levodopa available for transport to the brain.
Levodopa: Precursor of dopamine, which is deficient in parkinsonism patients.
Entacapone: Inhibits the enzyme that metabolizes levodopa (catechol-O-methyltransferase [COMT]), which increases and prolongs levodopa plasma levels.

Indications Treatment of idiopathic Parkinson disease: 1) to substitute (with equivalent strength of each of the 3 immediate-release components) for the previously administered individual products, 2) to replace immediate-release carbidopa/levodopa therapy (without entacapone) when patients experience signs and symptoms of end-of-dose "wearing-off" (only for patients taking a total daily dose of levodopa of 600 mg or less and not experiencing dyskinesias).

Contraindications Narrow-angle glaucoma; nonselective monoamine oxidase (MAO) inhibitors (eg, phenelzine) should be discontinued at least 2 wk prior to initiating therapy with carbidopa/levodopa/entacapone; patients with history of melanoma or suspicious undiagnosed skin lesions; hypersensitivity to any component of the product.

Route/Dosage
ADULTS: PO 1 tablet should be administered at each dosing interval. The product is available in 3 strengths, each in a 1:4 ratio of carbidopa to levodopa and combined with 200 mg of entacapone. Generally, the product should be used to substitute for patients already stabilized on a given dose of carbidopa, levodopa, and entacapone. However, some patients stabilized on a given dose of carbidopa/levodopa may be treated with this product if a decision to add entacapone has been made. The optimum daily dosage must be determined by careful titration

in each patient. Therapy should be individualized and adjusted according to the desired therapeutic response.

Interactions

Antihypertensive agents: Symptomatic postural hypotension may occur when adding carbidopa/levodopa; therefore, be prepared to adjust antihypertensive therapy as needed.

Dopamine D2 receptor antagonists (eg, phenothiazines, risperidone), isoniazid, papaverine, phenytoin: May reduce the therapeutic effects of levodopa.

Drugs known to interfere with biliary excretion, glucuronidation, and intestinal betaglucuronidase (eg, ampicillin, cholestyramine, chloramphenicol, erythromycin, probenecid, rifampin): Because entacapone is excreted via the bile, drugs known to interfere with biliary excretion, glucuronidation, and intestinal betaglucuronidase should be used with caution.

Drugs metabolized by COMT (eg, alphamethyldopa, bitolterol, dobutamine, dopamine, epinephrine, isoproterenol): Increased heart rate, possible arrhythmia, and excessive BP changes may occur.

Iron salts: May reduce the bioavailability of levodopa; however, the clinical importance is unclear.

MAO inhibitors: Concurrent therapy with non-selective MAO inhibitors (eg, phenelzine) is contraindicated. Therapy with MAO inhibitors should be discontinued 2 wk prior to starting carbidopa/levodopa/entacapone.

Metoclopramide: May increase levodopa bioavailability by increasing gastric emptying and because of its dopamine receptor antagonistic properties; metoclopramide may also adversely affect disease control.

Pyridoxine: Pyridoxine in doses of 10 to 25 mg may reverse the effects of levodopa; however, carbidopa inhibits this effect of levodopa. Therefore, supplemental pyridoxine can be given concurrently.

Tricyclic antidepressants (TCA [eg, amitriptyline]): Rare reports of adverse reactions, including hypertension and dyskinesia, have been noted with concomitant use of levodopa/carbidopa and TCA.

Lab Test Interferences False-positive reactions for urinary ketone bodies may occur when a test tape is used for ketonuria determination; false-positive Coombs test results may occur; because falsely diagnosed pheochromocytoma has occurred, exercise caution when interpreting plasma and urine levels of catecholamines and their metabolites.

Adverse Reactions

CV:

Carbidopa/Levodopa – Cardiac irregularities, hypotension, orthostatic effects (including orthostatic hypotension, hypertension, syncope, phlebitis, palpitation); MI (levodopa).

Entacapone – Dyspnea (3%).

CNS:

Carbidopa/Levodopa – Dyskinesias (including choreiform, dystonic, and other involuntary movements), psychotic episodes (including delusions, hallucinations, paranoid ideation), neuroleptic malignant syndrome, bradykinetic episodes ("on-off" phenomenon), confusion, agitation, dizziness, somnolence, dream abnormalities, insomnia, paresthesia, headache, depression with or without development of suicidal tendencies, dementia, increased libido, convulsions (carbidopa/levodopa); fatigue, ataxia, extrapyramidal disorder, anxiety, gait abnormalities, nervousness, decreased mental acuity, memory impairment, disorientation, euphoria, blepharospasm, trismus, increased tremor, numbness, muscle twitching, activation of latent Horner syndrome, peripheral neuropathy (levodopa).

Entacapone – Dyskinesia (25%); hyperkinesia (10%); hypokinesia (9%); agitation (1%).

DERM:

Carbidopa/Levodopa – Rash, increased sweating, alopecia, dark sweat; malignant melanoma, flushing (levodopa).

EENT:

Levodopa – Oculogyric crisis; diplopia; blurred vision; dilated pupils.

GI:

Carbidopa/Levodopa – Nausea, dark saliva, GI bleeding, duodenal ulcer, anorexia, vomiting, diarrhea, constipation, dyspepsia, dry mouth, taste alteration; GI pain, dysphagia, sialorrhea, flatulence, bruxism, burning sensation of the tongue, heartburn, hiccups (levodopa).

Entacapone – Nausea (14%); diarrhea (10%); abdominal pain (8%); constipation (6%); vomiting (4%); dry mouth (3%); dyspepsia, flatulence (2%); gastritis, nonspecific GI disorders (1%).

GU:

Carbidopa/Levodopa – UTI, urinary frequency, dark urine; urinary retention, urinary incontinence, priapism (levodopa).

Entacapone – Urine discoloration (10%); renal toxicity.

HEMA:

Carbidopa/Levodopa – Agranulocytosis; hemolytic and nonhemolytic anemia; thrombocytopenia; leukopenia.

METAB:

Levodopa – Edema; weight gain; weight loss.

RESP:

Carbidopa/Levodopa – Dyspnea, upper respira-

tory tract infection; pharyngeal pain, cough (levodopa).
Entacapone – Purpura (2%).
OTHER:
Carbidopa/Levodopa – Chest pain, asthenia, angioedema, urticaria, pruritus, Henoch-Schönlein purpura, bullous lesions (including pemphigus-like reactions), back pain, shoulder pain, muscle cramps, decreased hemoglobin and hematocrit, abnormalities in alkaline phosphatase, ALT, AST, lactic dehydrogenase, bilirubin, BUN, and Coombs test, elevated serum glucose, bacteria, and blood in the urine (carbidopa/levodopa); abdominal pain and distress, leg pain, bizarre breathing patterns, faintness, hoarseness, malaise, hot flashes, sense of stimulation, decreased WBC, decreased serum potassium, increased serum creatinine and uric acid, protein and glucose in urine (levodopa).
Entacapone – Fatigue (6%); back pain (4%); asthenia, increased sweating (2%); bacterial infection (1%); aggravation of Parkinson disease symptoms.

Precautions

Pregnancy: Category C.
Lactation: Undetermined.
Children: Safety and efficacy not established.
Hepatic function impairment: Use with caution; AUC and C_{max} of entacapone approximately doubled.
Special risk patients: Use with caution in patients with severe cardiovascular or pulmonary disease, bronchial asthma, biliary obstruction, renal, hepatic or endocrine disease, administer cautiously to patients with history of MI who have residual atrial, nodal, or ventricular arrhythmias and to patients with wide-angle glaucoma.
Blepharospasm: May be an early sign of excessive dosage, which may indicate the need for dosage reduction.
Dyskinesia: Entacapone may potentiate the dopaminergic side effects of levodopa; exacerbating preexisting dyskinesia; dosage reduction may be required.
Fibrotic complications: Cases of retroperitoneal fibrosis, pulmonary infiltrates, pleural effusion, and pleural thickening have been reported.
Hallucinations: Dopaminergic therapy has been associated with hallucinations.
Hormone levels: Prolactin secretion may be decreased while growth hormone levels may be increased.
Hyperpyrexia/confusion: Elevated temperature, muscular rigidity, altered consciousness, and elevated CPK have been reported with rapid dose reduction or withdrawal of other dopaminergic drugs.
Mental disturbances: Observe carefully for the development of depression with concomitant suicidal tendencies, or with past or current psychosis.
Neuroleptic malignant syndrome: A symptom complex resembling neuroleptic malignant syndrome has been reported in association with dose reductions or withdrawal of carbidopa/levodopa therapy.
Peptic ulcer: The risk of upper GI hemorrhage may be increased.
Rhabdomyolysis: Severe cases have been reported in patients receiving entacapone in combination with levodopa.

Overdosage: Signs and Symptoms

Dopaminergic overstimulation, CNS disturbances, cardiovascular disturbances (eg, hypotension, tachycardia), severe psychiatric problems, rhabdomyolysis, transient renal insufficiency, COMT inhibition.

PATIENT CARE CONSIDERATIONS

Administration/Storage

- Discontinue MAO inhibitors at least 14 days before initiating therapy.
- Administer prescribed dose without regard to meals. Administer with food if GI upset occurs, however, do not administer with high-protein foods because they reduce absorption of medication.
- Administer only 1 tablet at each dosing interval. If an increased dose is needed, a different tablet strength will need to be administered.
- Store at controlled room temperature (59° to 86°F).

Assessment/Interventions

- Obtain patient history, including drug history and any known allergies. Note history of kidney or liver disease, biliary obstruction, asthma, endocrine disease, severe cardiovascular or pulmonary disease, arrhythmias, peptic ulcer disease, glaucoma, melanoma, or undiagnosed skin lesions.
- Note concurrent or recent (within 2 wk) MAO-inhibitor therapy or concurrent use of drugs metabolized by COMT (eg, alpha-methyl dopa).
- Do not administer any other antiparkinsonian medication unless advised by health care provider.
- Assess parkinsonian symptoms before and periodically during therapy.
- Ensure that liver, cardiovascular, hematopoietic, and renal function are assessed before and periodically during therapy.
- Assess neurologic status before and during treatment. Observe for involuntary body and facial movements, depression, hallucinations,

or dizziness. Inform health care provider if noted.
• Monitor BP and pulse routinely during therapy. Inform health care provider if significant changes in BP or orthostatic symptoms are noted.

Patient/Family Education
• Explain name, dose, action, and potential side effects of drug.
• Advise patient, family, or caregiver that medication is not a cure for the disease but may help reduce symptoms.
• Advise patient, family, or caregiver that medication is started at a low dose and gradually increased to achieve maximum benefit.
• Caution patient, family, or caregiver that only 1 tablet should be taken at each dosing interval and that no more than 8 tablets should be taken in any 24-hr period.
• Advise patient, family, or caregiver that medication can be taken without regard to meals but to take with food if GI upset occurs. However, caution against taking medication with high-protein foods because they reduce absorption and effectiveness of medication.
• Caution patient, family, or caregiver that tablets should never be cut, split, or crushed.
• Advise patient, family, or caregiver that medication should be taken as prescribed and to not stop taking or change the dose unless advised by health care provider. Emphasize that medication must be taken at regular intervals to obtain maximum benefit.
• Advise patient, family, or caregiver that if a dose is missed it should be taken as soon as remembered but to never double the dose to catch up or take more than the prescribed total daily dose.
• Caution patient, family, or caregiver not to take any other antiparkinsonian medications unless advised by health care provider.
• Caution patient to avoid sudden position changes to prevent orthostatic hypotension (dizziness or faintness when arising suddenly from a sitting or lying position).
• Advise patient that the drug may cause dizziness or other nervous system disorders and to use caution while driving or performing other tasks requiring mental alertness until tolerance is determined.
• Advise patient, family, or caregiver that medication may cause a red, brown, or black discoloration of saliva, urine, or sweat that is not harmful but may discolor clothing or bedding.
• Advise patient family or caregiver to report any of the following to health care provider: worsening of Parkinson symptoms before next dose ("wearing off" effect); persistent or frequent nausea or vomiting; involuntary body or facial movements; mood or mental changes; hallucinations; or any unexplained symptom or problem.
• Advise women to notify health care provider if pregnant, planning to become pregnant, or breastfeeding.
• Warn patient, family, or caregiver not to take any prescription or OTC drugs or dietary supplements without consulting health care provider.
• Advise patient, family, or caregiver that follow-up visits will be necessary to monitor therapy and to keep appointments.

Carbinoxamine Maleate

(car-bih-NOCK sah-meen MAL-ee-ate)

Class Antihistamine

How Supplied
Histex CT Tablets, timed-release 8 mg • *Histex Pd* Liquid 4 mg/5 mL • *Pediatex* Liquid 1.75 mg/5 mL

Action
PHARMACOLOGY: Competitively antagonizes histamine at H_1 receptor sites.
PHARMACOKINETICS/DYNAMICS:
Excretion: The t½ is 10 to 20 hr. No intact drug is excreted in the urine.

Indications Relief of nasal and nonnasal symptoms of seasonal and perennial allergic rhinitis.

Contraindications MAO inhibitor therapy; patients with narrow-angle glaucoma, urinary retention, or breathing problems such as emphysema or chronic bronchitis; hypersensitivity to any component of the product.

Route/Dosage
HISTEX CT TABLETS
ADULTS AND CHILDREN (12 YR AND OVER): PO 8 mg q 12 hr.
CHILDREN (6 TO 12 YR): PO 4 mg q 12 hr.
HISTEX PD LIQUID
ADULTS AND CHILDREN (6 YR AND OVER): PO 5 mL qid.
CHILDREN (18 MO TO 6 YR): PO 2.5 mL qid.
CHILDREN (9 TO 18 MO): PO 1.25 to 2.5 mL qid.
PEDIATEX
ADULTS AND CHILDREN (6 YR AND OVER): PO 10 mL qid.
CHILDREN (18 MO TO 6 YR): PO 5 mL qid.
CHILDREN (9 TO 18 MO): PO 3.75 to 5 mL qid.
CHILDREN (6 TO 9 MO): PO 3.75 mL qid.

CHILDREN (3 TO 6 MO): **PO** 2.5 mL qid.
CHILDREN (1 TO 3 MO): **PO** 1.25 mL qid.

Interactions
Alcohol, barbiturates (eg, phenobarbital), tricyclic antidepressants (eg, amitriptyline), other CNS depressants: Effects may be enhanced by carbinoxamine.
MAO inhibitors: May prolong and intensify the effects of carbinoxamine.

Lab Test Interferences May interfere with diagnostic test results for skin tests using allergen extracts.

Adverse Reactions
CNS: Sedation; dizziness; headache; nervousness; nausea; anorexia; heartburn; weakness; excitability in children.
EENT: Diplopia.
GI: Vomiting; diarrhea; dry mouth.
GU: Polyuria.

Precautions
Pregnancy: Category C.
Lactation: Undetermined; use with caution.

Overdosage: Signs and Symptoms
In young children, predominant symptoms include the following: excitation, hallucination, ataxia, incoordination, tremors, flushed face, fever, convulsions, fixed and dilated pupils, coma, death; in adults, predominant symptoms include the following: fever, flushing, excitement, convulsions, postictal depression preceded by drowsiness and coma, respiratory depression.

PATIENT CARE CONSIDERATIONS

Administration/Storage
- Give ½ or 1 tablet q 12 hr as prescribed without regard to meals. Give with food if GI upset occurs.
- Tablet can be broken in half without affecting release of medication. Tablets or half-tablets should not be crushed or chewed.
- Give liquid dose 4 times/day as prescribed without regard to meals. Give with food if GI upset occurs.
- Use caution when administering liquid. Note that there are 2 concentrations (1.75 mg/5 mL and 4 mg/5 mL) available. Administering the wrong liquid can result in an overdose or underdose.
- Use dosing spoon or syringe to measure liquid dose.
- Store liquid at controlled room temperature (59° to 86°F).

Assessment/Interventions
- Obtain patient history, including drug history, and any known allergies. Note history of narrow angle glaucoma, stenosing peptic ulcer, pyloric obstruction, prostatic hypertrophy, bladder neck obstruction, asthma, emphysema, chronic bronchitis, and concurrent or recent use of MAO inhibitors or oral anticoagulants.
- Ensure that orders for liquid carbinoxamine contain the concentration (ie, 1.75 mg/5 mL or 4 mg/5 mL) of the liquid to be administered.
- Assess for allergy symptoms (eg, rhinitis, nasal congestion, sneezing, itching, watery eyes) before and periodically throughout therapy.
- Monitor patient for dizziness and excessive drowsiness. If noted, hold therapy and notify health care provider.
- Monitor patient for CNS, GI, and general body side effects. Inform health care provider if noted and significant.

Patient/Family Education
- Explain name, dose, action, and potential side effects of drug.
- Advise patient to take ½ or 1 tablet q 12 hr as prescribed without regard to meals, but to take with food if GI upset occurs.
- Advise patient, parent, or caregiver that tablets or half-tablets should not be crushed or chewed but should be swallowed whole.
- Advise patient, parent, or caregiver that liquid medication is taken 4 times/day as prescribed.
- Advise patient, parent, or caregiver to use dosing spoon or syringe to measure liquid dose.
- Advise patient, parent, or caregiver that if allergy symptoms are not controlled not to increase the dose of medication or frequency of use but to inform their health care provider. Inform patient that larger or more frequent dosing does not increase effectiveness and may cause drowsiness.
- Advise patient that medication may cause drowsiness or dizziness and to not drive or perform other activities requiring mental alertness until tolerance is determined.
- Caution patient that alcohol and other CNS depressants (eg, sedatives) will have additional sedative effects if taken with carbinoxamine.
- Caution patient not to take any OTC antihistamines while taking this medication unless advised by their health care provider.
- Advise patient to take sips of water, suck on ice chips or sugarless hard candy, or chew sugarless gum if dry mouth occurs.
- If patient is to have allergy skin testing, advise to not take the medication for at least 7 days before the skin testing.

- Advise women to notify health care provider if pregnant, plan on becoming pregnant, or breastfeeding.
- Instruct patient to stop taking drug and immediately report any of these symptoms to health care provider: dizziness, excessive drowsiness.
- Caution patient to not take any prescription or OTC medications, or dietary supplements unless advised to do so by health care provider.

Carbinoxamine Maleate/ Pseudoephedrine Hydrochloride/ Dextromethorphan HBr

(car-bih-NOCK sah-meen MAL-ee-ate/SUE-doe-eh-FED-rin HIGH-droe-KLOR-ide/DEX-troe-meth-OR-fan HIGH-droe-BROE-mide)

Class Antihistamine/Decongestant/Antitussive

How Supplied
Cardec DM Syrup 4 mg carbinoxamine, 60 mg pseudoephedrine, 15 mg dextromethorphan per 5 mL, Drops 2 mg carbinoxamine, 25 mg pseudoephedrine, 4 mg dextromethorphan per dropperful (1 mL)

Action
PHARMACOLOGY:
Carbinoxamine: Competitively antagonizes histamine at H_1 receptor sites.
Pseudoephedrine: Causes vasoconstriction and subsequent shrinkage of nasal mucous membranes by alpha-adrenergic stimulation, which promotes nasal drainage.
Dextromethorphan: Suppresses cough by central action on cough center in medulla.

Indications Relief of coughs and upper respiratory tract symptoms, including nasal congestion, associated with allergy or the common cold.

Contraindications Hypersensitivity or idiosyncratic reaction to any ingredients of product; severe hypertension; severe coronary artery disease; narrow-angle glaucoma; urinary retention; peptic ulcer; asthma attack; MAO inhibitor therapy or for 2 wk after stopping MAO inhibitor therapy.

Route/Dosage
SYRUP
CHILDREN 9 TO 18 MO: **PO** 1 dropperful (1 mL) qid.
CHILDREN 6 TO 9 MO: **PO** ¾ dropperful (¾ mL) qid.
CHILDREN 3 TO 6 MO: **PO** ½ dropperful (½ mL) qid.
CHILDREN 1 TO 3 MO: **PO** ¼ dropperful (¼ mL) qid.

DROPS
ADULTS AND CHILDREN 6 YR AND OVER: **PO** 1 tsp (5 mL) qid.

CHILDREN 18 MO TO 6 YR: **PO** ½ tsp (2.5 mL) qid.

Interactions
Alcohol, barbiturates (eg, phenobarbital), tricyclic antidepressants (eg, amitriptyline), other CNS depressants: Effects may be enhanced by carbinoxamine.
MAO inhibitors (eg, isocarbozazid): May prolong and intensify the effects of carbinoxamine and increase the effects of pseudoephedrine. Dextromethorphan is contraindicated with MAO inhibitors.
Mecamylamine, methyldopa, reserpine, veratrum alkaloids: Antihypertensive effects may be reduced by pseudoephedrine.
Narcotic antitussives (eg, codeine): May increase the cough suppressant effects of dextromethorphan.

Lab Test Interferences May interfere with diagnostic test results for skin tests using allergen extracts.

Adverse Reactions
CV:
Pseudoephedrine – Cardiac arrhythmia; increased heart rate; increased BP.
CNS:
Carbinoxamine – Sedation; dizziness; headache; nervousness; excitability in children (rare).
Pseudoephedrine – Convulsions; CNS stimulation; hallucinations; tremors; nervousness; insomnia.
Dextromethorphan – Drowsiness; dizziness.
EENT:
Carbinoxamine – Diplopia.
GI:
Carbinoxamine – Vomiting; diarrhea; dry mouth; nausea; anorexia; heartburn.
Dextromethorphan – GI disturbance.
GU:
Carbinoxamine – Polyuria; dysuria; urinary retention in patients with prostatic hypertrophy.
Pseudoephedrine – Dysuria.
RESP:
Pseudoephedrine – Respiratory difficulties.
OTHER:
Carbinoxamine – Weakness.
Pseudoephedrine – Pallor; weakness.

Precautions
Pregnancy: Category C.
Lactation: Undetermined.
Elderly: Patients 60 yr and older are more likely to exhibit adverse effects.

Special risk patients: Use with caution in patients with hypertension, heart disease, asthma, hyperthyroidism, increased intraocular pressure, diabetes mellitus, or prostatic hypertrophy.

PATIENT CARE CONSIDERATIONS
Administration/Storage
- Give prescribed dose q 4 to 6 hr as needed, up to qid.
- Use supplied dropper to measure dose.
- Give with food if GI upset occurs.
- Store syrup at controlled room temperature (59° to 86°F). Keep tightly closed.

Assessment/Interventions
- Obtain patient history, including drug history and any known allergies. Note history of peptic ulcer disease, diabetes, hypertension, hyperthyroidism, enlarged prostate, asthma, narrow angle glaucoma, urinary retention, severe hypertension, coronary artery disease, or concurrent use of or within 2 wk of stopping MAO inhibitor therapy.
- Assess for allergy symptoms (eg, cough, rhinitis, nasal congestion, sneezing, itching, watery eyes) before and periodically throughout therapy.
- Monitor pulse and BP periodically during therapy.
- Monitor patient for nervousness, dizziness, and insomnia. If noted, hold therapy and notify health care provider.

Patient/Family Education
- Explain name, dose, action, and potential side effects of drug.
- Advise caregiver to administer prescribed dose q 4 to 6 hr as needed, up to qid.
- Caution caregiver to use supplied dropper to measure each dose.
- Advise caregiver to administer with food if GI upset occurs.
- Advise caregiver to administer last dose late in the afternoon or early evening to reduce chance of drug causing sleeplessness.
- Advise caregiver that if a dose is missed to take as soon as remembered unless it is nearing time for the next dose. Caution caregiver to not double the dose to catch up.
- Advise caregiver that if allergy symptoms are not controlled not to increase the dose of medication but to inform health care provider.
- Caution caregiver that drug may cause drowsiness.
- Advise caregiver to avoid administering alcohol and other CNS depressants because of risk of excessive sedation.
- Caution caregiver not to administer any OTC antihistamines or decongestants while taking this medication unless advised by health care provider.
- If patient is to have allergy skin testing, advise not to take the medication for at least 6 days before the skin testing.
- Instruct caregiver to stop administering drug and immediately report any of the following symptoms to health care provider: nervousness, dizziness, sleeplessness.
- Caution caregiver not to administer any prescription or OTC medications or dietary supplements unless advised by health care provider.

Carboplatin

(car-boe-PLATT-in)

Class Alkylating agent

How Supplied
Paraplatin Lyophilized powder for injection 50 mg vial, Lyophilized powder for injection 150 mg vial, Lyophilized powder for injection 450 mg vial, Injection 10 mg/mL
✤ *Paraplatin-AQ*

Action
PHARMACOLOGY: Platinum coordination compound that produces predominantly interstrand DNA cross-links causing equivalent lesions and biological effects.

PHARMACOKINETICS/DYNAMICS:
Distribution: Carboplatin is not protein bound; platinum from carboplatin is irreversibly protein bound. Vd is 16 L.

Metabolism: Aquated to produce the active species.

Excretion: Initial t½ is 1.1 to 2 hr. Postdistribution t½ is 2.6 to 5.9 hr. Cl is 4.4 L/hr. 71% is excreted in the urine in 24 hr.

Special Populations:
Renal Function Impairment – In those with Ccr less than 60 mL/min, the total body and renal Cl decreases as the Ccr decreases. Dosage reduction is recommended.

Indications
Adults: Initial treatment of advanced ovarian carcinoma in combination with other chemotherapy agents. Secondary treatment for palliative treatment of patients with ovarian carcinoma recurrent after prior chemotherapy.
Unlabeled use(s): Small cell and non-small cell lung, head, neck, and testicular cancer.

Contraindications History of severe allergic reactions to cisplatin or other platinum compounds or mannitol; severe bone marrow depression; significant bleeding.

Route/Dosage

Ovarian Carcinoma (Single-Agent Therapy)
ADULTS: **IV** 360 mg/m^2 on day 1 q 4 wk if neutrophil count is at least 2,000/mm^3 and platelet count is at least 100,000/mm^3.

Ovarian Carcinoma (Combination Therapy with Cyclophosphamide)
ADULTS: **IV** Carboplatin 300 mg/m^2 plus cyclophosphamide 600 mg/m^2, both on day 1 q 4 wk for 6 cycles. Do not repeat intermittent courses of the combination until the neutrophil count is at least 2,000/mm^3 and the platelet count is at least 100,000/mm^3.

Calvert Formula Dosing
ADULTS: **IV** Carboplatin may be dosed to achieve a target AUC based on the patient's glomerular filtration rate (GFR) using the Calvert formula. The desired target AUC depends on the disease and the patient's treatment status. The Calvert formula calculates the carboplatin dose in mg as follows: Total dose (mg) = target AUC (mg/mL•min) × (GFR [mL/min] + 25).

Dosage Adjustments Based on Lowest Post-treatment Blood Counts
ADULTS: **IV** If platelets above 100,000/mm^3 and neutrophils above 2,000/mm^3, then give 125% of adjusted dose from prior course. If platelets are 50,000 to 100,000/mm^3 and neutrophils are 500 to 2,000/mm^3, no dosage adjustment is necessary. If platelets below 50,000/mm^3 and neutrophils below 500/mm^3, then give 75% of adjusted dose from prior course. Doses above 125% of the starting dose are not recommended.

Renal Function Impairment (Dosage Adjustment)
ADULTS: **IV** Baseline Ccr is 41 to 59 mL/min, the recommended dose on day 1 is 250 mg/m^2; 16 to 40 mL/min is 200 mg/m^2; below 15 mL/min, data too limited to permit a recommendation for treatment.

Interactions

Aminoglycosides: Concomitant use may increase risk of nephrotoxicity or ototoxicity.
Phenytoin: Serum concentrations may be decreased, resulting in a loss of therapeutic effect.

Lab Test Interferences
Abnormal LFTs; alkaline phosphatase; AST; total bilirubin.

Adverse Reactions
Percentages are for carboplatin single agent therapy.
CV: CV events (11%); fatal CV events including cardiac failure, embolism, cerebrovascular accidents (less than 1%); hypertension (postmarketing).
CNS: Asthenia (23%); peripheral neuropathies including mild paresthesias (6%); central neurotoxicity (5%); ototoxicity (1%); malaise (postmarketing).
DERM: Alopecia (3%).
EENT: Reversible vision loss.
ELECDIST: Sodium loss (47%); magnesium loss (43%); calcium loss (31%); potassium loss (28%).
GI: Nausea and vomiting (92%); vomiting (81%); other GI side effects (21%); anorexia (postmarketing).
GU: Elevated BUN (22%); elevated serum creatinine (10%).
HEPA: Elevated alkaline phosphatase (37%); elevated AST (19%); elevated bilirubin (5%).
HEMA/LYMPH: Anemia (90%); leukopenia (85%); neutropenia (67%); thrombocytopenia (62%); infections, bleeding (5%).
HYPERSEN: Allergic reaction (2%).
LOCAL: Pain, redness, swelling (postmarketing).
RESP: Respiratory (6%).
OTHER: Pain (23%); mucositis (1%).

> **WARNING:**
>
> *Anemia:* May be cumulative and transfusions required.
>
> *Bone marrow suppression:* Leukopenia, neutropenia, and thrombocytopenia are dose dependent and are the dose-limiting toxicities; they may result in infection or bleeding.
>
> *Emesis:* Vomiting is another frequent drug-related side-effect and usually ceases within 24 hr of treatment. The incidence and intensity of emesis have been reduced by antiemetic premedication.
>
> *Hypersensitivity:* Anaphylactic-like reactions may occur within minutes of administration. Epinephrine, corticosteroids, and antihistamines may alleviate symptoms.

Precautions

Pregnancy: Category D.
Lactation: Undetermined. Because of possibility of toxicity in nursing infants, discontinue breastfeeding.
Children: Safety and efficacy not established.
Renal function impairment: Patients with impaired kidney function (Cr below 60 mL/min) are at increased risk of severe bone marrow suppression.
Peripheral neurotoxicity: Infrequent, but its incidence is increased in patients older than 65 yr of age and in patients previously treated with cisplatin.

Renal toxicity: Limited, but cotreatment with aminoglycosides has resulted in increased renal or audiologic toxicity. Exercise caution when patient receives both drugs.

PATIENT CARE CONSIDERATIONS
Administration/Storage
- May be used alone or in combination with cyclophosphamide.
- Do not administer to patient with Ccr less than 15 mL/min.
- For IV infusion only. Not for intradermal, subcutaneous, IM, IV bolus, intra-arterial, or oral administration.
- Diligently follow institutional and NIH procedures for handling, administration, and disposal of anticancer drugs. Wear appropriate protective equipment when preparing and administering carboplatin.
- Do not use needles or IV administration sets containing aluminum parts that could come in contact with carboplatin during preparation or administration. Aluminum can react with carboplatin, causing precipitation and loss of potency.
- Reconstitute powder for injection with sterile water for injection, 5% dextrose in water, or 0.9% sodium chloride injection. Add 5 mL of diluent to 50 mg vial, 15 mL of diluent to 150 mg vial, or 45 mL of diluent to 450 mg vial to produce solution with a final concentration of 10 mg/mL.
- Reconstituted solution, or premixed aqueous solution, may be further diluted with 5% dextrose in water or 0.9% sodium chloride injection.
- Do not administer if discoloration, particulate matter, or cloudiness is noted.
- Administer prescribed dose by IV infusion over at least 15 minutes. Infusion may be lengthened to 24 hr, or total dose given as 5 consecutive daily pulse doses, for patient who experiences significant emesis.
- Administer antiemetic as prescribed before administering carboplatin.
- Store aqueous solution and powder for injection at controlled room temperature (59° to 86°F). Protect from light. Reconstituted solution is stable for 8 hr at controlled room temperature (77°F). Reconstituted solution does not contain a preservative and any unused solution must be discarded 8 hr after reconstitution. Do not save any unused solution for future use. Carboplatin aqueous solution multidose vials are stable at room temperature (77°F) for up to 14 days following initial needle entry.

Overdosage: Signs and Symptoms
Bone marrow suppression, hepatic toxicity.

Assessment/Interventions
- Obtain patient history, including drug history and any known allergies. Note bone marrow depression, significant bleeding, history of severe allergic reaction to cisplatin or other platinum compounds or mannitol, or concurrent treatment with aminoglycoside.
- Ensure women of childbearing potential are not pregnant before starting therapy and use effective contraception during treatment.
- Ensure Ccr is determined before starting therapy and that initial dose of carboplatin is reduced in patient with renal failure: 250 mg/m^2 with baseline Ccr of 41 to 59 mL/min; 200 mg/m^2 with baseline Ccr of 16 to 40 mL/min. Adjust subsequent doses based on degree of bone marrow suppression.
- Consider formula dosing of carboplatin based on estimated GFR in elderly patient to minimize risk of toxicity.
- Ensure CBC with differential and platelet count are monitored frequently (at least weekly) during treatment and, when appropriate, until recovery is achieved. Ensure that carboplatin dose is adjusted based on lowest posttreatment platelet or neutrophil value following manufacturer's guidelines.
- Notify health care provider immediately if neutropenia and/or thrombocytopenia develops. Be prepared to withhold therapy until bone marrow recovery occurs (ie, neutrophil count is at least 2,000 cells/mm^3 and platelet count is at least 100,000/mm^3).
- Notify health care provider if anemia develops. Be prepared to transfuse patient during prolonged therapy.
- Monitor patient for signs or symptoms of infection or bleeding. Inform health care provider immediately if noted and be prepared to treat appropriately (eg, IV antibiotics, colony stimulating factors, transfusions).
- Monitor patient for signs of anaphylactic or serious allergic reactions. Discontinue therapy and immediately notify health care provider if noted. Be prepared to treat appropriately.
- Ensure electrolytes are evaluated before starting therapy and periodically thereafter during prolonged treatment. Be prepared to treat abnormalities if clinically indicated.
- Monitor patient for CNS, GI, HEMA, and general body side effects, and injection site

reactions. Report to health care provider if noted and significant.

Patient/Family Education
* Explain name, action, and potential side effects of the treatment regimen. Review the treatment regimen including dosing schedule, duration of treatment, and monitoring that will be required.
* Advise patient, family, or caregiver that medication will be prepared and administered by health care professionals in a health care setting.
* Advise patient, family, or caregiver that medication may be used in combination with other agents to achieve max benefit possible.
* Advise patient, family, or caregiver that medication may cause hair loss but that this is reversible when therapy is stopped.
* Advise patient, family, or caregiver to immediately report any of the following to health care provider: rash; hives; difficulty breathing or unexplained shortness of breath; fever, chills, or other signs of infection; sores in mouth; loss of vision; pain redness, or swelling at injection site.
* Advise patient, family, or caregiver to report any of the following to health care provider: persistent nausea, vomiting, or appetite loss; persistent or worsening general body weakness; changes in hearing or ringing in the ears; abnormal skin sensations; any other unexplained sensation.
* Instruct patient not to take any prescription or OTC medications, herbal preparations, or dietary supplements unless advised by health care provider.
* Caution female patient of childbearing potential to avoid becoming pregnant during therapy.
* Advise women to notify health care provider if pregnant, planning to become pregnant, or breastfeeding.
* Advise patient that frequent follow-up visits and laboratory tests will be required to monitor therapy and to keep appointments.

Carisoprodol

(car-eye-so-PRO-dole)

Class Skeletal muscle relaxant/Centrally acting

How Supplied
Soma Tablets 350 mg

Action
PHARMACOLOGY: Produces skeletal muscle relaxation, probably as result of its sedative properties.
PHARMACOKINETICS/DYNAMICS:
Metabolism: Metabolized in the liver.
Excretion: Eliminated via the urine.
Onset: 30 min.
Duration: 4 to 6 hr.

Indications Adjunctive treatment of acute, painful musculoskeletal conditions (eg, muscle strain).

Contraindications Acute intermittent porphyria; hypersensitivity to related compounds such as meprobamate; suspected porphyria.

Route/Dosage
ADULT: **PO** 350 mg tid or qid.

Interactions
Alcohol and other CNS depressants: May cause additive CNS depression.

Lab Test Interferences None well documented.

Adverse Reactions
CV: Tachycardia; orthostatic hypotension; facial flushing.
CNS: Dizziness; drowsiness; vertigo; ataxia; tremor; agitation; irritability; headache; depressive reactions; syncope; insomnia.
GI: Nausea; vomiting; hiccoughs; epigastric distress.
OTHER: Allergic or idiosyncratic reactions within first to fourth doses, including skin rash, erythema multiforme, pruritus, eosinophilia, and fixed drug eruption; severe reactions include asthma, fever, weakness, dizziness, angioneurotic edema, hypotension, and anaphylactoid shock.

Precautions
Pregnancy: Undetermined.
Lactation: Excreted in breast milk.
Children: Not recommended in children under 12 yr.
Renal function impairment: Use with extreme caution.
Hepatic function impairment Use with extreme caution.
Tartrazine sensitivity: Some products contain tartrazine, which may cause allergic reactions (including bronchial asthma) in susceptible individuals. Such patients often also have aspirin hypersensitivity.
Drug dependency: Use with caution in addiction-prone patients.

Overdosage: Signs and Symptoms
Stupor, coma, shock, respiratory depression.

PATIENT CARE CONSIDERATIONS
Administration/Storage
- Give with food or milk if GI upset occurs.
- Administer last dose at bedtime.
- Store in tightly closed container in cool, dry place.

Assessment/Interventions
- Obtain patient history, including drug history and any known allergies. Note history of porphyria and hypersensitivity or allergy to meprobamate or carisoprodol.
- Obtain baseline LFTs, serum BUN, and creatinine.
- Note history of drug dependence.
- Monitor for signs of idiosyncratic response: disorientation, agitation, vision disturbances, impaired verbal communication, extreme weakness, transient quadriplegia, dizziness, ataxia, euphoria. These reactions may appear within minutes or hours of first dose. Symptoms usually subside over several hours. If such reactions occur, withhold drug and notify health care provider.
- Monitor LFTs, BUN, and creatinine.
- Notify health care provider if patient experiences hiccough, hives, or shortness of breath.

Patient/Family Education
- Instruct patient to take last daily dose at bedtime.
- Tell patient to take medication with meals if GI upset occurs.
- Instruct patient to report these symptoms to health care provider: palpitations, tremors, hiccough, ataxia.
- Advise patient to avoid intake of alcoholic beverages or other CNS depressants.
- Caution patient that drug may cause drowsiness and to use caution while driving or performing other tasks requiring mental alertness.

Carisoprodol/Aspirin/Codeine Phosphate

(car-eye-so-PRO-dole/ASS-pihr-in/KOE-deen FOSS-fate)

Class Skeletal muscle relaxant/Analgesic/Narcotic analgesic

How Supplied
Soma compound with codeine Tablets 200 mg carisoprodol, 325 mg aspirin, 16 mg codeine

Action
PHARMACOLOGY:
Carisoprodol: Produces skeletal muscle relaxation, probably as a result of its sedative properties.
Aspirin: Inhibits prostaglandin synthesis, resulting in analgesia, anti-inflammatory activity, and inhibition of platelet aggregation.
Codeine: Stimulates opiate receptors in the CNS.

Indications Adjunct to rest, physical therapy, and other measures for the relief of pain, muscle spasm, and limited mobility associated with acute, painful musculoskeletal conditions.

Contraindications Acute intermittent porphyria; bleeding disorders; allergic or idiosyncratic reactions to any component of product.

Route/Dosage
ADULTS AND CHILDREN (AT LEAST 12 YR): PO 1 or 2 tablets qid.

Interactions
Ammonium chloride: By lowering the urinary pH, agents such as ammonium chloride can elevate plasma salicylate levels.
Antacids: By raising urinary pH, antacids may increase salicylate elimination, decreasing plasma salicylate levels; conversely, discontinuing antacid therapy may increase levels.
Anticoagulants (eg, warfarin): Aspirin may enhance the potential for bleeding in patients on anticoagulants.
Antidiabetic drugs (oral): May enhance hypoglycemia.
Corticosteroids: Salicylate plasma levels may be decreased.
Ethyl alcohol: Increased risk of aspirin-induced fecal blood loss.
Methotrexate: Increased risk of methotrexate toxicity.
Probenecid, sulfinpyrazone: Uricosuric effect of these agents may be decreased by large doses of aspirin, in addition, renal excretion of salicylate may be reduced.

Lab Test Interferences
Aspirin: May cause false-positive reading of urine glucose by copper reduction method (*Clinitest*) and false-negative readings by glucose oxidase method (*Clinistix*); may interfere with urine tests of 5-hydroxyindoleacetic acid, ketone, phenolsulfonphthalein, and vanillymandelic acid.
Codeine: May interfere with amylase and lipase determinations for up to 24 hr after administration.

Adverse Reactions
CV:
Carisoprodol – Tachycardia; postural hypotension; facial flushing.
CNS:
Carisoprodol – Drowsiness; dizziness; vertigo; ataxia; tremor; agitation; irritability; headache; depression; syncope; insomnia.

Codeine – Sedation; dizziness.
DERM:
Aspirin – Rash; pruritus; urticaria.
EENT:
Aspirin – Tinnitus.
Codeine – Miosis.
GI:
Carisoprodol – Nausea; vomiting; epigastric distress; hiccup.
Aspirin – Nausea; vomiting; gastritis; occult bleeding; constipation; diarrhea; gastric erosion.
Codeine – Nausea; vomiting; constipation.
HEMA:
Carisoprodol – Leukopenia; pancytopenia.
RESP:
Aspirin – Asthma.
OTHER:
Carisoprodol – Idiosyncratic reactions (including extreme weakness, transient quadriplegia, dizziness, ataxia, temporary loss of vision, diplopia, mydriasis, dysarthria, agitation, euphoria, confusion, disorientation); allergic reactions (including skin rash, erythema multiforme, pruritus, eosinophilia, and fixed drug eruptions.
Aspirin – Angioedema; aspirin intolerance (including rhinorrhea, shortness of breath, edema).

Precautions

Pregnancy: Category C.
Lactation: Carisoprodol, aspirin, and codeine are excreted in breast milk.
Children: Safety and efficacy in children less than 12 yr not established.
Special risk patients: Use with caution in patients with compromised renal or hepatic function, in elderly or debilitated patients, patients with a history of gastritis or peptic ulcer, and addiction-prone individuals.
Drug dependence: Drug dependence of the morphine type may result.
Idiosyncratic reactions: Rarely first dose may cause idiosyncratic reactions (eg, extreme weakness, transient quadriplegia, dizziness, ataxia, temporary loss of vision, confusion, disorientation).
Sodium metabisulfite: Contains metabisulfite, a sulfite that may cause allergic-type reactions, including anaphylactic symptoms and life-threatening or less severe asthmatic episodes in susceptible patients.

Overdosage: Signs and Symptoms

Carisoprodol: Stupor, coma, shock, respiratory depression, rarely death.
Aspirin: Headache, tinnitus, hearing difficulty, dim vision, dizziness, lassitude, hyperpnea, rapid breathing, thirst, nausea, vomiting, sweating, occasionally diarrhea, hyperthermia, dehydration, delirium, mental disturbances, skin eruptions, GI hemorrhage, pulmonary edema; CNS stimulation followed by increasing depression, stupor, coma.
Codeine: Pinpoint pupils, CNS depression, coma, respiratory failure, cardiovascular collapse.

PATIENT CARE CONSIDERATIONS

Administration/Storage

- Administer 1 to 2 tablets as prescribed up to qid if needed.
- Administer without regard to meals, but administer with food if GI upset occurs.
- Store at controlled room temperature (59° to 86°F). Protect from moisture.

Assessment/Interventions

- Obtain patient history, including drug history and any known allergies. Note history of addiction, sulfite sensitivity, bleeding or coagulation disorders, hepatic or renal impairment, peptic ulcer or other serious GI lesions, porphyria, or the syndrome of nasal polyps, rhinitis, and bronchospastic reactivity to aspirin or other NSAIDs.
- Assess musculoskeletal symptoms before starting therapy and periodically during treatment.
- Monitor for signs of idiosyncratic reaction: extreme weakness, transient quadriplegia, dizziness, ataxia, double vision or temporary loss of vision, slurred speech, agitation, confusion, disorientation. Discontinue therapy and notify health care provider immediately if noted.
- Monitor patient for CNS, GI, and general body side effects. Report to health care provider if noted and significant.
- Monitor for signs of allergic reaction, unusual bleeding or bruising, shortness of breath, black or tarry stools, vomiting of blood or coffee ground-like material.

Patient/Family Education

- Explain name, dose, action, and potential side effects of drug.
- Advise patient to take 1 to 2 tablets as prescribed, up to qid if needed for muscle pain, muscle spasm, or limited mobility.
- Advise patient to take without regard to meals but to take with food if GI upset occurs.
- Instruct patient to avoid alcoholic beverages and other depressants while taking this medication.
- Advise patient that drug may impair judgment, thinking, or motor skills, or cause drowsiness. Use caution while driving or performing other tasks requiring mental alertness until tolerance is determined.

- Advise patient to stop taking the drug and notify health care provider if any of the following symptoms occur: allergic reaction, unusual bleeding or bruising, shortness of breath, black or tarry stools, vomiting of blood or coffee ground-like material, excessive sedation, extreme weakness, paralysis, dizziness, stumbling, double vision or temporary loss of vision, slurred speech, agitation, confusion, disorientation.
- Advise women to notify health care provider if pregnant, planning to become pregnant, or breastfeeding.
- Warn patient not to take any prescription or OTC drugs or dietary supplements without consulting health care provider.
- Advise patient that follow-up visits may be necessary to monitor therapy and to keep appointments.

Carmustine

(CAR-muss-teen)

Class Alkylating agent/Nitrosoureas

How Supplied
BiCNU Powder for injection 100 mg ♦ Gliadel Wafer 7.7 mg

Action
PHARMACOLOGY: Carmustine alkylates DNA and RNA and also inhibits several enzymes by carbamoylation of amino acids in proteins. Antineoplastic and toxic activities may be caused by metabolites.

PHARMACOKINETICS/DYNAMICS:
Absorption:
IV – Vd is 3.25 L/kg. Crosses the blood-brain barrier.

Excretion:
IV – The t½ is 22 min. Cl is 56 mL/min/kg. Approximately 60% is excreted in the urine; 6% is expired as CO_2.

Indications Brain tumors, multiple myeloma, Hodgkin and non-Hodgkin lymphomas; adjunct to surgery and radiation in newly diagnosed high-grade malignant glioma patients and as an adjunct in recurrent glioblastoma multiforme patients (wafer). **Unlabeled use(s):** Mycosis fungoides.

Contraindications Standard considerations.

Route/Dosage
Brain Tumors, Multiple Myeloma, Hodgkin and Non-Hodgkin Lymphomas (Single Agent in Previously Untreated Patients)
ADULTS: **IV** 150 to 200 mg/m² q 6 wk, as a single dose or divided into 2 successive daily infusions.

Dosage Reduction
ADULTS: **IV** Compromised bone marrow function or therapy with other myelosuppressive drugs requires a reduction in dose. Do not administer repeat courses until acceptable leukocyte and platelet counts have recovered (usually greater than 4000/mm³ and 100,000/mm³, respectively). Subsequent doses are determined by the clinical and hematologic tolerance of the previous dose. The following leukocyte and platelet counts refer to the levels reached at nadir after prior dose. Give 100% of the prior dose given if the leukocytes are greater than 3000 cells/mm³ and the platelets are greater than 75,000 cells/mm³. Give 70% of the prior dose given if the leukocytes are 2000 to 2999 cells/mm³ and the platelets are 25,000 to 74,999 cells/mm³. Give 50% of the prior dose given if the leukocytes are less than 2000 cells/mm³ and the platelets are less than 25,000 cells/mm³.

Adjunct To Surgery And Radiation In Newly Diagnosed High-Grade Malignant Glioma Patients And As An Adjunct In Recurrent Glioblastoma Multiforme Patients
ADULTS: **Wafer for implantation** 8 wafers placed in the resection cavity, for a total dose of 61.6 mg. If the cavity size and shape will not accommodate this, use the greatest number of wafers that will fit.

Interactions
Cimetidine: Cimetidine may enhance the myelosuppressive effects of carmustine.
Digoxin, phenytoin: Digoxin and phenytoin serum levels may be reduced by carmustine.

Lab Test Interferences None well documented.

Adverse Reactions
CV:
Wafer – Deep thrombophlebitis (10%); pulmonary embolus (8%); hemorrhage (7%).
CNS:
Wafer – Depression (16%); intracranial hypertension (9%); anxiety, facial paralysis (7%); ataxia, hypesthesia (6%); dizziness, hallucinations, seizures (5%); headache (28%); meningitis; abscess; asthenia; confusion; somnolence; brain edema; intracranial infection.
DERM: Rash (wafer) (12%); local burning pain at the injection site; intense flushing of the skin.
GI: Constipation (19%); abdominal pain, diarrhea (5%), (wafer); nausea (22%); vomiting (21%).

GU: UTI (8%; wafer); amenorrhea; male infertility.
HEMA: Bone marrow suppression; myelosuppression.
HEPA: Transient LFT elevations; hepatic necrosis and veno-occlusive disease after bone marrow transplantation.
METAB: Diabetes mellitus (wafer).
RENAL: Dose-related, delayed-onset, progressive renal failure.
RESP: Early pulmonary toxicity; delayed pulmonary fibrosis.
SPEC SENSE: Retinitis; optic neuritis; suffusion of the conjunctiva.
OTHER:
Wafer – Surgical wound healing abnormalities (16%); fever (12%); back pain, pain (7%); face edema (6%); abscess, chest pain (5%); CSF leak; subdural fluid collection; subgaleal or wound effusion; wound breakdown.

> **WARNING:**
>
> Bone marrow suppression (notably thrombocytopenia and leukopenia): May contribute to bleeding and infections. Toxicity is cumulative, thus adjust dose based on nadir counts from prior doses. Do not repeat doses more frequently than q 6 wk. Perform weekly complete blood cell counts for 6 wk postdose.
>
> Hematologic: The most frequent and serious toxic effect of injectable carmustine is delayed myelosuppression.
>
> Pulmonary fibrosis: Delayed onset pulmonary fibrosis has occurred up to 17 yr after treatment and has been reported in patients who received injectable carmustine in childhood and early adolescence.
>
> Pulmonary toxicity: Pulmonary toxicity from injectable carmustine appears to be dose-related. Patients receiving more than 1400 mg/m^2 cumulative dose are at significantly higher risk than those receiving less. Other risk factors include history of lung disease and duration of treatment. Cases of fatal pulmonary toxicity have occurred.

Precautions
Pregnancy: Category D.
Lactation: Undetermined.
Children: Safety and efficacy not established.
Mutagenesis: Long-term use of nitrosoureas has been reported to be associated with the development of secondary malignancies.
Fertility impairment: There have been reports of persistent testicular damage causing infertility with injectable carmustine.
Brain edema: Brain edema was noted in 4% of patients treated with the wafer.
Brain herniation: Cases of intracerebral mass effect unresponsive to corticosteroids have been described in patients treated with the wafer.
GI: Nausea and vomiting after IV administration. This dose-related toxicity appears within 2 hr of dosing and lasts 4 to 6 hr.
Healing abnormalities: The majority of these events were mild to moderate in severity.
Hepatic toxicity: Reversible hepatic toxicity, manifested by increased transaminase, alkaline phosphatase, and bilirubin levels, has occurred in a small percentage of patients using injectable carmustine.
Intracranial infection: Intracranial infection (eg, meningitis, abscess) occurred in 4% to 5% of patients treated with the wafer.
Obstructive hydrocephalus: Avoid communication between the surgical resection cavity and the ventricular system to prevent the wafers from migrating into the ventricular system and causing obstructive hydrocephalus.
Ocular: Toxicity manifested as nerve fiber-layer infarcts and retinal hemorrhages has been associated with high dose injectable carmustine therapy.
Renal toxicity: Decrease in kidney size, progressive azotemia, and renal failure have occurred in patients.
Seizures: The majority of seizures in the placebo vs wafer study were mild or moderate in severity.
Wafer remnants: Remnants of implanted wafers may be observed on brain imaging scans or during later operations even though all components are extensively degraded. Remnants removed from 2 patients after 64 and 92 days contained less than 0.0004% and 0.034%, respectively, of the original carmustine content. Remnants may persist for up to 232 days after implantation.

PATIENT CARE CONSIDERATIONS
Administration/Storage
- Administer by IV infusion or intracranial implantation.
- Follow procedures for proper handling and disposal of chemotherapy drugs. Wear gloves and avoid skin exposure and inhalation of fumes.

IV:
- Refrigerate vials of the dry powder. Protect from light.

- The reconstituted solution is administered by IV drip over 1 to 2 hr. Shorter infusion times may produce intense pain and burning at the site of injection.
- Store unopened vials of the dry powder in a refrigerator. After reconstitution, the solution is stable for 8 hr at room temperature protected from light. Vials further diluted to a concentration of 0.2 mg/mL should be utilized within 8 hr at room temperature in glass protected from light.
- Temperatures of 30.5°C (86°F) or more cause carmustine to decompose and appear oily; discard these vials. The drug can still be used if it appears as dry flakes or as a dry, congealed mass when viewed under a bright light.
- Dissolve 1 vial with 3 mL of the dehydrated alcohol diluent, followed by 27 mL of sterile water for injection for a final concentration of 3.3 mg/mL in 10% alcohol. This solution may be further diluted with 5% dextrose for a concentration of 0.2 mg/mL in glass containers.
- Carmustine is preservative-free and should be used as a single-dose vial. The possibility of microbial contamination of reconstituted solutions must be considered.
- Accidental contact of carmustine with skin can cause temporary hyperpigmentation; wear gloves when handling. Double gloving is recommended.
- When administered with polyvinyl chloride tubing, longer infusion times may result in unacceptable drug loss. To avoid drug loss, polyethylene tubing, such as nitroglycerin tubing, can be utilized for infusions of carmustine.

Wafer:
- Oxidized regenerated cellulose (*Oxycel, Surgicel*) may be placed on top of the wafers to secure them against the cavity surface.
- Avoid communication between the resection cavity and the ventricular system to prevent wafers from migrating and causing obstructive hydrocephalus.
- Open the foil pouches containing the wafer in the operating room immediately prior to implantation.
- Store wafers for implantation in the freezer.
- Unopened foil pouches are stable at room temperature for up to 6 hr at a time. Administer by intracranial implantation.
- Wafers may be used if broken in half. Do not use if broken in more than 2 pieces; dispose of as a hazardous chemical waste.
- Use a dedicated surgical instrument for handling the wafers during implantation.
- Wafers may overlap slightly and should cover as much of the resection cavity as possible.

Assessment/Interventions
IV:
- When preparing high doses of carmustine larger than 900 mg/m^2, only 50% of the alcohol will be used to reconstitute carmustine powder. Reconstituted carmustine is further diluted with 500 mL of 5% dextrose and infused over 2 hr.
- Because of delayed bone marrow suppression, monitor blood counts weekly for at least 6 wk after a dose.
- Conduct baseline pulmonary function studies and frequent pulmonary function tests during treatment. Patients with a baseline less than 70% of predicted forced vital capacity (FVC) or carbon monoxide diffusing capacity (DL$_{co}$) are at particular risk. Monitor liver and renal function tests periodically.
- Delayed myelosuppression usually occurs 4 to 6 wk after administration and is dose related. Thrombocytopenia occurs at about 4 wk postadministration and persists for 1 to 2 wk. Leukopenia occurs at 5 to 6 wk after a dose and persists for 1 to 2 wk. Thrombocytopenia generally is more severe than leukopenia.

Wafer:
- Monitor patients undergoing craniotomy for malignant glioma and implantation of the wafer closely for known complications of craniotomy, including seizures, intracranial infections, abnormal wound healing, and brain edema.

Patient/Family Education
- Contraceptive measures are recommended during therapy.

Carteolol Hydrochloride

(CAR-tee-oh-lahl HIGH-droe-KLOR-ide)
Class Beta-adrenergic blocker
How Supplied
Cartrol Tablets 2.5 mg ♦ *Cartrol* Tablets 5 mg ♦ *Ocupress* Solution 1%

Action
PHARMACOLOGY: Blocks beta-receptors, primarily affecting cardiovascular system (eg, decreases heart rate, cardiac contractility, BP) and lungs (promotes bronchospasm). Ophthalmic use reduces IOP, probably by decreasing aqueous production.

CARTEOLOL HYDROCHLORIDE

PHARMACOKINETICS/DYNAMICS:
Absorption:
Oral – Well absorbed. T_{max} is 1 to 3 hr. Bioavailability is about 85%.

Distribution:
Oral – 23% to 30% protein bound.

Metabolism:
Oral – Metabolized to 8-hydroxycarteolol (active) and glucuronide conjugates.

Excretion:
Oral – The t½ is about 6 hr (carteolol) and about 8 to 12 hr (8-hydroxycarteolol). About 50% to 70% is excreted unchanged by the kidneys.

Special Populations:
Renal Function Impairment –
Oral: The t½ may be prolonged and elimination decreased. Dosage adjustment may be needed.

Indications Management of hypertension. Ophthalmic preparation for control of intraocular hypertension and lowering of IOP in chronic open-angle glaucoma. **Unlabeled use(s):** Treatment of angina.

Contraindications Hypersensitivity to beta-blockers; persistently severe bradycardia; greater than first-degree AV block; CHF unless secondary to tachyarrhythmia treatable with beta-blockers; overt cardiac failure; sinus bradycardia; cardiogenic shock; bronchial asthma or bronchospasm, including severe COPD.

Route/Dosage
ADULTS: **PO** 2.5 to 10 mg qd.
Ophthalmic use – 1 drop bid in affected eye(s). Consider concomitant therapy if IOP is not at satisfactory level.

Interactions
Clonidine: May enhance or reverse antihypertensive effect; may cause potentially life-threatening increases in BP, especially on simultaneous discontinuation of both drugs.
Epinephrine: May cause initial hypertensive episode followed by bradycardia.
Ergot derivatives: May cause peripheral ischemia with cold extremities. Peripheral gangrene possible.
NSAIDs: May impair antihypertensive effect.
Prazosin: May increase orthostatic hypotension.
Systemic beta-blocker: When coadministered with ophthalmic carteolol hydrochloride solution, may cause additive effects and toxicity.
Theophyllines: May reduce elimination of theophylline. May cause pharmacologic antagonism, reducing effects of one or both drugs.
Verapamil: May increase effects of both drugs.

Lab Test Interferences None well documented.

Adverse Reactions
CV: Hypotension; bradycardia; CHF; cold extremities; first-, second-, or third-degree atrioventricular block; arrhythmias; syncope.
CNS: Insomnia; fatigue; dizziness; depression; lethargy; drowsiness; forgetfulness; headache.
DERM: Rash; hives; alopecia.
EENT: Dry eyes; blurred vision; tinnitus; slurred speech; dry mouth; sore throat. Eye discomfort or stinging; tearing; keratitis; drooping eyelids; visual disturbances; diplopia; ptosis (ophthalmic use).
GI: Nausea; vomiting; diarrhea; constipation.
GU: Impotence; painful, difficult, or frequent urination.
HEMA: Agranulocytosis; thrombocytopenic purpura.
METAB: Hyperglycemia; hypoglycemia; unstable diabetes mellitus; hypercholesterolemia; hyperlipidemia; increased LDH.
RESP: Bronchospasm; shortness of breath; wheezing.
OTHER: Weight changes; fever; facial swelling; cramps; muscle weakness. Antinuclear antibodies may develop.

Precautions
Pregnancy: Category C.
Lactation: Excreted in breast milk.
Children: Safety and efficacy not established.
Renal function impairment: Requires dosage adjustment.
Hepatic function impairment: Requires dosage adjustment.
Cessation of therapy: Discontinue therapy gradually, over about 2 wk, with careful observation of patient and limited physical activity.
CHF: Administer cautiously in patients with CHF treated with digitalis and diuretics.
Diabetes mellitus: Drug may mask signs and symptoms of hypoglycemia (eg, tachycardia, BP changes). May potentiate insulin-induced hypoglycemia.
Peripheral vascular disease: Drug may precipitate or aggravate symptoms of arterial insufficiency.
Thyrotoxicosis: May mask clinical signs of developing or continuing hyperthyroidism (eg, tachycardia). Abrupt withdrawal may exacerbate symptoms of hyperthyroidism, including thyroid storm.

Overdosage: Signs and Symptoms
Bradycardia, cardiac failure, hypotension, bronchospasm, hypoglycemia.

PATIENT CARE CONSIDERATIONS
Administration/Storage
- For ophthalmic solution, pull out lower lid to create pocket, administer drop without touching eye, release lower lid, close eye, and apply gentle pressure on inner canthus of eye to avoid systemic absorption.
- Store at room temperature.

Assessment/Interventions
- Obtain patient history, including drug history and any known allergies. Note history of CHF, asthma, diabetes, hypertension, or sensitivity to sulfite preservatives, which may be present in ophthalmic solution.
- Determine baseline serum lipids and glucose before initiating treatment with systemic medication.
- Perform measurements of IOP on regular basis to assess therapeutic effect of ophthalmic medication.
- At end of drug regimen, taper dosage slowly under health care provider supervision to prevent rebound symptoms and adverse effects.
- In patients with diabetes, closely monitor blood glucose and diabetic medications. Changes in diabetic medications may be required.
- Monitor BP and pulse frequently when starting oral medication or when dosage is changed.
- Note that ophthalmic solution may produce same adverse reactions as oral form because of absorption.
- Be aware that systemic medication may mask signs of hyperthyroidism.
- If signs of anaphylactic reaction are noted, withhold drug and notify health care provider.
- Notify health care provider at first sign or symptom of CHF or unexplained respiratory problem.
- Observe patient for the following signs of withdrawal syndrome: hypertension, tachycardia, anxiety, angina, MI.

Patient/Family Education
- Instruct patient in proper method of instilling eye drops.
- Teach patient how to monitor pulse before taking oral medication and to notify health care provider if pulse remains less than 50 bpm after taking drug and if fatigue and dizziness occur.
- Instruct patient to inform health care provider of any scheduled surgery or dental work; dosage may need to be gradually tapered (and ophthalmic solution discontinued) before surgery or treatment.
- Caution patient not to discontinue medication without consulting health care provider.
- Instruct diabetic patient to monitor blood glucose closely because carteolol hydrochloride may mask signs of hypoglycemia.
- Inform patient that ophthalmic solution may cause burning or stinging when first instilled in eye.
- Instruct patient to report these symptoms to health care provider: CHF, dizziness, decreased pulse, confusion, shortness of breath, rash, any unusual bleeding.
- Advise patient that drug may cause drowsiness and to use caution while driving or performing other tasks requiring mental alertness.
- Instruct patient not to take otc medications without consulting health care provider.

Carvedilol

(CAR-veh-DILL-ole)

Class Alpha-adrenergic blocker/Beta-adrenergic blocker

How Supplied
Coreg Tablets 3.125 mg, Tablets 6.25 mg, Tablets 12.5 mg, Tablets 25 mg

Action
PHARMACOLOGY: Blocks alpha-1 receptors and nonselective beta-receptors to decrease BP.

PHARMACOKINETICS/DYNAMICS:

Absorption: Rapidly and extensively absorbed. Bioavailability is approximately 25% to 35% because of first-pass metabolism. Food decreases the rate of absorption. Take with food.

Distribution: More than 98% protein bound, primarily to albumin. Lipophilic, with a Vd of about 115 L. Plasma Cl is 500 to 700 mL/min.

Metabolism: Undergoes first-pass metabolism. Metabolized by aromatic ring oxidation and glucuronidation; 3 active metabolites are formed, 1 of which is about 13 times more potent than carvedilol. CYP450 enzymes are involved in carvedilol metabolism.

Excretion: The $t_{½}$ is 7 to 10 hr. Less than 2% is excreted unchanged in urine. Metabolites are excreted via the bile into feces.

Special Populations:
Renal Function Impairment – Plasma concentrations may be higher (40% to 50% in those with moderate to severe renal impairment).
Hepatic Function Impairment – Cirrhotic liver disease patients have a 4- to 7-fold increase in concentrations. Use in patients with hepatic

impairment is not recommended.
Elderly – Plasma levels are about 50% higher in the elderly.
CHF – AUC and C_{max} are increased.

Indications Management of essential hypertension; treatment of mild to severe heart failure of ischemic or cardiomyopathic origin. Reduce cardiovascular mortality in clinically stable patients who have survived the acute phase of MI and have a left ventricular ejection fraction of 40% or less. **Unlabeled use(s):** Angina pectoris.

Contraindications Decompensated cardiac failure requiring use of IV inotropic therapy; bronchial asthma or related bronchospastic conditions; second- or third-degree AV block; sick sinus syndrome (unless a permanent pacemaker is in place); cardiogenic shock; severe bradycardia; hypersensitivity to the drug.

Route/Dosage
Individualize dose and monitor during up-titration.

Essential Hypertension
ADULTS: **PO** Start with 6.25 mg bid, then if tolerated (based on standing BP about 1 hr after dosing), maintain the dose for 7 to 14 days; then increase to 12.5 mg bid, if tolerated, maintain the dose for 7 to 14 days; then increase to 25 mg bid if tolerated and needed (max, 50 mg/day).

CHF
ADULTS: **PO** Start with 3.125 mg bid for 14 days, then, if tolerated, dose may be increased to 6.25 mg bid; dosing may be doubled q 2 wk to the highest amount tolerated by patient (max, 25 mg bid/patients less than 85 kg [187 lbs]; 50 mg bid/patients over 85 kg).

Left Ventricular Dysfunction Following MI
ADULTS: **PO** Start treatment once patient is stable and fluid retention is minimized. The recommended starting dose is 6.25 mg bid and increased to 12.5 mg bid after 3 to 10 days, based on tolerability. The dose may be increased again to the target dose of 25 mg bid. A lower starting dose may be used (3.125 mg bid) and/or, the rate of up-titration may be slowed if clinically indicated (eg, because of low BP, heart rate, or fluid retention). Patients may be maintained at lower dose if higher doses are not tolerated. The recommended dosing regimen need not be altered in patients receiving treatment with an IV or oral β-blocker during the acute phase of the MI.

Interactions
Antidiabetic agents (insulin and oral agents): Blood glucose-lowering effect may be enhanced.
Calcium channel blockers (eg diltiazem): Conduction disturbances may occur and BP may be altered.
Catecholamine-depleting agents (eg, reserpine): Monitor for hypotension or severe bradycardia.
Clonidine: Heart rate and BP-lowering effects may be potentiated.
Cyclosporine, digoxin: Plasma levels may be elevated by carvedilol, increasing the therapeutic and adverse effects.
Inhibitors of CYP2D6 (eg, fluoxetine, paroxetine, propafenone, quinidine) poor metabolizers of debrisoquine: Expected to increase carvedilol blood levels.
Rifampin: May reduce carvedilol plasma levels, decreasing the pharmacologic effect.

Lab Test Interferences None well documented.

Adverse Reactions
CV: Hypotension (14%); bradycardia (10%); syncope (8%); angina pectoris (6%); cerebrovascular accident, fluid overload, postural hypotension, aggravated angina pectoris, AV block, palpitation, hypertension (1% to 3%).
CNS: Dizziness (32%); fatigue (24%); headache (8%); lung edema (for treatment of LVD following MI [more than 3%]); somnolence, vertigo, hypesthesia, paresthesia, depression, insomnia (1% to 3%).
DERM: Purpura (1% to 3%).
EENT: Abnormal vision (5%); blurred vision, pharyngitis (1% to 3%).
GI: Diarrhea (12%); nausea (9%); vomiting (6%); melena, periodontitis, GI pain (1% to 3%).
GU: Impotence, renal insufficiency, albuminuria, hematuria, UTI (1% to 3%).
HEMA: Anemia (for treatment of LVD following MI [more than 3%]); prothrombin decreased, thrombocytopenia (1% to 3%); leukopenia; aplastic anemia (postmarketing).
HEPA: ALT and AST increased (1% to 3%).
METAB: Hyperglycemia, weight increase (12%); peripheral edema (7%); BUN and NPN increase (6%); hypercholesterolemia (4%); hyperuricemia, hypoglycemia, hyponatremia, increase alkaline phosphatase, glycosuria, hypervolemia, diabetes mellitus, GGT increased, weight loss, hyperkalemia, creatinine increased, hypertriglyceridemia (1% to 3%).
RESP: Upper respiratory tract infection (18%); increased cough (8%); sinusitis, bronchitis (5%); rales (4%); dyspnea (for treatment of LVD following MI [more than 3%]).
OTHER: Asthenia (11%); pain (9%); edema generalized, arthralgia (6%) edema dependent (4%); allergy, malaise, hypovolemia, fever, leg

edema, infection, viral infection, back pain muscle cramps, arthritis, hypotonia, flu syndrome, peripheral vascular disorder (1% to 3%).

Precautions

Pregnancy: Category C.
Lactation: Undetermined.
Children: Safety and efficacy not established.
Elderly: Carvedilol plasma levels average 50% higher in elderly compared with young subjects; however, there were no notable differences in efficacy or adverse events.
Renal function impairment: May result in deterioration of renal function.
Special risk patients: Use with caution in patients with pheochromocytoma, CHF, or Prinzmetal variant angina.
Anaphylactic reaction: Patients receiving a β-blocking agent and who have a history of severe anaphylactic reaction to a variety of allergens may be more reactive to repeated challenge. Such patients may be unresponsive to the usual doses of epinephrine used to treat allergic reactions.
Anesthesia and major surgery: If carvedilol is continued perioperatively, use with caution with anesthetic agents that depress myocardial function (eg, ether).
Bronchial asthma: Death in patients with status asthmaticus has occurred.
Diabetes and hypoglycemia: May mask symptoms of hypoglycemia, particularly tachycardia; may potentiate insulin-induced hypoglycemia and delay recovery of serum glucose levels.

Discontinuation: Because carvedilol has β-blocking activity, do not discontinue abruptly. Severe exacerbation of angina and occurrence of MI and ventricular arrhythmias have been reported. Discontinue over 1 or 2 wk.
Hepatic toxicity: Mild hepatocellular injury may occur. Perform laboratory testing at first signs or symptoms of liver dysfunction. If there is laboratory evidence of liver injury or jaundice, carvedilol therapy should be stopped and not restarted.
Nonallergic bronchospasm: In general, patients with bronchospastic disease should not receive β-blocker therapy. In patients who do not respond to, or cannot tolerate other antihypertensive agents, carvedilol may be used with caution and in the smallest effective dose so that inhibition of endogenous or exogenous β-agonists is minimized.
Peripheral vascular disease: Because symptoms of arterial insufficiency may be aggravated or precipitated in patients with peripheral vascular disease, use with caution in such patients.
Thyrotoxicosis: May mask signs of hyperthyroidism, such as tachycardia; abrupt withdrawal may exacerbate symptoms of hyperthyroidism and precipitate thyroid storm.

Overdosage: Signs and Symptoms

Severe hypotension, bradycardia, cardiac insufficiency, cardiogenic shock, cardiac arrest, respiratory problems, bronchospasms, vomiting, lapses of consciousness, generalized seizures.

PATIENT CARE CONSIDERATIONS

Administration/Storage

- Give each dose with food to minimize risk of orthostatic hypotension.
- Do not chew or crush. Instruct patient to swallow tablet whole.
- Store tablets at controlled room temperature (59° to 86°F). Protect from moisture.

Assessment/Interventions

- Obtain patient history, including drug history and any known allergies. Note history of asthma, AV block, sick sinus syndrome, bradycardia, or liver disease.
- Monitor CHF patient for orthostatic hypotension (eg, dizziness, lightheadedness, change in BP) for 1 hr after first dose and at initiation of each dose increase.
- Monitor and record BP and pulse in hypertensive patient. Should hypotension result, hold medication.
- Take safety precautions if orthostatic hypotension occurs.
- Monitor weight and respiratory status in CHF patients.
- Monitor blood sugar in diabetic patient when drug is started or dose is changed.

Patient/Family Education

- Explain name, dose, action, and potential side effects of drug.
- Advise patient that medication is started at a low dose and gradually increased as needed and tolerated.
- Instruct patient not to interrupt therapy or discontinue drug abruptly.
- Remind patient to take each dose with food to reduce risk of orthostatic hypotension.
- Caution patient to avoid sudden position changes to prevent orthostatic hypotension.
- Instruct patient to lie or sit down if experiencing dizziness or lightheadedness when standing.
- Instruct patient in BP and pulse measurement skills.
- Instruct CHF patient to measure and record BP, pulse, weight, and symptoms qd and to report abnormal measurements. Take record to each follow-up office visit.

- Emphasize importance of other modalities on BP (eg, weight control, regular exercise, smoking cessation, moderate intake of alcohol and salt) to hypertensive patient.
- Advise women to notify health care provider if pregnant, planning to become pregnant, or breastfeeding.
- Instruct diabetic patient to monitor blood glucose more frequently when dose is changed or drug is stopped. Patient should inform health care provider of significant changes in readings.
- Advise patients who wear contact lenses that drug may cause decreased tearing and dry eyes.
- Instruct patient to report any of these symptoms to health care provider: dark urine, persistent anorexia, pruritus, right upper quadrant tenderness, unexplained flu-like symptoms, bradycardia, fainting or persistent dizziness when arising from a sitting or lying position, weight gain, swelling of feet or ankles, increasing shortness of breath, or fatigue.
- Caution patient that drug may cause dizziness or fainting and to avoid situations such as driving or performing other hazardous tasks until tolerance is determined.
- Caution patient not to take any prescription or OTC medications or dietary supplements unless advised by health care provider.
- Remind CHF patients that they should be seen by health care provider before each dose change and to keep appointments.

Caspofungin Acetate

(KASS-poe-FUN-jin ASS-eh-tate)

Class Anti-infective/Antifungal

How Supplied
Cancidas Powder for injection, lyophilized 50 mg, Powder for injection, lyophilized 70 mg

Action
PHARMACOLOGY: Inhibits synthesis of β-(1,3)-D-glucan, an integral component of fungal cell wall.

PHARMACOKINETICS/DYNAMICS:
Distribution: About 97% protein bound (albumin).
Metabolism: Slowly metabolized by hydrolysis and N-acetylation and also undergoes spontaneous chemical degradation.
Excretion: The t½ is 9 to 11 hr (beta phase) and 40 to 50 hr (gamma phase). 35% is excreted in feces and 41% in urine (about 1.4% as unchanged drug). Renal Cl is about 0.15 mL/min. Total Cl is 12 mL/min. Not dialyzable.

Special Populations:
Renal Function Impairment – AUC is increased 30% to 49% in those with Ccr up to 49 mL/min. No dosage adjustment is needed.
Hepatic Function Impairment –
Mild: AUC is increased about 55%. No dosage adjustment is needed.
Moderate: AUC is increased 76%. Dosage reduction is recommended.
Elderly – AUC is increased about 28%. No dosage adjustment is needed.

Indications Treatment of invasive aspergillosis in patients refractory to or intolerant of other antifungal therapies.

Contraindications Standard considerations.

Route/Dosage
ADULTS: IV
Loading dose: 70 mg given by slow infusion of about 1 hr on day 1.
Maintenance dose: 50 mg daily by slow infusion of about 1 hr thereafter.

Interactions
Cyclosporine: Avoid concurrent use if possible because caspofungin levels may be elevated, increasing the risk of side effects.
Inducers or mixed inducers/inhibitors of drug clearance (eg, carbamazepine, dexamethasone, efavirenz, nelfinavir, nevirapine, phenytoin, rifampin): Caspofungin blood levels may be decreased, reducing the efficacy.
Tacrolimus: Tacrolimus blood levels may be decreased, reducing the efficacy.
INCOMPATIBILITIES: Do not mix or coinfuse with other medications.

Lab Test Interferences None well documented.

Adverse Reactions
CV: Vein complications; phlebitis; thrombophlebitis; tachycardia; vasculitis.
CNS: Headache; insomnia; paresthesia; tremor.
DERM: Flushing; erythema; induration; pruritus; rash; sweating.
GI: Nausea; vomiting; abdominal pain; anorexia; diarrhea.
HEMA: Eosinophilia; anemia; decreased hematocrit, hemoglobin, neutrophils, WBC count, and platelet count; increased prothrombin time.
HEPA: Increased bilirubin, ALT, and AST.
METAB: Edema; increased serum bicarbonate, potassium, and uric acid.
OTHER: Myalgia; back pain; musculoskeletal pain; asthenia; fatigue; fever; chills; flu-like illness; malaise; pain; warm sensation; anaphylaxis; hypersensitivity; tachypnea.

Precautions
Pregnancy: Category C.
Lactation: Undetermined.
Children: Safety and efficacy not established.

PATIENT CARE CONSIDERATIONS

Administration/Storage

- Follow manufacturer's instructions for reconstitution and administration. Use 0.9% Sodium Chloride Injection. Do not reconstitute with diluents containing glucose.
- Allow refrigerated vial of caspofungin powder to warm to room temperature before reconstituting.
- Do not administer reconstituted solution directly into patient. Reconstituted solution must be transferred to IV bag or bottle containing 0.9% Sodium Chloride for Injection.
- Use aseptic technique while handling medication.
- Do not mix or coinfuse with other medications.
- Do not administer if particulate matter, discoloration, or cloudiness are noted.
- Administer once daily by slow IV infusion of about 1 hr.
- Store unused vials in refrigerator. Reconstituted solution may be stored at temperature less than 77°F for up to 1 hr prior to preparation of patient infusion solution. Final patient infusion solution in the IV bag or bottle can be stored for up to 24 hr at a temperature less than 77°F.

Assessment/Interventions

- Obtain patient history, including drug history and any known allergies. Note history of liver disease.
- Complete CBC and blood chemistry tests prior to initiating therapy.
- Obtain fungal culture as needed before onset of therapy.
- Monitor IV infusion site for signs of reaction or phlebitis.
- Assess patient for CNS, GI, cardiovascular, hematological, musculoskeletal, and dermatologic side effects. Notify health care provider if these effects occur.
- Monitor laboratory values, including liver enzymes and serum potassium, during therapy.
- Monitor temperature during and after administration. Fever is common.
- Notify health care provider if severe side effects or signs of anaphylactic reaction occur; stop infusion.

Patient/Family Education

- Explain name, dose, action, and potential side effects of drug.
- Instruct patient to report any discomfort at injection site immediately.
- Instruct patient to report any of the following symptoms to the health care provider: fever, chills, nausea, headache.

Cefaclor

(SEFF-uh-klor)

Class Antibiotic/Cephalosporin

How Supplied

Ceclor Powder for Oral Suspension 125 mg/5 mL, Powder for Oral Suspension 187 mg/5 mL, Powder for Oral Suspension 250 mg/5 mL, Powder for Oral Suspension 375 mg/5 mL ◆ *Ceclor Pulvules* Capsules 250 mg, Capsules 500 mg ❋ *Apo-Cefaclor* ◆ *Novo-Cefaclor* ◆ *Nu-Cefaclor* ◆ *PMS-Cefaclor*

Action

PHARMACOLOGY: Inhibits mucopeptide synthesis in bacterial cell wall.

PHARMACOKINETICS/DYNAMICS:
Absorption:
Extended-Release (375 to 500 mg with food) – C_{max} is 3.7 to 8.2 mcg/mL, T_{max} is 2.5 to 2.7 hr, AUC is 9.9 to 18.1 mcg•hr/mL.
Immediate-Release (500 mg without food) – C_{max} is 16.8 mcg/mL, T_{max} is 0.9 hr, AUC is 19.2 mcg•hr/mL.

Food – The AUC and C_{max} are greater when the extended-release tablets are taken with food. The C_{max} is decreased when the immediate-release capsules are taken with food.

Distribution: Cefaclor is 25% protein bound.

Metabolism: No evidence of metabolism.

Excretion: Plasma t½ is about 1 hr. About 60% to 85% is excreted unchanged in the urine within 8 hr.

Special Populations:
Renal Function Impairment – The t½ is slightly prolonged. In those with complete absence of renal function, t½ is 2.3 to 2.8 hr.

Indications Treatment of infections of respiratory tract, urinary tract, skin and skin structures; treatment of otitis media caused by susceptible strains of specific microorganisms.

Contraindications Hypersensitivity to cephalosporins.

Route/Dosage

ADULTS: **PO** 250 to 500 mg q 8 hr.
CHILDREN: **PO** 20 to 40 mg/kg/day in divided

doses q 8 hr (for otitis media and pharyngitis, q 12 hr) (max 1 g/day).

Acute Bacterial Exacerbations of Chronic Bronchitis
ADULTS:
Extended-release: **PO** 500 mg/day for 7 days.

Secondary Bacterial Infection of Acute Bronchitis
ADULTS: **PO** 500 mg/12 hr for 7 days.

Pharyngitis or Tonsillitis
ADULTS: **PO** 375 mg/12 hr for 10 days.

Uncomplicated Skin and Skin Structure Infections
ADULTS: **PO** 375 mg/12 hr for 7 to 10 days.

Interactions
Probenecid: Inhibition of renal excretion of cefaclor.

Lab Test Interferences May cause false-positive urine glucose test results with *Benedict's* solution, *Fehling's* solution, or *Clinitest* tablets but not with enzyme-based tests (eg, *Clinistix, Tes-tape*); false-positive test results for proteinuria with acid and denaturization-precipitation tests; false-positive direct *Coombs'* test results in certain patients (eg, those with azotemia); false elevations in urinary 17-ketosteroid values.

Adverse Reactions
GI: Nausea; vomiting; diarrhea; anorexia; abdominal pain or cramps; flatulence; colitis, including pseudomembranous colitis.
GU: Pyuria; renal dysfunction; dysuria; reversible interstitial nephritis; hematuria; toxic nephropathy.
HEMA: Eosinophilia; neutropenia; lymphocytosis; leukocytosis; thrombocytopenia; decreased platelet function; anemia; aplastic anemia; hemorrhage.
HEPA: Hepatic dysfunction, abnormal LFT results.
OTHER: Hypersensitivity, including Stevens-Johnson syndrome, erythema multiforme and toxic epidermal necrolysis; serum sickness–like reactions (eg, skin rash, polyarthritis, arthralgia, fever); candidal overgrowth.

Precautions
Pregnancy: Category B.
Lactation: Excreted in breast milk.
Children: In infants, consider benefits relative to risks. Safety and efficacy in children under 1 mo not established.
Hypersensitivity: Reactions range from mild to life-threatening. Administer drug with caution to penicillin-sensitive patients because of possible cross-reactivity.
Renal function impairment: Use drug with caution in patients with renal impairment. Dosage adjustment based on renal function may be required.
Pseudomembranous colitis: Consider in patients in whom diarrhea develops.
Superinfection: May result in bacterial or fungal overgrowth of nonsusceptible microorganisms.

Overdosage: Signs and Symptoms
Seizures.

PATIENT CARE CONSIDERATIONS
Administration/Storage
- Administer with food or milk if GI upset occurs.
- Tablets, extended-release: Administer with food to enhance absorption. Do not crush or chew.
- After reconstitution, oral suspension must be refrigerated and will remain stable for up to 14 days. Do not freeze. Shake well before use. Do not administer if solution is cloudy or precipitate is present.

Assessment/Interventions
- Obtain patient history, including drug history and any known allergies. Note renal impairment and allergy to cephalosporins or penicillins.
- Obtain specimens for culture and sensitivity before beginning therapy and periodically during treatment.
- Monitor renal function carefully during treatment.
- Monitor for signs of infection, especially fever, and for positive response to antibiotic therapy.
- Assess for signs and symptoms of anaphylaxis (eg, shortness of breath, wheezing, laryngeal spasm). Have resuscitation equipment available.
- Assess for symptoms of superinfection, such as vaginitis or stomatitis.
- Assess for severe diarrhea with blood or pus, which may be symptom of pseudomembranous colitis. Symptoms may occur after antibiotic treatment.

Patient/Family Education
- Instruct patient to complete full course of therapy.
- Instruct patient to check body temperature daily. If fever persists for more than a few days or if high fever (greater than 102°F) or shaking chills are noted, notify health care provider immediately.

- Advise patient to maintain normal fluid intake while using this medication.
- Advise diabetic patient to use enzyme-based tests (eg, *Clinistix*, *Testape*) for monitoring urine glucose because drug may give false results with other tests.
- Instruct patient to report these symptoms to health care provider: nausea, vomiting, diarrhea, skin rash, hives, muscle or joint pain.
- Advise patient to report signs of superinfection: Black "furry" tongue, white patches in mouth, foul-smelling stools, vaginal itching or discharge.
- Warn patient that diarrhea that contains blood or pus may be a sign of serious disorders. Tell patient to seek medical care and not to treat at home.
- Instruct patient to seek emergency care immediately if wheezing or difficulty in breathing occurs.

Cefadroxil

(SEFF-uh-DROX-ill)

Class Antibiotic/Cephalosporin

How Supplied

Duricef Capsules 500 mg (as monohydrate), Tablets 1 g (as monohydrate), Powder for Oral Suspension 125 mg/5 mL, Powder for Oral Suspension 250 mg/5 mL, Powder for Oral Suspension 500 mg/5 mL

♣ *Apo-Cefadroxil* ♦ *Novo-Cefadroxil*

Action

PHARMACOLOGY: Inhibits mucopeptide synthesis in bacterial cell wall.

PHARMACOKINETICS/DYNAMICS:

Absorption: Rapidly absorbed. C_{max} is about 16 mcg/mL (500 mg dose) and 28 mcg/mL (1000 mg dose).

Distribution: 20% protein bound.

Excretion: More than 90% is excreted in the urine as unchanged drug within 24 hr; $t_{1/2}$ is 78 to 96 min.

Special Populations:
Renal Function Impairment – The $t_{1/2}$ is increased. Adjust dose.

Indications Treatment of infections of urinary tract, skin and skin structures; treatment of pharyngitis and tonsillitis caused by susceptible strains of specific microorganisms.

Contraindications Hypersensitivity to cephalosporins.

Route/Dosage

ADULTS: **PO** 1 to 2 g/day in single dose or 2 divided doses.

CHILDREN: **PO** 30 mg/kg/day in single dose or 2 divided doses.

Interactions

Probenecid: Inhibition of renal excretion of cefadroxil.

Lab Test Interferences May cause false-positive urine glucose test results with Benedict's solution, Fehling's solution, or *Clinitest* tablets but not with enzyme-based tests (eg, *Clinistix*, *Tes-tape*); false-positive test results for proteinuria with acid and denaturization-precipitation tests; false-positive direct *Coombs'* test results in certain patients (eg, those with azotemia); false elevations in urinary 17-ketosteroid values.

Adverse Reactions

GI: Nausea; vomiting; diarrhea; anorexia; abdominal pain or cramps; flatulence; colitis, including pseudomembranous colitis.

GU: Pyuria; renal dysfunction; dysuria; reversible interstitial nephritis; hematuria; toxic nephropathy.

HEMA: Eosinophilia; neutropenia; lymphocytosis; leukocytosis; thrombocytopenia; decreased platelet function; anemia; aplastic anemia; hemorrhage.

HEPA: Hepatic dysfunction, abnormal LFT results.

OTHER: Hypersensitivity, including Stevens-Johnson syndrome, erythema multiforme and toxic epidermal necrolysis; serum sickness–like reactions (eg, skin rash, polyarthritis, arthralgia, fever); candidal overgrowth.

Precautions

Pregnancy: Category B.
Lactation: Excreted in breast milk.
Children: In infants, consider benefits relative to risks. Drug may accumulate in newborns.
Hypersensitivity: Reactions range from mild to life-threatening. Administer drug with caution to penicillin-sensitive patients because of possible cross-reactivity.
Renal function impairment: Use drug with caution in patients with renal impairment. Dosage adjustment based on renal function may be required.
Superinfection: May result in bacterial or fungal overgrowth of nonsusceptible microorganisms.
Pseudomembranous colitis: Consider in patients in whom diarrhea develops.

Overdosage: Signs and Symptoms

Seizures.

PATIENT CARE CONSIDERATIONS

Administration/Storage
- Administer with food or milk if GI upset occurs.
- Oral suspension must be refrigerated and will remain stable for up to 14 days. Do not freeze. Shake well before use.

Assessment/Interventions
- Obtain patient history, including drug history and any known allergies. Note renal impairment and allergy to cephalosporins or penicillins.
- Obtain specimens for culture and sensitivity before beginning therapy and periodically during treatment.
- Monitor renal function carefully during treatment.
- Monitor for signs of infection, especially fever, and for positive response to antibiotic therapy.
- Assess for signs and symptoms of anaphylaxis (eg, shortness of breath, wheezing, laryngeal spasm). Have resuscitation equipment available.
- Assess for symptoms of superinfection, such as vaginitis or stomatitis.
- Assess for severe diarrhea with blood or pus, which may be symptom of pseudomembranous colitis. Symptoms may occur after antibiotic treatment.

Patient/Family Education
- Instruct patient to complete full course of therapy.
- Instruct patient to check body temperature daily. If fever persists more than a few days or if high fever (greater than 102°F) or shaking chills are noted, notify health care provider immediately.
- Advise patient to maintain normal fluid intake while using this medication.
- Advise diabetic patient to use enzyme-based tests (eg, *Clinistix*, *Testape*) for monitoring urine glucose because drug may give false results with other tests.
- Instruct patient to report these symptoms to health care provider: nausea, vomiting, diarrhea, skin rash, hives, muscle or joint pain.
- Instruct patient to report signs of superinfection: black "furry" tongue, white patches in mouth, foul-smelling stools, vaginal itching or discharge.
- Warn patient that diarrhea that contains blood or pus may be a sign of serious disorders. Tell patient to seek medical care and not to treat at home. Instruct patient to seek emergency care immediately if wheezing or difficulty in breathing occurs.

Cefamandole Nafate

(SEFF-uh-MAN-dahl NA-fate)

Class Antibiotic/Cephalosporin

How Supplied
Mandol Powder for Injection 1 g, Powder for Injection 2 g

Action
PHARMACOLOGY: Inhibits mucopeptide synthesis in bacterial cell wall.

PHARMACOKINETICS/DYNAMICS:
Absorption:
IM – C_{max} is 13 mcg/mL (500 mg dose) and 25 mcg/mL (1 g dose). T_{max} is 30 to 120 min.
IV – C_{max} is 139 to 533 mcg/mL (1 to 3 g doses). T_{max} is 10 min.

Distribution: Therapeutic levels are reached in pleural and joint fluids and in bile.

Excretion: The t½ is 32 min (IV) and 60 min (IM); 65% to 85% is excreted by the kidneys within 8 hr.

Indications Treatment of infections of lower respiratory tract, urinary tract, skin and skin structures, bone and joint; treatment of mixed infections; treatment of septicemia and peritonitis caused by susceptible strains of specific microorganisms; perioperative prophylaxis.

Contraindications Hypersensitivity to cephalosporins.

Route/Dosage
ADULTS: **IV/IM** 500 mg 1 g q 4 to 8 hr (life-threatening infections or infections caused by less susceptible organisms: up to 2 g q 4 hr) (max, 12 g/day).
CHILDREN OVER 1 MO: **IV/IM** 50 to 150 mg/kg/day in equally divided doses q 4 to 8 hr (max, 12 g/day).

Perioperative Prophylaxis
Adults – **IV/IM** 1 to 2 g 30 min to 1 hr prior to surgical procedure followed by 1 to 2 g q 6 hr for 24 to 48 hr.
Children 3 mo and over: **IV/IM** 50 to 100 mg/kg/day in equally divided doses q 6 hr for 24 to 48 hr.

Interactions
Alcohol: May cause acute alcohol intolerance (eg, disulfiram-like reaction); reaction may occur up to 3 days after last dose of cefamandole nafate.
Aminoglycosides: May increase risk of nephrotoxicity.
Anticoagulants, oral: May increase anticoagulant effect; may cause bleeding complications.

Probenecid: Inhibition of renal excretion of cefamandole.

INCOMPATIBILITIES:

Aminoglycosides: Do not add aminoglycosides to cefamandole solutions because inactivation of both drugs may result; administer at separate sites if concurrent therapy is indicated.

Lab Test Interferences May cause false-positive urine glucose test results with *Benedict's* solution, *Fehling's* solution, or *Clinitest* tablets but not with enzyme-based tests (eg, *Clinistix*, *Tes-tape*); false-positive test result for proteinuria with acid and denaturization-precipitation tests; false-positive direct *Coombs'* test result in certain patients (eg, those with azotemia); false elevations in urinary 17-ketosteroid values.

Adverse Reactions

GI: Nausea; vomiting; diarrhea; anorexia; abdominal pain or cramps; flatulence; colitis, including pseudomembranous colitis.

GU: Pyuria; renal dysfunction; dysuria; reversible interstitial nephritis; hematuria; toxic nephropathy.

HEMA: Eosinophilia; neutropenia; lymphocytosis; leukocytosis; thrombocytopenia; decreased platelet function; anemia; aplastic anemia; hemorrhage.

HEPA: Hepatic dysfunction and cholestatic jaundice; abnormal LFTs.

OTHER: Hypersensitivity, including Stevens-Johnson syndrome, erythema multiforme, toxic epidermal necrolysis; candidal overgrowth; serum sickness–like reactions (eg, skin rash, polyarthritis, arthralgia, fever); phlebitis, thrombophlebitis, and pain at injection site.

Precautions

Pregnancy: Category B.
Lactation: Excreted in breast milk.
Children: Safety and efficacy in children under 1 mo not established.
Renal function impairment: Use drug with caution. Dosage adjustment based on renal function may be required.
Superinfection: Drug may cause bacterial or fungal overgrowth of nonsusceptible microorganisms.
Coagulation abnormalities: Cefamandole nafate may interfere with hemostasis. There is increased risk of bleeding abnormalities associated with hepatic and renal dysfunction, thrombocytopenia and concomitant use of anticoagulants or other drugs that affect hemostasis (eg, aspirin).
Pseudomembranous colitis: Consider in patients in whom diarrhea develops.

Overdosage: Signs and Symptoms

Seizures.

PATIENT CARE CONSIDERATIONS

Administration/Storage

- For IM administration, dilute in ratio of 1 g/3 mL of Sterile Water for Injection, Bacteriostatic Water for Injection, 0.9% Sodium Chloride for Injection, or Bacteriostatic Sodium Chloride. Shake well until dissolved.
- For IV administration, reconstitute in ratio of 1 g/10 mL of Sterile Water for Injection, D5W, or 0.9% Sodium Chloride for Injection.
- Administer IV or inject deep into large muscle mass to minimize pain.
- Store open vials at room temperature.
- May store drug at room temperature for 24 hr after reconstitution. Do not administer if solution is cloudy or precipitate is present.
- May refrigerate reconstituted drug for 96 hr.
- When drug is administered for perioperative prophylaxis, administration is usually discontinued 24 to 48 hr after surgical procedure but can be continued for up to 3 to 5 days postoperatively following complicated surgical procedures.

Assessment/Interventions

- Obtain patient history, including drug history and any known allergies. Note allergy to cephalosporins and penicillins.
- Obtain specimens for culture and sensitivity before beginning therapy.
- Monitor renal function.
- Monitor for coagulation abnormalities. Elevated prothrombin time or abnormal platelet count may occur. If bleeding occurs and PT is prolonged, vitamin K may be indicated.
- Monitor for signs of infection, especially fever, and for positive response to antibiotic therapy.
- Assess for signs and symptoms of anaphylaxis (eg, shortness of breath, wheezing, laryngeal spasm). Have resuscitation equipment available.
- Assess for signs of superinfection, such as vaginitis or stomatitis.
- Assess for diarrhea with blood or pus, which may be symptom of pseudomembranous colitis. Symptoms may occur after antibiotic treatment.
- Monitor IV site for infiltration, infection, and thrombophlebitis.

Patient/Family Education

- Instruct patient to check body temperature daily. If fever persists for more than a few days or if high fever (greater than 102°F) or shaking chills are noted, notify health care provider immediately.

- Advise patient to maintain normal fluid intake while using this medication.
- Advise patient not to drink alcoholic beverages or take alcohol-containing medications while taking this medication and for several days after discontinuing it.
- Instruct patient to report any increase in ecchymoses, petechiae, nose bleeds.
- Advise patient to report signs of superinfection: black "furry" tongue, white patches in mouth, foul-smelling stools, vaginal itching or discharge.
- Instruct patient in good personal hygiene (especially mouth and perineal area care).
- Instruct patient to eat/drink 4 oz of yogurt or buttermilk a day as a prophylaxis against intestinal superinfection.
- Advise diabetic patient to use enzyme-based tests (eg. *Clinistix* , *Testape*) for monitoring urine glucose because drug may give false results with other tests.
- Instruct patient to report these symptoms to health care provider: nausea, vomiting, diarrhea, skin rash, hives, sore throat, bruising, bleeding, muscle or joint pain.
- Warn patient that diarrhea that contains blood or pus may be a sign of serious disorders. Tell patient to seek medical care and not to treat at home.
- Instruct patient to seek emergency care if wheezing or difficulty breathing occurs.

Cefazolin Sodium

(seff-UH-zoe-lin SO-dee-uhm)

Class Antibiotic/Cephalosporin

How Supplied
Ancef Injection 500 mg (2.1 mEq sodium/g), Injection 1 g (2.1 mEq sodium/g), Powder for Injection 500 mg (2.1 mEq sodium/g), Powder for Injection 1 g (2.1 mEq sodium/g), Powder for Injection 5 g (2.1 mEq sodium/g), Powder for Injection 10 g (2.1 mEq sodium/g) ♦ *Zolicef* Powder for Injection 500 mg (2.1 mEq sodium/g), Powder for Injection 1 g (2.1 mEq sodium/g)

Action
PHARMACOLOGY: Inhibits mucopeptide synthesis in bacterial cell wall.

PHARMACOKINETICS/DYNAMICS:
Absorption:
IV – C_{max} is about 185 mcg/mL.

Distribution: 80% to 86% protein bound. Crosses the placenta. Very low concentrations are found in breast milk.

Excretion: The t½ is approximately 1.8 hr (IV) and approximately 2 hr (IM). 70% to 80% is excreted unchanged in the urine.

Special Populations:
Renal Function Impairment – The t½ is increased. Dosage adjustment is needed.

Indications Treatment of infections of respiratory tract, genitourinary tract, skin and skin structures, biliary tract, bone and joint; perioperative prophylaxis; treatment of septicemia and endocarditis caused by susceptible strains of specific microorganisms.

Contraindications Hypersensitivity to cephalosporins.

Route/Dosage
ADULTS: **IV/IM** 250 mg to 1.5 g q 6 to 12 hr (severe infections: up to 12 g/day).
CHILDREN OVER 1 MO: **IV/IM** 25 to 50 mg/kg/day in 3 to 4 equal divided doses q 6 to 8 hr (severe infections: up to 100 mg/kg/day).

Perioperative Prophylaxis
Adults – **IV/IM** 1 g 30 min to 1 hr prior to surgery; 0.5 to 1 g at appropriate intervals (at least 2 hr) during surgery; 0.5 to 1 g q 6 to 8 hr for 24 hr (up to 5 days) after surgery.
Children over 1 mo – **IV/IM** 25 to 50 mg/kg/day divided into 3 to 4 equal doses; (max, 100 mg/kg/day).

Interactions
Aminoglycosides: May increase risk of nephrotoxicity.
Probenecid: Inhibition of renal excretion of cefazolin.
INCOMPATIBILITIES:
Aminoglycosides: Do not add aminoglycosides to cefazolin solutions because inactivation of both drugs may result; administer at separate sites if concurrent therapy is indicated.

Lab Test Interferences May cause false-positive urine glucose test results with Benedict's solution, Fehling's solution, or *Clinitest* tablets but not with enzyme-based tests (eg, *Clinistix*, *Tes-tape*); false-positive test results for proteinuria with acid and denaturization-precipitation tests; false-positive direct *Coombs'* test result in certain patients (eg, those with azotemia); false elevations in urinary 17-ketosteroid values.

Adverse Reactions
GI: Nausea; vomiting; diarrhea; anorexia; abdominal pain or cramps; colitis, including pseudomembranous colitis.
GU: Renal dysfunction; anal pruritus.
HEPA: Hepatic dysfunction; abnormal LFT results.
HEMA: Eosinophilia; neutropenia; lymphocytosis; leukocytosis; thrombocytopenia; thrombocythemia; decreased platelet function; anemia; aplastic anemia; hemorrhage.

OTHER: Hypersensitivity, including Stevens-Johnson syndrome, erythema multiforme, toxic epidermal necrolysis; candidal overgrowth; serum sickness–like reactions (eg, skin rash, polyarthritis, arthralgia, fever); phlebitis, thrombophlebitis, and pain at injection site.

Precautions
Pregnancy: Category B.
Lactation: Excreted in breast milk.
Children: Safety and efficacy in children under 1 mo not established.
Renal function impairment: Use drug with caution. Dosage adjustment based on renal function may be needed.
Superinfection: May cause bacterial or fungal overgrowth of nonsusceptible microorganisms.
Pseudomembranous colitis: Consider in patients in whom diarrhea develops.

Overdosage: Signs and Symptoms
Seizures.

PATIENT CARE CONSIDERATIONS

Administration/Storage
- For IM administration, dilute in ratio of 1 g/3 mL of Sterile Water for Injection, Bacteriostatic Water for Injection, 0.9% Sodium Chloride for Injection or Bacteriostatic Sodium Chloride. Shake well until dissolved. Inject deep into large muscle mass to minimize pain.
- For IV administration, reconstitute in ratio of 1 g/10 mL of Sterile Water for Injection, D5W, or 0.9% Sodium Chloride for Injection. Solution can be frozen in original container for up to 12 wk. Thaw premixed frozen solution at room temperature. May store at room temperature for 48 hr after thawing or may refrigerate for 10 days. Do not refreeze. Do not administer if solution is cloudy or precipitate is present.
- Store unopened vials at room temperature.
- May be stored at room temperature for 24 hr after reconstitution.
- May refrigerate reconstituted drug for 96 hr.
- Reconstituted solution should be light yellow to amber. Do not administer if solution is cloudy or precipitate is present.
- When drug is administered for perioperative prophylaxis, administration is usually discontinued 24 hr postoperatively but can be continued for up to 3 to 5 days following complicated surgical procedures.

Assessment/Interventions
- Obtain patient history, including drug history and any known allergies. Note allergy to cephalosporins and penicillins.
- Obtain specimens for culture and sensitivity before beginning therapy and periodically during treatment.
- Monitor for signs of infection, especially fever, and for positive response to antibiotic therapy.
- Assess for signs and symptoms of anaphylaxis (eg, shortness of breath, wheezing, laryngeal spasm). Have resuscitation equipment available.
- Assess for signs of superinfection, such as vaginitis or stomatitis.
- Assess for diarrhea with blood or pus, which may be symptom of pseudomembranous colitis. Symptoms may occur after antibiotic treatment.
- Monitor IV site for infiltration, infection, and thrombophlebitis.
- Monitor for coagulation abnormalities. Elevated prothrombin time or abnormal platelet count may occur. If bleeding occurs and PT is prolonged, vitamin K may be indicated.

Patient/Family Education
- Instruct patient to check body temperature daily. If fever persists for more than a few days or if high fever (greater than 102°F) or shaking chills are noted, notify health care provider immediately.
- Advise patient to maintain normal fluid intake while using this medication.
- Advise patient to report signs of superinfection: black "furry" tongue, white patches in mouth, foul-smelling stools, vaginal itching or discharge.
- Instruct patient in good personal hygiene (especially mouth and perineal care).
- Advise patient to report any increase in ecchymoses, petechiae, nose bleeds.
- Instruct patient to eat/drink 4 oz of yogurt or buttermilk a day as a prophylaxis against intestinal superinfection.
- Advise diabetic patient to use enzyme-based tests (eg, *Clinistix*, *Testape*) for monitoring urine glucose because drug may give false results with other tests.
- Instruct patient to report these symptoms to health care provider: nausea, vomiting, diarrhea, skin rash, hives, sore throat, bruising, bleeding, muscle or joint pain.
- Warn patient that diarrhea that contains blood or pus may be a sign of serious disorders. Tell patient to seek medical care and not to treat at home.
- Instruct patient to seek emergency care if wheezing or difficulty in breathing occurs.

Cefdinir

(SEFF-dih-ner)

Class Antibiotic/Cephalosporin

How Supplied
Omnicef Capsules 300 mg, Oral Suspension 125 mg/5 mL

Action
PHARMACOLOGY: Inhibits mucopeptide synthesis in bacterial cell wall.

PHARMACOKINETICS/DYNAMICS:
Absorption: T_{max} is 2 to 4 hr. Bioavailability is 21% (capsules) and 25% (suspension). For the capsules, the C_{max} is about 1.6 to 2.87 mcg/mL and the AUC is about 7.05 to 11.1 mcg•hr/mL.

Distribution: Vd is about 0.35 L/kg. 60% to 70% protein bound.

Metabolism: Not appreciably metabolized.

Excretion: The t½ is about 1.7 hr. Renally eliminated with 11.6% to 18.4% excreted unchanged in the urine. Renal Cl is about 2 mL/min/kg. Oral Cl is about 11.6 to 15.5 mL/min/kg. Cefdinir is dialyzable.

Special Populations:
Renal Function Impairment – Cl is reduced. Dosage adjustment is recommended in patients with Ccr less than 30 mL/min.
Elderly – C_{max} is increased 44% and AUC by 86%. No dosage adjustment is required.

Indications Treatment of community-acquired pneumonia, acute exacerbations of chronic bronchitis, acute maxillary sinusitis, pharyngitis and tonsillitis, uncomplicated skin and skin structure infections, and otitis media (pediatric patients only) caused by susceptible strains of specific microorganisms.

Contraindications Hypersensitivity to cephalosporins.

Route/Dosage
ADULTS AND CHILDREN OVER 13 YR: **PO** 600 mg for 10 days (5 to 10 for pharyngitis/tonsillitis).
CHILDREN 6 MO TO 12 YR: **PO** 14 mg/kg (max, 600 mg).

Renal Impairment (Ccr less than 30 mL/min)
ADULTS AND CHILDREN OVER 13 YR: **PO** 300 mg/day.
CHILDREN 6 MO TO 12 YR: **PO** 7 mg/kg (max, 300 mg).

PATIENT CARE CONSIDERATIONS
Administration/Storage
* After mixing the suspension can be stored at room temperature or in the refrigerator. Keep the containers tightly closed, and shake the suspension well before each administration. Discard after 10 days.

Interactions
Aluminum- or magnesium-containing antacids: Concurrent administration reduced absorption of cefdinir (separate doses by 2 hr).
Probenecid: Inhibition of renal excretion of cefdinir.
Iron supplements and vitamins with iron: Concurrent administration reduces absorption of cefdinir (separate doses by 2 hr).

Lab Test Interferences May cause false-positive urine ketone test results when using nitroprusside reagent, but nor with nitroferricyanide-based tests; may cause false positive urine glucose test results with *Benedict's* solution, *Fehling's* solution, or *Clinitest* tablets but not with enzyme-based tests (eg, *Clinistix*, *Tes-Tape*); false-positive direct *Coombs'* test result in certain patients (eg, those with azotemia); false elevations in urinary 17-ketosteroid values.

Adverse Reactions
CNS: Headache.
DERM: Rash; cutaneous moniliasis.
GI: Diarrhea; nausea; vomiting; abdominal pain.
GU: Vaginitis.
OTHER: Elevated liver enzymes; proteinuria; RBCs in urine; eosinophilia; elevated urine pH.

Precautions
Pregnancy: Category B.
Lactation: Undetermined.
Children: Safety and efficacy in children under 6 mo not established.
Hypersensitivity: Reactions range from mild to life-threatening. Administer drug with caution to penicillin-sensitive patients because of possible cross-reactivity.
Renal function impairment: Use drug with caution in patients with renal impairment. Dosage adjustment is recommended in patients with Ccr less than 30 mL/min.
Superinfection: May result in bacterial or fungal overgrowth of nonsusceptible microorganisms.
Pseudomembranous colitis: Consider possibility in patients in whom diarrhea develops.
Hemodialysis patients: A single dose of 300 mg or 7 mg/kg (max, 300 mg) may be administered at the end of each dialysis session. Subsequent doses are then administered every other day.

Overdosage: Signs and Symptoms
Seizures.

- Administer without regard to food.
- Administer 2 hr before or after iron supplements or antacids.
- Administer cautiously to penicillin-sensitive patients as cross-allergic reactions, although rare, can occur. Do not administer to patients with a history of severe reaction to penicillin.
- Do not administer prior to hemodialysis, as dialysis removes cefdinir from the body. Follow recommended administration schedule for patients on dialysis.
- Note dosage adjustments for patients with renal function impairment.
- Store capsules at room temperature. Protect from moisture.

Assessment/Interventions
- Obtain patient history and drug history especially any known allergies to cephalosporins and penicillins.
- Obtain specimens for culture and sensitivity.
- Ensure adequate fluid intake.
- Assess renal function and monitor during therapy. Patients with renal insufficiency must receive reduced dosages to prevent accumulation to toxic levels.
- Monitor patient for signs of infection, fever, and clinical response to treatment (eg, breath sounds, heart sounds, appearance of stools and urine).
- Review laboratory tests (including CBC, x-rays) as soon as possible.
- Assess for signs of superinfections (eg, vaginitis, stomatitis, oral or vaginal white plaques, red raised rash, diarrhea).
- Assess for diarrhea with blood or pus, which may be symptomatic of pseudomembranous colitis. Symptoms may occur after antibiotic treatment is stopped.

Patient/Family Education
- Provide patient information pamphlet.
- Instruct patient to complete full course of therapy.
- If GI upset occurs, patient should take oral preparation with food.
- Inform diabetic patients to use an enzyme-based test as medication can cause false positive test reaction for urine glucose.
- Inform diabetic patients to use an enzyme-based test as medication can cause a false positive test reaction for urine glucose.
- Instruct patient to take cefdinir 2 hr before or after iron supplements or antacids.
- Remind patient to monitor body temperature daily. If fever persists for more than a few days, or if high fever (greater than 102° F) or shaking chills present, notify health care provider immediately.
- Encourage patient to report any symptoms of nausea, vomiting, diarrhea, skin rash, sore throat, bruising, hives, muscle or joint pain to their primary care provider.
- Instruct patient to report signs of superinfection, which often occurs with prolonged or multiple drug therapy. These include vaginal itching or discharge, white or gray patches in the mouth, furry tongue, red raised rash, or foul-smelling stools.
- Warn the patient that diarrhea containing pus or blood may indicate a serious disorder and they should seek immediate treatment.
- Teach patient to identify signs of hypersensitivity that might occur during the course of therapy (eg, urticaria, rash, hypotension, difficulty in breathing, wheezing). Patient should discontinue drug immediately and seek emergency therapy if wheezing or difficulty breathing occurs.

Cefditoren Pivoxil

(SEFF-dih-TORE-ehn pih-VOX-ill)

Class Antibiotic/Cephalosporin

How Supplied
Spectracef Tablets 200 mg

Action
PHARMACOLOGY: Inhibits mucopeptide synthesis in bacterial cell wall.

PHARMACOKINETICS/DYNAMICS:
Absorption: C_{max} is about 1.8 mcg/mL. T_{max} is 1 to 3 hr. Cefditoren dipivoxil is about 14% bioavailable.
Food – Administration following a high-fat meal increased AUC 70% and C_{max} 50%.

Distribution: Vd is about 9.3 L (at steady state). About 88% protein bound, primarily to albumin.

Metabolism: Hydrolyzed to cefditoren by esterases.

Excretion: The $t_{½}$ is about 1.6 hr. Eliminated by excretion into the urine. Renal Cl is about 4 to 5 L/hr.

Special Populations:
Renal Function Impairment –
Moderate impairment (Ccr 30 to 49 mL/min/ 1.73 m^2): Unbound C_{max} is 90% higher, AUC is 232% higher, and $t_{½}$ is 2.7 hr.
Severe impairment (Ccr less than 30 mL/min/ 1.73 m^2): Unbound C_{max} is 114% higher, AUC is 324% higher, and $t_{½}$ is 4.7 hr. Dosage adjustment is recommended.

Elderly – C_{max} is increased 26% and AUC 33%, t½ is 16% to 26% longer, and renal Cl is 20% to 24% lower. No dosage adjustment is needed.

Indications Treatment of mild to moderate infections of acute bacterial exacerbation of chronic bronchitis, pharyngitis/tonsillitis, and uncomplicated skin and skin-structure infections caused by susceptible strains of specific microorganisms.

Contraindications Hypersensitivity to cephalosporins or milk protein; carnitine deficiency or inborn errors of metabolism that result in clinically important carnitine deficiency.

Route/Dosage
Acute Bacterial Exacerbation of Chronic Bronchitis
ADULTS AND CHILDREN (12 YR AND OVER): PO 400 mg bid for 10 days.

Pharyngitis/Tonsillitis and Uncomplicated Skin and Skin-Structure Infections
ADULTS AND CHILDREN (12 YR AND OVER): PO 200 mg bid for 10 days.

Renal Insufficiency
ADULTS AND CHILDREN (12 YR AND OVER): Mild renal impairment (Ccr 50 to 80 mL/min/ 1.73 m^2): PO No dosage adjustment is necessary.
Moderate renal impairment (Ccr 30 to 49 mL/ min/1.73 m^2): PO less than 200 mg bid.
Severe renal impairment (Ccr less than 30 mL/ min/1.73 m^2): PO 200 mg daily.
End-stage renal disease: PO Dose not determined.

Interactions
Antacids, H$_2$-receptor antagonists (eg, famotidine): May decrease cefditoren plasma levels, possibly reducing the efficacy.
Probenecid: May increase plasma levels and the duration of activity of cefditoren.

Lab Test Interferences May cause false-positive direct *Coombs* test; may cause false-positive urine glucose test results with *Benedict* or *Fehling* solution or *Clinitest* tablets but not with enzyme-based tests (eg, *Clinistix, Tes-Tape*); may cause false-negative test in the ferricyanide test for blood glucose but not the glucose oxidase or hexokinase methods of determination.

Adverse Reactions
CNS: Headache; reversible hyperactivity; seizures.
DERM: Stevens-Johnson syndrome; erythema multiforme; toxic epidermal necrolysis.
GI: Diarrhea; nausea; abdominal pain; dyspepsia; vomiting; pseudomembranous colitis; colitis.
GU: Vaginal moniliasis; hematuria; increased urine WBC; renal dysfunction; toxic nephropathy.
HEMA: Decreased hematocrit; aplastic anemia; hemolytic anemia; hemorrhage; pancytopenia; neutropenia; agranulocytosis.
HEPA: Hepatic dysfunction (eg, cholestasis).
METAB: Increased glucose.
OTHER: Allergic reactions; anaphylaxis; drug fever; hypertonia; superinfection; serum sickness-like reaction.

Precautions
Pregnancy: Category B.
Lactation: Undetermined.
Children: Safety and efficacy not determined in children under 12 yr.
Elderly: Because elderly patients are more likely to have decreased renal function, select dose with caution.
Hypersensitivity: Reactions range from mild to life-threatening. Administer drug with caution to penicillin-sensitive patients because of possible cross-reactivity.
Renal function impairment: Dosage adjustment is necessary.
Superinfection: Drug may cause bacterial or fungal overgrowth of nonsusceptible microorganisms.
Pseudomembranous colitis: Consider pseudomembranous colitis as a possibility in patients who develop diarrhea.

Overdosage: Signs and Symptoms
Nausea, vomiting, epigastric distress, diarrhea, convulsions.

PATIENT CARE CONSIDERATIONS
Administration/Storage
- Medication is usually administered twice daily.
- Administer each dose with food to increase absorption.
- Administer reduced dose to patient with renal impairment.
- Store tablets at controlled room temperature (59° to 86°F). Protect from light and moisture.

Assessment/Interventions
- Obtain patient history, including drug history and any known allergies. Note history of allergy to penicillins, cephalosporins or milk protein, renal impairment, severe hepatic impairment, carnitine deficiency, or inborn errors of metabolism that may result in carnitine deficiency.
- Review results of culture and sensitivity testing as available.

- Monitor for signs of infection, especially fever, and for positive response to antibiotic therapy.
- Monitor patient for signs of anaphylaxis or severe allergic reaction. Discontinue therapy and immediately notify health care provider if noted. Be prepared to treat appropriately.
- Monitor patient for GI side effects. Report to health care provider if noted and significant.

Patient/Family Education
- Explain name, dose, action, and potential side effects of drug.
- Review dosing schedule and prescribed length of therapy with patient.
- Instruct patient to take each dose with food to enhance absorption.
- Instruct patient not to take antacids or other acid-suppressive therapy (eg, H_2-receptor antagonists, proton pump inhibitors) concomitantly with this medication.
- Remind patient, family, or caregiver to complete entire course of therapy, even if symptoms of infection have disappeared.
- Advise patient, family, or caregiver to discontinue therapy and contact the health care provider immediately if skin rash, hives, itching, or shortness of breath occurs.
- Advise patient, family, or caregiver to report the following signs of superinfection to health care provider: black "furry" tongue, white patches in mouth, foul-smelling stools, vaginal itching or discharge.
- Warn patient, family, or caregiver that diarrhea containing blood or pus may be a sign of a serious disorder and to seek medical care if noted and not to treat at home.
- Instruct patient not to take any prescription or otc medications or dietary supplements unless advised to do so by the health care provider.
- Advise patient, family, or caregiver that follow-up examinations and lab tests may be required to monitor therapy and to be sure and keep appointments.

Cefepime

(SEFF-eh-pim)

Class Antibiotic/Cephalosporin

How Supplied
Maxipime Powder for Injection 500 mg, Powder for Injection 1 g, Powder for Injection 2 g

Action
PHARMACOLOGY: Inhibits mucopeptide synthesis in bacterial cell wall.

PHARMACOKINETICS/DYNAMICS:
Absorption:
IV (500 mg to 2 g doses) – C_{max} is 39.1 to 163.9 mcg/mL. AUC is about 70.8 to 284.8 hr•mcg/mL.
IM (500 mg to 2 g doses) – C_{max} is about 13.9 to 57.5 mcg/mL. AUC is about 60 to 262 hr•mcg/mL. T_{max} is about 1.4 to 1.6 hr.

Distribution: Vd is about 18 L (at steady state). About 20% protein bound. Excreted in human milk; crosses the inflamed blood-brain barrier.

Metabolism: Metabolized to N-methylpyrrolidine, which is then converted to the N-oxide.

Excretion: About 85% is excreted unchanged in the urine; t½ is 102 to 138 min.

Special Populations:
Renal Function Impairment – Total body clearance is decreased proportionally with Ccr. Dosage adjustment is recommended.
Elderly – Total body clearance is decreased. Adjust dose if Ccr is less than or equal to 60 mL/min.

Indications Treatment of pneumonia and infections of the skin and skin structures and urinary tract caused by susceptible strains of specific microorganisms. Treatment of empiric therapy for febrile neutropenic patients as monotherapy. Treatment for complicated intra-abdominal infections in combination with metronidazole.

Contraindications Hypersensitivity to cephalosporins, penicillins, or other beta-lactam antibiotics.

Route/Dosage
Mild to Moderate Uncomplicated or Complicated Urinary Tract Infections
ADULTS: IV/IM 0.5 to 1 g q 12 hr for 7 to 10 days.

Severe Uncomplicated or Complicated Urinary Tract Infections
ADULTS: IV 2 g q 12 hr for 10 days.

Moderate to Severe Pneumonia
ADULTS: IV 1 to 2 g q 12 hr for 10 days.

Moderate to Severe Uncomplicated Skin and Skin Structure Infections
ADULTS: IV 2 g q 12 hr for 10 days
CHILDREN UNDER 40 KG: 50 mg/kg/dose q 12 hr (q 8 hr for febrile neutropenic patients) for 7 to 10 days. Do not exceed the recommended adult dose.

Renal Impairment (Children)
Data not available; however, changes in dosing regimen similar to those in adults are recommended.

Interactions
Aminoglycosides: Increased risk of nephrotoxicity and ototoxicity.

INCOMPATIBILITIES: Metronidazole, vancomycin, gentamicin, tobramycin, netilmicin, aminophylline, and ampicillin (greater than 40 mg/mL).

Lab Test Interferences May cause false-positive reaction for glucose in the urine when using *Clinitest* tablets but not with tests based on enzymatic glucose oxidase reactions (eg, *Clinistix*).

Adverse Reactions
CNS: Headache.
GI: Nausea; vomiting; diarrhea; colitis; including pseudomembranous colitis; oral moniliasis.
DERM: Rash; pruritus; urticaria.
OTHER: Hypersensitivity, including Stevens-Johnson syndrome; erythema multiforme; toxic epidermal necrolysis; candidal overgrowth; serum sickness–like reactions (eg, skin rashes, polyarthritis, arthralgia, fever); phlebitis; pain or inflammation at injection site; fever.

PATIENT CARE CONSIDERATIONS
Administration/Storage
- IM rate indicated only for mild to moderate, uncomplicated, or complicated UTIs caused by *Escherichia coli*.
- Inject IM preparations deep into large muscle groups.
- Dilute IV preparations with 50 to 100 mL of compatible IV fluid and administer over 30 min.
- Do not administer if particulate matter is noted in reconstituted solution.
- Store unopened vials at room temperature (68° to 77°F). Store reconstituted solutions at room temperature (68° to 77°F) for up to 24 hr or refrigerated (36° to 46°F) for up to 7 days.
- Protect from light.

Assessment/Interventions
- Obtain patient history, including drug history and any known allergies. Note allergy to cephalosporins and penicillins.
- Obtain specimens for culture and sensitivity before beginning therapy and periodically during treatment.
- Monitor for signs of infection, especially fever, and for positive response to antibiotic therapy.
- Assess for signs and symptoms of anaphylaxis (eg, shortness of breath, wheezing, laryngeal spasm). Have resuscitation equipment available.
- Assess for signs of superinfection, such as vaginitis or stomatitis.
- Assess for diarrhea with blood or pus, which may be a symptom of pseudomembranous colitis. Symptoms may occur after antibiotic treatment.

Precautions
Pregnancy: Category B.
Lactation: Excreted in breast milk.
Children: Safety and efficacy in children under 12 yr have not been established.
Hypersensitivity: Reactions range from mild to life-threatening. Administer drug with caution to penicillin-sensitive patients because of possible cross-sensitivity.
Renal function impairment: Dosage adjustment is necessary in patients with Ccr less than 60 mL/min.
Superinfection: Drug may cause bacterial or fungal overgrowth of nonsusceptible microorganisms.
Pseudomembranous colitis: Consider in patients in whom diarrhea develops.

Overdosage: Signs and Symptoms
Seizures, encephalopathy, neuromuscular excitability.

- Monitor IV site for infiltration, infection, and thrombophlebitis.

Patient/Family Education
- Instruct patient to check body temperature daily. If fever persists for more than a few days or if high fever (greater than 102°F) or shaking chills are noted, notify health care provider immediately.
- Advise patient to maintain normal fluid intake while using this medication.
- Advise patient to report signs of superinfection: black "furry" tongue, white patches in mouth, foul-smelling stools, vaginal itching or discharge.
- Instruct patient in good personal hygiene (especially mouth and perineal care).
- Advise patient to report any increase in ecchymoses, petechiae, or nose bleeds.
- Advise patient to eat/drink 4 oz of yogurt or buttermilk a day as a prophylaxis against intestinal superinfection.
- Advise diabetic patient to use enzyme-based tests (eg, *Clinistix*, *Testape*) for monitoring urine glucose because drug may give false results with other tests.
- Instruct patient to report these symptoms to health care provider: nausea, vomiting, diarrhea, skin rash, hives, sore throat, bruising, bleeding, muscle or joint pain.
- Warn patient that diarrhea containing blood or pus may be a sign of serious disorders.
- Tell patient to seek medical care for symptoms and not to treat at home. Instruct patient to seek emergency care if wheezing or difficulty in breathing occurs.

Cefixime

(SEFF-IKS-eem)

Class Antibiotic/Cephalosporin

How Supplied
Suprax Oral suspension 100 mg per 5 mL, Tablets 400 mg

Action
PHARMACOLOGY: Inhibits mucopeptide synthesis in bacterial cell wall.

PHARMACOKINETICS/DYNAMICS:
Absorption: About 40% to 50% is absorbed. C_{max} following 200 mg and 400 mg doses of oral suspension are 3 mcg/mL and 4.6 mcg/mL, respectively. T_{max} occurs between 2 and 6 hr following administration of 400 mg and between 2 and 5 hr after a 200 mg dose.

Distribution: Protein binding is about 65%.

Excretion: About 50% of absorbed dose is excreted unchanged in the urine in 24 hr. Serum t½ averages 3 to 4 hr but may be as long as 9 hr in some normal subjects.

Indications Treatment of uncomplicated UTIs, otitis media, pharyngitis, tonsillitis, acute bronchitis, acute exacerbations of chronic bronchitis, and uncomplicated gonorrhea caused by susceptible strains of specific organisms.

Contraindications Allergy to cephalosporin group of antibiotics.

Route/Dosage
Infection
ADULTS AND CHILDREN (WEIGHING MORE THAN 50 KG OR OLDER THAN 12 YR OF AGE): **PO** 400 mg daily.
CHILDREN 6 MO TO 12 YR OF AGE: **PO** 8 mg/kg/day as a single daily dose or in 2 divided doses of 4 mg/kg q 12 hr.

Uncomplicated Gonorrhea
ADULTS: **PO** 400 mg as a single dose.

Dose Adjustment for Renal Function Impairment
Ccr between 21 to 60 mL/min or on hemodialysis, give 75% of dose (300 mg/day). Ccr less than 20 mL/min or on continuous peritoneal dialysis, give 50% of dose (200 mg/day).

Interactions
Carbamazepine: Plasma concentrations may be elevated by cefixime, increasing the risk of side effects.
Warfarin: Increased PT, with and without bleeding, may occur.

Lab Test Interferences May cause false-positive urine glucose test results with Benedict solution, Fehling solution, or *Clinitest* tablets but not with enzyme-based tests (eg, *Clinistix, Testape*); false-positive test results for ketones in the urine may occur with tests using nitroprusside but not nitroferricyanide; false-positive direct Coombs test.

Adverse Reactions
CNS: Headaches, dizziness, seizures (less than 2%).
DERM: Toxic epidermal necrolysis (less than 2%).
GI: Diarrhea (16%); nausea (7%); loose or frequent stools (6%); flatulence (4%); abdominal pain, dyspepsia (3%); vomiting (less than 2%).
GU: Genital pruritus, vaginitis, candidiasis (less than 2%).
HEMA/LYMPH: Transient thrombocytopenia, leukopenia, neutropenia, eosinophilia, prolongation in PT (less than 2%); pancytopenia, agranulocytosis.
HEPA: Transient elevations in ALT, AST, alkaline phosphatase, hepatitis, jaundice (less than 2%).
HYPERSEN: Anaphylactic/anaphylactoid reactions (including shock and death); skin rashes, urticaria, drug fever, pruritus, angioedema, facial edema, erythema multiforme, Stevens-Johnson syndrome, serum sickness-like reactions (less than 2%).
LABTESTABS: Hyperbilirubinemia (less than 2%).
RENAL: Transient elevations in BUN or creatine, acute renal failure (less than 2%).

Precautions
Pregnancy: Category B.
Lactation: Undetermined.
Children: Safety and efficacy not established in children under 6 mo of age.
Hypersensitivity: If administered to penicillin-allergic patients, use with caution because cross-sensitivity has been documented and may occur in up to 10% of patients with penicillin allergy.
Renal function impairment: Use with caution in patients with renal impairment. Dosage adjustment based on renal function may be required.
Superinfection: May result in bacterial or fungal overgrowth of nonsusceptible microorganisms.
GI disease: Use with caution, especially for colitis.
Pseudomembranous colitis: Consider possibility if diarrhea develops.

PATIENT CARE CONSIDERATIONS
Administration/Storage
- Tablets should not be substituted for oral suspension in the treatment of otitis media because of lack of bioequivalence.
- Administer prescribed dose without regard to meals, but administer with food if GI upset occurs.
- Administer tablets with a full glass of water.
- Shake suspension well before measuring dose.
- Measure and administer prescribed dose of suspension using dosing syringe, dosing spoon, or medicine cup.
- Store tablets at controlled room temperature (68° to 77°F). Store oral suspension at controlled room temperature or under refrigeration (36° to 46°F) for up to 14 days. Keep tightly closed. Discard unused portion after 14 days.

Assessment/Interventions
- Obtain patient history, including drug history and any known allergies. Note renal impairment, or history of allergy or intolerance to penicillin or cephalosporin antibiotics.
- Ensure that reduced dose is administered to patient with renal impairment (Ccr less than 60 mL/min) following manufacturer's guidelines.
- Review results of culture and sensitivity testing as appropriate.
- Monitor patient's response to therapy. Notify health care provider if infection does not appear to be improving or is worsening.
- Monitor patient for signs of allergic reaction. Discontinue therapy and immediately notify health care provider if noted. Be prepared to treat appropriately.
- Monitor patient for GI, CNS, general body side effects, and signs of superinfection. Report to health care provider if noted and significant. Immediately report severe diarrhea, diarrhea containing blood or pus, or severe abdominal cramping.

Patient/Family Education
- Explain name, dose, action, and potential side effects of drug.
- Review dosing schedule and prescribed length of therapy with patient.
- Instruct patient using tablets to take dose with a full glass of water.
- Instruct patient or caregiver using oral suspension to shake well before measuring dose and to measure and administer prescribed dose using dosing spoon, dosing syringe, or medicine cup.
- Advise patient to take without regard to meals but to take with food if GI upset occurs.
- Instruct patient to complete entire course of therapy even if symptoms of infection have disappeared.
- Advise patient to discontinue therapy and contact health care provider immediately if skin rash, hives, itching, or shortness of breath occur.
- Advise women to notify health care provider if pregnant, planning to become pregnant, or breastfeeding.
- Advise patient to report the following signs of superinfection to health care provider: black "furry" tongue, white patches in mouth, foul-smelling stools, vaginal itching or discharge.
- Warn patient that diarrhea containing blood or pus may be a sign of a serious disorder and to seek medical care if noted and not treat at home.
- Caution patient not to take any prescription or OTC medications, dietary supplements, or herbal preparations unless advised by health care provider.
- Advise patient that follow-up examinations and lab tests may be required to monitor therapy and to keep appointments.

Cefmetazole Sodium

(seff-MET-uh-zole)

Class Antibiotic/Cephalosporin

How Supplied
Zefazone Powder for Injection 1 g (2 mEq sodium/g), Powder for Injection 2 g (2 mEq sodium/g), Injection 1 g/50 mL (2.7 mEq sodium/g), Injection 2 g/50 mL (2.7 mEq sodium/g)

Action
PHARMACOLOGY: Inhibits mucopeptide synthesis in bacterial cell wall.

PHARMACOKINETICS/DYNAMICS:
Absorption:
IV – C_{max} is 143 mcg/mL (2 g dose).
IM – C_{max} is 34 mcg/mL (1 g dose). T_{max} is about 1.5 hr.

Distribution: 65% protein bound.

Excretion: The t½ is about 1.2 hr (IV) and about 1.5 hr (IM). Plasma clearance is 121 mL/min. About 85% is excreted unchanged in the urine over 12 hr.

Special Populations:
Renal Function Impairment – Cl is decreased and t½ is prolonged. Dosage adjustment is recommended.

Indications Treatment of infections of urinary tract, lower respiratory tract, skin and skin structure; treatment of intra-abdominal infections caused by susceptible microorganisms; perioperative prophylaxis.

Contraindications Hypersensitivity to cephalosporins.

Route/Dosage
ADULTS: **IV** 2 g q 6 to 12 hr.

Perioperative Prophylaxis
ADULTS: **IV** 1 to 2 g at specified times prior to surgery.

Abdominal Hysterectomy/Cholecystectomy (High-Risk)
ADULTS: **IV** 1 g 30 to 90 min before surgery and repeated 8 hr and 16 hr later.

Cesarean Section
ADULTS: **IV** 2 g after clamping cord or 1 g after clamping cord and repeated 8 and 16 hr later.

Colorectal Surgery/Vaginal Hysterectomy
ADULTS: **IV** 2 g 30 to 90 min before surgery or 1 to 2 g 30 to 90 min before surgery and repeated 8 and 16 hr later.

Interactions
Alcohol: May cause acute alcohol intolerance (eg, disulfiram-like reaction); reaction may occur several days after last dose of cefmetazole.
Aminoglycosides: May increase risk of nephrotoxicity.
Anticoagulants, oral: May increase anticoagulant effects; may cause bleeding complications.
Probenecid: Inhibition of renal excretion of cefmetazole.
INCOMPATIBILITIES:
Aminoglycosides: Do not add aminoglycosides to cefmetazole solutions because inactivation of both drugs may result; administer at separate sites if concurrent therapy is indicated.

Lab Test Interferences May cause false-positive urine glucose test results with *Benedict's* solution, *Fehling's* solution, or *Clinitest* tablets but not with enzyme-based tests (eg, *Clinistix*, *Tes-tape*); false-positive test results for proteinuria with acid and denaturization-precipitation tests; false-positive direct *Coombs'* test results in certain patients (eg, those with azotemia); false elevations in urinary 17-ketosteroid values.

Adverse Reactions
CV: Hypotension; shock.
CNS: Headache; hot flashes.
GI: Nausea; vomiting; diarrhea; abdominal pain or cramps; flatulence; colitis, including pseudomembranous colitis.
GU: Renal dysfunction; increased BUN; increased creatinine.
HEMA: Eosinophilia; neutropenia; lymphocytosis; leukocytosis; thrombocytopenia; decreased platelet function; anemia; aplastic anemia; hemorrhage.
HEPA: Hepatic dysfunction; abnormal LFT results.
RESP: Shortness of breath; pleural effusion.
OTHER: Hypersensitivity, including Stevens-Johnson syndrome, erythema multiforme, toxic epidermal necrolysis; candidal overgrowth; serum sickness–like reactions (eg, skin rash, polyarthritis, arthralgia, fever); phlebitis, thrombophlebitis, and pain at injection site.

Precautions
Pregnancy: Category B.
Lactation: Excreted in breast milk.
Children: Safety and efficacy not established.
Renal function impairment: Use drug with caution. Dosage adjustment based on renal function may be required.
Superinfection: Drug may cause bacterial or fungal overgrowth of nonsusceptible microorganisms.
Pseudomembranous colitis: Consider in patients in whom diarrhea develops.

Overdosage: Signs and Symptoms
Seizures.

PATIENT CARE CONSIDERATIONS

Administration/Storage
- Administer IV.
- Reconstitute in ratio of 1 g/10 mL of Sterile Water for Injection, D5W, or 0.9% Sodium Chloride for Injection.
- May store drug at room temperature for 24 hr after reconstitution. Reconstituted drug is stable for 7 days if refrigerated and for 6 wk if frozen. Do not use if solution is cloudy or precipitate is present.

Assessment/Interventions
- Obtain patient history, including drug history and any known allergies. Note allergy to cephalosporins or penicillins.
- Obtain specimens for culture and sensitivity before beginning therapy and during treatment.
- Monitor renal function during therapy.
- Monitor IV site during infusion.
- Monitor for signs of infection, especially fever, and for positive response to antibiotic therapy.
- Assess for signs and symptoms of anaphylaxis (eg, shortness of breath, wheezing, laryngeal spasm). Have resuscitation equipment available.
- Assess for signs of superinfection, such as vaginitis or stomatitis.
- Assess for diarrhea with blood or pus, which

may be a symptom of pseudomembranous colitis. Symptoms may occur after antibiotic treatment.
- Monitor IV site for infiltration, infection, and thrombophlebitis.

Patient/Family Education
- Instruct patient to check body temperature daily. If fever persists for more than a few days or if high fever (greater than 102°F) or shaking chills are noted, notify health care provider immediately.
- Advise patient to maintain normal fluid intake while using this medication.
- Advise diabetic patient to use enzyme-based tests (eg, *Clinistix*, *Tes-tape*) for monitoring urine glucose because drug may give false results with other tests.
- Instruct patient to report these symptoms to health care provider: nausea, vomiting, diarrhea, skin rash, hives, sore throat, bruising, bleeding, muscle or joint pain.
- Instruct patient to report signs of superinfection: black "furry" tongue, white patches in mouth, foul-smelling stools, vaginal itching or discharge.
- Warn patient that diarrhea that contains blood or pus may be a sign of serious disorders. Tell patient to seek medical care and not to treat at home.
- Instruct patient to seek emergency care if wheezing or difficulty in breathing occurs.
- Advise patient not to drink alcoholic beverages or to take alcohol-containing medications while receiving cefmetazole and for several days after discontinuing drug.

Cefoperazone Sodium

(SEFF-oh-PURR-uh-zone SO-dee-uhm)

Class Antibiotic/Cephalosporin

How Supplied
Cefobid Powder for Injection 1 g (1.5 mEq sodium/g. Also may contain dextrose hydrous.), Powder for Injection 2 g (1.5 mEq sodium/g. Also may contain dextrose hydrous.), Injection 1 g (1.5 mEq sodium/g. Also may contain dextrose hydrous.), Injection 2 g (1.5 mEq sodium/g. Also may contain dextrose hydrous.), Injection 10 g (1.5 mEq sodium/g. Also may contain dextrose hydrous.)

Action
PHARMACOLOGY: Inhibits mucopeptide synthesis in bacterial cell wall.

PHARMACOKINETICS/DYNAMICS:
Distribution: Cefoperazone is 82% to 93% protein bound. CSF levels are relatively low.

Excretion: The t½ is about 2 hr. Cefoperazone is extensively excreted in bile; 20% to 30% is recovered unchanged in the urine.

Special Populations:
Hepatic Function Impairment – The t½ increased 2- to 4-fold in patients with hepatic disease or biliary obstruction.

Indications Treatment of infections of respiratory tract, urinary tract, skin and skin structures; treatment of pelvic inflammatory disease, endometritis, and other female genital tract infections; treatment of septicemia and peritonitis caused by susceptible microorganisms.

Contraindications Hypersensitivity to cephalosporins.

Route/Dosage
ADULTS: **IV/IM** 2 to 4 g/day in equally divided doses q 12 hr (severe infections: 6 to 12 g/day in equally divided doses [1.5 to 4 g/dose] q 6, 8, or 12 hr).

Interactions
Alcohol: May cause acute alcohol intolerance (disulfiram-like reaction); reaction may occur up to 3 days after last dose of cefoperazone.
Aminoglycosides: May increase risk of nephrotoxicity.
Anticoagulants, oral: May increase anticoagulant effect; bleeding complications may occur.
INCOMPATIBILITIES:
Aminoglycosides: Do not add aminoglycosides to cefoperazone solutions because inactivation of both drugs may result; administer at separate sites if concurrent therapy is indicated.

Lab Test Interferences May cause false-positive urine glucose test results with *Benedict's* solution, *Fehling's* solution, or *Clinitest* tablets but not with enzyme-based tests (eg, *Clinistix*, *Tes-tape*); false-positive test result for proteinuria with acid and denaturization-precipitation tests; false-positive direct *Coombs'* test result in certain patients (eg, those with azotemia); false elevations in urinary 17-ketosteroid values.

Adverse Reactions
GI: Nausea, vomiting, diarrhea; pseudomembranous colitis.
GU: Renal dysfunction; elevation in serum creatinine.
HEMA: Eosinophilia; neutropenia; lymphocytosis; leukocytosis; thrombocytopenia; decreased platelet function; anemia; aplastic anemia; hemorrhage.

HEPA: Hepatitis; abnormal LFT results.
OTHER: Hypersensitivity, including Stevens-Johnson syndrome, erythema multiforme, toxic epidermal necrolysis; candidal overgrowth; serum sickness–like reactions (eg, skin rashes, polyarthritis, arthralgia, fever); phlebitis, thrombophlebitis, and pain at injection site.

Precautions
Pregnancy: Category B.
Lactation: Small quantities may be excreted in breast milk.
Children: Safety and efficacy in children not established.
Hypersensitivity: Reactions range from mild to life-threatening. Administer drug with caution to penicillin-sensitive patients because of possible cross-reactivity.

Hepatic function impairment: Since cefoperazone is extensively excreted in bile, serum concentrations may be elevated; monitor levels at doses above 4 g.
Superinfection: May result in bacterial or fungal overgrowth of nonsusceptible microorganisms.
Coagulation abnormalities: Cefoperazone may interfere with hemostasis. Bleeding abnormalities are greater risk in presence of hepatic and renal dysfunction, thrombocytopenia, concomitant use of anticoagulants or other drugs that affect hemostasis (eg, aspirin) and in elderly, malnourished, or debilitated patients.
Pseudomembranous colitis: Consider in patients in whom diarrhea develops.

Overdosage: Signs and Symptoms
Seizures.

PATIENT CARE CONSIDERATIONS

Administration/Storage
- If drug is administered IM with concentration greater than 250 mg/mL, give with 0.5% lidocaine or any other suitable diluent.
- For IV infusion, dilute reconstituted drug in 50 to 100 mL 0.9% sodium chloride or D5W and infuse over 30 min.
- For IM administration, inject deeply within body of large muscle (eg, gluteus muscle).
- May freeze medication. Thaw at room temperature and discard unused portions. Do not refreeze.
- Before reconstitution, protect from light and store at cool temperature.
- Solutions are stable for 24 hr at room temperature and 5 days if refrigerated. Do not administer if solution is cloudy or precipitate is present.

Assessment/Interventions
- Obtain patient history, including drug history and any known allergies. Note allergy to cephalosporins and penicillins.
- Obtain specimens for culture and sensitivity before beginning therapy and periodically during treatment.
- Monitor renal function carefully during treatment.
- Monitor for signs of infection, especially fever, and for positive response to antibiotic therapy.
- Assess for signs and symptoms of anaphylaxis (eg, shortness of breath, wheezing, laryngeal spasm). Have resuscitation equipment available.
- Assess for signs of superinfection, such as vaginitis or stomatitis.
- Assess for diarrhea with blood or pus, which may be a symptom of pseudomembranous colitis. Symptoms may occur after antibiotic treatment.
- Monitor IV site for infiltration, infection, and thrombophlebitis.
- Monitor for coagulation abnormalities. Elevated prothrombin time or abnormal platelet count may occur. If bleeding occurs and PT is prolonged, vitamin K may be indicated.

Patient/Family Education
- Instruct patient to check body temperature daily. If fever persists for more than a few days or if high fever (greater than 102°F) or shaking chills are noted, notify health care provider immediately.
- Advise patient to maintain normal fluid intake while using this medication.
- Advise diabetic patient to use enzyme-based tests (eg, *Clinistix* , *Testape*) for monitoring urine glucose because drug may give false results with other tests.
- Instruct patient to report these symptoms to health care provider: nausea, vomiting, diarrhea, skin rash, hives, sore throat, bruising, bleeding, muscle or joint pain.
- Warn patient that diarrhea that contains blood or pus may be a sign of serious disorders. Tell patient to seek medical care and not to treat at home.
- Instruct patient to seek emergency care if wheezing or difficulty in breathing occurs.
- Advise patient to report signs of superinfection: black "furry" tongue, white patches in mouth, foul-smelling stools, vaginal itching or discharge.
- Instruct patient not to drink alcoholic beverages or to take alcohol-containing medications while taking this medication and for several days after discontinuing it.

Cefotaxime Sodium

(seff-oh-TAX-eem SO-dee-uhm)
Class Antibiotic/Cephalosporin

How Supplied
Claforan Powder for Injection 500 mg (2.2 mEq sodium/g), Powder for Injection 1 g (2.2 mEq sodium/g), Powder for Injection 2 g (2.2 mEq sodium/g), Powder for Injection 10 g (2.2 mEq sodium/g), Injection 1 g (2.2 mEq sodium/g), Injection 2 g (2.2 mEq sodium/g)

Action
PHARMACOLOGY: Inhibits mucopeptide synthesis in bacterial cell wall.

PHARMACOKINETICS/DYNAMICS:
Absorption:
IM – C_{max} is 11.7 mcg/mL (500 mg dose) and 20.5 mcg/mL (1 g dose). T_{max} is about 1 hr.

Distribution: Cefotaxime is 30% to 40% protein bound.

Metabolism: Cefotaxime is metabolized to desacetyl derivative (active).

Excretion: About 60% is recovered in the urine in 6 hr; about 20% to 36% is excreted as unchanged cefotaxime and 15% to 25% as desacetyl derivative. The t½ is 60 min.

Special Populations:
Renal Function Impairment – The t½ is prolonged. Dosage adjustment is recommended.

Indications
Treatment of infections of lower respiratory tract including pneumonia, urinary tract, skin and skin structures, bone and joints; treatment of bacteremia/septicemia, CNS infections, intra-abdominal infections and gynecological infections including pelvic inflammatory disease, endometritis and pelvic cellulitis caused by susceptible strains of specific microorganisms; perioperative prophylaxis.

Contraindications
Hypersensitivity to cephalosporins.

Route/Dosage
Infection
ADULTS: **IV/IM** Up to 12 g/day in divided doses (from q 4 hr for septicemia to q 12 hr for uncomplicated infection) usually for 7 to 10 days. IV route is preferable for severe infections.
CHILDREN 1 MO TO 12 YR: **IV/IM** 50 to 180 mg/kg/day in 4 to 6 divided doses.
INFANTS 1 TO 4 WK: **IV** 50 mg/kg q 8 hr.
NEWBORNS UNDER 1 WK: **IV** 50 mg/kg q 12 hr.

Gonorrhea
ADULTS: **IM** 1 g as single dose.

Perioperative Prophylaxis
ADULTS: **IV/IM** 1 g 30 to 90 min prior to surgery.

Cesarean Section
ADULTS: **IV** 1 g as soon as umbilical cord is clamped; second and third dose IV/IM at 6- and 12-hr intervals after first dose.

Interactions
Aminoglycosides: Increased risk of nephrotoxicity.
INCOMPATIBILITIES: Do not add aminoglycosides to cefotaxime solutions because inactivation of both drugs may result; administer at separate sites if concurrent therapy is indicated.

Lab Test Interferences May cause false-positive urine glucose test results with *Benedict's* solution, *Fehling's* solution or *Clinitest* tablets but not with enzyme-based tests (eg, *Clinistix*, *Testape*); false-positive test result for proteinuria with acid and denaturization-precipitation tests; false-positive direct *Coombs'* test results in certain patients (eg, those with azotemia); false elevations in urinary 17-ketosteroid values.

Adverse Reactions
CNS: Headache; dizziness; fatigue; paresthesia; confusion; nervousness; sleeplessness.
GI: Nausea; vomiting; diarrhea; anorexia; abdominal pain or cramps; flatulence; colitis, including pseudomembranous colitis.
GU: Pyuria; renal dysfunction; transient elevations in BUN and creatinine; dysuria; reversible interstitial nephritis; hematuria; toxic nephropathy.
HEMA: Eosinophilia; neutropenia; lymphocytosis; leukocytosis; thrombocytopenia; decreased platelet function; anemia; aplastic anemia; hemorrhage.
HEPA: Hepatic dysfunction; abnormal LFT results.
OTHER: Hypersensitivity, including Stevens-Johnson syndrome, erythema multiforme, pruritus, fever, toxic epidermal necrolysis; candidal overgrowth; serum sickness-like reactions (eg, skin rashes, polyarthritis, arthralgia, fever); phlebitis, thrombophlebitis, and pain at injection site.

Precautions
Pregnancy: Category B.
Lactation: Excreted in breast milk.
Children: Cephalosporins may accumulate in newborns.
Hypersensitivity: Reactions range from mild to life-threatening. Administer drug with caution to penicillin-sensitive patients because of possible cross-reactivity.

Renal function impairment: Use drug with caution in patients with renal impairment. Dosage adjustment based on renal function may be required.

Hepatic function impairment: Use drug with caution in patients with hepatic impairment. Dosage adjustment based on hepatic function may be required.

PATIENT CARE CONSIDERATIONS
Administration/Storage
- Reconstituted solution should be light yellow to amber. Do not administer if solution is cloudy or precipitate is present.
- When giving by IM route, inject deeply into large muscle (eg, upper outer quadrant of gluteus muscle or lateral thigh). Massage well.
- Divide IM 2 g dose and administer in 2 separate sites.
- When giving by IV route, administer slowly over 3 to 5 min. Reconstituted drug may be diluted in 50 to 100 mL D5W or 0.9% Sodium Chloride Injection and infused over 20 to 30 min. Change IV sites q 48 to 72 hr.
- For perioperative surgical prophylaxis, administer cefotaxime 30 to 90 min before surgical incision.
- Store sterile powder at room temperature and protect from light.
- Reconstituted solutions are stable at room temperature for 24 hr.

Assessment/Interventions
- Obtain patient history, including drug history and any known allergies. Note allergy to cephalosporins or penicillins.
- Obtain specimens for culture and sensitivity before beginning therapy and periodically during treatment. Repeat cultures are indicated if resistance is suspected.
- Monitor renal function carefully during treatment.
- Monitor for signs of infection, especially fever, and for positive response to antibiotic therapy.
- Assess for signs and symptoms of anaphylaxis (eg, shortness of breath, wheezing, laryngeal spasm). Have resuscitation equipment available.

Superinfection: May result in bacterial or fungal overgrowth of nonsusceptible microorganisms.
Pseudomembranous colitis: Consider in patients in whom diarrhea develops.

Overdosage: Signs and Symptoms
Seizures, acute renal failure, acidosis, hypernatremia.

- Assess for signs of superinfection, such as vaginitis or stomatitis.
- Assess for severe diarrhea with blood or pus, which may be a symptom of pseudomembranous colitis. Symptoms may occur after antibiotic treatment.
- Monitor IV site for infiltration, infection, and thrombophlebitis.

Patient/Family Education
- Instruct patient to check body temperature daily. If fever persists for more than a few days or if high fever (greater than 102°F) or shaking chills are noted, notify health care provider immediately.
- Advise patient to maintain normal fluid intake while using this medication.
- Advise diabetic patient to use enzyme-based tests (eg, *Clinistix* , *Tes-tape*) for monitoring urine glucose because drug may give false results with other tests.
- Instruct patient to report these symptoms to health care provider: nausea, vomiting, diarrhea, skin rash, hives, sore throat, bruising, bleeding, muscle or joint pain.
- Warn patient that diarrhea that contains blood or pus may be a sign of serious disorders. Tell patient to seek medical care and not to treat at home.
- Instruct patient to seek emergency care if wheezing or difficulty in breathing occurs.
- Instruct patient to report signs of superinfection: black "furry" tongue, white patches in mouth, foul-smelling stools, vaginal itching or discharge.

Cefotetan Disodium

(SEFF-oh-tee-tan die-SO-dee-uhm)

Class Antibiotic/Cephalosporin

How Supplied
Cefotan Powder for Injection 1 g (3.5 mEq sodium/g), Powder for Injection 2 g (3.5 mEq sodium/g), Powder for Injection 10 g (3.5 mEq sodium/g), Injection 1 g/50 mL, Injection 2 g/50 mL

Action
PHARMACOLOGY: Inhibits mucopeptide synthesis in bacterial cell wall.

PHARMACOKINETICS/DYNAMICS:
Distribution: Cefotetan is 88% protein bound.

Metabolism: No active metabolites are detected; however, less than 7% may be converted to the tautomer (active).

Excretion: The $t_{1/2}$ is 3 to 4.6 hr; 51% to 81% is excreted unchanged by the kidneys in 24 hr.

Special Populations:
Renal Function Impairment – The t½ is prolonged. Dosage adjustment is recommended.

Indications Treatment of infections of urinary tract, lower respiratory tract, skin and skin structures, bone and joint; treatment of gynecological infections; treatment of intra-abdominal infections caused by susceptible strains of specific microorganisms; perioperative prophylaxis.
Concomitant antibiotic therapy: If cefotetan and an aminoglycoside are to be used concomitantly, carefully monitor renal function, especially if higher dosages of the aminoglycoside are to be administered or if therapy is to be prolonged, because of the potential nephrotoxicity and ototoxicity of aminoglycosides.

Contraindications Hypersensitivity to cephalosporins.

Route/Dosage
Infection
ADULTS: **IV/IM** 1 to 2 g q 12 hr (life-threatening infections: up to 3 g q 12 hr) for 7 to 10 days.

Urinary Tract Infection
ADULTS: **IV/IM** 500 mg q 12 hr, 1 or 2 g q 24 hr, 1 or 2 g ever 12 hr.

Perioperative Prophylaxis
ADULTS: **IV** 1 to 2 g 30 to 60 min prior to surgery. In Cesarean section, give dose as soon as umbilical cord is clamped.

Interactions
Alcohol: Acute alcohol intolerance (disulfiram-like reaction) may occur up to 3 days after last dose of cefotetan.
Aminoglycosides: Increased risk of nephrotoxicity.
Anticoagulants, oral: Increased anticoagulant effect; bleeding complications may occur.
INCOMPATIBILITIES:
Aminoglycosides: Do not add aminoglycosides to cefotetan solutions because inactivation of both drugs may result; administer at separate sites if concurrent therapy is indicated.

Lab Test Interferences May cause false-positive urine glucose test results with *Benedict's* solution, *Fehling's* solution, or *Clinitest* tablets but not with enzyme-based tests (eg, *Clinistix*, *Tes-tape*); false-positive test result for proteinuria with acid and denaturization-precipitation tests; false-positive direct *Coombs'* test results in certain patients (eg, those with azotemia); false elevations in urinary 17-ketosteroid values. High concentrations may interfere with creatinine concentrations measured by the Jaffe reaction, producing false results; do not analyze serum samples for creatinine if obtained within 2 hr of drug administration.

Adverse Reactions
GI: Nausea; vomiting; diarrhea; anorexia; abdominal pain or cramps; flatulence; colitis, including pseudomembranous colitis.
GU: Pyuria; renal dysfunction; dysuria; reversible interstitial nephritis; hematuria; toxic nephropathy.
HEMA: Eosinophilia; neutropenia; lymphocytosis; leukocytosis; thrombocytopenia; decreased platelet function; anemia; aplastic anemia; hemorrhage.
HEPA: Hepatic dysfunction; abnormal LFT results.
OTHER: Hypersensitivity, including Stevens-Johnson syndrome, erythema multiforme, toxic epidermal necrolysis; candidal overgrowth; serum sickness–like reactions (eg, skin rashes, polyarthritis; arthralgia, fever); phlebitis, thrombophlebitis, and pain at injection site.

Precautions
Pregnancy: Category B.
Lactation: Excreted in breast milk.
Children: Safety and efficacy in children not established.
Hypersensitivity: Reactions range from mild to life-threatening. Administer drug with caution to penicillin-sensitive patients because of possible cross-reactivity.
Renal function impairment: Use drug with caution in patients with renal impairment. Dosage adjustment based on renal function may be required.
Superinfection: May result in bacterial or fungal overgrowth of nonsusceptible microorganisms.
Pseudomembranous colitis: Consider in patients who develop diarrhea.

Overdosage: Signs and Symptoms
Seizures.

PATIENT CARE CONSIDERATIONS
Administration/Storage
- Reconstituted solution may be light yellow to amber. Do not administer if solution is cloudy or precipitate is present.
- For IM injection, drug may be reconstituted with 0.5% or 1% lidocaine without epinephrine to minimize pain on injection.
- When giving by IM route, inject deeply into large muscle (eg, upper outer quadrant of gluteus muscle or lateral thigh). Massage well.
- When giving by IV route, administer slowly over 3 to 5 min. Reconstituted drug may be diluted in 50 to 100 mL of D5W or 0.9% sodium chloride and infused over 20 to 30 min. Change IV sites q 48 to 72 hr.

- For perioperative prophylaxis, administer cefotetan 50 to 120 min before surgical incision.
- Store sterile powder at room temperature and protect from light.

Assessment/Interventions
- Obtain patient history, including drug history and any known allergies. Note allergy to cephalosporins or penicillins.
- Obtain specimens for culture and sensitivity before beginning therapy and periodically during treatment.
- Monitor renal function carefully during treatment.
- This is particularly important if cefotetan is administered concomitantly with an aminoglycoside because of potential nephrotoxicity and ototoxicity.
- Monitor for coagulation abnormalities. Elevate prothrombin time or abnormal platelet count may occur. If bleeding occurs and PT is prolonged, vitamin K may be indicated.
- Monitor for signs of infection, especially fever, and for positive response to antibiotic therapy.
- Assess for signs and symptoms of anaphylaxis (eg, shortness of breath, wheezing, laryngeal spasm). Have resuscitation equipment available.
- Assess for signs of superinfection, such as vaginitis or stomatitis.
- Assess for diarrhea with blood or pus, which may be a symptom of pseudomembranous colitis. Symptoms may occur after antibiotic treatment.
- Monitor IV site for infiltration, infection, and thrombophlebitis.

Patient/Family Education
- Instruct patient to check body temperature daily. If fever persists for more than a few days or if high fever (greater than 102°F) or shaking chills are noted, notify health care provider immediately.
- Advise patient to maintain normal fluid intake while using this medication.
- Advise patient not to drink alcoholic beverages or take alcohol-containing medications while taking cefamandole nafate and for several days after discontinuing drug.
- Advise diabetic patient to use enzyme-based tests (eg, *Clinistix*, *Testape*) for monitoring urine glucose because drug may give false results with other tests.
- Instruct patient to report these symptoms to health care provider: nausea, vomiting, diarrhea, skin rash, hives, sore throat, bruising, bleeding, muscle or joint pain.
- Warn patient that diarrhea that contains blood or pus may be a sign of serious disorders. Tell patient to seek medical care and not to treat at home.
- Instruct patient to seek emergency care if wheezing or difficulty in breathing occurs.
- Instruct patient to report signs of superinfection: black "furry" tongue, white patches in mouth, foul-smelling stools, vaginal itching or discharge.

Cefoxitin Sodium

(seff-OX-ih-tin SO-dee-uhm)

Class Antibiotic/Cephalosporin

How Supplied
Mefoxin Powder for Injection 1 g (2.3 mEq sodium/g), Powder for Injection 2 g (2.3 mEq sodium/g), Powder for Injection 10 g (2.3 mEq sodium/g), Injection 1 g, Injection 2 g

Action
PHARMACOLOGY: Inhibits mucopeptide synthesis in bacterial cell wall.

PHARMACOKINETICS/DYNAMICS:
Absorption:
IV – C_{max} is 110 mcg/mL (1 g dose). T_{max} is 5 min.

Distribution: Passes into pleural and joint fluids and is detectable in antibacterial concentrations in the bile. Excreted in human milk (low concentrations).

Excretion: The t½ is 41 to 59 min (IV). About 85% is excreted unchanged by the kidneys in 6 hr.

Special Populations:
Renal Function Impairment – The t½ is increased. Dosage adjustment is recommended.

Indications Treatment of infections of lower respiratory tract, urinary tract, skin and skin structures, bone and joint; treatment of intraabdominal infections, gynecological infections, and septicemia caused by susceptible microorganisms; perioperative prophylaxis. Many infections caused by gram-negative bacteria resistant to some cephalosporins and penicillins respond to cefoxitin.

Contraindications Hypersensitivity to cephalosporins.

Route/Dosage
Infection
ADULTS: **IV/IM** 1 to 2 g q 6 to 8 hr.
CHILDREN 3 MO AND OVER: **IV/IM** 80 to 160 mg/kg/day in divided doses q 4 to 6 hr (max, 12 g/day).

Surgical Prophylaxis
ADULTS: **IV/IM** 2 g just prior to surgery, then 2 g q 6 hr for 24 hr.

CHILDREN 3 MO AND OVER: **IV/IM** 30 to 40 mg/kg just prior to surgery, then 30 to 40 mg/kg q 6 hr for 24 hr.

Interactions
Aminoglycosides: May increase risk of nephrotoxicity.
Probenecid: Inhibition of renal excretion of cefoxitin.
INCOMPATIBILITIES:
Aminoglycosides: Do not add aminoglycosides to cefoxitin solutions because inactivation of both drugs may result; administer at separate sites if concurrent therapy is indicated.

Lab Test Interferences
May cause false-positive urine glucose test results with *Benedict's* solution, *Fehling's* solution, or *Clinitest* tablets but not with enzyme-based tests (eg, *Clinistix, Tes-tape*); false-positive test result for proteinuria with acid and denaturization-precipitation tests; false-positive direct *Coombs'* test result in certain patients (eg, those with azotemia); false elevations in urinary 17-ketosteroid values. High concentrations may interfere with creatinine concentrations measured by the Jaffe reaction, producing false results; do not analyze serum samples for creatinine if obtained within 2 hr of drug administration.

Adverse Reactions
CV: Hypotension.
GI: Nausea; vomiting; diarrhea; colitis, including pseudomembranous colitis.
GU: Renal dysfunction; elevated renal function tests; pyuria; dysuria; reversible interstitial nephritis; hematuria; toxic nephropathy.
HEMA: Eosinophilia; neutropenia; lymphocytosis; leukocytosis; thrombocytopenia; decreased platelet function; anemia; hemolytic anemia; aplastic anemia; hemorrhage.
HEPA: Hepatic dysfunction; jaundice; abnormal LFT results.
OTHER: Hypersensitivity, including Stevens-Johnson syndrome, erythema multiforme, toxic epidermal necrolysis; candidal overgrowth; serum sickness–like reactions (eg, skin rashes, polyarthritis; arthralgia, fever); phlebitis, thrombophlebitis, and pain at injection site.

Precautions
Pregnancy: Category B.
Lactation: Excreted in breast milk.
Children: In children 3 mo and over, high doses of cefoxitin have been associated with increased incidence of eosinophilia and elevated AST.
Hypersensitivity: Reactions range from mild to life-threatening. Administer drug with caution to penicillin-sensitive patients because of possible cross-reactivity.
Renal function impairment: Use drug with caution. Dosage adjustment based on renal function may be required.
Superinfection: May result in bacterial or fungal overgrowth of nonsusceptible microorganisms.
Pseudomembranous colitis: Consider in patients in whom diarrhea develops.

Overdosage: Signs and Symptoms
Seizures.

PATIENT CARE CONSIDERATIONS
Administration/Storage
- For IM administration reconstitute each gram with 2 mL of Sterile Water for Injection or 2 mL of 0.5% lidocaine without epinephrine to minimize discomfort. Inject deeply into large muscle (eg, gluteus or lateral thigh).
- For IV use, reconstitute each gram with 10 mL of Sterile Water for Injection. Administer slowly over 3 to 5 min. Reconstituted drug may be diluted in 50 to 100 mL of 0.9% Sodium Chloride or D5W and infused over 30 min.
- Change IV sites q 48 to 72 hr.
- Solutions are stable for 24 hr at room temperature and for 1 wk if refrigerated.
- May freeze medication. Thaw at room temperature. After thawing, discard unused portion. Do not refreeze. Do not administer if solution is cloudy or precipitate is present.

Assessment/Interventions
- Obtain patient history, including drug history and any known allergies. Note allergy to cephalosporins and penicillins.
- Obtain specimens for culture and sensitivity before beginning therapy and periodically during treatment.
- Monitor renal function carefully during treatment.
- Monitor for signs of infection, especially fever, and for positive response to antibiotic therapy.
- Monitor for coagulation abnormalities. Elevated prothrombin time or abnormal platelet count may occur. If bleeding occurs and PT is prolonged, vitamin K may be indicated.
- Assess for signs and symptoms of anaphylaxis (eg, shortness of breath, wheezing, laryngeal spasm). Have resuscitation equipment available.
- Assess for signs of superinfection, such as vaginitis or stomatitis.
- Assess for diarrhea with blood or pus, which may be symptom of pseudomembranous colitis. Symptoms may occur after antibiotic treatment.
- Monitor IV site for vein irritation, infiltration, infection and thrombophlebitis.

Patient/Family Education
- Instruct patient to check body temperature daily. If fever persists for more than a few days or if high fever (greater than 102°F) or shaking chills are noted, notify health care provider immediately.
- Advise patient to maintain normal fluid intake while using this medication.
- Advise diabetic patient to use enzyme-based tests (eg, *Clinistix*, *Testape*) for monitoring urine glucose because drug may give false results with other tests.
- Warn patient to report these symptoms to health care provider: nausea, vomiting, diarrhea, skin rash, hives, sore throat, bruising, bleeding, muscle or joint pain.
- Instruct patient to report signs of superinfection: black "furry" tongue, white patches in mouth, foul-smelling stools, vaginal itching or discharge.
- Warn patient that diarrhea that contains blood or pus may be a sign of serious disorders. Tell patient to seek medical care and not to treat at home.
- Instruct patient to seek emergency care if he or she experiences wheezing or difficulty breathing.

Cefpodoxime Proxetil

(SEF-pode-OX-eem PROX-uh-til)

Class Antibiotic/Cephalosporin

How Supplied
Vantin Tablets 100 mg, Tablets 200 mg, Granules for Suspension 50 mg/5 mL, Granules for Suspension 100 mg/5 mL

Action
PHARMACOLOGY: Inhibits mucopeptide synthesis in bacterial cell wall.

PHARMACOKINETICS/DYNAMICS:
Absorption: About 50% absorbed.
Tablets – C_{max} is 1.4 to 3.9 mcg/mL (100 to 400 mg dose). T_{max} is about 2 to 3 hr.
Suspension – C_{max} is about 1.5 mcg/mL (100 mg dose).
Food – AUC and C_{max} are increased when tablets are taken with food. T_{max} is increased 48% when suspension is taken with food.

Distribution: 21% to 29% plasma protein bound.

Metabolism: Cefpodoxime proxetil is a prodrug and de-esterified to cefpodoxime (active).

Excretion: About 29% to 33% of the absorbed dose is excreted unchanged in the urine in 12 hr. The t½ is 2.09 to 2.84 hr.

Special Populations:
Renal Function Impairment – Elimination is reduced in those with Ccr less than 50 mL/min. Dosage adjustment is recommended.
Elderly – The t½ is increased to about 4.2 hr. Dosage adjustment is recommended in those with diminished renal function.

Indications
Treatment of infections of respiratory tract, urinary tract, skin and skin structures; treatment of sexually transmitted diseases caused by susceptible strains of specific microorganisms.

Contraindications
Hypersensitivity to cephalosporins.

Route/Dosage
ADULTS: **PO** 100 to 400 mg q 12 hr.
CHILDREN 6 MO TO 12 YR: **PO** 10 mg/kg/day in divided doses q 12 hr (max 200 mg/dose).

Interactions
Probenecid: Inhibition of renal excretion of cefpodoxime.

Lab Test Interferences
May cause false-positive urine glucose test results with *Benedict's* solution, *Fehling's* solution, or *Clinitest* tablets but not with enzyme-based tests (eg, *Clinistix*, *Tes-tape*); false-positive test results for proteinuria with acid and denaturization-precipitation tests; false-positive direct *Coombs'* test result in certain patients (eg, those with azotemia); false elevations in urinary 17-ketosteroid values.

Adverse Reactions
GI: Nausea; vomiting; diarrhea; anorexia; abdominal pain or cramps; flatulence; colitis, including pseudomembranous colitis.
GU: Pyuria; renal dysfunction; dysuria; reversible interstitial nephritis; hematuria; toxic nephropathy.
HEMA: Eosinophilia; neutropenia; lymphocytosis; leukocytosis; thrombocytopenia; decreased platelet function; anemia; aplastic anemia; hemorrhage.
HEPA: Hepatic dysfunction; abnormal LFT results.
OTHER: Hypersensitivity, including Stevens-Johnson syndrome, erythema multiforme, toxic epidermal necrolysis; serum sickness–like reactions (eg, skin rashes, polyarthritis, arthralgia, fever); candidal overgrowth.

Precautions
Pregnancy: Category B.
Lactation: Excreted in breast milk.
Children: Consider benefits relative to risks. Safety and efficacy in children under 6 mo not established.
Hypersensitivity: Reactions range from mild to life-threatening. Administer drug with caution

to penicillin-sensitive patients because of possible cross-reactivity.
Renal function impairment: Use drug with caution in patients with renal impairment. Dosage adjustment based on renal function may be required.
Superinfection: May result in bacterial or fungal overgrowth of nonsusceptible microorganisms.
Pseudomembranous colitis: Consider in patients in whom diarrhea develops.

Overdosage: Signs and Symptoms
Seizures.

PATIENT CARE CONSIDERATIONS
Administration/Storage
- Administer with food to enhance absorption.
- Oral suspension must be refrigerated and will remain stable for up to 14 days. Do not freeze. Shake well before use.

Assessment/Interventions
- Obtain patient history, including drug history and any known allergies. Note renal impairment and allergy to cephalosporins or penicillins.
- Obtain specimens for culture and sensitivity before beginning therapy and periodically during treatment.
- Monitor renal function carefully during treatment.
- Monitor for signs of infection, especially fever, and for positive response to antibiotic therapy.
- Assess for signs and symptoms of anaphylaxis (eg, shortness of breath, wheezing, laryngeal spasm). Have resuscitation equipment available.
- Assess patient for symptoms of superinfection, vaginitis or stomatitis.
- Assess for diarrhea with blood or pus, which may be a symptom of pseudomembranous colitis. Symptoms may occur after antibiotic treatment.

Patient/Family Education
- Instruct patient to complete full course of therapy.
- Advise patient to take with food to enhance absorption.
- Remind patient to check body temperature daily. If fever persists for more than a few days or if high fever (greater than 102°F) or shaking chills are noted, notify health care provider immediately.
- Advise patient to maintain normal fluid intake while using this medication.
- Advise diabetic patient to use enzyme-based tests (eg, *Clinistix* , *Testape*) for monitoring urine glucose because drug may give false results with other tests.
- Instruct patient to report these symptoms to health care provider: nausea, vomiting, diarrhea, skin rash, hives, muscle or joint pain.
- Instruct patient to report signs of superinfection: black "furry" tongue, white patches in mouth, foul-smelling stools, vaginal itching or discharge.
- Warn patient that diarrhea that contains blood or pus may be a sign of serious disorders. Tell patient to seek medical care and not to treat at home.
- Instruct patient to seek emergency care immediately if wheezing or difficulty breathing occurs.

Cefprozil

(SEFF-pro-zill)

Class Antibiotic/Cephalosporin

How Supplied
Cefzil Tablets 250 mg (as anhydrous), Tablets 500 mg (as anhydrous), Powder for Oral Suspension 125 mg/5 mL (as anhydrous). Contains sucrose, aspartame, 28 mg/5 mL phenylalanine, Powder for Oral Suspension 250 mg/5 mL (as anhydrous). Contains sucrose, aspartame, 28 mg/5 mL phenylalanine

Action
PHARMACOLOGY: Inhibits mucopeptide synthesis in bacterial cell wall.

PHARMACOKINETICS/DYNAMICS:
Absorption: Cefprozil is about 95% absorbed. Food increased T_{max} 0.25 to 0.75 hr. T_{max} is about 1.5 hr. C_{max} is 18.3 mcg/mL.

Distribution: Vd is about 0.23 L/kg. Cefprozil is about 36% protein bound.

Excretion: Plasma $t_{½}$ is 1.3 hr. Total body Cl is about 3 mL/min/kg. Renal Cl is about 2.3 mL/min/kg. The 8-hr urinary excretion accounted for 54% to 62% of the dose.

Special Populations:
Renal Function Impairment – The $t_{½}$ may be up to 5.2 hr.
Hepatic Function Impairment – The $t_{½}$ increases to about 2 hr.
Elderly – AUC is about 35% to 60% higher.

Indications Treatment of infections of skin and skin structures, bronchitis, pharyngitis, tonsillitis, and otitis media caused by susceptible strains of specific microorganisms.

Contraindications Hypersensitivity to cephalosporins.

Route/Dosage
ADULTS: PO 250 to 500 mg q 12 to 24 hr.
CHILDREN 6 MO TO 12 YR: PO 7.5 to 15 mg/kg q 12 hr.

Interactions
Probenecid: Inhibition of renal excretion of cefprozil.

Lab Test Interferences May cause false-positive urine glucose test results with *Benedict's* solution, *Fehling's* solution, or *Clinitest* tablets but not with enzyme-based tests (eg, *Clinistix*, *Tes-tape*); false-positive test results for proteinuria with acid and denaturization-precipitation tests; false-positive direct *Coombs'* test result in certain patients (eg, those with azotemia); false elevations in urinary 17-ketosteroid values.

Adverse Reactions
CNS: Headache; dizziness; fatigue; paresthesia; confusion; nervousness; sleeplessness; insomnia.
GI: Nausea; vomiting; diarrhea; abdominal pain or cramps; flatulence; colitis, including pseudomembranous colitis.
GU: Genital pruritus; vaginitis; renal dysfunction.
HEMA: Eosinophilia; neutropenia; lymphocytosis; leukocytosis; thrombocytopenia; decreased platelet function; anemia; aplastic anemia; hemorrhage.
HEPA: Hepatic dysfunction; cholestatic jaundice; abnormal LFT results.
OTHER: Hypersensitivity, including Stevens-Johnson syndrome, erythema multiforme, toxic epidermal necrolysis; candidal overgrowth; serum sickness–like reactions (eg, skin rashes, polyarthritis, arthralgia, fever).

Precautions
Pregnancy: Category B.
Lactation: Excreted in breast milk.
Children: Safety and efficacy in children under 6 mo not established.
Hypersensitivity: Reactions range from mild to life-threatening. Administer drug with caution to penicillin-sensitive patients because of possible cross-reactivity.
Renal function impairment: Use drug with caution in patients with renal impairment. Dosage adjustment based on renal function may be required.
Superinfection: May result in bacterial or fungal overgrowth of nonsusceptible microorganisms.
Pseudomembranous colitis: Consider in patients in whom diarrhea develops.

Overdosage: Signs and Symptoms
Seizures.

PATIENT CARE CONSIDERATIONS

Administration/Storage
- May be given without regard to meals. Administer with food or milk if GI upset occurs. Food slows but does not decrease absorption.
- Administer after hemodialysis because drug is partially removed by dialysis.
- After reconstitution, oral suspension must be refrigerated. Solution may be stored for up to 14 days in refrigerator. Do not freeze. Shake well before use.
- Store tablets at room temperature.

Assessment/Interventions
- Obtain patient history, including drug history and any known allergies. Note renal or hepatic impairment and allergy to cephalosporins or penicillins.
- Obtain specimens for culture and sensitivity before beginning therapy and periodically during treatment.
- Monitor renal function carefully during treatment.
- Monitor for signs of infection, especially fever, and for positive response to antibiotic therapy.
- Assess for signs and symptoms of anaphylaxis (eg, shortness of breath, wheezing, laryngeal spasm). Have resuscitation equipment available.
- Assess for signs of superinfection, such as vaginitis or stomatitis.
- Assess for severe diarrhea with blood or pus, which may be symptom of pseudomembranous colitis. Symptoms may occur after antibiotic treatment.

Patient/Family Education
- Instruct patient to complete full course of therapy.
- Remind patient to check body temperature daily. If fever persists for more than a few days or if high fever (greater than 102°F) or shaking chills are noted, notify health care provider immediately.
- Advise patient to maintain normal fluid intake while using this medication.
- Remind diabetic patient to use enzyme-based tests (eg, *Clinistix*, *Testape*) for monitoring urine glucose because drug may give false results with other tests.
- Advise patient to report these symptoms to health care provider: nausea, vomiting, diarrhea, skin rash, hives, muscle or joint pain.
- Instruct patient to report signs of superinfection: black "furry" tongue, white patches in mouth, foul-smelling stools, vaginal itching or discharge.
- Warn patient that diarrhea that contains

blood or pus may be a sign of serious disorders. Tell patient to seek medical care and not to treat at home.
- Instruct patient to seek emergency care immediately if he or she experiences wheezing or difficulty breathing.
- Caution patient to avoid alcohol intake while taking medication.

Ceftazidime

(seff-TAZE-ih-deem)
Class Antibiotic/Cephalosporin

How Supplied
Ceptaz Powder for Injection 1 g (as pentahydrate w/ L-arginine), Powder for Injection 2 g (as pentahydrate w/ L-arginine) ♦ *Fortaz* Powder for Injection 500 mg (2.3 mEq sodium/g), Powder for Injection 1 g (2.3 mEq sodium/g), Powder for Injection 2 g (2.3 mEq sodium/g), Powder for Injection 6 g (2.3 mEq sodium/g), Injection 1 g with 2.2 g dextrose hydrous, Injection 2 g with 1.6 g dextrose hydrous ♦ *Tazicef* Powder for Injection 1 g (2.3 mEq sodium/g), Powder for Injection 2 g (2.3 mEq sodium/g), Powder for Injection 6 g (2.3 mEq sodium/g), Injection 1 g, Injection 2 g ♦ *Tazidime* Powder for Injection 500 mg (as pentahydrate w/ L-arginine), Powder for Injection 1 g (as pentahydrate w/ L-arginine), Powder for Injection 2 g (as pentahydrate w/ L-arginine), Powder for Injection 6 g (as pentahydrate w/ L-arginine)

Action
PHARMACOLOGY: Inhibits mucopeptide synthesis in bacterial cell wall.

PHARMACOKINETICS/DYNAMICS:
Absorption:
IV – C_{max} is 45 to 90 mcg/mL (500 mg and 1 g doses).
IM – C_{max} is 17 to 39 mcg/mL (500 mg and 1 g doses). T_{max} is about 1 hr.
Distribution: Ceftazidime is less than 10% protein bound. It is excreted in human milk in low concentrations.

Excretion: The t½ is about 1.9 to 2 hr. About 80% to 90% is excreted unchanged by the kidneys. Renal Cl is about 100 mL/min. Plasma Cl is about 115 mL/min.

Special Populations:
Renal Function Impairment – The t½ is significantly prolonged. Dosage adjustments are recommended.

Indications
Treatment of infections of lower respiratory tract, skin and skin structures, urinary tract, bone and joint; treatment of gynecological infections; treatment of intra-abdominal infections; treatment of septicemia and CNS infections including meningitis caused by susceptible strains of specific microorganisms; concomitant antibiotic therapy.

Contraindications
Hypersensitivity to cephalosporins.

Route/Dosage
ADULTS: **IV/IM** 250 mg to 2 g q 8 to 12 hr.
CHILDREN 1 MO TO 12 YR: **IV** 30 to 50 mg/kg q 8 hr (max, 6 g/day).
NEWBORNS UNDER 4 WK: **IV** 30 mg/kg q 12 hr.

Interactions
Aminoglycosides: Increased risk of nephrotoxicity.
INCOMPATIBILITIES:
Aminoglycosides: Do not add aminoglycosides to ceftazidime solutions because inactivation of both drugs may result; administer at separate sites if concurrent therapy is indicated.
Sodium bicarbonate: Do not dilute ceftazidime with sodium bicarbonate.

Lab Test Interferences
May cause false-positive urine glucose test results with *Benedict's* solution, *Fehling's* solution, or *Clinitest* tablets but not with enzyme-based tests (eg, *Clinistix*, *Tes-Tape*); false-positive test results for proteinuria with acid and denaturization-precipitation tests; false-positive direct *Coombs'* test result in certain patients (eg, those with azotemia); false elevations in urinary 17-ketosteroid values.

Adverse Reactions
GI: Nausea; vomiting; diarrhea; anorexia; abdominal pain or cramps; flatulence; colitis, including pseudomembranous colitis.
GU: Pyuria; renal dysfunction; dysuria; reversible interstitial nephritis; hematuria; toxic nephropathy.
HEMA: Eosinophilia; neutropenia; lymphocytosis; leukocytosis; thrombocytopenia; thrombocytosis; decreased platelet function; anemia; aplastic anemia; hemorrhage.
HEPA: Hepatic dysfunction; cholestatic jaundice; abnormal LFT results.
OTHER: Hypersensitivity, including Stevens-Johnson syndrome, erythema multiforme, toxic epidermal necrolysis; candidal overgrowth; serum sickness–like reactions (eg, skin rashes, polyarthritis, arthralgia, fever); phlebitis; thrombophlebitis, and pain at injection site.

Precautions
Pregnancy: Category B.
Lactation: Excreted in breast milk.
Hypersensitivity: Reactions range from mild to life-threatening. Administer drug with caution to penicillin-sensitive patients because of possible cross-reactivity.

Renal function impairment: Use drug with caution in patients with renal impairment. Dosage adjustment based on renal function may be required.

Superinfection: May result in bacterial or fungal overgrowth of nonsusceptible microorganisms.

Pseudomembranous colitis: Consider in patients in whom diarrhea develops.

Overdosage: Signs and Symptoms

Neuromuscular excitability, asterixis, seizures, encephalopathy.

PATIENT CARE CONSIDERATIONS

Administration/Storage

- Administer by parenteral route (IV or IM) only.
- Follow manufacturer's instructions for reconstitution and dilution.
- Reconstituted solution should be light yellow to amber; darkened solution or powder does not indicate altered potency. Do not administer if solution is cloudy or precipitate is present.
- When giving by IM route, add 3 mL diluent to 1 g vial to yield 280 mg/mL. Inject deeply into large muscle (eg, upper outer quadrant of gluteus muscle or lateral thigh); massage well.
- When giving by IV route, add 10 mL Sterile Water for Injection to 1 g vial to yield 280 mg/mL. Administer slowly over 3 to 5 min. Change IV sites q 48 to 72 hr.
- For intermittent infusions, reconstituted solution can be further diluted with 50 to 100 mL of D5W or 0.9% Sodium Chloride and infused over 30 min.
- Store sterile powder at room temperature and protect from light.
- When reconstituted with Sterile Water for Injection, solution is stable for 7 days if refrigerated and for 18 to 24 hr when stored at room temperature. If frozen immediately after reconstitution, solution is stable for 3 mo. Completely thaw frozen preparation at room temperature before use. After thawing, solution may be stored for 18 to 24 hr at room temperature or 4 days in refrigerator. Do not refreeze.

Assessment/Interventions

- Obtain patient history, including drug history and any known allergies. Note renal impairment and allergy to cephalosporins or penicillins.
- Obtain specimens for culture and sensitivity before beginning therapy and periodically during treatment.
- Monitor renal function carefully during treatment.
- Monitor for signs of infection, especially fever, and for positive response to antibiotic therapy.
- Assess for signs and symptoms of anaphylaxis (eg, shortness of breath, wheezing, laryngeal spasm). Have resuscitation equipment available.
- Assess for signs of superinfection, such as vaginitis or stomatitis.
- Assess for diarrhea with blood or pus, which may be a symptom of pseudomembranous colitis. Symptoms may occur after antibiotic treatment.
- Monitor IV site for infiltration, infection, thrombophlebitis, and bleeding.

Patient/Family Education

- Remind patient to check body temperature daily. If fever persists for more than a few days or if high fever (greater than 102°F) or shaking chills are noted, notify health care provider immediately.
- Advise patient to maintain normal fluid intake while using this medication.
- Remind diabetic patient to use enzyme-based tests (eg, *Clinistix*, *Tes-Tape*) for monitoring urine glucose because drug may give false results with other tests.
- Advise patient to report these symptoms to health care provider: nausea, vomiting, diarrhea, skin rash, hives, sore throat, bruising, bleeding, muscle or joint pain.
- Instruct patient to report signs of superinfection: black "furry" tongue, white patches in mouth, foul-smelling stools, vaginal itching or discharge.
- Warn patient that diarrhea that contains blood or pus may be a sign of serious disorders. Tell patient to seek medical care and not to treat at home.
- Instruct patient to seek emergency care immediately if wheezing or difficulty breathing occurs.
- Advise patient not to drink alcoholic beverages or to take alcohol-containing medications while taking this medication and for several days after discontinuing it.

Ceftibuten

(seff-TIE-byoo-ten)

Class Antibiotic/Cephalosporin

How Supplied
Cedax Capsules 400 mg, Powder for Oral Suspension 90 mg/5 mL, Powder for Oral Suspension 180 mg/5 mL

Action
PHARMACOLOGY: Inhibits mucopeptide synthesis in bacterial cell wall.

PHARMACOKINETICS/DYNAMICS:
Absorption:
Capsules – C_{max} is 17.9 mcg/mL.
Suspension – C_{max} is about 15 mcg/mL. T_{max} is about 2.6 hr. AUC is about 73.7 mcg•hr/mL.
Food –
Capsules: T_{max} is increased 1.75 hr. C_{max} is decreased 18%. AUC is decreased 8%.
Suspension: C_{max} is decreased 17% to 26%. AUC is decreased 12% to 17%. Take on an empty stomach.

Distribution: Vd is about 0.21 L/kg (capsules) and 0.5 L/kg (suspension).

Excretion: The t½ is about 2.4 hr. Cl is about 1.3 mL/min/kg. About 56% is excreted in the urine and 39% in the feces.

Special Populations:
Renal Function Impairment – The t½ is increased and Cl decreased. Dosage adjustment is recommended.
Elderly – Drug accumulation in the plasma was increased to 40%. Dosage adjustment may be needed.

Indications
Treatment of pharyngitis/tonsillitis caused by *Streptococcus pyogenes*, otitis media caused by *Moraxella catarrhalis*, *Haemophilus influenzae* (including beta-lactamase-producing strains) or *S. pyogenes*, and acute bacterial exacerbation of chronic bronchitis caused by *Streptococcus pneumoniae* (penicillin-susceptible strains), *H. influenzae* (including betalactamase-producing strains) or *M. catarrhalis* (including beta-lactamase-producing strains).

Contraindications
Hypersensitivity to cephalosporins.

Route/Dosage
ADULTS AND CHILDREN 12 YR AND OVER: PO 400 mg qd for 10 days.
CHILDREN UNDER 12 YR: PO 9 mg/kg qd (max 400 mg) for 10 days. Give suspension 2 hr before or 1 hr after a meal.

Interactions None well documented.

Lab Test Interferences May cause false-positive urine glucose test results with *Benedict's* solution, *Fehling's* solution or *Clinitest* tablets, but not with enzyme-based tests (eg, *Clinistix*, *Test-tape*); false-positive test results for proteinuria with acid and denaturization-precipitation tests; false-positive direct *Coombs'* test results in certain patients (eg, those with azotemia); false elevations in urinary 17-ketosteroid values.

Adverse Reactions
GI: Nausea; vomiting; diarrhea; anorexia; abdominal pain or cramps; flatulence; colitis.
GU: Pyuria; dysuria; renal dysfunction; reversible interstitial nephritis; hematuria; toxic nephropathy.
HEMA: Eosinophilia; neutropenia; lymphocytosis; leukocytosis; thrombocytopenia; decreased platelet function; anemia; aplastic anemia; hemorrhage.
HEPA: Hepatic dysfunction; abnormal LFT results.
OTHER: Hypersensitivity, including Stevens-Johnson syndrome, erythema multiforme, and toxic epidermal necrolysis; serum sickness–like reactions (eg, skin rash, polyarthritis, arthralgia, fever); candidal overgrowth.

Precautions
Pregnancy: Category B.
Lactation: Undetermined.
Children: In infants consider benefits relative to risks. Safety and efficacy in children under 6 mo not established.
Hypersensitivity: Reactions range from mild to life-threatening. Administer drug with caution to penicillin-sensitive patients because of possible cross-sensitivity.
Renal function impairment: Use drug with caution in patients with renal impairment. Dosage adjustment based on renal function may be required.
Superinfection: May result in bacterial or fungal overgrowth on nonsusceptible microorganisms.
Pseudomembranous colitis: Consider possibility in patients in whom diarrhea develops.
Hemodialysis patients: A single 400 mg capsule or 9 mg/kg (max, 400 mg) dose may be administered at the end of each hemodialysis session.

Overdosage: Signs and Symptoms
Seizures.

PATIENT CARE CONSIDERATIONS
Administration/Storage
- Administer oral suspension 2 hr before or 1 hr after meal.
- After mixing, the suspension may be kept for 14 days stored in refrigerator. Keep tightly closed. Shake well before use. Capsules may

be stored at room temperature.

Assessment/Interventions
- Assess for hypersensitivity reaction or previous penicillin allergy.
- Assess renal function prior to starting therapy.
- Obtain specimens for culture and sensitivity before beginning therapy and periodically during treatment.
- Monitor for signs of infection, especially fever, and for positive response to antibiotic therapy.
- Assess for signs and symptoms of anaphylaxis. Have resuscitation equipment available.
- Assess for signs of superinfection, such as vaginitis or stomatitis.
- Assess for severe diarrhea with blood or pus, which may be symptom of pseudomembranous colitis. Symptoms may occur after antibiotic treatment is discontinued.

Patient/Family Education
- Inform diabetic patients that oral suspension contains 1 g sucrose/teaspoon of suspension.
- Instruct patient to complete full course of therapy.
- Have patient take drug with food or milk to avoid GI upset.
- Notify healthcare provider if patient has penicillin allergy or cephalosporin allergy.
- Notify healthcare provider of nausea, vomiting or diarrhea, especially if severe or contains blood, mucus or pus.
- Remind diabetic patient to use an enzyme-based test for urine glucose or may otherwise obtain a false-positive result.
- Remind patient to check body temperature daily. If fever persists for more than a few days or if high fever (greater than 102°F) or shaking chills are noted, notify health care provider.
- Instruct patient to report signs of superinfection: black "furry" tongue, white patches in mouth, foul-smelling stools, vaginal itching or discharge.
- Instruct patient to seek emergency care if he or she experiences wheezing or difficulty breathing.

Ceftizoxime Sodium

(SEFF-tih-ZOX-eem SO-dee-uhm)

Class Antibiotic/Cephalosporin

How Supplied
Cefizox Powder for Injection 500 mg (2.6 mEq sodium/g), Powder for Injection 1 g (2.6 mEq sodium/g), Powder for Injection 2 g (2.6 mEq sodium/g), Powder for Injection 10 g (2.6 mEq sodium/g), Injection 1 g as sodium, Injection 2 g as sodium

Action
PHARMACOLOGY: Inhibits mucopeptide synthesis in bacterial cell wall.

PHARMACOKINETICS/DYNAMICS:
Distribution: Ceftizoxime is 30% protein bound. It achieves therapeutic levels in various body fluids (eg, CSF in those with inflamed meninges) and body tissues. It is excreted in human milk in low concentrations.

Metabolism: Ceftizoxime is not metabolized.

Excretion: The t½ is about 1.7 hr. Ceftizoxime is excreted unchanged by the kidneys in 24 hr.

Special Populations:
Renal Function Impairment – The t½ is prolonged. Dosage adjustment is recommended.

Indications Treatment of infections of lower respiratory tract, urinary tract, skin and skin structures, bone and joint; treatment of intra-abdominal infections, pelvic inflammatory disease, gonorrhea, septicemia, and meningitis caused by susceptible microorganisms.

Contraindications Hypersensitivity to cephalosporins.

Route/Dosage
ADULTS: **IV/IM** 1 to 2 g q 8 to 12 hr (life-threatening infections: IV up to 2 g q 4 hr or 3 to 4 g q 8 hr).
CHILDREN OVER 6 MO: **IV/IM** 50 mg/kg q 6 to 8 hr up to 200 mg/kg/day (max, 12 g/day).

Interactions
Aminoglycosides: Increased risk of nephrotoxicity.
Probenecid: Inhibition of renal excretion of ceftizoxime.
INCOMPATIBILITIES:
Aminoglycosides: Do not add aminoglycosides to ceftizoxime solutions because inactivation of both drugs may result; administer at separate sites if concurrent therapy is indicated.

Lab Test Interferences May cause false-positive urine glucose test results with *Benedict's* solution, *Fehling's* solution, or *Clinitest* tablets but not with enzyme-based tests (eg, *Clinistix*, *Tes-tape*); false-positive test results for proteinuria with acid and denaturization-precipitation tests; false-positive direct *Coombs'* test results in certain patients (eg, those with azotemia); false elevations in urinary 17-ketosteroid values.

Adverse Reactions
GI: Nausea; vomiting; diarrhea; anorexia; abdominal pain or cramps; flatulence; colitis, including pseudomembranous colitis.

GU: Pyuria; renal dysfunction; dysuria; reversible interstitial nephritis; hematuria; toxic nephropathy.
HEMA: Eosinophilia; neutropenia; lymphocytosis; leukocytosis; thrombocytopenia; decreased platelet function; anemia; aplastic anemia; hemorrhage.
HEPA: Hepatic dysfunction; abnormal LFT results.
OTHER: Hypersensitivity, including Stevens-Johnson syndrome, erythema multiforme, toxic epidermal necrolysis; candidal overgrowth; serum sickness–like reactions (eg, skin rashes, polyarthritis, arthralgia, fever); phlebitis; thrombophlebitis and pain at injection site.

Precautions
Pregnancy: Category B.
Lactation: Excreted in breast milk.

Children: Safety and efficacy in infants under 6 mo not established. In infants, consider benefits relative to risks.
Hypersensitivity: Reactions range from mild to life-threatening. Administer drug with caution to penicillin-sensitive patients because of possible cross-reactivity.
Renal function impairment: Use drug with caution in patients with baseline renal impairment. Dosage adjustment based on renal function may be required.
Superinfection: May result in bacterial or fungal overgrowth of nonsusceptible micro-organisms.
Pseudomembranous colitis: Consider in patients who develop diarrhea.

Overdosage: Signs and Symptoms
Seizures.

PATIENT CARE CONSIDERATIONS
Administration/Storage
- IV route may be preferable for life-threatening infections.
- Administer after hemodialysis, because drug is partially removed by dialysis.
- When giving by IM route, inject deeply into large muscle (eg, upper outer quadrant of gluteus muscle or lateral thigh); massage well. For amounts greater than 2 g, divide dose and administer in different muscle masses.
- Reconstituted solution should be light yellow to amber. Do not administer if solution is cloudy or precipitate is present.
- When giving by IV route, administer slowly over 3 to 5 min using direct (bolus) injection. Change IV sites q 48 to 72 hr.
- When drug is administered by intermittent IV infusion, reconstituted solution can be further diluted with 50 to 100 mL of 0.9% Sodium Chloride or D5W and infused over 30 min.
- Completely thaw frozen preparations at room temperature before use. Do not introduce additives. After thawing, solution is stable for 24 hr at room temperature or for 10 days if refrigerated. Do not refreeze.
- Store sterile powder at room temperature and protect from light.
- Reconstituted solution is stable for 96 hr if refrigerated and 24 hr when stored at room temperature.

Assessment/Interventions
- Obtain patient history, including drug history and any known allergies. Note renal impairment and allergy to cephalosporins or penicillins.
- Obtain specimens for culture and sensitivity before beginning therapy and periodically during treatment.
- Monitor renal function carefully during treatment.
- Monitor for signs of infection, especially fever, and for positive response to antibiotic therapy.
- Assess for signs and symptoms of anaphylaxis (eg, shortness of breath, wheezing, laryngeal spasm). Have resuscitation equipment available.
- Assess for signs of superinfection, such as vaginitis or stomatitis.
- Assess for severe diarrhea with blood or pus, which may be symptom of pseudomembranous colitis. Symptoms may occur after antibiotic treatment.
- Monitor IV site for infiltration, infection, thrombophlebitis, and bleeding.

Patient/Family Education
- Remind patient to check body temperature daily. If fever persists for more than a few days or if high fever (greater than 102°F) or shaking chills are noted, notify health care provider immediately.
- Advise patient to maintain normal fluid intake while using this medication.
- Instruct diabetic patient to use enzyme-based tests (eg, *Clinistix*, *Testape*) for monitoring urine glucose because drug may give false results with other tests.
- Advise patient to report these symptoms to health care provider: nausea, vomiting, diarrhea, sore throat, bruising, bleeding, hives, bone or joint pain.
- Instruct patient to report signs of superinfection: black "furry" tongue, white patches in

mouth, foul-smelling stools, vaginal itching or discharge.
- Warn patient that diarrhea that contains blood or pus may be a sign of serious disorders. Tell patient to seek medical care and not to treat at home.
- Instruct patient to seek emergency care immediately if wheezing or difficulty in breathing occurs.
- Advise patient to avoid ingesting alcohol.

Ceftriaxone Sodium

(SEFF-TRY-AXE-own SO-dee-uhm)

Class Antibiotic/Cephalosporin

How Supplied
Rocephin Powder for Injection 250 mg (3.6 mEq sodium/g), Powder for Injection 500 mg (3.6 mEq sodium/g), Powder for Injection 1 g (3.6 mEq sodium/g), Powder for Injection 2 g (3.6 mEq sodium/g), Powder for Injection 10 g (3.6 mEq sodium/g), Injection 1 g (3.6 mEq sodium/g), Injection 2 g (3.6 mEq sodium/g)

Action
PHARMACOLOGY: Inhibits mucopeptide synthesis in bacterial cell wall.

PHARMACOKINETICS/DYNAMICS:
Absorption:
IM – Ceftriaxone is completely absorbed. T_{max} is 2 to 3 hr.

Distribution: Vd is 5.78 to 13.5 L. Ceftriaxone is 85% to 95% protein bound.

Excretion: 33% to 67% is excreted in urine as unchanged drug and the remainder in feces; t½ is 5.8 to 8.7 hr. Plasma Cl is 0.58 to 1.45 L/hr. Renal Cl is 0.32 to 0.73 L/hr.

Indications Treatment of infections of lower respiratory tract, skin and skin structures, bone and joint, urinary tract; treatment of pelvic inflammatory disease, intra-abdominal infections, gonorrhea, meningitis, and septicemia caused by susceptible microorganisms; preoperative prophylaxis. **Unlabeled use(s):** Treatment of Lyme disease in patients refractory to penicillin G.

Contraindications Hypersensitivity to cephalosporins.

Route/Dosage
Infection
ADULTS: **IV/IM** 1 to 2 g/day or in equally divided doses q 12 hr (max, 4 g/day).
CHILDREN: **IV/IM** 50 to 75 mg/kg/day in equally divided doses q 12 hr (max, 2 g/day).

Uncomplicated Gonococcal Infections
ADULTS: **IM** 250 mg as single dose.

Surgical Prophylaxis
ADULTS: **IV/IM** 1 g as single dose 30 min to 2 hr before surgery.

Pediatric Meningitis
CHILDREN: **IV/IM** 75 mg/kg as loading dose then 100 mg/kg/day in divided doses q 12 hr (max, 4 g/day).

Interactions
Aminoglycosides: Increased risk of nephrotoxicity.
INCOMPATIBILITIES: Other antimicrobial drugs.

Lab Test Interferences May cause false-positive urine glucose test result with *Benedict's* solution, *Fehling's* solution, or *Clinitest* tablets but not with enzyme-based tests (eg, *Clinistix*, *Tes-tape*); false-positive test results for proteinuria with acid and denaturization-precipitation tests; false-positive direct *Coombs'* test results in certain patients (eg, those with azotemia); false elevations in urinary 17-ketosteroid values.

Adverse Reactions
GI: Nausea; vomiting; diarrhea; colitis, including pseudomembranous colitis.
GU: Renal dysfunction; pyuria; dysuria; reversible interstitial nephritis; hematuria; toxic nephropathy, urinary casts.
HEMA: Eosinophilia; neutropenia; lymphocytosis; leukocytosis; thrombocytopenia; decreased platelet function; anemia; aplastic anemia; hemorrhage.
HEPA: Hepatic dysfunction; jaundice; abnormal LFT results.
OTHER: Hypersensitivity, including Stevens-Johnson syndrome, erythema multiforme, toxic epidermal necrolysis; candidal overgrowth; serum sickness–like reactions (eg, skin rashes, polyarthritis; arthralgia, fever); phlebitis, thrombophlebitis, and pain at injection site.

Precautions
Pregnancy: Category B.
Lactation: Excreted in breast milk.
Children: Cephalosporins may accumulate in newborns.
Hypersensitivity: Reactions range from mild to life-threatening. Administer drug with caution to penicillin-sensitive patients because of possible cross-reactivity.
Superinfection: May result in bacterial or fungal overgrowth of nonsusceptible microorganisms.
Pseudomembranous colitis: Consider in patients in whom diarrhea develops.

Overdosage: Signs and Symptoms
Seizures.

PATIENT CARE CONSIDERATIONS
Administration/Storage
- Reconstituted solution should be light yellow to amber. Do not administer if solution is cloudy or precipitate is present.
- When giving by IM route, inject deeply into large muscle (eg, upper outer quadrant of gluteus muscle or lateral thigh); massage well.
- When giving by IV route, administer slowly over 3 to 5 min. Change IV sites q 48 to 72 hr.
- Reconstituted drug should not be mixed with other antibiotics.
- For piggyback infusion, reconstituted solution may be diluted with D5W or 0.9% Sodium Chloride infused over 30 to 60 min.
- For preoperative surgical prophylaxis, administer ceftriaxone 50 to 120 min before surgical incision.
- When reconstituted with 250 mL of diluent, use within 24 hr when stored at room temperature and within 3 days if refrigerated.
- When reconstituted with 100 mL of Sterile Water for Injection, 0.9% Sodium Chloride, or 5% Dextrose, use within 3 days when stored at room temperature and within 10 days if refrigerated.
- Completely thaw frozen preparations at room temperature before use; do not refreeze.
- Store sterile powder at room temperature and protect from heat or light.

Assessment/Interventions
- Obtain patient history, including drug history and any known allergies. Note allergy to cephalosporins or penicillins.
- Obtain specimens for culture and sensitivity before beginning therapy and periodically during treatment.
- Monitor renal function carefully during treatment.
- Monitor for signs of infection, especially fever, and for positive response to antibiotic therapy.
- Assess for signs and symptoms of anaphylaxis (eg, shortness of breath, wheezing, laryngeal spasm). Have resuscitation equipment available.
- Assess for signs of superinfection, such as vaginitis or stomatitis.
- Assess for diarrhea with blood or pus, which may be a symptom of pseudomembranous colitis. Symptoms may occur after antibiotic treatment.
- Monitor for coagulation abnormalities. Elevated prothrombin time or abnormal platelet count may occur. If bleeding occurs and PT is prolonged, vitamin K may be indicated.
- Monitor IV site for infiltration, infection, thrombophlebitis, and bleeding.

Patient/Family Education
- Remind patient to check body temperature daily. If fever persists for more than a few days or if high fever (greater than 102°F) or shaking chills are noted, notify health care provider immediately.
- Advise patient to maintain normal fluid intake while using this medication.
- Instruct diabetic patient to use enzyme-based tests (eg, *Clinistix*, *Testape*) for monitoring urine glucose because drug may give false results with other tests.
- Instruct patient to report these symptoms to health care provider: nausea, vomiting, diarrhea, skin rash, hives, sore throat, bruising, bleeding, muscle or joint pain.
- Advise patient to report signs of superinfection: black "furry" tongue, white patches in mouth, foul-smelling stools, vaginal itching or discharge.
- Warn patient that diarrhea that contains blood or pus may be a sign of serious disorders. Tell patient to seek medical care and not to treat at home.
- Instruct patient to seek emergency care immediately if wheezing or difficulty in breathing occurs.

Cefuroxime

(SEFF-yur-OX-eem)

Class Antibiotic/Cephalosporin

How Supplied
Ceftin Tablets 125 mg, Tablets 250 mg, Tablets 500 mg, Suspension 125 mg/5 mL, Suspension 250 mg/5 mL ◆ *Zinacef* Powder for Injection 750 mg (2.4 mEq sodium/g), Powder for Injection 1.5 g (2.4 mEq sodium/g), Powder for Injection 7.5 g (2.4 mEq sodium/g), Injection 750 mg (2.4 mEq sodium/g), Injection 1.5 g (2.4 mEq sodium/g)

❖ *Apo-Cefuroxime*

Action
PHARMACOLOGY: Inhibits mucopeptide synthesis in bacterial cell wall.

PHARMACOKINETICS/DYNAMICS:
Absorption:
Tablets – C_{max} is 2.1 mcg/mL (125 mg dose) to 13.6 mcg/mL (1000 mg dose). T_{max} is 2.2 to 3 hr. AUC is 6.7 mcg•hr/mL (125 mg dose) to

50 mcg•hr/mL (1000 mg dose).
Suspension (10 to 20 mg/kg) – C_{max} is 3.3 to 7 mcg/mL. T_{max} is 2.7 to 3.6 hr. AUC is 12.4 to 32.8 mcg•hr/mL.
IM (750 mg dose) – C_{max} is 27 mcg/mL. T_{max} is about 45 min.
IV – C_{max} is about 50 mcg/mL (750 mg dose) and about 100 mcg/mL (1.5 g dose). T_{max} is 15 min.

Distribution: Cefuroxime is detectable in therapeutic concentrations in pleural and joint fluid, bile, sputum, bone, aqueous humor, and CSF (in those with meningitis). It is 50% protein bound.

Excretion: The t½ is 1.2 to 1.3 hr (tablets), 1.4 to 1.9 hr (suspension), and about 80 min (IV/IM). About 50% is excreted unchanged in the urine within 12 hr (tablets/suspension) and about 89% over 8 hr (IV/IM).

Special Populations:
Renal Function Impairment – The t½ is prolonged. Dosage reduction is recommended.

Indications
Oral form: Treatment of infections of lower respiratory tract, urinary tract, skin and skin structures; treatment of uncomplicated gonorrhea, otitis media, pharyngitis, and tonsillitis caused by susceptible strains of specific microorganisms. Treatment of early Lyme disease, pharyngitis/tonsillitis, and impetigo.
Parenteral form: Treatment of infections of lower respiratory tract, urinary tract, skin and skin structures, bone and joint; preoperative prophylaxis; treatment of septicemia, gonorrhea, and meningitis caused by susceptible strains of specific microorganisms.

Contraindications Hypersensitivity to cephalosporins.

Route/Dosage
Infection
ADULTS AND CHILDREN 12 YR AND OVER: **PO** 125 to 500 mg bid. **IV/IM** 750 mg to 1.5 g q 8 hr.
CHILDREN UNDER 12 YR: **PO** 125 to 250 mg bid.
INFANTS AND CHILDREN OVER 3 MO: **IV/IM** 50 to 150 mg/kg/day (not to exceed adult dose) in equally divided doses q 6 to 8 hr.

Bacterial Meningitis
ADULTS AND CHILDREN 12 YR AND OVER: **IV/IM** Up to 3 g q 8 hr.
INFANTS AND CHILDREN 3 MO TO 12 YR: **IV/IM** 200 to 240 mg/kg/day in divided doses q 6 to 8 hr.

Uncomplicated Gonorrhea
ADULTS AND CHILDREN 12 YR AND OVER: **PO** 1 g as single dose. **IM** 1.5 g as single dose.

Preoperative Prophylaxis
ADULTS: **IV/IM** 1.5 g 30 min to 1 hr before surgery then 750 mg q 8 hr for duration of surgery.

Interactions
Aminoglycosides: Increased risk of nephrotoxicity with parenteral cefuroxime.
Probenecid: Inhibition of renal excretion of cefuroxime.
INCOMPATIBILITIES:
Aminoglycosides: Do not add aminoglycosides to cefuroxime solutions because inactivation of both drugs may result; administer at separate sites if concurrent therapy is indicated.

Lab Test Interferences May cause false-positive urine glucose test results with *Benedict's* solution, *Fehling's* solution, or *Clinitest* tablets but not with enzyme-based tests (eg, *Clinistix*, *Tes-tape*); false-positive test results for proteinuria with acid and denaturization-precipitation tests; false-positive direct *Coombs'* test results in certain patients (eg, those with azotemia); false elevations in urinary 17-ketosteroid values; false-negative reaction in ferricyanide test for blood glucose.

Adverse Reactions
GI: Nausea; vomiting; diarrhea; anorexia; abdominal pain or cramps; flatulence; colitis, including pseudomembranous colitis.
GU: Pyuria; renal dysfunction; dysuria; reversible interstitial nephritis; hematuria; toxic nephropathy.
HEMA: Eosinophilia; neutropenia; lymphocytosis; leukocytosis; thrombocytopenia; decreased platelet function; anemia; aplastic anemia; hemorrhage.
HEPA: Hepatic dysfunction; abnormal LFT results.
OTHER: Hypersensitivity, including Stevens-Johnson syndrome, erythema multiforme, toxic epidermal necrolysis; candidal overgrowth; serum sickness–like reactions (eg, skin rashes, polyarthritis, arthralgia, fever); phlebitis, thrombophlebitis, and pain at injection site.

Precautions
Pregnancy: Category B.
Lactation: Excreted in breast milk.
Children: Safety and efficacy in children under 3 mo not established.
Hypersensitivity: Reactions range from mild to life-threatening. Administer drug with caution to penicillin-sensitive patients because of possible cross-reactivity.
Renal function impairment: Use drug with caution in patients with renal impairment. Dosage adjustment based on renal function may be required.

Superinfection: May result in bacterial or fungal overgrowth of nonsusceptible microorganisms.
Pseudomembranous colitis: Consider in patients in whom diarrhea develops.

PATIENT CARE CONSIDERATIONS
Administration/Storage
- Sodium salt is for parenteral administration. Axetil salt is for oral administration.
- Administer oral form with food to enhance absorption.
- May crush and mix with food or beverages; however, crushed tablets have strong, persistent bitter taste. Consider alternative therapy if children cannot swallow whole tablets.
- Reconstituted solution should be light yellow to amber. Do not administer if solution is cloudy or precipitate is present.
- When giving by IM route, shake IM suspension gently before administration. Aspirate to prevent injection into blood vessel. Inject deeply into large muscle (eg, upper outer quadrant of gluteus muscle or lateral thigh); massage well. Rotate injection sites.
- When giving by IV route, use direct intermittent infusion. Administer slowly over 3 to 5 min. Change IV sites q 48 to 72 hr.
- For intermittent IV infusion with Y-type administration set, administer over 30 min. and temporarily stop other solutions at Y-site.
- For continuous infusion, reconstituted solution may be further diluted with D5W or 0.9% Sodium Chloride.
- Reconstituted solution is stable for 24 hr at room temperature. When refrigerated, solution in vials is stable for 48 hr; IV solution is stable for 7 days when refrigerated.
- Completely thaw frozen solution at room temperature before use; do not refreeze.
- Do not add supplementary medication to premixed solution.
- Store sterile powder at room temperature and protect from light.
- Store tablets at room temperature.

Assessment/Interventions
- Obtain patient history, including drug history and any known allergies. Note renal impairment and allergy to cephalosporins or penicillins.
- Obtain specimens for culture and sensitivity before beginning therapy and periodically during treatment.
- Monitor renal function carefully during treatment.
- Monitor for signs of infection, especially fever, and for positive response to antibiotic therapy.
- Assess for signs and symptoms of anaphylaxis (eg, shortness of breath, wheezing, laryngeal spasm). Have resuscitation equipment available.
- Assess for signs of superinfection, such as vaginitis or stomatitis.
- Assess for diarrhea with blood or pus, which may be symptom of pseudomembranous colitis. Symptoms may occur after antibiotic treatment.
- Monitor IV site for infiltration, infection and thrombophlebitis.

Patient/Family Education
- Instruct patient to complete full course of therapy.
- Advise patient to take with meals to enhance absorption. If tablet must be crushed, mix with food or beverage.
- Advise parent to contact health care provider if child is unable to tolerate crushed tablet with food or beverage.
- Remind patient to check body temperature daily. If fever persists for more than a few days or if high fever (greater than 102°F) or shaking chills are noted, notify health care provider immediately.
- Advise patient to maintain normal fluid intake while using this medication.
- Advise diabetic patient to use enzyme-based tests (eg, *Clinistix, Testape*) for monitoring urine glucose because drug may give false results with other tests.
- Instruct patient to report these symptoms to health care provider: nausea, vomiting, diarrhea, skin rash, sore throat, bruising, hives, muscle or joint pain.
- Instruct patient to report signs of superinfection: black "furry" tongue, white patches in mouth, foul-smelling stools, vaginal itching or discharge.
- Warn patient that diarrhea that contains blood or pus may be a sign of serious disorders. Tell patient to seek medical care and not to treat at home.
- Instruct patient to seek emergency care immediately if wheezing or difficulty breathing occurs.

Overdosage: Signs and Symptoms
Seizures.

Celecoxib

(sel-eh-cox-ib)
Class COX-2 inhibitor
How Supplied
Celebrex Capsules 100 mg, Capsules 200 mg
Action
PHARMACOLOGY: Reduces inflammation (eg, pain, redness, swelling, heat), fever, and pain by inhibiting chemicals in the body that cause inflammation, fever, and pain. This is probably caused by the inhibition of prostaglandin synthesis, primarily via inhibition of cyclooxygenase-2 (COX-2) isoenzyme.

PHARMACOKINETICS/DYNAMICS:
Absorption: T_{max} is about 3 hr.
Food – T_{max} increased about 1 to 2 hr and AUC increased 10% to 20% when taken with a high-fat meal.
Distribution: Celecoxib is about 97% protein bound. Vd is about 400 L.
Metabolism: Metabolized in the liver; primarily mediated via CYP2C9 to inactive metabolites.
Excretion: Less than 3% is excreted unchanged in the urine and feces. About 57% is excreted in feces and 27% in urine. The t½ is about 11 hr. Cl is about 500 mL/min.

Special Populations:
Renal Function Impairment – AUC is about 40% lower in those with Ccr 35 to 60 mL/min.
Hepatic Function Impairment – AUC is increased about 40% in mild impairment and 180% in moderate impairment. Reduce dosage.
Elderly – C_{max} is 40% higher and AUC is 50% higher. Dosage adjustment generally is not necessary.
Race – AUC is about 40% higher in blacks vs Caucasians.

Indications Relief of symptoms of osteoarthritis; relief of symptoms of rheumatoid arthritis in adults; management of acute pain in adults; treatment of primary dysmenorrhea; reduction of the number of adenomatous colorectal polyps in familial adenomatous polyposis (FAP), as an adjunct to usual care (eg, endoscopic surveillance, surgery).

Contraindications Allergy to celecoxib or any of its ingredients; allergy to sulfonamides; aspirin triad (eg, asthma, nasal polyps, allergy to aspirin); previous allergic reactions following aspirin or other NSAID use (eg, asthma, hives, rash).

Route/Dosage
Osteoarthritis
ADULTS: **PO** 200 mg/day administered as a single dose or as 100 mg bid.

Rheumatoid Arthritis
ADULTS: **PO** 100 to 200 mg bid.
Acute Pain, Primary Dysmenorrhea
ADULTS: **PO** 400 mg initially followed by an additional 200 mg dose on day 1, if needed, then 200 mg twice daily as needed.
FAP
ADULTS: **PO** Continue usual medical care for FAP patients while on celecoxib. To reduce the number of adenomatous colorectal polyps in patients with FAP, the recommended dose is 400 mg (2 × 200 mg capsules) bid. Take with food.

Interactions
ACE inhibitors: NSAIDs may diminish the antihypertensive effect of ACE inhibitors.
Aspirin: Coadministration with celecoxib may result in an increased rate of GI ulceration or other complications.
Fluconazole: Increase in celecoxib plasma concentration may occur because of inhibition of celecoxib metabolism.
Furosemide: NSAIDs can reduce the natriuretic effect of furosemide and thiazides in some patients.
Lithium: Mean steady-state lithium plasma levels increased about 17% in subjects receiving lithium with celecoxib.
P450 2C9 inhibitors: There is a potential for an in vivo drug interaction with drugs that are metabolized by P450 2D6.
Warfarin: Monitor anticoagulant activity, particularly in the first few days, after initiating or changing celecoxib therapy in patients receiving warfarin or similar agents because these patients are at an increased risk of bleeding complications.

Lab Test Interferences None well documented.

Adverse Reactions
CV: Aggravated hypertension; angina pectoris; coronary artery disorder; MI; palpitations; tachycardia.
CNS: Dizziness; insomnia; fatigue; migraine; anxiety; anorexia; increased appetite; depression; nervousness; somnolence.
DERM: Rash; alopecia; dermatitis; nail disorder; photosensitivity; pruritus; erythematous rash; maculopapular rash; skin disorder; dry skin; increased sweating; urticaria; contact dermatitis; injection site reaction; skin nodule; cellulitis.
EENT: Rhinitis; sinusitis; esophagitis; deafness; ear abnormality; earache; tinnitus; laryngitis; taste perversion; blurred vision; cataracts; conjunctivitis; eye pain; glaucoma.
GI: Abdominal pain; diarrhea; dyspepsia; flatulence; constipation; diverticulitis; dysphagia;

eructation; gastritis; gastroenteritis; gastroesophageal reflux; hemorrhoids; hiatal hernia; melena; dry mouth; stomatitis; tenesmus; tooth disorder; vomiting.
GU: Breast fibroadenosis; breast neoplasm; breast pain; dysmenorrhea; menstrual disorder; vaginal hemorrhage; vaginitis; prostatic disorder; albuminuria; cystitis; dysuria; hematuria; micturition frequency; renal calculus; urinary incontinence; urinary tract infection.
HEMA: Ecchymosis; epistaxis; thrombocythemia; anemia.
HEPA: Abnormal hepatic function; elevated AST and ALT.
METAB: Increased BUN, CPK, creatinine, nonprotein nitrogen, and alkaline phosphatase; diabetes mellitus; hypercholesterolemia; hypokalemia; weight gain.
RESP: Pharyngitis; upper respiratory tract infection; bronchitis; bronchospasm; aggravated bronchospasm; coughing; dyspnea; pneumonia.
OTHER: Peripheral edema; accidental injury; allergic reaction; asthenia; chest pain; generalized edema; facial edema; fever; hot flushes; flu-like symptoms; pain; peripheral pain; leg cramps; hypertonia; hypesthesia; neuralgia; neuropathy; paresthesia; vertigo; arthralgia; arthrosis; bone disorder; accidental fracture; myalgia; neck stiffness; synovitis; tendonitis.

Precautions

Pregnancy: Category C.
Lactation: Undetermined.
Children: Safety and effectiveness in patients under 18 yr not established.
Elderly: Initiate therapy with lowest recommended dose.
Asthma: Use with caution in patients with pre-existing asthma.
GI effects: Serious GI toxicity (eg, bleeding, ulcerations, perforations) can occur at any time, with or without warning symptoms.

Overdosage: Signs and Symptoms

Lethargy, drowsiness, nausea, vomiting, epigastric pain, GI bleeding, hypertension, acute renal failure, respiratory depression, coma.

PATIENT CARE CONSIDERATIONS

Administration/Storage

- Store at room temperature 25°C (77°F); excursions permitted to 15° to 30°C (59° to 86°F).
- Do not administer to patient who has experienced asthma, urticaria, or hypersensitivity reactions after taking aspirin or other NSAIDs.
- Do not administer to pregnant women or nursing mothers.
- Administer the lowest therapeutic dose possible as prescribed for each patient.
- Do not administer to patients with hypersensitivity to sulfonamides, NSAIDs, aspirin, celecoxib, or any of their ingredients.
- Administer to adults older than 18 yr.

Assessment/Interventions

- Assess for signs and symptoms of hypersensitivity.
- Take a complete drug history and monitor potential drug/drug interactions and contraindications that should be reported to the primary care provider.
- Monitor for signs of GI bleeding, adverse CNS symptoms, and any other adverse events.
- Monitor for signs of skin rash.
- Monitor for the following signs and symptoms of decreased renal function: serum creatinine, BUN, unexpected weight gain, edema.
- Monitor for signs of hypophosphatemia and hyperchloremia.
- Monitor hepatic function, as decreased hepatic function may require a reduced dose.

Patient/Family Education

- Instruct patient to take medication as prescribed.
- Advise patient to inform primary care provider if taking or planning to take any OTC medications, as there is potential for drug interactions.
- Advise patient with sensitive stomach to take medication with food to help avoid GI distress.
- Instruct patient to promptly report signs or symptoms of GI ulceration or bleeding, skin rash, unexplained weight gain, or edema to primary care provider.
- Inform patient of the warning signs and symptoms of hepatotoxicity (eg, nausea, fatigue, lethargy, pruritus, jaundice, right upper quadrant tenderness, flu-like symptoms) and to stop therapy and contact the primary care provider should any of these occur.
- Instruct patient to seek immediate emergency help in case of an anaphylactoid reaction.
- Warn women with childbearing potential to avoid becoming pregnant and apprise them of the potential hazard to the fetus, especially in the third trimester.
- Warn nursing mothers of the danger of transferring the drug to the baby through the mother's milk. Make a decision to discontinue the drug or nursing in collaboration with the primary health care provider.
- Instruct patient to report any unusual reaction or concern to the primary care provider.

Cephalexin

(seh-fuh-LEX-in)

Class Antibiotic/Cephalosporin

How Supplied
Biocef Capsules 500 mg, Powder for Oral Suspension 125 mg/5 mL, Powder for Oral Suspension 250 mg/5 mL ◆ *Keflex* Capsules 250 mg, Capsules 500 mg, Powder for Oral Suspension 125 mg/5 mL, Powder for Oral Suspension 250 mg/5 mL ◆ *Keftab* Tablets 500 mg (as hydrochloride monohydrate)
🍁 *APO-Cephalex* ◆ *Novo-Lexin* ◆ *Nu-Cephalex*

Action

PHARMACOLOGY: Inhibits mucopeptide synthesis in bacterial cell wall.

PHARMACOKINETICS/DYNAMICS:

Absorption: Cephalexin is rapidly absorbed. C_{max} is about 9 to 32 mcg/mL (250 mg to 1 g doses). T_{max} is 1 hr.

Distribution: Cephalexin is 10% protein bound.

Excretion: More than 90% is excreted unchanged in the urine within 8 hr. The $t_{½}$ is 50 to 80 min.

Indications Treatment of infections of respiratory tract, urinary tract, skin and skin structures and bone; treatment of otitis media caused by susceptible strains of specific microorganisms.

Contraindications Hypersensitivity to cephalosporins.

Route/Dosage
ADULTS: **PO** 1 to 4 g/day in divided doses (max, 4 g/day).
CHILDREN: **PO** (cephalexin monohydrate only) 25 to 100 mg/kg/day in divided doses.

Interactions
Probenecid: Inhibition of renal excretion of cephalexin.

Lab Test Interferences May cause false-positive urine glucose test results with *Benedict's* solution, *Fehling's* solution, or *Clinitest* tablets but not with enzyme-based tests (eg, *Clinistix*, *Tes-tape*); false-positive test results for proteinuria with acid and denaturization-precipitation tests; false-positive direct *Coombs'* test results in certain patients (eg, those with azotemia); false elevations in urinary 17-ketosteroid values.

Adverse Reactions
GI: Nausea; vomiting; diarrhea; anorexia; abdominal pain or cramps; flatulence; colitis, including pseudomembranous colitis.
GU: Pyuria; renal dysfunction; dysuria; reversible interstitial nephritis; hematuria; toxic nephropathy.
HEMA: Eosinophilia; neutropenia; lymphocytosis; leukocytosis; thrombocytopenia; decreased platelet function; anemia; aplastic anemia; hemorrhage.
HEPA: Hepatic dysfunction; abnormal LFT results.
OTHER: Hypersensitivity, including Stevens-Johnson syndrome, erythema multiforme, toxic epidermal necrolysis; candidal overgrowth; serum sickness–like reactions (eg, skin rash, polyarthritis, arthralgia, fever).

Precautions
Pregnancy: Category B.
Lactation: Excreted in breast milk.
Children: Safety and efficacy of cephalexin hydrochloride monohydrate (*Keftab*) in children not established. Cephalosporins may accumulate in newborns.
Hypersensitivity: Reactions range from mild to life-threatening. Administer drug with caution to penicillin-sensitive patients because of possible cross-reactivity.
Renal function impairment: Use drug with caution in patients with renal impairment. Dosage adjustment based on renal function may be required.
Superinfection: May result in bacterial or fungal overgrowth of nonsusceptible microorganisms.
Pseudomembranous colitis: Consider in patients in whom diarrhea develops.

Overdosage: Signs and Symptoms
Seizures.

PATIENT CARE CONSIDERATIONS

Administration/Storage

- Administer with food or milk if GI upset occurs. Food slows but does not decrease absorption.
- Shake oral suspension well before administering. Space doses evenly around clock.
- Oral suspension is stable up to 14 days after reconstitution when refrigerated.
- Store capsules and tablets at room temperature.

Assessment/Interventions

- Obtain patient history, including drug history and any known allergies. Note renal impairment and allergy to cephalosporins or penicillins.
- Obtain specimens for culture and sensitivity before beginning therapy and periodically during treatment.
- Monitor renal function carefully during treatment.

- Monitor for signs of infection, especially fever, and positive response to antibiotic therapy.
- Assess for signs and symptoms of anaphylaxis (eg, shortness of breath, wheezing, laryngeal spasm). Have resuscitation equipment available.
- Assess for signs of superinfection, such as vaginitis or stomatitis.
- Assess for diarrhea with blood or pus, which may be symptom of pseudomembranous colitis. Symptoms may occur after antibiotic treatment.

Patient/Family Education
- Instruct patient to complete full course of therapy.
- Advise patient to take with food or milk if GI distress occurs.
- Remind patient to check body temperature daily. If fever persists for more than a few days or if high fever (greater than 102°F) or shaking chills are noted, notify health care provider immediately.
- Advise patient to maintain normal fluid intake while using this medication.
- Advise diabetic patient to use enzyme-based tests (eg, *Clinistix*, *Testape*) for monitoring urine glucose because drug may give false results with other tests.
- Instruct patient to report these symptoms to health care provider: nausea, vomiting, diarrhea, skin rash, hives, muscle or joint pain.
- Instruct patient to report signs of superinfection: black "furry" tongue, white patches in mouth, foul-smelling stools, vaginal itching or discharge.
- Warn patient that diarrhea that contains blood or pus may be a sign of serious disorders. Tell patient to seek medical care and not to treat at home.
- Instruct patient to seek emergency care immediately if wheezing or difficulty breathing occurs.

Cephradine

(SEFF-ruh-deen)

Class Antibiotic/Cephalosporin

How Supplied
Velosef Capsules 250 mg, Capsules 500 mg, Powder for Oral Suspension 125 mg/5 mL, Powder for Oral Suspension 500 mg/5 mL

Action
PHARMACOLOGY: Inhibits mucopeptide synthesis in bacterial cell wall.

PHARMACOKINETICS/DYNAMICS:
Absorption: Cephradine is rapidly absorbed. C_{max} is about 9 mcg/mL (250 mg) to 24.2 mcg/mL (1 g). T_{max} is 1 hr. Food delays absorption.

Distribution: 8% to 17% protein bound.

Excretion: More than 90% is excreted unchanged in the urine. The t½ is 48 to 80 min.

Special Populations:
Renal Function Impairment – The t½ is prolonged. Dosage adjustment is recommended.

Indications Treatment of infections of respiratory tract, urinary tract, skin and skin structure; treatment of otitis media caused by susceptible strains of microorganisms.

Contraindications Hypersensitivity to cephalosporins.

Route/Dosage
ADULTS: PO 250 mg to 1 g q 6 to 12 hr.
CHILDREN: PO 25 to 100 mg/kg/day in equally divided doses q 6 to 12 hr (max, 4 g/day).

Interactions
Probenecid: Inhibition of renal excretion of cephradine.

Lab Test Interferences May cause false-positive urine glucose test results with *Benedict's* solution, *Fehling's* solution, or *Clinitest* tablets but not with enzyme-based tests (eg, *Clinistix*, *Testape*); false-positive test results for proteinuria with acid and denaturization-precipitation tests; false-positive direct *Coombs'* test result in certain patients (eg, those with azotemia); false elevations in urinary 17-ketosteroid values; false-positive reactions in urinary protein tests that use sulfosalicylic acid.

Adverse Reactions
GI: Nausea; vomiting; diarrhea; colitis, including pseudomembranous colitis.
GU: Renal dysfunction; pyuria; dysuria; reversible interstitial nephritis; hematuria; toxic nephropathy.
HEMA: Eosinophilia; neutropenia; lymphocytosis; leukocytosis; decreased platelet function; anemia; aplastic anemia.
HEPA: Hepatic dysfunction; abnormal LFT results.
OTHER: Hypersensitivity, including Stevens-Johnson syndrome, erythema multiforme, toxic epidermal necrolysis; candidal overgrowth; serum sickness–like reactions (eg, skin rashes, polyarthritis, arthralgia, fever).

Precautions
Pregnancy: Category B.

Lactation: Excreted in breast milk.
Children: Safety and efficacy for infants under 9 mo not established.
Hypersensitivity: Reactions range from mild to life-threatening. Administer drug with caution to penicillin-sensitive patients because of possible cross-reactivity.
Renal function impairment: Use drug with caution in patients with renal impairment. Monitor renal function and dosage adjusted.
Superinfection: Drug may result in bacterial or fungal overgrowth of nonsusceptible microorganisms.
Pseudomembranous colitis: Consider in patients in whom diarrhea develops.

Overdosage: Signs and Symptoms
Seizures.

PATIENT CARE CONSIDERATIONS
Administration/Storage
- May administer without regard to meals. Administer with food or milk if GI upset occurs. Food slows but does not decrease absorption.
- Reconstituted oral suspension may be stored at room temperature for up to 7 days or in refrigerator for 14 days. Shake well before pouring.
- When drug is stored at room temperature, protect from light.

Assessment/Interventions
- Obtain patient history, including drug history and any known allergies. Note renal impairment and allergy to cephalosporins or penicillins.
- Obtain specimens for culture and sensitivity before beginning therapy and periodically during treatment.
- Monitor renal function carefully during therapy.
- Monitor for signs of infection, especially fever, and for positive response to antibiotic therapy.
- Assess for signs and symptoms of anaphylaxis (eg, shortness of breath, wheezing, laryngeal spasm). Have resuscitation equipment available.
- Assess for signs and symptoms of superinfection, such as vaginitis or stomatitis.
- Assess for diarrhea with blood or pus, which may be a symptom of pseudomembranous colitis. Symptoms may occur after antibiotic treatment.

Patient/Family Education
- Instruct patient to complete full course of therapy.
- Advise patient to take with food or milk if GI distress occurs.
- Remind patient to check body temperature daily. If fever persists for more than a few days or if high fever (higher than 102°F) or shaking chills are noted, notify health care provider immediately.
- Advise patient to maintain normal fluid intake while using this medication.
- Remind diabetic patient to use enzyme-based tests (eg, *Clinistix* or *Testape*) for monitoring urine glucose because drug may give false results with other tests.
- Instruct patient to report these symptoms to health care provider: nausea, vomiting, diarrhea, skin rash, muscle or joint pain.
- Advise patient to report signs of superinfection: black "furry" tongue, white patches in mouth, foul-smelling stools, vaginal itching or discharge.
- Warn patient that diarrhea that contains blood or pus may be sign of serious disorders. Tell patient to seek medical care and not to treat at home.
- Instruct patient to seek emergency care immediately if wheezing or difficulty in breathing occurs.

Cetirizine
(seh-TEER-ih-zeen)
Class Antihistamine

How Supplied
Zyrtec Tablets 5 mg, Tablets 10 mg, Tablets, chewable 5 mg, Tablets, chewable 10 mg, Syrup 5 mg per 5 mL
✤ *Apo-Cetirizine* ♦ *Reactine*

Action
PHARMACOLOGY: Competitively antagonizes histamine at the H_1-receptor site.

PHARMACOKINETICS/DYNAMICS:
Absorption: Rapidly absorbed. T_{max} is about 1 hr. C_{max} is 311 ng/mL.
Food – T_{max} is delayed 1.7 hr, and C_{max} is decreased 23%.

Distribution: 93% protein bound.

Metabolism: Cetirizine has a low degree of first-pass metabolism. It also is metabolized by oxidative O-dealkylation to an inactive metabolite.

Excretion: 70% is excreted in the urine (50% as unchanged drug) and 10% in the feces. The t½ is 8.3 hr. Cl is about 53 mL/min.

Onset: 20 to 60 minute.

Duration: At least 24 hr.

Special Populations:
Renal Function Impairment –
Moderate impairment (Ccr 11 to 31 mL/min): The t½ is increased 3-fold, and Cl is decreased 70%. Dosage adjustment is recommended in those with moderate or severe impairment.
Hepatic Function Impairment – The t½ is increased 50%, and Cl is decreased 40%. Dosage adjustment is recommended.
Elderly – The t½ is prolonged 50%, and Cl is 40% lower. Dosage adjustment is recommended.
Children – Cl is increased, and t½ is decreased.

Indications Symptomatic relief of symptoms (eg, nasal, nonnasal) associated with seasonal and perennial allergic rhinitis; treatment of uncomplicated skin manifestations of chronic idiopathic urticaria.

Contraindications Hypersensitivity to any components of the product or to hydroxyzine.

Route/Dosage

ADULTS AND CHILDREN 6 YR OF AGE AND OVER: **PO** 5 or 10 mg/day.

CHILDREN 2 TO 5 YR OF AGE: **PO** 2.5 mg once daily (max, 5 mg/day as 5 mg once daily or 2.5 mg q 12 hr).

CHILDREN 6 MO TO LESS THAN 2 YR OF AGE: **PO** 2.5 mg once daily. The dose in 12 to 23 mo of age may be increased to a max dose of 5 mg once daily or 2.5 mg q 12 hr.

ELDERLY (77 YEARS OF AGE AND OLDER): **PO** 5 mg/day.

Hepatic Impairment
PO 5 mg/day (do not administer to children younger than 6 yr of age with hepatic impairment).

Renal Impairment
CCR (11 TO 31 ML/MIN OR HEMODIALYSIS): **PO** 5 mg/day. (Do not administer to children younger than 6 yr of age with renal impairment.)

Interactions None well documented.

Lab Test Interferences May prevent or diminish otherwise positive reactions to skin tests.

Adverse Reactions

CV: Palpitations, tachycardia, hypertension, cardiac failure, syncope; severe hypotension (postmarketing).

CNS: Somnolence, headache (14%); fatigue (6%); dizziness (2%); paresthesia, confusion, hyperkinesia, hypertonia, migraine, tremor, vertigo, ataxia, dystonia, abnormal coordination, hyperesthesia, hypoesthesia, myelitis, paralysis, twitching, insomnia, sleep disorder, nervousness, depression, emotional lability, impaired concentration, anxiety, depersonalization, paroniria, abnormal thinking, agitation, amnesia, decreased libido, euphoria, dysphonia, ptosis (less than 2%); convulsions, hallucinations, orofacial dyskinesia, suicidal ideation (postmarketing).

DERM: Pruritus, dry skin, urticaria, acne, dermatitis, erythematous rash, increased sweating, alopecia, angioedema, furunculosis, bullous eruption, eczema, hyperkeratosis, hypertrichosis, photosensitivity reaction, maculopapular rash, seborrhea, purpura, skin disorder, skin nodule, photosensitivity toxic reaction (less than 2%).

EENT: Pharyngitis (6%); epistaxis (4%); visual field defect, earache, blindness, loss of accommodation, eye pain, conjunctivitis, xerophthalmia, glaucoma, ocular hemorrhage, tinnitus, deafness, sinusitis, nasal polyp, parosmia, ototoxicity, periorbital edema (less than 2%).

GI: Abdominal pain (6%); dry mouth (5%); nausea, diarrhea, vomiting (3%); anorexia, salivation, increased appetite, dyspepsia, flatulence, constipation, stomatitis, ulcerative stomatitis, aggravated tooth caries, tongue discoloration, tongue edema, gastritis, rectal hemorrhage, hemorrhoids, melena, eructation, enlarged abdomen, taste perversion, taste loss (less than 2%).

GU: Urinary retention, polyuria, cystitis, dysuria, UTI, hematuria, micturition frequency, urinary incontinence, dysmenorrhea, female breast pain, intermenstrual bleeding, leukorrhea, menorrhagia, vaginitis (less than 2%); glomerulonephritis (postmarketing).

HEMA: Hemolytic anemia, thrombocytopenia (postmarketing).

HEPA: Abnormal hepatic function (less than 2%); cholestasis, hepatitis (postmarketing).

METAB: Thirst, dehydration, diabetes mellitus, weight gain (less than 2%).

MUSC: Myalgia, arthralgia, arthrosis, arthritis, muscle weakness.

RESP: Coughing, epistaxis (4%); bronchospasm (3%); bronchitis, rhinitis, dyspnea, upper respiratory tract infection, hyperventilation, increased sputum, pneumonia, respiratory disorder (less than 2%).

OTHER: Flushing, edema (face, leg, peripheral, and generalized), lymphadenopathy, back pain, malaise, fever, asthenia, rigors, pain, chest pain, leg cramps, increased weight, pallor, hot flashes (less than 2%); anaphylaxis, stillbirth, suicide (postmarketing).

Precautions

Pregnancy: Category B.
Lactation: Excreted in breast milk.
Children: Safety and efficacy not established in children younger than 6 mo of age.

Renal function impairment: Dosage adjustment may be needed.
Hepatic function impairment: Dosage adjustment may be needed.

PATIENT CARE CONSIDERATIONS
Administration/Storage
- Do not administer to patient younger than 6 yr of age with renal or hepatic impairment.
- Administer prescribed dose without regard to meals. Administer with food if GI upset occurs.
- Administer chewable tablets with or without water.
- Measure and administer prescribed dose of syrup using dosing spoon, syringe, or cup.
- Store tablets, chewable tablets, and syrup at controlled room temperature (59° to 86°F). Syrup also can be stored in refrigerator (36° to 46°F). Keep container tightly closed.

Assessment/Interventions
- Obtain patient history, including drug history and any known allergies. Note hepatic impairment, renal impairment, or history of sensitivity to hydroxyzine.
- Ensure that daily dose does not exceed 5 mg in patient 77 yr of age or older.
- Ensure that daily dose does not exceed 5 mg in patient 6 yr of age or older with hepatic impairment, decreased renal function (Ccr less than 31 mL/min), or on hemodialysis.
- Assess patient for allergy symptoms (eg, rhinitis, nasal congestion, sneezing, itching, watery eyes, hives) before starting therapy, and periodically throughout therapy. Notify health care provider if symptoms do not improve or worsen.

Patient/Family Education
- Explain name, dose, action, and potential side effects of drug.
- Advise patient to take each dose without regard to meals but to take with food if stomach upset occurs.
- Advise patient or caregiver using syrup to measure and administer each dose using a dosing spoon, syringe, or cup.

Overdosage: Signs and Symptoms
Somnolence, restlessness, irritability, drowsiness.

- Advise patient using chewable tablet that tablet may be taken with or without water.
- Advise patient that if allergy symptoms are not controlled not to increase the dose of medication or frequency of use but to inform health care provider. Inform patient that larger doses or more frequent dosing does not increase effectiveness and may cause excessive drowsiness or other side effects.
- Caution patient not to take any OTC antihistamines while taking this medication unless advised by health care provider.
- Caution patient to avoid alcohol and other CNS depressants (eg, sedatives) while using this medication.
- Caution patient that drug may cause drowsiness and to use caution driving or performing other tasks requiring mental alertness until tolerance is determined.
- Advise patient that medication may cause sensitivity to sunlight and to avoid unnecessary exposure to UV light (sunlight, tanning booths) and to use sunscreen and wear protective clothing until tolerance is determined.
- Advise patient to take frequent sips of water, suck on ice chips or sugarless hard candy, or chew sugarless gum if dry mouth occurs.
- Advise patient having allergy skin testing not to take cetirizine for at least 4 days before the skin testing.
- Advise women to notify health care provider if pregnant, planning to become pregnant, or breastfeeding.
- Instruct patient to stop taking drug and report persistent dizziness or excessive drowsiness to health care provider.
- Caution patient not to take any prescription or OTC medications, herbal preparations, or dietary supplements unless advised by health care provider.

Cetuximab

(seh-TUCKS-ih-mab)

Class Antineoplastic/Monoclonal antibody

How Supplied
Erbitux Injection 100 mg (2 mg/mL)

Action
PHARMACOLOGY: Competitively inhibits binding of epidermal growth factor (EGF) to receptors, which blocks phosphorylation and activation of receptor-associated kinases, resulting in inhibition of cell growth.

PHARMACOKINETICS/DYNAMICS:

Absorption: C_{max} about 184 mcg/mL. Steady-state peak and trough values range from 168 to 235 mcg/mL and 41 to 85 mcg/mL, respectively.

Distribution: Vd is approximately 2 to 3 L/m^2.

Excretion: Mean t½ is about 114 hr. The elimination t½ is approximately 97 hr.

Indications Use alone and in combination

with irinotecan for treatment of EGF receptor expressing, metastatic colorectal carcinoma in patients intolerant or refractory to irinotecan.

Contraindications Standard considerations.

Route/Dosage

ADULTS: **IV** 400 mg/m^2 as an initial loading dose administered as a 120-min infusion (max rate of infusion, 5 mL/min). The weekly maintenance dose is 250 mg/m^2 infused over 60 min (max rate of infusion, 5 mL/min).

Dose Modification
ADULTS:

Infusion Reactions: **IV** Permanently reduce the infusion rate 50% in patients experiencing mild or moderate (grade 1 or 2) infusion reactions; permanently discontinue in patients experiencing severe (grade 3 or 4) infusion reactions.
Dermatologic Toxicity: **IV** If patient experiences severe acneform rash: First occurrence: Delay infusion 1 to 2 wk and, if improvement occurs, continue at 250 mg/m^2. Discontinue if no improvement. Second occurrence: Delay infusion 1 to 2 wk and, if improvement occurs, reduce dose to 200 mg/m^2. Discontinue if no improvement. Third occurrence: Delay infusion 1 to 2 wk and, if improvement occurs, reduce dose to 150 mg/m^2. Discontinue if no improvement. Fourth occurrence: Discontinue.

Interactions None well documented.

Lab Test Interferences None well documented.

Adverse Reactions Percentages for adverse reactions are for grades 1 to 4 toxicity with cetuximab monotherapy.
CNS: Headache (25%); insomnia (10%); depression (9%).
DERM: Acneform rash (90%); nail disorder (16%); pruritus (10%); alopecia, skin disorder (5%).
EENT: Conjunctivitis (7%).
GI: Nausea (29%); constipation, diarrhea (28%); abdominal pain, vomiting, anorexia (25%); stomatitis (11%); dyspepsia (7%).
HEMA/LYMPH: anemia (10%); leukopenia (1%).
METAB: Peripheral edema (10%); weight loss, dehydration (9%).
RENAL: Kidney failure (2%).
RESP: Dyspnea (20%); increased cough (10%); pulmonary embolus (1%).
OTHER: Asthenia/malaise (49%); fever (33%); infusion reaction (25%); pain (19%); infection, back pain (11%); sepsis (3%).

> **WARNING:**
> Severe infusion reactions, characterized by rapid onset of airway obstruction, urticaria, and hypotension, may occur in approximately 3% of patients and are rarely fatal. About 90% were associated with first infusion. Severe infusion reactions require immediate interruption of infusion and permanent discontinuation from treatment.

Precautions

Pregnancy: Category C.
Lactation: Undetermined.
Children: Safety and efficacy not established.
Hypersensitivity: Use with caution in patients hypersensitive to cetuximab, murine proteins, or any component of this product.
Dermatologic toxicity: Reactions including acneform rash, skin drying and fissuring, and inflammatory and infectious sequelae may occur.
Pulmonary toxicity: Interstitial lung disease has been reported.
Sun exposure: Because sunlight can exacerbate any skin reactions, patients should wear sunscreen and hats and limit sun exposure.

PATIENT CARE CONSIDERATIONS

Administration/Storage

- May be used alone or in combination with irinotecan.
- For IV infusion only. Not for IV bolus or push, intradermal, SC, IM, or intra-arterial administration.
- Follow institutional procedures for handling, administration, and disposal of anticancer drugs.
- Premedicate patient with antihistamine (eg, diphenhydramine IV) as ordered.
- Do not shake or dilute.
- Do not mix with any other medications.
- Do not administer if cloudiness or discoloration is noted. A small amount of white amorphous particulates is normal.
- Administer prescribed dose using syringe pump or infusion pump following manufacturer's recommendations.
- Administer with use of low protein binding 0.22 mcm in-line filter placed as proximal to the patient as possible.
- Administer initial loading dose by IV infusion over 120 min (max infusion rate, 5 mL/min).
- Administer weekly maintenance doses by IV infusion over 60 min (max infusion rate, 5 mL/min).
- Flush IV line with 0.9% saline solution at end of infusion.
- Discard unused portions of vial. Do not save any unused portions for future use.
- Store unopened vials in refrigerator (36° to

46°F). Do not freeze. Preparations of cetuximab in infusion containers are stable for up to 8 hr at controlled room temperature (68° to 77°F) or 12 hr if refrigerated (36° to 46°F). Discard any remaining solution in infusion container after 8 hr at controlled room temperature or after 12 hr if refrigerated.

Assessment/Interventions
- Obtain patient history, including drug history and any known allergies. Note hypersensitivity to murine proteins or previous infusion-related reaction to cetuximab.
- Ensure that patient who has experienced a severe reaction receives no further treatments with cetuximab.
- Ensure that premedication with IV antihistamine (eg, diphenhydramine) has been ordered for each infusion.
- Closely monitor patient during, and for 1 hr following, each infusion for signs and symptoms of infusion reaction (eg, bronchospasm, stridor, hoarseness, hives, hypotension). If noted and severe, immediately discontinue infusion, notify health care provider, and be prepared to treat appropriately (eg, epinephrine, corticosteroids, IV antihistamines, bronchodilators, oxygen).
- Ensure that slower infusion rates (50% reduction) and continued use of antihistamines is used in subsequent doses of cetuximab in patient who experienced mild to moderate infusion reaction during previous infusion.
- Monitor patient for dermatological toxicity (eg, acneform rash, skin drying and fissuring, inflammation, infection). Inform health care provider if noted. Be prepared to treat infectious sequelae with topical and/or oral antibiotics.
- Ensure that dosage adjustments are made for patient experiencing severe acneform rash following manufacturer's guidelines.
- Monitor patient for signs and symptoms of interstitial lung disease (eg, acute onset or worsening of pulmonary symptoms). Interrupt therapy if noted and inform health care provider.
- Ensure that women of childbearing potential are not pregnant or attempting to become pregnant.
- Assess patient for GI, CNS, and general body side effects. Report to health care provider if noted and significant.

Patient/Family Education
- Explain name, action, and potential side effects of drug.
- Advise patient, family, or caregiver that medication will be prepared and administered by health care provider in a health care setting.
- Review dosing schedule with patient, family, or caregiver.
- Advise patient, family, or caregiver to immediately report any of the following to health care provider: acne-like rash, skin drying or splitting, inflammation or infection; unexplained shortness or breath or difficulty breathing; fever.
- Advise patient, family, or caregiver to report any of the following to health care provider: persistent nausea, vomiting, diarrhea, or appetite loss; sores in mouth; persistent or worsening general body weakness or fatigue.
- Advise patient to avoid unnecessary exposure to sunlight or tanning lamps and to use sunscreen and wear protective clothing to reduce risk of worsening cetuximab-induced skin reactions.
- Caution women of childbearing potential to avoid becoming pregnant during therapy.
- Advise women to notify health care provider if pregnant, planning to become pregnant, or breastfeeding.
- Instruct patient not to take any prescription or OTC medications or dietary supplements unless advised by health care provider.
- Advise patient, family, or caregiver that frequent follow-up visits and laboratory tests will be required to monitor therapy and to keep appointments.

Cevimeline Hydrochloride

(seh-vih-MEH-leen)
Class Cholinergic agonist
How Supplied
Evoxac Gelatin capsules 30 mg

Action
PHARMACOLOGY: Cevimeline is a cholinergic agonist that binds to muscarinic receptors. Muscarinic agonists in sufficient dosage can increase secretion of exocrine glands, such as salivary and sweat glands, and increase tone of the smooth muscle in the GI and urinary tracts.

PHARMACOKINETICS/DYNAMICS:
Absorption: Cevimeline is rapidly absorbed. T_{max} is 1.5 to 2 hr. Food decreases the rate of absorption and C_{max} (by 17.3%).

Distribution: Vd is about 6 L/kg. Cevimeline is less than 20% protein bound. It is extensively bound to tissues.

Metabolism: Cevimeline is metabolized by CYP2D6 and CYP3A3/4.

Excretion: After 24 hr, 84% is excreted in the urine (16% as unchanged drug). The t½ is about 5 hr.

Indications Relieves dry mouth in patients with Sjogren syndrome.

Contraindications Patients with uncontrolled asthma, hypersensitivity to cevimeline, or any condition in which miosis could be harmful (eg, acute iritis, narrow-angle glaucoma).

Route/Dosage
Dry Mouth with Sjogren Syndrome
ADULTS: PO 30 mg tid.

Dosage Adjustments
ADULTS: PO Because cevimeline is eliminated extensively in the urine, dosage adjustments may be required for patients with severe renal failure. However, specific recommendations are not established.

Interactions
Anticholinergic medications (eg, atropine, ipratropium bromide, phenothiazines, tricyclic antidepressants): Cevimeline antagonizes the pharmacologic effects of these medications.
Beta-adrenergic blockers (eg, levobunolol): Cardiac conduction disturbances possible. Use caution during concomitant therapy.
CYP450 system: Drugs that inhibit CYP2D6 and CYP3A3/4 also inhibit the metabolism of cevimeline. Use with caution in individuals known or suspected to be deficient in CYP2D6.
Drugs that induce CYP3A3/4 (eg, aminoglutethimide, barbiturates, carbamazepine, dexamethasone, griseofulvin, modafinil, nafcillin, phenytoin, primidone, rifabutin, rifampin): Increased cevimeline metabolism; reduced cevimeline concentrations and efficacy possible.
Drugs that inhibit CYP2D6 (eg, amiodarone, fluoxetine, paroxetine, quinidine, ritonavir) or CYP3A3/4 (eg, diltiazem, erythromycin, itraconazole, ketoconazole, verapamil): Reduced cevimeline metabolism; increased cevimeline concentrations and toxicity possible.
Food: Absorption of cevimeline is decreased when administered with food.
Parasympathomimetics (eg, bethanecol, donepezil, galantamine, neostigmine, physostigmine, pilocarpine, pyridostigmine, rivastigmine, tacrine): Additive pharmacologic effects and increased toxicity possible.

Lab Test Interferences None well documented.

PATIENT CARE CONSIDERATIONS
Administration/Storage
- Store at room temperature.
- Administer PO.
- May be taken with or without food. However, food reduces cevimeline absorption.

Adverse Reactions
CNS: Dizziness; fatigue.
DERM: Excessive sweating.
GI: Nausea; vomiting; diarrhea; dyspepsia.
GU: UTI.
MUSC: Back pain; arthralgia.
RESP: Sinusitis; upper respiratory tract infection; rhinitis; cough.
SPEC SENSE: Conjunctivitis; excessive salivation; blurred vision; decreased visual acuity; impaired depth perception.
OTHER: Drugs that inhibit CYP2D6 and CYP3A3/4 also inhibit the metabolism of cevimeline. Use with caution in individuals known or suspected to be deficient of CYP2D6 activity.

Precautions
Pregnancy: Category C.
Lactation: Undetermined.
Children: Safety and efficacy not established.
Elderly: Exercise special care when cevimeline treatment is initiated in an elderly patient, considering the greater frequency of decreased hepatic, renal, or cardiac function, and of concomitant disease or other drug therapy in the elderly.
Biliary tract: Administer with caution to patients with a history of nephrolithiasis.
CV: Cevimeline can potentially alter cardiac conduction or heart rate. Use with caution in patients with a history of CV disease evidenced by angina pectoris or MI.
Ocular: Ophthalmic formulations of muscarinic agonists have been reported to cause visual blurring that may result in decreased visual acuity (especially at night and in patients with central lens changes) and impairment of depth perception. Advise caution while driving at night or performing hazardous activities in reduced lighting.
Pulmonary: Cevimeline can potentially increase airway resistance, bronchial smooth muscle tone, and bronchial secretions. Administer with caution to patients with asthma, chronic bronchitis, or COPD.
Renal colic: Administer with caution to patients with a history of nephrolithiasis.

Overdosage: Signs and Symptoms
Headache, visual disturbance, lacrimation, sweating, respiratory distress, GI spasm, nausea, vomiting, diarrhea, AV block, tachycardia, bradycardia, hypotension, hypertension, shock, mental confusion, cardiac arrhythmia, and tremors.

Assessment/Interventions
- Obtain patient history, including drug history and any known allergies. Note history of asthma, COPD, significant cardiovascular disease, narrow angle glaucoma, nephrolithiasis, and cholelithiasis.

- Monitor patient for signs of improvement after therapy is started.
- Monitor patient for excessive parasympathomimetic, GI, RESP, CNS, and general body side effects. Notify health care provider if noted and significant.

Patient/Family Education
- Inform patient that cevimeline may cause visual disturbances, especially at night, that could impair their ability to drive safely.
- If a patient sweats excessively while taking cevimeline, consult health care provider and advise the patient to drink extra water as dehydration may develop.

Charcoal, activated

(CHAR-kole)

Class Antidote

How Supplied
Actidose-Aqua Liquid 208 mg/mL ♦ *Actidose with Sorbitol* Liquid 208 mg/mL ♦ *CharcoAid* Suspension 15 g, Suspension 30 g ♦ *CharcoAid 2000* Liquid 15 g, Liquid 50 g, Granules 15 g ♦ *Liqui-Char* Liquid 208 mg/mL
🌼 *Charcodote* ♦ *Charcodote Aqueous* ♦ *Charcodote TFS*

Action
PHARMACOLOGY: Inhibits GI absorption.

Indications Emergency treatment of poisoning by most drugs and chemicals. **Unlabeled use(s):** Treatment of diarrhea, stomach gas, and excessive flatulence.

Contraindications None known. Ineffective for poisonings by cyanide, mineral acids and alkalis. Not particularly effective for poisonings by ethanol, methanol, and iron salts.

Route/Dosage
Acute Intoxication
PO/Gavage tube 30 to 100 g (or 1 g/kg or about 5 to 10 times amount of poison ingested) as suspension (mixed with 6 to 8 oz water).

GI Dialysis
PO/Gavage tube 20 to 40 q 6 hr for 1 to 2 days; alternate aqueous suspension and sorbitol suspension.

Interactions
Food (eg, milk, ice cream, sherbet): Decrease the absorptive capacity of drug.
Other medications: May have decreased effectiveness because of absorption by activated charcoal (eg, oral acetylcysteine used as antidote for acetaminophen overdose).
Syrup of ipecac: Inactivated because of absorption by activated charcoal. Do not administer together.

Lab Test Interferences None well documented.

Adverse Reactions
GI: Vomiting; constipation or diarrhea; black stools. Sorbitol may cause loose stools and vomiting.

Precautions
Pregnancy: Pregnancy category undetermined.
Lactation: Undetermined.
Children: Use under health care provider's supervision so fluid and electrolyte balance can be monitored properly.

PATIENT CARE CONSIDERATIONS

Administration/Storage
- When inducing vomiting, do so before giving activated charcoal. When large doses of drugs have been ingested, remove as much of ingested poison as possible by gastric lavage.
- Note that patient may be intolerant of activated charcoal for 1 to 2 hr after ipecac-induced vomiting.
- Administer orally to conscious patients only.
- For comatose patients or patients with altered mental status, administer via nasogastric tube.
- Mix 30 to 100 g as a slurry with 6 to 8 oz water or use premixed solution with 12.5 to 50 g in sorbitol suspension.
- In acute poisoning, administer as soon as possible. Drug is most effective when given within 30 min of poisoning.
- Store in tightly closed container. Premixed suspension can be stored for up to 1 yr.

Assessment/Interventions
- Obtain patient history, including drug history and any known allergies, and note which medications were ingested and amounts ingested, if syrup of ipecac was given and if ingested material was acidic.
- Obtain a toxicology screen of urine and serum.

- Assess and monitor vital signs and neurologic signs.
- Assess mental status and LOC.
- Monitor airway, ECG, and I&O.
- Observe for vomiting or diarrhea.
- Keep patient well hydrated.

Patient/Family Education
- This drug should not be used as antidote in home.
- Advise patient that stools will be black for several days.
- Advise patient that diarrhea may continue for 24 to 48 hr.

Chloral Hydrate

(KLOR-uhl HIGH-drate)
Class Sedative/Hypnotic/Nonbarbiturate

How Supplied
Aquachloral Supprettes Suppositories 324 mg, Suppositories 648 mg
❋ PMS-Chloral Hydrate

Action
PHARMACOLOGY: Exact mechanism is unknown; can produce mild CNS depression.
PHARMACOKINETICS/DYNAMICS:
Absorption: Readily absorbed.
Distribution: 35% to 41% protein bound (trichloroethanol). Excreted in breast milk.
Metabolism: Metabolized to trichloroethanol (active), which is then converted in liver and kidney to trichloroacetic acid (inactive).
Excretion: The t½ is 7 to 10 hr (trichloroethanol). Metabolites are excreted in urine and bile.

Indications Management of short-term insomnia; sedation; adjunctive to anesthesia, analgesia; prevention or suppression of alcohol withdrawal symptoms (rectal). **Unlabeled use(s):** Conscious sedation in pediatric dentistry.

Contraindications Hypersensitivity to chloral derivatives; severe renal or hepatic impairment; gastritis (oral forms); severe cardiac disease.

Route/Dosage
Insomnia
ADULTS: PO/PR 500 mg to 1 g 15 to 30 min before bedtime.
CHILDREN: PO/PR 50 mg/kg/day (up to 1 g per dose) for sleep.

Premedication
ADULTS: PO 500 mg to 1 g 30 min before surgery.

Sedation
ADULTS: PO 250 mg tid after meals.
CHILDREN: PO/PR 25 mg/kg/day; may be given in divided doses.

Dental Sedation
CHILDREN: 75 mg/kg; supplementation with nitrous oxide may provide better sedation than manufacturer's recommended dosage.

Interactions
Alcohol and other CNS depressants: May produce additive CNS depression.
Furosemide (IV): Administration within 24 hr of chloral hydrate may lead to diaphoresis, hot flashes, tachycardia, and hypertension.
Oral anticoagulants: Anticoagulant effects may be increased, especially during first 2 wk.
Phenytoin: May reduce effects of phenytoin.

Lab Test Interferences May cause false-positive urine glucose test results with *Benedict's* solution or cupric sulfide tablets (eg, *Clinitest*), but not with enzyme-based tests (eg, *Clinistix, Tes-tape*); altered urinary 17-ketosteroid values when using the Reddy, Jenkins, and Thorn procedure; false-positive phentolamine test results; results of fluorometric tests for urine catecholamines may be altered (do not administer chloral hydrate 48 hr before this test).

Adverse Reactions
CNS: Somnambulism; ataxia; dizziness; headache; "hangover" effect.
GI: Stomach pain; nausea; vomiting; diarrhea; flatulence; unpleasant taste in mouth.
HEMA: Leukopenia; eosinophilia.
RESP: Respiratory depression.
OTHER: Hypersensitivity (eg, rash, itching, erythema multiforme, fever).

Precautions
Pregnancy: Category C.
Lactation: Excreted in breast milk.
Tartrazine sensitivity: Some products contain tartrazine, which can cause allergic-type reactions in some individuals.
Acute intermittent porphyria: Attacks may be precipitated in susceptible patients.
Drug dependency: May be habit forming. Use with caution in patients with history of drug or alcohol addiction.
GI disorders: Avoid use in patients with esophagitis, gastritis or gastric or duodenal ulcers.
Skin/Mucous membrane irritation: Irritates skin and mucous membranes.

Overdosage: Signs and Symptoms
Stupor, coma, pinpoint pupils, hypotension, slow or rapid and shallow respirations, hypothermia, muscle flaccidity; also: nausea, vomiting, gastritis, hemorrhagic gastritis, and gastric necrosis caused by drug's corrosive action.

PATIENT CARE CONSIDERATIONS
Administration/Storage
- Administer syrup or capsules with full glass of water or fruit juice to help prevent GI or renal problems. Chilling of syrup may lessen its unpleasant taste.
- Store at room temperature in tightly closed, light-resistant container.

Assessment/Interventions
- Obtain patient history, including drug history and any known allergies. Note history of drug abuse; allergic or hypersensitivity responses to chloral hydrate, tartrazine, or aspirin; and history of cardiac or GI disease.
- Institute safety precautions (eg, use of siderails and having call bell within patient's reach).
- If signs of gastric, liver, or renal dysfunction occur, notify health care provider.
- Observe patient for signs of alertness and signs of psychologic or physical dependence.

Patient/Family Education
- Instruct patient to take medication exactly as prescribed. Warn that taking doses too close together could result in overdose. Omit missed doses.
- Inform patient that effects of medication may not be noted until after 48 hr.
- Advise that medication will be discontinued gradually to prevent withdrawal symptoms, including CNS excitation with tremor, anxiety, hallucinations or delirium.
- Instruct patient to report these symptoms to health care provider: visual changes, irregular heartbeats or palpitations, yellowing of skin or eyes, rash or unusual bleeding or bruising, abdominal pains or gastrointestinal problems.
- Advise patient that drug may cause drowsiness or dizziness and to use caution when driving or performing other tasks requiring mental alertness.
- Caution patient to avoid intake of alcoholic beverages and other CNS depressants such as barbiturates and narcotics.
- Instruct patient not to take otc medications without consulting health care provider.

Chlorambucil

(klor-AM-byoo-sill)

Class Alkylating agent/Nitrogen mustard

How Supplied
Leukeran Tablets 2 mg

Action
PHARMACOLOGY: Chlorambucil is a bifunctional alkylating agent of the nitrogen mustard type. A cell cycle nonspecific drug, chlorambucil interacts with cellular DNA to produce a cytotoxic cross-linkage.

PHARMACOKINETICS/DYNAMICS:
Absorption: Rapidly and completely absorbed. T_{max} is within 1 hr. C_{max} is about 1 mcg/mL.
Distribution: 99% protein bound (albumin). Crosses the placenta.
Metabolism: Rapidly and extensively metabolized in the liver to phenylacetic acid mustard (active).
Excretion: The t½ is 1.5 hr (chlorambucil) and 2.4 hr (phenylacetic acid mustard). 15% to 60% is excreted in urine after 24 hr (less than 1% as chlorambucil or phenylacetic acid mustard).

Indications
Chronic lymphatic leukemia; malignant lymphomas including lymphosarcoma, giant follicular lymphoma, and Hodgkin disease. **Unlabeled use(s):** Ovarian and testicular carcinoma, non-Hodgkin lymphoma, Waldenström macroglobulinemia.

Contraindications
Prior resistance or hypersensitivity.

Route/Dosage
Initial Treatment
ADULTS: **PO** 0.1 to 0.2 mg/kg/day (4 to 10 mg/day) for 3 to 6 wk. Hodgkin disease usually requires 0.2 mg/kg/day, whereas lymphomas or chronic lymphocytic leukemia usually require 0.1 mg/kg/day.

Maintenance
ADULTS: **PO** Doses should not exceed 0.1 mg/kg/day and may be as low as 0.03 mg/kg/day. Doses of 2 to 4 mg/day are typical.

Interactions
None well documented.

Lab Test Interferences
None well documented.

Adverse Reactions
CNS: Confusion; agitation; ataxia; hallucinations; tremors; muscular twitching; flaccid paresis; peripheral neuropathy; seizures; myoclonia.
DERM: Rash; urticaria; skin hypersensitivity (including rare reports of skin rash progressing to erythema multiforme, toxic epidermal necrolysis, and Stevens-Johnson syndrome).
GI: Nausea; vomiting; diarrhea; oral ulceration; mucositis.
GU: Sterile cystitis; reversible and permanent sterility.
HEMA: Bone marrow suppression; leukemia.
HEPA: Hepatotoxicity; jaundice.
HYPERSEN: Angioedema.
RESP: Interstitial pneumonia; pulmonary fibrosis.
OTHER: Acute myelogenous leukemia; drug fever; secondary malignancies.

> **WARNING:**
>
> *Bone marrow damage:* Chlorambucil can severely suppress bone marrow function.
>
> *Carcinogenesis:* Because of its carcinogenic properties, do not give to patients with conditions other than chronic lymphatic leukemia or malignant lymphomas.
>
> *Fertility:* Chlorambucil has caused chromatid or chromosome damage in men. Reversible and permanent sterility have occurred in men and women.
>
> *Mutagenicity and teratogenicity:* Probable in humans.

Precautions
Pregnancy: Category D.
Lactation: Undetermined.
Children: Safety and efficacy not established.
Elderly: Use with caution because of the greater frequency of decreased hepatic, renal, or cardiac function, and concomitant diseases or other drug therapy.
Chromosome damage: Chromosome or chromatid damage may occur.
Dermatologic: Skin rash progressing to erythema multiforme, toxic epidermal necrolysis, or Stevens-Johnson syndrome may occur.
Radiation and chemotherapy: Do not give a full dosage before 4 wk after a full course of radiation therapy or chemotherapy because of the vulnerability of the bone marrow to damage under these conditions.
Seizures: Rare, focal, or generalized seizures have occurred in adults and children at therapeutic daily doses, pulse dosing regimens, and in acute overdosage. Exercise caution when administering chlorambucil to patients with a history of seizure disorders, head trauma, or to patients receiving other potentially epileptogenic drugs.

Overdosage: Signs and Symptoms
Reversible pancytopenia, neurological toxicity ranging from agitated behavior and ataxia to multiple grand mal seizures.

PATIENT CARE CONSIDERATIONS
Administration/Storage
- Dose, frequency of administration, and duration of therapy vary with condition being treated and clinical situation.
- Diligently follow institutional and NIH procedures for handling, administration, and disposal of anticancer drugs.
- Prescribed dose may be given at one time.
- Administer without regard to meals but administer with food if GI upset occurs.
- Store tablets in refrigerator (36° to 46°F).

Assessment/Interventions
- Obtain patient history, including drug history and any known allergies. Note recent (within 4 wk) full course of radiation therapy or chemotherapy, hypersensitivity to other alkylating agents, nephrotic syndrome, history of seizure disorder or head trauma, concurrent therapy with potentially epileptogenic drugs.
- Ensure women of childbearing potential are not pregnant when therapy is initiated and are using effective contraception during treatment.
- Document total cumulative dose.
- Ensure hemoglobin levels, total and differential leukocyte counts, and quantitative platelet counts are determined before starting therapy and then weekly thereafter, and, during the first 3 to 6 wk of therapy, perform WBC 3 to 4 days after each of the weekly complete blood counts.
- Ensure dose is reduced when an abrupt fall in WBC is noted.
- Ensure that reduced dose is administered during first 4 wk following full course of radiation therapy or chemotherapy, or if pretherapy leukocyte or platelet counts are depressed from bone marrow disease process prior to institution of therapy.
- Ensure that daily dose does not exceed 0.1 mg/kg in patient with confirmed hypoplastic bone marrow or bone marrow infiltration.
- Implement infection control measures if WBC drops; implement bleeding precautions if platelet count drops.
- Monitor patient for signs of anaphylactic or serious allergic reactions. Discontinue therapy and immediately notify health care provider if noted. Be prepared to treat appropriately.
- Monitor patient for CNS, GI, DERM, and general body side effects. Report to health care provider if noted and significant.
- Monitor patient for signs and symptoms of bacterial, viral, or fungal infection. Report to health care provider immediately if noted.

Patient/Family Education
- Explain name, action, and potential side effects of the treatment regimen. Review the treatment regimen including dosing schedule, duration of treatment, and monitoring that will be required.
- Review benefits of therapy and risks, including potential infertility, leukemia, or secondary malignancies.
- Advise patient, family, or caregiver to immediately report any of the following to health

care provider: skin rash; difficulty breathing; fever, chills, or other signs of infection; bleeding or unusual or bruising; seizures; yellow discoloration of skin or eyes; unusual lumps or masses.
- Advise patient, family, or caregiver to report any of the following to health care provider: persistent nausea, vomiting, or diarrhea; persistent cough; loss of menstruation.
- Instruct patient not to take any prescription or OTC medications, herbal preparations, or dietary supplements unless advised by health care provider.
- Caution women of childbearing potential to avoid becoming pregnant during therapy.
- Advise women of childbearing potential to notify health care provider if pregnant, planning to become pregnant, or breastfeeding.
- Advise men that therapy may temporarily or permanently impair their fertility.
- Advise patient, family, or caregiver that follow-up visits and laboratory tests will be required to monitor therapy and to keep appointments.

Chloramphenicol

(KLOR-am-FEN-ih-kahl)

Class Antibiotic

How Supplied
Chloromycetin Sodium Succinate Powder for Injection 100 mg/mL (as base) when reconstituted
✤ *Pentamycetin*

Action
PHARMACOLOGY: Interferes with or inhibits microbial protein synthesis.

PHARMACOKINETICS/DYNAMICS:
Absorption:
Oral – Chloramphenicol is rapidly absorbed and 75% to 90% bioavailable. C_{max} is 11.2 mcg/mL. T_{max} is 1 hr. Therapeutic concentrations are 10 to 20 mcg/mL (peak) and 5 to 10 mcg/mL (trough).

Distribution: Chloramphenicol diffuses rapidly; highest concentrations are found in the liver and kidney and lowest concentrations are found in the brain and CSF. It also is found in pleural and ascitic fluid, saliva, milk, and aqueous and vitreous humors. It crosses the placenta and is about 60% protein bound.

Metabolism: Chloramphenicol or sodium succinate is hydrolyzed to active chloramphenicol base.

Excretion: 68% to 99% is excreted in the urine. 8% to 12% is excreted as free chloramphenicol; the remainder is excreted as inactive metabolites. Small amounts are found in bile and feces. The t½ is about 1.5 to 4 hr.

Special Populations:
Renal Function Impairment – Metabolism and excretion may be reduced. Dosage adjustment is recommended.
Hepatic Function Impairment – Metabolism and excretion may be reduced. Dosage adjustment is recommended.

Indications Treatment of infections caused by susceptible strains of specific microorganisms; serious systemic infections for which less potentially dangerous drugs are ineffective or contraindicated.

Contraindications Trivial infections (eg, colds, influenza, throat infections) or infections other than indicated; prophylaxis of systemic bacterial infections; hypersensitivity to product.

Route/Dosage
Systemic Infections
ADULTS: **IV** 50 mg/kg/day in divided doses q 6 hr; may require up to 100 mg/kg/day initially for infections caused by moderately resistant organisms.
CHILDREN: **IV** 50 mg/kg/day in 4 doses q 6 hr; 50 to 100 mg/kg/day for severe infections (eg, bacteremia, meningitis).
INFANTS AND CHILDREN WITH IMMATURE METABOLIC PROCESSES: **IV** 25 mg/kg/day.
NEWBORNS: **IV** Usually 25 mg/kg/day in 4 doses q 6 hr.
NEWBORNS OVER 14 DAYS (OVER 2 KG): **IV** up to 50 mg/kg/day in 4 doses q 6 hr.
NEWBORNS UNDER 2 KG AND BIRTH TO 14 DAYS (OVER 2 KG): **IV** 25 mg/kg qd.

Interactions
Agents that suppress bone marrow: Risk or severity of bone marrow suppression may be increased.
Anticoagulants: May enhance anticoagulation action.
Barbiturates: May reduce effectiveness of chloramphenicol while barbiturate effects may be enhanced; effects may last days after barbiturates are withdrawn.
Ferrous salts: May increase serum iron levels.
Hydantoins (eg, phenytoin): May increase serum hydantoin levels, with possible toxicity; chloramphenicol levels may increase or decrease.
Rifampin: May reduce chloramphenicol serum levels; effect may last days after rifampin is withdrawn.
Sulfonylureas: May cause clinical manifestations of hypoglycemia.

Vitamin B$_{12}$: May decrease hematologic effects of vitamin B$_{12}$ in patients with pernicious anemia.

Lab Test Interferences None well documented.

Adverse Reactions

CNS: Headache; mental confusion; delirium; mild depression; optic neuritis; peripheral neuritis.

GI: Diarrhea; nausea; vomiting; glossitis; stomatitis; enterocolitis.

HEMA: Bone marrow depression; aplastic anemia; hypoplastic anemia; thrombocytopenia; granulocytopenia.

OTHER: Hypersensitivity reactions (eg, fever, rash, angioedema, urticaria, anaphylaxis); Gray syndrome.

> **WARNING:**
> Probably mutagenic and teratogenic in humans.

Precautions

Pregnancy: Category C.
Lactation: Excreted in breast milk.
Children: Use drug with caution and in reduced dosages in premature and term infants and children with immature metabolic functions to avoid Gray syndrome toxicity (eg, toxic and potentially fatal reaction in premature infants and newborns). Symptoms of Gray syndrome generally appear in this sequence: abdominal distention with or without emesis; progressive pallid cyanosis; vasomotor collapse, frequently accompanied by irregular respiration; death within a few hours of onset (death occurs in 40% of patients within 2 days of initial symptoms). Other initial symptoms of Gray syndrome may include refusal to suck, loose green stools, flaccidity, ashen gray color, decreased temperature, and refractory lactic acidosis.

Renal function impairment: Excessive blood levels of drug may occur; dosage adjustment may be required.

Hepatic function impairment: Excessive blood levels of drug may occur; dosage adjustment may be required. Pre-existing liver dysfunction may be significant risk factor for Gray syndrome.

Special risk patients: Use drug with caution in patients with acute intermittent porphyria or G-6-PD deficiency.

Superinfection: Use of antibiotics may result in bacterial or fungal overgrowth.

Blood dyscrasias: Serious and fatal blood dyscrasias can occur.

Overdosage: Signs and Symptoms

Nausea, vomiting, unpleasant taste, diarrhea, bone marrow suppression.

PATIENT CARE CONSIDERATIONS

Administration/Storage

- For IV use only; it is less effective when given via IM route.
- Give direct IV as 10% solution in water for injection or 5% dextrose injection over at least 1 min. Do not administer if cloudy.
- Substitute oral dosage form of another appropriate antibiotic as soon as possible.

Assessment/Interventions

- Obtain patient history, including drug history and any known allergies. Note any renal or hepatic impairment.
- Determine baseline of infectious state: measure temperature; assess vital signs; examine appearance of wound, eye, ear, urine, and stool; perform blood studies.
- Confirm diagnosis from cultures prior to administration of drug.
- Determine baseline CBC and platelet count and monitor q 2 days.
- Avoid concurrent therapy with other drugs that suppress bone marrow.
- Avoid repeat course of therapy if possible.
- Monitor serum levels of medication weekly. Therapeutic level peak is 10 to 20 mcg/mL; if level is higher, notify health care provider.
- If signs of anemia, leukopenia, reticulocytopenia, or thrombocytopenia develop, notify health care provider.
- Observe patient daily for signs of bone marrow depression (eg, fatigue, sore throat, bleeding, aplastic anemia, hypoplastic anemia, thrombocytopenia, agranulocytosis) and Gray syndrome in infants.
- Discontinue drug at first sign of hematologic disorders attributable to chloramphenicol.

Patient/Family Education

- Emphasize importance of follow-up examinations because of possible complications from drug that can occur up to months after therapy is completed.
- Instruct patient that bitter taste that occurs after IV administration will subside 2 to 3 min after injection.
- Instruct patient to report these symptoms to health care provider: bleeding, fever, sore throat, itching, nausea, vomiting, diarrhea, bruising, numbness, weakness of hands or feet.
- Advise parents to report these symptoms to health care provider if they occur in infants:

failure to feed, abdominal distention, drowsiness, blue or gray skin color, any problems in breathing.

- Instruct patient to report signs of further infection or worsening of current infection to health care provider.

Chlordiazepoxide

(klor-DIE-aze-ee-POX-ide)
Class Antianxiety/Benzodiazepine

How Supplied
Librium Capsules 5 mg, Capsules 10 mg, Capsules 25 mg, Powder for Injection 100 mg
✦ *Apo-Chlordiazepoxide*

Action
PHARMACOLOGY: Potentiates action of GABA to produce CNS depression.

PHARMACOKINETICS/DYNAMICS:
Absorption: T_{max} is 0.5 to 4 hr.
Distribution: 96% protein bound.
Metabolism: Metabolized in the liver to the major metabolite desmethylchlordiazepoxide and to several inactive intermediate metabolites.
Excretion: The t½ is 5 to 30 hr. Excreted in the urine, with 1% to 2% as unchanged drug and 3% to 6% as a conjugate.

Indications
Management of anxiety disorders; relief of acute alcohol withdrawal symptoms; relief of preoperative apprehension and anxiety.
Unlabeled use(s): Treatment of irritable bowel syndrome.

Contraindications
Hypersensitivity to benzodiazepines; psychoses; acute narrow-angle glaucoma; shock; coma.

Route/Dosage
Individualize dosage. Acute symptoms may be rapidly controlled IM or IV, with subsequent oral treatment (max, 300 mg/day).
CHILDREN OVER 6 YR: **PO** 5 mg bid to qid; may be increased to 10 mg bid to tid.
CHILDREN OVER 12 YR: **IM** 25 to 50 mg

Mild to Moderate Anxiety
ADULTS: **PO** 5 to 10 mg tid or qid.

Severe Anxiety
ADULTS: **PO** 20 to 25 mg tid or qid.
Initial dose: **IM/IV** 50 to 100 mg, then 25 to 50 mg tid or qid.
ELDERLY OR DEBILITATED PATIENTS: **PO** 5 mg bid to qid. **IM/IV** 25 to 50 mg.

Preoperative Apprehension/Anxiety
ADULTS: **PO** 5 to 10 mg tid or qid on days preceding surgery. **IM** 50 to 100 mg 1 hr prior to surgery.

Acute Alcohol Withdrawal
ADULTS: **IM/IV** 50 to 100 mg; repeat q 2 to 4 hr prn. **PO** 50 to 100 mg, repeat prn (max oral or parenteral dose is 300 mg/day).

Interactions
Alcohol and CNS depressants: Additive CNS depressant effects are possible.
Azole antifungal agents (eg, itraconazole, ketoconazole), fluvoxamine, isoniazid, nefazodone, protease inhibitors (eg, indinavir): May increase chlordiazepoxide plasma concentrations.
Cigarette smoking, theophyllines: May antagonize sedative effects.
Cimetidine, oral contraceptives, disulfiram, omeprazole: May increase effects of chlordiazepoxide with excessive sedation and impaired psychomotor function.
Digoxin: May increase serum digoxin concentrations.
Rifamycins: May decrease chlordiazepoxide plasma concentrations.

Lab Test Interferences
None well documented.

Adverse Reactions
CV: CV collapse; hypotension; hypertension; tachycardia; bradycardia; edema; phlebitis or thrombosis at IV sites.
CNS: Drowsiness; confusion; ataxia; dizziness; fatigue; apathy; memory impairment; disorientation; anterograde amnesia; restlessness; headache; slurred speech; loss of voice; stupor; coma; euphoria; irritability; vivid dreams; psychomotor retardation; paradoxical reactions (eg, anger, hostility, mania, insomnia, muscle spasms); syncope; extrapyramidal symptoms.
DERM: Rash.
EENT: Visual or auditory disturbances; depressed hearing; blurred vision.
GI: Constipation; diarrhea; dry mouth; coated tongue; nausea; anorexia; vomiting.
GU: Menstrual irregularities; increase or decrease in libido.
HEMA: Blood dyscrasias including agranulocytosis; anemia; thrombocytopenia; leukopenia; neutropenia.
HEPA: Abnormal LFTs; hepatic dysfunction including hepatitis and jaundice.
OTHER: Dependency/withdrawal syndrome.

Precautions
Pregnancy: Category D. Avoid especially in first trimester because of possible increased risk of congenital malformations.
Lactation: Excreted in breast milk.
Children: Initial dose should be small and gradually increased. Oral form not recommended in children under 6 yr; parenteral form not recommended in children under 12 yr.
Elderly: Initial dose should be small and gradu-

ally increased. Use with caution in patients with limited pulmonary reserve.
Renal function impairment: Observe caution to avoid accumulation of drug.
Hepatic function impairment: Observe caution to avoid accumulation of drug.
Debilitated patients: Initial dose should be small and gradually increased. Use with caution in patients with limited pulmonary reserve.
Drug dependency: Prolonged use can lead to dependency. Withdrawal syndrome has occurred within 4 to 6 wk of treatment, especially if drug is abruptly discontinued. For discontinuation after long-term treatment, use caution and taper dosage.

Psychiatric disorders: Not intended for patients with primary depressive disorder, psychosis, or disorders in which anxiety is not prominent.
Parenteral administration: Reserved primarily for acute states.
Suicide: Use with caution in patients with suicidal tendencies; do not allow access to large quantities of drug.

Overdosage: Signs and Symptoms
Drowsiness, confusion, somnolence, impaired coordination, diminished reflexes, lethargy, ataxia, hypotonia, hypotension, hypnosis, coma, death.

PATIENT CARE CONSIDERATIONS
Administration/Storage
- Administer prescribed dose without regard to meals but administer with food if GI upset occurs.
- Store capsules and powder for injection at controlled room temperature (59° to 86°F).
- Do not exceed 300 mg in any 24-hr period.

Injection:
- For IM or IV administration only. Not for intradermal, SC, or intra-arterial administration.
- Reconstitute powder for injection immediately before administration. Do not administer if particulate matter, cloudiness, or discoloration noted. Discard any unused solution. Do not save for future use.
- For IM administration, reconstitute powder for injection using supplied special diluent and following manufacturer's guidelines. Do not use diluent if it is opalescent or hazy.
- Administer deep IM injection slowly into upper outer quadrant of gluteus muscle.
- Do not administer solution prepared with IM diluent via IV route because of bubbles that form during reconstitution.
- For IV administration reconstitute powder for injection using 5 mL sterile normal saline for injection or sterile water for injection.
- Administer IV injection slowly over 1 min.
- Do not administer solution prepared for IV injection via IM route because of pain on injection.

Assessment/Interventions
- Obtain patient history, including drug history and any known allergies. Note hepatic or renal impairment, pulmonary disease, depression, psychosis, suicidal tendency, seizure disorder, history of drug abuse or sensitivity to other benzodiazepines, or concurrent use of other psychotropic medications or CNS depressants.
- Ensure that reduced dose and slower dose escalation is used in elderly patient or patient with debilitating disease.
- Ensure that women of childbearing potential are not pregnant when therapy is initiated.
- Closely observe patient who has received parenteral therapy for at least 3 hr, preferably at bed rest. Use side rails and be prepared to assist patient with ambulation if necessary.
- Ensure that CBC with differential and liver enzymes are evaluated periodically in patient on prolonged therapy.
- Frequently assess patient for response to treatment. Notify health care provider if condition does not appear to be improving or is worsening.
- Ensure that therapy is periodically reviewed to determine if therapy needs to be continued without change or if a dose change (eg, increase, decrease, discontinuation) is indicated.
- If treatment is to be discontinued, or the dose reduced, gradually taper the dose and monitor patient for withdrawal symptoms. If significant withdrawal symptoms develop (eg, increased anxiety, tremor, muscle or abdominal cramps, sweating) reinstitute previous dosing schedule and attempt a less rapid tapering regimen after patient has stabilized.
- Monitor patient for CNS, GI, psychiatric, and general body side effects and injection site reactions. Report to health care provider if noted and significant. Implement safety precautions if excessive drowsiness or dizziness occurs.

Injection:
- Ensure that a benzodiazepine-receptor antagonist (eg, flumazenil), oxygen, and resuscitation and intubation equipment are available when medication is administered by IV injection.

Patient/Family Education
- Explain name, dose, action, and potential side effects of drug.
- Advise patient or caregiver to read the *Patient Information* leaflet before starting therapy and with each refill.
- Advise patient that medication is usually started at a low dose and then gradually increased until maximum benefit is obtained.
- Caution patient that medication may be habit forming and to take as prescribed and not to stop taking or change the dose unless advised to do so by health care provider.
- Advise patient to take each dose without regard to meals but to take with food if stomach upset occurs.
- Advise patient that if a dose is missed to skip that dose and take the next dose at the regularly scheduled time. Caution patient to never take 2 doses at the same time.
- Advise patient that if medication needs to be discontinued it will be slowly withdrawn unless safety concerns (eg, rash) require a more rapid withdrawal.
- Instruct patient to avoid alcoholic beverages and other depressants while taking this medication.
- Advise patient with anxiety to take medication as needed and to seek alternative methods for controlling or preventing anxiety (eg, stress reduction, counseling).
- Instruct patient to contact health care provider if symptoms do not appear to be getting better, are getting worse, or if bothersome side effects (eg, drowsiness, memory impairment) occur.
- Advise patient that drug may cause drowsiness or impair judgment, thinking, or reflexes and to use caution while driving or performing other tasks requiring mental alertness until tolerance is determined.
- Advise women to notify health care provider if pregnant, planning to become pregnant, or breastfeeding.
- Warn patient not to take any prescription or OTC drugs or dietary supplements without consulting health care provider.
- Advise patient that follow-up visits and lab tests may be necessary to monitor therapy and to keep appointments.

Injection:
- Advise patient or caregiver that medication will be prepared by a health care provider and administered in a health care setting under close observation when oral therapy is not feasible.

Chlordiazepoxide/ Amitriptyline

(klor-DIE-aze-ee-POX-ide/am-ee-TRIP-tih-leen)

Class Psychotherapeutic combination

How Supplied
Limbitrol DS 10-25 Tablets 10 mg chlordiazepoxide and 25 mg amitriptyline

Action
PHARMACOLOGY: Amitriptyline blocks reuptake of serotonin and norepinephrine in CNS. Chlordiazepoxide potentiates effects of GABA in CNS.

Indications Treatment of moderate to severe depression associated with moderate to severe anxiety.

Contraindications Hypersensitivity to chlordiazepoxide or other benzodiazepines; hypersensitivity to amitriptyline or other tricyclic antidepressants; concomitant MAO inhibitor use; acute recovery phase of MI.

Route/Dosage
PO 1 tablet (10 mg chlordiazepoxide with 25 mg amitriptyline) tid or qid. May increase to 6 tablets daily if needed; some patients may respond to 1 tablet bid.

Interactions
Cimetidine, fluoxetine, haloperidol, phenothiazine antipsychotic compounds, oral contraceptives: May cause increased amitriptyline blood levels.
Cimetidine, oral contraceptives, disulfiram, fluoxetine, isoniazid, ketoconazole, metoprolol, propoxyphene, propranolol, valproic acid: May increase chlordiazepoxide effects.
Clonidine: May result in hypertensive crisis.
CNS depressants, alcohol: Depressant effects may be additive.
Digoxin: May increase digoxin serum levels.
Guanethidine: May diminish antihypertensive effects.
MAO inhibitors: May result in hypertensive crises, convulsions, and death.
Oral anticoagulants: May result in increased anticoagulant effect.

Lab Test Interferences None well documented.

Adverse Reactions
CV: Hypotension; hypertension; tachycardia; palpitations; MI; arrhythmias; heart block; ECG changes; stroke.
CNS: Hallucinations; hypomania; delusions; poor concentration; incoordination; tingling and paresthesias of extremities; extrapyramidal symptoms; syncope; changes in EEG patterns; dizzi-

ness; sedation; drowsiness; headache; lethargy; fatigue.
DERM: Rash; urticaria; photosensitivity; edema of face and tongue; pruritus.
EENT: Pupil dilation; blurred vision; nasal stuffiness; alteration in taste perception; parotid swelling.
GI: Nausea; epigastric distress; vomiting; anorexia; diarrhea; black tongue; bloating; dry mouth; constipation.
GU: Testicular swelling; decreased urinary frequency; menstrual irregularities; loss of bladder function; change in sex drive.
HEMA: Bone marrow depression including agranulocytosis; eosinophilia; purpura; thrombocytopenia.
HEPA: Jaundice; hepatic dysfunction; increased AST, ALT, alkaline phosphatase.
METAB: Elevation or depression of glucose levels.
RESP: Difficult breathing.
OTHER: Weight gain or loss; paradoxical sweating; gynecomastia; breast enlargement and galactorrhea (women); SIADH.

PATIENT CARE CONSIDERATIONS
Administration/Storage
* If patient has been taking MAO inhibitor, wait 2 wk before beginning limbitrol therapy. Cautiously begin treatment with reduced dosage.
* Therapy may begin with 1 tablet at bedtime with dosage titrated upward as tolerance to CNS depressant effect develops.
* Administer with food or water to reduce gastric irritation.
* Give larger portion of total daily dose at bedtime.
* Store in moisture-resistant container at room temperature.

Assessment/Interventions
* Obtain patient history, including drug history and any known allergies, especially to drug, amitriptyline or other benzodiazepines.
* Evaluate medical history for potential risk of drug or alcohol abuse or suicide.
* If elective surgery is planned, discontinue drug several days before surgical procedure.
* If patient is addiction-prone or suicidal, remain with patient while patient takes tablet. Observe for signs of hoarding.
* Closely monitor patients with history of hyperthyroidism or patients taking thyroid medication.

Precautions
Pregnancy: Pregnancy category undetermined.
Lactation: Excreted in breast milk.
Children: Not recommended in children under 12 yr.
Elderly: Unit dosage to smallest effective amount to decrease risk of ataxia, oversedation, confusion, or anticholinergic effects.
Special risk patients: Use with caution in patients with history of seizures, urinary retention, urethral spasm, angle-closure glaucoma or increased intraocular pressure, cardiovascular disorders and hepatic or renal impairment; hyperthyroid patients or those receiving thyroid medication; schizophrenic or paranoid patients.
Debilitated patients: Unit dosage to smallest effective amount to decrease risk of ataxia, oversedation, confusion, or anticholinergic effects.

Overdosage: Signs and Symptoms
Drowsiness, temporary confusion, visual hallucinations, hypothermia, tachycardia, arrhythmias, CHF, dilated pupils, convulsions, hypotension, stupor, coma, agitation, hyperactive reflexes, muscle rigidity, vomiting, hyperpyrexia.

* Monitor BP and pulse during initial therapy.
* If patient is undergoing long-term treatment, perform periodic blood counts and liver function studies.

Patient/Family Education
* Instruct patient to avoid intake of alcoholic beverages and other CNS depressants because additive effects can cause dangerous level of sedation and CNS depression.
* Advise patient that drug may cause drowsiness and to use caution while driving or performing other tasks requiring mental alertness.
* Instruct patient not to discontinue medication abruptly or change dosage without consulting with health care provider because withdrawal symptoms can occur.
* Caution patient to avoid excessive exposure to sunlight and to use sunscreen or wear protective clothing to avoid photosensitivity reaction.
* Advise patient that dry mouth may occur and that it may be relieved by taking sips of water frequently or sucking on hard sugarless candy or gum.
* Caution patient not to take any *otc* medications without consulting health care provider.

Chlorhexidine Gluconate

(klor-HEX-ih-deen GLUE-koe-nate)

Class Antiseptic/Germicide

How Supplied
Bactoshield Solution 4% with 4% isopropyl alcohol, Foam 4% with 4% isopropyl alcohol ♦ *Bactoshield 2* Solution 2% with 4% isopropyl alcohol ♦ *Betasept* Liquid 4% with 4% isopropyl alcohol ♦ *Dyna-Hex 2 Skin Cleanser* Liquid 2% with 4% isopropyl alcohol ♦ *Dyna-Hex Skin Cleanser* Liquid 4% with 4% isopropyl alcohol ♦ *Exidine-2 Scrub* Solution 2% with 4% isopropyl alcohol ♦ *Exidine-4 Scrub Care* Solution 4% with 4% isopropyl alcohol ♦ *Exidine Skin Cleanser* Liquid 4% with 4% isopropyl alcohol ♦ *Hibiclens* Sponge/Brush 4% with 4% isopropyl alcohol ♦ *Hibiclens Antiseptic/Antimicrobial Skin Cleanser* Liquid 4% with 4% isopropyl alcohol ♦ *Hibistat Germicidal Hand Rinse* Rinse 0.5% with 70% isopropanol and emollients ♦ *Hibistat Towelettes* Wipes 0.5% with 70% isopopranolol ♦ *Peridex* Oral Rinse 0.12% ♦ *PerioChip* Chip 2.5 mg ♦ *PerioGard* Oral Rinse 0.12%

❉ *Apo-Chlorhexidine*

Action
PHARMACOLOGY: Provides antimicrobial effect against a wide range of microorganisms.

Indications Surgical scrub; skin cleanser; preoperative skin preparation; skin wound cleanser; hand rinse; oral rinse for gingivitis; an adjunct to scaling and root planning procedures for reduction of pocket depth in adults with periodontitis. **Unlabeled use(s):** Treatment of acne vulgaris. Amelioration of oral mucositis associated with cytoreductive therapy for bone marrow transplant candidates.

Contraindications Standard considerations.

Route/Dosage

Skin Use
5 mL is applied to skin and worked into lather.

Periodontitis
2.5 mg (1 chip) inserted into periodonted pocket with probing depth at least 5 mm.

Oral Rinse for Gingivitis
15 mL (1 capful) bid for 30 sec, morning and evening after brushing teeth. Expectorate after rinsing; do not swallow.

Interactions None well documented.

Lab Test Interferences None well documented.

Adverse Reactions
DERM: Irritation; dermatitis; photosensitivity; sensitization and generalized allergic reactions, especially in genital area.
EENT: Deafness; transient parotitis; altered taste perception.
OTHER: Staining of teeth and oral surfaces; increased calculus formation; minor irritation and superficial desquamation of oral mucosa.

Precautions
Pregnancy: Category B (oral rinse). Pregnancy category undetermined for skin use.
Lactation: Undetermined.

Overdosage: Signs and Symptoms
Gastric distress, alcohol intoxication.

PATIENT CARE CONSIDERATIONS

Administration/Storage
- For surgical wash, scrub, or bacteriostatic cleansing: wet hands with warm water and squeeze 5 mL into palm, add water, work up lather, apply lather to area being cleansed, rinse thoroughly.
- For oral rinse: swish in mouth for 30 sec after brushing teeth and expectorate.
- For surgical hand scrub: wet hands and use nail cleaner under fingernails and to clean cuticles. Wet hands and forearms to elbows with warm water, apply lather, scrub for 3 min, and rinse thoroughly. Scrub for additional 3 min, rinse and dry hands and forearms with sterile towel.
- Keep medication out of ears, eyes, and mouth. Serious and permanent eye injury and deafness may occur if used improperly.
- Do not use this medication routinely on wounds involving more than superficial layers of skin.
- Avoid contact with meninges.
- Do not freeze.
- Store at room temperature (store *PerioChip* in the refrigerator).
- Prolonged direct exposure to strong light may cause brownish surface discoloration but does not affect action.
- Shake to disperse color.

Assessment/Interventions
- Obtain patient history, including drug history and any known allergies.
- Monitor for allergic reactions (eg, urticaria, bronchospasm, cough, shortness of breath).
- Monitor skin and mouth for irritation.

Patient/Family Education
- Inform patient that staining of teeth, dental work, tongue and oral tissue may occur. Staining does not adversely affect health and can usually be removed by professional techniques.

- Caution patient that taste perception may be altered during treatment; permanent taste alteration has not been noted.
- Inform patient that oral rinse contains alcohol.
- Instruct patient to avoid having medication come into contact with ears and eyes, which could cause permanent damage.
- Instruct patient not to swallow product but to expectorate after oral rinsing.
- Advise patient to avoid eating 2 to 3 hr after treatment.
- Advise patients to avoid dental floss at the site of chip insertion for 10 days after placement because flossing might dislodge the chip.
- Instruct patient to notify dentist promptly if chip dislodges.
- Advise patient that although mild to moderate sensitivity is normal during the first week after placement of the chip, notify dentist if pain, swelling, or other problems occur.

Chloroquine

(KLOR-oh-kwin)

Class Anti-infective/Antimalarial

How Supplied

Chloroquine Phosphate
Aralen Phosphate Tablets 500 mg (equivalent to 300 mg base)

Chloroquine Hydrochloride
Aralen Hydrochloride Injection 50 mg (equivalent to 40 mg base)/mL

 Aralen

Action

PHARMACOLOGY: Inhibits parasite growth, possibly by concentrating within parasite acid vesicles, raising pH.

PHARMACOKINETICS/DYNAMICS:

Absorption: Rapidly and almost completely absorbed from the GI tract.

Distribution: About 55% bound to nondiffusable plasma constituents. Distributed considerably into tissues (ie, liver, spleen, kidney, lung) and to a lesser extent into brain and spinal cord.

Metabolism: The main metabolite is desethylchloroquine.

Excretion: Slowly excreted, but increased by acidification of the urine. A small amount is excreted in the feces. About 25% of the dose is excreted in urine as desethylchloroquine. More than 50% of urinary drug product is unchanged chloroquine.

Indications Prophylaxis and treatment of acute attacks of malaria caused by *Plasmodium vivax, P. malariae, P. ovale*, and susceptible strains of *P. falciparum*; extraintestinal amebiasis.

Unlabeled use(s): Treatment of rheumatoid arthritis, systemic and discoid lupus erythematosus, porphyria cutanea tarda, scleroderma, pemphigus, lichen planus, polymyositis and sarcoidosis.

Contraindications Retinal or visual field changes.

Route/Dosage
Doses are listed in base equivalents. (Chloroquine phosphate, 500 mg equals 300 mg base; chloroquine hydrochloride, 50 mg equals 40 mg base.)

Acute Malaria
CHLOROQUINE PHOSPHATE:
Adults: PO Initial dose is 600 mg, then 300 mg 6 hr later and 300 mg qd for 2 days.
Children: PO Initial dose is 10 mg/kg, then 5 mg/kg 6 hr later and 5 mg/kg qd for 2 days.
CHLOROQUINE HYDROCHLORIDE:
Adults: IM Initial dose is 160 to 200 mg; repeat dose in 6 hr if needed (max, 800 mg base total dose in first 24 hr).
Children: 5 mg/kg/dose; repeat dose in 6 hr (max, 10 mg base/kg/24 hr; do not exceed 5 mg/kg as single parenteral dose).

Malaria Suppression
Adults – PO 300 mg base.
Children – 5 mg/kg/dose (max 300 mg base) weekly. Begin 1 to 2 wk prior to exposure and continue for 4 wk after leaving endemic area. If suppressive therapy is not begun prior to exposure, double initial loading dose and give in 2 divided doses 6 hr apart.

Extraintestinal Amebiasis
CHLOROQUINE PHOSPHATE:
Adults: PO 600 mg base/day for 2 days, then 300 mg base/day for 2 to 3 wk.
CHLOROQUINE HYDROCHLORIDE:
Adults: IM 4 to 5 mL (160 to 200 mg base)/day for 10 to 12 days.

Interactions
Cimetidine: May increase chloroquine serum concentration.
Kaolin aluminum or magnesium trisilicate antacids: May decrease GI absorption of chloroquine.
Rabies vaccine: Concomitant administration of intradermally administered rabies vaccine and chloroquine may result in diminished antibody response to vaccine. In this situation CDC recommends administering rabies vaccine IM.

Lab Test Interferences
None well documented.

Adverse Reactions
CV: Hypotension; ECG changes.
CNS: Headache; neuropathy; seizures; psychotic episodes.
DERM: Pruritus; pigment changes; skin eruptions.
EENT: Visual disturbances; retinal damage and deafness with prolonged high-dose use; tinnitus.
GI: Anorexia; nausea; vomiting; diarrhea; abdominal cramps.
HEMA: Agranulocytosis; blood dyscrasias; aplastic anemia.
HEPA: Hepatitis.
OTHER: Muscle weakness.

Precautions
Pregnancy: Category D.
Lactation: Excreted in breast milk.

PATIENT CARE CONSIDERATIONS

Administration/Storage
- Administer with food or milk.
- If taken once weekly, take on same day of week.
- Store in airtight, light-resistant container at room temperature.

Assessment/Interventions
- Obtain patient history, including drug history and any known allergies.
- Review history for blood disorders, eye or vision problems, G-6-PD deficiency, liver disease, alcoholism, porphyria, or psoriasis.
- Arrange for a complete eye examination to establish baseline values.
- Perform baseline assessment for signs and symptoms of infection.
- Provide small, frequent meals if GI distress occurs.
- Arrange for and monitor periodic CBCs.
- If sore throat, fever, weakness, fatigue, or unusual bleeding or bruising occurs, notify health care provider.
- Perform periodic neuromuscular examinations

Children: Especially sensitive to adverse effects; do not exceed recommended dose.
Special risk patients: Monitor patients with hepatic disease or alcoholism or taking other hepatotoxic medications for evidence of worsening liver function such as bleeding.
G-6-PD deficiency: May induce hemolysis in presence of infection or stressful condition.
Muscular weakness: May need to discontinue therapy if muscle weakness occurs.
Psoriasis or porphyria: May be exacerbated.
Retinopathy: Irreversible retinal damage has occurred.

Overdosage: Signs and Symptoms
Headache, drowsiness, visual disturbances, cardiovascular collapse, seizures, respiratory and cardiac arrest, death.

and notify patient if knee and ankle reflexes are weak.

Patient/Family Education
- Remind patient to take medication with food to minimize GI irritation.
- Stress importance of compliance with full course of therapy. If used for suppression, drug must be taken ≥ 1 wk before entering and for 4 wk after leaving endemic area.
- Caution patient to drink alcoholic beverages sparingly because of increased GI irritation and higher risk of liver damage.
- Stress importance of eye examinations q 3 to 6 mo during prolonged daily therapy.
- Inform patient that drug may cause rusty or brown discoloration of urine.
- Advise use of dark glasses in bright light to reduce risk of ocular damage.
- Instruct patient to report these symptoms to health care provider: blurring or change in vision, buzzing or difficulty hearing, muscle weakness, rash, vomiting or stomach pain, difficulty breathing or swallowing.

Chlorothiazide

(klor-oh-THIGH-uh-zide)

Class Thiazide diuretic

How Supplied
Diuril Tablets 250 mg, Tablets 500 mg, Oral Suspension 250 mg/5 mL, Powder for Injection, lyophilized 500 mg (as sodium) ♦ *Diurigen* Tablets 500 mg

Action
PHARMACOLOGY: Enhances excretion of sodium, chloride, and water by interfering with transport of sodium ions across renal tubular epithelium.

PHARMACOKINETICS/DYNAMICS:
Distribution: Chlorothiazide crosses the placenta but not the blood-brain barrier.

Metabolism: Chlorothiazide is not metabolized.

Excretion: Excreted by the kidney. Plasma t½ 45 to 120 min. Following IV administration, 96% is excreted unchanged in the urine within 23 hr.

Onset: Within 2 hr after oral administration; within 15 min after IV administration.

Peak: Approximately 4 hr after oral administration; approximately 30 min after IV administration.

Duration: Approximately 6 to 12 hr after oral administration.

Indications Adjunctive treatment in edema associated with CHF, hepatic cirrhosis, and corticosteroid and estrogen therapy; edema caused by various forms of renal dysfunction such as nephrotic syndrome, acute glomerulonephritis, and chronic renal failure (oral and IV); management of hypertension (oral).

Contraindications Anuria, hypersensitivity to sulfonamide-derived drugs or any component of this product.

Route/Dosage

Diuresis and Control of Hypertension
CHILDREN YOUNGER THAN 6 MO (SEE PRECAUTIONS): **PO** 30 mg/kg in 2 divided doses may be required.
CHILDREN 6 MO TO 2 YR (SEE PRECAUTIONS): **PO** 10 to 20 mg/kg/day in single or 2 divided doses (max, 375 mg/day).
CHILDREN 2 TO 12 YR (SEE PRECAUTIONS): **PO** 1 g/day.

Edema
ADULTS: **PO** 500 to 1000 mg qd or bid. Many patients respond to intermittent therapy (alternate day therapy or administration on 3 to 5 days each wk). **IV** Should be reserved for patients unable to take oral medication or for emergency situations. Individualize dosage according to patient response, using the smallest dosage necessary.

Hypertension
ADULTS: **PO** 500 to 1000 mg as a single or divided dose. Increase or decrease dose according to BP response. Rarely, some patients may require up to 2 g/day in divided doses.

Interactions

Alcohol, barbiturates, narcotics: May potentiate orthostatic hypotension.
Bile acid sequestrants: May reduce thiazide absorption; give thiazide at least 2 hr before bile acid sequestrants.
Diazoxide: May cause hyperglycemia.
Digitalis glycosides: Diuretic-induced hypokalemia and hypomagnesemia may precipitate digitalis-induced arrhythmias.
Lithium: May decrease renal excretion of lithium.
Loop diuretics: Synergistic effects may result in profound diuresis and serious electrolyte abnormalities.
Sulfonylureas, insulin: May decrease hypoglycemic effect of sulfonylureas. Because chlorothiazide may elevate blood glucose levels, may need to increase dosage of sulfonylureas or insulin.

Lab Test Interferences May produce false-negative results with the phentolamine and tyramine tests; may interfere with the phenolsulfonphthalein test because of decreased excretion; may cause diagnostic interference of serum electrolyte levels, blood and urine glucose levels, and a decrease in serum protein-bound iodine levels without signs of thyroid disturbance.

Adverse Reactions

CV: Hypotension; orthostatic hypotension.
CNS: Vertigo; paresthesia; dizziness; headache; restlessness.
DERM: Erythema multiforme (including Stevens-Johnson syndrome); exfoliative dermatitis (including toxic epidermal necrolysis); alopecia.
EENT: Transient blurred vision; xanthopsia.
GI: Pancreatitis; diarrhea; vomiting; sialoadenitis; cramping; constipation; gastric irritation; nausea; anorexia.
GU: Impotence.
HEPA: Jaundice (intrahepatic cholestatic).
HEMA/LYMPH: Aplastic anemia; agranulocytosis; leukopenia; hemolytic anemia; thrombocytopenia.
HYPERSEN: Anaphylactic reactions; necrotizing angiitis (vasculitis and cutaneous vasculitis); respiratory distress including pneumonitis and pulmonary edema; photosensitivity; fever; urticaria; rash; purpura.
METAB: Hyperglycemia; glycosuria; hyperuricemia.
MUSC: Weakness; muscle spasm.
RENAL: Renal failure; renal dysfunction; interstitial nephritis.

Precautions

Pregnancy: Category C.
Lactation: Excreted in breast milk.
Children: Safety and efficacy not established. Oral dosing recommendation is supported by empiric use in pediatric patients and published literature regarding the treatment of hypertension.
Hypersensitivity: May occur in patients with or without history of allergy or bronchial asthma; cross-sensitivity with sulfonamides also may occur.
Renal function impairment: Drug may precipitate azotemia; use drug with caution.
Hepatic function impairment: Minor alterations of fluid and electrolyte balance may precipitate hepatic coma; use with caution.
Diabetes mellitus: May become manifest.
Electrolytes: Increased urinary excretion of sodium, potassium, or magnesium may occur; decreased urinary excretion of calcium may occur.

Hyperuricemia: May occur or frank gout may be precipitated.
Lupus erythematosus: Exacerbation or activation may occur.
Postsympathectomy patients: Antihypertensive effects may be enhanced.

PATIENT CARE CONSIDERATIONS
Administration/Storage
- Store tablets and suspension at controlled room temperature (59° to 86°F). Protect from freezing. Store powder for injection in refrigerator (36° to 46°F) or at controlled room temperature.

Tablets and Suspension:
- Administer qd or bid as prescribed without regard to meals. Administer with food if GI upset occurs.
- Administer alone or in combination with other antihypertensives.
- Shake suspension well before measuring dose. Use dosing syringe, spoon, or cup to measure prescribed dose of suspension.

Injection:
- Administer by IV route only. Not for intradermal, SC, or IM administration.
- Reconstitute powder for injection following manufacturer's recommendations using sterile water for injection.
- Do not administer if particulate matter, cloudiness, or discoloration is noted.
- Administer by slow IV injection or IV infusion as ordered. Take special precautions to avoid extravasation.
- Discard any unused portion of vial. Do not save for future use.

Assessment/Interventions
- Obtain patient history, including drug history and any known allergies. Note liver or kidney disease, diabetes, lupus erythematosus, anuria, or allergy to sulfonamides.
- Ensure that serum electrolytes, BUN, creatinine, and uric acid are monitored periodically.
- Monitor and record BP and pulse. Should hypotension result, hold medication and notify health care provider.
- Take safety precautions if orthostatic hypotension occurs.
- Monitor blood sugar in diabetic patient when drug is started or dose is changed. Report significant changes to health care provider.
- Monitor patient for GI, CV, CNS, and general body side effects. Inform health care provider if paresthesia, weakness, fatigue, confusion, hypotension, tachycardia, or other significant effects are noted.

Overdosage: Signs and Symptoms
Electrolyte depletion (hypokalemia, hypochloremia, hyponatremia), dehydration; hypokalemia may accentuate cardiac arrhythmias if digitalis is being administered.

Patient/Family Education
- Explain name, dose, action, and potential side effects of drug.

Injection:
- Advise patient that medication will be prepared by a health care professional and administered in a health care setting.

Tablets and Suspension:
- Advise patient to take prescribed dose qd or bid without regard to meals but to take with food if stomach upset occurs.
- Advise patient or caregiver using suspension to shake well before measuring dose and to use dosing spoon, syringe, or cup to measure prescribed dose.
- Advise patient that medication will initially increase urination, but that this should go away after a few weeks of treatment.
- Advise patient if a dose is missed to skip that dose and take the next dose at the regularly scheduled time. Caution patient not to double the dose to catch up.
- Inform patient that drug controls but does not cure hypertension and to continue taking medication as prescribed even when BP is not elevated.
- Caution patient not to change the dose or stop taking unless advised by health care provider.
- Instruct patient to continue taking other BP medications as prescribed by health care provider.
- Instruct patient in BP and pulse measurement skills.
- Advise patient to monitor and record BP and pulse at home and to inform health care provider should abnormal measurements be noted. Also advise patient to take record of BP and pulse to each follow-up visit.
- Instruct patient to lie or sit down if experiencing dizziness or lightheadedness when standing.
- Caution patient that inadequate fluid intake, excessive perspiration, diarrhea, or vomiting can lead to excessive fall in BP, resulting in lightheadedness or fainting.

- Instruct diabetic patient to monitor blood glucose more frequently when drug is started or dose is changed and to inform health care provider of significant changes in readings.
- Caution patient to avoid unnecessary exposure to UV light (sunlight, tanning booths) and to use sunscreen and wear protective clothing when exposed to UV light until tolerance is determined.
- Emphasize to hypertensive patient importance of the following modalities on BP: weight control, regular exercise, smoking cessation, moderate intake of alcohol and salt.
- Advise women to notify health care provider if pregnant, planning to become pregnant, or breastfeeding.
- Instruct patient to inform health care provider if any of the following occur: muscle pain, weakness, or cramps; persistent nausea or vomiting; excessive thirst; unexplained tiredness; drowsiness; increased heart rate; unexplained joint pain; abnormal skin sensations.
- Caution patient not to take any prescription or OTC medications or dietary supplements unless advised by health care provider.
- Advise patient that follow-up visits and lab tests may be required to monitor therapy and to keep appointments.

Chlorpheniramine Maleate

(klor-fen-AIR-uh-meen MAL-ee-ate)

Class Antihistamine/Alkylamine

How Supplied
Aller-Chlor Tablets 4 mg, Syrup 2 mg/5 mL ◆ *Allergy* Tablets 4 mg ◆ *Chlo-Amine* Tablets, chewable 2 mg ◆ *Chlor-Trimeton Allergy 8 Hour* Tablets, extended-release 8 mg ◆ *Chlor-Trimeton Allergy 12 Hour* Tablets, extended-release 12 mg ◆ *Efidac 24* Tablet, extended-release 16 mg ❋ *Chlor-Tripolon*

Action
PHARMACOLOGY: Competitively antagonizes histamine at H_1 receptor sites.

PHARMACOKINETICS/DYNAMICS:
Absorption: Readily absorbed.
Distribution: 72% protein bound.
Metabolism: Metabolized predominantly in the liver, but also in the lung and kidneys.
Excretion: Renally eliminated, mostly as metabolites within 24 hr.

Indications
Temporary relief of sneezing, itchy, watery eyes, itchy nose or throat, and runny nose caused by hay fever (allergic) rhinitis or other respiratory allergies.

Contraindications
Hypersensitivity to antihistamines; narrow-angle glaucoma; stenosing peptic ulcer; symptomatic prostatic hypertrophy; asthmatic attack; bladder neck obstruction; pyloroduodenal obstruction; MAO therapy; use in newborn or premature infants and in nursing mothers.

Route/Dosage
Symptomatic Allergic Conditions
ADULTS AND CHILDREN OVER 12 YR: **PO** 4 mg q 4 to 6 hr (immediate-release form) or 8 to 12 mg at bedtime or q 8 to 12 hr (sustained-release form) (max, 24 mg/24 hr). *Efidac:* 16 mg q 24 hr (max, 16 mg/24 hr). **SC/IM/IV** 5 to 20 mg as single dose (max, 40 mg/24 hr).
CHILDREN 6 TO 12 YR: **PO** 2 mg q 4 to 6 hr (immediate-release form) or 8 mg at bedtime or during day as indicated (sustained-release form) (max, 12 mg/24 hr).
CHILDREN 2 TO 6 YR: **PO** (only tablet or syrup; sustained-release not recommended) 1 mg q 4 to 6 hr (max, 4 mg/24 hr).

Allergic Reactions to Blood or Plasma
ADULTS: **SC/IM/IV** 10 to 20 mg as single dose (max, 40 mg/24 hr).

Anaphylaxis
ADULTS: **IV** 10 to 20 mg as single dose.

Interactions
Alcohol and CNS depressants: May cause additive CNS depressant effects.
MAO Inhibitors: May increase anticholinergic effects of chlorpheniramine.

Lab Test Interferences
Skin testing procedures: Antihistamines may prevent or diminish otherwise positive reaction to dermal reactivity indicators.

Adverse Reactions
CV: Orthostatic hypotension; palpitations; bradycardia; tachycardia; reflex tachycardia; extrasystoles; faintness.
CNS: Drowsiness (often transient); sedation; dizziness; faintness; disturbed coordination; nervousness; restlessness.
GI: Dry mouth; epigastric distress; anorexia; nausea; vomiting; diarrhea; constipation; change in bowel habits.
GU: Urinary frequency or retention; dysuria.
HEMA: Hemolytic anemia; thrombocytopenia; agranulocytosis.
METAB: Increased appetite; weight gain.
RESP: Thickening of bronchial secretions; chest tightness; wheezing; nasal stuffiness; dry nose and throat; sore throat; respiratory depression.

OTHER: Hypersensitivity reactions; photosensitivity.

Precautions
Pregnancy: Category B. Do not use during third trimester.
Lactation: Contraindicated in nursing mothers.
Children: Overdosage may cause hallucinations, convulsions, and death. Antihistamines may diminish mental alertness. In young child, they may produce paradoxical excitation. Contraindicated in newborn or premature infants. Sustained-release form not recommended in children less than 6 yr.
Elderly: Greater likelihood of dizziness, excessive sedation, syncope, toxic confusional states and hypotension in patients greater than 60 yr. Dosage reduction may be required.

Hypersensitivity: May occur. Have epinephrine 1:1000 immediately available.
Hepatic function impairment: Use drug with caution in patients with cirrhosis or other liver disease.
Special risk patients: Use drug with caution in patients with predisposition to urinary retention, history of bronchial asthma, increased IOP, hyperthyroidism, cardiovascular disease, or hypertension. Avoid in patients with sleep apnea.
Respiratory disease: Generally not recommended to treat lower respiratory tract symptoms including asthma.

Overdosage: Signs and Symptoms
Diminished mental alertness, ataxia, hallucinations, convulsions, death.

PATIENT CARE CONSIDERATIONS
Administration/Storage
- Administer with food or milk to decrease GI upset.
- Instruct patient not to chew or crush sustained-release tablets; have patient swallow tablet whole.
- Instruct patient to chew chewable tablets and not to swallow tablet whole.
- Administer 10 mg/mL solution IV, IM, or SC.
- Administer 100 mg/mL solution IM or SC only; do not administer IV.
- Administer IV solution undiluted in 10 mg dose over at least 1 min.
- Store at room temperature. Protect syrup and injectable forms from light.

Assessment/Interventions
- Obtain patient history, including drug history and any known allergies.
- Note baseline vital signs and monitor throughout therapy.
- Monitor I&O. Note any urinary retention or problems with voiding.
- Notify health care provider if patient has history of asthma.
- If signs of allergy or difficulty breathing occur, notify health care provider.
- Monitor breath sounds and report abnormalities to health care provider.

Patient/Family Education
- Caution patient to avoid intake of alcoholic beverages or other CNS depressants.
- Instruct patient to notify health care provider if blurred vision occurs.
- Advise patient to use good oral hygiene, to take sips of water frequently, suck on ice chips or sugarless hard candy, or chew sugarless gum if dry mouth occurs.
- Advise patient that coadministration of MAO inhibitors may prolong and intensify effects of medication.
- Instruct patient to maintain adequate fluid intake to avoid thickening of respiratory secretions.
- Caution patient to avoid exposure to sunlight and to use sunscreen or wear protective clothing to avoid photosensitivity reaction.
- Advise patient that drug may cause drowsiness and to use caution while driving or performing other tasks requiring mental alertness.
- Advise patient to carry *Medi-Alert* identification noting allergic condition.

Chlorpheniramine Maleate/ Phenylephrine Hydrochloride/ Methscopolamine Nitrate

(klor-fen-AIR-uh-meen MAL-ee-ate/Fen-ill-EFF-rin HIGH-droe-KLOR-ide/meth-skoe-PAHL-uh-meen NYE-trate)

Class Antihistamine/Decongestant/Anticholinergic

How Supplied

AH-chew Tablets 10 mg phenylephrine, 2 mg chlorpheniramine, 1.25 mg methscopolamine ♦ *D.A. Chewable* Tablets 10 mg phenylephrine, 2 mg chlorpheniramine, 1.25 mg methscopolamine ♦ *Dallergy* Syrup 10 mg phenylephrine, 2 mg chlorpheniramine, 0.625 mg methscopolamine, Tablets 10 mg phenylephrine, 4 mg chlorpheniramine, 1.25 mg methscopolamine, Tablets 20 mg phenylephrine, 12 mg chlorpheniramine, 2.5 mg methscopolamine ♦ *Dehistine* Syrup 10 mg phenylephrine, 2 mg chlorpheniramine, 1.25 mg methscopolamine ♦ *DriHist SR* Tablets 20 mg phenylephrine, 8 mg chlorpheniramine, 2.5 mg methscopolamine ♦ *Duradryl* Syrup 10 mg phenylephrine, 2 mg chlorpheniramine, 1.25 mg methscopolamine ♦ *Ex-Histine* Syrup 10 mg phenylephrine, 2 mg chlorpheniramine, 1.25 mg methscopolamine ♦ *Extendryl* Chewable Tablets 10 mg phenylephrine, 2 mg chlorpheniramine, 1.25 mg methscopolamine, SR Capsules 20 mg phenylephrine, 8 mg chlorpheniramine, 2.5 mg methscopolamine, Syrup 10 mg phenylephrine, 2 mg chlorpheniramine, 1.25 mg methscopolamine ♦ *Hista-Vent DA* Tablets 20 mg phenylephrine, 8 mg chlorpheniramine, 2.5 mg methscopolamine ♦ *Omnihist L.A.* Tablets 20 mg phenylephrine, 8 mg chlorpheniramine, 2.5 mg methscopolamine ♦ *Pre-Hist-D* Tablets 20 mg phenylephrine, 8 mg chlorpheniramine, 2.5 mg methscopolamine

Action

PHARMACOLOGY:

Chlorpheniramine: Competitively antagonizes histamine at H_1 receptor sites.
Phenylephrine: Stimulates postsynaptic alpha-receptors, resulting in vasoconstriction, which reduces congestion.
Methscopolamine: Competitively inhibits action of acetylcholine at muscarinic receptors.

Indications Temporary relief of symptoms of allergic rhinitis, vasomotor rhinitis, sinusitis, and the common cold.

Contraindications Hypersensitivity or idiosyncratic reaction to any ingredients of product; severe hypertension; severe coronary artery disease; narrow-angle glaucoma; urinary retention; hyperthyroidism; peptic ulcer; asthma attack; MAO inhibitor therapy or for 2 wk after stopping MAO inhibitor therapy.

Route/Dosage

EXTENDED-RELEASE FORMULATIONS
ADULTS AND CHILDREN (12 YR AND OLDER): PO 1 tablet/capsule q 12 hr.
CHILDREN 6 TO 12 YR: PO ½ tablet/capsule q 12 hr.

CHEWABLE TABLETS
ADULTS AND CHILDREN (12 YR AND OLDER): PO 1 to 2 tablets q 4 hr.
CHILDREN 6 TO 12 YR: PO 1 tablet q 4 hr.
CHILDREN LESS THAN 6 YR: PO As recommended by health care provider.

SYRUP
ADULTS: PO 1 to 2 tsp (5 to 10 mL) q 3 to 4 hr.
CHILDREN 6 TO 12 YR: PO ½ to 1 tsp (2.5 to 5 mL), depending on weight of child; may repeat q 4 hr.
CHILDREN LESS THAN 6 YR: PO As recommended by health care provider.

PREHIST-D/HISTA-VENT DA
ADULTS AND CHILDREN 12 YR AND OLDER: PO 1 tablet q 12 hr.
CHILDREN 6 TO 12 YR: PO ½ tablet q 12 hr.

Interactions

Alcohol, barbiturates (eg, phenobarbital), tricyclic antidepressants (eg, amitriptyline), other CNS depressants: Effects may be enhanced by chlorpheniramine.
MAO inhibitors (eg, isocarboxazid): May prolong and intensify the effects of chlorpheniramine and increase the effects of phenylephrine.
Mecamylamine, methyldopa, reserpine, veratrum alkaloids: Antihypertensive effects may be reduced by phenylephrine.

Lab Test Interferences May interfere with diagnostic test results for skin tests using allergen extracts.

Adverse Reactions

CV:
Phenylephrine – Tachycardia; palpitations; arrhythmias; cardiovascular collapse; hypotension.
CNS:
Chlorpheniramine – Drowsiness; dizziness.
Phenylephrine – Nervousness; insomnia; restlessness; headache; fear; anxiety; tremor; weakness; insomnia; hallucinations; convulsions; CNS

depression; irritability; tenseness.
DERM:
Phenylephrine – Pallor.
EENT:
Chlorpheniramine – Blurred vision; nose, throat, and mouth dryness.
GI:
Phenylephrine – Gastric irritation and irritability.
GU:
Chlorpheniramine – Urinary retention.
Phenylephrine – Dysuria; urinary retention.
RESP:
Phenylephrine – Respiratory difficulty.

Precautions

Pregnancy: Category C.
Lactation: Undetermined.

Children: Safety and efficacy in children less than 6 yr not established. Antihistamines may cause excitability in children.
Elderly: Patients 60 yr and older more likely to exhibit adverse effects.
Special risk patients: Use with caution in patients with hypertension, heart disease, asthma, hyperthyroidism, increased IOP, diabetes mellitus, and prostatic hypertrophy.

Overdosage: Signs and Symptoms

Dry mouth, dilated pupils, hallucinations, severe hypertension, ventricular extrasystoles, short paroxysms of ventricular tachycardia, CNS depression, CNS stimulation, somnolence, convulsions, shock, death.

PATIENT CARE CONSIDERATIONS

Administration/Storage

Syrup:
- Give prescribed dose q 3 to 4 hr as needed.
- Give with food or milk if GI upset occurs.
- Use dosing spoon or syringe for pediatric doses of syrup.
- Store at controlled room temperature. Keep syrup tightly capped and protect from freezing.

Chewable tablets:
- Give prescribed dose q 4 hr as needed.
- Give with food or milk if GI upset occurs.
- Store at controlled room temperature (69° to 77°F).

Extended-release formulations:
- Give prescribed dose q 12 hr as needed.
- Caplets may be broken in half but should not be crushed or chewed.
- Give with food or milk if GI upset occurs.
- Store at controlled room temperature (69° to 77°F).

Assessment/Interventions

- Obtain patient history, including drug history and any known allergies. Note history of peptic ulcer disease, diabetes, hypertension, hyperthyroidism, enlarged prostate, asthma, narrow angle glaucoma, urinary retention, severe hypertension or coronary artery disease, or concurrent use of or within 2 wk of stopping MAO inhibitor therapy.
- Assess for allergy symptoms (eg, rhinitis, nasal congestion, sneezing, itching, watery eyes) before and periodically throughout therapy.
- Monitor children for antihistamine-induced excitability.
- Monitor pulse and BP periodically during therapy.
- Monitor patient for nervousness, dizziness, and insomnia. If noted, hold therapy and notify health care provider.

Patient/Family Education

- Explain name, dose, action, and potential side effects of drug.
- Review dosing schedule for prescribed dose form (eg, syrup, chewable tablet, extended-release tablet).
- Advise caregiver to use dosing spoon or syringe when giving syrup to children.
- Caution patient that extended-release tablet can be broken in half but that dose should be swallowed whole and not crushed or chewed.
- Advise patient to take with food or milk if GI upset occurs.
- Advise patient to take last dose late in the afternoon or early evening to reduce chance of drug causing sleeplessness.
- Advise patient that if a dose is missed to take as soon as remembered unless it is nearing time for the next dose. Caution patient to not double the dose to catch up.
- Advise patient that if allergy symptoms are not controlled, not to increase the dose of medication but to inform health care provider.
- Caution patient that drug may cause drowsiness and to use caution while driving or performing other tasks requiring mental alertness until tolerance is determined.
- Advise patient to avoid alcohol and other CNS depressants because of risk of excessive sedation.
- Caution patient not to take any OTC antihistamines or decongestants while taking this medication unless advised by health care provider.
- If patient is to have allergy skin testing, advise to not take the medication for at least 6 days before the skin testing.

- Advise women to notify health care provider if pregnant, planning to become pregnant, or breastfeeding.
- Instruct patient to stop taking drug and immediately report any of the following symptoms to health care provider: nervousness, dizziness, sleeplessness.
- Caution patient to not take any prescription or OTC medications or dietary supplements unless advised by health care provider.

Chlorpheniramine Maleate/ Pseudoephedrine Hydrochloride/Codeine Phosphate

(klor-fen-AIR-uh-meen MAL-ee-ate/SUE-doe-eh-FED-rin HIGH-droe-KLOR-ide/KOE-deen FOSS-fate)

Class Antihistamine/Decongestant/Antitussive

How Supplied
Decohistine DH Liquid 10 mg codeine phosphate, 2 mg chlorpheniramine maleate, 30 mg pseudoephedrine hydrochloride ◆ *Dihistine DH* Elixir 10 mg codeine phosphate, 2 mg chlorpheniramine maleate, 30 mg pseudoephedrine hydrochloride ◆ *Ryna-C* Liquid 10 mg codeine phosphate, 2 mg chlorpheniramine maleate, 30 mg pseudoephedrine hydrochloride

Action
PHARMACOLOGY:
Chlorpheniramine: Competitively antagonizes histamine at H_1 receptor sites.
Pseudoephedrine: Causes vasoconstriction and subsequent shrinkage of nasal mucous membranes by alpha-adrenergic stimulation, which promotes nasal drainage.
Codeine: Suppresses cough reflex.

Indications
Temporary relief of runny nose, sneezing, and itchy, watery eyes due to hay fever (allergic rhinitis); temporary relief of cough due to minor bronchial irritation and nasal congestion caused by common cold; temporary relief of sinus congestion and pressure.

Contraindications
Hypersensitivity or idiosyncratic reaction to any ingredients of product; severe hypertension; severe coronary artery disease; narrow-angle glaucoma; urinary retention; peptic ulcer; asthma attack; MAO inhibitor therapy or for 2 wk after stopping MAO inhibitor therapy.

Route/Dosage
ADULTS AND CHILDREN 12 YR AND OLDER: **PO** 2 tsp (10 mL) q 6 hr, not exceeding 4 doses/24 hr.
CHILDREN 6 TO UNDER 12 YR: **PO** 1 tsp (5 mL) q 6 hr, not exceeding 4 doses/24 hr.
CHILDREN LESS THEN 6 YR: Consult health care provider.

Interactions
Alcohol, barbiturates (eg, phenobarbital), tricyclic antidepressants (eg, amitriptyline), other CNS depressants: Effects may be enhanced by carbinoxamine.
MAO inhibitors (eg, isocarboxazid): May prolong and intensify the effects of chlorpheniramine and increase the effects of pseudoephedrine.
Mecamylamine, methyldopa, reserpine, veratrum alkaloids: Antihypertensive effects may be reduced by pseudoephedrine.

Lab Test Interferences May interfere with diagnostic test results for skin tests using allergen extracts.

Adverse Reactions
CV:
Pseudoephedrine – Cardiac arrhythmia; increased heart rate; increased BP.
CNS:
Chlorpheniramine – Sedation; dizziness; headache; nervousness; rare excitability in children.
Pseudoephedrine – Convulsions; CNS stimulation; hallucinations; tremors; nervousness; insomnia.
Codeine – Lightheadedness; disorientation; drowsiness; dizziness.
EENT:
Codeine – Miosis.
GI:
Chlorpheniramine – Vomiting; diarrhea; dry mouth; nausea; anorexia; heartburn.
Codeine – Nausea; vomiting; constipation; abdominal pain; anorexia; biliary tract spasm.
GU:
Chlorpheniramine – Polyuria; dysuria; urinary retention in patients with prostatic hypertrophy.
Pseudoephedrine – Dysuria.
RESP:
Pseudoephedrine – Respiratory difficulties.
OTHER:
Pseudoephedrine – Pallor.

Precautions
Pregnancy: Consult health care provider before use.
Lactation: Consult health care provider before use.
Special risk patients: Use with caution in patients with hypertension, heart disease, asthma, hyperthyroidism, increased IOP, diabetes mellitus, prostatic hypertrophy.

Overdosage: Signs and Symptoms
Chlorpheniramine: Decreased mental alertness, ataxia, hallucinations, convulsions, death.
Pseudoephedrine: Somnolence, sedation, profuse sweating, hypotension, shock, coma, elderly

patients may experience hallucinations, seizures, CNS depression, death.
Codeine: Miosis, respiratory and CNS depression, circulatory collapse, seizures, cardiopulmonary arrest, death.

PATIENT CARE CONSIDERATIONS
Administration/Storage
- Give prescribed dose q 6 hr as needed, up to 4 doses/day.
- Give with food or milk if GI upset occurs.
- Use dosing spoon or syringe for pediatric doses.
- Store elixir at controlled room temperature (68° to 77°F). Keep tightly capped.

Assessment/Interventions
- Obtain patient history, including drug history and any known allergies. Note history of peptic ulcer disease, diabetes, hypertension, hyperthyroidism, enlarged prostate, asthma, narrow angle glaucoma, urinary retention, severe hypertension or coronary artery disease, or concurrent use of or within 2 wk of stopping MAO inhibitor therapy.
- Assess for allergy symptoms (eg, cough, rhinitis, nasal congestion, sneezing, itching, watery eyes) before and periodically throughout therapy.
- Monitor pulse and BP periodically during therapy.
- Monitor patient for nervousness, dizziness, and insomnia. If noted, hold therapy and notify health care provider.

Patient/Family Education
- Explain name, dose, action, and potential side effects of drug.
- Advise patient to take prescribed dose q 6 hr as needed, up to qid.
- Advise caregiver to use dosing spoon or syringe when giving elixir to children.
- Advise patient to take with food or milk if GI upset occurs.
- Advise patient to take last dose late in the afternoon or early evening to reduce chance of drug causing sleeplessness.
- Advise patient that if a dose is missed to take as soon as remembered unless it is nearing time for the next dose. Caution patient to not double the dose to catch up.
- Advise patient that if allergy symptoms are not controlled, not to increase the dose of medication but to inform health care provider.
- Caution patient that drug may cause drowsiness and to use caution while driving or performing other tasks requiring mental alertness until tolerance is determined.
- Advise patient to avoid alcohol and other CNS depressants due to risk of excessive sedation.
- Caution patient not to take any OTC antihistamines or decongestants while taking this medication unless advised by health care provider.
- If patient is to have allergy skin testing, advise to not take the medication for at least 6 days before the skin testing.
- Advise women to notify health care provider if pregnant, planning to become pregnant, or breastfeeding.
- Instruct patient to stop taking drug and immediately report any of the following symptoms to health care provider if occurring: nervousness, dizziness, sleeplessness.
- Caution patient to not take any prescription or OTC medications or dietary supplements unless advised by health care provider.

Chlorpromazine Hydrochloride

(klor-PRO-muh-zeen HIGH-droe-KLOR-ide)

Class Antipsychotic/Phenothiazine/Antiemetic

How Supplied
Chlorpromazine Hydrochloride Tablets 10 mg, Oral concentrate 100 mg/mL ◆ *Thorazine* Tablets 25 mg, Tablets 50 mg, Tablets 100 mg, Tablets 200 mg, Suppositories 100 mg as base, Injection 25 mg/mL
✤ *Largactil*

Action
PHARMACOLOGY: Effects apparently caused by dopamine receptor blockade in CNS.

PHARMACOKINETICS/DYNAMICS:
Absorption: About 32% bioavailable. T_{max} is 1 to 4 hr. C_{max} is 25 to 150 ng/mL.

Distribution: 95% to 98% protein bound. Vd is about 21 L/kg. Excreted in breast milk.

Metabolism: Metabolized in the liver to 7-hydroxychlorpromazine (active) and chlorpromazine N-oxide.

Excretion: The $t_{½}$ is about 30 hr. Less than 1% is excreted in urine. Cl is about 8.6 mL/min/kg.

Indications Management of manic phase of manic-depressive disorder; treatment of schizophrenia; relief of anxiety and restlessness prior to surgery; adjunct in treatment of tetanus; management of acute intermittent porphyria, severe behavioral and conduct disorders in children; control of nausea and vomiting; relief of intractable hiccoughs. **Unlabeled use(s):** Treatment of migraine headaches (IM or IV forms).

Contraindications Comatose or severely depressed states; allergy to product or other phenothiazines; presence of large amounts of other CNS depressants.

Route/Dosage
ADULTS:
Psychiatric (outpatient): **IM** 25 mg for prompt control; may repeat in 1 hr. **PO** 25 to 50 mg tid after initial regimen. May initiate oral dosing with 10 mg tid to qid or 25 mg bid or tid.
Psychiatric (inpatient): **PO** 25 mg tid; increase prn; usually 400 mg/day. **IM** 25 mg initially; may give additional 25 to 50 mg in 1 hr. Increase gradually until controlled. Up to 2,000 mg/day may be needed but generally not for extended periods.
Acute Intermittent Porphyria: **PO** 25 to 50 mg tid or qid; **IM** 25 mg tid to qid.
Tetanus: **IM** 25 to 50 mg tid to qid; **IV** 25 to 50 mg diluted to greater than or equal to 1 mg/mL and administered at rate of 1 mg/min.
Nausea and Vomiting: **PO** 10 to 25 mg q 4 to 6 hr prn. **PR** 100 mg q 6 to 8 hr prn. **IM** 25 mg. If no hypotension, may give 25 to 50 mg q 4 to 6 hr prn.
During surgery: **IM** 12.5 mg; repeat in 0.5 hr if necessary and if no hypotension. **IV** 2 mg per fractional injection, at 2-min intervals (max, 25 mg). Dilute to 1 mg/mL (1 mL [25 mg]) mixed with 24 mL of saline.
Presurgical apprehension: **PO** 25 to 50 mg 2 to 3 hr prior to surgery. **IM** 12.5 to 25 mg 1 to 2 hr before surgery.
Intractable Hiccoughs: **PO** 25 to 50 mg tid to qid. **IM** May give 25 to 50 mg if symptoms persist 2 to 3 days. **IV** May use slow infusion if hiccoughs persist.
CHILDREN OLDER THAN 6 MO OF AGE:
Psychiatric (Outpatient): **PO** 0.5 mg/kg q 4 to 6 hr prn; **PR** 1 mg/kg q 6 to 8 hr prn; **IM** 0.5 mg/kg q 6 to 8 hr prn.
Psychiatric (Inpatient): **PO** Start low and increase gradually; 50 to 100 mg/day may be needed in severe cases or 200 mg/day or more in older children. **IM** Up to 5 yr of age: Do not exceed 40 mg/day. 5 to 12 yr of age: Do not exceed 75 mg/day if possible.
Tetanus: **IM/IV** 0.5 mg/kg q 6 to 8 hr. When giving IV, dilute to at least 1 mg/mL and administer at rate of 1 mg/2 min. In children 23 kg or under, do not exceed 40 mg/day; 23 to 45 kg, do not exceed 75 mg/day if possible.
Nausea and Vomiting: **PO** 0.55 mg/kg q 4 to 6 hr. **PR** 1.1 mg/kg q 6 to 8 hr prn. **IM** 0.55 mg/kg q 6 to 8 hr prn. Do not exceed 40 mg/day if younger than 5 yr of age or 75 mg/day if 5 to 12 yr of age.
Presurgical apprehension: **PO** 0.55 mg/kg 2 to 3 hr before surgery. **IM** 0.55 mg/kg 1 to 2 hr before surgery.

Interactions
Alcohol and other CNS depressants: May cause increased CNS depression and may precipitate extrapyramidal reaction.
Anticholinergics: May reduce therapeutic effects of and increase anticholinergic effects of chlorpromazine; may lead to tardive dyskinesia.
Barbiturate anesthetics: May increase frequency and severity of neuromuscular excitation and hypotension.
Beta-blockers: May result in increased plasma levels of beta-blocker and chlorpromazine.
Cisapride, sparfloxacin: The risk of life-threatening cardiac arrhythmias, including torsades de pointes, may be increased.
Epinephrine, norepinephrine: Actions of these drugs may be decreased or reversed.
Guanethidine: The hypotensive effect of guanethidine may be inhibited.
Lithium: May cause disorienting unconsciousness and extrapyramidal effects.
Meperidine: May result in excessive sedation and hypotension.
Metrizamide: Risk of seizure may increase.
Paroxetine: Plasma levels of chlorpromazine may be elevated, increasing the risk of side effects.

Lab Test Interferences Chlorpromazine may discolor urine (pink to red-brown). False-positive pregnancy test results may occur (less likely with a serum test). Increases in protein-bound iodine have been reported. False-positive phenylketonuria test results may occur.

Adverse Reactions
CV: Orthostatic hypotension; hypertension; tachycardia; bradycardia; syncope; cardiac arrest; circulatory collapse; ECG changes.
CNS: Faintness; drowsiness; dystonias; dizziness; extrapyramidal side effects (eg, pseudoparkinsonism, tardive dyskinesia); muscle spasms; motor restlessness; headache; weakness; tremor; fatigue; slurring; insomnia; vertigo; seizures; sedation; neuroleptic malignant syndrome; cerebral edema.
DERM: Photosensitivity; skin pigmentation; dry skin; exfoliative dermatitis; urticarial rash; maculopapular hypersensitivity reaction; seborrhea; eczema; contact dermatitis.
EENT: Pigmentary retinopathy; glaucoma; photophobia; blurred vision; increased IOP; mydriasis; nasal congestion; miosis.
GI: Dry mouth; dyspepsia; constipation; adynamic ileus (with possible complications result-

ing in death); nausea; atonic colon; obstipation.
GU: Urinary retention and hesitancy; impotence; sexual dysfunction; menstrual irregularities; lactation; moderate breast engorgement; priapism; breast enlargement; galactorrhea.
HEMA: Agranulocytosis; eosinophilia; leukopenia; hemolytic anemia; thrombocytopenic purpura; pancytopenia.
HEPA: Jaundice.
METAB: Altered cholesterol levels.
RESP: Laryngospasm; bronchospasm; dyspnea, aspiration pneumonia; asthma; laryngeal edema.
OTHER: Increased appetite and weight; polydipsia; heat stroke/hyperpyrexia; sudden death; angioneurotic edema; anaphylactoid reactions; systemic lupus erythematosus-like syndrome; increased prolactin levels.

Precautions

Pregnancy: Safety not established.
Lactation: Excreted in breast milk.
Children: Do not use in children under 6 mo unless considered life-saving. Do not use in conditions for which specific children's dosage not established.
Elderly: More susceptible to enhanced effects; consider lower dose.
Special risk patients: Use caution in patients with CV disease or mitral insufficiency, history of glaucoma, EEG abnormalities or seizure disorders, prior brain damage, or hepatic or renal impairment, or who will be exposed to extreme heat.
Abrupt withdrawal: Abrupt withdrawal of high-dose therapy may cause symptoms resembling physical dependence such as gastritis, nausea, vomiting, dizziness, and tremulousness.

Antiemetic effect: May mask the signs and symptoms of overdosage of other drugs and obscure the diagnosis and treatment of other conditions such as intestinal obstruction, brain tumor, or Reye syndrome.
Aspiration: As result of suppression of cough reflex, aspiration of vomitus possible.
Bone marrow suppression: Patients with bone marrow depression or who have previously demonstrated a hypersensitivity reaction with a phenothiazine should not receive chlorpromazine unless, in the judgment of the physician, the potential benefits outweigh the possible risks.
CNS effects: May impair mental or physical abilities, especially during the first few days of therapy.
Hepatic effects: Jaundice usually occurs between 2nd and 4th weeks of treatment; considered hypersensitivity reaction. Usually reversible.
Neuroleptic malignant syndrome: Has occurred with agents of this class; is potentially fatal. Signs and symptoms are hyperpyrexia, muscle rigidity, altered mental status, irregular pulse, irregular BP, tachycardia, and diaphoresis.
Tardive dyskinesia: Syndrome of potentially irreversible involuntary body and facial movements may develop. Prevalence highest in the elderly, especially women. Use smallest effective dose.

Overdosage: Signs and Symptoms

CNS depression, hypotension, extrapyramidal symptoms, agitation, restlessness, convulsions, fever, hypothermia, hyperthermia, coma, autonomic reactions, ECG changes, cardiac arrhythmias.

PATIENT CARE CONSIDERATIONS

Administration/Storage

- Dose and frequency of administration are variable, depending on condition being treated.
- Administer tablets as prescribed, without regard to meals. Administer with food if GI upset occurs.
- Measure prescribed dose of oral concentrate using calibrated dropper supplied with medication.
- Oral concentrate should be mixed with semisolid foods (eg, soup, pudding) or diluted with 2 oz of water, coffee, tea, tomato or fruit juice, orange syrup, or carbonated beverages just prior to administration. Do not prepare dilutions ahead of time and store.
- Undiluted injection is for IM administration only. Inject prescribed dose slowly, deep into outer quadrant of buttock.
- Injection must be diluted, following manufacturer's guidelines, before administering IV.

- Injection is not for intradermal or SC administration.
- Do not administer injection if particulate matter or marked discoloration noted. A slight yellowish discoloration is normal and will not alter potency.
- If oral concentrate or injection is spilled on skin or clothing, rinse area immediately with water to prevent contact dermatitis.
- Store tablets, suppositories, and injection at controlled room temperature (59° to 86°F). Store oral solution below 77°F. Protect oral solution and injection from light.

Assessment/Interventions

- Obtain patient history, including drug history and any known allergies. Note allergy to chlorpromazine or other phenothiazines, sulfite sensitivity, previous episode of jaundice with phenothiazine therapy, renal impairment, hepatic impairment, ischemic heart disease, heart failure, arrhythmias, cerebrovas-

CHLORPROMAZINE HYDROCHLORIDE 383

cular disease, asthma, emphysema, narrow-angle glaucoma, epilepsy, mitral insufficiency, pheochromocytoma, prostatic hypertrophy, condition predisposing to hypotension (eg, dehydration, hypovolemia), concomitant use of antihypertensive drugs, or previous episodes of neuroleptic malignant syndrome.
- Ensure that medication is discontinued at least 48 hr before myelography and not resumed until at least 24 hr after procedure to reduce chance of seizures occurring.
- Frequently assess patient for response to treatment. Notify health care provider if condition being treated is not improving or is worsening.
- Ensure that therapy is periodically reviewed to determine if it needs to be continued without change or if a dose change (eg, increase, decrease, discontinuation) is indicated.
- Avoid sudden discontinuation of therapy if possible. Attempt to gradually reduce dose if decision to discontinue medication is made.
- Inform health care provider immediately if hyperpyrexia, muscle rigidity, altered mental status, irregular pulse and BP, tachycardia, and diaphoresis develop.
- Notify health care provider immediately if palpitations or syncope occur.
- Assess neurologic status before and during treatment. Observe for involuntary body and facial movements, excessive drowsiness, agitation, tremor, or anxiety. Inform health care provider if noted.
- Administer IM dose to patient who is bedfast. Keep patient lying down for at least 30 min after injection to minimize hypotensive effects.
- Monitor patient for CNS, CV, GI, GU, PSYCH, MUSC, and general body side effects. Inform health care provider if noted and significant.
- Assess medication compliance.

Patient/Family Education

- Explain name, dose, action, and potential side effects of drug.
- Advise patient, family, or caregiver that dose will be adjusted periodically until maximum benefit has been obtained.
- Advise patient, family, or caregiver not to change the dose or stop taking unless advised by health care provider.
- Instruct patient, family, or caregiver to measure prescribed dose of oral concentrate using calibrated dropper supplied with medication.
- Advise patient, family, or caregiver that oral concentrate should be mixed with semisolid foods (eg, soup, pudding) or diluted with 2 oz of water, coffee, tea, tomato or fruit juice, orange syrup, or carbonated beverages just prior to administration. Caution patient, family, or caregiver to not prepare dilutions ahead of time and store.
- Instruct patient not to stop taking chlorpromazine when feeling better.
- Instruct patient, family, or caregiver to immediately report fainting or loss of consciousness, palpitations, dizziness, high fever, muscle rigidity, altered mental status, irregular pulse, sore throat, unusual bruising, yellowing of the skin or eyes.
- Advise patient, family, or caregiver to notify health care provider of any of the following: excessive drowsiness, increased agitation or anxiety, involuntary body or facial movements.
- Advise patient to avoid strenuous activity during periods of high temperature or humidity.
- Instruct patient to avoid alcoholic beverages and other depressants while taking this medication.
- Instruct patient to get up slowly from lying or sitting position and to avoid sudden position changes to prevent postural hypotension. Advise patient to report dizziness with position changes to health care provider. Caution patient that hot tubs and hot showers or baths may make dizziness worse.
- Advise patient to take sips of water, suck on ice chips or sugarless hard candy, or chew sugarless gum if dry mouth occurs.
- Advise patient that drug may cause drowsiness, impaired judgment or thinking skills, and to use caution while driving or performing other tasks requiring mental alertness until tolerance is determined.
- Caution patient that medication may cause sensitivity to sunlight and to avoid unnecessary exposure to UV light (sunlight, tanning booths) and to use sunscreen and wear protective clothing when exposed to UV light until tolerance is determined.
- Advise women to notify health care provider if pregnant, planning to become pregnant, or breastfeeding.
- Instruct patient not to take any prescription or OTC medications, herbal preparations, or dietary supplements unless advised by health care provider.
- Advise patient that follow-up visits may be required to monitor therapy and to keep appointments.

Chlorpropamide

(klor-PRO-puh-mide)

Class Antidiabetic/Sulfonylurea

How Supplied
Diabinese Tablets 100 mg, Tablets 250 mg
✤ *APO-Chlorpropamide*

Action

PHARMACOLOGY: Decreases blood glucose by stimulating insulin release from pancreas.

PHARMACOKINETICS/DYNAMICS:

Absorption: Rapidly absorbed. T_{max} is 2 to 4 hr. C_{max} is 30 mcg/mL.

Distribution: Excreted in breast milk.

Metabolism: Metabolized in the liver.

Excretion: The t½ is about 36 hr. 80% to 90% is excreted in urine within 96 hr (as unchanged drug and as hydroxylated or hydrolyzed metabolites).

Onset: Within 1 hr.

Peak: 3 to 5 hr.

Duration: 24 to 60 hr.

Special Populations:
Renal Function Impairment – The t½ is prolonged. Dosage adjustment may be needed.

Indications Adjunct to diet to lower blood glucose in patients with non-insulin-dependent diabetes mellitus (type II) whose hyperglycemia cannot be controlled by diet alone. **Unlabeled use(s):** Control of neurogenic diabetes insipidus.

Contraindications Hypersensitivity to sulfonylureas; diabetes complicated by ketoacidosis with or without coma; sole therapy for insulin-independent (type I) diabetes mellitus; diabetes when complicated by pregnancy.

Route/Dosage

ADULTS:
Initial dose: **PO** 250 mg/day in single dose.

ELDERLY:
Initial dose: **PO** 100 to 125 mg/day in single dose.

MAINTENANCE: **PO** 100 to 250 mg/day in single dose.

SEVERELY DIABETIC ADULTS: **PO** up to 500 mg/day; avoid doses above 750 mg/day.

Interactions

Androgens, anticoagulants, chloramphenicol, clofibrate, fenfluramine, methyldopa, MAO inhibitors, phenylbutazone, probenecid, salicylates, sulfonamides, tricyclic antidepressants, urinary acidifiers: May increase hypoglycemic effect.

Beta-blockers, corticosteroids, diazoxide, hydantoins, rifampin, thiazide diuretics, urinary alkalinizers: May decrease hypoglycemic effect.

Lab Test Interferences

LFTs: Drug causes elevated results.

BUN and creatinine: Drug causes mild to moderate elevations.

Adverse Reactions

CV: Increased risk of cardiovascular mortality when compared with patients treated with diet alone.

CNS: Dizziness; vertigo.

DERM: Allergic skin reactions; eczema; pruritus; erythema; urticaria; morbilliform or maculopapular eruptions; lichenoid reactions; photosensitivity.

EENT: Tinnitus.

GI: GI disturbances (eg, nausea, epigastric fullness, heartburn).

HEMA: Leukopenia; thrombocytopenia; aplastic anemia; agranulocytosis; hemolytic anemia; pancytopenia; hepatic porphyria.

HEPA: Cholestatic jaundice; elevated LFTs.

METAB: Hypoglycemia; SIADH with water retention and dilutional hyponatremia, especially in patients with CHF or hepatic cirrhosis.

OTHER: Disulfiram-like reaction; weakness; paresthesia; fatigue; malaise.

Precautions

Pregnancy: Category C. Insulin is recommended to maintain blood glucose levels during pregnancy. Prolonged severe neonatal hypoglycemia can occur if sulfonylureas are administered at time of delivery. If administering to pregnant patient, discontinue 2 days to 4 wk before expected date of delivery.

Lactation: Excreted in breast milk.

Children: Safety and efficacy not established.

Elderly: Particularly susceptible to hypoglycemic action. Hypoglycemia can be difficult to recognize in elderly patients.

Renal function impairment: Use drug with caution and monitor renal function frequently.

Hepatic function impairment: Use drug with caution and monitor liver function frequently.

Debilitated patients: Particularly susceptible to hypoglycemic action.

Disulfiram-like syndrome: A sulfonylurea-induced facial flushing reaction may occur when administered with alcohol.

Overdosage: Signs and Symptoms

Hypoglycemia, tingling of lips and tongue, hunger, nausea, lethargy, confusion, agitation, nervousness, tachycardia, sweating, tremor, convulsions, stupor, coma.

PATIENT CARE CONSIDERATIONS

Administration/Storage
* Administer once a day.
* Give with food or 30 min before meal if drug causes GI upset.
* When discontinuing chlorpropamide and switching to another oral hypoglycemic agent, exercise caution for 2 wk; prolonged action of chlorpropamide may provoke hypoglycemia.
* Store in cool environment in tightly closed container.

Assessment/Interventions
* Obtain patient history, including drug history and any known allergies. Note presence of hepatic or renal impairment and nature of patient's diabetic illness.
* Check blood sugar levels frequently and observe for symptoms of hypoglycemia or hyperglycemia and report to health care provider.
* Be aware that hypoglycemia may be difficult to recognize in elderly patients or patients taking beta-blockers.
* When patients with impaired liver or renal function are receiving this drug, check liver and renal function test results frequently.
* Observe for evidence of possible water retention (especially in patients with CHF) and report to health care provider.
* If cholestatic jaundice occurs, discontinue drug and notify health care provider.

Patient/Family Education
* Explain that this medication will not cure disease.
* Emphasize that drug must be taken on daily basis and should not be discontinued abruptly.
* Tell patient that drug may cause GI upset and to take it with food if GI upset occurs.
* Teach patient to self-monitor blood glucose.
* Inform patient to contact health care provider if symptoms of hypoglycemia occur (eg, fatigue, excessive hunger, profuse sweating, numbness of extremities).
* Instruct patient to notify health care provider if symptoms of hyperglycemia occur (eg, excessive thirst or urination, urinary glucose, or ketones).
* Tell patient to report constipation, nausea, vomiting, drowsiness, dizziness, fever, sore throat, rash, or unusual bruising or bleeding to health care provider.
* Inform patient that this drug is not a substitute for exercise and diet control; patient must follow prescribed regimens of diet, exercise and personal hygiene.
* Instruct patient to inform all health care providers involved in patient's care that this drug is being taken.
* Advise patient not to take any medication (including *otc*) or drink alcoholic beverages without consulting health care provider; flushing has been reported with chlorpropamide.
* Caution patient to avoid exposure to sunlight and to use sunscreen or wear protective clothing to avoid photosensitivity reaction.
* Advise patient that drug can cause dizziness and to use caution while driving or performing other tasks requiring mental alertness.
* Remind patient to wear *Medi-Alert* identification.

Chlorthalidone
(klor-THAL-ih-dohn)

Class Thiazide diuretic

How Supplied
Hygroton Tablets 25 mg, Tablets 50 mg, Tablets 100 mg ♦ *Thalitone* Tablets 15 mg, Tablets 25 mg ♦ *Apo-Chlorthalidone*

Action
PHARMACOLOGY: Inhibits reabsorption of sodium and chloride in proximal portion of distal convoluted tubules.

PHARMACOKINETICS/DYNAMICS:
Absorption: 64% absorbed.
Distribution: Excreted in breast milk.
Excretion: The t½ is 40 hr.
Onset: 2 to 3 hr.
Peak: 2 to 6 hr.
Duration: 24 to 72 hr.

Indications Reduction of edema associated with CHF, hepatic cirrhosis, renal dysfunction, corticosteroid and estrogen therapy; management of hypertension. **Unlabeled use(s):** Treatment of calcium nephrolithiasis, osteoporosis, diabetes insipidus.

Contraindications Hypersensitivity to thiazides, related diuretics, or sulfonamide-derived drugs; anuria; renal decompensation.

Route/Dosage
Edema
ADULTS: **PO** 50 to 200 mg daily or on alternate days.

Hypertension
ADULTS: **PO** 25 to 100 mg daily. Doses above 25 mg/day potentiate potassium excretion but do

not benefit sodium excretion or BP reduction.

Interactions
Allopurinol: Concurrent use may increase incidence of hypersensitivity reactions to allopurinol.
Amphotericin B, corticosteroids: May intensify potassium depletion.
Anticholinergics: May increase chlorthalidone absorption.
Anticoagulants: May diminish anticoagulant effects.
Bile acid sequestrants: May reduce chlorthalidone absorption. Give chlorthalidone at least 2 hr before bile acid sequestrant.
Calcium salts: Hypercalcemia may develop.
Diazoxide: May cause hyperglycemia.
Digitalis glycosides: Diuretic-induced hypokalemia and hypomagnesemia may precipitate digitalis-induced arrhythmias.
Lithium: May decrease renal excretion of lithium.
Loop diuretics: Synergistic effects may result in profound diuresis and serious electrolyte abnormalities.
Methenamines, NSAIDs: May decrease effectiveness of chlorthalidone.
Sulfonylureas, insulin: May decrease hypoglycemic effect of sulfonylureas.

Lab Test Interferences
Increased serum bilirubin levels. Serum magnesium levels in uremic patients may be increased.

Adverse Reactions
CNS: Dizziness; lightheadedness; vertigo; headache; paresthesias; weakness; restlessness; insomnia.
DERM: Purpura; photosensitivity; rash; urticaria; necrotizing angiitis; vasculitis; cutaneous vasculitis; exfoliative dermatitis; toxic epidermal necrolysis.
EENT: Xanthopsia (yellow vision).
GI: Anorexia; gastric irritation; nausea; vomiting; abdominal pain or cramping; bloating; diarrhea; constipation; pancreatitis.
GU: Impotence; reduced libido.
HEMA: Leukopenia; thrombocytopenia; agranulocytosis; aplastic or hypoplastic anemia.
HEPA: Jaundice.
METAB: Hyperglycemia; glycosuria; hyperuricemia; fluid and electrolyte imbalances.
OTHER: Muscle cramps or spasms.

Precautions
Pregnancy: Category B.
Lactation: Excreted in breast milk.
Children: Safety and efficacy not established.
Hypersensitivity: May occur in patients with or without history of allergy or bronchial asthma; cross-sensitivity with sulfonamides also may occur.
Renal function impairment: May precipitate azotemia; use with caution.
Hepatic function impairment: Minor alterations of fluid and electrolyte balance may precipitate hepatic coma; use with caution.
Lipids: May cause increased concentrations of total serum cholesterol, total triglycerides and LDL in some patients.
Postsympathectomy patients: Antihypertensive effects may be enhanced.

Overdosage: Signs and Symptoms
Orthostatic hypotension, dizziness, drowsiness, syncope, potassium depletion, nausea, vomiting, lethargy, coma, GI irritation, GI hypermotility, seizures.

PATIENT CARE CONSIDERATIONS

Administration/Storage
- Administer drug early in the morning so that diuresis will occur during day rather than night.
- Give with meals or milk to avoid GI upset.

Assessment/Interventions
- Obtain patient history, including drug history and any known allergies.
- Assess serum electrolytes and digitalis level (if appropriate) periodically.
- Closely monitor blood sugar, CBC, and platelets.
- Review triglyceride and cholesterol levels periodically.

Patient/Family Education
- Teach patient signs and symptoms of hypokalemia (eg, weakness, cramps, nausea, dizziness), especially if patient is taking digitalis.
- Explain diuretic effects of drug so patient is aware of expected and potential outcomes.
- Instruct patient to follow low-sodium diet to enhance action of medication.
- If high-potassium diet is recommended by health care provider, help patient identify appropriate meal plans or potassium supplements.
- Teach patient to record weight daily at a consistent time and to notify health care provider if weight fluctuates ± 5 pounds.
- Tell patient to notify health care provider of salt or water retention occurs (eg, swelling of feet, ankles, calves).
- Caution patient to avoid exposure to sunlight and to use sunscreen or wear protective clothing to avoid photosensitivity reaction.
- Advise patient to avoid sudden position changes to prevent orthostatic hypotension.

Have patient get up slowly and dangle feet before getting out of bed.

Chlorzoxazone

(klor-ZOX-uh-zone)

Class Skeletal muscle relaxant, centrally acting

How Supplied
Paraflex Caplets 250 mg ♦ *Parafon Forte DSC* Caplets 500 mg ♦ *Remular-S* Tablets 250 mg

Action
PHARMACOLOGY: Action may be related to its sedative properties or to inhibition of reflex arcs at spinal cord and subcortical levels of brain.

PHARMACOKINETICS/DYNAMICS:
Absorption: T_{max} is 1 to 2 hr.
Metabolism: Rapidly metabolized.
Excretion: Excreted in the urine as glucuronide conjugate. Less than 1% is excreted in the urine as unchanged drug. The t½ is about 60 min.
Onset: 1 hr.
Duration: 3 to 4 hr.

Indications Relief of discomfort associated with painful musculoskeletal conditions.

Contraindications Standard considerations.

Route/Dosage
ADULTS: PO Initial (for acute pain): 500 mg tid to qid; increase to 750 mg if needed. As improvement occurs, reduce dose; 250 mg tid to qid is usually sufficient.

PATIENT CARE CONSIDERATIONS

Administration/Storage
- Give with meals to avoid GI upset.
- Discuss dosage adjustments with health care provider according to patient's response.

Assessment/Interventions
- Notify health care provider if patient is pregnant or nursing.
- Obtain patient history, including drug history and any known allergies.
- Monitor skin and sclera for jaundice.
- Monitor liver function throughout therapy.
- Report signs of liver dysfunction to health care provider.

Patient/Family Education
- Instruct patient to inform health care provider of any urticaria, redness or itching.
- Tell patient to report to health care provider

- Caution patient not to take any *otc* medications without consulting health care provider.

Interactions
Alcohol and other CNS depressants: Additive CNS depressant effects may occur.

Lab Test Interferences None well documented.

Adverse Reactions
CNS: Drowsiness; dizziness; lightheadedness; malaise; overstimulation.
DERM: Allergic-type skin rashes; petechiae.
GI: GI disturbances.
GU: Urine discoloration (orange or purple red).
HEPA: Drug-induced hepatitis.
OTHER: Hypersensitivity (eg, angioneurotic edema); anaphylaxis).

Precautions
Pregnancy: Pregnancy category undetermined.
Lactation: Undetermined.
Hepatic function impairment: Avoid use in patients with liver impairment; discontinue if signs of dysfunction occur.
Hazardous tasks: May impair ability to perform tasks requiring mental or physical coordination or dexterity, including driving. Drowsiness is very common.

Overdosage: Signs and Symptoms
Nausea, vomiting, diarrhea, drowsiness, dizziness, lightheadedness, malaise, sluggishness, loss of muscle tone, decreased deep tendon reflex, respiratory depression.

any yellowing of skin or eyes.
- Advise patient that drug may cause drowsiness and to use caution while driving or performing other tasks that require mental alertness.
- Advise patient to avoid intake of alcoholic beverages and other medications that cause drowsiness while taking product.
- Advise patient to notify health care provider before discontinuing medication.
- Inform patient to take a missed dose as soon as possible, unless several hours have passed. Advise patient not to double doses.
- Inform patient urine may turn orange or purple-red while taking this medication.
- Instruct patient to take with meals to avoid GI upset.

Cholestyramine

(koe-less-TIE-ruh-meen)

Class Antihyperlipidemic/Bile acid sequestrant

How Supplied
LoCHOLEST Powder for Suspension 4 g anhydrous cholestyramine resin/9 g powder ♦ *LoCHOLEST Light* Powder for Suspension 4 g anhydrous cholestyramine resin/5.7 g powder ♦ *Prevalite* Powder 4 g (as anhydrous cholestyramine resin)/5.5 g powder ♦ *Questran* Powder for Suspension 4 g anhydrous cholestyramine resin/9 g powder, Tablets 1 g anhydrous cholestyramine resin ♦ *Questran Light* Powder 4 g (as anhydrous cholestyramine resin)/5 g powder ❦ *Novo-Cholamine* ♦ *Novo-Cholamine Light*

Action
PHARMACOLOGY: Increases removal of bile acids from body by forming insoluble complexes in intestine, which are then excreted in feces. As body loses bile acids, it converts cholesterol from blood to bile acid, thus lowering serum cholesterol.

PHARMACOKINETICS/DYNAMICS:
Absorption: Not absorbed.
Onset: LDL reductions are noticed in 4 to 7 days and serum cholesterol reductions are evident by 1 mo.
Duration: After discontinuation, serum cholesterol usually returns to baseline within 1 mo.

Indications
Reduction of serum cholesterol in patients with primary hypercholesterolemia; relief of pruritus associated with partial biliary obstruction. **Unlabeled use(s):** Treatment of antibiotic-induced pseudomembranous colitis, bile salt-mediated diarrhea and digitalis toxicity.

Contraindications
Hypersensitivity to bile acid sequestering resins; complete biliary obstruction.

Route/Dosage
ADULTS: PO 4 g 1 to 6 times/day; generally given 3 to 4 times/day.

Interactions
Acetaminophen, amiodarone, corticosteroids, digitalis glycosides, HMG-CoA reductase inhibitors (eg, fluvastatin), methotrexate, some NSAIDs (eg, piroxicam), propranolol, thiazide diuretics, ursodiol, warfarin, and other drugs: Cholestyramine may interfere with the absorption of many drugs, especially those listed.
Fats and fat-soluble vitamins A, D, E, and K: Cholestyramine may interfere with normal fat absorption and digestion; consider supplementation with these vitamins and with folic acid.
Iopanoic acid: Coadministration may result in abnormal cholecystography.

Lab Test Interferences
Increased serum phosphorus and chloride; decreased serum sodium and potassium.

Adverse Reactions
DERM: Rash; irritation of skin, tongue, and perianal area.
GI: Constipation (can be severe and at times accompanied by fecal impaction); aggravation of hemorrhoids; abdominal pain and distention; bleeding; belching; flatulence; nausea; vomiting; diarrhea; heartburn; anorexia; steatorrhea.
HEMA: Bleeding tendencies related to vitamin K deficiency; folic acid deficiency.
METAB: Fat-soluble vitamin deficiencies; hyperchloremic acidosis and increased urinary calcium excretion; osteoporosis.

Precautions
Pregnancy: Safety not established.
Lactation: Undetermined.
Children: Safety and efficacy not established.
Carcinogenesis: Incidence of intestinal tumors in studies was greater in cholestyramine-treated rats than in controls; relevance to clinical practice is not known.

Overdosage: Signs and Symptoms
GI obstruction.

PATIENT CARE CONSIDERATIONS

Administration/Storage
- Administer cholestyramine separate from other drugs. Give other drugs 1 hr before or 4 to 6 hr after cholestyramine.
- In general, give medication before meals.
- Never administer dry powder without liquid. Use any noncarbonated fluid.
- Instruct patient to chew tablets thoroughly. Follow with full glass of water.

Assessment/Interventions
- Obtain patient history, including drug history and any known allergies.
- Document serum cholesterol and triglycerides levels.
- Monitor electrolyte balance, and notify health care provider of increased serum phosphorus and chloride, or decreased serum sodium and potassium.

Patient/Family Education
- In general, instruct patient to take medication before meals.
- Advise patient to take any other medications, including otc medications, 1 hr before or 4 to 6 hr after taking cholestyramine.

- Instruct patient to use dry powder form to mix with fluid (2 to 6 oz) according to packet directions.
- Teach patient how to implement any vitamin and mineral supplementation recommended by the health care provider.
- Help patient identify appropriate meal plans that supply adequate sodium and potassium and are low in phosphorus.
- Tell patient to take prune juice, fruits and vegetables, and good fluid intake on a regular basis to avoid constipation. If constipation or other GI upset occurs, instruct patient to notify health care provider.
- Advise patient to follow regular exercise routine.
- Instruct patient to adhere to a diet low in fats and to participate in a weight management program, if appropriate.
- Advise patients with phenylketonuria that a 5 g dose of *Questran Light* contains aspartame equivalent to 16.8 mg of phenylalanine.
- Instruct patient to report the following symptoms to the health care provider: constipation, flatulence, nausea, heartburn, abnormal bleeding.

Chorionic Gonadotropin

(core-ee-AHN-ik goe-NAD-oh-troe-pin)

Class Sex hormones/Ovulation stimulant

How Supplied
Chorex-10 Powder for injection 10,000 units/vial with 10 mL diluent (to make 1000 units/mL), Powder for injection 20,000 units/vial with 10 mL diluent (to make 2000 units/mL) ◆ *Chorionic Gonadotropin* Powder for injection 5000 units/vial with 10 mL diluent (to make 500 units/mL), Powder for injection 10,000 units/vial with 10 mL diluent (to make 1000 units/mL) ◆ *Novarel* Powder for injection 10,000 units/vial with 10 mL diluent (to make 1000 units/mL) ◆ *Pregnyl* Powder for injection 10,000 units/vial with 10 mL diluent (to make 1000 units/mL) ◆ *Profasi* Powder for injection 5000 units/vial with 10 mL diluent (to make 500 units/mL), Powder for injection 10,000 units/vial with 10 mL diluent (to make 1000 units/mL)

Action
PHARMACOLOGY: Stimulates production of gonadal steroid hormones by stimulating interstitial cells (Leydig cells) of the testis to produce androgens and corpus luteum of the ovary to produce progesterone.

PHARMACOKINETICS/DYNAMICS:
Absorption: A detectable rise in human chorionic gonadotropin (hCG) is seen in 2 hr; peak levels are reached in 6 hr and remain at this level for 36 hr.
Excretion: hCG levels begin to decline at 48 hr and approach baseline at 72 hr.

Indications Prepubertal cryptorchidism not caused by anatomical obstruction; selected cases of hypogonadotropic hypogonadism (eg, hypogonadism secondary to pituitary deficiency) in men; induction of ovulation in anovulatory, infertile women in whom the cause of anovulation is secondary and not caused by primary ovarian failure and who have been appropriately pretreated with human menotropins.

Contraindications Precocious puberty; prostatic carcinoma or other androgen-dependent neoplasm; prior allergic reaction to hCG.

Route/Dosage
Prepubertal Cryptorchidism
CHILDREN (4 YR AND OLDER):
Various authorities have advocated the following regimens: **IM** (1) 4000 USP U 3 times/wk for 3 wk, (2) 5000 USP U qod for 4 injections, (3) 15 injections of 500 to 1000 USP U over a period of 6 wk, or (4) 500 USP U 3 times/wk for 4 to 6 wk (if not successful, another course is begun 1 mo later using 1000 USP U/injection).

Hypogonadotropic Hypogonadism in Men
ADULTS:
Various authorities have advocated the following regimens: **IM** 500 to 1000 USP U 3 times/wk for 3 wk, followed by same dose twice a week for 3 wk, or 4000 USP U 3 times/wk for 6 to 9 mo, following which the dosage may be reduced to 2000 USP U 3 times/wk for an additional 3 mo.

Interactions None well documented.

Lab Test Interferences Interference with radioimmunoassay for gonadotropins, particularly luteinizing hormone.

Adverse Reactions
CNS: Headache; irritability; restlessness; depression; fatigue.
GU: Precocious puberty; gynecomastia.
METAB: Edema.
OTHER: Pain at injection site.

Precautions
Pregnancy: Category C.
Lactation: Undetermined.
Children: Safety and efficacy in children less than 4 yr not established.
Special risk patients: Because chorionic gonadotropin may cause fluid retention, use with caution in patients with cardiac or renal disease, epilepsy, migraine, or asthma.
Health care provider use: Use in conjunction with human menopausal gonadotropins only by

health care provider experienced with infertility problems.

PATIENT CARE CONSIDERATIONS
Administration/Storage
- Follow manufacturer's instructions for reconstituting the Powder for Injection.
- Do not administer if particulate matter or discoloration noted.
- Administer only by IM injection. Not for ID, SC, or IV administration.
- With patient lying down or sitting, administer drug by IM injection. Rotate injection sites.
- To minimize bleeding, do not rub site after injection.
- Discard any unused reconstituted material.
- Store vials at controlled room temperature (59° to 86°F). Store reconstituted solution in refrigerator (36° to 46°F) and use within 30 or 60 days per manufacturer's recommendations.

Assessment/Interventions
- Obtain patient history, including drug history and any known allergies.
- Review patient's health history for any condition that could contraindicate chorionic gonadotropin (eg, previous allergic reaction to chorionic gonadotropin, precocious puberty, prostatic carcinoma, other androgen-dependent neoplasm).
- Ensure that women have had a thorough gynecological and endocrinological evaluation before starting therapy.

Precocious puberty: May induce precocious puberty in patients treated for cryptorchidism.

- Ensure that men have had a thorough medical and endocrinological evaluation before starting therapy.
- Monitor women for signs of overstimulation of the ovary (eg, difficulty breathing, severe pelvic pain, nausea, vomiting, weight gain, stomach pain or bloating, diarrhea, infrequent urination) and report to health care provider immediately if noted.

Patient/Family Education
- Explain name, dose, action, and potential side effects of drug. Review the treatment regimen including duration and monitoring that will be required.
- If patient will be administering at home, teach patient how to store, prepare, and administer the dose, and dispose of used equipment and supplies.
- Warn women that close monitoring for overstimulation of the ovary is required and to report any of the following immediately to health care provider: difficulty breathing, severe pelvic pain, nausea, vomiting, weight gain, stomach pain or bloating, diarrhea, or infrequent urination.
- Advise patient that follow-up visits and laboratory tests will be required to monitor therapy and to be sure to keep appointments.

Chromic Phosphate P 32

(KROME-ik FOSS-fate)

Class Radiopharmaceuticals

How Supplied
Phosphocol P 32 Suspension 15 mCi with a concentration of up to 5 mCi/mL

Action
PHARMACOLOGY: Local irradiation by beta emission. Chromic phosphate P32 decays by beta emission with a physical half-life of 14.3 days.

Indications
Adults: Treatment of peritoneal or pleural effusions caused by metastatic disease, cancer.

Contraindications
Presence of ulcerative tumors; administration in exposed cavities or where there is evidence of loculation unless its extent is determined.

Route/Dosage
Treatment of Peritoneal or Pleural Effusions Caused by Metastatic Disease, Cancer
ADULTS (ABOUT 70 KG): **Intraperitoneal** 10 to 20 mCi.

ADULTS (ABOUT 70 KG): **Intrapleural** 6 to 12 mCi.

ADULTS (ABOUT 70 KG): **Interstitial** 0.1 to 0.5 mCi/g of estimated weight of tumor.

Interactions
None well documented.

Lab Test Interferences
None well documented.

Adverse Reactions
GI: Nausea; abdominal cramping.
OTHER: Transitory radiation sickness; bone marrow depression; pleuritis; peritonitis.

Precautions
Pregnancy: Category C.
Lactation: Use only when clearly needed.

Benzyl alcohol: This product contains benzyl alcohol, which has been associated with fatal "gasping syndrome" in preterm infants.
Intracavitary use: Not for intravascular use.
Large tumor masses: When other forms of treatment fail to control effusion, chromic phosphate P 32 may be used.
Radioactive materials: Ensure minimum radiation exposure to the patient and occupational workers consistent with proper patient management.

PATIENT CARE CONSIDERATIONS
Administration/Storage
- Consult manufacturer product information for specific calibration and dosimetry information.
- For interstitial or intracavitary use only. Measure dose by suitable radioactivity calibration system immediately prior to use.

Assessment/Interventions
- Careful intracavitary instillation is required to avoid placing the dose of chromic phosphate P 32 into intrapleural or intraperitoneal loculations, bowel lumen, or the body wall. Intestinal fibrosis or necrosis and chronic fibrosis or the body wall have resulted from unrecognized misplacement of the therapeutic agent.

Patient/Family Education
- Explain name, dose, action, and potential side effects of drug.
- Advise patient, family, or caregiver that medication will be prepared and administered by health care provider in a health care setting.
- Advise patient, family, or caregiver that medication may be used in combination with other agents to achieve maximum benefit possible.
- Advise patient, family, or caregiver that medication is usually administered one time only.
- Advise patient, family, or caregiver to immediately report any of the following to health care provider: difficulty breathing or severe chest pain caused by breathing; fever, chills or other signs of infection; sores in mouth; unusual bleeding or bruising.
- Advise patient, family, or caregiver to report any of the following to health care provider: persistent nausea or vomiting or appetite loss; any other unexplained sensation.
- Instruct patient to not take any prescription or *otc* medications or dietary supplements unless advised to do so by health care provider.
- Instruct women of childbearing potential to notify health care provider if becoming pregnant, planning on becoming pregnant, or are breastfeeding.
- Advise patient that frequent follow-up visits and laboratory tests will be required to monitor therapy and to be sure to keep appointments.

Chromium

(KROE-mee-uhm)

Class Trace Metal

How Supplied
Chromic Chloride Injection 4 mcg/mL (as 20.5 mcg chromic chloride hexahydrate), Injection 20 mcg/mL (as 102.5 mcg chromic chloride hexahydrate) ◆ *Chromium Chloride* Injection 4 mcg/mL (as 20.5 mcg chromic chloride hexahydrate) ◆ *Chroma-Pak* Injection 4 mcg/mL (as 20.5 mcg chromic chloride hexahydrate), Injection 20 mcg/mL (as 102.5 mcg chromic chloride hexahydrate)

Action
PHARMACOLOGY: Helps maintain normal glucose metabolism and peripheral nerve function.

PHARMACOKINETICS/DYNAMICS:
Absorption: Typical blood levels range from 1 to 5 mcg/L.
Excretion: Primarily via the kidney.

Indications Use as a supplement to IV solutions given for total parenteral nutrition (TPN) to prevent depletion of endogenous stores and subsequent deficiency symptoms.

Contraindications Direct IM or IV injection.

Route/Dosage
Trace Metal for TPN
ADULTS: **TPN Additive** 10 to 15 mcg/day. Metabolically stable adults with intestinal fluid loss may require 20 mcg/day.
CHILDREN: **TPN Additive** 0.14 to 0.20 mcg/kg/day.

Interactions None well documented.

Lab Test Interferences None well documented.

Adverse Reactions None known.

Precautions
Pregnancy: Category C.
Lactation: Undetermined.
Children: Safety and efficacy not established (see Route/Dosage).
Renal function impairment: Dosage may need to be adjusted or omitted.
General: Use only in conjunction with a

pharmacy-directed admixture program using aseptic technique in a laminar flow environment.

PATIENT CARE CONSIDERATIONS
Administration/Storage
- For admixture in TPN solution only. Not for intradermal, SC, IM, or direct IV administration.
- Add prescribed additive dose to TPN solution using aseptic technique, preferably under a laminar flow hood.
- Do not administer if particulate matter, cloudiness, or discoloration are noted.
- Discard any unused solution in the single-dose vial. Do not save for future use.
- Store vials at controlled room temperature (59° to 86°F).

Assessment/Interventions
- Obtain patient history, including drug history and any known allergies. Note renal impairment.

Overdosage: Signs and Symptoms
Nausea, vomiting, GI ulcers, renal and hepatic damage, convulsions, coma.

- Ensure that renal function is evaluated before starting therapy and periodically during treatment.
- Frequently assess vascular access site for signs of inflammation or infection. Inform health care provider if noted.

Patient/Family Education
- Explain name, action, and potential side effects of drug.
- Advise patient, family, or caregiver that medication will be added to TPN solution.
- Advise patient to report pain, redness, warmth, or swelling of TPN access site.
- Advise patient that follow-up visits and lab tests will be required to monitor therapy and to keep appointments.

Ciclopirox
(sigh-kloe-PEER-ox)
Class Topical anti-infective/Antifungal

How Supplied
Loprox Cream 0.77%, Suspension, topical 0.77%, Gel 0.77%, Shampoo 1% ♦ *Penlac Nail Lacquer* Solution, topical 8%

Action
PHARMACOLOGY: Broad-spectrum, antifungal agent with an unknown mechanism of action.

PHARMACOKINETICS/DYNAMICS:
Absorption: Absorption is 1.3% with topical application followed by occlusion for 6 hr.
Excretion: The primary route of metabolism is glucuronidation. The t½ is 1.7 hr with excretion primarily via the kidney.

Indications
Loprox:
Shampoo/Gel – Topical treatment of seborrheic dermatitis of the scalp in adults.
Gel – Interdigital tinea pedis and tinea corporis caused by *T. rubrum*, *T. mentagroyphytes*, or *E. floccosum*.
Cream/Suspension – Tinea pedis (athlete's foot), tinea cruris (jock itch), and tinea corporis (ringworm) caused by *T. rubrum*, *T. mentagrophytes*, *E. floccosum*, and *M. canis*; cutaneous candidiasis (moniliasis) caused by *C. albicans*; tinea (pityriasis) versicolor caused by *M. furfur*.
Penlac: As a component of a comprehensive management program for topical treatment in immunocompetent patients with mild to moderate onychomycosis of fingernails and toenails without lunula involvement, caused by *T. rubrum*.

Contraindications Standard considerations.

Route/Dosage
LOPROX SHAMPOO
ADULTS AND CHILDREN 16 YR AND OLDER:
Topical Wet hair and apply approximately 1 tsp (5 mL) to the scalp. Up to 2 tsp (10 mL) may be used for long hair. Lather and leave on hair and scalp for 3 min. Rinse off. Repeat treatment 2 times/wk for 4 wk, with a minimum of 3 days between applications. If no improvement after 4 wk of treatment, reevaluate the diagnosis.

LOPROX CREAM/SUSPENSION
ADULTS AND CHILDREN 10 YR AND OLDER:
Topical Gently massage cream into the affected and surrounding skin areas bid, morning and evening. If no improvement after 4 wk of treatment, reevaluate the diagnosis.

LOPROX GEL
ADULTS AND CHILDREN 16 YR AND OLDER:
Topical Gently massage gel into affected skin areas of scalp areas bid, morning and evening. If no improvement after 4 wk of treatment, reevaluate the diagnosis.

PENLAC
ADULTS: **Topical** Apply qd, at bedtime or 8 hr before washing, to all affected nails with the provided applicator. Apply evenly over the entire nail plate. If possible, apply to nail bed, hyponychium, and the under surface of the nail plate when it is free of the nail bed (eg, onycholysis). Do not remove product on a daily

basis. Make daily applications over the previous coat and remove with alcohol q 7 days, repeating this cycle throughout the duration of therapy. As a comprehensive management program for onychomycosis, removal of the unattached, infected nail, as frequently as monthly, by a health care professional, weekly trimming by the patient, and daily application of the medication are integral parts of therapy.

Interactions None well documented.

Lab Test Interferences None well documented.

Adverse Reactions
CV: Ventricular tachycardia (*Loprox* shampoo).
DERM: Pruritus at application site, worsening of clinical signs and symptoms, burning (*Loprox* cream); skin burning sensation upon application (34% of patients with seborrheic dermatitis; 7% with tinea pedis); periungual erythema and erythema of the proximal nail fold (5%); contact dermatitis, pruritus (1% to 5%); dry skin, acne, rash, alopecia, pain upon application, eye pain, facial edema (less than 1%; *Loprox* gel); pruritus, burning (*Loprox* suspension); increased itching, application site reactions (eg, burning, erythema, itching), nail disorders (eg, shape change, irritation), application site reactions and/or burning of the skin (1%); seborrhea, rash, headache, skin disorder (*Loprox* shampoo); mild rash (*Penlac* topical solution).

Precautions
Pregnancy: Category B.
Lactation: Undetermined.
Children:
Loprox shampoo/gel – Safety and efficacy not established in children under 16 yr.
Loprox cream/suspension – Safety and efficacy not established in children under 10 yr.
Penlac – Safety and efficacy not established.
Application: For external use only, avoid contact with the eyes.
Sensitivity: If sensitivity or chemical irritation occurs, discontinue treatment and institute appropriate therapy.

PATIENT CARE CONSIDERATIONS

Administration/Storage
- For topical use only. Not for ophthalmic, otic, oral, or intravaginal use.
- Cream, gel, and suspension should be applied topically to skin lesions bid. Wash and dry areas to be treated; gently massage small amount into the affected and surrounding skin areas. Do not use occlusive wraps or dressings on treated areas.
- Topical solution is applied to affected nails qd at bedtime or 8 hr before washing. Apply small amount of solution to affected nails and skin immediately surrounding the treated nails using applicator brush supplied with bottle; apply solution under surface of nail when it is free of the nail bed; daily applications should be made over the previous coat and then removed with alcohol q 7 days following which the nails should be trimmed and loose nail material filed away with emery board. The cycle is then repeated.
- Shampoo is used 2 times/wk, with a minimum of 3 days between applications. Wet hair; apply approximately 1 tsp (up to 2 tsp for long hair) of shampoo to scalp; lather and leave on hair and scalp for 3 min then rinse hair and scalp. Avoid contact with eyes. If contact occurs, rinse thoroughly with water.
- Store cream, gel, solution, suspension, and shampoo at room temperature (59° to 86°F). Discard any unused shampoo 8 wk after opening. Protect solution from light and away from heat and flame. Keep solution tightly capped and stored in original carton after each use.

Assessment/Interventions
- Obtain patient history, including drug history and any known allergies.
- Assess the skin or nails, as appropriate, and identify areas where medication is to be applied.
- Assess and document skin or nail condition before initial application and periodically throughout treatment.
- Monitor for application site reactions, including redness, itching, burning, blistering, swelling, or oozing. Inform health care provider if noted and significant.

Patient/Family Education
- Explain name, action, and potential side effects of drug.
- Advise patient that improvement in symptoms may take a week or longer to occur but to notify health care provider if symptoms have not improved after 4 wk of continuous use.
- Instruct patient to use medication for the full treatment time even if symptoms have improved.
- Advise patient that shampoo is used 2 times/wk, with a minimum of 3 days between applications.
- Advise patient that cream, gel, or suspension should be applied topically to skin lesions bid.
- Advise patient that topical solution is applied to affected nails qd at bedtime or 8 hr before washing.
- Teach patient proper technique for applying cream, suspension, or gel: wash hands; wash

and dry areas to be treated; gently massage small amount into the affected and surrounding skin areas. Wash hands after applying medication.
- Inform patient that a sensation of burning or stinging may be felt shortly after application of the gel and that this is expected and should be of no concern.
- Caution patient to avoid using occlusive dressings or wraps following application of cream, gel, or suspension.
- Teach patient proper technique for applying shampoo: wet hair; apply approximately 1 tsp (up to 2 tsp for long hair) of shampoo to scalp; lather and leave on hair and scalp for 3 min then rinse hair and scalp. Avoid contact with eyes; if contact occurs, rinse thoroughly with water.
- Teach patient proper technique for applying topical solution: review Patient Information and Instructions sheet provided with medication; wash hands; apply small amount of solution to affected nails and skin immediately surrounding the treated nails using applicator brush supplied with bottle; apply solution under surface of nail when it is free of the nail bed; daily applications should be made over the previous coat and then removed with alcohol q 7 days following which the nails should be trimmed and loose nail material filed away with emery board. The cycle is then repeated. Professional removal of unattached infected nails should be performed as frequently as monthly by health care provider.
- Caution diabetic patient using solution to talk with health care provider before trimming or removing any nail material.
- Advise patient using solution on nails not to use nail polish or other nail cosmetic products on treated nails.
- Caution patient using solution to avoid use near open flame because product is flammable.
- Advise patient that if application site of any of these products shows signs of increased irritation (eg, redness, itching, burning, blistering, swelling, oozing) to stop using the medication and contact health care provider.
- Advise women to notify health care provider if pregnant, planning to become pregnant, or breastfeeding.
- Warn patient not to take any prescription or OTC drugs or dietary supplements without consulting health care provider.
- Advise patient that follow-up visits to examine the skin or nail lesions may be necessary and to keep appointments.

Cidofovir

(sigh-DAH-fah-vihr)

Class Anti-infective/Antiviral

How Supplied
Vistide Injection 75 mg/mL

Action

PHARMACOLOGY: Inhibits viral DNA synthesis by interfering with viral DNA polymerase.

PHARMACOKINETICS/DYNAMICS:

Absorption: Based on administration with probenecid, C_{max} is about 9.8 to 19.6 mcg/mL and AUC is about 25.7 to 40.8 mcg•hr/mL.

Distribution: Vd is about 410 mL/kg (at steady state). Less than 6% protein bound.

Excretion: Cl is about 148 mL/min/1.73 m^2. Renal Cl is about 98.6 mL/min/1.73 m^2.

Special Populations:
Renal Function Impairment – Cl decreases proportionally with Ccr. Dosage adjustment is recommended.

Indications Treatment of CMV retinitis in patients with AIDS.

Contraindications History of clinically severe hypersensitivity to probenecid or other sulfa-containing medications; direct intraocular injection. Patients receiving agents with a nephrotoxic potential must discontinue use of such agents at least 1 wk prior to beginning therapy. Initiation of therapy in patients with a serum creatinine greater than 1.5 mg/dL, a calculated Ccr of less than or equal to 55 mL/min, or a urine protein at least 100 mg/dL.

Route/Dosage

ADULT:

Induction: **IV** 5 mg/kg once weekly for 2 consecutive weeks.

Maintenance dose: **IV** 5 mg/kg once q 2 wk.
Nephrotoxicity – Reduce the dose of cidofovir to 3 mg/kg for increases in serum creatinine (0.3 to 0.4 mg/dL).

Probenecid – Administer probenecid orally with each dose of cidofovir. Probenecid 2 g given 3 hr prior to the cidofovir dose and 1 g administered 2 hr and again at 8 hr after completion of the cidofovir infusion.

Interactions
Nephrotoxic agents (eg, aminoglycosides, amphotericin B, foscarnet, IV pentamidine): Risk of nephrotoxicity is increased.

Lab Test Interferences
None well documented.

Adverse Reactions
CV: Hypotension; postural hypotension; pallor; syncope; tachycardia.

CNS: Headache; amnesia; anxiety; confusion; convulsion; depression; dizziness; abnormal gait; hallucinations; insomnia; neuropathy; paresthesia; somnolence; vasodilation.

DERM: Alopecia; rash; acne; skin discoloration; dry skin; herpes simplex; pruritus; sweating; urticaria.

EENT: Amblyopia; conjunctivitis; eye disorder; iritis; retinal detachment; uveitis; abnormal vision; hypotonia.

GI: Nausea; vomiting; diarrhea; anorexia; abdominal pain; colitis; constipation; tongue discoloration; dyspepsia; dysphagia; flatulence; gastritis; melena; oral candidiasis; rectal disorder; stomatitis; aphthous stomatitis; mouth ulceration; dry mouth; taste perversion.

GU: Renal toxicity; proteinuria; elevated creatinine and decreased Ccr; glycosuria; hematuria; urinary incontinence; urinary tract infection.

HEMA: Thrombocytopenia; neutropenia; anemia.

HEPA: Hepatomegaly; abnormal LFTs; increased AST; increased ALT.

METAB: Dehydration; hyperglycemia; hyperlipidemia; hypocalcemia; hypokalemia; metabolic acidosis; increased alkaline phosphatase; weight loss.

RESP: Asthma; bronchitis; coughing; dyspnea; hiccough; increased sputum; lung disorder; pharyngitis; pneumonia; rhinitis; sinusitis.

OTHER: Allergy; edema; malaise; back pain; chest pain; neck pain; sarcoma; sepsis; arthralgia; asthenia; myasthenia; myalgia; fever; chills; infection.

PATIENT CARE CONSIDERATIONS
Administration/Storage
- For IV infusion only. Do not administer by direct intraocular injection.
- Follow National Institutes of Health guidelines for handling and disposal of this mutagenic agent.
- Inspect vial for particulate matter and discoloration. Do not use if noted.
- Prescribed dose must be withdrawn from vial and diluted in 100 mL of Normal Saline before IV administration.
- Administer diluted solution over 1 hr using infusion pump.
- Patient should receive 1 L of Normal Saline

> **WARNING:**
> *Animal data:* Carcinogenic and teratogenic effects and impaired fertility reported.
> *Nephrotoxicity:* Major toxicity occurs. Cases of acute renal failure resulting in dialysis and/or contributing to death occurred with as few as 1 or 2 doses. Reduce possible nephrotoxicity with IV prehydration (normal saline) and administration of probenecid. Monitor serum creatinine and urine protein within 48 hr prior to each dose. Dose adjustment required for changes in renal function.
> *Neutropenia:* May occur; monitor neutrophil count.

Precautions
Pregnancy: Category C.
Lactation: Undetermined.
Children: Safety and efficacy not established.
Elderly: Because elderly individuals frequently have reduced glomerular filtration, assess renal function before and during cidofovir therapy.
Renal function impairment: Cidofovir administration is not recommended if serum creatinine greater than 1.5 mg/dL or Ccr less than or equal to 55 mL/min.
Monitoring: Monitor serum creatinine, urine protein, and WBC with differential prior to each dose.
Contraception: Women of childbearing potential should use effective contraception during and for 1 mo following treatment. Men should use a barrier contraceptive during and for 3 mo following treatment.
Intraocular pressure: May be associated with decreases in intraocular pressure and impairment of vision.
Direct intraocular injection: May be associated with iritis, ocular hypotony, and permanent impairment of vision.
Metabolic acidosis: Decreased serum bicarbonate associated with proximal tubule injury and renal wasting syndrome may occur.
Uveitis/Iritis: Uveitis/Iritis has been reported.

infused over a 1- to 2-hr period immediately before the cidofovir infusion.
- Administer a second liter of Normal Saline at the start of the cidofovir infusion or immediately afterward if the patient can tolerate it, and infuse over 1 to 3 hr.
- Unopened vial can be stored at room temperature (68° to 77°F).
- Discard any unused medication remaining in vial.
- IV admixtures may be stored for 24 hr under refrigeration (36° to 46°F).
- Warm IV solution to room temperature before administration.

Assessment/Interventions
- Obtain patient history, including drug history and any known allergies.
- Report any suspected side effects to health care provider.
- Ensure that serum creatinine, urine protein, and WBC are obtained prior to each dose. If proteinuria is noted, administer IV hydration and repeat the test.
- If patient is taking zidovudine, ensure that zidovudine is discontinued or reduce dose by 50% on days of cidofovir infusion.
- Ensure that IOP, visual acuity, and ocular symptoms are periodically monitored.
- Administer 2 g probenecid 3 hr before IV dose, and 1 g at 2 and 8 hr after the dose. Administer with food if patient experiences probenecid-induced nausea or vomiting. If nausea or vomiting persist, notify health care provider. An antiemetic may need to be prescribed.
- Administer 1 L of Normal Saline over a 1 to 2 hr period immediately before cidofovir dose. Ensure that a second liter of Normal Saline is infused during or after the cidofovir dose if the patient can tolerate it.
- Monitor patient for allergic reaction to probenecid. Notify health care provider if suspected. Prophylactic antihistamine may be needed.

Patient/Family Education
- Advise patient that this medication does not cure CMV retinitis and that progression of retinitis during and following treatment may be experienced.
- Instruct patient to continue taking the antiretroviral therapy. However, if patient is taking zidovudine, to either reduce the dose by ½ or stop on days of cidofovir administration.
- Instruct patient taking oral cidofovir that it is essential to take a full course of probenecid with each dose (2 g 3 hr before and 1 g 2 hr and 8 hr after completing the infusion).
- Inform patient that taking the probenecid after a meal or the use of antiemetics may decrease nausea.
- Instruct patient of childbearing potential that cidofovir is embryotoxic and that appropriate contraceptive methods should be used by women during treatment and for 1 mo after treatment is completed. Men should use barrier contraceptive during and for 3 mo following completion of therapy.
- Advise patient that regular eye examinations will be necessary and to keep appointments.
- Advise patient to report any suspected side effects to health care provider.
- Inform patient of the major toxicities of cidofovir, ie, renal impairment, and that dose modification, including reduction, interruption, and discontinuation may be necessary.
- Advise patient that cidofovir causes tumors (eg, mammary adenocarcinomas) in rats and should be considered a potential carcinogen in humans.

Cilostazol

(sigh-low-stay-zol)

Class Antiplatelet

How Supplied
Pletal Tablets 50 mg, Tablets 100 mg

Action
PHARMACOLOGY: Quinolinone derivative that inhibits cellular phosphodiesterase and exhibits a higher specificity for phosphodiesterase III.

PHARMACOKINETICS/DYNAMICS:
Absorption: A high-fat meal increases C_{max} about 90% and AUC 25%.
Distribution: 95% to 98% protein bound, predominantly to albumin.
Metabolism: Extensively metabolized in the liver by CYP3A4 and, to a lesser extent, CYP2C19. Two of the metabolites are active.
Excretion: The $t_½$ is about 11 to 13 hr. About 74% is excreted in the urine and 20% in the feces as metabolites.

Special Populations:
Renal Function Impairment – The free fraction of cilostazol was 27% higher.
Smoking – Smoking decreased exposure by about 20%.

Indications Reduction of symptoms of intermittent claudication as indicated by an increased walking distance.

Contraindications CHF of any severity; hypersensitivity to any components of the product. Cilostazol and several of its metabolites are inhibitors of phosphodiesterase III. Several drugs with this pharmacologic effect have caused decreased survival compared with placebo in patients with class III to IV CHF.

Route/Dosage
Intermittent Claudication
PO 100 mg twice daily, taken at least 30 min before or 2 hr after breakfast and dinner. Consider a dose of 50 mg twice daily during coadministration of such inhibitors of CYP3A4 and CYP2C19.

Interactions
Aspirin: Short-term (up to 4 days) coadministration of aspirin with cilostazol showed a 23% to 35% increase in inhibition of ADP-induced ex vivo platelet aggregation compared with aspirin alone.
Diltiazem: Diltiazem increased cilostazol plasma concentrations by about 53%. Initiate therapy at half the recommended dose.
Macrolides: Erythromycin increased cilostazol C_{max} by 47% and AUC by 73%. Other macrolide antibiotics would be expected to have similar effects. Initiate therapy at half the recommended dose.
Omeprazole: Coadministration of omeprazole did not significantly affect the metabolism of cilostazol, but the systemic exposure to 3,4-dehydro-cilostazol was increased by 69%, probably the result of omeprazole's potent inhibition of CYP2C19. Initiate therapy at half the recommended dose.
P450 system: Cilostazol could have pharmacokinetic interactions because of effects of other drugs on its metabolism by CYP3A4 or CYP2C19.
Platelet function inhibitors: Cilostazol could have pharmacodynamic interactions with other platelet function inhibitors.

Lab Test Interferences
None well documented.

Adverse Reactions
CV: Palpitations; tachycardia.
CNS: Dizziness; vertigo.
GI: Abnormal stool; diarrhea; dyspepsia; flatulence; nausea.
RESP: Increased cough; pharyngitis; rhinitis.
OTHER: Abdominal pain; back pain; headache; infection; myalgia; peripheral edema.

> **WARNING:**
> CHF: Contraindicated for use in CHF patients of any severity. Cilostazol and metabolites are inhibitors of phosphodiesterase III. Such activity has been shown to decrease survival of patients with class III to IV CHF.

Precautions
Pregnancy: Category C.
Lactation: Undetermined.
Children: Safety and efficacy in children have not been established.

PATIENT CARE CONSIDERATIONS

Administration/Storage
- Store at room temperature in a nonmoist environment (59° to 86°F).
- Administer 30 min before or 2 hr after meals.
- Do not administer with grapefruit juice. Avoid concurrent use because of food/drug interaction.
- Do not administer to patient with any type of CHF.
- Do not administer to patient with a hypersensitivity to cilostazol or any of its active ingredients.
- Administer with caution to patients with renal, liver, or coagulation impairment.
- Administer with caution to patients on other anticoagulant medications.

Assessment/Interventions
- Obtain a complete drug history of prescription and nonprescription drugs.
- Assess patient for potential drug interactions especially with those drugs metabolized by the P450 enzyme system especially CYP3A4 and 2C19 (eg, erythromycin, fluconazole, ketoconazole, itraconazole, omeprazole).
- Monitor patient for signs of hypersensitivity, adverse, and therapeutic reactions.
- Assess smokers for signs of therapy effectiveness.
- Assess patient for adverse cardiac signs and symptoms and signs of CHF.
- Monitor patient for signs and symptoms of bleeding, especially those concurrently on other anticoagulants.

Patient/Family Education
- Instruct patient to take cilostazol as directed and to read the patient package insert before starting therapy or restarting therapy.
- Advise patient to inform primary care provider if taking or planning to take any *otc* medications, as there is potential for drug interactions.
- Advise patient that beneficial effects of cilostazol may not be immediate as relief of symptoms may require greater than 2 to 12 wk.
- Instruct patient to avoid consuming grapefruit juice to avoid drug/food interactions.
- Advise smokers of risks, including potential

interaction with the drug, and the benefits of not smoking.
- Warn patient of the uncertainty concerning the cardiovascular risk with long-term use or for the patient with underlying heart disease. Instruct patient to report adverse cardiac symptoms immediately to primary care provider before continuing next dose
- Advise patient not to take aspirin or any other NSAID without informing the primary care provider
- Instruct patient to inform the primary caregiver of any adverse reactions.
- Warn women with childbearing potential to avoid becoming pregnant and apprise them of the potential hazard to the fetus.
- Warn nursing mothers of the danger of transferring the drug to the baby through mother's milk and possible infant effects. Make a decision to discontinue the drug or nursing in collaboration with the health care provider.
- Instruct patient to report any unusual reaction or concern to the primary care provider.

Cimetidine

(sigh-MET-ih-deen)

Class Histamine H_2 antagonist

How Supplied
Tagamet Tablets 200 mg, Tablets 300 mg, Tablets 400 mg, Tablets 800 mg, Liquid 300 mg (as hydrochloride)/5 mL, Injection 300 mg (as hydrochloride)/2 mL, Injection, premixed 300 mg (as hydrochloride) in 50 mL 0.9% sodium chloride ♦ *Tagamet HB* Tablets 100 mg ❋ *Apo-Cimetidine* ♦ *Gen-Cimetidine* ♦ *Novo-Cimetine* ♦ *Nu-Cimet*

Action
PHARMACOLOGY: Reversibly and competitively blocks histamine at H_2 receptors, particularly those in gastric parietal cells, leading to inhibition of gastric acid secretion.

PHARMACOKINETICS/DYNAMICS:
Absorption:
Oral – Rapidly absorbed. T_{max} is 45 to 90 min. 60% to 70% bioavailable.

Distribution: 13% to 25% protein bound. Vd is 0.8 to 1.2 L/kg. Crosses the placenta and is excreted in breast milk.

Metabolism: Following oral administration, cimetidine is extensively metabolized with the sulfoxide being the major metabolite.

Excretion: The t½ is about 2 hr.
Oral – 48% is excreted unchanged in the urine.
IV/IM – About 75% is excreted unchanged in the urine.

Special Populations:
Renal Function Impairment – Drug accumulation may occur in those with severe renal failure. Dosage adjustment may be necessary.

Indications
Management of duodenal ulcer; treatment of gastroesophageal reflux disease (GERD), including erosive esophagitis; therapy for benign gastric ulcer; treatment of pathologic hypersecretory conditions; prevention of upper GI bleeding. **Unlabeled use(s):** Prevention of aspiration pneumonia and stress ulcers; herpes virus infection; chronic idiopathic urticaria; anaphylaxis (relieves dermatologic symptoms only); dyspepsia; used before anesthesia to prevent aspiration pneumonitis; treatment of hyperparathyroidism and control of secondary hyperparathyroidism in chronic hemodialysis patient; treatment of chronic viral warts in children.

Contraindications
Hypersensitivity to cimetidine or other H_2 antagonists.

Route/Dosage
Duodenal Ulcer (Active)
ADULTS: **PO** 800 mg at bedtime for 4 to 6 wk.
ALTERNATE REGIMENS: **PO** 300 mg qid with meals and at bedtime or 400 mg bid.
MAINTENANCE THERAPY: **PO** 400 mg at bedtime.

Active Benign Gastric Ulcer
ADULTS: **PO** 800 mg at bedtime.

GERD
ADULTS: **PO** 1600 mg daily in divided doses (800 mg or 400 mg) for 12 wk, although some patients may require chronic therapy.

Pathologic Hypersecretory Conditions
ADULTS: **PO** 300 mg qid w/meals and at bedtime. If needed, 300 mg doses may be given more often (max, 2400 mg/day).

Prevention of Upper GI Bleeding
ADULTS: Continuous IV infusion of 50 mg/hr. For hospitalized patients with pathologic hypersecretory conditions or intractable ulcers, or patients unable to take PO medication. Usual dose: **IM/IV** 300 mg q 6 h to 8 h (max 2400 mg/day).

Interactions
Antacids, anticholinergics, metoclopramide: May decrease absorption of cimetidine.
Benzodiazepines, caffeine, calcium channel blockers, carbamazepine, chloroquine, labetalol, lidocaine, metoprolol, metronidazole, moricizine, pentoxifylline, phenytoin, propranolol, quinidine, quinine, sulfonylureas, theophyllines, triamterene, tricyclic antidepressants, warfarin: Cimetidine may reduce metabolism and increase serum concentration and pharmacologic/toxic effects of these drugs.

Carmustine: Bone marrow toxicity may be enhanced.
Cigarette smoking: Reversed cimetidine's effects on suppression of nocturnal gastric secretion.
Ferrous salts, indomethacin, fluconazole, ketoconazole, tetracyclines: Cimetidine may decrease absorption of these drugs.
Hydantoins: Hydantoin levels may increase.
Narcotic analgesics: Toxic effects (eg, respiratory depression) may be increased.
Procainamide: Levels of procainamide and its active metabolite may increase.
Tocainide: Cimetidine may decrease the pharmacologic effects of tocainide.

Lab Test Interferences None well documented.

Adverse Reactions
CV: Cardiac arrhythmias.
CNS: Headache; somnolence; fatigue; dizziness; confusional states; hallucinations.
DERM: Exfoliative dermatitis or erythroderma; alopecia; rash; erythema multiforme; epidermal necrolysis.
GI: Diarrhea.
GU: Impotence; loss of libido.
RESP: Bronchospasm.
OTHER: Gynecomastia; hypersensitivity reactions; transient pain at injection site; reversible exacerbation of joint symptoms with pre-existing arthritis, including gouty arthritis.

Precautions
Pregnancy: Category B.
Lactation: Excreted in breast milk.
Children: Safety and efficacy not established.
Elderly: May have reduced renal function; decreased Cl may occur.
Hypersensitivity: Rare cases of anaphylaxis have occurred as well as rare episodes of hypersensitivity.
Renal function impairment: Decreased Cl may occur; reduced dosage may be needed.
Hepatic function impairment: Use caution; decreased clearance may occur.
Gastric malignancy: Symptomatic relief with cimetidine does not preclude gastric malignancy.
Antiandrogenic effect: Gynecomastia may occur, especially in patients treated for pathologic hypersecretory states.
Rapid IV administration: Has been followed by rare instances of cardiac arrhythmias and hypotension.
Reversible CNS effects: Mental confusion, agitation, psychosis, depression, anxiety, hallucinations, and disorientation have occurred, predominantly in severely ill patients. Advanced age and pre-existing liver or renal disease appear to be contributing factors.

PATIENT CARE CONSIDERATIONS

Administration/Storage
- Administer medication with or before meals and at bedtime for max effect.
- Administer IM dose undiluted. Dilute IV dose (300 mg) in 0.9% Normal Saline, D5W, or other compatible solution to a total of 20 mL. Inject slowly over at least 5 min.
- For intermittent IV infusion, dilute 300 mg in at least 50 mL of compatible solution; infuse over at least 20 min (continuous IV infusion is usually preceded by a loading dose).
- Do not add drugs or additives to mixture. Stop other inline drugs while administering, and flush lines before and after administration.
- Do not allow equipment containing aluminum to come in contact with the solution.
- Use only compatible solutions for admixture: 0.9% Normal Saline, 5% and 10% Dextrose in Water, lactated Ringer's solution, 5% Sodium Bicarbonate.
- Product may be added to standard TPN solutions.
- Store premixed products at room temperature. Discard any unused mixed solutions after 48 hr.

Assessment/Interventions
- Obtain patient history, including drug history and any known allergies.
- Establish baseline vital signs.
- Avoid administering antacids within 1 hr of medication.
- Review periodic monitoring of serum concentrations and clinical effects for other drugs affected by cimetidine.
- Renal/Liver function studies and blood counts are all especially important in elderly.
- Assess patient for abdominal pain, confusion and GI bleeding (eg, blood in stools, emesis).
- Assess gastric pH q 8 hr, when possible.

Patient/Family Education
- Counsel patients to stop smoking, since smoking reduces ulcer-healing efficacy of cimetidine.
- Instruct patients to keep appointments for laboratory testing and health care provider follow-up.
- Advise patients not to take *otc* medications without consulting health care provider.
- Instruct patients to report to health care provider immediately any black tarry stools,

coffee-ground emesis, abdominal pain or confusion.
- Counsel patients regarding need for life-style changes, stress reduction programs and dietary modifications (eg, avoid spicy foods and alcohol).

Cinacalcet Hydrochloride

(sin-a-KAL-set HIGH-dore-KLOR-ide)

Class Calcimimetic

How Supplied
Sensipar Tablets 30 mg, Tablets 60 mg, Tablets 90 mg

Action
PHARMACOLOGY: Lowers parathyroid hormone (PTH) levels by increasing sensitivity of calcium sensing receptor to extracellular calcium.

PHARMACOKINETICS/DYNAMICS:
Absorption: C_{max} approximately 2 to 6 hr. Steady state achieved within 7 days.

Distribution: Vd is approximately 1,000 L. Protein binding is 93% to 97%.

Metabolism: Metabolized by cytochrome P450 (CYP) 3A4, CYP2D6, and CYP1A2.

Excretion: Terminal t½ 30 to 40 hr. Approximately 80% of a dose is recovered in the urine and 15% in the feces.

Special Populations:
Hepatic Function Impairment – In patients with moderate or severe hepatic impairment, the AUCs were 2.4 and 4.2 times higher, respectively, than in normal subjects; the t½ is prolonged 33% and 70%, respectively.

Indications Treatment of secondary hyperparathyroidism in patients with chronic kidney disease on dialysis; hypercalcemia in patients with parathyroid carcinoma.

Contraindications Standard considerations.

Route/Dosage
Secondary Hyperparathyroidism in Patients with Chronic Kidney Disease on Dialysis
ADULTS: **PO** Start with 30 mg daily. Titrate dose q 2 to 4 wk through sequential doses of 60, 90, 120, and 180 mg daily based on target intact PTH.

Parathyroid Carcinoma
ADULTS: **PO** Start with 30 mg bid. Titrate q 2 to 4 wk through sequential doses of 30, 60, and 90 mg bid, and 90 mg tid or qid as needed to normalize serum calcium levels.

Interactions
Drugs metabolized by CYP2D6 (eg, flecainide, thioridazine): Plasma levels may be elevated by cinacalcet, increasing the pharmacologic and adverse effects.

Strong inhibitors of CYP3A4 (eg, erythromycin, ketoconazole, itraconazole): May elevate cinacalcet concentrations, increasing the pharmacologic and adverse effects.

Lab Test Interferences None well documented.

Adverse Reactions
CV: Hypertension (7%).
CNS: Dizziness (10%).
GI: Nausea (31%); vomiting (27%); diarrhea (21%); anorexia (6%).
MUSC: Myalgia (15%).
OTHER: Asthenia (7%); non-cardiac chest pain (6%); access infection (5%).

Precautions
Pregnancy: Category C.
Lactation: Undetermined.
Children: Safety and efficacy not established.
Hepatic function impairment: Closely monitor PTH and serum calcium concentrations throughout therapy in patients with moderate or severe hepatic impairment.
Adynamic bone disease: May occur if intact PTH levels are suppressed below 100 picograms/mL.
Hypocalcemia: May occur; closely monitor.
Parathyroid carcinoma patients: Measure serum calcium within 1 wk after starting or adjusting the dose of cinacalcet; once maintenance dose levels are established, serum calcium should be measured q 2 mo.
Seizures: Seizures may occur. Closely monitor serum calcium levels, particularly in patients with a history of seizures.

Overdosage: Signs and Symptoms
Hypocalcemia.

PATIENT CARE CONSIDERATIONS

Administration/Storage
- Can be used alone or in combination with vitamin D and/or phosphate binders.
- Administer prescribed dose with food or shortly after a meal. Instruct patient to swallow tablets whole and not to chew or divide.
- Store tablets at ambient room temperature (59° to 86°F).

Assessment/Interventions
- Obtain patient history, including drug history and any known allergies. Note hepatic impairment, seizure disorder, history of seizures, concurrent use of medications known to be metabolized by CYP2D6 (eg, flecainide, tricyclic antidepressants), or concurrent use of strong inhibitors of CYP3A4 (eg, ketoconazole).

- Ensure that serum calcium and phosphorus are measured within 1 wk of initiating therapy or dose adjustment and then monthly (2 mo in patient with parathyroid carcinoma) once maintenance dose has been established.
- Ensure that intact PTH is measured 1 to 4 wk after initiating therapy or dose adjustment and then q 1 to 3 mo once maintenance dose has been established.
- Ensure that therapy is not started in patient whose baseline serum calcium is less than 8.4 mg/dL.
- Carefully monitor patient for signs and symptoms of hypocalcemia (eg, paresthesias, myalgia, cramping, tetany, convulsions). Immediately inform health care provider if noted.
- Be prepared to administer calcium-containing phosphate binders and/or vitamin D to patient who develops symptoms of hypocalcemia, or whose serum calcium level falls below 8.4 mg/dL but is above 7.5 mg/dL.
- Ensure that cinacalcet is temporarily discontinued in patient whose serum calcium falls below 7.5 mg/dL or if symptoms of hypocalcemia persist and the dose of vitamin D cannot be increased. Therapy can be reinstituted using next lowest dose when serum calcium level reaches 8 mg/dL and/or symptoms of hypocalcemia have resolved.
- Ensure that dose of cinacalcet and/or vitamin D is reduced if intact PTH levels decrease to less than 150 picograms/mL.
- Assess patient for GI and general body side effects. Inform health care provider if noted and significant.

Patient/Family Education
- Explain name, dose, action, and potential side effects of drug.
- Advise patient to take prescribed dose with food or shortly after a meal. Caution patient to swallow tablets whole and not to chew, divide, or crush.
- Caution patient not to change the dose or stop taking unless advised by health care provider.
- Instruct patient to continue taking other medications (eg, vitamin D and/or phosphate binders) as prescribed by health care provider for controlling calcium levels.
- Instruct patient to immediately inform health care provider if the following signs or symptoms of hypocalcemia develop: abnormal skin sensations, muscle aches, muscle cramping or spasm, seizure activity.
- Advise women to notify health care provider if pregnant, planning to become pregnant, or breastfeeding.
- Caution patient not to take any prescription or OTC medications, dietary supplements, or herbal preparations unless advised by health care provider.
- Advise patient that follow-up visits and lab tests will be required to monitor therapy and to keep appointments.

Ciprofloxacin

(sip-ROW-FLOX-uh-sin)

Class Antibiotic/Fluoroquinolone

How Supplied

Ci*pro* Tablets 100 mg, Tablets 250 mg, Tablets 500 mg, Tablets 750 mg, Powder for oral suspension 250 mg/5 mL (5%) (when reconstituted), Powder for oral suspension 500 mg/5 mL (10%) (when reconstituted) ♦ *Cipro* XR Tablets, extended-release 500 mg, Tablets, extended-release 1000 mg ♦ *Cipro* IV Injection 200 mg, Injection 400 mg ♦ *Ciloxan* Solution 3.5 mg/mL (equivalent to 3 mg base), Ointment 3.33 mg/g (equivalent to 3 mg base)

Action

PHARMACOLOGY: Interferes with microbial DNA synthesis.

PHARMACOKINETICS/DYNAMICS:

Absorption:
Oral – Rapidly and well absorbed. Bioavailability is about 70%. T_{max} is 1 to 2 hr. C_{max} is 1.2 to 5.4 mcg/mL (250 to 1000 mg).
IV – C_{max} is 2.1 to 4.6 mcg/mL.

Distribution: 20% to 40% protein bound. Widely distributed and excreted in breast milk. Diffuses into the CSF, but concentrations are less than 10% that of peak serum concentrations.

Metabolism:
Oral – Four metabolites are identified that account for about 15% of the dose; they are less active than the parent compound.
IV – Three metabolites are identified that account for about 10% of the dose.

Excretion:
Oral – About 40% to 50% is excreted unchanged in urine; 20% to 35% is recovered in feces. The t½ is about 4 hr. Cl is about 300 mL/hr. Renal Cl is about 22 L/hr.
IV – About 50% to 70% is excreted unchanged in urine; about 15% is recovered in feces. The t½ is about 5 to 6 hr. Cl is about 35 L/hr. Renal Cl is about 22 L/hr.

Special Populations:
Renal Function Impairment – The t½ is prolonged. Dosage adjustments are recommended.
Elderly – C_{max} increased 16% to 40%, AUC

increased about 30%, and t½ increased about 20%. Differences are not considered clinically significant.

Indications Treatment of infections of lower respiratory tract, skin and skin structure, bones and joints, urinary tract; gonorrhea, chancroid, and infectious diarrhea caused by susceptible strains of specific organisms; typhoid fever; uncomplicated cervical and urethral gonorrhea; women with acute uncomplicated cystitis; acute sinusitis; nosocomial pneumonia; chronic bacterial prostatitis; complicated intra-abdominal infections; reduction of incidence or progression of inhalational anthrax following exposure to aerosolized *Bacillus anthracis*.
Cipro IV: Empirical therapy for febrile neutropenic patients.
Cipro XR: Uncomplicated and complicated UTIs, acute uncomplicated pyelonephritis.
Ophthalmic use: Treatment of corneal ulcers and conjunctivitis caused by susceptible organisms.
Unlabeled use(s): Treatment of pulmonary exacerbations associated with cystic fibrosis; management of malignant external otitis, traveler's diarrhea, mycobacterial infections.

Contraindications Hypersensitivity to fluoroquinolones or quinolones.

Route/Dosage
Acute Sinusitis
ADULTS: **PO** 500 mg or **IV** 400 mg q 12 hr for 10 days.

Acute Uncomplicated Pyelonephritis
ADULTS: **PO** (*Cipro XR*) 1000 mg q 24 hr for 7 to 14 days.

Bones and Joints
ADULTS:
Mild/Moderate: **PO** 500 mg or **IV** 400 mg q 12 hr for at least 4 to 6 wk.
Severe/Complicated: **PO** 750 mg q 12 hr or **IV** 400 mg q 8 hr for at least 4 to 6 wk.

Chronic Bacterial Prostatitis
ADULTS: **PO** 500 mg or **IV** 400 mg q 12 hr for 28 days.

Empirical Therapy for Febrile Neutropenic Patients
ADULTS: **IV** 400 mg ciprofloxacin q 8 hr plus 50 mg/kg piperacillin (not to exceed 24 g/day) q 4 hr for 7 to 14 days.

Infectious Diarrhea
ADULTS: **PO** 500 mg q 12 hr for 5 to 7 days.

Inhalational Anthrax (Postexposure)
ADULTS: **PO** 500 mg q 12 hr for 60 days or **IV** 400 mg q 12 hr for 60 days.
CHILDREN: **PO** 15 mg/kg/dose (max, 500 mg dose) q 12 hr for 60 days or **IV** 10 mg/kg/dose (max, 400 mg dose) q 12 hr for 60 days.

Intra-abdominal
ADULTS:
Complicated: **PO** 500 mg or **IV** 400 mg q 12 hr for 7 to 14 days.

Lower Respiratory Tract
ADULTS:
Mild/Moderate: **PO** 500 mg or **IV** 400 mg q 12 hr for 7 to 14 days.
Severe/Complicated: **PO** 750 mg q 12 hr or **IV** 400 mg q 8 hr for 7 to 14 days.

Nosocomial Pneumonia
ADULTS: **IV** 400 mg q 8 hr for 10 to 14 days.

Ocular Infections
ADULTS:
Corneal ulcers: **Topical** 2 drops in affected eye q 15 min for 6 hr, then 2 drops q 30 min for remainder of 1st day. Day 2: two drops q hr. Days 3 through 14: two drops q 4 hr. May continue treatment after 14 days if corneal re-epithelialization has not occurred.
Conjunctivitis: **Ointment** Apply half-inch ribbon into conjunctival sac tid for 5 days. **Solution** 1 to 2 drops q 2 hr while awake for 2 days, then 1 to 2 drops q 4 hr while awake for 5 days.

Skin and Skin Structure
ADULTS:
Mild/Moderate: **PO** 500 mg or **IV** 400 mg q 12 hr for 7 to 14 days.
Severe/Complicated: **PO** 750 mg q 12 hr or **IV** 400 mg q 8 hr for 7 to 14 days.

Tuberculosis
ADULTS: **PO** 1000 to 1500 mg/day (max, 1500 mg/day).

Typhoid Fever
ADULTS: **PO** 500 mg q 12 hr for 10 days.

Urethral/Cervical Gonococcocal Infections
ADULTS: **PO** 250 mg as a single dose.

UTIs
ADULTS:
Acute Uncomplicated: **PO** 100 to 250 mg q 12 hr for 3 days.
Mild/Moderate: **PO** 250 or **IV** 200 mg q 12 hr for 7 to 14 days.
Severe/Complicated: **PO** 500 mg or **IV** 400 mg q 12 hr for 7 to 14 days.
Cipro XR:
Acute Uncomplicated
PO 500 mg q 24 hr for 3 days.
Complicated
PO 1000 mg q 24 hr for 7 to 14 days.

Interactions
Antacids, didanosine, iron salts, sucralfate, calcium, zinc salts: May decrease oral absorption of fluoroquinolone. Stagger administration times.
Anticoagulants: May increase effect of warfarin; monitor PT.

Antineoplastic agents: Fluoroquinolone serum levels may be decreased by cyclophosphamide, cytarabine, daunorubicin, doxorubicin, mitoxantrone, and vincristine.
Azlocillin: Decreased Cl of ciprofloxacin.
Caffeine: Cl of caffeine is reduced.
Cimetidine: May interfere with fluoroquinolone elimination and increase effect.
Cyclosporine: Nephrotoxic effects of cyclosporine may be increased; monitor renal function.
Probenecid: Decreased ciprofloxacin renal Cl.
Sulfonylurea glyburide: Coadministration has resulted in severe hypoglycemia. Fatalities have been reported.
Theophylline: Decreased Cl and increased plasma levels of theophylline may result in toxicity; monitor theophylline level.

Lab Test Interferences Increased ALT, AST, LDH, alkaline phosphatase, serum bilirubin; increased serum creatinine and BUN; increased triglycerides and cholesterol.

Adverse Reactions

CV: Hypotension, PT prolongation (postmarketing).
CNS: Headache, restlessness (1%); agitation, confusion, delirium, toxic psychosis (postmarketing).
DERM: Rash (1%); erythema multiforme, exfoliative dermatitis, Stevens-Johnson syndrome, toxic epidermal necrolysis (postmarketing).
EENT: Lid margin crusting, foreign body sensation, itching, conjunctival hyperemia, sensitivity reaction (eg, transient irritation, burning, stinging, inflammation, angioneurotic edema, dermatitis), decreased vision (ophthalmic); taste loss, anosmia, nystagmus (postmarketing).
GI: Nausea (5%); diarrhea, vomiting, abdominal pain/discomfort (2%); constipation, flatulence, dyspepsia, pseudomembranous colitis (postmarketing).
GU: Candiduria, vaginal candidiasis, albuminuria, renal calculi (postmarketing).
HEMA: Agranulocytosis, hemolytic anemia, methemoglobinemia (postmarketing).
HEPA: Hepatic necrosis, jaundice, (postmarketing).
LABTESTABS: Elevations of ALT; AST; alkaline phosphatase; LDH; serum bilirubin; eosinophilia; leukopenia; decreased blood platelets; elevated blood platelets; pancytopenia; elevated serum creatinine and BUN.
METAB: Elevated cholesterol, glucose, potassium, and triglyceride (postmarketing).
MUSC: Myalgia, myasthenia gravis, myoclonus, tendonitis, tendon rupture (postmarketing).
OTHER: Anaphylactic reactions, dysphagia, pancreatitis, vasculitis (postmarketing).

Precautions

Pregnancy: Category C.
Lactation: Excreted in breast milk.
Children: Do not use tablets, oral suspension, or IV ciprofloxacin in children under 18 yr, except for inhalational anthrax. Do not use ophthalmic solution in children below the age of 1 yr, or ointment in children below the age of 2 yr.
Hypersensitivity: Serious and potentially fatal reactions have occurred. Discontinue drug if allergic reaction occurs.
Renal function impairment: Reduced Cl may occur; adjust dose downward accordingly in patients with Ccr less than 50 mL/min. Refer to manufacturer's package insert for dose calculations.
Superinfection: Use of antibiotics may result in bacterial or fungal overgrowth. Do not use topically in deep-seated ocular infections.
Photosensitivity: Moderate to severe reactions have occurred with some fluoroquinolones; avoid excessive sunlight and discontinue therapy if phototoxicity occurs.
Convulsions: CNS stimulation can occur; use with caution in patients with known or suspected CNS disorders.
Crystalline precipitate: A white crystalline precipitate in superficial portion of corneal defect may occur; reaction is generally self-limiting and does not appear to affect outcome.
Pseudomembranous colitis: Consider possibility in patients with diarrhea.
Tendon ruptures: Achilles and other tendon ruptures requiring surgical repair or prolonged disability have been reported.

Overdosage: Signs and Symptoms

Acute renal failure.

PATIENT CARE CONSIDERATIONS

Administration/Storage

- Route of administration, dose, and duration of therapy are dependent on condition being treated.

Tablets and Suspension:

- Extended-release tablets and immediate-release tablets are not interchangeable.
- Extended-release tablets are administered qd.
- Administer tablets with a full glass of water without regard to meals. Administer with food if GI upset occurs.
- Administer extended-release tablets whole. Do not split, crush, or chew.
- Do not administer with dairy products or calcium-fortified juices unless they are part of a meal.
- Administer ciprofloxacin either 2 hr before or 6 hr after: magnesium/aluminum antacids;

didanosine buffered tablets or pediatric powder; other products containing calcium, iron, or zinc.
- Shake suspension well for 15 sec before measuring dose.
- Administer prescribed dose of suspension using dosing spoon, syringe, or cup. Caution patient not to chew the microcapsules in the suspension.
- Suspension cannot be administered through feeding tube.
- Store tablets at room temperature (59° to 86°F). Store suspension in refrigerator (36° to 46°F) or at room temperature (47° to 86°F). Protect suspension from freezing. Discard any unused suspension after 14 days.

Ophthalmic Solution and Ointment:
- For ophthalmic use only. Not for use on the skin or for injection into eye.
- Instill prescribed number of drops or ribbon of ointment into affected eye(s) as ordered.
- If using other topical ophthalmic drugs, separate each medication by at least 5 min. Instill ointment last.
- Store ophthalmic solution in refrigerator (36° to 46°F) or at room temperature (47° to 86°F). Store ophthalmic ointment in refrigerator or at controlled room temperature (47° to 77°F). Keep container tightly closed.

Injection:
- For IV infusion only.
- Dilute aqueous concentrate, following manufacturer's instructions, before administration.
- Diluted solution is stable for up to 14 days in refrigerator or at room temperature.
- Inspect solution visually before administration. Do not administer if solution is cloudy, discolored, or contains particulate matter.
- Infuse prescribed dose over 60 min in large vein to reduce risk of venous irritation.
- If other drugs are being administered through same IV line, administer each medication separately.
- Store vials below 86°F. Store flexible containers below 77°F. Protect from light, excessive heat, and freezing.

Assessment/Interventions

- Obtain patient history, including drug history and any known allergies. Note renal impairment, epilepsy, predisposition to convulsions, cerebral arteriosclerosis, or allergy to fluoroquinolone antibiotics.
- Review results of culture and sensitivity testing as available.
- Ensure that reduced dose is administered to patient with renal impairment following manufacturer's guidelines.
- Ensure that extended-release tablets are not used to treat infections other than UTIs.
- Ensure that patient on parenteral therapy is switched to oral therapy as soon as condition warrants.
- Ensure that CBC (including platelets and differential), renal function, and liver enzymes are evaluated before starting therapy and periodically thereafter during prolonged therapy.
- Monitor for signs of infection, especially fever, and for positive response to antibiotic therapy.
- Ensure that patient is well hydrated to prevent formation of concentrated urine.
- Monitor patient for signs of allergic reaction. Discontinue therapy and immediately notify health care provider if noted. Be prepared to treat appropriately.
- Monitor patient for GI, CNS, general body side effects, and injection site reaction. Report to health care provider if noted and significant.

Ophthalmic Solution and Ointment:
- Monitor patient's response to therapy. Notify health care provider if eye or eyelid inflammation is noted or if symptoms do not improve or worsen.

Patient/Family Education

- Advise patient to read *Patient Information Leaflet* before starting therapy and with each refill.
- Explain name, dose, action, and potential side effects of drug.
- Review dosing schedule and prescribed length of therapy with patient.
- Remind patient to complete entire course of therapy, even if symptoms of infection have disappeared.
- Advise patient to drink fluids liberally (eg, eight 8 oz glasses of water daily) while taking this medication.
- Advise patient to discontinue therapy and contact health care provider immediately if skin rash, hives, itching, shortness of breath, palpitations, fainting, or pain, tenderness, or rupture of tendon occurs.
- Advise patient to report any of the following signs of superinfection to health care provider: black "furry" tongue, white patches in mouth, foul-smelling stools, vaginal itching or discharge.
- Warn patient that diarrhea containing blood or pus may be a sign of a serious disorder and to seek medical care if noted and not to treat at home.
- Caution patient that drug may cause dizziness and to use caution while driving or performing other tasks requiring mental alertness

until tolerance is determined.
- Advise patient to avoid unnecessary exposure to sunlight or tanning lamps and to use sunscreen and wear protective clothing to avoid photosensitivity reactions.
- Advise women to notify health care provider if pregnant, planning to become pregnant, or breastfeeding.
- Instruct patient not to take any prescription or OTC medications or dietary supplements unless advised by health care provider.
- Advise patient that follow-up examinations and lab tests may be required to monitor therapy and to keep appointments.

Tablets and Suspension:
- Instruct patient to take tablets with a full glass of water.
- Advise patient that medication can be taken without regard to meals but to take with food if GI upset occurs.
- Caution patient not to take with dairy products or calcium-fortified juices unless they are part of a meal.
- Caution patient taking extended-release tablet to swallow whole and not to chew, crush, or split the tablet.
- Instruct patient using suspension to shake well for 15 sec before measuring dose and to use dosing spoon, syringe, or cup. Caution patient not to chew the microcapsules in the suspension.
- Advise patient to take ciprofloxacin either 2 hr before or 6 hr after: magnesium/aluminum antacids; didanosine buffered tablets or pediatric powder; other products containing calcium, iron, or zinc.
- Advise patient that if a dose is missed to take as soon as remembered. However, if it is nearing the time for the next dose to skip the dose and take the next dose at the regularly scheduled time. Caution patient taking extended-release tablets to never take more than 1 tablet per day, even if a dose is missed.

Ophthalmic Solution and Ointment:
- Remind patient that eye drops or ointment are for use in the eye only.
- Teach patient proper technique for instilling eye drops: wash hands; do not allow dropper to touch eye. Tilt head back, look up; pull lower eyelid down; instill prescribed number of drops. Close eye for 1 to 2 min and apply gentle pressure to bridge of nose for 3 to 5 min. Do not rub eye.
- Teach patient, family, or caregiver proper technique for instilling ointment: wash hands; do not allow tip of tube to touch eye, eyelid, fingers, or any other surface. Tilt head back, look up; pull lower eyelid down to form pocket; place prescribed amount of ointment in the pocket. Look downward before closing eye. Do not rub eye.
- Advise patient that if more than 1 topical ophthalmic drug is being used, administer the drugs at least 5 min apart. Administer ointment last.
- Inform patient that temporary blurred vision, eye pain, or eye discomfort are the most common side effects and to contact health care provider if they occur and are bothersome.
- Advise patient to contact eye doctor if eye or eyelid inflammation is noted, or if eye symptoms do not improve or worsen.
- Instruct patient not to wear contact lenses during treatment.

Ciprofloxacin Hydrochloride/ Hydrocortisone

(Sip-ROW-FLOX-uh-sin HIGH-droe-KLOR-ide/HIGH-droe-core-tih-sone)

Class Antibiotic/Corticosteroid

How Supplied
Cipro HC Otic Suspension 2 mg ciprofloxacin, 10 mg hydrocortisone/mL

Action

PHARMACOLOGY:
Ciprofloxacin: Interferes with microbial DNA synthesis.
Hydrocortisone: Depresses formation, release, and activity of endogenous mediators of inflammation as well as modifying body's immune response.

Indications Treatment of acute otitis externa in adults and pediatric patients caused by susceptible strains of *Pseudomonas aeruginosa*, *Staphylococcus aureus*, and *Proteus mirabilis*.

Contraindications Viral infections of the external canal, including varicella and herpes simplex infections; perforated tympanic membrane; hypersensitivity to hydrocortisone, ciprofloxacin, or any member of the quinolone class of antimicrobial agents.

Route/Dosage

ADULTS AND CHILDREN (1 YR AND OLDER):
OTIC Instill 3 drops of suspension into affected ear bid for 7 days.

Interactions None well documented.

Lab Test Interferences None well documented.

Adverse Reactions
CNS: Headache; migraine.
DERM: Pruritus; fungal dermatitis; rash; alopecia; urticaria.
RESP: Cough.
OTHER: Hypesthesia; paresthesia.

Precautions
Pregnancy: Category C.
Lactation: Ciprofloxacin and hydrocortisone are excreted in breast milk following oral administration.
Children: Safety and efficacy in pediatric patients 2 yr and older have been established; although no data are available on patients less than 2 yr, there are no known safety concerns or differences in the disease process in this population that would preclude use in patients 1 yr and older.
Hypersensitivity: Serious and occasionally fatal hypersensitivity (anaphylactic) reactions, some following the first dose, have been reported in patients receiving systemic quinolones.
Superinfection: Prolonged use may result in bacterial or fungal overgrowth of nonsusceptible microorganisms.
Bacterial resistance: Bacterial resistance to components of the product may develop.

PATIENT CARE CONSIDERATIONS
Administration/Storage
- For otic use only. Not for oral, nasal, or ocular use.
- Hold bottle in hand for 1 to 2 min to warm suspension.
- Shake well immediately before using.
- Instill prescribed number of drops into external ear canal bid as directed using supplied dropper.
- Do not touch ear with dropper.
- Do not rinse dropper after use.
- Store below 77°F. Avoid freezing. Protect from light.

Assessment/Interventions
- Obtain patient history, including drug history and any known allergies. Note presence of perforated tympanic membrane or viral infection of the external ear canal.
- Monitor patient for improvement of symptoms of infection.
- Monitor patient for sensitization or irritation and report to health care provider if noted.

Patient/Family Education
- Explain name, dose, action, and potential side effects of medication.
- Remind patient, family, or caregiver that medication is for use in the ear only.
- Teach patient proper technique for instilling ear drops: Wash hands; warm solution by holding bottle in hand for 1 to 2 min; shake well. Tilt head to side or lie on side with affected ear upward; instill prescribed number of drops and maintain position for 30 to 60 sec to allow drops to penetrate ear canal. Repeat, if necessary, for the opposite ear. Do not allow dropper to touch ear; replace dropper.
- Advise patient, family, or caregiver to only use supplied dropper and not to rinse dropper after use.
- Advise patient, family, or caregiver to notify health care provider if symptoms do not improve or if irritation, inflammation, or itching of ear canal is noted.
- Advise patient, family, or caregiver that follow-up examinations may be required to monitor therapy and to keep appointments.

Cisatracurium Besylate
(sis-ah trah-CURE-ee-uhm BESS-ih-late)

Class Nondepolarizing neuromuscular blocking agent

How Supplied
Nimbex Injection 2 mg/mL, Injection 10 mg/mL

Action
PHARMACOLOGY: Binds competitively to cholinergic receptors on motor end-plate to antagonize action of acetylcholine, resulting in block of neuromuscular transmission.

PHARMACOKINETICS/DYNAMICS:
Metabolism: Degradation is mainly caused by hepatic metabolism.
Excretion: Metabolites are eliminated primarily by the liver and kidney.
Special Populations: The times to maximum block were approximately 1 min faster in liver transplant patients compared with healthy adults. The times to 90% block were approximately 1 min slower in patients with end-stage renal disease.

Indications
Intermediate-onset/intermediate-duration neuromuscular blockade for inpatients and outpatients as adjunct to general anesthesia, to facilitate tracheal intubation and to provide skeletal muscle relaxation during surgery or mechanical ventilation.

Contraindications
Hypersensitivity to bis-

benzylisoquinolinium agents or any component of the product.

Route/Dosage
Use of a peripheral nerve stimulator will permit the most advantageous use of cisatracurium and will minimize the possibility of overdosage or underdosage and assist in the evaluation of recovery.
ADULTS: **IV** 0.15 and 0.2 mg/kg, as components of a propofol/nitrous oxide/oxygen induction-intubation technique, may produce generally good or excellent conditions for tracheal intubation in 2 and 1.5 min, respectively.
ELDERLY AND RENAL FUNCTION IMPAIRMENT: **IV** Recommended dose is 0.03 mg/kg for maintenance of neuromuscular block during prolonged surgery, which sustains neuromuscular block for approximately 20 min. Maintenance dosing is generally required 40 to 50 min after an initial dose of 0.15 mg/kg and 50 to 60 minutes following an initial dose of 0.2 mg/kg.
CHILDREN 2 TO 12 YR: **IV** Recommended dose is 0.1 mg/kg over 5 to 10 sec during either halothane or opioid anesthesia. When given during stable opioid/nitrous oxide/oxygen anesthesia, 0.1 mg/kg produces maximum neuromuscular block in an average of 2.8 min and clinically effective block for 28 min.

Continuous Infusion
ADULTS AND CHILDREN (2 YR AND OLDER): **IV** Adjust rate of administration according to the patient's response as determined by peripheral nerve stimulation. Initiate the infusion only after early evidence of spontaneous recovery from the initial bolus dose.

Infusion in ICU or Operating Room
ADULTS: **IV** Approximately 3 mcg/kg/min should provide adequate neuromuscular block. Following recovery from neuromuscular block, readministration of a bolus dose may be necessary to quickly re-establish neuromuscular block prior to reinstitution of the infusion.

Interactions
Antibiotics (eg, aminoglycoside antibiotics [eg, kanamycin], bacitracin, clindamycin, lincomycin, polymyxins, sodium colistimethate, tetracyclines), lithium, local anesthetics, magnesium salts, procainamide, quinidine: May enhance the neuromuscular blocking action of cisatracurium.
Carbamazepine, phenytoin: Resistance to neuromuscular blocking action of cisatracurium may occur.
Nitrous oxide/oxygen with either enflurane or isoflurane: May prolong the clinically effective duration of action of initial and maintenance doses of cisatracurium and decrease the required infusion rate.

Succinylcholine: Time of onset of maximum block following cisatracurium is approximately 2 min faster with prior administration of succinylcholine.
INCOMPATIBILITIES: Alkaline solutions with a pH greater than 8.5 (eg, barbiturate solutions); propofol or ketorolac for Y-side administration.

Lab Test Interferences None well documented.

Adverse Reactions
CV: Bradycardia, hypotension.
DERM: Rash.
RESP: Bronchospasm.
OTHER: Flushing.

Precautions
Pregnancy: Category B.
Lactation: Undetermined.
Children: Safety and efficacy not established in children under 2 yr.
Elderly: The time of maximum block is approximately 1 min slower in patients over 65 yr.
Renal function impairment: The onset time was approximately 1 min faster in patients with end-stage liver disease and approximately 1 min slower in patients with renal dysfunction compared with healthy adults.
Hepatic function impairment: The onset time was approximately 1 min faster in patients with end-stage liver disease and approximately 1 min slower in patients with renal dysfunction compared with healthy adults.
Administration: Use under the supervision of experienced clinicians who are familiar with cisatracurium action and complications. Personnel and facilities for resuscitation and life support and an antagonist of cisatracurium should be immediately available.
Benzyl alcohol: The 10 mL multiple-dose vial contains benzyl alcohol, which has been associated with neurological and other complications that are sometimes fatal in neonates.
Endotracheal intubation: Because of intermediate onset, not recommended for use.
Malignant hyperthermia: May occur.
Patient distress: Because cisatracurium does not affect consciousness, pain threshold, or cerebration, do not induce neuromuscular block before unconsciousness.
Special populations: May have profound effect in patients with neuromuscular disease (eg, myasthenia gravis). Patients with burns, hemiparesis, or paraparesis may have resistance to cisatracurium. Acid-base or serum electrolyte imbalance may potentiate or antagonize the action of cisatracurium.

Overdosage: Signs and Symptoms
Prolonged neuromuscular block.

PATIENT CARE CONSIDERATIONS
Administration/Storage
- For IV administration only. Do not administer intradermal, IM, or SC.
- Follow manufacturer's instructions for preparation and storage of solutions for continuous IV infusion.
- Inspect solution visually before administration. Solution may have a slightly yellow or greenish-yellow color. Do not administer if solution is cloudy, discolored, or contains particulate matter.
- Store vials in refrigerator (36° to 46°F) in original carton. Do not freeze. May be removed from refrigerator and stored at controlled room temperature (59° to 86°F) but injection must be used within 21 days even if rerefrigerated.

Assessment/Interventions
- Obtain patient history, including drug history and any known allergies. Note history of hypersensitivity to benzyl alcohol.
- Have tracheal intubation equipment, oxygen, suction equipment, and mechanical ventilator available for respiratory support.
- Ensure that peripheral nerve stimulator is used to monitor neuromuscular function during administration in order to monitor effectiveness of dosing, need for additional doses, and to confirm recovery from neuromuscular blockade.
- Ensure that patient is unconscious before administering cisatracurium.
- Administer reduced dose to patient with neuromuscular disease (eg, myasthenia gravis).
- To avoid inaccurate dosing in patient with hemiparesis or paraparesis, monitor neuromuscular function on a nonparetic limb.
- Provide total care for immobilized patient.
- Check mechanical ventilator settings frequently.
- Assess respiratory status frequently. Inform health care provider immediately if deterioration in respiratory status or blood gases are noted.
- Monitor vital signs frequently. Inform health care provider immediately if cardiovascular instability is noted.

Patient/Family Education
- Explain name, action, and potential side effects of drug.
- Advise patient, family, or caregiver that medication will be prepared and administered by a health care provider in a health care setting.
- Reassure patient, family, or caregiver that breathing will be closely monitored and supported while medication is being administered and that breathing and muscle function will return to normal after medication has been discontinued.

Cisplatin
(SIS-plat-in)

Class Alkylating agent

How Supplied
Platinol AQ Solution for injection 1 mg/mL, Powder for injection 1 mg/mL

Action
PHARMACOLOGY: The antitumor effect of cisplatin has been correlated with binding to DNA, production of intrastrand crosslinks, and formation of DNA adducts.

PHARMACOKINETICS/DYNAMICS:
Distribution: Vd is about 11 to 12 L/m^2 (steady state). Platinum is 90% protein bound. Cisplatin is excreted in breast milk.

Excretion: The t½ is about 20 to 30 min (cisplatin) and at least 5 days (platinum-albumin complexes). Cl is about 15 to 16 L/hr/m^2. Renal Cl is 50 to 62 mL/min/m^2. Cisplatin is 90% excreted in urine and less than 10% removed by biliary excretion.

Indications Metastatic testicular or ovarian tumors, advanced bladder cancer. **Unlabeled use(s):** Squamous cell carcinoma of the head and neck and of the cervix; lung carcinomas, osteogenic sarcoma, brain tumors; advanced esophageal, adrenal cortex, breast, endometrial, and liver carcinoma, bone marrow transplantation.

Contraindications Pre-existing renal impairment; myelosuppression; hearing impairment; history of allergic reactions to cisplatin or other platinum-containing compounds.

Route/Dosage
Metastatic Testicular Tumors
ADULTS: **IV** Cisplatin 20 mg/m^2/day IV for 5 days q 3 wk for 3 courses (combination regimen). Single doses of cisplatin up to 120 mg/m^2 in combination with other antineoplastics have been used.

Metastatic Ovarian Tumors (Cyclophosphamide Combination Therapy)
ADULTS: **IV** Cisplatin 75 to 100 mg/m^2 once

q 4 wk. Cyclophosphamide 600 mg/m² once q 4 wk (day 1).

Metastatic Ovarian Tumors (Single Agent Therapy)
ADULTS: **IV** Administer as a single agent of 100 mg/m² IV/cycle once q 4 wk.

Advanced Bladder Cancer
ADULTS: **IV** Administer as a single agent. Give 50 to 70 mg/m² once q 3 to 4 wk, depending on prior radiation therapy or chemotherapy. For heavily pretreated patients, give an initial dose of 50 mg/m²/cycle repeated q 4 wk.

Repeat Courses
ADULTS: **IV** Do not give a repeat course until serum creatinine is below 1.5 mg/dL or BUN is below 25 mg/dL or until circulating blood elements are at an acceptable level (platelets at least 100,000/mm³, WBC at least 4000/mm³). Do not give subsequent doses until an audiometric analysis indicates that auditory acuity is within normal limits.

Renal Impairment
ADULTS: **IV** The manufacturer does not recommend the use of cisplatin in patients with renal impairment. Some clinicians recommend not giving cisplatin to patients with a Ccr below 30 mL/min.

Interactions
Aminoglycosides: Potentiation of nephrotoxicity is possible.
Lithium: Cisplatin may transiently decrease lithium serum levels.
Loop diuretics (eg, furosemide): Potentiation of ototoxicity is possible.
Paclitaxel: Paclitaxel clearance decreases when cisplatin is given immediately prior to paclitaxel, resulting in increased hematologic toxicity.
Phenytoin: Cisplatin may decrease absorption or increase metabolism, resulting in lower serum levels of phenytoin.

Lab Test Interferences None well documented.

Adverse Reactions
CV: MI; cerebrovascular accident; cerebral arteritis; thrombotic microangiopathy.
CNS: Peripheral sensory neuropathy with a glove-and-stocking distribution.
GI: Nausea; vomiting; anorexia; transient LFT elevations.
HEMA: Bone marrow suppression.
HYPERSEN: Anaphylactic reaction.
METAB: Hypomagnesemia; hypocalcemia; hypokalemia; SIADH.
RENAL: Dose-related and cumulative renal tubular damage.
SPEC SENSE: Tinnitus; high frequency hearing loss.

> **WARNING:**
> *Overdose/confusion with carboplatin:* Doses above 100 mg/m²/cycle once every 3 to 4 wk rarely used. Avoid confusion with carboplatin or prescribing practices that fail to differentiate daily doses from total dose per cycle.
>
> *GI:* Marked nausea and vomiting occur in almost all patients and are occasionally so severe that the drug must be discontinued.
>
> *Hematologic:* Myelosuppression occurs in 25% to 30% of patients. Leukopenia and thrombocytopenia are more pronounced at doses above 50 mg/m². Anemia (decrease of 2 g hemoglobin/dL) occur at the same frequency and with the same timing as leukopenia and thrombocytopenia.
>
> *Hypersensitivity:* Anaphylactic-like reactions have occurred.
>
> *Ototoxicity:* Has occurred in no more than 31% of patients given a single dose of 50 mg/m². It is manifested by tinnitus or loss of high frequency hearing, and occasionally deafness. May be pronounced in children.
>
> *Renal toxicity:* Dose-related and cumulative renal insufficiency is the major dose-limiting toxicity. This is manifested by elevations in BUN and creatinine, serum uric acid, or a decrease in Ccr. Renal toxicity becomes more severe and prolonged with repeated courses; therefore, renal function must return to normal before another dose can be given. Amifostine can be used to reduce renal toxicity in patients with advanced ovarian cancer receiving repeated doses of cisplatin.

Precautions
Pregnancy: Category D.
Lactation: Reported to be found in breast milk. Do not breastfeed.
Children: Safety and efficacy not established.
Electrolyte disturbances: Hypomagnesemia, hypocalcemia, hyponatremia, hypokalemia, and hypophosphatemia have occurred and are probably related to renal tubular damage.
Extravasation risk: Local irritation or phlebitis may occur. Refer to your institution specific protocol.
Hepatotoxicity: Transient elevations of liver enzymes, especially AST, as well as bilirubin have been reported.

High/Cumulative doses: Muscle cramps, defined as localized painful, involuntary skeletal muscle contractions of sudden onset and short duration, have occurred.

Hyperuricemia: Occurs at about the same frequency as increase in BUN and serum creatinine. It is more pronounced after doses above 50 mg/m^2.

Neuropathies: Neurotoxicity, usually characterized by peripheral neuropathy, have occurred. Severe neuropathies have occurred in patients receiving higher doses of cisplatin or greater dose frequencies than those recommended, or after prolonged therapy. Discontinue therapy when symptoms are observed.

Ophthalmic effects: Optic neuritis, papilledema, and cerebral blindness have occurred infrequently in patients receiving recommended cisplatin doses.

Vascular toxicities: These events are rare and coincident with the use of cisplatin in combination with other antineoplastic agents. These events may include MI, cerebrovascular accident, thrombotic microangiopathy, or cerebral arteritis.

Overdosage: Signs and Symptoms

Kidney failure, liver failure, deafness, ocular toxicity, significant myelosuppression, intractable nausea and vomiting, neuritis, death.

PATIENT CARE CONSIDERATIONS

Administration/Storage

- Store at 15° to 25°C. Protect unopened container from light. Do not refrigerate. The cisplatin remaining in the amber vial following initial entry is stable for 28 days protected from light or for 7 days under fluorescent room light.
- Cisplatin powder reconstituted with Bacteriostatic Water for Injection is chemically stable for 3 days at room temperature with protection from light.
- If not protected from light, reconstituted cisplatin solution is stable for 6 hr at room temperature.
- Administer by IV over 6 to 8 hr. More rapid administration rates (30 min to 2 hr) are commonly used
- Cisplatin degrades and forms a black precipitate on contact with aluminum. Although needles and administration sets rarely contain aluminum, consider this interaction if a black precipitate is observed.
- Reconstitute powder with 50 mL of sterile Water for Injection or Bacteriostatic Water for Injection for a final concentration of 1 mg/mL. The resulting solution should be clear and colorless.
- Skin reactions associated with accidental exposure may occur. Use gloves. If solution contacts skin or mucosa, wash immediately and thoroughly with soap and water and flush mucosa with water.
- Cisplatin and fluorouracil admixtures are stable in 0.9% Normal Saline for 1 hr.
- The manufacturer recommends further dilution in 2 L of solution containing 37.5 g mannitol, using 5% Dextrose with 0.45% Sodium Chloride. More concentrated solutions, up to a max concentration of 0.7 mg/mL have been used. Cisplatin (up to 200 mg) may also be diluted in 500 mL of 0.9% Sodium Chloride with 12.5 to 25 g mannitol.
- Exercise caution to prevent inadvertent cisplatin overdose. Doses above 100 mg/m^2/cycle once q 3 to 4 wk are rarely used. Care must be taken to avoid cisplatin overdose because of confusion with carboplatin or prescribing practices that fail to differentiate daily doses from total dose per cycle.
- The administration of cisplatin using a 6- to 8-hr infusion with IV hydration and mannitol has been used to reduce nephrotoxicity.

Pretreatment hydration:

- Adequately hydrate patients before and for 24 hr after administration of cisplatin to increase urine output and minimize nephrotoxicity. The manufacturer recommends hydrating patients with 1 to 2 L of fluid infused for 8 to 12 hr before cisplatin administration. Patients may be given 1 L of 0.9% Sodium Chloride (with or without Potassium Chloride) over 2 to 4 hr prior to cisplatin administration to establish good urine output.

Assessment/Interventions

- Monitor serum uric acid. Minimize effects with hydration, urinary alkalinization, and allopurinol.
- Monitor peripheral blood counts weekly and liver function periodically. Measure serum creatinine, BUN, Ccr, magnesium, sodium, calcium, and potassium levels prior to initiating therapy and to each subsequent course. Do not give more frequently than once q 3 to 4 wk at the recommended dosage.
- Perform neurologic and auditory examinations regularly. Carefully perform audiometry before starting therapy and prior to subsequent doses.
- Delayed emesis typically occurs 24 to 72 hr after cisplatin administration. Severity may be reduced by administration of a prophylactic regimen of dexamethasone in combination with metaclopramide or prochlorperazine.

Begin prophylactic therapy 16 to 24 hr after cisplatin administration and continue for a total of 4 days. Add additional antiemetics if breakthrough nausea and vomiting occur.
• Amifostine may decrease the risk of cumulative renal toxicity with repeated courses in ovarian cancer patients.

Patient/Family Education
• Explain name, dose, action, and potential side effects of drug.
• Advise patient, family, or caregiver that medication will be prepared and administered by health care provider in a health care setting.
• Advise patient, family, or caregiver that medication may be used in combination with other agents to achieve maximum benefit possible.
• Review dosing schedule with patient, family, or caregiver.
• Advise patient, family, or caregiver to immediately report any of the following to health care provider: rash; hives; difficulty breathing; fever, chills or other signs of infection; sores in mouth; unusual bleeding or bruising.
• Advise patient, family, or caregiver to report any of the following to health care provider: persistent nausea, vomiting or appetite loss; persistent or worsening general body weakness; changes in hearing or ringing in the ears; dizziness or feeling of whirling motion; abnormal skin sensations; any other unexplained sensation; pain, redness or swelling at injection site.
• Instruct patient to not take any prescription or otc medications or dietary supplements unless advised by the health care provider.
• Instruct women of childbearing potential to notify the health care provider if becoming pregnant, planning on becoming pregnant, or are breastfeeding.
• Advise patient that frequent follow-up visits, hearing tests and laboratory tests will be required to monitor therapy, and to keep appointments.

Citalopram

(sye-TAL-oh-pram)
Class Antidepressant/Selective serotonin reuptake inhibitor

How Supplied
Celexa Tablets 20 mg, Tablets 40 mg, Oral solution 10 mg/mL peppermint flavor

Action
PHARMACOLOGY: Inhibits the CNS neuronal uptake of serotonin, potentiating serotonergic activity.

PHARMACOKINETICS/DYNAMICS:
Absorption: T_{max} is about 4 hr. About 80% bioavailable.
Distribution: Vd is about 12 L/kg. About 80% bound to plasma proteins.
Metabolism: Metabolized in the liver; CYP3A4 and CYP2C19 are the primary isozymes involved in N-demethylation of citalopram. Metabolites are demethylcitalopram (DCT), didemethylcitalopram (DDCT), citalopram-N-oxide, and deaminated propionic acid derivative.
Excretion: About 10% is excreted in urine as citalopram. Systemic Cl is 330 mL/min (about 20% is due to renal Cl). The t½ is about 35 hr.
Special Populations:
Renal Function Impairment – Oral Cl decreased by 17%.
Hepatic Function Impairment – Oral Cl decreased by 37% and t½ doubled.
Elderly –
Single-dose: AUC increased 30% and t½ increased 50%.
Multiple-dose: AUC increased 23% and t½ increased 30%.

Indications Treatment of major depression as defined in the DSM-III and DSM-III-R category of major depressive disorders.

Contraindications Standard considerations; concomitant use of MAO inhibitors.

Route/Dosage
ADULTS: PO Initiate with 20 mg once daily and titrate up to 40 mg/day; max, 60 mg/day.
ELDERLY: PO Initiate with 20 mg once daily; titrate up to 40 mg/day, if needed.
Hepatic Impairment
ADULTS: PO Initiate with 20 mg once daily; titrate up to 40 mg/day, if needed.
Maintenance: Periodically reevaluate long-term usefulness if used for extended periods.
MAO Inhibitor Therapy
Allow at least 14 days between starting or stopping either agent.

Interactions
Beta Blockers (ie, carvedilol, metoprolol, propranolol): Inhibition of metabolism of the beta blocker may occur, resulting in excessive beta blockade (eg, bradycardia).
Cimetidine: Serum levels of citalopram may be increased 40%.
Cyproheptadine: May decrease the pharmacologic effect of citalopram.

Lithium: Lithium may enhance the serotonergic effects of citalopram; use caution if coadministered.

MAO inhibitors: Do not administer with citalopram.

Sumatriptan: Rare postmarketing reports of weakness, hyperreflexia, and incoordination following coadministration.

Metoprolol: Coadministration with citalopram has increased plasma levels of metoprolol 2-fold.

Lab Test Interferences None well documented.

Adverse Reactions

CNS: Dizziness, insomnia, somnolence, agitation, anxiety, anorexia, decreased libido, yawning, tremor.

GI: Nausea, vomiting, dry mouth, diarrhea, dyspepsia.

GU: Dysmenorrhea, ejaculation disorder, impotence.

OTHER: Asthenia, arthralgia, fatigue, fever, myalgia, sweating.

Precautions

Pregnancy: Category C.

Lactation: Excreted in breast milk; may affect infant.

Children: Safety and efficacy not established.

Elderly: May require lower dose.

Renal function impairment: Use with caution.

Mania/Hypomania: May activate hypomania or mania. Use cautiously in patients with history of mania.

Cognitive and motor performance: Patients should use caution in operating potentially hazardous machinery (eg, driving) until they know whether the drug impairs their ability; avoid use of alcohol.

PATIENT CARE CONSIDERATIONS

Administration/Storage

- Do not administer with or within 14 days of MAO inhibitor administration.
- Administer dose qd, in the morning or evening, without regard to meals.
- Store tablets and oral solution at controlled room temperature (59° to 86°F).

Assessment/Interventions

- Obtain patient history, including drug history and any known allergies.
- Determine whether any MAO inhibitors have been used in the past 14 days.
- Note history of liver or kidney disease or seizure disorder.
- Continue suicide monitoring of high-risk patients.
- Observe for signs of mood change and report to health care provider.
- Monitor patient for CNS, GI, psychiatric, musculoskeletal, and general body side effects. Report to health care provider if noted and significant.

Patient/Family Education

- Explain name, dose, action, and potential side effects of drug.
- Advise patient to take qd without regard to meals.
- Inform patient that it may take 1 to 4 wk to note improvement in symptoms and to continue with the prescribed therapy once improvement has been noted.
- Advise patient to take frequent sips of water, suck on ice chips or sugarless hard candy, or chew sugarless gum if dry mouth occurs.
- Advise patient to avoid alcoholic beverages.
- Advise patient that drug may cause drowsiness or dizziness and to use caution while driving or performing other tasks requiring mental alertness until tolerance is determined.
- Advise patient to contact the health care provider if experiencing the following side effects: unusual sweating, headache, drowsiness, insomnia, nausea, tremors, or changes in sexual function.
- Advise patient that drug may cause photosensitivity and to avoid unnecessary exposure to the sun and other UV light (eg, tanning booths). Advise patient to use sunscreens and wear protective clothing until tolerance is determined.
- Instruct patient not to take prescription or OTC drugs or dietary supplements without consulting with the health care provider.
- Advise women to notify their health care provider if pregnant, planning to become pregnant, or breastfeeding.

Cladribine

(KLAD-rih-BEAN)
Class Antimetabolite/Pyrimidine

How Supplied
Leustatin Solution for injection 1 mg/mL, 10 mL single-use vials

Action
PHARMACOLOGY: The selective toxicity of cladribine toward certain normal and malignant lymphocyte and monocyte populations is based on the relative activities of deoxycytidine kinase, deoxynucleotidase, and adenosine deaminase. In cells with a high ratio of deoxycytidine kinase to deoxynucleotidase, cladribine passively crosses the cell membrane. Cladribine is cytotoxic to actively dividing and quiescent lymphocytes and monocytes, inhibiting DNA synthesis and repair.

PHARMACOKINETICS/DYNAMICS:
Distribution: Vd is about 4.5 L/kg. About 20% protein bound.

Excretion: The t½ is about 5.4 hr. Cl is about 978 mL/hr/kg.

Indications
Adult: Hairy cell leukemia. **Unlabeled use(s):** Chronic lymphocytic leukemia, non-Hodgkin lymphoma, acute myeloid leukemia.

Contraindications
Standard considerations.

Route/Dosage
Hairy Cell Leukemia
ADULTS: **Continuous IV infusion** 0.09 mg/kg/day for 7 days, single course. For patients weighing more than 85 kg, preparation of a single dose for administration over 7 days is not advised because solutions may be inadequately preserved because of increased dilution of benzyl alcohol.

Interactions
None well documented.

Lab Test Interferences
None well documented.

Adverse Reactions
CNS: Fatigue; headache; dizziness; insomnia.
DERM: Rash; injection site reactions.
GI: Nausea; vomiting.
HEMA: Bone marrow suppression; decreased CD4 count.
MUSC: Myalgia; arthralgia.
OTHER: Fever.

> WARNING:
>
> *Bone marrow suppression:* Severe bone marrow suppression, including neutropenia, anemia, and thrombocytopenia, has been observed in patients treated with cladribine, especially at high doses.
>
> *Nephrotoxicity:* Associated with high dose and concurrent nephrotoxic drugs.
>
> *Neurotoxicity:* Severe cases more common with continuous high-dose infusions. Serious neurological toxicity (including irreversible paraparesis and quadraparesis) has been reported with doses 4 to 9 times the recommended dose for hairy-cell leukemia. Severe neurological toxicity has been rarely reported with standard dosing regimens.

Precautions
Pregnancy: Category D.
Lactation: Undetermined.
Children: Safety and efficacy not established.
Fever: Fever 37.8°C (at least 100°F) was associated with the use of cladribine in about 66% of patients in the first month of therapy.
Extravasation risk: Local irritation or phlebitis may occur. Refer to the institution's specific protocol.

Overdosage: Signs and Symptoms
Irreversible neurologic toxicity (paraparesis/quadraparesis); acute nephrotoxicity; severe bone marrow suppression resulting in neutropenia, anemia, and thrombocytopenia.

PATIENT CARE CONSIDERATIONS

Administration/Storage
- Store vials in refrigerator and protect from light. May be frozen. If frozen, allow to thaw at room temperature. Do not heat, microwave, or refreeze. After dilution, cladribine solution may be stored in the refrigerator for up to 8 hr prior to administration.
- Cladribine is administered as a 7-day continuous infusion. It can be prepared each day as a 24-hr infusion or as a single dose to infuse over 7 days in an ambulatory infusion pump.
- Avoid mixing with 5% Dextrose because increased degradation may occur.
- Administer by IV infusion daily or continuously for 7 days.
- The use of disposable gloves and protective garments is recommended.

Daily infusion:
- Mix calculated dose of cladribine in 500 mL

0.9% Sodium Chloride solution prior to infusion.
- Solutions diluted in 0.9% Sodium Chloride are stable for at least 24 hr at room temperature in PVC containers.

7-day infusion:
- Diluted solutions prepared in 0.9% Bacteriostatic Sodium Chloride (with benzyl alcohol) are stable for at least 7 days at room temperature.

Assessment/Interventions
- Monitor CBC at baseline and for 4 to 8 wk after therapy.
- Perform baseline neurologic exam and monitor for 4 to 12 wk after therapy.
- Assess renal function at baseline and throughout therapy.
- Hyperuricemia may occur because of rapid cell lysis; monitor serum uric acid. Minimize effects of hyperuricemia with hydration, urinary alkalinization, and allopurinol.

Patient/Family Education
- Explain name, dose, action, and potential side effects of drug.
- Advise patient, family, or caregiver that medication will be prepared and administered by health care provider in a health care setting.
- Review dosing schedule with patient, family, or caregiver.
- Advise patient, family, or caregiver to carefully follow instructions for supplemental therapies designed to protect the kidneys from excessive uric acid (eg, increased fluid intake, allopurinol, urinary alkalinizing agents).
- Advise patient, family, or caregiver to immediately report any of the following to health care provider: rash; hives; difficulty breathing; fever, chills, or other signs of infection; sore throat; unusual bleeding or bruising.
- Advise patient, family, or caregiver to report any of the following to the health care provider: persistent nausea, vomiting or appetite loss; persistent fatigue; injection site reaction.
- Instruct patient to not take any prescription or *otc* medications or dietary supplements unless advised by health care provider.
- Instruct women of childbearing potential to notify health care provider if becoming pregnant, planning on becoming pregnant, or are breastfeeding.
- Advise patient that frequent follow-up visits and laboratory tests will be required to monitor therapy, and to keep appointments.

Clarithromycin

(kluh-RITH-row-MY-sin)

Class Antibiotic/Macrolide

How Supplied
Biaxin Tablets 250 mg, Tablets 500 mg, Granules for oral suspension 125 mg per 5 mL after reconstitution, Granules for oral suspension 250 mg per 5 mL after reconstitution ♦ *Biaxin XL* Tablets, extended release 500 mg
✤ *Biaxin BID*

Action
PHARMACOLOGY: Inhibits microbial protein synthesis.

PHARMACOKINETICS/DYNAMICS:

Absorption: Rapidly absorbed. Bioavailability is about 50%. T_{max} is 2 to 3 hr.

Distribution: Widely distributed. 40% to 70% protein bound.

Metabolism: Metabolized to 14-OH clarithromycin (active).

Excretion: The t½ is about 3 to 4 hr (250 mg) and 5 to 7 hr (500 mg). 20% to 40% is excreted in urine as unchanged drug; 10% to 15% is excreted as 14-OH clarithromycin.

Indications Treatment of infections of respiratory tract, skin and skin structure; treatment of disseminated atypical mycobacterial infections caused by susceptible strains of specific microorganisms. Prevention of disseminated *Mycobacterium avium* complex disease in patients with advanced HIV infection. Clarithromycin in combination with omeprazole is indicated for the treatment of patients with an active duodenal ulcer associated with *Helicobacter pylori* infection.

Children: Acute otitis media.

Contraindications Hypersensitivity to erythromycin or any macrolide antibiotic. Patients receiving terfenadine who have preexisting cardiac abnormalities or electrolyte disturbances.

Route/Dosage

Acute Maxillary Sinusitis
ADULTS: PO Extended-release two 500 mg tablets q 24 hr for 14 days.

Acute exacerbation of chronic bronchitis caused by H. influenzae, H. parainfluenzae, M. catarrhalis, S. pneumoniae
ADULTS: PO Extended-release two 500 mg tablets q 24 hr for 7 days.

Community-acquired pneumonia caused by C. pneumoniae, H. influenzae, H. parainfluenzae, M. catarrhalis, S. pneumoniae
ADULTS: PO Extended-release two 500 mg tablets q 24 hr for 7 days.

Mycobacterial infections
ADULTS AND CHILDREN 12 YR OF AGE AND OLDER: **PO** 250 to 500 mg q 12 hr for 7 to 14 days; use 500 mg q 12 hr for prevention and treatment of mycobacterial infections.
CHILDREN: **PO** 7.5 mg/kg q 12 hr for 10 days. Maximum dose for treatment and prevention of mycobacterial infections is 500 mg bid.

Active Duodenal Ulcer Associated with H. pylori Infection
ADULTS: **PO** 500 mg clarithromycin and 40 mg omeprazole tid for days 1 to 14 and omeprazole 20 mg daily for days 15 to 28.

Interactions
Benzodiazepines metabolized by oxidation (eg, midazolam): Increased and prolonged CNS effects.

Buspirone, cilostazol, corticosteroids (eg, methylprednisolone): Plasma levels of buspirone may be elevated, increasing the pharmacologic and adverse effects.

Carbamazepine: May increase blood level concentrations of carbamazepine; recommend monitoring levels.

Cisapride, pimozide: Elevated plasma levels of cisapride and increased risk of serious cardiotoxicity, including arrhythmias and death.

Cyclosporine: Elevated cyclosporine levels with increased risk of toxicity.

Digoxin: Elevated serum digoxin levels.

Ergot derivatives (eg, ergotamine): The risk of acute ergotism (eg, peripheral ischemia) may be increased.

HMG-CoA reductase inhibitors (eg, lovastatin): Increased risk of myopathy and rhabdomyolysis.

Rifamycins (eg, rifabutin): Antimicrobial effects of clarithromycin may be decreased, while adverse effect of rifamycins may be increased.

Tacrolimus: Increased plasma levels with increased risk of toxicity.

Theophylline: May increase theophylline plasma concentration; recommend monitoring levels.

Warfarin: The anticoagulant effect may be increased, increasing the risk of hemorrhage.

Lab Test Interferences None well documented.

Adverse Reactions
CV: Ventricular arrhythmias.
CNS: Headache; dizziness; insomnia; nightmares; vertigo.
DERM: Rash.
EENT: Hearing loss; tinnitus; abnormal sense of smell.
GI: Diarrhea; nausea; vomiting; abnormal taste; dyspepsia; abdominal pain/discomfort; glossitis; stomatitis; oral moniliasis; vomiting.
GU: Elevated BUN.
HEMA: Elevated PT.
HEPA: Hepatitis; jaundice.
OTHER: Urticaria; hypersensitivity; anaphylaxis; Stevens-Johnson syndrome.

Precautions
Pregnancy: Category C.
Lactation: Undetermined. Other drugs of this class are excreted in breast milk.
Children: Safety and efficacy in children under 6 mo not established. Indicated for use in children only for mycobacterial infections; safety in children younger than 20 mo of age not established.
Renal function impairment: Use cautiously and adjust dose in patients with severe renal impairment.
Hepatic function impairment: No dosage adjustment necessary if patient has impaired hepatic function but normal renal function.
Pseudomembranous colitis: Consider possibility in patients in whom diarrhea develops.

Overdosage: Signs and Symptoms
Nausea, vomiting, diarrhea.

PATIENT CARE CONSIDERATIONS

Administration/Storage
* Administer with full glass of water.
* Give drug at evenly spaced intervals.
* Do not store liquid preparation in refrigerator. Discard 14 days after reconstitution.

Assessment/Interventions
* Obtain patient history, including drug history and any known allergies. Consider cross-sensitivity with other macrolides.
* Monitor serum levels of theophylline and carbamazepine, because clarithromycin may increase these drug levels.
* Notify health care provider if patient develops headache, abdominal pain, abnormal taste, diarrhea, nausea, or vomiting.

Patient/Family Education
* Instruct patient not to take non-sedating antihistamines unless discussed with health care provider or pharmacist.
* Tell patient that if dose is missed not to double dose and to continue on schedule. If more than 1 dose is missed, tell patient to contact health care provider.
* Instruct patient to report the following symptoms to health care provider: diarrhea, stomach pain.

Clemastine Fumarate

(KLEM-ass-teen FEW-muh-rate)

Class Antihistamine/Ethanolamine

How Supplied
Dayhist-1 Tablets 1.34 mg as fumarate (equiv. to 1 mg clemastine) ♦ *Tavist Allergy* Tablets 1.34 mg as fumarate (equiv. to 1 mg clemastine) ♦ *Clemastine Fumarate* Tablets 2.68 mg (equiv. to 2 mg clemastine), Syrup 0.67 mg/5 mL (equiv. to 0.5 mg clemastine)

Action
PHARMACOLOGY: Competitively antagonizes histamine at H_1 receptor sites.

PHARMACOKINETICS/DYNAMICS:
Absorption: Well absorbed. T_{max} is 2 to 5 hr.
Distribution: Small amounts excreted in breast milk.
Metabolism: Metabolized in the liver by mono- and didemethylation and glucuronide conjugation.
Excretion: Excreted mainly via urine.
Peak: 5 to 7 hr.
Duration: 10 to 12 hr, possibly up to 24 hr.

Indications
Relief of symptoms associated with allergic rhinitis or other upper respiratory allergies, such as sneezing, rhinorrhea, pruritus, and lacrimation; relief of mild, uncomplicated allergic skin manifestation of urticaria and angioedema.

Contraindications
Hypersensitivity to antihistamines; narrow-angle glaucoma; stenosing peptic ulcer; symptomatic prostatic hypertrophy; asthmatic attack; bladder neck obstruction; pyloroduodenal obstruction; MAO inhibitor therapy; use in newborn or premature infants and in nursing women.

Route/Dosage
ADULTS AND CHILDREN OVER 12 YR: **PO** 1.34 mg bid to 2.68 mg tid (max, 8.04 mg/day).
CHILDREN 6 TO 12 YR: **PO** (syrup only) 0.67 to 1.34 mg bid (max, 4.02 mg/day).

Interactions
Alcohol, CNS depressants: May cause additive CNS depressant effects.
MAO Inhibitors: May increase anticholinergic effects of clemastine fumarate.

Lab Test Interferences
Skin testing procedures: Drug may prevent or diminish otherwise positive reaction to dermal reactivity indicators.

Adverse Reactions
CV: Orthostatic hypotension; palpitations; bradycardia; tachycardia; arrhythmias.
CNS: Drowsiness (often transient); sedation; dizziness; faintness; disturbed coordination.
EENT: Blurred vision; tinnitus.
GI: Epigastric distress; nausea; vomiting; diarrhea; constipation.
HEMA: Hemolytic anemia; thrombocytopenia; agranulocytosis.
METAB: Increased appetite; weight gain.
RESP: Thickening of bronchial secretions; chest tightness; wheezing; nasal stuffiness; dry mouth, nose and throat; sore throat; respiratory depression.
OTHER: Hypersensitivity reactions; photosensitivity.

Precautions
Pregnancy: Category B.
Lactation: Contraindicated in nursing mothers.
Children: Safety and efficacy in children less than 12 yr not established.
Elderly: Elderly and debilitated patients are at an increased risk of dizziness, excessive sedation, syncope, toxic confusional states, and hypotension. Dosage reduction may be required.
Hepatic function impairment: Use with caution in patients with cirrhosis or other liver disorders.
Special risk patients: Use drug with caution in patients predisposed to urinary retention, history of bronchial asthma, increased intraocular pressure, hyperthyroidism, cardiovascular disease, or hypertension. Avoid use in patients with history of sleep apnea.

Overdosage: Signs and Symptoms
CNS depression, hallucinations, convulsions, cardiovascular collapse.

PATIENT CARE CONSIDERATIONS

Administration/Storage
- Administer drug whole. If patient cannot take whole tablet, administer syrup form.
- Administer drug with food to avoid GI irritation.
- Store at room temperature.

Assessment/Interventions
- Obtain patient history, including drug history and any known allergies, especially to antihistamines.
- Determine whether there is history of glaucoma, ulcer, asthma, or urinary tract obstruction.
- Notify health care provider if patient has history of hypertension or other cardiovascular disorders or is taking an MAO inhibitor.

Patient/Family Education
- Instruct patient not to take drug for 4 days before allergy testing.
- Caution elderly patients that signs of CNS depression will be more pronounced.
- Instruct patient to report the following symptoms to health care provider: difficulty breathing or problems voiding.
- Advise patient to take sips of water frequently, suck on ice chips or sugarless hard candy, or chew sugarless gum if dry mouth occurs.
- Instruct patient to avoid intake of alcoholic beverages or other CNS depressants.
- Advise patient that drug may cause drowsiness and to use caution while driving or performing other tasks requiring mental alertness.
- Caution patient to avoid exposure to sunlight and to use sunscreen or wear protective clothing to avoid photosensitivity reaction.

Clindamycin

(KLIN-duh-MY-sin)
Class Antibiotic/Lincosamide

How Supplied

Clindamycin Phosphate
Cleocin Vaginal ovules 100 mg, Vaginal cream 2% ♦ Cleocin T Gel 1%, Lotion 1%, Solution, topical 1% ♦ Clindets Suspension, topical 1% ♦ ClindaMax Gel 1% ♦ ClindaMax Lotion Suspension, topical 1% ♦ Clindagel Gel 1% ♦ Cleocin Phosphate Injection 150 mg (as phosphate) per mL

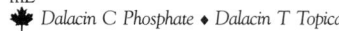 Dalacin C Phosphate ♦ Dalacin T Topical

Clindamycin Hydrochloride
Cleocin Capsules 75 mg (as hydrochloride), Capsules 150 mg (as hydrochloride), Capsules 300 mg (as hydrochloride)

Clindamycin Palmitate Hydrochloride
Cleocin Pediatric Granules for Oral Solution 75 mg per 5 mL (as palmitate)
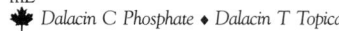 Dalacin C ♦ ratio-Clindamycin

Action
PHARMACOLOGY: Suppresses bacterial protein synthesis.

PHARMACOKINETICS/DYNAMICS:
Absorption:
Oral – Rapidly absorbed. C_{max} is 2.5 mcg/mL. T_{max} is 45 min. Bioavailability is 90%.
IM – T_{max} is 3 hr (adults) and 1 hr (children).
IV – C_{max} is 7 to 14 mcg/mL.
Vaginal – About 5% is absorbed.

Distribution: Widely distributed (including bones); no significant levels attained in CSF. Excreted in breast milk.

Metabolism: Rapidly converted to active clindamycin.

Excretion: The t½ is 2.4 to 3.2 hr. About 10% of bioactivity is excreted in the urine and 3.6% in the feces; the remainder is excreted as inactive metabolites.

Special Populations:
Renal Function Impairment – The t½ is increased slightly. Dosage adjustment is not usually needed.
Hepatic Function Impairment – The t½ is increased slightly. Dosage adjustment is not usually needed.
Elderly – The t½ is increased slightly. Dosage adjustment is not usually needed.

Indications Treatment of serious infections caused by susceptible strains of specific microorganisms; treatment of acne vulgaris (topical use); treatment of bacterial vaginosis (vaginal use).

Contraindications Hypersensitivity to lincosamides or any product component; history of regional enteritis, ulcerative colitis, or antibiotic-associated colitis.

Route/Dosage
ADULTS: **PO** 150 to 450 mg q 6 hr. **IM/IV** 0.6 to 2.7 g/day divided into 2 to 4 equal doses. For more serious infections, these doses may need to be increased. Do not use more than 600 mg in single IM injection.
CHILDREN:
Clindamycin hydrochloride: **PO** 8 to 20 mg/kg/day divided into 3 to 4 doses.
Clindamycin palmitate hydrochloride: **PO** 8 to 25 mg/kg/day divided into 3 to 4 doses.
CHILDREN OVER 1 MO OF AGE: **IM/IV** 20 to 40 mg/kg/day divided into 3 to 4 equal doses.
NEWBORNS UNDER 1 MO OF AGE: **IM/IV** 15 to 20 mg/kg/day divided into 3 to 4 equal doses.

Acne
ADULTS: **Topical** Apply thin film to affected area bid.

Acute Pelvic Inflammatory Disease
ADULTS: **IV** 900 mg q 8 hr with gentamicin loading dose 2 mg/kg IV or IM, followed by 1.5 mg/kg 8 hr. Parenteral therapy may be discontinued after 24 hr. After discharge from

hospital, continue with doxycycline 100 mg bid for 10 to 14 days or oral clindamycin 450 mg qid for 10 to 14 days.

Vaginosis
ADULTS: **Intravaginal cream** 1 applicatorful, preferably at bedtime, for 3 or 7 consecutive days in nonpregnant patients and 7 days in pregnant patients. **Intravaginal suppositories** Insert 1 suppository per day, preferably at bedtime, for 3 consecutive days.

Interactions
Erythromycin: May cause antagonism.
Kaolin-pectin antidiarrheals: May delay absorption of clindamycin.
Nondepolarizing neuromuscular blockers: May enhance actions of neuromuscular blocking agents.
INCOMPATIBILITIES: Ampicillin, phenytoin sodium, barbiturates, aminophylline, magnesium sulfate, calcium gluconate.

Lab Test Interferences
None well documented.

Adverse Reactions
CV: Hypotension; cardiopulmonary arrest.
DERM: Hypersensitivity (eg, skin rash, urticaria, vesiculobullous rash, erythema multiforme, some cases resembling Stevens-Johnson syndrome), burning, itching, dryness, erythema, oiliness/oily skin, peeling, pruritus (topical).
GI: Colitis, including pseudomembranous colitis (0.01% to 10%, more frequent with oral administration); diarrhea; nausea; vomiting; abdominal pain; esophagitis; anorexia.
GU: Azotemia; oliguria; proteinuria; cervicitis or vaginitis, vulvovaginal disorder, vaginal pain, vaginal moniliasis (with intravaginal form of drug).
HEMA: Neutropenia; leukopenia; agranulocytosis; thrombocytopenia; eosinophilia.
HEPA: Jaundice; LFT abnormalities.
OTHER: Pain after injection; induration and sterile abscess after IM injection; thrombophlebitis after IV infusion; anaphylaxis. Topical or vaginal use may theoretically produce adverse effects seen with systemic use as a result of absorption.

> WARNING:
> These agents can cause severe and possibly fatal colitis, characterized by severe persistent diarrhea, severe abdominal cramps, and possibly the passage of blood and mucus. When significant diarrhea occurs, discontinue the drug or, if necessary, continue only with close observation of the patient. Large bowel endoscopy is recommended. Promptly manage moderate to severe cases with fluid, electrolyte, and protein supplements as indicated. Systemic corticosteroids and corticosteroid retention enemas may help relieve the colitis. Reserve for serious infections in which less toxic antimicrobial agents are inappropriate. Do not use in patients with nonbacterial infections (most upper respiratory tract infections).

Precautions
Pregnancy: Category B. Clindamycin does cross the placenta.
Lactation: Excreted in breast milk.
Children: Monitor organ system functions in newborns and children (16 yr of age and younger); parenteral form may contain benzyl alcohol, which can cause gasping syndrome in premature infants.
Intravaginal – Safety and efficacy not established.
Topical – Safety and efficacy not established in children under 12 yr of age.
Elderly: May not tolerate diarrhea well (dehydration).
Hypersensitivity: Use drug with caution in patients with asthma or significant allergies or who are atopic.
Renal function impairment: Use drug with caution in patients with severe renal disease with severe metabolic aberrations. Dosage modifications may be necessary.
Hepatic function impairment: Use drug with caution in patients with severe hepatic disease with severe metabolic aberrations.

Superinfection: May result in bacterial or fungal overgrowth of nonsusceptible organisms.
Tartrazine sensitivity: Some products contain tartrazine, which may cause allergic-type reactions in susceptible individuals.
Debilitated patients: May not tolerate diarrhea well (dehydration).
Meningitis: Drug does not diffuse into CSF. Do not use to treat meningitis.
Mineral oil: Vaginal cream contains mineral oil, which may weaken latex rubber condoms or diaphragms.

PATIENT CARE CONSIDERATIONS

Administration/Storage

- Route of administration, dose, and dosing frequency are variable, depending on condition being treated.
- Store capsules, oral solution, injection, and topical gel, lotion, and solution at controlled room temperature (68° to 77°F). Do not refrigerate oral solution (causes thickening) and discard any unused oral solution after 14 days. Store vaginal cream at controlled room temperature. Protect from freezing. Store vaginal ovules at ambient room temperature (59° to 86°F). Avoid high humidity and temperature greater than 86°F.

Capsule and oral solution:

- Administer without regard to meals but administer with food if GI upset occurs.
- Administer capsules with a full glass of water to reduce esophageal irritation.
- Administer prescribed dose of oral solution using dosing spoon or dosing syringe.

Vaginal cream and ovules:

- For intravaginal use only. Not for ophthalmic, dermal, or oral administration.
- Administer cream using disposable applicator provided with medication.
- Administer ovule using reusable applicator.
- If accidental contact of vaginal cream with the eye(s) occurs, rinse the eye(s) with large amounts of cool tap water.

Topical gel, solution, and lotion:

- For topical use only. Not for ophthalmic, vaginal, or oral administration.
- Cleanse areas to be treated before applying medication. Apply a thin film of medication bid to entire affected areas.
- Shake lotion well just before use.
- If using topical solution pledget, remove pledget from foil just before use. Do not use if seal is broken. Discard pledget after single use.
- Topical solution contains an alcohol base and will cause burning and irritation if applied to sensitive surfaces. Avoid contact with the eyes, mucous membranes, and abraded skin. If accidental contact with the eye(s), mucus membrane, or abraded skin occurs, rinse with large amounts of cool tap water.

Injection:

- For IV infusion or IM administration only. Not for intradermal, subcutaneous, or intraarterial administration.
- To minimize injection site reactions, administer by deep IM injection and avoid prolonged use of indwelling IV catheters.
- Do not administer doses greater than 600 mg by IM injection. Rotate injection sites.
- Do not administer undiluted solution by IV bolus. Infuse over at least 10 to 60 min. Follow manufacturer's guidelines for recommended dilutions and infusion rates.
- Follow manufacturer's recommendations for reconstituting clindamycin when using the ADD-Vantage System.
- Do not administer if particulate matter, cloudiness, or discoloration noted. Gently squeeze premixed IV solution bag before administration. Discard if leaks are detected.
- For IV infusion, the concentration of clindamycin should not exceed 18 mg/mL. Infusion rates should not exceed 30 mg per minute.
- Do not add other drugs to the clindamycin infusion bag.
- Do not use plastic IV containers in series connections because of risk of air embolism.

Assessment/Interventions

- Obtain patient history, including drug history and any known allergies. Note liver disease, atrophic history, history of GI disease (eg, colitis, regional enteritis), history of antibiotic-associated colitis, sensitivity to lincomycin or tartrazine, or concurrent use of neuromuscular blocking agents.
- Review results of culture and sensitivity testing as available.
- Monitor for signs of infection, especially fever, and for positive response to antibiotic therapy.
- Ensure that blood counts, liver enzymes, and renal function are determined periodically during prolonged therapy.
- Monitor patient for GI, DERM, general body side effects, and signs of superinfection. Report to health care provider if noted and significant. Immediately report severe diarrhea, diarrhea containing blood or pus, or severe abdominal cramping.

Patient/Family Education

- Explain name, dose, action, and potential side effects of drug.
- Instruct patient to take exactly as prescribed

and not to change the dose or discontinue therapy unless advised by health care provider.
• Instruct patient to complete entire course of therapy, even if symptoms of infection have disappeared.
• Instruct patient to notify health care provider if infection does not appear to be improving or appears to be getting worse.
• Advise patient to report the following signs of superinfection to health care provider: black "furry tongue," white patches in mouth, foul-smelling stools, vaginal itching or discharge.
• Warn patient that diarrhea containing blood or pus may be a sign of a serious disorder and to seek medical care if noted and not treat at home. Caution patient that this may occur even weeks after completing therapy.
• Advise patient to report any other bothersome side effect to health care provider.
• Advise women to notify health care provider if pregnant, planning to become pregnant, or breastfeeding.
• Instruct patient not to take any prescription or OTC medications, dietary supplements, or herbal preparations unless advised by health care provider.
• Advise patient that follow-up examinations and lab tests may be required to monitor therapy and to keep appointments.

Capsules and oral solution:
• Advise patient or caregiver that capsules and oral solution can be taken without regard to meals but to take with food if stomach upset occurs.
• Advise patient to take capsules with a full glass of water.
• Advise patient or caregiver that oral solution should be administered using a dosing spoon or syringe.

Vaginal cream and ovules:
• Remind patient using ovules that they are for intravaginal use only and not to take by mouth.
• For patient using vaginal cream, review instructions for filling applicator and administering medication. Advise patient that applicator is disposable and not to reuse.
• For patient using vaginal ovules, review instructions for loading and administering applicator and cleaning applicator for reuse. Advise patient that ovule can also be inserted directly using fingers.
• Advise patient using vaginal cream that if accidental contact with the eye(s) occurs, rinse the eye(s) with large amounts of cool tap water. Advise patient to notify health care provider if eye irritation persists after rinsing.
• Advise patient to avoid vaginal intercourse or use other vaginal products (eg, tampons, douches) during treatment with either product.
• Caution patient that vaginal cream contains mineral oil and vaginal ovule contains an oil-type base that can weaken latex or rubber products such as condoms and vaginal contraceptive diaphragms, and to not use such products within 72 hr following treatment with the vaginal cream.
• Advise patient to discontinue use and notify health care provider if vaginal irritation develops while using the medication.

Topical gel, solution, and lotion:
• Advise patient to cleanse areas to be treated before applying medication, then apply a thin film of medication bid to entire affected areas.
• Advise patient using lotion to shake well just before use.
• Advise patient using topical solution pledget to remove pledget from foil just before use and then discard pledget after using. Caution patient not to use pledget if seal is broken.
• Advise patient using topical solution that it contains an alcohol base and will cause burning and irritation if applied to sensitive surfaces. Caution patient to avoid contact with the eyes, mucous membranes, and abraded skin. Advise patient that if accidental contact with the eye(s), mucus membrane, or abraded skin occurs to rinse with large amounts of cool tap water.
• Advise patient that if local irritation occurs to apply the medication less frequently. If irritation persists, advise patient to discontinue use and notify health care provider.

Injection:
• Advise patient, family, or caregiver that medication will be prepared and administered by a health care provider in a health care setting.
• Advise patient to report injection site pain or redness.

Clobetasol Propionate

(kloe-BEE-tah-sahl PRO-pee-oh-nate)
Class Corticosteroid/Topical
How Supplied
Clobex Lotion 0.05%, Shampoo 0.05% ◆ *Cormax* Ointment 0.05% ◆ *Embeline* Cream 0.05%, Gel 0.05%, Ointment 0.05%, Scalp application 0.05% ◆ *Embeline E* Cream 0.05% ◆ *Olux* Foam 0.05% ◆ *Temovate* Cream 0.05%, Gel 0.05%, Ointment 0.05%, Scalp application 0.05% ◆ *Temovate Emollient* Cream 0.05%
❀ *Dermovate* ◆ *Gen-Clobetasol Cream/Ointment* ◆ *Gen-Clobetasol Scalp Application* ◆ *Novo-Clobetasol*

Action
PHARMACOLOGY: Topical glucocorticoid with anti-inflammatory, antipruritic, and vasoconstrictive properties. Thought to act by inducing phospholipase A_2 inhibitory proteins, thus controlling biosynthesis of potent mediators of inflammation.
Indications Relief of inflammatory and pruritic manifestations of corticosteroid-responsive dermatoses; moderate to severe plaque-type psoriasis (*Olux* foam, *Clobex* lotion, *Temovate E* cream).
Contraindications Primary scalp infections (scalp application formulation). Standard considerations.

Route/Dosage
ADULTS AND CHILDREN OVER 12 YR OF AGE:

Topical Apply thin film to affected area bid. When using the foam, apply directly to the affected area. Treatment (except psoriasis) should be limited to 2 consecutive wk and less than 50 g/wk or 50 mL/wk. In psoriasis, no more than 4 consecutive wk and less than 50 g/wk.
Interactions None well documented.
Lab Test Interferences None well documented.
Adverse Reactions
DERM: Burning; stinging; pruritus; irritation; erythema; folliculitis; cracking, fissuring, and numbness of fingers; elbow tenderness; skin atrophy; telangiectasia; hypertrichosis.
Precautions
Pregnancy: Category C.
Lactation: Undetermined.
Children: Not recommended in children under 12 yr of age. Children are at higher risk than adults of HPA axis suppression and Cushing syndrome when they are treated with topical corticosteroids.
General: Not for use in treating rosacea or perioral dermatitis; should not be used on face, groin, or axillae.
Occlusive dressings: Do not use gel or scalp application with occlusive dressings.
Systemic: Systemic absorption may produce HPA axis suppression and systemic side effects; HPA axis suppression shown at doses as low as 2 g/day.

PATIENT CARE CONSIDERATIONS

Administration/Storage
- For topical use only. Not for ophthalmic, oral, or intravaginal use.
- Do not apply to face, groin, or axillae.
- Apply cream, ointment, gel, lotion, or scalp application sparingly, but in sufficient quantity, to cover affected areas; rub in gently.
- Apply cream, ointment, lotion, or gel bid as prescribed.
- Apply scalp application to affected scalp areas bid, once in the morning and once at night. Do not use near open flame.
- Apply foam to affected area(s) bid, once in the morning and once at night, gently massaging into affected area until foam disappears. Hold can upside down and depress applicator to squirt a small amount of foam into the cap of the can, a saucer, or other cool surface, or on the affected skin area. Do not squirt foam directly into hand (unless hand is affected area) because the foam will begin to melt right away on contact with warm skin.
- Avoid contact with the eyes. If medication does come into contact with the eyes, wash the eye(s) with large amounts of cool water. Notify health care provider if eye irritation occurs.
- Store cream and ointment at controlled room temperature (59° to 86°F). Do not refrigerate cream. Store gel in refrigerator (36° to 46°F) or at controlled room temperature. Store scalp application between 39° and 77°F. Do not use near open flame. Store lotion and foam at controlled room temperature (68° to 77°F). Avoid fire, flame, or smoking during and immediately following application of foam.

Assessment/Interventions
- Therapy should be discontinued when control has been achieved. If no improvement is seen within 2 wk, reassessment of the diagnosis may be necessary.
- Obtain patient history, including drug history and any known allergies. Note primary infection of scalp (scalp application only).

- Ensure that appropriate antifungal or antibacterial therapy is used in patient who has a concomitant skin infection.
- Assess and document skin condition before initial application and periodically throughout treatment. Inform health care provider if condition does not improve, worsens, or if application site reactions develop.
- Ensure that patient applying medication to a large surface area or to areas under occlusion is periodically evaluated for evidence of hypothalamic-pituitary axis suppression (eg, adrenocorticotropic hormone stimulation, AM plasma cortisol, urinary free cortisol tests).

Patient/Family Education
- Explain name, action, and potential side effects of drug.
- Teach patient or caregiver proper technique for applying cream, ointment, lotion, gel, scalp application, or foam: wash hands; apply sufficient cream or ointment to cover affected areas sparingly and gently massage into skin; wash hands after applying cream or ointment.
- Advise patient to apply medication bid as directed by health care provider.
- Advise patient that if a dose is missed to apply it as soon as remembered and then continue on regular schedule. If it is almost time for the next application, instruct patient to skip the dose and continue on regular schedule. Caution patient not to apply double doses.
- Caution patient not to apply to face, underarms, or groin area unless directed by health care provider.
- Caution patient not to bandage, cover, or wrap treated skin areas or use cosmetics or other skin products over treated areas unless advised by health care provider.
- Caution patient to avoid contact with the eyes. Advise patient that if medication does come into contact with the eyes, to wash eyes with large amounts of cool water and contact health care provider if eye irritation occurs.
- Advise patient that symptoms should begin to improve fairly soon after starting treatment and to notify health care provider if condition does not improve, worsens, or if application site reactions (eg, burning, stinging, redness, itching) develop.
- Advise patient that therapy is usually discontinued when control has been achieved.
- Advise women to notify health care provider if pregnant, planning to become pregnant, or breastfeeding.
- Caution patient not to take any prescription or OTC drugs, dietary supplements, or herbal preparations without consulting health care provider.
- Advise patient that follow-up visits to monitor response to treatment may be required and to keep appointments.

Clomiphene Citrate

(KLOE-mih-feen SIH-trate)

Class Ovulation stimulant

How Supplied
Clomid Tablets 50 mg ◆ *Milophene* Tablets 50 mg ◆ *Serophene* Tablets 50 mg

Action
PHARMACOLOGY: Induces ovulation in selected anovulatory women.
PHARMACOKINETICS/DYNAMICS:
Absorption: Readily absorbed.
Excretion: About 42% is excreted in feces; about 8% is excreted in urine. May still be detectable in feces 6 weeks after administration. May exhibit enterohepatic recycling.

Indications Treatment of ovulatory failure in women desiring pregnancy when partner is fertile and potent. **Unlabeled use(s):** Treatment of male infertility.

Contraindications Liver disease; history of liver dysfunction; abnormal bleeding of undetermined origin; pregnancy.

Route/Dosage
INITIAL THERAPY: **PO** 50 mg/day for 5 days.
SECOND AND THIRD COURSES: **PO** 100 mg/day for 5 days.

Interactions None well documented.

Lab Test Interferences None well documented.

Adverse Reactions
CV: Vasomotor flushes.
CNS: Headache, dizziness; lightheadedness.
EENT: Visual symptoms; blurring spots or flashes; diplopia; photophobia.
GI: Abdominal pain/discomfort; distension; bloating; nausea; vomiting.
HEPA: Sulfobromophthalein retention.
GU: Abnormal uterine bleeding; abnormal ovarian enlargement, luteal cyst formation.
OTHER: Breast tenderness.

Precautions
Pregnancy: Category X.
Lactation: Undetermined.

Multiple pregnancy: May increase chance for multiple pregnancies.

PATIENT CARE CONSIDERATIONS
Administration/Storage
- Administer initially over 5 days at approximately 50 mg/day. Follow with second course of 100 mg/day for 5 days.

Assessment/Interventions
- Obtain patient history, including drug history and any known allergies.
- Monitor LFTs before beginning therapy and throughout therapy in patients at risk for hepatotoxicity.
- Notify health care provider if patient experiences abdominal pain, abnormal uterine bleeding, visual changes, or jaundice.

Patient/Family Education
- Caution patient that this medication must not be taken during pregnancy or when pregnancy is possible. Advise patient to use reliable form of birth control while taking this drug.
- Counsel patient and partner in purpose of scheduling clomiphene citrate, sexual intercourse and ovulation time to be successful in achieving pregnancy.
- Advise women that increased midcycle ovarian discomfort may be experienced and can assist in planning intercourse.
- Instruct patient of importance of well-balanced diet, mild exercise routine, and avoidance of drugs, caffeine and alcohol while attempting to achieve pregnancy.
- Inform patient of possibility for multiple pregnancies.
- Explain that medication may cause dizziness, hot flashes, headache, nausea and weight gain but that these effects will subside after medication is stopped.
- Instruct patient to report these symptoms to health care provider: abnormal uterine bleeding, yellowish skin or eyes, blurred vision.
- Advise patient to use caution while driving or using heavy equipment because blurring of vision can occur.

Ophthalmologic effects: May cause blurring of vision.

Clomipramine Hydrochloride

(kloe-MIH-pruh-meen HIGH-droe-KLOR-ide)

Class Tricyclic antidepressant

How Supplied
Anafranil Capsules 25 mg, Capsules 50 mg, Capsules 75 mg

🍁 *Apo-Clomipramine* ♦ *Gen-Clomipramine* ♦ *Novo-Clopamine*

Action
PHARMACOLOGY: Inhibits reuptake of serotonin in CNS.

PHARMACOKINETICS/DYNAMICS:

Absorption: C_{max} is about 92 ng/mL (single 50 mg dose). T_{max} is about 4.7 hr (single 50 mg dose). C_{max} at steady state is about 218 ng/mL (multiple 150 mg doses). Concentrations and AUC are not dose-proportional. Time to steady state is 7 to 14 days.

Distribution: Distributes into CSF, brain, and breast milk. About 97% protein bound, principally to albumin.

Metabolism: Extensively biotransformed to desmethylclomipramine (active) and other metabolites.

Excretion: The t½ is 19 to 37 hr. Metabolites are excreted in the urine and feces following biliary elimination.

Indications
Relief of obsessive-compulsive disorder. **Unlabeled use(s):** Treatment of panic disorder or chronic pain (eg, migraine, chronic tension headache, diabetic neuropathy, tic douloureux, cancer pain, peripheral neuropathy, postherpetic neuralgia, arthritic pain).

Contraindications
Hypersensitivity to any tricyclic antidepressant. Not to be given in combination with or within 14 days of treatment with MAO inhibitors. Not to be given during acute recovery phases of MI

Route/Dosage
ADULTS:

Initial dose: **PO** 25 mg/day; gradually increase dose to 100 mg/day during first 2 wk. Dose may then be gradually increased to max of 250 mg/day.

CHILDREN (10 YR AND UNDER):

Initial dose: **PO** 25 mg/day; gradually increase dose to 3 mg/kg/day or 100 mg/day (whichever is less) during first 2 wk; then slowly increase dose to max 3 mg/kg/day or 200 mg/day (whichever is less).

Interactions
Anticholinergics: Effects may be increased.
Barbiturates, charcoal: May increase effects of clomipramine.
Cimetidine, fluoxetine, haloperidol, phenothiazine antipsychotics, oral contraceptives: May increase effects of clomipramine.
Clonidine: May result in hypertensive crisis.

CNS depressants: Depressant effects may be additive.
Guanethidine: Antihypertensive effects may be decreased.
MAO inhibitors: Sweating, convulsions, and death may occur.

Lab Test Interferences None well documented.

Adverse Reactions
CV: Orthostatic hypotension; hypertension; tachycardia; palpitations; arrhythmias; ECG changes.
CNS: Hyperthermia; confusion; hallucinations; delusions; nervousness; restlessness; agitation; panic; insomnia; nightmares; mania; exacerbation of psychosis; drowsiness; dizziness; weakness; fatigue; emotional lability; aggressive reaction; seizures.
DERM: Rash; pruritus; photosensitivity; dry skin; acne; itching; dermatitis.
EENT: Conjunctivitis; blurred vision; dilated pupils; increased intraocular pressure; tinnitus; nasal congestion; peculiar taste in mouth.
GI: Nausea; vomiting; anorexia; GI distress; diarrhea; flatulence; dry mouth; constipation.
GU: Impotence; sexual dysfunction; ejaculation failure; urinary tract infection; vaginitis; cystitis; dysmenorrhea; amenorrhea; urinary retention or hesitancy.
HEMA: Bone marrow depression including agranulocytosis; eosinophilia; purpura; thrombocytopenia; leukopenia; anemia.
HEPA: Hepatitis; elevated LFTs.
METAB: Elevation or depression of glucose levels.
RESP: Pharyngitis; rhinitis; sinusitis; laryngitis; cough.
OTHER: Numbness; tremors; breast enlargement; nonpuerperal lactation; extrapyramidal symptoms (pseudoparkinsonism, movement disorders, akathisia); vestibular disorder; muscle weakness; significant weight gain; hypothyroidism.

Precautions
Pregnancy: Category C. Neonatal withdrawal symptoms have been reported.
Lactation: Excreted in breast milk.
Children: Not recommended for children under 10 yr.
Special risk patients: Use with caution in patients with history of seizures, urinary retention, urethral or ureteral spasm, angle-closure glaucoma or increased IOP, hepatic or renal impairment, or cardiovascular disorders; hyperthyroid patients or those receiving thyroid medication; and schizophrenic or paranoid patients.

Overdosage: Signs and Symptoms
Confusion, hallucinations, agitation, cardiac arrhythmias, dilated pupils, seizures, flushing, dry mouth, fever, tachycardia, cardiac arrest, coma, respiratory depression, cyanosis, hypotension, shock, sweating.

PATIENT CARE CONSIDERATIONS
Administration/Storage
- During titration phase administer drug in divided doses daily with meals to lessen GI side effects.
- After titration, give daily dose at bedtime with large glass of water to minimize daytime sedation.
- Do not administer drug to patients who have taken MAO inhibitors within past 14 days.
- Supervise medication intake when prescribed for psychiatric patients.
- Store at room temperature. Protect from moisture.

Assessment/Interventions
- Obtain patient history, including drug history and any known allergies.
- Assess patient's physical and psychological condition monthly.
- Dosage must be gradually decreased before discontinuation.
- Monitor liver function, ECG, blood sugars (in patients with diabetes), and blood counts (CBC with differential) as needed.
- Monitor body weight monthly.
- Watch for anticholinergic effects: flushing, dry mouth, dilated pupils, hyperpyrexia.
- If there is urinary elimination problem, signs of neuroleptic malignant syndrome or drop in BP of 20 mm Hg, withhold medication and notify health care provider.
- If arrhythmia or increase in heart rate develops, notify health care provider.
- Discontinue medication immediately if patient demonstrates increased agitation or paranoid delusions.

Patient/Family Education
- Instruct patient to keep weekly record of weight and to decrease caloric intake if necessary.
- Teach patient how to monitor BP and heart rate.
- Instruct patient on oral hygiene habits to prevent and treat dry mucous membranes.
- Advise patient to increase fluid intake.
- Instruct patient not to discontinue taking drug abruptly.
- Inform men of possible impotence or ejaculation failure.
- Caution patient to avoid sudden position changes to prevent orthostatic hypotension.

- Instruct patient to avoid intake of alcoholic beverages or other CNS depressants.
- Advise patient that drug may cause drowsiness and to use caution while driving or performing other tasks requiring mental alertness.
- Caution patient to avoid exposure to sunlight and to use sunscreen or wear protective clothing to avoid photosensitivity reaction.
- Instruct patient not to take OTC medications without notifying health care provider.

Clonazepam

(kloe-NAY-ze-pam)
Class Anticonvulsant/Benzodiazepine
How Supplied
Klonopin Tablets 0.5 mg, Tablets 1 mg, Tablets 2 mg, Tablets, orally disintegrating 0.125 mg, Tablets, orally disintegrating 0.25 mg, Tablets, orally disintegrating 0.5 mg, Tablets, orally disintegrating 1 mg, Tablets, orally disintegrating 2 mg

✺ *Apo-Clonazepam* ♦ *Gen-Clonazepam* ♦ *Novo-Clonazepam* ♦ *Nu-Clonazepam* ♦ *PMS-Clonazepam* ♦ *ratio-Clonazepam* ♦ *Rivotril* ♦ *Rhoxal-clonazepam*

Action
PHARMACOLOGY: Potentiates action of GABA, inhibitory neurotransmitter, resulting in increased neuronal inhibition and CNS depression, especially in limbic system and reticular formation.

PHARMACOKINETICS/DYNAMICS:
Absorption: Rapidly absorbed. About 90% bioavailable. T_{max} is 1 to 4 hr.
Distribution: About 85% protein bound.
Metabolism: Highly metabolized in the liver; CYP450, including CYP3A4, may play a major role in oxidation and reduction of clonazepam.
Excretion: The t½ is 30 to 40 hr. Less than 2% is excreted in urine as unchanged drug.

Indications Treatment of Lennox-Gastaut syndrome; management of akinetic and myoclonic seizures and absence seizures unresponsive to succinimides; panic disorders. **Unlabeled use(s):** Treatment of restless legs syndrome, parkinsonian dysarthria, acute manic episodes of bipolar affective disorder, multifocal tic disorders and neuralgias; adjunctive therapy for schizophrenia.

Contraindications Hypersensitivity to benzodiazepines; psychoses; acute narrow-angle glaucoma; significant liver disease; shock; coma; acute alcohol intoxication.

Route/Dosage
Panic Disorder
ADULTS: **PO** Start with 0.25 mg bid. An increase to the target dose for most patients of 1 mg/day may be made after 3 days. Dose may be increased in increments of 0.125 to 0.25 mg bid q 3 days until panic disorder is controlled or side effects make further increases undesired (max, 4 mg/day).

Seizure Disorders
ADULTS:
Initial dose: **PO** 1.5 mg/day in 3 divided doses. Increase by 0.5 to 1 mg q 3 days until seizures are adequately controlled (max, 20 mg/day).
INFANTS AND CHILDREN (10 YR OR YOUNGER; 30 KG OR LESS):
Initial dose: **PO** 0.01 to 0.03 mg/kg/day in 2 to 3 divided doses. Increase by 0.25 to 0.5 mg q 3 days until maintenance dose of 0.1 to 0.2 mg/kg has been reached.

Interactions
Alcohol and CNS depressants: May cause additive CNS depressant effects.
Carbamazepine, phenytoin, rifampin: May reduce clonazepam serum concentrations, decreasing the clinical effect.
Cimetidine, oral contraceptives, disulfiram: May cause effects of clonazepam to increase, with excessive sedation and impaired psychomotor function.
Digoxin: May increase serum digoxin concentrations.
Theophyllines: May antagonize sedative effects.

Lab Test Interferences None well documented.

Adverse Reactions
CV:
Seizure disorders – CV collapse; hypotension; phlebitis or thrombosis at IV sites.
CNS:
Panic disorder – Somnolence (50%); dizziness (12%); abnormal coordination (9%); ataxia, depression (8%); memory disturbance (5%); nervousness, reduced intellectual ability, dysarthria (4%); decreased libido (3%); emotional lability, confusion (2%).
Seizure disorders – Drowsiness (50%); ataxia (30%); confusion; dizziness; lethargy; fatigue; apathy; memory impairment; disorientation; anterograde amnesia; restlessness; headache; slurred speech; aphonia; stupor; coma; euphoria; irritability; vivid dreams; psychomotor retardation; paradoxic reactions (eg, anger, hostility, mania, insomnia, muscle spasms).

DERM:
Seizure disorders – Rash.
EENT:
Panic disorder – Pharyngitis, blurred vision (3%).
Seizure disorders – Visual and auditory disturbances; depressed hearing.
GI:
Panic disorder – Constipation (5%); decreased appetite (3%); abdominal pain (2%).
Seizure disorders – Constipation; diarrhea; dry mouth; coated tongue; excessive salivation; nausea; anorexia; vomiting.
GU:
Panic disorder – Dysmenorrhea (6% [women]); colpitis (4% [women]); impotence (men); micturition frequency, delayed ejaculation (2% [men]), UTI (2%).
Seizure disorders – Dysuria; enuresis; nocturia; urinary retention.
HEMA:
Seizure disorders – Blood dyscrasias including agranulocytosis; anemia; thrombocytopenia; leukopenia; neutropenia.
HEPA:
Seizure disorders – Hepatic dysfunction, including hepatitis and jaundice; elevated LDH, ALT, AST, and alkaline phosphatase.
RESP:
Panic disorder – Upper respiratory tract infection (10%); sinusitis (8%); rhinitis, coughing (4%); bronchitis (2%).
OTHER:
Panic disorder – Fatigue (9%); influenza (5%); allergic reaction, myalgia (4%).
Seizure disorders – Dependence/withdrawal syndrome (eg, confusion, abnormal perception of movement, depersonalization, muscle twitching, psychosis, paranoid delusions, seizures).

Precautions
Pregnancy: Category D.
Lactation: Excreted in breast milk.
Children:
Panic disorder – Safety and efficacy not established.
Seizure disorders – Initial dose should be small and gradually increased. Long-term use may cause adverse effects such as possibly delayed mental or physical development.
Renal function impairment: Use drug with caution to avoid accumulation.
Hepatic function impairment: Use drug with caution to avoid accumulation.
Dependence: Withdrawal symptoms of the barbiturate type may occur.
Elderly or debilitated patients: Initial dose should be small and gradually increased. Give drug with extreme care to elderly or very ill patients with limited respiratory reserve.
Hypersalivation: Because an increase in salivation may occur, use with caution in patients who have difficulty handling secretions or those with chronic respiratory disease.
Psychiatric disorders: Not intended for use in patients with primary depressive disorder, psychosis, or disorders in which anxiety is not prominent.
Seizure: In patients with multiple seizure types, drug may increase incidence or precipitate onset of grand mal seizures.
Suicide: Use drug with caution in patients with suicidal tendencies; do not allow patient access to large quantities.
Withdrawal: Abrupt discontinuation, particularly in patients on long-term, high-dose therapy, may precipitate status epilepticus.

Overdosage: Signs and Symptoms
Somnolence, confusion, diminished reflexes, coma.

PATIENT CARE CONSIDERATIONS

Administration/Storage

- May be used alone or in combination with other antiepileptic drugs when treating seizure disorder.
- May be administered without regard to meals. Administer with food if GI upset occurs.

Tablets:
- Administer prescribed dose with water. Have patient swallow whole. Do not crush, chew, divide, or break tablet.

Orally disintegrating tablet:
- Do not open pouch until immediately before dose is to be administered.
- Open pouch and peel back foil on blister. Do not push tablet through foil. Immediately upon opening the blister, using dry hands, remove the tablet and place in mouth. Tablet disintegrates rapidly in saliva and may be swallowed with or without water.
- Store tablets and orally disintegrating tablets at ambient room temperature (59° to 86°F).

Assessment/Interventions

- Obtain patient history, including drug history and any known allergies. Note hepatic or renal impairment, pulmonary disease, acute narrow-angle glaucoma, history of drug abuse, sensitivity to other benzodiazepines, or concurrent use of other psychotropic medications or CNS depressants.
- Ensure that reduced dose and slower dose escalation are used in elderly patient or patient with debilitating disease.

- Ensure that women of childbearing potential are not pregnant when therapy is initiated.
- Ensure that CBC with differential and liver enzymes are evaluated periodically in patient on prolonged therapy.
- Frequently assess patient for response to treatment. Notify health care provider if condition does not appear to be improving or is worsening.
- Implement seizure precautions as warranted.
- Ensure that therapy is periodically reviewed to determine if it needs to be continued without change or if a dose change (eg, increase, decrease, discontinuation) is indicated.
- If treatment is to be discontinued or the dose reduced, gradually taper the dose and monitor patient for withdrawal symptoms. If significant withdrawal symptoms develop (eg, increased anxiety, tremor, muscle or abdominal cramps, sweating), reinstitute previous dosing schedule and attempt a less rapid tapering regimen after patient has stabilized.
- Monitor patient for CNS, PSYCH, GI, RESP, and general body side effects. Report to health care provider if noted and significant. Implement safety precautions if excessive drowsiness or dizziness occurs.

Patient/Family Education

- Explain name, dose, action, and potential side effects of drug.
- Advise patient or caregiver to read the *Patient Information* leaflet before starting therapy and with each refill.
- Advise patient that medication is usually started at a low dose and then gradually increased until max benefit is obtained.
- Caution patient that medication may be habit forming, to take as prescribed, and not to stop taking or change the dose unless advised by health care provider.
- Advise patient to take each dose without regard to meals but to take with food if stomach upset occurs.
- Advise patient taking tablets to take each dose with water and to swallow whole. Caution patient not to crush, chew, or break tablet.
- Advise patient taking orally disintegrating tablets to open pouch, peel back foil on blister, and, using dry hands, immediately remove the tablet and place in mouth. Advise patient that tablet disintegrates rapidly in saliva and may be swallowed with or without water. Caution patient not to open pouch until just before dose is needed.
- Advise patient that if a dose is missed to skip that dose and take the next dose at the regularly scheduled time. Caution patient to never take 2 doses at the same time.
- Advise patient that if medication needs to be discontinued, it will be slowly withdrawn unless safety concerns (eg, rash) require a more rapid withdrawal.
- Instruct patient to avoid alcoholic beverages and other depressants while taking this medication.
- Instruct patient to contact health care provider if symptoms (eg, panic attacks, seizures) do not appear to be getting better or are getting worse, or if bothersome side effects (eg, drowsiness, memory impairment) occur.
- Advise patient that drug may cause drowsiness or impair judgment, thinking, or reflexes and to use caution while driving or performing other tasks requiring mental alertness until tolerance is determined.
- Encourage patient with seizure disorder to carry identification (eg, *Medi-Alert*) indicating condition and medication being used to treat.
- Advise women to notify health care provider if pregnant, planning to become pregnant, or breastfeeding.
- Warn patient not to take any prescription or OTC drugs or dietary supplements without consulting health care provider.
- Advise patient that follow-up visits and lab tests may be necessary to monitor therapy and to keep appointments.

Clonidine Hydrochloride

(KLOE-nih-DEEN HIGH-droe-KLOR-ide)

Class Antihypertensive/Antiadrenergic/ Centrally acting analgesic

How Supplied

Catapres Tablets 0.1 mg, Tablets 0.2 mg, Tablets 0.3 mg ♦ *Catapres-TTS-1* Transdermal System 2.5 mg ♦ *Catapres-TTS-2* Transdermal System 5 mg ♦ *Catapres-TTS-3* Transdermal System 7.5 mg ♦ *Duraclon* Injection 100 mcg/mL, Injection 500 mcg/mL

🍁 APO-Clonidine ♦ Dixarit ♦ Novo-Clonidine ♦ Nu-Clonidine

Action

PHARMACOLOGY: Stimulates central alpha-adrenergic receptors to inhibit sympathetic cardioaccelerator and vasoconstrictor centers.

PHARMACOKINETICS/DYNAMICS:

Absorption:

Oral – T_{max} is about 3 to 5 hr.
Epidural – C_{max} is about 4.4 ng/mL. T_{max} is about 19 min.
Transdermal – Therapeutic levels are achieved in 2 to 3 days.

Distribution: Vd is about 2.1 L/kg. Clonidine is 20% to 40% protein bound.
IV – Distribution t½ is about 11 min.

Metabolism: About 50% metabolized in the liver. The major metabolite is p-hydroxychlonidine.

Excretion:
Oral – The t½ is 12 to 16 hr. 40% to 60% is excreted unchanged in urine in 24 hr.
IV – The t½ is about 9 hr. 72% is excreted in urine in 96 hr (40% to 50% as unchanged drug). Renal Cl is about 133 mL/min. Cl is about 219 mL/min.
Epidural – The t½ is about 22 hr. Cl is about 190 min.
Transdermal – After removal, therapeutic levels persist for about 8 hr and decline slowly over several days.

Onset:
Oral – 30 to 60 min.

Peak:
Oral – 2 to 4 hr.

Special Populations:
Renal Function Impairment – The t½ increases up to 41 hr in those with severe renal impairment. Dosage adjustment is recommended.

Indications Management of hypertension. Used in combination with opiates for epidural use for relief of cancer pain. **Unlabeled use(s):** Treatment of constitutional growth delay in children; diabetic diarrhea; Gilles de la Tourette syndrome; hypertensive urgencies; menopausal flushing; postherpetic neuralgia; diagnosis of pheochromocytoma; ulcerative colitis; reduction of allergen-induced inflammatory reactions in patients with extrinsic asthma; facilitation of smoking cessation; alcohol withdrawal; methadone/opiate detoxification.

Contraindications Hypersensitivity to clonidine or any component of adhesive layer of transdermal system.
Injection: In the presence of an injection site infection; patients on anticoagulant therapy; patients with a bleeding diathesis; administration above the C4 dermatome because there are not adequate safety data to support such use.

Route/Dosage
Hypertension
ADULTS:
Initial dose: **PO** 0.1 mg bid; maintenance dose: increase by increments of 0.1 to 0.2 mg/day until desired response is achieved (max, 2.4 mg/day in divided doses). **SL** 0.2 to 0.4 mg/day.
Transdermal 0.1 mg patch weekly initially; titrate to determine best response. Dosage greater than two 0.3 mg patches does not improve efficacy.
CHILDREN: **PO** 5 to 25 mcg/kg/day in divided doses given q 6 hr; increase dose as necessary at 5 to 7 day intervals.

Pain Relief
ADULTS: **Epidural infusion** 30 mcg/hr as starting dose. Dosage may be titrated up or down depending on pain relief and occurrence of adverse events. Experience with dosage rates greater than 40 mcg/hr is limited.

Interactions
Alcohol, CNS depressants: Clonidine may enhance depressant effects.
Beta-adrenergic blocking agents: May increase potential for rebound hypertension when clonidine therapy is discontinued.
Local anesthetics: Epidural clonidine may prolong the duration of pharmacologic effects of epidural local anesthetics, including sensory and motor blockade.
Narcotic analgesics: May potentiate the hypotensive effects of clonidine.
Tricyclic antidepressants: May reduce effect of clonidine.

Lab Test Interferences None well documented.

Adverse Reactions
CV: CHF; orthostatic symptoms; palpitations; tachycardia; bradycardia.
CNS: Drowsiness; dizziness; sedation; nightmares; insomnia; nervousness or agitation; headache; fatigue; hypotension (epidural only); confusion (epidural only).
DERM: Rash; urticaria; erythema (with transdermal form); transient localized skin reactions; pruritus.
EENT: Itching, burning, or dry eyes; retinal degeneration; dry nasal polyps.
GI: Dry mouth; constipation; anorexia; nausea; vomiting.
GU: Impotence; decreased libido; nocturia; difficulty in micturition; urinary retention.
METAB: Weight gain; gynecomastia; transient elevations in blood glucose or serum creatinine phosphokinase.
OTHER: Increased sensitivity to alcohol; pallor; muscle weakness; muscle or joint pain; cramps of lower limbs; weakly positive *Coombs'* test.

> **WARNING:**
> Not recommended for obstetrical, postpartum, or perioperative pain management as the risk of hemodynamic instability (eg, hypotension, bradycardia) may be unacceptable in this population. Dilute the 500 mcg/mL strength prior to use.

Precautions
Pregnancy: Category C.
Lactation: Excreted in breast milk.
Children: Restrict the use of clonidine to pediatric patients with severe intractable pain from malignancy that is unresponsive to epidural or spinal opiates or other more conventional analgesia techniques. Select the starting dose on a per kilogram basis (0.5 mcg/kg/hr) and cautiously adjust based on clinical response.
Elderly: Reduced dosage may be required.
Labor and delivery: Use of epidural clonidine during labor and delivery is not indicated.
Debilitated patients: Reduced dosage may be required.
Cardiac effects: Clonidine frequently causes decreases in heart rate. Rarely, AV block greater than first degree has been reported. Clonidine does not alter the hemodynamic response to exercise but may mask the increase in heart-associated hypovolemia.
Depression: Depression is commonly seen in cancer patients and may be exacerbated by clonidine treatment.
Hypotension: Because severe hypotension may follow clonidine administration, use with caution in all patients. It is not recommended in most patients with severe cardiovascular disease or in those who are otherwise hemodynamically unstable. Balance the benefit of administration in these patients against the potential risks resulting from hypotension. Monitor vital signs frequently, especially during the first few days of epidural administration. When clonidine is infused into the upper thoracic spinal segments, more pronounced decreases in BP may be seen.
Perioperative considerations: Continue clonidine therapy to within 4 hr of surgery and resume as soon as possible thereafter.
Rebound hypertension: Discontinue therapy by reducing dose gradually over 2 to 4 days to avoid rapid increase in BP.
Respiratory depression and sedation: Clonidine administration may result in sedation. High clonidine doses cause sedation and ventilatory abnormalities that are usually mild. Tolerance to these effects can develop with chronic administration.
Sensitization to transdermal clonidine: Generalized skin rash may develop in patients with localized reaction to patch if they are switched to oral clonidine.

Overdosage: Signs and Symptoms
Bradycardia, hypotension, CNS depression, respiratory depression, constricted pupils, seizures, lethargy, agitation, vomiting, hypothermia, drowsiness, decreased or absent reflexes, irritability.

PATIENT CARE CONSIDERATIONS
Administration/Storage
Oral:
* Administer in divided doses q 12 hr.
* Store tablets in tightly closed light-resistant container at room temperature.

Transdermal:
* Each transdermal system has 2 parts: (1) patch containing active drug, and (2) adhesive overlay. Apply patch to hairless area of intact skin on upper arm or torso as directed. Then apply adhesive overlay to ensure good adhesion of patch.
* Do not alter or trim patch.
* Change patch q 7 days.
* Alternate sites of patch application to prevent skin irritation.
* Before discarding old patch, fold adhesive edges together.

Epidural:
* The recommended starting dose for continuous epidural infusion is 30 mcg/hr. May be titrated up or down depending on pain relief and occurrence of adverse events. Experience with dosage rates greater than 40 mcg/hr is limited.
* Dilute the 500 mcg/mL product in 0.9% sodium chloride injection to a final concentration of 100 mcg/mL.
* Must not be used with a preservative.
* Store at controlled room temperature 15° to 30°C (50° to 86°F). Discard any unused portion.

Assessment/Interventions
* Obtain patient history, including drug history and any known allergies.
* Assess BP and apical pulse before administering drug. If systolic BP is less than 90 mm Hg or pulse is less than 60 bpm, withhold drug and notify health care provider.
* Weigh patient daily and record weight.
* Note any rash or skin irritation when removing patch.
* Observe for fluid retention and weight gain.

- In diabetic patients, monitor blood glucose levels.
- Monitor BP and pulse during initial therapy.
- If drug is being given to patients who have undergone prior beta-blocker therapy, be alert for signs of rebound hypertensive crisis (eg, agitation, headache, tachycardia, sweating, flushing).

Epidural:
- Implantable epidural catheters are associated with a risk of catheter-related infections. Evaluation of fever in a patient receiving epidural clonidine should include the possibility of a catheter-related infection such as meningitis or epidural abscess.
- Sudden cessation of clonidine treatment, regardless of the route of administration, has, in some cases, resulted in symptoms of nervousness, agitation, headache, and tremor, accompanied or followed by a rapid rise in BP. Reactions appear to be greater after administration of higher doses with concomitant beta-blocker treatment. Special caution is advised in these situations.
- Rare instances of hypertensive encephalopathy, cerebrovascular accidents, and death have been reported after abrupt clonidine withdrawal. Patients with a history of hypertension or other underlying cardiovascular conditions may be at particular risk of the consequences of abrupt discontinuation of clonidine.
- When discontinuing therapy with epidural clonidine, gradually reduce the dose over 2 to 4 days to avoid withdrawal symptoms. If therapy is to be discontinued in patients receiving a beta-blocker and clonidine concurrently, discontinue the beta-blocker several days before the gradual discontinuation of epidural clonidine.
- Caused by the possibility of severe hypotension, monitor signs frequently, especially during the first few days of epidural clonidine therapy. When clonidine is infused into the upper thoracic spinal segments, more pronounced decreases in BP may be seen.
- Monitor for signs and symptoms of depression, especially in patients with a known history of affective disorders.
- May produce drowsiness.

Clonidine Hydrochloride/Chlorthalidone

(KLOE-nih-DEEN HIGH-droe-KLOR-ide/klor-THAL-ih-dohn)

Class Antihypertensive/Diuretic

How Supplied
Clorpres Tablets 0.1 mg clonidine and 15 mg chlorthalidone, Tablets 0.2 mg clonidine and 15 mg chlorthalidone, Tablets 0.3 mg clonidine and 15 mg chlorthalidone

Action
PHARMACOLOGY:
Clonidine: Stimulates central alpha-adrenergic receptors to inhibit sympathetic cardioaccelerator and vasoconstrictor centers.
Chlorthalidone: Inhibits reabsorption of sodium and chloride in the proximal portion of the distal convoluted tubules.

Indications
Treatment of hypertension; not indicated for initial therapy.

Contraindications
Known hypersensitivity to any component of product or sulfonamide derived drugs.

Route/Dosage
ADULTS: **PO** Once or twice/day from a minimum dose of 0.1 mg clonidine plus 15 mg chlorthalidone to a maximum dose of 0.6 mg clonidine plus 30 mg chlorthalidone.

Interactions
Alcohol, barbiturates, other sedatives: CNS depressive effects may be enhanced with clonidine.
Antihypertensive agents: Action may be increased or potentiated by chlorthalidone.
Insulin, sulfonylureas (eg, chlorpropamide): Hypoglycemic effect may be decreased by chlorthalidone, necessitating an increase in dosage.
Lithium: Because renal excretion of lithium may be reduced, avoid use if possible.
Norepinephrine: Arterial responsiveness to norepinephrine may be decreased.
Tricyclic antidepressants: Effects on clonidine may be reduced.

Lab Test Interferences
Chlorthalidone may decrease serum protein bound iodine levels without signs of thyroid disturbance.

Adverse Reactions
CV:
Clonidine – Orthostatic hypotension; palpitations; tachycardia; bradycardia; Raynaud phenomena; CHF; ECG abnormalities; arrhythmias.
Chlorthalidone – Orthostatic hypotension.
CNS: Drowsiness; dizziness; sedation
Clonidine – Malaise; agitation; nervousness; depression; headache; insomnia; vivid dreams; nightmares; restlessness; anxiety; visual and auditory hallucinations; delirium; fatigue; vertigo.
Chlorthalidone – Dizziness; paresthesias; headache; xanthopsia.
DERM:
Clonidine – Rash; pruritus; hives; angioneurotic edema; urticaria; alopecia.

Chlorthalidone – Purpura; photosensitivity; rash; urticaria; niacinitis; toxic epidermal necrolysis.
EENT:
Clonidine – Dryness and burning of eyes; blurred vision; dryness of nasal mucosa.
GI: Dry mouth; constipation.
Clonidine – Nausea; vomiting; anorexia.
Chlorthalidone – Anorexia; gastric irritation; nausea; vomiting; cramping; diarrhea; constipation; jaundice; pancreatitis.
GU:
Clonidine – Decreased sexual activity; impotence; loss of libido; nocturia; micturition; urinary retention.
Chlorthalidone – Hyperuricemia; impotence.
HEMA:
Chlorthalidone – Leukopenia; agranulocytosis; thrombocytopenia; aplastic anemia.
HEPA:
Clonidine – Transient abnormalities in LFTs.
METAB:
Clonidine – Weight gain.
Chlorthalidone – Hyperglycemia; hyperuricemia.
OTHER:
Clonidine – Weakness; discontinuation syndrome; muscle and joint pain; cramps of the lower limbs; pallor; weakly positive Combs test; muscle spasm.
Chlorthalidone – Weakness; restlessness.

Precautions
Pregnancy: Category C.
Lactation: Excreted in breast milk.
Children: Safety and efficacy not established.

PATIENT CARE CONSIDERATIONS
Administration/Storage
- Give qd or bid as prescribed, with or without food.
- Administer alone or in combination with other antihypertensives.
- Store tablets at controlled room temperature (59° to 86°F). Protect from moisture.

Assessment/Interventions
- Obtain patient history, including drug history and any known allergies. Note history of diabetes, gout, anuria, lupus erythematosus, kidney or liver disease, cerebrovascular disease, severe coronary insufficiency, recent MI, or allergy to any other sulfonamide-derived medications.
- Ensure that serum electrolytes and renal function are monitored before starting therapy and periodically thereafter.
- Monitor and record BP and pulse. Should hypotension result, hold medication and notify health care provider.
- Take safety precautions if orthostatic hypotension occurs.

Renal function impairment: Use with caution in patients with severe renal disease.
Hepatic function impairment: Use with caution, minor alterations of fluid and electrolyte balance may precipitate hepatic coma.
Coronary insufficiency: Use with caution in patients with severe coronary insufficiency, recent MI, or cerebral vascular disease.
Electrolyte abnormalities: Hypokalemia and other electrolyte abnormalities, including hyponatremia and hypochloremic alkalosis, are common while receiving chlorthalidone.
Perioperative use: Continue clonidine therapy to within 4 hr of surgery and resume as soon as possible thereafter.
Sensitization to transdermal clonidine: General skin rash may develop in patients with localized reaction to the patch if they are switched to oral clonidine.
Systemic lupus erythematosus: May be activated or exacerbated.
Uric acid: Hyperuricemia may occur, or frank gout may be precipitated.
Withdrawal: Discontinue therapy by reducing the dose gradually over 2 to 4 days to avoid rapid increase in BP.

Overdosage: Signs and Symptoms
Clonidine: Hypotension, bradycardia, lethargy, irritability, weakness, somnolence, diminished or absent reflexes, miosis, vomiting, hypoventilation, arrhythmias, apnea, seizures, transient hypertension.
Chlorthalidone: Nausea, weakness, dizziness, disturbances of electrolyte balance.

- Ensure that if medication is discontinued that it is slowly tapered over 2 to 4 days to avoid withdrawal symptoms (eg, nervousness, agitation, headache, rapid rise in BP).
- Monitor blood sugar in diabetic patient when drug is started or dose is changed. Report significant changes to health care provider.
- Monitor patient for CNS, CV, GI, GU, and general body side effects. Inform health care provider if noted and significant.

Patient/Family Education
- Explain name, dose, action, and potential side effects of drug.
- Advise patient to take qd or bid as prescribed, without regard to meals.
- Advise patient to try to take each dose at about the same time qd.
- Inform patient that drug controls, but does not cure hypertension and to continue taking drug as prescribed even when BP is not elevated.
- Caution patient not to change the dose or

stop taking unless advised by health care provider.
- Caution patient that if medication is ever stopped, slowly reduce dose over 2 to 4 days. Advise patient that sudden discontinuation may result in withdrawal symptoms, including nervousness, agitation, headache, and rapid rise in BP.
- Instruct patient to continue taking other BP medications as prescribed by health care provider.
- Advise patient to monitor and record BP and pulse at home and to inform health care provider if abnormal measurements are noted. Also advise patient to bring record of BP and pulse to each follow-up visit.
- Caution patient to avoid sudden position changes to prevent orthostatic hypotension.
- Instruct patient to lie or sit down if experiencing dizziness or lightheadedness when standing.
- Caution patient that alcohol ingestion, inadequate fluid intake, excessive perspiration, diarrhea, or vomiting can lead to excessive fall in BP, resulting in lightheadedness or fainting.
- Instruct diabetic patient to monitor blood glucose more frequently when drug is started or dose is changed and to inform health care provider of significant changes in readings.
- Advise patient that drug may impair judgment, thinking, or motor skills, or cause drowsiness. Use caution while driving or performing other tasks requiring mental alertness until tolerance is determined.
- Caution patient to avoid unnecessary exposure to UV light (eg, sunlight, tanning booths) and to use sunscreen and wear protective clothing when exposed to UV light to avoid photosensitivity reaction.
- Emphasize to hypertensive patient importance of other modalities on BP: weight control, regular exercise, smoking cessation, and moderate intake of alcohol and salt.
- Advise women to notify health care provider if pregnant, planning to become pregnant, or breastfeeding.
- Instruct patient to report any of these symptoms to health care provider: excess thirst, unexplained tiredness, drowsiness or restlessness, muscle pains or cramps, nausea, vomiting, or increased heart rate.
- Caution patient to not take any prescription or OTC medications or dietary supplements unless advised by health care provider.
- Advise patient that follow-up visits and lab tests may be required to monitor therapy and to keep appointments.

Clopidogrel

(kloh-PID-oh-grel)

Class Antiplatelet/Aggregation inhibitor

How Supplied
Plavix Tablet 75 mg (as base)

Action

PHARMACOLOGY: Clopidogrel is a thienopyridine derivative, chemically related to ticlopidine, that inhibits platelet aggregation. It acts by irreversibly modifying the platelet ADP receptor. Therefore, platelet aggregation is inhibited for both ADP-mediated and ADP-amplified (by other agonists) platelet activation. Consequently, platelets exposed to clopidogrel are affected for the remainder of their lifespan.

PHARMACOKINETICS/DYNAMICS:
Absorption: Rapidly absorbed. T_{max} is about 1 hr. C_{max} is about 3 mg/L.

Distribution: 98% reversibly bound to plasma proteins; active metabolite is 94% reversibly bound to plasma proteins.

Metabolism: Extensively metabolized in the liver; undergoes rapid hydrolysis to carboxylic acid derivative (active).

Excretion: 50% excreted in urine. 46% excreted in feces. The $t_{1/2}$ of active metabolite is 8 hr.

Onset: 2 hr.

Peak: 3 to 7 days.

Duration: About 5 days.

Indications Reduction of atherosclerotic events (eg, MI, stroke, vascular death) in patients with atherosclerosis documented by recent stroke, recent MI, or established peripheral arterial disease. Treatment of acute coronary syndrome (unstable angina/non-Q-wave MI), including patients managed medically and those managed with percutaneous coronary intervention (with or without stent) or coronary artery bypass graft.

Contraindications Hypersensitivity to any component of the product; active pathological bleeding such as peptic ulcer or intracranial hemorrhage.

Route/Dosage

Acute Coronary Syndrome (Unstable Angina/Non-Q-Wave MI)
ADULTS: **PO** Start with a 300 mg loading dose, then continue at 75 mg once daily, initiating and continuing aspirin (75 to 325 mg/day) in combination with clopidogrel.

Recent MI, Recent Stroke, or Established Peripheral Arterial Disease
PO 75 mg once daily with or without food.

Interactions Clopidogrel inhibits P450 2C9. Accordingly, clopidogrel may interfere with the metabolism of phenytoin, tamoxifen, tolbutamide, warfarin (prolongs bleeding time), torsemide, fluvastatin, and many NSAIDs, but there are no data with which to predict the magnitude of these interactions. Use with caution when administering clopidogrel with any of these drugs.

Lab Test Interferences None well documented.

Adverse Reactions
CV: Hypertension, edema (4%).
CNS: Headache (8%); dizziness (6%); depression (4%); confusion, hallucinations (postmarketing).
DERM: Rash (4%); pruritus (3%); angioedema, erythema multiforme (postmarketing).
EENT: Conjunctival, ocular, and retinal bleeding (postmarketing).
GI: Abdominal pain (6%); dyspepsia, diarrhea (5%); nausea (3%); colitis (including ulcerative or lymphocytic), taste disorders (postmarketing).
GU: UTI (3%); glomerulopathy, abnormal creatinine levels (postmarketing).
HEMA: Purpura/bruise (5%); epistaxis (3%); bleeding (including intracranial, GI and retroperitoneal hemorrhage), agranulocytosis, aplastic anemia/pancytopenia, thrombotic thrombocytopenic purpura (postmarketing).

HEPA: Abnormal LFTs, hepatitis (postmarketing).
METAB: Hypercholesterolemia (4%).
MUSC: Arthralgia, back pain (6%); vasculitis (postmarketing).
RESP: Upper respiratory tract infection (9%); dyspnea (5%); rhinitis, bronchitis (4%); coughing (3%); bronchospasm (postmarketing).
OTHER: Chest pain, accidental injury, influenza-like symptoms (8%); pain (6%); fatigue (3%); hypersensitivity reactions, anaphylactoid reactions (postmarketing).

Precautions
Pregnancy: Category B.
Lactation: Undetermined.
Children: Safety and efficacy not established.
Renal function impairment: Use with caution.
Hepatic function impairment: Use with caution in patients with severe hepatic disease who may have bleeding diathesis.
Bleeding risk: Use with caution in patients with increased bleeding from trauma, surgery, or other pathological conditions. If undergoing surgery and antiplatelet effect is not desired, discontinue clopidogrel 7 days prior.
GI bleeding: Clopidogrel prolongs bleeding time. Use with caution in patients who have lesions with a propensity to bleed (eg, ulcers). Cautiously use drugs that might increase such lesions (eg, aspirin, NSAIDs).
Thrombotic thrombocytopenic purpura: May occur, sometimes after short-term exposure (less than 2 wk).

PATIENT CARE CONSIDERATIONS
Administration/Storage
- Administer prescribed dose daily without regard to meals. Administer with food if GI upset occurs.
- Store at controlled room temperature (59° to 86°F).

Assessment/Interventions
- Obtain patient history, including drug history and any known allergies. Note renal impairment, hepatic disease with bleeding diathesis, pathological bleeding (eg, peptic ulcer, intracranial hemorrhage), propensity to bleed, or concurrent use of medications that can cause hemorrhagic lesions (eg, NSAIDs).
- Monitor patient for bleeding or unusual bruising and report to health care provider if noted.
- Monitor patient for GI, CNS, CV, MUSC, and general body side effects. Report to health care provider if noted and significant.
- Ensure that clopidogrel is discontinued 5 days prior to elective surgery in patient in whom an antiplatelet effect is not desired.

Patient/Family Education
- Explain name, dose, action, and potential side effects of drug.
- Advise patient that each dose may be taken without regard to meals but to take with food if stomach upset occurs.
- Advise patient that if a dose is missed to skip that dose and take the next dose at the regularly scheduled time.
- Instruct patient not to change the dose or stop taking unless advised by health care provider.
- Inform patient that it may take longer than usual to stop bleeding while taking clopidogrel and to report bleeding or unusual bruising to health care provider without delay.
- Advise patient to inform health care providers about use of this drug before undergoing surgical or dental procedures and before any new drug is taken.
- Advise women to notify health care provider if pregnant, planning to become pregnant, or breastfeeding.

- Caution patient not to take any prescription or OTC medication, dietary supplements, or herbal preparations unless advised by health care provider.
- Advise patient that follow-up visits and laboratory tests may be required to monitor therapy and to keep appointments.

Clorazepate Dipotassium

(klor-AZE-uh-PATE DIE-poe-TASS-ee-uhm)

Class Antianxiety/Benzodiazepine

How Supplied
Tranxene T-tab Tablets 3.75 mg, Tablets 7.5 mg, Tablets 15 mg ♦ *Tranxene-SD* Tablets 11.25 mg, Tablets 22.5 mg, Tablets, extended-release 22.5 mg ♦ *Tranxene-SD Half Strength* Tablets, extended-release 11.25 mg

♣ *Apo-Clorazepate* ♦ *Novo-Clopate*

Action
PHARMACOLOGY: Potentiates action of GABA, inhibitory neurotransmitter, resulting in increased neuronal inhibition and CNS depression, especially in limbic system and reticular formation.

PHARMACOKINETICS/DYNAMICS:

Absorption: T_{max} is 1 to 2 hr.

Distribution: 97% to 98% protein bound.

Metabolism: Rapidly metabolized in the liver to nordiazepam.

Excretion: About 80% excreted in urine and feces. The t½ is 40 to 50 hr.

Indications
Management of anxiety disorders; relief of acute alcohol withdrawal symptoms; adjunctive therapy in management of partial seizures. **Unlabeled use(s):** Treatment of irritable bowel syndrome.

Contraindications
Hypersensitivity to benzodiazepines; psychoses; acute narrow-angle glaucoma.

Route/Dosage

Acute Alcohol Withdrawal
ADULTS:
Day 1: **PO** Initial dose is 30 mg, then 30 to 60 mg in divided doses.
Day 2: 45 to 90 mg in divided doses.
Day 3: 22.5 to 45 mg in divided doses.
Day 4: 15 to 30 mg in divided doses. Then gradually reduce to 7.5 to 15 mg/day; discontinue when patient is stable.

Anxiety
ADULTS: **PO** 15 to 60 mg/day in divided doses. Single bedtime dosing: **PO** Initial dose is 15 mg.

Elderly or Debilitated Patients
Initial dose – **PO** 7.5 to 15 mg/day.

Maintenance
ADULTS: **PO** 22.5 mg/day as single dose alternative once patient is stabilized with 7.5 mg tid; do not use 22.5 mg in single dose to initiate therapy. The 11.25 mg tablet may be given as single dose q 24 hr.

Partial Seizures
ADULTS AND CHILDREN OVER 12 YR: Maximum initial dose: 7.5 mg tid; increase by no more than 7.5 mg/wk (max, 90 mg/day).
CHILDREN 9 TO 12 YR: Maximum initial dose: 7.5 mg bid; increase by no more than 7.5 mg/wk (max, 60 mg/day).

Interactions
Alcohol and CNS depressants: Possible additive CNS depressant effects.

Azole antifungal agents (eg, itraconazole, ketoconazole), fluvoxamine, isoniazid, macrolide antibiotics (eg, erythromycin), nefazodone, nonnucleoside reverse transcriptase inhibitors (eg, delavirdine, efavirenz), protease inhibitors (eg, indinavir): May increase diazepam plasma concentrations.

Cimetidine, oral contraceptives, disulfiram: May increase effects of clorazepate, with excessive sedation and impaired psychomotor function.

Digoxin: May increase serum digoxin concentrations.

Omeprazole: May increase clorazepate serum levels and enhance effects.

Rifamycins: May decrease diazepam plasma concentrations.

Theophyllines: May antagonize sedative effects of clorazepate.

Lab Test Interferences
None well documented.

Adverse Reactions
CV: CV collapse; hypotension.
CNS: Drowsiness; confusion; ataxia; dizziness; lethargy; fatigue; apathy; memory impairment; disorientation; anterograde amnesia; restlessness; nervousness; headache; slurred speech; loss of voice; stupor; coma; euphoria; irritability; vivid dreams; psychomotor retardation; paradoxical reactions (eg, anger, hostility, mania, insomnia, muscle spasms); depression; tremor.
DERM: Rash.
EENT: Blurred vision; diplopia.
GI: Constipation; diarrhea; dry mouth; coated tongue; nausea; anorexia; vomiting.
HEMA: Blood dyscrasias.
HEPA: Hepatic dysfunction, including hepatitis and jaundice; elevated LDH, alanine amino-

transferase, aspartate aminotransferase, and alkaline phosphatase.
OTHER: Dependence/withdrawal syndrome.

Precautions
Pregnancy: Category D.
Lactation: Excreted in breast milk.
Children: Initial dose should be small and gradually increased. Not recommended in children under 9 yr.
Elderly: Initial dose should be small and gradually increased.
Renal function impairment: Observe caution to avoid accumulation of drug.
Hepatic function impairment: Observe caution to avoid accumulation of drug.
Debilitated patients: Initial dose should be small and gradually increased.
Drug dependency: Prolonged use may lead to dependence. Withdrawal syndrome has occurred within 4 to 6 wk of treatment, especially if abruptly discontinued. Use caution and taper dosage.
Psychiatric disorders: Not intended for use in patients with primary depressive disorder, psychosis, or disorders in which anxiety is not prominent.
Seizures: May occur during abrupt drug discontinuation or dose reduction.

Overdosage: Signs and Symptoms
Drowsiness, confusion, somnolence, impaired coordination, diminished reflexes, lethargy, ataxia, hypotonia, hypotension, hypnosis, coma.

PATIENT CARE CONSIDERATIONS

Administration/Storage
- Administer in combination with other anticonvulsant medications when treating seizure disorder.
- Extended-release tablets are intended for conversion from stabilized immediate-release regimen and should not be used to initiate therapy.
- Administer prescribed dose without regard to meals but administer with food if GI upset occurs.
- Administer extended-release tablets qd. Have patient swallow whole. Do not crush, chew, divide, or break tablet.
- Store tablets below 77°F. Protect from moisture.

Assessment/Interventions
- Obtain patient history, including drug history and any known allergies. Note hepatic or renal impairment, depression, acute narrow-angle glaucoma, suicidal tendency, seizure disorder, history of drug abuse or sensitivity to other benzodiazepines, or concurrent use of other psychotropic medications or CNS depressants.
- Ensure that reduced dose and slower dose escalation are used in elderly patient or patient with debilitating disease.
- Ensure that women of childbearing potential are not pregnant when therapy is initiated.
- Ensure that CBC with differential and liver enzymes are evaluated periodically in patient on prolonged therapy.
- Frequently assess patient for response to treatment. Notify health care provider if condition does not appear to be improving or is worsening.
- Ensure that therapy is periodically reviewed to determine if it needs to be continued without change or if a dose change (eg, increase, decrease, discontinuation) is indicated.
- If treatment is to be discontinued, or the dose reduced, gradually taper the dose. Monitor patient for withdrawal symptoms (eg, increased anxiety, tremor, muscle or abdominal cramps, sweating). If significant withdrawal symptoms develop, reinstitute previous dosing schedule and attempt a less rapid tapering regimen after patient has stabilized.
- Monitor patient for CNS, GI, and general body side effects. Report to health care provider if noted and significant. Implement safety precautions if excessive drowsiness or dizziness occurs.

Patient/Family Education
- Explain name, dose, action, and potential side effects of drug.
- Advise patient or caregiver to read the *Patient Information* leaflet before starting therapy and with each refill.
- Instruct patient with seizure disorder to continue to take other medications for the condition unless advised otherwise by health care provider.
- Advise patient that medication is usually started at a low dose and then gradually increased until maximum benefit is obtained.
- Caution patient that medication may be habit forming and to take as prescribed and not to stop taking or change the dose unless advised by health care provider.
- Advise patient to take each dose without regard to meals but to take with food if stomach upset occurs.
- Advise patient using extended-release tablets to take prescribed dose qd. Caution patient to swallow tablets whole and not to crush, chew, divide, or break the tablet.
- Advise patient that if a dose is missed to skip that dose and take the next dose at the regu-

larly scheduled time. Caution patient to never take 2 doses at the same time.
- Advise patient that if medication needs to be discontinued it will be slowly withdrawn unless safety concerns (eg, rash) require a more rapid withdrawal.
- Instruct patient to avoid alcoholic beverages and other depressants while taking this medication.
- Advise patient with anxiety to take as needed and to seek alternative methods for controlling or preventing anxiety (eg, stress reduction, counseling).
- Instruct patient to contact health care provider if symptoms (eg, anxiety, panic attacks, seizures) do not appear to be getting better, are getting worse, or if bothersome side effects (eg, drowsiness, memory impairment) occur.
- Advise patient that drug may cause drowsiness or impair judgment, thinking, or reflexes and to use caution while driving or performing other tasks requiring mental alertness until tolerance is determined.
- Encourage patient with seizure disorder to carry identification (eg, *Medi-Alert*) indicating condition and medication being used to treat.
- Advise women to notify health care provider if pregnant, planning to become pregnant, or breastfeeding.
- Warn patient not to take any prescription or OTC drugs or dietary supplements without consulting health care provider.
- Advise patient that follow-up visits may be necessary to monitor therapy and to keep appointments.

Clotrimazole

(kloe-TRIM-uh-zole)

Class Topical/Antifungal

How Supplied
Cruex Cream 1% ♦ *Desenex* Cream 1% ♦ *Gyne-Lotrimin 3* Vaginal suppositories 200 mg, Vaginal cream 2% ♦ *Gyne-Lotrimin 3 Combination Pack* Vaginal suppositories 200 mg, Topical cream 1% ♦ *Gyne-Lotrimin 7* Vaginal cream 1% ♦ *Lotrimin AF* Cream 1%, Solution, topical 1%, Lotion 1% ♦ *Mycelex* Troches 10 mg ♦ *Mycelex-7* Vaginal cream 1% ♦ *Mycelex-7 Combination Pack* Vaginal suppositories 100 mg, Topical cream 1% ✣ *Canesten*

Action
PHARMACOLOGY: Inhibits yeast growth by increasing cell membrane permeability in susceptible fungi.

PHARMACOKINETICS/DYNAMICS:
Absorption: After oral administration, the mean serum concentrations were about 4.98 and 3.23 ng/mL at 30 and 60 min, respectively. Minimally absorbed following topical and vaginal administration.

Indications
Topical use: Treatment of tinea pedis (athlete's foot), tinea cruris (jock itch), tinea corporis (ringworm), candidiasis, and tinea versicolor.
Oral use (troche): Treatment of oropharyngeal candidiasis; prophylaxis of oropharyngeal candidiasis in specific groups of immunocompromised patients.
Vaginal use: Treatment of vulvovaginal candidiasis.

Contraindications Standard considerations.

Route/Dosage
Oropharyngeal Candidiasis
ADULTS AND CHILDREN OVER 3 YR: **PO** One 10 mg troche (lozenge) dissolved slowly in the mouth 5 times/day for 14 days.

Prophylaxis
PO One 10 mg troche dissolved slowly in the mouth tid.

Dermal Infections
Topical cream Apply thin layer to affected and surrounding areas bid in the morning and evening. **Topical lotion** Apply thin layer to affected areas bid.

Vaginal Infections
WOMEN AND GIRLS OVER 12 YR: **Intravaginal** Insert 1 applicatorful (5 g) of cream or one suppository at bedtime for 7 to 14 days (treatment for 14 days may yield higher cure rate).
Gyne-Lotrimin Combination Pack: Insert suppository intravaginally at bedtime for 7 consecutive days. Apply topical cream to affected areas bid (morning and evening) for 7 consecutive days.
Mycelex 7 Combination Pack: Insert suppository intravaginally at bedtime for 7 consecutive days. Apply topical cream to affected area bid (morning and evening) for 7 consecutive days.

Interactions None well documented.

Lab Test Interferences None well documented.

Adverse Reactions
DERM: Pruritus; erythema, stinging, blistering, peeling, edema, urticaria, burning, general skin irritation, rash (topical and vaginal products).
EENT: Unpleasant mouth sensations (troche).
GI: Nausea, vomiting (troche).
HEPA: Abnormal LFT results (troche).

Precautions
Pregnancy: Category C (troches); Category B (topical and vaginal use).
Lactation: Undetermined.
Children:
Oral (troches) – Safety not established in children under 3 yr.

Topical – Safety and efficacy not established in children under 2 yr.
Recurrent infections: May indicate underlying medical cause, including diabetes or HIV infection.
Systemic or ophthalmic infections: Do not use for these conditions.

PATIENT CARE CONSIDERATIONS
Administration/Storage
Topical Cream, Lotion, Solution:
- For topical use only. Not for ophthalmic use.
- Avoid contact with eyes. If eye contact occurs, flush immediately and thoroughly with water.
- Shake lotion well before application.
- Use gloves if applying cream, lotion, or solution on patient; thoroughly massage cream or lotion into the affected and surrounding skin areas bid.
- Store cream and lotion in refrigerator (36° to 46°F) or at controlled room temperature (59° to 86°F). Keep tightly capped.

Vaginal Cream and Vaginal Tablets:
- For vaginal use only. Not for oral or ophthalmic use.
- Insert 1 vaginal suppository or applicator full of cream into vagina qd, preferably at bedtime.
- Store vaginal cream and tablets at controlled room temperature (less than 86°F). Protect from freezing.

Oral Troche:
- For treatment of oropharyngeal infections only. Not for intravaginal use or to treat systemic fungal infections.
- Have patient slowly dissolve troche in mouth. Instruct patient not to chew or swallow troche and to retain saliva as long as possible before swallowing.
- Store troches at controlled room temperature (below 86°F). Protect from freezing.

Assessment/Interventions
- Obtain patient history, including drug history and any known allergies. Note condition(s) that may predispose to recurrent infection (eg, diabetes, concurrent antibiotic therapy, immunosuppression, HIV, AIDS) or liver disease (oral troche).
- Ensure that transaminases are determined periodically during prolonged therapy with oral troches, especially in patient with pre-existing hepatic impairment.
- Ensure that appropriate microbiological studies are completed before starting therapy and repeated to confirm diagnosis and rule out other pathogens before instituting another course of antimycotic therapy.
- Monitor patient's response to therapy. Notify health care provider if symptoms do not improve or worsen.
- Notify health care provider if skin inflammation, irritation, or sensitization are noted at cream, lotion, or solution application site(s).
- Notify health care provider if patient using oral troche develops nausea, vomiting, abdominal cramps or discomfort, or unpleasant mouth sensations.

Patient/Family Education
- Explain name, dose, action, and potential side effects of drug.
- Instruct patient using OTC products to carefully read and follow the instructions that come with each package.
- Caution patient or caregiver to avoid contact with eyes and that if accidental eye contact occurs to immediately flush the eyes with water to remove medication. Advise patient or caregiver to notify health care provider if eye irritation or sensitivity follows exposure to the eyes.
- Advise patient or caregiver that follow-up visits may be necessary and to keep appointments.

Topical Cream, Solution, or Lotion:
- Teach patient or caregiver proper technique for applying cream, lotion, or solution: wash hands; use gloves if applying to another person; thoroughly massage medication into affected and surrounding skin areas.
- Advise patient that improvement in symptoms may take up to a week to occur and to notify health care provider if there is no improvement after 4 wk.
- Advise patient to use medication for the full treatment time even if symptoms have improved.
- Advise patient to notify health care provider if application site shows signs of increased irritation (redness, itching, burning, itching, blistering, swelling, oozing).

Vaginal Cream and Vaginal Tablets:
- Teach patient proper technique for inserting vaginal cream or suppository. Advise patient that cream may also be applied to irritated

area(s) of vulva to relieve external vaginal itching.
- Caution patient that cream may reduce the effectiveness of vaginal spermicides and may damage condoms and diaphragms, causing them to fail. Advise patient to use another method of birth control while using vaginal cream.
- Advise patient to avoid using tampons while infection is being treated with this medication.
- Advise patient to notify health care provider if any of the following occur: symptoms do not improve after 3 days of treatment or persist for more than 7 days; stomach or pelvic pain; fever; foul-smelling discharge; infection returns within 2 mo.

Oral Troche:
- Teach patient proper technique for using oral troche as follows: slowly dissolve troche in mouth and retain saliva as long as possible before swallowing. Caution patient not to chew or swallow the troche.
- Advise patient to notify health care provider if any of the following occur: nausea, vomiting, abdominal cramps or discomfort, unpleasant mouth sensations, symptoms do not improve or worsen.

Clozapine

(KLOE-zuh-PEEN)
Class Antipsychotic
How Supplied
Clozapine Tablets 12.5 mg ◆ *Clozaril* Tablets 25 mg, Tablets 100 mg
✤ Rhoxal-clozapine

Action

PHARMACOLOGY: Interferes with dopamine binding at D_1, D_2, D_3, and D_5 receptors in CNS; antagonizes adrenergic, cholinergic, histaminergic, and serotonergic neurotransmission.

PHARMACOKINETICS/DYNAMICS:
Absorption: C_{max} is about 319 ng/mL (at steady state). T_{max} is about 2.5 hr.
Distribution: About 97% protein bound.
Metabolism: Extensively metabolized.
Excretion: The t½ is about 8 hr (single dose) and about 12 hr (steady state). About 50% is excreted in urine and 30% in feces as metabolites.

Indications Management of severely and chronically mentally ill schizophrenic patients who have not responded to or cannot tolerate standard antipsychotic drug treatment; to reduce risk of recurrent suicidal behavior in patients with schizophrenia or schizoaffective disorder who are judged to be at chronic risk for reexperiencing suicidal behavior.

Contraindications History of clozapine-induced agranulocytosis or severe granulocytopenia; myeloproliferative disorders; simultaneous administration with other agents known to cause bone marrow suppression; severe CNS depression or comatose states; uncontrolled epilepsy; hypersensitivity to product.

Route/Dosage
Cautious titration and divided dosage schedules are recommended.
ADULTS:
Initial dose: **PO** 12.5 mg daily or bid; increase by 25 to 50 mg daily up to 300 to 450 mg daily within 2 wk. May then increase dose in increments not to exceed 100 mg once or twice a wk. Usual dosage: 300 to 600 mg daily (max, 900 mg daily).

Interactions

Agents that suppress bone marrow: Risk or severity of bone marrow suppression may be increased.
Anticholinergics: Anticholinergic effects may be potentiated.
Antihypertensives: Hypotensive effects may be potentiated.
Barbiturates (eg, phenobarbital), nicotine, phenytoin, rifampin: May decrease blood levels of clozapine.
Caffeine, cimetidine, erythromycin, ritonavir, serotonin reuptake inhibitors (eg, fluoxetine): May increase blood levels of clozapine.
CNS drugs (eg, carbamazepine, benzodiazepines, tricyclic antidepressants) and alcohol: Use with caution because of CNS effects of clozapine.
Type 1C antiarrhythmics (eg, propafenone, flecainide): Use with caution.

Lab Test Interferences None well documented.

Adverse Reactions

CV: Tachycardia (25%); hypotension (9%); hypertension (4%); chest pain/angina, ECG change/cardiac abnormality (1%); cardiomyopathy; myocarditis, atrial or ventricular fibrillation, periorbital edema (postmarketing).
CNS: Drowsiness/sedation (39%); dizziness/

vertigo (19%); headache (7%); tremor, syncope (6%); disturbed sleep/nightmares, restlessness, hypokinesia/akinesia, agitation (4%); seizures, rigidity, akathisia, confusion (3%); fatigue, insomnia (2%); hyperkinesia, weakness, lethargy, ataxia, slurred speech, epileptiform movements/myoclonic jerks, depression, anxiety (1%); delirium, abnormal EEG, exacerbation of psychosis, myoclonus, paresthesia, mild cataplexy, status epilepticus (postmarketing).
DERM: Rash (2%); erythema multiforme, Stevens-Johnson syndrome (postmarketing).
EENT: Visual disturbances (5%); throat discomfort, nasal congestion (1%); narrow-angle glaucoma (postmarketing).
GI: Salivation (31%); constipation (14%); dry mouth (6%); nausea (5%); abdominal discomfort/heartburn (4%); nausea/vomiting (3%); diarrhea (2%); liver test abnormality, anorexia (1%); acute pancreatitis, dysphagia, fecal impaction, intestinal obstruction/paralytic ileus, salivary gland swelling (postmarketing).
GU: Urinary abnormalities (2%); incontinence, abnormal ejaculation, urinary urgency/frequency, urinary retention (1%); acute interstitial nephritis, priapism (postmarketing).
HEMA: Leukopenia/decreased WBC/neutropenia (3%); agranulocytosis, eosinophilia (1%); deep vein thrombosis, elevated hemoglobin/hematocrit, erythrocyte sedimentation rate increase, pulmonary embolism, sepsis, thrombocytosis, thrombocytopenia (postmarketing).
HEPA: Cholestasis, hepatitis, jaundice (postmarketing).
METAB: Weight gain (4%); hyperglycemia, hyperuricemia, hyponatremia, weight loss (postmarketing).
RESP: Dyspnea (1%); aspiration, pleural effusion (postmarketing).
OTHER: Sweating (6%); fever (5%); muscle weakness, pain (back, neck, legs), muscle spasm, muscle pain/ache, tongue numb/sore (1%); hypersensitivity reactions; photosensitivity, vasculitis, myasthenic syndrome, rhabdomyolysis, CPK elevation (postmarketing).

> **WARNING:**
>
> *Agranulocytosis:* Life-threatening adverse event. Monitor WBC and differential count before initiation of treatment and at least weekly for the first 6 mo and for 4 wk after discontinuation of treatment. Do not initiate therapy if WBC is less than $3,500/mm^3$ or if patient has a history of myeloproliferative disease.
>
> *CV and respiratory effects:* Orthostatic hypotension can occur. Rarely, collapse can be profound and accompanied by respiratory and/or cardiac arrest. Orthostatic hypotension is more likely to occur during initial dose titration in association with rapid dose escalation. Caution is advised with use of psychotropics or benzodiazepines as reports of collapse, respiratory arrest, and cardiac arrest have been reported.
>
> *Myocarditis:* Increased risk of fatal myocarditis, especially during the first month of therapy. Promptly discontinue clozapine if myocarditis is suspected.
>
> *Seizures:* Associated with therapy; use caution when administering to patients with a history of seizures or other predisposing factors. High clozapine dosage appears to be an important predictor of seizures.

Precautions
Pregnancy: Category B.
Lactation: Undetermined.
Children: Safety and efficacy not established.
Elderly: Lower doses required; high risk for anticholinergic and hypotensive effects. Approach dose selection with caution, taking into consideration decreased renal, hepatic, and cardiac function, and other concomitant disease and drug therapy.

Hepatic function impairment: Use caution when administering clozapine to patients who have concurrent hepatic disease. Hepatitis has been reported in patients with normal and preexisting liver function abnormalities.

Special risk patients: Use great caution in patients with renal or cardiac disease, narrow-angle glaucoma, enlarged prostate, or history of seizures. Greater likelihood of seizure at higher doses.

Cognitive and motor performance: Because of initial sedation, mental and/or physical abilities may be impaired, especially during the first few days of therapy.

Debilitated patients: Lower doses required; high risk for anticholinergic and hypotensive effects.

ECG changes: Some patients experience ECG repolarization changes during treatment. Several have experienced significant cardiac events including ischemic changes, MI, nonfatal arrhythmias, and sudden, unexplained death.

Fever: May experience transient temperature elevations above 100.4°F with peak incidence within first 3 wk of treatment.

General anesthesia: Because of the CNS effects of clozapine, caution is advised in patients receiving general anesthesia.

GI: Varying degrees of impairment of intestinal peristalsis, ranging from constipation to intestinal obstruction; fecal impaction and paralytic ileus have been associated with clozapine use.

Hyperglycemia and diabetes mellitus: Severe hyperglycemia possibly leading to ketoacidosis has been reported. Monitor patients with established diagnosis of diabetes mellitus regularly for worsening of glucose control.

Neuroleptic malignant syndrome (NMS): This potentially fatal condition has been reported in association with antipsychotic drugs. Signs and symptoms include hyperpyrexia, muscle rigidity, altered mental status, irregular pulse or BP, tachycardia, diaphoresis, and cardiac arrhythmias.

Pulmonary embolism: Consider the possibility in patients who present with deep vein thrombosis, acute dyspnea, chest pain, or other respiratory signs or symptoms.

Tardive dyskinesia: This syndrome of potentially irreversible, involuntary dyskinetic movements has occurred with other antipsychotic agents. Incidence is highest among elderly, especially women.

Withdrawal of medication: For planned discontinuation of therapy, gradually reduce dosage over 1 to 2 wk. If abrupt discontinuation is required (eg, leukopenia), carefully observe the patient for recurrence of psychotic symptoms and symptoms of cholinergic rebound (eg, headache, nausea, vomiting).

Overdosage: Signs and Symptoms

Excessive salivation, hypotension, drowsiness, delirium, coma, seizures, tachycardia, respiratory depression or failure, aspiration pneumonia, cardiac arrhythmias, seizures.

PATIENT CARE CONSIDERATIONS

Administration/Storage

- Only available through a distribution system that ensures monitoring of WBC counts.
- Administer prescribed dose without regard to meals.
- Administer with food if GI upset occurs.
- Store tablets at controlled room temperature (59° to 86°F).

Assessment/Interventions

- Obtain patient history, including drug history and any known allergies. Note history of clozapine-induced agranulocytosis, granulocytopenia or myocarditis, myeloproliferative disorder, liver disease, CV disease, pulmonary disease, narrow-angle glaucoma, previous episodes of NMS, seizures or conditions that predispose to seizures (eg, Alzheimer disease), conditions that would predispose to hypotension (eg, dehydration, hypovolemia, treatment with antihypertensive medications), or coadministration of a benzodiazepine or any other psychotropic medication, CYP450 inducer (eg, phenytoin), or CYP450 inhibitor (eg, macrolides antibiotics).
- Ensure that WBC and differential are determined prior to, weekly for the first 6 mo of treatment, and then every other week for duration of treatment. WBC and differential should be determined weekly for 4 wk following discontinuation of treatment.
- Do not initiate treatment if WBC is less than 3,500/mm^3.
- Repeat WBC count and differential if, after initial treatment, the total WBC count has dropped below 3,500/mm^3, or it has dropped a substantial amount (single drop of 3,000 or more in the WBC count or a cumulative drop of 3,000 or more within 3 wk) from baseline, even if the WBC count is above 3,500/mm^3, or if immature forms are present. If subsequent WBC counts are between 3,000 and 3,500/mm^3 and the ANC is above 1,500/mm^3, increase WBC and differential counts to twice weekly.
- Withhold therapy if WBC count falls below 3,000/mm^3 or the ANC falls below 1,500/mm^3. Repeat WBC count and differential daily and closely monitor patient for symp-

toms of infection. Consider reinstituting clozapine if no symptoms of infection develop, and if the total WBC count returns to levels greater than 3,000/mm^3 and the ANC returns to levels above 1,500/mm^3. Continue to monitor WBC counts and differential twice weekly until total WBC counts return to levels above 3,500/mm^3.
* Ensure WBC counts and differential are performed daily and bone marrow aspiration is considered if the total WBC count falls below 2,000/mm^3 or the ANC falls below 1,000/mm^3.
* Ensure that appropriate cultures are obtained and appropriate antibiotics are started if patient develops signs or symptoms of infection.
* Ensure that clozapine therapy is not restarted in patient whose total WBC count falls below 2,000/mm^3 or the ANC falls below 1,000/mm^3.
* Take safety precautions if orthostatic hypotension occurs.
* Monitor blood sugar in diabetic patient when drug is started or dose is changed. Report significant changes to health care provider.
* Ensure that fasting blood glucose is evaluated before starting therapy and periodically thereafter during therapy in patient with risk factors for diabetes mellitus (eg, obesity, family history of diabetes).
* Inform health care provider immediately if hyperpyrexia, muscle rigidity, altered mental status, irregular pulse and BP, tachycardia, and diaphoresis develop.
* Notify health care provider immediately if lethargy, weakness, sore throat, or other signs of infection occur.
* Notify health care provider if any of the following develop: excessive drowsiness, dizziness, persistent nausea or vomiting, constipation, symptoms of hyperglycemia (polyuria, polydipsia, polyphagia), unexplained fatigue, dyspnea, fever, chest pain, palpitations, tachycardia.
* Assess baseline neurologic status and during treatment observe for involuntary body and facial movements, drowsiness, agitation, anxiety, aggressive reaction, or seizure activity.
* Frequently assess patient for response to treatment. Notify health care provider if condition does not appear to be improving or is worsening.
* Ensure that therapy is periodically reviewed to determine if it needs to be continued without change or if a dose change (eg, increase, decrease, discontinuation) is indicated.
* Avoid sudden discontinuation of therapy if possible. Attempt to gradually reduce dose over a period of 1 to 2 wk if decision to discontinue medication is made.
* Monitor patient for suicidal tendencies often associated with schizophrenia.
* Assess medication compliance.

Patient/Family Education
* Explain name, dose, action, and potential side effects of drug.
* Instruct patient to take prescribed dose without regard to meals but to take with food if GI upset occurs.
* Advise patient that dose will be started low and then increased until max benefit is obtained.
* Instruct patient not to change the dose or stop taking unless advised by health care provider.
* Advise patient that if a dose is missed to take it as soon as possible and then return to the normal schedule. Instruct patient that if a dose is skipped not to double the dose to catch up. Caution patient that if medication has not been taken for more than 2 days not to restart medication but to contact health care provider for new dosing instructions.
* Advise patient that if medication needs to be discontinued it will be slowly withdrawn over a period of 1 to 2 wk unless safety concerns (eg, low WBC count) require a more rapid withdrawal.
* Instruct patient not to stop taking clozapine when feeling better.
* Instruct diabetic patient to monitor blood glucose more frequently when drug is started or dose is changed and to inform health care provider of significant changes in readings.
* Tell patient to immediately report lethargy, weakness, sore throat, or other signs of infection, muscle rigidity, altered mental status, rapid or irregular heartbeat, sweating, seizures, chest pain, unexplained fatigue, swelling of feet or ankles, rapid or difficult breathing, unquenchable thirst, or frequent urination to health care provider.
* Advise patient to notify health care provider of the following: excessive drowsiness, weight gain, involuntary body or facial movements, rapid pulse, change in personality or mood.
* Advise patient to avoid strenuous activity during periods of high temperature or humidity.
* Instruct patient to avoid alcoholic beverages and sedatives (eg, diazepam) while taking clozapine.
* Instruct patient to get up slowly from lying or sitting position and to avoid sudden position changes to prevent postural hypotension.

Advise patient to report dizziness with position changes to health care provider. Caution patient that hot tubs and hot showers or baths may make dizziness worse.
* Advise patient taking antihypertensives to monitor BP at regular intervals.
* Advise patient that drug may impair judgment, thinking, or motor skills or cause drowsiness and to use caution while driving or performing other tasks requiring mental alertness until tolerance is determined.
* Advise patient with history of seizures that drug may cause seizures and not to engage in any activity in which sudden loss of consciousness could cause serious risk to patient or others (eg, driving, swimming, climbing).
* Advise women to notify health care provider if pregnant, planning to become pregnant, or breastfeeding.
* Instruct patient not to take any prescription or OTC medications, dietary supplements, or herbal preparations unless advised by health care provider.
* Advise patient that follow-up visits and weekly blood cell counts will be required to monitor therapy and to keep appointments.

Codeine

(KOE-deen)

Class Narcotic analgesic/Antitussive

How Supplied
Available as generic only
✤ Codeine Contin ◆ ratio-Codeine

Action
PHARMACOLOGY: Stimulates opiate receptors in the CNS; also causes respiratory depression, peripheral vasodilation, inhibition of intestinal peristalsis, stimulation of the chemoreceptors that cause vomiting, increased bladder tone, and suppression of cough reflex.

PHARMACOKINETICS/DYNAMICS:
Metabolism: Metabolized in the liver by undergoing O-demethylation, N-demethylation, and partial conjugation.

Excretion: Excreted in the urine, largely as inactive metabolites, and small amounts of free and conjugated morphine. The t½ is 3 hr.

Onset:
Oral/SC – 15 to 30 min.

Peak:
Oral – 60 min.

Duration:
Oral/SC – 4 to 6 hr.

Indications Relief of mild to moderate pain; cough suppression.

Contraindications Hypersensitivity to opiates; upper airway obstruction; respiratory compromise; acute asthma; diarrhea caused by poisoning or toxins.

Route/Dosage
ANALGESIC
ADULTS: **IM/slow IV/PO/SC** 15 to 60 mg q 4 to 6 hr (max, 360 mg/day).
CHILDREN 1 YR AND OVER: **IM/PO/SC** 0.5 mg/kg q 4 to 6 hr.

ANTITUSSIVE
ADULTS: **PO** 10 to 20 mg q 4 to 6 hr (max, 120 mg/day).
CHILDREN 6 TO 12 YR: **PO** 5 to 10 mg q 4 to 6 hr (max, 60 mg/day).
CHILDREN 2 TO 6 YR: **PO** 2.5 to 5 mg q 4 to 6 hr (max, 30 mg/day).

Interactions
CNS depressants, (eg, tranquilizers, sedatives, and alcohol): Causes additive CNS depression.
Quinidine: May decrease the analgesic effect of codeine by interference with metabolism of codeine to morphine.

Lab Test Interferences Amylase and lipase determination: Increased levels for up to 24 hr after administration.

Adverse Reactions
CV: Hypotension; orthostatic hypotension; bradycardia; tachycardia; shock.
CNS: Lightheadedness; dizziness; sedation; disorientation; incoordination; euphoria; delirium.
DERM: Sweating; pruritus; urticaria.
EENT: Miosis.
GI: Nausea; vomiting; constipation; abdominal pain; anorexia; biliary tract spasm.
GU: Urinary retention or hesitancy.
RESP: Laryngospasm; depression of cough reflex; respiratory depression.
OTHER: Tolerance; psychological and physical dependence with chronic use.

Precautions
Pregnancy: Category C. Therapeutic doses of codeine have increased duration of labor.
Lactation: Excreted in breast milk.
Children: Do not give IV to children under 12 yr. Children are more sensitive to effects of drug. Safety and efficacy not established in newborn infants.
Elderly: More sensitive to effects of drug.
Renal function impairment: Duration of action may be prolonged; may need to reduce dose.
Hepatic function impairment: Duration of action may be prolonged; may need to reduce dose.
Special risk patients: Use with caution in patients with myxedema, acute alcoholism, history of drug abuse potential, acute abdominal conditions, ulcerative colitis, decreased respiratory reserve,

head injury or increased intracranial pressure, hypoxia, supraventricular tachycardia, depleted blood volume, circulatory shock, hypothyroidism, and urinary/bowel elimination problems.
Drug dependency: Codeine has abuse potential.

PATIENT CARE CONSIDERATIONS
Administration/Storage
- Administer oral medication with food or milk to avoid GI irritation.
- Protect injectable forms from excessive exposure to light.
- Codeine is two-thirds as effective given orally as parenterally.

Assessment/Interventions
- Obtain patient history, including drug history and any known allergies. Patients with sulfite sensitivity have increased risk of allergy with certain injectable codeine products.
- Assess degree of pain before and after administration.
- Monitor pulmonary status and heart rhythm after administration.
- Monitor bowel movements and inform health care provider of significant pattern change.
- If respiratory compromise or increased sedation develop, withhold medication and notify health care provider.

Overdosage: Signs and Symptoms
Miosis, respiratory and CNS depression, circulatory collapse, seizures, cardiopulmonary arrest, death.

Patient/Family Education
- Instruct patient on self-assessment of pain and on how and when to administer medication.
- Advise patient to increase fluid intake to relieve constipation and to take stool softener or mild laxative as needed.
- Advise patient to take medication with food if GI upset occurs and to monitor for GI irritation.
- Explain that codeine may be habit forming.
- Caution patient to avoid sudden position changes to prevent orthostatic hypotension.
- Instruct patient to avoid intake of alcoholic beverages or other CNS depressants.
- Advise patient that drug may cause drowsiness and to use caution while driving or performing other tasks requiring mental alertness.
- Instruct patient not to take OTC medications without contacting health care provider.

Codeine Polistirex/ Chlorpheniramine Polistirex
(KOE-deen pahl-ee-STIE-rex/klor-fen-AIR-uh-meen pahl-ee-STIE-rex)

Class Narcotic analgesic/Antitussive/Antihistamine/Alkylamine

How Supplied
Codeprex Suspension, extended-release 20 mg codeine and 4 mg chlorpheniramine maleate per 5 mL

Action
PHARMACOLOGY:
Codeine: Stimulates opiate receptors in the CNS; also causes respiratory depression, peripheral vasodilation, inhibition of intestinal peristalsis, stimulation of chemoreceptors that cause vomiting, increased bladder tone, and suppression of cough reflex.
Chlorpheniramine: Competitively antagonizes histamine at H_1 receptor sites.

Indications Temporary relief of cough; temporary relief of runny nose, sneezing, itching of the nose or throat, and itching watery eyes caused by hay fever, upper respiratory allergies, or allergic rhinitis.

Contraindications Hypersensitivity to certain other opioids or any component of the product.

Route/Dosage
ADULTS AND CHILDREN 12 YR OF AGE AND OLDER: PO 2 tsp (10 mL) q 12 hr (max, 4 tsp [20 mL] in 24 hr).
CHILDREN 6 TO UNDER 12 YR OF AGE: PO 1 tsp (5 mL) q 12 hr (max, 2 tsp [10 mL] in 24 hr).

Interactions
Anticholinergics: Additive adverse effects, resulting from cholinergic blockade (eg, xerostomia, blurred vision, constipation) may occur.
Antidepressants (eg, tricyclic antidepressants, MAO inhibitors): Effects of antidepressants or codeine may be increased.
CNS depressants (eg, opioids, antihistamines, alcohol): Additive CNS depressant effects may occur.
CYP3A4 inducers, CYP2D6 inhibitors: May decrease plasma levels of the active metabolites of codeine, morphine, and morphine-6-glucuronide).
Phenytoin: Chlorpheniramine may inhibit the hepatic metabolism of phenytoin, increasing phenytoin serum levels and toxicity.

Lab Test Interferences Codeine may produce spasm of sphincter of Oddi, resulting in elevation of plasma amylase and lipase and causing determination of these enzyme levels to be unreliable.

Adverse Reactions
CV: Fast, slow, or pounding heartbeat; hypertension; hypotension; orthostatic hypotension; palpitation; shock-like state; syncope.
CNS: Asthenia; confusion; dizziness; depression; drowsiness; sedation; headache; euphoria; facial dyskinesia; false sense of well-being; feeling faint; lightheadedness; general feeling of discomfort or illness; excitability; nervousness; agitation; restlessness; minimal sedation; somnolence; insomnia; dyskinesia; irritability; tremor.
DERM: Redness or flushing of face; dermatitis; excessive perspiration; urticaria; erythema; pruritus; rash.
EENT: Blurred or double vision, or other visual disturbances; nasal stuffiness; labyrinthitis; tinnitus; vertigo; farsightedness; increased lacrimation; mydriasis; photophobia.
GI: Abdominal distension; abdominal pain; acute pancreatitis; constipation; diarrhea; dry mouth; dyspepsia; epigastric distress; loss of appetite; nausea; vomiting; decreased gastric motility; esophageal reflux.
ENDO: Changes in glucose utilization; decreased lactation; early menses; glycosuria; hypoglycemia; increased appetite; increased libido; pheochromocytoma stimulation.
GU: Dysuria; irritative bladder symptoms; urinary frequency; urinary hesitancy; urinary retention; gynecomastia; ureteral spasm.
HYPERSEN: Allergic laryngospasm; atelectasis; bronchospastic allergic reaction; hives; itching; swelling of face.
RESP: Dryness of pharynx and respiratory passages; laryngismus; wheezing; troubled breathing; respiratory depression.
OTHER: Feeling of relaxation; unusual tiredness or weakness.

Precautions
Pregnancy: Category C.
Lactation: Codeine and its metabolite morphine as well as chlorpheniramine are excreted in breast milk.
Children: Safety and efficacy not established in children under 6 yr of age.
Elderly: Use with caution because of the greater frequency of decreased hepatic, renal, or cardiac function, and concomitant diseases or other drug therapy.
Acute abdominal conditions: Diagnosis or clinical course of patients with acute abdominal conditions may be obscured.
Head injury or increased intracranial pressure: Opioids may elevate cerebrospinal fluid pressure, which may be markedly exaggerated in the presence of head injury, other intracranial lesions or a preexisting increase in intracranial pressure.
Obstructive bowel disease – Opioids may result in obstructive bowel disease, especially in patients with underlying intestinal motility disorder.
Respiratory depression – Pediatric patients may be more susceptible to respiratory depressant effects of codeine, including respiratory arrest, coma, and death.
Special risk patients – Use with caution in patients with persistent or chronic cough, narrow-angle glaucoma, asthma, prostatic hypertrophy, hepatic or renal function impairment, hypothyroidism, Addison disease, prostatic hypertrophy, or urethral stricture.

Overdosage: Signs and Symptoms
Codeine: Respiratory depression, extreme somnolence progressing to stupor or coma, miosis, skeletal muscle flaccidity, cold and clammy skin, bradycardia, hypotension, apnea, circulatory collapse, cardiac arrest, death.
Chlorpheniramine: CNS effects ranging from depression to stimulation (central toxic effects characterized by agitation, anxiety, delirium, disorientation, hallucinations, hyperactivity, sedation, seizures), coma, medullary paralysis, death, hypertension, tachycardia, dysrhythmias, vasodilation, hyperpyrexia, mydriasis, urinary retention, decreased GI motility, dry mouth, pharynx, bronchi and nasal passages, impaired secretion from the sweat glands predisposing to hyperthermia.

PATIENT CARE CONSIDERATIONS
Administration/Storage
- Shake suspension well before measuring dose.
- Measure and administer prescribed dose using dosing spoon, syringe, or cup.
- Do not dilute suspension with other fluids or mix with other medications.
- Administer prescribed dose q 12 hr as needed, without regard to meals. Administer with food if GI upset occurs.
- Store suspension at controlled room temperature (less than 77°F). Protect from light.

Assessment/Interventions
- Obtain patient history, including drug history and any known allergies. Note severe renal or hepatic impairment, pulmonary disease (eg, COPD, asthma), shortness of breath, head injury or intracranial lesion, acute abdominal condition, obstructive bowel disease, enlarged prostate, narrow angle glaucoma, hypothyroidism, Addison disease, or hypersensitivity to any opioid.
- Assess symptoms (eg, cough, rhinitis, nasal congestion, sneezing, watery eyes, itching nose, throat, or eyes) before starting therapy and periodically during therapy. Notify health care provider if symptoms are not improving or are getting worse.

- Monitor patient for GI, CNS, RESP, GU, and general body side effects. Inform health care provider if noted and significant.

Patient/Family Education
- Explain name, dose, action, and potential side effects of drug.
- Advise patient to take prescribed dose q 12 hr as needed.
- Advise patient or caregiver to shake suspension well before measuring dose and to use dosing spoon, syringe, or cup to measure and administer dose.
- Advise patient to take without regard to meals but to take with food if stomach upset occurs.
- Caution patient or caregiver not to dilute or mix with other medications.
- Advise patient that if symptoms are not controlled, not to increase the dose of medication but to inform health care provider.
- Caution patient that drug may cause drowsiness and to use caution while driving or performing other tasks requiring mental alertness until tolerance is determined.
- Advise patient to avoid alcohol and other CNS depressants while taking this medication because of risk of excessive sedation.
- Caution patient not to take any OTC antihistamines or decongestants while taking this medication unless advised by health care provider.
- If patient is to have allergy skin testing, advise patient not to take the medication for at least 6 days before the skin testing.
- Advise women to notify health care provider if pregnant, planning to become pregnant, or breastfeeding.
- Caution patient not to take any prescription or OTC medications, herbal preparations, or dietary supplements unless advised by health care provider.

Colchicine

(KOHL-chih-seen)

Class Analgesic/Gout

How Supplied
Colchicine Tablets 0.6 mg, Injection 0.5 mg/mL
✤ ratio-Colchicine

Action
PHARMACOLOGY: Inhibits inflammation and reduces pain and swelling associated with gouty arthritis.

PHARMACOKINETICS/DYNAMICS:
Absorption: Rapidly absorbed. T_{max} is 0.5 to 2 hr.
Distribution: Large amounts present in bile and intestinal secretions. High concentrations also found in kidney, liver, and spleen. About 50% protein bound. Vd is 1 to 3 L/kg.
Metabolism: Undergoes enterohepatic recirculation. Deacetylated primarily by the liver.
Excretion: Plasma t½ 10 to 60 min. Excreted via biliary and renal routes; 10% to 20% excreted unchanged in urine.

Indications Treatment and relief of pain in attacks of acute gouty arthritis; regular prophylaxis between attacks and is often effective in aborting an attack when taken at the first sign of articular discomfort; colchicine IV is used when rapid response is desired or if GI side effects interfere with oral use. **Unlabeled use(s):** Familial Mediterranean fever; hepatic cirrhosis; primary biliary cirrhosis; treatment of Behcet disease; scleroderma; Sweet syndrome

Contraindications Serious GI, renal, hepatic, or cardiac disorders; blood dyscrasias.

Route/Dosage
Acute Gouty Arthritis
ADULTS: Initial dose (give at first sign of attack) PO 1.2 mg; then 0.6 q hr or 1.2 mg q 2 hr until pain is relieved or diarrhea ensues. Total dose is usually 4 to 8 mg. Wait 3 days before initiating a second course of therapy. **IV** Initial dose 2 mg; then 0.5 mg q 6 hr until satisfactory response is achieved (max, 4 mg/24 hr or 1 course of treatment).

Prophylaxis
ADULTS: PO 0.6 mg/day for 3 to 4 days/wk if fewer than 1 attack/yr; if more than 1 attack/yr, 0.6 mg/day. Severe cases may require 1.2 to 1.8 mg/day.

Prophylaxis or Maintenance of Recurrent or Chronic Gouty Arthritis
ADULTS: **IV** 0.5 to 1 mg 1 or 2 times/day; however, oral form is preferable, usually in conjunction with a uricosuric agent.

Surgical Patients
ADULTS: PO 0.6 mg tid for 3 days before and 3 days after surgery.

Interactions None well documented.
INCOMPATIBILITIES: Do not dilute with 5% Dextrose in water.

Lab Test Interferences May cause false-positive results in urine tests for RBCs and hemoglobin.

Adverse Reactions
DERM: Dermatoses; purpura; alopecia.
GI: Nausea; vomiting; diarrhea; abdominal pain.
HEMA: Bone marrow depression with aplastic anemia; agranulocytosis, leukopenia or thrombo-

cytopenia (long-term therapy).
HEPA: Elevated alkaline phosphatase and AST.
OTHER: Reversible azoospermia; myopathy; peripheral neuritis.

Precautions
Pregnancy: Category C (oral). Category D (parenteral).
Lactation: Undetermined.
Children: Safety and efficacy not established.
Elderly: Administer with great caution to elderly and debilitated patients.
Hepatic function impairment: Increased colchicine toxicity may occur.
GI effects: Drug may cause nausea, vomiting, diarrhea, and abdominal pain that may aggravate pre-existing peptic ulcer or spastic colon. Discontinue drug if these symptoms appear.

PATIENT CARE CONSIDERATIONS

Administration/Storage
Parenteral:
- Reconstitute with 0.9% Sodium Chloride (without preservatives) only.
- Administer parenterally via IV route only. Considerable irritation and tissue damage may occur if leakage into surrounding tissue occurs.

Oral:
- Store tablets in airtight, light-resistant container.

Assessment/Interventions
- Obtain patient history, including drug history and any known allergies.
- Monitor serum uric acid and creatinine throughout therapy.
- Check blood counts periodically in patients undergoing long-term therapy.
- Monitor for phlebitis and extravasation.
- Assess for signs of toxicity (eg, abdominal pain, alopecia, nausea, vomiting, diarrhea, myopathy, peripheral neuritis). Notify health care provider immediately if these signs occur.
- Assess for signs of vitamin B_{12} deficiency (eg, anemia, paresis of extremities).

Injection: Severe local irritation occurs if drug is given by SC or IM route.
Myopathy and neuropathy: Myoneuropathy may occur and cause weakness in patients with impaired kidney function; serum creatine kinase may be elevated. Usually resolves in 3 to 4 wk after drug withdrawal.
Vitamin B_{12} malabsorption: Colchicine induces reversible malabsorption of vitamin B_{12} with long-term use.

Overdosage: Signs and Symptoms
Nausea, severe abdominal pain, vomiting, diarrhea, shock, ST segment elevation, paralysis, respiratory failure, liver damage, renal failure, leukopenia, thrombocytopenia, coagulopathy, alopecia, stomatitis.

Patient/Family Education
- Instruct patient to take colchicine regularly to prevent acute attacks.
- Instruct patient not to exceed 8 mg in course of therapy for acute attack. To minimize cumulative toxicity, patient should wait 3 days before starting second course.
- Advise patient with gout to drink at least 2000 mL of fluid daily, unless contraindicated.
- Reinforce health care provider's instructions about weight loss, diet, and alcohol intake.
- Advise patient to have extra supply of drug on hand in case health care provider gives instructions to increase dosage.
- Instruct patient to stop taking drug if nausea, vomiting, diarrhea, or abdominal pain occurs, especially if patient has history of spastic colon or ulcers.

Colesevelam Hydrochloride

(koe-leh-SEV-eh-lam HIGH-droe-KLOR-ide)
Class Antihyperlipidemic/Bile acid sequestrant

How Supplied
Welchol Tablets 625 mg

Action
PHARMACOLOGY: Increases removal of bile acids from the body by binding bile acids in the intestine, impeding their reabsorption. As the bile acid pool becomes depleted, the conversion of cholesterol to bile acids is increased, which decreases serum cholesterol.

PHARMACOKINETICS/DYNAMICS:
Absorption: Colesevelam is not absorbed from the GI tract.

Indications Adjunctive therapy to diet and exercise given alone or with an HMG-CoA reductase inhibitor for the reduction of elevated LDL cholesterol in patients with primary hypercholesterolemia (Fredrickson type IIa).

Contraindications Bowel obstruction; hypersensitivity to any component of the product.

Route/Dosage
ADULTS:
Monotherapy: PO 1875 mg (3 tablets) bid with meals or 3750 mg (6 tablets) qd with a meal. Depending upon the desired effect the dose can be increase to 4375 mg/day (7 tablets).
Combination therapy: PO 2500 to 3750 mg (4 to 6 tablets) qd.

Interactions None well documented.

Lab Test Interferences None well documented.

Adverse Reactions
GI: Constipation; dyspepsia.
RESP: Pharyngitis.
OTHER: Accidental injury; asthenia; myalgia.

PATIENT CARE CONSIDERATIONS

Administration/Storage

* Administer qd or bid as prescribed with liquid and food.
* May be used alone or in combination with an HMG-CoA reductase inhibitor.
* Store at controlled room temperature (59° to 86°F). Protect from moisture.

Assessment/Interventions

* Obtain patient history, including drug history and any known allergies. Note history of bowel obstruction, vitamin K or fat soluble vitamin deficiencies, dysphagia, swallowing disorder, major GI surgery, or severe GI motility disorder.
* Ensure that total-C, LDL-C, and triglycerides are determined before starting therapy and periodically thereafter.
* Ensure that diseases that can contribute to increased cholesterol (eg, hypothyroidism, diabetes mellitus) have been investigated and treated before initiating therapy.
* Ensure that patient is receiving a low cholesterol, high fiber diet.
* Assess patient for GI side effects. Inform health care provider if noted and significant.

Precautions
Pregnancy: Category B.
Children: Safety and efficacy not established.
Special risk patients: Use with caution in patients with vitamin A, D, or K deficiencies, dysphagia, swallowing disorders, severe GI motility disorders, or major GI tract surgery.

Patient/Family Education

* Explain name, dose, action, and potential side effects of drug.
* Advise patient to take prescribed dose qd or bid with liquid and food.
* Instruct patient to take as prescribed and to not change the dose or stop taking unless advised by health care provider.
* Instruct patient about life-style changes (eg, low fat-high fiber diet, regular exercise, smoking cessation) that facilitate cholesterol/triglyceride control.
* Advise patient to take vitamin supplements as recommended by health care provider.
* Advise patient to notify health care provider if GI side effects occur and become bothersome.
* Advise women to notify health care provider if pregnant, planning to become pregnant, or breastfeeding.
* Instruct patient to not take any prescription or OTC medications or dietary supplements unless advised by health care provider.
* Advise patient that follow-up visits and lab tests will be required to monitor therapy and to keep appointments.

Colestipol Hydrochloride

(koe-LESS-tih-pole HIGH-droe-KLOR-ide)
Class Antihyperlipidemic/Bile acid sequestrant

How Supplied
Colestid Tablets 1 g, Granules 5 g colestipol hydrochloride/dose, Granules 5 g colestipol hydrochloride/7.5 g powder

Action
PHARMACOLOGY: Increases removal of bile acids from body by forming insoluble complexes in intestine, which are then excreted in feces. As body loses bile acids, it converts cholesterol from blood to bile acids, thus lowering serum cholesterol.

PHARMACOKINETICS/DYNAMICS:
Absorption: Not absorbed.
Excretion: Less than 0.17% is excreted in the urine.

Onset: Decline in serum cholesterol is evident by 1 mo.

Duration: Cholesterol levels usually return to baseline levels within 1 mo.

Indications Reduction of cholesterol in patients with primary hypercholesterolemia who do not respond adequately to diet. **Unlabeled use(s):** Treatment of digitalis toxicity.

Contraindications Hypersensitivity to bile acid sequestering resins; complete biliary obstruction.

Route/Dosage
ADULTS:
Tablets: **PO** 2 to 16 g/day given once or in divided doses. Start with 2 g once or twice daily and increase in amounts of 2 g once or twice daily at 1- or 2-mo intervals
Granules: **PO** 5 to 30 g/day given once or in divided doses. Start with 5 g once or twice daily

and increase in amounts of 5 g daily over 1 to 2 mo intervals.

Interactions
Digitalis glycosides, furosemide, gemfibrozil, hydrocortisone, penicillin G, phosphate supplements, propanolol, tetracyclines, thiazide diuretics, fat soluble vitamins (ie, A, D, E, K): Absorption of these drugs may be decreased.

Lab Test Interferences
None well documented.

Adverse Reactions
DERM: Rash; urticaria.
EENT: Difficulty swallowing.
GI: Constipation; abdominal pain and cramping; intestinal bloating; flatulence; indigestion; heartburn; diarrhea; nausea; vomiting; bloody hemorrhoids and stools; esophageal obstruction.
HEMA: Bleeding tendencies related to vitamin K deficiency.
HEPA: Elevated LFTs.
METAB: Fat-soluble vitamin deficiencies.

Precautions
Pregnancy: Category undetermined.
Lactation: Undetermined.
Children: Safety and efficacy not established.

Overdosage: Signs and Symptoms
GI obstruction.

PATIENT CARE CONSIDERATIONS

Administration/Storage
- Administer before meals.
- Do not administer simultaneously with other medicines. Administer other medications 1 hr before or 4 to 6 hr after colestipol.
- Tablets are large and may be difficult to swallow.
- Swallow each tablet whole. Do not cut, crush or chew tablets.
- Drink plenty of fluids as the tablets are swallowed.
- Granulated form of medication should not be taken dry. Mix well in at least 90 mL of liquids of any type (except alcoholic beverages), soups, cereal, or pulpy fruits. Colestipol will not dissolve.
- Rinse glass with small amount of beverage to ensure that all the medication is consumed.
- Store granules and tablets at room temperature.

Assessment/Interventions
- Obtain patient history.
- Monitor for signs of increased bleeding tendencies, such as swollen joints, ecchymotic areas, and petechiae.
- Assess for bowel function, particularly pre-existing problems with constipation that may worsen with its use.
- Document serum cholesterol and triglyceride levels.
- Provide diet high in fiber; increase fluids to 2 to 3 L unless contraindicated. If constipation develops, notify health care provider.
- Obtain baseline serum total and LDL cholesterol and triglyceride levels.

Patient/Family Education
- Instruct patient to take medication before meals.
- Advise patient to take any other medications, including OTC medications, 1 hr before or 4 to 6 hr after taking colestipol.
- Advise patient regarding proper mixing of granules.
- Advise patient to implement any vitamin and mineral supplementation recommended by healthcare provider.
- Advise patient to drink prune juice, eat fruit and vegetables, and maintain good fluid intake on a regular basis to avoid constipation.
- Advise patient to notify healthcare provider if GI side effects (eg, constipation, cramping, heartburn, bloating, gas) become bothersome.
- Instruct patient in life-style changes (eg, low fat diet, regular exercise, weight reduction) that facilitate cholesterol/triglyceride control.
- Advise patient that lab tests will be required to monitor therapy. Be sure to keep appointments.

Colistin Sulfate/Neomycin Sulfate/Thonzonium Br/ Hydrocortisone Acetate

(koe-LISS-tin SULL-fate/NEE-oh-MY-sin SULL-fate/thahn-ZOE-nee-uhm BROE-mide/ HIGH-droe-core-tih-sone ASS-uh-TATE)

Class Antibiotic/Corticosteroid

How Supplied
Coly-Mycin S Otic Suspension 1% hydrocortisone, 4.71 mg neomycin sulfate (equiv. to 3.3 mg neomycin base), 3 mg colistin (as sulfate), and 0.05% thonzonium Br/mL ♦
Cortisporin-TC Otic Suspension 1% hydrocortisone, 3.3 mg neomycin sulfate, 3 mg colistin (as sulfate), and 0.5 mg thonzonium Br

Action
PHARMACOLOGY:
Colistin: Bactericidal agent against most gram-negative organisms, particularly, *Pseudomonas aeruginosa*.
Neomycin: Inhibits protein synthesis by binding to ribosomal RNA, causing bacterial genetic code misreading.
Thonzonium: Surface-active agent that promotes tissue contact by dispersion and penetration of the cellular debris and exudates.
Hydrocortisone: Depresses formation, release, and activity of endogenous mediators of inflammation as well as modifying body's immune response.

Indications
Treatment of superficial bacterial infections of the external auditory canal caused by susceptible organisms; treatment of infection of mastoidectomy and fenestration cavities caused by susceptible organisms.

Contraindications
Sensitivity to any component of the product; external auditory canal disorder caused by cutaneous viral infections (eg, herpes simplex virus, varicella zoster virus).

Route/Dosage
ADULTS: **Otic** Thoroughly clean external auditory canal and dry with sterile cotton applicator. Using the calibrated dropper, instill 5 drops of the suspension into affected ear tid or qid.

PEDIATRICS: **Otic** Thoroughly clean external auditory canal and dry with sterile cotton applicator. Using the calibrated dropper, instill 4 drops of the suspension into affected ear tid or qid. Alternatively, a cotton wick may be inserted into the canal and then saturated with the suspension. The wick may be kept moist by adding additional solution q 4 hr. Replace wick at least once q 24 hr.

Interactions
None well documented.

Lab Test Interferences
None well documented.

Adverse Reactions
DERM: Cutaneous sensitization (particularly neomycin).

Precautions
Superinfection: Prolonged use may result in bacterial or fungal overgrowth of nonsusceptible microorganisms.
Bacterial resistance: Bacterial resistance to components of the product may develop.
Cross allergy: Allergic cross-sensitivity may occur, which could prevent future use of the following antibiotics: kanamycin, paromomycin, streptomycin, and possibly gentamicin.
Perforated eardrum/Chronic otitis media: Use with caution because of possibility of neomycin-induced ototoxicity.

PATIENT CARE CONSIDERATIONS

Administration/Storage
- For otic use only. Not for oral, nasal, or ocular use.
- Cleanse external ear canal and dry with sterile cotton applicator before instilling drops.
- Hold bottle in hand for 1 to 2 min to warm suspension.
- Shake well immediately before using.
- Instill prescribed number of drops into external ear canal tid to qid as directed using supplied dropper, or insert cotton wick into the canal and then saturate the cotton with suspension q 4 hr.
- If using cotton wick, replace wick at least once q 24 hr.
- Do not touch ear with dropper.
- Do not rinse dropper after use.
- Store at controlled room temperature (59° to 86°F).

Assessment/Interventions
- Obtain patient history, including drug history and any known allergies. Note presence of perforated tympanic membrane or viral infection of the external ear canal.
- Monitor patient for improvement of symptoms of infection.
- Monitor patient for sensitization or irritation and report to health care provider if noted.

Patient/Family Education
- Explain name, dose, action, and potential side effects of medication.
- Remind patient, family, or caregiver that medication is for use in the ear only.
- Teach patient proper technique for instilling ear drops: wash hands; thoroughly clean external ear canal and dry with sterile cotton applicator. Warm solution by holding bottle in hand for 1 to 2 min; shake well. Tilt head to side or lie on side with affected ear upward; instill prescribed number of drops and maintain position for 5 min to allow drops to penetrate ear canal. Repeat, if necessary, for the opposite ear. Do not allow dropper to touch ear; replace dropper.
- If preferred, a cotton wick may be placed in the ear canal and then saturated with suspension q 4 hr. Instruct patient to replace wick at least once q 24 hr.
- Advise patient, family, or caregiver to use only supplied dropper and to not rinse dropper after use.
- Advise patient, family, or caregiver to notify health care provider if symptoms do not improve or if irritation, inflammation, or itch-

ing of ear canal is noted.
- Advise patient, family, or caregiver that follow-up examinations may be required to monitor therapy and to keep appointments.

Contraceptives, Oral (Combination Products)

(kon-tra-SEP-tiv, OR-al)

Class Hormone/Contraceptive

How Supplied

Alesse Tablets 20 mcg ethinyl estradiol/0.1 mg levonorgestrel ◆ *Apri* Tablets 30 mcg ethinyl estradiol/0.15 mg desogestrel ◆ *Aviane* Tablets 20 mcg ethinyl estradiol/0.1 mg levonorgestrel ◆ *Brevicon* Tablets 35 mcg ethinyl estradiol/0.5 mg norethindrone ◆ *Cryselle* Tablets 30 mcg ethinyl estradiol/0.3 mg norgestrel ◆ *Cyclessa* Tablets Phase 1: 0.1 mg desogestrel/25 mcg ethinyl estradiol. Phase 2: 0.125 mg desogestrel/25 mcg ethinyl estradiol. Phase 3: 0.15 mg desogestrel/25 mcg ethinyl estradiol. ◆ *Demulen 1/35* Tablets 35 mcg ethinyl estradiol/1 mg ethynodiol diacetate ◆ *Demulen 1/50* Tablets 50 mcg ethinyl estradiol/1 mg ethynodiol diacetate ◆ *Desogen* Tablets 30 mcg ethinyl estradiol/0.15 desogestrel ◆ *Enpresse* Tablets Phase 1: 0.05 mg levonorgestrel/30 mcg ethinyl estradiol. Phase 2: 0.075 mg levonorgestrel/40 mcg ethinyl estradiol. Phase 3: 0.125 mg levonorgestrel/30 mcg ethinyl estradiol. ◆ *Estrostep 21* Tablets Phase 1: 1 mg norethindrone acetate/20 mcg ethinyl estradiol. Phase 2: 1 mg norethindrone acetate/30 mcg ethinyl estradiol. Phase 3: 1 mg norethindrone acetate/35 mcg ethinyl estradiol. ◆ *Estrostep Fe* Tablets Phase 1: 1 mg norethindrone acetate/20 mcg ethinyl estradiol. Phase 2: 1 mg norethindrone acetate/30 mcg ethinyl estradiol. Phase 3: 1 mg norethindrone acetate/35 mcg ethinyl estradiol. ◆ *Jenest-28* Tablets Phase 1: 0.5 mg norethindrone/35 mcg ethinyl estradiol. Phase 2: 1 mg norethindrone/35 mcg ethinyl estradiol ◆ *Kariva* Tablets 20 mcg ethinyl estradiol (white tablets)/10 mcg ethinyl estradiol (lt. blue tablets)/0.15 mg desogestrel (white tablets only) ◆ *Lessina* Tablets 20 mcg ethinyl estradiol/0.1 mg levonorgestrel ◆ *Levlen* Tablets 30 mcg ethinyl estradiol/0.15 mg levonorgestrel ◆ *Levlite* Tablets 20 mcg ethinyl estradiol/0.1 mg levonorgestrel ◆ *Levora 0.15/30* Tablets 30 mcg ethinyl estradiol/0.15 mg levonorgestrel ◆ *Loestrin 21 1/20* Tablets 20 mcg ethinyl estradiol/1 mg norethindrone acetate ◆ *Loestrin 21 1.5/30* Tablets 30 mcg ethinyl estradiol/1.5 mg norethindrone acetate ◆ *Loestrin Fe 1/20* Tablets 20 mcg ethinyl estradiol/1 mg norethindrone acetate ◆ *Loestrin Fe 1.5/30* Tablets 30 mcg ethinyl estradiol/1.5 mg norethindrone acetate ◆ *Lo/Ovral* Tablets 30 mcg ethinyl estradiol/0.3 mg norgestrel ◆ *Low-Ogestrel* Tablets 30 mcg ethinyl estradiol/0.3 mg norgestrel ◆ *Microgestin Fe 1/20* Tablets 20 mcg ethinyl estradiol/1 mg norethindrone acetate ◆ *Microgestin Fe 1.5/30* Tablets 30 mcg ethinyl estradiol/1.5 mg norethindrone acetate ◆ *Mircette* Tablets Phase 1: 0.15 mg desogestrel/20 mcg ethinyl estradiol. Phase 2: 0.01 mg ethinyl estradiol. ◆ *Modicon* Tablets 35 mcg ethinyl estradiol/0.5 mg norethindrone ◆ *Mononessa* Tablets 35 mcg ethinyl estradiol/0.25 mg norgestimate ◆ *Necon 0.5/35* Tablets 35 mcg ethinyl estradiol/0.5 mg norethindrone ◆ *Necon 1/35* Tablets 35 mcg ethinyl estradiol/1 mg norethindrone ◆ *Necon 1/50* Tablets 50 mcg mestranol/1 mg norethindrone ◆ *Necon 10/11* Tablets Phase 1: 0.5 mg norethindrone/35 mcg ethinyl estradiol. Phase 2: 1 mg norethindrone/35 mcg ethinyl estradiol. ◆ *Nordette* Tablets 30 mcg ethinyl estradiol/0.15 mg levonorgestrel ◆ *Norinyl 1 + 35* Tablets 35 mcg ethinyl estradiol/1 mg norethindrone ◆ *Norinyl 1 + 50* Tablets 50 mcg mestranol/1 mg norethindrone ◆ *Nortrel 0.5/35* Tablets 35 mcg ethinyl estradiol/0.5mg norethindrone ◆ *Nortrel 1/35* Tablets 35 mcg ethinyl estradiol/ 1 mg norethindrone ◆ *Ogestrel 0.5/50* Tablets 50 mcg ethinyl estradiol/0.5 mg norgestrel ◆ *Ortho-Cept* Tablets 30 mcg ethinyl estradiol/0.15 mg desogestrel ◆ *Ortho-Cyclen* Tablets 35 mcg ethinyl estradiol/0.25 mg norgestimate ◆ *Ortho-Novum 1/50* Tablets 50 mcg mestranol/1 mg norethindrone ◆ *Ortho-Novum 1/35* Tablets 35 mcg ethinyl estradiol/1 mg norethindrone ◆ *Ortho-Novum 7/7/7* Tablets Phase 1: 0.5 mg norethindrone/35 mcg ethinyl estradiol. Phase 2: 0.75 mg norethindrone/35 mcg ethinyl estradiol. Phase 3: 1 mg norethindrone/35 mcg ethinyl estradiol. ◆ *Ortho-Novum 10/11* Tablets Phase 1: 0.5 mg norethindrone/35 mcg ethinyl estradiol. Phase 2: 1 mg norethindrone/35 mcg ethinyl estradiol. ◆ *Ortho Tri-Cyclen* Tablets Phase 1: 0.18 mg norgestimate/35 mcg ethinyl estradiol. Phase 2: 0.215 mg norgestimate/35 mcg ethinyl estradiol. Phase 3: 0.25 mg norgestimate/35 mcg ethinyl estradiol. ◆ *Ortho Tri-Cyclen Lo* Tablets Phase 1: 0.18 mg norgestimate/25 mcg ethinyl estradiol. Phase 2: 0.215 mg norgestimate/25 mcg ethinyl estradiol. Phase 3: 0.25 mg norgestimate/25 mcg ethinyl estradiol. ◆ *Ovcon-35* Tablets 35 mcg ethinyl estradiol/0.4 mg norethindrone ◆ *Ovcon-50* Tablets 50 mcg ethinyl estradiol/1 mg norethindrone ◆ *Ovral-28* Tablets 50 mcg ethinyl estradiol/0.5 mg norethindrone ◆ *Portia* Tablets 30 mcg ethinyl estradiol/0.15 mg levonorgestrel ◆ *Seasonale* Tablets 30 mcg ethinyl estradiol/0.15 mg levonorgestrel ◆ *Sprintec* Tablets 35 mcg ethinyl estradiol/0.25 mg norgestimate ◆ *Tri-Levlen* Tablets Phase 1: 0.05 mg levonorgestrel/30 mcg ethinyl estradiol. Phase 2: 0.075 mg levonorgestrel/40 mcg ethinyl estradiol. Phase 3: 0.125 mg levonorgestrel/30 mcg ethinyl estradiol. ♦ *Tri-Norinyl* Tablets Phase 1: 0.5 mg norethindrone/35 mcg ethinyl estradiol. Phase 2: 1 mg norethindrone/35 mcg ethinyl estradiol. Phase 3: 0.5 mg norethindrone/35 mcg ethinyl estradiol. ♦ *Triphasil* Tablets Phase 1: 0.05 mg levonorgestrel/30 mcg ethinyl estradiol. Phase 2: 0.075 mg levonorgestrel/40 mcg ethinyl estradiol. Phase 3: 0.125 mg levonorgestrel/30 mcg ethinyl estradiol. ♦ *Trivora-28* Tablets Phase 1: 0.05 mg levonorgestrel/30 mcg ethinyl estradiol. Phase 2: 0.075 mg levonorgestrel/40 mcg ethinyl estradiol. Phase 3: 0.125 mg levonorgestrel/30 mcg ethinyl estradiol. ♦ *Yasmin* Tablets 30 mcg ethinyl estradiol/3 mg drospirenone ♦ *Zovia 1/35E* Tablets 35 mcg ethinyl estradiol/1 mg ethynodiol diacetate ♦ *Zovia 1/50E* Tablets 50 mcg ethinyl estradiol/1 mg ethynodiol diacetate

Action
PHARMACOLOGY: Inhibits ovulation by suppressing gonadotropins, follicle-stimulating hormone and luteinizing hormone.

Indications Prevention of pregnancy.
Unlabeled use(s): Postcoital contraceptive.

Contraindications Thrombophlebitis; thromboembolic disorders; history of deep vein thrombophlebitis; cerebral vascular disease; MI; coronary artery disease; known or suspected breast carcinoma or estrogen-dependent neoplasia; past or present benign or malignant liver tumors that developed during use of estrogen-containing products; past or present angina pectoris; undiagnosed abnormal genital bleeding; known or suspected pregnancy; cholestatic jaundice of pregnancy or jaundice with prior pill use.

Route/Dosage
SUNDAY-START PACKAGING
ADULTS: **PO** 1 tablet daily beginning on first Sunday after menstruation begins. If menstruation begins on Sunday, take first tablet on that day.

21-DAY REGIMEN
ADULTS: **PO** 1 tablet daily for 21 days, beginning on day 5 of cycle. Take no tablets for 7 days; then start new course of 21-day regimen.

28-DAY REGIMEN
ADULTS: **PO** 1 tablet daily.

Interactions
Barbiturates, carbamazepine, felbamate, modafinil, oxcarbazine, protease inhibitors, St. John's wort, hydantoins, rifampin, griseofulvin, penicillin, tetracyclines: Decreased effectiveness of oral contraceptive. Use additional form of birth control during concomitant therapy.
Benzodiazepines, caffeine, corticosteroids, cyclosporine, metoprolol, selegiline, theophylline, tricyclic antidepressants: Effects may be increased by oral contraceptives, increasing the risk of toxicity.
Lamotrigine: Concentration may be decreased, reducing the therapeutic effect.

Lab Test Interferences May cause increases in sulfobromophthalein retention; factors II, VII, VIII, IX, X; plasminogen, fibrinogen; norepinephrine-induced platelet aggregation; thyroid-binding globulin, leading to increased total thyroid hormone measurements; transcortin; corticosteroid levels; triglycerides and phospholipids; ceruloplasmin; aldosterone; amylase; gamma-glutamyl transpeptidase; iron-binding capacity; transferrin; prolactin; renin activity; vitamin A. May cause decreases in anti-thrombin III; free T_3 resin uptake; pregnanediol excretion; response to metyrapone test; folate; glucose tolerance; albumin; cholinesterase; haptoglobin; zinc; vitamin B_{12}.

Adverse Reactions
CV: Coronary thrombosis; MI; hypertension.
CNS: Cerebral thrombosis; cerebral hemorrhage; migraine; mental depression.
DERM: Melasma; rash; photosensitivity.
EENT: Steepening of corneal curvature; contact lens intolerance.
GI: Nausea and vomiting; abdominal cramps; bloating; mesenteric thrombosis.
GU: Renal artery thrombosis; break-through bleeding; spotting; change in menstrual flow; dysmenorrhea; amenorrhea; temporary infertility after discontinuation; change in cervical erosion and cervical secretions; endocervical hyperplasia; increase in size of uterine leiomyomata; vaginal candidiasis.
HEMA: Thrombophlebitis and thrombosis; arterial thromboembolism.
HEPA: Cholestatic jaundice; gallbladder disease.
RESP: Pulmonary embolism.
OTHER: Raynaud disease; congenital anomalies; liver tumors; hepatocellular carcinoma; breast tenderness, enlargement, secretion, diminished lactation; edema; weight change; reduced carbohydrate tolerance; prolactin-secreting pituitary tumors; increased prevalence of cervical chlamydia trachomatous.

> **WARNING:**
> *Smoking:* Cigarette smoking increases the risk of serious cardiovascular side effects. The risk increases with age (older than 35 yr) and heavy smoking (at least 15 cigarettes/day). Smoking is not recommended during therapy.

Precautions
Pregnancy: Category X.

Lactation: Excreted in breast milk. Defer use until infant weaned.

Tartrazine sensitivity: Some products may contain tartrazine, which may cause allergic-type reaction in susceptible individuals.

Acute intermittent porphyria: May be precipitated by estrogen therapy in susceptible individuals.

Carbohydrate and lipid metabolism: Glucose tolerance may decrease; triglycerides and total phospholipids may increase. Progestins may elevate LDL levels.

Depression: Use drug with caution in patients with history of depression.

Fibroids: Oral contraceptives may cause an increase in size of preexisting uterine leiomyomata (fibroids).

Fluid retention: Use drug with caution in patients with hypertension; convulsive disorders; migraines; asthma; cardiac, hepatic, or renal dysfunction.

Liver dysfunction: May impair metabolism of oral contraceptives.

Pyridoxine deficiency: May occur due to disturbance in normal tryptophan metabolism.

Serum folate: May be depressed by oral contraceptive therapy.

Overdosage: Signs and Symptoms
Withdrawal bleeding.

PATIENT CARE CONSIDERATIONS
Administration/Storage
- Give at same time each day. Efficacy depends on strict adherence to dosage schedule.
- May be given with or without food.

Assessment/Interventions
- Obtain patient medical history, including drug history and any known allergies.
- Monitor blood glucose levels in patients with diabetes.
- If spotting or breakthrough bleeding continues past second month, notify health care provider.
- Do not administer oral contraceptives to induce withdrawal bleeding as test for pregnancy.

Patient/Family Education
- Advise patient to use additional method of birth control until after first week of administration in initial cycle.
- Advise patient what to do if dose is missed: (1) if missed 1, take when remember or take 2 the next day; (2) if missed 2, take 2 on 2 consecutive days; (3) if missed at least 3, stop pills; (4) use alternative form of birth control in all cases.
- Advise patient to take multiple daily vitamin.
- Encourage patient who smokes to stop. Cardiovascular dysfunction and thromboembolic disease have been associated with use of oral contraceptives in patients who smoke.
- Advise patient that oral contraceptives may change the fit of rigid contact lenses.
- Caution patient to avoid prolonged exposure to sunlight, and to use sunscreen or wear protective clothing to avoid photosensitivity reaction.
- Advise patient to wait at least 3 mo after discontinuing oral contraceptives to try to become pregnant.
- Caution patient that antibiotics may decrease effectiveness of oral contraceptives and to use a nonhormonal form of contraception while taking antibiotics and for 7 days after stopping antibiotics.
- Instruct patient to report symptoms of blood clots (eg, pain, numbness, shortness of breath, visual disturbances).
- Teach patient routine breast self-examination technique.
- Warn patient that side effects such as nausea and breakthrough bleeding are common at first.

Contraceptives, Oral (Progestin-Only Products)

(kon-tra-SEP-tiv, OR-al)

Class Hormone/Contraceptive

How Supplied
Micronor Tablets 0.35 mg norethindrone ♦ *Nor-Q.D.* Tablets 0.35 mg norethindrone ♦ *Ovrette* Tablets 0.075 mg norgestrel

Action
PHARMACOLOGY: Alters cervical mucus, interferes with implantation and may suppress ovulation.

Indications Prevention of pregnancy.

Contraindications Thrombophlebitis; thromboembolic disorders; history of deep vein thrombophlebitis; cerebral vascular disease; MI; coronary artery disease; known or suspected breast carcinoma; impaired liver function or disease; undiagnosed abnormal genital bleeding; known or suspected pregnancy; as diagnostic test for pregnancy.

Route/Dosage
ADULTS: PO 1 tablet daily, starting on first day of menstruation.

Interactions
Hydantoins (eg, phenytoin): May reduce plasma levels and pharmacologic effect of levonorgestrel and norgestrel.
Rifampin: Reduced plasma levels and pharmacologic effects of norethindrone.
Lab Test Interferences Results of LFTs, coagulation tests (increased prothrombin, factors VII, VIII, IX and X), thyroid function tests, metyrapone test, and endocrine function tests may be altered. Pregnanediol determination may be altered.
Adverse Reactions
CV: Thrombophlebitis; cerebrovascular disorders.
CNS: Depression; tiredness; fatigue.
DERM: Rash with and without pruritus; acne; melasma or chloasma; photosensitivity.
EENT: Retinal thrombosis.
GU: Breakthrough bleeding; spotting; hypomenorrhea; amenorrhea; changes in cervical erosion and cervical secretions.
HEPA: Cholestatic jaundice.
RESP: Pulmonary embolism.
OTHER: Breast changes; masculinization of female fetus; edema; weight change.

Precautions
Pregnancy: Category X.
Lactation: Excreted in breast milk.
Tartrazine sensitivity: Some products may contain tartrazine, which may cause allergic-type reaction in susceptible individuals.
Depression: Use drug with caution in patients with history of depression.
Fluid retention: Use with caution in patients with hypertension; convulsive disorders;, migraines; asthma; cardiac, hepatic, or renal dysfunction.
Lipid disorders: Progestins may elevate LDL levels.

Overdosage: Signs and Symptoms
Nausea.

PATIENT CARE CONSIDERATIONS

Administration/Storage
- Administer at same time each day.
- Start on first day of menstruation.
- If GI upset occurs, administer with food.

Assessment/Interventions
- Obtain patient history, including drug history and any known allergies.
- Perform baseline physical examination before beginning therapy.
- If spotting or breakthrough bleeding continues past second month, notify health care provider.
- Do not administer oral contraceptives to induce withdrawal bleeding as test for pregnancy.

Patient/Family Education
- Advise patient to use additional method of birth control until after first wk of administration in initial cycle.
- Teach patient what to do if dose is missed. If 1 tablet is missed, take as soon as remembered and then take next tablet at regular time. If 2 consecutive tablets are missed; do not take missed tablets; discard and take next tablet at regular time. Use additional form of contraception until pregnancy is ruled out or menses occurs. If 3 consecutive tablets are missed, discontinue drug immediately. Use additional form of contraception until pregnancy is ruled out or menses occurs.
- Encourage patient who smokes to stop. Cardiovascular dysfunction and thromboembolic disease have been associated with use of oral contraceptives in patients who smoke.
- Advise patient that oral contraceptives may change fit of rigid contact lenses.
- Caution patient to avoid prolonged exposure to sunlight, and to use sunscreen or wear protective clothing to avoid photosensitivity reaction.
- Advise patient to wait at least 3 mo after discontinuing oral contraceptives before trying to become pregnant.
- Instruct patient to report symptoms of blood clots (eg, pain, numbness, shortness of breath, visual disturbances).

Corticotropin (Adrenocorticotropic hormone; ACTH)

(core-tih-koe-TROE-pin)
Class Adrenal cortical steroid

How Supplied
ACTH Powder for Injection 40 units/vial ♦
Acthar Powder for Injection 25 units/vial, Powder for Injection 40 units/vial

Action
PHARMACOLOGY: Stimulates adrenal cortex to produce and secrete adrenocortical hormones (eg, corticosteroids, glucocorticoids).
PHARMACOKINETICS/DYNAMICS:
Absorption: T_{max} is within 1 hr.
Excretion: Plasma concentrations begin to decrease after 2 to 4 hr.
Onset: Rapid.
Indications Diagnostic testing of adrenocorti-

cal function; include diuresis or remission of proteinuria in the nephrotic syndrome without uremia of the idiopathic type or that caused by lupus erythematosus; treatment of nonsuppurative thyroiditis, hypercalcemia associated with cancer, acute exacerbations of multiple sclerosis, tuberculous meningitis when accompanied by antituberculous chemotherapy, trichinosis with neurologic or myocardial involvement, and treatment of glucocorticoid responsive rheumatic, collagenous, dermatologic, allergic, ophthalmic, respiratory, hematologic, neoplastic, and GI diseases. **Unlabeled use(s):** Treatment of infantile spasms.

Contraindications Scleroderma; osteoporosis; systemic fungal infections; ocular herpes simplex; recent surgery; history or presence of peptic ulcer; CHF; hypertension; sensitivity to porcine proteins; conditions accompanied by primary adrenocortical insufficiency or adrenocortical hyperfunction. IV administration is contraindicated, except in treatment of idiopathic thrombocytopenic purpura or diagnostic testing of adrenocortical function.

Route/Dosage
Repository Injection
IM/SC 40 to 80 U q 24 to 72 hr. Not suitable for IV use.

Acute Exacerbations of Multiple Sclerosis
IM 80 to 120 U/day for 2 to 3 wk.

Interactions
Anticholinesterases: Effects of these agents may be antagonized in myasthenia gravis.
Barbiturates: May decrease effects of corticotropin.

Lab Test Interferences May decrease I^{131} uptake; possible suppression of skin test reactions; falsely decreased urinary estradiol and estriol concentrations with Brown method; falsely decreased urinary estrogen concentrations with colorimetry and fluorometry.

Adverse Reactions
CV: Hypertension; CHF; necrotizing angiitis.
CNS: Convulsions; vertigo; headache; increased intracranial pressure with papilledema; pseudotumor cerebri.
DERM: Impaired wound healing; petechiae and ecchymoses; increased sweating; hyperpigmentation; thin, fragile skin; facial erythema; acne.

EENT: Posterior subcapsular cataracts; increased IOP; glaucoma with possible optic nerve damage; exophthalmos.
GI: Pancreatitis; ulcerative esophagitis; abdominal distention; peptic ulcer.
METAB: Negative nitrogen balance because of protein catabolism; fluid and electrolyte disturbances (eg, sodium and fluid retention, potassium and calcium loss, hypokalemic alkalosis); antibody production and loss of stimulatory effect of ACTH with prolonged use.
OTHER: Infection; musculoskeletal disturbances (eg, weakness, myopathy, loss of muscle mass, osteoporosis, vertebral compression fractures, pathologic fracture of long bones, aseptic necrosis of femoral and humeral heads); endocrine abnormalities (eg, menstrual irregularities, growth suppression in children, hirsutism, cushingoid state, glucose intolerance, decreased carbohydrate tolerance, increased requirement for insulin or oral hypoglycemic agent in diabetic patients, secondary adrenocortical, pituitary unresponsiveness.

Precautions
Pregnancy: Category C.
Lactation: Undetermined.
Children: Because prolonged use inhibits skeletal growth, careful monitoring is necessary.
Fluid and electrolyte balance: Drug may elevate BP, cause salt and water retention, and increase potassium and calcium excretion.
Immunosuppression: Live vaccine immunization is usually contraindicated, especially with high doses of corticotropin.
Infection: Drug may mask signs of infection; resistance to infection may be decreased.
Long-term administration: May lead to irreversible adverse effects. Complications are dependent on dose and duration of treatment. Prolonged use increases risk of hypersensitivity reactions and ocular effects.
Sensitivity to porcine proteins: Perform skin testing in patients with suspected sensitivity to porcine proteins. Observe for sensitivity reactions during or after administration.
Stress: Increased dosage of rapid-acting corticosteroid may be needed before, during, and after stressful situations.

PATIENT CARE CONSIDERATIONS
Administration/Storage
- Medication may be given via IM or SC route. Do not use IV route.
- If patient is sensitive to porcine proteins, skin tests must be performed before administration.
- Standard tests for adrenal responsiveness to corticotropin are performed via same route that will be used for administration of drug.

Corticotropin repository injection:
- Note that this form is for IM or SC use only, not for IV administration.
- Store repository corticotropin injection in refrigeration.

Assessment/Interventions
- Obtain patient history, including drug history and any known allergies.
- Observe patient for possible hypersensitivity reaction. Have epinephrine 1:1000 available for emergency use.
- Take patient's vital signs and monitor throughout therapy.
- Monitor I&O and weight.
- Monitor serum potassium and sodium levels.
- In patients with diabetes, monitor blood glucose frequently because dosage of insulin or oral hypoglycemic agent may need to be increased.
- Assess for recurrent symptoms that may result from sudden withdrawal of medication after prolonged use.
- If any of these signs occur, report them to health care provider: fluid retention; muscle weakness; abdominal pain; seizures; headache; adrenal insufficiency (eg, fatigue, anorexia, nausea, vomiting, diarrhea, weight loss, weakness, dizziness); visual disturbances; cushingoid symptoms.

Patient/Family Education
- Counsel patient to follow dietary regimen carefully (eg, salt restriction, potassium supplementation).
- Advise patient to avoid receiving live virus vaccinations while taking this medication.
- Instruct patient to have periodic eye examinations while taking medication as long-term therapy.
- If patient has diabetes, instruct to monitor blood glucose regularly throughout therapy since dosage of insulin or oral hypoglycemic agent may need to be increased.
- Advise patient to contact health care provider before discontinuing medication.
- Instruct patient to notify health care provider at first sign of infection: prolonged cold symptoms, sore throat, weight gain, GI upset, heart irregularities, delayed wound healing or changes in mood behavior.
- Tell patient to report these symptoms to health care provider: fluid retention, muscle weakness, abdominal pain, seizures, headaches.
- Instruct patient not to take OTC medications without consulting health care provider.

Cortisone (Cortisone Acetate)

(CORE-tih-sone)

Class Corticosteroid

How Supplied
Cortone Acetate Tablets 25 mg, Injection 50 mg/mL

Action
PHARMACOLOGY: As short-acting glucocorticoid; depresses formation, release and activity of endogenous mediators of inflammation; has some salt-retaining properties.

PHARMACOKINETICS/DYNAMICS:
Distribution: Crosses the placenta and is excreted in breast milk.

Excretion: The t½ is 30 min.

Indications Treatment of primary or secondary adrenal cortex insufficiency; rheumatic disorders; collagen diseases; dermatologic diseases; allergic states; allergic and inflammatory ophthalmic processes; respiratory diseases; hematologic disorders; neoplastic diseases; edematous states (caused by nephrotic syndrome); GI diseases; multiple sclerosis; tuberculous meningitis; trichinosis with neurologic or myocardial involvement.

Contraindications Systemic fungal infections; administration of live virus vaccines in patients receiving immunosuppressive doses.

Route/Dosage
ADULTS: **PO** 25 to 300 mg/day. Use lowest possible effective dose.

ALTERNATE-DAY THERAPY: Provides greater than or equal to twice usual daily dosage of short- to intermediate-acting medication.

ADULTS: **IM** 20 to 300 mg/day. In less severe cases less than 20 mg/day may be sufficient, in severe cases greater than 300 mg/day may be required.

Interactions
Anticholinesterases: Drug may antagonize anticholinesterase effects in myasthenia gravis.
Anticoagulants, oral: Drug may increase or decrease anticoagulant dose requirements.
Barbiturates: May decrease pharmacologic effect of cortisone.
Phenytoin: May decrease therapeutic efficacy of cortisone.

Rifampin: May decrease therapeutic efficacy of cortisone.
Salicylates: Drug may reduce serum levels and efficacy of salicylates.
Troleandomycin: May increase effects of cortisone.

Lab Test Interferences False-negative nitroblue tetrazolium test.

Adverse Reactions
CV: Thromboembolism or fat embolism; thrombophlebitis; necrotizing angiitis; cardiac arrhythmias or ECG changes; syncopal episodes; hypertension; myocardial rupture after recent MI; CHF.
CNS: Convulsions; increased intracranial pressure with papilledema; vertigo; headache; neuritis/paresthesias; psychosis; fatigue; insomnia.
DERM: Impaired wound healing; petechiae and ecchymoses; erythema; lupus erythematosus–like lesions; suppression of skin test reactions; SC fat atrophy; purpura; hirsutism; acneiform eruptions; allergic dermatitis; urticaria; angioneurotic edema; perineal irritation; hyperpigmentation or hypopigmentation.
EENT: Cataracts; increased IOP; glaucoma; exophthalmos.
GI: Pancreatitis; abdominal distention; ulcerative esophagitis; nausea; vomiting; increased appetite and weight gain; peptic ulcer; small bowel and large bowel perforation, especially in inflammatory bowel disease.
GU: Increased or decreased motility and number of spermatozoa.
HEMA: Leukocytosis.
METAB: Sodium and fluid retention; hypokalemia; hypokalemic alkalosis; metabolic alkalosis; increased serum cholesterol; hypocalcemia; hypothalamicpituitary-axis suppression; endocrine abnormalities (decreased T_3, T_4 and ^{131}I uptake, menstrual irregularities, cushingoid state, growth suppression in children, increased sweating, decreased carbohydrate tolerance, hyperglycemia, glycosuria, increased insulin or sulfonylurea requirements, manifestations of latent diabetes mellitus, negative nitrogen balance because of protein catabolism, hirsutism).
OTHER: Musculoskeletal effects (eg, muscle weakness, myopathy, tendon rupture, osteoporosis, aseptic necrosis of femoral and humeral heads, spontaneous fractures; anaphylactoid reactions, aggravation or masking of infections; malaise.

Precautions
Pregnancy: Pregnancy category undetermined.
Lactation: Excreted in breast milk.
Children: Observe growth and development of infants and children undergoing prolonged therapy.
Elderly: May require lower doses.
Hypersensitivity: Anaphylactoid reactions have occurred rarely.
Hepatic function impairment: Use cautiously.
Adrenal suppression: Prolonged therapy may lead to HPA suppression. Withdraw gradually after prolonged therapy.
Cardiovascular disease: Use with caution in patients with recent MI.
Fluid and electrolyte balance: Drug can cause elevated BP, salt and water retention, increased potassium and calcium excretion. Dietary salt restriction and potassium supplementation may be necessary.
Hepatitis: Drug may be harmful in chronic active hepatitis that is positive for hepatitis B surface antigen.
Infections: Drug may mask signs of infection and decrease host-defense mechanisms that prevent dissemination of infection.
Ocular effects: Use cautiously in ocular herpes simplex because of possible corneal perforation.
Peptic ulcer: Drug may contribute to peptic ulceration, especially in large doses.
Stress: Increased dosage of rapid-acting corticosteroid may be needed before, during and after stressful situations.

Overdosage: Signs and Symptoms
Acute adrenal insufficiency caused by too-rapid withdrawal: fever, myalgia, arthralgia, malaise, anorexia, nausea, desquamation of skin, orthostatic hypotension, dizziness, fainting, dyspnea, hypoglycemia. Cushingoid changes from chronic use of too large dose: moonface, central obesity, striae, hirsutism, acne, ecchymoses, fluid and electrolyte imbalance, hypertension, osteoporosis, myopathy, sexual dysfunction, diabetes, hyperlipidemia, peptic ulcer.

PATIENT CARE CONSIDERATIONS

Administration/Storage
Oral only:
- Administer with meals or snacks to avoid GI irritation.
- Give single daily dose or alternate-day dose before 9 AM to obtain maximum benefit.
- Space multiple doses evenly throughout day.
- When giving large doses of cortisone, administer antacids between meals.

Oral and injection:
- Store at room temperature in tightly closed container. Protect from heat and freezing.

Assessment/Interventions
- Obtain patient history, including drug history and any known allergies.

- Note any sensitivity to sulfites, tartrazine, and aspirin.
- Be prepared for emergency treatment of hypersensitivity reaction.
- Obtain baseline weight, vital signs, chemistry profile, 2 hr postprandial blood glucose and chest x-ray.
- Monitor I&O and weight daily. Observe for edema, and report steady weight gain to health care provider.
- Monitor renal function throughout therapy.
- Monitor for development of steroid psychosis, manifested by changes in mood behavior.
- If patient has diabetes, monitor blood glucose frequently.
- Monitor drug withdrawal carefully. Drug must be discontinued gradually to avoid adrenal insufficiency.
- Observe for signs of infection: depression, malaise, anorexia, and delayed healing.
- Observe growth and development of infants and children undergoing prolonged therapy.
- Report signs of adrenal insufficiency to health care provider: fatigue, anorexia, nausea, vomiting, diarrhea, weight loss, weakness, and dizziness.
- Report signs of cushingoid symptoms to health care provider.
- Monitor patient closely for signs that might require dosage adjustments, including changes as a result of remissions or exacerbations of the disease, individual drug responsiveness, and the effect of stress.

Injection only:

- After a favorable initial response, determine the proper maintenance dosage by decreasing the initial dosage in small amounts to the lowest dosage that maintains adequate clinical response.

Patient/Family Education

- Instruct patient to take with meals to avoid GI upset.
- Tell patient to take single daily dose before 9 AM.
- Instruct patient to monitor weight daily and to report steady gain to health care provider.
- Inform patients with diabetes to monitor blood glucose regularly.
- Instruct elderly patients undergoing long-term therapy to have BP, blood glucose and electrolytes checked q 6 mo.
- Advise patient to avoid receiving live virus vaccine during therapy.
- Instruct patients undergoing long-term therapy to have an annual eye examination and to carry ID card.
- For discontinuation after long-term therapy, instruct patient to adhere to tapering schedule.
- Advise patient to notify health care provider before discontinuing medication.
- Instruct patient to report these symptoms to health care provider: cold, infection or prolonged sore throat; change in vision; swelling of extremities; weakness; black tarry stools; irregular heartbeat; menstrual irregularities; changes in mood or behavior; fatigue; anorexia; nausea; vomiting; diarrhea; weight loss.

Cosyntropin (Synthetic Corticotropin, Synthetic ACTH)

(koe-sin-TROE-pin)

Class Adrenal cortical steroid

How Supplied
Cortrosyn Powder for Injection 0.25 mg

Action
PHARMACOLOGY: Exhibits full corticosteroidogenic activity of natural ACTH, stimulating adrenal cortex to produce and secrete adrenocortical hormones.

Indications Diagnostic testing of adrenal function.

Contraindications Standard considerations.

Route/Dosage
ADULTS: **IM/IV (direct injection)** 0.25 to 0.75 mg. IV infusion 0.25 mg in D5W or 0.9% saline administered at 0.04 mg/hr over 6 hr.
CHILDREN 2 YR AND UNDER: **IM/IV** 0.125 mg often will be sufficient.

Interactions
Anticholinesterases: May antagonize anticholinesterase effects in myasthenia gravis.
Barbiturates: May decrease pharmacologic effect of cosyntropin.
Hydantoins: May increase clearance and decrease therapeutic efficacy of cosyntropin.

Lab Test Interferences None well documented.

Adverse Reactions
OTHER: Rare hypersensitivity.

Precautions
Pregnancy: Category C.
Lactation: Undetermined.
Hypersensitivity: Exhibits slight immunologic activity but is less likely to cause reactions than natural ACTH.

PATIENT CARE CONSIDERATIONS
Administration/Storage
- Before administration, be prepared to treat possible acute hypersensitivity reaction.
- Administer by IM route, direct IV injection or IV infusion.
- Reconstitute 0.25 mg vial with 1 mL of 0.9% Sodium Chloride for Injection.
- Administer reconstituted drug via IM route or by direct IV injection over 2 min or further dilute in D5W or normal saline and infuse over 4 to 8 hr.
- Do not allow cosyntropin to mix with blood or plasma infusions.
- Reconstituted preparations should not be retained.

Assessment/Interventions
- Obtain patient history, including drug history and any known allergies. Note hypersensitivity to natural corticotropin.
- Measure plasma cortisol concentrations prior to and 30 to 60 min after administration. Collect blood sample of 6 to 7 mL in heparinized tube.
- Alternatively, measure urinary steroids before and after IV infusion.

Patient/Family Education
- Explain purpose of the test.
- Emphasize importance of lab tests.
- Instruct patients taking corticosteroids or aldosterone to omit doses on day of test.

Cromolyn Sodium (Disodium Cromoglycate)

(KROE-moe-lin SO-dee-uhm)

Class Respiratory inhalant

How Supplied
Crolom Solution, ophthalmic 4% ♦ *Gastrocrom* Oral concentrate 5 mg/100 mL ♦ *Intal* Solution 20 mg/amp (for nebulizer only), Aerosol spray 800 mcg/actuation ♦ *Nasalcrom* Nasal Solution 40 mg/mL (each actuation delivers 5.2 mg)
❧ *Apo-Cromolyn Nasal Spray* ♦ *Apo-Cromolyn Sterules* ♦ *Nalcrom* ♦ *Nu-Cromolyn*

Action
PHARMACOLOGY: Stabilizes mast cells, which release histamine and other mediators of allergic reactions.

PHARMACOKINETICS/DYNAMICS:
Absorption:
Inhalation – 8% absorbed from the lungs.
Oral – Up to 1% absorbed.

Excretion:
Inhalation – After 8% is absorbed from the lung, it is rapidly excreted unchanged in bile and urine. The remainder is either exhaled or swallowed and excreted via the alimentary tract.
Oral – 0.28% to 0.5% of the dose is excreted in the urine.

Indications
Inhalation: Prophylaxis of severe bronchial asthma; prevention of exercise-induced asthma; prevention of acute bronchospasm induced by environmental pollutants and known antigens.
Nasal solution: Prevention and treatment of allergic rhinitis.
Oral: Treatment of mastocytosis.
Ophthalmic: Treatment of vernal keratoconjunctivitis, vernal conjunctivitis, and vernal keratitis.

Unlabeled use(s):
Oral – Symptoms of food allergies; eczema; dermatitis; ulceration; urticaria pigmentosa; chronic urticaria; hay fever; and postexercise bronchospasm.

Contraindications Standard considerations.

Route/Dosage
Bronchial Asthma
ADULTS AND CHILDREN (5 YR OR UNDER FOR CAPSULES, AT LEAST 2 YR FOR SOLUTION): **Nebulization** Initially 20 mg inhaled qid at regular intervals.
ADULTS AND CHILDREN (OVER 5 YR): **Aerosol** 2 metered sprays (1600 mcg) inhaled qid at regular intervals.

Prevention of Acute Bronchospasm
ADULTS: 2 metered dose sprays or 20 mg via inhaled capsule or nebulizer (10 to 15 min but no longer than 60 min) before exposure to precipitating factor.

Seasonal or Perennial Rhinitis
ADULTS AND CHILDREN (OVER 6 YR): **Nasal solution with spray device** Begin treatment prior to contact with allergen and continue throughout exposure period. One spray (5.2 mg) in each nostril 3 to 6 times/day at regular intervals.

Mastocytosis
ADULTS: **PO** 200 mg qid 30 min before meals and at bedtime.
CHILDREN (2 TO 12 YR): **PO** 100 mg qid 30 min before meals and at bedtime (max, 40 mg/kg/day). Dosage maintenance levels are decreased gradually, except with major complication. Abrupt withdrawal may result in increased asthma symptoms.
TERM INFANTS TO 2 YR: **PO** 20 mg/kg/day in 4 divided doses (max, 20 mg/kg/day).

PREMATURE TO TERM INFANTS: Not recommended.

Vernal Keratoconjunctivitis, Vernal Conjunctivitis, and Vernal Keratitis
ADULTS: **Solution** 1 or 2 drops in each eye 4 to 6 times/day at regular intervals.

Interactions None well documented.

Lab Test Interferences None well documented.

Adverse Reactions
CNS: Dizziness; headache.
DERM: Rash; urticaria; angioedema.
EENT: Lacrimation; nasal stinging, burning, or irritation; sneezing; nasal congestion; bad taste; swollen parotid gland; dry or irritated throat.
GI: Nausea; substernal burning; diarrhea (oral form).
GU: Dysuria; urinary frequency.
OPHTH: Stinging; burning; watery eyes; itchy eyes; dryness around the eye; puffy eyes; eye irritation; styes.
RESP: Cough; wheezing; bronchospasm.
OTHER: Joint pain and swelling.

Precautions
Pregnancy: Category B.
Lactation: Undetermined.

Children:
Aerosol – Safety and efficacy not established in children less than 5 yr.
Inhalation solution – Safety and efficacy not established in children less than 2 yr.
Nasal – Do not use in children less than 2 yr unless directed by health care provider.
Oral – In term infants up to 6 mo, data suggest the dose not exceed 20 mg/kg/day. Reserve use in children less than 2 yr for patients with severe disease in which potential benefits clearly outweigh risks.
Hypersensitivity: Severe anaphylactic reactions may occur.
Renal function impairment: Decreased dose is recommended.
Hepatic function impairment: Decreased dose is recommended.
Acute asthma: Do not use for acute asthma attack. Effects depend on regular administration.
Aerosol: Use with caution in patients with coronary artery disease or cardiac arrhythmias because of propellants in this preparation.
Bronchospasm: Cough or bronchospasm may follow inhalation.
Eosinophilic pneumonia: If signs of this condition occur, therapy will need to be discontinued.

PATIENT CARE CONSIDERATIONS

Administration/Storage
Oral:
- Open and dissolve capsule contents completely in ½ glass of hot water. While stirring, add equal amount of cold water. Administer all of liquid. Do not mix with juice, milk, or foods.
- Administer 30 min before meals and at bedtime.
- Do not use oral capsules for inhalation.
- Store in airtight, light-resistant container at room temperature (59° to 86°F).

Inhalation:
- Administer when patient's airway is clear for inhalation. Do not administer during acute asthmatic attack.

Nebulizer solution/inhalation capsules:
- Instruct patient to close eyes during inhalation to prevent accidental contact with eyes.
- If bronchodilating inhalant is also prescribed, give bronchodilator 5 to 15 min before cromolyn to enhance drug delivery. Have patient exhale completely, place mouthpiece between lips, inhale deeply and rapidly, hold breath for few seconds, remove mouthpiece, then exhale. Repeat until entire dose is taken.

Aerosol:
- Store away from heat and direct sunlight. Protect from freezing. Do not puncture, break or burn container.
- Use spacer (eg, Aero chamber) to enhance delivery of drug.

Inhalation capsules:
- Store in tight, light-resistant container. Avoid storing in moist environment (eg, bathroom).

Nasal:
- Clear patient's nasal passages before administering spray. Have patient inhale medication through nose.
- Hold container upright. Use pumping motion to force solution mist into nasal passages.
- Store in airtight, light-resistant container.

Ophthalmic solution:
- The effectiveness of cromolyn therapy is dependent on its administration at regular intervals, as directed.
- Patient may experience a transient stinging or burning sensation following instillation of cromolyn.

Assessment/Interventions
- Obtain patient history, including drug history and any known allergies.
- Evaluate therapeutic effectiveness by decrease in frequency or severity of clinical symptoms or decrease in need for cotherapy over period of 4 wk.
- Notify health care provider if the following symptoms occur: wheezing or coughing after inhalation or stinging effect after nasal instil-

lation; joint pain; severe wheezing, difficulty breathing, chills, sweating, or chest pain, which may indicate eosinophilic pneumonia.

Patient/Family Education
- Explain that cromolyn is used for prevention, not treatment, of acute asthma attacks.
- Give patient clear instructions about what to do during an acute asthma attack.
- Teach patient correct use of administration device (see instructions in package). Have patient demonstrate its use.
- Emphasize that inhalation capsules are not to be swallowed.
- Explain that oral capsules are oversized to prevent powder from spilling when capsule is opened. Remind patient to dissolve powder in water only and to drink entire contents of solution.
- Advise patient to minimize exposure to known allergens or precipitating factors.
- Instruct patient with cold- or exercise-induced asthma to use medication at least 10 to 15 min before exposure but no longer than 1 hr.
- Advise patient to rinse mouth or gargle after oral inhalation to prevent throat irritation.
- If patient is taking concurrent bronchodilators or corticosteroids, stress importance of not discontinuing abruptly, particularly systemic corticosteroids.
- Advise patient that effectiveness of therapy is dependent on administration at regular intervals. Maximum effectiveness may take 4 wk.
- Caution patient not to discontinue abruptly unless advised by health care provider.
- Instruct patient to report the following symptoms to health care provider: increased difficulty in breathing, increased wheezing, difficulty in swallowing, joint pain or swelling, severe headache.
- Advise patient to not wear contact lenses while using cromolyn ophthalmic solution.

Crotamiton
(kroe-TAM-ih-tuhn)
Class Scabicide
How Supplied
Eurax Cream 10%, Lotion 10%

Action
PHARMACOLOGY: Undetermined.

Indications Eradication of scabies (*Sarcoptes scabiei*) and symptomatic treatment of pruritic skin.

Contraindications Primary irritation response to topical medications; hypersensitivity to any component of the product.

Route/Dosage
Scabies
ADULTS: **Topical** Thoroughly massage into the skin of whole body from chin down, paying particular attention to all folds and creases. A second application is advisable 24 hr later. Change clothing and bed linen the next morning. A cleansing bath should be taken 48 hr after last application.
Pruritus
ADULTS: **Topical** Massage gently into affected areas until medication is completely absorbed. Repeat as needed.

Interactions None well documented.

Adverse Reactions
DERM: Primary irritation, including dermatitis, pruritus, and rash.
OTHER: Allergic sensitivity.

Precautions
Pregnancy: Category C.
Lactation: Not stated.
Children: Safety and efficacy not established.
Hypersensitivity: Sensitization or severe irritation may occur. May cause irritation when applied to eyes or mouth.

PATIENT CARE CONSIDERATIONS
Administration/Storage
- For topical use only. Not for ophthalmic, oral, or intravaginal use.
- Do not apply to skin that has open wounds, cuts, or sores, or is inflamed.
- Avoid contact with eyes or mouth. If eye or mouth contact occurs, flush immediately and thoroughly with water.
- Shake lotion well before applying.

Scabies:
- Have patient take bath or shower, then thoroughly massage cream or lotion into the skin from the chin down, paying particular attention to all folds and creases. Trim fingernails short and put cream or lotion under fingernails using toothbrush. Wrap used toothbrush in paper and discard in trash. Repeat application in 24 hr then have patient take a cleansing bath 48 hr after the last application.
- Change linen and bed clothing the day after each application.

Pruritus:
- Massage lotion or cream into affected area(s) until medication is completely absorbed. Repeat as needed.
- Store lotion and cream at controlled room

temperature (59° to 86°F). Keep tightly capped.

Assessment/Interventions
- Obtain patient history, including drug history and any known allergies.
- Identify areas where medication is to be applied and areas with inflammation, cuts, open wounds, or sores that should be avoided.
- Assess and document skin condition before initial application and periodically throughout treatment.
- Discontinue use and notify health care provider if irritation or sensitization occurs, or if condition does not improve or worsens.

Patient/Family Education
- Explain name, dose, action, and potential side effects of drug.
- Caution patient or caregiver not to apply to skin areas that have open wounds, cuts, or sores, or is inflamed.
- Caution patient or caregiver to avoid contact with eyes or mouth and that if accidental eye or mouth contact occurs to immediately flush the eyes with water to remove medication. Advise patient or caregiver to notify health care provider if eye or mouth irritation or sensitivity follows accidental exposure.
- Teach patient or caregiver proper technique for applying lotion or cream for treatment of scabies: take shower or bath; use gloves if applying to another person; thoroughly massage cream or lotion (shake lotion well before applying) into the skin from the chin down, paying particular attention to all folds and creases. Trim fingernails short and put cream or lotion under fingernails using toothbrush. Wrap used toothbrush in paper and discard in trash. Repeat application in 24 hr then take a cleansing bath 48 hr after the last application.
- Advise patient or caregiver that all recently used clothing, underwear, pajamas, bed sheets, pillows, and towels should be washed in very hot water or dry cleaned to prevent re-exposure.
- Teach patient or caregiver proper technique for applying lotion or cream for treatment of pruritus as follows: massage lotion (shake well before applying) or cream into affected area(s) until medication is completely absorbed; repeat as needed.
- Advise patient or caregiver to stop using and notify health care provider if irritation or sensitization occurs or if condition does not improve or worsens.
- Advise patient or caregiver that follow-up visits may be necessary and to keep appointments.

Cyanocobalamin (Vitamin B$_{12}$)

(sigh-an-oh-koe-BAL-uh-min)

Class Blood modifier/Vitamin

How Supplied
Big Shot B-12 Tablets 5000 mcg ♦ *Crystamine* Injection 1000 mcg/mL ♦ *Crysti 1000* Injection 1000 mcg/mL ♦ *Cyanoject* Injection 1000 mcg/mL ♦ *Cyomin* Injection 1000 mcg/mL ♦ *Nascobal* Gel, intranasal 500 mcg/0.1 mL ♦ *Rubesol-1000* Injection 1000 mcg/mL

Action

PHARMACOLOGY: Involved in protein synthesis; essential to growth, cell reproduction, hematopoiesis, and nucleoprotein and myelin synthesis.

PHARMACOKINETICS/DYNAMICS:
Absorption:
IM – T$_{max}$ is 1 hr.
Intranasal – T$_{max}$ is 1 to 2 hr. C$_{max}$ is about 1414 pg/mL.
Oral – Bound to intrinsic factor during transit through the stomach; separation occurs in the presence of calcium and vitamin B$_{12}$ enters the mucosal cells for absorption.

Distribution: Distributed and stored primarily in the liver and bone marrow. In the blood, it is bound to trancobalam II.

Excretion: Unbound vitamin B$_{12}$ is rapidly eliminated in the urine.
IM – 50% to 98% is excreted in the urine within 48 hr.

Indications Treatment of vitamin B$_{12}$ deficiency caused by inadequate utilization of vitamin B$_{12}$; dietary deficiency of vitamin B$_{12}$ occurring in strict vegetarians; malabsorption syndrome of various causes (eg, pernicious anemia, GI pathology, fish tapeworm infestation, malignancy of pancreas or bowel, gluten enteropathy, small bowel bacterial overgrowth, gastrectomy, accompanying folic acid deficiency); supplementation because of increased requirements (eg, associated with pregnancy, thyrotoxicosis, hemolytic anemia, hemorrhage, malignancy, hepatic and renal disease); vitamin B$_{12}$ absorption test (eg, Schilling test).

Contraindications Hypersensitivity to cobalt, vitamin B$_{12}$, or any component of these medications; hereditary optic nerve atrophy.

Route/Dosage

Recommended Dietary Allowance
ADULTS: **PO** 2 mcg/day.
CHILDREN: **PO** 0.3 to 2 mcg/day.

Vitamin B$_{12}$ Deficiency
ADULTS: PO 25 to 1000 mcg/day. **IM or deep SC** 30 mcg/day for 5 to 10 days followed by 100 to 200 mcg/mo. **Intranasal** 500 mcg once weekly after malabsorption is in remission following injectable therapy.

Addisonian Pernicious Anemia
ADULTS: **IM or deep SC** 100 mcg/day for 6 to 7 days. If reticulocyte response occurs, give 100 mcg qod for 7 doses, then give 100 mcg q 3 to 4 days for 2 to 3 wk. After this regimen, give 100 mcg/mo for life.

Shilling Test Flushing Dose
ADULTS: **IM** 1000 mcg (z-tract method preferred).

Interactions
Chloramphenicol: Decreases hematologic effects of vitamin B$_{12}$ in patients with pernicious anemia.

Colchicine, excessive alcohol intake (more than 2/wk) neomycin, time-released potassium, para-aminosalicylic acid: Decreases GI absorption of vitamin B$_{12}$.

Lab Test Interferences
Methotrexate, pyrimethamine and most antibiotics: May invalidate vitamin B$_{12}$ diagnostic microbiological blood assays.

Adverse Reactions With parenteral/intranasal administration:
CV: Pulmonary edema; CHF; peripheral vascular thrombosis.
DERM: Itching; transitory exanthema; urticaria.
EENT: Severe and rapid optic nerve atrophy.
GI: Mild transient diarrhea.
OTHER: Hypersensitivity; pain at injection site; sensation of body swelling; hypokalemia; polycythemia vera; asthenia, headache, infection, glossitis, nausea, paresthesia, rhinitis (intranasal).

Precautions
Pregnancy: Category A (Category C in doses that exceed the RDA).
Lactation: Excreted in breast milk.
Children: Some products contain benzyl alcohol, which has been associated with fatal "gasping syndrome" in premature infants.
Hypersensitivity: Anaphylactic shock and death have been associated with parenteral use.
Hypokalemia:: Possibly fatal hypokalemia could occur as result of increased erythrocyte potassium requirements in severe megaloblastic anemia intensely treated with vitamin B$_{12}$.

PATIENT CARE CONSIDERATIONS
Administration/Storage
- If patient is sensitive to cobalamins, perform an intradermal skin test prior to administering drug.
- Give IM injection or deep SC injection in large muscle mass.
- Parenteral administration is required in treatment of pernicious anemia.
- Prime intranasal gel dispenser prior to initial use.
- Protect parenteral and intranasal vitamin B$_{12}$ from light. Do not freeze.

Assessment/Interventions
- Obtain patient history, including drug history and any known allergies. Note any history of Leber disease or sensitivity to cobalt and vitamin B$_{12}$.
- Obtain baseline reticulocyte counts, hematocrit, vitamin B$_{12}$, iron and folic acid levels, and then repeat tests between 5th and 7th days of treatment.
- Obtain periodic hematology tests as long as patient is on therapy.
- Monitor serum potassium levels during the first 48 hr of treatment.
- Throughout treatment, monitor and report vision changes to health care provider.
- Report signs of hypersensitivity (eg, urticaria, redness, itching) and hypokalemia (eg, muscle weakness, heart irregularity) to health care provider.

Patient/Family Education
- Instruct patient with pernicious anemia of need to continue therapy throughout lifetime.
- Advise patient to administer intranasal gel at least 1 hr before or 1 hr after ingestion of hot foods or liquids.
- Advise patient with nasal congestion, allergic rhinitis, or upper respiratory tract infections to defer treatment with intranasal gel until symptoms have subsided.
- Teach patient of need to maintain well-balanced diet. Remind patient of the following good sources of vitamin B$_{12}$: seafood, egg yolks, organ meats, fortified breakfast cereals, meat, cheeses, milk, other dairy products.
- Advise patient that folic acid is not substitute for vitamin B$_{12}$ but may be taken concurrently.
- Instruct vegetarians who do not use animal products of need for daily oral vitamin B$_{12}$.

- Inform patient with pernicious anemia of need to have periodic GI evaluations.
- Instruct patient to report the following symptoms to health care provider: muscle weakness, shortness of breath, heart irregularity, vision disturbances.

Cyclobenzaprine Hydrochloride

(SIGH-kloe-BEN-zuh-preen HIGH-droe-KLOR-ide)

Class Skeletal muscle relaxant/Centrally acting

How Supplied
Flexeril Tablets 5 mg, Tablets 10 mg
🍁 Apo-Cyclobenzaprine ◆ Gen-Cyclobenzaprine ◆ Novo-Cycloprine ◆ Nu-Cyclobenzaprine ◆ ratio-Cyclobenzaprine

Action
PHARMACOLOGY: Relieves skeletal muscle spasms of local origin without interfering with muscle function by acting within CNS at brain stem. Structurally and pharmacologically related to tricyclic antidepressants.

PHARMACOKINETICS/DYNAMICS:
Absorption: Well absorbed. T_{max} is 4 to 6 hr.
Distribution: Highly bound to plasma proteins.
Metabolism: Extensively metabolized, primarily to glucuronide-like conjugates.
Excretion: Excreted primarily via kidneys. The t½ is 1 to 3 days.
Onset: 1 hr.
Duration: 12 to 24 hr.

Indications Relief of muscle spasms associated with acute painful musculoskeletal conditions.
Unlabeled use(s): Treatment of fibrositis.

Contraindications Use of MAO inhibitors or within 14 days of their discontinuation; acute recovery phase of MI; arrhythmias; heart block or conduction disturbances; CHF; hyperthyroidism.

PATIENT CARE CONSIDERATIONS
Administration/Storage
- Give with meals to avoid GI irritation.
- Do not give concomitantly with MAO inhibitors or within 14 days of last dose of MAO inhibitors.

Assessment/Interventions
- Obtain patient history, including drug history and any known allergies.
- Record any sensitivity to tricyclic antidepressants and cyclobenzaprine.
- Take vital signs as needed.
- Monitor for development of psychotic symptoms (eg, disorientation, depressed mood, anxiety, hallucinations).
- Obtain ECG if heart arrhythmia develops.

Route/Dosage
ADULTS: PO 10 mg tid (max, 60 mg/day). Do not use longer than 3 wk.

Interactions
Alcohol and other CNS depressants: May cause additive CNS depression.
MAO inhibitors: May cause hyperpyretic crisis, severe convulsions, and death.

Lab Test Interferences None well documented.

Adverse Reactions
CV: Tachycardia; syncope; arrhythmias; vasodilation; palpitation; hypertension.
CNS: Drowsiness; dizziness; fatigue; asthenia; headache; nervousness; convulsions; confusion.
DERM: Sweating; skin rash; urticaria.
EENT: Blurred vision.
GI: Dry mouth; nausea; constipation; dyspepsia; unpleasant taste.
HEMA: Purpura; bone marrow depression; leukopenia; eosinophilia; thrombocytopenia.
METAB: Hypoglycemia; hyperglycemia.

Precautions
Pregnancy: Category B.
Lactation: Undetermined.
Children: Safety and efficacy in children under 15 yr not established.
Anticholinergic effects: Use with caution in patients with urinary retention, angle-closure glaucoma, and increased IOP.

Overdosage: Signs and Symptoms
Confusion, agitation, visual hallucinations, arrhythmia, CHF, hyperpyrexia, hyperactive reflexes, vomiting, drowsiness, stupor, coma, hypothermia, tachycardia, dilated pupils, seizures, hypotension.

Patient/Family Education
- Inform patient that this medication makes injury temporarily feel better. Caution patient not to rush recovery and to avoid lifting or exercising too soon, which may further damage muscles.
- Caution patient to rise slowly from a sitting or standing position to avoid injury.
- Instruct patient to report these symptoms to health care provider: shortness of breath, palpitations, weight gain, heart irregularities, confusion, yellowing of skin or eyes, fever or difficulty urinating.
- Advise patient to take sips of water frequently, suck on ice chips or sugarless hard

candy or chew sugarless gum if dry mouth occurs.
- Instruct patient to avoid intake of alcoholic beverages or other CNS depressants.
- Advise patient that drug may cause drowsiness and to use caution while driving or performing other tasks requiring mental alertness.
- Instruct patient not to take OTC medications without consulting health care provider.

Cyclopentolate Hydrochloride/ Phenylephrine Hydrochloride

(SIGH-kloe-pen-TOLL-ate HIGH-droe-KLOR-ide/fen-ill-EFF-rin HIGH-droe-KLOR-ide)

Class Anticholinergic/Decongestant/Mydriatic

How Supplied
Cyclomydril Solution 0.2% cyclopentolate hydrochloride, 1% phenylephrine hydrochloride

Action
PHARMACOLOGY:
Cyclopentolate: Inhibits action of acetylcholine at muscarinic receptors.
Phenylephrine: Stimulates postsynaptic alpha-receptors, resulting in vasoconstriction.

Indications For production of mydriasis.

Contraindications Untreated narrow-angle glaucoma; untreated anatomically narrow angles; hypersensitivity to any component of product.

Route/Dosage
ADULTS AND CHILDREN: **Ophthalmic** 1 drop each eye q 5 to 10 min.

Interactions
Carbachol, pilocarpine, ophthalmic cholinesterase inhibitors: Cyclopentolate may interfere with antihypertensive action of these agents.

Lab Test Interferences None well documented.

Adverse Reactions
CV: Tachycardia; vasodilation.
CNS: Psychotic reactions and behavioral disturbances in children including ataxia, incoherent speech, restlessness, hallucinations, hyperactivity, seizures, disorientation as to time and place, and failure to recognize people.
EENT: Increased IOP; burning/irritation upon instillation; photophobia; blurred vision; superficial punctate keratitis; decreased secretion in salivary glands, pharynx, and nasal passages.
GI: Decreased GI motility.
GU: Urinary retention.
RESP: Decreased secretion in bronchi.
OTHER: Hyperpyrexia; decreased secretion in sweat glands.

Precautions
Pregnancy: Category C.
Lactation: Undetermined.
Children: Psychotic reactions and behavioral disturbances may occur in children. Signs and symptoms include ataxia, incoherent speech, restlessness, hallucinations, hyperactivity, seizures, disorientation as to time and place, and failure to recognize people.

Overdosage: Signs and Symptoms
Behavioral disturbances, tachycardia, hyperpyrexia, hypertension, elevated intraocular pressure, vasodilation, urinary retention, diminished GI motility, decreased secretion in salivary and sweat glands, pharynx, bronchi, and nasal passages, coma, medullary paralysis, death.

PATIENT CARE CONSIDERATIONS

Administration/Storage
- For ophthalmic use only. Not for use in the ears or on the skin.
- Instill 1 drop into affected eye(s) q 5 to 10 min as prescribed.
- Do not allow tip of dropper bottle to touch eye, eyelid, fingers, or any other surface.
- Compress lacrimal sac for 2 to 3 min following instillation to reduce systemic absorption.
- If using other topical ophthalmic medications, instill drops first, wait at least 5 min, and instill ointment last.
- Store solution at controlled room temperature (40° to 80°F). Keep bottle tightly capped.

Assessment/Interventions
- Obtain patient history, including drug history and any known allergies. Note history of untreated narrow-angle glaucoma, coronary artery disease, hypertension, hyperthyroidism, or Down syndrome.
- Observe infants for 30 min following instillation for CNS and cardiopulmonary side effects. Discontinue therapy and inform health care provider immediately if noted and significant.

Patient/Family Education
- Explain name, dose, action, and potential side effects of drug.
- Teach patient, parent or caregiver proper technique for instilling eye drops: wash hands; do not allow tip of dropper bottle to touch eye, eyelid, fingers, or any other surface. Tilt head back, look up; pull lower eyelid down to form pocket; place prescribed number of drops

in the pocket. Look downward before closing eye; apply pressure to lacrimal sac for 2 to 3 min. Do not rub eye. Wash hands (and child's hands) after instillation.
- Advise parent or guardian to withhold feeding for 4 hr following installation of drops.
- Advise parent or guardian to discontinue therapy and notify health care provider immediately if any of the following occur after instilling drops: stumbling, speech changes, changes in thinking or behavior, rapid heart rate, fever.
- Warn patient that sensitivity to light may be experienced, and to protect eyes in bright illumination while pupils are dilated.
- Caution patient to avoid driving or engaging in hazardous activities while pupils are dilated.
- Inform patient that blurred vision, stinging or burning, and sensitivity to light are the most common side effects and to contact health care provider if they occur and are bothersome.
- Advise patient that follow-up visits and eye examinations may be necessary following therapy and to keep appointments.

Cyclophosphamide

(sigh-kloe-FOSS-fuh-mide)
Class Alkylating agent/Nitrogen mustard
How Supplied
Cytoxan Lyophilized powder for injection 100 mg, Lyophilized powder for injection 200 mg, Lyophilized powder for injection 500 mg, Lyophilized powder for injection 1 g, Lyophilized powder for injection 2 g, Tablets 25 mg, Tablets 50 mg ♦ *Neosar* Dry powder for injection 100 mg, Dry powder for injection 200 mg, Dry powder for injection 500 mg, Dry powder for injection 1 g, Dry powder for injection 2 g
🍁 *Procytox*

Action
PHARMACOLOGY: Cyclophosphamide is first hydroxylated by hepatic microsomal enzymes to the intermediate metabolites 4-hydroxycyclophosphamide and aldophosphamide. These are oxidized to the active antineoplastic alkylating compounds acrolein and phosphoramide mustard. The mechanism of action of the active metabolites is thought to involve cross-linking of DNA, which interferes with growth of susceptible neoplasms and normal tissues.

PHARMACOKINETICS/DYNAMICS:
Absorption: Well absorbed orally. T_{max} is 2 to 3 hr for metabolites (IV dose).
Distribution: More than 75% bioavailable after oral administration. More than 60% of metabolites are bound to plasma proteins. Low protein binding for cyclophosphamide.
Metabolism: Converted to active alkylating metabolites in the liver.
Excretion: The $t_{½}$ is 3 to 12 hr (unchanged drug). Eliminated primarily as metabolites. 5% to 25% is excreted in urine as unchanged drug.

Special Populations:
Renal Function Impairment – Metabolites may be elevated but increased toxicity has not been seen.

Indications
Adult: Lymphomas, multiple myeloma, leukemias, disseminated neuroblastoma, ovarian adenocarcinoma, retinoblastoma, breast carcinoma, mycosis fungoides.
Pediatric: Lymphomas, multiple myeloma, leukemias, disseminated neuroblastoma, ovarian adenocarcinoma, retinoblastoma, breast carcinoma, mycosis fungoides. **Unlabeled use(s):** Bronchogenic, small-cell lung, cervical, endometrial, prostate, and testicular carcinomas; sarcomas, bone marrow transplantation; systemic lupus erythematosus, vasculitis, rheumatoid arthritis, and other autoimmune diseases.

Contraindications Previous hypersensitivity to the drug; continued use in severely depressed bone marrow function.

Route/Dosage
Lymphomas, Multiple Myeloma, Leukemias, Disseminated Neuroblastoma, Ovarian Adenocarcinoma, Retinoblastoma, Breast Carcinoma, Mycosis Fungoides
ADULTS: **PO/IV** Dosage regimens that include cyclophosphamide are too numerous to list. Usual doses range from 500 to 1500 mg/m² per course of therapy. In myelosuppressed patients, reduce initial loading dose by 33% to 50%.**PO** 60 to 120 mg/m²/day for initial and maintenance therapy.

Dosage Adjustment (Hepatic Dysfunction Reduction)
ADULTS: **PO/IV** If LFTs show bilirubin 3.1 to 5 mg/dL or AST greater than 180 units/L, administer 75% of dose. If bilirubin is greater than 5 mg/dL, no dose is to be given.

Lymphomas, Multiple Myeloma, Leukemias, Ovarian Adenocarcinoma, Retinoblastoma, Breast Carcinoma, Mycosis Fungoides
PEDIATRIC: **PO/IV** Doses are similar to those used in adult regimens and calculated based on BSA. Usual doses range from 500 to 1500 mg/m^2 per course of therapy. Follow dosage adjustment guidelines recommended for adults.**PO** 60 to 120 mg/m^2/day for initial and maintenance therapy.

Neuroblastoma
PEDIATRIC: **IV** 3000 mg/m^2/day for 2 days or 2000 mg/m^2/day for 3 consecutive days.

Interactions
Anticoagulants: Increased hypoprothrombinemic effect may occur.
Barbiturates, other enzyme inducers: May increase the rate of active cyclophosphamide metabolite formation and possibly increase neutropenic effects.
Chloramphenicol, other enzyme inhibitors: May inhibit cyclophosphamide's antineoplastic activity by decreasing rate of active metabolite formation.
Digoxin: May cause decreased serum levels of digoxin.
Oral quinolone antibiotics: May cause decreased GI absorption of quinolone antibiotics.
Succinylcholine and possibly mivacurium: Prolongation of neuromuscular blockade by cyclophosphamide's inhibition of pseudocholinesterase may occur.

Lab Test Interferences
None well documented.

Adverse Reactions
CV: Acute hemorrhagic myocarditis; CHF; cardiac necrosis.
DERM: Alopecia; skin and fingernail hyperpigmentation; palmar-plantar erythrodysesthesia.
ENDO: SIADH.
GI: Nausea; vomiting; diarrhea; mucositis.
GU: Hemorrhagic cystitis; amenorrhea; reversible oligospermia and azoospermia; sterility.
HEMA: Bone marrow suppression.
HYPERSEN: Cross-sensitivity with other alkylating agents.
OTHER: Secondary malignancy; bladder carcinoma; hemorrhagic cystitis; myeloproliferative malignancy; lymphoproliferative malignancy.
RENAL: Renal tubular necrosis.
RESP: Interstitial pulmonary fibrosis.

Precautions
Pregnancy: Category D.
Lactation: Cyclophosphamide is excreted in breast milk.
Hypersensitivity: Hypersensitivity reactions (type I) have occurred.
Renal function impairment: Use cautiously. There is no evidence indicating a need for modified dosage in these patients.
Hepatic function impairment: Use cautiously. There is no evidence indicating a need for modified dosage in these patients.
Carcinogenesis: Secondary neoplasia has developed with cyclophosphamide alone or with other antineoplastic drugs or radiation therapy. These most frequently have been urinary bladder, myeloproliferative, and lymphoproliferative malignancies.
Fertility impairment: Cyclophosphamide interferes with oogenesis and spermatogenesis. It may cause sterility in men and women. Amenorrhea associated with decreased estrogen and increased gonadotropin secretion develops in a significant proportion of women treated with cyclophosphamide.
Special risk patients: Give cautiously to patients with leukopenia, thrombocytopenia, tumor cell infiltration of bone marrow, previous radiation therapy, or previous cytotoxic therapy.
Adrenalectomy patients: Adjustment of the doses of both replacement steroids and cyclophosphamide may be necessary for the adrenalectomized patient.
Cardiac toxicity: Few instances of cardiac dysfunction have occurred. No causal relationship has been established. Cardiotoxicity has been observed in some patients receiving high doses of cyclophosphamide ranging from 120 to 270 mg/kg administered over a period of a few days.
GU: Acute hemorrhagic cystitis occurs in 7% to 12% of patients, although some report an occurrence of up to 40%, and is probably caused by urinary metabolites. Ample fluid intake and frequent voiding help to prevent cystitis. A formalin (37% formaldehyde solution diluted to a 1% solution) bladder instillation has successfully controlled the cystitis. Complications may occur with the 10% solution; there appears to be no additional value in using greater than 4% solutions. The use of mesna has reduced the incidence of cyclophosphamide-induced cystitis.
Hematologic: Leukopenia of less than 2000 cells/mm^3 develops commonly in patients treated with an initial loading dose of the drug. Thrombocytopenia or anemia develop occasionally. Recovery from leukopenia usually begins in 7 to 10 days after cessation of therapy.
Hyperuricemia: May occur because of rapid cell lysis; monitor serum uric acid. Minimize effects of hyperuricemia with hydration, urinary alkalinization, and allopurinol.
Immunosuppression: May cause significant suppression of immune responses. Serious, sometimes fatal infections may develop in severely

immunosuppressed patients.
Renal effects: SIADH has occurred with IV doses greater than 50 mg/kg. It is both a limitation to and consequence of fluid loading. Hemorrhagic ureteritis and renal tubular necrosis have occurred.
Wound healing: May interfere with normal wound healing.

PATIENT CARE CONSIDERATIONS
Administration/Storage
- Store tablets or powder for injection at room temperature.
- Reconstitute powder for injection with Sterile Water or Bacteriostatic Water (with parabens only) for Injection, shaking the vial to dissolve the powder.
- Reconstitute cyclophosphamide according to the following guidelines: 100 mg vial with 5 mL diluent; 200 mg vial with 10 mL; 500 mg vial with 25 mL (20 to 25 mL for Cytoxan lyophilized powder); 1000 mg vial with 50 mL; 2000 mg vial with 100 mL (80 to 100 mL for Cytoxan lyophilized powder).
- Reconstituted solutions may be further diluted with: 5% Dextrose, 5% Dextrose with 0.9% Sodium Chloride, or 0.45% Sodium Chloride. The maximum concentration of cyclophosphamide for IV infusion is 20 mg/mL.
- For use in bone marrow transplantation regimens, reconstitute powder with Sterile Water for Injection. The reconstituted 20 mg/mL solution may be infused without further dilution.
- Solutions prepared with Sterile Water for Injection are preservative free. Discard preservative-free cyclophosphamide solutions within 24 hr of preparation.
- Administer by oral, IV infusion, or IV/IM injection.
- Vigorous hydration and frequent urination reduces the risk of hemorrhagic cystitis. Patients may be hydrated with 1.5 to 2 L of fluids for 3 hr prior to cyclophosphamide to ensure adequate urine output. Encourage patients to drink extra fluids (especially water) during the next 24 hr to maintain urine output.
- Oral tablets should be taken on an empty stomach.
- Follow safe handling procedures when dispensing and disposing oral chemotherapy. Wear gloves and avoid skin exposure and inhalation of fumes.

IV infusion:
- Cyclophosphamide may be infused over 1 to 2 hr.

Extemporaneous oral solution:
- Oral solutions may be prepared from powder for injection (dry or lyophilized) by dissolving the powder in *Aromatic Elixir* NF to a concentration of 1 to 5 mg/mL. It is stable for up to 14 days in glass bottles under refrigeration.

Cytoxan:
- Solutions prepared with Bacteriostatic Water for Injection are stable for 48 hr at room temperature or up to 28 days under refrigeration.

Neosar:
- Solutions prepared with Bacteriostatic Water for Injection are stable for 24 hr at room temperature or up to 6 days under refrigeration.

Assessment/Interventions
- During treatment, monitor the patient's hematologic profile (particularly neutrophils and platelets) regularly to determine the degree of hematopoietic suppression. Examine urine regularly for red cells, which may precede hemorrhagic cystitis.

Mesna treatment:
- Cotreatment with mesna (a uroprotectant) may be required to prevent hemorrhagic cystitis in patients receiving high doses of cyclophosphamide. Consider mesna prophylaxis when cyclophosphamide doses greater than 1000 mg/m^2 are administered.

Patient/Family Education
- Take tablets preferably on an empty stomach. If GI upset is severe, take with food.
- Notify health care provider if the following symptoms occur: unusual bleeding or bruising, fever, chills, sore throat, cough, shortness of breath, seizures, lack of menstrual flow, unusual lumps or masses, flank or stomach pain, joint pain, sores in the mouth or on the lips, yellow discoloration of the skin or eyes.
- Contraceptive measures are recommended during therapy for men and women.

Cycloserine
(sigh-kloe-SER-een)
Class Anti-infective/Antitubercular
How Supplied
Seromycin Pulvules Capsules 250 mg

Action
PHARMACOLOGY: Inhibits cell wall synthesis in susceptible strains of certain microorganisms.
PHARMACOKINETICS/DYNAMICS:
Absorption: Readily absorbed. T_{max} is 4 to 8 hr.
Distribution: Widely distributed in tissues (eg,

Cycloserine

CSF, pleural fluid).
Metabolism: 35% metabolized to unknown metabolites.
Excretion: About 65% of a single dose is excreted in urine within 72 hr. Maximum excretion rate occurs 2 to 6 hr after dose, with 50% eliminated in 12 hr.

Indications Treatment of active pulmonary and extrapulmonary tuberculosis when organisms are susceptible (after failure of adequate treatment with primary medications); treatment of UTIs caused by susceptible bacteria when conventional therapy has failed; treatment of Gaucher disease.

Contraindications Epilepsy; depression; severe anxiety or psychosis; severe renal insufficiency; excessive concurrent use of alcohol.

Route/Dosage
ADULTS: **PO** 250 to 500 mg q 12 hr; start with 250 mg q 12 hr for first 2 wk (max, 1 g/day).
CHILDREN: **PO** 15 to 20 mg/kg/day administered in 2 equally divided doses (max, 1 g/day).

Interactions
Alcohol: Increases possibility and risk of epileptic episodes. Do not use together.
Isoniazid: May increase cycloserine CNS side effects (eg, dizziness).

PATIENT CARE CONSIDERATIONS
Administration/Storage
- Administer with meals if GI irritation occurs.
- Store in airtight, light-resistant container at room temperature.

Assessment/Interventions
- Obtain patient history, including drug history and any known allergies.
- Review history for epilepsy, depression, severe anxiety or psychosis, renal insufficiency, or excessive alcohol use.
- Review liver function, BUN, creatinine, and CBC before beginning therapy.
- Obtain culture before treatment and verify susceptibility when results are available.
- Perform baseline assessment of signs and symptoms of infection.
- If patient has active and infectious tuberculosis, institute infection control measures.
- Monitor serum cycloserine levels at least weekly in patients receiving more than 500 mg/day and in patients with reduced renal function or symptoms of toxicity. Blood levels should remain less than 30 mcg/mL.
- Monitor CBC and liver and renal function studies.

Lab Test Interferences None well documented.

Adverse Reactions
CV: CHF.
CNS: Convulsions; drowsiness; somnolence; headache; tremor; dysarthria; vertigo; confusion; loss of memory; psychoses with suicidal tendencies, behavior changes, hyperirritability, aggression, paresis; hyperreflexia; paresthesias; major and minor clonic seizures; coma; dizziness.
DERM: Rash.
HEPA: Elevated hepatic transaminase.

Precautions
Pregnancy: Category C.
Lactation: Undetermined.
Children: Safety and dosage not well established.
Renal function impairment: Determine weekly blood levels of drug and adjust dosage to keep blood levels below 30 mcg/mL.
CNS toxicity: Discontinue drug or decrease dosage if symptoms of CNS toxicity develop. May be increased with excessive alcohol consumption. Pyridoxine 200 to 300 mg/day may be given to prevent neurotoxic effects.

Overdosage: Signs and Symptoms
CNS depression, drowsiness, mental confusion, headache, vertigo, hyperirritability, paresthesias, dysarthrias, psychosis, paresis, convulsions, coma.

- If allergic dermatitis or symptoms of CNS toxicity, convulsions, psychosis, depression, headache, tremor, vertigo, paresis, or dysarthria develop, withhold medication and notify health care provider.
- If CNS alterations occur, institute safety precautions.
- In patients with tuberculosis, assess for therapeutic effectiveness by monitoring clinical signs and symptoms, sputum cultures, or smears for acid-fast bacilli and chest x-rays.
- In patients with UTIs, assess for therapeutic effectiveness by monitoring clinical signs and symptoms and urine cultures.

Patient/Family Education
- Instruct patient that if depression or suicidal thoughts occur, notify health care provider immediately.
- Stress importance of regular follow-up visits to health care provider for ongoing assessment.
- If patient does not have adequate family support system, refer patient to community health organization for monitoring and support.

- Instruct patient to report the following symptoms to health care provider: rash, anxiety, restlessness, confusion or tremor.
- Caution patient to avoid intake of alcoholic beverages because of increased risk of seizures.
- Advise patient that drug may cause drowsiness and to use caution while driving or performing other tasks requiring mental alertness.

Cyclosporine (Cyclosporin A)

(SIGH-kloe-spore-EEN)

Class Immunosuppressive

How Supplied
Sandimmune Capsules, soft gelatin 25 mg, Capsules, soft gelatin 50 mg, Capsules, soft gelatin 100 mg, Oral solution 100 mg/mL, IV solution 50 mg/mL ♦ Neoral Capsules, soft gelatin, for microemulsion 25 mg, Capsules, soft gelatin, for microemulsion 50 mg, Oral solution for microemulsion 100 mg/mL ♦ SangCya Oral solution 100 mg/mL

🍁 Rhoxal-cyclosporine ♦ Sandimmune

Action
PHARMACOLOGY: Suppresses cell-mediated immune reactions and some humoral immunity, but exact mechanism is not known.

PHARMACOKINETICS/DYNAMICS:
Absorption:
Oral – Absorption is incomplete and variable. Bioavailability is less than 10% in liver transplant patients (Sandimmune), up to 89% in renal transplant patients (Sandimmune), and about 30% for the oral solution. T_{max} is 1.5 to 2 hr (Neoral) and 3.5 hr (Sandimmune). Food decreases the AUC and C_{max}.

Distribution: Vd is 3 to 5 L/kg at steady state (IV). Cyclosporine is 90% protein bound (primarily lipoprotein) and is excreted in human milk.

Metabolism: Extensively metabolized by CYP3A in the liver and to a lesser degree in the GI tract and kidney.

Excretion: Eliminated primarily in the bile; 6% is excreted unchanged in the urine (0.1% as unchanged drug). The t½ is about 8.4 hr (Neoral) and about 19 hr (Sandimmune). Blood Cl is about 5 to 7 mL/min/kg (IV).

Indications Prophylaxis of organ rejection in kidney, liver, and heart allogeneic transplants in conjunction with adrenal corticosteroid therapy; treatment of chronic rejection in patients previously treated with other immunosuppressive agents. Increase tear production in patients whose tear production is presumed to be suppressed because of ocular inflammation associated with keratoconjunctivitis sicca (ophthalmic emulsion). **Unlabeled use(s):** Prophylaxis in other transplant procedures; treatment of aplastic anemia, atopic dermatitis, Behcet disease, biliary cirrhosis, Crohn disease, rheumatoid arthritis, severe psoriasis, nephrotic syndrome, pulmonary sarcoidosis, pyoderma gangrenosum, ulcerative colitis, alopecia areata.

Contraindications Hypersensitivity to polyoxyethylated castor oil, which is present in concentrate for injection. Active ocular infections (ophthalmic emulsion)

Route/Dosage
ADULTS AND CHILDREN: **PO** 15 mg/kg/day (range, 14 to 18 mg/kg/day) beginning 4 to 12 hr before transplantation. Continue for 1 to 2 wk postoperatively, then taper dose by 5%/wk to maintenance level of 5 to 10 mg/kg/day. Lower doses may be used on basis of patient response, rejection rate, and cyclosporine plasma concentrations.
IV 5 to 6 mg/kg/day as single IV dose starting 4 to 12 hr before transplantation. Switch to oral form as soon as patient can tolerate.

Interactions
Aminoglycosides, amphotericin B, NSAIDs, trimethoprim-sulfamethoxazole, melphalan, quinolones: Additive nephrotoxicity possible.
Amiodarone, diltiazem, fluconazole, imipenem-cilastatin, ketoconazole, macrolide antibiotics (eg, erythromycin), nicardipine: May increase cyclosporine concentrations.
Azathioprine, corticosteroids, cyclophosphamide, verapamil: May cause additive immunosuppression, increasing risk of infection and malignancy.
Carbamazepine, hydantoins, phenobarbital, rifampin, rifabutin: May decrease cyclosporine effects.
Digoxin: May cause elevated digoxin concentrations and toxicity.
Etoposide: May increase etoposide concentrations.
Lovastatin: May cause severe myopathy or rhabdomyolysis; avoid concurrent use.
Metoclopramide: Increases absorption of cyclosporine.
Potassium-sparing diuretics: Causes hyperkalemic effects; avoid concomitant use.

Lab Test Interferences None well documented.

Adverse Reactions
CV: Hypertension; MI.
CNS: Tremor; convulsions; headache; confusion; flushing; ataxia; hallucinations; mania; depression; encephalopathy.
DERM: Hirsutism; acne; brittle fingernails.
GI: Gingival hyperplasia; diarrhea; nausea; vomiting; abdominal discomfort; anorexia; gas-

tritis; peptic ulcer; hiccoughs.
GU: Renal dysfunction.
HEMA: Lymphoma; hemolytic anemia; leukopenia; anemia; thrombocytopenia.
HEPA: Hepatotoxicity.
METAB: Hyperglycemia; hyperkalemia; hyperuricemia.
OTHER: Paresthesia; gynecomastia; allergic reactions including anaphylaxis; cramps.

> **WARNING:**
> Only physicians experienced in immunosuppressive therapy and managing organ transplant patients should prescribe cyclosporine. Manage patients in facilities equipped and staffed with adequate lab and supportive medical resources.
>
> Administer with adrenal corticosteroids but not with other immunosuppressants. Cyclosporine for microemulsion (*Neoral*) may be given with other immunosuppressants.
>
> *Sandimmune* capsules and oral solution have decreased bioavailability compared with *Neoral*. Oral absorption during chronic *Sandimmune* use is erratic. Monitor cyclosporine blood levels during oral therapy at repeated intervals and make dose adjustments to avoid toxicity or possible organ rejection. For a given trough concentration, cyclosporine exposure will be greater with *Neoral* than with *Sandimmune*. If a patient who is receiving exceptionally high doses of *Sandimmune* is converted to *Neoral*, use particular caution. *Neoral* and *Sandimmune* are not bioequivalent and cannot be used interchangeably.
>
> Risks of neoplasia and susceptibility to infection are increased with cyclosporine use.
>
> Psoriasis patients have an increased risk of developing skin malignancies if previously treated with PUVA, methotrexate, other immunosuppressants, UVB, coal tar, or radiation therapy.
>
> Renal dysfunction, including structural kidney damage, is a potential consequence of therapy. Monitor renal function during therapy.

Precautions
Pregnancy: Category C.
Lactation: Excreted in breast milk.
Children: Although safety and efficacy have not been established, patients as young as 6 mo have received drug. May require higher doses than adults.
Renal function impairment: Requires close monitoring and possible dosage adjustment.
Absorption: Absorption during long-term use is erratic. Patients with malabsorption may have difficulty achieving therapeutic concentrations with oral use.
Anaphylactic reactions: Occur rarely with IV use. Have epinephrine 1:1000 and oxygen readily available.
Convulsions: Have occurred, particularly in combination with high-dose methylprednisolone.
Nephrotoxicity: Common adverse effect; may respond to decreased dose.

Overdosage: Signs and Symptoms
Hepatotoxicity, nephrotoxicity.

PATIENT CARE CONSIDERATIONS
Administration/Storage
- Give with adrenal corticosteroids but not with other immunosuppressive agents.

IV:
- Dilute parenteral solution immediately before use. Dilute each 1 mL (50 mg) concentrate in 20 to 100 mL of 0.9% Sodium Chloride for Injection or D5W. Observe for particulate matter and discoloration. Give IV infusion slowly over 2 to 6 hr.
- Store in glass container at room temperature. Protect from light. Solutions diluted with D5W are stable for 24 hr.

Oral:
- Use calibrated pipettes for oral doses. Prepare solution in glass container just before administering to patient.
- Prepare with room-temperature white or chocolate milk or orange juice to improve flavor. Stir well and give to patient to drink. Do not use plastic utensils (drug binds to plastics). Do not allow mixture to stand before administering.
- Do not refrigerate or freeze. Use within 2 mo after opening.

Assessment/Interventions
- Obtain patient history, including drug history and any known allergies. Note hypersensitivity to cyclosporine or polyoxyethylated castor oil.
- Perform renal and hepatic function tests in conjunction with potassium and lipid level determinations before beginning treatment

and periodically repeat tests during drug therapy.
- Assess vital signs initially and note hypertension, especially with children.
- Note any signs of infection (eg, fever, sore throat, tiredness), unusual bleeding, hematuria, or bruising.
- Have emergency equipment available for IV drug administration and assess vital signs frequently (eg, q 5 to 10 min × 4) or according to hospital policy.
- Ensure medical asepsis and eliminate any potential sources of environmental contamination.
- Weigh patient daily and monitor I&O.

Patient/Family Education
- Instruct patient on necessity for frequent laboratory monitoring while taking medication.
- Instruct patient on proper technique for self-monitoring of BP and vital signs.
- Instruct patient to report any adverse reactions: infection (eg, fever, sore throat, fatigue, frequency, dysuria, cloudy urine), unusual bleeding (eg, hematuria, bleeding of gums, bruising), chest pain, headache, tremors, or liver dysfunction (eg, abdominal pain, jaundice, dark urine, pruritus, light-colored stools).
- Direct patient to avoid contact with others who may have infections.
- Caution patient to avoid any trauma.
- Advise patient to use soft toothbrush, practice frequent oral hygiene, and have regular dental checkups.
- Counsel patient on need for balanced diet and fluid intake according to specific health care provider orders.
- Advise patient to consult health care provider before any vaccinations.

Cyproheptadine Hydrochloride

(sip-row-HEP-tuh-deen HIGH-droe-KLOR-ide)

Class Antihistamine

How Supplied
Periactin Tablets 4 mg, Syrup 2 mg/5 mL

Action
PHARMACOLOGY: Competitively antagonizes histamine at H_1 receptor sites. Also exhibits antiserotonin activity.

PHARMACOKINETICS/DYNAMICS:
Metabolism: The principal metabolite found in the urine is the quaternary ammonium glucuronide conjugate of cyproheptadine.
Excretion: 2% to 20% is excreted in the feces, of which 34% (5.7% of the dose) is unchanged drug. At least 40% is excreted in the urine.

Indications Symptomatic relief of perennial and seasonal allergic rhinitis, vasomotor rhinitis, allergic conjunctivitis; amelioration of allergic reactions to blood or plasma; management of allergic pruritic symptoms, mild skin manifestations of uncomplicated urticaria and angioedema, and cold urticaria.

Contraindications Hypersensitivity to antihistamines; newborn or premature infants; nursing mothers; narrow-angle glaucoma; stenosing peptic ulcer; symptomatic prostatic hypertrophy; asthmatic attack; bladder neck obstruction; pyloroduodenal obstruction; MAO therapy.

Route/Dosage
ADULTS: **PO** 4 mg q 8 hr then 4 to 20 mg/day; not to exceed 0.5 mg/kg/day.
CHILDREN 7 TO 14 YR: **PO** 4 mg bid or tid (max, 16 mg/day).
CHILDREN 2 TO 6 YR: **PO** 2 mg bid or tid (max, 12 mg/day). (**PO** Total daily dosage 0.25 mg/kg or 8 mg/m^2.)

Interactions
Alcohol, CNS depressants: May cause additive CNS depressant effects.
Fluoxetine: Effects of fluoxetine may be reversed.
MAO inhibitors: Anticholinergic effects of cyproheptadine may increase.

Lab Test Interferences In skin testing procedures, antihistamines may prevent or diminish otherwise positive reaction to dermal reactivity indicators.

Adverse Reactions
CV: Orthostatic hypotension; palpitations; tachycardia; reflex tachycardia; extrasystoles; faintness.
CNS: Drowsiness (often transient); sedation; dizziness; faintness; disturbed coordination; confusion; restlessness; excitement; nervous tremor; paresthesias; convulsions; hallucinations.
DERM: Photosensitivity; rash.
EENT: Dry mouth, nose, and throat; sore throat.
GI: Epigastric distress; nausea; vomiting; diarrhea; anorexia; constipation; change in bowel habits.
HEMA: Hemolytic anemia; thrombocytopenia; agranulocytosis.
HEPA: Jaundice.
RESP: Thickening of bronchial secretions; chest tightness; wheezing; nasal stuffiness; respiratory depression.

Precautions
Pregnancy: Category B.
Lactation: Contraindicated in nursing women.
Children: Safety and efficacy in children younger than 2 yr not established.
Elderly: Dosage reduction may be required.
Hepatic function impairment: Use drug with caution in patients with cirrhosis or other liver disease.
Special risk patients: Use drug with caution in patients with predisposition to urinary retention, history of bronchial asthma, increased IOP, hyperthyroidism, cardiovascular disease, or hypertension.

Respiratory disease: Generally not recommended for treatment of lower respiratory tract symptoms including asthma.
Sedatives/CNS depressants: Avoid in patients with history of sleep apnea.

Overdosage: Signs and Symptoms
CNS depression, cardiovascular collapse, cardiovascular stimulation, seizures, hypotension, anticholinergic effects (eg, dilated pupils, dry mouth, flushing), hyperthermia (especially in children), dystonic reactions, dizziness, ataxia, blurred vision.

PATIENT CARE CONSIDERATIONS
Administration/Storage
- Administer dose bid to tid as prescribed, without regard to meals.
- Administer with food if GI upset occurs.
- Store tablets and syrup at controlled room temperature (59° to 86°F). Keep container tightly closed.

Assessment/Interventions
- Obtain patient history, including drug history and any known allergies. Note asthma, untreated hyperthyroidism, hypertension, cardiovascular disease, glaucoma, stenosing peptic ulcer, symptomatic prostatic hypertrophy, bladder neck obstruction, pyloroduodenal obstruction, debilitation, or coadministration of MAO inhibitor.
- Assess for allergy symptoms (eg, rhinitis, nasal congestion, sneezing, itching, watery eyes) before and periodically throughout therapy.
- Monitor patient for dizziness and excessive drowsiness. If noted, hold therapy and notify health care provider.

Patient/Family Education
- Explain name, dose, action, and potential side effects of drug.
- Advise patient to take dose bid to tid as prescribed and not to stop taking or change the dose unless advised by health care provider.
- Advise patient that if allergy symptoms are not controlled not to increase the dose of medication or frequency of use but to inform health care provider. Inform patient that larger or more frequent dosing does not increase effectiveness and may cause drowsiness.
- Caution patient not to take any OTC antihistamines while taking this medication unless advised by health care provider.
- Caution patient to avoid alcohol and other CNS depressants (eg, sedatives) while using this medication.
- Caution patient that drug may cause drowsiness and to use caution while driving or performing other tasks requiring mental alertness until tolerance is determined.
- Advise patient that medication may cause sensitivity to sunlight and to avoid unnecessary exposure to UV light (sunlight, tanning booths), use sunscreen, and wear protective clothing until tolerance is determined.
- Advise patient to take frequent sips of water, suck on ice chips or sugarless hard candy, or chew sugarless gum if dry mouth occurs.
- If patient is to have allergy skin testing, advise not to take the medication for at least 4 days before the skin testing.
- Advise women to notify health care provider if pregnant, planning to become pregnant, or breastfeeding.
- Instruct patient to stop taking drug and immediately report any of the following symptoms to health care provider: dizziness, excessive drowsiness.
- Caution patient not to take any prescription or OTC medications or dietary supplements unless advised by health care provider.

Cytarabine

(SITE-ah-rah-been)
Class Pyrimidine antimetabolite
How Supplied
Cytosar-U Sterile powder for reconstitution 100 mg, 500 mg, 1 g, 2 g vials

♣ Cytosar

Action
PHARMACOLOGY: Cytarabine exhibits cell-phase specificity, primarily killing cells undergoing DNA synthesis (S-phase) and under certain conditions, blocking the progression of cells from the G_1-phase to the S-phase.

Pharmacokinetics/Dynamics:
Distribution: Distribution t½ is about 10 min.

Metabolism: Metabolized by deoxycytidine kinase and other nucleotide kinases to nucleotide triphosphate (active). Inactivated by a pyrimidine nucleotide deaminase to nontoxic uracil derivative.

Excretion: Elimination t½ is about 1 to 3 hr. About 80% is excreted in the urine within 24 hr (90% of which is excreted as ara-U).

Indications Acute lymphocytic leukemia, acute and chronic myelocytic leukemia, meningeal leukemia, erythroleukemia, non-Hodgkin lymphoma. **Unlabeled use(s):** Hodgkin disease, bone marrow transplantation.

Contraindications Standard considerations.

Route/Dosage
Acute Leukemia Induction
ADULTS: **Continuous IV infusion or rapid injection** 100 to 200 mg/m^2/day or 3 mg/kg/day as a continuous IV infusion over 24 hr or in divided doses by rapid injection for 5 to 10 days with the courses repeated about q 2 wk.

PEDIATRIC: **Continuous IV infusion or rapid injection** 100 to 200 mg/m^2/day as a continuous IV infusion over 24 hr or in divided doses by rapid injection for 5 to 10 days with the courses repeated about q 2 wk.

Acute Leukemia Maintenance
ADULTS: **SC** 1 mg/kg/dose 1 or 2 times/wk.

PEDIATRIC: **SC or IM** 1 to 1.5 mg/kg/dose q 1 to 4 wk.

Alternate maintenance regimen: 70 to 200 mg/m^2/day IV for 2 to 5 days repeated q mo.

Acute Nonlymphocytic Leukemia (Combination with Other Chemotherapeutic Drugs)
ADULTS: **Continuous infusion** 100 mg/m^2/day on days 1 through 7, or 100 mg/m^2 q 12 hr for 7 days.

Alternate regimen: Cytarabine 10 mg/m^2/dose SC bid for 7 to 14 days in combination with other chemotherapeutic drugs.

PEDIATRIC: **Continuous infusion** 100 mg/m^2/day on days 1 through 7, or 100 mg/m^2 q 12 hr for 7 days.

Refractory Acute Leukemia or Lymphomas
ADULTS:
High-dose cytarabine: **IV** 2000 to 3000 mg/m^2 q 12 hr for 2 to 6 days. Suspend or modify the dose of cytarabine if ANC is less than 1000/mm^3 or the platelet count is less than 50,000/mm^3.

PEDIATRIC:
High-dose cytarabine: **IV** 1000 to 3000 mg/m^2 q 12 hr for 2 to 6 days. Suspend or modify the dose of cytarabine if ANC is less than 1000/mm^3 or the platelet count is less than 50,000/mm^3.

Adjustment in Hepatic Insufficiency
ADULTS: May require dosage reduction; specific guidelines not established.

PEDIATRIC: Follow dosage adjustment guidelines recommended for adults.

Meningeal Leukemia
ADULTS: **Intrathecally** to 75 mg/m^2 at intervals ranging from once a day for 4 days to once q 4 days (range, 2 to 7 days).

PEDIATRIC: **Intrathecally** to 75 mg/m^2 at intervals ranging from once a day for 4 days to once q 4 days (range, 2 to 7 days). Many clinicians recommend dosing intrathecal cytarabine by the child's age.

Pretreatment Regimen
Prophylactic use of corticosteroid eye drops decreases the risk of conjunctivitis or keratitis. Begin prophylactic therapy prior to chemotherapy and continue for 48 hr after the last dose of cytarabine.

Interactions
L-asparaginase: Prior therapy with L-asparaginase may increase the risk of acute pancreatitis.

Digoxin: Oral absorption of digoxin may be decreased.

Gentamicin: Gentamicin effectiveness against *Klebsiella pneumoniae* strains may be decreased.

Quinolone antibiotics: Cytarabine may decrease the oral absorption of quinolone antibiotics.

Lab Test Interferences
None well documented.

Adverse Reactions
CNS: Headache, dizziness; seizures, cerebral or cerebellar dysfunction presenting as personality changes, somnolence, coma, ataxia, dysarthria, and nystagmus (high dose); sensory neuropathy (high dose); necrotizing leukoencephalopathy with intrathecal cytarabine and cranial radiation.

DERM: Rash; cellulitis; thrombophlebitis; palmar-plantar erythrodysesthesia; severe rash with desquamation (high dose).

GI: Nausea; vomiting; anorexia; mucositis; diarrhea; transient elevation of LFTs; neutropenic colitis; severe GI ulceration (high dose).

HEMA: Bone marrow suppression.

RESP: Pulmonary edema, diffuse interstitial pneumonitis (high dose).

OTHER: Cytarabine syndrome; arthralgias; myalgias; chest pain; fever; general feeling of discomfort or weakness; reddened eyes; skin rash.

SPEC SENSE: Hemorrhagic conjunctivitis, corneal toxicity, photophobia (high dose).

> **WARNING:**
> For induction therapy, treat patients in a facility with laboratory and supportive resources sufficient to monitor drug tolerance and protect and maintain a patient compromised by drug toxicity. Less serious toxicity includes nausea, vomiting, diarrhea, abdominal pain, oral ulceration, and hepatic dysfunction. The physician must judge possible benefit to the patient against known toxic effects of the drug in considering the advisability of therapy.
>
> Anemia, leukopenia, thrombocytopenia, megaloblastosis, and reduced reticulocytes can be expected. The severity of these reactions is dose- and schedule-dependent.

Precautions

Pregnancy: Category D.
Lactation: Undetermined.
Children: Conventional cytarabine is indicated for use in children.
Hypersensitivity: Cases of anaphylaxis have occurred resulting in acute cardiopulmonary arrest which required resuscitation. This occurred immediately after IV administration.
Renal function impairment: Patients with renal function impairment may have a higher likelihood of CNS toxicity after high-dose cytarabine. Use the drug with caution and possibly at reduced doses in patients with poor kidney function.
Hepatic function impairment: Patients with hepatic function impairment may have a higher likelihood of CNS toxicity after high-dose cytarabine. Use the drug with caution and possibly at reduced doses in patients with poor liver function.
Benzyl alcohol: Benzyl alcohol is contained in the diluent for some conventional cytarabine products. Benzyl alcohol has been reported to be associated with a fatal "gasping syndrome" in premature infants. Do not use conventional cytarabine injection with benzyl alcohol intrathecally.
Extravasation risk: May cause local irritation or phlebitis. Refer to your institution specific protocol.
Infection: Viral, bacterial, fungal, parasitic, or saprophytic infections in any location in the body may be associated with the use of cytarabine alone or in combination with other immunosuppressive agents.
Intrathecal use: If used intrathecally, do not use a diluent with benzyl alcohol.
Neuropathies: Peripheral motor and sensory neuropathies have occurred.
Neurotoxicity: Enhanced neurotoxicity has been associated with concurrent use of intrathecal cytarabine and other cytotoxic agents administered intrathecally.

PATIENT CARE CONSIDERATIONS

Administration/Storage

- Store at room temperature.
- When reconstituted with Bacteriostatic Water for Injection (with benzyl alcohol), cytarabine is stable for 2 days at room temperature. Use preservative-free cytarabine solutions within 24 hr of reconstitution. Discard if solution appears hazy.
- Diluted cytarabine solutions (concentration 0.5 mg/mL) are stable for 8 days at room temperature when diluted with Sterile Water, 0.9% Sodium Chloride, or 5% Dextrose.
- Administer by SC/IM injection, by IV injection or infusion, or intrathecally.
- Rotate injection sites for SC/IM administration.

IV Infusion:

- Reconstitute with Bacteriostatic Water for Injection (with 0.9% benzyl alcohol). May be further diluted with greater than 50 mL of 0.9% Sodium Chloride for IV infusion.
- Give by bolus injection over 1 to 3 min through a running IV line; infuse IV over 15 min in greater than 50 mL of 0.9% Sodium Chloride; continuous IV infusion over 5 days. Cytarabine doses are often infused over 30 min.

Intrathecal:

- Dilute with an isotonic buffered diluent without preservative such as Lactated Ringer's injection or 0.9% Sodium Chloride.

High dose:

- Dilute with preservative-free 0.9% Sodium Chloride.
- Give IV infusion over 1 to 3 hr.

SC/IM:

- Smaller volumes of diluent can be used to prepare a 100 mg/mL solution for SC/IM injection.

Assessment/Interventions

- Hyperuricemia may occur because of rapid cell lysis; monitor serum uric acid. Minimize effects of hyperuricemia with hydration, urinary alkalinization, and allopurinol.
- During induction therapy, perform leukocyte and platelet counts daily. Perform bone marrow examinations frequently after blasts have disappeared from the peripheral blood.
- Suspend or modify therapy when drug-

induced marrow depression results in a platelet count less than 50,000/mm^3 or a polymorphonuclear granulocyte count less than 1000/mm^3.
♦ Perform periodic checks of bone marrow, liver, and kidney functions.
♦ Observe patients on high-dose cytarabine for neuropathy.

Patient/Family Education
♦ Inform patients about the expected adverse events of headache, nausea, vomiting, and fever, and about the early signs and symptoms of neurotoxicity. Instruct patients to seek medical attention if signs or symptoms of neurotoxicity develop, or if oral dexamethasone is not well tolerated.

Cytarabine Liposomal
(SITE-ah-rah-been)
Class Pyrimidine antimetabolite
How Supplied
DepoCyt Suspension equivalent to 10 mg/mL cytarabine
Action
PHARMACOLOGY: Cytarabine exhibits cell-phase specificity, primarily killing cells undergoing DNA synthesis (S-phase) and under certain conditions, blocking the progression of cells from the G$_1$ phase to the S-phase.
PHARMACOKINETICS/DYNAMICS:
Absorption: T$_{max}$ is within 5 hr for free cytarabine in both the ventricle and the lumbar sac.
Metabolism: Intracellularly converted to cytarabine-5'-triphosphate (ara-CTP), which is the active metabolite. Metabolism to ara-U (inactive) is primary route of elimination.
Excretion: ara-U is excreted in the urine. Biphasic elimination; terminal t½ is 100 to 263 hr (12.5 to 75 mg).
Indications
Adult: Lymphomatous meningitis.
Contraindications Active meningeal infection hypersensitivity to cytarabine or any other ingredient in the formulation.
Route/Dosage
LIPOSOMAL CYTARABINE DOSE
The dose of liposomal cytarabine is different from the dose of conventional cytarabine.
Induction Therapy
ADULTS: **Intrathecally** 50 mg q 14 days for 2 doses, during weeks 1 and 3.
Consolidation Therapy
ADULTS: **Intrathecally** 50 mg q 14 days for 3 doses, during weeks 5, 7, and 9. Then, give an additional 50 mg dose during week 13.
Maintenance Regimen
ADULTS: **Intrathecally** 50 mg q 28 days for 4 doses, during weeks 17, 21, 25, and 29.
Dosage Adjustment for Neurologic Toxicity
ADULTS: **Intrathecally** If neurologic toxicity occurs, reduce the dose to 25 mg. Discontinue if toxicity persists.

Pretreatment Regimen
ADULTS: **Intrathecally** To reduce the incidence of chemical arachnoiditis, treat all patients with 4 mg dexamethasone orally or IV twice daily for 5 days starting the day of liposomal cytarabine administration. Inject via an intraventricular reservoir or directly into the lumbar sac. The patient should lie flat for at least 1 hr after the injection. Do not use in-line filters.
Interactions
Antineoplastics: Coadministration may increase the risk of neurotoxicity.
Gentamicin: Gentamicin effectiveness against *Klebsiella pneumoniae* strains may be decreased.
Lab Test Interferences Because liposomal cytarabine particles are similar in size and appearance to white blood cells, take care in interpreting CSF examinations following liposomal cytarabine administration.
Adverse Reactions
CNS: Headache; asthenia; confusion; somnolence; Transient elevations in CSF protein and WBC; encephalopathy; gait disturbance; neurotoxicity; meningismus; paresthesia.
GI: Nausea; vomiting; constipation.
HEMA: Neutropenia; thrombocytopenia.
MUSC: Myelopathy; back pain; pain.
OTHER: Chemical arachnoiditis syndrome; nausea; vomiting; headache; fever; neck rigidity; neck pain; meningismus; back pain; CSF pleocytosis.
Precautions
Pregnancy: Category D.
Children: Safety and efficacy have not ben established.
Hypersensitivity: Cases of anaphylaxis have occurred resulting in acute cardiopulmonary arrest which required resuscitation. This occurred immediately after IV administration.
Renal function impairment: Patients with renal function impairment may have a higher likelihood of CNS toxicity after high-dose cytarabine. Use the drug with caution and possibly at reduced doses in patients with poor kidney function.
Hepatic function impairment: Patients with hepatic function impairment may have a higher likelihood of CNS toxicity after high-dose

cytarabine. Use the drug with caution and possibly at reduced doses in patients with poor kidney function.

Chemical arachnoiditis: A syndrome manifested primarily by nausea, vomiting, headache, and fever has been a common adverse event in all studies. If left untreated, chemical arachnoiditis may be fatal. The incidence and severity of chemical arachnoiditis can be reduced by coadministration of dexamethasone.

CSF examination interpretation: Liposomal cytarabine particles and white blood cells are similar in appearance and size. Use caution when interpreting CSF examinations after administration of liposomal cytarabine.

Extravasation risk: Liposomal cytarabine is an irritant and can cause local irritation or phlebitis. Refer to your institution specific protocol.

Infection: Viral, bacterial, fungal, parasitic, or saprophytic infections in any location in the body may be associated with the use of cytarabine alone or in combination with other immunosuppressive agents.

Intrathecal use: If used intrathecally, do not use a diluent with benzyl alcohol.

Myelosuppression/Hematologic: Anemia, leukopenia, thrombocytopenia, megaloblastosis, and reduced reticulocytes can be expected. The severity of these reactions is dose- and schedule-dependent.

Neuropathies: Peripheral motor and sensory neuropathies have occurred.

Neurotoxicity: Enhanced neurotoxicity has been associated with concurrent use of intrathecal cytarabine and other cytotoxic agents administered intrathecally.

PATIENT CARE CONSIDERATIONS

Administration/Storage
- Refrigerate unopened vials; do not freeze. Avoid shaking vials vigorously. Unopened vials are stable at room temperature for up to 72 hr.
- Warm the vial to room temperature. Gently swirl or invert the vial to suspend the particles.
- Do not dilute.
- Liposomal cytarabine is preservative-free. Use the suspension within 4 hr after removing it from the vial.
- Administer by intrathecal injection over 1 to 5 min.

Assessment/Interventions
- Monitor neurologic function at baseline and periodically throughout treatment.
- During induction therapy, perform leukocyte and platelet counts daily. Perform bone marrow examinations frequently after blasts have disappeared from the peripheral blood.
- Suspend or modify therapy when drug-induced marrow depression results in a platelet count less than $50,000/mm^3$ or a polymorphonuclear granulocyte count less than $1000/mm^3$.
- Perform periodic checks of bone marrow, liver, and kidney functions.
- Observe patients in high-dose cytarabine for neuropathy.

Patient/Family Education
- Inform patients about the expected adverse events of headache, nausea, vomiting and fever, and about the early signs and symptoms of neurotoxicity.
- Emphasize the importance of dexamethasone coadministration at the initiation of each cycle of liposomal cytarabine treatment. Instruct patients to seek medical attention if signs or symptoms of neurotoxicity develop, or if oral dexamethasone is not well tolerated.

Dacarbazine

(da-CAR-buh-zeen)

Class Alkylating agent/Triazine

How Supplied
DTIC-Dome Powder for injection 100 mg, Powder for injection 200 mg

Action

PHARMACOLOGY: Exact mechanism is unknown. Three mechanisms are hypothesized: 1) inhibition of DNA synthesis by acting as a purine analog; 2) action as an alkylating agent; and 3) interaction with sulfhydryl groups.

PHARMACOKINETICS/DYNAMICS:
Distribution: Vd exceeds total body water content, suggesting localization in some body tissue, probably liver. Not appreciably bound to proteins.
Metabolism: Extensive major metabolite is 5-amino-imidazole-4 carboxamide.
Excretion: Biphasic, initial t½ is 19 min and terminal t½ is 5 hr; 40% excreted unchanged in urine in 6 hr.

Special Populations:
Hepatic Function Impairment – Initial t½ increased to 55 min and terminal t½ increased to 7.2 hr in a patient with renal and hepatic impairment.

Indications Treatment of metastatic malignant melanoma; in combination with other agents as second-line therapy for Hodgkin disease. **Unlabeled use(s):** In combination with cyclophosphamide and vincristine for malignant pheochromocytoma; in combination with other agents for treatment of advanced metastatic soft tissue sarcoma; alone or in combination with other agents for management of Kaposi sarcoma.

Contraindications Standard considerations.

Route/Dosage

Malignant Melanoma
ADULTS: **IV** 2 to 4.5 mg/kg/day for 10 days is recommended; may be repeated at 4 wk intervals. Alternatively, administer 250 mg/m^2 daily for 5 days; may be repeated q 3 wk.

Hodgkin Disease
ADULTS: **IV** 150 mg/m^2 daily for 5 days in combination with other effective drugs is recommended; may be repeated q 4 wk. Alternatively, 375 mg/m^2 on day 1 in combination with other effective drugs, repeated q 15 days.

Interactions None well documented.

Lab Test Interferences None well documented.

Adverse Reactions

DERM: Alopecia; facial flushing; erythematous and urticarial rashes.
GI: Anorexia, nausea, vomiting (over 90% with initial few doses).
HEMA: Bone marrow suppression.
LABTESTABS: Abnormal liver or renal function tests.
MUSC: Myalgia.
OTHER: Flu-like syndrome; malaise; facial paresthesia.

> WARNING:
> Administer under supervision of a qualified physician experienced in use of cancer chemotherapeutic agents; hemopoietic depression is most common toxicity; hepatic necrosis has been reported; carcinogenic and teratogenic effects demonstrated in animals; weigh possibility of achieving therapeutic benefit against risk of toxicity when treating patient.

Precautions

Pregnancy: Category C.
Lactation: Undetermined.
Hemopoietic depression: Hemopoietic depression is the most common toxicity and involves primarily leukocytes and platelets, although anemia sometimes occurs. Leukopenia and thrombocytopenia may be severe enough to cause death. Possible bone marrow suppression requires careful monitoring of RBC, WBC, and platelets.
Hepatotoxicity: Hepatotoxicity, accompanied by hepatic vein thrombosis and hepatocellular necrosis resulting in death, may occur.

Overdosage: Signs and Symptoms
Bone marrow suppression.

PATIENT CARE CONSIDERATIONS

Administration/Storage

- For IV administration only. Not for intradermal, subcutaneous, IM, intra-arterial, or oral administration.
- Dose and frequency of administration vary with condition being treated and clinical situation.
- Follow institutional and NIH procedures for handling, administration, and disposal of anticancer drugs.
- Reconstitute 100 mg vial with 9.9 mL sterile water for injection. Reconstitute 200 mg vial with 19.7 mL sterile water for injection.

Resulting solution contains 10 mg/mL of dacarbazine.
- Reconstituted solution may be further diluted with 5% dextrose injection or sodium chloride injection for administration as an IV infusion.
- Do not administer if particulate matter, cloudiness, or discoloration is noted.
- To reduce GI side effects, restrict the patient's food intake for 4 to 6 hr prior to treatment if possible.
- Store unopened vials in refrigerator (36° to 46°F). Protect from light. Store reconstituted solution in vial at 39.2°F for up to 72 hr or at normal room conditions for up to 8 hr. If reconstituted solution is further diluted with 5% dextrose injection or sodium chloride injection, store diluted solution at 39.3°F for up to 24 hr or at normal room conditions for up to 8 hr.

Assessment/Interventions
- Obtain patient history, including drug history and any known allergies.
- Ensure that CBC with differential and platelet count is evaluated before starting therapy and then frequently during therapy.
- Implement infection control measures if WBC drops; implement bleeding precautions if platelet count drops.
- Monitor patient for signs of anaphylactic or serious allergic reactions. Discontinue therapy and immediately notify health care provider if noted. Be prepared to treat appropriately.
- Assess injection site frequently for signs or symptoms of extravasation (eg, burning, pain, induration). Discontinue infusion immediately if suspected and notify health care provider. Be prepared to apply hot packs to minimize local reaction.
- Monitor patient for GI, DERM, and general body side effects. Report to health care provider if noted and significant. Consider using phenobarbital and/or prochlorperazine for recurrent or prolonged vomiting.
- Monitor patient for signs and symptoms of bacterial, viral, or fungal infection. Report to health care provider immediately if noted.

Patient/Family Education
- Explain name, action, and potential side effects of drug.
- Advise patient, family, or caregiver that medication will be prepared and administered by health care providers in a health care setting.
- Advise patient, family, or caregiver that medication may be used in combination with other agents, including antiemetics and sedatives, to achieve max benefit possible.
- Advise patient, family, or caregiver that restricting food intake for 4 to 6 hr before treatment may help reduce nausea and vomiting.
- Advise patient, family, or caregiver to immediately report any of the following to health care provider: rash; hives; difficulty breathing; fever, chills, or other signs of infection; unusual bleeding or bruising; pain, redness, or swelling at injection site.
- Advise patient, family, or caregiver to report any of the following to health care provider: persistent nausea, vomiting, diarrhea, or appetite loss; persistent or worsening general body weakness.
- Advise patient, family, or caregiver that hair loss is a common side effect of therapy, but that this is usually reversible after therapy has been completed.
- Instruct patient not to take any prescription or OTC medications, herbal preparations, or dietary supplements unless advised by health care provider.
- Caution women of childbearing potential to avoid becoming pregnant during therapy.
- Advise women to notify health care provider if pregnant, planning to become pregnant, or breastfeeding.
- Advise patient, family, or caregiver that frequent follow-up visits and laboratory tests will be required to monitor therapy and to keep appointments.

Daclizumab

(da-KLIZ-uh-mab)
Class Immunosuppressive
How Supplied
Zenapax Injection 25 mg per 5 mL
Action
PHARMACOLOGY: Binds with high-affinity to the Tac subunit of the high-affinity interleukin-2 (IL-2) complex and inhibits IL-2 binding, thereby impairing the response of the immune system to antigenic challenges.

PHARMACOKINETICS/DYNAMICS: At recommended doses, the Tac subunit of the IL-2 receptor is saturated for about 90 and 120 days posttransplant in pediatric and adult patients, respectively.

Indications Prophylaxis of acute organ rejection in patients receiving renal transplants.
Contraindications Standard considerations.

Route/Dosage
ADULTS AND CHILDREN 11 MO OF AGE AND OLDER: **IV** 1 mg/kg for 5 doses as part of an immunosuppressive regimen that contains cyclosporine and corticosteroids. Give the first dose no more than 24 hr before transplantation and the remaining 4 doses at intervals of 14 days.

Interactions None well documented.

Lab Test Interferences None well documented.

Adverse Reactions The safety of daclizumab was determined in patients receiving concomitant cyclosporine and corticosteroids.
CV: Hypertension, hypotension, aggravated hypertension, tachycardia (at least 5%).
CNS: Tremor, headache, dizziness, insomnia (at least 5%); depression, anxiety (2% to less than 5%).
DERM: Impaired wound healing without infection, acne (at least 5%); pruritus, hirsutism, rash, night sweats, increased sweating, application site reaction (2% to less than 5%).
EENT: Pharyngitis, rhinitis, blurred vision (2% to less than 5%).
GI: Constipation, nausea, diarrhea, vomiting, abdominal pain, pyrosis, dyspepsia, abdominal distention, epigastric pain (at least 5%); flatulence, gastritis, hemorrhoids (2% to less than 5%).
GU: Oliguria, dysuria, renal tubular necrosis (at least 5%); renal damage, hydronephrosis, urinary tract bleeding, urinary tract disorder, renal insufficiency, urinary retention (2% to less than 5%).
HEMA/LYMPH: thrombosis, bleeding, lymphocele (at least 5%).
M/N: Edema of the extremities, edema (at least 5%); fluid overload, diabetes mellitus, dehydration (2% to less than 5%).
MUSC: Muscular pain, back pain (at least 5%); leg cramps, arthralgia, myalgia (2% to less than 5%).
RESP: Dyspnea, pulmonary edema, coughing (at least 5%); atelectasis, congestion, hypoxia, rales, abnormal breath sounds, pleural effusion (2% to less than 5%).
OTHER: Posttraumatic pain, chest pain, fever, pain, fatigue (at least 5%); shivering, generalized weakness, prickly sensation (2% to less than 5%).

> **WARNING:**
> Only physicians experienced with immunosuppressive therapy and management of organ transplant patients should prescribe daclizumab. Daclizumab should be given by health care personnel trained in the administration of the drug and who have available laboratory and supportive medical resources.

Precautions
Pregnancy: Category C.
Lactation: Undetermined.
Children: Safety and efficacy not established in children younger than 11 mo of age.
Elderly: Use with caution.
Hypersensitivity: Anaphylactic reactions can occur.
Immune system: It is not known if there will be a long-term effect on the ability of the immune system to respond to antigens first encountered during daclizumab-induced immunosuppression.

PATIENT CARE CONSIDERATIONS
Administration/Storage
- Administer in combination with immunosuppressive regimen that includes cyclosporine and corticosteroids.
- Concentrate must be diluted before administering to patient.
- For IV infusion only. Not for IV bolus, intradermal, subcutaneous, IM, or intra-arterial administration.
- Add prescribed amount of concentrate to 50 mL sterile 0.9% sodium chloride injection. Mix by gently inverting IV bag to avoid foaming. Do not shake.
- Discard any remaining concentrate in vial. Do not save unused concentrate for later use.
- Do not administer if solution is discolored, cloudy, or if particulate matter is noted.
- Administer infusion solution within 4 hr of preparation or within 24 hr if stored in refrigerator.
- Administer prescribed dose by IV infusion over 15 minutes. Dose is usually repeated q 14 days for total of 5 doses.
- Do not mix with other IV substances or additives or infuse simultaneously through the same IV line. If the same IV line is used for sequential infusion of different medications, flush line with saline solution.
- Store unopened vials in refrigerator (36° to 46°F). Do not freeze or shake. Protect from direct light. Diluted infusion solution is stable for 4 hr at room temperature or for 24 hr if refrigerated.

Assessment/Interventions
- Obtain patient history, including drug history and any known allergies.
- Ensure that women of childbearing potential use effective contraception before beginning therapy, during therapy, and for 4 mo following completion of daclizumab therapy.

- Monitor patient for signs of allergic reaction. Discontinue therapy and immediately notify health care provider if noted. Be prepared to treat serious allergic events appropriately.
- Monitor patient for signs and symptoms of bacterial, viral, or fungal infection. Report to health care provider immediately if noted or suspected.
- Monitor patient for GI, CNS, CV, RESP, DERM, GU, and general body side effects. Report to health care provider if noted and significant.

Patient/Family Education
- Explain name, action, and potential side effects of drug.
- Advise patient, family, or caregiver that medication will be prepared and administered by health care provider in a health care setting with close monitoring.
- Review dosing schedule with patient, family, or caregiver.
- Advise patient, family, or caregiver that medication will be used in combination with other agents, including cyclosporine and corticosteroids, to achieve max benefit possible.
- Instruct patient to continue to take other medications prescribed for preventing organ transplant rejection.
- Instruct patient to seek medical attention if any of the following occur: skin rash; hives; rapid heart beat; difficulty breathing; unexplained shortness of breath; fever, chills, or other signs of infection.
- Advise patient to notify health care provider if bothersome side effects occur.
- Caution patient that medication may cause dizziness or blurred vision and to use caution when driving or performing other tasks that require mental alertness, coordination, or physical dexterity until tolerance is determined.
- Caution women of childbearing potential to use effective contraception before starting therapy, during therapy, and for 4 mo following completion of treatment with daclizumab.
- Advise women to notify health care provider if pregnant, planning to become pregnant, or breastfeeding.
- Caution patient not to take any prescription or OTC medications, herbal preparations, or dietary supplements unless advised by health care provider.
- Advise patient, family, or caregiver that frequent follow-up visits and laboratory tests will be required to monitor therapy and to keep appointments.

Dactinomycin

(DAK-tih-no-MY-sin)

Class Antineoplastic antibiotic

How Supplied
Cosmegen Lyophilized powder for reconstitution 500 mcg vial with 20 mg of mannitol.

Action

PHARMACOLOGY: Dactinomycin is the principal component of the mixture of actinomycins produced by *Streptomyces parvullus*. It inhibits messenger RNA synthesis.

PHARMACOKINETICS/DYNAMICS:
Distribution: Concentrated in nucleated cells. Does not penetrate blood-brain barrier.
Metabolism: Minimally metabolized.
Excretion: Approximately 30% recovered in urine and feces in 1 wk; t½ approximately 36 hr.

Indications Treatment of Wilms tumor, childhood rhabdomyosarcoma, Ewings sarcoma, and metastatic nonseminomatous testicular cancer as part of combination chemotherapy and/or multimodality treatment regimen; palliative and/or adjunctive treatment of locally recurrent or locoregional solid malignancies as a component of regional perfusion; treatment of gestational trophoblastic neoplasia as a single agent or as part of a combination chemotherapy regimen.

Contraindications If given at or about the time of infection with chicken pox or herpes zoster, a severe generalized disease may occur, which could result in death.

Route/Dosage

ADULTS AND CHILDREN: IV The dosage varies depending on the tolerance of the patient, the size and location of the neoplasm, and the use of other forms of therapy. The dose intensity per 2-wk cycle for adults and children should not exceed 15 mcg/kg/day or 400 to 600 mcg/m^2/day for 5 days. Calculate the dosage for obese or edematous patients on the basis of surface area to more closely relate dosage to lean body mass.

Interactions No specific drug interactions reported.

Lab Test Interferences Bioassay procedures for the determination of antibacterial drug levels.

Adverse Reactions
CNS: Fatigue; lethargy; malaise.
DERM: Acne; alopecia; edema; epidermolysis; erythema; extravasation; flare-up of erythema; skin eruptions; increased pigmentation of previously irradiated skin.
EENT: Pharyngitis.

GI: Abdominal pain; anorexia; cheilitis; diarrhea; dysphagia; esophagitis; GI ulceration; nausea; ulcerative stomatitis; vomiting.
GU: Proctitis.
HEMA/LYMPH: Agranulocytosis; anemia; aplastic anemia; leukopenia; pancytopenia; reticulocytopenia; thrombocytopenia.
HEPA: Hepatomegaly; hepatic veno-occlusive disease; hepatitis; abnormal LFTs; liver toxicity including ascites.
LABTESTABS: Hypercalcemia.
METAB: Growth retardation.
MUSC: Myalgia.
RESP: Pneumonitis.
OTHER: Fever; infection.

> **WARNING:**
> Dactinomycin is extremely corrosive to soft tissue. If extravasation occurs during IV use, severe damage to soft tissues will occur. In at least one instance, this has led to contracture of the arms. Avoid use in pregnancy. Dactinomycin is also carcinogenic, mutagenic, and teratogenic.

Precautions
Pregnancy: Category D.
Lactation: Undetermined.
Children: Toxicity is increased in infants. Avoid use in infants younger than 6 to 12 mo of age.
Elderly: Use with caution because of the greater frequency of decreased hepatic, renal, or cardiac function, and concomitant diseases or other drug therapy.
Chicken pox or herpes zoster: Do not give at or about the time of infection with chicken pox or herpes zoster; severe generalized disease may occur.
GI toxicity and marrow suppression: Increased incidence.
Radiation: With combined dactinomycin-radiation therapy, the normal skin, as well as the buccal and pharyngeal mucosa, may show early erythema. A smaller than usual x-ray dose, when given with dactinomycin, causes erythema and vesiculation, which progress more rapidly through the tanning and desquamation stages. Erythema from previous x-ray therapy may be reactivated by dactinomycin alone, even when irradiation occurred many months earlier, and especially when the interval between the 2 forms of therapy is brief. When the nasopharynx is irradiated, the combination may produce severe oropharyngeal mucositis. Severe reactions may appear if high doses are used or if the patient is particularly sensitive to such combined therapy.
Second primary tumors: Increased incidence.

PATIENT CARE CONSIDERATIONS
Administration/Storage
- May be used alone or in combination with other chemotherapeutic agents and/or radiotherapy.
- For IV or regional perfusion only. Not for intradermal, subcutaneous, IM, intra-arterial, or oral administration.
- Dose, frequency of administration, and duration of therapy vary with condition being treated, tolerance of the patient, size and location of the neoplasm, and the use of other forms of therapy.
- Dosage schedules and perfusion techniques vary for regional perfusion of locally recurrent and locoregional solid malignancies.
- Dactinomycin is highly toxic. Handle and administer powder and reconstituted solution with extreme care. Diligently follow institutional and NIH procedures for handling, administration, and disposal of anticancer drugs. Wear appropriate protective equipment when preparing and administering dactinomycin. Avoid inhalation of dust or vapors and contact with skin, mucus membranes, and eyes.
- If accidental skin or mucus membrane contact occurs, immediately irrigate affected area with copious amounts of water for at least 15 minutes while removing contaminated clothing and shoes. Seek medical attention immediately. Destroy contaminated clothing and thoroughly clean shoes before reuse.
- If accidental eye contact occurs, immediately institute irrigation with copious amounts of water, normal saline or a balanced salt ophthalmic irrigating solution for at least 15 minutes. Prompt ophthalmic evaluation should follow irrigation.
- Reconstitute powder for injection with 1.1 mL sterile water for injection (without preservative). Mix thoroughly to obtain complete dissolution. Resulting solution contains 500 mcg/mL (0.5 mg/mL) of dactinomycin.
- Do not reconstitute powder for injection using diluents with preservatives that can cause precipitation of dactinomycin.
- Do not administer if particulate matter or cloudiness is noted. Reconstituted solution should be a clear, golden-colored solution.
- Add prescribed dose or reconstituted solution directly to infusion solution of 5% dextrose or sodium chloride injection or to the tubing of a running IV infusion.
- If medication is to be given directly into a vein without the use of an infusion, use the "2-needle technique" to reduce risk of tissue

damage. Reconstitute and withdraw the calculated dose from the vial with one sterile needle. Use another sterile needle for direct injection into the vein.
- Do not use inline filters made of cellulose which can remove dactinomycin.
- Store powder for injection at room temperature (59° to 86°F). Protect from light and humidity. Dactinomycin is stable after reconstitution but does not contain a preservative. Use reconstituted solution as soon as possible. Discard any unused solution. Do not save any unused solution for future use.

Assessment/Interventions

- Obtain patient history, including drug history and any known allergies. Note current or recent infection with chicken pox or herpes zoster, and previous radiation therapy.
- Ensure women of childbearing potential are not pregnant before starting therapy and use effective contraception during treatment.
- Ensure liver function (ie, transaminases, bilirubin) and renal function (ie, Scr, BUN) are evaluated before starting therapy and frequently thereafter during treatment. Notify health care provider if abnormalities develop.
- Note that toxic effects (with exception of nausea and vomiting) usually do not become apparent until 2 to 4 days after a course of therapy is stopped, and may not peak until 1 to 2 wk have elapsed.
- Ensure CBC with differential and platelet count are evaluated daily. Notify health care provider immediately if neutropenia and/or thrombocytopenia develops. Be prepared to withhold therapy until bone marrow recovery occurs, which may take up to 3 wk.
- Monitor patient for signs or symptoms of infection or bleeding. Inform health care provider immediately if noted and be prepared to treat appropriately (eg, IV antibiotics, colony stimulating factors, transfusions).
- Monitor patient closely for toxic side effects of therapy, especially when multiple chemotherapy is being used. Inform health care provider if stomatitis, nausea, vomiting, or diarrhea develop. Be prepared to withhold therapy until patient has recovered.
- Monitor patient for signs of anaphylactic or serious allergic reactions. Discontinue therapy and immediately notify health care provider if noted. Be prepared to treat appropriately.
- Monitor IV injection site for signs or symptoms of extravasation. If noted, immediately discontinue infusion and restart in another vein. Be prepared to treat extravasation site with intermittent ice packs (15 minutes qid for 3 days) and extremity elevation. Frequently examine extravasation site and immediately inform health care provider if pain, erythema, edema, or vesiculation is noted or if patient reports persistent pain.
- Monitor patient for GI, DERM, and general body side effects, and injection site reactions. Report to health care provider if noted and significant.

Patient/Family Education

- Explain name, action, and potential side effects of the treatment regimen. Review the treatment regimen including dosing schedule, duration of treatment, and monitoring that will be required.
- Review benefits of therapy and risks, including reactivation of erythema from previous radiation therapy, and potential of developing secondary primary tumors.
- Advise patient, family, or caregiver that medication will be prepared and administered by health care professionals in a health care setting.
- Advise patient, family, or caregiver that medication may be used in combination with other agents to achieve max benefit possible.
- Advise patient, family, or caregiver that medication may cause hair loss but that this is reversible when therapy is stopped.
- Advise patient, family, or caregiver to immediately report any of the following to health care provider: rash; hives; difficulty breathing or unexplained shortness of breath; fever, chills, or other signs of infection; sores in mouth; pain, redness, or swelling at injection site.
- Advise patient, family, or caregiver to report any of the following to health care provider: persistent nausea, vomiting, or appetite loss; persistent or worsening general body weakness; skin changes; nail changes.
- Instruct patient not to take any prescription or OTC medications, herbal preparations, or dietary supplements unless advised by health care provider.
- Caution women of childbearing potential to avoid becoming pregnant during therapy.
- Advise women to notify health care provider if pregnant, planning to become pregnant, or breastfeeding.
- Advise patient that frequent follow-up visits and laboratory tests will be required to monitor therapy and to keep appointments.

Dalteparin Sodium

(dal-TEH-puh-rin SO-dee-uhm)

Class Anticoagulant

How Supplied
Fragmin Injection 2500 IU (16 mg/0.2 mL), Injection 5000 IU (32 mg/0.2 mL), Injection 10,000 IU (64 mg/mL)

Action
PHARMACOLOGY: Inhibits reactions that lead to clotting.

PHARMACOKINETICS/DYNAMICS:
Absorption: Bioavailability is approximately 87%.
T_{max} is approximately 4 hr.
Distribution: Vd is 40 to 60 mL/kg.
Excretion:
SC – t½ is 3 to 5 hr.

Indications Prophylaxis of deep vein thrombosis (DVT), which may lead to pulmonary embolism, in patients undergoing hip replacement surgery or in patients undergoing abdominal surgery who are at risk for thromboembolic complications; prophylaxis of ischemic complications in unstable angina and non-Q-wave MI in patients on aspirin therapy.

Contraindications Active major bleeding, thrombocytopenia, hypersensitivity to heparin or pork products; patients undergoing regional anesthesia for unstable angina or non-Q-wave MI.

Route/Dosage

DVT Prophylaxis (Abdominal Surgery)
ADULTS: SC 2500 units starting 1 to 2 hr before surgery and continuing qd for 5 to 10 days. Do not give IM.

DVT Prophylaxis (Hip Replacement Surgery)
ADULTS: SC If started postoperatively, 2500 units within 4 to 8 hr after surgery, followed by 5000 units/day for 5 to 10 days; if started preoperatively on day of surgery, 2500 units within 2 hr before surgery, followed by 2500 units 4 to 8 hr after surgery and continued at 5000 units/day for 5 to 10 days; if started preoperatively on the evening before surgery, 5000 units 10 to 14 hr before surgery, followed by 5000 units 4 to 8 hr after surgery and continued at 5000 units/day for 5 to 10 days.

Unstable Angina/Non-Q-Wave MI
ADULTS: SC 120 units/kg of body weight (max, 10,000 units) q 12 hr with aspirin (75 to 165 mg/day, unless contraindicated) therapy. Continue treatment until patient is clinically stabilized, usually 5 to 8 days.

Interactions
Anticoagulants; platelet inhibitors: Increased risk of bleeding.

Lab Test Interferences
Aminotransferase (AST and ALT): Drug caused increased concentrations.

Adverse Reactions
HEMA: Thrombocytopenia; hematoma; bleeding.
HEPA: Serum transaminase elevation rarely associated with increased bilirubin.
OTHER: Injection site pain/hematoma; allergic reactions (eg, pruritus, rash, fever); skin necrosis; anaphylactoid reactions.

> WARNING:
> *Spinal/Epidural hematomas:* Risk of spinal/epidural hematoma increased in patients receiving neuraxial anesthesia or spinal puncture and are anticoagulated with LMWH or heparinoids. Other risk factors include indwelling epidural catheters, repeated/traumatic epidural/spinal puncture, or other drugs affecting hemostasis (eg, NSAIDs, platelet inhibitors, anticoagulants). Risk of long-term or permanent paralysis. Frequently monitor for signs or symptoms of neurological impairment.

Precautions
Pregnancy: Category B.
Lactation: Undetermined.
Children: Safety and efficacy not established.
Thrombocytopenia: Use very cautiously in patients with history of heparin-induced thrombocytopenia.
Interchangeability with heparin: Cannot be exchanged on a unit per unit basis with other types of heparin.
Bleeding risk: Avoid use in patients at risk for bleeding (eg, severe hypertension, severe liver or kidney disease, platelet defects, recent GI bleeding) or shortly after brain, spinal, or ophthalmological surgery.
Benzyl alcohol: The multiple-dose vial of dalteparin contains benzyl alcohol as a preservative, which has been associated with fatal "gasping syndrome" in premature infants.

Overdosage: Signs and Symptoms
Hemorrhagic complications.

PATIENT CARE CONSIDERATIONS

Administration/Storage
- Do not mix with other injections or infusions until compatibility is determined.
- Do not administer by IM injection.
- Inspect all preparations for particulate matter prior to administration.
- Vary injection site daily.
- Store at room temperature.

Assessment/Interventions
- Obtain patient history.
- Assess for signs of bleeding or bruising.
- Assess patient for signs of renal or hepatic insufficiency.
- During the course of treatment, monitor complete blood counts, including platelet count and stool occult blood tests.

Patient/Family Education
- Instruct patient to report any signs of bleeding immediately.

Danazol

(DAN-uh-ZOLE)

Class Hormone

How Supplied
Danocrine Capsules 50 mg, Capsules 100 mg, Capsules 200 mg
✤ *Cyclomen*

Action
PHARMACOLOGY: Suppresses pituitary-ovarian axis by inhibiting output of pituitary gonadotropins; has weak, dose-related androgenic activity with no estrogenic or progestational activity.

PHARMACOKINETICS/DYNAMICS:
Absorption: Extent of availability and C_{max} increase 3- to 4-fold, respectively, following food. T_{max} delayed by 30 min after food.

Indications
Treatment of endometriosis; symptomatic treatment of fibrocystic breast disease; prevention of attacks of hereditary angioedema. **Unlabeled use(s):** Treatment of precocious puberty, gynecomastia, and menorrhagia; treatment of idiopathic immune thrombocytopenia, lupus-associated thrombocytopenia, and autoimmune hemolytic anemia.

Contraindications
Pregnancy; lactation; undiagnosed abnormal genital bleeding; markedly impaired hepatic, renal, or cardiac function.

Route/Dosage

Endometriosis
ADULTS: PO 800 mg/day in 2 divided doses.

Fibrocystic Breast Disease
ADULTS: PO 100 to 400 mg/day in 2 divided doses.

Hereditary Angioedema
ADULTS: PO 200 mg bid to tid.

Interactions
Anticoagulants: May increase anticoagulant effects.
Carbamazepine: May increase carbamazepine concentration.
Cyclosporine: May increase cyclosporine levels, thus increasing risk of nephrotoxicity.
Insulin: Diabetic patients may need increased insulin doses.

Lab Test Interferences May interfere with tests for determination of testosterone, androstenedione, and dehydroepiandrosterone levels.

Adverse Reactions
DERM: Acne; mild hirsutism; oily skin or hair.
GI: Gastroenteritis.
HEPA: Jaundice; elevated LFT results; hepatic dysfunction.
OTHER: Edema; decreased breast size; deepening of voice; weight gain; flushing; sweating; vaginitis; nervousness; emotional lability; amenorrhea; anovulation; breakthrough bleeding.

> **WARNING:**
>
> *Pregnancy:* Contraindicated in pregnancy. Negative pregnancy test must be obtained immediately prior to therapy. Nonhormonal method of contraception is recommended during therapy.
>
> *Intracranial hypertension:* Benign intracranial hypertension (Pseudotumor cerebri) has been reported. Screen for early signs of intracranial hypertension (eg, headache, nausea, vomiting, visual disturbances).
>
> *Peliosis hepatitis and benign hepatic adenoma:* Peliosis hepatitis and benign hepatic adenoma have been observed with long-term use.
>
> *Thromboembolism and thrombotic events:* Thromboembolism and thrombotic events have been reported, including life-threatening or fatal strokes.

Precautions
Pregnancy: Category X.
Lactation: Drug contraindicated in nursing women.
Children: Safety and efficacy not established.
Hepatic function impairment: Hepatic dysfunc-

tion may occur; observe patient; monitor LFTs periodically.
Androgenic effects: May not be reversible even when drug is discontinued.
Carcinoma of breast: Exclude before treatment of fibrocystic breast disease.
Fluid retention: Carefully observe patients who cannot tolerate edema (eg, those with epilepsy, cardiac/renal dysfunction, migraine).
Long-term experience: Limited. Similar drugs have been associated with serious toxicity (eg, cholestatic jaundice, peliosis hepatitis). Use lowest effective dose and consider decreasing dose or withdrawing therapy periodically.

PATIENT CARE CONSIDERATIONS

Administration/Storage
- Initiate therapy during menstruation or after negative pregnancy test result.
- Give medication with food or milk to minimize GI irritation.
- When treating endometriosis, titrate dosage down to lowest dose sufficient to maintain amenorrhea and therapeutic response.
- Store drug in closed, light-resistant container at room temperature.

Assessment/Interventions
- Obtain patient history, including drug history and any known allergies.
- Review pregnancy test results to be certain that pregnancy has been ruled out before starting drug therapy.
- Perform CBC and serum electrolytes before drug therapy is initiated.
- Monitor patient closely for masculinizing effects and changes in sexuality pattern.
- Monitor patient for signs of liver dysfunction (eg, LFT changes, jaundice, nausea, vomiting, dark amber urine).
- Monitor patient's mental status for the following: mood or behavioral changes, aggression, sleep disturbances, depression.
- Check semen for volume, viscosity, sperm count, and motility q 3 to 4 mo.
- Perform ongoing assessment of patient's fluid balance (eg, I&O, daily weight). Note edema or weight gain more than 2 lb/wk. Report findings to health care provider.
- Observe for signs of hypercalcemia: GI symptoms, polydipsia, polyuria, increased calcium levels, decreased muscle tone.

Patient/Family Education
- Caution patient that this medication must not be taken during pregnancy or when pregnancy is possible. Advise patient to use reliable form of birth control while taking this drug.
- Remind patient to take medication with food or milk to minimize GI upset.
- Instruct patient to notify health care provider if masculinizing effects occur (eg, abnormal facial hair or other fine body hair growth, deepening of voice, acne, clitoral enlargement, testicular atrophy, decrease in breast size). Inform patient that most of these side effects will cease after drug is discontinued; however, some changes may be irreversible (eg, permanent voice changes have occurred because of structural changes in larynx).
- Inform patient to notify health care provider if change in libido occurs because this may indicate toxicity.
- Instruct patient to eat low-sodium diet to prevent fluid retention and to notify health care provider of any signs of edema.
- Advise women being treated for fibrocystic breast disease to notify health care provider of any nodule that persists or enlarges during treatment. Review proper technique for breast self-examination.
- Caution patient not to discontinue drug abruptly.
- Advise patient to notify health care provider of irregular menses. Explain that amenorrhea usually occurs but that menstruation usually resumes 2 to 3 mo after termination of therapy.
- Explain that drug-induced anovulation is reversible within 2 to 3 mo of discontinuation of therapy.

Dantrolene Sodium

(dan-troe-LEEN SO-dee-uhm)
Class Skeletal muscle relaxant/direct acting

How Supplied
Dantrium Capsules 25 mg, Capsules 50 mg, Capsules 100 mg ♦ *Dantrium Intravenous* Powder for Injection 20 mg/vial (approximately 0.32 mg/mL after reconstitution)

Action
PHARMACOLOGY: Affects contraction of muscle at site beyond myoneural junction and directly on muscle itself; believed to interfere with calcium release from sarcoplasmic reticulum. Affects CNS, causing drowsiness, dizziness, and generalized weakness.

Pharmacokinetics/Dynamics:

Absorption:
Oral – Absorption is incomplete and slow, but consistent.

Distribution: Significantly protein bound, mostly albumin.

Metabolism: Metabolized in the liver to the major metabolites 5-hydroxy dantrole and an acetylamino metabolite.

Excretion: t½ is 4 to 8 hr (IV), 9 hr (oral).

Indications Control of spasticity associated with spinal cord injury, stroke, cerebral palsy or multiple sclerosis; prophylaxis, treatment and postcrisis therapy of malignant hyperthermia.

Unlabeled use(s): Management of exercise-induced muscle pain, neuroleptic malignant syndrome, heat stroke.

Contraindications Active hepatic disease; muscle spasm resulting from rheumatic disorders; where spasticity is used to sustain upright posture and balance in locomotion or to obtain or maintain increased function.

Route/Dosage

Chronic Spasticity

ADULTS: **PO** Initial dose 25 mg q day; increase at 4 to 7 day intervals to 25 mg bid to qid, up to max 100 mg bid to qid if necessary.

CHILDREN: **PO** Initial dose 0.5 mg/kg bid; increase to 0.5 mg/kg tid to qid, then by increments of 0.5 mg/kg, up to 3 mg/kg bid to qid, if necessary. Max 100 mg qid.

Malignant Hyperthermia

ADULTS AND CHILDREN:

Preoperative prophylaxis: **PO** 4 to 8 mg/kg/day in 3 or 4 divided doses for 1 or 2 days prior to surgery with last dose given 3 to 4 hr before surgery or **IV** 2.5 mg/kg approximately 75 min before anesthesia. Infused over 1 hr. May repeat during surgery, if needed.

Treatment: **IV** 1 mg/kg by continuous rapid push; evaluate and repeat as needed until cumulative total dose is up to 10 mg/kg.

Postcrisis follow-up: **PO** 4 to 8 mg/kg/day in 4 divided doses for 1 to 3 days to prevent recurrence. If IV route must be utilized, start with at least 1 mg/kg, as needed.

Interactions

Clofibrate: Plasma protein binding of dantrolene reduced.

Estrogens: Women receiving these may be at increased risk for hepatotoxicity.

Verapamil: Hyperkalemia and myocardial depression possible.

Warfarin: Plasma protein binding of dantrolene reduced.

Lab Test Interferences None well documented.

Adverse Reactions Caused by oral administration except where otherwise indicated.

CV: Tachycardia; erratic BP; phlebitis.

CNS: Drowsiness; dizziness; weakness; general malaise; fatigue; speech disturbances; seizures; headache; lightheadedness; insomnia, mental depression or confusion; increased nervousness.

DERM: Abnormal hair growth; acne-like rash; pruritus; urticaria (IV); eczematoid eruption; sweating; erythema (IV).

EENT: Visual disturbance, diplopia, alteration of taste.

GI: Diarrhea; constipation; bleeding; anorexia; dysphagia; gastric irritation; abdominal cramps.

GU: Increased urinary frequency; hematuria; crystalluria; difficult erection; urinary incontinence; nocturia; dysuria; urinary retention.

HEPA: Hepatitis.

RESP: Pleural effusion with pericarditis; pulmonary edema (IV).

OTHER: Myalgia; backache; chills; fever; feeling of suffocation; excessive tearing; thrombophlebitis (IV).

> **WARNING:**
> Should not be used in conditions other than those recommended.
> *Hepatotoxicity:* The incidence of symptomatic (fatal and nonfatal) hepatitis is lower with doses up to 400 mg/day compared with 800 mg/day or greater. Overt hepatitis was most frequent during the third and twelfth mo but may occur at anytime. Risk is higher in females, patients older than 35 yr, and with concurrent therapy. Use only in conjunction with liver monitoring.

Precautions

Pregnancy: Category C (parenteral).

Lactation: Do not use in nursing women.

Children: Safety in children younger than 5 yr not established.

Hepatic function impairment: Fatal and nonfatal liver disorders may occur; use drug with caution in patients with pre-existing hepatic impairment and in women and patients older than 35 yr.

Special risk patients: Use drug with caution in patients with impaired pulmonary function (especially COPD) or cardiac function.

Photosensitivity: Photosensitization may occur.

Extravasation: Because of the high pH of the IV formulation, prevent extravasation into the surrounding tissue.

IV Dantrolene: IV dantrolene is also associated with the loss of grip strength and weakness in the legs.

Long-term use: Safety and efficacy not established; use only if significant pain or disability is present or nursing care is reduced. Consider carcinogenicity risk and liver damage with long-term use. Discontinue therapy if no benefit within 45 days.

PATIENT CARE CONSIDERATIONS
Administration/Storage
- Ensure good IV site using large peripheral vein; medication is very irritating to tissues.
- Reconstitute powder for IV infusion in 60 mL of sterile water without bacteriostatic agent.
- Shake until solution is clear.
- Store at room temperature for up to 6 hr. Protect from direct light.

Assessment/Interventions
- Obtain patient history, including drug history and any known allergies.
- Assess neuromuscular status before and during therapy.
- Assess family's anesthesia history. Ask specifically about crises or deaths in operating room.
- Assess for constipation, and auscultate bowel sounds regularly.
- Encourage patient to increase fluid and fiber intake during therapy.
- Keep emergency equipment nearby to treat respiratory depression.
- Measure and document intake and output.
- Monitor infusion site regularly for potential complications.
- If weakness or dizziness develops, keep side rails up and supervise ambulation.

Malignant hyperthermia: Supportive care should be foremost in treatment (ie, concurrent with dantrolene therapy).

- If difficulty swallowing develops, implement safety precautions with meals and medications.

Patient/Family Education
- Teach patient and family the name, action, administration, and side effects of dantrolene.
- Emphasize importance of follow-up exams and laboratory work to monitor drug therapy.
- Instruct patient to report these symptoms to health care provider: weakness, malaise, fatigue, nausea, diarrhea, skin rash, itching, bloody or black tarry stools, yellowish discoloration of skin.
- Instruct patient to avoid intake of alcoholic beverages or other CNS depressants.
- Advise patient that drug may cause drowsiness and to use caution while driving or performing other tasks requiring mental alertness.
- Caution patient to avoid exposure to sunlight and to use sunscreen or wear protective clothing to avoid photosensitivity reaction.
- Caution patient that dantrolene may decrease grip strength and increase weakness of leg muscles especially when walking down stairs.
- Advise patients to exercise caution in eating on day of administration because difficulty swallowing and choking is possible.

Dapsone

(DAP-sone)

Class Anti-infective/Leprostatic

How Supplied
Dapsone Tablets 25 mg, Tablets 100 mg

Action
PHARMACOLOGY: Mechanism of action is unknown; however, dapsone is bactericidal and bacteriostatic against *Mycobacterium leprae*.

PHARMACOKINETICS/DYNAMICS:

Absorption: Rapidly and nearly completely absorbed from the GI tract, reaching peak plasma concentrations in 4 to 8 hr. Administration of 200 mg/day for 8 days achieves plateau levels of 0.1 to 7 mcg/mL.

Distribution: Approximately 70% to 90% bound to plasma protein. The main metabolite, monoacetyl dapsone, is nearly 100% protein bound.

Metabolism: Dapsone is acetylated in the liver, the degree of which is genetically determined.

Excretion: The plasma t½ ranges from 10 to 50 hr. Approximately 70% to 85% is excreted in the urine as conjugates and unidentified metabolites. Enterohepatic circulation accounts for appreciable tissue levels 3 wk after discontinuation of therapy.

Indications Treatment of dermatitis herpetiformis; leprosy.

Contraindications Standard considerations.

Route/Dosage
Dermatitis Herpetiformis
ADULTS AND CHILDREN: PO Start with 50 mg/day in adults and correspondingly smaller doses in children. If full control is not achieved with 50 to 300 mg/day, higher doses may be tried. Reduce dose to minimum maintenance level as soon as possible. The time for dosage reduction is 8 mo (range 4 mo to 2½ yr) and for dosage elimination 29 mo (range 6 mo to 9 yr).

Leprosy
ADULTS AND CHILDREN: PO 100 mg/day in adults and correspondingly smaller doses in children without interruption in therapy with at least 1 antileprosy drug.

Interactions
Didanosine: Absorption of dapsone may be decreased, resulting in a loss of efficacy.
Trimethoprim: Plasma concentrations of both dapsone and trimethoprim may be elevated, increasing the pharmacologic and toxic effects.

Lab Test Interferences None well documented.

Adverse Reactions
CV: Tachycardia.
CNS: Peripheral neuropathy; motor loss; muscle weakness; insomnia; headache; psychosis.
EENT: Blurred vision; tinnitus.
GI: Nausea; vomiting; abdominal pains; pancreatitis; vertigo.
GU: Albuminuria; nephrotic syndrome; renal papillary necrosis; male infertility.
HEMA: Hemolysis; increased reticulocyte count; shortened red cell life span; rise in methemoglobin.
RESP: Pulmonary eosinophilia.
OTHER: Fever; phototoxicity; hypoalbuminemia; lupus erythematosus; infectious mononucleosis-like syndrome.

Precautions
Pregnancy: Category C.
Lactation: Excreted in breast milk.
Children: Children are treated on the same schedule as adults but with correspondingly smaller doses. Dapsone is generally not considered to have an effect on the later growth and functional development of the child.

PATIENT CARE CONSIDERATIONS
Administration/Storage
- Administer prescribed dose daily.
- Administer each dose without regard to meals. Administer with food if GI upset occurs.
- Store tablets at controlled room temperature (59° to 86°F).

Assessment/Interventions
- Obtain patient history, including drug history and any known allergies. Note history of G6PD deficiency, methemoglobin reductase deficiency, hemoglobin M, or anemia.
- Ensure that CBC and differential are performed and evaluated prior to starting therapy, weekly for the first month of therapy, then monthly for 6 mo, and then every 6 mo thereafter during treatment.
- Ensure that liver enzymes are determined and evaluated prior to starting therapy and periodically during treatment.
- Ensure that 1 or more other antileprosy agents are being used concurrently in patient being treated for leprosy.

Hypersensitivity: Serious cutaneous reactions (eg, erythema multiforme, toxic epidermal necrolysis) resulting from hypersensitivity may occur. In addition, sulfone syndrome, a potentially fatal hypersensitivity with symptoms of fever, malaise, jaundice with hepatic necrosis, exfoliative dermatitis, lymphadenopathy, methemoglobinemia, and hemolytic anemia may occur.
Hepatic function impairment: Toxic hepatitis or cholestatic jaundice reported and hyperbilirubinemia may occur more frequently in patients with G-6-PD deficiency.
Hematologic: Deaths caused by agranulocytosis, aplastic anemia, and other blood dyscrasias occurred. Treat severe anemia prior to initiation of dapsone therapy.
Hemolysis: Because hemolysis and Heinz body formation may be exaggerated in individuals with glucose-6-phosphate dehydrogenase (G-6-PD) deficiency, methemoglobin reductase deficiency or hemoglobin M, give dapsone with caution to patients with these conditions or patients exposed to other agents or conditions (eg, diabetic ketosis) capable of producing hemolysis.

Overdosage: Signs and Symptoms
Nausea, vomiting, hyperexcitability, methemoglobin-induced depression, convulsions or severe cyanosis, severe anoxia (with retinal and optic nerve damage).

- Monitor patient for GI, CNS, and general body side effects. Inform health care provider if noted and significant.

Patient/Family Education
- Explain name, dose, action, and potential side effects of drug.
- Review dosing schedule and prescribed length of therapy with patient.
- Advise patient that medication may be started at a low dose and then gradually increased to provide maximum benefit.
- Instruct patient to continue to take other prescribed medications while taking dapsone.
- Emphasize to patient that treatment will be lengthy and that the entire course of treatment must be completed to avoid relapse or development of resistance.
- Advise patient to take each dose with food if GI upset occurs.
- Instruct patient to stop using and notify health care provider immediately if any of the following symptoms occur: skin rash, sore throat, fever, paleness, purple discoloration of

skin, yellowing of skin or eyes, muscle weakness.
- Advise women to notify health care provider if pregnant, planning to become pregnant, or breastfeeding.
- Advise patient that drug may cause blurred vision or dizziness and to use caution while driving or performing other tasks requiring mental alertness until tolerance is determined.
- Instruct patient to not take any prescription or OTC medications or dietary supplements unless advised by health care provider.
- Advise patient that follow-up visits and lab tests will be required to monitor therapy and to keep appointments.

Daptomycin

(DAP-toe-MY-sin)

Class Anti-infective/Lipopeptide

How Supplied
Cubicin Powder for injection, lyophilized 250 mg, Powder for injection, lyophilized 500 mg

Action
PHARMACOLOGY: Binds to bacterial membranes and causes a rapid depolarization of membrane potential, which inhibits protein, DNA, and RNA synthesis, resulting in bacterial cell death.

PHARMACOKINETICS/DYNAMICS:

Absorption: At a dose of 4 mg/kg, steady-state concentrations are achieved by the third daily dose. The mean steady-state trough concentration (days 4 to 8) is 5.9 mcg/mL.

Distribution: The mean serum protein binding is approximately 92% following a dose of 4 mg/kg.

Excretion: Primarily excreted by the kidney (78%).

Special Populations:
Renal function – Dosage adjustment is needed in patients with severe renal insufficiency (Ccr less than 30 mL/min).

Indications Treatment of complicated skin and skin structure infections caused by susceptible strains of Gram-positive microorganisms.

Contraindications Standard considerations.

Route/Dosage
Complicated Skin and Skin Structure Infections
ADULTS: **IV** 4 mg/kg/day administered over a 30-min infusion.

Renal Impairment
ADULTS: **IV** Ccr less than 30 mL/min, including hemodialysis or continuous ambulatory peritoneal dialysis. Administer 4 mg/kg q 48 hr.

Interactions None well documented.

Incompatibilities: Do not mix with dextrose-containing diluents.

Lab Test Interferences None well documented.

Adverse Reactions
CV: Hypotension (2%); cardiac failure (1% to 2%); hypertension (1%).
CNS: Headache, insomnia (5%); dizziness (2%); anxiety, confusion (1% to 2%).
DERM: Rash (4%); pruritus (3%).
EENT: Sore throat (1% to 2%).
GI: Constipation, nausea (6%); diarrhea (5%); vomiting (3%); abdominal pain (1% to 2%); dyspepsia (1%).
GU: UTI, renal failure (2%).
HEMA: Anemia (2%); leukocytosis, thrombocytopenia, thrombocytosis, eosinophilia, increased international normalized ratio (less than 1%).
LABTESTABS: Abnormal LFTs, elevated CPK (2%).
METAB: Edema; hypoglycemia, hyperglycemia, hypokalemia (1% to 2%).
MUSC: Limb pain (2%); arthralgia (1%).
RESP: Dyspnea (2%); cough (1% to 2%).
OTHER: Injection site reactions (6%); fungal infections (3%); fever (2%); cellulitis, decreased appetite, chest pain, back pain, *Candida* infections (1% to 2%).

Precautions
Pregnancy: Category B.
Lactation: Undetermined.
Children: Safety and efficacy not established.
Renal function impairment: Dosage adjustment is needed in patients with severe renal insufficiency (Ccr less than 30 mL/min).
Lab test abnormalities: Elevated serum CPK may occur, including symptoms of muscle pain or weakness.
Superinfection: May result in bacterial or fungal overgrowth of nonsusceptible microorganisms.
Pseudomembranous colitis: Consider the possibility in patients who develop diarrhea.

PATIENT CARE CONSIDERATIONS

Administration/Storage
- Administer by IV route only. Not for intradermal, SC, or IM administration.
- Administer prescribed dose by 30 min IV infusion q 24 hr.
- Reconstitute powder using 0.9% sodium

chloride injection. Add 5 mL to 250 mg vial or 10 mL to 500 mg vial.
- Reconstituted solution must be further diluted in 0.9% sodium chloride for injection before infusing.
- Do not administer if particulate matter, cloudiness, or discoloration noted. Reconstituted solution may have a pale yellow to light brown color, which is normal and of no concern.
- If other drugs are being administered through same IV line, flush IV line before and after infusion of daptomycin with 0.9% sodium chloride injection or lactated Ringer's injection.
- Store vials in refrigerator (36° to 46°F). Reconstituted solution is stable for 12 hr at room temperature (68° to 77°F) or up to 48 hr if stored under refrigeration. The diluted solution is stable for 12 hr at room temperature or up to 48 hr if stored under refrigeration. The combined time (reconstituted vial and infusion bag) at room temperature should not exceed 12 hr; the combined time (reconstituted vial and infusion bag) under refrigeration should not exceed 48 hr.

Assessment/Interventions
- Obtain patient history, including drug history and any known allergies. Note renal impairment, severe hepatic impairment, and concurrent use of medications known to cause rhabdomyolysis (eg, HMG-CoA reductase inhibitors).
- Review results of culture and sensitivity testing as available.
- Ensure that dosing frequency is adjusted, following manufacturer's recommendations, for patient with severe renal impairment (Ccr less than 30 mL/min).
- Consider temporarily discontinuing, if possible, any other medication known to cause rhabdomyolysis (eg, HMG-CoA reductase inhibitor) until therapy with daptomycin has been completed.
- Ensure that CPK is determined weekly during therapy with daptomycin. Assess patient who develops unexplained elevation of CPK more frequently for signs and symptoms of myopathy. Ensure that medication is discontinued in patient with unexplained signs and symptoms of myopathy and CPK elevation greater than 1000 IU/L or in patient without symptoms but with CPK elevation greater than 2000 IU/L.
- Monitor for signs of infection, especially fever, and for positive response to antibiotic therapy.
- Monitor patient for signs of allergic reaction. Discontinue therapy and immediately notify health care provider if noted.
- Monitor patient for GI, CNS, musculoskeletal, and general body side effects. Report to health care provider if noted and significant. Immediately report any signs or symptoms of myopathy or neuropathy.

Patient/Family Education
- Explain name, dose, action, and potential side effects of drug.
- Advise patient, family, or caregiver that medication will be prepared and administered by a health care provider in a health care setting.
- Advise patient to report injection site pain or redness, muscle weakness, pain, or tenderness, or abnormal sensations in the legs or arms (eg, pain, numbness) to health care provider.
- Advise patient to report signs of superinfection to health care provider: black furry tongue, white patches in mouth, foul-smelling stools, vaginal itching or discharge.
- Warn patient that diarrhea containing blood or pus may be a sign of a serious disorder and to seek medical care if noted and not to treat at home.
- Advise patient that follow-up examinations and lab tests may be required to monitor therapy and to keep appointments.

Darbepoetin Alfa

(dahr-bee-POE-eh-tin AL-fah)

Class Recombinant human erythropoietin

How Supplied
Aranesp Solution for injection 25 mcg/mL, Solution for injection 40 mcg/mL, Solution for injection 60 mcg/mL, Solution for injection 100 mcg/mL, Solution for injection 150 mcg/0.75 mL, Solution for injection 200 mcg/mL, Solution for injection 300 mcg/mL, Solution for injection 500 mcg/mL

Action
PHARMACOLOGY: Stimulates red blood cell production.

PHARMACOKINETICS/DYNAMICS:
Absorption:
SC – Absorption is slow and rate-limiting. T_{max} is approximately 34 hr. Bioavailability is approximately 37%.

Distribution: Confined to vascular space (approximately 60 mL/kg). Distribution t½ approximately 1.4 hr (IV).

Excretion: t½ is approximately 21 hr (IV) and approximately 49 hr (SC).

Onset: Increased hemoglobin levels are observed in 2 to 6 wk.

Indications Treatment of anemia associated with chronic renal failure, whether or not the patient is on dialysis. Treatment of anemia in patients with nonmyeloid malignancies where anemia is caused by coadministered chemotherapy.

Contraindications Uncontrolled hypertension; hypersensitivity to the active substance or the excipients.

Route/Dosage

Anemia Associated with Chronic Renal Failure
ADULTS: IV/SC Initial dose 0.45 mcg/kg once weekly. Maintenance: Individually titrate to a target hemoglobin not to exceed 12 g/dL.

Conversion from Epoetin Alfa
ADULTS: IV/SC If weekly epoetin dose is less than 2500 units/wk, start with darbepoetin 6.25 mcg/wk; if weekly epoetin dose is 2500 to 4999 units/wk, start with darbepoetin 12.5 mcg/wk; if weekly epoetin dose is 5000 to 10,999 units/wk, start with darbepoetin 25 mcg/wk; if weekly epoetin dose is 11,000 to 17,999 units/wk, start with darbepoetin 40 mcg/wk; if weekly epoetin dose is 18,000 to 33,999 units/wk, start with darbepoetin 60 mcg/wk; if weekly epoetin dose is 34,000 to 89,999 units/wk, start with darbepoetin 100 mcg/wk; if weekly epoetin dose is greater than 90,000 units/wk, start with darbepoetin 200 mcg/wk. Maintenance: Individually titrate to a target hemoglobin not to exceed 12 g/dL.

Dosage Adjustment
Do not increase dose of darbepoetin alfa more frequently than once a month. If the hemoglobin is increasing and approaching 12 g/dL, reduce dose approximately 25%. If hemoglobin continues to increase, withhold doses temporarily until hemoglobin begins to decrease, then reinstate dose approximately 25% below the previous dose. If hemoglobin increases by more than 1 g/dL in a 2-wk period, decrease dose approximately 25%.

Cancer Patients Receiving Chemotherapy
ADULTS: SC Initial dose: 2.25 mcg/kg/wk.

PATIENT CARE CONSIDERATIONS

Administration/Storage

- Do not shake or vigorously agitate medication vial to prevent inactivation of medication.
- Do not administer if particulate matter, cloudiness, or discoloration are noted.
- Withdraw prescribed dose into syringe for injection. Do not dilute solution.

Maintenance: Individually titrate to achieve a target hemoglobin. If there is less than a 1 g/dL increase in hemoglobin after 6 wk of therapy, increase the dose up to 4.5 mcg/kg. If hemoglobin increases more than 1 g/dL in a 2-wk period or if the hemoglobin exceeds 12 g/dL, reduce the dose approximately 25%. If the hemoglobin exceeds 13 g/dL, temporarily withhold doses until the hemoglobin falls to 12 g/dL. Reinitiate therapy at a dose approximately 25% below the previous dose.

Interactions None well documented.

Lab Test Interferences None well documented.

Adverse Reactions
CV: Thrombosis, CHF; cardiac arrhythmias; hypertension; hypotension; cardiac arrest; angina pectoris; cardiac chest pain; stroke; acute MI; transient ischemic attack.
CNS: Headache; dizziness; seizure.
DERM: Pruritus.
GI: Diarrhea; nausea; vomiting; abdominal pain; constipation.
RESP: Upper respiratory tract infection; dyspnea; cough; bronchitis.
OTHER: Sepsis; infection; myalgia; fever; chest pain; arthralgia; limb pain; back pain; peripheral edema; fatigue; injection site pain; fluid overload; access infection; flu-like symptoms; access hemorrhage; asthenia; death.

Precautions
Pregnancy: Category C.
Lactation: Undetermined.
Children: Safety and efficacy not established.
Hypersensitivity: Anaphylactic reactions, skin rashes, and urticaria may occur.
Dialysis management: Increased red blood cell production and decreased plasma volume because of darbepoetin treatment may reduce dialysis efficiency; it may be necessary to adjust the dialysis prescription in patients who are marginally dialyzed.
Seizures: Seizures may occur; however, relationship to drug is uncertain.

Overdosage: Signs and Symptoms
Polycythemia.

- Vials contain no preservative. Discard any unused portion. Do not combine unused portions.
- Administer via IV or SC route only.
- Do not administer in conjunction with other drug solutions.
- Prescribed dose is administered once weekly.

- Rotate SC injection sites.
- Dose will be slowly adjusted based on hemoglobin levels.
- Store vials in refrigerator (36° to 46°F). Do not freeze or shake. Protect from light.

Assessment/Interventions
- Obtain patient history, including drug history and any known allergies. Note uncontrolled hypertension.
- Ensure that BP is controlled in hypertensive patients before initiating therapy.
- Ensure that hemoglobin is determined weekly until stable when initiating therapy or changing the dose.
- Ensure that serum ferritin or transferrin saturation is determined before and during therapy.
- Closely monitor BP during therapy. Report elevations in BP to health care provider.
- Monitor patient for signs and symptoms of anaphylactic or serious allergic reactions. Be prepared to treat appropriately.
- Assess patient for CV, CNS, GI, RESP, musculoskeletal, and general body side effects. Report to health care provider if noted and significant.

Patient/Family Education
- Explain name, dose, action, and potential side effects of drug. If patient or caregiver will be administering at home, review Information for Patients and Caregivers insert with the patient or caregiver. Ensure that the patient or caregiver understands how to store, prepare, and administer the dose, and dispose of used equipment and supplies.
- Remind patient that injection is administered once a week.
- Advise patient that dose will be adjusted based upon measured hemoglobin level.
- Advise patient to continue to follow their dietary and dialysis prescriptions while taking this medication.
- Advise patient to notify the health care provider immediately if any of the following occur: rash; hives; shortness of breath; swelling of the eyes, mouth, or throat; palpitations; severe headache; signs of infection (eg, fever, chills); swelling of feet or ankles; intolerable GI effects (eg, nausea, vomiting, diarrhea).
- Instruct women to notify health care provider if pregnant, planning on becoming pregnant, or breastfeeding.
- Instruct patient not to take any prescription or OTC medications or dietary supplements unless advised by the health care provider.
- Remind patient that office visits and laboratory tests will be required to monitor therapy and to keep appointments.

Daunorubicin Citrate Liposomal

(DAW-no-RUE-bih-sin SIH-trate LIP-oh-sohm-ul)

Class Antineoplastic/Anthracycline antibiotic

How Supplied
DaunoXome Solution for injection 2 mg/mL (equivalent to 50 mg daunorubicin base)

Action
PHARMACOLOGY: Anthracycline antibiotic formulated to increase selectivity for solid tumors in situ.

PHARMACOKINETICS/DYNAMICS:
Distribution: Vd is approximately 6.4 L. Distribution t½ approximately 4.41 hr.

Metabolism: Metabolized to daunorubicinol (active).

Excretion: The t½ is 4.4 hr. Plasma Cl approximately 17.3 mL/min.

Indications Advanced HIV-associated Kaposi sarcoma.

Contraindications Standard considerations.

Route/Dosage

Advanced HIV-Associated Kaposi Sarcoma
ADULTS: IV 40 mg/m^2/dose (of daunorubicin base) administered over 1 hr q 2 wk. The dose of daunorubicin citrate liposomal is different from the dose of daunorubicin hydrochloride.

Dosage Adjustment for Renal or Hepatic Function
If serum bilirubin is 1.2 to 3 mg/dL, then give 75% of adjusted dose from prior course. If serum bilirubin is more than 3 mg/dL or serum creatinine is more than 3 mg/dL, then give 50% of adjusted dose from prior course.

Interactions
Quinolones (eg, ciprofloxacin): Antimicrobial effects may be reduced.
Lab Test Interferences None well documented.
Adverse Reactions
CV: Hot flashes, hypertension, palpitation, syncope, tachycardia (at least 5%).
CNS: Fatigue (43%); headache (22%); neuropathy (13%); malaise (9%); dizziness (8%); depression (7%); insomnia (6%); amnesia, anxiety, ataxia, confusion, convulsions, emotional lability, abnormal gait, hallucination, hyperkinesias, hypertonia, meningitis, somnolence, abnormal thinking, tremor (at least 5%).
DERM: Alopecia (8%); pruritus (7%); folliculitis, seborrhea, dry skin (at least 5%).
EENT: Rhinitis (12%); abnormal vision (3%); conjunctivitis, deafness, earache, eye pain, taste perversion, tinnitus (at least 5%).
GI: Nausea (51%); diarrhea (34%); anorexia (21%); vomiting, abdominal pain (20%); stomatitis (9%); constipation (7%); tenesmus (4%); increased appetite, dysphagia, GI hemorrhage, gastritis, gingival bleeding, hemorrhoids, hepatomegaly, melena, dry mouth, tooth caries (at least 5%).
GU: Dysuria, nocturia, polyuria (at least 5%).
HEMA/LYMPH: Neutropenia (less than 1,000 cells/mm^3 [36%]); neutropenia (less than 500 cells/mm^3 [15%]); lymphadenopathy, splenomegaly (at least 5%).
LOCAL: Injection site inflammation (at least 5%).
M/N: Dehydration, thirst (at least 5%).
MUSC: Rigors (19%); back pain (16%); arthralgia, myalgia (7%).
RESP: Cough (26%); dyspnea (23%); sinusitis (8%); hemoptysis, hiccups, pulmonary infiltration, increased sputum (at least 5%).
OTHER: Fever (42%); opportunistic infection (40%); allergic reactions (21%); triad of back pain, flushing, and chest tightness (14%); increased sweating (12%); edema, chest pain (9%); flu-like symptoms (5%).

PATIENT CARE CONSIDERATIONS
Administration/Storage
- For IV infusion only. Not for intradermal, subcutaneous, IM, IV bolus, or intra-arterial administration.
- Follow institutional procedures for handling, administration, and disposal of anticancer drugs.
- Injection must be diluted prior to administration. Dilute injection concentrate 1:1 with 5% dextrose injection. Resulting solution contains 1 mg daunorubicin/mL.

> **WARNING:**
> *Cardiotoxicity:* Cumulative dose related.
> *Decreased left ventricular ejection fraction (LVEF):* Anthracycline-induced cardiomyopathy is associated with decreased LVEF.
> *Hepatic impairment:* Assess hepatic function before initiating therapy; adjust dose as necessary. Reduce dosage for hepatic function impairment.
> *Infusion reaction:* Back pain, flushing, and chest tightness can occur. Usually occurs within first 5 min of infusion and subsides with infusion interruption. Does not usually recur if infusion is restarted at a slower rate. Appears to be related to lipid component.
> *Myelosuppression:* The primary toxicity of daunorubicin is myelosuppression, especially of the granulocytic series, which may be severe, with much less marked effects on the platelets and erythroid series.

Precautions
Pregnancy: Category D.
Lactation: HIV-infected mothers should not breastfeed infants.
Children: Safety and efficacy not established.
Renal function impairment: Assess renal function before initiating therapy; adjust dose as necessary. Reduce dosage for renal function impairment.
Daunorubicin dose: The dose of daunorubicin citrate liposomal is different from the dose of daunorubicin hydrochloride.
Extravasation risk: Local irritation or phlebitis may occur. Refer to your institution-specific protocol.

Overdosage: Signs and Symptoms
Symptoms of acute overdosage are increased severities of the observed dose-limiting toxicities of therapeutic doses, myelosuppression (especially granulocytopenia), fatigue, nausea, and vomiting.

- Discard unused portions of vial. Do not save any unused portions for future use.
- Do not mix with any other IV solution than 5% dextrose nor mix with any other medication.
- Do not administer if solution is opaque or contains particulate matter. Solution will have a red discoloration and disperse light to some degree. This is normal and of no concern.
- Administer prescribed dose over a 60-min

period into free-flowing IV, taking precautions to avoid extravasation. Do not use an in-line filter.
- Store vials in refrigerator (36° to 46°F). If not used immediately, store diluted solution in refrigerator for up to 6 hr. Do not freeze. Protect from light.

Assessment/Interventions
- Obtain patient history, including drug history and any known allergies. Note renal or hepatic impairment, bone marrow suppression, cardiac disease, concomitant or previous radiation to mediastinal-pericardial area, and history of prior anthracycline therapy.
- Ensure cardiac function is evaluated and documented by a history and physical examination before starting therapy and before each course of therapy. Ensure that LVEF is determined at a total cumulative dose of 320 mg/m^2 and every 160 mg/m^2 thereafter in patient with no prior therapy with anthracyclines, no evidence of cardiac disease, and no prior radiotherapy encompassing the heart. Ensure that LVEF is determined before starting therapy and at every total cumulative dose of 160 mg/m^2 in patient with prior therapy with anthracyclines (doxorubicin dose greater than 300 mg/m^2 or equivalent), preexisting cardiac disease, or prior radiotherapy encompassing the heart.
- Ensure CBC with differential is evaluated prior to starting therapy and before each dose. Withhold therapy if absolute neutrophil count is less than 750 cells/mm^3.
- Ensure reduced dose is administered to patient with renal (Ccr greater than 3 mg/dL) or hepatic impairment (bilirubin greater than 1.2 mg/dL) following manufacturer's guidelines.
- Ensure women of childbearing potential are not pregnant before starting therapy and use effective contraception during treatment.
- Monitor patient for infusion-related reaction (eg, back pain, flushing, chest tightness). If noted, be prepared to temporarily discontinue infusion and resume at lower rate once symptoms have subsided.
- Monitor patient for signs or symptoms of infection. Inform health care provider immediately if noted, and be prepared to treat appropriately.
- Monitor IV infusion site for signs or symptoms of extravasation. If noted, immediately discontinue infusion and restart in another vein.
- Assess patient for GI, CNS, DERM, RESP, MUSC, and general body side effects. Report to health care provider if noted and significant.

Patient/Family Education
- Explain name, action, and potential side effects of drug.
- Advise patient, family, or caregiver that medication will be prepared and administered by health care provider in a health care setting.
- Review dosing schedule with patient, family, or caregiver.
- Advise patient, family, or caregiver that medication may cause a red coloration of the urine. Advise that this is not a problem and is expected because the medication is being eliminated in the urine.
- Advise patient, family, or caregiver to immediately report any of the following to health care provider: rash; hives; difficulty breathing; chest pain; fever, chills, or other signs of infection; unusual bleeding or bruising; pain, redness, or swelling at injection site.
- Advise patient, family, or caregiver to report any of the following to health care provider: persistent nausea, vomiting or appetite loss; persistent or worsening general body weakness.
- Advise patient, family, or caregiver that hair loss is a common side effect of therapy, but that this is usually reversible after therapy has been completed.
- Caution women of childbearing potential to avoid becoming pregnant during therapy.
- Advise women to notify health care provider if pregnant, planning to become pregnant, or breastfeeding.
- Instruct patient not to take any prescription or OTC medications, herbal preparations, or dietary supplements unless advised by health care provider.
- Advise patient that follow-up visits, heart function tests, and laboratory tests will be required to monitor therapy and to keep appointments.

Daunorubicin Hydrochloride
(DAW-no-RUE-bih-sin)

Class Antineoplastic/Anthracycline antibiotic

How Supplied
Cerubidine Lyophilized powder for injection 20 mg vial with 100 mg mannitol added, Solution for injection 5 mg/mL, 4 mL vial

Action
PHARMACOLOGY: Antimitotic and cytotoxic activity.

PHARMACOKINETICS/DYNAMICS:
Distribution: Extensive and rapid protein binding. Highest concentrations in spleen, kidneys, liver, lungs, and heart.
Metabolism: Extensively metabolized in liver and other tissues to daunorubicinol (active).
Excretion: t½ is 18.5 hr (daunorubicin) and 26.7 hr (daunorubicinol). Approximately 25% excreted in active form in the urine and 40% by biliary excretion.

Indications Acute lymphocytic leukemia.
Unlabeled use(s): Chronic myelogenous leukemia, Kaposi sarcoma.

Contraindications None well documented.

Route/Dosage
Acute Nonlymphocytic Leukemia (Combination Therapy)
ADULTS (UNDER 60 YR): **IV** Daunorubicin 45 mg/m^2/day on days 1 to 3 of first course and days 1 to 2 of subsequent courses. May require up to 3 courses.
ADULTS (OVER 60 YR): **IV** Daunorubicin 30 mg/m^2/day on days 1 to 3 of first course and days 1 to 2 of subsequent courses. May require 3 courses.

Acute Lymphocytic Leukemia (Combination Therapy)
ADULTS: **IV** Daunorubicin 45 mg/m^2/day on days 1 to 3.

Acute Lymphocytic Leukemia
CHILDREN (AT LEAST 2 YR): **IV** Daunorubicin 25 mg/m^2 on day 1 q wk with vincristine and oral prednisone. Generally, complete remission will be obtained with 4 courses of therapy. If after 4 courses the patient is in partial remission, an additional 1 or, if necessary, 2 courses may be given.
CHILDREN (UNDER 2 YR OR UNDER 0.5 M^2 BSA): **IV** Calculate dosage on the basis of weight (mg/kg) instead of BSA.

Dosage Adjustment for Renal or Hepatic Function
If serum bilirubin is 1.2 to 3 mg/dL, then give 75% of adjusted dose from prior course. If serum bilirubin is above 3 mg/dL or serum creatinine is above 3 mg/dL, then give 50% of adjusted dose from prior course.

Lifetime Cumulative Doses Above Which Frequency of Cardiotoxicity Increases
ADULTS: **IV** No more than 550 mg/m^2.
ADULTS HAVING RECEIVED MEDIASTINAL RADIATION: **IV** No more than 400 mg/m^2.
CHILDREN (AT LEAST 2 YR): **IV** No more than 300 mg/m^2.
CHILDREN (UNDER 2 YR): **IV** No more than 10 mg/m^2.

Interactions
Cyclophosphamide: May result in increased daunorubicin toxicity.
Hepatotoxic medications: May impair liver function and increase the risk of toxicity.
Myelosuppressive agents: Dosage reduction of daunorubicin may be required.
Quinolone antibiotics: Daunorubicin may decrease the oral absorption of quinolone antibiotics.

Lab Test Interferences
Hyperuricemia: May be induced secondary to a rapid lysis of leukemic cells. As a precaution, administer allopurinol prior to initiating antileukemic therapy.

Adverse Reactions
CV: Delayed dose-related cardiomyopathy; acute arrhythmias.
DERM: Alopecia; rash; contact dermatitis; urticaria; radiation recall; nail hyperpigmentation.
GI: Nausea; vomiting; mucositis; esophagitis; diarrhea; abdominal pain.
HEMA: Bone marrow suppression.
HYPERSEN: Anaphylaxis.
OTHER: Fever; chills.

Precautions
Pregnancy: Category D.
Lactation: Advise mothers to discontinue nursing.
Children: Cardiotoxicity may be more frequent and occur at lower cumulative doses.
Elderly: Cardiotoxicity may be more frequent. Use caution in patients who have inadequate bone marrow reserves because of old age.
Renal function impairment: Some health care providers recommend not giving daunorubicin to patients with a bilirubin above 5 mg/dL. Reduce dose.
Hepatic function impairment: Some health care providers recommend not giving daunorubicin to patients with a bilirubin above 5 mg/dL. Reduce dose.
Extravasation risk: Local irritation of phlebitis may occur. Refer to the institution's specific protocol.
Health care provider administration: It is recom-

mended that daunorubicin be administered only by health care providers who are experienced in leukemia chemotherapy.

Myelosuppression: Occurs when used in therapeutic doses; this may lead to infection or hemorrhage.

Myocardial toxicity: Potentially fatal CHF may occur when total cumulative dosage exceeds 400 to 550 mg/m^2 in adults, 300 mg/m^2 in children above 2 yr, or 10 mg/kg in children under 2 yr. This may occur during therapy or several months to years after therapy.

Previous cumulative dose: Do not use in patients who have previously received the recommended maximum cumulative dose of either doxorubicin or daunorubicin.

Secondary leukemias: There have been reports of secondary leukemias in patients exposed to daunorubicin when used in combination with other antineoplastic agents or radiation therapy.

PATIENT CARE CONSIDERATIONS
Administration/Storage

- Store powder at room temperature (59° to 86°F). Protect from light.
- Refrigerate unopened vials of solution. Protect from light.
- Reconstitute vials of powder with Sterile Water for Injection for a final concentration of 5 mg/mL. Shake vial gently to dissolve contents. Maximum concentration of daunorubicin for administration is 5 mg/mL; more concentrated solutions are hyperosmolar.
- Withdraw the desired dose into a syringe containing 10 to 15 mL of normal saline; inject into a rapidly flowing IV infusion of 5% glucose or normal saline solution.
- Although reconstituted solution is chemically stable under refrigeration longer, it contains no preservative; use within 24 hr. Protect from sunlight.
- Color change of solution from red to blue-purple indicates decomposition.
- Administer by IV push or IV infusion.
- Dilute 5 mg/mL solution with 10 to 15 mL of 0.9% Sodium Chloride. Give by direct IV injection or by IV side arm.
- Reconstituted solution has also been diluted in 100 mL of 5% Dextrose or 0.9% Sodium Chloride and infused IV over 30 to 45 min. However, many health care providers consider the risk of extravasation unacceptable unless infused through a central venous catheter.
- Do not mix with other drugs or heparin.

Assessment/Interventions

- Attaining a normal appearing bone marrow may require no more than 3 courses of induction therapy. Evaluate bone marrow following recovery from the previous induction course to determine the need for a further course of induction treatment.
- Monitor ECG and systolic ejection fraction as the maximum cumulative lifetime dose approaches. Certain ECG changes and a decrease in the systolic injection fraction from pretreatment baseline may aid in recognizing those patients at greatest risk. A decrease of at least 30% in limb lead QRS voltage has been associated with significant risk of drug-induced cardiomyopathy. Perform an ECG or determine systolic ejection fraction before each course.
- Assess hepatic and renal function prior to each course of therapy.
- Observe patient closely and monitor chemical and laboratory tests extensively.
- Monitor serum uric acid. Minimize effects of hyperuricemia with hydration, urinary alkalinization, and allopurinol.
- Urine discoloration (red) may occur.

Patient/Family Education

- Explain name, action, and potential side effects of drug.
- Advise patient, family, or caregiver that medication will be prepared and administered by health care provider in a health care setting.
- Advise patient, family, or caregiver that medication may be used in combination with other agents to achieve maximum benefit possible.
- Review dosing schedule with patient, family, or caregiver.
- Advise patient, family, or caregiver that medication will usually cause a red coloration of the urine. Advise that this is not a problem and is expected because the medication is being eliminated in the urine.
- Advise patient, family, or caregiver that medication may cause hair loss but that this is reversible when therapy is stopped.
- Advise patient, family, or caregiver to immediately report any of the following to health care provider: rash; hives; difficulty breathing; chest pain; fever, chills, or other signs of infection; sores in mouth; unusual bleeding or bruising; pain, redness or swelling at injection site.
- Advise patient, family, or caregiver to report any of the following to health care provider: persistent nausea, vomiting or appetite loss; persistent or worsening general body weakness.
- Instruct patient to not take any prescription or *otc* medications or dietary supplements unless advised by health care provider.

- Caution women of childbearing potential to avoid becoming pregnant while being treated.
- Instruct women of childbearing potential to notify health care provider if becoming pregnant, planning on becoming pregnant, or are breastfeeding.
- Advise patient that following discharge from the hospital that frequent follow-up visits, ECGs, or heart function tests, and laboratory tests will be required to monitor therapy and to keep appointments.

Delavirdine Mesylate

(Dell-ah-ver-deen MEH-sih-late)

Class Antiretroviral/Non-nucleoside reverse transcriptase inhibitor

How Supplied
Rescriptor Tablets 100 mg

Action

PHARMACOLOGY: Inhibits replication of HIV-1 infection by interfering with DNA synthesis.

PHARMACOKINETICS/DYNAMICS:

Absorption: Rapidly absorbed. T_{max} approximately 1 hr. C_{max} approximately 35 mcM. AUC approximately 180 mcM•hr.

Distribution: Approximately 98% protein bound, primarily albumin.

Metabolism: Primarily metabolized by CYP3A and possibly CYP2D6 to several inactive metabolites.

Excretion: Approximately 44% excreted in feces and approximately 51% in urine (less than 5% as unchanged drug). t½ is approximately 5.8 hr.

Indications Treatment of HIV-1 infection in combination with appropriate antiretroviral agents when therapy is warranted.

Contraindications Standard considerations.

Route/Dosage

ADULTS AND CHILDREN OLDER THAN 16 YR: PO 400 mg tid in combination with appropriate antiretroviral therapy.

Interactions

Antacids: Antacids reduce absorption of delavirdine. Separate doses by at least 1 hr.
Anticonvulsants (eg, carbamazepine, phenobarbital, phenytoin): Induce hepatic metabolism of delavirdine resulting in decreased plasma concentrations.
Benzodiazepines (eg, alprazolam, midazolam, triazolam): Delavirdine may increase blood levels of these drugs, which may produce extreme sedation and respiratory depression.
Cisapride, dapsone, ergot derivatives, quinidine, rifabutin, warfarin: Delavirdine may elevate blood levels of these drugs, which may increase the risk of arrhythmias or other potentially serious side effects.
Clarithromycin: Coadministration may increase blood levels of delavirdine or clarithromycin.
Didanosine: Separate administration of didanosine and delavirdine by at least 1 hr; coadministration results in a 20% reduction in systemic exposure of both drugs.
Dihydropyridine calcium channel blockers (eg, nifedipine): Delavirdine may elevate blood levels, which may increase toxicity.
Fluoxetine, ketoconazole: Increased delvirdine plasma concentrations.
H_2 antagonists (eg, cimetidine): Concurrent use may reduce absorption of delavirdine. Chronic use of these drugs with delavirdine is not recommended.
Indinavir: Delavirdine inhibits metabolism of indinavir. Consider indinavir dosage reduction if coadministered with delavirdine.
Rifabutin, rifampin: Induce hepatic metabolism of delavirdine resulting in decreased plasma concentrations. These agents should not be coadministered with delavirdine.
Saquinavir: Delavirdine inhibits metabolism of saquinavir. Monitor hepatocellular enzymes frequently if coadministered.

Lab Test Interferences None well documented.

Adverse Reactions

CV: Fatigue; tachycardia; bradycardia; pallor; palpitation; postural hypotension; syncope; vasodilation.
CNS: Lethargy; headache; migraine; abnormal coordination; agitation; amnesia; anxiety; change in dreams; cognitive impairment; confusion; depression; disorientation; dizziness; emotional lability; hallucination; hyperesthesia; impaired concentration; insomnia; manic symptoms; nervousness; neuropathy; nightmares; paranoid symptoms; paresthesia; restlessness; somnolence; tingling; tremor; vertigo.
DERM: Rash; pruritus; angioedema; dermal leukocytoclastic vasculitis; dermatitis; desquamation; sweating; dry skin; erythema; erythema multiforme; folliculitis; fungal dermatitis; alopecia; nail disorder; petechial rash; seborrheic; skin nodule; Stevens-Johnson syndrome; urticaria; vesiculobullous rash; bruise; ecchymosis; petechia; purpura.
EENT: Nystagmus; blepharitis; conjunctivitis; diplopia; dry eyes; photophobia; tinnitus; ear pain; esophagitis; laryngismus; pharyngitis; sinusitis; rhinitis; epistaxis.
GI: Nausea; diarrhea; vomiting; abdominal cramps; distention; pain; lip edema; anorexia; aphthous stomatitis; bloody stool; colitis; consti-

pation; decreased appetite; diverticulitis; duodenitis; dry mouth; dyspepsia; dysphagia; enteritis; fecal incontinence; flatulence; gagging; gastritis; gastroesophageal reflux; GI bleeding; gingivitis; gum hemorrhage; increased appetite; increased saliva; thirst; mouth ulcer; pancreatitis; rectal disorder; sialadenitis; stomatitis; tongue edema; ulceration; taste perversion.
GU: Decreased libido; breast enlargement; kidney calculi; epididymitis; hematuria; hemospermia; impotence; kidney pain; metrorrhagia; nocturia; polyuria; proteinuria; vaginal moniliasis.
HEMA: Anemia; eosinophilia; granulocytosis; neutropenia; pancytopenia; prolonged partial thromboplastin; spleen disorder; thrombocytopenia.
HEPA: Increased ALT; increased AST; hepatitis.
METAB: Bilirubinemia; hyperkalemia; hyperuricemia; hypocalcemia; hyponatremia; hypophosphatemia; increased gamma glutamyl transpeptidase, lipase, serum alkaline phosphatase, serum amylase, serum creatinine phosphokinase, or serum creatinine; peripheral edema.
RESP: Upper respiratory infection; bronchitis; chest congestion; cough; dyspnea.
OTHER: Asthenia; back pain; chest pain; flank pain; chills; edema; fever; flu-like syndrome; lethargy; weakness; malaise; neck rigidity; sebaceous and epidermal cysts; muscle cramps; paralysis; weight increase or decrease; arthralgia; arthritis; bone disorder; bone pain; myalgia; tendon disorder; tenosynovitis; tetany.

Precautions

Pregnancy: Category C.
Lactation: Undetermined. HIV infected mothers should not breastfeed their infants.
Children: Safety and efficacy in children younger than 16 yr not established.
Hepatic function impairment: Delavirdine is metabolized primarily by the liver. Use with caution in patients with impaired hepatic function.
Rash: Rash is the most common side effect and may range from minor to severe.
Resistance: Resistant virus emerges rapidly when delavirdine is administered as monotherapy. Always use in combination with appropriate antiretroviral therapy.

PATIENT CARE CONSIDERATIONS

Administration/Storage

- Administer with or without food.
- Administer with an acidic beverage (eg, orange or cranberry juice) if patient has achlorhydria.
- May disperse tablets in water prior to administration. Add tablets to at least 3 oz of water. Stir until uniformly dispersed and administer promptly. Rinse glass and have patient swallow the rinse to ensure the entire dose is consumed.
- If patient also takes antacids, separate doses by at least 1 hr.
- Store at controlled room temperature in tightly closed container. Protect from high humidity.

Assessment/Interventions

- Obtain patient history, including drug history and any known allergies. Note hepatic function impairment.
- Ensure that patient is also receiving concurrent antiretroviral therapy.
- If used in combination with saquinavir, ensure that hepatocellular enzymes are monitored frequently.
- Monitor patient for development of severe rash or rash accompanied by symptoms of fever, blistering, oral lesions, conjunctivitis, swelling, or muscle or joint aches. If any occur, discontinue therapy and notify health care provider.

Patient/Family Education

- Advise patient to take medication with or without food exactly as prescribed.
- If patient has difficulty swallowing tablets, instruct patient in proper method for dispersing tablets in water.
- Advise patients with achlorhydria to take each dose with an acidic beverage (eg, orange or cranberry juice).
- Advise patients who are also taking antacids or didanosine to separate doses by ≥ 1 hr.
- Warn patient not to alter dose or discontinue the medication without consulting health care provider.
- Advise patient that if dose is missed, take as soon as possible and return to normal dose. However, if a dose is skipped, do not double the next dose.
- Instruct patient not to take any other medications (including OTC), without checking with the health care provider. This medication interacts with a wide range of medications.
- Explain to the patient to have frequent follow-up blood and urine tests during the course of treatment and to keep appointments.
- Inform patients that this medication is not a cure for HIV infection and they may continue to acquire secondary illnesses associated with the disease.

- Emphasize to patient, family, and significant others that this medication does not reduce the risk of transmitting HIV to others through sexual contact or blood contamination.
- Inform patient that rash is the most common adverse effect and advise patient to promptly notify the health care provider should rash occur.
- Advise patient to discontinue therapy and contact the health care provider immediately should any of the following occur: severe rash; rash accompanied by fever, blistering, oral lesions, conjunctivitis, swelling, muscle or joint aches.
- Inform patient to report serious or bothersome side effects to the health care provider.
- Explain that the long-term effects of this medication are not known at this time.

Demeclocycline

(DEH-meh-kloe-sigh-cleen)
Class Antibiotic/Tetracycline

How Supplied
Declomycin Tablets 150 mg, Tablets 300 mg

Action
PHARMACOLOGY: Inhibits bacterial protein synthesis.

PHARMACOKINETICS/DYNAMICS:

Absorption: Peak concentration is reached in about 4 hr. The mean concentrations 1 and 3 hr after 150 mg oral dose are 0.46 and 1.22 mcg/mL, respectively.

Distribution: Penetrates well into various body fluids and tissues. Protein binding is about 40%.

Excretion: Concentrated in the liver and excreted into the bile. Renal Cl is about 35 mL/min/1.73 m^2. In data from a small number of patients, approximately 44% is excreted in the urine, and 13% to 46% is excreted in feces.

Indications
Treatment of infections caused by susceptible strains of gram-positive and gram-negative microorganisms.

Contraindications
Hypersensitivity to any tetracycline and any component of the product.

Route/Dosage
ADULTS: **PO** 150 mg qid or 300 mg bid.
CHILDREN OLDER THAN 8 YR: **PO** Usual dose is 7 to 13 mg/kg/day divided into 2 to 4 doses (max, 600 mg/day).

Gonorrhea
ADULTS: **PO** 600 mg followed by 300 mg q 12 hr for 4 days (total 3 g).

Interactions
Antacids containing aluminum, calcium, or magnesium, iron-containing products, dairy products: May decrease the absorption of demeclocycline.
Anticoagulants: Effect of anticoagulant may be enhanced, necessitating a downward adjustment in dosage.
Methoxyflurane: Increased potential for life-threatening renal toxicity.
Oral contraceptives: May reduce the effectiveness of oral contraceptives.
Penicillins: The bactericidal action may be decreased by tetracyclines.

Lab Test Interferences None well documented.

Adverse Reactions
CNS: Pseudotumor cerebri; bulging fontanels (in infants); dizziness; headache; myasthenic syndrome.
DERM: Maculopapular and erythematous rashes; erythema multiforme; exfoliative dermatitis; fixed drug eruptions; Stevens-Johnson syndrome; pigmentation of skin and mucous membranes; lesions on the glans penis causing balanitis; phototoxicity.
EENT: Esophageal ulcerations; tinnitus; visual disturbances.
GI: Anorexia; nausea; vomiting; diarrhea; glossitis; dysphagia; enterocolitis; pancreatitis; inflammatory lesions in the anogenital region (eg, monilial overgrowth); tooth discoloration (children under 8 yr).
HEMA: Hemolytic anemia; thrombocytopenia; neutropenia; eosinophilia.
HEPA: Increased liver enzymes; hepatic toxicity; hepatitis; liver failure.
RENAL: Acute renal toxicity; increased BUN; nephrogenic diabetes insipidus.
OTHER: Hypersensitivity (including urticaria, angioneurotic edema, polyarthralgia, anaphylaxis, anaphylactoid purpura, pericarditis, exacerbation of SLE, lupus-like syndrome, pulmonary infiltrates with eosinophilia); brown-black thyroid gland discoloration.

Precautions
Pregnancy: Category D.
Lactation: Excreted in breast milk.
Children: Safety and efficacy not established in children under 8 yr because abnormal bone formation and discoloration of teeth may occur.
Renal function impairment: May lead to excessive accumulation of the drug and possible liver toxicity; dosage reduction may be required.
Hazardous tasks: Patients experiencing CNS symptoms should be cautioned about driving vehicles or using dangerous machinery.
Superinfection: Prolonged use may result in bacterial or fungal overgrowth.

Photosensitivity: May manifest as exaggerated sunburn.
Diabetes insipidus syndrome: May occur.

Pseudotumor cerebri (benign intracranial hypertension): Has been reported.

PATIENT CARE CONSIDERATIONS
Administration/Storage
- Administer each dose with a full glass of water.
- Administer prescribed dose on an empty stomach at least 1 hr before or 2 hr after meals.
- Administer antacids containing aluminum, calcium, or magnesium, or preparations containing iron at least 2 hr before or after the demeclocycline.
- Store tablets at controlled room temperature (68° to 77°F).

Assessment/Interventions
- Obtain patient history, including drug history and any known allergies. Note renal or hepatic impairment, history of allergy, or intolerance to other tetracycline antibiotics.
- Review results of culture and sensitivity testing as appropriate.
- Ensure that women are not pregnant or breastfeeding.
- Ensure that CBC, liver enzymes, and renal function are periodically evaluated during prolonged therapy.
- Monitor patient's response to therapy. Notify health care provider if infection does not appear to be improving or is worsening.
- Monitor patient for signs of allergic reaction. Discontinue therapy and immediately notify health care provider if noted. Be prepared to treat appropriately.
- Monitor patient for GI, CNS, DERM, and general body side effects. Report to health care provider if noted and significant.

Patient/Family Education
- Explain name, dose, action, and potential side effects of drug.
- Review dosing schedule and prescribed length of therapy with patient. Advise patient that dose and duration of therapy are dependent on site and cause of infection.
- Instruct patient to take prescribed dose with a full glass of water at least 1 hr before or 2 hr after meals.
- Advise patient taking iron-containing products or antacids containing aluminum, calcium, or magnesium to take these products either 2 hr before or after the demeclocycline.
- Instruct patient to complete entire course of therapy, even if symptoms of infection have disappeared.
- Advise patient that diarrhea, headache, and nausea are most common side effects and to inform health care provider if they occur and are intolerable.
- Advise patient to discontinue therapy and contact health care provider immediately if skin rash, hives, itching, shortness of breath, headache, blurred vision, unexplained weakness or thirst, or frequent urination occur.
- Advise patient to avoid unnecessary exposure to sunlight or tanning lamps and to use sunscreens and wear protective clothing to avoid photosensitivity reactions.
- Caution women taking oral contraceptives that demeclocycline may make birth control pills less effective and to use nonhormonal forms of contraception during treatment.
- Advise women to notify health care provider if pregnant, planning to become pregnant, or breastfeeding.
- Caution patient that drug may cause dizziness, lightheadedness, or blurred vision and to use caution while driving or performing other hazardous tasks until tolerance is determined.
- Advise patient to report the following signs of superinfection to health care provider: black furry tongue, white patches in mouth, foul-smelling stools, vaginal itching or discharge.
- Warn patient that diarrhea containing blood or pus may be a sign of a serious disorder and to seek medical care if noted and to not treat at home.
- Instruct patient not to take any prescription or OTC medications or dietary supplements unless advised by health care provider.
- Advise patient to discard any unused demeclocycline by the expiration date noted on the label.
- Advise patient that follow-up examinations and lab tests may be required to monitor therapy and to keep appointments.

Denileukin Diftitox

(duh-nih-LOO-kin DIFF-tih-tox)

Class Biologic response modifier

How Supplied
Ontak Frozen, solution for injection 150 mcg/mL

Action
PHARMACOLOGY: Denileukin, a recombinant DNA-derived cytotoxic protein fused to diphtheria toxin fragments A and B, is designed to direct the cytocidal action of diphtheria toxin to cells that express the IL-2 receptor.

PHARMACOKINETICS/DYNAMICS:
Distribution: Distribution t½ approximately 2 to 5 min. Vd is 0.06 to 0.08 L/kg.

Metabolism: Metabolized by proteolytic degradation.

Excretion: Terminal t½ approximately 70 to 80 min. Cl approximately 1.5 to 2 mL/min/kg. Excreted material is less than 25% of the dose and consisted of metabolites.

Indications Cutaneous T-cell lymphoma.

Contraindications Standard considerations.

Route/Dosage
Cutaneous T-Cell Lymphoma
ADULTS: IV 1 treatment cycle is 9 or 18 mcg/kg/day administered for 5 consecutive days q 21 days. Infuse over at least 15 min.
PRETREATMENT REGIMEN:
Adults: Give acetaminophen 650 mg (**PO** or **rectal**) and diphenhydramine 25 to 50 mg (**PO** or **IV**) 30 to 60 min before administering denileukin diftitox.
DOSAGE ADJUSTMENTS:
Adults: Delay therapy in patients with serum albumin below 3 g/dL.

Interactions
Beta blockers, other antihypertensives: May exacerbate denileukin diftitox-induced hypotension.

Lab Test Interferences None well documented.

PATIENT CARE CONSIDERATIONS

Administration/Storage
* Administer by IV use only. Do not administer as a bolus injection. Do not physically mix with other drugs. Do not administer through an in-line filter.
* Dilute the desired dose with 0.9% Sodium Chloride for a final concentration of at least 15 mcg/mL. The denileukin diftitox concentration should not be less than 15 mcg/mL at any time during product preparation. Swirl vial gently to mix the solution. Do not shake vial.

Adverse Reactions
CV: Capillary leak syndrome; hypotension; edema; chest pain; tachycardia; thrombotic events; MI.
CNS: Asthenia; headache; dizziness; paresthesia; nervousness; confusion; insomnia.
DERM: Rash; pruritus; injection site irritation.
ENDO: Hypoalbuminemia; infection; impaired immune function; hypocalcemia; albuminuria.
GI: Nausea; vomiting; elevated LFTs; anorexia; diarrhea; constipation; weight loss; dysphagia.
GU: Hematuria; pyuria.
HEMA: Anemia; thrombocytopenia; leukopenia.
HYPERSEN: Hypotension; dyspnea; vasodilation; rash; pruritus; anaphylaxis.
METAB: Dehydration.
MUSC: Myalgia; arthralgia; pain.
RENAL: Hematuria; pyuria; increased serum creatinine.
RESP: Dyspnea; cough increase; pharyngitis; rhinitis.
OTHER: Chills; fever.

Precautions
Pregnancy: Category C.
Lactation: Undetermined. Patients receiving denileukin should discontinue nursing.
Children: Safety and efficacy not established.
Elderly: Anorexia, hypotension, anemia, confusion, rash, nausea, or vomiting tended to be more frequent or severe in patients at least 65 yr.
Hypersensitivity: Acute hypersensitivity reactions were reported in 69% of patients during or within 24 hr of infusion; about 50% of the events occurred on the first day of dosing regardless of the treatment cycle.
Vascular leak syndrome: Occurs within 2 wk after starting therapy. Take special caution in patients with preexisting cardiovascular disease.

* Administer prepared solutions within 6 hr, using a syringe pump or IV infusion bag.
* Discard unused portions immediately.
* Store frozen at no more than -10°C (14°F). Must be brought to room temperature, at no more than 25°C (77°F), before preparing the dose. The vials may be thawed in the refrigerator at 2° to 8°C (36° to 46°F) for no more than 24 hr or at room temperature for 1 to 2 hr. Do not heat denileukin. Do not refreeze.
* Do not use glass IV containers.

Assessment/Interventions
- Denileukin diftitox should be used only by health care providers experienced in the use of antineoplastic therapy and management of patients with cancer. Manage patients treated with denileukin diftitox in a facility equipped and staffed for cardiopulmonary resuscitation and where the patient can be closely monitored for an appropriate period based on his or her health status.
- Prior to administration of this product, test the patient's malignant cells for CD25 expression.
- Perform a CBC and a blood chemistry panel, including liver and renal function and serum albumin levels, prior to initiation of treatment and weekly during therapy.
- Monitor serum albumin levels prior to the initiation of each treatment course. Delay administration until serum albumin levels are at least 3 g/dL.
- Carefully monitor weight, edema, BP, urine output, and serum albumin levels on an outpatient basis.
- Carefully monitor patients for infections.

Patient/Family Education
- Explain name, action, and potential side effects of drug.
- Advise patient, family, or caregiver that medication will be prepared and administered by health care provider in a health care setting.
- Review dosing schedule with patient, family, or caregiver.
- Advise patient, family, or caregiver that home blood pressure measurements and weighing may be necessary. Instruct patient, family, or caregiver in proper technique if necessary.
- Advise patient, family, or caregiver to immediately report any of the following to health care provider: rash; hives; flushing; difficulty breathing; chest pain or tightness; back pain; difficulty swallowing; fainting; swelling; fever, chills, or other signs of infection; sores in mouth; unusual bleeding or bruising.
- Advise patient, family, or caregiver to report any of the following to health care provider: persistent nausea, vomiting, diarrhea or appetite loss; persistent or worsening general body weakness; pain, redness, or swelling at injection site.
- Instruct patient to not take any prescription or otc medications or dietary supplements unless advised to do so by health care provider.
- Instruct women of childbearing potential to notify health care provider if becoming pregnant, planning on becoming pregnant, or are breastfeeding.
- Advise patient that frequent follow-up visits and laboratory tests will be required to monitor therapy and to keep appointments.

Desipramine Hydrochloride

(dess-IPP-ruh-meen HIGH-droe-KLOR-ide)

Class Tricyclic antidepressant

How Supplied
Norpramin Tablets 10 mg, Tablets 25 mg, Tablets 50 mg, Tablets 75 mg, Tablets 100 mg, Tablets 150 mg
✤ *Apo-Desipramine* ♦ *Novo-Desipramine* ♦ *Nu-Desipramine* ♦ *PMS-Desipramine* ♦ *ratio-Desipramine*

Action
PHARMACOLOGY: Inhibits reuptake of norepinephrine and serotonin in CNS.

PHARMACOKINETICS/DYNAMICS:
Absorption: Rapidly absorbed.

Metabolism: Metabolized in the liver.

Excretion: Approximately 70% excreted in the urine. t½ is 12 to 24 hr.

Onset: 2 to 5 days.

Peak: 2 to 3 wk.

Special Populations:
Elderly – Rate of metabolism is slower. Dosage adjustment recommended.

Indications Relief of symptoms of depression.
Unlabeled use(s): Facilitation of cocaine withdrawal; treatment of panic and eating disorders (eg, bulimia nervosa).

Contraindications Hypersensitivity to any tricyclic antidepressant. Not to be given in combination with or within 14 days of treatment with an MAOI; cross-sensitivity may occur across the dibenzazepines. Do not give during acute recovery phases of MI.

Route/Dosage
ADULTS: **PO** 100 to 300 mg/day. May be given in divided doses or once daily at bedtime.
ELDERLY AND ADOLESCENT PATIENTS: **PO** 25 to 150 mg/day.

Interactions
Barbiturates, carbamazepine, charcoal: May decrease desipramine effects.
Cimetidine, fluoxetine, haloperidol, quinidine, oral contraceptives, phenothiazine antipsychotics: May increase desipramine effects.
Clonidine: May result in hypertensive crisis.
CNS depressants: CNS and respiratory effects may be increased.
MAOIs: Hyperpyretic crises, severe convulsions

and death may occur if administered together or within 14 days of each other.

Lab Test Interferences None well documented.

Adverse Reactions

CV: Orthostatic hypotension; hypertension; tachycardia; palpitations; arrhythmias; ECG changes; hypertensive episodes during surgery; stroke; heartblock; CHF.
CNS: Confusion; disturbed concentration; hallucinations; delusions; nervousness; numbness; tremors; extrapyramidal symptoms (pseudoparkinsonism; movement disorders; akathisia); restlessness; agitation; panic; insomnia; nightmares; mania; exacerbation of psychosis; drowsiness; dizziness; weakness; fatigue; emotional lability; seizures.
DERM: Rash; pruritus; photosensitivity reaction; dry skin; acne; itching; sweating.
EENT: Conjunctivitis; blurred vision; increased intraocular pressure; mydriasis; tinnitus; nasal congestion; peculiar taste in mouth.
GI: Nausea; vomiting; anorexia; GI distress; diarrhea; flatulence; dry mouth; constipation.
GU: Impotence; sexual dysfunction; nocturia; urinary frequency; urinary tract infection; vaginitis; cystitis; urinary retention or hesitancy.
HEPA: Hepatitis; jaundice.
HEMA: Bone marrow depression including agranulocytosis; eosinophilia; purpura; thrombocytopenia; leukopenia.
METAB: Elevation or depression of blood sugar levels.
RESP: Pharyngitis; rhinitis; sinusitis; bronchospasm; cough.
OTHER: Breast enlargement.

Precautions

Pregnancy: Category C.
Lactation: Excreted in breast milk.
Children: Not recommended in children younger than 12 yr.
Special risk patients: Use drug with caution in patients with history of seizures, urinary retention, urethral or ureteral spasm, angle-closure glaucoma, increased intraocular pressure, or cardiovascular disorders; in patients receiving thyroid medication and in patients who have hepatic or renal impairment, schizophrenia, or paranoia.

Overdosage: Signs and Symptoms

Confusion, agitation, hallucinations, seizures, status epilepticus, clonus, choreoathetosis, hyperactive reflexes, positive Babinski signs, coma, cardiac arrhythmias, renal failure, flushing, dry mouth, dilated pupils, hyperpyrexia.

PATIENT CARE CONSIDERATIONS

Administration/Storage

* Administer in equal doses or one dose at bedtime.

Assessment/Interventions

* Obtain patient history, including drug history and any known allergies.
* Document serum bilirubin, alkaline phosphatase, and blood glucose levels throughout therapy.
* Assess and document baseline behaviors and psychological status.
* Notify health care provider and discontinue medication immediately if patient has increased agitation or paranoid delusions.
* Document body weight monthly.
* Notify health care provider and withhold medication if there is a BP drop of 20 mm Hg or if heart arrhythmia or increase in heart rate develops.
* Inform health care provider if patient has urinary elimination problems.

Patient/Family Education

* Warn patient of risk of seizure.
* Instruct patient to keep weekly record of weight.
* Teach patient how to take BP and heart rate.
* Explain missed medication procedure: less than 2 hr, take medication; more than 2 hr, wait until next scheduled dose. Do not double doses.
* Teach proper techniques for oral hygiene to help prevent/treat dry mucous membranes.
* Tell patient to increase fluid intake.
* Inform men of possible sexual dysfunction.
* Tell patient of possible difficult urination.
* Instruct patient to avoid intake of alcoholic beverages or other CNS depressants.
* Advise patient that drug may cause drowsiness and to use caution while driving or performing other tasks requiring mental alertness.
* Advise patient to complete full course of therapy; may take 4 to 6 wk to see full benefits.

Desirudin

(deh-SIHR-uh-din)

Class Anticoagulants

How Supplied

Iprivask Powder for injection, lyophilized 15 mg

Action

PHARMACOLOGY: Binds to thrombin, blocking the thrombogenic activity of thrombin, thereby prolonging the clotting time of human plasma. Activated partial thromboplastin time (aPTT) is a measure of the anticoagulant activity of desirudin.

PHARMACOKINETICS/DYNAMICS:

Absorption: Following SC administration of 0.3 or 0.5 mg/kg, absorption is complete. C_{max} is reached 1 and 3 hr after single SC doses of 0.1 to 0.75 mg/kg, respectively.

Distribution: Binds directly to thrombin.

Metabolism: Metabolized and eliminated by the kidney with 40% to 50% excreted unchanged.

Excretion: Mean terminal elimination t½ is approximately 2 hr.

Special Populations:

Renal Function Impairment – Elimination t½ is prolonged in severe renal insufficiency up to 12 hr. Dose adjustments are recommended in certain circumstances based on degree of impairment or aPTT measurements.

Elderly – Because elderly patients are more likely to have decreased renal function, care should be taken in dose selection. Dosage adjustment in patients with moderate and severe renal impairment is necessary.

Indications Prophylaxis of deep vein thrombosis, which may lead to pulmonary embolism, in patients undergoing elective hip replacement surgery.

Contraindications Hypersensitivity to natural or recombinant hirudins; patients with active bleeding and/or irreversible coagulation disorders.

Route/Dosage

ADULTS: SC 15 mg q 12 hr with the initial dose given up to 5 to 15 min before surgery, but after induction of regional block anesthesia if used.

Renal Function Impairment

ADULTS: SC *Moderate impairment (Ccr 31 to 60 mL/min/1.73 m²)* - Initiate therapy at 5 mg q 12 hr. If aPTT exceeds 2 times control, interrupt therapy until the value returns to less than 2 times control, then resume therapy at a reduced dose based on the initial degree of aPTT abnormality. *Severe impairment (Ccr less than 31 mL/min/1.73 m²)* - Initiate therapy at 1.7 mg q 12 hr and monitor aPTT and serum creatinine at least daily. If aPTT exceeds 2 times control, interrupt therapy until the value returns to less than 2 times control; then consider further dose reductions based on the initial degree of aPTT abnormality.

Interactions

Agents that enhance risk of hemorrhage (eg, anticoagulants, Dextran 40, systemic glucocorticoids, thrombolytics): Discontinue prior to initiation of desirudin therapy.

INCOMPATIBILITIES: Do not mix with other injections, solvents, or infusions.

Lab Test Interferences None well documented.

Adverse Reactions

CV: Thrombosis, hypotension, cerebrovascular disorder (less than 2%).

GI: Nausea (2%); vomiting, hematemesis (less than 2%).

OTHER: Hemorrhage (30%); hematomas (6%); injection site mass, wound secretion (4%); serious hemorrhage, anemia (3%); deep thrombophlebitis (2%); hypersensitivity, leg edema, fever, decreased hemoglobin, hematuria, dizziness, epistaxis, impaired healing (less than 2%); major hemorrhage (less than 1%, also reported rarely in postmarketing but sometimes fatal); anaphylactic/anaphylactoid (postmarketing).

> WARNING:
>
> *Spinal/Epidural hematomas:* Neuraxial anesthesia (epidural/spinal anesthesia) or spinal puncture in patients anticoagulated with selective inhibitors of thrombin, such as desirudin, may increase the risk of developing an epidural or spinal hematoma, which can result in long-term or permanent paralysis. The risk of these events may be increased by use of indwelling spinal catheters for analgesia administration or by concurrent use of drugs affecting hemostasis (eg, nonsteroidal anti-inflammatory drugs, platelet inhibitors, or other anticoagulants). The risk appears to be increased by traumatic or repeated epidural or spinal puncture. Patients should be monitored frequently for signs and symptoms of neurological impairment. If neurological compromise is noted, urgent treatment is necessary.

Precautions

Pregnancy: Category C.

Lactation: Undetermined.

Children: Safety and efficacy not established.
Elderly: Use with caution because of increased likelihood of decreased renal function.
Renal function impairment: Use with caution, adjusting the dose as indicated.
Hepatic function impairment: Use with caution.
Antibodies/Re-exposure: Antibodies have been reported in patients treated with hirudin. Do not exclude potential for cross-sensitivity to hirudin products.
Hemorrhagic events: Use with caution in patients with increased risk of hemorrhage (eg, recent major surgery, organ biopsy, or puncture of a noncompressible vessel within the last month, history of hemorrhagic stroke, intracranial or intraocular bleeding, recent ischemic stroke, severe uncontrolled hypertension, bacterial endocarditis, known hemostatic disorder, history of GI or pulmonary bleeding within the past 3 mo).
Laboratory tests: Monitor aPTT daily in patients with increased risk of bleeding and/or renal impairment. Monitor serum creatinine daily in patients with renal impairment.
Switching from oral anticoagulants: Greater inhibition of hemostasis measured by aPTT, PT, and INR occurs. Monitor anticoagulant activity in evaluation of overall coagulation status of the patient during the switch.

Overdosage: Signs and Symptoms
Hemorrhagic complications.

PATIENT CARE CONSIDERATIONS
Administration/Storage
- For SC administration only. Not for intradermal, IM, or IV administration.
- Prescribed dose is administered q 12 hr.
- Rotate injection sites between left and right anterolateral or posterolateral thigh or abdominal wall.
- Administer initial dose 5 to 15 min before surgery but after induction of regional block anesthesia, if used.
- Follow manufacturer's instructions for reconstitution of powder. Do not use any diluent other than that supplied with the powder.
- Inspect solution visually before administration. Do not administer if solution is cloudy, discolored, or contains particulate matter.
- Use reconstituted solution immediately if possible. Reconstituted solution may be stored for up to 24 hr at room temperature and protected from light. Discard any unused solution or solution that has been stored for over 24 hr.
- Do not mix with other injections, solvents, or infusions.
- Desirudin cannot be used interchangeably with other hirudins.
- Store unopened vials at controlled room temperature (59° to 86°F). Protect from light.

Assessment/Interventions
- Obtain patient history, including drug history and any known allergies. Note history of renal impairment, liver disease, recent puncture of organ or noncompressible vessel, severe uncontrolled hypertension, hemorrhagic stroke, recent ischemic stroke, intracranial or intraocular bleeding including hemorrhagic diabetic retinopathy, intracerebral surgery or other neuraxial procedures, bacterial endocarditis, recent major bleeding, hemostatic defect, GI or pulmonary bleeding within past 3 mo, and concurrent therapy with agents that may increase the risk of hemorrhage (eg, *Dextran 40*, glucocorticoids, thrombolytics, anticoagulants, platelet inhibitors).
- Note any condition that would contraindicate use of desirudin, including active bleeding and/or irreversible coagulation disorder.
- Ensure that patient is evaluated for bleeding risk before initiating therapy.
- Discontinue any agent that could increase risk of hemorrhage prior to initiating desirudin therapy (eg, *Dextran 40*, glucocorticoids, thrombolytics, anticoagulants, platelet inhibitors). If coadministration cannot be avoided, ensure patient is monitored closely with clinical assessment for bleeding and laboratory analysis of coagulation status (eg, aPTT).
- Ensure that renal function is assessed in elderly patient.
- Ensure that aPTT is monitored daily in patient with increased risk of bleeding and/or renal impairment. If peak aPTT exceeds 2 times control, interrupt therapy until aPTT is less than 2 times control, then resume therapy with reduced dose.
- Ensure that serum creatinine is monitored daily in patient with moderate or severe renal impairment. Follow manufacturer's guidelines for dosage reduction in patient with renal impairment.
- Ensure that baseline hematocrit or hemoglobin, platelet count, and aPTT ratio (patient aPTT over aPTT reference value) are performed and evaluated prior to starting therapy.
- If patient has concurrent epidural spinal anesthesia/analgesia, ensure catheter is placed prior to initiating desirudin therapy and is removed when the anticoagulant effect of desirudin is low. Frequently assess patient with

- epidural catheter for signs or symptoms of spinal hematoma (eg, midline back pain, numbness or weakness in lower extremities, bowel and/or bladder dysfunction). Notify health care provider immediately if spinal hematoma is suspected.
- Monitor patient for signs of bleeding throughout therapy. If bleeding develops (eg, epistaxis, hematuria, hematemesis, bloody or black, tarry stools) or is suspected (eg, unexplained fall in hematocrit or BP or any unexplained symptoms), notify health care provider immediately.
- Monitor patient for signs of anaphylaxis or severe allergic reaction. Discontinue therapy and immediately notify health care provider if noted. Be prepared to treat appropriately.

Patient/Family Education
- Explain name, action, and potential side effects of drug.
- Advise patient, family, or caregiver that medication will be prepared and administered by a health care professional in a hospital setting.
- Instruct patient or family member to report any signs of bleeding or allergic reaction immediately.
- Instruct patient with epidural catheter to immediately report any of the following: midline back pain, numbness or weakness in lower extremities, bowel and/or bladder dysfunction.

Desloratadine

(dess-lore-AT-ah-deen)

Class Antihistamine

How Supplied
Clarinex Tablets 5 mg ♦ Clarinex RediTabs Tablets, rapidly disintegrating 5 mg
 Aerius

Action
PHARMACOLOGY: Long-acting histamine antagonist with selective H_1-receptor histamine antagonist activity.

PHARMACOKINETICS/DYNAMICS:

Absorption: T_{max} approximately 3 hr. C_{max} approximately 4 ng/mL. AUC approximately 56.9 ng•hr/mL.

Distribution: 82% to 87% protein bound.

Metabolism: Metabolized to 3-hydroxydesloratadine (active).

Excretion: The t½ is 27 hr. Approximately 87% excreted in urine and feces.

Onset: 1 hr.

Duration: 24 hr.

Special Populations:
Renal Function Impairment – AUC and C_{max} are increased. Dosage adjustment is recommended.
Hepatic Function Impairment – AUC and t½ are increased. Dosage adjustment is recommended.
Elderly – C_{max} and AUC are 20% greater. The t½ is 33.7 hr.

Indications Relief of nasal and nonnasal symptoms of seasonal and perennial allergic rhinitis; in chronic idiopathic urticaria for relief of symptoms of pruritus and reduction in number and size of hives.

Contraindications Hypersensitivity to any components of the product or to loratadine.

Route/Dosage
ADULTS AND CHILDREN 12 YR OF AGE AND OLDER: PO 5 mg once daily.
Renal/Hepatic impairment – PO 5 mg every other day.

Interactions None well documented.

Lab Test Interferences May prevent or diminish otherwise positive reactions to skin tests.

Adverse Reactions
CV: Tachycardia, palpitations (postmarketing).
CNS: Headache (14%); fatigue (5%); dizziness (4%); somnolence (2%).
EENT: Pharyngitis (4%); dry mouth (3%).
GI: Nausea (5%); dyspepsia (3%).
GU: Dysmenorrhea (2%).
OTHER: Myalgia (3%); hypersensitivity (including rash, pruritus, urticaria, edema, dyspnea, anaphylaxis [postmarketing]).

Precautions
Pregnancy: Category C.
Lactation: Excreted in breast milk.
Children: Safety and efficacy not established in children younger than 12 yr of age.
Elderly: Select dose with caution, reflecting greater frequency of decreased hepatic, renal, or cardiac function and comorbidity.
Renal function impairment: Dosage adjustment is recommended.
Hepatic function impairment: Dosage adjustment is recommended.

Overdosage: Signs and Symptoms
Increased heart rate and corrected QT interval.

PATIENT CARE CONSIDERATIONS
Administration/Storage
- Do not administer orally disintegrating tablet to patient with phenylketonuria without first discussing with health care provider.
- Administer prescribed dose daily without regard to meals.
- Administer with food if GI upset occurs.
- Remove orally disintegrating tablet from blister just before administration. Have patient place on tongue and allow tablet to dissolve. May administer with or without water.
- Store tablets and orally disintegrating tablets at controlled room temperature (59° to 86°F). Do not remove orally disintegrating tablet from blister until just prior to administration.

Assessment/Interventions
- Obtain patient history, including drug history and any known allergies. Note renal impairment, hepatic impairment, phenylketonuria, or hypersensitivity to loratadine.
- Administer reduced dose (every-other-day dosing) to patient with liver or kidney disease.
- Assess patient for allergy symptoms (eg, rhinitis, nasal congestion, sneezing, itching, watery eyes, hives) before starting therapy and periodically throughout therapy. Notify health care provider if symptoms are not controlled or worsen.
- Monitor patient for dizziness and excessive drowsiness. If noted, hold therapy and notify health care provider.

Patient/Family Education
- Explain name, dose, action, and potential side effects of drug.
- Advise patient to take dose daily as prescribed and not to stop taking or change the dose unless advised by health care provider.
- Ensure patient understands how to store and take the orally disintegrating tablet.
- Advise patient to take without regard to meals but to take with food if stomach upset occurs.
- Advise patient that if allergy symptoms are not controlled, not to increase the dose of medication or frequency of use but to inform health care provider. Inform patient that larger or more frequent dosing does not increase effectiveness and may cause drowsiness.
- Caution patient not to take any OTC antihistamines while taking this medication unless advised by health care provider.
- Caution patient to avoid alcohol and other CNS depressants (eg, sedatives) while using this medication.
- Caution patient that drug may cause drowsiness and to use caution while driving or performing other tasks requiring mental alertness until tolerance is determined.
- Advise patient to take frequent sips of water, suck on ice chips or sugarless hard candy, or chew sugarless gum if dry mouth occurs.
- If patient is to have allergy skin testing, advise not to take the medication for at least 4 days before the skin testing.
- Advise women to notify health care provider if pregnant, planning to become pregnant, or breastfeeding.
- Instruct patient to stop taking drug and report persistent dizziness or excessive drowsiness to health care provider.
- Caution patient not to take any prescription or OTC medications, herbal preparations, or dietary supplements unless advised by health care provider.

Desmopressin Acetate (1-Deamino-8-D-Arginine Vasopressins)

(DESS-moe-PRESS-in ASS-uh-TATE)

Class Posterior pituitary hormone

How Supplied
DDAVP Tablets 0.1 mg, Tablets 0.2 mg, Nasal Solution 0.1 mg (0.1 mg/mL equals 400 IU arginine vasopressin), Injection 4 mcg/mL, Injection 15 mcg/mL ♦ *Stimate* Nasal Solution 1.5 mg/mL, Injection 4 mcg/mL
✤ *Apo-Desmopressin* ♦ *DDAVP Rhinyle Nasal Solution* ♦ *Minirin* ♦ *Octostim* ♦ *Octostim Spray*

Action
PHARMACOLOGY: Has antidiuretic effect that decreases urinary volume and increases urine osmolality.

PHARMACOKINETICS/DYNAMICS:
Absorption:
Oral – T_{max} is 0.9 hr.
Intranasal – T_{max} is 1.5 hr.

Excretion: $t_{½}$ is 1.5 to 2.5 hr (oral), 7.8 and 75.5 min for the fast and slow phases, respectively (IV and intranasal).

Onset: Approximately 1 hr (oral), within 30 min to increase Factor VIII (IV and intranasal).

Peak: 4 to 7 hr (oral), 1.5 to 2 hr to increase Factor VIII (IV and intranasal).

Duration: 8 to 12 hr (oral).

Indications Control of primary nocturnal

enuresis; control of central cranial diabetes insipidus; maintenance of hemostasis in patients with hemophilia A and type I von Willebrand disease during surgery and postoperatively.

Unlabeled use(s): Treatment of chronic autonomic failure.

Contraindications Standard considerations.

Route/Dosage

Central Cranial Diabetes Insipidus

ADULTS AND CHILDREN 12 YR AND OLDER: **Intranasal** 0.1 to 0.4 qd. **IV/SC** 0.5 to 1 mL qd in 2 divided doses. **PO** 0.05 mg bid adjusted for adequate diurnal rhythm (range 0.1 to 1.2 mg/day divided).

CHILDREN 3 MO TO 12 YR: **Intranasal** 0.05 to 0.3 mL qd, either as a single dose or 2 divided doses. **PO** Begin dosing with 0.05 mg. Careful fluid intake restrictions in children is required to prevent hyponatremia and water intoxification.

Hemophilia A, Type I von Willebrand Disease

ADULTS AND CHILDREN: **IV** Administer 0.3 mcg/kg diluted in sterile physiologic saline infused slowly over 15 to 30 min. In patients weighing more than 10 kg, use 50 mL diluent; in children weighing up to 10 kg, use 10 mL. **Intranasal** Administer by nasal insufflation, 1 spray per nostril, to provide a total dose of 300 mcg. In patients weighing less than 50 kg, 150 mcg administered as a single spray provided the expected effect on Factor VIII coagulant activity, Factor VIII ristocetin cofactor activity, and skin bleeding time.

Primary Nocturnal Enuresis

ADULTS AND CHILDREN 6 YR AND OLDER: **Intranasal** 20 mcg (0.2 mL) at bedtime.

Interactions

Carbamazepine; chlorpropamide: May potentiate antidiuretic effects of desmopressin.

Lab Test Interferences
None well documented.

Adverse Reactions

CV: Slight elevation in BP, facial flushing (intranasal); chest pain, palpitations, tachycardia, edema (*Stimate*).
CNS: Headache (intranasal); somnolence, dizziness, insomnia, agitation (*Stimate*).
DERM: Local erythema, swelling, pain (injection).
EENT: Rhinitis, nosebleed, sore throat (intranasal); itchy or light-sensitive eyes (*Stimate*).
GI: Nausea, mild abdominal cramps (intranasal); dyspepsia, vomiting (*Stimate*).
GU: Vulval pain (intranasal); balanitis (*Stimate*).
HEPA: Elevated LFT (injection).
RESP: Cough, upper respiratory infection (intranasal).
OTHER: Chills, warm feeling, pain (*Stimate*).

Precautions

Pregnancy: Category B.
Lactation: Undetermined.
Children: Infants and children require careful fluid intake restriction to prevent possible hyponatremia and water intoxication. Safety and efficacy of intranasal form have not been established in children younger than 11 mo. Safety and efficacy of parenteral form for control of diabetes insipidus have not been established for children younger than 12 yr.
Elderly: Elderly patients should ingest only enough fluid to satisfy thirst; water intoxication and hyponatremia are possible.
Hypersensitivity: Rare severe allergic reactions have been reported. Anaphylaxis has occurred with IV administration.
Special risk patients: Use drug with caution in patients with coronary artery insufficiency or hypertensive cardiovascular disease. Use with caution in patients with conditions associated with fluid and electrolyte imbalance (eg, cystic fibrosis). These patients are prone to hyponatremia. Use with caution in patients predisposed to thrombus formation. Rare thrombotic events have occurred in these patients.
Decrease in plasma osmolality: An extreme decrease in plasma osmolality occurs rarely and may result in seizures and coma.

Overdosage: Signs and Symptoms
Headache, abdominal cramps, nausea, facial flushing.

PATIENT CARE CONSIDERATIONS

Administration/Storage

- For intranasal administration, ensure that nasal passages are intact, clean, and free of obstruction before administration of drug. Calibrated plastic tube is provided in nasal tube delivery system. Draw solution up into this tube and insert into nostril. Place opposite end of tube in mouth and blow into tube to deliver medication.
- Cranial surgery, changes in nasal mucosa, and nasal packing can compromise intranasal delivery. In this situation, parenteral therapy should be considered.
- If used preoperatively, administer injection 30 min prior to procedure; administer intranasally 2 hr before.
- The nasal spray pump only delivers doses of 10 mcg (*DDAVP*) or 150 mcg (*Stimate*). If doses other than these are required, consider nasal tube delivery or injection.

- The *Stimate* pump must be primed prior to the first use. To prime pump, press down 4 times. Discard the bottle after 25 doses because the amount delivered thereafter per spray may be substantially less than 150 mcg.
- Refrigerate nasal solution. Nasal solution will maintain stability for up to 3 wk when stored at room temperature.
- Refrigerate injectable solution at 2° to 8°C (36° to 46°F).

Assessment/Interventions
- Obtain patient history, including drug history and any known allergies.
- Obtain baseline and ongoing measurements of both urine and plasma osmolality when treating patient with diabetes insipidus.
- Monitor BP and pulse during infusion.
- Check coagulation status prior to treating patients with hemophilia A and type I von Willebrand disease. Coagulation testing may include Factor VIII coagulant activity, Factor VIII antigen, ristocetin cofactor, activated PTT, and skin bleeding time.
- Monitor I&O closely and accurately when drug is administered to very young and elderly patients. Fluid restriction in infants, children, and elderly is required to prevent possible hyponatremia and water intoxication.
- Continually assess patient for signs of fluid intoxication including lungs, extremities (edema), weight, or jugular venous distention.
- Check for nasal mucosa changes (eg, edema, discharge, congestion, scarring), transphenoidal hypophysectomy, and nasal packing because they may compromise intranasal delivery; consider IV method.
- Occasional change in response to IV desmopressin occurs with time, usually longer than 6 mo.

Patient/Family Education
- Instruct patient on proper intranasal administration techniques and have patient or family demonstrate ability to perform.
- Remind patient receiving drug intranasally to frequently inspect nasal passages.
- Explain that it is important to reduce fluid intake when therapy is initiated to decrease chance of water intoxication.
- Instruct patient to report the following symptoms to health care provider: headache, shortness of breath, heartburn, nausea, abdominal cramps, vulvar pain.
- Inform patients that *DDAVP* nasal spray accurately delivers 25 or 50 doses. Discard any solution remaining after the 25 or 50 doses because the amount delivered thereafter may be substantially less than prescribed.

Desonide

(DESS-oh-nide)

Class Corticosteroid/Topical

How Supplied
DesOwen Cream 0.05%, Ointment 0.05%, Lotion 0.05% ◆ *Tridesilon* Cream 0.05%, Ointment 0.05%, Lotion 0.05%
 Desocort

Action
PHARMACOLOGY: Low-potency topical corticosteroid that depresses formation, release, and activity of endogenous mediators of inflammation including prostaglandins, kinins, histamine, liposomal enzymes and complement system; modifies body's immune response.

Indications
Relief of inflammatory and pruritic manifestations of corticosteroid-responsive dermatoses.

Contraindications
Hypersensitivity to other corticosteroids; monotherapy in primary bacterial infections; ophthalmic use.

Route/Dosage
ADULTS AND CHILDREN: **Topical** Apply sparingly to affected area bid to tid.

Interactions None well documented.

Lab Test Interferences None well documented.

Adverse Reactions
DERM: Burning; itching; irritation; dryness; folliculitis; hypertrichosis; acneiform eruptions; hypopigmentation; perioral dermatitis; allergic contact dermatitis; skin maceration; secondary infection; skin atrophy; striae; miliaria.
EENT: Cataracts; glaucoma.

Precautions
Pregnancy: Category C.
Lactation: May be excreted in breast milk.
Children: May be more susceptible to topical corticosteroid-induced HPA axis suppression and Cushing syndrome; conditions that may augment systemic absorption include use over large body surface areas, prolonged use, and occlusive dressings.
Systemic effects: Systemic absorption may produce reversible HPA axis suppression, manifestations of Cushing syndrome, hyperglycemia, and glucosuria.

Desoximetasone

(dess-OX-ee-MET-ah-sone)

Class Corticosteroid/Topical

How Supplied
Topicort Ointment 0.25%, Cream 0.25%, Gel 0.05% ♦ *Topicort LP* Cream 0.05%

 Desoxi

Action
PHARMACOLOGY: High-potency topical corticosteroid that depresses formation, release, and activity of endogenous mediators of inflammation including prostaglandins, kinins, histamine, liposomal enzymes, and complement system; modifies the body's immune response.

Indications Relief of inflammation and pruritic manifestations of corticosteroid-responsive dermatoses.

Contraindications Hypersensitivity to other corticosteroids; monotherapy in primary bacterial infections; ophthalmic use.

Route/Dosage
ADULTS AND CHILDREN OLDER THAN 10 YR OF AGE: **Topical** Apply sparingly to affected areas bid.

Interactions None well documented.

Lab Test Interferences None well documented.

Adverse Reactions
DERM: Burning; itching; irritation; dryness; folliculitis; hypertrichosis; acneiform eruptions; hypopigmentation; perioral dermatitis; allergic contact dermatitis; maceration of the skin; secondary infection; skin atrophy; striae; miliaria.
EENT: Cataracts; glaucoma.

Precautions
Pregnancy: Category C.
Lactation: May be excreted in breast milk.
Children: Safety and efficacy is not determined in children younger than 10 yr of age. Children may be more susceptible to topical corticosteroid-induced hypothalamic-pituitary-adrenal (HPA) axis suppression and Cushing syndrome; conditions that may augment systemic absorption include use over large body surface areas, prolonged use, and occlusive dressings.
Infections: Use with appropriate antimicrobials in the presence of skin infections.
Occlusive dressings: Adverse effects are more common when occlusive dressings are used.
Systemic: Systemic absorption may produce reversible HPA axis suppression, manifestations of Cushing syndrome, hyperglycemia, and glucosuria.

PATIENT CARE CONSIDERATIONS

Administration/Storage
- For topical use only. Not for ophthalmic, oral, or intravaginal use.
- Apply cream, ointment, or gel sparingly but in sufficient quantity to cover affected areas; rub in gently.
- Apply bid as prescribed.
- Avoid contact with the eyes.
- Store cream, ointment, and gel at ambient room temperature (59° to 86°F). Keep tube tightly capped.

Assessment/Interventions
- Obtain patient history, including drug history and any known allergies.
- Ensure that appropriate antifungal or antibacterial therapy is used in patient who has a concomitant skin infection.
- Assess and document skin condition before initial application and periodically throughout treatment. Inform health care provider if condition does not improve, worsens, or if application site reactions develop.
- Ensure that patient applying medication to a large surface area or to areas under occlusion is periodically evaluated for evidence of HPA axis suppression (eg, adrenocorticotropic hormone [ACTH] stimulation, morning plasma cortisol, urinary free cortisol tests).

Patient/Family Education
- Explain name, action, and potential side effects of drug.
- Teach patient or caregiver proper technique for applying cream, ointment, or gel: Wash hands; apply sufficient cream or ointment to cover affected areas sparingly and then gently massage into skin; wash hands after applying cream, ointment, or gel.
- Advise patient to apply cream, ointment, or gel to affected areas bid as directed by health care provider.
- Advise patient that if a dose is missed, to apply it as soon as remembered and then continue on the regular schedule. If it is almost time for the next application, instruct patient to skip the dose and continue on the regular schedule. Caution patient not to apply double doses.
- Caution patient not to apply to face, underarms, or groin area unless directed by health care provider.
- Caution patient not to bandage, cover, or wrap treated skin areas, or use cosmetics or

other skin products over treated areas unless advised by health care provider.
- Caution patient to avoid contact with eyes. Advise patient that if cream does come into contact with the eyes, to wash them with large amounts of cool water and contact health care provider if eye irritation occurs.
- Caution parents of pediatric patients not to use tight-fitting diapers or plastic pants on child being treated in the diaper area.
- Advise patient that symptoms should begin to improve fairly soon after starting treatment and to notify health care provider if condition does not improve, worsens, or if application site reactions (eg, burning, stinging, redness, itching) develop.
- Advise patient that therapy is usually discontinued when control has been achieved.
- Advise women to notify health care provider if pregnant, planning to become pregnant, or breastfeeding.
- Warn patient not to take any prescription or OTC drugs, dietary supplements, or herbal preparations without consulting health care provider.
- Advise patient that follow-up visits to monitor response to treatment may be required and to keep appointments.

Dexamethasone

(DEX-uh-METH-uh-sone)
Class Corticosteroid

How Supplied
Aeroseb-Dex Aerosol 0.01% ♦ *Decadron* Tablets 0.5 mg, Tablets 0.75 mg, Tablets 4 mg, Elixir 0.5 mg/5 mL ♦ *Decaspray* Aerosol 0.04% ♦ *Dexameth* Tablets 0.5 mg, Tablets 0.75 mg, Tablets 1.5 mg, Tablets 4 mg ♦ *Dexone* Tablets 0.5 mg, Tablets 0.75 mg, Tablets 1.5 mg, Tablets 4 mg ♦ *Hexadrol* Tablets 1.5 mg, Tablets 4 mg, Tablets therapeutic pack, Elixir 0.5 mg/5 mL ♦ *Maxidex* Suspension 0.1%

Dexamethasone Acetate
Dalalone DP Injection 16 mg/mL suspension ♦ *Dalalone LA* Injection 8 mg/mL suspension ♦ *Decadron-LA* Injection 8 mg/mL suspension ♦ *Decaject-L.A.* Injection 8 mg/mL suspension ♦ *Dexasone-L.A.* Injection 8 mg/mL suspension ♦ *Dexone LA* Injection 8 mg/mL suspension ♦ *Solurex LA* Injection 8 mg/mL suspension

Dexamethasone Sodium Phosphate
AK-Dex Solution 0.1% ♦ *Dalalone* Injection 4 mg/mL ♦ *Decadron Phosphate* Cream 0.1%, Injection 4 mg/mL, Injection 24 mg/mL, Ointment 0.05%, Solution 0.1% ♦ *Decaject* Injection 4 mg/mL ♦ *Dexasone* Injection 4 mg/mL ♦ *Dexone* Injection 4 mg/mL ♦ *Hexadrol Phosphate* Injection 4 mg/mL, Injection 10 mg/mL, Injection 20 mg/mL ♦ *Solurex* Injection 4 mg/mL
🍁 *Dexair* ♦ *PMS-Dexamethasone* ♦ *ratio-Dexamethasone*

Action
PHARMACOLOGY: Synthetic long-acting glucocorticoid that depresses formation, release and activity of endogenous mediators of inflammation including prostaglandins, kinins, histamine, liposomal enzymes and complement system. Also modifies body's immune response.

PHARMACOKINETICS/DYNAMICS:
Metabolism: Metabolized in the liver by CYP3A4.
Excretion: The t½ 1.8 to 3.5 hr.
Onset: Rapid (injection).
Duration: Short (injection).

Indications Testing of adrenal cortical hyperfunction; management of primary or secondary adrenal cortex insufficiency, rheumatic disorders, collagen diseases, dermatologic diseases, allergic states, allergic and inflammatory ophthalmic processes, respiratory diseases, hematologic disorders, neoplastic diseases, cerebral edema associated with primary or metastatic brain tumor, craniotomy or head injury, edematous states (caused by nephrotic syndrome), GI diseases, multiple sclerosis, tuberculous meningitis, trichinosis with neurologic or myocardial involvement.
Intralesional administration: Treatment for such conditions as keloids, psoriatic plaques, discoid lupus erythematosus, alopecia areata.
Intra-articular or soft tissue administration: Short-term adjunctive treatment for such conditions as synovitis of osteoarthritis, rheumatoid arthritis, acute gouty arthritis, posttraumatic osteoarthritis.
Topical: Treatment of inflammatory and pruritic manifestations of corticosteroid-responsive dermatoses.
Oral inhalation: Treatment of corticosteroid-responsive and bronchial asthma bronchospastic states.
Intranasal: Treatment of allergic or inflammatory nasal conditions, nasal polyps (excluding those originating within sinuses).
Ophthalmic: Treatment of steroid-responsive inflammatory conditions of palpebral and bulbar conjunctiva, lid, cornea, and anterior segment of globe. **Unlabeled use(s):** Treatment of acute

mountain sickness, bacterial meningitis, bronchopulmonary dysplasia in preterm infants; diagnosis of depression; treatment of hirsutism; and use as antiemetic.

Contraindications Systemic fungal infections; IM use in idiopathic thrombocytopenic purpura; administration of live virus vaccines; topical monotherapy in primary bacterial infections; intranasal use in untreated localized infections involving nasal mucosa; ophthalmic use in acute superficial herpes simplex keratitis, fungal diseases of ocular structures, vaccinia, varicella, and ocular tuberculosis.

Route/Dosage
All dosages shown are for adults unless indicated otherwise.

DEXAMETHASONE
Initial dose – **PO** 0.75 to 9 mg/day.
Suppression Tests –
Cushing syndrome: **PO** 1 mg at 11 PM or 0.5 mg q 6 hr for 48 hr.
To distinguish Cushing syndrome-caused pituitary ACTH excess from other causes: **PO** 2 mg q 6 hr for 48 hr.
Acute Mountain Sickness – **PO** 4 mg q 6 hr.
Antiemetic – **PO** 16 to 20 mg.
Diagnosis of Depression – **PO** 1 mg.
Hirsutism – **PO** 0.5 to 1 mg/day.

DEXAMETHASONE ACETATE
Systemic – **IM** 8 to 16 mg; may repeat in 1 to 3 wk.
Interlesional – **IM** 0.8 to 1.6 mg.
Intra-Articular and Soft Tissue – **IM** 4 to 16 mg; may repeat at 1 to 3 wk intervals.

DEXAMETHASONE SODIUM PHOSPHATE
Systemic – **IV/IM** 0.5 to 9 mg/day.
Cerebral Edema – **IV** 10 mg, then IM 4 mg q 6 hr until max response.
Brain Tumors – **IV/IM** 2 mg bid to tid.
Unresponsive shock – **IV** 1 to 6 mg/kg as single injection; or 40 mg followed by repeated IV injections q 2 to 6 hr.
Bacterial meningitis – **IV** 0.15 mg/kg q 6 hr.
Bronchopulmonary dysplasia in preterm infants – **IV** 0.5 mg/kg.
Intra-Articular, Intralesional, or Soft Tissue – Large joints 2 to 4 mg; small joints 0.8 to 1 mg; bursae 2 to 3 mg; tendon sheaths 0.4 to 1 mg; soft tissue infiltration 2 to 6 mg; ganglia 1 to 2 mg.
Topical – Apply sparingly to affected areas bid to qid.
Oral Inhalation –
Adults: 3 inhalations tid to qid.
Children: 2 inhalations tid to qid.
Intranasal –
Adults: 2 sprays (168 mcg) into each nostril bid to tid.
Children 6 to 12 yr: 1 or 2 sprays (84 to 168 mcg) into each nostril bid.
Ophthalmic solution – Instill 1 to 2 drops into conjunctival sac q 1 hr during day and q 2 hr during night.
Ophthalmic ointment – Apply thin coating in lower conjunctival sac tid to qid.

Interactions
Aminoglutethimide: May decrease dexamethasone-induced adrenal suppression.
Anticholinesterases: May antagonize anticholinesterase effects in myasthenia gravis.
Anticoagulants, oral: May alter anticoagulant dose requirements.
Barbiturates: May decrease effects of dexamethasone.
Hydantoins: May increase clearance and decrease therapeutic efficacy of dexamethasone.
Rifampin: May increase clearance and decrease therapeutic efficacy of dexamethasone.
Salicylates: May reduce serum levels and efficacy of salicylates.
Troleandomycin: May increase dexamethasone effects.

Lab Test Interferences May cause increased urine glucose and serum cholesterol; decreased serum levels of potassium, T_3 and T_4; decreased uptake of thyroid ^{131}I; false-negative nitroblue-tetrazolium test; altered brain scan results; suppression of skin test reactions.

Adverse Reactions
CV: Thromboembolism or fat embolism; thrombophlebitis; necrotizing angiitis; cardiac arrhythmias or ECG changes; syncopal episodes; hypertension; myocardial rupture; CHF.
CNS: Convulsions; increased intracranial pressure with papilledema (pseudotumor cerebri); vertigo; headache; neuritis; paresthesias; psychosis.
DERM: Impaired wound healing; thin fragile skin; petechiae and ecchymoses; erythema; lupus erythematosus–like lesions; subcutaneous fat atrophy; striae; hirsutism; acneiform eruptions; allergic dermatitis; urticaria; angioneurotic edema, perineal irritation; hyperpigmentation or hypopigmentation. Burning; itching; irritation; erythema; dryness; folliculitis; hypertrichosis; pruritus; perioral dermatitis; allergic contact dermatitis; stinging, cracking and tightening of skin; secondary infections; skin atrophy; striae; miliaria; telangiectasia (topical).
EENT: Posterior subcapsular cataracts; increased IOP; glaucoma; exophthalmos. Dry mouth; throat irritation; hoarseness; dysphonia; coughing (oral inhalation). Nasal irritation; burning; stinging; dryness; epistaxis or bloody mucus; rebound congestion; sneezing, rhinorrhea; anosmia; loss of sense of taste; throat discomfort

(intranasal). Glaucoma with optic nerve damage; visual acuity and field defects; posterior subcapsular cataract formation; secondary ocular infections; transient stinging or burning (ophthalmic).
GI: Pancreatitis; abdominal distension; ulcerative esophagitis; nausea; vomiting; increased appetite and weight gain; peptic ulcer with perforation and hemorrhage; bowel perforation.
GU: Increased or decreased number and motility of spermatozoa.
HEMA: Leukocytosis.
METAB: Sodium and fluid retention; hypokalemia; hypokalemic alkalosis; metabolic alkalosis; hypocalcemia.
RESP: Wheezing (oral inhalation).
OTHER: Musculoskeletal effects (eg, weakness, myopathy, muscle mass loss, osteoporosis, spontaneous fractures); endocrine abnormalities (eg, menstrual irregularities, cushingoid state, growth suppression in children sweating, decreased carbohydrate tolerance, hyperglycemia, glycosuria, increased insulin or sulfonylurea requirements in diabetics, anaphylactoid or hypersensitivity reactions); aggravation or masking of infections; malaise; leukocytosis; fatigue; insomnia. Osteonecrosis; tendon rupture; infection; skin atrophy; postinjection flare; hypersensitivity; facial flushing (intra-articular). Topical use may theoretically produce adverse reactions seen with systemic use because of absorption.

Precautions
Pregnancy: Pregnancy category undetermined (systemic use); Category C (topical uses).
Lactation: Excreted in breast milk.
Children: May be more susceptible to adverse reactions from topical use than are adults. Observe growth and development of infants and children on prolonged therapy.
Elderly: May require lower doses.

PATIENT CARE CONSIDERATIONS
Administration/Storage
- For IM injection, inject dexamethasone acetate deep into gluteal muscle. Avoid injection into deltoid, and rotate injection sites. Do not use SC route.
- Refer to package insert for directions on how to store particular form of dexamethasone.
- If ordered PO, administer in morning to coincide with body's normal secretion of cortisol.

Assessment/Interventions
- Obtain patient history, including drug history and any known allergies.
- Obtain baseline weight and vital signs.
- Assess involved system before and periodically during therapy.
- When used in child, periodically assess child's growth.

Renal function impairment: Use cautiously; monitor renal function.
Sulfite sensitivity: Some products may contain sodium bisulfite, which may cause allergic-type reactions in some individuals.
Adrenal suppression: Prolonged therapy may lead to hypothalamic-pituitary-adrenal suppression.
Fluid and electrolyte balance: Can cause elevated BP, salt and water retention, and increased potassium and calcium excretion. Dietary salt restriction and potassium supplementation may be needed.
Hepatitis: May be harmful in chronic active hepatitis B surface antigen.
Infections: May mask signs of infection. May decrease host-defense mechanisms to prevent dissemination of infection.
Ocular effects: Use systemically with caution in ocular herpes simplex because of possible corneal perforation.
Ophthalmic use: Prolonged use may result in glaucoma or other complications.
Peptic ulcer: May contribute to peptic ulceration, especially in large doses.
Stress: Increased dosage of rapidly acting corticosteroid may be needed before, during and after stressful situations.
Withdrawal: Abrupt discontinuation may result in adrenal insufficiency. Discontinue gradually.

Overdosage: Signs and Symptoms
Fever, myalgia, arthralgia, malaise, anorexia, nausea, skin desquamation, orthostatic hypotension, dizziness, fainting, dyspnea, hypoglycemia (acute overdose); moonface central obesity, striae, hirsutism, acne, ecchymoses, hypertension, osteoporosis, myopathy, sexual dysfunction, diabetes, hyperlipidemia, peptic ulcer, infection, electrolyte and fluid imbalance (chronic cushingoid changes).

- Monitor intake and output.
- Assess patient regularly for signs of infection (eg, delayed wound healing, WBC count) because steroids can mask other common signs of infection such as fever, swelling and redness.
- Notify health care provider if signs of fluid overload develop (eg, peripheral edema, weight gain, rales/crackles, dyspnea).
- If emotional changes occur, such as depression, take safety measures such as suicide precautions.
- If side effects develop with long-term therapy, expect to change to alternate-day therapy. Check medication record and document well.

Patient/Family Education
- Caution patient that stopping drug abruptly is

- dangerous and may cause adrenal insufficiency.
- Explain rationale for tapering off medication when that time comes.
- Teach patient or family procedures for correctly administering specific form of drug (eg, ophthalmic, inhalation, topical).
- Caution patient against receiving immunizations while drug is being taken.
- Advise patient on long-term therapy to carry medication identification card or to wear bracelet. In case of emergency, this information is important for treatment.
- Instruct patient to avoid people with infections, particularly respiratory.
- If form patient is receiving is intranasal, instruct patient to clear nasal passages of secretions before administering drug.
- If topical, advise patient not to use occlusive dressings such as plastic wrap more than 12 hr a day. Occlusion may lead to sweat retention and bacterial and fungal infections. Remember that tight-fitting plastic diapers on infants may also be occlusive.
- Teach patient to take oral forms with meals or snacks if GI irritation occurs.
- Review guidelines for missed doses of particular product with patient.
- Teach patient on long-term therapy how to keep a weight record.
- Instruct patient to inform other health care providers if taking a steroid.
- Review signs of infection and remind patient that fever, swelling, and redness may be masked in infection.
- Review possible side effects of dexamethasone with patient and to report these to health care provider.

Dexamethasone/Tobramycin

(DEX-uh-METH-uh-sone/TOE-bruh-MY-sin)

Class Ophthalmic/Antibiotic/Corticosteroid

How Supplied
TobraDex Ointment 0.1% dexamethasone/0.3% tobramycin, Ophthalmic Suspension 0.1% dexamethasone/0.3% tobramycin

Action
PHARMACOLOGY: Tobramycin inhibits bacterial protein synthesis, causing death; dexamethasone suppresses inflammatory response.

Indications Superficial bacterial ocular infection or risk of bacterial ocular infection; inflammatory conditions of palpebral and bulbar conjunctiva, cornea, and anterior segment of globe where inherent risk of steroid use in certain infective conjunctivitis is accepted to obtain a diminution of edema and inflammation; chronic anterior uveitis and corneal injury from chemical, radiation, or thermal burns, or penetration of foreign bodies; risk of superficial ocular infection is high or is an expectation or potentially dangerous numbers of bacteria will be present in the eye.

Contraindications Epithelial herpes simplex keratitis (dendritic keratitis), vaccinia, varicella, and many other viral diseases of the cornea and conjunctiva; mycobacterial infection of the eye; fungal diseases of ocular structure; hypersensitivity to a component of the product.

Route/Dosage
SOLUTION
ADULTS: **Ophthalmic** Start with 1 or 2 drops instilled into conjunctival sac(s) q 4 to 6 hr during first 24 to 48 hr; dosage may be increased to 1 or 2 drops q 2 hr.

OINTMENT
ADULTS AND CHILDREN 2 YR AND OLDER: **Ophthalmic** Apply small amount (approximately 0.5-inch ribbon) into conjunctival sac(s) up to 3 or 4 times daily.

Interactions None well documented.

Lab Test Interferences None well documented.

Adverse Reactions
EENT: Localized ocular toxicity (eg, lid itching, swelling, conjunctival erythema); elevated IOP (with possible glaucoma); infrequent optic nerve damage; posterior subcapsular cataract formation; delayed wound healing; secondary infection (eg, corneal fungal infections); secondary bacterial ocular infection.
OTHER: Hypersensitivity.

Precautions
Pregnancy: Category C.
Lactation: Tobramycin: Undetermined; dexamethasone: Excreted in breast milk.
Children: Ophthalmic solution: Safety and efficacy not established; ophthalmic ointment: safety and efficacy not established in children younger than 2 yr.
Hypersensitivity: Sensitivity to topically applied aminoglycosides and cross-sensitivity to other aminoglycosides may occur.
Fungal infections: Consider possibility of fungal infections with long-term steroid dosing; prolonged use may result in overgrowth of nonsusceptible organisms, including fungi.

Overdosage: Signs and Symptoms
Punctate keratitis, erythema, increased lacrimation, edema, lid itching.

PATIENT CARE CONSIDERATIONS

Administration/Storage
- Shake suspension well before use.
- Instill prescribed number of drops of suspension q 2 to 6 hr as ordered.
- Instill prescribed amount of ointment 3 to 4 times a day as ordered.
- If using other topical ophthalmic drugs, separate each medication by at least 5 min.
- Store at controlled room temperature. Keep suspension upright. Keep container tightly closed.

Assessment/Interventions
- Obtain patient history, including drug history and any known allergies. Note history of viral, fungal, or mycobacterial infection of the eye.
- Monitor patient's response to therapy.

Patient/Family Education
- Explain name, dose, action, and potential side effects of drug.
- Review prescribed dosing schedule with patient.
- Teach patient proper technique for instilling eye drops: Wash hands; do not allow dropper to touch eye. Tilt head back, look up; pull lower eyelid down; instill prescribed number of drops. Close eye for 1 to 2 min and apply gentle pressure to bridge of nose for 3 to 5 min. Do not rub eye.
- Teach patient proper technique for instilling ointment: Wash hands; do not allow tip of tube to touch eye. Tilt head back, look up; pull lower eyelid down to form pocket; place prescribed amount of ointment in the pocket. Look downward before closing eye. Do not rub eye.
- Advise patient that if > 1 topical ophthalmic drug is being used, administer the drugs at least 5 min apart.
- Inform patient that temporary blurred vision and stinging of the eye are the most common side effects and to contact the health care provider if they occur and are bothersome.
- Advise patient to contact the eye doctor if eye or eyelid inflammation is noted or if eye symptoms worsen or do not improve.
- Advise patient that the entire course of therapy must be completed to ensure maximal benefit and to complete full course of therapy even if symptoms have resolved.
- Instruct patient not to wear contact lenses during treatment.
- Remind patient that follow-up eye examinations may be necessary while using this medication and to keep appointments.

Dexchlorpheniramine Maleate

(dex-klor-fen-AIR-uh-meen MAL-ee-ate)

Class Antihistamine

How Supplied
Dexchlorpheniramine maleate Tablets, extended-release 4 mg, Tablets, extended-release 6 mg

Action
PHARMACOLOGY: Competitively antagonizes histamine H_1 at receptor sites.

PHARMACOKINETICS/DYNAMICS:
Absorption: C_{max} approximately 7 ng/mL. T_{max} approximately 3 hr.
Distribution: 69% to 72% protein bound.
Metabolism: Extensively metabolized.
Excretion: t½ is 20 to 24 hr. Approximately 19% of dose is excreted in urine as parent drug and metabolites in 24 hr.

Indications Treatment of perennial and seasonal allergic rhinitis; vasomotor rhinitis; allergic conjunctivitis; mild, uncomplicated allergic skin manifestations of urticaria and angioedema; amelioration of allergic reactions to blood or plasma; dermographism; and adjunctive anaphylactic therapy.

Contraindications Treatment of lower respiratory tract symptoms; MAO inhibitor therapy; any component of the product or other antihistamines of similar chemical structure.

Route/Dosage
ADULTS AND CHILDREN (12 YR AND OLDER): PO 6 mg at bedtime or q 8 to 10 hr.

Interactions
Alcohol, other sedative:: Will potentiate the sedative effects of dexchlorpheniramine.
MAO inhibitors:: May cause severe hypotension.

Lab Test Interferences May interfere with diagnostic test results for skin tests using allergen extracts.

Adverse Reactions
CV: Palpitations; tachycardia; extrasystoles; hypotension.
CNS: Drowsiness; headache; sedation; dizziness; vertigo; disturbed coordination; fatigue; confusion; restlessness; excitation; nervousness; tremor; irritability; insomnia; euphoria; paresthesia; hysteria; neuritis; convulsions.

DERM: Urticaria; drug rash.
EENT: Tinnitus; acute labyrinthitis; blurred vision; nasal stuffiness.
GI: Dryness of mouth, nose and throat; epigastric distress; anorexia; nausea; vomiting; diarrhea; constipation.
GU: Urinary frequency; difficult urination; urinary retention; early menstruation.
HEMA: Hemolytic anemia; hypoplastic anemia; thrombocytopenia; agranulocytosis.
RESP: Thickening of bronchial secretions; tightness of chest; wheezing.
OTHER: Anaphylactic shock; photosensitivity; excessive perspiration; chills.

PATIENT CARE CONSIDERATIONS

Administration/Storage
- Give 1 to 3 times daily as prescribed without regard to meals. Give with food if GI upset occurs.
- Store tablets at controlled room temperature (36° to 77°F).

Assessment/Interventions
- Obtain patient history, including drug history and any known allergies. Note history of narrow angle glaucoma, stenosing peptic ulcer, pyloric obstruction, prostatic hypertrophy, bladder neck obstruction, hyperthyroidism, asthma, hypertension, cardiovascular disease, and concurrent or recent use of MAO inhibitors or oral anticoagulants.
- Assess for allergy symptoms (eg, rhinitis, nasal congestion, sneezing, itching, watery eyes) before and periodically throughout therapy.
- Monitor patient for dizziness and excessive drowsiness. If noted hold therapy and notify health care provider.
- Monitor patient for CNS, CV, GI, RESP, and general body side effects. Inform health care provider if noted and significant.

Patient/Family Education
- Explain name, dose, action, and potential side effects of drug.
- Advise patient to take as prescribed without regard to meals, but to take with food if GI upset occurs.
- Advise patient that if allergy symptoms are not controlled not to increase the dose of medication or frequency of use but to inform health care provider. Inform patient that larger or more frequent dosing does not increase effectiveness and may cause drowsiness.
- Advise patient that medication may cause drowsiness or dizziness and to not drive or perform other activities requiring mental alertness until tolerance is determined.
- Caution patient that alcohol and other CNS depressants (eg, sedatives) will have additional sedative effects if taken with dexclorpheniramine.
- Caution patient not to take any OTC antihistamines while taking this medication unless advised by health care provider.
- Advise patient to take sips of water, suck on ice chips or sugarless hard candy, or chew sugarless gum if dry mouth occurs.
- Caution patient that medication may cause sensitivity to sunlight and to avoid excessive exposure to the sun or UV light (eg, tanning booths), and to use protective clothing and sunscreens until tolerance is determined.
- If patient is to have allergy skin testing, advise to not take the medication for at least 7 days before the skin testing.
- Advise women to notify health care provider if pregnant, planning to become pregnant, or breastfeeding.
- Instruct patient to stop taking drug and immediately report any of the following symptoms to health care provider: dizziness or excessive drowsiness.
- Caution patient to not take any prescription or OTC medications or dietary supplements unless advised by health care provider.

Precautions
Pregnancy: Category B.
Lactation: Undetermined.
Children: Safety and efficacy not established in children under 12 yr.
Special risk patients: Use with caution in patients with hypertension, heart disease, asthma, hyperthyroidism, increased intraocular pressure, diabetes mellitus, prostatic hypertrophy, bronchial asthma.

Overdosage: Signs and Symptoms
CNS depression and stimulation (particularly in children), death, dizziness, tinnitus, ataxia, blurred vision, hypotension.

Dexmethylphenidate Hydrochloride

(DEX-meth-ill-FEN-ih-date HIGH-droe-KLOR-ide)

Class Psychotherapeutic/CNS stimulant

How Supplied
Focalin Tablets 2.5 mg, Tablets 5 mg, Tablets 10 mg

Action
PHARMACOLOGY: Exact mechanism of action is unknown; however, may block the reuptake of norepinephrine and dopamine into presynaptic neurons and increase release of these monoamines into extraneuronal spaces.

PHARMACOKINETICS/DYNAMICS:
Absorption: Readily absorbed. T_{max} is 1 to 1.5 hr.
Food – High-fat food increased T_{max} to 2.9 hr.
Metabolism: Metabolized by de-esterification to d-ritalinic acid (inactive).
Excretion: Approximately 90% recovered in urine (approximately 80% as ritalinic acid). t½ approximately 2.2 hr.

Indications Treatment of attention deficit hyperactivity disorder (ADHD).

Contraindications Marked anxiety, tension, agitation; glaucoma; motor tics; family history or diagnosis of Tourette syndrome; MAOI treatment and within 14 days following discontinuation of an MAOI; hypersensitivity to methylphenidate or other components of product.

Route/Dosage
Patients New To Methylphenidate
ADULTS AND CHILDREN OLDER THAN 6 YR: **PO** 2.5 mg bid; adjust dose in 2.5 to 5 mg increments at weekly intervals (max, 10 mg bid).

Patients Currently Receiving Methylphenidate
ADULTS AND CHILDREN OLDER THAN 6 YR: **PO** 50% the dose of racemic methylphenidate initially (max, 10 mg bid).

Interactions
Antihypertensive agents, pressor agents (eg, dopamine): Effects may be decreased by dexmethylphenidate.
Coumarin anticoagulants (eg, warfarin), anticonvulsants (eg, phenytoin), tricyclic antidepressants (eg, amitriptyline), selective serotonin reuptake inhibitors (eg, fluoxetine): Effects may be increased by dexmethylphenidate, necessitating a decrease in dosage.
MAOIs (eg, phenelzine): Discontinue MAOI therapy at least 14 days before starting dexmethylphenidate.

Lab Test Interferences None well documented.

Adverse Reactions
CV: Tachycardia; angina; arrhythmia; palpitations; increased or decreased pulse; increased or decreased blood pressure; cerebral arteritis or occlusion.
CNS: Twitching; insomnia; nervousness; dizziness; drowsiness; dyskinesia; headache; Tourette syndrome; toxic psychosis; depressed mood; neuroleptic malignant syndrome
DERM: Skin rash; urticaria; exfoliative dermatitis; erythema multiforme with necrotizing vasculitis; thrombocytopenia purpura; alopecia.
GI: Anorexia; abdominal pain; nausea; loss of appetite.
HEMA: Leukopenia; anemia.
HEPA: Abnormal liver function.
METAB: Weight loss.
OTHER: Fever; arthralgia.

Precautions
Pregnancy: Category C.
Lactation: Undetermined.
Children: Safety and efficacy not established in children younger than 6 yr.
Depression or fatigue: Do not administer.
Drug dependence: Use with caution in patients with a history of drug dependence or alcoholism.
Psychosis: Symptoms of behavior disturbance and thought disorder might be exacerbated in psychotic children.
Seizures: May lower convulsive threshold in patients with history of seizures.
Hypertension: Use with caution, monitoring BP.
Cardiovascular conditions: Use with caution.
Visual disturbances: Blurring of vision and difficulties with accommodation may occur.

Overdosage: Signs and Symptoms
Vomiting, agitation, tremors, hyperreflexia, muscle twitching, convulsions, euphoria, confusion, hallucinations, delirium, sweating, flushing, headache, hyperpyrexia, tachycardia, palpitations, cardiac arrhythmias, hypertension, mydriasis, dryness of mucous membranes, coma.

PATIENT CARE CONSIDERATIONS

Administration/Storage
- Discontinue MAOI at least 14 days before initiating therapy.
- Administer prescribed dose twice daily, at least 4 hr apart.
- Administer last dose at least 8 hr before bed-

time to avoid sleeplessness.
- Administer without regard to food.
- Dosage adjustments may be made at weekly intervals.
- Store at controlled room temperature (59° to 86°F).

Assessment/Interventions
- Obtain patient history, including drug history and any known allergies. Note history of marked anxiety, tension, and agitation; glaucoma; motor tics; Tourette syndrome; family history of Tourette syndrome; seizures; history of drug dependence or alcoholism.
- Ensure medication is used as part of a total treatment program for ADHD that may include psychological, educational, and social interventions.
- Monitor patient for response to therapy.
- Monitor height and weight in children before starting therapy and periodically during therapy.
- Monitor CBC, differential, and platelet count periodically during long-term treatment.
- Monitor patient for CNS, CV, GI, and general body side effects. Report to health care provider if noted and significant.
- Discontinue medication periodically to assess behavior and determine need to continue therapy.

Patient/Family Education
- Explain name, dose, action, and potential side effects of drug.
- Advise patient or caregiver to read "Patient Information" sheet provided with medication.
- Advise patient or caregiver that doses should be separated by at least 4 hr.
- Advise patient or caregiver that last dose should be taken at least 8 hr before bedtime to avoid sleeplessness.
- Advise patient or caregiver that this drug is part of a total treatment program for ADHD that should also include psychological, educational, and social interventions.
- Advise patient that the health care provider may periodically change the dose to obtain maximal benefit and to take as prescribed and not to stop taking or change the dose unless advised to do so by the health care provider.
- Advise patient or caregiver that health care provider may discontinue medication periodically to assess behavior and determine need to continue therapy.
- Caution patient that drug may impair their ability to drive or perform other tasks requiring mental alertness.
- Advise patient or caregiver to notify health care provider if appetite loss, nervousness, or difficulty sleeping occur and are bothersome.
- Advise patient or caregiver to notify health care provider if any unusual or unexplained symptoms are noted.
- Advise female patient to inform the health care provider if becoming pregnant, planning on becoming pregnant, or are breastfeeding.
- Warn patient or caregiver not to take any prescription or *otc* drugs or dietary supplements without consulting the health care provider.
- Advise patient or caregiver that follow-up visits and lab tests may be necessary to monitor therapy and to be sure to keep appointments.

Dexrazoxane

(dex-ray-ZOX-ane)
Class Cardioprotectant
How Supplied
Zinecard Powder for injection, lyophilized 250 mg (10 mg/mL reconstituted), Powder for injection, lyophilized 500 mg (10 mg/mL reconstituted)

Action
PHARMACOLOGY: Dexrazoxane is a potent intracellular chelating agent. The mechanism by which dexrazoxane exerts its cardioprotective activity is not fully understood.

PHARMACOKINETICS/DYNAMICS:
Absorption: C_{max} is 36.5 mcg/mL (at end of infusion).

Distribution: Vd approximately 22 L/m^2. Not bound to plasma proteins.

Metabolism: Metabolized to a diacid-diamide cleavage product and 2 monoacid-monoamide ring products.

Excretion: Elimination t½ is 2.1 to 2.5 hr. Plasma Cl is 6.25 to 7.88 L/hr/m^2. Renal Cl is 3.35 L/hr/m^2; 42% excreted in urine.

Indications Reduce incidence and severity of cardiomyopathy in female breast cancer patients who have received a cumulative doxorubicin dose of 300 mg/m^2 and who may benefit from additional doxorubicin therapy. It is not recommended for use with the initiation of doxorubicin therapy. **Unlabeled use(s):**
Cardioprotectant for other anthracyclines.

Contraindications Do not use with chemotherapy regimens that do not contain an anthracycline.

Route/Dosage
Cardiomyopathy
ADULTS: **IV** The recommended IV dosage ratio of dexrazoxane:doxorubicin is 10:1 (eg, 500 mg/m^2 dexrazoxane would be given with 50 mg/m^2 doxorubicin). Doxorubicin must be administered within 30 min of starting the dexrazoxane infusion.

Interactions
Other chemotherapeutic agents: May increase the myelosuppressive effects of other chemotherapeutic agents.
INCOMPATIBILITIES: Do not mix with other drugs.

Lab Test Interferences
None well documented.

Adverse Reactions
DERM: Alopecia; urticaria; streaking/erythema; recall skin reaction.
CNS: Fatigue; malaise; neurotoxicity.
GI: Nausea; vomiting; dysphagia; stomatitis; diarrhea; elevated transaminases; anorexia; esophagitis.
HEMA: Dose-related additive myelosuppression; leukopenia; thrombocytopenia; granulocytopenia.
OTHER: Pain on injection; sepsis; phlebitis; hemorrhage; infection; fever.

Precautions
Pregnancy: Category C.
Lactation: Undetermined.
Children: Safety and efficacy not established.
Hepatic function impairment: Dose reduction is recommended.
Fertility impairment: Testicular atrophy.
Anthracycline-induced cardiac toxicity: Carefully monitor cardiac function.
Antitumor interference: The use of dexrazoxane concurrently with the initiation of fluorouracil, doxorubicin, cyclosporine (FAC) therapy may interfere with the antitumor efficacy of the regimen; this use is not recommended.
Carcinogenesis: Secondary malignancies (primarily acute myeloid leukemia) have been reported in patients treated chronically with razoxane.
Extravasation risk: Local irritation or phlebitis may occur. Refer to institution-specific protocol.

PATIENT CARE CONSIDERATIONS
Administration/Storage
- Only for use in combination with chemotherapy regimens containing anthracyclines.
- For IV administration only. Not for intradermal, subcutaneous, IM, or intra-arterial administration.
- Follow institutional procedures for handling, administration, and disposal of anticancer drugs. Use caution in preparing and handling the reconstituted solution; use of gloves is recommended. If dexrazoxane powder or solution contact the skin or mucosa, immediately wash exposed area(s) with soap and water.
- Reconstitute powder for injection using the provided sodium lactate solution to give a dexrazoxane concentration of 10 mg/mL. This solution may be administered without further dilution or further diluted with 5% dextrose injection or 0.9% sodium chloride injection to provide a final dexrazoxane concentration of 1.3 to 5 mg/mL.
- Do not administer if cloudiness or particulate matter is noted.
- Do not mix dexrazoxane with other drugs.
- Administer prescribed dose by either slow IV push or rapid IV infusion.
- Administer the IV injection of doxorubicin after completing the dexrazoxane infusion and prior to a total elapsed time of 30 min from the beginning of the dexrazoxane infusion.
- Store powder for injection at controlled room temperature (59° to 86°F). Reconstituted and diluted solutions are stable for 6 hr at controlled room temperature or under refrigeration (36° to 46°F). Discard any unused solution.

Assessment/Interventions
- Obtain patient history, including drug history and any known allergies. Note liver impairment and previous treatment and cumulative dose of doxorubicin.
- Ensure that reduced dose is administered to patient with hepatic function impairment.
- Ensure that CBC with differential is evaluated before starting therapy and frequently during treatment.
- Ensure that cardiac function is closely monitored in patient who has previously received anthracycline-containing chemotherapy.
- Monitor patient for signs or symptoms of infection or bleeding. Inform health care provider immediately if noted and be prepared to treat appropriately.
- Assess patient for GI, DERM, HEMA, and general body side effects. Report to health care provider if noted and significant.

Patient/Family Education
- Explain name, action, and potential side effects of drug.
- Advise patient, family, or caregiver that medication will be prepared and administered by

- health care provider in a health care setting.
- Review dosing schedule with patient, family, or caregiver.
- Advise patient, family, or caregiver to immediately report any of the following to health care provider: rash; hives; flushing; fever, chills, or other signs of infection; sores in mouth; unusual bleeding or bruising.
- Advise patient, family, or caregiver to report any of the following to health care provider: persistent nausea, vomiting, diarrhea, or appetite loss; persistent or worsening general body weakness; pain, redness, or swelling at injection site; streaking or redness of skin.
- Instruct patient not to take any prescription or OTC medications, dietary supplements, or herbal preparations unless advised by health care provider.
- Advise women to notify health care provider if pregnant, planning to become pregnant, or breastfeeding.
- Advise patient that frequent follow-up visits and laboratory tests will be required to monitor therapy and to keep appointments.

Dextroamphetamine Saccharate/Amphetamine Aspartate Monohydrate/ Dextroamphetamine Sulfate/ Amphetamine Sulfate

(DEX-troe-am-FET-uh-meen SACK-uh-rate/ am-FET-uh-meen ass-PAR-tate MAH-no-HIGH-drate/DEX-troe-am-FET-uh-meen SULL-fate/am-FET-uh-meen SULL-fate)

Class CNS stimulant/Amphetamine

How Supplied
Adderall Tablets 5 mg (1.25 mg dextroamphetamine sulfate, 1.25 mg dextroamphetamine saccharate, 1.25 mg amphetamine aspartate monohydrate, 1.25 mg amphetamine sulfate), Tablets 7.5 mg (1.875 mg dextroamphetamine sulfate, 1.875 mg dextroamphetamine saccharate, 1.875 mg amphetamine aspartate monohydrate, 1.875 mg amphetamine sulfate), Tablets 10 mg (2.5 mg dextroamphetamine sulfate, 2.5 mg dextroamphetamine saccharate, 2.5 mg amphetamine aspartate monohydrate, 2.5 mg amphetamine sulfate), Tablets 12.5 mg (3.125 mg dextroamphetamine sulfate, 3.125 mg dextroamphetamine saccharate, 3.125 mg amphetamine aspartate monohydrate, 3.125 mg amphetamine sulfate), Tablets 15 mg (3.75 mg dextroamphetamine sulfate, 3.75 mg dextroamphetamine saccharate, 3.75 mg amphetamine aspartate monohydrate, 3.75 mg amphetamine sulfate), Tablets 20 mg (5 mg dextroamphetamine sulfate, 5 mg dextroamphetamine saccharate, 5 mg amphetamine aspartate monohydrate, 5 mg amphetamine sulfate), Tablets 30 mg (7.5 mg dextroamphetamine sulfate, 7.5 mg dextroamphetamine saccharate, 7.5 mg amphetamine aspartate monohydrate, 7.5 mg amphetamine sulfate) ◆ Adderall XR Capsules 10 mg (2.5 mg dextroamphetamine sulfate, 2.5 mg dextroamphetamine saccharate, 2.5 mg amphetamine aspartate monohydrate, 2.5 mg amphetamine sulfate), Capsules 20 mg (5 mg dextroamphetamine sulfate, 5 mg dextroamphetamine saccharate, 5 mg amphetamine aspartate monohydrate, 5 mg amphetamine sulfate), Capsules 30 mg (7.5 mg dextroamphetamine sulfate, 7.5 mg dextroamphetamine saccharate, 7.5 mg amphetamine aspartate monohydrate, 7.5 mg amphetamine sulfate)

Action
PHARMACOLOGY: Activates nonadrenergic neurons, causing CNS and respiratory stimulation. Stimulates satiety center in brain, causing appetite suppression.

Indications Narcolepsy (Adderall), treatment of attention deficit hyperactivity disorder.

Contraindications Advanced arteriosclerosis, symptomatic cardiovascular disease; moderate to severe hypertension; hyperthyroidism; glaucoma; known hypersensitivity or idiosyncrasy to sympathomimetics amines; agitated states; history of drug abuse; during or within 14 days following the administration of MAO inhibitors.

Route/Dosage
ADDERALL
Attention Deficit Disorder with Hyperactivity
CHILDREN 3 TO 5 YR: **PO** Start with 2.5 mg/day, increasing the daily dose in increments of 2.5 mg at weekly intervals until optimal response is obtained.

CHILDREN OLDER THAN 6 YR: **PO** Start with 5 mg qd or bid, increasing the daily dose in increments of 5 mg at weekly intervals until optimal response is obtained. Rarely will it be necessary to exceed 40 mg/day. Administer first dose on awakening; 1 or 2 additional doses at intervals of 4 to 6 hr.

Narcolepsy
Narcolepsy seldom occurs in children younger than 12 yr; however, when it does, dextroamphetamine may be administered.

CHILDREN OLDER THAN 12 YR: **PO** Start with 10 mg, increasing the daily dose in increments of 10 mg at weekly intervals until optimal response is obtained.

CHILDREN 6 TO 12 YR: **PO** Start with 5 mg

daily, increasing the daily dose in increments of 5 mg at weekly intervals until optimal response is obtained.

ADDERALL XR
Attention Deficit Disorder with Hyperactivity
CHILDREN 6 YR OF AGE AND OLDER: **PO** Start with 10 mg qd in the morning; daily dose may be increased in 10 mg increments at weekly intervals (max, 30 mg/day).

Interactions
Adrenergic blocking agents: Effect may be inhibited by amphetamines.
Antihistamines, antihypertensives (eg, guanethidine), veratrum alkaloids: Effects may be antagonized by amphetamines.
Chlorpromazine, haloperidol, lithium, methenamine: May inhibit the CNS stimulant effects of amphetamines.
Ethosuximide: Amphetamines may delay absorption.
Furazolidone: May cause hypertensive crisis and intracranial hemorrhage.
GI acidifying agents (eg, ascorbic acid, fruit juices, glutamic acid, guanethidine, reserpine): Decreased amphetamine absorption, reducing plasma levels and therapeutic effects.
GI alkalinizing agents (eg, sodium bicarbonate): Increased amphetamine absorption, increasing plasma levels, and pharmacologic and adverse effects.
Meperidine, norepinephrine: Amphetamines potentiate their effects.
MAO inhibitors (eg, phenelzine): May slow amphetamine metabolism, increasing plasma levels and potentiating the effects. May cause hypertensive crisis and intracranial hemorrhage.
Phenobarbital, phenytoin: Absorption may be delayed by amphetamines; coadministration with amphetamines may produce a synergistic anticonvulsant action.
Propoxyphene: Propoxyphene overdose may potentiate amphetamine CNS stimulation, leading to fatal convulsions.
Tricyclic antidepressants (eg, desipramine): Activity of both agents may be increased; cardiovascular effects may be potentiated.
Urinary acidifiers (eg, ammonium chloride, sodium acid phosphate): Increased amphetamine urinary excretion, decreasing plasma levels and therapeutic effects.

Urinary alkalinizers (eg, acetazolamide): Decreased amphetamine urinary excretion, increasing plasma levels as well as pharmacologic and adverse effects.

Lab Test Interferences Plasma and urinary steroid levels may be altered.

Adverse Reactions
CV: Palpitations; tachycardia; hypertension; cardiomyopathy.
CNS: Psychotic episodes; overstimulation; restlessness; dizziness; nervousness; insomnia; emotional lability; depression; euphoria; dyskinesia; dysphoria; tremor; headache; exacerbation of motor and phonic tics and Tourette syndrome; changes in libido.
DERM: Urticaria.
GI: Dry mouth; unpleasant taste; diarrhea; dyspepsia; nausea; vomiting; constipation; anorexia; weight loss; loss of appetite; GI disturbances.
GU: Impotence; changes in libido.
METAB: Weight loss.
OTHER: Abdominal pain; accidental injury; asthenia; fever; infection; viral infection; allergy.

Precautions
Pregnancy: Category C.
Lactation: Excreted in breast milk.
Children: Safety and efficacy not established in children younger than 3 yr (*Adderall*). Safety and efficacy not established in children less than 6 yr (*Adderall XR*).
Elderly: Safety and efficacy in geriatric population not established (*Adderall XR*).
Drug dependence: Has high potential for dependence and abuse.
Hypertension: Use with caution.
Psychosis: Symptoms of behavior disturbance and thought disorder may be exacerbated.
Tics: Motor and phonic tics and Tourette syndrome may be exacerbated.
Tolerance: May occur; do not exceed recommended dose.

Overdosage: Signs and Symptoms
Restlessness, tremor, hyperreflexia, rapid respiration, confusion, assaultiveness, hallucination, panic states, hyperpyrexia, rhabdomyolysis, CNS stimulation, arrhythmias, hypertension, hypotension, circulatory collapse, fatigue, depression, nausea, vomiting, diarrhea, abdominal cramps, convulsions, coma, death.

PATIENT CARE CONSIDERATIONS
Administration/Storage
- Discontinue MAO inhibitors at least 14 days before initiating therapy.
- Administer prescribed dose early in the morning to reduce potential for insomnia.
- Swallow capsules whole. Do not crush or chew.
- Capsules also can be opened and the entire

contents sprinkled on applesauce. The applesauce mixture must be consumed immediately and not stored for future use. The applesauce must be swallowed in its entirety without chewing.
• Store at controlled room temperature (59° to 86°F).

Assessment/Interventions
• Obtain patient history, including drug history and any known allergies. Note history of advanced coronary artery disease, moderate to severe hypertension, hyperthyroidism, sensitivity to sympathomimetic amines, motor tics, Tourette syndrome, glaucoma, agitation, history of drug abuse, or concurrent or recent MAO inhibitor therapy.
• With parental permission, consult with school personnel regarding drug effectiveness.
• Discontinue drug periodically to assess behavior and to determine need for continued therapy.
• Monitor height and weight in children.
• Promote total treatment program (eg, psychological, educational, social) when treating attention-deficit disorder with hyperactivity.
• Monitor patient for CV, CNS, GI, and general body side effects. Report to health care provider if noted and significant.

Patient/Family Education
• Explain name, dose, action, and potential side effects of drug.
• Caution patient or caregiver to swallow capsules whole and not to crush or chew the capsules.
• Advise patient or caregiver that capsules may be opened and the entire contents sprinkled on applesauce. The applesauce mixture must be consumed immediately and not stored for future use. The applesauce must be swallowed in its entirety without chewing.
• Advise patient, family, or caregiver that medication is started at a low dose and gradually increased as needed and tolerated.
• Advise patient, family, or caregiver to take medication as prescribed and not to stop taking or change dosage unless advised by health care provider.
• Advise patient, family, or caregiver that the drug is part of a total treatment program that should also include psychological, educational, and social interventions.
• Advise parents to inform school or daycare personnel about drug use and administration.
• Caution patient that drug may impair the ability to drive or perform other tasks requiring mental alertness.
• Advise women to notify health care provider if pregnant, planning to become pregnant, or breastfeeding.
• Warn patient, family, or caregiver not to take any prescription or OTC drugs or dietary supplements without consulting health care provider.
• Advise patient, family, or caregiver that follow-up visits may be necessary to monitor therapy and to keep appointments.

Dextroamphetamine Sulfate

(DEX-troe-am-FET-uh-meen SULL-fate)
Class CNS stimulant/Amphetamine

How Supplied
Dexedrine Tablets 5 mg • *Dexedrine Spansules* Capsules, sustained-release 5 mg, Capsules, sustained-release 10 mg, Capsules, sustained-release 15 mg • *Dextrostat* Tablets 5 mg

Action
PHARMACOLOGY: Activates noradrenergic neurons causing CNS and respiratory stimulation; stimulates satiety center in brain causing appetite suppression.

PHARMACOKINETICS/DYNAMICS:
Absorption: Well absorbed. T_{max} approximately 3 hr (IR tablets) and approximately 8 hr (SR capsules).

Distribution: Widely distributed with high concentrations in the brain.

Metabolism: Metabolized in the liver by hydroxylation, N-deakylation and deamination.

Excretion: t½ approximately 12 hr (urine pH less than 5.6, t½ is 7 to 8 hr; urine pH alkaline, t½ is 18.6 to 33.6 hr).

Indications Treatment of narcolepsy, attention-deficit disorder with hyperactivity; adjunct therapy for short-term (ie, few weeks) exogenous obesity when alternative therapy has been ineffective.

Contraindications Advanced arteriosclerosis; symptomatic cardiovascular disease; moderate to severe hypertension; hyperthyroidism; hypersensitivity or idiosyncratic reactions to sympathomimetic amines; glaucoma; agitated states; history of drug abuse; concurrent use or within 14 days of MAOI use.

Route/Dosage
Narcolepsy
ADULTS (OLDER THAN 12 YR): **PO** 10 mg/day; may increase weekly by 10 mg to max 60 mg/day in divided doses.

CHILDREN (6 TO 12 YR): **PO** 5 mg/day; may increase weekly by 5 mg to max 60 mg/day in divided doses.

Attention Deficit Disorder
CHILDREN 6 YR OR OLDER: **PO** 5 mg/day; may increase weekly by 5 mg to max 40 mg/day in divided doses. Usual range is 0.1 to 0.5 mg/kg/dose q morning.
CHILDREN 3 TO 5 YR: **PO** 2.5 mg/day; may increase weekly by 2.5 mg. Usual range is 0.1 to 0.5 mg/kg/dose q morning.

Exogenous Obesity
ADULTS 12 YR OR OLDER: **PO** 5 to 10 mg 30 to 60 min before meals, up to 30 mg/day. For long-acting form, 10 to 15 mg q morning.

Interactions
Guanethidine: Amphetamines may decrease effectiveness.
MAOIs, furazolidone: Hypertensive crisis and intracranial hemorrhage may occur.
Tricyclic antidepressants: May decrease amphetamine effect.
Urinary acidifiers (eg, ammonium chloride, ascorbic acid): May decrease amphetamine levels.
Urinary alkalinizers (eg, acetazolamide, sodium bicarbonate): May increase amphetamine levels.

Lab Test Interferences
Plasma and urinary steroid levels may be altered.

Adverse Reactions
CV: Palpitations; tachycardia; hypertension; arrhythmias.
CNS: Nervousness; tremors; dizziness; insomnia, euphoria; headache.
DERM: Urticaria.
EENT: Dry mouth; unpleasant taste.
GI: Diarrhea; constipation; anorexia.
GU: Impotence.

> **WARNING:**
> Drug dependence may develop with chronic use. Avoid prolonged periods of use.
> High abuse/diversion potential.
> Prescribe/dispense sparingly because of high diversion potential.

Precautions
Pregnancy: Category C.
Lactation: Excreted in breast milk.
Children: Do not use as anorectic agent in children younger than 12 yr. Not recommended for attention-deficit disorder in children younger than 3 yr.
Tartrazine sensitivity: Some products contain tartrazine, which may cause allergic reactions in susceptible individuals.
Tolerance: Tolerance may occur; do not exceed recommended dose to overcome this.

Overdosage: Signs and Symptoms
Restlessness, tremor, hyperreflexia, confusion, hallucinations, panic, fatigue, depression, convulsions, coma, arrhythmias, hypertension, hypotension, circulatory collapse, nausea, vomiting, diarrhea, abdominal cramps.

PATIENT CARE CONSIDERATIONS
Administration/Storage
- Limit patient's access to medication.
- Give medication 30 to 45 min before meals. Give sustained-release tablets once daily in morning.
- Do not crush or open sustained-release tablets.

Assessment/Interventions
- Obtain patient history, including drug history and any known allergies.
- Assess baseline nutritional status.
- Document any abnormal behavior.
- Document monthly measurement of physical growth in children.
- Document weight weekly.
- Notify health care provider and withhold medication if BP increases by 20 mm Hg or if heart arrhythmias or increase in heart rate develops.

Patient/Family Education
- Instruct patient to take medication early in morning and, if possible, to take last dose at bedtime.
- Tell patient to record body weight weekly.
- Instruct patient/family to measure height monthly if patient is child.
- Tell patient to limit intake of coffee, tea, cocoa, chocolate, and caffeinated soft drinks.
- Explain importance of good oral hygiene to prevent or treat dry mouth and changes in breath odor.
- Instruct patient to be aware of increased agitation, palpitations, and dizziness, and to take precautions while performing tasks that require physical coordination or mental alertness.

Dextromethorphan Hydrobromide

(DEX-troe-meth-OR-fan HIGH-droe-BROE-mide)

Class Antitussive/Nonnarcotic

How Supplied
Benylin Adult Liquid 15 mg/5 mL ◆ *Benylin DM* Syrup 10 mg/5 mL ◆ *Benylin Pediatric* Liquid 7.5 mg/5 mL ◆ *Creo-Terpin* Liquid 10 mg/15 mL (3.33 mg/ 5 mL) ◆ *Delsym* Liquid, sustained-action Dextromethorphan polistirex equivalent to 30 mg dextromethorphan HBr/5 mL. ◆ *Diabetes CF* Syrup 10 mg/5 mL ◆ *Drixoral Cough Liquid Caps* Capsules 30 mg ◆ *Hold DM* Lozenges 5 mg ◆ *Pediatric Vicks 44d Dry Hacking Cough and Head Congestion* Syrup 15 mg/15 mL (1 mg/mL ◆ *Pertussin CS* Liquid 3.5 mg/5 mL ◆ *Pertussin ES* Liquid 15 mg/5 mL ◆ *Robitussin Cough Calmers* Lozenges 5 mg ◆ *Robitussin Pediatric* Liquid 7.5 mg/5 mL ◆ *Scot-Tussin DM Cough Chasers* Lozenges 2.5 mg ◆ *Silphen DM* Syrup 10 mg/5 mL ◆ *St. Joseph Cough Suppressant* Liquid 7.5 mg/5 mL ◆ *Sucrets 4-hr Cough* Lozenges 15 mg ◆ *Sucrets Cough Control* Lozenges 5 mg ◆ *Suppress* Lozenges 7.5 mg ◆ *Trocal* Lozenges 7.5 mg ◆ *Vicks Dry Hacking Cough* Liquid 15 mg/5 mL

🍁 *Balminil DM* ◆ *Balminil DM Children* ◆ *Benylin DM* ◆ *Benylin DM for Children* ◆ *Benylin DM 12 Hour* ◆ *Benylin DM for Children 12 Hour* ◆ *Koffex DM* ◆ *Robitussin Children's* ◆ *Robitussin Honey Cough DM*

Action

PHARMACOLOGY: Suppresses cough by central action on cough center in medulla.

PHARMACOKINETICS/DYNAMICS:
Absorption: Rapidly absorbed.
Metabolism: Metabolized in the liver.
Excretion: Excreted in the urine as unchanged drug and demethylated metabolites.

Indications Management of nonproductive cough.

Contraindications Standard considerations.

Route/Dosage

GELCAPS
ADULTS AND CHILDREN (AT LEAST 12 YR): PO 30 mg q 6 to 8 hr (max, 120 mg/day).

LOZENGES
ADULTS AND CHILDREN (AT LEAST 12 YR): PO 5 to 15 mg q 1 to 4 hr (max, 120 mg/day).
CHILDREN (6 TO UNDER 12 YR): PO 5 to 10 mg q 1 to 4 hr (max, 60 mg/day).

LIQUID AND SYRUP
ADULTS AND CHILDREN (AT LEAST 12 YR): PO 10 to 20 mg q 4 hr or 30 mg q 6 to 8 hr (max, 120 mg/day).
CHILDREN (6 TO UNDER 12 YR): PO 15 mg q 6 to 8 hr (max, 60 mg/day).
CHILDREN (2 TO UNDER 6 YR): PO 7.5 mg q 6 to 8 hr (max, 30 mg/day).

EXTENDED-RELEASE SUSPENSION
ADULTS AND CHILDREN (AT LEAST 12 YR): PO 60 mg q 12 hr (max, 120 mg/day).
CHILDREN (6 TO UNDER 12 YR): PO 30 mg q 12 hr (max, 60 mg/day).
CHILDREN (2 TO UNDER 6 YR): PO 15 mg q 12 hr (max, 30 mg/day).

Interactions
MAO Inhibitors: Hypotension, hyperpyrexia, nausea, myoclonic jerks, and coma may develop after coadministration.

Lab Test Interferences None well documented.

Adverse Reactions Nausea, drowsiness, dizziness.

Precautions
Pregnancy: Category C.
Lactation: Undetermined.
Chronic cough: Do not use for persistent or chronic cough (eg, smoking, asthma, emphysema) or when cough is accompanied by excessive secretions. People with high fever, rash, persistent headache, nausea, or vomiting should use only under medical supervision.
Drug abuse and dependence: Anecdotal reports of abuse have increased. However, abuse and dependency potential is undetermined.

Overdosage: Signs and Symptoms

Ataxia, respiratory depression, convulsions (children); altered sensory perception, dysphoria, slurred speech (adults).

PATIENT CARE CONSIDERATIONS

Administration/Storage
◆ Store liquids, lozenges, and syrups at room temperature and out of reach of children.

Assessment/Interventions
◆ Obtain patient history, including drug history and any known allergies. Note any respiratory problems and smoking history.
◆ Assess type of cough (dry or productive), severity, and progression.
◆ Assess baseline vital signs including fever.
◆ Do not administer for persistent or chronic cough, longer than 7 days, or when cough is

accompanied by excessive secretions.
- Monitor blood glucose levels in diabetic patients.

Patient/Family Education
- Alert patient that many products contain alcohol.
- Instruct patient to notify health care provider before taking medication with other prescriptions (eg, MAOIs).
- Inform diabetic patients that base may contain sucrose or other sugars.
- Encourage increased fluid intake to thin secretions.
- Teach patients how to cough and breathe deeply to maximize respiratory efforts.
- Explain to parents not to give lozenges to young children.

Dextromethorphan Hydrobromide/Benzocaine

(DEX-troe-meth-OR-fan HIGH-droe-BROE-mide/BEN-zoe-caine)

Class Antitussive/Anesthetic

How Supplied
Cough-X Lozenges 5 mg dextromethorphan and 2 mg benzocaine ◆ *Tetra-Formula* Lozenges 10 mg dextromethorphan and 15 mg benzocaine

Action
PHARMACOLOGY: Suppresses cough by central action on cough center in medulla.

Indications Temporary relief of minor sore throat; temporary reduction in cough caused by minor throat and bronchial irritation.

Contraindications MAOI therapy or for 2 wk after stopping MAOI therapy; allergy to local anesthetics (eg, butacaine, procaine) or any component of this product.

Route/Dosage
COUGH-X
ADULTS AND CHILDREN 6 YR AND OLDER: **PO** 1 lozenge q 2 hr as needed (max, 12 lozenges/24 hr), or as directed by a physician.
CHILDREN (2 TO 6 YR): **PO** 1 lozenge q 4 hr (max, 6 lozenges/24 hr), or as directed by a physician.
TETRA-FORMULA
ADULTS AND CHILDREN 6 YR AND OLDER: **PO** Dissolve 1 lozenge slowly in the mouth, do not chew. May be repeated q 4 hr or as directed by a physician.

Interactions
MAOIs (eg, isocarboxazid): Dextromethorphan is contraindicated with MAOIs.

Lab Test Interferences None well documented.

Adverse Reactions
CNS: Drowsiness; dizziness.
GI: Nausea.

Precautions
Pregnancy: Consult physician before use.
Lactation: Consult physician before use.

Overdosage: Signs and Symptoms
Respiratory depression.

PATIENT CARE CONSIDERATIONS

Administration/Storage
- Slowly dissolve lozenge in the mouth. Lozenges should not be chewed or swallowed whole.
- Give lozenge every 2 to 4 hr as prescribed.
- Store lozenges at controlled room temperature (59° to 86°F). Protect from moisture.

Assessment/Interventions
- Obtain patient history, including drug history and any known allergies. Note history of allergy to local anesthetics and concurrent or recent use of MAOIs or oral anticoagulants.
- Assess patient's response to therapy. Notify health care provider if symptoms (eg, cough, sore throat) persist despite therapy.

Patient/Family Education
- Explain name, dose, action, and potential side effects of drug.
- Advise patient to take as directed on the package insert or as advised by their health care provider.
- Advise patient that if symptoms are not controlled not to increase the dose of medication or frequency of use but to inform their health care provider.
- Instruct patient to notify their health care professional if any of the following occur: cough persists for longer than 1 wk or tends to recur; severe sore throat persists for more than 2 days, or if cough or sore throat is accompanied by fever, persistent headache, rash, swelling, nausea, or vomiting.
- Advise women to notify physician if pregnant, plan on becoming pregnant, or breastfeeding.
- Caution patient to not take any prescription or OTC medications, or dietary supplements unless advised to do so by health care provider.

Dextromethorphan HBr/ Phenylephrine Hydrochloride/ Chlorpheniramine Maleate

(DEX-troe-meth-OR-fan HIGH-droe-BROE-mide/fen-ill-EFF-rin HIGH-droe-KLOR-ide/klor-fen-AIR-uh-meen MAL-ee-ate)

Class Antitussive/Decongestant/Antihistamine

How Supplied
Alka-Seltzer Plus Cold & Cough Tablets 10 mg dextromethorphan, 5 mg phenylephrine, 2 mg chlorpheniramine ♦ *Ameriruss AD* Liquid 15 mg dextromethorphan, 10 mg phenylephrine, 3 mg chlorpheniramine ♦ *Father John's Medicine Plus* Liquid 1.66 mg dextromethorphan, 1.66 mg phenylephrine, 0.66 mg chlorpheniramine ♦ *Norel DM* Liquid 15 mg dextromethorphan, 10 mg phenylephrine, 4 mg chlorpheniramine

Action
PHARMACOLOGY:
Dextromethorphan: Suppresses cough by central action on cough center in medulla.
Phenylephrine: Stimulates postsynaptic alpha-receptors, resulting in vasoconstriction, which reduces nasal congestion.
Chlorpheniramine: Competitively antagonizes histamine at H_1 receptor sites.

Indications
Temporary relief of coughs and upper respiratory symptoms, including nasal congestion, associated with allergy or common cold.

Contraindications
Hypersensitivity to any ingredients of product; bronchial asthma; severe hypertension; severe coronary artery disease; narrow-angle glaucoma; urinary retention; peptic ulcer; MAO-inhibitor therapy or for 2 wk after stopping MAO-inhibitor therapy.

Route/Dosage
LIQUID DOSEFORMS
ADULTS AND CHILDREN OVER 12 YR: PO 2 tsp (10 mL) q 6 hr.
CHILDREN 6 TO 12 YR: PO 1 tsp (5 mL) q 6 hr.
CHILDREN 2 TO 6 YR: PO ½ tsp (2.5 mL) q 6 hr.
CHILDREN LESS THAN 2 YR: PO as directed by health care prover (max, 4 doses/24 hr).

TABLETS
ADULTS AND CHILDREN 12 YR AND OLDER: 2 tablets fully dissolved in 4 oz of water q 4 hr (max, 8 tablets/24 hr).

PATIENT CARE CONSIDERATIONS
Administration/Storage
- Give prescribed dose q 6 hr as needed, up to qid for liquid doseforms.
- Dissolve 2 effervescent tablets in 4 oz water q 4 hr. Do not exceed 8 tablets in 24 hr.

CHILDREN LESS THAN 12 YR: Consult health care provider.

Interactions
CNS depressants (eg, hypnotics, sedatives, tranquilizers, antianxiety agents): Effects of these agents may be enhanced.
MAO inhibitors (eg, isocarboxazid): Hypertensive crisis may occur. Do not use in patients receiving MAO-inhibitor therapy or within 14 days of stopping such treatment. May prolong and intensify the effects of chlorpheniramine.

Lab Test Interferences
May interfere with diagnostic test results for skin tests using allergen extracts.

Adverse Reactions
CV: Hypotension; hypertension; cardiac arrhythmias.
CNS: Sedation; dizziness; disturbed coordination; tremor; irritability; insomnia; weakness; nervousness; convulsions; headache; euphoria; dysphoria.
DERM: Urticaria; rash; photosensitivity; pruritus.
EENT: Dryness of nose and throat; thickening of bronchial secretions; visual disturbances.
GI: Dryness of mouth; epigastric discomfort; anorexia; nausea; vomiting; diarrhea; constipation.
GU: Urinary frequency; difficult urination.
HEMA: Hemolytic anemia; thrombocytopenia; agranulocytosis.
RESP: Tightness of chest; wheezing; shortness of breath.

Precautions
Pregnancy: Category C.
Lactation: Undetermined.
Children: Safety and efficacy in children less than 2 yr not established.
Sodium and phenylalanine: Each effervescent Alka-Seltzer Plus Cold & Cough tablet contains sodium 504 mg and phenylalanine 11 mg.

Overdosage: Signs and Symptoms
Dextromethorphan: Drowsiness, ataxia, nystagmus, opisthotonos, convulsive seizures.
Phenylephrine: Hypertension, headache, convulsions, cerebral hemorrhage, vomiting.
Chlorpheniramine: CNS depression (eg, sedation, apnea, diminished mental alertness, cardiovascular collapse), CNS stimulation (eg, insomnia, hallucinations, tremors, convulsions), death.

- Give with food or milk if GI upset occurs.
- Use dosing spoon or syringe for pediatric doses.
- Store syrup at controlled room temperature (68° to 77°F).

Assessment/Interventions
- Obtain patient history, including drug history and any known allergies. Note history of peptic ulcer disease, diabetes, hypertension, hyperthyroidism, enlarged prostate, asthma, narrow angle glaucoma, urinary retention, severe hypertension, coronary artery disease, concurrent use of or within 2 wk of stopping MAO inhibitor therapy, or allergy to alkylamine antihistamines (eg, triprolidine) or sympathomimetic amines.
- Assess for allergy symptoms (eg, cough, rhinitis, nasal congestion, sneezing, itching, watery eyes) before and periodically throughout therapy.
- Monitor pulse and BP periodically during therapy.
- Monitor patient for nervousness, dizziness, and insomnia. If noted, hold therapy and notify health care provider.

Patient/Family Education
- Explain name, dose, action, and potential side effects of drug.
- Advise patient to take dose q 6 hr as needed, up to qid, as prescribed for liquid doseforms.
- Advise patient to dissolve 2 effervescent tablets in 4 oz of water q 4 hr and not to exceed 8 tablets in 24 hr, or as prescribed.
- Advise caregiver to use dosing spoon or syringe for children's doses.
- Advise patient to take with food or milk if GI upset occurs.
- Advise patient to take last dose late in the afternoon or early evening to reduce chance of drug causing sleeplessness.
- Advise patient that if a dose is missed to take as soon as remembered unless it is nearing time for the next dose. Caution patient to not double the dose to catch up.
- Advise patient that if allergy symptoms are not controlled, not to increase the dose of medication but to inform health care provider.
- Advise patient that each effervescent tablet contains sodium 504 mg and phenylalanine 11 mg.
- Caution patient that drug may cause drowsiness and to use caution while driving or performing other tasks requiring mental alertness until tolerance is determined.
- Advise patient to avoid alcohol and other CNS depressants due to risk of excessive sedation.
- Caution patient not to take any OTC antihistamines or decongestants while taking this medication unless advised by health care provider.
- If patient is to have allergy skin testing, advise to not take the medication for at least 6 days before the skin testing.
- Advise women to notify health care provider if pregnant, planning to become pregnant, or breastfeeding.
- Instruct patient to stop taking drug and immediately report any of the following symptoms to health care provider: nervousness, dizziness, sleeplessness.
- Caution patient to not take any prescription or OTC medications or dietary supplements unless advised by health care provider.

Diazepam

(DIE-aze-uh-pam)

Class Antianxiety/Benzodiazepine/Anticonvulsant

How Supplied
Diastat Gel, rectal 2.5 mg (pediatric), Gel, rectal 10 mg, Gel, rectal 15 mg (adult), Gel, rectal 20 mg (adult) ♦ *Diazepam* Solution, oral 1 mg/mL, Injection 5 mg/mL ♦ *Diazepam Intensol* Solution (intensol) 5 mg/mL ♦ *Valium* Tablets 2 mg, Tablets 5 mg, Tablets 10 mg
🍁 *Apo-Diazepam* ♦ *Diazemuls* ♦ *Valium Roche Oral*

Action
PHARMACOLOGY: Potentiates action of GABA, inhibitory neurotransmitter, resulting in increased neural inhibition and CNS depression, especially in limbic system and reticular formation.

PHARMACOKINETICS/DYNAMICS:
Absorption:
IM – Slow and erratic absorption unless administered in the deltoid muscle; C_{max} is lower than oral or IV administration.
Rectal – T_{max} is 1.5 hr. Bioavailability is 90%.
Oral – T_{max} is 0.5 to 2 hr.

Distribution: 95% to 98% protein bound. Highly lipophilic. Crosses the placenta and is excreted in breast milk.

Metabolism: Metabolized in the liver (involving CYP2C19 and CYP3A4) to desmethyldiazepam (active) and 2 minor active metabolites.

Excretion: The t½ is 20 to 80 hr.

Onset: Rapid.

Special Populations:
Hepatic Function Impairment – The t½ is prolonged and Cl decreased in those with alcoholic cirrhosis.

Elderly – The t½ is increased and Cl is decreased.
Children – The t½ is longer in neonates and children under 2 yr; t½ is shorter in children 2 to 16 yr.

Indications Management of anxiety disorders; relief of acute alcohol withdrawal symptoms; relief of preoperative apprehension and anxiety and reduction of memory recall; treatment of muscle spasms, convulsive disorders (used adjunctively), and status epilepticus. **Unlabeled use(s):** Treatment of irritable bowel syndrome; relief of panic attack.

Contraindications Hypersensitivity to benzodiazepines; psychoses; acute narrow-angle glaucoma; use in children younger than 6 mo; lactation.

Route/Dosage
Individualize dosage; increase cautiously.
ADULTS AND CHILDREN: Usual recommended dose **IM/IV** 2 to 20 mg, depending on indication and severity. In acute conditions injection may be repeated within 1 hr, but q 3 to 4 hr is usually satisfactory. Dosage and route vary with indication and age.
CHILDREN 6 MO AND OLDER: Usual daily dose **PO** 1 to 2.5 mg tid or qid initially; increase gradually as needed and tolerated.

Acute Alcohol Withdrawal
ADULTS: **PO** 10 mg tid to qid first 24 hr, then 5 mg tid to qid prn. **IM/IV** 10 mg initially, then 5 to 10 mg in 3 to 4 hr if needed.

Anticonvulsant Adjunct
ADULTS: **PO** 2 to 10 mg bid to qid.
ELDERLY OR DEBILITATED PATIENTS: **PO** Initial dose 2 to 2.5 mg qd to bid; increase gradually.

Anxiety
ADULTS: **PO** 2 to 10 mg bid to qid. **IM/IV** 2 to 10 mg; repeat in 3 to 4 hr if needed.

Cardioversion (Anxiety and Tension)
ADULTS: **IM/IV** 5 to 15 mg 5 to 10 min before procedure.

Endoscopic Procedures
IM/IV 10 to 20 mg IV or 5 to 10 mg IM approximately 30 min prior to procedure.

Preoperative (Anxiety and Tension)
ADULTS: **IM** 10 mg before surgery.

Sedation/Muscle Relaxation
ADULTS: **IM/IV** 2 to 10 mg/dose q 3 to 4 hr prn.
CHILDREN 6 MO AND OLDER: **PO** 0.12 to 0.8 mg/kg/day in divided doses. **IM/IV** 0.04 to 0.2 mg/kg/dose q 2 to 4 hr (max, 0.6 mg/kg in 8-hr period).

Skeletal Muscle Spasm
ADULTS: **PO** 2 to 10 mg tid to qid. **IM/IV** 5 to 10 mg initially, then 5 to 10 mg in 3 to 4 hr if needed. Larger doses may be necessary in tetanus.

Status Epilepticus and Severe Recurrent Convulsive Disorders
ADULTS: **IM/IV** (IV preferred) 5 to 10 mg initially; then 5 to 10 mg at 10 to 15 min intervals (max total dose, 30 mg). If needed, repeat in 2 to 4 hr.
CHILDREN 5 YR AND OLDER: **IM/IV** 1 mg q 2 to 5 min (max total dose, 10 mg). If needed, repeat in 2 to 4 hr.
INFANTS AND CHILDREN 1 MO TO 5 YR: **IM/IV** 0.2 to 0.5 mg slowly q 2 to 5 min (max total dose, 5 mg).

Tetanus
CHILDREN 5 YR AND OLDER: **IM/IV** 5 to 10 mg; repeat q 3 to 4 hr prn.
INFANTS AND CHILDREN 1 MO TO 5 YR: **IM/IV** 1 to 2 mg slowly; repeat q 3 to 4 hr prn.

RECTAL GEL
CHILDREN 2 TO 5 YR: **Rectal** 0.5 mg/kg.
CHILDREN 6 TO 11 YR: **Rectal** 0.3 mg/kg.
ADULTS AND CHILDREN 12 YR AND OLDER: **Rectal** 0.2 mg/kg.
A second dose, when required, may be given 4 to 12 hr after the first dose.

Interactions
Azole antifungal agents (eg, itraconazole, ketoconazole), diltiazem, fluvoxamine, isoniazid, macrolide antibiotics (eg, erythromycin), nefazodone, non-nucleoside reverse transcriptase inhibitors (eg, delavirdine, efavirenz), protease inhibitors (eg, indinavir): May increase diazepam plasma concentrations.
Cimetidine, oral contraceptives, disulfiram: May increase effects of diazepam with excessive sedation and impaired psychomotor function.
Digoxin: May increase serum digoxin concentrations.
Omeprazole: May increase diazepam levels and enhance effects.
Rifamycins: May decrease diazepam plasma concentrations.
Theophyllines: May antagonize sedative effects of diazepam.
INCOMPATIBILITIES: Diazepam interacts with plastic containers and IV tubing, significantly decreasing availability of drug delivered. Do not mix or dilute with other solutions or drugs in a syringe or infusion container.

Lab Test Interferences None well documented.

Adverse Reactions
CV: CV collapse; bradycardia; tachycardia; hypertension; palpitations; edema; hypotension; phlebitis or thrombosis at IV sites.
CNS: Drowsiness; confusion; ataxia; dizziness;

lethargy; fatigue; apathy; memory impairment; disorientation; anterograde amnesia; restlessness; headache; slurred speech; loss of voice; stupor; coma; euphoria; irritability; vivid dreams; psychomotor retardation; paradoxical reactions (eg, anger, hostility, mania, insomnia, muscle spasms); depression; dysarthria; hypoactivity; tremor; vertigo.
DERM: Urticaria; skin rash.
EENT: Visual or auditory disturbances; depressed hearing; blurred vision; diplopia; nystagmus.
GI: Constipation; diarrhea; dry mouth; coated tongue; nausea; anorexia; vomiting.
GU: Incontinence; changes in libido; urinary retention.
HEMA: Blood dyscrasias including agranulocytosis, anemia, thrombocytopenia, leukopenia, neutropenia.
HEPA: Hepatic dysfunction including hepatitis and jaundice; abnormal LFTs.
OTHER: Dependency/withdrawal symptoms.

Precautions
Pregnancy: Category D. Avoid drug especially during first trimester because of possible increased risk of congenital malformations.
Lactation: Excreted in breast milk.
Children: Oral form not recommended in patients younger than 6 mo; parenteral form not recommended in infants younger than 30 days.
Elderly: Initial dose should be small and gradually increased. Give with extreme care to elderly patients with limited pulmonary reserve.
Renal function impairment: Observe caution to avoid accumulation of drug.
Hepatic function impairment: Observe caution to avoid accumulation of drug.
Dependency: Prolonged use can lead to dependency. Withdrawal syndrome has occurred within 4 to 6 wk of treatment, especially if abruptly discontinued. For discontinuation after long-term treatment, use caution and taper dosage.
Parenteral administration: Reserved primarily for acute states.
Psychiatric disorders: Not intended for use in patients with primary depressive disorder, psychosis, or disorders in which anxiety is not prominent.
Seizures: Tonic status epilepticus has been precipitated in patients treated with IV for petit mal or variant status.
Suicide: Use drug with caution in patients with suicidal tendencies; do not allow access to large quantities of drug.

Overdosage: Signs and Symptoms
Hypotension, respiratory or cardiac arrest, drowsiness, confusion, somnolence, impaired coordination, diminished reflexes, lethargy, ataxia, hypotonia, hypnosis, coma, death.

PATIENT CARE CONSIDERATIONS
Administration/Storage
- Administer in combination with other anticonvulsant medications when treating seizure disorder.
- Administer prescribed dose without regard to meals but administer with food if GI upset occurs.
- Store tablets, oral solution, and injection at controlled room temperature (59° to 86°F). Protect from light. Protect tablets from moisture.

Oral Solution:
- Use caution to make sure proper oral solution is being used (regular oral solution or concentrated oral solution).
- Use calibrated dropper to measure prescribed dose of concentrated oral solution. Add prescribed dose to a liquid (eg, juice, water, soda) or semisolid food (eg, applesauce, pudding); stir for a few seconds then immediately administer entire amount of mixture. Do not prepare and store doses for future use.

Injection:
- For IM or IV administration only. Not for intradermal, SC, or intra-arterial administration.
- Do not administer if particulate matter, cloudiness, or discoloration is noted.
- For IM administration, inject deeply into muscle.
- To reduce risk of IV injection site reactions (eg, venous thrombosis, phlebitis, local irritation) administer IV injection slowly (no more than 5 mg/min) directly into large vein. Do not administer using small veins (eg, dorsum of hand, wrist).
- To reduce risk of apnea and hypersomnolence in children, administer prescribed IV dose over 3 min.
- Do not mix or dilute with other solutions or medications in syringe or infusion flask. If direct IV injection is not feasible, inject slowly through infusion tubing as close as possible to the vein insertion.

Assessment/Interventions
- Obtain patient history, including drug history and any known allergies. Note hepatic or renal impairment, pulmonary disease, acute narrow-angle glaucoma, depression, psychosis, suicidal tendency, seizure disorder, history of drug abuse, sensitivity to other benzodiazepines, or concurrent use of other psychotropic medications or CNS depressants.

- Ensure that reduced dose and slower dose escalation is used in elderly patient or patient with debilitating disease.
- Ensure that women of childbearing potential are not pregnant when therapy is initiated.
- Closely observe patient who has received parenteral therapy for at least 3 hr, preferably at bed rest. Use side rails and be prepared to assist patient with ambulation if necessary.
- Ensure that CBC with differential and liver enzymes are evaluated periodically in patient on prolonged therapy.
- Frequently assess patient for response to treatment. Notify health care provider if condition does not appear to be improving or is worsening.
- Ensure that therapy is periodically reviewed to determine if it needs to be continued without change or if a dose change (eg, increase, decrease, discontinuation) is indicated.
- If treatment is to be discontinued, or the dose reduced, gradually taper the dose and monitor patient for withdrawal symptoms. If significant withdrawal symptoms develop (eg, increased anxiety, tremor, muscle or abdominal cramps, sweating), reinstitute previous dosing schedule and attempt a less rapid tapering regimen after patient has stabilized.
- Monitor patient for CNS, GI, psychiatric, or general body side effects and injection site reactions. Report to health care provider if noted and significant. Implement safety precautions if excessive drowsiness or dizziness occurs.

Injection:
- Ensure that a benzodiazepines-receptor antagonist (eg, flumazenil), oxygen, and resuscitation and intubation equipment are available when medication is administered by IV injection.

Patient/Family Education

- Explain name, dose, action, and potential side effects of drug.
- Advise patient or caregiver to read the *Patient Information* leaflet before starting therapy and with each refill.
- Advise patient that medication is usually started at a low dose and then gradually increased until maximum benefit is obtained.
- Caution patient that medication may be habit forming, to take as prescribed, and not to stop taking or change the dose unless advised by health care provider.
- Advise patient to take each dose without regard to meals but to take with food if stomach upset occurs.
- Advise patient or caregiver using concentrated oral solution to measure prescribed dose using calibrated dropper and then add solution to a liquid (eg, juice, water, soda) or semisolid food (eg, applesauce, pudding); stir for a few seconds then immediately take (give) the entire mixture. Caution patient or caregiver not to prepare mixtures ahead of time and store.
- Advise patient that if a dose is missed to skip that dose and take the next dose at the regularly scheduled time. Caution patient to never take 2 doses at the same time.
- Advise patient if medication needs to be discontinued, it will be slowly withdrawn unless safety concerns (eg, rash) require a more rapid withdrawal.
- Instruct patient to avoid alcoholic beverages and other depressants while taking this medication.
- Advise patient with anxiety to take medication as needed and to seek alternative methods for controlling or preventing anxiety (eg, stress reduction, counseling).
- Instruct patient to contact health care provider if symptoms (eg, anxiety, panic attacks, seizures) do not appear to be getting better, are getting worse, or if bothersome side effects (eg, drowsiness, memory impairment) occur.
- Advise patient that drug may cause drowsiness or impair judgment, thinking, or reflexes and to use caution while driving or performing other tasks requiring mental alertness until tolerance is determined.
- Encourage patient with seizure disorder to carry identification (eg, *Medi-Alert*) indicating condition and medication being used to treat.
- Advise women to notify health care provider if pregnant, planning to become pregnant, or breastfeeding.
- Warn patient not to take any prescription or OTC drugs or dietary supplements without consulting health care provider.
- Advise patient that follow-up visits and lab tests may be necessary to monitor therapy and to keep appointments.

Injection:
- Advise patient or caregiver that medication will be prepared by a health care provider and administered in a health care setting under close observation, when oral therapy is not feasible.
- Caution patient who receives parenteral therapy as an outpatient (eg, outpatient surgery) to use caution while ambulating, avoid ingestion of alcohol or other sedatives, and avoid driving or other hazardous activities for 24 to 48 hr.

Diazoxide, Oral

(DIE-aze-OX-ide)

Class Glucose-elevating agent

How Supplied
Proglycem Capsules 50 mg; Oral suspension 50 mg/mL

Action
PHARMACOLOGY: Produces prompt dose-related increase in blood glucose by inhibiting pancreatic insulin release.

PHARMACOKINETICS/DYNAMICS:
Distribution: 90% protein bound. Crosses the placenta.
Excretion: t½ is 24 to 36 hr. Excreted by kidneys.
Onset: Within 1 hr.
Duration: Less than 8 hr.
Special Populations:
Renal Function Impairment – t½ is prolonged.

Indications Management of hypoglycemia caused by hyperinsulinism in adults with inoperable islet cell adenoma or carcinoma or extrapancreatic malignancy, in infants and children with leucine sensitivity, islet cell hyperplasia, nesidioblastosis, extrapancreatic malignancy, islet cell adenoma or adenomatosis.

Contraindications Hypersensitivity to thiazides; functional hypoglycemia.

Route/Dosage
ADULTS AND CHILDREN: **PO** 3 to 8 mg/kg/day in 2 to 3 equal doses q 8 to 12 hr.
INFANTS AND NEWBORNS: **PO** 8 to 15 mg/kg/day in 2 to 3 equal doses q 8 to 12 hr.

Interactions
Antihypertensive agents: Enhanced antihypertensive effect.
Hydantoins: Possible loss of seizure control.
Sulfonylureas: Decreased pharmacologic effects of both drugs.
Thiazide diuretics: Increased hyperglycemic and hyperuricemic effects of diazoxide; hypotension.

Lab Test Interferences Hypoglycemia and hyperuricemia produced by diazoxide may affect assessment of these metabolic states. Increased renin secretion and IgG concentrations and decreased cortisol secretion may occur. False-negative insulin response to glucagon may occur.

Adverse Reactions
CV: Tachycardia; palpitations; hypotension; transient hypertension; chest pain.
CNS: Headache; weakness; malaise; anxiety; dizziness; insomnia; polyneuritis; paresthesia; extrapyramidal signs; fever.
DERM: Hirsutism of lanugo type on forehead, back and limbs; skin rash; pruritus; monilial dermatitis; herpes; loss of scalp hair.
EENT: Transient cataracts; subconjunctival hemorrhage; ring scotoma; blurred vision; diplopia; lacrimation.
GI: Anorexia; nausea; vomiting; abdominal pain; ileus; diarrhea; transient loss of taste; acute pancreatitis; pancreatic necrosis.
GU: Azotemia; decreased Ccr; reversible nephrotic syndrome; decreased urinary output; hematuria; albuminuria; glycosuria.
HEMA: Thrombocytopenia with or without purpura; transient neutropenia; eosinophilia; decreased hemoglobin or hematocrit; excessive bleeding; decreased IgG.
METAB: Hyperglycemia; increased serum uric acid; gout; galactorrhea; breast lump enlargement; increased AST and alkaline phosphatase.
OTHER: Sodium and fluid retention; advance in bone age.

Precautions
Pregnancy: Category C.
Lactation: Undetermined.
Labor and delivery: May cause cessation of uterine contractions.
Renal function impairment: May have decreased protein binding of diazoxide resulting in increased hypotensive effect.
Blood levels: May be higher with liquid than with capsule formulation; use caution when changing dosage forms.
Fluid retention: May precipitate CHF in patients with compromised cardiac reserve.
Ketoacidosis and nonketotic hyperosmolar coma: May occur with recommended doses.

Overdosage: Signs and Symptoms
Hypotension, hyperglycemia.

PATIENT CARE CONSIDERATIONS

Administration/Storage
- Shake oral suspension well before administering.
- Store at room temperature. Protect suspension from light.

Assessment/Interventions
- Obtain patient history, including drug history and any known allergies. Note cardiac or renal impairment.
- Ensure that baseline laboratory tests have been obtained before beginning therapy.
- Monitor BP (lying, standing) for hypotensive effect, especially if patient is taking antihypertensive agent.
- Monitor blood and urine glucose and ketones carefully until stabilized, usually within 1 wk.

- Monitor I&O and weight at least weekly to monitor fluid retention.
- Monitor for signs of CHF: peripheral edema, dyspnea, rales/crackles, fatigue, weight gain, jugular vein distention. Notify health care provider immediately if these occur.
- Observe for signs of hirsutism.
- If ecchymosis, petechiae or hemorrhage occur, notify health care provider immediately. Drug may need to be discontinued.

Patient/Family Education
- Instruct patient to take medicine as directed at the same time each day. Warn patient not to switch from capsule to suspension without notifying health care provider.
- Review symptoms of hypoglycemia and hyperglycemia with patient and family.
- Advise patient to follow prescribed diet, medication and exercise regimen to prevent hypoglycemic or hyperglycemic reactions.
- Instruct patient to monitor blood glucose, urine glucose and ketones daily.
- Instruct patient to report these symptoms to health care provider: bruising, bleeding, fluid retention.
- Caution patient to avoid sudden position changes to prevent orthostatic hypotension. Inform patient that hirsutism is common side effect but should be reversed when drug is discontinued.
- Instruct patient not to take *otc* medications without consulting health care provider.

Diazoxide, Parenteral

(DIE-aze-OX-ide)

Class Agent for hypertensive emergencies

How Supplied
Hyperstat IV Injection 15 mg/mL

Action
PHARMACOLOGY: Relaxes smooth muscle in peripheral arterioles, thus reducing BP.

PHARMACOKINETICS/DYNAMICS:
Distribution: Greater than 90% protein bound. Crosses placenta.
Excretion: t½ approximately 28 hr.
Onset: 1 min.
Peak: 2 to 5 min.
Duration: Less than 12 hr.

Indications Short-term emergency reduction of BP in severe, nonmalignant, and malignant hypertension in hospitalized patients.

Contraindications Dissecting aortic aneurysm; hypersensitivity to thiazides or other sulfonamide derivatives; treatment of compensatory hypertension, such as that associated with aortic coarctation or arteriovenous shunt. Diazoxide is ineffective against hypertension caused by pheochromocytoma.

Route/Dosage
ADULTS: **IV** 1 to 3 mg/kg (max 150 mg in single injection) by rapid injection. May repeat at 5 to 15 min intervals until satisfactory reduction in BP. May repeat at intervals of 4 to 24 hr until oral therapy can be initiated. Do not use for longer than 10 days.

Interactions
Antihypertensive agents: Enhanced antihypertensive effect.
Highly protein-bound agents: Higher blood levels of these agents may occur as a result of displacement by diazoxide.
Hydantoins: Possible loss of seizure control.
Sulfonylureas: Hyperglycemia may occur.
Thiazide diuretics: May increase hyperuricemic, hyperglycemic, and antihypertensive effects of diazoxide.

Lab Test Interferences Hyperglycemia and hyperuricemia produced by diazoxide may affect assessment of these metabolic states. Increased renin secretion and IgG concentrations and decreased cortisol secretion may occur. May cause false-negative insulin response to glucogon.

Adverse Reactions
CV: Sodium and water retention; hypotension to shock levels; CHF; edema; myocardial ischemia (eg, angina, arrhythmias, ECG changes); supraventricular tachycardia; palpitations; bradycardia.
CNS: Dizziness; weakness; cerebral ischemia; cerebral infarction (eg, unconsciousness, convulsions, paralysis, confusion, focal neurologic deficit); sweating; flushing and feelings of warmth; transient neurologic findings (eg, headache, lethargy, somnolence, euphoria, ringing in the ears, momentary hearing loss).
DERM: Cellulitis or phlebitis at site of extravasation; warmth or pain along course of injected vein.
GI: Nausea; vomiting; acute pancreatitis (rare); diarrhea; abdominal discomfort.
METAB: Hyperglycemia; hyperosmolar coma; hyperuricemia.
OTHER: Hypersensitivity reactions; papilledema.

Precautions
Pregnancy: Category C.
Lactation: Undetermined.
Special risk patients: Diabetic patients may need treatment for hyperglycemia. Use with care in patients with impaired cerebral or cardiac circulation in whom rapid reduction in BP might be

deleterious. Observe caution when reducing severely elevated BP.
Fluid and electrolyte balance: Because of sodium and water retention, with possible edema and CHF, concomitant use of diuretic may be needed. However, thiazide diuretics may potentiate diazoxide's antihypertensive, hyperglycemic, and hyperuricemic actions.

Overdosage: Signs and Symptoms
Hypotension, hyperglycemia.

PATIENT CARE CONSIDERATIONS

Administration/Storage
- Administer IV, not SC or IM, over no longer than 30 sec.
- Have patient remain supine during IV administration.
- Protect liquid solution from light. Do not freeze.

Assessment/Interventions
- Obtain patient history, including drug history and any known allergies.
- Obtain baseline BP and pulse before therapy. Monitor BP and pulse frequently.
- Monitor for hyperglycemia in the diabetic patient.
- If signs of cerebral ischemia occur such as slowed mental processes or anxiety, help patient into supine position, elevate patient's legs and notify health care provider.
- If signs of CHF (eg, edema, dyspnea, weight gain, jugular vein distention) occur, notify health care provider.
- If headache occurs, administer analgesics as prescribed by health care provider.
- If nausea or vomiting occurs, offer small frequent feedings and fluids. Give antiemetic if ordered.

Patient/Family Education
- Emphasize importance of follow-up exams and blood testing to assure effectiveness and to minimize adverse reactions.
- Tell patient to report adverse reactions to health care provider.
- Caution patient to avoid sudden position changes to prevent orthostatic hypotension.
- Instruct patient not to take *otc* medications without consulting health care provider.

Diclofenac
(die-KLOE-fen-ak)
Class Analgesic/NSAID

How Supplied
Cataflam Tablets 50 mg (as potassium) ◆ *Solaraze* Gel 3% (1 g contains 30 mg diclofenac sodium) ◆ *Voltaren* Tablets, delayed-release 25 mg (as sodium), Tablets, delayed-release 50 mg (as sodium), Tablets, delayed-release 75 mg (as sodium), Solution 0.1% ◆ *Voltaren-XR* Tablets, delayed-release 100 mg (as sodium)
✤ *Apo-Diclo* ◆ *Apo-Diclo Rapide* ◆ *Apo-Diclo SR* ◆ *Novo-Difenac* ◆ *Novo-Difenac K* ◆ *Novo-Difenac SR* ◆ *Nu-Diclo* ◆ *Nu-Diclo-SR* ◆ *PMS-Diclofenac* ◆ *PMS-Diclofenac SR* ◆ *Voltaren Ophtha* ◆ *Voltaren Rapide*

Action
PHARMACOLOGY: Decreases inflammation, pain, and fever, probably through inhibition of cyclo-oxygenase activity and prostaglandin synthesis.

PHARMACOKINETICS/DYNAMICS:
Absorption: Bioavailability approximately 50% because of first-pass metabolism. Food decreases T_{max} and C_{max}.
Diclofenac potassium (50 mg dose) – AUC approximately 1309 ng•hr/mL, C_{max} approximately 1312 ng/mL, T_{max} approximately 1 hr.
Diclofenac sodium extended-release (100 mg dose) – AUC approximately 2079 ng•hr/mL, C_{max} approximately 417 ng/mL, T_{max} approximately 5.25 hr.
Diclofenac sodium delayed-release (50 mg dose) – AUC approximately 1429 ng•hr/mL, C_{max} approximately 1417 ng/mL, T_{max} approximately 2.22 hr.

Distribution: More than 99% protein bound (albumin). Vd approximately 1.4 L/kg.

Metabolism: Undergoes first-pass metabolism; metabolized to inactive metabolites.

Excretion: Approximately 65% excreted in urine and 35% in the bile. The $t_{½}$ is 2 hr.

Indications Treatment of rheumatoid arthritis, ankylosing spondylitis, and osteoarthritis. Potassium salt is approved for management of mild to moderate pain and primary dysmenorrhea when prompt pain relief is needed.
Ophthalmic: Treatment of postoperative inflammation after cataract removal; temporary relief of pain and photophobia following corneal refractive surgery.
Topical: Treatment of actinic keratosis.

Unlabeled use(s): Treatment of biliary colic, enuresis, glomerular disease, gout, migraine headache, and renal colic.

Contraindications Sensitivity to aspirin or any NSAID; soft contact lenses (ophthalmic); sensitivity to diclofenac, benzyl alcohol, polyethylene glycol monomethyl ether 350, and hyaluronate sodium (topical).

Route/Dosage
Actinic Keratosis
ADULT: **Topical** Apply gel to lesions bid.

Analgesia and Primary Dysmenorrhea (Potassium Salt Only)
PO 50 mg tid; may give initial dose of 100 mg if needed.

Ankylosing Spondylitis
PO 100 to 125 mg/day in divided doses; may give additional 25 mg at bedtime.

Osteoarthritis
PO 100 to 150 mg/day in divided doses.

Rheumatoid Arthritis
PO 100 to 200 mg/day in divided doses.

OPHTHALMIC

Cataract Surgery – 1 drop of 0.1% solution in affected eye qid beginning 24 hr after cataract surgery and continuing during the first 2 wk of postoperative period.

Corneal Refractive Surgery – 1 or 2 drops within the hour prior to corneal refractive surgery; then, within 15 min after surgery, 1 or 2 drops applied to the operative eye and continued qid for up to 3 days.

Interactions
Cyclosporine: May increase nephrotoxicity.
Digoxin: May increase digoxin serum concentrations.
Diuretics: May inhibit diuretic and antihypertensive effects.
Lithium: May decrease lithium clearance.
Methotrexate: May increase methotrexate levels.
Warfarin: May increase risk of gastric erosion and bleeding.

Lab Test Interferences May prolong bleeding time.

Adverse Reactions
CV:
Topical – Hypertension, phlebitis, migraine (greater than 1%).
CNS:
Oral – Dizziness, headache (1% to 10%).
Ophthalmic – Dizziness, headache, insomnia (3% or less).
Topical – Headache, anxiety, dizziness, hypokinesia (greater than 1%).
DERM:
Oral – Pruritus, rash (1% to 10%).
Topical – Acne, alopecia, contact dermatitis, dry skin, edema, exfoliation, hyperesthesia, pain, paresthesia, photosensitivity, pruritus, rash, vesiculobullous rash, macular rash, skin carcinoma, skin nodule, skin ulcer (greater than 1%).
EENT:
Oral – Tinnitus (1% to 10%).
Ophthalmic – Lacrimation complaints (30%), keratitis (28%), elevated IOP, transient ocular burning and stinging (15%), abnormal vision, acute elevated IOP, blurred vision, conjunctivitis, corneal deposits, corneal edema, corneal opacity, corneal lesions, discharge, eyelid swelling, injection, iritis, irritation, itching, lacrimation disorder, ocular allergy (5% or less), rhinitis (3% or less), corneal erosion, corneal infiltrates, corneal perforation, corneal thinning, corneal ulceration, epithelial breakdown, superficial punctuate keratitis (postmarketing).
Topical – Pharyngitis, rhinitis, conjunctivitis, eye pain (greater than 1%).
GI:
Oral – Abdominal pain, constipation, diarrhea, dyspepsia, flatulence, gross bleeding/perforation, heartburn, nausea, GI ulcers (gastric/duodenal), vomiting (1% to 10%).
Ophthalmic – Abdominal pain, nausea, vomiting (3% or less).
Topical – Abdominal pain, constipation, diarrhea, dyspepsia (greater than 1%).
GU:
Topical – Hematuria (greater than 1%).
HEPA:
Oral – Elevated liver enzymes (1% to 10%).
Topical – Increased AST or ALT (greater than 1%).
HEMA/LYMPH:
Oral – Anemia, increased bleeding time (1% to 10%).
M/N:
Oral – Edema (1% to 10%).
Topical – Increased creatine phosphokinase, increased creatinine, edema, hypercholesterolemia, hyperglycemia (greater than 1%).
MUSC:
Topical – Arthralgia, arthrosis, myalgia (greater than 1%).
RENAL:
Oral – Abnormal renal function (1% to 10%).
RESP:
Topical – Asthma, dyspnea, pneumonia, sinusitis (greater than 1%).
OTHER:
Ophthalmic – Asthenia, chills, fever, pain, viral infection, facial edema (3% or less).
Topical – Accidental injury, allergic reaction, asthenia, back pain, chest pain, chills, flu-like syndrome, neck pain, pain (greater than 1%).

Precautions
Pregnancy: Category C. Category B (topical).
Lactation: Undetermined.
Children: Safety and efficacy not established.
Elderly: Increased risk of adverse reactions.
Renal function impairment: Acute renal insufficiency, interstitial nephritis, hyperkalemia, hyponatremia, and renal papillary necrosis may occur.
Special risk patients: Use with caution in patients with fluid retention, hypertension, or heart failure.
Anaphylactoid reactions: Diclofenac should not

be given to patients with the aspirin triad, which typically occurs in asthmatic patients who experience rhinitis with or without nasal polyps, or who exhibit severe, potentially fatal bronchospasm after taking aspirin or other NSAIDs. *GI effects:* Serious GI toxicity (eg, bleeding, ulceration, perforation) can occur at any time, with or without warning symptoms.

Overdosage: Signs and Symptoms
Acute renal failure, nausea, vomiting, drowsiness.

PATIENT CARE CONSIDERATIONS
Administration/Storage
- Different tablet formulations of diclofenac are not necessarily bioequivalent.

Immediate-release, delayed-release, and extended-release tablets:
- Administer prescribed dose without regard to meals. Administer with food, milk, or antacids if GI upset occurs.
- Administer immediate-release and delayed-release tablets bid, tid, or qid as prescribed. Have patient swallow whole. Do not break, cut, crush, or chew tablet.
- Administer extended-release tablets qd as prescribed. Have patient swallow whole. Do not break, cut, crush, or chew tablet.
- Store tablets at ambient room temperature (59° to 86°F). Protect from moisture.

Gel:
- For dermatological use only. Not for ophthalmic, intravaginal, or oral use.
- Using gloves, gently smooth onto affected skin bid. Apply gel to adequately cover each lesion.
- Avoid contact with the eyes, mouth, and other mucus membranes.
- Do not apply occlusive dressings unless ordered by health care provider.
- Do not apply other topical products unless advised by health care provider.
- Store gel at ambient room temperature (59° to 86°F). Protect from heat. Avoid freezing. Keep tube tightly capped.

Ophthalmic Solution:
- For ophthalmic use only. Not for use on the skin or for injection into eye.
- Have patient tilt head back and instill prescribed number of drops into affected eye(s) as ordered. Have patient close eye(s) for 2 to 3 min and apply light finger pressure to lacrimal sac for 1 to 2 min after installation. Do not touch top of dropper bottle to eye, fingers, or other surface.
- If using other topical ophthalmic drugs, separate each medication by at least 5 min. Instill ophthalmic ointment last.
- Store ophthalmic solution at controlled room temperature (59° to 86°F). Keep tightly capped and protect from light.

Assessment/Interventions
- Obtain patient history, including drug history and any known allergies. Note renal or hepatic impairment, dehydration, hypertension, heart failure, fluid retention, asthma, history of GI bleeding or ulcers, coagulation disorder, allergic reaction to aspirin or other NSAIDs, renal or hepatic impairment, or hypersensitivity to benzyl alcohol (gel only).
- Obtain baseline assessments of pain and ability to perform activities of daily living.
- Ensure that CBC, serum electrolytes, and serum transaminases are evaluated periodically during prolonged therapy.
- Ensure that renal function has been assessed prior to initiating therapy and periodically during therapy in patient with renal impairment.
- Notify health care provider if indigestion, epigastric pain, unusual bleeding or bruising, or dark tarry stools occur.
- Monitor patient for signs and symptoms of liver dysfunction (eg, flu-like symptoms, persistent nausea, fatigue, right upper quadrant abdominal pain, yellowing of skin or eyes, dark urine). If noted, discontinue therapy immediately and inform health care provider.
- Monitor patient for GI, CNS, CV, RESP, and general body side effects. Report to health care provider if noted and significant.

Gel:
- Assess the skin and identify areas where medication is to be applied and areas that should be avoided (eg, open skin wounds, infected skin, skin that is scaling).
- Assess and document skin condition before initial application and periodically throughout treatment. Inform health care provider if condition does not improve, worsens, or if application site reactions occur and are bothersome.

Ophthalmic Solution:
- Monitor patient's response to therapy. Notify health care provider if eye or eyelid inflammation is noted or if symptoms do not improve or worsen.

Patient/Family Education
- Explain name, dose, action, and potential side effects of drug.
- Advise patient that dose is individualized based upon severity of symptoms and response to therapy.

- Advise patient to take prescribed dose without regard to meals but to take with food, milk, or antacids if stomach upset occurs.
- Advise patient not to cut, crush, chew, or break tablets and to swallow whole with a full glass of water.
- Caution patient to avoid smoking, alcohol, and aspirin-containing medications while taking this drug.
- Advise patient that if a dose is missed, to take it as soon as possible, but if close to the next dose, do not double up and take the next dose as scheduled.
- Advise patient to discontinue drug and notify health care provider if any of the following occur: persistent or recurrent GI upset, skin rash, itching, visual disturbances, black stools, weight gain or edema, changes in urine patterns, joint pain, fever, unusual bleeding or bruising, persistent nausea, fatigue, yellowing of skin or eyes.
- Advise patient to avoid unnecessary exposure to sunlight or tanning lamps and to use sunscreen and wear protective clothing to avoid photosensitivity reactions.
- Advise women to notify health care provider if pregnant, planning to become pregnant, or breastfeeding.
- Instruct patient not to take any prescription or OTC medications or dietary supplements unless advised by health care provider.
- Advise patient that follow-up examinations and lab tests may be required to monitor therapy and to keep appointments.

Gel:
- Advise patient that gel will not work immediately but to expect a slow improvement over several weeks. Inform patient that gel is usually applied daily for 60 to 90 days and that complete healing of the lesion(s) may not be evident for up to 30 days following cessation of therapy.
- Advise patient to gently smooth gel onto skin lesions bid as directed by health care provider.
- Teach patient or caregiver proper technique for applying gel: wash hands; gently smooth enough gel onto affected skin to adequately cover each lesion; wash hands after applying gel.
- Caution patient not to apply gel to open skin wounds, infected skin, or skin that is scaling.
- Caution patient to avoid contact with eyes. Advise patient that if gel does come into contact with eyes to wash them with large amounts of cool water and contact health care provider if eye irritation occurs.
- Advise patient to talk to health care provider before using any other topical agents (eg, medicated soaps, astringents, cosmetics) on treated skin.
- Caution patient that drug may cause drowsiness or dizziness and to use caution while driving or performing other tasks requiring mental alertness until tolerance is determined.
- Advise patient that avoiding ultraviolet light is an important part of therapy and to avoid exposure to sunlight or tanning lamps and to use sunscreen and wear protective clothing during treatment.
- Advise patient to notify health care provider if condition does not improve, worsens, or if application site reactions (eg, rash, dry skin, scaling, redness, irritation) develop and are bothersome.
- Advise patient that follow-up examinations will be required to monitor therapy and to keep appointments.

Ophthalmic Solution:
- Remind patient that eye drops are for use in the eye only.
- Teach patient proper technique for instilling eye drops: wash hands; do not allow dropper to touch eye. Tilt head back, look up; pull lower eyelid down; instill prescribed number of drops. Close eye for 2 to 3 min and apply gentle pressure to bridge of nose for 1 to 2 min. Do not rub eye.
- Advise patient not to touch top of dropper bottle to eye, fingers, or other surface.
- Advise patient that if more than 1 topical ophthalmic drug is being used, administer the drugs at least 5 min apart. Administer ointment last.
- Inform patient that temporary stinging or burning are the most common side effects and to contact health care provider if these occur and are bothersome.
- Advise patient to contact eye doctor if eye or eyelid inflammation is noted or if eye symptoms do not improve or worsen.
- Instruct patient wearing contact lenses to remove lenses when instilling eye drops.

Diclofenac Sodium/ Misoprostol

(die-KLOE-fen-ak SO-dee-uhm my-so-PRAHST-ole)

Class Analgesic/Nonnarcotic analgesic combination

How Supplied
Arthrotec Tablets 50 gm diclofenac sodium/200 mcg misoprostol, Tablets 75 mg diclofenac sodium/200 mcg misoprostol

Action
PHARMACOLOGY: Diclofenac, a nonsteroidal anti-inflammatory drug, decreases inflammation, pain, and fever, probably through inhibition of cyclooxygenase activity and prostaglandin synthesis. Misoprostol, a GI mucosal protective prostaglandin E_1 analog, provides gastric antisecretory, and mucosal protective properties.

Indications Treatment of signs and symptoms of osteoarthritis and rheumatoid arthritis in patients at high risk of developing NSAID-induced gastric and duodenal ulcers and their complications.

Contraindications Pregnancy; sensitivity to aspirin or any NSAID; sensitivity to misoprostol or other prostaglandins; history of asthma, urticaria, or other allergic-type reactions after taking aspirin or other NSAIDs.

Route/Dosage
Osteoarthritis
ADULTS: PO 50/200 (50 mg diclofenac/200 mg misoprostol) tid, or 50/200 bid or 75/200 (75 mg diclofenac/200 mg misoprostol) bid for patients experiencing intolerance. Take with meals.

Rheumatoid Arthritis
ADULTS: PO 50/200 tid, qid, or 50/200 bid or 75/200 bid for patients experiencing intolerance. Take with meals.

Interactions
Antihypertensive agents: May inhibit activity of antihypertensives.
Aspirin: May reduce serum diclofenac concentrations.
Cyclosporine: May increase nephrotoxicity.
Digoxin: May increase serum digoxin concentrations.
Lithium: May decrease lithium clearance, increasing lithium concentrations.
Magnesium-containing antacids: May increase incidence of diarrhea.
Methotrexate: May increase methotrexate levels.
Warfarin: May increase risk of gastric erosion and bleeding.

Lab Test Interferences May prolong bleeding time.

Adverse Reactions
GI: Abdominal pain; diarrhea; dyspepsia; nausea; flatulence.
GU: Postmenopausal vagina. bleeding (misoprostol).

Precautions
Pregnancy: Category X.
Lactation: Diclofenac — Excreted in breast milk. Misoprostol — Undetermined.
Children: Safety and efficacy in children younger than 18 yr not established.
Elderly: Increased risk of adverse reactions.
Renal function impairment: NSAIDs may cause further decrease in renal function in patients with preexisting renal impairment. Use is not recommended in patients with advanced kidney disease.
Hepatic function impairment. Diclofenac can cause hepatitis, usually within the first 2 mo of therapy. Monitor liver enzymes within 4 to 8 wk after initiating treatment.
Women of childbearing potential: Contraindicated in pregnant women because of abortifacient properties. Avoid in women of childbearing potential unless patient requires NSAIDs and is at high risk of complications from gastric ulcers associated with use of NSAIDs. If used in women of childbearing potential the following criteria should be met: patient is capable of complying with effective contraceptive measures; received verbal and written warnings of the hazards of misoprostol, risk of possible contraception failure, and the danger to other women of childbearing potential should drug be taken by mistake; negative serum pregnancy test within 2 wk prior to starting therapy; and will begin therapy only on the second or third day of the next menstrual period.
GI effects: NSAIDs may cause serious GI toxicity (eg, bleeding, ulceration, perforation) which can occur at any time, with or without warning symptoms.
Asthma: NSAIDs may precipitate bronchospasm in some patients with asthma.
Hematologic disorders: NSAIDs interfere with platelet function and vascular response to bleeding; use with caution in patients with coagulation disorders or receiving anticoagulants.
Fluid retention: NSAIDs may cause fluid retention and edema; use with caution in patients with fluid retention, hypertension, or heart failure.

Overdosage: Signs and Symptoms
Acute renal failure, drowsiness, nausea, vomiting (diclofenac); abdominal pain, bradycardia, diarrhea, dyspnea, fever, hypotension, palpitations, sedation, seizure, tremor (misoprostol).

PATIENT CARE CONSIDERATIONS
Administration/Storage
- Administer tablet whole; do not crush or dissolve.
- Administer with meals.
- Do not coadminister with magnesium-containing antacids to minimize incidence of diarrhea.
- Do not give to pregnant or nursing women. Do not use routinely in women of childbearing age, unless benefits outweigh the risks.
- Store tablets at room temperature. Protect from moisture.

Assessment/Interventions
- Review patient history, including drug history.
- If woman is of childbearing age, determine the following: if the patient is willing and able to comply with effective contraceptive measures; if the patient has had a negative serum pregnancy test within 2 wk, prior to beginning treatment; if the patient has received both written and verbal warnings of the hazards of misoprostol, risk of possible contraception failure, and danger to other women of childbearing age if the medicine is taken by mistake; if the patient will begin therapy on the second or third day of her next normal menstrual period.
- Note possible drug interactions and take appropriate action.
- Do not administer if patient is allergic to NSAIDs or aspirin.
- Do not administer to patients with aspirin-sensitive asthma or hepatic porphyria. Administer with caution to patients with pre-existing asthma.
- Assess hydration status of patient, rehydrate before beginning therapy.
- Assess patients for signs and symptoms of decreased renal blood flow (eg, decreased urine output, increased serum creatine), which might precipitate renal decompensation. Patients at greater risk include those with impaired renal function, heart failure, impaired liver function, those taking diuretics and ACE inhibitors, and the elderly.
- Monitor chemistry profile and CBC of patients on long-term therapy.
- Assess patient on long-term therapy for anemia. If symptoms are present, hemoglobin and hematocrit should be checked and appropriate therapy instituted.
- Carefully monitor patients with coagulation disorders or those on anticoagulants for signs of bleeding or bruising.
- Administer with caution to any patient with a history of cardiac decompensation, hypertension, or other conditions predisposing to fluid retention. Assess patient for signs of edema or fluid retention (eg, pulmonary rales, dyspnea, weight gain, swelling).

Patient/Family Education
- Provide patient information pamphlet.
- Caution women not to take this medicine if they are pregnant and to take measures to prevent pregnancy while they are on this drug. If a patient suspects she is pregnant, she should stop taking the drug and contact her primary care giver immediately.
- Instruct patient to report any signs or symptoms of GI ulceration or bleeding, skin rash, weight gain, or swelling.
- Instruct patient not to take drug and seek immediate medical attention if signs of liver toxicity occur, including nausea, fatigue, lethargy, itching, jaundice, right upper quadrant tenderness, or flu-like symptoms.
- Caution nursing mothers to discontinue breastfeeding because of potential harm to the baby.
- Tell patient that diarrhea, abdominal pain, upset stomach, and nausea may develop during first few weeks of therapy and usually stop after approximately 1 wk of continued treatment. To minimize diarrhea, take with meals and avoid antacids containing magnesium. If difficulty persists for more than 7 days or if symptoms become severe, patient should notify primary care giver.
- Instruct patients to swallow pill whole; do not crush, chew, or dissolve.

Dicloxacillin Sodium

(DIE-klox-uh-SILL-in SO-dee-uhm)
Class Antibiotic/Penicillin

How Supplied
Dicloxacillin Sodium Capsules 250 mg, Capsules 500 mg

Action
PHARMACOLOGY: Inhibits bacterial cell wall mucopeptide synthesis.

PHARMACOKINETICS/DYNAMICS:
Absorption: Rapid and incomplete absorption. T_{max} is 1 to 1.5 hr. C_{max} is 10 to 17 mcg/mL. Food delays absorption; take on empty stomach.

Distribution: Approximately 98% protein bound, mainly to albumin. Excreted in breast milk and crosses the placenta. Low CSF penetration.

Excretion: Rapidly eliminated, primarily as unchanged drug in the urine. Nonrenal elimination includes hepatic inactivation and excretion in bile. t½ approximately 0.7 hr.

Indications Treatment of infections caused by penicillinase-producing staphylococcal infection; initial therapy of suspected staphylococcal infection.

Contraindications Hypersensitivity to penicillins.

Route/Dosage
ADULTS AND CHILDREN WEIGHING GREATER THAN 40 KG: **PO** 125 to 250 mg q 6 hr.
CHILDREN WEIGHING LESS THAN 40 KG: **PO** 12.5 to 25 mg/kg/day divided in equal doses q 6 hr.

Interactions
Contraceptives, oral: May reduce efficacy of oral contraceptives.
Food: Antibacterial action may be reduced.
Tetracyclines: May impair bactericidal effects of dicloxacillin.

Lab Test Interferences May cause false-positive urine glucose test results with *Benedict's Solution, Fehling's Solution,* or *Clinitest* tablets but not with enzyme-based tests (eg, *Clinistix, Testape*); false-positive direct *Coombs'* test results in certain patient groups; false-positive protein reactions with sulfosalicylic acid and boiling test, acetic acid test, biuret reaction and nitric acid test but not with bromphenol blue test (*Multistix*).

Adverse Reactions
CNS: Dizziness; fatigue; insomnia; reversible hyperactivity; seizures.
DERM: Urticaria; dermatitis; vesicular eruptions; erythema multiforme; rashes.
EENT: Laryngospasm; laryngeal edema; itchy eyes.
GI: Glossitis; stomatitis; gastritis; sore mouth or tongue; dry mouth; furry tongue; "black hairy" tongue; abnormal taste sensation; anorexia; nausea; vomiting; abdominal pain or cramps; diarrhea or bloody diarrhea; rectal bleeding; flatulence; enterocolitis; pseudomembranous colitis.
GU: Interstitial nephritis (eg, oliguria, proteinuria, hematuria, hyaline casts, pyuria); nephropathy.
HEMA: Anemias; thrombocytopenia; eosinophilia; leukopenia; granulocytopenia; neutropenia; bone marrow depression; agranulocytosis; reduced hemoglobin or hematocrit; prolonged bleeding and prothrombin time; altered lymphocyte count; increased monocytes, basophils, platelets.
HEPA: Transient hepatitis; cholestatic jaundice.
METAB: Elevated serum alkaline phosphatase and hypernatremia; reduced serum potassium, albumin, total proteins and uric acid.
OTHER: Hypersensitivity reactions that may lead to death; vaginitis; hyperthermia.

Precautions
Pregnancy: Category B.
Lactation: Excreted in breast milk.
Hypersensitivity: Reactions range from mild to life-threatening. Administer cautiously to cephalosporin-sensitive patients because of possible crossreactivity.
Superinfection: May result in bacterial or fungal overgrowth of nonsusceptible organisms.
Pseudomembranous colitis: Consider possibility in patients with diarrhea.

PATIENT CARE CONSIDERATIONS
Administration/Storage
- Obtain specimens for culture before initiating antibiotic therapy.
- Capsules can be opened and contents mixed with small amount of food or fluid, but patient may experience bad taste.
- Give on empty stomach (30 min to 1 hr before meal or 2 hr after a meal).
- Give with full glass of water, not juice or carbonated beverage.
- If stored at room temperature, discard reconstituted oral solution after 7 days; discard after 14 days if refrigerated. Do not freeze.
- Always give in divided doses throughout day to maintain steady state.

Assessment/Interventions
- Obtain patient history, including drug history and any known allergies.
- Assess signs of infection before and during therapy (eg, fever, vital signs, appearance of wounds, WBC).
- If signs of anaphylaxis (eg, rash, pruritus, laryngeal edema, wheezing) occur, discontinue drug and notify health care provider immediately.

Patient/Family Education
- Instruct patient to take antibiotic on empty stomach before (30 min to 1 hr) meals or after (2 hr) meals with full glass of water.
- Explain that doses should be evenly spaced throughout day and night to maintain adequate drug levels.
- Teach patient signs of sensitivity reaction and appropriate steps to take if occurring.
- Tell patient to discard any liquid solution after 7 days when stored at room temperature or after 14 days of refrigeration.
- Instruct patient to shake bottle before measur-

ing pediatric suspension and to use a medication cup or other calibrated device for accurate dosing.
♦ Teach patient signs of superinfection, which can occur with any antibiotic (eg, black, furry tongue, vaginal itching) and tell patient to notify health care provider if any occur.
♦ Instruct patient never to share antibiotic prescriptions with others.
♦ Advise patient to follow complete course of therapy, even if feeling better.

Dicyclomine Hydrochloride

(die-SIGH-kloe-meen HIGH-droe-KLOR-ide)

Class Anticholinergic/Antispasmodic

How Supplied
Antispas Injection 10 mg/mL ♦ *Bemote* Capsules 10 mg, Tablets 20 mg ♦ *Bentyl* Capsules 10 mg, Tablets 20 mg, Syrup 10 mg/5 mL, Injection 10 mg/mL ♦ *Byclomine* Capsules 10 mg, Tablets 20 mg ♦ *Dibent* Injection 10 mg/mL ♦ *Dilomine* Injection 10 mg/mL ♦ *Di-Spaz* Capsules 10 mg, Injection 10 mg/mL ♦ *Or-Tyl* Injection 10 mg/mL
✻ *Bentylol* ♦ *Lomine*

Action
PHARMACOLOGY: Relieves smooth muscle spasm of GI tract through anticholinergic effects and direct action on GI smooth muscle.

PHARMACOKINETICS/DYNAMICS:
Absorption: Rapidly absorbed. T_{max} is 60 to 90 min (oral).

Distribution: Vd approximately 3.65 L/kg.

Excretion: 79.5% excreted in the urine and 8.4% in feces. t½ approximately 1.8 hr.

Indications Treatment of functional bowel/irritable bowel syndrome (eg, irritable colon, spastic colon, mucous colitis). **Unlabeled use(s):** Intestinal colic in children older than 6 mo.

Contraindications Narrow angle glaucoma; adhesions between iris and lens; obstructive uropathy; obstructive disease of GI tract; paralytic ileus; intestinal atony of elderly or debilitated patient; severe ulcerative colitis; toxic megacolon complicating ulcerative colitis; hepatic or renal disease; tachycardia; myocardial ischemia; unstable cardiovascular status in acute hemorrhage; myasthenia gravis; infants younger than 6 mo.

Route/Dosage
ADULTS: **PO** 80 mg/day in 4 equally divided doses. Increase to 160 mg/day in 4 equally divided doses.
IM 80 mg/day in 4 divided doses.

Interactions
Amantadine, tricyclic antidepressants: May cause increased anticholinergic side effects.
Atenolol, digoxin: May increase pharmacologic effects of these drugs.
Phenothiazines: May reduce antipsychotic effectiveness.

Lab Test Interferences None well documented.

Adverse Reactions
CV: Palpitations; tachycardia.
CNS: Headache; flushing; nervousness; drowsiness; weakness; dizziness; confusion; insomnia; fever (especially in children); mental confusion or excitement (especially in elderly, even with small doses); CNS stimulation (restlessness, tremor); light-headedness.
DERM: Severe allergic reactions including anaphylaxis, urticaria and dermal manifestations; local irritation following injection.
EENT: Blurred vision; mydriasis; photophobia; cycloplegia; increased IOP; dilated pupils; nasal congestion.
GI: Dry mouth; altered taste perception; nausea; vomiting; dysphagia; heartburn; constipation; bloated feeling; paralytic ileus.
GU: Urinary hesitancy and retention; impotence.
OTHER: Suppression of lactation; decreased sweating.

Precautions
Pregnancy: Category B.
Lactation: Excreted in breast milk.
Children: Safety and efficacy have not been established. Contraindicated in infants younger than 6 mo. In infants, serious respiratory symptoms, seizures, syncope, pulse rate fluctuation, muscular hypotonia, coma, and death have been reported.
Elderly: Elderly patients may react with excitement, agitation, drowsiness, and other untoward manifestations to even small doses.
Special risk patients: Use with caution in patients with autonomic neuropathy, hyperthyroidism, hypertension, coronary heart disease, CHF, hiatal hernia, prostatic hypertrophy.
Anticholinergic psychosis: Reported in sensitive individuals and may include confusion, disorientation, short-term memory loss, hallucinations, dysarthria, ataxia, coma, euphoria, decreased anxiety, fatigue, insomnia, agitation and mannerisms, and inappropriate affect.
Diarrhea: Diarrhea may be symptom of incomplete intestinal obstruction, especially in patients with ileostomy or colostomy. Treatment of diarrhea with drug is inappropriate and possibly harmful.

Gastric ulcer: May delay gastric emptying rate and complicate therapy.
Heat prostration: Can occur in presence of high environmental temperature.

Overdosage: Signs and Symptoms
Circulatory failure, vomiting, abdominal distention, muscle weakness, anxiety, stupor, blurred vision, photophobia, dilated pupils, urinary retention.

PATIENT CARE CONSIDERATIONS
Administration/Storage
- For parenteral administration, give only IM. Drug is not for IV use.
- Administer drug 30 min before meals.
- Store in tightly closed container at room temperature and protect from light. Injection fluid should be clear.

Assessment/Interventions
- Obtain patient history, including drug history and any known allergies.
- Assess baseline vital signs.
- Monitor I&O.
- Ask patient if difficulty in voiding is a problem.
- Assess hydration status (eg, skin turgor, mucous membranes, stool consistency, frequency) and bowel sounds.
- Monitor patient for changes in vital signs and sensorium (eg, fever, tachycardia, confusion, anxiety).

Patient/Family Education
- Instruct patient not to take any otc medications without consulting health care provider.
- Advise contact lens wearers to use lubricating solutions.
- Warn patients to avoid direct sunlight and any heat extremes (eg, exercise in hot weather, saunas, prolonged activity in hot weather).
- Instruct patient to take sips of water frequently, suck on ice chips or sugarless hard candy, or chew sugarless gum if dry mouth occurs.
- Alert patients to pay special attention to fever, decreased ability to sweat and changes in bowel or bladder habits.
- Advise elderly patients to report eye pain to health care provider or ophthalmologist and to undergo testing for glaucoma.
- Advise patient that drug may cause drowsiness and to use caution while driving or performing other tasks requiring mental alertness.
- Tell patient to report any difficulty in swallowing to health care provider.

Didanosine (ddl; dideoxyinosine)
(die-DAN-oh-SEEN)

Class Antiretroviral/Nucleoside reverse transcriptase inhibitor

How Supplied
Videx Tablets, buffered, chewable/dispersible 25 mg, Tablets, buffered, chewable/dispersible 50 mg, Tablets, buffered, chewable/dispersible 100 mg, Tablets, buffered, chewable/dispersible 200 mg, Powder for Oral Solution, buffered 100 mg, Powder for Oral Solution, buffered 250 mg, Powder for Oral Solution, pediatric 2 g, Powder for Oral Solution, pediatric 4 g ♦ *Videx EC* Capsules, delayed-release (with enteric-coated beadlets) 125 mg, Capsules, delayed-release (with enteric-coated beadlets) 200 mg, Capsules, delayed-release (with enteric-coated beadlets) 250 mg, Capsules, delayed-release (with enteric-coated beadlets) 400 mg

Action
PHARMACOLOGY: Inhibits replication of HIV by interfering with DNA synthesis.

PHARMACOKINETICS/DYNAMICS:
Absorption: T_{max} is 0.25 to 1.5 hr (buffered formulation), 2 hr (delayed-release). Bioavailability approximately 42% (buffered formulation). Food decreases the C_{max} and AUC approximately 55% of the buffered formulation and decreases the C_{max} and AUC of the delayed-release capsules approximately 46% and 19%, respectively. Take on an empty stomach.

Distribution: Less than 5% protein bound. Vd approximately 1.08 L/kg.

Metabolism: Intracellularly converted by enzymes to dideoxyadenosine 5′-triphosphate (active).

Excretion: t½ approximately 1.5 hr (buffered formulation). Approximately 18% recovered in the urine (buffered formulation). Renal clearance approximately 5.5 mL/min/kg (buffered formulation).

Special Populations:
Renal Function Impairment – t½ is increased and clearance is decreased. Dosage reduction recommended in those with Ccr less than 60 mL/min.

Indications
Didanosine (Videx): Treatment of HIV-1 infection in combination with other antiretrovirals.
Didanosine EC (Videx EC): In combination with other antiretroviral agents for the treatment of HIV-1 infection in adults who require

once-daily administration of didanosine or an alternative didanosine formulation.

Contraindications Standard considerations.

Route/Dosage
Didanosine EC (*Videx EC*) has not been studied in pediatric patients. Children's dosage recommendations are for didanosine (*Videx*).

ADULTS LESS THAN 60 KG: **PO** 125 mg (as 2 tablets) or 167 mg (powder for suspension) q 12 hr or 250 mg qd (capsules).

ADULTS MORE THAN 60 KG: **PO** 200 mg (as 2 tablets) or 250 mg (powder for suspension) q 12 hr or 400 mg qd (capsules).

CHILDREN: **PO** 120 mg/m^2 bid.

Interactions
Allopurinol: Because allopurinol may cause increased didanosine plasma levels, do not coadminister.

Antacids: Aluminum or magnesium containing antacids may potentiate adverse events associated with the antacid component of didanosine chewable or dispersible tablets and pediatric powder.

Antiretroviral agents: Antiretroviral agents have caused fatal lactic acidosis in women when coadministered with didanosine.

Delavirdine, indinavir: Administer 1 hr prior to didanosine to avoid decreasing plasma levels of delavirdine or indinavir.

Drugs that cause peripheral neuropathy or pancreatitis: Increased risk of these toxicities.

Food: Reduces absorption of didanosine by as much as 50%.

Fluoroquinolones, tetracyclines: Do not administer within 2 hr of didanosine.

Ganciclovir: When coadministered with didanosine, an increase in didanosine plasma levels and a decrease in ganciclovir concentrations may occur.

Itraconazole, ketaconazole, dapsone, and other drugs whose absorption can be affected by gastric acidity: Administer at least 2 hr before didanosine.

Methadone: May decrease didanosine plasma levels.

Lab Test Interferences None well documented.

Adverse Reactions
CNS: Peripheral neuropathy; asthenia; headache; pain; seizure.
DERM: Rash; pruritus; alopecia.
EENT: Retinal depigmentation.
GI: Pancreatitis; diarrhea; abdominal pain; nausea; vomiting; anorexia; dry mouth.
HEMA: Leukopenia, thrombocytopenia, granulocytopenia.
HEPA: Hepatic failure; elevated LFTs.
OTHER: Myopathy; chills, fever.

Precautions
Pregnancy: Category B.

Lactation: Undetermined. HIV-infected mothers should not breastfeed their infants.

Children: Safety and efficacy of didanosine EC (*Videx EC*) not established.

Renal function impairment: Dosage reduction is recommended with Ccr less than 60 mL/min.

Hepatic function impairment: Dosage may need to be reduced. Hepatic failure has occurred in pediatric patients.

Mutagenesis: May be genotoxic.

Hepatomegaly with steatosis: Fatal cases of severe hepatomegaly with steatosis have been reported.

Lactic acidosis: Fatal cases of lactic acidosis have been reported. Use with caution in pregnancy.

Pancreatitis: Major toxicity; has been fatal. Should be considered if patient develops abdominal pain, nausea, vomiting, or lab test abnormalities.

Peripheral neuropathy: Occurs frequently; may be dose-related.

Retinal changes and optic neuritis: Retinal changes and optic neuritis have been reported in adult and pediatric patients.

Special diets: Each tablet contains 36.5 mg phenylalanine; single-dose powder packet contains 1380 mg sodium.

PATIENT CARE CONSIDERATIONS

Administration/Storage
- Give on an empty stomach.
- Have patients chew or manually crush tablets or disperse tablets in water (2 tablets/1 oz water).
- When dispersing tablets in water, stir until uniform dispersion occurs, then have patient drink entire amount immediately.
- When preparing buffered powder for oral suspension, do not use fruit juice or other acid-containing liquid. Stir until completely dissolved in 4 oz liquid, then have patient drink entire amount immediately.
- Pediatric powder for oral suspension is first mixed with purified water to obtain concentration of 20 mg/mL, then mixed with antacid to obtain final concentration of 10 mg/mL.
- Pediatric oral solution admixture may be stored for up to 30 days if refrigerated. Shake well before use.

Assessment/Interventions
- Obtain patient history, including drug history and any known allergies. Note renal or liver

impairment, history of pancreatitis, and prior response to zidovudine therapy.
- Ensure that liver and renal function tests are obtained before beginning drug therapy and repeat periodically.
- Notify health care provider if diarrhea develops in patient receiving oral solution. Switching to tablets may alleviate symptoms.
- If patient has abdominal pain, nausea, or vomiting, or has elevated amylase or LFT results, contact health care provider and withhold drug until pancreatitis can be excluded.
- Observe for symptoms of peripheral neuropathy (eg, distal numbness, tingling, pain in feet or hands) or evidence of opportunistic infections. Notify health care provider if these occur.
- Monitor uric acid levels closely for possible asymptomatic hyperuricemia.
- Monitor body temperature to detect possible infection.
- Perform periodic retinal examinations for retinal changes and optic neuritis.
- Document any change in vision in pediatric patients. Perform dilated examination q 6 mo.

Patient/Family Education
- Advise patient to take drug on empty stomach and to chew or crush tablets.
- Inform patient that drug does not completely eliminate HIV virus and, therefore, does not reduce risk of transmitting HIV. Appropriate precautions must be continued.
- Emphasize that drug does not cure AIDS or AIDS-related complex (ARC) and to report significant changes in health to health care provider.
- Instruct patient to report these symptoms to health care provider: abdominal pain, diarrhea, nausea, vomiting, tingling pain or numbness in hands or feet, fever, sore throat, flu-like symptoms.
- Advise patient to alcoholic beverages or taking OTC medications without first notifying health care provider.

Diethylpropion Hydrochloride

(die-ETH-uhl-PRO-pee-ahn HIGH-droe-KLOR-ide)

Class CNS stimulant/Anorexiant

How Supplied
Tenuate Tablets 25 mg ◆ *Tenuate Dospan* Tablets, sustained-release 75 mg

Action
PHARMACOLOGY: Stimulates satiety center in brain, causing appetite suppression.

PHARMACOKINETICS/DYNAMICS:
Absorption: Rapidly absorbed.

Distribution: Crosses the blood-brain barrier and the placenta.

Metabolism: Extensively metabolized, involving N-dealkylation and reduction, to many active metabolites.

Excretion: 75% to 100% excreted in the urine. Plasma t½ of aminoketone metabolites is 4 to 6 hr.

Indications Short-term (few weeks) adjunct to diet plan to reduce weight.

Contraindications Advanced arteriosclerosis; symptomatic cardiovascular disease; moderate to severe hypertension; hyperthyroidism; hypersensitivity to sympathomimetic amines; glaucoma; agitated states; history of drug abuse; concurrent use with or within 14 days of MAOI; coadministration with other CNS stimulants.

Route/Dosage
ADULTS: **PO** Immediate-release tablets 25 mg tid, 1 hr before meals; Sustained-release tablets 75 mg once daily, in mid-morning.

Interactions
Guanethidine: May decrease hypotensive effect.
MAOIs, furazolidone: Hypertensive crisis and intracranial hemorrhage may occur.
Selective serotonin reuptake inhibitors: Sympathomimetic effects of diethylpropion may be increased; increased risk of "serotonin syndrome."
Tricyclic antidepressants: May decrease anorexiant effect.

Lab Test Interferences None well documented.

Adverse Reactions
CV: Palpitations; tachycardia; arrhythmias; hypertension; hypotension.
CNS: Overstimulation; dizziness; insomnia; euphoria; tremor; headache.
DERM: Excessive sweating; flushing.
EENT: Mydriasis; blurred vision.
GI: Dry mouth; unpleasant taste; nausea; diarrhea; constipation; stomach pain.
GU: Dysuria; urinary frequency; impotence; menstrual disturbances.
HEMA: Bone marrow depression; agranulocytosis; leukopenia.

OTHER: Hair loss; myalgia; gynecomastia; allergic reactions (eg, urticaria; rash; erythema).

Precautions

Pregnancy: Category B.
Lactation: Excreted in breast milk.
Children: Not recommended in children younger than 16 yr.
Cardiovascular effects: Diethylpropion may cause or aggravate hypertension or arrhythmias.
Convulsions: Diethylpropion may aggravate convulsions; dose titration or discontinuance may be necessary.
Drug dependence: Related to amphetamine; has abuse potential.
Tolerance: Tolerance may occur.

Overdosage: Signs and Symptoms

Restlessness, tremor, hyperreflexia, fever, tachypnea, dizziness, panic, aggression, hallucinations, seizure, coma, arrhythmias, hypotension, hypertension, death.

PATIENT CARE CONSIDERATIONS

Administration/Storage

- Give medication 1 hr before meals. Give sustained-release tablets once daily at midmorning.
- Do not crush or open sustained-release tablets.

Assessment/Interventions

- Obtain patient history, including drug history and any known allergies.
- Assess physical and psychological status throughout therapy.
- Measure patient's weight weekly.
- Notify health care provider and withhold medication if there is a BP increase of 20 mm Hg or if heart dysrhythmia or increase in heart rate develop.

Patient/Family Education

- Explain potential for increased agitation, palpitations, and dizziness, and identify precaution to take when performing tasks that require physical coordination or mental concentration.
- Tell patient to record weight weekly.
- Explain that drug will make patient feel less hungry and thus make it easier to adhere to diet but that weight loss will occur only with calorie reduction and increased physical activity.
- Instruct patient on missed medication procedure: if less than 2 hr, take medication; if more than 2 hr, wait until next scheduled dose. Do not double up on medication.
- Advise patient to limit intake of coffee, tea, cocoa, chocolate, and caffeinated soft drinks.
- Identify techniques to prevent or treat dry mouth.

Diflorasone Diacetate

(die-FLORE-ah-sone die-ASS-eh-tate)

Class Anti-inflammatory agent/Corticosteroid/Topical

How Supplied

Psorcon E Cream 0.05%, Ointment 0.05%

Action

PHARMACOLOGY: Therapeutic effects are caused by anti-inflammatory activity which are nonspecific (ie, they act against most causes of inflammation including mechanical, chemical, microbiological, and immunological).

Indications Relief of the anti-inflammatory and pruritic manifestations of corticosteroid responsive dermatoses.

Contraindications Standard considerations.

Route/Dosage

Occlusive dressings may be used for certain conditions.

CREAM

ADULT: **Topical** Apply sparingly to affected area 1 to 3 times/day

OINTMENT

ADULT: **Topical** Apply sparingly to affected area 1 to 4 times/day

Interactions None well documented.

Lab Test Interferences None well documented.

Adverse Reactions These may occur more frequently with occlusive dressings.

DERM: Burning; itching; irritation; dryness; folliculitis; hypertrichosis; acneiform eruptions; hypopigmentation; perioral dermatitis; allergic contact dermatitis; skin maceration; secondary infection; skin atrophy; striae; miliaria.
OTHER: Systemic absorption may produce reversible hypothalamic pituitary adrenal (HPA) axis suppression, manifestations of Cushing syndrome, hyperglycemia, and glycosuria.

Precautions

Pregnancy: Category C.
Lactation: Use with caution. It is not known whether topical corticosteroids could result in sufficient systemic absorption to produce adverse effects in infants.
Children: Children may be more susceptible to

topical corticosteroid-induced HPA axis suppression and Cushing syndrome than adults because of larger skin surface area to body weight ratio.
Systemic effects: Systemic absorption of topical corticosteroids has produced reversible HPA axis suppression, Cushing syndrome, hyperglycemia, and glycosuria. Conditions that may augment systemic absorption include use over large body surface areas, prolonged use, and occlusive dressings.

Diflunisal

(die-FLOO-nih-sal)

Class Analgesic/Salicylate

How Supplied
Dolobid Tablets 25 mg, Tablets 50 mg
❈ *Apo-Diflunisal* ♦ *Novo-Diflunisal* ♦ *Nu-Diflunisal*

Action
PHARMACOLOGY: Decreases inflammation and relieves pain by inhibiting prostaglandin synthesis and release.

PHARMACOKINETICS/DYNAMICS:
Absorption: Rapidly and completely absorbed. T_{max} is 2 to 3 hr. C_{max} approximately 41 to 124 mcg/mL (250 to 1000 mg single doses).

Distribution: Greater than 99% protein bound. Excreted in breast milk.

Metabolism: Metabolized to glucuronide conjugates.

Excretion: $t_{½}$ is 8 to 12 hr. Approximately 90% excreted in the urine as two soluble glucuronide conjugates.

Onset: 1 hr.

Peak: 2 to 3 hr.

Indications Relief of mild to moderate pain, rheumatoid arthritis, and osteoarthritis.

Contraindications Hypersensitivity to NSAIDs or aspirin.

Route/Dosage
Mild to Moderate Pain
ADULTS: PO 500 to 1000 mg for first dose, then 250 to 500 mg q 8 to 12 hr.

Arthritis
ADULTS: PO 250 to 500 mg bid. Max dose 750 mg bid.

Interactions
Antacids: Decreased plasma concentration of diflunisal.
Cyclosporine: Increased nephrotoxic effect of cyclosporine possible.
Methotrexate: Life-threatening methotrexate toxicity possible.
Warfarin: Prothrombin time may increase; increased risk of bleeding.

Lab Test Interferences May falsely elevate salicylate serum concentrations.

Adverse Reactions
CV: Peripheral edema.
CNS: Headache; somnolence; insomnia; dizziness.
DERM: Rash; erythema multiforme; photosensitivity.
EENT: Angioedema; tinnitus.
GI: Nausea; dyspepsia; GI pain; diarrhea; GI bleeding.
GU: Renal impairment; interstitial nephritis; dysuria.
HEMA: Thrombocytopenia; agranulocytosis; hemolytic anemia.
HEPA: Jaundice.
RESP: Bronchospasm.
OTHER: Anaphylaxis; hypersensitivity syndrome (eg, fever, chills, rash, liver or kidney dysfunction, leukopenia, thrombocytopenia, eosinophilia, DIC).

Precautions
Pregnancy: Category C.
Lactation: Excreted in breast milk.
Children: Not recommended for children younger than 12 yr. May increase risk of Reye syndrome; do not use if varicella infection or flu symptoms are suspected.
Fluid retention: Use with caution in patients with CHF, hypertension, or other conditions associated with fluid retention.
History of peptic ulcer: Use carefully and closely monitor for GI bleeding or peptic ulcer; closely monitor patients with GI disease.

Overdosage: Signs and Symptoms
Drowsiness, vomiting, nausea, diarrhea, hyperventilation, tachycardia, sweating, tinnitus, disorientation, decreased urine output, cardiorespiratory arrest, stupor and coma; may lead to death.

PATIENT CARE CONSIDERATIONS

Administration/Storage
♦ Do not crush or allow patient to chew tablets.
♦ Administer with milk or food to minimize gastric irritation, give patient generous amounts of water or other fluids to increase gastric emptying.

Assessment/Interventions
♦ Obtain patient history, including drug history and any known allergies.
♦ Assess pain prior to and after administration of medication.

- Monitor I&O. Notify health care provider if signs of renal dysfunction occur (eg, decreased urine output, elevated BUN, elevated creatinine).
- Include hepatic function in each assessment and notify health care provider if any signs or symptoms of hepatic dysfunction are noted (eg, fatigue, jaundice, abdominal pain, elevated liver enzymes, dark urine).

Patient/Family Education
- Advise patient to swallow tablets whole and not to chew or crush them.
- Explain that relief of arthritis may not occur for 1 wk to several weeks.
- Caution patients against taking products with aspirin or acetaminophen concurrently with diflunisal unless directed by health care provider.
- Warn patient that this medication can precipitate Reye syndrome.
- Advise patients to avoid exposure to sunlight and to use sunscreens or wear protective clothing to avoid photosensitivity reaction until tolerance is determined.
- Inform patients that first dose tends to have slower onset of pain relief than other drugs with comparable effects.
- Instruct patients to report immediately any signs of nephrotoxicity including decreased urine output, weight gain, edema, anorexia, nausea, and vomiting.
- Advise patients with history of GI problems to notify health care provider if abdominal pain, melena, or hematemesis develops during therapy.
- Advise patient to report degree of pain relief to health care provider.

Digoxin

(dih-JOX-in)

Class Cardiac glycoside

How Supplied
Digitek Tablets 0.125 mg, Tablets 0.25 mg ♦ *Lanoxicaps* Capsules 0.05 mg, Capsules 0.1 mg, Capsules 0.2 mg ♦ *Lanoxin* Tablets 0.125 mg, Tablets 0.25 mg, Elixir, pediatric 0.05 mg/mL, Injection 0.25 mg/mL, Injection, pediatric 0.1 mg/mL

Action

PHARMACOLOGY: Increases force and velocity of myocardial systolic contraction (positive inotropic action), slows heart rate, and decreases conduction through atrioventricular node.

PHARMACOKINETICS/DYNAMICS:

Absorption:
Bioavailability – 100% (IV), 90% to 100% (capsules), 70% to 85% (elixir), 60% to 80% (tablets). T_{max} is 1 to 3 hr (oral). Food slows the rate of absorption after oral administration.

Distribution: 6 to 8 hr tissue distribution phase. Large apparent Vd. Crosses blood-brain barrier and placenta. Excreted in breast milk. Approximately 25% protein bound.

Metabolism: Approximately 16% metabolized; metabolites formed by hydrolysis, oxidation, and conjugation.

Excretion: Elimination follows first-order kinetics. 50% to 70% excreted unchanged in the urine (after IV administration). $t_{½}$ is 1.5 to 2 days.

Onset: 0.5 to 2 hr (oral), 5 to 30 min (IV).

Peak: 2 to 6 hr (oral), 1 to 4 hr (IV).

Special Populations:
Renal Function Impairment – Clearance correlates with Ccr. Dosage adjustment recommended.

Indications Treatment of CHF, atrial fibrillation, atrial flutter, paroxysmal atrial tachycardia, cardiogenic shock.

Contraindications Ventricular fibrillation; ventricular tachycardia except in certain cases; digitalis toxicity; beriberi heart disease; hypersensitivity to digoxin; some cases of hypersensitive carotid sinus syndrome.

Route/Dosage

Rapid digitalization with loading dose
ADULTS: **IV** 0.4 to 0.6 mg or **PO** tablets 0.5 to 0.75 mg or capsules 0.4 to 0.6 mg in previously undigitalized patients; additional doses may be given cautiously at 6 to 8 hr intervals (**IV** 0.1 to 0.3 mg or **PO** tablets 0.125 to 0.375 mg or capsules 0.1 to 0.3 mg) until clinical response is achieved; thereafter adjust dosage based on levels (usual range 0.125 to 0.5 mg/day as single daily dose). In previously digitalized patients, adjust dosage in proportion to ratio of desired vs current serum levels.

INFANTS AND CHILDREN: Individualize dosage. Usual pediatric doses are listed at end of section.

Interactions

Amiodarone, anticholinergics, bepridol, benzodiazepines, ACE inhibitors, clarithromycin, cyclosporine, diltiazem, erythromycin, indomethacin, itraconazole, propafenone, quinidine, quinine, tetracycline, verapamil: May increase digoxin serum levels.

Antacids, antineoplastics, cholestyramine, colestipol, kaolin/pectin, metoclopramide: May decrease absorption and effect of digoxin.
Penicillamine: May decrease effect of digoxin.
Potassium-sparing diuretics: May alter effect of digoxin.
Thiazide or loop diuretics: May increase effect of digoxin.
St. John's wort, thyroid hormones, thioamines: May decrease effect of digoxin.

Lab Test Interferences None well documented.

Adverse Reactions
CV: Arrhythmias (supraventricular arrhythmias are more common in infants and children), including ventricular tachycardia and premature ventricular contractions.
CNS: Headache; weakness; apathy; drowsiness; mental depression; confusion; disorientation.
EENT: Visual disturbances (eg, blurred vision, halo effect).
GI: Anorexia; nausea; vomiting; diarrhea.

Precautions
Pregnancy: Category C.
Lactation: Excreted in breast milk.
Children: Newborns show varying tolerance. Premature and immature infants are particularly sensitive; reduce and individualize dose as needed.
Elderly: Use with caution; renal clearance likely to be reduced.
Renal function impairment: Excretion may be decreased, leading to digoxin accumulation and toxicity; adjust dosage.
Cardiovascular disease: Electrical conversion of arrhythmias may require dose reduction.
Digitalis toxicity: Anorexia, nausea, and vomiting may be associated with toxicity or CHF. Arrhythmias for which digoxin is indicated may also be a reflection of toxicity.
Electrolyte imbalance: Maintain normal serum potassium, calcium, and magnesium levels.
Lanoxicaps: Lanoxicaps have greater bioavailability than standard tablets. The 0.2 mg capsule is equivalent to 0.25 mg tablet; the 0.1 mg capsule to 0.125 mg tablet; the 0.05 mg capsule to 0.0625 mg tablet.

Usual Pediatric Digitalizing and Maintenance Dosages with Normal Renal Function Based on Lean Body Weight

Age	Digitalizing Dose (mcg/kg) PO	Digitalizing Dose (mcg/kg) IV	Daily Maintenance Dose as % of Loading Dose (mcg/kg in 2 to 3 divided doses)
Premature	20 to 30	15 to 25	20% to 30%
Term	25 to 35	20 to 30	25% to 35%
1 to 24 mo	35 to 60	30 to 50	25% to 35%
2 to 5 yr	30 to 40	25 to 35	25% to 35%
5 to 10 yr	20 to 35	15 to 30	25% to 35%
> 10 yr	10 to 15	8 to 12	25% to 35%

Overdosage: Signs and Symptoms
GI tract (eg, anorexia, nausea, vomiting, diarrhea); nervous system (eg, headache, weakness, apathy, drowsiness, visual disturbances such as blurred, yellow or green vision, halo effect), depression, confusion, restlessness, disorientation, seizures, EEG abnormalities, delirium, hallucinations, neuralgia and psychosis; cardiovascular system (eg, ventricular tachycardia, PVCs, paroxysmal and nonparoxysmal nodal rhythms, AV dissociation, accelerated nodal rhythm and premature atrial contraction with block, atrial fibrillation, ECG changes, al. alterations in cardiac rate and rhythm). Conduction disturbances are common manifestations of toxicity in children.

PATIENT CARE CONSIDERATIONS

Administration/Storage
- Administer IM doses deep into gluteal muscles and massage well to reduce painful, local reactions. IM route should be avoided; use only when other routes not available.
- If dilution for IV administration is desired, do not use solutions that are discolored or contain precipitate.
- For IV administration, digoxin injection may be diluted (up to 4-fold) with normal saline, D5W, or Sterile Water for Injection. Infuse slowly, over 5 min or longer.
- Do not mix digoxin solution with other drugs.
- Before administering loading dose, determine if patient has taken digoxin or other digitalis

preparation in past 2 wk.

Assessment/Interventions
- Obtain patient history, including drug history and any known allergies.
- Monitor apical pulse for 1 full min before administering. Withhold dose and notify health care provider if pulse rate is less than 60 bpm in adult, less than 70 bpm in child, or less than 90 bpm in infant.
- Assess for peripheral edema and auscultate lungs for rales/crackles before and throughout therapy.
- Plan for dosage adjustments when changing from parenteral to oral (and vice versa) route of administration.
- Notify health care provider if signs of toxicity occur (eg, abdominal pain, anorexia, nausea, vomiting, visual disturbance, bradycardia, ECG changes, arrhythmias, headache, seizure). Be prepared to administer digoxin antibodies (digoxin-immune Fab) for severe overdose toxicity.
- Measure and record patient's daily weight and I&O.
- Monitor serum electrolyte levels, renal and hepatic function studies, and digoxin serum levels and report changes to health care provider.

Patient/Family Education
- Instruct patient to take digoxin at same time each day to ensure steady-state dosing and to contact health care provider for instructions if dose is missed.
- Teach patient and family name, action, administration, side effects, and toxic effects of particular digoxin preparation.
- Emphasize importance of regular follow-up exams to determine effectiveness and to monitor for toxicity.
- Caution patient to avoid taking otc medications without consulting health care provider. Antacids and antidiarrheals, for example, slow absorption of digoxin.
- Teach patient and family to take pulse and to seek health care provider's advice for rates less than 60 bpm or greater than 100 bpm (adults).
- If patient is directed by health care provider, help identify ways to supplement potassium intake.

Dihydroergotamine Mesylate

(DIE-high-droe-err-GOT-uh-meen MEH-sih-LATE)

Class Analgesic/Migraine/Ergotamine derivative

How Supplied
D.H.E. 45 Injection 1 mg/mL • *Migranal* Spray, nasal 4 mg/mL. With 10 mg caffeine and 50 mg dextrose.

Action
PHARMACOLOGY: Constricts peripheral and cranial blood vessels, depresses central vasomotor centers, and reduces extracranial blood flow.

PHARMACOKINETICS/DYNAMICS:
Distribution: 93% protein bound. Vd approximately 800 L.

Metabolism: Four metabolites identified, with one being equivalent to dihydroergotamine in potency.

Excretion: Major elimination route is via the bile in the feces. 6% to 7% excreted unchanged in the urine after IM injection. Renal clearance is 0.1 L/min. t½ approximately 9 hr.

Onset: 15 to 30 min (IM).

Duration: 3 to 4 hr (IM).

Indications Acute treatment of migraine headaches with or without aura; acute treatment of cluster headache episodes (injection).

Contraindications Hypersensitivity to ergot alkaloids; hepatic or renal impairment; severe pruritus; coronary artery disease; uncontrolled peripheral vascular disease; hypertension; sepsis; use during pregnancy, lactation or in women who may become pregnant; concurrent vasoconstrictor therapy. CYP3A4 inhibitors (eg, macrolide antibiotics [eg, erythromycin], protease inhibitors [eg, ritonavir]).

Route/Dosage
ADULTS: **Intranasal** 1 spray (0.5 mg) in each nostril; administer an additional spray (0.5 mg) in each nostril 15 min later for a total dosage of 4 sprays (2 mg).

IM/IV/SC Administer 1 mL (1 mg); repeat dose as needed at 1-hr intervals to a total dose of 3 mL (3 mg) for IM or SC administration or 2 mL (2 mg) for IV administration in a 24-hr period (max, 6 mL/wk).

Interactions
Beta-blockers, vasoconstrictors (eg, epinephrine): Can increase peripheral ischemia, cyanosis, and numbness caused by ergot alkaloids.
CYP3A4 inhibitors (eg, macrolide antibiotics [eg, erythromycin], protease inhibitors [eg, ritonavir]): May increase the risk of life-threatening peripheral ischemia.
Nitrates (eg, nitroglycerin): May oppose effects of nitrates.

Lab Test Interferences None well documented.

Adverse Reactions
CV: Pulselessness; precordial distress or pain; transient tachycardia or bradycardia; raised arterial pressure; coronary vasoconstriction.
GI: Nausea; vomiting; abdominal pain.
OTHER: Numbness and tingling of fingers and toes; muscle pain in extremities; weakness in legs; localized edema; itching. Drug has oxytocic and spasmolytic properties.

Precautions
Pregnancy: Category X.
Lactation: Excreted in breast milk and may inhibit lactation. Drug can cause symptoms of ergotism in infant.
Children: Safety and efficacy not established.
Dependence/Withdrawal syndrome: Dependence/withdrawal has occurred with other ergot alkaloids; therefore, recommended dosage should not be exceeded.

Overdosage: Signs and Symptoms
Nausea, vomiting, leg weakness, pain in limb muscles, numbness and tingling of toes, precordial pain, changes in heart rate and BP, localized edema, itching, peripheral ischemia, gangrene, confusion, depression, drowsiness, convulsions.

PATIENT CARE CONSIDERATIONS
Administration/Storage
- IM route is preferred. Do not mix with any other drug in syringe or solution.
- For IM administration, inject at first sign of headache. To determine minimal effective dose, adjust dose for several headaches and then use minimal effective dose at onset of subsequent attacks.
- For rapid effect, administer IV. May be given undiluted; give 1 mg or fraction thereof over 1 min.
- After drug is administered, have patient lie supine and relax for few minutes, preferably in quiet, darkened room.
- Avoid prolonged administration or excessive dosage because of danger of ergotism and gangrene.
- Protect ampules from light and heat.

Assessment/Interventions
- Obtain patient history, including drug history and any known allergies.
- Determine history of hypersensitivity to dihydroergotamine and ergotamine derivatives.
- Obtain baseline vital signs, with special attention to pulse and BP.
- Evaluate mental status and peripheral neurocirculatory status (eg, sensation, edema, color, weakness).
- Prepare drug in syringe that is free of other drugs and solutions and administer drug undiluted.
- Obtain baseline assessment of pain severity.
- Monitor for changes in vital signs, especially pulse and BP.
- Monitor for changes in mental status (eg, confusion, drowsiness).
- Monitor for effectiveness of headache relief with pain assessments q 15 min and for minimal effective dose.
- Check neurocirculatory status of extremities, especially distally (eg, pulse, warmth, color).

Patient/Family Education
- Caution patient that this medication must not be taken during pregnancy or when pregnancy is possible. Advise patient to use reliable form of birth control while taking this drug.
- Teach patient to measure or rate drug effectiveness (eg, use analog or other validated rating scale).
- Instruct patient to take drug at first sign of impending headache and not to exceed maximum dosage.
- Advise patient to relax in supine position in quiet, darkened room after drug administration.
- Tell patient to inform health care provider if diagnosed with any peripheral vascular disease.
- Instruct patient to report the following symptoms to health care provider: pain, itching, weakness, tingling, edema, pallor, coolness, numbness (especially in distal extremities), chest discomfort, pain or any change in mental status (eg, drowsiness, light-headedness, syncope, seizures).
- Advise patient to avoid intake of alcoholic beverages, smoking, and exposure to cold because these vasoconstrictors may further impair peripheral circulation and cause or aggravate migraine headache.

Diltiazem Hydrochloride

(dill-TIE-uh-zem HIGH-droe-KLOR-ide)

Class Calcium channel blocker

How Supplied

Cardizem Tablets 30 mg, Tablets 60 mg, Tablets 90 mg, Tablets 120 mg, Powder for injection 25 mg, Injection 5 mg/mL ◆ *Cardizem CD* Capsules, extended-release 120 mg, Capsules, extended-release 180 mg, Capsules, extended-release 240 mg, Capsules, extended-release 300 mg, Capsules, extended-release 360 mg ◆ *Cardizem LA* Tablets, extended-release 120 mg, Tablets, extended-release 180 mg, Tablets, extended-release 240 mg, Tablets, extended-release 300 mg, Tablets, extended-release 360 mg, Tablets, extended-release 420 mg ◆ *CartiaXT* Capsules, extended-release 120 mg, Capsules, extended-release 180 mg, Capsules, extended-release 240 mg, Capsules, extended-release 300 mg ◆ *Dilacor XR* Capsules, extended-release 120 mg, Capsules, extended-release 180 mg, Capsules, extended-release 240 mg ◆ *Diltia XT* Capsules, extended-release 120 mg, Capsules, extended-release 180 mg, Capsules, extended-release 240 mg ◆ *Diltiazem Hydrochloride Extended Release* Capsules, extended-release 60 mg, Capsules, extended-release 90 mg ◆ *Taztia XT* Capsules, extended-release 120 mg, Capsules, extended-release 180 mg, Capsules, extended-release 240 mg, Capsules, extended-release 300 mg, Capsules, extended-release 360 mg ◆ *Tiazac* Capsules, extended-release 120 mg, Capsules, extended-release 180 mg, Capsules, extended-release 240 mg, Capsules, extended-release 300 mg, Capsules, extended-release 360 mg, Capsules, extended-release 420 mg

❀ *Apo-Diltiaz* ◆ *Apo-Diltiaz CD* ◆ *Apo-Diltiaz Injectable* ◆ *Apo-Diltiaz SR* ◆ *Gen-Diltiazem* ◆ *Novo-Diltiazem* ◆ *Novo-Diltiazem SR* ◆ *Nu-Diltiaz* ◆ *Nu-Diltiaz-CD* ◆ *ratio-Diltiazem CD* ◆ *Rhoxal-diltiazem CD*

Action

PHARMACOLOGY: Inhibits movement of calcium ions across cell membrane in systemic and coronary vascular smooth muscle; slows calcium ion movement across cell membranes in both cardiac muscle and cardiac pacemaker cells, decreasing sinoatrial and atrioventricular (AV) conduction.

PHARMACOKINETICS/DYNAMICS:

Absorption:
IV – T_{max} is 2 to 3 hr.
Extended release (ER) – T_{max} is 10 to 14 hr.
Immediate release (IR) – T_{max} is 2 to 4 hr.

Distribution: Vd approximately 305 L. 70% to 80% protein bound (approximately 40% to α_1-acid glycoprotein and approximately 30% to albumin). Excreted in breast milk.

Metabolism: Metabolized in the liver (including via CYP450) to several metabolites; desacetyl diltiazem is 25% to 50% as potent as diltiazem. Undergoes first-pass metabolism after oral administration.

Excretion: The t½ is approximately 3.4 hr (IV), 4 to 9 hr (ER), and 3 to 4.5 hr (IR). 2% to 4% excreted unchanged in urine (oral). Systemic Cl approximately 65 L/hr (IV).

Peak: 2 to 5 min (IV).

Special Populations:
Hepatic Function Impairment – Bioavailability is increased, and t½ is prolonged.

Indications

Oral: Treatment of angina pectoris caused by coronary artery spasm; chronic stable angina (classic effort-associated angina); essential hypertension (extended- and sustained-release forms only).

Parenteral: Treatment of atrial fibrillation or flutter; paroxysmal supraventricular tachycardia.

Contraindications Sick sinus syndrome; second- or third-degree AV block; except with functioning pacemaker; hypotension with systolic pressure less than 90 mm Hg; acute MI; pulmonary congestion; hypersensitivity to the drug; ventricular tachycardia (IV); atrial fibrillation or atrial flutter associated with an accessory bypass tract (IV); IV diltiazem and IV beta-blockers administered together (within a few hours).

Route/Dosage

Dosage regimens should be individualized.

Angina

ADULTS: **PO**

Cardizem: Start with 30 mg qid before meals and at bedtime. Gradually increase dosage at 1- to 2-day intervals until optimum response (average optimum dose range 180 to 360 mg/day).

Cardizem CD and *Cartia XT:* Start with 120 to 180 mg once daily. Some patients may respond to doses up to 480 mg once daily. When necessary, titrate the dose over 7 to 14 days.

Cardizem LA: Start with 180 mg once daily. Some patients may respond to doses up to 360 mg once daily. Titrate dose over 7 to 14 days.

Dilacor XR and *Diltia XT:* Start with 120 mg once daily. Some patients may respond to doses up to 480 mg once daily. When necessary, titrate the dose over 7 to 14 days.

Tiazac: Start with 120 to 180 mg once daily. Some patients may respond to doses up to 540 mg once daily. When necessary, titrate the dose over 7 to 14 days.

Atrial Fibrillation/Flutter/Paroxysmal Supraventricular Tachycardia
ADULTS: **Parenteral**
Direct IV single bolus injection: Initial dose is 0.25 mg/kg as a bolus administered over 2 min (reasonable dose is 20 mg for average patient). If response is inadequate after 15 min, administer as a second 0.35 mg/kg over 2 min (reasonable dose is 25 mg for average patient). Individualize subsequent IV doses. Dose low body weight patients on a mg/kg basis. Although the duration of action may be shorter, some patients may respond to an initial dose of 0.15 mg/kg. Continuous IV infusion: For continued reduction of heart rate (up to 24 hr) in patients with atrial fibrillation or atrial flutter, IV infusion may be administered. Immediately following administration of a bolus dose of 20 mg (0.25 mg/kg) or 25 mg (0.35 mg/kg) and reduction of heart rate, begin an IV infusion. The recommended initial infusion rate is 10 mg/hr; however, some patients may maintain response to an initial rate of 5 mg/hr. The infusion rate may be increased in 5 mg/hr increments up to 15 mg/hr as needed, if further reduction in heart rate is necessary. The infusion may be maintained for up to 24 hr (max, 24 hr and 15 mg/hr).

Hypertension
ADULTS: **PO**
Extended-release capsules: Start with 60 to 120 mg bid or 180 to 240 mg once daily. Max antihypertensive effect usually occurs by 14 days of chronic therapy (optimum dose range 240 to 360 mg once daily, but some patients respond to lower doses or higher doses up to 480 mg once daily).

Cardizem CD and Cartia XT
180 to 240 mg once daily; however, some patients may respond to lower doses. Maximum effect is usually achieved by 14 days of chronic therapy. Usual range is 240 to 360 mg once daily. Some patients may respond to doses up to 480 mg once daily.

Cardizem LA
Start with 180 to 240 mg once daily; however, some patients may respond to lower doses. Max effect is usually achieved by 14 days of chronic therapy. Dose range studied in clinical trials was 120 to 540 mg once daily (max, 540 mg daily).

Dilacor XR and Diltia XT
180 to 240 mg once daily (usual dose range, 180 to 480 mg once daily). Individual patients, particularly those 60 yr of age and older, may respond to lower doses of 120 mg once daily. Some patients may require doses up to 540 mg once daily.

Tiazac
Start with 120 to 240 mg once daily. Max effect is usually achieved by 14 days of chronic therapy. Usual dose range is 120 to 540 mg once daily.

Interactions
Anesthetics: Depression of cardiac contractility, conductivity, and automaticity as well as vascular dilation associated with anesthetics may be potentiated.

Benzodiazepines (eg, midazolam, triazolam), carbamazepine, cyclosporine, digitalis, encainide, lovastatin: Plasma levels of these agents may be elevated by diltiazem, increasing the pharmacologic and toxic effects.

Beta-blockers: May have additive negative inotropic and chronotropic effects.

Cimetidine, ranitidine: Diltiazem levels may be increased.

Other antihypertensive agents. May have additive effects.

Rifampin: Coadministration lowered diltiazem plasma concentrations to undetectable levels.

INCOMPATIBILITIES: Do not mix with furosemide.

Lab Test Interferences
None well documented.

Adverse Reactions
CV: Bradycardia (4%); first-degree AV block (3%); angina, arrhythmia, AV block (second- or third-degree), bundle branch block, CHF, ECG abnormalities, hypotension, palpitations, syncope, tachycardia, ventricular extrasystoles (less than 2%); peripheral edema, asystole, MI (postmarketing).

CNS: Dizziness (6%); headache, fatigue (5%); asthenia (3%); abnormal dreams, amnesia, depression, gait abnormalities, hallucinations, insomnia, nervousness, paresthesia, personality change, somnolence, tremor (less than 2%); lightheadedness; weakness; shakiness; extrapyramidal symptoms (postmarketing).

DERM: Rash (1%); petechiae, photosensitivity, pruritus, ecchymosis (less than 2%); alopecia, erythema multiforme (including Stevens-Johnson syndrome), toxic epidermal necrolysis, exfoliative dermatitis, purpura, generalized rash (postmarketing).

EENT: Amblyopia, epistaxis, eye irritation, nasal congestion, rhinitis, tinnitus (less than 2%); retinopathy (postmarketing).

GI: Nausea (1%); anorexia, constipation, diarrhea, dry mouth, dysgeusia, thirst, vomiting (less than 2%); abdominal discomfort; cramps; dyspepsia; gingival hyperplasia (postmarketing).

GU: Albuminuria, crystalluria, hyperuricemia, impotence, nocturia, polyuria, sexual difficulties, gynecomastia (less than 2%).

HEMA/LYMPH: Hemolytic anemia, increased bleeding time, leukopenia, thrombocytopenia (postmarketing).

LABTESTABS: Mild elevations of ALT, AST, LDH, and alkaline phosphatase, CPK increase (less than 2%).
M/N: Hyperglycemia, weight gain (less than 2%).
MUSC: Muscle cramps, neck rigidity, osteoarticular pain (less than 2%); joint pain.
RESP: Cough (2%); dyspnea (less than 2%).
OTHER: Lower limb edema (7%); edema (5%); flushing (1%); allergic reactions, pain (less than 2%); angioedema (postmarketing).

Precautions
Pregnancy: Category C.
Lactation: Excreted in breast milk.
Children: Safety and efficacy not established.
Elderly: Use with caution because of the greater frequency of decreased hepatic, renal, or cardiac function, and concomitant diseases or other drug therapy.
Renal function impairment: Use with caution. Dosage may need to be decreased.
Hepatic function impairment: Use with caution. Dosage may need to be decreased.
Acute hepatic injury: Mild elevations of transaminases with and without concomitant elevation in alkaline phosphatase and bilirubin have been observed. These elevations were usually transient and often resolved with continued treatment.
Cardiac conduction: Prolongs AV node refractory periods without prolonging sinus node recovery time, except in patients with sick sinus syndrome. This may rarely cause abnormally slow heart rates, particularly in patients with sick sinus syndrome, or second- or third-degree AV block.
CHF: Use with caution.
Withdrawal syndrome: Abrupt withdrawal may cause increased frequency and duration of angina. Dosage is tapered gradually.

Overdosage: Signs and Symptoms
Bradycardia, hypotension, high-degree AV block, heart failure.

PATIENT CARE CONSIDERATIONS

Administration/Storage
* May be used alone or in combination with other CV medications for the treatment of hypertension and angina.

Immediate-release tablets:
* Administer dose tid to qid as prescribed without regard to meals. Administer with food if GI upset occurs.

Extended-release tablets and capsules:
* Administer prescribed dose once daily without regard to meals. Administer with food if GI upset occurs.
* Swallow tablets and capsules whole. Do not crush, chew, or break.
* Store tablets and capsules at controlled room temperature (59° to 86°F). Protect from moisture.

Injection:
* For administration by IV bolus or infusion only. Not for intradermal, subcutaneous, IM, or intra-arterial administration.
* Follow manufacturer's recommendations for reconstituting powder for injection.
* Administer IV bolus dose over 2 min. A second dose may be administered 15 min later if response to first dose is inadequate.
* For IV infusion, add prescribed dose to prescribed volume of 0.9% sodium chloride, 5% dextrose in water, or 5% dextrose in 0.45% sodium chloride following manufacturer's dilution charts.
* Discard any unused solution. Do not save for future use.
* Store vials for injection in refrigerator (36° to 46°F). May store vials for injection at room temperature for up to 1 mo, but any unused injection must be destroyed after 1 mo.
* Store syringes and vials of powder for injection at room temperature (59° to 86°F). Do not freeze. Use reconstituted solution immediately or store for up to 24 hr at controlled room temperature.

Assessment/Interventions
* Obtain patient history, including drug history and any known allergies. Note renal or hepatic impairment, sick sinus syndrome, second or third degree AV block, CHF, or acute MI with pulmonary congestion.
* Ensure renal function (eg, BUN, serum creatinine) and liver enzymes are periodically evaluated during long-term treatment.
* Monitor and record BP and pulse frequently during treatment. Hold medication and notify health care provider if hypotension and/or bradycardia develop.
* Implement safety precautions if orthostatic hypotension occurs.
* Monitor patient for CV, GI, CNS, and general body side effects. Report to health care provider if noted and significant.

Injection:
* Review patient's history for any of the following conditions that could contraindicate the use of IV diltiazem: atrial fibrillation or flutter associated with accessory bypass tract, concurrent or recent use of IV beta-blockers, ventricular tachycardia.
* Ensure that a defibrillator and emergency

resuscitation equipment are readily available.
- Continuously monitor ECG during administration.
- Monitor BP frequently during administration. Be prepared to treat hypotension (eg, IV fluids, Trendelenburg position).

Patient/Family Education
- Explain name, dose, action, and potential side effects of drug.
- Advise patient or caregiver that IV diltiazem will be prepared and administered by health care professionals in a medical setting.
- Advise patient that dose of medication may be adjusted to obtain max benefit.
- Advise patient taking immediate-release tablets to take tid to qid as prescribed. Advise patient to take each dose without regard to meals but to take with food if stomach upset occurs.
- Advise patient taking extended-release products to take once daily as prescribed, without regard to meals. Advise patient to take with food if stomach upset occurs.
- Caution patient to swallow extended-release products whole and not to crush or chew.
- Advise patient to try to take each dose at about the same time each day.
- Inform patient that drug controls, but does not cure, hypertension or angina and to continue taking as prescribed even when BP is not elevated or angina symptoms are not present.
- Caution patient not to change the dose or stop taking unless advised by health care provider.
- Instruct patient to continue taking other BP or angina medications as prescribed by health care provider.
- Instruct patient being treated for angina to notify health care provider if frequency or severity of chest pain or need for sublingual nitroglycerin appears to be increasing.
- Instruct patient in BP and pulse measurement skills.
- Advise patient to monitor and record BP and pulse at home and to inform health care provider if abnormal measurements are noted. Also advise patient to take record of BP and pulse to each follow-up visit.
- Instruct patient to lie or sit down if experiencing dizziness or lightheadedness when standing.
- Advise patient to notify health care provider if any of the following occur: frequent episodes of dizziness when arising; slow heart beat; persistent fatigue; any other unusual or unexplained symptom or sign.
- Emphasize to hypertensive patient importance of other modalities on BP: weight control, regular exercise, smoking cessation, moderate intake of alcohol and salt.
- Advise women to notify health care provider if pregnant, planning to become pregnant, or breastfeeding.
- Caution patient not to take any prescription or OTC medications, herbal preparations, or dietary supplements unless advised by health care provider.
- Advise patient that follow-up visits and lab tests may be required to monitor therapy and to keep appointments.

Dimenhydrinate

(die-men-HIGH-drih-nate)

Class Antiemetic/Antivertigo/Anticholinergic

How Supplied
Calm-X Tablets 50 mg ◆ Children's Dramamine Liquid 12.5 mg/5 mL ◆ Dimetabs Tablets 50 mg ◆ Dinate Injection 50 mg/mL ◆ Dramamine Liquid 15.62mg/5 mL, Liquid 12.5 mg/4 mL, Tablets 50 mg, Tablets, chewable 50 mg ◆ Dramanate Injection 50 mg/mL ◆ Dymenate Injection 50 mg/mL ◆ Hydrate Injection 50 mg/mL ◆ Triptone Tablets 50 mg/mL
✤ Apo-Dimenhydrinate ◆ Gravol

Action
PHARMACOLOGY: Directly inhibits labyrinthine stimulation for up to 3 hr.

PHARMACOKINETICS/DYNAMICS:
Distribution: Small amounts excreted in breast milk.

Excretion: Renally eliminated.
Onset: 20 to 30 min (IM).
Duration: 3 to 6 hr.

Indications Prevention and treatment of motion sickness, dizziness, nausea, vomiting.
Unlabeled use(s): Treatment of Meniere disease, nausea and vomiting of pregnancy, postoperative nausea, and vomiting.

Contraindications Use in newborns; allergic reactions to diphenhydramine.

Route/Dosage
Motion Sickness
ADULTS: **PO** 50 to 100 mg 30 min prior to travel, followed by 50 to 100 mg q 4 to 6 hr (max 400 mg/day). **IM** 50 mg prn. **IV** 50 mg in 10 mL of Sodium Chloride for Injection administered over 2 min.
CHILDREN (6 TO 12 YR): **PO** 25 to 50 mg q 6 to 8 hr (max 150 mg/day). **IM** 1.25 mg/kg qid (max 300 mg/day).

CHILDREN (2 TO 6 YR): **PO** Up to 12.5 to 25 mg q 6 to 8 hr (max 75 mg/day). **IM** 1.25 mg/kg qid (max 300 mg/day).

Interactions
Alcohol, CNS depressants: Enhances CNS depressant effects.
Aminoglycosides: May mask signs of aminoglycoside-related ototoxicity.
Anticholinergic drugs: Causes additive anticholinergic effects.
INCOMPATIBILITIES: Ammonium chloride, amobarbital, butorphanol, chlorpromazine, glycopyrrolate, heparin, hydrocortisone, hydroxyzine, midazolam, pentobarbital, phenobarbital, phenytoin, prednisolone, prochlorperazine, promethazine, tetracycline, theophylline, thiopental, trifluoperazine.

Lab Test Interferences May cause false elevation in serum theophylline levels.

Adverse Reactions
CV: Palpitations; hypotension; tachycardia.
CNS: Sedation; hallucinations; delirium; drowsiness; confusion, nervousness; restlessness; headache; insomnia; tingling, heaviness and weakness of hands; vertigo; dizziness; lassitude; excitation.
DERM: Fixed drug eruption; photosensitivity.
EENT: Diminished night vision; decreased color discrimination; exacerbation of narrow-angle glaucoma; blurred vision; diplopia; nasal stuffiness; dryness of nose and throat.
GI: Nausea; vomiting; diarrhea; GI distress; constipation; anorexia; dry mouth.
GU: Prostatic enlargement; difficult or painful urination.
RESP: Tightness of chest; wheezing; thickening of bronchial secretions.
OTHER: Anaphylaxis.

Precautions
Pregnancy: Category B.
Lactation: Excreted in breast milk.
Children: Safety and efficacy in children younger than 2 yr not established.
Hypersensitivity: Previous reactions to diphenhydramine.
Special risk patients: Use caution in patients with asthma, prostatic hypertrophy, narrow-angle glaucoma, stenosing peptic ulcer, cardiac arrhythmias.

Overdosage: Signs and Symptoms
Drowsiness, hallucinations, convulsions, coma, respiratory depression.

PATIENT CARE CONSIDERATIONS
Administration/Storage
- Administer with food or milk to minimize nausea or GI distress.
- When administering drug IM, use Z-track method to avoid SC irritation.
- When administering drug IV, confirm correct catheter or needle placement. Note that this drug should never be given intra-arterially.

Assessment/Interventions
- Obtain patient history, including drug history and any known allergies.
- Assess drug history for concomitant use of other CNS depressants, alcohol and nonprescription CNS depressants, which could have additive effect.
- Take safety precautions if drowsiness or dizziness occurs.
- Assess patient's nutritional status, weigh patient daily and monitor I&O if drug is given to stop or prevent nausea and vomiting.
- If a paradoxical effect occurs (eg, insomnia, CNS stimulation), notify health care provider.
- If visual or auditory disturbances occur (eg, blurred vision/tinnitus, hearing loss), notify the health care provider.

Patient/Family Education
- Advise patient to take medication 30 to 60 min before activity that may produce nausea or motion sickness.
- Instruct patient to report these symptoms to health care provider: drowsiness, nervousness, dry mouth, insomnia, constipation, blurred vision.
- If dimenhydrinate is being given as antiemetic, instruct patient to report nausea and vomiting to the health care provider.
- Instruct patient to take sips of water frequently, suck on ice chips or sugarless hard candy, or chew sugarless gum if dry mouth occurs and to relieve constipation with increased fiber in diet and good hydration.
- Caution patient to avoid intake of alcoholic beverages or other CNS depressants.
- Advise patient that drug may cause drowsiness and to use caution while driving or performing other tasks requiring mental alertness.

Dinoprostone (PGE2; Prostaglandin E2)

(DIE-no-PROSTE-ohn)

Class Prostaglandin/Cervical ripening/Abortifacient

How Supplied
Cervidil Vaginal insert 10 mg ♦ *Prepidil* Gel 0.5 mg ♦ *Prostin E2* Vaginal suppository 20 mg

Action
PHARMACOLOGY: Stimulates gravid uterus to contract; also stimulates smooth muscle of GI tract.

PHARMACOKINETICS/DYNAMICS:

Absorption: T_{max} is 0.5 to 0.75 hr (gel). C_{max} approximately 484 pg/mL (gel).

Metabolism: Rapidly metabolized in the local tissue. Systemically absorbed drug is extensively metabolized in the lungs, liver, and kidney.

Excretion: $t_{½}$ is 2.5 to 5 min. Metabolites excreted in the urine.

Indications
Gel: Cervical ripening in pregnant women at or near term with need for labor induction.
Vaginal suppositories: Termination of pregnancy from 12 to 20 wk.

Contraindications Hypersensitivity to prostaglandins; patients in whom oxytocic drugs are contraindicated or when prolonged contractions of uterus are considered inappropriate; ruptured membranes; placenta previa; unexplained vaginal bleeding during current pregnancy; when vaginal delivery is not indicated; acute pelvic inflammatory disease; active cardiac, pulmonary, renal or hepatic disease.

Route/Dosage
Cervical Ripening
ADULTS: **Intravaginal Gel** 0.5 mg (contents of one syringe); may repeat dose 6 hr later if necessary (max dose 1.5 mg (3 syringes/24 hr). **Intravaginal Insert** 10 mg (1 insert). Releases approximately 0.3 mg/hr over 12 hr. Remove insert upon onset of active labor or 12 hr after insertion.

Termination of Pregnancy
ADULTS: **Intravaginal** 1 suppository (20 mg) high into vagina. Repeat at 3 to 5 hr intervals until abortion occurs. Do not give continuously for longer than 2 days.

Interactions
Oxytocic agents: May augment effect of other oxytocic agents; avoid concomitant use.

Lab Test Interferences None well documented.

Adverse Reactions
CV: Transient fall in BP; syncope; dizziness; arrhythmias.
CNS: Headache; flushing; anxiety; tension; hot flashes; paresthesia; weakness.
EENT: Blurred vision; eye pain.
GI: Anorexia; nausea; vomiting; diarrhea.
GU: Uterine contractile abnormality; endometritis; uterine rupture; uterine pain; amnionitis; premature rupture of membranes; vaginal pain; warm feeling in vagina.
RESP: Bronchospasm; coughing; dyspnea; wheezing.
OTHER: Back pain; muscular cramps; fever; chills; joint inflammation; breast tenderness; diaphoresis; rash; leg cramps; dehydration. Fetal effects: Fetal heart rate abnormalities; bradycardia; deceleration; sepsis; depression (1 min Apgar less than 7); acidosis.

> **WARNING:**
> *Experienced physician/equipped facility:*
> Use only with strict adherence to recommended dosages by medically trained personnel that can provide immediate intensive care in acute surgical facilities.

Precautions
Pregnancy: Category C. Contraindicated if fetus in utero has reached viability stage except when cervical ripening is indicated.
Lactation: Undetermined.
Special risk patients: Use with caution in patients with asthma, glaucoma, or raised IOP, hypotension or hypertension, cardiovascular or renal or hepatic dysfunction, anemia, jaundice, diabetes, epilepsy, compromised uterus, infected endocervical lesions; acute vaginitis.

Overdosage: Signs and Symptoms
Uterine hypercontractility, uterine hypertonus.

PATIENT CARE CONSIDERATIONS
Administration/Storage
- Store suppository and insert in freezer. Store gel in refrigerator. Bring both to room temperature just prior to use, do not use external sources of heat (eg, hot water bath, microwave oven) to decrease warming time.
- Carefully examine vagina to determine degree of effacement and appropriate length of endocervical catheter to be used for application of gel (10 mm if 50% effaced, 20 mm if no effacement).
- Patient should be in dorsal position for administration and remain supine for 15 to 30 min after administration.
- Prevent contact of this drug with skin. Use of latex gloves followed by thorough hand wash-

ing with soap and water are recommended.
- Use drug in hospital setting only.

Assessment/Interventions
- Obtain patient history, including drug history and any known allergies.
- Perform physical assessment to determine baseline vital signs and fetopelvic relationships.
- Perform careful uterine and fetal monitoring throughout use of dinoprostone.
- Wait at least 6 to 12 hr after administration of gel before using IV oxytocin, a dosing interval of at least 30 mins is recommended after removal of insert.
- Monitor patient closely for adverse reactions including nausea, vomiting, or diarrhea.
- Monitor vital signs frequently during administration, noting especially any increase in temperature and hypertension or hypotension.
- Monitor for hypersensitivity reactions such as bronchospasms, cardiac arrhythmias or seizures. Notify health care provider should any of these symptoms occur.

Patient/Family Education
- Inform patient of expected action and possible adverse reactions with drug.
- Inform patient that uterine contractions are expected and that if pain from contractions becomes severe, health care provider will be notified to obtain order for analgesic.
- Instruct patient to report these symptoms to nurse immediately: nausea, vomiting, difficulty breathing, chest pain, headache.

Diphenhydramine Hydrochloride

(die-fen-HIGH-druh-meen HIGH-droe-KLOR-ide)

Class Antihistamine/Ethanolamine

How Supplied
40 Winks Tablets 50 mg ♦ *Allergy Medication* Liquid 12.5 mg/5 mL ♦ *AllerMax* Tablets 50 mg ♦ *AllerMax Allergy and Cough Formula* Liquid 6.25 mg/5 mL ♦ *Banophen* Capsules 25 mg ♦ *Benadryl* Injection 50 mg/mL ♦ *Benadryl Allergy* Capsules, soft-gels 25 mg, Tablets 25 mg, Tablets, chewable 12.5 mg, Liquid 12.5 mg/5 mL ♦ *Benadryl Allergy Ultratabs* Tablets 25 mg ♦ *Benadryl Dye Free* Liquid 12.5 mg/5 mL ♦ *Benadryl Dye Free Allergy Liqui Gels* Capsules, soft gels 25 mg ♦ *Bydramine Cough* Syrup 12.5 mg/5 mL ♦ *Compoz Gel Caps* Capsules 25 mg ♦ *Compoz Nighttime Sleep Aid* Tablets 50 mg ♦ *Diphen AF* Liquid 6.25 mg/5 mL ♦ *Diphen Cough* Syrup 12.5 mg/5 mL ♦ *Diphenhist* Solution 12.5 mg/5 mL ♦ *Diphenhist Captabs* Tablets 25 mg ♦ *Dormin* Tablets 25 mg, Capsules 25 mg ♦ *Genahist* Liquid 12.5 mg/5 mL ♦ *Hyrexin-50* Injection 50 mg/mL ♦ *Maximum Strength Nytol* Tablets 50 mg ♦ *Maximum Strength Sleepinal Capsules and Soft Gels* Capsules 50 mg ♦ *Maximum Strength Unisom SleepGels* Capsules 50 mg/mL ♦ *Midol PM* Tablets 50 mg ♦ *Miles Nervine* Tablets 25 mg ♦ *Nighttime Sleep Aid* Tablets 50 mg ♦ *Nytol* Tablets 25 mg ♦ *Scot-Tussin Allergy DM* Liquid 12.5 mg/5 mL ♦ *Siladryl* Elixir 12.5 mg/5 mL ♦ *Silphen DM* Syrup 10 mg/5 mL ♦ *Sleep-Eze 3* Tablets 25 mg ♦ *Sleepwell 2-nite* Tablets 25 mg ♦ *Snoozefast* Tablets 50 mg ♦ *Sominex* Tablets 25 mg, Tablets 50 mg ♦ *Sylphen Cough* Syrup 12.5 mg/5 mL ♦ *Tusstat* Syrup 12.5 mg/5 mL ♦ *Twilite* Tablets 50 mg ♦ *Uni-Bent Cough* Syrup 12.5 mg/5 mL*Wehdryl*

🌺 *Allerdryl* ♦ *Allernix* ♦ *Nytol Extra Strength* ♦ *PMS-Diphenhydramine* ♦ *Simply Sleep* ♦ *Unisom Extra Strength* ♦ *Unisom Extra Strength Sleepgels*

Action

PHARMACOLOGY: Competitively antagonizes histamine at H_1 receptor sites.

PHARMACOKINETICS/DYNAMICS:
Absorption: T_{max} is 1 to 4 hr (oral).

Distribution: Widely distributed, including the CNS. Excreted in breast milk. 98% to 99% protein bound.

Metabolism: Metabolized in the liver.

Excretion: A portion of the drug excreted unchanged in the urine. $t_{1/2}$ is 1 to 4 hr.

Onset: Rapid onset (IV or IM).

Duration: 6 to 8 hr.

Indications Symptomatic relief of perennial and seasonal allergic rhinitis, vasomotor rhinitis and allergic conjunctivitis; temporary relief of runny nose and sneezing caused by common cold; relief of allergic and nonallergic pruritic symptoms; treatment of urticaria and angioedema; amelioration of allergic reactions to blood or plasma; adjunct to epinephrine and other standard measures in anaphylaxis; relief of uncomplicated allergic conditions of immediate type when oral therapy is impossible or contraindicated (parenteral form); treatment and prophylactic treatment of motion sickness; nighttime sleep aid; management of parkinsonism (including drug-induced) in elderly who are intolerant of more potent agents, in mild cases in other age groups and in combination with centrally acting anticholinergics; control of cough from colds or allergy (syrup formulations).

Contraindications Hypersensitivity to antihistamines; narrow-angle glaucoma; stenosing peptic ulcer; symptomatic prostatic hypertrophy;

asthmatic attack; bladder neck obstruction; pyloroduodenal obstruction; MAOI therapy; history of sleep apnea; use in newborn or premature infants and in nursing women.

Route/Dosage

Hypersensitivity Reactions, Type 1/Antiparkinsonism/Motion Sickness
ADULTS: **PO** 25 to 50 mg q 4 to 6 hr (max, 300 mg/day). **IV/IM** 10 to 100 mg (rate not exceeding 25 mg/min or deep IM; max, 400 mg/day).
CHILDREN (6 TO UNDER 12 YR): **PO** 12.5 to 25 mg q 4 to 6 hr (max, 150 mg). **IV/IM** 5 mg/kg/day or 150 mg/m^2/day (max, 300 mg divided into 4 doses at a rate not exceeding 25 mg/min or deep IM).

Nighttime Sleep Aid
ADULTS: **PO** 50 mg at bedtime.

Cough Suppressant (Syrup)
ADULTS: **PO** 25 mg q 4 hr (max, 150 mg/24 hr).
CHILDREN (6 TO 12 YR): **PO** 12.5 mg q 4 hr (max, 75 mg/24 hr).
CHILDREN (2 TO 6 YR): **PO** 6.25 mg q 4 hr (max, 25 mg/24 hr).

Interactions

Alcohol, CNS depressants: May cause additive CNS depression.
MAOIs: May increase anticholinergic effects.
INCOMPATIBILITIES: Injectable form is incompatible with dexamethasone sodium phosphate, furosemide, iodipamide meglumine, parenteral barbiturates, and phenytoin.

Lab Test Interferences

Skin tests: Antihistamines may prevent or diminish otherwise positive reaction to dermal reactivity indicators.

Adverse Reactions

CV: Orthostatic hypotension; palpitations; bradycardia; tachycardia; reflex tachycardia; extrasystoles; faintness.
CNS: Drowsiness (often transient); sedation; dizziness; faintness; disturbed coordination.
EENT: Nasal stuffiness; dry mouth, nose and throat; sore throat.
GI: Epigastric distress; nausea; vomiting; diarrhea; constipation; change in bowel habits.
HEMA: Hemolytic anemia; thrombocytopenia; agranulocytosis.
METAB: Increased appetite, weight gain.
RESP: Thickening of bronchial secretions; chest tightness; wheezing; respiratory depression.
OTHER: Hypersensitivity reactions; photosensitivity.

Precautions

Pregnancy: Category B.
Lactation: Excreted in breast milk.
Children: Contraindicated in newborn and premature infants. Overdosage may cause hallucinations, convulsions, and death. Antihistamines may diminish mental alertness. In young children drug may produce paradoxical excitation. Use with caution in children younger than 2 yr.
Elderly: Greater risk of dizziness, excessive sedation, syncope, toxic confusional states, and hypotension in patients older than 60 yr. Dosage reduction may be required.
Hypersensitivity: May occur. Have epinephrine 1:1000 immediately available.
Hepatic function impairment: Use with caution in patients with cirrhosis or other liver diseases.
Special risk patients: Use with caution in patients predisposed to urinary retention, prostatic hypertrophy, history of bronchial asthma, increased intraocular pressure, hyperthyroidism, cardiovascular disease, or hypertension.
Sulfite sensitivity: Some diphenhydramine products may contain sulfites as preservatives and aspartame as sweetener. Avoid in sulfite-allergic patients and in patients with phenylketonuria, respectively.
Respiratory disease: Generally not recommended to treat lower respiratory tract symptoms including asthma.

Overdosage: Signs and Symptoms

Circulatory collapse; cardiac arrest; respiratory depression or arrest; toxic psychosis; coma; stupor; seizures; ataxia; anxiety; incoherence; hyperactivity; combativeness; anhidrosis; fever; hot, dry, or flushed skin; dry mucous membranes; dysphagia; decreased bowel sounds; dilated and sluggish pupils.

PATIENT CARE CONSIDERATIONS

Administration/Storage

♦ If patient is prone to excessive salivation (eg, postencephalitic patients), administer drug after meals. If mouth dries excessively, administer drug before meals.
♦ Syrup formulations are used only for control of cough.
♦ If drug is prescribed for motion sickness, administer first dose 30 min prior to exposure to motion.
♦ Give IM injection deep in muscle.
♦ Do not administer drug for at least 2 days before skin allergy testing.
♦ Store in tightly closed containers at room temperature.
♦ Store injection formulation in light-resistant container and protect from light.

Assessment/Interventions

♦ Obtain patient history, including drug history and any known allergies. Be alert for conditions that may place patient at greater risk for

adverse effects (eg, bronchial asthma, glaucoma, prostatic hypertrophy).
- Be prepared to institute supportive treatment (eg, advanced life support) in event of severe adverse reaction or overdose.
- Observe patient for adverse reactions to medication such as dry mouth, headaches, disorientation, drowsiness, tachycardia, shortness of breath, nausea, skin rash, urinary retention, constipation, or increase in BP.
- If administering medication to children or elderly, be alert to fact that they are more likely to experience side effects and paradoxical reactions such as excitement, irritability, sleeplessness.
- Explain that drowsiness may occur at first but will lessen or disappear during long-term therapy.

Patient/Family Education
- Instruct patient not to discontinue long-term therapy without consulting health care provider.
- Warn patient using topical medication to avoid excessive application to skin eruptions.
- Instruct patient to report these symptoms to health care provider: excessive drowsiness or dry mouth, GI upset, constipation, blurred vision, rash, hives, difficulty breathing, difficulty urinating, confusion, fainting, irregular heart rate.
- Encourage patient to take sips of water frequently, suck on ice chips or sugarless hard candy, or chew sugarless gum if dry mouth occurs.
- Instruct patient to avoid intake of alcoholic beverages or other CNS depressants.
- Advise patient that drug may cause drowsiness and to use caution while driving or performing other tasks requiring mental alertness.

Diphenoxylate Hydrochloride/Atropine Sulfate

(die-fen-OX-ih-late HIGH-droe-KLOR-ide/ AT-troe-peen SULL-fate)

Class Antidiarrheal

How Supplied
Logen Tablets 2.5 mg diphenoxylate hydrochloride and 0.025 mg atropine sulfate ♦ *Lomanate* Liquid 2.5 mg diphenoxylate hydrochloride and 0.025 mg atropine sulfate per 5 mL ♦ *Lomotil* Liquid 2.5 mg diphenoxylate hydrochloride and 0.025 mg atropine sulfate per 5 mL, Tablets 2.5 mg diphenoxylate hydrochloride and 0.025 mg atropine sulfate ♦ *Lonox* Tablets 2.5 mg diphenoxylate hydrochloride and 0.025 mg atropine sulfate

Action
PHARMACOLOGY: Diphenoxylate, related to meperidine, decreases motility of GI tract. Atropine discourages deliberate overdosage of diphenoxylate.

Indications Adjunctive therapy in treatment of diarrhea.

Contraindications Obstructive jaundice; diarrhea associated with pseudomembranous enterocolitis or enterotoxin-producing bacteria; narrow-angle glaucoma; use in children younger than 2 yr.

Route/Dosage
ADULTS: Initial dose: PO 5 mg qid. Individualize dose.
CHILDREN 2 TO 12 YR: PO 0.3 to 0.4 mg/kg/day in 4 divided doses.

Interactions
Alcohol, barbiturates, CNS depressants, tranquilizers: May increase depressant action
MAOIs: May precipitate hypertensive crisis.

Lab Test Interferences None well documented.

Adverse Reactions
CV: Tachycardia.
CNS: Dizziness; drowsiness; sedation; headache; malaise; lethargy; restlessness; euphoria; depression; numbness of extremities; confusion.
DERM: Pruritus; angioneurotic edema; urticaria; dry skin and mucous membranes; flushing.
GI: Dry mouth; anorexia; nausea; vomiting; abdominal discomfort; paralytic ileus; toxic megacolon; pancreatitis; constipation.
GU: Urinary retention.
OTHER: Swelling of gums; anaphylaxis; hyperthermia.

Precautions
Pregnancy: Category B.
Lactation: Excreted in breast milk.
Children: Contraindicated in children younger than 2 yr. Greater risk of atropinism, especially with Down syndrome.
Hepatic function impairment: Use with extreme caution; may precipitate hepatic coma.
Diarrhea: Do not give for diarrhea associated with organisms that penetrate the intestinal mucosa (ie, Salmonella, Shigella), acute Crohn disease or pseudomembranous colitis caused by antibiotic therapy. Notify health care provider and discontinue therapy for abdominal distention or other untoward symptoms.
Fluid/electrolyte imbalance: Dehydration may contribute to adverse effects, especially in young

children. If dehydration or electrolyte imbalance occurs, may need to discontinue therapy until condition is corrected.

Overdosage: Signs and Symptoms
Dry skin and mucous membranes, mydriasis, restlessness, flushing, hyperthermia, tachycardia, lethargy, coma, nystagmus, pinpoint pupils, respiratory depression.

PATIENT CARE CONSIDERATIONS
Administration/Storage
- May administer drug with food if GI irritation occurs.
- Administer liquid form to children 2 to 12 yr.
- Tablets may be crushed and administered with fluid.
- Store in tightly closed, light-resistant container at room temperature.

Assessment/Interventions
- Obtain patient history, including drug history and any known allergies. Note if patient is currently using MAOIs (discontinuation may be necessary).
- Assess frequency and consistency of stools before and throughout therapy.
- Assess skin turgor and monitor fluid and electrolyte status during therapy.
- If signs of dehydration occur (eg, poor skin turgor, decreased urine output, orthostatic hypotension, pulse changes, weight loss), notify health care provider.
- If signs and symptoms of toxic megacolon occur (eg, abdominal pain, distention), notify health care provider.

Patient/Family Education
- Advise patient to continue taking drug until diarrhea has stopped for 24 to 36 hr. Discontinuing medication earlier may result in relapse or return of diarrhea.
- Instruct patient to notify health care provider if fever and palpitations occur or when diarrhea persists or becomes malodorous or bloody.
- Tell patient to take sips of water frequently, suck on ice chips or sugarless hard candy, or chew sugarless gum if dry mouth occurs.
- Instruct patient to avoid intake of alcoholic beverages or other CNS depressants.
- Advise patient that drug may cause drowsiness and to use caution while driving or performing other tasks requiring mental alertness.

Diphtheria and Tetanus Toxoids and Acellular Pertussis Adsorbed, Hepatitis B (Recombinant) and Inactivated Poliovirus Vaccine Combined

(diff-THEER-ee-uh and TET-ah-nus TOX-oyds and ay-SELL-you-luhr per-TUSS-iss absorbed, hep-uh-TIGHT-iss B (recombinant) and Inactivated poe-lee-oh-VYE-russ vaccine combined)

Class Vaccine, inactivated

How Supplied
Pediarix Injection 25 Lf diphtheria toxoid, 10 Lf tetanus toxoid, 25 mcg inactivated pertussis toxin (PT), 25 mcg filamentous hemagglutinin (FHA), 8 mcg pertactin, 10 mcg hepatitis B surface antigen (HBsAg), 40 D-antigen units (DU) Type 1 poliovirus, 8 DU Type 2 poliovirus, and 32 DU Type 3 poliovirus per 0.5 mL

Action
PHARMACOLOGY: Diphtheria and tetanus toxoids induce antibodies against toxins made by *Corynebacterium diphtheriae* and *Clostridium tetani*; pertussis vaccine protects against *Bordetella pertussis*; hepatitis B vaccine induces specific antibodies against hepatitis B virus; poliovirus vaccine induces protective antipoliovirus antibodies, reducing pharyngeal excretion of poliovirus types 1, 2, and 3.

Indications Active immunization against diphtheria, tetanus, pertussis, all known types of hepatitis B virus and poliomyelitis (caused by types 1, 2, and 3).

Contraindications Use of this vaccine after a serious allergic reaction temporally associated with a previous dose of the vaccine or with any components of this vaccine; encephalopathy (eg, coma, decreased level of consciousness, prolonged seizures) within 7 days of administration of a previous dose of a pertussis-containing vaccine that is not attributable to another identifiable cause; progressive neurologic disorder (including infantile spasms, uncontrolled epilepsy or progressive encephalopathy) until a treatment regimen has been established and the condition has stabilized; hypersensitivity to any component of the vaccine (including yeast, neomycin, and polymyxin B).

Route/Dosage
Primary immunization
CHILDREN (AT LEAST 6 WK): **IM** 3 doses of 0.5 mL at 6- to 8-wk intervals (preferably 8 wk); customary age for the first dose is 2 months.

Children Previously Vaccinated with Hepatitis B Vaccine
CHILDREN (BORN OF HBsAg-NEGATIVE MOTHERS AND WHO HAVE RECEIVED A DOSE OF HEPATITIS B AT OR SHORTLY AFTER BIRTH): **IM** 3 doses of 0.5 mL according to the recommended schedule.

Children Previously Vaccinated with Infanrix
CHILDREN: **IM** *Pediarix* may be used to complete the first 3 doses of the DTaP series in infants who have received 1 or 2 doses of *Infanrix* and also are scheduled to receive the other vaccine components of *Pediarix*.

Children Previously Vaccinated with Inactivated Poliovirus Vaccine (IPV)
CHILDREN: **IM** *Pediarix* may be used to complete the first 3 doses of the IPV series in infants who have received 1 or 2 doses of IVP and who are also scheduled to receive the other vaccine components of *Pediarix*.

Interchangeability of Pediarix and Licensed DTaP, IPV, or Recombinant Hepatitis B Vaccines
It is recommended that *Pediarix* be given for all 3 doses because data are limited regarding the safety and efficacy of using acellular pertussis vaccines from different manufacturers for successive doses of the pertussis vaccination series. Because of a lack of data, *Pediarix* is not recommended for completion of a DTaP vaccination series initiated with a DTaP vaccine from a different manufacturer. However, *Pediarix* may be used to complete hepatitis B vaccination series initiated with a licensed hepatitis B (recombinant) vaccine from a different manufacturer and may be used complete the first 3 doses of the IPV vaccination series initiated with IPV from a different manufacturer.

Additional Dosing Information
If any recommended dose of pertussis vaccine cannot be given, DT (for pediatric use), hepatitis B (recombinant) and IPV should be given as needed to complete the series. Children who have received a 3-dose primary series of *Pediarix* should be given a fourth dose of IPV at 4 to 6 yr of age and a fourth dose DTaP vaccine at 15 to 18 mo of age.

Interactions
Immunosuppressive agents (large amounts of corticosteroids, antimetabolites, alkylating agents, cytotoxic agents): Children may not respond optimally to active immunization.
Other vaccines: Do not mix other vaccine in the same syringe or vial.

Lab Test Interferences
None well documented.

Adverse Reactions
CV: Cyanosis; edema; pallor.
CNS: Seizure (including febrile seizure, infantile spasms); sleeping more than usual; convulsive disorder; demyelinating diseases of the CNS; peripheral and cranial mononeuropathy; lethargy; convulsions; encephalopathy; headache; hypotension; hypotonic-hyporesponsive episode; somnolence; crying; irritability.
DERM: Alopecia; erythema; erythema multiforme; petechiae; pruritus; rash; urticaria.
EENT: Ear pain.
GI: Loss of appetite; abdominal pain; anorexia; diarrhea; intussusception; nausea; vomiting.
HEMA: Idiopathic thrombocytopenia purpura; lymphadenopathy; thrombocytopenia.
HEPA: Jaundice; LFT abnormalities.
RESP: Respiratory tract infection.
OTHER: Injection site reactions (eg, pain, redness or swelling); fussiness/restlessness; fever; swelling; congenital immunodeficiency with sepsis; sudden infant death (causal relationship not established); anaphylactic reaction (including, hives, swelling of the mouth, difficulty breathing, hypotension, or shock); arthus-type hypersensitivity reactions (characterized by severe local reactions); asthenia; malaise; angioedema; cellulitis; arthralgia; limb swelling.

Precautions
Pregnancy: Category C.
Children: Safety and efficacy not established in children under 6 wk. *Pediarix* is not recommended for people 7 yr or older.
Elderly: Not recommended for use in the adult population.
Special risk patients: Use with caution and consider the benefits and risks in the following conditions: temperature of 40.5°C (105°F) within 48 hr not due to an identifiable cause; collapse or shock-like state within 48 hr; persistent, inconsolable crying lasting at least 3 hr, occurring with 48 hr; seizures with or without fever occurring within 3 days.
Bleeding disorders: Use with caution in children with bleeding disorders (eg, hemophilia or thrombocytopenia) with steps taken to avoid the risk of hematoma following the injection.

PATIENT CARE CONSIDERATIONS
Administration/Storage
- For IM injection only. Not for IV, SC, or intradermal administration.
- Do not administer to infants less than 6 wk or individuals 7 yr or older.
- Vaccination regimen consists of 3 doses, at 6- to 8-wk intervals (preferably 8 wk). First dose is usually administered at 2 mo but can be given as young as 6 wk.
- Interruption of recommended schedule with a delay between doses does not interfere with development of final immunity. There is no need to start the series over again.
- Use vaccine as supplied; no dilution or reconstitution is necessary.
- Shake vial or syringe vigorously immediately prior to use to obtain a uniform suspension. Do not use if vaccine cannot be resuspended.
- Examine vial or syringe after shaking. Suspension should be homogeneous and white. Do not use if particulate matter or discoloration are noted of if vaccine cannot be resuspended.
- Administer immediately after drawing vaccine into syringe.
- Administer IM in anterolateral thigh in infants or the deltoid muscle of the upper arm in toddlers and young children. Avoid injection into gluteal area or areas where there may be a major nerve trunk or blood vessel. Gluteal injections may result in a suboptimal hepatitis B immune response.
- Use separate syringes and different sites for concomitant administration of other vaccines.
- Always record manufacturer's name and vaccine lot number in patient's permanent medical record file along with date of administration, and name and title of person administering vaccine.
- Store vials in refrigerator (36° to 46°F). Do not freeze. Discard if vaccine has been frozen.

Assessment/Interventions
- Obtain patient history, including drug history and any known allergies. Note history of: previous serious reaction to this vaccine or with any component of this vaccine; progressive neurologic disorder; encephalopathy within 7 days of administration of previous dose of pertussis-containing vaccine; latex sensitivity; anticoagulant therapy; bleeding disorder; thrombocytopenia.
- Check patient's immunization history to verify that administration regimen is being followed.
- Consider delaying immunization during course of moderate or severe acute febrile illness.
- Monitor patient for signs of anaphylaxis or severe allergic reaction. Discontinue therapy and immediately notify health care provider if noted. Be prepared to treat appropriately.
- When child returns for next dose in series, question child's parent or guardian about serious side effects with previous dose. If any side effects that would contraindicate additional pertussis vaccine are noted, inform child's health care provider. Continue immunization series with DT, hepatitis B and IPV vaccines to complete series.

Patient/Family Education
- Explain name, action, and potential side effects of vaccine.
- Provide and review Vaccine Information Sheet prior to immunization.
- Review immunization schedule and advise parent or guardian that entire series must be completed to provide maximum benefit.
- Provide parent or guardian with immunization history record.
- Advise parent or guardian to use OTC analgesics (eg, acetaminophen or ibuprofen) for fever, pain, or discomfort at injection site.
- Advise parent or guardian to notify health care provider if bothersome side effects last more than 24 hr.

Diphtheria/Tetanus Toxoids/Acellular Pertussis Vaccine (DTaP)

(diff-THEER-ee-uh/TET-ah-nus toxoids/ay-SELL-you-luhr per-TUSS-iss vaccine)

Class Vaccine, inactivated bacteria

How Supplied
Daptacel Injection 15 Lf diphtheria toxoid, 5 Lf tetanus toxoid, 10 mcg pertussis toxoid, 5 mcg FHA, 3 mcg pertactin, 5 mcg fimbriae types 2 and 3 per 0.5 mL ♦ *Infanrix* Injection 25 Lf units diphtheria, 10 Lf units tetanus toxoid, 25 mcg pertussis toxin, 25 mcg FHA, 8 mcg pertactin per 0.5 mL ♦ *Tripedia* Injection 6.7 Lf units diphtheria toxoid, 5 Lf units tetanus toxoid, 46.8 mcg pertussis antigens (approximately 23.4 mcg each of inactivated pertussis toxin and FHA) per 0.5 mL

Action
PHARMACOLOGY: Diphtheria and tetanus toxoids induce antibodies against toxins made by *Corynebacterium diphtheriae* and *Clostridium tetani*. Pertussis vaccine protects against *Bordetella pertussis*.

Indications Active immunization against diphtheria, tetanus, and pertussis in infants and children 6 wk through 6 yr of age (prior to seventh birthday).

Contraindications Adults and children 7 yr and older; encephalopathy within 7 days of previous administration of DTP or DTaP that is not attributable to another cause; progressive neurologic disorders (eg, infantile spasms, uncontrolled epilepsy, progressive encephalopathy) in addition, pertussis vaccine should not be administered to individuals with these conditions until a treatment regimen has been established and condition has stabilized; if contraindication to pertussis-vaccine component occurs, substitute diphtheria and tetanus toxoids for pediatric use (DT) for each remaining doses; defer elective immunization procedures during outbreak of poliomyelitis because of risk of provoking paralysis; hypersensitivity to any component of the vaccine; history of serious allergic reaction temporarily associated with a previous dose of vaccine or any component of the vaccine.

Route/Dosage
It is recommended that the same brand of DTaP be given for all doses in the immunization series because no data exist on the interchangeability of DTaP vaccines.

DAPTACEL

CHILDREN: **IM** Immunization is 4 doses of 0.5 mL at 2, 4, and 6 mo of age, at intervals of 6 to 8 wk and at 17 to 20 mo of age. The interval between the third and fourth dose should be at least 6 mo.

INFANRIX

CHILDREN: **IM** Primary immunization series is 3 doses at 0.5 mL at 4- to 8-wk intervals (preferably 8 wk). Customarily, the first dose is 2 mo of age (but may be given at 6 wk of age). A fourth dose (booster immunization) is recommended at 15 to 20 mo of age (interval between third and fourth dose at least 6 mo). A fifth dose is recommended at 4 to 6 yr of age in those who received all 4 doses by the fourth birthday. If the fourth dose is given after the fourth birthday, a fifth dose prior to school entry is not necessary.

TRIPEDIA

CHILDREN: **IM** Primary immunization series is 3 doses of 0.5 mL at 4- to 8-wk intervals. A fourth dose is recommended at 15 to 20 mo of age (interval between third and fourth dose at least 6 mo). A fifth dose is recommended at 4 to 6 yr of age, preferably prior to school entry. If the fourth dose is given after the fourth birthday, a fifth dose prior to school entry is not necessary.

Interactions
Anticoagulants: Give DTaP with caution to patients on anticoagulant therapy.
Immunosuppressants: May reduce vaccine's effectiveness.
Influenza vaccine: To attribute causality of adverse reactions, do not give influenza vaccine within 3 days of pertussis vaccination.

Lab Test Interferences None well documented.

Adverse Reactions
CNS: Drowsiness; brachial neuritis; Guillain-Barré syndrome; neurological complications (including cochlear lesions, brachial plexus neuropathies, paralysis of radial nerve, paralysis of recurrent nerve, accommodation paresis, EEG disturbances with encephalopathy); convulsions, hypotonia, hypotonic-hyporesponsive episode, irritability, somnolence (postmarketing).
DERM: Erythema, pruritus, rash, urticaria (postmarketing).
EENT: Ear pain (postmarketing).
GI: Anorexia; vomiting; diarrhea, intussusception (postmarketing).
HEMA/LYMPH: Idiopathic thrombocytopenic purpura, lymphadenopathy, thrombocytopenia (postmarketing).
HYPERSEN: Anaphylactic reactions; arthus-type hypersensitivity.
LOCAL: Redness; swelling; pain.
RESP: Respiratory tract infection (postmarketing).
OTHER: Fever; crying (for 3 hr or more); irritability; fussiness; cellulitis, cyanosis, injection site reactions, limb swelling, sudden infant death (postmarketing).

Precautions
Pregnancy: Category C.
Lactation: Undetermined.
Children: Contraindicated for children less than 6 wk or 7 yr or older.
Special risk patients: If any of the following occurs in temporal relation with receipt of either whole-cell pertussis DTP or DTaP, carefully consider decision to administer subsequent doses of vaccine containing pertussis component: temperature of at least 40.5°C (105°F) within 48 hr, not caused by another identifiable cause; collapse or shock-like state (hypotonic-hyporesponsive episode) within 48 hr; persistent inconsolable crying lasting at least 3 hr, occurring within 48 hr; or convulsions, with or without fever, occurring within 3 days. If the decision is made to withhold pertussis component, continue immunization with DT. If Guillain-Barré syndrome occurs within 6 wk of receipt of prior vaccine containing tetanus toxoid, base decision to give subsequent doses of DTaP or any vaccine containing tetanus toxoid on potential benefits versus risks.
Convulsions: When given whole-cell pertussis

DTP vaccine, infants and children with a history of convulsions in first-degree family members (parents, siblings) may have an increased risk of neurologic events compared with those without such histories.

Febrile illness or acute infection: Defer immunization during course of illness. Minor respiratory illness, such as mild upper respiratory tract infection, is usually not reason to defer immunization.

Immunodeficiency: Defer immunization, if possible, until immunocompetency is restored.

Latex sensitivity: Stoppers for *Daptacel* and *Tripedia* vials and tip cap and rubber plunger of *Infanrix* needleless prefilled syringes contain dry natural latex rubber that may cause allergic reactions in latex sensitive individuals.

Thrombocytopenia or coagulation disorder that would contraindicate IM injection: Give vaccine with caution.

PATIENT CARE CONSIDERATIONS
Administration/Storage

- For IM injection only. Not for IV, SC, or intradermal administration.
- Do not administer to infants younger than 6 wk or individuals 7 yr or older.
- Attempt to use the same brand of vaccine for the entire series. However, when this is not possible, use any DTaP vaccine to continue or complete the series.
- Interruption of recommended schedule with a delay between doses does not interfere with development of final immunity. There is no need to start the series over again.
- Use vaccine as supplied; no dilution or reconstitution is necessary. Do not mix with any other vaccine in the same vial or syringe.
- Shake vial or syringe vigorously immediately prior to use to obtain a uniform suspension. Rotate vial or syringe in palm to bring contents to room temperature.
- Examine vial or syringe after shaking. Suspension should be homogeneous and white. Do not use if particulate matter or discoloration are noted or if vaccine cannot be resuspended.
- Administer immediately after drawing vaccine into syringe from vial. Discard any vaccine remaining in the vial.
- Administer IM in anterolateral thigh in infants (younger than 1 yr) or the deltoid muscle of the upper arm (for older children). Avoid injection into gluteal area or areas where there may be a major nerve trunk or blood vessel.
- May administer vaccine in conjunction with injectable polio, *Haemophilus influenzae* type b, hepatitis B, varicella, and measles, mumps, pneumococcal conjugate, and rubella virus vaccines.
- Use separate syringes and different sites for coadministration of other vaccines.
- Always record manufacturer's name and vaccine lot number in patient's permanent medical record file along with date of administration and name and title of person administering vaccine.
- Store vials and syringes in refrigerator (36° to 46°F). Do not freeze. Discard if vaccine has been frozen.

Assessment/Interventions

- Obtain patient history, including drug history and any known allergies. Note history of seizure disorder or risk factors for seizures, family member with seizure disorder, latex sensitivity, immunosuppression, anticoagulant therapy, bleeding disorder, or thrombocytopenia.
- Review patient's medical history for any condition that would contraindicate use of DTaP: previous serious reaction to this vaccine or with any component of this vaccine; progressive neurologic disorder; encephalopathy within 7 days of administration of previous dose of pertussis-containing vaccine.
- Review patient's history to determine if any of the following occurred in a temporal relationship to any previous dose of pertussis-containing vaccine: temperature of at least 105°F within 48 hr; collapse or shock-like state within 48 hr; persistent inconsolable crying lasting at least 3 hr; convulsions, with or without fever, occurring within 3 days. If noted, carefully consider decision to administer subsequent doses of pertussis-containing vaccine.
- Check patient's immunization history to verify that administration regimen is being followed.
- Consider delaying immunization during course of moderate or severe illness with or without fever. Minor respiratory illness such as mild upper respiratory infection is not usually a reason to defer immunization.
- Monitor patient for signs of anaphylaxis or severe allergic reaction. Immediately notify health care provider if noted. Be prepared to treat appropriately.
- When child returns for next dose in series, question parent or guardian about serious side effects with previous dose. If any side effects that would contraindicate additional pertussis vaccine are noted, inform child's health care provider. Continue immunization series with DT to complete series.
- If any event listed in the Vaccine Injury

Table or other serious side effects occur, report them through the Vaccine Adverse Event Reporting System (VAERS) per organizational policy.

Patient/Family Education
- Explain name, action, and potential side effects of vaccine.
- Provide and review the *Vaccine Information Statements* prior to immunization.
- Review immunization schedule and advise parent or guardian that entire series must be completed to obtain max benefit.
- Provide parent or guardian with immunization history record and record this immunization.
- Advise parent or guardian of child with history of seizures, or family member with seizure disorder, that controlling fever after vaccination is very important. Advise parent or guardian to give the child an aspirin-free pain reliever (eg, acetaminophen or ibuprofen) when the shot is given and for the next 24 hr, following package instructions.
- Advise parent or guardian that the following problems occur frequently soon after vaccination but are generally mild: fever, redness, swelling, soreness, tenderness at injection site. Advise patient that these occur more commonly after the fourth and fifth dose.
- Advise parent or guardian that the following problems occur frequently within 1 to 3 days after vaccination but are generally mild: fussiness, tiredness, poor appetite, vomiting.
- Advise parent or guardian to use aspirin-free OTC analgesics (eg, acetaminophen, ibuprofen) for fever, pain, or discomfort at injection site.
- Instruct parent or guardian to immediately notify health care provider if: child develops fever of 105°F or more; faints or persistently cries for more than 3 hr within 48 hr of receiving vaccine; has a seizure, with or without fever, within 3 days of receiving vaccine.
- Instruct parent or guardian to immediately notify health care provider if change in mental alertness, unresponsiveness, or seizures occur within 7 days of receiving vaccination.

Dipivefrin Hydrochloride

(die-PIHV-eh-FRIN HIGH-droe-KLOR-ide)

Class Sympathomimetic

How Supplied
Propine Solution 0.1%

Action
PHARMACOLOGY: Dipivefrin is a prodrug of epinephrine and is converted to epinephrine in the eye by hydrolysis. It exerts its action by decreasing aqueous production and enhancing outflow facility.

PHARMACOKINETICS/DYNAMICS:
Absorption: Absorbed into the eye.
Metabolism: Metabolized by hydrolysis to epinephrine.
Onset: About 30 min.
Peak: Approximately 1 hr.

Indications Control of IOP in chronic open-angle glaucoma.

Contraindications Narrow-angle glaucoma; hypersensitivity to any component of the product.

Route/Dosage
ADULTS: **Ophthalmic** 1 gtt in affected eye(s) q 12 hr.

Interactions None well documented.

Lab Test Interferences None well documented.

Adverse Reactions
CV: Tachycardia; arrhythmias; hypertension.
CNS: Headache.
EENT: Burning, stinging (6%); follicular conjunctivitis; eye pain; mydriasis; blurry vision; eye pruritus.
OTHER: Allergy.

Precautions
Pregnancy: Category B.
Lactation: Undetermined.
Children: Safety and efficacy not established.
Aphakic patients: Macular edema occurred in up to 30% of aphakic patients treated with epinephrine.

PATIENT CARE CONSIDERATIONS

Administration/Storage
- For topical ophthalmic use only. Not for injection or oral use.
- Usual dose is 1 drop in affected eye(s) q 12 hr.
- Do not allow tip of container to touch any surface, the eyelids, or surrounding areas.
- If using other topical ophthalmic drugs, separate each medication by at least 5 min.
- Store at controlled room temperature (59° to 77°F). Keep container tightly closed and protected from light.

Assessment/Interventions
- Obtain patient history, including drug history and any known allergies. Note narrow angles or aphakia (absence of lens).
- Ensure that IOPs are measured and docu-

mented in the patient's record before starting therapy and periodically during therapy.
* Monitor patient for ocular (eg, redness, burning, stinging) and systemic reactions (eg, headaches). Inform health care provider if noted and significant.

Patient/Family Education
* Explain name, dose, action, and potential side effects of drug.
* Advise patient that usual dose is 1 drop in the affected eye(s) bid.
* Caution patient not to change the dose or discontinue therapy unless advised by health care provider.
* Teach patient proper technique for instilling eye drops: Wash hands; do not allow dropper to touch eye; tilt head back, look up; pull lower eyelid down; instill prescribed number of drops; close eye for 1 to 2 min and apply gentle pressure to bridge of nose for 3 to 5 min; do not rub eye.
* Advise patient that if more than 1 topical ophthalmic drug is being used to wait at least 5 min before instilling the second medication.
* Advise patient that if a dose is missed to skip that dose. Caution patient not to try to catch up on the missed dose by instilling more than 1 dose at a time.
* Inform patient that burning or stinging of the eye are the most common side effects and to contact health care provider if these occur and are bothersome.
* Advise patients who wear contact lenses to remove lenses before instilling this medicine and to wait at least 15 min after instilling eye drop before inserting lenses.
* Advise patient to contact eye doctor if eye or eyelid inflammation is noted and of any eye injury or eye surgery.
* Advise women to notify health care provider if pregnant, planning to become pregnant, or breastfeeding.
* Instruct patient not to take any prescription or OTC medications, dietary supplements, or herbal preparations unless advised by health care provider.
* Remind patient that eye examinations and measurement of IOP will be necessary while using this medication and to keep appointments.

Dipyridamole

(DIE-pih-RID-uh-mole)
Class Antiplatelet/Diagnostic agent

How Supplied
Persantine Tablets 25 mg, Tablets 50 mg, Tablets 75 mg ♦ *Dipyridamole* Injection 5 mg/mL

Action
PHARMACOLOGY: Lengthens abnormally shortened platelet survival time in a dose-dependent manner by inhibiting platelet aggregation in response to various stimuli, such as platelet activating factor, collagen, and adenosine diphosphate. Vasodilation may result from inhibition of adenosine uptake, which is an important mediator of coronary vasodilation.

PHARMACOKINETICS/DYNAMICS:

Absorption: Two minutes after a 4 min IV infusion, the mean serum level is 4.6 mcg/mL.

Distribution: Highly bound to plasma protein (99%). Vd is 1 to 2.5 L/kg.

Metabolism: Metabolized in the liver (conjugated as a glucuronide).

Excretion: Excreted in the bile. Average total body Cl is 2.3 to 3.5 mL/min/kg. The alpha t½ (initial decline following C_{max}) is about 40 min, while the beta t½ (terminal decline in plasma level) is approximately 10 hr (oral).

Triexponential: the t½ range is 3 to 13 min, 33 to 62 min, and 11.6 hr (IV).

Peak: The average time to C_{max} is about 75 min.

Indications Adjunct to coumarin anticoagulants in prevention of postoperative thromboembolic complication of cardiac valve replacement (oral). Alternative to exercise in thallium myocardial perfusion imaging for evaluating coronary artery disease in patients who cannot exercise adequately (IV).

Contraindications Standard considerations.

Route/Dosage

Adjunctive Use in Prophylaxis of Thromboembolism after Cardiac Valve Replacement
ADULTS AND CHILDREN 12 YR AND OLDER: **PO** 75 to 100 mg qid is recommended as an adjunct to the usual warfarin therapy.

Adjunct to Thallium Myocardial Perfusion Imaging
ADULTS: **IV** 0.142 mg/kg/min (0.57 mg/kg total) infused over 4 min is recommended. Total doses exceeding 60 mg are not needed for any patient.

Interactions
Adenosine: Plasma levels of adenosine may be elevated, increasing the CV effects.
Cholinesterase inhibitors: Anticholinesterase effects may be counteracted by dipyridamole, potentially aggravating myasthenia gravis.

Theophyllines, xanthine derivatives (eg, caffeine): May abolish coronary vasodilation induced by IV dipyridamole.

Lab Test Interferences None well documented.

Adverse Reactions
CV: **Oral** Angina pectoris; hypotension, palpitation, tachycardia (postmarketing). **IV** Chest pain, angina pectoris (20%).
CNS: **Oral** Dizziness (14%); headache (2%); fatigue, malaise, (postmarketing). **IV** Headache, dizziness (12%); paresthesia, fatigue (1%).
DERM: **Oral** Rash (2%); pruritus; alopecia (postmarketing).
EENT: **Oral** Larynx edema (postmarketing).
GI: **Oral** Abdominal distress (6%); diarrhea; vomiting; nausea, dyspepsia (postmarketing). **IV** Nausea (5%); dyspepsia (1%).
HEPA: **Oral** Hepatic failure; elevated liver enzymes; hepatitis, cholelithiasis (postmarketing).
HEMA/LYMPH: Thrombocytopenia (postmarketing).
LABTESTABS: **IV** ECG abnormalities/ST-T changes (8%); ECG abnormalities/extrasystoles, hypotension (5%); ECG abnormalities/tachycardia (3%); BP lability, hypertension (2%).

PATIENT CARE CONSIDERATIONS
Administration/Storage
Tablets:
- Administer concurrently with warfarin therapy in patient with cardiac valve replacement.
- Administer prescribed dose without regard to meals. Administer with food if GI upset occurs.
- Store tablets at controlled room temperature (59° to 86°F).

Injection:
- For IV infusion only.
- Dilute prescribed dose, following manufacturer's instructions, before administration.
- Do not mix with other drugs in same syringe or infusion container.
- Inspect solution visually before administration. Do not administer if solution is cloudy, discolored, or contains particulate matter.
- Infuse prescribed dose over 4 min.
- Thallium-201 should be injected within 5 min of completion of the 4-min infusion of dipyridamole.
- If other drugs are being administered through same IV line, administer each medication separately.
- Discard any unused solution. Do not save for future use.

MUSC: **Oral** Myalgia (postmarketing).
RESP: **IV** Dyspnea (3%).
OTHER: **Oral** Flushing; hypersensitivity (including rash, urticaria, severe bronchospasm, angioedema), arthritis, paresthesia (postmarketing). **IV** Flushing, unspecific pain (3%).

Precautions
Pregnancy: Category B.
Lactation: Excreted in breast milk.
Children: Safety and efficacy not established in children under 12 yr (oral). Safety and efficacy not established (IV).
Coronary artery disease: Because dipyridamole has a vasodilatory effect, use with caution in patients with severe coronary artery disease.
Hypotension: Because dipyridamole can produce peripheral vasodilation, use with caution in patients with hypotension.
Serious adverse reactions: Administration of IV dipyridamole has been associated with cardiac death, fatal and nonfatal MI, ventricular fibrillation, symptomatic ventricular tachycardia, stroke, transient cerebral ischemia, seizures, anaphylactoid reaction, and bronchospasm.

Overdosage: Signs and Symptoms
Warm feeling, flushes, sweating, restlessness, feeling of weakness, dizziness.

- Store injection at controlled room temperature (59° to 77°F). Protect from light and freezing.

Assessment/Interventions
- Obtain patient history, including drug history and any known allergies. Note hypotension, unstable angina, recent MI, asthma, myasthenia gravis, or concurrent therapy with xanthine derivatives (eg, caffeine, theophylline).

Tablets:
- Ensure that patient is receiving warfarin therapy concurrently.
- Ensure that patient is not taking aspirin concurrently.
- Assess patient for CV, GI, CNS, and general body side effects. Inform health care provider if noted and significant.

Injection:
- Ensure that parenteral aminophylline and sublingual nitroglycerin are available before administering infusion.
- Monitor vital signs and ECG during and for 10 to 15 min after infusion has been completed. Be prepared to treat hypotension, bronchospasm, or ischemic chest pain.

Patient/Family Education
- Explain name, action, and potential side effects of drug.

Tablets:
- Advise patient to take as prescribed without regard to meals but to take with food if stomach upset occurs.
- Advise patient that if a dose is missed to take as soon as remembered unless it is nearing time for the next dose. Caution patient not to double the dose to catch up.
- Advise patient not to stop taking or change the dose unless advised by health care provider.
- Caution patient that drug may cause dizziness and to use caution while driving or performing other tasks requiring mental alertness until tolerance is determined.
- Advise patient to notify health care provider immediately if any of the following occur: rash or hives, difficulty breathing, persistent dizziness when arising from a sitting or lying position, fainting, yellowing of the skin or eyes.
- Advise patient to notify health care provider if bothersome side effects occur.
- Advise women to notify health care provider if pregnant, planning to become pregnant, or breastfeeding.
- Caution patient not to take any prescription or OTC medications or dietary supplements unless advised by health care provider.
- Advise patient that follow-up examinations and lab tests may be required to monitor therapy and to keep appointments.

Injection:
- Advise patient that medication will be prepared and administered by a health care provider in a health care setting.

Dipyridamole/Aspirin

(dye-peer-ID-a-mole/ASS-pihr-in)

Class Antiplatelet

How Supplied
Aggrenox Capsules 200 mg dipyridamole, extended-release/25 mg aspirin

Action
PHARMACOLOGY: Antithrombotic action resulting from additive antiplatelet effects.

Indications Reduce the risk of stroke in patients who have had transient ischemia of the brain or complete ischemic stroke caused by thrombosis.

Contraindications Hypersensitivity to dipyridamole, aspirin, or other components of product; allergy to NSAIDs; patients with asthma, rhinitis, and nasal polyps; children or teenagers with viral infections, with or without fever (Reye syndrome).

Route/Dosage
ADULTS: **PO** 1 capsule (200 mg extended-release dipyridamole/25 mg aspirin) bid, 1 in morning and 1 in evening. Do not crush or chew.

Interactions
Adenosine: Metabolism of adenosine may be inhibited by dipyridamole, producing profound bradycardia.
Cholinesterase inhibitors (eg, tacrine): Dipyridamole may counteract anticholinesterase effect, potentially aggravating myasthenia gravis.
ACE inhibitors (eg, captopril), beta blockers (eg, propranolol), diuretics (eg, furosemide), uricosuric agents (eg, probenecid): The effects of these agents may be decreased by aspirin.
Acetazolamide, anticoagulants (eg, warfarin), anticonvulsants (eg, valproic acid), methotrexate, NSAIDs (eg, ibuprofen), oral hypoglycemic agents (eg, chlorpropamide): The pharmacologic and toxic effects of these agents may be increased by aspirin.

Lab Test Interferences None well documented.

Adverse Reactions
CV: Cardiac failure; arrhythmia; supraventricular tachycardia.
CNS: Headache; amnesia; convulsions; anorexia; somnolence; confusion; coma; cerebral, subarachnoid, and intracranial hemorrhage.
DERM: Stevens-Johnson syndrome.
GI: Abdominal pain; dyspepsia; nausea; vomiting; diarrhea; melena; rectal hemorrhage; GI hemorrhage; hemorrhoids; perforation; Reye syndrome.
HEMA: Hemorrhage; epistaxis; anemia; purpura.
HEPA: Hepatic failure.
RESP: Coughing; upper respiratory infection.
OTHER: Arthralgia; arthritis; myalgia; arthrosis; pain; fatigue; back pain; asthenia; neoplasm; malaise; syncope; anaphylaxis; laryngeal edema; rhabdomyolysis.

Precautions
Pregnancy: Category D (aspirin); Category B (dipyridamole).
Lactation: Excreted in breast milk.
Children: Safety and efficacy not established.
Renal function impairment: Avoid in patients with severe renal failure (ie, glomerular filtration rate less than 10 mL/min).
Alcohol: Concurrent consumption of alcohol may increase risk of bleeding.

Coagulation: Platelet function may be inhibited, increasing the risk of bleeding.
Coronary artery disease: Use with caution.
Hypotension: Use with caution.

Overdosage: Signs and Symptoms
Dipyridamole: warm feeling, flushes, sweating, restlessness, weakness, dizziness, hypotension, tachycardia. Aspirin: tinnitus, nausea, vomiting, dizziness, respiratory alkalosis, metabolic acidosis, hemorrhage, convulsions. Significant overdose (4 to 10 g aspirin) is a medical emergency.

PATIENT CARE CONSIDERATIONS

Administration/Storage
- Do not chew or crush. Instruct patient to swallow capsule whole.
- Give twice daily, morning and evening with a full glass of water.
- Store at controlled room temperature. Protect from excessive moisture.

Assessment/Interventions
- Obtain patient history, including drug history and any known allergies. Note history of peptic ulcer disease, bleeding disorders, severe kidney, liver or heart disease, or syndrome of asthma, rhinitis, and nasal polyps.
- Monitor patient for GI, CNS, and musculoskeletal side effects. Report to health care provider if noted and significant.
- Monitor patient for rash, urticaria, dyspnea, or anaphylactic reaction. If any occur notify health care provider immediately.
- Monitor patient for signs and symptoms of cerebral ischemia. If any occur notify health care provider immediately.

Patient/Family Education
- Explain name, dose, action, and potential side effects of drug.
- Advise patient to not crush or chew medication and to swallow the capsule whole with a full glass of water two times a day.
- Advise patient regarding risks of drinking alcohol while taking this medication.
- Advise patient to report any of the following to their health care provider immediately: recurrent signs or symptoms of cerebral ischemia, unusual bleeding, rash, hives, or difficulty breathing.
- Advise patients to inform their health care provider if they experience bothersome side effects such as headache, indigestion, stomach pain, nausea, dizziness, or excessive bruising while taking this medication.

Dirithromycin

(die-RITH-row-MY-sin)

Class Antibiotic/Macrolide

How Supplied
Dynabac Tablets, enteric coated 250 mg

Action
PHARMACOLOGY: Interferes with microbial protein synthesis.

PHARMACOKINETICS/DYNAMICS:
Absorption: Rapidly absorbed and converted by nonenzymatic hydrolysis to erythromycylamine (active). For erythromycylamine, the C_{max} is approximately 0.3 to 0.4 mcg/mL. T_{max} approximately 3.9 to 4.1 hr. AUC approximately 0.9 to 1.8 mcg•hr/mL.

Distribution: For erythromycylamine, the protein binding is 15% to 30% and the Vd is 800 L.

Excretion: 81% to 97% excreted in the feces and approximately 2% eliminated through the kidneys. For erythromycylamine, the plasma t½ is approximately 8 hr, the terminal t½ is approximately 44 hr, and the Cl is approximately 23 L/hr.

Special Populations:
Renal Function Impairment – C_{max} and AUC are increased. No dosage adjustment necessary.
Hepatic Function Impairment – In those with mild hepatic impairment, the C_{max}, AUC, and Vd are increased. No dosage adjustment necessary.
Elderly – C_{max} and AUC increase with age. No dosage adjustment necessary.

Indications Treatment of acute bacterial infection of chronic bronchitis, secondary bacterial infection of acute bronchitis, community-acquired pneumonia, pharyngitis/tonsillitis, and uncomplicated skin and skin structure infections caused by susceptible organisms.

Contraindications Hypersensitivity to erythromycin or any macrolide antibiotic.

Route/Dosage
ADULTS AND CHILDREN 12 YR AND OLDER: **PO** 500 mg once daily for 7 to 14 days.

Interactions
Terfenadine: Since cardiotoxicity and death have occurred with other macrolide antibiotics, monitor patient during concurrent use; however, available clinical data indicate that there is no interaction.
Theophylline: Slight decrease in theophylline serum concentrations may occur.

Lab Test Interferences None well documented.

Adverse Reactions
CNS: Headache; dizziness; vertigo; insomnia.
DERM: Rash; pruritus; urticaria.
GI: Abdominal pain; nausea; diarrhea; vomiting; dyspepsia; flatulence.
HEMA: Increased platelet count; eosinophilia; increased segmented neutrophils.
METAB: Decreased bicarbonate.
RESP: Increased cough; shortness of breath.
OTHER: Increased serum potassium; pain; weakness; increased CPK.

Precautions
Pregnancy: Category C.

PATIENT CARE CONSIDERATIONS
Administration/Storage
- Take tablets with food or within 1 hr after eating. Food helps increase absorption.
- Swallow each tablet whole. Do not cut, crush, or chew tablets.
- Drink plenty of fluids as tablets are swallowed.
- Store at room temperature.

Assessment/Interventions
- Obtain patient history.
- Obtain baseline lab work including albumin, CBC, WBC with diff, platelet count, and total protein.
- Monitor for signs and symptoms of superinfections.
- Monitor for diarrhea, nausea, vomiting, and abdominal cramping.

Lactation: Undetermined.
Children: Safety and efficacy in children younger than 12 yr not established.
Pseudomembranous colitis: Consider possibility in patients who develop diarrhea.
Superinfection: Prolonged use of antibiotics may result in bacterial or fungal overgrowth of nonsusceptible microorganisms.

Overdosage: Signs and Symptoms
Nausea, vomiting, epigastric distress, diarrhea.

- Assess infection for indications of effectiveness of medication.

Patient/Family Education
- Instruct patient to take medication with food or within 1 hr after meals.
- Instruct patient to notify healthcare provider if rash develops or difficulty breathing occurs.
- Stress to patient that entire course of therapy must be completed, and not to stop taking medication when feeling better.
- Warn patient that if infection does not seem to improve after 5 days, to notify healthcare provider.
- Instruct patient to drink 2 to 3 liters of fluid per day while taking oral antibiotics.

Disopyramide
(DIE-so-PIR-uh-mide)

Class Antiarrhythmic

How Supplied
Norpace Capsules 100 mg, Capsules 250 mg as phosphate ♦ *Norpace CR* Capsules, extended-release 100 mg, Capsules, extended-release 250 mg as phosphate
✠ *Rythmodan* ♦ *Rythmodan-LA*

Action
PHARMACOLOGY: Decreases rate of diastolic depolarizations rate; decreases upstroke velocity; increases action potential duration; prolongs refractory period.

PHARMACOKINETICS/DYNAMICS:
Absorption:
IR – Rapidly and almost completely absorbed. T_{max} is 2 hr.
ER (300 mg dose) – C_{max} approximately 3.23 mcg/mL. T_{max} approximately 2.5 hr.

Distribution: 50% to 65% protein bound (concentration dependent). Excreted in human milk.

Excretion: t½ approximately 6.7 hr (IR) and approximately 11.65 hr (ER). Approximately 50% excreted unchanged in the urine and approximately 30% as metabolites.

Special Populations:
Renal Function Impairment – Because more than 50% excreted in the urine, dosage reduction recommended.
Hepatic Function Impairment – t½ increased. Dosage reduction recommended.
Heart failure – T_{max} and C_{max} increased. t½ also prolonged.
Heart disease – t½ slightly prolonged to approximately 7.8 hr.

Indications Suppression and documented prevention of ventricular arrhythmias considered to be life threatening. **Unlabeled use(s):** Treatment of paroxysmal supraventricular tachycardia.

Contraindications Cardiogenic shock; pre-existing second- or third-degree atrioventricular block (if no pacemaker present); congenital QT prolongation; sick sinus syndrome.

Route/Dosage
ADULTS: PO 400 to 800 mg/day in 4 divided, evenly spaced doses.
CHILDREN (12 TO 18 YR): PO 6 to 15 mg/kg/day in divided doses.

CHILDREN (4 TO 12 YR): **PO** 10 to 15 mg/kg/day in divided doses.
CHILDREN (1 TO 4 YR): **PO** 10 to 20 mg/kg/day in divided doses.
CHILDREN (YOUNGER THAN 1 YR): **PO** 10 to 30 mg/kg/day in divided doses.

Severe Refractory Ventricular Tachycardia
May give **PO** up to 400 mg q 6 hr.

With Cardiomyopathy or Cardiac Decompensation
Limit to **PO** 100 mg q 6 to 8 hr initially.

Renal/Hepatic Impairment
ADULTS: **PO** 100 mg q 6 hr; increase to q 8 to 24 hr for patients with deteriorating renal function.

Interactions
Antiarrhythmic agents: May cause widened QRS and prolonged QT.
Erythromycin: May cause increased disopyramide plasma levels.
Hydantoins: May decrease disopyramide serum levels, half-life, and bioavailability.
Rifampin: May decrease disopyramide serum levels.

Lab Test Interferences
None well documented.

Adverse Reactions
CV: Hypotension; CHF; edema; shortness of breath; syncope; chest pain.
CNS: Dizziness; fatigue; headache; nervousness.
DERM: Rash; dermatoses; itching.
EENT: Blurred vision; dry nose, eyes, throat.
GI: Nausea; pain; bloating; gas; anorexia; vomiting; diarrhea; dry mouth; constipation.
GU: Urinary retention, frequency and urgency; impotence; urinary hesitancy.
OTHER: Muscle weakness; malaise; aches and pains; hypokalemia; weight gain; elevated cholesterol and triglycerides; hypoglycemia.

Precautions
Pregnancy: Category C.
Lactation: Excreted in breast milk.
Renal function impairment: Dosage should be reduced.
Hepatic function impairment: Dosage should be reduced.
Anticholinergic activity: Use with extreme caution in patients with urinary retention, glaucoma, or myasthenia gravis.
Conduction abnormalities: Use with caution in patients with bundle branch block or Wolff-Parkinson-White syndrome.
Heart block: Reduce dose if first-degree block occurs; drug may need to be discontinued if heart block continues.
Heart failure/hypotension: May cause or aggravate CHF or produce severe hypotension, especially in patients with depressed systolic function.
Potassium imbalance: Disopyramide may be ineffective in hypokalemia and have enhanced toxicity in hyperkalemia.

Overdosage: Signs and Symptoms
Loss of consciousness, cardiac arrhythmias, loss of spontaneous respiration, death.

PATIENT CARE CONSIDERATIONS

Administration/Storage
- Have patient swallow capsules whole.
- Administer doses 6 hr apart (12 hr apart for extended-release form).
- Adjust dosage according to physiologic effect and serum levels.
- Store capsules in light-resistant container.

Assessment/Interventions
- Obtain patient history, including drug history and any known allergies.
- Assess apical/radial heart rate.
- Obtain baseline 12-lead ECG.
- Correct hypokalemia before giving drug.
- Assess I&O.
- Monitor patient weight daily.
- Monitor plasma levels and therapeutic response.
- Monitor serum electrolytes.
- If BP drop of 20 mm Hg occurs, notify health care provider immediately.
- If heart arrhythmia or increase in heart rate develops, notify health care provider immediately.
- If serum potassium level is higher than recommended level, notify health care provider.
- If serum level of drug is higher than therapeutic level, notify health care provider.
- If patient has urinary elimination problems, notify health care provider.

Patient/Family Education
- Instruct patient how to take own BP and heart rate.
- Tell patient to keep weekly record of weight and report any change of 2 lb or more to health care provider.
- Instruct patient to increase roughage in diet.
- Inform patient about possibility of urinary elimination problems and instruct to notify health care provider if problems persist.
- Instruct patient not to crush or chew capsules.
- Advise patient about possibility of hypoglycemia and to be alert for cold sweats, drowsiness, confusion, anxiety, and cool, pale skin.
- Instruct patient to take sips of water frequently, suck on ice chips or sugarless hard

candy, or chew sugarless gum if dry mouth occurs.
* Caution patient to avoid sudden position changes to prevent orthostatic hypotension.
* Instruct patient to avoid intake of alcoholic beverages or other CNS depressants.
* Advise patient that drug may cause drowsiness and to use caution while driving or performing other tasks requiring mental alertness.

Disulfiram

(die-SULL-fih-ram)
Class Antialcoholic agent

How Supplied
Antabuse Tablets 250 mg

Action
PHARMACOLOGY: Produces intolerance to alcohol by blocking oxidation of acetaldehyde by enzyme aldehyde dehydrogenase, resulting in high blood levels of acetaldehyde and unpleasant physical symptoms.

PHARMACOKINETICS/DYNAMICS:
Absorption: Slowly absorbed from the GI tract.
Metabolism: Ultimately metabolized to carbon disulfide and diethylamine.
Excretion: Slowly eliminated with approximately 20% of the drug remaining in the body after 1 wk.
Peak: 12 hr.
Duration: 1 to 2 wk.

Indications
Aid in management of alcoholism in selected patients who want to remain in state of enforced sobriety.

Contraindications
Hypersensitivity to thiuram derivatives used in pesticides and rubber vulcanization; severe myocardial disease or coronary occlusion; psychoses; patients receiving or who have recently received metronidazole, paraldehyde, alcohol, or alcohol-containing products.

Route/Dosage
ADULTS: PO
Initial dose: 500 mg qd (single dose) initially for 1 to 2 wk.
Maintenance dose: 125 to 500 mg qd (max, 500 mg/day).

Interactions
Alcohol: Causes severe alcohol-intolerance reaction. Symptoms include flushing, throbbing in head and neck, respiratory difficulty, nausea, vomiting, sweating, thirst, chest pain, palpitations, shortness of breath, tachycardia, hypotension, syncope, weakness, vertigo, blurred vision, and confusion. In severe reactions, there may be respiratory depression, cardiovascular collapse, unconsciousness, convulsions, and death.
Anticoagulants: Disulfiram may increase anticoagulant effect.
Antidepressants, tricyclic: May produce acute organic brain syndrome.
Benzodiazepines: Disulfiram decreases plasma clearance of benzodiazepines metabolized by oxidation, possible increase in CNS side effects.
Chlorzoxazone: CNS side effects of chlorzoxazone may be increased.
Cocaine: CV side effects of cocaine may be increased.
Hydantoins: Disulfiram may increase serum hydantoin levels.
Isoniazid: Acute behavioral and coordination changes.
Metronidazole: May cause patients to exhibit acute toxic psychosis or confusional state. One or both agents may need to be discontinued.
Theophyllines: Disulfiram may inhibit metabolism and increase effect of theophyllines.

Lab Test Interferences
None well documented.

Adverse Reactions
CNS: Drowsiness; fatigue; headache; psychotic reactions.
DERM: Skin eruptions; allergic dermatitis; acneform eruptions.
EENT: Metallic or garlic-like aftertaste.
HEPA: Hepatotoxicity; hepatitis (including cholestatic and fulminant).
OTHER: Peripheral neuropathy; polyneuritis; optic or peripheral neuritis; impotence.

> WARNING:
> *Counseling:* Never administer to patient in a state of alcohol intoxication or without patient's full knowledge. Instruct patient's relatives accordingly.

Precautions
Pregnancy: Category C.
Lactation: Undetermined.
Hypersensitivity: Evaluate patients with history of rubber contact dermatitis for hypersensitivity to thiuram derivatives.
Special risk patients: Use with caution in patients with diabetes mellitus, hypothyroidism, epilepsy, cerebral damage, chronic and acute nephritis, and hepatic cirrhosis or insufficiency.
Disulfiram-alcohol reaction: Avoid alcohol in all forms, including alcoholic beverages, vinegars, liquid medications such as cough syrups or tonic, some sauces, and aftershave products. Do not give disulfiram within 12 hr of drinking

alcohol. Reactions can occur up to 2 wk after discontinuing disulfiram.

Ethylene dibromide: Patients receiving disulfiram should not be exposed to ethylene dibromide or its vapors; toxic interaction resulting in tumors and death has occurred in research animals.

Hepatic toxicity: Hepatic toxicity, including hepatic failure resulting in transplantation or death, has been reported.

PATIENT CARE CONSIDERATIONS

Administration/Storage

- Do not administer until patient has abstained from alcohol for at least 12 hr.
- May crush or mix tablets with liquid.
- May administer at bedtime if sedative effect is experienced.
- Store tablets at controlled room temperature (59° to 86°F).
- Administer prescribed dose qd without regard to meals. Administer with food if GI upset occurs.

Assessment/Interventions

- Obtain patient history, including drug history and any known allergies. Note kidney or liver disease, diabetes, hypothyroidism, epilepsy, CV disease, cerebral vascular disease, psychosis, current or recent use of metronidazole or alcohol-containing preparations (eg, cough syrup, tonic), or history of rubber contact dermatitis.
- Ensure that transaminases are determined before and 10 to 14 days after starting therapy and then periodically during treatment.
- Ensure that serum electrolytes, renal function, and CBC are determined before and q 6 mo during treatment.
- Evaluate history to ensure patient has not ingested any form of alcohol within 12 hr prior to initiation of therapy (including cough syrups, tonics, vinegars).
- Monitor patient for disulfiram-alcohol reaction. Notify health care provider immediately and be prepared to treat appropriately.
- Perform psychosocial assessment to determine patient's readiness to initiate and follow through with this type of therapy.
- Monitor patient for CNS, GI, and general body side effects. Inform health care provider if noted and significant.

Patient/Family Education

- Explain that disulfiram will not cure alcohol dependence and should be used in conjunction with psychotherapy.
- Advise patient that even trace amounts of alcohol in some food products or alcohol absorbed through skin (eg, aftershave lotion) can precipitate reaction.
- Inform patient of all effects that will occur if alcohol is ingested while taking this medication.
- Advise patient and family that some alcohol-disulfiram reactions can have serious effects on heart and respiratory system that may require immediate emergency treatment.
- Instruct patients to read all product labels or consult pharmacist about alcohol content of all liquid medications before choosing one.
- Instruct patient to carry *Medi-Alert* identification while taking this drug. Information should include health care provider's phone number or name of medical facility that should be contacted in case of reaction.
- Caution patient that prolonged disulfiram therapy does not produce tolerance to alcohol but increased sensitivity.
- Advise patient that drug may cause drowsiness and to use caution while driving or performing other tasks requiring mental alertness.
- Explain that alcohol-disulfiram reactions may occur for several weeks after discontinuation of therapy.
- Explain name, dose, action, and potential side effects of drug.
- Caution patient not to change the dose or stop taking unless advised by health care provider.
- Instruct patient to immediately notify health care provider or seek medical care if disulfiram-alcohol reaction occurs.
- Advise women to notify health care provider if pregnant, planning to become pregnant, or breastfeeding.
- Instruct patient not to take any prescription or OTC medications or dietary supplements unless advised by health care provider.
- Advise patient that follow-up visits may be required to monitor therapy and to keep appointments.

Dobutamine

(doe-BYOOT-uh-meen)

Class Vasopressor

How Supplied
Dobutrex Injection 12.5 mg/mL

Action
PHARMACOLOGY: Stimulates $beta_1$-receptors in heart, causing more complete and forceful contractions (inotropy) without significantly increasing heart rate or BP.
PHARMACOKINETICS/DYNAMICS:
Metabolism: Methylation and conjugation.
Excretion: t½ is 2 min. Urinary excretion of metabolites.
Onset: 1 to 2 min.
Peak: Up to 10 min.

Indications Treatment of cardiac decompensation caused by organic heart disease or cardiac surgical procedures. **Unlabeled use(s):** Congenital heart disease in children undergoing diagnostic cardiac catheterization.

Contraindications Idiopathic hypertrophic subaortic stenosis.

Route/Dosage
ADULTS: **IV infusion** 2.5 to 10 mcg/kg/min; titrate to desired response; increase in heart rate more than 10% may develop in rate greater than 20 mcg/kg/min; rates up to 40 mcg/kg/min are rarely used. Duration of therapy up to 72 hr without decrease in clinical effectiveness may be used.

Interactions
Beta-blockers: May antagonize beta receptor-stimulating activity of dobutamine.
Furazolidone, methyldopa, rauwolfia alkaloids: Hypertension may result.
Guanethidine: May increase pressor response.
Halogenated hydrocarbon anesthetics: May increase risk of arrhythmias by sensitizing cardiac tissue to sympathomimetic agents.
Tricyclic antidepressants: May potentiate effect of dobutamine; use combination with caution.
INCOMPATIBILITIES: Chemically incompatible with sodium bicarbonate or other alkaline solutions.

Lab Test Interferences None well documented.

Adverse Reactions
CV: Increased systolic BP; increased heart rate; chest pain; increased number of premature ventricular beats.
CNS: Headache; tingling sensations; paresthesia.
GI: Nausea; vomiting.
RESP: Dyspnea.
OTHER: Phlebitis; local inflammation after infiltration; leg cramps.

Precautions
Pregnancy: Safety not established.
Lactation: Undetermined.
Children: Safety and efficacy not established.
Special risk patients: Use with extreme caution after myocardial ischemia. Avoid use in uncorrected hypovolemic states unless used as temporary emergency measure to maintain coronary and cerebral flow.
Sulfite sensitivity: Use caution in sulfite-sensitive individuals; some preparations contain sodium bisulfite.
Cardiovascular effects: May greatly increase BP and heart rate, especially with preexisting hypertension. Dose reduction may reverse effects. May precipitate or exacerbate ventricular ectopic activity.
Hypokalemia: Mild hypokalemia may occur.

Overdosage: Signs and Symptoms
Excessive hypertension, tachycardia, nausea, vomiting, tremor, headache, chest pain.

PATIENT CARE CONSIDERATIONS

Administration/Storage
- Administer by IV infusion only. Use electronic infusion device to monitor infusion rate.
- Reconstitution/dilution is done in two stages.
- First, more concentrated solution can be kept under refrigeration for 48 hr or at room temperature for 6 hr.
- Before administration, solution is further diluted to typical concentration of 0.25 to 1 mg/mL (250 to 1000 mcg/mL). Final concentration should not exceed 5 mg/mL. This solution should be used within 24 hr.
- Solution may have pink color, because of slight oxidation, but this effect does not indicate loss of potency.

- Do not freeze solution because crystallization may occur.

Assessment/Interventions
- Obtain patient history, including drug history and any known allergies.
- Monitor vital signs, ECG, cardiac output, pulmonary capillary wedge pressure, central venous pressure and urinary output carefully throughout infusion.
- Monitor potassium levels to detect possible hypokalemia.
- Monitor patency and placement of IV catheter to reduce risk of extravasation and phlebitis.
- If patient has diabetes, monitor blood glucose level. Report significant increase to health care provider.

Patient/Family Education
- Instruct patient to report these symptoms to health care provider: pain or discomfort at IV site, any anginal pain.

Docetaxel

(doe-seh-TAX-ehl)
Class Mitotic inhibitor

How Supplied
Taxotere Injection 20 mg, Injection 80 mg

Action
PHARMACOLOGY: Docetaxel acts by disrupting cells' microtubular network that is essential for mitotic and interphase cellular functions. Docetaxel binds to free tubulin and promotes the assembly of tubulin into stable microtubules while simultaneously inhibiting their disassembly.

PHARMACOKINETICS/DYNAMICS:
Distribution: Approximately 94% to 97% protein bound. Vd is 113 L (at steady-state)
Metabolism: Metabolized by CYP3A4 to 1 major and 3 minor metabolites.
Excretion: The t½ is 4 min (alpha phase), 36 min (beta phase), and 11.1 hr (gamma phase). Cl is 21 L/h/m^2. Approximately 6% excreted in urine and approximately 75% in the feces (less than 8% as unchanged drug).

Indications Locally advanced or metastatic breast cancer; locally advanced or metastatic non-small cell lung cancer. **Unlabeled use(s):** Ovarian cancer.

Contraindications History of severe hypersensitivity reactions to docetaxel or to other drugs formulated with polysorbate 80; neutrophil counts of less than 1500 cells/mm^3.

Route/Dosage
Locally Advanced or Metastatic Breast Cancer
ADULTS: IV 60 to 100 mg/m^2 administered over 1 hr q 3 wk.

Dosage Adjustment for Breast Cancer
ADULTS:
Initial dose (100 mg/m^2): Adjust dose to 75 mg/m^2 in patients who experience febrile neutropenia, neutrophils less than 500 cells/mm^3 for longer than 1 wk, severe or cumulative cutaneous reactions, or severe peripheral neuropathy. If reactions continue, decrease the dosage to 55 mg/m^2 or discontinue treatment.
Initial dose (60 mg/m^2): Patients who do not experience these symptoms may tolerate higher doses. Discontinue docetaxel treatment entirely if patients develop at least grade 3 peripheral neuropathy.

Locally Advanced or Metastatic Non-Small Cell Lung Cancer
ADULTS: IV 70 mg/m^2 administered over 1 hr q 3 wk.

Dosage Adjustments for Non-Small Cell Lung Cancer
ADULTS:
Initial dose (75 mg/m^2): Withhold treatment in patients who experience febrile neuropenia, neutrophils less than 500 cells/mm^3 for longer than 1 wk, severe or cumulative cutaneous reactions, or other grade 3 and 4 nonhematological toxicities during treatment until resolution of the toxicity, and then resume at 55 mg/m^2. Discontinue docetaxel treatment entirely if patients develop at least grade 3 peripheral neuropathy.

Locally Advanced or Metastatic Non-Small Cell Lung Cancer Not Previously Treated with Chemotherapy
ADULTS: **IV** Docetaxel 75 mg/m^2 over 1 hr immediately followed by cisplatin 75 mg/m^2 over 30 to 60 min q 3 wk. In patients who are dosed initially at 75 mg/m^2 of docetaxel in combination with cisplatin, and whose nadir platelet count during the previous course of therapy is less than 25,000 cells/mm^3, in patients who experience febrile neutropenia, and in patients with serious nonhematologic toxicities, reduce the docetaxel dose to 65 mg/m^2 in subsequent cycles. In patients who require a further dose reduction, a dose of 50 mg/m^2 is recommended. For cisplatin dosage adjustments, see manufacturer's prescribing information.

Dosage Adjustments in Hepatic Dysfunction
ADULTS: **IV** Avoid use in patients with bilirubin above the upper limit of normal, AST or ALT greater than 1.5 times the upper limit of normal concomitant with alkaline phosphatase greater than 2.5 times the upper limit of normal.

Pretreatment Regimen
To reduce the severity of hypersensitivity reactions and fluid retention, premedicate with 8 mg dexamethasone orally twice daily for 3 days starting the day before docetaxel administration.

Interactions
CYP450: Docetaxel is metabolized by cytochrome P450 3A. Potential exists for significant drug interactions between docetaxel and agents that inhibit or induce cytochrome P450 enzymes (eg, rifampin, phenobarbital, erythromycin, ketoconazole).

Lab Test Interferences
None well documented.

Adverse Reactions
CV: Edema; weight gain; pleural effusion; pericardial effusion or ascites; hypotension.
CNS: Peripheral neuropathies.
DERM: Alopecia; localized edema; desquamation of extremities; rash with pruritus; hypo- or hyperpigmentation of nails; onycholysis; pain of nails.
GI: Nausea; vomiting; diarrhea; stomatitis; elevated LFTs.
HEMA: Bone marrow suppression.
HYPERSEN: Hypotension; bronchospasm; generalized rash; erythema; flushing; rash with or without pruritus; chest tightness; back pain; dyspnea; drug fever; chills.
MUSC: Arthralgia, myalgia.

WARNING:

Fluid retention: Severe fluid retention has occurred.

Hypersensitivity: Severe hypersensitivity reactions may be characterized by hypotension or bronchospasm, or generalized rash/erythema. May occur within a few minutes following initiation of infusion and despite dexamethasone pretreatment. Severe reactions should not receive rechallenge. Do not administer to patients with prior severe hypersensitivity reactions or to other drugs formulated with polysorbate 80.

Increased mortality: Increased mortality in patients with liver dysfunction, receiving higher doses, with non-small cell lung carcinoma, and prior platinum therapy receiving 100 mg/m^2 of docetaxel.

Neutropenia: Neutropenia (less than 2000 neutrophils/mm^3) occurs in virtually all patients given 60 to 100 mg/m^2 of docetaxel, and grade 4 neutropenia (less than 500 cells/mm^3) occurs in 85% of patients given 100 mg/m^2 and 75% of patients given 60 mg/m^2. Do not administer to patients with neutrophils less than 1500 cells/mm^3.

Special risk patients: In general, do not give docetaxel to patients with bilirubin greater than the upper limit of normal (ULN) or to patients with AST or ALT greater than 1.5 × ULN concomitant with alkaline phosphatase (AP) greater than 2.5 × ULN. These patients are at increased risk for the development of grade 4 neutropenia, febrile neutropenia, infections, severe thrombocytopenia, severe stomatitis, severe skin toxicity, and toxic death.

Precautions
Pregnancy: Category D.
Lactation: Undetermined.
Children: Safety and efficacy not established in children less than 16 yr.
Asthenia: Severe asthenia has been reported in 14.9% of metastatic breast cancer patients.

Dermatologic: Reversible cutaneous reactions characterized by a rash, including localized eruptions, mainly on the feet or hands, but also on the arms, face, or thorax, usually associated with pruritus, have been observed. Localized erythema of the extremities with edema followed by desquamation has been observed. Severe nail disorders have been reported also.

Extravasation risk: Local irritation or phlebitis may occur. Refer to your institution-specific protocol.

PATIENT CARE CONSIDERATIONS
Administration/Storage
* Refrigerate and protect from light. Reconstituted 10 mg/mL solution is stable for 8 hr at room temperature or stored in the refrigerator. Diluted 0.3 to 0.9 mg/mL solution is stable at room temperature for 4 hr under normal room lighting.
* Allow to stand at room temperature for 5 min before reconstitution.
* Withdraw diluent and add to the docetaxel vial. This results in a 10 mg/mL solution. Gently rotate vial for 15 sec to mix.
* After reconstitution, dilute with 0.9% Sodium Chloride or 5% Dextrose to a final docetaxel concentration of 0.3 to 0.74 mg/mL.
* Diluted solutions may leach DEHP from polyvinyl chloride (PVC) infusion sets or bags. Use glass, polypropylene, or polyolefin containers and polyethylene-lined administration sets.
* Administer by IV infusion over 1 hr.

Assessment/Interventions
* Monitor CBC at baseline and throughout therapy. Docetaxel is contraindicated in patients with neutrophil counts less than 1500/mm^3.

Neurologic: Severe neurosensory symptoms (eg, paresthesia, dysesthesia, pain) were observed in 5.5% of metastatic breast cancer patients. Dosage must be adjusted. If symptoms persist, discontinue treatment.

Overdosage: Signs and Symptoms
Bone marrow suppression, peripheral neurotoxicity, mucositis.

* Closely monitor patients with preexisting effusions from the first dose for the possible exacerbation of the effusions.
* Observe patients closely for hypersensitivity reactions, especially during the first and second infusions.
* Obtain bilirubin, AST, or ALT, and alkaline phosphatase values prior to each cycle of docetaxel therapy.

Patient/Family Education
* Advise patients to call health care provider immediately if a fever over 100°F occurs. Tell doctor about symptoms of infection, such as a sore throat or cough or a burning sensation while urinating.
* Advise patients to tell health care provider if a warm sensation, difficulty in breathing, itching, flushing, or rash during or shortly after treatment occur.
* Advise patients to tell health care provider if any signs of fluid retention, shortness of breath, swelling of feet or hands, or unexplained weight gain occur.
* Advise patients to notify health care provider if muscle or joint pain occur.

Docusate

(DOCK-you-sate)

Class Laxative/Fecal softener

How Supplied

Docusate Sodium (Dioctyl Sodium Sulfosuccinate; DSS)
Colace Capsules 50 mg, Capsules 100 mg, Liquid 150 mg/15 mL, Syrup 60 mg/15 mL ♦ *Diocto* Liquid 150 mg/15 mL, Syrup 60 mg/15 mL ♦ *Docu* Liquid 150 mg/15 mL, Syrup 20mg/5 mL ♦ *D.O.S* Capsules, soft-gel 100 mg, Capsules, soft-gel 250 mg ♦ *D-S-S* Capsules 100 mg ♦ *ex-lax Stool Softener* Tablets 100 mg ♦ *Genasoft* Capsules, soft-gel 100 mg ♦ *Non-Habit Forming Stool Softener* Capsules 100 mg ♦ *Phillips' Liqui-Gels* Capsules, soft-gel 100 mg ♦ *Regulax SS* Capsules 100 mg ♦ *Silace* Syrup 60 mg/15 mL ♦ *Stool Softener* Capsules 100 mg, Capsules 250 mg

♣ *Selax* ♦ *Soflax* ♦ *ratio-Docusate Sodium*

Docusate Calcium (Dioctyl Calcium Sulfosuccinate)
DC Softgels *Stool Softener* *Stool Softener DC* *Surfak Liquigels*
♣ *ratio-Docusate Calcium*

Docusate Potassium (Dioctyle Potassium Sulfosuccinate)
Dialose *Diocto-K* *Kasof* *Perestan*

Action

PHARMACOLOGY: Facilitates stool softening by detergent activity.

PHARMACOKINETICS/DYNAMICS:
Onset: 12 to 72 hr.

Indications Short-term treatment of constipation; prophylaxis in patients who should not strain during defecation (eg, after anorectal surgery, MI); to evacuate the colon for rectal and bowel examinations; prevention of dry, hard stools.

Contraindications Nausea, vomiting or other symptoms of appendicitis; acute surgical abdomen; fecal impaction; intestinal obstruction; undiagnosed abdominal pain; coadministration with mineral oil.

Route/Dosage

DOCUSATE SODIUM
ADULTS AND CHILDREN OLDER THAN 12 YR: **PO** 50 to 500 mg.
CHILDREN 6 TO 12 YR: **PO** 40 to 120 mg.
CHILDREN 3 TO 6 YR: **PO** 20 to 60 mg.
CHILDREN YOUNGER THAN 3 YR: **PO** 10 to 40 mg.

DOCUSATE CALCIUM
ADULTS: **PO** 240 mg.
CHILDREN 6 YR AND OLDER AND ADULTS WITH MINIMAL NEEDS: **PO** 50 to 150 mg.

DOCUSATE POTASSIUM
ADULTS: **PO** 100 to 300 mg.
CHILDREN 6 YR AND OLDER: **PO** 100 mg at bedtime.

Interactions

Mineral oil: Docusate may increase absorption of mineral oil from GI tract, leading to toxicity.

PATIENT CARE CONSIDERATIONS

Administration/Storage

- Administer each dose with full glass of water.
- Do not open or otherwise alter capsules.
- Do not give within 1 hr of other drugs or antacids, milk or histamine H_2 blockers.
- Do not administer for more than 1 wk without follow-up evaluation.
- Store capsules at room temperature. Protect liquid preparations from light.

Assessment/Interventions

- Obtain patient history, including drug history and any known allergies.
- Assess patient's bowel regimen to determine nonpharmacologic interventions for bowel evacuation.
- Review patient's diet history for medical restriction of sodium. If sodium restriction is present, docusate sodium should not be used.
- Document daily I&O.
- Evaluate and document patient's response to stool softener, noting and reporting any adverse reactions such as nausea, vomiting,

Lab Test Interferences None well documented.

Adverse Reactions

CV: Palpitations.
CNS: Dizziness; fainting.
GI: Excessive bowel activity (griping, diarrhea, nausea, vomiting); perianal irritation; bloating; flatulence; abdominal cramping.
OTHER: Sweating; weakness.

Precautions

Pregnancy: Category C.
Lactation: Undetermined.
Abuse/dependence: Long-term use may lead to laxative dependence, fluid and electrolyte imbalances, steatorrhea, osteomalacia, and vitamin and mineral deficiencies.
Fluid and electrolyte imbalance: Excessive laxative use may lead to significant fluid and electrolyte imbalance.
Rectal bleeding or failure to respond: May indicate serious condition that may require further medical attention.
Concomitant laxative use: Do not use other laxatives, especially during the initial phase of therapy for portal-systemic encephalopathy; the resulting loose stools may falsely suggest adequate lactulose dosage.

---

abdominal cramping, or diarrhea.
- Monitor patient frequently for signs and symptoms of dehydration and electrolyte imbalance such as weakness, dizziness, confusion, palpitations, thirst, or decreased urine output.

Patient/Family Education

- Tell patient to drink full glass of water with each dose.
- Instruct patient to swallow tablets whole and not to chew them.
- Instruct patient not to use mineral oil while taking this drug.
- Teach patient other methods of stimulating regular bowel evacuation: attempt to evacuate bowels at same time each day; drink 6 to 8 full glasses of water; eat high-fiber diet; exercise daily; respond to urge for bowel movement as soon as possible.
- Explain that liquid forms, excluding syrup, may be mixed with fruit juice or milk to mask unpleasant taste.

Dofetilide

(doe-FEH-till-ide)

Class Antiarrhythmic

How Supplied
Tikosyn Capsules 125 mcg, Capsules 250 mcg, Capsules 500 mcg

Action
PHARMACOLOGY: Blockade of the cardiac ion channel carrying the rapid component of the delayed rectifier potassium currents.

PHARMACOKINETICS/DYNAMICS:
Absorption: Bioavailability greater than 90%. T_{max} is 2 to 3 hr.
Distribution: 60% to 70% protein bound. Vd is 3 L/kg.
Metabolism: Metabolized by N-delkylation and N-oxidation, and to a lesser extent by CYP3A4.
Excretion: t½ approximately 10 hr. Approximately 80% excreted in urine of which approximately 80% is unchanged drug.
Special Populations:
Renal Function Impairment – Clearance is decreased and t½ is prolonged. Dosage adjustment recommended.
Gender – Women have approximately 12% to 18% lower clearance.

Indications Maintenance of normal sinus rhythm (delay in time to recurrence of atrial fibrillation/atrial flutter [AF/AFl]) in patients with AF/AFl of more than 1 wk duration who have been converted to normal sinus rhythm; conversion of AF/AFl to normal sinus rhythm.
Unlabeled use(s): Ventricular arrhythmias.

Contraindications Hypersensitivity to drug; congenital or acquired long QT syndromes; baseline QT interval of QTc greater than 440 msec (500 msec in patients with ventricular conduction abnormalities); severe renal impairment (Ccr less than 20 mL/min); concurrent use of cimetidine, ketoconazole, trimethoprim (alone or in combination with sulfamethoxazole), or verapamil; concomitant use of known inhibitors of renal cation transport (eg, megestrol, prochlorperazine).

Route/Dosage
ADULTS: **PO** The dose must be individualized according to calculated Ccr and QTc. Use the QT interval if the heart rate is less than 60 bpm. There are no data on use if the heart rate is less than 50 bpm. The usual recommended dose is 500 mcg bid, as modified by the dosing algorithm described in the manufacturer's prescribing information.

Interactions
Cimetidine, inhibitors of renal cationic exchange (eg, megestrol, phenothiazines), ketoconazole, trimethoprim (alone or in combination with sulfamethoxazole), verapamil: Are contraindicated.
Drugs actively secreted by renal cationic secretion (eg, amiloride, metformin, triamterene), inhibitors of CYP3A4 isozymes (eg, amiodarone, azole antifungal agents, cannabinoids, diltiazem, grapefruit juice, macrolide antibiotics, nefazodone, norfloxacin, protease inhibitors, quinine, serotonin reuptake inhibitors, zafirlukast): May increase dofetilide levels; use with caution.
Class I (eg, quinidine) or Class III (eg, sotalol) antiarrhythmics: Withhold for at least 3 half-lives prior to dosing with dofetilide.
Drugs that prolong the QT interval (eg, bepridil, cisapride, phenothiazines, tricyclic antidepressants, erythromycin): Concurrent use not recommended.

Lab Test Interferences None well documented.

Adverse Reactions
CV: Ventricular tachyarrhythmia; chest pain; torsades de pointes; AV block; bundle branch block; heart block; angioedema; bradycardia; cerebral ischemia; cerebrovascular accident; cardiac arrest; MI; syncope.
CNS: Headache; dizziness; insomnia; migraine.
DERM: Rash.
EENT: Increased cough.
GI: Diarrhea; abdominal pain.
HEPA: Liver damage.
RESP: Respiratory tract infection; dyspnea.
OTHER: Flu syndrome; back pain; edema; facial paralysis; paralysis; paresthesia; sudden death.

> WARNING:
>
> *Equipped facility:* Administer in an equipped facility that can provide Ccr calculations, continuous ECG monitoring, and resuscitation for at least 3 days when therapy is initiated or restarted.
>
> *Restricted distribution:* Restrict distribution to facilities/prescribers who have received approved educational program.

Precautions
Pregnancy: Category C.
Lactation: Undetermined.
Children: Safety and efficacy not established.
Elderly: Select dose with caution, reflecting the greater frequency of decreased renal function.

Renal function impairment: Plasma concentrations of dofetilide may be increased; dosage must be adjusted based on Ccr.
Hepatic function impairment: Use with caution in patients with severe hepatic impairment.
Potassium levels: Should be within normal range prior to and during administration of drug.
Torsades de pointes: Risk may be reduced by controlling plasma concentrations of dofetilide by dosing according to Ccr and monitoring ECG.

Overdosage: Signs and Symptoms
Prolongation of the QT interval, ventricular fibrillation, cardiac arrest.

PATIENT CARE CONSIDERATIONS

Administration/Storage
- Administer first 3 days of therapy to patient who is on continuous ECG monitoring.
- May administer without regard to meals.
- Give reduced dose to patient with decreased renal function or if QTc prolongs after first dose.
- Do not administer if QTc greater than 500 msec anytime after the second dose.
- If a dose is missed do NOT double up. Give next dose at scheduled time.
- Store capsules at controlled room temperature. Protect from moisture.

Assessment/Interventions
- Obtain patient history, including drug history and any known allergies. Note history of congenital or acquired long QT syndrome, severe renal impairment (CrCl less than 20 mL/min), severe hepatic impairment, or concurrent use of cimetidine, trimethoprim, verapamil, or ketaconazole.
- Ensure that Ccr has been calculated and the QTc interval and serum potassium have been determined before initiating therapy and periodically (at least q 3 mo) during treatment.
- Ensure that patient is under continuous ECG monitoring for at least the first 3 days of therapy.
- Determine QTc interval 2 to 3 hr after first dose and note change from baseline QTc interval. Notify health care provider if it has increased more than 15% or is greater than 500 msec.
- Monitor ECG for arrhythmias and conduction changes.
- Monitor patient for CNS, GI, and general body side effects. Report to health care provider if noted and significant.

Patient/Family Education
- Explain name, dose, action, and potential side effects of drug.
- Advise patient that each dose may be taken without regard to meals.
- Instruct patient that if a dose is missed, do not double up. Advise patient to take the next dose at the usual time.
- Caution patient NOT to change the dose or discontinue therapy unless advised to do so by health care provider.
- Instruct patient in BP and pulse measurement skills.
- Instruct patient to immediately report any of these symptoms to health care provider: dizziness or weakness associated with change in pulse; excessive or prolonged diarrhea, sweating or vomiting; loss of appetite or thirst.
- Instruct patient to not take any prescription or *otc* medications or dietary supplements unless advised to do so by health care provider.
- Instruct patient to notify health care provider if they are hospitalized or prescribed a new medication for any condition.
- Instruct women to notify health care provider if they become pregnant, plan on becoming pregnant, or are breastfeeding.
- Advise patient that follow-up visits and laboratory tests will be required to monitor therapy and to be sure and keep appointments.

Dolasetron Mesylate

(dahl-AH-set-rahn)

Class Antiemetic/Antinauseant

How Supplied
Anzemet Injection 20 mg/mL, Tablets 50 mg, Tablets 100 mg

Action
PHARMACOLOGY: Selective serotonin (5-HT$_3$) receptor antagonist that inhibits serotonin receptors in the GI tract and chemoreceptor zone.

PHARMACOKINETICS/DYNAMICS:
Absorption: Parent drug rapidly eliminated and completely metabolized to hydrodolasetron (active). T_{max} for hydrodolasetron is approximately 1 hr (oral) and approximately 0.6 hr (IV). Bioavailability is approximately 75% (determined by hydrodolasetron).

Distribution: Vd approximately 5.8 L/kg (hydrodolasetron). Hydrodolasetron is 69% to 77% protein bound.

Metabolism: Reduced to hydrodolasetron by carbonyl reductase. Subsequent hydroxylation due to CYP2D6 and N-oxidation due to CYP3A and flavin monooxygenase.

Excretion: Approximately 67% of dose recovered in the urine (61% as hydrodolasetron) and approximately 33% recovered in the feces.

$t_{½}$ less than 10 min for dolasetron (IV), approximately 7.3 hr for hydrodolasetron (IV), and approximately 8.1 hr (oral).

Cl approximately 9.4 mL/min/kg (IV) and approximately 13.4 mL/min/kg (oral) for hydrodolasetron.

Indications
Parenteral or oral: Prevention of nausea and vomiting associated with initial and repeat courses of emetogenic chemotherapy; prevention of postoperative nausea and vomiting in patients at risk.

Parenteral only: Treatment of postoperative nausea and vomiting. **Unlabeled use(s):** Radiotherapy-induced nausea and vomiting.

Contraindications
Standard considerations.

Route/Dosage
Prevention of Chemotherapy-Induced Nausea and Vomiting
ADULTS AND CHILDREN OLDER THAN 16 YR: **PO** 100 mg within 1 hr before chemotherapy. **IV** 1.8 mg/kg (or 100 mg) infused rapidly over 30 sec or diluted and infused over 15 min, 30 min before chemotherapy.

CHILDREN 2 TO 16 YR: **PO** 1.8 mg/kg (max 100 mg) within 1 hr before chemotherapy. **IV** 1.8 mg/kg (max 100 mg) infused rapidly over 30 sec or diluted and infused over 15 min, 30 min before chemotherapy.

Prevention of Postoperative Nausea and Vomiting in Patients at Risk
ADULTS AND CHILDREN OLDER THAN 16 YR: **PO** 100 mg within 2 hr before surgery. **IV** 12.5 mg 15 min before cessation of anesthesia.
CHILDREN 2 TO 16 YR: **PO** 1.2 mg/kg (max of 100 mg) within 2 hr before surgery. **IV** 0.35 mg/kg (max of 12.5 mg) 15 min before cessation of anesthesia.

Treatment of Postoperative Nausea and Vomiting
ADULTS AND CHILDREN OLDER THAN 16 YR: **IV** 12.5 mg as a single dose as soon as nausea and vomiting presents.
CHILDREN 2 TO 16 YR: **IV** 0.35 mg/kg as a single dose as soon as nausea and vomiting present.

Interactions
Drugs that prolong the QTc interval (eg, quinidine, etc.): Additive effects on conduction.
Atenolol: Increased serum levels of active metabolite (IV only).
Cimetidine: Increased serum levels of active metabolite.
Rifampin: Decreased serum levels of active metabolite.

Lab Test Interferences None well documented.

Adverse Reactions
CV: Tachycardia; bradycardia; flushing; hypertension; hypotension.
CNS: Headache; vertigo; dizziness agitation; drowsiness; sleep disorder; depersonalization.
DERM: Rash; itching; sweating.
GI: Abdominal pain; constipation; diarrhea; dyspepsia; anorexia; taste perversion; abnormal liver function.
GU: Oliguria; urinary retention.
OTHER: Fever; fatigue; pain; chills; shivering.

Precautions
Pregnancy: Category B.
Lactation: Undetermined.
Children: Safety and efficacy in children younger than 2 yr not established.
Conditions predisposing to prolongation of cardiac conduction intervals (eg, electrolyte abnormalities, class 1A antiarrhythmias): Use with caution.
ECG Changes: Can cause ECG interval change (PR, QTc, JT) prolongation and QRS widening) which could cause cardiovascular consequences, including heart block and arrhythmias. These changes are related in magnitude and frequency to the active metabolite.

PATIENT CARE CONSIDERATIONS
Administration/Storage
- Administer oral dose without regard to food.
- Dolasetron injection may be mixed with apple or apple-grape juice for oral administration in pediatric patients. Use within 2 hrs of dilution.
- Dolasetron injection can be infused IV as rapidly as 100 mg/30 sec or diluted in 50 mL of a compatible IV solution and infused over a period of up to 15 min.
- Compatible IV fluids include: 0.9% Sodium Chloride, 5% Dextrose, 5% Dextrose and 0.45% Sodium Chloride, 5% Dextrose and Lactated Ringer's Injection, Lactated Ringer's Injection and 10% Mannitol Injection.
- Do not mix dolasetron injection with solution for which compatibility has not been established.
- Do not mix dolasetron injection with other drugs.
- Flush infusion line before and after administration of dolasetron injection.
- Inspect injectable solutions for particulate matter or discoloration before use.

- Diluted injection is stable for 24 hr at room temperature or for 48 hr if refrigerated.
- Store tablets and undiluted injection at room temperature protected from light.

Assessment/Interventions
- Obtain patient history, including drug history and any known allergies. Note risk factors that can cause ECG interval changes.
- Assess patient for nausea, vomiting, and side effects.
- Monitor I&O carefully.
- Be prepared to give additional IV fluids to patient who is vomiting but do not overhydrate.

Patient/Family Education
- Advise patient that headache is common side effect.
- Advise patient that medication will greatly reduce likelihood of nausea and vomiting but that these are still possible

Donepezil

(Dawn-epp-uh-zill)
Class Reversible cholinesterase inhibitor
How Supplied
Aricept Tablets 5 mg, Tablets 10 mg

Action
PHARMACOLOGY: Increases acetylcholine by inhibiting acetylcholinesterase, thereby increasing cholinergic function.

PHARMACOKINETICS/DYNAMICS:
Absorption: Bioavailability is 100%. T_{max} is 3 to 4 hr.

Distribution: Vd is 12 L/kg (at steady state). Approximately 96% protein bound (75% to albumin and 21% alpha-$_1$ acid glycoprotein)

Metabolism: Metabolized by CYP 2D6 and 3A4 and undergoes glucuronidation to 4 major metabolites (2 active) and several minor metabolites.

Excretion: t½ approximately 70 hr. Cl is 0.13 L/hr/kg. Approximately 57% recovered in urine and 15% in feces; approximately 17% of dose recovered unchanged in urine.

Special Populations:
Hepatic Function Impairment – Clearance decreased in patients with stable alcoholic cirrhosis.

Indications Treatment of mild to moderate dementia of the Alzheimer type.

Contraindications Hypersensitivity to donepezil or piperidine derivatives.

Route/Dosage
ADULTS: PO 5 mg once daily. May increase to 10 mg qd after 4 to 6 wk.

Interactions
Anticholinergic drugs: Possible reduction of anticholinergic effects.

Cholinesterase inhibitors/Cholinomimetics: Synergistic effects may occur.

Lab Test Interferences None well documented.

Adverse Reactions
CV: Syncope; chest pain; hypertension; hypotension; vasodilation; atrial fibrillation; hot flashes; delusions; tremor; irritability; paresthesia; aggression; vertigo; ataxia; increased libido; restlessness; abnormal crying; nervousness; aphasia.
CNS: Depression; abnormal dreams; somnolence; insomnia; fatigue; dizziness.
DERM: Diaphoresis; urticaria; pruritus.
EENT: Cataract; eye irritation; blurred vision.
GI: Nausea; diarrhea; vomiting; anorexia; fecal incontinence; GI bleeding; bloating; epigastric pain.
GU: Frequent urination; urinary incontinence; nocturia.
HEMA: Anemia; thrombocytopenia; eosinophilia.
METAB: Weight decrease; dehydration.
RESP: Dyspnea; sore throat; bronchitis.
OTHER: Muscle cramps; arthritis; tooth pain.

Precautions
Pregnancy: Category C.
Lactation: Undetermined.
Children: Safety and efficacy not established.
Concomitant medical conditions: Increases cholinergic activity and therefore can affect other organ systems, possibly leading to bradycardia, bladder outflow obstruction, increased gastric acid secretion, or bronchoconstriction. Use drug with caution in patients susceptible to these effects.

Overdosage: Signs and Symptoms
Cholinergic crisis (eg, severe nausea, vomiting, salivation, sweating, bradycardia, hypotension, respiratory depression, muscle weakness, collapse, convulsions).

PATIENT CARE CONSIDERATIONS
Administration/Storage
- Available only in PO form at this time.
- Administer as a single dose daily, in the evening, just before retiring.
- Store at room temperature (59° to 86°F).
- May be administered with or without food.

Assessment/Interventions
- Obtain complete patient history, including drug history and any known allergies. Note

current cardiac, GI, GU, or pulmonary conditions.
- Evaluate patient's mental status and function prior to initiation of therapy.
- Monitor patient for signs of improvement after therapy is started.
- Monitor patient for side effects of drug. Report any to health care provider.

Patient/Family Education
- Advise patient, family, or caregivers that this drug does not alter the Alzheimer process and that the effectiveness of the medication may lessen over time.
- Advise patient's family or caregivers that side effects tend to diminish as therapy continues.
- Advise patient, family, or caregivers to not discontinue the drug or change the dose unless advised to do so by the health care provider.

Dopamine Hydrochloride

(DOE-puh-meen HIGH-droe-KLOR-ide)

Class Vasopressor

How Supplied
Dopamine Hydrochloride Injection 40 mg/mL, Injection 80 mg/mL, Injection 160 mg/mL ♦
Dopamine Hydrochloride in 5% Dextrose Injection 80 mg/100 mL (0.8 mg/mL), Injection 160 mg/100 mL (1.6 mg/mL), Injection 320 mg/100 mL (3.2 mg/mL)

Action
PHARMACOLOGY: Stimulates beta$_1$ receptors in heart, causing more complete and forceful contractions (inotropy). Also acts on alpha receptors (dose dependent) and has dopaminergic effects.

PHARMACOKINETICS/DYNAMICS:
Distribution: Widely distributed; does not cross the blood-brain barrier to a significant extent.
Metabolism: Metabolized in the liver, kidney, and plasma by MAO and catechol-O-methyltransferase to inactive compounds. Approximately 25% of dose is taken up in the adrenergic nerve terminals where it is hydrolyzed to norepinephrine.
Excretion: t½ approximately 2 min.
Approximately 80% excreted in the urine within 24 hr as metabolites; a very small amount excreted unchanged.
Onset: Within 5 min.
Duration: Less than 10 min.

Indications Correction of hemodynamic imbalances present in shock syndrome after MI, trauma, endotoxic septicemia, surgery and renal failure or imbalances in conditions of chronic refractory cardiac decompensation (eg, CHF).

Contraindications Pheochromocytoma; uncorrected tachyarrhythmias; ventricular fibrillation.

Route/Dosage
ADULTS: **IV** Initial dose 2 to 5 mcg/kg/min with incremental changes of 5 to 10 mcg/kg/min at 10 to 15 min intervals until adequate response is noted. Most patients are maintained at less than 20 mcg/kg/min. If dosage exceeds 50 mcg/kg/min, assess renal function frequently.

Interactions
Furazolidone, methyldopa, rauwolfia alkaloids: Hypertension may result.
Guanethidine: Antihypertensive effects of guanethidine may be negated.
MAOIs: May greatly increase pressor response from dopamine.
Phenytoin: Severe hypotension and bradycardia may result after concomitant administration with dopamine.
Tricyclic antidepressants: May decrease pressor response from dopamine.
INCOMPATIBILITIES: Chemically incompatible with alkaline solutions (drug is inactivated).

Lab Test Interferences None well documented.

Adverse Reactions
CV: Ectopic beats; tachycardia; anginal pain; palpitation; hypotension; vasoconstriction; ventricular arrhythmias (at high doses); hypertension.
CNS: Headache; anxiety.
EENT: Dilated pupils (at high doses).
GI: Nausea; vomiting.
GU: Decreased urine output.
RESP: Dyspnea.
OTHER: Gangrene of extremities.

Precautions
Pregnancy: Category C.
Lactation: Undetermined.
Children: Safety and efficacy not established.
Special risk patients: Do not give in presence of uncorrected tachyarrhythmias or ventricular fibrillation.
Sulfite sensitivity: Use caution in sulfite-sensitive individuals; some commercial preparations contain sodium bisulfite.
Extravasation: Avoid by infusing into large vein and monitoring infusion carefully.

Overdosage: Signs and Symptoms
Hypertension.

PATIENT CARE CONSIDERATIONS
Administration/Storage
- Administer by IV infusion only. Metering device is essential for controlling rate of flow.
- Dopamine is potent drug. Dilute before use if not prediluted.
- Dilute medication just prior to administration. Solution is stable for 24 hr after dilution.
- Do not use if solution is discolored.
- Store at room temperature and protect from light. Discard dissolved solution.

Assessment/Interventions
- Obtain patient history, including drug history and any known allergies.
- Monitor vital signs and ECG closely throughout therapy.
- Monitor I&O regularly. Notify health care provider promptly if urine output decreases.
- Monitor IV rate for free flow throughout administration.
- Monitor central venous pressure or pulmonary wedge pressure if possible during infusion.
- Observe infusion site for extravasation. If extravasation occurs, treat by infiltrating the area with 10 to 15 mL of normal saline containing 5 to 10 mg of phentolamine.
- Notify health care provider immediately if these signs occur: significant changes in vital signs, ECG changes (eg, arrhythmias, tachycardia); deterioration of peripheral pulses, and cold, mottled extremities.

Patient/Family Education
- Instruct patient to inform nurse immediately if these signs occur: chest pain, dyspnea, numbness, tingling or burning of extremities, and discomfort at IV site.

Dornase Alfa (Recombinant Human Deoxyribonuclease; DNase)
(DOR-nace AL-fuh)

Class Respiratory inhalant/enzyme

How Supplied
Pulmozyme Solution for inhalation 1 mg/mL

Action
PHARMACOLOGY: Cleaves DNA released by neutrophils that are mobilized to respiratory tract in response to infection, reducing viscoelasticity of purulent lung secretions, increasing airflow, and decreasing risk of infection.

Indications
Treatment of cystic fibrosis.

Contraindications
Hypersensitivity to Chinese hamster ovary cell products.

Route/Dosage
ADULTS AND CHILDREN OLDER THAN 5 YR:
Inhalation 2.5 mg once daily by oral inhalation via nebulizer; patients older than 21 yr and those with baseline forced vital capacity more than 85% benefit from 2.5 mg bid.

Interactions
None well documented.

Lab Test Interferences
None well documented.

Adverse Reactions
CV: Chest pain.
DERM: Rash.
EENT: Conjunctivitis; sore throat; voice alterations; hoarseness.
RESP: Hoarseness; pharyngitis; laryngitis.

Precautions
Pregnancy: Category B.
Lactation: Undetermined.
Children: Safety and efficacy in children younger than 5 yr not established.

PATIENT CARE CONSIDERATIONS
Administration/Storage
- Use in conjunction with standard therapies for cystic fibrosis.
- Discard solution if cloudy or discolored.
- Discard unused portions of ampules.
- Do not dilute or mix drug with other drugs in nebulizer.
- Keep refrigerated and protected from strong light. Storing at room temperature for less than 24 hr does not adversely affect product.

Assessment/Interventions
- Obtain patient history, including drug history and any known allergies.
- Assess patient's ability to clear secretions. Provide assistance with coughing, positioning (semi-Fowler's or sitting upright) and suctioning.
- Provide hydration to liquefy secretions and replace fluids.
- Perform auscultation to determine quality of breath sounds. Note characteristics of cough and sputum.
- Perform chest physiotherapy (percussion and postural drainage) as ordered.

Patient/Family Education
- Teach patient to follow manufacturer's instructions on use and maintenance of nebulizer and compression system.
- Instruct patient in proper administration and storage of drug.
- Tell patient that drug may cause sore throat, voice alterations or hoarseness and to inform health care provider if these or any other symptoms become bothersome.
- Inform patient that benefits of treatment may not become apparent for months.
- Emphasize importance of avoiding contraction of respiratory infections.

Dorzolamide

(dore-ZOLE-uh-mide)

Class Carbonic anhydrase inhibitor

How Supplied
Trusopt Solution 2%

Action
PHARMACOLOGY: Inhibits carbonic anhydrase enzyme, reducing rate of aqueous humor formation and thus lowering IOP.

Indications Treatment of elevated IOP in patients with ocular hypertension or open-angle glaucoma.

Contraindications Hypersensitivity to other sulfonamides.

Route/Dosage
ADULTS: **Ophthalmic** One drop in affected eye(s) tid.

Interactions None well documented.

Lab Test Interferences None well documented.

Adverse Reactions
CNS: Headache.
EENT: Ocular burning, stinging or discomfort; superficial punctate keratitis; blurred vision; tearing; conjunctivitis; ocular dryness; photophobia; ocular allergic reaction.
OTHER: Nausea; bitter taste.

Precautions
Pregnancy: Category C.
Lactation: Unknown.
Children: Safety and efficacy not established.
Renal function impairment: Not recommended for use in patients with severe renal impairment.
Hepatic function impairment: Use with caution.
Bacterial keratitis: Can occur by using contaminated eye drops.
Concomitant use of oral carbonic anhydrase inhibitors: Not recommended.
Contact lenses: Do not administer while wearing soft contact lenses; preservative may be absorbed by soft contact lenses.

Overdosage: Signs and Symptoms
Electrolyte imbalance, acidotic state, possible CNS effects.

PATIENT CARE CONSIDERATIONS

Administration/Storage
- Wash hands before and after using.
- To avoid contamination, do not touch tip of container to any surface or to eye structures.
- Administer only to affected eye.
- Gently apply pressure over nasolacrimal drainage system for 1 to 2 min after administration.
- Replace cap after administration and keep tightly closed when not in use.
- If used concomitantly with other topical ophthalmic drug products, wait 10 min between administering medications.
- Do not use with soft contact lenses. They may absorb the preservative.
- Other therapeutic interventions should be used in conjunction with dorzolamide in the treatment of acute narrow angle glaucoma.
- Store at room temperature, protected from light.

Assessment/Interventions
- Obtain patient history.
- Obtain baseline lab work including electrolytes and RBCs.
- Note baseline intraocular pressure before starting medication.

Patient/Family Education
- Instruct patient in proper administration of eye drop medications.
- Instruct patient about the need to keep the tip of the dropper clean to prevent eye infections.
- Inform patient that eye drops commonly produce transient stinging or discomfort upon administration, and to notify healthcare provider if they are severe.
- Stress need to return to healthcare provider frequently for monitoring of eye pressure.
- Inform patient not to wear soft contact lenses while using this medication.
- Inform patient that they may experience a bitter taste in mouth immediately after administration.
- Explain the need to be cautions when driving

or participating in activities requiring close hand-eye coordination.
- Instruct patient to notify the healthcare provider if any symptoms of eye infection (ie, burning, redness, itching, possible discharge) occur.

Dorzolamide Hydrochloride/ Timolol Maleate

(dore-ZOLE-uh-mide/TI-moe-lahl MAL-ee-ate)

Class Carbonic anhydrase inhibitor/Beta adrenergic blocker

How Supplied
Cosopt Solution 2% dorzolamide, 0.5% timolol

Action
PHARMACOLOGY: Inhibits carbonic anhydrase enzyme, reducing rate of aqueous humor formation thus lowering IOP (dorzolamide); reduces elevated and normal IOP via decreasing production of aqueous humor or increasing flow (timolol).

Indications Reduction of IOP in patients with ocular hypertension or open-angle glaucoma.

Contraindications Bronchial asthma; history of bronchial asthma; severe chronic obstructive pulmonary disease; sinus bradycardia; second or third degree atrioventricular block; overt cardiac failure; cardiogenic shock; hypersensitivity to any component of product.

Route/Dosage
ADULTS: **Ophthalmic** 1 drop in affected eye(s) bid.

Interactions
Acid-base disturbances: Although not reported with ophthalmic use of dorzolamide, oral administration has caused acid-base and electrolyte disturbances, which may interfere with renal elimination of certain drugs (eg, salicylates).
Beta-adrenergic blocking agents: Potential additive effect on beta blockade.
Calcium antagonists: Possible increased risk of atrioventricular conduction disturbances, left ventricular failure, and hypotension.
Carbonic anhydrase inhibitors: Potential additive effect on patients receiving an oral carbonic anhydrase inhibitor.
Catecholamine-depleting drugs (eg, reserpine): Possible additive effect with timolol, producing hypotension and bradycardia, which may result in vertigo, syncope, and postural hypotension.
Clonidine: Increased risk of rebound hypertension following clonidine withdrawal may be exacerbated.
Digitalis and calcium antagonists: With these agents, timolol has an additive effect in prolonging atrioventricular conduction.
Quinidine: Systemic effect of timolol may be potentiated because of increased plasma levels (eg, decreased heart rate).

Lab Test Interferences None well documented.

Adverse Reactions
CV: Hypertension; bradycardia; cardiac failure; cerebral vascular accident; chest pain; hypotension; MI; arrhythmias, syncope, heart block, cerebral ischemia, worsening of angina pectoris, palpitations, cardiac arrest, edema, claudication (timolol).
CNS: Dizziness; headache; depression; fatigue; signs and symptoms of myasthenia gravis, somnolence, insomnia, nightmares, behavioral changes, psychic disturbances (eg, confusion), hallucinations, anxiety, disorientation, nervousness, memory loss (timolol).
DERM: Contact dermatitis (dorzolamide); alopecia, psoriasiform rash, exacerbation of psoriasis, pruritus, urticaria (timolol).
EENT: Ocular burning and stinging; conjunctival hyperemia; blurred vision; superficial punctate keratitis; eye itching; blepharitis; cloudy vision; conjunctival discharge, edema, follicles, or infection; conjunctivitis; corneal erosion; corneal staining; cortical lens opacity; cough; dry eyes; eye debris, discharge, pain, tearing, or edema; eyelid erythema, exudates, scales, pain or discomfort; foreign body sensation; glaucomatous cupping; lens nucleus coloration; lens opacity; nuclear lens opacity; pharyngitis; post-subcapsular cataract; sinusitis; visual field defect; vitreous detachment; throat irritation, eyelid crusting, transient myopia (dorzolamide); ptosis, decreased corneal sensitivity, cystoid macular edema, visual disturbances (eg, refractive changes, diplopia), pseudopemphigoid, choroidal detachment after filtration surgery, tinnitus (timolol).
GI: Bitter, sour, or unusual taste; abdominal pain; dyspepsia; nausea; anorexia (timolol).
GU: Urinary tract infection; urolithiasis; retroperitoneal fibrosis, impotence, Peyronie disease (timolol).
RESP: Bronchitis; influenza; upper respiratory infection; respiratory failure; pulmonary edema, bronchospasm (timolol).
OTHER: Back pain; allergic hypersensitivity, asthenia (dorzolamide/timolol); systemic lupus erythematosus, Reynaud phenomenon, cold hands and feet, decreased libido (timolol).

Precautions
Pregnancy: Category C.
Lactation:
Dorzolamide – Undetermined.
Timolol – Excreted in breast milk.
Children: Safely and efficacy not established.
Cardiac failure: Inhibition of beta-adrenergic receptor blockade may precipitate more severe cardiac failure in patients with diminished myocardial contractility.
Diabetes mellitus: Use with caution; beta-adrenergic blocking agents may mask the signs and symptoms of acute hypoglycemia.
Major surgery: Some patients receiving beta-adrenergic receptor blocking agents have experienced protracted severe hypotension during surgery.
Thyrotoxicosis: Beta-adrenergic blocking agents may mask certain signs of hyperthyroidism (eg, tachycardia); abrupt withdrawal of agent may precipitate thyroid storm.

Overdosage: Signs and Symptoms
Electrolyte imbalance, acidotic state, dizziness, headache, shortness of breath, bradycardia, bronchospasm; cardiac arrest, possible CNS effects.

PATIENT CARE CONSIDERATIONS

Administration/Storage
- Sulfonamide allergy: discontinue if signs of hypersensitivity reaction occurs.
- Instill 1 drop bid.
- If using other topical ophthalmic drugs, separate each medication by at least 5 min.
- Store at controlled room temperature. Keep container tightly closed and protected from light.

Assessment/Interventions
- Obtain patient history, including drug history and any known allergies. Note history of asthma, severe COPD, bradycardia, AV block, CHF, or renal or hepatic impairment.
- Ensure that IOPs have been measured and documented in the patient's record.

Patient/Family Education
- Explain name, dose, action, and potential side effects of drug.
- Advise patient that usual dose is 1 drop in the affected eye(s) bid.
- Teach patient proper technique for instilling eye drops: wash hands; do not allow dropper to touch eye. Tilt head back, look up; pull lower eyelid down; instill prescribed number of drops. Close eye for 1 to 2 min and apply gentle pressure to bridge of nose for 3 to 5 min. Do not rub eye.
- Advise patient that if more than 1 topical ophthalmic drug is being used, administer the drugs at least 10 min apart.
- Inform patients that taste abnormalities (eg, bitter, sour, unusual taste) and burning or stinging of the eye are the most common side effects. Inform patients to contact their health care provider if side effects occur and are bothersome.
- Advise patients who wear contact lenses to remove their lenses before instilling this medicine and to wait at least 15 min after instilling eye drop before inserting their lenses.
- Advise patients to contact their eye care physician if eye or eyelid inflammation is noted or if they injure their eye or are going to have surgery on their eye.
- Remind patient that eye examinations and measurement of IOP will be necessary while using this medication and to be sure to keep appointments.

Doxapram Hydrochloride

(DOX-uh-pram HIGH-droe-KLOR-ide)
Class CNS stimulant/Analeptic

How Supplied
Dopram Injection 20 mg/mL

Action
PHARMACOLOGY: Increases depth of respirations (tidal volume) by stimulating respiratory center in CNS; respiratory rate may increase slightly. May elevate BP by increasing cardiac output. Respiratory depression from opiates is reversed without affecting pain relief.

PHARMACOKINETICS/DYNAMICS:
Metabolism: Extensively metabolized.
Excretion: Metabolites and a small amount of unchanged drug excreted in urine. t½ is 2.4 to 4.1 hr.

Onset: 20 to 40 sec.

Peak: 1 to 2 min.

Duration: 5 to 12 min.

Indications Reversal of respiratory depression caused by anesthesia (other than muscle relaxants) or drug overdose; temporary measure for acute respiratory failure in patients with COPD who are not undergoing mechanical ventilation.
Unlabeled use(s): Low doses of doxapram have been used in the treatment of apnea of prematurity when methylxanthines have failed.

Contraindications Use in newborns (contains benzyl alcohol); seizures; muscle paresis; epilepsy or other convulsive states; flail chest;

head injury; pneumothorax; acute asthma; pulmonary fibrosis; other conditions that restrict chest wall, respiratory muscles or alveolar expansion; severe hypertension; CVA.

Route/Dosage

Anesthesia-induced Respiratory Depression
ADULTS: **Bolus IV injection** 0.5 to 1 mg/kg (single dose not to exceed 1.5 mg/kg). Can be given as multiple IV injections q 5 min (not to exceed total dose of 2 mg/kg). **IV infusion** Initial rate 5 mg/min until satisfactory respiratory response is noted. Maintenance rate: 1 to 3 mg/min. Max total infusion dose is 4 mg/kg.

Drug-induced CNS Depression
ADULTS: Max daily dose is 3 g. **Bolus IV injection** Priming dose is 2 mg/kg. Repeat in 5 min. Depending on response, may give q 1 to 2 hr. **Intermittent IV infusion** Priming dose is 2 mg/kg. If respirations improve, give by IV infusion at 1 to 2 mg/min. Discontinue after 2 hr or if patient awakens.

Acute Hypercapnia from COPD
ADULTS: **IV infusion** 2 mg/mL with initial rate of 1 to 2 mg/min; may increase to max 3 mg/min; discontinue after 2 hr.

Interactions

Cyclopropane, enflurane, halothane: To prevent arrhythmias, wait at least 10 min after stopping these anesthetics before giving doxapram.
MAOIs, sympathomimetics: Increased risk of hypertension.
Muscle relaxants: Residual effects may be temporarily masked by doxapram.
INCOMPATIBILITIES: Do not add to or give with alkaline solutions such as aminophylline, thiopental, or sodium bicarbonate.

Lab Test Interferences None well documented.

Adverse Reactions

CV: Arrhythmias; tachycardia; increased BP; tightness in chest; chest pain; phlebitis.
CNS: Seizures; paresthesia; increased reflexes; disorientation; dizziness; involuntary movements.
EENT: Mydriasis.
GI: Nausea; vomiting; diarrhea; desire to defecate.
GU: Urinary incontinence and retention; elevation of BUN.
HEMA: Hemolysis (with rapid infusion).
RESP: Laryngospasm; bronchospasm; rebound hypoventilation; cough; hiccoughs; dyspnea.
OTHER: Flushing; feelings of warmth; sweating.

Precautions

Pregnancy: Category B.
Lactation: Undetermined.
Children: Safety and efficacy not established in children younger than 12 yr. Doxapram contains benzyl alcohol, which has been associated with fatal "gasping syndrome" in premature infants.
COPD patients: Do not increase infusion rate in severely ill patients; drug may increase work of breathing.
Drug-induced CNS and respiratory depression: Used as adjunct to supportive care.
Postanesthesia: Do not use as antidote for opiates or neuromuscular blockers.

Overdosage: Signs and Symptoms

Severe hypertension, tachycardia, hyperactive reflexes, seizures.

PATIENT CARE CONSIDERATIONS

Administration/Storage

- Ensure that patent airway has been established before administration.
- Do not give in conjunction with mechanical ventilation.
- Have readily available oxygen, IV barbiturates (eg, Valium) and resuscitative equipment.
- Allow 10 min after administration of anesthetic before starting infusion.
- Rotate injection sites to avoid skin irritation.
- For intermittent infusion, dilute 250 mg in 250 mL of D5W, D10W, or 0.9% normal saline for concentration of 1 mg/mL. Dilute 400 mg in 180 mL of IV fluid for 2 mg/mL concentration.
- Store at room temperature.

Assessment/Interventions

- Obtain patient history, including drug history and any known allergies. Note any history of seizure disorder.
- Assess BP, pulse, deep tendon reflexes, neurologic status, ECG, and ABGs before infusion and q 30 min during infusion.
- Institute seizure precautions before administering drug.
- Assess for poststimulation respiratory depression for at least 30 min to 1 hr after patient becomes alert.
- Monitor respiratory status Position patient on side in slightly elevated position to prevent aspiration.
- Monitor BP and deep tendon reflexes to prevent overdosage.
- Monitor patient's CBC; rapid infusion can cause hemolysis.
- If ABGs deteriorate, notify health care provider immediately. Drug may need to be discontinued and mechanical ventilation started.
- Check infusion site regularly for extravasation, skin irritation, and signs of thrombophlebitis.

Patient/Family Education
- Instruct patient/family to notify health care provider immediately if shortness of breath worsens.

Doxazosin Mesylate

(DOX-uh-ZOE-sin MEH-suh-late)

Class Antihypertensive/Antiadrenergic, peripherally acting

How Supplied
Cardura Tablets 1 mg, Tablets 2 mg, Tablets 4 mg, Tablets 8 mg
🍁 Apo-Doxazosin ♦ Cardura-1 ♦ Cardura-2 ♦ Cardura-4 ♦ Gen-Doxazosin ♦ Novo-Doxazosin ♦ ratio-Doxazosin

Action
PHARMACOLOGY: Selectively blocks postsynaptic alpha$_1$-adrenergic receptors, resulting in dilation of arterioles and veins.

PHARMACOKINETICS/DYNAMICS:
Absorption: T_{max} is 2 to 3 hr. Bioavailability approximately 65%. Enterohepatic recycling. Food decreases C_{max} 18% and AUC 12%.

Metabolism:
Liver – First-pass metabolism; extensively metabolized by O-demethylation or hydroxylation to several active metabolites.

Excretion: The t½ is approximately 22 hr.
Feces – 63% of dose; 4.8% as unchanged drug.
Urine – 9% of dose; trace amount as unchanged drug. Elimination is biphasic.

Special Populations:
Cirrhosis patients – 40% increase in exposure.

Indications Treatment of hypertension, alone or in combination with other agents; treatment of benign prostatic hyperplasia (BPH).

Contraindications Hypersensitivity to doxazosin, prazosin, or terazosin.

Route/Dosage
Hypertension
ADULTS: PO
Initial dose: 1 mg qd.
Maintenance: Based on standing BP response, may increase to 2 mg and thereafter to 4, 8, and 16 mg.

Benign Prostatic Hyperplasia
ADULTS: PO
INITIAL DOSE: 1 mg/day.
MAINTENANCE: Increase to 2 mg, and thereafter to 4 and 8 mg qd, which is the max dose for BPH. Recommended titration interval is 1 to 2 wk.

PATIENT CARE CONSIDERATIONS

Administration/Storage
- Administer prescribed dose qd, morning or evening, without regard to meals or food. Administer with food if GI upset occurs.

Interactions
Cimetidine: 10% increase in mean AUC of doxazosin.

Lab Test Interferences None well documented.

Adverse Reactions
CV: Hypotension, palpitation (2%); arrhythmia, hypotension (1%).
CNS: Dizziness (19%); headache (14%); fatigue/malaise (12%); somnolence (5%); vertigo, nervousness (2%); anxiety, kinetic disorders, ataxia, hypertonia, muscle cramps, insomnia, depression (1%).
EENT: Abnormal vision (2%); tinnitus, conjunctivitis, eye pain (1%).
GI: Nausea (3%); dry mouth, diarrhea (2%); constipation, dyspepsia, flatulence (1%).
GU: Sexual dysfunction, polyuria (2%); urinary incontinence (1%).
METAB: Edema (4%); face edema (1%).
MUSC: Arthralgia/arthritis, muscle weakness, myalgia (1%).
RESP: Dyspnea, rhinitis (3%); respiratory disorder (1%).
OTHER: Pain, chest pain (2%); flushing, rash, pruritus (1%).

Precautions
Pregnancy: Category C.
Lactation: Undetermined.
Children: Safety and efficacy not established.
Hepatic function impairment: Use drug with extreme caution.
"First-dose" effect: Marked hypotension (especially orthostatic) and syncope may occur 2 to 6 hr after first few doses, after reintroduction, with rapid increase in dosing or after addition of another antihypertensive.
Leukopenia/Neutropenia: Mean WBC and neutrophil counts decreased by 2.4% and 1%, respectively. No patients became symptomatic as a result of the low WBC or neutrophil count.
Lipids: Slight decrease in total serum cholesterol and LDL may occur as well as increase in HDL.
Priapism: Occurs rarely, may lead to permanent impotence if not promptly treated.
Prostate cancer: Rule out before starting therapy.

Overdosage: Signs and Symptoms
Hypotension.

- Use alone or in combination with other antihypertensives when treating hypertension.
- Store at controlled room temperature (59° to 86°F).

Assessment/Interventions

- Obtain patient history, including drug history and any known allergies. Note hypersensitivity to quinazolines (eg, prazosin, terazosin) or hepatic impairment.
- Ensure that therapy is initiated with 1 mg dose and then gradually increased q 2 wk until max benefit has been achieved.
- Monitor BP and pulse, and patient for evidence of postural hypotension, for 6 hr after the initial dose and after the first dose of a dosage increase. If syncope occurs, place patient in recumbent position and treat with supportive measures. Notify health care provider if symptomatic orthostatic hypotension is noted.
- Implement safety precautions for patients who experience dizziness.
- Monitor and record BP and pulse periodically during treatment in hypertensive patient. If hypotension results, hold medication and notify health care provider. Inform health care provider if BP is not adequately controlled.
- Assess changes in urinary symptoms such as frequency, hesitancy, weak stream, volume, dribbling, and nocturia.
- Monitor patient for GI, CNS, GU, CV, and general body side effects. Report to health care provider if noted and significant.

Patient/Family Education

- Explain name, dose, action, and potential side effects of drug.
- Advise patient to take prescribed dose qd, morning or evening, without regard to meals but to take with food if stomach upset occurs.
- Advise patient that medication will be started at a low dose and then gradually increased as tolerated until max benefit is obtained.
- Caution patient not to change the dose or stop taking unless advised by health care provider.
- Inform hypertensive patient that drug controls but does not cure hypertension and to continue taking drug as prescribed even when BP is not elevated.
- Instruct hypertensive patient to continue taking other BP medications as prescribed by health care provider.
- Emphasize to hypertensive patient importance of the following modalities on BP: weight control, regular exercise, smoking cessation, and moderate intake of alcohol and salt.
- Instruct hypertensive patient in BP and pulse measurement skills.
- Advise hypertensive patient to monitor and record BP and pulse at home and to inform health care provider if abnormal measurements are noted. Also advise patient to take record of BP and pulse to each follow-up visit.
- Caution patient to avoid sudden position changes to prevent orthostatic hypotension.
- Caution patient that drug may cause dizziness or fainting and to avoid driving or performing hazardous tasks for 24 hr after the first dose, after a dosage increase, and after interruptions of therapy when treatment is resumed.
- Advise patient that drug may cause drowsiness and to use caution while driving or performing other tasks requiring mental alertness until tolerance is determined.
- Advise patient with BPH to contact health care provider if urinary symptoms do not improve or if they worsen while taking this medication.
- Instruct patient to report the following symptoms to health care provider: dizziness, fainting, prolonged or painful erection, or bothersome side effects.
- Advise women to notify health care provider if pregnant, planning to become pregnant, or breastfeeding.
- Caution patient not to take any prescription or OTC drugs or dietary supplements unless advised by health care provider.
- Advise patient that follow-up visits may be necessary to monitor therapy and to keep appointments.

Doxepin Hydrochloride

(DOX-uh-pin HIGH-droe-KLOR-ide)

Class Antianxiety/Tricyclic antidepressant

How Supplied

Sinequan Capsules 10 mg, Capsules 25 mg, Capsules 50 mg, Capsules 75 mg, Capsules 100 mg, Capsules 150 mg ♦ *Zonalon* Cream 5%
✤ *Apo-Doxepin* ♦ *Novo-Doxepin*

Action

PHARMACOLOGY: Moderately blocks reuptake of norepinephrine and weakly blocks reuptake of serotonin; also produces antihistaminic and anticholinergic activity.

PHARMACOKINETICS/DYNAMICS:
Absorption: T_{max} is 2 to 8 days (steady-state).

Metabolism: Metabolized in the liver to desmethyldoxepin (active).

Excretion: Urinary excretion; t½ is 8 to 24 hr (oral), 28 to 52 hr (topical).

Indications Treatment of psychoneurotic patients with depression and/or anxiety; depression and/or anxiety associated with alcoholism (not to be taken concomitantly with alcohol); depression and/or anxiety associated with organic disease (the possibility of drug interaction should be considered if the patient is receiving other drugs concomitantly); psychotic depressive disorders with associated anxiety including involutional depression and manic-depressive disorders; moderate pruritus with atopic dermatitis or lichen simplex chronicus (topical). **Unlabeled use(s):** Neurogenic pain, peptic ulcer disease.

Contraindications Hypersensitivity to tricyclic antidepressants; use during acute recovery phase after MI; glaucoma; risk of urinary retention; concomitant use with MAO inhibitor; dibenzoxepines may produce cross-sensitivity.

Route/Dosage

Depression and/or Anxiety

ADULTS: **PO** Initial dose 75 mg/day, increasing as tolerated (max, 300 mg/day). May be given qd or on a divided dosage schedule. If given qd, the max recommended dose is 150 mg/day.
For Mild Cases with Organic Diseases – **PO** 25 to 50 mg/day.

Pruritus

ADULTS: **Topical** Apply thin film qid with at least 3 to 4 hr between applications. Not recommended for more than 8 days.

Interactions

Alcohol/CNS depressants: CNS and respiratory depression may be potentiated.
Cimetidine: May inhibit metabolism of doxepin, leading to increased concentrations.
Clonidine: Concurrent use may lead to loss of BP control and possibly dangerous increases in BP.
Guanethidine: Hypotensive action may be inhibited.
MAO inhibitors: Concurrent use may lead to severe seizures, hyperpyretic crisis, and fatal reactions. Generally, allow 7 to 10 days between discontinuation of 1 drug and start of another.
SSRIs (eg, fluoxetine): May increase serum concentrations of doxepin; effect may occur up to 5 wk after discontinuation of fluoxetine.
Sympathomimetics (eg, dopamine, epinephrine): Pressor response may increase or decrease; arrhythmias may occur.
Type IC antiarrhythmics (eg, propafenone, flecainide): May inhibit metabolism of doxepin, leading to increased concentrations.

Lab Test Interferences None well documented.

Adverse Reactions

CV: Orthostatic hypotension; hypertension; fainting; tachycardia.
CNS: Dizziness; drowsiness; headache; confusion; weakness; tremors; convulsions; fatigue; disorientation; hallucinations; numbness; paresthesias; ataxia; extrapyramidal symptoms; tardive dyskinesia.
DERM: Skin rash; edema; photosensitization; pruritus. Topical use: Local burning or stinging; dry or tight skin.
EENT: Mydriasis; photophobia; blurred vision; tinnitus.
GI: Nausea; constipation; dry mouth; paralytic ileus; vomiting; indigestion; taste perversion; diarrhea; anorexia; aphthous stomatitis.
GU: Urinary retention; nocturia; altered libido; testicular swelling, gynecomastia (males); enlargement of breasts, galactorrhea (females).
HEPA: Jaundice.
HEMA: Agranulocytosis; eosinophilia; purpura; thrombocytopenia; leukopenia.
METAB: Weight gain; syndrome of inappropriate secretion of antidiuretic hormone; raising or lowering of blood sugar levels.
RESP: Exacerbation of asthma.
OTHER: Hyperthermia; alopecia; sweating; chills.

Precautions

Pregnancy: Category C (oral form); category B (topical).
Lactation: Excreted in breast milk.
Children: Not recommended for children younger than 12 yr.
Special risk patients: Use drug with caution in patients with history of seizures, urinary retention, urethral spasm, angle-closure glaucoma or increased IOP, cardiovascular disorders, hyperthyroidism (or those receiving thyroid medication), hepatic or renal impairment, schizophrenia, or paranoia.
Contact sensitization: Use of cream can cause Type IV hypersensitivity reactions.
Suicide: Use drug with caution in patients with suicidal tendencies; do not allow access to large quantities of drug.
Topical use: For external use only; do not use ophthalmically, orally, or intravaginally. Because of absorption of drug, drowsiness often occurs.

Overdosage: Signs and Symptoms

Confusion, agitation, transient visual hallucinations, seizures, hyperactive reflexes, coma, cardiac arrhythmias, dilated pupils, hyperpyrexia, severe hypotension, CNS depression, ECG changes (QRS axis or width), disturbed concentration, stupor, drowsiness, muscle rigidity, vomiting, hypothermia.

PATIENT CARE CONSIDERATIONS

Administration/Storage
* Do not administer with or within 14 days of MAO inhibitor administration.
* Administer prescribed dose without regard to meals. Administer with food if GI upset occurs.
* Store capsules below 86°F.
* The 150 mg capsule strength is intended for maintenance therapy only and is not recommended for initiation of treatment.

Assessment/Interventions
* Obtain patient history, including drug history and any known allergies. Note kidney or liver disease, glaucoma, urinary retention, seizure disorder, sensitivity to other tricyclic antidepressants, concurrent or recent (eg, within 14 days) use of MAO inhibitor, or concurrent use of selective serotonin reuptake inhibitor (SSRI).
* Ensure that reduced initial dose and slower dose escalation are used in elderly patient.
* Continue suicide monitoring of high-risk patients.
* Frequently assess patient for response to treatment. Notify health care provider if condition does not appear to be improving or is worsening.
* Ensure that therapy is periodically reviewed to determine if it needs to be continued without change or if a dose change (eg, increase, decrease, discontinuation) is indicated.
* Observe for signs of mood change and report to health care provider.
* If treatment is to be discontinued, or the dose reduced, gradually taper the dose and monitor patient for withdrawal symptoms (eg, dizziness, abnormal skin sensations, agitation, anxiety, nausea, sweating). If significant withdrawal symptoms develop, reinstitute previous dosing schedule and attempt a less rapid tapering regimen after patient has stabilized.
* Monitor patient for CNS, GI, psychiatric, MUSC, GU, and general body side effects. Report to health care provider if noted and significant.

Patient/Family Education
* Explain name, dose, action, and potential side effects of drug.
* Advise patient to read *Patient Information* leaflet before starting therapy and with each refill.
* Advise patient that medication is usually started at a low dose and then gradually increased as tolerated until max benefit is obtained.
* Advise patient to take prescribed dose without regard to meals, but to take with food if stomach upset occurs.
* Advise patient not to change the dose or stop taking unless advised by health care provider.
* Inform patient that it may take 2 to 6 wk to note improvement in symptoms and to continue with the prescribed therapy once improvement has been noted.
* Instruct patient to contact health care provider if symptoms do not appear to be getting better, are getting worse, or if bothersome side effects (eg, unusual sweating, urination difficulty, drowsiness, dizziness, constipation, changes in sexual function) occur.
* Advise patient to take frequent sips of water, suck on ice chips or sugarless hard candy, or chew sugarless gum if dry mouth occurs.
* Instruct patient to avoid alcoholic beverages and other depressants while taking this medication.
* Advise patient that drug (oral and topical) may cause drowsiness, dizziness, or impair reflexes and to use caution while driving or performing other tasks requiring mental alertness until tolerance is determined.
* Instruct patient not to take prescription or OTC drugs or dietary supplements without consulting health care provider.
* Caution patient to avoid unnecessary exposure to UV light (sunlight, tanning booths) and to use sunscreen and wear protective clothing when exposed to UV light until tolerance is determined.
* Advise women to notify health care provider if pregnant, planning to become pregnant, or breastfeeding.
* Advise patient that follow-up visits may be necessary to monitor therapy and to keep appointments.

Doxorubicin, Conventional

(DOX-oh-ROO-bih-sin)

Class Antineoplastic/Anthracycline antibiotic

How Supplied
Adriamycin RDF Preservative-free solution for injection 2 mg/mL, Lyophilized powder for injection 10 mg, 20 mg, 50 mg, 100 mg, and 150 mg vials, Aqueous injection 2 mg/mL 5 mL, 10 mL, and 25 mL vials ◆ *Adriamycin PFS* Preservative-free solution for injection 2 mg/mL, 5 mL, 10 mL, 25 mL, and 100 mL vials, Aqueous injection 2 mg/mL 5 mL, 10 mL, and 25 mL vials ◆ *Rubex* Preservative-free solution for injec-

tion 2 mg/mL, Aqueous injection 2 mg/mL 5 mL, 10 mL, and 25 mL vials.
✤ Caelyx ◆ Myocet

Action
PHARMACOLOGY: Cells treated with doxorubicin have been shown to manifest the characteristic morphologic changes associated with apoptosis or programmed cell death. Doxorubicin-induced apoptosis may be an integral component of the cellular mechanism of action relating to therapeutic effects, toxicities, or both.

PHARMACOKINETICS/DYNAMICS:

Distribution: Distribution t½ approximately 5 min. Vd greater than 20 to 30 L/kg (at steady state). 74% to 76% protein bound.

Metabolism: Metabolized to doxorubicinol (active).

Excretion: t½ is 20 to 48 hr. Cl is 8 to 20 mL/min/kg. Approximately 40% appears in the bile and 5% to 12% in the urine in 5 days.

Special Populations:
Hepatic Function Impairment – Excretion is slower, resulting in increased retention and accumulation. Reduce dose in those with elevated bilirubin.

Indications
Adult: Leukemias, lymphomas, soft tissue and bone sarcomas; breast, ovarian, transitional cell bladder, thyroid, bronchogenic, and gastric carcinoma.
Children: Leukemias, lymphomas, Wilms tumor, neuroblastoma, bone sarcomas. **Unlabeled use(s):** Refractory multiple myeloma; endometrial, islet cell, and lung carcinomas; AIDS-related Kaposi sarcoma.

Contraindications
Marked myelosuppression induced by previous treatment with other antitumor agents or by radiotherapy; history of hypersensitivity reactions to conventional or liposomal doxorubicin or their components; previous treatment with complete cumulative doses of doxorubicin, daunorubicin, idarubicin, or other anthracyclines and anthracenes.

Route/Dosage
Single Agent Therapy
ADULTS: **IV** 60 to 75 mg/m^2 as a single dose q 21 days. Alternative regimens are 30 mg/m^2/day for 3 successive days q 4 wk; or 20 mg/m^2 once weekly. Give the lower dose to patients with inadequate marrow reserves because of old age, prior therapy, or neoplastic marrow infiltration.

Intravesical Instill 50 mg in the bladder q 3 to 4 wk, retaining the solution in the bladder for 30 to 120 min.
CHILDREN: **IV** 35 to 75 mg/m^2, as a single dose q 21 days. Alternative regimens are 20 mg/m^2 once weekly for 3 wk or 20 mg/m^2/day for 3 successive days q 3 to 4 wk.

Combination Therapy
ADULTS: **IV** 40 to 60 mg/m^2 as a single dose q 21 to 28 days. Give the lower dose to patients with inadequate marrow reserves because of old age, prior therapy, or neoplastic marrow infiltration.

Patients with Elevated Bilirubin
Dosage reduction – If serum bilirubin is 1.2 to 3 mg/dL, give 50% of adjusted dose from prior course. If serum bilirubin is 3.1 to 5 mg/dL, give 25% of adjusted dose from prior course.

Dosage Reduction in Hepatic Insufficiency
If serum bilirubin is 1.2 to 3 mg/dL, give 50% of adjusted dose from prior course. If serum bilirubin is above 3 mg/dL, give 25% of adjusted dose from prior course.

Lifetime Cumulative Doses Above Which Frequency of Cardiotoxicity Increases
ADULTS AND CHILDREN: **IV** No more than 500 mg/m^2.
ADULTS AND CHILDREN WHO HAVE RECEIVED MEDIASTINAL RADIATION: **IV** No more than 400 mg/m^2.
ADULTS OLDER THAN 70 YR WITH OR WITHOUT MEDIASTINAL RADIATION: **IV** No more than 300 mg/m^2.

Interactions
Digoxin: Doxorubicin may decrease oral absorption of digoxin tablets.

Lab Test Interferences None well documented.

Adverse Reactions
CV: Acute arrhythmias; cardiomyopathy.
DERM: Alopecia; facial flushing; hyperpigmentation of nail beds and dermal creases; onycholysis; radiation recall; palmar-plantar erythrodysesthesia; urticaria; vein itching or streaking.
GI: Nausea; vomiting; mucositis; necrotizing colitis.
HEMA: Bone marrow suppression.
HYPERSEN: Anaphylaxis; cross-sensitivity to lincomycin.
OTHER: Fever; chills.

> **WARNING:**
>
> *Cardiac toxicity:* Potentially fatal CHF may occur during therapy or months to years after termination of therapy. The risk of developing CHF increases rapidly with increasing total cumulative doses of doxorubicin in excess of 450 mg/m^2. This toxicity may occur at lower cumulative doses in patients with prior mediastinal irradiation or on concurrent cyclophosphamide therapy or with preexisting heart disease. Pediatric patients are at increased risk for developing delayed cardiotoxicity.
>
> *Extravasation risk:* Local irritation may occur. Refer to institution-specific protocol.
>
> *Hepatic dysfunction:* Reduce dose.
>
> *Myelosuppression:* Severe myelosuppression may occur. Leukopenia is usually transient, reaching its nadir 10 to 14 days after treatment, with recovery usually by day 21. Expect white blood cell counts as low as 1000/mm^3 during treatment.

Precautions

Pregnancy: Category D.

Lactation: Discontinue nursing.

Children: Children are at increased risk for developing delayed cardiotoxicity. Doxorubicin may contribute to prepubertal growth failure. It also may contribute to gonadal impairment, which is usually temporary.

Elevated bilirubin: Some clinicians recommend not giving doxorubicin to patients with a bilirubin above 5 mg/dL.

Necrotizing colitis: Manifested by typhlitis (eg, cecal inflammation, bloody stools, severe and sometimes fatal infections).

Radiation: Radiation-induced toxicity to the myocardium, mucosa, skin, and liver have been increased.

Overdosage: Signs and Symptoms

Acute overdosage enhances the toxic effects of mucositis, leukopenia, pancytopenia, and thrombocytopenia. Chronic overdosage increases the risk of cardiomyopathy and resultant CHF.

PATIENT CARE CONSIDERATIONS

Administration/Storage

- Give by IV push injection or IV side arm into a running infusion.
- Dilute the 10 mg vial with 5 mL, the 20 mg vial with 10 mL, the 50 mg vial with 25 mL, and the 150 mg vial with 75 mL of 0.9% Sodium Chloride for a final concentration of 2 mg/mL. Bacteriostatic diluents are not recommended.
- Extravasation may occur with or without an accompanying burning or stinging sensation. Immediately terminate the injection or infusion and restart in another vein. If extravasation is suspected, intermittent application of ice to the site for 15 min qid for 3 days may be helpful.
- Infusion reactions appear to occur with the first infusion and do not appear to occur with later infusions if not present initially. In most patients, these reactions resolve over the course of several hours to a day once the infusion is terminated. In some patients, slowing the rate of infusion resolves the reaction.
- Phlebosclerosis may occur when small veins or a single vein is used for repeated administration; facial flushing may occur if injection is too rapid.
- Incompatible with heparin, fluorouracil, cephalothin, and dexamethasone sodium phosphate.
- A color change in doxorubicin from red to blue-purple, which denotes decomposition, occurs with aminophylline and 5-fluorouracil. Do not mix doxorubicin with other drugs.
- Store lyophilized powder at room temperature and protect from sunlight.
- Refrigerate preservative-free solution and protect from light.
- Store Bedford aqueous injection in the refrigerator.
- Reconstituted solution is stable for 7 days at room temperature (59° to 86°F) and under normal room light (100 foot-candles) and 15 days under refrigeration (2° to 8°C; 36° to 46°F). Protect from sunlight. Discard any of the unused solution from the 10, 20, and 50 mg single-dose vials. Discard unused solutions of the multiple-dose vial remaining beyond the recommended storage times.
- For intravesical instillation in the bladder, doxorubicin may be diluted in 50 to 150 mL of sterile water or 0.9% Sodium Chloride.

IV infusion:

- Administer slowly into a freely running IV infusion of NaCl Injection or 5% Dextrose

Injection. Attach tubing to a butterfly needle inserted into a large vein. Avoid veins over joints or in extremities with compromised venous or lymphatic drainage. Administer over at least 3 to 5 min. Local erythematous streaking along the vein as well as facial flushing may indicate too rapid administration.

Assessment/Interventions

- Initial treatment requires close patient observation and extensive laboratory monitoring. Hospitalize patients at least during the first phase of treatment. Initial treatment requires observation of the patient and periodic monitoring of CBCs, hepatic function tests, and radionuclide left ventricular ejection fraction.
- Monitor ECG and systolic ejection fraction as the maximum cumulative lifetime dose approaches.
- Assess hepatic function prior to therapy.
- Doxorubicin may cause red discoloration of the urine for 1 to 2 days after administration.
- Mucositis may occur 5 to 10 days after administration, leading to ulceration, and represent a site or origin for severe infections. Incidence and severity of mucositis is greater with the 3 successive daily dosage regimen. Ulceration and necrosis of the colon, especially the cecum, may occur leading to bleeding or severe infections that can be fatal.
- Administration of live vaccines to immunosuppressed patients may be hazardous.

Hyperuricemia:

- Monitor serum uric acid. Minimize effects of hyperuricemia with hydration, urinary alkalinization, and allopurinol.

Patient/Family Education

- Doxorubicin imparts a red color to the urine for 1 to 2 days after administration; advise patients to expect this during active therapy.
- Explain name, action, and potential side effects of drug.
- Advise patient, family, or caregiver that medication will be prepared and administered by health care provider in a health care setting.
- Advise patient, family, or caregiver that medication may be used in combination with other agents to achieve maximum benefit possible.
- Review dosing schedule with patient, family, or caregiver.
- Advise patient, family, or caregiver that medication will usually cause a red coloration of the urine for 1 to 2 days after administration. Advise that this is not a problem and is expected because the medication is being eliminated in the urine.
- Advise patient, family, or caregiver that medication may cause hair loss but that this is reversible when therapy is stopped.
- Advise patient, family, or caregiver to immediately report any of the following to health care provider: rash; hives; difficulty breathing; chest pain; fever, chills, or other signs of infection; sores in mouth; unusual bleeding or bruising; pain, redness, or swelling at injection site.
- Advise patient, family, or caregiver to report any of the following to health care provider: persistent nausea, vomiting, diarrhea or appetite loss; persistent or worsening general body weakness.
- Instruct patient to not take any prescription or otc medications or dietary supplements unless advised by health care provider.
- Caution women of childbearing potential to avoid becoming pregnant while being treated.
- Instruct women of childbearing potential to notify health care provider if becoming pregnant, planning on becoming pregnant, or are breastfeeding.
- Advise patient that following discharge from the hospital that frequent follow-up visits, ECGs, or heart function tests, and laboratory tests will be required to monitor therapy and to keep appointments.

Doxorubicin, Liposomal

(DOX-oh-ROO-bih-sin)

Class Antineoplastic/Anthracycline antibiotic encapsulated in *Stealth* liposomes

How Supplied

Doxil Solution for injection equivalent to 2 mg/mL doxorubicin hydrochloride in 10 mL single-use vials.

Action

PHARMACOLOGY: Binds DNA and inhibits nucleic acid synthesis. Cell structure studies have demonstrated rapid cell penetration and perinuclear chromatin binding, rapid inhibition of mitotic activity and nucleic acid synthesis, and induction of mutagenesis and chromosomal aberrations.

PHARMACOKINETICS/DYNAMICS:

Absorption: C_{max} approximately 4.12 to 8.34 mcg/mL. AUC approximately 277 to 590 mcg/mL•hr.

Distribution: Vd approximately 2.72 to 2.83 L/m² (at steady-state).

Metabolism: Metabolized to doxorubicinol.

Excretion: t½ approximately 4.7 to 5.2 hr (first phase) and approximately 52.3 to 55 hr (second phase). Plasma clearance approximately 0.041 to 0.056 L/hr/m^2

Indications AIDS-related Kaposi sarcoma; refractory metastatic ovarian carcinoma.

Contraindications None well documented.

Route/Dosage

Kaposi Sarcoma
ADULTS: Note: The dose of liposomal doxorubicin is different from the dose of conventional doxorubicin. **IV** 20 mg/m^2/dose over 30 min q 3 wk, for as long as the patient responds satisfactorily and tolerates treatment. Do not administer as a bolus injection or an undiluted solution. Rapid infusion may increase the risk of infusion-related reactions.

Paclitaxel- and Platinum-Refractory Metastatic Ovarian Cancer
ADULTS: **IV** 50 mg/m^2/dose over 1 hr q 4 wk. Give minimum of 4 courses, continuing therapy until disease progression occurs.

Alternative dose schedules:
ADULTS: **IV** Alternative dosing schedules are recommended for patients with palmar-plantar erythrodysesthesia, hematologic toxicity, or stomatitis.

Dosage Adjustment for Impaired Hepatic Function
If serum bilirubin is 1.2 to 3 mg/dL, give 50% of adjusted dose from prior course. If serum bilirubin is greater than 3 mg/dL, give 25% of adjusted dose from prior course.

Lifetime Cumulative Doses Above Which Frequency of Cardiotoxicity Increases
ADULTS: **IV** up to 500 mg/m^2.
ADULTS WHO HAVE RECEIVED MEDIASTINAL RADIATION OR OTHER CARDIOTOXIC DRUGS: **IV** up to 400 mg/m^2.
ADULTS OLDER THAN 70 YR WITH OR WITHOUT MEDIASTINAL RADIATION: **IV** up to 300 mg/m^2.

Interactions

Digoxin: Doxorubicin may decrease oral absorption of digoxin tablets.

Lab Test Interferences None well documented.

Adverse Reactions

CV: Cardiomyopathy; chest pain; hypotension; tachycardia.
CNS: Asthenia; headache; dizziness; somnolence; emotional lability.
DERM: Palmar-plantar skin eruptions; alopecia; rash; itching; radiation recall reactions.
ENDO: Hyperglycemia; albuminuria.
GI: Nausea; vomiting; elevated LFTs; diarrhea; stomatitis; glossitis; oral moniliasis; constipation; anorexia; abdominal pain.
HEMA: Bone marrow suppression.
MUSC: Back pain.
RESP: Dyspnea.
OTHER: Flushing; shortness of breath; facial swelling; headache; chills; back pain; chest or throat tightness; hypotension.

> **WARNING:**
>
> *Acute infusion-associated reactions:* Serious and sometimes life-threatening or fatal allergic/anaphylactoid-like infusion reactions have been reported in up to 10% of patients. Flushing, shortness of breath, facial swelling, headache, chills, back pain, tightness in the chest or throat, and hypotension have occurred. In most patients, these reactions resolve over the course of several hours to a day once the infusion is terminated. In some patients, the reaction resolves by slowing the infusion rate.
>
> *Hepatic function impairment:* Assess hepatic function before initiating therapy. Reduce dosage in patients with impaired hepatic function.
>
> *Myelosuppression:* Severe myelosuppression may occur. It appears to be dose-limiting. Leukopenia, anemia, and thrombocytopenia can also be expected.
>
> *Myocardial toxicity:* Serious irreversible myocardial toxicity with delayed CHF often unresponsive to supportive therapy may occur as total dosage of liposomal doxorubicin approaches 550 mg/m^2. Prior use of other anthracyclines or anthracenediones will reduce the total dose of doxorubicin hydrochloride that can be given without cardiac toxicity. Cardiac toxicity also may occur at lower cumulative doses in patients with prior mediastinal irradiation or who are receiving concurrent cyclophosphamide therapy.
>
> *Substitution of liposomal doxorubicin:* Accidental substitution of liposomal doxorubicin for conventional doxorubicin has resulted in severe side effects. Do not substitute on a mg per mg basis.

Precautions

Pregnancy: Category D.
Lactation: Discontinue nursing prior to taking this drug.
Children: Safety and efficacy not established.
Renal function impairment: Assess renal function before initiating therapy.
Doxorubicin liposomal dose: The dose of liposomal doxorubicin is different from the dose of conventional doxorubicin.

Extravasation risk: Local irritation or phlebitis may occur. Refer to your institution-specific protocol.
Mucositis: May occur 5 to 10 days after administration.
Palmar-plantar erythrodysesthesia: Generally seen after at least 6 wk of treatment.
Radiation therapy: Recall of skin reaction.

Overdosage: Signs and Symptoms
Acute overdosage enhances the toxic effects of mucositis, leukopenia, and thrombocytopenia.

PATIENT CARE CONSIDERATIONS
Administration/Storage
- Refrigerate unopened vials. Prolonged freezing (longer than 1 mo) can adversely affect the drug.
- Dilute the desired dose of liposomal doxorubicin (max 90 mg) in 250 mL of 5% Dextrose before administration. Do not use with in-line filters.
- Refrigerate diluted solutions at 2° to 8°C (36° to 46°F), and administer within 24 hr. Avoid freezing. Short-term freezing (less than 1 mo) does not appear to have a deleterious effect on liposomal doxorubicin.
- Diluted solutions are preservative-free. Discard within 24 h of preparation.
- Administer by IV infusion over 30 to 60 min. Do not administer via small peripheral veins.
- Do not mix with other drugs. Do not use with any diluent other than 5% Dextrose Injection. Do not use any bacteriostatic agents, such as benzyl alcohol.
- For ovarian carcinoma, initiate the infusion at a rate of 1 mg/min to reduce the risk of infusion reactions.

Assessment/Interventions
- Infusion reactions have occurred with liposomal doxorubicin, usually during the first dose. They do not appear to occur with later infusions if not present initially. Infusion reactions usually subside within several hours to days after stopping the infusion. In some patients, the reaction ceases when the infusion rate is decreased. They presumably represent a reaction to liposomal doxorubicin.
- Consider measuring left ventricular ejection fraction (LVEF) as the patient approaches the max cumulative total doxorubicin dose.
- Obtain a CBC, including platelet counts, frequently and at a minimum prior to each dose.
- Monitor white blood cell and platelet counts and Hbg/Hct. Hematologic toxicity may require dose reduction or suspension or delay of liposomal doxorubicin therapy. Persistent severe myelosuppression may result in superinfection or hemorrhage.
- Prior to dosing, evaluate hepatic function using clinical laboratory tests such as AST, ALT, alkaline phosphatase, and bilirubin.
- Acute left ventricular failure has occurred, particularly in patients who have received total dosage exceeding the recommended limit of 550 mg/m^2. This limit appears to be lower (400 mg/m^2) in patients who received radiotherapy to the mediastinal area. Take into account the total dose of drug of any previous or concomitant therapy with other potentially cardiotoxic agents such as cyclophosphamide or daunorubicin. Cardiomyopathy or CHF may occur several weeks after drug discontinuation and is often unresponsive to medical or physical therapy. A baseline cardiac evaluation with an ECG, LVEF), and an echocardiogram (ECHO) or multigated radionuclide (MUGA) scans, is recommended especially in patients with risk factors for increased cardiac toxicity (eg, pre-existing heart disease, mediastinal irradiation, concurrent cyclophosphamide therapy). Obtain subsequent evaluation at a cumulative dose of doxorubicin of at least 400 mg/m^2 and periodically thereafter during the course of therapy. Pediatric patients are at increased risk for developing delayed cardiotoxicity following doxorubicin administration. Doxorubicin cardiomyopathy is associated with persistent reduction in voltage of the QRS wave, prolongation of the systolic time interval, and reduction of ejection fraction. In adults, a 10% decline in LVEF to below the lower limit of normal, an absolute LVEF of 45%, or a 20% decline in LVEF at any level is indicative of deterioration in cardiac function. In pediatric patients, a drop in fractional shortening (FS) by an absolute value of 10 or more percentile units or less than 29% and a decline in LVEF of 10 percentile units or an LVEF up to 55%. Preliminary evidence suggests cardiotoxicity may be reduced and total dosage safely increased by giving the drug on a weekly schedule or as a prolonged (48 to 96 hr) continuous infusion.
- Extravasation at injection site with or without a stinging or burning sensation may occur. If any signs of extravasation occur, terminate the infusion immediately and restart in another vein. The application of ice over the site of extravasation for approximately 30 min may be helpful in alleviating the local reac-

tion. Do not give IM or SC.
- Administration of live vaccines to immunosuppressed patients may be hazardous.

Patient/Family Education
- Doxorubicin may cause red discoloration of the urine for 1 to 2 days after administration.

Doxycycline

(DOX-ee-SIGH-kleen)
Class Antibiotic/Tetracycline

How Supplied
Adoxa Tablets 50 mg (as monohydrate), Tablets 75 mg (as monohydrate), Tablets 100 mg (as monohydrate) ◆ *Atridox* Injection 42.5 mg (as hyclate, 10%) ◆ *Doryx* Capsules, coated pellets 75 mg (as hyclate), Capsules, coated pellets 100 mg (as hyclate) ◆ *Doxy 100* Powder for Injection, lyophilized 100 mg (as hyclate) ◆ *Doxy 200* Powder for Injection, lyophilized 200 mg (as hyclate) ◆ *Monodox* Capsules 50 mg (as monohydrate), Capsules 100 mg (as monohydrate) ◆ *Periostat* Tablets 20 mg (as hyclate) ◆ *Vibramycin* Capsules 50 mg (as hyclate), Capsules 100 mg (as hyclate), Powder for Injection 100 mg (as hyclate), Powder for Oral Suspension 25 mg (as monohydrate) per 5 mL when reconstituted, Syrup 50 mg per 5 mL (as calcium) ◆ *Vibra-Tabs* Tablets 100 mg (as hyclate) ❋ *Apo-Doxy* ◆ *Apo-Doxy-Tabs* ◆ *Doxycin* ◆ *Novo-Doxylin* ◆ *Nu-Doxycycline* ◆ *ratio-Doxycycline*

Action
PHARMACOLOGY: Inhibits bacterial protein synthesis.

PHARMACOKINETICS/DYNAMICS:
Absorption: Well absorbed. T_{max} is 2 hr (oral). C_{max} is 2.6 mcg/mL (200 mg oral dose), 2.5 to 3.6 mcg/mL (100 to 200 mg IV dose). Absorption may be decreased by 20% when given with food or milk.

Distribution: Bound to plasma proteins. Crosses the placenta; excreted in breast milk.

Excretion: Approximately 40% excreted by the kidneys in 72 hr. The t½ is 18 to 22 hr.

Special Populations:
Renal Function Impairment – Excretion by the kidneys may fall as low as 1% to 5% in 72 hr in those with Ccr less than 10 mL/min.

Indications Treatment of infections caused by susceptible strains of gram-positive and gram-negative bacteria (eg, *Rickettsia*, *Mycoplasma pneumoniae*); treatment of trachoma and susceptible infections when penicillins are contraindicated; treatment of acute intestinal amebiasis; uncomplicated gonorrhea in adults; prophylaxis of malaria caused by *Plasmodium falciparum*; anthrax (including inhalational anthrax); severe acne.

Periodontitis:
Tablet – Adjunct treatment to scaling and root planing to promote attachment level gain and reduce pocket depth.
Subgingival injection – For chronic adult periodontitis for a gain in clinical attachment, reduction in probing depth, and reduction in bleeding on probing.

Contraindications Hypersensitivity to tetracyclines; nursing mothers, infants, and children (*Periostat*).

Route/Dosage

Acute Epididymo-Orchitis Caused by Neisseria Gonorrhoeae or Chlamydia Trachomatis
ADULTS: PO 100 mg bid for at least 10 days.

Chlamydia Infections
ADULTS AND CHILDREN 8 YR OF AGE AND OLDER: PO 100 mg bid for 7 days.

Epididymitis Most Likely Caused by Gonococcal or Chlamydial Infection
ADULTS: PO 100 mg bid for 10 days plus a single dose of 250 mg ceftriaxone IM.

Infection
ADULTS AND CHILDREN OLDER THAN 8 YR OF AGE AND WEIGHING MORE THAN 45 KG: PO 200 mg on the first day (100 mg q 12 hr) then 100 mg/day. For more severe infections (particularly chronic UTI), administer 100 mg q 12 hr. IV 200 mg on the first day (as 1 or 2 infusions) then 100 to 200 mg/day, depending upon the severity of infections, with 200 mg administered in 1 or 2 infusions.
CHILDREN OLDER THAN 8 YR OF AGE AND WEIGHING 45 KG OR LESS: PO 4.4 mg/kg divided into 2 doses on day 1 followed by 2.2 mg/kg/day as a single dose or divided into 2 doses on subsequent day. For more severe infections, 4.4 mg/kg may be used. IV 4.4 mg/kg on day 1 (in 1 or 2 infusions) followed with 2.2 to 4.4 mg/kg given as 1 or 2 infusions, depending on the severity of the infection.

Lymphogranuloma Venereum and Granuloma Inguinale
ADULTS: PO 100 mg bid for at least 21 days.

Malaria Prophylaxis
ADULTS: PO 100 mg daily, beginning 1 to 2 days before travel and continuing for 4 wk after leaving area.
CHILDREN OLDER THAN 8 YR OF AGE: PO 2 mg/kg daily up to 100 mg per day. Begin 1 to 2 days before travel and continue for 4 wk after leaving area.

Nongonococcal Urethritis
ADULTS: **PO** 100 mg bid for 7 days.

Pelvic Inflammatory Disease
ADULTS: **PO/IV** 100 mg q 12 hr plus 2 g cefotetan IV q 12 hr or 2 g cefoxitin IV q 6 hr. Parenteral therapy may be discontinued after 24 hr; continue oral therapy with doxycycline for a total of 14 days.

Periodontitis (Periostat, Atridox)
ADULTS: **PO** 20 mg bid as an adjunct following scaling and root planing for up to 9 mo. Administer tablets at least 2 hr before or after meals.
ADULTS: **Subgingival Injection** Variable dose, depending on the size, shape, and number of pockets being treated (see product information for preparation and administration).

Sexual Assault Prophylaxis
ADULTS: **PO** 100 mg bid for 7 days plus ceftriaxone and metronidazole.

Syphilis
Early (except Adoxa, Doryx, Monodox) – **PO** 100 mg bid for 14 days.
More than 1 yr duration (except Adoxa, Doryx, Monodox) – 100 mg bid for 28 days.
Primary and secondary (Adoxa, Doryx, Monodox) – 300 mg/day in divided doses for at least 10 days.

Uncomplicated Gonococcal Infection (Except Anorectal Infections in Men)
ADULTS: **PO** 100 mg bid for at least 7 days. Single visit dose: 300 mg immediately followed with 300 mg in 1 hr.

Uncomplicated Urethral, Endocervical, or Rectal Infections Caused by C. Trachomatis
ADULTS: **PO** 100 mg bid for at least 7 days.

Inhalation Anthrax (Post-exposure)
ADULTS AND CHILDREN (100 LB [45 KG] OR MORE): **PO** 100 mg bid for 60 days.
CHILDREN (LESS THAN 100 LB [45 KG]): **PO** 2.2 mg/kg bid for 60 days.

Interactions
Antacids (containing aluminum, calcium, or magnesium), bismuth salts, divalent/trivalent cations, zinc salts: May decrease oral absorption of doxycycline.
Barbiturates, carbamazepine, hydantoins: May increase metabolism of and decrease effect of doxycycline.
Cholestyramine, colestipol: May decrease absorption of doxycycline.
Digoxin: May increase digoxin serum levels.
Iron salts: May decrease absorption of doxycycline.
Isotretinoin: Because the risk of pseudotumor cerebri may be increased, avoid isotretinoin administration shortly before, during, or after doxycycline therapy.
Methoxyflurane: Increased potential for nephrotoxicity exists; do not use together.
Milk and dairy products: Although the effects of milk and dairy products on doxycycline absorption are less than observed with other tetracycline derivatives, avoid the administration of milk or dairy products with all tetracycline derivatives.
Oral contraceptives: May decrease contraceptive efficacy.
Penicillins: May interfere with bactericidal action of penicillins.
Warfarin: Anticoagulant effect may be increased; dose may need to be decreased.

Lab Test Interferences False elevations of urinary catecholamine levels may occur because of interference with fluorescence test.

Adverse Reactions
CNS: Dizziness; headache; pseudotumor cerebri (manifested by headache and blurred vision).
DERM: Maculopapular and erythematous rashes; exfoliative dermatitis; photosensitivity.
GI: Anorexia; nausea; vomiting; diarrhea; glossitis; dysphagia; enterocolitis; inflammatory lesions (with monilial overgrowth) in anogenital area; abdominal pain or discomfort; bulky loose stools; sore throat.
GU: Increase BUN.
HEMA/LYMPH: Hemolytic anemia; thrombocytopenia; neutropenia; eosinophilia.
HEPA: Hepatotoxicity.
HYPERSEN: Hypersensitivity (including urticaria, angioneurotic edema, anaphylaxis, anaphylactoid reactions, purpura, pericarditis, exacerbation of SLE).
OTHER: Bulging fontanels (infants); benign intracranial hypertension (adults).

Precautions
Pregnancy: Category D.
Lactation: Excreted in breast milk.
Children: Not recommended in children younger than 8 yr of age; abnormal bone formation and tooth discoloration may result.
Renal function impairment: Dosage reduction may be required.
Hepatic function impairment: Doses greater than 2 g/day associated with liver failure; monitor function and avoid other hepatotoxic drugs.
Superinfection: Prolonged use may result in bacterial or fungal overgrowth.
Photosensitivity: Photosensitivity may occur; avoid exposure to sunlight or ultraviolet light.
Outdated product: Do not use; degradation products of drug are highly nephrotoxic.
Prolonged IV use: May result in thrombophlebitis; use oral form whenever reasonable.
Special considerations: Doxycycline periodontal injection has not been clinically evaluated for

use in the regeneration of alveolar bone, use in immunocompromised patients, or for use in patients with conditions involving extremely severe periodontal defects with very little remaining periodontium.

PATIENT CARE CONSIDERATIONS
Administration/Storage
- Route of administration, dose, and dosing frequency are variable, depending on condition being treated.

Oral:
- Administer *Periostat* 1 hr before or 2 hr after meals.
- Administer other oral doxycycline products without regard to meals but administer with food if GI upset occurs.
- Administer tablets or capsules with a full glass of water.
- Shake suspension well before measuring dose.
- Administer prescribed dose of suspension or syrup using dosing syringe, dosing spoon, or medicine cup.
- Administer *Periostat* 2 hr before or 2 hr after antacids containing aluminum, calcium, or magnesium; preparations containing iron or zinc; or dairy products (eg, milk, cheese, ice cream).
- Administer other oral doxycycline products 1 hr before or 2 hr after antacids containing aluminum, calcium, or magnesium, or preparations containing iron or zinc.
- Store tablets, capsules, syrup, and oral suspension at controlled room temperature (59° to 86°F).

Injection:
- For IV infusion only. Not for intradermal, subcutaneous, IM, intra-arterial, or IV bolus administration.
- Because of the risk of thrombophlebitis, use parenteral therapy only when oral therapy is not indicated. Institute oral therapy as soon as possible.
- Follow manufacturer's guidelines for reconstituting and further diluting the powder for injection.
- Do not administer if particulate matter, cloudiness, or discoloration noted.
- Protect diluted solutions from direct sunlight during storage and infusion.
- For solutions diluted with lactated Ringer's injection or 5% dextrose in lactated Ringer's, complete infusion within 6 hr of reconstitution. Discard any remaining solution after 6 hr.
- Solutions diluted with other IV infusion solutions may be stored for up to 72 hr prior to start of infusion if refrigerated (36° to 46°F) and protected from sunlight and artificial light. Infusion must be completed within 12 hr. Discard any remaining solution after 12 hr.
- Store lyophilized powder at controlled room temperature at or below 77°F.

Subgingival Injection:
- *Atridox* is for instillation into periodontal pockets. Not for intradermal, subcutaneous, IM, IV, or intra-arterial administration.
- Prepare injection solution using supplied syringes following manufacturer's directions.
- Injection solution will be instilled by a dental professional.
- Store unopened *Atridox* pouch in refrigerator (36° to 46°F). Pouch can be removed from refrigerator 15 min before mixing. Coupled syringes can be stored in the resealable pouch for up to 3 days at room temperature.

Assessment/Interventions
- Obtain patient history, including drug history and any known allergies. Note renal or hepatic impairment, sulfite sensitivity (oral syrup only), or history of allergy or intolerance to other tetracycline antibiotics.
- Ensure that expiration date has not been exceeded.
- Review results of culture and sensitivity testing as appropriate.
- Ensure that women are not pregnant or breastfeeding.
- Ensure that CBC, liver enzymes, and renal function are periodically evaluated during prolonged therapy.
- Monitor patient's response to therapy. Notify health care provider if infection does not appear to be improving or is worsening.
- Monitor patient for signs of allergic reaction. Discontinue therapy and immediately notify health care provider if noted. Be prepared to treat appropriately.
- Monitor patient for GI, CNS, DERM, general body side effects, and signs of superinfection. Report to health care provider if noted and significant. Immediately report severe diarrhea, diarrhea containing blood or pus, or severe abdominal cramping.

Patient/Family Education
- Explain name, dose, action, and potential side effects of drug.
- Review dosing schedule and prescribed length of therapy with patient. Advise patient that dose and duration of therapy are dependent on site and cause of infection.

- Instruct patient using tablets or capsules to take prescribed dose with a full glass of water.
- Instruct patient or caregiver using syrup or oral suspension to measure and administer prescribed dose using dosing spoon, dosing syringe, or medicine cup.
- Advise patient to take without regard to meals but to take with food if GI upset occurs.
- Advise patient using other oral doxycycline products to take 1 hr before or 2 hr after antacids containing aluminum, calcium, or magnesium, or preparations containing iron or zinc.
- Instruct patient to complete entire course of therapy, even if symptoms of infection have disappeared.
- Instruct patient taking doxycyline for malaria prophylaxis to take daily, beginning 1 to 2 days prior to arrival in malaria-infected area, while in the malaria-infected area, and for 28 days after leaving the malaria-infected area. Advise patient that medication is not 100% effective and that protective clothing, insect repellants, and bednets are important components of malaria prophylaxis.
- Advise patient to discontinue therapy and contact health care provider immediately if skin rash, hives, itching, shortness of breath, headache, or blurred vision occur.
- Advise patient that medication may cause photosensitivity (sensitivity to sunlight) and to avoid unnecessary exposure to sunlight or tanning lamps and to use sunscreens and wear protective clothing to avoid photosensitivity reactions.
- Caution women taking oral contraceptives that doxycycline may make birth control pills less effective and to use nonhormonal forms of contraception during treatment.
- Advise women to notify health care provider if pregnant, planning to become pregnant, or breastfeeding.
- Caution patient that drug may cause dizziness, light-headedness, or blurred vision and to use caution while driving or performing other hazardous tasks until tolerance is determined.
- Advise patient to report the following signs of superinfection to health care provider: black "furry" tongue, white patches in mouth, foul-smelling stools, vaginal itching or discharge.
- Warn patient that diarrhea containing blood or pus may be a sign of a serious disorder and to seek medical care if noted and not treat at home.
- Caution patient not to take any prescription or OTC medications, dietary supplements, or herbal preparations unless advised by health care provider.
- Advise patient to discard any unused doxycycline by the expiration date noted on the label.
- Advise patient that follow-up examinations and lab tests may be required to monitor therapy and to keep appointments.

Periostat:
- Inform patient that this antibiotic will be taken daily for up to 9 mo to help treat periodontitis.
- Warn patient that although this is a tetracycline antibiotic, the dose is too small to treat infections and should not be used for that purpose.
- Instruct patient to take 1 hr before or 2 hr after meals with a full glass of water.
- Advise patient to take either 2 hr before or 2 hr after antacids containing aluminum, calcium, or magnesium, preparations containing iron or zinc, or dairy products (eg, milk, cheese, ice cream).

Subgingival Injection:
- Caution patient to avoid any mechanical oral hygiene procedure (eg, tooth brushing, flossing) on any treated areas for 7 days after application.

Dronabinol

(droe-NAB-ih-nahl)

Class Antiemetic/Antivertigo/Appetite stimulant

How Supplied
Marinol Capsules, gelatin 2.5 mg, Capsules, gelatin 5 mg, Capsules, gelatin 10 mg

Action
PHARMACOLOGY: Principal psychoactive substance derived from cannabis (marijuana); mechanism by which it prevents nausea and vomiting is unknown.

PHARMACOKINETICS/DYNAMICS:
Absorption: 90% to 95% absorbed. T_{max} approximately 2 to 4 hr.

Distribution: 10% to 20% reaches systemic circulation. Vd approximately 10 L/kg. Approximately 97% protein bound.

Metabolism:
Liver – Extensive first-pass metabolism yielding active and inactive metabolites.

Excretion: Initial t½ approximately 4 hr. Terminal t½ is 25 to 36 hr. Clearance is 0.2 L/kg/hr.
Feces – Approximately 50% of dose; less than 5% unchanged drug.

Urine – 10% to 15%.
Onset: 0.5 to 1 hr.
Peak: 2 to 4 hr.
Duration: 4 to 6 hr (psychoactive effects), 24 hr or longer (appetite stimulant).

Indications Control of chemotherapy-induced nausea and vomiting unresponsive to other antiemetics; appetite stimulation in AIDS cachexia.

Contraindications Hypersensitivity to marijuana or sesame oil.

Route/Dosage
Antiemetic
ADULTS AND CHILDREN: **PO** 5 mg/m^2 1 to 3 hr before chemotherapy and q 2 to 4 hr after chemotherapy. Can give 4 to 6 doses/day and increase by 2.5 mg/m^2/dose; do not exceed 15 mg/m^2/dose.

Appetite Stimulation
ADULTS: **PO** 2.5 mg bid. Can give single daily dose of 2.5 mg to patients in whom adverse effects develop. Can increase by 2.5 mg/day; do not exceed 20 mg/day.

Interactions
Amphetamines, cocaine, sympathomimetics: Hypertension; tachycardia.
CNS depressants: Increased CNS adverse effects.

Lab Test Interferences None well documented.

Adverse Reactions
CV: Tachycardia; hypotension.
CNS: Euphoria; dizziness; paranoid reaction; somnolence; seizures in patients with existing seizure disorders.
OTHER: Tolerance, psychological and physical dependence with chronic use.

Precautions
Pregnancy: Category B.
Lactation: Excreted in breast milk.
Children: Not recommended in children with AIDS cachexia.
Elderly: More sensitive to psychoactive effects.
Drug dependence: Drug has abuse potential.

Overdosage: Signs and Symptoms
Drowsiness, euphoria, heightened sensory awareness, altered time perception, reddened conjunctiva, dry mouth, tachycardia (mild intoxication). Memory impairment, depersonalization, mood alteration, urinary retention, reduced bowel motility (moderate intoxication). Decreased motor coordination, lethargy, slurred speech, postural hypotension (severe intoxication). Apprehensive patients may experience panic reactions. Patients with seizure disorder may experience seizures.

PATIENT CARE CONSIDERATIONS

Administration/Storage
* When given as appetite stimulant, administer bid before lunch and supper.
* Refrigerate capsules; do not freeze.

Assessment/Interventions
* Obtain patient history, including drug history and any known allergies. Note history of drug or alcohol abuse.
* Assess for nausea, vomiting, appetite, bowel sounds, and abdominal pain before and after drug is administered.
* Monitor BP and pulse rate during therapy, especially in patients with hypotension or cardiac disease.
* Monitor I&O, hydration, nutritional status, and weight regularly.
* Monitor side effects, which vary with each patient and are usually dose related. Side effects may be exacerbated in elderly, manic, depressive, or schizophrenic patients.
* Administer IV fluids as ordered for severe nausea and vomiting.
* Assess for signs of withdrawal syndrome, including: irritability, restlessness, insomnia, hot flashes, sweating, rhinorrhea, loose stools, hiccoughs, anorexia.
* Limit quantity of drug available to patient to amount necessary for single cycle of chemotherapy.
* Assist patient with ambulation. Implement safety measures (eg, side-rails) to prevent falls, especially in elderly patients.

Patient/Family Education
* Instruct patient to take drug exactly as ordered by health care provider.
* Discuss psychoactive symptoms with patient and family. Symptoms may be minimized by providing quiet, supportive environment.
* Explain that signs of overdose (eg, mood changes, confusion, hallucinations, depression, nervousness, fast or pounding heartbeat) may occur with increased doses.
* Instruct patient to make position changes slowly to prevent orthostatic hypotension.
* Advise patient and family that adult supervision is necessary as patient may experience drowsiness, dizziness, difficulty concentrating, and perceptual and coordination impairment.
* Instruct patient to avoid intake of alcoholic beverages, barbiturates, and other CNS depressants.
* Advise patient that drug may cause drowsiness and to use caution while driving or performing other tasks requiring mental alertness.

Droperidol

(dro-PER-i-dahl)

Class General anesthetic

How Supplied
Inapsine Injection 2.5 mg/mL

Action

PHARMACOLOGY: Produces tranquilization, sedation and antiemetic effects, as well as mild alpha-adrenergic blockade, resulting in hypotension and decreased peripheral vascular resistance.

PHARMACOKINETICS/DYNAMICS:
Distribution: Vd is 1.5 L/kg (at steady-state). Biphasic distribution with a t½ of approximately 1.4 min (rapid phase) and approximately 14.3 min (slower phase).

Metabolism: Extensively metabolized.

Excretion:
IM – Approximately 75% excreted in the urine (1% as unchanged drug) and 22% excreted in feces. t½ approximately 134 min.

Onset: 3 to 10 min.

Peak: 30 min.

Duration: 2 to 4 hr.

Indications Reduction of incidence of nausea and vomiting in surgical and diagnostic procedures. **Unlabeled use(s):** Antiemetic in cancer chemotherapy.

Contraindications Known or suspected QT prolongation (ie, QTc interval greater than 440 msec for men or greater than 450 msec for women), including patients with congenital long QT syndrome. Hypersensitivity to butyrophenones.

Route/Dosage

ADULTS: **IM** or slow **IV** 2.5 mg max recommended initial dose; additional 1.25 mg doses may be administered to achieve desired effect.
CHILDREN (2 TO 12 YR): **IM/IV** 0.1 mg/kg max recommended initial dose, taking into account age and other clinical factors.

Interactions

CNS depressants: Additive CNS depression may result.
Diuretics, drugs known to increase the QT interval (eg, cisapride, pimozide): Risk of life-threatening arrhythmias, including torsades de pointes, may be increased.
INCOMPATIBILITIES: Barbiturates are physically incompatible with droperidol.

Lab Test Interferences None well documented.

Adverse Reactions

CV: QT interval prolongation; torsades de pointes; cardiac arrest; ventricular tachycardia; hypotension.
CNS: Postoperative drowsiness; extrapyramidal effects (eg, dystonia, akathisia and oculogyric crisis); restlessness; hyperactivity; anxiety; dizziness; postoperative hallucinations; mental depression.
RESP: Respiratory depression; bronchospasm; laryngospasm.
OTHER: Muscular rigidity; chills or shivering.

> **WARNING:**
>
> *Contraindications:* Contraindicated in patients with known or suspected QT prolongation.
>
> *QT prolongation/torsades de pointes:* Have been reported at or below recommended doses. Some cases have been in patients without known risk factors for QT prolongation. Some cases have been fatal. Perform baseline 12-lead ECG prior to initiation of therapy. Do not administer if QTc is greater than 440 msec in men or 450 msec in women. Use with extreme caution in patients at risk of developing prolonged QT syndrome (eg, CHF, bradycardia, diuretic use, cardiac hypertrophy, hypokalemia, hypomagnesemia, drugs that prolong QT interval, older than 65 yr, alcohol abuse, or taking benzodiazepines, volatile anesthetics, or IV opiates).
>
> *Refractory disease:* Reserve treatment in refractory disease because of serious proarrhythmic effects.

Precautions

Pregnancy: Category C.
Lactation: Undetermined.
Children: Safety and efficacy in children less than 2 yr not established.
Special risk patients: Decreased dose may be necessary. Use drug with caution in elderly, debilitated, and hepatically or renally impaired patients.
Neuroleptic malignant syndrome: Rare cases of neuroleptic malignant syndrome (eg, altered consciousness, muscle rigidity, autonomic instability) have been reported.

Overdosage: Signs and Symptoms

Extension of pharmacologic effects, including QT prolongation, serious arrhythmias (eg, torsades de pointes), sedation, and hypotension.

PATIENT CARE CONSIDERATIONS
Administration/Storage
- If direct IV has been ordered, administer at slow rate (do not exceed 10 mg/30 to 60 sec).
- Administer with caution to patients at risk for development of prolonged QT syndrome (eg, CHF, bradycardia, use of a diuretic, cardiac hypertrophy, other drugs known to prolong the QT interval, cardiac disease, electrolyte imbalance).
- Store at room temperature and protect from light. Solution remains stable for 7 to 10 days.
- Compatible when mixed in syringe with atropine, butorphanol, chlorpromazine, fentanyl, glycopyrrolate, hydroxyzine, morphine, meperidine, perphenazine, promazine, promethazine, or scopolamine.

Assessment/Interventions
- Obtain patient history, including drug history and any known allergies.
- Obtain a 12-lead ECG prior to administration of droperidol to determine if a prolonged QT interval (ie, QTc greater than 440 msec for men or greater than 450 msec for women) is present. If prolonged QT interval is present, do not administer droperidol.
- Monitor ECG prior to treatment and continue for 2 to 3 hr after completing treatment to monitor for arrhythmias if the potential benefit outweighs the risk of potentially serious arrhythmias.
- Assess patient's respiratory status continuously. If patient is receiving narcotic analgesic concurrently, respiratory depression may occur.
- If patient experiences drowsiness, keep siderails up and assist with ambulation.
- If extrapyramidal symptoms (eg, dystonia, hyperactivity, neck extension) occur, notify health care provider immediately.

Patient/Family Education
- Caution patient to avoid sudden changes in position to prevent orthostatic hypotension.
- Instruct patient to call for help before rising from bed.
- Advise patient to avoid intake of alcoholic beverages or other CNS depressants for greater than or equal to 24 hr after treatment.

Drotrecogin Alfa (Activated)
(droh-truh-KO-jin AL-fah)
Class Thrombolytic agent/Recombinant human activated protein C

How Supplied
Xigris Powder for infusion, lyophilized 5 mg, Powder for infusion, lyophilized 20 mg

Action
PHARMACOLOGY: Exerts antithrombotic effect by inhibiting Factors Va and VIIIa.

PHARMACOKINETICS/DYNAMICS:
Absorption: Steady-state concentration of 45 ng/mL attained within 2 hr.
Excretion: Cl approximately 40 L/hr.
Special Populations:
Severe sepsis – Clearance is approximately 50% higher. Dosage adjustment not required.

Indications Reduction of mortality in adult patients with severe sepsis who have a high risk of death.

Contraindications Patients with the following situations in whom bleeding could be associated with a high risk of death or important morbidity: active internal bleeding; recent (within 3 mo) hemorrhagic stroke; recent (within 2 mo) intracranial or intraspinal surgery or severe head trauma; trauma with an increased risk of life-threatening bleeding; presence of an epidural catheter; intracranial neoplasm, mass lesion, or evidence of cerebral herniation. Hypersensitivity to drotrecogin alfa (activated) or any component of the product.

Route/Dosage
ADULTS: IV 24 mcg/kg/hr for a total infusion duration of 96 hr. If infusion is interrupted, restart at the 24 mcg/kg/hr infusion rate.

Interactions
Aspirin, oral anticoagulants (eg, warfarin), glycoprotein IIb/IIIa inhibitors: Increased risk of bleeding.
INCOMPATIBILITIES: Administer through a dedicated line or dedicated lumen of a multilumen central venous catheter. Only 0.9% Sodium Chloride for Injection, Lactated Ringer's injection, dextrose, or dextrose and saline mixtures can be administered through the same line as drotrecogin alfa (activated).

Lab Test Interferences Because drotrecogin alfa may variably prolong the activated partial thromboplastin time (aPTT), aPTT cannot be reliably used to assess the status of coagulopathy during drotrecogin alfa administration; drotrecogin alfa present in plasma samples may interfere with 1-stage coagulation assay based on the aPTT (eg, factor VIII, IX, and XI) assays.

Adverse Reactions
HEMA: Bleeding/hemorrhage (eg, GI, intra-abdominal, intrathoracic, retroperitoneal, intracranial, GU, skin/soft tissue, other sites).

Precautions
Pregnancy: Category C.
Lactation: Undetermined.
Children: Safety and efficacy not established.
Bleeding: Severe bleeding may occur.

PATIENT CARE CONSIDERATIONS
Administration/Storage
- Administer by IV infusion only.
- Reconstitute powder using Sterile Water for Injection. Slowly add 2.5 mL to 5 mg vial or 10 mL to 20 mg vial. Swirl vial gently to dissolve. Do not shake or invert vial.
- Reconstituted solution must be further diluted in 0.9% Sodium Chloride for Injection. Slowly withdraw prescribed amount of reconstituted drotrecogin alfa and add to infusion bag of 0.9% Sodium Chloride for Injection by directing the stream to the side of the infusion bag to minimize agitation. Gently invert the infusion bag to mix. Do not agitate the infusion solution or transport using mechanical delivery systems.
- Vials contain no preservative. Discard any unused portion. Do not combine unused portions.
- Reconstituted solution should be immediately diluted for IV infusion. If not diluted immediately it may be stored at controlled room temperature (59° to 86°F) for up to 3 hr. IV administration must be completed within 12 hr after the IV solution is prepared.
- Administer infusion solution via dedicated IV line or dedicated lumen of a multilumen central venous catheter using IV infusion pump or syringe pump.
- Usual infusion rate is 24 mcg/kg/hr for 96 hr.
- Do not administer if particulate matter, cloudiness, or discoloration is noted.
- Do not mix with other drug solutions. Lactated Ringer's Injection, 0.9% Sodium Chloride Injection, dextrose, or dextrose and saline mixtures are the only solutions that can be administered through the same IV line as drotrecogin alfa.
- Avoid exposing infusion solution to heat and direct sunlight.

Immunogenicity: As with all therapeutic proteins, immunogenicity may occur.

Overdosage: Signs and Symptoms
Monitor closely for hemorrhagic complications.

- Store vials in refrigerator (36° to 46°F). Do not freeze. Protect unreconstituted vials from light. Retain in carton until time of use. Do not use beyond expiration date stamped on vial.

Assessment/Interventions
- Obtain patient history, including drug history and any known allergies.
- Review patient's health history for any condition that could contraindicate drotrecogin alfa (previous allergic reaction to drotrecogin alfa; active internal bleeding; recent [within 3 mo] hemorrhagic stroke; recent [within 2 mo] intracranial or intraspinal surgery or severe head trauma; trauma with increased risk of life-threatening bleeding; presence of epidural catheter; intracranial neoplasm or mass lesion with evidence of cerebral herniation).
- Discontinue infusion 2 hr before performing invasive procedures or procedures with inherent risk of bleeding. When adequate hemostasis has been achieved, the infusion may be restarted 12 hr after major invasive procedures or surgery or immediately after uncomplicated, less invasive procedures.
- Monitor patient for signs of bleeding. If clinically important bleeding is noted, immediately stop the infusion solution and notify health care provider.

Patient/Family Education
- Explain name, dose, action, and potential side effects of drug.
- Advise patient or family that medication will be prepared and administered by health care provider while the patient is in the intensive care unit.

Duloxetine Hydrochloride
(doo-LOX-eh-teen HIGH-droe-KLOR-ide)
Class Antidepressant

How Supplied
Cymbalta Capsule 22.4 mg (equiv. to 20 mg duloxetine), Capsule 33.7 mg (equiv. to 30 mg duloxetine), Capsule 67.3 mg (equiv. to 60 mg duloxetine)

Action
PHARMACOLOGY: Unknown; however, potentiation of serotonergic and noradrenergic activity in the CNS is suspected.

PHARMACOKINETICS/DYNAMICS:
Absorption: Well absorbed. C_{max} occurs 6 hr postdose. Steady-state reached after 3 days.

Distribution: Vd about 1,640 L. Protein binding is greater than 90%.

Metabolism: Hepatic metabolism by CYP1A2 and CYP2D6 to numerous metabolites

Excretion: Elimination t½ approximately 12 hr. Less than 1% excreted unchanged in the urine. Of the administered dose, 70% appears in the urine as metabolites and 20% in the feces.

Special Populations:
Hepatic Function Impairment – The t½ is about 3 times longer in cirrhotic patients. Not recommended in patients with any degree of hepatic insufficiency.
Renal insufficiency – Use not recommended in patients with end stage renal disease.

Indications Treatment of major depressive disorder.

Contraindications Uncontrolled narrow-angle glaucoma; MAO inhibitor therapy; hypersensitivity to any component of product.

Route/Dosage
ADULTS: **PO** 40 mg daily (given as 20 mg bid) to 60 mg daily (given once a day or as 30 mg bid) without regards to meals.

Interactions
CNS active drugs: Use with caution because of possible additive effects.
Drugs affecting gastric acidity: Because duloxetine is enteric coated, drugs that raise GI pH may lead to earlier release of duloxetine. However, aluminum- and magnesium-containing antacids or famotidine have no significant effect on rate or extend of duloxetine absorption.
Drugs with a narrow therapeutic index and extensively metabolized by CYP2D6 (amitriptyline, desipramine, flecainide imipramine, nortriptyline, propafenone): Plasma concentrations of these agents may be elevated, increasing the risk of side effects. Avoid thioridazine because of possible serious ventricular arrhythmias and sudden death resulting from elevated plasma levels.
Inhibitors of CYP1A2 (eg, fluvoxamine, some quinolone antibiotics), inhibitors of CYP2D6 (eg, fluoxetine, paroxetine, quinidine): Duloxetine plasma levels may be elevated, increasing the risk of side effects.
MAO inhibitors (eg, isocarboxazid): Concurrent use with duloxetine is contraindicated. Because duloxetine is an inhibitor of serotonin and norepinephrine reuptake, it is recommended that duloxetine not be use in combination with and MAO inhibitor, or within 14 days of discontinuing treatment with an MAO inhibitor. Allow at least 5 days after stopping duloxetine before starting an MAO inhibitor.

Lab Test Interferences None well documented.

Adverse Reactions
CV: Hot flushes (2%).
CNS: Insomnia (11%); dizziness (9%); fatigue (8%); somnolence (7%); tremor, anxiety, decreased libido, abnormal orgasm (3%); initial insomnia, irritability, lethargy, nervousness, nightmare, restlessness, sleep disorder (at least 1%).
DERM: Increased sweating (6%); night sweats, pruritus, rash (at least 1%).
EENT: Blurred vision (4%).
GI: Nausea (20%); dry mouth (15%); constipation (11%); diarrhea (8%); vomiting (5%); gastritis (at least 1%).
GU: Erectile dysfunction (4%); delayed ejaculation, ejaculation dysfunction (3%); dysuria (at least 1%).
M/N: Decreased appetite (8%); decreased weight (2%).

Precautions
Pregnancy: Category C.
Lactation: Undetermined.
Children: Safety and efficacy not established.
Hepatic function impairment: Because greatly increased exposure to duloxetine occurs in patients with hepatic insufficiency, do not administer duloxetine to these patients.
Discontinuation of therapy: A gradual reduction in dose rather than abrupt discontinuation of therapy is recommended in order to minimize discontinuation symptoms (eg, dizziness, headache, paresthesia, nightmares).
Hepatotoxicity: The risk of elevated transaminase levels may be increased.
Special risk patients: Use with caution in patients with history of seizures or mania or with controlled narrow-angle glaucoma.
Suicide: Supervise depressed patients at risk during initial therapy. Prescribe the smallest quantity consistent with good patient management in order to reduce the risk of overdose.

PATIENT CARE CONSIDERATIONS
Administration/Storage
- Do not administer with or within 14 days of MAO inhibitor administration.
- Administer prescribed dose without regard to meals. Administer with food if GI upset occurs.
- Advise patient to swallow capsule whole and not to crush, chew, or open the capsule.
- Store capsules at controlled room temperature (59° to 86°F).

Assessment/Interventions
- Obtain patient history, including drug history and any known allergies. Note renal or hepatic impairment, narrow angle glaucoma, mania or history of mania, seizures or history of seizure disorder, alcohol consumption, con-

dition associated with delayed gastric emptying, history of drug abuse, concurrent or recent (eg, within 14 days) use of MAO inhibitor, concurrent use of strong inhibitor of CYP1A2 or CYP2D6, or concurrent use of drug extensively metabolized by CYP2D6.
- Ensure that BP is monitored before starting therapy and periodically during prolonged treatment. Inform health care provider if persistent elevations in BP are noted.
- Frequently assess patient being treated for depression for clinical worsening and suicidality, especially when initiating therapy, or when the escitalopram dose is increased or decreased. Immediately notify health care provider if depression worsens or suicidal ideation or behavior are noted.
- Ensure that therapy is periodically reviewed to determine if therapy needs to be continued without change or if a dose change (eg, increase, decrease, discontinuation) is indicated.
- If treatment is to be discontinued, or the dose reduced, gradually taper the dose and monitor patient for withdrawal symptoms (eg, irritability, dizziness, abnormal skin sensations, nausea, vomiting, headaches, nightmares). If significant withdrawal symptoms develop, reinstitute previous dosing schedule and attempt a less rapid tapering regimen after patient has stabilized.
- Monitor patient for CNS, GI, GU, PSYCH, and general body side effects. Report to health care provider if noted and significant.

Patient/Family Education

- Explain name, dose, action, and potential side effects of drug.
- Advise patient to read *Patient Information Leaflet* before starting therapy and with each refill.
- Advise patient to take prescribed dose without regard to meals but to take with food if stomach upset occurs.
- Caution patient not to crush or chew the capsule nor open the capsule and sprinkle the contents on food or mix with liquids.
- Advise patient not to change the dose or stop taking unless advised by health care provider.
- Inform patient that it may take 1 to 4 wk to note improvement in symptoms and to continue with the prescribed therapy once improvement has been noted.
- Instruct patient to notify health care provider if symptoms do not appear to be getting better, are getting worse, or if bothersome side effects (eg, unusual sweating, headache, drowsiness, insomnia, nausea, diarrhea, nervousness, changes in sexual function) occur.
- Advise patient being treated for depression, and family or caregiver of patient, to be alert for abnormal changes in mood or thinking and to immediately report any of the following to health care provider: anxiety, agitation, panic attacks, irritability, hostility or aggressiveness, impulsivity, suicidal thoughts or behavior.
- Instruct patient in BP and pulse measurement skills.
- Advise patient to periodically monitor and record BP and pulse at home and to inform health care provider if abnormal measurements are noted. Also, advise patient to take record of BP and pulse to each follow-up visit.
- Advise patient that if medication needs to be discontinued it will be slowly withdrawn unless safety concerns (eg, rash) require a more rapid withdrawal.
- Advise patient to take frequent sips of water, suck on ice chips or sugarless hard candy, or chew sugarless gum if dry mouth occurs.
- Advise patient to avoid alcoholic beverages and other depressants while taking duloxetine.
- Advise patient that drug may impair judgment, thinking, or motor skills, or cause drowsiness or dizziness, and to use caution while driving or performing other tasks requiring mental alertness or coordination until tolerance is determined.
- Instruct patient not to take any prescription or OTC drugs, herbal preparations, or dietary supplements without consulting health care provider.
- Advise women to notify health care provider if pregnant, planning to become pregnant, or breastfeeding.
- Advise patient that follow-up visits may be necessary to monitor therapy and to keep appointments.

Dutasteride

(Doo-TASS-teer-ide)

Class Androgen hormone inhibitor

How Supplied
Avodart Capsules 0.5 mg

Action
PHARMACOLOGY: Inhibits the conversion of testosterone to 5-alpha-dihydrotestosterone, a potent androgen.

PHARMACOKINETICS/DYNAMICS:
Absorption: T_{max} is 2 to 3 hr; bioavailability is approximately 60%; administration with food decreased C_{max} 10% to 15%.
Distribution: Vd is 300 to 500 L; highly protein bound.
Metabolism: Metabolized by CYP3A4.
Excretion: Mainly excreted in feces (approximately 5% as unchanged dutasteride and approximately 40% as metabolites). The t½ is approximately 5 wk.

Indications Treatment of symptomatic benign prostatic hyperplasia in men with an enlarged prostate.

Contraindications Women; children; hypersensitivity to 5-alpha-reductase inhibitors or any component of the product.

Route/Dosage
ADULTS: PO 0.5 mg once daily.

Interactions
Cytochrome P450 3A4 inhibitors (eg, cimetidine, ciprofloxacin, diltiazem, ketoconazole, ritonavir, verapamil): Plasma concentrations of dutasteride may be elevated, increasing the risk of side effects.

Lab Test Interferences Decreased prostate-specific antigen levels.

Adverse Reactions
GU: Impotence; decreased libido; ejaculation disorder; gynecomastia.

Precautions
Pregnancy: Category X.
Lactation: Undetermined.
Children: Safety and efficacy not established.
Hepatic function impairment: Use with caution.
Obstructive uropathy: Carefully monitor patients with large residual urine volume or severely diminished urinary flow.

PATIENT CARE CONSIDERATIONS

Administration/Storage
- Not for use in women.
- Do not handle dutasteride capsules if pregnant or possibly pregnant.
- Women who are not pregnant should use caution whenever handling dutasteride capsules. If contact is made with leaking capsules, wash the contacted area immediately with soap and water.
- Administer as prescribed once daily without regard to meals.
- Swallow capsules whole. Do not crush, cut, or chew.
- Do not use capsules that are cracked or leaking.
- Store at controlled room temperature (59° to 86°F). Protect from light.

Assessment/Interventions
- Obtain patient history, including drug history and any known allergies. Note history of liver disease.
- Ensure that patient has had complete physical examination to rule out causes of urinary tract symptoms other than BPH.
- Ensure that baseline PSA level is determined before starting therapy and periodically thereafter during therapy.
- Monitor urine volume and frequency for evidence of improvement in symptoms.

Patient/Family Education
- Explain name, dose, action, and potential side effects of drug.
- Advise patient to read the "Patient Information" leaflet before starting dutasteride and with each refill.
- Advise patient that prescribed dose is to be taken once daily without regard to meals and to try to take the dose at about the same time each day.
- Advise patient that if a dose is missed to take as soon as remembered but to never take 2 doses the same day.
- Advise patient that drug does not work immediately and that it may take 3 to 6 mo to experience maximum benefit.
- Advise patient that ejaculate volume may be decreased during treatment but that this decrease does not interfere with normal sexual function.
- Instruct patient to not stop taking dutasteride when symptoms have improved.
- Caution patient that women who are or may be pregnant should not handle the medication because of risk of absorption though the skin and risk to developing male fetus.
- Caution patient that a woman who is not pregnant can handle the capsules with caution but if contact is made with a leaking

- capsule to wash the contacted area immediately with soap and water.
- Advise patient that impotence, decreased libido, and ejaculation disorder may occur with therapy but that these symptoms should lessen as treatment continues.
- Advise patient against donating blood for at least 6 mo following discontinuation of therapy to prevent pregnant women from receiving dutasteride through a blood transfusion.
- Instruct patient to not take any prescription or OTC medications or dietary supplements unless advised by health care provider.
- Advise patient that follow-up visits and lab tests will be required to monitor therapy and to keep appointments.

Dyphylline

(DIE-fih-lin)

Class Bronchodilator/Xanthine derivative

How Supplied
Lufyllin Tablets 200 mg, Tablets 400 mg, Elixir 100 mL/15 mL (33.3 mg/5 mL), Injection 250 mg/mL ♦ *Dilor* Elixir 160 mg/15 mL (53.3 mg/5 mL), Injection 250 mg/mL

Action
PHARMACOLOGY: Relaxes bronchial smooth muscle and stimulates central respiratory drive.

PHARMACOKINETICS/DYNAMICS:

Absorption: Rapidly absorbed, reaching a mean C_{max} of 17.1 mcg/mL in about 45 min.

Metabolism: Not metabolized.

Excretion: Unchanged by the kidney. Elimination t½ is approximately 2 hr.

Indications
Relief of acute bronchial asthma and for reversible bronchospasm associated with chronic bronchitis and emphysema.

Contraindications
Hypersensitivity to any component of the product or related xanthine compounds.

Route/Dosage
ADULT: **PO** Usual dose up to 15 mg/kg q 6 hr. Elixir: 200 to 400 mg (2 to 4 Tbsp) q 6 hr. Dose should be titrated to severity of condition and response of patient.

Interactions
Probenecid: May increase the plasma t½ of dyphylline.

Sympathomimetic bronchodilators: Synergistic pharmacologic effect may occur.

Lab Test Interferences None well documented.

Adverse Reactions
CV: Palpitation; tachycardia; extrasystoles; flushing; hypotension; circulatory failure; ventricular arrhythmias.
CNS: Headache; irritability; restlessness; insomnia; hyperexcitability; agitation; muscle twitching; generalized clonic and tonic convulsions.
GI: Nausea; vomiting; epigastric pain; hematemesis; diarrhea.
METAB: Hyperglycemia; inappropriate antidiuretic hormone syndrome.
RENAL: Albuminuria; gross and microscopic hematuria; diuresis.
RESP: Tachypnea.

Precautions
Pregnancy: Category C.
Lactation: Excreted in breast milk.
Children: Safety and efficacy not established.
Renal function impairment: Cl is reduced in patients with impaired renal function.
Special risk patients: Use with caution in patients with severe cardiac disease, hypertension, hyperthyroidism, acute myocardial injury, or peptic ulcer.

Overdosage: Signs and Symptoms
Restlessness, anorexia, nausea, vomiting, diarrhea, insomnia, irritability, headache, agitation, severe vomiting, dehydration, excessive thirst, tinnitus, cardiac arrhythmias, hyperthermia, diaphoresis, generalized clonic and tonic convulsions, seizures, CV collapse, death.

Econazole Nitrate

(ee-CON-uh-zole NYE-trate)

Class Topical/Antifungal

How Supplied
Spectazole Cream 1%
❦ *Ecostatin*

Action
PHARMACOLOGY: Increases cell membrane permeability in susceptible fungi.

Indications Treatment of tinea pedis (athlete's foot), tinea cruris (jock itch), tinea corporis (ringworm), cutaneous candidiasis, tinea versicolor.

Contraindications Standard considerations.

Route/Dosage
Tinea Pedis, Tinea Cruris, Tinea Corporis, and Tinea Versicolor
ADULTS AND CHILDREN: **Topical** Apply sufficient quantity to cover affected areas qd. Treat tinea versicolor, tinea cruris, and tinea corporis for 2 wk and tinea pedis for 1 mo.

Cutaneous Candidiasis
ADULTS AND CHILDREN: **Topical** Apply bid morning and evening for 2 wk.

Interactions None well documented.

Lab Test Interferences None well documented.

Adverse Reactions
DERM: Burning, itching, stinging, erythema (3%).

Precautions
Pregnancy: Category C.
Lactation: Undetermined.

PATIENT CARE CONSIDERATIONS

Administration/Storage
- For topical use only. Not for ophthalmic, oral, or intravaginal use.
- Thoroughly dry affected areas of skin before application of cream.
- Apply cream in sufficient quantity to cover affected areas qd or bid as prescribed.
- Avoid contact with the eyes.
- Store cream at controlled room temperature (below 86°F). Keep tube tightly capped.

Assessment/Interventions
- Obtain patient history, including drug history and any known allergies. Note pregnancy or breastfeeding.
- Assess and document skin condition before initial application and periodically throughout treatment. Inform health care provider if condition does not improve, worsens, or if application site reactions are bothersome.

Patient/Family Education
- Explain name, action, and potential side effects of drug.
- Advise patient to try to keep affected areas as dry as possible because moist skin favors growth of fungi.
- Advise patient being treated for tinea cruris (jock itch) to avoid over-bathing, to dust drying powder into involved areas with excessive perspiration or skin folds caused by obesity, and to wear loose-fitting underwear.
- Advise patient being treated for tinea pedis (athlete's foot) to carefully dry between the toes after showering or bathing, apply drying and dusting powders as necessary, and change socks frequently.
- Teach patient or caregiver proper technique for applying cream: wash hands; apply sufficient cream to cover affected areas and gently massage into skin. Wash hands after applying cream.
- Advise patient to apply cream to affected areas qd or bid as directed by health care provider.
- Caution patient to avoid contact with eyes. Advise patient that if cream does come into contact with the eyes to wash eyes with large amounts of cool water and contact health care provider if eye irritation occurs.
- Advise patient that symptoms should begin to improve soon after starting treatment but to continue applying cream as directed for full treatment period to prevent recurrence of infection.
- Advise patient to notify health care provider if condition does not improve, worsens, or if application site reactions (eg, burning, stinging, redness, itching) develop and are bothersome.
- Advise women to notify health care provider if pregnant, planning to become pregnant, or breastfeeding.
- Warn patient not to take any prescription or OTC drugs or dietary supplements without consulting health care provider.
- Advise patient that follow-up visits to monitor response to treatment may be required and to keep appointments.

Edetate Calcium Disodium (Calcium EDTA)

(EH-duh-tate KAL-see-uhm die-SO-dee-uhm)

Class Antidote

How Supplied
Calcium Disodium Versenate Injection 200 mg/mL

Action

PHARMACOLOGY: Calcium is displaced by heavy metals, such as lead, to form stable EDTA complexes that are excreted in urine.

PHARMACOKINETICS/DYNAMICS:

Absorption: Poorly absorbed from the GI tract.

Distribution: Does not penetrate cells; distributed in the extracellular fluid with approximately 5% found in spinal fluid.

Metabolism: Not metabolized.

Excretion: The $t_{1/2}$ is 20 to 60 min. Excreted primarily by the kidneys, with about 50% excreted in 1 hr and more than 95% within 24 hr.

Indications Treatment of acute and chronic lead poisoning and lead encephalopathy.

Contraindications Anuria; active renal disease; hepatitis.

Route/Dosage

ASYMPTOMATIC ADULTS: **IV** 5 mL ampule diluted with 250 to 500 mL normal saline or D5W. Administer dilution over 1 hr or more bid for up to 5 days. Interrupt therapy for 2 days; follow with 5 additional days if needed (max 50 mg/kg/day).

SYMPTOMATIC ADULTS: **IV** 5 mL ampule diluted with 250 to 500 mL normal saline or D5W. Administer dilution over 2 hr. Give second daily infusion 6 hr or more after first.

CHILDREN AND PATIENTS WITH OVERT OR INCIPIENT LEAD ENCEPHALOPATHY: **IM** 35 mg/kg bid q 8 to 12 hr for 3 to 5 days; give second course no sooner than 4 days later. Procaine or lidocaine may be added (for concentration of up to 0.5%) to minimize pain on injection.

Interactions None well documented.

Lab Test Interferences None well documented.

Adverse Reactions
GU: Renal tubular necrosis.

Precautions
Pregnancy: Safety not established.
Lactation: Undetermined.
Hydration: Patients may be dehydrated from vomiting. Because drug is excreted in urine, establish urine flow by IV infusion before administering first dose; then restrict IV fluid to basal water and electrolyte requirements.
Lead encephalopathy: Rapid infusion may be lethal in patients with cerebral edema, because of sudden increases in intracranial pressure. IM route is preferred.
Renal damage: Discontinue if urinalysis reveals large renal epithelial cells, increasing numbers of red blood cells in urinary sediment or greater proteinuria.

Overdosage: Signs and Symptoms
Cerebral edema, renal tubular necrosis.

PATIENT CARE CONSIDERATIONS

Administration/Storage

- Dilute 5 mL ampule in 250 to 500 mL of normal saline or D5W for IV administration.
- Use infusion pump to control rate of infusion. Infuse over 1 hr or more for asymptomatic adults. Infuse over 2 hr or more for symptomatic adults.
- Administer second daily infusion 6 hr or more after first dose.
- Administer IM if patient is child or has lead encephalopathy. Inject deep into well-developed muscle, and rotate injection sites. Use procaine or lidocaine to minimize pain at injection site.
- Administer dimercaprol in separate injection site if used concurrently with edetate calcium disodium.
- Administer in courses of 3 to 5 days, with second course given 2 days or more later if given IV or 4 days later if given IM.

Assessment/Interventions

- Obtain patient history, including drug history and any known allergies.
- Assess renal function prior to and during administration, including frequent urinalysis, BUN and creatinine.
- Document serum lead level prior to and during administration.
- Assess hydration status prior to administering drug.
- Assess for signs of increased intracranial pressure prior to and during IV administration.
- Obtain baseline and periodic ECG.
- Hydrate patient with IV infusion prior to administration because patient may be dehydrated from vomiting, and then reduce rate to basal fluid and electrolyte requirements.
- Maintain strict I&O measurement and daily weights. Do not administer unless patient has

adequate urine output. Discontinue drug and notify health care provider if anuria develops.
- Monitor vital signs and assess for paresthesia, hypotension, arrhythmias, febrile reactions and histamine-like reaction including flushing, headache, sweating, sneezing, congestion, and tachycardia.
- Wait 1 hr after administering dose before drawing serum lead sample.
- Notify health care provider and discontinue drug if urinalysis reveals renal damage, including large epithelial cells, increased protein, RBCs, or BUN.
- Rehydrate in event of anuria and continue drug once urine flow resumes.
- Discontinue IV administration and notify health care provider if signs of increased intracranial pressure develop.
- Obtain ECG if patient complains of palpitations or heart rate irregularities.

Patient/Family Education
- Explain method of administration and potential side effects.
- Instruct patient to notify health care provider immediately if side effects occur.
- Explain rationale for strict I&O measurement and how to assist.
- Refer to public health agency regarding potential sources of lead poisoning and assistance for family in proper removal.
- Provide appropriate referrals for child who has learning deficits resulting from lead poisoning.
- Teach signs of lead poisoning, including metallic taste in mouth, abdominal cramping, GI upset, decreased urine output, alteration in mentation, blue-black line along gum, paresthesia, seizures, and coma. Instruct to notify health care provider if any of these signs appear.
- Counsel family in low-fat diet with adequate calcium, magnesium, zinc, iron, and copper to prevent binding and storage of lead in body.
- Review follow-up schedule of appointments to monitor serum lead levels.

Edetate Disodium (EDTA)

(EH-duh-tate die-SO-dee-uhm)

Class Cardiovascular

How Supplied
Endrate Injection 150 mg/mL

Action
PHARMACOLOGY: Forms chelates with polyvalent metals, especially calcium, thus increasing their urinary excretion.

PHARMACOKINETICS/DYNAMICS:
Excretion: The chelate formed is excreted in the urine.

Indications Emergency treatment of hypercalcemia; control of ventricular arrhythmias associated with digitalis toxicity.

Contraindications Anuria.

Route/Dosage
ADULTS: **IV** 50 mg/kg/day (max 3 g/day). Usually administered in 5 consecutive daily doses followed by 2 days without medication, with repeated courses prn, for total of 15 doses.
CHILDREN: **IV** 40 mg/kg/day (max 70 mg/kg/day) or 15 to 50 mg/kg/day (max 3 g/day) with 5 days between courses.

Interactions None well documented.

Lab Test Interferences None well documented.

Adverse Reactions
CV: Transient drop in BP; adverse effects on myocardial contractility; thrombophlebitis.
CNS: Transient circumoral paresthesia; numbness; headache.
DERM: Exfoliative dermatitis; toxic skin and mucous membrane reactions.
GI: Nausea; vomiting; diarrhea.
GU: Nephrotoxicity; damage to reticuloendothelial system.
HEMA: Thrombophlebitis; anemia.
METAB: Electrolyte imbalances including hypocalcemia, hypokalemia, and hypomagnesemia; hyperuricemia.
OTHER: Febrile reactions.

Precautions
Pregnancy: Category C.
Lactation: Undetermined.
Special risk patients: Use drug cautiously in patients with limited cardiac reserve or incipient congestive failure.
Diabetic patients: Blood sugar and insulin requirements may be lower in insulin-dependent diabetic patients.
IV infusion: Rapid IV infusion or high serum concentrations can cause a precipitous and potentially fatal drop in serum calcium. Do not exceed maximum dose or rate.

Overdosage: Signs and Symptoms
Drop in serum calcium.

PATIENT CARE CONSIDERATIONS

Administration/Storage
- Do not confuse edetate disodium with edetate calcium disodium.
- Adults: Dissolve 50 mg/kg dose in 500 mL of D5W or 0.9% Sodium Chloride for Injection. Infuse over 3 hr or more.
- Children: Dissolve drug in sufficient volume of D5W or 0.9% Sodium Chloride for Injection to bring final concentration to 3% or less. Infuse over 3 hr or more.
- Store at room temperature.

Assessment/Interventions
- Obtain patient history, including drug history and any known allergies. Note previous history of renal disease or CHF.
- Because of potential for electrolyte disturbances, obtain appropriate laboratory determinations (eg, electrolytes, calcium, renal function test).
- Adequately hydrate patient before administration.
- Assess patency of IV site frequently during therapy.
- Assist patient with ambulation.
- After infusion, have patient remain supine for short period because of possible orthostatic hypotension.
- Assess for these allergic reactions: rash, urticaria. Withhold drug and notify health care provider if these signs occur.
- Monitor vital signs and I&O.
- Monitor rate of infusion closely.
- If signs or symptoms of hypocalcemia occur (eg, circumoral numbness/tingling, positive Chvostek's or Trousseau's signs, tetany), notify health care provider.
- If signs or symptoms of cardiac dysfunction occur (eg, tachycardia, arrhythmias, hypotension), notify health care provider.

Patient/Family Education
- Advise patient to remain recumbent for 30 min after infusion because of possibility of orthostatic hypotension.
- Inform patient that breath may be odorous.

Edrophonium Chloride

(eh-droe-FOE-nee-uhm KLOR-ide)

Class Cholinergic muscle stimulant/Anticholinesterase

How Supplied
Enlon Injection 10 mg/mL ♦ *Reversol* Injection 10 mg/mL ♦ *Tensilon* Injection 10 mg/mL

Action
PHARMACOLOGY: Facilitates myoneural junction impulse transmission by inhibiting acetylcholine destruction by cholinesterase.

PHARMACOKINETICS/DYNAMICS:
Onset: 30 to 60 sec.
Duration: 10 min.

Indications
Differential diagnosis of myasthenia gravis; adjunct in evaluating treatment of myasthenia gravis; evaluation of emergency treatment of myasthenic crises; reversal of neuromuscular blockade by curare gallamine or tubocurarine; treatment of respiratory depression caused by curare overdose.

Contraindications
Hypersensitivity to anticholinesterases; mechanical intestinal and urinary obstruction.

Route/Dosage
Diagnosis of Myasthenia Gravis
ADULTS: **IM/IV** 10 mg.
CHILDREN 34 KG OR LESS: **IV** 2 mg. If no response after 45 sec, may titrate up to 10 mg in increments of 1 mg q 30 to 45 sec. or IM 5 mg as single dose.
CHILDREN MORE THAN 34 KG: **IV** 1 mg. If no response after 45 sec, may titrate up to 5 mg in increments of 1 mg q 30 to 45 sec or **IM** 2 mg as single dose.
INFANTS: **IV** 0.5 mg.

Crisis Test
ADULTS: **IV** When respiration is adequate, give 1 mg initially. If after 1 min patient is not further impaired, give additional 1 mg.

Curare Antagonist
ADULTS: **IV** 10 mg over 30 to 45 sec. Repeat prn up to max total dose of 40 mg.

Evaluation of Myasthenia Gravis Treatment
ADULTS: **IV** 1 to 2 mg 1 hr after ingestion of treatment drug.

Interactions
Corticosteroids: May antagonize anticholinesterases in myasthenia gravis, producing profound muscular depression.
Succinylcholine: Neuromuscular blockade produced by succinylcholine may be either prolonged or antagonized.

Lab Test Interferences
None well documented

Adverse Reactions
CV: Arrhythmia (especially bradycardia); hypotension; tachycardia; atrioventricular block; nodal rhythm; non-specific ECG changes; car-

diac arrest; syncope.
CNS: Convulsions; dysarthria; dysphonia; dizziness; loss of consciousness; drowsiness; headache.
DERM: Rash; urticaria; flushing.
EENT: Lacrimation; miosis; spasm of accommodation; diplopia; conjunctival hyperemia; visual changes.
GI: Increased salivary, gastric and intestinal secretions; nausea; vomiting; dysphagia; increased peristalsis; diarrhea; abdominal cramps; flatulence.
GU: Urinary urgency, frequency and incontinence.
RESP: Increased tracheobronchial secretions; laryngospasm; bronchiolar constriction; respiratory paralysis; dyspnea; respiratory depression; respiratory arrest; bronchospasm.
OTHER: Allergy and anaphylaxis; weakness; fasciculations; muscle cramps and spasms; arthralgia; diaphoresis.

Precautions
Pregnancy: Undetermined.
Lactation: Undetermined.
Special risk patients: Use with caution in patients with bronchial asthma, epilepsy, bradycardia, recent coronary occlusion, vagotonia, hyperthyroidism, cardiac arrhythmias, or peptic ulcer.
Anticholinesterase insensitivity: May develop.

Overdosage: Signs and Symptoms
Increasing parasympathomimetic action, cholinergic crisis, nausea, vomiting, diarrhea, sweating, increased bronchial and salivary secretions with resulting bronchial obstruction, bradycardia.

PATIENT CARE CONSIDERATIONS

Administration/Storage
- Given IM or IV only.
- Store at room temperature.

Assessment/Interventions
- Obtain patient history, including drug history and any known allergies.
- Assess neuromuscular status before and frequently during therapy.
- Obtain baseline ECG and vital signs before therapy and monitor throughout administration.
- If ECG changes develop (supraventricular tachycardia), notify health care provider immediately.
- Take seizure precautions.
- Keep atropine available in syringe as antidote.
- Have respiratory support equipment available.

Patient/Family Education
- Teach patient and family name, desired action, method of administration and potential side effects of edrophonium.
- Inform patient that effects of medication last up to 30 min after IM administration.
- Show patient and family how to assess and record changes in muscle strength.
- Advise patient that urinary urgency and frequency and increased GI motility and secretion will occur and should be reported to health care provider.

Efalizumab

(eh-fah-lih-ZOO-mab)

Class Immunosuppressive

How Supplied
Raptiva Powder for injection, lyophilized 150 mg (designed to deliver 125 mg/1.25 mL)

Action
PHARMACOLOGY: Inhibits binding of leukocyte function antigen-1 to intercellular adhesion molecule-1, thereby interfering with the adhesion of leukocytes to other cell types.

PHARMACOKINETICS/DYNAMICS:
Absorption: Bioavailability following SC administration is 50%. Steady-state trough concentrations are about 9 mcg/mL.

Excretion: Mean steady-state Cl is 24 mL/kg/day; mean time to elimination following the last steady-state dose is 25 days.

Indications Treatment of chronic moderate to severe plaque psoriasis in adult patients who are candidates for systemic therapy or phototherapy.

Contraindications Standard considerations.

Route/Dosage
ADULTS: SC Single 0.7 mg/kg conditioning dose followed by weekly doses of 1 mg/kg (max single dose, 200 mg).

Interactions
Immunosuppressive agents: Do not use efalizumab with other immunosuppressive agents.
Live vaccines (eg, acellular, Lve, live-attenuated): Do not use during efalizumab therapy.

Lab Test Interferences Increased lymphocyte counts related to pharmacologic action are frequently observed.

Adverse Reactions
CNS: Headache (32%).
DERM: Acne (4%); psoriasis (1% or 2% greater than placebo).
GI: Nausea (11%).

LAB TESTS ABS: Thrombocytopenia, lymphocytosis (40%); leukocytosis (26%); elevated alkaline phosphatase (4%); elevated LFTs.
MUSC: Myalgia (8%); arthralgia (1% or 2% greater than placebo).
OTHER: Infection (29%); chills (13%); pain (10%); flu-like syndrome, fever (7%); back pain (4%); asthenia, peripheral edema, hypersensitivity (1% or 2% greater than placebo).

Precautions
Pregnancy: Category C.
Lactation: Undetermined.
Children: Safety and efficacy not established.
Elderly: Use with caution because of increased incidence of infections in the elderly.
Infections: The risk of infection and reactivation of latent, chronic infections may be increased.
Malignancies: Because many immunosuppressants have the potential to increase the risk of malignancies, use with caution in patients at high risk for malignancy or history of malignancy.
Thrombocytopenia: May occur.
Worsening of psoriasis: May occur during or after discontinuation of efalizumab.
First-dose reaction: The conditioning dose is recommended to reduce the incidence and severity of reactions associated with initiation of therapy (eg, headache, fever, nausea, vomiting).

Overdosage: Signs and Symptoms
Vomiting.

PATIENT CARE CONSIDERATIONS
Administration/Storage
- For SC administration only. Not for intradermal, IM, or IV administration.
- Reconstitute powder for injection following manufacturer's guidelines using the prefilled diluent syringe provided with medication.
- Do not shake the vial during reconstitution or reconstitute with diluents other than those supplied or add other medications to vial.
- Reconstituted solution should be administered immediately after reconstitution but can be stored, if necessary, for up to 8 hr at room temperature.
- Dose is usually administered every week.
- Do not administer if particulate matter, cloudiness, or discoloration noted.
- Rotate injection sites (thigh, buttocks, abdomen, upper arm). Give new injections at least 1 inch from previous site and never into areas where the skin is tender, bruised, red, or hard.
- Discard any unused solution or reconstituted solution that is not used within 8 hr of dilution. Do not save for future administration.
- Store vials in refrigerator (36° to 46°F). Store in original carton until time of use. Protect from light.

Assessment/Interventions
- Obtain patient history, including drug history and any known allergies. Note history of the following: recurrent infections, conditions predisposing to infections, prior malignancy, or concurrent treatment with immunosuppressive agents or phototherapy.
- Ensure that patient does not have an active infection prior to starting therapy.
- Ensure that first dose is a conditioning dose to reduce risk of first-dose reactions (eg, headache, chills, fever, nausea, vomiting, myalgia).
- Monitor patient for signs and symptoms of infection and immediately report to health care provider if noted. Be prepared to discontinue efalizumab if infection is determined to be serious.
- Monitor patient for signs and symptoms of anaphylactic or serious allergic reactions. Be prepared to treat appropriately if noted.
- Ensure that platelet counts are determined before starting therapy and periodically during treatment. Be prepared to discontinue efalizumab if thrombocytopenia develops or signs or symptoms of thrombocytopenia (eg, petechiae, easy bruising or bleeding) are noted.
- Monitor patient for CNS, GI, respiratory, and general body side effects, and injection site reactions. Report to health care provider if noted and significant.
- Assess patient's response to therapy. Inform health care provider if psoriasis does not appear to be improving or is worsening.
- Do not administer live virus vaccines while patient is on efalizumab therapy.

Patient/Family Education
- Explain name, dose, action, and potential side effects of drug.
- Advise patient to read the patient package insert before starting therapy and with each refill.
- Ensure that the patient or caregiver understands how to store, prepare, and administer the dose, and dispose of used equipment and supplies if administering at home. The first injection should be performed under the supervision of a qualified health professional.
- Advise patient that if a dose is missed to contact health care provider to find out when the next dose should be taken and what schedule to follow after that.
- Advise patient to notify health care provider if psoriasis is not improving or appears to be

worsening. Caution patient not to change the dose or stop taking unless advised by health care provider.
* Instruct patient to continue taking other psoriasis medications as prescribed by health care provider.
* Advise patient to report any of the following to health care provider: intolerable injection site reactions, fever or other signs of infection, sore throat, rash, itching, hives, unexplained shortness of breath or difficulty breathing, easy bleeding from gums, unexplained bruising, small purple spots under the skin.
* Advise women to notify health care provider if pregnant, planning to become pregnant, or breastfeeding.
* Instruct patient not to take any prescription or OTC medications or dietary supplements unless advised by health care provider.
* Remind patient that office visits and laboratory tests will be required to monitor therapy and to keep appointments.

Efavirenz

(EH-fah-VIE-renz)

Class Antiretroviral/Non-nucleoside reverse transcriptase inhibitor

How Supplied
Sustiva Capsules 50 mg, Capsules 100 mg, Capsules 200 mg, Tablets 600 mg

Action
PHARMACOLOGY: Noncompetitive inhibition of HIV-1 reverse transcriptase.

PHARMACOKINETICS/DYNAMICS:
Absorption: C_{max} is 1.6 to 9.1 mcM. T_{max} is 3 to 5 hr. Food significantly increases the AUC and C_{max}. Take on empty stomach.
Distribution: Approximately 99.5% is protein bound, predominantly albumin.
Metabolism: Metabolized in the liver by CYP450 (primarily CYP3A4 and CYP2B6) to inactive metabolites.
Excretion: The t½ is 52 to 76 hr (single-dose) and 40 to 55 hr (multiple doses). Approximately 14% to 34% is excreted in the urine (less than 1% as unchanged drug), and 16% to 61% is excreted in the feces.

Indications Treatment of HIV-1 infection in combination with other antiretroviral agents.

Contraindications Concomitant use with cisapride, ergot derivatives, midazolam, or triazolam; hypersensitivity to product.

Route/Dosage
ADULTS: PO 600 mg/day in combination with other antiretroviral agents.
CHILDREN 10 TO LESS THAN 15 KG: PO 200 mg/day in combination with other antiretroviral agents.
CHILDREN 15 TO LESS THAN 20 KG: PO 250 mg/day in combination with other antiretroviral agents.
CHILDREN 20 TO LESS THAN 25 KG: PO 300 mg/day in combination with other antiretroviral agents.
CHILDREN 25 TO LESS THAN 32.5 KG: PO 350 mg/day in combination with other antiretroviral agents.
CHILDREN 32.5 TO LESS THAN 40 KG: PO 400 mg/day in combination with other antiretroviral agents.
CHILDREN AT LEAST 40 KG: PO 600 mg/day in combination with other antiretroviral agents.

Interactions
Alprazolam, midazolam, triazolam: May increase blood levels of these drugs, which may produce extreme sedation and respiratory depression. Do not administer concurrently.
Clarithromycin, indinavir, methadone, saquinavir: Efavirenz may decrease plasma concentrations, which could reduce activity of these agents.
Cisapride, ergot derivatives: May elevate levels of these drugs, which may increase the risk of arrhythmias, hematologic abnormalities, or other potentially serious adverse effects. Do not coadminister.
Ethinyl estradiol, nelfinavir, ritonavir: Efavirenz may increase plasma concentrations, which could increase activity or toxicity of these agents.
Phenytoin, carbamazepine, phenobarbital: Plasma concentrations of the anticonvulsant or efavirenz may decrease.
Rifampin: May decrease plasma levels of efavirenz, which may reduce antiviral activity.
Ritonavir: May increase efavirenz plasma level, which could increase side effects.
St. John's wort: May reduce efavirenz plasma concentrations, which may decrease the clinical efficacy.
Warfarin: Plasma concentrations may be increased or decreased.

Lab Test Interferences False-positive urine assay screening test for cannabinoid may occur.

Adverse Reactions
CV: Flushing; palpitations.
CNS: Dizziness (28.1%); fatigue; headache; hypesthesia; impaired concentration (8.3%); insomnia (16.3%); abnormal dreams (6.2%); somnolence (7%); depression; anorexia; nervousness; ataxia; confusion; impaired coordination; paresthesia; neuropathy; tremor; agitation;

emotional lability; hallucination; psychosis.
DERM: Maculopapular rash; rash (26.3%; eg, blistering, desquamation, mucosal involvement, fever); pruritus; increased sweating.
EENT: Abnormal vision; tinnitus.
GI: Nausea; vomiting; diarrhea; dyspepsia; abdominal pain.
HEPA: Hepatitis; LFT elevation.
METAB: Increased total cholesterol; increased amylase.
RESP: Cough; dyspnea.
OTHER: Arthralgia; myalgia; asthenia; fever; pain.

Precautions
Pregnancy: Category C.
Lactation: HIV-infected mothers should not breastfeed their infants.
Children: Ongoing study.

CNS symptoms: Reported in 53% of patients.
Hepatitis: Monitor liver enzymes in patients with known or suspected history of hepatitis B or C infection and in patients receiving medication associated with liver toxicity.
Monotherapy: Resistant virus may emerge rapidly.
Psychiatric symptoms: Serious adverse psychiatric experiences have been reported. Patients with a prior history of psychiatric disorders may be at greater risk. There have been occasional reports of death by suicide, delusions, and psychosis-like behavior.
Skin rash: Reported in 26% of adults and 46% of pediatric patients.

Overdosage: Signs and Symptoms
Increased CNS symptoms, muscle contractions.

PATIENT CARE CONSIDERATIONS

Administration/Storage
* Store oral capsules and tablets at room temperature (77°F); excursions permitted (59° to 86°F).
* Administer on an empty stomach.
* Avoid high-fat meal, as it may increase absorption.
* Administer at bedtime initially and when CNS symptoms are present to improve tolerance of these symptoms.
* Always give in combination with other antiviral agents.
* Do not administer to nursing women.

Assessment/Interventions
* Obtain patient history, including drug history and any known allergies.
* Monitor for signs of hypersensitivity (eg, fever, rash, fatigue, nausea, vomiting, diarrhea, abdominal pain, malaise, lethargy, myalgia, arthralgia, edema, shortness of breath, paresthesia); discontinue use immediately if signs of hypersensitivity are present and notify primary health care provider.
* Monitor for adverse reactions, the most significant of which are CNS symptoms and rash.
* Monitor liver enzymes in patients with hepatitis B or C infections and in patients treated with other medications with known liver toxicity.
* Conduct pregnancy test prior to initial administration of efavirenz.

Patient/Family Education
* Instruct patient to take efavirenz at the same time each day as prescribed in combination with other antiviral drugs and not to skip doses, which could increase the viral load.
* Inform patient not to alter the dose or discontinue therapy without consulting health care provider.
* Inform patient that efavirenz may cause dizziness, impaired concentration, or drowsiness, and to avoid potentially hazardous tasks such as driving or operating machinery if experiencing these symptoms.
* Inform patient that dosing at bedtime improves the tolerability of CNS symptoms.
* Alert patient to the potential for additive CNS effects when efavirenz is used concomitantly with alcohol or psychoactive drugs.
* Instruct patient to avoid OTC medications unless prescribed by primary health care provider.
* Caution patient or family that long-term effects and adverse effects are not known. Therefore, report any problems to the primary care provider.
* Warn patient of the potential adverse effects and drug/drug interactions.
* Instruct patient to notify health care provider immediately if signs of rash or rash accompanied by fever, blistering, oral lesions, conjunctivitis, swelling, muscle or joint aches, general malaise, infection such as a sore throat, fever, cough, or respiratory congestion occur.
* Instruct patient to notify health care provider immediately if symptoms of serious psychiatric adverse experiences occur.
* Inform patient of potential false-positive urine cannabinoid test results.
* Inform patient that efavirenz has not been shown to reduce the risk of passing HIV to others through sexual contact or blood contamination. Encourage abstinence or practicing safe sex and not sharing needles.
* Advise women to use barrier contraception in

combination with other methods of contraception (eg, oral or other hormonal contraceptives).
* Caution mothers to discontinue nursing while receiving efavirenz as there is potential for adverse effects from the drug in nursing infants and transmission of the HIV virus.
* Advise women to inform health care provider if pregnant, planning to become pregnant, or breastfeeding.
* Stress the importance of regular exams and laboratory work.

Eletriptan Hydrobromide
(ell-eh-TRIP-tan HIGH-droe-BROE-mide)
Class Analgesic/Migraine
How Supplied
Relpax Tablets 24.2 mg, Tablets 48.5 mg
Action
PHARMACOLOGY: Selective agonist for vascular serotonin (5-HT$_1$) receptor subtype, causing vasoconstriction of cranial arteries.
PHARMACOKINETICS/DYNAMICS:
Absorption: Eletriptan is well absorbed, reaching a peak plasma level in approximately 1.5 hr. The mean absolute bioavailability is approximately 50%.
Distribution: Eletriptan is approximately 85% protein bound. The Vd is 138 L after IV injection.
Metabolism: The N-demethylated metabolite is active.
Excretion: The terminal elimination t½ is approximately 4 hr. The mean renal Cl is 3.9 L/hr after oral administration. Non-renal Cl accounts for about 90% of total Cl.
Special Populations:
Hepatic Function Impairment – Mild to moderate impairment results in an increase in both AUC (34%) and t½, while the peak plasma level increased 18%.
Elderly – Increased t½ from about 4.4 to 5.7 hr in elderly (65 to 93 yr of age).
Age: Increased t½ from about 4.4 to 5.7 hr in younger subjects (18 to 45 yr of age).
Indications Acute treatment of migraine with or without aura.
Contraindications Ischemic heart disease (eg, angina pectoris); symptoms or findings consistent with ischemic heart disease; coronary artery vasospasm (including Prinzmetal variant angina); significant underlying CV disease; cerebrovascular syndromes (including strokes of any type or transient ischemic attacks); peripheral vascular disease (including ischemic bowel disease); uncontrolled hypertension; hemiplegic or basilar migraine; severe hepatic impairment; hypersensitivity to any component of the product; within 24 hr of treatment with another 5-HT$_1$ agonist or an ergotamine-containing or ergot-type medication (eg, methysergide).

Route/Dosage
ADULTS: **PO** 20 to 40 mg single dose. If required, a second dose may be taken at least 2 hr after the initial dose (max, 80 mg/day).
Interactions
Ergot derivatives (eg, dihydroergotamine): Risk of vasospastic reactions may be increased. Concomitant use within 24 hr of eletriptan is not recommended.
Other 5-HT$_1$ agonists: Concomitant use of other 5-HT$_1$ agonists within 24 hr of eletriptan is not recommended.
Potent cytochrome P450 3A4 inhibitors (eg, clarithromycin, itraconazole, ketoconazole, nefazodone, nelfinavir, ritonavir, troleandomycin): Eletriptan should not be used within 72 hr of drugs that are potent CYP3A4 inhibitors.
Lab Test Interferences None well documented.
Adverse Reactions
CV: Palpitation (at least 1%); coronary artery vasospasm; transient myocardial ischemia; MI; ventricular tachycardia; ventricular fibrillation.
CNS: Dizziness, somnolence (7%); headache (4%); hypertonia, hypesthesia, paresthesia, vertigo (at least 1%).
DERM: Sweating (at least 1%).
GI: Nausea (8%); dry mouth (4%); dyspepsia, dysphagia (eg, throat tightness, difficulty swallowing) (2%).
RESP: Pharyngitis (at least 1%).
OTHER: Asthenia (10%); pain, tightness, or pressure of chest (4%); stomach pain, cramps, or pressure, abdominal pain or discomfort (2%); back pain, chills (at least 1%).
Precautions
Pregnancy: Category C.
Lactation: Excreted in breast milk.
Children: Safety and efficacy not established.
Elderly: There is an increased t½ (from about 4.4 to 5.7 hr) in the elderly (65 to 93 yr of age).
CV/Cardiac events: It is recommended that eletriptan not be given to patients in whom unrecognized coronary artery disease (CAD) is predicted based on the presence of risk factors (eg, hypertension, hypercholesterolemia, smoker, obesity, diabetes, strong family history of CAD, women with surgical or physiological menopause, men over 40 yr of age). Serious adverse cardiac events, including MI, life-threatening

disturbances of cardiac rhythm, and death have been reported within a few hours of administration of a 5-HT$_1$ agonist.

Cerebrovascular events: Cerebral hemorrhage, subarachnoid hemorrhage, stroke, and other cerebrovascular events have been reported with 5-HT$_1$ agonists.

Hypertensive crisis: Elevation in BP, including hypertensive crisis, have been reported with administration of 5-HT$_1$ agonists.

Overdosage: Signs and Symptoms

Hypertension or other more serious CV symptoms may occur.

PATIENT CARE CONSIDERATIONS

Administration/Storage

- Administer prescribed dose at onset of migraine symptoms.
- Administer without regard to meals.
- Do not administer within 72 hr of treatment with ketoconazole, itraconazole, nefazodone, troleandomycin, clarithromycin, ritonavir, nelfinavir, or other potent CYP3A4 inhibitors.
- Do not administer within 24 hr of treatment with another 5-HT$_1$ agonist or ergot-containing or ergot-type medication.
- If headache recurs after initial relief, a second tablet may be administered, provided there is an interval of at least 2 hr between doses.
- If first dose is ineffective, do not administer a second dose unless prescribed by health care provider.
- Do not administer greater than 80 mg per 24-hr period.
- Store at ambient room temperature (59° to 86°F).

Assessment/Interventions

- Obtain patient history, including drug history and any known allergies. Note history of ischemic or vasospastic CAD, previous MI, uncontrolled hypertension, peripheral vascular disease, ischemic bowel disease, stroke, transient ischemic attacks, hemiplegic or basilar migraine, or severe hepatic impairment.
- Note recent (within 24 hr) use of other 5-HT$_1$ agonists or ergotamine-containing or ergot-type drugs.
- Note recent (within 72 hr) use of the following: ketoconazole, itraconazole, nefazodone, troleandomycin, clarithromycin, ritonavir, nelfinavir, any other potent CYP3A4 inhibitor.
- Assess pain location, intensity, duration, and associated symptoms of migraine attack and response to treatment.
- Provide quiet, calm environment. Decrease stimuli, noise, and light.
- Ensure that patients with potential for CAD, including postmenopausal women, men over 40 yr of age, patients with risk factors for CAD (eg, hypertension, hypercholesterolemia, obesity, diabetes, smokers, family history), undergo a CV evaluation before initiating therapy.
- Administer first dose in physician's office or other adequately staffed medical facility to patient with potential for CAD whose CV evaluation provided clinical evidence that patient is reasonably free of coronary artery and ischemic myocardial disease or other significant underlying CV disease. Consider obtaining an ECG during the interval immediately following administration of the first dose of medication to patient with potential for CAD.
- Monitor patient for signs of allergic reaction. Discontinue therapy and immediately notify health care provider if noted. Be prepared to treat appropriately.
- Ensure that patient who is a long-term user of triptans, such as eletriptan, undergoes periodic CV evaluation.
- Monitor patient for CNS, CV, GI, and general body side effects. Report to health care provider if noted and significant.

Patient/Family Education

- Explain name, dose, action, and potential side effects of drug.
- Advise patient to read the *Patient Information* leaflet before starting therapy and again with each refill.
- Explain that drug is to be used only during migraine and does not prevent or reduce the number of attacks. Emphasize that drug is used only to treat actual migraine attack and should not be used to prevent migraine headaches or treat headaches caused by other conditions.
- Advise patient that drug is to be taken as soon as symptoms of migraine appear. A second dose may be taken if symptoms return, but no sooner than 2 hr following the first dose. For a given attack, if there is no response to the first tablet, do not take a second tablet without first consulting with health care provider. Do not take more than 2 tablets in any 24-hr period.
- Advise patient that safety of treating more than 3 headaches in a 30-day period has not been established and to inform health care

provider if headaches are occurring more frequently.
- Advise patient to immediately notify health care provider if any of the following occur after taking a dose of frovatriptan: severe chest pain or chest pain that does not go away; sudden and/or severe stomach pain; shortness of breath; wheezing; swelling of eyelids, face, or lips.
- Advise patient that if tightness, pain, pressure or heaviness in chest, throat, neck, or jaw occurs when using sumatriptan, to discuss these symptoms with health care provider before using again.
- Advise patient to notify health care provider if feelings of tingling, heat, flushing, tiredness, dizziness, heaviness, or pressure after treatment occur.
- Advise patient that drug may cause fatigue or dizziness and to use caution while driving or performing other activities requiring mental alertness.
- Advise patient to avoid unnecessary exposure to sunlight or tanning lamps and to use sunscreen and wear protective clothing to avoid photosensitivity reactions.
- Instruct patient to continue to take migraine prophylactic medications daily as directed.
- Advise patient not currently taking a migraine prophylactic drug to discuss the use of such drugs with health care provider.
- Advise women to notify health care provider if pregnant, planning to become pregnant, or breastfeeding.
- Warn patient not to take any prescription or OTC drugs, dietary supplements, or herbal preparations without consulting health care provider.
- Advise patient that follow-up visits may be necessary to monitor therapy and to keep appointments.

Emtricitabine

(Em-try-SIGH-tah-bean)

Class Antiviral

How Supplied
Emtriva Capsule 200 mg

Action

PHARMACOLOGY: Inhibits activity of HIV-1 reverse transcriptase by competing with the natural substrate deoxycytidine 5′-triphosphate and by being incorporated into nascent viral DNA, resulting in chain termination.

PHARMACOKINETICS/DYNAMICS:

Absorption: Rapidly and extensively absorbed after oral administration. Absolute bioavailability is about 93%. Postdose C_{max} about 1 to 2 hr. Steady-state C_{max} is about 1.8 mcg/mL. AUC is about 10 mcg/mL•hr. Mean steady state trough plasma concentration 24 hr postdose is 0.09 mcg/mL.

Excretion: Plasma t½ is approximately 10 hr. Eliminated in the urine (86% with 13% as putative metabolites) and feces (14%).

Indications In combination with other antiretroviral agents for the treatment of HIV-1 infections in adults.

Contraindications Standard considerations.

Route/Dosage
ADULTS: PO 200 mg qd.

Renal impairment
ADULTS: PO Ccr at least 50 mL/min administer 200 mg q 24 hr; Ccr 30 to 49 mL/min administer 200 mg q 48 hr; Ccr 15 to 29 mL/min administer 200 mg q 72 hr; Ccr less than 15 mL/min (including hemodialysis patients) 200 mg q 96 hr (if dosing on day of dialysis, give dose after dialysis).

Interactions None well documented.

Lab Test Interferences None well documented.

Adverse Reactions
CNS: Headache (13%); insomnia (7%); depressive disorders (6%); paresthesia (5%); dizziness, neuropathy/peripheral neuritis (4%); abnormal dreams (2%).
DERM: Rash; skin discoloration (hyperpigmentation on palms and/or soles); rash event (including rash, pruritus, maculopapular rash, urticaria, vesiculobullous rash, pustular rash, allergic reaction [17%]).
EENT: Rhinitis (18%).
GI: Diarrhea (23%); nausea (18%); vomiting (9%); dyspepsia (4%).
RESP: Increased cough (14%).
OTHER: Asthenia (16%); abdominal pain (8%); arthralgia (3%); myalgia (4%).

> WARNING:
> *Lactic acidosis/severe hepatomegaly with stenosis:* Lactic acidosis and severe hepatomegaly with stenosis, including fatal cases, have been reported with use of nucleoside analogues alone and in combination with other antiretroviral agents.

Precautions
Pregnancy: Category B.
Lactation: Undetermined. HIV-infected mothers should not breastfeed their infants.

Children: Safety and efficacy not established.
Elderly: Use with caution because of the greater frequency of decreased hepatic, renal, or cardiac function, and concomitant diseases or other drug therapy.
Fat redistribution: Redistribution and accumulation of body fat including central obesity, dorsocervical fat enlargement (buffalo hump), peripheral wasting, facial wasting, breast enlargement, and cushingoid appearance have occurred in patients receiving antiretroviral therapy.

Hepatitis B: Exacerbations of hepatitis B have been reported after discontinuation of emtricitabine. It is recommended that all patients with HIV be tested for chronic hepatitis B virus (HBV) before initiating antiretroviral therapy. Patients co-infected with HIV and HBV should be closely monitored with both clinical and laboratory follow-up for at least several months after stopping treatment.
Impaired renal function: Dosage adjustment is recommended.

PATIENT CARE CONSIDERATIONS
Administration/Storage
- Administer prescribed dose qd.
- May be administered without regard to meals. Administer with food if GI upset occurs.
- Store capsules at controlled room temperature (59° to 86°F).

Assessment/Interventions
- Obtain patient history, including drug history and any known allergies. Note renal impairment.
- Ensure that medication is used in combination with other antiretroviral agents.
- Ensure that the dosing interval is adjusted in patient with renal impairment (Ccr less than 50 mL/min).
- Ensure that patient is tested for presence of chronic hepatitis B infection before initiating therapy.
- Monitor patient for signs of lactic acidosis. If patient develops profound weakness or tiredness, unexpected stomach discomfort, feeling cold, dizzy, or lightheaded, or slow or irregular heartbeat, withhold drug and contact health care provider.
- Assess patient for GI, CNS, musculoskeletal, and general body side effects. Inform health care provider if noted and significant.

Patient/Family Education
- Advise patient to read the "Patient Information" leaflet before starting therapy and with each refill.
- Explain name, dose, action, and potential side effects of drug.
- Warn patient that this drug is not to be used by itself but is combined with other antiviral agents and to not change the dose or stop taking any of the antiviral agents unless advised by health care provider.
- Advise patient to take prescribed dose qd without regard to meals but to take with food if stomach upset occurs.
- Advise patient that if a dose is missed to take the dose as soon as possible and then return to their normal schedule. However, if it is within 6 hr of the next dose to skip the dose and take the next dose at the regular time. If a dose is skipped caution patient to not double the dose to catch up but to continue with their normal schedule unless advised by health care provider.
- Instruct patient to report these symptoms immediately to health care provider: persistent nausea or vomiting, profound weakness or tiredness, unexpected stomach discomfort, difficulty breathing.
- Inform patient that drug does not completely eliminate HIV virus and, therefore, does not reduce risk of transmitting HIV to others. Appropriate precautions must still be followed.
- Advise patient that the drug is not a cure for HIV infection and illnesses associated with HIV infection, including opportunistic infections, as they may continue to be acquired. Patient should remain under the care of health care provider.
- Instruct patient not to take any prescription or OTC medications or dietary supplements unless advised by health care provider.
- Advise women to notify health care provider if pregnant, planning to become pregnant, or breastfeeding. Caution HIV-infected mother that breastfeeding could cause HIV infection in the baby.
- Remind patient that examinations and laboratory tests will be required to monitor therapy and to keep appointments.

Emtricitabine/Tenofovir Disoproxil Fumarate

(em-try-SIGH-tah-bean/teh-NOE-fo-veer DIE-so-prox-ill FYU-mah-rate)

Class Antiretroviral combination

How Supplied
Truvada Tablets 200 mg emtricitabine/300 mg tenofovir disoproxil fumarate (equiv. to 245 mg tenofovir disoproxil)

Action
PHARMACOLOGY:
Emtricitabine: Inhibits activity of HIV-1 reverse transcriptase by competing with the natural substrate deoxycytidine 5-triphosphate and by being incorporated into nascent viral DNA, resulting in chain termination.
Tenofovir disoproxil fumarate: Tenofovir disoproxil fumarate is a prodrug of tenofovir, which inhibits the activity of HIV-1 reverse transcriptase by competing with deoxyadenosine 5-triphosphate and by DNA chain termination after incorporation into DNA.

Indications Treatment of HIV-1 infection in combination with other antiretroviral agents.

Contraindications Standard considerations.

Route/Dosage
ADULTS: **PO** 200 mg emtricitabine/300 mg tenofovir disoproxil fumarate once daily.

Renal Impairment
ADULTS: **PO** Ccr 50 mL/min or more give dose q 24 hr. Ccr 30 to 49 mL/min give dose q 48 hr. Ccr less than 30 mL/min do not administer.

Interactions
Atazanavir, lopinavir/ritonavir: Tenofovir concentrations may be elevated, increasing the risk of adverse effects. The AUC and C_{min} of atazanavir may be decreased.
Didanosine: AUC and C_{max} of didanosine may be elevated, increasing the risk of adverse effects (eg, pancreatitis, neuropathy).
Drugs that reduce renal function or compete for active tubular secretion (eg, acyclovir, ganciclovir): May increase serum concentrations of emtricitabine or tenofovir.

Lab Test Interferences None well documented.

Adverse Reactions
CNS:
Emtricitabine – Asthenia, headache, dizziness (more than 5%); abnormal dreams, depressive disorder, insomnia, neuropathy, peripheral neuritis, paresthesia.
Tenofovir – Headache, depression (more than 5%); asthenia, dizziness, insomnia, abnormal dreams, paresthesia, peripheral neuropathy.
DERM:
Emtricitabine – Rash including pruritus, maculopapular, urticaria, vesiculobullous, pustular (more than 5%).
Tenofovir – Rash including pruritus, maculopapular rash, urticaria, vesiculobullous rash, pustular rash, sweating.
EENT:
Emtricitabine – Rhinitis.
GI:
Emtricitabine – Abdominal pain, diarrhea, nausea, vomiting (more than 5%); dyspepsia.
Tenofovir – Nausea, vomiting, diarrhea, vomiting (more than 5%); abdominal pain, flatulence, anorexia, dyspepsia; pancreatitis (postmarketing).
GU:
Tenofovir – Renal insufficiency, renal failure, acute renal failure, Fanconi syndrome, proximal tubulopathy, proteinuria, increased creatinine, acute tubular necrosis (postmarketing).
HYPERSEN:
Tenofovir – Allergy (postmarketing).
LABTESTABS:
Emtricitabine – Elevated ALT, AST, bilirubin, creatine kinase, decreased neutrophils, pancreatic amylase, serum amylase, serum glucose, serum lipase, triglycerides.
M/N:
Tenofovir – Weight loss; hypophosphatemia, lactic acidosis (postmarketing).
MUSC:
Emtricitabine – Arthralgia, myalgia.
Tenofovir – Back pain, arthralgia, myalgia.
RESP:
Emtricitabine – Cough.
Tenofovir – Pneumonia; dyspnea (postmarketing).
OTHER:
Tenofovir – Pain, chest pain, fever.

> **WARNING:**
> Lactic acidosis and hepatomegaly with steatosis (including fatal cases) have been reported with use of nucleoside analogues alone and in combination with other antiretroviral agents. *Truvada* is not indicated for the treatment of chronic hepatitis B virus (HBV) infection and the safety and efficacy have not been established in patients co-infected with HBV and HIV.

Precautions
Pregnancy: Category B.
Lactation: Undetermined. HIV-infected mothers should not breastfeed infants.
Children: Safety and efficacy not established.
Elderly: Use with caution because of greater

frequency of decreased hepatic, renal, or cardiac function, and concomitant diseases or other drug therapy.
Bone effects: Decreases from baseline bone mineral density at the lumbar spine and hip have been seen.
Fat redistribution: Redistribution and accumulation of body fat including central obesity, dorsocervical fat enlargement (buffalo hump), peripheral wasting, facial wasting, breast enlargement, and cushingoid appearance may occur.

Hepatitis B: Exacerbations of hepatitis B have been reported after discontinuation of emtricitabine. It is recommended that all patients with HIV be tested for chronic hepatitis B virus (HBV) before initiating antiretroviral therapy. Patients co-infected with HIV and HBV should be closely monitored with both clinical and laboratory follow-up for at least several months after stopping treatment.
Impaired renal function: Dosage adjustment is recommended.

PATIENT CARE CONSIDERATIONS
Administration/Storage
- For use in combination with other antiretroviral medications.
- Administer 1 tablet once daily without regard to meals. Administer with food if GI upset occurs.
- If coadministering with didanosine enteric-coated tablets, administer with a light meal or under fasted conditions. If coadministering with didanosine buffered tablet, administer under fasted conditions.
- Store tablets at controlled room temperature (59° to 86°F).

Assessment/Interventions
- Obtain patient history, including drug history and any known allergies. Note renal or hepatic impairment, osteopenia or osteoporosis, or concurrent use of nephrotoxic agents.
- Ensure that medication is not coadministered with emtricitabine, tenofovir, or other drugs containing lamivudine.
- Ensure that medication is used in combination with other antiretroviral agents.
- Ensure that renal function is evaluated before starting therapy and repeated periodically during prolonged treatment, especially in patient at risk for, or with a history of renal dysfunction. Ensure that medication is not used in patient with Ccr less than 30 mL/min and dosing interval is adjusted to q 48 hr in patient with Ccr between 30 and 49 mL/min.
- Ensure that liver enzymes are evaluated before starting therapy and periodically thereafter during prolonged treatment.
- Ensure that patient has been tested for hepatitis B virus (HBV) before starting therapy. In patient co-infected with HBV and HIV, closely monitor patient with clinical and laboratory follow-up for at least several months after discontinuation of tenofovir because of risk of potential exacerbation of HBV.
- Ensure that bone density monitoring is performed in HIV-infected patient with history of pathologic bone fracture or at substantial risk for osteopenia.
- Ensure that supplementation with calcium and vitamin D has been considered in patients with HIV-associated osteopenia or osteoporosis.
- Monitor patient for GI, CNS, and general body side effects. Notify health care provider if noted and significant.
- Monitor patient for signs of lactic acidosis. Withhold drug and notify health care provider immediately of any of the following: profound weakness or tiredness; unexpected stomach discomfort; fatty diarrhea; feeling cold, dizzy, or lightheaded; slow or irregular heartbeat.

Patient/Family Education
- Explain name, dose, action, and potential side effects of drug.
- Advise patient or caregiver to review the *Patient Information Leaflet* before starting therapy and with each refill.
- Advise patient to take 1 tablet once daily without regard to meals but to take with food if stomach upset occurs.
- Instruct patient if a dose is missed to take it as soon as possible and then take the next dose at the regularly scheduled time. If it is almost time for the next dose, advise patient not to take the missed dose and wait and take the next dose as scheduled. Caution patient not to double the next dose to catch up.
- Warn patient that this drug is not to be used by itself but is combined with other antiviral agents.
- Instruct patient to report the following symptoms immediately to health care provider: abdominal swelling or enlargement; fatty diarrhea; profound weakness or tiredness; unexpected stomach discomfort; feeling cold, dizzy, or lightheaded; slow or irregular heartbeat.
- Inform patient that drug does not completely eliminate HIV virus and, therefore, does not reduce risk of transmitting HIV to others. Appropriate precautions must still be followed.

- Advise patient that drug is not a cure for HIV infection and that they may continue to acquire illnesses associated with HIV infection (including opportunistic infections) and should remain under a physician's care.
- Advise patient with HIV-associated osteopenia or osteoporosis to discuss need for supplementation with calcium and vitamin D with health care provider
- Advise women to notify health care provider if pregnant, planning to become pregnant, or breastfeeding. Advise HIV-infected mothers not to breastfeed to prevent infecting infants with HIV.
- Instruct patient not to take any prescription or OTC medications, herbal preparations, or dietary supplements unless advised by health care provider.
- Remind patient that follow-up visits and laboratory tests will be required to monitor therapy and to keep appointments.

Enalapril Maleate

(EH-NAL-uh-prill MAL-ee-ate)
Class Antihypertensive/ACE inhibitor

How Supplied
Vasotec Tablets 2.5 mg, Tablets 5 mg, Tablets 10 mg, Tablets 20 mg ♦ *Vasotec IV* Injection 1.25 mg enalaprilat/mL

Action
PHARMACOLOGY: Competitively inhibits angiotensin I-converting enzyme, preventing conversion of angiotensin I to angiotensin II, a potent vasoconstrictor that also stimulates release of aldosterone. Results in decrease in BP, reduced sodium absorption, and potassium retention.

PHARMACOKINETICS/DYNAMICS:
Absorption: Bioavailability is approximately 60%. T_{max} is within 1 hr (enalapril); 3 to 4 hr (enalaprilat).
Distribution: Enalapril crosses the blood-brain barrier poorly, if at all. Enalaprilat does not cross the blood-brain barrier.
Metabolism: Enalapril is a prodrug and is hydrolyzed to enalaprilat (more potent than enalapril).
Excretion: Intact enalapril and approximately 40% of the dose as enalaprilat is excreted in the urine. Approximately 94% is recovered in the urine and feces. The t½ is 1.3 hr (enalapril). Enalaprilat is dialyzable.
Onset: 1 hr.
Peak: 4 to 6 hr.
Duration: At least 24 hr.
Special Populations:
Renal Function Impairment – In those with glomerular filtration rate 30 mL/min or less, the peak and trough enalaprilat levels increase, T_{max} increases, and time to steady state may be delayed. Dosage adjustment recommended.

Indications Treatment of hypertension and symptomatic CHF in combination with diuretics and digitalis and asymptomatic left ventricular dysfunction. **Unlabeled use(s):** Treatment of diabetic nephropathy, childhood hypertension, hypertension related to scleroderma, and renal crisis scleroderma.

Contraindications History of angioedema related to previous treatment with an ACE inhibitor and in patients with hereditary or idiopathic angioedema; hypersensitivity to ACE inhibitors.

Route/Dosage
Heart Failure
ADULTS: **PO** Initial dose: 2.5 mg bid. Usual dose: 2.5 to 20 mg/day in 2 divided doses (max, 40 mg/day). Titrate doses upward as tolerated over a period of a few days or weeks. The max daily dose is 40 mg in divided doses.

High-Risk Patients
ADULTS: **IV** Hypertensive patients at risk (eg, those with heart failure, hyponatremia, high-dose diuretic therapy, recent intensive diureses or increase in diuretic dose, renal dialysis, or severe volume or salt depletion of any etiology) have potential for extremely hypotensive response. Initiate therapy under very close medical supervision. The starting dose should be 0.625 mg or less administered IV over a period of 5 min or more and preferably longer (up to 1 hr).

Hypertension
ADULTS: **PO** Initial dose: 2.5 to 5 mg/day. Titrate to desired BP control. Usual maintenance dose: 10 to 40 mg/day in single or twice daily doses. **IV** 1.25 mg over a 5-min period q 6 hr. For patients with Ccr of 30 mL/min or less, the dose is 0.625 mg. Dose may be repeated if after 1 hr the clinical response is inadequate. Additional doses of 1.25 mg may be administered at 6-hr intervals. For dialysis patients, the initial dose is 0.625 mg or less given over 5 min or preferably longer (up to 1 hr).
CHILDREN: **PO** Initial dose: 0.08 mg/kg (up to 5 mg) qd. Adjust dose according to BP response. Doses above 0.58 mg/kg (or in excess of 40 mg) have not been studied in pediatric patients.

Left Ventricular Dysfunction
ADULTS: **PO** Initial dose: 2.5 mg bid. Titrate to targeted daily dose of 20 mg in divided doses.

Renal Function Impairment
ADULTS: PO Titrate dosage upward until BP is controlled or until a max dosage of 40 mg/day is reached. Use an initial dosage of 5 mg/day in normal renal function and mild impairment (Ccr more than 30 mL/min); 2.5 mg/day in moderate to severe renal impairment (Ccr 30 mL/min or less); and 2.5 mg on the day of dialysis in dialysis patients (adjust dosage on nondialysis days based on BP response).

Interactions
Allopurinol: Greater risk of hypersensitivity possible with coadministration.
Antacids: Enalapril bioavailability may be decreased. Separate administration times by 1 to 2 hr.
Capsaicin: Cough may be exacerbated.
Digoxin: May increase or decrease plasma levels of digoxin.
Indomethacin, salicylates (eg, aspirin): Hypotensive effects may be reduced, especially in low-renin or volume-dependent hypertensive patients.
Lithium: Increased lithium levels and symptoms of lithium toxicity may occur.
Phenothiazines: May increase pharmacologic effect of enalapril.
Potassium preparations, potassium-sparing diuretics: May increase serum potassium levels.
Rifampin: Pharmacologic effects of enalapril may be decreased.

Lab Test Interferences False elevation of liver enzymes or serum bilirubin may occur.

Adverse Reactions
CV: Hypotension (7%); angina, chest pain, orthostatic hypotension, syncope (2%); myocardial infarction (1%); tachycardia (less than 1%).
CNS: Headache (5%); dizziness (4%); fatigue (3%); vertigo (2%); asthenia (1%).
DERM: Rash (1%); photosensitivity (less than 1%).
GI: Abdominal pain, diarrhea (2%); nausea, vomiting (1%).
GU: UTI (1%).
HEMA: Decreased hemoglobin and hematocrit, neutropenia, agranulocytosis, thrombocytopenia, pancytopenia, eosinophilia.
METAB: Hyperkalemia.
RESP: Bronchitis, cough, dyspnea (1%).

PATIENT CARE CONSIDERATIONS
Administration/Storage
- Administer alone or in combination with other antihypertensives.
- Do not administer to pregnant women during second and third trimesters as fetal and neonatal morbidity and death can occur.
- Follow manufacturer's recommendations when converting from IV to PO therapy or from PO to IV therapy.

Tablets:
- Give prescribed dose without regard to meals. Administer with food if GI upset occurs.
- Store tablets at controlled room temperature (59° to 89°F). Protect from moisture.

Suspension:
- Tablets may be mixed with *Bicitra* and *Ora-*

> **WARNING:**
> *Pregnancy:* Use in second and third trimesters may cause injury and death to fetus.

Precautions
Pregnancy: Category D (second, third trimester); Category C (first trimester).
Lactation: Excreted in breast milk.
Children: Safety and efficacy not established in pediatric patients younger than 1 mo of age, neonates, or pediatric patients with glomerular filtration rate less than 30 mL/min/1.73 m^2 (oral). Safety and efficacy not established (IV).
Renal function impairment: Reduce dose and give less frequently. In renal insufficiency, stable elevations in BUN and serum creatinine may occur because of inadequate renal perfusion; monitor renal function during first few weeks of therapy and adjust dosage.
Angioedema: May occur. Use drug with extreme caution in patients with hereditary angioedema.
Aortic stenosis/hypertrophic cardiomyopathy: As with other vasodilators, enalapril should be used with caution in patients with obstruction in the outflow tract of the left ventricle.
Cough: Chronic dry cough may occur during treatment; higher incidence in women.
Hepatic failure: Rarely, ACE inhibitors have been associated with a syndrome that starts with cholestatic jaundice and progresses to fulminant hepatic necrosis and sometimes death.
Hypotension/first-dose effect: Significant decreases in BP may occur after first dose, especially in severely salt- or volume-depleted patients or in those with heart failure; monitor closely for 2 hr or more after initial dose and during first 2 wk of therapy. Minimize risk by discontinuing diuretics, decreasing dose, or increasing salt intake approximately 1 wk prior to initiating enalapril.
Neutropenia and agranulocytosis: Have occurred; risk appears greater with renal dysfunction, heart failure, or immunosuppression; monitor WBC counts frequently.

Overdosage: Signs and Symptoms
Hypotension.

Sweet SF, following manufacturer's guidelines, to form a suspension.
- Shake well before measuring dose.
- Administer prescribed dose using cup, spoon, or syringe.
- Store suspension in refrigerator (36° to 46°F). Discard any unused suspension after 30 days.

Injection:
- For IV administration only when oral therapy is not practical. Not for intradermal, subcutaneous, or IM administration.
- May be administered undiluted or mixed with up to 50 mL of D5W, NS, D5WNS, or D5W in Lactated Ringer's injection. Dilution is stable for up to 24 hr at room temperature.
- Do not administer if particulate matter, cloudiness, or discoloration is noted.
- Administer prescribed dose by slow IV infusion over 5 min.
- Store injection at controlled room temperature (59° to 89°F).

Assessment/Interventions

- Obtain patient history, including drug history and any known allergies. Note renal or hepatic impairment, conditions predisposing to volume depletion (eg, prolonged diuretic therapy), diabetes, heart failure, anuria, hereditary or idiopathic angioedema, lupus erythematosus, left ventricular outflow obstruction, allergy to any other ACE inhibitor, and concurrent use of potassium-containing salt substitutes, potassium supplements, or potassium-sparing diuretics.
- Ensure that small initial dose and gradual escalation of dose are used in patient with heart failure or severe renal impairment (Ccr less than 30 mL/min).
- Ensure that volume and/or salt depletion have been corrected before initiating therapy.
- Ensure that serum electrolytes and renal function are monitored periodically.
- Ensure that CBC with differential are evaluated prior to starting therapy, at 2 wk intervals for 3 mo, and periodically thereafter in patient with renal impairment.
- Monitor and record BP and pulse. Should symptomatic hypotension occur, hold medication and notify health care provider.
- Take safety precautions if orthostatic hypotension occurs.
- Assess heart failure patient for evidence of worsening failure (eg, daily weights, evaluation of peripheral edema, shortness of breath). Inform health care provider if rapid weight gain (eg, 2 pounds in 1 day or 5 pounds in 1 wk) is noted or if patient is experiencing worsening edema or other symptoms of heart failure (eg, worsening shortness of breath).
- Monitor for signs of hypersensitivity including angioedema involving swelling of the face, lips, eyelids, and tongue. Discontinue medication and notify health care provider immediately if noted. Be prepared to treat appropriately.
- Assess patient for GI, CNS, and general body side effects. Inform health care provider if noted and significant.

Patient/Family Education

- Explain name, dose, action, and potential side effects of drug.

Injection:
- Advise patient that medication will be prepared and administered by a health care professional in a medical setting.

Tablets and Suspension:
- Advise patient to take prescribed dose without regard to meals but to take with food if stomach upset occurs.
- Advise patient to try to take each dose at about the same time each day.
- Advise patient or caregiver to shake suspension well before measuring each dose.
- Inform hypertensive patient that drug controls, but does not cure, hypertension and to continue taking drug as prescribed even when BP is not elevated.
- Caution patient not to change the dose or stop taking unless advised by health care provider.
- Instruct patient to continue taking other medications for the condition as prescribed by health care provider.
- Instruct patient in BP and pulse measurement skills.
- Advise patient to monitor and record BP and pulse at home and to inform health care provider if abnormal measurements are noted. Also advise patient to take record of BP and pulse to each follow-up visit.
- Caution patient to avoid sudden position changes to prevent orthostatic hypotension.
- Instruct patient to lie or sit down if experiencing dizziness or lightheadedness when standing.
- Emphasize to hypertensive patient the importance of other modalities on BP control: weight control, regular exercise, smoking cessation, and moderate intake of alcohol and salt.
- Emphasize to heart failure patient the importance of other modalities that can help control heart failure symptoms: weight control, progressive exercise program, smoking cessation, and moderate intake of alcohol and salt.
- Advise heart failure patient to weigh daily, keep a record of daily weights, and notify

health care provider if rapid weight gain (eg, 5 pounds in 1 wk) is noted or if edema or shortness of breath are getting worse.
- Caution patient that inadequate fluid intake, excessive perspiration, diarrhea, or vomiting can lead to excessive fall in BP resulting in lightheadedness or fainting.
- Advise patient that medication may cause dizziness or lightheadedness and to use caution while driving or performing other tasks requiring mental alertness until tolerance is determined.
- Caution patient to avoid unnecessary exposure to UV light (sunlight, tanning booths) and to use sunscreen and wear protective clothing when exposed to UV light to avoid photosensitivity reaction.
- Instruct women to inform health care provider if pregnant, planning to become pregnant, or breastfeeding.
- Instruct patient to stop taking drug and immediately report any of these symptoms to health care provider: sore throat, fever, swelling of the hands or feet, irregular heartbeat, chest pains, fainting, swelling of the face, lips, eyelids, or tongue, difficulty breathing.
- Instruct patient to inform health care provider if a persistent cough develops while taking this medication.
- Caution patient not to take any prescription or OTC medications, potassium-containing salt substitutes, potassium supplements, or dietary supplements unless advised by health care provider.
- Advise patient that follow-up visits and lab tests will be required to monitor therapy and to keep appointments.

Enalapril Maleate/ Felodipine

(EH-NAL-uh-prill MAL-ee-ate/feh-LOW-dih-peen)

Class Antihypertensive combinations

How Supplied
Lexxel Extended-release tablets enalapril maleate 5 mg/felodipine 2.5 mg, Extended-release tablets enalapril maleate 5 mg/felodipine 5 mg

Action
PHARMACOLOGY: The 2 components have complementary antihypertensive actions. Enalapril suppresses the renin-angiotension-aldosterone system. Felodipine dihydropyridine calcium channel blocker produces peripheral vasodilation.

Indications
Hypertension: Not indicated for initial treatment of hypertension.

Contraindications History of angioedema.

Route/Dosage
ADULT: **PO** 1 tablet qd for patients whose BP is not adequately controlled with felodipine or enalapril monotherapy. If inadequate BP control persists beyond 1 to 2 wk, increase to 2 tablets/day.

Interactions
Allopurinol: Enalapril may increase risk of hypersensitivity.
Antacids: Enalapril bioavailability may be decreased. Separate administration times by 1 to 2 hr.
Barbiturates: Effects of felodipine may be decreased.
Capsaicin: Enalapril-induced cough may be exacerbated.
Carbamazepine: Plasma levels of felodipine may be decreased, reducing effect.
CYP3A4 inhibitors (eg, erythromycin): Increased effect of felodipine.
Diuretics: Excessive reduction in BP may occur.
Food: Effects of felodipine may increase if given with grapefruit juice.
Hydantoins: Serum felodipine levels may be decreased, reducing effects.
Indomethacin: Hypotensive effects may be reduced, especially in low-renin or volume-dependent hypertensive patients.
Lithium: Increased lithium levels and symptoms of lithium toxicity may occur.
Phenothiazine: Enalapril may increase pharmacological effect of phenothiazines.
Potassium preparations, potassium-sparing diuretics: Enalapril may increase serum potassium levels.
Rifampin: Pharmacologic effects of enalapril may be decreased.

Lab Test Interferences None well documented.

Adverse Reactions
CV: Peripheral edema (4%); angina; arrhythmias; AV block; chest pain; hypotension; MI; orthostatic hypotension; palpitation; syncope; tachycardia; vasculitis.
CNS: Headache (10%); dizziness (4%); asthenia, fatigue (2%); anxiety; insomnia; irritability; lightheadedness; nervousness; paresthesias; psychiatric disturbances; somnolence; vertigo.
DERM: Flushing (2%); pruritus; rash.
GI: Abdominal discomfort; constipation; cramps; diarrhea; dry mouth; dyspepsia; flatulence; nausea; thirst; vomiting.
GU: Micturition disorders; sexual difficulties; UTI.
HEMA: Agranulocytosis; decreased hemoglobin

and hematocrit; eosinophilia; epistaxis; neutropenia; pancytopenia; thrombocytopenia.
HEPA: Hepatic failure.
RESP: Cough (2%); bronchitis; dyspnea; nasal or chest congestion; pharyngitis; respiratory infections; rhinitis; shortness of breath; sinusitis; sneezing; wheezing.
OTHER: Arthralgia; arthritis; fever; gingival hyperplasia; hyperkalemia; muscle cramps; myalgia; pain; inflammation.

> **WARNING:**
> When used in pregnancy during the second and third trimesters, ACE inhibitors can cause injury and even death to the developing fetus.

Precautions
Pregnancy: Category C (first trimester); Category D (second and third trimesters).
Lactation: Secreted into breast milk.
Children: Safety and efficacy have not been determined.
Elderly: May have greater hypotensive effects and increased risk of peripheral edema with higher doses.
Renal function impairment: Reduce dose and give less frequently. Dose reduction or discontinuation may be necessary. Monitor renal function during first few weeks of therapy and adjust dosage.
Hepatic function impairment. Use with caution in patients with impaired hepatic function or reduced hepatic blood flow.
Angioedema: Angioedema may occur; use is contraindicated in patients with history of angioedema.
Aortic stenosis/Hypertrophic cardiomyopathy: Use with caution.
CHF: Use felodipine with caution. Transient hypotension may occur.
Cough: Chronic dry cough may occur during treatment; higher incidence in women.
Neutropenia and agranulocytosis: Neutropenia and agranulocytosis have occurred; risk appears greater with renal dysfunction and collagen vascular disease; monitor WBC counts frequently.
Surgery/Anesthesia: During major surgery or anesthesia, with agents that produce hypotension, enalapril may block angiotensin II formation secondary to compensatory renin release. If hypotension occurs and is considered to be caused by this mechanism, it can be corrected by volume expansion.
Withdrawal effects: Abrupt withdrawal of calcium channel blockers may cause increased frequency and duration of angina. Taper dose gradually.

PATIENT CARE CONSIDERATIONS
Administration/Storage
- Administer qd as prescribed without regard to meals. Administer with food if GI upset occurs.
- Have patient swallow whole. Do not crush, chew, or divide.
- Administer alone or in combination with other antihypertensives.
- Do not administer to pregnant women as fetal and neonatal morbidity and death can occur.
- Administer with caution and reduced dosage in patients with possible depletion of intravascular volume.
- Store tablets at controlled room temperature (59° to 86°F). Protect from moisture and light.

Assessment/Interventions
- Obtain patient history, including drug history and any known allergies. Note history of angioedema with previous ACE inhibitor therapy, renal or hepatic impairment, heart failure, hypotension, hypertrophic cardiomyopathy, lupus erythematosus, or allergy to any other ACE inhibitor or sulfonamide-derived medications. Note concurrent use of potassium-containing salt substitutes, potassium supplements, potassium-sparing diuretics, or potent inhibitors of CYP3A4 (eg, itraconazole).
- Ensure that serum electrolytes and renal function are evaluated before starting therapy and periodically during treatment.
- Ensure that volume and/or salt depletion have been corrected before initiating therapy.
- Monitor and record BP and pulse. Should hypotension result, hold medication and notify health care provider.
- Take safety precautions if orthostatic hypotension occurs.
- Monitor for signs of hypersensitivity, including angioedema involving swelling of the face, lips, eyelids, and tongue. Discontinue medication and notify health care provider immediately if noted. Be prepared to treat appropriately.
- Assess patient for CV, GI, CNS, and general body side effects. Report to health care provider if noted and significant.

Patient/Family Education
- Explain name, dose, action, and potential side effects of drug.

- Advise patient that medication will be started at a low dose and then gradually increased as tolerated until max benefit has been obtained.
- Advise patient to take qd as prescribed at about the same time each day.
- Instruct patient to swallow tablets whole and to not crush, chew, or divide the tablets.
- Advise patient to take without regard to meals but to take with food if GI upset occurs.
- Inform patient that drug controls, but does not cure, hypertension and to continue taking drug as prescribed even when BP is not elevated.
- Caution patient not to change the dose or stop taking unless advised by health care provider.
- Instruct patient to continue taking other BP medications as prescribed by health care provider.
- Instruct patient in BP and pulse measurement skills.
- Advise patient to monitor and record BP and pulse at home and to inform health care provider should abnormal measurements be noted. Also advise patient to take record of BP and pulse to each follow-up visit.
- Caution patient to avoid sudden position changes to prevent orthostatic hypotension.
- Instruct patient to lie or sit down if experiencing dizziness or lightheadedness when standing and to inform health care provider if this happens frequently.
- Caution patient that inadequate fluid intake, excessive perspiration, diarrhea, or vomiting can lead to excessive fall in BP resulting in lightheadedness or fainting.
- Emphasize to hypertensive patient importance of other modalities on BP: weight control, regular exercise, smoking cessation, and moderate intake of alcohol and food.
- Inform patient that swelling of the gums can occur but that good oral hygiene will help prevent this from occurring or keep it from becoming severe.
- Advise women to notify health care provider if pregnant, planning to become pregnant, or breastfeeding.
- Instruct patient to stop taking drug and immediately report any of these symptoms to health care provider: fainting, swelling of the face, lips, eyelids, or tongue, difficulty breathing, sore throat, fever or other signs of infection, yellowing of the skin or eyes.
- Instruct patient to inform health care provider if a persistent cough or other bothersome side effects develop while taking this medication.
- Caution patient not to take any prescription or OTC medications, potassium-containing salt substitutes, potassium supplements, or dietary supplements unless advised by health care provider.
- Advise patient that follow-up visits and lab tests may be required to monitor therapy and to keep appointments.

Enalapril Maleate/Hydrochlorothiazide

(EH-NAL-uh-prill MAL-ee-ate high-droe-klor-oh-THIGH-uh-zide)

Class Antihypertensive

How Supplied
Vaseretic 5-12.5 Tablets 12.5 mg hydrochlorothiazide, 5 mg enalapril maleate ♦ Vaseretic 10-25 Tablets 25 mg hydrochlorothiazide, 10 mg enalapril maleate

Action
PHARMACOLOGY: Enalapril causes vasodilation and decreased BP; hydrochlorothiazide causes loss of body water and increases urine output.

Indications Treatment of hypertension.

Contraindications Hypersensitivity to any component or to other sulfonamide-derived drugs; history of angioedema related to previous treatment with ACE inhibitor; anuria.

Route/Dosage
ADULTS: PO 1 to 2 tablets (each containing 10 mg enalapril maleate and 25 mg hydrochlorothiazide) per day.

Interactions
Cholestyramine and colestipol resins: May bind to hydrochlorothiazide and decrease its bioavailability.
Diazoxide: Hyperglycemia may occur.
Digitalis glycosides: Arrhythmias may occur.
Indomethacin: Hypotensive effects may be reduced.
Lithium: Toxicity risk is greater; avoid use.
Loop diuretics: Synergistic effects may cause profound diuresis and electrolyte abnormalities.
Potassium preparations, potassium-sparing diuretics: May increase serum potassium levels.
Sulfonylureas: May require dose adjustment.

Lab Test Interferences PBI levels may be decreased without signs of thyroid disturbances; diagnostic interference with serum electrolyte levels, blood and urinary glucose levels, serum bilirubin levels and serum uric acid levels.

Adverse Reactions
CV: Hypotension; orthostatic effects; palpitations; tachycardia; chest pain.

DERM: Rash, pruritus.
CNS: Dizziness; headache; insomnia; nervousness; paresthesia; somnolence; vertigo; syncope.
EENT: Tinnitus; dry mouth.
GI: Nausea; diarrhea; abdominal pain; vomiting; dyspepsia; constipation; flatulence.
GU: Impotence; decreased libido; urinary tract infections.
HEMA: Neutropenia; agranulocytosis.
METAB: Hyperkalemia; hyponatremia; hypercalcemia; hypochloremic alkalosis; hypokalemia; gout; hypomagnesemia; hyperglycemia; increased triglyceride and cholesterol levels.
RESP: Chronic cough; dyspnea.
OTHER: Angioedema; fatigue; weakness; muscle cramps; back pain; sweating.

Precautions

Pregnancy: Category D (second, third trimester); Category C (first trimester).
Lactation: Excreted in breast milk.
Children: Safety and efficacy not established.
Renal function impairment: Use drug with caution in patients with renal disease and monitor renal function periodically; may precipitate azotemia; may alter renal function in susceptible individuals (including those with severe CHF). Use drug with caution in patients with impaired hepatic function or progressive liver disease, because changes in fluid and electrolyte balance can precipitate hepatic coma.
Hepatic function impairment: Use drug with caution in patients with renal disease and monitor renal function periodically; may precipitate azotemia; may alter renal function in susceptible individuals (including those with severe CHF). Use drug with caution in patients with impaired hepatic function or progressive liver disease, because changes in fluid and electrolyte balance can precipitate hepatic coma.
Angioedema: Angioedema of face, extremities, lips, tongue, glottis, or larynx has been reported in patients treated with enalapril. Discontinue drug.
Bone marrow depression: Other ACE inhibitors have caused bone marrow depression, particularly in patients with renal impairment and collagen vascular disease. Monitor hematopoietic system.
Diabetes: Monitor closely, because adjustments may be needed in hypoglycemic agents.
Systemic lupus erythematosus: May be activated or exacerbated.

Overdosage: Signs and Symptoms

Hypotension, orthostatic hypotension, dizziness, drowsiness, syncope, electrolyte abnormalities, hemoconcentration, confusion, muscular weakness, nausea, vomiting, depressed respiration, lethargy, coma.

PATIENT CARE CONSIDERATIONS

Administration/Storage

- If patient is receiving diuretics keep patient under medical supervision for 2 hr after initial dose. Continue to monitor patient until BP is stable for 1 hr.
- Give with food or milk if nausea occurs.
- Store at room temperature in sealed container.

Assessment/Interventions

- Obtain patient history, including drug history and any known allergies.
- Obtain baseline vital signs.
- Review baseline creatinine, BUN, magnesium, glucose, triglyceride, cholesterol, serum electrolytes, and LFT results.
- After initial dose, monitor vital signs for 2 hr until vital signs are stable for 1 hr.
- Assist patient with postural changes, and monitor orthostatic BP frequently during initial therapy and regularly thereafter.
- In diabetic patients, monitor blood glucose closely.
- Monitor I&O, serum electrolytes, LFT results, glucose, and CBC.
- Assess for vertigo, somnolence, headache, nausea, and abdominal pain.
- Notify health care provider if severe hypotension, chest pain, or arrhythmia occur.

Patient/Family Education

- Advise patient to take with food or milk if nausea occurs.
- Caution patient that medication increases urination and to take as early in day as possible.
- Advise patient that lethargy may be experienced until body adjusts.
- Caution patient to take missed dose as soon as possible but not to take missed dose with next dose. If 1 or more doses is missed, tell patient to contact health care provider.
- Advise patient not to use salt substitutes unless approved by health care provider.
- Instruct patient to report these symptoms to health care provider: weakness, muscle cramps, dizziness, nausea, neck or facial swelling, faintness on standing, sore throat or dry, persistent cough.

Enfuvirtide

(en-FYOO-veer-tide)
Class Antiretroviral/Fusion inhibitor

How Supplied
Fuzeon Injection 90 mg/mL

Action
PHARMACOLOGY: Interferes with entry of HIV-1 into cells by inhibiting fusion of viral and cellular membranes.

PHARMACOKINETICS/DYNAMICS:
Absorption: Following a 90 mg SC injection, the mean C_{max} was 4.59 mcg/mL, AUC was 55.8 mcg•h/mL, and median t_{max} was 8 hr. The absolute bioavailability was 84.3%.

Distribution: After IV administration, the mean V_d was 5.5 L. Enfuvirtide is approximately 92% protein bound.

Metabolism: Enfuvirtide is expected to undergo catabolism to its constituent amino acids, with subsequent recycling into the body pool.

Excretion: The elimination $t_{½}$ is 3.8 hr and the mean apparent clearance is 24.8 mL/hr/kg.

Special Populations:
Gender – Clearance is 20% lower in women than men; however, no dose adjustment is recommended for gender.

Indications
In combination with other antiretroviral agents for the treatment of HIV-1 infection in treatment-experienced patients with evidence of HIV-1 replication despite ongoing antiretroviral therapy.

Contraindications
Standard considerations.

Route/Dosage
ADULTS: **SC** 90 mg bid.
CHILDREN 6 YR AND OLDER: **SC** 2 mg/kg bid (max, 90 mg bid).

Interactions None well documented.

Lab Test Interferences None well documented.

Adverse Reactions
CNS: Fatigue; peripheral neuropathy; taste disturbances; insomnia; depression; anxiety; decreased appetite; Guillain-Barre syndrome; sixth nerve palsy.
DERM: Injection site reactions (including erythema, induration, nodules or cysts, abscess, cellulitis, pain, discomfort, pruritus, ecchymosis); skin papilloma.
EENT: Conjunctivitis.
GI: Diarrhea; nausea; anorexia; constipation; upper abdominal pain; pancreatitis.
GU: Renal insufficiency (glomerulonephritis); renal failure.
HEMA: Lymphadenopathy; thrombocytopenia; neutropenia.
METAB: Weight decrease; hyperglycemia.
RESP: Cough; sinusitis; pneumonia.
OTHER: Herpes simplex; influenza; flu-like symptoms; myalgia; fever.

Precautions
Pregnancy: Category B.
Lactation: Undetermined; however, HIV-infected mothers should not breastfeed their infants.
Children: Safety and efficacy not established in children less than 6 yr of age.
Hypersensitivity: May occur and recur on rechallenge.
Pneumonia: An increased incidence of bacterial pneumonia observed.

PATIENT CARE CONSIDERATIONS

Administration/Storage
- For SC administration only. Not for intradermal, IM, or IV administration.
- Inject prescribed dose bid into upper arm, anterior thigh, or abdomen.
- Administer each injection at a site different from the preceding injection site and only where there is no current injection site reaction from an earlier dose.
- Do not inject into moles, scar tissue, bruises, or the navel.
- Follow manufacturer's instructions for reconstitution and administration. Use Sterile Water for Injection for reconstitution.
- Do not administer if particulate matter, bubbles, cloudiness, or discoloration noted.
- Do not mix other medications in same syringe.
- Reconstituted solution should be injected immediately or kept refrigerated in original vial for up to 24 hr. Refrigerated solution should be allowed to come to room temperature before injection and inspected visually again to ensure that the contents are fully dissolved in solution and that the solution is clear, colorless, and without bubbles or particulate matter.
- Discard any unused solution. Do not save unused solution for later administration.
- Store unopened vials at controlled room temperature (59° to 86°F). Reconstituted solution should be stored under refrigeration (36° to 46°F) and used within 24 hr.

Assessment/Interventions
- Obtain patient history, including drug history and any known allergies.

- Follow manufacturer's dosing chart for pediatric use.
- Assess patient for CNS, psychiatric, respiratory, GI, and general body side effects. Inform health care provider if noted and significant.
- Monitor patient for signs and symptoms of pneumonia. Inform health care provider if cough with fever, unexplained rapid breathing, or shortness of breath are noted.
- Assess injection sites for reactions. Inform health care provider if noted and significant or if cellulitis is suspected.

Patient/Family Education
- Explain name, dose, action, and potential side effects of drug.
- If patient or caregiver will be administering at home, review "Patient Package Insert" and "Injection Instructions" with the patient or caregiver. Ensure that the patient or caregiver understands how to store, prepare, and administer the dose, and dispose of used equipment and supplies. The first injection should be performed under the supervision of a qualified health professional.
- Instruct patient or caregiver to administer prescribed dose bid.
- Advise patient that if a dose is missed to take it as soon as remembered. However, if it is close to the time for the next scheduled dose, wait and take the next dose as scheduled. Caution patient not to administer 2 doses at the same time.
- Warn patient that this drug is not to be used by itself but is combined with other antiretroviral agents.
- Advise patient not to change the dose or dosing schedule of this medication or any other antiretroviral medication unless advised by health care provider.
- Advise patient that injection site reactions are common and analgesics (eg, acetaminophen, ibuprofen) may be used to manage pain but to notify health care provider if multiple injection site reactions develop or if reactions are intolerable.
- Instruct patient to report the following symptoms immediately to health care provider: allergic reaction, fever, chills, persistent nausea or vomiting, signs of pneumonia (cough with fever, unexplained rapid breathing or shortness of breath), or signs of infection at injection site (eg, oozing, swelling, redness, pain, increasing heat).
- Inform patient that drug does not completely eliminate HIV virus and, therefore, does not reduce risk of transmitting HIV. Appropriate precautions must still be followed.
- Advise patient that drug is not a cure for HIV infection and that patient may continue to acquire illnesses associated with HIV infection, including opportunistic infections and to remain under a health care provider's care.
- Advise patient that drug may cause dizziness and to use caution while driving or performing other tasks requiring mental alertness until tolerance is determined.
- Instruct patient not to take any prescription or OTC medications or dietary supplements unless advised by health care provider.
- Advise women to notify health care provider if pregnant, planning to become pregnant, or breastfeeding.
- Remind patient that examinations and laboratory tests will be required to monitor therapy and to keep appointments.

Enoxaparin Sodium

(eh-NOX-uh-par-in SO-dee-uhm)

Class Anticoagulant

How Supplied
Lovenox Injection 30 mg/0.3 mL, Injection 40 mg/0.4 mL, Injection 60 mg/0.6 mL, Injection 80 mg/0.8 mL, Injection 100 mg/mL, Injection 120 mg/0.8 mL, Injection 150 mg/mL, Injection 300 mg/3 mL

🍁 *Lovenox HP*

Action
PHARMACOLOGY: Causes higher anti-factor Xa to antithrombin activities (anti-factor IIa) ratio than heparin, which may prevent thrombosis.

PHARMACOKINETICS/DYNAMICS:
Absorption: Bioavailability is 92%.

Distribution: Vd is approximately 6 L (for anti-factor Xa activity).

Excretion: Cl is approximately 15 mL/min. The $t_{1/2}$ is 4.5 hr (based on anti-factor Xa activity).

Peak: 3 to 5 hr.

Special Populations:
Renal Function Impairment – Cl is approximately 30% lower in those with severe renal impairment (Ccr less than 30 mL/min).

Indications Prevention of deep vein thrombosis (DVT), which may lead to pulmonary embolism (PE) in patients undergoing hip or knee replacement surgery or abdominal surgery; in conjunction with warfarin sodium for inpatient treatment of acute DVT with and without PE or outpatient treatment of acute DVT without PE; prevention of ischemic complications of unstable and non-Q-wave MI when coadministered with aspirin. In medical patients who are at risk for thromboembolic complications due to severely restricted mobility during acute illness.

Contraindications Hypersensitivity to enoxaparin, heparin, or pork products; active major bleeding; thrombocytopenia associated with positive in vitro test for antiplatelet antibody in presence of enoxaparin.

Route/Dosage

Hip or Knee Replacement Surgery
ADULTS: **SC** 30 mg bid, with initial dose given within 12 to 24 hr postoperatively, provided hemostasis has been established. Average duration of administration is 7 to 10 days, up to 14 days. For hip replacement surgery, 40 mg qd, given initially 9 to 15 hr prior to surgery; continue prophylaxis for 3 wk.

Abdominal Surgery
ADULTS: **SC** 40 mg/day with the initial dose given 2 hr prior to surgery. Usual duration of administration is 7 to 10 days; up to 12 days.

Acute Illness
ADULTS: **SC** 40 mg qd for 6 to 11 days, up to 14 days, in patients at risk for thromboembolic complications caused by severely restricted mobility during acute illness.

DVT/PE Treatment
Outpatient – **SC** 1 mg/kg q 12 hr.
Inpatient – **SC** 1 mg/kg q 12 hr or 1.5 mg/kg qd (same time each day).
Outpatient and inpatient – Initiate warfarin therapy when appropriate (usually within 72 hr of enoxaparin). Continue enoxaparin for a minimum of 5 days and until a therapeutic anticoagulant effect has been achieved. The average duration is 7 days; up to 17 days has been well tolerated.

Unstable Angina/Non-Q-Wave MI
ADULTS: **SC** 1 mg/kg q 12 hr in conjunction with oral aspirin therapy (100 to 325 mg qd); usual duration of treatment is 2 to 8 days, up to 12.5 days.

Thromboembolic Recurrence/Prophylaxis
ADULTS: **SC** 40 mg qd.

Interactions

Anticoagulants, NSAIDs, platelet inhibitors: Use enoxaparin with care because of increased risk of hemorrhagic reactions.
INCOMPATIBILITIES: Do not mix enoxaparin with other injections or infusions.

Lab Test Interferences

Transaminase determinations: Drug causes asymptomatic elevations in AST and ALT.

Adverse Reactions

DERM: Local erythema and ecchymosis.
HEMA: Hemorrhage; thrombocytopenia; anemia.
OTHER: Local irritation and pain; hematoma; nausea; confusion; fever; edema; peripheral edema.
Postmarketing – Dyspnea; injection site hemorrhage; hematuria; epidural or spinal hematoma; systemic allergic reactions (ie, pruritus, urticaria, anaphylactoid reactions); vesiculobullous rash, purpura, thrombocytosis; hyperlipidemia.

> **WARNING:**
>
> *Spinal/Epidural hematomas:* Risk of spinal/epidural hematoma increased in patients receiving neuraxial anesthesia or spinal puncture and are anticoagulated with LMWH or heparinoids. Other risk factors include indwelling epidural catheters, repeated/traumatic epidural/spinal puncture or other drugs affecting hemostasis (eg, NSAIDs, platelet inhibitors, anticoagulants). Risk of long term or permanent paralysis. Monitor frequently for signs/ symptoms of neurological impairment.

Precautions

Pregnancy: Category B.
Lactation: Undetermined.
Children: Safety and efficacy not established.
Elderly: Delayed elimination of drug possible. Use with caution.
Renal function impairment: Delayed elimination of drug may occur. Use with caution.
Special risk patients: Use drug with caution in patients with diabetic retinopathy, bleeding diathesis, uncontrolled arterial hypertension, or history of recent GI ulceration and hemorrhage.
Benzyl alcohol: Multiple-dose vials contain benzyl alcohol as a preservative; has been associated with a fatal "gasping syndrome" in premature neonates.
Hemorrhage: Use drug with extreme caution in patients with conditions associated with increased risk of hemorrhage.
Interchangeability with heparin: Cannot be used interchangeably (unit for unit) with heparin or other low molecular weight heparins.
Prosthetic heart valves: Use is not recommended for thromboprophylaxis in patients with prosthetic heart valves.
Teratogenesis: There have been reports of congenital anomalies in infants born to women who received enoxaparin during pregnancy including cerebral anomalies, limb anomalies, hypospadias, peripheral vascular malformation, fibrotic dysplasia, and cardiac defects. A cause and effect relationship has not been established.
Thrombocytopenia: Use with extreme caution in

patients who have a history of heparin-induced thrombocytopenia. Closely monitor any degree of thrombocytopenia.

PATIENT CARE CONSIDERATIONS
Administration/Storage
- Administer only by deep SC injection; enoxaparin cannot be administered via IM or IV injection.
- With patient lying down, administer drug by SC injection. Alternate administration between left and right anterolateral and posterolateral abdominal wall. Introduce whole length of needle into skinfold held between thumb and forefinger; hold skinfold throughout injection.
- Do not aspirate into syringe; do not rub site after injection. These activities may cause tissue damage and SC bleeding.
- Store at room temperature (59° to 86°F). Do not freeze.

Assessment/Interventions
- Obtain patient history, including drug history and any known allergies.
- Review patient's health history for any condition that could contraindicate enoxaparin (eg, active major bleeding, thrombocytopenia, hypersensitivity to enoxaparin, heparin, or pork products).
- Review patient's medication record for use of drugs that present special risks when used with enoxaparin (eg, anticoagulants, platelet inhibitors).

Overdosage: Signs and Symptoms
Hemorrhage.

- Obtain bleeding disorder laboratory tests before administering enoxaparin.
- Monitor patient for signs of bleeding throughout therapy.
- Perform periodic CBCs (including platelet count) and stool occult blood tests during course of treatment.
- If bleeding develops (eg, epistaxis, hematuria, hematemesis, bloody or black, tarry stools), notify health care provider immediately.
- If laboratory studies for coagulation and bleeding are abnormal, notify health care provider.

Patient/Family Education
- Teach patient and family the name, action, administration, and side effects of enoxaparin.
- Instruct patient to report any signs of bleeding immediately.
- Explain to patient the rationale for follow-up examinations and laboratory studies to ensure effectiveness of medication and to monitor for side effects.
- If patient has home therapy, teach patient or family proper SC injection technique.
- Caution patient to take safety precautions to prevent cuts and bruising (eg, use electric razor, soft toothbrush, handrails).

Entacapone

(en-TACK-ah-pone)
Class Antiparkinson
How Supplied
Comtan Tablets 200 mg

Action
PHARMACOLOGY: The exact mechanism of action is unknown. Inhibits catechol-O-methyl transferase (COMT) thus blocking the degradation of catechols including dopamine and levodopa. This may lead to more sustained levels of dopamine and consequently a more prolonged antiparkinson effect.

PHARMACOKINETICS/DYNAMICS:

Absorption: Rapidly absorbed. T_{max} is approximately 1 hr. C_{max} is approximately 1.2 mcg/mL (single 200 mg dose).

Distribution: Vd is 20 L (IV). 98% is protein bound, mainly to albumin.

Metabolism: Almost completely metabolized; inactive metabolites formed by isomerization and glucuronidation.

Excretion: Approximately 10% is excreted in the urine (0.2% as unchanged drug) and 90% in feces.

Special Populations:
Hepatic Function Impairment – AUC and C_{max} are approximately 2-fold higher in those with a a history of alcoholism and hepatic impairment.

Indications As an adjunct to levodopa/carbidopa for the treatment of idiopathic Parkinson disease in patients who experience signs and symptoms of end-of-dose "wearing-off."

Contraindications Standard considerations.

Route/Dosage
ADULTS: **PO** 200 mg concomitantly with each levodopa/carbidopa dose to max 8 times/day.

Interactions
Ampicillin, cholestyramine, chloramphenicol, erythromycin, probenecid, rifampin: May interfere with biliary excretion or metabolism of entacapone.

Apomorphine, bitolterol, dobutamine, dopamine, epinephrine, isoetherine, isoproterenol, methyldopa, norepinephrine: Excessive changes in BP, increased heart rate, and arrhythmias may occur.

Lab Test Interferences May decrease iron stores by chelation of iron.

Adverse Reactions
CNS: Dyskinesia; hyperkinesia; hypokinesia; dizziness; anxiety; somnolence; agitation; hallucinations.
EENT: Taste perversion.
GI: Nausea; diarrhea; abdominal pain; constipation; vomiting; dry mouth; dyspepsia; flatulence; gastritis.
GU: Urine discoloration.
HEMA: Purpura.
RESP: Dyspnea.
OTHER: Sweating; back pain; fatigue; asthenia.

Precautions
Pregnancy: Category C.
Lactation: Undetermined.
Children: Safety and efficacy not established.
Hepatic impairment or biliary obstruction: Use with caution.
Hyperpyrexia and confusion: Exercise caution. Rhabdomyolysis and symptom complex resembling neuroleptic malignant syndrome reported in association with therapy.
MAOIs: Avoid concurrent use of non-selective MAOIs (ie, isocarboxazid, phenelzine, tranylcypromine). Administration of MAOIs may result in inhibition of the majority of pathways for catecholamine metabolism.

Overdosage: Signs and Symptoms
Abdominal pain, loose stools.

PATIENT CARE CONSIDERATIONS

Administration/Storage
- Store at room temperature in tightly closed containers. Excursions permitted to 15° to 30° C (59° to 86°F).
- Always administer in association with levodopa/carbidopa as entacapone has no antiparkinson effect on its own.
- Administer with or without food.
- Withdraw treatment slowly as rapid withdrawal could lead to signs and symptoms of Parkinson disease or hyprexia and confusion.
- If patient is also taking drugs metabolized by COMT enzyme system (eg, catecholamines, epinephrine, dopamine), administer with caution as their interaction could result in increased heart rates, arrhythmias, and excessive changes in BP.

Assessment/Interventions
- Obtain patient history, including drug history and any known allergies.
- Anticipate a decreased dose of levodopa if patient has been taking either high doses of levodopa or experiencing moderate or severe dyskinesia before taking entacapone.
- Monitor patient for dyskinesia/hyperkinesia, nausea, urine discoloration, hallucinations, abdominal pain, loose stools, and (rarely) signs and symptoms of rhabdomyolysis.
- Monitor patient closely if the dose has been abruptly reduced or discontinued for high fever or severe rigidity as these are symptoms of hyperpyrexia and confusion, a complex syndrome resembling neuroleptic malignant syndrome.
- Monitor patient closely if the decision has been made to discontinue entacapone, as other antiparkinson medications will need to be adjusted.

Patient/Family Education
- Inform patient that entacapone is not a cure for Parkinson disease, but should help reduce the symptoms and decrease the need for higher doses of their other medications.
- Instruct patient to take entacapone only as prescribed.
- Advise patient that hallucinations can occur.
- Advise patient that postural (orthostatic) hypotension with or without symptoms such as dizziness, nausea, syncope, and sweating may develop. Hypotension may occur more frequently during initial therapy.
- Caution patient against rising rapidly, especially after prolonged periods of sitting or lying down.
- Caution patient about possible additive sedative effects when taking other CNS depressants in combination with entacapone.
- Caution patient to neither drive a car, operate other complex machinery, or engage in any hazardous activity until sure entacapone does not affect mental or motor performance.
- Inform patient that nausea or hypotension may occur, especially at the initiation of treatment.
- Advise patients of the possibility of an increase in dyskinesia.
- Inform patient that treatment with entacapone may cause a change in urine color to a brownish orange in approximately 10% of people, but that it will not cause harm should it occur.
- Advise patient to notify primary caregiver if becoming pregnant, planning to become pregnant, or breastfeeding.

Ephedrine

(eh-FED-rin)

Class Vasopressor/Decongestant

How Supplied
Pretz-D Solution 0.25% ephedrine sulfate

Action

PHARMACOLOGY: Stimulates both alpha-and beta-receptors, causing increased heart rate, unchanged or augmented stroke volume, enhanced cardiac output, and increased BP. Causes relaxation of smooth muscle of bronchi and GI tract, stimulation of cerebral cortex, and pupil dilation.

PHARMACOKINETICS/DYNAMICS:

Distribution: Excreted in breast milk.

Metabolism: Small amounts are slowly metabolized in the liver.

Excretion: Renally eliminated and mostly as unchanged drug. The $t_{1/2}$ is approximately 3 to 6 hr (dependent on urinary pH).

Onset: Immediate (IV). More than 20 min (SC). 10 to 20 min (IM). 15 to 60 min (oral).

Duration: 1 hr (parenteral). 3 to 5 hr (oral).

Indications

IM/IV/SC: Treatment of acute hypotensive states; treatment of Adams-Stokes syndrome with complete heart block; stimulation of CNS to combat narcolepsy and depressive states; treatment of acute bronchospasm; treatment of enuresis; treatment of myasthenia gravis; allergic disorders, such as bronchial asthma.

Nasal: Treatment of nasal congestion; promotion of nasal or sinus drainage; relief of eustachian tube congestion.

PO: Temporary relief of shortness of breath, tightness of chest, and wheezing caused by bronchial asthma. Eases breathing for asthma patients by reducing spasms of bronchial muscles.

Contraindications Angle-closure glaucoma; patients anesthetized with cyclopropane or halothane; cases in which vasopressor drugs are contraindicated (eg, thyrotoxicosis, diabetes mellitus, hypertension of pregnancy); MAOI therapy; narrow-angle glaucoma; nonanaphylactic shock during general anesthesia with halogenated hydrocarbons or cyclopropane.

Route/Dosage

Asthma

ADULTS AND CHILDREN 12 YR AND OLDER: **PO** 12.5 to 25 mg q 4 hr, not to exceed 150 mg in 24 hr.

ADULTS: **SC/IM/IV** 25 to 50 mg SC or IM, or 5 to 25 mg administered by slow IV, repeated q 5 to 10 min, if necessary.

CHILDREN: **SC/IM** 0.5 to 0.75 mg/kg or 16.7 to 25 mg/m^2 q 4 to 6 hr.

Hypotension

ADULTS: **SC** 25 to 50 mg.(IM/IV if rapid effect is needed) 10 to 25 mg may be given by IV push; may give additional doses at 5 to 10 min intervals (max, 150 mg/24 hr).

CHILDREN: **IV/SC** 3 mg/kg/day or 25 to 100 mg/m^2/day in 4 to 6 divided doses.

Labor

ADULTS: **SC/IV/IM** prn to maintain BP 130/80 mm Hg or less.

Nasal Congestion

ADULTS: **Nasal** Dose is product specific. See labeling.

Interactions

Alpha-adrenergic blockers (eg, phentolamine): Vasoconstricting and hypertensive effects are antagonized.

Diuretics: Vascular response may be decreased.

General anesthetics (eg, halothane, cyclopropane), cardiac glycosides: The potential for the myocardium to be sensitized to the effects of sympathomimetic amines is increased. Arrhythmias may result with coadministration and may respond to beta blockers.

Guanethidine: May negate antihypertensive effects.

MAOIs: Increases pressor response from vasopressors significantly; hypertensive crisis and intracranial hemorrhage are possible.

Rauwolfia alkaloids, methyldopa, furazolidone: May result in hypertension.

Tricyclic antidepressants: May potentiate pressor response.

Urinary acidifiers: May increase elimination of ephedrine.

Urinary alkalinizers: May decrease elimination of ephedrine.

INCOMPATIBILITIES: Ephedrine is chemically incompatible with sodium bicarbonate; avoid admixture.

Lab Test Interferences

Amphetamine enzyme-multiplied immunoassay test (EMIT) assay: False-positive results may occur.

Adverse Reactions

CV: Palpitation; tachycardia; precordial pain; cardiac arrhythmias; hypertension.

CNS: Headache; insomnia; sweating; nervousness; vertigo; confusion; delirium; restlessness; anxiety; tension; tremor; weakness; dizziness; hallucinations.

EENT: Local irritation, sneezing, rebound congestion (nasal use).

GI: Nausea; vomiting; anorexia; dry mouth.

GU: Difficult and painful urination; urinary

retention in men with prostatism; decreased urine formation (initial parenteral use).
RESP: Shortness of breath.
OTHER: Pallor.

Precautions

Pregnancy: Category C. Parenteral administration of ephedrine to maintain BP during low or other spinal anesthesia for delivery can cause acceleration of fetal heart rate; do not use in obstetrics when maternal BP exceeds 130/80.
Lactation: Undetermined.
Asthma: Use drug with caution.
Hypertension: Drug may cause severe hypertension, resulting in intracranial hemorrhage, angina, or potentially fatal arrhythmias, especially in patients with organic heart disease or those receiving drugs that sensitize myocardium.
Labor: Do not use when maternal BP exceeds 130/80 mmHg; use during delivery may cause acceleration of fetal heart rate.
Sulfite sensitivity: Use nasal decongestant form of drug with caution.

Overdosage: Signs and Symptoms

Convulsions, nausea, vomiting, chills, cyanosis, irritability, nervousness, fever, suicidal behavior, tachycardia, dilated pupils, blurred vision, opisthotonos, spasms, pulmonary edema, gasping respirations, coma, respiratory failure, personality changes, hypertension with anuria.

PATIENT CARE CONSIDERATIONS

Administration/Storage

- For nasal spray, have patient keep head upright. Instruct patient to sniff hard for few min after administration.
- Protect from light. Do not give unless solution is clear. Discard any unused medication.

Assessment/Interventions

- Obtain patient history, including drug history and any known allergies. Note any hypersensitivity to epinephrine or sulfites.
- Obtain baseline assessment of vital signs and monitor frequently.
- Determine baseline glucose for patients with diabetes mellitus.
- Monitor for nervousness and agitation.
- Monitor for nasal congestion.

Patient/Family Education

- Caution patient to use topical decongestants only in acute states and not to use for > 3 to 5 days.
- Inform patient that nasal burning or stinging may occur with nasal drops or spray.
- Caution patient not to share nasal spray container with others.
- Advise patient to notify health care provider if symptoms do not improve after 7 days.
- With topical decongestant form of drug, instruct patient to report the following symptoms to health care provider: headache, palpitations, tremors, sweating, faintness, insomnia, weakness.
- With SC form of drug, advise patient to notify health care provider of syncope, palpitations, weakness, agitation, dizziness, or chest pain.
- Instruct patient to take sips of water frequently, suck on ice chips or sugarless hard candy, or chew gum if dry mouth occurs.
- Caution patient not to take *otc* medications without consulting health care provider.

Epinastine Hydrochloride

(epp-ih-NAS-teen HIGH-droe-KLOR-ide)
Class Antihistamine

How Supplied
Elestat Ophthalmic solution 0.05%

Action
PHARMACOLOGY: Direct H_1-receptor antagonist that inhibits release of histamine from the mast cell.

PHARMACOKINETICS/DYNAMICS:
Absorption: Low systemic exposure.
Distribution: Plasma protein binding approximately 64%.
Metabolism: Less than 10% metabolized.
Excretion: Terminal plasma elimination t½ is about 12 hr. Mainly excreted unchanged (after IV dosing about 55% in urine and 30% in feces). Renal elimination via active tubular secretion.

Indications Prevention of itching associated with allergic conjunctivitis.

Contraindications Standard considerations.

Route/Dosage
ADULTS AND CHILDREN 3 YR AND OLDER: Ophthalmic 1 gtt in each eye bid, continuing treatment throughout the period of exposure (until pollen season is over or until exposure to offending allergen is terminated) even when symptoms are absent.

Interactions None well documented.

Lab Test Interferences None well documented.

Adverse Reactions
CNS: Headache (1% to 3%).
EENT: Burning sensation in eye, folliculosis,

hyperemia, pruritus (1% to 10%); rhinitis, sinusitis, pharyngitis (1% to 3%).
RESP: Upper respiratory infection (10%); increased cough (1% to 3%).
OTHER: Symptoms of cold (10%).

PATIENT CARE CONSIDERATIONS

Administration/Storage
- For topical ophthalmic use only. Not for injection or oral use.
- Instill 1 gtt into affected eyes bid.
- Do not allow tip of container to touch any surface, the eyelids, or surrounding areas.
- If using other topical ophthalmic drugs, separate each medication by at least 10 min.
- Store ophthalmic solution at controlled room temperature (59°F to 77°F). Keep tightly closed.

Assessment/Interventions
- Obtain patient history, including drug history and any known allergies.
- Assess ophthalmic symptoms (eg, itching) before and periodically throughout therapy. Notify health care provider if symptoms are not controlled with medication.
- Monitor patient for ocular (eg, burning, stinging) and systemic (eg, headaches) reactions. Inform health care provider if noted and significant.

Patient/Family Education
- Advise patient to read patient instruction sheet that accompanies each bottle of azelastine.
- Explain name, dose, action, and potential side effects of drug.
- Advise patient that usual dose is 1 gtt instilled into the affected eyes bid.
- Teach patient proper technique for instilling eye drops: wash hands; do not allow dropper tip to touch eye. Tilt head back, look up; pull lower eyelid down; instill prescribed number of gtt. Close eye for 1 to 2 min and apply gentle pressure to bridge of nose for 3 to 5 min. Do not rub eye.
- Advise patient that medication should be used daily during the period of exposure to allergens in order to prevent symptoms from recurring.
- Advise patient that if symptoms are not controlled not to increase the dose but to inform health care provider.
- Advise patient that if more than 1 topical ophthalmic drug is being used, to administer the drugs at least 10 min apart.
- Advise patient who wears contact lenses not to wear lenses if eyes are red.
- Advise patient who wears contact lenses, and whose eyes are not red, to remove lenses before instilling this medicine and to wait at least 10 min after instilling eye drops before inserting lenses.
- Inform patient that temporary redness, itching, burning, or stinging of the eye are the most common side effects and to contact health care provider if they occur and are bothersome.
- Advise women to notify health care provider if pregnant, planning to become pregnant, or breastfeeding.
- Caution patient not to take any prescription or OTC medications or dietary supplements unless advised by health care provider.

Precautions
Pregnancy: Category C.
Lactation: Undetermined.
Children: Safety and efficacy not established in children under 3 yr.

Epinephrine
(epp-ih-NEFF-rin)

Class Alpha agonist/Beta agonist

How Supplied
Adrenalin Chloride Solution for injection 1 mg/mL (1:1,000) as hydrochloride, Solution for injection 10 mg/mL (1:100) as hydrochloride ◆ *EpiPen* Solution 1 mg/mL (1:1,000) ◆ *EpiPen Jr.* Solution 0.5 mg/mL (1:2,000) ◆ *microNefrin* Solution for inhalation 2.25% racepinephrine hydrochloride ◆ *Primatene Mist* Aerosol 0.22 mg epinephrine per spray ◆ *S2* Solution for inhalation 2.25% racepinephrine hydrochloride
✤ *Adrenalin* ◆ *Vaponefrin*

Action
PHARMACOLOGY: Stimulates alpha- and beta-receptors (alpha-receptors at high doses; beta$_1$- and beta$_2$-receptors at moderate doses) within sympathetic nervous system. Relaxes smooth muscle of bronchi and iris and is antagonist of histamine.

PHARMACOKINETICS/DYNAMICS:

Metabolism: Inactivated by enzymatic transformation to metabephrine or normetanephrine; these are subsequently conjugated and excreted in the urine.

Excretion: Mostly excreted in urine as inactive metabolites; remainder excreted as unchanged drug or conjugated.

Onset: 5 to 10 minutes (subcutaneous), 1 to 5 minutes (inhalation).

Duration: 4 to 6 hr (subcutaneous), 1 to 4 hr (IM), 1 to 3 hr (inhalation).

Indications Treatment and prophylaxis of cardiac arrest and attacks of transitory AV heart block; treatment of Adams-Stokes syndrome; treatment of hay fever; relief of bronchial asthma; treatment of syncope caused by heart block or carotid sinus hypersensitivity; symptomatic relief of serum sickness, urticaria, and angioedema; relaxation of uterine musculature; anaphylaxis; allergic reactions (eg, bronchospasm, urticaria, pruritus, angioneurotic edema, swelling of the lips, eyelids, tongue, and nasal mucosa) because of anaphylactic shock caused by stinging insects (primarily of the order Hymenoptera, which includes bees, wasps, hornets, yellow jackets, bumble bees, and fire ants); severe allergic or anaphylactoid reactions caused by allergy injections; exposures to pollens, dusts molds, foods, drugs; exercise; unknown substances (so-called idiopathic anaphylaxis); severe, life-threatening asthma attacks characterized by wheezing, dyspnea, and inability to breathe.
Nasal solution: Treatment of nasal congestion; relief of eustachian tube congestion.
Inhalation: Temporary relief from acute paroxysms of bronchial asthma and other states; treatment of postintubation and infectious croup.

Contraindications Hypersensitivity to epinephrine; narrow-angle glaucoma; concomitant use during general anesthesia with halogenated hydrocarbons or cyclopropane; cerebral arteriosclerosis or organic brain damage; use with anesthesia for fingers and toes; use during labor; phenothiazine-induced circulatory collapse; MAO inhibitor therapy; nonanaphylactic shock during general anesthesia with halogenated hydrocarbons or cyclopropane; organic heart disease; cardiac dilation and coronary insufficiency.

Route/Dosage
Cardiac Arrest
ADULTS: **IV/Intracardiac** 0.5 to 1 mg (5 to 10 mL of 1:10,000 solution) q 5 minute as needed. Myocardial injection usually given in left ventricular chamber by trained personnel at dose of 0.3 to 0.5 mg.

Other IV Uses
ADULTS: **IV** 1 mg in 250 mL of D5W (4 mcg/mL) for infusion at 1 to 4 mcg/min (15 to 60 mL/hr).

Intraspinal Use
ADULTS: **Intraspinal** 0.2 to 0.4 mL of 1:1,000 solution added to anesthetic spinal fluid mixture. Epinephrine 1:100,000 to 1:200,000 is usual concentration employed with local anesthetics.

Allergic Emergencies
ADULTS: **IM** (*Epipen*) Usual dose is 0.3 mg.
CHILDREN: **IM** (*Epipen* or *Epipen Jr*) 0.01 mg/kg is recommended.

Nasal Congestion
ADULTS AND CHILDREN 6 YR OF AGE AND OLDER: **Nasal** Apply as drops, spray, or with sterile swab as required.

Asthma
ADULTS AND CHILDREN 4 YR OF AGE AND OLDER: **Inhalation** *Hand pump nebulizer:* Place 0.5 mL (approximately 8 to 10 drops) of racemic epinephrine into nebulizer reservoir. Squeeze bulb 1 to 3 times in partially opened mouth. If relief does not occur within 2 to 3 minutes, administer 2 to 3 additional inhalations. Do not administer more often than q 3 hr. *Aerosol-nebulizer:* Add 0.5 mL (approximately 10 drops) racemic epinephrine to 3 mL of diluent or 0.2 to 0.4 mL (approximately 4 to 8 drops) of *MicroNefrin* to 4.6 to 4.8 mL water. Administer for 15 minutes q 3 to 4 hr. *Aerosol:* Start with 1 inhalation, then wait at least 1 minute; repeat once more if needed. Do not use again for at least 3 hr.
ADULTS: **Subcutaneous/IM** *Solution (1:1,000):* 0.2 to 1 mL (0.2 to 1 mg); repeat q 4 hr. **IV** *Solution (1:10,000):* 0.1 to 0.25 mg (1 to 2.5 mL) injected slowly.

INFANTS AND CHILDREN: **Subcutaneous** *Solution (1:1,000):* 0.01 mL/kg or 0.3 mL/m^2 (0.01 mg/kg or 0.3 mg/m^2); repeat q 20 minutes to 4 hr. Do not exceed 0.5 mL (0.5 mg) in single dose. **IV** *Solution (1:10,000):* 0.01 mg/kg to 0.05 mg repeated at 20 to 30 minute intervals.

Interactions
Alpha-adrenergic blockers (eg, phentolamine): Vasoconstricting and hypertensive effects are antagonized.
Antihistamines: Epinephrine effects may be potentiated.
Beta-blocking agents: May decrease effects of these agents, resulting in hypertension.
Diuretics: Vascular response may be decreased.
Ergot alkaloids, phenothiazines, nitrates: Pressor effects of epinephrine may be reversed.
Furazolidone, methyldopa, Rauwolfia alkaloids: May cause hypertension.
General anesthetics (eg, halothane, cyclopropane), cardiac glycosides: The potential for the myocardium to be sensitized to the effects of sympathomimetic amines is increased.
Arrhythmias may result with coadministration and may respond to beta-blockers.
Guanethidine: May increase pressor response.
Levothyroxine: Epinephrine effects may be potentiated.
Oxytoxic drugs: May cause severe persistent hypertension.
Tricyclic antidepressants: May potentiate epinephrine's vasopressive effects.
INCOMPATIBILITIES: Epinephrine is unstable in

alkaline solutions (eg, sodium bicarbonate); avoid admixture.

Lab Test Interferences None well documented.

Adverse Reactions

CV: Cardiac arrhythmias and excessive hypertension; palpitations (especially in hyperthyroid and hypertensive patients); tachycardia; anginal pain in predisposed patients; cerebral and subarachnoid hemorrhage; flushing.
CNS: Anxiety; headache; restlessness; tremor; weakness; hemiplegia; dizziness; insomnia.
EENT: Nasal use: Local irritation; sneezing; rebound congestion.
GI: Nausea; vomiting.
GU: Decreased urine formation with initial parenteral use.
RESP: Shortness of breath.
OTHER: Severe metabolic acidosis; pallor; urticaria; wheal and hemorrhage at site of injection; necrosis at injection site following repeated injections; sweating; transient elevations of blood glucose; elevated serum lactic acid.

Precautions

Pregnancy: Category C.
Lactation: Excreted in breast milk.
Children: Administer drug with caution. Syncope has occurred in asthmatic children.
Labor and delivery: Do not use when maternal BP exceeds 130/80 mm Hg; may delay second stage or induce uterine atony.
Special risk patients: Use drug with caution in elderly patients, patients with CV disease, pulmonary edema, hypertension, hyperthyroidism, diabetes, psychoneurotic illness, asthma, prefibrillatory rhythm, or anesthetic cardiac accidents.
Sulfite sensitivity: Some products contain sulfites; use drug with caution in sulfite-sensitive individuals.
Bronchial asthma/Emphysema: Administer with extreme caution to patients with long-standing bronchial asthma and emphysema who develop degenerative heart disease.
Cerebrovascular hemorrhage: May result from overdosage or inadvertent IV injection.
Fatalities: Death may result from pulmonary edema because of peripheral constriction and cardiac stimulation produced.
Pulmonary edema: May cause fatalities because of peripheral constriction or cardiac stimulation.

Overdosage: Signs and Symptoms

Precordial distress, vomiting, headache, shortness of breath, unusually elevated BP, cerebrovascular hemorrhage, pulmonary arterial hypertension, pulmonary edema, ventricular hyperirritability, bradycardia, tachycardia, arrhythmias, extreme pallor, cold skin, metabolic acidosis, kidney failure.

PATIENT CARE CONSIDERATIONS

Administration/Storage

- Multiple concentrations and dosage forms are available. Ensure the proper concentration and dose form is being used.

Injection:

- Do not administer if particulate matter, cloudiness, or discoloration noted.
- Preferred route of administration is subcutaneous or IM. IV administration is usually used for medical emergencies (eg, cardiac arrest, life-threatening bronchospasm, anaphylaxis). Injection solution also can be administered via endotracheal tube directly into bronchial tree, if ordered, when using for cardiac resuscitation.
- Rotate subcutaneous administration sites to reduce chance of injection-site reaction.
- Auto-injectors are for patients to use for self-treatment of anaphylactic reactions.
- Discard any unused solution when using single-dose vials or ampules.

Solution for Inhalation:

- Dosage is individualized.
- Dilute with normal saline or water as ordered. Administer via nebulizer over 15 minutes q 3 to 4 hr as needed.
- Do not use if solution is pinkish or darker than slightly yellow, or if it contains a precipitate.

Inhalation Aerosol:

- Have patient inhale 1 spray. Repeat 1 time if symptoms are not relieved after 1 minute.
- Do not administer more than 2 inhalations q 3 or more hr.

Topical Solution:

- Apply locally as drops, spray, or directly on mucosal surface with sterile swab, as directed.
- Store inhalation solution and inhalation aerosol at controlled room temperature (68° to 77°F). Store all other dose forms at controlled room temperature (59° to 86°F). Protect from light, extreme heat, and freezing. Do not remove ampules or syringes from carton until ready to use.

Assessment/Interventions

- Obtain patient history, including drug history and any known allergies. Note hypersensitivity to sympathomimetic amines, narrow-angle glaucoma, organic brain damage, hyperthyroidism or thyrotoxicosis, toxemia, hyperten-

sion, cardiac arrhythmias, CV disease, diabetes, prostatic hypertrophy, or sulfite sensitivity (topical solution, solution for inhalation, and injection only).
- Monitor patient for CV, CNS, general body side effects, and injection site reactions. Inform health care provider if noted and significant.

Inhalation Solution and Aerosol:
- Ensure baseline pulmonary function tests have been completed.
- Note frequency and severity of asthma attacks.
- Monitor pulse, BP, RR, and lung sounds before and after treatment. Notify health care provider of unexpected or unusual findings.
- Monitor patient's respiratory status during each treatment. If bronchospasm worsens during a treatment, discontinue the treatment and notify health care provider immediately.
- Notify health care provider if patient needs treatments on an increasingly frequent basis.

Topical Solution:
- Monitor response to therapy. Notify health care provider if mucosal congestion does not improve or worsens.

Injection:
- Do not use during general anesthesia with halogenated hydrocarbons or cyclopropane because of risk of arrhythmias, or with local anesthesia to fingers or toes caused by risk of vasoconstriction producing sloughing of tissue.

Patient/Family Education
- Explain name, dose, action, and potential side effects of drug.

Injection:
- Advise patient, family, or caregiver that medication (other than that delivered by auto-injector) will be prepared and administered by a health care provider in a medical setting.
- Ensure patient using auto-injector understands how to store, prepare the auto-injector, administer the injection, and dispose of used equipment.
- Ensure patient using auto-injector understands how and when to use oral medications for allergic reactions (eg, antihistamines, corticosteroids) if prescribed or recommended by health care provider.

Inhalation Solution and Aerosol:
- If using solution for inhalation, ensure patient or caregiver can prepare, use, and clean the nebulizer without difficulty. If using the aerosol, ensure patient understands how to store and use the inhaler properly.
- Instruct patient not to mix with other nebulizer medications unless advised by health care provider.
- Instruct patient not to exceed prescribed dose or frequency of use. Advise patient to contact health care provider if this medication no longer seems to control asthma symptoms or if increasing doses of the medicine are needed. This may indicate worsening asthma.
- Advise patients using more than 1 inhaled medication to use this medication first if needed. Inhaled corticosteroids or other inhaled controller medications should be taken last.
- Advise patient that if breathing symptoms worsen during or immediately after using this medication to stop using it and inform health care provider immediately.
- Caution patient not to use solution if it is pinkish or darker than slightly yellow, or if it contains a precipitate.
- Caution patient not to puncture canister, dispose of used aerosol canister in incinerator, or store canister near open flame or heat above 120°F.

Topical Solution:
- Ensure patient or caregiver understands how and when to apply topical solution as drops, spray, or directly on mucosal surface with sterile swab, as directed.
- Advise patient or caregiver not to increase the frequency of use if symptoms of congestion do not improve or worsen but to notify health care provider.

Epirubicin Hydrochloride

(EH-pih-ROO-bih-sin HIGH-droe-KLOR-ide)

Class Antineoplastic antibiotic/Anthracycline

How Supplied
Ellence Solution for injection 2 mg/mL
❖ *Pharmorubicin PFS*

Action
PHARMACOLOGY: Epirubicin is a cell cycle phase, nonspecific anthracycline. It forms a complex with DNA by intercalation of its planar rings between nucleotide base pairs, with consequent inhibition of nucleic acid (DNA and RNA) and protein synthesis.

PHARMACOKINETICS/DYNAMICS:
Absorption: C_{max} is 5.3 to 9.3 mcg/mL. AUC is 1.6 to 4.2 mcg•hr/mL (dose dependent).

Distribution: Rapidly and widely distributed into tissues. Approximately 77% is protein bound (predominantly albumin).

Metabolism: Extensively and rapidly metabolized by liver and also by other organs and cells, including RBC.

Excretion: Parent and metabolites eliminated through biliary, and to a lesser extent, urinary. Triphasic elimination with alpha t½ is approximately 3 minutes, beta t½ is 2.5 hr, and gamma t½ is approximately 33 hr. Cl is 65 to 83 L/hr.

Special Populations:
Hepatic Function Impairment – Cl is reduced.

Indications Breast cancer with axillary node involvement. **Unlabeled use(s):** Small-cell lung cancer, nonsmall-cell lung cancer, Hodgkin lymphoma, non-Hodgkin lymphoma.

Contraindications Baseline neutrophil count less than 1,500 cells/mm^3; severe myocardial insufficiency or recent MI; severe arrhythmias; previous treatment with anthracyclines up to the max cumulative dose; hypersensitivity to epirubicin, other anthracyclines, or anthracenediones; severe hepatic dysfunction.

Route/Dosage

Epirubicin is given in repeated 3- to 4-wk cycles. The total dose may be given on day 1 of each cycle or divided equally and given on days 1 and 8 of each cycle.

Breast Cancer, Combination Therapy

ADULTS: **IV** Recommended starting dose is 100 to 120 mg/m^2. Make dosage adjustments after the first treatment cycle based on hematologic and nonhematologic toxicities. Patients experiencing nadir platelet counts less than 50,000/mm^3, absolute neutrophil counts (ANC) less than 250/mm^3, neutropenic fever, or grades 3/4 nonhematologic toxicity after the first treatment cycle should have the day 1 dose in subsequent cycles reduced 75% of the day 1 dose given in the current cycle. Delay day 1 chemotherapy in subsequent courses until platelet counts are at least 100,000/mm^3, ANC at least 1,500/mm^3, and nonhematologic toxicities have recovered to grade 1 or less. For patients receiving a divided dose (ie, day 1 and day 8), the day 8 dose should be 75% of day 1 if platelet counts are 75,000 to 100,000/mm^3 and ANC is 1,000 to 1,499 mm^3. If day 8 platelet counts are less than 75,000/mm^3, ANC less than 1,000/mm^3, or grade 3/4 nonhematologic toxicity has occurred, omit the day 8 dose.

Bone Marrow Dysfunction

ADULTS: **IV** Consider a lower starting dose (75 to 90 mg/m^2) for heavily pretreated patients, patients with preexisting bone marrow depression, or in the presence of neoplastic bone marrow infiltration.

Hepatic Dysfunction

Definitive recommendations are not available because patients with hepatic abnormalities were excluded from adjuvant trials. If bilirubin is 1.2 to 3 mg/dL or AST is 2 to 4 ULN, give ½ of recommended starting dose. If bilirubin is greater than 3 mg/dL or AST is greater than 4 times the ULN, give ¼ of recommended starting dose. Patients with severe hepatic impairment should not receive epirubicin.

Renal Dysfunction

Because of limited available data, no specific recommendations can be made; however, consider lower doses in patients with severe renal impairment (serum creatinine greater than 5 mg/dL).

Interactions

Cimetidine: Cimetidine increases the AUC of epirubicin 50%. Stop cimetidine treatment during treatment with epirubicin.

Lab Test Interferences None well documented.

Adverse Reactions Adverse reactions listed occurred in patients receiving combination therapy with epirubicin, cyclophosphamide, and fluorouracil.

CV: Delayed dose-related cardiomyopathy; acute arrhythmias. Previous therapy with other anthracyclines may increase risk of cardiotoxicity.

DERM: Alopecia (96%); rash; contact dermatitis; urticaria; radiation recall; nail hyperpigmentation.

ENDO: Hot flashes.

GI: Moderate to high potential for nausea and vomiting; mucositis within 5 to 10 days of administration; diarrhea.

GU: Amenorrhea.

HEMA: Dose-limiting bone marrow suppression, leukocyte nadir at 10 to 14 days and recovery by day 21; thrombocytopenia and anemia also may occur with nadirs at 14 to 20 days and 7 to 14 days, respectively.

SPEC SENSE: Conjunctivitis; keratitis.

OTHER: Acute leukemia and malignant tumors observed.

WARNING:
IV route only. Do not administer via IM or subcutaneous route.

Hepatic function impairment: Reduce dose of epirubicin in patients with impaired hepatic function. Evaluate serum total bilirubin and AST levels before and during treatment with epirubicin. Lower doses are recommended in patients with elevated bilirubin or AST. Patients with severe hepatic impairment should not use epirubicin.

Extravasation: Local irritation or phlebitis may occur. Severe local tissue necrosis will occur in there is extravasation. Refer to your institution-specific protocol.

Myocardial toxicity: May occur either during therapy with epirubicin or months to years after termination of therapy.

Secondary, acute, myelogenous leukemia (AML): AML has been reported in patients with breast cancer treated with anthracyclines, including epirubicin. Secondary leukemia is more common when such drugs are given in combination with DNA-damaging antineoplastic agents when patients have been heavily pretreated with cytotoxic drugs, or when doses of the anthracyclines have been escalated. These leukemias can have a short latency period.

Myelosuppression: Severe myelosuppression may occur.

Precautions
Pregnancy: Category D.
Lactation: Undetermined. Mothers should discontinue nursing prior to taking this drug.
Children: Safety and efficacy in pediatric patients not established.
Renal function impairment: Reduce dose of epirubicin in patients with impaired renal function. Dosage adjustment is necessary in patients with serum creatinine more than 5 mg/dL.
Hepatic function impairment: Evaluate serum total bilirubin and AST levels before and during treatment with epirubicin. Lower doses are recommended in patients with elevated bilirubin or AST. Patients with severe hepatic impairment should not use epirubicin. Specific guidelines are not available for dosage reduction in renal dysfunction.
Concurrent cytotoxic therapy: May show on-treatment additive toxicity, especially hematologic and GI effects.
Flushing/local streaking: Facial flushing or local erythematous streaking along the vein may be indicative of excessively rapid administration and may precede local phlebitis or thrombophlebitis.
Hematologic: A dose-dependent, reversible leukopenia and/or neutropenia. The WBC nadir is reached 10 to 14 days from drug administration. It is usually transient, returning to normal values by day 21 after drug administration. Severe thrombocytopenia and anemia also may occur. Clinical consequences of severe myelosuppression include fever, infection, septicemia, septic shock, hemorrhage, tissue hypoxia, symptomatic anemia, or death.
Radiation therapy: Previous radiation therapy may induce an inflammatory recall reaction at the site of irradiation.
Secondary leukemia: The occurrence with or without preleukemic phase has been reported in patients treated with anthracyclines.
Thromboembolic phenomenon: Thrombophlebitis and thromboembolic phenomenon, including pulmonary embolism, have been reported.
Tumor lysis syndrome: Epirubicin may induce hyperuricemia.

Overdosage: Signs and Symptoms
Bone marrow aplasia, grade 4 mucositis, GI bleeding, hyperthermia, multiple organ failure (respiratory and renal), acute lactic acidosis, increased lactate dehydrogenase, anuria, death.

PATIENT CARE CONSIDERATIONS
Administration/Storage
- Used in combination with other antineoplastic medications.
- For IV infusion only. Not for IV bolus, intradermal, subcutaneous, IM, or intra-arterial administration.
- Do not allow pregnant staff members to work with epirubicin.
- Diligently follow institutional and NIH procedures for handling, administration, and disposal of anticancer drugs. Wear appropriate protective equipment when preparing and administering epirubicin. Discard all items used for reconstitution, administration, or cleaning in high-risk, waste-disposal bags for high temperature incineration.
- Treat spillage or leakage with dilute sodium hypochlorite (1% available chlorine), preferably by soaking, and then water. Place all contaminated and cleaning materials in high-risk, waste-disposal bags for incineration.
- Avoid exposure to direct contact of the skin, mucous membranes, and eyes. If accidental skin or mucus membrane contact occurs,

wash thoroughly with soap and water or sodium bicarbonate solution. If accidental eye contact occurs, immediately institute vigorous irrigation.
- Do not administer if particulate matter or cloudiness is noted. Solution has a red-orange color, which is normal and of no concern.
- Administer antiemetic as prescribed before administering epirubicin.
- Administer prescribed dose slowly (over 3 to 20 minutes) into freely flowing IV infusion of 0.9% sodium chloride injection or 5% dextrose in water injection. Attach tubing to butterfly needle or other suitable device and insert into large vein. Take precautions to avoid extravasation. A burning or stinging sensation may be indicative of perivenous infiltration; immediately terminate infusion and restart in another vein.
- Do not mix with any other medications. Flush infusion line with D5W or 0.9% sodium chloride injection prior to administration of any concomitant medication.
- Store vials in refrigerator (36° to 46°F). Protect from light and freezing. Use within 24 hr of first penetration of the rubber stopper. Discard any unused solution. Do not save unused portions for later use.

Assessment/Interventions

- Obtain patient history, including drug history and any known allergies. Note renal or hepatic impairment, bone marrow suppression, cardiac disease, anemia, infection, leukemic pericarditis and/or myocarditis, concomitant or previous radiation to mediastinal-pericardial area, coadministration of cimetidine or drugs with potential to suppress myocardial contractility, or history of prior anthracycline or anthracenedione therapy.
- Review patient's health history for any of the following conditions that would contraindicate epirubicin therapy: baseline neutrophil count less than 1,500 cells/mm^3; severe myocardial insufficiency; recent MI; severe arrhythmias; previous treatment with anthracyclines up to maximum cumulative dose; severe hepatic dysfunction; hypersensitivity to epirubicin, other anthracyclines, or anthracenediones.
- Ensure that women of childbearing potential are not pregnant before starting therapy and use effective contraception during treatment.
- Ensure that men undergoing epirubicin therapy use effective contraceptive methods.
- Ensure that lower starting dose (eg, 75 to 90 mg/m^2) has been considered for patient who has been heavily pretreated with cytotoxic drugs, has preexisting bone marrow depression, or neoplastic bone marrow infiltration.
- Ensure that active infection has been controlled before initiating or resuming therapy with epirubicin.
- Document total cumulative dose. Ensure that dosing beyond 900 mg/m^2 is only attempted after careful evaluation of the patient and clinical situation.
- Ensure that CBC with differential, absolute neutrophil count, and platelet count, renal function (eg, Scr), hepatic function (eg, AST, bilirubin), and cardiac function (eg, ECG, LVEF measured by MUGA scan or ECHO) are evaluated before and during each cycle of epirubicin therapy.
- Ensure that reduced dose is administered to patient with renal impairment (Ccr greater than 5 mg/dL), or hepatic impairment (bilirubin greater than 1.2 mg/dL or AST 2 to 4 times ULN), following manufacturer's guidelines.
- Discontinue therapy at the first sign of impaired cardiac function and resume therapy only after careful evaluation of the risk vs benefit of continued therapy.
- Adjust dose following first treatment cycle based on hematologic and nonhematologic toxicity following manufacturer's guidelines.
- Evaluate risk of developing hyperuricemia before starting therapy and initiate hypouricemic therapy, including adequate fluid intake, and monitoring of uric acid, before starting treatment in patient determined to be at risk for developing hyperuricemia and urate precipitation.
- Monitor patient for signs or symptoms of infection or bleeding. Inform health care provider immediately if noted and be prepared to treat appropriately (eg, IV antibiotics, colony stimulating factors, transfusions).
- Monitor IV infusion site for signs or symptoms of extravasation. If noted, immediately discontinue infusion and restart in another vein. Frequently examine extravasation site and immediately inform health care provider if pain, erythema, edema, or vesiculation is noted or if patient reports persistent pain.
- Monitor toxicity when administered to women at least 70 years of age.
- Monitor patient for signs of anaphylactic or serious allergic reactions. Discontinue therapy and immediately inform health care provider if noted. Be prepared to treat appropriately.
- Monitor patient for CV, CNS, GI, RESP, HEMA, DERM, and general body side effects. Report to health care provider if noted and significant.

Patient/Family Education
- Explain name, action, and potential side effects of the treatment regimen. Review the treatment regimen including dosing schedule, duration of treatment, and monitoring that will be required.
- Review benefits of therapy and risks, including potential of developing secondary acute myelogenous leukemia, irreversible amenorrhea, or premature menopause.
- Advise patient, family, or caregiver that medication will be prepared and administered by health care professionals in a health care setting.
- Advise patient, family, or caregiver that medication will be used in combination with other agents to achieve maximum benefit possible.
- Advise patient, family, or caregiver that medication may cause a red coloration of the urine but that this is not a problem and is expected.
- Advise patient, family, or caregiver that medication may cause hair loss but that this is reversible when therapy is stopped.
- Advise patient, family, or caregiver to immediately report any of the following to health care provider: rash; hives; difficulty breathing; chest pain; palpitations; swelling or rapid weight gain; fever, chills, or other signs of infection; sores in mouth; bleeding or unusual bruising; pain, redness, or swelling at injection site.
- Advise patient, family, or caregiver to report any of the following to health care provider: persistent nausea, vomiting, or appetite loss; persistent or worsening general body weakness.
- Instruct patient not to take any prescription or OTC medications, herbal preparations, or dietary supplements unless advised by health care provider.
- Caution men undergoing epirubicin therapy to use effective contraceptive methods during treatment.
- Caution women of childbearing potential to avoid becoming pregnant during therapy.
- Advise women to notify health care provider if pregnant, planning to become pregnant, or breastfeeding.
- Advise patient that following discharge from the hospital that frequent follow-up visits, electrocardiograms, heart function tests, and laboratory tests will be required to monitor therapy and to keep appointments.

Eplerenone

(eh-PLER-en-ohn)

Class Antihypertensive/Selective aldosterone receptor antagonists

How Supplied
Inspra Tablets 25 mg, Tablets 50 mg

Action
PHARMACOLOGY: Binds to mineralocorticoid receptor, blocking the binding of aldosterone.

PHARMACOKINETICS/DYNAMICS:
Absorption: T_{max} is 1.5 hr.

Distribution: Approximately 50% is protein bound (primarily to alpha 1-acid glycoprotein). The Vd is 43 to 90 L (at steady state).

Metabolism: Metabolized by CYP3A4; no active metabolites formed.

Excretion: The elimination $t_{½}$ is approximately 4 to 6 hr. Approximately 32% is excreted in feces and approximately 67% is excreted in urine. Less than 5% is excreted as unchanged drug. The plasma Cl is approximately 10 L/hr.

Special Populations:
Renal Function Impairment – AUC and C_{max} increased 38% and 24%, respectively, in those with severe renal impairment.
Hepatic Function Impairment – C_{max} and AUC increased 3.6% and 42%, respectively, in those with moderate hepatic impairment.
Elderly – C_{max} increased 22% and AUC increased 45%.
Race – C_{max} decreased 19% and AUC decreased 26% in black patients.

Indications Treatment of hypertension; improve survival of stable patients with left ventricular systolic dysfunction and clinical evidence of CHF after an acute MI.

Contraindications Patients with serum potassium greater than 5.5 mEq/L, type 2 diabetes with microalbuminuria, serum creatinine greater than 2 mg/dL in men or greater than 1.8 mg/dL in women, Ccr 30 mL/min or less, patients treated concurrently with potassium supplements, potassium-sparing diuretics (eg, spironolactone), or strong inhibitors of CYP3A4 (eg, ketoconazole).

Route/Dosage
CHF Post-MI
ADULTS: **PO** Start with 25 mg qd and titrate to target dose of 50 mg qd within 4 wk as tolerated by the patient.

Dosage Adjustment in CHF
ADULTS: **PO** If serum potassium is less than 5 mEq/L, increase dose from 25 mg qd to 50 mg qd; if potassium levels are between 5 and 5.4 mEq/L, maintain dose; if potassium levels are between 5.5 and 5.9 mEq/L, decrease dose from 50 mg qd to 25 mg qd, or 25 mg qd to 25 mg qod, or 25 mg qod to withhold; if potassium

levels are 6 mEq/L or greater, withhold the dose. When potassium levels have fallen below 5.5 mEq/L, restart dose at 25 mg qod.

Hypertension
ADULTS: PO Initial dose 50 mg qd. The full therapeutic effect is seen within 4 wk. Patients with an inadequate BP response to 50 mg qd may be increased to 50 mg bid (max, 100 mg/day). Patients receiving weak CYP3A4 inhibitors (eg, saquinavir) start with 25 mg qd.

Interactions
ACE inhibitors and angiotensin II receptor antagonists: May increase the risk of hyperkalemia.
CYP3A4 inhibitors (eg, clarithromycin, nefazodone, ritonavir): Elevated plasma levels of eplerenone, increasing the risk of side effects.
St. John's wort: Reduced plasma levels of eplerenone, decreasing the therapeutic effect.

Adverse Reactions
CV: Angina pectoris; MI.
CNS: Headache; dizziness; fatigue.
GI: Diarrhea; abdominal pain.
GU: Albuminuria; abnormal vaginal bleeding; mastodynia, gynecomastia (men).
METAB: Hyponatremia; hypercholesterolemia; hypertriglyceridemia; increased BUN; increased uric acid; increase serum creatinine; increased ALT; hyperkalemia.
RESP: Coughing.
OTHER: Flu-like symptoms.

Precautions
Pregnancy: Category B.
Lactation: Undetermined.
Children: Safety and efficacy not established.
Hyperkalemia: Hyperkalemia may occur. Risk can be minimized by patient selection, avoidance of certain drugs, and monitoring.

Overdosage: Signs and Symptoms
Hypotension, hyperkalemia.

PATIENT CARE CONSIDERATIONS
Administration/Storage
- May be used alone for the treatment of hypertension or in combination with other antihypertensive agents.
- Administer with or without food. Administer with food if GI upset occurs.
- Administer 50 mg dose qd. Administer 100 mg dose as 50 mg bid.
- Store tablets at ambient room temperature (59° to 86°F).

Assessment/Interventions
- Obtain patient history, including drug history and any known allergies.
- Review health history for any of the following conditions that would contraindicate eplerenone therapy: serum potassium greater than 5.5 mEq/L at initiation of therapy; Ccr less than 30 mL/min; or concurrent use of strong inhibitors of CYP3A4 (eg, ketoconazole).
- Review health history for any of the following conditions that would contraindicate eplerenone therapy for treatment of hypertension: type 2 diabetes with microalbuminuria; serum creatinine greater than 1.8 mg/dL in women or 2 mg/dL in men; Ccr less than 50 mL/min; or concurrent use of potassium supplements, potassium-sparing diuretics, or potassium-containing salt substitutes.
- Ensure that reduced starting dose is administered to patient who is concurrently receiving a weak CYP3A4 inhibitor (eg, erythromycin).
- Ensure that serum potassium is determined before starting therapy, within the first week, and at 1 mo after the start of therapy or dose adjustment. Periodically assess serum potassium thereafter.
- Ensure that dose is adjusted, following manufacturer's guidelines, based on serum potassium.
- Monitor and record BP and pulse. Should hypotension result, hold medication and notify health care provider.
- Take safety precautions if orthostatic hypotension occurs.
- Assess patient for GI and general body side effects. Inform health care provider if noted and significant.

Patient/Family Education
- Explain name, dose, action, and potential side effects of drug.
- Advise patient to take qd as prescribed, without regard to meals. Advise patient to take with food if GI upset occurs.
- Advise patient to try to take each dose at about the same time each day.
- Inform patient that drug controls but does not cure hypertension and to continue taking it as prescribed even when BP is not elevated.
- Caution patient not to change the dose or stop taking unless advised by health care provider.
- Instruct patient to continue taking other BP medications as prescribed by health care provider.
- Instruct patient in BP and pulse measurement skills.
- Advise patient to monitor and record BP and pulse at home and to inform health care pro-

- vider should abnormal measurements be noted. Also advise patient to take record of BP and pulse to each follow-up visit.
- Instruct patient to lie or sit down if experiencing dizziness or lightheadedness when standing.
- Emphasize to hypertensive patient importance of the following other modalities on BP: weight control, regular exercise, smoking cessation, moderate intake of alcohol and salt.
- Advise women to notify health care provider if pregnant, planning to become pregnant, or breastfeeding.
- Caution patient not to take any prescription or OTC medications, salt substitutes, potassium supplements, or dietary supplements unless advised by health care provider.
- Advise patient that follow-up visits and lab tests may be required to monitor therapy and to keep appointments.

Epoetin Alfa (Erythropoietin; EPO)

(eh-POE-eh-tin AL-fuh)

Class Recombinant human erythropoietin

How Supplied
Epogen Injection 2000 units/mL, Injection 3000 units/mL, Injection 4000 units/mL, Injection 10,000 units/mL, Injection 20,000 units/mL, Injection 40,000 units/mL ♦ *Procrit* Injection 2000 units/mL, Injection 3000 units/mL, Injection 4000 units/mL, Injection 10,000 units/mL, Injection 20,000 units/mL, Injection 40,000 units/mL

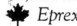 *Eprex*

Action
PHARMACOLOGY: Stimulates red blood cell production.

PHARMACOKINETICS/DYNAMICS:
Absorption: T_{max} is 5 to 24 hr (SC).

Excretion: Administered IV, epoetin alfa is eliminated via first-order kinetics with a circulating $t_{1/2}$ approximately 4 to 13 hr.

Indications Treatment of anemia related to chronic renal failure, zidovudine therapy in HIV-infected patients and nonmyeloid malignancies. Reduction of allogenic blood transfusions in surgery patients.

Contraindications Hypersensitivity to mammalian cell-derived products or human albumin; uncontrolled hypertension.

Route/Dosage
Chronic Renal Failure
ADULTS: **IV/SC** *Initial dose:* 50 to 100 units/kg 3 times/wk. *Maintenance:* Individually titrate.
CHILDREN (1 MO AND OLDER): **IV/SC** 50 units/kg 3 times/wk.
Do not adjust dose more frequently than once/month, unless clinically indicated. After any dose adjustment, determine the hematocrit twice/wk for at least 2 to 6 wk. If the hematocrit is increasing and approaching 36%, reduce the dose to maintain the suggested target hematocrit range. If the reduced dose does not stop the rise in hematocrit and it exceeds 36%, temporarily withhold doses until the hematocrit begins to decrease, then reinitiate at a lower dose. At any time, if the hematocrit increases by more than 4 points in a 2-wk period, immediately decrease the dose. After the dose reduction, monitor hematocrit twice/wk for 2 to 6 wk. If a hematocrit increase of 5 to 6 points is not achieved after an 8-wk period and iron stores are adequate, the dose may be incrementally increased. Further increases may be made at 4- to 6-wk intervals until the desired response is attained.

Zidovudine-Treated HIV-Infected Patients
ADULTS: **IV/SC** *Initial dose:* 100 units/kg 3 times/wk for 8 wk; increase by 50 to 100 units/kg 3 times/wk until appropriate maintenance dose is reached.
If hematocrit exceeds 40%, stop the dose until hematocrit drops to 36%. When resuming treatment, reduce the dose by 25%, then titrate to maintain desired hematocrit.

Nonmyeloid Malignancies
ADULTS: **SC** *Initial dose:* 150 units/kg 3 times/wk for 8 wk; if response not satisfactory, may increase up to 300 units/kg 3 times/wk.
If hematocrit exceeds 40%, hold the dose until it falls to 36%. Reduce the dose by 25% when treatment is resumed and titrate to maintain desired hematocrit. If initial dose causes an increase of more than 4% in any 2-wk period of the hematocrit, reduce the dose.

Surgery
ADULTS: **SC** 300 units/kg/day for 10 days before surgery, on the day of surgery and for 4 days after surgery. *Alternate dose schedule:* **SC** 600 units/kg once/wk doses (21, 14, and 7 days before surgery) plus a fourth dose on the day of surgery.

Interactions None well documented.
INCOMPATIBILITIES: Do not give with other drug solutions.

Lab Test Interferences None well documented.

Adverse Reactions
CV: Hypertension; tachycardia; clotted vascular access.

CNS: Headache; seizures; insomnia.
GI: Nausea; vomiting; diarrhea; constipation; dyspepsia.
RESP: Shortness of breath; cough.
OTHER: Allergy, including anaphylaxis, skin rashes and urticaria; fever; paresthesia; arthralgia; edema; pruritus.
Postmarketing – Antibody-induced pure red cell aplasia.

Precautions
Pregnancy: Category C.
Lactation: Undetermined.
Children: Safety and efficacy not established in children younger than 1 mo.
Hypersensitivity: Anaphylactoid reactions, mild and transient skin rashes and urticaria may occur.
Anemia: Because epoetin alfa may obviate the need for maintenance transfusion, it is not intended for chronic renal failure patients who require correction of severe anemia or for anemia in HIV-infected or cancer patients caused by other factors (eg, iron or folate deficiencies, hemolysis, or GI bleeding).
Benzyl alcohol: Benzyl alcohol preservative present in some of these products has been associated with a fatal "gasping syndrome" in premature infants.
Dialysis management: Epoetin alfa may result in an increase in hematocrit and a decrease in plasma volume that could affect dialysis efficiency. This does not appear to adversely affect dialyzer function or efficiency of high-flux hemodialysis. Increased anticoagulation with heparin may be required to prevent clotting of the artificial kidney.
Diet: Patients may experience an improved sense of well being as the hematocrit increases. Reinforce the importance of compliance with dietary guidelines and frequency of dialysis.
Drug abuse/dependence: Deaths have resulted from use of epoetin alfa by athletes to enhance performance by increasing hemoglobin ("blood doping").
Growth factor: Epoetin alfa can act as a growth factor for any type of tumor, particularly myeloid malignancies.
Hematology: Elevated bleeding time characteristic of chronic renal failure decreases toward normal after correction of anemia in epoetin alfa-treated patients.
Hypertension: Not for use in patients with uncontrolled hypertension; control BP adequately before initiation of therapy.
Pure red cell aplasia (PRCA): Observed in patients treated with recombinant erythropoietins in association with neutralizing antibodies to native erythropoietin. Reported primarily in patients with chronic renal failure. Discontinue epoetin alfa in any patient with evidence of PRCA and evaluate for the presence of binding and neutralizing antibodies to epoetin alfa, native erythropoietin, and any other recombinant erythropoietin the patient received.
Seizures: May occur; relationship to drug uncertain.
Thrombotic events: During hemodialysis, patients may need increased anticoagulation to prevent clotting of vascular access. Epoetin alfa also appears to increase the risk of thrombotic events in patients at risk.

Overdosage: Signs and Symptoms
Polycythemia.

PATIENT CARE CONSIDERATIONS
Administration/Storage
- Administer via IV or SC route only.
- Prescribed dose is administered 2 to 3 times/wk.
- Do not shake or vigorously agitate medication vial to prevent inactivation of medication.
- Do not administer if particulate matter or discoloration noted.
- Withdraw prescribed dose into syringe for injection.
- IV dose is administered as bolus.
- Rotate SC injection sites.
- Single-dose vials contain no preservative. Discard any unused portion. Do not combine unused portions.
- Do not administer in conjunction with other drug solutions. However, before SC administration may admix with bacteriostatic 0.9% sodium chloride with benzyl alcohol. Benzyl alcohol acts as a local anesthetic to reduce SC injection site discomfort.
- Dose will be slowly adjusted based on hematocrit levels.
- Store vials in refrigerator (36° to 46°F). Do not freeze or shake. Multidose vials may be stored for up to 21 days in refrigerator after initial use.

Assessment/Interventions
- Obtain patient history, including drug history and any known allergies. Note uncontrolled hypertension and history of allergy to human albumin or mammalian cell-derived products.
- Ensure that BP is controlled in hypertensive patient before initiating therapy.
- Ensure that hematocrit is determined twice/wk for 2 to 6 wk, or until stable, following initiation of therapy or changing the dose in patient with chronic renal failure. Be prepared to adjust the dose or withhold therapy based on changes in hematocrit.

- Ensure that hematocrit is determined weekly until stable following initiation of therapy or changing the dose in zidovudine-treated HIV-infected patient or cancer patient. Be prepared to adjust the dose or withhold therapy based on changes in hematocrit.
- Notify health care provider if hematocrit increases by more than 4 points in a 2-wk period, does not increase 5 to 6 points after 8 wk of therapy, or exceeds target value.
- Ensure that serum ferritin and transferrin saturation is determined before and during therapy.
- Ensure that iron supplementation is provided if transferring saturation is less than 20%.
- Closely monitor BP during therapy. Report elevations in BP to health care provider. Be prepared to adjust dose of antihypertensive agent(s).
- Ensure that renal function and fluid and electrolyte balance is monitored closely in patient with chronic renal failure.
- Ensure that CBC with differential and platelet counts are performed regularly in patient with chronic renal failure.
- Monitor patient for signs and symptoms of anaphylactic or serious allergic reactions. Notify health care provider immediately if noted and be prepared to treat appropriately.
- Assess patient for CV, CNS, GI, respiratory, musculoskeletal, and general body side effects. Report to health care provider if noted and significant.

Patient/Family Education

- Explain name, dose, action, and potential side effects of drug. If patient or caregiver will be administering at home, review "Information for Patients and Caregivers" insert with the patient or caregiver. Ensure that the patient or caregiver understands how to store, prepare, and administer the dose, and dispose of used equipment and supplies.
- Review injection schedule with patient or caregiver.
- Advise patient that dose will be adjusted based upon measured hematocrit level.
- Advise patient to continue following dietary and dialysis prescriptions while taking this medication.
- Advise patient that iron supplementation will probably be needed and to take iron supplement as prescribed.
- Advise patient to have BP checked regularly.
- Advise patient to notify health care provider immediately if any of the following occur: rash, hives, shortness of breath, swelling of the eyes, mouth, or throat, palpitations, severe headache, swelling of feet or ankles, intolerable GI effects (eg, nausea, vomiting, diarrhea), intolerable injection-site reaction.
- Inform patient that drug may be associated with risk of seizures during first 90 days of treatment and to avoid driving or performing other hazardous tasks during this period.
- Advise women to notify health care provider if pregnant, planning to become pregnant, or breastfeeding.
- Instruct patient not to take any prescription or OTC medications or dietary supplements unless advised by health care provider.
- Remind patient that office visits and laboratory tests will be required to monitor therapy and to keep appointments.

Epoprostenol Sodium

(EH-poe-PROSTE-eh-nole SO-dee-uhm)

Class Antihypertensive

How Supplied
Flolan Powder for reconstitution 0.5 mg, Powder for reconstitution 1.5 mg

Action
PHARMACOLOGY: Direct vasodilation of pulmonary and systemic arterial vascular beds; inhibition of platelet aggregation.

PHARMACOKINETICS/DYNAMICS:
Metabolism: Rapidly hydrolyzed at neutral pH in blood and also undergoes entymatic defradation. Metabolized to 2 primary active metabolites and several inactive metabolites.

Excretion: The $t_{1/2}$ is approximately 6 min. Excreted mostly in the urine and a small amount in the feces.

Indications Long-term IV treatment of primary pulmonary hypertension in NYHA Class III and IV patients.

Contraindications Chronic use in patients with CHF caused by severe left ventricular systolic dysfunction.

Route/Dosage
ADULTS: ACUTE DOSE RANGING: **IV** Mean max dose that did not elicit dose-limiting pharmacological effects is 8.6 ng/kg/min.

CONTINUOUS CHRONIC INFUSION: **IV** Initiate chronic infusions at 4 ng/kg/min less than the maximum tolerated infusion (MTI) rate determined during the acute dose ranging. If the MTI is less than 5 ng/kg/min, start chronic infusion at one-half the MTI rate.

INCREMENTS: Increase infusion by 1 to 2 ng/kg/

min increments at intervals sufficient to allow assessment of clinical response (15 min or more).
DECREMENTS: Gradually make 2 ng/kg/min decrements q 15 min or longer until dose-limiting effects resolve.

Interactions
Antiplatelet drugs, anticoagulants: May increase risk of bleeding.
Diuretics, antihypertensives, vasodilators: May cause additional reductions in BP.
INCOMPATIBILITIES: Reconstitute with sterile epoprostenol diluent. Do not reconstitute or mix with any other parenteral medications or solutions.

Lab Test Interferences
None well documented.

Adverse Reactions
CV: Hypotension (acute and chronic dosing); chest pain (acute and chronic dosing); tachycardia; flushing (acute and chronic dosing); syncope; arrhythmia; bradycardia (acute and chronic dosing); supraventricular tachycardia; pallor cyanosis; palpitations; cerebrovascular accident; hemorrhage.
CNS: Headache (acute and chronic dosing); anxiety (acute and chronic dosing); nervousness (acute and chronic dosing); agitation (acute dose ranging); tremor; dizziness (acute and chronic dosing); hypesthesia; hyperesthesia; paresthesia convulsions.
DERM: Pruritus; rash; sweating.
EENT: Amblyopia; vision abnormality.
GI: Nausea (acute and chronic dosing); vomiting (acute and chronic dosing); diarrhea; abdominal pain; constipation.
METAB: Hypokalemia; weight reduction; weight gain.
RESP: Hypoxia; cough increase; dyspnea (acute and chronic dosing); epistaxis; pleural effusion.
OTHER: Jaw pain; myalgia; musculoskeletal pain; chills; fever; sepsis; flu-like symptoms; arthralgia; chest pain; asthenia; local infection; pain at injection site.

Precautions
Pregnancy: Category B.
Lactation: Undetermined.
Children: Safety and efficacy not established.
Elderly: Use caution in dose selection, reflecting greater frequency of decreased hepatic, renal or cardiac function and concomitant disease or other drug therapy.
Abrupt withdrawal: May result in symptoms associated with rebound pulmonary hypertension, including dyspnea, dizziness, and asthenia.
Pulmonary edema: May result during dose ranging in patients with primary pulmonary hypertension. If this occurs, discontinue medication.

Overdosage: Signs and Symptoms
Flushing, headache, hypotension, tachycardia, nausea, vomiting, diarrhea.

PATIENT CARE CONSIDERATIONS
Administration/Storage
- Available for IV administration only.
- Store unopened vials at room temperature (59° to 77° F), protected from light.
- Reconstitute as directed using sterile diluent for epoprostenol.
- Must not be mixed with other medications or solutions.
- Reconstituted medication may be stored for up to 40 hr in refrigerator (36° to 46° F). Do not freeze. Protect from light.
- Discard any solution that has been refrigerated for more than 48 hr or has been frozen.
- A single dose can be administered over 8 hr at room temperature, then must be discarded.
- Cold pouch administration can be used up to 24 hr.
- Do not expose to direct sunlight. Insulate solution from temperature higher than 77° and lower than 32° F.
- Must be administered through a central venous catheter only. Temporary peripheral IV infusions may be used until central access is established.
- Avoid abrupt withdrawal of the medication to prevent rebound pulmonary hypertension.

Assessment/Interventions
- Obtain patient history, including drug history and any known allergies.
- Monitor BP and pulse frequently during initial dosage adjustment period and periodically throughout therapy.
- Monitor patient for signs and symptoms of adverse effects. Notify health care provider if noted. Be prepared to adjust infusion rate if indicated.
- Perform routine catheter care per policy. Closely observe catheter site for evidence of infection or inflammation.
- Ensure that infusion is not interrupted except for replacement of infusion pouch.

Patient/Family Education
- Instruct patient and family that therapy for PPH may be required for months and even years and that commitment is required for drug reconstitution, drug administration and proper care of the permanent central venous catheter.
- Instruct patients that the medication is infused continuously through a permanent

- indwelling central venous catheter by an infusion pump.
- Warn patient that even brief interruptions in the delivery of the medication will result in rapid return of symptoms.
- Provide appropriate instructions for home administration (eg, mixing, administration, rate, catheter care).
- Instruct patient and family that therapy for PPH may be required for months or even years and that commitment to required for drug reconstitution, drug administration and proper care of the permanent central venous catheter.
- Advise patient that this therapy is added to, and does not replace other therapy that has been prescribed for PPA.
- Advise patient to not change the dose or discontinue therapy unless advised to do so by their health care provider.
- Advise patient to not take any other medications (prescription, *otc* , natural product) without consulting with their health care provider.

Eprosartan Mesylate

(eh-pro-SAHR-tan MAL-ee-ate)

Class Antihypertensive/Angiotensin II antagonist

How Supplied
Teveten Tablets 400 mg, Tablets 600 mg

Action
PHARMACOLOGY: Antagonizes the effect of angiotensin II (vasoconstriction and aldosterone secretion) by blocking the angiotensin II receptor (AT_1 receptor) in vascular smooth muscle and the adrenal gland, producing decreased BP.

PHARMACOKINETICS/DYNAMICS:
Absorption: Bioavailability is approximately 13%. T_{max} is 1 to 2 hr.
Distribution: Approximately 98% is protein bound. Vd is 308 L (at steady state).
Metabolism: Metabolized to inactive metabolites.
Excretion: The $t_{1/2}$ is 5 to 9 hr. Approximately 90% recovered in the urine and approximately 7% in the urine (80% as unchanged drug). Cl is approximately 48.5 L/hr.
Onset: 1 to 2 hr.
Peak: 2 to 3 wk.

Special Populations:
Renal Function Impairment – AUC increased approximately two-fold, and C_{max} increased 50% and 30% in those with moderate or severe renal impairment, respectively. Unbound fraction increased by 35% and 59%. No dosage adjustment needed.
Hepatic Function Impairment – AUC increased approximately 40%. No dosage adjustment needed.
Elderly – AUC, C_{max}, and T_{max} increased approximately two-fold. No dosage adjustment needed.

Indications Treatment of hypertension.
Contraindications Standard considerations.

Route/Dosage
ADULTS: PO 400 to 800 mg/day; usual starting dose 600 mg/day.

Interactions None well documented.

Lab Test Interferences
Lithium: Plasma concentrations may be increased by eprosartan, resulting in an increase in the pharmacologic and adverse effects of lithium.

Adverse Reactions
CV: Abnormal ECG; extrasystoles; atrial fibrillation.
CNS: Fatigue; depression.
GI: Abdominal pain.
GU: UTI.
METAB: Hypertriglyceridemia; hyperkalemia; hypokalemia.
RESP: Upper respiratory tract infection; rhinitis; pharyngitis; coughing.
OTHER: Arthralgia.

> **WARNING:**
> *Pregnancy:* Use in second and third trimesters may cause injury and death to fetus.

Precautions
Pregnancy: Category C (first trimester); Category D (second and third trimesters).
Lactation: Undetermined.
Children: Safety and efficacy not established.
Renal function impairment: Use with caution in patients whose renal function may depend on the activity of the renin-angiotensin-aldosterone system (eg, patients with severe CHF), use may be associated with oliguria, progressive azotemia, acute renal failure, and death.

PATIENT CARE CONSIDERATIONS

Administration/Storage
- Store at room temperature in a tightly closed container.
- Administer alone or in combination with other antihypertensives such as diuretic and calcium channel blocker.
- Assess patient status and do not administer to patients with intravascular volume depletion until the condition has been corrected.

Assessment/Interventions
- Obtain patient history, including drug history and any known allergies.
- Monitor BP and pulse.
- Should hypotension, tachycardia, or bradycardia occur, withhold the medication and notify the health care provider.
- Monitor patient for signs of hypersensitivity including angioedema involving swelling of the face, lips, and tongue, or difficulty breathing.

Patient/Family Education
- Instruct patient to take the medication as prescribed at the same time each day.
- Inform patient that eprosartan controls but does not cure hypertension.
- Caution patient to take the dose exactly as prescribed and not to stop taking the medication even if feeling better.
- Instruct patient not to increase or decrease the dosage.
- Instruct patient that achievement of maximum BP reduction will usually take about 2 to 3 wk.
- Instruct family and patient in BP and pulse measurement skills.
- Caution patient to call primary health care provider should abnormal measurements occur.
- Instruct patient in methods of fall prevention including rising slowly and sitting on the side of the bed before standing, especially early in therapy.
- Inform patient of the importance of adjunct therapies such as dietary planning, regular exercise program, weight reduction, low sodium diet, alcohol reduction, smoking cessation, and stress management.
- Instruct patient to report symptoms of weakness, fatigue, dizziness, or lightheadedness to health care provider.
- Caution patient to notify health care provider or dentist of eprosartan use prior to surgery or treatment.
- Advise women to contact health care provider if pregnant, planning on becoming pregnant, or breastfeeding.

Eptifibatide
(epp-tih-FYE-bah-tide)

Class Antiplatelet

How Supplied
Integrilin Injection for solution 0.75 mg/mL, Injection for solution 2 mg/mL

Action
PHARMACOLOGY: Inhibits platelet aggregation by preventing the binding of fibrinogen, von Willebrand factor, and other adhesive ligands to glycoprotein IIb/IIIa.

PHARMACOKINETICS/DYNAMICS:

Distribution: Approximately 25% is protein bound.

Excretion: The $t_{1/2}$ is approximately 2.5 hr. Majority excreted in the urine as eptifibatide and metabolites. Cl is 55 to 58 mL/kg/hr. Renal clearance is approximately 50% of the total body clearance.

Indications Treatment of acute coronary syndrome, including patients managed medically and those undergoing percutaneous coronary intervention (PCI); treatment of PCI, including patients undergoing intracoronary stenting.

Contraindications History of bleeding diathesis; evidence of active abnormal bleeding within previous 30 days; severe hypertension (systolic BP greater than 200 mmHg or diastolic BP greater than 110 mmHg); major surgery within preceding 6 wk; history of stroke within 30 days; history of hemorrhagic stroke; current or planned administration of another parenteral glycoprotein IIb/IIIa inhibitor; dependence on renal dialysis; hypersensitivity to any component of the product.

Route/Dosage

Acute Coronary Syndrome

ADULTS: Serum creatinine less than 2 mg/dL: **IV bolus** 180 mcg/kg as soon as possible after diagnosis followed immediately by continuous infusion of 2 mcg/kg/min until hospital discharge or initiation of coronary artery bypass graft surgery, up to 72 hr. If patient is to undergo PCI while receiving eptifibatide, continue infusion up to discharge, or up to 18 to 24 hr after procedure, whichever occurs first, allowing for 96 hr of therapy. Patients weighing more than 121 kg should receive a max bolus of 22.6 mg followed by a max infusion rate of 15 mg/hr.

ADULTS: Serum creatine 2 to 4 mg/dL: **IV bolus** 180 mcg/kg as soon as possible after diagnosis followed by continuous infusion of 1 mcg/

kg/min. Patients weighing more than 121 kg should receive a max bolus of 22.6 mg followed by a max infusion rate of 7.5 mg/hr.

Percutaneous Coronary Intervention
ADULTS: Serum creatinine less than 2 mg/dL: **IV bolus** 180 mcg/kg immediately before initiation of PCI followed by continuous infusion of 2 mcg/kg/min and a second 180 mcg/kg bolus 10 min after the first bolus. Continue infusion until hospital discharge or up to 18 to 24 hr, whichever occurs first. A min of 12 hr of infusion is recommended. Patients weighing more than 121 kg should receive a max bolus of 22.6 mg followed by a max infusion rate of 15 mg/hr. Serum creatinine 2 to 4 mg/dL: **IV bolus** 180 mcg/kg immediately before initiation of PCI, immediately followed by continuous infusion of 1 mcg/kg/min and a second 180 mcg/kg bolus 10 min after the first bolus. Patients weighing more than 121 kg should receive a max bolus of 22.6 mg followed by a max infusion rate of 7.5 mg/hr.

Interactions
Dipyridamole, nonsteroidal anti-inflammatory agents, oral anticoagulants, thrombolytics: Use with caution because eptifibatide inhibits platelet aggregation.

Inhibitors of platelet receptor glycoprotein IIb/IIIa inhibitors: Avoid because of additive pharmacologic effects with eptifibatide.

Lab Test Interferences None well documented.

Adverse Reactions
EENT: Oropharyngeal bleeding.
GI: Bleeding.
GU: Bleeding.
HEMA: Intracranial hemorrhage; spontaneous gross hematuria; spontaneous hematemesis; major bleeding; minor bleeding; bleeding at femoral artery access site.
OTHER: Retroperitoneal bleeding.

Precautions
Pregnancy: Category B.
Lactation: Undetermined.
Children: Safety and efficacy not established.
Bleeding: Take special care to minimize risk of bleeding.
Platelet count: Use with caution in patients with a platelet count less than 100,000/mm^3.
Trauma: Minimize use of arterial or venous punctures, IM injections, use of urinary catheters, nasotracheal intubation, and nasogastric tubes.

PATIENT CARE CONSIDERATIONS

Administration/Storage
- For IV use only. Not for intra-arterial, SC, IM, or ID administration.
- Eptifibatide is administered as an IV bolus dose (180 mcg/kg, not to exceed 22.6 mg) followed immediately by an IV infusion (2 mcg/kg/min, not to exceed 15 mg/hr.)
- Administer reduced infusion dose (1 mcg/kg/min, not to exceed 7.5 mg/hr) to patient with serum creatinine between 2 to 4 mg/dL.
- Withdraw bolus dose from 10 mL vial into a syringe. Administer the bolus dose by IV push.
- Administer continuous infusion undiluted directly from 100 mL vial via IV infusion pump using vented infusion set.
- Administer IV infusion in same IV line with 0.9% Sodium Chloride or 0.9% Sodium Chloride with 5% Dextrose.
- May be administered in same IV line with potassium chloride, alteplase, atropine, dobutamine, heparin, lidocaine, meperidine, metoprolol, midazolam, morphine, nitroglycerin, or verapamil.
- Do not administer in IV line containing furosemide.
- Discontinue eptifibatide infusion prior to coronary artery bypass graft surgery.
- Do not administer if particulate matter or discoloration is noted.
- Store vials in refrigerator (36° to 46°F). May be transferred for storage at controlled room temperature (59° to 86°F) for up to 2 mo. Protect from light until administration.

Assessment/Interventions
- Obtain patient history, including drug history and any known allergies. Note history of bleeding disorders; evidence of active abnormal bleeding within previous 30 days; uncontrolled severe hypertension; major surgery within preceding 6 wk; history of stroke within 30 days or any history of hemorrhagic stroke; dependency on renal dialysis; current or planned administration of another parenteral GP IIb/IIIa inhibitor; or concurrent use of thrombolytic agent, oral anticoagulant, non-steroidal anti-inflammatory drug, or dipyridamole.
- Administer appropriate doses of heparin and aspirin concomitantly if indicated.
- Ensure that baseline hematocrit or hemoglobin, platelet count, serum creatinine, and PT/aPTT are performed and evaluated prior to starting therapy. Perform an activated clotting time (ACT) and evaluate prior to starting therapy in patients undergoing PCI.
- Maintain aPTT between 50 to 70 sec in patients treated concurrently with heparin unless PCI is to be performed. Maintain ACT between 200 to 300 sec during PCI.

- Determine aPTT or ACT prior to removal of arterial sheath. Do not remove sheath until aPTT is less than 45 sec or ACT is less than 150 sec.
- Monitor patient for unusual bleeding or bruising, especially at vascular access sites, and report to health care provider if noted.
- Discontinue eptifibatide and heparin if platelet count decreases to less than 100,000/mm^3.
- Minimize arterial and venous punctures, IM injections, and use of urinary catheters, nasotracheal intubation, and nasogastric tubes while patient is receiving eptifibatide.
- Avoid IV access through noncompressible sites (eg, subclavian or jugular veins).
- Monitor patient for evidence of ongoing myocardial ischemia or hemodynamic instability. Report to health care provider if noted.

Patient/Family Education
- Explain name, action, and potential side effects of drug.
- Advise patient, family, or caregiver that medication will be prepared and administered by health care provider in a health care setting.
- Advise patient, family, or caregiver that medication may be used in combination with other agents, including aspirin and heparin, to achieve maximum benefit possible.
- Review dosing schedule with patient, family, or caregiver.
- Advise patient, family, or caregiver to report any unusual bleeding or bruising to health care provider while medication is being administered.

Ergoloid Mesylates (Dihydrogenated Ergot Alkaloids; Dihydroergotoxine)

(err-GO-loyd- MEH-suh-lates)

Class Psychotherapeutic

How Supplied
Gerimal Tablets, oral 1 mg, Tablets, sublingual 0.5 mg, Tablets, sublingual 1 mg ♦ *Hydergine* Liquid 1 mg/mL, Tablets, oral 1 mg, Tablets, sublingual 0.5 mg, Tablets, sublingual 1 mg

Action
PHARMACOLOGY: Unknown; may increase brain metabolism, possibly increasing cerebral blood flow.

PHARMACOKINETICS/DYNAMICS:

Absorption: Approximately 25% is absorbed; approximately 50% is removed by the first-pass metabolism. T_{max} is 1.5 to 3 hr.

Distribution: Excreted in breast milk.

Metabolism: Undergoes first-pass metabolism.

Excretion: The t½ is approximately 2.6 to 5.1 hr (unchanged ergoloid in the plasma).

Indications
Treatment of age-related decline in mental capacity, primary progressive dementia, Alzheimer dementia, multi-infarct dementia and senile onset.

PATIENT CARE CONSIDERATIONS

Administration/Storage
- Instruct patient to allow sublingual tablets to completely dissolve under tongue; do not allow patient to swallow, crush, or chew tablet.
- Do not permit patient to eat, drink, or smoke while sublingual tablet is dissolving.
- Store in tightly closed, light-resistant container at room temperature.

Contraindications
Hypersensitivity to ergoloid mesylates or other ergot alkaloids; acute or chronic psychosis.

Route/Dosage
ADULTS: **PO/SL** 1 to 2 mg tid (up to 12 mg/day has been used).

Interactions None well documented.

Lab Test Interferences None well documented.

Adverse Reactions
CV: Orthostatic hypotension; bradycardia.
DERM: Rash.
GI: Transient nausea; GI disturbances; sublingual irritation.

Precautions
Pregnancy: Pregnancy category undetermined.
Lactation: Undetermined.
Children: Safety and efficacy not established.
Hepatic function impairment: Elimination of drug may be affected.
Special risk patients: Administer drug with caution to patients with history of bradycardia or hypotension.

Overdosage: Signs and Symptoms
Headache, flushing, anorexia nausea, vomiting, abdominal cramps, nasal congestion, impaired vision, dizziness, fainting.

Assessment/Interventions
- Obtain patient history, including drug history and any known allergies.
- Potentially reversible and treatable conditions should be ruled out prior to use of ergoloid

mesylates in treating age-related decline of mental capacity.
- Assess patient's mental status (eg, alertness, memory, orientation, mood, emotional liability, self-care) prior to and during administration of drug.
- Monitor BP and pulse rate prior to initiation of therapy and at periodic intervals during therapy.
- Take appropriate safety measures if lightheadedness, weakness, or changes in mental status develop.

Patient/Family Education
- Teach patient how to decrease effects of orthostatic hypotension by rising slowly from supine position and dangling feet for few min before standing.
- Instruct patient to avoid alcohol consumption, which may enhance hypotensive effect.
- Caution patient not to take OTC cough, cold and allergy preparations that contain alcohol.
- Instruct patient to avoid excessive exposure to cold since temperature regulation may be impaired.
- Instruct patient to notify health care provider if adverse reactions occur.
- Advise patient/family that it may require 3 to 4 wk and up to 6 mo to determine clinical effectiveness of drug.

Ergonovine Maleate

(ehr-go-NO-veen MAL-ee-ate)
Class Oxytocic

How Supplied
Ergotrate Tablets 0.2 mg

Action
PHARMACOLOGY: Increases strength, duration, and frequency of uterine contractions and decreases uterine bleeding.

PHARMACOKINETICS/DYNAMICS:
Onset: Produces a firm tetanic contraction of postpartum uterus within 6 to 15 min that, in the course of about 90 min, gradually changes to a series of clonic contractions that persist for 90 min or more.

Indications Prevention and treatment of postpartum and postabortal hemorrhage caused by uterine atony. **Unlabeled use(s):** Oxytocin challenge test.

Contraindications Induction of labor; threatened spontaneous abortion; previous allergic or idiosyncratic reactions to drug.

Route/Dosage
ADULTS: **PO** Immediate postpartum dose 0.2 mg. To minimize late postpartum bleeding, 0.2 to 0.4 mg bid to qid (q 6 to 12 hr) until danger of uterine atony has passed (usually 48 hr).

Interactions
Inhibitors of metabolism (eg, protease inhibitors [eg, ritonavir]): Increased risk of ergot toxicity (eg, peripheral vasospasm, ischemia of extremities).
Sympathomimetics: Possible hypertension caused by additive vasoconstriction.

Lab Test Interferences None well documented.

Adverse Reactions
CV: Increased BP (sometimes extreme).
GI: Nausea, vomiting, cramping.
OTHER: Allergy (including shock), ergotism.

Precautions
Pregnancy: Category X. Contraindicated during pregnancy.
Lactation: Ergot alkaloids are excreted in breast milk.
Labor and delivery: Because of the high uterine tone produced, ergonovine is not recommended for routine use prior to the delivery of the placenta, unless the surgeon is familiar with the technique described by Davis and others and has adequate facilities and personnel at his or her disposal.
Calcium deficiency: Hypocalcemia may affect response to drug.
Duration: Avoid prolonged use and discontinue if symptoms of ergotism appear.
Severe cramping: This is evidence of effectiveness but may justify reduction in dosage.
Special risk patients: Use with caution in patients with hypertension, heart disease, venoatrial shunts, mitral-valve stenosis, obliterative vascular disease, sepsis, hepatic impairment, or renal impairment.
Uterine effects: Hyperstimulation of uterus may lead to uterine tetany and impairment of uteroplacental blood flow, uterine rupture, cervical and perineal lacerations, amniotic fluid embolism, and trauma to infant (eg, intracranial hemorrhage).

Overdosage: Signs and Symptoms
Convulsions, gangrene, chest pain, diarrhea, dizziness, dyspnea, hypercoagulability, loss of consciousness, numbness and coldness of extremities, increase or decrease in BP, tingling, vomiting, weak pulse.

PATIENT CARE CONSIDERATIONS

Administration/Storage
- Administer prescribed dose by mouth or sublingually q 6 to 12 hr as ordered.
- Administer without regard to meals but administer with food if GI upset occurs.
- Store tablets at controlled room temperature (59° to 86°F).

Assessment/Interventions
- Obtain patient history, including drug history and any known allergies. Note renal or hepatic impairment, hypertension, heart disease, venoatrial shunt, mitral valve stenosis, obliterative vascular disease, sepsis, threatened spontaneous abortion, concurrent use of regional anesthesia, previous administration of a vasoconstrictor, or concurrent use of a protease inhibitor.
- Obtain baseline vital signs, with special attention to pulse and BP. Closely monitor BP during treatment. Notify health care provider immediately if BP becomes elevated. Be prepared to discontinue therapy and treat appropriately.
- Monitor and document uterine response during and after administration. Notify health care provider if uterine contractions are not maintained or if cramping is severe.
- Note character and amount of vaginal bleeding.
- Closely monitor patient for signs and symptoms of ergotism (eg, intense vasoconstriction, coldness of the extremities, chest pain, gangrene). Immediately discontinue therapy and inform health care provider if noted or suspected.
- Monitor patient for CV, GI, and general body side effects. Report to health care provider if noted and significant.

Patient/Family Education
- Explain name, dose, action, and potential side effects of drug.
- Advise patient that medication will usually be administered by a health care professional in a medical setting.
- Advise patient to take prescribed dose either orally or sublingually as ordered.
- Caution patient not to change the dose or take for longer period than prescribed.
- Advise patient to stop taking the medication and notify health care provider immediately if any of the following occur: numbness, tingling, coldness, or paleness in the fingers or toes; muscle pain in arms or legs; weakness in the legs; chest pain, tightness, or pressure; changes in heart rate.
- Advise patient to report excessive or severe uterine cramping.
- Warn patient not to take any prescription or OTC drugs, herbal preparations, or dietary supplements without consulting health care provider.
- Advise patient that follow-up visits will be necessary to monitor therapy and to keep appointments.

Ergotamine Tartrate

(ehr-GOT-ah-meen TAR-trate)

Class Ergotamine derivatives

How Supplied
Ergomar Tablets, sublingual 2 mg

Action
PHARMACOLOGY: Reduces extracranial blood flow, causes decline in amplitude of pulsation in the cranial arteries and decreases hyperperfusion of the territory of the basilar artery; produces constriction of both arteries and veins.

PHARMACOKINETICS/DYNAMICS:
Absorption: Poorly absorbed following GI and SL administration.
Metabolism: Metabolized by the liver.
Excretion: $T_{1/2}$ is approximately 2 hr; 90% of metabolites are excreted in the bile. Unmetabolized ergotamine is erratically excreted in the saliva and trace amounts are excreted in the feces and urine.

Indications Abort or prevent vascular headache (eg, migraine).

Contraindications Peripheral vascular disease; coronary heart disease; hypertension; impaired hepatic or renal function; severe pruritus; sepsis; hypersensitivity to any component of the product; pregnancy.

Route/Dosage
SL 2 mg under tongue at first sign of attack or to relieve symptoms after onset of an attack; another tablet should be taken at 30–min intervals thereafter, if necessary (max, 6 mg/24 hr and 10 mg in any 1 wk).

Interactions
Troleandomycin: May elevate ergotamine plasma levels, increasing the pharmacologic and adverse effects.

Lab Test Interferences None well documented.

Adverse Reactions

CV: Transient changes in heart rate.
GI: Nausea; vomiting.
OTHER: Weakness of legs, limb muscle pain; numbness and tingling of the fingers and toes; precordial pain; localized edema; itching.

Precautions

Pregnancy: Category X.
Lactation: Excreted in breast milk.
Ergotism: Signs and symptoms are rare; however, remain within limits of recommended dosage.
Dependency: Prolonged use may result in dependency and increase the dose requirement for relief of vascular headaches and to prevent dysphoria following withdrawal of the drug.

Overdosage: Signs and Symptoms

Nausea, vomiting, weakness of the legs, pain in limb muscles, numbness, itching of fingers and toes, precordial pain, tachycardia, bradycardia, hypertension, hypotension, localized edema, itching together with signs and symptoms of ischemia caused by vasoconstriction of peripheral arteries and arterioles, cold, pale and numb feet and hands, muscle pain while walking and later at rest, gangrene, confusion, depression, drowsiness, convulsions.

PATIENT CARE CONSIDERATIONS

Administration/Storage

- For sublingual administration only. Do not crush, chew, or swallow tablet.
- Place 1 tablet under the tongue at the first sign of migraine attack or to relieve symptoms after onset of attack.
- May repeat dose at 30-min intervals if necessary, but total dose should not exceed 3 tablets in any 24-hr period or 5 tablets in any 1 wk.
- Administer without regard to meals.
- Do not administer within 24 hr of treatment with another 5-HT$_1$ agonist or other ergot-containing or ergot-type drug (eg, methysergide).
- Store at controlled room temperature (59° to 86°F). Protect from light and heat.

Assessment/Interventions

- Obtain patient history, including drug history and any known allergies. Note history of peripheral vascular disease, ischemic or vasospastic coronary artery disease, hypertension, hepatic or renal impairment, childbearing potential, hemiplegic or basilar migraine.
- Note recent (within 24 hr) use of 5-HT$_1$ agonists or other ergotamine-containing or ergot-type drugs (eg, methysergide).
- Ensure that women of childbearing potential are not pregnant before administering medication.
- Assess pain location, intensity, duration, and associated symptoms of migraine attack.
- Obtain baseline vital signs, with special attention to pulse and BP.
- Provide quiet, calm environment. Decrease stimuli, noise, and light.
- Monitor patient for effectiveness of headache relief and minimal effective dose.
- Monitor patient for CNS, CV, GI, musculoskeletal, and general body side effects. Report to health care provider if noted and significant.
- Discontinue therapy and notify health care provider immediately if any of the following occur: numbness, tingling, coldness, or paleness in the fingers or toes; muscle pain in arms or legs; weakness in the legs; chest pain, tightness or pressure; changes in heart rate; sudden worsening of headache; swelling; itching.

Patient/Family Education

- Explain name, dose, action, and potential side effects of drug.
- Explain that drug is to be used only during migraine and does not prevent or reduce the number of attacks. Emphasize that drug is used only to treat actual migraine attack.
- Instruct patient in proper use of sublingual tablet. Caution patient not to chew, crush, or swallow tablet.
- Advise patient that drug is to be taken as soon as symptoms of migraine appear, and that the dose may be repeated q 30 min if needed but that no more than 3 tablets should be used in any 24-hr period or 5 tablets used in any 1-wk period.
- Caution patient not to exceed the dosing guidelines because of the risk of toxic effects developing.
- Advise patient to stop taking the drug and notify their health care provider if any of the following occur: numbness, tingling, coldness, or paleness in the fingers or toes; muscle pain in arms or legs; weakness in the legs; chest pain, tightness or pressure; changes in heart rate; sudden worsening of headache; swelling; itching.
- Instruct patient that if they have migraine prophylactic medications prescribed to take daily as directed.
- Advise patient that if not currently taking a migraine prophylactic drug to discuss the use of such drugs with health care provider.
- Advise women to inform health care provider

if pregnant, planning to become pregnant, or breastfeeding.
• Warn patient not to take any prescription or OTC drugs or dietary supplements without consulting health care provider.
• Advise patient that follow-up visits may be necessary to monitor therapy and to keep appointments.

Ertapenem

(Err-tah-PEN-em)
Class Anti-infective/Carbapenem
How Supplied
Invanz Powder, lyophilized 1.046 g ertapenem sodium (equivalent to 1 g ertapenem)
Action
PHARMACOLOGY: Inhibits cell wall synthesis.
PHARMACOKINETICS/DYNAMICS:
Absorption: Bioavailability for IM dose is approximately 90%. T_{max} is approximately 2.3 hr (IM).
Distribution: Approximately 85% to 95% is protein bound (concentration dependent). Vd is approximately 8.2 L (at steady state).
Metabolism: Major metabolite is the inactive ring-opened derivative formed by hydrolysis of the beta-lactam ring.
Excretion: The $t_{1/2}$ is approximately 4 hr. Approximately 80% excreted in urine (approximately 38% as unchanged drug) and 10% in feces.
Special Populations:
Renal Function Impairment – Unbound AUC increased 1.5-fold and 2.3-fold in those with mild and moderate renal insufficiency, respectively. No dosage adjustment necessary. Unbound AUC increased 4.4-fold and 7.6-fold in those with advanced and end-stage renal insufficiency, respectively. Dosage adjustment required.
Elderly – The total and unbound AUC increased 37% and 67%, respectively.
Indications Treatment of moderate to severe complicated intra-abdominal infections, complicated skin and skin structure infections, community-acquired pneumonia, complicated urinary tract infections (UTIs) (including pyelonephritis), and acute pelvic infections (including postpartum endomyometritis, septic abortion, and postsurgical gynecologic infections) caused by susceptible microorganisms.
Contraindications Hypersensitivity to any component of this product or to other drugs in the same class, patients who have demonstrated anaphylactic reactions to beta-lactams; because of the lidocaine diluent, patients with known sensitivity to local anesthetics of the amide type.
Route/Dosage
Complicated Intra-Abdominal Infections
ADULTS: **IV/IM** 1 g/day for 5 to 14 days.

Complicated Skin and Skin Structure Infections
ADULTS: **IV/IM** 1 g/day for 7 to 14 days.
Community-Acquired Pneumonia or Complicated UTIs
ADULTS: **IV/IM** 1 g/day for 10 to 14 days.
Acute Pelvic Infections
ADULTS: **IV/IM** 1 g/day for 3 to 10 days.
Renal Insufficiency
ADULTS: **IV/IM** Ccr less than 30 mL/min: 500 mg/day.
Hemodialysis
ADULTS: **IV/IM** 500 mg within 6 hr prior to hemodialysis and a supplemental dose of 150 mg following the hemodialysis session.
Interactions
Probenecid: Inhibits renal excretion of ertapenem; coadministration is not recommended.
INCOMPATIBILITIES: Do not mix or co-infuse with other medications; do not use diluents containing dextrose.
Lab Test Interferences None well documented.
Adverse Reactions
CV: Chest pain; hypertension; hypotension; tachycardia.
CNS: Headache; altered mental status; anxiety; dizziness; insomnia; fatigue.
DERM: Erythema; extravasation; infused vein complication; phlebitis/thrombophlebitis; pruritus; rash.
EENT: Pharyngitis.
GI: Diarrhea; nausea; abdominal pain; acid regurgitation; constipation; oral candidiasis; vomiting.
GU: Vaginitis; increased serum creatinine.
HEMA: Increased eosinophils; decreased hematocrit, hemoglobin, and platelets.
HEPA: Increased ALT, AST, and bilirubin.
METAB: Increased serum glucose and serum potassium; decreased serum potassium.
RESP: Cough; dyspnea; rales/rhonchi; respiratory distress.
OTHER: Asthenia; edema/swelling; fever; leg pain.
Precautions
Pregnancy: Category B.
Lactation: Excreted in breast milk.
Children: Safety and efficacy not established.
Elderly: Because elderly are more likely to have decreased renal function, select dose with caution.

Hypersensitivity: Hypersensitivity reactions may occur; do not administer to patients who have demonstrated anaphylactic reactions to beta-lactams, carbapenams, or penicillin.
Renal function impairment: Adjust dose accordingly.
Superinfection: May result in bacterial or fungal overgrowth of nonsusceptible organisms.

CNS: Seizures and other CNS adverse effects may occur.
Pseudomembranous colitis: Consider possibility in patients with diarrhea.

Overdosage: Signs and Symptoms
Nausea, diarrhea, dizziness.

PATIENT CARE CONSIDERATIONS
Administration/Storage
- For IV or IM administration only. Do not administer SC.
- Administer prescribed dose once daily.
- Administer reduced dose to patients with renal impairment.
- For IV infusion, reconstitute with 10 mL of compatible diluent (Water for Injection, 0.9% Sodium Chloride Injection, or Bacteriostatic Water for Injection). Do not use diluents containing dextrose. Shake well to dissolve powder and immediately transfer contents of the reconstituted vial to 50 mL of 0.9% Sodium Chloride Injection. Infuse prescribed dose over 30 min. Complete infusion within 6 hr of reconstitution. Do not mix or co-infuse with other medications.
- Do not administer if reconstituted solution is cloudy, discolored, or contains particulate matter.
- For IM administration, reconstitute with 3.2 mL of 1% Lidocaine Hydrochloride Injection (without epinephrine). Shake vial thoroughly to form clear solution. Immediately withdraw contents of vial and administer by deep IM injection into large muscle mass. Do not administer IV. Use reconstituted IM solution within 1 hr after preparation.
- Reconstituted solution may exhibit a pale yellow color, which is normal and does not affect potency.
- If other drugs are being administered through same IV line, flush IV line before and after infusion of ertapenem with 0.9% Sodium Chloride Injection.
- Store lyophilized powder lower than 77°F. Reconstituted solution for IV administration, diluted in 0.9% Sodium Chloride Injection, may be stored at room temperature and used within 6 hr or stored under refrigeration for 24 hr and used within 4 hr after removal from refrigeration. Protect from freezing. Use reconstituted solution for IM administration within 1 hr of preparation.

Assessment/Interventions
- Obtain patient history, including drug history and any known allergies, especially to amide type local anesthetics, penicillin and beta-lactam antibiotics. Note history of renal impairment, seizures, or brain lesions.
- Review results of culture and sensitivity testing as available.
- Monitor for signs of infection, especially fever, and for positive response to antibiotic therapy.
- Monitor patient for signs of anaphylaxis or severe allergic reaction. Discontinue therapy and immediately notify health care provider if noted. Be prepared to treat appropriately.
- Monitor patient for GI, CNS, and general body side effects. Report to health care provider if noted and significant.
- If seizure occurs, withhold drug, institute safety measures, and notify health care provider.
- Withhold drug and notify health care provider if any of the following occurs: severe diarrhea; loose, foul-smelling stools; vaginal itching or discharge.

Patient/Family Education
- Explain name, dose, action, and potential side effects of drug. Explain to patient that medication will be prepared and administered by a health care provider.
- Review dosing schedule and prescribed length of therapy with patient. Advise patient that dose and duration of therapy are dependent on site and cause of infection and response to therapy.
- Instruct patient to report the following to health care provider: itching; rash; hives; difficulty breathing; diarrhea; black furry tongue; loose, foul-smelling stools; vaginal itching or discharge.

Erythromycin

(eh-RITH-row-MY-sin)

Class Antibiotic/Macrolide

How Supplied

A/T/S Gel 2%, Solution 2% ♦ Akne-mycin Ointment 2%, Solution 2% ♦ Del-Mycin Solution 2% ♦ E-Base Tablets, enteric coated 333 mg, Tablets, enteric coated 500 mg ♦ E-Mycin Tablets, enteric coated 250 mg, Tablets, enteric coated 333 mg ♦ E.E.S. 200 Suspension 200 mg/5 mL as ethylsuccinate ♦ E.E.S. 400 Tablets 400 mg as ethylsuccinate, Suspension 400 mg/5 mL as ethylsuccinate ♦ E.E.S. Granules Powder for oral suspension 200 mg/5 mL when reconstituted as ethylsuccinate ♦ Emgel Gel 2%, Ointment 2% ♦ Ery-Tab Tablets, enteric coated 250 mg, Tablets, enteric coated 333 mg, Tablets, enteric coated 500 mg ♦ Eryc Capsules, delayed release 250 mg ♦ Erycette Solution 2% ♦ Eryderm Solution 2% ♦ Erymax Solution 2% ♦ EryPed Tablets, chewable 200 mg as ethylsuccinate ♦ EryPed 200 Suspension 200 mg/5 mL as ethylsuccinate ♦ EryPed 400 Suspension 400 mg/5 mL as ethylsuccinate ♦ EryPed Drops Suspension 100 mg/2.5 mL as ethylsuccinate ♦ Erythra-Derm Solution 2% ♦ Erythrocin Stearate Tablets, film coated 250 mg, Tablets, film coated 500 mg as stearate ♦ Ilosone Capsules 250 mg as estolate, Suspension 125 mg/5 mL, Suspension 250 mg/5 mL as estolate, Tablets 500 mg as estolate ♦ Ilotycin Ointment 5% ♦ Ilotycin Gluceptate Injection 1 g/vial as gluceptate ♦ PCE Dispertab Tablets with polymer coated particles 333 mg, Tablets with polymer coated particles 500 mg ♦ Theramycin Z Solution 2%

❀ Apo-Erythro Base ♦ Apo-Erythro E-C ♦ Apo-Erythro-ES ♦ Apo-Erythro-S ♦ EES 600 ♦ Erybid ♦ Novorythro Encap ♦ Nu-Erythromycin-S ♦ PMS-Erythromycin

Action

PHARMACOLOGY: Interferes with microbial protein synthesis.

Indications

Oral/IV use: Treatment of infections of respiratory tract, skin and skin structure, and sexually transmitted diseases caused by susceptible organisms; treatment of pertussis, diphtheria, erythrasma, intestinal amebiasis, conjunctivitis of newborn, and Legionnaire disease; prevention of attacks of rheumatic fever; prevention of bacterial endocarditis.
Ophthalmic use: Treatment of superficial ocular infections caused by strains of susceptible organism.
Topical use: Treatment of acne vulgaris.
Unlabeled use(s): Treatment of *Neisseria gonorrhoeae* in pregnancy; treatment of diarrhea caused by *Campylobacter jejuni*; as alternative to penicillin in selected infections, *Treponema pallidum*, *Lymphogranuloma venereum*, *Granuloma inguinale*, *Haemophilus ducreyi* (chancroid). Other uses as alternative to penicillins include the following: anthrax, Vincent gingivitis, erysipeloid, tetanus, actinomycosis, *Nocardia* infections (with a sulfonamide), *Eikenella corrodens* infections, *Borrelia* infections (including early Lyme disease).

Contraindications
Hypersensitivity to erythromycin or any macrolide antibiotic; pre-existing liver disease (with estolate salt); epithelial herpes simplex keratitis; fungal disease of eye; vaccinia or varicella (ophthalmic use).

Route/Dosage

Systemic Use
ADULTS: **PO** 250 to 500 mg of base (400 to 800 mg ethylsuccinate) q 6 hr or 500 mg q 12 hr or 333 mg q 8 hr. **IV** 15 to 20 mg/kg/day; up to 4 g/day in very severe infections.
CHILDREN: **PO** 30 to 50 mg/kg/day in divided doses.

Acute Ocular Infection
ADULTS AND CHILDREN: **Ophthalmic** 0.5-inch ribbon of ointment placed in eye q 3 to 4 hr.

Mild to Moderate Ocular Infection
ADULTS AND CHILDREN: **Ophthalmic** 0.5-inch ribbon of ointment placed in eye bid to tid.

Prophylaxis of Neonatal Gonococcal or Chlamydia Conjunctivitis
NEWBORNS: **Ophthalmic** 0.2 to 0.4 inch ribbon of ointment placed in each conjunctival sac at time of delivery.

Skin Infections
ADULTS AND CHILDREN: **Topical** Apply qd to qid to affected area.

Acne Vulgaris
ADULTS AND CHILDREN: **Topical** Apply bid, morning and evening.

Interactions

Anticoagulants: May increase anticoagulant effects.
Antihistamines, non-sedating (eg, astemizole, terfenadine): May increase antihistamine levels and cause serious adverse cardiovascular events, including ventricular arrhythmias and death.
Bromocriptine: May increase serum bromocriptine levels.
Carbamazepine: May result in serious carbamazepine toxicity.
Clindamycin, topical: Antagonism may occur with topical erythromycin.
Cyclosporine: May cause increased cyclosporine levels with renal toxicity.
Digoxin: May cause increased digoxin levels.

Lovastatin: Severe myopathy or rhabdomyolysis may occur.
Methylprednisolone: May decrease Cl of methylprednisolone.
Theophyllines: May increase theophylline plasma concentration.

Lab Test Interferences None well documented.

Adverse Reactions
DERM: Rash; photosensitivity; erythema and peeling (topical use).
GI: Diarrhea; nausea; vomiting abdominal pain/cramping.
GU: Vaginitis.
HEPA: Hepatotoxicity (primarily with estolate salt).
OTHER: Venous irritation or phlebitis with IV administration.

Precautions
Pregnancy: Category B.
Lactation: Excreted in breast milk.
Children:
Topical – Safety and efficacy not established.

Hypersensitivity: Serious reactions, including anaphylaxis, have occurred.
Hepatic function impairment: Use drug cautiously. Hepatic dysfunction, with or without jaundice, has occurred. Cholestatic hepatitis has occurred.
Superinfection: Prolonged use of antibiotics may result in bacterial or fungal overgrowth of nonsusceptible microorganisms.
Acne therapy: Cumulative irritant effect may occur.
Ophthalmic ointments: May slow corneal epithelial healing.
Ototoxicity: May occur, especially in patients with renal or hepatic insufficiency and elderly patients and with administration of large doses.
Pseudomembranous colitis: Consider possibility in patients in whom diarrhea develops.

Overdosage: Signs and Symptoms
Severe nausea, vomiting, diarrhea, epigastric distress, hearing loss, vertigo.

PATIENT CARE CONSIDERATIONS
Administration/Storage
Oral:
- Administer with full glass of water 1 hr before or 2 hr after meals. If GI upset is significant, give with food or milk. Do not crush tablets or allow patient to chew them.

Parenteral:
- Use only sterile water for injection for reconstitution. Do not use diluents containing preservatives or organic salts.
- Dilute reconstituted drug in 1 to 5 mg/mL in 0.9% sodium chloride. If D5W is used, buffer solution with sodium bicarbonate or neutralize (add 1 mL/100 mL of solution).
- Administer IV infusion at slow rate over 30 to 60 min to reduce venous irritation.
- Piggyback vial must be used within 8 hr of preparation if stored at room temperature or 24 hr if refrigerated.
- Frozen solution may be stored for 30 days. Thaw in refrigerator and use within 8 hr after thawing. Do not refreeze thawed solution.

Topical:
- With topical use, cleanse affected area with 0.9% sodium chloride before application.
- For ophthalmic use, have patient tilt head back, pull lid down, place medication in conjunctival sac, and have patient close eyes. Take care not to touch lids.

Assessment/Interventions
- Obtain patient history, including drug history and any known allergies. Note any hypersensitivity to macrolide antibiotics and history of liver disease, fungal disease, or colitis.
- Culture and sensitivity testing should be done to determine organism sensitivity.
- Obtain baseline LFTs and CBC.
- Monitor LFTs routinely.
- Monitor I&O.
- Monitor for signs and symptoms of superinfection (eg, thrush, vaginal yeast, perianal irritation, vaginal discharge, black furry tongue).
- Monitor for diarrhea, nausea, vomiting, or abdominal discomfort. Contact health care provider if these symptoms are persistent.
- If skin rash, respiratory distress, or urticaria occur, stop infusion immediately and notify health care provider.
- Monitor IV site if using IV route. Change IV heparin locks q 3 days or per institution guidelines.
- If patient is undergoing oral anticoagulant therapy, monitor PT.

Patient/Family Education
- Advise patient to take medication with full glass of water 1 hr before or 2 hr after meals. If extreme GI distress occurs, drug may be taken with food or milk.
- Inform patient that following ophthalmic administration, temporary blurring of vision or stinging may occur. Advise patient to notify health care provider if redness, irritation, or pain persists or worsens. Instruct patient to use medication 1 hr before driving.
- Instruct patient to notify health care provider

if nausea, vomiting, diarrhea, abdominal pain, jaundice, dark urine, pale stools, unusual fatigue, or signs of superinfection occur.
- Instruct patient to follow complete course of therapy.
- When used topically for treatment of acne vulgaris, caution patient not to use OTC peeling, abrasive agents, or abrasive sponges because cumulative irritant effect may occur.
- When drug is used topically, advise patient to avoid exposure to sunlight, use sunscreen, or wear protective clothing to avoid photosensitivity reaction.

Erythromycin/Benzoyl Peroxide

(eh-RITH-row-MY-sin/BEN-zoe-il)
Class Anti-infective
How Supplied
Benzamycin
Action
PHARMACOLOGY: Exact mechanism not known, however, in part, due to antibacterial effect of erythromycin. The keratoyltic and desquamative effects of benzoyl peroxide may also be beneficial.
Indications Topical treatment of acne vulgaris.
Contraindications Standard considerations.
Route/Dosage
ADULTS AND CHILDREN OLDER THAN 12 YR:

Topical Twice daily, morning and evening, or as directed by physician, to affected areas after skin is thoroughly washed with warm water and patted dry.
Interactions None well documented.
Adverse Reactions
DERM: Dry skin; urticarial reaction; skin irritation and peeling; itching; burning sensation; erythema; inflammation of the face, eyes, and nose; eye irritation; skin discoloration; skin oiliness and tenderness.
Precautions
Pregnancy: Category C.
Lactation: Undetermined; however, erythromycin is excreted in breast milk after oral and parenteral administration.
Children: Safety and efficacy unknown in children.

PATIENT CARE CONSIDERATIONS

Administration/Storage
- For topical use only. Avoid contact with eyes, nose, mouth, and all mucus membranes.
- Gel is usually applied to affected areas bid, usually in the morning and evening.
- Thoroughly wash the affected areas with a mild or soapless cleanser, rinse with warm water, and pat dry before applying gel.
- Apply a thin film of gel to cover the affected area(s).
- Store in refrigerator. Do not freeze. Keep container tightly capped. Discard any unused gel after 3 mo.

Assessment/Interventions
- Obtain patient history, including drug history and any known allergies.
- Assess the skin and identify areas where medication is to be applied. Avoid areas that are sunburned, have eczema, abrasions, or cuts.
- Monitor for side effects, including redness, scaling, dryness, persistent itching, or burning.

Patient/Family Education
- Explain name, dose, action, and potential side effects of drug to the patient.
- Advise patient that gel is applied topically to skin lesions bid, usually in the morning and evening.
- Teach patient proper technique for applying gel: wash hands; cleanse area with mild or soapless cleanser. Rinse and pat dry. Apply a thin film of gel to cover affected skin areas. Wash hands after applying gel.
- Warn patient that applying gel more often than prescribed or in excessive quantities will not produce more rapid improvement or better results but will result in greater side effects (eg, redness, scaling, drying).
- Warn patient to avoid contact with the eyes, nose, mouth, and all mucous membranes.
- Advise patient to avoid areas where eczema, abrasions, or cuts exist.
- Caution patient that gel may bleach hair or colored fabric.
- Advise patient to talk to a health care provider before using any other topical agents (eg, medicated soaps, astringents, cosmetics, other acne products) on treated skin.
- Advise patient that if severe dermal reactions occur to stop using the gel and contact health care provider.
- Advise patient that follow-up visits to examine the skin lesions may be necessary and make sure to keep appointments.

Erythromycin Ethylsuccinate/Sulfisoxazole

(eh-RITH-row-MY-sin ETH-il-SUX-inate/
sul-fih-SOX-uh-zole)

Class Anti-infective

How Supplied
Eryzole Granules for oral suspension Erythromycin ethylsuccinate (equivalent to 200 mg erythromycin activity) and sulfisoxazole acetyl (equivalent to 600 mg sulfisoxazole) per 5 mL when reconstituted ◆ *Pediazole* Granules for oral suspension Erythromycin ethylsuccinate (equivalent to 200 mg erythromycin activity) and sulfisoxazole acetyl (equivalent to 600 mg sulfisoxazole) per 5 mL when reconstituted

Action

PHARMACOLOGY: Erythromycin suppresses bacterial protein synthesis; sulfonamides interfere with bacterial folic acid synthesis.

PHARMACOKINETICS/DYNAMICS:

Absorption: C_{max} is 0.3 to 2 mcg/mL. T_{max} is 1.6 hr.

Distribution: Largely bound to plasma proteins. Diffuses into most body fluids. Passage across the blood-brain barrier increases in meningitis. Crosses the placenta and is excreted in breast milk.

Metabolism: Metabolized in the liver by demethylation.

Excretion: Mostly excreted in the bile; less than 5% recovered in the active form in the urine.

Indications Treatment of acute otitis media in children caused by susceptible strains of *Haemophilus influenzae*.

Contraindications Hypersensitivity to chemically related drugs (eg, sulfonylureas, thiazide and loop diuretics, carbonic anhydrase inhibitors, sunscreens containing PABA, local anesthetics) or salicylates; patients taking terfenadine or astemizole; porphyria; use in infants younger than 20 mo, pregnant women at term and women nursing infants younger than 2 mo.

Route/Dosage
CHILDREN: **PO** 50 mg/kg/day erythromycin and 150 mg/kg/day (max 6 gm/day) sulfisoxazole in equally divided doses qid for 10 days.

Interactions
Anticoagulants: May increase anticoagulant effects.
Antihistamines, non-sedating (eg, astemizole, terfenadine): Erythromycin significantly alters metabolism of terfenadine. Rare cases of serious cardiovascular events including death have been reported.
Astemizole, bromocriptine, carbamazepine, disopyramide, hexobarbital, methylprednisolone, phenytoin: May cause decreased metabolism and increased concentrations of these drugs.
Cyclosporine: Erythromycin may interfere with metabolism while sulfonamides may decrease cyclosporine levels; both increase risk of nephrotoxicity.
Digoxin: May increase digoxin levels.
Lovastatin: Severe myopathy or rhabdomyolysis may occur.
Methotrexate: Sulfonamides can displace methotrexate from protein-binding sites and increase free methotrexate levels.
Sulfonylureas: Sulfisoxazole may potentiate hypoglycemic effects.
Theophyllines: May increase theophylline plasma concentrations.
Thiopental: May enhance anesthetic effects of thiopental.

Lab Test Interferences
Sulfosalicylic acid turbidity test for urinary protein: Sulfisoxazole may produce false-positive results.
Urinary glucose test: Sulfonamides may produce false-positive results when performed by Benedict's method.
Urobilistix test: Sulfisoxazole may interfere with test results.

Adverse Reactions
CNS: Headache; peripheral neuropathy; dizziness; psychosis; hallucinations; depression; convulsions.
DERM: Urticaria; skin eruptions; pruritus; photosensitivity; anaphylaxis; erythema multiforme; toxic epidermal necrolysis; exfoliative dermatitis; angioedema; arteritis; vasculitis.
EENT: Hearing loss (associated with high doses erythromycin and renal insufficiency).
GI: Nausea; vomiting; abdominal pain/cramping; diarrhea; anorexia.
GU: Crystalluria; hematuria; increased BUN and creatinine; nephritis; toxic nephrosis with oliguria.
HEPA: Hepatic dysfunction; abnormal LFT results; pseudomembranous colitis; GI hemorrhage; pancreatitis.
HEMA: Leukopenia; agranulocytosis; aplastic anemia; thrombocytopenia; hemolytic anemia; purpura; eosinophilia; clotting disorders; methemoglobinemia.
OTHER: Fever; chills; arthralgias; myalgias; periarteritis nodosum; systemic lupus erythematosus; serum sickness.

Precautions
Pregnancy: Category C.
Lactation: Both erythromycin and sulfisoxazole are excreted in breast milk.

Children: Do not expose children younger than 2 mo (directly or through breast milk) to sulfonamides because of risk of kernicterus.
Renal function impairment: Use drug with caution in patients with renal or hepatic impairment. Hepatotoxicity has been associated with erythromycin.
Hepatic function impairment: Use drug with caution in patients with renal or hepatic impairment. Hepatotoxicity has been associated with erythromycin.
Special risk patients: May aggravate weakness in patients with myasthenia gravis. Use drug with caution in patients with severe allergies or bronchial asthma. Dose-related hemolytic anemia may occur in patients with G-6-PD deficiency.
Superinfection: Prolonged use may result in bacterial or fungal overgrowth of nonsusceptible microorganisms.

Fatalities: Rare fatalities from severe reactions associated with hypersensitivity, agranulocytosis, aplastic anemia, blood dyscrasias, renal and hepatic damage, irreversible neuromuscular and CNS changes, and fibrosing alveolitis have been reported with sulfonamides.
Ototoxicity: May occur, especially in patients with renal or hepatic insufficiency and elderly patients and with administration of large doses.
Pseudomembranous colitis: Consider possibility in patients with diarrhea.

Overdosage: Signs and Symptoms
Nausea, vomiting, diarrhea, hearing loss, vertigo, dizziness, headache, drowsiness, unconsciousness, toxic fever, acidosis, hemolytic anemia.

PATIENT CARE CONSIDERATIONS
Administration/Storage
- Give with full glass of water 1 hr before or 2 hr after meals.
- If GI upset is significant, administer with food or milk.
- Shake oral suspension well. Refrigerate after opening. Discard unused portion after 14 days.

Assessment/Interventions
- Obtain patient history, including drug history and any known allergies. Note any hypersensitivity to erythromycin or macrolide antibiotics and history of liver disease, fungal disease or colic.
- Obtain baseline CBC, BUN, creatinine, and LFTs and monitor throughout therapy.
- Obtain culture and sensitivity before instituting drug regimen.
- Monitor for diarrhea, nausea, vomiting, and abdominal discomfort. If severe, contact health care provider.
- Monitor I&O. Encourage oral intake of fluids.
- Monitor for signs and symptoms of superinfection: perianal irritation, black furry tongue, vaginal discharge.
- Notify health care provider of tachycardia, palpitations, syncope, cyanosis, seizures, and hallucinations or any change in hearing.
- Notify health care provider if urticaria or anemia occur.

Patient/Family Education
- Instruct patient/family to follow complete course of therapy.
- Advise patient to shake suspension well before using and refrigerate after opening.
- Tell patient to take drug with full glass of water 1 hr before or 2 hr after meals. If GI distress occurs, take with food or milk.
- Instruct patient to report these symptoms to health care provider: tachycardia, palpitations, syncope, cyanosis, seizures, hallucinations, shortness of breath, rash, bleeding, diarrhea, inability to void, urticaria, abdominal pain, signs of superinfection.
- Caution patient to avoid exposure to sunlight and to use sunscreen or wear protective clothing to avoid photosensitivity reaction.
- Instruct patient not to take otc medications without consulting health care provider.

Escitalopram Oxalate
(ESS-sigh-TAL-oh-pram OX-ah-late)
Class Antidepressant/Selective serotonin reuptake inhibitor
How Supplied
Lexapro Tablets 5 mg, Tablets 10 mg, Tablets 20 mg, Oral solution 5 mg per 5 mL

Action
PHARMACOLOGY: Inhibits the CNS neuronal uptake of serotonin, potentiating serotonergic activity.

PHARMACOKINETICS/DYNAMICS:
Absorption: T_{max} is approximately 5 hr. Bioavailability is approximately 80%.
Distribution: Vd is approximately 12 L/kg. Approximately 56% is protein bound.
Metabolism: Metabolized in the liver to 2 metabolites (minimally active); CYP3A4 and CYP2C19 involved in N-demethylation.
Excretion: The $t_{½}$ is approximately 27 to 32 hr. Approximately 8% is recovered in the urine as escitalopram and 10% as a metabolite. Cl is

600 mL/min (approximately 7% caused by renal Cl).

Special Populations:
Renal Function Impairment – Oral Cl decreased 17% in those with mild to moderate renal function impairment.
Hepatic Function Impairment – Oral Cl was reduced 37% and t½ was doubled in these patients.
Elderly – AUC and t½ increased approximately 50%.

Indications Treatment of major depressive disorders and generalized anxiety as defined in DSM-IV.

Contraindications Standard consideration; concurrent use of MAO inhibitors or within 14 days of discontinuing MAO inhibitor treatment.

Route/Dosage
Generalized Anxiety Disorder
ADULTS: **PO** Start with 10 mg once daily. The dose may be increased to 20 mg once daily after 1 wk.

Major Depressive Disorder
ADULTS: **PO** Start with 10 mg once daily. The dose may be increased to 20 mg after 1 wk. However, 20 mg has not shown a clinical benefit over 10 mg.

Elderly/Hepatic Function Impairment
ADULTS: **PO** 10 mg per day.

Interactions
Alcohol: May potentiate the effects of alcohol; use of alcohol is not recommended.
Aspirin, NSAIDs (eg, ibuprofen): The risk of bleeding may be increased.
Carbamazepine: Consider possibility of decreased escitalopram serum concentrations and reduced efficacy.
Cimetidine: Serum levels may be increased by cimetidine.
CNS drugs: Use with caution.
Cyproheptadine: May decrease the pharmacologic effect of escitalopram.
Ketoconazole: Plasma concentrations may be reduced by escitalopram, decreasing the therapeutic effect of ketoconazole.
Lithium: Serotonergic effects of escitalopram may be enhanced; use with caution.
MAO inhibitors: Do not use in patients receiving MAO inhibitor therapy or within 14 days of stopping treatment.
Metoprolol: Serum levels may be increased by escitalopram.
Sumatriptan: Rare postmarketing reports of weakness, hyperreflexia, and incoordination following coadministration with selective serotonin reuptake inhibitors have been reported.

Lab Test Interferences None well documented.

Adverse Reactions
CV: Palpitation, hypertension (at least 1%); QT prolongation, torsades de pointes (postmarketing).
CNS: Headache (24%); insomnia (14%); somnolence (13%); decreased libido, dizziness (7%); decreased appetite, abnormal dreaming, lethargy (3%); paresthesia, yawning (2%); lightheadedness, migraine, increased appetite, irritability, impaired concentration (at least 1%); grand mal seizures (postmarketing).
DERM: Rash (at least 1%); toxic epidermal necrolysis (postmarketing).
EENT: Rhinitis (5%); nasal congestion, blurred vision, tinnitus (at least 1%).
GI: Nausea (18%); diarrhea (14%); dry mouth (9%); constipation, indigestion (6%); vomiting (3%); abdominal pain, flatulence, toothache (2%); heartburn, abdominal cramp, gastroenteritis (at least 1%); GI hemorrhage, pancreatitis (postmarketing).
GU: Ejaculation disorder (14%); anorgasmia (6%); impotence (3%); menstrual disorder (2%); menstrual cramps, menstrual disorder, urinary frequency, UTI (at least 1%); acute renal failure (postmarketing).
HEMA: Thrombocytopenia (postmarketing).
M/N: Increased weight (at least 1%).
MUSC: Neck/shoulder pain (3%); limb pain, arthralgia, myalgia (at least 1%); rhabdomyolysis (postmarketing).
RESP: Sinusitis (2%); bronchitis, sinus congestion, coughing, sinus headache (at least 1%).
OTHER: Fatigue, increased sweating (8%); influenza-like symptoms, fatigue (5%); allergy, fever, hot flushes, chest pain (at least 1%); angioedema, neuroleptic malignant syndrome, serotonin syndrome (postmarketing).

Precautions
Pregnancy: Category C.
Lactation: Excreted in breast milk.
Children: Safety and efficacy not established.
Abnormal bleeding: Bleeding episodes have been reported in patients treated with drugs that interfere with serotonin reuptake.
Cognitive and motor performance: Patients should use caution in operating potentially hazardous machinery or driving until they know whether the drug impairs their ability.
Concomitant illness: Use with caution in patients with concurrent systemic illness.
Discontinuation: When discontinuing treatment, taper the dose to avoid adverse effects.
Hyponatremia: Cases of hyponatremia or SIADH have been reported.

Mania/Hypomania: May activate hypomania or mania.
Seizures: Initiate therapy with caution in patients with history of seizure disorders.
Suicide: Supervise depressed patients at risk during initial therapy. Prescribe the smallest quantity consistent with good patient management in order to reduce the risk of overdose.

PATIENT CARE CONSIDERATIONS
Administration/Storage
- Do not administer with or within 14 days of MAO inhibitor administration.
- Do not administer concurrently with citalopram.
- Administer prescribed dose once daily, in the morning or evening, without regard to meals. Administer with food if GI upset occurs.
- Use dosing spoon, cup, or syringe to measure and administer prescribed dose or oral solution.
- Store tablets and oral solution at controlled room temperature (59° to 86°F).

Assessment/Interventions
- Obtain patient history, including drug history and any known allergies. Note hypersensitivity to citalopram, renal or hepatic impairment, mania or history of mania, seizure disorder or history of seizure, concurrent or recent (eg, within 14 days) use of MAO inhibitor, or concurrent use of aspirin, NSAIDs, or other medications that can affect coagulation.
- Ensure that reduced dose is used in elderly patient, or patient with hepatic impairment or severe renal impairment.
- Frequently assess patient being treated for depression for clinical worsening and suicidality, especially when initiating therapy, or when the escitalopram dose is increased or decreased. Immediately notify health care provider if depression worsens or suicidal ideation or behavior are noted.
- Ensure that therapy is periodically reviewed to determine if it needs to be continued without change or if a dose change (eg, increase, decrease, discontinuation) is indicated.
- If treatment is to be discontinued or the dose reduced, gradually taper the dose and monitor patient for withdrawal symptoms (eg, dysphoric mood, irritability, agitation, dizziness, abnormal skin sensations, anxiety, confusion, nausea, sweating). If significant withdrawal symptoms develop, reinstitute previous dosing schedule and attempt a less rapid tapering regimen after patient has stabilized.
- Monitor patient for CNS, GI, GU, PSYCH, MUSC, and general body side effects. Report to health care provider if noted and significant.

Overdosage: Signs and Symptoms
Dizziness, sweating, nausea, vomiting, tremor, somnolence, sinus tachycardia, convulsions, amnesia, confusion, coma, hyperventilation, cyanosis, rhabdomyolysis, ECG changes (including QTc prolongation, nodal rhythm, ventricular arrythmia, and 1 possible case of torsades de pointes).

Patient/Family Education
- Explain name, dose, action, and potential side effects of drug.
- Advise patient to read patient information leaflet before starting therapy and with each refill.
- Advise patient that medication is usually started at a low dose and then gradually increased until max benefit is obtained.
- Advise patient to take prescribed dose once daily, in the morning or evening, without regard to meals but to take with food if stomach upset occurs.
- Advise patient, family, or caregiver to use dosing spoon, cup, or syringe to measure and administer prescribed dose of oral solution.
- Advise patient not to change the dose or stop taking unless advised by a health care provider.
- Inform patient that it may take 1 to 4 wk to note improvement in symptoms and to continue with the prescribed therapy once improvement has been noted.
- Instruct patient to notify health care provider if symptoms do not appear to be getting better, are getting worse, or if bothersome side effects (eg, unusual sweating, headache, drowsiness, insomnia, nausea, diarrhea, nervousness, changes in sexual function) occur.
- Advise patient being treated for depression, and family or caregiver of patient, to be alert for abnormal changes in mood or thinking. The following symptoms should be reported immediately to health care provider: anxiety, agitation, panic attacks, irritability, hostility or aggressiveness, impulsivity, suicidal thoughts or behavior.
- Advise patient that if medication needs to be discontinued it will be slowly withdrawn unless safety concerns (eg, rash) require a more rapid withdrawal.
- Advise patient to take frequent sips of water, suck on ice chips or sugarless hard candy, or chew sugarless gum if dry mouth occurs.

- Advise patient to avoid alcoholic beverages and other depressants while taking escitalopram.
- Advise patient that drug may impair judgment, thinking, or reflexes and to use caution while driving or performing other tasks requiring mental alertness until tolerance is determined.
- Instruct patient not to take any prescription or OTC drugs, herbal preparations, or dietary supplements without consulting with a health care provider.
- Advise women to notify a health care provider if pregnant, planning to become pregnant, or breastfeeding.
- Advise patient that follow-up visits may be necessary to monitor therapy and to keep appointments.

Esmolol Hydrochloride

(ESS-moe-lahl HIGH-droe-KLOR-ide)

Class Beta-adrenergic blocker

How Supplied
Brevibloc Injection 10 mg/mL, Injection 250 mg/mL

Action
PHARMACOLOGY: Blocks beta-receptors primarily affecting cardiovascular system (eg, decreases heart rate, contractility, BP) and lungs (promoting bronchospasm).

PHARMACOKINETICS/DYNAMICS:
Distribution: Distribution $t_{1/2}$ is approximately 2 min. 55% is protein bound.

Metabolism: Rapidly metabolized by the esterases in the cytosol of red blood cells to an acid metabolite and methanol.

Excretion: The $t_{1/2}$ is approximately 9 min. Less than 2% excreted unchanged in the urine.

Indications Short-term management of supraventricular tachyarrhythmias and noncompensatory sinus tachycardia. **Unlabeled use(s):** Treatment of caffeine toxicity; attenuation of cardiovascular responses to electroconvulsive therapy or induction of anesthesia; adjunct therapy for acute MI and unstable angina; treatment of thyroid storm.

Contraindications Sinus bradycardia; second- or third-degree heart block; CHF unless secondary to tachyarrhythmia treatable with beta-blockers; overt cardiac failure; cardiogenic shock.

Route/Dosage
ADULTS: Usual: **IV** 500 mcg/kg/min for 1 min; then infusion of 50 to 200 mcg/kg/min, which has been titrated to desired endpoint (eg, heart rate, BP) in 50 mcg/kg/min increments.

Interactions
Clonidine: May enhance or reverse antihypertensive effect; potentially life-threatening increases in BP may occur, especially on withdrawal.

NSAIDs: Some agents may impair antihypertensive effect.

Prazosin: Potential for and degree of orthostatic hypotension may be increased.

Verapamil: Effects of both drugs may be increased.

INCOMPATIBILITIES: 5% Sodium Bicarbonate Injection.

Lab Test Interferences Antinuclear antibodies may develop; usually reversible on discontinuation. May interfere with glucose or insulin tolerance test results. May cause changes in serum lipid levels.

Adverse Reactions
CV: Hypotension; bradycardia; CHF; cold extremities; pallor; second or third-degree heart block.
CNS: Insomnia; fatigue; dizziness; depression; lethargy; drowsiness; forgetfulness.
DERM: Rash; hives; fever; alopecia.
EENT: Dry eyes; blurred vision; tinnitus; slurred speech; sore throat.
GI: Nausea; vomiting; diarrhea; dry mouth.
GU: Impotence; painful, difficult, or frequent urination.
HEMA: Agranulocytosis; thrombocytopenia purpura.
RESP: Bronchospasm; shortness of breath; wheezing.
OTHER: Weight changes; facial swelling; muscle weakness; inflammation at infusion site.

Precautions
Pregnancy: Category C.
Lactation: Undetermined.
Children: Safety and efficacy not established.
Renal function impairment: Reduced daily dose advised.
Hepatic function impairment: Reduced daily dose advised.
Anaphylaxis: Deaths have occurred; aggressive therapy may be required.
CHF: Administer drug in patients with CHF controlled by digitalis and diuretics. Notify health care provider at first sign or symptom of CHF or other unexplained respiratory symptoms.
Diabetes mellitus: May mask signs and symptoms of hypoglycemia (eg, tachycardia, BP changes). May potentiate insulin-induced hypoglycemia.
Nonallergic bronchospasm (eg, chronic bronchitis, emphysema): Use caution in patients with bronchospastic diseases.
Peripheral vascular disease: May precipitate or

aggravate symptoms of arterial insufficiency.
Thyrotoxicosis: May mask clinical signs (eg, tachycardia) of developing or continuing hyperthyroidism. Abrupt withdrawal may exacerbate symptoms of hyperthyroidism, including thyroid storm.

PATIENT CARE CONSIDERATIONS
Administration/Storage
- Avoid concentrations over 10 mg/min in order to minimize venous irritation.
- 10 mg/mL vial does not need further dilution.
- Do not administer through butterfly needles.
- For IV administration, use 250 mg/mL solution diluted in 5% Dextrose Injection and 0.9% or 0.45% Sodium Chloride Injection, Lactated Ringer's Injection, and Potassium Chloride (40 mEq/L) in 5% Dextrose Injection or 0.9% or 0.45% Sodium Chloride Injection. To prepare solution remove 20 mL from 500 mL bottle of suitable infusion fluid and add 2 amps of 250 mg/mL solution of esmolol. Final concentration is 10 mg/mL.
- Do not mix with sodium bicarbonate.
- Store diluted solution at room temperature or under refrigeration. Discard after 24 hr.
- Use of esmolol infusion up to 24 hr is well documented. Limited data indicate that esmolol is well tolerated up to 48 hr.
- When converting patient to another agent, reduce esmolol infusion rate by 50% 30 min after first dose of new drug. After second dose of new drug, if patient is stable for 1 hr, discontinue esmolol infusion.

Assessment/Interventions
- Obtain patient history, including drug history and any known allergies.

Overdosage: Signs and Symptoms
Hypotension, bradycardia, intraventricular conduction disturbances, shock.

- Obtain baseline ECG and measure QT interval.
- Obtain baseline vital signs and weight.
- Auscultate and document baseline heart and lung sounds and monitor throughout therapy.
- Monitor vital signs frequently.
- Monitor I&O, BUN, creatinine, serum glucose, CBC, LFTs, and bilirubin throughout therapy.
- Assess patient for rashes, urticaria, shortness of breath, arthralgia, and systemic lupus erythematosus syndrome.
- If reaction develops at infusion site, use alternative site.
- Notify health care provider if vomiting, abdominal distention, vertigo, bradycardia, new ventricular arrhythmia, shock symptoms, or signs of CHF occur.
- If patient is receiving digoxin, monitor digoxin levels and observe patient for digoxin toxicity.

Patient/Family Education
- Caution patient to notify health care provider of any urticaria, shortness of breath, vertigo, syncope, or inability to void.
- Advise diabetic patient to notify health care provider of hypoglycemic reaction symptoms.

Esomeprazole Magnesium
(es-om-ME-pray-zol mag-NEE-zhum)
Class Gastrointestinal/Proton Pump Inhibitor
How Supplied
Nexium Capsules, delayed-release 20 mg, Capsules, delayed-release 40 mg

Action
PHARMACOLOGY: Suppresses gastric acid secretion by blocking proton pump within gastric parietal cells.

PHARMACOKINETICS/DYNAMICS:
Absorption: T_{max} is 1.5 hr. Bioavailability is approximately 90% (repeated once-daily dosing) and 64% (single dose). Food decreases AUC 33% to 53%. Take at least 1 hr before meals.
Distribution: 97% is protein bound. Vd is approximately 16 L (at steady state).
Metabolism: Metabolized in the liver by CYP2C19 and CYP3A4 to inactive metabolites.
Excretion: The $t_{1/2}$ is approximately 1 to 1.5 hr. Less than 1% of parent drug excreted in urine; approximately 80% is excreted as inactive metabolites in the urine, and the remainder is found in feces.

Special Populations:
Elderly – AUC and C_{max} were increased 25% and 18%, respectively. No dosage adjustment needed.

Indications Treatment of heartburn and other symptoms of gastroesophageal reflux disease (GERD); short-term treatment in healing and symptomatic resolution of erosive esophagitis; maintain symptom resolution and healing of erosive esophagitis; in combination with amoxicillin and clarithromycin for treatment of *Helicobacter pylori* infection and duodenal ulcer disease to eradicate *H. pylori*.

Contraindications Standard considerations.

Route/Dosage

Healing of Erosive Esophagitis
ADULTS: PO 20 or 40 mg once daily for 4 to 8 wk.

Maintenance of Healing of Erosive Esophagitis
ADULTS: PO 20 mg once daily.

Symptomatic GERD
ADULTS: PO 20 mg once daily for 4 wk.

H. pylori Eradication to Reduce Risk of Duodenal Ulcer Recurrence
ADULTS: PO 40 mg once daily for 10 days in combination with amoxicillin 1000 mg bid and clarithromycin 500 mg bid for 10 days.

Interactions

Drugs dependent on gastric pH for bioavailability (eg, ketoconazole, iron salts, digoxin): Absorption of these drugs may be affected.

Lab Test Interferences None well documented.

Adverse Reactions

CNS: Headache.
EENT: Dry mouth.
GI: Diarrhea; nausea; flatulence; abdominal pain; constipation.

Precautions

Pregnancy: Category B.
Lactation: Undetermined.
Children: Safety and efficacy not determined.

Overdosage: Signs and Symptoms

Confusion, drowsiness, blurred vision, tachycardia, nausea, diaphoresis, flushing, headache, dry mouth.

PATIENT CARE CONSIDERATIONS

Administration/Storage

- Do not crush or chew; swallow capsule whole. If patient has difficulty swallowing capsule whole, open the capsule and gently mix the pellets with 1 tablespoon of cool or cold applesauce in a small bowl. Swallow mixture immediately without chewing. Do not crush or chew the pellets. Discard remaining pellet/applesauce mixture.
- Administer once daily 1 hr or more before meals.
- Store at controlled room temperature. Keep container tightly closed.

Assessment/Interventions

- Obtain patient history, including drug history and any known allergies. Note history of liver disease.
- Assess for bloody or coffee ground emesis and black tarry stools.
- Assess for symptoms of esophageal reflux (eg, heart burn, acid regurgitation) or peptic ulcer activity (eg, indigestion, abdominal pain, nausea).
- Assess for headache and dry mouth.
- Monitor elimination patterns, and document any problems such as constipation or diarrhea.

Patient/Family Education

- Explain name, dose, action, and potential side effects of drug.
- Instruct patient to not crush or chew medication and to swallow the capsule whole.
- Advise patient that if experiencing difficulty swallowing the capsule, to open the capsule and gently mix the pellets with 1 tablespoon of cool or cold applesauce and then immediately swallow the mixture without chewing. Remind patient that pellets should not be crushed or chewed and that the pellet/applesauce mixture should not be stored for future use.
- Instruct patient to take each dose at least 1 hr before meals.
- Inform patient that antacids may be taken concurrently with esomeprazole.
- Remind patient that esomeprazole should be taken daily and not "as needed" or only when symptoms are present.
- Instruct patient to notify health care provider if pregnant, planning on becoming pregnant, or breastfeeding.
- Advise patient to report any of the following symptoms to the health care provider: bloody or coffee ground emesis, black tarry stools, recurrent heart burn, recurrent indigestion or abdominal pain, increasing need for antacid use.

Estazolam

(ess-TAZZ-OH-lam)

Class Sedative/Hypnotic/Benzodiazepine

How Supplied
ProSom Tablets 1 mg, Tablets 2 mg

Action

PHARMACOLOGY: Potentiates action of GABA, an inhibitory neurotransmitter, resulting in increased neuronal inhibition and CNS depression, especially in limbic system and reticular formation.

PHARMACOKINETICS/DYNAMICS:
Distribution: Plasma protein binding is 93%.
Metabolism: Extensively metabolized (4-hydroxy estazolam is the major metabolite).

Excretion: Metabolites primarily excreted in the urine with less than 5% of an administered dose excreted unchanged in the urine. Only 4% of the dose appears in the feces. Mean elimination t½ varies from 10 to 24 hr.

Indications Short-term management of insomnia characterized by difficulty in falling asleep, frequent nocturnal awakenings, and/or early morning awakenings.

Contraindications Pregnancy; hypersensitivity to benzodiazepines.

Route/Dosage

ADULTS: **PO** Start with 1 mg at bedtime; however, some patients may need a 2 mg dose.

Interactions

Alcohol, anticonvulsants, antihistamines, barbiturates, MAO inhibitors, narcotics, phenothiazines, psychotropic drugs: May potentiate the CNS depressant effects of estazolam.

Azole antifungal agents (eg, ketoconazole), cimetidine, disulfiram, oral contraceptives, protease inhibitors (eg, indinavir): Estazolam plasma levels may be elevated, increasing the pharmacologic and adverse effects.

Digoxin: May increase serum digoxin concentrations.

Rifamycins (eg, rifampin): Estazolam plasma levels may be reduced, decreasing the pharmacologic effects.

Theophyllines: May antagonize sedative effects of estazolam.

Lab Test Interferences None well documented.

Adverse Reactions

CNS: Somnolence (42%); hypokinesia (8%); dizziness (7%); abnormal coordination (4%); hangover (3%); confusion (2%); abnormal thinking (2%); anxiety (at least 1%).
DERM: Pruritus (1%); Stevens-Johnson syndrome (postmarketing).
GI: Constipation, dry mouth (at least 1%).
HEMA: Agranulocytosis (postmarketing).
OTHER: Asthenia (11%); lower extremity pain (3%); photosensitivity (postmarketing).

Precautions

Pregnancy: Category X.
Lactation: Undetermined.
Children: Safety and efficacy not established.
Elderly: Use with caution in small or debilitated elderly patients.
Amnesia: As with other benzodiazepines, amnesia may occur.
Debilitated patients: Increased side effects; start with lowest dose.
Depression: Use with caution in patients exhibiting signs and symptoms of depression. Suicidal tendencies may be present in such patients. The least amount of drug that is feasible should be dispensed.
Paradoxical reactions: Paradoxical reactions (eg, excitement, agitation) may occur.
Respiratory depression: Patients with compromised respiratory function may be at increased risk of respiratory depression.
Withdrawal: Signs and symptoms may occur following rapid or abrupt discontinuation.

Overdosage: Signs and Symptoms

Somnolence, respiratory depression, confusion, impaired coordination, slurred speech, coma.

PATIENT CARE CONSIDERATIONS

Administration/Storage

- Administer prescribed dose 30 min before bedtime.
- Administer prescribed dose without regard to meals but administer with food if GI upset occurs.
- Store tablets at controlled room temperature (below 86°F).

Assessment/Interventions

- Obtain patient history, including drug history and any known allergies. Note hepatic or renal impairment, pulmonary disease, acute narrow angle glaucoma, depression, suicidal tendency, seizure disorder, history of drug abuse or sensitivity to other benzodiazepines, or concurrent use of other psychotropic medications or CNS depressants.
- Ensure that reduced dose and slower dose escalation is used in elderly patient or patient with debilitating disease.
- Ensure that women of childbearing potential are not pregnant when therapy is initiated.
- Ensure that CBC with differential, urinalysis, and blood chemistries are evaluated periodically in patient on prolonged therapy.
- Frequently assess patient for response to treatment. Notify health care provider if condition does not appear to be improving or is worsening.
- Ensure that therapy is periodically reviewed to determine if it needs to be continued without change or if a dose change (eg, increase, decrease, discontinuation) is indicated.
- If treatment is to be discontinued or the dose reduced after prolonged therapy, gradually taper the dose. Monitor patient for withdrawal symptoms (eg, increased anxiety, tremor, muscle or abdominal cramps, sweating). If significant withdrawal symptoms develop, reinstitute previous dosing schedule and attempt a less rapid tapering regimen after patient has stabilized.

- Monitor patient for CNS, PSYCH, GI, and general body side effects. Report to health care provider if noted and significant. Implement safety precautions if excessive drowsiness or dizziness occurs.

Patient/Family Education
- Explain name, dose, action, and potential side effects of drug.
- Advise patient or caregiver to read the *Patient Information* leaflet before starting therapy and with each refill.
- Advise patient that medication may be started at a low dose and then gradually increased as tolerated until maximum benefit is obtained.
- Caution patient that medication may be habit forming and to take as prescribed and not to stop taking or change the dose unless advised by health care provider.
- Advise patient to take prescribed dose at bedtime with or without food but to take with food if stomach upset occurs.
- Advise patient that if medication needs to be discontinued, it will be slowly withdrawn unless safety concerns (eg, rash) require a more rapid withdrawal.
- Instruct patient to avoid alcoholic beverages and other depressants while taking this medication.
- Instruct patient to contact health care provider if sleep disorder does not appear to be getting better, is getting worse, or if bothersome side effects (eg, drowsiness, memory impairment) occur.
- Advise patient that drug may cause drowsiness or impair judgment, thinking, or reflexes and to use caution while driving or performing other tasks requiring mental alertness until tolerance is determined. Caution patient that there may be residual daytime effects on performance from the dose taken the night before.
- Advise women of childbearing potential to use effective contraception while using this medication.
- Advise women to notify health care provider if pregnant, planning to become pregnant, or breastfeeding.
- Warn patient not to take any prescription or OTC drugs or dietary supplements without consulting health care provider.
- Advise patient that follow-up visits may be necessary to monitor therapy and to keep appointments.

Esterified Estrogens/ Methyltestosterone

(ess-TER-ih-fide ESS-truh-janz/METH-ill-tess-TAHS-ter-ohn)

Class Sex hormones

How Supplied
Estratest Tablets 1.25 mg esterified estrogens and 2.5 mg methyltestosterone ◆ *Estratest HS* Tablets 0.625 mg esterified estrogens and 1.25 mg methyltestosterone

Action

PHARMACOLOGY:

Esterified Estrogens: Promotes growth and development of female reproductive system and secondary sex characteristics; affects release of pituitary gonadotropins; inhibits ovulation and prevents postpartum breast engorgement; conserves calcium and phosphorous and encourages bone formation; overrides stimulatory effects of testosterone.

Methyltestosterone: Promotes growth and development of male reproductive organs; maintains secondary sex characteristics; increases protein anabolism; decreases protein catabolism.

Indications Treatment of moderate to severe vasomotor symptoms associated with the menopause in patients not improved by estrogens alone.

Contraindications Known or suspected cancer of the breast except in appropriately selected patients being treated for metastatic disease; known or suspected estrogen-dependent neoplasia; known or suspected pregnancy; undiagnosed abnormal genital bleeding; active thrombophlebitis or thromboembolic disorders; past history of thrombophlebitis, thrombosis, or thromboembolic disorders associated with previous estrogen use except when treating breast malignancy. In addition, methyltestosterone should not be used in the presence of severe liver damage, pregnancy, and breastfeeding mothers because of the possibility of masculinization of the female fetus or breast-fed infant.

Route/Dosage
ADULTS: **PO** Usual dose range is 1 tablet (*Estratest*) or 1 to 2 tablets (*Estratest HS*) daily.

Interactions
Anticoagulants (eg, Coumadin): The hypoprothrombinemic effect of oral anticoagulants is potentiated by 17-alkyl androgens. Oral anticoagulant dose requirements will be reduced. Estrogens affect several coagulation and fibrinolysis tests and at high doses, could increase the risk of thromboembolism. The benefit from oral anticoagulants could be diminished by estrogen.
Insulin: Blood glucose may be reduced, decreasing the insulin requirements.
Oxyphenbutazone: Serum levels of oxyphen-

butazone may be elevated, increasing the risk of side effects.

Lab Test Interferences Increased sulfobromophthalein retention; increased prothrombin and factors VII, VIII, IX and X; decreased antithrombin; increased norepinephrine-induced platelet aggregability; impaired glucose tolerance; decreased pregnanediol excretion; increased thyroxine-binding globulin (TBG), leading to increased circulating total thyroid hormone as measured by protein bound iodine, T4 by column, or T4 by radioimmunoassay; free T3 resin uptake is decreased (reflecting the elevated TBG); reduced response to metyrapone test; reduced serum folate concentration; increase serum triglyceride and phospholipid concentrations.

Adverse Reactions
CNS: Headache; migraine; dizziness; mental depression; chorea; changes in libido; anxiety; generalized paresthesia.
DERM: Chloasma; melasma; erythema multiforme; erythema nodosum; hemorrhagic eruption; loss of scalp hair; hirsutism; male pattern baldness; acne.
EENT: Steepening of corneal curvature; intolerance to contact lenses.
GI: Nausea; vomiting; abdominal cramps; bloating.
GU: Breakthrough bleeding; spotting; change in menstrual flow; dysmenorrhea; premenstrual-like syndrome; amenorrhea during and after treatment; increase in size of uterine fibromyomata; vaginal candidiasis; change in cervical erosion and degree of cervical secretion; cystitis-like syndrome; breast tenderness, enlargement, and secretion; menstrual irregularities; inhibition of gonadotropin secretion and virilization (including deepening of voice and clitoral enlargement).
HEMA: Suppression of clotting factors II, V, VII, and X; polycythemia.
HEPA: Cholestatic jaundice; alterations in LFTs; hepatocellular neoplasms (rarely); peliosis hepatitis (rarely).
METAB: Increase or decrease in weight; reduced carbohydrate tolerance; edema; retention of sodium, chloride, water, potassium, calcium, and inorganic phosphates; increased serum cholesterol.
OTHER: Aggravation of porphyria; anaphylactoid reactions.

PATIENT CARE CONSIDERATIONS
Administration/Storage
♦ Administer prescribed dose once daily as ordered.
♦ Administer without regard to meals. Adminis-

Precautions
Pregnancy: Category X.
Lactation: Undetermined.
Elderly: Risk for development of prostatic hypertrophy or prostatic carcinoma may be increased.
Special risk patients: Use with caution in patients with impaired liver function, renal insufficiency, metabolic bone diseases associated with hypercalcemia, and in young patients in whom bone growth is not complete.
Depression: Carefully observe patients with history of depression.
Elevated blood pressure: Increased BP during estrogen replacement during menopause has been reported.
Fluid retention: Use with careful observation when conditions that might be affected by fluid retention are present (eg, asthma, cardiac or renal dysfunction, epilepsy).
Gallbladder disease: Risk of gallbladder disease may increase in women receiving postmenopausal estrogens.
Glucose tolerance: A worsening of glucose tolerance has been observed. Diabetic patients should be carefully monitored while receiving estrogens.
Hepatic conditions: Benign hepatic adenomas and hepatocellular carcinoma appear to be associated with oral contraceptive use. Prolonged use of high doses of androgens has been associated with peliosis hepatitis and hepatic neoplasms. Cholestatic hepatitis and jaundice have been reported. Patients with history of jaundice during pregnancy have an increased risk of recurrence while receiving estrogen-containing oral contraceptive therapy.
Hypercalcemia: In patients with breast cancer or bone metastases, severe hypercalcemia has occurred with estrogen therapy.
Induction of malignant neoplasm: May increase risk of endometrial or other carcinomas.
Thromboembolic disease: Risk of various thromboembolic and thrombotic vascular diseases (eg, pulmonary embolism, stroke, MI, retinal thrombosis) are increased.
Uterine bleeding: Certain patients may develop abnormal uterine bleeding.
Uterine leiomyomata: Preexisting uterine leiomyomata may increase in size during estrogen use.

Overdosage: Signs and Symptoms
Nausea, withdrawal bleeding.

ter with food if GI upset occurs.
♦ Store tablets at controlled room temperature (59° to 86°F).

Assessment/Interventions

- Obtain patient history, including drug history and any known allergies. Note history of: breast nodules, fibrocystic disease, abnormal mammograms, family history of breast disease, hypertension, diabetes, breast cancer with bone metastases, metabolic bone disease other than osteoporosis, liver disease, renal disease, cardiac disease, epilepsy, migraine headaches, jaundice during pregnancy, asthma.
- Review patient's health history for any condition that could contraindicate therapy (previous allergic reaction to either drug, known or suspected pregnancy, known or suspected cancer of the breast, known or suspected estrogen-dependent cancer, undiagnosed abnormal uterine bleeding, active or past history of thromboembolic disorders or stroke, or liver dysfunction or disease).
- Ensure that breast, abdominal, and pelvic examination and Pap smear have been completed and documented before starting therapy.
- Ensure that a progestin is used to prevent endometrial hyperplasia in women with an intact uterus.
- Monitor blood sugar in diabetic patient when drug is started or dose is changed. Report significant changes to health care provider.
- Assess BP at beginning of therapy and periodically during treatment.
- Monitor patient for GI, GU, and general body side effects. Inform health care provider if noted and significant.
- Notify health care provider if any of the following are noted: pain, swelling, redness or warmth in calves; sudden severe headache; visual disturbances; weakness or numbness of arms or legs; signs of liver dysfunction (eg, dark urine, jaundice); abdominal pain, tenderness, or swelling; nausea; vomiting; ankle swelling; hoarseness; acne; increased facial hair; signs of depression.
- Ensure that, if feasible, therapy is discontinued at least 4 wk before surgery of the type associated with an increased risk of thromboembolism or during periods of prolonged immobilization.
- Ensure that attempts are made to discontinue or taper the medication at 3 to 6 mo intervals.
- Obtain LFTs and check hemoglobin and hematocrit periodically.

Patient/Family Education

- Explain name, dose, action, and potential side effects of drug
- Advise patient to read "Information for Patient" leaflet before starting therapy and with each refill.
- Instruct patient to take as prescribed and not to change the dose or stop taking unless advised to do so by health care provider.
- Advise patient that medication can be taken without regard to meals, but to take with food if GI upset occurs.
- Instruct diabetic patient to monitor blood glucose more frequently when drug is started or dose is changed and to inform health care provider of significant changes in readings.
- Review nonhormonal modalities that help prevent osteoporosis: 1500 mg/day of calcium; vitamin D supplementation; exercise.
- Instruct patient to report these symptoms to health care provider: pain in groin or calves; sharp chest pain or sudden shortness of breath; abnormal vaginal bleeding; breast lumps; sudden severe headache; dizziness or fainting; vision or speech problems; weakness or numbness of arms or legs; severe abdominal pain; yellowing of skin or eyes; abdominal pain, tenderness, or swelling; nausea, vomiting, or ankle swelling; hoarseness; acne; increased facial hair; or signs of depression.
- Advise women to notify health care provider if pregnant, planning to become pregnant, or breastfeeding.
- Teach patient proper method of breast self-examination.
- Advise patient that follow-up visits and examinations, including Pap smear, at least once a year will be required to monitor therapy and to keep appointments.

Estradiol

(ESS-truh-DIE-ole)

Class Estrogens

How Supplied

Alora Transdermal System 0.77 mg, Transdermal System 1.5 mg, Transdermal System 2.3 mg, Transdermal System 3.1 mg ♦ *Climara* Transdermal System 2 mg, Transdermal System 2.85 mg, Transdermal System 3.8 mg, Transdermal System 4.55 mg, Transdermal System 5.7 mg, Transdermal System 7.6 mg ♦ *Esclim* Transdermal System 5 mg, Transdermal System 7.5 mg, Transdermal System 10 mg, Transdermal System 15 mg, Transdermal System 20 mg ♦ *Estrace* Tablets 0.5 mg micronized estradiol, Tablets 1 mg micronized estradiol, Tablets 2 mg micronized estradiol ♦ *Estraderm* Transdermal

System 4 mg, Transdermal System 8 mg ♦ *Estrasorb* Topical Emulsion 2.5 mg estradiol hemihydrate/g ♦ *Estring* Ring 2 mg ♦ *Gynodiol* Tablets 0.5 mg micronized estradiol, Tablets 1 mg micronized estradiol, Tablets 1.5 mg micronized estradiol, Tablets 2 mg micronized estradiol ♦ *Vivelle* Transdermal System 3.28 mg, Transdermal System 4.33 mg, Transdermal System 6.57 mg, Transdermal System 8.66 mg ♦ *Vivelle-Dot* Transdermal System 0.39 mg, Transdermal System 0.585 mg, Transdermal System 0.78 mg, Transdermal System 1.17 mg, Transdermal System 1.56 mg

✤ *Estraderm 25* ♦ *Estradot*

Estradiol Valerate
Delestrogen Injection 10 mg/mL, Injection 20 mg/mL, Injection 40 mg/mL

Estradiol Cypionate
Depo-Estradiol Injection 5 mg/mL

Action
PHARMACOLOGY: Promotes growth and development of female reproductive system and secondary sex characteristics; affects release of pituitary gonadotropins; inhibits ovulation and prevents postpartum breast engorgement; conserves calcium and phosphorous and encourages bone formation; overrides stimulatory effects of testosterone.

PHARMACOKINETICS/DYNAMICS:
Absorption: Well absorbed through the skin, mucous membranes, and GI tract.
Distribution: Approximately 80% is bound to sex hormone-binding globulin; most of the rest is loosely bound to albumin, and approximately 20% is unbound. Crosses the placenta.
Metabolism: Orally administered estradiol undergoes first-pass effect. Metabolic conversion occurs primarily in the liver but also at local target tissue sites. Also undergoes enterohepatic recirculation.
Excretion: A certain portion is excreted in the bile and then reabsorbed from the intestine. Excreted in the urine as conjugates.

Indications Management of moderate to severe vasomotor symptoms associated with menopause, female hypogonadism, female castration, primary ovarian failure, postpartum breast engorgement, and atrophic conditions caused by deficient endogenous estrogen production; atrophic urethritis; palliative treatment of metastatic breast or prostate cancer in selected women and men; prevention and treatment of osteoporosis; abnormal uterine bleeding caused by hormonal imbalance in the absence of organic pathology and only when associated with a hypoplastic or atrophic endometrium.

Contraindications Breast cancer (except in patients being treated for metastatic disease); estrogen-dependent neoplasia; undiagnosed abnormal genital bleeding; thrombophlebitis or thromboembolic disorders associated with previous estrogen use; known or suspected pregnancy; active deep vein thrombosis, pulmonary embolism, or history of these conditions; active or recent (eg, within past year) arterial thromboembolic disease (eg, MI, stroke); liver dysfunction or disease.

Route/Dosage
Breast Cancer
ADULTS:
Estradiol: **PO** 10 mg tid for 3 mo or more.
Ethinyl Estradiol: **PO** 1 mg tid.

Female Hypogonadism
ADULTS:
Estradiol: **PO** 1 to 2 mg/day. Adjust to control symptoms.
Valerate Injection: **IM** 10 to 20 mg q 4 wk given cyclically.
Cypionate Injection: **IM** 1.5 to 2 mg q mo given cyclically.
Ethinyl Estradiol: **PO** 0.05 mg qd to tid during first 2 wk of theoretical menstrual cycle given cyclically.

Osteoporosis Prevention
ADULTS:
Estradiol: **PO** 0.5 mg/day (3 wk on, 1 wk off). **Transdermal** 0.025 to 0.1 mg. Start with 0.025 mg system applied to skin twice/wk and adjust dose as necessary to control symptoms.

Prostatic Carcinoma
ADULTS:
Estradiol: **PO** 1 to 2 mg tid.
Valerate Injection: **IM** 30 mg or more q 1 to 2 wk.
Ethinyl Estradiol: **PO** 0.15 to 2 mg/day.

Vasomotor Symptoms
ADULTS:
Estradiol: **PO** 1 to 2 mg/day, adjust to control symptoms; cyclic therapy recommended. **Transdermal** 0.025 to 0.1 mg. Start with 0.025 mg system applied to skin once or twice/wk and adjust dose as necessary to control symptoms. **Topical** Application of two 1.74-g pouches/day (*Estrasorb*).
Valerate Injection: **IM** 10 to 20 mg q 4 wk.
Cypionate Injection: **IM** 1 to 5 mg q 3 to 4 wk.
Ring: Start at lowest dose. Press into an oval and insert as deeply as possible into the upper 1/3 of the vaginal vault. The ring is to remain in place continuously for 3 mo, then removed

and, if appropriate, replaced by a new ring. If the ring is removed or falls out during the 90-day treatment, rinse it in lukewarm water and reinsert.

Vulva/Vaginal Atrophy Associated with Menopause, Female Castration, Primary Ovarian Failure
ADULTS:
Estradiol: **PO** 1 to 2 mg/day; adjust to control symptoms; cyclic therapy recommended. **Transdermal** 0.025 to 0.1 mg. Start with 0.025 mg system applied to skin twice weekly and adjust dose as necessary to control symptoms. Give continuously in women without intact uterus; otherwise give cyclically. **Intravaginal** Insert 2 to 4 g/day for 1 to 2 wk. **Ring** Start at lowest dose. Press into an oval and insert as deeply as possible into the upper 1/3 of the vaginal vault. The ring is to remain in place continuously for 3 mo, then removed and, if appropriate, replaced by a new ring. If the ring is removed or falls out during the 90-day treatment, rinse it in lukewarm water and reinsert.
Valerate Injection: **IM** 10 to 20 mg q 4 wk.
Cypionate Injection (vulva/vaginal atrophy): **IM** 1 to 1.5 mg q 3 to 4 wk.

Interactions
Anticoagulants: Estrogens may reduce the effect of anticoagulants.
Antidepressants, tricyclic: Estradiol may alter effects and increase toxicity of these agents.
Barbiturates, modafinil, rifampin, St. John's wort, topiramate: May decrease estradiol concentration.
Corticosteroids: An increase in the pharmacologic and toxicologic effects of corticosteroids may occur.
CYP3A4 inhibitors (eg, erythromycin, clarithromycin, ketoconazole, itraconazole, ritonavir, grapefruit juice): May increase plasma concentrations of estrogens.
Hydantoins: Loss of seizure control or decreased estrogenic effects may occur.
Thyroid hormones: Increased serum thyroxine-binding globulin concentrations; thyroid hormone requirements may need to be increased.

Lab Test Interferences
Endocrine and LFT results may be affected; possible decreased PT and increased platelet aggreability; decreased antithrombin III activity; increased thyroid-binding globulin and total T_4; impaired glucose tolerance; decreased serum folate concentration; increased serum triglyceride and phospholipid concentrations; increased corticosteroid binding globulin and sex-hormone binding globulin; increased plasma HDL concentrations; reduced LDL cholesterol concentrations; increased triglyceride levels; reduced response to metyrapone test.

Adverse Reactions
CV: Thrombosis; thrombophlebitis; MI; elevated BP; pulmonary embolism; stroke.
CNS: Headache; migraine; dizziness; depression; insomnia; anxiety; emotional lability; chorea; nervousness; mood disturbance; irritability; somnolence; exacerbation of epilepsy.
DERM: Chloasma; melasma; erythema nodosum or multiforme; scalp hair loss; hirsutism; urticaria; dermatitis; skin hypertrophy; pruritus; hemorrhagic eruption.
EENT: Intolerance to contact lenses; retinal vascular thrombosis; steepening of corneal curvature.
GI: Nausea; vomiting; abdominal cramps; bloating; colitis; acute pancreatitis; diarrhea; dyspepsia; flatulence; gastritis; gastroenteritis; enlarged abdomen; hemorrhoids; increased incidence of gallbladder disease.
GU: Increased risk of endometrial carcinoma; breakthrough bleeding; dysmenorrhea; amenorrhea; vaginal candidiasis; premenstrual-like syndrome; increased size of uterine fibromyomata; hemolytic uremic syndrome; UTI; vaginitis; vaginal discomfort/pain; cystitis; dysuria; genital pruritus; urinary incontinence; change in amount of cervical secretion; changes in cervical ectropion; ovarian cancer; endometrial hyperplasia.
HEPA: Cholestatic jaundice.
METAB: Hyperglycemia; hypercalcemia.
RESP: Upper respiratory tract infection; sinusitis; rhinitis; pharyngitis; flu-like symptoms; allergy; bronchitis; chest pain.
OTHER: Pain at injection site; redness and irritation at site of transdermal system; increase/decrease in weight; reduced carbohydrate tolerance; edema; changes in libido; breast tenderness; acute intermittent porphyria; vaginal bleeding; hypersensitivity reactions; back pain; arthritis; arthralgia; hot flushes; leg edema; otitis media; toothache; breast enlargement and pain; nipple discharge; galactorrhea; fibrocystic breast changes; breast cancer; increased triglycerides.

> **WARNING:**
> Estrogens increase the risk of endometrial cancer. Close clinical surveillance of all women taking estrogen is important. Compared with placebo, increased risks of MI, stroke, deep vein thrombosis, pulmonary emboli, and invasive breast cancer were reported in postmenopausal women during 5-yr treatment with conjugated estrogens combined with medroxyprogesterone acetate.

Precautions
Pregnancy: Category X.
Lactation: Excreted in breast milk.
Children: Safety and efficacy not established.
Hepatic function impairment: Metabolism may be impaired; use drug with caution.
Special risk patients: Because asthma, diabetes melitus, epilepsy, migraine, porphyria, systemic lupus erythematosus, and hepatic hemangiomas may be exacerbated by estrogens, use with caution.
Tartrazine sensitivity: Some products contain tartrazine, which may cause allergic reaction in susceptible patients.
Breast cancer: Estrogen has been associated with an increased risk of breast cancer.
Calcium and phosphorus metabolism: Use drug with caution in patients with metabolic bone diseases.
Elevated BP: BP increases during estrogen replacement therapy usually return to normal upon discontinuation of the drug. BP should be monitored during estrogen use. Elevation of BP in previously normotensive or hypertensive patients should be evaluated and estrogen therapy may have to be stopped.
Endometriosis: May be exacerbated with administration of estrogens.
Fluid retention: Use drug with careful observation when conditions that might be affected by this factor are present (eg, asthma, cardiac or renal dysfunction, epilepsy).
Gallbladder disease: Risk of gallbladder disease may increase in women receiving postmenopausal estrogens.
Hypercoagulability: Estrogen therapy may promote hypercoagulability, primarily related to decreased antithrombin activity.
Hypothyroidism: Estrogen administration may lead to increased thyroid-binding globulin (TBG) levels.
Induction of malignant neoplasms: May increase risk of endometrial or other carcinomas (endometrial, breast).
Familial hyperlipoproteinemia: May be associated with massive elevations of plasma triglycerides.
Uterine leiomyomata: Pre-existing uterine leiomyomata may increase in size during estrogen use.
Unopposed estrogen administration (eg, without progesterone): Increases risk of uterine cancer. Therefore, when using estrogens on long-term basis in a woman with intact uterus, consider cyclic therapy with progesterone (eg, estrogen on days 1 to 25 of mo with progesterone added for last 12 days) or daily coadministration of estrogen plus progesterone on daily basis. In a woman without uterus, use of cyclic therapy and/or therapy with progesterone is not necessary.
Visual abnormalities: Retinal vascular thrombosis has been reported in patients receiving estrogen.

Overdosage: Signs and Symptoms
Nausea, withdrawal bleeding in women.

PATIENT CARE CONSIDERATIONS
Administration/Storage
Tablets:

* Administer prescribed dose without regard to meals. Administer with food if GI upset occurs.
* Store tablets at controlled room temperature (59° to 86°F).

Transdermal System:

* Open pouch; remove protective liner from patch, and immediately apply patch to clean, dry skin on lower abdomen or upper quadrant of buttock. Do not apply patch to breasts; skin areas that are oily, damaged, or irritated, which have had powder, lotion, or moisturizer applied, or where clothing or sitting could dislodge patch.
* Press firmly with palm of hand for approximately 10 sec. Be sure good contact is made, especially at edges. If patch falls off, attempt to reapply. Apply new patch to different site if necessary.
* Rotate application sites so that no site is used more than once a week.
* Store patches at controlled room temperature (59° to 86°F). Do not remove from pouch until just immediately before application.

Estradiol Ring:

* Remove vaginal ring from protective pouch; press opposite sides of ring together and have patient insert into the vagina. If patient has difficulty inserting ring, health care provider can insert ring. If patient feels discomfort gently push ring further into the vagina.
* Store vaginal ring at controlled room temperature (59° to 86°F). Do not remove ring from pouch until immediately before insertion.

Topical Emulsion:

* Emulsion is applied qd in the morning, while in a comfortable seated position, to skin on both legs that is clean, dry, and not irritated.
* Cut or tear first pouch at notches indicated near the top of the pouch; push the entire contents from the bottom of the pouch through the neck of the pouch to the left thigh. Have patient use 1 or both hands to rub the emulsion into the entire left thigh and calf for 3 min until thoroughly absorbed; have patient rub any excess emulsion remaining on hands on the buttocks. Repeat this

process using the second pouch and the right thigh and calf, including rubbing any remaining emulsion on the hands on the buttocks. Have patient wash hands with soap and water to remove any residual medication.
- Instruct patient to allow application areas to dry thoroughly before covering with clothing to avoid transfer to other individuals.
- Store pouches at controlled room temperature (59° to 86°F).

Injection:
- For IM administration only. Not for intradermal, SC, or IV administration.
- Inspect solution visually before administration. Do not administer if solution is cloudy, discolored, or contains particulate matter. Crystals may form if solution is stored at low temperature but will dissolve readily when solution is warmed.
- Administer prescribed dose by deep IM injection into upper outer quadrant of gluteal muscle.
- Store injection at controlled room temperature (68° to 77°F).

Assessment/Interventions

- Obtain patient history, including drug history and any known allergies. Note history of breast nodules, fibrocystic breast disease, abnormal mammogram, strong family history of breast cancer, cerebral vascular disease, coronary artery disease, diabetes, epilepsy, migraine headaches, heart failure, jaundice during previous pregnancy or past estrogen use, liver or kidney impairment, endometriosis, porphyria, gallbladder disease, or hypothyroidism.
- Review patient's health history for any condition that could contraindicate estradiol (eg, previous allergic reaction to estrogen, known or suspected pregnancy, known or suspected cancer of the breast except in patient being treated for metastatic disease, known or suspected estrogen-dependent cancer, undiagnosed abnormal uterine bleeding, active or past history of thromboembolic disorders, MI, stroke).
- Ensure that breast, abdominal, and pelvic examinations and Pap smear have been completed and documented before starting therapy and annually thereafter during prolonged therapy.
- Ensure that progestin therapy is utilized in women with intact uterus to prevent endometrial hyperplasia.
- Monitor blood sugar in diabetic patient when drug is started or dose is changed. Report significant changes to health care provider.
- Assess BP at beginning of therapy and periodically during treatment.
- Assess patient for GU, GI, CNS, DERM, and general body side effects. Inform health care provider if noted and significant.
- Notify health care provider of pain, swelling, redness, or warmth in calves; sudden severe headache; visual disturbances; weakness or numbness of arms or legs; signs of liver dysfunction (eg, dark urine, jaundice); abdominal pain or tenderness; abdominal mass; or signs of depression.
- Consider discontinuing therapy during periods of prolonged immobilization and, if possible, 4 to 6 wk before surgery that is associated with an increased risk of thromboembolic disease.
- Ensure that attempts are made q 3 to 6 mo to discontinue therapy or reduce the dose of medication.

Estradiol ring:
- Assess patient's tolerance to ring. Patient should not feel the ring when in place nor should it interfere with sexual intercourse. Have patient reposition ring if necessary. Notify health care provider if repositioning ring does not resolve abnormal sensations.
- If ring is totally expelled from vagina, rinse it in lukewarm water and reinsert.
- If vaginal infection develops during use of ring, determine if ring can be left in place during treatment or removed until after the infection has been treated.
- Note date of initial insertion. Ring should be removed and replaced by new ring 3 mo after initial insertion.

Patient/Family Education

- Advise patient to review *Patient Information* leaflet before starting therapy and with each refill.
- Instruct patient to take (or use) as prescribed and not to change the dose or stop taking unless advised by health care provider.
- Advise patient taking tablets that medication can be taken without regard to meals, but to take with food if GI upset occurs.
- Instruct diabetic patient to monitor blood glucose more frequently when drug is started or dose is changed and to inform health care provider of significant changes in readings.
- Review the following nonhormonal modalities that help prevent osteoporosis: 1500 mg/day of calcium, vitamin D supplementation, exercise.
- Instruct patient to report the following symptoms to health care provider: pain in groin or calves, sharp chest pain or sudden shortness of breath, abnormal vaginal bleeding, breast

lumps, sudden severe headache, dizziness or fainting, vision or speech problems, weakness or numbness of arms or legs, severe abdominal pain or swelling, yellowing of skin or eyes, severe depression.
* Advise women to notify health care provider if pregnant, planning to become pregnant, or breastfeeding.
* Teach patient proper method of breast self-examination.
* Advise patient that follow-up visits and examinations, including Pap smear, at least once a year will be required to monitor therapy and to keep appointments.

Transdermal system:
* Advise patient not to apply patch to breasts, or to skin areas that are oily, damaged, or irritated, which have had powder, moisturizer, or lotion applied, or to where clothing or sitting could dislodge patch.
* Teach patient proper procedure for applying patch as follows: open pouch, remove protective liner from patch, and immediately apply patch to clean, dry skin on lower abdomen or upper quadrant of buttock. Press firmly with palm of hand for approximately 10 sec. Be sure good contact is made, especially at edges.
* Advise patient that if patch falls off, it should be reapplied to a different site. If patch cannot be reapplied, instruct patient to apply a new patch at a different site but to continue to follow the original dosing scheduled.
* Teach patient proper procedure for changing patch as follows: slowly peel off used patch, fold in half, and discard in trash. Apply new patch at different site. Instruct patient to rotate application sites so that no site is used more than once a week.
* Advise patient that if scheduled patch change is missed to remove the old patch and apply a new patch to a different site but to continue to follow the original application schedule.
* Advise patient to notify health care provider if skin irritation or persistent redness or itching occur at application site.

Estradiol ring:
* Teach patient proper procedure for inserting or replacing ring as follows: wash hands before and after insertion; remove vaginal ring from protective pouch, press opposite sides of ring together, and insert into the vagina. If patient has difficulty inserting ring, health care provider can insert it. If ring causes discomfort, gently push it further into the vagina.
* Advise patient that the ring should not be felt when in place, nor should it interfere with sexual intercourse; repositioning the ring should result in resolution of any abnormal sensation. Advise patient to notify health care provider if repositioning ring does not resolve abnormal sensations.
* Advise patient that if ring is totally expelled from vagina, to clean the it in warm water and reinsert.
* Remind patient that ring should be removed and replaced by a new ring q 3 mo in order to maintain beneficial effects.

Topical Emulsion:
* Advise patient to apply emulsion qd in the morning to skin on both legs that is clean and dry.
* Caution patient not to apply emulsion to any skin area that appears to be red or irritated.
* Teach patient proper procedure for applying emulsion as follows: cut or tear first pouch at notches indicated near the top of the pouch; while in a comfortable seated position push the entire contents from the bottom of the pouch through the neck of the pouch onto the left thigh; using 1 or both hands, rub the emulsion into the entire left thigh and calf for 3 min until thoroughly absorbed; rub any excess emulsion remaining on hands on the buttocks; repeat this process using the second pouch and the right thigh and calf including rubbing any remaining emulsion on the hands on the buttocks; wash hands with soap and water to remove any residual medication.
* Instruct patient to allow application areas to dry thoroughly before covering with clothing to avoid transfer to other individuals.
* Advise patient that if application of the emulsion in the morning is missed, to apply it as soon as remembered and to never apply the emulsion more than once each day.

Injection:
* Advise patient that medication will be prepared and administered by a health care professional in a medical setting on a scheduled basis.

Estradiol Cypionate/ Medroxyprogesterone Acetate

(ESS-truh-DIE-ole SIP-ee-oh-nate/Meh-DROX-ee-por-JESS-tuh-rone ASS-uh-TATE)

Class Estrogen/Progestin

How Supplied
Lunelle Injection 5 mg estradiol and 25 mg medroxyprogesterone/0.5 mL

Action
PHARMACOLOGY:
Estradiol: Inhibits ovulation.
Medroxyprogesterone: Inhibits secretion of pituitary gonadotropins, thereby preventing follicular maturation and ovulation.

Indications Prevention of pregnancy.

Contraindications Known or suspected pregnancy; thrombophlebitis or thromboembolic disorders; past history of deep-vein thrombophlebitis or thromboembolic disorders; cerebral vascular or coronary artery disease; undiagnosed abnormal genital bleeding; liver dysfunction or disease (such as history of hepatic adenoma or carcinoma) history of cholestatic jaundice or pregnancy or jaundice with prior hormonal contraceptive use (including severe pruritus of pregnancy); carcinoma of the endometrium, breast or other known or suspected estrogen-dependent neoplasia; heavy smoking (at least 15 cigarettes/day) and age over 35 yr; severe hypertension; diabetes with vascular involvement; headaches with focal neurological symptoms; valvular heart disease with complication; known hypersensitivity to any ingredient of product.

Route/Dosage
ADULTS (WOMEN AND POSTPUBERTAL ADOLESCENT FEMALES): **IM** 0.5 mL administered by IM injection into the deltoid, gluteus maximus, or anterior thigh. Give first injection within first 5 days of onset of normal menstrual period, within 5 days of complete first trimester abortion, or no earlier than 4 wk postpartum if not breastfeeding (no earlier than 6 wk postpartum if breastfeeding). Give subsequent injections monthly (28 to 30 days) after previous injection, not to exceed 33 days.

Interactions
Acetaminophen, ascorbic acid: Estrogen plasma levels may be elevated, increasing the risk of side effects.
Antibiotics (eg, tetracycline), anticonvulsants (eg, carbamazepine, phenytoin), phenylbutazone, rifampin, St. John's wort: Contraceptive efficacy may be reduced.
Clofibric acid, morphine, salicylic acid, temazepam: Plasma levels of these agents may be reduced, decreasing their therapeutic effect.
Cyclosporine, prednisolone, theophylline: Plasma levels of these agents may be elevated, increasing the risk of side effects.

Lab Test Interferences Endocrine and liver function test results may be affected; possible increased PT and increased platelet aggregability; increased thyroid-binding globulin and total T_4; impaired glucose tolerance; decreased serum triglyceride and phospholipid concentrations; increased corticosteroid binding globulin and sex-hormone-binding globulin; increased plasma HDL concentration; reduced LDL cholesterol concentrations; increased triglyceride levels; reduced response to metyrapone test; reduced folate concentration.

Adverse Reactions
CV: Arterial thromboembolism; cerebral hemorrhage; cerebral thrombosis; hypertension; MI; pulmonary embolism; thrombophlebitis; mesenteric thrombosis; retinal thrombosis.
CNS: Depression; headache; dizziness; nervousness; migraine; emotional lability; change in appetite; asthenia.
DERM: Acne; alopecia; erythema multiforme; erythema nodosum; hirsutism.
EENT: Corneal curvature changes (eg, steepening); intolerance to contact lenses; cataract.
GI: Nausea; colitis; abdominal pain; enlarged abdomen.
GU: Amenorrhea; dysmenorrhea; menorrhagia; metrorrhagia; breast tenderness; breast pain; vaginal spotting; decreased libido; vaginal moniliasis; vulvovaginal disorder; breast changes (eg, enlargement, secretion); cervical changes; temporary infertility after treatment discontinuation; diminution in lactation when given immediately postpartum; changes in libido; PMS; vaginitis; cystitis-like syndrome; impaired renal function; gallbladder disease.
HEMA: Hemolytic uremic syndrome; porphyria; hemorrhagic eruption.
HEPA: Hepatic adenoma or benign liver tumor; cholestatic jaundice; Budd-Chiari syndrome.
METAB: Weight gain or decrease; reduced carbohydrate tolerance; edema.
OTHER: Hypersensitivity (eg, anaphylactic reactions, rash); persistent melasma.

> **WARNING:**
> Cigarette smoking increases the risk of serious cardiovascular side effects from contraceptives containing estrogen. This risk increases with age and with heavy smoking (15 or more cigarettes/day) and is quite marked in women over 35 yr. Women using this injection are strongly advised not to smoke.

Precautions
Pregnancy: Category X.
Lactation: Undetermined.
Children: Use of this product before menarche is not indicated.
Special risk patients: Contraceptive use is associated with increased risks of MI, thromboembolism, stroke, hepatic neoplasm, and gallbladder disease.
Anaphylaxis and anaphylactoid reactions: May occur.
Bone mineral density changes: Use of injectable progestogen-only methods is among the risk factors for development of osteoporosis.
Cigarette smoking: May increase risk of serious cardiovascular side effects from contraceptives containing estrogen. These risks increase with age (women more than 35 yr) and with smoking more than 15 cigarettes/day.
Depression: Carefully observe patients with history of depression.
Elevated BP: Increased BP during estrogen replacement has been attributed to idiosyncratic reactions.
Familial hyperlipoproteinemia: May be associated with massive elevations of plasma triglycerides.
Fluid retention: Use with careful observation when conditions that might be affected by fluid retention are present (eg, asthma, cardiac or renal dysfunction, epilepsy).
Headache: Development of headache or onset or exacerbation of migraine with a new pattern that is recurrent, persistent, or severe requires evaluation of the cause before further injection of product.
Hypercalcemia: In patients with breast cancer or bone metastases, severe hypercalcemia has occurred with estrogen therapy.
Induction of malignant neoplasm: May increase risk of endometrial or other carcinomas.
Lipid disorders: Because some progestogens may elevate LDL, monitor closely women who are being treated for hyperlipidemias.
Uterine bleeding: Certain patients may develop abnormal uterine bleeding.
Visual abnormalities: Retinal thrombosis has been associated with oral contraceptive use. Discontinue medication if there are any sudden changes in vision, sudden onset of proptosis, diplopia, migraine, papilledema, or retinal vascular lesions.

Overdosage: Signs and Symptoms
Nausea, vomiting, vaginal bleeding, menstrual irregularities.

PATIENT CARE CONSIDERATIONS
Administration/Storage
- For IM injection only. Not for intradermal, SC, or intra-arterial administration.
- Inject prescribed dose q 28 to 30 days.
- Inject first dose during first 5 days of normal menstrual cycle.
- Store at controlled room temperature (59° to 86°F).
- When switching from oral contraceptives, the first injection should be given within 7 days after the last active pill was taken.

Assessment/Interventions
- Obtain patient history, including drug history and any known allergies.
- Review patient's health history for any condition that would contraindicate use of conjugated estrogens/progesterone: previous allergic reaction to either drug; known or suspected pregnancy; known or suspected cancer of the breast; known or suspected estrogen-dependent cancer; undiagnosed abnormal uterine bleeding; active or past history of thromboembolic disorders or stroke; liver dysfunction or disease; heavy smoking and age greater than 35 yr; severe hypertension; diabetes with vascular involvement; headaches with focal neurological symptoms; valvular heart disease with complications.
- Ensure that breast, abdominal, and pelvic examination and Pap smear have been completed and documented before starting therapy.
- Document time of last injection. If less than 28 days or more than 33 days, notify health care provider before administering.
- Monitor blood sugar in diabetic patient when therapy is started. Report significant changes to health care provider.
- Assess BP at beginning of therapy and periodically during treatment.
- Assess patient for GI, CNS, GU, and general body side effects. Inform health care provider if noted and significant.
- Notify health care provider immediately if any of the following are noted: pain in groin or calves; sharp chest pain, coughing blood, or sudden shortness of breath; crushing chest pain or heaviness in chest; abnormal vaginal bleeding; breast lumps; sudden severe headache; dizziness or fainting; vision or speech

problems; weakness or numbness of arms or legs; severe abdominal pain; symptoms of depression; yellowing of skin or eyes.

Patient/Family Education
- Explain name, dose, action, and potential side effects of drug.
- Advise patient that medication will be prepared and administered by a health care provider in a medical setting.
- Advise patient that medication must be administered q 28 to 30 days but no later than 33 days following the last injection.
- Instruct diabetic patient to monitor blood glucose more frequently when drug is started and to inform health care provider of significant changes in readings.
- Caution patient that this medication does not protect against HIV infection or other sexually transmitted diseases.
- Instruct patient to immediately report these symptoms to health care provider: pain in groin or calves; sharp chest pain, coughing blood, or sudden shortness of breath; crushing chest pain or heaviness in chest; abnormal vaginal bleeding; breast lumps; sudden severe headache; dizziness or fainting; vision or speech problems; weakness or numbness of arms or legs; severe abdominal pain; yellowing of skin or eyes; depression; persistent pain, pus, or bleeding at injection site.
- Instruct patient to notify health care provider if any of the following occur: missed menstrual period; persistent or bothersome altered menstrual bleeding; excessive weight gain; intolerance to contact lenses or change in vision while wearing contact lenses; swelling of fingers or ankles; other bothersome effects.
- Advise women to notify health care provider if pregnant, planning to become pregnant, or breastfeeding.
- Teach patient proper method of breast self-examination.
- Advise patient that follow-up visits and examinations, including Pap smear at least once a year, will be required to monitor therapy and to keep appointments.

Estradiol/Norethindrone Acetate

(ESS-truh-DIE-ole/NOR-eth-IN-drone ass-SUH-tate)

Class Estrogen and progestin combined

How Supplied
CombiPatch Transdermal patch 0.05 mg estradiol/0.14 mg norethindrone acetate/day, Transdermal patch 0.05 mg estradiol/0.25 mg norethindrone acetate/day

Action
PHARMACOLOGY: Estrogens are essential in developing and maintaining female reproductive system and secondary sex characteristics. Progestins transform proliferative endometrium into secretory endometrium.

Indications Treatment of moderate to severe vasomotor symptoms associated with menopause; vulvar and vaginal atrophy; hypoestrogenism caused by hypogonadism, castration, or primary ovarian failure.

Contraindications Known or suspected pregnancy, including use for or as a diagnostic test for pregnancy. Known or suspected cancer of the breast. Known or suspected estrogen-dependent neoplasia. Undiagnosed abnormal genital bleeding. Active thrombophlebitis, thromboembolic disorders, or stroke.

Route/Dosage
CONTINUOUS COMBINED REGIMEN

ADULTS: **Transdermal** Apply twice weekly. One 0.05 mg estradiol/0.14 mg norethindrone acetate patch applied to the lower abdomen. A dose of 0.05 mg estradiol/0.25 mg norethindrone acetate may be used if a greater progestin dose is desired.

CONTINUOUS SEQUENTIAL REGIMEN

ADULTS: **Transdermal** Apply twice weekly. May be applied as a sequential regimen in combination with an estradiol-only transdermal delivery system.

Interactions None well documented.

Lab Test Interferences
Increased: Prothrombin time, activated partial thromboplastin time, and platelet aggregation time; increased platelet count; increased factors II, VII antigen, VIII antigen, VIII coagulation activity, IX, X, XII, VII-X complex, II-VII-X complex, and beta-thromboglobulin; increased levels of fibrinogen activity; increased plasminogen antigen and activity; increased thyroid-binding globulin (TBG) leading to increased circulating total thyroid hormone, as measured by protein-bound iodine; increased corticosteroid binding globulin; increased angiotensinogen/renin substrate, alpha-1-antitrypsin, ceruloplasmin; increased TG and levels of various other lipids and lipoproteins may be affected; increased sulfobromophthalein retention.

Decreased: Decreased levels of anti-Factor Xa and antithrombin III; decreased antithrombin III activity; T3 resin uptake is decreased, reflecting elevated TBG; reduced response to metyrapone test; reduced serum folate concentration.

Adverse Reactions
CNS: Asthenia; depression; dizziness; headache; insomnia; nervousness.
DERM: Acne; irritation at application site; rash.
GI: Constipation; diarrhea; dyspepsia; flatulence; nausea; tooth disorder; abdominal pain.
RESP: Bronchitis; pharyngitis; respiratory disorder; rhinitis; sinusitis.
OTHER: Accidental injury; arthralgia; back pain; breast pain; influenza syndrome; leukorrhea; menstrual disorders; pain; peripheral edema; suspicious pap smear; vaginal hemorrhage; vaginitis; dysmenorrhea; menorrhagia.

Precautions
Pregnancy: Category X.
Lactation: Secreted into breast milk.
Hepatic function impairment: Metabolism may be impaired; use drug with caution.
Breast cancer: Moderately increased risk of developing breast cancer. Increased risk of hypercalcemia in patients with breast cancer and bone metastases.
Calcium/Phosphorus metabolism: Use drug with caution in patients with metabolic bone diseases.
Cardiovascular disease: Increased risk with large doses of estrogen (5 mg conjugated estrogens/day).
Elevated BP: May increase; attributed to idiosyncratic reactions to estrogen.
Familial hyperlipoproteinemia: May be associated with massive elevations of plasma triglycerides, possibly leading to pancreatitis and other complications.
Fluid retention: Use with careful observation when conditions that might be affected by this factor are present (eg, asthma, migraine, cardiac or renal dysfunction, seizure disorder).
Gallbladder disease: Risk of gallbladder disease may increase in women receiving postmenopausal estrogens.
Hypercoagulability: Increased risk, primarily related to decreased antithrombin activity.
Induction of malignant neoplasia: May increase risk of endometrial or other carcinomas.

PATIENT CARE CONSIDERATIONS

Administration/Storage
- This product is to be used in women with an intact uterus.
- May be used alone or in combination with estradiol-only transdermal system.
- Patch is applied twice weekly.
- Open pouch, remove one side of protective liner from patch, taking care not to touch adhesive part of patch, and immediately apply patch to clean, smooth (fold-free), dry skin on lower abdomen. Remove the second side of the protective liner and press firmly with palm of hand for approximately 10 sec. Be sure good contact is made, especially at edges. If patch falls off, attempt to reapply to another area of the lower abdomen. If necessary, a new transdermal system may be applied, in which case the original treatment schedule should be continued.
- Do not apply patch on or near the breasts, skin areas that are oily, damaged or irritated, or skin areas that have had powder, lotion, or moisturizer applied, or to skin areas where clothing or sitting could dislodge patch.
- Rotate application sites so that no site is used more than once weekly.
- Store patches at controlled room temperature (below 77°F) for up to 6 mo. Protect from extreme temperatures. Do not remove from pouch until just immediately before application.

Assessment/Interventions
- Obtain patient history, including drug history and any known allergies. Note asthma, epilepsy, migraine headaches, cardiovascular disease, hepatic impairment, renal impairment, and familial hyperlipoproteinemia.
- Review patient's health history for any condition that could contraindicate use of the estradiol/norethindrone transdermal system (previous allergic reaction to either drug or component of the patch, known or suspected pregnancy, known or suspected cancer of the breast, known or suspected estrogen-dependent cancer, undiagnosed abnormal uterine bleeding, or active or past history of thromboembolic disorders or stroke).
- Ensure that breast, abdominal, and pelvic examination and Pap smear have been completed and documented before starting therapy and are repeated periodically during therapy (at least once a year).
- Ensure that therapy is reevaluated q 3 to 6 mo to determine if changes in hormone replacement therapy or if continued hormone replacement therapy is appropriate.
- Monitor blood sugar more frequently in diabetic patient when therapy is started or dose is changed. Report significant changes to health care provider.
- Assess BP at beginning of therapy and periodically during treatment.

- Notify health care provider immediately of the following: pain, swelling, redness, or warmth in calves; sudden, severe headache; visual disturbances; weakness or numbness of arms or legs; signs of liver dysfunction (eg, dark urine, jaundice); signs of depression.
- Monitor patient for application site reactions and CNS, GI, GU, and general body side effects. Inform health care provider if noted and significant.

Patient/Family Education

- Advise patient to review patient information insert before using for the first time and with each refill.
- Explain name, dosing schedule, and potential side effects of drug.
- Teach patient proper method of applying patch. Open pouch, remove one side of protective liner from patch, taking care not to touch adhesive part of patch, and immediately apply patch to clean, smooth (fold-free), dry skin on lower abdomen. Remove the second side of the protective liner and press firmly with palm of hand for approximately 10 sec. Be sure good contact is made, especially at edges.
- Caution patient not to apply patch on or near the breasts, skin areas that are oily, damaged, or irritated, or skin areas that have had powder, lotion, or moisturizer applied, or to skin areas where clothing or sitting could dislodge patch.
- Advise patient that if patch falls off to attempt to reapply to another area of the lower abdomen. If that fails, a new transdermal system may be applied, in which case, the original treatment schedule should be continued.
- Instruct patient to rotate application sites so that no site is used more than once weekly.
- Advise patient that patch may cause reactions at application site and to inform health care provider if this occurs and is bothersome.
- Advise patient not to expose patch to direct sunlight for long periods of time (eg, sunbathing).
- Instruct diabetic patient to monitor blood glucose more frequently when drug is started or dose is changed and to inform health care provider of significant changes in readings.
- Review nonhormonal modalities that help prevent osteoporosis: 1500 mg/day of calcium, vitamin D supplementation, exercise.
- Instruct patient to immediately report the following symptoms to health care provider: pain in groin or calves, sharp chest pain or sudden shortness of breath, abnormal vaginal bleeding, breast lumps, sudden severe headache, dizziness or fainting, vision or speech problems, weakness or numbness of arms or legs, severe abdominal pain, yellowing of skin or eyes, severe depression.
- Advise women to notify health care provider if pregnant, planning to become pregnant, or breastfeeding.
- Teach patient proper method of breast self-examination.
- Advise patient that follow-up visits and examinations, including breast exam and Pap smear, will be required at least once a year to monitor therapy and to keep appointments.
- Tell patient that bathing, swimming, or showering should not affect the patch.
- Advise patient that a new patch is applied q 3 to 4 days and to change the patch on the same days of the week.
- Advise patient that removal of the patch should be done carefully to avoid irritation of the skin. If any adhesive remains on skin, allow area to dry and rub with an oil-based cream or lotion to remove residue.

Estramustine Phosphate Sodium

(ESS-truh-muss-TEEN)

Class Estrogens/Alkylating agent

How Supplied

Emcyt Capsules for oral use 140 mg estramustine phosphate.

Action

PHARMACOLOGY: Estramustine appears to act as a relatively weak alkylating agent and imparts a weak estrogenic activity. The estrogenic portion of the molecule acts as a carrier to facilitate selective uptake of the drug into estrogen receptor-positive cells. Because of the selective steroidal uptake, the alkylating effect of the nitrogen mustard is enhanced in these cells. Estramustine phosphate is readily dephosphorylated during absorption, and the major metabolites in plasma are estromustine, the estrone analog, estradiol, and estrone. Terminal half-life of estramustine phosphate is approximately 20 hr and mainly excreted in the stool.

PHARMACOKINETICS/DYNAMICS:

Metabolism: Readily dephosphorylated during absorption; major metabolites in plasma are estromustine, the estrone analog, estradiol, and estrone.

Excretion: The $t_{1/2}$ is approximately 20 hr. Majority excreted in the feces.

Special Populations:
Hepatic Function Impairment – May be poorly metabolized in these patients.

Indications Palliative therapy of metastatic or progressive prostate cancer. **Unlabeled use(s):** Metastatic renal cell carcinoma.

Contraindications Hypersensitivity to estradiol or nitrogen mustard; active thrombophlebitis or thromboembolic disorders, except where the actual tumor mass is the cause of the thromboembolic phenomenon and the benefits of therapy outweigh the risks.

Route/Dosage
Prostate Cancer
ADULTS: **PO** 14 mg/kg/day (range, 10 to 16 mg/kg/day) in 3 to 4 divided doses for 30 to 90 days before assessing for continuation of therapy. Continue therapy as long as response is favorable.

Interactions
Food: Milk, milk products, and calcium-rich foods or antacids may impair the absorption of estramustine.

Lab Test Interferences Abnormalities of hepatic enzymes and of bilirubin have occurred but have seldom required cessation of therapy. Perform such tests at appropriate intervals during therapy and repeat after the drug has been withdrawn for 2 mo.

Adverse Reactions
CV: Hypertension; CHF; edema; increased risk of cerebrovascular accident; MI, thrombosis.
CNS: Lethargy; emotional lability; insomnia.
DERM: Rash; pruritus; dry skin; easy bruising.
ENDO: Decreased glucose tolerance; breast tenderness or enlargement.
GI: Nausea; vomiting; diarrhea; anorexia; flatulence; elevated LFTs.
GU: Decreased glucose tolerance; gonadal suppression; breast tenderness; breast enlargement.
HEMA: Leukopenia and thrombocytopenia have been reported in a small number of patients.
MUSC: Leg cramps.
RESP: Dyspnea.

Precautions
Children: Safety and efficacy not established.
Hepatic function impairment: Estramustine may be poorly metabolized in patients with impaired liver function.
Mutagenesis: Both estradiol and nitrogen mustard are mutagenic. Advise use of contraceptive measures.
Thrombosis: The risk of thrombosis including nonfatal MI, increases in men receiving estrogens for prostate cancer. Use with caution in patients with a history of thrombophlebitis, thrombosis, or thromboembolic disorders, especially if associated with estrogen therapy. Use with caution in patients with cerebral vascular or coronary artery disease.
Glucose tolerance: Tolerance to glucose may be decreased.
Elevated BP: BP elevation may occur.
Fluid retention: Exacerbation of preexisting or incipient peripheral edema or CHD may occur.
Calcium/Phosphorus metabolism: Calcium/phosphorus metabolism may be influenced. Use with caution in patients with metabolic bone disease associated with hypercalcemia or in patients with renal insufficiency.

PATIENT CARE CONSIDERATIONS
Administration/Storage
- Refrigerate. Capsules may be stored at room temperature for 24 to 48 hr without affecting potency. Protect from light.
- Administer PO with water 1 hr or more before or 2 hr after meals.
- Follow procedures for proper handling and disposal of anticancer drugs. Wear gloves and avoid skin exposure and inhalation of fumes.

Assessment/Interventions
- Monitor LFTs at appropriate intervals during therapy and repeat for 2 mo after the drug has been withdrawn.
- Monitor BP periodically while on estramustine.
- Monitor diabetic patients' glucose tolerance carefully while receiving estramustine.

Patient/Family Education
- Use contraceptive measures during therapy because of the possibility of mutagenic effects.
- Milk, milk products, and calcium-rich foods or antacids may impair the absorption of estramustine.
- Take with water at least 1 hr before or 2 hr after meals.

Estrogens, Conjugated or Esterified

(ESS-truh-janz)
Class Estrogens

How Supplied

Esterified Estrogen
Menest Tablets 0.3 mg, Tablets 0.625 mg, Tablets 1.25 mg, Tablets 2.5 mg

Conjugated Estrogen
Premarin Tablets 0.3 mg, Tablets 0.45 mg, Tablets 0.625 mg, Tablets 0.9 mg, Tablets 1.25 mg, Tablets 2.5 mg ♦ Premarin IV Injection 25 mg
❖ C.E.S. ♦ Congest

Action

PHARMACOLOGY: Promotes growth and development of female reproductive system and secondary sex characteristics; affects release of pituitary gonadotropins; inhibits ovulation and prevents postpartum breast engorgement; conserves calcium and phosphorous and encourages bone formation; overrides stimulatory effects of testosterone.

PHARMACOKINETICS/DYNAMICS:
Absorption: Well absorbed from GI tract. The tablets slowly release the drug over several hours.

Distribution: Bound to sex hormone-binding globulin and albumin. Widely distributed and generally found in higher concentration in the sex hormone target organs. Crosses the placenta.

Metabolism: Metabolized in the liver and undergoes enterohepatic recirculation. Estradiol is converted reversibly to estrone, and both can be converted to estriol (major urinary metabolite).

Excretion: Estradiol, estrone, and estriol are excreted in the urine along with glucuronide and sulfate conjugates.

Indications

Management of moderate to severe vasomotor symptoms associated with menopause; treatment of atrophic vaginitis, kraurosis vulvae, female hypogonadism, symptoms of female castration, and primary ovarian failure; prevention and treatment of osteoporosis (conjugated estrogens); palliative treatment of metastatic breast or prostate cancer in selected women and men; treatment of postpartum breast engorgement and abnormal uterine bleeding (parenteral form).

Contraindications

Breast cancer (except in patients being treated for metastatic disease); estrogen-dependent neoplasia; undiagnosed abnormal genital bleeding; thrombophlebitis or thromboembolic disorders associated with previous estrogen use; known or suspected pregnancy.

Route/Dosage

Vasomotor Symptoms
ADULTS: PO 1.25 mg/day.

Female Castration, Primary Ovarian Failure
ADULTS: PO 0.3 to 1.25 mg/day (3 wk on estrogen, 1 wk off).

Atrophic Vaginitis, Atrophic Urethritis, Kraurosis Vulvae
ADULTS: PO 0.3 to 1.25 mg or more/day (3 wk on estrogen, 1 wk off). **Intravaginal** 0.5 to 2 g/day (3 wk on estrogen, 1 wk off).

Female Hypogonadism
ADULTS: PO 2.5 to 7.5 mg/day in divided doses for 20 days, followed by 10-day rest period.

Prostatic Carcinoma
ADULTS: PO 1.25 to 2.5 mg tid.

Breast Cancer
ADULTS: PO 10 mg tid for 3 mo or more.

Osteoporosis
ADULTS: PO 0.625 mg/day (3 wk on conjugated estrogen, 1 wk off).

Postpartum Breast Engorgement
ADULTS: PO 3.75 mg q 4 hr for 5 doses, or 1.25 mg q 4 hr for 5 days.

Abnormal Uterine Bleeding
ADULTS: **IV/IM** 25 mg; may repeat in 6 to 12 hr.

Interactions

Antidepressants, tricyclic: Estrogens may alter effects and increase toxicity of these agents.
Barbiturates, modafinil, topiramate, St. John's wort, rifampin: May decrease estrogen concentration.
Corticosteroids: An increase in pharmacologic and toxicologic effects of corticosteroids may occur.
Hydantoins: Loss of seizure control or decreased estrogenic effects may occur.
INCOMPATIBILITIES: Infusion of conjugated estrogen with other agents is not recommended. Solution is compatible with normal saline, dextrose, and invert sugar solutions. It is not compatible with any solution with acidic pH.

Lab Test Interferences

Endocrine and LFT results may be affected; possible decreased PT and increased platelet aggregability; increased thyroid-binding globulin and total T_4; impaired glucose tolerance; decreased serum folate concentration; increased serum triglyceride and phospholipid concentrations; increased corticosteroid binding globulin and sex-hormone binding globulin; increased plasma HDL concentrations; reduced LDL cholesterol concentrations; increased triglyceride levels.

Adverse Reactions

CV: Thrombosis; thrombophlebitis; pulmonary embolism; MI; elevated BP.

CNS: Headache; migraine; dizziness; depression; anxiety; emotional lability.
DERM: Chloasma; melasma; erythema nodosum/multiforme; scalp hair loss; hirsutism; urticaria; dermatitis; skin hypertrophy; pruritus.
EENT: Intolerance to contact lenses.
GI: Nausea; vomiting; abdominal cramps; bloating; colitis; acute pancreatitis; diarrhea; dyspepsia; flatulence; gastritis; gastroenteritis; enlarged abdomen; hemorrhoids.
GU: Increased risk of endometrial carcinoma; breakthrough bleeding; dysmenorrhea; amenorrhea; vaginal candidiasis; premenstrual-like syndrome; increased size of uterine fibromyomata; hemolytic uremic syndrome; UTI; vaginitis; vaginal discomfort/pain; cystitis; dysuria; genital pruritus; urinary incontinence.
HEPA: Cholestatic jaundice.
METAB: Hyperglycemia; hypercalcemia.
RESP: Upper respiratory tract infection; sinusitis; rhinitis; pharyngitis; flu-like symptoms; allergy; bronchitis; chest pain.
OTHER: Increase or decrease in weight; reduced glucose tolerance; edema; changes in libido; breast tenderness; acute intermittent porphyria; vaginal bleeding; hypersensitivity reactions; back pain; arthritis; arthralgia; hot flushes; leg edema; otitis media; toothache.

Precautions

Pregnancy: Category X.
Lactation: Excreted in breast milk.
Children: Safety and efficacy not established.
Hepatic function impairment: Metabolism may be impaired; use drug with caution.
Cardiovascular and other risks: Compared with placebo, increased risks of MI, stroke, deep vein thrombosis, pulmonary emboli, and invasive breast cancer were reported in postmenopausal women during 5 yr of treatment with conjugated equine estrogens combined with medroxyprogesterone acetate. Other combinations of estrogens and progestins were not studied; however, in the absence of comparable data, assume these risks to be similar.
Calcium/phosphorus metabolism: Use drug with caution in patients with metabolic bone diseases.
Fluid retention: Use with careful observation when conditions that might be affected by this factor are present (eg, asthma, cardiac or renal dysfunction, epilepsy).
Gallbladder disease: Risk of gallbladder disease may increase in women receiving postmenopausal estrogens.
Induction of malignant neoplasms: May increase risk of endometrial or other carcinomas.
Familial hyperlipoproteinemia: May be associated with massive elevations of plasma triglycerides.
Uterine leiomyomata: Preexisting uterine leiomyomata may increase in size.
Unopposed estrogen administration (eg, without progesterone): Increases risk of uterine cancer. Therefore, when using estrogens on long-term basis in a woman with intact uterus, consider cyclic therapy with progesterone (eg, estrogen on days 1 to 25 of mo with progesterone added for last 12 days) or daily coadministration of estrogen plus progesterone on daily basis. In a woman without a uterus, use of cyclic therapy or therapy with progesterone is not necessary.

Overdosage: Signs and Symptoms
Nausea, withdrawal bleeding in women.

PATIENT CARE CONSIDERATIONS
Administration/Storage
Conjugated Estrogen:
- Administer IM injection deeply into muscle.
- Administer IV injection slowly to avoid flushing.
- Insert vaginal cream high in vagina (approximately ⅔ length of applicator).
- Store vials for parenteral administration in refrigerator.
- Use reconstituted solution within a few hr.
- Reconstituted solution can be stored for 60 days in refrigerator.
- Do not use parenteral preparation if darkening or precipitation is noted.

Esterified Estrogen:
- Administer as prescribed without regard to meals.
- Administer with food if GI upset occurs.
- Store at controlled room temperature (59° to 86°F).

Assessment/Interventions
- Obtain patient history, including drug history and any known allergies. Note history of endometriosis, breast nodules, fibrocystic breast disease, abnormal mammogram, strong family history of breast cancer, cerebral vascular disease, CAD, epilepsy, migraine headache, heart failure, depression, jaundice during previous pregnancy, liver or kidney impairment, metabolic bone disease, or gallbladder disease.
- Monitor blood glucose level in diabetic patients.
- Note history of breast nodules, fibrocystic breast disease, abnormal mammogram, strong family history of breast cancer, cerebral vascular disease, coronary artery disease, epilepsy, migraine headaches, heart failure, depression, jaundice during previous pregnancy, liver, or kidney impairment, metabolic bone disease, or gallbladder disease.

- Include in physical assessment thorough documentation of BP; breast, abdomen, and pelvic examination; review results of Pap smear, which should be conducted at least annually.

Esterified Estrogens:
- Review patient's health history for any condition that could contraindicate esterified estrogen (previous allergic reaction to either drug, known or suspected pregnancy, known or suspected cancer of the breast except in patient being treated for metastatic disease, known or suspected estrogen-dependent cancer, undiagnosed abnormal uterine bleeding, active or history of thromboembolic disorders or stroke, or liver dysfunction or disease).
- Ensure that breast, abdominal and pelvic examination and Pap smear have been completed and documented before starting therapy and annually thereafter during prolonged therapy.
- Ensure that progestin therapy is utilized in women with intact uterus to prevent endometrial hyperplasia.
- Assess BP at beginning of therapy and periodically during treatment.
- Assess patient for GU, GI, CNS, DERM, and general body side effects. Inform health care provider if noted and significant.
- Notify health care provider of pain, swelling, redness, or warmth in calves; sudden severe headache; visual disturbances; weakness or numbness of arms or legs; signs of liver dysfunction (eg, dark urine, jaundice); abdominal pain or tenderness, abdominal mass or signs of depression.
- Consider discontinuing therapy during periods of prolonged immobilization and, if possible, 4 wk before surgery that is associated with an increased risk of thromboembolic disease.

Patient/Family Education
- Explain name, dose, action, and potential side effects of drug.
- Advise patient to review Patient Information leaflet before starting therapy and with each refill.
- Instruct patient to take as prescribed and to not change the dose or stop taking unless advised to do so by health care provider.
- Advise patient that medication can be taken without regard to meals, but to take with food if GI upset occurs.
- Instruct diabetic patient to monitor blood glucose more frequently when drug is started or dose is changed and to inform health care provider of significant changes in readings.
- Review nonhormonal modalities that help prevent osteoporosis: 1500 mg/day of calcium; vitamin D supplementation; exercise.
- Caution patient that this medication must not be taken during pregnancy or when pregnancy is possible. Advise patient to use reliable form of birth control while taking this drug.
- Advise women to notify health care provider if pregnant, planning to become pregnant, or breastfeeding.
- Advise patient regarding importance of smoking cessation or reduction of intake to less than 15 cigarettes/day because of risk of cardiovascular complications.
- Teach patient proper method of performing breast self-examination.
- Advise patient to avoid exposure to sunlight or other sources of UV light. Sunscreens and/or protective clothing should be used until sun tolerance is determined.
- Instruct patient to report these symptoms to health care provider: pain in groin or calves; sharp chest pain or sudden shortness of breath; abnormal vaginal bleeding; breast lumps; sudden severe headache; dizziness or fainting; vision or speech problems; weakness or numbness in arm or leg; severe abdominal pain; yellowing of skin or eyes; severe depression.
- Remind patient to have Pap smear q 6 to 12 mo while undergoing therapy.

Estrogens, Synthetic Conjugated, A or B

(ESS-truh-janz, sin-THE-tik KAHN-juh-gay-tuhd, A or B)

Class Estrogens

How Supplied
Cenestin Tablets 0.3 mg (synthetic conjugated estrogens, A), Tablets 0.45 mg (synthetic conjugated estrogens, A), Tablets 0.625 mg (synthetic conjugated estrogens, A), Tablets 0.9 mg (synthetic conjugated estrogens, A), Tablets 1.25 mg (synthetic conjugated estrogens, A) ◆ *Enjuvia* Tablets 0.625 mg (synthetic conjugated estrogens, B), Tablets 1.25 mg (synthetic conjugated estrogens, B)

Action
PHARMACOLOGY: Estrogens are responsible for the development and maintenance of the female reproductive system and secondary sexual characteristics. Circulating estrogens modulate the pituitary secretion of the gonadotropins luteinizing hormone (LH) and follicle stimulating hormone (FSH) through a negative feed-

back mechanism and estrogen replacement therapy acts to reduce the elevated levels of these hormones seen in postmenopausal women.

Indications Treatment of moderate to severe symptoms associated with menopause (synthetic conjugated estrogens, A or B); vulvar and vaginal atrophy (synthetic conjugated estrogens, A only).

Contraindications Known or suspected pregnancy; undiagnosed abnormal genital bleeding; known or suspected cancer of the breast (except in appropriately selected patients being treated for metastatic disease); known or suspected estrogen-dependent neoplasia; active thrombophlebitis or thromboembolic disorder; liver dysfunction or disease; hypersensitivity to estrogens.

Route/Dosage
Menopause
ADULTS: PO Synthetic conjugated estrogens, A: Start with 0.625 mg/day and titrate up to 1.25 mg/day based on response. Synthetic conjugated estrogens, B: Start with 0.625 mg/day, titrated dose based on patient response.

Vulvar and Vaginal Atrophy
ADULTS: PO Synthetic conjugated estrogens, A: 0.3 mg/day.

Interactions None well documented.

Lab Test Interferences Accelerated PT, PTT, and platelet aggregation with increased clotting factor activity; increased thyroid-binding globulin (TBG) with increased total circulating thyroid hormone; increased plasma HDL, reduced LDL cholesterol, and increased triglycerides; impaired glucose tolerance; reduced response to metyrapone test.

Adverse Reactions
CV: Palpitation.
CNS: Depression, dizziness, hypertonia, insomnia, nervousness, paresthesia, vertigo, headache, asthenia.
GI: Abdominal pain, constipation, diarrhea, dyspepsia, flatulence, nausea, vomiting.
GU: Breast pain, dysmenorrhea, vaginitis, metrorrhagia.
METAB: Peripheral edema.
MUSC: Arthralgia, myalgia.
RESP: Cough, pharyngitis, rhinitis, bronchitis, sinusitis.
OTHER: Back pain, fever, infection, pain, accidental injury, flu syndrome, leg cramps.

> **WARNING:**
> Estrogens increase the risk of endometrial cancer. Close clinical surveillance of all women taking estrogen is important.
>
> Compared with placebo, an increased risk of MI, stroke, deep vein thrombosis, pulmonary emboli, and invasive breast cancer were reported in postmenopausal women during 5 yr treatment with conjugated estrogens combined with medroxyprogesterone acetate.
>
> An increased risk of developing dementia was reported in postmenopausal women (65 yr of age or older) during 4 yr of treatment with oral conjugated estrogens plus medroxyprogesterone acetate compared with placebo. It is not known if these findings apply to younger postmenopausal women or women taking estrogens alone.

Precautions
Pregnancy: Not indicated during pregnancy or immediate postpartum period.
Lactation: May reduce quantity and quality of breast milk.
Children: Safety not established.
Special risk patients: Because asthma, diabetes mellitus, epilepsy, migraine, porphyria, systemic lupus erythematosus, and hepatic hemangiomas may be exacerbated by estrogens, use with caution.
Cancer: Increased frequency of carcinomas of breast, uterus, cervix, vagina, liver, and testis. Use of a progestin may reduce risk of endometrial hyperplasia.
Cardiovascular: Large doses may increase risk of MI, pulmonary embolism, and thrombophlebitis.
Cholestatic jaundice history: Use with caution and discontinue if there is recurrence.
Elevated BP: Substantial increases in BP have been attributed to idiosyncratic reactions to estrogens.
Endometriosis: May be exacerbated with administration of estrogens.
Fluid retention: Because estrogens may cause fluid retention, carefully monitor patients with conditions influenced by fluid retention (eg, cardiac or renal dysfunction).

Gallbladder: Increased risk of gallbladder disease requiring surgery.
Hypercalcemia: Estrogen administration may lead to severe hypercalcemia in patients with breast cancer and bone metastases.
Hypertriglyceridemia: Increased triglycerides in familial hyperlipoproteinemia.
Hypocalcemia: Use with caution.
Hypothyroidism: Estrogen administration leads to increased thyroid-binding globulin levels.
Impaired liver function: Estrogens may be poorly metabolized in patients with impaired liver function.
Ovarian cancer: Estrogen plus progestin has been reported to increase the risk of cancer.
Visual abnormalities: Retinal vascular thrombosis may occur, leading to loss of vision, sudden onset of proptosis, diplopia, or migraine.

PATIENT CARE CONSIDERATIONS

Administration/Storage

- Administer prescribed dose once daily without regard to meals.
- Administer with food if GI upset occurs.
- Store at controlled room temperature (59° to 86°F).

Assessment/Interventions

- Obtain patient history, including drug history and any known allergies. Note history of endometriosis, breast nodules, fibrocystic breast disease, abnormal mammogram, strong family history of breast cancer, cerebral vascular disease, coronary artery disease, epilepsy, asthma, hypertension, diabetes, hyperlipidemia, tobacco use, obesity, migraine headache, systemic lupus erythematosus, heart failure, hypothyroidism, depression, jaundice during previous pregnancy, liver or kidney impairment, metabolic bone disease, porphyria, hypocalcemia, gallbladder disease, or hypothyroidism.
- Review patient's health history for any condition that could contraindicate synthetic conjugated estrogens (eg, previous allergic reaction to either drug, known or suspected pregnancy, known or suspected cancer of the breast, known or suspected estrogen-dependent cancer, undiagnosed abnormal uterine bleeding, active or history of thromboembolic disorders or stroke, liver dysfunction or disease).
- Ensure breast, abdominal, and pelvic examination and Pap smear have been completed and documented before starting therapy and annually thereafter during prolonged therapy.
- Ensure progestin therapy is used in women with intact uterus to prevent endometrial hyperplasia.
- Monitor blood sugar in diabetic patient when drug is started or dose is changed. Report significant changes to health care provider.
- Assess BP at beginning of therapy and periodically during treatment.
- Assess patient for GU, GI, CNS, DERM, and general body side effects. Inform health care provider if noted and significant.
- Notify health care provider of pain, swelling, redness, or warmth in calves; sudden severe headache; visual disturbances; weakness or numbness of arms or legs; signs of liver dysfunction (eg, dark urine, jaundice); abdominal pain or tenderness, abdominal mass; or signs of depression.
- Consider discontinuing therapy during periods of prolonged immobilization and, if possible, 4 wk before surgery that is associated with an increased risk of thromboembolic disease.
- Ensure attempts are made q 3 to 6 mo to discontinue therapy or reduce the dose of medication.

Patient/Family Education

- Explain name, dose, action, and potential side effects of drug.
- Advise patient to review *Patient Information* leaflet before starting therapy and with each refill.
- Advise patient that dose may be adjusted periodically to obtain max benefits.
- Instruct patient to take as prescribed and to not change the dose or stop taking unless advised by health care provider.
- Advise patient that medication can be taken without regard to meals, but to take with food if GI upset occurs.
- Instruct diabetic patient to monitor blood glucose more frequently when drug is started or dose is changed and to inform health care provider of significant changes in readings.
- Advise patient that if a dose is missed, to take it as soon as remembered. However, if it is nearing time for the next dose, skip the missed dose and take only the next regularly scheduled dose. Advise patient to not double the dose to catch up.
- Instruct diabetic patient to monitor blood glucose more frequently when drug is started or dose is changed, and to inform health care provider of significant changes in readings.
- Review nonhormonal modalities that help prevent osteoporosis: 1,500 mg/day of calcium; vitamin D supplementation; exercise.
- Instruct patient to report the following symptoms to health care provider: pain in groin or calves; sharp chest pain or sudden shortness of breath; abnormal vaginal bleeding; breast lumps; sudden severe headache; dizziness or

fainting; vision or speech problems; weakness or numbness in arm or leg; severe abdominal pain; yellowing of skin or eyes; severe depression.
- Advise women to notify health care provider if pregnant, planning to become pregnant, or breastfeeding.
- Teach patient proper method of performing breast self-examination.
- Advise patient that follow-up visits and examinations, including Pap smear, at least once a year will be required to monitor therapy and to keep appointments.

Estrogens, Conjugated/ Medroxyprogesterone Acetate

(ESS-truh-janz, KAHN-juh-gay-tuhd/meh-DROX-ee-pro-JESS-tuh-rone a-sah-tate)

Class Sex hormones

How Supplied
Premphase Tablets 0.625 mg conjugated estrogens and 0.625 mg conjugated estrogens/5 mg medroxyprogesterone acetate ◆ Prempro Tablets 0.625 mg conjugated estrogens/5 mg medroxyprogesterone acetate, Tablets 0.625 mg conjugated estrogens/2.5 mg medroxyprogesterone acetate

Action
PHARMACOLOGY: Conjugated estrogens: promotes growth and development of female reproductive system and secondary sex characteristics; affects release of pituitary gonadotropins; inhibits ovulation and prevents postpartum breast engorgement; conserves calcium and phosphorous and encourages bone formation; overrides stimulatory effects of testosterone; progesterone: inhibits secretion of pituitary gonadotropins, thereby preventing follicular maturation and ovulation (contraceptive effect); inhibits spontaneous uterine contraction; transforms proliferative endometrium into secretory endometrium.

Indications Treatment of moderate-to-severe vasomotor symptoms associated with menopause; treatment of vulval and vaginal atrophy; osteoporosis prevention. **Unlabeled use(s):** Treatment of hypercholesterolemia in postmenopausal women.

Contraindications Do not use combined estrogens/progestins in conditions or circumstances of: 1) known or suspected pregnancy; 2) known or suspected cancer of the breast; 3) known or suspected estrogen-dependent neoplasm; 4) undiagnosed abnormal genital bleeding; 5) active or past history of thrombophlebitis; thromboembolic disorders, or stroke; 6) liver dysfunction or disease; 7) hypersensitivity to ingredients of tablets.

Route/Dosage
Menopause and Vulval/Vaginal Atrophy
Revaluate patient at 3- to 6-mo intervals to determine need for continued treatment.

Osteoporosis
Monitor women with intact uterus closely for signs of endometrial cancer, evaluate recurrent or persistent abnormal vaginal bleeding to rule out malignancy.

PREMPRO
ADULTS: PO One 0.625 mg conjugated estrogen/2.5 mg medroxyprogesterone once daily.

PREMPHASE
ADULTS: PO One 0.625 mg conjugated estrogen once daily on days 1 through 14 and one 0.625 mg conjugated estrogen/5 mg medroxyprogesterone once daily on days 15 through 28.

Interactions
Conjugated estrogens:
Barbiturates; rifamycins (eg, rifampin) – May decrease estrogen levels.
Corticosteroids – Pharmacologic and adverse effects of corticosteroids may be increased.
Hydantoins (eg, phenytoin) – Loss of seizure control or decreased estrogenic effects may occur.
Tricyclic antidepressants – Estrogens may alter effects and increase toxicity.
Medroxyprogesterone:
Aminoglutethimide – May increase metabolism and decrease effect of medroxyprogesterone.

Lab Test Interferences Endocrine and liver function test results may be affected; possible increased PT and increased platelet aggregability; increased thyroid binding globulin and total T_4; impaired glucose tolerance; increased corticosteroid binding globulin and sex-hormone binding globulin; increased plasma HDL concentration; reduced LDL cholesterol concentrations; increased triglyceride levels; reduced response to metyrapone test; reduced folate concentration.

Adverse Reactions
CV: Change in BP; thrombophlebitis; cerebral thrombosis and embolism; pulmonary embolism.
CNS: Headache; depression; dizziness; hypertonia; nervousness; migraine; chorea; insomnia; somnolence; change in libido.
DERM: Pruritus; rash; chloasma; erythema multiforme; erythema nodosum; hemorrhagic eruption; alopecia; hirsutism; itching; urticaria; acne.
EENT: Pharyngitis; rhinitis; sinusitis; retinal

thrombosis; optic neuritis; contact lenses intolerance.
GI: Abdominal pain and cramps; diarrhea; dyspepsia; flatulence; nausea; changes in appetite; vomiting; bloating.
GU: Breast pain; cervix disorder; dysmenorrhea; leukorrhea; vaginal hemorrhage; vaginitis; abnormal withdrawal bleeding or flow; breakthrough bleeding; spotting; changes in cervical secretion; premenstrual-like syndrome; cystitis-like syndrome; vaginal candidiasis; amenorrhea; changes in cervical erosion; breast tenderness and enlargement; galactorrhea.
HEPA: Cholestatic jaundice.
METAB: Peripheral edema; increase or decrease in weight; edema; reduced carbohydrate tolerance.
OTHER: Accidental injury; back pain; flu-like syndrome; infection; pain; pelvic pain; arthralgia; leg cramps; gallbladder disease; pancreatitis; fatigue; aggravation of porphyria; anaphylactoid reaction; anaphylaxis.

Precautions
Pregnancy: Category X.
Lactation: Excreted in breast milk.
Elevated blood pressure: Increased blood pressure during estrogen replacement has been attributed to idiosyncratic reactions.
Hypercalcemia: In patients with breast cancer or bone metastases, severe hypercalcemia has occurred with estrogen therapy.
Induction of malignant neoplasm: May increase risk of endometrial cancer or other carcinomas.
Gallbladder disease: Risk of gallbladder disease may increase in women receiving postmenopausal estrogens.
Visual abnormalities: Discontinue medication if there are any sudden changes in vision, sudden onset of proptosis, diplopia, migraine, papilledema, or retinal vascular lesions.
Fluid retention: Use with caution when conditions that might be affected by fluid retention are present (eg, asthma, cardiac, or renal dysfunction, epilepsy).
Uterine bleeding: Certain patients may develop abnormal uterine bleeding.
Familial hyperlipoproteinemia: May be associated with massive elevations of plasma triglycerides.
Depression: Carefully observe patients with history of depression.

Overdosage: Signs and Symptoms
Nausea, vomiting, withdrawal bleeding.

PATIENT CARE CONSIDERATIONS
Administration/Storage
- This product is to be used only in women with an intact uterus.
- Administer 1 tablet as prescribed every day, without regard to meals.
- Remove 1 tablet at a time from provided dispensing dial. When dial is empty, begin new dial the following day.
- Store at controlled room temperature. Do not remove tablet from dispensing dial until ready to administer.

Assessment/Interventions
- Obtain patient history, including drug history and any known allergies.
- Review patient's health history for any condition that could contraindicate conjugated estrogens/progesterone (previous allergic reaction to either drug, known or suspected pregnancy, known or suspected cancer of the breast, known or suspected estrogen-dependent cancer, undiagnosed abnormal uterine bleeding, active or past history of thromboembolic disorders or stroke, or liver dysfunction or disease).
- Ensure that breast, abdominal, and pelvic examination and Pap smear have been completed and documented before starting therapy.
- Monitor blood sugar in diabetic patient when drug is started or dose is changed. Report significant changes to health care provider.
- Assess BP at beginning of therapy and periodically during treatment.
- Notify health care provider of pain, swelling, redness, or warmth in calves; sudden severe headache; visual disturbances; weakness or numbness of arms or legs; signs of liver dysfunction (eg, dark urine, jaundice); or signs of depression.

Patient/Family Education
- Explain name, dose, action, and potential side effects of drug.
- Instruct patient to take 1 tablet every day from the dispensing dial.
- Advise patient that medication can be taken without regard to meals, but to take with food if GI upset occurs.
- Caution patient not to take tablets out of sequence and when dispensing dial is empty, to begin a new cycle of tablets the next day.
- Advise patient to keep tablets in provided plastic dispensing device until dose is needed.
- Caution patient to not change brands without consulting health care provider. Products made by different companies may not be equally effective.
- Instruct diabetic patient to monitor blood glucose more frequently when drug is started or dose is changed and to inform health care provider of significant changes in readings.
- Review nonhormonal modalities, which help

prevent osteoporosis: 1500 mg/day of calcium; vitamin D supplementation; and exercise.
* Instruct patient to report these symptoms to health care provider: pain in groin or calves; sharp chest pain or sudden shortness of breath; abnormal vaginal bleeding; breast lumps; sudden severe headache; dizziness or fainting; vision or speech problems; weakness or numbness of arms or legs; severe abdominal pain; yellowing of skin or eyes; or severe depression.
* Instruct patients to notify health care provider if they become pregnant, plan on becoming pregnant, or are breastfeeding.
* Teach patient proper method of breast self-examination.
* Advise patient that follow-up visits and examinations, including Pap smear, at least once a year will be required to monitor therapy and to keep appointments.

Estropipate (Piperazine Estrone Sulfate)

(ESS-troe-PIH-pate)

Class Estrogens

How Supplied
Ogen Tablets 0.625 mg, Tablets 1.25 mg, Tablets 2.5 mg sodium estrone sulfate ♦ *Ortho-Est* Tablets 0.625 mg, Tablets 1.25 mg sodium estrone sulfate

Action
PHARMACOLOGY: Promotes growth and development of female reproductive system and secondary sex characteristics; affects release of ovulation and prevents postpartum breast engorgement; conserves calcium and phosphorous and encourages bone formation; overrides stimulatory effects of testosterone.

PHARMACOKINETICS/DYNAMICS:
Absorption: Well absorbed from the GI tract.
Distribution: Largely bound to sex hormone-binding globulin and albumin. Crosses the placenta.
Metabolism: Undergoes first-pass metabolism. Metabolic conversion occurs primarily in the liver, but also at local target tissue sites. Also undergoes enterohepatic recirculation.
Excretion: A certain portion is excreted into the bile and then reabsorbed from the intestine. Excreted in the urine as conjugates.

Indications Management of moderate to severe vasomotor symptoms associated with menopause; female hypogonadism, female castration, primary ovarian failure, and atrophic conditions caused by deficient endogenous estrogen production; prevention and treatment of osteoporosis.

Contraindications Breast cancer; estrogen-dependent neoplasia; undiagnosed abnormal genital bleeding; thrombophlebitis or thromboembolic disorders associated with previous estrogen use; known or suspected pregnancy.

Route/Dosage
Dosage is calculated as estrone sulfate.

Vasomotor Symptoms
ADULTS: PO 0.625 to 5 mg/day given cyclically.
Female Hypogonadism, Female Castration, Primary Ovarian Failure
ADULTS: PO 1.25 to 7.5 mg/day for 3 wk followed by 8 to 10 day drug-free period.

Osteoporosis
ADULTS: PO 0.625 mg/day for 25 days of 31-day cycle.

Atrophic Vaginitis, Kraurosis Vulvae
ADULTS: PO 0.625 to 5 mg/day. Give cyclically.
Intravaginal 2 to 4 g/day. Give cyclically.

Interactions
Antidepressants, tricyclic: Estrogens may alter effects and increase toxicity of these agents.
Barbiturates, modafinil, rifampin, St. John's wort, topiramate: May decrease estropipate concentration.
Corticosteroids: An increase in the pharmacologic and toxicologic effects of corticosteroids may occur.
Hydantoins: Loss of seizure control or decreased estrogenic effects may occur.

Lab Test Interferences Endocrine and LFT results may be affected; possible decreased PT and increased platelet aggregability; increased thyroid-binding globulin and total T_4; impaired glucose tolerance; decreased serum folate concentration; increased serum triglyceride and phospholipid concentrations; increased corticosteroid binding globulin and sex-hormone binding globulin; increased plasma HDL concentrations; reduced LDL cholesterol concentrations; increased triglyceride levels.

Adverse Reactions
CV: Thrombosis; thrombophlebitis; increased BP; pulmonary embolism; MI.
CNS: Headache; migraine; dizziness; depression; insomnia; anxiety; emotional lability.
DERM: Chloasma; melasma; erythema nodosum/multiforme; scalp hair loss; hirsutism; urticaria; dermatitis; skin hypertrophy; pruritus.
EENT: Intolerance to contact lenses.
GI: Nausea; vomiting; abdominal cramps; bloating; colitis; acute pancreatitis; diarrhea; dyspep-

sia; flatulence; gastritis; gastroenteritis; enlarged abdomen; hemorrhoids.

GU: Increased risk of endometrial carcinoma; breakthrough bleeding; dysmenorrhea; amenorrhea; vaginal candidiasis; premenstrual-like syndrome; increased size of uterine fibromyomata; hemolytic uremic syndrome; urinary tract infection; vaginitis; vaginal discomfort/pain; cystitis; dysuria; genital pruritus; urinary incontinence.

HEPA: Cholestatic jaundice.

METAB: Hyperglycemia; hypercalcemia.

RESP: Upper respiratory tract infection; sinusitis; rhinitis; pharyngitis; flu-like symptoms; allergy; bronchitis; chest pain.

OTHER: Increase or decrease in weight; edema; changes in libido; breast tenderness; acute intermittent porphyria; vaginal bleeding; hypersensitivity reactions; back pain; arthritis; arthralgia; hot flushes; otitis media; toothache.

Precautions

Pregnancy: Category X.

Lactation: Excreted in breast milk.

Children: Safety and efficacy not established.

Hepatic function impairment: Metabolism may be impaired; use drug with caution.

Calcium and phosphorus metabolism: Use drug with caution in patients with metabolic bone diseases.

Cardiovascular and other risks: Compared with placebo, increased risks of MI, stroke, deep vein thrombosis, pulmonary emboli, and invasive breast cancer were reported in postmenopausal women during 5 yr of treatment with conjugated equine estrogens combined with medroxyprogesterone acetate. Other combinations of estrogens and progestins were not studied; however, in the absence of comparable data, assume these risks to be similar.

Fluid retention: Use drug with careful observation when conditions that might be affected by this factor are present (eg, asthma, cardiac or renal dysfunction, epilepsy).

Gallbladder disease: Risk of gallbladder disease may increase in women receiving postmenopausal estrogens.

Induction of malignant neoplasms: May increase risk of endometrial or other carcinomas.

Familial hyperlipoproteinemia: May be associated with massive elevations of plasma triglycerides.

Uterine leiomyomata: Preexisting uterine leiomyomata may increase in size.

Unopposed estrogen administration (eg, without progesterone): Increases risk of uterine cancer. Therefore, when using estrogens on long-term basis in a woman with intact uterus, consider cyclic therapy with progesterone (eg, estrogen on days 1 to 25 of mo with progesterone added for last 12 days) or daily coadministration of estrogen plus progesterone on daily basis. In a woman without uterus, use of cyclic therapy and/or therapy with progesterone is not necessary.

Overdosage: Signs and Symptoms

Nausea, withdrawal bleeding in women.

PATIENT CARE CONSIDERATIONS

Administration/Storage

- Administer vaginal cream high in vagina (approximately ⅔ length of applicator).
- Give tablets with meal to decrease GI upset.

Assessment/Interventions

- Obtain patient history, including drug history and any known allergies.
- Include in physical assessments BP measurements, and examination of breasts, abdomen, and pelvic organs. Review results of Pap test, which should be conducted at least annually.
- Monitor blood sugar in diabetic patients and report changes to health care provider.
- Be alert for changes in LFT results and possible decreased PT.

Patient/Family Education

- Caution patient that this medication must not be taken during pregnancy or when pregnancy is possible. Advise patient to use reliable form of birth control while taking this drug.
- Instruct patient to report these symptoms to health care provider: pain in groin or calves; sharp chest pain or sudden shortness of breath; abnormal vaginal bleeding; breast lumps; sudden severe headache; dizziness or fainting; vision or speech problems; weakness or numbness of arms or legs; severe abdominal pain; yellowing of skin or eyes; or severe depression.
- Advise patient to stop smoking or to reduce number of cigarettes smoked to less than 15/day because of increased risk of cardiovascular complications.
- Remind patient to have Pap smear q 6 to 12 mo while undergoing therapy.
- Teach patient proper method of breast self-examination.
- Advise patient to avoid prolonged exposure to sunlight or other sources of UV light. Sunscreens and protective clothing should be used until tolerance is determined.

Etanercept

(EE-tan-err-sept)

Class Immunomodulator

How Supplied
Enbrel Powder for injection, lyophilized 25 mg

Action
PHARMACOLOGY: Binds specifically to tumor necrosis factor (TNF), blocks its interaction with cell surface TNF receptors, and modulates biological responses that are induced or regulated by TNF.

PHARMACOKINETICS/DYNAMICS:

Absorption: C_{max} is approximately 1.1 mcg/mL. T_{max} is approximately 69 hr (single dose). C_{max} increases 2- to 7-fold, while AUC increases approximately 4-fold with repeated dosing.

Excretion: The t½ is approximately 102 hr. Cl is approximately 160 mL/hr.

Special Populations:
Children –
4 to 8 yr: Cl is slightly reduced.

Indications
Reducing signs and symptoms and inhibiting the progression of structural damage in moderately to severely active rheumatoid arthritis; reducing signs and symptoms of moderately to severely active polyarticular-course juvenile rheumatoid arthritis (JRA) in patients responding inadequately to 1 or more disease-modifying antirheumatic drugs; reducing signs and symptoms of psoriatic arthritis; reducing signs and symptoms in patients with active ankylosing spondylitis. May be used in combination with methotrexate (MTX) in patients who do not respond adequately to MTX alone in the treatment of rheumatoid or psoriatic arthritis.

Unlabeled use(s): Psoriasis; treatment of Wegener granulomatosis (orphan status).

Contraindications Sepsis; hypersensitivity to etanercept or to any of its components.

Route/Dosage
ADULTS: SC 50 mg/wk, given as two 25 mg injections at separate sites on the same day or 3 or 4 days apart.

CHILDREN (4 TO 17 YR): SC 0.8 mg/kg (max, 50 mg) per wk given. For patients weighing more than 31 kg, give the weekly dose as 2 injections, either on the same day or separated by 3 or 4 days.

Interactions None well documented. However, a 7% rate of serious infections was observed in a 24-wk study with patients receiving etanercept and anakinra therapy.

Lab Test Interferences None well documented.

Adverse Reactions
CV: Heart failure; MI; myocardial ischemia; hypertension; hypotension; deep vein thrombosis; thrombophlebitis.
Postmarketing – Chest pain vasodilation (flushing); new-onset CHF.
CNS: Headache (24%); dizziness (8%); hydrocephalus; seizure; stroke; cerebral ischemia; multiple sclerosis; depression.
JRA patients – Personality disorder; aseptic meningitis.
Postmarketing – Paresthesias; isolated demyelinating conditions (eg, transverse myelitis, optic neuritis).
DERM: Rash (14%); alopecia (6%).
JRA patients – Cutaneous ulcer.
Postmarketing in pediatric patients – Cutaneous vasculitis.
Postmarketing – Cutaneous vasculitis; pruritus; SC nodules; urticaria.
EENT: Rhinitis (16%); pharyngitis (7%); sinusitis (5%).
Postmarketing in pediatric patients – Optic neuritis.
Postmarketing – Dry eyes; ocular inflammation.
GI: Nausea (15%); dyspepsia (11%); abdominal pain (10%); mouth ulcer (6%); vomiting (5%); GI bleeding; cholecystitis; pancreatitis; GI hemorrhage.
JRA patients – Gastroenteritis; esophagitis/gastritis.
Postmarketing – Anorexia; altered sense of taste; diarrhea; dry mouth; intestinal perforation.
GU: Membranous glomerulonephropathy.
Postmarketing in pediatric patients – UTI.
HEMA/LYMPH: Pancytopenia.
Postmarketing in pediatric patients – Coagulopathy.
Postmarketing – Adenopathy; anemia; aplastic anemia; leukopenia; neutropenia; thrombocytopenia.
LABTESTSABS:
Postmarketing in pediatric patients – Transaminase elevations.
LOCAL: Injection site reactions (37%).
M/N:
JRA patients – Type I diabetes mellitus.
Postmarketing – Weight gain.
MUSC: Bursitis; polymyositis.
Postmarketing – Joint pain; lupus-like syndrome.
RESP: Upper respiratory tract infections (31%); cough (6%); respiratory disorder (5%); pulmonary embolism; dyspnea.
Postmarketing – Interstitial lung disease; pulmonary disease; worsening of prior lung disorder.
OTHER: Non-upper respiratory tract infections (51%); asthenia (11%); peripheral edema (8%).
JRA patients – Group A streptococcal septic

shock; soft tissue and postoperative wound infection; varicella infection.
Postmarketing in pediatric patients: Abscess with bacteremia; tuberculous arthritis.
Postmarketing: Angioedema; fatigue; fever; flu-like symptoms; generalized pain; sepsis; death.

Precautions

Pregnancy: Category B.
Lactation: Undetermined.
Children: Safety and efficacy not established in children younger than 4 yr.
Elderly: Because there is a higher incidence of infection in the elderly, use with caution.
Autoimmunity: Formation of autoantibodies (eg, ANA, new positive anti-double-stranded DNA) and, rarely, development of lupus-like syndrome may occur.
Heart failure: Worsening of CHF, with and without identifiable precipitating factors, has been reported postmarketing.
Immunizations: If possible, JRA patients should be brought up-to-date with all immunizations in agreement with current guidelines prior to initiating therapy. Patients with significant exposure to varicella virus should temporarily discontinue therapy and be considered for prophylactic treatment with varicella zoster immune globulin.
Benzyl alcohol: The diluent preservative contains benzyl alcohol, which has been associated with fatal gasping syndrome in premature infants.
Hematologic: Rare and sometimes fatal cases of pancytopenia, including aplastic anemia, reported.
Infections: Serious infections and sepsis, including death, may occur. Do not initiate treatment in patients with active infections, including chronic or localized infections. Rare cases of tuberculosis (TB) have been observed.
Injection site reactions: Mild to moderate injection site reactions (eg, erythema, itching, swelling) may occur.
Neurologic events: Agents that inhibit TNF have been associated with rare cases of new-onset or exacerbation of CNS demyelinating disorders, some presenting with mental status changes and some associated with permanent disability; transverse myelitis, optic neuritis, multiple sclerosis, and new onset or exacerbation of seizure disorders have been observed.
Vaccinations: Do not give live virus vaccines concomitantly with etanercept.

PATIENT CARE CONSIDERATIONS

Administration/Storage

- Administer via SC route only. Not for intradermal, IM, or IV administration.
- Administer dose for adult or pediatric patient weighing more than 68 pounds as 2 injections at separate sites. Injections can either be given together on the same day once weekly, or as single injections separated by 3 or 4 days.
- Administer dose for pediatric patient weighing 68 pounds or less as a single injection once weekly.
- Reconstitute powder following manufacturer's instructions using supplied diluent only. To prevent excessive foaming, inject diluent slowly into medication vial and swirl gently to dissolve. Do not shake or vigorously agitate medication vial. Complete dissolution may take up to 10 min.
- Reconstituted solution should be clear and colorless and administered within 14 days of reconstitution.
- Do not administer if particulate matter, cloudiness, or discoloration is noted.
- Withdraw prescribed dose into syringe for injection. Do not filter reconstituted solution. Do not mix contents with or transfer to another vial of etanercept.
- Rotate injection sites (eg, thigh, abdomen, upper arm). Give new injections at least 1 inch or more from old site and never into areas where the skin is tender, bruised, red, or hard.
- Do not add other medications to etanercept nor reconstitute with other diluents.
- MTX, glucocorticoids, salicylates, NSAIDs, and analgesics may be continued during treatment with etanercept.
- Store etanercept dose tray in refrigerator (36° to 46°F). Do not freeze. Use reconstituted solution immediately or store in refrigerator for up to 14 days. Discard solution if not used within 14 days.

Assessment/Interventions

- Obtain patient history, including drug history and any known allergies. Note any findings suggestive of active infection. Note history of recurrent infections, poorly controlled diabetes, hematologic abnormalities, tuberculosis, heart failure, immunosuppression, or preexisting or recent onset of CNS demyelinating disorder.
- Document baseline disease state activity (eg, number of tender or swollen joints, pain, disability). Reassess periodically to document response to therapy.
- Ensure that patients with JRA are brought up-to-date with all immunizations in agreement with current guidelines prior to initiating therapy if possible.

- Monitor patient for signs and symptoms of blood dyscrasias or infection (eg, persistent fever, sore throat, unusual bruising, bleeding, pallor). Immediately report to health care provider if noted.
- Monitor patient for signs and symptoms of anaphylactic or serious allergic reactions. Be prepared to treat appropriately.
- Monitor patient for CNS, GI, RESP, CV, general body side effects, and injection-site reactions. Report to health care provider if noted and significant.
- Do not administer live virus vaccines to patient receiving etanercept.

Patient/Family Education
- Advise patient, family, or caregiver to read *Patient Information* brochure before starting therapy and with each refill.
- Explain name, dose, action, and potential side effects of drug. If patient or caregiver will be administering at home, review *How to Use Enbrel* and *Instructions for Preparing and Giving an Injection* insert with the patient or caregiver. Ensure that the patient or caregiver understands how to store, prepare, and administer the dose, and how to dispose of used equipment and supplies. Perform the first injection under the supervision of a qualified health care professional.
- Caution patient not to change the dose or discontinue therapy unless advised by health care provider.
- Advise patient that if a dose is missed to contact health care provider for instructions about when to take the next dose.
- Advise patient to continue other arthritis medications as recommended by health care provider.
- Advise patient to immediately report any of the following symptoms to health care provider: fever or other signs of infection, sore throat, unusual bruising or bleeding.
- Advise patient to report intolerable injection site reactions or unusual symptoms to health care provider.
- Advise women to notify health care provider if pregnant, planning to become pregnant, or breastfeeding.
- Instruct patient not to take any prescription or OTC medications or dietary supplements unless advised by health care provider.
- Advise patient that office visits and laboratory tests will be required to monitor therapy and to keep appointments.

Ethacrynic Acid (Ethacrynate)

(eth-uh-KRIN-ik acid)

Class Loop diuretic

How Supplied
Edecrin Tablets 25 mg, Tablets 50 mg ◆ *Edecrin Sodium* Powder for injection 50 mg (as ethacrynate sodium) per vial

Action
PHARMACOLOGY: Inhibits reabsorption of sodium and chloride in proximal and distal tubules and in loop of Henle.

PHARMACOKINETICS/DYNAMICS:
Absorption: Approximately 100% bioavailable.
Excretion: The $t_{1/2}$ is 60 to 90 min (oral).
Onset: Within 30 min (oral), 5 min (IV).
Peak: 2 hr (oral), 15 to 30 min (IV).
Duration: 6 to 8 hr (oral), 30 to 60 min (IV).

Indications Treatment of edema associated with CHF, hepatic cirrhosis, or renal disease; treatment of ascites, congenital heart disease, nephrotic syndrome. **Unlabeled use(s):** Treatment of glaucoma; treatment of nephrogenic diabetes insipidus, hypercalcemia.

Contraindications Anuria; infants; increasing azotemia; severe diarrhea; dehydration; electrolyte imbalance; hypotension.

Route/Dosage
ADULTS: **PO** 50 to 200 mg qd. **IV** 50 mg (0.5 to 1 mg/kg) qd.
CHILDREN: **PO** 25 mg qd.

Interactions
Aminoglycosides: May increase auditory toxicity.
Cisplatin: May cause additive ototoxicity.
Digitalis glycosides: Electrolyte disturbances may predispose to digitalis-induced atrial and ventricular arrhythmias.
Lithium: May increase plasma lithium levels and toxicity.
NSAIDs: May decrease effects of ethacrynic acid.
Salicylates: May impair diuretic response in patients with cirrhosis and ascites.
Thiazide diuretics: Synergistic effects may result in profound diuresis and serious electrolyte abnormalities.

Lab Test Interferences None well documented.

Adverse Reactions
CV: Orthostatic hypotension; emboli.
CNS: Apprehension; confusion; fatigue; malaise; vertigo; headache; dysphagia.
DERM: Rash.
EENT: Blurred vision; sense of ear fullness; tinnitus; hearing loss.

GI: Anorexia; nausea; vomiting; diarrhea; pancreatitis; discomfort; pain; sudden watery, profuse diarrhea; bleeding.
GU: Hematuria.
HEMA: Neutropenia; thrombocytopenia; agranulocytosis; hyponatremia; hypokalemia; hypomagnesemia; hypocalcemia; hypercalciuria; hypovolemia.
HEPA: Jaundice; abnormal LFTs.
METAB: Acute gout; hyperuricemia; hyperglycemia.
OTHER: Fever; chills; local irritation and pain with parenteral administration.

Precautions
Pregnancy: Category B.
Lactation: Undetermined.
Children: Safety and efficacy not established in infants (see Contraindications) and in children (IV).
Photosensitivity: May occur.

Dehydration: Excessive diuresis may cause dehydration and decreased blood volume with circulatory collapse and possible vascular thrombosis and embolism, especially in elderly.
Electrolyte imbalance: May be more likely in patients receiving large doses with restricted salt intake.
Hepatic cirrhosis and ascites: Sudden alterations of electrolyte balance may precipitate hepatic encephalopathy and coma.
Ototoxicity: Associated with rapid injection, very large doses or concurrent use of other ototoxic drugs.
Systemic lupus erythematosus: May be exacerbated or activated.

Overdosage: Signs and Symptoms
Water loss, volume depletion, electrolyte depletion, circulatory collapse, vascular thrombosis and embolism, weakness, dizziness, confusion, anorexia, lethargy, vomiting, cramps.

PATIENT CARE CONSIDERATIONS
Administration/Storage
- Administer drug PO or IV only. SC or IM injection causes local pain and irritation.
- To prepare IV solution, add 50 mL of D5W or normal saline. If solution is hazy or opalescent, do not use.
- For IV dose, administer drug slowly. Rotate injection sites to avoid thrombophlebitis.
- Discard reconstituted solution if not used within 24 hr.
- Do not administer drug with other drugs or with blood products.
- Do not give with other ototoxic drugs.
- Give oral medication after meal or with food to prevent GI upset.
- Avoid administering within 6 to 8 hr of bedtime to avoid nocturia.

Assessment/Interventions
- Obtain patient history, including drug history and any known allergies.
- Obtain baseline BUN, creatinine, potassium, and sodium chloride, and monitor daily.
- Closely monitor blood glucose.
- Monitor I&O and obtain daily weight.
- Assess patient for signs of GI bleeding.
- Monitor CBC and differential daily.
- Obtain BP and pulse before and during treatment, observing for orthostatic hypotension.
- Assess neurologic status prior to administering drug and during treatment.
- If severe, watery diarrhea occurs, report to health care provider.

- If signs of ototoxicity (eg, ear fullness, tinnitus, vertigo, hearing loss) occur, slow rate of IV injection.
- If patient develops anuria, hematuria, increases in BUN or creatinine or significant changes in electrolytes, report to health care provider.
- If signs of dehydration develop (eg, hypotension, tachycardia, postural hypotension, rapid weight loss, decreased filling pressures), notify health care provider.
- If patient shows change in LOC or mentation, notify health care provider.
- If patient is elderly or debilitated, observe for possible dehydration.

Patient/Family Education
- Tell patient to take drug with food or milk.
- Instruct patient to take drug in morning.
- Advise patient to avoid exposure to sunlight or UV light and to use sunscreen or wear protective clothing to avoid photosensitivity reaction.
- Caution patient to avoid sudden position changes to prevent orthostatic hypotension.
- Instruct patient to report these symptoms to health care provider: confusion or mood changes, increased thirst, dizziness, irregular heart beat, weakness or increased tiredness, diarrhea, blood in urine or stool, muscle weakness or cramps, sudden joint pain or any changes in hearing.
- Advise patients with diabetes mellitus to monitor blood glucose levels closely.

Ethambutol Hydrochloride

(eth-AM-byoo-tahl HIGH-droe-KLOR-ide)

Class Anti-infective/Antitubercular

How Supplied
Myambutol Tablets 100 mg, Tablets 400 mg

Action
PHARMACOLOGY: Inhibits synthesis of 1 or more metabolites, causing impairment of cell metabolism, arrest of multiplication, and cell death.

PHARMACOKINETICS/DYNAMICS:
Absorption: The T_{max} is reached in 2 to 4 hr.
Metabolism: Primarily metabolized in the liver to a dicarboxylic acid derivative.
Excretion: Approximately 50% excreted unchanged in the urine; 8% to 15% excreted as metabolites; 20% to 22% excreted unchanged in the feces.

Indications
Treatment of pulmonary tuberculosis in combination with 1 or more other antituberculous agents.

Contraindications
Patients with known optic neuritis; hypersensitivity to any component of the product.

Route/Dosage
ADULTS AND CHILDREN (13 YR AND OLDER): PO In patients not previously treated with antituberculous therapy, administer 15 mg/kg as a single dose every 24 hr. In patients who have received previous antituberculous treatment, administer 25 mg/kg as a single dose every 24 hr.

Interactions
Aluminum salts (eg, aluminum hydroxide): The absorption of ethambutol may be delayed or reduced; separate the administration times by several hours.

Lab Test Interferences None well documented.

Adverse Reactions
CNS: Malaise; headache; dizziness; mental confusion; disorientation; possible hallucinations; numbness and tingling of extremities.
EENT: Decreased visual acuity.
GI: Anorexia; nausea; vomiting; GI upset; abdominal pain.
HEMA: Eosinophilia.
HEPA: Transient liver function impairment.
METAB: Elevated serum uric acid; precipitation of acute gout.
RESP: Pulmonary infiltrates.
OTHER: Hypersensitivity (including anaphylactoid reactions; dermatitis; pruritus); fever; joint pain.

Precautions
Pregnancy: Category B.
Children: Safety and efficacy not established in children under 13 yr.
Renal function impairment: Reduced dosage is necessary.
Visual effects: Unilateral or bilateral changes in visual acuity may occur. Evaluation of changes is more difficult in patients with visual defects such as cataracts, diabetic retinopathy, or optic neuritis.

PATIENT CARE CONSIDERATIONS

Administration/Storage
- Administer prescribed dose once daily without regard to meals.
- Administer with food if GI upset occurs.
- Directly observe that patient swallows prescribed dose.
- Store tablets at controlled room temperature (59° to 86°F).

Assessment/Interventions
- Obtain patient history, including drug history and any known allergies. Note history of renal impairment or optic neuritis.
- Assess mycobacterial studies and susceptibility tests before and periodically throughout therapy to detect possible resistance.
- Ensure that a reduced dose is administered based on serum levels in patients with renal impairment.
- Ensure that 1 or more other antituberculosis agents are being used concurrently.
- Ensure that ophthalmoscopy, finger perimetry, and color discrimination are evaluated prior to and periodically during therapy.
- Ensure that renal function, liver enzymes, and CBC are determined prior to starting therapy and periodically thereafter.
- Monitor patient for GI, CNS, and general body side effects. Inform health care provider if noted and significant.

Patient/Family Education
- Explain name, dose, action, and potential side effects of drug.
- Review dosing schedule and prescribed length of therapy with patient.
- Emphasize to patient that treatment will be lengthy and that the entire course of treatment must be completed to avoid relapse or development of resistance.
- Advise patient to take each dose without regard to meals, but to take with food if GI upset occurs.
- Instruct patient to immediately report the following to health care provider: change in vision, visual abnormalities.

- Advise women to contact health care provider if pregnant, planning to become pregnant, or breastfeeding.
- Instruct patient to not take any prescription or OTC medications or dietary supplements unless advised by health care provider.
- Advise patient that follow-up visits and lab tests will be required to monitor therapy and to keep appointments.

Ethchlorvynol

(eth-klor-VIH-nahl)

Class Sedative and hypnotic/Nonbarbiturate

How Supplied
Placidyl Capsules 200 mg, Capsules 500 mg, Capsules 750 mg

Action
PHARMACOLOGY: Unknown; produces CNS depressant effects similar to those of barbiturates.

PHARMACOKINETICS/DYNAMICS:
Absorption: Rapidly adsorbed. T_{max} is within 2 hr.
Distribution: Distributed extensively to tissues, particularly adipose. Also detected in liver, kidneys, spleen, brain, bile, and CSF.
Metabolism: Major metabolite is secondary alcohol of ethchlorvynol. Undergoes enterohepatic recirculation.
Excretion: Plasma $t_{1/2}$ is approximately 10 to 20 hr. 33% excreted in the urine, mostly as metabolites.
Onset: Within 15 min to 1 hr.
Duration: 5 hr.

Indications Short-term therapy in management of insomnia (up to 1 wk). **Unlabeled use(s):** Sedation.

Contraindications Porphyria.

Route/Dosage
ADULTS: **PO** 500 to 1000 mg at bedtime. If patient awakens in early morning, give additional 200 mg.

Interactions
Alcohol and CNS depressants: Enhances CNS depressant effects.
Anticoagulants: May decrease anticoagulant activity.

Lab Test Interferences None well documented.

PATIENT CARE CONSIDERATIONS
Administration/Storage
- Obtain baseline vital signs before administering drug. If respiratory rate is lower than 12 to 14 breaths/min, do not administer medication.
- Administer with snack and full glass of water, milk, or fruit juice to reduce potential giddiness and ataxia.

Adverse Reactions
CV: Hypotension.
CNS: Dizziness; facial numbness; paradoxical reaction (eg, excitement, restlessness).
EENT: Blurred vision.
GI: Nausea; vomiting; gastric upset; unpleasant taste in mouth.
HEMA: Thrombocytopenia.
OTHER: Hangover; muscle weakness; symptoms of acute toxicity (eg, low body temperature, shortness of breath, slow heart beat); symptoms of chronic toxicity (eg, confusion, slurred speech, double vision, tingling, trembling, staggering); hypersensitivity reactions (eg, rash, itching, cholestatic jaundice).

Precautions
Pregnancy: Category C.
Lactation: Undetermined.
Children: Safety and efficacy not established.
Elderly: Should receive smallest effective dose.
Renal function impairment: Use with caution.
Hepatic function impairment: Use with caution.
Tartrazine sensitivity: Some products contain tartrazine, which may cause allergic-type reactions in susceptible individuals.
Dependency: Do not administer for periods over 1 wk. Prolonged use may lead to tolerance or physical and psychological dependence; withdrawal symptoms (eg, intoxication, tremors, slurred speech, diplopia, muscle weakness) may occur after prolonged use. Use with caution or avoid in patients with history of drug/alcohol abuse.
Mental depression: Use with caution in depressed patients with or without suicidal tendencies.

Overdosage: Signs and Symptoms
Respiratory depression, hypotension, somnolence, confusion, shock, constricted pupils, tachycardia, edema, hepatic dysfunction, coma.

- Instruct patient to swallow capsule whole and not to chew.
- Supplemental dose of 200 mg may be given if patient reawakens during early morning hrs following bedtime dose.
- Store in tightly closed, light-resistant container at room temperature.

Assessment/Interventions

- Obtain patient history, including drug history and any known allergies. Note use of CNS depressants or anticoagulants, drug or alcohol abuse, depression, suicidal tendencies, porphyria, renal or liver disease, and hypersensitivity reactions, especially to ethchlorvynol, aspirin, and tartrazine.
- Assess usual sleep patterns, nature of sleep disturbance and drug effectiveness.
- Provide pain-relieving measures prior to administering drug to patient experiencing pain.
- Adjust dosage of anticoagulants at initiation and discontinuance of treatment.
- Enhance effectiveness of drug by encouraging usual sleep patterns and routines.
- Provide relaxing environment that facilitates sleep induction.
- Eliminate stimuli that inhibit sleep.
- Utilize safety precautions to prevent injury such as keeping bed in low position with siderails up.
- Inform patient to call for assistance when getting up in the night because patient may experience dizziness.
- Monitor coagulation laboratory results if patient is taking anticoagulants.
- Observe for side effects such as hypotension, dizziness, weakness, unpleasant aftertaste, hangover, vomiting, or paradoxical reaction.
- In patients receiving daytime sedation, report appearance of mental confusion, hallucinations or drowsiness to health care provider.

Patient/Family Education

- Instruct patient that drug is for short-term use only and that its use can lead to tolerance and physical and psychological dependency.
- Warn patient that if drug is taken for more than 2 wk, withdrawal symptoms may be experienced.
- Instruct patient on how drug should be taken and that it should be taken in prescribed dose only.
- Inform patient that some side effects can be reduced if drug is taken with food.
- If medication is to be taken at bedtime, remind patient to take before midnight. Explain that if medication is being used as sedative it should not be taken in middle of night or early in morning.
- Instruct patient to report these symptoms to health care provider: visual changes, irregular heart beats, chest pains, yellowing of skin and eyes, rash, unusual bleeding or bruising.
- Instruct patient to avoid intake of alcoholic beverages or other CNS depressants.
- Advise patient that drug may cause drowsiness and to use caution while driving or performing other tasks requiring mental alertness.

Ethinyl Estradiol/Levonorgestrel

(ETH-in-ill ess-trah-DIE-ole/LEE-voe-nor-JESS-truhl)

Class Contraceptive/Hormone

How Supplied
Preven Tablets Ethinyl estradiol 0.05 mg; levonorgestrel 0.25 mg

Action
PHARMACOLOGY: Inhibits ovulation. May also impair tubal transport of sperm or ova (inhibiting fertilization) or altering the endometrium (inhibiting implantation). Not effective for a woman who is already pregnant.

Indications Prevention of pregnancy in women after known or suspected contraceptive failure or unprotected intercourse.

Contraindications The following contraindications for daily cyclical oral contraceptives may or may not apply to emergency contraception: known or suspected pregnancy; current or history of pulmonary embolism; current or history of ischemic heart disease; history of cerebrovascular accidents; valvular heart disease with complications; severe hypertension; diabetes mellitus with vascular involvement; headaches with focal neurological symptoms; major surgery with prolonged immobilization; known or suspected carcinoma of the breast or personal history of breast cancer; benign or malignant liver tumors; or active liver disease.

Route/Dosage
ADULT AND POSTPUBERTAL FEMALES: Pregnancy test is used to verify presence or absence of pregnancy. Medication is not given if the patient is already pregnant. PO 2 tablets as soon as possible but within 72 hr of unprotected intercourse. Repeat with the remaining 2 tablets in 12 hr. May be used at any time during the menstrual cycle.

Interactions None well documented.

Lab Test Interferences None well documented.

Adverse Reactions
CNS: Headache; dizziness.
GI: Nausea; vomiting; abdominal pain or cramps.
GU: Menstrual irregularities; breast tenderness.

Precautions
Pregnancy: No significant effects on fetal development associated with long-term use before

pregnancy or when taken inadvertently during early pregnancy.
Lactation: Secreted into breast milk.
Children: Use before menarche not recommended.

Ethionamide

(eh-THIGH-ohn-ah-mide)
Class Anti-infective/Antitubercular
How Supplied
Trecator-SC Tablets 250 mg

Action
PHARMACOLOGY: Inhibition of peptide synthesis in susceptible organisms is suspected.

PHARMACOKINETICS/DYNAMICS:
Absorption: Essentially completely absorbed.
Distribution: Ethionamide is approximately 30% bound to plasma protein. It is widely distributed into tissues and fluids with significant concentrations found in cerebrospinal fluid. Concentrations approximating the therapeutic range are usually seen within 2 hr following doses of 250 to 500 mg.
Metabolism: Ethionamide is extensively metabolized in the liver to active and inactive metabolites.
Excretion: The plasma elimination t½ is approximately 2 hr. Less than 1% is excreted unchanged in the urine.

Indications Treatment of tuberculosis, in combination with other agents, in patients with *Mycobacterium tuberculosis* resistant to isoniazid or rifampin, or when there is intolerance to other antituberculous agents.

Contraindications Severe hepatic impairment; hypersensitivity to any component of the product.

Route/Dosage
ADULTS: **PO** 15 to 20 mg/kg taken once daily (max, 1 g/day). To reduce GI intolerance, initiate therapy with 250 mg/day and titrate to optimal dose as tolerated (eg, 250 mg/day for 1 or 2 days, followed by 250 mg bid for 1 or 2 days, subsequently increasing the dose to 1 g in 3 or 4 divided doses).
CHILDREN 12 YR AND OLDER: **PO** 10 to 20 mg/kg/day in 2 to 3 divided doses given after meals or 15 mg/kg q 24 hr as a single daily dose.

PATIENT CARE CONSIDERATIONS
Administration/Storage
- Administer with or after meals to reduce GI side effects.
- Directly observe that patient swallows prescribed dose.

Special risk patients: Do not use for ongoing pregnancy protection or as a routine form of contraception. Complications of emergency contraception are not well documented.

Interactions
Antituberculous agents (eg, cycloserine): Adverse effects may be potentiated.
Cycloserine: Risk of occurrence of adverse effects or convulsions may be increased.
Ethanol: Risk of occurrence of psychotic reactions may be increased.
Isoniazid: Transient increases in isoniazid serum levels may occur.

Lab Test Interferences None well documented.

Adverse Reactions
CNS: Psychotic disturbances; depression; drowsiness; dizziness; headache; restlessness; peripheral neuritis.
DERM: Rash; acne.
EENT: Blurred vision; diplopia; optic neuritis.
GI: Nausea; vomiting; diarrhea; abdominal pain; excessive salivation; metallic taste; stomatitis; anorexia.
GU: Gynecomastia; impotence.
HEMA: Thrombocytopenia; purpura.
HEPA: Transient increases in serum bilirubin, AST and ALT; hepatitis (with or without jaundice).
METAB: Weight loss; hypoglycemia; difficulty in managing diabetes mellitus.
OTHER: Postural hypotension; photosensitivity; pellagra-like syndrome.

Precautions
Pregnancy: Category C.
Lactation: Undetermined.
Children: Safety and efficacy not established. Do not administer to patients less than 12 yr unless organisms are definitely resistant to primary therapy and systemic dissemination of the disease, or other life-threatening complications or tuberculosis are judged imminent.
Monitoring: Determine serum transaminases (ie, AST, ALT) prior to therapy and monthly during therapy; monitor blood glucose and perform ophthalmologic examinations prior to therapy and periodically during therapy.
Resistance: Use of ethionamide alone may result in rapid development of resistance.

- Store tablets at controlled room temperature (59° to 86°F).

Assessment/Interventions
- Obtain patient history, including drug history and any known allergies. Note history of liver impairment.

- Assess mycobacterial studies and susceptibility tests before and periodically throughout therapy to detect possible resistance.
- Ensure that 1 or more other antituberculosis agents are being used concurrently.
- Ensure that liver enzymes are determined prior to starting therapy and monthly during therapy.
- Ensure that ophthalmologic examinations are performed prior to starting therapy and periodically during therapy.
- Ensure that blood glucose and thyroid function tests are determined prior to starting therapy and periodically during therapy.
- Monitor diabetic patient for hypoglycemia. Be prepared to treat appropriately if noted.
- Consider coadministration of pyridoxine to prevent or treat neurotoxic side effects.
- Monitor patient for GI, CNS, and general body side effects. Inform health care provider if noted and significant.
- If GI side effects occur and are bothersome, change time of drug administration, administer in divided doses after meals, administer reduced dose if ordered, or obtain order for antiemetic therapy.

Patient/Family Education
- Explain name, dose, action, and potential side effects of drug.
- Review dosing schedule and prescribed length of therapy with patient.
- Emphasize to patient that treatment will be lengthy and that the entire course of treatment must be completed to avoid relapse or development of resistance.
- Advise patient to take each dose with food to prevent or reduce GI side effects.
- Advise diabetic patient to monitor blood sugar throughout therapy and to be alert for episodes of hypoglycemia. Ensure that patient has a plan for treating hypoglycemic events should they occur and to inform health care provider should this occur.
- Instruct patient to report the following to health care provider: intolerable GI side effects, changes in thinking or mood, dizziness, blurred vision or loss of vision, with or without eye pain.
- Instruct women to notify health care provider if pregnant, planning to become pregnant, or breastfeeding.
- Advise patient that drug may cause drowsiness or dizziness and to use caution while driving or performing other tasks requiring mental alertness until tolerance is determined.
- Instruct patient to not take any prescription or OTC medications or dietary supplements unless advised by health care provider.
- Advise patient that follow-up visits and lab tests will be required to monitor therapy and to keep appointments.

Ethosuximide

(ETH-oh-SUX-ih-mide)
Class Anticonvulsant/Succinimide

How Supplied
Zarontin Capsules 250 mg, Syrup 250 mg/5 mL

Action
PHARMACOLOGY: Elevates seizure threshold and suppresses paroxysmal spike and wave activity associated with lapses of consciousness common in absence (petit mal) seizures.

PHARMACOKINETICS/DYNAMICS:
Absorption: T_{max} is 3 to 7 hr.

Metabolism: Extensively metabolized to inactive metabolites.

Excretion: Approximately 20% is excreted unchanged by the kidneys. The $t_{1/2}$ is approximately 60 hr (adults), 30 hr (children).

Indications Control of absence (petit mal) seizures.

Contraindications Hypersensitivity to succinimides.

Route/Dosage
ADULTS AND CHILDREN 6 YR. AND OLDER: PO 500 mg/day. Optimal dose for most children is 20 mg/kg/day. Maintenance therapy: Individualize dose. Increase daily dose slowly by 250 mg q 4 to 7 days until control is achieved with minimal side effects. Administered doses exceeding 1.5 g/day in divided doses under strict medical supervision.

CHILDREN 3 TO 6 YR: INITIAL DOSE: PO 250 mg/day.

Interactions
Hydantoins: May increase serum hydantoin levels.

Primidone: Lower primidone and phenobarbital levels may occur.

Lab Test Interferences None well documented.

Adverse Reactions
CNS: Drowsiness; headache; dizziness; euphoria; hiccups; irritability; hyperactivity; lethargy; fatigue; ataxia; psychological disturbances such as sleep disorders; night terrors; poor concentration; aggressiveness.

DERM: Urticaria; Stevens-Johnson syndrome; systemic lupus erythematosus; pruritic erythematous rash; hirsutism.
EENT: Myopia.
GI: Anorexia; GI upset; nausea; vomiting; cramps; epigastric and abdominal pain; weight loss; gum hypertrophy; tongue swelling.
GU: Vaginal bleeding; microscopic hematuria.
HEMA: Leukopenia; agranulocytosis; pancytopenia; bone marrow suppression; eosinophilia.

Precautions

Pregnancy: Anticonvulsant drugs have been observed to increase the incidence of birth defects.
Renal function impairment: Use caution and perform periodic function tests.
Hepatic function impairment: Use caution and perform periodic function tests.

Hematologic effects: Blood dyscrasias, including fatal cases, have occurred. Periodic blood counts should be done.
Lupus: Cases of systemic lupus erythematosus have occurred.
Withdrawal: Do not withdraw drug abruptly as this may precipitate absence (petit mal) status; proceed slowly when increasing or decreasing dose.

Overdosage: Signs and Symptoms

Acute overdose: Confusion; sleepiness; unsteadiness; flaccid muscles; coma with slow, shallow respiration; nausea and vomiting. Chronic overdose: Skin rash; confusion; ataxia; dizziness; drowsiness; irritability; poor judgment; periorbital edema; proteinuria; hepatic dysfunction; fatal bone marrow aplasia; hematuria; nephrosis.

PATIENT CARE CONSIDERATIONS

Administration/Storage

- Dosage should be increased in small increments.
- If GI upset occurs, give with food or milk.
- Store capsules in tight containers and syrup in light-resistant containers at room temperature. Avoid freezing.

Assessment/Interventions

- Obtain patient history, including drug history and any known allergies.
- Assess location, duration, and characteristics of seizure activity.
- Document baseline CBC, hepatic function, and urinalysis, and monitor routinely throughout course of therapy.
- Observe frequently for occurrence of seizure activity and report findings to health care provider.
- Ensure that patient is protected from injury. Supervise and assist with ambulation if dizziness and drowsiness are problems. Pad side rails and head of bed with towels or blanket for patients who experience seizures during night.
- Assess patient's mood, behavior patterns, and facial expressions. Patients with history of psychiatric disorders have an increased risk of developing behavioral changes.
- Observe for GI symptoms, drowsiness, ataxia, dizziness, and other neurologic side effects.

Patient/Family Education

- Instruct patient to take medication with food to minimize GI upset.
- Advise patient to carry wallet identification card or *Medi-Alert* bracelet, describing disease process and medication regimen, health care provider's name and telephone number.
- Emphasize importance of follow-up exams to monitor progress and side effects.
- Explain that medication may change color of urine to pink, red, or red-brown, and assure that this is not harmful.
- Instruct patient to report these symptoms to health care provider: skin rash, sore throat, fever, unusual bleeding or bruising, swollen glands, pregnancy.
- Tell patient to avoid intake of alcoholic beverages or other CNS depressants.
- Advise patient that drug may cause drowsiness and to use caution while driving or performing other tasks requiring mental alertness.
- Instruct patient not to take otc medications without consulting health care provider.

Ethotoin

(ETH-oh-toyn)

Class Anticonvulsant/Hydantoin

How Supplied
Peganone Tablets 250 mg

Action

PHARMACOLOGY: May act at motor cortex to inhibit spread of seizure activity. Possibly works by promoting sodium efflux from neurons, thereby stabilizing threshold against hyperexcitability. Also, decreases posttetanic potentiation at synapse.

PHARMACOKINETICS/DYNAMICS:
Absorption: Fairly rapidly absorbed.

Metabolism: Major metabolites are to N-deethyl and p-hydroxyl-ethotoin.

Excretion: Elimination t½ ranges from 3 to 9 hr.

Indications Control of tonic-clonic (grand

mal) and complex partial (psychomotor) seizures.

Contraindications Patients with hepatic abnormalities or hematologic disorders.

Route/Dosage

ADULTS: PO Start with 1 g/day or less (in 4 to 6 divided doses daily), with subsequent gradual dosage increases over a period of several days. Optimum dosage is based on individual response. Usual maintenance dose is 2 to 3 g/day. Doses less than 2 g have not been found to be effective in most adults.

CHILDREN: PO Dose depends on age and weight of patient. Do not start with more than 750 mg/day. Usual maintenance dose ranges from 500 mg to 1 g; although occasionally 2 g or, rarely, 3 g may be necessary.

Interactions

Coumarin anticoagulants: Anticoagulant effect may be decreased.
Drugs known to adversely affect the hematopoietic system: Avoid coadministration.

Lab Test Interferences None well documented.

Adverse Reactions

CNS: Ataxia; dizziness; headache; insomnia; fatigue.
DERM: Skin rash.
EENT: Nystagmus; diplopia.
GI: Gingival hyperplasia; vomiting, nausea; diarrhea.
LYMPH: Lymphadenopathy.
OTHER: Systemic lupus erythematosus; chest pain; fever; numbness.

Precautions

Pregnancy: Category C.
Lactation: Excreted in breast milk.
Blood dyscrasias: May occur. In addition, there is some evidence that hydantoin-like compounds may interfere with folic acid metabolism, precipitating megaloblastic anemia.

Overdosage: Signs and Symptoms

Drowsiness, visual disturbances, nausea, ataxia, coma.

PATIENT CARE CONSIDERATIONS

Administration/Storage

- May be used alone or in combination with other antiepileptic drugs (AEDs).
- Medication is administered in divided doses as regularly spaced as possible.
- Administer prescribed dose after food.
- Store tablets at controlled room temperature (below 77°F).

Assessment/Interventions

- Obtain patient history, including drug history and any known allergies. Note hepatic impairment, hematologic disorder, or history of sensitivity to other hydantoins (eg, phenytoin).
- Ensure that folic acid levels are periodically evaluated during prolonged therapy. Be prepared to supplement folic acid to prevent megaloblastic anemia.
- Ensure that urinalysis and CBC with differential are performed before starting therapy and at monthly intervals for several months during therapy.
- Ensure that medication is discontinued in patients who develop hepatic dysfunction, marked depression of blood count, or lymphadenopathy.
- Frequently assess patient for response to treatment. Notify health care provider if seizures do not improve or appear to worsen.
- Ensure that therapy is periodically reviewed to determine if it needs to be continued without change or if a dose change (eg, increase, decrease, discontinuation) is indicated.
- Avoid sudden discontinuation of therapy if possible. Attempt to gradually reduce dose over a period of several weeks if decision to discontinue medication is made.
- Monitor patient for skin rash, fever, or other signs of infection; sores in the mouth; unusual bruising or bleeding; petechiae. Notify health care provider immediately if noted.
- Monitor patient for GI, CNS, and general body side effects. Report to health care provider if noted and significant.
- Implement safety precautions for patients who experience dizziness or ataxia.

Patient/Family Education

- Explain name, dose, action, and potential side effects of drug.
- Instruct patient to continue to take other antiepileptic medications as prescribed by health care provider.
- Advise patient to read the *Patient Information* leaflet before starting therapy and with each refill.
- Instruct patient to take exactly as prescribed and to not change the dose or discontinue unless advised by health care provider.
- Advise patient that dose is gradually increased as tolerated until maximum benefit has been obtained.
- Advise patient that each dose should be taken after food.
- Advise patient that if a dose is missed to take it as soon as remembered but if several hours have passed, or it is nearing the time for the next scheduled dose, to skip that dose and take the next dose at the regularly scheduled

time. Caution patient to never double the dose to catch up.
- Advise patient that if medication needs to be discontinued it will be slowly withdrawn over a period of several weeks unless safety concerns (eg, rash) require a more rapid withdrawal.
- Caution patient that drug may cause dizziness and to use caution while driving or performing other tasks requiring mental alertness until tolerance is determined.
- Advise women of childbearing potential to use effective contraception during treatment with ethotoin.
- Advise women to notify health care provider if pregnant, planning to become pregnant, or breastfeeding.
- Instruct patient to contact health care provider immediately if skin rash, fever, sore throat or other signs of infection, yellowing of skin or eyes, easy or unusual bruising, bleeding, or swollen lymph glands develop.
- Instruct patient to inform health care provider if seizures get worse or if new types of seizures occur.
- Advise patient to carry identification (eg, Medi-Alert) indicating epilepsy and medication use.
- Advise patient not to take any prescription or OTC medications or dietary supplements unless advised by health care provider.
- Advise patient that laboratory tests and follow-up visits will be required to monitor therapy and to keep appointments.

Etidronate Disodium

(eh-TIH-DROE-nate die-SO-dee-uhm)

Class Hormone/Biphosphonates

How Supplied
Didronel Tablets 200 mg, Tablets 400 mg ♦
Didronel IV Injection 30 mg/mL

Action
PHARMACOLOGY: Inhibits normal and abnormal bone resorption; reduces bone formation.

PHARMACOKINETICS/DYNAMICS:
Absorption: Approximately 3% is absorbed.
Distribution: Approximately 50% of the absorbed dose is distributed to bone compartments. Does not cross blood-brain barrier.
Metabolism: Not metabolized.
Excretion: The $t_{1/2}$ is 1 to 6 hr. Bone clearance is 165 days. Unabsorbed drug excreted in feces. Approximately 50% of the absorbed dose is excreted in the urine within 24 hr.

Indications Treatment of symptomatic Paget disease; prevention and treatment of heterotopic ossification; treatment of hypercalcemia of malignancy. **Unlabeled use(s):** Treatment of postmenopausal osteoporosis.

Contraindications Hypersensitivity to biphosphonates; patients with class Dc and higher renal functional impairment (serum creatinine greater than 5 mg/dL).

Route/Dosage
Paget Disease
ADULTS: **PO** Initial treatment is 5 to 10 mg/kg/day (not to exceed 6 mo) or 11 to 20 mg/kg/day (not to exceed 3 mo). Reserve doses greater than 10 mg/kg/day for specific situations. For retreatment, initiate only after etidronate-free period of at least 90 days and if there is evidence of active disease.

Heterotopic Ossification from Spinal Cord Injury
ADULTS: **PO** 20 mg/kg/day for 2 wk followed by 10 mg/kg/day for 10 wk; total treatment period is 12 wk.

Heterotopic Ossification Complicating Total Hip Replacement
ADULTS: **PO** 20 mg/kg/day for 1 mo preoperatively followed by 20 mg/kg/day for 3 mo postoperatively.

Hypercalcemia
ADULTS: **IV** 7.5 mg/kg/day for 3 successive days given by slow infusion (over a period of at least 2 hr). Retreatment may be needed; wait at least 7 days between courses. Adjust dose for renal impairment. Regimen of oral etidronate (20 mg/kg/day for 30 days) may be started after last infusion.

Interactions None well documented.

Lab Test Interferences
Calcium supplements, antacids, foods: Products containing calcium and other multi-valent cations interfere with etidronate absorption.

Adverse Reactions
EENT: Metallic or altered taste; loss of taste.
GI: Diarrhea; nausea; constipation; stomatitis; diarrhea in enterocolitis patients.
GU: Abnormal elevations of serum creatinine and BUN; mild to moderate abnormalities in renal function.
OTHER: Hypersensitivity (eg, angioedema, urticaria, rash, pruritus); increased or recurrent bone pain in Paget disease; hypocalcemia; fractures with excessive doses; convulsions; hypophosphatemia; hypomagnesemia.

Precautions
Pregnancy: Category C.
Lactation: Undetermined.
Children: Safety and efficacy not established.

GI disorders: Use this drug with caution in patients with active upper GI problems such as dysphagia (difficulty swallowing); symptomatic esophageal diseases; gastritis; duodenitis or ulcers.
Paget disease: Response may be slow and may continue for months after treatment has been discontinued. Dosage must not be prematurely increased or treatment prematurely reinitiated until patient has had at least 90-day etidronate-free interval.

Overdosage: Signs and Symptoms
Diarrhea, vomiting, hypocalcemia.

PATIENT CARE CONSIDERATIONS

Administration/Storage
- Have patient take drug on empty stomach 2 hr before meals.
- Administer oral medication as a single dose. If GI upset occurs, dose may be divided.
- To maximize absorption of drug, have patient avoid food high in calcium (eg, milk and milk products), vitamins with mineral supplements and antacids high in metals within 2 hr of dosing.
- Dilute daily IV dose in at least 250 mL of sterile normal saline.
- Slow IV infusion is important. Infuse diluted dose over 2 hr or more.
- Store diluted dose at room temperature no longer than 48 hr.
- Store IV medication away from excessive heat.

Assessment/Interventions
- Obtain patient history, including drug history and any known allergies. Note any hypersensitivity to biphosphonates.
- Record dates of any previous treatments with etidronate.
- Treatment of hypocalcemia includes IV calcium administration.
- Monitor serum calcium, phosphate, potassium, BUN, and creatinine.
- Monitor renal status throughout treatment.

Patient/Family Education
- Instruct patient to avoid eating 2 hr before and 2 hr after taking medication because absorption of drug is reduced by food.
- Advise patient to avoid vitamins, mineral supplements, and antacids that are high in metals, especially calcium, iron, magnesium, and aluminum.
- Instruct patient to maintain adequate intake of foods containing calcium and vitamin D within 2 hr of taking eticronate.
- Inform patient of transient effect of metallic or altered taste or loss of taste.
- Tell patient to report the following symptoms to health care provider: rash, respiratory difficulty, GI upset, visual disturbances, jaundice.
- Instruct patient not to take any OTC medications without consulting the health care provider.

Etodolac

(EE-toe-DOE-lak)

Class Analgesic/NSAID

How Supplied
Lodine Capsules 200 mg, Capsules 300 mg, Tablets 400 mg, Tablets 500 mg ♦ *Lodine XL* Tablets, extended-release 400 mg, Tablets, extended-release 500 mg, Tablets, extended-release 600 mg ❀ Apo-Etodolac ♦ Ultradol

Action
PHARMACOLOGY: Decreases inflammation, pain and fever, probably through inhibition of cyclooxygenase activity and prostaglandin synthesis.

PHARMACOKINETICS/DYNAMICS:
Absorption: Well-absorbed. Bioavailability is 80% or more. C_{max} is approximately 14 to 37 mcg/mL. T_{max} is approximately 1.4 hr (IR), 6.7 hr (ER). Food decreases C_{max} approximately 50% and increases T_{max} by 1.4 to 3.8 hr.

Distribution: Vd is approximately 362 mL/kg (IR), 566 mL/kg (ER). More than 99% protein bound.

Metabolism:
Liver – Extensively metabolized.

Excretion: Distribution $t_{1/2}$ is approximately 0.71 hr. Terminal $t_{1/2}$ is approximately 7.3 hr (IR), 8.4 hr (ER). Cl is approximately 47 mL/h/kg/ Approximately 72% is recovered in the urine, with 1% as unchanged drug. 16% is excreted in feces. Not dialyzable.

Onset: 0.5 hr (IR).

Peak: 1 to 2 hr (IR).

Duration: 4 to 6 hr (IR).

Special Populations:
Elderly – Clearance is reduced approximately 15%. No dosage adjustment is necessary.

Indications Management of pain (*Lodine* only); management of signs and symptoms of osteoarthritis and rheumatoid arthritis.

Unlabeled use(s): Control of symptoms of rheumatoid arthritis; treatment of temporal arteritis.

Contraindications Patients in whom aspirin, iodides or any NSAID has caused allergic-type reactions.

Route/Dosage

Analgesia
ADULTS: PO 200 to 400 mg q 6 to 8 hr prn. Do not exceed 1200 mg/day. Do not exceed 20 mg/kg in patients 60 kg or less.

Osteoarthritis/Rheumatoid Arthritis
ADULTS: PO 300 mg bid, tid, or 400 mg or 500 mg bid. The dose may be increased to 1200 mg/day when a higher level of therapeutic activity is required.

Interactions

Anticoagulants: May increase prothrombin time. Watch for signs and symptoms of bleeding.
Beta-blockers: May decrease antihypertensive effect of beta-blockers.
Lithium: May increase lithium levels and effects.
Loop diuretics: May decrease diuretic effect.
Methotrexate: May increase methotrexate levels.
Salicylates: Plasma concentrations of NSAIDs may be decreased when taken with salicylates. There is no therapeutic advantage to this combination, but adverse GI effects may be increased.

Lab Test Interferences

Serum uric acid levels: Drug may cause small decrease.
Urinary bilirubin test: Drug may cause false-positive results.
Urinary dipstick tests: Drug may cause results that are false positive for ketones.

Adverse Reactions

CV: Fluid retention; edema; hypertension; flushing; CHF; syncope; palpitations.
CNS: Dizziness; headaches; drowsiness; insomnia; asthenia; malaise; depression; nervousness.
DERM: Rash; pruritus; Stevens-Johnson syndrome; hyperpigmentation; urticaria; purpura.
EENT: Blurred vision; photophobia; visual changes; tinnitus.
GI: Dyspepsia; nausea; vomiting; diarrhea; indigestion; heartburn; abdominal pain; constipation; flatulence; gastritis; melena; dry mouth; anorexia; stomatitis; peptic ulcers.
GU: Urinary frequency; dysuria.
HEMA: Anemia; leukopenia; pancytopenia; thrombocytopenia; increased bleeding time; agranulocytosis; hemolytic anemia; neutropenia.
HEPA: Jaundice; cholestatic jaundice; hepatitis.
METAB: Weight gain; hypouricemia.
RESP: Asthma.
OTHER: Chills; fever.

Precautions

Pregnancy: Category C.
Lactation: Undetermined.
Children: Safety and efficacy not established.
Elderly: Increased risk of adverse reactions.
Hypersensitivity: May occur; use caution in aspirin sensitive individuals because of possible cross-sensitivity.
Renal function impairment: Assess renal function before and during therapy. Acute renal insufficiency, interstitial nephritis, hyperkalemia, hyponatremia, and renal papillary necrosis may occur.
GI effects: Serious GI toxicity (eg, bleeding, ulceration, perforation) can occur at any time, with or without warning symptoms.

Overdosage: Signs and Symptoms

Respiratory depression, hypotension, epigastric pain, drowsiness, lethargy, GI irritation/bleeding, nausea, vomiting, tinnitus, sweating, acute renal failure.

PATIENT CARE CONSIDERATIONS

Administration/Storage

- Do not give more than 20 mg/kg to patients weighing 60 kg or less.
- Food delays peak action of medication by 1 to 4 hr.
- Give with food, milk or antacids if stomach upset occurs.
- Store at room temperature in tightly closed container. Protect from moisture.

Assessment/Interventions

- Obtain patient history, including drug history and any known allergies, especially to aspirin, iodides or other NSAIDs. Note history of GI bleeding.
- Assess location, duration and intensity of pain before and 60 min after administration.
- Monitor hematocrit and hemoglobin levels in patients on long-term therapy.
- Monitor for signs of agranulocytosis (eg, sore throat, fever).
- Monitor renal function.
- Monitor for edema and weight gain in patients with CHF and renal impairment.
- Monitor PT/APTT levels of patients taking anticoagulants.
- Monitor elderly patients carefully for possible adverse reactions.
- Review LFT results, and report signs of hepatic dysfunction to the health care provider.
- Discontinue drug if hypersensitivity develops.
- Inform health care provider of decreased renal function, hyponatremia, and hyperkalemia

laboratory values.
Extended-release:
- After satisfactory response is achieved, usually after 1 to 2 wk, assess patient to determine if dose needs to be adjusted.

Patient/Family Education
- Advise patient to take medication with full glass of water and to remain upright for 15 to 30 min after administration.
- Encourage patient on long-term therapy to have regular eye examinations.
- Advise patient to inform health care provider or dentist of medication regimen before treatment or surgery.
- Instruct patient to report these symptoms to health care provider: rash, stomach problems, tinnitus, dizziness or visual disturbances, black tarry stools, increased bruises or bleeding.
- Caution patient not to use aspirin or other otc medications or drink alcoholic beverages while taking this medication.
- Advise patient that drug may cause drowsiness and to use caution while driving or performing tasks requiring mental alertness.
- Caution patient to avoid exposure to sunlight and to use sunscreen or wear protective clothing to avoid photosensitivity reaction.

Etoposide

(EH-toe-POE-side)
Class Podophyllotoxin derivative
How Supplied
VePesid Concentrate for injection 20 mg/mL, Liquid-filled capsules for oral use 50 mg ♦
Toposar Concentrate for injection 20 mg/mL, Liquid-filled capsules for oral use 50 mg ♦
Etopophos Powder for injection 100 mg vial

Action
PHARMACOLOGY: Etoposide's main effect appears to be at the G_2 portion of the cell cycle. At high concentrations (10 mcg/mL or more), lysis of cells entering mitosis is seen; at low concentrations (0.3 to 10 mcg/mL), cells are inhibited from entering prophase. Predominant macromolecular effect appears to be DNA synthesis inhibition.

PHARMACOKINETICS/DYNAMICS:
Absorption: Bioavailability is approximately 50% (oral).
Distribution: Distribution $t_{1/2}$ is approximately 1.5 hr. Vd is approximately 18 to 29 L (at steady state). 97% is protein bound.
Metabolism: Etoposide phosphate is rapidly dephosphonylate to etoposide in the plasma. Etoposide is extensively metabolized in the liver (including CYP3A4).
Excretion: The $t_{1/2}$ is approximately 4 to 11 hr. Cl is 33 to 48 mL/min. 42 to 67% is excreted in the urine and 0 to 16% is excreted in the feces. Less than 50% is excreted in the urine and less than 6% is excreted in bile as etoposide.
Special Populations:
Renal Function Impairment – Total body clearance is reduced, AUC is increased, and Vd is lower.

Indications Refractory testicular tumors, small-cell lung cancer. **Unlabeled use(s):** Bladder carcinoma, lymphomas, leukemias, Ewing sarcoma, Kaposi sarcoma, brain tumors, gestational trophoblastic tumors, ovarian germ cell tumors, refractory breast tumors, rhabdomyosarcomas, Wilms tumor, bone marrow transplantation.

Contraindications Standard considerations.
Route/Dosage
Testicular Cancer
ADULTS: **IV** 50 to 100 mg/m^2/day for 3 to 5 days every 3 to 4 wk.
Small-Cell Lung Cancer
ADULTS: **IV** 35 to 50 mg/m^2/day IV for 4 to 5 days every 3 to 4 wk. **PO** 2 times the IV dose, rounded to nearest 50 mg, given orally for 21 days. Alternately, 50 mg/m^2/day orally for 21 days has been given. Repeat regimen after a 1- to 2-wk rest period. Oral bioavailability of the capsules is erratic, averaging 50% (range, 25% to 75%).

DOSAGE ADJUSTMENT
ADULTS: Hold etoposide if the platelet count is less than 50,000/mm^3 or the absolute neutrophil count is less than 500/mm^3.

ADJUSTMENT IN HEPATIC INSUFFICIENCY
ADULTS: Dosage reduction may be warranted; specific guidelines are not available.

ADJUSTMENT IN RENAL INSUFFICIENCY
ADULTS: For patients with Ccr of 16 to 50 mL/min, give 75% of the usual dose. Consider further dose reduction for those with Ccr 15 mL/min or less.

Interactions
Warfarin: Etoposide may increase the hypoprothrombinemic effects of warfarin.

Lab Test Interferences None well documented.

Adverse Reactions
CV: Hypotension.
DERM: Alopecia; radiation recall.
GI: Nausea and vomiting; abdominal pain;

anorexia; diarrhea; mucositis with high doses or prior radiation to head and neck; elevation of LFTs; hepatocellular necrosis.
GU: Amenorrhea.
HEMA: Bone marrow suppression, granulocyte nadir at 7 to 14 days, platelet nadir at 9 to 16 days.
HYPERSEN: Acute anaphylactoid reaction.
OTHER: Increased risk of acute nonlymphocytic leukemia.

> **WARNING:**
>
> *Myelosuppression:* Severe cases with resulting infection or bleeding may occur. Dose-limiting bone marrow suppression is the most significant toxicity.

PATIENT CARE CONSIDERATIONS
Administration/Storage
- Follow procedures for proper handling and disposal of anticancer drugs. Wear gloves and avoid skin exposure and inhalation of fumes.
- Administer by oral or IV infusion.

Vials:
- Store at room temperature. At room temperature, 0.2 mg/mL solution is stable for 96 hr, 0.4 mg/mL solution is stable for 48 hr.

Capsules:
- Refrigerate; can be stored at room temperature for 3 mo.

IV:
- Dilute prior to use with 5% Dextrose or 0.9% Sodium Chloride to final concentration of 0.2 or 0.4 mg/mL. Concentrations less than 0.4 mg/mL may precipitate.
- Infuse over 30 to 60 min. Do not give by rapid IV injection because of the risk of hypotension.

Extemporaneous oral solution:
- Etoposide solution for injection can be mixed to a final concentration 0.4 mg/mL or less with orange juice, apple juice, or lemonade for oral administration.
- Stable for 3 hr at room temperature.

Precautions
Pregnancy: Category D.
Lactation: Undetermined.
Children: Safety and efficacy in children not established.
Anaphylaxis: Anaphylaxis manifested by chills, fever, tachycardia, bronchospasm, dyspnea, facial flushing, hypertension, or hypotension may occur.
Hypotension: Administer by slow IV infusion because hypotension may occur with rapid IV injection.
Extravasation: Can cause local irritation or phlebitis. Refer to your institution-specific protocol.

Overdosage: Signs and Symptoms
Bone marrow suppression.

Assessment/Interventions
- Monitor BP before and after infusion.
- Perform at the start of therapy and prior to each subsequent dose: platelet count, hemoglobin, white blood cell count and differential. A platelet count less than 50,000/mm^3 or an absolute neutrophil count less than 500/mm^3 is an indication to withhold further therapy until the blood counts have sufficiently recovered.
- Carefully monitor renal and hepatic function tests prior to and during therapy.

Patient/Family Education
- Contraceptive measures are recommended during treatment.
- Notify health care provider of any of the following: fever; chills; rapid heartbeat; difficult breathing.

Exemestane

(ex-e-MES-tane)
Class Steroidal irreversible aromatase inhibitor
How Supplied
Aromasin Tablets for oral use 25 mg
Action
PHARMACOLOGY: An irreversible, steroidal aromatase inactivator. It lowers circulating estrogen concentrations in postmenopausal women. Exemestane is 90% bound to plasma proteins. Exemestane is extensively metabolized.

PHARMACOKINETICS/DYNAMICS:
Absorption: Rapidly absorbed. At least 42% if the dose is absorbed. T_{max} is 1.2 hr (women with breast cancer) and 2.9 hr (healthy women). When taken after a high-fat breakfast, the plasma levels increased approximately 40%.

Distribution: 90% protein bound.

Metabolism: Extensively metabolized. CYP3A4 is the principal isoenzyme involved in the oxidation of exemestane. The metabolites are inactive or inhibit aromatase with decreased potency compared to exemestane.

Excretion: The $t_{1/2}$ is 24 hr. Approximately 42% is excreted in the urine and approximately 42% is excreted in the feces. Less than 1% is excreted unchanged in the urine.

Special Populations:
Renal Function Impairment – AUC is about 3 times higher in those with moderate or severe renal insufficiency. No dosage adjustment necessary.
Hepatic Function Impairment – AUC increased approximately 3 times in those with moderate or sever hepatic insufficiency. No dosage adjustment necessary.

Indications Advanced breast cancer in postmenopausal women with disease progression following tamoxifen therapy. **Unlabeled use(s):** Prevention of prostate cancer.

Contraindications Standard considerations.

Route/Dosage
Breast Cancer
ADULTS: **PO** 25 mg once daily.

Interactions
Agents that inhibit or induce cytochrome P4503A4 (eg, rifampin, phenobarbital, erythromycin, ketoconazole, and others): A possible decrease of exemestane by agents which inhibit or induce cytochrome P450 3A4 (eg, rifampin, phenobarbital, erythromycin, ketoconazole).

Lab Test Interferences None well documented.

PATIENT CARE CONSIDERATIONS

Administration/Storage
- Store at controlled room temperature.
- Take after a meal.

Assessment/Interventions
- Rule out pregnancy prior to starting exemestane.

Adverse Reactions
CV: Chest pain; hypertension; peripheral edema.
CNS: Fatigue; depression; insomnia; anxiety; headache; dizziness.
DERM: Rash; increased sweating; androgenic effects reported including hypertrichosis, hair loss, and acne.
ENDO: Hot flushes; weight gain.
GI: Low potential for nausea and vomiting; abdominal pain; anorexia; constipation; diarrhea; and increased appetite.
HEMA: Lymphopenia.
MUSC: Musculoskeletal pain; arthralgia.
RESP: Dyspnea; coughing.
OTHER: Flu-like symptoms with fever; hoarseness.

Precautions
Pregnancy: Category D.
Lactation: Undetermined.
Children: Safety and efficacy not established in patients younger than 18 yr.
Endocrine effects: Increases in testosterone and androstenedione levels observed.
Premenopausal women: Do not administer exemestane tablets to premenopausal women.
Lymphocytopenia: Approximately 20% of patients receiving exemestane in clinical studies experienced common toxicity criteria. Grade 3 or 4 lymphocytopenia.

Patient/Family Education
- Androgenic effects have been reported with exemestane. Inform patients that hypertrichosis, hair loss, acne, or hoarseness may occur.

Ezetimibe

(Ezz-ET-ih-mibe)

Class Antihyperlipidemic

How Supplied
Zetia Tablets 10 mg

Action
PHARMACOLOGY: Inhibits absorption of cholesterol by the small intestine.

PHARMACOKINETICS/DYNAMICS:
Absorption: C_{max} is 3.4 to 5.5 ng/mL (ezetimibe) and 45 to 71 ng/mL (metabolite). T_{max} is 4 to 12 hr (ezetimibe) and 1 to 2 hr (metabolite).
Distribution: More than 90% protein bound.
Metabolism: Metabolized (active) in small intestine and liver to ezetimibe glucuronide.
Excretion: The t½ is approximately 22 hr. Approximately 78% is excreted in feces and 11% in urine.

Special Populations:
Renal Function Impairment – AUC increased approximately 1.5-fold in those with severe renal disease (Ccr up to 30 mL/min).
Hepatic Function Impairment – AUC increased approximately 1.7-fold in those with mild insufficiency, 3- to 4-fold in moderate insufficiency and 5- to 6-fold in severe impairment.
Elderly – Plasma concentrations are approximately 2-fold higher.

Indications Administration alone or with HMG-CoA reductase inhibitors as adjunctive therapy to diet for reduction of elevated total cholesterol, low density lipoprotein cholesterol (LDL), and apolipoprotein in patients with primary hypercholesterolemia; with atorvastatin or simvastatin for the reduction of elevated total cholesterol and LDL levels in patients with homozygous familial hypercholesterolemia as an adjunct to other lipid-lowering treatments or if such treatments are unavailable; as adjunctive therapy to diet for the reduction of elevated sitosterol and campesterol levels in patients with homozygous familial sitosterolemia.

Contraindications Ezetimibe is contraindicated in combination with HMG-CoA reductase inhibitors in patients with active liver disease or unexplained persistent elevations in serum transaminases; hypersensitivity to any component of the product.

Route/Dosage
ADULTS AND CHILDREN OVER 10 YR: PO 10 mg once daily.

Interactions
Antacids: Aluminum- and magnesium-containing antacids decrease the peak concentration of ezetimibe but not the AUC.
Cholestyramine: The AUC of ezetimibe may be decreased.
Cyclosporine, fibric acid derivatives (eg, fenofibrate, gemfibrozil): Concentrations of ezetimibe may be increased.

Lab Test Interferences None well documented.

Adverse Reactions
CNS: Fatigue; headache; dizziness.
EENT: Sinusitis; pharyngitis.
GI: Diarrhea; abdominal pain.
RESP: Coughing; upper respiratory tract infection.
OTHER: Back pain; arthralgia; viral infection; myalgia; chest pain.

Precautions
Pregnancy: Category C.
Lactation: Undetermined.
Children: Safety and efficacy not established in children under 10 yr.
Hepatic function impairment: Use not recommended because of unknown effects on liver.
Secondary causes of hyperlipidemia: Ruled out or treat secondary causes of hyperlipidemia before starting treatment with ezetimibe.

PATIENT CARE CONSIDERATIONS

Administration/Storage
- Give prescribed dose once daily with or without food.
- Administer alone or in combination with other lipid-lowering therapy.
- May be administered at the same time as an HMG-CoA reductase inhibitor.
- Administer 2 hr before or 4 hr after a bile acid sequestrant.
- Store tablets at controlled room temperature (59° to 86°F). Protect from moisture.

Assessment/Interventions
- Obtain patient history, including drug history and any known allergies. Note presence of active liver disease or moderate to severe hepatic insufficiency.
- Ensure that patient is on a cholesterol-lowering diet.
- Ensure that lipids are measured before therapy is started and periodically during therapy.
- Assess patient for GI, musculoskeletal, respiratory, and general body side effects. If noted and significant, inform health care provider.

Patient/Family Education
- Explain name, dose, action, and potential side effects of drug.
- Advise patient to review "Patient Information about *Zetia*" before starting the medication and each time when refilling the medication.
- Advise patient to take once daily as prescribed, without regard to meals.
- Advise patient to try to take each dose at about the same time each day.
- Inform patient that drug helps control, but not does cure, cholesterol abnormality and to continue taking drug as prescribed if cholesterol levels are lowered.
- Caution patient not to change the dose or stop taking unless advised by health care provider.
- Advise patient that if a dose is missed to take as soon as remembered but to never take more than 1 dose of medicine a day.
- Instruct patient to continue taking other cholesterol-lowering medications as prescribed by health care provider.
- Emphasize to patient importance of the following other modalities on cholesterol control: dietary changes (eg, reduced saturated fat intake, increase soluble fiber intake); weight control, regular exercise, and smoking cessation.
- Advise women to contact health care provider if pregnant, planning to become pregnant, or breastfeeding.
- Caution patient to not take any prescription or OTC medications or dietary supplements unless advised by health care provider.

- Instruct patient to notify health care provider if experiencing any unexplained muscle pain, tenderness, or weakness or noting any other unusual feelings.
- Advise patient that follow-up visits and lab tests will be required to monitor therapy and to keep appointments.

Ezetimibe/Simvastatin

(ezz-ET-ih-mibe/SIM-vah-STAT-in)

Class Antihyperlipidemic combination

How Supplied
Vytorin 10/10 Tablets 10 mg ezetimibe/10 mg simvastatin ◆ Vytorin 10/20 Tablets 10 mg ezetimibe/20 mg simvastatin ◆ Vytorin 10/40 Tablets 10 mg ezetimibe/40 mg simvastatin ◆ Vytorin 10/80 Tablets 10 mg ezetimibe/80 mg simvastatin

Action

PHARMACOLOGY:

Ezetimibe: Inhibits absorption of cholesterol by the small intestine.

Simvastatin: Increases rate at which body removes cholesterol from blood and reduces production of cholesterol by inhibiting enzyme that catalyzes early rate-limiting step in cholesterol synthesis.

Indications Adjunctive treatment to diet for reduction of elevated total-cholesterol, LDL cholesterol, triglycerides, non-HDL cholesterol, and apolipoprotein B (Apo B), and to increase HDL cholesterol in patients with primary hypercholesterolemia or mixed hyperlipidemia; as an adjunct to other lipid-lowering treatment for the reduction of total cholesterol and LDL cholesterol in patients with homozygous familial hypercholesterolemia.

Contraindications Active liver disease or unexplained persistent elevations in serum transaminases; pregnancy and lactation; hypersensitivity to any component of the product.

Route/Dosage

Primary Hypercholesterolemia

ADULTS: **PO** Dosage range is 10 mg ezetimibe/10 mg simvastatin through 10/80 mg daily. Start with 10/20 mg daily. Lipid levels may be analyzed after 2 or more wk and dosage adjusted. For patients requiring a large reduction in LDL cholesterol (greater than 55%), therapy may be started at 10/40 mg daily.

Homozygous Familial Hypercholesterolemia

ADULTS: **PO** 10/40 mg daily or 10/80 mg daily in the evening. Use as an adjunct to other lipid lowering treatments.

Interactions

Amiodarone, verapamil: Risk of myopathy/rhabdomyolysis may be increased. Dose of ezetimibe/simvastatin should not exceed 10/20 mg daily.

Bile acid sequestrant (eg, cholestyramine): Ezetimibe concentrations may be reduced, decreasing the therapeutic effect. Give at least 2 hr before or 4 hr after the bile acid sequestrant.

Cyclosporine: Exposure to ezetimibe may be increased, especially in patients with severe renal insufficiency. Dose of ezetimibe/simvastatin should not exceed 10/10 mg daily.

Digoxin: Digoxin plasma concentrations may be slightly elevated.

Fibrates (eg, fenofibrate, gemfibrozil): Ezetimibe concentrations may be increased.

Potent inhibitors of CYP3A4 (eg, clarithromycin, cyclosporine, erythromycin, HIV protease inhibitors, itraconazole, ketoconazole, nefazodone, large quantities of grapefruit juice [greater than 1 quart daily]): May reduce the elimination of simvastatin, increasing the risk of myopathy.

Propranolol: Simvastatin peak plasma concentrations may be reduced.

Warfarin: The anticoagulant effect, as measured by the INR, may be modestly potentiated.

Lab Test Interferences None well documented.

Adverse Reactions The incidence stated for the following adverse reaction were reported with Vytorin (ezetimibe/simvastatin) administration. Adverse reactions occurring with administration of either ezetimibe or simvastatin can be found listed in their respective monographs.
CNS: Headache (7%).
MUSC: Myalgia (4%); pain in extremity (2%).
PULM: Upper respiratory tract infection (4%).
OTHER: Influenza (3%).

Precautions

Pregnancy: Category X.
Lactation: Undetermined.
Children: Safety and efficacy not established.
Hepatic function impairment: Use is not recommended in patients with moderate or severe hepatic insufficiency.

Liver dysfunction: Use with caution in patients who consume substantial quantities of alcohol or who have history of liver disease. Marked, persistent increases in serum transaminases can occur.

Secondary causes of hyperlipidemia: Rule out or treat secondary causes of hyperlipidemia before starting treatment.

Skeletal muscle effects: Rhabdomyolysis with renal dysfunction secondary to myoglobinuria has occurred with statin administration. Consider myopathy in any patient with diffuse myalgias, muscle tenderness or weakness, or marked CPK elevation.

PATIENT CARE CONSIDERATIONS

Administration/Storage

- May be used alone or in combination with other cholesterol-lowering medications.
- Administer prescribed dose once daily in the evening without regard to meals. Administer with food if GI upset occurs.
- Administer ezetimibe/simvastatin at least 2 hr before or 4 hr after administration of a bile acid sequestrant (eg, cholestyramine).
- Store tablets at controlled room temperature (68° to 77°F).

Assessment/Interventions

- Obtain patient history, including drug history and any known allergies. Note active liver disease or past history of liver disease, unexplained elevations of serum transaminases, severe renal insufficiency, pregnancy, breast feeding, alcohol consumption, concurrent use of potent inhibitors of CYP3A4 (eg, cyclosporine, ketoconazole), and concurrent therapy with medications known to increase the risk of myopathy (eg, fibrates, niacin, amiodarone, verapamil).
- Ensure that dose does not exceed 10/10 mg/day in patient taking cyclosporine, or 10/20 mg/day in patient taking verapamil or amiodarone.
- Ensure that secondary causes of hypercholesterolemia (eg, poorly controlled diabetes, hypothyroidism, drugs that increase LDL-C and decrease HDL-C) are excluded or, if appropriate, treated before starting therapy.
- Ensure that patient is on a cholesterol-lowering diet before starting therapy and that diet is continued during treatment.
- Ensure that lipid levels are measured before therapy is started, at least 2 wk after starting ezetimibe/simvastatin therapy or changing the dose, and then periodically thereafter.
- Ensure that therapy is temporarily withheld in patient with an acute, serious condition suggestive of myopathy or predisposing to the development of renal failure secondary to rhabdomyolysis (eg, sepsis, hypotension, major surgery).
- Ensure that serum transaminases are determined before starting therapy and periodically thereafter as clinically indicated. For patient being titrated to 10/80 mg dose, ensure that transaminases are determined before titration, 3 mo after titration to 10/80 mg dose, and periodically thereafter (eg, q 6 mo) for first year of treatment.
- If elevated serum transaminase levels develop during treatment, repeat levels more frequently. If transaminase levels rise to 3 times upper limit of normal or greater and persist, notify health care provider. Be prepared to discontinue therapy.
- Monitor patient for symptoms of myopathy (muscle pain, tenderness, weakness) when medication is started and when dose is increased. Discontinue therapy and immediately notify health care provider if myopathy suspected.
- Assess patient for GI, CNS, and general body side effects. Inform health care provider if noted and significant.

Patient/Family Education

- Explain name, dose, action, potential side effects of medication, and LDL-C goal.
- Advise patient that dose of medication may change, based on results of cholesterol blood tests, in an effort to reach LDL-C goal.
- Review other substances (eg, grapefruit juice) and medications (eg, potent CYP3A4 inhibitors, fibrates) that should not be taken with this medication.
- Advise patient to take prescribed dose once daily in the evening without regard to meals, but to take with food if stomach upset occurs.
- Advise patient that if a dose is missed to take as soon as remembered but to never take more than 1 dose of medicine a day.
- Caution patient not to change the dose or stop taking unless advised by health care provider.
- Advise patient that drug helps control, but does not cure, cholesterol abnormality and to continue taking drug as prescribed when LDL-C goal has been met.

- Instruct patient to continue taking other cholesterol-lowering medications as prescribed by health care provider.
- Advise patient who is also taking a bile acid sequestrant (eg, cholestyramine) to take the ezetimibe/simvastatin at least 2 hr before or 4 hr after the sequestrant.
- Instruct patient to immediately notify health care provider if experiencing any unexplained muscle pain, tenderness, and/or weakness, or if they note any other unusual feelings.
- Emphasize to patient importance of other modalities on cholesterol control: dietary changes (reduced saturated fat intake, increase soluble fiber intake), weight control, regular exercise, smoking cessation.
- Advise women of childbearing potential to use effective contraception during treatment with ezetimibe/simvastatin.
- Advise women to notify health care provider if pregnant, planning to become pregnant, or breastfeeding.
- Caution patient not to take any prescription or OTC medications, herbal preparations, or dietary supplements unless advised by health care provider.
- Advise patient that follow-up visits and lab tests will be required to monitor therapy and to keep appointments.

Factor IX Concentrates

Class Antihemophilic

How Supplied
AlphaNine SD Concentrate Dried plasma fraction of Factors II, VII, IX, and X ◆ *Konyne 80* Concentrate Dried plasma fraction of coagulation Factors II, VII, IX, and X ◆ *Profilnine SD* Concentrate Dried plasma fraction of coagulation Factors II, VII, IX, and X ◆ *Proplex T* Concentrate Dried plasma fraction of coagulation Factors II, VII, IX, and X ◆ *BeneFix* Concentrate Nonpyrogenic lyophilized powder preparation. Purified protein produced by recombinant DNA for use in therapy of Factor IX deficiency. ◆ *Hemonyne* Concentrate Dried plasma fraction of coagulation Factors II, VII, IX, and X ◆ *Mononine* Concentrate 100 IU Factor IX with non-detectable levels of Factors II, VII, and X per mL when reconstituted
✤ *Immunine* VH

Action
PHARMACOLOGY: Restores hemostasis in patients with Factor IX deficiency.

PHARMACOKINETICS/DYNAMICS:
Excretion: The t½ is about 21 hr.

Indications Management of Factor IX deficiency (hemophilia B, Christmas disease), bleeding episodes in patients with inhibitors to Factor VIII; reversal of coumarin anticoagulant hemorrhage; prevention or control of bleeding in patients with Factor VII deficiency (*Proplex T* only).

Contraindications Treatment of Factor VII deficiency (except for *Proplex T*); liver disease with signs of intravascular coagulation or fibrinolysis.

PATIENT CARE CONSIDERATIONS

Administration/Storage

- Use powder and diluent at room temperature when reconstituting.
- Gently swirl solution during reconstitution to prevent foaming. Infuse within 3 hr of reconstitution.
- Administer by IV infusion only.
- Start infusion within 3 hr after reconstitution.
- Maintain prescribed rate of infusion, (eg, *Konyne-80*, 100 U/min; *Profilnine SD*, less than 10 mL/min; *Proplex T*, less than 3 mL/min.)
- Store powdered form of drug in refrigerator. Do not freeze.
- Do not refrigerate reconstituted solution.

Route/Dosage
ADULTS AND CHILDREN: IV Dose based on patient condition, degree of deficiency and desired level of Factor IX to be achieved.
Dosing guideline: 1 U/kg times body weight (kg) times desired increase (% of normal).
Factor VII deficiency: 0.5 U/kg times body weight (kg) times desired increase (% of normal), repeated q 4 to 6 h prn.
Hemarthroses – In hemophiliacs with inhibitors to Factor VIII, IV 75 IU/kg.
Maintenance: Usually, IV 10 to 20 IU/kg/day.
Hemophilia A patients with inhibitors to Factor VIII: IV 75 IU/kg as single dose followed by second dose in 12 hr if necessary.

Prophylaxis
In patients with hemophilia B, IV 10 to 20 IU/kg 1 to 2 times/wk.

Interactions
Aminocaproic acid: May increase risk of thrombosis.

Lab Test Interferences None well documented.

Adverse Reactions
CV: Thrombosis or DIC; changes in BP; MI (with high doses).
CNS: Headache.
DERM: Flushing; urticaria.
GI: Nausea; vomiting.
RESP: Pulmonary embolism.
OTHER: Pyrogenic reactions (eg, fever and chills); tingling.

Precautions
Pregnancy: Category C.
Hepatitis and HIV infection: Some risk because of preparation from pooled units of plasma.
Intravascular coagulation: If signs of DIC occur, stop infusion promptly.

Assessment/Interventions

- Obtain patient history, including drug history and any known allergies. Note hepatitis B vaccination.
- In patients with major bleeding or those being prepared for surgery, monitor Factor VII or IX assays daily prior to infusion.
- In patients receiving Factor IX for prolonged periods, monitor Factors II, IX, and X daily.
- Assess BP and heart rate prior to and during infusion.
- Observe for signs of DIC, MI, pulmonary embolus, and venous thrombosis.
- Monitor I&O and observe for hemolytic reaction.

- Stop infusion and notify health care provider if any of the following develops: tingling, urticaria, chills, fever, headache, flushing, nausea or vomiting, change in heart rate, BP. Infusion may be restarted at a slower rate when symptoms subside.
- Discontinue infusion if signs of DIC (eg, petechiae, oozing from puncture sites), tachycardia, tachypnea, or joint pain develop, and notify health care provider.

Patient/Family Education
- Instruct patient to report any chills, headache, urticaria, tingling, flushing, nausea, and vomiting to nurse or health care provider.
- Tell patient to immediately report any chest pain/pressure or difficulty breathing.
- Caution patient to avoid activities that could lead to injury or bleeding.
- Instruct patient to report any signs of bleeding (eg, petechiae, purpura, bleeding gums or rectum, blood in urine).
- Discuss questions concerning HIV and hepatitis risk.
- Instruct patient to report any signs or symptoms of AIDS or hepatitis.
- Review methods of preventing and stopping bleeding.
- Advise patient to carry identification/information regarding bleeding tendency.

Famciclovir

(fam-SYE-kloe-veer)
Class Anti-infective/Antiviral

How Supplied
Famvir Tablets 125 mg, Tablets 250 mg, Tablets 500 mg

Action
PHARMACOLOGY: Converts to penciclovir, which inhibits viral DNA replication by interfering with viral DNA polymerase.

PHARMACOKINETICS/DYNAMICS:
Absorption: Bioavailability is about 77%. T_{max} is 0.9 hr. $AUC_{0-\infty}$ is 2.24 to 8.95 depending on dose. C_{max} is 0.8 to 3.3 mcg/mL depending on the dose.
Distribution: Vd is about 1.08 L/kg; 20% bound to plasma proteins.
Metabolism: Route is the liver; deacetylated and oxidized to form inactive penciclovir metabolites.
Excretion: Cl is about 36.6 L/hr; about 75% is renally cleared. The t½ is about 2 to 3 hr.
Special Populations:
Renal Function Impairment – With Ccr 40 to 59 mL/min, Cl_R is about 13 L/hr and t½ is about 3.4 hr. With Ccr 20 to 39 mL/min, Cl_R is about 4.24 L/hr and t½ is about 6.2 hr. With Ccr less than 20 mL/min, Cl_R is about 1.64 L/hr and t½ is about 13.4 hr.
Hepatic Function Impairment – Penciclovir C_{max} decreased 44%; T_{max} increased by 0.75 hr.

Indications Treatment of acute herpes zoster; treatment or suppression of recurrent genital herpes in immunocompetent patients; treatment of recurrent mucocutaneous herpes simplex infections in HIV-infected patients.

Contraindications Hypersensitivity to famciclovir, other components of the formulation, or penciclovir cream.

Route/Dosage
Herpes zoster
ADULTS: **PO** 500 mg q 8 hr for 7 days. Initiate treatment immediately after diagnosis.
Herpes Simplex
ADULTS:
Recurrent Genital Herpes: **PO** 125 mg bid for 5 days. Initiate treatment at the first sign of recurrence.
ADULTS:
Suppression Of Recurrent Genital Herpes: **PO** 250 mg bid for up to 1 year.
HIV-Infected Patients
ADULTS:
Recurrent orolabial or genital herpes: **PO** 500 mg bid for 7 days.
Renal Impairment
ADULTS:
Herpes Zoster: Ccr 60 mL/min or more - 500 mg q 8 hr; Ccr 40 to 59 mL/min - 500 mg q 12 hr; Ccr 20 to 39 mL/min - 500 mg q 24 hr; Ccr less than 20 mL/min - 250 mg q 24 hr.
ADULTS:
Recurrent Genital Herpes: Ccr 40 or more - 125 mg q 12 hr; Ccr 20 to 39 - 125 mg q 24 hr; Ccr less than 20 - 125 mg q 24 hr.

Interactions
Digoxin: Famciclovir may increase digoxin serum concentration.
Probenecid or other drugs significantly eliminated by active renal tubular secretion: May increase famciclovir (penciclovir) serum concentrations.

Lab Test Interferences None well documented.

Adverse Reactions
CNS: Headache (39%); paresthesia, migraine (3%); confusion, delirium, disorientation, confusional state (postmarketing).
DERM: Pruritus (4%); rash (3%); urticaria (postmarketing).
GI: Nausea (13%); diarrhea (9%); abdominal pain (8%); vomiting, flatulence (5%).

GU: Dysmenorrhea (8%).
HEMA: Anemia, leukopenia, neutropenia (postmarketing).
LABTESTABS: Elevated AST, ALT, total bilirubin, serum creatine, amylase, lipase (postmarketing).
OTHER: Fatigue (5%).

Precautions
Pregnancy: Category B.
Lactation: Undetermined.
Children: Safety and efficacy not established.
Renal function impairment: Dosage adjustment is recommended when Ccr is 60 mL/min or less.
Genital herpes: Sexual intercourse must be avoided when lesions are present. Use of famciclovir does not prevent transmission.

PATIENT CARE CONSIDERATIONS

Administration/Storage
- Administer prescribed dose without regard to meals. Administer with food if GI upset occurs.
- Dose and duration of therapy is dependent on condition being treated.
- Store tablets at controlled room temperature (59° to 86°F).

Assessment/Interventions
- Obtain patient history, including drug history and any known allergies. Note impaired renal function.
- Ensure that reduced dose is administered to patient with renal impairment (Ccr less than 60 mL/min.
- For herpes zoster (shingles) assess for history of present illness and time of rash onset. Start treatment no later than 72 hr after onset of rash.
- For genital herpes, assess for history of present illness and time of onset of symptoms. Start treatment no later than 6 hr after onset of symptoms of recurrent episode.
- For recurrent genital herpes, assess history of frequency of recurrence.
- Monitor for effectiveness of treatment.
- Monitor patient for CNS, GI, and general body side effects. Report to health care provider if noted and significant.

Patient/Family Education
- Explain name, dose, action, and potential side effects of drug.
- Review dose and appropriate dosing schedule depending on condition being treated (shingles, cold sores, or recurrent genital herpes). Instruct patient to take medication exactly as prescribed and not to stop taking or change the dose unless advised by health care provider.
- Advise patient that medication can be taken without regard to meals but to take with food if stomach upset occurs.
- Remind patient using medication for recurrent episodes of genital herpes to initiate therapy at the first sign or symptom or recurrence and that medication may not be effective if started more than 6 hr after onset of signs or symptoms of recurrence.
- Advise patient with genital herpes that this drug is not a cure for genital herpes and does not prevent transmission of virus. Instruct patient to avoid sexual intercourse when lesions and/or symptoms are present to avoid infecting partner.
- Advise patient to contact health care provider if medication does not seem to be controlling lesions and/or symptoms or if intolerable side effects develop.
- Advise women to notify health care provider if pregnant, planning to become pregnant, or breastfeeding.
- Instruct patient to not take any prescription or OTC medications or dietary supplements unless advised by health care provider.
- Advise patient that follow-up visits may be necessary to monitor therapy and to keep appointments.

Famotidine

(fuh-moE-tih-deen)
Class Histamine H_2 antagonist

How Supplied
Pepcid Tablets 20 mg, Tablets 40 mg, Powder for Oral Suspension 40 mg/5 mL when reconstituted, Injection 10 mg/mL, Injection, pre-mixed 20 mg/50 mL in 0.9% NaCl ♦ *Pepcid AC* Tablets, chewable 10 mg ♦ *Pepcid AC* Tablets 10 mg ♦ *Pepcid AC* Gelcaps 10 mg ♦ *Pepcid RPD* Tablets, orally disintegrating 20 mg, Tablets, orally disintegrating 40 mg

🍁 *Apo-Famotidine* ♦ *Gen-Famotidine* ♦ *Novo-Famotidine* ♦ *Nu-Famotidine* ♦ *Pepcid IV* ♦ *ratio-Famotidine* ♦ *Rhoxal-famotidine*

Action
PHARMACOLOGY: Reversibly and competitively blocks histamine at H_2 receptors, particularly those in gastric parietal cells, leading to inhibition of gastric acid secretion.

PHARMACOKINETICS/DYNAMICS:
Absorption: Bioavailability is 40% to 45%; T_{max} is 1 to 3 hr; C_{max} is 0.076 to 0.1 mcg/mL (dose dependent).

Distribution: Protein binding is 15% to 20% and Vd is 1.1 to 1.4 L/kg.

Metabolism: The major metabolite is S-oxide.

Excretion: The $t_{1/2}$ is 2.5 to 3.5 hr and 25% to 30% of the oral dose and 65% to 70% of the IV dose is excreted unchanged in the urine.

Special Populations:
Renal Function Impairment – The $t_{1/2}$ is increased.

Indications Short-term treatment and maintenance therapy for duodenal ulcer, gastroesophageal reflux disease (GERD, including erosive or ulcerative disease), benign gastric ulcer, treatment of pathologic hypersecretory conditions. **Unlabeled use(s):** Treatment of upper GI bleeding; prevention of stress ulcers; prior to anesthesia for prevention of pulmonary aspiration of gastric acid.

Contraindications Hypersensitivity to other H_2 antagonists.

Route/Dosage
Duodenal Ulcer (Active) – **PO** 40 mg at bedtime or 20 mg bid for 6 to 8 wk.
Maintenance: 20 mg at bedtime.
Benign Gastric Ulcer (Acute) – **PO** 40 mg at bedtime.

GERD
ADULTS: 20 mg bid (max 6 wk). For esophagitis and accompanying symptoms caused by GERD, 20 to 40 mg bid (max 12 wk).

Pathologic Hypersecretory Conditions
ADULTS: Start at 20 mg q 6 hr, continued as clinically indicated; doses up to 160 mg q 6 hr have been used.

Moderate or Severely Impaired Renal Function
(Ccr less than 10 mL/min) May need to reduce to half the dose or increase dosing interval to 36 to 48 hr.

For Hospitalized Patients with Pathologic Hypersecretory Conditions or Intractable Ulcers, or Patients Unable to Take Orally
Parenteral – 20 mg **IV** q 12 hr. Parenteral use in GERD not established.

Interactions
Ketoconazole: Effects of ketoconazole may be decreased.

Lab Test Interferences None well documented.

Adverse Reactions
CV: Palpitations.
CNS: Headache; somnolence; fatigue; dizziness; confusion; hallucinations; agitation or anxiety; depression; insomnia; paresthesias.
DERM: Alopecia; rash; pruritus; urticaria; acne; dry skin; flushing.
EENT: Tinnitus; taste disorder; orbital edema; conjunctival injection.
GI: Diarrhea; constipation; nausea; vomiting; abdominal discomfort; anorexia; dry mouth.
GU: Impotence; loss of libido.
HEMA: Thrombocytopenia.
RESP: Bronchospasm.
OTHER: Arthralgia; transient pain at injection site; fever.

Precautions
Pregnancy: Category B.
Lactation: Undetermined.
Children: Safety and efficacy not established.
Elderly: May have reduced renal function; decreased clearance may occur.
Hypersensitivity: Rare cases of anaphylaxis have occurred.
Renal function impairment: Decreased clearance may occur; reduced dose may be needed.
Hepatic function impairment: Use caution; decreased clearance may occur.
Gastric malignancy: Symptomatic response to famotidine does not preclude gastric malignancy.

PATIENT CARE CONSIDERATIONS
Administration/Storage
- To prepare for IV push, dilute 2 mL famotidine (solution containing 10 mg/mL) with 0.9% Sodium Chloride for Injection in 5 to 10 mL volume. Administer over 2 min.
- To prepare IV infusion, dilute 2 mL famotidine (solution containing 10 mg/mL) with 100 mL 5% Dextrose. Other diluents that may be used include 0.9% Sodium Chloride for Injection, 10% Dextrose, Lactated Ringer's Injection, or 5% sodium bicarbonate. Infuse over 15 to 30 min.
- Keep powder vials away from heat. After reconstitution, store in the refrigerator, but do not freeze. Discard after 30 days.
- Store parenteral solutions in refrigerator. When mixed in polyvinyl chloride minibags, stability is 14 days in refrigerator; if frozen, solution remains stable for 28 days and for 48 hr at room temperature.
- Administer with antacids if necessary.
- Medication may be mixable with TPN. Stability depends on solution used.

Assessment/Interventions
- Obtain patient history, including drug history and any known allergies.
- Monitor renal and hepatic function in elderly patients. Notify health care provider of any changes in hepatic or renal function.
- Monitor fluid I&O for possible dosage adjustment.
- Give with antacids if necessary.

Patient/Family Education
- Instruct patient not to double up on medication if dose is missed, but to wait and take next scheduled dose on time.
- Tell patient to notify health care provider immediately of any black, tarry stool or "coffee-ground" vomit.
- Tell patient to notify health care provider of any shortness of breath, GI disturbances, bleeding, rash, dizziness, or fever.
- Tell patient to shake suspension well before taking.

Felbamate

(FELL-buh-MATE)

Class Anticonvulsant

How Supplied
Felbatol Tablets 400 mg, Tablets 600 mg, Suspension 600 mg/5 mL

Action
PHARMACOLOGY: May reduce seizure spread in generalized tonic-clonic or partial seizures and may increase seizure threshold in absence seizures.

PHARMACOKINETICS/DYNAMICS:

Distribution: Vd is about 756 mL/kg and the drug is 22% to 25% bound to plasma proteins.

Metabolism: About 40% to 50% is excreted unchanged in the urine.

About 40% is unidentified metabolites and conjugates and about 15% is parahydroxy-felbamate, 2-hydroxyfelbamate, and felbamate monocarbamate; none have significant anticonvulsant activity.

Excretion: The t½ is 20 to 23 hr. Cl is about 30 mL/hr/kg.

Special Populations:
Renal Function Impairment – Decreased felbamate Cl and increased t½ were associated with diminishing renal function.

Indications
Monotherapy or adjunctive therapy in treatment of partial seizures with and without generalization in epileptic adults. Adjunctive therapy in treatment of partial and generalized seizures associated with Lennox-Gastaut syndrome in children.

Contraindications
Hypersensitivity to felbamate or ingredients of this product; hypersensitivity reactions to other carbamates; history of any blood dyscrasia or hepatic dysfunction.

Route/Dosage
Because of reports of aplastic anemia, it has been recommended to stop use of this drug unless health care provider decides that withdrawal would cause greater risk.

Initial Monotherapy
ADULTS AND ADOLESCENTS 14 YR AND OLDER: PO 1200 mg/day in 3 or 4 divided doses; increase in 600 mg increments q 2 wk to 2400 mg/day and then 3600 mg/day if indicated.

Conversion to Monotherapy
ADULTS AND ADOLESCENTS 14 YR AND OLDER: Initial dose: PO 1200 mg/day in 3 or 4 divided doses, reducing dose of other antiepileptic drugs by ⅓. At wk 2, increase felbamate to 2400 mg/day and at week 3, increase to 3600 mg/day; continue to reduce dose of other antiepileptic drugs as indicated.

Adjunctive Therapy
ADULTS AND ADOLESCENTS 14 YR AND OLDER: Initial dose: PO 1200 mg/day in 3 or 4 divided doses; reduce original dose of other antiepileptic drugs by 20% to 33% for 1 wk. At week 2, increase felbamate to 2400 mg/day and at week 3, increase to 3600 mg/day if needed; reduce dosage of other antiepileptic drugs as clinically indicated.

CHILDREN 2 TO 14 YR WITH LENNOX-GASTAUT SYNDROME: PO 15 mg/kg/day in 3 or 4 divided doses while reducing other antiepileptic drugs at least 20%. Increase felbamate by 15 mg/kg/day increments at weekly intervals up to 45 mg/kg/day; continue to reduce dosage of other antiepileptic drugs as needed.

Interactions
Antiepileptic drugs: Felbamate may increase blood levels of phenytoin and valproic acid and decrease blood levels of carbamazepine. Phenytoin or carbamazepine may increase clearance of felbamate.

Lab Test Interferences
None well documented.

Adverse Reactions
CNS: Insomnia; headache; anxiety; somnolence; dizziness; nervousness; tremor; abnormal gait; depression; paresthesia; ataxia; dry mouth; stupor; thinking abnormalities; emotional lability.
DERM: Acne; rash; pruritus.
EENT: Diplopia; abnormal vision; miosis; otitis media; rhinitis; sinusitis; taste perversion; pharyngitis.
GI: Dyspepsia; vomiting; constipation; diarrhea; nausea; anorexia; abdominal pain; hiccoughs.
GU: Urinary incontinence; intramenstrual bleeding; UTI.
HEMA: Aplastic anemia; purpura; leukopenia.
HEPA: Increased ALT and AST; acute liver failure.

RESP: Upper respiratory tract infection; coughing.
OTHER: Fatigue; weight decrease; facial edema; fever; chest pain; pain; hypophosphatemia; myalgia.

> **WARNING:**
>
> *Hematological:* Aplastic anemia associated with use. Risk 100-fold in felbamate-treated patients compared to untreated population. May be fatal. Use only in patients with severe epilepsy in which risk of aplastic anemia is acceptable.
>
> *Hepatotoxicity:* Acute liver failure reported with use, initiate use in patients with normal liver function. Monitor ALT, AST, and bilirubin at baseline and at 1- to 2-wk intervals. Discontinue if AST or ALT increase is greater than or equal to 2 times the upper limit of normal.

PATIENT CARE CONSIDERATIONS
Administration/Storage
- Instruct patient to take tablet whole with full glass of water; do not crush.
- May administer tablet with food.
- Administer suspension if patient is unable to swallow tablets.
- Shake suspension prior to administration.
- Do not discontinue administration suddenly because of the possibility of increased frequency of seizures.
- Store at room temperature in tightly closed container away from excessive heat, direct sunlight, and moisture.

Assessment/Interventions
- Obtain patient history, including drug history and any known allergies. Note current status and frequency of seizures and use of other antiepileptic drugs, nonprescription drugs, and social drugs (alcohol).
- Assess baseline data on patient's weight and hematologic and hepatic functions.
- Monitor for effectiveness; note any changes in seizure patterns and frequency.
- If seizures occur, protect patient from injury.
- Weigh patient weekly and record weight.
- Monitor serum levels of felbamate or other antiepileptic drugs as necessary.

Precautions
Pregnancy: Category C.
Lactation: Excreted in breast milk.
Children: Safety and efficacy not established other than for adjunctive therapy of Lennox-Gastaut syndrome.
Elderly: Use caution and start with low doses. Clinical experience is limited.
Hypersensitivity: Administer drug with caution to patients with prior hypersensitivity reactions to carbamates.
Carcinogenesis: Drug may have carcinogenic potential.
Discontinuation: Withdraw drug slowly to avoid increased seizure frequency.
Pre-existing liver failure: 8 cases of acute liver failure have occurred, including 4 deaths, in association with the use of felbamate. Evaluate patients prior to treatment initiation for evidence of pre-existing liver damage; avoid use in patients with pre-existing liver pathology. Immediately withdraw the drug in patients who develop lab findings indicating liver injury.

Patient/Family Education
- Instruct patient to drink at least 1 full glass of water with each dose.
- Remind patient to take tablet whole; do not crush.
- Inform patient that tablet may be taken with food.
- Caution patient to not stop taking this medication suddenly because of possibility of increasing seizure frequency.
- Advise patient to avoid exposure to sunlight or sunlamps and to use sunscreen or wear protective clothing to avoid photosensitivity reaction.
- Instruct patient and family that if seizures occur, they should protect patient from injury.
- Inform patient to report these symptoms to health care provider: loss of appetite, nausea, vomiting, indigestion, constipation, diarrhea, weight loss/gain, anxiety, nervousness, tremors, dizziness, depression, chest pain, fever, headache, poor coordination, drowsiness, sleeplessness, edema (fluid retention), intramenstrual bleeding (women), dry mouth, vision problems and any changes in seizure activity.
- Advise patient that drug may cause drowsiness, dizziness, and vision problems, and to use caution while driving or performing other tasks requiring mental alertness.

Felodipine

(feh-LOW-dih-peen)
Class Calcium channel blocker

How Supplied
Plendil Tablets, extended release 2.5 mg, Tablets, extended release 5 mg, Tablets, extended release 10 mg
✤ *Renedil*

Action
PHARMACOLOGY: Inhibits movement of calcium ions across cell membrane in systemic and coronary vascular smooth muscle, altering contractile process.

PHARMACOKINETICS/DYNAMICS:

Absorption: Systemic bioavailability is about 20% and T_{max} is 2.5 to 5 hr. C_{max} is increased by about 60% and AUC is unchanged with a high fat or carbohydrate meal.

Distribution: Vd is about 40 L/kg and it is greater than 99% bound to plasma proteins.

Metabolism: Extensive first pass metabolism; 6 metabolites account for 23% of activity.

Excretion: The $t_½$ is 11 to 16 hr; 70% of the drug is eliminated in the urine and 10% in the feces.

Onset: 2 to 5 hr.

Duration: 24 hr (during chronic administration).

Special Populations:
Hepatic Function Impairment – About 40% reduction in clearance.

Indications
Treatment of hypertension.

Contraindications
Sick sinus syndrome; second- or third-degree AV block except with functioning pacemaker; hypotension with systolic BP less than 90 mm Hg.

Route/Dosage
PO 2.5 to 10 mg once daily. Max 20 mg once daily. Elderly rarely require more than 10 mg qd.

Interactions
Barbiturates: Effects of felodipine may be decreased.
Carbamazepine: Plasma levels of felodipine may be decreased, reducing effect.
Food: Effects of felodipine may increase if given with grapefruit juice.
Histamine H_2-antagonists: Cimetidine may increase effects of felodipine.
Hydantoins: Serum felodipine levels may be decreased, reducing effects.
Other antihypertensive agents: May have additive effects.

Lab Test Interferences
None well documented.

Adverse Reactions
CV: Peripheral edema; hypotension; syncope; AV block; MI; arrhythmias; angina; tachycardia.
CNS: Headache; dizziness; lightheadedness; nervousness; psychiatric disturbances; paresthesias; somnolence; asthenia; insomnia; anxiety; irritability.
GI: Nausea; diarrhea; constipation; abdominal discomfort; cramps; dyspepsia; vomiting; dry mouth; thirst; flatulence.
GU: Micturition disorders; sexual difficulties.
HEMA: Epistaxis.
RESP: Nasal or chest congestion; sinusitis; rhinitis; pharyngitis; shortness of breath; wheezing; cough; sneezing; respiratory infections.
OTHER: Muscle cramps, pain, or inflammation; gingival hyperplasia.

Precautions
Pregnancy: Category C.
Lactation: Undetermined.
Children: Safety and efficacy not established.
Elderly: May have greater hypotensive effects and increased risk of peripheral edema when dosage exceeds 20 mg/day. Monitor closely; doses more than 10 mg usually not needed.
Hepatic function impairment: Use with caution in patients with impaired hepatic function or reduced hepatic blood flow.
CHF: Use with caution.
Withdrawal syndrome: Abrupt withdrawal may cause increased frequency and duration of angina. Taper dose gradually.

Overdosage: Signs and Symptoms
Hypotension, bradycardia, nausea, weakness, dizziness, slurred speech.

PATIENT CARE CONSIDERATIONS

Administration/Storage
♦ Do not crush tablet or allow patient to chew it.
♦ Give with food if patient experiences GI upset.

Assessment/Interventions
♦ Obtain patient history, including drug history and any known allergies.
♦ Monitor BP frequently during dosage adjustment, especially for patients more than 65 yr and patients with liver dysfunction.

Patient/Family Education
♦ Instruct patient not to crush or chew tablets.
♦ Teach patient and family member correct method of measuring BP.
♦ Explain that mild peripheral edema may

occur within 2 to 3 wk after beginning therapy.
- Advise patient that drug may cause drowsiness and dizziness. Use caution while driving or performing other tasks requiring mental alertness.
- Instruct patient to avoid sudden position changes to prevent postural hypotension.
- Explain importance of proper oral hygiene and regular dental examinations to prevent gum disease.
- Tell patient not to double up medication if dose is missed, but to wait and take next scheduled dose on time.
- Instruct patient to report the following symptoms to health care provider: irregular heart beat, increased frequency or severity of angina, shortness of breath, swelling of hands and feet, dizziness, constipation, nausea, unusual bleeding or bruising, hypotension.

Fenofibrate

(FEN-oh-fih-brate)

Class Antihyperlipidemic

How Supplied
Lofibra Capsules 67 mg, Capsules 134 mg, Capsules 200 mg ◆ *Tricor* Tablets 54 mg, Tablets 160 mg
❀ *Apo-Fenofibrate* ◆ *Apo-Feno-Micro* ◆ *Gen-Fenofibrate Micro* ◆ *Lipidil Micro* ◆ *Lipidil Supra* ◆ *Nu-Fenofibrate* ◆ *PMS-Fenofibrate Micro*

Action
PHARMACOLOGY: Mechanism not well established. Apparently decreases plasma levels of triglycerides by decreasing their synthesis. Also reduces plasma levels of very low density lipoproteins (VLDL) cholesterol by reducing their release into the circulation and increasing catabolism. Reduces serum uric acid levels by increasing urinary excretion of uric acid.

PHARMACOKINETICS/DYNAMICS:
Absorption: Well absorbed; absorption increased about 35% with food. T_{max} is 6 to 8 hr.

Distribution: About 99% bound to plasma proteins; Vd is about 30 L. Steady state is achieved within 5 days of dosing.

Metabolism: Hydrolyzed by esterases to the active metabolite of fenofibric acid. Fenofibric acid is conjugated with glucuronic acid and then excreted.

Excretion: Excretion is 60% in the urine in the form of metabolites; 25% excreted in the feces. The t½ is 20 hr, and Cl is 1.1 L/hr.

Special Populations:
Renal Function Impairment – With severe renal impairment of Ccr less than 50 mL/min, rate of Cl is greatly reduced. Minimize dosage.

Indications
Adjunctive therapy to diet for treatment of hypertriglyceridemia in adult patients with type 4 or 5 hyperlipidemia who are at risk of pancreatitis; adjunctive therapy to diet for the reduction of LDL cholesterol, total cholesterol, triglycerides, and apolipoprotein B, and to increase HDL cholesterol in adults with primary hypercholesterolemia or mixed dyslipidemia (Fredrickson types IIa and IIb).

Contraindications
Hepatic or severe renal dysfunction, including primary biliary cirrhosis; patients with unexplained persistent liver function abnormality; preexisting gallbladder disease; hypersensitivity to fenofibrate.

Route/Dosage
ELDERLY: **PO** 67 mg/day.

Hypertriglyceridemia
ADULTS: **PO** *Tricor* Start with 54 to 160 mg/day (max, 160 mg/day). *Lofibra:* 67 to 200 mg/day (max, 200 mg/day).

Primary Hypercholesterolemia/Mixed Hyperlipidemia
ADULTS: **PO** *Tricor* Initial dose is 160 mg/day. *Lofibra:* 200 mg/day.

Renal Function Impairment
ADULTS: **PO** 67 mg/day.

Interactions
Bile acid sequestrants (eg, cholestyramine): Reduces absorption of fenofibrate.
Cyclosporine (eg, Sandimmune): Increases risk of nephrotoxicity.
HMG-CoA reductase inhibitors (eg, lovastatin): Increased risk of severe myopathy, rhabdomyolysis, and acute renal failure.
Oral anticoagulants (eg, warfarin): Anticoagulant effect may be increased.

Lab Test Interferences
None well documented.

Adverse Reactions
CV: Arrhythmia.
CNS: Dizziness; insomnia; paresthesia; headache; fatigue; asthenia.
DERM: Rash; pruritus; urticaria.
EENT: Eye irritation; blurred vision; conjunctivitis; eye floaters; earache; rhinitis.
GI: Dyspepsia; nausea; vomiting; diarrhea; constipation; abdominal pain; flatulence; eructation; increased appetite; pancreatitis.
GU: Decreased libido; polyuria; vaginitis.
HEMA: Anemia; leukopenia; mild to moderate hemoglobin, hematocrit, and WBC decreases.
HEPA: Elevated liver enzymes.

LABTESTABS: Increased AST, ALT, and creatine phosphokinase.
RESP: Rhinitis; sinusitis; cough; respiratory disorder.
OTHER: Flu syndrome; arthralgia; back pain; hypersensitivity reactions (including severe skin rashes, Stevens-Johnson syndrome, toxic epidermal necrolysis); myositis; myopathy; rhabdomyolysis.

Precautions
Pregnancy: Category C.
Lactation: Do not use in nursing women. Discontinue drug or discontinue nursing.
Children: Safety and efficacy not established.
Renal function impairment: When Ccr is below 50 mL/min, initiate therapy at 67 mg/day and increase only after evaluation of the effects on renal function and triglyceride levels at this dose.
Hepatic function impairment: Drug can cause significant increases in serum transaminases. Perform regular periodic monitoring of liver function for duration of therapy; discontinue therapy if enzyme levels persist more than 3 times the normal limit.
Monitoring: Evaluate serum lipids periodically (eg, 4 to 8 wk) during initial therapy to determine lowest effective dose; withdraw therapy if an adequate response is not achieved after 2 mo of treatment with the max dose. Perform periodic blood counts during first 12 mo of therapy to detect rare episodes of thrombocytopenia and granulocytopenia.
Cholelithiasis: May increase cholesterol secretion into the bile, leading to cholelithiasis. If cholelithiasis is suspected, gallbladder studies are indicated. Discontinue therapy if gallstones are found.
Myopathy/Myositis: Can be used by fibrates alone or in combination with HMG-CoA reductase inhibitors. Consider in any patient with diffuse myalgia, muscle tenderness or weakness, or marked CPK elevations. Discontinue therapy if myopathy/myositis is suspected or diagnosed.
Pancreatitis: Has been reported in patients taking fenofibrate.

PATIENT CARE CONSIDERATIONS
Administration/Storage
- May be used alone or in combination with other lipid-lowering therapy.
- Administer prescribed dose with food to increase absorption.
- Administer prescribed dose 1 hr before or 4 to 6 hr after a bile acid sequestrant (eg, cholestyramine).
- Store capsules at controlled room temperature (68° to 77°F). Protect from moisture.

Assessment/Interventions
- Obtain patient history, including drug history and any known allergies. Note renal or hepatic impairment, persistent liver function abnormality, or gallbladder disease.
- Ensure secondary causes of hypercholesterolemia (eg, poorly controlled diabetes, hypothyroidism) and hypertriglyceridemia (eg, excess alcohol, medications) are excluded before starting therapy.
- Ensure patient is on a lipid-lowering diet before starting therapy and that diet is continued during treatment.
- Ensure lowest starting dose and slower dose escalation is used in patient with severe renal impairment (Ccr less than 50 mL/min).
- Ensure serum lipids are measured before therapy is started and periodically thereafter.
- Ensure serum transaminases are determined before starting therapy and periodically thereafter during prolonged treatment. If elevated serum transaminase levels develop during treatment, repeat levels more frequently. If transaminase levels rise to 3 times upper limit of normal and persist, notify health care provider. Be prepared to discontinue therapy.
- Ensure CBC with differential and platelet count is evaluated before starting therapy and periodically thereafter during the first 12 mo of therapy. Notify health care provider if abnormalities noted.
- If muscle pain, tenderness, and/or weakness develop during therapy, notify health care provider immediately. Be prepared to determine CPK levels and discontinue therapy if myopathy or myositis is suspected or diagnosed.
- Assess patient for GI, MUSC, and general body side effects. Inform health care provider if noted and significant.

Patient/Family Education
- Explain name, dose, action, and potential side effects of drug.
- Advise patient to take each dose with food to increase absorption and lipid-lowering effectiveness.
- Advise patient who is also taking a bile acid resin (eg, cholestyramine) to take the fenofibrate 1 hr before or 4 to 6 hr after the resin.
- Advise patient to try to take each dose at about the same time each day.
- Inform patient that drug helps control, but not does cure, lipid abnormality and to con-

tinue taking drug as prescribed if lipid levels are lowered.
* Caution patient not to change the dose or stop taking unless advised by health care provider.
* Advise patient if a dose is missed to take as soon as remembered but to never take more than 1 dose of fenofibrate a day.
* Instruct patient to continue taking other cholesterol-lowering medications as prescribed by health care provider.
* Emphasize to patient importance of the following other modalities on cholesterol control: dietary changes (reduced saturated fat intake, increase soluble fiber intake, weight control, regular exercise, smoking cessation).
* Advise women of childbearing potential to notify health care provider if pregnant, planning to become pregnant, or breastfeeding.
* Caution patient not to take any prescription or OTC medications, herbal preparations, or dietary supplements unless advised by health care provider.
* Instruct patient to immediately notify health care provider if they experience any unexplained muscle pain, tenderness and/or weakness, or severe stomach pain associated with nausea and vomiting.
* Advise patient that follow-up visits and lab tests will be required to monitor therapy and to keep appointments.

Fenoprofen Calcium

(FEN-oh-PRO-fen KAL-see-uhm)
Class Analgesic/NSAID

How Supplied
Nalfon Pulvules Capsules 200 mg, Capsules 300 mg

Action
PHARMACOLOGY: Decreases inflammation, pain and fever, probably through inhibition of cyclooxygenase activity and prostaglandin synthesis.

PHARMACOKINETICS/DYNAMICS:
Absorption: T_{max} is 2 hr; C_{max} is 50 mcg/mL.
Distribution: Fenoprofen is about 99% protein bound.
Metabolism: Major urinary metabolites are fenoprofen glucuronide and 4′-hydroxyfenoprofen glucuronide.
Excretion: The t½ is 3 hr; about 90% is renally eliminated.

Indications Symptomatic relief for rheumatoid arthritis, osteoarthritis, mild to moderate pain. **Unlabeled use(s):** Symptomatic relief for juvenile rheumatoid arthritis; migraine prophylaxis and treatment.

Contraindications Sensitivity to aspirin or other NSAIDs; preexisting renal disease.

Route/Dosage
Rheumatoid Arthritis/Osteoarthritis
PO 300 to 600 mg tid to qid; do not exceed 3.2 g/day.

Mild/Moderate Pain
PO 200 mg q 4 to 6 h prn.

Interactions
Anticoagulants: May increase risk of bleeding caused by gastric erosion.
Methotrexate: May increase methotrexate levels.
Phenobarbital: Phenobarbital, an enzyme inducer, may decrease fenoprofen half-life. Dosage adjustments of fenoprofen may be required if phenobarbital is added or withdrawn.

Lab Test Interferences False elevation in free and total serum T_3 as measured by *Amerlex-M* kit.

Adverse Reactions
CV: CHF; hypotension; hypertension; peripheral edema; fluid retention; vasodilation.
CNS: Dizziness; drowsiness; headaches; nervousness; anxiety; confusion; somnolence.
DERM: Pruritus; erythema; urticaria.
EENT: Visual disturbances; tinnitus; dry eyes.
GI: Heartburn; dyspepsia; nausea; vomiting; diarrhea; constipation; increased or decreased appetite; indigestion; GI bleeding; ulceration; abdominal distress/pain; flatulence; occult blood in stool.
GU: Hematuria; proteinuria; renal insufficiency; glomerular and interstitial nephritis; acute renal failure with preexisting renal dysfunction.
HEMA: Bone marrow depression; neutropenia; leukopenia; hypocoagulability.
METAB: Hyperglycemia; hypoglycemia; hyponatremia.
RESP: Bronchospasm; laryngeal edema; hemoptysis; shortness of breath.

Precautions
Pregnancy: Category B.
Lactation: Undetermined.
Children: Safety and efficacy not established.
Elderly: Increased risk of adverse reactions.
Hypersensitivity: Use caution in aspirin-sensitive individuals because of possible cross-sensitivity.
Renal function impairment: Acute renal insufficiency, interstitial nephritis, hyperkalemia, hyponatremia, and renal papillary necrosis may occur.
GI effects: Serious GI toxicity (eg, bleeding, ulceration, perforation) can occur at any time, with or without warning symptoms.

GU effects: GU tract problems have occurred (most frequently dysuria, cystitis, hematuria, nephrotic syndrome). This may be preceded by fever, rash, arthralgia, oliguria, and azotemia, and may progress to anuria. Rapid recovery followed early recognition and drug withdrawal.

PATIENT CARE CONSIDERATIONS
Administration/Storage
- Give with food, milk, or antacids if GI upset occurs.

Assessment/Interventions
- Obtain patient history, including drug history and any known allergies.
- Assess baseline renal function, BP, blood glucose levels, PT, and CBC prior to beginning therapy and monitor periodically during therapy.
- Monitor blood glucose closely in patients with diabetes.
- Assess for any visual disturbances. Notify health care provider if any visual changes occur.
- Assess auditory function during prolonged therapy in patients with impaired hearing.
- Report any CNS or respiratory disturbances to health care provider.
- Monitor PT if patient is concurrently taking anticoagulants.
- Evaluate for signs and symptoms of ulceration and bleeding if patient is on prolonged therapy.

Patient/Family Education
- Instruct patient to take with food, milk, or antacids if GI symptoms occur (eg, pain, nausea, anorexia). If symptoms persist, report to health care provider.
- Advise patient that improvement may occur in 2 to 3 days but 2 to 3 wk may be required.
- Inform patient taking anticoagulant concurrently to watch for signs and symptoms of bleeding or unusual bruising and report immediately to health care provider.
- Instruct patient to call health care provider if headaches or other CNS disturbances occur. If headaches persist despite dosage reduction, drug may be discontinued.
- Advise patient to avoid aspirin and alcoholic beverages while taking medication.
- Instruct patient that drug may cause drowsiness and to use caution while driving or performing other tasks requiring mental alertness, coordination, and dexterity.
- Instruct patient to report to health care provider any fever, rash, joint pain, or any changes in urinary elimination including those associated with pain, discoloration, or decreased amount.
- Advise patient to minimize exposure to sun and to use sunscreen or wear protective clothing outdoors until tolerance is determined.

Overdosage: Signs and Symptoms
Drowsiness, dizziness, mental confusion, disorientation, lethargy, paresthesias, numbness, vomiting, gastric irritation, nausea, abdominal pain, headache, tinnitus, sweating, convulsions, blurred vision, elevations in serum creatine and BUN, hypotension, tachycardia.

Fentanyl Citrate

(FEN-tuh-nill)

Class Narcotic analgesic

How Supplied
Sublimaze Injection 0.05 mg base (as citrate)/mL
- *Fentanyl Oralet* Lozenges 100 mcg, Lozenges 200 mcg, Lozenges 300 mcg, Lozenges 400 mcg
- *Actiq* Lozenge on a stick 200 mcg, Lozenge on a stick 400 mcg, Lozenge on a stick 600 mcg, Lozenge on a stick 800 mcg, Lozenge on a stick 1200 mcg, Lozenge on a stick 1600 mcg

Action
PHARMACOLOGY: A potent, short-acting, rapid-onset opiate agonist that relieves pain by stimulating opiate receptors in CNS; also causes respiratory depression, peripheral vasodilation, inhibition of intestinal peristalsis, sphincter of Oddi spasm, stimulation of chemoreceptors that cause vomiting, and increased bladder tone.

PHARMACOKINETICS/DYNAMICS:
Absorption: Absolute bioavailability is 50% total between transmucosal and GI absorption. C_{max} is 0.39 to 2.51 ng/mL; T_{max} is 20 to 480 minutes.

Distribution: Highly lipophilic. It is 80% to 85% protein bound. Vd_{ss} is 4 L/kg.

Metabolism: Metabolized in the liver and intestinal mucosa to the active metabolite norfentanyl by cytochrome P450 3A4.

Excretion: Total plasma clearance is 0.5 L/hr/kg; $t_{½}$ is about 7 hr. More than 7% is excreted unchanged in the urine and about 1% is excreted unchanged in feces. Inactive metabolites are primarily excreted in the urine.

Onset: 7 to 8 min.

Duration: 1 to 2 hr. Therapeutic concentration

for analgesia at 1 to 2 ng/mL, for surgical anesthesia and profound respiratory depression at 10 to 20 ng/mL.

Special Populations:
Renal Function Impairment – Alters kinetics because of alterations in clearance and plasma proteins. Individualize dose and use caution.
Hepatic Function Impairment – Alters kinetics because of alterations in clearance and plasma proteins. Individualize dose and use caution.

Indications Short-term analgesia before, during, and after anesthesia; supplement to general or regional anesthesia; for administration with neuroleptic during anesthesia; anesthesia with oxygen for high-risk patients.

Contraindications Known intolerance to fentanyl.

Route/Dosage
Premedication
ADULTS: **IM** 0.05 to 0.1 mg 30 to 60 min before surgery. Elderly patients may need reduced dose.

Postoperative (Recovery Room)
IM/IV 0.05 to 0.1 mg for pain control, tachypnea, or emergent delirium. May repeat in 1 to 2 hr.

Adjunct to Regional Anesthesia
IM/IV 0.05 to 0.1 mg; dose administered over 1 to 2 min prn.

Adjunct to General Anesthesia
See dosage information in table below.

General Anesthesia
IV 0.05 to 0.1 mg/kg with oxygen and muscle relaxant. Max IV 0.15 mg/kg.
CHILDREN 2 TO 12 YR: For induction and maintenance, reduce dose as low as IV 2 to 3 mcg/kg.

Interactions
Amiodarone: Profound bradycardia, sinus arrest, and hypotension may occur.
Barbiturate anesthetics, other CNS depressants: May have additive effects. Dose of fentanyl required will be less than usual.
Diazepam: Diazepam may produce cardiovascular depression when given with high doses of fentanyl.
Droperidol: May cause hypotension and decrease pulmonary arterial pressure.
Nitrous oxide: Nitrous oxide may cause cardiovascular depression with high-dose fentanyl.
Protease inhibitors: Monitor for increased CNS and respiratory depression.

Lab Test Interferences Increased amylase and lipase may occur up to 24 hr after dose.

Adverse Reactions
CV: Hypotension; hypertension; bradycardia; tachycardia; chest wall rigidity.
CNS: Lightheadedness; dizziness; sedation; disorientation; incoordination; seizures.
DERM: Sweating; pruritus; urticaria.
GI: Nausea; vomiting; constipation; abdominal pain.
GU: Urinary retention or hesitancy.
RESP: Laryngospasm; depression of cough reflex; respiratory depression; rebound respiratory depression postoperatively.
OTHER: Skeletal muscle rigidity; tolerance; psychological and physical dependence with chronic use.

Precautions
Pregnancy: Category C. Fentanyl has been shown to impair fertility and to have an embryocidal effect in rats at doses 0.3 times the upper human dose for 12 days. The use of fentanyl is not recommended in labor.
Lactation: Excreted in breast milk.
Children: Not recommended for children less than 2 yr.
Renal function impairment: Duration of action may be prolonged; may need to reduce dose.
Hepatic function impairment Duration of action may be prolonged; may need to reduce dose.
Special risk patients: Use with caution in elderly patients and patients with myxedema, acute alcoholism, acute abdominal conditions, ulcerative colitis, decreased respiratory reserve, head injury or increased intracranial pressure, hypoxia, bradycardia, supraventricular tachycardia, depleted blood volume, circulatory shock.
Hypoventilation: Naloxone and intubation equipment must be available.
Skeletal muscle rigidity: Fentanyl may cause skeletal muscle rigidity, particularly of the truncal muscles.

Adjunct to General Anesthesia

Depth of anesthesia	Total dose	Maintenance*
Low	0.002 mg/kg	Usually not needed
Moderate	0.002 to 0.02 mg/kg	0.025 to 0.1 mg IV/IM
High	0.02 to 0.05 mg/kg	0.025 mg to 50% of induction dose

*Given when vital signs indicate surgical stress/lightening of anesthesia.

Overdosage: Signs and Symptoms
Miosis, respiratory depression, CNS depression, circulatory collapse, seizures, cardiopulmonary arrest, death.

PATIENT CARE CONSIDERATIONS
Administration/Storage
- Use medication immediately after dilution.
- Check calculated dose volume carefully.
- Administer IV dose slowly over 1 to 2 min.
- Store at room temperature and protect from light.

Assessment/Interventions
- Obtain patient history, including drug history and any known allergies.
- Assess pain type and intensity prior to administration; assess effectiveness of pain relief shortly after administration.
- Assess respiratory rate, heart rate, and BP frequently. Report significant changes to health care provider.
- Assess for confusion; implement safety precautions as needed.
- Monitor GI, urinary, and bowel function (urinary retention commonly occurs).
- Take precautions to prevent falls secondary to lightheadedness, dizziness, confusion, and/or hypotension.
- Ensure that naloxone and intubation/airway management equipment are available in event of overdose.

Patient/Family Education
- Instruct patient about adverse effects, and identify signs and symptoms that should be reported.
- Explain that lightheadedness and dizziness are frequently experienced and that transfer assistance should be used as needed.
- Instruct patient to avoid use of other CNS depressants or alcohol and to avoid driving after administration.
- Explain potential for tolerance with continued use.

Fentanyl Transdermal System

(FEN-tuh-nill)

Class Narcotic analgesic

How Supplied
Duragesic-25 Transdermal System 2.5 mg ♦
Duragesic-50 Transdermal System 5 mg ♦
Duragesic-75 Transdermal System 7.5 mg ♦
Duragesic-100 Transdermal System 10 mg
🍁 *Duragesic*

Action
PHARMACOLOGY: A potent, short-acting, rapid-onset opiate agonist that relieves pain by stimulating opiate receptors in CNS; also causes respiratory depression, peripheral vasodilation, inhibition of intestinal peristalsis, sphincter of Oddi spasm, stimulation of chemoreceptors that cause vomiting, and increased bladder tone.

PHARMACOKINETICS/DYNAMICS:
Absorption: T_{max} is 24 to 72 hr; C_{max} is about 0.6 to 2.5 ng/mL (dose-dependent).

Excretion: Mean t½ is 17 hr (after removal).

Indications Management of chronic pain refractory to less potent agents.

Contraindications Hypersensitivity to fentanyl or adhesives.

Route/Dosage
PATIENTS WHO HAVE NOT TAKEN ANOTHER OPIATE CHRONICALLY (ADULTS): Give lowest dose (25 mcg/hr) initially.
ELDERLY: May need reduced dose.
PATIENTS WHO HAVE RECEIVED ANOTHER OPIATE CHRONICALLY (ADULTS): Calculate dose based on previous day's opiate requirement. Maximum pain relief does not occur until 24 hr after application; a short-acting opiate may be needed for breakthrough pain. Initial dose can be increased after 3 days. Further dosage increases should occur at least 6-day intervals. Replace patches q 3 days; some patients require new patch q 2 days.

Interactions
Amiodarone: Profound bradycardia, sinus arrest, and hypotension may occur.
Barbiturate anesthetics, other CNS depressants: May have additive effects. Dosage of fentanyl required will be less than usual.

Lab Test Interferences None well documented.

Adverse Reactions
CV: Hypotension; orthostatic hypotension; hypertension; bradycardia; tachycardia; chest pain.
CNS: Lightheadedness; dizziness; sedation; disorientation; incoordination; headache; hallucinations; euphoria; depression; seizures.
DERM: Sweating; pruritus; urticaria; exfoliative dermatitis.
GI: Nausea; vomiting; constipation; abdominal pain; diarrhea; dyspepsia; dry mouth.
GU: Urinary retention or hesitancy.
RESP: Laryngospasm; depression of cough reflex; dyspnea; hypoventilation.
OTHER: Tolerance; psychological and physical dependence with chronic use.

FENTANYL TRANSDERMAL SYSTEM

> **WARNING:**
> Only for chronic pain in patients who are already receiving continuous opioid therapy and cannot be managed by lesser means. Risk of potentially fatal hypoventilation contraindicates use in acute or postoperative pain, intermittent pain responsive to prn or non-opioid therapy.

Precautions
Pregnancy: Category C.
Lactation: Excreted in breast milk.
Children: Do not use in children less than 12 yr, or less than 18 yr who weigh less than 50 kg.
Renal function impairment: Use with caution because fentanyl is renally and hepatically excreted.
Hepatic function impairment: Use with caution because fentanyl is renally and hepatically excreted.
Special risk patients: Use with caution in elderly patients or patients with myxedema, acute alcoholism, acute abdominal conditions, ulcerative colitis, decreased respiratory reserve, head injury or increased intracranial pressure, hypoxia, supraventricular tachycardia, depleted blood volume, or circulatory shock
Exposure to external heat: Direct contact with heating pads, electric blankets, saunas, or hot tubs could increase fentanyl absorption.
Fever: May increase absorption of fentanyl; monitor for adverse reactions.

Overdosage: Signs and Symptoms
Miosis, respiratory depression, CNS depression, hypoventilation, circulatory collapse, seizures, cardiopulmonary arrest, death.

PATIENT CARE CONSIDERATIONS
Administration/Storage
- Select dry, flat surface on chest or back for application. If excessive body hair is present, clip hair in affected area. Do not shave.
- Avoid applying to any irritated body area.
- After removing wrap, apply to skin using firm pressure for about 20 sec. Be certain that edges are sealed. If gel accidentally comes in contact with skin, wash area with water.
- Remove after 72 hr; fold adhesive side in on itself and discard in toilet.
- Rotate application sites.
- If patch becomes loose, reinforce edges with tape. Do not completely cover patch with another occlusive dressing.

Assessment/Interventions
- Obtain patient history, including drug history and any known allergies.
- Assess respiratory rate, heart rate, and BP prior to administration and frequently during therapy, especially after dosage adjustment. Report significant alterations to health care provider.
- Assess pain type and intensity prior to administration and 24 hr after administration. Assess need for intermittent short-term analgesia until adequate pain control is achieved.
- Reassess 72 hr after administration to determine effectiveness of initial dose and after every dosage adjustment.
- Assess for signs of developing tolerance.
- Monitor GI, urinary, and bowel function.
- Take precautions to prevent falls, especially with initial dosages.
- If adverse reactions occur, remove patch and notify health care provider. Continue to monitor patient frequently for at least 12 hr.
- Assure that naloxone and intubation/airway management equipment are available.

Patient/Family Education
- Inform patient that maximal effect is not achieved for 3 days after initial application, and that supplemental analgesia may be needed.
- Instruct patient to self-monitor effectiveness of medication regularly and to report any significant change. Inform patient that tolerance may develop.
- Advise patient that patches are generally changed q 3 days, but that in some cases a change q 2 days is more effective.
- Explain adverse reactions, and identify signs and symptoms that should be reported. Inform patient that adverse reactions can persist for several hours after removal of patch.
- Explain measures to reduce constipation if present.
- Instruct patient to avoid driving or other potentially hazardous activities unless tolerant to the effects of the drug.
- Caution patient to avoid intake of alcoholic beverages or other CNS depressants.
- Explain potential for tolerance and abuse.
- Inform patient that withdrawal symptoms may be experienced when drug is discontinued and not to discontinue unless advised by health care provider.

Ferrous Salts

(FER-uhs salts)

Class Iron product

How Supplied

DexFerrum Injection 50 mg iron/mL as dextran ◆ *ED-IN-SOL* Drops 75 mg per 0.6 mL (15 mg iron/0.6 mL) as ferrous sulfate ◆ *Fe^{50}* Caplets, extended release 160 mg (50 mg iron) as ferrous sulfate exsiccated ◆ *Femiron* Tablets 63 mg (20 mg iron) as ferrous fumarate ◆ *Feosol* Elixir 220 mg per 5 mL (44 mg iron per 5 mL) as ferrous sulfate, Tablets 50 mg as carbonyl iron, Tablets 200 mg (65 mg iron) as ferrous sulfate exsiccated ◆ *Feostat* Tablets, chewable 100 mg (33 mg iron) as ferrous fumarate, Suspension 100 mg per 5 mL (33 mg iron per 5 mL) as ferrous fumarate, Drops 45 mg per 0.6 mL (15 mg iron per 0.6 mL) as ferrous fumarate ◆ *Feratab* Tablets 187 mg (60 mg iron) as ferrous sulfate exsiccated ◆ *Fer-gen-sol* Drops 75 mg/0.6 mL (15 mg iron/0.6 mL) as ferrous sulfate ◆ *Fergon* Tablets 240 mg (27 mg iron) as ferrous gluconate ◆ *Fer-In-Sol* Syrup 90 mg per 5 mL (18 mg iron per 5 mL) as ferrous sulfate, Drops 75 mg per 0.6 mL (15 mg iron per 0.6 mL) as ferrous sulfate ◆ *Fer-Iron* Drops 75 mg per 0.6 mL (15 mg iron per 0.6 mL) as ferrous sulfate ◆ *Ferrex 150* Capsules 150 mg iron as polysaccharide-iron complex ◆ *Ferro-Sequels* Tablets, timed-release 50 mg iron as ferrous fumarate ◆ *Hemocyte* Tablets 324 mg (106 mg as iron) as ferrous fumarate ◆ *Hytinic* Capsules 150 mg iron as polysaccharide-iron complex ◆ *Icar* Suspension 15 mg carbonyl iron per 1.25 mL ◆ *Ircon* Tablets 200 mg (66 mg iron) as ferrous fumarate ◆ *Nephro-Fer* Tablets 350 mg (115 mg iron) as ferrous fumarate ◆ *Niferex* Tablets 50 mg iron as polysaccharide-iron complex, Elixir 100 mg iron per 5 mL as polysaccharide-iron complex ◆ *Niferex–150* Capsules 150 mg iron as polysaccharide-iron complex ◆ *Nu-Iron* Elixir 100 mg iron per 5 mL as polysaccharide-iron complex ◆ *Nu-Iron 150* Capsules 150 mg iron as polysaccharide-iron complex ◆ *Slow-FE* Tablets, slow-release 160 mg (50 mg iron) as ferrous sulfate exsiccated ◆ *Vitron-C* Tablets 200 mg (66 mg iron) as ferrous fumarate

✤ *Apo-Ferrous Sulfate* ◆ *Ferodan* ◆ *Palafer*

Action

PHARMACOLOGY: Iron is a major factor in oxygen transport and an essential mineral component of hemoglobin, myoglobin, and several enzymes.

PHARMACOKINETICS/DYNAMICS:

Absorption: Primary site of absorption is the duodenum and upper jejunum. Food decreases absorption 40% to 66%.

Excretion: Daily loss of iron from urine, sweat, and sloughing of intestinal mucosal cells equals about 0.5 to 1 mg in healthy men and about 1 to 2 mg in menstruating women.

Indications Prevention and treatment of iron-deficiency anemia. **Unlabeled use(s):** Use with epoetin to ensure hematologic response to epoetin.

Contraindications Hypersensitivity to any ingredient, hemosiderosis, hemolytic anemia.

Route/Dosage

Stated iron dose is for elemental iron. Dosage must be calculated based on salt form. Ferrous sulfate is 20% elemental iron. Ferrous sulfate, exsiccated, is approximately 30% elemental iron. Ferrous gluconate is about 12% elemental iron. Ferrous fumarate is 33% elemental iron.

ADULT MEN: **PO** 10 mg.
WOMEN 11 TO 50 YR OF AGE: **PO** 15 mg.
WOMEN 51 YR OF AGE OR MORE: **PO** 10 mg.
PREGNANCY: 30 mg.
LACTATION: 15 mg.

Iron Replacement in Deficiency States

ADULTS: **PO** 100 to 200 mg tid.
CHILDREN (2 TO 12 YR OF AGE): 3 mg/kg/day in 3 to 4 divided doses.
CHILDREN (6 MO TO 2 YR OF AGE): Up to 6 mg/kg/day in 3 to 4 divided doses.
INFANTS: 10 to 25 mg once daily in 3 to 4 divided doses.

Interactions

Antacids: May decrease iron absorption.
Chloramphenicol: May increase serum iron concentrations.
Food: May decrease iron absorption; eggs and milk decrease iron absorption.
Levodopa: Effects of levodopa may be decreased.
Penicillamine: Decreased absorption of penicillamine.
Quinolones: Iron may decrease quinolone absorption.
Tetracyclines: Absorption of both drugs may be decreased.

Lab Test Interferences None well documented.

Adverse Reactions

GI: Irritation; anorexia; nausea; vomiting; diarrhea; constipation; dark stool.
OTHER: Teeth staining with liquid formulation.

Precautions

Tartrazine sensitivity: Some products contain tartrazine, which may cause allergic-type reactions in susceptible individuals.
Sulfite sensitivity: Some products contain sulfites, which cause allergic-type reactions in susceptible individuals.

GI effects: Discomfort, such as nausea, may be minimized by taking with food.

Overdosage: Signs and Symptoms
Lethargy, nausea, vomiting, abdominal pain, tarry stool, weak/rapid pulse, hypotension, dehydration, acidosis, coma, diffuse vascular congestion, pulmonary edema, shock, acidosis, convulsions, anuria, hypothermia, pyloric or antral stenosis, hepatic cirrhosis, CNS damage.

PATIENT CARE CONSIDERATIONS

Administration/Storage
- Administer drug orally only.
- Do not crush sustained-release tablets.
- Administer between meals for maximum absorption. Give with food or meals if GI upset occurs.
- When giving liquid preparation, dilute to decrease staining of teeth. Patient may drink through straw to avoid staining.

Assessment/Interventions
- Obtain patient history, including drug history and any known allergies.
- Document baseline Hbg, Hct, bilirubin, and reticulocyte count and monitor at regular intervals.
- Monitor color of stool.
- If anorexia, nausea, vomiting, constipation, or diarrhea develops, report to health care provider.
- Test stool for occult blood if bleeding is suspected.

Patient/Family Education
- Tell patient to take drug on an empty stomach unless GI upset develops. Instruct patient to then take drug after meals or with food, but not to take with eggs or milk.
- Advise patient taking sustained release preparation not to chew, open, or crush drug.
- Advise patient to dilute liquid iron preparations in water or juice, to drink through a straw, and to rinse mouth after taking.
- Instruct patient not to take drug with antacids.
- Tell patient that drug may cause black stools, constipation, or diarrhea, and to report anorexia, nausea, vomiting, or pronounced diarrhea or constipation.
- Identify foods to include for iron-rich diet.
- Warn patient that iron poisoning may occur if more than prescribed amount of medication is taken.

Fexofenadine Hydrochloride
(fex-oh-FEN-ah-deen HIGH-droe-KLOR-ide)

Class Antihistamine

How Supplied
Allegra Tablets 30 mg, Tablets 60 mg, Tablets 180 mg, Capsules 60 mg
🍁 *Allegra 12 Hour* ♦ *Allegra 24 Hour*

Action
PHARMACOLOGY: Competitively antagonizes histamine at the H_1-receptor site.

PHARMACOKINETICS/DYNAMICS:
Absorption: T_{max} is 2.6 hr; C_{max} is 131 ng/mL.
Distribution: 60% to 70% is bound to plasma proteins. The drug does not cross the blood-brain barrier.
Metabolism: About 5% is metabolized.
Excretion: Mean $t_½$ is 14.4 hr. About 80% is excreted in the feces and 11% in the urine.
Onset: 1 hr.
Peak: 2 to 3 hr.
Duration: 8 to 12 hr.
Special Populations:
Renal Function Impairment – Mild to moderate with a Ccr of 41 to 80 mL/min has an 87% increase in C_{max} and a 59% longer $t_½$. Severe with a Ccr of 11 to 40 mL/min has a 111% increase in C_{max} and a 72% longer $t_½$.
Elderly – C_{max} is increased 99%.
Children – AUC increased 56%.
Hemodialysis – With Ccr 10 mL/min or less, C_{max} is increased 82% and $t_½$ is 31% longer.

Indications Symptomatic relief of symptoms (nasal and nonnasal) associated with seasonal allergic rhinitis; treatment of uncomplicated skin manifestations of chronic idiopathic urticaria.

Contraindications Standard considerations.

Route/Dosage
Seasonal Allergic Rhinitis
ADULTS AND CHILDREN 12 YR OF AGE AND OLDER: PO 60 mg bid or 180 mg once daily.
CHILDREN 6 TO 11 YR OF AGE: PO 30 mg bid.

Chronic Idiopathic Urticaria
ADULTS AND CHILDREN 12 YR OF AGE AND OLDER: PO 60 mg bid.
CHILDREN 6 TO 11 YR OF AGE: PO 30 mg bid.

Renal Function Impairment
ADULTS AND CHILDREN 12 YR OF AGE AND OLDER: PO 60 mg once daily, as a starting dose.
CHILDREN 6 TO 11 YR OF AGE: PO 30 mg once daily as a starting dose.

Interactions
Aluminum/Magnesium antacids: Taken concomitantly, fexofenadine AUC decreased 41%, and C_{max} decreased 43%.
Erythromycin: Increased plasma levels of fexofenadine.
Ketoconazole: Increased plasma levels of fexofenadine.

Lab Test Interferences May prevent or diminish otherwise positive reactions to skin tests.

Adverse Reactions
CNS: Headache (11%); drowsiness, dizziness (2%); fatigue (1%).
EENT: Coughing (4%); otitis media, sinusitis (2%).
GI: Nausea (2%); dyspepsia (1%).
GU: Dysmenorrhea (2%).
RESP: Upper respiratory tract infection (4%).
OTHER: Viral infection (cold, flu); accidental injury, back pain (3%); fever, pain (2%).

Precautions
Pregnancy: Category C.
Lactation: Undetermined.
Children: Safety and efficacy not established in children younger than 6 yr of age.
Renal function impairment: Use lower starting dose.

Overdosage: Signs and Symptoms
Dizziness, drowsiness, dry mouth.

PATIENT CARE CONSIDERATIONS

Administration/Storage
- Administer prescribed dose without regard to meals.
- Administer with food if GI upset occurs.
- Store tablets and capsules at controlled room temperature (68° to 77°F). Protect foil-backed blister packs containing capsules and all tablet packaging from excessive moisture.

Assessment/Interventions
- Obtain patient history, including drug history and any known allergies. Note renal impairment.
- Ensure reduced dose (once daily) is used in patient with renal impairment.
- Assess for allergy symptoms (eg, rhinitis, nasal congestion, sneezing, itching, watery eyes) before starting therapy and periodically throughout therapy. Notify health care provider if symptoms do not improve or worsen.
- Monitor patient for dizziness and excessive drowsiness. If noted, hold therapy and notify health care provider.

Patient/Family Education
- Explain name, dose, action, and potential side effects of drug.
- Advise patient to take without regard to meals but to take with food if stomach upset occurs.
- Advise patient that if allergy symptoms are not controlled not to increase the dose of medication or frequency of use but to inform health care provider.
- Inform patient that larger doses or more frequent dosing does not increase effectiveness and may cause drowsiness.
- Caution patient not to take any OTC antihistamines while taking this medication unless advised by health care provider.
- Caution patient to avoid alcohol and other CNS depressants (eg, sedatives) while using this medication.
- If patient is to have allergy skin testing, advise not to take the medication for at least 4 days before the skin testing.
- Caution patient that drug may cause drowsiness and to use caution driving or performing other tasks requiring mental alertness until tolerance is determined.
- Advise women to notify health care provider if pregnant, planning to become pregnant, or breastfeeding.
- Instruct patient to stop taking drug and report any symptoms of persistent dizziness or excessive drowsiness to health care provider.
- Caution patient not to take any prescription or OTC medications, herbal preparations, or dietary supplements unless advised by health care provider.
- Caution patient not to take aluminum/magnesium antacids together at the same time.

Fexofenadine Hydrochloride/ Pseudoephedrine Hydrochloride

(fex-oh-FEN-ah-deen HIGH-droe-KLOR-ide/ SUE-doe-eh-FED-rin)

Class Antihistamine/Decongestant

How Supplied
Allegra-D Tablets 120 mg pseudoephedrine/ 60 mg fexofenadine

Action
PHARMACOLOGY:
Fexofenadine: Competitively antagonizes histamine at the H_1-receptor site.
Pseudoephedrine: Causes vasoconstriction and subsequent shrinkage of nasal mucous membranes by alpha-adrenergic stimulation, promoting nasal drainage.

Indications Relief of symptoms associated with seasonal allergic rhinitis.

Contraindications Hypersensitivity to any ingredient of the product; patients with narrow-angle glaucoma, urinary retention, severe hypertension, or severe coronary artery disease; MAO inhibitor therapy; idiosyncratic reactions to adrenergic agents.

Route/Dosage
ADULTS AND CHILDREN 12 YR AND OLDER: **PO** 1 tablet (60 mg fexofenadine/120 mg pseudoephedrine) bid.

Interactions Because the following interactions may occur with the components of this product, take into consideration these interactions when administering the agents that are listed.
Fexofenadine:
Erythromycin, ketoconazole – Plasma levels of fexofenadine may be increased.
Pseudoephedrine:
MAO inhibitors – Contraindicated in patients taking MAO inhibitors and for 14 days after stopping use of an MAO inhibitor.
Antihypertensive agents that interfere with sympathetic activity (eg, mecamylamine, methyldopa, reserpine, veratrum alkaloids) – Antihypertensive effect of these agents may be reduced.

Digitalis – Increased ectopic pacemaker activity may occur.

Lab Test Interferences May diminish or prevent positive reactions to skin tests.

Adverse Reactions
CV: Palpitations; tachycardia, pressor activity, cardiac arrhythmias, cardiovascular collapse (pseudoephedrine).
CNS: Headache; insomnia; dizziness; agitation; nervousness; anxiety; excitability, restlessness, weakness, drowsiness, fear, tenseness, hallucinations, seizures (pseudoephedrine).
DERM: Pallor.
EENT: Throat irritation.
GI: Nausea; dry mouth; dyspepsia; abdominal pain.
GU: Dysuria.
RESP: Upper respiratory infection; respiratory difficulties.
OTHER: Back pain.

Precautions
Pregnancy: Category C.
Lactation:
Fexofenadine – Undetermined.
Pseudoephedrine – Excreted in breast milk.
Children: Safety and efficacy not established in children less than 12 yr.
Elderly: Use lower starting dose, reflecting increased incidence of adverse reaction due to decreased hepatic, renal, or cardiac function and comorbidity.
Special risk patients: Use with caution in patients with hyperthyroidism, severe hypertension, diabetes, cardiovascular disease, increased intraocular pressure, or prostatic hypertrophy.
Sympathomimetic amines (eg, pseudoephedrine): May cause CNS stimulation with convulsions or cardiovascular collapse with accompanying hypotension.

Overdosage: Signs and Symptoms
Dizziness, drowsiness, dry mouth, giddiness, headache, nausea, vomiting, sweating, thirst, tachycardia, precordial pain, palpitations, difficulty in micturition, muscular weakness and tension, anxiety, restlessness insomnia, toxic psychosis with delusions and hallucinations, cardiac arrhythmias, circulatory collapse, convulsions, coma, respiratory failure.

PATIENT CARE CONSIDERATIONS

Administration/Storage
- Give twice daily on an empty stomach, 1 hr before or 2 hr after eating.
- Start patients with reduced renal function on 1 tablet daily.
- Store tablets at controlled room temperature.

Keep container tightly closed.

Assessment/Interventions
- Obtain patient history, including drug history and any known allergies. Note history of renal impairment, narrow-angle glaucoma, urinary retention, severe hypertension or

coronary artery disease, or concurrent use of or within 2 wk of stopping MAO inhibitor therapy.
* Assess for allergy symptoms (eg, rhinitis, nasal congestion, sneezing, itching, watery eyes) before and periodically throughout therapy.
* Monitor pulse and BP periodically during therapy.
* Monitor patient for nervousness, dizziness, and insomnia. If noted, hold therapy and notify health care provider.

Patient/Family Education
* Explain name, dose, action, and potential side effects of drug.
* Advise patient to take bid as prescribed, on an empty stomach, 1 hr before or 2 hr after eating.
* Advise patient to take last dose late in the afternoon or early evening to reduce chance of drug causing sleeplessness.
* Caution patient not to break, chew, or crush tablet and to swallow whole.
* Advise patient that if allergy symptoms are not controlled, not to increase the dose of medication but to inform the health care provider.
* Do not take this medication for 4 days or longer if having an allergy skin test.
* Instruct women to notify health care provider if they become pregnant, plan on becoming pregnant, or are breastfeeding.
* Instruct patient to stop taking the drug and immediately report any of the following symptoms to health care provider: nervousness, dizziness, or sleeplessness.
* Caution patient to not take any prescription or otc medications, or dietary supplements unless advised by health care provider.

Filgrastim (G-CSF)

(fill-GRAH-stim)

Class Colony-stimulating factor

How Supplied
Neupogen Injection 300 mcg/mL

Action
PHARMACOLOGY: Stimulates neutrophil production within bone marrow.

PHARMACOKINETICS/DYNAMICS:
Absorption: C_{max} is 4 to 49 ng/mL (SC); T_{max} is 2 to 8 hr (SC).

Distribution: Vd is about 150 mL/kg.

Excretion: t½ is about 3.5 hr and Cl is 0.5 to 0.7 mL/min/kg.

Indications Decrease incidence of infection, manifested by febrile neutropenia, in patients with nonmyeloid malignancies receiving myelosuppressive anticancer drugs; cancer patients receiving myelosuppressive chemotherapy; cancer patients receiving bone-marrow transplant; patients with severe chronic neutropenia (SCN); peripheral blood progenitor cell (PBPC) collection and therapy in cancer patients. **Unlabeled use(s):** Filgrastim may be beneficial in AIDS, drug-induced and congenital agranulocytosis, alloimmune neonatal neutropenia.

Contraindications Hypersensitivity to *Escherichia coli*-derived proteins.

Route/Dosage
Myelosuppressive chemotherapy – **IV/SC** 5 mcg/kg/day as a single daily injection; may increase in increments of 5 mcg/kg for each chemotherapy cycle.

Bone marrow transplant
IV/SC 10 mcg/kg/day given as an IV infusion of 4 or 24 hr or as a continuous 24 hr SC infusion.

Severe chronic neutropenia
Congenital neutropenia –
Starting dose: 6 mcg/kg twice daily SC qd.
Idiopathic or cyclic neutropenia –
Starting dose: 5 mcg/kg as a single injection SC qd.
Dose adjustments: Chronic daily administration is required to maintain clinical benefit. Do not use ANC as the sole indication of efficacy. Individually adjust the dose based on the patients' clinical course as well as ANC. In the Phase III study, the target ANC was 1500 to 10,000/mm^3. However, patients may experience clinical benefit with ANCs below this target range. Reduce the dose if the ANC is persistently more than 10,000/mm^3.

Interactions Drugs that may potentiate the release of neutrophils, such as lithium, should be used with caution.

INCOMPATIBILITIES: Precipitate may form if diluted with saline.

Lab Test Interferences None well documented.

Adverse Reactions
HEMA: Leukocytosis.
OTHER: Bone pain; reversible elevations in uric acid, LDH, and alkaline phosphatase.

Precautions
Pregnancy: Category C.
Lactation: Undetermined.
Cardiac events: Monitoring patients with preexisting cardiac conditions is recommended.
Chronic administration: Safety and efficacy not established.

Hematologic effects: Regular monitoring of hematocrit and platelet count recommended because of possible increased risk of thrombocytopenia or anemia.

PATIENT CARE CONSIDERATIONS
Administration/Storage
- Do not give filgrastim 24 hr before or 24 hr after cytotoxic chemotherapy.
- Do not shake medication.
- Warm to room temperature before injection. Use within 24 hr.
- Use only 1 dose per vial, and do not reenter vial.
- Do not dilute with saline.
- Give IV injection, diluted in D5W, over 15 to 30 min.
- Store in refrigerator, but do not freeze. Discard any unused vial left at room temperature more than 6 hr.

Assessment/Interventions
- Obtain complete patient history, including drug history and any known allergies.
- Monitor hematocrit, CBC, and platelet count 2 to 3 times/wk.

Overdosage: Signs and Symptoms
Leukocytosis.

- Document any hypotensive effects.
- Document CBC and platelet counts prior to chemotherapy and twice/wk during therapy.
- Inform health care provider and discontinue dose if absolute neutrophil count more than 10,000/mm^3.

Patient/Family Education
- Instruct in proper techniques for administration and storage.
- Explain that most common adverse effect is bone pain.
- Explain importance of follow-up laboratory work as directed.
- Counsel patient on signs of thrombocytopenia (eg, bruising, petechiae, ecchymosis, epistaxis, bleeding from mucus membranes) and ways to avoid infection.

Finasteride

(fih-NASS-teer-IDE)

Class Androgen hormone inhibitor

How Supplied
Propecia Tablets 1 mg ♦ *Proscar* Tablets 5 mg

Action
PHARMACOLOGY: Inhibits conversion of testosterone into 5-alpha-dihydrotestosterone, a potent androgen.

PHARMACOKINETICS/DYNAMICS:
Absorption: Mean bioavailability is 65% (range, 26% to 170%). C_{max} at steady state is 4.9 to 13.7 ng/mL (mean, 9.2 ng/mL) (*Propecia*). C_{max} is 37 ng/mL (range, 27 to 49 ng/mL) (*Proscar*). T_{max} is 1 to 2 hr. AUC_{0-24} is 20 to 154 ng•hr/mL (mean, 53 ng•hr/mL).

Distribution: Vd_{ss} is 44 to 96 L (mean, 76 L) and it is about 90% bound to plasma proteins. The drug crosses the blood-brain barrier but does not appear to distribute preferentially to the CSF.

Metabolism: Extensively metabolized in the liver, primarily via the cytochrome P450 3A4 enzyme subfamily. Two metabolites have been identified: t-butyl side chain monohydroxylated and monocarboxylic acid; each possesses no more than 20% activity.

Excretion: Plasma Cl is 70 to 279 mL/min (mean, 165 mL/min). Mean t½ is 4.8 hr (range, 3.3 to 13.4 hr) (*Propecia*). Mean t½ is 6 hr (range 3 to 16 hr) (*Proscar*); 32% to 46% is excreted in the urine as metabolites, and 51% to 64% is excreted in the feces.

Special Populations:
Elderly – Mean t½ increases to 8 hr (70 yr of age and older). Mean AUC_{0-24} increases 15%.

Indications
Propecia: Treatment of male pattern hair loss (androgenic alopecia) in men only.
Proscar: Treatment of symptomatic benign prostatic hyperplasia (BPH) in men with enlarged prostate; in combination with doxazosin to reduce the risk of symptomatic progression of BPH.

Contraindications Use during pregnancy; use in women or children.

Route/Dosage
ADULTS: PO *Propecia*: 1 mg daily. *Proscar*: 5 mg daily.

Interactions None well documented.

Lab Test Interferences Decreased prostate-specific antigen levels.

Adverse Reactions
CV: *Proscar*: Postural hypotension (9%); hypotension (1%).
CNS: *Propecia*: Decreased libido (2%). *Proscar*: Decreased libido (10%); dizziness (7%); headache, somnolence (2%).
GU: *Propecia*: Erectile dysfunction, ejaculation disorders (1%); breast tenderness/enlargement in men (postmarketing). *Proscar*: Impotence

(19%); abnormal ejaculation (7%); decreased volume of ejaculate (4%); abnormal sexual function (3%); breast enlargement in men (2%).
HYPERSEN: Pruritus, urticaria, swelling of lips and face, testicular pain (postmarketing).
METAB: Proscar: Peripheral edema (1%).
RESP: Proscar: Rhinitis (1%).
OTHER: Proscar: Asthenia (5%).

Precautions
Pregnancy: Category X.
Lactation: Undetermined.
Children: Safety and efficacy not established.
Hepatic function impairment: Use with caution.

Carcinogenesis: Based on animal studies, may have carcinogenic or mutagenic potential.
Duration of therapy: Minimum 6 mo therapy may be necessary to see effect (*Proscar*). Minimum 3 mo therapy may be necessary to see effect (*Propecia*).
Obstructive uropathy: Carefully monitor patients with large residual urine volume or severely diminished urinary flow.
Prostate-specific antigen (PSA) levels: Carefully evaluate any increase in PSA level, consider noncompliance with therapy.

PATIENT CARE CONSIDERATIONS
Administration/Storage
- Not indicated for use in women or children.
- May be used alone or in combination with doxazosin (alpha$_1$-adrenergic blocker) for treatment of prostatic hypertrophy.
- Administer prescribed dose daily without regard to meals. Administer with food if GI upset occurs.
- Do not allow women who are pregnant or may be pregnant to handle crushed or broken finasteride tablets. Intact coating on tablet will prevent contact with finasteride during normal handling.
- Store tablets at controlled room temperature (59° to 86°F). Protect from light.

Assessment/Interventions
- Obtain patient history, including drug history and any known allergies. Note hepatic impairment or liver function abnormalities.
- Before starting therapy, ensure that patient being treated for BPH has been evaluated for other conditions (eg, infection, prostate cancer, neurogenic disorder) that could mimic BPH.
- Ensure that patient with BPH is evaluated for possible prostate cancer (eg, digital rectal exam, PSA level) before starting therapy and periodically during prolonged treatment.
- Assess urinary symptoms (eg, frequency, nocturia, need to strain, volume, dribbling) in patient being treated for BPH before starting therapy and periodically during treatment. Notify health care provider if symptoms do not improve or appear to worsen.
- Carefully monitor patient with large residual urinary volume or severely diminished urinary flow for obstructive uropathy. Notify health care provider immediately if obstructive uropathy is suspected.
- Monitor patient for GU, CV, CNS, and general body side effects. Report to health care provider if noted and significant.

Patient/Family Education
- Explain name, dose, action, and potential side effects of drug.
- Advise patient to read *Patient Information* insert before starting therapy and with each refill.
- Advise patient to take prescribed dose once daily without regard to meals but to take with food if stomach upset occurs.
- Caution patient that female companion of childbearing potential should not handle crushed or broken tablets.
- Advise patient being treated for BPH that although symptoms may improve early in treatment, it may take 6 to 12 mo for full benefit to be noted.
- Advise patient being treated for male pattern baldness that it may take 3 mo or more of daily therapy before improvement is noted and that continued use is required to maintain benefit. Advise patient that stopping therapy will result in reversal of effect within 12 mo.
- Advise patient being treated for BPH to notify health care provider if urinary symptoms do not improve or worsen while taking this medication.
- Advise patient that volume of ejaculate may be decreased but that this does not appear to interfere with normal sexual function in most patients. Advise patient to notify health care provider if sexual dysfunction (eg, decreased libido, impotence) develops while taking finasteride.
- Instruct patient to immediately report breast lumps, breast pain, or nipple discharge.
- Caution patient not to take any prescription or OTC drugs, dietary supplements, or herbal preparations unless advised by health care provider.
- Advise patient that follow-up visits may be necessary to monitor therapy and to keep appointments.

Flavocoxid

(FLAY-voh-cox-id)

Class Nutritional supplement

How Supplied
Limbrel Capsule 250 mg

Action

PHARMACOLOGY: Inhibition of prostaglandin synthesis by inhibition of cyclo-oxygenase. Also, flavocoxid may act as an antioxidant, reducing reactive oxygen species including hydroxyl radical, superoxide anion radical, and hydrogen peroxide. Flavocoxid reduces pro-inflammatory cytokine interleukin-1-beta and tumor necrosis factor alpha in vitro.

PHARMACOKINETICS/DYNAMICS:

Absorption: Ingestion with or 1 hr before or after food may modestly inhibit absorption.

Metabolism: Primarily by glucuronidation and sulfation with little hepatic metabolism involving CYP isoenzymes.

Indications Dietary management of osteoarthritis, including associated inflammation.

Contraindications Standard considerations.

Route/Dosage

ADULTS: PO 250 mg q 12 hr. Larger doses should only be taken under a physician's direction.

Interactions None well documented.

Lab Test Interferences None well documented.

Adverse Reactions

CV: Hypertension (at least 2%).
DERM: Psoriasis (at least 2%).
OTHER: Varicose veins, fluid accumulation in the knee (at least 2%).

Precautions

Pregnancy: Use not recommended.
Lactation: Undetermined.
Children: Safety and efficacy not established.
Gastrointestinal: GI side effects such as bleeding, ulceration, and stomach perforation can occur at any time, with or without symptoms.

PATIENT CARE CONSIDERATIONS

Administration/Storage

- Administer prescribed dose 1 hr before or after meals.
- Store capsules at controlled room temperature (59° to 86°F). Protect from light and moisture.

Assessment/Interventions

- Obtain patient history, including drug history and any known allergies. Note history of GI bleeding or ulcers or current or previous use of NSAIDs or COX-2 inhibitors.
- Obtain baseline assessments of pain and ability to perform activities of daily living in patient with osteoarthritis. Periodically reassess response to therapy. Notify health care provider if symptoms do not appear to be improving or worsen.
- Notify health care provider if indigestion, epigastric pain, unusual bleeding, bruising, or dark tarry stools occur.
- Monitor patient for GI, CNS, and general body side effects. Report to health care provider if noted and significant.

Patient/Family Education

- Explain name, dose, action, and potential side effects of drug.
- Instruct patient to take exactly as prescribed and not to change the dose or stop taking unless advised by health care provider.
- Advise patient to take each dose 1 hr before or after a meal.
- Advise patient that dose is individualized based upon severity of symptoms and response to therapy.
- Advise patient to continue other arthritis medications as recommended by health care provider.
- Advise patient that if a dose is missed, take it as soon as possible. If close to the next dose, do not double up; take the next dose as scheduled.
- Advise patient to notify health care provider if arthritis symptoms do not appear to be getting better or worsen.
- Instruct patient to discontinue drug and notify health care provider if any of the following occur: persistent GI upset or nausea, skin rash, itching, black stools.
- Advise women to notify health care provider if pregnant, planning to become pregnant, or breastfeeding.
- Instruct patient not to take any prescription or OTC medications, herbal preparations, or dietary supplements unless advised by health care provider.
- Advise patient that follow-up examinations and lab tests may be required to monitor therapy and to keep appointments.

Flavoxate

(flay-voke-sate)

Class Urinary tract antispasmodic/Alkalinizer

How Supplied
Urispas Tablets 100 mg

Action
PHARMACOLOGY: Counteracts smooth muscle spasms of urinary tract.
PHARMACOKINETICS/DYNAMICS:
Absorption: Well absorbed from GI tract.
Excretion: 10% to 30% excreted renally within 6 hr; 57% excreted in 24 hr.
Onset: 55 min.
Peak: 112 min.

Indications Symptomatic relief of dysuria, urgency, nocturia, suprapubic pain, frequency and incontinence associated with cystitis, prostatitis, urethritis, urethrocystitis/urethrotrigonitis.

Contraindications Pyloric or duodenal obstruction; obstructive intestinal lesions or ileus; achalasia; GI hemorrhage; obstructive uropathies of lower urinary tract.

Route/Dosage
ADULTS AND CHILDREN (MORE THAN 12 YR): PO 100 to 200 mg 3 to 4 times/day.

Interactions None well documented.

Lab Test Interferences None well documented.

Adverse Reactions
CV: Tachycardia; palpitations.
CNS: Nervousness; headache; drowsiness; mental confusion.
DERM: Urticaria and other dermatoses.
EENT: Vertigo; blurred vision, ocular tension; disturbances in accommodation.
GI: Nausea; vomiting; dry mouth.
GU: Dysuria.
HEMA: Eosinophilia; leukopenia.
OTHER: High fever.

Precautions
Pregnancy: Category B.
Lactation: Undetermined.
Children: Safety and efficacy in children less than 12 yr not established.
Glaucoma: Give cautiously to patients with suspected glaucoma.

PATIENT CARE CONSIDERATIONS

Administration/Storage
- Administer drug orally only.

Assessment/Interventions
- Obtain patient history, including drug history and any known allergies.
- Assess baseline mental status and monitor during therapy.
- Carefully monitor patients with glaucoma.
- Report to health care provider any problems such as visual disturbances, nausea or vomiting, dysuria, high fever, tachycardia, palpitations, or mental status changes.

Patient/Family Education
- Caution patient against performing potentially hazardous activities until effects of product are well-tolerated.
- Instruct patient to take sips of water frequently, suck on ice chips or sugarless hard candy, or chew sugarless gum if dry mouth occurs.
- Advise patient to report these symptoms to health care provider: persistent or worsening dry mouth, hives, rash, nausea or vomiting, unusual nervousness, vertigo, headache, drowsiness, confusion, high fever, dysuria, tachycardia, palpitations, vision problems.

Flecainide Acetate

(fleh-CANE-ide ASS-uh-TATE)

Class Antiarrhythmic

How Supplied
Tambocor Tablets 50 mg, Tablets 100 mg, Tablets 150 mg

Action
PHARMACOLOGY: Produces a dose-related decrease in intracardiac conduction in all parts of the heart; also has local anesthetic activity.
PHARMACOKINETICS/DYNAMICS:
Absorption: About 100% absorbed. T_{max} is 1 to 6 hr.
Distribution: About 40% protein bound.
Metabolism: There are 2 major metabolites: meta-o-dealkylated flecainide (active, but about ⅓ as potent) and meta-o-dealkylated lactam of flecainide (nonactive).
Excretion: The $t_{½}$ is 12 to 27 hr; 10% to 50% is excreted in the urine as unchanged drug.
Hemodialysis – About 1% of unchanged drug is removed by hemodialysis.
Special Populations:
Renal Function Impairment – The $t_{½}$ is prolonged.
Children –
At birth: The $t_{½}$ is up to 29 hr.

At 3 mo of age: The t½ is 11 to 12 hr.
At 1 to 12 yr of age: The t½ is 6 to 8 hr.
CHF (NYHA Class III) – The t½ is increased.

Indications Prevention of paroxysmal atrial fibrillation/flutter (PAF) associated with disabling symptoms; paroxysmal supraventricular tachycardias (PSVTs), including AV nodal reentrant tachycardia and AV reentrant tachycardia; prevention of documented life-threatening ventricular arrhythmias, such as sustained ventricular tachycardia (VT).

Contraindications Preexisting second- or third-degree AV block; right bundle branch block when associated with a left hemiblock (unless a pacemaker is present); presence of cardiogenic shock; hypersensitivity to the drug.

Route/Dosage
PSVT, PAF
ADULTS:
Initial dose: **PO** 50 mg q 12 hr, increasing 50 mg bid q 4 days until efficacy is achieved. Max, 300 mg/day.

Sustained VT
ADULTS:
Initial dose: **PO** 100 mg q 12 hr, increasing 50 mg bid q 4 days until efficacy is achieved. Max, 400 mg/day.

Children
YOUNGER THAN 6 MO OF AGE: **PO** 50 mg/m^2 divided into 2 or 3 equally spaced doses.
OLDER THAN 6 MO OF AGE: **PO** 100 mg/m^2/day. The maximum recommended dose is 200 mg/m^2/day.

Renal Function Impairment
When Ccr is less than 35 mL/min, the initial dose is 100 mg once daily (or 50 mg bid).

Administration with Amiodarone
Reduce dose of flecainide 50% when given with amiodarone.

Interactions
Amiodarone: Increased flecainide plasma levels; reduce dose of flecainide 50%.
Cimetidine: Increased bioavailability and half-life of flecainide.
Cisapride, disopyramide, verapamil: Has negative inotropic effects; administer with flecainide only if benefit outweighs the risks. Coadministration with flecainide is not recommended because of the increased risk of life-threatening cardiac arrhythmias.
Digoxin: Increased digoxin plasma levels.
Drugs that inhibit CYP2D6 (eg, quinidine, ritonavir): Flecainide plasma concentrations may be elevated, increasing the risk of toxicity.
Propranolol: Levels of either drug may be increased; additive negative inotropic effects.
Smoking: Increased dosage may be required.

Urinary acidifiers: Effects of flecainide may be decreased.
Urinary alkalinizers: Effects of flecainide may be increased.

Lab Test Interferences None well documented.

Adverse Reactions
CV: Palpitation (6%); chest pain (5%); tachycardia (1% to less than 3%); sinus bradycardia, sinus pause, sinus arrest (1%); new or worsening arrhythmia, unresuscitatable VT or ventricular fibrillation, new or worsening CHF, second- or third-degree AV block.
CNS: Dizziness including lightheadedness, faintness, unsteadiness, and near syncope (19%); headache (10%); fatigue (8%); asthenia, tremor (5%); hypoesthesia, paresthesia, paresis, ataxia, flushing, increased sweating, vertigo, syncope, somnolence, anxiety, insomnia, depression, malaise (1% to less than 3%).
DERM: Rash (1% to less than 3%).
EENT: Visual disturbances including blurred vision, difficulty focusing, spots before eyes (16%); tinnitus, diplopia (1% to less than 3%).
GI: Nausea (9%); constipation (4%); abdominal pain (3%); vomiting, diarrhea, dyspepsia, anorexia (1% to less than 3%).
RESP: Dyspnea (10%).
OTHER: Edema (4%); fever (1% to less than 3%).

> **WARNING:**
>
> *Mortality:* An excessive mortality or nonfatal cardiac arrest rate was observed in patients with nonlife-threatening ventricular arrhythmias who had a recent MI.
>
> Ventricular pro-arrhythmic effects have been observed in patients with atrial fibrillation/flutter. This drug is not recommended in patients with chronic atrial fibrillation.

Precautions
Pregnancy: Category C.
Lactation: Excreted in breast milk.
Children: Safety and efficacy not established.
Hepatic function impairment: Do not use in patients with hepatic impairment unless benefits outweigh risks.
CV disorders: Use with caution in patients with arrhythmias, CHF, cardiomyopathy, low ejection fraction, and conduction abnormalities. Use with extreme caution in patients with sick sinus syndrome, because drug may cause sinus bradycardia, sinus pause, or sinus arrest.
Conduction disturbance: Flecainide slows cardiac conduction in most patients to produce a dose-related increase in PR, QRS, and QT intervals.

Pacemaker threshold: Flecainide increases endocardial pacing thresholds and may suppress ventricular escape rhythms in patients with pacemakers.

Potassium imbalances: Effect of flecainide may be altered in patients with hypokalemia or hyperkalemia; correct condition before administering flecainide.

PATIENT CARE CONSIDERATIONS

Administration/Storage
- May be used alone or in combination with other antiarrhythmic medications.
- Initiate therapy for sustained VT in-hospital with close monitoring of cardiac rhythm.
- Administer dose q 8 or 12 hr as prescribed without regard to meals. Administer with food if GI upset occurs.
- Do not increase dose more often than q 4 days during dosage titration as optimal effect may not be achieved during the first 2 to 3 days following initiation of therapy or dose increase.
- Store tablets at controlled room temperature (59° to 86°F).

Assessment/Interventions
- Obtain patient history, including drug history and any known allergies. Note renal or hepatic impairment; heart failure or myocardial dysfunction; sick sinus syndrome; chronic atrial fibrillation; permanent pacemaker; temporary pacing electrodes; or concurrent therapy with amiodarone, CYP450 2D6 inhibitors (eg, quinidine), or medications with negative inotropic effects (eg, disopyramide).
- Review patient's health history and current situation for any of the following conditions that would contraindicate flecainide therapy: hypersensitivity to flecainide, pre-existing second- or third-degree AV block, right bundle branch block associated with left hemiblock (bifasicular block) unless pacemaker is present, severe cardiogenic shock.
- Ensure renal function (BUN, Scr) and liver enzymes are evaluated before initiating therapy and periodically thereafter during long-term treatment.
- Review baseline ECG. Monitor cardiac rhythm while initiating therapy or when adjusting dose. Notify health care provider immediately of increase in ventricular rate, new or worsening premature ventricular contractions, VT, or ventricular fibrillation. Be prepared to treat appropriately.
- Measure PR, QRS, and QT intervals before initiating therapy and closely thereafter while adjusting dose. Notify health care provider immediately of significant prolongation.

Overdosage: Signs and Symptoms
Nausea and vomiting, convulsions, hypotension, bradycardia, syncope, extreme widening of the QRS complex, widening of the QT interval, widening of the PR interval, VT, AV nodal block, asystole, bundle branch block, cardiac failure, cardiac arrest, death.

- Ensure pre-existing hypo- or hyperkalemia has been corrected before initiating therapy.
- Ensure pacing threshold is determined before starting therapy, after 1 wk of therapy, and at regular intervals thereafter in patient with pacemaker.
- Ensure reduced initial dose, slower dose titration, and frequent plasma level monitoring (to guide dosage adjustment) are used in patients with renal impairment or significant hepatic impairment.
- Ensure flecainide dose is reduced 50% and plasma level monitoring is used to guide flecainide dosage when coadministering with amiodarone.
- Ensure reduced initial dose, careful dose titration, and plasma level monitoring (to guide dosage adjustment) are used in patient with history of heart failure or myocardial dysfunction. Ensure therapy for maintenance of cardiac function (eg, digitalis, diuretics) has been optimized.
- Ensure reduced dose and plasma level monitoring (to guide dosage adjustment) are used in infant if milk is removed from diet (eg, gastroenteritis, weaning).
- Monitor and record BP and pulse frequently during treatment. Notify health care provider of any significant changes.
- Monitor patient with heart failure or myocardial dysfunction for evidence of worsening heart failure (eg, new or worsening shortness of breath, peripheral edema, rapid weight gain). Inform health care provider if noted or suspected.
- Monitor patient for CV, GI, CNS, OPHTH, and general body side effects. Inform health care provider if noted and significant.

Patient/Family Education
- Explain name, dose, action, and potential side effects of drug.
- Advise patient that dose of medication will be changed periodically to obtain max benefit.
- Caution patient to take prescribed dose q 8 or 12 hr exactly as ordered. Advise patient that serious heart disturbances can result from missing doses.

- Advise patient to take each dose without regard to meals but to take with food if stomach upset occurs.
- Caution patient not to change the dose or stop taking unless advised by health care provider. Advise patient that serious side effects can result from increasing or decreasing the dose without medical supervision.
- Inform patient that drug controls, but does not cure, abnormal heart rhythm and to continue taking as prescribed once heart rhythm has been controlled.
- Instruct patient to continue taking other heart medications as prescribed by health care provider.
- Instruct patient in BP and pulse measurement skills.
- Advise patient to monitor and record BP and pulse at home and to inform health care provider if abnormal measurements are noted. Also advise patient to take record of BP and pulse to each follow-up visit.
- Advise patient with heart failure, or those taking other medications with negative inotropic effect, to monitor and record weight on a daily basis and inform health care provider if noting unexplained or rapid weight gain
- Instruct patient to lie or sit down if experiencing dizziness or lightheadedness when standing.
- Advise patient to notify health care provider if any of the following occur: frequent episodes of dizziness or lightheadedness, persistent fatigue, persistent headache, nausea, any other unusual or unexplained symptom or sign.
- Instruct patient to immediately report fainting, pounding in chest, new or worsening shortness of breath, change in pulse or heart rhythm, swelling in feet or ankles, or rapid weight gain to health care provider.
- Caution patient that drug may cause dizziness or drowsiness and to use caution while driving or performing other tasks requiring mental alertness or coordination until tolerance is determined.
- Advise patient to carry medical identification (eg, *Medi-Alert*) describing cardiac condition and medication regimen.
- Advise women to notify health care provider if pregnant, planning to become pregnant, or breastfeeding.
- Caution patient not to take any prescription or OTC medications, herbal preparations, or dietary supplements unless advised by health care provider.
- Offer family instruction in basic life support.
- Advise patient that follow-up visits and lab tests will be required to monitor therapy and to keep appointments.

Floxuridine

(flox-YOUR-ih-deen)

Class Pyrimidine antimetabolite

How Supplied

FUDR Powder for injection 500 mg, Solution for injection 100 mg/mL

Action

PHARMACOLOGY: The primary effect is to interfere with the synthesis of deoxyribonucleic acid (DNA) and to a lesser extent inhibit the formation of ribonucleic acid (RNA).

PHARMACOKINETICS/DYNAMICS:

Metabolism: When given by rapid intra-arterial injection, floxuridine is rapidly catabolized to 5-fluorouracil. When given by continuous intra-arterial infusion, direct anabolism to floxuridine-monophosphate is enhanced. Floxuridine is metabolized in the liver.

Excretion: The drug is excreted intact as urea, fluorouracil, alpha-fluoro-beta-ureidopropionic acid, dihydrofluorouracil, alpha-fluoro-beta-guanidopropionic acid, and alpha-fluoro-beta alanine in the urine. It also is expired as respiratory carbon dioxide.

Indications Palliative management of GI adenocarcinoma metastatic to the liver administered by continuous regional intra-arterial infusion as long as cancer does not extend beyond area perfused by a single artery. **Unlabeled use(s):** Tumors of the liver, gallbladder, bile ducts, or kidneys.

Contraindications Patients in a poor nutritional state, those with depressed bone marrow function or those with potentially serious infections.

Route/Dosage

Hepatic Artery Infusion

ADULTS: **Implantable pump** Using an implantable pump, administer 0.1 to 0.6 mg/kg/day for 1 to 6 wk, followed by a 14-day rest period between courses. Repeat cycles as long as response continues.

Solid Tumors

ADULTS: **IV infusion** 0.5 to 1 mg/kg/day for 6 to 15 days or until toxicity occurs.

Interactions

Cimetidine: Cimetidine may increase the bioavailability of floxuridine.

Lab Test Interferences None well documented.

Adverse Reactions
CV: Arterial aneurysm; ischemia; thrombosis; embolism; fibromyositis.
DERM: Localized erythema; alopecia; rash.
GI: Nausea and vomiting; diarrhea; enteritis; mucositis; duodenal ulcers; elevated LFTs; hepatic necrosis; hepatic abscesses; intra- and extrahepatic biliary sclerosis; acalculous cholecystitis.
HEMA: Bone marrow suppression, nadir at 9 to 14 days; bleeding at the catheter site.
OTHER: Fever and malaise; infection of the catheter site.

> **WARNING:**
> Hospitalization recommended for first course of therapy due to the possibility of severe toxic reactions.

Precautions
Pregnancy: Category D.
Lactation: Undetermined.
Children: Safety and efficacy not established.

Special risk patients: Use with extreme caution in poor-risk patients who have had high-dose pelvic irradiation or previous use of alkylating agents, who have wide-spread involvement of bone marrow by metastatic tumors, or impaired hepatic or renal function.

Discontinue use: According to product labeling, promptly discontinue floxuridine if any of the following occur: myocardial ischemia, mucositis or esophagopharyngitis, leukopenia with WBC less than 3500/mm^3, intractable vomiting, frequent diarrhea, GI ulcer or bleeding, thrombocytopenia with platelets less than 100,000/mm^3, or hemorrhage from any site.

Extravasation: Local irritation or phlebitis may occur. Refer to your institution-specific protocol.

Overdosage: Signs and Symptoms
Nausea, vomiting, diarrhea, GI ulceration and bleeding, bone marrow depression (eg, thrombocytopenia, leukopenia, agranulocytosis).

PATIENT CARE CONSIDERATIONS

Administration/Storage
- Store powder for injection at room temperature. Protect from light. Refrigerate reconstituted solutions. Floxuridine is chemically stable for up to 2 wk under refrigeration. Use preservative-free solutions of floxuridine within 24 hr of reconstitution.
- Reconstitute each vial of powder with 5 mL Sterile Water for Injection for a floxuridine concentration of 100 mg/mL.
- Further dilute the calculated daily dose with 5% Dextrose or 0.9% Sodium Chloride to an appropriate volume for infusion pump delivery.
- For intra-arterial administration, infuse with an appropriate pump to overcome pressure in large arteries.
- Heparin may be added to floxuridine infusions to prevent thrombotic complications.

Assessment/Interventions
- Careful monitoring of the WBC and platelet count is recommended.

Patient/Family Education
- Contraceptive measures are recommended for men and women during therapy.
- Notify health care provider if chills, nausea, vomiting, unusual bleeding or bruising, yellowing of skin or eyes, abdominal pain, flank or joint pain, or swelling of feet or legs occurs.
- Notify health care provider if the following become pronounced: diarrhea, fever, weakness
- Drink plenty of liquids while taking this drug.
- Inform patients of expected toxic effects, particularly oral manifestations.
- Alert patient to the possibility of alopecia as a result of therapy, and inform patient that alopecia is usually a transient effect.

Fluconazole

(flew-KOE-nuh-zole)

Class Anti-infective/Antifungal

How Supplied
Diflucan Tablets 50 mg, Tablets 100 mg, Tablets 150 mg, Tablets 200 mg, Powder for Oral Suspension 10 mg/mL when reconstituted, Powder for Oral Suspension 40 mg/mL when reconstituted, Injection 2 mg/mL
✤ *Apo-Fluconazole* ♦ *Apo-Fluconazole-150* ♦ *Diflucan-150*

Action
PHARMACOLOGY: Interferes with the formation of fungal cell membrane, causing leakage of cellular contents and cell death.

PHARMACOKINETICS/DYNAMICS:
Absorption: Bioavailability is more than 90%. T_{max} is 1 to 2 hr.

Distribution: Apparent Vd is 0.65 L/kg, and it is 11% to 12% protein bound. Ratio of tissue (fluid) concentrations to concurrent plasma concentrations is as follows: CSF 0.5 to 0.9, saliva 1, sputum 1, blister fluid 1, urine 10, normal skin 10, nails 1, blister skin 2, vaginal tissue 1, and vaginal fluid 0.4 to 0.7.

Excretion: Mean body Cl is 0.23 mL/min/kg; t½ is 20 to 50 hr. The drug is cleared primarily by renal excretion, about 80% in urine as unchanged drug and 11% excreted in urine as metabolites.

Hemodialysis – A 3-hr session decreases plasma concentrations about 50%.

Special Populations:

Renal Function Impairment – Pharmacokinetics are markedly affected; there is an inverse relationship between t½ and Ccr.

Children –

9 mo to 15 yr: Mean Cl is 0.4 to 0.66 mL/min/kg; t½ is 15.2 to 25 hr. C_{max} is 2.9 to 14.1 mcg/mL; Vd_{ss} is 0.722 to 1.069.

Neonates (gestational age 26 to 29 wk): Mean Cl is 0.18 to 0.333 mL/min/kg (increases with time after birth); t½ is 73.6 to 46.6 hr (decreases with time after birth).

Indications Oropharyngeal and esophageal candidiasis; vaginal candidiasis; prevention of candidiasis in bone marrow transplant; *Cryptococcal meningitis*.

Contraindications Coadministration of cisapride; hypersensitivity to any component of the product.

Route/Dosage

Candidemia and Disseminated Candida Infections

CHILDREN: **PO/IV** 6 to 12 mg/kg/day.

C. meningitis: 12 mg/kg on first day, followed by 6 mg/kg/day (or 12 mg/kg/day based on medical judgment of patient's response). Recommended duration is 10 to 12 wk after CSF becomes culture negative.

NEWBORNS: Experience is limited to pharmacokinetic studies in premature newborns. Prolonged t½ has been noted. These children, in the first 2 wk of life, should receive the same mg/kg dosage as other children, but administered q 72 hr. After the first 2 wk, dose qd.

Cryptococcal Meningitis

ADULTS: **PO/IV** 400 mg first day, followed by 200 mg qd thereafter (400 mg may be used) for 10 to 12 wk after CSF culture is negative for initial meningitis; 200 mg qd for suppression of relapse of cryptococcal meningitis.

Oropharyngeal or Esophageal Candidiasis

ADULTS: **PO/IV** 200 mg first day, followed by 100 mg qd thereafter for minimum of 2 wk for oropharyngeal candidiasis, or for 3 wk and at least 2 wk following resolution of symptoms for esophageal candidiasis.

CHILDREN: **PO/IV** 6 mg/kg on first day, followed by 3 mg/kg qd thereafter for minimum of 2 wk for oropharyngeal candidiasis or 3 wk (at least 2 wk after symptom resolution) for esophageal candidiasis.

Prevention of Candidiasis in Bone Marrow Transplant

ADULTS: **PO/IV** 400 mg qd; in patients with anticipated severe granulocytopenia (less than 500 neutrophils/mm³), start fluconazole several days before anticipated onset and continue 7 days after neutrophil count rises more than 1000 cells/mm³.

Systemic Candida Infections

ADULTS: Optimal therapeutic dosage and duration not established; however, in noncomparative studies of small numbers of patients, doses up to 400 mg/day have been used.

UTIs and Peritonitis

ADULTS: Daily doses of 50 to 200 mg have been used in open, noncomparative studies of small numbers of patients.

Vaginal Candidiasis

ADULTS: **PO** 150 mg single dose.

Interactions

Alfentanil, benzodiazepines (eg, midazolam), buspirone, corticosteroids (eg, prednisone), losartan, nisoldipine, sulfonylureas (eg, glyburide), tacrolimus, theophylline, tricyclic antidepressants, vinca alkaloids (eg, vincristine), zidovudine, zolpidem: Levels may be elevated by fluconazole, increasing the risk of side effects and toxicity.

Anticoagulants (eg, warfarin): Anticoagulant effect may be increased.

Cimetidine, rifamycins (eg, rifampin): Fluconazole plasma levels may be reduced, decreasing therapeutic effects.

Cisapride: Contraindicated; increased cisapride plasma levels with cardiotoxicity may occur.

Cyclosporine: Increased cyclosporine concentrations.

Hydantoins (eg, phenytoin): Increased hydantoin levels.

Hydrochlorothiazide: May increase fluconazole levels, increasing side effects.

Lab Test Interferences None well documented.

Adverse Reactions

CV: QT prolongation (including torsades de pointes).

CNS: Headache (2%).

DERM: Skin rash (2%); exfoliative skin disorders (including Stevens-Johnson syndrome and toxic epidermal necrolysis).

GI: Nausea (4% [children 2%]); vomiting (2% [children 5%]); abdominal pain (2% [children 3%]); diarrhea (2%).

HEMA: Leukopenia (including neutropenia and agranulocytosis); thrombocytopenia.

HEPA: Hepatitis; cholestasis; fulminant hepatitis.

Precautions
Pregnancy: Category C.
Lactation: Excreted in breast milk.
Children: An open-label, randomized, controlled trial has shown fluconazole to be effective in children 6 mo to 13 yr. Efficacy has not been established in infants younger than 6 mo.
Renal function impairment: Dosage reduction based on Ccr may be necessary.

Anaphylaxis: Anaphylaxis occurred rarely.
Dermatologic changes: Exfoliative skin disorders reported.
Hepatic injury: Monitor patients with abnormal LFT results for development of more severe hepatic injury.
Immunocompromised patients: To prevent relapse, patients with AIDS and cryptococcal meningitis usually require maintenance therapy.

Overdosage: Signs and Symptoms
Hallucinations, paranoid behavior.

PATIENT CARE CONSIDERATIONS

Administration/Storage
- No dosage adjustment is necessary when switching from IV to oral therapy.
- Dose and duration of therapy are dependent on condition being treated.

Tablets:
- Administer tablets with a full glass of water without regard to meals. Administer with food if GI upset occurs.
- Store tablets at controlled room temperature (below 86°F).

Suspension:
- Shake well before measuring dose.
- Measure prescribed dose using dosing cup, spoon, or syringe.
- Store dry powder below 86°F. Store reconstituted suspension between 41° and 86°F. Protect from freezing. Discard any unused suspension after 2 wk.

Injection:
- For IV infusion only. Not for intradermal, intrathecal, intraperitoneal, SC, or IM administration.
- Inspect solution visually before administration. Do not administer if solution is cloudy, discolored, contains particulate matter, or if the flexible container has any leaks.
- Infuse prescribed dose at rate not exceeding 200 mg/hr.
- Do not add other medications or additives to injection bag.
- If other drugs are being administered through same IV line, administer each medication separately and flush IV line with compatible solution before and after infusion of fluconazole.
- Premixed flexible containers and glass bottles are for single use only; discard any unused solution.
- Do not use flexible containers in series connections because of risk of air embolism.
- Store flexible injection bags between 41° and 77°F. Protect from freezing. Store glass bottles between 41° and 86°F. Protect from freezing.

Assessment/Interventions
- Obtain patient history, including drug history and any known allergies. Note renal or hepatic impairment, structural heart disease, electrolyte abnormalities, allergy to azole antifungal agents, or concurrent use of cisapride, medications metabolized by CYP3A4 and CYP2C9, or medications with potential to prolong the QT interval.
- Ensure that necessary fungal cultures have been obtained before beginning therapy.
- Review results of culture and sensitivity testing as available.
- Administer reduced dose to patient with renal impairment (Ccr less than 50 mL/min) following manufacturer's guidelines.
- Ensure that renal function and liver enzymes are determined before starting therapy and periodically during prolonged treatment.
- Monitor patient's response to therapy. Inform health care provider if infection does not improve or worsens.
- Monitor patient for signs of allergic reaction. Discontinue therapy and immediately notify health care provider if noted. Be prepared to treat appropriately.
- Monitor patient for signs and symptoms of hepatic injury (eg, right upper quadrant abdominal pain, persistent nausea, vomiting, dark urine, yellowing of skin or eyes). Inform health care provider if noted and be prepared to discontinue therapy.
- Monitor patient for GI, CNS, CV, DERM, and general body side effects. Report to health care provider if noted and significant. If patient develops skin rash, monitor closely and be prepared to discontinue the medication if lesions progress.

Patient/Family Education
- Explain name, dose, action, and potential side effects of drug.
- Advise patient to read *Patient Information* leaf-

let before starting therapy and with each refill.
- Review dosing schedule and prescribed length of therapy with patient. Advise patient that treatment may be prolonged (eg, several weeks or months) and to continue medication until advised to stop using by health care provider.

Tablets and Suspension:
- Advise patient that tablets can be taken with a full glass of water without regard to meals but to take with food if GI upset occurs.
- Advise patient using suspension that the suspension can be taken without regard to meals but to take with food if GI upset occurs.
- Advise patient or caregiver to shake suspension well before measuring dose and to measure prescribed dose of suspension using dosing cup, spoon, or syringe.
- Advise patient that if a dose is missed, to take as soon as remembered. However, if it is nearing the time for the next dose, to skip the dose and take the next dose at the regularly scheduled time.
- Remind patient to complete entire course of therapy, even if symptoms of infection have disappeared.
- Advise patient to inform health care provider if infection does not improve or worsens.
- Advise patient to contact health care provider immediately if skin rash, persistent nausea or vomiting, dark urine, or yellowing of skin or eyes occur.
- Advise women to notify health care provider if pregnant, planning to become pregnant, or breastfeeding.
- Instruct patient not to take any prescription or OTC medications or dietary supplements unless advised by health care provider.
- Advise patient that follow-up examinations and lab tests may be required to monitor therapy and to keep appointments.

Injection:
- Advise patient that medication will be prepared and administered by a health care professional in a health care setting when oral therapy is not feasible, but that the patient will be switched to oral therapy when health care provider believes it is appropriate.

Flucytosine

(flew-SITE-oh-seen)

Class Anti-infective/Antifungal

How Supplied
Ancobon Capsules 250 mg, Capsules 500 mg

Action
PHARMACOLOGY: Exact mechanism is unknown; interferes with DNA and RNA synthesis. Active against *Candida* and *Cryptococcus*.

PHARMACOKINETICS/DYNAMICS:

Absorption: Bioavailability is 78% to 89%. C_{max} is 30 to 40 mcg/mL; T_{max} is 1 to 2 hr.

Distribution: The drug is 2.9% to 4% protein bound. It readily penetrates the blood-brain barrier achieving clinically significant concentrations in the CSF.

Excretion: Primarily renally excreted via glomerular filtration. The $t_{½}$ is 2.4 to 4.8 hr. More than 90% is excreted in the urine unchanged and about 1% in the urine as metabolite (α-fluoro-β-ureido-propionic acid).

Special Populations:
Renal Function Impairment – Prolonged $t_{½}$ (29.9 to 250 hr in anuric or nephrectomized patients).

Indications Treatment of serious infections caused by susceptible strains of *Candida* or *Cryptococcus*. **Unlabeled use(s):** Treatment of chromomycosis.

Contraindications Standard considerations.

Route/Dosage
ADULTS AND CHILDREN MORE THAN 50 KG: PO 50 to 150 mg/kg/day in divided doses q 6 hr.

Interactions
Amphotericin B: Increased therapeutic action and toxicity of flucytosine.
Cytosine: Inactivates antifungal activity of flucytosine.

Lab Test Interferences Interferes with creatinine value determinations with dry-slide enzymatic method (Kodak Ektachem analyzer); use Jaffe method.

Adverse Reactions
CV: Cardiac arrest.
CNS: Ataxia; hearing loss; headache; sedation; confusion; fatigue; weakness; dizziness; vertigo, paresthesia; parkinsonism; peripheral neuropathy; pyrexia; hallucinations; psychosis.
DERM: Rash; pruritus; urticaria; photosensitivity.
GI: Nausea; emesis; abdominal pain; diarrhea; anorexia; duodenal ulcer; GI hemorrhage.
GU: Azotemia; creatinine and BUN elevation; crystalluria; renal failure; dry mouth.
HEMA: Anemia; agranulocytosis; aplastic anemia; eosinophilia; leukopenia; pancytopenia; thrombocytopenia.
HEPA: Hepatic dysfunction; jaundice; ulcerative colitis; increased bilirubin; elevated hepatic enzymes.

METAB: Hypoglycemia; hypokalemia.
RESP: Respiratory arrest; chest pain; dyspnea.

> **Warning:**
> Use with extreme caution in patients with renal impairment. Close monitoring of hematologic, renal, and hepatic function is essential.

Precautions
Pregnancy: Category C.
Lactation: Undetermined.
Children: Safety and efficacy not established.

PATIENT CARE CONSIDERATIONS
Administration/Storage
- Administer capsules a few at a time over 15 min to minimize GI upset.

Assessment/Interventions
- Obtain patient history, including drug history and any known allergies.
- Ensure that baseline LFTs, BUN, and creatinine, electrolytes, and glucose have been obtained before beginning therapy, and monitor at regular intervals.
- Obtain baseline CBC with differential and repeat daily. Assess for bone marrow depression.
- Obtain specimens for culture and sensitivity before beginning therapy.
- Monitor BP at regular intervals during therapy. Assess for cardiovascular collapse.
- Monitor blood levels of drug closely in patient with impaired renal function.
- If patient has ataxia, hearing loss, headache, paresthesia, peripheral neuropathy, pyrexia, hallucinations, psychosis, laboratory evidence of liver or renal dysfunction, chest pain, or respiratory distress, notify health care provider immediately.

Hepatic function impairment: Adjust dose according to blood levels and monitor hepatic function.
Bone marrow depression: Use with extreme caution in patients with bone marrow depression or those at risk (eg, hematologic disease, radiation treatment, other bone marrow suppressant drugs).

Overdosage: Signs and Symptoms
Nausea, vomiting, diarrhea, CNS changes, leukopenia, thrombocytopenia, hepatitis.

Patient/Family Education
- Instruct patient to take capsules a few at a time over a 15-min period with food.
- Instruct diabetic patients to monitor glucose closely.
- Instruct patient to report the following symptoms to health care provider: sore throat, cough, unusual bleeding or bruising, petechiae, blood in urine, bleeding gums, abdominal pain, nausea, vomiting, change in color or consistency of stools, fever, yellow skin/eyes, ataxia, hearing loss, paresthesia, shaking, tingling, altered sensation, parkinsonism, peripheral neuropathy, hallucinations or psychosis, anorexia, increased fatigue, rash or itching.
- Warn patient to seek emergency care if respiratory distress or chest pain occur.
- Advise patient that drug may cause dizziness or vertigo and to use caution while driving or performing other tasks requiring mental alertness.
- Caution patient to avoid unnecessary exposure to sunlight and to use sunscreen and wear protective clothing to avoid photosensitivity reaction.

Fludarabine Phosphate
(flew-DAR-uh-BEAN)
Class Purine antimetabolite
How Supplied
Fludara Powder for injection 50 mg
Action
PHARMACOLOGY: Fludarabine is a fluorinated nucleotide analog of the antiviral agent vidarabine. Fludarabine's metabolite appears to act by inhibiting DNA polymerase alpha, ribonucleotide reductase, and DNA primase, thus inhibiting DNA synthesis.

PHARMACOKINETICS/DYNAMICS:
Absorption: Fludarabine is rapidly converted to the active metabolite, 2-fluoro-ara-A, within minutes after IV infusion.

Distribution: In vitro, plasma protein binding of fludarabine ranged between 19% and 29%.
Metabolism: The t½ of 2-fluoro-ara-A is approximately 20 hr.
Excretion: Renal Cl represents approximately 40% of the total body Cl.

Indications Refractory or progressive chronic B-cell lymphocytic leukemia. **Unlabeled use(s):** Leukemias, non-Hodgkin lymphoma.

Contraindications Standard considerations.
Route/Dosage
Chronic Lymphocytic Leukemia
ADULTS: IV 25/m²/day over approximately 30 min daily for 5 consecutive days. Each 5-day course should commence q 28 days.

Renal Insufficiency
ADULTS: IV Reduce dose 20% in moderate

renal impairment (Ccr 30 to 70 mL/min/ 1.73 m^2). Do not administer in patients with severely impaired renal function (Ccr less than 30 mL/min/1.73 m^2).

Interactions
Pentostatin: Concomitant therapy may cause severe or fatal pulmonary toxicity.

Lab Test Interferences None well documented.

Adverse Reactions
CV: Deep venous thrombosis, phlebitis (at least 1%); aneurysm; angina; arrhythmia; cerebrovascular accident; CHF; MI; supraventricular tachycardia; transient ischemic attack.
CNS: Weakness (65%); fatigue (38%); paresthesia (12%); malaise (8%); agitation; coma; confusion; headache; weakness.
DERM: Rash (15%); diaphoresis (13%); pruritus (at least 1%); alopecia; seborrhea.
EENT: Visual disturbances (15%); hearing loss, sleep disorder (at least 1%); cerebellar syndrome; depression; impaired mentation.
GI: Nausea/vomiting (36%); anorexia (34%); diarrhea (15%); GI bleeding (13%); constipation (at least 1%); dysphagia; esophagitis; mucositis; stomatitis.
GU: Dysuria, hematuria; urinary infection (at least 1%); abnormal renal function test; hemorrhagic cystitis; proteinuria; renal failure; urinary hesitancy.
HEMA/LYMPH: Anemia (60%); neutropenia (59%); thrombocytopenia (55%); autoimmune hemolytic anemia; pancytopenia (postmarketing).
HEPA: Abnormal LFTs (at least 1%); cholelithiasis; liver failure.
HYPERSEN: Anaphylaxis.
M/N: Hyperglycemia (at least 1%); tumor lysis syndrome (including hyperuricemia, hyperphosphatemia, hypocalcemia, metabolic acidosis, hyperkalemia, hematuria, urate crystalluria, renal failure).
MUSC: Myalgia (16%); arthralgia; osteoporosis.
RESP: Cough (44%); dyspnea, pneumonia (22%); hemoptysis, upper respiratory tract infections (at least 1%); allergic pneumonitis; bronchitis; epistaxis; hypoxia; pharyngitis; pulmonary hypersensitivity; sinusitis; respiratory distress, pulmonary hemorrhage, pulmonary fibrosis, respiratory failure (postmarketing).
OTHER: Fever (69%); infection (44%); pain (22%); chills, edema (19%); dehydration; hemorrhage.

> **WARNING:**
> Neurotoxicity associated with high doses in dose ranging studies in acute leukemia. Autoimmune hemolytic anemia reported after at least 1 cycle. Concurrent use with pentostatin not recommended, based on increased incidence of fatal pulmonary toxicity. Severe CNS toxicity occurred in 36% patients receiving doses approximately 4 times greater than the recommended dose. (96 mg/m^2/day for 5 to 7 days). At recommended doses, severe CNS toxicity is rare.
>
> *Bone marrow suppression:* Severe bone marrow suppression, notably anemia, thrombocytopenia, and neutropenia, occurred.

Precautions
Pregnancy: Category D.
Lactation: Undetermined.
Children: Safety and efficacy not established.
Renal function impairment: Administer cautiously.
Dose-dependent toxicity: There are clear dose-dependent toxic effects seen with fludarabine.
Transfusion: Transfusion-associated graft/host disease may occur after transfusion of nonirradiated blood.
Tumor lysis syndrome: Tumor lysis syndrome has occurred.

Overdosage: Signs and Symptoms
Irreversible CNS toxicity characterized by delayed blindness, coma, and death; severe thrombocytopenia and neutropenia.

PATIENT CARE CONSIDERATIONS
Administration/Storage
- Do not administer to patient with severe renal impairment (Ccr less than 30 mL/min) or in combination with pentostatin.
- For IV administration only. Not for intradermal, subcutaneous, IM, intra-arterial, or oral administration.
- Diligently follow institutional and NIH procedures for handling, administration, and disposal of anticancer drugs. Wear appropriate protective equipment when preparing and administering fludarabine. Avoid exposure by inhalation or by direct contact of the skin, mucous membranes, and eyes.
- If accidental skin or mucus membrane contact occurs, wash thoroughly with soap and water. If accidental eye contact occurs, immediately institute copious irrigation with plain water.
- Reconstitute powder for injection with 2 mL sterile water for injection. Gently agitate vial to dissolve drug. Resulting solution contains 25 mg/mL of fludarabine.
- Prior to administration further dilute reconsti-

tuted solution in 100 to 125 mL D5W or 0.9% sodium chloride injection.
- Do not administer if particulate matter, cloudiness, or discoloration is noted.
- Administer prescribed dose by IV infusion over 30 minutes.
- Store unopened vials in refrigerator (36° to 46°F). Reconstituted solution contains no preservative and should be used within 8 hr of reconstitution.

Assessment/Interventions
- Obtain patient history, including drug history and any known allergies. Note renal impairment, bone marrow impairment, or concurrent treatment with pentostatin.
- Ensure that women of childbearing potential are not pregnant when therapy is initiated and use effective contraception during treatment.
- To prevent graft/host disease ensure that irradiated blood products are used in patient requiring transfusion during treatment with fludarabine.
- Evaluate risk of developing hyperuricemia before starting therapy and initiate hypouricemic therapy, including adequate fluid intake, and monitoring of uric acid before starting treatment in patient determined to be at risk for developing hyperuricemia and urate precipitation.
- Evaluate CBC with differential and platelet count, and renal function before starting therapy, and then frequently during therapy.
- Implement infection control measures if WBC drops; implement bleeding precautions if platelet count drops.
- Reduce dose or delay therapy in patient exhibiting hematologic or nonhematologic toxicity.
- Reduce fludarabine dose 20% in patient with moderate renal impairment (Ccr between 30 and 70 mL/min).
- Monitor patient for signs and symptoms of hemolysis (unexplained fatigue, jaundice, splenomegaly). Notify health care provider if suspected.
- Monitor patient for signs of anaphylactic or serious allergic reactions. Discontinue therapy and immediately notify health care provider if noted. Be prepared to treat appropriately.
- Monitor patient for HEMA, CNS, GI, CV, DERM, and general body side effects. Report to health care provider if noted and significant. If neurotoxicity develops ensure drug is discontinued or further administration is delayed.
- Monitor patient for signs and symptoms of bacterial, viral, or fungal infection. Report to health care provider immediately if noted.

Patient/Family Education
- Explain name, action, and potential side effects of the treatment regimen. Review the treatment regimen including dosing schedule, duration of treatment, and monitoring that will be required.
- Advise patient, family, or caregiver that medication will be prepared and administered by health care providers in a health care setting.
- Advise patient, family, or caregiver that medication may be used in combination with other agents to achieve maximum benefit possible.
- Advise patient, family, or caregiver to immediately report any of the following to health care provider: rash; hives; difficulty breathing; fever, chills, or other signs of infection; bleeding or unusual bruising; sores in mouth; dark urine; yellowing of skin or eyes; pain, redness, or swelling at injection site.
- Advise patient, family, or caregiver to report any of the following to health care provider: persistent nausea, vomiting, diarrhea, or appetite loss; persistent or worsening general body weakness.
- Instruct patient not to take any prescription or OTC medications, herbal preparations, or dietary supplements unless advised by health care provider.
- Caution women of childbearing potential to avoid becoming pregnant during therapy.
- Advise women to notify health care provider if pregnant, planning to become pregnant, or breastfeeding.
- Advise patient, family, or caregiver that following discharge frequent follow-up visits and laboratory tests will be required to monitor therapy and to keep appointments.

Fludrocortisone Acetate

(flew-droe-CORE-tih-sone ASS-uh-TATE)
Class Mineralocorticoid
How Supplied
Florinef Acetate Tablets 0.1 mg

Action
PHARMACOLOGY: Exerts salt-retaining (mineralocorticoid) activity by acting on renal distal tubules to enhance reabsorption of sodium and increasing urinary excretion of potassium, hydrogen, and magnesium ions.

Pharmacokinetics/Dynamics:
Absorption: Fludrocortisone is rapidly absorbed from the GI tract. T_{max} is 1.7 hr.
Excretion: The plasma t½ is about 3.5 hr. The biological t½ is 18 to 36 hr.

Indications Partial replacement therapy for primary and secondary adrenocortical insufficiency in Addison disease; treatment of salt-losing adrenogenital syndrome. **Unlabeled use(s):** Treatment of severe orthostatic hypotension.

Contraindications Systemic fungal infections.

Route/Dosage
Addison Disease
ADULTS: **PO** 0.05 to 0.1 mg/day (range, 0.1 mg 3 times/wk to 0.2 mg/day).

Salt-Losing Adrenogenital Syndrome
ADULTS: **PO** 0.1 to 0.2 mg/day.

Interactions
Amphotericin, potassium-losing diuretics: May increase potassium loss.
Anticholinesterase agents (eg, neostigmine): May antagonize the effects of anticholinesterase agents in myasthenia gravis.
Anticoagulants (eg, warfarin): Dose requirement of anticoagulant may be reduced or effect opposed.
Barbiturates, hydantoins (eg, phenytoin), rifampin: Decreased fludrocortisone activity.
Salicylates: Serum levels may be reduced by corticosteroids, decreasing the effectiveness; in addition, the ulcerogenic effects of both agents may be increased.

Lab Test Interferences None well documented.

Adverse Reactions
CV: Edema; hypertension; CHF; heart enlargement.
DERM: Bruising; increased sweating; hives; rash.
OTHER: Hypokalemic alkalosis. May also cause adverse reactions associated with glucocorticoids (eg, dexamethasone).

Precautions
Pregnancy: Category C.
Lactation: Excreted in breast milk.
Children: Safety and efficacy not established.
Addison disease: Patients with Addison disease may exhibit exaggerated side effects; monitor closely for development of edema, significant weight gain, or increases in BP.
Adrenal insufficiency: Adrenal insufficiency may occur. Increased doses may be needed before, during, or after stressful situations.
Electrolyte disturbances: Sodium retention and potassium loss are increased by high sodium intake. Sodium restriction and potassium supplementation may be necessary.
GI: Use with caution in patients with nonspecific ulcerative colitis if there is a possibility of impending perforation, abscess or other pyogenic infection, diverticulitis, fresh intestinal anastomoses, or peptic ulcer.
Infections: Drug may mask signs of infection and may decrease host-defense mechanisms to prevent dissemination of infection.
Immunizations: Because of possible hazards of neurological complications and a lack of antibody response, do not vaccinate patients against smallpox while receiving corticosteroid therapy or undertake other immunization procedures.
Ocular effects: Prolonged use may produce posterior subcapsular cataracts and glaucoma with possible damage to the optic nerves and may enhance the establishment of secondary ocular infections caused by fungi or viruses.
Supplemental measures: Patients receiving fludrocortisone may need supplemental measures (eg, glucocorticoids, electrolyte control) for optimal control of symptoms.

Overdosage: Signs and Symptoms
Hypertension, edema, hypokalemia, excessive weight gain, increase in heart size.

PATIENT CARE CONSIDERATIONS
Administration/Storage
- Store in tightly closed container at room temperature (68° to 77°F). Protect from light.

Assessment/Interventions
- Obtain patient history, including drug history and any known allergies. Note cardiovascular disorders and recent or present fungal infection or other systemic infections.
- Assess baseline psychological status before beginning therapy.
- Take pulse and BP and monitor daily during therapy.
- Ensure that chest x-ray and serum electrolyte levels have been obtained before beginning therapy, and monitor frequently during treatment.
- Monitor weight gain and I&O during therapy.
- If signs of concurrent infection, significant increase in weight or BP, signs of hypokalemic alkalosis, dizziness, or severe headache occur, notify health care provider.

Patient/Family Education
- Instruct patient to take medication exactly as prescribed. If dose is missed, it should be taken as soon as possible. Do not double up if within several hours of next dose. Caution

patient not to stop medication abruptly. Instruct patient to notify health care provider if greater than 1 dose is missed or a dosage cannot be taken because of nausea or vomiting.
- Advise patient to reduce dietary sodium, which accelerates potassium loss, and to eat foods rich in potassium.
- Tell patient to notify health care provider when experiencing a stressful situation (eg, emotional upheavals, dental extractions, trauma, surgery, illness) as increased dosage may be needed.
- Instruct patient to report the following symptoms to health care provider: increased or irregular heart beat, high BP, fluid retention, joint pain, muscle weakness, headache, dizziness, fever, unusual weight gain.
- Instruct patient to report euphoria, depression, or other changes in mental status.
- Tell patient to be alert for spontaneous fractures and impaired wound healing.
- Advise patient of the importance of keeping follow-up visits.

Flumazenil

(flew-MAZ-ah-nil)

Class Antidote

How Supplied
Romazicon Injection 0.1 mg/mL
♣ Anexate

Action
PHARMACOLOGY: Antagonizes actions of benzodiazepines on CNS by blocking receptors.

PHARMACOKINETICS/DYNAMICS:
Absorption: Mean C_{max} is 24 ng/mL (range, 11 to 43 ng/mL); mean AUC was 15 ng•hr/mL (range, 10 to 22 ng•hr/mL).

Distribution: Initial distribution t½ is 7 to 15 min. $VD_{initial}$ is 0.5 L/kg; Vd_{ss} is 0.177 to 1.60 L/kg. Protein binding is about 50%.

Metabolism: Primarily hepatically metabolized and dependent on hepatic blood flow (highly extracted).

Excretion: Terminal t½ is 41 to 79 min. Total clearance is 0.7 to 1.3 L/hr/kg (increases by 50% during ingestion of food). Less than 1% is excreted unchanged in the urine; 90% to 95% is excreted in urine and 5% to 10% in feces.

Onset: 1 to 2 min.

Peak: 6 to 10 min.

Duration: Related to the plasma concentration of the benzodiazepine as well as the dose of flumazenil.

Special Populations:
Hepatic Function Impairment –
Moderate: Mean total clearance decreased 40% to 60%; t½ increases to 1.3 hr.
Severe: Mean total clearance decreased 75%; t½ increases to 2.4 hr.
Children –
1 to 17 yr: The t½ is shorter and more variable, ranging 20 to 75 min.

Indications Complete or partial reversal of sedative effects of benzodiazepines where general anesthesia induced or maintained with benzodiazepines, where sedation produced with benzodiazepines for diagnostic or therapeutic procedures, and for the management of benzodiazepine overdose.

Contraindications Hypersensitivity to flumazenil or benzodiazepines; in patients given benzodiazepines for control of a potentially life-threatening condition (eg, status epilepticus); in patients showing signs of serious cyclic antidepressant overdose.

Route/Dosage
Reversal of Conscious Sedation or in General Anesthesia
ADULTS: **IV** 0.2 mg over 15 sec. If desired level of consciousness is not achieved in 45 sec, additional 0.2 mg doses can be administered at 60 sec intervals (max, 1 mg). In event of resedation, repeat doses (0.2 mg/min to max 1 mg) at 20 min intervals as needed (max, 3 mg/hr).

Management of Suspected Benzodiazepine Overdose
ADULTS: **IV** 0.2 mg over 30 sec. If desired level of consciousness is not achieved in 30 sec, an additional dose of 0.3 mg over 30 sec can be administered. Further doses of 0.5 mg over 30 sec can be administered at 1 min intervals as needed (max, 3 mg).

Interactions Toxic effects of other drugs taken in toxic doses may emerge with reversal of benzodiazepine effect.

Lab Test Interferences None well documented.

Adverse Reactions
CV: Cutaneous vasodilation (eg, sweating, flushing, hot flushes); palpitations.
CNS: Convulsions; headache; dizziness; agitation; emotional lability; fatigue; paresthesia; insomnia; dyspnea; hypoesthesia.
DERM: Sweating.
EENT: Visual field defect; diplopia; blurred vision.
GI: Nausea; vomiting.
RESP: Hyperventilation.

OTHER: Injection site pain; injection site reaction; dry mouth.

Precautions

Pregnancy: Category C.
Labor and delivery – Not recommended; effects on newborn are unknown.
Lactation: Undetermined.
Children: Safety and efficacy not determined.
Hepatic function impairment: Elimination of flumazenil is reduced in patients with liver disease.
Ambulatory: The effects of flumazenil may wear off before a long-acting benzodiazepine is completely cleared from the body.
Benzodiazepine tolerance: Flumazenil may cause benzodiazepine withdrawal symptoms in individuals who have been taking benzodiazepines long enough to have some degree of tolerance or physical dependence.
Drug/alcohol dependence: Use with caution in patients with alcoholism and other drug dependencies because of the increased frequency of benzodiazepine tolerance and dependence observed in these patient populations.
Head injury: Use with caution in patients with head injury because of risk of precipitating convulsions or altering cerebral blood flow in patients receiving benzodiazepines.

Intensive care unit: Use of flumazenil to diagnose benzodiazepine-induced sedation in the ICU is not recommended because of the risk of adverse effects.
Neuromuscular blocking agents: Do not use flumazenil until effects of neuromuscular blocking agents have been fully reversed.
Overdose situations: Flumazenil is intended as an adjunct to, not a substitute for, proper management of overdose patients (eg, airway maintenance, decontamination).
Psychiatric: Flumazenil may provoke panic attacks in patients with a history of panic disorder.
Resedation/Hypoventilation: Flumazenil may not fully reverse postoperative airway problems or ventilatory insufficiency induced by benzodiazepines; its effects may wear off before the effects of many benzodiazepines.
Seizures: Reversal of benzodiazepine effects may be associated with the onset of seizures in certain high-risk populations including the following: Concurrent major sedative-hypnotic drug withdrawal; recent therapy with repeated doses of parenteral benzodiazepines; myoclonic jerking or seizure activity prior to flumazenil in overdose cases; concurrent cyclic antidepressant poisoning.

PATIENT CARE CONSIDERATIONS

Administration/Storage

- For IV use only.
- Compatible with D5W, LR, and NS.
- Administer through a freely flowing IV in a large vein.
- In high-risk patients, administer smallest amount effective. Wait 6 to 10 min between trial dose administration in high-risk patients.
- Do not rush administration. Secure airway and IV access.
- If patient does not respond after 5 min of a cumulative dose of 5 mg, sedation is probably not caused by benzodiazepines.
- Do not use if solution is discolored or has particulate matter.
- Stable for 24 hr at room temperature after mixing. Best if used just after mixing.

Assessment/Interventions

- Obtain patient history.
- Determine reason for use prior to administration (eg, benzodiazepine overdose, reverse anesthesia, sedation). Use this information to select the proper dosing strategy.
- Monitor level of consciousness during and after administration.
- Resedation may take place in 15 to 30 min because half-life of many benzodiazepines is longer than flumazenil.
- Monitor patient during and after administration for seizure activity and respiratory or cardiac arrest.
- Monitor patient for confusion, agitation, emotional lability, and perceptual distorting after administration.

Patient/Family Education

- Instruct patient that flumazenil does not reverse amnesia. Repeat patient instructions in post-procedure period.
- Warn patient that despite feelings of alertness at time of discharge, effects of benzodiazepines may reoccur, affecting memory and judgment.
- Instruct patient to avoid activities requiring complete alertness, such as operating hazardous machinery or driving, for at least 18 to 24 hr after discharge.
- Warn patients to avoid alcohol or over-the-counter drugs for at least 18 to 24 hr after discharge.

Flunisolide

(flew-NISS-oh-lide)
Class Corticosteroid

How Supplied
AeroBid Aerosol approximately 250 mcg/actuation ◆ AeroBid-M Aerosol approximately 250 mcg/actuation ◆ *Nasarel* Nasal spray 0.025% (25 mcg/actuation)
🍁 *Apo-Flunisolide* ◆ *ratio-Flunisolide*

Action

PHARMACOLOGY: Has local anti-inflammatory activity on lung or nasal mucosa with minimal systemic effect. May decrease number and activity of cells involved in inflammatory response and enhance effect of other drugs or endogenous substances that aid in bronchodilation.

PHARMACOKINETICS/DYNAMICS:
Absorption: Systemic bioavailability is 40% (oral inhalation) and 50% (nasal inhalation).
Metabolism: Converted to the 6β-OH metabolite and water-soluble conjugates in the liver.
Excretion: The $t_{½}$ is 1.8 hr.

Indications

Inhalation: Maintenance treatment of asthma for patients requiring chronic treatment with corticosteroids.
Intranasal: Symptoms of perennial or seasonal rhinitis.

Contraindications Primary treatment of status asthmaticus or acute asthma when intensive measures are required (inhalation use); untreated local infection of the nasal mucosa (intranasal use); hypersensitivity to any component of the product.

Route/Dosage

ADULTS AND CHILDREN 6 TO 15 YR OF AGE:
Inhalation 2 inhalations (500 mcg) bid.
Adults: Do not exceed 4 inhalations bid (2 mg/day).
Children: Do not exceed 2 inhalations bid (1 mg/day).
ADULTS:
Initial dose: **Intranasal** 2 sprays (50 mcg) in each nostril bid (200 mcg/day).
Max: 8 sprays in each nostril daily (400 mcg/day).
CHILDREN 6 TO 14 YR OF AGE:
Initial dose: **Intranasal** 1 spray (25 mcg) in each nostril tid or 2 sprays in each nostril bid.
Max: 4 sprays in each nostril daily (200 mcg/day).

Interactions None well documented.

Lab Test Interferences None well documented.

Adverse Reactions

CV:
Oral inhalation – Palpitations (3% to 9%); hypertension, tachycardia (1% to 3%).
CNS:
Oral inhalation – Headache (25%); dizziness, irritability, nervousness, shakiness (3% to 9%); anxiety, depression, faintness, fatigue, hyperactivity, hypoactivity, insomnia, moodiness, numbness, vertigo (1% to 3%).
DERM:
Oral inhalation – Eczema, itching, rash (3% to 9%); acne, hives, urticaria (1% to 3%).
EENT:
Oral inhalation – Sore throat (20%); rhinitis, sinus congestion, sinus drainage, sinus infection, sinusitis, ear infection, loss of smell or taste (3% to 9%); dry throat, glossitis, pharyngitis, throat irritation, phlegm, nasal irritation and discomfort, blurred vision, earache, eye discomfort, eye infection (1% to 3%).
Nasal spray – Burning and stinging (13%); epistaxis, nasal dryness, pharyngitis (greater than 1%).
GI:
Oral inhalation – Nausea/vomiting (25%); diarrhea, upset stomach, unpleasant taste (10%); abdominal pain, heartburn, *Candida* infection (3% to 9%); constipation, dyspepsia, gas, mouth irritation (1% to 3%).
Nasal spray – Aftertaste (17%); nausea (greater than 1%).
GU:
Oral inhalation – Menstrual disturbances (3% to 9%).
HEMA/LYMPH:
Oral inhalation – Capillary fragility, enlarged lymph nodes (1% to 3%).
M/N:
Oral inhalation – Weight gain (1% to 3%).
RESP:
Oral inhalation – Upper respiratory tract infection (25%); cold symptoms, nasal congestion (15%); chest congestion, cough, hoarseness, sneezing, sputum, wheezing (3% to 9%); bronchitis, chest tightness, dyspnea, epistaxis, head stuffiness, laryngitis, pleurisy, pneumonia (1% to 3%).
Nasal spray – Increased cough (greater than 1%).
OTHER:
Oral inhalation – Flu (10%); chest pain, decreased appetite, edema, fever (3% to 9%); chills, peripheral edema, sweating, weakness, malaise, increased appetite (1% to 3%).

Precautions

Pregnancy: Category C.
Lactation: Undetermined. Because other

corticosteroids are excreted in human milk, use caution.

Children: Safety and efficacy in children less than 6 yr of age not established. Oral corticosteroids may suppress growth in children and adolescents, particularly with higher doses over extended periods.

Hypersensitivity: Immediate and delayed reactions have occurred.

Special risk patients: Use inhaled corticosteroids with caution in patients with active or quiescent tuberculosis infection, untreated systemic fungal, bacterial, parasitic or viral infections, or ocular herpes simplex.

Acute asthma: Not indicated for rapid relief of bronchospasm.

Fungal infections: Antifungal therapy and discontinuance of steroid may be necessary.

Immunology: Patients receiving immunosuppressant agents are more susceptible to infections than healthy adults. If a patient is exposed to measles or chickenpox, appropriate prophylaxis and treatment may be indicated.

Systemic effects: Transfer from oral to inhaled corticosteroids has resulted in death because of adrenal insufficiency related to a lower systemic availability. Use cautiously in patients taking alternate-day prednisone; may increase likelihood of HPA suppression. Exceeding recommended dose may cause systemic effects.

PATIENT CARE CONSIDERATIONS

Administration/Storage

Inhalation Aerosol:

- May be administered alone or in combination with systemic corticosteroids.
- For oral inhalation only. Avoid spraying into the nose or eyes.
- If patient is also receiving bronchodilators by inhalation, administer bronchodilator 5 min before flunisolide to enhance penetration of latter drug into bronchial tree.
- Thoroughly shake inhaler before each inhalation. Have patient exhale as completely as possible and place inhaler in mouth and close lips around mouthpiece, keeping tongue below mouthpiece. Tilt patient's head back slightly. Instruct patient to take slow, deep breath while inhaler is being activated and to hold breath for 5 to 10 sec and then breathe out slowly. A spacing device (eg, Aerochamber) may be used to enhance delivery of medication. Have patient rinse mouth after inhalations are complete.
- If more than 1 spray/dose is ordered, administer each spray individually, waiting a few seconds between sprays.
- Store inhalation aerosol at ambient room temperature (59° to 86°F) away from heat or open flame. Do not puncture or discard pressurized canister in incinerator.

Nasal Inhalation:

- For intranasal use only. Avoid spraying into the eyes, mouth, or directly into the nasal septum.
- Shake well before each use.
- To prime before first use, actuate the pump 5 to 6 times, or until a fine mist appears. If pump has not been used for 5 consecutive days, reprime the pump until a fine mist appears.
- Clear nasal passages of secretions prior to use. If patient is congested, use topical, short-acting decongestant just before administration to ensure adequate penetration of spray. Saline nasal lavage may help remove secretions.
- Place nasal adapter into 1 nostril and gently close other nostril with finger. While inhaling from nostril, activate canister. Repeat process on other side.
- Do not blow nose immediately after administration.
- If 2 sprays per dose are ordered, administer 1 spray in each nostril, wait a few seconds, and administer second spray into each nostril.
- Store nasal spray at ambient room temperature (59° to 86°F). Protect from freezing. Discard bottle when labeled number of sprays have been used, even if bottle is not completely empty.

Assessment/Interventions

- Obtain patient history, including drug history and any known allergies. Note hepatic impairment, diabetes, osteoporosis, glaucoma, cataracts, peptic ulcer disease, untreated fungal, bacterial, or systemic viral infection, active or quiescent tuberculosis, ocular herpes simplex, recent nasal surgery or trauma, or septal ulcers (intranasal only).
- If change is made from systemic (oral) corticosteroids to inhaled or intranasal corticosteroids, observe patient carefully for signs of adrenal insufficiency (eg, nausea, fatigue, dizziness, hypotension, depression, or abdominal, joint, or muscle pain). Notify health care provider if these signs occur. Deaths caused by adrenal insufficiency have occurred during and after converting to aerosol corticosteroids.
- Assess patient's symptoms before initiating therapy and periodically during treatment. Notify health care provider if symptoms do not improve or worsen.

- Plot growth pattern in children on prolonged therapy. Inform health care provider if abnormalities are noted.
- Notify health care provider if oral, nasal, or pharyngeal irritation occurs.

Patient/Family Education
- Explain name, dose, action, and potential side effects of drug.
- Advise patient to read the *Patient Information* leaflet before starting therapy and again with each refill.
- Advise patient that dose may be changed periodically, depending on how well symptoms are controlled.
- Explain that effects of drug are not immediate. Benefit requires daily use as instructed and usually begins to occur within 1 or 2 days, but full benefit may take 1 to 2 wk, depending on the condition being treated and the dose and route of administration of medication being used.
- Caution patient not to decrease the dose or stop taking unless advised by health care provider.
- Caution patient not to increase dose if symptoms do not seem to be improving or are worsening and to notify health care provider.
- If patient is being converted from oral to inhaled or intranasal corticosteroids, review signs and symptoms of adrenal insufficiency, which may occur days or weeks after conversion is complete. Advise patient to carry Medi-Alert card indicating possible need of supplemental systemic corticosteroids during periods of stress or a severe asthma attack.
- Instruct diabetic patient to monitor blood glucose more frequently when drug is started or dose is changed and to inform health care provider of significant changes in readings.
- Advise patient to avoid exposure to chickenpox and measles and to seek medical advice immediately if exposed.
- Advise women to notify health care provider if pregnant, planning to become pregnant, or breastfeeding.
- Caution patient not to take any prescription or OTC medications, dietary supplements, or herbal preparations unless advised by health care provider.
- Advise patient that follow-up visits may be required to monitor therapy and to keep appointments.
- Instruct patient not to stop the medication once symptoms have been controlled. Continued daily use is necessary to control symptoms.

Inhalation Aerosol:
- Warn patient that drug is an asthma controller and is not to treat an acute asthma attack. Advise patient to use rescue medication (bronchodilator) to obtain rapid relief of asthma symptoms.
- Advise patient to discard the inhaler when labeled number of doses has been used.
- Instruct patient to carry Medi-Alert card if experiencing acute severe asthma attacks requiring rapid systemic treatment.
- Advise patient to report the following symptoms to health care provider: sore throat or mouth, cough, dry mouth, rash, facial swelling, worsening asthma symptoms (increasing need for bronchodilator).

Nasal Inhalation:
- Review proper administration technique. Have patient demonstrate technique to ensure effective use of the nasal spray.
- Instruct patient to use with caution if sores develop or injuries occur in nasal passages. Drug may prevent or slow proper healing.
- Advise patient to report the following symptoms to health care provider: sneezing, nasal irritation, nosebleed.
- Advise patient to discard bottle when labeled number of sprays has been used even if bottle is not completely empty.

Fluocinolone Acetonide

(floo-oh-SIN-oh-lone ah-SEE-toe-nide)

Class Corticosteroid/Topical

How Supplied
Synalar Cream 0.025%, Ointment 0.025%, Solution, topical 0.01%
✤ *Fluoderm*

Action
PHARMACOLOGY: High-potency topical corticosteroid that depresses formation, release, and activity of endogenous mediators of inflammation including prostaglandins, kinins, histamine, liposomal enzymes, and complement system; modifies body's immune response.

Indications Relief of the inflammatory and pruritic manifestations of corticosteroid-responsive dermatoses.

Contraindications Hypersensitivity to other corticosteroids; monotherapy in primary bacterial infections; ophthalmic use.

Route/Dosage
ADULTS: **Topical** Apply sparingly to affected areas 2 to 4 times/day.

Interactions None well documented.

Lab Test Interferences None well documented.

Adverse Reactions

DERM: Burning; itching; irritation; dryness; folliculitis; hypertrichosis; acneiform eruptions; hypopigmentation; perioral dermatitis; allergic contact dermatitis; maceration of the skin; secondary infection; skin atrophy; striae; miliaria.
EENT: Cataracts; glaucoma.
OTHER: Systemic absorption may produce reversible hypothalamic pituitary adrenal (HPA) axis suppression, manifestations of Cushing syndrome, hyperglycemia, and glycosuria.

Precautions

Pregnancy: Category C.
Lactation: Undetermined.
Children: May be more susceptible to topical corticosteroid-induced HPA axis suppression and Cushing syndrome; conditions that may augment systemic absorption include use over large body surface areas, prolonged use, and occlusive dressings.

Fluocinonide

(flew-oh-SIN-oh-nide)

Class Corticosteroid

How Supplied
Lidex Cream 0.05%, Gel 0.05%, Ointment 0.05%, Topical Solution 0.05% ♦ Lidex-E Cream 0.05%
❋ Tiamol ♦ Topsyn

Action

PHARMACOLOGY: Depresses formation, release, and activity of endogenous mediators of inflammation such as prostaglandins, kinins, histamine, liposomal enzymes, and complement system.

Indications Relief of inflammatory and pruritic manifestations of corticosteroid-responsive dermatoses.

Contraindications Standard considerations.

Route/Dosage
Apply to the affected area as a thin film 2 to 4 times/day depending on the severity of the condition.

Interactions None well documented.

Lab Test Interferences None well documented.

Adverse Reactions

DERM: Burning, itching, irritation, dryness, folliculitis, hypertrichosis, acneiform eruptions, hypopigmentation, perioral dermatitis, allergic contact dermatitis, maceration of the skin, skin atrophy, striae, miliaria; secondary infection

Precautions

Pregnancy: Category C.
Lactation: Unknown whether topical administration could result in sufficient systemic absorption to produce detectable quantities in human breast milk. Exercise caution when topical corticosteroids are administered to a nursing woman.
Children: May demonstrate greater susceptibility to topical corticosteroid-induced HPA axis suppression and Cushing syndrome.

Fluorometholone/ Sulfacetamide

(flure-oh-METH-oh-LONE/sull-fah-SEE-tah-mide)

Class Corticosteroid/Anti-inflammatory/Anti-infective

How Supplied
FML-S Ophthalmic Suspension 0.1% fluorometholone and 10% sodium sulfacetamide

Action

PHARMACOLOGY:
Fluorometholone: Depresses formation, release, and activity of endogenous mediators of inflammation as well as modifying body's immune response.
Sulfacetamide: Competitively antagonizes PABA, an essential component of folic acid synthesis.

Indications Treatment of steroid-responsive inflammatory ocular conditions for which a corticosteroid is indicated and where superficial bacterial ocular infection or a risk of bacterial ocular infection exists. Ocular steroids are indicated in inflammatory conditions of the palpebral and bulbar conjunctiva, cornea, and anterior segment of the globe, where the inherent risk of steroid use in certain infective conjunctivitides is accepted to obtain a diminution in edema and inflammation. They are also indicated in chronic anterior uveitis and corneal injury from chemical, radiation, or thermal burns or penetration of foreign bodies. Use of corticosteroids in combination with an anti-infective agent is indicated where the risk of superficial ocular infection is high or where there is an expectation that potentially dangerous numbers of bacteria will be present.

Contraindications Epithelial herpes simplex

keratitis (dendritic keratitis) and vaccinia; varicella, mycobacterial infection, and fungal diseases of the ocular structure; hypersensitivity to any component of this product.

Route/Dosage

ADULTS: **Topical** Instill 1 gtt into the conjunctival sac qid, taking care not to discontinue therapy prematurely.

Interactions None well documented.
INCOMPATIBILITIES: Silver preparations.

Lab Test Interferences None well documented.

Adverse Reactions

EENT: Local irritation; elevation in IOP with possible development of glaucoma; optic nerve damage; posterior subscapular cataract formation; delayed wound healing.
HEMA: Agranulocytosis; aplastic anemia and other blood dyscrasias.
HEPA: Fulminant hepatic necrosis.
OTHER: Allergic sensitization; Stevens-Johnson syndrome; toxic epidermal necrolysis; secondary infections (including fungal).

Precautions

Pregnancy: Category C.
Lactation: Undetermined; however, systemic hydrocortisone is excreted in breast milk.
Children: Safety and efficacy not established.
Hypersensitivity: Deaths associated with sulfonamide administration have been reported rarely from hypersensitivity reactions, Stevens-Johnson syndrome, toxic epidermal necrolysis, agranulocytosis, aplastic anemia, and other blood dyscrasias. Early indications of serious blood disorders include sore throat, fever, pallor, purpura, or jaundice.
Herpes simplex: Use corticosteroid with caution in patients with a history of herpes simplex.
Long-term use: Long-term use of topical corticosteroids may cause corneal and scleral thinning, possibly leading to perforation.
Ocular damage: Prolonged use may result in glaucoma with damage to the optic nerve, defects in visual acuity, fields of vision, and in posterior subcapsular cataract formation.
Secondary infection: Prolonged use may result in bacterial or fungal overgrowth of nonsusceptible microorganisms.
Sensitivity: May occur irrespective of the route of administration.

PATIENT CARE CONSIDERATIONS

Administration/Storage

- For ophthalmic use only. Not for use in the ears or on the skin.
- Do not use if suspension is dark brown.
- Shake well before instilling gtt.
- Instill 1 gtt into conjunctival sac(s) qid as prescribed.
- If using other topical ophthalmic medications, instill gtt first, wait at least 5 min, and instill ointment last.
- Store suspension at controlled room temperature (59° to 86°F). Keep bottle tightly capped and protect from freezing and light.

Assessment/Interventions

- Obtain patient history, including drug history and any known allergies. Note history of viral, mycobacterial, or fungal infection of the eye(s), and sensitivity to sulfonamides.
- Monitor patient's response to therapy. Notify health care provider if eye or eyelid inflammation is noted or if symptoms do not improve or worsen.
- Ensure that intraocular pressure is measured if therapy is continued beyond 10 days.

Patient/Family Education

- Explain name, dose, action, and potential side effects of drug.
- Review prescribed dosing schedule with patient, family, or caregiver.
- Remind patient, family, or caregiver that suspension is for use in the eye only.
- Teach patient, family, or caregiver proper technique for instilling suspension: wash hands; do not allow tip of dropper bottle to touch eye, eyelid, fingers, or any other surface. Tilt head back, look up; pull lower eyelid down to form pocket; place prescribed number of gtt in the pocket. Look downward before closing eye. Do not rub eye.
- Advise patient, family, or caregiver that if more than 1 topical ophthalmic drug is being used, instill eye gtt first, wait at least 5 min, and then instill ointment last.
- Inform patient that temporary blurred vision and stinging of the eye are the most common side effects and to contact health care provider if they occur and are bothersome.
- Advise patient to contact eye doctor if eye or eyelid inflammation is noted or if eye symptoms do not improve or worsen.
- Advise patient that the entire course of therapy must be completed to ensure maximal benefit and to complete full course of therapy even if symptoms have resolved.
- Instruct patient not to wear contact lenses during treatment.
- Remind patient, family, or caregiver that follow-up eye examinations may be necessary while using this medication and to keep appointments.

Fluorouracil

(FLURE-oh-YOUR-uh-sill)

Class Pyrimidine antimetabolite

How Supplied
Adrucil Injection 50 mg/mL ♦ *Carac* Cream 0.5%
♦ *Efudex* Cream 5%, Solution 2%, Solution 5%
♦ *Fluoroplex* Cream 1%, Solution 1%

Action

PHARMACOLOGY: The metabolism of fluorouracil in the anabolic pathway blocks the methylation reaction of deoxyuridylic acid to thymidylic acid. In this manner, fluorouracil interferes with the synthesis of DNA and to a lesser extent inhibits the formation of RNA.

PHARMACOKINETICS/DYNAMICS:

Distribution: Fluorouracil distributes into tumors, intestinal mucosa, bone marrow, liver, CSF, and brain tissue.

Metabolism: Metabolization takes place primarily in the liver; catabolic metabolism results in inactive degradation products.

Excretion: The parent drug is excreted unchanged (7% to 20%) in the urine in 6 hr. The mean $t_{½}$ is about 16 min (range, 8 to 20 min) and is dose dependent.

Indications Colon, rectum, breast, gastric, and pancreatic carcinoma (injection); multiple actinic or solar keratoses, superficial basal cell carcinoma (topical). **Unlabeled use(s):** Ovarian, cervical, bladder, hepatic, islet cell, prostate, endometrial, esophageal, and head and neck carcinoma.

Contraindications Poor nutritional status; depressed bone marrow function; potentially serious infections; hypersensitivity to fluorouracil or product components; pregnancy (topical); dihydropyrimidine dehydrogenase enzyme (DPD) deficiency (*Carac*).

Route/Dosage

Colon, Rectum, Breast, Gastric, and Pancreatic Carcinomas
ADULTS: **IV** Individualize dosage based on actual body weight. Use lean body weight if patient is obese or has abnormal fluid retention. Initial dose: 12 mg/kg/day for 4 days. Do not exceed 800 mg/day. If no toxicity is observed, give 6 mg/kg on days 6, 8, 10, and 12. No therapy is given on days 5, 7, 9, or 11. Discontinue at end of day 12, even with no apparent toxicity.

In poor risk patients and those with inadequate nutritional status: 6 mg/kg/day for 3 days. If no toxicity is observed, give 3 mg/kg on days 5, 7, and 9. Give no therapy on days 4, 6, or 8. Do not exceed 400 mg/day.

Maintenance therapy: Start maintenance therapy 30 days after the last dose. If no toxicity is observed with the first course of therapy, repeat that dose of fluorouracil at 30-day intervals. If toxicity is observed with the first course of therapy, after the patient has recovered from initial toxicity, use a single weekly dose of 10 to 15 mg/kg. Do not exceed a weekly maintenance dose of 1000 mg. Poor risk patients may require a reduced maintenance dose.

Multiple Actinic or Solar Keratoses
ADULTS: **Topical** Apply enough medication to cover affected areas bid for 2 to 6 wk. Complete healing may not occur until 1 to 2 mo after therapy is stopped. Continue medication until the inflammatory response reaches the erosion stage.

Carac: The 0.5% cream is only indicated for the face and anterior scalp areas. Using fingertips, apply qd to cover lesions with a thin film. Do not apply near eyes, nostrils, or mouth. Apply 10 min after thoroughly washing, rinsing, and drying the entire area. After application, wash hands thoroughly. Continued treatment up to 4 wk results in greater lesion reduction.

Superficial Basal Cell Carcinoma (5% Strength Only)
ADULTS: **Topical** Apply a sufficient amount to cover the lesions bid for 3 to 6 wk. Treatment may be required for 10 to 12 wk.

Interactions

Cimetidine: May increase serum concentrations of fluorouracil and potentially increase toxicity.
Leucovorin: Leucovorin may enhance GI toxicity of fluorouracil. Fatalities have occurred because of severe toxic enterocolitis.

Lab Test Interferences None well documented.

Adverse Reactions

CV:
Adrucil – Myocardial ischemia, angina.
CNS:
Adrucil – Acute cerebellar syndrome (may persist following discontinuation treatment); nystagmus; headache; disorientation; confusion; euphoria.
Carac – Headache (3%).
DERM:
Adrucil – Alopecia; dermatitis (pruritic maculopapular rash usually appearing on extremities and less frequently on the trunk); dry skin; fissuring; photosensitivity (erythema or increased pigmentation of the skin); vein pigmentation; palmar-plantar erythrodysesthesia syndrome (tingling of the hands and feet followed by pain, erythema, and swelling).
Carac – Application site reaction (95%); erythema (93%); dryness (83%); burning (75%); erosion, pain (44%); irritation (1%).

Efudex – Ulceration (most frequent); burning; crusting; allergic contact dermatitis; erosions; erythema; hyperpigmentation; irritation; pain; photosensitivity; pruritus; scarring; rash; soreness.
Fluoroplex – Pain; pruritus; burning; irritation; inflammation; allergic contact dermatitis; telangiectasia.
EENT:
Adrucil – Lacrimal duct stenosis; visual changes; lacrimation; photophobia.
Carac – Eye irritation (5%); sinusitis (2%).
GI:
Adrucil – Stomatitis; esophagopharyngitis (which may lead to sloughing and ulceration), diarrhea; anorexia; nausea; emesis (most common); GI ulceration; bleeding.
HEMA:
Adrucil – Leukopenia (lowest WBC counts most commonly seen between the 9th and 14th days after first course of treatment, maximal depression may be delayed for as long as 20 days, count usually returns to normal by the 30th day); pancytopenia; thrombocytopenia; agranulocytosis; anemia.
Efudex – Leukocytosis (frequent); eosinophilia; thrombocytopenia; toxic granulation (infrequent).
HYPERSEN:
Adrucil – Anaphylaxis; generalized allergic reactions.
OTHER:
Adrucil – Thrombophlebitis; epistaxis; mail changes (including loss of nails).
Carac – Edema (35%); common cold (2%); allergy (1%).
Efudex – Cases of miscarriage/birth defect (ventricular septal defect) when applied to mucous membranes.

> **WARNING:**
> Hospitalization recommended for first course of injection therapy because of the possibility of severe toxic reactions.

Precautions
Pregnancy: Category D (injection); Category X (topical).
Lactation: Undetermined.

Children: Safety and efficacy not established.
Hypersensitivity: The potential for delayed hypersensitivity exists (topical).
Special risk patients: Use with extreme caution in poor-risk patients who have had high-dose pelvic irradiation or previous use of alkylating agents, who have widespread involvement of bone marrow by metastatic tumors, or impaired hepatic or renal function.
Photosensitivity: Avoid exposure to UV rays because the intensity of the reaction may be increased.
Discontinue use: Discontinue if the following signs of toxicity occur: stomatitis or esophagopharyngitis (at first visible sign); rapidly falling WBC count; leukopenia (WBC less than 3500/mm^3); intractable vomiting; diarrhea or frequent bowel movements; GI ulceration and bleeding; thrombocytopenia (platelets less than 100,000/mm^3); hemorrhage.
DPD deficiency (Carac and Adrucil): Rarely, severe toxicity (eg, stomatitis, diarrhea, neutropenia, neurotoxicity) has been attributed to DPD deficiency.
Extravasation: Can cause local irritation or phlebitis. Refer to your institution-specific protocol.
Hand-foot syndrome (injection): May occur; characterized as a tingling sensation of hands and feet which progress over the next few days to pain when holding objects or walking. Interruption of therapy is followed by gradual resolution over 5 to 7 days.
Obese/Edematous patients: Base dose on body surface area in obese or edematous patients.
Topical use: Avoid application to mucous membranes because of possibility of local inflammation and ulceration. Occlusive dressing may increase the incidence of inflammatory reactions.
Toxicity: Severe toxicity, including hematologic, GI hemorrhage, and death, have occurred.

Overdosage: Signs and Symptoms
Nausea, vomiting, diarrhea, GI ulceration and bleeding, bone marrow depression (including thrombocytopenia, leukopenia, agranulocytosis).

PATIENT CARE CONSIDERATIONS

Administration/Storage
Injection:
- Follow institutional procedures for handling, administration, and disposal of anticancer drugs.
- Give IV; avoid extravasation. No dilution required.
- Do not administer if particulate matter or cloudiness is noted. Slight discoloration is normal and of no concern.
- Store injection at controlled room temperature (59° to 86°F). Protect from light. A precipitate may form if stored at low temperature but warming the injection to 140°F and shaking vigorously will resolubilize the medication.

Topical Solution and Creams:
- Do not apply 0.5% cream to areas other than face and anterior scalp.

- Avoid contact with eyes, nostrils, mouth, mucus membranes, and ulcerated or inflamed skin.
- Apply to affected areas bid using nonmetal applicator or suitable glove. If applied with fingers, wash hands immediately after applying.
- Do not cover with occlusive dressings. A porous gauze dressing may be applied for cosmetic reasons.
- Store topical solutions and creams at controlled room temperature (59° to 86°F). Protect from freezing.

Assessment/Interventions

- Obtain patient history, including drug history and any known allergies. Note liver or kidney impairment, pregnancy, DPD deficiency, malnutrition, depressed bone marrow function or widespread involvement of bone marrow by metastatic tumors, active infection, history of high-dose pelvic irradiation, or previous exposure to alkylating agents.
- Ensure that women are not pregnant, planning to become pregnant, or breastfeeding.
- To rule out the presence of a frank neoplasm, a biopsy should be made of those areas failing to respond to treatment or recurring after treatment.

Injection:

- Ensure that CBC with differential and platelet count is determined before starting therapy and before each dose during treatment. Discontinue therapy if WBC is less than 3500/mm^3 or platelet count is less than 100,000/mm^3.
- Monitor patient for development of hand-and-foot syndrome (eg, redness, swelling, numbness, discomfort of the hands and feet), stomatitis, nausea, vomiting, or bleeding. Inform health care provider if noted.
- Monitor patient for CNS, GI, DERM, and general body side effects. Report to health care provider if noted and significant.

Topical Cream or Solution:

- Assess and document skin condition and response to therapy.
- Monitor the inflammatory reaction and when it reaches the erosion, ulceration, and necrosis stages, drug should be terminated.

Patient/Family Education

- Explain name, dose, action, and potential side effects of drug.
- Caution women of childbearing potential to avoid becoming pregnant while being treated.
- Advise women to notify health care provider if pregnant, planning to become pregnant, or breastfeeding.
- Instruct patient not to take any prescription or OTC medications or dietary supplements unless advised by health care provider.
- Advise patient that follow-up visits will be required to monitor therapy and to keep appointments.

Injection:

- Advise patient that medication will usually be prepared and administered by a health care professional in a health care setting but that home administration may be possible in some situations.
- If administering at home, ensure that the patient or caregiver understands how to store, prepare, and administer the dose and dispose of used equipment and supplies.
- Advise patient to notify health care provider if any of the following occur: diarrhea with 4 to 6 stools per day or diarrhea at night; sores in the mouth; persistent vomiting; redness, swelling, and pain of the hands or feet; fever, chills, or other signs of infection.
- Advise patient that hair loss and skin reactions (dermatitis) occur frequently during treatment but that these effects are reversible once therapy has been discontinued.

Topical Solution and Cream:

- Teach patient or caregiver proper technique for applying solution or cream.
- Instruct patient, unless advised differently by health care provider, to apply bid until ulceration of application site occurs and then discontinue use of solution or cream.
- Advise patient or caregiver that response to therapy is slow and may take several weeks with complete healing taking up to 1 to 2 mo to occur following discontinuation of therapy.
- Advise patient or caregiver that most common side effects are application site reactions (eg, burning, swelling, irritation) and to inform health care provider if reaction occurs and is intolerable.
- Advise patient or caregiver that treated areas may be unsightly during therapy and for several weeks following therapy and that area may be covered with a gauze wrap for cosmetic reasons. Caution patient not to cover area with an occlusive wrap.
- Caution patient to avoid prolonged or unnecessary exposure to UV light (eg, sunlight, tanning booths) while under treatment with fluorouracil to prevent increasing intensity of skin reaction to medication.
- Instruct patient to avoid contact with eyes, nose, mouth, and mucus membranes, or inflamed skin.
- Instruct patient to wash hands immediately after applying topical medication.

Fluorescein Sodium/ Proparacaine Hydrochloride

(FLURE-eh-seen SO-dee-uhm /pro-PAR-ah-cane HIGH-droe-KLOR-ide)

Class Disclosing agent/Local anesthetic

How Supplied
Fluoracaine Solution 0.5% proparacaine hydrochloride and 0.25% fluorescein sodium

Action
PHARMACOLOGY:
Fluorescein: Diagnostic aid (corneal trauma indicator)
Proparacaine: Stabilizes neuronal membranes by inhibiting the ionic fluxes required for the initiation and conduction of impulses, thereby effecting local anesthetic action.

Indications Procedures requiring a disclosing agent in combination with an anesthetic agent (eg, tonometry, gonioscopy, removal of corneal foreign bodies and other short corneal or conjunctival procedures).

Contraindications Known hypersensitivity to any component of the product.

Route/Dosage
Removal of Foreign Bodies and Sutures and for Tonometry
ADULTS: **Topical** Single instillation of 1 to 2 drops in each eye before operating.
Deep Ophthalmic Anesthesia
ADULTS: **Topical** Instill 1 drop in each eye q 5 to 10 min for 5 to 7 doses.

Interactions None well documented.

Lab Test Interferences None well documented.

Adverse Reactions
CNS: Stimulation followed by depression.
EENT: Temporary stinging; burning; conjunctival redness; immediate-type hyperallergic corneal reaction (with acute, intense, and diffuse epithelial keratitis, gray, ground glass appearance, sloughing of large areas of necrotic epithelium corneal filaments and sometimes, iritis with descemetitis).
DERM: Allergic contact dermatitis (with drying and fissuring of the fingertips).

Precautions
Pregnancy: Category C.
Lactation: Undetermined.
Children: Safety and efficacy not established.
Special risk patients: Use with caution in patients with known allergies, cardiac disease, or hyperthyroidism.
Prolonged use: Not recommended; may cause permanent corneal opacification with visual loss and delay wound healing.

PATIENT CARE CONSIDERATIONS

Administration/Storage

- For ophthalmic use only. Not for use in the ears or on the skin.
- Instill 1 to 2 drops into affected eye(s) before procedure. May repeat 1 drop q 5 to 10 min for deep ophthalmic anesthesia.
- Do not allow tip of eye dropper to touch eye, eyelid, fingers or any other surface.
- If using other topical ophthalmic medications, instill drops first, wait at least 5 min and instill ointment last.
- Store solution in refrigerator (36° to 46°F). Keep bottle tightly capped and protect from light.

Assessment/Interventions

- Obtain patient history, including drug history and any known allergies. Note history of coronary artery disease or hyperthyroidism.
- Ensure that patient's eye(s) are protected from irritating chemicals, foreign bodies, and rubbing during the period of anesthesia. An eye patch is recommended for this protection.
- Monitor patient's response to therapy. Notify health care provider if eye or eyelid irritation or inflammation is noted.

Patient/Family Education

- Explain name, dose, action, and potential side effects of drug.
- Advise patient that medication will be prepared and administered by a health care professional in a medical setting to obtain short-term anesthesia of the eye(s).
- Caution patient to avoid rubbing or touching the eye(s) until the anesthesia has worn off.
- Inform patient that temporary blurred vision, stinging or burning, or redness of the eye are the most common side effects and to contact their health care provider if they occur and are bothersome.
- Advise patient that follow-up visits and eye examinations may be necessary following therapy and to be sure and keep appointments.

Fluoxetine Hydrochloride

(flew-OX-uh-teen HIGH-droe-KLOR-ide)http://www.fda.gov/medwatch/SAFETY/2004/safety04.htm#antidepressants

Class Antidepressant

How Supplied
Prozac Tablets 10 mg, Pulvules 10 mg, Pulvules 20 mg, Solution, oral 20 mg/5 mL ♦ *Prozac Weekly* Capsules, delayed-release 90 mg ♦ *Sarafem* Pulvules 10 mg, Pulvules 20 mg ♣ *Apo-Fluoxetine* ♦ *CO Fluoxetine* ♦ *Gen-Fluoxetine* ♦ *Novo-Fluoxetine* ♦ *Nu-Fluoxetine* ♦ *PMS-Fluoxetine* ♦ *ratio-Fluoxetine* ♦ *Rhoxal-fluoxetine* ♦ *STCC-Fluoxetine*

Action
PHARMACOLOGY: Blocks reuptake of serotonin, enhancing serotonergic function.

PHARMACOKINETICS/DYNAMICS:
Absorption: T_{max} is 6 to 8 hr; C_{max} is 15 to 55 ng/mL. Bioavailability is 94%.

Distribution: Protein binding is about 94.5%.

Metabolism: The major metabolite is norfluoxetine (active) formed by demethylation. The primary route is hepatic.

Excretion: The t½ is 1 to 384 hr (including active metabolite). The primary route is renal excretion of inactive metabolites.

Special Populations:
Hepatic Function Impairment – The t½ is prolonged for fluoxetine and norfluoxetine. Use a lower or less frequent dose in these patients.

Indications
Prozac: Depression as defined in the DSM-IV; obsessive-compulsive disorder (OCD) as defined in the DSM-III-R; bulimia nervosa, panic disorder as defined in the DSM-III-R.
Sarafem: Premenstrual dysphoric disorder (PMDD). **Unlabeled use(s):** Alcoholism; anorexia nervosa; attention deficit hyperactivity disorder; bipolar II disorder; borderline personality disorder; chronic rheumatoid pain; diabetic peripheral neuropathy; kleptomania; levodopa-induced dyskinesia; migraine, chronic daily headaches, and tension-type headache; narcolepsy; schizophrenia; social phobia; trichotillomania.

Contraindications
Concurrent use with, or within 14 days of discontinuation of, MAO inhibitors.

Route/Dosage
PROZAC
Depression
ADULTS: **PO** 20 to 80 mg/day. Weekly dosing (90 mg delayed-release capsule) may be started 7 days after last 20 mg/day dose. If response is not satisfactory, consider reestablishing daily dosage regimen.
CHILDREN 8 TO 18 YR: **PO** Start with 10 or 20 mg/day. After 1 wk at 10 mg/day, increase the dose to 20 mg/day. In lower-weight children, a starting and target dose may be 10 mg/day. A dose increase to 20 mg/day may be considered after several weeks if insufficient clinical improvement is observed.

OCD
ADULTS: **PO** 20 to 80 mg/day.
CHILDREN 8 TO 18 YR: **PO** Start with 10 mg/day. After 2 wk, increase the dose to 20 mg/day. Additional dose increases may be considered after several more weeks if insufficient clinical improvement is observed (dose range, 20 to 60 mg/day).

Bulimia Nervosa
PO 60 mg/day administered in morning.

Panic Disorder
ADULTS: **PO** Start with 10 mg/day. After 1 wk, increase the dose to 20 mg/day. A dose increase may be considered after several weeks if no clinical improvement is observed. Doses above 60 mg/day have not been systematically evaluated.

SARAFEM
PMDD
ADULTS: **PO** 20 mg/day every day of menstrual cycle or daily starting 14 days prior to anticipated onset of menstruation through the first full day of menses and repeating for each new cycle (max dose, 80 mg/day).

Interactions
5-HT$_1$ agonists (eg, naratriptan, rizatriptan, sumatriptan, zolmitriptan): Weakness, hyperreflexia, and incoordination have been reported rarely.
Benzodiazepines: Coadministration of alprazolam and fluoxetine has resulted in increased alprazolam levels and decreased psychomotor performance. Half the initial alprazolam dose and titrate to lowest effective dose.
Beta Blockers: Excessive beta blockade (bradycardia) may occur with certain beta blockers (eg, carvedilol, metoprolol, propranolol).
Buspirone: Effects of buspirone may be decreased.
Carbamazepine: Increased carbamazepine levels, causing toxicity.
Clozapine: Elevated serum clozapine levels have occurred. Closely monitor patients on coadministration.
Cyclosporine: Concentrations of cyclosporine may be elevated, increasing the risk of toxicity.
Cyproheptadine: Decreased or reversed effects of fluoxetine.
Haloperidol: Serum concentrations of haloperi-

dol may be increased; recall memory and attentional function tests may be delayed.
Hydantoins (eg, phenytoin): Increased hydantoin levels, causing toxicity.
Lithium: Lithium levels may be increased or decreased by fluoxetine with possible neurotoxicity and increased serotonergic effects.
MAO Inhibitors: Combination may lead to serious, possibly fatal, reactions. Discontinue MAO inhibitor at least 14 days before starting fluoxetine; discontinue fluoxetine at least 5 wk before starting MAO inhibitor.
Sympathomimetics (eg, amphetamine): Sensitivity of sympathomimetics and risk of "serotonin syndrome" may be increased.
Tricyclic antidepressants: Increased toxic effects of tricyclic antidepressant.

Lab Test Interferences None well documented.

Adverse Reactions
CV: Hot flashes; palpitations; angina; heart block; cerebral ischemia; MI; ventricular arrhythmias.
CNS: Agitation; anxiety; nervousness; headache; insomnia; abnormal dreams; drowsiness; dizziness; tremor; fatigue; decreased libido; decreased concentration; seizures; delusions; hallucinations; coma.
DERM: Increased sweating; rash; itching; erythema multiforme.
EENT: Visual disturbances.
GI: Nausea; vomiting; diarrhea; dry mouth; anorexia; upset stomach; constipation; abdominal pain; change in taste.
GU: Painful menstruation; sexual dysfunction (decreased libido); frequent micturition; urinary tract infection.
HEMA: Blood dyscrasias; leukopenia; petechiae; purpura; altered platelet function.
METAB: Weight loss; hypoglycemia; hyponatremia.
RESP: Flu-like symptoms; bronchitis; rhinitis; yawning; coughing; asthma; pneumonia; apnea; lung edema; pleural effusion.
OTHER: Weakness; chills; joint or muscle pain; fever; hypersensitivity reaction.

Precautions
Pregnancy: Category C.
Lactation: Excreted in breast milk.
Children: Safety and efficacy not established.
Renal function impairment: Use with caution. A lower or less-frequent dosing schedule may be required.
Hepatic function impairment: Use with caution. A lower or less-frequent dosing schedule may be required.
Anorexia: Weight loss and decreased appetite are more likely to occur with fluoxetine than with tricyclic antidepressants.
Diabetes mellitus: May alter glycemic control. Insulin dosing may need adjustment.
Dose changes: The long elimination half-life of fluoxetine means that changes in dose will not be fully reflected in plasma for several weeks, affecting titration to final dose and withdrawal from treatment.
Mania/Hypomania: Fluoxetine may precipitate mania/hypomania in susceptible patients.
Seizures: Use with caution in patients with a history of seizures.
Suicide: Supervise depressed patients at risk during initial drug therapy.

Overdosage: Signs and Symptoms
Nausea, vomiting, agitation, restlessness, hypomania, seizures.

PATIENT CARE CONSIDERATIONS

Administration/Storage
- Administer oral medication with food to minimize GI upset.
- Ensure that patient swallows capsule to avoid hoarding for suicide attempt.
- Capsules may be emptied and mixed with food or juice if patient has difficulty swallowing.
- Administer medication at least 6 hr before bedtime to prevent insomnia. Morning and early afternoon administration is advised.
- Store at room temperature. Avoid heat and moisture.

Assessment/Interventions
- Obtain patient history, including drug history and any known allergies. Note recent use of MAO inhibitors or history of drug or alcohol abuse.
- Assess vital signs and weight before beginning therapy and at regular intervals thereafter.
- Assess mental status, mood changes, affect, and suicidal tendencies daily.
- In patients with diabetes, monitor blood glucose levels before beginning and periodically during therapy.
- Assess for the following symptoms of blood dyscrasias: fever, sore throat, malaise, unusual bleeding, excessive bruising.
- Determine whether suicide precautions are advisable and implement them as necessary.
- Assist patient to ambulate and change positions to prevent postural hypotension.
- Weigh patient several times/week on same scale at same time of day.
- Monitor I&O and evaluate bowel elimination.

Sarafem:
- Reassess periodically to determine need for continued treatment.

Patient/Family Education
- Instruct patient not to skip or double up on doses. Advise patient not to change dose except as directed by health care provider.
- Explain that improvement in mood and functioning may not be noted for several weeks after initiation of drug therapy. Discuss fact that dosage may be increased or decreased by health care provider in effort to achieve optimal outcome.
- Instruct patient to avoid taking medication within 6 hr of bedtime as it may cause insomnia.
- Tell patient that doses over 20 mg can be taken as single dose or split into morning and noontime doses.
- Advise patient to take sips of water frequently, suck on ice chips or sugarless hard candy, or chew sugarless gum if dry mouth occurs.
- Instruct patient to avoid sudden position changes to prevent orthostatic hypotension.
- Advise patients with diabetes that drug may cause loss of glycemic control.
- Instruct patient to report the following symptoms to health care provider: fever, malaise, unusual bleeding, excessive bruising, sore throat, persistent nausea or vomiting, severe headache, tachycardia, severe anorexia, weight loss.
- Advise patient to avoid caffeine, as this may increase stimulant effect of drug.
- Advise patient to avoid intake of alcoholic beverages or other CNS depressants (eg, analgesics, sedatives, antihistamines).
- Warn patient that drug may cause drowsiness and to use caution while driving or performing other tasks requiring mental alertness.
- Instruct patient not to take OTC medications without consulting health care provider.
- Advise patient to carry Medi-Alert information at all times describing medications being taken.

Fluoxymesterone

(flew-ox-ee-MESS-teh-rone)

Class Androgen

How Supplied
Fluoxymesterone Tablets 10 mg

Action

PHARMACOLOGY: Promotes growth and development of male reproductive organs, maintains secondary sex characteristics, increases protein anabolism, and decreases protein catabolism.

Indications Replacement therapy in conditions associated with symptoms of deficiency or absence of endogenous testosterone; delayed puberty (men); palliation of androgen-responsive recurrent mammary cancer in women who are more than 1 yr but less than 5 yr postmenopausal (women).

Contraindications Men with carcinoma of the breast; men with known or suspected carcinoma of the prostate gland; women known or suspected to be pregnant; patients with serious cardiac, hepatic, or renal disease; hypersensitivity to any component of the product.

Route/Dosage

Delayed Puberty (Men)
ADULTS: PO Titrate dose utilizing a low dose, appropriate skeletal monitoring, and by limiting the duration of therapy to 4 to 6 mo.

Inoperable Carcinoma of the Breast (Women)
ADULTS: PO 10 to 40 mg/day, in divided doses, for palliative therapy.

Male Hypogonadism
ADULTS: PO 5 to 20 mg/day, for complete replacement.

Interactions

Insulin: Blood glucose levels may be reduced by fluoxymesterone, decreasing insulin requirements.

Oral anticoagulants (eg, warfarin): Effects of oral anticoagulant may be increased. Dosage reduction may be required.

Lab Test Interferences Thyroxine-binding globulin levels may be decreased; however, thyroid hormone levels remain unchanged and there is no clinical evidence of thyroid dysfunction.

Adverse Reactions

CNS: Increased or decreased libido; headache; anxiety; depression; generalized paresthesia.
DERM: Hirsutism; male pattern baldness; seborrhea; acne.
GI: Nausea.
GU: Amenorrhea and other menstrual irregularities, inhibition of gonadotropin secretion, virilization including deepening of voice, clitoral enlargement (women); gynecomastia, excessive frequency and duration of penile erection, oligospermia (men).
HEMA: Suppression of clotting factors II, V, VII, and X; polycythemia.
HEPA: Cholestatic jaundice; altered LFTs; hepatocellular neoplasms, peliosis hepatitis.
METAB: Sodium, chloride, water, potassium, calcium, and inorganic phosphate retention.
OTHER: Allergic hypersensitivity (including

skin manifestations and anaphylactoid reactions).

Precautions

Pregnancy: Category X.

Lactation: Undetermined.

Children: Use with caution and only by specialists aware of the adverse effects on bone maturation.

Elderly: Elderly men may be at increased risk of developing prostatic hypertrophy or carcinoma.

Athletic performance: Abuse of this agent to enhance athletic performance has potential risk of serious side effects.

Breast cancer and immobilized patients: May cause hypercalcemia.

Delayed puberty: Because bone maturation without compensatory linear growth can occur, use with caution in males with delayed puberty.

Edema: Use with caution in patients with conditions that might be affected by fluid retention (eg, renal, hepatic, or cardiac disease).

Gynecomastia: May occur and persist in patients being treated for hypogonadism.

Hepatic effects: Cholestatic hepatitis and jaundice may occur. Prolonged use of high doses may result in hepatic adenomas, hepatocellular carcinoma, and peliosis hepatitis.

Oligospermia and reduced ejaculatory volume: May occur after prolonged use or excessive dosage.

Priapism: May be indicative of excessive dosage.

Urethral obstruction: May develop in patients with benign prostatic hypertrophy.

Virilization: May occur in women using high-dose androgens.

PATIENT CARE CONSIDERATIONS

Administration/Storage

- Dose will vary depending on the individual, the condition being treated, and its severity.
- Administer prescribed dose without regard to meals. Administer with food if GI upset occurs.
- Store tablets at controlled room temperature (68° to 77°F).

Assessment/Interventions

- Obtain patient history, including drug history and any known allergies. Note renal or hepatic impairment, cardiac disease, prostatic hypertrophy, known or suspected carcinoma of prostate gland, breast carcinoma in men, known or suspected pregnancy, or tartrazine sensitivity.
- Ensure that women are not pregnant, planning to become pregnant, or breastfeeding.
- Ensure that liver enzymes, lipid profile, and hemoglobin and hematocrit levels are determined before starting and periodically during treatment.
- Ensure that serum and urinary calcium levels are frequently determined in women being treated for disseminated breast cancer.
- Ensure that prostate-specific antigen is determined in men before starting and periodically during treatment.
- Ensure that X-ray examinations of bone age are made q 6 mo during treatment of prepubertal male.
- Monitor blood sugar in diabetic patient when drug is started or dose is changed. Report significant changes to health care provider.
- Assess patient for GU, GI, CNS, DERM, and general body side effects. Report to health care provider if noted and significant. Immediately report hoarseness, deepening of voice, increase in facial hair, acne, or menstrual irregularities in women, and too frequent or persistent erections in men.
- Ensure that therapy is periodically reviewed to determine if therapy needs to be continued without change or if a dose change (eg, increase, decrease, discontinuation) is indicated.

Patient/Family Education

- Explain name, dose, action, and potential side effects of drug.
- Instruct patient, family, or caregiver to take (give) exactly as prescribed and to not change the dose or discontinue therapy unless advised by health care provider.
- Advise patient, family, or caregiver that each dose may be taken without regard to meals but to take with food if stomach upset occurs.
- Instruct patient, family, or caregiver that if a dose is missed to skip that dose and not to double the next dose.
- Advise patient that medication does not enhance athletic performance and not to use for this purpose because of potential serious adverse health risks.
- Instruct diabetic patient to monitor blood glucose more frequently when drug is started or dose is changed and to inform health care provider of significant changes in readings.
- Instruct patient, family, or caregiver to discontinue therapy and immediately contact health care provider if any of the following occur: persistent nausea or vomiting, yellowing of skin or eyes, swelling of feet or ankles.
- Instruct men to report too frequent or persistent erections to health care provider.
- Instruct women to report hoarseness, acne, changes in menstrual periods, or increase in

facial hair to health care provider.
- Caution women of childbearing potential to avoid becoming pregnant while being treated.
- Advise women to notify health care provider if pregnant, planning to become pregnant, or breastfeeding.
- Advise patient, family, or caregiver not to take (give) any prescription or OTC medications or dietary supplements unless advised by health care provider.
- Advise patient, family, or caregiver that laboratory tests and follow-up visits will be required to monitor therapy and to keep appointments.

Fluphenazine

(flew-FEN-uh-zeen)

Class Antipsychotic/Phenothiazine

How Supplied

Fluphenazine Hydrochloride
Fluphenazine Hydrochloride Tablets 1 mg, Tablets 2.5 mg, Tablets 5 mg, Tablets 10 mg
✤ Apo-Fluphenazine ◆ Fluphenazine Omega ◆ Moditen Hydrochloride

Fluphenazine Decanoate
Prolixin Decanoate Injection 25 mg/mL
✤ Apo-Fluphenazine Decanoate Injection ◆ Modecate ◆ Modecate Concentrate ◆ PMS-Fluphenazine Decanoate

Action

PHARMACOLOGY: Blocks dopamine receptor in CNS.

PHARMACOKINETICS/DYNAMICS:
Absorption: T_{max} is 24 to 72 hr (decanoate).
Metabolism: Primary site is the liver.
Excretion: The $t_{½}$ is 6.8 to 9.6 days (single dose of decanoate).
Onset: 24 to 72 hr (decanoate).
Duration: At least 4 wk (decanoate).

Indications

Fluphenazine hydrochloride: Management of psychotic disorders.
Fluphenazine decanoate: Long-acting parenteral depot products for long-term antipsychotic therapy. **Unlabeled use(s):** Nausea/vomiting.

Contraindications
Allergy to any phenothiazine; comatose or severely depressed states; concurrent use of large doses of other CNS depressants; bone marrow depression or blood dyscrasias; liver damage; cerebral arteriosclerosis; coronary artery disease; severe hypotension or hypertension; subcortical brain damage.

Route/Dosage

FLUPHENAZINE HYDROCHLORIDE
ADULTS: **PO** Initially, 2.5 to 10 mg/day in divided doses at 6 to 8 hr intervals. When symptoms are controlled, gradually reduce dosage to 1 to 5 mg/day.

FLUPHENAZINE DECANOATE
ADULTS: **IM/SC**
Initial dose: 12.5 to 25 mg. Do not exceed 100 mg/dose.
Usual dosing interval: 1 to 4 wk and as long as 6 wk in some patients.

Interactions
Alcohol and other CNS depressants: Increased CNS depression; may precipitate extrapyramidal reaction.
Anticholinergics: Reduced therapeutic effects and increased anticholinergic side effects of fluphenazine; may lead to tardive dyskinesia.
Barbiturate anesthetics: Increased frequency and severity of neuromuscular excitation and hypotension.
Beta-blockers: Increased plasma levels of both drugs.
Bromocriptine: Effectiveness of bromocriptine may be reduced.
Cisapride, sparfloxacin: The risk of life-threatening cardiac arrhythmias, including torsades de pointes, may be increased.
Guanethidine: Hypotensive action may be inhibited.
Hydantoins (eg, phenytoin): Increase or decrease in phenytoin levels.
Lithium: May result in disorientation, unconsciousness, and extrapyramidal symptoms.
Metrizamide: Increased seizure risk.
Paroxetine: Plasma levels of fluphenazine may be elevated, increasing the risk of side effects.

Lab Test Interferences
False-positive pregnancy tests may occur but are less likely with serum test. Increases in protein-bound iodine have been reported. Increased cephalin flocculation accompanied by altered LFTs has been reported with fluphenazine enanthate. Pink to red-brown urine discoloration.

Adverse Reactions
CV: Orthostatic hypotension; hypertension; tachycardia; bradycardia; syncope; cardiac arrest; circulatory collapse; ECG changes; arrhythmias; CHF.
CNS: Pseudoparkinsonism; dyskinesia; motor restlessness; oculogyric crises; opisthotonos; hyperreflexia; tardive dyskinesia; headache;

weakness; tremor; fatigue; slurring; insomnia; vertigo; seizures; drowsiness; hallucinations; lethargy; increased libido; lightheadedness; faintness; dizziness.

DERM: Photosensitivity; skin pigmentation; dry skin; exfoliative dermatitis; urticarial rash; maculopapular hypersensitivity reaction; seborrhea; eczema; jaundice; perspiration; erythema.

EENT: Pigmentary retinopathy; glaucoma; photophobia; blurred vision; miosis; mydriasis; increased IOP; dry mouth or throat; nasal congestion.

GI: Nausea; dyspepsia; constipation; salivation; fecal impaction; paralytic ileus; adynamic ileus (may result in death).

GU: Menstrual irregularities; urinary hesitancy and retention; impotence; sexual dysfunction; bladder paralysis; abnormal lactation; dysmenorrhea; breast enlargement; galactorrhea.

HEMA: Agranulocytosis; eosinophilia; leukopenia; hemolytic anemia; thrombocytopenic purpura; nonthrombocytopenic purpura; pancytopenia.

HEPA: Jaundice.

METAB: Decreased cholesterol; weight change.

RESP: Laryngospasm; bronchospasm; dyspnea; acute fulminating pneumonia or pneumonitis.

OTHER: Increases in appetite and weight; polydipsia; increased prolactin levels; neuroleptic malignant syndrome; loss of appetite; peripheral edema; sudden unexpected and unexplained death.

Precautions

Pregnancy: Pregnancy category undetermined.
Lactation: Undetermined.
Children: Not recommended in children younger than 12 yr.
Elderly: More susceptible to effects; consider reduced dose.
Special risk patients: Use with caution in patients with CV disease or mitral insufficiency, pheochromocytoma, history of glaucoma, EEG abnormalities or seizure disorders, prior brain damage, hepatic or renal impairment, and patients exposed to extreme heat or phosphorous insecticides.

Abrupt withdrawal: Although this drug is not known to cause psychological or physical dependence, abrupt discontinuation of high-dose therapy has been associated with withdrawal symptoms (eg, nausea, vomiting, dizziness, headache, insomnia, tremulousness).

Adolescents: More susceptible to effects; consider reduced dose.

Debilitated patients: More susceptible to effects; consider reduced dose.

Hepatic effects: Jaundice usually occurs between 2nd and 4th weeks of treatment; considered hypersensitivity reaction. Usually reversible.

Neuroleptic malignant syndrome: Potentially fatal condition that has occurred, most often with fluphenazine decanoate. Signs and symptoms include hyperpyrexia, muscle rigidity, altered mental status, irregular pulse, fluctuating BP, tachycardia, and diaphoresis.

Pulmonary effects: Cases of bronchopneumonia, some fatal, have occurred.

Sudden death: Has been reported; predisposing factors may be seizures or previous brain damage. Flare-up of psychotic behavior may precede death.

Tardive dyskinesia: Syndrome of potentially irreversible, involuntary body and facial movements may develop. Prevalence highest in elderly, especially women. Use smallest effective doses for shortest possible time period.

Overdosage: Signs and Symptoms

Somnolence, coma, extrapyramidal symptoms, cardiac arrhythmias, fever, hypotension, seizures.

PATIENT CARE CONSIDERATIONS

Administration/Storage

- Dose and frequency of administration are variable, depending on condition being treated.
- Administer tablets as prescribed, without regard to meals. Administer with food if GI upset occurs.
- Injection is for IM or SC administration only. Not for intradermal or IV administration.
- Use dry syringe and needle to withdraw and administer IM or SC dose.
- Do not administer injection if particulate matter or marked discoloration is noted.
- Store tablets and injection at controlled room temperature (59° to 86°F). Protect from light. Do not freeze injection.

Assessment/Interventions

- Obtain patient history, including drug history and any known allergies. Note allergy to fluphenazine or other phenothiazines, previous episode of jaundice with phenothiazine therapy, bone marrow depression or blood dyscrasias, hepatic impairment, ischemic heart disease, cerebrovascular disease, narrow-angle glaucoma, epilepsy, mitral insufficiency, pheochromocytoma, prostatic hypertrophy, condition predisposing to hypotension (eg, dehydration, hypovolemia), concomitant use of antihypertensive drugs, or previous episodes of neuroleptic malignant syndrome.
- Ensure that medication is discontinued at least 48 hr before myelography and not

resumed until at least 24 hr after procedure to reduce chance of seizures occurring.
- Frequently assess patient for response to treatment. Notify health care provider if condition being treated is not improving or is worsening.
- Ensure that therapy is periodically reviewed to determine if it needs to be continued without change or if a dose change (eg, increase, decrease, discontinuation) is indicated.
- Avoid sudden discontinuation of therapy if possible. Attempt to gradually reduce dose if decision to discontinue medication is made.
- Inform health care provider immediately if hyperpyrexia, muscle rigidity, altered mental status, irregular pulse and BP, tachycardia, or diaphoresis develop.
- Notify health care provider immediately if palpitations or syncope occur.
- Assess neurologic status before and during treatment. Observe for involuntary body and facial movements, excessive drowsiness, agitation, tremor, or anxiety. Inform health care provider if noted.
- Monitor patient for CNS, CV, GI, GU, psychiatric, musculoskeletal, and general body side effects. Inform health care provider if noted and significant.
- Assess medication compliance.

Patient/Family Education
- Explain name, dose, action, and potential side effects of drug.
- Advise patient, family, or caregiver that dose will be adjusted periodically until maximum benefit has been obtained.
- Advise patient, family, or caregiver not to change the dose or stop taking unless advised by health care provider.
- Instruct patient not to stop taking fluphenazine when feeling better.
- Instruct patient, family, or caregiver to immediately report fainting or loss of consciousness, palpitations, dizziness, high fever, muscle rigidity, altered mental status, irregular pulse, or yellowing of the skin or eyes.
- Advise patient, family, or caregiver to notify health care provider of the following: excessive drowsiness, increased agitation or anxiety, involuntary body or facial movements.
- Advise patient to avoid strenuous activity during periods of high temperature or humidity.
- Instruct patient to avoid alcoholic beverages and other depressants while taking this medication.
- Instruct patient to get up slowly from a lying or sitting position and to avoid sudden position changes to prevent postural hypotension. Advise patient to report dizziness with position changes to health care provider. Caution patient that hot tubs and hot showers or baths may make dizziness worse.
- Advise patient to take sips of water, suck on ice chips or sugarless hard candy, or chew sugarless gum if dry mouth occurs.
- Advise patient that drug may cause drowsiness and impaired judgment or thinking skills and to use caution while driving or performing other tasks requiring mental alertness until tolerance is determined.
- Caution patient that medication may cause sensitivity to sunlight and to avoid unnecessary exposure to UV light (sunlight, tanning booths), use sunscreen, and wear protective clothing when exposed to UV light until tolerance is determined.
- Advise women to notify health care provider if pregnant, planning to become pregnant, or breastfeeding.
- Instruct patient not to take any prescription or OTC medications or dietary supplements unless advised by health care provider.
- Advise patient that follow-up visits may be required to monitor therapy and to keep appointments.

Flurazepam Hydrochloride
(flure-AZE-uh-pam HIGH-droe-KLOR-ide)
Class Sedative and hypnotic/Benzodiazepine
How Supplied
Dalmane Capsules 15 mg, Capsules 30 mg
♣ *Apo-Flurazepam* ♦ *Novo- Flupam*
Action
PHARMACOLOGY: Potentiates action of gamma-aminobutyric acid, an inhibitory neurotransmitter, resulting in increased neural inhibition and CNS depression, especially in limbic system and reticular formation.

PHARMACOKINETICS/DYNAMICS:
Absorption: T_{max} is 0.5 to 1 hr (parent) and 7.6 to 13.6 hr (active metabolite). It is rapidly and completely absorbed.

Distribution: Protein binding is 97%. Flurazepam crosses the placenta and is secreted into breast milk. It has a high lipid:water distribution coefficient in the nonionized form.

Metabolism: The major metabolite is N-desalkylflurazepam (active).

Excretion: The t½ is 2 to 3 hr and 47 to 100 hr for the active metabolite. Less than 1% is excreted unchanged in the urine.

FLURAZEPAM HYDROCHLORIDE

Indications Treatment of insomnia.
Contraindications Hypersensitivity to benzodiazepines; pregnancy.

Route/Dosage
ADULTS: PO 15 to 30 mg at bedtime.
ELDERLY: PO 15 mg until individual response is determined.
DEBILITATED PATIENTS: PO 15 mg until individual response is determined.

Interactions
Alcohol, other CNS depressants: Additive CNS depressant effects; may continue several days after discontinuation.
Cimetidine, disulfiram, oral contraceptives, isoniazid, omeprazole: Increased effects of flurazepam.
Digoxin: Serum digoxin concentrations may increase.
Phenytoin: Serum concentrations may be increased.
Rifampin: Decreased effects of flurazepam.
Theophyllines: May antagonize sedative effects.

Lab Test Interferences None well documented.

Adverse Reactions
CV: Palpitations; chest pains; tachycardia; hypotension (rare).
CNS: Dizziness; drowsiness; lightheadedness; staggering; ataxia; falling; lethargy; confusion; impaired memory; headache; weakness; paradoxical excitement; talkativeness; euphoria; apprehension; irritability; hallucinations; slurred speech; depression.
DERM: Pruritus; rash.
EENT: Difficulty focusing; blurred vision; burning of eyes; taste alterations.
GI: Heartburn; nausea and vomiting; diarrhea; constipation; anorexia; upset stomach; GI pain; dry mouth.
GU: Urinary incontinence; urinary retention, hesitancy, or urgency.
HEMA: Leukopenia; granulocytopenia.
HEPA: Elevated AST, ALT, bilirubin and alkaline phosphatase; hepatitis.
RESP: Shortness of breath.
OTHER: Tolerance; physical and psychological dependence; body and joint pains; sweating; flushing.

Precautions
Pregnancy: Contraindicated.
Lactation: Excreted in breast milk.
Children: Not recommended in children less than 15 yr.
Elderly: Increased side effects; start with lowest dose.
Renal function impairment: Use with caution. Abnormal LFTs and blood dyscrasias have occurred.
Hepatic function impairment: Use with caution. Abnormal LFTs and blood dyscrasias have occurred.
Debilitated patients: Increased side effects; start with lowest dose.
Anterograde amnesia: Has occurred with similar drugs. Alcohol may increase risk.
Depression: Administer with caution to severely depressed patients or those with suicidal tendencies. Signs and symptoms of depression may be intensified.
Withdrawal: Withdrawal symptoms may occur after discontinuation of higher doses taken over long periods.

Overdosage: Signs and Symptoms
Somnolence, confusion, respiratory depression, apnea, hypotension, impaired coordination, slurred speech, seizures, coma.

PATIENT CARE CONSIDERATIONS

Administration/Storage
- Administer at bedtime with fluid.
- Store at room temperature in light-resistant container.

Assessment/Interventions
- Obtain patient history, including drug history and any known allergies.
- Perform baseline neuro assessment and reassess with initiation of drug.
- Ensure that side rails are raised after administration.
- Assist patient with ambulation after drug administration.
- Assess vision before beginning drug therapy and monitor during initial treatment period.
- Ensure that baseline CBC, LFTs, and kidney function tests have been obtained before beginning therapy, and monitor at regular intervals.
- Assess for signs of bleeding (eg, petechiae, bruising, oozing at puncture sites).
- Assess for right upper quadrant abdominal tenderness or jaundice.

Patient/Family Education
- Caution patient that this medication must not be taken during pregnancy or when pregnancy is possible. Advise patient to use reliable form of birth control while taking this drug.
- Tell patient to take drug with full glass of water at bedtime.
- Emphasize importance of not exceeding recommended dosage. If symptoms do not improve within 2 to 3 days of beginning drug

therapy, or if tolerance develops, notify health care provider.
- Tell patient not to stop taking drug abruptly to avoid withdrawal symptoms. Explain that nighttime sleep may be disturbed for 1 to 2 nights after gradual discontinuation.
- Instruct patient to monitor weight and to report any excessive gain or loss.
- Advise patient to report the following symptoms to health care provider: palpitations or chest pain, signs of bleeding, abdominal pain, jaundice, shortness of breath, rash, confusion, dizziness, nausea, vomiting.
- Instruct patient to take sips of water frequently, suck on ice chips or sugarless hard candy, or chew sugarless gum if dry mouth occurs.
- Advise patient to avoid intake of alcoholic beverages or other CNS depressants.
- Advise patient that drug may cause drowsiness and to use caution while driving or performing other tasks requiring mental alertness.

Flurbiprofen

(FLURE-bih-PRO-fen)
Class Analgesic/NSAID

How Supplied
Ansaid Tablets 50 mg, Tablets 100 mg
✤ *Apo-Flurbiprofen* ◆ *Froben* ◆ *Froben SR* ◆ *Novo-Flurbiprofen* ◆ *Novo-Flurprofen* ◆ *Nu-Flurbiprofen* ◆ *ratio-Flurbiprofen*

Flurbiprofen Sodium
Ocufen Solution 0.03%

Action
PHARMACOLOGY: Decreases inflammation, pain, and fever, probably through inhibition of cyclooxygenase activity and prostaglandin synthesis.

PHARMACOKINETICS/DYNAMICS:
Absorption: T_{max} is about 1.5 hr (range, 0.5 to 4 hr).
Distribution: Flurbiprofen is more than 99% protein bound. Vd is 0.1 to 0.2 L/kg.
Metabolism: The major metabolite is 4′-hydroxy-flurbiprofen.
Excretion: The t½ is about 6 hr; Cl is 1.13 L/hr. The drug is excreted in the urine as conjugates, about 50% as hydroxylated metabolites.

Indications
Systemic: Treatment of rheumatoid arthritis and osteoarthritis.
Ophthalmic: Inhibition of intraoperative miosis.
Unlabeled use(s): Treatment of juvenile rheumatoid arthritis; migraine; dysmenorrhea; sunburn; mild to moderate pain; acute gout; ankylosing spondylitis; tendonitis; bursitis; inflammation after cataract surgery; uveitis.

Contraindications
Systemic/ophthalmic: Patients in whom aspirin, iodides, or any NSAID has caused allergic-type reactions; dendritic keratitis.
Ophthalmic: Epithelial herpes simplex keratitis.

Route/Dosage
Rheumatoid Arthritis or Osteoarthritis
ADULTS: **PO** 200 to 300 mg in divided doses bid to qid; do not exceed 300 mg/day.

Dysmenorrhea
ADULTS: **PO** 50 mg qid.

Inhibition of Intraoperative Miosis
ADULTS: **Topical** 1 drop of 0.03% solution q 30 min beginning 2 hr before surgery.

Interactions
Beta-blockers: Decreased antihypertensive effect of beta-blocker.
Cyclosporine: Increased risk of nephrotoxicity.
Lithium: Increased levels and effects of lithium.
Loop diuretics: Decreased diuretic effect.
Methotrexate: Increased methotrexate levels.
Salicylates: Increased risk of GI toxicity.
Warfarin: Increased risk of gastric erosion and bleeding.

Lab Test Interferences May prolong bleeding time.

Adverse Reactions
CV: CHF; hypotension; hypertension; peripheral edema; fluid retention; vasodilation.
CNS: Dizziness; drowsiness; vertigo; headaches; nervousness; migraine; anxiety; confusion.
DERM: Pruritus; erythema; photosensitivity; urticaria.
EENT: Blurred vision, changes in color vision, hearing disturbances, taste changes (systemic use); ocular irritation, transient stinging and burning of eyes (ophthalmic use).
GI: Heartburn; dyspepsia; nausea; vomiting; anorexia; diarrhea; constipation; increased or decreased appetite; indigestion; GI bleeding; ulceration.
GU: Hematuria; proteinuria; renal insufficiency; glomerular and interstitial nephritis; acute renal failure with pre-existing renal dysfunction.
HEMA: Anemia; bone marrow depression; neutropenia; leukopenia; hypocoagulability.
RESP: Bronchospasm; laryngeal edema; dyspnea; hemoptysis; shortness of breath.
OTHER: Hyperglycemia; hypoglycemia; hyponatremia.

Precautions
Pregnancy: Category B (flurbiprofen); Category C (flurbiprofen sodium).
Lactation: Excreted in breast milk.
Children: Safety and efficacy not established.

Elderly: Increased risk of adverse reactions.
Hypersensitivity: May occur; use caution in aspirin-sensitive individuals because of possible cross-sensitivity.
Renal function impairment: Assess function before and during therapy, because NSAID metabolites are eliminated renally. Acute renal insufficiency, interstitial nephritis, hyperkalemia, hyponatremia, and renal papillary necrosis may occur.

GI effects: Serious GI toxicity (eg, bleeding, ulceration, perforation) can occur at any time, with or without warning symptoms.

Overdosage: Signs and Symptoms
Drowsiness, dizziness, mental confusion, disorientation, lethargy, numbness, vomiting, nausea, gastric upset, abdominal pain, headache, convulsions, renal failure, coma.

PATIENT CARE CONSIDERATIONS
Administration/Storage
- Give with food, milk, or antacids.
- Have patient remain in an upright position for 15 to 30 min after administration, if possible.
- Store at room temperature in tightly closed, light-resistant container.

Assessment/Interventions
- Obtain patient history, including drug history and any known allergies. Note hypersensitivity to aspirin products, renal impairment, ulcer disease or bleeding disorders.
- Monitor effectiveness of drug therapy by evaluating joint symptoms and pain regularly.
- For patients undergoing prolonged or high-dose therapy, monitor hemoglobin and renal and hepatic function.
- Be aware that effects of this drug may mask signs and symptoms of infection.

Patient/Family Education
- Instruct patient to take medication as prescribed, not to skip a dose, and not to double up doses if close to next dose.
- Advise diabetic patient to monitor blood glucose levels carefully during treatment.
- Warn patients about the potential for bleeding and the need to notify other health care professionals that drug is being taken.
- Instruct patient using ophthalmic preparation to use great care to prevent contamination of solution.
- Instruct patient to report the following symptoms to health care provider: bleeding, bruising, dyspnea, edema (oral drug); burning or stinging, tearing, photophobia (ophthalmic drug).
- Advise patient that drug may cause drowsiness and to use caution while driving or performing other tasks requiring mental alertness.
- Tell patient to avoid intake of alcoholic beverages, aspirin or other *otc* medications without consulting health care provider.

Flutamide
(FLEW-tuh-mide)

Class Antiandrogen/Antineoplastic hormone

How Supplied
Eulexin Capsules for oral use 125 mg
✤ *Apo-Flutamide* ♦ *Euflex* ♦ *Novo-Flutamide* ♦ *PMS-Flutamide*

Action
PHARMACOLOGY: Flutamide inhibits androgen uptake or inhibits nuclear binding of androgen in target tissues or both.

PHARMACOKINETICS/DYNAMICS:
Absorption: Flutamide is rapidly and completely absorbed. T_{max} is approximately 2 hr (for the active metabolite).

Distribution: The parent drug and the active metabolite are 94% to 96% and 92% to 94% protein bound at steady state, respectively.

Metabolism: Flutamide is rapidly and extensively metabolized to at least 6 metabolites. The active metabolite is hydroxyflutamide.

Excretion: The t½ is about 6 hr (active metabolite). The drug is excreted primarily in the urine with 4.2% excreted in feces.
Hemodialysis – The parent drug and active metabolite are not well dialyzed.

Special Populations:
Renal Function Impairment – The t½ is slightly prolonged. No dosage adjustment is necessary.
Elderly – The t½ and T_{max} are slightly prolonged.

Indications Metastatic prostate cancer, combination therapy with a luteinizing hormone-releasing hormone (LHRH) analog (eg, goserelin, leuprolide). **Unlabeled use(s):** Treatment of hirsutism in women (250 mg/day).

Contraindications Patients with severe hepatic impairment.

Route/Dosage
Prostate Cancer
ADULTS: PO 250 mg (2 capsules) q 8 hr.
Stage B_2-C Prostatic Carcinoma
ADULTS: PO Start treatment at 8 wk prior to initiating radiation therapy and continue during radiation therapy.
Stage D_2 Metastatic Carcinoma
ADULTS: PO Initiate flutamide capsules with the LHRH agonist and continue until progression.

Interactions Prothrombin time may increase when flutamide therapy is initiated in patients stabilized on chronic warfarin therapy.

Lab Test Interferences Elevated AST, ALT, bilirubin, SGGT, BUN, and serum creatinine.

Adverse Reactions
CNS: Decreased libido.
ENDO: Hot flashes, gynecomastia.
GI: Low potential for nausea and vomiting; diarrhea; hepatocellular necrosis; cholestatic jaundice; elevated LFTs.
GU: Impotence; reduced sperm count.

PATIENT CARE CONSIDERATIONS
Administration/Storage
- Store capsules in refrigerator or at room temperature; protect from moisture.
- For PO administration.
- For patients unable to swallow capsules, open the capsule and mix the contents with applesauce, pudding, or other semi-solid foods. Administer immediately.

Assessment/Interventions
- Monitor serum transaminase levels at baseline and monthly during the first 4 mo of treatment. Monitor periodically during continued treatment, especially if the patient experiences signs and symptoms of liver dysfunction. Immediately discontinue flutamide if ALT increases more than 2 times above the upper limit of normal.

> **WARNING:**
> *Hepatic injury:* Hospitalization and rarely death from liver failure. Evidence of hepatic injury included elevated serum transaminase levels, jaundice, hepatic encephalopathy, and death related to acute hepatic failure. The hepatic injury was reversible after discontinuation of therapy in some patients. Approximately 50% of the reported cases occurred within the initial 3 mo of treatment.

Precautions
Pregnancy: Category D.
Aniline exposure: A metabolite of flutamide, 4-nitro-3-fluoro-methylaniline, may cause methemoglobinemia, hemolytic anemia, and cholestatic jaundice in patients treated with flutamide.
Women: Flutamide is used only in men.

Overdosage: Signs and Symptoms
Hypoactivity; piloerection; slow respiration; ataxia; lacrimation; anorexia; tranquilization; emesis; methemoglobinemia.

- Monitor methemoglobin levels in patients susceptible to aniline toxicity (eg, people with glucose-6-phosphate dehydrogenase deficiency or hemoglobin M disease as well as patients who smoke).
- Regular assessment of serum prostate specific antigen (PSA) may be helpful in monitoring the patient's response.

Patient/Family Education
- The urine was noted to change to an amber or yellow-green appearance.
- Photosensitization may occur.
- Flutamide and LHRH-agonists should be administered concomitantly; and do not interrupt dosing or stop taking these medications without consulting the health care provider.

Fluticasone Propionate
(flew-TICK-ah-SONE PRO-pee-oh-nate)
Class Corticosteroid
How Supplied
Flonase Nasal spray 50 mcg/actuation ◆ *Flovent* Aerosol 44 mcg/actuation, Aerosol 110 mcg/actuation, Aerosol 220 mcg/actuation ◆ *Flovent Diskus* Powder for inhalation 50 mcg/actuation, Powder for inhalation 100 mcg/actuation, Powder for inhalation 250 mcg/actuation ◆ *Flovent Rotadisk* Powder for inhalation 50 mcg/actuation, Powder for inhalation 100 mcg/actuation, Powder for inhalation 250 mcg/actuation
🍁 *Florinef* ◆ *Floven HFA*

Action
PHARMACOLOGY: Exerts potent anti-inflammatory effect on nasal passages.

PHARMACOKINETICS/DYNAMICS:
Absorption: C_{max} is 0.1 to 1 ng/mL. Systemic bioavailability is about 13.5% for the powder and 30% for the aerosol.

Distribution: The average Vd is 4.2 L/kg, and the drug is about 91% protein bound.

Metabolism: The major metabolite is a 17-βcarboxylic acid derivative metabolized in the liver via the cytochrome P450 3A4 pathway.

Excretion: The t½ is about 7.8 hr. It is primarily excreted in the feces as parent drug and metabolites, with less than 5% excreted in the urine as metabolites.

Peak: At least 1 to 2 wk.

Indications Management of the nasal symptoms of seasonal and perennial allergic and nonallergic rhinitis in adults and pediatric patients 4 yr and older (*Flonase*); patients requiring oral corticosteroid therapy for asthma (*Flovent, Flovent Rotadisk, Flovent Diskus*); maintenance treatment of asthma as prophylactic therapy in patients 4 yr and older (*Flovent Diskus, Flovent Rotadisk*) and 12 yr and older (*Flovent*).

Contraindications Hypersensitivity (*Flonase*); primary treatment of status asthmaticus or other acute episodes of asthma in which intensive measures are required (*Flovent*); hypersensitivity to the drug or any component of the product.

Route/Dosage

FLONASE

ADULTS: **Nasal Inhalation** Starting dose is 2 sprays in each nostril qd (total daily dose, 200 mcg). Same dose divided into 100 mcg bid also is effective. After the first few days, dosage may be reduced to 100 mcg (1 spray each nostril daily) for maintenance therapy. Max daily dose, 200 mcg.

CHILDREN 4 YR OF AGE AND OLDER: Starting dose is 1 spray in each nostril qd (total daily dose, 100 mcg). May be increased to 200 mcg/day (2 sprays in each nostril) if not adequately responding. Depending on response, dosage may be decreased to 100 mcg/day. Max daily dose, 200 mcg.

FLOVENT

Individuals will experience variable time to onset and degree of symptom relief. Improvement can occur within 24 hr of starting treatment; although, maximum benefit may take 1 to 2 wk or longer. After achieving stability, titrate to the lowest effective dose to reduce side effects.

ADULTS AND CHILDREN 12 YR OF AGE AND OLDER: **Inhalation Aerosol** For patients not responding adequately to the starting dose after 2 wk, higher doses may provide additional asthma control. The recommended starting doses, based on prior antiasthma therapy are: 1) bronchodilators alone – start with 88 mcg bid (max, 440 mcg bid); 2) inhaled corticosteroids – start with 88 to 220 mcg bid (max, 440 mcg bid); and 3) oral corticosteroids – start with 880 mcg bid (max, 880 mcg bid). Starting doses above 88 mcg bid may be considered for patients with poorer asthma control or who have previously required doses of inhaled corticosteroids in the higher range for that specific agent.

ADULTS: **Inhalation Powder** The recommended starting doses, based on prior antiasthma therapy are: 1) bronchodilators alone – start with 100 mcg bid (max, 500 mcg bid); 2) inhaled corticosteroids – start with 100 to 250 mcg bid (max, 500 mcg bid); 3) oral corticosteroids – start with 500 (designated with *Flovent Diskus*) to 1000 mcg bid (max, 1000 mcg bid).

CHILDREN 4 TO 11 YR OF AGE: **Inhalation Powder** The recommended starting doses, based on prior antiasthma therapy are: 1) bronchodilators alone – start with 50 mcg bid (max, 100 mcg bid); and 2) inhaled corticosteroids – start with 50 mcg bid (max, 100 mcg bid). Because individual responses may vary, children previously maintained on *Flovent Rotadisk* 50 or 100 mcg bid may require dosage adjustments upon transfer to *Flovent Diskus*. Starting doses above 100 mcg bid for adults and adolescents and 50 mcg bid for children 4 to 11 yr of age may be considered for patients with poorer asthma control or who have previously required doses of inhaled corticosteroids that are in the higher range for that specific agent.

Chronic Oral Corticosteroid Therapy

Prednisone should be reduced no faster than 2.5 mg/day on a weekly basis, beginning after at least 1 wk of therapy with *Flovent* inhalation aerosol or powder.

Interactions

Ketoconazole: Concomitant use may increase fluticasone concentrations and reduce plasma cortisol AUC.

Ritonavir: Can significantly increase plasma fluticasone exposure, resulting in significantly reduced serum cortisol concentrations. Systemic effects including Cushing syndrome and adrenal suppression have been reported.

Lab Test Interferences None well documented.

Adverse Reactions

CV: Flovent inhalation powder: Palpitation (1% to 3%).

CNS: Flonase: Headache (16%); dizziness (1% to 3%); *Flovent* inhalation aerosol: headache (22%); giddiness (1% to 3%); dizziness; *Flovent* inhalation powder: headache (14%); dizziness, sleep disorders, migraines, paralysis of cranial nerves, mood disorders, malaise, fatigue (1% to 3%).

DERM: Flovent inhalation aerosol: Dermatitis, rash, skin eruption (1% to 3%); *Flovent* inhalation powder: rash, urticaria, photodermatitis,

dermatitis, dermatosis, viral skin infections, eczema, fungal infections, acne, pruritus, folliculitis (1% to 3%).
EENT: *Flonase*: Pharyngitis (8%); nosebleed (7%); nasal burning/irritation (3%); blood in nasal mucus, runny nose (1% to 3%); alteration or loss of sense of taste or smell, glaucoma, increased IOP, cataracts; *Flovent* inhalation aerosol: nasal congestion (16%); pharyngitis (14%); dysphonia (8%); sinusitis (6%); nasal discharge, allergic rhinitis, oral candidiasis (5%); nasal sinus pain, rhinitis, eye irritation (1% to 3%); *Flovent* inhalation powder: throat irritation (22%); sinusitis/sinus infection (10%); oral candidiasis (9%); rhinitis (4%); ear signs and symptoms, rhinorrhea/postnasal drip, hoarseness/dysphonia, epistaxis, tonsillitis, nasal signs and symptoms, laryngitis, unspecified oropharyngeal plaques, otitis, ear/nose/throat/tonsil signs and symptoms, ear/nose/throat polyps, allergic ear/nose/throat disorders, throat constriction, keratitis, conjunctivitis, blepharoconjunctivitis (1% to 3%).
ENDO: *Flovent* inhalation powder: Fluid disturbances, weight gain, goiter, disorders of uric acid metabolism, appetite disturbances (1% to 3%).
GI: *Flonase*: Nausea, vomiting (5%); abdominal pain, diarrhea (1% to 3%); *Flovent* inhalation aerosol: nausea, vomiting diarrhea, dyspepsia, stomach disorder (1% to 3%); *Flovent* inhalation powder: nausea, vomiting (8%); viral infection (5%); discomfort/pain (4%); diarrhea, GI signs and symptoms, oral ulcerations, dental discomfort and pain, gastroenteritis, infection abdominal discomfort and pain, oral erythema and rashes, mouth and tongue disorders, oral discomfort and pain, tooth decay (1% to 3%).
GU: *Flovent* inhalation aerosol: Dysmenorrhea (1% to 3%); *Flovent* inhalation powder: bacterial reproductive infections, UTI (3% to 15%).
HEPA: *Flovent* inhalation powder: Cholecystitis (1% to 3%).
MUSC: *Flovent* inhalation aerosol: pain joint, sprain/strain, aches, pains, pain in limb (1% to 3%); *Flovent* inhalation powder: muscle injury/pain (5%); arthralgia, articular rheumatism, muscle cramps and spasms, inflammation (1% to 3%).
RESP: *Flonase*: Asthma symptoms (7%); cough (4%); bronchitis (1% to 3%); *Flovent* inhalation aerosol: upper respiratory tract infection (22%); influenza (8%); bronchitis, chest congestion (1% to 3%); *Flovent* inhalation powder: upper respiratory tract infection (21%); bronchitis (8%); lower respiratory infection, cough (5%); upper respiratory inflammation (4%).
OTHER: *Flonase*: Fever, flu-like symptoms, aches and pains (1% to 3%); hypersensitivity (including angioedema, anaphylaxis/anaphylactoid reactions); growth suppression; *Flovent* inhalation aerosol: fever, dental problems (1% to 3%); immediate and delayed hypersensitivity, including urticaria, rash, angioedema, and bronchospasm (2% or less); *Flovent* inhalation powder: fever (7%); viral infection (5%); immediate and delayed hypersensitivity reactions, including rash, angioedema, and bronchospasm (less than 2%); soft tissue injury, contusions, hematomas, wounds, lacerations, postoperative complications, burns, poisoning and toxicity, pressure-induced disorders, chest symptoms, pain edema, swelling, bacterial infections, fungal infections, mobility disorders, cysts, lumps, masses (1% to 3%).

Precautions

Pregnancy: Category C.
Lactation: Undetermined.
Children:
Flonase, Flovent inhalation powder – Safety and efficacy not established for children younger than 4 yr.
Flovent inhalation aerosol – Safety and efficacy not established for children younger than 12 yr.
Hypersensitivity: Reactions, including anaphylaxis, may occur.
Adrenal suppression: Prolonged therapy may lead to hypothalamic-pituitary-adrenal suppression.
Fungal infections: Local fungal infections have rarely developed. Antifungal treatment or discontinuance of drug may be necessary.
General: Rare instances of wheezing, nasal septum perforation, cataracts, glaucoma, and increased IOP may occur.
Growth velocity: A reduction in growth velocity may occur as a result of inadequate control of chronic diseases such as asthma or from use of corticosteroids for treatment.
Infections: Drug may mask signs of infection and may decrease host-defense mechanisms.
Route change: Particular caution is needed when transferring patient from systemically active corticosteroids to fluticasone inhaler because deaths caused by adrenal insufficiency have occurred in asthmatic patients during and after transfer from systemic to aerosol corticosteroids.
Withdrawal: Because deaths caused by adrenal insufficiency have occurred in patients with asthma during and after transfer from systemic corticosteroids to less systemically available inhaled corticosteroids, particular care is needed for patients who are transferred from systemically active corticosteroids to *Flovent*. After withdrawal from systemic corticosteroids, a number of months are needed for recovery of hypothalamic-pituitary-adrenal (HPA) function. Patients maintained on prednisone, 20 mg/day or more (or its equivalent), may be most susceptible, especially when the systemic corticosteroid is almost completely withdrawn.

PATIENT CARE CONSIDERATIONS
Administration/Storage
- May be administered alone or in combination with systemic corticosteroids.

Oral inhalation of aerosol:
- For oral inhalation only. Avoid spraying into the nose or eyes.
- Shake well before each use.
- If patient also receiving bronchodilators by inhalation, administer bronchodilator 5 min before fluticasone to enhance penetration of latter drug into bronchial tree.
- Before oral inhalation, give patient drink of water to moisten throat. Place inhaler mouthpiece 2 fingerbreadths away from patient's mouth. Tilt patient's head back slightly. Instruct patient to take slow, deep breaths while inhaler is being activated and to hold breath for 5 to 10 sec and then breathe out slowly. A spacing device (eg, *Aerochamber*) may be used to enhance delivery of medication. Have patient rinse mouth after inhalations are complete.
- If more than 1 spray/dose is ordered, administer each spray individually, waiting a few seconds between sprays.
- Store at controlled room temperature (36° to 86°F). Protect from freezing and direct sunlight. Store pressurized canister with nozzle end down. Store at room temperature while using aerosol.
- Do not puncture or discard pressurized canister in incinerator.

Oral inhalation of dry powder:
- For oral inhalation only.
- Activate and use the inhalation device in a level, horizontal position. Do not shake inhalation device before or during inhalation.
- Prepare dose by activating inhalation device immediately prior to administration. Have patient exhale fully then place inhaler mouthpiece between lips. Do not close teeth. Instruct patient to take slow, deep breath and to hold breath for 5 to 10 sec and then breathe out slowly. Have patient rinse mouth after inhalations are complete.
- Do not use with a spacer device (eg, *Aerochamber*). Do not exhale into the inhalation device, wash, or attempt to take the inhalation device apart.
- Store at controlled room temperature (68° to 77°F) in a dry place. Protect from direct heat or sunlight. Discard 50 mcg strength *Diskus* 6 wk (or 100 and 250-mcg strength 2 mo) after removal from moisture-protective foil overwrap or when the dose indicator reads "0." Discard *Rotadisk* blisters 2 mo after opening moisture-protective foil overwrap or before expiration date, whichever comes first.

Nasal inhalation:
- Shake well before each use.
- Actuate the pump 6 times to prime before first use or after a period of nonuse of more than 1 wk.
- Before nasal inhalation, instruct patient to blow nose gently to clear nasal passages. If needed, a topical decongestant may be used 5 to 10 min before administration to ensure adequate tissue penetration. Nasal lavage with saline may also help remove secretions. Clean outer portion of nose with a damp tissue. Wash and dry hands.
- Insert nozzle into patient's nostril. Use finger to keep other nostril closed. Instruct patient to inhale through nostril while you activate the spray pump. Repeat with other nostril.
- If 2 sprays/dose are ordered, administer 1 spray in each nostril, wait a few seconds and administer second spray into each nostril.
- Store at controlled room temperature (39° to 86°F). Protect from freezing. Discard bottle when labeled number of sprays have been used.

Assessment/Interventions
- Obtain patient history, including drug history and any known allergies.
- If change is made from systemic (oral) corticosteroids to inhaled or intranasal corticosteroids, observe patient carefully for signs of adrenal insufficiency (eg, nausea, fatigue, dizziness, hypotension, depression, or abdominal, joint or muscle pain). Notify health care provider if these signs occur. Deaths caused by adrenal insufficiency have occurred during and after converting to aerosol corticosteroids.
- Assess patient's symptoms before initiating therapy and periodically during treatment. Notify health care provider if symptoms do not improve or worsen.
- Notify health care provider if oral, nasal, or pharyngeal irritation occurs or if symptoms worsen.

Patient/Family Education
- Explain name, dose, action, and potential side effects of drug.
- Advise patient to read the Patient's Instructions for Use before starting therapy and again with each refill.
- Advise patient to continue taking other medications for same condition as prescribed by health care provider.
- Review proper administration technique. Have patient demonstrate technique.

- Advise patient that dose may be changed periodically depending on how well symptoms are controlled.
- Instruct patient not to exceed prescribed dose.
- Explain that effects of drug are not immediate. Benefit requires daily use as instructed and usually occurs after 1 to 2 days but full relief may take 1 to 2 wk.
- Instruct patient not to stop the medication once symptoms have been controlled. Continued daily use is necessary to continue to control symptoms.
- Advise patient not to increase dose and to inform health care provider if symptoms do not improve or worsen.
- If patient is being converted from oral corticosteroids to inhaled or intranasal corticosteroids, review signs and symptoms of adrenal insufficiency, which may occur days or weeks after conversion is complete. Advise patient to carry Medi-Alert card indicating they may need supplemental systemic corticosteroids during periods of stress or a severe asthma attack.
- Advise patient to discard the aerosol canister or nasal spray bottle when the labeled number of doses has been used. Advise patient using dry powder inhalation device on storage and expiration dates once device or blisters are removed from moisture-protective foil overwrap.
- Advise patient to avoid exposure to chickenpox and measles and to seek medical advice immediately if exposed.
- Advise women to notify health care provider if pregnant, planning to become pregnant, or breastfeeding.
- Caution patient not to take any prescription or OTC medications, or dietary supplements unless advised by health care provider.
- Advise patient that follow-up visits may be required to monitor therapy and to keep appointments.

Oral inhalation (dry powder or aerosol):

- Warn patient that drug is an "asthma controller" and is not to be used to treat an acute asthma attack. They must use their "rescue medication" (bronchodilator) to obtain rapid relief of asthma symptoms.
- Instruct patient to carry Medi-Alert card if experiencing acute severe asthma attacks requiring rapid systemic treatment.
- Advise patient to rinse mouth with water after inhalations are complete. Instruct patient to spit rinse water out and not to swallow rinse water.
- Advise patient to report the following symptoms to health care provider: sore throat or mouth, cough, dry mouth, rash, facial swelling, or worsening asthma symptoms (eg, increasing need for bronchodilator).

Nasal inhalation:

- Instruct patient to use with caution if sores develop or injuries occur in nasal passages. Drug may prevent or slow proper healing.
- Advise patient to report the following symptoms to health care provider: sneezing, nasal irritation, nosebleed.

Fluticasone Propionate/Salmeterol

(flew-TICK-ah-SONE PRO-pee-oh-nate/sal-MEET-ah-rahl)

Class Respiratory inhalant combination

How Supplied
Advair Diskus Powder for inhalation 100 mcg fluticasone propionate, 50 mcg salmeterol, Powder for inhalation 250 mcg fluticasone propionate, 50 mcg salmeterol, Powder for inhalation 500 mcg fluticasone propionate, 50 mcg salmeterol

Action
PHARMACOLOGY:

Fluticasone: Inhibits multiple cell types (eg, mast cells) and mediator production or secretion (eg, histamine) involved in the asthmatic response.

Salmeterol: Produces bronchodilation by relaxing bronchial smooth muscle through beta-2-receptor stimulation.

PHARMACOKINETICS/DYNAMICS:

Absorption: Peak plasma levels of fluticasone are achieved in 1 to 2 hr, and those of salmeterol are achieved in about 5 min. Mean peak steady-state plasma level of fluticasone following administration of *Advair Diskus* 500/50 was 57 pg/mL.

Excretion: The terminal $t_{½}$ of fluticasone averaged 5.33 to 7.65 hr when administered as *Advair Diskus*.

Indications Long-term maintenance treatment of asthma; COPD associated with chronic bronchitis.

Contraindications Primary treatment of status asthmaticus or other acute episodes of asthma in which intensive measures are required; hypersensitivity to any component of the product.

Route/Dosage
Advair Diskus is available in 3 strengths, containing 100, 250, and 500 mcg of fluticasone propionate each in combination with 50 mcg of salmeterol.

ADULTS AND CHILDREN 12 YR OF AGE AND OLDER: **Inhalation** 1 inhalation bid (morning and evening, approximately 12 hr apart). For patients not currently on an inhaled corticosteroid, the recommended starting dose is fluticasone/salmeterol 100/50 bid. For patients on an inhaled corticosteroid, the recommended starting dose of fluticasone/salmeterol varies from 100/50 to 500/50 bid, depending on the concomitant inhaled corticosteroid and the dose.

CHILDREN 4 TO 11 YR OF AGE (SYMPTOMATIC ON INHALED CORTICOSTEROIDS): **Inhalation** 100/50 mcg bid (morning and evening, approximately 12 hr apart).

COPD Associated with Chronic Bronchitis
ADULTS: **Inhalation** 1 inhalation (250/50 mcg) bid (morning and evening, approximately 12 hr apart).

Interactions

Beta-adrenergic blocking agents (eg, propranolol): May block the pulmonary effect of salmeterol.
Inhibitors of cytochrome P450 3A4 (eg, ketoconazole, ritonavir): Plasma levels of fluticasone may be increased and plasma cortisol AUC may be reduced.
Long-acting beta$_2$-agonists: Because this product already contains salmeterol, do not use other long-acting inhaled beta$_2$-agonists for prevention of exercise-induced bronchospasm or maintenance treatment of asthma.
Loop diuretics (eg, furosemide), thiazide diuretics (eg, hydrochlorothiazide): ECG changes and hypokalemia may be worsened.
MAO inhibitors (eg, isocarboxazid), tricyclic antidepressants (eg, amitriptyline): Use with extreme caution in patients receiving these agents or within 2 wk of discontinuation.

Lab Test Interferences None well documented.

Adverse Reactions The following adverse reactions occurred at a rate of at least 1% and were more common than in the placebo group.
CV: Palpitations.
CNS: Headache; sleep disorders; tremors; hypnagogic effects; compressed nerve symptoms.
DERM: Hives; urticaria; skin flakiness; acquired ichthyosis; sweating; disorders of sweat and sebum.
EENT: Pharyngitis (including localized infection of pharynx with *Candida albicans*); sinusitis; hoarseness; rhinorrhea; postnasal drip; ear, nose, and throat infections; ear signs and symptoms; nasal signs and symptoms; nasal sinus disorders; rhinitis; sneezing; nasal irritation; blood in nasal mucosa; keratitis; conjunctivitis; viral eye infections; eye redness; congestion.
GI: Oral candidiasis; nausea; vomiting; GI discomfort and pain; diarrhea; GI infections (including viral); dental discomfort and pain; GI signs and symptoms; gastroenteritis; GI disorders; oral ulcerations; oral erythema and rashes; constipation; appendicitis; unusual taste.
HEMA: Eosinophilia; lymphatic signs and symptoms.
HEPA: Abnormal LFTs.
METAB: Hypokalemia; changes in blood glucose; candidiasis; musculoskeletal pain; fluid retention.
RESP: Upper respiratory tract inflammation and infection; viral respiratory infections; bronchitis; cough; pneumonia; lower respiratory signs and symptoms; lower respiratory tract infections.
OTHER: Muscle injuries; fractures; wounds; lacerations; contusions; hematoma; burns; arthralgia; articular rheumatism; muscle stiffness; tightness and rigidity; bone and cartilage disorders; allergies and allergic reactions; viral and bacterial infections; pain; chest symptoms; wheezing.

> **WARNING:**
> When added to usual asthma therapy, there may be a small increase in asthma-related deaths in patients receiving salmeterol compared with placebo. The risk may be greater in black patients compared with white patients.

Precautions

Pregnancy: Category C.
Lactation:
Fluticasone – Undetermined; however, other corticosteroids are excreted in breast milk.
Salmeterol – Undetermined.
Children: Safety and efficacy not established in children with asthma younger than 4 yr of age.
Elderly: Use with caution in geriatric patients who have concurrent cardiovascular disease.
Hypersensitivity: Immediate hypersensitivity reactions may occur.
Adrenal suppression: Hypothalamic-pituitary-adrenal suppression may occur.
Cardiovascular disorders: Use with caution in patients with cardiovascular disease, especially coronary insufficiency, cardiac arrhythmias, and hypertension.
Immunosuppression: Patients receiving immunosuppressive therapy may be more susceptible to infection than healthy individuals.
Increased use: If therapy becomes less effective, this may be a marker of destabilization of asthma, which requires reevaluation.
Paradoxical bronchospasm: May occur and be life-threatening.
Special warnings: Do not use for transferring patients from systemic corticosteroid therapy; not to be initiated in patients during rapidly deteriorating or potentially life-threatening epi-

sodes of asthma; not for use in treating acute asthma symptoms; do not exceed recommended dose.

Upper airway symptoms: Laryngeal spasm, irritation, or swelling (eg, stridor, choking) may occur.

Overdosage: Signs and Symptoms

Fluticasone: Hypercorticism.
Salmeterol: Excessive beta-adrenergic stimulation or occurrence or exaggeration of adverse effects (eg, seizures, angina, hypertension, hypotension, tachycardia, arrhythmias, nervousness, headache, tremor, muscle cramps, dry mouth, palpitation, nausea, dizziness, fatigue, malaise, insomnia), prolongation of the QTc interval, hypokalemia, hyperglycemia, cardiac arrest, death.

PATIENT CARE CONSIDERATIONS

Administration/Storage

- May be administered alone or in combination with systemic corticosteroids.
- Have patient take 1 inhalation bid, morning and evening, as prescribed.
- If patient is also receiving short-acting bronchodilator by inhalation, administer bronchodilator 5 min before fluticasone/salmeterol to enhance penetration of latter drugs into bronchial tree.
- Have patient rinse mouth with water without swallowing after inhalation is complete.
- Discard delivery device 30 days after removing from foil pouch or after every blister has been used and dose indicator reads "0."
- Store delivery device at controlled room temperature (68° to 77°F) in a dry place away from direct heat or sunlight.

Assessment/Interventions

- Obtain patient history, including drug history and any known allergies. Note history of hepatic impairment, coronary artery disease, arrhythmias, hypertension, hyperthyroidism, or seizures.
- If change is made from systemic (oral) corticosteroids to inhaled corticosteroids observe patient carefully for signs of adrenal insufficiency (eg, nausea; fatigue; dizziness; hypotension; depression; abdominal, joint, or muscle pain). Notify health care provider if these signs occur. Deaths caused by adrenal insufficiency have occurred during and after converting to inhaled corticosteroids.
- Ensure therapy is not initiated in patient who is experiencing rapidly deteriorating or potentially life-threatening episode of asthma.
- Ensure patient is not receiving another inhaled, long-acting bronchodilator (eg, formoterol) simultaneously.
- Ensure baseline pulmonary function tests have been completed.
- Ensure eye examinations are performed regularly during prolonged therapy.
- Ensure bone mineral density (BMD) is assessed prior to starting therapy and periodically thereafter in patient with risk factors for decreased BMD being treated for COPD. Be prepared to introduce therapy to treat or prevent osteoporosis if indicated.
- Frequently assess patient for response to treatment. Notify health care provider if condition does not appear to be improving or worsens.
- Ensure therapy is periodically reviewed in patient with COPD associated with chronic bronchitis for periods longer than 6 mo to assess the continuing benefits and potential risks of treatment.
- Assess patient for RESP, CNS, CV, GI, and general body side effects. Inform health care provider if noted and significant.

Patient/Family Education

- Explain name, dose, action, and potential side effects of drug.
- Instruct patient to continue using other medications for asthma or COPD as prescribed by health care provider.
- Instruct patient on the proper storage, handling, and use of the dry powder inhaler, referring to the *Patient's Instructions for Use* instruction sheet included with the medication.
- Advise patient that medication should never be administered with a spacer device.
- Caution patient not to exceed prescribed dose of 1 inhalation bid, morning and evening, and to rinse mouth with water, without swallowing, after each dose.
- Caution patient not to use salmeterol or other long-acting bronchodilators (eg, formoterol) for prevention of exercise-induced asthma or for maintenance treatment of asthma.
- Warn patient that drug is an asthma controller and is not to be used to treat an acute asthma attack. Rescue medication (bronchodilator) must be used to obtain rapid relief of asthma symptoms.
- Explain that effects of drug are not immediate. Benefit requires daily use as instructed and may occur after 30 min but may take 1 wk or more.
- Advise patient that they may or may not feel or taste a dose of medicine during inhalation. Caution patient not to exceed the prescribed

dose of 1 inhalation bid if delivered dose.
- Advise patient not to increase dose and to inform health care provider if symptoms do not improve or worsen, if more short-acting bronchodilator than usual is needed, or if the short-acting bronchodilator appears to become less effective.
- If patient is being converted from oral corticosteroids, review signs and symptoms of adrenal insufficiency, which may occur days or weeks after conversion is complete. Advise patient to carry *Medi-Alert* card indicating that supplemental systemic corticosteroids may be needed during periods of stress or a severe asthma attack.
- Advise patient to carry *Medi-Alert* card if experiencing acute severe asthma attacks requiring rapid systemic treatment.
- Advise patient to report the following symptoms to health care provider: sore throat or mouth, persistent cough, palpitations, chest pain, rapid heart rate, tremor, nervousness.
- Advise patient to avoid exposure to chickenpox and measles and to seek medical advice immediately if exposed.
- Advise women to notify health care provider if pregnant, planning to become pregnant, or breastfeeding.
- Caution patient not to take any prescription or OTC medications, herbal preparations, or dietary supplements unless advised by health care provider.
- Advise patient that follow-up visits may be required to monitor therapy and to keep appointments.

Fluvastatin

(FLEW-vah-stat-in)

Class Antihyperlipidemic/HMG-CoA reductase inhibitor

How Supplied
Lescol Capsules 20 mg, Capsules 40 mg ◆ *Lescol XL* Tablets, extended-release 80 mg

Action
PHARMACOLOGY: Increases rate at which body removes cholesterol from blood and reduces production of cholesterol in body by inhibiting enzyme that catalyzes early rate-limiting step in cholesterol synthesis; increases HDL; reduces LDL, VLDL, and triglycerides.

PHARMACOKINETICS/DYNAMICS:
Absorption: Absolute bioavailability is 9% to 50%. The relative bioavailability for the extended-release form is 9% to 66%. T_{max} is less than 1 hr. C_{max} is 48.9 to 990 ng/mL.
Immediate release – Administration with food at steady state increases T_{max} and decreases C_{max}.
Extended release – Administration with a high-fat meal increases bioavailability by about 50%.

Distribution: Fluvastatin is 98% protein bound. The mean Vd_{ss} is about 0.35 L/kg.

Metabolism: No active metabolites are present systemically. The drug is metabolized in the liver primarily via hydroxylation; oxidation occurs via CYP2C9 isozyme systems (75%), 3A4 (about 20%), and 2C8 (about 5%).

Excretion: About 90% is excreted in the feces as metabolites and less than 2% is unchanged. The t½ is less than 3 hr.

Special Populations:
Hepatic Function Impairment – AUC and C_{max} increase 2.5-fold.

Indications
Atherosclerosis: To slow the progression of coronary atherosclerosis.
Hypercholesterolemia: Reduction of elevated total cholesterol, LDL, apo-B, and triglyceride cholesterol levels and to increase HDL levels.
Secondary prevention of coronary events: To reduce the risk of undergoing coronary revascularization procedures in patients with coronary heart disease.

Contraindications Active liver disease or unexplained persistent elevations of LFTs; pregnancy; lactation.

Route/Dosage
ADULTS: PO 20 to 80 mg qd.

Interactions
Azole antifungal agents (eg, fluconazole), cyclosporine, gemfibrozil, macrolide antibiotics (eg, erythromycin), niacin: Severe myopathy or rhabdomyolysis may occur with coadministration.
Cholestyramine: Reduced absorption of fluvastatin if taken with or up to 4 hr after cholestyramine.
Cimetidine, ranitidine, omeprazole: Fluvastatin serum levels may be increased.
Diclofenac, digoxin, glyburide, hydantoins: Serum levels of these agents may be increased.
Rifampin: Fluvastatin serum levels may be reduced.
Warfarin: Anticoagulant effect of warfarin may be increased.

Lab Test Interferences None well documented.

Adverse Reactions
CNS: Headache (9%); fatigue, insomnia (3%).
EENT: Sinusitis (4%).
GI: Dyspepsia (8%); diarrhea, abdominal pain (5%); nausea, flatulence (3%).

GU: UTI (3%).
MUSC: Myalgia (5%).
RESP: Bronchitis (3%).
OTHER: Flu-like symptoms (7%); accidental trauma (5%).

Precautions
Pregnancy: Category X.
Lactation: Excreted in breast milk; do not breastfeed while taking.
Children: Safety and efficacy in children younger than 18 yr not established.
Endocrine effects: Use caution when administering HMG-CoA reductase inhibitors with drugs that affect steroid levels or activity.
LFTs: Perform LFTs before initiating therapy, and at 12 wk (or elevation in dose).
Liver dysfunction: Use with caution in patients who consume substantial quantities of alcohol or who have a history of liver disease.
Skeletal muscle effects: Rhabdomyolysis with renal dysfunction secondary to myoglobinuria has been reported with other drugs in this class. Temporarily withhold therapy in any patient experiencing an acute or serious condition predisposing to the development of renal failure secondary to rhabdomyolysis (eg, sepsis, hypotension). The risk of myopathy with other drugs in this class was found to be increased if therapy with either cyclosporine, gemfibrozil, erythromycin, or niacin is administered concurrently. Consider myopathy in any patient with diffuse myalgias, muscle tenderness or weakness, or marked elevations of CPK.

PATIENT CARE CONSIDERATIONS
Administration/Storage
- Administer alone or in combination with other lipid-lowering therapy.
- Administer prescribed dose without regard to meals, but administer with food if GI upset occurs.
- Have patient swallow extended-release tablets whole. Do not cut, crush, or chew tablet
- Administer bile acid resin (eg, cholestyramine) at least 2 hr before fluvastatin.
- Store capsules and tablets at controlled room temperature (59° to 86°F). Protect from light.

Assessment/Interventions
- Obtain patient history, including drug history and any known allergies. Note active liver disease, unexplained elevations of serum transaminases, alcohol consumption, and concurrent therapy with medications known to increase the risk of myopathy (eg, cyclosporine, gemfibrozil).
- Ensure that secondary causes of hypercholesterolemia (eg, poorly controlled diabetes, hypothyroidism) are excluded before starting therapy.
- Ensure that patient is on a cholesterol-lowering diet before starting therapy and that diet is continued during treatment.
- Ensure that therapy is temporarily withheld in patient with an acute, serious condition suggestive of myopathy or predisposing to the development of renal failure secondary to rhabdomyolysis (eg, sepsis, hypotension).
- Ensure that serum cholesterol and triglycerides are measured before therapy is started and not less than 4 wk of starting therapy or changing the fluvastatin dose and then periodically thereafter.
- Ensure that LFTs (transaminases) are determined before and 12 wk following initiation of therapy, or after increase in dose, and periodically thereafter (eg, q 6 mo).
- If elevated serum transaminase levels develop during treatment, repeat levels more frequently. If transaminase levels rise to 3 times upper limit of normal and persist, notify health care provider. Be prepared to reduce dose or discontinue therapy if ordered.
- If muscle tenderness and/or weakness develops during therapy, determine CPK levels. Notify health care provider if CPK levels are markedly increased or if muscle symptoms continue or worsen.
- Assess patient for GI, CNS, MUSC, and general body side effects. If noted and significant, inform health care provider.

Patient/Family Education
- Explain name, dose, action, and potential side effects of drug
- Advise patient to take prescribed dose without regard to meals but to take with food if stomach upset occurs.
- Caution patient to swallow extended-release tablet whole and not to cut, chew, or crush the tablet.
- Advise patient who is also taking a bile acid resin (eg, cholestyramine) to take the resin at least 2 hr before fluvastatin.
- Advise patient to try to take each dose(s) at about the same time each day.
- Inform patient that drug helps control, but does not cure, cholesterol abnormality and to continue taking drug as prescribed if cholesterol levels are lowered.
- Caution patient not to change the dose or stop taking unless advised by health care provider.
- Advise patient that if a dose is missed to take it as soon as remembered but never take more

- than 1 dose of medicine a day.
- Instruct patient to continue taking other cholesterol-lowering medications as prescribed by health care provider.
- Emphasize to patient importance of the following other modalities on cholesterol control: dietary changes (reduced saturated fat intake, increase soluble fiber intake); weight control, regular exercise, and smoking cessation.
- Advise women of childbearing potential to use effective contraception during treatment with fluvastatin.
- Advise women to notify health care provider if pregnant, planning to become pregnant, or breastfeeding.
- Caution patient not to take any prescription or OTC medications or dietary supplements unless advised by health care provider.
- Instruct patient to notify health care provider if experiencing any unexplained muscle pain, tenderness, and/or weakness, or any other unusual feelings.
- Advise patient that follow-up visits and lab tests will be required to monitor therapy and to keep appointments.

Fluvoxamine Maleate

(flu-VOX-uh-meen MAL-ee-ate)

Class Antidepressant/Selective serotonin inhibitor

How Supplied
Luvox Tablets 25 mg, Tablets 50 mg, Tablets 100 mg

✤ *Apo-Fluvoxamine* ◆ *Novo-Fluvoxamine* ◆ *Nu-Fluvoxamine* ◆ *PMS-Fluvoxamine* ◆ *ratio-Fluvoxamine*

Action
PHARMACOLOGY: Inhibits neuronal reuptake of serotonin in brain.

PHARMACOKINETICS/DYNAMICS:

Absorption: Absolute bioavailability is 53%. At steady-state, T_{max} is 3 to 8 hr and C_{max} is 88 to 546 ng/mL.

Distribution: Mean apparent Vd is about 25 L/kg and fluvoxamine is about 80% protein bound.

Metabolism: Fluvoxamine is extensively metabolized by the liver. The main routes are oxidative demethylation and deamination of 9 metabolites; the major metabolite is fluvoxamine acid.

Excretion: About 2% is excreted unchanged in the urine. Mean t½ is 15.6 hr at steady-state.

Special Populations:
Hepatic Function Impairment – 30% decrease in Cl.

Indications Treatment of obsessive-compulsive disorder as defined in DSM-III-R.

Contraindications Do not use within 14 days of starting or stopping MAO inhibitors or in combination with cisapride or pimozide.

Route/Dosage
ADULTS: **PO** 50 mg as a single dose at bedtime initially.
Usual range: 100 to 300 mg/day. Increase dose in 50-mg increments q 4 to 7 days, as tolerated, until max therapeutic benefit is achieved (max, 300 mg/day). Give total daily doses more than 100 mg in 2 divided doses; if doses are unequal, give larger dose at bedtime.
Maintenance: Dosage is adjusted to maintain patient on lowest effective dosage. Periodically reassess need to continue treatment.
CHILDREN (8 TO 17 YR): **PO** Start with 25 mg as a single daily dose at bedtime.
Usual range: 50 to 200 mg/day. Increase dose in 25-mg increments q 4 to 7 days, as tolerated, until max therapeutic benefit is achieved (max, 200 mg/day). Give total daily doses of more than 50 mg in 2 divided doses; if doses are unequal, give larger dose at bedtime.

Interactions
5-HT$_1$ agonists (eg, naratriptan, rizatriptan, sumatriptan, zolmitriptan): Weakness, hyperreflexia, and incoordination have been reported rarely.
Cisapride, pimozide: Increased plasma concentrations of cisapride cause QT prolongation and have been associated with sometimes fatal torsades de pointes-type ventricular tachycardia.
Cyproheptadine: May antagonize the effects of fluvoxamine.
Lithium, tryptophan: May enhance serotonergic effects of fluvoxamine.
MAO inhibitors: Similar selective serotonin inhibitors can cause serious (sometimes fatal) reactions. Do not give fluvoxamine in combination with MAO inhibitors or less than 14 days of discontinuation of MAO inhibitors. After stopping fluvoxamine, wait at least 2 wk before starting MAO inhibitors.
Smoking: Increases metabolism of fluvoxamine.
Sympathomimetics (eg, amphetamine), St. John's wort: May increase the risk of serotonin syndrome.
Warfarin, clozapine, tricyclic antidepressants, benzodiazepines (eg, alprazolam, diazepam, midazolam, triazolam), carbamazepine, methadone, metoprolol, propranolol, theophylline, tacrine, cyclosporine: Plasma levels of these drugs may be increased.

Lab Test Interferences None well documented.

Adverse Reactions

CV: Palpitations, vasodilation (eg, feeling warm or flushed) (3%).
CNS: Headache, somnolence (22%); insomnia (21%); nervousness (12%); dizziness (11%); tremor, anxiety (5%); hypertonia, agitation, decreased libido, depression, stimulation (2%).
DERM: Sweating (7%).
EENT: Taste perversion, amblyopia (3%).
GI: Nausea (40%); dry mouth (14%); diarrhea (11%); constipation, dyspepsia (10%); anorexia (6%); vomiting (5%); flatulence (4%); tooth discoloration (3%); dysphagia (2%).
GU: Abnormal ejaculation (8%); urinary frequency (3%); impotence, anorgasmia (2%); urinary retention (1%).
METAB: Hyponatremia.
RESP: Upper respiratory tract infection (9%); dyspnea, yawn (2%).
OTHER: Asthenia (14%); flu-like syndrome (3%); chills (2%).

Precautions

Pregnancy: Category C.
Lactation: Excreted in breast milk.
Children: Safety and efficacy in patients less than 8 yr have not been established.
Elderly: Because of decreased drug Cl, reduce initial dose and titrate slowly.
Hepatic function impairment: Because of decreased drug Cl, reduce initial dose and titrate slowly.
Cognitive and motor performance: Caution patients in operating potentially hazardous machinery (eg, driving) until they know whether the drug impairs their ability. Avoid use of alcohol.
Concomitant illness: Caution is advised in patients with diseases or conditions that could affect hemodynamic responses or metabolism (eg, liver dysfunction).
Mania/Hypomania: Fluvoxamine may activate hypomania or mania. Use cautiously in patients with history of mania.
Seizures: Use with caution in patients with history of seizures. Seizures have been reported in small numbers of patients given this drug.
Suicide: Supervise depressed patients at risk during initial therapy. Prescribe the smallest quantity consistent with good patient management in order to reduce the risk of overdose.

Overdosage: Signs and Symptoms

Drowsiness, vomiting, diarrhea, dizziness, coma, tachycardia, bradycardia, hypotension, ECG abnormalities, liver function abnormalities, convulsions, complications such as aspiration pneumonitis, respiratory difficulties, or hypokalemia caused by unconsciousness or vomiting.

PATIENT CARE CONSIDERATIONS

Administration/Storage

- Do not administer with or within 14 days of MAO inhibitor administration.
- Administer prescribed dose qd, preferably at bedtime. Administer without regard to meals but administer with food if GI upset occurs.
- Administer total daily doses greater than 100 mg in 2 divided doses. If doses are not equal, administer larger dose at bedtime.
- Increase dose no more often than q 4 to 7 days. Do not exceed 300 mg/day.
- Store tablets at controlled room temperature (59° to 86°F). Protect from moisture.

Assessment/Interventions

- Obtain patient history, including drug history and any known allergies. Note mania, liver disease, seizure disorder, concurrent or recent (eg, within 14 days) use of MAO inhibitor, or concurrent use of terfenadine, astemizole, cisapride, or pimozide.
- Ensure that reduced initial dose and slower dose escalation are used in elderly patient or patient with liver dysfunction.
- Ensure that serum electrolytes, BUN, and creatinine are regularly evaluated in patient with SIADH, edema, adrenal disease, or condition associated with fluid loss.
- Continue suicide monitoring of high-risk patient.
- Ensure that growth and weight are monitored in pediatric patient on long-term therapy.
- Frequently assess patient for response to treatment. Notify health care provider if condition does not appear to be improving or is worsening.
- Ensure that therapy is periodically reviewed to determine if therapy needs to be continued without change or if a dose change (eg, increase, decrease, discontinuation) is indicated.
- Observe for signs of mood change and report to health care provider.
- Monitor patient for CNS, GI, psychiatric, MUSC, GU, and general body side effects. Report to health care provider if noted and significant.

Patient/Family Education

- Explain name, dose, action, and potential side effects of drug.
- Advise patient to read *Patient Information* leaflet before starting therapy and with each refill.
- Advise patient that medication is usually started at a low dose and then gradually increased until max benefit is obtained.

- Advise patient taking qd dose to take at bedtime.
- Advise patient to take prescribed dose without regard to meals, but to take with food if stomach upset occurs.
- Advise patient to not change the dose or stop taking unless advised by health care provider.
- Inform patient that it may take 1 to 4 wk to note improvement in symptoms and to continue with the prescribed therapy once improvement has been noted.
- Instruct patient to contact health care provider if symptoms do not appear to be getting better, are getting worse, or if bothersome side effects (eg, unusual sweating, headache, drowsiness, insomnia, nausea, diarrhea, nervousness, changes in sexual function) occur.
- Advise patient to take frequent sips of water, suck on ice chips or sugarless hard candy, or chew sugarless gum if dry mouth occurs.
- Instruct patient to avoid alcoholic beverages and other depressants while taking this medication.
- Advise patient that drug may impair judgment, thinking, or reflexes and to use caution while driving or performing other tasks requiring mental alertness until tolerance is determined.
- Instruct patient not to take prescription or OTC drugs or dietary supplements without consulting with health care provider.
- Advise women to notify health care provider if pregnant, planning to become pregnant, or breastfeeding.
- Advise patient that follow-up visits may be necessary to monitor therapy and to keep appointments.

Folic Acid

(FOE-lik AH-sid)

Class Vitamin

How Supplied
Folvite Tablets 0.4 mg, Tablets 0.8 mg, Tablets 1 mg, Injection 5 mg/mL
✢ *Apo-Folic*

Action

PHARMACOLOGY: Required for nucleoprotein synthesis and maintenance of normal erythropoiesis; precursor of tetrahydrofolic acid, which is necessary for tranformylation reactions in the biosynthesis of purines and thymidylates of nucleic acids.

PHARMACOKINETICS/DYNAMICS:

Absorption: T_{max} occurs within 1 hr. Absorption occurs primarily in the proximal portion of the small intestine.

Metabolism: Folic acid is metabolized in the liver to 7,8-dihydrofolic acid and eventually to 5,6,7,8-tetrahydrofolic acid.

Excretion: Up to 90% is excreted in the urine and small amounts in the feces.
Therapeutic concentrations – Normal serum levels of folate are about 5 to 15 ng/mL; the CSF levels are about 16 to 21 ng/mL.

Special Populations:
Lactation – Folic acid is excreted in breast milk.

Indications Megaloblastic anemia caused by folic acid deficiency as may be seen in tropical or nontropical sprue in anemias of nutritional origin, pregnancy, infancy, or childhood.

Contraindications Treatment of pernicious anemia and other megalobastic anemias where vitamin B_{12} is deficient (not effective).

Route/Dosage

Therapeutic Dose
ADULTS AND CHILDREN: PO/IV/IM/SC Up to 1 mg/day. May need to be increased in alcoholism, hemolytic anemia, anticonvulsant therapy, or chronic infection.

Maintenance Dose
ADULTS AND CHILDREN AT LEAST 4 YR: PO/IV/IM/SC 0.4 mg/day.
PREGNANT AND LACTATING WOMEN: 0.8 mg/day
CHILDREN LESS THAN 4 YR: PO/IV/IM/SC Up to 0.3 mg/day.
INFANTS: PO/IV/IM/SC 0.1 mg/day.

Interactions

Aminosalicylic acid: Reduced folic acid levels.
Folic acid antagonists (eg, methotrexate): Reduced effect of folic acid.
Phenytoin: Reduced effect due to folic acid.
Sulfasalazine: May reduce absorption of folic acid.

Lab Test Interferences None well documented.

Adverse Reactions Adverse effects are rare.
HYPERSEN: Hypersensitivity reactions rarely have occurred and have included erythema, skin rash, itching, general malaise, and bronchospasm.

Precautions

Pregnancy: Category A. Folic acid is recommended for women who are contemplating pregnancy or who are pregnant to avoid birth defects due to deficiency.
Lactation: Secreted into breast milk.
Special risk patients: May obscure signs of pernicious anemia.
Alcoholism: Dosage may need to be increased.

Folic Acid/Cobalamin/Pyridoxine Hydrochloride

(FOLE-ic acid//koe-BAL-uh-min/peer-ih-DOX-een HIGH-droe-KLOR-ide)

Class Nutritional combination

How Supplied
Foltx Tablets 25 mg vitamin B_6, 1 mg vitamin B_{12}, 2.5 mg folic acid

Action
PHARMACOLOGY:
Folic acid and cobalamin: Reduces homocysteine by metabolizing it to methionine.
Pyridoxine: Facilitates breakdown of homocysteine to cysteine and other byproducts.

Indications For nutritional requirement of patients with end-stage renal failure, dialysis, hyperhomocysteinemia, homocystinuria, nutrient malabsorbtion or inadequate dietary intake, particularly for patients with or at risk for cardiovascular disease, cerebrovascular disease, peripheral vascular disease, arteriosclerotic vascular disease, neurological disorders, Alzheimer disease, and renal disease.

Contraindications Standard considerations.

Route/Dosage
ADULTS: **PO** 1 tablet qd or as directed by health care provider.

PATIENT CARE CONSIDERATIONS

Administration/Storage
- Administer prescribed dose qd without regard to meals. Administer with food if GI upset occurs.
- Store tablets at controlled room temperature (59° to 86°F). Protect from light and moisture.

Assessment/Interventions
- Obtain patient history, including drug history and any known allergies.
- Monitor patient for GI, CNS, and general body side effects. Inform health care provider if noted and significant.

Patient/Family Education
- Explain name, dose, action, and potential side effects of drug.

Interactions
Hydantoins (eg, phenytoin): Pharmacologic effect of hydantoins may be decreased.
Levodopa: Pharmacologic activity of levodopa may be antagonized (interaction does not occur with levodopa/carbidopa combination with pyridoxine).

Lab Test Interferences
Pyridoxine: May result in false-positive urobilinogen in the spot test using Ehrlich's reagent.

Adverse Reactions
CV: Peripheral vascular thrombosis.
CNS: Paresthesia; somnolence.
DERM: Itching; transitory exanthema.
GI: Mild transient diarrhea.
HEMA: Polycythemia vera.
OTHER: Allergy; feeling of body swelling.

Precautions
Lactation:
Folic acid – Excreted in breast milk.
Cobalamin – Excreted in breast milk.
Pyridoxine – Excreted in breast milk and may inhibit lactation.
Pernicious anemia: Folic acid may obscure pernicious anemia; however, cyanocobalamin present in product should address this precaution.

Overdosage: Signs and Symptoms
Pyridoxine: Ataxia, sensory neuropathy.

- Instruct patient to take prescribed dose qd.
- Advise patient that medication can be taken without regard to meals, but to take with food if GI upset occurs.
- Caution patient not to change the dose or stop taking unless advised by health care provider.
- Advise patient to notify health care provider if any of the following are noted: rash, itching, drowsiness, abnormal skin or body sensations, diarrhea.
- Caution patient not to take any prescription or OTC medications or dietary supplements unless advised by health care provider.
- Advise patient that follow-up visits may be necessary and to keep appointments.

Follitropin Alfa

(fole-lih-TROE-pin AL-fah)

Class Sex hormone/Ovulation stimulant

How Supplied
Gonal-f Powder for injection, lyophilized 82 units follicle-stimulating hormone (FSH) activity (to deliver 75 units), Powder for injection, lyophilized 600 units FSH activity (to deliver 450 units), Powder for injection, lyophilized 1,200 units FSH activity (to deliver 1,050 units) ◆ *Gonal-f RFF Pen* Injection 415 units FSH activity (to deliver at least 300 units per 0.05 mL), Injection 568 units FSH activity (to deliver at least 450 units per 0.75 mL), Injection 1,026 units FSH activity (to deliver at least 900 units per 1.5 mL)

Action

Pharmacology: Stimulates ovarian follicular growth in women who do not have primary ovarian failure.

Pharmacokinetics/Dynamics:

Absorption: T_{max} is about 25 hr for an IM dose and about 16 hr for a subcutaneous dose. AUC is about 206 units•hr/L for an IM dose and about 176 units•hr/L for a subcutaneous dose. C_{max} is about 3 units/L and about 9 units/L at steady state. Bioavailability is about 76% for IM dosing and about 66% for subcutaneous dosing.

Distribution: Mean Vd is 10 L.

Excretion: Total Cl is 0.6 L/hr for an IV dose. The t½ is about 50 hr for an IM dose and about 24 hr for a subcutaneous dose.

Indications
Induction of ovulation and pregnancy in anovulatory infertile patients in whom the cause of infertility is functional and not caused by primary ovarian failure; to stimulate development of multiple follicles in ovulatory patients undergoing assisted reproductive therapy (ART [eg, in vitro fertilization]); induction of spermatogenesis in men with primary and secondary hypogonadotropic hypogonadism in whom the cause of infertility is not primary testicular failure (except prefilled pen).

Contraindications
Women and men who exhibit the following: 1) prior hypersensitivity to recombinant FSH preparations or 1 of their excipients; 2) high levels of FSH indicating primary ovarian failure; 3) uncontrolled thyroid or adrenal dysfunction; 4) an organic intracranial lesion such as a pituitary tumor; 5) sex hormone-dependent tumors of the reproductive tract and accessory organs; and in women who exhibit: 6) abnormal uterine bleeding of undetermined origin; 7) ovarian cyst or enlargement of undetermined origin; and 8) pregnancy.

Route/Dosage

Ovulation Induction
ADULTS: **Subcutaneous** Initial dose of first cycle is 75 units/day; an incremental dosage adjustment of up to 37.5 units may be considered after 14 days. Further dose increases of 37.5 units may be made q 7 days if necessary. Treatment duration should not exceed 35 days unless serum estradiol increase indicates imminent follicular development. To complete follicular development and effect ovulation in the absence of an endogenous LH surge, administer 5,000 units human chorionic gonadotropin (hCG) 1 day after last dose of follitropin alfa. Withhold hCG if serum estradiol is over 2,000 pg/mL. In subsequent cycles, individualize initial dose for each patient. Max daily dose is 300 units.

Follicle Stimulation
ADULTS: **Subcutaneous** 150 units/day started in early follicular phase (cycle day 2 or 3) until sufficient follicular development is attained (in most cases therapy should not exceed 10 days). In patients undergoing ART whose endogenous gonadotropin levels are suppressed, initiate follitropin alfa at a dose of 150 units/day (under 35 yr of age) or 225 units/day (35 yr of age and older). Continue treatment until adequate follicular development is indicated as determined by ultrasound in combination with serum estradiol level measurements. Consider adjusting the dose after 5 days based on patients response; adjust subsequent dosages q 3 to 5 days and by no more than 75 to 150 units additionally at each adjustment (max, 450 units/day). Administer hCG (5,000 to 10,000 units) once adequate follicular development is evident.

Spermatogenesis
ADULTS: Pretreat with hCG alone (1,000 to 2,250 units 2 to 3 times/wk). Continue hCG for a period sufficient to achieve serum testosterone levels within normal range, which may take 3 to 6 mo. It may be necessary to increase the hCG dose to achieve normal testosterone levels. After normal testosterone levels are reached, follitropin alfa may be administered. **Subcutaneous** 150 units follitropin alfa 3 times/wk and hCG 1,000 units 3 times/wk. If azoospermia persists, the follitropin alfa dose may be increased to a max of 300 units 3 times/wk. It may be necessary to administer therapy for up to 18 mo to achieve adequate spermatogenesis.

Interactions
None well documented.

Lab Test Interferences
None well documented.

Adverse Reactions
CV: Palpitation (2%).
CNS: Headache (22%); emotional lability (5%); migraine (4%); dizziness (3%); anorexia, anxiety, somnolence, fatigue (2%).
DERM: Acne (4%); injection site pain (3%); pruritus (2%).
EENT: Rhinitis (7%); pharyngitis (3%).
GI: Nausea (14%); abdominal pain (9%); diarrhea (8%); flatulence (7%); vomiting (3%); dyspepsia, paresthesia, constipation, ulcerative stomatitis (2%).
GU: Ovarian cyst (15%); intermenstrual bleeding (9%); ovarian hyperstimulation (7%); female breast pain, vaginal hemorrhage (4%); dysmenorrhea, cervix lesion, genital moniliasis, menstrual disorder (3%); genital pruritus, leukorrhea, UTI, ovarian disorder, micturition frequency (2%).
METAB: Weight increase (4%).
RESP: Upper respiratory tract infection (12%); sinusitis (5%); coughing, dyspnea (2%).
OTHER: Pain (6%); back pain (5%);

influenza-like symptoms, fever (4%); enlarged abdomen, chest pain, tooth disorder, thirst, myalgia, hot flashes, malaise (2%); hemoptysis; pilonidal cyst; lymphadenopathy; spontaneous abortion; ectopic pregnancy; premature labor; postpartum fever.

Precautions
Pregnancy: Category X.
Lactation: Undetermined.
Children: Safety and efficacy not established.
Health care provider use: Follitropin alfa should be used only by health care providers thoroughly familiar with infertility problems and their management.
Multiple births: In ovulation induction trials, 12.3% of live births were multiple births; in in vitro fertilization clinical trials, 44% of live births were multiple births.
Ovarian enlargement: Mild to moderate uncomplicated ovarian enlargement may occur in about 20% of women treated and generally regresses without treatment within 2 to 3 wk.
Ovarian hyperstimulation syndrome (OHSS): Warning signs include difficulty breathing, severe pelvic pain, nausea, vomiting, rapid weight gain, stomach pain or bloating, diarrhea, and infrequent urination. May progress within 24 hr to several days to become a serious medical event. Treatment must be stopped and patient hospitalized.
Pulmonary and vascular complications: Intravascular thrombosis and embolism can reduce blood flow to critical organs (eg, pulmonary infarct, cerebral vascular occlusion) or the extremities (may cause loss of limbs).

Overdosage: Signs and Symptoms
OHSS, multiple gestations.

PATIENT CARE CONSIDERATIONS
Administration/Storage
- Follitropin alfa stimulates ovarian follicular growth and must be used in conjunction with hCG, which induces ovulation.
- Follitropin alfa must be used in conjunction with hCG to stimulate spermatogenesis.
- Dose and duration of therapy are variable, depending on indication for use and patient response.
- For subcutaneous administration only. Not for intradermal, IM, or IV administration.
- Follow manufacturer's instructions for reconstituting the powder for injection in single- or multi-dose vials using supplied diluent.
- If using prefilled pen, prepare the pen following manufacturer's instructions. Select prescribed dose by turning dosage dial to the proper dose mark on the dial in front of the arrow mark. Load the pen by pulling on injection button and check red dosage confirmation scale on injection button before administering dose.
- If using prefilled pen or multidose vial that has been stored in refrigerator, allow solution to adjust to room temperature before administering dose.
- Do not administer if solution is discolored or cloudy, or if particulate matter is noted.
- Store unopened single-dose ampules in refrigerator (36° to 46°F) or at controlled room temperature (68° to 77°F). Protect from light. Use immediately after reconstitution. Discard any unused solution.
- Store unopened multidose vials in refrigerator or at controlled room temperature. Store reconstituted solution in refrigerator or at controlled room temperature. Protect from light and freezing. Discard any unused solution after 28 days.
- Store prefilled injection pen in refrigerator until dispensed. Upon dispensing, store pen in refrigerator until expiration date, or at controlled room temperature for up to 1 mo or until the expiration date, whichever occurs first. After the first injection, store pen in refrigerator or at controlled room temperature for up to 28 days. Protect from light. Do not freeze. Discard any unused solution after 28 days.

Assessment/Interventions
- Obtain patient history, including drug history and any known allergies.
- Review patient's health history for any condition that could contraindicate follitropin alfa (previous allergic reaction to follitropin alfa, high levels of FSH, uncontrolled thyroid or adrenal dysfunction, intracranial lesion, sex hormone dependent tumors, and in women, abnormal uterine bleeding of undetermined origin, ovarian cyst or enlargement not caused by polycystic ovary syndrome, or pregnancy).
- Ensure women have had a thorough gynecological and endocrinologic evaluation before starting therapy.
- Ensure men have had a thorough medical and endocrinologic evaluation before starting therapy.
- Ensure women and their partners have been advised of the potential risk of multiple births before treatment for ovulation induction or follicle stimulation is started.
- To reduce risk of overstimulation of the ovary in women, ensure ovarian response to therapy is closely monitored (eg, serum estradiol levels and ultrasonography). Do not administer hCG to patient if serum estradiol level is

greater than 2,000 pg/mL. If the ovaries are abnormally enlarged or abdominal pain occurs, discontinue follitropin alfa therapy, do not administer hCG, and caution patient to avoid intercourse.
- Monitor women for signs and symptoms of overstimulation of the ovary (eg, dyspnea, severe pelvic pain, nausea, vomiting, diarrhea, rapid weight gain, abdominal pain or distension, oliguria) during therapy and for 2 wk after hCG has been discontinued. Report to health care provider immediately if noted or suspected.
- Monitor patient for signs and symptoms of thromboembolic events (eg, venous thrombophlebitis, pulmonary embolism, pulmonary infarction, stroke, arterial occlusion). Report to health care provider immediately if noted or suspected.
- Assess patient for CNS, GU, GI, RESP, and general body side effects and injection site reactions. Inform health care provider if noted and significant.

Patient/Family Education
- Explain names, actions, and potential side effects of the treatment regimen, including risk of multiple births. Review the treatment regimen, including duration of treatment and monitoring that will be required.
- If patient will be administering at home, teach patient how to store, prepare, and administer the dose, and dispose of used equipment and supplies. Advise patient to review the *Patient Education Leaflet* that comes with the multidose vials or, if using the prefilled syringe, the *Patient Information Leaflet* that comes with the prefilled pen, before starting therapy.
- Advise patient that if medication has been stored in refrigerator to allow solution to warm to room temperature before administering dose.
- Caution patient not to change the dose or stop taking unless advised by health care provider.
- Caution patient that if a dose is missed not to double the dose to catch up. Advise patient to contact health care provider for further instructions.
- Remind women that drug is administered to promote follicular growth and egg production, and that hCG will need to be administered to induce ovulation.
- Remind men that drug is administered to promote sperm development and that hCG will need to also be administered to normalize testosterone levels.
- Encourage women receiving drug for infertility to have intercourse daily, beginning on the day prior to administration of hCG until ovulation has become apparent.
- Warn women that close monitoring for overstimulation of the ovary is required and to report any of the following immediately to health care provider: difficulty breathing, severe pelvic pain, nausea, vomiting, rapid weight gain, stomach pain or bloating, diarrhea, or infrequent urination.
- Advise patient to inform health care provider of any side effects, symptoms, or physical changes, or bothersome injection site reactions.
- Instruct patient not to take any prescription or OTC medications, herbal preparations, or dietary supplements unless advised by health care provider.
- Advise patient that follow-up visits and laboratory tests will be required to monitor therapy and to keep appointments.

Follitropin Beta

(fole-lih-TROE-pin BAY-tah)

Class Sex hormones/Ovulation stimulation

How Supplied
Follistim Powder for injection, lyophilized 75 IU IFS activity
✤ *Puregon*

Action

PHARMACOLOGY: Stimulates ovarian follicular growth in women who do not have primary ovarian failure.

PHARMACOKINETICS/DYNAMICS:
Absorption: The mean C_{max} is about 4.3 to 11.3 IU/L with IM dosing and about 4.3 to 13.9 IU/L with SC dosing.

Excretion: Mean $t_{1/2}$ is about 26.9 to 43.9 hr and is dose dependent.

Indications For development of multiple follicles in ovulatory patients participating in an assisted reproductive technology (ART) program; for induction of ovulation and pregnancy in anovulatory infertile patients in whom the cause of infertility is functional and not caused by primary ovarian failure.

Contraindications Prior hypersensitivity to recombinant human follicle-stimulating hormone products; high circulating FSH level (indicating primary ovarian failure); uncontrolled thyroid or adrenal dysfunction; tumor of the ovary, breast, uterus, hypothalamus, or pituitary gland; pregnancy; heavy or irregular vaginal bleeding of undetermined origin; ovarian cysts or enlargement not caused by polycystic ovary syndrome.

Route/Dosage
Follicle Stimulation (ART)
ADULTS: **IM/SC** 150 to 225 IU/day for first 4 days of treatment, then adjust dose upon patient's ovarian response. Daily maintenance dosages ranging from 75 to 300 IU for 6 to 12 days is usually sufficient; although longer treatment may be necessary. However, in low or poor responders, maintenance doses of 375 to 600 IU have been administered (max, 600 IU/day). The final maturation of the follicles is induced by administering human chorionic gonadotropin (hCG) at a dose of 5000 to 10,000 IU.

Ovulation Induction
ADULTS: **IM/SC** There are various treatment protocols. In studies using a gradually increasing dosing scheme, treatment was initiated with 75 IU/day for up to 14 days, then the dose was increased 37.5 IU at weekly intervals until follicular growth or serum estradiol levels indicate an adequate response (max, 300 IU). Continue treatment until ultrasonic visualization or serum estradiol determinations indicate pre-ovulatory conditions at least those of normal individuals followed by hCG, 5000 to 10,000 IU. If the ovaries are abnormally enlarged on the last day, hCG must be withheld during this course of treatment.

Interactions None well documented.

Lab Test Interferences None well documented.

Adverse Reactions
CV: Vascular complications (eg, venous thrombosis, cerebral vascular accident, arterial occlusion); tachycardia.
CNS: Dizziness.
DERM: Dry skin; rash; hair loss; hives.
GI: Abdominal discomfort; lower abdominal pain; abdominal pain.
GU: Miscarriage; ovarian hyperstimulation syndrome; ovarian cyst; ectopic pregnancy; vaginal hemorrhage; breast tenderness; ovarian neoplasm (benign and malignant).
RESP: Pulmonary complication (eg, atelectasis, acute respiratory distress syndrome); dyspnea; tachypnea.
OTHER: Injection site pain; hemoperitoneum; adnexal torsion; febrile reactions; flu-like symptoms (eg, fever, chills, musculoskeletal aches, joint pain, nausea, headache, malaise).

Precautions
Pregnancy: Category X.
Lactation: Undetermined.
Children: Safety and efficacy not established.
Elderly: Safety and efficacy in subjects 65 yr and older not established.
Physician use: Product should be used only by physicians experienced in infertility treatment.
Multiple births: In clinical trials, multiple gestation rates were 31% in follicle stimulation (ie, ART) and 8% in ovulation induction.
Ovarian enlargement: To minimize hazards associated with abnormal ovarian enlargement, use the lowest effective dose.
Ovarian hyperstimulation syndrome: Warning signs include pelvic pain, nausea, vomiting, distention, and weight gain. May progress within 24 hr to several days to become a serious medical event.
Pulmonary and vascular complications: May occur, resulting in intravascular thrombosis and embolism, which may reduce blood flow to critical organs (may result in pulmonary infarct) or extremities (which may cause loss of limbs).

Overdosage: Signs and Symptoms
Ovarian hyperstimulation syndrome, multiple gestations.

PATIENT CARE CONSIDERATIONS
Administration/Storage
- Follow manufacturer's instructions for reconstituting the Powder for Injection. Administer prescribed dose immediately after reconstitution.
- Do not administer if particulate matter or discoloration noted.
- Administer only by IM or SC injection. Not for IV administration.
- With patient lying down or sitting, administer drug by SC or IM injection. Rotate injection sites.
- To minimize bleeding do not rub site after injection.
- Discard any unused reconstituted material.
- Store vials in refrigerator or at controlled room temperature (59° to 86°F). Protect from light.

Assessment/Interventions
- Obtain patient history, including drug history and any known allergies.
- Review patient's health history for any condition that could contraindicate follitropin beta (previous allergic reaction to other recombinant hFSH products, high levels of FSH, uncontrolled thyroid or adrenal dysfunction, intracranial lesion, sex hormone dependent tumors, abnormal uterine bleeding of undetermined origin, ovarian cyst or enlargement of undetermined origin, pregnancy).
- Ensure that patient has had a thorough gynecological and endocrinological evaluation

before starting therapy.
- Monitor patient for signs of overstimulation of the ovary (eg, difficulty breathing, severe pelvic pain, nausea, vomiting, weight gain, stomach pain or bloating, diarrhea, infrequent urination) and report to health care provider immediately if noted.

Patient/Family Education
- Explain name, dose, action, and potential side effects of drug. Review the treatment regimen including duration and monitoring that will be required.
- If patient will be administering at home, teach how to store, prepare, and administer the dose, and dispose of used equipment and supplies.
- Remind patient that drug is administered to promote follicular growth and egg production, and that hCG will need to be administered to induce ovulation.
- Encourage patient receiving drug for infertility to have intercourse daily, beginning on the day prior to administration of hCG until ovulation has become apparent.
- Warn patient that close monitoring for overstimulation of the ovary is required and to report any of the following immediately to health care provider: difficulty breathing, severe pelvic pain, nausea, vomiting, weight gain, stomach pain or bloating, diarrhea, infrequent urination.
- Advise patient that follow-up visits and laboratory tests will be required to monitor therapy and to keep appointments.

Fondaparinux Sodium

(fon-dah-PAH-rin-uck SO-dee-uhm)

Class Anticoagulant

How Supplied
Arixtra Injection 2.5 mg

Action

PHARMACOLOGY: Selective inhibition of antithrombin III (ATIII), which potentiates the innate neutralization of factor Xa by ATIII. Neutralization of factor Xa interrupts the blood coagulation cascade and inhibits thrombin formation and thrombus development.

PHARMACOKINETICS/DYNAMICS:

Absorption: Following SC administration, rapidly and completely absorbed. C_{max} is 0.34 mg/L and is reached in about 2 hr. Peak steady-state plasma level is 0.39 to 0.5 mg/L and is reached approximately 3 hr postdose.

Distribution: Distributes primarily in the blood and to a minor extent in extravascular fluid. Protein binding is at least 94%, specifically to ATIII and does not bind significantly to other plasma protein.

Metabolism: Because the majority of the drug is eliminated unchanged in the urine, the metabolism has not been studied.

Excretion: Up to 77% of an administered dose is eliminated unchanged in the urine within 72 hr. Elimination t½ is 17 to 21 hr.

Special Populations:
Renal Function Impairment – Elimination is prolonged.
Elderly – Elimination is prolonged in patients over 75 yr.
Weight – Total Cl is decreased approximately 30% in patients weighing less than 50 kg.

Indications Prophylaxis of deep vein thrombosis, which may lead to pulmonary embolism in patients undergoing hip fracture surgery, hip replacement surgery, or knee replacement surgery.

Contraindications Patients with severe renal impairment (Ccr less than 30 mL/min); body weight less than 50 kg; active major bleeding, bacterial endocarditis, thrombocytopenia associated with positive in vitro test for antiplatelet antibody in the presence of fondaparinux; hypersensitivity to any component of the product.

Route/Dosage

ADULTS: **SC** 2.5 mg qd. After hemostasis is established, give the initial dose 6 to 8 hr after surgery. Usual duration of therapy is 5 to 9 days.

Interactions

Agents that increase the risk of hemorrhage: Discontinue prior to administration of fondaparinux.

Lab Test Interferences None well documented.

Adverse Reactions

CV: Hypotension (4%).
CNS: Insomnia (5%); dizziness (4%); confusion (3%); headache (2%).
DERM: Rash (8%); purpura (4%); bullous eruption (3%); injection site bleeding; pruritus.
GI: Nausea (11%); constipation (9%); vomiting (6%); diarrhea (3%); dyspepsia (2%).
GU: UTI (4%); urinary retention (3%).
HEMA: Anemia (20%); major bleeding, minor bleeding (3%); postoperative hemorrhage (2%); reoperation caused by bleeding (0.3%); thrombocytopenia.
LABTESTABS: Asymptomatic elevations in ALT (3%) and AST (2%).
METAB: Edema (9%); hypokalemia (4%).
OTHER: Fever (14%); increased wound drainage (5%); hematoma (3%); pain (2%).

> **WARNING:**
> When epidural/spinal anesthesia or spinal puncture is employed in patients anticoagulated with fondaparinux, the risk of developing an epidural or spinal hematoma, which can result in long-term or permanent paralysis, is increased.

Precautions
Pregnancy: Category B.
Lactation: Undetermined.
Children: Safety and efficacy not established.
Elderly: Use with caution.
Renal function impairment: Risk of hemorrhage increases with increasing renal impairment.
Special risk patients: Use with caution in the elderly and in patients with bleeding diathesis, uncontrolled arterial hypertension, history of recent GI ulceration, diabetic retinopathy, hemorrhage, history of heparin-induced thrombocytopenia.
Lab test abnormalities: Discontinue if unexpected changes in coagulation parameters or major bleeding occur; periodic, routine CBCs (including platelet count), serum creatinine level and stool occult blood tests are recommended.
Hemorrhage: Use with caution in conditions of increased risk of hemorrhage (eg, congenital bleeding disorder, active ulcerative GI disease).
Thrombocytopenia: Can occur.

Overdosage: Signs and Symptoms
Hemorrhagic complications

PATIENT CARE CONSIDERATIONS
Administration/Storage
- For SC administration only. Not for intradermal, IM, or IV administration.
- Prescribed dose is administered q 24 hr.
- Rotate injection sites between left and right anterolateral or posterolateral abdominal wall.
- Administer initial dose 6 to 8 hr after surgery.
- Inspect solution visually before administration. Do not administer if solution is cloudy, discolored, or contains particulate matter.
- Follow manufacturer's instructions for preparing syringe, administering dose, and discarding the prefilled syringe.
- Do not expel air bubble from syringe before administration.
- Do not mix with other injections or infusions.
- Fondaparinux cannot be used interchangeably with heparin, low molecular weight heparins, or heparinoids.
- Store syringes at controlled room temperature (59° to 86°F).

Assessment/Interventions
- Obtain patient history, including drug history and any known allergies. Note body weight, renal impairment, recent puncture of organ or noncompressible vessel, congenital or acquired bleeding disorder, active ulcerative or angiodysplastic GI disease, hemorrhagic stroke, uncontrolled hypertension, diabetic retinopathy, recent intracerebral, spinal or ophthalmological surgery, bacterial endocarditis, recent major bleeding, concurrent therapy with agents that may increase the risk of hemorrhage (eg, Dextran 40, thrombolytics, anticoagulants, platelet inhibitors), and history of heparin-induced thrombocytopenia.
- Note any condition that would contraindicate use of fondaparinux (Ccr less than 30 mL/min, body weight less than 50 kg, active major bleeding, bacterial endocarditis, thrombocytopenia with antiplatelet antibody in presence of fondaparinux).
- Ensure that patient is evaluated for bleeding risk before initiating therapy.
- Ensure that first dose is administered no less than 6 hr following surgery.
- Discontinue any agent that could increase risk of hemorrhage prior to initiating fondaparinux therapy (eg, Dextran 40, thrombolytics, anticoagulants, platelet inhibitors). If coadministration cannot be avoided, ensure that patient is monitored closely with clinical assessment for bleeding.
- Ensure that renal function is periodically assessed during therapy. Discontinue fondaparinux immediately if severe renal impairment (Ccr less than 30 mL/min) or labile renal function is noted.
- Ensure that CBC and platelet count is assessed periodically during therapy. Discontinue fondaparinux if platelet count falls below 100,000/mm^3.
- If patient has concurrent epidural spinal anesthesia/analgesia, ensure that catheter is placed prior to initiating fondaparinux therapy and is removed when the anticoagulant effect of fondaparinux is low. Frequently assess patient with epidural catheter for signs or symptoms of spinal hematoma (midline back pain, numbness or weakness in lower extremities, bowel and/or bladder dysfunction). Notify health care provider immediately if spinal hematoma is suspected.
- Monitor patient for signs of bleeding throughout therapy. If bleeding develops (epistaxis, hematuria, hematemesis, bloody or black, tarry stools) or is suspected (unexplained fall in hematocrit or BP or any unexplained

symptoms), notify health care provider immediately.
* Assess patient for GI, CNS, and general body side effects. Inform health care provider if noted and significant.

Patient/Family Education
* Explain name, action, and potential side effects of drug.
* Advise patient, family, or caregiver that medication will be prepared and administered by a health care professional in a hospital setting.
* Instruct patient or family member to report any signs of bleeding or allergic reaction immediately.
* Instruct patient with epidural catheter to immediately report any of the following: midline back pain, numbness or weakness in lower extremities, bowel and/or bladder dysfunction.

Formoterol Fumarate

(fore-MOE-ter-ole FEW-mah-rate)

Class Bronchodilator/Sympathomimetic

How Supplied
Foradil Aerolizer Inhalation powder in capsules 12 mcg (as fumarate)
✤ *Oxeze Turbuhaler*

Action
PHARMACOLOGY: Relaxes bronchial smooth muscles.

PHARMACOKINETICS/DYNAMICS:
Absorption: C_{max} is 92 pg/mL and T_{max} is 5 min.
Distribution: Protein binding is 61% to 64%.
Metabolism: Formoterol is primarily metabolized by direct glucuronidation and o-demethylation by cytochrome P450 2D6, 2C19, 2C9, and 2A6 isozymes.
Excretion: About 10% is excreted unchanged in the urine and about 15% to 18% is excreted in the urine as conjugates. The mean t½ is 10 hr.
Duration: 12 hr.
Special Populations:
Children – About 6% is excreted unchanged and 6.5% to 9% as conjugates in the urine.
COPD – About 7% excreted unchanged in urine and 6% to 9% as conjugates.

Indications Long-term maintenance treatment of asthma; prevention of bronchospasms; prevention of exercise-induced bronchospasm; concomitant therapy with short-acting beta$_2$-agonists, inhaled or systemic corticosteroids, and theophylline therapy; long-term administration in the maintenance of bronchoconstriction in patients with chronic obstructive pulmonary disease (COPD), including chronic bronchitis and emphysema.

Contraindications Standard considerations.

Route/Dosage
Maintenance Treatment of Asthma
ADULTS AND CHILDREN AT LEAST 5 YR: Inhalation 12 mcg q 12 hr.

Prevention of Exercise-Induced Bronchospasm
ADULTS AND CHILDREN AT LEAST 12 YR: Inhalation 12 mcg 15 min prior to exercise given on an occasional, as-needed basis.

Maintenance Treatment of COPD
ADULTS: Inhalation 12 mcg q 12 hr (max, 24 mcg/24 hr).

Interactions
Diuretics, steroids, xanthine derivatives: May potentiate the hypokalemic effect of formoterol.
Nonpotassium sparing diuretics (eg, loop or thiazide diuretics): ECG changes and hypokalemia may be worsened by formoterol.
MAOIs, tricyclic antidepressants, drugs known to prolong the QT_c interval: Formoterol may potentiate these agents, increasing the risk of cardiac arrhythmia.
Beta blockers: Effects of both agents may be inhibited.

Lab Test Interferences None well documented.

Adverse Reactions
CV: Angina; hypertension; hypotension; tachycardia; arrhythmias; palpitations.
CNS: Nervousness; headache; tremor; dizziness; fatigue; malaise; insomnia; dysphoria.
EENT: Rhinitis; tonsillitis.
GI: Dry mouth; nausea; gastroenteritis; abdominal pain; dyspepsia.
METAB: Hypokalemia; hyperglycemia; metabolic acidosis.
OTHER: Muscle cramps; chest infection; viral infection.

Precautions
Pregnancy: Category C.
Lactation: Undetermined.
Children: Safety and efficacy in children less than 5 yr not established.
Cardiovascular effects: Because formoterol can produce clinically important cardiovascular effects, use with caution in patients with cardiovascular disorders, especially coronary insufficiency, cardiac arrhythmia, and hypertension.
Paradoxical bronchospasm: If paradoxical bronchospasm occurs, discontinue formoterol and institute alternative therapy.

Acute worsening or deteriorating asthma: Use of formoterol in these conditions is inappropriate.

Overdosage: Signs and Symptoms
Angina, hypertension, hypotension, tachycardia, arrhythmias, nervousness, headache, tremor, seizures, muscle cramps, dry mouth, palpitation, nausea, dizziness, fatigue, malaise, hypokalemia, hyperglycemia, insomnia, metabolic acidosis, cardiac arrest, death.

PATIENT CARE CONSIDERATIONS

Administration/Storage
- This medication is available only as a dry powder for oral inhalation.
- Administer only with supplied inhaler.
- Do not use a spacer with the inhalation powder. Keep inhaler dry and never wash. Store medication-filled capsules in their blisters and only remove immediately before using. Capsules are for inhalation only and should not be swallowed.
- Store capsules in blisters at controlled room temperature. Protect from heat and moisture.

Assessment/Interventions
- Obtain patient history, including drug history and any known allergies. Note history of coronary artery disease, arrhythmias, hypertension, or seizures.
- Ensure that baseline pulmonary function tests have been completed.
- Note frequency and severity of asthma attacks.

Patient/Family Education
- Explain name, dose, action, and potential side effects of drug.
- Instruct patient on the proper storage and use of the dry powder inhaler, referring to the instruction sheet included with the medication.
- Remind patient that capsules should only be used with the *Aerolizer Inhaler* and should not be taken by mouth.
- Inform patient to never wash the *Aerolizer Inhaler* and to have dry hands when handling the capsules containing the medication.
- Advise patient using more than 1 inhaled medication to use short-acting bronchodilator medication first if needed and then use this medicine. Take inhaled corticosteroids or other inhaled controller medications last.
- Remind patient that this medicine should not be used more frequently than bid (morning and evening) for maintenance treatment of asthma.
- Remind patient that if using this medicine to prevent exercise-induced bronchospasm, to use at least 15 min before exercise and not to take additional doses for at least 12 hr.
- Remind patient that this medication is not a "rescue medication" and is not to be used for the treatment of acute or deteriorating asthma.
- Advise patient if asthma symptoms worsen immediately after using this medication, to stop using it and inform health care provider immediately.
- Inform patient that formoterol is not a substitute for inhaled or oral corticosteroids and not to stop or reduce the dose of their corticosteroid medication.
- Advise patient to contact health care provider if medication no longer seems to control asthma symptoms or if increasing doses of the short-acting bronchodilator ("rescue" medicine) are needed. This may indicate worsening asthma.

Fosamprenavir Calcium
(FOSS-am-PREN-ah-veer KAL-see-uhm)

Class Antiviral

How Supplied
Lexiva Tablets 700 mg (equivalent to 600 mg amprenavir)

Action
PHARMACOLOGY: Fosamprenavir is a prodrug of amprenavir that inhibits HIV protease, the enzyme required to form functional proteins in HIV-infected patients.

PHARMACOKINETICS/DYNAMICS:
Absorption: As fosamprenavir is absorbed, it is rapidly hydrolyzed to amprenavir by enzymes in the gut epithelium. T_{max} is between 1.5 and 4 hr. C_{max} is about 4.82 mcg/mL. AUC is approximately 33 mcg•hr/mL. C_{min} is approximately 0.35 mcg/mL.

Distribution: Approximately 90% protein bound, primarily to alpha$_1$-acid glycoprotein.

Metabolism: After oral administration, fosamprenavir is rapidly and almost completely hydrolyzed to amprenavir, which is metabolized in the liver by CYP3A4.

Excretion: Approximately 1% excreted unchanged in the urine. About 14% and 75% (with more than 90% as metabolites) of an administered dose of amprenavir excreted in the urine and feces, respectively. The t½ is approximately 7.7 hr.

Special Populations:

Hepatic Function Impairment – Moderate cirrhosis increases AUC, while severe cirrhosis increases AUC and C_{max}. Patients with impaired hepatic function may require dosage reduction.

Indications Treatment of HIV infections in combination with other antiretroviral agents.

Contraindications Coadministration with drugs highly dependent on CYP3A4 for clearance and for which elevated plasma concentrations are associated with serious and/or life-threatening events (eg, ergot derivatives [eg, ergonovine]), GI motility agent, neuroleptic agent (eg, pimozide), and sedative/hypnotics (eg, midazolam, triazolam); when administered with ritonavir, flecainide and propafenone are contraindicated; hypersensitivity to any component of this product or to amprenavir.

Route/Dosage

Therapy-Naïve Patients

ADULTS: PO 1400 mg bid without ritonavir; 1400 mg qd plus 200 mg ritonavir qd; 700 mg bid plus ritonavir 100 mg bid.

Protease Inhibitor-Experienced Patients

ADULTS: PO 700 mg bid plus ritonavir 100 mg bid. Once-daily administration of fosamprenavir plus ritonavir is not recommended in protease inhibitor-experienced patients.

Hepatic Impairment

ADULTS: PO In patients with mild or moderate hepatic impairment receiving fosamprenavir without ritonavir reduce dosage to 700 mg bid. Do not use in patients with severe hepatic impairment.

Interactions

Amiodarone, bepridil, systemic lidocaine, quinidine, tricyclic antidepressants (eg, amitriptyline): Plasma levels of these drugs may be increased, resulting in serious and/or life-threatening drug interactions.

Atorvastatin, benzodiazepines (eg, alprazolam, clorazepate, diazepam, flurazepam), calcium channel blockers (eg, amlodipine, diltiazem, felodipine, isradipine, nicardipine, nifedipine, nimodipine, nisoldipine, verapamil), cyclosporine, itraconazole, ketoconazole, oral contraceptives (eg, ethinyl estradiol/norethindrone), rapamycin, rifamycins (eg, rifabutin), tacrolimus: Plasma levels of these agents may be elevated by fosamprenavir, increasing the risk of adverse reactions.

Carbamazepine, corticosteroids (eg, dexamethasone), efavirenz, histamine H_2-receptor antagonists (eg, cimetidine), lopinavir/ritonavir combination, nevirapine, phenobarbital, phenytoin, proton pump inhibitors (eg, omeprazole), saquinavir: Amprenavir plasma levels may be reduced, leading to a decrease in virologic response.

Delavirdine: May lead to loss of virologic response and possible resistance to delavirdine.

Drugs highly dependent on CYP3A4 for clearance (eg, ergot derivatives [eg, dihydroergotamine, ergotamine, ergonovine, methylergonovine]), GI motility agent, neuroleptic agent (eg, pimozide), and sedative/hypnotics (eg, midazolam and triazolam): Administration of these agents with fosamprenavir is contraindicated because of the potential for serious and/or life-threatening reactions.

Flecainide, propafenone: These agents are contraindicated when fosamprenavir is administered with ritonavir.

HMG-CoA reductase inhibitors metabolized by CYP3A4 (eg, lovastatin, simvastatin): Coadministration is not recommended because the risk of myopathy, including rhabdomyolysis, may be increased.

Indinavir, nelfinavir: Amprenavir plasma levels may be elevated, leading to an increase in adverse reactions.

Methadone: Plasma levels may be reduced by fosamprenavir, resulting in a loss of pharmacologic response.

Phosphodiesterase inhibitors (eg, sildenafil, vardenafil): Plasma levels may be increased by amprenavir, increasing the risk of side effects.

Rifampin: Because amprenavir plasma levels may be reduced about 90%, avoid coadministration.

St. John's wort (hypericum perforatum): Amprenavir plasma concentrations may be reduced by St. John's wort, decreasing the clinical efficacy; may lead to loss of virologic response and possible resistance to fosamprenavir or to the class of protease inhibitors.

Warfarin: Because warfarin concentrations may be altered, monitoring of international normalized ratio is recommended.

Lab Test Interferences None well documented.

Adverse Reactions

CNS: Headache (19%); depressive/mood disorders (8%); paresthesia (2%).
DERM: Rash (35%); pruritus (7%); Stevens-Johnson syndrome.

GI: Nausea (39%); diarrhea (34%); vomiting (16%); abdominal pain (5%).
HEMA/LYMPH: Neutropenia (3%); acute hemolytic anemia.
LABTESTABS: Increased serum lipase (8%); increased ALT and AST (6%).
OTHER: Fatigue (10%).

Precautions
Pregnancy: Category C.
Lactation: HIV-infected mothers should not breastfeed their infants.
Children: Safety and efficacy not established.
Elderly: Select dose with caution, reflecting greater frequency of decreased hepatic, renal, or cardiac function and comorbidity.
Hepatic function impairment: Because patients with impaired hepatic function may require dosage reduction, use with caution.

Cross-resistance/Resistance: It is not known what effect fosamprenavir therapy will have on the subsequent administration of protease inhibitors.
Diabetes mellitus/Hyperglycemia: New onset and exacerbation of preexisting diabetes mellitus and hyperglycemia have been reported.
Fat redistribution: Redistribution and accumulation of body fat have been observed in patients receiving fosamprenavir. A causal relationship has not been established.
Hemophilia: Spontaneous bleeding has been reported in patients with hemophilia A and B treated with protease inhibitors.
Sulfa allergy: Because fosamprenavir contains a sulfonamide moiety, use with caution in patients with sulfa allergy.

PATIENT CARE CONSIDERATIONS

Administration/Storage
- Administer prescribed dose without regard to meals. Administer with food if GI upset occurs.
- Store tablets at controlled room temperature (59° to 86°F). Keep tightly capped.

Assessment/Interventions
- Obtain patient history, including drug history and any known allergies. Note sulfonamide allergy, hepatic or renal impairment, diabetes, concurrent infection with hepatitis B or C, hemophilia, concurrent use of medications metabolized by CYP3A (eg, midazolam), concurrent use of medications that induce (eg, rifampin) or inhibit CYP3A4 (eg, St. John's wort), or concurrent use of ergot derivatives, pimozide, midazolam, or triazolam.
- Ensure that medication is used in combination with other antiretroviral agents.
- Review medication history to be sure that patient is currently not taking amprenavir or any medication that would contraindicate the use of fosamprenavir.
- Ensure that reduced dose is administered to patient with moderate hepatic insufficiency.
- Ensure that liver enzymes are determined before starting therapy and periodically during therapy in patient with history of hepatitis B or C infection.
- Ensure that triglycerides and cholesterol are evaluated prior to starting therapy and periodically during treatment.
- Monitor blood sugar in diabetic patient when drug is started or dose is changed. Report significant changes to health care provider.
- Assess patient for GI, CNS, DERM, musculoskeletal, and general body side effects. Inform health care provider if noted and significant.

Patient/Family Education
- Advise patient to read the *Patient Information* leaflet before starting therapy and with each refill.
- Explain name, dose, action, and potential side effects of drug.
- Warn patient that this drug is not to be used by itself but is combined with other antiviral agents and not to change the dose or stop taking any of the antiviral agents unless advised by health care provider.
- Advise patient to take prescribed dose without regard to meals but to take with food if GI upset occurs.
- Advise patient that if a dose is missed by more than 4 hr, to wait and take the next dose at the regular time. If a dose is missed by less than 4 hr, take the missed dose right away and then take the next dose at the regular time. If a dose is skipped, caution patient not to double the dose to catch up but to continue with normal schedule.
- Instruct patient to report the following symptoms immediately to health care provider: rash; persistent nausea, vomiting, or diarrhea; any unusual symptom.
- Inform patient that the drug does not completely eliminate HIV virus and therefore does not reduce risk of transmitting HIV to others. Appropriate precautions must still be taken.
- Advise patient that the drug is not a cure for HIV infection and that illnesses associated with HIV infection (including opportunistic infections) may continue to be acquired. Patients should remain under a physician's care.
- Instruct patient not to take any prescription

or OTC medications or dietary supplements unless advised by health care provider.
- Instruct diabetic patient to monitor blood glucose more frequently when drug is started or dose is changed and to inform health care provider of significant changes in readings.
- Caution women using hormonal contraceptives to use alternative contraceptive measures during therapy because hormonal contraceptive effectiveness may be reduced.
- Advise women to notify health care provider if pregnant, planning to become pregnant, or breastfeeding. Caution HIV-infected mother that breastfeeding can cause HIV infection in the baby.
- Remind patient that examinations and laboratory tests will be required to monitor therapy and to keep appointments.

Foscarnet Sodium (Phosphonoformic Acid)

(foss-CAR-net SO-dee-uhm)

Class Anti-infective/Antiviral

How Supplied
Foscavir Injection 24 mg/mL

Action
PHARMACOLOGY: Inhibits replication of all known herpes viruses, including cytomegalovirus (CMV), herpes simplex virus types 1 and 2 (HSV-1, HSV-2), human herpes virus 6 (HHV-6), Epstein-Barr virus (EBV) and varicella-zoster virus (VZV).

PHARMACOKINETICS/DYNAMICS:
Absorption: C_{max} is about 589 to 623 mcmol. C_{min} is about 63 to 114 mcmol.

Distribution: Protein binding is 14% to 17%. The drug deposits into the bone. Vd is about 0.41 to 0.52 L/kg.

Excretion: Terminal $t_{½}$ is about 87.5 hr. Systemic clearance is about 6.2 to 7.1 L/hr and Cl_R is about 5.6 to 6.4 L/hr. Plasma $t_{½}$ is about 4 hr.

Special Populations:
Renal Function Impairment – Ccr of 50 to 80 mL/min has a Cl of about 1.33 mL/min/kg and a plasma $t_{½}$ of about 3.35 hr. Ccr of 25 to 49 mL/min has a Cl of about 0.46 mL/min/kg and a plasma $t_{½}$ of about 13 hr. Ccr of 10 to 24 mL/min has a Cl of 0.43 mL/min/kg and plasma $t_{½}$ about 25.3 hr.

Indications Treatment of CMV retinitis in patients with AIDS; treatment of acyclovir-resistant mucocutaneous HSV infections in immunocompromised patients; combination therapy with ganciclovir for patients who have relapsed after monotherapy with either drug.

Contraindications Standard considerations.

Route/Dosage
CMV *Retinitis*
ADULTS: IV
Initial dose: 60 mg/kg/dose at constant rate over at least 1 hr q 8 hr for 2 to 3 wk. Adjust for clinical response and renal function.
Maintenance dose: 90 mg/kg/day infused over 2 hr, individualized; max maintenance dose is 120 mg/kg/day.

HSV Infections
ADULTS: IV
Initial dose: 40 mg/kg/dose (min, 1 hr infusion) q 8 or 12 hr for 2 to 3 wk or until healed.
Maintenance: 90 mg/kg/day given as an IV infusion over 2 hr, individualized; max maintenance dose is 120 mg/kg/day.

Interactions
Nephrotoxic drugs: Elimination of foscarnet may be impaired by drugs that inhibit renal tubular secretion. Increased potential for nephrotoxicity with aminoglycosides, amphotericin B, and IV pentamidine.
Pentamidine: Concomitant IV pentamidine may cause hypocalcemia.
Zidovudine: Increased risk of anemia.
INCOMPATIBILITIES: Do not give other drugs or supplements via same IV catheter.

Lab Test Interferences None well documented.

Adverse Reactions
CV: Hypertension; palpitations; ECG abnormalities including sinus tachycardia, first-degree heart block, nonspecific ST-T segment changes; hypotension; flushing; cerebrovascular disorder.
CNS: Headache; paresthesia; dizziness; involuntary muscle contractions; hypoesthesia; neuropathy; seizures; depression; confusion; anxiety;

tremor; ataxia; dementia; stupor; generalized spasms; sensory disturbances; meningitis; aphasia; abnormal coordination; leg cramps; EEG abnormalities; insomnia; somnolence; nervousness; amnesia; agitation; aggressive reaction; hallucination.
DERM: Rash; increased sweating; pruritus; skin ulceration; seborrhea; erythematous or maculopapular rash; skin discoloration; facial edema.
EENT: Vision abnormalities; eye pain; conjunctivitis; sinusitis; rhinitis; taste perversions; pharyngitis.
GI: Anorexia; nausea; diarrhea; vomiting; abdominal pain; constipation; dysphagia; dyspepsia; rectal hemorrhage; dry mouth; melena; flatulence; ulcerative stomatitis; pancreatitis.
GU: Alterations in renal function, including decreased Ccr, abnormal renal function; albuminuria; dysuria; polyuria; urethral disorder; urinary retention; UTI; acute renal failure; nocturia; abnormal albumin-globulin ratio; increased AST and ALT.
HEMA: Anemia; bone marrow suppression; granulocytopenia; leukopenia; thrombocytopenia; platelet abnormalities; thrombosis; WBC abnormalities; lymphadenopathy.
METAB: Mineral and electrolyte imbalances, including hypo- or hypercalcemia, hypokalemia, hypomagnesemia, hypo- or hyperphos-phatemia, hyponatremia; decreased weight; increased alkaline phosphatase, LDH, BUN; acidosis.
RESP: Coughing; dyspnea; pneumonia; respiratory disorders or insufficiency; pulmonary infiltrates; stridor; pneumothorax; hemoptysis; bronchospasm.
OTHER: Fever; fatigue; rigors; asthenia; malaise; arthralgia or myalgia; cachexia; thirst; infection; sepsis; death; back or chest pain; edema; influenza-like symptoms; abscess; lymphoma-like disorders; sarcoma; injection site pain or inflammation.

> **WARNING:**
>
> *Nephrotoxicity:* Major toxicity. Frequent serum creatinine monitoring with dose adjustments for changes in renal function and adequate hydration is essential.
>
> Seizures related to levels of minerals and electrolytes. May require supplementation.

Precautions
Pregnancy: Category C.
Lactation: Undetermined.
Children: Safety and efficacy not studied. Drug is deposited in teeth and bone.
Renal function impairment: If Ccr drops below 0.4 mL/min/kg, discontinue drug.
Mineral and electrolyte imbalances: Patients, especially those on concomitant drugs known to influence serum minerals or electrolytes or those with cardiac or neurological abnormalities, may experience changes in electrolytes (eg, calcium, potassium, magnesium, phosphate) that could cause cardiac disturbances or seizures. Replacement therapy may be needed.
Toxicity/local irritation: Infuse into veins with adequate blood flow to permit rapid dilution and distribution and avoid local irritation. Drug is excreted in urine and may cause irritation or ulceration of penile or vulvovaginal epithelium.

Overdosage: Signs and Symptoms
Electrolyte disturbances, paresthesia, renal dysfunction, seizures, coma.

PATIENT CARE CONSIDERATIONS
Administration/Storage
- Administer by IV infusion only, at rate not to exceed 1 mg/kg/min. Use infusion pump to prevent rapid or bolus injection.
- When administering through central vein, 24 mg/mL solution may be used. In peripheral veins, dilute with D5W or normal saline to 12 mg/mL.
- Administer only with normal saline or D5W; incompatible with many drugs and supplements.
- Do not use same tubing or catheter for any other drug or IV solution.
- Prehydrate patient with 0.9% Sodium Chloride to decrease chance of renal damage.
- Use prepared solutions within 24 hr of first entry into sealed bottle.

Assessment/Interventions
- Obtain patient history, including drug history and any known allergies. Note cardiac, neurologic, or renal disorders.
- Ensure that baseline serum electrolyte levels (eg, calcium, magnesium, potassium, phosphate) have been obtained before beginning therapy, and repeat 2 to 3 times/wk during induction therapy and 1 to 2 times/wk during maintenance therapy.
- Ensure that baseline renal function tests have been obtained before beginning therapy, and repeat 2 to 3 times/wk during induction therapy and 1 to 2 times/wk during maintenance therapy. Dosage will be adjusted or drug discontinued if Ccr decreases.

- Assess renal function before and after administration in elderly patients.
- Monitor I&O and ensure that patient is well hydrated. Note urine pH.
- Monitor for anemia; obtain CBC frequently.
- Monitor for seizures, especially in patients with CNS disorder such as toxoplasmosis or HIV encephalopathy.
- Observe for fever, nausea, diarrhea, vomiting, and headache. Report these and other common side effects to health care provider.
- If symptoms of electrolyte imbalance, such as complaints of perioral tingling, numbness in extremities, or paresthesia occur, notify health care provider immediately. Infusion may need to be discontinued and electrolyte supplementation initiated.

Patient/Family Education
- Emphasize that drug does not cure CMV retinitis but may help prevent worsening of symptoms.
- Explain that good hygiene and drinking plenty of fluids may help reduce risk of genital irritation or ulceration.
- Instruct patient to report the following symptoms to health care provider: perioral tingling, numbness in extremities, paresthesia, fever, nausea, diarrhea, vomiting, headache, increased or decreased frequency or amount of urination, other bothersome side effects.
- Caution patient not to take any otc medications without consulting health care provider. Explain that serious drug interactions may result.

Fosfomycin Tromethamine
(foss-foe-MY-sin troe-METH-ah-meen)

Class Antibiotic

How Supplied
Monurol Granules 3 g

Action
PHARMACOLOGY: Interferes with bacterial cell wall biosynthesis.

PHARMACOKINETICS/DYNAMICS:
Absorption: Absolute bioavailability is 37% while fasting; it is reduced 30% with food. C_{max} is about 26 mcg/mL while fasting; about 17.6 mcg/mL with a high-fat meal. T_{max} is 2 hr, about 4 hr with a high-fat meal.

Distribution: Mean Vd_{ss} is about 136 L. Fosfomycin is 0% protein bound. It distributes to the kidneys, bladder wall, prostate, seminal vesicles, and crosses the placental barrier.

Excretion: About 38% is excreted in urine unchanged and about 18% from the feces. Mean $t_{½}$ is about 5.7 hr.

Special Populations:
Renal Function Impairment – The $t_{½}$ is 40 hr in hemodialysis patients. Patients with Ccr 7 to 54 mL/min have a $t_{½}$ of 11 to 50 hr, and urinary excretion decreases to 11%.

PATIENT CARE CONSIDERATIONS
Administration/Storage
- Never take in dry form; always mix with water.
- Pour the entire contents of the single-dose sachet into 3 to 4 oz of water and stir to dissolve.
- Do not use hot water.
- Administer immediately after mixing.
- May be taken with or without food.

Indications Treatment of uncomplicated UTI (acute cystitis) in women caused by susceptible strains of specific microorganisms.

Contraindications Standard considerations.

Route/Dosage
ADULT WOMEN: **PO** One 3 g sachet dissolved in 3 to 4 oz of cool water.

Interactions
Metoclopramide: May decrease serum concentrations and urinary excretion of fosfomycin.

Lab Test Interferences None well documented.

Adverse Reactions
CNS: Headache; dizziness.
DERM: Rash.
EENT: Rhinitis; pharyngitis.
GI: Diarrhea; nausea; dyspepsia; abdominal pain.
GU: Vaginitis; dysmenorrhea.
OTHER: Asthenia; back pain; pain.

Precautions
Pregnancy: Category B.
Lactation: Undetermined.
Children: Safety and efficacy not established.
Elderly: No dosage adjustment necessary.
Single dose: Do not use more than 1 single dose to treat a single episode of infection.

- Store dry powder at room temperature (59° to 86° F).

Assessment/Interventions
- Obtain patient history, including drug history and any known allergies.
- Obtain urine for C&S prior to starting therapy.
- Obtain results of CBC and other lab tests ordered by health care provider.

- Obtain vital signs. Monitor weight and I&O.
- Evaluate for signs of infection (eg, fever, chills, burning, frequency).
- Monitor patient for side effects of drug. Report any to the health care provider.

Patient/Family Education
- Instruct patient in proper preparation of medication.
- Inform patient that this is a single-dose treatment and repeated doses do not improve the clinical success.
- Advise patient that symptoms should improve in 2 to 3 days after taking drug. If symptoms do not improve, instruct patient to contact health care provider.
- Increase fluid intake to 2,000 to 3,000 mL/day.
- Instruct the patient on proper personal hygiene to help prevent recurrence of infections.

Fosinopril Sodium

(FAH-sin-oh-PRILL SO-dee-uhm)
Class Antihypertensive/ACE inhibitor

How Supplied
Monopril Tablets 10 mg, Tablets 20 mg, Tablets 40 mg

Action
PHARMACOLOGY: Competitively inhibits angiotensin I-converting enzyme, preventing conversion of angiotensin I to angiotensin II, a potent vasoconstrictor that also stimulates release of aldosterone. Results in decrease in BP, reduced sodium reabsorption, and potassium retention.

PHARMACOKINETICS/DYNAMICS:

Absorption: Absolute bioavailability averages 36%. T_{max} is about 3 hr.

Distribution: Protein binding is about 99.4%. Fosinopril does not cross the blood-brain barrier.

Metabolism: The major active metabolite is fosinoprilat.

Excretion: There is approximately equal elimination between the liver and the kidney. The t½ is about 12 hr (fosinoprilat). Cl in hemodialysis is about 2% and about 7% with peritoneal dialysis.

Onset: 1 hr.

Peak: 2 to 12 hr.

Duration: 24 hr.

Indications
Hypertension; heart failure.

Contraindications
Hypersensitivity to ACE inhibitor; history of angioedema related to previous treatment with an ACE inhibitor and in patients with hereditary or idiopathic angioedema.

Route/Dosage
Heart Failure
ADULTS: PO
Initial dose: 10 mg qd. Increase over several weeks. Usual range is 20 to 40 mg/day. Do not exceed 40 mg/day.

Hypertension
ADULTS: PO
Initial dose: 10 mg qd.
Maintenance dose: 20 to 80 mg/day; if inadequate response, consider dividing into 2 doses.
CHILDREN (WEIGHING MORE THAN 50 KG): PO
5 to 10 mg qd as monotherapy.

Interactions
Allopurinol: Increased risk of hypersensitivity reactions.
Antacids: May decrease effects of fosinopril.
Capsaicin: Cough may be exacerbated.
Digoxin: May increase or decrease levels of digoxin.
Indomethacin, salicylates (eg, aspirin): Hypotensive effects may be reduced, especially in low-renin or volume-dependent hypertensive patients.
Lithium: Increased lithium levels and symptoms of lithium toxicity may occur.
Phenothiazines: May increase pharmacologic effect of fosinopril.
Potassium preparations, potassium-sparing diuretics: May increase serum potassium levels.

Lab Test Interferences Measurement of serum digoxin with *DigiTab RIA* kit may be falsely low. False elevation of liver enzymes or serum bilirubin may occur.

Adverse Reactions
CV: Hypotension (4%); orthostatic hypotension (2%); subjective cardiac rhythm disturbance (1%).
CNS: Dizziness (12%); weakness (1%).
GI: Diarrhea (2%); nausea, vomiting (1%).
HEMA: Transient hemoglobin decrease; neutropenia; leukopenia; eosinophilia.
METAB: Hyperkalemia; hyponatremia.
MUSC: Pain (3%).
RESP: Cough (10%); upper respiratory tract infection (2%).
OTHER: Chest pain (2%).

> **WARNING:**
> *Pregnancy:* Use in second and third trimesters may cause injury and death to fetus.

Precautions

Pregnancy: Category D (second, third trimester); Category C (first trimester).
Lactation: Excreted in breast milk.
Children: Safety and efficacy not established in children weighing less than 50 kg.
Elderly: Use with caution, usually starting at the low end of the dose range, because of the greater frequency of decreased hepatic, renal, or cardiac function, and concomitant diseases or other drug therapy.
Renal function impairment: Reduce dose and give less frequently. In renal insufficiency, stable elevations in BUN and serum creatinine may occur because of inadequate renal perfusion; monitor renal function during first few weeks of therapy and adjust dosage.
Hepatic function impairment: May result in elevated plasma levels; monitor carefully; reduce doses.
Angioedema: May occur. Use extreme caution in patients with hereditary angioedema.

PATIENT CARE CONSIDERATIONS

Administration/Storage

- Administer alone or in combination with other antihypertensives.
- Do not administer to pregnant women during second and third trimesters as fetal and neonatal morbidity and death can occur.
- Give prescribed dose without regard to meals. Administer with food if GI upset occurs.
- Store tablets at controlled room temperature (59° to 89°F). Protect from moisture.

Assessment/Interventions

- Obtain patient history, including drug history and any known allergies. Note renal or hepatic impairment, conditions predisposing to volume depletion (eg, prolonged diuretic therapy), diabetes, heart failure, anuria, hereditary or idiopathic angioedema, lupus erythematosus, left ventricular outflow obstruction, allergy to any other ACE inhibitor, and concurrent use of potassium-containing salt substitutes, potassium supplements, or potassium-sparing diuretics.
- Ensure that small initial dose and gradual escalation of dose are used in patient with heart failure and moderate to severe renal impairment (Ccr less than 50 mL/min) or following vigorous diuresis.
- Ensure that volume and/or salt depletion have been corrected before initiating therapy.
- Ensure that serum electrolytes and renal function are monitored periodically.
- Ensure that CBC with differential are evaluated prior to starting therapy, at 2 wk intervals for 3 mo, and periodically thereafter in patient with renal impairment.

Hepatic failure: Rarely, ACE inhibitors have been associated with a syndrome that starts with cholestatic jaundice and progresses to fulminant hepatic necrosis and sometimes death.
Hypotension/First-dose effect: Significant decreases in BP may occur after first dose, especially in severely salt- or volume-depleted patients or those with heart failure; monitor closely for at least 2 hr after initial dose and during first 2 wk of therapy. Minimize risk by discontinuing diuretics, decreasing dose, or increasing salt intake about 1 wk prior to initiating fosinopril.
Neutropenia and agranulocytosis: Have occurred; risk appears greater in patients with renal dysfunction, heart failure, or immunosuppression; monitor WBC counts frequently.
Proteinuria: May occur, especially in patients with prior renal disease or those receiving high doses; generally within 6 mo.

Overdosage: Signs and Symptoms
Hypotension.

- Monitor and record BP and pulse. Should symptomatic hypotension occur, hold medication and notify health care provider.
- Take safety precautions if orthostatic hypotension occurs.
- Assess heart failure patient for evidence of worsening failure (eg, daily weights, evaluation of peripheral edema, shortness of breath). Inform health care provider if rapid weight gain (eg, 2 pounds in 1 day or 5 pounds in 1 wk) is noted or if patient is experiencing worsening edema or other symptoms of heart failure (eg, worsening shortness of breath).
- Monitor for signs of hypersensitivity including angioedema involving swelling of the face, lips, eyelids, and tongue. Discontinue medication and notify health care provider immediately if noted. Be prepared to treat appropriately.
- Assess patient for GI, CNS, and general body side effects. Inform health care provider if noted and significant.

Patient/Family Education

- Explain name, dose, action, and potential side effects of drug.
- Advise patient to take prescribed dose without regard to meals but to take with food if stomach upset occurs.
- Advise patient to try to take each dose at about the same time each day.
- Inform hypertensive patient that drug controls, but does not cure, hypertension and to continue taking drug as prescribed even when BP is not elevated.
- Caution patient not to change the dose or

stop taking unless advised by health care provider.
* Instruct patient to continue taking other medications for the condition as prescribed by health care provider.
* Instruct patient in BP and pulse measurement skills.
* Advise patient to monitor and record BP and pulse at home and to inform health care provider should abnormal measurements be noted. Also advise patient to take record of BP and pulse to each follow-up visit.
* Caution patient to avoid sudden position changes to prevent orthostatic hypotension.
* Instruct patient to lie or sit down if experiencing dizziness or lightheadedness when standing.
* Emphasize to hypertensive patient the importance of other modalities on BP control: weight control, regular exercise, smoking cessation, and moderate intake of alcohol and salt.
* Emphasize to heart failure patient the importance of other modalities that can help control heart failure symptoms: weight control, progressive exercise program, smoking cessation, and moderate intake of alcohol and salt.
* Advise heart failure patient to weigh daily, keep a record of daily weights, and notify health care provider if rapid weight gain (eg, 2 pounds in 1 day or 5 pounds in 1 wk) is noted or if edema or shortness of breath are getting worse.
* Caution patient that inadequate fluid intake, excessive perspiration, diarrhea, or vomiting can lead to excessive fall in BP, resulting in lightheadedness or fainting.
* Advise patient that medication may cause dizziness or lightheadedness and to use caution while driving or performing other tasks requiring mental alertness until tolerance is determined.
* Caution patient to avoid unnecessary exposure to UV light (sunlight, tanning booths) and to use sunscreen and wear protective clothing when exposed to UV light to avoid photosensitivity reaction.
* Instruct women to inform health care provider if pregnant, planning to become pregnant, or breastfeeding.
* Instruct patient to stop taking drug and immediately report any of the following symptoms to health care provider: sore throat, fever, swelling of the hands or feet, irregular heartbeat, chest pains, fainting, swelling of the face, lips, eyelids, or tongue, difficulty breathing.
* Instruct patient to inform health care provider if a persistent cough develops while taking this medication.
* Caution patient not to take any prescription or OTC medications, potassium-containing salt substitutes, potassium supplements, or dietary supplements unless advised by health care provider.
* Advise patient that follow-up visits and lab tests will be required to monitor therapy and to keep appointments.

Fosphenytoin

(FOSS-FEN-ih-toe-in)

Class Anticonvulsant/Hydantoin

How Supplied

Cerebyx Injection 150 mg (100 mg phenytoin sodium), Injection 750 mg (500 mg phenytoin sodium)

Action

PHARMACOLOGY: Fosphenytoin is a prodrug, which is converted to the active metabolite phenytoin. Appears to act at motor cortex by inhibiting spread of seizure activity. Possibly works by promoting sodium efflux from neurons, thereby stabilizing threshold against hyperexcitability.

PHARMACOKINETICS/DYNAMICS:
Absorption: T_{max} is about 30 min. Bioavailability is 100% with IM dosing.
Distribution: Protein binding is 95% to 99%, about 88% for phenytoin. Vd is 4.3 to 10.8 L.
Metabolism: Fosphenytoin converts to phenytoin by hydrolysis. Phenytoin is extensively metabolized in the liver.
Excretion: The $t_{½}$ is about 15 min; the mean $t_{½}$ is 12 to 28.9 hr (phenytoin). Fosphenytoin is primarily excreted in the urine as metabolites.

Special Populations:
Renal Function Impairment – Increased fraction of unbound phenytoin may occur.
Hepatic Function Impairment – Increased fraction of unbound phenytoin may occur.
Elderly – Cl decreases about 20% in patients over 70 yr.
Hypoalbuminemia – Increased fraction of unbound phenytoin may occur.

Indications Short-term parenteral administration when other means of phenytoin administration are unavailable, inappropriate, or less advantageous; treatment of generalized convulsive status epilepticus; prevention and treatment of seizures occurring during neurosurgery; short-term substitution for oral phenytoin.

Contraindications Hypersensitivity to phenytoin or other hydantoins; patients with sinus bradycardia, sino-atrial block, second- and third-degree AV block, and Adams-Stokes syndrome.

Route/Dosage
To avoid the need to perform molecular weight-based adjustments when converting between fosphenytoin and phenytoin sodium, the fosphenytoin dose is expressed as phenytoin sodium equivalents (PE).

Status Epilepticus
ADULTS: **IV**
Initial/Loading dose: 15 to 20 mg PE/kg.

Maintenance and Non-Emergent Dose
ADULTS: **IV/IM**
Loading dose: 10 to 20 mg PE/kg
Maintenance dose: 4 to 6 PE/kg/day.

Interactions
Amiodarone, benzodiazepines, chloramphenicol, cimetidine, disulfiram, estrogens, felbamate, fluconazole, fluoxetine, isoniazid, oxyphenbutazone, phenacemide, phenylbutazone, succinimides, sulfonamides: May increase phenytoin serum concentrations and effects.

Antineoplastic drugs, carbamazepine, diazoxide, enteral nutritional therapy, rifabutin, rifampin, sucralfate: May decrease serum phenytoin concentrations and effects.

Corticosteroids, coumarin anticoagulants, doxycycline, estrogens, felodipine, levodopa, loop diuretics, methadone, oral contraceptives, mexiletine, quinidine, rifabutin, rifampin: The effects of these agents may be impaired.

Cyclosporine: Cyclosporine concentrations may be decreased.

Disopyramide: Disopyramide concentrations and bioavailability may be decreased, while anticholinergic actions may be enhanced.

Divalproex sodium, phenobarbital, sodium valproate, valproic acid: May increase or decrease phenytoin concentrations and effects.

Folic acid: May cause folic acid deficiency.

Itraconazole: Effects of itraconazole may be decreased, while those of phenytoin may be increased.

Metyrapone: Phenytoin may cause subnormal response to metyrapone.

Non-depolarizing muscle relaxants: May cause these agents to have shorter duration or decreased effects.

Primidone: May increase concentrations of primidone and metabolites, increasing the effects.

PATIENT CARE CONSIDERATIONS
Administration/Storage
- Do not administer solution if particulate matter or discoloration is noted.
- May use D5W or NS for dilution prior to administration.

Sympathomimetics (eg, dopamine): May cause profound hypotension and possibly cardiac arrest.

Theophyllines: Effects of either agents may be decreased.

INCOMPATIBILITIES: Do not mix with other drugs.

Lab Test Interferences
Fosphenytoin may interfere with metapyrone and dexamethasone tests, causing inaccurate results because of increased metabolism of these agents. Drug may cause decrease in serum levels of protein-bound iodine. It may cause increased levels of glucose, alkaline phosphatase, and gamma glutamyl-transpeptidase.

Adverse Reactions
CV: CV collapse; hypotension; vasodilation; tachycardia; atrial and ventricular conduction depression; ventricular fibrillation; hypertension.
CNS: Nystagmus; headache; dizziness; somnolence; ataxia; stupor; incoordination; paresthesia; extrapyramidal syndrome; tremor; agitation; hypesthesia; dysarthria; vertigo; brain edema.
DERM: Pruritus; rash; ecchymosis (IM).
EENT: Diplopia; amblyopia; tinnitus; deafness.
GI: Nausea; vomiting; constipation; tongue disorder; taste perversion; dry mouth.
METAB: Hypokalemia.
RESP: Pneumonia.
OTHER: Pelvic and back pain; weakness; asthenia; myasthenia; fever; chills; face edema; injection site inflammation.

Precautions
Pregnancy: Category D.
Lactation: Undetermined.
Children: Safety and efficacy not established.
Special risk patients: Use drug with caution with hepatic or renal impairment, hypotension, severe myocardial insufficiency, alcohol abuse, and porphyria.
Age: Age does not affect fosphenytoin pharmacokinetics. Phenytoin dosing requirements are variable and should be individualized.
Withdrawal: Abrupt withdrawal may precipitate status epilepticus. Dosage must be reduced or other anticonvulsant medicine substituted gradually.

Overdosage: Signs and Symptoms
Nystagmus, ataxia, dysarthria, hypotension, diminished mental capacity, coma, unresponsive pupils, respiratory and cardiovascular depression.

- Avoid administering with other IV solutions or medication; fosphenytoin is incompatible with most.
- Administer IV medication no faster than 150 mg/min to prevent hypotension.

- Store in refrigerator at 36° to 46° F. Do not keep at room temperature for more than 48 hr.

Assessment/Interventions
- Obtain patient history, including drug history and any known allergies. Note hepatic impairment and cardiac disease.
- Before initiation of therapy, assess the patient for hepatic or renal disorders, hypotension, alcohol abuse, or porphyria.
- Monitor the BP and ECG continuously during IV administration.
- Observe for side effects including nystagmus, ataxia, drowsiness, nausea, or vomiting, and report to health care provider.

Patient/Family Education
- Explain to family and patient that the medication is a short-term substitute for the regular use of phenytoin.
- Explain to family that sedation or drowsiness might occur as a result of the medication.
- Avoid alcohol or other CNS drugs while taking this medication.
- Never suddenly discontinue the medication; may lead to status epilepticus.
- Instruct patient what to do in case of a missed dose.

Frovatriptan Succinate

(froe-va-TRIP-tan)

Class Analgesic/Migraine

How Supplied
Frova Tablets 2.5 mg (as base)

Action
PHARMACOLOGY: Selectively agonizes 5-hydroxy-tryptamine$_1$ (5-HT$_{1B/1D}$) receptor, inhibiting excessive dilation of extracerebral and intracranial arteries in migraine.

PHARMACOKINETICS/DYNAMICS:
Absorption: T$_{max}$ is about 2 to 4 hr. Bioavailability is about 20% in men and about 30% in women.

Distribution: Protein binding is about 15%. Mean Vd$_{ss}$ is 4.2 L/kg in men and 3 L/kg in women.

Metabolism: Cytochrome P450 1A2 is the major enzyme involved.

Excretion: About 32% is excreted in urine and 62% in feces. Mean Cl is 220 mL/min in men and 130 mL/min in women. Mean t½ is about 26 hr.

Special Populations:
Hepatic Function Impairment – In mild (Child-Pugh class 5 to 6) to moderate (Child-Pugh class 7 to 9) hepatic impairment, AUC increased 2 times that of healthy subjects.
Elderly – AUC was 1.5- to 2-fold higher in elderly subjects.

Indications Acute treatment of migraine attacks with or without aura in adults.

Contraindications Patients with ischemic heart disease (eg, angina pectoris, history of MI, documented silent ischemia); history of symptoms or findings consistent with ischemic heart disease, coronary artery vasospasm, including Prinzmetal variant angina or other underlying CV disease; cerebrovascular syndromes (eg, strokes of any type, transient ischemic attacks); peripheral vascular disease (eg, ischemic bowel disease); uncontrolled hypertension; hemiplegic or basilar migraine; within 24 hr of another 5-HT$_1$ agonist, and ergotamine-containing or ergot-type medication (eg, dihydroergotamine); hypersensitive to frovatriptan or any inactive ingredient in the tablet.

Route/Dosage
ADULTS: PO 2.5 mg with fluids; if headache recurs after initial relief, a second 2.5-mg tablet may be taken provided the interval is at least 2 hr between doses (max, three 2.5 mg tablets/day).

Interactions
Contraceptives, oral and propranolol: May increase frovatriptan plasma concentrations.
Ergotamine-containing or ergot-type drugs (eg, methysergide): May reduce frovatriptan plasma levels; additive prolonged vasospastic reactions may occur.
Other 5-HT$_1$ agonists (eg, sumatriptan): Contraindicated within 24 hr of frovatriptan administration.
SSRIs (eg, fluoxetine): May cause weakness, hyperreflexia, and incoordination when given concurrently.

Lab Test Interferences None well documented.

Adverse Reactions
CV: Flushing (4%); palpitations (at least 1%).
CNS: Dizziness (8%); fatigue (5%); headache, paresthesia (4%); dysesthesia, hypoesthesia, insomnia, anxiety (at least 1%).
DERM: Increased sweating (at least 1%).
EENT: Abnormal vision, tinnitus (at least 1%).
GI: Dry mouth (3%); dyspepsia (2%); vomiting, abdominal pain, diarrhea (at least 1%).
MUSC: Skeletal pain (3%).
RESP: Sinusitis, rhinitis (at least 1%).
OTHER: Hot or cold sensation (3%); chest

pain (2%); pain (at least 1%).

Precautions
Pregnancy: Category C.
Lactation: Undetermined.
Children: Safety and efficacy not established.
CV events: Serious cardiac events, including acute MI, life-threatening cardiac arrhythmias, and death may occur.
Cerebrovascular events: Stroke, cerebral hemorrhage, subarachnoid hemorrhage, and other cerebrovascular events may occur.
Vasospastic events: Vasospastic-related reactions (eg, peripheral vascular ischemia, colonic ischemia) may occur.

PATIENT CARE CONSIDERATIONS

Administration/Storage
- Administer prescribed dose at onset of migraine symptoms.
- Administer without regard to meals.
- Do not administer within 24 hr of treatment with another $5\text{-}HT_1$ agonist or ergot-containing drug.
- If headache recurs after initial relief, a second tablet may be administered, providing there is an interval of at least 2 hr between doses.
- If first dose is ineffective, do not administer a second dose unless prescribed by health care provider.
- Do not administer more than 3 doses per 24-hr period.
- Store at ambient room temperature (59° to 86°F) protected from light and moisture.

Assessment/Interventions
- Obtain patient history, including drug history and any known allergies. Note history of ischemic or vasospastic coronary artery disease, uncontrolled hypertension, peripheral vascular disease, ischemic bowel disease, stroke, transient ischemic attacks, or hemiplegic or basilar migraine.
- Note recent (within 24 hr) use of other $5\text{-}HT_1$ agonists or ergotamine-containing or ergot-type drugs.
- Assess pain location, intensity, duration, and associated symptoms of migraine attack and response to treatment.
- Provide quiet, calm environment. Decrease stimuli, noise, and light.
- Ensure that patients with potential for coronary artery disease (CAD), including postmenopausal women and men older than 40 yr of age, and patients with risk factors for CAD (eg, hypertension, hypercholesterolemia, obesity, diabetes, smokers, family history) undergo a CV evaluation before initiating therapy.
- Administer first dose in physician's office or other adequately staffed medical facility to patient with potential for CAD whose CV evaluation provided clinical evidence that patient is reasonably free of coronary artery and ischemic myocardial disease or other significant underlying CV disease. Consider obtaining an ECG during the interval immediately following administration of the first dose of medication to patient with potential for CAD.
- Monitor patient for signs of allergic reaction. Discontinue therapy and immediately notify health care provider if noted. Be prepared to treat appropriately.
- Ensure that patient who is a long-term user of triptans, such as frovatriptan, undergoes periodic CV evaluation.
- Monitor patient for CNS, CV, GI, and general body side effects. Report to health care provider if noted and significant.

Patient/Family Education
- Explain name, dose, action, and potential side effects of drug.
- Advise patient to read the *Patient Information* leaflet before starting therapy and again with each refill.
- Explain that drug is to be used only during migraine and does not prevent or reduce the number of attacks. Emphasize that drug is used only to treat actual migraine attack and should not be used to prevent migraine headaches or treat headaches caused by other conditions.
- Advise patient that drug is to be taken as soon as symptoms of migraine appear. A second dose may be taken if symptoms return, but no sooner than 2 hr following the first dose. For a given attack, if there is no response to the first tablet, do not take a second tablet without first consulting health care provider. Do not take more than 3 tablets in any 24-hr period.
- Advise patient that safety of treating more than 4 headaches in a 30-day period has not been established and to inform health care provider if headaches are occurring more frequently.
- Advise patient to immediately notify health care provider if any of the following occur after taking a dose of frovatriptan: severe chest pain or chest pain that does not go away; sudden and/or severe stomach pain; shortness of breath; wheezing; swelling of eyelids, face, or lips.
- Advise patient that if tightness, pain, pressure, or heaviness in chest, throat, neck, or jaw occur when using sumatriptan, to discuss

these symptoms with health care provider before using again.
- Advise patient to notify health care provider if feelings of tingling, heat, flushing, tiredness, dizziness, heaviness, or pressure occur after treatment.
- Advise patient that drug may cause fatigue or dizziness and to use caution while driving or performing other activities requiring mental alertness.
- Advise patient to avoid unnecessary exposure to sunlight or tanning lamps and to use sunscreen and wear protective clothing to avoid photosensitivity reactions.
- Instruct patient to continue to take migraine prophylactic medications daily as directed.
- Advise patient not currently taking a migraine prophylactic drug to discuss the use of such drugs with health care provider.
- Advise women to notify health care provider if pregnant, planning to become pregnant, or breastfeeding.
- Warn patient not to take any prescription or OTC drugs, dietary supplements, or herbal preparations without consulting health care provider.
- Advise patient that follow-up visits may be necessary to monitor therapy and to keep appointments.

Fulvestrant

(fool-VESS-trant)

Class Antiestrogen

How Supplied
Faslodex Solution for injection 50 mg/mL

Action
PHARMACOLOGY: Fulvestrant competitively binds to the estrogen receptor and downregulates the estrogen receptor protein in human breast cancer cells.

PHARMACOKINETICS/DYNAMICS:
Absorption: C_{max} is about 8.5 ng/mL and about 15.8 ng/mL at steady state. T_{max} is 7 days. C_{min} is about 2.6 ng/mL and about 7.4 ng/mL at steady state. AUC is about 131 ng•day/mL and about 328 ng•day/mL at steady state.
Distribution: Apparent Vd_{ss} is 3 to 5 L/kg. Protein binding is 99%.
Metabolism: Metabolism takes place in the liver by oxidation via cytochrome P450 3A4 isoenzyme, aromatic hydroxylation, and conjugation with glucuronic acid and/or sulphate.
Excretion: The t½ is about 40 days. Cl is about 690 mL/min. Fulvestrant is cleared by the hepatobiliary route; renal elimination is less than 1%. It is primarily excreted in the feces (about 90%).

Indications Treatment of hormone receptor-positive metastatic breast cancer in postmenopausal women with disease progression following antiestrogen therapy.

Contraindications Pregnancy; hypersensitivity to the drug or any component of the product.

Route/Dosage
ADULTS: **IM** 250 mg into buttock at 1-mo intervals.

Interactions None well documented.

Lab Test Interferences None well documented.

Adverse Reactions
CNS: Headache; dizziness; insomnia; paresthesia; depression; anxiety.
DERM: Rash; sweating.
EENT: Pharyngitis.
GI: Nausea; vomiting; constipation; diarrhea; abdominal pain; anorexia.
GU: Urinary tract infection.
HEMA: Anemia.
RESP: Dyspnea; increased cough.
OTHER: Back pain; hot flushes; bone pain; arthritis; asthenia; pain; transient pain and inflammation at injection site; vasodilation; pelvic pain; peripheral edema; chest pain; flu-like syndrome; fever; accidental injury.

Precautions
Pregnancy: Category D.
Lactation: Undetermined.
Children: Safety and efficacy not established.

PATIENT CARE CONSIDERATIONS

Administration/Storage
- For IM administration only. Not for IV, SC, or ID administration.
- Administer prescribed dose once monthly using prefilled syringe(s) and supplied safety needle(s).
- Administer as single 5 mL injection or concurrent 2.5 mL injections into buttock.
- Administer injection slowly.
- Do not administer if cloudiness or particulate matter is noted.
- Store prefilled syringes in refrigerator (36° to 46°F).

Assessment/Interventions
- Obtain patient history, including drug history and any known allergies. Note history of liver function impairment, bleeding diatheses,

thrombocytopenia, or concurrent use of anticoagulants.
- Ensure that patient has negative pregnancy test before starting therapy.
- Monitor patient for GI, CNS, general body side effects, and injection site reactions. Inform health care provider if noted and significant.

Patient/Family Education
- Explain name, dose, action, and potential side effects of drug.
- Advise patient that medication will be prepared and administered by health care provider in a health care setting on a monthly basis.
- Instruct patient to inform health care provider if any of the following symptoms occur: intolerable nausea, vomiting, constipation, diarrhea, stomach pain, headache, hot flushes, injection site pain or inflammation.
- Instruct patient to not take any prescription or otc medications or dietary supplements unless advised by health care provider.
- Instruct women to notify health care provider if they become pregnant, plan on becoming pregnant, or are breastfeeding.
- Advise patient that follow-up visits and laboratory tests will be required to monitor therapy and to be sure to keep appointments.

Furosemide

(fyu-ROH-se-mide)
Class Loop diuretic

How Supplied
Lasix Tablets 20 mg, Tablets 40 mg, Tablets 80 mg, Oral solution 10 mg/mL, Injection 10 mg/mL

✤ *Apo-Furosemide* ◆ *Furosemide Special* ◆ *Lasix Special*

Action
PHARMACOLOGY: Inhibits reabsorption of sodium and chloride in proximal and distal tubules and loop of Henle.

PHARMACOKINETICS/DYNAMICS:
Absorption: Mean bioavailability is 64% with the tablet and 60% with the oral solution.
Distribution: Protein binding is 91% to 99%.
Metabolism: The major metabolite is furosemide glucuronide.
Excretion: The t½ is about 2 hr; furosemide is excreted in the urine.
Onset: 1 hr.
Peak: 1 to 2 hr.
Duration: 6 to 8 hr.

Indications Treatment of edema associated with CHF, hepatic cirrhosis, and renal disease; hypertension.

Contraindications Hypersensitivity to sulfonylureas; anuria.

Route/Dosage
Edema
ADULTS: **PO** 20 to 80 mg/day as a single dose; may titrate up to 600 mg/day. **IV/IM** 20 to 40 mg qd or bid.

Hypertension
ADULTS: **PO** 40 mg bid.
Max dose: 6 mg/kg.

CHF and Chronic Renal Failure
ADULTS: **PO** Up to 2 to 2.5 g/day. **IV** Up to 2 to 2.5 g/day.
Max IV bolus: 1 g/day over 30 min.

Acute Pulmonary Edema
ADULTS: **IV** 40 mg (over 1 to 2 min). If response not satisfactory within 1 hr, increase to 80 mg.
INFANTS AND CHILDREN: **PO**
Usual dose: 0.5 to 2 mg/kg qd or bid.
Max dose: 6 mg/kg. **IV/IM**
Usual dose: 1 mg/kg
Max dose: 6 mg/kg.

Interactions
Aminoglycosides: May increase auditory toxicity.
Charcoal: May reduce absorption of furosemide.
Cisplatin: May cause additive ototoxicity.
Digitalis glycosides: Electrolyte disturbances may predispose to digitalis-induced arrhythmias.
Lithium: May increase plasma lithium levels and toxicity.
NSAIDs: May decrease effects of furosemide.
Phenytoin: May reduce diuretic effects of furosemide.
Salicylates: May impair diuretic response in patients with cirrhosis and ascites.
Thiazide diuretics: Synergistic effects that may result in profound diuresis and serious electrolyte abnormalities.
INCOMPATIBILITIES: Gentamicin, milrinone, or netilmicin in D5W or NS: Do not add to furosemide solution; precipitate forms. Highly acidic solutions of pH less than 5.5: Do not mix with furosemide solution.

Lab Test Interferences None well documented.

Adverse Reactions
CV: Orthostatic hypotension; thrombophlebitis; chronic aortitis.
CNS: Vertigo; headache; dizziness; paresthesia; restlessness; fever.

DERM: Photosensitivity; urticaria; pruritus; necrotizing angiitis (eg, vasculitis, cutaneous vasculitis); exfoliative dermatitis; erythema multiforme; rash; occasionally, local irritation and pain with parenteral use.
EENT: Blurred vision; xanthopsia (yellow vision); tinnitus; hearing impairment.
GI: Anorexia; nausea; vomiting; diarrhea; oral and gastric irritation; cramping; constipation; pancreatitis.
GU: Urinary bladder spasm; interstitial nephritis; glycosuria.
HEMA: Anemia; leukopenia; purpura; aplastic anemia; thrombocytopenia; agranulocytosis.
HEPA: Jaundice; ischemic hepatitis.
METAB: Hyperuricemia; hyperglycemia; hypokalemia; metabolic alkalosis.
OTHER: Muscle spasm; weakness.

Precautions

Pregnancy: Category C.
Lactation: Excreted in breast milk.
Children: May increase incidence of patent ductus arteriosus in premature infants with respiratory distress syndrome, especially in first few weeks of life.
Hypersensitivity: Patients with known sulfonamide sensitivity may show allergic reactions to furosemide.

Renal function impairment: If severe effects occur, may need to discontinue. If high-dose parenteral therapy is used, controlled IV infusion is advised.
Photosensitivity: Photosensitization may occur.
Dehydration: Excessive diuresis may cause dehydration and decreased blood volume with circulatory collapse and possible vascular thrombosis and embolism, especially in elderly.
Diarrhea: Furosemide solution vehicle contains sorbitol and may induce diarrhea, especially in children.
Hepatic cirrhosis and ascites Sudden alterations of electrolyte balance may precipitate hepatic encephalopathy and coma; monitor carefully.
Ototoxicity: Associated with rapid injection, severe renal impairment, very large doses, or concurrent use of other ototoxic drugs.
Systemic lupus erythematosus: May be exacerbated or activated.

Overdosage: Signs and Symptoms

Acute profound water loss, volume and electrolyte depletion, dehydration, reduction of blood volume, circulatory collapse with possibility of vascular thrombosis and embolism.

PATIENT CARE CONSIDERATIONS

Administration/Storage

- Administer oral medication with food to prevent GI irritation.
- Administer qd dose in morning and bid doses at 8 am and 2 pm to avoid nocturia and sleep disturbance.
- Do not exceed infusion rate of 4 mg/min in adults.
- Use infusion solutions mixed with cefoperazone sodium in D5W within 24 hr if stored at room temperature and within 5 days if kept refrigerated.
- Do not use if discolored.
- Store medication at room temperature; avoid excessive exposure to light.

Assessment/Interventions

- Obtain patient history, including drug history and any known allergies. Note renal or hepatic impairment, systemic lupus erythematosus, hearing impairment, or hypersensitivity to sulfonamides.
- Obtain baseline hearing evaluation.

- Ensure that baseline BP; atypical pulse; weight; serum electrolyte, calcium, glucose, uric acid, CO_2, BUN and serum creatine levels; CBC; and liver and renal function tests have been obtained before beginning therapy and monitor regularly.
- Monitor I&O and weigh patient daily.
- Monitor renal function and notify health care provider if increasing azotemia, oliguria, or increases in BUN or creatinine occur.
- Notify health care provider if sudden alteration in fluid and electrolyte status is noted.
- Monitor for signs and symptoms of hypokalemia.

Patient/Family Education

- Instruct patient to take medication early in day to avoid disruption of sleep from increased urination and to take with food or milk to avoid GI upset.
- Teach patient to take and monitor pulse daily, especially if patient is taking cardiac drugs in addition to furosemide.

- Advise patient to eat diet high in potassium. Provide list of suggested foods (eg, baked potato, bananas, cantaloupe, avocados, dates, raisins, orange juice, peaches, watermelon).
- Emphasize importance of follow-up visits and frequent assessment of BP while taking drug.
- Advise patient to control hypertension through weight loss, sodium restriction, and exercise.
- Explain to diabetic patients that drug may increase blood glucose levels and affect urine glucose test results, and that glucose levels should be monitored carefully.
- For patients taking furosemide to lower BP, explain that they may feel fatigued during the first few weeks of therapy. Instruct patient to continue taking drug, but to consult with health care provider if problem persists.
- Instruct patient to report the following symptoms to health care provider: indication of weakness, dizziness, mental confusion, anorexia, lethargy, vomiting, cramps, persistent headache or fever, abdominal pain, diarrhea, rapid or irregular heart beat, yellowing of skin or eyes, dyspnea.
- Caution patient to avoid sudden position changes to prevent orthostatic hypotension.
- Advise patient to avoid exposure to sunlight and to use sunscreens or wear protective clothing to avoid photosensitivity reaction.
- Instruct patient not to take aspirin or otc medications without consulting health care provider.

Gabapentin

(GAB-uh-PEN-tin)

Class Anticonvulsant

How Supplied
Neurontin Capsules 100 mg, Capsules 300 mg, Capsules 400 mg
🍁 Apo-Gabapentin ♦ Novo-Gabapentin ♦ PMS-Gabapentin

Action
PHARMACOLOGY: Mechanism unknown; gabapentin-binding sites have been found in neocortex and hippocampus areas of the brain.

PHARMACOKINETICS/DYNAMICS:
Absorption: Bioavailability is approximately 60%.
Distribution: Less than 3% bound to plasma proteins. Vd is about 58 L.
Metabolism: Not significantly metabolized in humans.
Excretion: Excreted unchanged in urine. T½ is 5 to 7 hr.

Special Populations:
Renal Function Impairment – In Ccr less than 30 mL/min, t½ is about 52 hr.
Hemodialysis – T½ is about 132 hr on nondialysis days; gabapentin is significantly removed by hemodialysis.

Indications Adjunctive therapy in treatment of partial seizures with or without secondary generalization in patients above 12 yr with epilepsy; adjunctive therapy for partial seizures in children 3 to 12 yr; management of postherpetic neuralgia in adults.

Contraindications Standard considerations.

Route/Dosage
Epilepsy
ADULTS AND CHILDREN ABOVE 12 YR: **PO** 900 to 1800 mg/day in divided doses tid. Initial dose: 300 mg on day 1 and titrate upward rapidly. To minimize CNS side effects, administer initial dose on day 1 at bedtime.

CHILDREN 3 TO 12 YR: **PO** Initiate therapy at 10 to 15 mg/kg/day in divided doses (ie, tid) and titrate dose upward over a period of about 3 days to the effective dose.

CHILDREN AT LEAST 5 YR: **PO** The effective dose is 25 to 35 mg/kg/day in divided doses (ie, tid).

CHILDREN 3 TO 4 YR: **PO** The effective dose is 40 mg/kg/day in divided doses (ie, 3 times/day).

Postherpetic Neuralgia
ADULTS: **PO** Start with a single 300 mg dose on day 1, 600 mg on day 2 (divided bid), and 900 mg on day 3 (divided tid). Subsequently, titrate the dose upward as needed for pain relief to a daily dose of 1800 mg (divided tid).

Interactions
Antacids: May reduce bioavailability of gabapentin.
Cimetidine: Reduces renal clearance of gabapentin.

Lab Test Interferences False-positive readings for Ames N-Multistix SG dipstick test when gabapentin is added to other antiepileptic drugs. Sulfosalicylic acid precipitation procedure is recommended instead.

Adverse Reactions
CV: Hypertension.
CNS: Somnolence; dizziness; ataxia; tremor; nervousness; dysarthria; amnesia; depression; abnormal thinking; twitching; abnormal coordination; vertigo; hyperkinesia; paresthesia; reflex abnormality; hostility; anxiety.
DERM: Pruritus; abrasion; purpura.
EENT: Diplopia; amblyopia nystagmus; abnormal vision; gingivitis.
GI: Dyspepsia; dry mouth or throat; constipation; dental abnormalities; increased appetite; anorexia; flatulence.
RESP: Rhinitis; pharyngitis; coughing; pneumonia.
OTHER: Fatigue; weight increase; back pain; peripheral edema; impotence; leukopenia; vasodilation; asthenia; malaise; facial edema; arthralgia.

Precautions
Pregnancy: Category C.
Lactation: Secreted in breast milk.
Children: Safety and efficacy in children below 3 yr not established; safety and efficacy in management of postherpetic neuralgia in pediatric patients not established.
Elderly: Because of age-related renal impairment, dosage adjustment may be required.
Renal function impairment: Dose reduction recommended.
Carcinogenesis: May have carcinogenic potential.
Serious adverse effects: During clinical trials, some patients experienced status epilepticus, and 8 sudden, unexplained deaths occurred. The association of these events with gabapentin use is unclear.
Withdrawal: Do not discontinue antiepileptic drugs abruptly because of possible increased seizure frequency from drug withdrawal.

Overdosage: Signs and Symptoms
Ataxia, labored breathing, ptosis, sedation, hypoactivity or excitation, double vision, slurred speech, drowsiness, lethargy, diarrhea.

PATIENT CARE CONSIDERATIONS

Administration/Storage
- Administer medication with or without food and at least 2 hr after antacid administration.
- Administer initial dose on day 1 at bedtime to minimize CNS side effects.
- Titrate to effective dose given tid up to 1800 mg/day; maximum time between doses in tid schedule should not exceed 12 hr.
- Discontinue medication gradually over minimum of 1 wk.
- Store medication in tightly sealed container.

Assessment/Interventions
- Obtain patient history, including drug history and any known allergies. Note compromised renal and cardiovascular function and seizure pattern.
- Assess baseline vital signs.
- Evaluate for reduced renal clearance when administered concurrently with cimetidine.
- Withdraw medication gradually to avoid the possibility of increasing seizure frequency.

Patient/Family Education
- Instruct patient to take medication at least 2 hr after taking antacid.
- Explain that missed dose should be taken as soon as remembered but that 2 doses should not be taken together. Instruct patient to call health care provider if at least 2 doses are missed.
- Instruct patient to report the following symptoms to health care provider: excessive fatigue or weakness, dizziness, somnolence, incoordination, tremor or other symptoms of CNS depression, change in normal behavior, weight gain, back pain, alterations in GI system, alteration in skin or mucous membranes, fluid retention, general body discomfort, anorexia, visual disturbances, impotence.
- Advise patient that drug may cause drowsiness and to use caution while driving or performing other tasks requiring mental alertness.

Galantamine Hydrobromide

(gah-LAN-tah-meen HIGH-droe-BRO-mide)http://www.fda.gov/medwatch/SAFETY/2004/safety04.htm#Reminyl

Class Cholinesterase inhibitor

How Supplied
Reminyl Tablets 4 mg (as base), Tablets 8 mg (as base), Tablets 12 mg (as base), Oral Solution 4 mg/mL

Action
PHARMACOLOGY: May enhance cholinergic function by increasing acetylcholine.

PHARMACOKINETICS/DYNAMICS:

Absorption: Absolute bioavailability is about 90%. T_{max} is about 1 hr. Food decreases C_{max} by 25% and delayed T_{max} by 1.5 hr.

Distribution: Mean Vd is 175 L. Protein binding is 18%.

Metabolism: Metabolized by hepatic cytochrome P450 2D6 and 3A4 enzymes and glucuronidated.

Excretion: $T_{½}$ is about 7 hr. Approximately 95% is excreted in urine and 5% in feces.

Peak: Approximately 1 hr.

Special Populations:
Renal Function Impairment – AUC increased 37% and 67% in moderate and severe renal impairment.

Hepatic Function Impairment – Cl decreased by about 25% in moderate (Child-Pugh 7 to 9) hepatic impairment.

Elderly – Decreased concentrations.

CYP2D6 poor metabolizers – Approximately 35% increase in AUC of unchanged drug and 25% decrease in median Cl.

Indications Treatment of mild to moderate dementia of the Alzheimer type.

Contraindications Standard considerations.

Route/Dosage
ADULTS: PO 4 mg bid. May increase to 8 mg bid after 4 wk. A further increase to 12 mg bid may be attempted after min 4 wk at previous dose.

Interactions
Bethanechol, succinylcholine: May act synergistically with galantamine.

Erythromycin; ketoconazole; paroxetine: May elevate galantamine levels, increasing the risk of side effects.

Lab Test Interferences None well documented.

Adverse Reactions
CV: Syncope; bradycardia; chest pain; hypertension.
CNS: Dizziness; fatigue; headache; tremor; depression; insomnia; somnolence; agitation; confusion; anxiety; hallucinations.
DERM: Purpura.
GI: Nausea; vomiting; anorexia; diarrhea; abdominal pain; dyspepsia; constipation; flatulence.
GU: UTI; hematuria; urinary incontinence.
HEMA: Anemia.
METAB: Weight decrease.

RESP: Rhinitis; upper respiratory tract infection; bronchitis; coughing.
OTHER: Injury; back pain; peripheral edema; asthenia; falling.

Precautions
Pregnancy: Category B.
Lactation: Undetermined.
Children: Safety and efficacy not established.
Renal function impairment: Use with caution in patients with moderately impaired function; not recommended in severe impairment.
Hepatic function impairment: Use with caution in patients with moderately impaired function; not recommended in severe impairment.
Concomitant medical conditions: As a result of increased cholinergic activity, other organ systems may be affected, possibly leading to bradycardia, obstructed bladder outflow, increased gastric acid secretion, or bronchoconstriction. Use with caution in patients susceptible to these effects.

Overdosage: Signs and Symptoms
Cholinergic crisis (eg, severe nausea, vomiting, salivation, sweating, bradycardia, hypotension, respiratory depression, muscle weakness, collapse, convulsions).

PATIENT CARE CONSIDERATIONS
Administration/Storage
- Administer twice daily, preferably with morning and evening meal.
- Store at controlled room temperature (59° to 86°F). Keep container tightly closed.

Assessment/Interventions
- Obtain patient history, including drug history and any known allergies.
- Note current cardiac, GI, GU, or pulmonary conditions and history of liver disease or renal disease.
- Evaluate patient's mental status and function prior to initiation of therapy.
- Monitor patient for signs of improvement after therapy is started.
- Monitor patient for side effects of drug. Report any to health care provider.

Patient/Family Education
- Explain name, dose, action, and potential side effects of drug.
- Advise patient, family or caregiver that this drug does not alter the Alzheimer process and that the effectiveness of the medication may lessen over time.
- Advise patient or caregiver that medication is taken twice daily, preferably with the morning and evening meal.
- Advise patient or caregiver that medication is started at a low dose and gradually increased (up to q 4 wk) as tolerated.
- Caution patient or caregiver that if medication has been stopped for several days or longer that the medication must be restarted at the lowest dose and gradually increased to the current dose.
- Advise patient or caregiver that nausea and vomiting are the most common side effects and that taking the medication with food and ensuring adequate fluid intake reduces these side effects. If nausea and vomiting become a problem, the patient or caregiver should inform the prescribing health care provider.
- Advise patient, family, or caregiver to not discontinue the drug or change the dose unless advised to do so by the health care provider.

Gallium Nitrate

(GAL-ee-uhm NYE-trate)
Class Hypocalcemic agent
How Supplied
Ganite Injection 25 mg/mL

Action
PHARMACOLOGY: Exerts hypocalcemic effect by inhibiting calcium resorption from bone, possibly by stabilizing bone matrix, thereby reducing increased bone turnover.

PHARMACOKINETICS/DYNAMICS:
Absorption: Steady state is achieved in 24 to 48 hr.
Distribution: Vd is 1.27 L/kg.
Excretion: Plasma Cl is 0.12 to 0.2 L/hr/kg. The t½ is 24 to 115 hr. Major route of elimination is kidney.
Duration: Median is 6 to 8 days.

Indications Treatment of symptomatic, cancer-related hypercalcemia unresponsive to adequate hydration.

Contraindications Severe renal impairment (serum creatinine more than 2.5 mg/dL).

Route/Dosage
ADULTS: **IV** 100 to 200 mg/m^2/day for 5 consecutive days.

Interactions
Nephrotoxic drugs (eg, aminoglycosides, amphotericin B): May increase risk for development of renal insufficiency.

Lab Test Interferences None well documented.

Adverse Reactions
CV: Tachycardia; lower extremity edema; asymptomatic hypotension.
CNS: Lethargy, confusion, dreams, hallucinations, paresthesia.
EENT: Acute optic neuritis; visual impairment; tinnitus; decreased hearing.
GI: Nausea or vomiting; diarrhea; constipation.
GU: Increased BUN and creatinine (13%); acute renal failure.
HEMA: Anemia; leukopenia.
METAB: Mild to moderate transient hypophosphatemia (79%); decreased serum bicarbonate concentrations (50%); hypocalcemia.
RESP: Shortness of breath; rales and rhonchi; pleural effusion; pulmonary infiltrates.
OTHER: Hypothermia; fever; skin rash.

> **WARNING:**
> Concomitant use of gallium nitrate and potentially nephrotoxic drugs (eg, aminoglycosides, amphotericin B) may increase the risk for developing severe renal insufficiency in patients with cancer-related hypocalcemia. If use of potentially nephrotoxic drugs is indicated, discontinue gallium and continue hydration for several days after administration of the potentially nephrotoxic agent.

Precautions
Pregnancy: Category C.
Lactation: Undetermined.
Children: Safety and efficacy not established.
Renal function impairment: Hypercalcemia in cancer patients is commonly associated with impaired renal function.
Asymptomatic or mild to moderate hypocalcemia: Occurs frequently.
Visual and auditory disturbances: Acute optic neuritis and decreased hearing have occurred in some patients treated with multiple high doses of gallium combined with investigational anticancer drugs.

Overdosage: Signs and Symptoms
Nausea, vomiting, renal insufficiency.

PATIENT CARE CONSIDERATIONS

Administration/Storage
- For IV infusion only. Not for IV bolus, intradermal, subcutaneous, IM, or intra-arterial administration.
- Dilute prescribed dose in 1 L 0.9% sodium chloride injection or 5% dextrose injection.
- Infuse over 48 hr using infusion control device.
- Do not administer if particulate matter or cloudiness is noted.
- Discard unused portions of vial. Do not save any unused portions for future use.
- Store unopened vials at controlled room temperature (68° to 77°F). Diluted solutions can be stored for up to 48 hr at ambient room temperature (59° to 86°F) or 7 days if stored under refrigeration (36° to 46°F).

Assessment/Interventions
- Obtain patient history, including drug history and any known allergies. Note renal impairment, CV disease, or concurrent use of diuretics or potentially nephrotoxic medications (eg, aminoglycosides, amphotericin B).
- Do not administer to patient with serum creatinine greater than 2.5 mg/dL.
- Ensure that patient is adequately hydrated using oral and/or IV fluids (preferably saline) and that a satisfactory urine output (eg, 2 L/day) is established before beginning therapy. Ensure that adequate hydration is maintained during therapy but avoid overhydration in patient with compromised CV function.
- Ensure that gallium is temporarily discontinued in patient who requires therapy with a potentially nephrotoxic drug. Continue hydration for several days following administration of the potentially nephrotoxic drug before restarting gallium. Closely monitor serum creatinine and urine output during and after this period.
- Assess vital signs and visual, auditory, and neurologic status before starting therapy and frequently during treatment. Notify health care provider if abnormalities or significant changes are noted.

- Ensure that renal function (BUN, creatinine) is evaluated before starting therapy and frequently during therapy. Discontinue therapy if creatinine level exceeds 2.5 mg/dL.
- During therapy, ensure that serum calcium and phosphorous is determined before starting therapy and then daily for calcium, and twice weekly for phosphorous. If direct measurement of free-ionized calcium is not available, measure serum albumin concentration and correct serum calcium.
- Frequently assess patient for signs or symptoms of hypercalcemia (eg, anorexia, lethargy, fatigue, nausea, vomiting, constipation, impaired mental status) and hypocalcemia (eg, muscle cramps, positive Chvostek or Trousseau sign, paraesthesia of lips or extremities). Inform health care provider if noted. Be prepared to discontinue gallium infusion and administer calcium supplement if hypocalcemia develops.
- Assess patient for CV, CNS, GI, and general body side effects. Report to health care provider if noted and significant.

Patient/Family Education
- Explain name, action, and potential side effects of drug.
- Advise patient or caregiver that medication will be prepared and administered by health care provider in a health care setting.
- Review dosing schedule with patient or caregiver.
- Advise patient to report any of the following to health care provider: abnormal dreams, chills, difficulty breathing, fast heartbeat, hallucinations, change in vision or hearing, weakness, mouth sores, muscle cramps or spasms, numbness or tingling around lips, abnormal skin sensations, confusion, constipation or diarrhea, swelling of ankles or feet, nausea, vomiting, rash.

Ganciclovir (DHPG)

(gan-SIGH-kloe-VIHR SO-dee-uhm)
Class Anti-infective/Antiviral

How Supplied
Cytovene Capsules 250 mg, Capsules 500 mg, Powder for Injection, lyophilized 500 mg (as sodium)/vial ♦ *Vitrasert* Implant 4.5 mg

Action
PHARMACOLOGY: Inhibits cytomegalovirus (CMV) and other virus replication by competitive inhibition of viral DNA polymerases and direct incorporation into viral DNA.

PHARMACOKINETICS/DYNAMICS:
Absorption: AUC_{0-24} is approximately 15.9 mcg•hr/mL (oral); approximately 22.1 to 26.8 mcg•hr/mL (IV). Fasting absolute bioavailability is approximately 5%. Absolute bioavailability following food is 6% to 9%. C_{max} is approximately 1.02 to 1.18 mcg/mL (oral); approximately 8.27 to 9 mcg/mL (IV). Time to steady state is 24 hr.

Distribution: Approximately 1% to 2% bound to plasma proteins. Vd_{ss} is about 0.74 L/kg.

Excretion: Major route is renal excretion of unchanged drug by glomerular filtration and active tubular secretion. T½ is about 3.5 to 4.8 hr. Systemic Cl is about 3.52 mL/min/kg. Hemodialysis reduces plasma concentration by about 50%.

Special Populations:
Renal Function Impairment –
Ccr 25 to 49 mL/min: Cl is about 57 mL/min; t½ is about 4.4 hr.
Ccr less than 25 mL/min: Cl is about 30 mL/min; t½ is about 10.7 hr.
Children –
9 mo to 12 yr: Vd_{ss} was about 0.64 L/kg; C_{max} was about 7.9 mcg/mL; systemic Cl was about 4.7 mL/min/kg; t½ was about 2.4 hr.
Neonates (2 to 49 days): C_{max} was about 5.5 to 7 mcg/mL; systemic Cl was about 3.14 to 3.56 mL/min/kg; t½ was about 2.4 hr.
Race – Black/Hispanic patients trend toward a lower AUC_{0-8} and steady-state C_{max}.

Indications
IV: Treatment of CMV retinitis in immunocompromised patients, including patients with AIDS; prevention of CMV disease in organ transplant patients at risk for CMV.
Oral: Alternative to the IV formulation for maintenance treatment of CMV retinitis in immunocompromised patients, including patients with AIDS, in whom retinitis is stable following appropriate induction therapy and for whom the risk of more rapid progression is balanced by the benefit associated with avoiding daily IV infusions; prevention of CMV disease in solid organ transplant recipients and in individuals with advanced HIV infection at risk for developing CMV disease. **Unlabeled use(s):** Treatment of other CMV infections (eg, pneumonitis, gastroenteritis, hepatitis) in some immunocompromised patients.

Contraindications Hypersensitivity to acyclovir.

Route/Dosage
CMV Retinitis
ADULTS: IV Induction: 5 mg/kg over 1 hr q 12 hr for 14 to 21 days. Maintenance: 5 mg/kg over 1 hr qd or 6 mg/kg over 1 hr/day 5 days/wk

(max 6 mg/kg over 1 hr). **PO** Following induction treatment, the recommended maintenance dose of oral ganciclovir is 1000 mg 3 times/day with food. Alternatively, the dosing regimen of 500 mg 6 times/day q 3 hr with food, during waking hours, may be used.

CMV Prevention in Transplant Recipients
ADULTS: **IV** 5 mg/kg over 1 hr q 12 hr for 7 to 14 days, followed by 5 mg/kg once daily 7 days/wk or 6 mg/kg once daily 5 days/wk. **PO**

CMV Prevention in Advanced HIV Infection
ADULTS: **PO** 1000 mg 3 times daily with food.

Decreased Renal Function
ADULTS: **IV** Induction: 5 mg/kg q 12 hr (Ccr at least 70 mL/min); 2.5 mg/kg q 12 hr (Ccr 50 to 69 mL/min); 2.5 mg/kg q 24 hr (Ccr 25 to 49 mL/min); 1.25 mg/kg q 24 hr (Ccr 10 to 24 mL/min); 1.25 mg/kg 3 times a week following hemodialysis (Ccr less than 10 mL/min). Maintenance: 5 mg/kg q 24 hr (Ccr at least 70 mL/min); 2.5 mg/kg q 24 hr (Ccr 50 to 69 mL/min); 1.25 mg/kg q 24 hr (Ccr 25 to 49 mL/min); 0.625 mg/kg q 24 hr (Ccr 10 to 24 mL/min); 0.625 mg/kg 3 times a week following hemodialysis (Ccr less than 10 mL/min). **PO** 1000 mg tid or 500 mg q 3 h, 6 times/day (Ccr at least 70 mL/min); 1500 mg qd or 500 mg tid (Ccr 50 to 69 mL/min); 1000 mg qd or 500 mg bid (Ccr 25 to 49 mL/min); 500 mg qd (Ccr 10 to 24); 500 mg 3 times/wk, following hemodialysis (less than 10 mL/min).

Interactions
Amphotericin B, cyclosporine, nephrotoxic drugs: May increase serum creatinine.
Cytotoxic drugs: May cause added toxicity.
Didanosine: Ganciclovir may increase didanosine plasma levels. Ganciclovir levels may be decreased when administered 2 hr after didanosine but not when given simultaneously.
Imipenem-cilastatin: May cause generalized seizures.
Probenecid: May reduce renal clearance and increase serum levels of ganciclovir.
Zidovudine: Zidovudine and ganciclovir can cause granulocytopenia; combination therapy at full dose may not be tolerated.
INCOMPATIBILITIES: Do not mix with other drugs.

PATIENT CARE CONSIDERATIONS
Administration/Storage
IV:
- Reconstitute with 10 mL of Sterile Water for Injection (do not use bacteriostatic water or other solutions), and shake well to dissolve drug.
- Prepare infusion solution by mixing with 0.9% Sodium Chloride for Injection, D5W, Ringer's Injection, or Lactated Ringer's Injection.
- Wear gloves, gown, and mask while preparing solution.
- Use caution during administration to prevent personal exposure.

Lab Test Interferences None well documented.

Adverse Reactions
CNS: Headache; confusion.
DERM: Rash; phlebitis or pain at injection site.
GU: Renal toxicity.
HEMA: Granulocytopenia; thrombocytopenia; anemia.
HEPA: Abnormal LFT results.
OTHER: Sepsis; fever.

> **WARNING:**
> *Animal data:* Aspermatogenesis, carcinogenic, teratogenic.
> *Hematological:* Granulocytopenia, anemia, and thrombocytopenia.
> *Oral capsules:* Associated with risk of rapid rate of CMV retinitis progression and should be used as maintenance therapy only in patients who benefit from avoiding daily IV infusions.

Precautions
Pregnancy: Category C.
Lactation: Undetermined.
Children: Safety and efficacy not established.
Renal function impairment: Use drug cautiously and adjust dose. Carefully monitor renal function, especially when other nephrotoxic drugs are given.
Carcinogenesis: Ganciclovir is potentially carcinogenic.
Cytopenia: Use drug with caution in patients with preexisting cytopenias; granulocytopenia is common.
Hydration: Accompany administration by adequate hydration because ganciclovir is excreted by the kidneys.
Retinal detachment: Has occurred; relationship to drug undetermined.

Overdosage: Signs and Symptoms
Neutropenia, emesis, hypersalivation, anorexia, bloody diarrhea, inactivity, cytopenia, elevated LFT results, elevated BUN and serum creatinine, testicular atrophy, death.

- Do not infuse at concentrations above 10 mg/mL.
- Use infusion pump to prevent rapid or bolus injection.
- Administer only into veins that permit rapid dilution and distribution.
- Do not administer to patients with absolute neutrophil count of less than 500/mm^3 or platelet count of less than 50,000/mm^3.
- Refrigerate infusion solution until use but not for more than 24 hr.
- Discard reconstituted drug if vial has particulate matter or is discolored.
- Reconstituted solution in vial is stable at room temperature for 12 hr; do not refrigerate.
- Dispose of unused drug with appropriate precautions for nucleoside analog cytotoxic agents.

Assessment/Interventions
- Obtain patient history, including drug history and any known allergies. Note history of cytopenia or impaired renal function.
- Obtain neutrophil and platelet counts before starting therapy, q 2 days during twice-daily dosing and weekly thereafter.
- Obtain daily neutrophil counts in patients with history of drug-induced leukopenia or in whom neutrophil counts are less than 1000/mm^3 at initiation of treatment.
- Obtain serum creatinine or measure Ccr at least q 2 wk.
- Be especially attentive to renal function of elderly.
- Be alert for evidence of new infection and report to health care provider.

Patient/Family Education
- Give patient and family members instructions regarding handling of ganciclovir and proper disposal techniques when drug is to be administered at home.
- Inform patient that it is important to drink plenty of fluids.
- Teach patient for CMV retinitis that drug is not a cure, but it may help to keep symptoms from getting worse.
- Advise CMV retinitis patients to have regular ophthalmologic examinations at least q 6 wk during treatment.
- Instruct patients to use barrier form of contraception for at least 90 days after treatment because ganciclovir is potentially teratogenic.
- Explain to men that drug may cause temporary or permanent male infertility.
- Tell patient to avoid crowds and people with infections.
- Instruct patient to report the following symptoms to health care provider: headache, mental status changes, rash, pain at injection site, fever, nausea, unusual bleeding or bruising, black tarry stools, other physical complaints.

Gatifloxacin

(ga-ti-FLOKS-a-sin)

Class Antibiotic/Fluoroquinolone

How Supplied
Tequin Tablets 200 mg, Tablets 400 mg, Solution for injection (single-use vials) 400 mg, Solution for injection (premix) 200 mg, Solution for injection (premix) 400 mg ◆ *Zymar* Ophthalmic solution 3 mg/mL

Action
PHARMACOLOGY: Treatment of infections caused by susceptible strains of the designated microorganism.

PHARMACOKINETICS/DYNAMICS:

Absorption: Bioavailability is about 96%. C_{max} is about 2 to 4.2 mcg/mL (dose-proportional). T_{max} is about 1 hr (about 1.5 hr after multiple doses). AUC is about 14.2 mcg•hr/mL after a 200 mg dose and about 33 mcg•hr/mL after a 400 mg dose.

Distribution: Protein binding is about 20%. Mean Vd_{ss} 1.5 to 2 L/kg.

Metabolism: Limited.

Excretion: Mean t½ ranges from 7 to 14 hr. Renal Cl ranges from 124 to 161 mL/min. Less than 1% excreted in urine as ethylenediamine and methylethylenediamine metabolites. Primarily renally excreted as unchanged drug via glomerular filtration and tubular secretion. May also undergo minimal biliary and/or intestinal elimination.

Special Populations:
Renal Function Impairment –
Moderate renal impairment (Ccr 30 to 49 mL/min): 57% decrease in total clearance. AUC increased by 2 times.
Severe renal impairment (Ccr less than 30 mL/min): 77% decrease in total clearance. AUC increased by 4 times. Dosage reduction recommended with a Ccr less than 40 mL/min.
Hepatic Function Impairment – In patients with moderate (Child-Pugh B) hepatic impairment, C_{max} increased 32% and $AUC_{0-\infty}$ increased 23%. No dosage adjustment is necessary.

Indications For treatment of bacterial infections, including chronic bronchitis; acute sinusitis; community-acquired pneumonia; uncomplicated and complicated UTIs; pyelonephritis;

uncomplicated urethral and cervical gonorrhea; uncomplicated skin and skin structure infections; uncomplicated rectal infections in women; bacterial conjunctivitis (ophthalmic).
Unlabeled use(s): Atypical pneumonia; chronic prostatitis.

Contraindications Standard considerations.

Route/Dosage

Acute Bacterial Exacerbation of Chronic Bronchitis
PO/IV 400 mg q 24 hr for 5 days.

Acute Pyelonephritis
PO/IV 400 mg q 24 hr for 7 to 10 days.

Acute Sinusitis
PO/IV 400 mg q 24 hr for 10 days.

Bacterial Conjunctivitis
Ophthalmic Days 1 and 2, instill 1 drop in affected eye(s) q 2 hr while awake, up to 8 times/day. Days 3 through 7, instill 1 drop up to qid while awake.

Complicated UTIs
PO/IV 400 mg q 24 hr for 7 to 10 days.

Community-Acquired Pneumonia
PO/IV 400 mg q 24 hr for 7 to 14 days.

Uncomplicated Skin and Skin Structure Infections
PO/IV 400 mg q 24 hr for 7 to 10 days.

Hemodialysis; Continuous Peritoneal Dialysis
PO/IV 400 mg initial dose then subsequent dose of 200 mg PO/IV q 24 hr (on day 2 of dosing).

Renal Impairment
ADULTS:
Ccr more than 40 mL/min: **PO/IV** 400 mg initial dose then subsequent dose of 400 mg.
PO/IV q 24 hr (on day 2 of dosing).
Ccr less than 40 mL/min: **PO/IV** 400 mg initial dose then subsequent dose of 200 mg. **PO/IV** q 24 hr (on day 2 of dosing).

Uncomplicated Urethral Gonorrhea in Men; Endocervical and Rectal Gonorrhea in Women
PO/IV 400 mg q 24 hr in a single dose.

Uncomplicated UTIs (Cystitis)
PO/IV 400 or 200 mg q 24 hr. Single dose for 3 days.

Interactions

Aluminum- and magnesium-containing antacids, didanosine-buffered tablets, iron, or zinc salts: May decrease the bioavailability of gatifloxacin.
Antiarrhythmic agents (ie, class IA [eg, procainamide, quinidine], class III [eg, amiodarone, sotalol]), antipsychotics, cisapride, erythromycin, tricyclic antidepressants, any other drug known to prolong the QTc interval: May increase the risk of life-threatening cardiac arrhythmias, including torsades de pointes.
Digoxin: Plasma level of digoxin may be elevated, increasing the risk of toxicity.
NSAIDs: Coadministration may increase the risks of CNS stimulation and convulsions.
Probenecid: Renal clearance of gatifloxacin may be decreased, prolonging the t½ and increasing plasma levels of gatifloxacin.
INCOMPATIBILITIES: Amphotericin B; amphotericin B cholesteryl sulfate; cefoperazone sodium; cefonicid; cefozitin sodium; diazepam; furosemide; heparin sodium; mezlocillin disodium; phenytoin sodium; piperacillin sodium/tazobactam sodium; potassium phosphates; vancomycin in 5% dextrose injection.

Lab Test Interferences None well documented.

Adverse Reactions

CV: Palpitations; hypertension.
CNS: Abnormal dream; insomnia; paresthesia; tremors; vasodilation; vertigo; agitation; anxiety; confusion; headache; dizziness; asthenia.
DERM: Rash; sweating; pruritus; dry skin.
EENT: Abnormal vision; tinnitus.
Ophthalmic – Conjunctival irritation; increased lacrimation; keratitis; papillary conjunctivitis; chemosis; conjunctival hemorrhage; dry eye; eye discharge; eye irritation; eye pain; eyelid edema.
GI: Abdominal pain; constipation; dyspepsia; glossitis; oral moniliasis; stomatitis; mouth ulcer; vomiting; nausea; diarrhea; anorexia.
GU: Dysuria; hematuria.
METAB: Peripheral and face edema; hyperglycemia.
RESP: Dyspnea; pharyngitis.
OTHER: Allergic reaction; chills; fever; back pain; chest pain; taste perversion.

Precautions

Pregnancy: Category C.
Lactation: Not known if excreted in human milk.
Children:
PO/IV – Safety and efficacy not established in patients less than 18 yr.
Ophthalmic – Safety and efficacy not established in patients less than 1 yr.
Hypersensitivity: Mild to life-threatening. Discontinue drug at first sign of hypersensitivity reaction.
Special risk patients: Renal insufficiency.
Superinfection: Use of antibiotics may result in bacterial or fungal overgrowth.
Convulsions/Toxic psychosis: CNS stimulation, lowering of the seizure threshold, and psychotic reactions have been reported with similar agents. Use with caution in patients with seizures or CNS disorders.
Pseudomembraneous colitis: Consider possibility in patients with diarrhea.
QT effects: Gatifloxacin may prolong the QT interval and should be avoided in patients with a history of prolongation of the QTc interval,

uncorrected electrolyte disorder (eg, hypokalemia, hypomagnesemia), and in patients receiving drugs that prolong the QTc interval.
Tendonitis: Inflammation and rupture of tendons

PATIENT CARE CONSIDERATIONS
Administration/Storage
Oral:
- Administer oral gatifloxacin more than 4 hr before the administration of ferrous sulfate, dietary supplements containing zinc, magnesium, or iron (eg, multivitamins); aluminum/magnesium-containing antacids, didanosine-buffered tablets, buffered solution, buffered powder, or oral suspension.
- Administer without regard to food, including milk and dietary supplements containing calcium, and without regard to age (over 18 yr) or gender.
- Store tablets at room temperature (59° to 86°F).

IV:
- Administer injection by IV infusion only.
- Administer by IV over a period of 60 min. Avoid rapid or bolus IV infusion.
- Store at room temperature; do not freeze.
- Single-use vials require dilution prior to administration.
- When switching from IV to oral administration, no dosage adjustment is necessary. Patients whose therapy is started with the injection may be switched to tablets when clinically indicated.

Ophthalmic solution:
- For topical instillation into eye(s) only.
- Instill 1 drop into affected eye(s) every 2 hr while awake (up to 8 times/day) for first 2 days then 1 drop up to qid for 5 days.
- Have patient tilt head back, pull lower lid out to make pocket, and instill medication into conjunctival sac. Have patient close eyes and apply light finger pressure to bridge of nose for 1 to 2 min. Advise patient not to blink or rub eyes.
- If using other topical ophthalmic drugs, separate each medication by at least 5 min.
- Store at controlled room temperature (59° to 77°F). Protect from freezing. Keep container tightly closed.

Assessment/Interventions
- Obtain patient history, including drug history and any known allergies.
- Monitor patient during first dose, as many adverse reactions, including hypersensitivity, can occur at this time.
- Monitor for symptoms of superinfections (eg, vaginitis, stomatitis, diarrhea). Notify health care provider if symptoms occur.

have been associated with the use of fluoroquinolone antibiotics.

Overdosage: Signs and Symptoms
Possible QTc prolongation.

- Monitor patient for convulsions, dizziness, confusion, tremors, hallucinations, depression, or suicidal thoughts; if occurring, discontinue medication and refer for appropriate treatment.
- Monitor for signs of arthropathy, pain, inflammation, or rupture of a tendon; if present, discontinue medication.
- Monitor for ECG changes.
- Notify health care provider if symptoms of pseudomembranous colitis occur (eg, loose or foul-smelling stools).

Ophthalmic solution:
- Monitor patient for signs and symptoms of ocular side effects (eg, burning, stinging pain, irritation) and improvement in conjunctivitis. Notify health care provider if conjunctivitis is not improving or is worsening or if intolerable side effects occur.

Patient/Family Education
- Instruct patient that gatifloxacin should be taken 4 hr before any aluminum or magnesium based antacids, ferrous sulfate, and multi-vitamins.
- Instruct patient to stop treatment and inform health care provider if experiencing pain, inflammation, or rupture of tendon, and to rest or refrain from exercise until diagnosis of tendonitis or tendon rupture has been excluded.
- Instruct patient that drug may be taken with or without food and to drink fluids liberally.
- Instruct patient regarding the signs and symptoms of hypersensitivity; discontinue the medication at once and seek treatment immediately if occurring.
- Instruct patient to inform health care provider of any personal or family history of QTc prolongation or proarrhythmic conditions such as recent hypokalemia, significant bradycardia, acute myocardial ischemia, or history of convulsions.
- Instruct patient to inform health care provider of any prescription or OTC medications concurrently being taken.
- Inform patient of the additive effects of other drugs such as cisapride, erythromycin, antipsychotics, and tricyclic antidepressants to further QTc prolongation.
- Instruct patient to contact primary caregiver if experiencing palpitations or fainting spells.
- Inform patient that drug may cause dizziness

and lightheadedness and not to drive an automobile, operate dangerous machinery, or engage in activities that require mental alertness and coordination.
- Instruct patient to complete full course of therapy, even if symptoms of infection have resolved.

Ophthalmic solution:
- Remind patients not to wear contact lenses if signs and symptoms of bacterial conjunctivitis occur.
- Review dosing regimen with patient.
- Teach patient proper technique for instilling eye drops: wash hands; do not allow dropper to touch eye. Tilt head back and look up; pull lower eyelid down; instill prescribed number of drops. Close eye for 1 to 2 min and apply gentle pressure to bridge of nose. Do not rub eye.
- Advise patient that if more than 1 topical ophthalmic drug is being used to administer the drugs at least 5 min apart.
- Advise patient to inform health care provider if ocular side effects occur and become bothersome or if infection is not improving.

Gemcitabine Hydrochloride

(JEM-sit-ah-BEAN)

Class Nucleoside analog

How Supplied
Gemzar Lyophilized powder for injection 200 mg, Lyophilized powder for injection 1000 mg

Action
PHARMACOLOGY: Gemcitabine exhibits cell phase specificity, primarily killing cells undergoing DNA synthesis in the S-phase. It also blocks the progression of cells through the G1/S-phase boundary.

PHARMACOKINETICS/DYNAMICS:
Distribution: Protein binding is negligible. Vd is 50 L/m^2 (short infusion), 370 L/m^2 (long infusion).

Metabolism: To inactive metabolite uracil metabolite (dFdU).

Excretion: Cl is 75.7 to 92.2 L/hr/m^2 (male); 57 to 69.4 L/hr/m^2 (female). Primary route is renal. Short infusion t½ is 32 to 94 min. Long infusion t½ is 245 to 638 min.

Special Populations:
Elderly – Cl is 55.1 L/hr/m^2 (male) and 41.5 L/hr/m^2 (female); t½ is 61 min (male) and 73 min (female).

Indications Locally advanced or metastatic pancreatic adenocarcinoma in patients previously treated with 5-fluorouracil; locally advanced or metastatic non-small cell lung cancer. **Unlabeled use(s):** Bladder cancer; biliary cancer; metastatic breast cancer; relapsed or refractory testicular cancer; squamous cell carcinoma of the head and neck; ovarian cancer.

Contraindications Standard considerations.

Route/Dosage
Pancreatic Adenocarcinoma
ADULTS: IV
Cycle 1: 1000 mg/m^2 once weekly for 7 wk followed by 1 wk of rest.
Subsequent cycles: Give the same dose once weekly for 3 consecutive wk followed by 1 wk of rest. After at least 7 doses (1 cycle), the dose may be increased to 1250 mg/m^2 once weekly for 3 wk, followed by 1 wk of rest, if the following criteria are met:
- Nonhematologic toxicity is no greater than WHO Grade 1,
- Platelet nadirs are greater than 100,000 x 10^6/L,
- The absolute neutrophil count nadir is more than 1500 x 10^6/L. If the patient still meets the above criteria after receiving 3 doses of the higher regimen, the gemcitabine dose may be increased to 1500 mg/m^2 IV once weekly for 3 wk, followed by 1 wk of rest.

Non-Small Cell Lung Cancer
ADULTS: IV In combination with cisplatin, 1000 mg/m^2 gemcitabine on days 1, 8, and 15 of each 28-day cycle. Alternatively, 1250 mg/m^2 gemcitabine may be given IV on days 1 and 8 of a 21-day cycle.

Dosage Adjustment
ADULTS: Reduce or delay the gemcitabine dose in patients with neutropenia or thrombocytopenia on the day of treatment. On the day of the scheduled dose, if the absolute granulocyte count is 500 to 99 x 10^6/L or the platelet count is 50,000 to 99,999 x 10^6/L, then give 75% of the prior dose. If the absolute granulocyte count is less than 500 x 10^6/L or the platelet count is less than 50,000 x 10^6/L, then hold dose. For grade 3 or 4 nonhematologic toxicity, hold gemcitabine or reduce the dose by 50% in patients with non-small cell lung cancer. Dosage reduction is not required for severe alopecia or nausea and vomiting. Dosage reduction may be necessary in impaired renal or hepatic function. Use additional caution in these patients.

Interactions No specific drug interactions have been reported.

Lab Test Interferences None well documented.

Adverse Reactions
CV: MI, arrhythmia, and hypertension have occurred in patients with a past history of cardiovascular disease.
CNS: Headache; mild paresthesias.
DERM: Minimal alopecia; rash (usually maculopapular and pruritic).
GI: Moderate-to-low potential for severe nausea and vomiting; mild nausea and vomiting; diarrhea; stomatitis; elevated liver function tests.
GU: Proteinuria and hematuria.
HEMA: Myelosuppression (eg, anemia, leukopenia, granulocytopenia, thrombocytopenia) is the dose-limiting adverse effect with a nadir at 8 to 15 days.
RESP: Dyspnea.
OTHER: Flu-like syndrome (eg, fever, asthenia, anorexia, headache, cough, chills, myalgia).

Precautions
Pregnancy: Category D.
Lactation: Undetermined.

PATIENT CARE CONSIDERATIONS
Administration/Storage
- Store at controlled room temperature. Reconstituted solutions are stable for up to 24 hr at controlled room temperature. Do not refrigerate reconstituted product as crystals may form in the bag or bottle.
- Reconstitute with preservative-free 0.9% Sodium Chloride.
- Reconstituted solution may be administered directly or it may be further diluted with 0.9% Sodium Chloride to a final gemcitabine concentration at least 0.1 mg/mL.
- Administer by IV infusion over 30 min.
- Prolonging infusions past 60 min increases the risk of myelosuppression.

Assessment/Interventions
- Monitor complete blood counts at baseline

Children: Safety and efficacy not established.
Renal function impairment: Mild proteinuria and hematuria were commonly reported. Renal failure may not be reversible even with discontinuation of therapy, and dialysis may be required.
Hepatic function impairment: Gemcitabine was associated with transient elevations of serum transaminases in about 70% of patients.
Extravasation: Local irritation or phlebitis may occur. Refer to your institution-specific protocol.
Fever: The overall incidence of fever was 41%.
Rash: Rash was reported in 30% of patients. The rash was typically a macular or finely granular maculopapular pruritic eruption of mild-to-moderate severity involving the trunk and extremities. Pruritus was reported in 13% of patients.

Overdosage: Signs and Symptoms
Myelosuppression, paresthesias, and severe rash.

and prior to each gemcitabine dose.
- Monitor renal and hepatic function at baseline and periodically throughout therapy.
- Female patients and the elderly may eliminate gemcitabine more slowly, increasing the risk of adverse effects.

Patient/Family Education
- Contact health care provider if any of the following occurs: a temperature greater than 100.4°F or shaking chills; unusual bruising or bleeding; pain around an infusion site; sore mouth or throat; prolonged or uncomfortable swelling; severe diarrhea; severe constipation; numbness or tingling in the hands or feet; vomiting for more than 24 hr after the treatment; any changes in the skin.

Gemfibrozil

(gem-FIE-broe-ZILL)
Class Antihyperlipidemic
How Supplied
Lopid Tablets 600 mg
🍁 *Apo-Gemfibrozil* ♦ *Gen-Gemfibrozil* ♦ *Novo-Gemfibrozil* ♦ *Nu-Gemfibrozil* ♦ *PMS-Gemfibrozil*

Action
PHARMACOLOGY: Decreases blood levels of triglycerides and VLDL by decreasing their production. Also decreases cholesterol and increases HDL.

PHARMACOKINETICS/DYNAMICS:
Absorption: Bioavailability is 100%. T_{max} is 1 to 2 hr.
Food – Max rate of absorption and a 50% to 60% increase in C_{max} when administered 30 min before meals vs with meals or fasting.
Distribution: Protein binding is high.
Metabolism: Mainly undergoes oxidation to form a hydroxymethyl and a carboxyl metabolite.
Excretion: Plasma t½ is 1.5 hr, biological t½ is longer because of enterohepatic circulation and reabsorption in the GI tract. Approximately 70% excreted in urine (about 2% as unchanged); 6% excreted in feces.

Indications
Treatment of hypertriglyceridemia in adult patients with type IV or V hyperlipidemia that presents risk of pancreatitis and does not respond to diet; reduction of coronary heart disease risk in type IIb patients who have low HDL levels (in addition to elevated LDL and

triglycerides) and have not responded to other measures.

Contraindications Hepatic or severe renal dysfunction, including primary biliary cirrhosis; preexisting gallbladder disease.

Route/Dosage
ADULTS: **PO** 600 mg bid 30 min before morning and evening meals.

Interactions
Lovastatin: Increases risk of rhabdomyolysis.
Oral anticoagulants (eg, warfarin): Anticoagulant effect may be increased.

Lab Test Interferences None well documented.

Adverse Reactions
CV: Atrial fibrillation.
CNS: Fatigue; vertigo; headache.

PATIENT CARE CONSIDERATIONS

Administration/Storage
- Administer 30 min before breakfast and supper.
- Store at room temperature in a tightly closed container.

Assessment/Interventions
- Obtain patient history, including drug history and any known allergies. Note preexisting kidney, liver, or gallbladder disease or diabetes.
- Assess dietary intake of fats.
- Perform periodic blood counts during first 12 mo of administration.
- Obtain periodic determinations of serum lipids.
- Monitor liver studies.
- Assess for side effects, particularly abdominal

DERM: Eczema; rash.
EENT: Blurred vision.
GI: Dyspepsia; abdominal pain; diarrhea; nausea; vomiting; constipation; acute appendicitis.
GU: Impotence.
HEMA: Anemia; leukopenia; bone marrow hypoplasia; eosinophilia.
HEPA: Elevated LFT results; cholestatic jaundice.
METAB: Mild hyperglycemia.
OTHER: Muscle pain or weakness; myositis; rhabdomyolysis; taste perversions.

Precautions
Pregnancy: Category B.
Lactation: Undetermined.
Children: Safety and efficacy not established.
Cholelithiasis: Drug may increase cholesterol excretion into the bile, leading to cholelithiasis.

pain, nausea, and vomiting.

Patient/Family Education
- Inform patient of need to restrict dietary intake of fats; teach patient dietary restrictions to follow.
- Emphasize importance of the following increased cardiac risk factors: smoking, alcohol consumption, lack of exercise.
- Instruct patient to report the following symptoms to health care provider: abdominal pain, persistent nausea and vomiting, bleeding, and irregular heartbeat.
- Advise patient that drug may cause dizziness or blurred vision and to use caution while driving or performing other tasks requiring mental alertness.

Gemifloxacin Mesylate

(jeh-mih-FLOKS-ah-sin MEH-sih-LATE)

Class Antibiotic/Fluoroquinolone

How Supplied
Factive Tablets 320 mg

Action
PHARMACOLOGY: Interferes with microbial DNA synthesis.

PHARMACOKINETICS/DYNAMICS:
Absorption: Rapidly absorbed from the GI tract. Bioavailability is approximately 71%. C_{max} is about 1.61 mcg/mL, and the AUC is about 9.93 mcg•hr/mL.

Distribution: Protein binding ranges from 55% to 73%. Mean Vd_{ss} is 4.18 L/kg.

Metabolism: Metabolized to a limited extent by the liver.

Excretion: 61% in the feces and 36% in the urine as unchanged drug and metabolites. The t½ is approximately 7 hr. The mean renal Cl following multiple doses was approximately 11.6 L/hr.

Special Populations:
Renal Function Impairment – Average increase in AUC of approximately 70% in patients with renal insufficiency.

Indications Treatment of acute bacterial exacerbation of chronic bronchitis and community-acquired pneumonia (mild to moderate) caused by susceptible strains of designated microorganisms.

Contraindications Standard considerations.

Route/Dosage
Acute Bacterial Exacerbation of Chronic Bronchitis
ADULTS: **PO** 320 mg/day for 5 days.

Community-Acquired Pneumonia (Mild to Moderate Severity)
ADULTS: PO 320 mg/day for 7 days.

Renal impairment
ADULTS (CCR 40 ML/MIN OR LESS): PO 160 mg q 24 hr. Patients requiring routine hemodialysis or continuous ambulatory peritoneal dialysis should receive 160 mg q 24 hr.

Interactions
Antacids containing aluminum, magnesium, and calcium; drug formulations containing divalent and trivalent cations (eg, didanosine); metal cations (eg, iron); multivitamins containing iron or zinc: May decrease the bioavailability of gemifloxacin.
Probenecid: The renal clearance of gemifloxacin may be decreased, increasing the bioavailability and AUC.
Sucralfate: May decrease the bioavailability of gemifloxacin. Take at least 2 hr before sucralfate.

Lab Test Interferences
None well documented.

Adverse Reactions
CNS: Headache, dizziness (1%).
DERM: Rash (3%).
GI: Diarrhea (4%); nausea (3%); vomiting, abdominal pain (1%).
HEPA: Increased ALT (2%) and AST (1%).

Precautions
Pregnancy: Category C.
Lactation: Undetermined; however, other fluoroquinolones have been shown to be excreted in breast milk.
Children: Safety and efficacy not established.
Hypersensitivity: Mild to life-threatening. Discontinue drug at first sign of hypersensitivity reaction.

Renal function impairment: Reduced clearance may occur; decrease the dose in patients with Ccr of 40 mL/min or less.
Superinfection: Use of antibiotics may result in bacterial or fungal overgrowth.
Photosensitivity: Photosensitivity reaction may occur.
CNS effects: Use with caution in patients with CNS disease (eg, epilepsy) or patients predisposed to convulsions.
Pseudomembranous colitis: Consider possibility in patients with diarrhea.
QT effects: Gemifloxacin may prolong the QT interval in some patients; avoid in patients with a history of prolongation of the QTc interval, patients with uncorrected electrolyte disorder (eg, hypokalemia or hypomagnesemia), and patients receiving class IA (eg, quinidine, procainamide) or class III (eg, amiodarone, sotalol) antiarrhythmic agents. Use gemifloxacin with caution in patients receiving drugs that prolong the QTc interval (eg, erythromycin, tricyclic antidepressants, antipsychotics) and in patients with ongoing proarrhythmic conditions (eg, clinically important bradycardia, acute MI).
Tendon and cartilage effects: Tendonitis and rupture of the shoulder, hand, and Achilles tendons, requiring surgical repair and resulting in prolonged disability, have been reported in patients receiving fluoroquinolones. The risk may be increased in patients receiving corticosteroids, especially in the elderly.

Overdosage: Signs and Symptoms
Possible QTc prolongation, tremor, convulsions.

PATIENT CARE CONSIDERATIONS
Administration/Storage
* Administer gemifloxacin either 2 hr before or 3 hr after sucralfate, antacids containing magnesium or aluminum, didanosine buffered tablets or pediatric powder, or other products containing iron or zinc.
* Administer prescribed dose qd with a full glass of water.
* Administer without regard to meals, but administer with food if GI upset occurs.
* Store tablets at room temperature (59° to 86°F). Protect from light.

Assessment/Interventions
* Obtain patient history, including drug history and any known allergies. Note renal impairment, uncorrected electrolyte disorder, concurrent use of drugs that prolong the QTc interval (eg, erythromycin), class IA (eg, quinidine) or class III (eg, amiodarone) antiarrhythmic agents, or history of prolongation of QTc interval, epilepsy, predisposition to convulsions, or allergy to fluoroquinolone antibiotics.
* Review results of culture and sensitivity testing as available.
* Ensure that reduced dose is administered to patient with Ccr less than 40 mL/min.
* Monitor for signs of infection, especially fever, and for positive response to antibiotic therapy.
* Monitor patient for evidence of CNS stimulation or psychiatric changes (eg, tremors, restlessness, lightheadedness, confusion, hallucinations, agitation, anxiety, or sleep disturbance). Inform health care provider if noted and be prepared to discontinue therapy.
* Ensure that patient is well hydrated to prevent formation of concentrated urine.
* Monitor patient for signs of allergic reaction.

Discontinue therapy and immediately notify health care provider if noted. Be prepared to treat appropriately.
• Monitor patient for GI, DERM, and general body side effects. Report to health care provider if noted and significant.

Patient/Family Education
• Explain name, dose, action, and potential side effects of drug.
• Advise patient to read *Patient Information* leaflet before starting therapy and with each refill.
• Review dosing schedule and prescribed length of therapy with patient.
• Instruct patient to take each dose with a full glass of water.
• Advise patient that medication can be taken without regard to meals, but to take with food if GI upset occurs.
• Advise patient that if a dose is missed to take as soon as remembered. However, if it is nearing the time for the next dose, to skip the dose and take the next dose at the regularly scheduled time. Caution patient not to take more than 1 dose of medication in a day.
• Remind patient to complete entire course of therapy, even if symptoms of infection have disappeared.
• Advise patient to inform health care provider if infection does not improve or worsens.
• Advise patient to drink fluids liberally (eg, eight 8 oz glasses of water daily) while taking this medication.
• Advise patient to discontinue therapy and contact health care provider immediately if skin rash, hives, itching, shortness of breath, palpitations, fainting, pain, tenderness, or rupture of tendon occur.
• Warn patient that diarrhea containing blood or pus may be a sign of a serious disorder and to seek medical care if noted and not to treat at home.
• Caution patient that drug may cause dizziness and to use caution while driving or performing other tasks requiring mental alertness until tolerance is determined.
• Advise patient to avoid unnecessary exposure to direct and indirect sunlight or tanning lamps and to use sunscreen and wear protective clothing to avoid photosensitivity reactions during therapy and for several days after stopping medication. Advise patient to discontinue therapy and notify health care provider if any of the following occur following exposure to sunlight or artificial UV light (eg, sunlamp): sensation of skin burning, redness, swelling, blistering, rash or itching.
• Inform patient not to take antacids containing magnesium and/or aluminum or products containing ferrous sulfate (iron), multivitamins containing zinc or other metal cations, or chewable buffered tablets (didanosine) within 3 hr before or 2 hr after taking gemifloxacin.
• Inform patient that gemifloxacin may produce prolongation of the QTc interval on an ECG.
• Instruct patient to inform health care provider of any personal or family history of QTc prolongation or proarrhythmic conditions such as recent hypokalemia, significant bradycardia, acute MI, or history of convulsions.
• Advise women to inform health care provider if breastfeeding.
• Instruct patient not to take any prescription or OTC medications or dietary supplements unless advised by health care provider.
• Advise patient that follow-up examinations and lab tests may be required to monitor therapy and to keep appointments.

Gemtuzumab Ozogamicin

(gem-TOO-ze-mab oh-ZOE-gam-ih-sin)

Class Humanized monoclonal anti-CD33 antibody conjugated to antitumor antibiotic.

How Supplied
Mylotarg Sterile Preservative-free Powder for Injection, Lyophilized 5 mg (protein equivalent) per vial

Action
PHARMACOLOGY: Chemotherapy agent composed of a recombinant humanized IgG_4 kappa antibody conjugated with a cytotoxic antitumor antibiotic, calicheamicin, isolated from fermentation of a bacterium. The antibody portion of gemtuzumab ozogamicin binds specifically to the CD33 antigen, which is expressed on the surface of leukemic blasts in patients with acute myeloid leukemia (AML), ultimately, resulting in DNA double-strand breaks and cell death.

PHARMACOKINETICS/DYNAMICS:
Absorption: AUC doubles after second dose.

Metabolism: Many metabolites found in liver microsomes, cytosol, and HL-60 promyelocytic leukemia cells.

Excretion: First dose $t_{½}$ is about 45 hr (total); 100 hr (unconjugated). Second dose $t_{½}$ is about 60 hr (total).

Indications CD33-positive AML in first relapse in patients at least 60 yr who are not candidates for other antineoplastics.

Contraindications Standard considerations.

Route/Dosage
CD33-positive Acute Myeloid Leukemia in First Relapse in Patients at Least 60 Yr Who Are Not Candidates for Other Antineoplastics
ADULTS: **IV** 9 mg/m^2/dose for a total of 2 doses, given on days 0 and 14. The second dose may be given in the absence of full hematologic recovery. Because the risk of prolonged severe myelosuppression increases when a third dose is given, do not administer more than 2 doses per treatment course.

Interactions Coadministration of drugs with similar pharmacologic effects may cause additive side effects, including toxicity.

Lab Test Interferences None well documented.

Adverse Reactions
CV: Peripheral edema; hypertension; hypotension.
CNS: Asthenia; headache; dizziness; insomnia.
DERM: Rash; petechiae.
GI: Moderate potential for nausea and vomiting; diarrhea; abdominal pain; mucositis; anorexia; constipation; transient increases in bilirubin, ALT, and AST. Veno-occlusive disease and fatal liver failure have been reported; risk may be increased in patients who undergo stem cell transplantation.
GU: May cause fetal harm. Decreased fetal weight, increased malformations, and increased fetal mortality seen in pregnant rats.
HEMA: Severe neutropenia and thrombocytopenia in most patients (98% to 99%), with recovery at a median of 40 days. Anemia is also common (47%).
HYPERSEN: Anaphylaxis.
METAB: Hypokalemia; hypomagnesia; hyperglycemia.
RESP: Dyspnea; cough; pharyngitis; rhinitis.
OTHER: Chills; fever; infection; pain.
Infusion reactions – Chills and fever reported in approximately 60% of patients within 24 hours after the initial infusion. Hypotension, hypertension, hypoxia, and dyspnea may also occur. Reactions are usually mild to moderate in severity and resolve after 2 to 4 hr. Provide supportive care as needed, such as diphenhydramine, acetaminophen, and IV fluids. The incidence of infusion reactions decreases with the second dose.

> WARNING:
>
> *Use as a single agent:* No studies demonstrating efficacy/safety in conjunction with other agents.
>
> *Hypersensitivity/anaphylaxis:* Postinfusion symptom complex of fever and chills, and less commonly hypotension and dyspnea may occur during the first 24 hr after administration. Grade 3 or 4 nonhematologic infusion-related adverse events include the following: chills, fever, hypotension, hypertension, hyperglycemia, hypoxia, dyspnea.
>
> Severe cases, including pulmonary events and infusion reactions may occur. Patients with high peripheral blast counts may be at greater risk for pulmonary events or tumor lysis syndrome. Consider leukoreduction prior to administration.
>
> *Hepatotoxicity:* Severe and sometimes fatal hepatic veno-occlusive disease has been reported with use. Increased risk in patients with hematopoietic stem-cell transplants, underlying liver disease or abnormal liver function, and in patients receiving adjunctive chemotherapy.
>
> *Myelosuppression:* Severe myelosuppression will occur in all patients given the recommended dose of this agent. Careful hematologic monitoring is required.

Precautions
Pregnancy: Category D.
Lactation: Because many drugs, including immunoglobulins, are excreted in breast milk, and because of the potential for serious adverse reactions in nursing infants from gemtuzumab ozogamicin, decide whether to discontinue nursing or to discontinue the drug, taking into account the importance of the drug to the mother.
Children: Safety and efficacy not studied.
Renal function impairment: Not studied in adult patients with renal dysfunction. Use with caution.
Hepatic function impairment: Not studied in patients with a bilirubin more than 2 mg/dL. Use with caution. Exercise caution when

administering in patients with hepatic impairment.

Tumor lysis syndrome: May be a consequence of leukemia treatment. Take appropriate measures (eg, hydration, allopurinol) to prevent hyperuricemia.

PATIENT CARE CONSIDERATIONS

Administration/Storage

- Refrigerate. Protect from sunlight and fluorescent light.
- Allow vial to warm to room temperature before reconstitution.
- Reconstitute vial aseptically with 5 mL of Sterile Water for Injection and swirl gently. The final gemtuzumab ozogamicin concentration will be 1 mg/mL.
- Withdraw appropriate dose from vial and dilute in 100 mL 0.9% Sodium Chloride. Visually inspect the solution for particulates.
- Protect reconstituted and diluted solutions from sunlight and unshielded fluorescent light. Turn off the light in the biologic safety hood during preparation; ambient room lights may be left on.
- Protect reconstituted and diluted solutions from sunlight and fluorescent light.
- Reconstituted solutions are preservative-free; refrigerate and use within 24 hr. The manufacturer recommends use within 8 hr.
- Use diluted solutions immediately.
- Administer by IV infusion. Do not administer as an IV push or bolus.
- Infuse over 2 hr. Observe patients for infusion-related symptoms (eg, fever, chills).
- Administer through a separate IV line with a low protein-binding 1.2 micron terminal filter.

Infusion reactions:

- The infusion may be slowed or continued at the same rate if the patient experiences a reaction. Interrupt the infusion for dyspnea or profound hypotension. Symptoms may be treated with diphenhydramine (eg, *Benadryl*), acetaminophen (eg, *Tylenol*), bronchodilators, or IV fluids. Monitor the patient until symptoms resolve completely. Patients who react to the initial infusion may receive a second dose. The infusion duration may be increased at the health care provider's discretion.

Assessment/Interventions

- Monitor vital signs (eg, heart rate, BP, respiratory rate, temperature) during the infusion and for 4 hr afterward.
- High peripheral blast counts may increase the risk of tumor lysis syndrome and pulmonary adverse events. Consider hydroxyurea or leukopheresis to reduce peripheral white count (less than 30,000 mcL) before therapy.

- Hyperuricemia may occur caused by rapid cell lysis; monitor serum uric acid. Minimize effects of hyperuricemia with hydration, urinary alkalinization, and allopurinol.
- Monitor CBC, differential, platelet count, electrolytes, renal function, and hepatic function at baseline and periodically during therapy.

Pretreatment regimens:

- Reduce incidence of infusion reactions with premedication. Give acetaminophen 650 to 1000 mg (oral or rectal) and diphenhydramine 50 mg (oral or IV) 60 min before administering gemtuzumab ozogamicin.

Patient/Family Education

- Explain name, action, and potential side effects of drug.
- Advise patient, family, or caregiver that medication will be prepared and administered by health care provider in a health care setting.
- Review dosing schedule with patient, family, or caregiver.
- Advise patient, family or caregiver that additional medications will be given before administration to reduce side effects of gemtuzumab.
- Advise patient, family, or caregiver to immediately report any of the following symptoms to health care provider: rash; difficulty breathing; fever, chills or other signs of infection; sores in mouth; unusual bleeding or bruising.
- Advise patient, family, or caregiver to report any of the following symptoms to health care provider: persistent nausea, vomiting, diarrhea or appetite loss; persistent or worsening general body weakness.
- Instruct patient to not take any prescription or *otc* medications or dietary supplements unless advised to do so by health care provider.
- Caution women of childbearing potential to avoid becoming pregnant while being treated.
- Instruct women of childbearing potential to notify health care provider if they become pregnant, plan on becoming pregnant, or are breastfeeding.
- Advise patient that frequent follow-up visits and laboratory tests will be required to monitor therapy and to be sure to keep appointments.

Gentamicin

(JEN-tuh-MY-sin)

Class Antibiotic/Aminoglycoside

How Supplied
Garamycin Ointment 3 mg/g (ophthalmic), Ointment 0.1% (as 1.7 mg sulfate/g), Cream 0.1% (as 1.7 mg sulfate/g), Solution 3 mg/mL (ophthalmic), Injection 40 mg/mL (as sulfate) ♦ *Gentak* Solution 3 mg/mL (ophthalmic), Ointment 3 mg/g (ophthalmic) ♦ *Genoptic* Solution 3 mg/mL (ophthalmic) ♦ *Genoptic S.O.P.* Ointment 3 mg/g (ophthalmic) ♦ *Gentacidin* Ointment 3 mg/g (ophthalmic), Solution 3 mg/mL (ophthalmic) ♦ *G-myticin* Ointment 1 mg base (as sulfate), Cream 1 mg base (as sulfate) ❧ *Gent-AK* ♦ *Minims Gentamicin* ♦ *ratio-Gentamicin*

Action
PHARMACOLOGY: Inhibits production of bacterial protein, causing bacterial cell death.

PHARMACOKINETICS/DYNAMICS:

Absorption: C_{max} is 4 to 8 mcg/mL (IV). T_{max} is 1 hr (IM). Oral absorption is poor.

Distribution: Vd is 0.2 to 0.4 L/kg. Protein binding is 0% to 10%. The t½ is 5 to 15 min. Distributed to extracellular ascitic, pericardial, pleural, synovial, lymphatic, and peritoneal fluids; body tissues; high concentrations in urine; low concentrations in breast milk, line spread function, and sputum. Crosses the placenta but does not cross the blood-brain barrier.

Excretion: The t½ is 2 hr. Peritoneal dialysis is 25% removed in 48 to 72 hr. Primary route is renal-glomerular filtration; 50% is removed during a 4 to 6 hr hemodialysis period.

Special Populations:
Renal Function Impairment – End-stage renal disease: t½ is 24 to 60 hr.
Children – In infants less than 1 wk old and less than 1500 g, Vd is up to 0.68 L/kg; more than 1500 g, Vd is up to 0.58 L/kg. The t½ is 5 to 8 hr.

Indications Short-term treatment of serious infections caused by susceptible strains of microorganisms, especially gram-negative bacteria; adjunct to systemic gentamicin in serious CNS infections (intrathecal); treatment of superficial ocular infections (ophthalmic); treatment of primary (eg, impetigo contagiosa) and secondary (eg, infectious eczemafoid dermatitis) skin infections; skin cysts and superficial skin infections, infection prophylaxis, and aid to healing (topical).

Contraindications Long-term therapy (parenteral); epithelial herpes simplex keratitis, vaccinia, varicella, mycobacterial infections, fungal diseases (ophthalmic); hypersensitivity to aminoglycosides.

Route/Dosage
ADULTS: **IM/IV** 3 to 5 mg/kg/day in divided doses. For obese patients, base dose on estimate of lean body weight.

CHILDREN: **IM/IV** 6 to 7.5 mg/kg/day (2 to 2.5 mg/kg q 8 hr).

INFANTS AND NEWBORNS: **IM/IV** 7.5 mg/kg/day (2.5 mg/kg q 8 hr).

PREMATURE OR TERM NEWBORNS (YOUNGER THAN 1 WK): **IM/IV** 5 mg/kg/day (2.5 mg/kg q 12 hr) or 2.5 mg/kg q 18 hr or 3 mg/kg q 24 hr.

Prevention of Bacterial Endocarditis
ADULTS: **IM/IV** 1.5 mg/kg with ampicillin 30 min before procedure (max 80 mg).
CHILDREN: **IM/IV** 2 mg/kg with ampicillin 30 min before procedure.

Superficial Skin Infections
ADULTS AND CHILDREN: **Topical** Apply tid to qid to infected area.

Ocular Infections
ADULTS AND CHILDREN: **Topical** Apply 0.5-inch ribbon of ointment in each eye bid or tid or 1 to 2 gtt 4 to 6 times/day.

Interactions
Drugs with nephrotoxic potential (eg, amphotericin, cephalosporins, enflurane, methoxyflurane, vancomycin): May increase risk of nephrotoxicity.

Loop diuretics: May increase risk of auditory toxicity.

Neuromuscular blocking agents: May enhance effects of these agents.

Polypeptide antibiotics: May increase risk of respiratory paralysis and renal dysfunction.

INCOMPATIBILITIES: Do not mix beta-lactam antibiotics (eg, penicillins, especially ticarcillin and carbenicillin, cephalosporins) in IV solutions.

Lab Test Interferences None well documented.

Adverse Reactions
CNS: Headache; dizziness; vertigo; encephalopathy; confusion; fever; lethargy; convulsions; muscle weakness and twitching; peripheral neuropathy; acute organic brain syndrome; depression; pseudotumor cerebri; increased CSF protein; arachnoiditis or burning at injection site after intrathecal administration.

DERM: Rash; urticaria; itching; anaphylaxis; photosensitivity (topical).

EENT: Blurred vision; tinnitus; hearing loss; mydriasis and conjunctival paresthesia (ophthalmic).

GI: Nausea; vomiting.

GU: Oliguria; proteinuria; increased serum cre-

atinine and BUN; casts; Fanconi-like syndrome.
HEMA: Anemia; eosinophilia; leukopenia; thrombocytopenia; granulocytopenia.
HEPA: Elevated LFT results.
RESP: Apnea; pulmonary fibrosis.
OTHER: Pain and irritation at injection site; splenomegaly; hypomagnesemia; hyponatremia; hypocalcemia; hypokalemia.

> **WARNING:**
>
> *Neurotoxicity:* Manifests as both auditory and vestibular ototoxicity, and primarily occurs in patients with pre-existing renal damage or in normal renal function with prolonged therapy. Partial or total irreversible deafness may continue to develop after drug is stopped. Other features of neurotoxicity include paresthesias, twitching, and seizures.
>
> *Nephrotoxicity:* Usually reversible.
>
> Teratogenic in pregnancy. Renal and eighth nerve function closely monitored in patients with suspected renal dysfunction. Monitor peak and trough concentrations. Dosage adjustments required in renal impairment.

Precautions
Pregnancy: Category D (parenteral). Category C (ophthalmic).
Lactation: Undetermined.
Children: Use cautiously in premature infants and newborns because of renal immaturity.
Elderly: Drug levels and renal function must be monitored closely.
Sulfite sensitivity: Some products contain sulfites. Do not use if there is history of hypersensitivity.
Burn patients: Pharmacokinetics may be altered; serum levels must be closely monitored for dosing.
Hypomagnesemia: Occurs often, especially in those with restricted diets or poor nutrition.
Neuromuscular blockade: Potential curare-like effects may aggravate muscle weakness or cause neurotoxicity. Use with caution with anesthesia or muscle relaxants; in patients with neuromuscular disorders, hypomagnesemia, hypocalcemia, and hypokalemia; and in newborns whose mothers received magnesium sulfate.

Overdosage: Signs and Symptoms
Nephrotoxicity, ototoxicity.

PATIENT CARE CONSIDERATIONS
Administration/Storage
- Do not premix with any other drugs; administer separately.
- For topical use, cleanse affected area of skin before applying ointment.
- For ophthalmic use, have patient tilt head back, place medication in conjunctival sac, and instruct patient to close eyes. Apply light finger pressure on lacrimal sac for 1 min after instillation.
- Store at room temperature (59° to 86°F).

Assessment/Interventions
- Obtain patient history, including drug history and any known allergies. Note sulfite sensitivity.
- Monitor renal function (eg, serum creatinine, BUN, Ccr) and 8th cranial nerve function.
- Evaluate peak and trough levels within 48 hr after initiating therapy and then q 3 to 4 days.
- If culture and sensitivity is ordered, obtain specimen prior to administration of drug.
- Keep patient well hydrated and monitor serum electrolytes.
- Withhold drug and notify health care provider if any of following symptoms occur: decreased urinary output, headache, dizziness, confusion, tinnitus, vertigo, hearing loss, vaginal itching, or discharge.

Patient/Family Education
- With parenteral administration, instruct patient to report any changes in urinary output (eg, decreased), hearing (eg, ringing in ears, hearing loss), dizziness, tingling or numbness in hands and feet, growth on tongue, and vaginal itch or discharge.
- For topical application, instruct patient to cleanse affected area of skin prior to application and to notify health care provider if rash or irritation develops or if condition worsens.
- For ophthalmic use, instruct patient in proper technique for instilling drops or ointment, emphasizing importance of avoiding contact between dispensing container and eyes. Inform patient that drug may cause temporary blurring of vision or stinging after administration. Advise patient to notify health care provider if stinging, itching, or burning

increase or if irritation or pain persists. Discard remaining ophthalmic preparation after completion of therapy.
♦ Instruct patient to continue using medication for prescribed time, even after signs and symptoms have been relieved, to prevent recurrence.
♦ Caution patient to avoid exposure to sunlight and to use sunscreen or wear protective clothing to avoid photosensitivity reaction.

Glatiramer Acetate

(glah-TEER-ah-mer ASS-eh-tate)
Class Immune modifier
How Supplied
Copaxone Injection 20 mg
Action
PHARMACOLOGY: Unknown. May modify the immune processes that are thought to be responsible for multiple sclerosis (MS).
Indications To reduce the frequency of relapses in patients with relapsing-remitting MS.
Contraindications Hypersensitivity to glatiramer acetate or mannitol.
Route/Dosage
ADULTS: **Subcutaneous** 20 mg q day.
Interactions None well documented.
Lab Test Interferences None well documented.
Adverse Reactions
CV: Vasodilation (27%); palpitation (17%); syncope, tachycardia (5%); hypertension (at least 1%); thrombosis, peripheral vascular disease, pericardial effusion, MI, deep thrombophlebitis, coronary occlusion, CHF, cardiomyopathy, cardiomegaly, arrhythmia, angina pectoris (postmarketing).
CNS: Asthenia (41%); anxiety (23%); hypertonia (22%); tremor (7%); vertigo (6%); migraine (5%); agitation (4%); foot drop (3%); confusion, nervousness, nystagmus, speech disorder (2%); abnormal dreams, emotional lability, stupor (at least 1%); meningitis, CNS neoplasm, cerebrovascular accident, brain edema, abnormal dreams, aphasia, convulsion, neuralgia, myelitis (postmarketing).
DERM: Pruritus, rash (18%); sweating (15%); erythema, herpes simplex, urticaria (4%); skin nodule (2%); eczema, herpes zoster, pustular rash, skin atrophy, warts (at least 1%).
EENT: Rhinitis (14%); eye pain (7%); eye disorder (4%); visual field changes (at least 1%); glaucoma, blindness, visual field defect (postmarketing).
GI: Nausea (22%); diarrhea (12%); anorexia (8%); vomiting (6%); GI disorder (5%); gastroenteritis (3%); bowel urgency, oral moniliasis, salivary gland enlargement, tooth caries and ulcerations (at least 1%); tongue edema, stomach ulcer, GI hemorrhage, eructation (postmarketing).
GU: Urinary urgency (10%); vaginal moniliasis (8%); dysmenorrhea (6%); amenorrhea, hematuria, impotence, menorrhagia, suspicious papanicolaou smear, urinary frequency, vaginal hemorrhage (at least 1%); urogenital neoplasm, urine abnormality, ovarian carcinoma, nephrosis, kidney failure, breast carcinoma, bladder carcinoma, urinary frequency (postmarketing).
HEMA/LYMPH: Lymphadenopathy (12%); ecchymosis (8%); thrombocytopenia, lymphoma-like reaction, acute leukemia (postmarketing).
HEPA: Abnormal liver function, liver damage, hepatitis, liver cirrhosis, cholelithiasis (postmarketing).
LOCAL: Injection site pain (73%); injection site erythema (66%); injection site Inflammation (49%); injection site pruritus (40%); injection site mass (27%); injection site induration (13%); injection site welt (11%); injection site hemorrhage, injection site urticaria (5%); injection site edema, atrophy, abscess or hypersensitivity (at least 1%).
M/N: Weight gain (3%); hypercholesterolemia (postmarketing).
MUSC: Arthralgia (24%); back pain (16%); neck pain (8%); rheumatoid arthritis, generalized spasm (postmarketing).
RESP: Dyspnea (19%); bronchitis (9%); Laryngismus (5%); hyperventilation; hay fever (at least 1%); pulmonary embolus, pleural effusion, lung carcinoma, (postmarketing).
OTHER: infection (50%); pain (28%); chest pain (21%); flu syndrome (19%); peripheral edema (7%); fever (8%); face edema (6%); bacterial infection (5%); chills (4%); edema (3%); cyst (2%); sepsis, lupus erythematosus syndrome, hydrocephalus, enlarged abdomen, allergic reaction, anaphylactoid reaction (postmarketing).
Precautions
Pregnancy: Category B.
Lactation: Undetermined.
Children: Safety and efficacy in children younger than 18 yr of age not established.
Immunity: Could possibly interfere with useful immune function (eg, decreased defense against infection or tumor surveillance).

Immediate postinjection reaction: Approximately 10% of patients experience a constellation of symptoms immediately after injection. Symptoms may include the following: flushing, chest pain, palpitations, anxiety, dyspnea, constriction of throat, urticaria. These symptoms are usually transient and self-limited and generally occur several months after starting therapy.

PATIENT CARE CONSIDERATIONS

Administration/Storage

- For subcutaneous administration only. Not for intradermal, IM, IV, or intra-arterial administration.
- Allow syringe to warm to room temperature before administering. This may take up to 20 min.
- Rotate injection sites (hips, thighs, abdomen, back of arms). Use a different area than where the last injection was administered. Do not inject into areas that are tender, bruised, red, or hard.
- Do not administer if particulate matter, cloudiness, or discoloration noted.
- Discard any unused solution. Do not save for future use.
- Store prefilled syringes in refrigerator (36° to 46°F). Protect from freezing and exposure to light. Discard any syringes that have been frozen. If a refrigerator is not available, the syringes may be stored at room temperature (59° to 86°F) for up to 7 days.

Assessment/Interventions

- Obtain patient history, including drug history and any known allergies.
- Assess patient for CV, CNS, GI, RESP, general body side effects and injection site reactions. Report to health care provider if noted and significant.

Patient/Family Education

- Explain name, dose, action, and potential side effects of drug.
- Advise patient, family, or caregiver that medication is not a cure for MS, but it may decrease the number of flare-ups and slow the development of some of the physical disabilities caused by MS.
- Advise patient or caregiver to review the *Patient Information* sheet before using the first time and with each refill.
- If patient or caregiver will be administering at home, ensure that the patient or caregiver has reviewed the *Patient Information* leaflet for self-injection procedure and understands how to store, prepare and administer the dose, and dispose of used equipment and supplies. The first injection should be performed under supervision of a qualified health care provider.
- Instruct patient to rotate injection sites as described in the *Patient Information* leaflet to reduce likelihood of severe injection site reactions developing.
- Advise patient not to change the dose or stop taking unless advised by health care provider.
- Instruct patient to notify health care provider immediately if any of the following occur: hives, skin rash with irritation, dizziness, sweating, chest pain, trouble breathing, or severe pain at injection site. Caution patient not to administer any more injections unless advised by health care provider.
- Patient may experience a short-term reaction right after injecting the glatiramer (flushing, chest pain tightness with heart palpitations, anxiety, trouble breathing). Advise patient that these symptoms appear a few minutes after an injection, last a few minutes, and go away by themselves without further problems. Instruct patient to discontinue use and immediately seek medical care if symptoms become severe and not to administer any more injections unless advised by health care provider.
- Advise patient that injection site reactions (redness, pain, swelling, itching, or lump at injection site) are the most common side effects and to inform health care provider if they occur and are bothersome.
- Advise patient to contact health care provider if experiencing bothersome side effects or experience any unusual problems.
- Caution patient that drug may cause dizziness and to use caution while driving or performing other tasks requiring mental alertness or coordination until tolerance is determined.
- Advise women to notify health care provider if pregnant, planning to become pregnant, or breastfeeding.
- Instruct patient not to take any prescription or OTC medications, herbal preparations, or dietary supplements unless advised by health care provider.
- Remind patient that office visits will be required to monitor therapy and to keep appointments.
- Instruct patient on proper self-injection techniques to ensure safe administration.

Glimepiride

(GLIE-meh-pie-ride)
Class Antidiabetic/Sulfonylurea

How Supplied
Amaryl Tablets 1 mg, Tablets 2 mg, Tablets 4 mg

Action
PHARMACOLOGY: Decreases blood glucose by stimulating insulin release from pancreas. May also decrease hepatic glucose production as well as increase sensitivity to insulin.

PHARMACOKINETICS/DYNAMICS:
Absorption: Bioavailability is 100%. C_{max} is about 103 to 591 ng/mL (dose-dependent). T_{max} is about 2 to 3 hr.
Food – T_{max} increased and C_{max} and AUC slightly decreased.
Distribution: Vd is 8.8 L. Protein binding is greater than 99.5%.
Metabolism: Completely metabolized by oxidation via cytochrome P450 2C9. Major metabolites are cyclohexyl hydroxy methyl (M1) (about ⅓ of the activity of the parent) and carboxyl (M2) derivatives.
Excretion: About 60% is excreted in urine and about 40% in feces as metabolites. T½ is about 5 to 9.2 hr.
Peak: 2 to 3 hr.
Duration: 24 hr.
Special Populations:
Renal Function Impairment – Serum levels decrease, M1 and M2 levels increase, and t½ for M1 and M2 increase.
Elderly – Mean AUC_{ss} was about 13% lower.

Indications
Adjunct to diet and exercise in type 2 diabetic patients whose hyperglycemia cannot be controlled by diet and exercise alone; in combination with insulin for type 2 diabetic patients with secondary failure to oral sulfonylureas.

Contraindications
Hypersensitivity to sulfonylureas; diabetic ketoacidosis with or without coma.

Route/Dosage
ADULTS: **PO** 1 to 2 mg qd with breakfast or the first main meal of the day. Increase by 1 to 2 mg/dose. Titrate at 1 to 2 wk intervals based on blood glucose response. Maintenance: 1 and 4 mg daily (max, 8 mg/day). Combination therapy with insulin is appropriate for secondary failure to oral sulfonylureas. The same dosing recommendations apply.

Interactions
Alcohol: Produces disulfiram-like reaction (eg, facial flushing, headache, breathlessness).
Chloramphenicol, clofibrate, fenfluramine, histamine H2 antagonists, miconazole, monoamine oxidase inhibitors, probenecid, salicylates, sulfinpyrazone, sulfonamides, tricyclic antidepressants, urinary acidifiers: May increase hypoglycemic effect.
Beta-blockers, cholestyramine, diazoxide, rifampin, thiazide diuretics, urinary alkalinizers: May decrease hypoglycemic effect.

Lab Test Interferences
None well documented.

Adverse Reactions
CV: Although issue is controversial, oral sulfonylureas may have increased risk of cardiovascular morbidity when compared with patients treated with diet alone.
CNS: Headache; dizziness.
DERM: Allergic skin reactions (eg, pruritus, erythema, urticaria, morbilliform or maculopapular rash); porphyria cutanea tarda; photosensitivity.
EENT: Blurred vision.
GI: Nausea; vomiting; GI pain; diarrhea.
HEMA: Leukopenia; agranulocytosis; thrombocytopenia; hemolytic anemia; aplastic anemia; pancytopenia.
HEPA: Cholestatic jaundice; elevated LFTs.
METAB: Hypoglycemia.
OTHER: Asthenia; hyponatremia with or without syndrome of inappropriate antidiuretic hormone (SIADH).

Precautions
Pregnancy: Category C. Insulin is recommended to maintain blood glucose levels during pregnancy. Prolonged severe neonatal hypoglycemia can occur if sulfonylureas are administered at time of delivery.
Lactation: Undetermined.
Children: Safety and efficacy not established.
Elderly: Increased risk for development of hypoglycemia. Hypoglycemia may be difficult to detect in elderly patients.
Renal function impairment: Use with caution; lower doses may be adequate.
Hepatic function impairment: Use with caution; lower doses may be adequate.

Overdosage: Signs and Symptoms
Hypoglycemia, tingling of lips and tongue, hunger, nausea, lethargy, tachycardia, sweating, confusion, tremor, convulsions, stupor, coma.

PATIENT CARE CONSIDERATIONS

Administration/Storage
- Give the dose with breakfast or the first meal of the day.
- Store at room temperature.

Assessment/Interventions
- Obtain patient history.
- Assess patient for evidence of hypoglycemic reaction; hypoglycemia may be difficult to detect in the elderly.
- Note hepatic or renal impairment.

Patient/Family Education
- Instruct patient in signs, symptoms, and treatment of hypoglycemic reaction.
- Review dietary and exercise guidelines for diabetes with patient.
- Instruct patient to take drug with breakfast.
- Teach patient to self-monitor urine or blood glucose.
- Instruct patients to inform health care provider that they are taking this drug and to carry medical identification (eg, *Medi-Alert* bracelet).
- Instruct patient to notify health care provider if symptoms of hypoglycemia occur (eg, fatigue, excessive hunger, profuse sweating, numbness of extremities) or if blood glucose is below 60 mg/dL.
- Tell patient to notify health care provider if symptoms of hyperglycemia occur (eg, excessive thirst or urination, urinary glucose or ketones).
- Instruct patient to report these symptoms to health care provider: nausea, vomiting, diarrhea, heartburn, sore throat, rash, unusual bleeding or bruising, other physical complaints.
- Advise patient not to take any medication, including *otc*, or alcohol without consulting health careprovider.
- Advise patient to avoid exposure to sunlight or sunlamps and to use sunscreen or wear protective clothing to avoid photosensitivity reaction.

Glipizide

(GLIP-ih-zide)

Class Antidiabetic/Sulfonylurea

How Supplied
Glucotrol Tablets 5 mg, Tablets 10 mg ♦ *Glucotrol XL* Tablets, extended release 5 mg, Tablets, extended release 10 mg

Action
PHARMACOLOGY: Decreases blood glucose by stimulating insulin release from pancreas and by increasing tissue sensitivity to insulin.

PHARMACOKINETICS/DYNAMICS:

Absorption: Bioavailability is 100% (immediate-release); 90% (extended-release). T_{max} is 1 to 3 hr (immediate-release); 6 to 12 hr (extended-release). Food delays absorption by about 40 min.

Distribution: The mean apparent Vd is about 10 L. Protein binding is 98% to 99%.

Metabolism: Hepatic.

Excretion: Mean t½ is 2 to 5 hr. Mean total Cl is about 3 L/hr. About 80% is excreted in urine and 10% in feces as metabolites.

Onset: 30 min.

Duration: 24 hr.

Indications Adjunct to diet to lower blood glucose in patients with non-insulin-dependent diabetes mellitus (type 2) whose hyperglycemia cannot be controlled by diet alone.

Contraindications Hypersensitivity to sulfonylureas; diabetes complicated by ketoacidosis, with or without coma; sole therapy of insulin-dependent (type 1) diabetes mellitus; diabetes when complicated by pregnancy.

Route/Dosage
ADULTS: PO 5 mg/day 30 min before breakfast. Adjust dose in 2.5 to 5 mg/day increments based on blood glucose response. Divided doses may be given (single daily dose max 15 mg; total daily dose max 40 mg).

ELDERLY OR PATIENTS WITH LIVER DISEASE: PO 2.5 mg/day initially.

Interactions
Alcohol: Produces disulfiram-like reactions (eg, facial flushing, headache, breathlessness).
Androgens, chloramphenicol, clofibrate, fenfluramine, fluconazole, gemfibrozil, histamine H_2 antagonists, magnesium salts, methyldopa, monoamine oxidase, oral anticoagulants, phenylbutazone, probenecid, salicylates, sulfinpyrazone, sulfonamides, tricyclic antidepressants, urinary acidifiers: Hypoglycemic effects may be increased.
Beta-blockers, cholestyramine, diazoxide, hydantoins, rifampin, thiazide diuretics, urinary alkalinizers: May decrease hypoglycemic effect.
Food: Absorption is delayed when taken with food. Give drug about 30 min before meal.

Lab Test Interferences Mild-to-moderate elevations in BUN and creatinine.

Adverse Reactions
CV: May have increased risk of cardiovascular mortality when compared with patients treated with diet alone.
CNS: Dizziness; vertigo.
DERM: Allergic skin reactions; eczema; pruritus; erythema; urticaria; morbilliform or maculopapular eruptions; lichenoid reactions; photosensitivity.
EENT: Tinnitus.
GI: GI disturbances (eg, nausea, epigastric fullness, heartburn); diarrhea.
GU: Mild diuresis; elevated BUN and creatinine.
HEPA: Cholestatic jaundice; elevated LFT results.
HEMA: Leukopenia; thrombocytopenia; aplastic anemia; agranulocytosis; hemolytic anemia; pancytopenia; hepatic porphyria.
METAB: Hypoglycemia.
OTHER: Disulfiram-like reaction; weakness; paresthesia; fatigue; malaise.

Precautions
Pregnancy: Category C. Insulin is recommended to maintain blood glucose levels during pregnancy. Prolonged severe neonatal hypoglycemia can occur if sulfonylureas are administered at time of delivery.
Lactation: Undetermined.
Children: Safety and efficacy not established.
Elderly: Elderly and debilitated patients are particularly susceptible to hypoglycemic action. Hypoglycemia may be difficult to recognize in elderly.
Renal function impairment: Use drug with caution and monitor renal function frequently.
Hepatic function impairment: Use drug with caution and monitor liver function frequently.

Overdosage: Signs and Symptoms
Prolonged hypoglycemia, tingling of lips and tongue, hunger, nausea, lethargy, yawning, confusion, agitation, nervousness, tachycardia, sweating, tremor, convulsions, stupor, coma.

PATIENT CARE CONSIDERATIONS
Administration/Storage
- Dose can be divided if single dose is not effective. Also divide doses if patient is taking more than 15 mg/day.
- Administer drug 30 min before meal; food delays absorption.
- If administering to pregnant patient, discontinue at least 1 mo before expected date of delivery.
- Store in tightly closed container at room temperature.

Assessment/Interventions
- Obtain patient history, including drug history and any known allergies. Note hepatic or renal impairment and nature of patient's diabetes (type 1 vs type 2).
- Check blood sugars frequently and observe for symptoms of hypoglycemia or hyperglycemia and report to health care provider.
- Test urine for glucose and acetone at least 3 times/day during titration period; report results to health care provider.
- When patients with impaired liver or renal function are receiving this drug, check liver and renal function tests frequently.

Patient/Family Education
- Remind patient to take medication on empty stomach 30 min before meals.
- Teach patient to self-monitor blood glucose.
- Emphasize importance of following diabetic diet.
- Inform patient that this drug is not substitute for exercise and diet control and that patient should follow prescribed regimens.
- Instruct patient to inform health care provider that they are taking this drug.
- Advise patient to carry identification stating that patient is diabetic.
- Inform patient to contact health care provider if symptoms of hypoglycemia occur (eg, fatigue, excessive hunger, profuse sweating, numbness of extremities).
- Tell patient to notify health care provider if symptoms of hyperglycemia occur (eg, excessive thirst or urination, urinary glucose or ketones).
- Instruct patient to report these symptoms to health care provider: nausea, vomiting, diarrhea, heartburn, sore throat, rash, unusual bruising or bleeding or other physical complaints.
- Advise patient not to take any medication (including *otc*) or alcohol without consulting health care provider.

Glipizide/Metformin Hydrochloride

(GLIP-ih-zide/met-FORE-min HIGH-droe-KLOR-ide)

Class Antidiabetic Combination/Sulfonylurea/Biguanide

How Supplied
Metaglip Tablets 2.5 mg/250 mg, Tablets 2.5 mg/500 mg, Tablets 5 mg/500 mg

Action
PHARMACOLOGY:
Glipizide: Decreases blood glucose by stimulating insulin release from pancreas and by increasing tissue sensitivity to insulin.
Metformin: Decreases blood glucose by reducing hepatic glucose production and may decrease intestinal absorption of glucose and increase response to insulin.

Indications Initial treatment as an adjunct to diet and exercise, to improve glycemic control in patients with type 2 diabetes whose hyperglycemia cannot be satisfactorily managed with diet and exercise alone; second-line therapy when diet, exercise, and initial treatment with a sulfonylurea or metformin do not result in adequate glycemic control in patients with type 2 diabetes.

Contraindications Patients with renal disease or renal dysfunction, which also may result from conditions such as CV collapse, acute MI, and septicemia; CHF requiring pharmacologic treatment; acute or chronic metabolic acidosis, with or without coma; known hypersensitivity to any component of the product.

Route/Dosage
Dosage must be individualized on the basis of both effectiveness and tolerance, while not exceeding the max recommended daily dose of 20 mg glipizide or 2000 mg metformin.
Initial Therapy
ADULTS: **PO** Recommended starting dose is 2.5 mg/250 mg qd with a meal. For patients whose fasting plasma glucose (FPG) is 280 to 320 mg/dL, consider a starting dose of 2.5 mg/500 mg bid. Make dosage increases, to achieve adequate glycemic control, in increments of 1 tablet/day q 2 wk to a max of 10 mg/1000 mg or 10 mg/2000 mg/day in divided doses. Efficacy in patients whose FPG is greater than 320 mg/dL has not been established.

Second-Line Therapy
ADULTS: **PO** Recommended starting dose is 2.5 mg/500 mg or 5 mg/500 mg bid with morning and evening meals. To avoid hypoglycemia, the starting dose should not exceed the daily doses of glipizide or metformin already being taken. Titrate the daily dose in increments of no more than 5 mg/500 mg up to the minimum effective dose that adequately controls blood glucose but not exceeding 20 mg/2000 mg/day. Patients previously treated with combination therapy of glipizide plus metformin may be switched to 2.5 mg/500 mg or 5 mg/500 mg; however, the starting dose should not exceed the daily dose of glipizide or equivalent dose of another sulfonylurea and metformin already being taken.

Interactions
Alcohol: The effects of metformin on lactate metabolism may be potentiated.
Beta adrenergic blocking agents, chloramphenicol, ciprofloxacin, coumarin anticoagulants, MAO inhibitors, miconazole, NSAIDs, probenecid, salicylates, sulfonamides: May potentiate the hypoglycemic action of glipizide.
Calcium channel blocking agents, corticosteroids, estrogens, isoniazid, nicotinic acid, oral contraceptives, phenothiazines, phenytoin, sympathomimetics, thiazides and other diuretics, thyroid products: These agents tend to produce hyperglycemia and may lead to loss of blood glucose control.
Furosemide: Metformin plasma levels may be elevated, while furosemide levels may be decreased.
Nifedipine: Metformin plasma levels may be increased.

Lab Test Interferences None well documented.

Adverse Reactions
CV: Hypertension (greater than 5%).
CNS: Dizziness, headache (greater than 5%).
GI: Diarrhea, nausea, vomiting, abdominal pain (greater than 5%).
GU: UTI (greater than 1%).
METAB: Hypoglycemia (greater than 5%).
RESP: Upper respiratory tract infections (greater than 5%).
OTHER: Musculoskeletal pain (greater than 5%).

> **WARNING:**
> Lactic acidosis is a rare, but serious metabolic complication that can occur because of metformin accumulation during treatment with glipizide/metformin. When it occurs, it is fatal in approximately 50% of cases.

Precautions
Pregnancy: Category C.
Lactation: Undetermined; however, some sulfo-

nylurea drugs are known to be excreted in breast milk.

Children: Safety and efficacy not established.

Elderly: In general, elderly patients are not titrated to the max dose because of age-related decreases in renal function.

Renal function impairment: Metabolism and excretion of glipizide may be slowed in patients with impaired renal or hepatic function. Decreased renal function results in decreased renal Cl and prolongation of the metformin t½. Concomitant medications that affect renal function may result in hemodynamic changes or interfere with disposition of metformin (eg, cationic drugs) and should be used with caution. Avoid metformin in patients whose serum creatinine levels exceed the upper limit of normal for their age or with clinical or laboratory evidence of hepatic disease.

Hepatic function impairment: Metabolism and excretion of glipizide may be slowed in patients with impaired renal or hepatic function. Decreased renal function results in decreased renal Cl and prolongation of the metformin t½. Concomitant medications that affect renal function may result in hemodynamic changes or interfere with disposition of metformin (eg, cationic drugs) and should be used with caution. Avoid metformin in patients whose serum creatinine levels exceed the upper limit of normal for their age or with clinical or laboratory evidence of hepatic disease.

CV mortality: Oral hypoglycemic agents have been associated with increased CV mortality compared with treatment with diet alone or diet plus insulin.

Iodinated contrast materials: Metformin therapy should be withheld at the time of or prior to parenteral contrast studies with iodinated materials. Reinstitute therapy 48 hr after the study and after renal function has been determined to be normal.

Lactic acidosis: Lactic acidosis can occur as a result of metformin accumulation (eg, renal impairment) or in pathophysiologic conditions associated with tissue hypoperfusion and hypoxia. The risk of lactic acidosis increases with the degree of renal dysfunction and the age of the patient.

Vitamin B_{12}: A decrease in vitamin B_{12} levels to subnormal may occur. Supplementation may be necessary.

Overdosage: Signs and Symptoms

Hypoglycemia, coma, seizures, neurological impairment (glipizide); lactic acidosis (metformin).

PATIENT CARE CONSIDERATIONS

Administration/Storage

- Do not administer to patients with renal impairment or type 1 diabetes mellitus.
- Administer dose bid as prescribed.
- Administer each dose with food to prevent GI distress.
- Store at controlled room temperature (59° to 86°F).

Assessment/Interventions

- Obtain patient history, including drug history and any known allergies. Note renal disease, liver disease, CHF, dehydration, chronic metabolic acidosis, or acute metabolic acidosis (eg, diabetic ketoacidosis).
- Ensure that renal function, hemoglobin, hematocrit, and RBC indices have been assessed prior to starting therapy and at least annually during therapy.
- Ensure that Ccr has been determined in patient older than 80 yr of age before initiating therapy.
- Check blood sugars frequently and observe for signs of hypoglycemia. Inform health care provider if blood sugar readings are outside target range or if hypoglycemic events are noted. Be prepared to treat hypoglycemic reactions.
- Ensure that medication is withheld before, and for 48 hr after, undergoing a radiologic study with intravascular administration of iodinated contrast material and is not restarted until renal function has been documented to be normal.
- Hold therapy in patient undergoing surgical procedure until oral intake has resumed and renal function has been documented to be normal.
- Monitor patient for signs or symptoms of metabolic acidosis (eg, malaise, myalgia, respiratory distress, unexplained drowsiness, nausea, vomiting, abdominal pain). Inform health care provider immediately if noted and be prepared to discontinue therapy.
- Assess patient for GI, CNS, and general body side effects. Inform health care provider if noted and significant.

Patient/Family Education

- Explain name, dose, action, and potential side effects of drug.
- Educate patient regarding diabetes and its management, including target ranges for blood sugar control. Advise patient that medication is not a substitute for diet and exercise and to continue to follow prescribed regimens.
- Educate patient or caregiver regarding poten-

tial long-term complications of diabetes and the need for regular physical and eye examinations.
- Advise patient to read *Patient Information* leaflet before starting therapy and with each refill.
- Advise patient to take prescribed dose bid and to take with food to decrease GI distress.
- Advise patient that dose may be gradually increased q 2 wk until max benefit is obtained.
- Advise patient to take as prescribed and not to stop taking or change the dose unless advised by health care provider.
- Ensure that patient understands how to use home glucose monitor and has a plan for monitoring and recording blood sugar measurements (eg, log). Advise patient to take log to each visit with health care provider.
- Educate patient regarding value of periodic hemoglobin A1c testing to confirm level of glucose control.
- Advise patient to discuss with health care provider a plan for managing each of the following situations: medication dosing during intercurrent conditions (eg, vomiting, infection, trauma, stress, sick days); accidental administration of too little or too much medication; missed dose; inadequate food intake or a skipped meal; travel across time zones; change in physical activity.
- Advise patient to carry medical identification of diabetes (eg, Medi-Alert).
- Caution patient to avoid excessive alcohol intake to reduce risk of lactic acidosis.
- Instruct patient to report any of the following to health care provider immediately: general body discomfort, muscle aches, unexplained rapid breathing or shortness of breath, unexplained drowsiness, nausea, vomiting, or abdominal pain.
- Review symptoms of hypoglycemia and hyperglycemia and action plans to undertake in the event either occur.
- Instruct patient to notify health care provider if experiencing hypoglycemic episodes or if measured blood sugars are outside target range.
- Advise women to notify health care provider if pregnant, planning to become pregnant, or breastfeeding.
- Instruct patient not to take prescription or OTC drugs or dietary supplements without consulting health care provider.
- Advise patient that follow-up visits and lab tests will be necessary to monitor therapy and to keep appointments.

Glucagon

(GLUE-kuh-gahn)

Class Glucose elevating agent

How Supplied
GlucaGen Powder for Injection 1 mg (1 unit) ◆ Glucagon Emergency Kit Powder for Injection 1 mg (1 unit) ◆ Glucagon Diagnostic Kit Powder for Injection 1 mg (1 unit)

Action
PHARMACOLOGY: Elevates blood glucose concentrations (by stimulating production from liver glycogen stores), relaxes smooth muscle of GI tract, decreases gastric and pancreatic secretions in GI tract, and increases myocardial contractility.

PHARMACOKINETICS/DYNAMICS:
Absorption: Mean C_{max} is 1,686 pg/mL (IM). Median T_{max} is 12.5 min (IM).
Metabolism: Degraded in liver, kidney, and plasma.
Excretion: Mean apparent $t_{½}$ 45 min (IM).
Onset: 10 min.
Peak: 30 min.

Indications Treatment of severe hypoglycemic reactions in diabetic patients when glucose administration is not possible or during insulin shock therapy in psychiatric patients; diagnostic aid in radiologic examination of stomach, duodenum, small bowel, and colon when diminished intestinal motility would be advantageous. GlucaGen: Treatment of severe hypoglycemic reactions that may occur in patients with diabetes treated with insulin; as a diagnostic aid during radiologic examinations to temporarily inhibit movement of the GI tract. **Unlabeled use(s):** Treatment of propranolol overdose, CV emergencies, and GI disturbances associated with spasms.

Contraindications Patients with pheochromocytoma or insulinoma; hypersensitivity to any component of the product.

Route/Dosage
Diagnostic Aid
ADULTS AND CHILDREN: **IM/IV** 0.25 to 2 mg, depending on procedure and desired length of smooth muscle relaxation.

Hypoglycemia
ADULTS AND CHILDREN MORE THAN 20 KG:
Subcutaneous/IM/IV 1 mg (1 unit). Do not use glucagon at concentrations above 1 mg/mL (1 unit/mL).
CHILDREN LESS THAN 20 KG: **Subcutaneous/IM/IV** 0.5 mg (0.5 unit) or a dose equivalent to 20 to 30 mcg/kg.
GLUCAGEN:
Adults and children weighing 25 kg or more: **Subcutaneous/IM/IV** 1 mg.
Children weighing less than 25 kg or younger than 8 yr of age: **Subcutaneous/IM/IV** 0.5 mg. Emergency assistance should be sought if patient fails to respond within 15 min after subcutaneous or IM injection of glucagon. The glucagon injection may be repeated while waiting for emergency assistance. IV glucose must be administered if patient fails to respond to glucagon. When the patient has responded, give oral carbohydrate to restore liver glycogen and prevent recurrence of hypoglycemia.

Insulin Shock Therapy
ADULTS: **Subcutaneous/IM/IV** 0.5 to 1 mg after 1 hr of coma (larger doses have been used to reverse coma). Patient will usually awaken in 10 to 25 min. If no response, may repeat dose.

Interactions
Anticoagulants, oral: May increase hypoprothrombinemic effects, possibly with bleeding.

PATIENT CARE CONSIDERATIONS
Administration/Storage
- Used in combination with supplemental carbohydrate administration when treating a severe hypoglycemic reaction.
- For subcutaneous, IM, or IV administration only. Not for intradermal or intra-arterial administration.
- Usual dose for treating hypoglycemia is 1 mg for adults and children weighing more than 55 pounds. Usual dose for children weighing less than 55 pounds is 0.5 mg (or 9 to 14 mg per pound).
- Reconstitute powder for injection using only supplied diluent (*GlucaGen*); may be reconstituted with supplied diluent or with 1 mL sterile water for injection. Roll vial gently until powder is completely dissolved and is free of particles.
- Administer solution immediately after reconstitution. Discard any unused solution. Do not save solution for future use.
- Do not administer glucagon if particulate matter, cloudiness, or discoloration is noted or if solution shows any signs of gel formation.
- Store unopened vials at controlled room temperature (68° to 77°F). Avoid freezing; protect from light.

Lab Test Interferences None well documented

Adverse Reactions
CV: Transient increase in BP and pulse rate; positive inotropic and chronotropic effects (tachycardia).
GI: Nausea; vomiting.
OTHER: Generalized allergic reactions, including urticaria, respiratory distress, and hypotension.

Precautions
Pregnancy: Category B.
Lactation: Undetermined.
Children:
Treatment of hypoglycemia – Glucagon has been shown to be safe and effective.
As diagnostic aid – Safety and efficacy not established.
Insulinoma/Pheochromocytoma: Administer cautiously to patient with history of insulinoma or pheochromocytoma.
Hypoglycemia: Glucagon is effective in treating hypoglycemia only if sufficient liver glycogen is present. Because glucagon is of little or no help in states of starvation, adrenal insufficiency, or chronic hypoglycemia, treat hypoglycemia in these conditions with glucose.

Overdosage: Signs and Symptoms
Nausea, vomiting, gastric hypotonicity, diarrhea without consequential toxicity, increased BP and pulse rate.

Assessment/Interventions
- Obtain patient history, including drug history and any known allergies. Note pheochromocytoma, insulinoma, prolonged fasting, starvation, adrenal insufficiency, chronic hypoglycemia, diabetes, or elderly patient with CV disease (GI examination only).
- When treating a patient with hypoglycemia, ensure that supplemental carbohydrates are given as soon as the patient awakens and is able to swallow.
- When using glucagon for radiologic examinations, ensure that patient is given oral carbohydrates as soon as the procedure has been completed.
- Monitor fingerstick blood sugars frequently in hypoglycemic patient until the patient is asymptomatic. Notify health care provider immediately if patient has not responded within 15 min of subcutaneous or IM dose of glucagon. Be prepared to administer IV glucose.
- Monitor BP and pulse after administering glucagon. Transient increases are not uncommon. Notify health care provider immediately if increase in BP is dramatic or patient experiences symptoms. Be prepared to administer

phentolamine to reduce BP in patient with pheochromocytoma or with coronary artery disease.
- Institute measures to protect airway in patient with decreased neurologic status who begins to vomit.
- Monitor patient for signs and symptoms of anaphylactic or serious allergic reactions. Be prepared to treat appropriately.

Patient/Family Education
- Explain name, dose, action, and potential side effects of drug.
- Advise patient and family members to read *Information for Patients* leaflet before using the first time and with each refill.
- Ensure that patient and family members understand how to store, prepare, and administer the dose of glucagon, and dispose of used equipment and supplies.
- Ensure that patient and family members can recognize symptoms of mild hypoglycemia and know how to treat it appropriately to prevent severe hypoglycemia from developing.
- Educate patient and family members regarding the risks of prolonged hypoglycemia and the need to arouse the hypoglycemic patient as rapidly as possible.
- Instruct patient or family members to monitor fingerstick blood sugars frequently when treating hypoglycemia until the patient is asymptomatic. Advise family members to call 911 if patient has not responded within 15 min of injection and to administer second dose of glucagon while awaiting emergency assistance.
- Instruct patient and family members that supplemental carbohydrates must be given as soon as the patient awakens and is able to swallow.
- Advise patient to inform health care provider when hypoglycemic reactions occur so that the treatment regimen may be adjusted if necessary.
- Instruct patient and family members regarding the following measures that may prevent or be used to rapidly treat hypoglycemic reactions caused by insulin: reasonable uniformity from day to day with regard to diet, insulin dose, and exercise; careful adjustment of insulin program; frequent monitoring of fingerstick blood sugars so that a change in insulin requirements can be foreseen; carrying sugar, candy, or other readily absorbable carbohydrate at all times so that it may be taken at the first warning of an oncoming hypoglycemic reaction.
- Caution patient not to take any prescription or OTC drugs, dietary supplements, or herbal preparations unless advised by health care provider.
- Advise patient that follow-up visits and lab tests may be necessary to monitor therapy and to keep appointments.

Glyburide

(glie-BYOO-ride)
Class Antidiabetic/Sulfonylurea

How Supplied
DiaBeta Tablets 1.25 mg, Tablets 2.5 mg, Tablets 5 mg ◆ *Glynase PresTab* Tablets, micronized 1.5 mg, Tablets, micronized 3 mg, Tablets, micronized 6 mg ◆ *Micronase* Tablets 1.25 mg, Tablets 2.5 mg, Tablets 5 mg

❋ Apo-Glyburide ◆ Diaβeta ◆ Euglucon ◆ Gen-Glybe ◆ Novo-Glyburide ◆ Nu-Glyburide ◆ ratio-Glyburide ◆ PMS-Glyburide

Action
PHARMACOLOGY: Decreases blood glucose by stimulating insulin release from pancreas. May also decrease hepatic glucose production or increased response to insulin.

PHARMACOKINETICS/DYNAMICS:
Absorption: Significantly absorbed. T_{max} is about 4 hr; about 2 to 3 hr (micronized). Mean C_{max} is 104 ng/mL; 106 ng/mL (micronized). Mean AUC is 746 ng•hr/mL; 568 ng•hr/mL (micronized).

Distribution: Protein binding is extensive.

Metabolism: The major metabolite is the 4-trans-hydroxy derivative (no significant activity). The minor metabolite is the 3-cis-hydroxy derivative (no significant activity).

Excretion: $T_{½}$ is about 10 hr, about 4 hr (micronized). Excreted as metabolites in the urine and feces equally.

Duration: 24 hr.

Indications Adjunct to diet to lower blood glucose in patients with non-insulin-dependent diabetes mellitus (type 2) whose hyperglycemia cannot be controlled by diet alone; in combination with metformin when diet and glyburide or diet and metformin alone do not result in adequate glycemic control.

Contraindications Hypersensitivity to sulfonylureas; diabetes complicated by ketoacidosis with or without coma; sole therapy of insulin-dependent diabetes mellitus (type 1); diabetes when complicated by pregnancy.

Route/Dosage
Nonmicronized Form
ADULTS: **PO** 2.5 to 5 mg/day with breakfast or first main meal.

Patients More Sensitive to Hypoglycemic Drugs (eg, elderly or patients with renal or hepatic dysfunction)
ADULTS: PO 1.25 mg/day initially. Maintenance: 1.25 to 20 mg daily in single or divided doses (patients receiving more than 10 mg/day may have better response to twice-daily dosing). Daily doses more than 20 mg are not recommended.

Micronized Form (Glynase Pres Tab)
ADULTS: PO 1.5 to 3 mg/day with breakfast or first main meal. Maintenance: 0.75 to 12 mg/day. Patients receiving more than 6 mg/day have more satisfactory response to twice-daily dosing. Daily doses more than 12 mg are not recommended.

Concomitant Metformin
ADULTS: PO Add micronized glyburide gradually to the dosing regimen of patients who have not responded to the maximum dose of metformin monotherapy after 4 wk.

Interactions
Alcohol: Produces disulfiram-like reaction (eg, facial flushing, headache, breathlessness).
Androgens, chloramphenicol, clofibrate, dicumarol, fenfluramine, fluconazole, gemfibrozil, histamine H_2 antagonists, magnesium salts, methyldopa, monoamine oxidase inhibitors, phenylbutazone, probenecid, salicylates, sulfinpyrazone, sulfonamides, tricyclic antidepressants, urinary acidifiers: May increase hypoglycemic effect.
Beta-blockers, cholestyramine, diazoxide, hydantoins, rifampin, thiazide diuretics, urinary alkalinizers: May decrease hypoglycemic effect.
Ciprofloxacin: A possible interaction between glyburide and ciprofloxacin has been reported, resulting in a potentiation of the hypoglycemic action.

Lab Test Interferences None well documented.

Adverse Reactions
CV: Although the issue is controversial, oral sulfonylureas may have increased risk of cardiovascular mortality when compared with patients treated with diet alone.
CNS: Dizziness; vertigo.
DERM: Allergic skin reactions; eczema; pruritus; erythema; urticaria; morbilliform or maculopapular eruptions; lichenoid reactions; photosensitivity.
EENT: Tinnitus.
GI: Nausea, epigastric fullness; heartburn.
GU: Mild diuresis; mild to moderate elevations in BUN and creatinine.
HEMA: Leukopenia; thrombocytopenia; aplastic anemia; agranulocytosis; hemolytic anemia; pancytopenia; hepatic porphyria.
HEPA: Cholestatic jaundice; elevated LFT results.
METAB: Hypoglycemia.
OTHER: Disulfiram-like reactions; weakness; paresthesia; fatigue; malaise.

Precautions
Pregnancy: Category B. Insulin is recommended to maintain blood glucose levels during pregnancy. Prolonged severe neonatal hypoglycemia can occur if sulfonylureas are administered at time of delivery.
Lactation: Undetermined.
Children: Safety and efficacy not established.
Elderly: Elderly and debilitated patients are particularly susceptible to the hypoglycemic action. Hypoglycemia may be difficult to recognize in elderly patients.
Renal function impairment: Use drug with caution; lower doses may be adequate.
Hepatic function impairment: Use drug with caution; lower doses may be adequate.
Bioavailability: Micronized glyburide (*Glynase Pres Tab*) and conventional (nonmicronized) glyburide formulations are not equivalent.

Overdosage: Signs and Symptoms
Hypoglycemia, tingling of lips and tongue, hunger, nausea, lethargy, yawning, confusion, agitation, nervousness, tachycardia, sweating, tremor, convulsions, stupor, coma.

PATIENT CARE CONSIDERATIONS
Administration/Storage
- Administer with first main meal of day; patients taking large doses may require twice-daily dosing.
- Dose must be readjusted when switching between micronized and conventional (nonmicronized) formulations; they are not bioequivalent.
- If administering to a pregnant patient, discontinue at least 1 mo before expected date of delivery.
- Store in tightly capped container, and keep out of reach of children.

Assessment/Interventions
- Obtain patient history, including drug history and any known allergies.
- Note hepatic or renal impairment and the nature of the patient's diabetes (type 1 vs type 2).
- Be aware that hypoglycemia may be difficult to recognize in elderly.
- Test urine for glucose and acetone at least 3 times daily during titration period, unless patient is already testing blood glucose. Report results to health care provider.

- When patients with impaired liver or renal function are receiving this drug, check liver and renal function tests frequently.
- Check blood sugars frequently and observe for symptoms of hypoglycemia or hyperglycemia and report to health care provider.

Patient/Family Education
- Review with patient dietary guidelines for diabetes.
- Instruct patient to take drug with meals.
- Teach patient to self-monitor urine or blood glucose.
- Inform patient that this drug is not substitute for exercise and diet control and that patient should follow prescribed regimens.
- Instruct patient to inform all health care providers involved in the patient's care that this drug is being taken and to carry medical identification (eg, *Medi-Alert* bracelet).
- Instruct patient to notify health care provider if symptoms of hypoglycemia occur (eg, fatigue, excessive hunger, profuse sweating, numbness of extremities) or if blood glucose is less than 60 mg/dL.
- Tell patient to notify health care provider if symptoms of hyperglycemia occur (eg, excessive thirst or urination, urinary glucose or ketones).
- Instruct patient to report these symptoms to health care provider: nausea, vomiting, diarrhea, heartburn, sore throat, rash, unusual bruising, or bleeding, other physical complaints.
- Advise patient not to take any medication (including *otc*) or alcohol without consulting health care provider.

Glyburide/Metformin Hydrochloride

(glie-BYOO-ride/met-FORE-min HIGH-droe-KLOR-ide)

Class Antidiabetic/Sulfonylurea/Biguanide

How Supplied
Glucovance Tablets 1.25 mg (glyburide)/250 mg (metformin), Tablets 2.5 mg (glyburide)/500 mg (metformin), Tablets 5 mg (glyburide)/500 mg (metformin)

Action
PHARMACOLOGY:
Glyburide: Decreases blood glucose by stimulating insulin release from pancreas and may decrease hepatic glucose production or increase response to insulin.
Metformin: Decreases blood glucose by decreasing hepatic glucose production and may decrease intestinal absorption of glucose and increase response to insulin.

Indications Adjunct to diet and exercise to improve glycemic control in patients with type 2 diabetes whose hyperglycemia cannot be satisfactorily managed by diet and exercise alone; second-line therapy when diet, exercise, and initial treatment with a sulfonylurea or metformin do not result in adequate glycemic control in patients with type 2 diabetes.

Contraindications Patients with renal disease or dysfunction, which may also result from conditions such as CV collapse, acute MI, and septicemia; CHF requiring pharmacologic treatment; acute or chronic metabolic acidosis (including diabetic ketoacidosis, with or without coma); known hypersensitivity to any component of product.

Route/Dosage
Initial Therapy
ADULTS: PO Starting dose 1.25 mg glyburide/250 mg metformin (1.25 mg/250 mg) qd with a meal; if glycosylated hemoglobin is greater than 9% or fasting plasma glucose is greater than 200 mg/dL, start with 1.25 mg/250 mg bid with morning and evening meals. Dosage increases may be made in increments of 1.25 mg/250 mg/day q 2 wk up to the minimum effective dose (there is no experience with daily doses greater than 10 mg glyburide/2000 mg metformin).

Second-Line Therapy
ADULTS: PO Start with 2.5 mg/500 mg or 5 mg/500 mg bid with morning and evening meals but not exceeding the daily dose of glyburide or metformin already being taken. Titrate the daily dose in increments of no more than 5 mg/500 mg up to the minimum effective dose (max, 20 mg glyburide/2000 mg metformin daily).

Interactions
Alcohol: The effects of metformin on lactate metabolism may be potentiated.
Beta adrenergic blocking agents, chloramphenicol, ciprofloxacin, coumarin anticoagulants, MAO inhibitors, NSAIDs, miconazole, probenecid, salicylates, sulfonamides: May potentiate the hypoglycemic action of glyburide.
Calcium channel blocking agents, corticosteroids, estrogens, isoniazid, nicotinic acid, oral contraceptives, phenothiazines, phenytoin, sympathomimetics, thiazides and other diuretics, thyroid products: These agents tend to produce hyperglycemia and may lead to loss of blood glucose control.
Furosemide: Metformin plasma levels may be elevated while furosemide levels may be decreased.

Nifedipine: Metformin plasma levels may be increased.

Lab Test Interferences None well documented.

Adverse Reactions
CNS: Headache, dizziness (greater than 5%).
GI: Diarrhea, nausea, vomiting, abdominal pain (greater than 5%).
METAB: Hypoglycemia (greater than 5%).
RESP: Upper respiratory tract infection (greater than 5%).

> **Warning:**
> Lactic acidosis is a rare, but serious metabolic complication that can occur caused by metformin accumulation during treatment with glyburide/metformin. When it occurs, it is fatal in approximately 50% of cases.

Precautions
Pregnancy: Category B.
Lactation: Undetermined.
Children: Safety and efficacy not established.
Elderly: In general, elderly patients are not titrated to the max dose because of age-related decreases in renal function.
Renal function impairment: Decreased renal function results in decreased renal Cl and prolongation of the metformin t½. Concomitant medications that affect renal function may result in hemodynamic changes or interfere with disposition of metformin (eg, cationic drugs) and should be used with caution.
CV mortality: The administration of oral hypoglycemic drugs has been reported to be associated with increased CV mortality as compared with treatment with diet alone or diet plus insulin.
Hepatic disease: Avoid metformin in patients with clinical or laboratory evidence of hepatic disease.
Iodinated contrast material: Withhold metformin therapy at time of or prior to parenteral contrast studies with iodinated materials. Reinstitute therapy 48 hr after the study and after renal function has been determined to be normal.
Lactic acidosis: Can occur as a result of metformin accumulation (eg renal impairment) or in pathophysiologic conditions associated with tissue hypoperfusion and hypoxia. The risk of lactic acidosis increases with the degree of renal dysfunction and the age of the patient.
Vitamin B_{12}: A decrease in vitamin B_{12} levels to subnormal may occur. Supplementation may be necessary.

Overdosage: Signs and Symptoms
Glyburide: Hypoglycemia, coma, seizures, neurological impairment.
Metformin: Lactic acidosis.

PATIENT CARE CONSIDERATIONS
Administration/Storage
- Do not administer to patients with renal impairment or to patients with type 1 diabetes mellitus.
- Administer dose bid as prescribed.
- Administer each dose with food to prevent GI distress.
- May be used in combination with a thiazolidinedione.
- Store at controlled room temperature (up to 77°F).

Assessment/Interventions
- Obtain patient history, including drug history and any known allergies. Note renal disease, liver disease, CHF, dehydration, chronic metabolic acidosis, or acute metabolic acidosis (eg, diabetic ketoacidosis).
- Ensure renal function, hemoglobin, hematocrit, and RBC indices have been assessed prior to starting therapy and at least annually during therapy.
- Ensure that Ccr has been determined in patient older than 80 yr before initiating therapy.
- Check blood sugars frequently and observe for signs of hypoglycemia. Inform health care provider if blood sugar readings are outside target range or if hypoglycemic events are noted. Be prepared to treat hypoglycemic reactions.
- Ensure that medication is withheld before, and for 48 hr after, undergoing a radiologic study with intravascular administration of iodinated contrast material and is not restarted until renal function has been documented to be normal.
- Hold therapy in patient undergoing surgical procedure until oral intake has resumed and renal function has been documented to be normal.
- Monitor patient for signs or symptoms of metabolic acidosis (eg, malaise, myalgia, respiratory distress, unexplained drowsiness, nausea, vomiting, abdominal pain). Inform health care provider immediately if noted and be prepared to discontinue therapy.
- Assess patient for GI, CNS, and general body side effects. Inform health care provider if noted and significant.

Patient/Family Education
- Explain name, dose, action, and potential side effects of drug.
- Educate patient regarding diabetes and its management, including target ranges for

blood sugar control. Instruct patient that medication is not a substitute for diet and exercise and to continue to follow prescribed regimens.
- Educate patient or caregiver regarding potential long-term complications of diabetes and need for regular general physical and eye examinations.
- Advise patient to read *Patient Information* leaflet before starting therapy and with each refill.
- Advise patient to take prescribed dose bid and to take with food to decrease GI distress.
- Advise patient that dose may be gradually increased q 2 wk until max benefit is obtained.
- Advise patient to take as prescribed and not to stop taking or change the dose unless advised by health care provider.
- Ensure that patient understands how to use home glucose monitor and has a plan for monitoring and recording blood sugar measurements (eg, log). Advise patient to take log to each visit with health care provider.
- Educate patient regarding value of periodic hemoglobin A1c testing to confirm level of glucose control.
- Advise patient to carry medical identification indicating diabetes (eg, *Medi-Alert*).
- Caution patient to avoid excessive alcohol intake to reduce risk of lactic acidosis.
- Instruct patient to report any of the following to health care provider immediately: general body discomfort, muscle aches, unexplained rapid breathing or shortness of breath, unexplained drowsiness, nausea, vomiting, abdominal pain.
- Review symptoms of hypoglycemia and hyperglycemia and action plans to undertake in the event either occur.
- Advise patient to discuss with health care provider a plan for managing each of the following situations: medication dosing during intercurrent conditions (eg, vomiting, infection, trauma, stress, sick days); accidental administration of too little or too much medication; missed dose; inadequate food intake or a skipped meal; travel across time zones; change in physical activity.
- Instruct patient to notify health care provider if experiencing hypoglycemic episodes or if measured blood sugars are outside target range.
- Advise women to notify health care provider if pregnant, planning to become pregnant, or breastfeeding.
- Instruct patient not to take prescription or OTC drugs or dietary supplements unless advised by health care provider.
- Advise patient that follow-up visits and lab tests will be necessary to monitor therapy and to keep appointments.

Glycerin (Glycerol)

(GLIH-suh-rin)
Class Osmotic diuretic/Laxative/Ophthalmic
How Supplied
Colace Suppositories glycerin ♦ *Fleet Babylax* Liquid 4 mL/applicator ♦ *Ophthalgan* Solution (ophthalmic) glycerin ♦ *Osmoglyn* Solution 50% (0.6 g glycerin/mL) ♦ *Sani-Supp* Suppositories glycerin
Action
PHARMACOLOGY: Reduces IOP by creating osmotic gradient between plasma and ocular fluids (oral form). Promotes bowel evacuation by local irritation and hyperosmotic actions (rectal form). Reduces edema and clears corneal haze by attracting water through semipermeable corneal epithelium (ophthalmic form).
PHARMACOKINETICS/DYNAMICS:
Excretion: Eliminated by the kidneys.
Indications
Oral: Control of acute attack of glaucoma; reduction of intraocular pressure prior to and after ocular surgery.
Rectal: Short-term treatment of constipation; to evacuate the colon for rectal and bowel examinations.
Ophthalmic: Clearance of edematous corneas to facilitate ophthalmoscopic and gonioscopic examination in acute glaucoma, bullous keratitis, and Fuchs' endothelial dystrophy. **Unlabeled use(s):** Reduction of intraocular and intracranial pressure via special IV preparations.
Contraindications
Oral form: Anuria, severe dehydration, frank or impending acute pulmonary edema, severe cardiac decompensation.
Rectal forms: Nausea, vomiting, acute surgical abdomen, fecal impaction, intestinal obstruction, undiagnosed abdominal pain.
Route/Dosage
ADULTS: **PO** 1 to 2 g/kg 1 to 90 min prior to surgery. **PR** Insert 1 suppository (3 g) or 5 to 15 mL as rectal enema and retain 15 min. Topical 1 to 2 gtt instilled in eye(s) prior to examination.
CHILDREN OLDER THAN 6 YR: **PR** Same as adults.
CHILDREN 2 TO 6 YR: **PR** 1 to 1.5 g suppository or 2 to 5 mL as rectal enema.

CHILDREN YOUNGER THAN 2 YR: Use only on advice of health care provider.

Interactions None well documented.

Lab Test Interferences None well documented.

Adverse Reactions
CV: Arrhythmias.
CNS: Headache; confusion; disorientation; weakness; dizziness; fainting.
DERM: Rectal form: Perianal irritation; sweating.
EENT: Ophthalmic solution: Ocular pain and irritation.
GI: Nausea; vomiting. Rectal form: Excessive bowel activity; abdominal cramps; bloating; flatulence.
METAB: Dehydration; hyperosmolar nonketotic coma.

Precautions
Pregnancy: Category C.
Lactation: Undetermined.
Children: Do not administer enemas or suppositories to children younger than 2 yr. Safety and efficacy of other forms undetermined.
Elderly: Use with caution.
Special risk patients: Use oral form with caution in patients with hypovolemia, confused mental states, CHF, diabetes mellitus, and severe dehydration.

PATIENT CARE CONSIDERATIONS

Administration/Storage
- Administer 50% oral solution with 0.9% Sodium Chloride flavored with orange, lemon, or lime juice or administer commercially prepared 50% or 75% flavored solution.
- Administer suppository high in rectum with patient lying on side; encourage patient to retain suppository in rectum for at least 15 min.
- To administer rectal liquid, have patient lie on left side, insert stem of applicator into rectum with tip pointing toward navel, squeeze unit until nearly all liquid has been dispensed, and remove applicator. Small amount of liquid may remain in unit.
- Ophthalmic solution may cause burning sensation in eye. Administer local anesthetic before instillation of drug.
- Store suppositories in cool location, but do not freeze. Other formulations may be stored at room temperature.

Assessment/Interventions
- Obtain patient history, including drug history and any known allergies.
- Assess for nausea, vomiting, headache, altered neurologic status, and dehydration.
- With ophthalmic form, assess for eye pain or discomfort.
- With rectal form, assess last bowel movement, use of laxatives, ability to retain suppository, and effectiveness of drug regimen.
- Monitor I&O.
- Systemic administration will cause diuresis and possibly hypotension with dizziness. Institute safety precautions in presence of neurologic manifestations. Have patient maintain supine position after administration.
- With oral or ophthalmic forms, do not give hypotonic solutions after drug is administered.
- With rectal form, encourage fluid intake, fiber in diet, and activity.

Patient/Family Education
- Inform patient of need to maintain supine position after administration of oral form of drug.
- With rectal form, advise patient about dangers associated with long-term laxative use. Instruct patient in alternative measures to encourage bowel movements (eg, increase fluid intake, increase intake of dietary fiber, increase activity). Instruct patient to avoid laxative use in presence of abdominal pain, vomiting, or nausea.

Glycopyrrolate

(glie-koe-PIE-row-late)

Class Anticholinergic/Antispasmodic

How Supplied
Robinul Tablets 1 mg, Injection 0.2 mg/mL ♦
Robinul Forte Tablets 2 mg

Action
PHARMACOLOGY: Exerts anticholinergic effects, resulting in GI smooth muscle relaxation, diminished volume and acidity of GI secretions, and reduced pharyngeal, tracheal, and bronchial secretions.

PHARMACOKINETICS/DYNAMICS:
Absorption: Absorption is poor and unreliable.
Distribution: Highly polar ammonium group of glycopyrrolate limits its passage across blood-brain barrier and other lipid membranes.
Onset: Within 1 min after IV injection.
Peak: 30 to 45 min after IM administration.

Duration: Vagal blocking effects persist for 2 to 3 hr. Antisialagogue effects persist up to 7 hours.

Indications

Oral: Adjunctive treatment of peptic ulcer.
Parenteral: Preoperative administration for reduction of salivary, tracheobronchial and pharyngeal secretions, reduction of volume and acidity of gastric secretions, and blockade of cardiac vagal inhibitory reflexes before and during induction of anesthesia and intubation; intraoperatively for counteraction of drug-induced or vagal traction reflexes with associated arrhythmias.

Contraindications

Narrow angle glaucoma; adhesions between iris and lens; obstructive uropathy; obstructive disease of GI tract; paralytic ileus; intestinal atony of elderly or debilitated patients; severe ulcerative colitis; toxic megacolon complicating ulcerative colitis; hepatic or renal disease; tachycardia; myocardial ischemia; unstable cardiovascular status in acute hemorrhage; myasthenia gravis.

Route/Dosage

Peptic Ulcer
ADULTS AND CHILDREN OLDER THAN 12 YR: **PO** 1 to 2 mg bid or tid. **IM/IV** 0.1 to 0.2 mg tid or qid.

Preanesthetic Medication
ADULTS: **IM** 0.004 mg/kg 20 min to 1 hr prior to anesthesia.
CHILDREN YOUNGER THAN 12 YR: **IM** 0.0044 to 0.0088 mg/kg.
CHILDREN YOUNGER THAN 2 YR: **IM** up to 0.0088 mg/kg.

Intraoperative Medication
ADULTS: **IV** 0.1 mg. May repeat at 2 to 3 min intervals.
CHILDREN: **IV** 0.004 mg/kg (max 0.1 mg in single dose); may repeat at 2 to 3 min intervals.

Reversal of Neuromuscular Blockade
ADULTS AND CHILDREN: **IV** 0.2 mg for each 1 mg neostigmine or 5 mg pyridostigmine. Administer simultaneously.

Interactions

Haloperidol: May cause decreased serum haloperidol levels, worsened schizophrenic symptoms, and tardive dyskinesia.
INCOMPATIBILITIES: Because stability of glycopyrrolate is questionable above pH of 6, do not combine in same syringe with methohexital sodium, chloramphenicol sodium succinate, dimenhydrinate, pentobarbital sodium, thiopental sodium, secobarbital sodium, sodium bicarbonate, diazepam, dexamethasone sodium phosphate, or buffered solution of Lactated Ringer's solution.

Lab Test Interferences
None well documented.

Adverse Reactions

CV: Palpitations; tachycardia; orthostatic hypotension.
CNS: Headache; flushing; nervousness; drowsiness; weakness; dizziness; confusion; insomnia; fever (especially in children); mental confusion or excitement (especially in elderly, even with small doses); CNS stimulation (restlessness, tremor, hallucinations).
DERM: Severe allergic reactions including anaphylaxis, urticaria, and dermal manifestations.
EENT: Blurred vision; mydriasis; photophobia; cycloplegia; increased intraocular pressure; dilated pupils; nasal congestion.
GI: Dry mouth; altered taste perception; nausea; vomiting; dysphagia; heartburn; constipation; bloated feeling; paralytic ileus.
GU: Urinary hesitancy and retention; impotence.
OTHER: Suppression of lactation; decreased sweating.

Precautions

Pregnancy: Category B.
Lactation: Undetermined.
Children: Not recommended for treatment of peptic ulcer in children younger than 12 yr.
Elderly: May react with excitement, agitation, drowsiness, and other untoward manifestations even with small doses.
Special risk patients: Use with caution in patients with autonomic neuropathy, hepatic or renal disease, ulcerative colitis, hyperthyroidism, coronary heart disease, CHF, cardiac tachyarrhythmias, hypertension, prostatic hypertrophy, hiatal hernia associated with reflux esophagitis.
Anticholinergic psychosis: Reported in sensitive individuals; may include confusion, disorientation, short-term memory loss, hallucinations, dysarthria, ataxia, coma, euphoria, anxiety, fatigue, insomnia, agitation, and inappropriate affect.
Diarrhea: May be symptom of incomplete intestinal obstruction, especially in patients with ileostomy or colostomy. Treatment of diarrhea with drug is inappropriate and possibly harmful.
Gastric ulcer: May delay gastric emptying rate and complicate therapy.
Heat prostration: Can occur in presence of high environmental temperature.

Overdosage: Signs and Symptoms

Dry mouth, thirst, vomiting, nausea, abdominal distention, difficulty swallowing, muscular weakness, paralysis, fever, coma, circulatory failure, rapid pulse and respiration, vasodilation, tachycardia with weak pulse, hypertension, hypotension, respiratory depression, palpitations.

PATIENT CARE CONSIDERATIONS
Administration/Storage
- For IM administration, give drug undiluted or mixed with D5W, D10W, or 0.9% Sodium Chloride.
- May administer undiluted drug IV.
- Do not administer parenteral solution if cloudy.
- Store parenteral and oral formulations at room temperature.

Assessment/Interventions
- Obtain patient history, including drug history and any known allergies.
- Assess bowel sounds and frequency of bowel movements.
- Monitor I&O.
- Monitor vital signs closely, particularly heart rate and BP, during parenteral administration.
- Assess for side effects: palpitations, neurologic alterations, GI alterations.
- Assess urinary output and signs and symptoms of urinary retention.
- Assess for presence of abdominal pain.

Patient/Family Education
- Instruct patient that constipation can occur and to institute preventive measures (eg, increase fluids, bulk in diet, and activity).
- Advise patient that urinary hesitancy or retention may be experienced. Instruct patient to assess urination patterns and to notify health care provider if urinary retention is experienced.
- Inform men that impotence is potential side effect and to report this symptom to health care provider.
- Because drug interferes with body's thermoregulation, instruct patient to avoid exposure to high environmental temperature to prevent heat prostration.
- Instruct patient to notify health care provider immediately if eye pain or increased sensitivity to light occurs. Emphasize importance of routine eye examinations throughout therapy.
- Inform patient that dry mouth is a normal side effect. Instruct patient to take sips of water frequently, suck on ice chips or sugarless hard candy, or chew sugarless gum if dry mouth occurs.
- Caution patient to avoid sudden position changes to prevent orthostatic hypotension.
- Advise patient that drug may cause drowsiness and blurred vision and to use caution while driving or performing other tasks requiring mental alertness.

Gold Sodium Thiomalate
(gold SO-dee-uhm thigh-oh-MAL-ate)

Class Anti-inflammatory/Antirheumatic/Gold compound

How Supplied
Aurolate Injection 50 mg/mL

Action
PHARMACOLOGY: Mechanism unknown; suppresses symptoms of rheumatoid arthritis and may slow progression of this disease.

PHARMACOKINETICS/DYNAMICS:
Absorption: Mean C_{ss} is 1 to 5 mcg/mL. T_{max} is 2 to 6 hr.
Distribution: Protein binding is 95% to 99%.
Excretion: Plasma $t_{1/2}$ is 3 to 27 d (single dose); 14 to 40 d (third dose); up to 168 d (11th dose). 70% is excreted in urine, 30% in feces.

Indications
Symptomatic relief of active adult and juvenile rheumatoid arthritis not adequately controlled by other therapies. **Unlabeled use(s):** Treatment of pemphigus and psoriatic arthritis.

Contraindications
Previous severe reaction to gold compounds or other heavy metals; uncontrolled diabetes mellitus or CHF; severe debilitation; kidney disease; liver disease; severe hypertension; agranulocytosis or bleeding disorder; recent radiation exposure; systemic lupus erythematosus; urticaria; eczema.

Route/Dosage
ADULTS: IM As weekly injections: First wk, 10 mg; second wk, 25 mg; third and following wks, 25 to 50 mg until major clinical improvement or toxicity occurs. If cumulative dose reaches 1 g without improvement, re-evaluate use of gold therapy. Once improvement occurs, dose may be decreased or dosing interval increased. Maintenance therapy: 25 to 50 mg every other wk for 2 to 20 wk. On basis of response, dosage interval may be increased to every third and subsequently fourth wk (maximum dose per injection: 100 mg).
CHILDREN: After test dose of 10 mg, give 1 mg/kg (maximum dose per injection: 50 mg). Dosage schedule similar to that for adults.

Interactions
Antimalarials, penicillamine: Safety of combination antirheumatic therapy is unknown.
Cytotoxic drugs, immunosuppressives (except steroids), phenylbutazone: May increase risk of blood dyscrasias.

Lab Test Interferences
None well documented.

Adverse Reactions
May occur months after therapy is discontinued.

DERM: Dermatitis; pruritus; exfoliative dermatitis; angioedema; chrysiasis (gray-blue skin pigmentation).
EENT: Stomatitis; corneal gold deposition; corneal ulceration; iritis; conjunctivitis; metallic taste. Children: Safety and efficacy in children younger than 6 yr have not been established.
GI: Diarrhea; nausea; cholestatic jaundice; ulcerative enterocolitis; GI bleeding; difficulty swallowing; abdominal pain and cramping.
GU: Nephrotic syndrome or glomerulitis with proteinuria and hematuria.
HEMA: Anemia; thrombocytopenia; leukopenia; aplastic anemia.
RESP: Interstitial pneumonitis; pulmonary fibrosis.
OTHER: Anaphylactoid reactions within minutes of injection, arthralgias for several days after injection, "nitritoid reaction" (eg, vasomotor reaction with flushing, fainting, weakness, dizziness, sweating, nausea, vomiting, malaise and headache).

Precautions
Pregnancy: Category C.
Lactation: Excreted in breast milk.
Elderly: Use with caution. Tolerance to gold decreases with age.
Special risk patients: Use with caution in patients with diabetes mellitus, CHF, history of blood dyscrasias, cardiovascular or cerebral circulation problems, skin rash, previous kidney or liver disease, marked hypertension, compromised circulation, or inflammatory bowel disease.
CNS: Confusion; hallucinations; seizures.

Overdosage: Signs and Symptoms
Hematuria, proteinuria, thrombocytopenia, granulocytopenia, fever, nausea, vomiting, diarrhea, skin lesions, urticaria, exfoliative dermatitis, severe pruritus.

PATIENT CARE CONSIDERATIONS
Administration/Storage
- Color of solution is pale yellow. Do not administer drug if it has darkened in color or contains precipitate.
- Mix contents of vial thoroughly before withdrawing into syringe.
- Administer drug only by IM injection into upper outer quadrant of gluteus maximus muscle.
- Instruct patient to remain lying down for 10 to 15 min after injection.
- Store in light-resistant containers at room temperature.

Assessment/Interventions
- Obtain patient history, including drug history and any known allergies.
- Review patient's history for indications of uncontrolled diabetes mellitus, systemic lupus erythematosus, renal disease, inflammatory bowel disease, liver disease, granulocytopenia, and previous hypersensitivity to medication.
- Review patient's laboratory values for indications of gold toxicity such as decreased hemoglobin, WBC less than 4000 mm^3, platelets less than 100,000 to 150,000/mm^3, granulocytes less than 1500/mm^3, proteinuria and elevated liver enzymes.
- Prior to each injection, assess patient for early signs and symptoms of toxicity: pruritus, dermatitis, stomatitis, metallic taste, indigestion, diarrhea.
- Collect urine to test for proteinuria and sediment changes prior to each injection.
- Assess patient for possible nitritoid reaction (eg, sweating, fainting, bradycardia, dizziness, flushing, nausea, vomiting, headaches, and weakness) and hypersensitivity of allergic reactions (eg, swelling of face, lips or eyelids, thickening of tongue, shortness of breath, rash, hypotension, tachycardia).
- If anaphylactic shock, syncope, bradycardia, thickening of the tongue, dysphagia, shortness of breath, or angioneurotic edema occur within minutes of injection, notify health care provider immediately.
- Exfoliative dermatitis, nephrosis, thrombocytopenia, and leukopenia require cessation of gold treatment.
- Order laboratory test for CBC including platelet estimation before every other injection throughout treatment.
- Monitor patients with GI symptoms for GI bleeding.

Patient/Family Education
- Explain that adverse reactions can occur any time during therapy, even months after drug has been discontinued.
- Caution patient to minimize exposure to sun and other sources of ultraviolet light (eg, sunlamp). Explain need to wear protective clothing outdoors.
- Advise patient of importance of continued assessment of disease status and monitoring of renal, hepatic, and hematologic functions.
- Teach patient to perform good oral hygiene, including use of soft toothbrush and daily flossing. If mild stomatitis develops, isotonic sodium chloride and sodium bicarbonate solution can be used. Advise patient to avoid strong commercial mouthwashes and spicy or acidic foods.
- Inform patient that joint pain may continue for 1 to 2 days after injection but will usually decrease after first few injections. Therapeutic

effects may not be seen until after 3 to 6 mo of treatment. Explain that drug will not reverse damage or cure disease but may slow or stop its progression.
- Instruct patient to report these symptoms to health care provider: dermatitis, pruritus, weakness, metallic taste, fatigue, hematuria, unusual bruising or ecchymosis, nose bleeds, sore mouth, dark-colored stools.

Gonadorelin Acetate

(go-NAD-oh-RELL-in ASS-uh-TATE)
Class Gonadotropin-releasing hormone

How Supplied
Lutrepulse Powder for Injection, lyophilized 0.8 mg, Powder for Injection, lyophilized 3.2 mg

Action
PHARMACOLOGY: Causes synthesis and release of luteinizing hormone and follicle-stimulating hormone.
PHARMACOKINETICS/DYNAMICS:
Metabolism: Rapid metabolism to various inactive peptide fragments.
Excretion: T½ is 10 to 40 min.
Peak: Mean time to peak is about 34 min (males, SC); about 27 min (males, IV); about 71.5 min (females, SC); about 36 min (females, IV).
Duration: 3 to 5 hr.

Indications
Treatment of infertility by induction of ovulation in women with primary hypothalamic amenorrhea.

Contraindications
Any condition that could be exacerbated by pregnancy; ovarian cysts or causes of anovulation other than of hypothalamic origin; hormonally dependent tumors.

Route/Dosage
ADULTS: IV 5 mcg over pulse period of 1 min and pulse frequency of 90 min delivered via gonadorelin pump. Pump also can be programmed to deliver 2.5 mcg, 10 mcg, and 20 mcg doses per pulse. Typically, patients are treated for 21 days. If ovulation occurs, therapy is continued for 2 wk to maintain corpus luteum.

Interactions
Ovulation stimulators: Do not use concomitantly.

Lab Test Interferences
None well documented.

Adverse Reactions
DERM: Local inflammation, hematoma at catheter site.
GU: Multiple pregnancy; ovarian hyperstimulation.
HEMA: Mild phlebitis.
OTHER: Anaphylaxis.

Precautions
Pregnancy: Category B.
Lactation: Undetermined.
Children: Safety and efficacy in children younger than 18 yr not established.
Multiple pregnancy: Multiple pregnancy is possible. Minimize risk by proper dosage and monitoring.
Ovarian hyperstimulation: Drug may cause sudden, abnormal ovarian enlargement.

Overdosage: Signs and Symptoms
Temporary reduction of pituitary responsiveness.

PATIENT CARE CONSIDERATIONS

Administration/Storage
- Reconstitute drug immediately prior to use.
- Dilute contents of vial with 8 mL of supplied diluent. Reconstituted solution should be clear, colorless, and free of particulate matter.
- After dilution, transfer solution to plastic pump reservoir.
- An 8 mL solution generally supplies 7 consecutive days.
- To avoid sepsis, carefully monitor infusion area and change IV site and cannula q 48 hr.
- Store unopened vials at room temperature.

Assessment/Interventions
- Obtain patient history, including drug history and any known allergies.
- Monitor for anaphylactic reaction.
- Assess for irritation or signs of infection at infusion site. Check pump to make sure that it is delivering medication correctly.
- If ovarian enlargement, ascites, pleural effusion, or phlebitis occurs, discontinue therapy and notify health care provider.
- Institute supportive therapy for local inflammation (ie, apply ice intermittently).

Patient/Family Education
- Advise patient of importance of repeated ovarian ultrasonographic examinations and continued treatment in event of pregnancy.
- When indicated, instruct patient regarding reconstitution of solution and use of pump.
- Instruct patient about potential side effects (eg, local inflammation) and supportive therapy that can be undertaken.
- Inform patient of signs and symptoms of ovarian enlargement, ascites, and pleural effusion and advise patient to notify health care provider immediately if these symptoms occur.

Goserelin Acetate

(GO-suh-REH-lin ASS-uh-TATE)
Class Gonadotropin-releasing hormone

How Supplied
Zoladex Implant 3.6 mg, Implant 10.8 mg
🍁 *Zoladex LA*

Action
PHARMACOLOGY: Synthetic analog of gonadotropin-releasing hormone (GnRH) that acts as potent inhibitor of pituitary gonadotropin secretion.

PHARMACOKINETICS/DYNAMICS:
Absorption: T_{max} for the 3.6 mg implant is 12 to 15 days in men and 8 to 22 days in women. T_{max} for the 10.8 mg implant is 2 hr in men. C_{max} for the 3.6 mg implant is about 1.46 ng/mL in women and 2.84 ng/mL in men and for the 10.8 mg is about 8 ng/mL in men.

Distribution: Vd is 44.1 L in men and 20.3 L in women. Protein binding is 27%.

Metabolism: Hydrolysis of the C-terminal amino acids.

Excretion: The t½ for the 3.6 mg implant is 4.2 hr in men and 2.3 hr in women. More than 90% is excreted in urine, 20% unchanged. Mean systemic Cl for the 3.6 mg implant is 111 mL/min in men and to 164 mL/min in women.

Onset: 1 wk.

Peak: 2 to 4 wk.

Special Populations:
Renal Function Impairment – In Ccr less than 20 mL/min, the t½ is 12.1 hr.
Increased body weight – A decline in AUC of about 1% to 2.5% was observed with a kg increase in body weight.

Indications
Goserelin 3.6 mg implant: Palliative treatment of advanced breast cancer in pre- and perimenopausal women; treatment of endometriosis; as an endometrial thinning agent prior to endometrial ablation for dysfunctional uterine bleeding.
Goserelin 3.6 and 10.8 mg implants: Palliative treatment of advanced carcinoma of the prostate; in combination with flutamide for management of locally confined Stage T2b-T4 (Stage B2-C) carcinoma of the prostate.

Contraindications Breastfeeding; women being treated for endometriosis or endometrial thinning who are or may become pregnant; known hypersensitivity to LHRH, LHRH agonist analogs, or any component of the product; 10.8 mg goserelin implant is not indicated in women.

Route/Dosage
ADULTS:
28 days: **Subcutaneous** 3.6 mg implant q 28 days into upper abdominal wall by sterile technique under health care provider's supervision.
ADULTS:
12 weeks: **Subcutaneous** 10.8 mg implant q 12 wk into upper abdominal wall by sterile technique under health care provider's supervision.

Advanced Breast Cancer
ADULTS: **Subcutaneous** (3.6 mg only). Intended for long-term administration unless clinically inappropriate.

Endometriosis
ADULTS: **Subcutaneous** (3.6 mg only). Current recommended duration of treatment is 6 mo.

Endometrial Thinning
ADULTS: **Subcutaneous** (3.6 mg only). Recommendation is 1 or 2 depots, given 4 wk apart. When 1 depot is administered, surgery should be at 4 wk. When 2 depots are administered, surgery should be within 2 to 4 wk following the second depot.

Prostatic Carcinoma
ADULTS: **Subcutaneous** (3.6 or 10.8 mg). Intended for long-term administration unless clinically inappropriate.

Stage B2 to C Prostatic Carcinoma
ADULTS: **Subcutaneous** (3.6 or 10.8 mg only). When given in combination with radiotherapy and flutamide, start treatment 8 wk prior to initiating radiotherapy and continue during radiation therapy. A regimen using goserelin 3.6 mg depot 8 wk before radiotherapy, followed in 28 days by the 10.8 mg depot, can be administered. Alternatively, 4 injections of 3.6 mg depot can be administered at 28 day intervals, 2 depots preceding the 2 during radiotherapy.

Interactions None well documented.

Lab Test Interferences
Diagnostic tests of pituitary-gonadotropic and gonadal functions: Results may be misleading.
Estrogen: Drug may cause initial transient increase in serum levels in women.
Hypercalcemia in patients with bone metastases: Drug may cause initial transient increase.
Testosterone: Drug may cause initial transient increases in serum levels in men.

Adverse Reactions
CV:
Women – Vasodilation (57%); migraine (7%); hypertension (6%); chest pain, hemorrhage, palpitations, tachycardia (at least 1%)
Men – CHF (5%); angina pectoris, arrhythmia, cerebral ischemia, cerebrovascular accident, chest pain, heart failure, hypertension, MI, peripheral vascular disorder, pulmonary embolus,

varicose veins (greater than 1% but less than 5%).

CNS:
Women – Headache (75%); emotional lability (60%); depression (54%); insomnia, asthenia (11%); dizziness (6%); fatigue, lethargy, malaise, nervousness (5%); hypertonia, abnormal thinking, anxiety, paresthesia somnolence (at least 1%).
Men – Lethargy (8%); dizziness, insomnia (5%); anxiety, depression, headache, paresthesia (greater than 1% but less than 5%).

DERM:
Women – Hot flashes (96%); sweating (45%); acne (42%); seborrhea (26%); hirsutism (7%); hair disorder (4%); pruritus (2%); alopecia, dry skin, ecchymosis, skin discoloration (at least 1%).
Men – Hot flashes (62%); rash, sweating (6%); herpes simplex, pruritus (greater than 1% but less than 5%).

EENT:
Women – Pharyngitis (6%); amblyopia, dry eyes (at least 1%).

GI:
Women – Nausea, abdominal pain (11%); vomiting (4%); increased appetite (2%); anorexia, constipation, diarrhea, dry mouth, dyspepsia, flatulence (at least 1%).
Men – Anorexia, nausea (5%); abdominal pain, constipation, diarrhea, hematemesis, ulcer, vomiting (greater than 1% but less than 5%).

GU:
Women – Vaginitis (75%); decreased libido (61%); breast atrophy (33%); breast enlargement, pelvic symptoms (18%); dyspareunia (14%); increased libido (12%); breast pain, dysmenorrhea (7%); uterine hemorrhage (6%); vulvovaginitis (5%); menorrhagia (4%); urinary frequency, UTI, vaginal hemorrhage (at least 1%).
Men – Sexual dysfunction (21%); decreased erections (18%); lower urinary tract infections (13%); bladder neoplasm, breast swelling and tenderness, hematuria, impotence, renal insufficiency, urinary obstruction, urinary frequency, urinary incontinence, urinary infrequency, urinary retention, urinary tract disorder, UTI (greater than 1% but less than 5%).

HEMA/LYMPH:
Men – Anemia (greater than 1% but less than 5%).

HYPERSEN: Anaphylaxis.

LOCAL:
Women – Elevated liver enzymes (ALT, AST) (at least 1%).

M/N:
Women – Weight gain (3%).
Men – Diabetes mellitus, gout, hyperglycemia, weight increase (greater than 1% but less than 5%); decreased bone mineral density and bony fracture in men, osteoporosis (postmarketing).

MUSC:
Women – Back pain (7%); myalgia (3%); leg cramps (2%); arthralgia, joint disorder (at least 1%).
Men – Back pain (greater than 1% but less than 5%).

RESP:
Women – Sinusitis (3%); bronchitis, epistaxis, increased cough, rhinitis (at least 1%).
Men – Upper respiratory infection (7%); chronic obstructive pulmonary disease (5%); dyspnea, increased cough, pneumonia (greater than 1% but less than 5%).

OTHER:
Women – Tumor flare (23%); peripheral edema (21%); pain (17%); infection (13%); flu syndrome (5%); voice alterations (3%), edema, fever (at least 1%).
Men – Pain, edema (8%); flu syndrome, sepsis, peripheral edema (greater than 1% but less than 5%).

Precautions

Pregnancy: Category D (breast cancer); Category X (endometriosis, endometrial thinning, 10.8 mg strength).

Lactation: Undetermined. Discontinue the drug prior to breastfeeding.

Children: Safety and efficacy not established.

Hypersensitivity: Antibody formation to goserelin has been observed. Anaphylactic reactions are possible.

Special risk patients: Isolated cases of spinal cord compression and ureteral obstruction have been reported in men. Use with caution in patients prone to these problems.

Bone mineral density changes: Decreases in vertebral trabecular bone mineral density have been observed; patients with certain risk factors (eg, alcohol or tobacco abuse, family history of osteoporosis) may be at additional risk.

Breast cancer worsening: Drug initially causes transient increase in estrogen. Worsening of signs and symptoms of breast cancer, such as bone pain, may occur during the first few weeks of treatment.

Prostatic cancer worsening: Drug initially causes transient increase in testosterone. Worsening of signs and symptoms of prostate cancer, such as bone pain, may occur during first few weeks of treatment.

10.8 mg implant: The 10.8 mg implant is not indicated in women as the data are insufficient to support reliable suppression of serum estradiol.

Hormone replacement therapy (HRT): Clinical studies suggest the addition of HRT (estrogens or progestins) to goserelin may decrease the occurrence of vasomotor symptoms and vaginal dryness associated with hypoestrogenism without compromising the efficacy of goserelin in relieving pelvic symptoms. The optimal drugs, dose, and duration of treatment not established.

Hypercalcemia: Hypercalcemia has occurred in some prostate and breast cancer patients with bone metastases after starting goserelin treatment.

Hypoestrogenism: Hypoestrogenism may be induced by goserelin, which results in loss of bone mineral density over the course of treatment and may be irreversible. Adverse events occurring with hypoestrogenism most frequently include hot flashes, headaches, vaginal dryness, emotional lability, changes in libido, depression, sweating, and change in breast size.

Pituitary gonadal axis: As with other hormonal interventions that disrupt pituitary-gonadal axis, some patients may experience a delay in return to menses and, rarely, patients may experience persistent amenorrhea.

Vaginal bleeding: Some women experience vaginal bleeding of variable duration and intensity. The bleeding represents estrogen withdrawal bleeding and is expected to stop spontaneously.

PATIENT CARE CONSIDERATIONS

Administration/Storage

- Dose (number or strength of implants), frequency of implantation, and duration of therapy are variable depending on condition being treated and clinical response.
- For subcutaneous implantation only. Not for intradermal, IM, or oral administration.
- Using preloaded syringe with attached needle, pellets are injected into the anterior abdominal wall below the navel line.
- Follow manufacturer's instructions regarding preparation of injection site, preparation of preloaded syringe, injection of implant, and disposal of used syringe.
- If blood appears in syringe, do not inject implant. Instead, withdraw needle and discard syringe. Use new syringe and inject implant at a different site.
- 3.6 mg pellet is generally implanted q 4 wk. 10.8 mg pellet is generally implanted q 12 wk.
- Pellets can be localized by ultrasound if surgical removal is necessary.
- Store preloaded syringe in foil pouch at controlled room temperature (less than 77°F). Do not remove syringe from foil pouch until just prior to use.

Assessment/Interventions

- Obtain patient history, including drug history and any known allergies. Note hypersensitivity to LHRH, LHRH agonist analogs, pregnancy, breastfeeding, undiagnosed abnormal vaginal bleeding, women (10.8 mg pellet only).
- Ensure women of childbearing potential are not pregnant before starting therapy and use effective nonhormonal contraception during treatment and continue until the return of menses or for at least 12 wk following the last pellet implantation.
- Ensure serum testosterone and prostatic acid phosphatase are periodically measured in patient being treated for prostate cancer to assess therapeutic response.
- Ensure serum calcium levels are monitored in patient being treated for prostate or breast cancer. Inform health care provider immediately if hypercalcemia is noted or patient develops signs or symptoms of hypercalcemia (eg, polyuria, confusion, drowsiness). Be prepared to treat appropriately (eg, 0.9% sodium chloride injection, furosemide).
- Monitor patient being treated for prostate or breast cancer for signs and symptoms of ureteral obstruction (eg, oliguria, lower abdominal or pelvic pain) or spinal cord compression (eg, paresthesias, numbness, tingling, loss of sphincter control, motor weakness). Inform health care provider immediately if suspected.
- Monitor women for signs and symptoms of estrogen deficiency. If symptoms develop, ensure that hormone replacement therapy is been considered to reduce symptoms.
- Ensure risks and benefits of therapy have been evaluated for patient with history of previous treatment with goserelin that may have resulted in bone mineral density loss, or in patient with major risk factors for decreased bone mineral density (ie, chronic alcohol or tobacco abuse, significant family history of osteoporosis, or chronic use of drugs that can reduce bone mineral density). Ensure that addition of hormone replacement therapy has been considered for patient at risk for osteoporosis who will receive goserelin.
- Monitor patient for signs of anaphylactic or serious allergic reactions. Discontinue therapy and immediately inform health care provider if noted. Be prepared to treat appropriately.
- Monitor patient for CNS, GI, GU, DERM, and general body side effects, and injection site reactions. Report to health care provider if noted and significant.

Patient/Family Education

- Explain name, action, and potential side

effects of the treatment regimen. Review the treatment regimen including dosing schedule, duration of treatment, and monitoring that will be required.
* Advise patient, family, or caregiver that medication will be prepared and administered by health care professionals in a health care setting.
* Advise patient, family, or caregiver that medication may be used in combination with other agents to achieve max benefit possible.
* Advise patient that pellet is biodegradable and will be absorbed by the body and does not have to be removed when next dose is due or when therapy is discontinued.
* Caution patient that missing 1 or more doses of goserelin may result in loss of beneficial effects and to be sure to return as scheduled for additional doses of medication.
* Advise patient being treated for prostate or breast cancer that temporary worsening of symptoms or additional signs and symptoms of the cancer may develop during the first few weeks of therapy but should improve once the medication begins to take effect.
* Advise women that the most common side effects of therapy are associated with estrogen deficiency (eg, change in breast size, reduction or loss of libido, depression, emotional lability, hot flashes or flushes, sweating, vaginal dryness). Advise patient to be prepared to discuss potential value of starting hormone replacement therapy with health care provider if estrogen deficiency symptoms occur and are intolerable.
* Advise patient, family, or caregiver to immediately report any of the following to health care provider: frequent urination or little or no urination; unexplained drowsiness; lower stomach or pelvic-area pain; abnormal skin sensations; numbness or tingling sensations; loss of sphincter control; unexplained weakness; rash or hives; difficulty breathing or unexplained shortness of breath; pain, redness, or swelling at injection site.
* Instruct patient not to take any prescription or OTC medications, herbal preparations, or dietary supplements unless advised to do so by health care provider.
* Advise women that menstruation should stop as a result of therapy with goserelin and to notify health care provider if regular menstruation continues. Caution patient that breakthrough menstrual bleeding and/or ovulation may occur if 1 or more does of goserelin are missed.
* Instruct women of childbearing potential to use effective nonhormonal contraception during treatment and until the return of menses or for at least 12 wk following the last pellet implantation.
* Advise women to notify health care provider if pregnant, planning to become pregnant, or breastfeeding.
* Advise patient that follow-up visits and laboratory tests will be required to monitor therapy and to keep appointments.

Granisetron Hydrochloride

(gran-IH-SEH-trahn)
Class Serotonin receptor blocker antiemetic
How Supplied
Kytril Injection 1 mg/mL, Tablets 1 mg
Action
PHARMACOLOGY: Selective 5-HT$_3$ receptor antagonists. Serotonin receptors of the 5-HT$_3$ type are located peripherally on vagal nerve terminals, enteric neurons in the GI tract, and centrally in the chemoreceptor trigger zone. During chemotherapy, mucosal enterochromaffin cells from the small intestine release serotonin, which stimulates the 5-HT$_3$ receptors. This evokes vagal afferent discharge, inducing vomiting. Clearance is predominantly by hepatic metabolism, and plasma protein binding is approximately 65%.

PHARMACOKINETICS/DYNAMICS:
Absorption: Mean C_{max} is 64 ng/mL.

Distribution: Vd is about 3 L/kg. Protein binding is 65%.

Excretion: Mean t½ is 5 hr. Mean Cl is 0.79 L/hr/kg.

Peak: 5 to 30 sec (injection).

Special Populations:
Hepatic Function Impairment – Total Cl decreased by about 50%.
Elderly – Mean C_{max} is 57 ng/mL. Mean t½ is 7.69 hr. Mean Cl is 0.44 L/hr/kg. Mean Vd is about 4 L/kg.
Cancer patients – C_{max} is 84 ng/mL. Mean t½ is 9 hr. Cl is 0.38 L/hr/kg.

Indications
Adults: Prevention of chemotherapy-induced nausea and vomiting; prevention of radiation-induced nausea and vomiting (oral only); postoperative nausea and vomiting (injection only).
Pediatric (2 to 16 yr): Prevention of chemotherapy-induced nausea and vomiting (injection only). Safety and efficacy not established in patients younger than 2 yr.

Contraindications Standard considerations.

Route/Dosage

Chemotherapy-Induced Nausea and Vomiting
ADULTS: IV 10 mcg/kg (commonly rounded to nearest 1 mg), given up to 30 min before starting chemotherapy. Give only on day(s) of chemotherapy.

Chemotherapy-Induced Nausea and Vomiting
ADULTS: PO 1 mg bid. Give the first oral dose up to 1 hr before chemotherapy and the second dose 12 hr later. Give granisetron only on day(s) of chemotherapy. Alternately, a single 2 mg dose may be given up to 1 hr before chemotherapy. PEDIATRIC: IV 10 mcg/kg, given up to 30 min before starting chemotherapy. Give only on day(s) of chemotherapy.

Radiation-Induced Nausea and Vomiting
ADULTS: PO 2 mg once daily. Give the dose up to 1 hr before radiation therapy. Give granisetron only on day(s) of radiation therapy.

Prevention/Treatment Postoperative Nausea and Vomiting
ADULTS: IV For prevention, use 1 mg undiluted, administered over 30 seconds, before induction of anesthesia or immediately before reversal of anesthesia. For treatment, use 1 mg undiluted, administered over 30 seconds, after surgery.

Interactions

Cytochrome P450 enzymes: Granisetron does not induce or inhibit the cytochrome P450 system; however, it is metabolized partially by cytochrome P450 3A enzymes. Medications that induce or inhibit cytochrome P450 3A isoenzymes may alter granisetron metabolism.

Lab Test Interferences
None well documented.

Adverse Reactions

CV: Hypertension; hypotension.
CNS: Headache; somnolence; agitation; anxiety; mood changes; insomnia.
DERM: Rash.
GI: Constipation; diarrhea; elevated AST and ALT; decreased appetite.
MUSC: Asthenia.
OTHER: Fever; taste disorder; shivers; alopecia.

Precautions

Pregnancy: Category B.
Lactation: Undetermined.
Children: Safety and efficacy of the injection in children younger than 2 yr not established.
Delayed nausea and vomiting: Granisetron is not consistently effective for treating delayed nausea and vomiting.

PATIENT CARE CONSIDERATIONS

Administration/Storage

- All dosage forms can be stored at room temperature or refrigerated. Protect granisetron injection from light.
- Administer by oral, IV push, or IV infusion.
- Undiluted granisetron may be given IV over 30 sec.
- Diluted granisetron solutions are infused over 5 min. Infuse admixtures containing granisetron and dexamethasone over 15 to 30 min.
- Oral solution and tablets are interchangeable.

Extemporaneous oral suspension:

- Granisetron 1 mg/5 mL oral suspension: Crush twelve 1 mg oral tablets completely and suspend in 30 mL of distilled water. Dilute with sufficient cherry syrup for a final total volume of 60 mL.
- The extemporaneous suspension is stable for up to 14 days when stored in amber plastic bottles.

IV:

- Dilute with 0.9% Sodium Chloride or 5% Dextrose to a total volume of 20 to 50 mL.

Assessment/Interventions

- Obtain patient history, including drug history, and any known allergies. Note history of prior use and effectiveness of antiemetic therapy.
- Monitor patient for antiemetic efficacy. Notify health care provider if nausea or vomiting are not prevented.
- Monitor patient for CNS, GI, and general body side effects. Inform health care provider if noted and significant.

Patient/Family Education

- Explain name, dose, action, and potential side effects of drug.
- Advise patient, family, or caregiver that IV medication will be prepared and administered by health care professional in a medical facility.
- Review dosing schedule with patient. Caution patient taking oral medication that tablets or solution must be taken no more than 1 hr before chemotherapy administration or radiation therapy to provide greatest protection against nausea and vomiting.
- Advise patient that medication will greatly reduce likelihood of nausea or vomiting but these are still possible.
- Instruct patient to inform health care provider if medication does not prevent nausea or vomiting.
- Advise patient to report any of the following to their health care provider: intolerable headache; persistent or intolerable constipation or diarrhea; persistent weakness.

- Instruct women to notify health care provider if pregnant, planning to become pregnant, or breastfeeding.
- Instruct patient to not take any prescription or OTC medications or dietary supplements unless advised by health care provider.

Griseofulvin

(griss-ee-oh-FULL-vin)

Class Anti-infective/Antifungal

How Supplied

Microsize

Grifulvin V Tablets 250 mg (as microsize), Tablets 500 mg (as microsize), Suspension, oral 125 mg/5 mL (as microsize) ♦ Grisactin 500 Tablets 500 mg (as microsize) ♦ Grisactin 250 Capsules 250 mg (as microsize)

Ultrasize

Fulvicin P/G Tablets 125 mg (as ultramicrosize), Tablets 165 mg (as ultramicrosize), Tablets 250 mg (as ultramicrosize), Tablets 330 mg (as ultramicrosize) ♦ Gris-PEG Tablets 125 mg (as ultramicrosize), Tablets 250 mg (as ultramicrosize) ♦ Grisactin Ultra Tablets 250 mg (as ultramicrosize)

Action

PHARMACOLOGY: Deposited preferentially into infected skin, which gradually sloughs off and is replaced by noninfected tissue; binds tightly to new keratin, which becomes highly resistant to fungal invasions.

PHARMACOKINETICS/DYNAMICS:

Absorption: C_{max} is 0.5 to 1.5 mcg/mL. T_{max} is about 4 hr.
Food – A high-fat meal may increase C_{max}. Microsize is 25% to 70% absorbed. Ultramicrosize is about 100% absorbed.

Distribution: Mainly deposited in the keratin layer of skin, hair, and nails.

Metabolism: Hepatic. Major metabolites are 6-methyl-griseofulvin and its glucuronide conjugate.

Excretion: T½ is about 24 hr. Primarily renal excretion. About 36% is excreted unchanged in the feces.

Indications Treatment of ringworm infections of skin, hair, and nails caused by susceptible fungi.

Contraindications Porphyria; hepatic disease.

Route/Dosage

ADULTS: **PO** 500 to 1000 mg microsize (330 to 750 mg ultramicrosize) in single or divided doses. May need to give for several weeks.

CHILDREN: **PO** 11 mg microsize/kg/day (125 to 500 mg) or 7.3 mg ultramicrosize/kg/day (82.5 to 330 mg).

Interactions

Alcohol: Effects of alcohol may be potentiated with tachycardia and flushing.
Anticoagulants: Anticoagulant effect may be decreased.
Barbiturates: May depress griseofulvin serum levels.
Contraceptives, oral: May cause loss of contraceptive effectiveness.

Lab Test Interferences False elevation of vanillylmandelic acid test assayed by photometric tests but not with gas or thin layer chromatography method.

Adverse Reactions

CNS: Headache; fatigue; dizziness; insomnia; confusion; paresthesias.
DERM: Rash; urticaria.
EENT: Oral thrush.
GI: Nausea; vomiting; epigastric distress; diarrhea; GI bleeding.
GU: Proteinuria.
HEMA: Leukopenia; granulocytopenia.
HEPA: Hepatic toxicity.
METAB: Interferes with porphyrin metabolism.
OTHER: Angioneurotic edema.

Precautions

Pregnancy: Category C.
Lactation: Undetermined.
Hypersensitivity: Drug may need to be discontinued. Also, penicillin cross-sensitivity is possible, although some penicillin-sensitive patients have used without difficulty.
Lupus: May exacerbate lupus or lupus-like syndrome.

PATIENT CARE CONSIDERATIONS

Administration/Storage

- Administer with or after meals, particularly with fatty foods if not contraindicated.
- Generally administered in conjunction with topical agent.
- Do not interchange griseofulvin microsize with ultramicrosize because dosage is different.
- Store at room temperature in tightly closed containers.

Assessment/Interventions

- Evaluate skin condition prior to and throughout therapy.
- Institute general supportive measures to maintain skin integrity.
- Observe for signs of infection or reinfection.
- Institute safety precautions if dizziness or other neurologic alterations occur.

Patient/Family Education
- Advise patient to inspect skin for signs of improvement of infection or re-infection.
- Explain importance of good hygiene, particularly to affected areas.
- Inform patient that beneficial effects of drug may not be observable for weeks to months.
- Emphasize importance of continued follow-up examinations.
- Instruct patient to report these symptoms to health care provider: fever, sore throat, skin rash.
- Caution patient to avoid intake of alcoholic beverages or other CNS depressants.
- Advise patient that drug may cause dizziness and to use caution while driving or performing other tasks requiring mental alertness.
- Caution patient to avoid exposure to sunlight and to use sunscreen or wear protective clothing to avoid photosensitivity reaction.

Guaifenesin (Glyceryl Guaiacolate)

(GWHY-fen-ah-sin)
Class Expectorant

How Supplied
Allfen Jr Tablets 400 mg ♦ *Anti-Tuss* Syrup 100 mg per 5 mL ♦ *Breonesin* Capsules 200 mg ♦ *Diabetic Tussin EX* Liquid 100 mg per 5 mL ♦ *Duratuss-G* Tablets 1,200 mg ♦ *Fenesin* Tablets, sustained-release 600 mg ♦ *Gee-Gee* Tablets 200 mg ♦ *Genatuss* Syrup 100 mg per 5 mL ♦ *GG-Cen* Capsules 200 mg ♦ *Glyate* Syrup 100 mg per 5 mL ♦ *Glycotuss* Tablets 100 mg ♦ *Glytuss* Tablets 200 mg ♦ *GuiaCough CF* Liquid 12.5 mg ♦ *GuiaCough PE* Liquid 100 mg ♦ *Guiafenex LA* Tablets, extended-release 600 mg ♦ *Guiatuss* Syrup 100 mg per 5 mL ♦ *Humibid LA* Tablets, sustained-release 600 mg ♦ *Humibid Sprinkle* Capsules, sustained-release 300 mg ♦ *Hytuss* Tablets 100 mg ♦ *Hytuss 2x* Capsules 200 mg ♦ *Liquibid* Tablets 400 mg, Tablets, sustained-release 600 mg ♦ *Monafed* Tablets, sustained-release 600 mg ♦ *Muco-Fen-LA* Tablets, sustained-release 600 mg ♦ *Mucinex* Tablets, extended-release 600 mg ♦ *Mytussin* Syrup 100 mg per 5 mL ♦ *Naldecon Senior EX* Liquid 200 mg per 5 mL ♦ *Organidin NR* Tablets 200 mg, Liquid 100 mg per 5 mL ♦ *Pneumomist* Tablets, sustained-release 600 mg ♦ *Robitussin* Syrup 100 mg per 5 mL ♦ *Scot-tussin Expectorant* Syrup 100 mg per 5 mL ♦ *Sinumist-SR Capsulets* Tablets, sustained-release 600 mg ♦ *Siltussin SA* Syrup 100 mg per 5 mL ♦ *Tussin* Syrup 100 mg per 5 mL ♦ *Tusibron* Syrup 100 mg per 5 mL ♦ *Uni-tussin* Syrup 100 mg per 5 mL
✤ *Balminil Expectorant* ♦ *Benylin E Extra Strength* ♦ *Robitussin Extra Strength*

Action
PHARMACOLOGY: May enhance output of respiratory tract fluid by reducing adhesiveness and surface tension, thus facilitating removal of viscous mucus and making nonproductive coughs more productive and less frequent. Efficacy not well documented.

PHARMACOKINETICS/DYNAMICS:
Absorption: Readily absorbed.
Excretion: The $t_{1/2}$ is 1 hr; renal excretion; major urinary metabolite is β-2-(methoxyphenoxy) lactic acid

Indications Temporary relief of cough associated with respiratory tract infections and related conditions such as sinusitis, pharyngitis, bronchitis, and asthma when these conditions are complicated by tenacious mucus or mucus plugs and congestion; effective for productive as well as nonproductive cough, particularly dry, nonproductive cough that tends to injure mucous membranes of the air passages; helps loosen phlegm and thin bronchial secretions in patients with stable chronic bronchitis.

Contraindications Standard considerations.

Route/Dosage
IMMEDIATE-RELEASE
ADULTS AND CHILDREN (AT LEAST 12 YR OF AGE): PO 200 to 400 mg q 4 hr (max, 2.4 g/day).
CHILDREN (6 TO UNDER 12 YR OF AGE): PO 100 to 200 mg q 4 hr (max, 1.2 g/day).
CHILDREN (2 TO UNDER 6 YR OF AGE): PO 50 to 100 mg q 4 hr (max, 600 mg/day). *Allfen Jr* is not recommended for use in children under 6 yr of age.
CHILDREN (6 MO TO UNDER 2 YR OF AGE): PO Individualize dose, 25 to 50 mg q 4 hr (max, 300 mg/day).

SUSTAINED- OR EXTENDED-RELEASE
ADULTS AND CHILDREN (AT LEAST 12 YR OF AGE): PO 600 mg to 1.2 g q 12 hr (max, 2.4 g/day).

Interactions None well documented.

Lab Test Interferences Guaifenesin may increase renal Cl for urate, which may lower serum uric acid levels; may produce an increase in urinary 5-hydroxyindoleacetic acid, which may interfere with interpretation of this test for diagnosis of carcinoid syndrome; may falsely elevate vanillymandelic acid in certain serotonin metabolite chemical tests because of color interference.

Adverse Reactions
CNS: Dizziness; headache.
DERM: Rash; urticaria.

GI: Nausea; vomiting.

Precautions
Pregnancy: Category C.
Lactation: Undetermined.
Persistent cough: May indicate serious condition.

PATIENT CARE CONSIDERATIONS

Administration/Storage
- Store liquid, syrup, capsules and immediate-release tablets at controlled room temperature (59° to 86°F).
- Store extended-release tablets at controlled room temperature (68° to 77°F).
- Protect from light. Protect capsules and tablets from moisture.

Syrup, liquid and immediate-release tablets and capsules:
- Administer prescribed dose q 4 hr as needed, up to 6 doses per day.
- Administer without regard to meals, but administer with food or milk if GI upset occurs.
- Measure and administer liquid or syrup dose using dosing spoon, syringe, or cup.

Extended-release tablets:
- Administer prescribed dose bid.
- Have patient swallow whole with a full glass of water. Caution patient not to chew, crush, or break tablet.
- Administer without regard to meals, but administer with food if GI upset occurs.

Assessment/Interventions
- Obtain patient history, including drug history and any known allergies
- Assess symptoms (eg, cough, sputum viscosity, color, volume) before and periodically throughout therapy.
- Maintain fluid intake of 2,000 mL/day if no contraindications exist.
- Notify health care provider if any of the following occur: persistent or recurrent cough; cough associated with fever, rash, or persistent headache.

Patient/Family Education
- Explain name, dose, action, and potential side effects of drug.
- Explain that expectorants are not usually used for chronic cough conditions such as those caused by smoking, asthma, chronic bronchitis, or emphysema, or when cough is accompanied by excessive secretions.
- Explain importance of maintaining increased fluid intake to help thin bronchial secretions.
- Advise patient using syrup, liquid, or immediate-release tablets or capsules, to take prescribed dose q 4 hr as needed, up to 6 times a day.
- Advise caregiver to use dosing spoon, syringe, or cup when giving liquid or syrup to children.
- Advise patient using extended-release tablets to take q 12 hr as needed, up to 2 times a day. Caution patient to swallow tablets whole with a full glass of water and not to chew, crush, or break the tablet.
- Advise patient or caregiver that medication can be taken without regard to meals, but to take with food if stomach upset occurs.
- Advise patient that if a dose is missed, to take as soon as remembered unless it is nearing time for the next dose, in which case the dose should be skipped and the next dose taken at the regularly scheduled time. Caution patient not to double the dose to catch up.
- Advise patient that if cough is not controlled, not to increase the dose of medication but to inform a health care provider.
- Instruct patient to inform health care provider if any of the following occur: cough persists for more than 1 wk; cough keeps coming back; cough is accompanied by high fever, skin rash, or headache.
- Advise women to notify health care provider if pregnant, planning to become pregnant, or breastfeeding.
- Caution patient not to take any prescription or OTC medications, herbal preparations, or dietary supplements unless advised by health care provider.

Notify health care provider, pharmacist, or nurse if cough persists for more than 1 wk, tends to recur, or is accompanied by high fever, rash, or persistent headache.

Guaifenesin/Codeine Phosphate

(GWHY-fen-ah-sin/KOE-deen FOSS-fate)
Class Expectorant/Analgesic/Antitussive

How Supplied
Guaitussin AC Syrup 10 mg codeine phosphate and 100 mg guaifenesin per 5 mL ◆ *Mytussin AC* Syrup 10 mg codeine phosphate and 100 mg guaifenesin per 5 mL ◆ *Romilar AC* Syrup 10 mg codeine phosphate and 100 mg guaifenesin per 5 mL

Action
PHARMACOLOGY:

Guaifenesin: May enhance output of respiratory tract fluid by reducing adhesiveness and surface

tension, enhancing removal of viscous mucus, and making nonproductive coughs more productive and less frequent.
Codeine: Stimulates opiate receptors in CNS; also causes suppression of cough.

Indications Temporary control of cough caused by minor throat and bronchial irritation as occurs with common cold or inhaled irritants; assists in loosening phlegm (mucus) and thins bronchial secretions to make cough more productive.

Contraindications Hypersensitivity to any component of product.

Route/Dosage
Administer with special measuring device for accurate dose.
ADULTS AND CHILDREN 12 YR AND OLDER: **PO** 1 tsp (5 mL) to 2 tsp (10 mL) q 4 to 6 hr (max, 12 tsp [60 mL] in 24 hr).
CHILDREN 6 TO UNDER 12 YR: **PO** ½ tsp (2.5 mL) to 1 tsp (5 mL) q 4 to 6 hr (max, 6 tsp [30 mL] in 24 hr).
CHILDREN UNDER 6 YR: **PO** As directed by health care provider.

Interactions
Antidepressants (eg, MAO inhibitors), sedatives (eg, barbiturates), tranquilizers (eg, benzodiazepines): May cause increased drowsiness.

Lab Test Interferences Guaifenesin may interfere with the interpretation of the test for urinary 5-hydroxyindoleacetic acid for the diagnosis of carcinoid syndrome.

Adverse Reactions
CV:
Codeine – Hypotension; orthostatic hypotension; bradycardia; tachycardia; shock.
CNS:
Guaifenesin – Dizziness; headache.
Codeine – Lightheadedness; dizziness; sedation; disorientation; incoordination; euphoria; delirium.
DERM:
Guaifenesin – Rash; urticaria.
Codeine – Sweating; pruritus; urticaria.
EENT:
Codeine – Miosis.
GI:
Guaifenesin – Nausea; vomiting.
Codeine – Nausea; vomiting; constipation; abdominal pain; anorexia; biliary tract spasm.
GU:
Codeine – Urinary retention or hesitancy.
RESP:
Codeine – Laryngospasm; depression of cough reflex; respiratory depression.
OTHER:
Codeine – Tolerance; psychological and physical dependence with chronic use.

Precautions
Children: Not recommended for children under 2 yr.
Dependence: Codeine has abuse potential; may be habit forming.
Persistent cough: Persistent cough may be a sign of a serious condition. Consult health care provider for a cough of more than 1 wk duration or for a cough accompanied by fever, rash, or persistent headache. Do not use for chronic or persistent cough, cough accompanied by excessive phlegm (mucus), shortness of breath, or chronic pulmonary disease without consulting health care provider.

Overdosage: Signs and Symptoms
Miosis, respiratory and CNS depression, circulatory collapse, seizures, cardiopulmonary arrest, death.

PATIENT CARE CONSIDERATIONS

Administration/Storage
- Give prescribed dose q 4 to 6 hr prn, up to 6 doses/day.
- Give with food or milk if GI upset occurs.
- Use dosing spoon or syringe for pediatric doses.
- Store liquid at controlled room temperature (59° to 86°F). Keep tightly capped.

Assessment/Interventions
- Obtain patient history, including drug history and any known allergies.
- Assess symptoms (eg, cough, sputum viscosity, color, volume) before and periodically throughout therapy.
- Notify health care provider if any of the following occur: persistent or recurrent cough, cough associated with fever, rash, or persistent headache.

Patient/Family Education
- Explain name, dose, action, and potential side effects of drug.
- Advise patient to take prescribed dose q 4 hr prn, up to 6 times/day.
- Advise caregiver to use dosing spoon or syringe when giving liquid to children.
- Advise patient to take with food or milk if GI upset occurs.
- Advise patient that if a dose is missed to take as soon as remembered unless it is nearing time for the next dose. Caution patient to not double the dose to catch up.
- Advise patient that if cough is not controlled,

not to increase the dose of medication but to inform health care provider.
- Caution patient that drug may cause drowsiness and to use caution while driving or performing other tasks requiring mental alertness until tolerance is determined.
- Advise patient to avoid alcohol and other CNS depressants because of risk of excessive sedation.
- Advise women to notify health care provider if pregnant, planning to become pregnant, or breastfeeding.
- Caution patient not to take any prescription or OTC medications or dietary supplements unless advised by health care provider.

Guanabenz Acetate
(GWAHN-uh-benz ASS-uh-TATE)

Class Antihypertensive/Antiadrenergic, centrally acting

How Supplied
Wytensin Tablets 4 mg, Tablets 8 mg

Action
PHARMACOLOGY: Appears to stimulate central alpha$_2$-adrenergic receptors, inhibiting sympathetic outflow from brain to peripheral circulation.

PHARMACOKINETICS/DYNAMICS:
Absorption: Bioavailability is about 75%.
Excretion: Less than 1% is excreted in the urine unchanged.
Onset: 60 min.
Peak: 2 to 4 hr.
Duration: 6 to 8 hr.

Indications
Treatment of hypertension alone or with a thiazide diuretic.

Contraindications
Standard considerations.

Route/Dosage
ADULTS: **PO** 4 mg bid initially; may increase by 4 to 8 mg daily q 1 to 2 wk; max dose 32 mg bid.

Interactions
CNS depressants: Increased sedation.

Lab Test Interferences
None well documented.

PATIENT CARE CONSIDERATIONS

Administration/Storage
- Administer with food or milk.
- Store in tightly closed container in cool environment.

Assessment/Interventions
- Obtain patient history, including drug history and any known allergies. Note any cardiovascular or cerebrovascular disease.
- Take patient's BP (lying, sitting, standing) and pulse before administering drug. Monitor periodically throughout therapy.

Adverse Reactions
CV: Chest pain; edema; arrhythmias; palpitations; atrioventricular dysfunction.
CNS: Drowsiness; sedation; dizziness; anxiety; ataxia; depression; sleep disturbances.
DERM: Rash; pruritus.
EENT: Blurred vision; nasal congestion.
GI: Dry mouth; constipation; diarrhea; nausea; vomiting; abdominal discomfort.
GU: Urinary frequency; disturbances of sexual function.
HEPA: Increased liver enzymes.
RESP: Dyspnea.
OTHER: Gynecomastia; muscle or joint pain; weakness; taste disorders.

Precautions
Pregnancy: Category C.
Lactation: Undetermined.
Children: Safety and efficacy in children younger than 12 yr not established.
Special risk patients: Use with caution in patients with severe coronary insufficiency, recent MI, or cerebrovascular disease.
Sedation: Occurs in large percentage of patients.
Withdrawal: Do not discontinue therapy without consulting health care provider; drug must be withdrawn gradually to avoid rapid rise in BP.

Overdosage: Signs and Symptoms
Marked hypotension, somnolence, lethargy, irritability, miosis, bradycardia.

- Assess for dry mouth and follow treatment measures as necessary.
- Report these signs to health care provider immediately: hypotension, chest pain, arrhythmias, edema, dyspnea.

Patient/Family Education
- Instruct patient and family member in proper technique for taking BP. Advise patient to check and record BP weekly.
- Advise patient to lie down if dizziness or blurred vision occurs.

- Explain that impotence may occur but is reversible. Tell patient to report to health care provider.
- Instruct patient not to discontinue drug abruptly.
- Counsel patient about benefits of weight reduction, exercise, reduction of alcohol and sodium, cessation of smoking.
- Instruct patient to report these symptoms to health care provider: headache, dizziness, weakness, blurred vision.
- Advise patient to take sips of water frequently, suck on ice chips or sugarless hard candy, or chew sugarless gum if dry mouth occurs.
- Caution patient to avoid sudden position changes to prevent orthostatic hypotension.
- Instruct patient to avoid intake of alcoholic beverages or other CNS depressants.
- Advise patient that drug may cause drowsiness and to use caution while driving or performing other tasks requiring mental alertness.
- Instruct patient not to take otc medications without consulting health care provider.

Guanadrel

(GWAHN-uh-drell)

Class Antihypertensive/Antiadrenergic, peripherally acting

How Supplied
Hylorel Tablets 10 mg, Tablets 25 mg

Action
PHARMACOLOGY: Inhibits vasoconstriction by restraining norepinephrine release from nerve storage sites; depletion of norepinephrine causes relaxation of vascular smooth muscle, decreasing total peripheral resistance, and venous return.

PHARMACOKINETICS/DYNAMICS:
Absorption: T_{max} is 1.5 to 2 hr.
Excretion: $T_{½}$ is about 10 hr. About 85% is excreted in the urine, about 40% as unchanged drug.

Special Populations:
Renal Function Impairment – Total Cl decreases and t½ is prolonged. Dosage adjustment may be necessary.

Indications Treatment of hypertension in patients not responding adequately to thiazide-type diuretics.

Contraindications Pheochromocytoma; concurrent use or use within 1 wk of MAOIs; frank CHF.

Route/Dosage
ADULTS: **PO** 10 mg/day (5 mg bid) initially. Maintenance dose: **PO** 20 to 75 mg/day, usually in 2 divided doses; tid or qid dosing may be needed. In patients with renal impairment, dosage adjustment may be necessary.

Interactions
Alpha-blockers, beta-blockers, reserpine: Effects of guanadrel may be potentiated, resulting in excessive orthostatic hypotension and bradycardia.
Indirect-acting sympathomimetics (eg, ephedrine): Reverse antihypertensive effect.
MAOIs, phenothiazines, tricyclic antidepressants: Inhibit antihypertensive effect.

Lab Test Interferences None well documented.

Adverse Reactions
CV: Palpitations; chest pain; peripheral edema; orthostatic hypotension; syncope.
CNS: Fatigue; headache; faintness; drowsiness; paresthesias; confusion; depression; sleep disorders.
EENT: Dilated pupils; visual disturbances; glossitis.
GI: Increased bowel movements; gas pain/indigestion; constipation; anorexia; nausea or vomiting; abdominal distress or pain.
GU: Nocturia; urination urgency or frequency; ejaculation disturbances; impotence; hematuria; decreased urine output.
RESP: Shortness of breath; coughing.
OTHER: Excessive weight loss or gain; aching limbs; leg cramps; back or neckache; joint pain or inflammation; gangrene.

Precautions
Pregnancy: Category B.
Lactation: Undetermined.
Children: Safety and efficacy not established.
Asthma: Drug may aggravate asthma because of depletion of catecholamines; drugs used to treat asthma may reduce hypotensive effect of guanadrel.
Surgery: Discontinue 48 to 72 hr before elective surgery to prevent vascular collapse during anesthesia; for emergency surgery, preanesthetic and anesthetic agents are administered in reduced dosage.

Overdosage: Signs and Symptoms
Marked dizziness, blurred vision, syncope, orthostatic hypotension.

PATIENT CARE CONSIDERATIONS

Administration/Storage
- Administer medication with food or milk.
- Store at room temperature.

Assessment/Interventions
- Obtain patient history, including drug history and any known allergies. Note any CHF, renal disease, asthma, and pheochromocytoma.
- Take patient's BP (lying, sitting, standing) and pulse before administering drug. Monitor periodically throughout therapy.
- Assess for symptoms of CHF: edema, dyspnea, wet rales.
- Notify health care provider if any of these signs occur: hypotension, chest pain, bradycardia, edema, dyspnea, coughing, confusion, syncope, nausea, oliguria, hematuria, excessive weight loss or gain.

Patient/Family Education
- Teach proper technique for taking BP. Advise patient to check BP weekly.
- Instruct patient not to discontinue drug abruptly.
- Advise patient about benefits of weight reduction, exercise, reduction of alcohol and sodium intake, cessation of smoking.
- Tell patient to lie down if dizziness or blurred vision occurs.
- Explain that impotence or ejaculation disturbance may occur but is reversible. Tell patient to report to health care provider.
- Instruct patient to report these symptoms to health care provider: headache, dizziness, myalgia, depression, chest pain, nausea, visual disturbances.
- Caution patient to avoid sudden position changes to prevent orthostatic hypotension.
- Caution patient to avoid intake of alcoholic beverages or other CNS depressants.
- Advise patient that drug may cause drowsiness and to use caution while driving or performing other tasks requiring mental alertness.
- Instruct patient not to take *otc* medications without consulting health care provider.

Guanethidine Monosulfate

(gwahn-ETH-ih-deen MAH-no-SULL-fate)

Class Antihypertensive/Antiadrenergic, peripherally acting

How Supplied
Ismelin Tablets 10 mg, Tablets 25 mg

Action
PHARMACOLOGY: Interferes with release or distribution of norepinephrine from nerve endings, resulting in reduction in total peripheral resistance and diastolic and systolic BP.

PHARMACOKINETICS/DYNAMICS:
Metabolism: Converted by the liver to 3 metabolites that are less active than the parent drug.
Excretion: Renal Cl is 56 mL/min. T½ is 1.5 to 8 d. Renal excretion.

Indications
Treatment of moderate and severe hypertension and renal hypertension, including that secondary to pyelonephritis, renal amyloidosis, and renal artery stenosis.

Unlabeled use(s): Reflex sympathetic dystrophy and causalgia.

Contraindications
Known or suspected pheochromocytoma; frank CHF not related to hypertension; use of MAOIs.

Route/Dosage
ADULTS:
Ambulatory: **PO** 10 mg qd initially; may increase by about 10 mg at 5 to 7 days; increase only if no decrease in standing BP is observed. Maintenance dose: 25 to 50 mg qd.
Hospitalized: **PO** 25 to 50 mg initially; increase by 25 or 50 mg/day or qod until desired response is obtained. Loading dose (for severe hypertension): Give at 6 hr intervals over 1 to 3 days, omitting nighttime dose.
Children: **PO** 0.2 mg/kg/24 hr (6 mg/m^2/24 hr) as single oral dose initially; increase by increment of 0.2 mg/kg/24 hr q 7 to 10 days. Max: 3 mg/kg/24 hr.

Interactions
Anorexiants: May reverse hypotensive effect of drug.
MAOIs: May decrease effectiveness of guanethidine; discontinue MAOIs more than 1 wk before starting guanethidine therapy.
Phenothiazines: May inhibit hypotensive effect.
Sympathomimetics (eg, ephedrine, epinephrine): May reverse hypotensive effect of guanethidine; guanethidine may potentiate effects of sympathomimetics.
Tricyclic antidepressants: May inhibit hypotensive effect of drug.

Lab Test Interferences
None well documented.

Adverse Reactions
CV: Bradycardia; orthostatic fluid retention; edema; angina.
CNS: Dizziness; weakness; lassitude; syncope; fatigue; muscle tremor; mental depression; chest paresthesias; ptosis; headache; confusion.

EENT: Blurred vision; nasal congestion.
GI: Nausea; vomiting; dry mouth; parotid tenderness; diarrhea (may be severe, requiring discontinuation of therapy); increase in bowel movements.
GU: Inhibition of ejaculation; nocturia; urinary incontinence; priapism.
HEMA: Anemia; thrombocytopenia.
RESP: Dyspnea; asthma in susceptible individuals.
OTHER: Myalgia; weight gain; dermatitis; scalp hair loss; leg cramps.

Precautions
Pregnancy: Category C.
Lactation: Excreted in breast milk.
Children: Safety and efficacy not established.
Elderly: More prone to side effects of guanethidine therapy, especially orthostatic hypotension.
Renal function impairment: Use very cautiously, because hypotension may worsen renal impairment.
Bronchial asthma: May aggravate the hypersensitive condition of asthmatics because of further catecholamine depletion.
Cardiovascular disease: Use cautiously in patients with coronary disease, recent MI, or cerebral vascular disease, especially with encephalopathy; avoid use in patients with severe cardiac failure.
Fever: May decrease dosage requirements.
Orthostatic hypotension: Occurs frequently, especially during initial treatment and with postural changes.
Peptic ulcer: Ulcers may be aggravated by relative increase in parasympathetic tone.
Preoperative withdrawal: Withdrawal is recommended 2 wk prior to surgery to reduce risk of vascular collapse and cardiac arrest during anesthesia; during emergency surgery administer preanesthetic and anesthetic agents cautiously in reduced dosages and prepare for possible vascular collapse.

Overdosage: Signs and Symptoms
Severe drowsiness, hypotension, bradycardia, severe diarrhea, nausea, vomiting, syncope.

PATIENT CARE CONSIDERATIONS

Administration/Storage
- Administer with food or milk.
- Store in tightly closed container at room temperature. Keep out of reach of children.

Assessment/Interventions
- Obtain patient history, including drug history and any known allergies. Note any cardiovascular, cerebrovascular or peptic ulcer disease, asthma, or pheochromocytoma.
- Take patient's BP (lying, sitting, standing) and pulse before administering drug. Monitor periodically throughout therapy.
- In patients with cardiac decompensation, monitor for weight gain and edema.
- Report these signs to health care provider immediately: hypotension, chest pain, edema, dyspnea, diarrhea, excessive weight loss or gain, CNS changes.

Patient/Family Education
- Instruct patient in proper technique for taking BP. Advise patient to check BP weekly.
- Caution patient not to get out of bed without help during period of dosage adjustment.
- Advise patient to lie down if dizziness or blurred vision occurs.
- Warn patient not to double up on doses.
- Instruct patient not to discontinue drug abruptly and not to stop taking drug because of improvement in symptoms.
- Counsel patient about benefits of weight reduction, exercise, reduction of alcohol and sodium intake, and cessation of smoking.
- Explain that impotence and ejaculation disturbances may occur but is reversible. Tell patient to report to health care provider.
- Instruct patient to report these symptoms to health care provider: dizziness, diarrhea, confusion, depression, fever, sore throat.
- Caution patient to avoid sudden position changes to avoid orthostatic hypotension.
- Instruct patient to avoid intake of alcoholic beverages or other CNS depressants.
- Advise patient that drug may cause drowsiness and to use caution while driving or performing other tasks requiring mental alertness.
- Instruct patient not to take *otc* medications without consulting health care provider.

Guanfacine Hydrochloride

(GWAHN-fay-seen HIGH-droe-KLOR-ide)

Class Antihypertensive/Antiadrenergic, centrally acting

How Supplied
Tenex Tablets 1 mg, Tablets 2 mg

Action
PHARMACOLOGY: Appears to stimulate central alpha$_2$-adrenergic receptors, with decreased sympathetic outflow causing decrease in peripheral vascular resistance and reduction in heart rate.

PHARMACOKINETICS/DYNAMICS:
Absorption: Absolute bioavailability is about 80%. T_{max} is 1 to 4 hr.
Distribution: Protein binding is about 70%. Mean Vd is 6.3 L/kg.
Excretion: T½ is 10 to 30 hr. About 50% is excreted in the urine as unchanged, the remainder as metabolites.

Special Populations:
Renal Function Impairment – Cl is reduced; plasma levels are only slightly increased.

Indications Treatment of hypertension.
Unlabeled use(s): Amelioration of heroin withdrawal symptoms.

Contraindications Standard considerations.

Route/Dosage
ADULTS: PO 1 mg daily at bedtime; may increase gradually up to 3 mg daily.

Interactions
Alcohol, CNS depressants: Increased CNS depression.
Barbiturates, phenytoin: Decreased guanfacine levels with loss of antihypertensive effect.

Lab Test Interferences None well documented.

Adverse Reactions
CV: Chest pain; bradycardia; palpitations.
CNS: Somnolence; drowsiness; dizziness; headache; sleep disturbances; insomnia; confusion; depression.
DERM: Dermatitis; pruritus; sweating.
EENT: Conjunctivitis; visual disturbance; tinnitus; rhinitis; taste perversion.
GI: Dry mouth; constipation; diarrhea; nausea; abdominal discomfort; dyspnea.
GU: Urinary incontinence; testicular disorder; decreased libido; impotence.
OTHER: Paresthesia; paresis; leg cramps; hypokinesia.

Precautions
Pregnancy: Category B.
Lactation: Excreted in breast milk.
Children: Safety and efficacy in children younger than 12 yr not established.
Special risk patients: Use with caution in patients with severe coronary insufficiency, recent MI, cerebrovascular disease, or chronic renal or hepatic impairment.
Sedation: Occurs in a large percentage of patients.
Withdrawal: Do not discontinue therapy without consulting health care provider; drug must be withdrawn gradually to avoid rapid rise in BP (rebound hypertension).

Overdosage: Signs and Symptoms
Severe drowsiness, hypotension, bradycardia.

PATIENT CARE CONSIDERATIONS

Administration/Storage
- Administer medication at bedtime.
- Give with food or milk if patient experiences stomach upset.
- Store in tightly closed container and protect from light.

Assessment/Interventions
- Obtain patient history, including drug history and any known allergies. Note cardiovascular, cerebrovascular, renal, or hepatic disease.
- Take patient's BP (lying, sitting, standing) and pulse before administering drug. Monitor periodically throughout therapy.
- Notify health care provider if these signs occur: hypotension, chest pain, palpitations, anemia, leukopenia, thrombocytopenia, edema, dyspnea, diarrhea.

Patient/Family Education
- Instruct patient to take medication at bedtime.
- Teach patient proper technique for taking BP. Advise patient to check BP weekly.
- Instruct patient not to discontinue drug abruptly.
- Advise patient on benefits of weight loss, exercise, reduction of alcohol and sodium intake and cessation of smoking.
- Instruct patient to lie down if dizziness or blurred vision occurs.
- Explain that impotence may occur but is reversible. Tell patient to report to health care provider.
- Instruct patient to report these symptoms to health care provider: dizziness, constipation, headache, insomnia, nausea, sweating, or weakness.
- Advise patient to take sips of water frequently, suck on ice chips or sugarless hard candy, or chew sugarless gum if dry mouth occurs.

- Caution patient to avoid sudden position changes to avoid orthostatic hypotension.
- Instruct patient to avoid intake of alcoholic beverages or other CNS depressants.
- Advise patient that drug may cause drowsiness and to use caution while driving or performing other tasks requiring mental alertness.
- Instruct patient not to take *otc* medications without consulting health care provider.

Guanidine

(GWAHN-ih-deen)

Class CNS agent/Cholinergic muscle stimulant

How Supplied
Guanidine Hydrochloride Tablets 125 mg

Action
PHARMACOLOGY: Enhances release of acetylcholine following a nerve impulse and appears to slow rates of depolarization and repolarization of muscle cell membranes.

Indications Reduce symptoms of muscle weakness and easy fatigability associated with Lambert-Eaton syndrome. **Unlabeled use(s):** Treatment of botulism.

Contraindications Standard considerations.

Route/Dosage
ADULTS: **PO** Start with 10 to 15 mg/kg/day in 3 or 4 divided doses, gradually increasing the dose to 35 mg/kg/day or up to the development of side effects.

Interactions None well documented.

Lab Test Interferences None well documented.

Adverse Reactions
CV: Palpitation; tachycardia; atrial fibrillation; hypotension.
CNS: Paresthesia of lips, face, hands, and feet; cold sensations in hands and feet; nervousness; lightheadedness; increased irritability; jitteriness; tremor; trembling sensations; ataxia; emotional lability; psychotic state; confusion; mood changes; hallucination.
DERM: Rash; flushing or pink complexion; folliculitis; petechiae; purpura; ecchymosis; sweating; skin eruptions; dryness and scaling of the skin.
EENT: Sore throat.
GI: Dry mouth; anorexia; gastric irritation; nausea; diarrhea; abdominal cramping.
GU: Uremia; chronic interstitial nephritis; renal tubular necrosis; acute interstitial nephritis.
HEMA: Serum creatinine elevation; bone marrow suppression with anemia, leukopenia, and thrombocytopenia.
LABTESTABS: Abnormal LFTs.
OTHER: Fever.

Precautions
Pregnancy: Safety for use in pregnancy not established.
Lactation: Excreted in breast milk.
Children: Safety and efficacy not established.
Renal function impairment: Renal function may be affected in some patients.
Bone marrow suppression: Dose-related fatal bone marrow suppression can occur. Avoid coadministration of other drugs that may cause bone marrow suppression.

Overdosage: Signs and Symptoms
Mild GI symptoms (eg, increased peristalsis, anorexia, diarrhea), slight numbness and tingling on the lips and fingertips, nervous hyperirritability, fibrillary tremors, convulsive muscle contractions, salivation, vomiting, hypoglycemia, circulatory disturbances.

PATIENT CARE CONSIDERATIONS

Administration/Storage
- Administer dose tid to qid as prescribed.
- Administer without regard to meals. Administer with food if GI upset occurs.
- Store tablets at controlled room temperature (59° to 86°F).

Assessment/Interventions
- Obtain patient history, including drug history and any known allergies. Note kidney disease or current use of medications known to suppress the bone marrow.
- Ensure that CBC with differential is obtained before starting therapy and repeated frequently during treatment. Be prepared to discontinue therapy if bone marrow suppression is noted.
- Ensure that renal function is evaluated before starting therapy and periodically during treatment.
- Ensure that parenteral atropine is available for emergency treatment of cholinergic crisis.
- Frequently assess muscle strength and function. Notify health care provider immediately of increasing muscle weakness and/or respiratory distress.
- Assess patient for CV, CNS, GI, muscle, and general body side effects. Inform health care provider if noted and significant.

Patient/Family Education
- Explain name, dose, action, and potential side effects of drug.
- Advise patient that dose and frequency of

administration may be adjusted to achieve maximum benefit.
- Advise patient to take exactly as prescribed and not to change the dose or stop taking unless advised by health care provider.
- Advise patient to take prescribed dose without regard to meals but to take with food if stomach upset occurs.
- Instruct patient to contact health care provider immediately if any of the following occur: worsening muscle weakness, difficulty breathing, rash or sore throat, fever, other signs of infection.
- Advise patient to inform health care provider if nervousness, tremor, or persistent nausea or diarrhea occur.
- Advise women to notify health care provider if pregnant, planning to become pregnant, or breastfeeding.
- Instruct patient not to take any prescription or OTC medications or dietary supplements unless advised by health care provider.
- Advise patient that follow-up visits will be required to monitor therapy and to keep appointments.

Haemophilus b Conjugate Vaccine

(hem-AHF-ill-us)

Class Vaccine, inactivated bacteria

How Supplied

ActHIB Powder for Injection, lyophilized 10 mcg purified capsular polysaccharide, 24 mcg tetanus toxoid/0.5 mL ♦ *Comvax* Injection 7.5 mcg *Haemophilus* b PRP purified capsular polysaccharide, 125 mcg *Neisseria meningitidis* OMPC, 5 mcg hepatitis B surface antigen, about 225 mcg aluminum, and 35 mcg sodium borate/ 0.5 mL ♦ *HibTITER* Injection 10 mcg purified *Haemophilus* b saccharide capsular oligosaccharide, about 25 mcg diphtheria CRM_{197} protein/ 0.5 mL dose ♦ *PedvaxHIB, Liquid* Injection 7.5 mcg *Haemophilus* b PRP, 125 mcg *Neisseria meningitidis* OMPC, and 225 mcg aluminum/ 0.5 mL

Action

PHARMACOLOGY: Induces specific protective antibodies against *Haemophilus influenzae* type b (Hib).

Indications Induction of active immunity against Hib infection. Routine immunization of all infants beginning at age 2 mo is recommended.

Contraindications Hypersensitivity to any product component (some products contain thimerosal).

Route/Dosage

HibTITER

PEDIATRIC: **IM** Beginning at 2 mo of age, give 3 doses, 2 mo apart, plus a booster dose at 15 mo.

ActHIB

PEDIATRIC: **IM** Beginning at 2 mo of age, give 3 doses, 2 mo apart, plus a booster dose at 15 to 18 mo.

PedvaxHIB

PEDIATRIC: **IM** Beginning at 2 mo of age, give 2 doses, 2 mo apart, plus a booster dose at 12 mo.

Interactions None well documented.

Lab Test Interferences Diagnostic value of antigen detection (eg, with latex agglutination kits) may be diminished in suspected Hib disease within few days to 2 wk after immunization.

Adverse Reactions

CNS: Irritability; fever; restless sleep; convulsions.
DERM: Rash; hives.
GI: Diarrhea; vomiting; loss of appetite.
GU: Renal failure.
OTHER: Guillain-Barre syndrome; local erythema; swelling; tenderness; induration.

Precautions

Pregnancy: Category C.
Lactation: Undetermined.
Children: HibTITER and PedvaxHIB are not recommended in children less than 6 wk.
Anticoagulant therapy: Administer Hib vaccine with caution to patients receiving anticoagulant therapy.
Interchange: In general, complete vaccination series begun with one brand of Hib vaccine with that brand unless specific information about interchangeability is available.

PATIENT CARE CONSIDERATIONS

Administration/Storage

- Administer IM in outer aspect of vastus lateralis, midthigh, or outer aspect of upper arm. Do not inject in gluteal area or near major nerve trunk.
- Do not inject via IV route.
- Inspect product for particulate matter or discoloration. If these conditions exist, do not administer vaccine.
- Keep vaccine refrigerated. Do not freeze.

Assessment/Interventions

- Obtain patient history, including drug history and any known allergies.
- Interview parent or guardian about child's current health. If any febrile illness or active infection is present, vaccine administration may need to be delayed until after recovery. Also question parent or guardian about any allergies the child might have, specifically to any component of vaccine or previous reactions to vaccine.
- Assess for possible anaphylaxis.

Patient/Family Education

- Advise that acetaminophen (appropriate for age) may be given q 4 hr for low-grade fever. Emphasize that aspirin should not be given to children.
- Instruct parent or guardian to report any adverse effects after vaccine administration.
- Remind parent to keep child's immunization record up to date.

Halcinonide

(hal-SIN-oh-nide)
Class Corticosteroid/Topical
How Supplied
Halog Ointment 0.1%, Cream 0.025, Cream 0.1%, Solution 0.1% ♦ *Halog-E* Cream 0.1%
Action
PHARMACOLOGY: Produces anti-inflammatory, antipruritic, and vasoconstrictive effects by an unknown mechanism.

Indications Relief of inflammation and pruritus caused by corticosteroid-responsive dermatoses.

Contraindications Standard considerations.
Route/Dosage
ADULTS AND CHILDREN: **Topical** Apply thin film to affected area bid to tid.

Interactions None well documented.

Lab Test Interferences None well documented.

Adverse Reactions
DERM: Burning, itching; irritation; dryness; folliculitis; hypertrichosis; acneiform eruptions; hypopigmentation; perioral dermatitis; allergic contact dermatitis; maceration of the skin; secondary infection; skin atrophy; striae; miliaria.

Precautions
Pregnancy: Category C.
Lactation: Undetermined.
Children: Pediatric patients may demonstrate greater susceptibility to topical corticosteroid-induced hypothalamic-pituitary-adrenal (HPA) axis suppression and Cushing syndrome than mature patients because of a larger skin surface area to body weight ratio.
Occlusive dressings: Adverse effects are more common when occlusive dressings are used.
Systemic absorption: Systemic absorption of topical corticosteroids has produced reversible HPA axis suppression, manifestations of Cushing syndrome, hyperglycemia, and glucosuria in some patients.

Halobetasol Propionate

(hal-oh-BAY-ta-sol)
Class Corticosteroid/Topical
How Supplied
Ultravate Cream 0.05%, Ointment 0.05%
Action
PHARMACOLOGY: Very high potency topical glucocorticoid with anti-inflammatory, antipruritic, and vasoconstrictive properties. Thought to act by inducing phospholipase A_2 inhibitory proteins, thus controlling biosynthesis of potent mediators of inflammation.

Indications Relief of inflammatory and pruritic manifestations of corticosteroid-responsive dermatoses.

Contraindications Standard considerations.
Route/Dosage
ADULTS AND CHILDREN (OLDER THAN 12 YR): **Topical** Apply to affected area once or twice daily. Not recommended for more than 2 consecutive wk or more than 50 g/wk.

Interactions None well documented.

Lab Test Interferences None well documented.

Adverse Reactions
DERM: Stinging; burning; itching.

Precautions
Pregnancy: Category C.
Lactation: Secreted into breast milk. Unknown effect.
Children: Not recommended for children younger than 12 yr.
Avoid use: For external use Not recommended for use on the face, groin, or axillae. Not recommended for rosacea or perioral dermatitis.
Skin infections: Use with appropriate antimicrobials in the presence of skin infections.
Systemic: Systemic absorption of topical corticosteroids has produced reversible HPA axis suppression. Pediatric patients may be more susceptible.

Haloperidol

(HAL-oh-pehr-i-dahl)
Class Antipsychotic/Butyrophenone
How Supplied
Haldol Tablets 0.5 mg, Tablets 1 mg, Tablets 2 mg, Tablets 5 mg, Tablets 10 mg, Tablets 20 mg, Concentrate 2 mg (as lactate)/mL, Injection 5 mg (as lactate)/mL
🍁 *Apo-Haloperidol* ♦ *Haloperidol-LA Omega* ♦ *Novo-Peridol* ♦ *PMS-Haloperidol LA* ♦ *ratio-Haloperidol*

Haloperidol Decanoate
Haldol Decanoate 50 Injection 50 mg (as 70.5 decanoate)/mL ♦ *Haldol Decanoate 100* Injection 100 mg (as 141.04 mg decanoate)/mL

✤ *Apo-Haloperidol Decanoate Injection*

Action
PHARMACOLOGY: Has antipsychotic effect, apparently caused by dopamine-receptor blockage in CNS.

PHARMACOKINETICS/DYNAMICS:
Absorption: When administered in sesame oil, it results in the slow and sustained release of haloperidol. T_{max} is 6 days after injection. Steady-state plasma concentrations are achieved after the third or fourth dose.

Distribution: The relationship between dose of haloperidol decanoate and plasma haloperidol concentration is roughly linear for doses below 450 mg.

Excretion: Apparent t½ is approximately 3 wk for the decanoate and 18 hr for oral.

Indications Management of psychotic disorders; control of Tourette disorder in children and adults; management of severe behavioral problems in children; short-term treatment of hyperactive children. Long-term antipsychotic therapy (haloperidol decanoate). **Unlabeled use(s):** Treatment of phencyclidine (PCP) psychosis; antiemetic; hiccoughs.

Contraindications Severe, toxic CNS depression or comatose states from any cause; Parkinson disease; hypersensitive to any component of the product.

Route/Dosage
Psychotic disorders
ADULTS: **PO** Moderate symptoms, geriatric or debilitated patients: 0.5 to 2 mg bid to tid. Severe symptoms, chronic or resistant patients: 3 to 5 mg bid to tid. Dosages up to 100 mg/day may be necessary in some patients. **IM** 2 to 5 mg for prompt control of acutely agitated schizophrenic patients with moderately severe to very severe symptoms. Depending on response, subsequent doses may be needed within 60 min; although 4 to 8 hr intervals may be satisfactory. CHILDREN 3 TO 12 YR (WEIGHT 15 TO 40 KG): **PO** Initial dose 0.5 mg/day. If needed, increase in 0.5 mg increments at 5 to 7 day intervals up to 0.15 mg/kg/day or until therapeutic effect is obtained. The dose may be divided and given bid to tid. **IM** Safety and efficacy not established in children.

Tourette disorder
ADULTS: **PO** Start with 0.5 to 1.5 mg tid (max, 10 mg/day).
CHILDREN 3 TO 12 YR (WEIGHT 15 TO 40 KG): **PO** 0.05 to 0.075 mg/kg/day. Severely disturbed psychotic children may require higher doses.

Behavioral disorders/hyperactivity
CHILDREN 3 TO 12 YR (WEIGHT 15 TO 40 KG): **PO** 0.05 to 0.075 mg/kg/day. Severely disturbed psychotic children may require higher doses. In severely disturbed, nonpsychotic children or in hyperactive children with conduct disorder, short-term administration may suffice. There is little evidence to support dosages greater than 6 mg/day.

HALOPERIDOL DECANOATE INJECTION
The dose should be individualized under close supervision during initiation and stabilization of therapy. The recommended interval between doses is monthly or q 4 wk, but variations in patient response may dictate a need for adjustments in dose or dosing interval.
ADULTS: **IM (deep injection)** Initial dose should not exceed 100 mg. If conversion from oral haloperidol to IM haloperidol decanoate requires more than 100 mg as an initial dose, administer that dose in 2 injections (max, 100 mg initially followed by balance in 3 to 7 days). In patients stabilized on low oral doses (10 mg or less/day), the initial recommended dose of haloperidol decanoate is 10 to 15 times the daily dose. In patients stabilized on higher oral doses, the recommended dose is 20 times the daily dose. Maintenance dosages should be titrated upward or downward based on therapeutic response.

Interactions
Anesthetics, opiates, alcohol: May increase CNS depressant effects.
Anticholinergics: May increase anticholinergic effects. May worsen schizophrenic symptoms, decrease haloperidol serum concentrations, and lead to tardive dyskinesia.
Azole antifungal agents (eg, itraconazole): Plasma levels of haloperidol may be elevated, increasing the risk of side effects.
Carbamazepine: May decrease effects of haloperidol.
Lithium: May induce disorientation, unconsciousness, and extrapyramidal symptoms.
Rifamycins (eg, rifampin): Plasma levels of haloperidol may be reduced, decreasing the clinical effectiveness.

Lab Test Interferences
Pregnancy tests: False-positive results may occur; less likely to occur with serum test.
Protein-bound iodine: Increases have been reported.

Adverse Reactions
CV: Orthostatic hypotension; hypertension; tachycardia; ECG changes.
CNS: Tardive dyskinesia; tardive dystonia; insomnia; restlessness; anxiety; euphoria; agitation; drowsiness; depression; lethargy; headache; confusion; vertigo; seizures; exacerbation of psychotic symptoms; pseudoparkinsonism (eg, mask-like face, drooling, pill rolling, shuffling

gait, inertia, tremors, cogwheel rigidity); muscle spasms; dyskinesia; akathisia; oculogyric crises; opisthotonos; hyperreflexia.
DERM: Maculopapular and acneiform skin reactions; photosensitivity; hair loss.
EENT: Cataracts; retinopathy; visual disturbances; mydriasis; increased IOP; nasal congestion.
GI: Dyspepsia; anorexia; diarrhea; hypersalivation; nausea; vomiting; dry mouth; elevated prolactin levels; adynamic ileus (may lead to death).
GU: Menstrual irregularities; breast enlargement; lactation; gynecomastia; impotence; sexual dysfunction; priapism; urinary hesitancy or retention.
HEMA: Agranulocytosis; leukopenia; leukocytosis; anemia.
HEPA: Jaundice; impaired liver function.
RESP: Laryngospasm; bronchospasm; increased depth of respiration; bronchopneumonia.
OTHER: Hyperglycemia; hypoglycemia; hyponatremia.

Precautions

Pregnancy: Safety not established.
Haloperidol decanoate – Category C.
Lactation: Excreted in breast milk.
Children: Do not use in children younger than 3 yr. Safety and efficacy of IM form not established.
Elderly: More susceptible to effects; consider lower dose.
Special risk patients: Use drug with caution in patients with CV disease or mitral insufficiency, history of glaucoma, EEG abnormalities or seizure disorders, prior brain damage, or hepatic or renal impairment.
Tartrazine sensitivity: Note that tartrazine may be a component of this product.
Abrupt withdrawal: Abrupt withdrawal in patients on maintenance therapy has been associated with transient dyskinetic signs, which may be indistinguishable from tardive dyskinesia.
Antiemetic effects: Caused by suppression of cough reflex, aspiration of vomitus possible.
CNS effects: May impair mental or physical abilities, especially during first few days of therapy.
Debilitated patients: More susceptible to effects; consider lower dose.
Hepatic effects: Jaundice usually occurs in 2 to 4 wk of treatment and is considered a hypersensitivity reaction. Usually reversible.
Neuroleptic malignant syndrome (NMS): Has occurred and is potentially fatal. Signs and symptoms are hyperpyrexia, muscle rigidity, altered mental status, irregular pulse, irregular BP, tachycardia, and diaphoresis.
Sensitivity to neuroleptic drugs: May require lower dosage.
Sudden death: Has been reported; predisposing factors may be seizures or previous brain damage. Flare up of psychotic behavior may precede death.
Tardive dyskinesia: Syndrome of potentially irreversible, involuntary dyskinetic movements may develop. Prevalence is highest in elderly, especially women. Use smallest effective dose for shortest period of time needed.

Overdosage: Signs and Symptoms

CNS depression, somnolence, hypotension, extrapyramidal symptoms, hypertension, shock-like state, coma, autonomic reactions, ECG changes associated with torsades de pointes, cardiac arrhythmias.

PATIENT CARE CONSIDERATIONS

Administration/Storage

- Dose and frequency of administration are variable, depending on condition being treated.
- Administer tablets as prescribed, without regard to meals. Administer with food if GI upset occurs.
- Measure prescribed dose of oral concentrate using calibrated dropper or dosing syringe.
- Oral concentrate can be mixed with semisolid foods (eg, soup, pudding) or diluted with 1 to 2 oz of water, coffee, tea, tomato or fruit juice just prior to administration. Do not prepare dilutions ahead of time and store.
- Injection is for IM administration only. Not for intradermal, SC, or IV administration.
- Double check injection dose form. Haloperidol decanoate is designed for monthly injection only.
- Inject prescribed dose slowly, deep into outer quadrant of buttock.
- Do not administer injection if particulate matter or marked discoloration noted. A slight yellowish discoloration is normal and will not alter potency.
- Store tablets, oral concentrate, and injection at controlled room temperature (59° to 86°F) protected from light. Do not freeze oral concentrate or injection.

Assessment/Interventions

- Obtain patient history, including drug history and any known allergies. Note CV disease, arrhythmias, cerebrovascular disease, narrow angle glaucoma, epilepsy, prostatic hypertrophy, condition predisposing to hypotension (eg, dehydration, hypovolemia), concomitant use of antihypertensive or anti-convulsant drugs, or previous episodes of Neuroleptic

Malignant Syndrome.
- Frequently assess patient for response to treatment. Notify health care provider if condition being treated is not improving or is worsening.
- Ensure that therapy is periodically reviewed to determine if therapy needs to be continued without change or if a dose change (eg, increase, decrease, discontinuation) is indicated.
- Avoid sudden discontinuation of therapy if possible. Attempt to gradually reduce dose if decision to discontinue medication is made.
- Inform health care provider immediately if hyperpyrexia, muscle rigidity, altered mental status, irregular pulse and BP, tachycardia, and diaphoresis develop.
- Assess neurologic status before and during treatment. Observe for involuntary body and facial movements, excessive drowsiness, agitation, tremor, or anxiety. Inform health care provider if noted.
- Monitor patient for CNS, CV, GI, GU, psychiatric, musculoskeletal, and general body side effects. Inform health care provider if noted and significant.
- Assess medication compliance.

Patient/Family Education
- Explain name, dose, action, and potential side effects of drug.
- Advise patient, family, or caregiver that dose will be adjusted periodically until maximum benefit has been obtained.
- Advise patient, family, or caregiver not to change the dose or stop taking unless advised by health care provider.
- Instruct patient, family, or caregiver to measure prescribed dose of oral concentrate using calibrated dropper or dosing syringe.
- Advise patient, family, or caregiver that oral concentrate can be mixed with semisolid foods (eg, soup, pudding) or diluted with 1 to 2 oz of water, coffee, tea, or tomato or fruit juice prior to administration. Caution patient, family, or caregiver not to prepare dilutions ahead of time and store.
- Instruct patient not to stop taking haloperidol when feeling better.
- Instruct patient, family, or caregiver to immediately report fainting or loss of consciousness, dizziness, high fever, muscle rigidity, or altered mental status to health care provider.
- Advise patient, family, or caregiver to notify health care provider of the following: excessive drowsiness, increased agitation or anxiety, or involuntary body or facial movements.
- Advise patient to avoid strenuous activity during periods of high temperature or humidity.
- Instruct patient to avoid alcoholic beverages and other depressants while taking this medication.
- Instruct patient to get up slowly from lying or sitting position and to avoid sudden position changes to prevent postural hypotension. Advise patient to report dizziness with position changes to health care provider. Caution patient that hot tubs and hot showers or baths may make dizziness worse.
- Advise patient to take sips of water, suck on ice chips or sugarless hard candy, or chew sugarless gum if dry mouth occurs.
- Advise patient that drug may cause drowsiness and impaired judgment or thinking skills and to use caution while driving or performing other tasks requiring mental alertness until tolerance is determined.
- Caution patient that medication may cause sensitivity to sunlight and to avoid unnecessary exposure to UV light (sunlight, tanning booths) and to use sunscreen and wear protective clothing when exposed to UV light until tolerance is determined.
- Advise women to notify health care provider if pregnant, planning to become pregnant, or breastfeeding.
- Instruct patient not to take any prescription or OTC medications or dietary supplements unless advised by health care provider.
- Advise patient that follow-up visits may be required to monitor therapy and to keep appointments.

Heparin

(HEP-uh-rin)

Class Anticoagulants

How Supplied
Heparin Sodium Injection 1000 units/mL, Injection 2000 units/mL, Injection 2500 units/mL, Injection 5000 units/mL, Injection 10,000 units/mL, Injection 20,000 units/mL, Injection 40,000 units/mL ◆ *Hep-Lock* Injection 10 units/mL, Injection 100 units/mL ◆ *Hep-Lock U/P* Injection 10 units/mL, Injection 100 units/mL
✤ *Hepalean* ◆ *Hepalean-Lok* ◆ *Heparin Leo* ◆ *Heparin Lock Flush*

Action
PHARMACOLOGY: Inhibits reactions that lead to clotting.

PHARMACOKINETICS/DYNAMICS:

Absorption: Heparin sodium is not absorbed from GI; must be given IV or SC. T_{max} is 2 to 4 hr (SC).

Distribution: Distribution is controlled by the liver; distributed in plasma and is extensively and nonspecifically protein bound.

Metabolism: The liver and the reticuloendothelial system are the sites of biotransformation.

Excretion: The average t½ is 30 to 180 min, and is dose-dependant and non-linear. Up to 50% is excreted in urine as unchanged.
Hemodialysis – Heparin is not removed.

Onset: Onset is immediate (IV) and 20 to 60 min (SC).

Special Populations:
Renal Function Impairment – The t½ may be increased.
Hepatic Function Impairment – The t½ may be increased.
Infection/malignancy/pulmonary embolism – The t½ may be decreased.
Obesity – The t½ may be increased.

Indications Prophylaxis and treatment of venous thrombosis and its extensions, pulmonary embolism (PE), peripheral arterial embolism, and atrial fibrillation with embolization; diagnosis and treatment of acute and chronic consumption coagulopathies (DIC); prevention of postoperative deep venous thrombosis (DVT), and PE. **Unlabeled use(s):** Prophylaxis of left ventricular thrombi and cerebrovascular accidents post-MI; treatment of myocardial ischemia; prevention of cerebral thrombosis in evolving strokes; adjunctive treatment of coronary occlusion with acute MI.

Contraindications Severe thrombocytopenia; uncontrolled bleeding (except because of DIC); patients in whom suitable blood coagulation tests cannot be performed.

Route/Dosage

ADULTS: **SC** 10,000 to 20,000 U as initial dose followed by 8000 to 20,000 U q 8 to 12 hr. **Intermittent IV** 10,000 U as initial dose followed by 5000 to 10,000 U q 4 to 6 hr. **IV infusion** 20,000 to 40,000 U/day.

CHILDREN: **Intermittent IV** 50 U/kg as initial dose followed by 100 U/kg q 4 hr. **IV infusion** 50 U/kg as initial dose followed by 20,000 U/m²/24 hr.

Low-dose Prophylaxis
SC 5000 U 2 hr before surgery and q 8 to 12 hr thereafter for 7 days or until patient is fully ambulatory, whichever is longer.

Surgery of Heart and Blood Vessels
ADULTS: 300 to 400 U/kg.

Blood Transfusion
Add 400 to 600 U/100 mL of whole blood.

Clearing Intermittent Infusion Sets
10 to 100 U/mL.

Laboratory Samples
Add 70 to 150 U/10 to 20 mL of whole blood.

Interactions

Dipyridamole, hydroxychloroquine, NSAIDs, salicylates: May cause increased risk of bleeding.
INCOMPATIBILITIES: Heparin is acidic and incompatible with many drugs.

Lab Test Interferences

Aminotransferase (AST and ALT): Drug causes increased concentrations.

Adverse Reactions

DERM: Necrosis; transient alopecia; urticaria.
HEMA: Hemorrhage; thrombocytopenia.
OTHER: Hypersensitivity (chills, fever, urticaria, asthma, rhinitis, lacrimation, headache, nausea, vomiting, shock); anaphylactoid reactions; allergic vasospastic reactions, including painful ischemia, cyanotic limbs; osteoporosis; priapism; rebound hyperlipidemia on discontinuation.

Precautions

Pregnancy: Category C.
Lactation: Not excreted in breast milk.
Elderly: Higher incidence of bleeding in women older than 60 yr.
Hypersensitivity: Generalized hypersensitivity can occur. Reactions range from mild to severe.
Benzyl alcohol sensitivity: Benzyl alcohol, used as preservative in some products, is associated with a fatal gasping syndrome in premature infants.
Debilitated patients: Higher incidence of bleeding in women older than 60 yr.
Hemorrhage: Hemorrhage can occur at virtually any site. Use heparin with extreme caution in patients at increased risk of hemorrhage.
Hyperlipidemia: Heparin administration may cause hyperlipidemia in patients with dysbetalipoproteinemia (type III).
IM use: Avoid IM use because of local irritation, erythema, pain, hematoma, or ulceration.

Overdosage: Signs and Symptoms

Bleeding, nosebleeds, hematuria, tarry stools, easy bruising, or petechiae.

PATIENT CARE CONSIDERATIONS
Administration/Storage
- Heparin is strongly acidic and is incompatible with many drugs. Avoid mixing any drug with heparin unless specifically advised by health care provider.
- Avoid IM administration.
- SC administration should be deep, preferably into fatty layers of abdomen. Use small-gauge needle to minimize tissue trauma. Bunch up tissue without pinching and insert needle at 90% angle to skin. Inject slowly.
- Do not aspirate patient to check entry into blood vessel. Apply gentle pressure to puncture site for approximately 1 min; do not massage. Rotate injection sites frequently and keep record.
- IV administration may be given undiluted over 1 min.
- For IV infusion, dilute prescribed amount in 0.9% Sodium Chloride for Injection, D5W, or Ringer's Injection solution. Use infusion pump to ensure accuracy.
- For heparin locks, inject diluted heparin solution of 10 to 100 U (0.5 to 1 mL).
- To prevent incompatibility of heparin with medication, flush heparin lock set with Sterile Water for Injection or 0.9% Sodium Chloride for Injection before and after medication is administered.
- Store at room temperature. Protect from freezing.
- Inspect all preparations for particulate matter prior to administration. Also inspect for discoloration; note that slight discoloration does not alter potency.

Assessment/Interventions
- Obtain patient history, including drug history and any known allergies.
- Monitor vital signs. Report fever, drop in BP, rapid pulse, and other signs and symptoms of hemorrhage to health care provider.
- Perform baseline blood coagulation tests, hemoglobin, hematocrit, RBC, and platelet counts before therapy is initiated.
- Monitor I&O during early therapy. Heparin may have diuretic effect beginning 36 to 48 hr after initial dose and last 36 to 48 hr after termination of therapy.
- Assess for signs of bleeding and hemorrhage. Venipuncture sites may require pressure to prevent bleeding and hematoma formation.
- Assess for evidence of additional or increased thrombosis.
- Observe injection sites for hematomas, ecchymosis, and inflammation.
- Activated partial thromboplastin time (aPTT) and activated coagulation time (ACT) are coagulation tests commonly used to monitor heparin therapy. Dosage is adjusted to keep aPTT between 1.5 and 2 times normal control level. ACT is ideally 2 to 3 times control value in sec.
- During dosage adjustment periods, draw blood for coagulation tests 30 min before each scheduled SC or intermittent IV dose.
- Follow agency protocol for heparin administration, particularly when "piggybacking" heparin with other drugs.
- Inform all personnel caring for patient that patient is receiving anticoagulant therapy.
- Avoid IM injections of other medication because hematomas may develop.
- In patients requiring long-term anticoagulation therapy, institute oral anticoagulation therapy. To ensure continuous anticoagulation, continue full heparin therapy for several days after PT has reached therapeutic range. Heparin can then be stopped without tapering.
- Monitor patient frequently for signs of infiltration, to see that tubing is not kinked, to ensure that tubing is properly positioned in pump, and to check all connections for leakage.
- Construct flow chart indicating dates, coagulation time determinations, Hct, leukocyte and platelet counts, heparin doses, and urine and stool tests for occult blood.
- Make accurate observations of clinical response.

Patient/Family Education
- Caution patient to avoid IM injections.
- Advise patient to avoid activities that carry risk of injury.
- Instruct patient to use soft toothbrush and electric razor.
- Caution patient to avoid aspirin and aspirin-containing medications.
- Advise patient to report unusual bruising or bleeding (eg, nosebleeds, bleeding gums) or tarry stools to health care provider immediately.
- Instruct patient to inform health care provider and dentist of use of this medication before treatment or surgery.
- Inform patient of potential for hair loss. Explain that this effect may occur several months after heparin therapy is started. Reassure patient that if alopecia occurs, hair growth will return after drug has been discontinued.
- Advise patient to carry identification card or

to wear a medication identification bracelet (ie, *Medi-Alert*) that indicates heparin therapy.
* Inform women that menstruation may be somewhat increased and prolonged. Usually this effect is not a contraindication to therapy if bleeding is not excessive and there is no underlying pathologic condition.
* Advise patient that smoking and alcohol may alter response to heparin, and therefore, are not advised.
* Inform patient that abrupt withdrawal of heparin may precipitate increased coagulability.

Hepatitis A Vaccine, Inactivated

(Hep-uh-TIGHT-iss)

Class Vaccine, inactivated virus

How Supplied
Havrix Suspension 720 EL.U/0.5 mL of viral antigen ◆ *Vaqta* Injectable 25 U/0.5 mL of HAV protein, Injectable 50 U/1 mL of HAV protein
❋ *Avaxim* ◆ *Avaxim Pediatric* ◆ *Epaxal Berna*

Action
PHARMACOLOGY: Provides active immunization.

Indications
Active immunization of patients 2 yr and older against disease caused by hepatitis A virus.

Contraindications
Hypersensitivity to any component of the vaccine.

Route/Dosage
ADULTS (19 YR AND OLDER): **IM (in the deltoid region)** *Havrix* 1440 EL.U (1 mL) or *Vaqta* 50 U (1 mL) in 2 doses at 0 and 6 to 12 mo later.
CHILDREN (2 TO 18 YR): **IM** *Havrix* 360 EL.U (0.5 mL) in 3 doses at 0, 1, and 6 to 12 mo later or *Havrix* 720 EL.U (0.5 mL) in 2 doses at 0 and 6 to 12 mo later or *Vaqta* 25 U (0.5 mL) in 2 doses at 0 and 6 to 18 mo later.

Interactions
Anticoagulants: Since bleeding may occur following IM administration, use with caution.
Immunosuppressants: May result in inadequate response to immunization; therefore, additional administration of vaccine may be required.
Immune Globulin (IG): Compared with giving hepatitis A vaccine alone, when coadministered with IG, lower antibody titers may be obtained. However, hepatitis A vaccine and IG may be given concurrently using different syringes and different injection sites.

Adverse Reactions
CNS: Headache; hypertonic episodes; insomnia; photophobia; vertigo; convulsions; encephalopathy; dizziness; neuropathy; myelitis; paresthesia; multiple sclerosis; Guillain-Barré syndrome; somnolence.
DERM: Pruritus; rash; urticaria; erythema multiforme; hyperhydrosis; generalized erythema; dermatitis; angioedema.
EENT: Pharyngitis; nasal congestion; eye irritation and itching.
GI: Anorexia; nausea; abdominal pain; diarrhea; dysgeusia; vomiting.
GU: Menstrual disorder.
HEPA: Jaundice; hepatitis.
RESP: Cough; upper respiratory tract infection; bronchial constriction; asthma; wheezing; dyspnea.
OTHER: Injection site soreness, pain, pruritus, and rash; tenderness; warmth; induration; redness; swelling; hematoma; ecchymosis; localized edema; arthralgia; myalgia; arm and back pain; stiffness; elevated creatine phosphokinase; fever; malaise; lymphadenopathy; congenital abnormality; syncope; anaphylaxis/anaphylactoid reactions; edema.

Precautions
Pregnancy: Category C.
Lactation: Undetermined.
Children: Safety and efficacy not established in children younger than 2 yr.
Anaphylaxis: There have been rare reports of anaphylaxis and anaphylactoid reactions.
Hepatitis: Hepatitis A vaccine will not prevent hepatitis caused by other agents, such as hepatitis B, C, or E virus or other pathogens that infect the liver.
Preexisting infection: Hepatitis A vaccine may not prevent hepatitis A infection in individuals who have an unrecognized hepatitis A infection at the time of vaccination; in addition, it may not prevent infection in individuals who do not achieve protective antibody titers.

PATIENT CARE CONSIDERATIONS
Administration/Storage
* For IM injection only. Not for IV, SC, or ID administration.
* Vaccination regimen consists of one primary dose and one booster dose. Booster dose is administered 6 to 18 mo after primary dose in patients 2 to 18 yr and 6 to 12 mo after primary dose in patients 19 yr.

- Shake vial or syringe well before use to maintain suspension of the vaccine.
- Examine vial or syringe after shaking. Suspension should be homogeneous and white. Discard if it appears otherwise.
- Use vaccine as supplied; no dilution or reconstitution is necessary.
- After removal of the appropriate volume from the single-dose vial, discard any remaining vaccine.
- Administer IM in deltoid region, or anterolateral thigh in toddlers and older children if deltoid muscle mass is inadequate. Avoid gluteal injection, which may result in less than optimal immune response.
- Record manufacturer's name and vaccine lot number in patient's permanent medical record file. Include date of administration, name, and title of person administering vaccine.
- Have epinephrine 1:1000 available in case of serious allergic reaction.
- Store vials and syringes in refrigerator. Do not freeze. Discard if vaccine has been frozen because freezing destroys potency.

Alternative vaccination regimen using 360 EL.U strength product in patients 2 to 18 yr:
- Three doses administered as primary dose, second dose 1 mo later, and third dose 6 to 12 mo later.

Interchangeability of booster dose:
- Products are interchangeable for booster dose (eg, Vaqta can be used for booster dose following primary dose of Havrix). Do not alternate between the 360 EL.U and 720 EL.U doses. Booster dose should be same strength as primary dose.

Assessment/Interventions
- Obtain patient history, including drug history and any known allergies. Note history of serious reactions to previous doses of hepatitis A vaccines, anticoagulant therapy, bleeding disorder, and thrombocytopenia.
- Check patient's immunization history to verify that administration regimen is being followed.
- Consider delaying immunization during course of moderate or severe acute febrile illness.
- Monitor patient for signs of anaphylaxis or severe allergic reaction. Discontinue therapy and immediately notify health care provider if noted. Be prepared to treat appropriately.

Missed booster dose:
- If booster dose is missed, administer as soon as possible. Do not restart the series. Delaying booster dose does not reduce final effectiveness of vaccine but may allow protective effect of primary dose to drop below protective levels until booster is administered.

Patient/Family Education
- Explain name, action, and potential side effects of vaccine.
- Advise patient that hepatitis A vaccine does not protect from other causes of food and waterborne diseases and to continue taking all necessary precautions to avoid contact with, or ingestion of, contaminated food and water.
- Review immunization schedule and advise patient that for vaccine to provide long-term protection, the booster dose needs to be administered as scheduled.
- Provide patient with immunization history record.
- Advise patient to use otc analgesics (eg, acetaminophen or ibuprofen) for fever or pain or discomfort at injection site.
- Advise patient to notify health care provider if bothersome side effects last more than 24 hr.

Hepatitis A Inactivated & Hepatitis B (Recombinant) Vaccine

(Hep-uh-TIGHT-iss)

Class Viral vaccine

How Supplied
Twinrix Injection at least 720 EL.U inactivated hepatitis A, 20 mcg recombinant HBsAg protein/mL

Action
PHARMACOLOGY: Provides active immunization.

Indications Active immunization of patients 18 yr or older against disease caused by hepatitis A and infection by all known subtypes of hepatitis B virus.

Contraindications Hypersensitivity to yeast or any other component of the vaccine or hypersensitivity after previous administration of this product or monovalent hepatitis A or hepatitis B vaccines.

Route/Dosage
ADULTS: **IM** 3 doses given on a 0-, 1-, and 6-mo schedule.

Interactions
Anticoagulants: Because bleeding may occur following IM administration, use with caution.
Immunosuppressants: May result in inadequate

Adverse Reactions
CNS: Headache; fatigue.
GI: Diarrhea; nausea; vomiting.
RESP: Upper respiratory tract infections.
OTHER: Local soreness, redness, induration, and swelling; fever.

Precautions
Pregnancy: Category C.
Lactation: Undetermined.
Children: Safety and efficacy not established in patients less than 18 yr.
Anaphylaxis: There have been rare reports of anaphylaxis and anaphylactoid reactions.

PATIENT CARE CONSIDERATIONS

Administration/Storage
- For IM injection only. Not for IV or ID administration.
- Primary immunizing regimen consists of 3 doses, given on a 0-, 1- and 6-month schedule.
- Shake vial or syringe well before use to maintain suspension of the vaccine.
- Examine vial or syringe after shaking. Suspension should be homogeneous and white. Discard if it appears otherwise.
- Use vaccine as supplied; no dilution or reconstitution is necessary.
- After removal of the appropriate volume from the single-dose vial, discard any vaccine remaining in the vial.
- Administer IM in deltoid region. Avoid gluteal injection, which may result in less than optimal immune response.
- Always record manufacturer's name and vaccine lot number in patient's permanent medical record file along with date of administration and name and title of person administering vaccine.
- Have epinephrine 1:1000 available in case of serious allergic reaction.
- Store vials and syringes in refrigerator. Do not freeze. Discard if vaccine has been frozen because freezing destroys potency.

Assessment/Interventions
- Obtain patient history, including drug history and any known allergies. Note history of the following: allergy to yeast; serious reactions to previous doses of hepatitis A or B vaccines; anticoagulant therapy; bleeding disorder; thrombocytopenia.
- Check patient's immunization history to verify that administration regimen is being followed.
- Consider delaying immunization during course of moderate or severe acute febrile illness.
- Monitor patient for signs of anaphylaxis or severe allergic reaction. Discontinue therapy and immediately notify health care provider if noted. Be prepared to treat appropriately.
- If a dose is missed, administer as soon as possible and resume schedule to complete series. Do not restart the series. Delaying immunization does not reduce effectiveness of vaccine but does delay time to achieve maximum protection.

Patient/Family Education
- Explain name, action, and potential side effects of vaccine.
- Advise patient that vaccine does not provide protection from other causes of food and waterborne diseases other than hepatitis A and to continue to take all necessary precautions to avoid contact with, or ingestion of, contaminated food and water.
- Review immunization schedule and advise patient that for vaccine to be effective, the complete series of 3 injections must be completed.
- Provide patient with immunization history record.
- Advise patient to use OTC analgesics (eg, acetaminophen, ibuprofen) for fever or pain or discomfort at injection site.
- Advise patient to notify health care provider if bothersome side effects last more than 24 hr.

Hepatitis B Immune Globulin (HBIG)

(hep-uh-TIGHT-iss)

Class Immune serum

How Supplied
BayHep B Injection 217 IU/mL ◆ *Nabi-HB* Injection 312 IU/mL

Action
PHARMACOLOGY: Directly neutralizes hepatitis B virus.

Indications For passive, transient prevention of hepatitis B infection after viral exposure via needlestick or mucous membrane contact; prevention of hepatitis B in infants born to HBsAg-positive mothers. Most effective when used within 7 days of exposure.

Contraindications None well documented.

Route/Dosage

ADULTS AND CHILDREN: **IM** 0.06 mL/kg (usually 3 to 5 mL). Administer as soon as possible after exposure and repeat 28 to 30 days later. NEWBORNS OF HBsAG-POSITIVE MOTHERS: **IM** 0.5 mL. Administer first HBIG dose as soon as possible, preferably less than 12 hr after birth. Also give hepatitis B vaccine. If hepatitis B vaccine is declined, repeat HBIG at 3 and 6 mo.

Interactions

Anticoagulants: Give HBIG with caution to people receiving anticoagulant therapy.

PATIENT CARE CONSIDERATIONS

Administration/Storage
- Inspect solution for particulate matter and discoloration before administration.
- Administer IM, preferably in gluteal or deltoid muscle in adults and children. In newborns, administer IM in anterolateral thigh. Do not give IV.
- Always record manufacturer's name and lot number on vial in patient's permanent record file along with date of administration, name and title of person administering injection.
- Refrigerate vials. Do not freeze.

Assessment/Interventions
- Obtain complete history, including drug history and any known allergies.
- Check patient's immunization history to verify that administration regimen is being followed.
- Review patient's medical history for history of serious adverse reactions to previous dose of HBIG.
- Monitor for hypersensitivity or anaphylaxis. Epinephrine should always be available to counteract any possible reactions.

Vaccines: To avoid inactivating vaccines containing live viruses (except measles vaccine) or bacteria, give live vaccines 3 mo after HBIG.

Lab Test Interferences None well documented.

Adverse Reactions

OTHER: Local pain and tenderness at injection site; urticaria; angioedema; anaphylactic reactions.

Precautions

Pregnancy: Category C.
Lactation: Undetermined.

Overdosage: Signs and Symptoms
Pain, tenderness.

Patient/Family Education
- Instruct parent to vaccinate all at-risk infants as soon after birth as possible and again at 3 mo.
- Instruct patient that therapy is useful as post-exposure prophylaxis as soon after exposure as possible (preferably within 7 days.)
- Provide patient or parent with immunization history record and record this injection in patient's medical records.
- Instruct patient to give analgesic for local pain. Avoid giving aspirin to children.
- Inform parent or patient of schedule for vaccination program if necessary.

Hepatitis B Vaccine

(hep-uh-TIGHT-iss)

Class Vaccine, inactivated virus

How Supplied

Engerix-B Injection (adult formulation) 20 mcg/mL hepatitis B surface antigen, Injection (pediatric formulation) 10 mcg/0.5 mL hepatitis B surface antigen ♦ *Recombivax HB* Injection (adult formulation) 10 mcg/mL hepatitis B surface antigen, Injection (pediatric/adolescent formulation) 5 mcg/0.5 mL hepatitis B surface antigen, Injection (dialysis formulation) 40 mcg/mL hepatitis B surface antigen

Action

PHARMACOLOGY: Induces specific antibodies against hepatitis B virus.

Indications Induction of active immunity against hepatitis B virus among people of all ages who are currently or who will be at increased risk of infection with this virus. Routine vaccination is recommended for infants and adolescents. All individuals not receiving the hepatitis B vaccine are recommended to be vaccinated at 11 to 12 yr. In addition, vaccination is recommended in older unvaccinated adolescents at high risk. Vaccination is also indicated for those at high risk of exposure to or development of hepatitis B virus, such as health care personnel (eg, dentists; dental hygienists; nurses; oral surgeons; health care providers; surgeons; podiatrists; paramedical and ambulance personnel; patients and staff in hemodialysis units and hematology/oncology units; hemodialysis patients and patients with early renal failure before they require hemodialysis; blood bank and plasma fractionation workers; laboratory personnel handling blood, its products, and patients' specimens; dental, medical, and nursing students); hospital cleaning staff who handle potentially infectious waste; patients requiring frequent or large-volume blood transfusions or clotting factor concentrates; residents and staff of institutions for mentally handicapped; household and other intimate contacts of people with persistent hepatitis B antigenemia; infants born to HBsAg-positive mothers; populations with high incidence of hepatitis B virus (eg, Alaskan Eskimos, Indochinese refugees, Haitian refugees); people at increased risk because of their sexual practices (eg, prostitutes; people who repeatedly contract STDs; homosexually active men; people with multiple sexual partners; international travelers; morticians; embalmers; prisoners; users of illicit injectable drugs; police and fire department personnel who render first aid or medical assistance.Risk factors for hepatitis C are similar to those for hepatitis B. Consequently, immunization with hepatitis B vaccine is recommended for individuals with chronic hepatitis C.

Revaccination (booster doses):
Adults and children with normal immune status – Antibody response lasts 10 yr or more.
Hemodialysis patients – Vaccine protection is less complete and may persist only as long as antibody levels remain more than 10 mIU/mL.
Vaccinated people who experience percutaneous or needle exposure to HBsAg-positive blood – Serological tests to assess immune status is recommended. If inadequate levels exist, treat with a booster dose of vaccine.
Nonresponders – Most people who do not initially respond to the primary series may develop adequate antibody concentrations after revaccination with a fourth or fifth dose or a new complete vaccine series.

Contraindications Hypersensitivity to yeast or any other component of vaccine.

Route/Dosage
ENGERIX-B
ADULTS 20 YR OR OLDER: **IM** 20 mcg at 0, 1, and 6 mo.
CHILDREN AND ADOLESCENTS 1 TO 19 YR: **IM** 10 mcg at 0, 1, and 6 mo.
INFANTS OF HBsAG-POSITIVE OR -NEGATIVE MOTHERS: **IM** 10 mcg at 0, 1, and 6 mo.
ADULT PREDIALYSIS AND DIALYSIS PATIENTS: **IM** 40 mcg at 0, 1, 2, and 6 mo.
ALTERNATE SCHEDULE: Designed for certain populations (eg, neonates born of hepatitis B-infected mothers, others who may have been recently exposed to the virus, certain travelers to high-risk areas).
Adults (Older than 19 Yr): **IM** 20 mcg at 0, 1, 2, 12 mo.
Adolescents (11 to 19 Yr): **IM** 20 mcg at 0, 1, 2, 12 mo, or 20 mcg at 0, 1, 6 mo.
Adolescents 11 to 16 Yr (For Whom an Extended Schedule is Acceptable Based on Risk of Exposure): **IM** 10 mcg at 0, 12, and 24 mo.
Children (Birth to 10 Yr): **IM** 10 mcg at 0, 1, 2, 12 mo.
Children 5 to 10 Yr (For Whom an Extended Schedule is Acceptable Based on Risk of Exposure): **IM** 10 mcg at 0, 12, and 24 mo.
Infants Born of HBsAG-Positive Mothers: **IM** 10 mcg at 0, 1, 2, and 12 mo.
REVACCINATION:
Hemodialysis patients: A booster dose may be considered for patients undergoing dialysis if anti-HBs level less than 10 mIU/mL 1 to 2 mo after third dose.
Other patients (when a booster dose is appropriate):
Adults and adolescents 11 to 19 yr
IM 20 mcg.
Children 10 yr or younger
IM 10 mcg.

RECOMBIVAX HB
Adults 20 yr or older – **IM** 10 mcg at 0, 1, and 6 mo.
Children and Adolescents 1 to 19 yr – **IM** 5 mcg at 0, 1, and 6 mo, alternatively.
Adolescents 11 to 15 yr – **IM** 10 mcg at 0 and 4 to 6 mo.
Infants of HBsAg-Positive or -Negative Mothers – **IM** 5 mcg at 0, 1, and 6 mo.
Adult Predialysis and Dialysis Patients – **IM** 40 mcg at 0, 1, and 6 mo.

Interactions
Anticoagulants: Use caution when administering to patients receiving anticoagulant therapy because coadministration may increase the immunization drug.
Immunosuppressants (including high-dose corticosteroids or radiation therapy): May result in an inadequate response to immunization.
Yellow fever vaccine: May reduce antibody titer otherwise expected from yellow fever vaccine. Separate these vaccines by 1 mo.

Lab Test Interferences None well documented.

Adverse Reactions
CNS: Fatigue; weakness; headache; malaise; dizziness.
DERM: Flushing; angioedema.
EENT: Earache; pharyngitis.
GI: Nausea; diarrhea.
RESP: Upper respiratory tract infection.
OTHER: Fever; pain; tenderness; pruritus; induration; erythema; ecchymosis; swelling; warmth or nodule formation at injection site; thrombocytopenia.

Precautions
Pregnancy: Category C. Problems have not been reported and are unlikely. Use if woman is likely to be exposed to hepatitis B virus during or after pregnancy.

Lactation: Undetermined.
Elderly: Hepatitis B immunogenicity may be reduced in patients older than 40 yr.
Hypersensitivity: Anaphylaxis and symptoms of immediate hypersensitivity have occurred within hours of administering vaccine.
Immunosuppressed patients: May require larger doses and may not respond to vaccine.
Infection: Delay use of hepatitis B vaccine in presence of serious active infection except when withholding vaccine entails greater risk.

Multiple sclerosis (MS): Although no casual relationship has been established, rare instances of MS exacerbation have been reported following administration of hepatitis vaccines and other vaccines.
Severely compromised cardiopulmonary status: Administer vaccine with caution.
Unrecognized hepatitis B infection: May be present at time of vaccination and vaccine may not prevent hepatitis B because of long incubation period.

PATIENT CARE CONSIDERATIONS

Administration/Storage
- Shake well before use to maintain suspension of the vaccine.
- Administer IM in deltoid muscle in adults. In infants and young children administer IM in anterolateral thigh. Avoid gluteal injection into buttock, which may result in less than optimal immune response.
- May administer vaccine SC in patients who are at risk of hemorrhage following IM injection (eg, people with hemophilia or thalassemia). However, SC route may produce less than optimal response and may lead to increased incidence of local reactions.
- Always record manufacturer's name and vaccine lot number in patient's permanent record file along with date of administration, name, and title of person administering vaccine.
- Have epinephrine 1:1000 available in case of laryngospasms.
- Use vaccine as supplied. No dilution or reconstitution is necessary. Note that vaccine is slightly opaque, white suspension.
- Refrigerate vials. Do not freeze. Freezing destroys potency.

Assessment/Interventions
- Obtain complete history, including drug history and any known allergies.
- Review patient's medical history for history of serious adverse reactions to previous dose of hepatitis B vaccine.
- Check patient's immunization history to verify that administration regimen is being followed.
- Consider delaying immunization during course of serious active infection.
- Monitor for hypersensitivity or anaphylaxis. Always have epinephrine available to counteract any possible reactions.

Patient/Family Education
- Instruct patient or parent to complete the series of injections for vaccine to be effective.
- Provide patient or parent with immunization history record and record of this immunization in patient's medical records.
- Instruct patient or parent to use antipyretics for fever or analgesics (eg, acetaminophen) for local pain.
- Inform patient or parent of immunization schedule.

Hetastarch (Hydroxyethyl Starch; HES)

(HET-uh-starch)

Class Plasma expander

How Supplied
Hespan Injection 6 g per 100 mL in 0.9% sodium chloride

Action
PHARMACOLOGY: Produces expansion of plasma volume. Does not have oxygen-carrying capacity or contain plasma protein, so it is not blood or plasma substitute.

PHARMACOKINETICS/DYNAMICS:
Excretion: Hetastarch is eliminated renally, and the mean t½ is 17 days.

Indications Adjunct therapy for plasma volume expansion in shock caused by hemorrhage, burns, surgery, sepsis, or other trauma; adjunct in leukapheresis to improve harvesting and increase yield of granulocytes.

Contraindications Severe bleeding disorders; severe cardiac failure; renal failure with oliguria or anuria.

Route/Dosage
Plasma Volume Expansion
ADULTS: IV 500 to 1000 mL/day; dosage does not usually exceed 1500 mL/day.

Leukapheresis
ADULTS: IV 250 to 700 mL.

Interactions None well documented.

Lab Test Interferences May alter coagulation and result in transient prolongation of prothrombin time (PT), partial thromboplastin time (PTT), bleeding and clotting times, decreased Hct and excessive plasma protein dilution; increases indirect bilirubin concentrations.

Adverse Reactions
CNS: Headache.
DERM: Itching.
EENT: Submaxillary and parotid glandular enlargement.
GI: Vomiting.
OTHER: Anaphylactoid reactions (eg, periorbital edema, urticaria, wheezing, mild temperature elevation); chills; mild influenza-like symptoms; muscle pain; peripheral edema of lower extremities.

Precautions
Pregnancy: Category C.
Lactation: Undetermined.
Children: No data available.
Hypersensitivity: May cause anaphylactoid reactions.
Special risk patients: Caused by possibility of circulatory overload, take special care when administering to patients with renal impairment, at risk of pulmonary edema, or with CHF.

PATIENT CARE CONSIDERATIONS

Administration/Storage
- Administer by IV infusion only.
- Store at room temperature.
- Do not use if solution is turbid deep brown or if crystalline precipitate forms.

Assessment/Interventions
- Obtain complete history, including drug history and any known allergies.
- Assess for bleeding disorders and severe cardiac failure with oliguria or anuria.
- Take baseline vital signs and hematologic parameters before administration of drug.
- Check vital signs q 5 min for first 30 min following administration.
- Monitor urinary output. If output does not increase, report to health care provider.
- Monitor CVP during infusion to assess for circulatory overload (eg, elevated CVP, rales/crackles, shortness of breath during and after administration).
- Report prolonged PT, PTT, bleeding and clotting times, decreased Hct, and decreased plasma proteins to health care provider.
- Report anaphylactoid reactions (eg, periorbital edema, urticaria, wheezing, fever), chills, muscle pain, peripheral edema to health care provider.
- During leukapheresis, monitor CBC, differential WBC count, Hgb, Hct, PT, and PTT.

Patient/Family Education
- Instruct patient to report these symptoms to health care provider: itching, dyspnea, chills, myalgia, headache, vomiting, glandular enlargement.

Hyaluronic Acid Derivatives

(high-uhl-yur-AHN-ick acid derivatives)
Class Physical adjunct

How Supplied
Hyalgan Solution 20 mg sodium hyaluronate per 2 mL ◆ Restylane Gel for injection 20 mg/mL ◆ Supartz Solution 25 mg sodium hyaluronate per 2.5 mL ◆ Synvisc Solution 16 mg hylan polymers (hylan G-F 20) per 2 mL

Action
PHARMACOLOGY: Improves elasticity and viscosity of synovial fluid.

Indications Treatment of pain of osteoarthritis of the knee. Mid to deep dermal implantation for correction of moderate to severe facial wrinkles and folds, such as nasolabial folds (Restylane).

Contraindications Infections or skin diseases in the area of the injection site; concomitant skin disinfectants containing quaternary ammonium salts; hypersensitivity to any component of the product. Severe allergies manifested by a history of anaphylaxis or history or presence of multiple allergies (Restylane); history of allergies to gram-positive bacterial proteins (Restylane); use in breast augmentation and for implantation into bone, tendon, ligament, or muscle (Restylane); implantation into blood or dermal vessels (Restylane).

Route/Dosage
HYALGAN; SUPARTZ
ADULTS: **Intra-articular** Give a total of 5 injections/treatment cycle (2 mL for Hyalgan and 2.5 mL for Supartz) at weekly intervals.

RESTYLANE
Correction of Severe Facial Wrinkles and Dermal Folds
ADULTS: **Dermal Implantation** Limit to 1.5 mL per treatment site.

SYNVISC
ADULTS: **Intra-articular** Give a total of 3 injections/treatment cycle (2 mL) at weekly intervals.

Interactions None well documented.

Adverse Reactions

CV:
Synvisc – Tachyrhythmia; phlebitis with varicosities.

CNS:
Hyalgan – Headache (18%).
Restylane – Depression; aggravated depression; headache.
Supartz – Headache (4%); dizziness (1% to 4%).
Synvisc – Headache, dizziness, chills, paresthesia, malaise (postmarketing).

DERM:
Restylane – Swelling (87%); redness (85%); bruising (52%); itching (30%); acne, contact dermatitis.
Synvisc – Rash on thorax and back, pruritus (2%); rash, itching hives (postmarketing).

EENT:
Restylane – Sinusitis.
Supartz – Sinusitis, rhinitis (1% to 4%).

GI:
Hyalgan – GI complaints (29%, severe in 2%).
Restylane – Tooth pain.
Supartz – Abdominal pain, diarrhea, dyspepsia, nausea (1% to 4%).
Synvisc – Nausea (postmarketing).

GU:
Restylane – Urinary incontinence.
Supartz – UTI (1% to 4%).

HEMA:
Restylane – Hypercholesterolemia.
Synvisc – Thrombocytopenia (postmarketing).

LOCAL:
Hyalgan – Injection site pain (23%); skin reaction (including ecchymosis and rash [14%]); joint pain, swelling (13%, severe in 1%); pruritus (7%); positive bacterial cultures of aspirated effusion for the treated knee (1%).
Supartz – Injection site reaction (including application/injection site inflammation and purpura [4%]); injection site pain (4%).
Synvisc – Knee pain or swelling (2%).

MUSC:
Restylane – Arthralgia.
Supartz – Arthralgia (18%); arthropathy/arthrosis/arthritis (11%).
Synvisc – Calf cramps; muscle pain; muscle cramps (postmarketing).

RESP:
Restylane – Upper respiratory tract infection; bronchitis; pneumonia.
Supartz – Upper respiratory tract infection, bronchitis (1% to 4%).
Synvisc – Respiratory difficulties (postmarketing).

OTHER:
Hyalgan – Fever, shock (postmarketing).
Restylane – Tenderness (78%); pain (57%); back pain; allergic reactions; osteoporosis; herpes simplex.
Supartz – Back pain, nonspecific pain (6%); flu-like symptoms, inflicted injury, leg pain and discomfort, fall (1% to 4%).
Synvisc – Ankle edema; low back sprain; hemorrhoid problems; fever, peripheral edema, flushing face edema, intra-articular infections (postmarketing).

Precautions

Pregnancy: Safety and efficacy not established.
Lactation: Undetermined.
Children: Safety and efficacy not established.
Hypersensitivity: Anaphylactoid reactions may occur.
Special risk patients: Use with caution in patients receiving immunosuppressive therapy; patients taking aspirin or NSAIDs may be at increased risk for bruising and bleeding (Restylane); use with caution in patients allergic to avian proteins, feathers, and egg products and when there is evidence of lymphatic or venous stasis in the leg (Synvisc).
Infection/inflammatory process: Defer treatment until inflammatory process or infection has been controlled; implantation carries risk of infection (Restylane).
Inflammatory arthritis: Transient increases in inflammation may occur in the injected knee.
Inflammatory reaction: Risk of inflammatory reaction may be increased if laser treatment, chemical peeling, or active dermal response is considered after Restylane.
Necrosis: Localized superficial necrosis may occur after injection in glabellar area (Restylane).
Quaternary ammonium salts: Because precipitation of drug may occur, avoid concomitant use of disinfectants or skin preparations containing quaternary ammonium salts.
Safety and efficacy: Long-term safety and efficacy (beyond 1 yr) has not been established (Restylane).

PATIENT CARE CONSIDERATIONS

Administration/Storage

Hyaluronic Acid Derivatives:
- For intra-articular administration into knee joint only. Not for intradermal, subcutaneous, IM, or IV administration, nor administration into any joint other than the knee.
- Dose is usually administered into affected knee once weekly for duration of treatment cycle. Treatment cycle depends on which product is being used.
- Inject subcutaneous lidocaine or similar local anesthetic prior to intra-articular injection of the hyaluronic acid derivative.
- Do not prepare injection site with skin disin-

fectants containing quaternary ammonium salts; precipitation of drug can occur.
- Do not administer other intra-articular drugs concomitantly.
- The vial/syringe is intended for single use only. Use immediately once package is opened. Discard any unused solution. Do not save unused solution for later administration.

Hyaluronic Acid:
- For mid to deep dermal implantation only. Not for intradermal, subcutaneous, IM, or IV administration, breast augmentation, nor administration into bone, tendon, ligament, or muscle.
- Carefully follow manufacturer's recommendations for assembly of needle to syringe and treatment procedure.
- The syringe is intended for single use only. Use immediately once package is opened. Discard any unused solution. Do not save unused solution for later administration.
- Do not use if contents of syringe show signs of separation and/or appear cloudy.
- Do not mix with other products prior to injection.
- Store *Hyalgan*, *Supartz*, and *Restylane* at controlled room temperature (less than 77°F). Store *Synvisc* at controlled room temperature (less than 86°F). Store in original package. Protect from light and freezing.

Assessment/Interventions

- Obtain patient history, including drug history and any known allergies. Note latex sensitivity and allergy to avian proteins, feathers, or egg products (hyaluronic acid derivatives only); severe allergies manifested by history of anaphylaxis, history or presence of multiple severe allergies, allergy to gram-positive bacterial proteins, susceptibility to keloid formation or hypertrophic scaring, or concomitant use of immunosuppressive therapy or medications that reduce coagulation (hyaluronic acid only).
- Assess injection site prior to administration. Avoid injecting into site with infection, skin disease, or active inflammatory process (eg, cysts, rash).
- Monitor patient for signs and symptoms of anaphylactic or serious allergic reactions. Be prepared to discontinue therapy and treat appropriately.
- Monitor patient for CNS, GI, general body side effects, and injection site reactions. Report to health care provider if noted and significant.

Hyaluronic Acid Derivatives:
- Ensure that joint effusions are removed prior to administering medication.

Patient/Family Education

- Explain name, dosing regimen, action, potential side effects, and expected response to treatment.
- Advise patient that medication will be prepared and administered in a health care setting by a health care provider.
- Advise patient to review *Patient Information* sheet before starting therapy.
- Advise women to notify health care provider if pregnant, planning to become pregnant, or breastfeeding.
- Instruct patient not to take any prescription or OTC medications, dietary supplements, or herbal preparations unless advised by health care provider.
- Remind patient that office visits will be required to monitor therapy and to keep appointments.

Hyaluronic Acid Derivatives:
- Explain importance of completing entire treatment cycle in order to obtain max benefit.
- Advise patient that transient pain and/or swelling of the injected joint may occur and to notify health care provider if this occurs and becomes intolerable or if the injection site becomes red and/or warm.
- Caution patient to avoid strenuous or prolonged (eg, more than 1 hr) weight-bearing activities (eg, jogging, tennis) for 48 hr after treatment.
- Instruct patient to continue taking other arthritis medications prescribed by health care provider.

Hyaluronic Acid:
- Advise patient that if treated area is swollen directly after the injection that an ice pack can be applied on the swollen site for a short period of time.
- Advise patient that mild to moderate injection-site reactions are common and should resolve in a few days but to notify health care provider if injection site reaction does not resolve or worsens.
- Caution patient to avoid exposing treated area to excessive sun and UV lamp and extreme cold weather until any initial swelling and redness have resolved.

Hydralazine Hydrochloride

(high-DRAL-uh-zeen HIGH-droe-KLOR-ide)

Class Antihypertensive/Vasodilator

How Supplied
Apresoline Tablets 25 mg, Tablets 50 mg, Tablets 100 mg, Injection 20 mg/mL
🍁 *Apo-Hydralazine* ♦ *Novo-Hylazin* ♦ *Nu-Hydral*

Action
PHARMACOLOGY: Directly relaxes vascular smooth muscle to cause peripheral vasodilation, decreasing arterial BP and peripheral vascular resistance.

PHARMACOKINETICS/DYNAMICS:

Absorption: Hydralazine is rapidly absorbed. T_{max} is 1 to 2 hr and bioavailability is 30% to 50%.

Distribution: Hydralazine is 87% protein bound.

Metabolism: Hydralazine is subject to polymorphic acetylation and undergoes extensive hepatic metabolism.

Excretion: Hydralazine is excreted in urine mainly in the form of metabolites. The t½ is 3 to 7 hr.

Onset: Onset is 10 to 20 min (parenteral).

Duration: Duration is 6 to 12 hr (oral) and 2 to 4 hr (parenteral).

Special Populations:
Slow acetylators – Slow acetylators generally have higher plasma levels of hydralazine and require lower doses to maintain control of BP.

Indications Treatment of essential hypertension (oral form). Treatment of severe essential hypertension (parenteral form). **Unlabeled use(s):** Reduction of overload in treatment of CHF, severe aortic insufficiency, and after valve replacement.

Contraindications Coronary artery disease; mitral valvular rheumatic heart disease.

Route/Dosage
Adjust individually.
ADULTS: **PO** Begin with 10 mg qid for 2 to 4 days; then 25 mg qid for 3 to 5 days; then 50 mg qid (max, 300 mg/day). **IV/IM** 20 to 40 mg repeated prn.
CHILDREN: **PO** 0.75 mg/kg/day in 4 divided doses initially; increase gradually over 3 to 4 wk to max 7.5 mg/kg/day or 200 mg/day. **IV/IM** 0.1 to 0.2 mg/kg/dose q 4 to 6 hr prn.

Interactions
Beta-blockers: May increase effect of hydralazine or effect of beta-blockers.
NSAIDs: Effects of hydralazine may be decreased.

Lab Test Interferences None well documented.

Adverse Reactions
CV: Palpitations; tachycardia; angina pectoris; edema.
CNS: Headache; peripheral neuritis with paresthesias, numbness and tingling; dizziness; tremors; depression; disorientation; anxiety.
EENT: Lacrimation; conjunctivitis.
GI: Anorexia; nausea; vomiting; diarrhea; constipation.
HEMA: Blood dyscrasias; decreased hemoglobin; decreased RBC; leukopenia; agranulocytosis.
OTHER: Hypersensitivity (eg, rash, urticaria, pruritus, fever, chills, arthralgia, eosinophilia); systemic lupus erythematosus.

Precautions
Pregnancy: Category C.
Lactation: Excreted in breast milk.
Children: Safety and efficacy have not been established by controlled clinical trials, but there is experience with its use.
Renal function impairment: Use drug with caution in patients with advanced renal damage.
Tartrazine sensitivity: Some of these products contain tartrazine, which can cause allergic-type reactions in susceptible individuals, especially those who have aspirin hypersensitivity.
Lupus erythematosus: Drug may produce clinical picture similar to that with systemic lupus erythematosus (eg, arthralgia, dermatoses, fever, splenomegaly), including glomerulonephritis, when more than 50 mg/day is given for long periods. Symptoms usually reverse when drug is discontinued, but treatment may be required.

Overdosage: Signs and Symptoms
Hypotension, tachycardia, headache, flushing, MI, myocardial ischemia, cardiac arrhythmias, profound shock.

PATIENT CARE CONSIDERATIONS

Administration/Storage
- Administer oral form of drug with food.
- Use parenteral form immediately after drawn into syringe.
- Parenteral solution discolors after contact with metal filter.
- Store at room temperature.

Assessment/Interventions
- Obtain complete history, including drug history and any known allergies. Note use of other medications (particularly beta-blockers and NSAIDs), coronary artery disease, mitral

valvular rheumatic heart disease, renal impairment, lupus erythematosus, pregnancy, or lactation.
- Monitor BP prior to and frequently during IV administration.
- Monitor CBC and antinuclear antibody titer.
- Monitor for orthostatic hypotension.
- If decreased hemoglobin or RBC, leukopenia, agranulocytosis, or purpura occur, report to health care provider.
- If symptoms of lupus erythematosus or positive antinuclear antibody titer occur, notify health care provider.
- If hypotension occurs during therapy, caution patient to sit or lie down (with head in low position). Discontinue drug and notify health care provider.

Patient/Family Education
- Instruct patient to take medication with meals to enhance absorption.
- Caution patient to avoid abrupt discontinuation of drug to prevent sudden increase in BP.
- Encourage patient to make lifestyle changes: weight reduction, sodium and alcohol restriction, discontinuance of smoking, regular exercise, behavior modification.
- Advise patient to monitor BP and weight regularly.
- Instruct patient to report sudden weight gain caused by fluid retention.
- Advise patient to follow health care provider's orders for monitoring of CBC and other laboratory values.
- Advise patient to avoid sudden changes in position or very hot baths to avoid orthostatic hypotension.
- Caution patient not to take otc medications without consulting health care provider.
- Instruct patient to report these symptoms to health care provider: prolonged tiredness, muscle or joint pain, chest pain, fever, numbness or tingling of hands or feet, rash.
- Explain that drug may cause drowsiness and to use caution when driving or performing other tasks requiring mental alertness.

Hydrochlorothiazide

(high-droe-klor-oh-THIGH-uh-zide)

Class Thiazide diuretic

How Supplied
Esidrix Tablets 25 mg, Tablets 50 mg ◆ *Ezide* Tablets 50 mg ◆ *Hydro-Par* Tablets 25 mg, Tablets 50 mg ◆ *Hydro-DIURIL* Tablets 25 mg, Tablets 50 mg, Tablets 100 mg ◆ *Microzide* Capsules 12.5 mg ◆ *Oretic* Tablets 25 mg, Tablets 50 mg ✣ *Apo-Hydro* ◆ *Urozide*

Action
PHARMACOLOGY: Enhances excretion of sodium, chloride, and water by interfering with transport of sodium ions across renal tubular epithelium.

PHARMACOKINETICS/DYNAMICS:
Absorption: Bioavailability is 65% to 75%, C_{max} is 70 to 490 ng/mL (dose dependent), and T_{max} is 1 to 5 hr. Food reduces the bioavailability 10% and the C_{max} 20%; increases the T_{max} from 1.6 to 2.9 hr. Plasma concentrations are linearly related to administration doses.
Distribution: Protein binding is 40% to 68% and crosses the placenta, but not the blood brain barrier. It is also excreted in breast milk.
Metabolism: Hydrochlorothiazide is not metabolized.
Excretion: Hydrochlorothiazide is eliminated primarily by renal pathways (as unchanged by the kidneys; 55% to 77% or the administration dose appear in urine with more than 95% of the absorbed dose excreted in urine unchanged). Plasma t½ is 5.6 to 14.8 hr.
Peak: The time to peak effect is about 4 hr.
Duration: Hydrochlorothiazide activity may persist for up to 24 hr.
Special Populations:
Renal Function Impairment – Hydrochlorothiazide plasma concentration is increased and the t½ is prolonged.

Indications Adjunctive therapy for edema associated with CHF, hepatic cirrhosis, renal dysfunction, and corticosteroid and estrogen therapy; treatment of hypertension. **Unlabeled use(s):** Prevention of formation and precurrence of calcium nephrolithiasis; therapy for nephrogenic diabetes insipidus.

Contraindications Hypersensitivity to thiazides, related diuretics, or sulfonamide-derived drugs; anuria; renal decompensation.

Route/Dosage
Edema
ADULTS: **PO** 25 to 100 mg/day. Rarely patients may require 200 mg/day.

Hypertension
ADULTS: **PO** 25 to 50 mg/day as single dose or 2 divided doses.
CHILDREN (2 TO 12 YR): **PO** 37.5 to 100 mg/day in 2 doses.
INFANTS (6 MO TO 2 YR): **PO** 12.5 to 37.5 mg/day in 2 doses.
INFANTS (YOUNGER THAN 6 MO): **PO** Up to 3.3 mg/kg/day in 2 doses.

Interactions
Bile acid sequestrants: May reduce thiazide absorption; give thiazide at least 2 hr before resin.
Diazoxide: May cause hyperglycemia.
Digitalis glycosides: Diuretic-induced hypokalemia and hypomagnesemia may precipitate digitalis-induced arrhythmias.
Lithium: May decrease renal excretion of lithium.
Loop diuretics: Synergistic effects may result in profound diuresis and serious electrolyte abnormalities.
Sulfonylureas, insulin: May decrease hypoglycemic effect of sulfonylureas. May need to increase dosage of sulfonylureas or insulin.

Lab Test Interferences Drug may decrease serum protein-bound iodine levels without signs of thyroid disturbance. May cause diagnostic interference of serum electrolyte levels, blood and urine glucose levels, serum bilirubin levels, and serum uric acid levels. Drug may increase serum magnesium levels in uremic patients. Drug may cause increased concentrations of total serum cholesterol, total triglycerides, and LDL.

Adverse Reactions
CV: Orthostatic hypotension.
CNS: Dizziness; lightheadedness; vertigo; headache; paresthesias; weakness; restlessness; insomnia.
DERM: Purpura; photosensitivity; rash; urticaria; necrotizing angitis, vasculitis, cutaneous vasculitis; alopecia; exfoliative dermatitis; toxic epidermal necrolysis; erythema multiforme; Stevens-Johnson syndrome.
EENT: Blurred vision; xanthopsia (yellow vision).
GI: Anorexia; gastric irritation; nausea; vomiting; abdominal pain or cramping; bloating; diarrhea; constipation; pancreatitis; sialadenitis.
GU: Impotence; reduced libido; interstitial nephritis.
HEMA: Leukopenia; thrombocytopenia; agranulocytosis; aplastic or hypoplastic anemia; hemolytic anemia.
HEPA: Jaundice.
METAB: Hyperglycemia; glycosuria; hyperuricemia; electrolyte imbalance.
RESP: Respiratory distress; pneumonitis; pulmonary edema.
OTHER: Muscle cramp or spasm; fever; anaphylactic reactions.

Precautions
Pregnancy: Category B.
Lactation: Excreted in breast milk.
Children: Safety and efficacy have not been established in controlled clinical studies.
Hypersensitivity: May occur in patients with or without history of allergy or bronchial asthma; cross-sensitivity with sulfonamides may also occur.
Renal function impairment: Drug may precipitate azotemia; use drug with caution.
Hepatic function impairment: Minor alterations of fluid and electrolyte balance may precipitate hepatic coma; use drug with caution.
Lupus erythematosus: Exacerbation or activation may occur.
Postsympathectomy patients: Drug may enhance antihypertensive effects.

Overdosage: Signs and Symptoms
Orthostatic or general hypotension, tachycardia, shock, weakness, syncope, confusion, dizziness, electrolyte abnormalities, potassium deficiency, vomiting, nausea, lethargy, cramps of calf muscles, thirst, polyuria, anuria.

PATIENT CARE CONSIDERATIONS
Administration/Storage
- If drug is administered as single dose, give in morning.
- Administer drug with food or milk to minimize GI irritation.
- Store tablets in tightly closed container at room temperature.

Assessment/Interventions
- Obtain patient history, including drug history and any known allergies. Note hypersensitivity to thiazides, oral antidiabetics, and sulfonamides.
- Weigh patient daily.
- Monitor I&O and check for fluid retention.
- Monitor BP lying and standing.
- Monitor serum potassium, sodium, calcium, magnesium, blood pH, ABGs, and uric acid.
- Monitor renal nonprotein nitrogen, BUN, creatinine, and LFTs (ALT, activated clotting time).
- Monitor blood and urine glucose levels of diabetic patients.
- Observe closely for anaphylaxis (eg, shortness of breath, rash, edema) after first dose.
- Report rising nonprotein nitrogen, BUN, creatinine, or liver enzyme levels to health care provider.
- Report muscle weakness, cramps, nausea, blurred vision, dizziness, and potassium levels less than 3.5 to health care provider.

Patient/Family Education
- Tell patient to take medication early in day with food or milk.
- Instruct patient to monitor weight daily.

- Advise patient to avoid exposure to sunlight and to use sunblock or wear protective clothing to avoid photosensitivity reaction.
- Instruct diabetic patients to report increased levels of blood glucose to health care provider.
- Caution patient to avoid intake of alcoholic beverages.
- Instruct patient not to take OTC medications without health care provider approval.
- Caution patient to rise slowly from lying or sitting position and to lie down if blurred vision or dizziness occurs.
- Tell patient to report these symptoms to health care provider: GI disturbances, decrease in urinary output, jaundice, muscle cramps, weakness, nausea, blurred vision, dizziness.
- Instruct patient to drink 2 to 3 L of fluids daily unless contraindicated by health care provider.
- Advise patient that drug may cause dizziness and blurred vision and to use caution while driving or performing other tasks requiring mental alertness.
- Tell patient that therapeutic effect may require 2 to 3 wk.

Hydrochlorothiazide/Lisinopril

(high-droe-klor-oh-THIGH-uh-zid/lie-SIN-oh-prille)

Class Antihypertensive combination

How Supplied

Prinzide Tablets 10 mg lisinopril/12.5 mg hydrochlorothiazide, Tablets 20 mg lisinopril/12.5 mg hydrochlorothiazide, Tablets 20 mg lisinopril/25 mg hydrochlorothiazide ♦ *Zestoretic* Tablets 10 mg lisinopril/12.5 mg hydrochlorothiazide, Tablets 20 mg lisinopril/12.5 mg hydrochlorothiazide, Tablets 20 mg lisinopril/25 mg hydrochlorothiazide

Action

PHARMACOLOGY: The 2 components have complementary antihypertensive actions. Lisinopril reduces blood pressure by inhibiting angiotensin-converting enzyme (ACE), thus preventing conversion of angiotensin I to angiotensin II, a potent vasoconstrictor. Hydrochlorothiazide produces a diuretic effect by increasing the elimination of sodium and chloride.

Indications Hypertension; combination not indicated for initial treatment of hypertension.

Contraindications History of angioedema related to an ACE inhibitor; anuria; hypersensitivity to other sulfonamide-related drugs.

Route/Dosage

ADULTS: PO Lisinopril 10 to 80 mg; hydrochlorothiazide 6.25 to 50 mg once daily.

Interactions

Alcohol, barbiturates, narcotics: Potentiation of orthostatic hypotension may occur.
Antacids: Lisinopril bioavailability may be decreased. Separate administration times by 2 hr.
Bile acid sequestrants: May reduce thiazide absorption; give thiazide 2 hr before resin.
Capsaicin: Lisinopril-induced cough may be exacerbated.
Diazoxide: Hydrochlorothiazide may have additive effects; hyperglycemia.
Digitalis glycosides: Hydrochlorothiazide-induced hypokalemia and hypomagnesemia may precipitate digitalis-induced arrhythmias.
Indomethacin: Reduced hypotensive effects, especially in low-renin or volume-dependent hypertensive patients.
Lithium: Hydrochlorothiazide may decrease renal excretion of lithium, increasing blood levels. Lisinopril may increase lithium levels and induce symptoms of lithium toxicity.
Loop diuretics: Synergistic effects with hydrochlorothiazide may result in profound diuresis and serious electrolyte abnormalities.
Potassium-sparing diuretics, potassium preparations: Lisinopril may increase serum potassium levels.
Skeletal muscle relaxants, depolarizing: May increase responsiveness to muscle relaxant.
Sulfonylureas, insulin: Hydrochlorothiazide may decrease hypoglycemic effect of sulfonylureas. May need to increase dosage of sulfonylureas or insulin.

Lab Test Interferences None well documented.

Adverse Reactions

CV: Orthostatic hypotension; chest pain; hypotension; angina.
CNS: Dizziness; lightheadedness; vertigo; headache; paresthesias; asthenia; weakness; restlessness; insomnia; dizziness; fatigue; depression.
DERM: Purpura; photosensitivity; rash; pruritus; urticaria; necrotizing angiitis; vasculitis; cutaneous vasculitis; alopecia; exfoliative dermatitis; toxic epidermal necrolysis; erythema multiforme; Stevens-Johnson syndrome.
EENT: Blurred vision; yellow vision.
GI: Anorexia; gastric irritation; nausea; vomiting; abdominal pain; bloating; diarrhea; constipation; pancreatitis; sialadenitis; dyspepsia.
GU: Impotence; reduced libido; interstitial nephritis.
HEMA: Leukopenia; thrombocytopenia; agranulocytosis; aplastic or hypoplastic anemia;

hemolytic anemia; decreases in hemoglobin and hematocrit; neutropenia; bone marrow depression; eosinophilia.
METAB: Hyperglycemia; glycosuria; hyperuricemia; electrolyte imbalance; hyperkalemia.
RESP: Respiratory distress; pneumonitis; pulmonary edema; cough (especially in females); upper respiratory symptoms; dyspnea.
OTHER: Muscle cramps or myalgia; fever; jaundice; angioedema; anaphylactic reactions.

Precautions
Pregnancy: Category C (first trimester), Category D (second and third trimesters). ACE inhibitors can cause fetal and neonatal morbidity and death when administered during pregnancy.
Lactation: Thiazides are secreted into breast milk. Avoid using in nursing women if possible.
Children: Safety and efficacy not established.
Elderly: May have higher blood levels and AUC than younger patients. Use caution when making dosage adjustments.
Renal function impairment: May need to reduce dose or discontinue diuretic. Loop diuretics are preferred to thiazides in some renal impairment.
Angioedema: Use with extreme caution in patients with history of angioedema.
Hypotension/First-dose effect: Significant decreases in blood pressure may occur after the first dose, especially in severely salt- or volume-depleted patients or those with heart failure. Minimize risk by discontinuing diuretics (switching to a single-entity antihypertensive), decreasing dose, or increasing salt intake prior to initiation of lisinopril.
Leukopenia/Neutropenia/Agranulocytosis: Risk is greater in patients with renal dysfunction, heart failure, immunosuppression, or collagen vascular disease.

Hydrochlorothiazide/Triamterene (HCTZ/Triamterene)

(high-droe-klor-oh-THIGH-uh-zide/try-AM-tur-een)

Class Diuretic combination

How Supplied
Maxzide-25MG Tablets 37.5 mg triamterene/25 mg hydrochlorothiazide ♦ *Dyazide* Capsules 37.5 mg triamterene/25 mg hydrochlorothiazide ♦ *Maxzide* Tablets 75 mg triamterene/50 mg hydrochlorothiazide
❀ *Apo-Triazide* ♦ *Novo-Triamzide* ♦ *Nu-Triazide*

Action
PHARMACOLOGY: Hydrochlorothiazide inhibits reabsorption of sodium and chloride in ascending loop of Henle and early distal tubules. Triamterene interferes with sodium reabsorption at distal tubule. Combination provides additive diuretic activity and antihypertensive effects and minimizes potassium depletion.

Indications Treatment of edema or hypertension in patients who have or are at risk of developing hypokalemia.

Contraindications Anuria; renal decompensation; severe hepatic disease; hypersensitivity to thiazides, triamterene, or sulfonamide-derived drugs; patients receiving spironolactone, amiloride, or potassium supplements; hyperkalemia; metabolic or respiratory acidosis.

Route/Dosage
ADULTS: PO 1 to 2 tablets or capsules daily.

Interactions
Angiotensin-converting enzyme inhibitors: May result in severely elevated serum potassium levels.
Allopurinol: May increase incidence of hypersensitivity reactions to allopurinol.
Amantadine: May increase amantadine plasma levels and risk for adverse effects.
Anticoagulants: May diminish anticoagulant effects.
Bile acid sequestrants: May reduce thiazide absorption; give thiazide at least 2 hr before sequestrant.
Diazoxide: May cause hyperglycemia.
Digitalis glycosides: Diuretic-induced hypokalemia and hypomagnesemia may precipitate digitalis-induced arrhythmias.
Indomethacin: May cause rapid progression into acute renal failure.
Lithium: May decrease renal excretion of lithium; monitor lithium levels.
Loop diuretics: May cause synergistic effects that may result in profound diuresis and serious electrolyte abnormalities.
Methenamines, NSAIDS: May decrease effectiveness of thiazide.
Potassium preparations: May severely increase serum potassium levels, possibly resulting in cardiac arrhythmias or cardiac arrest. Monitor serum potassium closely if potassium is coadministered.
Sulfonylureas, insulin: May decrease hypoglycemic effect of sulfonylureas. May need to adjust dosage of sulfonylureas or insulin.

Lab Test Interferences May interfere with the fluorescent measurement of quinidine serum levels. May decrease serum protein-bound iodine levels without signs of thyroid disturbance.

Adverse Reactions
CV: Orthostatic hypotension.

CNS: Dizziness; lightheadedness; vertigo; headache; paresthesias; weakness; restlessness; insomnia; fatigue.
DERM: Purpura; photosensitivity; rash; urticaria; necrotizing angitis, vasculitis, cutaneous vasculitis; alopecia; exfoliative dermatitis; toxic epidermal necrolysis; erythema multiforme; Stevens-Johnson syndrome.
EENT: Blurred vision; xanthopsia (yellow vision).
GI: Anorexia; gastric irritation; nausea; vomiting; abdominal pain or cramping; bloating; diarrhea; constipation; pancreatitis; sialadenitis; dry mouth.
GU: Impotence; reduced libido; interstitial nephritis; azotemia; elevated BUN and creatinine.
HEMA: Leukopenia; thrombocytopenia; agranulocytosis; aplastic or hypoplastic anemia; hemolytic anemia; megaloblastic anemia.
HEPA: Jaundice; liver enzyme abnormalities.
METAB: Hyperglycemia; glycosuria; hyperuricemia; hyperkalemia; electrolyte imbalance; hypochloremia; hyponatremia.
OTHER: Muscle cramp or spasm; fever; anaphylactic reactions.

Precautions

Pregnancy: Category C.
Lactation: Excreted in breast milk.
Children: Safety and efficacy have not been established.

Hypersensitivity: May occur in patients with or without history of allergy or bronchial asthma; cross-sensitivity with sulfonamides may also occur.
Renal function impairment: May precipitate azotemia or hypermagnesemia; use drug with caution.
Hepatic function impairment: Minor alterations of fluid and electrolyte balance may precipitate hepatic coma; use drug with caution.
Electrolyte imbalances and BUN increase: Hyperkalemia (serum potassium less than 5.5 mEq/L), hyponatremia, hypochloremia, and increases in BUN may occur.
Hematologic effects: Triamterene is a weak folic acid antagonist and may contribute to megaloblastosis.
Lipids: May affect total serum cholesterol, total triglycerides, and LDL in some patients.
Postsympathectomy: Antihypertensive effects may be enhanced.
Renal stones: Triamterene has been found in renal stones; use drug with caution in patients with histories of stone formation.

Overdosage: Signs and Symptoms

Orthostatic or general hypotension, tachycardia, syncope, electrolyte abnormalities, potassium deficiency, vomiting, nausea, shock, weakness, confusion, dizziness, cramps of calf muscles, thirst, polyuria, anuria, lethargy.

PATIENT CARE CONSIDERATIONS

Administration/Storage

- Administer as morning dose.
- Give with food or milk.
- Administer every other day to decrease electrolyte imbalance.
- Store in tightly closed container at room temperature.

Assessment/Interventions

- Obtain patient history, including drug history and any known allergies.
- Weigh patient daily.
- Measure I&O.
- Monitor patient's BP with patient lying down and standing.
- Monitor serum potassium, calcium, magnesium, sodium, ABGs, and uric acid.
- Monitor renal (eg, nonprotein nitrogen, BUN, creatinine) and LFTs (eg, ALT, AST).
- Monitor blood glucose levels in diabetic patients.
- Observe closely for anaphylaxis (eg, shortness of breath, rash, edema) after first dose.
- Report muscle weakness, cramps, nausea, blurred vision, or dizziness to health care provider.

Patient/Family Education

- Instruct patient to take medication early in day to avoid diuretic effect at night.
- Tell patient to take drug with food or milk and to report GI symptoms.
- Advise patient to limit sodium intake for optimal drug effect.
- Advise patient to limit exposure to sun and to use sunscreen or wear protective clothing to avoid photosensitivity reaction.
- Instruct diabetic patients to report increased levels of blood glucose.
- Caution patient to avoid sudden position changes to prevent orthostatic hypotension.
- Tell patient to report these symptoms to health care provider: decrease in urinary output, jaundice, muscle cramps, weakness, nausea, blurred vision, dizziness.
- Instruct patient to drink 2 to 3 L/day of water unless contraindicated.
- Advise patient that drug may cause drowsiness and to use caution while driving or performing other tasks requiring mental alertness.

Hydrocodone Bitartrate/Acetaminophen

(HIGH-droe-KOE-dohn by-TAR-trate/ass-eet-ah-MEE-noe-fen)

Class Narcotic analgesic

How Supplied

Anexsia 5/500 Tablets 5 mg hydrocodone bitartrate/500 mg acetaminophen ♦ *Anexsia 7.5/650* Tablets 7.5 mg hydrocodone bitartrate/650 mg acetaminophen ♦ *Anexsia 10/660* Tablets 10 mg hydrocodone bitartrate/660 acetaminophen ♦ *Bancap-HC* Capsules 5 mg hydrocodone bitartrate/500 mg acetaminophen ♦ *Ceta-Plus* Capsules 5 mg hydrocodone bitartrate/500 mg acetaminophen ♦ *Co-Gesic* Capsules 5 mg hydrocodone bitartrate/500 mg acetaminophen ♦ *Duocet* Tablets 5 mg hydrocodone bitartrate/500 mg acetaminophen ♦ *Dolacet* Capsules 5 mg hydrocodone bitartrate/500 mg acetaminophen ♦ *Duradyne DHC* Tablets 5 mg hydrocodone bitartrate/500 mg acetaminophen ♦ *Hydrocet* Capsules 5 mg hydrocodone bitartrate/500 mg acetaminophen ♦ *Hydrogesic* Capsules 5 mg hydrocodone bitartrate/500 mg acetaminophen ♦ *Hy-Phen* Tablets 5 mg hydrocodone bitartrate/500 mg acetaminophen ♦ *Lorcet 10/650* Tablets 10 mg hydrocodone bitartrate/650 mg acetaminophen ♦ *Lorcet-HD* Capsules 5 mg hydrocodone bitartrate/500 mg acetaminophen ♦ *Lorcet Plus* Tablets 7.5 mg hydrocodone bitartrate/650 mg acetaminophen ♦ *Lortab 5/500* Tablets 5 mg hydrocodone bitartrate/500 mg acetaminophen ♦ *Lortab 7.5/500* Tablets 7.5 mg hydrocodone bitartrate/500 mg acetaminophen ♦ *Lortab 10/500* Tablets 10 mg hydrocodone bitartrate/500 mg acetaminophen ♦ *Margesic H* Tablets 5 mg hydrocodone bitartrate/500 mg acetaminophen ♦ *Norco* Tablets 10 mg hydrocodone bitartrate/325 mg acetaminophen ♦ *Panacet 5/500* Tablets 5 mg hydrocodone bitartrate/500 mg acetaminophen ♦ *Stagesic* Capsules 5 mg hydrocodone bitartrate/500 mg acetaminophen ♦ *T-Gesic* Capsules 5 mg hydrocodone bitartrate/500 mg acetaminophen ♦ *Vicodin* Tablets 5 mg hydrocodone bitartrate/500 mg acetaminophen ♦ *Vicodin ES* Tablets 7.5 mg hydrocodone bitartrate/750 mg acetaminophen ♦ *Vicodin HP* Tablets 10 mg hydrocodone bitartrate/660 mg acetaminophen ♦ *Zydone* Tablets 7.5 mg hydrocodone bitartrate/400 mg acetaminophen, Tablets 10 mg hydrocodone bitartrate/400 mg acetaminophen

Action

PHARMACOLOGY: Inhibits synthesis of prostaglandins and binds to opiate receptors in CNS and peripherally blocks pain impulse generation; produces antipyresis by direct action on hypothalamic heat-regulating center; causes cough suppression by direct central action in medulla; may produce generalized CNS depression.

Indications Management of mild to moderate pain.

Contraindications Hypersensitivity to acetaminophen, hydrocodone, or similar compounds.

Route/Dosage

Varies according to product and strength.
ADULTS: **PO** 1 to 2 tablets or capsules (hydrocodone 2.5 to 10 mg; acetaminophen 500 to 1000 mg) q 4 to 6 hr or 5 to 10 mL (elixir, 15 mL) q 4 to 6 hr prn.
CHILDREN (YOUNGER THAN 12 YR): **PO** 10 to 15 mg acetaminophen/kg/dose q 4 hr to max 2.6 g/24 hr.

Interactions

Anticholinergics: May produce paralytic ileus.
Carbamazepine, hydantoins, sulfinpyrazone: May result in increased risk of hepatotoxicity from acetaminophen.
CNS depressants (eg, barbiturates, ethyl alcohol, other narcotics): May cause CNS toxicity.
MAO inhibitors: May cause additive CNS toxicity; may cause decreased BP.
Tricyclic antidepressants, phenzothiazines: May cause additive CNS toxicity.

Lab Test Interferences With *Chemstrip bG, Dextrostix,* and *Visidex II* home blood glucose systems, may cause false decrease in mean glucose values. May give false-positive urinary 5-hydroxyindoleacetic acid test. Amylase or lipase may be increased for 24 hr because of narcotic-induced increase in biliary tract pressure.

Adverse Reactions

CV: Hypotension; bradycardia.
CNS: Lightheadedness; dizziness; sedation; drowsiness; weakness; anxiety; fear; fatigue; dysphoria; psychological dependence; confusion.
GI: Nausea; vomiting; constipation.
GU: Decreased urination; urethral spasm.
RESP: Dyspnea; respiratory depression; irregular breathing.

Precautions

Pregnancy: Category C.
Lactation: Excreted in breast milk.
Children: Safety and effectiveness in children have not been established.
Hepatic function impairment: Chronic alcoholics should limit acetaminophen intake to less than 2 g/day.
Special risk patients: Closely monitor elderly, debilitated patients, and those with conditions accompanied by hypoxia or hypercapnia to avoid decrease in pulmonary ventilation. Also

use caution in patients sensitive to CNS depressants. Because of cough suppressant effects, exercise caution when using postoperatively or in patients with pulmonary disease.
Sulfite sensitivity: Use caution in sulfite-sensitive individuals; some commercial preparations contain sodium bisulfite.

PATIENT CARE CONSIDERATIONS
Administration/Storage
- Administer before pain becomes severe.
- Give medication with food.
- Store at room temperature and protect from light.

Assessment/Interventions
- Obtain complete patient history, including drug history and any known allergies.
- Assess vital signs before and periodically after administration. If hypotension, bradycardia, bradypnea, or difficulty in breathing occurs, notify health care provider.
- Monitor for orthostatic hypotension and supervise ambulation.
- Encourage coughing and deep breathing in patients with pulmonary problems.
- Monitor bowel and hepatic function. If decreased bowel sounds or abdominal distention, jaundice, or dark urine occurs, notify health care provider.
- If confusion or blurred vision occur, institute safety measures and notify health care provider.
- Check for reduced dosage if another CNS depressant medication is being administered concurrently.

Overdosage: Signs and Symptoms
Blood dyscrasias, respiratory depression, and hepatic necrosis (all may occur up to several days after overdose); renal tubular necrosis, hypoglycemic coma, nausea, vomiting, diaphoresis, malaise, somnolence, skeletal muscle flaccidity, bradycardia, hypotension, apnea, cardiac arrest.

Patient/Family Education
- Instruct patient to take before pain becomes severe.
- Advise patient to take with food or milk.
- When medication is being used for acute pain, advise patient of possible addiction and explain that drug should be used for short term only.
- Advise patient to change position slowly and to use caution when ambulating and performing other activities requiring mental alertness such as driving or operating machinery.
- Instruct patient to eat high-fiber diet, maintain adequate fluid intake, and use stool softener or bulk laxative to prevent constipation.
- Advise patient to avoid alcohol and any other drug that causes drowsiness such as sleeping aids and antihistamines.
- Instruct patient to discontinue drug and notify health care provider if blurred vision, rash, or yellowing of skin occurs.
- If lightheadedness, dizziness, drowsiness, nausea, or vomiting occur, advise patient to lie down until symptoms subside and to notify health care provider if symptoms persist.

Hydrocodone Bitartrate/ Chlorpheniramine Maleate

(HIGH-droe-KOE-dohn by-TAR-trate/klor-fen-AIR-uh-meen MAL-ee-ate)

Class Antitussive/Narcotic analgesic/Antihistamine

How Supplied
S-T Forte 2 Liquid 2.5 mg hydrocodone bitartrate and 2 mg chlorpheniramine maleate

Action
PHARMACOLOGY:
Hydrocodone: Suppresses cough reflex; stimulates opiate receptors in the CNS and peripherally blocks pain impulse generation.
Chlorpheniramine: Competitively antagonizes histamine at H_1 receptor sites.

Indications Provides relief of cough and rhinorrhea; symptomatic relief of stubborn cough and runny nose caused by cold or allergy.

Contraindications Hypersensitivity to any component of product.

Route/Dosage
ADULTS: PO 1 tsp (5 mL) tid or qid (max, 4 tsp [20 mL] in any 24 hr).
CHILDREN 6 TO 12 YR: PO ½ tsp (2.5 mL).
CHILDREN 1 TO 3 YR: PO 20 drops.
CHILDREN 6 MO TO 1 YR: PO 10 drops.

Interactions
Alcohol, CNS depressants, narcotic analgesics, phenothiazines or other tranquilizers, sedative-hypnotics: Increased CNS depression (eg, drowsiness) may occur.

Lab Test Interferences May interfere with diagnostic test results for skin tests using allergen extracts.

Adverse Reactions
CNS: Drowsiness.

GI: Nausea.

Precautions

Pregnancy: Consult health care provider before use.
Lactation: Consult health care provider before use.
Special risk patients: Use with caution in patients with hypertension, arteriosclerosis, or hyperthyroidism.

Hydrocodone: Excreted in breast milk.
Dependence: Hydrocodone has abuse potential; may be habit forming.

Overdosage: Signs and Symptoms

Respiratory and CNS depression, circulatory collapse, cardiopulmonary arrest, decreased mental alertness, ataxia, hallucinations, convulsions, death.

PATIENT CARE CONSIDERATIONS

Administration/Storage

- Give prescribed dose q 6 hr as needed, up to 4 doses/day.
- Give with food or milk if GI upset occurs.
- Use dosing spoon or syringe for pediatric doses.
- Store syrup at controlled room temperature (59° to 86°F). Keep tightly capped.

Assessment/Interventions

- Obtain patient history, including drug history and any known allergies. Note history of hypertension, hyperthyroidism, prostatic hypertrophy, narrow angle glaucoma, urinary retention, or coronary artery disease.
- Assess for allergy symptoms (eg, cough, rhinitis, nasal congestion, sneezing, itching, watery eyes) before and periodically throughout therapy.
- Monitor patient for excessive drowsiness or persistent nausea. If noted, hold therapy and notify health care provider.

Patient/Family Education

- Explain name, dose, action, and potential side effects of drug.
- Advise patient to take prescribed dose q 6 hr as needed, up to qid.
- Advise caregiver to use dosing spoon or syringe when giving syrup to children.
- Advise patient to take with food or milk if GI upset occurs.
- Advise patient that if a dose is missed to take as soon as remembered unless it is nearing time for the next dose. Caution patient not to double the dose to catch up.
- Advise patient that if allergy symptoms are not controlled, not to increase the dose of medication but to inform their health care provider.
- Caution patient that drug may cause drowsiness and to use caution while driving or performing other tasks requiring mental alertness until tolerance is determined.
- Advise patient to avoid alcohol and other CNS depressants because of risk of excessive sedation.
- Caution patient not to take any OTC antihistamines or decongestants while taking this medication unless advised by health care provider.
- If patient is to have allergy skin testing, advise not to take the medication for at least 6 days before the skin testing.
- Advise patient to notify health care provider if pregnant, planning to become pregnant, or breastfeeding.
- Instruct patient to stop taking drug and immediately report any of these symptoms to health care provider: persistent nausea or excessive drowsiness.
- Caution patient not to take any prescription or OTC medications, or dietary supplements unless advised by health care provider.

Hydrocodone Bitartrate/ Guaifenesin

(HIGH-droe-KOE-dohn by-TAR-trate/ GWHY-fen-ah-sin)

Class Analgesic/Antitussive/Expectorant

How Supplied

Pneumotussin 2.5 Cough Syrup 2.5 mg hydrocodone bitartrate and 200 mg guaifenesin ♦ *Pneumotussin* Tablets 2.5 mg hydrocodone bitartrate and 300 mg guaifenesin ♦ *Codiclear DH* Syrup 5 mg hydrocodone bitartrate and 100 mg guaifenesin ♦ *Hycosin Expectorant* Syrup 5 mg hydrocodone bitartrate and 100 mg guaifenesin ♦ *Hycotuss Expectorant* Syrup 5 mg hydrocodone bitartrate and 100 mg guaifenesin ♦ *Hydrocodone GF* Syrup 5 mg hydrocodone bitartrate and 100 mg guaifenesin ♦ *Kwelcof* Liquid 5 mg hydrocodone bitartrate and 100 mg guaifenesin ♦ *Vicodin Tuss* Syrup 5 mg hydrocodone bitartrate and 100 mg guaifenesin ♦ *Vitussin* Syrup 5 mg hydrocodone bitartrate and 100 mg guaifenesin

Action

PHARMACOLOGY:

Hydrocodone: Suppresses cough reflex; stimulates opiate receptors in the CNS and peripherally blocks pain impulse generation.
Guaifenesin: May enhance output of respiratory

tract fluid by reducing adhesiveness and surface tension, enhancing removal of viscous mucus, and making nonproductive coughs more productive and less frequent.

Indications Symptomatic relief of irritating nonproductive cough associated with upper and lower respiratory congestion.

Contraindications Hypersensitivity to any component of product; known hypersensitivity to other opioids; patients with increased intraocular pressure; depressed ventilatory function.

Route/Dosage
ADULT: PO 1 tsp (5 mL) after meals and at bedtime, not less than 4 hr apart (max, 6 tsp in 24 hr; max single dose, 3 tsp).
CHILDREN OVER 12 YR: PO Start with 1 tsp (max single dose, 2 tsp).
CHILDREN 6 TO 12 YR: PO Start with ½ tsp (max single dose, 1 tsp).

Interactions
Alcohol, CNS depressants, general anesthetics, other narcotic analgesics, phenothiazines, sedative-hypnotics, tranquilizers: CNS depression may be increased.

Lab Test Interferences Guaifenesin may interfere with the interpretation of the test for urinary 5-hydroxyindoleacetic acid for the diagnosis of carcinoid syndrome.

Adverse Reactions
CV: Hypertension; postural hypotension; palpitations.
CNS: Sedation; drowsiness; mental clouding; lethargy; impairment of mental performance; impairment of physical performance; anxiety; fear; dysphoria; dizziness; psychic dependence; mood change.
EENT: Blurred vision.
GI: Nausea; vomiting.
GU: Urethral spasms; spasm of vesical sphincters; urinary retention.
RESP: Respiratory depression.

Precautions
Pregnancy: Category C.
Lactation: Undetermined.
Children: Not recommended for children under 6 yr.
Dependence: Hydrocodone has abuse potential; may be habit forming.

Overdosage: Signs and Symptoms
Respiratory depression, extreme somnolence progressing to stupor and coma, skeletal muscle flaccidity, cold and clammy skin.

PATIENT CARE CONSIDERATIONS

Administration/Storage
- Give prescribed dose no more often than q 4 hr as needed for cough, not to exceed 6 doses/day.
- Give with food or milk if GI upset occurs.
- Use dosing spoon or syringe for pediatric doses.
- Store syrup at controlled room temperature (59° to 86°F). Keep tightly capped.

Assessment/Interventions
- Obtain patient history, including drug history and any known allergies. Note history of COPD, head trauma, increased intracranial pressure, or intracranial lesions.
- Assess symptoms (eg, cough, sputum viscosity, color, volume) before and periodically throughout therapy.
- Notify health care provider if any of the following occur: persistent or recurrent cough, cough associated with fever, rash, persistent headache, or bothersome side effects.

Patient/Family Education
- Explain name, dose, action, and potential side effects of drug.
- Advise patient to take prescribed dose up to q 4 hr as needed for cough, but to not take more than 6 times/day.
- Advise caregiver to use dosing spoon or syringe when giving liquid to children.
- Advise patient to take with food or milk if GI upset occurs.
- Advise patient that if a dose is missed to take as soon as remembered unless it is nearing time for the next dose. Caution patient not to double the dose to catch up.
- Advise patient that if cough is not controlled not to increase the dose of medication but to inform health care provider.
- Advise patient to inform health care provider if any of the following occur: cough associated with fever, rash, persistent headache, or bothersome side effects.
- Caution patient that drug may cause drowsiness and to use caution while driving or performing other tasks requiring mental alertness until tolerance is determined.
- Advise patient to avoid alcohol and other CNS depressants because of risk of excessive sedation.
- Advise women to notify health care provider if pregnant, planning to become pregnant, or breastfeeding.
- Caution patient to not take any prescription or OTC medications, or dietary supplements unless advised by health care provider.

Hydrocodone Bitartrate/ Homatropine Methylbromide

(HIGH-droe-KOE-dohn by-TAR-trate/hoe-MAT-troe-peen METH-ill-BROE-mide)

Class Analgesic/Antitussive/Anticholinergic

How Supplied
Hycodan Tablets, Syrup 5 mg hydrocodone bitartrate and 1.5 mg homatropine MBr ♦ *Tussigon* Tablets 5 mg hydrocodone bitartrate and 1.5 mg homatropine MBr

Action

PHARMACOLOGY:

Hydrocodone: Suppresses cough reflex; stimulates opiate receptors in the CNS and peripherally blocks pain impulse generation.
Atropine: Inhibits action of acetylcholine or other cholinergic stimuli at postganglionic cholinergic receptors.

Indications Symptomatic relief of cough.

Contraindications Hypersensitivity to any component of product.

Route/Dosage
ADULTS AND CHILDREN (12 YR AND OLDER): PO 1 tablet or 1 tsp (5 mL) of syrup q 4 to 6 hr (max, 6 tablets or 6 Tbsp in 24 hr).
CHILDREN 6 TO 12 YR: PO ½ tablet or ½ Tbsp (2.5 mL) q 4 to 6 hr (max, 3 tablets or 3 Tbsp in 24 hr).

Interactions
Alcohol, antianxiety agents, antihistamines, antipsychotic agents, CNS depressants, narcotics: CNS depressant effects may be increased.
MAO inhibitors, tricyclic antidepressants: Effects of these agents or hydrocodone may be increased.

Lab Test Interferences None well documented.

Adverse Reactions
CNS: Sedation; drowsiness; mental clouding; lethargy; impairment of mental and physical performance; anxiety; fear; dysphoria; dizziness; psychic dependence; mood change.
DERM: Skin rash; pruritus.
GI: Nausea; vomiting; constipation.
GU: Ureteral spasm; spasm of vesicle sphincters; urinary retention.
RESP: Dose-related respiratory depression.

Precautions
Pregnancy: Category C.
Lactation: Undetermined.
Children: Safety and efficacy in children under 6 yr not established.
Special risk patients: Use with caution in elderly or debilitated patients and in those with hepatic or renal dysfunction, hypothyroidism, Addison disease, prostatic hypertrophy or urethral stricture, asthma, and narrow-angle glaucoma.
Acute abdominal conditions: Diagnosis may be obscured.
Dependence: Hydrocodone has abuse potential; may be habit forming.
Head injury or increased intracranial pressure: Diagnosis of adverse reactions may be obscured; respiratory depression properties and capacity to elevate cerebrospinal fluid pressure of hydrocodone may be markedly exaggerated.

Overdosage: Signs and Symptoms
Respiratory depression, extreme somnolence progressing to stupor and coma, skeletal muscle flaccidity, cold and clammy skin, bradycardia, hypotension, apnea, circulatory collapse, cardiac arrest, death.

PATIENT CARE CONSIDERATIONS

Administration/Storage
- Give prescribed dose q 4 to 6 hr as needed for cough, not to exceed 6 doses per 24 hr.
- Give with food or milk if GI upset occurs.
- Use dosing spoon or syringe for pediatric doses of syrup.
- Tablets may be broken in half for pediatric dosing.
- Store tablets and syrup at controlled room temperature (59° to 86°F). Keep syrup tightly capped and protect from freezing.

Assessment/Interventions
- Obtain patient history, including drug history and any known allergies. Note history of head injury, intracranial lesions, increased intracranial pressure, acute abdominal conditions, COPD, hepatic or renal impairment, hypothyroidism, Addison disease, enlarged prostate or urethral stricture, asthma, or narrow angle glaucoma.
- Assess symptoms (eg, cough, sputum viscosity, color, volume) before and periodically throughout therapy.
- Notify health care provider if any of the following occur: persistent or recurrent cough, cough associated with fever, rash, persistent headache, or bothersome side effects.

Patient/Family Education
- Explain name, dose, action, and potential side effects of drug.
- Review dosing schedule for prescribed dose form (ie, syrup or tablet).
- Advise caregiver to use dosing spoon or syringe when giving syrup to children.

- Advise patient to take with food or milk if GI upset occurs.
- Advise patient that if a dose is missed to take as soon as remembered unless it is nearing time for the next dose. Caution patient not to double the dose to catch up.
- Advise patient that if cough is not controlled not to increase the dose of medication but to inform health care provider.
- Advise patient to inform health care provider if any of the following occur: cough associated with fever, rash, persistent headache, or bothersome side effects.
- Caution patient that drug may cause drowsiness and to use caution while driving or performing other tasks requiring mental alertness until tolerance is determined.
- Advise patient to avoid alcohol and other CNS depressants because of risk of excessive sedation.
- Advise women to notify health care provider if pregnant, planning to become pregnant, or breastfeeding.
- Caution patient not to take any prescription or OTC medications, or dietary supplements unless advised by health care provider.

Hydrocodone Bitartrate/Ibuprofen

(HIGH-droe-KOE-dohn by-TAR-trate/eye-BOO-pro-fen)

Class Analgesic/Antitussive/NSAID

How Supplied
Vicoprofen Tablets 7.5 mg hydrocodone bitartrate and 200 mg ibuprofen

Action
PHARMACOLOGY:
Hydrocodone: Suppresses cough reflex; stimulates opiate receptors in the CNS and peripherally blocks pain impulse generation.
Ibuprofen: Decreases inflammation, pain, and fever, probably through inhibition of cyclooxygenase activity and prostaglandin synthesis.

Indications Short-term (generally less than 10 days) management of acute pain. Not indicated for treatment of osteoarthritis or rheumatoid arthritis.

Contraindications Hypersensitivity to hydrocodone, other opioids, ibuprofen, or other NSAIDs; patients who have experienced asthma, urticaria, or allergic-type reactions after taking aspirin or other NSAIDs.

Route/Dosage
ADULTS AND CHILDREN (16 YR AND OLDER): PO 1 tablet q 4 to 6 hr (max, 5 tablets/24 hr period).

Interactions
ACE inhibitors (eg, Captopril): Antihypertensive effect may be decreased by ibuprofen.
Antianxiety agents, antihistamines, antipsychotic, CNS depressants (including alcohol), opioids: Possible additive CNS depression.
Anticholinergics: Increased risk of paralytic ileus.
Antidepressants (eg, MAO inhibitors, tricyclic antidepressants): The effect of either the antidepressant or hydrocodone may be increased.
Aspirin: Increased risk of side effects with coadministration of ibuprofen.
Lithium, methotrexate: Plasma levels may be increased by ibuprofen.
Loop diuretics (eg, furosemide), thiazide diuretics (eg, Chlorothiazide): Diuretic effects may be decreased by ibuprofen.
Warfarin: Risk of gastric erosion and bleeding may be increased.

Lab Test Interferences None well documented.

Adverse Reactions
CV:
Less than 3% – Palpitations, vasodilation.
Less than 1% – Arrhythmia, hypotension, tachycardia.
CNS: Headache (27%); somnolence (22%); dizziness (14%).
3 to 9% – Anxiety, insomnia, nervousness, paresthesia.
Less than 3% – Confusion, hypertonia, thinking abnormalities.
DERM:
3 to 9% – Pruritus, sweating.
EENT:
Less than 3% – Pharyngitis, rhinitis, tinnitus.
GI: Constipation (22%); nausea (21%); dyspepsia (12%).
3 to 9% – Diarrhea, dry mouth, flatulence, vomiting.
Less than 3% – Anorexia, gastritis, melena, mouth ulcer, thirst.
GU: Urinary frequency (less than 3%).
METAB: Edema (3 to 9%); liver enzyme elevation (less than 1%).
MUSC:
Less than 1% – Arthralgia, myalgia.
RESP:
Less than 3% – Dyspnea, hiccups.
Less than 1% – Pulmonary congestion, pneumonia.
OTHER:
3 to 9% – Abdominal pain, asthenia, infection.
Less than 3% – Fever, flu-like symptoms, pain. Allergic reaction (less than 1%).

Precautions

Pregnancy: Category C.
Lactation: Undetermined.
Children: Safety and efficacy in children below 16 yr not established.
Elderly: Use with caution because of possible increased sensitivity to renal and GI effects of ibuprofen, as well as increased respiratory depression with hydrocodone.
Renal function impairment: Use with caution and monitor kidney function in patients with advanced kidney disease.
Hepatic function impairment: As with other NSAIDs, ibuprofen has been reported to cause borderline elevations of one or more liver enzymes; this may occur in up to 15% of patients.
Special risk patients: Use with caution in elderly or debilitated patients and in those with hepatic or renal dysfunction, hypothyroidism, Addison disease, prostatic hypertrophy, or urethral stricture.
Acute abdominal conditions: Diagnosis may be obscured.
Aseptic meningitis: Aseptic meningitis with fever and coma has been observed on rare occasions in patients on ibuprofen therapy. If signs or symptoms of meningitis develop in a patient on Vicoprofen, the possibility of its being related to ibuprofen should be considered.
Cough reflex: Hydrocodone suppresses the cough reflex; as with opioids, caution should be exercised when Vicoprofen is used postoperatively and in patients with pulmonary disease.
Dependence: Hydrocodone has abuse potential; may be habit forming and cause physical dependence.
Effect on diagnostic signs: The antipyretic and anti-inflammatory activity of ibuprofen may reduce fever and inflammation, thus diminishing their utility as diagnostic signs in detecting complications of presumed noninfectious, noninflammatory painful conditions.
Fluid retention and edema: May occur, therefore, use with caution in patients with a history of cardiac decompensation, hypertension, or heart failure.
GI effects: Serious GI toxicity (eg, bleeding, ulceration, perforation) can occur at any time, with or without warning symptoms.
Head injury or increased intracranial pressure: Diagnosis of adverse reactions may be obscured; respiratory depression properties and capacity to elevate CSF pressure of hydrocodone may be markedly exaggerated.
Hematological effects: Ibuprofen, like other NSAIDs, can inhibit platelet aggregation but the effect is quantitatively less and of shorter duration than that seen with aspirin. Because this prolonged bleeding effect may be exaggerated in patients with underlying hemostatic defects, Vicoprofen should be used with caution in persons with intrinsic coagulation defects and those on anticoagulant therapy.
Preexisting asthma: Patients with asthma may have aspirin-sensitive asthma. The use of aspirin in patients with aspirin-sensitive asthma has been associated with severe bronchospasm, which may be fatal. Because cross-reactivity between aspirin and other NSAIDs has been reported in such aspirin-sensitive patients, Vicoprofen should not be administered to patients with this form of aspirin sensitivity and should be used with caution in patients with preexisting asthma.

Overdosage: Signs and Symptoms

Hydrocodone: Respiratory depression, extreme somnolence progressing to stupor or coma, skeletal muscle flaccidity, cold and clammy skin, bradycardia, hypotension, apnea, circulatory collapse, cardiac arrest, death.
Ibuprofen: GI irritation with erosion, hemorrhage or perforation, kidney, liver and heart damage, hemolytic anemia, meningitis, headache, dizziness, tinnitus, confusion, blurred vision, mental disturbances, skin rash, stomatitis, edema, reduced retinal sensitivity, corneal deposits, hyperkalemia.

PATIENT CARE CONSIDERATIONS

Administration/Storage

- Administer 1 tablet as prescribed q 4 to 6 hr if needed for pain.
- Do not exceed 5 tablets in 24 hr.
- Administer without regard to meals, but administer with food if GI upset occurs.
- Store at controlled room temperature (59° to 86°F).

Assessment/Interventions

- Obtain patient history, including drug history and any known allergies. Note history of addiction, COPD, bleeding or coagulation disorders, hepatic or renal impairment, peptic ulcer or other serious GI lesions, head injury, increased intracranial pressure or intracranial lesions, acute abdominal conditions, hypothyroidism, prostatic hypertrophy, urethral stricture, heart failure, hypertension, the syndrome of nasal polyps, rhinitis, and bronchospastic reactivity to aspirin or other NSAIDs.
- Assess pain before starting therapy and periodically during treatment.
- Monitor patient for CNS, GI, and general body side effects. Report to health care pro-

vider if noted and significant.
- Discontinue therapy and notify health care provider immediately if any of the following occur: allergic reaction, unusual bleeding or bruising, shortness of breath, black or tarry stools, vomiting of blood or coffee ground material.

Patient/Family Education
- Explain name, dose, action, and potential side effects of drug.
- Advise patient to take 1 tablet q 4 to 6 hr if needed for pain but to not take more than 5 tablets in 24 hr.
- Advise patient to take without regard to meals but to take with food if GI upset occurs.
- Advise patient that medication is intended to be used for short period of time (less than 10 days) for management of acute pain and is not for long-term use. If pain persists or is not controlled, advise patient to discuss other options for pain management with health care provider.
- Instruct patient to avoid alcoholic beverages and other depressants while taking this medication.
- Advise patient that drug may impair judgment, thinking, or motor skills or cause drowsiness and to use caution while driving or performing other tasks requiring mental alertness until tolerance is determined.
- Advise patient to stop taking the drug and notify health care provider if any of the following occur: allergic reaction, unusual bleeding or bruising, shortness of breath, black or tarry stools, vomiting of blood or coffee ground material, blurred vision, edema, excessive sedation.
- Advise women to notify health care provider if pregnant, planning to become pregnant, or breastfeeding.
- Warn patient not to take any prescription or OTC drugs or dietary supplements without consulting health care provider.
- Advise patient that follow-up visits may be necessary to monitor therapy and to keep appointments.

Hydrocodone Bitartrate/ Pseudoephedrine Hydrochloride

(HIGH-droe-KOE-dohn by-TAR-trate/SUE-doe-eh-FED-rin HIGH-droe-KLOR-ide)

Class Antitussive/Decongestant

How Supplied
Detussin Liquid 5 mg hydrocodone bitartrate and 60 mg pseudoephedrine hydrochloride ◆ *Histussin D* Liquid 5 mg hydrocodone bitartrate and 60 mg pseudoephedrine hydrochloride ◆ *P-V-Tussin* Tablets 5 mg hydrocodone bitartrate and 60 mg pseudoephedrine hydrochloride

Action
PHARMACOLOGY:
Hydrocodone: Suppresses cough reflex; stimulates opiate receptors in the CNS and peripherally blocks pain impulse generation.
Pseudoephedrine: Causes vasoconstriction and subsequent shrinkage of nasal mucous membranes by alpha-adrenergic stimulation, which promotes nasal drainage.

Indications Suppression of cough and relief of nasal congestion and other symptoms associated with the common cold, allergies, hay fever, sinusitis, and other respiratory illnesses.

Contraindications Hypersensitivity to any component of product, or hypersensitivity or idiosyncrasy to sympathomimetic amines which may be manifested by insomnia, dizziness, weakness, tremor, or arrhythmias. Patients known to be hypersensitive to other sympathomimetic amines may exhibit cross sensitivity with pseudoephedrine. Sympathomimetic amines are contraindicated in patients with severe hypertension, severe coronary artery disease, and patients on monoamine oxidase (MAO) inhibitor therapy. *P-V-Tussin* tablets are contraindicated in nursing mothers because of the higher than usual risk for infants from sympathomimetic amines.

Route/Dosage
LIQUID
ADULTS: **PO** 1 tsp (5 mL) qid.
TABLETS
ADULTS: **PO** 1 tablet q 4 to 6 hr (max, 4 in 24 hr).

Interactions
Alcohol, CNS depressants, narcotic analgesics, phenothiazines or other tranquilizers, sedative-hypnotics: Increased CNS depression (eg, drowsiness) may occur.

Lab Test Interferences None well documented.

Adverse Reactions
CV:
Hydrocodone – Hypotension; bradycardia.
Pseudoephedrine – Cardiac arrhythmia; increased heart rate; increased BP.
CNS:
Hydrocodone – Lightheadedness; dizziness; sedation; drowsiness; weakness; anxiety; fear; fatigue; dysphoria; psychological dependence; confusion.

Pseudoephedrine – Convulsions; CNS stimulation; hallucinations; tremors.
GI:
Hydrocodone – Nausea; vomiting; constipation.
GU:
Hydrocodone – Decreased urination; urethral spasm.
Pseudoephedrine – Dysuria.
RESP:
Hydrocodone – Dyspnea; respiratory depression; irregular breathing.
Pseudoephedrine – Respiratory difficulties.
OTHER:
Pseudoephedrine – Pallor.

Precautions
Pregnancy: Consult health care provider before use.
Lactation: Consult health care provider before use.
Hydrocodone – Excreted in breast milk.

Special risk patients: As with any narcotic, P-V-Tussin tablets should be given with caution to certain patients such as the elderly or debilitated and those with severe impairment of hepatic or renal function, hypothyroidism, Addison disease, prostatic hypertrophy or urethral stricture, asthma, and narrow angle glaucoma.
Dependence: Hydrocodone has abuse potential; may be habit forming.

Overdosage: Signs and Symptoms
Hydrocodone: Respiratory and CNS depression, circulatory collapse, cardiopulmonary arrest, death.
Pseudoephedrine: Cardiac arrhythmias, cerebral hemorrhage, pulmonary edema, palpitations, tremor, dizziness, vomiting, fear, labored breathing, headache, dryness of mouth, pallor, weakness, panic, anxiety, confusion, hallucination, delirium.

PATIENT CARE CONSIDERATIONS
Administration/Storage
- Give prescribed dose up to qid as needed.
- Give with food or milk if GI upset occurs.
- Use dosing spoon or syringe for pediatric doses.
- Store elixir at controlled room temperature (59° to 86°F). Keep tightly capped.

Assessment/Interventions
- Obtain patient history, including drug history and any known allergies. Note history of COPD, diabetes, hypertension, hyperthyroidism, enlarged prostate, narrow angle glaucoma, urinary retention, coronary artery disease, or concurrent use of or within 2 wk of stopping MAO inhibitor therapy.
- Assess for upper respiratory tract symptoms (eg, cough, rhinitis, nasal congestion) before and periodically throughout therapy.
- Monitor pulse and BP periodically during therapy.
- Monitor patient for nervousness, dizziness, and insomnia. If noted, hold therapy and notify health care provider.

Patient/Family Education
- Explain name, dose, action, and potential side effects of drug.
- Advise patient to take prescribed dose up to qid as needed.
- Advise caregiver to use dosing spoon or syringe when giving elixir to children.
- Advise patient to take with food or milk if GI upset occurs.
- Advise patient to take last dose late in the afternoon or early evening to reduce chance of drug causing sleeplessness.
- Advise patient that if a dose is missed to take as soon as remembered unless it is nearing time for the next dose. Caution patient not to double the dose to catch up.
- Advise patient that if symptoms are not controlled, not to increase the dose of medication but to inform health care provider.
- Caution patient that drug may cause drowsiness and to use caution while driving or performing other tasks requiring mental alertness until tolerance is determined.
- Advise patient to avoid alcohol and other CNS depressants because of risk of excessive sedation.
- Caution patient not to take any OTC decongestants while taking this medication unless advised by health care provider.
- Advise women to notify health care provider if pregnant, planning to become pregnant, or breastfeeding.
- Instruct patient to stop taking drug and immediately report any of the following symptoms to health care provider: nervousness, dizziness, sleeplessness.
- Caution patient not to take any prescription or OTC medications, or dietary supplements unless advised by health care provider.

Hydrocortisone (Cortisol)

(HIGH-droe-CORE-tih-sone)

Class Corticosteroid

How Supplied

Ala-Cort Cream 1%, Lotion 1% ◆ Ala-Scalp Lotion 1% ◆ Anusol-HC Cream 2.5% ◆ Cetacort Lotion 0.25%, Lotion 0.5%, Lotion 1% ◆ CortaGel, Extra Strength Gel 1% ◆ Cortaid Topical Spray Solution 1% ◆ Cort-Dome Cream 0.5%, Cream 1% ◆ Cortef Tablets 5 mg, Tablets 10 mg, Tablets 20 mg, Cream 0.5%, Oral Suspension 10 mg/5 mL hydrocortisone (as cypionate) ◆ Cortenema Enema 100 mg/60 mL unit ◆ Cortizone for Kids Cream 0.5% ◆ Cortizone-5 Cream 0.5%, Ointment 0.5% ◆ Cortizone-10 Cream 1%, Ointment 1% ◆ Cortizone 10 Quickshot Spray Solution 1% ◆ Cortizone–10 Plus Maximum Strength Cream 1% ◆ Dermacort Cream 0.5%, Lotion 1% ◆ Dermol HC Cream 1%, Cream 2.5%, Ointment 1% ◆ Dermtex HC Maximum Strength Spray Solution 1% ◆ Gynecort 10, Extra Strength Ointment 1% ◆ Hi-Cor 1.0 Cream 1% ◆ Hi-Cor 2.5 Cream 2.5% ◆ Hytone Cream 1%, Cream 2.5%, Lotion 1%, Lotion 2.5% ◆ KeriCort-10 Cream 1% ◆ LactiCare-HC Lotion 1%, Lotion 2.5% ◆ Lanacort 5 Ointment 0.5% ◆ Lanacort 10 Cream 1% ◆ Nutracort Cream 1%, Lotion 1%, Lotion 2.5% ◆ Penecort Solution 1% ◆ Proctocort Cream 1% ◆ ProctoCream-HC Cream 2.5% ◆ Scalpicin Liquid 1% ◆ S-T Cort Lotion 0.5% ◆ T/Scalp Liquid 1% ◆ Westcort Ointment 0.2%, Cream 0.2% ◆ U-Cort Cream 1%

❀ Aquacort ◆ Claritin Skin Itch Relief ◆ Cortoderm ◆ Emo-Cort ◆ Prevex HC ◆ Sarna HC ◆ Texacort

Hydrocortisone Acetate

Anucort-HC Suppositories 25 mg ◆ Anumed HC Suppositories 25 mg ◆ Anusol-HC Suppositories 25 mg ◆ Anusol HC-1 Hydrocortisone Anti-Itch Ointment 1% ◆ Caldecort Hydrocortisone Anti-Itch Cream 1% ◆ Cortaid with Aloe Ointment 0.5%, Cream 0.5% ◆ Cortaid, Maximum Strength Ointment 1%, Cream 1% ◆ Hemorrhoidal HC Suppositories 25 mg ◆ Hemril-HC Uniserts Suppositories 25 mg ◆ Lanacort Maximum Strength Cool Creme Cream 1% ◆ Proctocort Suppositories 30 mg

❀ Hyderm ◆ Uromol HC

Hydrocortisone Buteprate

Pandel Cream 0.1%, Cream 1%

Hydrocortisone Butyrate

Locoid Ointment 0.1%, Cream 0.1%, Solution 0.1%

Hydrocortisone Cypionate

Cortef Suspension, oral 10 mg/5mL

Hydrocortisone Phosphate

Hydrocortisone Phosphate Injection 50 mg/mL hydrocortisone (as sodium phosphate) solution

Hydrocortisone Sodium Succinate

A-Hydrocort Injection 100 mg/vial, Injection 250 mg/vial, Injection 500 mg/vial, Injection 1000 mg/vial ◆ Solu-Cortef Injection 100 mg/vial, Injection 250 mg/vial, Injection 500 mg/vial, Injection 1000 mg/vial

Hydrocortisone Valerate

Westcort Ointment 0.2%, Cream 0.2%

❀ HydroVal

Action

PHARMACOLOGY: Short-acting glucocorticoid that depresses formation, release, and activity of endogenous mediators of inflammation including prostaglandins, kinins, histamine, liposomal enzymes, and complement system. Also modifies body's immune response.

Indications Treatment of primary or secondary adrenal cortex insufficiency, rheumatic disorders, collagen diseases, dermatologic diseases, allergic states, allergic and inflammatory ophthalmic processes, respiratory diseases, hematologic disorders (idiopathic thrombocytopenic purpura), neoplastic diseases, edematous states (resulting from nephrotic syndrome), GI diseases (ulcerative colitis and sprue), multiple sclerosis, tuberculous meningitis, trichinosis with neurologic or myocardial involvement.

Intra-articular or soft tissue administration: Treatment of synovitis of osteoarthritis and symptoms of rheumatoid arthritis, bursitis, acute gouty arthritis, epicondylitis, acute nonspecific tenosynovitis, and post-traumatic osteoarthritis.

Intralesional administration: Treatment of keloids, lesions of lichen planus, psoriatic plaques, granuloma annulare, lichen simplex chronicus, discoid lupus erythematosus, necrobiosis lipoidica diabeticorum, alopecia areata, and cystic tumors of aponeurosis or tendon.

Topical administration: Treatment of inflammatory and pruritic manifestations of corticosteroid-responsive dermatoses, management of refractory lesions of psoriasis, and other deep-seated dermatoses.

Rectal administration: Relief of discomfort associated with hemorrhoids, perianal itching, or irritation.

Contraindications Systemic fungal infections; IM use in idiopathic thrombocytopenic purpura; administration of live virus vaccines in patients receiving immunosuppressive corticosteroid doses.

Route/Dosage

HYDROCORTISONE BUTEPRATE
ADULTS AND CHILDREN: **Topical** Apply thin film to affected area bid.

HYDROCORTISONE BUTYRATE
ADULTS AND CHILDREN: **Topical** Apply sparingly to affected areas bid to qid.

HYDROCORTISONE AND HYDROCORTISONE CYPIONATE
ADULTS AND CHILDREN: **PO** 20 to 240 mg/day.

HYDROCORTISONE SODIUM PHOSPHATE
ADULTS AND CHILDREN: **IV/IM/SC** 15 to 240 mg/day.

HYDROCORTISONE SODIUM SUCCINATE
ADULTS AND CHILDREN: **IV/IM** 100 to 500 mg q 2 to 6 hr.

HYDROCORTISONE ACETATE (INTRALESIONAL, INTRA-ARTICULAR OR SOFT TISSUE INJECTION ONLY)

Large Joints (Knee) and Bursae
Adults and Children: 25 to 37.5 mg.

Small Joints (Interphalangeal, Temporomandibular)
ADULTS AND CHILDREN: 10 to 25 mg.

Tendon Sheaths
ADULTS AND CHILDREN: 5 to 12.5 mg.

Soft Tissue Infiltration
ADULTS AND CHILDREN: 25 to 75 mg.

Ganglia
ADULTS AND CHILDREN: 12.5 to 25 mg.

Topical
ADULTS AND CHILDREN: Apply sparingly to affected areas bid to qid.

Interactions
Oral administration of hydrocortisone:

Anticholinesterases: May antagonize anticholinesterase effects in myasthenia gravis.
Anticoagulants, oral: May alter anticoagulant dose requirements.
Barbiturates: May decrease effect of hydrocortisone.
Cholestyramine: May decrease hydrocortisone levels.
Contraceptives (oral) estrogens: May decrease clearance of hydrocortisone.
Hydantoins, rifampin: May increase clearance and decrease therapeutic efficacy of hydrocortisone.
Salicylates: May reduce serum levels and efficacy of salicylates.
Troleandomycin: May increase effects of hydrocortisone.

Lab Test Interferences
May cause increased urine glucose and serum cholesterol, decreased serum levels of potassium, T_3 and T_4, decreased uptake of Thyroid I^{131}, false-negative nitroblue-tetrazolium test for bacterial infection, suppression of skin test reactions.

Adverse Reactions
CV: Thromboembolism or fat embolism; thrombophlebitis; necrotizing angitis; cardiac arrhythmias or ECG changes; syncopal episodes; hypertension; myocardial rupture; CHF.
CNS: Convulsions; increased intracranial pressure with papilledema (pseudotumor cerebri); vertigo; headache; neuritis; paresthesias; psychosis.
DERM: Impaired wound healing; thin, fragile skin; petechiae and ecchymoses; erythema; lupus erythematosus-like lesions; subcutaneous fat atrophy; striae; hirsutism; acneiform eruptions; allergic dermatitis; urticaria; angioneurotic edema; perineal irritation; hyperpigmentation or hypopigmentation. Topical application may cause burning; irritation; erythema; dryness; folliculitis; hypertrichosis; pruritus; perioral dermatitis; allergic contact dermatitis; stinging, cracking and tightening of skin; secondary infections; skin atrophy; striae; miliaria; telangiectasia.
EENT: Posterior subcapsular cataracts; increased IOP; glaucoma; exophthalmos.
GI: Pancreatitis; abdominal distension; ulcerative esophagitis; nausea; vomiting; increased appetite and weight gain; peptic ulcer with perforation and hemorrhage; bowel perforation.
GU: Increased or decreased motility and number of spermatozoa.
HEMA: Leukocytosis.
METAB: Sodium and fluid retention; hypokalemia; hypokalemic alkalosis; metabolic alkalosis; hypocalcemia.
OTHER: Musculoskeletal effects (eg, weakness, myopathy, muscle mass loss, osteoporosis, spontaneous fractures); endocrine abnormalities (eg, menstrual irregularities, cushingoid state, growth suppression in children, sweating, decreased carbohydrate tolerance, hyperglycemia, glycosuria, increased insulin or sulfonylurea requirements in diabetics); anaphylactoid or hypersensitivity reactions; aggravation or masking of infections; malaise; fatigue; insomnia. Topical use may cause same adverse reactions seen with systemic use because of possibility of absorption.

Precautions
Pregnancy: Safety not established (systemic use); Category C (topical).
Lactation: Excreted in breast milk.
Children: Children may absorb proportionally larger amounts of topical corticosteroids and thus be more susceptible to systemic toxicity. Observe growth and development of infants and children on prolonged therapy.

Elderly: May require lower doses.
Renal function impairment: Use cautiously; monitor renal function.
Adrenal suppression: Prolonged (daily systemic) therapy (more than 7 days) may lead to hypothalamic-pituitary-adrenal suppression.
Fluid and electrolyte balance: May cause elevation of BP, salt and water retention, and increased excretion of potassium and calcium. Dietary salt restriction and potassium supplementation may be needed.
Hepatitis: May be harmful in chronic active hepatitis positive for hepatitis B surface antigen.
Infections: May mask signs of infection. May decrease host-defense mechanisms.
Ocular effects: Use caution in patients with ocular herpes simplex because of possible corneal perforation.
Peptic ulcer: May contribute to peptic ulceration, especially in large doses.
Repository injections: Do not inject SC; avoid injection into deltoid and repeated IM injection into the same site.
Stress: Increased dosage of rapidly acting corticosteroid may be needed before, during, and after stressful situations.
Withdrawal: Abrupt discontinuation may result in adrenal insufficiency. Discontinue gradually; increase supplementation during times of stress.

Overdosage: Signs and Symptoms

Acute toxicity and death are rare. Acute adrenal insufficiency (caused by withdrawal after long-term use): Fever, myalgia, arthralgia, malaise, anorexia, nausea, shedding of skin, orthostatic hypotension, dizziness, fainting, dyspnea, hypoglycemia Cushingoid symptoms (caused by chronic large doses): Moonface, central obesity, striae, hirsutism, acne, ecchymoses, hypertension, osteoporosis, myopathy, sexual dysfunction, diabetes, hyperlipidemia, peptic ulcer, increased susceptibility to infection, electrolyte and fluid imbalance.

PATIENT CARE CONSIDERATIONS

Administration/Storage

- Give medication with food.
- With large doses, administer antacids between meals.
- For intra-articular injection, local anesthetic may be administered prior to or mixed in same syringe and used immediately. Discard unused portions of mixture.
- Shake optic solutions well prior to use.
- Apply topical doses sparingly.
- Topical absorption enhanced by heat, hydration, inflamed, denuded or thin skin surfaces, or occlusive dressings.
- Avoid mixing topical preparations with other agents.
- Avoid abrupt discontinuation of systemic preparations used for more than 7 days.

Assessment/Interventions

- Obtain patient history, including drug history and any known allergies. Note recent use of steroids.
- Monitor for covert infections.
- Monitor BP and body weight.
- Monitor routine laboratory studies including serum K^+ and Na^+.
- Monitor blood glucose.
- Monitor I&O for increased edema.
- Monitor growth and development in infants and children on prolonged therapy.
- Observe for signs of potassium depletion.
- Observe for signs of GI irritation.
- If local irritation occurs with topical use, discontinue and notify health care provider.
- Following dosage reduction or therapy withdrawal, monitor for signs of adrenal insufficiency, including fatigue, anorexia, nausea, vomiting, diarrhea, weight loss, weakness, dizziness, or low blood sugar.
- Notify health care provider of weight gain, swelling, muscle weakness, black tarry stools, hematemesis, facial puffiness, menstrual irregularities, prolonged sore throat, fever, cold, or signs of infection.

Patient/Family Education

- Advise patient to take oral medication with food to minimize GI upset.
- Warn patient not to stop taking drug abruptly.
- Caution diabetic patients that insulin or oral hypoglycemic agent needs may increase.
- Instruct elderly patient to have BP, blood glucose, and electrolytes monitored at least q 6 mo.
- Advise patient that sunglasses may reduce sensitivity to sunlight that occurs with optic administration.
- Caution against eye contact with topical agents.
- Instruct patient to wash or soak areas for topical administration prior to administration to increase absorption.
- Advise patient to apply topical agents sparingly, rubbing in lightly.
- Caution against covering topically treated areas unless specifically prescribed by health care provider.

- Advise against mixing topical agents with other products unless advised by health care provider.
- Instruct patient if topical dose is missed to apply as soon as remembered, but not to double doses.
- Teach patient using suppositories or other hemorrhoidal agents that appropriate diet, fluid intake, and adequate exercise are useful treatment adjuncts.
- Remind patient to wear *Medi-Alert* identification while taking this medication.
- Advise that temporary burning is common after administration of optic preparations.
- Caution patient that systemic reactions may occur with topical applications.

Hydrocortisone Acetate/ Pramoxine Hydrochloride

(HIGH-droe-core-tih-sone ASS-uh-TATE /pram-OX-een HIGH-droe-KLOR-ide)

Class Corticosteroid/Anesthetic

How Supplied

Analpram HC Cream 1% hydrocortisone acetate/1% pramoxine hydrochloride, Cream 2.5% hydrocortisone acetate/1% pramoxine hydrochloride ◆ *Enzone* Cream 1% hydrocortisone acetate/1% pramoxine hydrochloride ◆ *Pramosone* Ointment 1% hydrocortisone acetate/1% pramoxine hydrochloride, Ointment 2.5% hydrocortisone acetate/1% pramoxine hydrochloride, Cream 1% hydrocortisone acetate/1% pramoxine hydrochloride, Cream 2.5% hydrocortisone acetate/1% pramoxine hydrochloride, Lotion 1% hydrocortisone acetate/1% pramoxine hydrochloride, Lotion 2.5% hydrocortisone acetate/1% pramoxine hydrochloride ◆ *ProctoCream* HC Cream 1% hydrocortisone acetate/1% pramoxine hydrochloride, Cream 2.5% hydrocortisone acetate/1% pramoxine hydrochloride ◆ *ProctoFoam-HC* Aerosol Foam 1% hydrocortisone acetate/1% pramoxine hydrochloride ◆ *Zone-A Forte* Lotion 2.5% hydrocortisone acetate/1% pramoxine hydrochloride

✤ *Pramox HC*

Action

PHARMACOLOGY:

Hydrocortisone: Depresses formation, release and activity of endogenous mediators of inflammation, as well as modifying body's immune response.

Pramoxine: Stabilizes the neuronal membrane of nerve endings with which it comes in contact.

Indications Topical relief of the inflammatory and pruritic manifestations of corticosteroid-responsive dermatoses.

Contraindications History of hypersensitivity to any component of the product.

Route/Dosage

Topical:

Apply to the affected area as a thin film tid or qid, depending on severity of the condition. Administration of topical corticosteroids to children should be limited to the least amount compatible with an effective therapeutic regimen.

Interactions None well documented.

Lab Test Interferences None well documented.

Adverse Reactions

DERM: Burning; itching; irritation; dryness; folliculitis; hypertrichosis; acneiform eruptions; hyperpigmentation; perioral dermatitis; allergic contact dermatitis; maceration of the skin; secondary infection; skin atrophy; striae; miliaria.

Precautions

Pregnancy: Category C.

Lactation: Undetermined; however, systemic hydrocortisone is excreted in breast milk.

Children: Pediatric patients may demonstrate greater susceptibility to topical corticosteroids-induced hypothalamic-pituitary-adrenal (HPA) axis suppression and Cushing syndrome than mature patients because of a larger skin surface area to body weight ratio.

Topical absorption: Systemic absorption of topical corticosteroids can produce reversible HPA axis suppression, manifestations of Cushing syndrome, hyperglycemia, and glucosuria.

Overdosage: Signs and Symptoms

HPA axis suppression; manifestations of Cushing syndrome, hyperglycemia, and glucosuria, especially when large surface areas, prolonged use, or occlusive dressings are involved.

PATIENT CARE CONSIDERATIONS

Administration/Storage

- For topical use only. Not for ophthalmic or otic use.
- Apply a thin film to affected area(s) tid to qid as ordered. Use gloves or applicator as applicable.
- Do not apply an occlusive dressing unless ordered by health care provider.
- Store at controlled room temperature (59° to 86°F). Keep tube tightly closed.

Assessment/Interventions

- Obtain patient history, including drug history and any known allergies. Note history of bacterial, viral, fungal, or mycobacterial skin infections.

- Monitor patient's response to therapy. Notify health care provider if skin inflammation, irritation, or sensitization are noted or if symptoms do not improve or worsen.

Patient/Family Education
- Explain name, dose, action, and potential side effects of medication.
- Review prescribed dosing schedule with patient or caregiver.
- Remind patient or caregiver that cream is not to be used in the eye or ear.
- Teach patient or caregiver proper technique for applying product: wash hands; apply thin film to affected area(s) using fingers or applicator. Wash hands after applying product.
- Caution patient or caregiver to not cover area with an occlusive dressing unless advised by health care provider.
- Advise patient or caregiver to contact health care provider if local redness or swelling develops or if skin lesions do not improve or worsen.
- Remind patient or caregiver that follow-up examinations may be necessary while using this medication and to keep appointments.

Hydromorphone Hydrochloride

(HIGH-droe-moRE-phone HIGH-droe-KLOR-ide)

Class Narcotic/Analgesic

How Supplied
Dilaudid Tablets 1 mg, Tablets 2 mg, Tablets 3 mg, Tablets 4 mg, Tablets 8 mg, Injection 1 mg/mL, Injection 2 mg/mL, Injection 4 mg/mL, Suppositories 3 mg ◆ *Dilaudid-HP* Injection 10 mg/mL, Powder for Injection, lyophilized 250 mg
🍁 *Dilaudid-HP Plus* ◆ *Dilaudid Sterile Powder* ◆ *Dilaudid-XP* ◆ *Hydromorph Contin* ◆ *Hydromorphone HP 10* ◆ *Hydromorphone HP 20* ◆ *Hydromorphone HP 50* ◆ *Hydromorphone HP Forte* ◆ *PMS-Hydromorphone*

Action
PHARMACOLOGY: Relieves pain by stimulating opiate receptors in CNS; also causes respiratory depression, inhibition of cough reflex, peripheral vasodilation, inhibition of intestinal peristalsis, sphincter of Oddi spasm, stimulation of chemoreceptors that cause vomiting, and increased bladder tone.

PHARMACOKINETICS/DYNAMICS:

Distribution: The mean Vd is 91.5 L. Hydromorphone hydrochloride is rapidly removed from the bloodstream and distributed to skeletal muscles, kidneys, liver, intestinal tract, lungs, spleen, and brain. Hydromorphone also crosses placental membranes.

Metabolism: Hydromorphone is metabolized in the liver as glucuronidated conjugate (major metabolite) and 6-hydroxy (minor metabolite).

Excretion: The mean $t_{1/2}$ is approximately 2.64 hr. Hydromorphone is excreted primarily as the glucuronidated conjugate.

Onset: Onset of hydromorphone is 15 min (parentally) and 30 min (oral).

Peak: Time to peak effect is 0.5 to 1 hr.

Duration: Duration is longer than 5 hr.

Indications Relief of moderate to severe pain; control of persistent nonproductive cough.

Contraindications Hypersensitivity to similar compounds, depressed ventilatory function; acute asthma; diarrhea caused by poisoning or toxins; patients not already receiving large amounts of parenteral narcotics; patients with respiratory depression without access to resuscitative equipment; labor.

Route/Dosage
ADULTS: **PO/Tablet** 2 mg q 4 to 6 hr prn; at least 4 mg q 4 to 6 hr for more severe pain. **PO/Liquid** 2.5 to 10 mg q 4 to 6 hr. **SC/IM** 1 to 2 mg q 4 to 6 hr prn; 3 to 4 mg q 4 to 6 hr for more severe pain. **IV** May give slowly over 2 to 5 min. Use high potency (10 mg/mL) only for patients tolerant to other opiates. **PR** 3 mg q 6 to 8 hr.

Antitussive: **PO** 1 mg q 3 to 4 hr prn.

Interactions
CNS depressants (eg, tranquilizers, sedatives, alcohol): Additive CNS depression.
Barbiturate anesthetics: May have additive effects.

Lab Test Interferences Increased amylase and lipase may occur up to 24 hr after dose.

Adverse Reactions
CV: Hypotension; orthostatic hypotension; bradycardia; tachycardia.
CNS: Lightheadedness; dizziness; sedation; disorientation; incoordination; lethargy; anxiety.
DERM: Sweating; pruritus; urticaria.
GI: Nausea; vomiting; constipation; abdominal pain.
GU: Urinary retention or hesitancy.
RESP: Respiratory depression; laryngospasm; depression of cough reflex.
OTHER: Tolerance; psychological and physical dependence with chronic use.

Precautions
Pregnancy: Category C.

Lactation: Excreted in breast milk.
Children: Safety and efficacy not established.
Renal function impairment: May need to reduce dose.
Hepatic function impairment: May need to reduce dose.
Special risk patients: Use with caution in patients with myxedema, acute alcoholism, acute abdominal conditions, ulcerative colitis, decreased respiratory reserve, head injury or increased intracranial pressure, hypoxia, supraventricular tachycardia, depleted blood volume, or circulatory shock.
Drug dependence: Hydromorphone has abuse potential.

Overdosage: Signs and Symptoms
Miosis, respiratory and CNS depression, apnea, bradycardia, hypotension, circulatory collapse, seizures, cardiopulmonary arrest, death.

PATIENT CARE CONSIDERATIONS

Administration/Storage
- Administer before pain becomes severe.
- Give medication with food.
- If vomiting occurs, administer with antiemetic.
- Store at room temperature and protect from light.

Assessment/Interventions
- Obtain complete patient history, including drug history and any known allergies.
- Assess vital signs before and periodically after administration. If hypotension, bradycardia, bradypnea, or difficulty in breathing occurs, notify health care provider.
- Monitor I&O and check for urinary retention.
- Monitor for orthostatic hypotension and supervise ambulation.
- Encourage coughing and deep breathing in patients with pulmonary problems.
- Monitor bowel function. If decreased bowel sounds or abdominal distention occur, notify health care provider.
- Check for reduced dosage in patients with impaired renal and liver function.

Patient/Family Education
- Instruct patient to take medication before pain becomes severe.
- Advise patient to take medication with food or milk to decrease stomach upset.
- Advise patient that drug may cause drowsiness and to use caution while driving or performing other tasks requiring mental alertness.
- Advise patient to eat high-fiber diet and to maintain adequate fluid intake. A stool softener or bulk laxative may be recommended to prevent constipation.
- Instruct patient to avoid intake of alcoholic beverages or other CNS depressants.
- Instruct patient to discontinue drug and notify health care provider if difficulty in breathing or persistent nausea, vomiting or constipation occurs.
- When medication is used for acute pain, caution patient about potential for addiction and explain that medication should be for short-term use only.

Hydroxychloroquine Sulfate

(high-drox-ee-KLOR-oh-kwin SULL-fate)
Class Anti-infective/Antimalarial/Antirheumatic

How Supplied
Plaquenil Sulfate Tablets 200 mg (equivalent to 155 mg base)

Action
PHARMACOLOGY: May interfere with parasitic nucleoprotein (DNA/RNA) synthesis and parasite growth or cause lysis of parasite or infected erythrocytes. In rheumatoid arthritis, may suppress formation of antigens responsible for symptom-producing hypersensitivity reactions.

PHARMACOKINETICS/DYNAMICS:
Absorption: Hydroxychloroquine is readily absorbed from the GI tract. T_{max} is 1 to 3 hr.
Distribution: Hydroxychloroquine concentrates in the liver, spleen, kidney, heart, lungs, and brain.
Metabolism: It is partially hepatic to active de-ethylated metabolites.
Excretion: Approximately 50% of the unchanged drug is excreted in urine. Elimination in urine is very slow and may persist for months or years after discontinuation. Renal excretion is increased by acidification and decreased by alkalinization of the urine. The plasma t½ is approximately 32 days.

Special Populations:
Renal Function Impairment – Use with caution.
Hepatic Function Impairment – Use with caution.
Children – Use with caution. A number of fatalities have been reported following ingestion of chloroquines.

Indications
Prophylaxis and treatment of acute attacks of malaria caused by *Plasmodium vivax*, *Plasmodium malariae*, *Plasmodium ovale*, and susceptible strains of *Plasmodium falciparum*. Treatment of chronic discoid and systemic lupus

erythematosus (SLE) and acute or chronic rheumatoid arthritis in patients not responding to other therapies.

Contraindications Retinal or visual field changes caused by any 4-aminoquinoline compound; hypersensitivity to 4-aminoquinoline compounds; long-term therapy in children.

Route/Dosage

Acute Attack of Malaria
ADULTS: PO 800 mg (620 mg of base) followed by 400 mg in 6 to 8 hr and 400 mg on each of 2 consecutive days. Alternatively, a single 800 mg dose (620 mg of base) has proved effective.
CHILDREN: PO 10 mg/kg (base), up to adult dose; followed by 5 mg/kg (base), not exceeding 310 mg of base, 6 hr after first dose; followed in 18 hr after the second dose by 5 mg/kg (base). A fourth dose of 5 mg/kg (base) is given 24 hr after third dose.

Lupus Erythematosus
ADULTS: PO Initially 400 mg/day or bid. For prolonged therapy, reduce to 200 to 400 mg/day (155 to 310 mg of base).

Rheumatoid Arthritis
ADULTS:
Initial dose: PO 400 to 600 mg/day (310 to 465 mg of base) with food or milk.
Maintenance: PO After good response (usually 4 to 12 wk), reduce dosage 50% and continue at 200 to 400 mg/day (155 to 310 mg of base).

Suppression of Malaria
Begin 2 wk prior to exposure; continue for 8 wk after leaving area.
ADULTS: PO 400 mg (310 mg of base) weekly on same day each week.
CHILDREN: PO 5 mg/kg of base weekly on same day each week, up to max 400 mg (310 mg of base).

Interactions
Beta-blockers (eg, metoprolol): Plasma levels and CV effects of certain beta-blockers may be increased.
Cimetidine: Pharmacologic effect of hydroxychloroquine may be increased.
Cyclosporine: Serum levels may be increased by hydroxychloroquine, increasing the risk of nephrotoxicity.
Digoxin: May increase serum digoxin levels.
Hepatotoxic drugs: May increase potential for hepatotoxicity.
Magnesium sulfate: Absorption of hydroxychloroquine may be reduced, decreasing the pharmacologic effect; antacid activity of magnesium sulfate may be decreased.
Mefloquine: Coadministration may increase risk of seizures.

Lab Test Interferences None well documented.

Adverse Reactions
CV: Hypotension; ECG changes; cardiomyopathy (rare).
CNS: Headache; irritability; nervousness; emotional changes; nightmares; psychosis; dizziness; vertigo; nystagmus; nerve deafness; convulsions; ataxia.
DERM: Bleaching of hair; alopecia; pruritus; skin and mucosal pigmentation; skin eruptions; exacerbation of psoriasis.
EENT: Disturbance of accommodation with blurred vision; transient corneal edema; corneal opacities; decreased corneal sensitivity; retinal edema; retinal atrophy; abnormal retinal pigmentation; loss of retinal reflexes; optic disc pallor and atrophy; scotoma retinopathy; tinnitus.
GI: Anorexia; nausea; vomiting; diarrhea; abdominal cramps.
HEMA: Aplastic anemia; agranulocytosis; leukopenia; thrombocytopenia; hemolysis in G-6-PD deficiency; exacerbation of porphyria.
METAB: Weight loss.
OTHER: Immunoblastic lymphadenopathy; extraocular muscle palsies; skeletal muscle weakness; absent or hypoactive deep tendon reflexes.

Precautions
Pregnancy: Category C. Avoid use in pregnancy, except in suppression of malaria when benefit outweighs the possible hazard.
Lactation: Excreted in breast milk.
Children: Deaths have occurred following accidental ingestion of relatively small doses. Do not exceed recommended doses for children with malaria. Not indicated for juvenile rheumatoid arthritis.
Renal function impairment: Use with caution.
Hepatic function impairment: Use with caution. May increase risk of hepatotoxicity.
Special risk patients: May exacerbate psoriasis, porphyria, or other dermatitis; may cause hemolysis in patients with glucose-6-phosphate dehydrogenase (G-6-PD) deficiency.
Alcoholism: May increase risk of hepatotoxicity.
Muscular weakness: If weakness occurs, discontinue.
Ophthalmic effects: Irreversible retinal damage with long-term hydroxychloroquine therapy has been observed. Retinal changes and visual disturbances may progress after cessation of therapy.

Overdosage: Signs and Symptoms
Headache, drowsiness, visual disturbances, CV collapse, convulsions, respiratory and cardiac arrest, bradycardia, ventricular fibrillation.

PATIENT CARE CONSIDERATIONS
Administration/Storage
- Administer prescribed dose with food or milk to minimize GI side effects.
- Dose is administered once daily.
- Disease-modifying antirheumatic drugs, glucocorticoids, salicylates, NSAIDs, and analgesics may be continued during treatment of rheumatoid arthritis with hydroxychloroquine.
- Malaria treatment: Administer prescribed dose bid (separate doses by 6 to 8 hr) on 2 consecutive days.
- Malaria prophylaxis: Prescribed dose is taken once every 7 days, daily beginning 2 wk before entering a malaria-endemic area, while in the malaria-endemic area, and for 8 wk following return.
- Store tablets at controlled room temperature (up to 86°F).

Assessment/Interventions
- Obtain patient history, including drug history and any known allergies. Note renal or hepatic impairment, G-6-PD deficiency, porphyria, alcoholism, retinal or visual field changes attributable to any 4-aminoquinoline (eg, chloroquine), psoriasis, hypersensitivity to 4-aminoquinoline compound, or concurrent use of hepatotoxic medications.
- Ensure that ophthalmologic exam is obtained before starting therapy and periodically (eg, q 3 mo) thereafter during prolonged therapy.
- Ensure patient on long term therapy is periodically evaluated for development of muscular weakness. If weakness occurs, discontinue therapy and notify health care provider.
- Ensure CBC with differential and platelet count is evaluated before starting therapy and periodically thereafter during prolonged therapy. Inform health care provider if abnormalities noted. Be prepared to discontinue therapy if severe blood cell disorder develops.
- Document baseline disease state activity in patient being treated for rheumatoid arthritis or lupus erythematosus. Reassess periodically to document response to therapy.
- Ensure therapy is periodically reviewed to determine if therapy needs to be continued without change or if a dose change (eg, increase, decrease, discontinuation) is indicated.
- Monitor patient for CNS, GI, OPHTH, MUSC, DERM, and general body side effects. Report to health care provider if noted and significant. Immediately report any visual symptoms (eg, blurred vision, light flashes, streaks) to health care provider.

Patient/Family Education
- Explain name, dose, action, and potential side effects of drug.
- Advise patient to take each dose with milk or food to minimize stomach upset.
- Advise patient to continue other medications for arthritis or lupus as recommended by health care provider.
- Advise patient with arthritis that it may take several months of treatment before max benefit is seen. Advise patient to notify health care provider if symptoms have not improved after 6 mo of treatment or if symptoms appear to be getting worse.
- Instruct patient to take medication once weekly for malaria prophylaxis, beginning 2 wk prior to arrival in malaria-infected area, while in the malaria-infected area, and for 8 wk after leaving the malaria-infected area.
- Advise patient that protective clothing, insect repellants, and bednets are important components of malaria prophylaxis.
- Advise patient to immediately report any of the following to health care provider: any visual changes; muscle weakness; ringing in the ears or hearing loss; fever; sore throat; unusual bleeding or bruising; unusual pigmentation (eg, blue-black) of the skin; bleaching or loss of hair; mood or mental changes.
- Advise patient to notify health care provider if persistent or bothersome nausea, vomiting, diarrhea, stomach pain, or other symptoms develop.
- Advise patient that drug may cause dizziness and to use caution while driving or performing other tasks requiring mental alertness, coordination, or physical dexterity until tolerance is determined.
- Advise patient medication may cause photosensitivity (sensitivity to sunlight) and to avoid unnecessary exposure to sunlight or tanning lamps, and to use sunscreens and wear protective clothing to avoid photosensitivity reactions.
- Advise women to notify health care provider if pregnant, planning to become pregnant, or breastfeeding.
- Instruct patient not to take any prescription or OTC medications, herbal preparations, or dietary supplements unless advised by health care provider.
- Remind patient that office visits, eye exams, and laboratory tests will be required to monitor therapy and to keep appointments.

Hydroxyurea

(high-DROX-ee-you-REE-uh)

Class Antisickling/Substituted ureas/Antimetabolite

How Supplied
Droxia Capsules 200 mg, Capsules 300 mg, Capsules 400 mg ♦ *Hydrea* Capsules 500 mg ♦ *Mylocel* Tablets 1000 mg
✣ Gen-Hydroxyurea

Action
PHARMACOLOGY: Inhibits DNA synthesis, interferes with conversion of ribonucleotides to deoxyribonucleotides, and may inhibit incorporation of thymidine into DNA.

PHARMACOKINETICS/DYNAMICS:

Absorption: Hydroxyurea is rapidly absorbed. T_{max} is 1 to 4 hr, and the bioavailability is 79% to 100%.

Distribution: Hydroxyurea distributes rapidly and widely in the body, concentrates in leukocytes and erythrocytes, readily crosses blood brain barrier, and is secreted in breast milk. Vd is 0.65L/kg.

Metabolism: Up to 50% of oral dose undergoes conversion not fully characterized. In one minor route, hydroxyurea is degraded by urease in intestinal bacteria.

Excretion: Hydroxyurea is excreted by 2 nonlinear pathways, hepatic metabolism and first-order renal excretion. Approximately 40% to 80% is excreted in urine within 12 hr. Elimination t½ is approximately 2.8 to 4.5 hr.

Indications Reduce frequency of painful crises and need for blood transfusion in adults with sickle cell anemia with recurrent moderate to severe painful crises; treatment of melanoma; resistant chronic myelocytic leukemia (CML); recurrent, metastatic, or inoperable carcinoma of ovary; as an adjunct to irradiation in local control of primary squamous cell carcinomas of head and neck, excluding lip. **Unlabeled use(s):** Thrombocythemia; HIV; psoriasis; cervical carcinoma; polycythemia vera.

Contraindications Marked bone marrow suppression; severe anemia; hypersensitivity to product.

Route/Dosage
Base dosage on patient's actual or ideal weight, whichever is less.

Sickle Cell Anemia
ADULTS:
Initial dose: **PO** 15 mg/kg/day as a single dose. If blood counts are acceptable levels, dose may be increased by 5 mg/kg/day q 12 wk until max tolerated dose (highest dose not producing toxic blood counts over 24 consecutive wk), or 35 mg/kg/day is reached. Dose is not increased if blood counts are between acceptable and toxic levels. If blood counts are considered toxic, discontinue hydroxyurea until hematologic recovery, then resume therapy after reducing dose by 2.5 mg/kg/day from dose associated with hematologic toxicity. Then, titrate dose up or down q 12 wk in 2.5 mg/kg/day increments until patient is at a stable dose that does not result in hematologic toxicity for 24 wk. Any dose that produces hematologic toxicity twice should not be given again.

Solid Tumors
ADULTS:
Intermittent therapy: **PO** 80 mg/kg (2000 to 3000 mg/m^2) as a single dose every third day. Continuous therapy: **PO** 20 to 30 mg/kg as a single daily dose. Hold the dose if WBC decreases to less than 2500/mm^3 or platelet count less than 100,000/mm^3.

Concomitant Irradiation Therapy (Carcinoma of Head and Neck)
ADULTS: **PO** 80 mg/kg as a single dose every third day, beginning at least 7 days before initiation of irradiation and continue during radiotherapy and indefinitely afterwards, provided patient is adequately observed and exhibits no unusual or severe reactions.

Resistant CML
ADULTS: **PO** Continuous therapy of 20 to 30 mg/kg as a single daily dose.

Interactions
Antiretroviral agents (eg, didanosine, indinavir, stavudine): Hepatotoxicity, fatal hepatic failure, and severe neurotoxicity reported with concomitant use in HIV-positive patients.
Didanosine: Pancreatitis, occasionally resulting in death, reported with concomitant use in HIV-positive patients.
Fluorouracil: Coadministration may cause neurotoxicity.
Uricosuric agents (eg, probenecid): Hydroxyurea may increase serum uric acid levels.

Lab Test Interferences Serum uric acid, BUN, and creatinine levels may be increased.

Adverse Reactions
DERM: Hair loss; skin rash; black-pigmented nails; maculopapular rash; skin ulcers; dermatomyositis-like changes; peripheral and facial erythema; hyperpigmentation; skin and nail atrophy; scaling and violet papules; skin cancer.
GI: Stomatitis; anorexia; nausea; vomiting; diarrhea; constipation; increased LFTs.
HEMA: Neutropenia; low reticulocyte and platelet levels; bleeding; bone marrow suppres-

sion; leukopenia; anemia.
METAB: Weight gain.
RENAL: Temporary impairment of renal tubular function; uric acid nephropathy.
RESP: Pulmonary infiltrates and fibrosis.
OTHER: Fever; parvovirus B-19 infection; chills; malaise.

> **WARNING:**
> Treatment of patients with hydroxyurea capsules may be complicated by severe, sometimes life-threatening adverse effects. Hydroxyurea is mutagenic, clastogenic, and genotoxic. Secondary leukemias have been reported in patients receiving long-term hydroxyurea for myeloproliferative disorders.

Precautions
Pregnancy: Category D.
Lactation: Excreted in breast milk.
Children: Safety and efficacy not established.
Elderly: May be more sensitive to the effects of hydroxyurea and may require a lower dosage regimen.

Renal function impairment: May temporarily impair renal tubular function accompanied by elevated serum uric acid, BUN, and creatinine levels.
Bone marrow function: Because hydroxyurea is cytotoxic and myelosuppressive, do not administer if bone marrow function is markedly depressed.
Carcinogenesis: Hydroxyurea is presumed to be a human carcinogen.
Erythema: Patients who have received prior irradiation therapy may have an exacerbation of postirradiation erythema.
Erythrocytic abnormalities: Self-limiting megaloblastic erythropoiesis is often seen early in hydroxyurea therapy.

Overdosage: Signs and Symptoms
Mucocutaneous toxicity, soreness, violet erythema, edema on palms and soles followed by scaling of hands and feet, severe generalized hyperpigmentation of the skin, stomatitis.

PATIENT CARE CONSIDERATIONS
Administration/Storage
- Do not administer if WBC is under 2500/mm^3 or platelet count is under 100,000/mm^3.
- Do not administer if signs or symptoms of pancreatitis or hepatitis are noted.
- Administer prescribed number of capsules qd or every third day without regard to food, but administer in a consistent manner (either with or without food).
- Administer with food if GI upset occurs.
- If patient is unable to swallow capsules, the contents of the capsule can be emptied into a glass of water and swallowed immediately.
- Follow procedures for proper handling and disposal of anticancer drugs.
- If contents of capsule are spilled, wipe up immediately with a damp disposable towel and discard in a closed container, such as a plastic bag.
- Store capsules at controlled room temperature (59° to 86°F) in a tightly closed container.

Assessment/Interventions
- Obtain patient history, including drug history and any known allergies. Note history of renal or hepatic impairment, bone marrow depression, or previous treatment with radiotherapy or cytotoxic chemotherapy.
- Ensure that hemoglobin, WBC with differential, and platelet counts are determined before starting therapy and at least weekly during therapy.
- Ensure that baseline LFTs and kidney function are determined before starting therapy and periodically during therapy.
- Ensure that women of childbearing potential are not pregnant when therapy is started and use effective contraception during therapy.
- Monitor HIV-infected patient for signs and symptoms of pancreatitis (epigastric pain, nausea, vomiting, sweating, abdominal tenderness and distension) and hepatotoxicity (right upper quadrant pain, jaundice, dark urine) and report to health care provider if noted.
- Implement infection control measures if WBC drops; implement bleeding precautions if platelet count drops.
- Monitor patient for GI, CNS, and general body side effects. Report to health care provider if noted and significant.

Patient/Family Education
- Explain name, dose, action, and potential side effects of drug.
- Review dosing schedule with patient (qd or every third day).
- Advise patient that dose is individualized based upon condition being treated and size of the patient.
- Advise patient to take each dose either with or without food but to be consistent. Advise patient to take with food if stomach upset occurs.
- If patient unable to swallow capsules advise

patient that the contents of the capsule can be emptied into a glass of water and swallowed immediately.
* Advise patient that if a dose is missed, take it as soon as possible. If close to the next dose, do not double the dose to catch up and take the next dose as scheduled.
* Advise patient to immediately report any of the following to health care provider: fever, chills, or other signs of infection; sore throat, nausea, vomiting, or appetite loss; sores in the mouth or on the lips; unusual bruising or bleeding; skin rash.
* Advise HIV-infected patient to report any of the following to health care provider: epigastric pain, nausea, vomiting, sweating, abdominal tenderness or distension, right upper abdominal pain, yellowing of the skin or eyes, dark urine.
* Advise patient that medication may cause drowsiness, constipation, redness of the face, skin rash, itching, and hair loss and to notify health care provider if these occur and are bothersome or intolerable.
* Advise women of childbearing potential to use effective contraception during therapy.
* Advise women to notify health care provider if pregnant, planning to become pregnant, or breastfeeding.
* Advise patient that drug may cause drowsiness and to use caution while driving or performing other tasks requiring mental alertness until tolerance is determined.
* Instruct patient to not take any prescription or OTC medications or dietary supplements unless advised by health care provider.
* Advise patient that follow-up examinations and lab tests will be required to monitor therapy and to keep appointments.

Hydroxyzine

(high-DROX-ih-zeen HIGH-droe-KLOR-ide)
Class Antipsychotic/Antihistamine
How Supplied
Atarax Syrup 10 mg per 5 mL ♦ *Hydroxyzine Hydrochloride* Tablets 10 mg, Tablets 25 mg, Tablets 50 mg, Syrup 10 mg per 5 mL ♦ *Vistaril* Capsules 25 mg, Capsules 50 mg, Capsules 100 mg, Oral suspension 25 mg/5 mL, Injection 25 mg/mL
🍁 *Apo-Hydroxyzine* ♦ *Novo-Hydroxyzin* ♦ *Nu-Hydroxyzine* ♦ *PMS-Hydroxyzine*
Action
PHARMACOLOGY: May be caused by suppression of activity in subcortical areas of CNS.

PHARMACOKINETICS/DYNAMICS:
Absorption: Hydroxyzine is readily absorbed in the GI tract. T_{max} is approximately 3 hr and C_{max} is 82 ng/mL.
Metabolism: Hydroxyzine is metabolized by the liver.
Excretion: The mean t½ is 3 hr (reported to be up to 20 hr; may be longer in elderly).
Onset: Onset is 15 to 30 min (oral).
Peak: Time to peak is 1 to 2 hr.
Duration: Duration is 4 to 6 hr.
Indications Symptomatic relief of anxiety and tension associated with psychoneurosis; adjunct therapy in organic disease states with anxiety; management of pruritus caused by allergic conditions; sedative before and after general anesthesia (PO, IM).
IM route only: Relief of anxiety in acutely disturbed or hysterical patient; treatment of alcoholic delirium tremens or anxiety withdrawal symptoms; preoperative, postoperative, prepartum, and postpartum adjunctive medication to permit reduction in narcotic dosage; alleviation of anxiety; control of emesis; adjunctive therapy in asthma.

Contraindications Standard considerations.
Route/Dosage
Anxiety
ADULTS: PO/IM 50 to 100 mg qid.
CHILDREN OVER 6 YR: PO 50 to 100 mg/day in divided doses.
CHILDREN LESS THAN 6 YR: PO 50 mg/day in divided doses.

Nausea, Vomiting, and Analgesia (Adjunct)
ADULTS: IM 25 to 100 mg.
CHILDREN: IM 1.1 mg/kg.

Preoperative and Postoperative Administration
ADULTS: IM 25 to 100 mg.
CHILDREN: IM 1.1 mg/kg.

Prepartum and Postpartum Administration
ADULTS: IM 25 to 100 mg

Pruritus
ADULTS: PO/IM 25 mg tid to qid.
CHILDREN OVER 6 YR: PO 50 to 100 mg/day in divided doses.
CHILDREN LESS THAN 6 YR: PO 50 mg/day in divided doses.

Psychiatric and Emotional Emergencies (ie, acute alcoholism)
ADULTS: IM 50 to 100 mg stat and q 4 to 6 hr prn.

Sedation
ADULTS: PO/IM 50 to 100 mg.

CHILDREN: **PO/IM** 0.6 mg/kg.

Interactions
Alcohol and CNS depressants: CNS depressant effects may be increased.

Lab Test Interferences None well documented.

Adverse Reactions
CV: Chest tightness.
CNS: Transitory drowsiness; involuntary motor activity, including tremor and convulsions.
GI: Dry mouth.
RESP: Hypersensitivity reactions (eg, wheezing, shortness of breath).

Precautions
Pregnancy: Safety not established; avoid use.
Lactation: Undetermined.

Overdosage: Signs and Symptoms
Oversedation.

PATIENT CARE CONSIDERATIONS

Administration/Storage
- Administer prescribed dose without regard to meals. Administer with food if GI upset occurs.
- Shake suspension well before measuring dose.
- Measure dose of syrup or suspension using dosing cup, spoon, or syringe.

Injection:
- For IM administration only. Not for intradermal, SC, IV, or intra-arterial administration.
- Do not administer if particulate matter, cloudiness, or discoloration noted.
- Administer prescribed dose to adults by deep IM injection into the upper outer quadrant of the buttock or mid-lateral thigh.
- Administer prescribed dose to children by deep IM injection into mid-lateral muscles of the thigh. Avoid upper outer quadrant of gluteal region unless absolutely necessary (eg, burn patient).
- Store capsules, tablets, syrup, suspension, and injection at controlled room temperature (59° to 86°F).

Assessment/Interventions
- Obtain patient history, including drug history and any known allergies. Note coadministration of CNS depressants (eg, narcotics, barbiturates).
- Ensure that women of childbearing potential are not pregnant when therapy is initiated.
- Ensure that reduced dose and slower dose escalation is used in elderly patient.
- Frequently assess patient for response to treatment (eg, anxiety, pruritus). Notify health care provider if condition does not appear to be improving or is worsening.
- Ensure that therapy is periodically reviewed to determine if it needs to be continued without change or if a dose change (eg, increase, decrease, discontinuation) is indicated.
- Monitor patient for CNS, GI, and general body side effects. Report to health care provider if noted and significant. Implement safety precautions if excessive drowsiness or dizziness occurs.

Patient/Family Education
- Explain name, dose, action, and potential side effects of drug.
- Advise patient that medication is usually started at a low dose and then gradually increased until max benefit is obtained.
- Caution patient to take as prescribed and not to stop taking or change the dose unless advised by health care provider.
- Advise patient to take as prescribed without regard to meals but to take with food if stomach upset occurs.
- Instruct patient to contact health care provider if symptoms do not appear to be getting better, are getting worse, or if bothersome side effects (eg, drowsiness, dizziness) occur.
- Caution patient not to take any OTC antihistamines while taking this medication unless advised by health care provider.
- Caution patient to avoid alcohol and other CNS depressants (eg, sedatives) while using this medication.
- Caution patient that drug may cause drowsiness and to use caution driving or performing other tasks requiring mental alertness until tolerance is determined.
- Advise patient to take frequent sips of water, suck on ice chips or sugarless hard candy, or chew sugarless gum if dry mouth occurs.
- Advise women to notify health care provider if pregnant, planning to become pregnant, or breastfeeding.
- Caution patient to not take any prescription or OTC medications or dietary supplements unless advised by health care provider.
- Advise patient that follow-up visits may be necessary to monitor therapy and to keep appointments.

Hyoscyamine Sulfate

(hye-oh-SYE-a-mean)

Class Belladonna alkaloid

How Supplied

Anaspaz Tablets 0.125 mg ♦ *A-Spas S/L* Tablets, sublingual 0.125 mg ♦ *Cystospaz* Tablets 0.125 mg ♦ *Donnamar* Tablets 0.125 mg ♦ *ED-SPAZ* Tablets 0.125 mg ♦ *Gastrosed* Tablets 0.125 mg, Solution 0.125 mg/mL ♦ *Levbid* Tablets, extended-release 0.375 mg ♦ *Levsin* Tablets 0.125 mg, Elixir 0.125 mg/5 mL, Injection 0.5 mg/mL ♦ *Levsin Drops* Solution 0.125 mg/mL ♦ *Levsin/SL* Tablets, sublingual 0.125 mg ♦ *Levsinex Timecaps* Capsules, timed-release 0.375 mg ♦ *NuLev* Tablets, orally-disintegrating 0.125 mg

Action

PHARMACOLOGY: Inhibits the action of acetylcholine on structures innervated by postganglionic cholinergic nerves and on smooth muscles. These receptors are located in the autonomic effector cells of the smooth muscle, cardiac muscle, sinoatrial node, atrioventricular node, and exocrine glands. Inhibits GI propulsive motility and decreases gastric acid secretion. Controls excessive pharyngeal, tracheal, and bronchial secretions.

Indications To control gastric secretion, visceral spasm, hypermotility in spastic colitis, spastic bladder, cystitis, pylorospasm, and associated abdominal cramps; to reduce symptoms of functional intestinal disorders such as those seen with mild dysentery, diverticulitis, and acute enterocolitis; treatment of infant colic; as a "drying" agent in rhinitis; to reduce rigidity and tremors, and to control sialorrhea and hyperhidrosis of Parkinson disease; with morphine or other narcotics for symptomatic relief of biliary and renal colic; poisoning by anticholinesterase agents; adjunct in treatment of peptic ulcer, irritable bowel syndrome, functional GI disorders, neurogenic bladder, and neurogenic bowel disturbances; preoperative to reduce secretions; block cardiac vagal inhibitory reflexes during anesthesia induction and intubation.

Contraindications Glaucoma; obstructive uropathy; obstructive disease of the GI tract; paralytic ileus; intestinal atony in the elderly or debilitated; unstable cardiovascular status in acute hemorrhage; severe ulcerative colitis; toxic megacolon complicating ulcerative colitis; myasthenia gravis.

Route/Dosage

ADULTS: **PO** 0.125 to 0.25 mg q 4 hr or prn orally or sublingually (max, 12 tablets per 24 hr), 0.375 to 0.75 mg in sustained-release form q 12 hr (max, 4 tablets in 24 hr).

CHILDREN (2 TO 12 YR): **PO** (½ to 1 tablet) 0.0625 to 0.125 mg q 4 hr or prn (max, 6 tablets per 24 hr), 0.25 to 1 tsp (0.031 to 0.125 mg) of 0.125 mg/5 mL solution q 4 hr or prn (max, 12 mL in 24 hr).

CHILDREN (2 YR AND YOUNGER): **PO** Dosing of 0.125 mg/mL drops (as based on body weight) q 4 hr or prn (max, 6 doses in 24 hr) is:

CHILDREN'S DOSING IN RELATION TO BODY WEIGHT

Body weight	Usual dosage
2.3 kg (5 lb)	3 drops
3.4 kg (7.5 lb)	4 drops
5 kg (11 lb)	5 drops
7 kg (15 lb)	6 drops
10 kg (22 lb)	0.25 tsp (0.031 mg) or 8 drops
15 kg (33 lb)	11 drops
20 kg (44 lb)	0.5 tsp (0.063 mg)
40 kg (88 lb)	0.75 tsp (0.094 mg)
50 kg (110 lb)	1 tsp (0.125 mg)

ADULT: **SC/IM/IV** 0.25 to 0.5 mg bid to qid as needed.

Interactions

Antacids: Antacids may interfere with absorption of hyoscyamine.

Antimuscarinics, such as amantadine, haloperidol, phenothiazines, MAO inhibitors, tricyclic antidepressants, and some antihistamines: Additive anticholinergic effect when used with these drugs.

Lab Test Interferences None well documented.

Adverse Reactions

CNS: Headache; nervousness; drowsiness; weakness; dizziness; confusion, insomnia; fever; excitability; restlessness; tremor; speech disturbance.
CV: Palpitations; tachycardia.
DERM: Allergic reactions; urticaria; rash; flushing.
EENT: Nasal congestion; altered taste; mydriasis; cycloplegia; blurred vision; increased ocular tension.
GI: Xerostomia; nausea; vomiting; dysphagia;

heartburn constipation, bloated feeling; paralytic ileus.
GU: Urinary hesitancy and retention; impotence.
OTHER: Suppressed lactation; decreased sweating.

Precautions
Pregnancy: Category C.
Lactation: Excreted in human milk.
Children: Use cautiously in infants.
Special risk patients: Use cautiously in patients with autonomic neuropathy, hyperthyroidism, coronary artery disease, CHF, cardiac arrhythmias, tachycardia, hypertension, renal disease, and hiatal hernia associated with reflux esophagitis.
Drug-induced psychosis: Drug-induced psychosis has been reported in sensitive patients.
Diarrhea: Diarrhea may be an early sign of intestinal obstruction; hyoscyamine treatment would be inappropriate.
Heat prostration: Heat prostration may occur at high environmental temperatures.

Ibuprofen

(eye-BYOO-pro-fen)
Class Analgesic/NSAID

How Supplied
Advil Tablets 200 mg ♦ Advil Liqui-Gels Capsules 200 mg ♦ Advil Migraine Capsules 200 mg ♦ Children's Advil Tablets, chewable 50 mg, Suspension 100 mg/5 mL ♦ Children's Motrin Tablets, chewable 50 mg, Suspension 100 mg/5 mL ♦ Genpril Tablets 200 mg ♦ Haltran Tablets 200 mg ♦ Infant's Motrin Oral drops 40 mg/mL ♦ Junior Strength Advil Tablets, chewable 100 mg ♦ Junior Strength Motrin Tablets 100 mg, Tablets, chewable 100 mg ♦ Menadol Tablets 200 mg ♦ Midol Maximum Strength Cramp Formula Tablets 200 mg ♦ Motrin Tablets 400 mg, Tablets 600 mg, Tablets 800 mg ♦ Motrin IB Tablets 200 mg ♦ Motrin Migraine Pain Tablets 200 mg ♦ Nuprin Tablets 200 mg ♦ PediaCare Fever Suspension 100 mg/5 mL, Oral drops 40 mg/mL ♦ Pediatric Advil Drops Suspension 100 mg/2.5 mL ❈ Apo-Ibuprofen ♦ Motrin IB Extra Strength ♦ Motrin IB Super Strength ♦ Novo-Profen ♦ Nu-Ibuprofen

Action
PHARMACOLOGY: Decreases inflammation, pain, and fever, probably through inhibition of cyclooxygenase activity and prostaglandin synthesis.

PHARMACOKINETICS/DYNAMICS:
Absorption: T_{max} is 1 to 2 hr. Bioavailability is less than 80%.
Distribution: Vd is 0.15 L/kg. 99% protein bound.
Excretion: Plasma $t_{1/2}$ is 1.8 to 2 hr. 45% to 79% is eliminated through the urine. Cl is 3 to 35 L/hr.

Indications Relief of symptoms of rheumatoid arthritis, osteoarthritis, mild-to-moderate pain, primary dysmenorrhea, reduction of fever.
Unlabeled use(s): Symptomatic treatment of juvenile rheumatoid arthritis, sunburn, resistant acne vulgaris.

Contraindications Hypersensitivity to aspirin, iodides, or any other NSAID.

Route/Dosage
Rheumatoid Arthritis and Osteoarthritis
ADULTS: PO 300 to 800 mg tid to qid, not to exceed 3.2 g/day.

Mild-to-Moderate Pain
ADULTS: PO 400 mg q 4 to 6 hr prn.

Primary Dysmenorrhea
ADULTS: PO 400 mg q 4 hr prn.

Juvenile Arthritis
CHILDREN: PO 30 to 40 mg/kg/day in 3 to 4 divided doses.

Fever Reduction
CHILDREN 1 TO 12 YR: 39.2°C (102.5°F) and less recommended dose PO 5 mg/kg; more than 39.2°C (102.5°F) recommended dose PO 10 mg/kg; max daily dose 40 mg/kg.

OTC Use (Minor Aches/Pains, Dysmenorrhea, Fever Reduction)
PO 200 mg q 4 to 6 hr. Do not exceed 1.2 g in 24 hr or take for pain for more than 10 days or for fever for more than 3 days, unless directed by health care provider. Use smallest effective dose.

Interactions
Beta-blockers: Antihypertensive effect may be decreased.
Digoxin: Ibuprofen may increase digoxin serum levels.
Lithium: May increase lithium levels.
Loop diuretics: Diuretic effects may be decreased.
Methotrexate: May increase methotrexate levels.
Warfarin: May increase risk of gastric erosion and bleeding.

Lab Test Interferences None well documented.

Adverse Reactions
CV: Peripheral edema; water retention; worsening or precipitation of CHF.
CNS: Dizziness; lightheadedness; drowsiness; vertigo; headaches; aseptic meningitis.
DERM: Rash; pruritus; erythema.
EENT: Visual disturbances; photophobia; tinnitus.
GI: Gastric distress; occult blood loss; diarrhea; vomiting; nausea; heartburn; dyspepsia; anorexia; constipation; abdominal distress/cramps/pain; flatulence; indigestion; GI tract fullness.
GU: Menometrorrhagia; hematuria; cystitis; acute renal insufficiency; interstitial nephritis; hyperkalemia; hyponatremia; renal papillary necrosis.
OTHER: Muscle cramps.

Precautions
Pregnancy: Undetermined.
Lactation: Undetermined.
Children: Safety and efficacy not established.
Elderly: Increased risk of adverse reactions.
Renal function impairment: Increased risk of dysfunction in patients with preexisting renal disease.
GI effects: Serious GI toxicity (eg, bleeding, ulceration, perforation) can occur at any time, with or without warning symptoms.

Overdosage: Signs and Symptoms
Drowsiness, lethargy, GI irritation/bleeding, nausea, vomiting, tinnitus, sweating, acute renal failure, epigastric pain, metabolic acidosis.

PATIENT CARE CONSIDERATIONS

Administration/Storage
- Give medication soon after meals or with food, milk, or antacids to minimize GI irritation.

Assessment/Interventions
- Obtain complete patient history, including drug history and any known allergies.
- Notify health care provider if visual changes or indications of GI distress or liver or renal impairment occur.
- Monitor patient's following cardiac status: BP, pulse (eg, quality and rhythm), edema, tachycardia, palpitations.
- Assess renal function before and during therapy. Monitor serum creatinine, Ccr, and BUN in patients with renal impairment.
- Document any changes in liver function (AST, ALT), eye examinations, and Hgb and Hct in patients on long-term therapy.
- Notify health care provider if indigestion, epigastric pain, unusual bleeding or bruising, or dark tarry stools occur.

Patient/Family Education
- Tell patient to take medication soon after meals or with food, milk, or antacids.
- Tell patient to avoid alcohol and medications containing aspirin, such as cold remedies.
- Advise patient to discontinue drug and notify health care provider if any of the following occur: persistent GI upset or headache, skin rash, itching, visual disturbances, black stools, weight gain or edema, changes in urine pattern, joint pain, fever, blood in urine.
- Instruct patient not to take OTC preparation for more than 3 days for fever and more than 10 days for pain and to notify health care provider if condition does not improve.
- Advise patient that drug may cause drowsiness and to use caution while driving or performing other tasks requiring mental alertness.

Ibutilide Fumarate

(ih-BYOO-tih-lide FEW-muh-rate)

Class Antiarrhythmic

How Supplied
Corvert Solution 0.1 mg/mL

Action
PHARMACOLOGY: Prolongs atrial and ventricular action potential duration and refractoriness by activation of a slow inward current (predominantly sodium).

PHARMACOKINETICS/DYNAMICS:
Distribution: Vd_{ss} is approximately 11 L/kg. Approximately 40% is protein bound.
Metabolism: 8 metabolites are formed via oxidation. Only the -hydroxy metabolite possesses activity similar to ibutilide.
Excretion: Cl is 29 mL/min/kg. Approximately 82% is excreted in the urine (7% unchanged) and approximately 19% in feces. The mean $t_{1/2}$ is approximately 6 hr (range is 2 to 12 hr).

Indications
Rapid conversion of recent onset atrial fibrillation or atrial flutter to sinus rhythm.

Contraindications
Standard considerations.

Route/Dosage
ADULTS: **IV** Initial infusion: At least 60 kg (at least 132 lbs) 1 mg (1 vial) infused over 10 min; less than 60 kg (less than 132 lbs) 0.01 mg/kg (0.1 mL/kg) infused over 10 min. If the arrhythmia does not terminate within 10 min after the end of the initial infusion, a second 10 min infusion of equal strength may be administered 10 min after completion of the first infusion.

Interactions
Concomitant Class Ia and III antiarrhythmic agents (eg, amiodarone, disopyramide, procainamide, quinidine, sotalol): Do not give concurrently. Withhold for 5 half-lives prior to and for 4 hr after ibutilide infusion.
Medications that prolong the QT interval (eg, phenothiazines, tricyclic and tetracyclic antidepressants): Potential for proarrhythmia may be increased.
Digoxin: Cardiotoxicity (supraventricular arrhythmia) due to excessive digoxin concentrations may be masked.

Lab Test Interferences
None well documented.

Adverse Reactions
CV: Nonsustained monomorphic ventricular extrasystoles and ventricular tachycardia (VT); sinus; supraventricular sustained and nonsustained polymorphic VT; hypotension; postural hypotension; hypertension; bundle branch block; sustained polymorphic VT; AV block; sinus bradycardia; QT segment prolongation; palpitations.
CNS: Headache.
GI: Nausea.

WARNING:
Experienced physician/equipped facility. Potentially fatal arrhythmias have occurred and require administration in a setting of continuous ECG monitoring and personnel trained in identification and treatment of acute ventricular arrhythmias, particularly polymorphic ventricular tachycardia.

Patient selection: Patients with chronic atrial fibrillation have a strong tendency to revert after conversion to sinus rhythm, and treatment to maintain sinus rhythms carry risks. Patients for ibutilide therapy should be carefully selected.

Precautions
Pregnancy: Category C.
Lactation: Undetermined.
Children: Safety and efficacy not established.
Elderly: No age-related differences in safety and efficacy have been observed.
Hypokalemia/Hypomagnesemia: Correct hypokalemia/hypomagnesemia to reduce potential for proarrhythmia.
Anticoagulation: Patients with atrial fibrillation more than 2 to 3 days must be adequately anticoagulated, generally for at least 2 wk before attempted conversion.

Overdosage: Signs and Symptoms
CNS toxicity, rapid gasping breathing, convulsions, ventricular ectopy, ventricular tachycardia, AV block.

PATIENT CARE CONSIDERATIONS
Administration/Storage
- Available for IV administration only.
- Store unopened vials at room temperature (59° to 86°F).
- May be administered undiluted or further diluted in 50 mL of either Normal Saline (NS) or D5W.
- Diluted medication may be stored for up to 24 hr at room temperature (59° to 86°F), or for 48 hr refrigerated (36° to 46°F), following where any unused solution should be discarded.

Assessment/Interventions
- Obtain patient history, including drug history and any known allergies. Note use of antiarrhythmics (eg, Class Ia or III) or other agents (eg, phenothiazines, tricyclic antidepressants) that may increase arrhythmia risk.
- Obtain baseline 12-lead ECG, electrolytes, and LFTs prior to treatment.
- Ensure that potassium and magnesium serum levels are within normal levels.
- Ensure that any Class Ia or III antiarrhythmics have been discontinued for at least 5 half-lives.
- Observe patient with continuous ECG monitoring for at least 4 hours following infusion or until QTc has returned to baseline. Longer monitoring is required if any arrhythmic activity is noted or if patient has abnormal LFTs.
- Monitor blood pressure and pulse closely during administration.
- Have appropriate resuscitation equipment at bedside (eg, cardioverter/defibrillator, medications) during therapy.

Patient/Family Education
- Advise patient that this is a short-term treatment for arrhythmia, and long-term oral medications will likely be required for control if this therapy is successful.
- Teach patient and family how to take blood pressure and pulse for home management with medications.
- Advise patient to report any chest pain, shortness of breath, palpitations, fluttering in the chest, headache, or faintness immediately to the health care provider while the medication is infusing.

Idarubicin

(eye-DUH-RUE-bih-sin)

Class Antineoplastic antibiotic/Anthracycline

How Supplied

Idamycin PFS Solution for injection 1 mg/mL

Action

PHARMACOLOGY: Idarubicin is a DNA-intercalating analog of daunorubicin, which has an inhibitory effect on nucleic acid synthesis and interacts with the enzyme topoisomerase II.

PHARMACOKINETICS/DYNAMICS:

Distribution: Approximately 97% is protein bound, 94% (active metabolite).

Metabolism: The major metabolite is idarubicinol (active metabolite). Extensive extra hepatic metabolism.

Excretion: The t½ is approximately 22 hr. The t½ is at least 45 hr (active metabolite). Primarily excreted by biliary and, to a lesser extent, by renal excretion.

Special Populations:

Renal Function Impairment – Possible impaired metabolism and the disposition also may be affected. Consider dose reduction.

Hepatic Function Impairment – Possible impaired metabolism and the disposition may also be affected. Consider dose reduction.

Indications Acute myelocytic leukemia as part of a combination chemotherapy regimen.

Contraindications Standard considerations.

Route/Dosage

ADULTS: IV *Induction therapy in combination with other chemotherapeutic drugs*: Idarubicin 12 mg/m^2/day for 3 days by slow (10 to 15 minutes) IV injection in combination with cytarabine; may give second course if needed. Reduce dosage of subsequent courses 25% in patients experiencing severe mucositis. Delay therapy until recovery from mucositis occurs.

Interactions None well documented.

Lab Test Interferences None well documented.

Adverse Reactions

CV: CHF; serious arrhythmias (including atrial fibrillation); chest pain; MI; asymptomatic declines in left ventricular ejection fraction.
CNS: Headache (20%); neurologic involvement of peripheral nerves (7%); seizure (4%).
DERM: Hair loss (77%).
GI: Nausea/vomiting (82%); abdominal cramps/diarrhea (73%); mucositis (50%); severe enterocolitis with perforation (rare).
GU: Severe changes in renal function (1% or less).
HEPA: Changes in hepatic functions (less than 5%).
HEMA/LYMPH: Hemorrhage (63%); myelosuppression.
LOCAL: Hives.
RESP: Pulmonary allergy (2%).
OTHER: Infection (95%); fever (26%).

> WARNING:
>
> *IV use only:* Do not administer IM or subcutaneously.
>
> *Extravasation:* Local irritation or phlebitis may occur. Refer to your institution-specific protocol. Give idarubicin slowly into a freely flowing IV infusion; never give IM or subcutaneously. Extravasation may occur with or without an accompanying stinging or burning sensation even if blood returns well on aspiration of the infusion needle. If signs or symptoms of extravasation occur, terminate the injection or infusion immediately and restart in another vein.
>
> *Myocardial toxicity:* Idarubicin can cause myocardial toxicity, leading to potentially fatal CHF, acute life-threatening arrhythmias, or other cardiomyopathies. Cardiac toxicity is more common in patients who have received prior anthracyclines or who have preexisting cardiac disease.
>
> *Myelosuppression:* Severe myelosuppression occurs in all patients when idarubicin is used at therapeutic doses for induction, consolidation, or maintenance.

Precautions

Pregnancy: Category D.
Lactation: Undetermined. Discontinue nursing prior to taking this drug.
Children: Safety and efficacy not established.
Hepatic/Renal function impairment: Reduce dosage in patients with impaired hepatic or renal function. Do not administer if the bilirubin level is more than 5 mg/dL.
Bone marrow suppression: Idarubicin is a potent bone marrow suppressant. Do not give to patients with preexisting bone marrow suppression induced by previous drug therapy or radiotherapy unless the benefit warrants the risk.
Cardiac toxicity: Pre-existing heart disease and previous therapy with anthracyclines at high cumulative doses or other potentially cardiotoxic agents are co-factors for increased risk of idarubicin-induced cardiac toxicity.

Extravasation: Idarubicin can cause severe local tissue necrosis, which may occur with or without accompanying stinging or burning sensation.

PATIENT CARE CONSIDERATIONS
Administration/Storage
- Used in combination with other antileukemic medications.
- For IV infusion only. Not for IV bolus, intradermal, subcutaneous, IM, or intra-arterial administration.
- Diligently follow institutional and NIH procedures for handling, administration, and disposal of anticancer drugs. Wear appropriate protective equipment when preparing and administering idarubicin. Avoid exposure by direct contact of the skin, mucous membranes, and eyes.
- If accidental skin or mucus membrane contact occurs, wash thoroughly with soap and water. If accidental eye contact occurs, immediately institute standard irrigation techniques.
- Do not administer if particulate matter or cloudiness is noted. Solution has a red-orange color which is normal and of no concern.
- Administer prescribed dose slowly (over 10 to 15 minutes) into freely flowing IV infusion of 0.9% sodium chloride injection or 5% dextrose in water injection. Attach tubing to butterfly needle or other suitable device and insert into large vein. Take precautions to avoid extravasation.
- Discard unused portions of vial. Do not save any unused portions for future use.
- Do not mix with any other medications. Flush infusion line with D5W or 0.9% sodium chloride injection prior to administration of any concomitant medication.
- Store vials in refrigerator (36° to 46°F). Protect from light. Retain in original carton until time of use.

Assessment/Interventions
- Obtain patient history, including drug history and any known allergies. Note renal or hepatic impairment, bone marrow suppression, cardiac disease, anemia, infection, leukemic pericarditis and/or myocarditis, concomitant or previous radiation to mediastinal-pericardial area, or history of prior anthracycline therapy.
- Ensure active infection has been controlled before initiating or resuming therapy with idarubicin.
- Ensure cardiac function is evaluated and documented before starting therapy and periodically during treatment. Monitor patient for evidence of heart failure or arrhythmias during treatment and be prepared to treat appropriately.
- Ensure CBC with differential, liver enzymes, bilirubin, and renal function tests are done prior to and frequently during treatment.
- Ensure reduced dose is administered to patient with renal or hepatic impairment following manufacturer's guidelines and that medication is not administered to patient with bilirubin greater than 5 mg/dL.
- Ensure women of childbearing potential are not pregnant before starting therapy and use effective contraception during treatment.
- Ensure risk of developing hyperuricemia is evaluated before starting therapy and that hypouricemic therapy, including adequate fluid intake, and monitoring of uric acid, is initiated before starting treatment in patient determined to be at risk for developing hyperuricemia and urate precipitation.
- Monitor patient for signs or symptoms of infection or bleeding. Inform health care provider immediately if noted and be prepared to treat appropriately (eg, IV antibiotics, colony stimulating factors, transfusions).
- Monitor IV infusion site for signs or symptoms of extravasation. If noted, immediately discontinue infusion and restart in another vein. Be prepared to treat extravasation site with intermittent ice packs (½ hr immediately, then ½ hr qid for 3 days) and extremity elevation. Frequently examine extravasation site and immediately inform health care provider if pain, erythema, edema, or vesiculation is noted or if patient reports persistent pain.
- Monitor patient for CV, CNS, GI, RESP, HEMA, DERM, and general body side effects. Report to health care provider if noted and significant. Ensure that second course of therapy is withheld for patient who experienced severe mucositis until recovery has occurred and that subsequent doses are reduced 25%.

Patient/Family Education
- Explain name, action, and potential side effects of drug.
- Advise patient, family, or caregiver that medication will be prepared and administered by health care provider in a health care setting.
- Advise patient, family, or caregiver that medication will be used in combination with other agents to achieve max benefit possible.

Overdosage: Signs and Symptoms
Severe and prolonged myelosuppression. Possibly increased severity of GI toxicity.

- Review dosing schedule with patient, family, or caregiver.
- Advise patient, family, or caregiver that medication will usually cause a red coloration of the urine. Advise that this is not a problem and is expected because the medication is being eliminated in the urine.
- Advise patient, family, or caregiver that medication may cause hair loss but that this is reversible when therapy is stopped.
- Advise patient, family, or caregiver to immediately report any of the following to health care provider: rash; hives; difficulty breathing; chest pain; fever, chills or other signs of infection; sores in mouth; unusual bleeding or bruising; pain, redness, or swelling at injection site.
- Advise patient, family, or caregiver to report any of the following to health care provider: persistent nausea, vomiting, diarrhea, or appetite loss; persistent or worsening general body weakness.
- Instruct patient to not take any prescription or OTC medications, herbal preparations, or dietary supplements unless advised by health care provider.
- Advise women to notify health care provider if pregnant, planning to become pregnant, or breastfeeding.
- Advise patient that following discharge from the hospital that frequent follow-up visits, ECGs or heart function tests, and laboratory tests will be required to monitor therapy and to keep appointments.

Idoxuridine (IDU)

(EYE-dox-YOU-rih-deen)
Class Ophthalmic/Antiviral

How Supplied
Herplex Solution 0.1%
✤ *Herplex-D*

Action
PHARMACOLOGY: Blocks reproduction of herpes simplex virus by irreversibly inhibiting incorporation of thymidine into viral DNA.

Indications Treatment of herpes simplex keratitis.

Contraindications Standard considerations.

Route/Dosage
ADULTS: **Ophthalmic solution** Instill 1 gtt into infected eye(s) q hr during day and q 2 hr during night. Alternate schedule: Instill 1 gtt q 1 min for 5 min; repeat q 4 hr night and day.

Ointment Apply ointment to infected conjunctival sac q 4 hr (5 applications daily).

Interactions *Boric acid-containing solution:* May cause irritation; do not coadminister.

Lab Test Interferences None well documented.

Adverse Reactions
EENT: Ocular irritation, pain, pruritus, inflammation or edema; photophobia; corneal clouding; stippling; punctate defects in corneal epithelium; follicular conjunctivitis; puncta occlusion; conjunctival scarring.

Precautions
Pregnancy: Category C.
Lactation: Undetermined.
Children: Safety and efficacy not established.
Carcinogenesis: Based on animal studies, may be carcinogenic.
Recurrence: Continue medication for 5 to 7 days after epithelial healing to avoid recurrence.

PATIENT CARE CONSIDERATIONS

Administration/Storage
- For patient convenience, drops may be prescribed for waking hours and ointment for nighttime.
- Wash hands before and after instillation of solution or ointment.
- Do not mix with other topical eye medications.
- Store at room temperature and protect from light.

Assessment/Interventions
- Obtain complete patient history, including drug history and any known allergies.
- Assess for allergy, itching, lacrimation, redness, or swelling.
- Withhold drug and contact health care provider if unusual changes or inflammation of eye occur.

Patient/Family Education
- Demonstrate proper technique for instillation of drops or ointment, emphasizing importance of hand-washing and of not touching cap or tip of tube to eye, conjunctiva, fingers, or any unsterile object.
- Inform patient that vision may be hazy for short time after instillation.
- Explain importance of continuing medication for prescribed time even after healing has occurred, to avoid recurrence.
- Advise patient to wear sunglasses and to avoid prolonged exposure to bright light.
- Instruct patient to notify health care provider if condition worsens or if no improvement is noted in 2 wk. Contact health care provider if burning or stinging occurs.
- Caution patient not to use any other medica-

tions on eye such as boric acid.
- Warn patient not to use other peoples eye makeup, towels, washcloths, or eye medications; reinfection may occur.

- Instruct patient to report the following symptoms to health care provider: visual changes, pain, itching or swelling of eye.

Ifosfamide

(eye-FOSS-fuh-MIDE)
Class Alkylating agent/Nitrogen mustard
How Supplied
Ifex Powder for injection 1,000 mg, Powder for injection 3,000 mg

Action
PHARMACOLOGY: Ifosfamide requires metabolic activation by microsomal liver enzymes to produce biologically active metabolites. Enzymatic oxidation of the chloroethyl side chains and subsequent dealkylation produces the major urinary metabolites, dichloroethyl ifosfamide and dichloroethyl cyclophosphamide. The alkylated metabolites of ifosfamide interact with DNA.

PHARMACOKINETICS/DYNAMICS:
Metabolism: Requires metabolic activation by hydroxylation.

Excretion: Mean t½ is approximately 15 hr (at doses of 3.8 to 5 g/m^2). Mean t½ is approximately 7 hr (at doses of 1.6 to 2.4 g/m^2). 70% to 86% is excreted in the urine.

Indications Germ cell testicular cancer.
Unlabeled use(s): Soft-tissue, Ewing and osteogenic sarcomas; non-Hodgkin lymphomas; small cell lung, pancreatic, bladder, cervical, and ovarian carcinoma.

Contraindications Continued use in patients with severely depressed bone marrow function; hypersensitivity to ifosfamide.

Route/Dosage
Germ Cell Testicular Cancer
ADULTS: IV 1,200 mg/m^2/day for 5 days, repeating this course q 3 wk. Delay further courses until platelets are least 100,000/mm^3 and WBC at least 4,000/mm^3.

Germ Cell Testicular Cancer, Other Regimens
ADULTS: IV Other regimens use ifosfamide 2,000 mg/m^2/day on days 1 through 3 (MAID regimen, total dose is 6,000 mg/m^2 over 72 hr), or doses as high as 5,000 mg/m^2 continuous infusion for 24 hr in combination with other antineoplastics.

Interactions Ifosfamide may increase the hypoprothrombinemic effect of warfarin.
Lab Test Interferences None well documented.

Adverse Reactions
CNS: Somnolence; confusion; depression; hallucinations. CNS effects more common in patients with renal dysfunction, hypoalbuminemia, or receiving large single doses.
DERM: Alopecia.
GI: Moderate potential for nausea and vomiting; elevated liver function tests.
GU: Hematuria, dysuria, urinary frequency; hemorrhagic cystitis, which can be prevented with the administration of mesna.
HEMA: Bone marrow suppression, nadir at 7 to 14 days.
HYPERSEN: Allergic reactions observed with ifosfamide also can be attributed to mesna.
RENAL: Renal tubular acidosis; Fanconi-like syndrome.

> **WARNING:**
>
> *Urotoxic side effects:* Hemorrhagic cystitis frequently associated with ifosfamide. Obtain a urinalysis prior to each dose. Use ifosfamide with a protector, such as mesna, to prevent hemorrhagic cystitis.
>
> *Myelosuppression:* When given in combination with other chemotherapeutic agents, severe myelosuppression is frequent. It consisted mainly of leukopenia and, to a lesser extent, thrombocytopenia. A WBC count less than 3,000/mm^3 is expected in 50% of patients given ifosfamide alone at 1.2 g/m^2/day for 5 consecutive days. At this dose level, thrombocytopenia (platelets less than 100,000/mm^3) occurred in approximately 20% of patients. At total dosages of 10 to 12 g/m^2/cycle, 50% of the patients had a WBC count less than 1,000/mm^3 and 8% had platelet counts less than 50,000/mm^3. Myelosuppression is usually reversible, and treatment can be given q 3 to 4 wk. Close hematologic monitoring is recommended.
>
> *Neurologic manifestations:* Somnolence, confusion, hallucinations, and, in some instances, coma occurred.

Precautions
Pregnancy: Category D.
Lactation: Excreted in breast milk.
Children: Safety and efficacy not established.
Renal function impairment: Use with caution. Clinical signs (eg, elevation in BUN or serum

creatinine or decrease in Ccr) were usually transient and most likely related to tubular damage.
Hematuria: At doses of 1.2 g/m^2/day for 5 consecutive days without a protector, microscopic hematuria is expected in approximately 50% of the patients and gross hematuria in approximately 8% of patients. Dose fractionation, vigorous hydration and a protector (eg, mesna) can significantly reduce hematuria incidence, especially gross hematuria, associated with hemorrhagic cystitis.

PATIENT CARE CONSIDERATIONS
Administration/Storage
* Store powder at room temperature; avoid temperatures higher than 35°C.
* Reconstitute powder with sterile water for injection or bacteriostatic water for injection.
* Reconstitute 1,000 mg ifosfamide with 20 mL diluent for a final concentration of 50 mg/mL; 3,000 mg ifosfamide with 60 mL diluent for a final concentration of 50 mg/mL.
* Reconstituted 50 mg/mL solution may be further diluted to concentrations of 0.6 to 20 mg/mL with 5% dextrose, 0.9% sodium chloride, Lactated Ringer's solution, or sterile water for injection. Because stability is unchanged, other concentrations or mixtures of these solutions may be used, including 2.5% dextrose, 0.45% sodium chloride, or 5% dextrose with 0.9% sodium chloride.
* Ifosfamide, at a concentration of 100 mg/mL, is incompatible with bacteriostatic water for injection with benzyl alcohol. It is compatible at ifosfamide concentrations of up to 60 mg/mL.
* Solutions reconstituted with Bacteriostatic Water for Injection are stable for 1 wk at room temperature or 3 wk under refrigeration.
* Refrigerate solutions reconstituted with Sterile Water for Injection and use within 24 hr because they are preservative-free. The manufacturer recommends use within 6 hr of reconstitution.
* Diluted solutions are chemically stable for up to 1 wk at room temperature and for up to 6 wk under refrigeration in glass or plastic bags. Consider the possibility of microbial contamination of diluted solutions. Use preservative-free solutions within 24 hr.
* Administer by IV infusion, continuous IV infusion.
* Hydrate patient with at least 2 L/day of fluid, orally or IV, to reduce risk of ifosfamide-induced bladder toxicity.
* Slow IV infusion over at least 30 min.
* Give ifosfamide with mesna (a uroprotectant) to prevent hemorrhagic cystitis.

Assessment/Interventions
* Monitor WBC, platelet counts, and hemoglobin prior to each administration and at appropriate intervals. For WBC less than 2,000/mm^3 or platelet count less than 50,000/mm^3, give ifosfamide only in emergencies.
* Monitor urine for red blood cells and obtain urinalysis prior to each dose of ifosfamide. Withhold further therapy until complete resolution if microscopic hematuria occurs (more than 10 RBC/hpf).
* Monitor serum and urine chemistries including phosphorus, potassium, and alkaline phosphatase.

Patient/Family Education
* Notify health care provider of the following: unusual bleeding/bruising; fever; chills; sore throat; cough; shortness of breath; seizures; lack of menstrual flow; unusual lumps or masses; flank, stomach, or joint pain; sores in mouth or on lips; yellow discoloration of skin or eyes.
* Contraceptive measures are recommended during therapy for men and women.

Extravasation: Can cause local irritation or phlebitis. Refer to your institution-specific protocol.
Compromised bone marrow reserve: Administer cautiously to patients with leukopenia, granulocytopenia, extensive bone marrow metastases, prior therapy with radiation or other cytotoxic agents.
Wound healing: Ifosfamide may interfere with normal wound healing.

Imatinib

(eye-MAT-in-ib)
Class Tyrosine kinase inhibitor antineoplastic
How Supplied
Gleevec Tablets 100 mg, Tablets 400 mg
Action
PHARMACOLOGY: Imatinib inhibits proliferation and induces apoptosis in BCR-ABL positive cell lines as well as fresh leukemic cells from Philadelphia chromosome-positive (Ph+) chronic myeloid leukemia (CML). Imatinib inhibits tumor growth of BCR-ABL transfected murine myeloid cells and BCR-ABL positive leukemia lines derived from CML patients in blast crisis. It also inhibits the receptor tyrosine kinases for platelet-derived growth factor

(PDGF) and stem cell factor (SCF), c-Kit, and inhibits PDGF- and SCF-mediated cellular events.

PHARMACOKINETICS/DYNAMICS:
Absorption: T_{max} is 2 to 4 hr. Mean absolute bioavailability is 98% (capsule).

Distribution: Approximately 95% is protein bound.

Metabolism: In liver primarily via cytochrome P450 3A4 isoenzyme, minor: cytochrome P450 1A2, 2D6, 2C9, 2C19. Major metabolite is N-desmethyl derivative (active).

Excretion: The t½ is approximately 18 hr (parent drug) and 40 hr (major active metabolite); 68% is excreted in the feces and 13% in the urine primarily as metabolites. Cl increases with body weight: 50 kg = 8 L/hr and 100 kg = 14 L/hr.

Indications Treatment of newly diagnosed adult patients with Ph+ CML in chronic phase; patients with Ph+ CML in blast crisis, accelerated phase, or in chronic phase after failure of interferon-alpha treatment; children with Ph+ chronic phase CML whose disease has recurred after stem cell transplant or who are resistant to interferon-alpha therapy; treatment of gastrointestinal stromal tumors (GIST).

Contraindications Standard considerations.

Route/Dosage
Chronic Phase CML
ADULTS: PO 400 mg/day initially. Increase to 600 mg/day, as tolerated, in patients with disease progression, inadequate response to initial dose, or loss of previous hematologic response.
CHILDREN: PO 260 mg/m² daily initially. Increase to 340 mg/m² daily, as tolerated, in patients with disease progression, inadequate response to initial dose, or loss of previous hematologic response.

CML Treatment in Accelerated Phase, Blast Crisis, or Interferon-Refractory Chronic Phase
ADULTS: PO Continue imatinib as long as response is favorable. Assess therapeutic response after at least 3 mo of continued therapy.

CML in Accelerated Phase or Blast Crisis
ADULTS: PO 600 mg/day initially. Increase to 400 mg bid, as tolerated, in patients with disease progression, inadequate response to initial dose, or loss of previous hematologic response.

Dose Adjustments for Neutropenia and Thrombocytopenia in Patients with Accelerated Phase CML and Blast Crisis (starting dose 600 mg), Occurring After at Least 1 Month of Treatment
ADULTS: PO If absolute neutrophil count (ANC) is less than 0.5×10^9/L and/or platelets less than 10×10^9/L, check if cytopenia is related to leukemia by performing marrow aspirate or biopsy. If cytopenia is unrelated to imatinib, reduce dose to 400 mg. If cytopenia persists 2 wk, reduce dose to 300 mg. If cytopenia persists 4 wk and is still unrelated to leukopenia, stop imatinib until ANC is at least 1×10^9/L and platelets are at least 20×10^9/L, and then resume treatment at 300 mg.

Dose Adjustments for Neutropenia and Thrombocytopenia in Patients with Chronic Phase CML (starting dose 400 mg [adults] or 260 mg/m² [children]) or GIST (starting dose 400 or 600 mg)
ADULTS AND CHILDREN: PO If ANC less than 1×10^9/L and/or platelets less than 50×10^9/L, stop imatinib until ANC is at least 1.5×10^9/L and platelets are at least 75×10^9/L, then resume treatment at dose of 400 (children 260 mg) or 600 mg. If recurrence of ANC less than 1×10^9/L and/or platelets less than 50×10^9/L, stop imatinib until ANC is at least 1.5×10^9/L and platelets are at least 75×10^9/L, then resume at a reduced dose of 300 mg if starting dose was 400 mg (in children 200 mg/m² if starting dose was 260 mg/m²) or 400 mg if starting dose was 600 mg.

GISTs
ADULTS: PO 400 or 600 mg/day.

Hepatotoxicity or Severe Fluid Retention
ADULTS AND CHILDREN: PO If a severe nonhematologic adverse reaction develops (such as severe hepatotoxicity or severe fluid retention), withhold imatinib until the event has resolved. Thereafter, treatment can be resumed as appropriate depending on the initial severity of the event. If elevations in bilirubin are more than 3 times institutional upper limit of normal (IULN) or in liver transaminases more than 5 × IULN occur, withhold imatinib until bilirubin levels have returned to a less than 1.5 × IULN and transaminase levels to less than 2.5 × IULN. In adults, treatment with imatinib may then be continued at a reduced daily dose (ie, 400 to 300 mg or 600 to 400 mg). In children, daily doses can be reduced under the same circumstances from 260 to 200 mg/m²/day or from 340 to 260 mg/m²/day, respectively.

Interactions
Acetaminophen: Increased risk of hepatotoxicity.
Drugs that are metabolized by CYP2C9 (eg, fluvastatin, glimepiride, glipizide, glyburide, phenytoin, warfarin, some NSAIDs): Imatinib may reduce metabolism, resulting in increased concentrations and toxicity. Because warfarin if metabolized by CYP2C9 and CYP3A4, patients who require anticoagulation should receive low-

molecular weight or standard heparin.

Drugs that are metabolized by CYP2D6 (eg, propafenone, tricyclic antidepressants, some beta-adrenergic blockers, some SSRIs): Imatinib may reduce metabolism, resulting in increased concentrations and toxicity.

Drugs that induce CYP3A4 (eg, aminoglutethimide, barbiturates, carbamazepine, dexamethasone, griseofulvin, modafinil, nafcillin, phenytoin, primidone, rifabutin, rifampin, St. John's wort): Decreased imatinib concentrations and antineoplastic efficacy.

Drugs that inhibit CYP3A4 (eg, clarithromycin, diltiazem, erythromycin, itraconazole, ketoconazole, verapamil): Increased imatinib concentrations and toxicity.

Drugs that are metabolized by CYP3A4 (eg, simvastatin, cyclosporine, pimozide, triazolobenzodiazepines): Imatinib may reduce metabolism, resulting in increased concentrations and toxicity.

Lab Test Interferences None well documented.

Adverse Reactions Severity and frequency of adverse reactions vary with dose and duration of imatinib therapy.

CNS: Fatigue (48%); headache (36%); dizziness (16%); asthenia (15%); insomnia (14%); anxiety (8%); anorexia (7%); CNS hemorrhage (2%).
DERM: Rash (47%); pruritus (14%).
EENT: Nasopharyngitis (22%); pharyngolaryngeal pain (14%); lacrimation (11%).
GI: Nausea (63%); diarrhea (48%); vomiting (36%); dyspepsia (27%); flatulence (23%); constipation (9%); GI hemorrhage (2%).
HEMA/LYMPH: Neutropenia (48%); hemorrhage (30%).
HEPA: Liver toxicity (6%).
LABTESTABS: Elevated ALT, elevated alkaline phosphatase (6%); elevated AST, elevated bilirubin (4%); elevated creatinine (2%).
M/N: Increased weight (32%); hypokalemia (6%).
MUSC: Muscle cramps (62%); arthralgia (40%); musculoskeletal pain (38%); joint pain, myalgia (27%); back pain (11%); rigors (10%).
RESP: Cough (20%); upper respiratory tract infection, pneumonia (19%); dyspnea (12%); chest pain, sinusitis (11%).
OTHER: Fluid retention, superficial edema (76%); abdominal pain (32%); pyrexia (21%); night sweats (14%).

Precautions

Pregnancy: Category D.
Lactation: Undetermined.
Children: The safety and efficacy of imatinib in pediatric patients is not established except in children with Ph+ chronic phase CML whose disease recurred after stem cell transplantation or who are resistant to interferon-alpha therapy. No data in children under 3 yr of age.
Elderly: The efficacy of imatinib was similar in older and younger patients.
Dosage adjustment for hepatic dysfunction: Consider dosage reduction in patients with hepatic impairment at baseline.
Dosage adjustment for toxicity: Consider dosage reduction or temporary discontinuation for severe edema.
Fluid retention: Risk of severe edema increases with imatinib dose and in patients older than 65 yr of age. Edema may manifest as rapid weight gain and should be managed promptly with dose reduction, interruption of therapy, diuretics, or supportive care, as indicated.
GI irritation: Take with food and a large glass of water to minimize this problem.
Resistance: Resistance to imatinib has developed during continued therapy, usually in advanced-stage CML. In patients with blast crisis, resistance has occurred as soon as 42 days after starting therapy.

Overdosage: Signs and Symptoms
Experience with doses greater than 800 mg is limited.

PATIENT CARE CONSIDERATIONS

Administration/Storage

- Administer prescribed dose with a meal and large glass of water to minimize GI irritation.
- Administer doses of 400 to 600 mg as a single daily dose. Administer 800 mg dose as 400 mg bid.
- In children, medication can be administered as a single daily dose or, may be split into 2 doses (once in the morning and once in the evening).
- If patient is unable to swallow film-coated tablets, the tablets may be dispersed in a glass of water or apple juice. Place required number of tablets in a glass with appropriate volume of beverage (eg, 50 mL for 100 mg tablet, and 200 mL for 400 mg tablet) and stir with a spoon until the tablets have disintegrated. Immediately have patient swallow the suspension.
- Store tablets at controlled room temperature (59° to 86°F). Protect from moisture.

Assessment/Interventions

- Obtain patient history, including drug history and any known allergies. Note renal or hepa-

tic impairment, or concurrent use of potent CYP3A4 inducer (eg, rifampin, phenytoin) or inhibitor (eg, erythromycin, ketoconazole).
- Ensure women of childbearing potential are not pregnant when therapy is started and use effective contraception during treatment.
- Ensure CBC with differential and platelet count is evaluated before treatment is started, weekly for the first month, biweekly for the second month, and periodically thereafter as clinically indicated (eg, every 2 to 3 months) for duration of therapy.
- Ensure liver function (eg, transaminases, bilirubin, alkaline phosphatase) is evaluated before treatment is started and monthly, or as clinically indicated, thereafter for duration of therapy.
- Ensure medication is withheld and dose adjustments are made for hematologic and nonhematologic (eg, severe hepatotoxicity, severe fluid retention) toxicity following manufacturer's guidelines.
- Weigh patient before starting therapy and frequently during treatment. Monitor patient regularly for signs and symptoms of fluid retention. Notify health care provider of unexpected weight gain and/or signs and symptoms of fluid retention. Be prepared to treat appropriately.
- Monitor patient for signs or symptoms of infection or bleeding. Inform health care provider immediately if noted and be prepared to treat appropriately.
- Implement infection control measures if WBC drops; implement bleeding control measures if platelet count drops.
- Assess patient for CNS, DERM, GI, HEMA, MUSC, RESP, and general body side effects. Report to health care provider if noted and significant.

Patient/Family Education
- Explain name, dose, action, and potential side effects of drug.
- Review dosing schedule with patient.
- Advise patient that dose may be changed or medication temporarily stopped based upon results of lab tests, development of side effects, and response to therapy.
- Advise patient to take prescribed dose with food and large glass of water to minimize GI irritation.
- Caution patient to avoid grapefruit and grapefruit juice while taking imatinib.
- Advise patient that if a dose is missed, take it as soon as possible. If close to the next dose skip that dose and take the next dose at the regularly scheduled time. Caution patient not to double the dose to catch up.
- Advise patient to immediately report any of the following to health care provider: skin rash; swelling of the feet, ankles, legs, or around the eyes; rapid weight gain; bloating; shortness of breath or difficulty breathing; fever, chills, or other signs of infection; sore throat; persistent nausea, vomiting, or appetite loss; bleeding or unusual bruising.
- Advise patient that drug may cause dizziness and to use caution while driving or performing other tasks requiring mental alertness and coordination until tolerance is determined.
- Advise patient that medication may cause photosensitivity (sensitivity to sunlight or ultraviolet light) and to avoid unnecessary exposure to sunlight or tanning lamps and to use sunscreens and wear protective clothing until tolerance is determined.
- Caution women of childbearing potential to avoid becoming pregnant while being treated.
- Advise women to notify health care provider if pregnant, planning to become pregnant, or breastfeeding.
- Instruct patient not to take any prescription or OTC medications (eg, acetaminophen), herbal preparations, or dietary supplements (eg, St. John's wort) unless advised by health care provider.
- Advise patient that frequent follow-up examinations and lab tests will be required to monitor therapy and to keep appointments.

Imipenem-Cilastatin

(ih-mih-PEN-em-SIGH-luh-STAT-in)
Class Anti-infective/Carbapenem
How Supplied
Primaxin IV Powder for Injection 250 mg imipenem equivalent and 250 mg cilastatin equivalent. Contains 0.8 mEq sodium., Powder for Injection 500 mg imipenem equivalent and 500 mg cilastatin equivalent. Contains 1.6 mEq sodium. ◆ *Primaxin IM* Powder for Injection 500 mg imipenem equivalent and 500 mg cilastatin equivalent. Contains 1.4 mEq sodium., Powder for Injection 750 mg imipenem equivalent and 750 mg cilastatin equivalent. Contains 2.1 mEq sodium.

Action
PHARMACOLOGY: Imipenem inhibits bacterial cell wall synthesis. Cilastatin prevents metabolism of imipenem, resulting in increased urinary recovery and decreased renal toxicity.

Indications Treatment of serious infections of lower respiratory tract and urinary tract, intra-abdominal and gynecologic infections, bacterial septicemia, bone and joint infections, skin and skin structure infections, endocarditis, and polymicrobic infections due to susceptible microorganisms.

Contraindications IM use with hypersensitivity to local anesthetics of amide type or with severe shock or heart block. IV use with patients with meningitis (safety and efficacy have not been established).

Route/Dosage
ADULTS: **IV** 125, 250, or 500 mg dose over 20 to 30 min. Infuse a 750 mg or 1 g dose over 40 to 60 min. If nausea develops, slow the infusion rate. Max: 50 mg/kg/day or 4 g/day, whichever is lower.
ADULTS: **IM** 500 to 750 mg q 12 hr. Max: 1500 mg/day.
CHILDREN LESS THAN 40 KG: **IM** 60 mg/kg/day.
CHILDREN AT LEAST 40 KG: **IM** Adult dose.
PREMATURE INFANTS (AT LEAST 36 WK GESTATIONAL AGE): **IM** 20 mg/kg q 12 hr.

Interactions
Cyclosporine: CNS side effects (eg, myoclonia, seizures) may be increased.
Ganciclovir: Generalized seizures may occur; avoid use.
Probenecid: Minimal increases in imipenem levels and half-life; do not give probenecid concurrently.
INCOMPATIBILITIES: Do not physically mix imipenem-cilastatin with other antibiotics.

Lab Test Interferences May cause positive *Coombs* test results.

Adverse Reactions
CV: Hypotension; palpitations; tachycardia; phlebitis; thrombophlebitis.
CNS: Seizures.
GI: Nausea; diarrhea; vomiting; pseudomembranous colitis; hemorrhagic colitis; hepatitis.
GU: Presence of RBCs, WBCs, casts, and bacteria in urine; increased BUN and creatinine.
HEMA: Decreased Hgb and Hct; eosinophilia; increased or decreased WBCs and platelets; decreased erythrocytes.
HEPA: Increased AST, ALT, alkaline phosphatase, and bilirubin.
OTHER: Pain at injection site.

Precautions
Pregnancy: Category C.
Lactation: Undetermined.
Children: Safety and efficacy in children younger than 12 yr not established with IM use. IV use in newborns to 16 yr (with non-CNS infections) is supported by evidence from adequate and well-controlled studies. IV use is not recommended in pediatric patients with CNS infections because of the risk of seizures, or in pediatric patients less than 30 kg with impaired renal function as no data are available.
Hypersensitivity: Administer drug with caution to penicillin-sensitive patients due to possible cross-activity.
Renal function impairment: Dosage reduction or alteration of dosage interval is required.
Superinfection: May result in bacterial or fungal overgrowth of nonsusceptible organisms.
Benzyl alcohol: Benzyl alcohol as a preservative has been associated with toxicity in newborns, especially those younger than 3 mo. Do not use diluents containing benzyl alcohol when IV is constituted for administration to pediatric patients.
CNS: IV administration may result in myoclonic activity confusional states or seizures.
Pseudomembranous colitis: Consider possibility in patients with diarrhea.

Overdosage: Signs and Symptoms
Seizures.

PATIENT CARE CONSIDERATIONS
Administration/Storage
- Do not inject by direct IV bolus.
- For IV administration, reconstitute with 100 mL of compatible diluent. Shake until suspension is clear; add suspension to 100 mL of appropriate infusion solution. Then add 10 mL of infusion to vial; shake well to ensure that all medication is used and transfer resulting suspension to infusion solution. Color of solution may range from colorless to yellow. Solution is stable for 4 hr at room temperature and for 24 hr when refrigerated. Do not administer if solution is cloudy.
- Do not mix with or physically add to antibiotics. However, it may be administered concomitantly with other antibiotics (eg, aminoglycosides).
- Do not use IM preparation for IV administration.
- For IM administration, prepare with 1% lidocaine hydrochloride solution (without epinephrine). Prepare 500 mg vial with 2 mL and 750 mg vial with 3 mL of lidocaine. Agitate to form suspension. Color of solution may range from white to light tan. Withdraw and inject entire contents of vial IM. Use within 1 hr of preparation.
- Store unreconstituted powder less than 77°F.

Assessment/Interventions
- Obtain complete patient history, including drug history and any known allergies, espe-

cially to penicillin and beta-lactam antibiotics.
- Notify health care provider if signs of superinfection or resistance occur.
- Have epinephrine, antihistamines, and resuscitation equipment available in case of anaphylaxis.
- If seizure occurs, withhold drug, institute safety measures, and notify health care provider.
- If culture and sensitivity is ordered, obtain specimen prior to first dose.
- Withhold drug and notify health care provider if any of following occurs: fever, rash, hives, difficulty breathing, vaginitis, or severe diarrhea.
- Monitor vital signs, sputum, urine, stool, and WBC at beginning of and throughout therapy.

Patient/Family Education
- Instruct patient to report the following to health care provider: itching; rash; hives; difficulty breathing; diarrhea; black "furry" tongue; loose, foul-smelling stools; vaginal itching or discharge.

Imipramine Hydrochloride
(im-IPP-ruh-meen HIGH-droe-KLOR-ide)
Class Tricyclic antidepressant

How Supplied
Tofranil Tablets 10 mg, Tablets 25 mg, Tablets 50 mg
♣ *Apo-Imipramine* ◆ *Impril*

Imipramine Pamoate
Tofranil-PM Capsules 75 mg, Capsules 100 mg, Capsules 125 mg, Capsules 150 mg

Action
PHARMACOLOGY: Inhibits reuptake of norepinephrine and, to a lesser degree, serotonin in CNS.

PHARMACOKINETICS/DYNAMICS:
Absorption: T_{max} is 2 to 4 hr. Steady state is reached in 2 to 5 days.
Distribution: More than 90% is protein bound. Lipid soluble.
Metabolism: Significant first pass effect. Metabolism occurs in liver. Active metabolite is desipramine.
Excretion: The $t_{1/2}$ is 11 to 25 hr.
Peak: 2 to 4 weeks.

Indications Relief of symptoms of depression; treatment of enuresis in children 6 yr and older.
Unlabeled use(s): Treatment of chronic pain, panic disorder, eating disorders (bulimia nervosa), and facilitation of cocaine withdrawal.

Contraindications Hypersensitivity to any tricyclic antidepressant. Generally not to be given in combination with or within 14 days of treatment with MAO inhibitor or during acute recovery phase of MI; cross-sensitivity may occur among the dibenzazepines.

Route/Dosage
Depression
Use parenterally only in patients who are not able or not willing to take oral medication. Give via IM route. Do not administer IV. Up to 100 mg/day in divided doses may be given IM. Switch to oral as soon as possible.
ADULTS: PO 100 to 300 mg/day, in divided doses or once daily at bedtime.
ELDERLY & ADOLESCENTS: PO 30 to 40 mg/day; may increase up to 100 mg/day.
CHILDREN: PO 1.5 mg/kg/day in divided doses; up to maximum of 5 mg/kg/day.
CHILDHOOD ENURESIS (6 YR): PO 25 mg/day given 1 hr before bedtime; if response unsatisfactory after 1 wk, may increase to 50 mg in children younger than 12 yr. Children older than 12 yr may receive 75 mg/night. Do not exceed 2.5 mg/kg/day.

Interactions
Carbamazepine: Carbamazepine levels may increase; imipramine levels may decrease.
Cimetidine, fluoxetine: May cause increased imipramine blood levels and effects.
Clonidine: May result in hypertensive crisis.
CNS depressants: Depressant effects may be additive.
Dicumarol: Anticoagulant actions may increase.
Guanethidine: Hypotensive action may be inhibited.
MAO inhibitors: May cause hyperpyretic crises, severe convulsions, and death when given with imipramine.
Sympathomimetics: Pressor response may be decreased by indirect-acting sympathomimetics and increased by direct-acting ones.

Lab Test Interferences None well documented.

Adverse Reactions
CV: Orthostatic hypotension; hypertension; tachycardia; palpitations; arrhythmias; ECG changes; stroke; heartblock; CHF.
CNS: Confusion; hallucinations; delusions; nervousness; restlessness; agitation; panic; insomnia; nightmares; mania; exacerbation of psychosis; drowsiness; dizziness; weakness; numbness; extra-

pyramidal symptoms; emotional lability; seizures; tremors.
DERM: Rash; pruritus; photosensitivity reaction; dry skin; acne; itching.
EENT: Nasal congestion; tinnitus; conjunctivitis; mydriasis; blurred vision; increased IOP.
GI: Nausea; vomiting; anorexia; GI distress; diarrhea; flatulence; peculiar taste in mouth; dry mouth; constipation.
GU: Impotence; sexual dysfunction; nocturia; urinary frequency; UTI; vaginitis; cystitis; dysmenorrhea; amenorrhea; urinary retention and hesitancy.
HEMA: Bone marrow depression including agranulocytosis; eosinophilia; purpura; thrombocytopenia; leukopenia.
HEPA: Hepatitis; jaundice.
METAB: Elevation or depression of blood sugar.
RESP: Pharyngitis; rhinitis; sinusitis; laryngitis; coughing.
OTHER: Breast enlargement.

Precautions
Pregnancy: Category D.
Lactation: Excreted in breast milk.
Children: Safety and efficacy of imipramine as temporary adjunctive therapy for nocturnal enuresis in pediatric patients younger than 6 yr have not been established; chronic use in patients 6 yr and older has not been established. Do not exceed 2.5 mg/kg/day.
Special risk patients: Use with caution in patients with history of seizures, urinary retention, ureteral spasm, angle-closure glaucoma or increased IOP, conduction disorders, with hyperthyroid or those receiving thyroid medication, hepatic or renal impairment, schizophrenia or paranoia.
Hazardous tasks: Patients should use caution while performing tasks requiring alertness.
Cardiovascular disorders: Use with extreme caution in patients with cardiovascular disorders. These patients require cardiac surveillance at all dose levels of the drug.

Overdosage: Signs and Symptoms
Confusion, agitation, hallucinations, seizures, status epilepticus, clonus, choreoathetosis, hyperactive reflexes, positive Babinski sign, coma, cardiac arrhythmias, renal failure, flushing, dry mouth, dilated pupils, hyperpyrexia.

PATIENT CARE CONSIDERATIONS

Administration/Storage
- Do not give via IV route.
- Use IM form only for patients unwilling or unable to take oral form.
- Give IM form in divided doses during day.
- Immerse ampules in hot tap water for 1 min if crystals have formed during storage.

Assessment/Interventions
- Obtain complete patient history, including drug history and any known allergies.
- Review ECG for prolongation of QT interval prior to starting large doses and periodically thereafter.
- Be alert for signs of orthostatic hypotension and take orthostatic BPs. Document and report significant changes to health care provider.
- Observe for onset of therapeutic effect in depressed patients in 7 to 21 days and full response in up to 6 wk.
- Assess patients receiving IM form for ability to switch to oral administration.
- Assess elderly patients for signs and symptoms of confusion.
- Report drowsiness, dry mouth, constipation, or weight gain to health care provider.
- Watch for possible hypertension when coadministering clonidine.
- Be alert for possible drug interactions.

Patient/Family Education
- Warn patient of risk of seizure.
- Tell female patient to inform health care provider if becoming or intending to become pregnant.
- Explain that it may be several weeks before a response is noticed.
- Instruct patient to avoid intake of alcoholic beverages or other CNS depressants.
- Advise patient that drug may cause drowsiness and to use caution while driving or performing other tasks requiring mental alertness.
- Caution patient to avoid exposure to sunlight and to use sunscreen or wear protective clothing to avoid photosensitivity reaction.
- Teach patient to avoid sudden position changes to prevent orthostatic hypertension.
- Inform patient that dizziness, dry mouth (suggest taking frequent sips of water, sucking on ice chips, or sugarless hard candy or chewing sugarless gum), drowsiness, or constipation may occur, but that these side effects often subside with time.
- Instruct patient to report all problems to health care provider, including dizziness, drowsiness, dry mouth, constipation, or weight gain.

Imiquimod

(ih-mih-KWIH-mahd)
Class Immunomodulator
How Supplied
Aldara Cream 5%
Action
PHARMACOLOGY: Unknown; however, imiquimod induces mRNA encoding cytokines, including interferon-alpha at the treatment site.
PHARMACOKINETICS/DYNAMICS:
Absorption: Minimal percutaneous absorption.
Excretion: Less than 0.9% of topical dose excreted in urine and feces.
Indications Treatment of external genital and perianal warts/condyloma acuminata.
Contraindications Standard considerations.
Route/Dosage
ADULTS AND CHILDREN 12 YR AND OLDER:
Topical 3 times/wk (eg, Monday, Wednesday, Friday) and leave on skin for 6 to 10 hr. Remove cream by washing treated area with mild soap and water. Continue treatment until there is total clearance of genital/perianal warts or for a max of 16 wk. A rest period of several days may be taken if needed because of discomfort or severity of local skin reaction. Treatment may be resumed after reaction subsides.
Interactions None well documented.
Lab Test Interferences None well documented.
Adverse Reactions
CNS: Headache (5%); fatigue (greater than 1%).
DERM: Erythema (61%); itching (32%); erosion (30%); burning (26%); excoriation/flaking (25%); edema (17%); scabbing (13%); fungal infections (11%); pain (8%); induration (7%); ulceration (5%); vesicles, soreness (3%); wart site reactions (eg, hypopigmentation, irritation, rash, tenderness) (greater than 1%).
GI: Diarrhea (greater than 1%).
MUSC: Myalgia (1%).
OTHER: Flu-like symptoms (3%); bleeding, fever (greater than 1%).
Precautions
Pregnancy: Category B.
Lactation: Undetermined.
Children: Safety and efficacy not established in children under 12 yr.

PATIENT CARE CONSIDERATIONS

Administration/Storage
- For topical use only. Not for ophthalmic, oral, or intravaginal use.
- Cream is applied 3 times/wk, prior to normal sleeping hours.
- Wash hands before and after applying cream.
- Apply thin layer to wart area and rub in until cream is no longer visible. Leave on skin for 6 to 10 hr, then remove by washing treated area with mild soap and water.
- Do not cover with occlusive dressings. A porous gauze dressing or cotton underwear may be used in the management of skin reactions.
- Store cream below 77°F. Protect from freezing.

Assessment/Interventions
- Obtain patient history, including drug history and any known allergies. Note recent treatment of genital/perianal warts with other cutaneously applied drugs.
- Assess application site for evidence of irritation or inflammation from previous or current treatment. Avoid applying cream to these areas until tissue has healed.
- Assess application site and surrounding areas for local skin reaction (eg, erythema, erosion, excoriation, edema). If severe local skin reaction occurs, remove cream by washing with mild soap and water and inform health care provider.
- Periodically assess and document response to therapy.

Patient/Family Education
- Explain name, dose, action, and potential side effects of drug.
- Advise patient that medication is not a cure and that new warts may develop during or after therapy.
- Teach patient proper technique for applying cream.
- Caution women applying cream near opening of vagina to take special care not to accidentally apply to vaginal mucus membranes because of risk of severe tissue reaction.
- Remind patient that cream is applied 3 times/wk (eg, Monday, Wednesday, Friday) before bedtime and is removed by washing with mild soap and water after 6 to 10 hr.
- Advise patient that response to therapy is slow and may take several weeks to occur.
- Advise patient to continue therapy until there is total clearance of warts or for a max of 16 wk.
- Advise patient to temporarily discontinue application of cream if discomfort at application site occurs. Therapy can be restarted when reaction subsides.

- Instruct uncircumcised men treating warts under foreskin to retract the foreskin and clean the area daily.
- Caution patient not to cover application site with occlusive dressings. Advise patient that a porous gauze dressing or cotton underwear may be used to cover application site should local skin reactions occur.
- Caution patient that cream may weaken condoms and vaginal diaphragms and to use alternative methods of birth control while cream is on the skin.
- Advise patient to avoid sexual (genital, anal, oral) contact while cream is on the skin.
- Advise patient that most common side effects are application site reactions (eg, redness, swelling, erosion, excoriation) and to discontinue use and inform health care provider if severe reaction is noted.
- Advise women to notify health care provider if pregnant, planning to become pregnant, or breastfeeding.
- Instruct patient to not take any prescription or OTC medications or dietary supplements unless advised by health care provider.
- Advise patient that follow-up visits will be required to monitor therapy and to keep appointments.

Immune Globulin Intramuscular (IGIM; IG; Gamma Globulin; ISG)

(ih-MYOON GLAH-byoo-lin intramuscular)

Class Immune serum

How Supplied
BayGam Injection 151.515 mg/mL

Action
PHARMACOLOGY: Replaces normal human IgG antibodies.
PHARMACOKINETICS/DYNAMICS:
Excretion: The mean IgG $t_{1/2}$ is approximately 23 days.
Peak: The peak effect is 2 to 5 days.

Indications Passive immunization against or modification of hepatitis A. Prevention or modification of measles in susceptible persons exposed less than 6 days previously. Passive immunization against varicella in immunocompromised patients if varicella zoster immune globulin (VZIG) is not available and IGIM can be given promptly. IgG replacement therapy in certain persons with hypoglobulinemia or agammaglobulinemia.

Contraindications Immediate hypersensitivity to human antibody product or thimerosal; circulating anti-IgA antibodies; thrombocytopenia or any coagulation disorder.

Route/Dosage
Preexposure and Postexposure Hepatitis A Prophylaxis
ADULTS AND CHILDREN: **IM** 0.02 mL/kg. Preexposure hepatitis A prophylaxis for travelers to developing countries who will stay less than 3 mo. **IM** 0.06 mg/kg with booster doses q 4 to 6 mo throughout their stay.

Postexposure Measles Prophylaxis
ADULTS AND CHILDREN: **IM** 0.25 mL/kg.
SUSCEPTIBLE IMMUNOCOMPROMISED CHILDREN: **IM** 0.5 mL/kg (max, 15 mL).

Postexposure Varicella Prophylaxis
ADULTS AND CHILDREN: If VZIG is unavailable, **IM** 0.6 to 1.2 mL/kg.

Immunoglobulin Deficiency
ADULTS AND CHILDREN: **IM** 0.66 mL/kg (100 mg/kg) q 3 to 4 wk. Larger initial dose (eg, 1.2 mL/kg) is often given at onset of therapy. Patients who rapidly metabolize may require more frequent or larger doses.

Interactions
Live vaccines: To avoid inactivating vaccines containing live viruses or bacteria, give live vaccines 2 to 4 wk before or 3 to 6 mo after IGIU, depending on dose.

Lab Test Interferences None well documented.

Adverse Reactions
OTHER: Local pain and tenderness at injection site; urticaria; angioedema; anaphylactic reactions.

Precautions
Pregnancy: Category C.
Lactation: Undetermined.
Hypersensitivity: Hypersensitivity, including anaphylaxis, may occur. Administer drug with caution in patients with prior systemic allergic reactions to human immunoglobulins.
Special risk patients: Give drug cautiously to persons receiving anticoagulant therapy because of IM administration.

PATIENT CARE CONSIDERATIONS
Administration/Storage
- Administer via IM injection only; do not give by IV route.
- In adults, administer via IM injection, preferably in upper outer quadrant of gluteal region.
- In infants and children younger than 3 yr, administer IM in anterolateral thigh.
- Divide doses larger than 10 mL and inject

into several muscle sites to reduce local pain and discomfort.
* It is better not to inject more than 3 mL per injection site.
* Always record manufacturer's name and lot number of immune globulin in patient's permanent record file along with date of administration, name, address and title of person administering injection.
* Refrigerate vials. Do not freeze.

Assessment/Interventions
* Obtain patient history, including drug history and any known allergies.
* Monitor for hypersensitivity or anaphylaxis. Epinephrine should always be available to counteract any possible reactions.

Patient/Family Education
* Instruct patient to take analgesics (eg, acetaminophen) for local pain and tenderness at injection site if necessary.
* Provide patient or parent with immunization history record and record this injection in patient's medical records.

Immune Globulin IV (IGIV)
(ih-MYOON GLAH-byoo-lin)
Class Immune serum

How Supplied
Gamimune N Injection 5%, Injection 10% ♦ *Gammagard S/D* Powder for Injection (freeze-dried, solvent/detergent treated) 50 mg/mL ♦ *Gammar-P I.V.* Powder for Injection, lyophilized 5% IgG, 3% human albumin ♦ *Iveegam* Powder for Injection (freeze-dried) 50 mg/mL IgG ♦ *Polygam* Powder for Injection (freeze-dried) 50 mg/mL; 90% gammaglobulin ♦ *Polygam S/D* Powder for Injection (freeze-dried, solvent/detergent treated) 50 mg/mL; 90% gammaglobulin ♦ *Venoglobulin-I* Powder for Injection, lyophilized 50 mg/mL IgG ♦ *Venoglobulin-S* Solution for Injection (solvent/detergent treated) 5% immune globulin IV (human), Solution for Injection (solvent/detergent treated) 10% immune globulin IV (human)

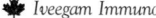 *Iveegam Immuno*

Action
PHARMACOLOGY: Replaces normal human IgG antibodies. Promotes opsonization, fixes complement, and neutralizes bacteria, viruses, fungi, and parasites, and their toxins.

PHARMACOKINETICS/DYNAMICS:
Excretion: Mean $t_{1/2}$ is approximately 40 days.

Indications Treatment of primary immunodeficiency states in patients unable to produce sufficient amounts of IgG antibodies; prevention of bacterial infections in patients with hypogamma globulinemia, recurrent bacterial infections associated with B-cell chronic lymphocytic leukemia or Kawasaki disease, children with AIDS, and bone-marrow transplant patients; treatment of immune thrombocytopenia purpura. **Unlabeled use(s):** Chronic fatigue syndrome; quinidine-induced thrombocytopenia.

Contraindications Immediate hypersensitivity to human antibody product; circulating anti-IgA antibodies; possible aseptic meningitis syndrome.

Route/Dosage
Immunodeficiency Syndrome
ADULTS AND CHILDREN: *Gammagard:* **IV** 200 to 400 mg/kg initially; then monthly doses of 100 mg/kg or more are recommended. *Gammar S/D:* **IV** Initial dose of 0.5 mL/kg/hr. Eventual: 5%: 4 mL/kg/hr; 10%: 8 mL/kg/hr. *Gammar-P I.V.:* **IV** Initial dose: 0.6 mL/kg/hr x 15 to 30 min. Eventual: 1.2 to 3.6 mL/kg/hr. *Gammar-IV* Initial loading dose of 200 mg/kg or more; then 100 to 200 mg/kg q 3 to 4 wk. *Gamimune N:* **IV** 100 to 200 mg/kg monthly. If clinical response or level of IgG is insufficient, increase dose to 400 mg/kg or repeat infusion more frequently. Pediatric HIV infection: 400 mg (8 mL/kg) q 28 days. *Iveegam:* **IV** 200 mg/kg monthly. If clinical response or level of IgG is insufficient, increase dose 4-fold or repeat infusion more frequently. Doses up to 800 mg/kg monthly have been tolerated. *Polygam:* **IV** 200 to 400 mg/kg recommended initially; then 100 mg/kg monthly. Doses based on monitoring clinical response. *Polygam S/D:* **IV** Initial: 0.5 mL/kg/hr. Eventual: 5%: 4 mL/kg/hr; 10%: 8 mL/kg/hr. *Sandoglobulin:* **IV** 200 mg/kg monthly. If clinical response or level of IgG is insufficient, increase dose to 300 mg/kg or repeat infusion more frequently. *Venoglobulin-I:* **IV** 200 mg/kg monthly. If clinical response or level of IgG is insufficient, increase dose to 300 to 400 mg/kg or repeat infusion more frequently.

Immune Thrombocytopenic Purpura
ADULTS AND CHILDREN: *Gammagard:* **IV** 1000 mg/kg. Give up to 3 doses on alternate days if required, based on clinical response and platelet count. *Gammagard S/D:* **IV** Initial dose of 0.5 mL/kg/hr. Eventual: 5%: 4 mL/kg/hr; 10%: 8 mL/kg/hr. *Gamimune N:* **IV** 400 mg/kg for 5 consecutive days. *Polygam:* IV 1000 mg/kg recommended initially; then additional doses determined by clinical response and platelet count.

Up to 3 doses may be given on alternate days if needed. *Polygam S/D:* **IV** Initial: 0.5 mL/kg/hr. Eventual: 5%: 4 mL/kg/hr; 10%: 8 mL/kg/hr. *Sandoglobulin:* **IV** 400 mg/kg for 2 to 5 consecutive days. *Venoglobulin-I:* IV Induction: 500 mg/kg/day for 2 to 7 consecutive days. Patients responding to induction therapy by manifesting platelet count of 30,000 to 50,000/mm^3 may be discontinued after 2 to 7 daily doses. Maintenance: If platelet count falls below 30,000/mm^3 or patient manifests significant bleeding, infuse 500 to 2000 mg/kg as single dose q 2 wk or less as needed to maintain platelet count above 30,000/mm^3 in children and 20,000/mm^3 in adults.

B-Cell Chronic Lymphocytic Leukemia
ADULTS AND CHILDREN: *Gammagard:* **IV** 400 mg/kg q 3 to 4 wk. *Polygam:* **IV** 400 mg/kg q 3 to 4 wk.

Interactions
Live vaccines: To avoid inactivating vaccines containing live viruses or bacteria, give live vaccines 2 to 4 wk before or 3 to 11 mo after IGIV depending on dose.

PATIENT CARE CONSIDERATIONS
Administration/Storage
- Administer via IV infusion only. Use separate IV line and electronic infusion device.
- Proceed with infusion only if reconstituted solution is clear and is at approximate body temperature.
- Store *Gamimune N* and *Iveegam* in refrigerator.
- Store *Sandoglobulin, Gammagard S/D, Gammar-P I.V., Polygam S/D,* and *Venoglobulin-I* at room temperature.
- Discard any unused solution.
- Avoid freezing. Do not use solution that has been frozen.

Assessment/Interventions
- Obtain patient history, including drug history

INCOMPATIBILITIES: Admixture: Do not mix IGIV with other medications.

Lab Test Interferences
Blood type: Blood-group antibodies may be transferred to IGIV recipients, causing confusion regarding recipient's blood type.

Adverse Reactions
CV: Palpitations; hypotension; hypertension.
CNS: Anxiety; dizziness; headache.
GI: Nausea; vomiting; abdominal cramps.
RESP: Shortness of breath; wheezing.
OTHER: Pallor; cyanosis; immediate anaphylactic and hypersensitivity reactions; back pain; chills; muscle or joint pain; arthralgia; malaise; flushing; chest tightness.

Precautions
Pregnancy: Category C.
Lactation: Undetermined.
Hypersensitivity: Hypersensitivity, including anaphylaxis, may occur.
Renal function impairment: Has been associated with renal dysfunction, acute renal failure, osmotic nephrosis, and death.

and any known allergies.
- Keep epinephrine (1:1000) and resuscitation equipment readily available.
- Monitor vital signs continuously and observe for adverse symptoms (eg, anaphylaxis, fever, chills, nausea, vomiting) throughout infusion.
- If adverse reactions such as fever, chills, nausea, or vomiting develop, slowing infusion rate will usually eliminate reaction.

Patient/Family Education
- Instruct patient to notify health care provider immediately of nausea, chills, shortness of breath, headache, and chest tightness during infusion.

Inamrinone

(in-AM-rih-nohn)
Class Cardiovascular/Positive inotropic

How Supplied
Inocor Injection 5 mg/mL (as lactate)

Action
PHARMACOLOGY: Positive inotropic agent with vasodilator activity.

PHARMACOKINETICS/DYNAMICS:
Distribution: Vd is 1.2 L/kg. 10 to 49% is protein bound. The t$_{1/2}$ is 4.6 min.
Metabolism: Several metabolites: N-glycolyl, N-acetate, O-glucuronide.

Excretion: The t$_{1/2}$ is 3.6 hr. The primary route is via the urine.
Peak: 10 minutes.
Duration: 30 min to 2 hr (dose-dependent)
Special Populations:
Children – There is increased Vd and decreased elimination t$_{1/2}$.
CHF – In CHF patients the mean elimination is t$_{1/2}$ of 5.8 hr. Monitor hemodynamic response or drug level.

Indications
Short-term management of CHF in patients whose condition can be closely monitored and who have not responded adequately to digitalis, diuretics, or vasodilators.

Contraindications Hypersensitivity to bisulfites.

Route/Dosage
ADULTS: **IV** *Initial dose:* 0.75 mg/kg bolus slowly over 2 to 3 min. *Maintenance:* 5 to 10 mcg/kg/min; additional 0.75 mg/kg bolus may be given 30 min after initiating therapy, not to exceed total daily dose of 10 mg/kg.

Interactions None well documented.
INCOMPATIBILITIES: Chemical interaction occurs slowly over 24 hr when mixed directly with dextrose-containing solutions. Do not inject furosemide into IV line containing inamrinone; immediate precipitate forms.

Lab Test Interferences None well documented.

Adverse Reactions
CV: Arrhythmia; hypotension.
GI: Nausea; vomiting.
HEMA: Thrombocytopenia.

Precautions
Pregnancy: Category C.
Lactation: Undetermined.
Children: Safety and efficacy not established.
Sulfite sensitivity: May cause allergic-type reaction in susceptible patients.
Arrhythmias: Supraventricular and ventricular arrhythmias have occurred.
Fluid balance: Vigorous diuretic therapy may cause inadequate response to inamrinone therapy; liberalization of fluids may be needed. CVP monitoring has been advocated.
Hepatotoxicity: Dose may be reduced or drug may be discontinued if there are alterations in liver enzymes; if alterations occur with clinical symptoms, drug is discontinued.
Post MI: Not recommended during acute phase.
Severe aortic or pulmonic valvular disease: Not recommended.
Thrombocytopenia: More common in patients on prolonged therapy.

Overdosage: Signs and Symptoms
Arrhythmias, excessive hypotension.

PATIENT CARE CONSIDERATIONS

Administration/Storage
IV infusion:
- Administer as supplied or dilute in 0.5% or 0.9% saline to a concentration of 1 to 3 mg/mL.
- Do not dilute in dextrose-containing solutions, although product may be injected into running dextrose infusion through Y-connector or directly into tubing. Do not infuse product and furosemide through same line.
- Administer maintenance infusion 5 to 10 g/kg/min, preferably with infusion pump; adjust rate according to patient response.
- Use diluted solutions within 24 hr.
- Protect ampules from light.
- Store at room temperature.

Assessment/Interventions
- Obtain patient history, including drug history and any known allergies. Determine presence or history of asthma.
- Review baseline ECG and assess ongoing cardiac monitoring. Notify health care provider of any arrhythmias.
- Assess cardiac rate and rhythm throughout therapy.
- Assess vital signs, especially BP and pulse, before and during therapy. Notify health care provider of excessive hypotension; slow or stop infusion.
- Monitor I&O, including changes (increase or decrease) in output.
- Monitor laboratory values for alterations in liver enzymes, renal function, platelets, and serum electrolytes. Notify health care provider of any changes.
- Monitor for nausea and vomiting and for signs of hepatotoxicity.

Patient/Family Education
- Instruct patient to avoid sudden position changes to prevent orthostatic hypotension.
- Advise patient to notify health care provider of shortness of breath and increased chest pain.

Indapamide
(IN-DAP-uh-mide)
Class Thiazide diuretic

How Supplied
Lozol Tablets 1.25 mg, Tablets 2.5 mg
✤ *Apo-Indapamide* ◆ *Gen-Indapamide* ◆ *Lozide* ◆ *Novo-Indapamide* ◆ *Nu-Indapamide* ◆ *PMS-Indapamide*

Action
PHARMACOLOGY: Enhances excretion of sodium, chloride, and water by interfering with transport of sodium ions across renal tubular epithelium.

PHARMACOKINETICS/DYNAMICS:
Absorption: C_{max} is approximately 115 to 260 ng/mL (dose-dependent). The T_{max} is 2 hr.
Distribution: 71% to 79% is protein bound.

Metabolism: Extensively metabolized.

Excretion: The $t_{1/2}$ is 26 hr. More than 70% is excreted in the urine, and 23% is excreted in the GI tract, probably including the biliary route.

Indications Treatment of edema associated with CHF, hepatic cirrhosis, renal dysfunction, and corticosteroid or estrogen therapy; management of hypertension. **Unlabeled use(s):** Treatment of calcium nephrolithiasis, osteoporosis, or diabetes insipidus.

Contraindications Hypersensitivity to thiazides, related diuretics, or sulfonamide-derived drugs; anuria.

Route/Dosage

ADULTS: PO 1.25 to 5 mg q morning. Maximum 5 mg/day.

Interactions

Bile acid sequestrants: May reduce thiazide absorption; give thiazide at least 2 hr before resin.

Diazoxide: Hyperglycemia may occur.

Digitalis glycosides: Diuretic-induced hypokalemia and hypomagnesemia may precipitate digitalis-induced arrhythmias.

Lithium: May decrease renal excretion of lithium; monitor lithium levels.

Loop diuretics: May result in synergistic effects and result in profound diuresis and serious electrolyte abnormalities.

Sulfonylureas, insulin: May decrease hypoglycemic effect of sulfonylureas. May need to adjust dosage of sulfonylureas or insulin.

Lab Test Interferences May decrease serum protein-bound iodine levels without signs of thyroid disturbance. May cause diagnostic interference of serum electrolyte levels, blood and urine glucose levels, serum bilirubin levels and serum uric acid levels. May increase serum magnesium levels in uremic patients.

Adverse Reactions

CV: Orthostatic hypotension; palpitations.
CNS: Dizziness; lightheadedness; vertigo; headache; weakness; restlessness; insomnia; drowsiness; fatigue; lethargy; anxiety; depression; nervousness.
DERM: Rash; necrotizing angiitis; vasculitis; cutaneous vasculitis; pruritus.
EENT: Blurred vision.
GI: Anorexia; gastric irritation; epigastric distress; nausea; vomiting; abdominal pain/cramping/bloating; diarrhea; constipation; dry mouth.
GU: Nocturia; impotence/reduced libido.
HEMA: Neutropenia.
METAB: Hyperglycemia; glycosuria; hyperuricemia.
RESP: Rhinorrhea.
OTHER: Muscle cramp or spasm; acute gout.

Precautions

Pregnancy: Category B.

Lactation: May be excreted in breast milk.

Hypersensitivity: May occur in patients with or without history of allergy or bronchial asthma; cross-sensitivity with sulfonamides may also occur.

Renal function impairment: May precipitate azotemia; use with caution.

Hepatic function impairment: Minor alterations of fluid and electrolyte balance may precipitate hepatic coma; use with caution.

Electrolyte balance: Severe hyponatremia and hypokalemia may infrequently occur with recommended doses; more common in elderly females.

Lipids: May cause increased concentrations of total triglycerides and LDL in some patients.

Lupus erythematosus: Exacerbation or activation may occur.

Postsympathectomy patients: Antihypertensive effects may be enhanced.

Overdosage: Signs and Symptoms

Orthostatic or general hypotension, syncope, electrolyte abnormalities, potassium deficiency, vomiting, respiratory depression, lethargy, shock, weakness, confusion, dizziness, cramps of calf muscles, thirst, polyuria, anuria.

PATIENT CARE CONSIDERATIONS

Administration/Storage

- Administer as morning dose to prevent nocturia.
- Give with food or milk if nausea occurs.
- Store in tightly closed, light-resistant container at room temperature.

Assessment/Interventions

- Obtain patient history, including drug history and any known allergies.
- Weigh patient daily.
- Assess feet, legs, and sacral area for edema daily.
- Measure I&O throughout therapy.
- Monitor BP, with patient lying and standing.
- Monitor renal function (eg, nonprotein nitrogen, BUN, creatinine, glomerular filtration) and serum potassium, sodium, calcium, magnesium, blood pH, and uric acid as ordered.
- Assess for signs of metabolic alkalosis and hypokalemia.
- Report to health care provider signs of renal dysfunction (eg, anuria, oliguria); liver dysfunction (eg, dark urine, jaundice, pruritus); gout (eg, rising serum uric acid, joint pain);

muscle weakness; cramps, nausea; dizziness; numbness; irregular heartbeat; irritability.

Patient/Family Education
* Tell patient to take medication early in day to prevent sleep problems.
* Instruct patient to take drug with food or milk to minimize GI irritation.
* Caution patient to avoid exposure to sunlight and to use sunscreen or wear protective clothing to avoid photosensitivity reaction.
* Instruct patients with diabetes to report increased blood glucose levels.
* Caution patients to avoid sudden position changes to prevent orthostatic hypotension.
* Advise patients to include in diet foods that are high in potassium (eg bananas, broccoli, dried fruits, grapefruit, lima beans, nuts, oranges).
* Tell patient to report decrease in urinary output, jaundice, muscle cramps, weakness, nausea, blurred vision, or dizziness.
* For patients being treated for hypertension, explain benefits of weight reduction, exercise, reduction of alcohol and sodium intake, cessation of smoking.

Indinavir Sulfate

(in-DIN-ah-veer SULL-fate)

Class Antiretroviral/Protease inhibitor

How Supplied
Crixivan Capsules 200 mg, Capsules 400 mg

Action
PHARMACOLOGY: Inhibits human immunodeficiency virus (HIV) protease, the enzyme that cleaves viral polyprotein precursors into functional proteins in HIV-infected cells. Inhibition of this enzyme by indinavir results in formation of immature noninfectious viral particles.

PHARMACOKINETICS/DYNAMICS:

Absorption: The T_{max} is approximately 0.8 hr (fasting). The C_{max} is approximately 12,617 nm. The AUC_{ss} is approximately 30,691 nm•hr. Administration is with a high calorie, fat, and protein meal. Reduction of approximately 77% in AUC and approximately 84% in C_{max}.

Distribution: 60% is protein bound.

Metabolism: There are 7 metabolites: 1 glucuronide conjugate and 6 oxidative metabolites. The major route is through the liver via cytochrome P450 3A4 for the formation of the oxidative metabolites.

Excretion: The $t_{1/2}$ is approximately 1.8 hr. Less than 20% is excreted unchanged in the urine. Approximately 83% is excreted in the urine and approximately 19% in the feces.

Special Populations:
Hepatic Function Impairment – Mild to moderate: decreased metabolism resulting in an approximate increase in AUC of 60% and increased $t_{1/2}$ to approximately 2.8 hr.
Children – AUC and C_{max} slightly increased and trough concentration were considerably lower.
Gender – Females have decreased AUC (13%) and decreased C_{max} (13%).

Indications Treatment of HIV infection in adults when antiretroviral therapy is warranted.

Contraindications Concomitant therapy with amiodarone, cisapride, ergot derivatives, midazolam, pimozide, or triazolam; hypersensitivity to any component of product.

Route/Dosage
ADULTS: PO 800 mg (two 400 mg capsules) q 8 hr.

Interactions
Cisapride, midazolam, triazolam: Concomitant use is contraindicated.
Delavirdine: Serum levels of indinavir may be increased; consider a dose reduction of indinavir to 600 mg q 8 hr when administering delavirdine 400 mg bid.
Didanosine: Separate administration by at least 1 hr. The buffers in didanosine preparations may interfere with indinavir's absorption.
Efavirenz: Serum levels of indinavir may be decreased; consider a dose increase of indinavir to 1000 mg q 8 hr.
Fentanyl: Indinavir may elevate plasma levels and prolong the half-life of fentanyl, increasing the risk of side effects.
Itraconazole: Serum levels of indinavir may be increased; consider a dose reduction of indinavir to 600 mg q 8 hr when administering ketoconazole.
Interleukins, ritonavir, sildenafil: Serum indinavir concentrations may be increased. Consider decreasing indinavir's dose.
Rifabutin: Serum concentrations of rifabutin may be increased. A 50% reduction in rifabutin dosage is recommended by the manufacturer.
Rifampin: May induce enzymes that metabolize indinavir; concomitant use not recommended.
Sildenafil: Ritonavir may elevate sildenafil plasma levels, increasing the risk of adverse

effects, including hypotension and visual changes.
St. John's wort: Serum levels of indinavir may be decreased, reducing the clinical effect.

Lab Test Interferences None well documented.

Adverse Reactions
CV: Palpitation; syncope.
CNS: Headache; insomnia; dizziness; somnolence; anxiety.
DERM: Rash; dry skin; pruritus.
EENT: Pharyngitis; altered taste; blurred vision.
GI: Nausea; vomiting; diarrhea; anorexia; acid reflux; dry mouth; abdominal pain; altered taste.
GU: Nephrolithiasis; dysuria; hematuria.
HEPA: Asymptomatic hyperbilirubinemia.
OTHER: Asthenia; fatigue; flank pain; back pain; chest pain; malaise; fever; flu-like symptoms.

Precautions
Pregnancy: Category C.
Lactation: Undetermined.
Children: Safety and efficacy not established.
Hepatic insufficiency/Cirrhosis: Lower indinavir doses may be required since indinavir is hepatically metabolized.

PATIENT CARE CONSIDERATIONS

Administration/Storage
- Administer drug without food but with water 1 hr before or 2 hr after a meal; alternatively, administer with other liquids (eg, skim milk, juice, coffee, tea) or a light meal (eg, dry toast with jelly, corn flakes with skim milk).
- The patient should drink 1.5 L (48 oz) of liquids in 24 hr.
- Store in a tightly closed container at room temperature, protected from moisture.

Assessment/Interventions
- Obtain patient history.
- Assess for evidence of hepatic insufficiency prior to starting therapy.
- Assess for nephrolithiasis during therapy.

Patient/Family Education
- Advise patient not to modify or discontinue treatment without first consulting the health care provider.
- Advise patient that this medicine must be taken at 8-hr intervals.
- If a dose is missed, the next dose should be taken as soon as possible but not doubled.
- If patient cannot take the drug with only water, the drug may be taken with other liquids or a light meal.
- Have patients store the drug in the original container to prevent moisture from affecting the drug.
- Advise patient that capsules should be used and stored in their original container.
- Inform patient that capsules are sensitive to moisture and the desiccant should remain in the bottle.
- Advise the patient that indinavir is not a cure for HIV, and that its long-term effects are unknown.
- Advise patient to contact health care provider if any of the following occurs: back/flank pain; pink or red-colored urine; yellowing of skin or eyes.

Indomethacin

(in-doe-METH-uh-sin)

Class Analgesic/NSAID

How Supplied
Indocin Capsules 25 mg, Capsules 50 mg, Oral Suspension 25 mg/5 mL, Suppositories 50 mg ◆ *Indocin SR* Capsules, sustained-release 75 mg
✥ *Apo-Indomethacin* ◆ *Indocid* ◆ *Novo-Methacin* ◆ *Nu-Indo* ◆ *ratio-Indomethacin* ◆ *Rhodacine*

Indomethacin Sodium Trihydrate
Indocin IV Injection 1 mg
✥ *Indocid P.D.A.*

Action
PHARMACOLOGY: Decreases inflammation, pain, and fever, probably through inhibition of cyclooxygenase activity and prostaglandin synthesis.

PHARMACOKINETICS/DYNAMICS:
Absorption: C_{max} is approximately 1 to 2 mcg/mL (dose-dependent). The T_{max} is approximately 2 hours. The bioavailability is approximately 100%.

Distribution: 99% is protein bound. Crosses blood-brain barrier and placenta.

Metabolism: Undergoes appreciable enterohepatic circulation. The metabolites are desmethyl, desbenzoyl, desmethyl-desbenzoyl.

Excretion: Eliminated via renal excretion, metabolism, and biliary excretion. The mean $t_{1/2}$ is approximately 4.5 hr. Approximately 60% is excreted in urine and 33% in feces.

Indications
Indomethacin: Symptomatic treatment of rheumatoid arthritis, osteoarthritis, ankylosing spondylitis, gouty arthritis, acute painful shoulder.
Indomethacin sodium trihydrate (IV): Closure of patent ductus arteriosus. **Unlabeled use(s):** Treatment of primary dysmenorrhea; migraine prophylaxis; treatment of cluster headache, poly-

hydramnios, sunburn; cystoid macular edema.

Contraindications Hypersensitivity to aspirin, iodides, or any NSAID. IV form is also contraindicated in the following cases: proven or suspected untreated infection, bleeding, thrombocytopenia, coagulation defects, necrotizing enterocolitis, significant renal impairment, congenital heart disease when patency of ductus arteriosus is necessary for satisfactory blood flow. Suppositories contraindicated in recent bleeding or proctitis history.

Route/Dosage

Rheumatoid Arthritis, Osteoarthritis, Ankylosing Spondylitis
ADULTS: **PO** 25 mg bid or tid up to maximum of 200 mg/day (or 75 mg sustained-release form 1 to 2 times daily)

Gouty Arthritis
ADULTS: **PO/PR** 50 mg tid; do not use sustained-release form.

Acute Painful Shoulder
ADULTS: **PO** 75 to 150 mg/day in divided doses for 7 to 14 days.

Patent Ductus Arteriosus
IV 3 doses total.
INFANTS YOUNGER THAN 2 DAYS: **IV** 0.2 mg/kg followed by 2 doses of 0.1 mg/kg 12 to 24 hr apart.
INFANTS 2 TO 7 DAYS: 3 doses of 0.2 mg/kg separated by 12 to 24 hr.
INFANTS OLDER THAN 7 DAYS: 0.2 mg/kg followed by 2 doses of 0.25 mg/kg separated by 12 to 24 hr.

Interactions

Anticoagulants: May increase risk of gastric erosion and bleeding.
Beta-blockers, ACE inhibitors: Antihypertensive effects may be decreased.
Diflunisal: Diflunisal may decrease the renal clearance and significantly increase indomethacin plasma concentrations that may produce toxicity.
Digoxin: May increase digoxin levels.
Lithium: May decrease lithium clearance.
Loop diuretics: May decrease diuretic effects.
Methotrexate: May increase methotrexate levels.

Penicillamine: Indomethacin may increase the bioavailability of penicillamine.
Potassium-sparing diuretics: Effects of potassium-diuretics may be decreased. Concomitant administration may increase serum potassium levels.
Sympathomimetics: Indomethacin and phenylpropanolamine coadministration may result in increased blood pressure.

Lab Test Interferences False-negative results may occur in dexamethasone suppression test.

Adverse Reactions

CV: Peripheral edema; water retention; worsening or precipitation of CHF.
CNS: Dizziness; headache; drowsiness; confusion.
EENT: Visual disturbances; tinnitus.
GI: Gastric distress; occult blood loss; nausea; diarrhea; vomiting; ulceration; perforation.
GU: Acute renal insufficiency; interstitial nephritis; hyponatremia; renal papillary necrosis.
HEMA: Leukopenia.
METAB: Hyperuricemia; hyperkalemia.

Precautions

Pregnancy: Safety not established.
Lactation: Undetermined.
Children: Safety and efficacy not established in children younger than 14 yr, except use of IV form in infants.
Renal function impairment: NSAIDs may worsen preexisting renal dysfunction.
CNS effects: May aggravate depression or other psychiatric disorders, epilepsy, or Parkinsonism; use with caution.
Electrolyte imbalance: IV indomethacin may suppress water excretion to greater extent than sodium excretion; monitor electrolytes and renal function.
GI effects: Usually not given to patients with active GI lesions or history of recurrent GI lesions.

Overdosage: Signs and Symptoms

Nausea, vomiting, headache, dizziness, mental confusion, disorientation, lethargy, paresthesias, numbness, convulsions, tinnitus.

PATIENT CARE CONSIDERATIONS

Administration/Storage

- Administer oral medication with food, milk, or antacids to minimize GI upset.
- Do not crush, break, or allow patient to chew sustained-release capsules.
- Shake suspension before giving; do not mix with antacid or any other liquid.
- Refrigerate oral suspension and suppositories. Protect oral suspension from freezing.

Rectal suppositories:
- Encourage patient to retain rectal suppositories for 1 hr.

IV for patent ductus:
- Dilute at least 1 mg/mL with normal saline or

Sterile Water for Injection without preservative. Administer over 5 to 10 sec. May also be given as retention enema or via orogastric tube.

Assessment/Interventions

- Obtain patient history, including drug history and any known allergies (especially allergy to aspirin).
- Observe for signs of rhinitis, asthma, and urticaria.
- Assess the following with arthritis patient: note type, location, and intensity of limitation of movement and pain before and 1 to 2 hr after administration of standard-release medication and 4 to 6 hr after sustained-release form.
- Monitor BUN, creatinine, CBC, serum potassium, AST, and ALT prior to therapy and periodically during long-term therapy. Urine glucose and protein concentrations may be increased; leukocyte and platelet count may be decreased; bleeding time may be prolonged for 1 day after discontinuation.
- Assess for blurred vision and tinnitus, which could indicate toxicity.
- Observe for signs of GI bleeding (eg, black stools, occult blood loss) throughout therapy.
- Assess for mood changes, depression, hallucinations, confusion.
- Report signs of adverse reactions to health care provider immediately, especially in elderly patients.

Patient/Family Education

- Tell patient to take medication with food, milk, or antacids if GI upset occurs. Inform health care provider if stomach distress continues.
- Caution patient to avoid aspirin, alcohol, and ibuprofen while taking this medication.
- Instruct patient to report the following symptoms to health care provider: skin rash, itching, black stools, unusual bruising or bleeding, visual disturbances, tinnitus, weight gain, edema, or persistent headache.
- Advise patient that drug may cause drowsiness and to use caution while driving or performing other tasks requiring mental alertness.
- Explain that therapeutic effects for rheumatoid arthritis may not be seen for up to 1 mo of drug use.
- Explain purpose of medication and, for parents of infant with ductus arteriosus, emphasize need for frequent monitoring.

Infliximab

(in-FLICK-sih-mab)

Class Monoclonal antibody

How Supplied

Remicade Powder for Injection 100 mg (500 mg sucrose)

Action

PHARMACOLOGY: Neutralizes the biological activity of tumor necrosis factor (TNFα) by binding to its soluble and transmembrane forms and inhibits TNFα receptor binding.

PHARMACOKINETICS/DYNAMICS:
Excretion: The t½ is 8 to 9.5 days.

Indications Reduce signs and symptoms and induce and maintain clinical remission of moderate to severe Crohn disease; reduce number of draining enterocutaneous and rectovaginal fistulas and maintain fistula closure in Crohn disease; in combination with methotrexate to reduce signs and symptoms, inhibit progression of structural damage, and improve physical function in patients with moderately to severely active rheumatoid arthritis who have had inadequate response to methotrexate. **Unlabeled use(s):** Treatment of plaque psoriasis, ankylosing spondylitis, ulcerative colitis, psoriatic arthritis, psoriasis, Behcet syndrome, uveitis, and juvenile arthritis.

Contraindications Hypersensitivity to murine proteins or other components of product; moderate or severe CHF.

Route/Dosage

Rheumatoid Arthritis
ADULTS: IV 3 mg/kg infusion followed by additional 3 mg/kg doses at 2 and 6 wk after the first infusion, then q 8 wk thereafter in combination with methotrexate. For patients with incomplete response, may give up to 10 mg/kg or treat as often as q 4 wk.

Moderate to Severe or Fistulizing Crohn Disease
ADULTS: IV 5 mg/kg as an induction regimen at 0, 2, and 6 wk, followed by a maintenance regimen of 5 mg/kg q 8 wk. In patients who respond and then lose their response, consider treatment with 10 mg/kg.

Interactions

Vaccines: Do not administer live vaccines concurrently.

INCOMPATIBILITIES: Do not infuse concomitantly with other agents in the same IV line.

Lab Test Interferences None well documented.

Adverse Reactions

CV: Hypertension (10%); chest pain (7%); hypotension; syncope; tachycardia; pulmonary embolism; deep thrombophlebitis; circulatory

failure; arrhythmia; bradycardia; cardiac arrest; myocardial infarction.
CNS: Headache (29%); depression (8%); insomnia (6%); dizziness; confusion; suicide attempt; meningitis; neuritis; peripheral neuropathy.
DERM: Rash (18%); pruritus (9%); urticaria; flushing; sweating; ulceration.
GI: Nausea (24%); diarrhea (19%); abdominal pain (17%); dyspepsia (10%); vomiting; intestinal obstruction, perforation, and stenosis; pancreatitis; proctalgia; constipation; GI hemorrhage; ileus; peritonitis.
GU: UTI (14%); renal failure; menstrual irregularity; renal calculus.
HEMA: Lymphoma; thrombocytopenia; anemia; leukopenia; lymphadenopathy; pancytopenia; hemolytic anemia.
HEPA: Elevated ALT and AST; biliary pain; cholecystitis; cholelithiasis; hepatitis.
METAB: Dehydration.
RESP: Upper respiratory tract infection (40%); sinusitis (20%); coughing (18%); pharyngitis (17%); rhinitis (14%); dyspnea (6%); adult respiratory distress syndrome; bronchitis; pleurisy; respiratory insufficiency.
OTHER: Infusion reactions (20%); fatigue; fever, back pain, arthralgia (13%); moniliasis (8%); abscess (6%); lupus-like syndrome; pain; infections; myalgia; tendon disorder; cellulitis; sepsis; cholecystitis; chills; allergic reaction; diaphragmatic hernia; edema; surgical/procedural sequela; intervertebral disk herniation; neoplasms (eg, blood cell, breast); serum sickness.
Postmarketing – Infections have been observed with various pathogens including viral, bacterial, fungal, and protozoal organisms and have been noted in all organ systems in patients receiving infliximab alone or in combination with immunosuppressive agents. Other adverse reactions reported during postmarketing experience include demyelinating disorders (eg, multiple sclerosis), Gullian-Barre syndrome, interstitial pneumonitis, fibrosis, neuropathies, hemolytic anemia, idiopathic thrombocytic purpura, thrombotic thrombocytopenic purpura, and transverse myelitis. Anaphylactic-like reactions, including laryngeal/pharyngitis edema, severe bronchospasm and seizure have been associated with infliximab administration.

PATIENT CARE CONSIDERATIONS
Administration/Storage
- Reconstitute powder using 10 mL of sterile water only. Gently swirl solution to dissolve. Do not shake vial. Allow reconstituted solution to sit for 5 min. Solution should be colorless to light yellow and opalescent.
- Do not use if reconstituted solution is discolored or contains opaque particles.

> **WARNING:**
> *Infection:* Serious infections, including tuberculosis (frequently disseminated or extrapulmonary), invasive fungal infections, sepsis, and other opportunistic infections may occur. Do not initiate treatment in patients with active infection; exercise caution in those with chronic infection or history of recurrent infection. Evaluate patients for latent tuberculosis infection with a tuberculin skin test.

Precautions
Pregnancy: Category B.
Lactation: Undetermined.
Children: Safety and efficacy not established.
Elderly: Use with caution because of higher incidence of infection in the elderly.
Hypersensitivity: Reactions vary in their time of onset. Urticaria, dyspnea, and hypotension have occurred during or within 2 hr of infliximab infusion; however, serum sickness-like reactions have been observed in Crohn disease patients 3 to 12 days after infliximab treatment.
Autoimmunity: May result in autoantibody formation and, rarely, development of a lupus-like syndrome.
CHF: Preliminary results of ongoing trials of patients with moderate to severe CHF have reported higher incidences of hospitalization and mortality for worsening heart failure in patients receiving infliximab. Do not administer doses greater than 5 mg/kg in patients with CHF.
Immunogenicity: Treatment can be associated with development of antibodies to infliximab. The incidence in patients given a 3-dose induction regimen followed by maintenance dosing is about 10%.
Malignancy: Patients with long duration of Crohn disease or rheumatoid arthritis and chronic exposure to immunosuppressant therapies are more prone to develop lymphomas.
Neurologic events: Rarely, optic neuritis, seizure, and new onset or exacerbation of clinical symptoms or radiographic evidence of CNS demyelinating disorders, including multiple sclerosis, may occur.

- Prepare infusion solution by further diluting to a total volume of 250 mL with 0.9% sodium chloride injection. Gently mix diluted solution.
- Use diluted solution within 3 hr of preparation.
- Administer via IV route only. Infuse slowly over a period of no less than 2 hr.

- Use in-line, sterile, low-protein binding filter of up to 1.2 mcm pore size.
- Do not infuse concomitantly in the same IV line with any other agents.
- Do not reuse or store any unused portion of the infusion solution.
- Store powder for injection in refrigerator. Do not freeze.
- Do not use beyond expiration date.

Assessment/Interventions
- Obtain patient history, including drug history and any known allergies. Note history of allergic reactions to rats or mice.
- Assess patient for evidence of active infection. Report to health care provider if noted.
- Monitor patient for hypersensitivity reactions during and shortly after infusion.

Patient/Family Education
- Explain name, dose, action, and potential side effects of drug.
- Advise patient to notify health care provider immediately if any of the following occur: rash; hives; shortness of breath; swelling of the eyes, mouth, or throat.
- Advise patient to notify health care provider if any of the following are noted: new or worsening joint or muscle pain; fever or other signs of infection; sore throat; difficulty swallowing; swelling of hands or face; headache.
- Advise women to notify health care provider if pregnant, planning to become pregnant, or breastfeeding.
- Warn patient not to receive live vaccines while taking this drug.
- Instruct patient not to take any prescription or OTC medications or dietary supplements unless advised by health care provider.
- Advise patient that follow-up visits for examinations, blood tests, and additional doses of medication will be required; remind patient to keep appointments.

Influenza Virus Vaccine

(in-flew-EN-zuh virus vaccine)

Class Vaccine, inactivated virus

How Supplied
FluMist Intranasal spray $10^{6.5-7.5}$ $TCID_{50}$ (median tissue culture infectious dose) each of [A/New Caledonia/20/99 (H1N1), A/Wyoming (H23N2), B/Jilin/20/2003] per 0.5 mL. ♦ *Fluvirin* Injection (purified split-virus) 15 mcg each: [A/Wyoming/3/2003/X-147 (A/Fujian/411/2003 (H3N2)-like), A/New Caledonia/20/99 IVR-116, and B/Jiangsu/10/2003 (B/Shanghai/361/2002-like)] per 0.5 mL. ♦ *Fluzone* Injection (purified split-virus) 15 mcg each: [A/Wyoming/03/2003 (H3N2) (A/Fujian/411/2002–like), A/New Caledonia/20/99 (H1N1), and B/Jiangsu/10/2003 (B/Shanghai/361/2002-like)] per 0.5 mL.

🍁 *Fluviral S/F* ♦ *Vaxigrip*

Action
PHARMACOLOGY: Induces formation of specific antibodies that protect against those strains of virus from which vaccine is prepared or closely related strains.

Indications Induction of active immunity against the specific influenza viruses corresponding to strains in current-year vaccine formula; prophylaxis for people at least 6 mo of age at increased risk of complications or exposure to influenza. *Fluvirin* is not indicated for children under 4 yr of age. *FluMist* is not indicated in patients under 5 yr of age or patients over 50 yr of age.

Contraindications Immediate hypersensitivity to product or other components; hypersensitivity to eggs, egg products, or chicken proteins; delayed immunization is recommended for people with active neurologic disorder characterized by changing neurologic findings; defer immunization during acute respiratory disease or other active infection or during acute febrile illness; known or suspected immune deficiency diseases.

FluMist: Do not administer parenterally; do not administer to children or adolescents 5 to 17 yr of age receiving aspirin; do not administer to patients with a history of Guillain-Barré syndrome (GBS); do not administer to patients with altered or compromised immune status as a consequence of treatment with systemic corticosteroids, alkylating drugs, antimetabolites, radiation, or other immunosuppressive therapies.

Route/Dosage
FLUZONE/FLUVIRIN

ADULTS AND CHILDREN AT LEAST 9 YR OF AGE: IM 0.5 mL 1 dose.

CHILDREN 3 TO 8 YR OF AGE (FLUVIRIN IS INDICATED ONLY IN CHILDREN 4 YR OF AGE AND OLDER): IM 0.5 mL 1 dose; however, if previously unvaccinated, give 2 doses at least 1 mo apart, administering the second dose before December if possible.

CHILDREN 6 TO 35 MO OF AGE (FLUVIRIN IS INDICATED ONLY IN CHILDREN 4 YR OF AGE AND OLDER): IM 0.25 mL 1 dose; however, if previously unvaccinated, give 2 doses at least 1 mo apart, administering the second dose before December if possible.

FluMist (nasal inhalational only)
Children and adults 9 through 49 yr of age: **Nasal** 0.5 mL/season.
Children 5 through 8 yr of age: **Nasal** 0.5 mL/season if previously vaccinated with *FluMist*; 2 doses of 0.5 mL/season, each 60 days apart, if not previously vaccinated with *FluMist*.

Interactions
Anticoagulants: As with other IM drugs, give with caution to patients receiving anticoagulant therapy.
Antivirals: Do not administer *FluMist* until 48 hr after cessation of antiviral therapy, and do not administer antivirals until 14 days after giving *FluMist*, unless medically indicated.
Aspirin: Contraindicated in children or adolescents receiving *FluMist*.
Immunosuppressant drugs (eg, high-dose corticosteroids), radiation therapy: May result in inadequate response to immunization.
Other vaccines: Do not administer *FluMist* concurrently with other vaccines.
Pertussis vaccine: In order to attribute causality of adverse reactions, do not give influenza vaccine within 3 days of pertussis vaccination.
Theophylline: Theophylline levels may be increased during first 24 hr following vaccination.

Lab Test Interferences
Nasopharyngeal secretions or swabs collected from individuals receiving *FluMist* may test positive for influenza virus for up to 3 wk.

Adverse Reactions
CNS: Headache (40% [*FluMist*]); tiredness/weakness (26%); irritability (20%).
DERM: Soreness at injection site (10% to 64% [parenteral]).
EENT: Runny nose, nasal congestion (48%); sore throat (28% [*FluMist*]).
RESP: Cough (39% [*FluMist*]).
OTHER: Muscle ache (17%); decreased activity (14% [*FluMist*]); chills (9%); fever, malaise, presumed allergic reactions (including hives, angioedema, allergic asthma, systemic anaphylaxis), myalgia (parenteral).

Precautions
Pregnancy: Category C.
Lactation:
Parenteral – Influenza vaccine does not affect the safety of breastfeeding for mothers or infants.
Inhalational – Undetermined.
Children: Safety and efficacy not established in children younger than 6 mo of age. Safety and efficacy of *Fluvirin* not established in children younger than 4 yr of age. Safety and efficacy of *FluMist* not established in children younger than 5 yr of age.
Deficient antibody production: An unexpected antibody response may occur with *Fluzone* administration to individuals deficient in producing antibodies, whether because of genetic defect, immunodeficiency disease, or immunosuppressive therapy.
Guillain-Barré syndrome: Do not administer *Fluzone* or *Flumist* to individuals with GBS. Avoid *Fluvirin* in patients known to have experienced GBS within 6 wk after a previous influenza vaccination.
Thrombocytopenia/coagulation disorder: Do not give injectable influenza virus vaccine to individuals with thrombocytopenia or any coagulation disorder that would contraindicate IM injection unless physician determines that benefit clearly outweighs the risk.

PATIENT CARE CONSIDERATIONS
Administration/Storage
Parenteral:
- For IM administration only. Not for intradermal, subcutaneous, IV or intraarterial administration.
- Do not administer to infants younger than 6 mo of age.
- May be administered concurrently with childhood vaccines.
- May be administered concurrently with pneumococcal vaccine, using separate syringes, and at different sites.
- Shake multidose vial well before withdrawing dose.
- Shake prefilled syringe well before administering dose.
- Do not administer if solution is discolored or if particulate matter is noted.
- Use deltoid muscle for adults and older children.
- Use anterolateral aspect of thigh for infants older than 6 mo of age and for young children.
- Store vials and prefilled syringes in refrigerator (36° to 46°F). Protect from freezing. Freezing destroys potency. Do not use vaccine if it has been frozen.

Intranasal Spray:
- For nasal use only. Not for parenteral administration.
- Do not administer to pregnant women or individuals 50 yr of age or older, or younger than 5 yr of age.
- Not to be administered by severely immunocompromised individuals.
- Avoid coadministration of other vaccines.

- Thaw vaccine following manufacturer's guidelines prior to administration.
- Administer one-half of dose (a single spray) into each nostril while the patient is in an upright position. Insert tip of sprayer just inside nostril and depress the plunger to spray. Remove the dose divider clip and administer second half of dose into the other nostril.
- Dispose of used sprayer following approved procedures for disposal of biohazardous waste.
- Store in non-frost-free freezer (at or below 5°F). Do not store in a frost-free freezer because temperature may cycle above 5°F, which can negatively impact the stability of the vaccine. Vaccine may be thawed by holding sprayer in palm of hand and supporting the plunger rod with the thumb; vaccine thawed in this manner must be administered immediately after thawing. Vaccine may also be thawed in refrigerator and stored (36° to 46°F) for no more than 60 hr prior to use. Do not refreeze after thawing.

Assessment/Interventions

- Report adverse events following immunization to the DHHS Vaccine Adverse Event Reporting System (VAERS).
- Monitor patient for signs of allergic reaction. Have epinephrine 1:1,000 readily available and be prepared to treat appropriately.
- Ensure that skin testing, using influenza virus vaccine as antigen, is performed prior to administering vaccine to patient suspected of being hypersensitive to egg protein. Do not administer vaccine to patient who reacts to skin test challenge.

Parenteral:

- Obtain patient history, including drug history and any known allergies. Note hypersensitivity to eggs, egg products, chicken feathers, chicken danderm, chicken protein, acute febrile illness, neurologic reaction to previous vaccine dose, history of GBS, thrombocytopenia, bleeding disorder, thimerosal sensitivity, or latex sensitivity (multidose vials only).
- Defer vaccination in patient with acute febrile illness for at least 72 hr and symptoms have abated.
- Delay immunization in patient with active neurologic disorder characterized by changing neurologic findings until stabilized.
- Monitor patient for CNS, local, and systemic side effects. Inform health care provider if noted and significant.

Intranasal spray:

- Obtain patient history, including drug history and any known allergies. Note hypersensitivity to eggs, egg products, chicken feathers, chicken dander, chicken protein, acute febrile or respiratory illness, history of GBS, or concurrent antiviral therapy.
- Review patient's health history for any condition that could contraindicate use of intranasal influenza vaccine: asthma or history of reactive airway disease, children and adolescents 5 to 17 yr of age receiving aspirin therapy or aspirin-containing therapy, pregnancy, chronic CV or pulmonary condition, chronic condition requiring regular medical follow-up (eg, metabolic condition, renal dysfunction, hemoglobinopathy), congenital or acquired immunosuppression caused by underlying disease of immunosuppressive therapy, HIV infection, malignancy, lymphoma, leukemia.
- Defer vaccination in patient with acute febrile illness and/or respiratory illness for at least 72 hr and until symptoms have abated.
- Do not administer with antiviral agents. Postpone administration of intranasal influenza vaccine for 48 hr after discontinuing antiviral therapy. Do not administer antiviral agents until 2 wk after administration of vaccine.
- Do not administer concomitantly with any other vaccine. Postpone administration of intranasal influenza vaccine for 1 mo following vaccination with live virus vaccine or 2 wk following vaccination with inactivated or subunit vaccine. Do not administer live virus vaccine for 1 mo or inactivated or subunit vaccine for 2 wk following administration of intranasal influenza vaccine.

Patient/Family Education

- Advise patient, parent, or caregiver that vaccine will be prepared and administered by a health care provider.
- Remind patient, parent, or caregiver that vaccine needs to be administered every year in order to provide ongoing protection.
- Advise patient, parent, or caregiver to report all adverse events after vaccine administration to health care provider.

Parenteral:

- Educate patient, parent, or caregiver that vaccine contains noninfectious killed viruses and cannot cause influenza but coincidental respiratory disease unrelated to influenza vaccine can occur after vaccination.
- Advise patient receiving parenteral vaccine that soreness at injection site is most common side effect and may last for up to 2 days.
- Advise patient, parent, or caregiver that fever, general body discomfort, and muscle pain can develop, and to use non-narcotic analgesic and antipyretic (eg, ibuprofen) for symptomatic relief. Advise patient, parent, or caregiver to report severe or persistent symptoms to

health care provider.
- Advise patient, parent, or caregiver to notify health care provider immediately if unusual neurologic reactions (eg, abnormal skin sensations, paralysis, unexplained change in thinking or behavior) are noted.
- Advise parent or guardian of child younger than 9 yr of age who has not previously received influenza vaccine that a second dose, at least 4 wk after the first dose, is required to obtain max protection.

Intranasal spray:
- Caution patient, parent, or caregiver that vaccine recipient should avoid close contact (eg, within same household) with immunocompromised individuals for at least 21 days following vaccination.
- Caution health care worker who receives vaccine to avoid contact with severely immunocompromised patients for 7 days following vaccination.
- Advise parent or guardian of child 5 to 8 yr of age who has not previously received intranasal flu vaccine that a second dose, at least 6 wk after the first dose, is required to obtain max protection.

Insulin

(IN-suh-lin)

Class Antidiabetic

How Supplied

Regular, Insulin Injection
Regular *Iletin II* Injection 100 units/mL purified pork ◆ *Humulin R* Injection 100 units/mL human insulin (rDNA) ◆ *Novolin R* Injection 100 units/mL human insulin (rDNA) ◆ *Velosulin BR* Injection 100 units/mL human insulin (semisynthetic)
❋ *Novolin ge Toronto*

NPH, Isophane Insulin Suspension
NPH *Iletin II* Injection 100 units/mL purified pork ◆ *Humulin N* Injection 100 units/mL human insulin (rDNA) ◆ *Novolin N* Injection 100 units/mL human insulin (rDNA)
❋ *Novolin ge 30/70* ◆ *Novolin ge 40/60* ◆ *Novolin ge 50/50* ◆ *Novolin ge NPH*

Insulin Zinc Suspension
Lente *Iletin II* Injection 100 units/mL purified pork ◆ *Humulin L* Injection 100 units/mL human insulin (rDNA) ◆ *Novolin L* Injection 100 units/mL human insulin (rDNA)
❋ *Novolin ge Lente* ◆ *Novolin ge Ultralente*

70% NPH, Human Insulin Isophane Suspension and 30% Regular, Human Insulin Injection ([rDNA] Origin)
Humulin 70/30 Injection 100 units/mL human insulin (rDNA) ◆ *Novolin 70/30* Injection 100 units/mL human insulin (rDNA)

Action

PHARMACOLOGY: Insulin and its analogs lower blood glucose levels by stimulating peripheral glucose uptake, especially by skeletal muscle and fat, and by inhibiting hepatic glucose production. Insulin inhibits lipolysis, proteolysis, and enhances protein synthesis. Insulin is composed of 2 amino acid chains (ie, A [acidic] and B [basic]) joined together by disulfide linkage. Human insulin has minor but important differences from animal insulin with respect to amino acid sequence on the B-chain. It is derived from a biosynthetic process with strains of *E. coli* (recombinant DNA [rDNA]) or yeast. In some patients, human insulin may have a more rapid onset and shorter duration of action than pork insulin. However, the bioavailability of the insulins is identical when given SC. Human insulin is slightly less antigenic than pork or beef insulins. Human insulin is also the insulin of choice for patients with insulin allergy, insulin resistance, all pregnant patients with diabetes, and any patient who uses insulin intermittently.

PHARMACOKINETICS/DYNAMICS:
Onset: 0.5 to 1 hr.
Duration: 8 to 12 hr.

Indications Management of type 1 diabetes mellitus (insulin-dependent) and type 2 diabetes mellitus (non-insulin-dependent) not properly controlled by diet, exercise, and weight reduction. In hyperkalemia, infusions of glucose and insulin lower serum potassium levels. IV or IM regular insulin may be given for rapid effect in severe ketoacidosis or diabetic coma. Highly purified (single component) and human insulins are used for treatment of local insulin allergy, immunologic insulin resistance, lipodystrophy at injection site, temporary insulin administration, and in newly diagnosed diabetic patients.

Contraindications Hypersensitivity to pork or mixed beef/pork insulin unless successful desensitization has been accomplished.

Route/Dosage
Insulin preparations are classified into 3 groups based on promptness, duration, and intensity of action following SC administration. These classifications are rapid-(*Regular* or *Semilente*), intermediate-(*Lente* or NPH) or long-(*Ultralente*) acting. Maintenance doses are given SC and must be individualized by monitoring patients closely. Consider following dosage guidelines.
CHILDREN AND ADULTS: SC 0.5 to 1 U/kg/day.
ADOLESCENTS (DURING GROWTH SPURT): SC 0.8 to 1.2 U/kg/day. Adjust doses to achieve

premeal and bedtime blood glucose levels of 80 to 140 mg/dL (children younger than 5 yr 100 to 200 mg/dL). Regular insulin is given **IV** or **IM** for severe ketoacidosis or diabetic coma.

Interactions

Alcohol, anabolic steroids, beta blockers, clofibrate, fenfluramine, guanethidine, MAO inhibitors, phenylbutazone, salicylates, sulfinpyrazone, tetracyclines: May increase hypoglycemic effects of insulin.

Contraceptives (oral), corticosteroids, dextrothyroxine, diltiazem, dobutamine, epinephrine, smoking, thiazide diuretics, thyroid hormone: May decrease hypoglycemic effects of insulin.

Lab Test Interferences
None well documented.

Adverse Reactions

DERM: Lipodystrophy (from repeated insulin injection into same site).
METAB: Hypoglycemia.
OTHER: Hypersensitivity reaction (eg, rash, shortness of breath, fast pulse, sweating, hypotension, anaphylaxis, angioedema); local reactions (eg, redness, swelling, itching at injection site).

Precautions

Pregnancy: Insulin is drug of choice for control of diabetes in pregnancy; supervise carefully.
Lactation: Not excreted in breast milk.
Breastfeeding may decrease insulin requirements despite increase in necessary caloric intake.
Changing insulin: Changes in purity, strength, brand, type, or species source of insulin may necessitate dosage adjustment. Make changes cautiously under medical supervision.
Diabetic ketoacidosis: May result from stress, illness, or insulin omission and may develop slowly after long period of poor insulin control. Condition is potentially life-threatening and requires prompt diagnosis and treatment.
Hypoglycemia: May result from excessive insulin dose, increased work or exercise without eating, or from illness with vomiting, fever, or diarrhea. May also occur when insulin requirements decline.
Insulin resistance: Requirements of more than 200 units/day of insulin for more than 2 days in absence of ketoacidosis or acute infection may occur, especially in obese patients, patients with acanthosis nigricans, patients with insulin receptor defects, or during infection.

Overdosage: Signs and Symptoms

Hypoglycemia (including fatigue, weakness, nervousness, confusion, headache, diplopia, convulsions, psychoses, dizziness, unconsciousness, rapid or shallow respiration, numb or tingling mouth, hunger, nausea, skin pallor, moist or dry skin).

PATIENT CARE CONSIDERATIONS

Administration/Storage

- For insulin suspension, ensure uniform dispersion by rolling vial gently between hands. Avoid vigorous shaking that may result in formation of air bubbles.
- When mixing insulins, draw regular insulin into syringe first.
- Use only insulin syringes.
- Select appropriate injection site according to patient history and needs; rotate administration sites to prevent lipodystrophy. SC insulin is absorbed most rapidly at abdominal injection sites, more slowly at sites on arms, and slowest at sites on anterior thigh.
- Administer insulin 30 min before meals.
- Store properly in accordance with patient's daily needs. Insulin remains stable for 1 mo at room temperature or 3 mo under refrigeration. Store extra bottle of insulin in refrigerator.
- Refrigerate prefilled plastic and glass syringes, which can be stored under refrigeration for up to 14 days.
- Do not freeze.
- Do not expose to extreme temperatures or sunlight.

Assessment/Interventions

- Obtain patient history, including drug history and any known allergies.
- Assess patient for signs of hypoglycemia (eg, anxiety, chills, confusion, cool and pale skin, drowsiness, excessive hunger, headache, irritability, nausea, rapid pulse, tremors).
- Observe patient for signs of ketoacidosis (eg, drowsiness, fruit-like breath odor, frequent urination, loss of appetite, thirst).
- Monitor blood glucose levels throughout course of therapy.
- Observe injection sites for signs of local hypersensitivity reaction (eg, redness, itching, burning).
- Notify health care provider if hypoglycemia or adverse reactions occur.
- If lipoatrophy or lipohypertrophy develops at injection site, use alternate sites or purified insulin.
- Document injection sites used.

Patient/Family Education

- Teach name, dose, action, and side effects of insulin.
- Tell patient not to change brand, strength, type, or dose without health care provider's knowledge.
- Dosage adjustments may be necessary when type of insulin is changed.

- Tell patient to consult health care provider for dosage changes during illness.
- Instruct patient to use same type and brand of syringe each time to prevent dosage errors.
- Explain potential long-term complications of diabetes, and encourage regular, general physical and eye examinations.
- Tell patient to report redness, swelling, or itching at injection site.
- Explain significance and importance of reporting the following side effects: visual changes; rash; infection that does not heal; increased thirst; increased urination; dry mouth; burning sensation in feet, legs, or hands; pain in legs after exercise; frequent episodes of low or high blood sugar levels.
- Show patient how to rotate injection sites to prevent scarring.
- Teach patient how to monitor blood glucose as directed.
- Identify source for obtaining medical ID (eg, Medi-Alert) and explain importance of information.
- Teach patient and family how to draw up and administer insulin.
- Demonstrate self-care techniques for patient using insulin pump.
- Emphasize importance of compliance with diet and exchange system for meals.
- Emphasize importance of regular exercise.
- Tell patient to carry source of sugar (eg, candy, sugar packets) to counteract hypoglycemia.

Insulin Analogs

(IN-suh-lin)

Class Antidiabetic

How Supplied

Insulin Aspart

NovoLog Injection 100 Units/mL human insulin aspart (rDNA) ◆ NovoLog Mix 70/30 Injection 100 Units/mL human insulin aspart

Insulin Glargine

Lantus Injection 100 Units/mL insulin glargine (rDNA)

Insulin Glulisine

Apidra Injection 100 Units/mL insulin glulisine

Insulin Lispro

Humalog Injection 100 Units/mL human insulin lispro (rDNA) ◆ Humalog Mix 75/25 Injection 100 Units/mL human insulin lispro

Action

PHARMACOLOGY: Insulin and its analogs lower blood glucose levels by stimulating peripheral glucose uptake, especially by skeletal muscle and fat, and by inhibiting hepatic glucose production. Insulin inhibits lipolysis and enhances protein synthesis. Insulin is composed of 2 amino acid chains (A [acidic] and B [basic]) joined together by disulfide linkage. Human insulin has minor but important differences from animal insulin with respect to amino acid sequence on the B-chain. It is derived from a biosynthetic process with strains of *Escherichia coli* (recombinant DNA [rDNA]) or yeast. In some patients, human insulin may have a more rapid onset and shorter duration of action than pork insulin. However, the bioavailability of the insulins is identical when given subcutaneously. Human insulin is slightly less antigenic than pork or beef insulins. Human insulin is also the insulin of choice for patients with insulin allergy or insulin resistance, all pregnant patients with diabetes, and any patient who uses insulin intermittently.

PHARMACOKINETICS/DYNAMICS:

Excretion:

Insulin Aspart – The t½ is 1.5 hr.
Indulin Glulisine – The t½ is 42 min.
Insulin Lispro – The t½ is 1 hr.

Onset:

Insulin Aspart – 0.25 hr.
Insulin Lispro – 0.25 hr.

Peak:

Insulin Aspart – 1 to 3 hr.
Insulin Glulisine – 55 min.
Insulin Lispro – 0.5 to 1.5 hr.

Duration:

Insulin Aspart – 3 to 5 hr.
Insulin Lispro – 3 to 5 hr.

Indications

Insulin aspart: Treatment of patients with diabetes mellitus for the control of hyperglycemia; however, because of rapid onset and short duration of action, insulin aspart should normally be used in regimens that include an intermediate- or long-acting insulin.

Insulin glargine: Treatment of adult and pediatric patients with type 1 or adult patients with type 2 diabetes mellitus who require long-acting insulin for control of hypoglycemia.

Insulin glulisine: Treatment of patients with diabetes mellitus for the control of hyperglycemia; however, because of the rapid onset and short duration of action, compared with regular human insulin, insulin glulisine should normally be used in regimens that include a longer-acting insulin or basal insulin analog.

Insulin lispro: Treatment of patients with diabetes mellitus for control of hyperglycemia. In patients with type 1 diabetes, use in regimens that include a longer-acting insulin. In patients with type 2 diabetes, may be used without longer-acting insulin when used concurrently with sulfonylureas.

Contraindications During episodes of hypoglycemia; hypersensitivity to any component.

Route/Dosage

INSULIN ASPART

ADULTS: **Subcutaneous** Individualized; determined by health care provider in accordance with patient's needs (usual requirement 0.5 to 1 units/kg/day). **Insulin pump** When used in the external insulin infusion pump, the initial pump programming is based on the total insulin dose of the previous regimen. Although there is interpatient variability, approximately 50% of the total dose is given as meal-related boluses, and the remainder as basal infusion.

INSULIN GLARGINE

ADULTS AND CHILDREN 6 YR OF AGE AND OLDER: **Subcutaneous** Start with 10 Units daily and adjust according to patient's need to a total daily dose ranging from 2 to 100 Units. Administer each day at the same time of day.

INSULIN GLULISINE

ADULTS: **Subcutaneous or external infusion pump** Administer within 15 min before a meal or within 20 min after starting a meal. Individualize dose based on health care provider's advice in accordance with the needs of the patient. Usually used in regimens that include a longer-acting insulin or basal insulin analog. Administer in abdominal wall, thigh, or deltoid by continuous subcutaneous infusion.

INSULIN LISPRO

Type 1 Diabetes
ADULTS: **Subcutaneous** Variable; determined by health care provider.

Type 2 Diabetes
ADULTS AND CHILDREN OLDER THAN 3 YR OF AGE (IN COMBINATION WITH SULFONYLUREAS): **Subcutaneous** Variable; determined by health care provider.

INSULIN LISPRO MIX

ADULTS: **Subcutaneous** Variable; determined by health care professional.

Interactions

Alcohol, angiotensin-converting enzyme inhibitors, beta-blockers, fibrates, fluoxetine, MAO inhibitors, oral hypoglycemic agents, pancreatic function inhibitors (eg, octreotide, salicylates, sulfa antibiotics), pentoxifylline, propoxyphene: May increase hypoglycemic effects of insulin lispro. Beta-blockers may mask the symptoms of hypoglycemia in some patients.

Atypical antipsychotics, corticosteroids, danazol, diazoxide, diuretics, estrogens, isoniazid, niacin, oral contraceptives, phenothiazines, protease inhibitors, somatropin, sympathomimetics, thyroid hormone: May decrease hypoglycemic effects of insulin lispro.

Lab Test Interferences None well documented.

Adverse Reactions

DERM: Lipodystrophy (from repeated insulin injection into same site); pruritus; rash.
METAB: Hypoglycemia; hypokalemia.
OTHER: Hypersensitivity reaction (eg, rash, shortness of breath, fast pulse, sweating, hypotension, anaphylaxis, angioedema); local reactions (eg, redness, swelling, itching at injection site).

Precautions

Pregnancy: Category B (insulin lispro); Category C (insulin aspart, insulin glargine, insulin glulisine).
Lactation: Undetermined.
Children:
Insulin aspart, insulin glulisine – Safety and efficacy not established.
Insulin glargine – Safety and efficacy not established in children younger than 6 yr of age with type 1 diabetes.
Insulin lispro – In combination with sulfonylureas, safety and efficacy not established in children up to 3 yr of age.
Insulin lispro mix – Safety and efficacy not established in children up to 18 yr of age.
Renal function impairment: Insulin lispro, insulin glargine, or insulin glulisine dose may need to be reduced.
Hepatic function impairment: Insulin lispro, insulin glargine, or insulin glulisine dose may need to be reduced.
Changing insulin: Changes in purity, strength, brand, type, species source, or method of manufacture (rDNA vs animal source) of insulin may necessitate dosage adjustment. Make changes cautiously under medical supervision.
Hypoglycemia: May result from excessive insulin dose, missed meals, increased work, or exercise without eating.

Overdosage: Signs and Symptoms

Hypoglycemia (including fatigue, weakness, nervousness, confusion, headache, diplopia, convulsions, psychosis, dizziness, unconsciousness, rapid or shallow respiration, numb or tingling mouth, hunger, nausea, skin pallor, moist or dry skin).

PATIENT CARE CONSIDERATIONS
Administration/Storage
Insulin aspart:
- For subcutaneous injection or subcutaneous infusion (insulin pump) only. Not to be administered intradermally, IM, IV, or intra-arterially.
- Do not administer insulin aspart if particulate matter, cloudiness, or discoloration is noted, or if solution has become viscous.
- Usually used in combination with an intermediate- or long-acting insulin when used by direct subcutaneous injection.
- Dose should be administered into abdominal wall, thigh, or deltoid. Rotate injection sites within same region.
- Administer prescribed dose immediately (5 to 10 min) before a meal.
- If mixing insulin aspart with NPH human insulin, draw insulin aspart into syringe first and then administer prescribed dose immediately after mixing.
- Do not mix insulin aspart with crystalline zinc insulin preparations (eg, *Lente*).
- Can be used alone when administered by subcutaneous infusion by external insulin pump.
- Infusion catheter should be placed in abdominal wall. Rotate infusion sites within same region.
- Do not mix or dilute insulin aspart with any other insulin or solution when used in an external insulin pump for subcutaneous infusion.
- Store unopened vials, cartridges, and prefilled syringes of insulin aspart in refrigerator (36° to 46°F). Protect from freezing. Discard if frozen or exposed to temperature exceeding 98.6°F. Store opened vials of insulin aspart in refrigerator or at temperature below 86°F. Do not refrigerate cartridges after insertion into pen. Infusion sets (reservoirs, tubing, catheters) and insulin aspart in reservoir should be discarded after no more than 48 hr or after exposure to temperatures greater than 98.6°F.

Insulin lispro:
- For subcutaneous injection only. Not to be administered intradermally, IM, IV, intra-arterially, or by insulin infusion pump.
- Do not administer insulin aspart if particulate matter, cloudiness, or discoloration is noted, or if solution has become viscous.
- Usually used in combination with an intermediate- or long-acting insulin when used in patient with type 1 diabetes.
- May be used without an intermediate- or long-acting insulin when used in patient with type 2 diabetes.
- Dose should be administered into abdominal wall, thigh, or deltoid. Rotate injection sites within same region.
- Administer prescribed dose immediately (within 15 min) before or immediately after a meal.
- If mixing insulin lispro with longer-acting insulin (eg, *Humulin N*), draw insulin lispro into syringe first and then administer prescribed dose immediately after mixing.
- Follow manufacturer's guidelines if diluting insulin lispro. Use on special "Sterile Diluent."
- Store unopened vials and cartridges of insulin lispro in refrigerator (36° to 46°F). Protect from freezing. Vial or cartridge in use can be stored in refrigerator or outside refrigerator at temperature less than 86°F and away from direct heat and light. Discard any unused insulin stored outside refrigerator after 28 days. Diluted insulin lispro may be used for up to 28 days if stored in refrigerator or for up to 14 days if stored at room temperature (below 86°F).

Insulin analog mixtures (eg, 70/30, 50/50):
- For subcutaneous injection only. Not to be administered intradermally, IM, IV, intra-arterially, or by insulin infusion pump.
- Do not mix with any other insulin product.
- Administer prescribed dose immediately (eg, 10 to 20 min) before a meal.
- Store unopened vials, cartridges, and prefilled syringes of insulin analog mixtures in refrigerator (36° to 46°F). Protect from freezing. Do not use if analog mixture has been frozen. Vial in use can be stored outside refrigerator at temperature less than 86°F and away from direct heat and light but discard any unused insulin after 28 days. Cartridges and prefilled syringes in use must not be stored in refrigerator. Cartridges and prefilled syringes in use can be used for up to 10 days (lispro mix) or 14 days (aspart mix) if stored at room temperature (below 86°F).

Insulin glargine:
- Administer insulin glargine by subcutaneous injection only. Not to be administered intradermally, IM, IV, intra-arterially, or by insulin infusion pump.
- Dose should be administered into abdominal wall, thigh, or deltoid. Rotate injection sites within same region.
- Administer prescribed dose of insulin glargine daily, without regard to meals, at the same time each day.
- Do not mix or dilute insulin glargine with any other insulin or solution.

- Do not administer insulin glargine if particulate matter, cloudiness, or discoloration is noted.
- Store unopened vials of insulin glargine in refrigerator (36° to 46°F). Protect from freezing. Discard vial if frozen. Store opened vials of insulin glargine in refrigerator or at room temperature (below 86°F). Protect from direct heat and light. Discard any unused insulin glargine 28 days after first use.

Insulin glulisine:
- For subcutaneous injection or subcutaneous infusion (insulin pump) only. Not to be administered intradermally, IM, IV, or intra-arterially.
- Do not administer insulin glulisine if particulate matter, cloudiness, or discoloration noted, or if solution has become viscous.
- Used in combination with an intermediate- or long-acting insulin when used by direct subcutaneous injection.
- Dose should be administered into abdominal wall, thigh, or deltoid. Rotate injection sites within same region.
- Administer prescribed dose 15 min before or within 20 min after starting a meal.
- If mixing insulin glulisine with NPH human insulin, draw insulin glulisine into syringe first and then administer prescribed dose immediately after mixing.
- Do not mix insulin glulisine with insulin preparations other than NPH.
- Insulin glulisine can be used alone when administered by subcutaneous infusion by external insulin pump.
- Do not mix or dilute insulin glulisine with any other insulin or solution when used in an external insulin pump for subcutaneous infusion.
- Infusion catheter should be placed in abdominal wall. Rotate infusion sites within same region.
- Store unopened vials of insulin glulisine in refrigerator (36° to 46°F). Protect from direct heat and light. Protect from freezing. Discard if frozen or exposed to temperature exceeding 98.6°F. Store opened vials of insulin aspart in refrigerator or at temperature below 77°F. Discard opened vial after 28 days. Infusion sets (reservoirs, tubing, catheters) and insulin glulisine in reservoir should be discarded after no more than 48 hr or after exposure to temperatures greater than 98.6°F.

Assessment/Interventions
- Obtain patient history, including drug history and any known allergies. Note renal or hepatic impairment or history of ketoacidosis.
- Ensure that injection sites are continuously rotated to reduce or prevent injection site reactions (eg, lipodystrophy, pain, inflammation). Do not inject or place infusion catheter into area that is erythematous, pruritic, or shows signs of lipodystrophy.
- Document injection sites used.
- Check blood sugar frequently and observe for signs of hypoglycemia and hyperglycemia. Inform health care provider if blood sugar readings are outside target range or if hypoglycemic events are noted. Be prepared to treat hypoglycemic reactions.
- Check urine for ketones in patient at risk for ketoacidosis and observe for signs and symptoms of ketoacidosis (eg, fruit-like breath, drowsiness, thirst, frequent urination).

Patient/Family Education
- Explain name, dose, action, and potential side effects of drug.
- Educate patient or caregiver regarding diabetes and its management, including target ranges for blood sugar control. Instruct patient that insulin is not a substitute for diet and exercise and to continue to follow prescribed regimens.
- Educate patient or caregiver regarding potential long-term complications of diabetes and need for regular general physical and eye examinations.
- Advise patient or caregiver to read *Patient Information* leaflets before using the first time and with each refill.
- Ensure that patient or caregiver understands how to store, prepare, and administer the insulin dose(s) and dispose of used equipment and supplies.
- Advise patient using pen administration system to read the *Information for the Patient* insert and user manual for the pen before first use and with each refill.
- Ensure that patient using external insulin pump has read both the *Patient Package Insert* for the appropriate insulin and also the pump manufacturer's manual. Ensure that patient understands how and when to rotate infusion sites, program the infusion pump, evaluate infusion pump for malfunction, and has a plan of action in the event of infusion pump malfunction.
- Advise patient using external insulin pump to keep extra insulin available for direct subcutaneous administration in the event of pump malfunction.
- Advise patient to continuously rotate injection sites (abdomen, thigh, upper arm) to reduce or prevent injection site reactions (eg, lipodystrophy, pain, inflammation). Caution patient not to inject or place infusion cath-

eter into skin sites that are reddened, itching, or show signs of lipodystrophy.
* Ensure that patient or caregiver understands how to use home glucose monitor and has a plan for monitoring and recording blood sugar measurements (eg, log). Advise patient to take log to each visit with health care provider.
* Advise patient that dose(s) of insulin will usually be adjusted based on the results of home glucose monitoring.
* Ensure that patient with type 1 diabetes understands how to monitor for ketones and has a plan of action should ketones be detected.
* Educate patient regarding value of periodic HbA1c testing to confirm level of glucose control.
* Review symptoms of hypoglycemia (low blood sugar) and hyperglycemia (high blood sugar) as well as action plans should either event occur.
* Advise patient to discuss with health care provider a plan for managing each of the following situations: insulin dosing during current conditions (eg, vomiting, infection, trauma, stress, sick days); accidental administration of too little or too much insulin; missed insulin dose; inadequate food intake or a skipped meal; travel across time zones; change in physical activity.
* Advise patient with diabetes to carry identification (eg, *Medi-Alert*) indicating condition.
* Instruct patient to notify health care provider if experiencing severe, continuous, or frequent hypoglycemic episodes, hypoglycemic episodes with few or no warning symptoms, continuous or severe hyperglycemia, or injection site reactions that do not go away after a few days or continue to occur.
* Advise women to notify health care provider if pregnant, planning to become pregnant, or breastfeeding.
* Instruct patient not to take prescription or OTC drugs, herbal preparations, or dietary supplements without consulting health care provider.
* Advise patient that follow-up visits and lab tests will be necessary to monitor therapy and to keep appointments.

Interferon Alfacon-I

(IN-ter-FEER-ahn AL-fuh-con-1)
Class Interferon/Immunomodulator
How Supplied
Infergen Injection 9 mcg, Injection 15 mcg
Action
PHARMACOLOGY: These small protein molecules bind to specific cell-surface receptors and initiate complex sequences of intracellular events, including production of enzymes and other products with antiviral, antiproliferative, and immunomodulatory effects.

PHARMACOKINETICS/DYNAMICS:
Absorption: The T_{max} is 24 to 36 hr (products).

Indications Treatment of chronic hepatitis C virus (HVC) infection in patients older than 18 yr of age with compensated liver disease who have anti-HCV serum antibodies and/or the presence of HCV RNA.

Contraindications Allergy to alpha-interferons, *Escherichia coli*-derived products, or any component of the product.

Route/Dosage
Initial Therapy
ADULTS: **Subcutaneous** 9 mcg 3 times/wk for 24 wk.

Nonresponders/Relapse
ADULTS: **Subcutaneous** 15 mcg 3 times/wk for up to 48 wk.

Dose Reduction
ADULTS: **Subcutaneous** Withhold dosage temporarily for patients who experience a severe adverse reaction. If the reaction does not become tolerable, discontinue therapy. Dose reduction to 7.5 mcg may be necessary following an intolerable adverse reaction.

Interactions
Agents metabolized by CYP pathway, myelosuppressive agents: Use interferon alfacon-1 with caution.

Lab Test Interferences None well documented.

Adverse Reactions
CV: Hypertension, palpitation (5%).
CNS: Headache (82%); insomnia (39%); nervousness (31%); depression (26%); dizziness (25%); abnormal thinking (20%); anxiety (19%); paresthesia (13%); emotional lability (12%); hypoesthesia, amnesia (10%); hypertonia, somnolence (7%); agitation (6%); confusion, hyperesthesia, decreased libido, apathy (5%).
DERM: Alopecia, pruritus (14%); rash, increased sweating (13%); erythema (9%); dry skin (6%); wound (4%).
EENT: Pharyngitis (34%); rhinitis (13%); conjunctivitis (8%); tinnitus (6%); earache, eye pain, abnormal vision (5%); otitis (3%).
ENDO: Abnormal thyroid test (9%).
GI: Abdominal pain (41%); nausea (40%);

diarrhea (29%); anorexia (24%); dyspepsia (21%); vomiting (13%); constipation (9%); flatulence (8%); toothache (7%); decreased salivation, hemorrhoids, ulcerative stomatitis (6%); gingivitis, taste perversion (5%).
GU: Dysmenorrhea (9%); vaginitis (8%); menstrual disorder (6%); menorrhagia, breast mass (5%); genital moniliasis, breast pain (2%).
HEMA/LYMPH: Granulocytopenia (42%); leukopenia (28%); thrombocytopenia (19%); lymphocytosis (11%); lymphadenopathy, ecchymosis, anemia (6%); increased PT (3%).
HEPA: Tender liver (6%); hepatomegaly (5%).
LABTESTABS: Decreased hemoglobin, hematocrit, WBC, and platelets; increased triglycerides.
LOCAL: Injection site erythema (23%); injection site pain (11%); injection site ecchymosis (6%).
M/N: Hypertriglyceridemia (6%); weight decrease (5%).
MUSC: Myalgia (58%); arthralgia (51%); back pain (42%); limb pain (26%); skeletal pain, neck pain (14%); musculoskeletal disorder (7%).
RESP: Upper respiratory tract infection (31%); cough (22%); sinusitis (17%); respiratory tract congestion (12%); upper respiratory tract congestion (10%); dyspnea, epistaxis (8%); bronchitis (6%).
OTHER: Fatigue (71%); rigors (66%); fever (61%); body pain (54%); flu-like symptoms (15%); chest pain (13%); hot flushes (13%); malaise (11%); asthenia (10%); peripheral edema (9%); access pain (8%); allergic reaction (7%); infection (6%).

> **WARNING:**
> *Neuropsychiatric, autoimmune, ischemic, and infectious disorders:* Interferons may cause or aggravate fatal or life-threatening disorders of this nature. Persistent severe or worsening signs or symptoms may necessitate discontinuation of therapy. Closely monitor patients with periodic clinical and laboratory evaluations.

Precautions
Pregnancy: Category C.
Lactation: Undetermined.
Children: Safety and efficacy in children younger than 18 yr of age not established.
Autoimmune disease: Do not use interferon alfacon-I in patients with autoimmune hepatitis, and use with caution in patients with other autoimmune disorders.
Bone marrow depression: Use with caution in patients with abnormally low peripheral blood cell counts or who are receiving agents known to cause myelosuppression.
Cardiac disease: Use with caution. Hypertension, supraventricular arrhythmias, chest pain, and MI have been associated with interferon therapies.
Decompensated hepatic disorder: Do not use in patients with decompensated hepatic disease. Discontinue use in patients who develop symptoms of hepatic decompensation (eg, jaundice, ascites, coagulopathy, decreased serum albumin).
Fever: May be related to flu-like symptoms associated with therapy. Rule out other possible causes if persistent fever occurs.
Ophthalmologic disorders: Decrease or loss of vision, retinopathy including macular edema, retinal hemorrhages, cotton wool spots, and retinal artery or vein thrombosis reported rarely. Optic neuritis or papilledema are induced or aggravated by treatment with alpha interferons.
Severe acute hypersensitivity: If hypersensitivity reactions occur (eg, anaphylaxis, angioedema, bronchoconstriction, urticaria), discontinue drug immediately.
Suicide/Mental disorders: Do not use in patients with history of severe psychiatric disorders. Discontinue use in patients developing severe depression, suicidal ideation, or other severe psychiatric disorders.
Thyroid disorders: Use has been associated with hypothyroidism requiring supplementation.

Overdosage: Signs and Symptoms
Anorexia, chills, fever, myalgia.

PATIENT CARE CONSIDERATIONS
Administration/Storage
- For subcutaneous administration only. Not for intradermal, IM, IV, or intra-arterial administration.
- Dose is usually administered 3 times/wk with at least 48 hr between doses.
- Administer at bedtime to reduce incidence and severity of flu-like symptoms.
- Do not administer if particulate matter, cloudiness, or discoloration noted.
- Rotate injection sites (eg, buttocks, thighs, abdomen, back of arms). Use a different area for each injection. Do not inject into areas where the skin is tender, bruised, red, or hard.
- Vials contain no preservative. Use only 1 dose per vial and do not re-enter the vial. Discard any unused portion. Do not save or combine unused portions for later use.

- Administer nonnarcotic analgesic (eg, acetaminophen, ibuprofen) as prescribed for treatment of flu-like symptoms (eg, fever, rigors, headache, myalgia, arthralgia).
- Store vials in refrigerator (36° to 46°F). Do not freeze. Avoid exposure to sunlight and vigorous shaking. May allow solution to come to room temperature just prior to injection.

Assessment/Interventions
- Obtain patient history, including drug history and any known allergies. Note cardiac disease, decompensated hepatic disease, autoimmune hepatitis, low peripheral blood cell count, immunosuppression, organ transplant, depression or history of depression, psychiatric disorder, concurrent therapy with myelosuppressive agents, or allergy to alpha interferons or products derived from *E. coli*.
- Ensure that CBC with differential, platelet count, serum creatinine, serum albumin, bilirubin, triglycerides, and thyroid function tests are evaluated before initiating therapy, 2 wk after initiating therapy, and periodically thereafter for duration of therapy.
- Implement infection control measures if neutrophil count drops; implement bleeding precautions if platelet count drops.
- Ensure that eye examination is performed in all patients before starting therapy and periodically during therapy in patient with preexisting ophthalmic disorder (eg, diabetic or hypertensive retinopathy).
- Assess patient for ocular symptoms periodically during therapy. If ocular symptoms are noted, ensure patient receives a prompt and complete eye examination. Be prepared to discontinue therapy in patient who develops new or worsening ophthalmic disorders.
- Ensure women of childbearing potential are not pregnant and take effective birth control measures when therapy is initiated.
- Ensure men use effective contraception while taking interferon alfacon-1.
- Monitor patient for signs or symptoms of depression and suicidal ideation. Implement appropriate precautions and immediately report to health care provider if noted.
- Monitor patient for signs and symptoms of anaphylactic or serious allergic reactions. Be prepared to treat appropriately.
- Assess patient for CV, CNS, PSYCH, GI, DERM, GU, RESP, MUSC, general body side effects, and injection site reactions. Report to health care provider if noted and significant. Be prepared to reduce or temporarily withhold dose or discontinue therapy, depending on severity of adverse effect.

Patient/Family Education
- Explain name, dose, action, and potential side effects of drug.
- Review *Medication Guide* if patient or caregiver will be administering at home. Ensure patient or caregiver understands how to store, prepare, and administer the dose, and how to dispose of used equipment and supplies. If possible, the first injection should be performed under supervision of a qualified health care professional.
- Review dosing schedule with patient or caregiver. Advise patient or caregiver to administer prescribed dose at bedtime to minimize flu-like side effects.
- Advise patient not to change the dose, stop taking, or change brand of drug unless advised by health care provider.
- Advise patient if a dose is missed to take it as soon as possible, and to schedule the next dose about 48 hr later.
- Instruct patient to rotate injection sites as described in the *Medication Guide* to minimize likelihood of severe injection site reactions.
- Advise patient that flu-like symptoms are common and nonnarcotic analgesics (eg, acetaminophen, ibuprofen) can be used to prevent or relieve fever, headache, and muscle and joint pain.
- Advise patient to notify health care provider immediately of any of the following: suicidal ideation, depressed mood, changes in thinking or behavior, vision changes, hives, shortness of breath or difficult breathing, persistent fever, sore throat, unusual bleeding or bruising, intolerable injection site reaction.
- Advise patient to contact health care provider if experiencing bothersome side effects or any unusual problems.
- Advise men and women of childbearing potential to use effective contraception during treatment.
- Advise women to notify health care provider if pregnant, planning to become pregnant, or breastfeeding.
- Advise patient that drug may cause drowsiness or dizziness, and to use caution while driving or performing other tasks requiring mental alertness until tolerance is determined.
- Instruct patient not to take any prescription or OTC medications, herbal preparations, or dietary supplements unless advised by health care provider.
- Remind patient that office visits and laboratory tests will be required to monitor therapy and to keep appointments.

Interferon Alfa-2a

(IN-ter-FEER-ahn AL-fuh-2a)
Class Biologic response modifier

How Supplied
Roferon-A Solution for injection 3 million IU/mL, 1 mL single-use vials (3 million IU/vial), Solution for injection 6 million IU/mL, 0.5 mL single-use prefilled syringes (3 million IU/syringe), Solution for injection 6 million IU/mL, 1 mL single-use vials (6 million IU/vial), Solution for injection 6 million IU/mL, 3 mL multiple-dose vials (18 million IU/vial), Solution for injection 10 million IU/mL, 0.9 mL multiple-dose vials (9 million IU/vial), Solution for injection 12 million IU/mL, 0.5 mL single-use prefilled syringes (6 million IU/syringe), Solution for injection 18 million IU/mL, 0.5 mL single-use prefilled syringes (9 million IU/syringe), Solution for injection 36 million IU/mL, 1 mL single-use vials (36 million IU/vial)

Action
PHARMACOLOGY: Interferon alfa-2a has antiproliferative and immunomodulatory activities. Its elimination half-life is 3.7 to 8.5 hr after IV infusion.

PHARMACOKINETICS/DYNAMICS:
Absorption: The mean T_{max} is 3.8 hr (IM) and 7.3 hr (SC). The mean C_{max} is 2020 pg/mL for IM and 1730 pg/mL for SC. The apparent bioavailability is more than 80% for IM.
Distribution: The Vd_{ss} is 0.223 to 0.748 L/kg.
Metabolism: Totally filtered through the glomeruli and undergoes rapid proteolytic degradation during tubular reabsorption. The hepatic metabolism has a minor pathway.
Excretion: The $t_{1/2}$ is 3.7 to 8.5 hr. The mean Cl is 2.79 mL/min/kg.

Indications
Adult: Hairy cell leukemia, AIDS-related Kaposi sarcoma, chronic myelogenous leukemia.
Pediatric: Chronic myelogenous leukemia.
Unlabeled use(s):
Adults – Bladder tumors, mycosis fungoides, essential thrombocythemia, non-Hodgkin lymphoma, ovarian and cervical cancer, renal cell carcinoma, melanoma.
Children – Hemangiomas of infancy, pulmonary hemangiomatosis.

Contraindications
Standard considerations.

Route/Dosage
Hairy Cell Leukemia
ADULTS: **IM or SC** *Induction:* 3 million IU (MIU)/day, for 16 to 24 wk; *Maintenance:* 3 million IU **IM or SC** 3 times/wk. Treat patients for about 6 mo before determining whether to continue therapy.

AIDS-Related Kaposi Sarcoma
ADULTS: **SC or IM** *Induction:* 36 MIU/day, for 10 to 12 wk. *Alternative induction:* 3 MIU for 3 days, then 9 MIU for 3 days, then 18 MIU for 3 days, then 36 MIU daily for a total of 10 to 12 wk. *Maintenance:* 36 MIU **SC or IM** 3 times/wk. Continue therapy until no evidence of tumor exists or rapid disease progression, severe opportunistic infection, or adverse effects require discontinuation.

Chronic Myelogenous Leukemia
ADULTS: **SC or IM** 9 MIU/day. *Alternative regimen:* 3 MIU/day for 3 days, then 6 MIU/day for 3 days, then 9 MIU/day for the duration of therapy. Treat patients for several months before determining whether to continue therapy.
PEDIATRIC: **IM** 2.5 to 5 MIU/m²/day. Treat patients for several months before determining whether to continue therapy; some patients may require therapy for up to 18 mo.

Hemangiomas of Infancy, Pulmonary Hemangiomatosis
PEDIATRIC: **SC** 1 to 3 MIU/m²/day once daily.

Interactions
Aldesleukin: There is an increased risk of renal failure when using aldesleukin with interferon alfa-2a.
Melphalan: Coadministration of melphalan and interferon alfa-2a may decrease serum levels of melphalan.
Theophylline and possibly barbiturates: Alfa-interferon may inhibit hepatic metabolism of theophylline and possibly barbiturates, leading to increased serum concentrations of theophylline or barbiturates.
Vidarabine: Alfa-interferon may potentiate neurotoxicity when administered with vidarabine.
Zidovudine, acyclovir: There are synergestic antiviral effects with alfa-interferon and zidovudine and acyclovir.

Lab Test Interferences
Leukopenia, neutropenia, thrombocytopenia, decreased hemoglobulin, severe anemia, severe cytopenias, AST, alkaline phosphatase, LDH, proteinuria, uric acid.

Adverse Reactions
CV: Edema; hypotension.
CNS: Perioral tingling; dizziness; depression and suicidal ideation; paresthesia; sleep disturbances; confusion; hallucination; seizures; encephalopathy; gait disturbance; ataxia; tremor.
DERM: Rash; transient alopecia or thinning of the hair; excessive sweating or night sweats.
ENDO: Hypothyroidism; hyperthyroidism.
GI: Moderate potential for nausea and vomiting; dysgeusia; diarrhea; dry mouth; gingivitis;

anorexia; weight loss; elevated LFTs.
HEMA: Neutropenia; thrombocytopenia.
HYPERSEN: Antinuclear antibodies; anaphylaxis; neutralizing antibody formation.
MUSC: Severe lower extremities myalgias in chronic myelogenous leukemia patients.
RENAL: Proteinuria; acute renal failure; nephrotic syndrome.
RESP: Dyspnea; cough; pharyngitis; sinusitis; drying of the oropharynx.
SPEC SENSE: Visual disturbance; ocular pain.
OTHER: Flu-like syndrome.

> **WARNING:**
> *Neuropsychiatric, autoimmune, ischemic, and infectious disorders:* Interferons may cause or aggravate fatal or life-threatening disorders of this nature. Persistent severe or worsening signs or symptoms may necessitate discontinuation of therapy. Closely monitor patients with periodic clinical and laboratory evaluations.

Precautions
Pregnancy: Category C.

PATIENT CARE CONSIDERATIONS
Administration/Storage
- Refrigerate all products; do not freeze or shake.
- Use multiple-dose vials within 30 days of vial entry.
- Administer by IM or SC injection. SC administration is suggested for patients who are thrombocytopenic or who are at risk for bleeding. Give prefilled syringes SC only because syringe needle included is ½-inch long.
- Pretreatment with a NSAID or acetaminophen may minimize the risk of developing fever or reduce its severity.
- Avoid intra-arterial administration of interferon alfa.

Assessment/Interventions
- Because interferon alfa-2a may cause or aggravate fatal or life-threatening neuropsychiatric, autoimmune, ischemic, and infectious disorders, closely monitor patients with periodic clinical and laboratory evaluations.

Lactation: Discontinue nursing or discontinue the drug.
Hypersensitivity: Avoid use in patients with hypersensitivity to mouse immunoglobulin.
Special risk patients: Administer with caution in patients with severe renal or hepatic disease, cardiac disease, seizure disorders, or compromised CNS function.
Anemia: Leukopenia and thrombocytopenia may occur.
Depression and suicidal behavior: Depression and suicidal behavior including suicidal ideation, suicidal attempts, and suicides reported in association with alfa-interferon treatment.
Dosage reduction: Dosage reduction by 50% or withholding therapy may be needed when severe adverse reactions occur.
Leukopenia and elevation of hepatic enzymes: Leukopenia and elevation of hepatic enzymes occurred frequently.
Neutralizing antibodies: Neutralizing antibodies can develop during alfa-interferon therapy and may contribute to therapeutic failure in some patients. In some studies, the development of neutralizing antibodies was more common with interferon alfa-2a than with interferon alfa-2b.

- Monitor serum uric acid. Minimize effects of hyperuricemia with hydration, urinary alkalinization, and allopurinol.
- Prior to therapy and periodically, monitor blood hemoglobin, platelets, granulocytes, hairy cell, and bone marrow hairy cells. If a patient does not respond within 6 mo, discontinue treatment.
- Perform periodic CBCs and LFTs during treatment.
- Those patients who have preexisting cardiac abnormalities or who are in advanced stages of cancer should have ECGs taken prior to and during the course of treatment.

Patient/Family Education
- Warn patients not to change brands of interferon; changes in dosage may be necessary.
- Well hydrate patients, especially during initial treatment.

Interferon Alfa-2b
(IN-ter-FEER-ahn AL-fuh-2b)
Class Biologic response modifier

How Supplied
Intron A Powder for Injection, lyophilized 3 million IU/vial with 1 mL diluent vial or syringe, Powder for Injection, lyophilized 5 million IU/vial with 1 mL diluent vial, Powder for Injection, lyophilized 10 million IU/vial with 2 mL diluent vial, Powder for Injection, lyophilized 25 million IU/vial with 5 mL diluent vial, Powder for Injection, lyophilized 18 million IU multiple-dose vial with 1 mL diluent vial, Powder for Injection, lyophilized 50 million IU/vial with 1 mL diluent vial, Solution for injection

3 million IU/0.5 mL vial, Solution for injection
5 million IU/0.5 mL vial, Solution for injection
10 million IU/1 mL vial, Solution for injection
18 million IU multiple-dose pen (actually contains 22.5 million IU/1.5 mL pen), Solution for injection 18 million IU multiple-dose vial (actually contains 22.8 million IU/3.8 mL vial), Solution for injection 25 million IU multiple-dose vial (actually contains 32 million IU/3.2 mL vial), Solution for injection 30 million IU multiple-dose pen (actually contains 37.5 million IU/1.5 mL pen), Solution for injection 60 million IU multiple-dose pen (actually contains 75 million IU/1.5 mL pen).

Action

PHARMACOLOGY: Inhibition of virus replication in virus-infected cells, suppression of cell proliferation and such immunomodulating activities as enhancement of the phagocytic activity of macrophages and augmentation of the specific cytotoxicity of lymphocytes for target cells.

PHARMACOKINETICS/DYNAMICS:
Absorption: The T_{max} is 3 to 12 hr (IM and SC) and 30 min (IV). The C_{max} is approximately 18 to 116 IU/mL (IM, SC) and 135 to 273 IU/mL (IV).

Metabolism: The kidney may be the main site for catabolism.

Excretion: The elimination $t_{1/2}$ is approximately 2 to 3 hr.

Indications Hairy cell leukemia; condylomata acuminata; AIDS-related Kaposi sarcoma; chronic hepatitis B; chronic non-A/non-B hepatitis (hepatitis C); malignant melanoma; follicular non-Hodgkin lymphoma. **Unlabeled use(s):** Bladder tumors; chronic myelogenous leukemia.

Contraindications Standard considerations.

Route/Dosage

Decreased Granulocyte or Platelet Counts
If granulocyte count is less than 750/mm^3 and the platelet count is less than 50,000/mm^3, then reduce dose 50%. If granulocyte count is less than 500/mm^3 and the platelet count is less than 30,000/mm^3, then interrupt dose. When platelet or granulocyte counts return to normal or baseline values, therapy can be reinstituted at up to 100% of initial dose.

Hairy Cell Leukemia
ADULTS: **IM** or **SC** Induction dose 2 million IU (MIU)/m^2, 3 times/wk. Treat patients for about 6 mo before determining whether to continue therapy.

Malignant Melanoma
ADULTS: **IV infusion**
Induction: 20 MIU/m^2 for 5 consecutive days each week for 4 wk.
Maintenance: 10 MIU/m^2 3 times/wk for 48 wk by **SC** injection. Discontinue treatment if disease progression occurs.

Condylomata Acuminata
ADULTS: **Intralesionally** 1 MIU/lesion 3 times/wk for 3 wk.

Chronic Hepatitis B
ADULTS: **SC** or **IM** 30 to 35 MIU/wk, either as 5 MIU/day or 10 MIU 3 times/wk for 16 wk.

Chronic Hepatitis C
ADULTS: **SC** or **IM** 3 MIU 3 times/wk. At 16 wk treatment, extend therapy to 18 to 24 mo at 3 MIU 3 times/wk to improve the sustained response. Consider discontinuing therapy in nonresponders after 16 wk.

Follicular Lymphoma
ADULTS: **SC** 5 MIU/m^2, 3 times/wk in combination with other antineoplastic agents. Continue therapy for up to 18 mo.

AIDS-Related Kaposi Sarcoma
ADULTS: **IM**, **IV**, or **SC** 30 MIU/m^2 3 times/wk. Use the 50 MIU vial.

Interactions

Melphalan: Coadministration of melphalan and interferon alfa-2a may decrease serum levels of melphalan.

Theophylline and possibly barbiturates: Alfa-interferon may inhibit hepatic metabolism of theophylline and possibly barbiturates, leading to increased theophylline or barbiturate serum concentrations.

Vidarabine: Alfa-interferon may potentiate neurotoxicity when administered with vidarabine.

Zidovudine, acyclovir: There are synergistic antiviral effects with alfa-interferon and zidovudine and acyclovir.

Lab Test Interferences A transient increase in ALT can occur and is more frequent in responders. Other abnormal lab values include the following: hemoglobin; WBC count; platelet count; serum creatinine; alkaline phosphatase; lactate dehydrogenase; serum urea nitrogen; AST; granulocyte count.

Adverse Reactions

CV: Edema; hypotension.
CNS: Perioral tingling; dizziness; depression; paresthesia; sleep disturbances; confusion; hallucination; seizures; encephalopathy; gait disturbance; ataxia; tremor.
DERM: Rash; transient alopecia or thinning of the hair; excessive sweating; night sweats.
ENDO: Hypothyroidism; hyperthyroidism.
GI: Nausea; vomiting; dysgeusia; diarrhea; dry mouth; gingivitis; anorexia; weight loss; elevated LFTs.
HEMA: Neutropenia, reversible and dose-

related; thrombocytopenia, reversible and dose-limiting.
HYPERSEN: Antinuclear antibodies; anaphylaxis; antibody formation.
MUSC: Severe lower extremities myalgias.
RENAL: Proteinuria; acute renal failure; nephrotic syndrome.
RESP: Dyspnea; cough; pharyngitis; sinusitis; drying of the oropharynx.
SPEC SENSE: Visual disturbance; ocular pain.
OTHER: Flu-like syndrome.

> **WARNING:**
> *Neuropsychiatric, autoimmune, ischemic, and infectious disorders:* Interferons may cause or aggravate fatal or life-threatening disorders of this nature. Persistent severe or worsening signs or symptoms may necessitate discontinuation of therapy. Closely monitor patients with periodic clinical and laboratory evaluations.

Precautions
Pregnancy: Category C.
Lactation: Discontinue nursing or discontinue the drug.
Hypersensitivity: Acute serious hypersensitivity reactions (eg, urticaria, angioedema, bronchoconstriction, anaphylaxis) have been observed in treated patients; if an acute reaction develops, discontinue the drug immediately, and institute appropriate medical therapy.
Hepatic function impairment: Do not treat patients with decompensated liver disease, autoimmune hepatitis, history of autoimmune disease, or immunosuppressed transplant recipients.

PATIENT CARE CONSIDERATIONS
Administration/Storage
- Refrigerate; do not freeze. Multiple-dose pens are stable for up to 2 days at room temperature.
- Do not shake.
- Reconstitute the lyophilized powder after adding diluent (Bacteriostatic Water for Injection); gently agitate the vial. No further dilution is required prior to administration. Commercially available solution does not require further dilution.
- The patient may self-administer the dose at bedtime.
- For IV infusion, the dose may be diluted with 100 mL of 0.9% Sodium Chloride, for a final concentration of at least 10 MIU/100 mL. Dilute immediately prior to use.
- Reconstituted solutions are stable under refrigeration for 30 days or at room temperature for 7 days.

Worsening liver disease, including jaundice, hepatic encephalopathy, hepatic failure, and death have occurred following therapy. Discontinue therapy for any patient developing signs and symptoms of liver failure.
Special risk patients: Administer with caution in patients with severe renal or hepatic disease, cardiac disease, seizure disorders, or compromised CNS function.
AIDS-related Kaposi sarcoma: Use only the 50 MIU vial size.
Dosage reduction: Dosage reduction by 50% or withholding therapy may be needed when severe adverse reactions occur.
Fever/"Flu-like" symptoms: Because of fever and other "flu-like" symptoms associated with this drug, use cautiously in debilitating medical conditions, such as those with a history of pulmonary disease (eg, chronic obstructive pulmonary disease) or diabetes mellitus prone to ketoacidosis. Observe caution in coagulation disorders (eg, thrombophlebitis, pulmonary embolism) or severe myelosuppression.
Malignant melanoma: Interferon solution for injection is not recommended for the IV treatment of malignant melanoma.
Neutralizing antibodies: May contribute to therapeutic failure in some patients.
Preexisting psychiatric condition/History of severe psychiatric disorder: Do not treat; discontinue therapy in any patient developing severe depression.
Thyroid abnormalities: Do not treat patients with preexisting thyroid abnormalities whose thyroid function cannot be maintained in the normal range by medication. Prior to initiation of therapy, evaluate serum TSH.

- Reconstituted solutions of 10 MIU/mL are stable frozen at temperatures of -10°C or less for 4 weeks in plastic syringes.
- Administer by IM or SC injection, IV infusion.
- SC administration is suggested for patients who are thrombocytopenic or who are at risk for bleeding.
- Administer IV infusion over 20 min.
- Pretreatment with NSAIDs or acetaminophen may minimize the risk of developing fever or its severity.
- Avoid intra-arterial administration of interferon alfa.

AIDS-related Kaposi sarcoma:
- 50 MIU vial administered IM, IV, or SC.

Condylomata acuminata:
- Use only 10 MIU vials because dilution of other strengths required for intralesional use

results in a hypertonic solution. Do not reconstitute 10 MIU vials with more than 1 mL diluent. Use tuberculin or a similar syringe and a 25- to 30-gauge needle. Do not go beneath the lesion too deeply or inject too superficially. As many as 5 lesions can be treated at 1 time. To reduce side effects, give in evening with acetaminophen. Direct the needle at the center of the base of the wart and at an angle almost parallel to the plane of the skin. This will deliver the interferon to the dermal core of the lesion, infiltrating the lesion and causing a small wheal.

Thrombocytopenia:

- Do not give IM to patients with platelet counts less than 60,000/mm^3. Instead, give SC.

Assessment/Interventions

- Since interferon alfa-2b may cause or aggravate fatal or life-threatening neuropsychiatric, autoimmune, ischemic, and infectious disorders, closely monitor patients with periodic clinical and laboratory evaluations.
- Monitor serum uric acid. Minimize effects of hyperuricemia with hydration, urinary alkalinization, and allopurinol.
- There may be synergistic adverse effects between interferon alfa-2b and zidovudine. Patients have had a higher incidence of neutropenia than that expected with zidovudine alone. Carefully monitor WBC count.
- Pulmonary infiltrates rarely occur. Take chest x-rays of any patient developing fever, cough, dyspnea, or other respiratory symptoms.
- Use therapy cautiously in patients with a history of MI or previous or current arrhythmic disorder who require therapy.
- Monitor any patient developing liver function abnormalities during treatment, and discontinue treatment if appropriate.
- Monitor any patient developing an autoimmune disorder during treatment. Discontinue treatment if appropriate.
- Symptomatic patients should have their blood glucose measured and followed up accordingly. Patients with diabetes mellitus may require adjustment of their antidiabetic regimen.
- In addition to tests normally required for monitoring patients, the following are recommended for all patients on interferon therapy, prior to beginning treatment and periodically thereafter: standard hematologic tests with CBCs and differential, platelet counts, blood chemistries, electrolytes, TSH, and LFTs. Patients with preexisting cardiac abnormalities, or in advanced stages of cancer, should have ECGs taken before and during treatments.
- Baseline chest x-rays are suggested; repeat if clinically indicated.
- For malignant melanoma patients, monitor differential WBC count and LFTs weekly during the induction phase of therapy and monthly during the maintenance phase of therapy.
- If increases in ALT occur during therapy for chronic hepatitis B, carefully monitor clinical symptomatology and LFTs, including ALT, prothrombin time, alkaline phosphatase, albumin, and bilirubin.
- Interferon may exacerbate preexisting psoriasis.

Chronic hepatitis B:

- Perform a liver biopsy to establish presence of chronic hepatitis and extent of liver damage. Establish that the patient has compensated liver disease.

Chronic hepatitis C:

- Perform a liver biopsy to establish diagnosis. Test for presence of antibody to HCV.

Retinal hemorrhages, cotton wool spots, and retinal artery or vein obstruction:

- Examine the eyes of any patient complaining of changes in visual acuity or visual fields or reporting any other ophthalmologic symptoms during treatment with interferon alfa-2b.

Patient/Family Education

- Photosensitivity may occur; therefore, caution patients to take protective measures (eg, sunscreens, protective clothing) against exposure to ultraviolet light or sunlight until tolerance is determined.
- May cause drowsiness or dizziness.
- Notify health care provider if hives, itching, tightness in the chest, cough, difficulty breathing, visual problems, wheezing, low blood pressure, or lightheadedness occurs.
- Contraceptive measures are recommended during therapy with interferon alfa-2b. Notify health care provider immediately if suspecting pregnancy.
- Store in the refrigerator at 2° to 8°C (36° to 46°F). Do not freeze or shake.
- Do not change brands of interferon; changes in dosage may be necessary.
- The most common adverse effects are "flu-like" symptoms, such as fever, headache, fatigue, anorexia, nausea, and vomiting. These appear to decrease in severity as treatment continues. Some of these "flu-like" symptoms may be minimized by bedtime doses. Use antipyretics to prevent or partially alleviate fever and headache.
- Hydrate patients well, especially during the initial stages of treatment.

Interferon Alfa-2b, Recombinant/Ribavirin

(IN-ter-FEER-ahn AL-fuh-2b/rhy-buh-VIE-rin)

Class Immunologic agent

How Supplied
Rebetron Injection/Capsules (Combination packages) 3 million IU interferon alfa-2b, recombinant/0.5 mL and 200 mg ribavirin

Action
PHARMACOLOGY: Interferon alfa-2b inhibits virus replication in virus-infected cells and suppresses cell proliferation; although the exact mechanism of action of ribavirin is not known, it has antiviral inhibitory activity against respiratory syncytial virus, influenza virus, and herpes simplex virus.

Indications Treatment of chronic hepatitis C in patients with compensated liver disease previously untreated with alpha interferon or who have relapsed after alpha interferon therapy.

Contraindications Women who are pregnant or men whose female partners are pregnant.

Route/Dosage
Administer interferon alfa-2b SC and ribavirin PO.

ADULTS 75 KG OR LESS: **SC** interferon alfa-2b 3 million IU 3 times/wk plus **PO** ribavirin 400 mg in morning and 600 mg in evening for 24 wk.

ADULTS MORE THAN 75 KG: **SC** interferon alfa-2b 3 million IU 3 times/wk plus **PO** ribavirin 600 mg in morning and evening for 24 wk.

Dose Modification
For patients with history of stable cardiovascular disease, a permanent dose reduction of interferon alfa-2b to **SC** 1.5 million IU 3 times/wk plus ribavirin to **PO** 600 mg/day is required if the hemoglobin decreases by at least 2 g/dL during any 4-wk period. In addition, for a cardiac history patient, if the hemoglobin remains below 12 g/dL after 4 wk on the reduced dose, discontinue combination therapy. It is recommended that patients whose hemoglobin level falls less than 10 g/dL have their ribavirin dose reduced to 200 mg in the morning and 400 mg in the evening. Permanently discontinue treatment in patients whose hemoglobin level falls below 8.5 g/dL from combination therapy. Reduce the interferon alfa-2b dose to 1.5 million IU 3 times/wk in patients whose WBC count is less than 1500/mm^3, neutrophil count is less than 750/mm^3, or platelet count is less than 50,000/mm^3. Permanently discontinue combination therapy in patients whose WBC count is less than 1000/mm^3, neutrophil count less than 500/mm^3, or platelet count less than 25,000/mm^3.

Interactions
Nucleoside analogs: Risk of lactic acidosis may be increased.

Lab Test Interferences None well documented.

Adverse Reactions
CNS: Insomnia; depression; irritability; suicidal behavior (eg, ideation, attempts); suicide; headache; vertigo; dizziness.
DERM: Alopecia; rash; pruritus.
EENT: Hearing loss; tinnitus; sinusitis; taste perversion.
GI: Nausea; anorexia; dyspepsia; vomiting.
HEMA: Hemolytic anemia; decreased hemoglobin.
RESP: Dyspnea.
OTHER: Inflammation at injection site; fatigue; rigors; fever; flu-like symptoms; asthenia; chest pain; myalgia; arthralgia; musculoskeletal pain.

> **WARNING:**
> *Neuropsychiatric, autoimmune, ischemic, and infectious disorders:* Interferons may cause or aggravate fatal or life-threatening disorders of this nature. Persistent severe or worsening signs or symptoms may necessitate discontinuation of therapy. Closely monitor patients with periodic clinical and laboratory evaluations.

Precautions
Pregnancy: Category X.
Lactation: Undetermined. Decide whether to discontinue nursing or to discontinue combination therapy.
Children: Safety and efficacy not established.
Elderly: Administer with caution, starting at the lower end of the dose range, reflecting the greater frequency of decreased renal, hepatic, and cardiac function as well as concomitant disease or drug therapy.
Bone marrow toxicity: Suppression of bone marrow function may occur, resulting in severe aplastic anemia.
Pulmonary disorders: Dyspnea, pulmonary infiltrates, pneumonitis, and pneumonia may occur.
Pancreatitis: Fatal and nonfatal pancreatitis may occur.
Diabetes: Diabetes mellitus and hyperglycemia may occur.
Ophthalmic disorders: Rarely, retinal hemorrhage, cotton wool spots, and retinal artery or vein obstruction may occur with interferon alpha.

PATIENT CARE CONSIDERATIONS
Administration/Storage
Ribavirin capsules:
- Administer prescribed number of capsules bid without regard to food, but administer in a consistent manner (ie, either with or without food).
- Administer reduced dose to patient with hemoglobin below 10 g/dL.

Interferon alfa-2b injection:
- Check doseform carefully. Available in single-use vial, multidose vial, and multidose pen.
- Administer prescribed dose 3 times/wk via SC route only.
- Administer reduced dose to patient if WBC is less than 1500/mm^3, absolute neutrophil count is less than 750/mm^3, or platelet count is less than 50,000/mm^3.
- Administer reduced dose to patient who develops moderate depression.
- Do not administer if particulate matter or discoloration noted.
- Store combination package (capsules and injection) in refrigerator. When separated, store injectable medication in refrigerator and capsules in refrigerator or at controlled room temperature. Interferon alfa-2b injection in vials is stable for 14 days or less at room temperature. Interferon alfa-2b injection in multidose pens is stable for 2 or less days at room temperature.

Assessment/Interventions
- Obtain patient history, including drug history and any known allergies. Note history of autoimmune hepatitis, autoimmune disorders, significant cardiovascular disease, hemoglobinopathies, cytopenia, psychiatric disorders, psoriasis, or impaired renal function.
- Ensure that female patient has negative pregnancy test before starting therapy, monthly during, and 6 mo following completion.
- Ensure that female partner of male patient is not pregnant before starting therapy.
- Ensure that female patient of childbearing potential and female partner of male patient are using 2 forms of effective contraception during and for 6 mo following completion of therapy.
- Ensure that baseline CBC and differential is determined before starting therapy, at 2 and 4 wk after starting therapy, and then periodically thereafter during therapy.
- Ensure that baseline LFTs and TSH are determined before starting therapy and periodically during therapy.
- Ensure that diabetic and hypertensive patients have a visual examination prior to starting therapy.
- Monitor blood sugar in diabetic patient when drug is started or dose is changed. Report significant changes to health care provider.
- Do not administer to patient if WBC is less than 1000/mm^3, absolute neutrophil count is less than 500/mm^3, platelet count is less than 25,000/mm^3, or hemoglobin is below 8.5 g/dL.
- Do not administer to patient who develops severe depression or suicidal ideation or attempt.
- Assess for flu-like symptoms (eg, fever, headache, fatigue, rigors, myalgia). If such symptoms occur, administer interferon alfa-2b in the evening and give nonnarcotic analgesics as prescribed.
- Monitor patient for evidence of CNS, GI, musculoskeletal, psychiatric, respiratory, visual, and general body side effects. If noted and significant, inform health care provider.
- If patient experiences adverse CNS symptoms (eg, dizziness), implement safety precautions such as lowering bed, putting side rails up, and supervising ambulation.
- Implement infection-control measures if WBC drops; implement bleeding precautions if platelet count drops.
- Monitor patient for signs of anaphylaxis or severe allergic reaction. Discontinue therapy and immediately notify health care provider if noted. Be prepared to treat appropriately.

Patient/Family Education
- Explain name, dose, action, and potential side effects of therapy. If patient will be administering interferon alfa-2b at home, review "Medication Guide" with the patient. Ensure that the patient understands how to store, prepare, and administer the dose, and dispose of used equipment and supplies.
- Review dosing schedule with patient. Caution patient that capsules and injection must be used as prescribed in order to achieve maximum benefit.
- Advise patient that capsules can be taken without regard to food but to be consistent (ie, either take with or without food).
- Warn female patient of childbearing potential and female partner of male patient that extreme care must be taken to avoid pregnancy during therapy and for 6 mo after completion of therapy because of significant risk of teratogenic and embryocidal effects. Instruct patient and partner to use 2 reliable forms of effective contraception during treatment and during the 6-mo posttreatment follow-up period.
- Advise female patient of childbearing potential that pregnancy tests will be performed

monthly during therapy and for 6 mo following completion of therapy.
- Instruct female patient or female partner of male patient to report suspected pregnancy immediately to health care provider.
- Instruct women to notify health care provider if pregnant, planning to become pregnant, or breastfeeding.
- Advise patient that flu-like symptoms (eg, headache, fatigue, myalgia, rigors, fever) are the most common side effects and may decrease in severity as treatment continues and that administering the interferon alfa-2b at bedtime may minimize these symptoms. Antipyretic analgesics (eg, acetaminophen, ibuprofen) can be used to alleviate headache, myalgia, and fever.
- Advise patient that it is not known if this therapy will prevent transmission of hepatitis C to others nor is it known if it can prevent cirrhosis, liver failure, or liver cancer that may develop as a result of hepatitis C infection.
- Advise patient to immediately report any of the following to the health care provider: fever or other signs of infection, sore throat, unusual bruising or bleeding.
- Instruct patient to not take any prescription or OTC medications or dietary supplements unless advised by the health care provider.
- Advise patient that laboratory tests and follow-up visits will be required to monitor therapy and to keep appointments.

Interferon Alfa-n3

(IN-ter-FEER-ahn AL-fuh-n 3)

Class Interferon/Immunomodulator

How Supplied
Alferon N Solution 5 million IU/mL

Action
PHARMACOLOGY: These small proteins bind to specific cell membranes and initiate complex sequences of intracellular events, including induction of certain enzymes that produce antiproliferative action against tumor cells and inhibit viral replication in virus-infected cells.

Indications Treatment of condyloma acuminatum.

Contraindications Known hypersensitivity to human interferon alpha proteins or any component of the product; anaphylactic sensitivity to mouse immunoglobulin, egg protein, or neomycin.

Route/Dosage
Condyloma Acuminatum
ADULTS: **Intralesional** 250,000 IU (0.05 mL) (max recommended dose per treatment session) injected into base of each wart. Administer twice weekly for up to 8 wk.

Interactions None well documented.

Lab Test Interferences None well documented.

PATIENT CARE CONSIDERATIONS

Administration/Storage
- Do not shake solution.
- Inject into base of each wart, preferably with 30-gauge needle.
- Store in refrigerator. Do not freeze.

Assessment/Interventions
- Obtain patient history, including drug history and any allergies.

Adverse Reactions
CV: Chest pain; hypotension; vasovagal response.
CNS: Headache; depression; fatigue; malaise; dizziness; insomnia; sleepiness.
DERM: Soreness at injection site; generalized pruritus; sweating.
EENT: Blurred vision; ocular rotation pain; sinus drainage; sore mouth; stomatitis; mucositis.
GI: Nausea; vomiting; dyspepsia; diarrhea; anorexia; dry mouth.
HEMA: Altered hemoglobin levels, WBC, platelet count, GGT.
HEPA: Altered AST, alkaline phosphatase, total bilirubin.
OTHER: Fever; chills; myalgias; arthralgia; back pain; flu-like syndrome.

Precautions
Pregnancy: Category C.
Lactation: Undetermined.
Children: Safety and efficacy not established in children younger than 18 yr.
Debilitating medical conditions: Fever and flu-like symptoms associated with drug may exacerbate medical conditions (eg, cardiovascular disease, pulmonary disease, diabetes mellitus with ketoacidosis, coagulation disorders, severe myelodepression, seizures).
Product interchange: Interferon products are not interchangeable because of manufacturing processes, strength, and type.

- Assess patient for side effects. If present, notify health care provider.
- Monitor hydration if patient experiences anorexia, nausea, or diarrhea. If vomiting and diarrhea occur frequently increase patient's fluid intake to 2 to 3 L/day.
- Monitor results of laboratory tests.
- Assess patient for symptoms of infection

because they may be masked by drug fever.
- If patient experiences adverse CNS symptoms (eg, LOC, mental status changes, dizziness, confusion), take safety precautions such as lowering bed, putting side rails up, and supervising ambulation.
- Discuss need for antiemetic with health care provider if patient develops nausea or vomiting.
- If flu-like symptoms occur, administer drug in evening, and administer acetaminophen as prescribed for fever and headache.

Patient/Family Education
- Stress importance of returning for follow-up blood tests.
- Teach infection control measures, bleeding precautions, and energy conservation measures.
- Emphasize importance of maintaining well-hydrated state.
- Caution patient not to change brand of drug because dosages vary among different forms.
- Advise patient to take medication at bedtime if flu-like symptoms occur, and to use acetaminophen as needed.
- Instruct patient to report the following symptoms that may represent side effects: hives, swollen ankles, dyspnea, chest pain, noisy breathing.
- Caution patient to take safety precautions and not to perform activities that require mental alertness if decreased mental status or dizziness occur.

Interferon Beta-1a

(In-ter-FEER-ahn BAY-tah 1a)

Class Interferon/Immunomodulator

How Supplied
Avonex Powder for injection, lyophilized 33 mcg (6.6 million IU) ◆ *Rebif* Powder for injection 22 mcg, Powder for injection 44 mcg

Action
PHARMACOLOGY: Has antiviral, antiproliferative, and immunoregulatory activities. Binds to specific cell membrane receptors that induce the expression of a number of gene products that mediate the biological actions of interferon beta-1a.

PHARMACOKINETICS/DYNAMICS:
Absorption: The T_{max} is 3 to 15 hr.
Excretion: The t½ is 10 hr.

Indications Treatment of relapsing forms of multiple sclerosis to slow accumulation of physical disability and decrease the frequency of clinical exacerbations.

Contraindications Hypersensitivity to natural or recombinant interferon beta, human albumin, or any other component of the formulation.

Route/Dosage
ADULTS: *Avonex*: **IM** 30 mcg once weekly. *Rebif*: **SC** 44 mcg 3 times/wk.

Interactions
Myelosuppressive agents: Because of potential to cause neutropenia and lymphopenia, monitor patients during concomitant therapy.

Lab Test Interferences None well documented.

Adverse Reactions
CV:
Avonex – Vasodilation (2%).
CNS:
Avonex – Headache (58%); depression (18%); dizziness (14%); migraine (5%); seizures (postmarketing).
Rebif – Headache (70%); fatigue (41%); depression (25%); hypertonia (7%); abnormal coordination, convulsions, somnolence (5%); suicidal ideation.
DERM:
Avonex – Alopecia (4%).
Rebif – Erythematous rash (7%); maculopapular rash (5%).
EENT:
Avonex – Sinusitis (14%); eye disorder (4%).
Rebif – Abnormal vision (13%); xerophthalmia (3%).
ENDO:
Avonex – Hyper- and hypothyroidism (postmarketing).
Rebif – Thyroid disorder (6%).
GI:
Avonex – Nausea (23%); abdominal pain (8%); toothache (3%).
Rebif – Abdominal pain (22%); dry mouth (5%).
GU:
Avonex – UTIs (17%); abnormal urine constituents (3%); meno- and metrorrhagia (postmarketing).
Rebif – Micturition frequency (7%); urinary incontinence (4%).
HEMA/LYMPH:
Avonex – Anemia (4%); idiopathic thrombocytopenia (postmarketing).
Rebif – Leukopenia (36%); lymphadenopathy

(12%); thrombocytopenia (8%); anemia (5%).
HEPA:
Avonex – Autoimmune hepatitis, elevated serum hepatic enzymes, hepatitis (postmarketing).
Rebif – Increased SGPT (27%); increased SGOT (17%); abnormal hepatic function (9%); bilirubinemia (3%).
LOCAL:
Avonex – Injection-site pain (8%); injection-site inflammation, injection-site ecchymosis (6%); injection-site reaction (3%).
Rebif – Injection-site reaction (92%); injection-site necrosis (3%).
MUSC:
Avonex – Myalgia (29%); arthralgia (9%).
Rebif – Myalgia, back pain (25%); skeletal pain (15%).
RESP:
Avonex – Upper respiratory tract infection (14%); bronchitis (8%).
OTHER:
Avonex – Flu-like symptoms (49%); asthenia (24%); pain (23%); fever (20%); chills (19%); infection (7%); chest pain (5%); anaphylaxis.
Rebif – Flu-like symptoms (59%); fever (28%); rigors (13%); chest pain (8%); malaise (5%); anaphylaxis.

Precautions
Pregnancy: Category C.
Lactation: Undetermined.
Children: Safety and efficacy in children younger than 18 yr not established.
Elderly: Use with caution because of greater frequency of decreased hepatic, renal, or cardiac function, and concomitant diseases or other drug therapy (*Rebif*).

PATIENT CARE CONSIDERATIONS
Administration/Storage
Rebif:
- Administer via SC route only. Not for intradermal, IM, or IV administration.
- Prescribed dose is administered 3 times/wk, at least 48 hr apart.
- Rotate injection sites (buttocks, thighs, abdomen, back of arms). Use a different area from where the last injection was administered. Do not inject into areas where the skin is tender, bruised, red, or hard.
- Do not mix with other drug solutions.
- Store prefilled syringes in refrigerator (36° to 46°F). Do not freeze. If a refrigerator is not available, prefilled syringes may be stored at temperatures less than 77°F for up to 30 days, away from heat and light.

Avonex:
- Administer via IM route only. Not for intradermal, SC, or IV administration.

Photosensitivity: May occur. Caution patient to use sunscreen (SPF 30 or more) and wear protective clothing until tolerance is determined.
Suicide/Depression: Suicide attempts occurred in clinical trials. Report depression and suicidal ideation immediately.
Seizures: Use caution when administering to patients with preexisting seizure disorder.
Cardiac disease: Interferon beta-1a-induced flu syndrome may prove stressful to patients with severe cardiac conditions (eg, CHF, arrhythmia, angina).
Albumin: Product contains albumin, a derivative of human blood; therefore, there is a remote risk for transmission of viral diseases.
Anaphylaxis: Anaphylaxis has been reported as a rare complication (*Rebif*).
Autoimmune disorders: Autoimmune disorders of multiple target organs have been reported including idiopathic thrombocytopenia, hyper- and hypothyroidism, and rare cases of autoimmune hepatitis. Monitor for signs of these disorders and implement appropriate treatment when observed.
Cardiomyopathy and CHF: Patients with cardiac disease, such as angina, CHF, or arrhythmia, should be closely monitored for worsening of clinical condition during initiation and continuation of treatment (*Avonex*).
Decreased peripheral blood counts: Decreased peripheral blood counts in all cell lines, including rare pancytopenia and thrombocytopenia, may occur.
Hepatic injury: Severe liver dysfunction, leading to hepatic failure requiring liver transplantation, may occur (*Rebif*).

- Prescribed dose is administered once weekly.
- Rotate injection sites (thighs and upper arms). Use a different area from where the last injection was administered. Do not inject into areas where the skin is infected, tender, bruised, red, or hard.
- Allow prefilled syringe to warm to room temperature before administering. Do not warm using external heat source (eg, hot water).
- Reconstitute powder for injection using supplied diluent only. Swirl vial gently to dissolve. Do not shake vial.
- Reconstituted solution should be clear to slightly yellow.
- Do not administer if particulate matter, cloudiness, or discoloration is noted.
- Withdraw prescribed dose into syringe for injection and administer immediately or within 6 hr if stored in refrigerator (36° to 46°F) after reconstitution.

- Vials contain no preservative. Discard any unused portion. Do not combine unused portions.
- Store prefilled syringes and unopened vials in refrigerator (36° to 46°F). Do not freeze. If a refrigerator is not available, unopened vials, but not prefilled syringes, may be stored at temperatures less than 77°F for up to 30 days, away from heat and light. Once warmed to room temperature, prefilled syringe must be used within 12 hr.

Assessment/Interventions
- Obtain patient history, including drug history and any known allergies. Note liver disease, depression or history of depression, alcohol abuse, seizure disorder, CV disease, or allergy to latex or human albumin.
- Ensure that hemoglobin, CBC with differential, platelet count, and blood chemistries, including LFTs, are performed before initiating therapy, at 1, 3, and 6 mo after starting therapy and then periodically thereafter.
- Ensure that thyroid function tests are performed before starting therapy and q 6 mo during therapy in patient with thyroid dysfunction.
- Administer acetaminophen or NSAIDs as prescribed for treatment of flu-like symptoms (fever, myalgia).
- Ensure that woman of childbearing potential is not pregnant when therapy is initiated and is using effective birth control measures.
- Assess injection sites for evidence of reactions. Notify health care provider if broken skin, blue-black discoloration, or drainage of fluid is noted at injection site.
- Monitor patient for signs or symptoms of depression and suicidal ideation. Implement appropriate precautions and report to health care provider if noted.
- Assess patient for CNS, GI, respiratory, musculoskeletal, and general body side effects. Report to health care provider if noted and significant.

Rebif:
- Ensure that reduced dose is administered to patient with ALT greater than 5 times upper limit of normal.

Patient/Family Education
- Explain name, dose, action, and potential side effects of drug.
- Advise patient, family, or caregiver that medication is not a cure for multiple sclerosis, but it may decrease the number of flare-ups and slow the development of some of the physical disabilities caused by multiple sclerosis.
- Advise patient or caregiver to review *Medication Guide* before using and with each refill.
- If patient or caregiver will be administering at home, ensure that the patient or caregiver understands how to store, prepare, and administer the dose and how to dispose of used equipment and supplies. If possible, the first injection should be performed under supervision of a qualified health professional.
- Advise patient not to change the dose or stop taking unless advised by health care provider.
- Advise patient that flu-like symptoms are common and that OTC fever and pain reducers (eg, acetaminophen, ibuprofen) can be used to relieve fever and muscle aches.
- Advise patient to notify health care provider immediately if any of the following occur: suicidal ideation, severely depressed mood, injection-site reaction with break in skin and blue-black discoloration, swelling, drainage of fluid.
- Advise patient to contact health care provider if experiencing bothersome side effects or experience any unusual problems.
- Advise women of childbearing potential to use effective contraception during treatment because of the abortifacient potential of these medications.
- Advise women to notify health care provider if pregnant, planning to become pregnant, or breastfeeding.
- Instruct patient not to take any prescription or OTC medications or dietary supplements unless advised by health care provider.
- Remind patient that office visits and laboratory tests will be required to monitor therapy and to keep appointments.

Rebif:
- Advise patient that if a dose is missed to take it as soon as possible and to schedule next dose approximately 48 hr later.
- Instruct patient to rotate injection sites as described in the *Medication Guide* to minimize likelihood of severe injection site reactions or tissue necrosis.

Avonex:
- Advise patient that if a dose is missed to take it as soon as possible and then continue regular schedule the following week.
- Instruct patient to rotate injection sites as described in the *Medication Guide* to minimize likelihood of severe injection-site reactions.

Interferon Beta-1b

(in-ter-FEER-ahn BAY-tah 1b)
Class Interferon/Immunomodulator

How Supplied
Betaseron Powder for injection, lyophilized 0.3 mg

Action
PHARMACOLOGY: Unknown; however, the biologic response-modifying properties are mediated through the interactions of interferon beta-1b with specific cell receptors found on the surface of human cells. Binding to these receptors induces the expression of a number of interferon-induced gene products that are believed to be mediators of the drug's biological action.

PHARMACOKINETICS/DYNAMICS:
Absorption: The T_{max} is 1 to 8 hr. The mean C_{max} is 40 IU/mL. The bioavailability is approximately 50% (SC).
Distribution: The mean Vd_{ss} is 0.25 to 2.88 L/kg.
Excretion: The mean t½ is 9 min to 4.3 hr.

Indications To reduce the frequency of clinical exacerbations of relapsing-remitting multiple sclerosis in ambulatory patients.

Contraindications History of hypersensitivity to natural or recombinant interferon beta, human albumin, or any other component of formulation.

Route/Dosage
ADULTS: **SC** 0.25 mg every other day.

Interactions
Zidovudine: Plasma levels of zidovudine may be elevated, increasing the pharmacologic and adverse effects.

Lab Test Interferences None well documented.

Adverse Reactions
CV: Peripheral edema (15%); vasodilation (8%); hypertension (7%); peripheral vascular disorder (6%); palpitation, tachycardia (4%); cardiomyopathy, deep vein thrombosis, pulmonary embolism (postmarketing).
CNS: Headache (57%); hypertonia (50%); dizziness, insomnia (24%); incoordination (21%); anxiety (10%); nervousness (7%); ataxia, confusion, convulsion, depersonalization, emotional lability, paresthesia (postmarketing).
DERM: Rash (24%); skin disorder (12%); sweating (8%); alopecia (4%); pruritus, skin discoloration, urticaria (postmarketing).
ENDO: Hypothyroidism, hyperthyroidism, thyroid dysfunction (postmarketing).
GI: Nausea (27%); constipation (20%); diarrhea (19%); dyspepsia (14%); pancreatitis, vomiting (postmarketing).
GU: Urinary urgency (13%); metrorrhagia (11%); impotence (9%); menorrhagia (8%); urinary frequency, dysmenorrhea (7%); prostatic disorder (3%); UTI, urosepsis (postmarketing).
HEMA/LYMPH: Decreased lymphocytes (88%); leukopenia (18%); decreased ANC, decreased WBC (14%); increased SGPT (10%); lymphadenopathy (8%); increased SGOT (3%); anemia; thrombocytopenia (postmarketing).
HEPA: Hepatitis (postmarketing).
LOCAL: Injection-site reaction (85%); injection-site inflammation (53%); injection-site pain (18%); injection-site necrosis (5%); hypersensitivity (3%).
METAB: Weight gain (7%); gamma GT increase, hypocalcemia, hyperuricemia, increased triglyceride (postmarketing).
MUSC: Myasthenia (46%); arthralgia (31%); myalgia (27%); leg cramps (4%).
RESP: Dyspnea (7%); bronchospasm, pneumonia (postmarketing).
OTHER: Asthenia (61%); flu-like symptoms (60%); pain (51%); chills (25%); abdominal pain (19%); chest pain (11%); malaise (8%); anaphylaxis (rare); fatal capillary leak syndrome (postmarketing).

Precautions
Pregnancy: Category C.
Lactation: Undetermined.
Children: Safety and efficacy not established.
Necrosis: Injection-site necrosis may occur within the first 4 mo of therapy at single- or multiple-injection sites.
Albumin: Product contains albumin, a derivative of human blood; therefore, there is a remote risk for transmission of viral diseases.
Anaphylaxis: Anaphylaxis has been reported as a rare complication of interferon beta-1b use.
Suicide/Depression: Suicide attempts and depression may occur with increased frequency.

PATIENT CARE CONSIDERATIONS
Administration/Storage
- Reconstitute powder using supplied diluent only. Swirl vial gently to dissolve. Do not shake vial.
- Reconstituted solution should be clear and colorless.
- Do not administer if particulate matter, cloudiness, or discoloration is noted.
- Administer immediately after reconstitution, or refrigerate and use within 3 hr.
- Withdraw prescribed dose into syringe for injection.

- Administer via SC route only.
- Prescribed dose is administered every other day.
- Rotate injection sites (eg, buttocks, thighs, abdomen, back of arms). Use a different area from where the last injection was administered. Do not inject into areas where the skin is tender, bruised, red, or hard.
- Vials contain no preservative. Discard any unused portion. Do not combine unused portions.
- Do not mix with other drug solutions.
- Administer acetaminophen as prescribed for treatment of flu-like symptoms (eg, fever, myalgia).
- Store unopened vials at controlled room temperature (59° to 86°F). May store reconstituted solution in refrigerator (36° to 46°F) for up to 3 hr. Do not freeze.

Assessment/Interventions
- Obtain patient history, including drug history and any known allergies. Note depression, history of depression, or allergy to human albumin.
- Ensure that hemoglobin, CBC with differential, platelet count, and blood chemistries, including LFTs, are performed before initiating therapy and periodically during therapy.
- Ensure that thyroid function tests are performed before starting therapy and q 6 mo during therapy in patient with thyroid dysfunction.
- Ensure that woman of childbearing potential is not pregnant when therapy is initiated and is using effective birth control measures because of the abortifacient potential of this medicine.
- Assess injection sites for evidence of reactions. Notify health care provider if broken skin, blue-black discoloration, or drainage of fluid is noted at injection site.
- Monitor patient for signs or symptoms of depression and suicidal ideation. Implement appropriate precautions and report to health care provider if noted.
- Assess patient for CV, CNS, GI, respiratory, musculoskeletal, and general body side effects. Report to health care provider if noted and significant.

Patient/Family Education
- Explain name, dose, action, and potential side effects of drug. If patient or caregiver will be administering at home, review *Betaseron Patient Information* sheet with the patient or caregiver. Ensure that the patient or caregiver understands how to store, prepare, and administer the dose, and how to dispose of used equipment and supplies. If possible, perform the first injection under supervision of a qualified health professional.
- Advise patient, family, or caregiver that medication is not a cure for multiple sclerosis, but it may decrease the number of flare-ups and slow the development of some of the physical disabilities caused by multiple sclerosis.
- Advise patient not to change the dose or stop taking unless advised by health care provider.
- Remind patient that injection is administered every other day.
- Advise patient that if a dose is missed to take it as soon as possible and to schedule next dose approximately 48 hr later.
- Instruct patient to rotate injection sites as described in the *Betaseron Patient Information* sheet to minimize likelihood of severe injection-site reactions or tissue necrosis.
- Advise patient that flu-like symptoms are common and that acetaminophen can be used to relieve fever and muscle aches.
- Advise patient to notify health care provider immediately if any of the following occur: suicidal ideation, severely depressed mood, injection-site reaction with break in skin and blue-black discoloration, swelling, drainage of fluid.
- Advise patient to contact health care provider if experiencing bothersome side effects or any unusual problems.
- Advise women of childbearing potential to use effective contraception during treatment because of abortifacient potential.
- Advise women to notify health care provider if pregnant, planning to become pregnant, or breastfeeding.
- Instruct patient not to take any prescription or OTC medications or dietary supplements unless advised by health care provider.
- Remind patient that office visits and laboratory tests will be required to monitor therapy and to keep appointments.

Interferon Gamma-1b

(IN-ter-FEER-ahn GAM-uh-1b)
Class Interferon/Immunomodulator

How Supplied
Actimmune Injection 100 mcg (2 million IU)/0.5 mL

Action

PHARMACOLOGY: Produces potent phagocyte-activating effects, including generation of toxic oxygen metabolites within phagocytes, which mediate killing of microorganisms. Activities include enhancement of oxidative metabolism of tissue macrophages and enhancement of antibody-dependent cellular cytotoxicity and natural killer (NK) cell activity.

PHARMACOKINETICS/DYNAMICS:
Absorption: The apparent bioavailability is more than 89% (IM, SC). The T_{max} is approximately 4 hr (IM) and 7 hr (SC).
Excretion: The mean $t_{1/2}$ is 38 min (IV), 2.9 hr (IM), and 5.9 hr (SC).

Indications Reduction of frequency and severity of serious infections associated with chronic granulomatous disease. **Unlabeled use(s):** Treatment of small-cell lung cancer, atopic dermatitis, trauma-related infections, metastatic renal-cell carcinoma, cutaneous T-cell lymphoma, asthma and allergies, refractory leishmaniasis, chronic myelogenous leukemia, and AIDS.

Contraindications Hypersensitivity to *E. coli*-derived products.

PATIENT CARE CONSIDERATIONS

Administration/Storage

- Discard unused portion of any vial. Product contains no preservative, and vials are only suitable for single dose.
- Refrigerate; do not freeze. Any unopened vial should not be left at room temperature for more than 12 hr. Do not shake vial.
- Administer by SC route only in right or left deltoid and anterior thigh.
- Give at bedtime with acetaminophen for fever and headache.

Assessment/Interventions

- Obtain patient history, including drug history and any known allergies.
- Obtain baseline CBC with differential, platelets, renal and hepatic studies, BUN, creatinine, ALT, and urinalysis. Monitor throughout therapy.
- Monitor results of laboratory tests.
- Assess patient for GI, CNS, cardiovascular,

Route/Dosage
ADULTS & CHILDREN: SC 50 mcg/m^2 (1.5 million U/m^2) if body surface area is more than 0.5 m^2 or 1.5 mcg/kg/dose if body surface area is 0.5 m^2 or less. Administer 3 times/wk (eg, Monday, Wednesday, Friday) into right or left deltoid or anterior thigh. If severe adverse reactions develop, reduced dosage or discontinuation of therapy may be necessary until those reactions subside.

Interactions
Live virus vaccines (eg, measles, mumps, polio, rubella): May inhibit antibody response after immunization; avoid concurrent use.
Myelosuppressive agents: Additive neutropenic effects are possible.

Lab Test Interferences None well documented.

Adverse Reactions
CNS: Decreased mental status; gait disturbance; dizziness; fatigue; headache.
GI: Diarrhea; vomiting; nausea.
GU: Proteinuria.
HEMA: Thrombocytopenia.
OTHER: Fever; chills; erythema or tenderness at injection site; myalgia; arthralgia.

Precautions
Pregnancy: Category C.
Lactation: Undetermined.
Children: Safety and efficacy in children younger than 1 yr not established.
Special risk patients: Exercise caution in patients with seizure disorders, compromised CNS function, cardiac disease, and myelosuppression.

dermatological, and hematological side effects. If present, notify health care provider.
- Monitor hydration if patient experiences anorexia, nausea, or diarrhea.
- If patient experiences adverse CNS symptoms, implement safety precautions such as lowering bed, putting side rails up, and supervising ambulation.
- Implement infection control measures if WBC drops; implement bleeding precautions if platelet count drops.
- Discuss need for antiemetic with health care provider if nausea or vomiting develops.
- If flu-like symptoms occur, administer drug in evening and give acetaminophen as prescribed.

Patient/Family Education

- Stress importance of returning for follow-up blood tests.
- Teach infection control measures, bleeding

precautions, and energy-conservation measures.
- Caution patient to use safety precautions and not to perform activities that require mental alertness if decreased mental status or dizziness occur.
- Advise patient to take medication at bedtime if flu-like symptoms occur, and to use acetaminophen as needed.
- Explain importance of adequate hydration.
- Teach patient or family to store, prepare, and administer drug SC.
- Provide puncture-resistant container for disposal of used syringes and needles.
- Instruct patient to report the following symptoms to health care provider: swollen ankles; dyspnea; chest pain; noisy breathing; flu-like symptoms; pain at injection site; headache; fever; fluid retention; pelvic pain; cysts; migraine headaches; pounding in chest; sleeplessness; menstrual problems; breast pain; frequent urination; hair loss; sweating; anxiety; confusion; joint and muscle aches; high blood pressure; sinus infection; difficulty breathing; laryngitis; convulsions.

Iodine

(EYE-uh-dine)

Class Thyroid/Trace metal/Antiseptic/Expectorant

How Supplied
Iodine Tincture Solution 2% iodine and 2.4% sodium iodide in 47% alcohol, purified water ♦ *Iodopen* Injection 100 mcg/mL (as 118 mcg sodium iodide) ♦ *SSKI* Solution 1 g/mL potassium iodide ♦ *Strong Iodine (Lugol's Solution)* Solution 5% iodine and 10% potassium iodide in water ♦ *Strong Iodine Tincture* Solution 7% iodine and 5% potassium iodide in 83% alcohol

Action
PHARMACOLOGY:
Antiseptic: Topical iodine possesses microbicidal properties.
Thyroid drug: Large doses of iodides inhibit thyroid hormone production and release into bloodstream.
Expectorant: Enhances secretion of respiratory fluids, decreasing mucus viscosity.

Indications
Antiseptic: Externally, to achieve broad microbicidal benefits.
Thyroid agent: As adjunct to antithyroid drug in hyperthyroid patients to prepare for thyroidectomy and to treat thyrotoxic crisis or neonatal thyrotoxicosis; thyroid blocking in radiation emergency.
Trace metal: Supplement to IV solutions given for TPN.
Expectorant: Treatment of chronic pulmonary diseases complicated by tenacious mucus, including bronchial asthma, chronic bronchitis, bronchiectasis, and pulmonary emphysema; adjunctive treatment in respiratory conditions such as cystic fibrosis and chronic sinusitis and to prevent atelectasis after surgery.

Contraindications Hypersensitivity to iodides; impaired renal function; acute bronchitis; hyperthyroidism; Addison disease; acute dehydration; heat cramps; hyperkalemia; iodism; tuberculosis.

Route/Dosage
Topical Antiseptic
Apply prn to intact skin.

Thyroid Agent Prior to Thyroidectomy
PO 2 to 6 drops of strong iodine solution (*Lugol's Solution*) tid for 10 days prior to surgery.

Thyroid Blocking in Radiation Emergency
Use at direction of state or local public health authorities.

Trace Metal for TPN (Supplied as Sodium Iodide)
METABOLICALLY STABLE ADULTS: 1 to 2 mcg/kg/day (normal adults, 75 to 150 mcg/day).
PREGNANT AND LACTATING WOMEN, GROWING CHILDREN: 2 to 3 mcg/kg/day.

Expectorant
ADULTS: PO 300 to 1000 mg initially after meals. If tolerated, 1 to 1.5 g tid.
CHILDREN: PO Half adult dose.

Interactions
Lithium: May have synergistic hypothyroid activity; may result in hypothyroidism.
Potassium-sparing diuretics: Increase risk of hyperkalemia, cardiac arrhythmias, and cardiac arrest.

Lab Test Interferences Potassium iodide may alter thyroid function test results.

Adverse Reactions
CV: Irregular heartbeat.
CNS: Confusion; unusual tiredness.
DERM: Rash; acne.
EENT: Swelling of neck, throat, or salivary glands.
GI: Bleeding.
METAB: Thyroid adenoma; goiter; myxedema; thyroid gland enlargement; acute parotitis.
OTHER: Hypersensitivity manifested by angioneurotic edema, cutaneous and mucosal hemorrhages, and symptoms resembling serum sickness (eg, fever, arthralgia, lymph node enlargement,

eosinophilia); numbness; tingling; pain or weakness in hands or feet; weakness or heaviness of legs; fever; iodism (eg, metallic taste, burning mouth and throat, sore teeth and gums, symptoms of head cold, stomach upset, diarrhea).

Precautions

Pregnancy: Category D (potassium iodide).
Lactation: Excreted in breast milk.
Children: Safety and efficacy not established.
Renal function impairment: Supplement dosage may be adjusted, reduced, or omitted.
Special risk patients: Pulmonary tuberculosis is considered a contraindication to use of iodides by some authorities; use with caution in such cases and in patients with cardiac disease, myotonia congenita, or renal impairment. Cystic fibrosis patients may have increased susceptibility to adverse effects.
GI effects: Nonspecific small bowel lesions have occurred with enteric-coated potassium salts.
Hypothyroidism (oral): Prolonged use can lead to hypothyroidism.
Topical: For external use only; highly toxic if ingested. Avoid contact with eyes and mucous membranes. Iodine preparations stain skin and clothing.

Overdosage: Signs and Symptoms

Iodine is corrosive; toxic symptoms are related primarily to local GI tract irritation; gastroenteritis, abdominal pain, and diarrhea (sometimes bloody) may be seen; fatalities may occur from circulatory collapse, because of shock, corrosive gastritis, or asphyxiation from swelling of glottis or larynx.

PATIENT CARE CONSIDERATIONS

Administration/Storage

- Do not give trace metal undiluted by direct injection into peripheral vein.
- Measure solutions carefully with calibrated dropper.
- Dilute expectorant in 60 mL of flavored beverages (eg, chocolate or plain milk, orange juice) to minimize bitter taste.
- Mix solutions in full glass of fruit juice, water, or milk.
- Administer after meals to minimize irritation.
- Have patient sip expectorant through straw to decrease burning sensation in mouth and to prevent discoloration of teeth.
- Store in airtight, light-resistant container at room temperature (59° to 86°F).

Assessment/Interventions

- Obtain patient history, including drug history and any known allergies.
- Assess for signs and symptoms of iodism (eg, metallic taste, stomatitis, skin lesions, cold symptoms).
- Monitor thyroid function before and periodically during course of therapy.
- Notify health care provider of any signs of hyperthyroidism (eg, tachycardia, palpitations, nervousness, insomnia, tremors, weight loss, diaphoresis).
- Report to health care provider any signs of iodism or sensitivity to drug.

Patient/Family Education

- Explain name, dose, action, and side effects of iodine product.
- Tell patient to discontinue use and notify health care provider if fever, rash, metallic taste, swelling of throat, burning of mouth and throat, sore gums and teeth, head cold symptoms, severe GI distress, or enlargement of thyroid gland (goiter) occur.
- Inform patient if replacement therapy is to be taken for life.
- Explain that sudden discontinuation of drug should not be performed without health care provider's guidance.
- Teach patient about foods that are high in iodine (eg, seafood, kale, turnips, iodized salt).
- Explain that darkening of solution does not affect potency.

Ipecac Syrup

(IPP-uh-kak syrup)

Class Antidote

How Supplied

Available as generic only Syrup Ipecac, USP

Action

PHARMACOLOGY: Produces vomiting by local irritant effect and stimulation of chemoreceptor trigger zone.

PHARMACOKINETICS/DYNAMICS:
Excretion: Eliminated very slowly. May be detected up to 60 days in urine.
Peak: Within 20 to 30 min.
Duration: 20 to 25 min.

Indications Treatment of drug overdose and certain poisonings.

Contraindications Do not use in semiconscious, unconscious, pregnant, or lactating persons; do not use if strychnine, corrosives (eg, alkalis, strong acids), or petroleum distillates have been ingested.

Route/Dosage

ADULTS: PO 15 to 30 mL followed by 3 to

4 glasses of water. May repeat dose within 20 min if vomiting does not occur.
CHILDREN YOUNGER THAN 1 YR: **PO** 5 to 10 mL followed by ½ glass of water.
CHILDREN 1 TO 12 YR: **PO** 15 mL followed by 1 to 2 glasses of water.

Interactions
Activated charcoal: Will absorb ipecac syrup. Give activated charcoal only after ipecac syrup has produced vomiting.
Milk or carbonated beverages: Do not administer with ipecac syrup.

Lab Test Interferences
None well documented.

Adverse Reactions
CV: Heart conduction disturbances; atrial fibrillation; fatal myocarditis.
CNS: Depression.
GI: Diarrhea.

Precautions
Pregnancy: Category C.
Lactation: Undetermined.
Abuse: Severe cardiomyopathies and death may occur in bulimic and anorexic persons abusing ipecac syrup.
Syrup/Fluid extract: Do not confuse ipecac syrup with ipecac fluid extract, which is 14 times stronger and has caused some deaths.

Overdosage: Signs and Symptoms
Cardiac conduction disturbances, bradycardia, atrial fibrillation, hypotension, fatal myocarditis.

PATIENT CARE CONSIDERATIONS

Administration/Storage
- Consult poison control center before administering, especially in children younger than 1 yr.
- Have patient sit upright with head forward before administering dose and for 30 min or more after administration.
- Follow administration with 3 to 4 glasses of water for adults and ½ to 2 glasses for children.
- If vomiting does not occur within 20 min, dose may be repeated.
- Do not administer with milk or carbonated beverages.
- Do not give to patient who is unconscious or convulsing.
- Do not give if patient has ingested caustic substances or oils.
- Administer activated charcoal only after vomiting has been induced and completed.

Assessment/Interventions
- Obtain patient history, including drug history and any known allergies. Determine what was ingested, paying particular attention to products for which ipecac is contraindicated (eg, caustic substances, oils).
- Assess patient's level of consciousness.
- Assess for adverse reactions such as CNS stimulation or depression, respiratory depression, prolonged vomiting, lethargy, or diarrhea.
- Assess effectiveness of drug shortly after administration.
- Assess respiratory rate and pattern, BP, and heart rate.
- Monitor for cardiac arrhythmias in patient receiving high doses of ipecac syrup, particularly if patient is very young (younger than 1 yr) or elderly.
- Notify health care provider if adverse reactions occur.
- Take the following safety precautions if sedation occurs: place bed in low position with head of bed elevated, put side rails up, and assist patient with ambulation.
- Repeat initial dose of ipecac syrup in 20 min if first dose was not effective.
- Inform health care provider frequently about effectiveness of drug (frequency and amount of vomiting).
- Save all emesis for laboratory identification of ingested poison.
- If patient experiences extreme vomiting, take measures to maintain hydration, such as IV fluid support including electrolytes.
- If vomiting does not occur within 30 min after second dose, perform gastric lavage.

Patient/Family Education
- Caution parents not to induce vomiting if child has swallowed caustic substance or petroleum product or if child is unconscious, semiconscious, or having convulsions.
- Instruct parents of children under 1 yr to keep small amount (one 30 mL bottle) on hand for emergencies.
- Instruct parents to always consult health care provider or poison control center before administration.
- Teach parents not to exceed recommended amounts.
- Teach families to give drug with adequate amounts of water, not milk or carbonated beverages.
- Advise parents that drug has shelf life of 1 yr and should be replaced yearly. Instruct parents to check expiration date before purchasing product.
- Do not give ipecac syrup to an unconscious

or drowsy child because vomited material may enter lungs and cause pneumonia.
- Teach parents to repeat dose if child does not vomit within 20 min and then to take child to emergency room, because gastric lavage may be necessary.

Ipratropium Bromide

(IH-pruh-TROE-pee-uhm BROE-mide)

Class Respiratory inhalant/Anticholinergic

How Supplied
Atrovent Aerosol Each actuation delivers 18 mcg, Solution for Inhalation 0.02% (500 mcg/vial), Nasal Spray 0.03%. Each spray delivers 21 mcg, Nasal Spray 0.06%. Each spray delivers 42 mcg
❀ *Apo-Ipravent* ♦ *Combivent Inhalation Solution* ♦ *Gen-Ipratropium* ♦ *Novo-Ipramide* ♦ *Nu-Ipratropium* ♦ *PMS-Ipratropium* ♦ *ratio-Ipratropium* ♦ *ratio-Ipratropium UDV*

Action

PHARMACOLOGY: Antagonizes action of acetylcholine on bronchial smooth muscle in lungs, causing bronchodilation.

PHARMACOKINETICS/DYNAMICS:
Absorption: Mean bioavailability is 7% (inhalation).
Distribution: 0 to 9% is protein bound.
Metabolism: Partially metabolized.
Excretion: The $t_{1/2}$ is approximately 1.6 hr (IV).

Indications

Bronchospasm: Maintenance treatment of bronchospasm associated with COPD, including chronic bronchitis and emphysema, used alone or in combination with other bronchodilators (especially beta-adrenergics).
Rhinorrhea: Symptomatic relief of rhinorrhea associated with allergic and nonallergic rhinitis and symptomatic relief of rhinorrhea associated with the common cold in patients 12 yr and older for aerosol and solution, 6 yr and older for 0.03% nasal spray, and 5 yr and older for 0.06% nasal spray.

Contraindications
Hypersensitivity to atropine or any anticholinergic derivatives or to soya lecithin or related food products.

Route/Dosage

ADULTS: **Aerosol/Inhalation** 2 inhalations (36 mcg) qid (max 12 inhalations/24 hr). Do not exceed 12 inhalations in 24 hours. **Solution:** 500 mcg (1 unit dose vial) administered 3 to 4 times a day by oral nebulization, with doses 6 to 8 hr apart. The solution can be mixed in the nebulizer with albuterol if used within 1 hr.
Spray 0.03 formulation: 2 sprays (42 mcg) per nostril 2 or 3 times daily (optimum dose varies). 0.06 formulation: 2 sprays (84 mcg) per nostril 3 or 4 times daily (optimum dose varies).

Interactions
Anticholinergics: There is some potential for additive anticholinergic effects when administered with other anticholinergic agents.

Lab Test Interferences
None well documented.

Adverse Reactions
CV: Palpitations; hypertension; aggravated hypertension.
RESP: Cough; exacerbation of symptoms.
CNS: Nervousness; dizziness; headache.
DERM: Rash.
EENT: Blurred vision; local irritation; epistaxis, nasal dryness, nasal congestion, taste perversion, nasal burning, conjunctivitis, hoarseness, pharyngitis (0.06 nasal spray formulation only).
GI: Nausea; dry mouth; GI distress; constipation.
OTHER: Arthritis.

Precautions
Pregnancy: Category B.
Lactation: Undetermined.
Children: Safety and efficacy in children younger than 12 yr not established for aerosol and solution; younger than 6 yr for 0.03% nasal spray; younger than 5 yr for 0.06% nasal spray.
Special risk patients: Use drug with caution in patients with narrow-angle glaucoma, prostatic hypertrophy, bladder neck obstruction due to increased risk for precipitation or worsening of underlying disease.
Acute bronchospasm: Not indicated for initial treatment of acute episodes of bronchospasm in which rapid response is required. For relief of bronchospasms in acute exacerbations of COPD, drugs with faster onset may be preferable as initial therapy. The combination of ipratropium and beta agonists in the relief of bronchospasms associated with COPD has not been demonstrated to be more efficacious than either drug alone.

PATIENT CARE CONSIDERATIONS
Administration/Storage
Inhalation:
- Store at room temperature. Avoid excessive humidity.
- Allow 1 to 2 min between inhalations.
- Shake inhaler well before administration.
- If patient is also receiving an inhaled beta$_2$-agonist, give beta$_2$-agonist before administering ipratropium.
- Use spacing device (eg, *Aerochamber*) to

facilitate intrapulmonary deposition.
- Have patient rinse mouth with water or mouthwash after each use.

Nasal spray:
- Initial pump priming: 7 actuations of the pump. For regular use, no further priming is required. If not used for more than 24 hr, 2 actuations are needed. If not used for more than 7 days, 7 actuations are needed.
- Store tightly between 59° and 86°F. Avoid freezing.

Solution:
- Store at room temperature. Protect from light. Store unused vials in the foil pouch.

Assessment/Interventions
- Obtain patient history, including drug history and any known allergies.
- Assess respiratory status before initiation of therapy and monitor after inhalation of ipratropium. Therapeutic response is demonstrated by patient's ability to breathe adequately.
- If exacerbation of symptoms occurs, notify health care provider.
- Give patient frequent sips of water and sugarless hard candy or gum to relieve dry mouth.
- Since drug tolerance may develop with long-term therapy, dosage may need to be increased.

Patient/Family Education
- Instruct patient on proper use of inhaler. Explain value of using spacing device.
- Instruct patient on proper sequencing and timing if using more than 1 inhaled agent.
- Teach patient how to determine when canister is empty and needs to be replaced.
- Teach patient how to properly use the nasal spray.
- Caution patient not to rely on ipratropium for acute bronchospasm.
- For relief of dry mouth, suggest use of saliva substitute, practice of good oral hygiene, rinsing of mouth after inhalation. Instruct patient to take sips of water frequently, suck on ice chips or sugarless hard candy, or chew sugarless gum.
- Caution patient to avoid spraying aerosol in eyes; temporary blurred vision may result.
- Advise patients using aerosol to seek immediate medical attention if recommended dosage does not provide relief or if symptoms worsen.
- Advise patients not to use other inhaled drugs unless prescribed while taking ipratropium inhalation aerosol.
- Use a nebulizer with a mouthpiece for the solution rather than a face mask to reduce the likelihood of the solution reaching the eyes.
- Instruct patient to notify health care provider if condition worsens or if the following symptoms occur: dizziness, nausea, headache, palpitations, or cough.
- Advise patient using nasal spray to avoid spraying in or around eyes. Patient should contact health care provider if experiencing eye pain, blurred vision, excessive nasal dryness, or nasal bleeding.
- Advise patient that drug may cause dizziness and to use caution while driving or performing other tasks requiring mental alertness.

Ipratropium Bromide/ Albuterol Sulfate

(IH-pruh-TROE-pee-umm BROE-mide al-BYOO-ter-ahl SULL-fate)

Class Bronchodilator

How Supplied
Combivent Aerosol 18 mcg ipratropium bromide and 103 mcg albuterol sulfate per actuation (equiv. to 90 mcg albuterol base) ◆ *DuoNeb* Inhalation solution 0.5 mg ipratropium bromide and 3 mg albuterol sulfate (equiv. to 2.5 mg albuterol base)

Action
PHARMACOLOGY:
Albuterol: Produces bronchodilation by relaxing bronchial smooth muscle through beta$_2$-receptor stimulation.
Ipratropium: Antagonizes action of acetylcholine on bronchial smooth muscle in lungs, causing bronchodilation.

Indications Treatment of bronchospasm associated with COPD in patients requiring more than 1 bronchodilator.

Contraindications History of hypersensitivity to soya lecithin or related food (eg, soybean, peanuts) (*Combivent* only) or to atropine and its derivatives.

Route/Dosage
COMBIVENT
ADULTS: **Inhalation** 2 inhalations qid (max, 12 inhalations per 24 hr).

DUONEB
ADULTS: **Inhalation** One 3 mL vial qid via nebulization with up to 2 additional 3 mL doses daily, if needed.

Interactions
Anticholinergic agents: Possible additive anticholinergic effects.
Beta-adrenergic agonists: Risk of adverse CV effects may be increased.
Beta-receptor blocking agents: These agents and

albuterol may inhibit the effect of each other.
Digoxin: Albuterol component may decrease serum digoxin concentrations and therapeutic effects.
Diuretics: Albuterol component may exaggerate ECG and/or hypokalemia from non-potassium-sparing diuretics.
MAO inhibitors, tricyclic antidepressants: Concomitant use of these agents or use within 2 wk of stopping such agents may potentiate the CV effects of albuterol.

Lab Test Interferences None well documented.

Adverse Reactions
CV: Hypertension, arrhythmia, palpitation, tachycardia, angina, hypotension (less than 2%).
CNS: Headache (6%); fatigue, dizziness, nervousness, tremor, paresthesia, insomnia (less than 2%); drowsiness, stimulation, coordination difficulty, weakness (postmarketing).
DERM: Alopecia (postmarketing).
EENT: Pharyngitis (4%); dysphonia (less than 2%); worsening of narrow-angle glaucoma, acute eye pain, blurred vision, nasal congestion, drying of secretions, mucosal ulcers (postmarketing).
GI: Nausea (2%); diarrhea, dry mouth, dyspepsia, vomiting, taste perversion (less than 2%); GI distress, constipation (postmarketing).
GU: UTI, dysuria (less than 2%); urinary difficulty (postmarketing).
MUSC: Arthralgia (less than 2%).
RESP: Bronchitis (12%); upper respiratory tract infection (11%); lung disease (6%); dyspnea (5%); coughing (4%); respiratory disorders (3%); sinusitis (2%); rhinitis, pneumonia (1%); paradoxical bronchospasm, wheezing, exacerbation of COPD symptoms (postmarketing).
OTHER: Pain, chest pain (3%); influenza, leg cramps (1%); allergic type reactions (including skin rash, angioedema of tongue, lips, and face, laryngospasm, anaphylaxis), edema, increased sputum (less than 2%); heartburn, itching, flushing (postmarketing).

Precautions
Pregnancy: Category C.
Lactation: Undetermined.
Children: Safety and efficacy not established.
Hypersensitivity: Immediate hypersensitivity reactions may occur.
Anticholinergic effects: Use with caution in patients with narrow-angle glaucoma, prostatic hypertrophy, or bladder neck obstruction.
CV effects: Toxic symptoms may occur in patients with CV disorders. Use with caution in patients with coronary insufficiency, arrhythmias, or hypertension.
CNS effects: CNS stimulation may occur; use cautiously in patients with history of seizures or hyperthyroidism.
Diabetes: Dosage adjustment of insulin may be required.
Excessive use: Death may occur with excessive use of inhaled sympathomimetic drugs in patients with asthma.
Hypokalemia: Transient decreases in potassium levels may occur.
Paradoxical bronchospasm: Life-threatening bronchospasms can occur, usually with the first use of a new container.

Overdosage: Signs and Symptoms
Tremor, palpitations, tachycardia, elevated BP, angina.

PATIENT CARE CONSIDERATIONS

Administration/Storage

* May be administered alone or in combination with inhaled or systemic corticosteroids.

Inhalation Aerosol:

* For oral inhalation only. Avoid spraying into the nose or eyes.
* Shake well before each use.
* Have patient exhale deeply through the mouth, place inhaler between lips, and take a slow, deep breath while inhaler is being activated. Have patient hold breath for 5 to 10 sec and then breathe out slowly. Wait 5 min before administering the second dose. A spacing device (eg, *Aerochamber*) may be used to enhance delivery of medication. Have patient rinse mouth after inhalations are complete.
* Store inhalation aerosol at ambient room temperature (59° to 86°F). Protect from excessive humidity. Store pressurized canister with nozzle end down, away from heat or open flame. Do not puncture or discard pressurized canister in incinerator.

Inhalation Solution:

* Administer only via nebulizer. Not for injection or oral use.
* Medication requires no dilution before administration and is added directly into the nebulizer reservoir.
* Discard solution if not colorless.
* Discard any unused solution.
* Do not mix with other nebulized medications unless ordered by health care provider.
* Store unused vials in protective foil pouch in refrigerator (36° to 46°F) or room temperature (less than 77°F). Protect vials from light.

Assessment/Interventions

* Obtain patient history, including drug history and any known allergies. Note renal or hepatic insufficiency, coronary artery disease, arrhythmias, hypertension, seizures, hyperthy-

roidism, diabetes or unusual sensitivity to sympathomimetic amines, narrow-angle glaucoma, prostatic hyperplasia, bladder neck obstruction, hypersensitivity to atropine or its derivatives (eg, ipratropium, tiotropium), hypersensitivity to soya lecithin, soybean, or peanuts (aerosol only), or concurrent or recent (within 2 wk) use of MAO inhibitor or tricyclic antidepressant.
• Monitor pulse, BP, respiratory rate, and lung sounds before and after treatment. Notify health care provider of unexpected or unusual findings.
• Monitor patient's respiratory status during each treatment. If bronchospasm worsens during or shortly after a treatment, discontinue the treatment and notify health care provider immediately.
• Assess patient's symptoms before initiating therapy and periodically during treatment. Notify health care provider if symptoms do not improve or worsen.
• Monitor patient for signs and symptoms of anaphylactic or serious allergic reactions. If noted, discontinue therapy and be prepared to treat appropriately.
• Monitor patient for signs and symptoms of acute narrow-angle glaucoma (eg, eye pain, blurred vision, visual halos, conjunctival congestion). If noted, discontinue therapy and inform health care provider immediately.
• Monitor patient for RESP, GI, and general body side effects. Inform health care provider if noted and significant.

Patient/Family Education
• Explain name, dose, action, and potential side effects of drug.
• Advise patient to continue taking other medications for same condition as prescribed by health care provider.
• Advise patient using inhalation solution for nebulizer to read the *Patient's Instructions for Use* before starting therapy and again with each refill.
• Ensure that patient using inhalation solution can prepare, use, and clean the nebulizer without difficulty.
• Review proper administration technique for patient using inhalation aerosol. Have patient demonstrate technique to ensure effective use of the MDI.
• Advise patient using inhalation aerosol to test-spray 3 times before using the first time or if the aerosol has not been used for more than 24 hr.
• Advise patient to discard the aerosol canister when the labeled number of doses has been used.
• Instruct patient not to exceed prescribed dose. Advise patient to inform health care provider if symptoms do not improve or worsen, if treatments are needed more often than usual, or if the medication appears to become less effective.
• Instruct patient not to stop the medication once symptoms have been controlled. Continued daily use is necessary to control symptoms.
• Advise patient to carry *Medi-Alert* card indicating COPD.
• Advise women to notify health care provider if pregnant, planning to become pregnant, or breastfeeding.
• Caution patient not to take any prescription or OTC medications, dietary supplements, or herbal preparations unless advised by health care provider.
• Advise patient that follow-up visits may be required to monitor therapy and to keep appointments.

Irbesartan

(ihr-beh-SAHR-tan)

Class Antihypertensive/Angiotensin II antagonist

How Supplied
Avapro Tablets 75 mg, Tablets 150 mg, Tablets 300 mg

Action
PHARMACOLOGY: Antagonizes the effect of angiotensin II (vasoconstriction and aldosterone secretion) by blocking the angiotensin II (AT1 receptor) in vascular smooth muscle and the adrenal gland, producing decreased BP.

PHARMACOKINETICS/DYNAMICS:
Absorption: The mean absolute bioavailability is 60% to 80%. The T_{max} is 1.5 to 2 hr.

Distribution: 90% is protein bound. The mean Vd is 53 to 93 L. Weakly crosses blood-brain barrier and placenta.

Metabolism: Less than 20% converted to metabolites, primarily via CYP2C9.

Excretion: Renal Cl is 3 to 3.5 mL/min. The mean t½ is 11 to 15 hr. Approximately, 20% is eliminated in the urine and 80% in the feces.

Peak: 4 hr.

Duration: 24 hr.

Indications Treatment of hypertension; nephropathy in type 2 diabetes.

Contraindications Standard considerations.

Route/Dosage
Hypertension
ADULTS: **PO** Start with 150 mg qd; then titrate to 300 mg qd as necessary.
CHILDREN (13 TO 16 YR): **PO** Start with 150 mg qd; then titrate patients requiring a further reduction in BP to 300 mg qd.
CHILDREN (6 TO 12 YR): **PO** Start with 75 mg qd; then titrate patients requiring a further reduction in BP to 150 mg qd.

Nephropathy in Type 2 Diabetes
ADULTS: **PO** Titrate dose to 300 mg qd.

Volume- and Salt-Depleted Patients
PO Start with 75 mg.

Interactions
Lithium: Plasma concentrations my be increased by irbesartan, resulting in an increase in the pharmacologic and adverse effects of lithium.

Lab Test Interferences None well documented.

Adverse Reactions
CV: Chest pain; tachycardia; edema.
CNS: Headache; anxiety/nervousness; dizziness.
GI: Diarrhea; dyspepsia/heartburn; abdominal pain; nausea/vomiting.
RESP: Upper respiratory tract infection; influenza; pharyngitis; rhinitis; sinus abnormality
OTHER: Musculoskeletal pain/trauma; fatigue; UTI; rash.

> **WARNING:**
> *Pregnancy:* Use in second and third trimesters may cause injury and death to fetus.

Precautions
Pregnancy: Category C (first trimester); Category D (second and third trimesters).
Lactation: Undetermined.
Children: Safety and efficacy not established in children younger than 6 yr.
Renal function impairment: Use with caution in patients whose renal function may depend on the activity of the renin-angiotensin-aldosterone system (eg, patients with severe CHF); use may be associated with oliguria, progressive azotemia, acute renal failure, and death.
Hypotension: Initiation of antihypertensive therapy may cause symptomatic hypotension in patients with intravascular volume or sodium-depletion.

PATIENT CARE CONSIDERATIONS
Administration/Storage
- Give prescribed dose qd with or without food.
- Administer alone or in combination with other antihypertensives.
- Do not administer to pregnant women because fetal and neonatal morbidity and death can occur.
- Administer with caution and reduced dosage in patients with possible depletion of intravascular volume or history of hepatic impairment.
- Store tablets at controlled room temperature (59° to 86°F).

Assessment/Interventions
- Obtain patient history, including drug history and any known allergies. Note history of anuria, lupus erythematosus, or kidney or liver disease.
- Ensure that serum electrolytes are monitored periodically.
- Monitor and record BP and pulse. Should hypotension result, hold medication and notify health care provider.
- Take safety precautions if orthostatic hypotension occurs.
- Monitor for signs of hypersensitivity including angioedema involving swelling of the face, lips, eyelids, and tongue. Discontinue medication and notify health care provider immediately if noted.

Patient/Family Education
- Explain name, dose, action, and potential side effects of drug.
- Advise patient to take prescribed dose once daily, without regard to meals.
- Advise patient to try to take each dose at about the same time each day.
- Inform patient that drug controls, but does not cure, hypertension, and to continue taking drug as prescribed even when BP is not elevated.
- Caution patient not to change the dose or stop taking unless advised by health care provider.
- Instruct patient in BP and pulse measurement skills.
- Advise patient to monitor and record BP and pulse at home and to inform health care provider should abnormal measurements be noted. Also advise patient to take record of BP and pulse to each follow-up visit.
- Caution patient to avoid sudden position changes to prevent orthostatic hypotension.
- Instruct patient to lie or sit down if they experience dizziness or lightheadedness when standing.
- Caution patient that inadequate fluid intake, excessive perspiration, diarrhea, or vomiting can lead to excessive fall in BP, resulting in lightheadedness or fainting.

- Emphasize to hypertensive patient importance of other modalities on BP: weight control, regular exercise, smoking cessation, moderate intake of alcohol and salt.
- Advise patient to contact health care provider if pregnant, planning to become pregnant, or breastfeeding.
- Instruct patient to stop taking drug and immediately report any of these symptoms to health care provider: fainting; swelling of the face, lips, eyelids, or tongue.
- Caution patient to not take any prescription or OTC medications, salt substitutes, or dietary supplements unless advised by health care provider.
- Advise patient that follow-up visits and lab tests may be required to monitor therapy and to keep appointments.

Irinotecan

(eye-rih-no-TEE-can)

Class Topoisomerase I inhibitor

How Supplied
Camptosar Injection 20 mg/mL, containing sorbitol 45 mg

Action
PHARMACOLOGY: Irinotecan is a derivative of camptothecin. Camptothecins interact specifically with the enzyme topoisomerase I, which relieves torsional strain in DNA by inducing reversible single-strand breaks.

PHARMACOKINETICS/DYNAMICS:
Absorption: T_{max} is 1 hr (active metabolite).
Distribution: 30 to 68% protein bound; approximately 95% of active metabolites protein bound.
Metabolism: SN-38 is the active metabolite. Metabolism occurs in the liver.
Excretion: The t½ is approximately 6 hr. Approximately 10 hr for the active metabolite. Primarily excreted in the urine.

Indications Metastatic cancer of the colon or rectum after standard treatment with fluorouracil. **Unlabeled use(s):** Cervical cancer, lung cancer (small cell or non-small cell), ovarian cancer.

Contraindications Standard considerations.

Route/Dosage
Colon or Rectal Cancer
ADULTS: **IV** Cycle 1: Irinotecan 125 mg/m^2 once weekly for 4 wk followed by 2 wk of rest. *Subsequent cycles:* Give irinotecan once weekly for 4 wk, followed by 2 wk of rest. Based on response and adverse effects, the dose may be adjusted in 25 to 50 mg/m^2 increments. The weekly dose may be increased to a max of 150 mg/m^2 or decreased to a min of 50 mg/m^2. *Alternate schedule:* Irinotecan 350 mg/m^2 **IV** once q 21 days. Give an initial dose of irinotecan 300 mg/m^2 **IV** q 21 days in patients at least 70 yr, patients with prior pelvic or abdominal radiation, or patients with a performance status of 2. Based on adverse effects, the dose may be decreased in 50 mg/m^2 increments to a min of 200 mg/m^2 (max, 350 mg/m^2).

Dosage Adjustment for Hepatic Dysfunction
ADULTS: **IV** *Once-daily regimen:* Dosage should be 125 mg/m^2 if serum bilirubin is less than 1 mg/dL. If bilirubin concentration is 1 to 2 mg/dL, dosage should be 100 mg/m^3. Irinotecan is not recommended if bilirubin is more than 2 mg/dL. *Every 21-day regimen:* Dosage should be 350 mg/m^2 if serum bilirubin is less than 1 mg/dL. If bilirubin concentration is 1 to 2 mg/dL, dosage should be 300 mg/m^2. Irinotecan is not recommended if bilirubin is more than 2 mg/dL.

Interactions
Antineoplastics: Irinotecan adverse effects (eg, myelosuppression, diarrhea) would possibly be exacerbated by other antineoplastics having similar adverse effects.
Dexamethasone: It is possible that coadministration of dexamethasone and irinotecan may enhance the likelihood of lymphocytopenia. Dexamethasone given as emetic prophylaxis can contribute to hyperglycemia in some patients.
Laxatives: Laxative therapy during irinotecan therapy may increase the severity of diarrhea, but this has not been studied.
Prochloperazine: The incidence of akathesia in clinical trials was greater (8.5%) when prochlorperazine was administered on the same day as irinotecan than when these drugs were given on separate days (1.3%).
Diuretics: The health care provider may wish to withhold diuretics during irinotecan dosing during periods of active vomiting or diarrhea because of the potential risk of dehydration secondary to irinotecan-induced vomiting and diarrhea.

Lab Test Interferences None well documented.

Adverse Reactions
CV: Flushing; edema.
CNS: Insomnia; headache; dizziness.
DERM: Alopecia; sweating; rash.
GI: Diarrhea ("early" occurring within 24 hr after infusion or "late" occurring an average of 11 to 18 days after infusion); moderate to high potential for nausea and vomiting; anorexia; constipation; flatulence; stomatitis; dyspepsia;

abdominal pain; increased LFTs.
HEMA: Leukopenia; lymphocytopenia; anemia; moderate to severe neutropenia. Neutrophil nadir occurs between days 15 to 27 with once weekly dosing and at days 8 to 9 with 21-day cycles.
RESP: Dyspnea; cough; rhinitis.
OTHER: Fever; pain; chills.

> **WARNING:**
> *Diarrhea:* Irinotecan injection can induce early and late forms of diarrhea, which may be severe and appear to be mediated by different mechanisms. May be life-threatening.
> *Myelosuppression:* Deaths caused by sepsis following severe myelosuppression have been reported in patients treated with irinotecan. Temporarily discontinue therapy if neutropenic fever occurs or if the absolute neutrophil count drops below 1000/mm^3.

Precautions
Pregnancy: Category D.
Lactation: Discontinue nursing when receiving therapy with irinotecan.
Children: Safety and efficacy not established.
Elderly: Exercise particular caution in monitoring the effects of irinotecan in the elderly (ie, at least 65 yr).
Hypersensitivity: Hypersensitivity reactions including severe anaphylactic or anaphylactoid reactions have been observed.
Renal function impairment: Rare cases of renal impairment and acute renal failure have been identified, usually in patients who became volume-depleted from severe vomiting or diarrhea.
Special risk patients: It has been noted that patients with modestly elevated baseline serum total bilirubin levels (1 to 2 mg/dL) have had a significantly greater likelihood of experiencing first-course grade 3 or 4 neutropenia than those with bilirubin levels that were less than 1 mg/dL.
Toxic deaths: Do not use in combination with the "Mayo Clinic" regimen of 5-FU/LV because of reports of increased toxicity, including toxic deaths. Use irinotecan as recommended.
Irradiation: Patients who have previously received pelvic/abdominal irradiation are at an increased risk of severe myelosuppression following irinotecan administration.
Extravasation: Local irritation or phlebitis may occur. Refer to the institution-specific protocol.
Adverse effects requiring irinotecan dosage modification: See manufacturer's recommendations.

PATIENT CARE CONSIDERATIONS
Administration/Storage
- Store solution for injection at room temperature and protect from light. Store in the protective packaging until just before use.
- Dilute to a final irinotecan concentration of 0.12 to 2.8 mg/mL before administration. The preferred diluent is 5% Dextrose, although 0.9% Sodium Chloride is acceptable. In most clinical trials, doses were diluted in 250 to 500 mL of 5% Dextrose.
- Diluted in 5% Dextrose, the final product is stable for up to 24 hr at ambient room temperature under fluorescent light. When refrigerated, the solution is stable for up to 48 hr. These solutions are preservative-free and should be used within 24 hr.
- When diluted with 0.9% Sodium Chloride, solutions may develop visible particulate matter if refrigerated. The manufacturer recommends using such solutions within 6 hr of preparation.
- IV infusion over 90 min. Shorter infusions (30 min) are associated with a higher incidence of myelosuppression.
- Do not begin a new course of therapy until the granulocyte count has recovered to at least 1500/mm^3 and the platelet count has recovered to at least 100,000/mm^3 and treatment-related diarrhea is fully resolved. Delay treatment 1 to 2 wk to allow recovery from treatment-related toxicities. If the patient has not recovered after a 2-wk delay, consider discontinuing therapy.
- Premedicate patients with antiemetic agents.

Assessment/Interventions
- Monitor the WBC with differential, hemoglobin, and platelet count before each irinotecan dose.

Patient/Family Education
- Instruct patients to call the health care provider if experiencing more than 3 days of diarrhea.
- Inform patients and caregivers of the expected toxic effects of irinotecan, particularly of its GI manifestations, such as nausea, vomiting, and diarrhea. Instruct each patient to have loperamide readily available and to begin treatment for late diarrhea (generally occurring more than 24 hr after administration) at the first episode of poorly formed or loose stools or the earliest onset of bowel movements more frequent than normally expected for the patient. One dosage regimen for loperamide is 4 mg at the first onset of late diarrhea and then 2 mg q 2 hr until the

patient is diarrhea-free for at least 12 hr. During the night, the patient may take 4 mg loperamide every 4 hr. Notify health care provider if diarrhea occurs. Premedication with loperamide is not recommended.
* Avoid the use of drugs with laxative properties because of the potential for exacerbation of diarrhea. Advise patients to contact the health care provider to discuss any laxative use.
* Consult health care provider if vomiting or fever occurs or evidence of infection develops, of if symptoms of dehydration, such as fainting, lightheadedness, or dizziness are noted following irinotecan therapy.

Iron Dextran

(iron DEX-tran)

Class Iron product

How Supplied

DexFerrum Injection 50 mg iron/mL (as dextran) ◆ *InFeD* Injection 50 mg iron/mL (as dextran)

 Dexiron ◆ *Infufer*

Action

PHARMACOLOGY: Replenishes Hgb and depleted iron stores.

PHARMACOKINETICS/DYNAMICS:

Absorption: Majority of IM injections are absorbed within 72 hr and then most of the remaining iron is absorbed over 3 to 4 wk.

Distribution: 90% or more is protein bound.

Metabolism: Removed from plasma by the reticuloendothelial system which splits the drug into its components.

Excretion: Removal by dialysis is negligible.

Onset: A few days.

Indications Treatment of iron deficiency anemia when oral administration of iron is unsatisfactory or impossible. **Unlabeled use(s):** Use with epoetin to ensure hematological response to epoetin.

Contraindications Anemia not associated with iron deficiency.

Route/Dosage

Prior to the first IV or IM iron dextran injection, give a 0.5 mL test dose by the same route, respectively. Anaphylactic reactions occurring following iron dextran injection are usually evident within a few minutes; however, at least 1 hr should elapse before the remainder of the therapeutic dose is given.

Iron Deficiency Anemia

ADULTS AND CHILDREN: **IM/IV** with dose based on formula to determine amount of iron required to restore hemoglobin to normal levels (max 2 mL/day undiluted iron dextran):

Mg iron = 0.3 x body weight in lb x $\dfrac{(100 - \text{Hgb [g/dL]} \times 100)}{14.8}$

Formula should not be used for patients weighing 30 lb or more.

Iron Replacement for Blood Loss

ADULTS AND CHILDREN: TEST DOSE: **IM/IV** with dose based on formula that 1 mL of normocytic, normochromic RBC cells contains 1 mg of elemental iron (maximum 2 mL/day undiluted iron dextran):

Mg iron – blood loss (mL) x Hct

Each day's dose should not exceed 0.5 mL (25 mg iron) for infants less than 10 lb or 1 mL (50 mg iron) for children less than 20 lb, or 2 mL (100 mg iron) for other patients.

Interactions

Chloramphenicol: May increase serum iron concentrations.

INCOMPATIBILITIES: Do not mix with other medications or add to parenteral nutrition solutions for IV infusions.

Lab Test Interferences

Serum bilirubin: Drug may cause falsely elevated values.

Serum calcium: Drug may cause falsely decreased values.

Adverse Reactions

CV: Hypotension; peripheral vascular flushing (IV).

CNS: Headache; dizziness; malaise; transitory paresthesias.

DERM: Brown skin discoloration at IM injection site.

GI: Nausea.

HEMA: Leukocytosis.

OTHER: Hypersensitivity (eg, fatal anaphylaxis, shortness of breath, urticaria, itching, arthralgia, myalgia, fever); pain and inflammation at injection site; sterile abscesses (IM); phlebitis at IV injection site; reactivation of arthritis in patients with inactive rheumatoid arthritis; backache; shivering. Delayed reactions may occur 1 to 2 days after administration.

> **WARNING:**
> Anaphylactic type reactions (sometimes fatal) have occurred with parenteral use of product. Reserve for use only in patients with lab-confirmed iron deficiency who are unable to take oral iron.

Precautions
Pregnancy: Safety not established. Based on animal studies, avoid if possible.
Lactation: Undetermined.
Children: Not recommended in children younger than 4 mo of age.
Hypersensitivity: Hypersensitivity, including anaphylaxis, may occur. Have epinephrine immediately available.
Hepatic function impairment: Use drug with extreme caution in severe hepatic impairment.

Allergies/Asthma: Use drug with caution in patients with history of significant allergies/asthma.
Arthritis: Patients with iron deficiency anemia and rheumatoid arthritis may have acute exacerbation of joint pain and swelling after IV administration.

Overdosage: Signs and Symptoms
Hemosiderosis.

PATIENT CARE CONSIDERATIONS
Administration/Storage
- Oral iron preparations should be discontinued before parenteral administration.
- Inject IM via Z-track technique into upper outer quadrant of buttock; never inject iron dextran into arm or other exposed areas. Use 2- to 3-inch 19- or 20-gauge needle.
- If patient is standing, weight should be placed on leg opposite injection site. If in bed, patient should be in lateral position with injection site uppermost.
- Change needles between withdrawal from container and injection to minimize staining of subcutaneous tissues. Stains usually are permanent.
- For IV administration, inject slowly at 1 mL/min or less.
- Store at room temperature.

Assessment/Interventions
- Obtain patient history, including drug history and any known allergies.
- Assess patient's nutritional status and dietary history to determine possible causes of anemia.
- Monitor Hgb, Hct, and reticulocyte values; transferrin, ferritin, total iron binding capacity; and plasma iron concentrations periodically during therapy.
- Assess patient for signs of anaphylaxis (eg, rash, pruritus, laryngeal edema, wheezing).
- Monitor BP and heart rate frequently during IV administration.
- Assess patient for symptoms of GI distress and constipation regularly throughout therapy.
- Provide diet high in iron (eg, organ meats; leafy, green vegetables; dried beans and peas; dried fruit; cereals).
- If constipation occurs, obtain order for laxative. Increase fiber and give additional fluids.

Patient/Family Education
- Teach family and patient the name, dose, action, and side effects of iron.
- Advise patient to take additional fluids to prevent constipation.
- Teach patient that certain foods, such as coffee, tea, eggs, and milk, interact with iron.
- Teach patient and family the daily iron requirements (children 6 mo to 10 yr of age: 10 mg; adolescents 11 to 18 yr of age, male: 12 mg; adolescents 11 to 18 yr of age, female: 15 mg; adult women, pregnant: 30 mg; adult women, nonpregnant: 15 mg; adult men: 10 mg).

Iron Sucrose
(I-ern SUE-krose)
Class Iron product

How Supplied
Venofer Injection 20 mg/mL

Action
PHARMACOLOGY: Replenishes Hgb and depleted iron stores.

PHARMACOKINETICS/DYNAMICS:
Distribution: The apparent Vd is 10 L and the Vd_{ss} is 7.9 L.

Metabolism: Dissociated into iron and sucrose by the reticuloendotherial system.

Excretion: Sucrose component mainly excreted in the urine. The $t_{1/2}$ is 6 hr. The Cl is 1.2 L/hr.

Indications
Treatment of iron deficiency anemia in patients undergoing chronic hemodialysis who are receiving erythropoietin therapy.

Contraindications
Iron overload; anemia not caused by iron deficiency.

Route/Dosage
ADULTS: IV 100 mg elemental iron (5 mL) directly into dialysis line by slow injection (ie, 20 mg [1 mL] undiluted solution/min) or by infusion (ie, 100 mg of elemental iron diluted in a max of 100 mL of 0.9% NaCl infused over 15 min or longer). Most patients will require 1000 mg of elemental iron, administered over 10 sequential dialysis sessions.

Interactions

Oral iron: Absorption of oral iron may be reduced.

INCOMPATIBILITIES: Do not mix with other medication or add to parenteral nutrition solutions for IV infusion.

Lab Test Interferences None well documented.

Adverse Reactions

CV: Hypotension; chest pain; hypertension; hypervolemia.
CNS: Headache; malaise; dizziness.
DERM: Pruritus; application site reaction.
GI: Nausea; vomiting; diarrhea; abdominal pain.
HEPA: Elevated liver enzymes.
RESP: Dyspnea; pneumonia; cough.
OTHER: Leg cramps; cramps; fever; pain; asthenia; musculoskeletal pain; hypersensitivity.

Precautions

Pregnancy: Category B.
Lactation: Undetermined.
Children: Safety and efficacy not established.
Elderly: Select dose with caution, reflecting greater frequency of decreased hepatic, renal, or cardiac function and comorbidity.
Hypersensitivity: Potentially fatal hypersensitivity reactions, including anaphylactic shock, may occur.
Iron overload: Exercise caution and withhold iron administration in the presence of evidence of tissue iron overload.
Hypotension: Hypotension related to the rate of administration and total dose administered may occur.

Overdosage: Signs and Symptoms

Hypotension, headache, vomiting, nausea, dizziness, joint aches, paresthesia, abdominal and muscle pain, edema, cardiovascular collapse, sedation, hypoactivity, bleeding in GI tract and lungs.

PATIENT CARE CONSIDERATIONS

Administration/Storage

- Discontinue oral iron preparations before administering parenteral iron products.
- Dose is administered 1 to 3 times/wk. Do not administer more than 3 times/wk.
- Administer by IV route only. Not for IM or SC administration.
- Administer prescribed dose directly into dialysis line either by slow injection or by infusion.
- For slow IV injection, administer undiluted solution at rate 1 mL/min or less. Max dose is 5 mL (1 vial).
- For IV infusion, dilute contents of 1 vial in 100 mL 0.9% NaCl immediately prior to infusion and infuse over 15 min. Discard any unused diluted solution.
- Do not mix with other IV medications or add to parenteral nutrition solutions.
- Do not administer if particulate matter or discoloration noted.
- Store vials at controlled room temperature. Protect from freezing.

Assessment/Interventions

- Obtain patient history, including drug history and any known allergies.
- Review patient's health history for any condition that could contraindicate iron sucrose: evidence of iron overload, anemia not caused by iron deficiency.
- Ensure that patient is also receiving erythropoietin therapy.
- Ensure that hemoglobin, hematocrit, serum ferritin, and transferrin saturation are determined before and periodically during treatment.
- Monitor BP during infusion. If hypotension occurs, slow infusion rate. If hypotension continues, discontinue infusion.
- Monitor patient for signs of anaphylactic reaction during and shortly after infusion. Be prepared to respond if a serious reaction occurs.

Patient/Family Education

- Explain name, dose, action, and potential side effects of drug.
- Advise patient that medication will be prepared and administered by health care provider during dialysis sessions and that medication will not be administered at home.
- Instruct patient to inform health care provider if noting any of the following symptoms during the administration of drug: anxiety, sweating, rapid heart beat, shortness of breath or difficulty breathing, swelling of the throat, rash, or itching.
- Advise patient that follow-up visits and laboratory tests will be required to monitor therapy, and to be sure to keep appointments.

Isocarboxazid

(eye-so-car-BOX-ah-zid)
Class Antidepressant/MAO inhibitor

How Supplied
Marplan Tablets 10 mg

Action
PHARMACOLOGY: Blocks activity of enzyme MAO, thereby increasing monoamine (eg, epinephrine, norepinephrine, serotonin) concentrations in CNS.

Indications Treatment of depression.

Contraindications Patients with known hypersensitivity to any component of the product; coadministration of MAO inhibitors, dibenzazepine derivatives, sympathomimetics (including amphetamines), some CNS depressants (including narcotics and alcohol), antihypertensives, diuretic, antihistaminic, anti-Parkinson drugs; sedative or anesthetic drugs, bupropion, buspirone, dextromethorphan, serotonin reuptake inhibitors (eg, fluoxetine); cheese or other foods high in tyramine content, excessive quantities of caffeine; patients with confirmed or suspected cerebrovascular defect, cardiovascular disease, hypertension, or history of headache, pheochromocytoma, history of liver disease, abnormal LFTs, severe renal impairment. Allow a medicine-free interval of at least 1 wk when transferring a patient to isocarboxazid from another MAO inhibitor or a dibenzazepine-related agent, then initiate therapy using ½ the normal starting dosage for at least the first week; similarly, allow 1 wk between discontinuing isocarboxazid and another MAO inhibitor or dibenzazepine-related agent, or readministration of isocarboxazid.

Route/Dosage
ADULTS AND CHILDREN 16 YR AND OLDER: PO Start with 10 mg bid. Dosage may be increased by 10 mg increments q 2 to 4 days to achieve a dosage of 40 mg by the end of the first week. Dosage can then be increased up to 20 mg/wk. Daily dosages should be divided into 2 to 4 doses (max, 60 mg/day).

Interactions
Amine-containing Foods: May cause severe hypertension or hemorrhagic strokes.
Anorexiants (eg, amphetamines): May cause exaggerated pharmacologic effects (eg, severe headaches, hypertension, hyperpyrexia) of anorexiant.
Antihypertensive agents (eg, thiazide diuretics): Potentiative hypotensive effects.
Antiparkinson agents (eg, levodopa): May cause hypertensive reactions.
Bupropion, buspirone, carbamazepine, CNS stimulants, cyclobenzaprine, guanethidine, maprotiline, serotonin reuptake inhibitors (fluoxetine), sympathomimetics, tricyclic antidepressants, tyramine: May lead to potentially fatal reactions, including seizures and hypertensive crisis; mental status changes, hyperthermia.
CNS depressants: May enhance CNS effects.
Dextromethorphan: Use has been associated with severe reactions (eg, hyperpyrexia, hypotension, death, psychosis, bizarre behavior).
Disulfiram: May cause convulsions and death.
Insulin, sulfonylureas (eg, chlorpropamide): May enhance hypoglycemic action.
Meperidine: May lead to severe reactions, including hypotension, convulsions, respiratory depression, and vascular collapse.
Selective 5-HT$_1$ receptor agonists (eg, sumatriptan): May increase the risk of cardiac toxicity (eg, coronary artery vasospasm).

Lab Test Interferences None well documented.

Adverse Reactions
CV: Orthostatic hypotension (4%); palpitations (2%).
CNS: Dizziness (29%); headache (15%); sleep disturbance (5%); drowsiness, insomnia, tremor (4%); anxiety, forgetfulness, hyperactivity, lethargy, sedation, myoclonic jerks, paresthesia (2%).
DERM: Sweating (2%).
GI: Nausea (10%); dry mouth (9%); constipation (7%); diarrhea (2%).
GU: Urinary hesitancy (4%); urinary frequency, impotence (2%).
OTHER: Chills, syncope, heavy feeling (2%).

Precautions
Pregnancy: Undetermined.
Lactation: Use not recommended.
Children: Safety and efficacy not established in children under 16 yr.
Elderly: Use with caution.
Renal function impairment: Use with caution.
Anginal pain: May be suppressed, masking a warning of MI.
Co-existing symptoms of depression: Symptoms, such as anxiety and agitation, may be aggravated.
Epilepsy: May lower seizure threshold.
Hyperactive or agitated patients: Use with caution.

Hypotension: Orthostatic hypotension is a significant side effect and may lead to falling and changes in heart rate.
Suicide: Strict supervision may be necessary in patients at risk.

PATIENT CARE CONSIDERATIONS
Administration/Storage
- Administer bid to qid as prescribed.
- Administer without regard to meals but give with food if GI upset occurs.
- Store tablets at controlled room temperature (59° to 86°F).

Assessment/Interventions
- Obtain patient history, including drug history and any known allergies. Note kidney disease, pheochromocytoma, heart failure, confirmed or suspected cerebrovascular disorder, CV disease, hypertension, headaches or history of headaches, diabetes, or seizure disorder.
- Before starting therapy, review medication and diet history for any medication or food that would be contraindicated during therapy with isocarboxazid. Ensure that adequate time elapses between discontinuing the interacting medication and starting isocarboxazid.
- Continue suicide monitoring of high-risk patients.
- Observe for signs of mood and behavior changes and report to health care provider.
- Monitor BP and pulse routinely during therapy. Inform health care provider if significant changes in BP or orthostatic symptoms are noted.
- Implement safety precautions for patient who experiences orthostatic hypotension.
- Monitor blood sugar in diabetic patient when drug is started or dose is changed. Report significant changes to health care provider.
- Assess patient for CNS, CV, GI, and general body side effects. Report to health care provider if noted and significant.
- Immediately notify health care provider if any of the following occur: palpitations, severe headache, unexplained rapid heartbeat, sweating, dizziness, neck stiffness, feeling of constriction in throat or chest, persistent nausea or vomiting, any other unusual symptom.
- Periodically attempt to reduce maintenance dose to lowest level that maintains therapeutic response.

Overdosage: Signs and Symptoms
Tachycardia, hypotension, coma, convulsions, respiratory depression, sluggish reflexes, pyrexia, diaphoresis.

Patient/Family Education
- Explain name, dose, action, and potential side effects of drug.
- Review foods, beverages, and medications that must be avoided during treatment and for at least 2 wk following discontinuation of therapy.
- Advise patient that medication will be started at a low dose and then increased as tolerated until max benefit is obtained.
- Inform patient that it may take 3 to 6 wk for symptoms to improve and to continue with the prescribed therapy once improvement has been noted.
- Advise patient to take prescribed dose without regard to meals but to take with food if GI upset occurs.
- Advise patient that if a dose is missed, to skip that dose and take the next dose at the regularly scheduled time. Caution patient never to take 2 doses at the same time.
- Caution patient not to change the dose or stop taking unless advised by health care provider.
- Advise patient to take frequent sips of water, suck on ice chips or sugarless hard candy, or chew sugarless gum if dry mouth occurs.
- Advise patient to avoid alcoholic beverages and tryptophan while taking isocarboxazid.
- Caution patient to avoid sudden position changes to prevent orthostatic hypotension (dizziness or faintness when arising suddenly from a sitting or lying position). Advise patient to sit or lie down if dizziness or faintness occurs and to notify health care provider if this persists or worsens.
- Instruct diabetic patient to monitor blood glucose more frequently when drug is started or dose is changed and to inform health care provider of significant changes in readings.
- Advise patient that drug may cause drowsiness or blurred vision and to use caution while driving or performing other tasks requiring mental alertness until tolerance is determined.

- Instruct patient to discontinue use and notify health care provider immediately if any of the following occur: pounding in the chest (palpitations), severe headache, unexplained rapid heartbeat, sweating, dizziness, neck stiffness, feeling of constriction in throat or chest, persistent nausea or vomiting, any other unusual symptom.
- Instruct patient not to take prescription or OTC drugs or dietary supplements unless advised by health care provider.
- Advise women to notify health care provider if pregnant, planning to become pregnant, or breastfeeding.
- Advise patient that follow-up visits will be necessary to monitor therapy and to keep appointments.

Isometheptene Mucate/ Dichloralphenazone/ Acetaminophen

(eye-so-meth-EPP-teen MYOO-kate/die-klor-uhl-FEN-uh-zone/ASS-et-ah-MEE-noe-fen)

Class Migraine

How Supplied
Isocom Capsules 65 mg isometheptene mucate, 100 mg dichloralphenazone, 325 mg APAP ♦
Isopap Capsules 65 mg isometheptene mucate, 100 mg dichloralphenazone, 325 mg APAP ♦
Midchlor Capsules 65 mg isometheptene mucate, 100 mg dichloralphenazone, 325 mg APAP ♦
Midrin Capsules 65 mg isometheptene mucate, 100 mg dichloralphenazone, 325 mg APAP ♦
Migratine Capsules 65 mg isometheptene mucate, 100 mg dichloralphenazone, 325 mg APAP

Action
PHARMACOLOGY: Isometheptene mucate acts as sympathomimetic to constrict dilated cranial and cerebral arterioles. Dichloralphenazone is a mild sedative that reduces emotional reaction to pain of vascular and tension headaches. Acetaminophen is a mild analgesic.

Indications Relief of tension and vascular headaches. FDA has classified drug as possibly effective in treatment of migraine headaches.

Contraindications Glaucoma; severe cases of renal disease; hypertension; organic heart disease; hepatic disease; MAO inhibitor therapy.

PATIENT CARE CONSIDERATIONS
Administration/Storage
- Administer at first sign of migraine headache.
- Administer with full glass of water.
- Store at room temperature in dry place in tightly closed container.

Assessment/Interventions
- Obtain patient history, including drug history and any known allergies.
- Assess frequency, duration, location, and characteristics of chronic headaches.
- Monitor BP and pulse periodically during therapy.
- Notify health care provider if hypertension occurs.

Route/Dosage
Migraine Headache
ADULTS: PO 2 capsules at once, followed by 1 capsule q hr until headache is relieved (max, 5 capsules in 12 hr period).

Tension Headache
ADULTS: PO 1 to 2 capsules q 4 hr (max, 8 capsules/day).

Interactions
MAO inhibitors: May result in severe headache, hypertension, hyperpyrexia, and possible hypertensive crisis.

Lab Test Interferences None well documented.

Adverse Reactions
CNS: Transient dizziness or drowsiness.
DERM: Rash.

Precautions
Pregnancy: Pregnancy category undetermined.
Lactation: Undetermined.
Children: Safety and efficacy not established.
Special risk patients: Observe caution in patients with hypertension or peripheral vascular disease and after recent CV attacks.
Hepatotoxicity: Can occur with chronic ingestion of acetaminophen. Chronic alcohol abusers are especially at risk.

Overdosage: Signs and Symptoms
Nausea; vomiting; drowsiness; confusion; liver tenderness; low or high BP; cardiac arrhythmias; jaundice; acute hepatic and renal failure.

- If relief from headache is not obtained, notify health care provider.

Patient/Family Education
- Instruct patient to take drug at first sign of impending headache.
- Encourage patient to rest in quiet, dark room after taking drug.
- Advise patient not to drink alcoholic beverages.
- Instruct patient to notify health care provider of dizziness or skin rash.
- Instruct patient to notify health care provider if headache persists.

Isoniazid (Isonicotinic Acid Hydrazide; INH)

(eye-so-NYE-uh-zid)

Class Anti-infective/Antitubercular

How Supplied
Nydrazid Injection 100 mg/mL ♦ *Isoniazid* Tablets 300 mg, Tablets 500 mg, Syrup 50 mg/5 mL
✤ *Isotamine* ♦ *PMS-Isoniazid*

Action
PHARMACOLOGY: Interferes with lipid and nucleic acid biosynthesis in actively growing tubercle bacilli.

PHARMACOKINETICS/DYNAMICS:
Absorption: T_{max} is 1 to 2 hr.

Distribution: Diffuses readily into cerebrospinal, pleural, and ascitic fluids, tissues, organs, saliva, sputum, feces, placental barrier, and in breast milk.

Metabolism: Primarily by acetylation and dehydrazination.

Excretion: 50% to 70% excreted in the urine in 24 hr.

Indications Treatment of all forms of tuberculosis. **Unlabeled use(s):** Improvement of severe tremor in multiple sclerosis.

Contraindications Previous isoniazid-associated hepatic injury, drug fever, chills, or arthritis; acute liver disease.

Route/Dosage
Tuberculosis
ADULTS: **PO/IM** 5 mg/kg/day as single daily dose (max, 300 mg/day) or 15 mg/kg 2 to 3 times/wk (max, 900 mg).
INFANTS AND CHILDREN: **PO/IM** 10 to 20 mg/kg/day in single daily dose (max, 300 mg/day) or 20 to 40 mg/kg 2 or 3 times/week (max, 400 mg).

Interactions
Aluminum salts: May reduce oral absorption of isoniazid; give isoniazid 1 to 3 hr before aluminum salts.

Carbamazepine: May result in carbamazepine toxicity or isoniazid hepatotoxicity. Monitor carbamazepine concentrations and liver function.

Disulfiram: May result in increased incidence of CNS effects (eg, coordination difficulties, confusion, irritability, aggressiveness).

Enflurane: May result in high-output renal failure in rapid acetylators. Monitor renal function.

Hydantoins: May increase serum hydantoin levels.

Rifampin: May result in higher rate of hepatotoxicity.

Lab Test Interferences None well documented.

Adverse Reactions
CNS: Peripheral neuropathy; convulsions; toxic encephalopathy; optic neuritis and atrophy; memory impairment; toxic psychosis.
DERM: Morbilliform, maculopapular, purpuric, or exfoliative skin eruptions.
GI: Nausea; vomiting; epigastric distress.
HEMA: Agranulocytosis; hemolytic, sideroblastic, or aplastic anemia; thrombocytopenia; eosinophilia.
HEPA: Hepatotoxicity, including elevated serum transaminase levels, bilirubinemia, bilirubinuria, jaundice, severe and sometimes fatal hepatitis.
METAB: Pyridoxine deficiency; pellagra; hyperglycemia; metabolic acidosis; hypocalcemia; hypophosphatemia.
OTHER: Gynecomastia; rheumatic syndrome; systemic lupus erythematosus-like syndrome; local irritation at IM injection site.

> **WARNING:**
> Severe and sometimes fatal hepatitis may occur during and many mo after treatment. Risk is related to age and increased with daily alcohol consumption. If reinitiated, start in small and gradual doses. Not for use in patients with active liver disease. Careful monitoring and monthly interviews are recommended.

Precautions
Pregnancy: Safety undetermined.
Lactation: Excreted in breast milk.
Hypersensitivity: Discontinue drug at first sign of hypersensitivity reaction. Restart only after symptoms have cleared.
Renal function impairment: Monitor patients with severe renal dysfunction carefully.
Hepatic function impairment: Common prodromal symptoms of hepatotoxicity include anorexia, nausea, vomiting, fatigue, malaise, and weakness. Patients with acute hepatic disease should have preventive tuberculosis treatment deferred. Incidence of hepatic reaction increases in patients older than 50 yr.
Pyridoxine administration: Prophylactic coadministration of pyridoxine (6 to 50 mg/day) is recommended in malnourished patients and those predisposed to neuropathy (eg, alcoholics, diabetics).

Overdosage: Signs and Symptoms
Nausea, vomiting, dizziness, slurring of speech, blurring of vision, visual hallucinations, respiratory distress, CNS depression, stupor, coma, severe seizures.

PATIENT CARE CONSIDERATIONS
Administration/Storage
- Oral form available in tablet and syrup forms.
- Administer oral medication on empty stomach 1 hr or more before or 2 hr after meals.
- If GI irritation becomes problematic, drug may be administered with food, although food decreases absorption of drug.
- Antacids may be given 1 hr before administration.
- Store at room temperature and protect from moisture.

Assessment/Interventions
- Obtain patient history, including drug history and any known allergies.
- Assess mycobacterial studies and susceptibility tests before and periodically throughout therapy to detect possible resistance.
- Evaluate hepatic function studies before and monthly during therapy (eg, AST, ALT) and serum bilirubin.
- Assess patient for the following adverse reactions: GI distress, peripheral neuritis, optic neuritis, or hypersensitivity reactions.
- If nausea, vomiting, anorexia, or diarrhea develop, obtain order for antiemetic or antidiarrheal medication and assess for hepatotoxicity.
- Take safety precautions if patient experiences adverse CNS symptoms such as confusion or incoordination.

Patient/Family Education
- Teach patient and family the name, dose, action, and side effects of isoniazid.
- Advise patient to minimize daily alcohol consumption while taking isoniazid because of the increased risk of hepatitis.
- Instruct patient to report the following symptoms to health care provider: weakness; fatigue; loss of appetite; nausea and vomiting; yellowing of skin or eyes; darkening of urine; numbness or tingling in hands or feet.
- Emphasize to patient that treatment will be lengthy and that patient must complete entire course of therapy. Relapse of tuberculosis is higher if chemotherapy is discontinued prematurely.
- Advise patient to return for laboratory follow-up.
- Caution patient not to perform activities that require mental alertness if adverse CNS symptoms occur.

Isoproterenol

(eye-so-pro-TER-uh-nahl)

Class Bronchodilator/Sympathomimetic

How Supplied
Isoproterenol Hydrochloride
Isuprel Injection (1:5000 solution) 0.2 mg/mL isoproterenol hydrochloride ♦ *Isoproterenol Hydrochloride* Injection (1:5000 solution) 0.2 mg/mL isoproterenol hydrochloride, Injection (1:50,000) 0.02 mg/mL isoproterenol hydrochloride

Isoproterenol Sulfate
Medihaler-ISO Aerosol Delivers 80 mcg isoproternol sulfate/actuation

Action
PHARMACOLOGY: Produces bronchodilation by relaxing bronchial smooth muscle through beta-2 receptor stimulation; increases heart rate and myocardial contractility by stimulating cardiac beta-1 receptors, which increases cardiac output.

PHARMACOKINETICS/DYNAMICS:
Onset: Within 5 minutes.
Peak: Five to 15 minutes.
Duration: Less than 3 hours.

Indications Management of bronchospasm during anesthesia; adjunctive treatment for shock.

Contraindications Cardiac arrhythmias associated with tachycardia; tachycardia or heart block caused by digitalis intoxication; angina; ventricular arrhythmias requiring inotropic therapy.

Route/Dosage
Bronchospasm during anesthesia
ADULTS: **IV** 0.01 to 0.02 mg. Repeat as necessary.

Shock and hypoperfusion
ADULTS: **IV** 0.5 mcg to 5 mcg/min. Rates over 30 mcg/min have been used in advanced stages of shock.

Heart block, Adams-Stokes attacks, and cardiac arrest
ADULTS: **Bolus IV** 0.02 mg to 0.06 mg initial dose with subsequent dose range of 0.01 mg to 0.2 mg; **IV infusion** 5mcg/min initial dose; **IM** 0.2 mg initial dose with a subsequent dose rang

of 0.02 mg to 1 mg; **SC** 0.2 mg initial dose of 0.2 mg with subsequent dose range of 0.15 mg to 0.2 mg; **Intracardiac** 0.02 mg initial dose. Subsequent dosage and administration method depend on ventricular rate and rapidity with which cardiac pacemaker can take over when drug is withdrawn.

Interactions
Cardiac glycosides: Arrhythmias may result with coadministration.
General anesthetics (eg, halothane, cyclopropane): Arrhythmias may result with coadministration.
Ergot alkaloids: Coadministration may result in additive peripheral vasoconstriction.

Lab Test Interferences Bilirubin may be falsely elevated if measured by sequential multiple analyzer. Urinary epinephrine values may be elevated.

Adverse Reactions
CV: Palpitations; tachycardia; blood pressure changes; arrhythmias; Adams-Stokes attacks; cardiac arrest.
CNS: Tremor; dizziness; nervousness; drowsiness; headache; insomnia.
GI: Nausea; GI distress.
RESP: Cough; throat irritation; bronchitis; sputum increase; pulmonary edema.
OTHER: Parotid gland swelling with prolonged use; saliva discoloration; sweating; skin flushing.

Precautions
Pregnancy: Category C.
Lactation: Undetermined.
Children: Safety and efficacy have not been established.
Elderly: Lower doses may be required.
Labor and delivery: May inhibit uterine contractions and delay preterm labor.
Cardiogenic shock: Isoproterenol hydrochloride injection, by increasing myocardial oxygen requirements while decreasing effective coronary perfusion, may have a deterious effect on the injured or failing heart. Most experts discourage its use as the initial agent in treating cardiogenic shock following myocardial infarction.
Cardiovascular disorders: Toxic symptoms in patients with cardiovascular disorders may occur. Doses sufficient to increase the heart rate more than 130 bpm may induce ventricular arrhythmias. Use with caution in patients with coronary artery disease, coronary insufficiency, diabetes, or hyperthyroidism, and in patients sensitive to sympathomimetic amines.
Hypovolemia: Adequate filling of the intravascular compartment by suitable volume expanders is of primary importance in most cases of shock and should precede the administration of vasoactive drugs.
Refractory asthmatic children: IV infusions of isoproterenol have caused clinical deterioration, myocardial necrosis, congestive heart failure, and death.

Overdosage: Signs and Symptoms
Tremor, palpitations, angina, arrhythmias, tachycardia, elevated or decreased blood pressure, seizures, nervousness, headache, dry mouth, nausea, dizziness, fatigue, malaise, insomnia.

PATIENT CARE CONSIDERATIONS

Administration/Storage
IV injection:
- Dilute 1 mL of 1:5000 solution to 10 mL with 5% Sodium Chloride or Dextrose Injection to achieve 1:50,000 solution.

IV infusion:
- Dilute 10 mL 1:5000 solution in 500 mL 5% Dextrose to produce 1:250,000 solution. Use microdrip or continuous infusion pump to prevent sudden influx of large amount of drug.

Metered dose inhaler:
- Shake container thoroughly to activate medication. Instruct patient in proper technique for use.

IPPB:
- Position patient properly for treatment, either sitting or in semi-Fowler position. Have patient rinse mouth after each session.

Nebulizer:
- Find location where patient can sit comfortably for 10 to 15 min. Do not mix different types of medication without consulting the package insert. Instruct patients to take slow, deep breaths and, if possible, hold breath for 10 sec before slowly exhaling. Continue until medication chamber is empty.
- Discard solution if precipitate or discoloration are present.
- Store in tight, light-resistant container at room temperature.

Assessment/Interventions
- Obtain patient history, including drug history and any known allergies.
- Monitor heart rate, respirations, BP, and urine output. Carefully monitor heart rate and rhythm and ECG pattern when used as treatment for shock.

Patient/Family Education
- Use verbal instructions and demonstrations to teach technique for inhalation therapy and explain that if more than 1 inhalation is necessary, patient should wait 3 to 5 min between doses.

- Tell patient to notify health care provider if no response to usual dose.
- Obtain patient history, including drug history and any known allergies.
- Monitor heart rate, respirations, BP, and urine output. Carefully monitor heart rate and rhythm and ECG pattern when used as treatment for shock.

Isosorbide Dinitrate

(EYE-sos-ORE-bide die-NYE-trate)

Class Antianginal

How Supplied
Dilatrate-SR Capsules, sustained-release 40 mg ♦ Isordil Tablets, sublingual 2.5 mg, Tablets, sublingual 5 mg, Tablets, sublingual 10 mg ♦ Isordil Titradose Tablets 5 mg, Tablets 10 mg, Tablets 20 mg, Tablets 30 mg, Tablets 40 mg ♦ Sorbitrate Tablets 5 mg, Tablets 10 mg, Tablets 20 mg, Tablets 30 mg, Tablets 40 mg, Tablets, chewable 5 mg, Tablets, chewable 10 mg
✣ APO-ISDN

Action
PHARMACOLOGY: Relaxation of smooth muscle of venous and arterial vasculature.

PHARMACOKINETICS/DYNAMICS:
Distribution: Approximately 60% protein bound.

Metabolism: Metabolized in the liver to 2- and 5-mononitrates, which are both active.

Onset: 2 to 5 min (SC); 4 to 6 hr (oral), 6 to 8 hr (oral, SR).

Indications Treatment and prevention of angina pectoris.

Contraindications Hypersensitivity to nitrates; severe anemia; closed-angle glaucoma; orthostatic hypotension; head trauma or cerebral hemorrhage.

Route/Dosage
Angina Pectoris
ADULTS: **SL** (sublingual tablets) 2.5 to 5 mg; **PO** (chewable tablets) 5 mg; **PO** (oral tablets) 5 to 40 mg q 6 hr; **PO** (sustained release tablets) 40 to 80 mg q 8 to 12 hr.

Acute Prophylaxis
ADULTS: **PO** (sublingual or chewable tablets) 5 to 10 mg q 2 to 3 hr.

Interactions
Alcohol: Severe hypotension and cardiovascular collapse.
Aspirin: Increased nitrate concentration and actions.
Dihydroergotamine: Increased systolic blood pressure and decreased antianginal effects.

Lab Test Interferences May cause false report of reduced serum cholesterol with *Zlatkis-Zak* color reaction.

Adverse Reactions
CV: Tachycardia; palpitations; hypotension; syncope; arrhythmias.
CNS: Headache; apprehension; weakness; vertigo; dizziness; agitation; insomnia.
DERM: Cutaneous vasodilation with flushing.
EENT: Blurred vision.
GI: Nausea; vomiting; diarrhea; dyspepsia.
GU: Dysuria; urinary frequency; impotence.
HEMA: Methemoglobinemia; hemolytic anemia.
RESP: Bronchitis; pneumonia.
OTHER: Arthralgia; perspiration; pallor; cold sweat; edema.

Precautions
Pregnancy: Category C.
Lactation: Undetermined.
Children: Safety and efficacy not established.
Special risk patients: Use with caution in patients with acute MI or CHF.
Angina: May aggravate angina caused by hypertrophic cardiomyopathy.
Orthostatic hypotension: May occur even with small doses; alcohol accentuates this reaction.
Tolerance: Tolerance to vascular and antianginal effects may develop.

Overdosage: Signs and Symptoms
Hypotension, tachycardia, flushing, diaphoresis, headache, vertigo, palpitations, visual disturbances, nausea, vomiting, confusion, dyspnea.

PATIENT CARE CONSIDERATIONS

Administration/Storage
- Sublingual tablets should be placed under tongue to dissolve. Do not swallow.
- Chewable tablets should be chewed and swallowed. Do not crush before administering.
- Oral dosage forms should be taken on empty stomach with full glass of water.
- Store at room temperature.

Assessment/Interventions
- Obtain patient history, including drug history and any known allergies.
- Monitor for headache, hypotension, tachycardia, decreased pulse rate, heart block, and decreased respiratory rate.
- Monitor hemoglobin levels.

Patient/Family Education
- Instruct patient not to chew sublingual tablets. Emphasize need to hold chewable tablets in mouth for 1 to 2 min and then chew thoroughly before swallowing, to allow for absorption.
- Advise patient not to stop taking medication suddenly; withdrawal syndrome may occur.
- Instruct patient to notify health care provider immediately or go to nearest hospital emergency department if chest pain persists or worsens after taking prescribed dose.
- Advise patient to notify health care provider if effectiveness of therapy decreases over time; tolerance may develop.
- Instruct patient to report the following symptoms to health care provider: Severe or persistent headache, blurred vision, dry mouth, dizziness, flushing.
- Caution patient to avoid sudden position changes to prevent orthostatic hypotension.
- Instruct patient to avoid intake of alcoholic beverages or alcohol-containing products.

Isosorbide Mononitrate

(EYE-sos-ORE-bide MAH-no-NYE-trate)

Class Antianginal

How Supplied
ISMO Tablets 20 mg ♦ *Imdur* Tablets, extended-release 30 mg, Tablets, extended-release 60 mg, Tablets, extended-release 120 mg ♦ *Monoket* Tablets 10 mg, Tablets 20 mg ♦ *Isotrate ER* Tablets, extended-release 60 mg

Action
PHARMACOLOGY: Relaxation of smooth muscle of venous and arterial vasculature.

PHARMACOKINETICS/DYNAMICS:

Absorption: The T_{max} is 30 min to 1 hr. The absolute bioavailability is approximately 100%.

Distribution: The Vd is 0.6 to 0.7 L/kg. Approximately 5% is protein bound.

Metabolism: Primarily metabolized by the liver. Five inactive metabolites.

Excretion: 96% excreted in the urine and approximately 1% in the feces. The mean plasma $t_{1/2}$ is approximately 5 hr.

Indications Prevention of angina pectoris.

Contraindications Hypersensitivity to nitrates; severe anemia; closed-angle glaucoma; orthostatic hypotension; head trauma or cerebral hemorrhage.

Route/Dosage
ADULTS: PO 20 mg bid, given 7 hr apart. Extended-release tablets are given as 30 (½ of 60 mg tablet) or 60 mg once daily. After several days dosage may be increased to 120 mg (given as two 60 mg tablets) once daily. Rarely, 240 mg may be required.

Interactions
Alcohol: Severe hypotension and cardiovascular collapse may occur.
Aspirin: Increased nitrate concentration and actions.
Calcium channel blockers: Symptomatic orthostatic hypotension.
Dihydroergotamine: Increased systolic BP and decreased antianginal effects may develop.

Lab Test Interferences May cause false report of reduced serum cholesterol with *Zlatkis-Zak* color reaction.

Adverse Reactions
CV: Tachycardia; palpitations; hypotension; syncope; arrhythmias.
CNS: Headache; apprehension; weakness; vertigo; dizziness; agitation; insomnia.
DERM: Cutaneous vasodilation with flushing.
EENT: Blurred vision.
GI: Nausea; vomiting; diarrhea; dyspepsia.
GU: Dysuria; urinary frequency; impotence.
HEMA: Methemoglobinemia; hemolytic anemia.
OTHER: Arthralgia; perspiration; pallor; cold sweat; edema.

Precautions
Pregnancy: Category C.
Lactation: Undetermined.
Special risk patients: Use with caution in patients with acute MI, CHF, glaucoma or angina caused by hypertrophic cardiomyopathy.
Acute angina: Not indicated for treatment of acute anginal episodes.
Orthostatic hypotension: May occur even with small doses; alcohol accentuates this reaction.
Tolerance: Tolerance to vascular and antianginal effects may develop.

Overdosage: Signs and Symptoms
Hypotension, tachycardia, flushing, diaphoresis, headache, vertigo, palpitations, visual disturbances, nausea, vomiting, confusion, dyspnea.

PATIENT CARE CONSIDERATIONS
Administration/Storage
- Administer first dose on awakening and second dose 7 hr later.
- Give on empty stomach with full glass of water.
- Tablets should not be crushed or chewed and

should be swallowed together.
- Store at cool temperature in tightly closed container.

Assessment/Interventions
- Obtain patient history, including drug history and any known allergies.
- Monitor for headache, hypotension, and tachycardia.

Patient/Family Education
- Instruct patient to take medication twice daily, with first dose in morning and second dose 7 hr later.
- Extended-release tablets should be taken in the morning on rising.
- Do not crush or chew tablets.
- Caution patient not to stop taking medication suddenly; withdrawal syndrome may occur.
- Advise patient to notify health care provider if effectiveness of therapy decreases over time; tolerance may develop.
- Instruct patient to report the following symptoms to health care provider: nausea, vomiting, abdominal pain, appetite loss, persistent headache, faintness, apprehension, restlessness, chest pain, flushing, excessive sweating, cold sweat, visual disturbances, fever, involuntary passing of urine and feces.
- Caution patient to avoid sudden position changes to prevent orthostatic hypotension.
- Instruct patient to avoid intake of alcoholic beverages or alcohol-containing products.

Isotretinoin (13-cis-Retinoic Acid)

(EYE-so-TREH-tih-NO-in)

Class Acne

How Supplied
Accutane Capsules 10 mg, Capsules 20 mg, Capsules 40 mg • *Claravis* Capsules 10 mg, Capsules 20 mg, Capsules 40 mg
✣ *Accutane Roche* • *Isotrex*

Action
PHARMACOLOGY: Reduces sebum secretion and sebaceous gland size, inhibits sebaceous gland differentiation, and alters sebum lipid composition.

PHARMACOKINETICS/DYNAMICS: The T_{max} is approximately 3 hr; 6 to 20 hr (metabolites). The mean C_{max} is 256 to 262 ng/mL; 87 to 399 ng/mL (metabolite). Absorption increases with food or milk.
99% is protein bound.
The major metabolite is 4-oxo-isotretinoin.
The $t_{1/2}$ is 10 to 20 hr; 17 to 50 hr (metabolite). 65 to 83% is excreted equally via the urine and feces.

Indications Treatment of severe recalcitrant cystic acne. **Unlabeled use(s):** Treatment of keratinization disorders, cutaneous T-cell lymphoma, leukoplakia; prevention of skin cancer in patients with xeroderma pigmentosum.

Contraindications Hypersensitivity to parabens; pregnancy.

Route/Dosage
ADULTS: **PO** 0.5 to 1 mg/kg/day divided into 2 doses with food for 15 to 20 wk. For severe cases, dose adjustments up to 2 mg/kg/day may be needed.

Interactions
Vitamin A: May increase toxic effects; do not take with isotretinoin.
Tetracycline/Minocycline: Have been associated with pseudotumor cerebri or papilledema in isotretinoin patients.
Carbamazepine: Coadministration has resulted in reduced carbamazepine plasma level.
Drug/Food interactions: When taken with food, the absorption of isotretinoin has increased.

Lab Test Interferences None well documented.

Adverse Reactions
CV: Transient chest pain; vasculitis; palpitation; tachycardia.
CNS: Fatigue; headache; pseudotumor cerebri (eg, benign intracranial hypertension with headache, visual disturbances, and papilledema); dizziness; drowsiness; insomnia; lethargy; malaise; nervousness; paresthesias; seizures; stroke; syncope; weakness; suicidal ideation; suicide attempts; suicide; psychosis; emotional instability; aggression; violent behaviors.
DERM: Cheilitis; skin fragility; dry skin; pruritus; facial skin desquamation dry mucous membranes; nail brittleness; rash; thinning of hair; skin infections; photosensitivity; palmoplantar desquamation; exaggerated healing response manifested by exuberant granulation tissue with crusting; pyogenic granuloma; petechiae; bruising; alopecia; eruptive xanthomas; flushing; hirsutism; hyperpigmentation and hypopigmentation; pyogenic granuloma; sweating; urticaria.
EENT: Conjunctivitis; corneal opacities; cataracts; visual disturbances; dry eyes; contact lens intolerance; decreased night vision; epistaxis; dry nose; impaired hearing; tinnitus.
GI: Dry mouth; nausea; vomiting; abdominal pain; nonspecific GI symptoms; anorexia;

inflammatory bowel disease; esophagitis/esophageal ulceration.
GU: WBC cells in urine; proteinuria; microscopic or gross hematuria; nonspecific urogenital findings; abnormal menses; glomerulonephritis.
HEMA: Anemia; decreased RBC parameters and WBC counts; elevated platelet counts; elevated sedimentation rate.
HEPA: Elevated liver enzymes; hepatitis.
HYPERSEN: Allergic reactions; systemic hypersensitivity.
LABTESTABS: Hypertriglyceridemia; elevated sedimentation rate; decreased red blood cell parameters and white blood cell counts, including severe neutropenia and rare reports of agranulocytosis; elevated platelet counts; decrease in serum HDL levels; elevations of serum cholesterol; increased alkaline phosphatase, AST, ALT, GGTP, and LDH; increased fasting blood sugar; hyperuricemia; thrombocytopenia; elevated CPK levels in patients who undergo vigorous physical activity.
METAB: Increased fasting serum glucose; hyperuricemia; elevated CPK levels after exercise.
MUSC: Arthralgia; bone, joint, and muscle pain and stiffness; calcification of tendons and ligaments; premature epiphyseal closure; arthritis; tendonitis; decreases in bone mineral density.
OPHTH: Photophobia; eyelid inflammation; color vision disorder; keratitis.
RESP: Bronchospasms, with or without a history of asthma; respiratory infections; voice alterations.
OTHER: Flushing; reversibly elevated triglycerides; increased cholesterol level; vasculitis (including Wegener's granulomatosis); lymphadenopathy; edema.

> **WARNING:**
>
> Isotretinoin must not be used by females who are pregnant. Major human fetal abnormalities related to isotretinoin administration in females have been documented. There is an increased risk of spontaneous abortion and premature births.
>
> Documented external abnormalities include the following: skull abnormality, ear abnormalities, eye abnormalities, facial dysmorphia, cleft palate. Documented internal abnormalities include the following: CNS abnormalities, cardiovascular abnormalities, thymus gland abnormality, parathyroid hormone deficiency.
>
> Cases of IQ scores less than 85 with or without obvious CNS abnormalities also have been reported.
>
> Isotretinoin is contraindicated in females of childbearing potential unless the patient meets all of the following conditions: must not be pregnant or breastfeeding, must be capable of complying with mandatory contraceptive measures required for isotretinoin therapy, must be reliable in understanding and carrying out instructions.
>
> *Accutane* must be prescribed under the System to Manage *Accutane*-Related Teratogenicity (SMART). Female patients must have had 2 negative urine or serum pregnancy tests and have committed to using 2 forms of effective contraception simultaneously. Patients must sign a patient information/consent form that contains warnings about the risk of potential birth defects if the fetus is exposed to isotretinoin. The yellow self-adhesive *Accutane* qualification sticker documents that the female patient is qualified and includes the date for qualification, patient gender, cut-off date for filling the prescription, and up to a 30-day supply limit with no refills. Prescribers are to report all cases of pregnancy to Roche at (800) 526-6367.
>
> *Information for pharmacists:* Isotretinoin must only be dispensed as follows: in no more than 30-day supply, only on presentation of an *Accutane* prescription with a yellow self-adhesive *Accutane* qualification sticker, prescription written within the previous 7 days, refills require a new prescription with a yellow self-adhesive *Accutane* qualification sticker, no telephone or computerized prescriptions are permitted. An *Accutane* medication guide must be given to the patient each time isotretinoin is dispensed, as required by law.

Precautions

Pregnancy: Category X. There is an extremely high risk of deformity to the infant if pregnancy occurs while taking this drug in any amount, even for short periods. Potentially, all exposed fetuses can be affected. Presently, there are no accurate means of determining after isotretinoin exposure which fetus has or has not been affected.

Lactation: Undetermined.
Children: Safety and efficacy not established in children under the age of 12 yr. Use with caution in children 12 to 17 yr of age, especially in those with known metabolic or structural bone disease.
Hypersensitivity: Anaphylactic reactions and other allergic reactions have been reported. Cutaneous allergic reactions and serious cases of allergic vasculitis, often with purpura, of the extremities and extracutaneous involvement (including renal) have been reported.
Hepatic function impairment: Clinical hepatitis possibly related to isotretinoin therapy has been reported. Mild to moderate elevations of liver enzymes have been seen.
Photosensitivity: May occur; avoid excessive sunlight and ultraviolet light.
Acne: Transient exacerbation of acne may occur, generally during initial therapy period.
Blood donation: Because of isotretinoin's teratogenic potential, patients receiving the drug should not donate blood for transfusion during treatment and for 1 mo after discontinuing therapy.
Diabetes: Certain patients have experienced problems in the control of their blood sugar. New cases of diabetes have been diagnosed during therapy.
Hearing impairment: Impaired hearing has been reported in patients taking isotretinoin.
Hypertriglyceridemia: Hypertriglyceridemia in excess of 800 mg/dL occurred in approximately 25% of patients; approximately 15% developed a decrease in high density lipoproteins (HDL) and approximately 7% showed an increase in cholesterol levels. Perform blood lipid determinations before isotretinoin is given and then at regular intervals.

PATIENT CARE CONSIDERATIONS
Administration/Storage
- Instruct patient to swallow capsules whole. Do not open or crush capsules.
- Give medication with meals.
- Second course of therapy may be initiated if needed after 2 mo off therapy.
- Store in tightly closed, light-resistant container at room temperature.

Assessment/Interventions
- Obtain patient history, including drug history and any known allergies. Note hypersensitivity to parabens.
- Obtain baseline lipid levels and then monitor q 2 wk for first month and then monitor monthly.

Inflammatory bowel disease: Inflammatory bowel disease, including regional ileitis, has been temporally associated with isotretinoin use.
Musculoskeletal effects: Decreases in lumbar spine and total hip bone mineral density have been observed. Osteoporosis, osteopenia, bone fracture, and delayed healing of bone fractures as well as premature epiphyseal closure have been seen in patients receiving isotretinoin.
Neutropenia/Agranulocytosis: Neutropenia and rare cases of agranulocytosis have been reported. Discontinue if clinically significant.
Pancreatitis: Acute pancreatitis has been reported with elevated or normal serum triglyceride levels. In rare cases, fatal hemorrhagic pancreatitis has been reported.
Pseudotumor cerebri (benign intracranial hypertension): Isotretinoin use has been associated with a number of cases of pseudotumor cerebri, some of which involved concomitant use of tetracyclines. Early signs and symptoms include papilledema, headache, nausea, vomiting, and visual disturbances.
Psychiatric disorders: May cause depression, psychosis, and rarely, suicidal ideation, suicide attempts, and suicide.
Visual impairment: Carefully monitor visual problems. If visual difficulties occur, discontinue the drug and have an ophthalmological examination. Corneal opacities have appeared in patients receiving isotretinoin for acne and more frequently in patients on higher dosages for keratinization disorders. Decreased night vision has occurred during therapy and in some cases persisted after therapy was discontinued.

Overdosage: Signs and Symptoms
Transient headache, vomiting, facial flushing, cheilosis, abdominal pain, dizziness, ataxia.

- Obtain LFTs at 2- to 3-wk intervals for first 6 mo and then every month throughout course of therapy.
- In diabetic patients, monitor glucose levels carefully.
- If increased triglyceride levels occur, discontinue drug immediately.
- Notify health care provider of signs and symptoms of decreased liver function (eg, dark urine, jaundice, pruritus), visual disturbances, nausea, vomiting, and headache.

Patient/Family Education
- Because of teratogenic effects, instruct patient to practice abstinence or use 2 reliable methods of birth control during therapy and for 1 mo before and after therapy.

- Advise patient to be seen by health care provider monthly and have a urine or serum pregnancy test performed each month to confirm negative pregnancy status.
- Instruct patient to notify health care provider immediately if pregnancy is suspected.
- Advise patient to take medication with meals.
- Instruct patient to discontinue any other acne medications (including OTC topical preparations) before starting therapy.
- Advise patient to control weight, decrease dietary fat, and restrict alcohol intake 36 hr before lipid determinations to avoid elevation in serum triglycerides.
- Caution patient against use of vitamin A, even in multivitamins, to avoid additive toxicity.
- Inform patient that contact lens tolerance may decrease.
- Suggest use of lubricant (eg, petroleum jelly) on lips to prevent cheilitis.
- Advise patient not to donate blood for at least 30 days after discontinuing therapy.
- Inform patient that transient exacerbations of acne may be experienced during first few weeks of therapy. Advise patient to continue drug therapy because this may be normal response.
- Caution patient that decreased night vision can occur and onset can be sudden. Advise patient to be cautious when driving or operating any vehicle at night.
- Advise patient to take sips of water frequently, suck on ice chips or sugarless hard candy, or chew sugarless gum if dry mouth occurs.
- Caution patient to avoid exposure to sunlight and to use sunscreen or wear protective clothing to avoid photosensitivity reactions.
- Caution patient that problems could arise in the control of blood sugar.
- Inform patient of availability of Patient Information leaflet, emphasizing the need to carefully review pregnancy warnings and fetal risks.
- Prior to use, have patient complete a consent form included with package insert.
- Instruct patient to immediately notify health care provider if any of the following symptoms occur: depression, visual disturbances, abdominal pain, rectal bleeding, severe diarrhea, difficulty in controlling blood sugar, decreased tolerance to contact lens.
- Inform patient to avoid wax epilation and skin resurfacing procedures (eg, dermabrasion, laser) during therapy and for at least 6 mo thereafter because of possible scarring.

Isoxsuprine Hydrochloride

(eye-SOX-you-preen HIGH-droe-KLOR-ide)

Class Peripheral vasodilator

How Supplied
Vasodilan Tablets 10 mg, Tablets 20 mg ♦
Voxsuprine Tablets 10 mg, Tablets 20 mg

Action
PHARMACOLOGY: Stimulates skeletal beta receptors to produce vasodilation; stimulates cardiac function (increased contractility, heart rate, and cardiac output) and relaxes uterus. At higher doses, inhibits platelet aggregation and decreases blood viscosity.

PHARMACOKINETICS/DYNAMICS:
Absorption: Well absorbed from the GI tract.
Metabolism: Partially conjugated in the blood.
Excretion: The $t_{1/2}$ is approximately 1.25 hr. Primarily excreted in the urine.
Onset: 1 hr (oral); 10 min (IV).
Special Populations:
Neonates – The $t_{1/2}$ is 1.5 to 3 hr (near term) and 6 to 8 hr (for less mature).

Indications Possibly effective for treatment of cerebral vascular insufficiency, peripheral vascular disease caused by arteriosclerosis obliterans, thromboangitis obliterans, Raynaud's disease.

Unlabeled use(s): Treatment of dysmenorrhea, premature labor.

Contraindications Arterial bleeding; use during immediate postpartum period.

Route/Dosage
ADULTS: **PO** 10 to 20 mg tid or qid.

Interactions None well documented.

Lab Test Interferences None well documented.

Adverse Reactions
CV: Hypotension; tachycardia; chest pain.
CNS: Dizziness; weakness.
DERM: Severe rash.
GI: Nausea; vomiting; abdominal distress.

Precautions
Pregnancy: Category C.
Lactation: Undetermined.

PATIENT CARE CONSIDERATIONS
Administration/Storage
- Store at room temperature in tightly closed container.

Assessment/Interventions
- Obtain patient history, including drug history and any known allergies. Note cardiovascular disease.
- Monitor for hypotension, tachycardia, and chest pain.
- If rash appears, withhold drug and notify health care provider.

Patient/Family Education
- Instruct patient to report the following symptoms to health care provider: Fast heartbeat, chest pain, pounding in chest, severe rash, flushing, weakness, nausea, vomiting, stomach pain.
- Caution patient to avoid sudden position changes to prevent orthostatic hypotension.

Isradipine
(iss-RAHD-ih-peen)

Class Calcium channel blocker

How Supplied
DynaCirc Capsules 2.5 mg, Capsules 5 mg ◆ DynaCirc CR Tablets, controlled-release 5 mg, Tablets, controlled-release 10 mg

Action
PHARMACOLOGY: Reduces systemic vascular resistance and BP by inhibiting movement of calcium ions across cell membrane in systemic and coronary vascular smooth muscle and myocardium.

PHARMACOKINETICS/DYNAMICS:

Absorption: The bioavailability is 15% to 24%. The C_{max} is approximately 1 ng/mL/mg (immediate release); 3 to 4 ng/mL (controlled release). The T_{max} is 1.5 hr (immediate release); 7 to 18 hr (controlled release). Increased bioavailability up to 25% with food.

Distribution: 95% is protein bound.

Metabolism: Completely metabolized by ring oxidation and ester cleavage primarily via cytochrome P450 3A4. Metabolites are inactive.

Excretion: The $t_{1/2}$ is approximately 8 hr. 60% to 65% is excreted in the urine, 25% to 30 % in the feces.

Special Populations:
Renal Function Impairment –
Mild (Ccr 30 to 80 mL/min): The AUC increases by 45%.
Severe (Ccr is less than 10 mL/min, hemodialysis): The AUC decreases by 20 to 50%.

Hepatic Function Impairment – The C_{max} increases by 32% and AUC increases by 52%.
Elderly – The AUC and C_{max} increases.

Indications Treatment of hypertension.

Contraindications Standard considerations.

Route/Dosage
ADULTS: PO 2.5 to 10 mg/day in 2 divided doses (max dose 20 mg/day).

Interactions None well documented.

Lab Test Interferences None well documented.

Adverse Reactions
CV: Peripheral edema; flushing; palpitations; angina; tachycardia; hypotension; syncope; CHF; MI; atrial or ventricular fibrillation.
CNS: Dizziness; lightheadedness; headache; fatigue; lethargy; weakness; shakiness; psychiatric disturbances.
DERM: Rash.
GI: Nausea; diarrhea; constipation; abdominal discomfort; cramps; dyspepsia; vomiting.
GU: Urinary frequency; micturition disorders; sexual difficulties.
RESP: Shortness of breath; dyspnea; wheezing.
OTHER: Transient ischemic attack; stroke.

Precautions
Pregnancy: Category C.
Lactation: Undetermined.
Children: Safety and efficacy not established.
CHF: Use with caution in patients with CHF.

Overdosage: Signs and Symptoms
Hypotension, dizziness, slurred speech, nausea, weakness, drowsiness, confusion.

PATIENT CARE CONSIDERATIONS
Administration/Storage
- May administer with or without food.
- Store in tightly closed container at room temperature. Protect from light.

Assessment/Interventions
- Obtain patient history, including drug history and any known allergies. Note cardiovascular disease.
- Monitor BP, cardiac, and respiratory function during therapy.
- Monitor for dizziness, headache, and peripheral edema.
- Assist patient with ambulation if dizziness occurs.

Patient/Family Education
- Explain that dosage will be tapered slowly

before stopping to avoid withdrawal symptoms. Warn patient that sudden discontinuation may cause serious chest pain.
* Tell patient to brush and floss teeth regularly to minimize gum changes (eg, overgrowth of gums).
* Instruct patient to report the following symptoms to health care provider: irregular heart beat, shortness of breath, swelling of hands or feet, pronounced dizziness, constipation, nausea, or hypotension.
* Advise patient that drug may cause dizziness and to use caution while driving or performing other tasks requiring mental alertness.

Itraconazole

(ih-truh-KAHN-uh-zole)

Class Anti-infective/Antifungal

How Supplied
Sporanox Capsules 100 mg, Oral Solution 10 mg/mL, Injection 10 mg/mL

Action
PHARMACOLOGY: Inhibits synthesis of ergosterol, which is a vital component of fungal cell membranes. Also inhibits endogenous respiration, causes accumulation of phospholipids and unsaturated fatty acids within fungal cells, and disrupts chitin synthesis.

PHARMACOKINETICS/DYNAMICS:

Absorption: The mean C_{max} at steady state is approximately 2856 ng/mL (IV) and 2010 ng/mL (oral). The mean C_{max} at steady state (active metabolites) is approximately 1906 ng/mL (IV) and 2614 ng/mL (oral). The mean T_{max} at steady state is approximately 1.08 hr (IV) and approximately 4 hr (oral). The mean T_{max} at steady state (active metabolites) is approximately 8.53 hr (IV) and approximately 6 hr (oral).

Distribution: 99.8% (itraconazole) and 99.5% (hydroxyitraconazole) are protein bound. The Vd is approximately 796 L (IV).

Metabolism: The active metabolite is hydroxyitraconazole. Metabolized predominantly by cytochrome P450 3A4 isoenzyme, resulting in several metabolites.

Excretion: The mean t½ at steady state is approximately 35 hr. Approximately 40% is excreted in the urine as metabolites, and 3 to 18% is excreted in the feces as the parent drug. The Cl is approximately 381 mL/min.

Special Populations:
Renal Function Impairment – If the Ccr is less than 19 mL/min, the Cl decreases 6-fold. Itraconazole injection should not be used with Ccr less than 30 mL/min.
Hepatic Function Impairment – Prolonged $t_{1/2}$. Monitor closely.

Indications
Injection: Treatment of aspergillosis, blastomycosis, febrile neutropenia, and histoplasmosis.
Capsules: Treatment of aspergillosis, blastomycosis, histoplasmosis, and onychomycosis.
Oral solution: Treatment of oropharyngeal or esophageal candidiasis and empiric treatment of febrile neutropenia. **Unlabeled use(s):** Treatment of other fungal infections [eg, superficial mycoses [eg, dermatophytoses]; systemic mycoses [eg, candidiasis, cryptococcus]; and miscellaneous fungal infections [eg, SC mycoses, cutaneous *Leishmaniasis*]).

Contraindications Coadministration with pimozide, quinidine, triazolam, or oral midazolam, HMG-CoA reductase inhibitors metabolized by the P450 3A enzyme system (eg, lovastatin, simvastatin); not for treatment of onychomycosis in pregnant women or women contemplating pregnancy; ventricular dysfunction such as CHF or history of CHF.

Route/Dosage

Blastomycosis, Aspergillosis, Histoplasmosis
ADULTS: **PO** 200 to 400 mg/day. Give doses over 200 mg in 2 divided doses. **IV** 200 mg bid for 4 doses, followed by 200 mg/day. Infuse over 1 hr. Continue **IV** for 14 days followed by **PO** for 3 mo or more and until clinical parameters and laboratory tests indicate active fungal infection has subsided. An inadequate treatment period may lead to recurrence.

Empiric Therapy in Febrile, Neutropenic Patients with Suspected Fungal Infections
ADULTS: **IV** 200 mg bid infused over 60 min for 4 doses, followed by 200 mg qd for up to 14 days; continue **PO** oral solution 200 mg bid until resolution of clinically important neutropenia (safety and efficacy over 28 days not established.)

Esophageal Candidiasis
ADULTS: **PO** 100 mg/day for a minimum of 3 wk. Continue treatment for 2 wk following resolution of symptoms. Doses up to 200 mg/day may be used based on medical judgment of the patient's response. Vigorously swish solution in mouth (10 mL at a time) for several seconds and swallow.

Onychomycosis, Fingernails Only
ADULTS: **PO** 2 treatment pulses separated by a 3-wk period without itraconazole. Each pulse consisting of 200 mg bid for 1 wk.

Onychomycosis, Toenails With or Without Fingernail Involvement
ADULTS: PO 200 mg/day for 12 wk.

Oropharyngeal Candidiasis
ADULTS: **PO, oral solution** 200 mg (20 mL)/day for 1 to 2 wk. Vigorously swish solution in mouth for several seconds and swallow.

Interactions

Alfentanil, carbamazepine, corticosteroids, haloperidol, protease inhibitors, rifamycins (eg, rifampin), sirolimus, tacrolimus, tolterodine, vinca alkaloids, warfarin, zolpidem: Levels may be elevated by itraconazole, increasing the risk of adverse effects.

Alprazolam, midazolam (oral), triazolam: Elevated plasma levels of these drugs; may potentiate and prolong their hypnotic and sedative effects. Sedative effects of parenteral midazolam may be prolonged.

Amphotericin B, oral contraceptives: Efficacy may be reduced by itraconazole.

Antacids, H_2-antagonists, nevirapine, phenobarbital, proton pump inhibitors: Reduced plasma itraconazole levels.

Buspirone, busulfan, docetaxel, dofetilide, haloperidol, itraconazole, methylprednisolone, trimetrexate: May elevate plasma concentrations. Adjust dose as needed.

Calcium blockers (eg, amlodipine, felodipine, nifedipine): Edema has occurred with concomitant dihydropyridine calcium blockers.

Cisapride, dofetilide, pimozide, quinidine: Increased levels may result in life-threatening cardiac dysrhythmias and death. Do not use with itraconazole.

Cyclosporine plus HMG-CoA reductase inhibitors: There are rare reports of rhabdomyolysis in renal transplant patients receiving this drug combination. Increased cyclosporine levels may occur. Monitor cyclosporine levels; reduce cyclosporine dose 50% when using itraconazole doses over 100 mg/day.

Didanosine: May decrease therapeutic effects of itraconazole. Administer itraconazole 2 hr or more before didanosine.

Digoxin: Increased digoxin levels. Monitor frequently.

Hypoglycemic agents: Hypoglycemia may occur. Monitor blood glucose.

Indinavir, ritonavir: Plasma levels of itraconazole may be decreased.

Macrolide antibiotics (eg, erythromycin): Plasma levels of itraconazole may be increased.

Phenytoin: Reduced plasma itraconazole levels; altered phenytoin metabolism.

Sulfonylurea: Hypoglycemia may occur.

Lab Test Interferences None well documented.

Adverse Reactions Incidence and type of reactions vary depending on usage and route of administration. In general, the adverse reactions listed occur in at least 1% of the patients treated.

CV: Hypertension; orthostatic hypotension; vasculitis.

CNS: Headache; dizziness; decreased libido; somnolence; vertigo; anxiety depression; abnormal dreaming.

DERM: Rash; pruritus; increased sweating.

GI: Nausea; vomiting; diarrhea; abdominal pain; anorexia; flatulence; constipation; dyspepsia; gingivitis; ulcerative stomatitis; gastritis; gastroenteritis; increased appetite; general GI disorders.

GU: Impotence; albuminuria; cystitis; abnormal renal function; menstrual disorders.

HEPA: Abnormal liver function; elevated liver enzyme; bilirubinemia; ALT increased; hepatic function abnormal; jaundice; AST increased.

METAB: Hypokalemia; alkaline phosphatase increased; BUN increased; hypomagnesemia.

RESP: Coughing; dyspnea; pneumonia; sinusitis; sputum increased; rhinitis; upper respiratory tract infection; pharyngitis.

OTHER: Edema; fatigue; fever; malaise; myalgia; bursitis; pain; injury; chest pain; back pain; *pneumocystis-carinii* infection; herpes zoster; application site reaction; vein disorder; asthenia; tremor; hypertriglyceridemia.

> **WARNING:**
> Not to be administered for treatment of onychomycosis patients with evidence of ventricular dysfunction (eg, CHF) or history of CHF. Monitor for signs and symptoms of CHF; discontinue if they develop. Coadministration of cisapride, dofetilide, pimozide, or quinidine is contraindicated.

Precautions

Pregnancy: Category C.

Lactation: Excreted in breast milk. Weigh benefits to mother against potential risk to infant.

Children: Safety and efficacy not established. Patients 6 mo to 16 yr have been treated with no serious adverse effects reported; however, the long-term effect in children is unknown.

Elderly: Use with caution because of the greater frequency of decreased hepatic, renal, or cardiac function, and concomitant diseases or other drug therapy.

Renal function impairment: Do not use injection in patients with severe renal dysfunction (Ccr less than 30 mL/min).
Hepatitis: Rare cases of hepatitis have been reported.

HIV-infected patients: Absorption may be decreased in HIV-infected individuals with hypochlorhydria.

PATIENT CARE CONSIDERATIONS

Administration/Storage

- Oral solution and capsules are not interchangeable.
- No dosage adjustment is necessary when switching from IV to oral therapy.
- Dose and duration of therapy are dependent on condition being treated.

Capsules:

- Administer capsules immediately after a full meal to ensure maximum absorption.
- Administer capsules with 8 oz of a cola beverage in HIV-infected patient or patient taking gastric acid suppressive therapy (eg, H_2 receptor antagonist, proton pump inhibitor).
- Administer antacids at least 1 hr before or 2 hr after administration of itraconazole capsules.
- Store capsules at controlled room temperature (59° to 77°F). Protect from light and moisture.

Oral Solution:

- Administer prescribed dose on an empty stomach to ensure maximum absorption.
- If treating oral or esophageal candidiasis, have patient vigorously swish the solution in mouth for several seconds and swallow.
- Measure prescribed dose using dosing cup, spoon, or syringe.
- Store oral solution below 77°F. Protect from freezing.

Injection:

- Do not administer parenteral itraconazole to patient with Ccr less than 30 mL/min.
- For IV infusion only. Not for intradermal, intrathecal, intraperitoneal, SC, IM, or IV bolus administration.
- Use only the components included in the injection kit. Do not substitute. Follow manufacturer's instructions for reconstituting and administering injectable itraconazole using kit components.
- Do not mix with any other diluent than 0.9% sodium chloride injection.
- Inspect solution visually before administration. Do not administer if solution is cloudy, discolored, or contains particulate matter.
- Do not add other medications or additives to injection bag or through same line used for itraconazole.

- Administer prescribed dose through dedicated infusion line over 60 min using filtered infusion set provided. Flush infusion set with 15 to 20 mL 0.9% sodium chloride injection over 30 sec to 15 minutes. Do not use bacteriostatic sodium chloride injection. Discard the entire infusion line after flushing with sodium chloride.
- Store infusion kit below 77°F. Protect from light and freezing. After reconstitution, store diluted itraconazole injection in refrigerator (36° to 46°F) or at controlled room temperature (59° to 77°F) for up to 48 hr if protected from light. Exposure to normal room light is acceptable during administration.

Assessment/Interventions

- Obtain patient history, including drug history and any known allergies. Note renal or hepatic impairment, CHF or history of CHF, allergy to azole antifungal agents, or concurrent use of cisapride, pimozide, dofetilide, quinidine, triazolam, oral midazolam, HMG-CoA reductase inhibitors metabolized by CYP3A4 (eg, lovastatin, simvastatin), other medications metabolized by CYP3A4, or potent CYP3A4 inducers or inhibitors.
- Ensure that necessary fungal cultures have been obtained before beginning therapy.
- Review results of culture and sensitivity testing as available.
- Ensure that women of child bearing potential are not pregnant when treatment for onychomycosis is initiated and that effective contraceptive measures are being used during treatment and for 2 mo following discontinuation of therapy.
- Ensure that renal function and liver enzymes are determined before starting therapy and periodically during prolonged treatment (ie, greater than 1 mo).
- Monitor patient's response to therapy. Inform health care provider if infection does not appear to be improving or is worsening.
- Monitor patient for signs of allergic reaction. Discontinue therapy and immediately notify health care provider if noted. Be prepared to treat appropriately.
- Monitor patient for signs and symptoms of CHF (eg, rapid weight gain, edema, shortness

of breath on exertion). Inform health care provider if noted and be prepared to discontinue therapy.
* Monitor patient for signs and symptoms of hepatic injury (fatigue, right upper quadrant abdominal pain, persistent appetite loss or nausea, vomiting, dark urine, yellowing of skin or eyes). Inform health care provider if noted and be prepared to discontinue therapy.
* Monitor patient for GI, CNS, DERM, RESP, and general body side effects. Report to health care provider if noted and significant.

Patient/Family Education
* Explain name, dose, action, and potential side effects of drug.
* Advise patient to read patient information leaflet before starting therapy and with each refill.
* Review dosing schedule and prescribed length of therapy with patient. Advise patient that treatment may be prolonged (eg, several weeks or months) and to continue medication until advised to stop using by health care provider.

Capsules and Oral Solution:
* Advise patient that capsules should be taken after a full meal to obtain maximum benefit.
* Administer HIV-infected patient or patient receiving gastric acid suppressive therapy (eg, H_2 receptor antagonist, proton pump inhibitor) to take capsules with 8 oz of a cola beverage to obtain maximum benefit.
* Advise patient using antacids to take the antacid at least 1 hr before or 2 hr after taking itraconazole capsules.
* Advise patient using oral solution to measure prescribed dose with dosing cup, spoon, or syringe and to take prescribed dose on an empty stomach to obtain maximum benefit.
* Advise patient using oral solution to treat oral or esophageal candidiasis to vigorously swish the solution in mouth for several seconds and then swallow.
* Advise patient that if a dose is missed to take as soon as remembered. However, if it is nearing the time for the next dose to skip the dose and take the next dose at the regularly scheduled time.
* Remind patient to complete entire course of therapy, even if symptoms of infection have disappeared.
* Advise patient to inform health care provider if infection does not improve or worsens.
* Advise patient to contact health care provider immediately of the following: swelling of feet, ankles, or legs; shortness of breath; skin rash; fatigue; persistent appetite loss; nausea; vomiting; dark urine; pale stool; yellowing of skin or eyes.
* Advise women of childbearing potential being treated for onychomycosis to use effective contraceptive measures during treatment and for 2 mo following discontinuation of therapy.
* Advise women to notify health care provider if pregnant, planning to become pregnant, or breastfeeding.
* Instruct patient not to take any prescription or OTC medications or dietary supplements unless advised by health care provider.
* Advise patient that follow-up examinations and lab tests will be required to monitor therapy and to keep appointments.

Injection:
* Advise patient that medication will be prepared and administered by a health care professional in a health care setting when oral therapy is not feasible but that the patient will be switched to oral therapy when health care provider believes it is appropriate.

Kanamycin Sulfate

(kan-uh-MY-sin SULL-fate)

Class Antibiotic/Aminoglycoside

How Supplied
Kantrex Capsules 500 mg, Injection 500 mg, Injection 1 g, Pediatric Injection 75 mg

Action
PHARMACOLOGY: Inhibits production of bacterial protein, causing cell death.

PHARMACOKINETICS/DYNAMICS:

Absorption: Rapidly absorbed after IM injection. T_{max} is approximately 1 hr. C_{max} is 22 mcg/mL (from the 7.5 mg/kg dose). Poorly absorbed from the normal GI tract (orally).

Distribution: Diffuses rapidly into most body fluids including synovial and peritoneal fluids and bile. Significant levels of drug appear in cord blood and amniotic fluid.

Metabolism: Little if any metabolic transformation occurs.

Excretion: Plasma t½ is 2 hr.
Excreted almost entirely by glomerular filtration and is not reabsorbed by the renal tubules. Renal excretion is extremely rapid. The unabsorbed portion is eliminated unchanged in the feces.

Duration: 48 to 72 hr

Special Populations:
Renal Function Impairment – Patients with renal function impairment or diminished glomerular pressure excrete kanamycin more slowly. May build up excessively high blood levels that lead to increased risk of ototoxic reactions.
Severely burned patients – In severely burned patients, t½ may significantly decrease. As result serum concentrations may be lower.

Indications
Parenteral: Short-term treatment of serious infections caused by susceptible strains of microorganisms, especially gram-negative bacteria.
Oral: Short-term adjunctive therapy for suppression of intestinal bacteria; treatment of hepatic coma.

Contraindications
Hypersensitivity to aminoglycosides; intestinal obstruction (oral). Generally not indicated for long-term therapy (more than 14 days) because of ototoxicity and nephrotoxicity.

Route/Dosage
Infection
ADULTS AND CHILDREN: **IM/IV** 15 mg/kg/day in 2 to 4 divided doses. Do not exceed 1.5 g/day.

Suppression of Intestinal Bacteria
ADULTS: **PO** 1 g qh for 4 hr, then 1 g q 6 hr for 36 to 72 hr.

Tuberculosis
ADULTS AND CHILDREN: **IM/IV** 15 to 30 mg/kg/day (max, 1 g/day).

Hepatic Coma
ADULTS: **PO** 8 to 12 g/day in divided doses.

Interactions
Beta-lactam antibiotics (eg, cephalosporins, penicillins): Do not mix in IV solutions.
Digoxin, methotrexate, vitamin A, vitamin K: Oral kanamycin may decrease absorption of these drugs.
Drugs with nephrotoxic potential (eg, amphotericin, cephalosporins, enflurane, methoxyflurane, vancomycin): Increased risk of nephrotoxicity.
Loop diuretics: Increased auditory toxicity.
Neuromuscular blocking agents: Enhanced effects of these agents.
Polypeptide antibiotics: Increased risk of respiratory paralysis and renal dysfunction.

Lab Test Interferences
None well documented.

Adverse Reactions
CNS: Neuromuscular blockade.
EENT: Hearing loss; deafness; loss of balance.
GI: Malabsorption syndrome (eg, increased fecal fat, decreased serum carotene, fall in xylose absorption); nausea; vomiting; diarrhea.
GU: Oliguria; proteinuria; elevated serum creatinine and BUN; granular casts; red and white cells in urine; decreased Ccr.
RESP: Apnea.
OTHER: Pain and irritation at injection site; acute muscular paralysis; hypomagnesemia.

> **WARNING:**
>
> *Neurotoxicity:* Manifests as both auditory and vestibular ototoxicity, and primarily occurs in patients with preexisting renal damage with prolonged therapy. Partial or total irreversible deafness may continue to develop after drug is stopped. Other features of neurotoxicity include paresthesia, twitching, and seizures.
>
> *Nephrotoxicity:* Usually reversible.
>
> Teratogenic in pregnancy.
>
> Closely monitor renal and eighth nerve function in patients with suspected renal dysfunction. Monitor peak and trough concentrations. Dosage adjustments are required in renal impairment.

Precautions
Pregnancy: Category D.
Lactation: Excreted in breast milk.
Children: Use cautiously in premature infants and newborns because of renal immaturity.
Neuromuscular blockade: Use with caution in patients with neuromuscular disorders, those receiving anesthesia or muscle relaxants, hypomagnesemia, hypocalcemia, hypokalemia, or in newborns whose mothers received magnesium sulfate.
Oral absorption: Increased absorption (and potential for toxicity) when intestinal mucosa is ulcerated or denuded.

Overdosage: Signs and Symptoms
Nephrotoxicity, auditory toxicity, vestibular toxicity, neuromuscular blockade, respiratory paralysis.

PATIENT CARE CONSIDERATIONS
Administration/Storage
- Do not mix with other antibacterial agents; administer separately.
- For IV administration, dilute each 500 mg with 100 to 200 mL or more of 0.9% Sodium Chloride or D5W. Give slowly over 30 to 60 min.
- Give IM injection deeply into upper outer quadrant of gluteal muscle.
- Store at room temperature. Darkening of vials during shelf life does not indicate loss of potency.

Assessment/Interventions
- Obtain patient history, including drug history and any known allergies. Note hypersensitivity to aminoglycosides.
- Ensure that culture and sensitivity, renal function tests, and serum electrolytes have been performed before beginning therapy and repeat periodically.
- Assess for superinfection (bacterial or fungal overgrowth).
- Assess for allergic-type reactions including anaphylactic symptoms and life-threatening or less severe asthmatic episodes in susceptible people (more frequent in asthmatic or atopic nonasthmatic persons).
- Keep patient well hydrated (especially important in elderly).
- Assess auditory function regularly.
- Monitor drug serum concentrations periodically.
- Monitor I&O.

Patient/Family Education
- Advise patient that drug may cause nausea, vomiting, or diarrhea.
- Instruct patient to drink plenty of fluids while taking medication.
- Emphasize importance of follow-up visits and serial audiograms, because ototoxicity may be asymptomatic.
- Instruct patient to report the following symptoms to health care provider: ringing in ears, hearing impairment, rash, difficulty urinating, or dizziness.

Kaolin/Pectin
(KAY-oh-lin/PECK-tin)
Class Antidiarrheal combination

How Supplied
Kao-Spen Suspension 5.2 g kaolin, 2 g pectin/30 mL ♦ *Kapectolin* Suspension 90 g kaolin, 2 g pectin/30 mL

Action
PHARMACOLOGY: Absorbs fluid, binds and removes digestive tract irritants.

PHARMACOKINETICS/DYNAMICS:
Absorption: Not absorbed.
Excretion: Up to 90% of pectin is decomposed in the GI tract.

Indications Symptomatic treatment of diarrhea.

Contraindications Use in infants and children younger than 3 yr of age without health care provider guidance; use for longer than 2 days or in presence of high fever; intestinal obstruction; colitis.

Route/Dosage
All doses are given after each loose bowel movement.
ADULTS: **PO** 60 to 120 mL (regular strength) or 45 to 90 mL (concentrate) after each loose bowel movement.
CHILDREN 6 TO 12 YR: **PO** 3 to 60 mL (regular strength) or 30 mL (concentrate) per dose.
CHILDREN 3 TO 5 YR: **PO** 15 to 30 mL (regular strength) or 15 mL (concentrate) per dose.

Interactions
Clindamycin, digoxin, lincomycin penicillamine (oral): Decreased absorption may occur; separate administration times by 2 to 4 hr.

Lab Test Interferences None well documented.

Adverse Reactions
GI: Constipation; fecal impaction (especially infants and elderly).

Precautions
Pregnancy: Category B.
Lactation: Kaolin and pectin are not absorbed

from GI tract; transfer into breast milk is not expected.

PATIENT CARE CONSIDERATIONS

Administration/Storage
- Administer after each loose bowel movement.
- Shake suspension well before pouring.

Assessment/Interventions
- Obtain patient history, including drug history and any known allergies. Note usual bowel patterns and onset of recent condition.
- Conduct complete abdominal assessment, including palpitation and auscultation.
- Assess for signs and symptoms of intestinal obstruction, fecal impaction, or dehydration; notify health care provider if present.
- Assess vital signs, especially temperature. Notify health care provider if increased.

Patient/Family Education
- Instruct patient to take medication after each diarrheal or loose stool.
- Advise patient to notify health care provider if diarrhea persists for longer than 48 hr or if fever develops.
- Caution patient not to exceed recommended dosage.

Overdosage: Signs and Symptoms
Constipation.

Ketamine Hydrochloride

(KEET-uh-MEEN HIGH-droe-KLOR-ide)

Class General anesthetic

How Supplied
Ketalar Injection 10 mg/mL, Injection 50 mg/mL, Injection 100 mg/mL

Action
PHARMACOLOGY: Produces rapid-acting anesthetic state with profound analgesia, normal pharyngeal-laryngeal reflexes, normal or slightly enhanced skeletal muscle tone, cardiovascular and respiratory stimulation, and, occasionally, transient and minimal respiratory depression.

PHARMACOKINETICS/DYNAMICS:
Absorption: Ketamine is rapidly absorbed. Mean C_{max} is 0.75 mcg/mL. T_{max} is 1 hr.
Distribution: Distribution t½ is approximately 10 to 15 min. Ketamine is rapidly distributed into body tissues, with high concentrations in body fat, liver, lungs, and brain. Protein binding with this drug is not significant.
Metabolism: Undergoes N-demethylation and hydroxylation of cyclohexone ring. The N-demethylated metabolite is less than ⅙ as potent and the demethyl cyclohexone derivative is less than ⅒ as potent as the drug.
Excretion: Elimination t½ is 2.5 hr. Approximately 91% is excreted in urine and 3% in feces.

Indications
Diagnostic and surgical procedures that do not require skeletal muscle relaxation; induction of anesthesia; supplementation of low-potency agents, such as nitrous oxide.

Contraindications
Patients in whom significant BP elevation would be a serious hazard; hypersensitivity to the drug.

Route/Dosage
ADULTS AND CHILDREN: INDUCTION OF ANESTHESIA: **IV** Initial: 1 to 4.5 mg/kg via slow infusion (over 60 sec); usual dose for 5 to 10 min anesthesia: 2 mg/kg. Maintenance: One-half to full induction dose, repeated as needed. Alternatively IV 0.1 to 0.5 mg/min infusion, augmented with diazepam IV 2 to 5 mg.
IM Initial: 6.5 to 13 mg/kg. Maintenance: One-half to full induction dose, repeated as needed.

Interactions
Halothane: Decreased cardiac output, BP, and pulse.
Tubocurarine and other nondepolarizing muscle relaxants: Increased neuromuscular effects, resulting in prolonged respiratory depression.
INCOMPATIBILITIES: Ketamine is physically incompatible with diazepam and barbiturates.

Lab Test Interferences
None well documented.

Adverse Reactions
CV: Hypertension; tachycardia; hypotension; bradycardia; arrhythmia.
CNS: Increased ICP. Emergence reaction: Vivid imagery; hallucinations; delirium; confusion; excitement; irrational behavior.
DERM: Transient erythema; morbilliform rash.
EENT: Diplopia; nystagmus; increased intraocular pressure.
GI: Anorexia; nausea; vomiting; hypersalivation.
RESP: Respiratory stimulation; severe respiratory depression; apnea after rapid injection; laryngospasm; other airway obstruction.

Precautions
Pregnancy: Category B.
Lactation: Undetermined.

Children: Safety and efficacy in children less than 16 yr have not been established.
Alcohol: Use with caution in chronic alcoholics and acutely alcohol intoxicated patients.
Cerebrospinal fluid pressure: Cerebrospinal fluid pressure increase has been reported following administration.
Hypertension or cardiac decompensation: In patients with these conditions, monitor function continuously during procedure.
Management: To terminate a severe emergence reaction, a small hypnotic dose of a short-acting or ultrashort-acting barbiturate may be required.
Preoperative preparation: Give atropine, scopolamine, or another drying agent at an appropriate interval prior to induction.

PATIENT CARE CONSIDERATIONS
Administration/Storage
- Premedicate patient with anticholinergic agent before giving anesthetic to prevent salivation.
- Administer slowly over 60 sec to prevent respiratory depression, unless otherwise indicated.

Assessment/Interventions
- Obtain patient history, including drug history and any known allergies. Note history of psychiatric disorders (schizophrenia or acute psychoses).
- Assess vital signs, especially BP, before administration.
- Place patient in quiet room with minimal stimulation to prevent recovery symptoms.

Respiratory effects: May occur with overdosage or too rapid a rate of administration.
Respiratory surgery/diagnostic procedures: Do not use in surgery or diagnostic procedures of the pharynx, larynx, or bronchial tree. Do not administer ketamine alone because pharyngeal and laryngeal reflexes are usually active. Muscle relaxants, with proper attention to respiration, may be required.
Visceral pain: In surgical procedures involving visceral pain pathways, supplement with an agent that obtunds visceral pain.

Overdosage: Signs and Symptoms
Respiratory depression.

- Observe patient for signs of delirium and hallucinations during recovery period.
- Check patient's airway regularly to prevent aspiration caused by hypersalivation.
- If respiratory, neurologic, or cardiovascular changes (eg, hypertension, tachycardia, hypotension, bradycardia, arrhythmia) occur, notify health care provider. Be prepared to support patient physically.

Patient/Family Education
- Advise patient that neurologic effects may persist for 24 hr after anesthesia. Advise patient to use caution during this period while driving or performing other tasks requiring mental alertness.

Ketoconazole
(KEY-toe-KOE-nuh-zole)
Class Anti-infective/Antifungal

How Supplied
Nizoral Tablets 200 mg, Cream 2% in an aqueous vehicle, Shampoo 2% in an aqueous suspension

✤ *Apo-Ketoconazole* ◆ *Novo-Ketoconazole*

Action
PHARMACOLOGY: Impairs synthesis of ergosterol, allowing increased permeability in fungal cell membrane and leakage of cellular components.

PHARMACOKINETICS/DYNAMICS:
Absorption: C_{max} is approximately equal to 3.5 mcg/mL (with a 200 mg dose taken with a meal). T_{max} is 1 to 2 hr. Requires acidity for dissolution and absorption. Absorbed in the GI.

Distribution: Approximately 99% protein bound (in vitro), mainly to the albumin fraction. Only a negligible proportion reaches the cerebrospinal fluid.

Metabolism: Major metabolic pathways are oxidation and degradation of the imidazole and piperazine, oxidative O-dealkylation, and aromatic hydroxylation. It is converted into several inactive metabolites.

Excretion: Approximately 13% of dose is excreted in urine; 2% to 4% is unchanged drug. The major route of excretion is through the bile into the intestinal tract. Plasma elimination is biphasic with $t_{½}$ of 2 hr during the first 10 hr and $t_{½}$ of 8 hr after 10 hr.

Indications Treatment of susceptible systemic and cutaneous fungal infections.
Topical: Seborrheic dermatitis; tinea corporis; tinea cruris; tinea pedis; tinea versicolor.

Contraindications Fungal meningitis.

Route/Dosage
ADULTS: PO 200 to 400 mg qd.
CHILDREN OLDER THAN 2 YR: PO 3.3 to 6.6 mg/kg/day. Treatment may last from 1 wk to 6 mo, depending on infection.
ADULTS: **Topical** Apply to affected and immediate surrounding area qd for 2 to 4 wk.

Interactions

Antacids: Increased gastric pH may inhibit ketoconazole absorption; separate administration by 2 hr or more.

Benzodiazepines (eg, midazolam): Plasma levels of benzodiazepines may be increased and prolonged.

Corticosteroids: Increased bioavailability and decreased clearance of corticosteroid.

Cyclosporine: Increased cyclosporine concentrations.

Didanosine, histamine H_2-receptor antagonists (eg, cimetidine), proton pump inhibitors (eg, omeprazole): May decrease ketoconazole absorption.

Dofetilide: Elevated plasma levels of dofetilide may increase the risk of life-threatening cardiac arrhythmia.

Nisoldipine, protease inhibitors (eg, indinavir), tacrolimus, tolterodine: Plasma levels may be elevated by ketoconazole, increasing the risk of side effects.

Rifampin: Decreased serum levels of either drug; avoid concomitant use.

Theophylline: Decreased theophylline serum concentrations.

Warfarin: Increased anticoagulant effect.

Lab Test Interferences None well documented.

PATIENT CARE CONSIDERATIONS

Administration/Storage

- Give oral drug with food to minimize GI upset. Administer 2 hr before antacid is given.
- Tablets can be crushed and mixed with small amount of food or fluid.
- In achlorhydria, dissolve tablet in 4 mL of 0.2 Normal Hydrochloride. Have patient use glass or plastic straw to avoid contact with teeth. Follow with glass of water.
- Apply topical medication once daily to cover affected and immediately surrounding area. Avoid contact with eyes.
- Store at room temperature in tightly closed container. Protect from light.

Assessment/Interventions

- Obtain patient history, including drug history, and any known allergies. Note hepatic impairment and sensitivity to antifungal agents.
- Ensure that LFTs have been obtained before beginning therapy, and monitor regularly during treatment.
- Assess for jaundice, anorexia, and hepatotoxicity. Notify health care provider immediately if these symptoms occur.
- Notify health care provider if severe irritation, itching, or stinging occurs after topical application.

Adverse Reactions

CNS: Headache; dizziness; somnolence.
DERM: Pruritus; urticaria; severe irritation, stinging, and itching (topical).
GI: Nausea; vomiting; abdominal pain.
GU: Oligospermia (with high doses); impotence; gynecomastia.
HEPA: Hepatitis.

> **WARNING:**
> Hepatotoxicity has included fatalities; use caution with other hepatotoxic drugs.

Precautions

Pregnancy: Category C.
Lactation: Undetermined.
Children: Safety and efficacy in children younger than 2 yr not established (PO). Safety and efficacy not established (topical).
Anaphylaxis: Has occurred after the first dose.
CNS infections: Drug penetrates CSF poorly. Although high doses have sometimes been used in CNS fungal infections, this is not the indicated use. Gastric acidity. Ketoconazole requires acid environment for dissolution and absorption.
Hormone levels: May lower serum testosterone or suppress adrenal corticosteroid secretion.

Patient/Family Education

- Instruct patient that if a dose is missed, take it as soon as possible. If several hours have passed or if close to the time of next dose, do not double up. Notify health care provider if more than 1 dose is missed.
- Advise patient not to take medication with antacids. If antacids are required, take ketoconazole 2 hr before antacid.
- Emphasize importance of completing full course of therapy, even if signs and symptoms resolve. Advise patient that maintenance therapy may be required for chronic infections.
- Instruct patient to notify health care provider if severe irritation, itching, or stinging occurs after application.
- Instruct patient to report the following symptoms to the health care provider: fatigue, loss of appetite, nausea, vomiting, yellowing of skin, dark urine, pale stools, abdominal pain, fever, diarrhea.
- Advise patient that drug may cause drowsiness and to use caution while driving or performing other tasks requiring mental alertness.
- Instruct patient not to take OTC medications, including antihistamine, without consulting health care provider.

Ketoprofen

(KEY-toe-PRO-fen)

Class Analgesic/NSAID

How Supplied

Orudis Capsules 25 mg, Capsules 50 mg, Capsules 75 mg ♦ Orudis KT Tablets 12.5 mg ♦ Oruvail Capsules, extended-release 100 mg, Capsules, extended-release 150 mg, Capsules, extended-release 200 mg

❖ APO-Keto ♦ APO-Keto-E ♦ APO-Keto SR ♦ Novo-Keto ♦ Novo-Keto-EC ♦ Nu-Ketoprofen ♦ Nu-Ketoprofen-SR ♦ Orudis SR ♦ Rhodis ♦ Rhodis-EC ♦ Rhodis SR ♦ Rhovail

Action

PHARMACOLOGY: Decreases inflammation, pain, and fever, probably through inhibition of cyclooxygenase activity and prostaglandin synthesis.

PHARMACOKINETICS/DYNAMICS:

Absorption: Immediate form is released in the stomach, T_{max} is 0.5 to 2 hr. Sustained form is released in the small intestine, T_{max} is 6 to 7 hr. Bioavailability is approximately 90%. Food does not change AUC, but the rate of absorption for either form is slowed.

Distribution: More than 99% protein bound, mainly to albumin. V_d is 0.1 L/kg.

Metabolism: Metabolic pathway is glucuronide conjugation. The metabolite is acylglucuronide which can be converted back to the parent drug. There are no known active metabolites.

Excretion: IV t½ is approximately 2.05 hr. Oral immediate release t½ is 2 to 4 hr. Sustained release t½ is approximately 5.4 hr. Cl is approximately 0.08 L/kg/hr.

Onset: Is within 30 min.

Duration: Persisted for up to 6 hr.

Special Populations:

Elderly – Plasma and renal clearance are reduced and the unbound fraction increases.

Hypoalbuminemia and renal function impairment – Patients with these conditions may be at greater risk of adverse effects due to increased fractions of free drug. It is recommended to give these patients lower doses of the drug and monitor them closely.

Indications Treatment of rheumatoid arthritis, osteoarthritis, mild to moderate pain, primary dysmenorrhea.

Sustained-release form only: Treatment of rheumatoid arthritis and osteoarthritis.

OTC use: Temporary relief of minor aches and pains associated with common cold, headache, toothache, muscular aches, backache, minor arthritis pain, menstrual cramps, and reduction of fever. **Unlabeled use(s):** Treatment of juvenile rheumatoid arthritis, sunburn, migraine prophylaxis.

Contraindications Patients in whom aspirin, iodides, or any NSAID have caused allergic-type reactions.

Route/Dosage

Rheumatoid or Osteoarthritis

ADULTS: **PO** 75 mg tid or 50 mg qid; do not exceed 300 mg/day. *Maintenance dose:* Reduce initial dosage to 75 to 150 mg/day in elderly or disabled patients or patients with renal impairment. *Sustained-release capsule:* 200 mg once daily can be used in patients already stabilized on that dose.

Mild to Moderate Pain, Primary Dysmenorrhea

ADULTS: **PO** 25 to 50 mg q 5 to 8 hr prn; do not exceed 300 mg/day.

Mild-To-Severe Renal Function Impairment

PO Maximum recommended total daily dose is 150 mg. In patients with a more severe renal impairment (GFR less than 25 mL/min or end-stage renal impairment), the max total daily dose should not exceed 100 mg.

Hepatic Function Impairment

PO For patients with impaired liver function and serum albumin concentration less than 3.5 g/dL, the max initial total daily dose should be 100 mg.

OTC Use

ADULTS: **PO** 12.5 mg with a full glass of liquid q 4 to 6 hr. If pain or fever persists after 1 hr, follow with 12.5 mg. Do not exceed 25 mg in a 4- to 6-hr period or 75 mg in a 24-hr period. Use the smallest effective dose.

CHILDREN: **PO** Do not give to those younger than 16 yr unless directed by a health care provider.

Interactions

Anticoagulants: Increased risk of gastric erosion and bleeding.

Aspirin: Additive GI toxicity.

Cyclosporine: Nephrotoxicity of both agents may be increased.

Lithium: Serum lithium levels may be increased.

Methotrexate: Increased methotrexate levels.

Lab Test Interferences May prolong bleeding time.

Adverse Reactions

CV: Peripheral edema; fluid retention; CHF.
CNS: Headache; dizziness; lightheadedness; drowsiness; vertigo.
DERM: Rash; pruritus.
EENT: Visual disturbances; stomatitis.
GI: Peptic ulcer; GI bleeding; dyspepsia; nausea; diarrhea; constipation; abdominal pain; flatulence; anorexia; vomiting.

GU: Menorrhagia.
RESP: Bronchospasm; laryngeal edema; rhinitis; dyspnea.

Precautions
Pregnancy: Category B.
Lactation: Excreted in breast milk.
Children: Safety and efficacy not established.
Elderly: Increased rate of adverse reactions.
Hypersensitivity: Hypersensitivity may occur; use caution in aspirin-sensitive individuals because of possible cross-sensitivity.
Renal function impairment: Lower doses may be necessary.

Hepatic function impairment: Avoid sustained-release product.
GI: Bleeding, ulceration or perforation can occur at any time, with or without warning symptoms.
GU: Acute renal insufficiency, interstitial nephritis, hyperkalemia, hyponatremia and renal papillary necrosis may occur.

Overdosage: Signs and Symptoms
Drowsiness, dizziness, confusion, disorientation, lethargy, numbness, vomiting, gastric irritation, nausea, abdominal pain, headache, tinnitus, convulsions, acute renal failure.

PATIENT CARE CONSIDERATIONS
Administration/Storage
- Do not crush capsules.
- Administer with food, milk, or antacids to minimize GI upset.
- Store at room temperature in tightly closed, light-resistant container.

Assessment/Interventions
- Obtain patient history, including drug history and any known allergies. Note renal or hepatic impairment or sensitivity to NSAIDs.
- Do not administer to patients in whom aspirin, iodides, or other NSAIDs have induced symptoms of asthma, rhinitis, urticaria, nasal polyps, angioedema, bronchospasm, and other symptoms of allergic or anaphylactoid reactions.
- Assess carefully for hypersensitivity (eg, fever, rash, abdominal pain, headache, nausea, vomiting, signs of liver damage) and for signs of infection (NSAIDs may mask the usual signs of infection).
- Monitor patients on long-term therapy for signs and symptoms of ulceration and bleeding of upper and lower GI tract.
- Monitor renal and hepatic function tests.
- If skin rash, diarrhea, weight gain, edema, black stools, constipation, persistent headache, blurred vision, dizziness, nervousness, ringing in the ears, taste changes, or changes in vision occur or are reported, discontinue use and notify health care provider.

Patient/Family Education
- Advise patient to take medication with food, milk, or antacids. Capsule should be swallowed whole, not chewed or crushed.
- Warn patient not to take aspirin or other NSAIDs.
- Caution patient to report changes in stool (eg, color, consistency, frequency), fluid retention and shortness of breath.
- Instruct patient to report the following symptoms to health care provider: skin rash, itching, visual disturbances, weight gain, edema, black stools, or persistent headache.
- Advise patient that drug may cause drowsiness and to use caution while driving or performing other tasks requiring mental alertness.
- Caution patient to avoid exposure to sunlight and other sources of ultraviolet light and to use sunscreen or wear protective clothing to avoid photosensitivity reaction.
- Instruct patient not to ingest alcohol or take *otc* medications without notifying health care provider.

Ketorolac Tromethamine
(KEY-TOR-oh-lak tro-METH-uh-meen)
Class Analgesic/NSAID

How Supplied
Acular Solution 0.5% ♦ *Acular LS* Solution 0.4% ♦ *Toradol* Tablets 10 mg, Injection 15 mg/mL, Injection 30 mg/mL
✤ *Apo-Ketorolac* ♦ *Apo-Ketorolac Injection* ♦ *Novo-Ketorolac* ♦ *Toradol IM*

Action
PHARMACOLOGY: Decreases inflammation, pain, and fever, probably through inhibition of cyclo-oxygenase activity and prostaglandin synthesis.

PHARMACOKINETICS/DYNAMICS:
Absorption: Bioavailability is 100%. T_{max} is approximately 44 min for oral 10 mg single dose, 33 min for IM, and 1.1 min for IV (15 mg). C_{max} is approximately 0.87 mcg/mL for oral single dose, 1.14 mcg/mL for IM, and 2.47 mcg/mL for IV.

Distribution: 99% protein bound. Nevertheless, even plasma concentrations as high as 10 mcg/mL will only occupy approximately 5% of the albumin binding sites. A decrease in serum albumin will lead to an increase in free drug concentrations. V_d is approximately 13 L.

Metabolism: Largely metabolized in the liver via hydroxylation and conjugation. A racemic mixture, with the S-form having analgesic activity.

Excretion: S-enantiomer is cleared 2 times faster than R-enantiomer. The t½ of S-enantiomer is approximately 2.5 hr and the t½ of R-enantiomer is approximately 5 hr. Some unchanged drug and 91% of metabolites excreted in the urine; 6% excreted in feces.

Onset: 30 min for injection.

Peak: 2 to 3 hr for injection.

Special Populations:
Renal Function Impairment – Ketorolac is contraindicated in patients with advanced renal impairment and in patients at risk for renal failure because of volume depletion.
Elderly – Adjust dosage for patients 65 yr and older.
Patients weighing less than 50 kg – Adjust dosage.
Active peptic ulcer disease – Ketorolac is contraindicated.

Indications
Oral and IM forms: Short-term management of moderately severe, acute pain.
Ophthalmic form: Relief of ocular itching caused by seasonal allergic conjunctivitis; treatment of postoperative inflammation in patients who have undergone cataract extraction.

Contraindications Patients in whom aspirin, iodides, or any NSAID have caused allergic-type reactions; active peptic ulcer disease, recent GI bleeding or perforation; advanced renal impairment and in patients at risk for renal failure because of volume depletion; suspected or confirmed cerebrovascular bleeding; hemorrhagic diathesis, incomplete hemostasis, and those at high risk of bleeding; as prophylactic analgesia before any major surgery and intraoperatively when hemostasis is critical; for intrathecal or epidural administration because of its alcohol content; in labor and delivery; in lactation; in concomitant use with aspirin or other NSAIDs; concomitant use with probenecid.
Ophthalmic use: Soft contact lens use.

Route/Dosage
Multiple Dose
ADULTS: **IM** Younger than 65 yr: 30 mg q 6 hr. Do not exceed 120 mg/day; older than 65 yr, renal impairment, or weight under 50 kg (110 lbs): 15 mg q 6 hr. Do not exceed 60 mg/day.

Single Dose
ADULTS: **IM** Younger than 65 yr: 60 mg; older than 65 yr, renal impairment, or weight under 50 kg (110 lbs): 30 mg. **IV** younger than 65 yr: 30 mg; older than 65 yr, renal impairment, or weight under 50 kg (110 lbs): 15 mg.
CHILDREN: **IM** 1 mg/kg up to 30 mg max. **IV** 0.5 mg/kg up to 15 mg max.

Transition from IV/IM to Oral
ADULTS: Younger than 65 yr: 20 mg as a first oral dose for patients who received 60 mg IM single dose, 30 mg IV single dose, or 30 mg multiple dose IV/IM, followed by 10 mg q 4 to 6 hr, not to exceed 40 mg/24 hr. Older than 65 years old, renal impairment, or weight under 50 kg (110 lbs): 10 mg as a first oral dose for patients who received a 30 mg IM single dose, 15 mg IV single dose, or 15 mg multiple dose IV/IM, followed by 10 mg q 4 to 6 hr, not to exceed 40 mg/24 hr.

Ophthalmic
1 gtt (0.25 mg) qid. For treatment of postoperative inflammation after cataract surgery, continue through first 2 wk of postoperative period.

Interactions
Anticoagulants: May increase risk of gastric erosion and bleeding.
Cyclosporine: Nephrotoxicity of both agents may be increased.
Lithium: Serum lithium levels may be increased.
Methotrexate: May increase methotrexate levels.
Salicylates: May cause additive GI toxicity.

Lab Test Interferences Drug may prolong bleeding time.

Adverse Reactions
CV: Edema (4%); hypertension (greater than 1%).
CNS: Headache (17%); dizziness (7%); drowsiness (6%); sweating (greater than 1%).
DERM: Pruritus, rash (greater than 1%).
EENT: Stomatitis (greater than 1%); Ophthalmic use: burning/stinging (40%); corneal edema, iritis, ocular inflammation/irritation, superficial keratitis, superficial ocular infections (1% to 10%); corneal erosion, corneal perforation, corneal thinning, epithelial breakdown (postmarketing).
GI: GI pain (13%); dyspepsia, nausea (12%); diarrhea (7%); constipation flatulence, GI fullness, vomiting (greater than 1%).
HEPA: Abnormal liver function test results.
RESP: Bronchospasm.
OTHER: Purpura, injection site pain (greater than 1%); muscle cramps; aseptic meningitis (postmarketing).

> **WARNING:**
> *Tablets, injection:* Limit therapy to 5 days.
> *GI effects:* Peptic ulcers, GI bleeding, and/or perforation. Contraindicated in patients with active or history of these states.
> *Renal effects:* Contraindicated in patients with advanced renal impairment or at risk of renal failure caused by volume depletion.
> Bleeding risk caused by platelet inhibition. Contraindicated as preoperative analgesic or as intra-operative analgesic when hemostasis is critical or in patients at high risk of bleeding. Intrathecal/epidural administration is contraindicated because of alcohol content.

Precautions

Pregnancy: Category C.
Lactation: Excreted in breast milk. Contraindicated.
Children:
IM/IV – Safety and efficacy not established in patients younger than 2 yr.
Ophthalmic – Safety and efficacy not established in patients younger than 3 yr.
Elderly: Increased risk of adverse reactions.
Hypersensitivity: Hypersensitivity may occur; use drug with caution in aspirin-sensitive individuals because of possible cross-sensitivity.
Renal function impairment: Assess function before and during therapy, because NSAID metabolites are eliminated renally. Dosage adjustments may be necessary.
Hepatic function impairment: May lead to liver enzyme elevations.
Photosensitivity: Drug can cause photosensitization.
Chronic use: IM drug is not intended for long-term use. Limit to short-term therapy (not longer than 5 days). Oral drug is intended for limited duration of use.
Ophthalmic use: Use of topical NSAIDs may result in keratitis. In some susceptible patients, continued use may result in epithelial breakdown, corneal thinning, corneal erosion, corneal ulceration, or corneal perforation. These events may be sight threatening. Patients with complicated ocular surgeries, corneal denervation, corneal epithelial defects, diabetes mellitus, ocular surface diseases, rheumatoid arthritis, or repeat ocular surgeries within a short period of time may be at increased risk for corneal adverse events. Use with caution in patients with known bleeding tendencies or who are receiving medications that may prolong bleeding time.
Renal effects: Acute renal insufficiency, interstitial nephritis, hyperkalemia, hyponatremia, and renal papillary necrosis may occur.

Overdosage: Signs and Symptoms

Drowsiness, dizziness, mental confusion, disorientation, lethargy, paresthesia, numbness, vomiting, gastric irritation, nausea, abdominal pain, intense headache, tinnitus, sweating, convulsions, blurred vision, elevations in serum creatinine and BUN.

PATIENT CARE CONSIDERATIONS

Administration/Storage

- The combined duration of ketorolac IV/IM and oral is not to exceed 5 days. Oral use is only indicated as continuation therapy to IV/IM.
- Do not mix IV/IM ketorolac in a small volume (eg, in a syringe) with morphine sulfate, meperidine hydrochloride, promethazine hydrochloride, or hydroxyzine hydrochloride; this will result in precipitation of ketorolac from solution.
- When administering IM/IV, the IV bolus must be given over no less than 15 sec. Give IM administration slowly and deeply into the muscle. The analgesic effect begins in 30 min with max effect in 1 to 2 hr after IV or IM dosing. Duration of the analgesic effect is usually 4 to 6 hr.
- If GI upset occurs, administer oral form with meals, milk, or antacids to decrease GI irritation.
- With IM administration, rotate injection sites.
- Wash hands before and after instillation.
- Lower doses may be necessary in patients with compromised renal or hepatic function.
- Store at room temperature (59° to 86°F). Protect from light.

Ophthalmic Solution:

- For ophthalmic use only. Not for use on the skin or for injection into eye.
- Have patient tilt head back and instill prescribed number of drops into affected eye(s) as ordered. Have patient close eye(s) for 2 to 3 min and apply light finger pressure to lacrimal sac for 1 to 2 min after instillation. Do not touch top of dropper bottle to eye, fingers, or other surface.
- If using other topical ophthalmic drugs, separate each medication by at least 5 min. Instill ophthalmic ointment last.

- Store ophthalmic solution at ambient temperature (59° to 86°F). Keep tightly capped and protect from light.

Assessment/Interventions
- Obtain patient history, including drug history and any known allergies.
- Assess degree, location, and type of pain before and after administration.
- Assess renal function before and during therapy. Monitor serum creatinine or Ccr.
- Monitor for hematomas and bleeding, especially with perioperative IM administration.
- Monitor LFTs. Notify health care provider if abnormal LFTs persist or worsen, if clinical signs and symptoms consistent with liver disease develop, or if systemic manifestations (eg, eosinophilia, rash) occur.
- Monitor patients with compromised cardiac function and hypertension for signs of fluid retention (eg, peripheral edema).
- Observe for signs of GI toxicity, especially in elderly patients.
- Observe for signs of infection because ketorolac may mask usual signs.
- Hypersensitivity reactions ranging from bronchospasm to anaphylactic shock have occurred; appropriate counteractive measures must be available when administering the first dose of ketorolac.

Ophthalmic Solution:
- Monitor patient's response to therapy. Notify health care provider if eye or eyelid inflammation is noted or if symptoms do not improve or worsen.

Patient/Family Education
- Instruct patient to take drug with food, milk, or antacid if GI upset occurs.
- Inform patient that drug is an NSAID and can cause serious side effects such as GI bleeding.
- Instruct patient to avoid alcohol, aspirin, and other NSAIDs.
- Advise patient to inform dentist and other health care providers of drug therapy before any treatment or surgery.
- Instruct patient to report the following symptoms to health care provider: skin rash, itching, visual disturbances, weight gain, edema, black stools, or persistent headache.
- Caution patient to avoid exposure to sunlight and other sources of UV light and to use sunscreen or wear protective clothing to avoid photosensitivity reaction.
- Advise patient that drug may cause drowsiness or dizziness and to use caution while driving or performing other tasks requiring mental alertness.
- Instruct patient not to take any OTC medications without consulting health care provider.

Ophthalmic Solution:
- Remind patient that eye drops are for use in the eye only.
- Teach patient proper technique for instilling eye drops: wash hands; do not allow dropper to touch eye. Tilt head back, look up; pull lower eyelid down; instill prescribed number of drops. Close eye for 1 to 2 min and apply gentle pressure to bridge of nose for 1 to 3 min. Do not rub eye.
- Advise patient not to touch top of dropper bottle to eye, fingers, or other surface.
- Advise patient that if more than 1 topical ophthalmic drug is being used, administer the drugs at least 5 min apart. Administer ointment last.
- Inform patient that temporary stinging or burning are the most common side effects and to contact health care provider if they occur and are bothersome.
- Advise patient to contact eye doctor if eye or eyelid inflammation is noted or if eye symptoms do not improve or worsen.
- Instruct patient wearing contact lenses to remove them when instilling eye drops.

Ketotifen Fumarate

(KEY-toe-TIF-fen FEW-mah-rate)
Class Ophthalmic antihistamine

How Supplied
Zaditor Solution 0.025%

Action
PHARMACOLOGY: Inhibits release of mediators from cells involved in hypersensitivity reactions.

PHARMACOKINETICS/DYNAMICS:
Absorption: Little systemic exposure following topical ocular administration.

Indications Temporary prevention of itching of eyes caused by allergic conjunctivitis.

Contraindications Standard considerations.

Route/Dosage
ADULTS AND CHILDREN 3 YR OF AGE AND OLDER: **Ophthalmic** 1 drop in affected eye(s) bid, q 8 to 12 hr.

Interactions None well documented.

Lab Test Interferences None well documented.

Adverse Reactions
CNS: Headache (10% to 25%).
EENT: Conjunctival injection, rhinitis (10% to 25%); ocular allergic reactions, burning or sting-

ing of eye, conjunctivitis, eye discharge, dry eye, eye pain, eyelid disorder, itching eye, keratitis, lacrimation disorder, mydriasis, photophobia, rash, pharyngitis (less than 5%).
OTHER: Flu syndrome (less than 5%).

PATIENT CARE CONSIDERATIONS
Administration/Storage
- For topical ophthalmic use only. Not for use on the skin, in the ear, or for injection into eye.
- Ask patient to tilt head back and instill prescribed number of drops into affected eye(s) as ordered. Ask patient to close eye(s) for 2 to 3 min and apply light finger pressure to lacrimal sac for 1 to 2 min after installation. Do not touch top of dropper bottle to eye, fingers, or any other surface.
- If using other topical ophthalmic medications, separate each medication by at least 5 min. Instill ophthalmic ointment last.
- Store ophthalmic solution between 39° and 77°F. Keep tightly capped.

Assessment/Interventions
- Obtain patient history, including drug history and any known allergies.
- Monitor patient's response to therapy. Notify health care provider if eye or eyelid inflammation is noted or if symptoms do not improve or worsen.

Patient/Family Education
- Remind patient that eye drops are for use in the eye only.
- Teach patient proper technique for instilling eye drops: Wash hands; do not allow dropper to touch eye; tilt head back and look up; pull lower eyelid down; instill prescribed number of drops; close eye for 1 to 2 min and apply gentle pressure to bridge of nose for 1 to 3 min; do not rub eye.
- Caution patient not to touch top of dropper bottle to eye, fingers, or any other surface.
- Advise patient that if more than 1 topical ophthalmic medication is being used to separate each medication by at least 5 min apart. Instill ophthalmic ointment last.
- Inform patient that eye redness, headaches, and runny nose are the most common side effects and to contact health care provider if they occur and are bothersome.
- Advise patient to contact eye doctor if eye or eyelid inflammation is noted or if eye symptoms do not improve or worsen.
- Instruct patient wearing contact lenses to remove lenses when instilling eye drops and, if wearing soft contact lenses, to wait 10 min after instilling drops before inserting lenses.
- Caution patient wearing contact lenses not to wear lenses if eyes are red.
- Advise patient that follow-up eye examinations may be necessary while using this medication and to keep appointments.

Precautions
Pregnancy: Category C.
Lactation: Undetermined.
Children: Safety and efficacy not established in children younger than 3 yr of age.

Labelol Hydrochloride

(la-BET-uh-lahl HIGH-droe-KLOR-ide)

Class Alpha-adrenergic blocker/Beta-adrenergic blocker

How Supplied
Normodyne Tablets 100 mg, Tablets 200 mg, Tablets 300 mg, Injection 5 mg/mL ♦ *Trandate* Tablets 100 mg, Tablets 200 mg, Tablets 300 mg, Injection 5 mg/mL
✤ *Apo-Labetalol*

Action
PHARMACOLOGY: Selectively blocks alpha-1 receptors and nonselectively blocks beta-receptors to decrease BP, heart rate, and myocardial oxygen demand.

PHARMACOKINETICS/DYNAMICS:
Absorption: Completely absorbed from the GI tract. T_{max} is 1 to 2 hr. Relative bioavailability is 100% (oral and solution). Absolute bioavailability for oral compared with IV is 25%. Absolute bioavailability increases when administered with food. Steady state levels are reached by about the third day of dosing.

Distribution: Crosses the placental barrier. Approximately 50% protein bound.

Metabolism: Mainly through conjugation to glucuronide metabolites.

Excretion: Plasma t½ is 6 to 8 hr (not altered in patient with decreased hepatic or renal function). Metabolites excreted in urine and via the bile into the feces. Approximately 55% to 60% appears in urine as conjugates or unchanged labetalol within 24 hr. Neither hemodialysis nor peritoneal dialysis removes a significant amount of labetalol from the general circulation.

Peak: 2 to 4 hr.

Duration: Lasting at least 8 hr following single oral dose of 100 mg and more than 12 hr after a 300 mg dose.

Special Populations:
Elderly – Elimination is reduced; lower maintenance dosage is generally required in elderly.

Indications
Management of hypertension.
Unlabeled use(s): Treatment of pheochromocytoma; management of clonidine-withdrawal hypertension.

Contraindications
Severe bradycardia; second- and third-degree heart block; heart failure; cardiogenic shock; bronchial asthma.

Route/Dosage
ADULTS: PO 100 mg bid initially; maintenance dose usually 200 to 400 mg bid. IV 20 mg over 2 min; then 40 to 80 mg q 10 min up to max of 300 mg. Infusions of 2 mg/min can be initiated and titrated to response.

Interactions
Beta-adrenergic agonists: Blunted bronchodilator effect.
Cimetidine: Increased bioavailability of labetalol.
Indomethacin: Impaired antihypertensive effect of labetalol.
Inhalation anesthetics: May exaggerate hypotension.
Nitroglycerin: Increased hypotension.
INCOMPATIBILITIES: Injection not compatible with 5% Sodium Bicarbonate.

Lab Test Interferences
Drug may cause false-positive increases in levels of urinary catecholamines.

Adverse Reactions
CV: Orthostatic hypotension; edema; flushing; ventricular arrhythmias; AV block; bradycardia; heart failure; chest pain.
CNS: Headache; fatigue; dizziness; depression; lethargy; drowsiness; forgetfulness; sleepiness; vertigo; paresthesia; nightmares.
DERM: Tingling of scalp; rash; facial erythema; alopecia; urticaria; pruritus; increased sweating.
EENT: Dry eyes; visual disturbances; altered taste perception.
GI: Nausea; vomiting; diarrhea; dyspepsia.
GU: Impotence; urinary retention; difficulty with urination; failure to ejaculate; priapism; Peyronie disease.
HEMA: Leukopenia.
HEPA: Elevated transaminases; jaundice; cholestasis.
METAB: Increases or decreases in serum glucose; increased creatinine and BUN.
RESP: Bronchospasm; shortness of breath; wheezing.
OTHER: Muscle cramps; systemic lupus erythematosus; increased hypoglycemic response to insulin; masking of hypoglycemic signs; asthenia.

Precautions
Pregnancy: Category C.
Lactation: Excreted in breast milk.
Children: Safety and efficacy not established.
Special risk patients: Use with caution in patients with diabetes mellitus, CHF, respiratory difficulties, or severely elevated BP.
Cardiac failure: Cardiac failure has been observed in patients with or without history.
Withdrawal: Do not discontinue abruptly. Abrupt discontinuation may worsen angina and precipitate ischemic event in susceptible individuals.

Overdosage: Signs and Symptoms
Excessive orthostatic hypotension, excessive bradycardia, cardiac failure, bronchospasm, seizures.

PATIENT CARE CONSIDERATIONS
Administration/Storage
- Administer oral form with food; tablets can be crushed.
- If nausea and dizziness occur with twice-daily dosing of oral form, same total daily dose can be administered as divided doses 3 times/day.
- Keep patient supine during IV administration and for 3 hr afterward.
- For repeated IV injection, give 20 mg dose slowly over 2 min.
- For slow, continuous infusion, dilute contents with compatible IV fluid and administer at a rate of 2 mg/min. Use controlled administration device. Once satisfactory response is obtained, infusion can be discontinued and treatment with oral labetalol can be initiated.
- Labetalol is compatible with following parenteral solutions: Ringer's, Lactated Ringer's, 5% Dextrose and Ringer's, 5% Lactated Ringer's and 5% Dextrose, 5% Dextrose, 0.9% Sodium Chloride, 5% Dextrose and 0.2% Sodium Chloride, 2.5% Dextrose and 0.45% Sodium Chloride, 5% Dextrose and 0.9% Sodium Chloride, and 5% Dextrose and 0.33% Sodium Chloride.
- Store at room temperature and protect from excessive moisture.
- Do not freeze injection vials. Protect from light. Parenteral solution is stable for 24 hr after dilution.

Assessment/Interventions
- Obtain patient history, including drug history and any known allergies.
- Measure vital signs and supine BP immediately before and at 5- to 10-min intervals after direct IV injection.
- Obtain renal and liver studies before therapy begins.
- Take safety precautions if orthostatic hypotension occurs.
- Closely monitor diabetic patients for signs of hypoglycemia.
- Assess skin turgor and dryness of mucous membranes for hydration status.

Patient/Family Education
- Caution patient to avoid sudden position changes to prevent orthostatic hypotension. Advise use of support hose.
- Advise patient to notify dentist and other health care providers of drug therapy before treatment or surgery.
- Caution diabetic patient to monitor serum glucose carefully.
- Instruct patient to not discontinue drug abruptly.
- Advise patient to carry identification (eg, Medi-Alert) indicating medical condition and drug regimen.
- Instruct patient how to measure BP and pulse.
- Emphasize importance of the following other modalities on BP: weight control, regular exercise, smoking cessation and moderate intake of alcohol and salt.
- Inform patient that transient scalp tingling may occur, especially when treatment is initiated.
- Instruct patient to report the following symptoms to health care provider: slow heart rate, dizziness, confusion, fever or depression, shortness of breath, fatigue, swelling of ankles and feet.
- Advise patient that drug causes dizziness and to use caution while driving or performing other tasks requiring mental alertness.
- Instruct patient not to take any OTC medications without consulting health care provider.

Lactulose

(LAK-tyoo-lohs)

Class Laxative

How Supplied
Cephulac Solution 10 g lactulose/15 mL (less than 1.6 g galactose, less than 1.2 g galactose, and up to 1.2 g of other sugars), ♦ *Cholac* Solution 10 g lactulose/15 mL (less than 1.6 g galactose, less than 1.2 g galactose, and up to 1.2 g of other sugars) ♦ *Chronulac* Solution 10 g lactulose/15 mL (less than 1.6 g galactose, less than 1.2 g galactose, and up to 1.2 g of other sugars) ♦ *Constilac* Solution 10 g lactulose/15 mL (less than 1.6 g galactose, less than 1.2 g galactose, and up to 1.2 g of other sugars) ♦ *Constulose* Solution 10 g lactulose/15mL (less than 1.6 g galactose, less than 1.2 g galactose, and up to 1.2 g of other sugars) ♦ *Duphalac* Solution 10 g lactulose/15 mL (less than 1.6 g galactose, less than 1.2 g galactose up to 1.2 g of other sugars) ♦ *Enulose* Solution 10 g lactulose per 15 mL (less than 1.6 g galactose, less than 1.2 g galactose, and up to 1.2 g of other sugars) ✤ *Apo-Lactulose* ♦ *Laxilose* ♦ *PMS-Lactulose* ♦ *ratio-Lactulose*

Action
PHARMACOLOGY: Produces increased osmotic pressure within colon and acidifies its contents, resulting in increased stool water content and

stool softening. Causes migration of ammonia from blood into colon, where it is converted to ammonium ion and expelled through laxative action.

Pharmacokinetics/Dynamics:
Absorption: Poorly absorbed from the GI tract when given PO and PR (no enzyme capable of hydrolysis of lactulose is present in GI tissue).

Metabolism: In the colon, lactulose is broken down primarily to lactic acid. Metabolized in the colon by bacteria.

Excretion: Less than 3% is excreted in the urine. Doses reach the colon virtually unchanged.

Onset: 24 to 48 hr.

Indications
Treatment of constipation; prevention and treatment of portal-systemic encephalopathy, including stages of hepatic precoma and coma.

Contraindications
Use in patients who require low-galactose diet.

Route/Dosage
Constipation (Chronulac, Constilac, Duphalac)
ADULTS: PO 15 to 30 mL (10 to 20 g lactulose) daily; may increase to 60 mL/day.

Portal-Systemic Encephalopathy (Cephulac, Cholac, Enulose)
ADULTS: PO 30 to 45 mL tid to qid. Adjust dosage to produce 2 to 3 soft stools/day. Hourly doses of 30 to 45 mL may be used for rapid laxation initially; once achieved, reduce to recommended daily dose. PR 300 mL with 700 mL water or physiologic saline solution via rectal balloon catheter; retain for 30 to 60 min. May repeat q 4 to 6 hr.

OLDER CHILDREN AND ADOLESCENTS: PO 40 to 90 mL/day in divided doses to produce 2 to 3 soft stools/day.

INFANTS: PO 2.5 to 10 mL/day in divided doses to produce 2 to 3 soft stools/day.

Interactions
Neomycin, other anti-infectives: May interfere with desired degradation of lactulose and prevent acidification of colonic contents.
Nonabsorbable antacids: May inhibit colonic acidification.

Lab Test Interferences
None well documented.

Adverse Reactions
GI: Gaseous distention with flatulence or belching, abdominal discomfort and cramping; diarrhea; nausea; vomiting.

Precautions
Pregnancy: Category B.
Lactation: Undetermined.
Children: Safety and efficacy not established. Administer with caution. Infants receiving lactulose may develop hyponatremia and dehydration.
Elderly: With long-term therapy (more than 6 mo) at increased risk of dehydration and electrolyte imbalance.
Concomitant laxative use: Do not use other laxatives, especially during initial phase of therapy. Resultant loose stools may falsely suggest adequate lactulose dosage.
Debilitated patients: With long-term therapy (more than 6 mo) at increased risk of dehydration and electrolyte imbalance.
Diabetic patients: Lactulose syrup contains galactose and lactose. Use with caution.
Electrocautery procedures: Although not reported for lactulose, theoretical hazard exists for patients being treated with lactulose who may undergo electrocautery procedures during proctoscopy or colonoscopy. Accumulation of hydrogen gas in presence of electrical spark may result in explosion. Therefore patients should have thorough bowel cleansing with nonfermentable solution before undergoing such procedures.

Overdosage: Signs and Symptoms
Diarrhea, abdominal cramps.

PATIENT CARE CONSIDERATIONS
Administration/Storage
- Mix with fruit juice, water, or milk to make more palatable.
- Administer with full glass of fruit juice, water, or milk.
- May administer to adults during impending coma or coma stage of portal-systemic encephalopathy as retention enema via rectal balloon catheter when danger of aspiration exists or when endoscopic or intubation procedures interfere with oral administration. Do not use cleansing enemas containing soapsuds or other alkaline agents. If enema is inadvertently evacuated too promptly, it may be repeated immediately.
- Store at room temperature; do not freeze.

Assessment/Interventions
- Obtain patient history, including drug history and any known allergies.
- Assess for abdominal distention and discomfort.
- Evaluate bowel sounds and bowel function.
- Assess consistency and frequency of stool produced.
- Do not use other laxatives.

- Encourage fluid intake.
- Keep patient clean and dry. Assess skin integrity frequently.
- Monitor electrolyte balance and liver function.
- Monitor I&O.
- In elderly or debilitated patients who receive lactulose more than 6 mo, measure serum electrolytes (eg, potassium, chloride) and carbon dioxide periodically.
- Monitor mental status (eg, orientation, lethargy, irritability) in portal-systemic encephalopathy patients.
- If concomitant oral anti-infectives are given, monitor patient closely.
- If diarrhea, rectal bleeding, nausea, vomiting, abdominal cramps, or distention occurs, discontinue medication and notify health care provider.

Patient/Family Education
- Advise patient that drug can be mixed with fruit juice, water, or milk to make it more palatable.
- Inform patient that drug may cause belching, flatulence, or abdominal cramps. Instruct patient to notify health care provider if these symptoms become bothersome or if diarrhea occurs.
- Instruct patient not to take other laxatives while receiving lactulose therapy.
- Encourage patient to increase dietary fiber and fluid intake and participate in regular exercise.

Lamivudine (3TC)

(la-MIH-view-deen)

Class Antiretroviral/Nucleoside reverse transcriptase inhibitor

How Supplied
Epivir Tablets 150 mg, Tablets 300 mg, Oral solution 10 mg/mL • *Epivir-HBV* Tablets 100 mg, Oral solution 5 mg/mL
🍁 Heptovir

Action
PHARMACOLOGY: Inhibits replication of HIV and hepatitis B virus (HBV)

PHARMACOKINETICS/DYNAMICS:
Absorption: C_{max} is approximately 1.28 mcg/mL (single dose of 100 mg). T_{max} is 0.5 to 2 hr. Absolute bioavailability is approximately 87%.

Distribution: Less than 36% protein bound. Vd is approximately 1.3 L/kg.

Metabolism: Metabolism of lamivudine is a minor route of elimination. The metabolite is trans-sulfoxide metabolite.

Excretion: The majority is eliminated unchanged in the urine. Mean t½ is 5 to 7 hr. Cl is approximately 398.5 mL/min.

Special Populations:
Renal Function Impairment – AUC, C_{max}, and t½ are increased. It is recommended that dosage be modified in these patients.

Indications
HIV infection:
Epivir – In combination with other antiretroviral agents for the treatment of HIV infection.
Chronic hepatitis B:
Epivir-HBV – Treatment of chronic hepatitis B associated with evidence of hepatitis B viral replication and active liver inflammation.

Contraindications Standard considerations.

Route/Dosage
HIV Infection
ADULTS: PO 150 mg bid or 300 mg/day in combination with other antiretroviral agents.
Ccr 30 to 49: PO 150 mg/day.
Ccr 15 to 29: PO 150 mg first dose, then 100 mg/day.
Ccr 5 to 14: PO 150 mg first dose, then 50 mg/day.
Ccr less than 5: PO 50 mg first dose, then 25 mg/day.
CHILDREN (3 MO TO 16 YR): PO 4 mg/kg bid (max, 150 mg bid) in combination with other antiretroviral agents. Dosage adjustment needed because of renal impairment.

Chronic Hepatitis B
ADULTS: PO 100 mg/day. Safety and efficacy of treatment older than 1 yr not established.
CHILDREN (2 TO 17 YR): PO 3 mg/kg/day (max, 100 mg/day). Safety and efficacy of treatment older than 1 yr not established.

Dosage Adjustments in Renal Impairment
ADULTS:
Ccr at least 50: PO 100 mg/day.
Ccr 30 to 49: PO 100 mg first dose then 50 mg/day.
Ccr 15 to 29: PO 100 mg first dose then 25 mg/day.
Ccr 5 to 14: PO 35 mg first dose then 15 mg/day.
Ccr less than 5: PO 35 mg first dose then 10 mg/day.

Interactions
Trimethoprim-sulfamethoxazole: May decrease clearance of lamivudine, increasing its serum concentration.
Zalcitabine: Lamivudine and zalcitabine may inhibit the intracellular phosphorylation of one

another. Use in combination is not recommended.

Lab Test Interferences None well documented.

Adverse Reactions
CNS: Headache; neuropathy; dizziness; sleep disturbances; depression; insomnia and other sleep disorders; depressive disorders.
DERM: Rash; alopecia; pruritus.
GI: Nausea; vomiting; diarrhea; anorexia; abdominal pain/cramps; dyspepsia; stomatitis.
HEMA: Anemia; neutropenia; hyperglycemia; weakness; lactic acidosis; lymphadenopathy; splenomegaly; lactic steatosis.
RESP: Nasal signs and symptoms; cough; paresthesia; abnormal breath sounds/wheezing.
OTHER: Malaise; fatigue; fever; chills; myalgia; arthralgia; pancreatitis; elevated liver enzymes; musculoskeletal pain; anaphylaxis; urticaria; rhabdomyolysis; peripheral neuropathy; hepatic steatosis; muscle weakness with CPK elevation; posttreatment exacerbation of hepatitis; redistribution/accumulation of body fat.

> **WARNING:**
> Lactic acidosis with hepatomegaly and steatosis (including fatal cases) has been reported with the use of nucleoside analogues alone or in combination.

PATIENT CARE CONSIDERATIONS
Administration/Storage
- Administer lamivudine in combination with other antiretroviral agents (ie, zidovudine).
- Adhere strictly to the prescribed dosage and schedule.
- A reduced dosage is recommended for patients with impaired renal function.
- Store tablets and oral solution at room temperature (59° to 86°F) in a tight, dry container.

Assessment/Interventions
- There is no known antidote.
- Obtain patient history.
- Monitor for signs and symptoms of infection or neurological changes.
- Monitor for emergence of resistance-associated HBV mutations.
- Assess patient for change in severity of symptoms.
- Monitor patient for signs and symptoms of pancreatitis, especially pediatric patients.
- Monitor BUN, serum creatinine, LFTs, amylase, and CBC during the course of therapy.
- If any clinical signs, symptoms, or laboratory tests suggest pancreatitis, notify health care provider immediately.

Precautions
Pregnancy: Category C.
Lactation: Excreted in breast milk. HIV-infected mothers should not breastfeed their infants.
Children:
Hepatitis B – Safety and efficacy in children under 2 yr not established.
HIV infection – Safety and efficacy in children under 3 mo not established.
Renal function impairment: Dosage adjustment recommended.
Exacerbation of hepatitis: Exacerbations of hepatitis has occurred after discontinuation of lamivudine.
Fat distribution: Accumulation/redistribution of body fat including central obesity, dorsocervical fat enlargement (buffalo hump), peripheral wasting, facial wasting, breast enlargement, and "cushingoid appearance" has occurred in patients receiving antiretroviral therapy. A causal relationship has not been established.
HIV-HBV coinfection: Epivir-HBV tablets and oral solution contain a lower dose of the same active ingredient as Epivir tablets and oral solution (and lamivudine/zidovudine tablets used to treat HIV infection). The formulation and dosage of lamivudine in Epivir-HBV are not appropriate for patients infected with HBV and HIV.
Pancreatitis: Reported in patients receiving lamivudine, particularly in HIV-infected pediatric patients with prior nucleoside exposure.

- In patients receiving lamivudine with zidovudine, monitor for increased risk of adverse effects including headache, fatigue, nausea, neuropathy, nasal signs and symptoms, cough, rash, and musculoskeletal pain.

Patient/Family Education
- Instruct patient that the lamivudine tablets and oral solution are for oral ingestion only and to take only as prescribed.
- Instruct patient to avoid OTC medications unless prescribed by health care provider.
- Instruct patient that lamivudine is not a cure for HIV or HBV infections and opportunistic infections and other complications of HIV and HBV infections may continue to develop.
- Caution patient or guardian that long-term effects of lamivudine and results from controlled clinical trials evaluating therapeutic and adverse effects are unknown.
- Inform patient of the potential adverse effects.
- Instruct patient to notify health care provider if signs of infection such as a sore throat, fever, cough, and respiratory congestion occur.
- Instruct family to notify health care provider of changes in neurological status such as memory loss or confusion.

- Advise patient that it may take at least 4 wk for max effect.
- Warn patient that the risk of transmission of HIV or HBV to others through sexual contact or exposure to the patient's blood is still present. Instruct patient in methods and precautions to prevent transmission of the HIV or HBV virus.
- Instruct parents or guardians to monitor patient, especially a pediatric patient, for signs and symptoms of pancreatitis.
- Caution mothers to discontinue breastfeeding if receiving lamivudine because of the potential for adverse effects from lamivudine in nursing infants as well as transmission of the HIV virus.
- Advise women to notify health care provider if pregnant or planning to become pregnant, as lamivudine is transferred to the fetus through the placenta.
- Stress the importance of regular exams and laboratory work. Encourage patient to comply with the treatment regimen.
- Advise patient that *Epivir-HBV* tablets and oral solution contain a lower dose of the same active ingredient as *Epivir* oral solution, tablets, and lamivudine/zidovudine tablets. Advise patient not to take *Epivir-HBV* concurrently with *Epivir* or lamivudine/zidovudine.
- Advise patients of the importance of taking lamivudine with combination therapy on a regular dosing schedule and to avoid missing doses.
- Inform patients that redistribution or accumulation of body fat may occur in patients receiving antiretroviral therapy.

Lamivudine/Zidovudine

(la-MIH-view-deen/zie-DOE-view-DEEN)

Class Antiviral combination

How Supplied
Combivir Tablets 150 mg lamivudine/300 mg zidovudine

Action
PHARMACOLOGY: Inhibits replication of HIV by incorporation into HIV DNA and producing an incomplete, nonfunctional DNA.

Indications Treatment of HIV infection.

Contraindications Hypersensitivity to any component of the product; use in patients requiring dosage adjustment (eg, renal function impairment with Ccr less than 50 mL/min, body weight less than 50 kg or 110 lb).

Route/Dosage
ADULTS AND CHILDREN AT LEAST 12 YR: PO One combination tablet bid.

Interactions
Ganciclovir, interferon-alpha, other bone marrow suppressives or cytotoxic agents: Increased hematologic toxicity of zidovudine. Note: Although pharmacokinetic interactions are reported with the following drugs, routine dose modification of lamivudine and zidovudine is not warranted: atovaquone, fluconazole, methadone, nelfinavir, probenecid, ritonavir, trimethoprim-sulfamethoxazole, valproic acid.

Lab Test Interferences None well documented.

Adverse Reactions
CNS: Headache; fatigue; neuropathy; insomnia; dizziness; depression.
DERM: Rash.
EENT: Nasal symptoms.
GI: Nausea; diarrhea; vomiting; anorexia; abdominal pain; abdominal cramps; dyspepsia.
HEMA: Anemia; neutropenia; thrombocytopenia.
HEPA: Elevated liver enzymes.
RESP: Cough.
OTHER: Malaise; fever; chills; myalgia; arthralgia; musculoskeletal pain.

Precautions
Pregnancy: Category C.
Lactation: Undetermined. HIV-infected mothers should not breastfeed infants.
Children: Not indicated in children less than 12 yr because it is a fixed-dose combination that prevents dosage adjustment.
Hepatic function impairment: Use with caution; suspend treatment in any patient who develops clinical or laboratory findings suggestive of lactic acidosis or hepatotoxicity.
Bone marrow suppression: Use with caution in patients who have bone marrow compromise evidenced by granulocyte count less than 1000 cells/cm or hemoglobin less than 9.5 g/dL.
Fixed-dose combination: Does not allow for dose reduction; do not use in patients requiring lamivudine or zidovudine dosage reduction (eg, children less than 12 yr; renal impairment with Ccr less than 50 mL/min; low body weight; or those patients experiencing dose-limiting side effects).
Monitoring: Frequent blood counts are recommended when using this drug combination in patients with advanced HIV disease; periodic blood counts are recommended when using in patients with asymptomatic or early HIV disease.

Overdosage: Signs and Symptoms
Nausea, vomiting, headache, dizziness, drowsiness, lethargy, confusion, grand mal seizure, hematologic changes (zidovudine).

PATIENT CARE CONSIDERATIONS
Administration/Storage
- Adhere strictly to the prescribed dosage schedule.
- Administer without regard to food.
- Store tablets and oral solution at room temperature (36° to 76°F) in a tight, dry container.

Assessment/Interventions
- Obtain patient history, including drug history.
- Assess for signs and symptoms of the major toxicities, including neutropenia and anemia, especially in patients with advanced disease.
- Administer with caution to patients with liver disease. Assess patient for clinical symptoms that might suggest the onset of lactic acidosis or severe hepatomegaly with steatosis (fatty degeneration).
- Monitor BUN, serum creatinine, LFTs, amylase, and CBC during the course of therapy.
- Monitor for signs and symptoms of infection or neurological changes. Assess patient for change in severity of symptoms.
- Monitor the patient for increased risk of adverse effects that included headache, fatigue, nausea, neuropathy, nasal signs and symptoms, cough, skin rashes, and musculoskeletal pain.

Patient/Family Education
- Provide patient information pamphlet.
- Teach patient that this medication is for oral use only and to take only as prescribed.
- Instruct the patient to avoid OTC medicines unless approved by health care provider.
- Stress the importance of regular exams and laboratory work.
- Inform patient that this medication is not a cure for the HIV infection and that the patient may continue to develop opportunistic infections and other complications of HIV infection. Patients will need to remain under the close observation of health care providers experienced in the treatment of patients with HIV-associated diseases.
- Caution patient not to discontinue use of drug even when feeling better.
- Caution patient that long-term effects of this medicine is not known.
- Instruct patient to notify health care provider of signs of infection, including sore throat, fever, cough, and respiratory congestion.
- Instruct family to notify health care provider of changes in neurological status such as memory loss or confusion.
- Advise patient that it may take at least 4 wk for maximum effect.
- Warn patient that the risk of transmission of HIV to others through sexual contact or exposure to the patient's blood is still present. Instruct patient in methods to prevent transmission of the HIV virus.
- Caution mothers to discontinue nursing if receiving this medication.
- Instruct women to inform health care provider immediately if suspecting pregnancy.
- Inform patient that the major toxicities are neutropenia and anemia and to have blood counts monitored closely.

Lamotrigine

(lah-MOE-trih-JEEN)

Class Anticonvulsant

How Supplied
Lamictal Tablets 25 mg, Tablets 100 mg, Tablets 150 mg, Tablets 200 mg ◆ *Lamictal Chewable Dispersible* Tablets, chewable 2 mg, Tablets, chewable 5 mg, Tablets, chewable 25 mg

Action
PHARMACOLOGY: Chemically unrelated to existing antiepileptic drugs (AEDs); precise mechanism(s) unknown. One proposed mechanism suggests inhibition of voltage-sensitive sodium channels, thereby stabilizing neuronal membranes, that modulates presynaptic transmitter release of excitatory amino acids (eg, glutamate, aspartate).

PHARMACOKINETICS/DYNAMICS:

Absorption: Rapidly and completely absorbed after oral administration. Absolute bioavailability is 98%; not affected by food. T_{max} is 1.4 to 4.8 hr. Chewable/dispersible tablets were found to be equivalent.

Distribution: Mean Vd is 0.9 to 1.3 L/kg independent of dose. Approximately 55% protein bound at concentrations from 1 to 10 mcg/mL.

Metabolism: Metabolized predominantly by glucuronic acid conjugation. Major metabolite is 2-N-glucuronide conjugate. Following multiple administration (150 mg bid), lamotrigine induced its own metabolism, resulting in a 25%

decrease in t½ and a 37% increase in Cl at steady state.

Excretion: Approximately 94% excreted in urine and 2% in feces.

Special Populations:
Renal Function Impairment – Plasma t½ is 42.9 hr in patients with Ccr of 13 mL/min. Reducing maintenance doses may be effective and is recommended.

Hepatic Function Impairment – The t½ is prolonged. Reduce initial, escalation, and maintenance doses approximately 50% in patients with moderate (Child-Pugh B) and 75% in patients with severe (Child-Pugh C) hepatic impairment.

Race – Oral Cl was 25% lower in nonwhite patients than in white patients.

Indications

Bipolar disorder: Maintenance treatment of bipolar I disorder to delay the time to occurrence of mood episodes in patients treated for acute mood episodes with standard therapy.
Epilepsy: Adjunctive therapy in the treatment of partial seizures in adults and as adjunctive therapy in the generalized seizures of Lennox-Gastaut syndrome in pediatric and adult patients. Conversion to monotherapy in adults with partial seizures who are receiving treatment with a single enzyme-inducing AED (EIAED).

Unlabeled use(s): May be useful in adults with generalized tonic-clonic, absence, atypical absence, and myoclonic seizures.

Contraindications Standard considerations.

Route/Dosage

AS ADD-ON THERAPY FOR EPILEPSY

Lamotrigine Plus AED Regimen Containing Valproic Acid

CHILDREN 2 TO 12 YR: **PO** Wk 1 and 2: 0.15 mg/kg/day in 1 to 2 divided doses. Wk 3 and 4: 0.3 mg/kg/day in 1 to 2 divided doses. Maintenance dose: 1 to 5 mg/kg/day (max, 200 mg/day in 1 to 2 divided doses).

ADULTS OLDER THAN 12 YR: **PO** Wk 1 and 2: 25 mg every other day. Wk 3 and 4: 25 mg/day. Maintenance dose: 100 to 400 mg/day in 1 to 2 divided doses. To achieve, escalate dose by 25 to 50 mg/day q 1 to 2 wk. In patients receiving valproic acid alone, maintenance doses as high as 200 mg/day have been used.

Lamotrigine Plus EIAEDs without Valproic Acid

CHILDREN 2 TO 12 YR: **PO** Wk 1 and 2: 0.6 mg/kg/day in 2 divided doses. Wk 3 and 4: 1.2 mg/kg/day in 2 divided doses.
Maintenance dose: 5 to 15 mg/kg/day (max, 400 mg/day in 2 divided doses).

ADULTS OLDER THAN 12 YR: **PO** Wk 1 and 2: 50 mg/day. Wk 3 and 4: 100 mg/day in 2 divided doses.
Maintenance dose: 300 to 500 mg/day in 2 divided doses. To achieve, escalate dose by 100 mg/day q 1 to 2 wk. Patients receiving multidrug regimens employing EIAEDs without valproic acid can have a maintenance dose of lamotrigine as high as 700 mg/day.

Conversion from a Single EIAED to Monotherapy with Lamotrigine

ADULTS AND CHILDREN AT LEAST 16 YR: **PO** 500 mg/day given as 2 divided doses. Begin conversion by titrating lamotrigine to the target dose (500 mg in 2 divided doses) while maintaining the dose of the EIAED at a fixed level, then withdraw concomitant EIAED by 20% decrements each wk over a 4-wk period.

ESCALATION REGIMEN FOR PATIENTS WITH BIPOLAR DISORDER

Patients Not Taking Carbamazepine (or Other Enzyme-Inducing Drugs) or Valproic Acid

ADULTS (AT LEAST 18 YR): **PO** Wk 1 and 2: 25 mg/day. Wk 3 and 4: 50 mg/day. Wk 5: 100 mg/day. Wk 6 and 7: 200 mg/day.

Patients Taking Valproic Acid

ADULTS (AT LEAST 18 YR): **PO** Wk 1 and 2: 25 mg every other day. Wk 3 and 4: 25 mg/day. Wk 5: 50 mg/day. Wk 6 and 7: 100 mg/day.

Patients Taking Carbamazepine (or Other Enzyme-Inducing Drugs) and Not Taking Valproic Acid

ADULTS (AT LEAST 18 YR): **PO** Wk 1 and 2: 50 mg/day. Wk 3 and 4: 100 mg/day in divided doses. Wk 5: 200 mg/day in divided doses. Wk 6: 300 mg/day in divided doses. Wk 7: up to 400 mg/day in divided doses.

LAMOTRIGINE DOSING ADJUSTMENTS FOR PATIENTS WITH BIPOLAR DISORDER FOLLOWING DISCONTINUATION OF PSYCHOTROPICS

After Discontinuation of Valproic Acid (Current Lamotrigine Dose 100 mg/day)

ADULTS (AT LEAST 18 YR): **PO** Wk 1: 150 mg/day. Wk 2: 200 mg/day. Wk 3 and onward: 200 mg/day.

After Discontinuation of Carbamazepine or Other Enzyme-Inducing Drugs (Current Lamotrigine Dose 400 mg/day)

ADULTS (AT LEAST 18 YR): **PO** Wk 1: 400 mg/day. Wk 2: 300 mg/day. Wk 3 and onward: 200 mg/day.

Interactions

Acetaminophen, carbamazepine, hydantoins (eg, phenytoin), oral contraceptives, oxcarbazepine, phenobarbital, primidone, progestins, rifamycins (eg, rifampin), succinimides (eg, methsuximide): Lamotrigine plasma levels may be reduced by these agents, decreasing the therapeutic effect.
Carbamazepine: The risk of carbamazepine toxicity may be increased.
Folate Inhibitors: Lamotrigine is an inhibitor of dihydrofolate reductase. Use caution with other agents that inhibit folate metabolism.
Valproic acid: Plasma levels may be reduced by lamotrigine, decreasing the therapeutic effect. Valproate increases lamotrigine levels.

Lab Test Interferences
None well documented.

Adverse Reactions

CV: Chest pain (25%).
CNS: Dizziness (38%); headache (29%); ataxia (22%); somnolence (14%); insomnia (10%); abnormal coordination (7%); xerostomia (6%); anxiety (5%); asthenia (at least 5%); tremor, depression (4%); convulsions, irritability, speech disorder (3%); concentration disturbance, seizure exacerbation (2%).
DERM: Rash (can be life-threatening) (10%); pruritus (3%).
EENT: Diplopia (28%); blurred vision (16%); nystagmus (at least 5%); abnormal vision (3%).
GI: Nausea (19%); vomiting (9%); dyspepsia (7%); abdominal pain, diarrhea (6%); constipation (5%); tooth disorder (3%); anorexia (2%).
GU: Dysmenorrhea (7%); vaginitis (4%); amenorrhea (2%).
RESP: Rhinitis (14%); pharyngitis (10%); increased cough (8%); sinusitis (at least 5%).
OTHER: Back pain, fatigue (8%); flu syndrome (7%); fever (6%); lymphadenopathy, infection, pain, weight decrease (at least 5%); neck pain, arthralgia (2%).

> **WARNING:**
> Serious rashes requiring hospitalization (including Stevens-Johnson syndrome) have occurred in 0.8% of pediatric patients and in 0.3% of adults. Toxic epidermal necrolysis may also occur. Almost all fatal cases have occurred within 2 to 8 wk of therapy.

Precautions

Pregnancy: Category C.
Lactation: Excreted in breast milk.
Children: For the treatment of partial seizures and for generalized seizures of Lennox-Gastaut syndrome, safety and efficacy not established for children under 2 yr. For other uses in epilepsy, safety and efficacy not established in children under 16 yr. Safety and efficacy have not been established in patients under 18 yr with bipolar disorder.
Hypersensitivity: Fatal or life-threatening hypersensitivity reactions may occur.
Renal function impairment: If significant impairment, reduce maintenance doses.
Hepatic function impairment: Reduce initial, escalation, and maintenance doses by approximately 50% in patients with moderate (Child-Pugh B) and 75% in patients with severe (Child-Pugh C) hepatic impairment.
Special risk patients: Use with caution in renal/hepatic/cardiac function impairment.
Photosensitivity: Photoallergy or phototoxicity may occur.
Acute multiorgan failure: Multiorgan failure, which in some cases has been fatal or irreversible, has been observed.
Blood dyscrasias: Blood dyscrasias have been reported that may or may not be associated with the hypersensitivity syndrome. These have included neutropenia, leukopenia, anemia, thrombocytopenia, pancytopenia, and, rarely, aplastic anemia and pure red cell aplasia.
Conversion from a single EIAED to monotherapy with lamotrigine: Effect the conversion to monotherapy under conditions that ensure adequate seizure control while mitigating the risk of serious rash associated with the rapid titration of lamotrigine.
Discontinuation strategy: Administer a stepwise reduction of dose (50%/wk) over a 2-wk period. Discontinuing an EIAED may prolong the t½ of lamotrigine; discontinuing valproic acid may shorten the t½ of lamotrigine.
Melanin-containing tissues: Lamotrigine binds to melanin and may cause toxicity with possibility of long-term ophthalmologic effects.
Suicide: Because of the possibility of suicide in patients with bipolar disorder, prescribe the smallest quantity of medication consistent with good patient management.
Withdrawal seizures: Do not abruptly discontinue AEDs because of possibility of increasing seizure frequency. Taper dose over a 2-wk period.

Overdosage: Signs and Symptoms
Ataxia, nystagmus, increased seizures, decreased levels of consciousness, coma, intraventricular conduction delay.

PATIENT CARE CONSIDERATIONS

Administration/Storage

- Tablets and chewable dispersible tablets are interchangeable on mg for mg basis.
- Dosing regimen is dependent on age of patient, condition being treated, and concurrent use of other antiepileptic or antipsychotic drugs.
- Administer prescribed dose without regard to meals. Administer with food if GI upset occurs.
- Tablets should be administered whole. Chewing tablet may leave a bitter taste.
- Chewable dispersible tablets may be administered by chewing, swallowing whole, or dispersing in water or diluted fruit juice. If chewed, provide a small amount of water or diluted fruit juice to aid in swallowing. Whole tablets and not fractions of tablets must be administered.
- To disperse chewable dispersible tablets, add prescribed number of tablets to a small amount (1 tsp or enough to cover tablets) of water or diluted fruit juice. Wait about 1 min for tablet to disperse then swirl solution and administer immediately. Do not attempt to administer partial quantities of the dispersed tablets.
- Store at controlled room temperature (59° to 86°F). Protect from moisture.

Assessment/Interventions

- Obtain patient history, including drug history and any known allergies. Note renal impairment, hepatic impairment, CV disease, concurrent use of valproic acid, or history of rash with previous lamotrigine treatment.
- Ensure that patient, family, or caregiver has reviewed the *Patient Information* leaflet before starting therapy.
- Follow manufacturer's recommendations for adding lamotrigine to a preexisting antiepileptic drug regimen or when converting from a single antiepileptic drug to monotherapy with lamotrigine.
- Follow manufacturer's recommendations for adding lamotrigine to a preexisting bipolar drug regimen or when withdrawing other antipsychotic agents from regimen containing lamotrigine.
- Ensure that reduced initial, escalation, and maintenance doses are administered to patient with moderate to severe hepatic impairment.
- Frequently assess patient for response to treatment. Notify health care provider if condition being treated is not improving or is worsening.
- Ensure that therapy is periodically reviewed to determine if it needs to be continued without change or if a dose change (eg, increase, decrease, discontinuation) is indicated.
- Avoid sudden discontinuation of therapy if possible. Attempt to gradually reduce dose over a period of 2 wk or more if decision to discontinue medication is made.
- Monitor patient for skin rash, fever, hives, sores in the mouth or around eyes, and lymphadenopathy. Immediately inform health care provider if noted and be prepared to discontinue therapy.
- Assess patient with bipolar disorder for suicide potential. Closely supervise high-risk patient during initial drug therapy.
- Monitor patient for GI, CNS, respiratory, GU, and general body side effects. Inform health care provider if noted and significant.
- Implement safety precautions for patients who experience dizziness or ataxia.

Patient/Family Education

- Explain name, dose, action, and potential side effects of drug.
- Advise patient, family, or caregiver to read the Patient Information leaflet before starting therapy and with each refill.
- Instruct patient, family, or caregiver to continue other medications for seizures or bipolar disorder unless advised to do otherwise by health care provider.
- Advise patient, family, or caregiver that medication will be started at a low dose and gradually increased as tolerated until max benefit has been obtained.
- Instruct patient, family, or caregiver to take exactly as prescribed and not to change the dose or discontinue therapy unless advised by health care provider.
- Advise patient to swallow tablet whole. Chewing the tablet may leave a bitter taste.
- Instruct patient, family, or caregiver in proper use of chewable dispersible tablets.
- Advise patient, family, or caregiver that each dose may be taken without regard to meals but to take with food if stomach upset occurs.
- Instruct patient, family, or caregiver that if a dose is missed to skip that dose and not to double up on the next dose.
- Instruct patient, family, or caregiver to discontinue therapy and contact health care provider immediately if any of the following occur: skin rash, hives, fever, swollen lymph glands, painful sores in the mouth or around the eyes, or swelling of the lips or tongue.
- Advise patient, family, or caregiver that if medication needs to be discontinued it will be slowly withdrawn over a period of 2 wk or

more unless safety concerns (eg, rash) require a more rapid withdrawal.
- Caution patient that drug may cause dizziness or drowsiness and to use caution while driving or performing other tasks requiring mental alertness until tolerance is determined.
- Advise women to notify health care provider if pregnant, planning to become pregnant, or breastfeeding.
- Caution patient, family, or caregiver that if medication is stopped for any reason to notify health care provider and not to restart the medication without instruction from health care provider because a dosage adjustment may be necessary if the medication is restarted.
- Instruct patient, family, or caregiver to contact health care provider if seizures get worse, if new types of seizures occur, or if bipolar symptoms do not improve or they worsen.
- Advise patient, family, or caregiver to contact health care provider if bothersome side effects occur.
- Advise patient, family, or caregiver not to take any prescription or OTC medications or dietary supplements unless advised by health care provider.
- Advise patient, family, or caregiver that laboratory tests and follow-up visits will be required to monitor therapy and to keep appointments.

Lansoprazole

(lan-SO-pruh-zole)
Class GI

How Supplied
Prevacid Tablets, orally disintegrating, delayed-release 15 mg, Tablets, orally disintegrating, delayed-release 30 mg, Capsules, delayed-release 15 mg, Capsules, delayed-release 30 mg, Enteric-coated granules for oral suspension, delayed-release 15 mg, Enteric-coated granules for oral suspension, delayed-release 30 mg ♦ *Prevacid I.V.* Injection 30 mg per vial

Action
PHARMACOLOGY: Suppresses gastric acid secretion by blocking "acid (proton) pump" within gastric parietal cells.

PHARMACOKINETICS/DYNAMICS:
Absorption: Absorption is rapid. T_{max} is approximately 1.7 hr. C_{max} and AUC are approximately proportional in doses from 15 to 60 mg single dose administration. Absolute bioavailability is over 80%. C_{max} and AUC decrease 50% if given 30 min after food.

Distribution: Protein binding (97%) is constant over the concentration range of 0.05 to 5 mcg/mL.

Metabolism: Extensively metabolized in the liver. Metabolites are hydroxylated sulfonyl and sulfone derivatives (very little activity).

Excretion: Significant biliary excretion of the metabolites. Mean t½ is 1.9 to 2.9 hr.

Special Populations:
Hepatic Function Impairment – Mean t½ prolonged to 3.2 to 7.2 hr and AUC increased up to 500%; dose reduction is recommended in severe hepatic disease.

Elderly – Cl is decreased with t½ increasing approximately 50% to 100%. Because mean t½ remains between 1.9 to 2.9 hr, repeated once daily dosing does not accumulate; no adjustment needed.

Indications Oral Short-term treatment of active duodenal ulcer; to maintain healing of duodenal ulcers; short-term treatment of all grades of erosive esophagitis; maintenance of healing of erosive esophagitis; long-term treatment of pathological hypersecretory conditions, including Zollinger-Ellison syndrome; in combination with amoxicillin plus clarithromycin or amoxicillin alone (in patients intolerant or resistant to clarithromycin) for the eradication of *H. pylori* in patients with active or recurrent duodenal ulcers; short-term treatment and symptomatic relief of active benign gastric ulcer (including NSAID-associated gastric ulcer in patients who continue NSAID use and for reducing risk of NSAID-associated gastric ulcer in patients with a history of NSAID-associated gastric ulcer); treatment of heartburn and other symptoms of gastroesophageal reflux disease (GERD). IV Short-term treatment (up to 7 days) of all grades of erosive esophagitis

Contraindications Standard considerations.

Route/Dosage
Duodenal Ulcer
ADULTS: **PO** 15 mg/day for 4 wk.

Duodenal Ulcer (Healed) Maintenance
ADULTS: **PO** 15 mg/day.

Erosive Esophagitis
ADULTS: **PO** 30 mg/day for up to 8 wk, an additional 8 wk may be helpful for patients who do not heal. For maintenance, use 15 mg/day.
IV 30 mg/day for up to 7 days.
CHILDREN 12 TO 17 YR OF AGE: **PO** 30 mg/day for up to 8 wk.
CHILDREN 1 TO 11 YR OF AGE: **PO** For children weighing over 30 kg, give 30 mg/day for up to 12 wk; for children weighing 30 kg or less, give 15 mg/day for up to 12 wk.

Gastric Ulcer
ADULTS: **PO** 30 mg/day for up to 8 wk.

GERD
ADULTS: **PO** 15 mg/day for up to 8 wk.
CHILDREN 12 TO 17 YR OF AGE: **PO** Nonerosive GERD: 15 mg once daily for up to 8 wk.
CHILDREN 1 TO 11 YR OF AGE: **PO** For children weighing over 30 kg, give 30 mg/day for up to 12 wk; for children weighing 30 kg or less, give 15 mg/day for up to 12 wk.

H. pylori
ADULTS: **PO** 30 mg lansoprazole plus 500 mg clarithromycin and 1 g amoxicillin bid for 10 to 14 days, or 1 g amoxicillin alone tid for 14 days.

Pathological Hypersecretory Conditions
ADULTS: **PO** Initial dose 60 mg/day. Dosages up to 90 mg bid have been administered. Divide daily doses of more than 120 mg.

Interactions
Digoxin: Increased digoxin absorption, leading to elevated levels and increased risk of toxicity may occur.
Ketoconazole: Effects may be decreased by lansoprazole.
Sucralfate: May delay and reduce absorption; give lansoprazole at least 30 min before sucralfate.

PATIENT CARE CONSIDERATIONS
Administration/Storage
- Dose, frequency of administration, and duration of therapy are dependent on condition being treated.
- Administer prescribed oral dose before a meal.
- Store delayed-release capsules, oral suspension, and orally disintegrating tablets at controlled room temperature (59° to 86°F).

Delayed-Release Capsule:
- The 15 mg delayed-release capsule contains phenylalanine. Do not administer to patient with phenylketonuria without first discussing with health care provider.
- Caution patient to swallow capsule whole and not crush or chew the capsule.
- If patient has difficulty swallowing capsule, the capsule may be opened and the contents sprinkled on 1 Tbsp applesauce, *Ensure* pudding, cottage cheese, yogurt, or strained pears. The mixture should be swallowed immediately without chewing the granules. The contents of the capsule may also be emptied into 2 oz apple juice, orange juice, or tomato juice, mixed briefly, then swallowed immediately without chewing the granules. The glass should be rinsed with 2 or more volumes of juice, and the contents swallowed immediately.
- Do not mix granules with any other food or liquid other than those noted above.

Lab Test Interferences
None well documented.

Adverse Reactions
CNS: Headache (more than 1%).
DERM: Erythema multiforme, Stevens-Johnson syndrome, toxic epidermal necrolysis (postmarketing).
EENT: Speech disorder (postmarketing).
GI: Diarrhea (4%); abdominal pain (2%); constipation, nausea (1%); pancreatitis, vomiting (postmarketing).
GU: Urinary retention (postmarketing).
HEPA: Hepatotoxicity (postmarketing).
HEMA/LYMPH: Agranulocytosis, aplastic anemia, hemolytic anemia, leukopenia, neutropenia, pancytopenia, thrombocytopenia, thrombotic thrombocytopenic purpura (postmarketing).
OTHER: Injection site pain/reaction (IV, 1%); anaphylactoid reactions (postmarketing).

Precautions
Pregnancy: Category B.
Lactation: Undetermined.
Children: Safety and efficacy not established in children younger than 1 yr of age. Safety and efficacy of lansoprazole IV has not been established in pediatric patients.
Hepatic function impairment: Consider dosage adjustment.

Delayed-Release Orally Disintegrating Tablet:
- Have patient place tablet on tongue and allow it to disintegrate, with or without water, until the particles can be swallowed. Caution patient not to chew the tablet or particles that are released.
- For patients having difficulty using the orally disintegrating tablet, the tablet can be placed in an oral syringe and mixed with 4 mL water (15 mg tablet) or 10 mL water (30 mg tablet). Shake syringe gently to allow for a quick dispersal and administer dispersed contents orally or via nasogastric tube (#8 French or greater) within 15 min. If dispersion was administered orally, refill syringe with 2 mL water (15 mg tablet) or 5 mL water (30 mg tablet), shake gently, and administer any remaining contents. If dispersion was administered via nasogastric tube, refill syringe with 5 mL water, shake gently, and flush the nasogastric tube.

Delayed-Release Oral Suspension:
- Open packet and empty contents into container containing 2 Tbsp water. Stir well and drink immediately without chewing granules. If any material remains after drinking, add more water, stir, and drink immediately.
- Do not mix oral suspension with any liquid other than water or with food.

- Do not administer oral suspension via enteral administration tubes.

IV:
- Reconstitute IV preparation with 5 mL sterile water for injection, then further dilute in 50 mL 0.9% sodium chloride injection, lactated Ringer's injection, or 5% dextrose injection.
- Administer once daily by infusing over a period of 30 min using the inline filter provided.
- Flush the IV line before and after administration with 0.9% sodium chloride injection, lactated Ringer's injection, or 5% dextrose injection.
- Do not administer with other drugs or diluents.
- Store the powder for injection at 77°F; protect from light. Store the reconstituted solution for up to 1 hr at 77°F. Store the admixture at 77°F for up to 24 hr (0.9% sodium chloride, lactated Ringer's injection) or up to 12 hr (5% dextrose injection).

Assessment/Interventions
- Obtain patient history, including drug history and any known allergies. Note phenylketonuria (15 mg delayed-release capsule only) or hepatic impairment.
- Assess for bloody or coffee ground emesis and black tarry stools. Inform health care provider immediately if noted.
- Assess for symptoms of esophageal reflux (eg, heart burn, acid regurgitation) or peptic ulcer activity (eg, indigestion, abdominal pain, nausea) before starting therapy and periodically thereafter. Inform health care provider if symptoms are not improving or appear to be worsening.
- Ensure therapy is periodically reviewed to determine if therapy needs to be continued without change or if a dose change (eg, increase, decrease, discontinuation) is indicated.
- Monitor patient for GI, CNS, and general body side effects. Inform health care provider if noted and significant.

Patient/Family Education
- Explain name, dose, action, and potential side effects of drug.
- Instruct patient to take each oral dose before a meal.
- Inform patients that antacids may be taken concurrently with lansoprazole.
- Remind patient that lansoprazole is to be taken every day as prescribed, not only when needed or symptoms are present.
- Advise patient not to change the dose or stop taking unless advised by health care provider.
- Advise patient to notify health care provider if symptoms do not improve or seem to be getting worse.
- Advise patient to immediately report bloody or coffee-ground-like vomit, or black tarry stools to health care provider.
- Instruct patient not to take any prescription or OTC drugs, herbal preparations, or dietary supplements without consulting health care provider.
- Advise women to notify health care provider if pregnant, planning to become pregnant, or breastfeeding.
- Advise patient that follow-up visits may be necessary to monitor therapy and to keep appointments.

Delayed-Release Capsule:
- Advise patient to swallow whole and not to crush or chew the capsule.
- Advise patient that if swallowing the capsule is difficult, the capsule may be opened and the contents sprinkled on 1 Tbsp applesauce, *Ensure* pudding, cottage cheese, yogurt, or strained pears. The mixture should be swallowed immediately without chewing the granules. Advise patient that the contents of the capsule may also be emptied into 2 oz apple juice, orange juice, or tomato juice, mixed briefly, then swallowed immediately without chewing the granules. Advise patient to then rinse the glass with 2 or more volumes of juice and swallow the contents immediately.
- Caution patient not to mix the contents of the capsule with any other food or liquid than those noted above.

Delayed-Release Orally Disintegrating Tablet:
- Instruct patient to place tablet on tongue and allow it to disintegrate, with or without water, until the particles can be swallowed. Caution patient not to chew the tablet or particles that are released.
- Advise patient or caregiver that if using the orally disintegrating tablet is difficult, the tablet can be placed in an oral syringe and mixed with 4 mL water (15 mg tablet) or 10 mL water (30 mg tablet). Advise patient or caregiver to shake syringe gently to allow for a quick dispersal and then administer the dispersed contents from the syringe within 15 min. Advise patient or caregiver to then refill the syringe with 2 mL water (15 mg tablet) or 5 mL water (30 mg tablet), shake gently, and administer any remaining contents.

Delayed-Release Oral Suspension:
- Advise patient to open packet and empty contents into container containing 2 Tbsp water. Ask patient to stir well and then drink immediately without chewing granules. If any material remains after drinking, advise patient to add more water, stir, and drink immediately.
- Caution patient not to mix oral suspension with any liquid other than water or with food.

Laronidase

(lare-AHN-ih-dase)

Class Enzyme replacement therapy

How Supplied
Aldurazyme Injection 2.9 mg laronidase/5 mL

Action
PHARMACOLOGY: Provides exogenous enzyme for uptake into lysosomes and increases the catabolism of glycosaminoglycans.

PHARMACOKINETICS/DYNAMICS:
Absorption: Mean AUC 4.5 to 6.9 mcg·hr/mL.
Distribution: Mean Vd 0.24 to 0.6 L/kg.
Excretion: Mean plasma clearance 1.7 to 2.7 mL/min/kg and elimination t½ 1.5 to 3.6 hr.

Indications Treatment of patients with Hurler and Hurler-Scheie forms of mucopolysaccharidosis I (MPS I); patients with Scheie form who have moderate to severe symptoms.

Contraindications Standard considerations.

Route/Dosage
ADULTS AND CHILDREN 5 YR AND OLDER: **IV** 0.58 mg/kg once/wk delivered over 3 to 4 hr.

Interactions None well documented.
INCOMPATIBILITIES: Do not mix with other medicinal products in the same infusion.

Lab Test Interferences None well documented.

PATIENT CARE CONSIDERATIONS
Administration/Storage
- For IV administration only. Do not administer intradermally, IM, or SC.
- Administer prescribed dose by IV infusion over 3 to 4 hr once/wk.
- Follow manufacturer's instructions for diluting the concentrated solution for infusion.
- Prepare infusion solution using PVC containers and administer with a PVC infusion set equipped with an in-line, low protein-binding 0.2 mcm filter.
- Do not shake or agitate vials during dilution. Do not use filter needles during preparation of infusion.
- Inspect solution visually before administration. Do not administer if solution is cloudy, discolored, or contains particulate matter.
- Discard any unused product. Vials are for single-use only. Do not save medication for future use.
- Initial IV infusion rate should be no more than 10 mcg/kg/hr. The initial infusion rate of 10 mcg/kg/hr may be incrementally increased every 15 min during first hour, as tolerated, until a max infusion rate of 200 mcg/kg/min is reached. The max rate is then maintained for remainder of the infusion.
- Do not administer in same IV line with other products.
- Store vials of concentrated solution in refrigerator (36° to 46°F). Do not freeze or shake. Use diluted infusion solution immediately. If immediate use is not possible, store the diluted infusion solution in refrigerator (36° to 46°F). Do not store diluted infusion solution longer than 36 hr from time of prepara-

Adverse Reactions
CV: Vein disorder (14%); hypotension (9%); dependent edema (9%).
CNS: Hyperreflexia (14%); paresthesia (14%).
DERM: Rash (36%).
EENT: Corneal opacity (9%).
HEMA: Thrombocytopenia (9%).
HEPA: Bilirubinemia (9%).
RESP: Upper respiratory tract infection (32%).
OTHER: Anaphylaxis; injection site reaction (18%); injection site pain (9%); infusion-related reactions (eg, flushing) (32%); chest pain (9%); abscess (9%); facial edema (9%); positive antibodies for laronidase (91%).

Precautions
Pregnancy: Category B.
Lactation: Undetermined.
Children: Safety and efficacy not studied in children under 5 yr.
Hypersensitivity/Infusion reactions: Infusion-related hypersensitivity reactions may occur. Because of increased prevalence of coronary artery disease in patients with MPS I, use epinephrine with caution. Prior to infusion, patients should receive antipyretics and/or antihistamines. If an infusion reaction occurs, decreasing the infusion rate, temporarily stopping the infusion, and/or administration of additional antipyretics and/or antihistamines may ameliorate the symptoms.

tion to completion of infusion.
Assessment/Interventions
* Obtain patient history, including drug history and any known allergies. Note previous allergic reaction to laronidase.
* Ensure that an antipyretic (eg, acetaminophen) or an antihistamine (eg, diphenhydramine) are administered 60 min prior to infusion to decrease or prevent infusion-associated reactions.
* Monitor patient for development of infusion reaction (eg, flushing, fever, headache, rash). If infusion reaction develops, be prepared to decrease the infusion rate, temporarily stop the infusion, or administer additional antipyretics or antihistamines.
* Assess patient for infusion site reactions, CNS, CV, and general body side effects. Inform health care provider if noted and significant.

Patient/Family Education
* Explain name, action, dosing regimen, and potential side effects of drug.
* Advise patient, family, or caregiver that medication will be prepared and administered by a health care provider in a health care setting.
* Advise patient, family, or caregiver that an antipyretic (eg, acetaminophen) and antihistamine (eg, diphenhydramine) will be administered before each treatment to prevent or reduce severity of infusion reactions.
* Advise patient, family, or caregiver to report any signs or symptoms of infusion reaction (eg, flushing, fever, headache, rash).
* Advise women to notify health care provider if pregnant, planning to become pregnant, or breastfeeding.
* Caution patient not to take any prescription or OTC medications or dietary supplements unless advised by health care provider.
* Encourage patient to enroll and participate in the MPS I (mucopolysaccharidosis I) registry as noted in the manufacturer's product information.
* Advise patient that follow-up visits may be necessary and to keep appointments.

Latanoprost

(lah-TAN-oh-prahst)
Class Ophthalmic prostaglandin agonist
How Supplied
Xalatan Ophthalmic solution 0.005% (50 mcg/mL)

Action
PHARMACOLOGY: Prostaglandin $F_{2\alpha}$ analog that reduces intraocular pressure (IOP) by increasing the output of aqueous humor.

Indications For reduction of elevated IOP in patients with open-angle glaucoma or ocular hypertension.

Contraindications Standard considerations.

Route/Dosage
1 drop (1.5 mcg) in the affected eye(s) qd in the evening.

Interactions
Thimerosal: Precipitation occurs when eye drops containing thimerosal are mixed with latanoprost. If such drugs are used, administer with an interval of at least 5 min between applications.

Lab Test Interferences None well documented.

Adverse Reactions
CV: Chest pain; angina pectoris.
DERM: Rash/allergic skin reaction.
RESP: Upper respiratory tract infection, cold, flu (4%).
SPEC SENSE: Blurred vision, burning, stinging, conjunctival hyperemia, foreign body sensation, itching, increased pigmentation of the iris, punctate epithelial keratopathy (5% to 15%); dry eye, excessive tearing, eye phobia, eye pain, lid crusting, lid edema, lid erythema, lid discomfort/pain, photophobia (1% to 4%).
OTHER: Muscle/joint/back pain.

Precautions
Pregnancy: Category C.
Lactation: Undetermined.
Children: Safety and efficacy not established.
Special risk patients: Use caution in patients with active intraocular inflammation (eg, iritis, uveitis).
Eye pigmentation: Changes to pigmented tissue (eg, iris, periorbital tissue [eyelid], eyelashes) may occur.
Macular edema: Macular edema, including cystoid macular edema, may occur.

PATIENT CARE CONSIDERATIONS
Administration/Storage
- Instill 1 drop into affected eye(s) qd, usually in the evening.
- If using other topical ophthalmic drugs, separate each medication by at least 5 min.
- Store unopened bottle in refrigerator. Once opened, bottle can be stored at room temperature up to 77°F for 6 wk. Keep container tightly closed and protected from light.

Assessment/Interventions
- Obtain patient history, including drug history and any known allergies.
- Ensure that IOP has been measured and documented in the patient's record.

Patient/Family Education
- Explain name, dose, action, and potential side effects of drug.
- Advise patient that usual dose is 1 drop in the affected eye(s) qd in the evening.
- Warn patient not to instill more often than qd. More frequent use may decrease effectiveness of the medication.
- Teach patient the following proper techniques for instilling eye drops: wash hands; do not allow dropper to touch eye; tilt head back and look up; pull lower eyelid down; instill prescribed number of drops. Close eye for 1 to 2 min and apply gentle pressure to bridge of nose. Do not rub eye.
- Advise patient wearing contact lenses to remove lenses before instilling this medicine and to wait at least 15 min after instilling eye drop before reinserting lenses.
- Advise patient that if more than 1 topical ophthalmic drug is being used, administer the drugs at least 5 min apart.
- Inform patient that this medication may cause a gradual increase in brown pigment in the pupil, which may slowly change eye color.
- Inform patient that this medication may also cause eyelid skin darkening and increases in length, thickness, color, and number of eyelashes.
- Advise patient to contact the eye doctor if eye or eyelid inflammation is noted, if eye injury occurs, or if planning eye surgery.
- Remind patient that eye examinations and measurement of IOP will be necessary while using this medication and to keep appointments.

Leflunomide

(leh-FLEW-nah-mide)

Class Antirheumatic agent

How Supplied
Arava Tablet 10 mg, Tablet 20 mg, Tablet 100 mg

Action
PHARMACOLOGY: An isoxazole immunomodulatory agent that inhibits dihydroorotate dehydrogenase and has antiproliferative and anti-inflammatory activity.

PHARMACOKINETICS/DYNAMICS:

Absorption: The T_{max} of active metabolite is 6 to 12 hr. Without a loading dose (100 mg/3 days), steady-state plasma concentration would require nearly 2 mo of dosing. Plasma levels are dose-proportional. High-fat food does not affect absorption.

Distribution: Vd_{ss} is 0.13 L/kg. Greater than 99.3% protein bound.

Metabolism: The specific site of metabolism is unknown. The major active metabolite responsible for all activity is A77#1726 (M1); 4-trifluor-methylaniline is the minor metabolite.

Excretion: The t½ is approximately 2 wk. Renally excreted as well as by direct biliary excretion. Renal excretion is more significant in the first 96 hr. Eliminated in urine (43%) and feces (48%). Primary urinary metabolites are leflunomide glucoronide and oxanilic acid derivative of M1. Primary fecal metabolite is M1.

Special Populations:
Hepatic Function Impairment – Studies have not been done; however, leflunomide is not recommended in these patients.
Tobacco use – Tobacco use has a 38% increase in Cl over nonsmokers; however, no difference in clinical efficacy was seen between smokers and nonsmokers.

Indications
Treatment of active rheumatoid arthritis (RA) to reduce signs and symptoms and to retard structural damage.

Contraindications
Pregnancy; standard considerations.

Route/Dosage
Loading dose:
PO 100 mg qd for 3 days.
Maintenance therapy:
PO 20 mg qd. If dosing at 20 mg/day is not well-tolerated, the dose may be decreased to 10 mg/day.

Interactions
Cholestyramine and charcoal: Decrease plasma leflunomide.
Hepatotoxic drugs: May potentiate the hepatotoxicity of leflunomide.
NSAIDs and tolbutamide: Free-fraction serum concentrations were increased by leflunomide.

Rifampin: May increase leflunomide serum levels.

Lab Test Interferences May cause hypophosphaturia. May cause an increase in uric acid excretion.

Adverse Reactions

CV: Hypertension; chest pain; palpitation; tachycardia; varicose vein; vasculitis; vasodilation.
CNS: Dizziness; headache; paresthesia; anxiety; depression; dry mouth; insomnia; neuralgia; neuritis; sleep disorder; vertigo; migraine.
DERM: Alopecia; eczema; pruritus; rash; dry skin; abscess; cyst; Stevens-Johnson syndrome and toxic epidermal necrolysis (rare, discontinue drug if symptoms occur).
ENDO: Diabetes mellitus; hyperthyroidism.
GI: Abdominal pain; anorexia; diarrhea; dyspepsia; gastroenteritis; nausea; mouth ulcer; vomiting.
GU: Albuminuria; cystitis; dysuria; hematuria; menstrual disorder; prostate disorder; urinary frequency; vaginal moniliasis.
HEMA/LYMPH: Anemia; ecchymosis.
HEPA: Abnormal liver enzymes.
HYPERSEN: Allergic reaction.
M/N: Increased CPK; hyperglycemia; hyperlipidemia; hypokalemia.
MUSC: Arthralgia; leg cramps; joint disorder; synovitis; tenosynovitis; arthrosis; bone necrosis; bone pain; bursitis; muscle cramps; myalgia; tendon rupture.
RESP: Bronchitis; increased cough; respiratory infection; pharyngitis; pneumonia; rhinitis; sinusitis; asthma; dyspnea; epistaxis; lung disorder.
SPEC SENSE: Blurred vision; cataract; conjunctivitis; eye disorder; taste perversion.
OTHER: Peripheral edema; weight loss; UTI; asthenia; flu syndrome; infection; injury; accident; pain; back pain; fever; hernia; malaise; neck pain; pelvic pain; increased sweating.

> **WARNING:**
> Contraindicated in pregnancy. Pregnancy must be excluded prior to initiation of therapy. Ensure reliable use of contraception in women with childbearing potential during therapy. Patient must avoid pregnancy prior to completion of the drug elimination procedure after leflunomide treatment.

Precautions

Pregnancy: Category X.
Lactation: Do not use in nursing mothers. It is not known if leflunomide is excreted in human milk.
Children: Not established.
Elderly: No dosage adjustment is needed in patients older than 65 yr.
Special risk patients: Renal impairment; immunocompromise; bone marrow dysplasia; severe, uncontrolled infections; pre-existing hepatic disease.
Drug elimination procedure: Without the drug elimination procedure, it may take up to 2 yr to reach plasma M1 metabolite levels less than 0.02 mg/L because of individual variation in drug Cl. Recommended to achieve nondetectable plasma levels (less than 0.02 mg/L) after stopping treatment:

- Administer cholestyramine 8 g 3 times daily for 11 days. (The 11 days do not need to be consecutive unless there is a need to lower the plasma level rapidly.)
- Verify plasma levels less than 0.02 mg/L by 2 separate tests at least 14 days apart. If plasma levels are more than 0.02 mg/L, consider additional cholestyramine treatment.

PATIENT CARE CONSIDERATIONS

Administration/Storage

- Administer qd without regard to meals.
- Do not administer until baseline liver enzymes have been evaluated.
- Do not administer to women of childbearing potential until negative pregnancy test has been obtained and patient is on reliable contraception.
- Store at controlled room temperature (59° to 86°F); protect from light.

Assessment/Interventions

- Obtain patient history, including drug history and any known allergies.
- Note history of kidney or liver disease and positive hepatitis B or C serology. Note presence of severe immunodeficiency state or severe, uncontrolled infection.
- Ensure that baseline liver enzymes (eg, ALT) are determined before starting therapy and periodically (eg, monthly) during therapy.
- Ensure that a woman of childbearing potential has a negative pregnancy test and is on reliable contraception before starting therapy.

Patient/Family Education

- Explain name, dose, action, and potential side effects of drug.
- Review usual dosing schedule with patient: 100 mg qd for 3 days (loading dose) then 20 mg qd for maintenance. Warn patient that taking more of the drug than prescribed can result in serious side effects, including liver damage.
- Advise patient that drug may be taken without regard to meals.

- Remind patient that other medications for RA may still be taken while taking this drug.
- Advise women that this drug may cause birth defects.
- Advise women to use effective contraception during treatment and not to attempt to become pregnant after stopping the drug until they have gone through the drug elimination procedure.
- Advise men wishing to father a child not to do so unless they have stopped the drug and have taken cholestyramine (part of drug elimination procedure) for 11 days.
- Advise patient to avoid live vaccines while taking this drug.
- Advise patient that diarrhea, nausea, indigestion, and headache are common side effects and to inform health care provider if they occur and are intolerable.
- Advise women to notify health care provider if pregnant, planning to become pregnant, or breastfeeding.
- Instruct patient not to take prescription or OTC medications or dietary supplements without consulting the health care provider.
- Remind patient that office visits and laboratory tests will be required to monitor therapy and to keep appointments.

Lepirudin

(LEP-ih-ruh-din)

Class Anticoagulant

How Supplied
Refludan Powder for Injection 50 mg

Action
PHARMACOLOGY: One molecule of lepirudin (rDNA) binds to 1 molecule of thrombin and blocks the thrombogenic activity of thrombin.

PHARMACOKINETICS/DYNAMICS:
Distribution: Following IV administration, distribution is confined to extracellular fluids and is characterized by an initial t½ of approximately 10 min.

Metabolism: Lepirudin is thought to be metabolized by release of amino acids via catabolic hydrolysis.

Excretion: Elimination follows first order kinetics and is characterized by a terminal t½ of approximately 1.3 hr. About 48% of the administered dose is excreted in the urine (35% unchanged).

Special Populations:
Renal Function Impairment – In patients with marked renal insufficiency (Ccr less than 15 mL/min) and on hemodialysis, the elimination t½ is prolonged up to 2 days.
Elderly – Systemic Cl is 20% lower in elderly than in younger patients.
Gender – Systemic Cl is about 25% lower in women than men.

Indications Anticoagulation in patients with heparin-induced thrombocytopenia and associated thromboembolic disease to prevent further thromboembolic complications. **Unlabeled use(s):** Adjunct therapy for treatment of unstable angina; acute MI without ST elevation; prevention of deep vein thrombosis; patients undergoing percutaneous coronary intervention.

Contraindications Hypersensitivity to hirudins or any component of the product.

Route/Dosage
Heparin-Induced Thrombocytopenia
ADULTS: **IV** 0.4 mg/kg (up to 110 kg body weight) slowly (eg, over 15 to 20 sec) as a bolus followed by 0.15 mg/kg (up to 110 kg/hr of body weight) as a continuous IV infusion for 2 to 10 days or longer if clinically needed.

Dose Modification
ADULTS: **IV** If the confirmed APTT ratio is below the target range, increase the infusion rate in steps of 20% and determine the APTT ratio again 4 hr later. Do not exceed an infusion rate of 0.21 mg/kg/hr without checking for coagulation abnormalities that might prevent an appropriate APTT response. If the confirmed APTT ratio is above the target range, stop the infusion for 2 hr. At restart, decrease the infusion 50% and determine the APTT ratio again 4 hr later.

Renal Function Impairment
ADULTS: **IV** Reduce the dose if there is known or suspected renal insufficiency (Ccr less than 60 mL/min or serum creatinine above 1.5 mg/dL). In addition to monitoring renal status, APTT monitoring should be used. In all patients with renal insufficiency, the bolus dose is to be reduced to 0.2 mg/kg. Reduce the standard initial infusion rate as follows – Ccr 45 to 60 mL/min or serum creatinine 1.6 to 2 mg/dL – Administer at 50% of the standard infusion rate (0.075 mg/kg/hr). Ccr 30 to 44 mL/min or serum creatinine 2.1 to 3 mg/dL – Administer at 30% of the standard infusion rate (0.045 mg/kg/hr). Ccr 15 to 29 mL/min or serum creatine 3.1 to 6 mg/dL – Administer at 15% of the standard infusion rate (0.0225 mg/kg/hr). Less than 15 mL/min or serum creatine greater than 6 mg/dL – Avoid or stop infusion.

Concomitant Use of Thrombolytic Therapy
ADULTS: **IV** Initial bolus of 0.2 mg/kg followed by continuous infusion of 0.1 mg/kg/hr.

Switching to Oral Anticoagulants
ADULTS: Gradually reduce the lepirudin dose to reach an APTT ratio just above 1.5 before initi-

ating oral anticoagulation. Initiate coumarin derivatives only when platelet counts are normalizing. Start maintenance dose with no loading dose. To avoid prothrombotic effects when initiating coumarin, continue parenteral anticoagulation for 4 to 5 days.

Interactions
Coumarin derivatives (eg, vitamin K antagonists), thrombolytics (eg, alteplase, streptokinase): Risk of bleeding may be increased.

Lab Test Interferences
None well documented.

Adverse Reactions
CV: Heart failure (2%).
DERM: Bleeding from puncture sites and wounds (11%); allergic skin reactions (4%).
EENT: Epistaxis (4%).
GI: GI and rectal bleeding (5%).
GU: Hematuria (4%); vaginal bleeding (2%).
HEMA: Anemia or isolated drop in hemoglobin (12%); sepsis (4%).
HEPA: Abnormal liver function (5%).
RENAL: Abnormal renal function (2%).
RESP: Pneumonia (4%).
OTHER: Hematoma or unclassified bleeding (11%); fever, multiorgan failure (4%); unspecified infections (2%); intracranial bleeding; allergic reactions (including cough, bronchospasm, stridor, dyspnea [1% to less than 10%]); anaphylactic reactions (postmarketing).

Precautions
Pregnancy: Category B.
Lactation: Undetermined.
Children: Safety and efficacy not established.
Hypersensitivity: Allergic and hypersensitivity reactions, including anaphylaxis (resulting in shock or death), can occur.
Renal function impairment: Adjust the dose as indicated.
Hepatic function impairment: May enhance the anticoagulant effect.
Hemorrhagic events: Hemorrhagic events may occur at any site.
Intracranial bleeding: Life-threatening intracranial bleeding may occur with coadministration of thrombolytic therapy (eg, alteplase, streptokinase).

Overdosage: Signs and Symptoms
Bleeding.

PATIENT CARE CONSIDERATIONS

Administration/Storage
- For IV administer only. Not for intradermal, IM, or SC administration.
- Follow manufacturer's instructions for reconstitution of powder and dilution of reconstituted solution.
- Use reconstituted solution immediately. Discard any unused infusion solution after 24 hr.
- Refer to manufacturer's insert for compatibility with IV fluids and other medications.
- Inspect solution visually before administration. Do not administer if solution is cloudy, discolored, or contains particulate matter.
- Warm solution to room temperature before administration.
- Administer initial dose as slow IV bolus over 15 to 20 sec. Follow bolus dose with continuous IV infusion as ordered.
- Store unopened vials in refrigerator (36° to 46°F) or at controlled room temperature (59° to 77°F). Reconstituted solution remains stable for up to 24 hr at room temperature (eg, during infusion).

Assessment/Interventions
- Obtain patient history, including drug history and any known allergies. Note history of the following: renal impairment, liver disease, recent puncture of large vessel or organ, severe uncontrolled hypertension, recent CVA, stroke, intracerebral surgery or other neuraxial procedures, recent major surgery, bacterial endocarditis, recent major bleeding, recent peptic ulcer, anomaly of blood vessels or organs, or hemostatic defect.
- Note coadministration of thrombolytic agent, vitamin K antagonist, or anti- platelet agent.
- Follow manufacturer's guidelines for administrating reduced bolus and maintenance doses to patient with renal impairment or to patient receiving thrombolytic therapy.
- Ensure that baseline hematocrit or hemoglobin, platelet count, and APTT ratio (patient APTT over APTT reference value) are performed and evaluated prior to starting therapy.
- Do not initiate therapy if baseline APTT ratio is 2.5 or greater.
- Ensure that APTT ratio is determined 4 hr after start of therapy and after every dosage adjustment, and at least q 24 hr thereafter during therapy.
- Ensure that dosage is adjusted to maintain APTT ratio between 1.5 and 2.5 following manufacturer's recommendations for dosage adjustments.
- Monitor patient for signs of bleeding throughout therapy. If bleeding develops (eg, epistaxis, hematuria, hematemesis, bloody or black, tarry stools) or is suspected (eg, unexplained fall in hematocrit or BP or any unexplained symptoms), notify health care provider immediately.

- Monitor patient for signs of anaphylaxis or severe allergic reaction. Discontinue therapy and immediately notify health care provider if noted. Be prepared to treat appropriately.

Patient/Family Education
- Explain name, action, and potential side effects of drug.
- Advise patient, family, or caregiver that medication will be prepared and administered by a health care professional in a hospital setting.
- Instruct patient, family member, or caregiver to report any signs of bleeding or allergic reaction immediately.

Letrozole

(let-ROW-zahl)

Class Nonsteroidal aromatase inhibitor

How Supplied
Femara Tablets 2.5 mg.

Action
PHARMACOLOGY: A nonsteroidal competitive inhibitor of the aromatase enzyme system; it inhibits the conversion of androgens to estrogens.

PHARMACOKINETICS/DYNAMICS:
Distribution: It is weakly protein bound.
Excretion: Renal excretion is the major pathway of letrozole clearance. Elimination t½ is approximately 2 days.

Indications
Advanced breast cancer in postmenopausal women with disease progression following antiestrogen therapy; first-line treatment of postmenopausal women with hormone receptor positive or hormone receptor unknown locally advanced or metastatic cancer.

Contraindications
Standard considerations.

Route/Dosage
Breast Cancer
ADULTS: PO 2.5 mg once daily (tablets).

Interactions
Contraceptives, oral: May alter the efficacy of oral contraceptives.
Tamoxifen: Plasma concentrations of letrozole may be decreased.

Lab Test Interferences
None well documented.

Adverse Reactions
CV: Chest pain; hypertension; peripheral edema.
CNS: Decreased appetite; fatigue; headache; insomnia; somnolence; dizziness; asthenia; weakness.
DERM: Rash; pruritus; alopecia.
GI: Nausea and vomiting; constipation; diarrhea; abdominal pain; anorexia; dyspepsia.
GU: Sexual inactivity; atrophy of the female reproductive organs; breast pain.
METAB: Hot flashes; weight gain; hypercholesterolemia; weight loss.
RESP: Dyspnea; coughing.
OTHER: Viral infections; musculoskeletal pain; arthralgia; flu-like symptoms.

Precautions
Pregnancy: Category D.
Lactation: Undetermined.
Children: Safety and efficacy not established.
Hepatic function impairment: Use caution in patients with severe hepatic dysfunction.

PATIENT CARE CONSIDERATIONS

Administration/Storage
- Store at controlled room temperature (59° and 86°F).
- Administer PO; may be taken without regard to meals.

Assessment/Interventions
- Obtain patient history, including drug history and any known allergies. Note history of liver disease.
- Monitor for GI, CNS, musculoskeletal, and general body side effects. Inform health care provide if noted and significant.

Patient/Family Education
- Explain name, dose, action, and potential side effects of drug.
- Review dosing schedule with patient.
- Advise patient that medication can be taken without regard to meals, but to take with food if GI upset occurs.
- Advise patient that if a dose is missed, take it as soon as possible, but if close to the next dose, do not double the dose to catch up and take the next dose as scheduled.
- Advise patient to report persistent or intolerable side effects to health care provider.
- Instruct patient to not take any prescription or OTC medications or dietary supplements unless advised to do so by the health care provider.
- Advise patient that follow-up examinations and lab tests will be required to monitor therapy and to keep appointments.

Leucovorin Calcium (Citrovorum Factor; Folinic Acid)

(loo-koe-VORE-in KAL-see-uhm)

Class Folic acid derivative

How Supplied
Wellcovorin Tablets 5 mg, Tablets 25 mg
🍁 *Lederle Leucovorin Calcium*

Action
PHARMACOLOGY: Acts as antidote to drugs that antagonize folic acid, such as methotrexate.

PHARMACOKINETICS/DYNAMICS:

Absorption: Following a 25-mg dose C_{max} is 393 ng/mL (160 to 550 ng/mL), T_{max} is 2.3 hr, and apparent bioavailability is 97% for 25-mg dose.

Metabolism: Metabolites are L-leucovorin, d-leucovorin, and 5-methyl-THF.

Excretion: Terminal $t_{½}$ is 5.7 hr.

Indications
Oral and parenteral: Treatment to diminish toxicity and counteract effect of overdosage of folic acid antagonists.

Parenteral: Treatment of megaloblastic anemia caused by folic acid deficiency when oral therapy is not feasible.

Contraindications
Pernicious anemia and other megaloblastic anemias secondary to vitamin B_{12} deficiency.

Route/Dosage

Colorectal Cancer
ADULTS: **IV** Either 200 mg/m^2 followed by 5-fluorouracil (5-FU) 370 mg/m^2 or 20 mg/m^2 followed by 5-FU 425 mg/m^2 qd for 5 days.

Leucovorin Rescue
ADULTS: **PO/IV/IM** 10 mg/m^2 q 6 hr for 10 doses.

Megaloblastic Anemia Caused by Folic Acid Deficiency
ADULTS: **IV/IM** 1 mg/day.

Interactions
Barbiturates, hydantoins (eg, phenytoin), primidone: May decrease anticonvulsant activity.
Fluorouracil: Enhances toxicity of fluorouracil.
Methotrexate: May decrease efficacy of intrathecal methotrexate.

Lab Test Interferences
None well documented.

Adverse Reactions
OTHER: Hypersensitivity, including anaphylaxis and urticaria. No other adverse reactions have been attributed to leucovorin alone.

Precautions
Pregnancy: Category C.
Lactation: Undetermined.
Benzyl alcohol: Present in 1 mL amp and some diluents. Benzyl alcohol has been associated with fatal "gasping syndrome" in premature infants.
5-FU toxicity: Leucovorin enhances toxicity of 5-FU; decrease dosage. Administer only under supervision of health care provider experienced in use of antimetabolite cancer chemotherapy.

PATIENT CARE CONSIDERATIONS

Administration/Storage
- When drug is given for leucovorin rescue after high-dose methotrexate therapy, administer first dose 24 hr after beginning methotrexate infusion.
- When drug is given as antidote for inadvertent overdosage of folic acid antagonists (eg, methotrexate), administer as soon as overdose is detected, preferably within first hour.
- Reconstitute parenteral solution using Bacteriostatic Water for Injection or Sterile Water for Injection. Bacteriostatic water mixtures must be used within 7 days; sterile water mixtures, immediately. If doses more than 10 mg/m^2 are needed, reconstitute with Sterile Water for Injection.
- Administer IV solution slowly, at rate of less than 160 mg/min, because of calcium content.
- If necessary, further dilution with 100 to 500 mL dextrose or saline solutions for intermittent infusion is possible.
- Tablets can be crushed if necessary.
- Store at room temperature and protect from light.

Assessment/Interventions
- Obtain patient history, including drug history and any known allergies.
- Ensure that baseline laboratory values, including liver and renal function tests, CBC, and platelet count, have been obtained before beginning therapy and monitor during treatment.
- Ensure that daily methotrexate levels are obtained when leucovorin is used for high-dose methotrexate rescue.
- Keep patient well hydrated. Carefully monitor I&O during treatment.

Patient/Family Education
- Instruct patient not to double up doses, and to notify health care provider if dose is missed.

- Instruct patient to report the following symptoms to health care provider: nausea, vomiting, diarrhea, sores in mouth, fatigue, difficulty breathing or skin disorders.
- Advise patient to notify health care provider if unable to keep dose down (ie, if vomiting occurs). Patient may need IM or IV therapy instead of oral medication.

Leuprolide Acetate

(loo-PRO-lide ASS-uh-TATE)

Class Gonadotropin-releasing hormone

How Supplied
Lupron Depot Microspheres for injection, lyophilized 3.75 mg, Microspheres for injection, lyophilized 7.5 mg/mL ♦ *Lupron Depot-3 Month* Microspheres for injection, lyophilized 11.25 mg, Microspheres for injection, lyophilized 22.5 mg ♦ *Lupron Depot-4 Month* Microspheres for injection, lyophilized 30 mg ♦ *Lupron Depot-Ped* Microspheres for injection, lyophilized 7.5 mg, Microspheres for injection, lyophilized 11.25 mg, Microspheres for injection, lyophilized 15 mg ♦ *Lupron for Pediatric Use* Injection 5 mg/mL ♦ *Viadur* Implant 72 mg

✤ *Lupron Depot 3.75 mg/11.25 mg* ♦ *Lupron/Lupron Depot 3.75 mg/7.5 mg* ♦ *Lupron/Lupron Depot 7.5 mg/22.5 mg/30 mg*

Action
PHARMACOLOGY: A synthetic luteinizing hormone-releasing hormone (LHRH) agonist of greater potency than naturally occurring gonadotropin-releasing hormone (GnRH). Occupies pituitary GnRH receptors and thus desensitizes them, inhibiting gonadotropin secretion required for gonadal production of testosterone and estrogen.

PHARMACOKINETICS/DYNAMICS:
Absorption:
Injection – Not active orally. Bioavailability SC is comparable to IV. C_{max} is 4.6 to 10.2 ng/mL. T_{max} is 4 hr.

Distribution:
Implant/Injection – Protein binding is 43% to 49%. Mean Vd_{ss} is 27 L.

Metabolism:
Implant – Major metabolite is pentapeptide (M-1).
Injection – Inactive metabolites: pentapeptide (metabolite I); tripeptides (metabolite II and III); dipeptide (metabolite IV).

Excretion:
Implant – Terminal t½ is 3 hr.
Injection – Plasma t½ is 3 hr.

Indications Palliative treatment of advanced prostatic cancer (alone or in combination with flutamide); management of endometriosis in women over 18 yr (depot preparation); treatment of children with central precocious puberty (CPP [pediatric injection or depot pediatric]); uterine leiomyomata (depot preparation).
Unlabeled use(s): Breast and ovarian carcinoma.

Contraindications Pregnancy; lactation; hypersensitivity to GnRH, GnRH agonist analogs, or product components; undiagnosed vaginal bleeding.

Route/Dosage
Advanced Prostate Cancer
ADULTS: SC 1 mg/day. IM 7.5 mg q mo (depot preparation).

CPP
ADULTS: **SC** Starting dose: 50 mcg/kg/day as single injection. Individualize dosage and titrate to response.

ADULTS: **IM** Starting dose: 0.3 mg/kg q 4 wk (minimum, 7.5 mg) as single injection (depot preparation). Must be administered by health care provider or designated health care provider.

Endometriosis
ADULTS: **IM** 3.75 mg as single monthly injection or 11.25 mg IM q 3 mo (depot preparation).

Uterine Leiomyomata
ADULTS: **IM** 3.75 mg as a single monthly injection or 11.25 mg IM q 3 mo.

Interactions None well documented.

Lab Test Interferences Diagnostic tests of pituitary gonadotropic and gonadal functions during treatment and up to 12 wk after discontinuing depot preparation may be misleading.

Adverse Reactions
CV: Arrhythmias; edema; angina or hypertension rarely.
CNS: Mental depression; headache; decreased libido.
DERM: Erythema; ecchymosis; irritation at injection site; acne.
ENDO: Hot flashes; gynecomastia.
GU: Vaginitis; vaginal dryness; impotence; testicular atrophy; amenorrhea; infertility.
MUSC: Decreased bone density; symptom flare, manifested by increased bone pain during first 1 to 2 wk of therapy in patients with bone metastases.

Precautions
Pregnancy: Category X. Use a nonhormonal method of contraception.
Lactation: Undetermined.
Children: Safety and efficacy of injection not

established; depot preparation recommended for CPP.

Hypersensitivity: Injection contains benzyl alcohol, which can cause local hypersensitivity reactions. Depot preparation is preservative-free.

Bone density changes: Use of depot preparation may result in decreased bone density. Decreased bone mineral content risk factors may cause additional bone loss with long-term use.

PATIENT CARE CONSIDERATIONS
Administration/Storage
- Use syringes included in the kit or low-dose insulin syringes (SC). Do not use needles smaller than 22-gauge (IM). Rotate injection sites.
- Reconstitute depot form only with diluent provided. Reconstituted suspension will appear milky. Suspension is stable for 24 hr after reconstitution.
- Store unreconstituted depot form at room temperature.
- Refrigerate injection (nondepot form) until used for first dose. May then be stored at room temperature until contents of vial have been administered. Protect from light.
- Store implant at room temperature.

Assessment/Interventions
- Obtain patient history, including drug history and any known allergies.
- Ensure that baseline laboratory tests (eg, testosterone, acid phosphase) have been obtained before beginning therapy and monitor periodically thereafter.
- Monitor I&O carefully and assess for bladder distention with prostate cancer. Transient exacerbation of symptoms (eg, urinary obstruction, hematuria) occurs in many patients during first week of therapy.

Patient/Family Education
- Caution patient that depot preparation must not be taken during pregnancy or when pregnancy is possible. Advise patient to use reliable form of birth control while taking this drug.
- Advise patient/family to follow prescribed regimen. Do not alter dose or discontinue therapy without consulting health care provider.
- Instruct patient on proper injection technique and have patient perform return demonstration.
- Advise patient to use nonhormonal forms of birth control because menstrual irregularities may occur.
- Inform patient that burning, itching, or swelling may develop at injection site, and to notify health care provider if these symptoms worsen.
- Advise patient that increased bone pain and difficulty urinating may occur in early treatment of prostate cancer.
- With patients receiving drug for CPP, inform family that menses or spotting may occur initially but to notify health care provider if symptoms continue beyond second month.
- Inform patients receiving drug for endometriosis/uterine leiomyomata that menstruation should stop and to notify health care provider if it persists.

Levalbuterol Hydrochloride

(lev-al-BYOO-ter-ol)

Class Bronchodilator/Sympathomimetic

How Supplied
Xopenex Solution for inhalation 0.31 mg levalbuterol per 3 mL, Solution for inhalation 0.63 mg levalbuterol per 3 mL, Solution for inhalation 1.25 mg levalbuterol per 3 mL

Action
PHARMACOLOGY: Produces bronchodilation by relaxing bronchial smooth muscles via beta$_2$-adrenergic receptor stimulation.

PHARMACOKINETICS/DYNAMICS:
Absorption: T_{max} is approximately 0.2 hr. C_{max} is approximately 1.1 to 4.5 ng/mL (dose-dependent). AUC is approximately 3.3 to 17.4 ng•hr/mL (dose dependent).

Excretion: The t½ is approximately 3 to 4 hr.
Onset: 17 min (0.63 mg); 10 min (1.25 mg).
Peak: Approximately 1.5 hr.
Duration: Approximately 5 to 8 hr.

Special Populations:
Children – AUC increases; use lower dose (children 6 to 11 yr of age).

Indications Treatment or prevention of bronchospasm in patients with reversible obstructive airway disease.

Contraindications Hypersensitivity to levalbuterol or racemic albuterol.

Route/Dosage
ADULTS AND CHILDREN AT LEAST 12 YR OF AGE: **Inhalation solution** Usual starting dose is 0.63 mg tid (q 6 to 8 hr) by nebulization. Patients with more severe asthma or patients who do not respond adequately to the 0.63 mg dose may benefit from 1.25 mg tid.

CHILDREN 6 THROUGH 11 YR OF AGE: **Inhalation solution** Recommended dose is 0.31 mg tid by nebulization (max, 0.63 mg tid).

Interactions
Beta-blockers (eg, propranolol): Severe bronchospasms may be produced in asthmatic patients taking levalbuterol.
Digoxin: Plasma digoxin levels may be decreased.
Diuretics (eg, loop [eg, furosemide] and thiazide [hydrochlorothiazide]): ECG changes and hypokalemia associated with diuretic therapy may be worsened by levalbuterol administration.
MAO inhibitors (eg, phenelzine), tricyclic antidepressants (eg, amitriptyline): The action of levalbuterol on the vascular system may be potentiated.

Lab Test Interferences
None well documented.

Adverse Reactions
CV: Tachycardia; migraine; abnormal ECG and ECG changes; hypertension; hypotension; syncope.
CNS: Dizziness, nervousness, tremor, anxiety, hypesthesia of the hand, insomnia, paresthesia; headache (children 6 to 11 yr of age).
DERM: Eczema, rash, urticaria (children 6 to 11 yr of age).
EENT: Rhinitis, sinusitis, turbinate edema, dry throat, eye itch; pharyngitis, otitis media (children 6 to 11 yr of age).
GI: Dyspepsia; diarrhea; dry mouth; gastroenteritis; nausea.
RESP: Increased cough; viral infection.
OTHER: Flu-like symptoms, accidental injury, pain, leg cramps, lymphadenopathy, myalgia; abdominal pain, asthma, fever (children 6 to 11 yr of age).

Precautions
Pregnancy: Category C.
Lactation: Undetermined.
Children: Safety and efficacy not established in children less than 6 yr of age.
Hypersensitivity: Immediate hypersensitivity reactions may occur.
Special risk patients: Use with caution in patients with CV disorders, convulsive disorders, hyperthyroidism, or diabetes, and in patients unusually responsive to sympathomimetic amines.
Bronchospasm: Life-threatening paradoxical bronchospasm may occur.
CV effects: Clinically important CV effects, as measured by pulse rate and BP, may occur; use with caution in patients with CV disorders, especially coronary insufficiency, cardiac arrhythmias, and hypotension.
CNS effects: CNS stimulation may occur; use with caution in patients with a history of seizures or hyperthyroidism.
Deterioration of asthma: A dosage requirement increase may indicate destabilization of asthma, requiring re-evaluation of the treatment regimen.
Diabetes mellitus: Use with caution.

Overdosage: Signs and Symptoms
Seizures, angina, hypertension, hypotension, tachycardia, arrhythmias, nervousness, headache, tremor, dry mouth, palpitation, nausea, dizziness, fatigue, malaise, sleeplessness, hypokalemia, cardiac arrest, death.

PATIENT CARE CONSIDERATIONS

Administration/Storage
- This medication is available only as an inhalation solution.
- Administer only via nebulizer. Not for injection or oral use.
- Administer prescribed dose q 6 to 8 hr as needed.
- Medication requires no dilution before administration and is added directly into the nebulizer reservoir.
- Once vial has been opened, administer immediately or discard.
- Discard solution if not colorless.
- Discard any unused solution.
- Do not mix with other nebulized medications unless ordered by health care provider.
- Store unused vials in protective foil pouch between 68° and 77°F. Once the foil pouch is opened, use vials within 2 wk. If vials are removed from pouch and not used immediately, use within 1 wk. Protect vials from light and excessive heat.

Assessment/Interventions
- Obtain patient history, including drug history and any known allergies. Note history of coronary artery disease, arrhythmias, hypertension, seizures, hyperthyroidism, diabetes, unusual sensitivity to sympathomimetic amines, or concurrent or recent (within 2 wk) use of MAO inhibitor or tricyclic antidepressant.
- Ensure that baseline pulmonary function tests have been completed.
- Note frequency and severity of asthma attacks.
- Monitor pulse, BP, respiratory rate, and lung sounds before and after treatment. Notify health care provider of unexpected or unusual findings.
- Monitor patient's respiratory status during

each treatment. If bronchospasm worsens during a treatment, discontinue the treatment and notify health care provider immediately.
* Notify health care provider if patient needs treatments on an increasingly frequent basis.
* Monitor patient for GI, CNS, CV, RESP, and general body side effects. Notify health care provider if noted and significant.

Patient/Family Education
* Explain name, dose, action, and potential side effects of drug.
* Advise patient to review illustrated *Patient's Instructions for Use*. Ensure that patient, family, or caregiver can prepare, use, and clean the nebulizer without difficulty.
* Instruct patient not to mix nebulizer medications unless advised by health care provider.
* Instruct patient to use nebulizer solution immediately after opening. If solution is not used immediately, advise patient to discard the solution.
* Advise patient to discard any unused nebulizer solution.
* Instruct patient not to exceed prescribed dose. Advise patient to contact health care provider if this medication no longer seems to control asthma symptoms or if increasing doses of the medicine are needed. These may indicate worsening asthma.
* Advise patients using more than 1 inhaled medication to use this medication first if needed. Take inhaled corticosteroids or other inhaled controller medications last.
* Advise patient that if breathing symptoms worsen during or immediately after using this medication, to stop using it and inform health care provider immediately.
* Inform patient that levalbuterol is not a substitute for inhaled or oral corticosteroids and not to stop or reduce the dose of corticosteroid medication.
* Instruct patient to discontinue use and immediately notify health care provider if eye pain or discomfort, blurred vision, vision halos, or colored images develop in association with red eyes. Advise patient that these symptoms may be associated with a serious problem that will require immediate medical care.
* Advise patient to carry Medi-Alert card indicating asthma or COPD.
* Advise women to notify health care provider if pregnant, planning to become pregnant, or breastfeeding.
* Caution patient not to take any prescription or OTC medications, dietary supplements, or herbal preparations unless advised by health care provider.
* Advise patient that follow-up visits will be required to monitor therapy and to keep appointments.

Levetiracetam

(lev-eh-TEER-ah-see-tam)

Class Anticonvulsant

How Supplied
Keppra Tablets 250 mg, Tablets 500 mg, Tablets 750 mg, Oral solution 100 mg/mL

Action
PHARMACOLOGY: Mechanism unknown; may selectively prevent hypersynchronization of epileptiform burst firing and propagation of seizure activity.

PHARMACOKINETICS/DYNAMICS:

Absorption: T_{max} is 1 hr. Oral bioavailability is 100%. Food does not affect the extent of absorption, but it can decrease C_{max} 20% and delay T_{max} 1.5 hr. Steady state is achieved after 2 days of multiple bid dosing.

Distribution: Linear kinetics over dose range 500 to 5,000 mg. Less than 10% protein bound.

Metabolism: Not extensively metabolized. Major metabolic pathway is the enzymatic hydrolysis of the acetamide group, which produces the carboxylic acid metabolite ucb L057.

Excretion: Plasma t½ is approximately 7 hr. It is eliminated from the systemic circulation by renal excretion as unchanged drug, which represents 66% of dose.

Special Populations:
Renal Function Impairment – Total body Cl decreases 40% in Ccr 50 to 80 mL/min patient. Total body Cl decreases 50% in Ccr 30 to 50 mL/min patient. Total body Cl decreases 60% in Ccr less than 30 mL/min patient. Dosage reduction recommended.
Hepatic Function Impairment –
Severe (Child-Pugh class C): Total body Cl decreases 50%. No dosage adjustment needed.
Elderly – Total body Cl decreased 38% and the t½ was 2.5 hr longer.
Children – Cl approximately 40% higher (children 6 to 12 yr of age).
Gender – C_{max} and AUC are 20% higher in women.

Indications Adjunctive therapy in partial onset seizures in adults with epilepsy.

Contraindications Standard considerations.

Route/Dosage
ADULTS: **PO** Initiate therapy with 500 mg bid; dose may be increased by 1,000 mg/day q 2 wk to a max daily dose of 3,000 mg.

Dosage Adjustment for Renal Impairment
For mild renal impairment (Ccr 50 to 80 mL/min), give 500 to 1,000 mg q 12 hr. For moderate impairment (Ccr 30 to 50 mL/min), give 250 mg to 750 mg q 12 hr. For severe impairment (Ccr less than 30 mL/min), give 250 to 500 mg q 12 hr. For patients on dialysis, give 500 to 1,000 mg q 12 hr (following dialysis, a 250 to 500 mg supplemental dose is recommended.

Interactions None well documented.

Lab Test Interferences None well documented.

Adverse Reactions The following adverse reaction figures were obtained when levetiracetam was added to concomitant antiepileptic drug therapy. The reported frequencies provide 1 basis to estimate the relative contribution to adverse event incidences.
CNS: Somnolence (15%); headache (14%); dizziness (9%); depression, nervousness (4%); ataxia, vertigo (3%); amnesia, anxiety, emotional lability, hostility, paresthesia (2%); confusion, convulsion, grand mal convulsion, insomnia, abnormal thinking, tremor (at least 1%).
DERM: Ecchymosis, rash (at least 1%).
EENT: Pharyngitis (6%); rhinitis (4%); sinusitis, diplopia (2%); amblyopia, otitis media (at least 1%).
GI: Anorexia (3%); constipation, diarrhea, dyspepsia, gastroenteritis, gingivitis, nausea, vomiting (at least 1%).
GU: UTI (at least 1%).
MUSC: Arthralgia (at least 1%).
RESP: Increased cough (2%); bronchitis (at least 1%).
OTHER: Asthenia (15%); infection (13%); pain (7%); abdominal pain, accidental injury, back pain, fever, flu syndrome, fungal infection, chest pain, weight gain (at least 1%).

Precautions
Pregnancy: Category C.
Lactation: Undetermined.
Children: Safety and efficacy not established in patients under 16 yr of age.
Renal function impairment: Use reduced doses.
Withdrawal seizures: Do not discontinue abruptly because of possible increased seizure frequency.
Dialysis patients: Administer supplemental doses because drug is removed during the treatment.
Hematologic abnormalities: Decreases in red blood cell count, hemoglobin, and hematocrit were seen.

Overdosage: Signs and Symptoms
Drowsiness.

PATIENT CARE CONSIDERATIONS
Administration/Storage
- Administer in combination with other antiepileptic drugs (AEDs).
- Administer prescribed dose bid.
- May be administered without regard to meals. Administer with food if GI upset occurs.
- Administer tablets whole. Caution patient not to break, chew, or crush the tablet.
- Administer oral solution using dosing syringe, medicine dropper, or medicine cup.
- Dose is gradually increased at 2-wk intervals.
- Store tablets and oral solution at controlled room temperature (59° to 86°F).

Assessment/Interventions
- Obtain patient history, including drug history and any known allergies. Note renal impairment.
- Ensure that patient has reviewed the *Patient Information* leaflet before starting therapy.
- Ensure that renal function studies are performed before starting therapy and periodically during therapy.
- Ensure that reduced dose is administered to patient with impaired renal function.
- Frequently assess patient for response to treatment. Notify health care provider if seizures do not improve or appear to worsen.
- Ensure that therapy is periodically reviewed to determine if it needs to be continued without change or if a dose change (eg, increase, decrease, discontinuation) is indicated.
- Avoid sudden discontinuation of therapy to minimize potential of increased seizure frequency. Attempt to gradually reduce dose over a period of several weeks if decision to discontinue medication is made.
- Monitor patient for GI, CNS, RESP, PSYCH, and general body side effects. Report to health care provider if noted and significant.
- Implement safety precautions for patients who experience dizziness or ataxia.

Patient/Family Education
- Explain name, dose, action, and potential side effects of drug.
- Advise patient to read the *Patient Information* leaflet before starting therapy and with each refill.
- Instruct patient, family, or caregiver to continue to take/give other medications for seizures unless advised to do otherwise by health care provider.
- Instruct patient to take exactly as prescribed and not to change the dose or discontinue unless advised by health care provider.

- Advise patient that dose may be gradually increased no more often than q 2 wk until max benefit has been obtained.
- Advise patient to swallow tablets whole and not crush, chew, or break.
- Advise patient using oral solution to measure dose using dosing syringe, dosing dropper, or medicine cup. Caution patient not to measure dose using spoon.
- Advise patient that each dose may be taken without regard to meals but to take with food if stomach upset occurs.
- Advise patient that the most common side effects of therapy are sleepiness, weakness, and dizziness, which can occur at any time but are most common during the first 4 wk of treatment.
- Advise patient that if medication needs to be discontinued, it will be slowly withdrawn over a period of several weeks unless safety concerns (eg, rash) require a more rapid withdrawal.
- Caution patient that drug may cause dizziness, drowsiness, or coordination problems and to use caution while driving or performing other tasks requiring mental alertness or coordination until tolerance is determined.
- Advise women to notify health care provider if pregnant, planning to become pregnant, or breastfeeding.
- Instruct patient to contact health care provider immediately if any of the following occur: extreme sleepiness, tiredness, and weakness; coordination problems; mood or behavior changes (eg, aggression, anger, depression, hostility, irritability, hallucinations, thoughts of suicide).
- Instruct patient to inform health care provider if seizures get worse or if new types of seizures occur.
- Advise patient not to take any prescription or OTC medications, dietary supplements, or herbal preparations unless advised by health care provider.
- Advise patient to carry identification (eg, *Medic Alert*) indicating medication usage and epilepsy.
- Advise patient that follow-up visits will be required to monitor therapy and to keep appointments.

Levobunolol

(LEE-voe-BYOO-no-lahl)

Class Ophthalmic/Glaucoma/Beta-adrenergic blocker

How Supplied
AK-Beta Solution 0.25%, Solution 0.5% ◆ *Betagan Liquifilm* Solution 0.25%, Solution 0.5% ✤ *Apo-Levobunolol* ◆ *Betagan* ◆ *Novo-Levobunolol* ◆ *PMS-Levobunolol* ◆ *ratio-Levobunolol*

Action
PHARMACOLOGY: Reduces IOP by reducing aqueous humor production.

PHARMACOKINETICS/DYNAMICS:
Onset: 1 hr after treatment.
Peak: 2 to 6 hr.
Duration: Up to 24 hr.

Indications
Treatment of IOP in chronic open-angle glaucoma or ocular hypertension.

Contraindications
Bronchial asthma; severe COPD; sinus bradycardia; second- and third-degree AV block; cardiac failure; cardiogenic shock.

Route/Dosage
ADULTS: **Topical** 1 drop in affected eye(s) qd or bid.

Interactions
Beta blockers, oral: Additive effects on systemic beta blockade.
Epinephrine, ophthalmic: Hypertension caused by unopposed alpha-adrenergic stimulation.

Lab Test Interferences None well documented.

Adverse Reactions
CV: Arrhythmia; bradycardia; hypotension; syncope; heart block; cerebrovascular accident; cerebral ischemia; CHF; cardiac arrest.
CNS: Headache; depression.
DERM: Rash.
EENT: Keratitis; blepharoptosis; visual disturbances; diplopia; ptosis; transient burning; stinging; blepharoconjunctivitis; decreased corneal sensitivity.
GI: Nausea.
RESP: Bronchospasm.

Precautions
Pregnancy: Category C.
Lactation: Undetermined.
Children: Safety and efficacy not established.
Special risk patients: Use with caution in patients with cerebrovascular insufficiency and bronchial diseases.
Sulfite sensitivity: Contains metabisulfite, which may cause allergic-type reactions in susceptible persons.
Diabetes mellitus: May mask hypoglycemic symptoms in patients with insulin-dependent diabetes. Use with caution.
Systemic absorption: Adverse effects like those seen with systemic beta-blockers may occur, due to absorption.

Thyroid disorders: May mask clinical signs of hyperthyroidism.

PATIENT CARE CONSIDERATIONS
Administration/Storage
- Position patient with head tilted back. Instruct patient to look upward. Gently depress conjunctival sac to create small area for medication administration.
- Instill medication from ½ to 1 inch from eye. Instilling from greater distance may cause pain and injury.
- Avoid eyelash and eyelid contamination of medication dispenser.
- Compress lacrimal sac for at least 1 min after administration to delay drainage of medication into nasolacrimal duct and to prevent systemic absorption.
- Wait at least 5 min before administering other types of ophthalmic solution.
- Discard medication that has become contaminated by foreign material.
- Store at room temperature. Protect from light.

Assessment/Interventions
- Obtain patient history, including drug history and any known allergies. Note history of cerebrovascular accident, cardiac disease, COPD, or diabetes mellitus.
- Monitor BP and pulse throughout course of therapy.
- Monitor IOP periodically during therapy to determine effectiveness of therapy.
- Observe for loss of corneal sensitivity.
- Be alert for systemic effects, including bradycardia, CHF, cardiac arrhythmias, bronchospasm, and dyspnea.

Overdosage: Signs and Symptoms
Bradycardia, hypotension, bronchospasm, heart failure.

Patient/Family Education
- Instruct patient in proper administration. Advise patient that if dose is missed, it should be administered as soon as possible unless close to time of next dose. Do not double up.
- Caution patient not to stop taking medication unless instructed to do so by health care provider.
- Emphasize importance of washing hands before drug administration and of not allowing dropper to come into contact with any surface including eyelashes.
- Instruct patient to report the following symptoms to health care provider: eye infection, inflammation, rash, itching or decreased vision.
- Instruct patient to notify health care provider immediately if severe or sudden eye pain occurs.
- Advise diabetic patient that drug may mask signs of hypoglycemia and to monitor glucose levels carefully.
- Instruct patient not to take OTC medications or allergy medications without consulting health care provider.
- Advise patient to inform health care provider or dentist of medication regimen before surgical or dental procedures. Gradual withdrawal of medication may be necessary before procedure.
- Explain importance of scheduling regular follow-up examinations while taking medication.

Levodopa

(LEE-voe-DOE-puh)
Class Antiparkinson

How Supplied
Dopar Capsules 100 mg, Capsules 250 mg, Capsules 500 mg

Action
PHARMACOLOGY: Crosses the blood-brain barrier and is converted to dopamine in basal ganglia and periphery.

PHARMACOKINETICS/DYNAMICS:
Absorption: Absorbed from the small bowel. T_{max} is 0.5 to 2 hr and may be delayed in presence of food. Rate of absorption is dependent upon rate of gastric emptying, pH of gastric juice, and length of time drug is exposed.

Distribution: Does not cross the blood-brain barrier.

Metabolism: Metabolites are dopamine and homovanillic acid (HVA). Extensively metabolized (greater than 95%) in the periphery and by the liver.

Excretion: Plasma t½ is 1 to 3 hr. Excreted primarily in the urine; 13% to 42% of HVA excreted in the urine within 24 hr.

Indications Treatment of idiopathic, postencephalitic, and symptomatic parkinsonism.
Unlabeled use(s): Relief of herpes zoster (shingles) pain and restless leg syndrome.

Contraindications Narrow-angle glaucoma; concomitant MAO inhibitor therapy (excluding MAO inhibitor-type B agents such as selegiline); history of or suspected melanoma.

Route/Dosage
ADULTS: **PO** 0.5 to 1 g/day in 2 to 4 divided doses initially. Increase dosage gradually in increments up to 0.75 g/day q 3 to 7 days as tolerated (max, 8 g/day).

Interactions
Anticholinergics, benzodiazepines, hydantoins, methionine, papaverine, pyridoxine, tricyclic antidepressants: May reduce the effectiveness of levodopa.
MAO inhibitors (except selegiline): Causes hypertensive reactions.

Lab Test Interferences
Antiglobulin Coombs' test: With extended therapy, drug may cause false-positive results.
Uric acid study: May result in elevated values with colorimetric method but not with uricase method.

Adverse Reactions
CV: Cardiac irregularity or palpitation; orthostatic hypotension; hypertension; phlebitis.
CNS: Ataxia; headache; dizziness; numbness; weakness; faintness; confusion; insomnia; nightmares; mental changes (eg, psychosis, paranoia, depression, dementia, hallucinations, delusions); agitation; anxiety; fatigue; euphoria; psychopathology; adventitious movements (eg, choreiform or dystonic movements); increased hand tremor; muscle twitching; trismus; bradykinesia ("on-off" phenomenon).
DERM: Flushing; skin rash; sweating.
EENT: Blepharospasm; diplopia; blurred vision; dilated pupils; impaired taste perception; oculogyric crisis.
GI: Anorexia; nausea; vomiting; abdominal pain; distress; dry mouth; dysphagia; excessive salivation; bruxism; GI bleeding; duodenal ulcer.
GU: Urine retention; urinary incontinence; priapism.
HEMA: Hemolytic anemia; anemia; agranulocytosis; leukopenia.
HEPA: Elevated AST, ALT LDH.
RESP: Bizarre breathing patterns.
OTHER: Malaise; hot flashes; weight gain or loss; dark sweat or urine; latent Horner's syndrome; elevated BUN, bilirubin, alkaline phosphatase, and protein-bound iodine; activation of malignant melanoma.

Precautions
Pregnancy: Pregnancy category undetermined.
Lactation: Undetermined. Do not use in nursing mothers.
Children: Safety and efficacy in children less than 12 yr not established.
Concomitant conditions: Use cautiously in patients with severe cardiovascular or pulmonary disease; renal, hepatic or endocrine disease; affective disorder; major psychosis; and cardiac arrhythmias.
Dosage reduction: Decrease levodopa dose 75% to 80% when used in combination with carbidopa.
MI: Administer cautiously to patients with history of MI who have residual arrhythmias. Administer drug in facility with coronary or intensive care unit.
Psychiatric patients: Use cautiously. Observe all patients for development of depression or suicidal ideation.
Upper GI hemorrhage: May occur in patients with prior history of peptic ulcer.

Overdosage: Signs and Symptoms
Shock, coma, blepharospasm, arrhythmias, seizures, CNS depression, muscle twitching.

PATIENT CARE CONSIDERATIONS
Administration/Storage
- Give medication with food to reduce nausea.
- Tablets can be crushed and capsules opened for mixing with small amount of fruit juice for patients being given tube feedings.
- Store at room temperature in light-resistant container.

Assessment/Interventions
- Obtain patient history, including drug history and any known allergies.
- Assess for skin lesions or history of malignant melanoma.
- Determine if patient is receiving MAO inhibitor. MAO inhibitor therapy must be discontinued at least 3 wk before levodopa regimen is instituted.
- Perform complete baseline assessment of parkinsonian signs and symptoms before instituting therapy.
- Monitor BP closely for hypotension if patient is taking antihypertensives concurrently.
- Assist with ambulation during initial phase of therapy because of dizziness caused by hypotension.
- Monitor protein intake because absorption of levodopa is decreased in the presence of high-protein foods.
- If uncontrollable movements, mental changes (eg, depression, paranoia), palpitations, difficult urination, or severe or persistent nausea and vomiting occur, notify health care provider.
- Offer support to patient and family because relief of parkinsonian symptoms may take several wk to mo after therapy is initiated.

Patient/Family Education
- Advise patient to take medication with food.
- Teach patient to avoid sudden position

changes to avoid orthostatic hypotension.
- Inform patient that fluctuation in effectiveness of levodopa sometimes occurs with long-term therapy. Instruct patient to notify health care provider if fluctuation in effectiveness is experienced.
- Advise patient to avoid use of OTC vitamins, fortified cereals and vitamin B_6, which reverse effects of levodopa.
- Warn patient not to increase dosage in an attempt to reduce parkinsonian symptoms more quickly. Noticeable lessening of symptoms may take more than 6 mo to occur.
- Advise patient to report the following symptoms to health care provider: uncontrolled movements, mood or mental changes, irregular heartbeats, difficulty in urination, severe or persistent nausea or vomiting, worsening of parkinsonian symptoms.
- Advise patient that levodopa may cause urine and perspiration to become dark, which is a harmless side effect.
- Inform patient that drug may cause drowsiness and to use caution while driving or performing tasks that require mental alertness.
- Instruct patient to take sips of water frequently, suck on ice chips or sugarless hard candy or chew sugarless gum if dry mouth occurs.

Levodopa/Carbidopa

(LEE-voe-DOE-puh/CAR-bih-doe-puh)

Class Antiparkinson

How Supplied
Sinemet 10/100 Tablets 10 mg carbidopa/100 mg levodopa ♦ *Sinemet 25/100 Tablets* 25 mg carbidopa/100 mg levodopa ♦ *Sinemet 25/250 Tablets* 25 mg carbidopa/250 mg levodopa ♦ *Sinemet CR Tablets,* sustained-release 25 mg carbidopa/100 mg levodopa, Tablets, sustained-release 50 mg carbidopa/200 mg levodopa
✤ *Apo-Levocarb* ♦ *Novo-Levocarbidopa* ♦ *Nu-Levocarb*

Action
PHARMACOLOGY: Levodopa is precursor of dopamine, which is deficient in parkinsonism patients. Carbidopa has no activity of its own but inhibits decarboxylation of levodopa, making it more available to brain.

Indications
Treatment of symptoms of idiopathic Parkinson disease (paralysis agitans), postencephalitic parkinsonism and symptomatic parkinsonism associated with carbon monoxide and manganese poisoning.

Contraindications
Narrow-angle glaucoma; undiagnosed skin lesions or prior history of suspected melanoma; concurrent use of or within 2 wk of MAO inhibitors.

Route/Dosage
Individualize by careful titration. Combination tablets are available in ratios of carbidopa to levodopa of 1:4 (25 mg/100 mg) and 1:10 (10 mg/100 mg; 25 mg/250 mg). Tablets of the 2 ratios may be administered separately or combined prn to provide optimum dosage. Provide at least 70 to 100 mg/day of carbidopa to reduce side effects.

IMMEDIATE-RELEASE TABLETS
ADULTS: **PO** Starting dose: 1 tablet of 25 mg carbidopa/100 mg levodopa tid or 10 mg carbidopa/100 mg levodopa tid to qid. Dosage may be increased by 1 tablet qd or qod prn (max, 8 tablets/day).

SUSTAINED-RELEASE TABLETS (50 MG CARBIDOPA/200 MG LEVODOPA)
ADULTS: **PO** Starting dose: 1 tablet at intervals at least 6 hr. Adjust dosage based on response. Usual range is 2 to 8 tablets/day in divided doses 4 to 8 hr while awake. Allow at least a 3-day interval between adjustments.

Interactions
Antihypertensive drugs: May cause symptomatic orthostatic hypotension.
MAO inhibitors: May result in hypertensive crisis. Use is contraindicated.
Phenothiazines, butyrophenones, phenytoin, and papaverine: May reduce levodopa efficacy.
Tricyclic antidepressants: Rare cases of hypertension and dyskinesia have occurred.

Lab Test Interferences May cause false-positive reaction for urinary ketone bodies (*Clinitest*) and false-negative test results with glucose-oxidase methods of testing for glucosuria (*Clinistix, Tes-tape*).

Adverse Reactions
CV: Cardiac irregularities; palpitations; hypertension; phlebitis; orthostatic hypotension.
CNS: Paranoid delusions; psychotic episodes; depression; suicidal ideation; dementia; convulsions; hallucinations; dizziness; choreiform; dystonic and other involuntary movements.
EENT: Diplopia; blurred vision.
GI: Nausea; anorexia; vomiting; GI distress; epigastric pain; GI bleeding; dry mouth; duodenal ulcer.
GU: Dark urine; urinary retention; urinary incontinence; priapism.
HEMA: Hemolytic and nonhemolytic anemia; thrombocytopenia; leukopenia; agranulocytosis.
HEPA: Elevated LFT results; hepatotoxicity.

OTHER: Positive *Coombs'* test; flushing; malaise.

Precautions
Pregnancy: Safety and effects unknown. Category C (sustained-release).
Lactation: Do not give to nursing mothers.
Special risk patients: Use drug with caution in patients with severe cardiovascular or pulmonary disease, bronchial asthma, or renal, hepatic, or endocrine disease.
Abrupt withdrawal: Rapid withdrawal of antiparkinson drugs may produce symptoms of neuroleptic malignant syndrome.
Dose conversion: Patients previously given levodopa alone should discontinue levodopa use at least 8 hr before starting carbidopa/levodopa. Eventually substitute combination drug at dosage providing about 25% of previous levodopa dose.
GI hemorrhage: Upper GI hemorrhage has been reported in patients with history of peptic ulcer.
MI: Patients with previous history of MI who have residual arrhythmias should have their cardiac function closely monitored on initiating drug dosage adjustment in facility with provisions for intensive cardiac care.
Neurologic/Psychiatric effects: Levodopa may cause involuntary movement and mental disturbances. Use drug with caution in patients with psychosis. Dyskinesias may occur at lower doses and sooner than with levodopa alone. Reduce dosages if necessary.

Overdosage: Signs and Symptoms
Muscle twitching, blepharospasm.

PATIENT CARE CONSIDERATIONS
Administration/Storage
- Do not crush or allow patient to chew sustained-release tablets; however, regular or sustained-release tablet may be cut in half.
- Scored immediate-release tablets may be crushed.
- Administer with food to reduce nausea.
- Do not administer with high-protein foods because they reduce absorption of medication.
- Discontinue levodopa at least 8 hr before initial dose of levodopa/carbidopa.
- Store at room temperature and protect from light.

Assessment/Interventions
- Obtain patient history, including drug history and any known allergies.
- Complete baseline assessment of parkinsonian symptoms before instituting therapy.
- Review baseline CBC and LFT results.
- Determine if patient has taken MAO inhibitors within 3 wk of beginning levodopa/carbidopa therapy.
- Assess for adverse reactions and drug interactions throughout course of therapy.
- Observe for therapeutic effects. Parkinsonian movements are reduced for about 5 hr after administration of medication and then gradually increase in intensity.
- Assess for orthostatic hypotension, dizziness, and mental changes during initial phase of therapy.
- Assist patient with position change and ambulation during initial therapy to prevent falling.
- Monitor BP and pulse routinely throughout therapy.
- Observe patients closely for possible depression or suicidal ideation.
- Monitor cardiac function closely, especially in patients with history of MI.
- Do not administer if significant changes in BP, pulse, or mental status occur. Notify health care provider.

Patient/Family Education
- Teach patient and family how to administer tablets correctly; do not crush or chew sustained-release tablets.
- Instruct patient to report the following symptoms to health care provider: uncontrollable movements, mood or mental changes, irregular heartbeat, difficult urination, severe or persistent nausea or vomiting, appetite loss, dry mouth, difficulty swallowing, or taste distortion.
- Instruct patient to avoid vitamin B_6 (pyridoxine), fortified cereals, and OTC vitamins because they reduce absorption of medication.
- Inform patient that drug may cause harmless darkening of sweat or urine.
- Advise patient that drug may cause drowsiness and to use caution while driving or performing other tasks requiring mental alertness.
- Instruct patient and family about longer onset of action (about 1 hr) during initial phase of therapy. Reduction of Parkinsonian symptoms may take several weeks to months to occur.
- Instruct patient to avoid sudden position changes to prevent orthostatic hypotension.

Levofloxacin

(lee-voe-FLOX-ah-sin)
Class Antibiotic/Fluoroquinolone
How Supplied
Levaquin Tablets 250 mg, Tablets 500 mg, Tablets 750 mg, Injection (concentrate) 500 mg (25 mg/mL), Injection (concentrate) 750 mg (25 mg/mL), Injection (premix) 250 mg (5 mg/mL), Injection (premix) 500 mg (5 mg/mL), Injection (premix) 750 mg (5 mg/mL) ♦ *Quixin* Solution, ophthalmic 0.5% (5 mg/mL)

Action

PHARMACOLOGY: Interferes with microbial DNA synthesis.

PHARMACOKINETICS/DYNAMICS:
Absorption:
Oral – T_{max} is 1 to 2 hr. Food slightly prolongs T_{max} (1 hr) and decreases C_{max} (14%). Can be administered with or without food. About 99% bioavailable. Steady state is reached within 48 hr following 500 mg dose. C_{max} is 5.7 mcg/mL and C_{min} is 0.5 mcg/mL following multiple oral doses of 500 mg.
Injection – C_{max} is about 6.2 mcg/mL after 500 mg dose infused over 60 min and about 11.5 mcg/mL after 750 mg dose infused over 90 min. Steady state is reached within 48 hr following a once-daily (500 or 750 mg) regimen. Oral and IV formulations are equivalent in AUC; therefore, route of administration is interchangeable.

Distribution:
Oral – Vd is 89 to 112 L. Protein binding is approximately 24% to 38%.
Injection – Vd is 74 to 112 L. Protein binding is approximately 24% to 38%.

Metabolism:
Oral – Undergoes limited metabolism.
Injection – Desmethyl and N-oxide, the only metabolites identified in humans, have little relevant pharmacological activity.

Excretion: Total body Cl is 144 to 226 mL/min. Renal Cl is 96 to 142 mL/min. Terminal t½ is 6 to 8 hr.
Oral – Primarily (87%) excreted as unchanged drug in urine, less than 4% in the feces.
Injection – About 87% of dose was recovered unchanged in urine within 48 hr. Less than 4% was recovered in feces in 72 hr. Hemodialysis and peritoneal dialysis do not remove levofloxacin from the body.

Special Populations:
Renal Function Impairment – Cl is reduced and t½ prolonged in patients with Ccr less than 50 mL/min. Dosage adjustment required.

Indications Treatment of acute maxillary sinusitis, acute bacterial exacerbation of chronic bronchitis, nosocomial pneumonia, community-acquired pneumonia, skin and skin structure infections, chronic bacterial prostatitis, UTI, and acute pyelonephritis caused by susceptible strains of specific microorganisms.
Ophthalmic use: Treatment of conjunctivitis caused by susceptible strains of aerobic gram-positive and aerobic gram-negative microorganisms.

Contraindications Hypersensitivity to fluoroquinolones, quinolone antibiotics, or any product component.

Route/Dosage
Acute Bacterial Exacerbation of Chronic Bronchitis
ADULTS: **PO/IV** 500 mg q 24 hr for 7 days.

Acute Maxillary Sinusitis
ADULTS: **PO/IV** 500 mg q 24 hr for 10 to 14 days.

Bacterial Conjunctivitis
ADULTS AND CHILDREN AT LEAST 1 YR:
Days 1 and 2: **Topical** Instill 1 to 2 gtt in affected eye(s) q 2 hr while awake, up to 8 times daily.
Days 3 through 7: **Topical** Instill 1 to 2 gtt in affected eye(s) q 4 hr while awake, up to qid.

Chronic Bacterial Prostatitis
ADULTS: **PO/IV** 500 mg q 24 hr for 28 days.

Community-Acquired Pneumonia
ADULTS: **PO/IV** 500 mg q 24 hr for 7 to 14 days.

Complicated Skin and Skin Structure Infections; Nosocomial Pneumonia
ADULTS: **PO/IV** 750 mg q 24 hr for 7 to 14 days.

Complicated UTIs; Acute Pyelonephritis
ADULTS: **PO/IV** 250 mg q 24 hr for 10 days.

Uncomplicated Skin and Skin Structure Infections
ADULTS: **PO/IV** 500 mg q 24 hr for 7 to 10 days.

Uncomplicated UTIs
ADULTS: **PO/IV** 250 mg q 24 hr for 3 days.

Interactions
Antacids, iron salts, sucralfate, zinc salts; didanosine chewable buffered tablets, multivitamins (oral only): May decrease oral absorption of levofloxacin. Stagger administration times.
Antiarrhythmic agents (class Ia [eg, quinidine] and class III [eg, amiodarone]): Because of increased risk of life-threatening cardiac arrhythmias, including torsades de pointes, avoid coadministration of levofloxacin.
Antidiabetic agents: Hyperglycemia or hypoglycemia may occur.

NSAIDs: May increase risk of CNS stimulation and convulsive seizures.

Lab Test Interferences None well documented.

Adverse Reactions

CV: Torsades de pointes, vasodilation (postmarketing).

CNS: Headache (6%); insomnia (5%); dizziness (3%); anxiety, fatigue (1%); abnormal EEG, encephalopathy (postmarketing).

DERM: Pruritus, rash (1%); erythema multiforme, Stevens-Johnson syndrome (postmarketing).

EENT: Sinusitis, rhinitis, pharyngitis (1%). Ophthalmic – Transient decreased vision, foreign body sensation, transient ocular burning, ocular pain or discomfort, photophobia (1% to 3%); lid edema, ocular dryness, ocular itching (less than 1%).

GI: Nausea (7%); diarrhea (6%); constipation, abdominal pain (3%); dyspepsia, vomiting (2%); flatulence (1%).

GU: Vaginitis (2%).

HEMA: Eosinophilia, hemolytic anemia, increased INR/PT (postmarketing).

LABTESTABS: Decreased glucose, decreased lymphocytes (2%).

RESP: Dyspnea (1%); allergic pneumonitis (postmarketing).

OTHER: Pain, chest pain, back pain (1%); anaphylactic shock, anaphylactoid reactions, dysphonia, multi-system organ failure, tendon rupture (postmarketing).

Precautions

Pregnancy: Category C.

Lactation: Undetermined; however, other drugs in this class are excreted in breast milk.

Children: Safety and efficacy in children younger than 18 yr (younger than 1 yr for ophthalmic) not established.

Hypersensitivity: Serious and potentially fatal reactions have occurred with drugs in this class. Discontinue drug if allergic reaction occurs.

Renal function impairment: Reduced Cl may occur; adjust dose downward accordingly in Ccr less than 50 mL/min. Refer to manufacturer's package insert for dose calculations.

Superinfection: Prolonged use may result in overgrowth of nonsusceptible organisms.

Photosensitivity: Moderate to severe reactions may occur; avoid excessive sunlight and ultraviolet light.

Arrhythmia: Levofloxacin has been associated with prolonged QT interval and infrequent cases of arrhythmia.

Blood glucose: Disturbances of blood glucose, including symptoms of hyperglycemia and hypoglycemia.

Convulsions: CNS stimulation can occur; use drug with caution in patients with known or suspected CNS disorders.

Pseudomembranous colitis: Consider possibility in patients who develop diarrhea.

Tendonitis: Ruptures of the shoulder, hand, or Achilles tendon may occur. The risk may be increased in patients receiving corticosteroids, especially in the elderly.

PATIENT CARE CONSIDERATIONS

Administration/Storage

Oral:

- Administer prescribed dose with a full glass of water.
- Administer without regard to meals but administer with food if GI upset occurs.
- Administer levofloxacin 2 hr before or after magnesium or aluminum antacids, sucralfate, iron supplement, multivitamin with minerals, or didanosine chewable/buffered tablets or oral solution.
- Store tablets at controlled room temperature (59° to 86°F). Protect from light.

Injection:

- For IV administration only. Not for intradermal, SC, IM, intrathecal, or intraperitoneal administration.
- Avoid rapid or bolus IV infusion. Infuse dose by slow IV infusion over 60 min (500 mg dose) or 90 min (750 mg dose) to prevent hypotensive reaction.
- Do not administer if particulate matter or discoloration noted. A slight yellow to greenish-yellow color is normal and of no concern.
- Dilute single-use vial (concentrate) before use, following manufacturer's guidelines.
- Premix solution requires no further dilution and can be administered directly.
- Check premix IV container for minute leaks by squeezing bag firmly. If leaks are detected or the seal is not intact, discard solution because sterility may be impaired.
- Do not use premix containers in series to reduce risk of air embolism.
- Discard any unused IV solution.
- Do not add other medications or additives to IV container or infuse simultaneously through same IV line.
- Flush IV line with compatible IV fluid before and after levofloxacin infusion if same IV line is used for sequential infusion of different drugs.
- Store injection concentrate at controlled room temperature (59° to 86°F). Protect

injection concentrate from light. Reconstituted injection can be stored for up to 72 hr at temperatures below 77°F, for up to 14 days if refrigerated (36° to 46°F), or up to 6 mo if frozen (-4°F). Thaw frozen container at room temperature (below 77°F) or under refrigeration. Do not force thawing by immersion in water or by microwave irradiation. Do not refreeze after initial thawing.

- Store premix below 77°F. Brief exposure up to 104°F does not adversely affect the product. Avoid excessive heat and protect from freezing and light.

Ophthalmic Solution:

- For topical instillation into eye(s) only.
- Instill 1 to 2 gtt into affected eye(s) q 2 hr while awake (up to 8 times/day) for first 2 days then 1 to 2 gtt up to qid for 5 days.
- Have patient tilt head back, pull lower lid out to make pocket, and instill medication into conjunctival sac. Have patient close eyes and apply light finger pressure to bridge of nose for 1 to 2 min. Advise patient to not blink or rub eyes.
- Do not touch top of dropper bottle to eye, fingers, or other surface.
- If using other topical ophthalmic drugs, separate each medication by at least 5 min.
- Store at controlled room temperature. Protect from freezing. Keep container tightly closed.

Assessment/Interventions

- Obtain patient history, including drug history and any known allergies. Note renal impairment, diabetes, uncorrected electrolyte disorder, bradycardia, cardiomyopathy, concurrent use of drugs that prolong the QTc interval (eg, erythromycin), class 1A (eg, quinidine) or class III (eg, amiodarone) antiarrhythmic agents, history of prolongation of QTc interval, epilepsy, predisposition to convulsions, or allergy to fluoroquinolone antibiotics.
- Review results of culture and sensitivity testing as available.
- Ensure that reduced dose is administered to patient with Ccr less than 50 mL/min.
- Monitor for signs of infection, especially fever, and for positive response to antibiotic therapy.
- Ensure that patient is well hydrated to prevent formation of concentrated urine.
- Monitor patient for signs of allergic reaction. Discontinue therapy and immediately notify health care provider if noted. Be prepared to treat appropriately.
- Monitor blood sugar more frequently in diabetic patient using insulin or oral hypoglycemic agents. Report significant changes to health care provider. If hypoglycemic event occurs, discontinue levofloxacin immediately and be prepared to treat appropriately.
- Monitor patient for GI, CNS, PSYCH, and general body side effects. Report to health care provider if noted and significant.
- If seizure occurs, withhold drug, institute safety measures, and notify health care provider.
- Withhold drug and notify health care provider if any of the following occurs: severe diarrhea; loose, foul-smelling stools; vaginal itching or discharge; pain, inflammation, or rupture of tendon.

Ophthalmic Solution:

- Monitor patient for signs and symptoms of ocular side effects (eg, burning, stinging, pain, irritation) and improvement in conjunctivitis. Notify health care provider if conjunctivitis is not improving or is worsening, or if intolerable side effects occur.

Patient/Family Education

- Explain name, dose, action, and potential side effects of drug.
- Review dosing schedule and prescribed length of therapy with patient.
- Remind patient to complete entire course of therapy, even if symptoms of infection have disappeared.
- Advise patient to contact health care provider if infection does not seem to improve or is worsening.
- Advise patient to drink fluids liberally (eg, eight 8 oz glasses of water daily) while taking this medication.
- Advise patient to discontinue therapy and contact health care provider immediately if skin rash, hives, itching, shortness of breath, palpitations, fainting, or pain, tenderness, or rupture of tendon occurs.
- Instruct diabetic patient using insulin or oral hypoglycemic agents to monitor blood glucose more frequently when drug is started and to inform health care provider of significant changes in readings. Advise patient that if a hypoglycemic event occurs to discontinue the levofloxacin immediately, treat the hypoglycemia, and notify health care provider.
- Warn patient that diarrhea containing blood or pus may be a sign of a serious disorder and to seek medical care if noted and to not treat at home.
- Caution patient that drug may cause dizziness or lightheadedness and to use caution while driving or performing other tasks requiring mental alertness until tolerance is determined.
- Advise patient to avoid unnecessary exposure to sunlight or tanning lamps and to use sunscreen and wear protective clothing to avoid photosensitivity reactions.

- Advise women to notify health care provider if pregnant, planning to become pregnant, or breastfeeding.
- Instruct patient not to take any prescription or OTC medications or dietary supplements unless advised by health care provider.
- Advise patient that follow-up examinations and lab tests may be required to monitor therapy and to keep appointments.

Oral:

- Advise patient or caregiver to read the *Patient Information* leaflet before starting therapy.
- Instruct patient to take each dose with a full glass of water.
- Advise patient that the medication can be taken without regard to meals but to take with food if GI upset occurs.
- Instruct patient to take levofloxacin 2 hr before or after magnesium or aluminum antacids, sucralfate, iron supplement, multivitamin with minerals, or didanosine chewable/buffered tablets or oral solution.

Injection:

- Explain to patient or caregiver that medication is usually prepared and administered by a health care provider in a health care setting but may be used at home in some situations if ordered by the patient's health care provider.
- If patient or caregiver is administering at home, ensure that the patient or caregiver understands how to store, prepare, and administer the dose, and dispose of used equipment and supplies. Perform the first injection under the supervision of a qualified health professional.
- Advise patient to contact health care provider if injection site reaction occurs.

Ophthalmic:

- Remind patient not to wear contact lenses if having signs and symptoms of bacterial conjunctivitis.
- Teach patient proper technique for instilling eye drops: wash hands; do not allow dropper to touch eye. Tilt head back, look up; pull lower eyelid down; instill prescribed number of drops. Close eye for 1 to 2 min and apply gentle pressure to bridge of nose. Do not rub eye.
- Advise patient not to touch top of dropper bottle to eye, fingers, or other surface.
- Advise patient that if more than 1 topical ophthalmic drug is being used, administer the drugs at least 5 min apart
- Advise patient to inform health care provider if ocular side effects occur and become bothersome or if infection is not improving.

Levonorgestrel

(LEE-voe-nor-JESS-truhl)

Class Contraceptive/Hormones

How Supplied

Mirena Levonorgestrel-releasing intrauterine system T-shaped unit containing a reservoir of 52 mg levonorgestrel covered by a silicone membrane ◆ *Norplant System* Levonorgestrel implants (subdermal) Set of 6 capsules each containing 36 mg levonorgestrel

Action

PHARMACOLOGY: Synthetic, biologically active progestin that transforms proliferative endometrium into secretory endometrium and inhibits secretion of pituitary gonadotropins, preventing follicular maturation and ovulation.

PHARMACOKINETICS/DYNAMICS:

Distribution: Unlike other oral contraceptives, plasma levels with the levonorgestrel-releasing intrauterine system do not display peaks and troughs. Primarily bound to proteins, mainly sex hormone–binding globulin.

Metabolism: Extensively metabolized to a large number of inactive metabolites.

Excretion: The $t_{\frac{1}{2}}$ is 17 hr. Both the parent drug and its metabolites are primarily excreted in urine.

Indications Prevention of pregnancy.

Contraindications

Subdermal implants: Active thrombophlebitis or thromboembolic disorders; undiagnosed abnormal genital bleeding; known or suspected pregnancy; acute liver disease; benign or malignant liver tumors; known or suspected breast carcinoma.

Intrauterine system: Pregnancy or suspicion of pregnancy; congenital or acquired uterine anomaly; acute pelvic inflammatory disease (PID) or history of PID unless there has been a subsequent intrauterine pregnancy; postpartum endometritis or infected abortion in past 3 mo; genital bleeding of unknown etiology; untreated acute cervicitis or vaginitis, including bacterial vaginosis or other lower genital tract infection until infection is controlled; woman or sexual partner with multiple sexual partners; conditions associated with increased susceptibility to infections with microorganisms (eg, leukemia, AIDS, IV drug use); genital actinomycosis; previously inserted IUD that has not been removed;

known or suspected carcinoma of the breast; history of ectopic pregnancy or condition that would predispose to ectopic pregnancy; hypersensitivity to any component of this product.

Route/Dosage

Intrauterine system

Adults: Insert into uterine cavity within 7 days of onset of menstruation or immediately after first trimester abortion. Replace q 5 yr.

Subdermal implants

Adults: 6 capsules inserted in midportion of upper arm during first 7 days of onset of menses. Remove after 5 yr.

Adults: PO 1 tablet (0.75 mg) within 72 hr after unprotected intercourse; second tablet (0.75 mg) 12 hr after the first dose.

Interactions

Carbamazepine: Reduced contraceptive efficacy.
Phenytoin: Reduced contraceptive efficacy.
Rifampin: Possible reduced contraceptive efficacy.

Lab Test Interferences
Endocrine tests may be affected. Sex hormone-binding globulin concentrations may be decreased; thyroxine concentrations may be slightly decreased and triiodothyronine uptake may be increased.

Adverse Reactions

CV: Syncope, bradycardia, hypertension (intrauterine system).
CNS: Headache; nervousness; dizziness; decreased libido (intrauterine system).
DERM: Dermatitis; acne; hirsutism; hypertrichosis; scalp hair loss; pain, itching, or infection near implant site.
GI: Nausea; change in appetite; abdominal discomfort.
GU: Prolonged, irregular, frequent, or scanty bleeding; spotting; amenorrhea; cervicitis; leukorrhea; vaginitis.
METAB: Weight gain.
RESP: Upper respiratory tract infection, sinusitis (intrauterine system).
OTHER: Adnexal enlargement; mastalgia; breast discharge; implant removal difficulty; musculoskeletal pain.

Precautions

Pregnancy: Category X.
Lactation: Excreted in breast milk.
Children: Safety and efficacy before menarche not established.
Bleeding irregularities: Most women can expect variation in menstrual bleeding patterns.
Delayed follicular atresia: Follicle may grow beyond usual size and may resemble ovarian cyst.
Ectopic pregnancies: Have occurred, although relationship to drug is not established.
Intrauterine pregnancy: Risk of septic abortion, miscarriage, sepsis, premature labor, and premature delivery may be increased with the intrauterine system.
Ocular lesions: Retinal thrombosis has occurred with oral contraceptives; consider possibility in levonorgestrel users.
Perforation: Perforation of the uterus and cervix by the intrauterine system may occur.
Thromboembolic disorders: Remove capsules if thrombophlebitis or thromboembolic disease occurs. Consider removal in patients immobilized for prolonged periods.
Valvular/Congenital heart disease: Patients with certain types of valvular or congenital heart disease and surgically constructed systemic-pulmonary shunts are at increased risk of infective endocarditis, and use of the intrauterine system may represent a potential source of septic emboli.

Overdosage: Signs and Symptoms
Fluid retention, uterine bleeding irregularities.

PATIENT CARE CONSIDERATIONS

Administration/Storage
- Capsules must be inserted only by health care provider trained in procedure.

Assessment/Interventions
- Obtain patient history, including drug history and any known allergies. Note pregnancy and lactation status, current or past thrombophlebitis, abnormal menstrual or vaginal bleeding, cervical cytology, any degree of immobility, liver disease, breast abnormalities, or hyperlipidemia.
- Ensure that complete physical examination is performed before insertion and repeated annually during use. Obtain baseline weight.
- After insertion, monitor site for healing and absence of infection.

Patient/Family Education
- Explain that contraceptive method will be effective for 5 yr; capsules should be removed after that period, but can be removed at any time; and that removal should be done by a health care provider trained in procedure.
- Encourage low-fat, low-cholesterol diet.
- Teach patient to identify and report signs of wound infection after insertion.
- Instruct patient to notify health care provider if capsule falls out.
- Instruct patient to report the following symptoms to health care provider: jaundice, fluid retention, depression, vision changes, abnormal bleeding, and weight gain.
- Emphasize that missed menstrual period is not

- an accurate indicator of pregnancy.
- Explain that menstrual irregularities are common, especially during first year of therapy.
- Emphasize importance of keeping follow-up visits to evaluate effectiveness of contraceptive therapy.

Levorphanol Tartrate

(lee-VORE-fah-nole TAR-trate)
Class Narcotic analgesic

How Supplied
Levo-Dromoran Tablets 2 mg, Injection 2 mg/mL

Action
PHARMACOLOGY: Acts at receptors in the gray matter in the brain and spinal cord to alter the transmission and perception of pain.

PHARMACOKINETICS/DYNAMICS:
Absorption: Steady-state plasma levels are reached by the third day of dosing. Well absorbed following oral administration, reaching the C_{max} in about 1 hr.
Distribution: Vd is 10 to 13 L/kg. Plasma protein binding is 40%.
Excretion: Terminal t½ is about 11 to 16 hr and Cl of 0.78 to 1.1 L/kg/hr.
Onset: Following IM administration, onset of effects appear to be within 15 to 30 min.

Indications
Management of moderate to severe pain or as a preoperative medication when opioid analgesia is appropriate.

Contraindications
Standard considerations.

Route/Dosage
ADULTS: **IV** Recommended starting dose is up to 1 mg given in divided doses, by slow injection. This may be repeated in 3 to 6 hr prn. Generally, total daily doses of more than 4 to 8 mg IV in 24 hr are not recommended. **IM/SC** Recommended starting dose is 1 to 2 mg. This may be repeated in 6 to 8 hr prn. Generally, total daily doses of more than 3 to 8 mg in 24 hr are not recommended. **PO** Recommended starting dose 2 mg. This may be repeated in 6 to 8 hr prn. If necessary, the dose may be increased to 3 mg q 6 to 8 hr. Generally, total oral daily doses of more than 6 to 12 mg in 24 hr are not recommended.

Chronic Pain
ADULTS: **PO** When converting a patient from morphine to levorphanol, the total daily dose of levorphanol should begin at approximately 1/15 to 1/12 of the total daily dose of oral morphine.

Perioperative Use
ADULTS: Dosage should be based on age, body weight, physical status, underlying pathological condition, other drug usage, type of anesthesia, surgical procedure, and severity of pain.

Premedication
ADULTS: **IM/SC** Usual dose 1 to 2 mg given 60 to 90 min before surgery. Elderly or debilitated patients usually require less drug.

Interactions
Agonist/antagonist opioid analgesics (eg, butorphanol, nalbuphine, pentazocine): Should not be administered to patients receiving levorphanol.
CNS depressants (eg, alcohol, hypnotics, sedatives, tranquilizers): Additive CNS depressant effects. Respiratory depression, hypotension, profound sedation, or coma may occur.
Incompatibilities: Do not mix with aminophylline, ammonium chloride, amobarbital, chlorothiazide, heparin, methicillin, nitrofurantoin, novobiocin, pentobarbital, perphenazine, phenobarbital, phenytoin, secobarbital, sodium bicarbonate, sodium iodide, sulfadiazine, sulfisoxazole, diethanolamine, or thiopental.

Lab Test Interferences
None well documented.

Adverse Reactions
CV: Cardiac arrest; shock; hypotension; arrhythmias (including bradycardia and tachycardia); palpitations; extra-systoles.
CNS: Coma; suicide attempt; convulsions; depression; dizziness; confusion; lethargy; abnormal dreams; abnormal thinking; nervousness; drug withdrawal; hypokinesia; dyskinesia; hyperkinesia; stimulation; personality disorder; amnesia; insomnia.
DERM: Sweating; pruritus; urticaria; rash; injection site reaction.
EENT: Abnormal vision; pupillary disorder; diplopia.
GI: Abdominal pain; dry mouth; nausea; vomiting; dyspepsia; biliary tract spasm.
GU: Kidney failure; urinary retention; difficulty urinating.
RESP: Apnea; cyanosis; hypoventilation.

Precautions
Pregnancy: Category C.
Lactation: Undetermined.
Children: Safety and efficacy not established.
Elderly: Initial dose should be reduced 50%.
Special risk patients: Use with caution and reduce initial dose in patients who are elderly or debilitated, or those who have severe hepatic or renal impairment, hypothyroidism, Addison disease, toxic psychosis, prostatic hypertrophy, urethral stricture, acute alcoholism, or delirium tremens.
Biliary surgery: May increase pressure in common bile duct when given in analgesic doses; use not recommended in biliary surgery.
CV effects: Because the effects on heart activity are unknown, limit levorphanol use in patients

with myocardial dysfunction, acute MI, or coronary insufficiency.

Drug dependence: Has abuse potential.

Head injury: Respiratory depressant effects may be markedly exaggerated in the presence of head injury, intracranial lesions, or preexisting increased intracranial pressure.

Hypotension: May cause severe hypotension in postoperative patients or in individuals whose ability to maintain BP is compromised (eg, volume depletion). May cause orthostatic hypotension in ambulatory patients.

Liver disease: Use with caution in patients with extensive liver disease.

Respiratory depression: May cause serious or potentially fatal respiratory depression if given in excessive dose, too frequently, or if given in full dosage to compromised patients. Use with caution in patients with impaired respiratory reserve or respiratory depression.

Withdrawal syndrome: Discontinuation after chronic use has been reported to result in withdrawal syndrome.

Overdosage: Signs and Symptoms
Respiratory depression, CV failure, CNS depression; extreme somnolence progressing to stupor or coma, skeletal muscle flaccidity, cold and clammy skin, constricted pupils, bradycardia, hypotension, apnea, circulatory collapse, cardiac arrest, death.

Levothyroxine Sodium (T_4; L-thyroxine)

(lee-voe-thigh-ROX-een SO-dee-uhm)

Class Thyroid hormone

How Supplied
Levothroid Tablets 0.025 mg, Tablets 0.05 mg, Tablets 0.075 mg, Tablets 0.088 mg, Tablets 0.1 mg, Tablets 0.112 mg, Tablets 0.125 mg, Tablets 0.137 mg, Tablets 0.15 mg, Tablets 0.175 mg, Tablets 0.2 mg, Tablets 0.3 mg, Powder for injection, lyophilized 200 mcg/vial, Powder for injection, lyophilized 500 mcg/vial ♦ *Levoxyl* Tablets 0.025 mg, Tablets 0.05 mg, Tablets 0.075 mg, Tablets 0.088 mg, Tablets 0.1 mg, Tablets 0.112 mg, Tablets 0.125 mg, Tablets 0.137 mg, Tablets 0.15 mg, Tablets 0.175 mg, Tablets 0.2 mg, Tablets 0.3 mg ♦ *Synthroid* Tablets 0.025 mg, Tablets 0.05 mg, Tablets 0.075 mg, Tablets 0.088 mg, Tablets 0.1 mg, Tablets 0.112 mg, Tablets 0.125 mg, Tablets 0.15 mg, Tablets 0.175 mg, Tablets 0.2 mg, Tablets 0.3 mg, Powder for injection, lyophilized 200 mcg/vial, Powder for injection, lyophilized 500 mcg/vial

Action
PHARMACOLOGY: Increases metabolic rate of body tissues; is needed for normal growth and maturation.

PHARMACOKINETICS/DYNAMICS:

Absorption: Bioavailability is 48% to 79%. Fasting increases absorption. Effective by parenteral route.

Distribution: More than 99% protein bound.

Excretion: The $t_{1/2}$ is 6 to 7 days for T_4.

Indications Replacement or supplemental therapy in hypothyroidism; TSH suppression (in thyroid cancer, nodules, goiters, and enlargement in chronic thyroiditis).

Contraindications Acute MI and thyrotoxicosis uncomplicated by hypothyroidism; coexistence of hypothyroidism and hypoadrenalism (Addison disease) unless treatment of hypoadrenalism with adrenocortical steroids precedes initiation of thyroid therapy.

Route/Dosage
Individualize dosage.

INFANTS AND CHILDREN: In infants with congenital or acquired hypothyroidism, institute therapy with full doses as soon as diagnosis is made. In children with chronic or severe hypothyroidism, an initial oral 25 mcg/day dose is recommended with increments of 25 mcg q 2 to 4 wk until desired effect is achieved. The following guidelines are recommended:

Children more than 12 yr (growth/puberty complete): PO 1.7 mcg/kg/day.
Children more than 12 yr (growth/puberty incomplete): PO 2 to 3 mcg/kg/day.
Children 6 to 12 yr: PO 4 to 5 mcg/kg/day.
Children 1 to 5 yr: PO 5 to 6 mcg/kg/day.
Children 6 to 12 mo: PO 6 to 8 mcg/kg/day.
Children 3 to 6 mo: PO 8 to 10 mcg/kg/day.
Children 0 to 3 mo: PO 10 to 15 mcg/kg/day.
Consider a lower starting dose (eg, 25 mcg/day) in infants at risk for cardiac failure, increasing the dose in 4- to 6-wk intervals based on clinical and laboratory response.

Hypothyroidism in Adults and Children in Whom Growth and Puberty are Complete
ADULTS AND CHILDREN: PO Average full replacement dose is approximately 1.7 mcg/kg/day (eg, 100 to 125 mcg/day for 70 kg adult). Older patients may require less than 1 mcg/kg/day. Doses greater than 200 mcg/day are seldom required. For most patients older than 50 yr or patients younger than 50 yr with underlying cardiac disease, an initial starting dose of 25 to 50 mcg/day is recommended, with gradual increments in dose at 6- to 8-wk intervals, as needed.

The recommended starting dose in elderly patients with cardiac disease is 12.5 to 25 mcg/day, with gradual dose increments at 4- to 6-wk intervals.

Severe Hypothyroidism
ADULTS: **PO** Recommended starting dose is 12.5 to 25 mcg/day with increases of 25 mcg/day q 2 to 4 wk, accompanied by clinical and laboratory assessment, until TSH level in normalized.
IV/IM May be substituted for oral form when oral ingestion is precluded for long periods of time. Initial parenteral dosage should be approximately 50% the previously established oral dosage. A daily maintenance dose of 50 to 100 mcg parenterally should maintain the euthyroid stat once established. Monitor the patient and adjust the dosage as needed.

Subclinical Hypothyroidism
ADULTS: **PO** If treated, a lower dose (eg, 1 mcg/kg/day) than that used for full replacement may be adequate to normalize serum TSH level.

Myxedema Coma
ADULTS: **IV** In myxedema coma or stupor, without concomitant severe heart disease, 200 to 500 mcg may be administered as a solution containing 100 mcg/mL. Full therapeutic effect may not be evident until the following day. An additional 100 to 300 mcg or more may be given on the second day if evidence of significant and progressive improvements has not occurred.

TSH Suppression in Well-Differentiated Thyroid Cancer and Thyroid Nodules
ADULTS: **PO** TSH suppression to less than 0.1 mU/L usually requires a levothyroxine dose greater than 2 mcg/kg/day; however, in patients with high-risk tumors, the target TSH suppression level may be less than 0.01 mU/L. In treatment of benign nodules and nontoxic multinodular goiter, TSH generally is suppressed to a higher target (eg, 0.1 to 0.5 mU/L or 1 mU/L) than that used for treatment of thyroid cancer.

Interactions
Anticoagulants, oral: May increase anticoagulant effects.
Cholestyramine, colestipol: May decrease thyroid hormone efficacy.
Digitalis glycosides: May reduce effects of glycosides.
Fasting: Increases absorption from GI tract.
Iron salts: May decrease efficacy of levothyroxine, resulting in hypothyroidism.
Theophyllines: Hypothyroidism; may cause decreased theophylline Cl; Cl may return to normal when euthyroid state is achieved.

Lab Test Interferences Consider changes in thyroxine binding globulin concentration when interpreting thyroxine (T_4) and triiodothyronine (T_3) values; medicinal or dietary iodine interferes with all in vivo tests of radioiodine uptake, producing low uptakes that may not reflect true decrease in hormone synthesis.

Adverse Reactions
CV: Palpitations; tachycardia; cardiac arrhythmias; angina pectoris; cardiac arrest.
CNS: Tremors; headache; nervousness; insomnia.
GI: Diarrhea; vomiting.
OTHER: Hypersensitivity; weight loss; menstrual irregularities; sweating; heat tolerance; fever; decreased bone density (in women using levothyroxine long term).

> **WARNING:**
> Not for use in obesity treatment. Ineffective for weight reduction indications and may produce life-threatening or serious consequences when used in large doses or in combination with other anorectics.

Precautions
Pregnancy: Category A.
Lactation: Minimal amounts excreted in breast milk.
Children: When drug is administered for congenital hypothyroidism, routine determinations of serum T_4 or TSH are strongly advised in newborns. In infants, excessive doses of thyroid hormone preparations may produce craniosynostosis. Children may experience transient partial hair loss in first few months of thyroid therapy.
Cardiovascular disease: Use caution when integrity of cardiovascular system, particularly coronary arteries, is suspect (eg, angina, elderly). Development of chest pain or worsening cardiovascular disease requires decrease in dosage.
Endocrine disorders: Therapy in patients with concomitant diabetes mellitus, diabetes insipidus, or adrenal insufficiency (Addison disease) exacerbates intensity of symptoms.
Therapy of myxedema coma requires simultaneous administration of glucocorticoids. In patients whose hypothyroidism is secondary to hypopituitarism, correct adrenal insufficiency, if present, with corticosteroids.
Hyperthyroid effects: Levothyroxine rarely may precipitate hyperthyroid state or may aggravate existing hyperthyroidism.
Infertility: Drug is unjustified for treatment of male or female infertility unless condition is accompanied by hypothyroidism.
Morphologic hypogonadism and nephrosis: Rule out before therapy.
Myxedema coma: Patients are particularly sensitive to thyroid preparations. Sudden administration of large doses is not without cardiovascular

risks. Small initial doses are indicated.

Overdosage: Signs and Symptoms

Symptoms of hyperthyroidism: headache, irritability, nervousness, sweating, tachycardia, increased bowel motility, menstrual irregularities, palpitations, vomiting, psychosis, seizure, fever, angina pectoris, CHF, shock, arrhythmias, thyroid storm.

PATIENT CARE CONSIDERATIONS

Administration/Storage

- Administer oral form once each day before breakfast. When given on empty stomach, absorption is increased. To maintain steady blood levels, be consistent in giving drug with or without food.
- Do not give sooner than 4 hr after administration of cholestyramine or colestipol. Cholestyramine or colestipol reduces effectiveness of levothyroxine.
- Do not switch from one brand to another without comparison studies of bioavailability.
- For infants and children who cannot swallow intact tablets, crush proper dose tablet and suspend freshly crushed tablet in small amount of formula or water; give by spoon or dropper. Do not store suspension for any period of time. Crushed tablet also may be sprinkled over small amount of food (eg, cooked cereal, applesauce).
- Parenteral therapy may be used when oral form of medication cannot be tolerated.
- IV therapy is preferred in emergency treatment of myxedema coma. Can be administered via nasogastric tube. Give no faster than 100 mcg/min. Too-rapid administration causes adverse cardiovascular reactions. Monitor closely during administration.
- Reconstitute injectable solution by adding 5 mL of 0.9% sodium chloride or bacteriostatic sodium chloride (benzyl alcohol). Shake vial to ensure complete dissolution.
- Administer via Y-tubing or 3-way stopcock. Do not add to IV infusion.
- Use IV solution immediately after reconstitution. Discard any unused portion.
- Store in tightly closed, light-resistant container at room temperature.

Assessment/Interventions

- Obtain patient history, including drug history and any known allergies.
- Prior to initial administration, obtain baseline data of TSH and T_4 levels.
- Successful therapy achieves euthyroid state. Expect responses to initial therapy to be diuresis, weight loss, increased sense of well-being, increased appetite and activity, increased energy, and return to normal texture of hair and skin.
- Monitor for signs and symptoms of thyroid deficit or excess.
- Do not give if pulse is greater than 100 bpm.
- In infants, monitor for normal growth, development, and intellectual functioning; monthly measurement of height is a good index.
- Compare laboratory tests of TSH and T_4 with baseline data; serum levels should return to normal. In some children TSH levels may remain abnormal.
- When given with oral anticoagulants, expect oral anticoagulant dosage to be reduced. Monitor more closely for bleeding.
- Give drug cautiously with catecholamines (eg, epinephrine, dopamine). When drug is given with catecholamines, monitor for cardiac arrhythmias.
- If patient is taking insulin, oral hypoglycemics, or digitalis, monitor effectiveness of these agents. Dosages of these agents may need to be altered. Monitor serum glucose levels, ECG, and pulse.
- Monitor thyroid function test results closely in patients over 65 yr; less levothyroxine is usually needed by elderly.

Patient/Family Education

- Explain to patient that medication will probably need to be taken for life. Instruct patient not to discontinue taking medication or change dosage without consulting health care provider.
- Instruct patient to take levothyroxine at same time each day, preferably in morning before breakfast.
- Instruct patient not to switch from one brand of medication to another unless advised to do so by health care provider.
- Teach patient how to monitor for signs and symptoms of thyroid deficit or excess. Instruct patient to notify health care provider of following persistent signs and symptoms: headache, nervousness, diarrhea, excessive sweating, heat intolerance, chest pain, increased pulse rate, palpitations.
- Teach patient to keep a record of signs and symptoms for health care provider review.
- Advise patient of importance of keeping appointments with health care provider for regular checkups.
- Caution patient not to take OTC or other prescribed medications without consulting health care provider.
- Advise patient to wear *Medi-Alert* bracelet or necklace and to carry *Medi-Alert* card in wallet.

- Caution patient not to take levothyroxine for weight control.
- Explain that partial hair loss may be experienced by children in first few months of therapy but that this side effect is transient.

Lidocaine Hydrochloride
(LIE-doe-cane HIGH-droe-KLOR-ide)
Class Antiarrhythmic/Local anesthetic
How Supplied
Anestacon Jelly 2% ♦ *Burn-o-Jel* Gel 0.5% ♦ *Dentipatch* Patch 23/2 cm² patch, Patch 46.1/2 cm² patch ♦ *DermaFlex* Gel 2.5% ♦ *Dilocaine* Injection 1%, Injection 2% ♦ *Duo-Trach Kit* Injection 4% ♦ *ELA-Max* Cream 4% ♦ *Lidocaine Hydrochloride for Cardiac Arrhythmias* Injection Direct IV administration - 1%, Injection Direct IV administration - 2%, Injection IV admixtures - 4%, Injection IV admixtures - 10%, Injection IV admixtures - 20% ♦ *Lidocaine Hydrochloride in 5% Dextrose* Injection 2 mg/mL, Injection 4 mg/mL, Injection 8 mg/mL ♦ *Lidoject-1* Injection 1% ♦ *Lidoject-2* Injection 2% ♦ *Lidopen Auto-Injector* Injection 300 mg/3 mL ♦ *Nervocaine* Injection 1% ♦ *Numby Stuff* Solution, Topical 2% ♦ *Octocaine* Injection 2% with 1:50,000 epinephrine, Injection 2% with 1:100,000 epinephrine ♦ *Solarcaine Aloe Extra Burn Relief* Cream 0.5%, Gel 0.5%, Spray 0.5% ♦ *Xylocaine* Solution 4%, Jelly 2% ♦ *Xylocaine Viscous* Solution 2% ♦ *Xylocaine Hydrochloride* Injection 0.5% with 1:200,000 epinephrine, Injection 1% with 1:100,000 epinephrine, Injection 1% with 1:200,000 epinephrine, Injection 2% with 1:50,000 epinephrine, Injection 2% with 1:100,000 epinephrine, Injection 2% with 1:200,000 epinephrine, Injection 1.5% with 7.5% dextrose ♦ *Xylocaine Hydrochloride IV for Cardiac Arrhythmias* Injection Direct IV administration - 2% ♦ *Xylocaine MPF* Injection 0.5%, Injection 1%, Injection 1.5%, Injection 2%, Injection 4%, Injection 1% with 1:200,000 epinephrine, Injection 1.5% with 1:200,000 epinephrine, Injection 2% with 1:200,000 epinephrine, Injection 5% with 7.5% glucose ♦ *Zilactin-L* Liquid 2.5%
♣ *Lidodan Endotracheal* ♦ *Lidodan Ointment* ♦ *Lidodan Viscous* ♦ *Xylocaine CO2* ♦ *Xylocaine Endotracheal* ♦ *Xylocaine 4% Sterile Solution* ♦ *Xylocaine Spinal 5%* ♦ *Xylocard*

Action
PHARMACOLOGY: Attenuates phase 4 diastolic depolarization, decreases automaticity, decreases action potential duration, and raises ventricular fibrillation threshold; inhibits conduction of nerve impulses from sensory nerves.

Indications Acute management of ventricular arrhythmias; topical anesthesia in local skin disorders; local anesthesia of accessible mucous membranes. **Unlabeled use(s):** Intraosseous or endotracheal administration to pediatric patients with cardiac arrest.

Contraindications Hypersensitivity to amide local anesthetics; Stokes-Adams syndrome; Wolff-Parkinson-White syndrome; severe degrees of sinoatrial, AV or intraventricular block in absence of pacemaker; ophthalmic use.

Route/Dosage
ADULTS: **IM** 300 mg. May be repeated after 60 to 90 min. **IV bolus** 50 to 100 mg at rate of 25 to 50 mg/min; may repeat, but do not exceed 200 to 300 mg/hr. **Continuous infusion** 1 to 4 mg/min. **Patch** Apply patch and allow to remain in place until the desired anesthetic effect is produced for up to 15 min. Use the lowest dosage for effectiveness.

CHILDREN: **IV bolus/intratracheal** 1 mg/kg/dose q 5 to 10 min (max dose, 5 mg/kg). Maintenance dose is 20 to 50 mcg/kg/min. **Topical** Apply as needed to affected area; use lowest dose possible when applying to mucous membranes.

Interactions
Beta-adrenergic blockers: Increased lidocaine levels.
Cimetidine: Decreased lidocaine clearance.
Class I antiarrhythmic agents (eg, tocainide, mexiletine): Toxic effects are additive and potentially synergistic.
Procainamide: Additive neurological and cardiac effects.
Succinylcholine: Prolongation of neuromuscular blockade.
INCOMPATIBILITIES: Amphotericin B, parenteral cephalosporins, doxycycline, epinephrine, isoproterenol, methohexital, nitroprusside, norepinephrine, phenytoin, sodium bicarbonate, sulfadiazine.

Lab Test Interferences IM administration may increase CPK levels.

Adverse Reactions
CV: Hypotension; bradycardia; cardiovascular collapse; cardiac arrest.
CNS: Dizziness; lightheadedness; nervousness; drowsiness; apprehension; confusion; mood changes; hallucinations; tremors.
EENT: Visual disturbances; diplopia; tinnitus.
GI: Nausea; vomiting.
RESP: Respiratory depression or arrest.
OTHER: Hypersensitivity reactions. Local reactions, including soreness at IM injection site; venous thrombosis or phlebitis; extravasation;

burning, stinging, sloughing, tenderness (with topical application). Difficulty in speaking, breathing, and swallowing; numbness of lips or tongue, and other paresthesias, including heat and cold.

Precautions

Pregnancy: Category B.
Lactation: Excreted in breast milk.
Children: Safety and efficacy not established. If used, reduce dose. IM autoinjector device not recommended in children less than 50 kg.
Hypersensitivity: May occur.
Renal function impairment: Use caution with repeated doses or prolonged use in patients with renal impairment.
Hepatic function impairment: Use caution with repeated doses or prolonged use in patients with hepatic impairment.
Cardiac effects: Use with caution and in lower doses in patients with CHF, reduced cardiac output, digitalis toxicity, and in the elderly.
IV use: May result in excessive depression of cardiac conductivity.
Malignant hyperthermia: Has been reported with administration of amide local anesthetics.
Methemoglobinemia: Do not use in patients with congenital oridiopathic methemoglobinemia or in infants less than 12 mo who are receiving methemoglobin-inducing drugs.
Oral use: May impair swallowing and enhance danger of aspiration; avoid food for 1 hr if used in mouth or throat.
Topical use: Systemic effects can occur following topical use; use lowest possible dose to avoid serious toxicity, shock, or heart block.

Overdosage: Signs and Symptoms

Confusion, drowsiness, unconsciousness, tremors, convulsions, hypotension, bradycardia, cardiovascular collapse, cardiac arrest, tinnitus, diplopia.

PATIENT CARE CONSIDERATIONS

Administration/Storage

IM:
- Use IM route for emergency situations (eg, no IV access, no ECG monitoring) only. Only use 10% solution for injection. Deltoid muscle is preferred IM site. Switch to IV route as soon as possible.

IV:
- When giving by IV route, use only 1% to 2% solutions of drug. Use only lidocaine specifically labeled for IV use (without preservatives or epinephrine). Do not administer with other agents.
- To initiate IV therapy, start IV of 5% Dextrose in Water at "keep vein open (KVO)" rate. Bolus loading dose of 50 to 100 mg may be given undiluted at rate of 25 to 50 mg/min. IV push is indicated for resuscitation situations.
- For continuous infusion, use prediluted solution or add 1 g of lidocaine to 500 mL of 5% Dextrose in Water to prepare 0.2% solution. Rate of administration should not exceed 1 to 4 mg/min. Adjust rate according to cardiac response.
- Use diluted solutions within 24 hr.
- When giving by topical route, apply thinly and to smallest area possible. Do not apply to abraded or otherwise injured areas of skin.
- Store all forms of drug at room temperature.
- For IV infusion, use microdropper and infusion pump or controller.

Patch:
- Gently dry the area of application with cotton gauze. Remove the clear protective liner and apply the patch.

Assessment/Interventions

- Obtain patient history, including drug history and any known allergies. Note renal, cardiac, or hepatic impairment and hypersensitivity to amide-type local anesthetics.
- Obtain baseline BP and ECG before administration.
- Monitor BP, ECG, and respirations during IV administration. Continuous ECG monitoring is essential for proper administration. Have resuscitative equipment and medication immediately available.
- Monitor serum levels of drug if given via IV for more than 24 hr. Therapeutic serum levels range from 1.5 to 6 mcg/mL; toxic levels are more than 6 to 10 mcg/mL.
- If serious adverse reactions occur, notify health care provider, but continue 5% Dextrose IV. Continue to monitor patient closely.
- Keep bolus dose of 100 mcg of lidocaine available at all times.
- For topical use, apply thinly and to smallest area possible. Do not apply to abraded or otherwise injured areas of skin.
- Assess for systemic toxicity, which can result if excessive amounts of topical drug are absorbed. Risk of toxicity is greatest when large surface area, mucous membranes, or abraded or otherwise injured skin is involved.
- If topical preparation is used during labor and delivery, monitor vital signs and level of consciousness of newborn and mother.
- Monitor activity and position of patient postanesthesia until senses of pain, pressure, and temperature return.

- Monitor I&O and voiding.
- When topical drug is applied to pharynx, maintain npo status until gag reflex returns. If tongue and oral mucosa are numb, do not permit patient to eat food or chew gum until sensation returns.

Patient/Family Education
- Explain that adverse reactions related to the CNS (eg, drowsiness, confusion, paresthesias, convulsions, respiratory arrest) can occur and are related to CNS toxicity.
- Emphasize importance of not allowing topical solution to come in contact with eyes or broken skin.
- Advise patient not to chew gum or eat food until 60 min after oral anesthetic has been administered.
- Advise patient that drug may cause dizziness or drowsiness and to avoid getting out of bed or walking without assistance.

Lidocaine Hydrochloride/ Epinephrine

(LIE-doe-cane HIGH-droe-KLOR-ide/epp-ih-NEFF-rin)

Class Local anesthetic/Vasopressor

How Supplied
Xylocaine with Epinephrine Injection 0.5% with 1:200,000 epinephrine, Injection 1% with 1:100,000 epinephrine, Injection 1% with 1:200,000 epinephrine, Injection 1.5% with 1:200,000 epinephrine, Injection 2% with 1:50,000 epinephrine, Injection 2% with 1:100,000 epinephrine, Injection 2% with 1:200,000 epinephrine

Action
PHARMACOLOGY:
Lidocaine: Stabilizes neuronal membranes by inhibiting the ionic fluxes required for the initiation and conduction of impulses, thereby effecting local anesthetic action.
Epinephrine: Stimulates both alpha- and beta-receptors within sympathetic nervous system; relaxes smooth muscle of bronchi and iris and is an antagonist of histamine.

Indications Production of local or regional anesthesia by infiltration techniques such as percutaneous injection, by peripheral nerve block techniques such as brachial plexus and intercostals, and by central neural techniques such as lumbar and caudal epidural blocks.

Contraindications History of hypersensitivity to local anesthetics of the amide type.

Route/Dosage
Dose determined by number of dermatomes to be anesthetized (2 to 3 mL/dermatome). The dose of local anesthetic administered varies with the procedure, vascularity of the tissues, depth of anesthesia, degree of required muscle relaxation, duration of anesthesia desired, and the physical condition of the patient. Reduce dosages for children, the elderly, debilitated patients, and patients with cardiac or liver disease. Consult individual prescribing information for dosage recommendations.

Interactions
Ergot derivatives (ergotamine), vasopressors: May cause severe persistent hypertension or cerebrovascular accidents.
MAO inhibitors (eg, isocarboxazid), tricyclic antidepressants (eg, amitriptyline): Severe prolonged hypertension may occur.
Phenothiazines (eg, thioridazine), butyrophenones (droperidol): May reduce or reverse the pressor effect of epinephrine.

Lab Test Interferences Lidocaine IM injection may increase creatine phosphokinase levels, which may compromise the diagnosis of acute MI.

Adverse Reactions
CV: Bradycardia; hypotension (3%); cardiovascular collapse; cardiac arrest.
CNS: Excitation; depression: lightheadedness; nervousness; apprehension; euphoria; confusion; dizziness; drowsiness; sensations of heat, cold, or numbness; twitching; tremors, convulsions, unconsciousness; positional headache (3%); shivering (2%).
EENT: Tinnitus; blurred or double vision; permanent injury to extraocular muscles.
GI: Vomiting; loss of bowel control.
GU: Loss of bladder control loss of sexual function.
RESP: Respiratory depression or arrest.
OTHER: Allergy (eg, cutaneous lesions, urticaria, edema, anaphylactoid reactions); backache.

Precautions
Pregnancy: Category B.
Lactation: Undetermined.
Children: Reduce dose; commensurate with age, body weight, and physical condition.
Special risk patients: Use with caution in areas of the body supplied by end arteries or having compromised blood supply, patients with neurological disease, spinal deformities, septicemia and severe hypertension, impaired cardiovascular function, or hepatic disease.
Peripheral or hypertensive vascular disease: May exhibit exaggerated vasoconstrictor response and ischemic injury or necrosis may result.

PATIENT CARE CONSIDERATIONS

Administration/Storage
- For local infiltration only. Not for intravascular administration.
- Multiple concentrations are available. Ensure that the proper concentration is being used.
- Do not administer if particulate matter, cloudiness, or discoloration noted.
- To avoid intravascular administration, aspirate injection site before anesthetic solution is injected.
- Do not use anesthetic solutions containing preservatives for epidural or spinal anesthesia.
- Discard any unused solution when using single dose vial or ampule.
- Store at controlled room temperature (59° to 86°F).

Assessment/Interventions
- Obtain patient history, including drug history and any known allergies. Note history of sulfite sensitivity and allergy to amide-type local anesthetics or parabens.
- Note the following conditions that may increase risk of side effects or toxicity: liver disease; existing neurological disease; heart block; spinal deformities; septicemia; severe hypertension; peripheral vascular disease; concurrent use of MAO inhibitors, tricyclic antidepressants, phenothiazines, butyrophenones, vasopressors, or ergot-type oxytocic drugs.
- Ensure that resuscitation equipment and trained personnel are available when medication is being administered.
- Administer reduced doses to debilitated, elderly, or acutely ill patients, and children.
- Monitor patient's vital signs and level of consciousness following each anesthetic injection. Notify health care provider immediately if any of the following are noted during or following injection: restlessness; anxiety; tinnitus; dizziness; blurred vision; drowsiness or change in mental status; change in heart rate; tachypnea; labile BP.
- Administer test dose during administration of epidural anesthesia and monitor patient for CNS and CV toxicity and unintended intrathecal administration.

Patient/Family Education
- Explain name, dose, action, and potential side effects of drug.
- Advise patient that medication will be prepared and administered by a health care provider in a medical setting.
- Caution patient that temporary loss of sensation and motor activity may be experienced.
- Instruct patient to inform health care provider if any of the following are experienced during or after the anesthetic injection: restlessness; anxiety; ringing in the ears; dizziness; blurred vision; drowsiness or change in mental status; rapid heart rate, rapid breathing or feeling of shortness of breath; hot or cold sensations.

Lidocaine Hydrochloride/ Prilocaine

(LIE-doe-cane HIGH-droe-KLOR-ide/PRILL-oh-cane)

Class Local anesthetic

How Supplied
EMLA Cream 2.5% lidocaine and 2.5% prilocaine, Anesthetic Disc 1 g EMLA emulsion (2.5% lidocaine, 2.5% prilocaine). Contact surface approximately 10 cm^2
❦ *EMLA Patch*

Action
PHARMACOLOGY: Stabilizes neuronal membranes by inhibiting the ionic fluxes required for the initiation and conduction of impulses, thereby effecting local anesthetic action.

Indications As a topical anesthetic for use on normal intact skin for local analgesia or genital mucous membranes for superficial minor surgery and as pretreatment for infiltration anesthesia.

Contraindications Sensitivity to local anesthetics of the amide type or any component of the product.

Route/Dosage

Minor Dermal Procedures
ADULTS: **TOPICAL** Apply 2.5 g of cream over 20 to 25 cm^2 of skin surface or 1 anesthetic disc (1 g over 10 cm^2) for at least 1 hr.

Major Dermal Procedures
ADULTS: **TOPICAL** Apply 2 g of the cream per 10 cm^2 of skin surface and allow to remain in contact with skin for at least 2 hr.

Male Genital Skin
ADULTS: **TOPICAL** As adjunct prior to local anesthetic infiltration, apply a thick layer of cream (1 g/10 cm^2) to the skin surface for 15 min. Perform local anesthetic infiltration immediately after removal of the cream.

Female Genital Mucous Membranes
ADULTS: **TOPICAL** Apply a thick layer (5 to 10 g) of cream for 5 to 10 min.

Pediatrics (Intact skin)
CHILDREN (0 TO 3 MO OR LESS THAN 5 KG): **TOPICAL** Apply 1 g per 10 cm^2 for a max of 1 hr.
CHILDREN (3 MO UP TO 12 MO AND MORE THAN 5 KG): **TOPICAL** Apply 2 g per 20 cm^2 for a max of 4 hr.
CHILDREN (1 YR TO 6 YR AND MORE THAN 10 KG): **TOPICAL** Apply 10 g per 100 cm^2 for a max of 4 hr.
CHILDREN (7 YR TO 12 YR AND MORE THAN 20 KG): **TOPICAL** Apply 20 g per 200 cm^2 for a max of 4 hr.
NOTE: If a patient is older than 3 mo and does not meet the min weight requirement, the max total dose should be restricted to that which corresponds to the patient's weight.

Interactions
Class I antiarrhythmic agents (eg, mexiletine, tocainide): Toxic effects may be additive or synergistic.
Methemoglobin-inducing agents: May increase risk of methemoglobinemia.

Lab Test Interferences
None well documented.

Adverse Reactions
CV: Bradycardia; hypotension, cardiovascular collapse leading to arrest.
CNS: CNS excitement or depression; lightheadedness; nervousness; apprehension; euphoria; confusion; dizziness; drowsiness; sensations of hot, cold, or numbness; twitching; tremors; convulsions, unconsciousness; respiratory depression and arrest.
DERM: Paleness (37%); erythema (30%); burning sensation (17%); edema (10%); alterations in temperature sensations (7%); itching (2%); discrete purpuric or petechial reactions at the site of application; hyperpigmentation (cream); redness; blistering of foreskin in neonates about to undergo circumcision.
EENT: Tinnitus; blurred or double vision.
GI: Vomiting.
OTHER: Allergic and anaphylactoid reactions (characterized by urticaria, angioedema, bronchospasm, and shock).

Precautions
Pregnancy: Category B.
Lactation: Lidocaine and probably prilocaine are excreted in human milk.
Children: Children under 7 yr have shown less overall benefit than older children or adults. Do not use in neonates with a gestational age of 37 wk or less.
Application: Application to larger areas or for longer than recommended could result in sufficient absorption causing serious adverse reactions.
Methemoglobinemia: Do not use in patients with congenital or idiopathic methemoglobinemia or in infants under 12 mo of age who are receiving treatment with methemoglobin-inducing agents (eg, acetaminophen, nitrates, phenytoin, sulfonamides).

Overdosage: Signs and Symptoms
Confusion, drowsiness, unconsciousness, tremors, convulsions, hypotension, bradycardia, cardiovascular collapse, cardiac arrest, tinnitus, diplopia.

PATIENT CARE CONSIDERATIONS
Administration/Storage
- For topical use only. Not for ophthalmic or otic use.
- Apply a thick layer as prescribed and cover with occlusive dressing for recommended amount of time before procedure or IV insertion. Use gloves or applicator as applicable.
- Dermal analgesia can be expected to increase for up to 3 hr under occlusive dressing and persist for 1 to 2 hr after removal of the cream.
- Store at controlled room temperature (59° to 86°F). Keep tube tightly closed.

Assessment/Interventions
- Obtain patient history, including drug history and any known allergies. Note history of the following: allergy to amide-type local anesthetics; liver disease; glucose-6-phosphate deficiency; congenital or idiopathic methemoglobinemia; concurrent treatment with methemoglobin-inducing drugs (eg, sulfonamides) in infants younger than 12 mo; concurrent treatment with Class I antiarrhythmic agents (eg, tocainide).
- Review manufacturer's dosing recommendations for infants and children before application. Ensure that cream is not applied to larger areas or for longer periods of time than recommended.
- Ensure that methemoglobin levels are determined before, during, and after application of cream in neonates and infants 3 mo or younger.
- Monitor patient's response to application. Remove cream and notify health care provider immediately if any of the following occur following application of cream: dizziness; excessive sleepiness; bluish discoloration of face or lips; agitation; twitching; tremors; serious reaction at application site.

Patient/Family Education
- Explain name, dose, action, and potential side effects of medication.
- Review "Instructions for Application" sheet

with patient, parent, or guardian.
- Review prescribed dosing schedule with patient, parent, or guardian.
- Caution parent or guardian to not exceed prescribed dose, area of application, nor duration of application when using in infants and young children.
- Caution patient, parent, or guardian that medication may block all skin sensations and to avoid trauma to the treated area by scratching, rubbing, or exposure to extreme hot or cold temperatures until complete sensation has returned.
- Caution patient, parent, or guardian not to apply near eyes or on open wounds.
- Advise patient, parent, or guardian to remove cream and contact health care provider immediately if any of the following occur following application of cream: dizziness; excessive sleepiness; bluish discoloration of face or lips; agitation; twitching; tremors; serious reaction at application site.
- Remind patient or caregiver that follow-up examinations may be necessary while using this medication and to keep appointments.

Lindane

(LIN-dane)

Class Scabicide/Pediculicide

How Supplied
Lindane Lotion 1%, Shampoo 1%
✤ Hexit ♦ PMS-Lindane

Action
PHARMACOLOGY: Exerts its action by being directly absorbed into the parasite and ova.

Indications
Lotion: Treatment of *Sarcoptes scabiei* (scabies) in patients who have failed to respond to adequate doses or are intolerant of other approved therapies.
Shampoo: Treatment of *Pediculus capitis* (head lice) and *Pediculus pubis* (crab lice) and their ova in patients who have failed to respond to adequate doses or are intolerant of other approved therapies.

Contraindications Premature neonates because their skin may be more permeable than full-term infants, and neonates' liver enzymes may not be sufficiently developed; patients with known seizure disorders; hypersensitivity to any component of the product.

Route/Dosage
Provide a patient medication guide each time lindane is dispensed.

LOTION
Apply a thin layer over all skin from neck down. Wash hands immediately after applying or use gloves. One ounce is sufficient for an average adult. Do not prescribe more than 2 oz for larger adults. Apply only once. Wash off in 8 to 12 hr (max, 12 hr). Do not retreat. Do not cover areas where medication is applied.

SHAMPOO
Apply shampoo directly to dry hair without adding water. Work thoroughly into hair and allow to remain in place for 4 min only. Special attention should be given to the fine hairs along the neck. After 4 min, add small quantities of water to hair until a good lather forms. Immediately rinse all lather away. Avoid unnecessary contact of lather with other body surfaces. Most patients will require only 1 oz; do not prescribe more than 2 oz for larger adults. Do not retreat.

Interactions
Drugs that may lower seizure threshold (eg, antipsychotics, antidepressants, centrally acting anticholinesterases): Because seizure threshold may be lowered, use with caution.
Oils: Oils may enhance absorption; therefore, avoid oil treatments and oil-based hair dressings or conditioners immediately before or after application of lindane shampoo.

Lab Test Interferences None well documented.

Adverse Reactions
CNS: Stimulation, dizziness, seizures/convulsions; headache (postmarketing).
DERM: Irritant dermatitis; alopecia, dermatitis, paresthesia, pruritus, urticaria (postmarketing).
OTHER: Death; pain (postmarketing).

> **WARNING:**
> Reserved for patients who are intolerant or failed first-line therapy. Contraindicated in premature infants and those with uncontrolled seizure disorders. Patient counseling in proper use is required.
>
> *Neurotoxicity:* Seizures and death have been reported with repeat or prolonged application and rarely with single application. Use with caution because of increased risk in infants, children, elderly, in those with other skin conditions, and in those who weigh less than 50 kg.

Precautions
Pregnancy: Category C.
Lactation: Excreted in breast milk in low concentrations.
Children: Pediatric patients have a higher surface to volume ratio and may be at risk of

greater systemic exposure when lindane is applied. Infants and children may be at even higher risk because of immaturity of organ systems such as skin and liver. Use with caution in patients weighing less than 50 kg and especially in infants.

Absorption: Lindane penetrates human skin and has the potential for CNS toxicity (eg, seizures).

PATIENT CARE CONSIDERATIONS
Administration/Storage
- For topical use only. Not for ophthalmic, oral, or intravaginal use.
- Do not apply to skin that has open wounds, cuts, or sores unless specifically directed by health care provider.
- Avoid contact with eyes. If eye contact occurs, flush immediately and thoroughly with water.

Lotion:
- Shake well; use gloves if applying to patient; apply prescribed amount to dry, affected skin in a thin layer and rub in thoroughly; trim nails and apply under nails with toothbrush (throw away toothbrush after use); leave lotion on for 8 to 12 hr (eg, overnight) then wash off with shower or bath.

Shampoo:
- Wash hair with regular shampoo (without conditioners), rinse, and dry thoroughly; use gloves if applying lindane shampoo to patient; shake well and apply prescribed amount of shampoo directly to dry hair without adding water; work thoroughly into hair and allow to remain in place for 4 min only; add small quantities of water to hair until a good lather forms then immediately rinse all lather away, avoiding unnecessary contact of lather with other body surfaces; towel dry hair briskly and remove nits with nit comb or tweezers.
- Store at controlled room temperature (59° to 86°F). Keep bottle tightly capped.

Assessment/Interventions
- Obtain patient history, including drug history and any known allergies. Note history of seizure disorder or diagnosis of Norwegian (encrusted) scabies.
- Identify areas where medication is to be applied and areas with cuts, open wounds, or sores that should be avoided.
- Assess and document skin condition before initial application and periodically throughout treatment.
- Ensure that pregnant patient receives no more than 2 treatments with lindane lotion during the pregnancy.

Toxic effects of topically applied lindane may be greater in the young.
External use: Avoid contact with eyes.
Reinfestation: Lindane does not prevent infestation or reinfestation and should not be used to ward off a possible infestation.

Overdosage: Signs and Symptoms
CNS excitation, seizures, convulsions.

Patient/Family Education
- Explain name, dose, action, and potential side effects of drug.
- Advise patient or caregiver to review Patient Directions for Use before applying medication.
- Caution patient or caregiver that medication has potential for causing serious harm and not to exceed prescribed dose or apply more frequently than prescribed by health care provider. Advise patient or caregiver not to reapply unless specifically advised by health care provider.
- Caution patient or caregiver to avoid contact with eyes, and if accidental eye contact occurs, immediately flush the eyes with water to remove medication. Advise patient or caregiver to notify health care provider if eye irritation or sensitivity follows exposure to the eyes.
- Teach patient or caregiver proper technique for applying lotion: shake well; wash hands; use gloves if applying to another person; apply prescribed amount to dry, affected skin in a thin layer and rub in thoroughly; trim nails and apply under nails with toothbrush (throw away toothbrush after use); wash hands after applying lotion; leave lotion on for 8 to 12 hr (eg, overnight) then wash off with shower or bath. Advise patient or caregiver that itching will continue for several weeks but that this is normal and does not require a second application.
- Advise patient or caregiver to avoid concurrent use of creams, ointments, or oils while using lindane lotion because of increased risk of absorption and toxicity.
- Teach patient or caregiver proper technique for applying shampoo: wash hair with regular shampoo (without conditioners), rinse, and dry thoroughly; use gloves if applying to another person; shake well and apply prescribed amount of shampoo directly to dry hair without adding water; work thoroughly into hair and allow to remain in place for 4 min only; add small quantities of water to

hair until a good lather forms then immediately rinse all lather away, avoiding unnecessary contact of lather with other body surfaces; towel dry hair briskly and remove nits with nit comb or tweezers.
- Advise patient or caregiver to avoid concurrent use of oil treatments or oil-based hair dressings or conditioners immediately before or after applying lindane shampoo because of increased risk of absorption and toxicity.
- Advise patient not to use any covering over the applied lotion that does not breathe, such as diapers with plastic lining, or plastic or tight clothes.
- Advise patient or caregiver that all recently used clothing, underwear, pajamas, bedclothes, pillows, and towels should be washed in hot water or dry cleaned to prevent reexposure.
- Advise nursing mother who is being treated that medication is probably safe but if there is any concern, use an alternate method of feeding for 4 days following application.
- Advise patient or caregiver that follow-up visits may be necessary and to keep appointments.

Linezolid

(lin-EH-zoe-lid)
Class Anti-infective/Antibiotic

How Supplied
Zyvox Tablets 400 mg (sodium content is 1.95 mg/400 mg tablet [0.1 mEq/tablet]), Tablets 600 mg (sodium content is 2.92 mg/600 mg tablet [0.1 mEq/tablet]), Powder for oral suspension 100 mg/5 mL (sodium content is 8.52 mg/5 mL [0.4 mEq/5 mL]), Injection 2 mg/mL (sodium content is 0.38 mg/mL [5 mEq/300 mL bag, 3.3 mEq/200 mL bag, 1.7 mEq/100 mL bag])
✤ Zyvoxam ◆ Zyvoxam IV

Action
PHARMACOLOGY: Prevents the formation of a functional 70S initiation complex, which is essential to the bacterial translation process.

PHARMACOKINETICS/DYNAMICS:
Absorption: Rapidly and extensively absorbed. T_{max} is 1 to 2 hr. Absolute bioavailability is about 100% (no dose adjustment needed from IV to oral). Food does not affect absorption; however, T_{max} is delayed from 1.5 to 2.2 hr and C_{max} is decreased 17% when high-fat food is given.

Distribution: Readily distributed to well-perfused tissues; 31% protein bound. Vd at steady state is 40 to 50 L.

Metabolism: Primarily metabolized by oxidation of the morpholine ring. Metabolites are aminoethoxyacetic acid (A) and hydroxyethyl glycine (B) metabolite.

Excretion: About 65% nonrenal Cl. Approximately 30% of dose appears in urine (40% as metabolite B, 10% as metabolite A). Renal Cl is 40 mL/min.

Indications
Treatment of vancomycin-resistant *Enterococcus faecium* infections; treatment of nosocomial pneumonia, complicated and uncomplicated skin and skin structure infections, and community-acquired pneumonia caused by susceptible strains of specific organisms.

Contraindications
Standard considerations.

Route/Dosage
No dosage adjustment is necessary when switching from IV to PO. Administer IV infusion over a period of 30 to 120 min.

Vancomycin-Resistant E. faecium Infections, Including Concomitant Bacteremia
ADULTS AND CHILDREN 12 YR AND OLDER: **PO** or **IV** 600 mg q 12 hr for 14 to 28 days.
CHILDREN (BIRTH THROUGH 11 YR): **PO** or **IV** 10 mg/kg q 8 hr for 14 to 28 days. Most preterm neonates younger than 7 days should start with 10 mg/kg q 12 hr. A dose of 10 mg/kg q 8 hr may be considered in neonates with a suboptimal response.

Nosocomial Pneumonia, Complicated Skin and Skin Structure Infections, Community-Acquired Pneumonia, Including Concomitant Bacteremia
ADULTS AND CHILDREN 12 YR AND OLDER: **PO** or **IV** 600 mg q 12 hr for 10 to 14 days.
CHILDREN BIRTH THROUGH 11 YR: **PO** or **IV** 10 mg/kg q 8 hr for 10 to 14 days. Most preterm neonates less than 7 days should start with 10 mg/kg q 12 hr. A dose of 10 mg/kg q 8 hr may be considered in neonates with a suboptimal response.

Uncomplicated Skin and Skin Structure Infections
ADULTS AND CHILDREN 12 YR AND OLDER: **PO** 400 mg q 12 hr for 10 to 14 days.
CHILDREN 5 TO 11 YR: **PO** 10 mg/kg q 12 hr for 10 to 14 days.
CHILDREN YOUNGER THAN 5 YR: **PO** 10 mg/kg q 8 hr for 10 to 14 days. Most preterm neonates younger than 7 days should start with 10 mg/kg q 12 hr. A dose of 10 mg/kg q 8 hr may be considered in neonates with a suboptimal response.

Interactions
Adrenergic agents (eg, dopamine, epinephrine): Effects may be enhanced by linezolid.

Serotonergic agents (eg, fluoxetine): Possible increased risk of serotonin syndrome.

Lab Test Interferences None well documented.

Adverse Reactions

CNS: Headache (7%); insomnia, convulsions (3%); dizziness (2%); vertigo (1%); neuropathy (postmarketing).
DERM: Rash (7%); skin disorder (2%).
EENT: Pharyngitis (3%).
GI: Diarrhea (11%); vomiting (9%); nausea (6%); generalized and localized abdominal pain, GI bleeding, loose stools, constipation, altered taste (2%); tongue discoloration, oral moniliasis (1%).
GU: Vaginal moniliasis (2%).
HEMA: Anemia (6%); thrombocytopenia (5%); thrombocythemia (3%); eosinophilia (1%); leukopenia, pancytopenia (postmarketing).
LABTESTABS: Abnormal LFTs (1%).
METAB: Hypokalemia (3%); generalized edema (2%); lactic acidosis (postmarketing).
RESP: Upper respiratory tract infection (4%); pneumonia, dyspnea (3%); cough, apnea (2%).
OTHER: Fever (14%); sepsis (8%); trauma, injection site reactions (3%); fungal infections, localized pain (2%).

Precautions

Pregnancy: Category C.
Lactation: Undetermined.
Children: See dosing recommendations.
Lactic acidosis: May occur.
Myelosuppression: Because myelosuppression has been reported, monitor CBC weekly in patients receiving linezolid.
Phenylketonurics: Oral suspension contains phenylalanine.
Pseudomembranous colitis: Consider pseudomembranous colitis in patients in whom diarrhea develops.

PATIENT CARE CONSIDERATIONS

Administration/Storage

- Do not administer suspension to patient with phenylketonuria without first discussing with health care provider.
- No dose adjustment is needed when switching from IV to oral tablets or suspension.
- Administer tablets and suspension without regard to meals.
- Gently mix suspension by inverting bottle 3 to 5 times before each dose. Do not shake suspension.
- Use suspension for adults who have difficulty swallowing.
- Store tablets, suspension, and IV solution at controlled room temperature (59° to 86°F). Protect infusion bags from freezing. Protect from light. Keep bottles tightly closed. Discard any unused suspension after 21 days.

IV administration:

- Keep infusion bag in protective overwrap until ready to administer.
- Before administering, check IV bag for minute leaks by firmly squeezing bag and visually inspect for particulate matter. Do not use if either is noted.
- Solution may exhibit a yellow color, which is normal and does not affect potency.
- Administer IV infusion over 30 to 120 min.
- Do not use IV infusion bag in series connections or add any other medications to bag.
- If other drugs are being administered through same IV line, flush line before and after infusion of linezolid with 5% dextrose injection, 0.9% sodium chloride injection, or lactated Ringer's injection.
- Injection is supplied in single-use, ready-to-use infusion bags.

Assessment/Interventions

- Obtain patient history, including drug history and any known allergies. Note hypertension, hepatic impairment, phenylketonuria, myelosuppression, or concurrent use of bone marrow suppressive therapy or serotonergic agents (eg, SSRIs).
- Review results of culture and sensitivity testing as available.
- Ensure that CBC is determined weekly during therapy with linezolid.
- Ensure that patient's diet contains no food with high tyramine content.
- Monitor for signs of infection, especially fever, and for positive response to antibiotic therapy.
- Monitor patient for signs of allergic reaction. Discontinue therapy and immediately notify health care provider if noted.
- Monitor patient for GI, CNS, and general body side effects. Report to health care provider if noted and significant.

Patient/Family Education

- Explain name, dose, action, and potential side effects of drug.
- Review dosing schedule and prescribed length of therapy with patient. Advise patient that dose and duration of therapy are dependent on site and cause of infection.
- Advise patient that medication may be taken without regard to meals.

- Instruct patient to complete entire course of therapy, even if symptoms of infection have disappeared.
- Instruct patient to avoid foods with high tyramine content. Review common foods known to have high tyramine content (eg, aged cheeses, soy sauce, fermented or air-dried meats, sauerkraut, tap beers, red wines).
- Advise patient that diarrhea, headache, and nausea are the most common side effects and to inform health care provider if these symptoms occur and are intolerable.
- Advise patient to discontinue therapy and contact health care provider immediately if skin rash, hives, itching, or shortness of breath occur.
- Advise patient to report the following signs of superinfection to health care provider: black, furry tongue; white patches in mouth; foul-smelling stools; vaginal itching or discharge.
- Warn patient that diarrhea containing blood or pus may be a sign of a serious disorder and to seek medical care if noted and not to treat at home.
- Caution patient not to take any OTC cold products or decongestants containing ephedrine or pseudoephedrine.
- Instruct patient not to take any prescription or OTC medications or dietary supplements unless advised by health care provider.
- Advise patient that follow-up examinations and lab tests may be required to monitor therapy and to keep appointments.

Liothyronine Sodium (T_3; triiodothyronine)

(lie-oh-THIGH-row-neen SO-deeuhm)

Class Thyroid hormone

How Supplied
Cytomel Tablets 5 mcg, Tablets 25 mcg, Tablets 50 mcg ◆ *Triostat* Injection 10 mcg/mL

Action
PHARMACOLOGY: Increases metabolic rate of body tissues; is needed for normal growth and maturation.

PHARMACOKINETICS/DYNAMICS:
Absorption: 95% absorbed.
Distribution: Protein binding is more than 99%.
Excretion: Biological t½ is 2.5 days.
Onset: Within a few hr.
Peak: Within 2 to 3 days.

Indications Replacement or supplemental therapy in hypothyroidism; TSH suppression for treatment or prevention of euthyroid goiters (eg, thyroid nodules, multinodular goiters, enlargement in chronic thyroiditis); diagnostic agent in suppression tests to differentiate suspected hyperthyroidism from euthyroidism; treatment of myxedema coma/precoma (IV).

Contraindications Acute MI and thyrotoxicosis uncomplicated by hypothyroidism; coexistence of hypothyroidism and hypoadrenalism (Addison disease), unless treatment of hypoadrenalism with adrenocortical steroids precedes initiation of thyroid therapy.

Route/Dosage
Individualize dosage.

Hypothyroidism
ADULTS: **PO** 25 mcg/day initially, increase by up to 25 mcg q 1 to 2 wk if needed.
CHILDREN: **PO** 5 mcg/day initially, increase by 5 mcg/day at 2 wk intervals, if needed.

Congenital Hypothyroidism
CHILDREN: **PO** 5 mcg/day initially; increase by 5 mcg/day every 3 to 4 days until desired response achieved. Infants a few mo of age may require only 20 mcg/day for maintenance; at 1 yr, 50 mcg/day may be required; and, above 3 yr, full adult dosage may be required.

Simple (Nontoxic) Goiter
ADULTS: **PO** 5 mcg/day initially, increase by 5 to 10 mcg q 1 to 2 wk. When 25 mcg/day is reached, increase by 12.5 to 25 mcg q 1 to 2 wk if needed.
CHILDREN: **PO** 5 mcg/day initially, increase by 5 mcg/day at 2-wk intervals, if needed.

Myxedema
ADULTS: **PO** 5 mcg/day initially, increase by 5 to 10 mcg q 1 to 2 wk. When 25 mcg/day is reached, increase by 12.5 to 25 mcg q 1 to 2 wk if needed.
CHILDREN: **PO** 5 mcg/day initially, increase by 5 mcg/day at 2-wk intervals, if needed.

Myxedema Coma/Precoma
ADULTS: **IV** 25 to 50 mcg initially. In patients with known or suspected cardiovascular disease, an initial dose of 10 to 20 mcg is suggested; however, base doses on continuous monitoring of the condition and response to therapy.

TSH Suppression Test
ADULTS: **PO** 75 to 100 mcg/day for 7 days.

Interactions
Anticoagulants, oral: May increase anticoagulant effects.
Beta blockers: May reduce effects of beta blockers.
Cholestyramine, colestipol: May decrease thyroid hormone efficacy.
Digitalis glycosides: May reduce effects of glycosides.

Theophyllines: Hypothyroidism; may cause decreased theophylline clearance; Cl may return to normal when euthyroid state is achieved.

Lab Test Interferences Consider changes in thyroxine-binding globulin concentration when interpreting thyroxine (T_4) and triiodothyronine (T_3) values; medicinal or dietary iodine interferes with all in vivo tests of radioiodine uptake, producing low uptakes that may not reflect true decrease in hormone synthesis.

Adverse Reactions
CV: Palpitations; tachycardia; cardiac arrhythmias; angina pectoris; cardiac arrest.
CNS: Tremors; headache; nervousness; insomnia.
GI: Diarrhea; vomiting.
OTHER: Hypersensitivity; weight loss; menstrual irregularities; sweating; heat intolerance; fever; decreased bone density (in women using drug long term).

> **WARNING:**
> Not for use in obesity treatment. Ineffective for weight reduction indications and may produce life-threatening or serious consequences when used in large doses or in combination with other anorectics.

Precautions
Pregnancy: Category A.
Lactation: Minimal amounts excreted in breast milk.
Children: When drug is administered for congenital hypothyroidism, routine determinations of serum T_4 or TSH are strongly advised in newborns. In infants, excessive doses of thyroid hormone preparations may produce craniosynostosis. Children may experience transient partial hair loss in first few months of thyroid therapy.
Elderly: Therapy should be started with 5 mcg q day and increased by 5 mcg increments at recommended intervals.
Cardiovascular disease: Use caution when integrity of cardiovascular system, particularly coronary arteries, is suspect (eg, angina, elderly). Development of chest pain or worsening cardiovascular disease requires decrease in dosage.
Endocrine disorders: Therapy in patients with concomitant diabetes mellitus, diabetes insipidus, or adrenal insufficiency (Addison disease) exacerbates intensity of their symptoms. Therapy of myxedema coma requires simultaneous administration of glucocorticoids. Use corticosteroids to correct adrenal insufficiency in patients whose hypothyroidism is secondary to hypopituitarism.
Hyperthyroid effects: Liothyronine may rarely precipitate hyperthyroid state or may aggravate existing hyperthyroidism.
Infertility: Drug is unjustified for treatment of male or female infertility unless condition is accompanied by hypothyroidism.
Morphologic hypogonadism and nephrosis: Rule out before therapy.
Myxedema coma: Patients are particularly sensitive to thyroid preparations. Sudden administration of large doses is not without cardiovascular risks. Small initial doses are indicated.

Overdosage: Signs and Symptoms
Symptoms of hyperthyroidism: Headache, irritability, nervousness, sweating, tachycardia, increased bowel motility, menstrual irregularities, palpitations, vomiting, psychosis, seizure, fever, angina pectoris, CHF, shock, arrhythmias, thyroid storm.

PATIENT CARE CONSIDERATIONS
Administration/Storage
- Administer once a day in the early morning to prevent sleep disturbances.
- Administer liothyronine injection IV only, do not give IM or SC.
- Administer with caution to patients with known cardiovascular disease.
- Administer cautiously to patients with possible thyroid gland autonomy as there is danger of an additive effect between the exogenous and endogenous sources.
- Administer only by injection to patients in myxedema coma and with precoma diagnoses.
- Ensure oral therapy is resumed as soon as patient is stabilized.
- Discontinue IV injection therapy gradually when switching to tablets. Expect a low dosage that will be increased gradually according to response.
- Administer cautiously to elderly patients and patients with known or suspected cardiovascular disease. Note contraindications in some serious cardiovascular conditions and thyrotoxicosis.
- Do not administer large doses of liothyronine with sympathomimetic amines, as serious and even life-threatening results can occur.
- Administer cholestyramine and thyroid hormones 4 to 5 hr apart.
- Store tablets in tightly closed container at room temperature; store injectable under refrigeration.

Assessment/Interventions
- Obtain patient history, including drug history and any known side effects.
- Prior to initial administration, obtain baseline data of TSH and T_4 levels.

- Monitor for signs and symptoms of thyroid deficit or excess.
- Periodically assess thyroid status by using the TSH suppression test.
- Monitor patients on anticoagulants for signs of bleeding.
- Monitor patients on insulin or oral hypoglycemics closely during initiation of thyroid replacement therapy. Increase in insulin or oral hypoglycemic dosage may be required.
- If patient is switching therapies, be aware that liothyronine has a rapid onset of action but residual effects of other thyroid preparations may persist for the first several weeks of therapy.
- Inform laboratory if patient is pregnant or taking androgens, corticosteroids, estrogens, oral contraceptives, preparations containing salicylates, iodine-containing preparations, or medicinal or dietary iodine, as these drugs are known to interfere with tests of patients on liothyronine therapy. Interacting medications may need to be held or discontinued prior to the test.
- Assess for side effects that can occur more rapidly with liothyronine because of its rapid onset.
- Monitor patient on digoxin for signs and symptoms of potential digitalis toxicity as thyroid hormone increases metabolic rate, which requires an increased digitalis dosage.

Patient/Family Education

- Instruct patient to take liothyronine as directed. Do not change or discontinue dosage without consulting health care provider. Explain that liothyronine does not cure hypothyroidism and that therapy will continue for rest of life.
- Instruct patient with diabetes mellitus to closely monitor urinary glucose levels. The daily dosage of antidiabetic medication may need readjustment as thyroid hormone replacement is achieved or if thyroid medication is stopped.
- Explain that partial hair loss may be experienced by children in first few months of therapy, but that this side effect is transient.
- Advise patient to wear *Medi-Alert* bracelet or necklace and to carry *Medi-Alert* card in wallet.
- Inform patient that liothyronine's effects are more rapid than levothyroxine, which requires several days before onset of action.
- Teach patient to take pulse and inform the health care provider if signs of tachycardia or dysrhythmias occur.
- Instruct patient to call the health care provider immediately if any adverse symptoms such as chest pain, palpitations, headaches, irritability, increased nervousness, diaphoresis, tachycardia, dysrhythmias, or heat intolerance occur.
- Inform patient of possible adverse reactions with other drugs or foods they may be taking. Caution patient to inform health care provider of any drugs, including OTC drugs, they may be taking or planning to take.
- Emphasize the importance of follow-up examinations and periodic laboratory tests.
- Caution patient not to take liothyronine for weight control.

Liotrix

(LIE-oh-trix)

Class Thyroid hormone

How Supplied

Thyrolar ¼ Tablets 3.1 mcg T_3/12.5 mcg T_4 (thyroid equivalent to 15) ♦ *Thyrolar* ½ Tablets 6.25 mcg T_3/25 mcg T_4 (thyroid equivalent to 30) ♦ *Thyrolar* 1 Tablets 12.5 mcg T_3/50 mcg T_4 (thyroid equivalent to 60) ♦ *Thyrolar* 2 Tablets 25 mcg T_3/100 mcg T_4 (thyroid equivalent to 120) ♦ *Thyrolar* 3 Tablets 37.5 mcg T_3/150 mcg T_4 (thyroid equivalent to 180)

Action

PHARMACOLOGY: Increases metabolic rate of body tissues; is needed for normal growth and maturation.

PHARMACOKINETICS/DYNAMICS:
Absorption: 40% to 80% of T_4 is absorbed; absorption is increased by fasting and decreased by certain foods. Approximately 95% of T_3 is absorbed in 4 hr.

Distribution: More than 99% is bound to serum proteins. Minimal amounts excreted in breast milk.

Metabolism: Approximately 80% of T_3 comes from monodeiodination of T_4. Conjugated hormone is found in the bile and gut where it may undergo enterahepatic circulation.

Excretion: Primarily eliminated by the kidneys. Approximately 20% of T_4 is excreted in feces.

Special Populations:
Age – T_4 absorption and urinary excretion are decreased with age.

Indications Replacement or supplemental therapy in hypothyroidism; pituitary TSH suppression in treatment or prevention of various types of euthyroid goiters, including thyroid nodules, subacute or chronic lymphocytic thyroiditis (Hashimoto's), multinodular goiter, and management of thyroid cancer; diagnostic agent in suppression tests to differentiate suspected and hyperthyroidism or thyroid gland autonomy.

Contraindications Diagnosed but uncorrected adrenal cortical insufficiency; untreated thyrotoxicosis; apparent hypersensitivity to any component of the product.

Route/Dosage
Hypothyroidism
Adults – **PO** Start with low doses, with increments depending on the cardiovascular status. Usual starting dose is 1 tablet of *Thyrolar* ½ with increments of 1 tablet of *Thyrolar* ¼ q 2 to 3 wk. In patients with long-standing myxedema, the recommended starting dose is 1 tablet daily of *Thyrolar* ¼ and reduce dosage if angina occurs. Readjust dosage within first 4 wk of therapy after proper clinical and laboratory evaluations, including serum levels of T_4 (bound and free) and TSH.

Congenital Hypothyroidism
CHILDREN (OVER 12 YR): **PO** More than 18.75 mcg of T_3 and 75 mcg T_4 daily.
CHILDREN (6 TO 12 YR): **PO** 12.5 mcg of T_3 and 50 mcg T_4 to 18.75 mcg of T_3 and 75 mcg T_4 daily.
CHILDREN (1 TO 5 YR): **PO** 9.35 mcg of T_3 and 37.5 mcg of T_4 to 12.5 mcg of T_3 and 50 mcg T_4 daily.
CHILDREN (6 MO TO 12 MO): **PO** 6.25 mcg of T_3 and 25 mcg of T_4 to 9.35 mcg of T_3 and 37.5 mcg of T_4 daily.
CHILDREN (0 MO TO 6 MO): **PO** 3.1 mcg of T_3 and 12.5 mcg of T_4 to 6.25 mcg of T_3 and 25 mcg of T_4 daily.

Thyroid Cancer
ADULTS: **PO** Larger amounts of thyroid hormone than those used for replacement therapy are required.

DIAGNOSTIC AGENT
ADULTS: **PO** Usual suppressive dose of T_4 is 1.56 mcg/kg/day for 7 to 10 days.

PATIENT CARE CONSIDERATIONS
Administration/Storage
- Administer prescribed dose once daily. When given on an empty stomach, absorption is increased. However, to maintain steady blood levels and effect, be consistent in administering drug with or without food.
- Store tablets in refrigerator (36° to 46°F).

Assessment/Interventions
- Obtain patient history, including drug history and any known allergies. Note history of uncorrected adrenocortical insufficiency, untreated thyrotoxicosis, angina pectoris, diabetes mellitus, diabetes insipidus, cardiovascular disease.

Interactions
Anticoagulants: May increase anticoagulant effect.
Cholestyramine, colestipol: Bind T_3 and T_4 in the intestine, impairing absorption.
Estrogens, oral contraceptives: Thyroid requirement may be increased in patients with nonfunctioning thyroid gland or receiving thyroid replacement therapy.
Insulin, oral hypoglycemics: Requirements of these agents may be increased by liotrix.

Lab Test Interferences Consider changes in thyroid binding globulin concentration when interpreting thyroxine (T_4) and triiodothyronine (T_3) values; medicinal or dietary iodine interferes with all in vivo tests of radioiodine uptake, producing low uptakes that may not reflect true decrease in hormone synthesis.

Adverse Reactions
METAB: Hypermetabolic state (indicative of hyperthyroidism).

Precautions
Pregnancy: Category A.
Lactation: Minimal amounts excreted in breast milk.
Children: When used for congenital hypothyroidism, routine determinations of serum T_4 or TSH are strongly advised in newborns.
Special risk patients: Use with great caution in patients with cardiovascular disease, especially if integrity of coronary arteries is suspected, including patients with angina pectoris or the elderly; may aggravate intensity of symptoms in patients with diabetes mellitus or insipidus or adrenal cortical insufficiency.
Myxedema coma: Requires simultaneous administration of glucocorticoids.
Weight reduction: Should not be used for weight reduction; may produce serious or life-threatening toxicity particularly when given with sympathomimetics or anorexiants.

Overdosage: Signs and Symptoms
Hypermetabolic state.

- Ensure that thyroid function tests (eg, TSH, T_4) are determined prior to starting therapy and periodically during treatment.
- Monitor height, weight, and intellectual function in children to document normal development.
- Monitor blood sugar in diabetic patient when drug is started or dose is changed. Report significant changes to health care provider.
- Notify health care provider if any of the following develops: chest pain, increased heart rate, palpitations, excessive sweating, heat intolerance, nervousness, tremors, other unusual events.

Patient/Family Education
- Explain name, dose, action, and potential side effects of drug.
- Instruct patient to take prescribed dose once daily.
- Advise patient to take each dose at about the same time each day and consistently with or without food.
- Advise patient that therapy will be started with a low dose and that the dose may be gradually increased until maximum benefit is obtained.
- Caution patient not to change the dose or stop taking unless advised to do so by health care provider.
- Inform patient that drug controls, but does not cure, symptoms of hypothyroidism, and to continue taking the drug as prescribed even when feeling better.
- Advise patient that thyroid replacement therapy is usually a life-long therapy.
- Advise patient to notify health care provider if any of the following are noted: chest pain, increased heart rate, palpitations, excessive sweating, heat intolerance, nervousness, tremors, other unusual events.
- Instruct diabetic patient to monitor blood glucose more frequently when drug is started or dose is changed and to inform health care provider of significant changes in readings.
- Explain to parent or guardian that partial hair loss may be experienced by child in first few months of therapy but that this side effect is usually reversible.
- Instruct women to notify health care provider if pregnant, planning to become pregnant, or breastfeeding.
- Instruct patient to not take any prescription or OTC medications or dietary supplements unless advised to do so by health care provider.
- Advise patient that follow-up visits and lab tests will be required to monitor therapy and to keep appointments.

Lisinopril

(lie-SIN-oh-prill)

Class Antihypertensive/ACE inhibitor

How Supplied
Prinivil Tablets 2.5 mg, Tablets 5 mg, Tablets 10 mg, Tablets 20 mg, Tablets 40 mg ♦ *Zestril* Tablets 2.5 mg, Tablets 5 mg, Tablets 10 mg, Tablets 20 mg, Tablets 30 mg, Tablets 40 mg ✤ *Apo-Lisinopril*

Action
PHARMACOLOGY: Competitively inhibits angiotensin I-converting enzyme (ACE), prevention of angiotensin I conversion to angiotensin II, a potent vasoconstrictor that also stimulates aldosterone secretion. Results in decrease in sodium and fluid retention, decrease in BP, and increase in diuresis.

PHARMACOKINETICS/DYNAMICS:
Absorption: T_{max} is about 7 hr.
Distribution: Does not appear to be bound to other serum proteins.
Metabolism: Does not undergo metabolism.
Excretion: The t½ is 12 hr. Excreted via the kidney; excreted unchanged entirely in the urine. Lisinopril can be removed by hemodialysis.
Onset: 1 hr.
Peak: 6 hr.
Duration: 24 hr.
Special Populations:
Renal Function Impairment – Decreased elimination when glomerular filtration rate is less than or equal to 30 mL/min.
Race – Black patients with hypertension had a smaller response to monotherapy of ACE inhibitor.
CHF (NYHA class II through IV) – Bioavailability decreases about 16% and Vd is slightly smaller.

Indications Treatment of hypertension; treatment of heart failure not responding to diuretics and digitalis; treatment of acute MI within 24 hr in hemodynamically stable patients.

Contraindications Hypersensitivity to ACE inhibitors and in patients with hereditary or idiopathic angioedema.

Route/Dosage
CHF
ADULTS:
Initial dose: **PO** 5 mg qd with diuretics and digitalis; reduce concomitant diuretic dose, if possible, to minimize hypovolemia. In patients with hyponatremia, initiate with 2.5 mg qd.
Usual dose: **PO** 5 to 20 mg/day.

Hypertension
ADULTS:
Initial dose: **PO** 10 mg qd.
Maintenance: **PO** 20 to 40 mg/day; may add diuretic if needed and decrease dose.
CHILDREN (6 YR AND OLDER): **PO** Start with 0.07 mg/kg qd (up to 5 mg). Adjust dose according to BP response. Doses above 0.61 mg/kg (or in excess of 40 mg) have not been studied.

MI
ADULTS:
Initial dose: **PO** 5 mg, then 5 mg after 24 hr, then 10 mg after 48 hr.

Maintenance: **PO** 10 mg/day for 6 wk. Patients should receive, as appropriate, the standard recommended treatments, such as thrombolytics, aspirin, and beta-blockers.

Interactions
Antacids: Lisinopril bioavailability may be decreased. Separate administration times by 1 to 2 hr.
Capsaicin: Cough may be exacerbated.
Digoxin: May increase or decrease plasma digoxin levels.
Indomethacin, salicylates (eg, aspirin): Reduced hypotensive effects, especially in low-renin or volume-dependent hypertensive patients.
Lithium: Increased lithium levels and symptoms of lithium toxicity.
Phenothiazines: May increase pharmacological effect of lisinopril.
Potassium-sparing diuretics, potassium preparations: May increase serum potassium levels.

Lab Test Interferences False elevation of liver enzymes or serum bilirubin may occur.

Adverse Reactions
CV: Hypotension (10%); orthostatic effects (1%); cardiac arrest.
CNS: Dizziness (12%); headache (6%); fatigue (3%).
DERM: Rash (2%).
GI: Diarrhea (4%); nausea (2%); vomiting (1%).
GU: Renal dysfunction (2%); impotence (1%).
HEMA: Bone marrow depression; hemolytic anemia; leukopenia/neutropenia; thrombocytopenia.
METAB: Hyperkalemia.
RESP: Cough (4%); upper respiratory tract infections (2%); common cold (1%).
OTHER: Chest pain (3%); abdominal pain (2%); asthenia (1%); anaphylactoid reactions.

> **WARNING:**
> *Pregnancy:* Use in second and third trimesters may cause injury and death to fetus.

Precautions
Pregnancy: Category D (second and third trimester); Category C (first trimester). Can cause injury or death to fetus if used during second or third trimester.
Lactation: Undetermined.
Children: Safety and efficacy not established in children younger than 6 yr.
Elderly: Reduced dosage may be necessary.
Renal function impairment: Reduce dose and give less frequently. In renal insufficiency, stable elevations in BUN and serum creatinine may occur because of inadequate renal perfusion; monitor renal function during first few weeks of therapy and adjust dosage carefully, especially if glomerular filtration rate less than 30 mL/min.
Angioedema: Use with extreme caution in patients with hereditary angioedema.
Aortic stenosis/hypertrophic cardiomyopathy: As with other vasodilators, lisinopril should be used with caution in patients with obstruction in the outflow tract of the left ventricle.
Hepatic failure: Rarely, ACE inhibitors have been associated with a syndrome that starts with cholestatic jaundice and progresses to fulminant hepatic necrosis and sometimes death.
Hypotension/first-dose effect: Significant decreases in BP may occur after first dose, especially in severely salt- or volume-depleted patients or those with heart failure. Minimize risk by discontinuing diuretics, decreasing dose, or increasing salt intake approximately 1 wk prior to initiating drug.
Neutropenia and agranulocytosis: May occur; risk appears greater in patients with renal dysfunction, heart failure, or immunosuppression.

Overdosage: Signs and Symptoms
Hypotension.

PATIENT CARE CONSIDERATIONS
Administration/Storage
- Administer alone or in combination with other antihypertensives.
- Do not administer to pregnant women during second and third trimesters as fetal and neonatal morbidity and death can occur.
- Give prescribed dose without regard to meals. Administer with food if GI upset occurs.
- Store tablets at controlled room temperature (59° to 89°F). Protect from moisture.

Suspension:
- Tablets may be mixed with *Bicitra* and *Ora-Sweet SF*, following manufacturer's guidelines, to form a suspension.
- Shake well before measuring dose.
- Administer prescribed dose using dosing cup, spoon, or syringe.
- Store suspension at controlled room temperature (below 77°F). Discard any unused suspension after 28 days.

Assessment/Interventions
- Obtain patient history, including drug history and any known allergies. Note renal or hepatic impairment, conditions predisposing to volume depletion (eg, prolonged diuretic therapy), diabetes, heart failure, anuria, hereditary or idiopathic angioedema, lupus erythematosus, left ventricular outflow

obstruction, allergy to any other ACE inhibitor, and concurrent use of potassium-containing salt substitutes, potassium supplements, or potassium-sparing diuretics.
- Ensure that small initial dose and gradual escalation of dose are used in patient with heart failure or moderate to severe renal impairment (Ccr less than 30 mL/min) or following vigorous diuresis.
- Ensure that patient at risk of excessive hypotension or complications from hypotension (eg, ischemic heart or cerebrovascular disease) are closely monitored for the first 2 wk after starting therapy and following dosing escalation.
- Ensure that volume and/or salt depletion have been corrected before initiating therapy.
- Ensure that serum electrolytes and renal function are monitored periodically.
- Ensure that CBC with differential are evaluated prior to starting therapy, at 2 wk intervals for 3 mo, and periodically thereafter in patient with renal impairment.
- Monitor and record BP and pulse. Should symptomatic hypotension occur, hold medication and notify health care provider.
- Take safety precautions if orthostatic hypotension occurs.
- Assess heart failure patient for evidence of worsening failure (eg, daily weights, evaluation of peripheral edema, shortness of breath). Inform health care provider if rapid weight gain (eg, 2 pounds in 1 day or 5 pounds in 1 wk) is noted or if patient is experiencing worsening edema or other symptoms of heart failure (eg, worsening shortness of breath).
- Monitor for signs of hypersensitivity including angioedema involving swelling of the face, lips, eyelids, and tongue. Discontinue medication and notify health care provider immediately if noted. Be prepared to treat appropriately.
- Assess patient for GI, CNS, and general body side effects. Inform health care provider if noted and significant.

Patient/Family Education

- Explain name, dose, action, and potential side effects of drug.
- Advise patient to take prescribed dose without regard to meals but to take with food if stomach upset occurs.
- Advise patient or caregiver to shake suspension well before measuring dose and administer prescribed dose using dosing cup, spoon, or syringe.
- Advise patient to try to take each dose at about the same time each day.
- Inform hypertensive patient that drug controls, but does not cure, hypertension and to continue taking drug as prescribed even when BP is not elevated.
- Caution patient not to change the dose or stop taking unless advised by health care provider.
- Instruct patient to continue taking other medications for the condition as prescribed by health care provider.
- Instruct patient in BP and pulse measurement skills.
- Advise patient to monitor and record BP and pulse at home and to inform health care provider should abnormal measurements be noted. Also advise patient to take record of BP and pulse to each follow-up visit.
- Caution patient to avoid sudden position changes to prevent orthostatic hypotension.
- Instruct patient to lie or sit down if experiencing dizziness or lightheadedness when standing.
- Emphasize to hypertensive patient the importance of other modalities on BP control: weight control, regular exercise, smoking cessation, and moderate intake of alcohol and salt.
- Emphasize to heart failure patient the importance of other modalities that can help control heart failure symptoms: weight control, progressive exercise program, smoking cessation, and moderate intake of alcohol and salt.
- Advise heart failure patient to weigh daily, keep a record of daily weights, and notify health care provider if rapid weight gain (eg, 5 pounds in 1 wk) is noted or if edema or shortness of breath are getting worse.
- Caution patient that inadequate fluid intake, excessive perspiration, diarrhea, or vomiting can lead to excessive fall in BP, resulting in lightheadedness or fainting.
- Advise patient that medication may cause dizziness or lightheadedness and to use caution while driving or performing other tasks requiring mental alertness until tolerance is determined.
- Caution patient to avoid unnecessary exposure to UV light (sunlight, tanning booths) and to use sunscreen and wear protective clothing when exposed to UV light to avoid photosensitivity reaction.
- Instruct women to inform health care provider if pregnant, planning to become pregnant, or breastfeeding.
- Instruct patient to stop taking drug and immediately report any of these symptoms to health care provider: sore throat, fever, swelling of the hands or feet, irregular heartbeat, chest pains, fainting, swelling of the face, lips,

eyelids, or tongue, difficulty breathing.
- Instruct patient to inform health care provider if a persistent cough develops while taking this medication.
- Caution patient not to take any prescription or OTC medications, potassium-containing salt substitutes, potassium supplements, or dietary supplements unless advised by health care provider.
- Advise patient that follow-up visits and lab tests will be required to monitor therapy and to keep appointments.

Lisinopril/ Hydrochlorothiazide

(Lie-SIN-oh-prill/high-droe-klor-oh-THIGH-uh-zide)

Class Antihypertensive combination

How Supplied
Prinzide 10/12.5 mg Tablets 10 mg lisinopril and 12.5 mg hydrochlorothiazide ♦ Prinzide 20/12.5 mg Tablets 20 mg lisinopril and 12.5 mg hydrochlorothiazide ♦ Prinzide 20/25 mg Tablets 20 mg lisinopril and 25 mg hydrochlorothiazide ♦ Zestoretic Tablets 12.5 mg hydrochlorothiazide and 10 mg lisinopril, Tablets 12.5 mg hydrochlorothiazide and 20 mg lisinopril, Tablets 25 mg hydrochlorothiazide and 20 mg lisinopril

Action

PHARMACOLOGY:

Lisinopril: Competitively inhibits angiotensin I-converting enzyme, prevention of angiotensin I conversion to angiotensin II, reversing the potassium loss associated with the diuretic.
Hydrochlorothiazide (HCTZ): Increases chloride, sodium, and water excretion by interfering with transport of sodium ions across renal tubular epithelium.

Indications Treatment of hypertension.

Contraindications History of angioedema related to previous treatment with an angiotensin converting enzyme inhibitor; hereditary or idiopathic angioedema; anuria; hypersensitivity to sulfonamide-derived drugs, hypersensitivity to any component of the product.

Route/Dosage
ADULTS: **PO** Using qd doses of lisinopril/HCTZ combination therapy in lisinopril doses of 10 to 80 mg and HCTZ doses of 6.25 to 50 mg, the antihypertensive response rates generally increase with increasing doses of either component. Do not use dosage higher than lisinopril 80 mg and HCTZ 50 mg.

Interactions
HCTZ:
Alcohol, barbiturates, narcotics – Increased risk of orthostatic hypotension.
Antidiabetic agents (oral agents and insulin) – Dosage adjustment of antidiabetic agent may be necessary.
Antihypertensive agent – Additive or potentiation of effects.
Cholestyramine, colestipol resins – Impaired absorption of HCTZ.
Corticosteroids, ACTH – Increased electrolyte depletion, increasing the risk of hypokalemia.
Lithium – Renal clearance of lithium may be reduced, increasing the risk of lithium toxicity.
Nondepolarizing skeletal muscle relaxants (eg, tubocurarine) – Increased effect of the muscle relaxant.
Nonsteroidal anti-inflammatory agents – The diuretic, natriuretic, and antihypertensive effects of loop, potassium-sparing, and thiazide diuretics may be reduced.
Pressor amines (eg, norepinephrine) – Decreased responsiveness to the pressor amine.
Lisinopril:
Diuretic therapy – Excessive reduction in BP after starting lisinopril therapy.
Nonsteroidal anti-inflammatory agents – Worsening of renal function in patients with compromised renal function; antihypertensive effects of lisinopril may be diminished.
Agents increasing serum potassium (eg, potassium-sparing diuretics [eg, spironolactone], potassium supplements, potassium-containing salt substitutes) – May lead to increases in serum potassium.
Lithium – Because of possible increased sodium elimination, the risk of lithium toxicity is increased.

Lab Test Interferences
HCTZ: May decrease serum protein-bound iodine levels without signs of thyroid disturbances. May cause diagnostic interference of serum electrolyte levels, blood and urine glucose levels, serum bilirubin levels, and serum uric acid levels.
Lisinopril: False elevation of liver enzymes, serum bilirubin, uric acid, or blood glucose may occur.

Adverse Reactions Adverse reactions have been limited to those that have been previously reported with lisinopril or HCTZ. The most frequently occurring adverse reactions reported with the combination include the following:
CV: Orthostatic effects; excessive hypotension; syncope; palpitation.
CNS: Dizziness; headache; fatigue; asthenia; paresthesia.
DERM: Rash.
GI: Diarrhea; nausea; vomiting; dyspepsia.
GU: Impotence.

RESP: Cough; upper respiratory infection.
OTHER: Muscle cramps; angioedema.

Precautions

Pregnancy: Category D (second and third trimesters); Category C (first trimester).
Lactation: Undetermined.
Children: Safety and efficacy not established.
Hypersensitivity: Angioedema, including swelling of the face, extremities, lips, tongue, glottis and/or larynx, has been reported rarely. Angioedema associated with laryngeal edema may be fatal; promptly discontinue drug.
Renal function impairment: Use with caution.
Hepatic function impairment: Use with caution. Minor alterations of fluid and electrolyte balance may precipitate hepatic coma.
Anaphylactoid reactions: ACE inhibitors affect the metabolism of eicosanoids and polypeptides, including endogenous bradykinin. Patients may be subject to a variety of adverse reactions, some of them serious.
Aortic stenosis/hypertrophic cardiomyopathy: Use with caution.
Cough: Persistent nonproductive cough has been reported; always resolves after discontinuation of therapy.
Fluid/Electrolyte imbalance: All patients receiving thiazide therapy should be observed for clinical signs of fluid or electrolyte imbalance, mainly hyperkalemia and hypokalemia, hypercalcemia, hyponatremia, and hypomagnesemia.
Glucose tolerance: Dosage adjustment of insulin or oral hypoglycemic agents may be required. Hyperglycemia may occur with thiazide diuretics.
Hyperuricemia: Hyperuricemia may occur or frank gout may be precipitated in certain patients receiving thiazide therapy.
Hypotension: Excessive hypotension may occur, especially in severely salt-or volume-depleted patients or those with severe CHF.
Lipids: Increases in cholesterol and triglyceride levels may be associated with thiazide diuretic therapy.
Neutropenia/Agranulocytosis: May occur more frequently in patients with renal impairment, especially if they also have collagen vascular disease.

Overdosage: Signs and Symptoms

Dehydration, electrolyte imbalance, hypotension.

PATIENT CARE CONSIDERATIONS

Administration/Storage

- Administer prescribed dose qd in the morning, with or without food.
- Administer with food if GI upset occurs.
- Administer alone or in combination with other antihypertensives.
- Do not administer to pregnant women as fetal and neonatal morbidity and death can occur.
- Store tablets at controlled room temperature (59° to 86°F). Keep container tightly closed. Protect from excessive light and moisture.

Assessment/Interventions

- Obtain patient history, including drug history and any known allergies. Note history of diabetes, anuria, lupus erythematosus, kidney or liver disease, hereditary or idiopathic angioedema, aortic stenosis, hypertrophic cardiomyopathy, or allergy to any other ACE inhibitor or sulfonamide-derived medications. Note concurrent use of potassium-containing salt substitutes, potassium supplements, or potassium-sparing diuretics.
- Ensure that serum electrolytes and renal function are monitored periodically.
- Ensure that volume and/or salt depletion have been corrected before initiating therapy.
- Monitor and record BP and pulse. Should hypotension result, hold medication and notify health care provider.
- Take safety precautions if orthostatic hypotension occurs.
- Monitor blood sugar in diabetic patient when drug is started or dose is changed. Report significant changes to health care provider.
- Monitor for signs of nonproductive cough and hypersensitivity, including angioedema involving swelling of the face, lips, eyelids, and tongue. Discontinue medication and notify health care provider immediately if noted. Be prepared to treat appropriately.

Patient/Family Education

- Explain name, dose, action, and potential side effects of drug.
- Advise patient to take prescribed dose qd, without regard to meals but to take with food if GI upset occurs.
- Advise patient to try to take each dose at about the same time each day.
- Inform patient that drug controls, but does not cure, hypertension and to continue taking drug as prescribed even when BP is not elevated.
- Caution patient not to change the dose or

- stop taking unless advised by health care provider.
- Instruct patient to continue taking other BP medications as prescribed by health care provider.
- Instruct patient in BP and pulse measurement skills.
- Advise patient to monitor and record BP and pulse at home and to inform health care provider if abnormal measurements are noted. Also advise patient to take record of BP and pulse to each follow-up visit.
- Caution patient to avoid sudden position changes to prevent orthostatic hypotension.
- Instruct patient to lie or sit down if experiencing dizziness or lightheadedness when standing.
- Caution patient that inadequate fluid intake, excessive perspiration, diarrhea, or vomiting can lead to excessive fall in BP resulting in lightheadedness or fainting.
- Instruct diabetic patient to monitor blood glucose more frequently when drug is started or dose is changed and to inform health care provider of significant changes in readings.
- Caution patient to avoid unnecessary exposure to UV light (eg, sunlight, tanning booths), to use sunscreen, and to wear protective clothing when exposed to UV light to avoid photosensitivity reaction.
- Emphasize to hypertensive patient importance of other modalities on BP: weight control, regular exercise, smoking cessation, moderate intake of alcohol and salt.
- Advise women to notify health care provider if pregnant, planning to become pregnant, or breastfeeding.
- Instruct patient to stop taking drug and immediately report any of these symptoms to health care provider: fainting; swelling of the face, lips, eyelids, or tongue; difficulty breathing; any indication of infection (eg, sore throat, fever).
- Instruct patient to inform health care provider if a persistent cough develops while taking this medication.
- Caution patient to not take any prescription or OTC medications, potassium-containing salt substitutes, potassium supplements, or dietary supplements unless advised by health care provider.
- Advise patient that follow-up visits and lab tests may be required to monitor therapy and to keep appointments.

Lithium

(LITH-ee-uhm)

Class Antipsychotic/Antimanic

How Supplied

Eskalith Capsules 300 mg lithium carbonate (8.12 mEq lithium), Tablets 300 mg lithium carbonate (8.12 mEq lithium) ♦ *Eskalith CR* Tablets, controlled-release 450 mg lithium carbonate (12.8 mEq lithium) ♦ *Lithobid* Tablets, slow-release 300 mg lithium carbonate (8.12 mEq lithium) ♦ *Lithonate* Capsules 300 mg lithium carbonate (8.12 mEq lithium) ♦ *Lithotabs* Tablets 300 mg lithium carbonate (8.12 mEq lithium) ✤ *Carbolith* ♦ *Duralith* ♦ *Lithane* ♦ *PMS-Lithium Carbonate* ♦ *PMS-Lithium Citrate*

Action

PHARMACOLOGY: Specific mechanism unknown; alters sodium transport in nerve and muscle cells and effects shift toward intraneuronal metabolism of catecholamines.

PHARMACOKINETICS/DYNAMICS:

Absorption: Readily absorbed from the GI tract. Absorption is not significantly impaired by food. T_{max} is 0.5 to 3 hr. Therapeutic serum level is 0.4 to 1 mEq/L. Steady state is reached in 5 to 7 days.

Distribution: Distribution space of lithium approximates that of total body water. Not protein bound. Distribution across the blood-brain barrier is slow; however, the CSF lithium level is about 40% of the plasma concentration.

Excretion: About 95% eliminated by the kidney; primarily excreted in the urine. Renal excretion is proportional to its plasma concentration. The t½ is about 24 hr (10 to 50 hr).

Special Populations:

Elderly – Decreases rate of excretion; increases incidence of toxic effects. Therefore, lower doses and more frequent monitoring are recommended.

Indications Management of bipolar disorder and manic episodes of manic-depressive illness.

Unlabeled use(s): Treatment of neutropenia; unipolar depression; schizoaffective disorder; prophylaxis of cluster headaches; premenstrual tension; tardive dyskinesia; hyperthyroidism; SIADH, postpartum affective psychosis; corticosteroid-induced psychosis.

Contraindications History of leukemia.

Route/Dosage

ADULTS: **PO** 900 to 1800 mg/day in 2 to 4 divided doses. Give regular capsules tid or qid; slow-release tablets bid or tid. Max dose, 2400 mg/day.

CHILDREN AT LEAST 12 YR: 15 to 20 mg/kg/day in 2 to 3 divided doses.

Interactions

Acetazolamide, osmotic diuretics, theophyllines, urinary alkalinizers: Increased renal excretion of lithium.
ACE inhibitors, fluoxetine, loop diuretics, NSAIDs, thiazide diuretics: Increased lithium serum levels.
Carbamazepine, haloperidol, methyldopa: Increased neurotoxic effects despite therapeutic serum levels and normal dosage range.
Iodide salts: Increased risk of hypothyroidism.
Neuromuscular blocking agents, tricyclic antidepressants: Increased pharmacological effects of additive drug.
Phenothiazines: Neurotoxicity, decreased phenothiazine concentrations, or increased lithium concentrations may occur.
Verapamil: Reductions in lithium levels and lithium toxicity have occurred.

Lab Test Interferences
None well documented.

Adverse Reactions

CV: Arrhythmias; hypotension; bradycardia; peripheral circulatory collapse.
CNS: Tremor; muscle hyperirritability; headache; fatigue; ataxia; dizziness; psychomotor retardation; confusion; dystonia; hallucinations; blackouts; seizures; pseudotumor cerebri; drowsiness; poor memory and intellectual function; muscular weakness; slurred speech.
DERM: Drying or thinning hair; dry skin; pruritus; exacerbation of psoriasis; acne.
EENT: Blurred vision; tinnitus.
GI: Anorexia; nausea; vomiting; diarrhea; sialorrhea; dry mouth; parotitis.
GU: Urinary urgency; stress incontinence; polyuria; albuminuria; sexual dysfunction; symptoms of nephrogenic diabetes; decreased Ccr.
HEMA: Leukocytosis; leukemia.
METAB: Hypothyroidism; hypercalcemia; hyperparathyroidism; hyponatremia; dehydration; weight gain.
OTHER: Taste distortion; thirst; fever; swollen joints.

> **WARNING:**
> Toxicity is closely related to serum concentrations and may occur at doses close to therapeutic levels. Equipped facilities should be identified prior to initiation of therapy to provide prompt and accurate serum concentration data.

Precautions

Pregnancy: Category D.
Lactation: Excreted in breast milk.
Children: Safety and efficacy not established in children less than 12 yr.
Renal function impairment: Chronic use may lead to nephrogenic diabetes insipidus. Patients who have reduced renal function, including elderly, should take lower doses.
Tartrazine sensitivity: Some products contain tartrazine, which may cause allergic-type reactions in susceptible individuals.
Encephalopathic syndrome: Encephalopathic syndrome has occurred in patients also taking a neuroleptic and may cause irreversible brain damage. Characterized by weakness, lethargy, fever, tremors, confusion, extrapyramidal symptoms, leukocytosis, and elevated serum enzymes, BUN, and fasting blood sugar.
Hypothyroidism: Has occurred with chronic use. Thyroid hormone replacement therapy may be required.
Infections: Reduction in dose or discontinuation may be required if patient has infection with fever, especially if accompanied by protracted sweating, vomiting, or diarrhea.
Sodium/Volume depletion: Because drug decreases renal sodium absorption, patients must maintain adequate salt and fluid intake.
Toxicity: Toxicity can occur even at therapeutic doses. Toxicity risk is greater in patients with renal or cardiovascular disease, debilitation, dehydration, or sodium depletion.

Overdosage: Signs and Symptoms

ECG changes, slurred speech, seizures, acute renal failure, coma, diarrhea, vomiting, drowsiness, muscle weakness, ataxia.

PATIENT CARE CONSIDERATIONS

Administration/Storage

- Administer with meals to minimize GI upset.
- Do not crush, chew, or break extended-release capsules or coated tablets.
- Observe carefully during administration to make sure patient swallows medication.
- Store at room temperature. Protect capsules from moisture.

Assessment/Interventions

- Obtain patient history, including drug history and any known allergies.
- Ensure that baseline renal and thyroid function studies and ECG have been obtained before beginning therapy.
- Assess mood and behavior before beginning medication and frequently, thereafter. Particu-

larly note the following: flight of ideas, elation, grandiosity, aggressiveness, and hyperactivity.
- Assess for lithium toxicity: Persistent nausea/vomiting, diarrhea, ataxia, blurred vision, tinnitus.
- Periodically assess thyroid and renal function.
- Ensure that weekly lithium blood levels are obtained until therapeutic level has been reached; obtain monthly levels thereafter.
- Monitor lithium level frequently while titrating, then periodically once dose is stable. Therapeutic doses are 1 to 1.5 mEq/L during acute manic attacks and 0.6 to 1.2 mEq/L for maintenance. Perform lithium serum testing as close as possible to 12 hr after last dose. Withhold dose and consult health care provider if blood level is greater than 1.5 mEq/L.
- Record I&O and weight daily. Report sudden changes to health care provider.
- Provide diet matching patient's normal sodium intake. Do not dramatically alter sodium intake from patient's usual amount.
- Encourage intake of 2500 to 3000 mL of fluids daily.
- If signs of neurological toxicity occur, withhold drug and notify health care provider.

Patient/Family Education
- Explain that therapeutic improvement will be noted in 1 to 3 wk.
- Instruct patient to take medication regularly even if feeling well. Symptoms may return if medication is discontinued.
- Advise patient not to decrease or increase dietary sodium intake.
- Tell patient to drink 8 to 10 glasses of water or other caffeine-free liquids daily.
- Caution patient to avoid excessive caffeine intake, as caffeine may increase urinary excretion of drug.
- Advise patient that thirst, frequent polyuria, taste distortion, and fine hand tremors are common side effects.
- Instruct patient to report the following symptoms to health care provider immediately: nausea, vomiting, diarrhea, muscular weakness, ataxia, blurred vision or tinnitus.
- Advise patient that drug may cause drowsiness and to use caution while driving or performing other tasks requiring mental alertness.
- Emphasize need for serum lithium level monitoring every 1 or 2 mo or as advised by health care provider.
- Encourage patient to wear a *Medi-Alert* tag at all times stating medication name and dosage.

Lomefloxacin Hydrochloride

(low-MUH-FLOX-uh-sin HIGH-droe-KLOR-ide)

Class Antibiotic/Fluoroquinolone

How Supplied
Maxaquin Tablets 400 mg

Action
PHARMACOLOGY: Interferes with microbial DNA synthesis.

PHARMACOKINETICS/DYNAMICS:
Absorption: 95% to 98% absorbed. T_{max} is 0.8 to 1.4 hr. C_{max} is 0.8 mcg/mL, and AUC is 5.6 mcg•hr/mL after 100 mg dose. Steady-state is achieved within 48 hr. Food delays rate of absorption of drug; T_{max} increased to 2 hr and AUC is decreased 12%.

Distribution: About 10% protein bound.

Metabolism: Minimally metabolized. Major metabolite is glucuronide (about 9% of administered dose).

Excretion: The t½ is about 8 hr. About 65% of an oral dose is excreted unchanged in the urine. Mean renal Cl is 145 mL/min. About 10% is excreted unchanged in the feces.

Special Populations:
Renal Function Impairment –
Ccr 10 to 40 mL/min/1.73 m^2: AUC is increased 335%; t½ is increased to 21 hr. Dose adjustment is warranted.
Ccr less than 10 mL/min/1.73 m^2: AUC is increased 700%; t½ is increased to 45 hr. Dose adjustment is warranted.

Indications Treatment of infections of the lower respiratory tract and urinary tract caused by susceptible organisms; prevention of UTIs in patients undergoing transurethral or transrectal procedures.

Contraindications Standard considerations.

Route/Dosage
ADULTS: PO 400 mg qd for 3 to 14 days.

Renal Function Impairment (Ccr 10 to 40 mL/min/1.73 m^2)
Initial dose: 400 mg. Maintenance dose: 200 mg qd.

Surgical Prophylaxis
ADULTS: PO (Transurethral surgical procedures) 400 mg 2 to 6 hr preoperatively.
ADULTS: PO (Transrectal prostate biopsy) 400 mg 1 to 6 hr prior to procedure.

Interactions

Antineoplastic agents: Decreased lomefloxacin serum levels.
Magnesium- or aluminum-containing antacids, iron salts, zinc salts, sucralfate, didanosine: Decreased oral absorption of lomefloxacin. Stagger administration times.
Probenecid: Decreased renal elimination of lomefloxacin.

Lab Test Interferences None well documented.

Adverse Reactions

CNS: Headache (4%); dizziness (2%).
DERM: Photosensitivity (2%).
GI: Nausea (4%); diarrhea, abdominal pain (1%).

Precautions

Pregnancy: Category C.
Lactation: Undetermined; however, other fluoroquinolones have been shown to be excreted in breast milk.
Children: Safety and efficacy not established.
Elderly: Cl may be decreased.
Hypersensitivity: Serious and potentially fatal reactions have occurred. Discontinue if allergic reaction occurs.
Renal function impairment: Reduced Cl may occur; adjust dose accordingly.
Superinfection: Use may result in bacterial or fungal overgrowth.
Chronic bronchitis: Not indicated for empiric treatment of acute bacterial exacerbation of chronic bronchitis when *Streptococcus pneumoniae* is the probable pathogen.
Convulsions: CNS stimulation can occur; use with caution in patients with known or suspected CNS disorders.
Phototoxic reaction: Moderate to severe phototoxic reactions have occurred when exposed to direct, indirect, and ultraviolet light.
Pseudomembranous colitis: Consider in patients who develop diarrhea.
Tendonitis: Ruptures of the shoulder, hand, or Achilles tendon may occur. The risk may be increased in patients receiving corticosteroids, especially in the elderly.

Overdosage: Signs and Symptoms

Renal failure (severely decreased urine output, weight gain, confusion, dry flaky skin), tremor, seizures, dyspnea.

PATIENT CARE CONSIDERATIONS

Administration/Storage

- Administer tablets with a full glass of water without regard to meals. Administer with food if GI upset occurs.
- Administer lomefloxacin either 2 hr before or 4 hr after sucralfate, antacids containing magnesium or aluminum, didanosine-buffered tablets or pediatric powder, or other products containing iron or zinc.
- Store tablets at controlled room temperature (59° to 77°F).

Assessment/Interventions

- Obtain patient history, including drug history and any known allergies. Note renal impairment, epilepsy, predisposition to convulsions, cerebral arteriosclerosis, or allergy to fluoroquinolone antibiotics.
- Review results of culture and sensitivity testing as available.
- Ensure that reduced dose is administered to patient with renal impairment (Ccr less than 40 mL/min) following manufacturer's guidelines.
- Monitor for signs of infection, especially fever, and for positive response to antibiotic therapy.
- Ensure that patient is well hydrated to prevent formation of concentrated urine.
- Monitor patient for signs of allergic reaction. Discontinue therapy and immediately notify health care provider if noted. Be prepared to treat appropriately.
- Monitor patient for evidence of CNS stimulation or psychiatric changes (eg, tremors, restlessness, lightheadedness, confusion, hallucinations, agitation, anxiety, sleep disturbance). Inform health care provider if noted and be prepared to discontinue therapy.
- Monitor patient for GI, DERM, and general body side effects. Report to health care provider if noted and significant.

Patient/Family Education

- Explain name, dose, action, and potential side effects of drug.
- Advise patient to read *Patient Information* leaflet before starting therapy and with each refill.
- Review dosing schedule and prescribed length of therapy with patient.
- Advise patient that medication can be taken with a full glass of water without regard to meals but to take with food if GI upset occurs.
- Advise patient to take each dose at least 12 hr before exposure to the sun to reduce risk of photosensitivity reaction.
- Advise patient that if a dose is missed to take as soon as remembered. However, if it is nearing the time for the next dose, to skip the

dose and take the next dose at the regularly scheduled time.
- Advise patient to take lomefloxacin either 2 hr before or 4 hr after sucralfate, antacids containing magnesium or aluminum, didanosine-buffered tablets or pediatric powder, or other products containing iron or zinc.
- Remind patient to complete entire course of therapy, even if symptoms of infection have disappeared.
- Advise patient to inform health care provider if infection does not appear to be improving or is getting worse.
- Advise patient to drink fluids liberally (eg, eight 8 oz glasses of water daily) while taking this medication.
- Advise patient to discontinue therapy and contact health care provider immediately if skin rash, hives, itching, shortness of breath, palpitations, fainting, or pain, tenderness or rupture of tendon occur.
- Advise patient to report the following signs of superinfection to health care provider: black furry tongue, white patches in mouth, foul-smelling stools, vaginal itching or discharge.
- Warn patient that diarrhea containing blood or pus may be a sign of a serious disorder and to seek medical care if noted and not treat at home.
- Caution patient that drug may cause dizziness and lightheadedness and to use caution while driving or performing other tasks requiring mental alertness until tolerance is determined.
- Advise patient to avoid unnecessary exposure to direct and indirect sunlight or tanning lamps, to use sunscreen, and wear protective clothing to avoid photosensitivity reactions during therapy and for several days after stopping medication. Advise patient to discontinue therapy and notify health care provider if any of the following occur following exposure to sunlight or artificial UV light (eg, sunlamp): sensation of skin burning, redness, swelling, blistering; rash or itching.
- Advise women to notify health care provider if pregnant, planning to become pregnant, or breastfeeding.
- Instruct patient not to take any prescription or OTC medications or dietary supplements unless advised by health care provider.
- Advise patient that follow-up examinations and lab tests may be required to monitor therapy and to keep appointments.

Lomustine

(LOW-muss-teen)
Class Alkylating agent/Nitrosoureas
How Supplied
CeeNU Capsules 10 mg, Capsules 40 mg, Capsules 100 mg

Action
PHARMACOLOGY: Its mechanism of action involves the inhibition of both DNA and RNA synthesis through DNA alkylation. Lomustine has been shown to affect a number of cellular processes including RNA, protein synthesis, and the processing of ribosomal and nucleoplasmic messenger RNA; DNA base component structure; the rate of DNA synthesis and DNA polymerase activity. It is cell cycle nonspecific.

PHARMACOKINETICS/DYNAMICS:
Absorption: Bioavailability is 100%.
Distribution: Vd is 3.25 L/kg. High lipid solubility; crosses blood-brain barrier readily. Levels of radioactivity in the CSF are at least 50% of those in plasma.
Metabolism: Readily degraded, apparently in the liver, to several cytotoxic metabolites.
Excretion: Plasma t½ of the metabolites is about 16 hr to 2 days. The average terminal t½ is 22 min. Cl is 56 mL/min/kg. 60% to 70% of the total dose is excreted in the urine in 96 hr and 6% is expired as CO_2.

Indications
Adults and children: Brain tumors, Hodgkin disease.

Contraindications Standard considerations.
Route/Dosage
Brain Tumors, Hodgkin Disease
ADULTS: **PO** 100 to 130 mg/m^2 administered as a single dose q 6 wk. Do not administer repeat doses of lomustine until leukocyte and platelet counts have recovered to acceptable levels (usually 4000/mm^3 and 100,000/mm^3, respectively). Reduce lomustine dose if administered with other myelosuppressive drugs. Give 100 mg/m^2 to patients with compromised bone marrow function. Some clinicians advocate dosage reductions of 25% when platelet nadirs are 50,000 to 74,999/mm^3, 50% when platelet nadirs are 25,000 to 49,999/mm^3, and 75% when platelet nadirs are less than 25,000/mm^3.
PEDIATRIC: **PO** 75 to 150 mg/m^2 administered as a single dose q 6 wk. Do not administer

repeat doses of lomustine until leukocyte and platelet counts have recovered to acceptable levels (usually 4000/mm^3 and 100,000/mm^3, respectively). Follow dosage adjustment guidelines recommended for adults.

Suggested Lomustine Dose Following Initial Dose

ADULTS: **PO** Give 100% of the prior dose if the leukocytes are greater than 3000 cells/mm^3 and the platelets are greater than 75,000 cells/mm^3. Give 70% of the prior dose if the leukocytes are 2000 to 2999 cells/mm^3 and the platelets are 25,000 to 74,999 cells/mm^3. Give 50% of the prior dose if the leukocytes are less than 2000 cells/mm^3 and the platelets less than 25,000 cells/mm.

Interactions

Alcohol: Lomustine is soluble in alcohol. Some sources recommend avoidance of alcohol on days that lomustine is administered to avoid possible effects on the absorption of lomustine, although there is no documentation of an interaction.

Lab Test Interferences None well documented.

Adverse Reactions

CNS: Disorientation; lethargy; ataxia; slurred speech.
GI: Very high potential for nausea and vomiting with doses at least 60 mg/m^2, moderate to high potential for nausea and vomiting with doses less than 60 mg/m^2; anorexia; transient elevation of LFTs.
HEMA: Bone marrow suppression, nadir at 4 to 6 wk.
RENAL: Renal failure associated with large cumulative dose.
OTHER: Acute leukemia and myelodysplastic disorders have occurred after long-term nitrosourea therapy.

PATIENT CARE CONSIDERATIONS

Administration/Storage

- Store in well-closed containers at room temperature. Lomustine capsules are stable for at least 2 yr when stored properly. Avoid excessive heat (greater than 40°C).
- Administer orally. Take lomustine on an empty stomach; avoid alcohol on that day.
- Follow procedures for proper handling and disposal of anticancer drugs. Wear gloves and avoid skin exposure and inhalation of fumes.

Assessment/Interventions

- Major toxicity is delayed bone marrow suppression; monitor blood counts weekly for 6 wk after a dose. Monitor liver and renal function periodically.

> **WARNING:**
> *Hematologic:* The most frequent and serious toxicity is delayed myelosuppression. It usually occurs 4 to 6 wk after drug administration and is dose-related. Thrombocytopenia occurs approximately 4 wk after a dose. Leukopenia occurs approximately 5 to 6 wk after a dose and persists for 1 to 2 wk. About 65% of patients develop WBC less than 5000/mm^3, and 36% of patients develop WBC less than 3000/mm^3. Thrombocytopenia is generally more severe than leukopenia. Anemia also occurs but is less frequent.

Precautions

Pregnancy: Category D.
Lactation: Undetermined.
Children: See Route/Dosage.
Fertility impairment: There have been reports of persistent testicular damage causing infertility.
Hepatic toxicity: A reversible type of hepatic toxicity manifested by increased transaminase, alkaline phosphatase, and bilirubin levels has occurred in a small percentage of patients.
Renal toxicity: Decreased kidney size, progressive azotemia, and renal failure have occurred in patients who received large cumulative doses after prolonged therapy.
Pulmonary toxicity: Pulmonary toxicity characterized by pulmonary infiltrates or fibrosis occurs rarely and appears to be dose-related. Onset of toxicity has occurred after an interval of at least 6 mo from start of therapy with cumulative doses usually greater than 1100 mg/m^2.
Secondary malignancies: Long-term use of nitrosoureas may be associated with development of secondary malignancies.

- Conduct baseline pulmonary function studies during treatment. Patients with a baseline less than 70% of the predicted forced vital capacity (FVC) or carbon monoxide diffusing capacity (DL$_{CO}$) are particularly at risk.
- Nausea and vomiting may occur 3 to 6 hr after an oral dose and usually last less than 24 hr. Antiemetics prior to dosing may diminish and sometimes prevent these effects. Also may be reduced by administration to fasting patients.

Patient/Family Education

- Notify health care provider if fever, chills, sore throat, unusual bleeding or bruising, shortness of breath, dry cough, swelling of feet or lower legs, yellowing of eyes and skin, con-

fusion, sores on the mouth or lips, or unusual tiredness occurs.
♦ Medication may cause loss of appetite; nausea; vomiting; hair loss; skin rash or itching (infrequent); notify health care provider if these reactions become pronounced.

♦ Take on an empty stomach to reduce nausea.
♦ Avoid alcohol for short periods after taking a dose of lomustine.
♦ Contraceptive measures are recommended during therapy.

Loperamide Hydrochloride

(low-PEHR-uh-mide HIGH-droe-KLOR-ide)
Class Antidiarrheal

How Supplied
Diar-aid Tablets 2 mg ♦ *Imodium* Capsules 2 mg ♦ *Imodium A-D* Tablets 2 mg, Liquid 1 mg/5 mL ♦ *Kaopectate II Caplets* Tablets 2 mg ♦ *Neo-Diaral* Capsules 2 mg ♦ *Pepto Diarrhea Control* Liquid 1 mg/ mL
✤ *Apo-Loperamide* ♦ *PMS-Loperamide Hydrochloride* ♦ *Rhoxal-loperamide*

Action
PHARMACOLOGY: Slows intestinal motility, affects water and electrolyte movement through intestine, inhibits peristalsis, reduces daily fecal volume, increases viscosity and bulk density of stool, diminishes loss of fluid and electrolytes.

PHARMACOKINETICS/DYNAMICS:
Absorption: T_{max} is 5 hr (capsule) and 2.5 hr (liquid). Bioavailability is 40%.
Excretion: Apparent t½ is 10.8 hr (9.1 to 14.4 hr). 25% is excreted unchanged in the feces; 1.3% is excreted in the urine unchanged and conjugated.

Indications
Control and symptomatic relief of acute nonspecific or chronic diarrhea; reduction in volume of ileostomy output.

Contraindications
Pseudomembranous colitis caused by antibiotic use; acute diarrhea associated with organisms that penetrate intestinal wall (eg, toxigenic *Escherichia coli*, *Salmonella*, *Shigella*); conditions in which constipation should be avoided; bloody diarrhea; fever; acute ulcerative colitis (potential for toxic megacolon).

Route/Dosage
Acute Diarrhea
ADULTS: **PO** 4 mg followed by 2 mg after each unformed stool, not to exceed 16 mg/24 hr.

CHILDREN 8 TO 12 YR (GREATER THAN 30 KG): 2 mg tid.
CHILDREN 6 TO 8 YR (20 TO 30 KG): 2 mg bid.
CHILDREN 2 TO 5 YR (13 TO 20 KG):
First day: 1 mg tid. May decrease to adjust for nutritional and hydration status after 24 hr; usually 0.1 mg/kg after each loose stool but do not exceed total first day dosing recommendations on any day.

Chronic Diarrhea
ADULTS: **PO** 4 to 8 mg qd or bid.

Interactions
None well documented.

Lab Test Interferences
None well documented.

Adverse Reactions
CNS: Fatigue; drowsiness; dizziness.
DERM: Rash.
GI: Abdominal pain; distention or discomfort; constipation; nausea; vomiting; dry mouth.

Precautions
Pregnancy: Category B.
Lactation: Undetermined.
Children: Not recommended for children less than 2 yr. Use with caution in young children.
Hepatic function impairment: Hepatic coma may be precipitated in patients with advanced hepatorenal disease or hepatic dysfunction.
Acute ulcerative colitis: Agents that inhibit intestinal motility or delay intestinal transit time may induce toxic megacolon. Discontinue if abdominal distention or other untoward symptoms occur.

Overdosage: Signs and Symptoms
Constipation, CNS depression, GI irritation.

PATIENT CARE CONSIDERATIONS

Administration/Storage
♦ Administer as ordered, usually after each unformed stool.
♦ Store at room temperature.

Assessment/Interventions
♦ Obtain patient history, including drug history and any known allergies.
♦ Assess frequency and consistency of stools.
♦ Assess bowel sounds before and throughout course of therapy.
♦ Monitor I&O, fluid and electrolyte balance, and skin turgor for signs of dehydration.

Patient/Family Education
- Instruct patient to record number and consistency of stools.
- Inform patient that medication may cause dry mouth. Encourage patient to drink plenty of clear fluids to help prevent dehydration that may accompany diarrhea.
- Advise patient to notify health care provider if diarrhea persists more than 48 hr or if fever develops.
- Inform patient that drug may cause drowsiness or dizziness and to use caution while driving or performing other tasks requiring mental alertness.

Lopinavir/Ritonavir

(loe-PIN-a-veer/ri-TOE-na-veer)

Class Antiviral

How Supplied
Kaletra Capsules, soft gelatin 133.3 mg lopinavir/33.3 mg ritonavir, Solution, oral 80 mg lopinavir/20 mg ritonavir per mL

Action
PHARMACOLOGY: Lopinavir inhibits HIV protease, the enzyme required to form functional proteins in HIV-infected patients. Ritonavir inhibits the cytochrome P450 (CYP) 3A-mediated metabolism of lopinavir, increasing lopinavir plasma concentrations.

Indications
Treatment of HIV infections in combination with other antiviral agents.

Contraindications
Coadministration with drugs that are highly dependent on CYP3A for Cl and for which elevated plasma levels are associated with serious or life-threatening reactions; hypersensitivity to any of its ingredients.

Route/Dosage
ADULTS: PO 400 mg/100 mg of lopinavir/ritonavir bid. When combined with efavirenz, amprenavir, nelfinavir, or nevirapine, consider a dose of 533 mg/133 mg of lopinavir/ritonavir bid.
CHILDREN 6 MO TO 12 YR: Dose based on lopinavir component of combination.

WITH EFAVIRENZ, NEVIRAPINE, OR AMPRENAVIR
CHILDREN 7 TO 14 KG: PO 13 mg/kg bid.
CHILDREN 15 TO 45 KG: PO 11 mg/kg bid.
CHILDREN GREATER THAN 45 KG: PO Adult dose.

WITHOUT EFAVIRENZ, NEVIRAPINE, OR AMPRENAVIR
CHILDREN 7 TO 14 KG: PO 12 mg/kg bid.
CHILDREN 15 TO 40 KG: PO 10 mg/kg bid.
CHILDREN GREATER THAN 40 KG: PO Adult dose.

Interactions
Amprenavir: Amprenavir concentrations may be increased while lopinavir concentrations may be decreased.
Antiarrhythmic agents (eg, amiodarone, bepridil, systemic lidocaine, quinidine), clarithromycin, dihydropyridine calcium channel blockers (eg, felodipine, nifedipine, nicardipine), HMG-CoA reductase inhibitors (eg, atorvastatin, lovastatin, simvastatin), immunosuppressants (eg, cyclosporine, sirolimus, tacrolimus, rapamycin), indinavir, itraconazole, ketoconazole, nelfinavir, rifabutin, saquinavir, sildenafil: Lopinavir/ritonavir may increase the effects of these agents.
Anticonvulsants (eg, carbamazepine, phenobarbital, phenytoin), corticosteroids (eg, dexamethasone), efavirenz, nevirapine, rifampin, St. John's wort: Effects of lopinavir/ritonavir may be decreased.
Atovaquone, methadone, oral contraceptives (eg, ethinyl estradiol): Lopinavir/ritonavir may decrease the efficacy of these agents.
Cisapride, ergot derivatives (eg, dihydroergotamine, ergonovine, ergotamine, methylergonovine), midazolam, pimozide, triazolam: Contraindicated because of potentially serious or life-threatening reactions.
Delavirdine: Lopinavir concentrations may be increased.
Didanosine: Because didanosine should be given on an empty stomach and lopinavir/ritonavir should be taken with food, didanosine should be given 1 hr before or 2 hr after lopinavir/ritonavir.
Disulfiram, metronidazole: Disulfiram-like reaction may occur because of alcohol present in lopinavir/ritonavir oral solution.
Warfarin: Because warfarin concentrations may be altered, monitor INR.

Lab Test Interferences
None well documented.

Adverse Reactions
CV: Atrial fibrillation, deep vein thrombosis, hypertension, migraine, palpitation, thrombophlebitis, varicose vein, vasculitis (less than 2%); bradyarrhythmias (postmarketing).
CNS: Headache, depression, insomnia (at least 2%); abnormal dreams, agitation, amnesia, anxiety, apathy, ataxia, confusion, convulsion, dizziness, dyskinesia, emotional lability, encephalopathy, facial paralysis, hypertonia, decreased libido, neuropathy, paresthesia, peripheral neuritis, som-

nolence, abnormal thinking, tremor (less than 2%).
DERM: Rash (at least 2%); acne, alopecia, dry skin, eczema, exfoliative dermatitis, furunculosis, maculopapular rash, nail disorder, pruritus, seborrhea, benign skin neoplasm, skin discoloration, skin ulcer, sweating (less than 2%).
EENT: Abnormal vision, eye disorder, otitis media, taste perversion, tinnitus (less than 2%).
GI: Abdominal pain, anorexia, diarrhea, dyspepsia, dysphagia, flatulence, nausea, vomiting (at least 2%); cholangitis, constipation, dry mouth, enlarged abdomen, enteritis, enterocolitis, eructation, esophagitis, fecal incontinence, gastritis, gastroenteritis, hemorrhagic colitis, increased appetite, mouth ulceration, pancreatitis, sialadenitis, stomatitis, ulcerative colitis (less than 2%).
ENDO: Cushing syndrome, diabetes mellitus, hypothyroidism (less than 2%).
GU: Abnormal ejaculation, gynecomastia, hypogonadism, kidney calculus, urine abnormality (less than 2%).
HEPA: Jaundice, cholecystitis (less than 2%).
HEMA/LYMPH: Anemia, leukopenia, lymphadenopathy (less than 2%).
LABTESTABS: Elevated glucose, uric acid, total bilirubin, AST, ALT, glucose tolerance test, total cholesterol, triglycerides, amylase, decreased inorganic phosphorus and neutrophils (at least 2%).
M/N: Avitaminosis, dehydration, edema, decreased glucose tolerance, lactic acidosis, obesity, peripheral edema, weight gain, weight loss.
MUSC: Arthralgia, arthrosis, myalgia (less than 2%).
RESP: Asthma, bronchitis, dyspnea, lung edema, pharyngitis, rhinitis, sinusitis (less than 2%).
OTHER: Asthenia, chills, fever (at least 2%); allergic reaction, back pain, chest pain (including substernal), cyst, face edema, flu syndrome, hypertrophy, bacterial infection, malaise, viral infection (less than 2%); redistribution/accumulation of body fat (postmarketing).

Precautions
Pregnancy: Category C.
Lactation: HIV-infected mothers should not breastfeed infants.
Children: Safety and efficacy not established in children less than 6 mo.
Elderly: Select dose with caution, reflecting greater frequency of decreased hepatic, renal, or cardiac function and comorbidity.
Hepatic function impairment Use with caution; decreased lopinavir/ritonavir Cl may occur.
Cross-resistance: Various degrees of cross-resistance among protease inhibitors have been observed.
Fat redistribution: Redistribution and accumulation of body fat has been observed.
Lipid elevations: Large increases in total cholesterol and triglycerides have resulted with treatment.
Pancreatitis: Fatalities have been associated with use.

Overdosage: Signs and Symptoms
Alcohol-related toxicity caused by 42.4% alcohol content of oral solution.

PATIENT CARE CONSIDERATIONS

Administration/Storage
- Administer prescribed dose bid.
- Administer each dose with food to enhance absorption.
- Use measuring cup, dosing spoon, or syringe to measure prescribed dose of oral solution.
- If patient is also taking didanosine, administer didanosine 1 hr before or 2 hr after lopinavir/ritonavir.
- Store capsule and oral solution in refrigerator (36° to 46°F) or at controlled room temperature (less than 77°F). Avoid exposure to excessive heat. Capsules and oral solution are stable until expiration date on label if stored in refrigerator. Discard any unused oral solution or capsules after 60 days if stored at room temperature.

Assessment/Interventions
- Obtain patient history, including drug history and any known allergies. Note hepatic impairment, concurrent infection with hepatitis B or C, elevated transaminase levels, history of pancreatitis, or hemophilia.
- Note concurrent therapy with any medication that is highly dependent on CYP3A4 for elimination and for which elevated plasma concentrations are associated with serious or life-threatening events (eg, lovastatin, sildenafil, flecainide, propafenone, dihydroergotamine, ergonovine, ergotamine, methylergonovine, pimozide, midazolam, cisapride, triazolam, astemizole, terfenadine).
- Ensure that medication is being administered in combination with other antiretroviral agents.
- Ensure that serum transaminases, cholesterol, and triglyceride levels are evaluated before starting therapy and periodically during therapy.
- Monitor blood sugar in diabetic patient when drug is started or dose is changed. Report significant changes to health care provider.

- Ensure that fasting blood glucose is evaluated before starting therapy and periodically thereafter during therapy in patient with risk factors for diabetes mellitus (eg, obesity, family history of diabetes).
- Ensure that women using estrogen-based hormonal contraceptive are using additional nonhormonal contraceptive measures.
- Monitor patient for signs or symptoms of opportunistic infections. Notify health care provider if suspected.
- Monitor patient for symptoms of pancreatitis (nausea, vomiting, abdominal pain). Inform health care provider if noted and be prepared to discontinue the medication.
- Monitor patient for GI, CNS, and general body side effects. Inform health care provider if noted and significant.

Patient/Family Education

- Explain name, dose, action, and potential side effects of drug.
- Advise patient to review *Patient Information* leaflet before starting therapy and with each refill of the medication.
- Review list of medications that must not be taken with lopinavir/ritonavir because of risk of very serious reactions.
- Instruct patient to continue to take other HIV medications as prescribed by health care provider while taking this medication.
- Advise patient taking didanosine to take the didanosine 1 hr before or 2 hr after the lopinavir/ritonavir.
- Caution patient not to change the dose or stop taking any of medications unless advised by health care provider.
- Advise patient to take prescribed dose bid.
- Advise patient or caregiver to use measuring cup, dosing spoon, or syringe to measure prescribed dose of oral solution.
- Advise patient to take each dose with food to increase absorption and effectiveness of the medication.
- Advise patient that if a dose is missed to take it as soon as possible and then return to the normal schedule. However, if it is almost time for the next dose, to skip the missed dose and take the next dose at the regularly scheduled time. Instruct patient that if a dose is skipped not to double the dose to catch up.
- Instruct diabetic patient to monitor blood glucose more frequently when drug is started or dose is changed and to inform health care provider of significant changes in readings.
- Instruct patient to report persistent nausea, vomiting, and abdominal pain, or frequent urination, thirst, and hunger to health care provider. Advise patient these symptoms could indicate a serious problem that will need medical care.
- Inform patient that drug does not completely eliminate HIV virus and therefore does not reduce risk of transmitting HIV. Appropriate precautions must still be followed.
- Advise patient that drug is not a cure for HIV infection and that illnesses associated with HIV infection, including opportunistic infections, may be acquired. Advise patient to remain under the health care provider's care.
- Caution patient taking sildenafil of increased risk of sildenafil-induced side effects (eg, low BP, visual changes, sustained erection) and to promptly report any symptoms to health care provider. Caution patient that an erection lasting longer than 4 hr requires medical help immediately to prevent permanent damage to the penis.
- Advise patient the medication may cause changes in body fat distribution and to inform health care provider if noted.
- Instruct patient not to take any prescription or OTC medications or dietary supplements (eg, St. John's wort) unless advised by health care provider.
- Advise women using estrogen-based hormonal contraceptive to use additional or alternative contraceptive measures while taking this medication.
- Advise women to notify health care provider if pregnant, planning to become pregnant, or breastfeeding. Advise HIV-infected mothers not to breastfeed infants to avoid risk of HIV transmission to the infant.
- Remind patient that examinations and laboratory tests will be required to monitor therapy and to keep appointments.

Loracarbef

(lor-a-KAR-bef)
Class Antibiotic/Cephalosporin
How Supplied
Lorabid Pulvules (capsules) 200 mg, Pulvules (capsules) 400 mg, Powder for oral suspension 100 mg/5 mL, Powder for oral suspension 200 mg/5 mL

Action
PHARMACOLOGY: Binds to proteins in bacterial cell wall, which inhibits cell wall synthesis.

PHARMACOKINETICS/DYNAMICS:

Absorption: About 90% absorbed from the GI tract. With food, C_{max} is increased 50% to 60%. C_{max} is approximately 8 to 14 mcg/mL (dose-dependent). T_{max} is 1.2 hr.

Distribution: Linear kinetics. 25% protein bound.

Excretion: Mean t½ is 1 hr.

Special Populations:
Renal Function Impairment –
Ccr 10 to 50 mL/min: Following a single 400 mg dose, plasma t½ is increased to 5.6 hr.
Ccr less than 10 mL/min: C_{max} is increased from 15.4 to 23 mcg/mL; t½ is increased to 32 hr.

Indications Treatment of otitis media, acute maxillary sinusitis, pharyngitis, tonsillitis, infections of lower respiratory tract, skin and skin structures, and urinary tract caused by susceptible strains of specific microorganisms.

Contraindications Hypersensitivity to cephalosporins or related antibiotics.

Route/Dosage

Lower Respiratory Tract Infections
ADULTS AND CHILDREN (AT LEAST 13 YR):
Secondary bacterial infection of acute bronchitis: **PO** 200 to 400 mg q 12 hr for 7 days.
Acute bacterial exacerbation of chronic bronchitis: **PO** 400 mg q 12 hr for 7 days.
Pneumonia: **PO** 400 mg q 12 hr for 14 days.

Upper Respiratory Tract Infections
ADULTS AND CHILDREN (AT LEAST 13 YR):
Pharyngitis/tonsillitis: **PO** 200 mg q 12 hr for 10 days.
Sinusitis: **PO** 400 mg q 12 hr for 10 days.
CHILDREN (6 MO TO 12 YR):
Acute otitis media/acute maxillary sinusitis: **PO** 30 mg/kg/day in divided doses q 12 hr for 10 days.
Pharyngitis/Tonsillitis: **PO** 15 mg/kg/day in divided doses q 12 hr for 10 days.

Skin and Skin Structures
ADULTS AND CHILDREN (AT LEAST 13 YR):
Uncomplicated skin and skin structure infections: **PO** 200 mg q 12 hr for 7 days.
CHILDREN (AT LEAST 6 MO TO 12 YR):
Impetigo: **PO** 15 mg/kg/day in divided doses q 12 hr for 7 days.

Urinary Tract Infections
ADULTS AND CHILDREN (AT LEAST 13 YR):
Uncomplicated cystitis: **PO** 200 mg q 24 hr for 7 days.
Uncomplicated pyelonephritis: **PO** 400 mg q 12 hr for 14 days.
Renal Impairment –
Ccr 10 to 49 mL/min: **PO** 50% recommended dose at usual dosage interval or normal recommended dose at twice the usual dosage interval.
Ccr less than 10 mL/min: **PO** Recommended dose q 3 to 5 days.
Hemodialysis: **PO** Administer another dose after dialysis.

Interactions
Probenecid: Inhibition of renal excretion of loracarbef.

Lab Test Interferences Increased prothrombin time; positive direct Coombs' test; elevated LDH; pancytopenia; neutropenia.

Adverse Reactions
CNS: Headache; somnolence.
DERM: Skin rash.
EENT: Rhinitis.
GI: Diarrhea; abdominal pain; nausea; vomiting; anorexia.
GU: Vaginitis; vaginal moniliasis.
OTHER: Hypersensitivity.

Precautions
Pregnancy: Category B.
Lactation: Undetermined.
Children: Safety and efficacy not established in children less than 6 mo.
Elderly: Evaluate renal function before use.
Hypersensitivity: Reactions may range from mild to life-threatening. Administer with caution to penicillin-sensitive patients because of possible cross-reactivity.
Renal function impairment: Use drug with caution. Dosage adjustment based on renal function may be necessary.
Superinfection: May result in bacterial or fungal overgrowth of nonsusceptible microorganisms.
Pseudomembranous colitis: Consider pseudomembranous colitis in patients who develop diarrhea.

Overdosage: Signs and Symptoms
Nausea, vomiting, epigastric distress, diarrhea.

PATIENT CARE CONSIDERATIONS

Administration/Storage
- Treat otitis media with suspension only. Do not substitute the capsule for the suspension when treating otitis media.
- Administer each dose on an empty stomach, at least 1 hr before or 2 hr after a meal.
- Shake suspension well before measuring dose.
- Use a medicine dropper or dosing spoon to administer suspension to children.
- Use suspension for adults who have difficulty swallowing.
- Administer reduced dose to patient with renal impairment.
- Store suspension and capsules at room temperature. Keep tightly closed. Discard any unused suspension after 14 days.

Assessment/Interventions
- Obtain patient history, including drug history and any known allergies. Note history of renal impairment and allergy to penicillins or cephalosporins.
- Review results of culture and sensitivity testing as available.
- Monitor for signs of infection, especially fever, and for positive response to antibiotic therapy.
- Monitor patient for signs of allergic reaction. Discontinue therapy and immediately notify health care provider if noted.
- Monitor patient for GI side effects. Report to health care provider if noted and significant.

Patient/Family Education
- Explain name, dose, action, and potential side effects of drug.
- Review dosing schedule and prescribed length of therapy with patient.
- Instruct patient to take each dose on an empty stomach, at least 1 hr before or 2 hr after a meal.
- Remind patient, family, or caregiver that patient should complete entire course of therapy, even if symptoms of infection have disappeared.
- Advise patient, family, or caregiver to have patient discontinue therapy and contact health care provider immediately if skin rash, hives, itching, or shortness of breath occurs.
- Advise patient, family, or caregiver to report signs of superinfection to health care provider: black "furry" tongue, white patches in mouth, foul-smelling stools, vaginal itching or discharge.
- Warn patient, family, or caregiver that diarrhea containing blood or pus may be a sign of a serious disorder and to seek medical care if noted and not to treat at home.
- Instruct patient not to take any prescription or OTC medications or dietary supplements unless advised to do so by health care provider.
- Advise patient, family, or caregiver that follow-up examinations and lab tests may be required to monitor therapy and to be sure and keep appointments.

Loratadine

(lore-AT-uh-DEEN)

Class Antihistamine

How Supplied
Alavert Tablets 10 mg, Tablets, orally disintegrating 10 mg ◆ *Claritin* Tablets 10 mg, Syrup 1 mg/mL ◆ *Claritin RediTabs* Tablets, rapidly disintegrating 10 mg ◆ *Tavist ND* Tablets 10 mg
❃ *Apo-Loratadine* ◆ *Claritin Kids*

Action
PHARMACOLOGY: Competitively antagonizes histamine at the H_1-receptor site.

PHARMACOKINETICS/DYNAMICS:
Absorption: Rapidly absorbed following oral administration. T_{max} is 1.3 hr for loratadine and 2.5 hr for its metabolite. Food increases bioavailability (AUC) by about 40%; however, T_{max} is delayed by 1 hr. Steady state is reached by about the fifth dosing day.

Distribution: 97% protein bound.

Metabolism: Metabolite is descarboethoxyloratadine. Metabolized by P450 3A4 and P450 2D6. Undergoes extensive first-pass metabolism.

Excretion: About 80% equally distributed between urine and feces in the form of metabolic products within 10 days. The t½ for loratadine is 8.4 hr (3 to 20 hr). The t½ for descarboethoxyloratadine is 28 hr (8.8 to 92 hr).

Onset: Rapid.

Special Populations:
Renal Function Impairment – With Ccr less than 30 mL/min, AUC and C_{max} are increased approximately 73% for loratadine and 120% for its metabolite.

Hepatic Function Impairment – AUC and C_{max} doubled for loratadine; t½ is 24 hr (loratadine) and 37 hr (metabolite).

Elderly – AUC and C_{max} are increased approximately 50%, and t½ ranged from 6.7 to 37 hr.

Indications
Temporarily relieves symptoms caused by hay fever or other upper respiratory allergies (runny nose, sneezing, itchy/watery eyes, itching of the nose or throat). **Unlabeled use(s):** Treatment of chronic idiopathic urticaria.

Contraindications
Standard considerations.

Route/Dosage
ADULTS AND CHILDREN AT LEAST 6 YR: **PO** 10 mg/day.
CHILDREN 2 TO 5 YR: **PO** 5 mg (5 mL) syrup qd.

Hepatic Impairment
ADULTS AND CHILDREN AT LEAST 6 YR: **PO** Start with 10 mg qod.
CHILDREN 2 TO 5 YR: **PO** 5 mg (5 mL) syrup qod.

Renal Impairment (Glomerular Filtration Rate Less Than 30 mL/min)
ADULTS AND CHILDREN AT LEAST 6 YR: **PO** Start with 10 mg qod.

CHILDREN 2 TO 5 YR: **PO** 5 mg (5 mL) syrup qod.

Interactions
Alcohol, CNS depressants: Additive CNS depressant effects.
Azole antifungals (eg, ketoconazole, itraconazole): Use of these agents with similar antihistamines has resulted in serious cardiac toxicity, including death.
Cimetidine: Concomitant use may increase plasma levels of loratadine.
Erythromycin: Loratadine plasma levels, including metabolite, may be increased.
Food: May increase absorption of loratadine.
MAO inhibitors: Concomitant use may prolong and intensify anticholinergic effects of loratadine and may result in hypotensive episodes.

Lab Test Interferences May prevent or diminish otherwise positive reactions to dermal reactivity indicators.

Adverse Reactions
CV: Hypotension; hypertension; palpitations; tachycardia; syncope.
CNS: Hyperkinesia; paresthesia; dizziness; migraine; tremor; vertigo; headache; somnolence; fatigue; impaired concentration; depression; agitation; nervousness; anxiety; confusion; insomnia.
DERM: Dermatitis; dry hair; dry skin; urticaria; rash; pruritus; purpura; photosensitivity; increased sweating.
EENT: Conjunctivitis; blurred vision; earache; eye pain; blepharospasm; dysphonia; altered taste.
GI: Anorexia; increased appetite and weight gain; nausea; vomiting; diarrhea; constipation; flatulence; gastritis; dyspepsia; dry mouth; thirst; abdominal pain; hiccough; stomatitis.
GU: Urinary discoloration; altered micturition; menstrual irregularities; impotence; vaginitis; urinary retention; urinary incontinence.
RESP: Nasal dryness; pharyngitis; epistaxis; nasal congestion; dyspnea; coughing; rhinitis; hemoptysis; sinusitis; sneezing; bronchospasm; bronchitis; laryngitis; wheezing; upper respiratory tract infection.
OTHER: Breast pain; arthralgia; myalgia; malaise; chest pain; leg cramps; asthenia; back pain; fever.

Precautions
Pregnancy: Category B.
Lactation: Excreted in breast milk.
Children: Safety and efficacy not established in children less than 6 yr (tablets) or under 2 yr (syrup).
Hypersensitivity: Hypersensitivity may occur.
Renal function impairment: Use drug with caution in patients with renal impairment.
Hepatic function impairment: Use drug with caution in patients with hepatic renal impairment.
Special risk patients: Use with caution in patients with a predisposition to urinary retention, history of bronchial asthma, increased IOP, hyperthyroidism, CV disease, or hypertension.

Overdosage: Signs and Symptoms
Somnolence, tachycardia, headache.

PATIENT CARE CONSIDERATIONS

Administration/Storage
- Administer on empty stomach 1 hr before or 2 hr after eating.
- Place rapidly disintegrating tablets on tongue; disintegration occurs rapidly. Administer with or without water.
- Use rapidly disintegrating tablets within 6 mo of opening foil pouch and immediately upon opening individual tablet blister.
- Store at room temperature (59° to 86°F).

Assessment/Interventions
- Obtain patient history, including drug history and any known allergies, especially to antihistamines.
- Obtain baseline BP, respirations, and pulse before beginning therapy.
- Monitor closely for signs of hypersensitivity if patient has history of allergic reactions to other antihistamines.
- Observe for dizziness, excessive sedation, syncope, confusion, and hypotension, especially in elderly patients.

Patient/Family Education
- Warn patient not to increase dose to obtain quicker relief of symptoms.
- If patient is to have allergy skin testing, advise to avoid taking medication for 4 days before test.
- Tell patient that drug may be used alone for symptoms of sneezing and runny nose with slight nasal congestion.
- Advise patient not to take any OTC medications and antihistamines without consulting health care provider.
- Instruct patient to maintain fluid intake of 1½ to 2 qt/day to decrease viscosity of secretions.
- Caution patient to avoid exposure to sunlight and to use sunscreen or wear protective clothing to avoid photosensitivity reaction.
- Instruct patient to avoid intake of alcoholic beverages or other CNS depressants (eg, sedatives, hypnotics, tranquilizers).
- Advise patient that drug may cause drowsi-

ness and to use caution while driving or performing other tasks requiring mental alertness until response to medication is known.
* Explain that rapidly disintegrating tablet will disintegrate on the tongue and may be administered with or without water.
* Advise patient to take frequent sips of water, suck on ice chips or sugarless hard candy, or chew sugarless gum if dry mouth occurs.
* Advise women to notify health care provider if pregnant, planning to become pregnant, or breastfeeding.

Loratadine/Pseudoephedrine Sulfate

(lore-AT-uh-DEEN/SUE-doe-eh-FED-rin)

Class Antihistamine/Decongestant

How Supplied
Claritin-D 12 Hour Tablets 120 mg pseudoephedrine sulfate and 5 mg loratadine ◆ *Claritin-D 24 Hour* Tablets 240 mg pseudoephedrine sulfate and 10 mg loratadine
✽ *Chlor-Tripolon N.D.* ◆ *Claritin Extra* ◆ *Claritin Liberator*

Action
PHARMACOLOGY:
Loratadine: Competitively antagonizes histamine at the H_1 receptor.
Pseudoephedrine: Causes vasoconstriction and subsequent shrinkage of nasal mucous membranes by alpha-adrenergic stimulation, promoting nasal drainage.

Indications Relief of symptoms of seasonal allergic rhinitis.

Contraindications Hypersensitivity to any ingredient of product; patients with narrow-angle glaucoma, urinary retention, severe hypertension, or severe coronary artery disease; MAO inhibitor therapy or within 14 days of stopping MAO inhibitor; idiosyncratic reactions to adrenergic agents.

Route/Dosage
ADULTS AND CHILDREN OLDER THAN 12 YR: PO 1 tablet qd (*Claritin-D 24 Hour*) or 1 tablet bid (*Claritin-D 12 Hour*).

Interactions
Loratadine:
Cimetidine, erythromycin, ketoconazole – May increase loratadine plasma levels.
Pseudoephedrine:
Antihypertensive agents that interfere with sympathetic activity (eg, beta-blockers, mecamylamine, methyldopa, reserpine, veratrum alkaloids) – Antihypertensive effect of these agents may be reduced.
Digitalis – Increased ectopic pacemaker activity may occur.
MAO inhibitors – Contraindicated in patients taking MAO inhibitors and for 14 days after stopping use of an MAO inhibitor.

Lab Test Interferences May diminish or prevent positive reactions to skin tests.

Adverse Reactions
CV: Hypertension; hypotension; palpitations; peripheral edema; syncope; tachycardia; ventricular extrasystoles.
CNS: Headache (19% for 12-hr tablet); insomnia (16% for 12-hr tablet; 5% for 24-hr tablet); somnolence (approximately 7%); nervousness, dizziness, fatigue (approximately 4%); aggressive reaction; agitation; anxiety; apathy; confusion; convulsions; decreased libido; depression; dysphonia; emotional lability; euphoria; hyperkinesia; hypertonia; impaired concentration; irritability; migraine; paresthesia; paroniria; tremors; vertigo.
DERM: Acne; bacterial skin infection; dry skin; eczema; epidermal necrolysis; erythema; flushing; hematoma; increased sweating; pruritus; rash; urticaria.
EENT: Pharyngitis (approximately 4%); abnormal lacrimation; abnormal vision; blurred vision; conjunctivitis; earache; ear infection; eye pain; mydriasis; photophobia; tinnitus.
GI: Dry mouth (14% for 12-hr tablet; 8% for 24-hr tablet); nausea (3%); anorexia (2%); dyspepsia (3% for 12-hr tablet); abdominal distension, distress, pain; altered taste; constipation; diarrhea; eructation; flatulence; gastritis; gingival bleeding; hemorrhoids; increased appetite; stomatitis; taste loss; tongue discoloration; tongue ulceration; toothache; vomiting.
GU: Dysmenorrhea (2%); dysuria; impotence; intermenstrual bleeding; micturition frequency; nocturia; oliguria; polyuria; urinary retention; UTI; vaginitis.
HEPA: Cholelithiasis; hepatic function abnormal.
METAB: Dehydration; edema; thirst; weight gain.
RESP: Coughing (3%); bronchitis; bronchospasm; chest congestion; dry throat; dyspnea; epistaxis; halitosis; hemoptysis; nasal congestion; nasal irritation; pleurisy; pneumonia; sinusitis; sneezing; sputum increased; upper respiratory infection; wheezing.
OTHER: Thirst (2%); abscess; arthralgia; asthenia; back pain; chest pain; facial edema; fever; flu-like symptoms; hypoesthesia; leg cramps; lymphadenopathy; malaise; musculoskeletal pain;

myalgia; rigors; tendinitis; torticollis; viral infection.

Precautions
Pregnancy: Category B.
Lactation: Excreted in breast milk.
Children: Safety and efficacy not established in children younger than 12 yr.
Special risk patients: Use with caution in patients with hypertension, hyperthyroidism, diabetes, cardiovascular disease, increased intraocular pressure, renal impairment, hepatic impairment, or prostatic hypertrophy.
Swallowing difficulty: Esophageal obstruction and perforation has been reported with product; therefore, should not be used by patients with history of difficulty in swallowing tablets or who have known upper GI narrowing or abnormal esophageal peristalsis.
Sympathomimetic amines (eg pseudoephedrine): May cause CNS stimulation with convulsions or cardiovascular collapse with accompanying hypotension.

Overdosage: Signs and Symptoms
Somnolence, tachycardia, headache, giddiness, nausea, vomiting, sweating, thirst, precordial pain, palpitations, difficulty in micturition, muscular weakness and tenseness, anxiety, restlessness, insomnia, toxic psychosis with delusions and hallucinations, cardiac arrhythmias, circulatory collapse, convulsions, coma, respiratory failure.

PATIENT CARE CONSIDERATIONS
Administration/Storage
- Give qd (*Claritin-D 24 Hour*) or bid (*Claritin-D 12 Hour*) with a full glass of water.
- Do not break, chew, or crush tablets.
- Patients with reduced renal function (Ccr less than 30 mL/min) should be started on 1 tablet q other day (*Claritin-D 24 Hour*) or 1 tablet qd (*Claritin-D 12 Hour*).
- Store tablets at controlled room temperature (59° to 77°F). Keep container tightly closed. Protect unit-dose hospital pack from light.

Assessment/Interventions
- Obtain patient history, including drug history and any known allergies. Note history of difficulty swallowing tablets, upper GI narrowing, abnormal esophageal peristalsis, narrow-angle glaucoma, urinary retention, severe hypertension or coronary artery disease, hepatic or renal dysfunction, or concurrent use of or within 2 wk of stopping MAO-inhibitor therapy.
- Assess for allergy symptoms (eg, rhinitis, nasal congestion, sneezing, itching, watery eyes) before and periodically throughout therapy.
- Monitor pulse and BP periodically during therapy.
- Monitor patient for nervousness, dizziness, and insomnia. If noted, hold therapy and notify health care provider.

Patient/Family Education
- Explain name, dose, action, and potential side effects of drug.
- Advise patient to take with a full glass of water.
- Advise patient to take last dose late in the afternoon or early evening to reduce chance of drug causing sleeplessness.
- Caution patient not to break, chew, or crush tablet and to swallow whole.
- Advise patient that if allergy symptoms are not controlled not to increase the dose of medication but to inform health care provider.
- Caution patient not to take any OTC antihistamines or decongestants while taking this medication unless advised by health care provider.
- If patient is to have allergy skin testing, advise patient not to take the medication for at least 6 days before the skin testing.
- Advise women to notify health care provider if pregnant, planning to become pregnant, or breastfeeding.
- Instruct patient to stop taking drug and immediately report any of these symptoms to health care provider: nervousness, dizziness, sleeplessness.
- Caution patient not to take any prescription or OTC medications, or dietary supplements unless advised by health care provider.

Lorazepam

(lore-AZE-uh-pam)

Class Antianxiety/Benzodiazepine

How Supplied

Ativan Injection 2 mg/mL, Injection 4 mg/mL ♦ *Lorazepam* Tablets 0.5 mg, Tablets 1 mg, Tablets 2 mg ♦ *Lorazepam Intensol* Oral Solution, Concentrated 2 mg/mL

🍁 *Apo-Lorazepam* ♦ *Novo-Lorazem* ♦ *Nu-Loraz*

Action

PHARMACOLOGY: Potentiates action of GABA, resulting in increased neuronal inhibition and CNS depression, especially in limbic system and reticular formation.

PHARMACOKINETICS/DYNAMICS:

Absorption: Absolute bioavailability is 90%. T_{max} is about 2 hr. C_{max} is 20 ng/mL after 2 mg dose (dose-dependent).

Distribution: 85% protein bound.

Metabolism: Rapidly conjugated at its 3-hydroxy group into lorazepam glucuronide.

Excretion: The t½ is approximately 12 hr for unconjugated lorazepam and approximately 18 hr for lorazepam glucuronide.

Indications

Treatment of anxiety, anxiety associated with depression (oral); preanesthetic medication for sedation/anxiety and decreased recall, status epilepticus (IV). **Unlabeled use(s):** Relief of chemotherapy-induced nausea and vomiting; acute alcohol withdrawal; psychogenic catatonia.

Contraindications

Acute narrow-angle glaucoma; intra-arterial administration (injection); hypersensitivity to benzodiazepines.

Route/Dosage

Antianxiety

ADULTS: **PO** *Usual dose:* 2 to 6 mg/day (range, 1 to 10 mg/day) in divided doses; largest dose at bedtime.

ELDERLY/DEBILITATED PATIENTS: Initial dose: 1 to 2 mg/day in divided doses; increase gradually.

Insomnia Caused By Anxiety or Transient Situational Stress

ADULTS: **PO** 2 to 4 mg at bedtime.

Preanesthesia

ADULTS: **IM** 0.05 mg/kg at least 2 hr before procedure (max, 4 mg).

Initial dose: **IV** 2 mg total or 0.044 mg/kg, whichever is smaller. Do not exceed in patients over 50 yr.

For increased lack of recall: 0.05 mg/kg (max, 4 mg), 15 to 20 min before procedure.

Status epilepticus

ADULTS: **IV** Recommended dose 4 mg given at rate of 2 mg/min. If seizures continue or recur after a 10- to 15-min observation period, an additional 4 mg IV may be administered slowly.

Interactions

Alcohol/CNS depressants: Additive CNS depressant effects.

Digoxin: Increased serum digoxin concentrations.

Oral contraceptives: Cl rate of lorazepam may be increased.

Rifampin: Pharmacologic effect of lorazepam may be decreased.

Scopolamine: May result in increased incidence of hallucinations, irrational behavior, and sedation.

Theophyllines: May antagonize sedative effects.

Lab Test Interferences None well documented.

Adverse Reactions

CV: CV collapse; hypotension; phlebitis or thrombosis at IV sites.

CNS: Drowsiness; confusion; ataxia; dizziness; lethargy; fatigue; apathy; memory impairment; disorientation; anterograde amnesia; restlessness; headache; slurred speech; aphonia; stupor; coma; euphoria; irritability; vivid dreams; psychomotor retardation; paradoxical reactions (eg, anger, hostility, mania, insomnia).

DERM: Rash.

EENT: Visual or auditory disturbances; depressed hearing.

GI: Constipation; diarrhea; dry mouth; coated tongue; nausea; anorexia; vomiting; difficulty swallowing.

HEMA: Leukopenia.

HEPA: Elevated LDH, ALT, AST, and alkaline phosphatase; hepatic dysfunction, including hepatitis and jaundice.

RESP: Partial airway obstruction (injection); respiratory depression.

OTHER: Dependence/withdrawal syndrome (eg, confusion, abnormal perception of movement, depersonalization, muscle twitching, psychosis, paranoid delusions, seizures); pain, burning, redness at IM injection site.

Precautions

Pregnancy: Category D. Avoid use, especially during first trimester because of possible increased risk of congenital malformations. Advise women of childbearing age to use effective contraceptive method. Not recommended during labor and delivery.

Lactation: Undetermined.

Children: Do not use in patients less than 18 yr (IM/IV); safety and efficacy in patients less than 12 yr not established (oral).

Renal function impairment: Injection is not recommended in these patients. Use oral form with caution.
Hepatic function impairment: Injection is not recommended in these patients. Use oral form with caution.
Benzyl alcohol: Solution for injection contains 2% benzyl alcohol; avoid use in infants because toxicity may occur.
Drug dependency: Prolonged use can lead to dependence.
Parenteral administration: Primarily for acute states. Keep patients under observation for up to 3 hr. Use with extreme care in elderly, very ill patients, or those with limited pulmonary reserve because of the possibility of apnea or cardiac arrest. Do not give to patients in shock or coma or those with acute alcohol intoxication.
Psychiatric disorders: Not intended for use in patients with primary depressive disorder, psychosis, or disorders in which anxiety is not prominent.
Suicide: Use with caution in patients with suicidal tendencies; do not allow access to large quantities of drug.

Overdosage: Signs and Symptoms
Ataxia, lethargy, slurred speech, hypotension, respiratory depression, coma, CNS depression.

PATIENT CARE CONSIDERATIONS
Administration/Storage
* Administer prescribed dose without regard to meals but administer with food if GI upset occurs.
* Tablets may be administered sublingually to patient who has difficulty swallowing tablets.
* Store tablets at controlled room temperature (59° to 86°F). Protect from moisture. Store injection and oral solution in refrigerator (36° to 46°F). Protect from light.

Oral Solution:
* Use calibrated dropper to measure prescribed dose of concentrated oral solution. Add prescribed dose to a liquid (eg, juice, water, soda) or semisolid food (eg, applesauce, pudding); stir for a few seconds then immediately administer entire amount of mixture. Do not prepare and store doses for future use.

Injection:
* For IM or IV administration only. Not for intradermal, SC, or intra-arterial administration.
* For IM administration, inject undiluted solution deeply into muscle.
* For IV administration, dilute with equal volume of compatible solution (eg, sterile water for injection, sodium chloride injection or 5% dextrose injection). Do not shake vigorously to avoid air entrapment. Administer directly into a vein or into tubing of existing IV infusion at rate not exceeding 2 mg/min.
* Do not administer if particulate matter, cloudiness, or discoloration is noted. Discard any unused solution. Do not save for future use.

Assessment/Interventions
* Obtain patient history, including drug history and any known allergies. Note hepatic or renal impairment, pulmonary disease, acute narrow-angle glaucoma, depression, psychosis, suicidal tendency, seizure disorder, history of drug abuse, sensitivity to other benzodiazepines, or concurrent use of other psychotropic medications or CNS depressants.
* Ensure that reduced dose and slower dose escalation is used in elderly patient or patient with debilitating disease.
* Ensure that women of childbearing potential are not pregnant when therapy is initiated.
* Ensure that CBC with differential and liver enzymes are evaluated periodically in patient on prolonged therapy.
* Frequently assess patient for response to treatment. Notify health care provider if condition does not appear to be improving or is worsening.
* Ensure that therapy is periodically reviewed to determine if therapy needs to be continued without change or if a dose change (eg, increase, decrease, discontinuation) is indicated.
* If treatment is to be discontinued, or the dose reduced, gradually taper the dose and monitor patient for withdrawal symptoms. If significant withdrawal symptoms develop (eg, increased anxiety, tremor, muscle or abdominal cramps, sweating) reinstitute previous dosing schedule and attempt a less rapid tapering regimen after patient has stabilized.
* Monitor patient for CNS, GI, psychiatric, and general body side effects and injection site reactions. Report to health care provider if noted and significant. Implement safety precautions if excessive drowsiness or dizziness occurs.

Injection:
* Ensure that a benzodiazepine-receptor antagonist (eg, flumazenil), oxygen, and resuscitation and intubation equipment are available when medication is administered by IV injection.

Patient/Family Education

- Explain name, dose, action, and potential side effects of drug.
- Advise patient or caregiver to read the *Patient Information* leaflet before starting therapy and with each refill.
- Advise patient that medication is usually started at a low dose and then gradually increased until maximum benefit is obtained.
- Caution patient that medication may be habit forming and to take as prescribed and not to stop taking or change the dose unless advised by health care provider.
- Advise patient to take each dose without regard to meals but to take with food if stomach upset occurs.
- Advise patient or caregiver using concentrated oral solution to measure prescribed dose using calibrated dropper and then add solution to a liquid (eg, juice, water, soda) or semisolid food (eg, applesauce, pudding); stir for a few seconds then immediately take (give) the entire mixture. Caution patient or caregiver not to prepare mixtures ahead of time and store.
- Advise patient that if a dose is missed to skip that dose and take the next dose at the regularly scheduled time. Caution patient to never take 2 doses at the same time.
- Advise patient that if medication needs to be discontinued it will be slowly withdrawn unless safety concerns (eg, rash) require a more rapid withdrawal.
- Instruct patient to avoid alcoholic beverages and other depressants while taking this medication.
- Advise patient with anxiety to take medication as needed and to seek alternative methods for controlling or preventing anxiety (eg, stress reduction, counseling).
- Instruct patient to contact health care provider if symptoms (eg, anxiety, panic attacks, seizures) do not appear to be getting better, are getting worse, or if bothersome side effects (eg, drowsiness, memory impairment) occur.
- Advise patient that drug may cause drowsiness or impair judgment, thinking, or reflexes and to use caution while driving or performing other tasks requiring mental alertness until tolerance is determined.
- Encourage patient with seizure disorder to carry identification (eg, *Medi-Alert*) indicating condition and medication being used to treat.
- Advise women to notify health care provider if pregnant, planning to become pregnant, or breastfeeding.
- Warn patient not to take any prescription or OTC drugs or dietary supplements without consulting health care provider.
- Advise patient that follow-up visits and lab tests may be necessary to monitor therapy and to keep appointments.

Injection:

- Advise patient or caregiver that medication will be prepared by a health care provider and administered in a health care setting under close observation when oral therapy is not feasible.
- Caution patient who receives parenteral therapy as an outpatient (eg, outpatient surgery) to use caution while ambulating, and to avoid ingestion of alcohol or other sedatives as well as driving or other hazardous activities for 24 to 48 hr.

Losartan Potassium

(low-SAHR-tan poe-TASS-ee-uhm)

Class Antihypertensive/Angiotensin II antagonist

How Supplied

Cozaar Tablets 25 mg, Tablets 50 mg, Tablets 100 mg

Action

PHARMACOLOGY: Antagonizes the effect of angiotension II (vasoconstriction and aldosterone secretion) by blocking the angiotensin II receptor (AT_1 receptor) in vascular smooth muscle and the adrenal gland, producing decreased BP.

PHARMACOKINETICS/DYNAMICS:

Absorption: Well absorbed. Food decreases absorption. Systemic bioavailability is about 33%. T_{max} is 1 hr (losartan) and 3 to 4 hr (metabolite). While C_{max} of drug and metabolite are equal, metabolite AUC is 4 times greater than that of losartan.

Distribution: Linear kinetics. Vd is 34 L (losartan) and 12 L (metabolite). Neither losartan nor metabolite accumulates in plasma upon repeated doses. Highly bound to plasma proteins.

Metabolism: Undergoes substantial first-pass metabolism by cytochrome P450 enzymes. The active metabolite, carboxylic acid, is responsible for most of the angiotensin II receptor antagonist activity. Fourteen percent of an oral dose is converted to active metabolite.

Excretion: The t½ is 2 hr (losartan) and 6 to 9 hr (metabolite). Renal Cl is 75 mL/min (losartan) and 25 mL/min (metabolite). Total plasma Cl is 600 mL/min (losartan) and 50 mL/min (metabolite). Biliary excretion contributes to the elimination of losartan and metabolite. About 4% is excreted unchanged in the urine.

Special Populations:
Renal Function Impairment – With Ccr less than 30 mL/min, AUC is approximately 50% increased. No dose adjustment is needed unless the patient is volume-depleted.
Hepatic Function Impairment – Plasma concentrations are increased and clearance decreased. A lower starting dose is recommended.

Indications Treatment of hypertension; nephropathy in type 2 diabetic patients; reduce risk of stroke in patients with hypertension and left ventricular hypertrophy.

Contraindications Standard considerations.

Route/Dosage
Hypertension
ADULTS:
Initial dose: **PO** 50 mg qd; 25 mg qd if volume depleted or history of hepatic impairment.
Maintenance: **PO** 25 to 100 mg/day.

Nephropathy in Type 2 Diabetes
ADULTS:
Initial dose: **PO** 50 mg qd; the dose may be increased to 100 mg qd based on BP response.

Hypertension in Patients with Left Ventricular Hypertrophy
ADULTS: **PO** 50 mg qd; add hydrochlorothiazide 12.5 mg/day and/or increase the dose of losartan to 100 mg/day followed by an increase in hydrochlorothiazide to 25 mg qd based on BP response.

Interactions
Fluconazole: Losartan plasma levels may be elevated, increasing the antihypertensive and adverse effects.
Indomethacin: The antihypertensive effect of losartan may be blunted.
Lithium: Plasma concentrations may be increased by losartan, resulting in an increase in the pharmacologic and adverse effects of lithium.
Potassium supplement: Concomitant use of potassium-sparing diuretics, potassium supplements, or salt substitutes containing potassium may lead to increases in serum potassium.

Lab Test Interferences None well documented.

Adverse Reactions
CNS: Dizziness; insomnia; headache.
EENT: Nasal congestion.
GI: Diarrhea; dyspepsia; abdominal pain; nausea.
RESP: Cough; sinusitis; upper respiratory infection; pharyngitis.
OTHER: Muscle cramps; myalgia; back pain; leg pain; chest pain; edema/swelling.

> **WARNING:**
> *Pregnancy:* Use in second and third trimesters may cause injury and death to fetus.

Precautions
Pregnancy: Category D (second and third trimester); Category C (first trimester).
Lactation: Undetermined.
Children: Safety and efficacy in children younger than 18 yr not established.
Hypersensitivity: Angioedema, including swelling of the larynx and glottis, causing airway obstruction and/or swelling of the face, lips, pharynx, and tongue have been reported rarely.
Renal function impairment: Use caution in treating patients whose renal function may depend on the activity of the renin-angiotension-aldosterone system (eg, patients with severe CHF).
Hepatic function impairment: Losartan total plasma clearance is lower (50%) and total bioavailability is higher (2-fold) in patients with hepatic insufficiency as compared with healthy subjects. A lower initial dose is recommended for patients with a history of hepatic impairment.
Hypotension/Volume-depleted patients: Symptomatic hypotension may occur after initiation of losartan in patients who are intravascularly volume depleted (eg, those treated with diuretics). Correct these conditions prior to administration of losartan or use a lower starting dose.
Black patients: Losartan may not be as effective in black patients.

Overdosage: Signs and Symptoms
Hypotension, tachycardia, bradycardia.

PATIENT CARE CONSIDERATIONS
Administration/Storage
- Administer alone or in combination with other antihypertensives.
- Administer with caution and reduce dosage in patients with possible depletion of intravascular volume or a history of hepatic impairment.
- Can be administered with or without food.
- Do not administer to pregnant women as fetal and neonatal morbidity and death can occur.
- Safety not established for nursing infants and children.
- Store in tightly closed, light-resistant container at room temperature (59° to 86°F).

Assessment/Interventions
- Obtain patient history.
- Monitor BP and pulse. Should hypotension, tachycardia, or bradycardia result, withhold the medication and notify the health care provider.
- Monitor for signs of hypersensitivity, including angioedema involving swelling of the face, lips, and tongue.

Patient/Family Education
- Instruct patient to take the medication as prescribed at the same time each day.
- Inform patient that losartan controls, but does not cure, hypertension.
- Caution patient to take the dose exactly as prescribed and not to stop taking the medication even if they feel better. Instruct patient not to decrease or increase the dosage.
- Instruct patient in BP and pulse measurement skills. Caution patient to call health care provider should abnormal measurements occur.
- Instruct patient in methods of fall prevention, including rising slowly and sitting on the side of the bed before standing, especially early in therapy.
- Inform patient of the importance of adjunct therapies such as dietary planning, regular exercise program, weight reduction, low sodium diet, smoking cessation program, alcohol reduction, and stress management.
- Instruct patient to report symptoms of weakness, fatigue, dizziness, or lightheadedness to health care provider.
- Caution patient to notify health care provider or dentist prior to surgery or treatment.
- Advise women to contact health care provider if pregnant, planning to become pregnant, or breastfeeding.
- Instruct patient not to use potassium supplements or salt substitutes containing potassium without consulting with their health care provider.

Losartan Potassium/ Hydrochlorothiazide

(low-SAHR-tan poe-TASS-ee-uhm/high-droe-klor-oh-THIGH-uh-zide)

Class Antihypertensive

How Supplied
Hyzaar Tablets 12.5 mg hydrochlorothiazide/ 50 mg losartan potassium, Tablets 25 mg hydrochlorothiazide/100 mg losartan potassium

Action
PHARMACOLOGY: Losartan antagonizes the effect of angiotensin II (vasoconstriction and aldosterone secretion) by blocking the angiotensin II receptor (AT1 receptor) in vascular smooth muscle and the adrenal gland, producing decreased BP; hydrochlorothiazide inhibits reabsorption of sodium and chloride in ascending loop of Henle and early distal tubules.

Indications
Hypertension.

Contraindications
Anuria; hypersensitivity to other sulfonamide-derivatives or any component of product.

Route/Dosage
ADULTS: PO 50 mg losartan/12.5 mg hydrochlorothiazide once daily is usual dose (max, 100 mg losartan/25 mg hydrochlorothiazide daily).

Interactions
Losartan potassium:
Fluconazole – Losartan plasma levels may be elevated, increasing the antihypertensive and adverse effects.
Lithium – Plasma levels of lithium may be elevated, increasing the pharmacologic and adverse effects.
Rifamycins (eg, rifampin) – Losartan plasma levels may be reduced, decreasing the antihypertensive effects.
Potassium-sparing diuretics (eg, spironolactone), potassium supplements, salt substitutes containing potassium – May lead to increased serum potassium.
Hydrochlorothiazide:
Alcohol, barbiturates, narcotics – Increased risk of orthostatic hypotension.
Antidiabetic agents – Dose adjustments of antidiabetic agent may be needed.
Antihypertensives – Actions of other antihypertensive agents may be potentiated.
Cholestyramine, colestipol resins – Absorption of hydrochlorothiazide may be impaired.
ACTH, corticosteroids – Increased risk of electrolyte depletion (eg, hypokalemia).
Pressor amines (eg, norepinephrine) – Decreased response to pressor amine.
Nondepolarizing skeletal muscle relaxants (eg, turbocurarine) – Responsiveness to muscle relaxant may be increased.
Lithium – Plasma levels of lithium may be elevated, increasing the risk of toxicity.
NSAIDs – Antihypertensive, diuretic, and natriuretic effects of hydrochlorothiazide may be reduced.

Lab Test Interferences Serum levels of protein-bound iodine may be decreased without signs of thyroid dysfunction.

Adverse Reactions
CV: Palpitations; orthostatic effects, angina pectoris, arrhythmias (eg, atrial fibrillation, sinus

bradycardia, tachycardia, ventricular tachycardia, ventricular fibrillation), CVA, hypotension, MI, second-degree AV block (losartan); orthostatic hypotension (hydrochlorothiazide).
CNS: Dizziness; syncope, anxiety, ataxia, confusion, depression, dream abnormality, hyperesthesia, insomnia, decreased libido, memory impairment, migraine, nervousness, panic disorder, paresthesia, peripheral neuropathy, sleep disorder, somnolence, tremor, vertigo (losartan); restlessness (hydrochlorothiazide).
DERM: Rash; alopecia, dermatitis, dry skin, ecchymosis, erythema, flushing, photosensitivity, pruritus, sweating, urticaria (losartan); photosensitivity, urticaria, necrotizing angiitis (vasculitis and cutaneous vasculitis), erythema multiforme (eg, Stevens-Johnson syndrome), exfoliative dermatitis (eg, toxic epidermal necrolysis), purpura (hydrochlorothiazide).
EENT: Sinusitis; cough; nasal congestion, angioedema, pharyngeal discomfort, rhinitis, blurred vision, burning/stinging in the eyes, conjunctivitis, decreased visual acuity, taste perversion, tinnitus (losartan); transient blurred vision, xanthopsia (hydrochlorothiazide).
GI: Abdominal pain; anorexia, constipation, dental pain, dry mouth, dyspepsia, flatulence, gastritis, vomiting (losartan); pancreatitis, sialadenitis, cramping, gastric irritation (hydrochlorothiazide).
GU: Impotence, nocturia, urinary frequency, UTI (losartan); glucosuria, renal failure, renal dysfunction, interstitial nephritis (hydrochlorothiazide).
HEMA: Anemia (losartan); aplastic anemia, agranulocytosis, leukopenia, hemolytic anemia, thrombocytopenia (hydrochlorothiazide).
HEPA: Jaundice (intrahepatic cholestatic jaundice) (hydrochlorothiazide).
METAB: Edema; gout (losartan); hyperglycemia, hyperuricemia (hydrochlorothiazide).
RESP: Upper respiratory tract infection; dyspnea, epistaxis, respiratory congestion (losartan); respiratory distress (eg, pneumonitis, pulmonary edema) (hydrochlorothiazide).
OTHER: Back pain; chest pain, facial edema, arm pain, arthralgia, arthritis, fibromyalgia, hip pain, joint swelling, knee pain, leg pain, muscle cramps, muscle weakness, musculoskeletal pain, myalgia, shoulder pain, stiffness (losartan); weakness, fever, muscle spasm (hydrochlorothiazide).

Precautions
Pregnancy: Category C (first trimester); category D (second and third trimester).
Lactation: Undetermined (losartan); excreted in breast milk (hydrochlorothiazide).
Children: Safety and efficacy not established.
Hypersensitivity: May occur in patients with or without history of allergy or bronchial asthma; cross-sensitivity with sulfonamides may also occur.
Renal function impairment: Use with caution.
Hepatic function impairment: Do not use.
Hypotension, volume-depleted patients: Correct condition before using drug.
Systemic lupus erythematosus Exacerbation or activation may occur with thiazide diuretics.

Overdosage: Signs and Symptoms
Hypotension. tachycardia, bradycardia, electrolyte depletion (eg, hypokalemia), dehydration.

PATIENT CARE CONSIDERATIONS
Administration/Storage
- Give once daily in the morning, with or without food.
- Administer alone or in combination with other antihypertensives.
- Do not administer to pregnant women as fetal and neonatal morbidity and death can occur.
- Administer with caution and reduce dosage in patients with possible intravascular volume depletion or history of hepatic impairment.
- Store tablets at controlled room temperature. Keep container tightly closed. Protect from light.

Assessment/Interventions
- Obtain patient history, including drug history and any known allergies. Note history of diabetes, anuria, lupus erythematosus, gout, or kidney or liver disease.
- Ensure that serum electrolytes are monitored periodically.
- Monitor and record BP and pulse. Should hypotension result, hold medication and notify health care provider.
- Take safety precautions if orthostatic hypotension occurs.
- Monitor blood sugar in diabetic patient when drug is started or dose is changed. Report significant changes to health care provider.
- Monitor for signs of hypersensitivity including angioedema involving swelling of the face, lips, eyelids, and tongue. Discontinue medication and notify health care provider immediately, if noted.

Patient/Family Education
- Explain name, dose, action, and potential side effects of drug.
- Advise patient to take every day as prescribed, without regard to meals.
- Advise patient to try to take at the same time each day.
- Inform patient that drug controls, but not

does cure, hypertension and to continue taking drug as prescribed even when BP is not elevated.
- Caution patient not to change the dose or stop taking unless advised to do so by health care provider.
- Instruct patient to continue taking other BP medications as prescribed by health care provider.
- Instruct patient in BP and pulse measurement skills.
- Advise patient to monitor and record BP and pulse at home and to inform health care provider should abnormal measurements be noted. Also advise patient to take record of BP and pulse to each follow-up visit.
- Caution patient to avoid sudden position changes to prevent orthostatic hypotension.
- Instruct patient to lie or sit down if they experience dizziness or lightheadedness when standing.
- Caution patient that inadequate fluid intake, excessive perspiration, diarrhea, or vomiting can lead to excessive fall in BP resulting in lightheadedness or fainting.
- Instruct diabetic patient to monitor blood glucose more frequently when drug is started or dose is changed and to inform health care provider of significant changes in readings.
- Caution patient to avoid unnecessary exposure to UV light (eg, sunlight, tanning booths) and to use sunscreen and wear protective clothing when exposed to UV light to avoid photosensitivity reaction.
- Emphasize to hypertensive patient importance of other modalities on BP: weight control, regular exercise, smoking cessation, and moderate intake of alcohol and salt.
- Instruct women to notify health care provider if they become pregnant, plan on becoming pregnant, or are breastfeeding.
- Instruct patient to stop taking drug and immediately report any of the following symptoms to health care provider: fainting or swelling of the face, lips, eyelids or tongue.
- Caution patient to not take any prescription or OTC medications, salt substitutes, or dietary supplements unless advised to do so by health care provider.
- Advise patient that follow-up visits and lab tests may be required to monitor therapy and to keep appointments.

Lovastatin

(LOW-vuh-STAT-in)

Class Antihyperlipidemic/HMG-CoA reductase inhibitor

How Supplied
Altoprev Tablets, extended-release 10 mg, Tablets, extended-release 20 mg, Tablets, extended-release 40 mg, Tablets, extended-release 60 mg ♦ *Mevacor* Tablets 10 mg, Tablets 20 mg, Tablets 40 mg
✤ *Apo-Lovastatin* ♦ *Gen-Lovastatin* ♦ *ratio-Lovastatin*

Action

PHARMACOLOGY: Increases rate at which body removes cholesterol from blood and reduces production of cholesterol in body by inhibiting enzyme that catalyzes early rate-limiting step in cholesterol synthesis; increases HDL; reduces LDL, VLDL, and triglycerides.

PHARMACOKINETICS/DYNAMICS:
Absorption: About 35% absorbed. T_{max} is 2 to 4 hr.

Distribution: More than 95% protein bound (highly selective for the liver; achieved substantially higher concentrations than nontarget tissue). Crosses the blood-brain and placental barriers.

Metabolism: Major metabolites are beta-hydroxyacid and 6'-hydroxy derivative. Undergoes extensive first-pass metabolism (CYP 3A4). Less than 5% of an oral dose reaches general circulation.

Excretion: 10% excreted in urine; 83% excreted in feces.

Special Populations:
Renal Function Impairment – For Ccr less than 30 mL/min, use doses over 20 mg/day with caution because of increased plasma concentration.

Indications To reduce elevated cholesterol and LDL cholesterol levels in patients with primary hypercholesterolemia (types IIa and IIb [immediate-release only]); to slow progression of coronary atherosclerosis in patients with coronary heart disease; to reduce risk of MI, unstable angina, and coronary revascularization procedures; as an adjunct to diet to reduce total and LDL cholesterol and apolipoprotein B levels in adolescent boys and girls (who are at least 1 yr postmenarche) 10 to 17 yr with heterozygous familial hypercholesterolemia (immediate-release only). As an adjunct to diet for reduction of elevated total and LDL cholesterol, apolipoprotein B, and triglycerides and to increase HDL cholesterol in patients with primary hypercholesterolemia (heterozygous familial and nonfamilial) and mixed dyslipidemia (Fredrickson types IIa and IIb) when response to diet restricted in saturated fat and cholesterol and to nonpharmacological measures alone has been inadequate (extended-release only).

Contraindications Active liver disease or unexplained persistent elevations of LFTs; pregnancy; lactation.

Route/Dosage
ADULTS:
Immediate-release: **PO** 10 to 80 mg/day in a single dose with evening meal or 2 divided doses.
Extended-release: **PO** 10 to 60 mg/day as a single dose in the evening at bedtime. Individualize dose according to recommended goal of therapy. For patients requiring a small reduction in cholesterol level, a starting dose of 10 mg may be considered.

Heterozygous Familial Hypercholesterolemia
ADOLESCENTS (10 TO 17 YR):
Immediate-release: **PO** 10 to 40 mg/day (max, 40 mg/day).

Interactions
Azole antifungal agents (eg, itraconazole), cyclosporine, danazol, gemfibrozil, grapefruit juice, macrolide antibiotics (eg, erythromycin), niacin, verapamil: Severe myopathy or rhabdomyolysis may occur with coadministration.
Isradipine: May increase the clearance of lovastatin and its metabolites by increasing hepatic blood flow.
Warfarin: Enhanced anticoagulant effect.

Lab Test Interferences
None well documented.

Adverse Reactions
CNS: Headache; dizziness; paresthesia; insomnia.
DERM: Rash; pruritus.
EENT: Blurred vision; dysfunction of certain cranial nerves (including alteration of taste, impairment of extraocular movement, facial paresis).
GI: Nausea; vomiting; diarrhea; abdominal pain; constipation; flatulence; heartburn; dyspepsia; pancreatitis.
HEPA: Hepatitis; cholestatic jaundice; fatty change in liver; cirrhosis; fulminant hepatic necrosis; hepatoma.
OTHER: Myalgia; muscle cramps; myopathy; rhabdomyolysis with increased CPK; arthralgias; hypersensitivity syndrome (eg, anaphylaxis, angioedema, lupus erythematosus–like syndrome, polymyalgia rheumatica, vasculitis, purpura, thrombocytopenia, leukopenia, hemolytic anemia, arthritis, arthralgia, urticaria, fever, chills, dyspnea, toxic epidermal necrolysis, erythema multiforme.)

Precautions
Pregnancy: Category X.
Lactation: Undetermined.
Children: Safety and efficacy not established in children under 18 yr.
Hepatic function impairment: Use with caution in patients who consume substantial quantities of alcohol or those with liver disease. Marked, persistent increases in serum transaminases have occurred during therapy.
Adults older than 70 yr: The AUC of lovastatin is increased.
Ophthalmologic effects: There was a high prevalence of baseline lenticular opacities during the early trials of lovastatin.
Skeletal muscle effects: Rhabdomyolysis with renal dysfunction secondary to myoglobinuria has been reported, mostly in those taking lovastatin concomitantly with cyclosporine, erythromycin, gemfibrozil, or nicotinic acid.
Immunosuppressants may increase active lovastatin metabolites, which are associated with myopathy, myalgia, and muscle weakness associated with markedly increased CPK levels.

Overdosage: Signs and Symptoms
No specific symptoms with overdose of up to 6 g.

PATIENT CARE CONSIDERATIONS
Administration/Storage
- Administer with meals. If given as a single dose, administer with evening meal.
- Store at room temperature in tightly closed, light-resistant container.

Assessment/Interventions
- Obtain patient history, including drug history and any known allergies. Note hepatic impairment, alcohol consumption, and other medications that may increase risk of myopathy.
- Ensure that blood cholesterol and triglyceride levels are assessed before beginning therapy and repeated periodically during treatment.
- Place patient on standard cholesterol-lowering diet before beginning therapy and continue diet during treatment.
- Ensure that LFTs are performed q 4 to 6 wk during first 3 mo of therapy, q 6 to 8 wk during next 18 mo, and q 6 mo thereafter.
- If elevated serum transaminase levels develop during treatment, repeat tests more frequently.
- If transaminase levels rise to 3 times upper limit of normal and are persistent, notify health care provider. Drug may be discontinued.
- If muscle tenderness or weakness develops during therapy, monitor CPK levels. Notify

health care provider if CPK levels are markedly increased or if symptoms continue.

Patient/Family Education
- Caution patient that this medication must not be taken during pregnancy or when pregnancy is possible. Advise patient to use reliable form of birth control while taking this drug.
- Advise patient to take medication with evening meal if possible.
- Explain importance of adhering to low-cholesterol, low-fat diet during treatment. Suggest consultation with nutritionist as needed.
- Instruct patient to report the following symptoms to health care provider: unexplained muscle pain, tenderness, or weakness, especially if accompanied by fever or malaise.
- Caution patient to avoid or decrease alcohol intake.
- Advise patient not to take any additional medications or supplementation without approval by health care provider.
- Emphasize importance of returning for follow-up LFTs and blood cholesterol tests as instructed.
- Explain that this treatment must be continued over years.

Loxapine

(LOX-ah-peen)

Class Antipsychotic

How Supplied
Loxitane Capsule 5 mg, Capsule 10 mg, Capsule 25 mg, Capsule 50 mg
✤ *Apo-Loxapine* ♦ *Loxapac* ♦ *Nu-Loxapine* ♦ *PMS-Loxapine*

Action
PHARMACOLOGY: Unknown. Changes level of excitability of subcortical inhibitory areas in some animals.

PHARMACOKINETICS/DYNAMICS:
Absorption: Systemic bioavailability is one third of IM dose. T_{max} is 1 hr.
Distribution: Widely distributed in the tissues; 91% to 99% protein bound. Highly lipophilic.
Metabolism: First-pass metabolism. Metabolites found in serum are 8-hydroxyloxapine and 8-hydroxydesmethylloxapine. Extensively metabolized.
Excretion: The apparent t½ is 4 hr (1 to 14 hr). Approximately 40% is recovered in urine as metabolites.
Onset: 20 to 30 min.
Peak: 1.5 to 3 hr.
Duration: 12 hr.

Indications Treatment of schizophrenia.

Contraindications Comatose or severe drug-induced depressed states (eg, barbiturates); hypersensitivity to dibenzoxazepines.

Route/Dosage
ADULTS:
Initial dose: **PO** 10 mg bid, up to 50 mg/day, titrated fairly rapidly over first 7 to 10 days until symptoms are controlled.
Maintenance dose: Reduce dosage to lowest amount compatible with symptom control. Usual range is 60 to 100 mg/day; many patients have been maintained satisfactorily at a dosage range of 20 to 60 mg/day. Dosages higher than 250 mg/day are not recommended.

Interactions
Lorazepam: Respiratory depression, stupor, and hypertension may occur.

Adverse Reactions
CV: Tachycardia; hypotension; hypertension; orthostatic hypotension; lightheadedness; syncope.
CNS: Extrapyramidal effects; transient drowsiness; sedation; dizziness; faintness; staggering gait; shuffling gait; muscle twitching; weakness; insomnia; agitation; tension; seizures; akinesia; slurred speech; numbness; mental confusion; neuroleptic malignant syndrome (NMS); dystonic (eg, muscle spasms of the neck and face) and dyskinetic reactions (eg, choreoathetoid movements); tardive dyskinesia; headache.
DERM: Edema; pruritus; rash; alopecia; seborrhea.
EENT: Nasal congestion; blurred vision.
GI: Dry mouth; constipation; paralytic ileus; nausea; vomiting.
GU: Urinary retention; amenorrhea; gynecomastia; menstrual irregularity.
HEMA: Agranulocytosis; thrombocytopenia; leukopenia.
HEPA: Hepatocellular injury; jaundice; hepatitis.
METAB: Weight gain/loss.
RESP: Dyspnea.
OTHER: Hyperpyrexia; facial flushing; paresthesia; ptosis; polydipsia; prolactin levels increased.

Precautions
Pregnancy: Undetermined.
Lactation: Undetermined.
Children: Safety and efficacy not established.
Special risk patients: Use with extreme caution in patients with a history of convulsive disorders, CV disease, glaucoma, or tendency to urinary retention.
NMS: This potentially fatal condition has been reported in association with antipsychotic

agents. Signs and symptoms include hyperpyrexia, muscle rigidity, altered mental status, irregular pulse or BP, tachycardia, diaphoresis, cardiac arrhythmias.

Ocular toxicity: Carefully observe patient for pigmentary retinopathy and lenticular pigmentation.

Tardive dyskinesia: This syndrome of potentially irreversible, involuntary, dyskinetic movements has occurred with other antipsychotic agents. Incidence appears to be highest among the elderly.

Overdosage: Signs and Symptoms
CV and CNS depression, profound hypotension, respiratory depression, unconsciousness, extrapyramidal symptoms, convulsive seizures, renal failure.

PATIENT CARE CONSIDERATIONS
Administration/Storage
- Administer bid to qid as prescribed without regard to meals.
- Administer with food if GI upset occurs.
- Store at controlled room temperature (59° to 86°F).

Assessment/Interventions
- Obtain patient history, including drug history and any known allergies. Note history of CV disease, glaucoma, urinary retention, prostatic hypertrophy, previous episodes of NMS, seizures, or conditions that predispose to seizures (eg, Alzheimer disease).
- Inform health care provider immediately if hyperpyrexia, muscle rigidity, altered mental status, irregular pulse and BP, tachycardia, or diaphoresis develop.
- Assess baseline neurologic status and, during treatment, observe for involuntary body and facial movements and excessive drowsiness. Inform health care provider if noted.
- Assess and document effect of medication on psychotic symptoms.
- Monitor patient for CV, GI, CNS, and general body side effects. Inform health care provider if noted and significant.
- Assess medication compliance.
- Ensure that therapy is periodically reviewed to determine if therapy needs to be continued without change or if a dose change (eg, increase, decrease, discontinuation) is indicated.
- Avoid sudden discontinuation of therapy if possible. Attempt to gradually reduce dose if decision to discontinue medication is made.

Patient/Family Education
- Explain name, dose, action, and potential side effects of drug.
- Advise patient that dose will be started low and then increased until max benefit is achieved; advise patient not to take more than prescribed or increase the dose more rapidly than advised.
- Instruct patient not to change the dose or stop taking unless advised by health care provider.
- Instruct patient not to stop taking loxapine when symptoms have improved.
- Tell patient to immediately report high fever, muscle rigidity, involuntary body or facial movements, altered mental status, irregular pulse, or sweating to health care provider.
- Advise patient to avoid strenuous activity during periods of high temperature or humidity.
- Instruct patient to avoid alcohol and other CNS depressant medications.
- Advise patient to take sips of water, suck on ice chips or sugarless hard candy, or chew sugarless gum if dry mouth occurs.
- Advise patient that drug may cause drowsiness and to use caution while driving or performing other tasks requiring mental alertness until tolerance is determined.
- Advise women to notify health care provider if pregnant, planning to become pregnant, or breastfeeding.
- Advise patient to notify health care provider if excessive drowsiness occurs.
- Instruct patient not to take any prescription or OTC medications or dietary supplements unless advised by health care provider.
- Advise patient that follow-up visits will be required to monitor therapy and to keep appointments.

Lymphocyte Immune Globulin

(lim-fo-site ih-MYOON GLAH-byoo-lin)
Class Equine polyclonal antibody
How Supplied
Atgam Solution for injection 50 mg/mL

Action
PHARMACOLOGY: Antilymphocytic effect is believed to reflect an alteration of the function of the T lymphocytes.

PHARMACOKINETICS/DYNAMICS:
Absorption: T_{max} is 5 days
Excretion: Mean t½ is 5.7 days (2.7 to 8.7 days).

Onset: Rapid.

Indications Moderate to severe aplastic anemia; treatment of acute allograft rejection in renal transplantation. **Unlabeled use(s):** Immunosuppressant in course of liver, bone-marrow, heart, and other organ transplants; treatment of multiple sclerosis, myasthenia gravis, pure red-cell aplasia, and scleroderma.

Contraindications Hypersensitivity to lymphocyte immune globulin or any other equine gamma globulin preparation.

Route/Dosage

Aplastic Anemia
ADULTS: **IV** 10 to 20 mg/kg/day for 8 to 14 days; additional doses may be given every other day for a total of 21 doses (inclusive).

Renal Allograft Recipients
ADULTS: **IV** 10 to 30 mg/kg/day.
CHILDREN: **IV** 5 to 25 mg/kg/day.

Delaying the Onset of Renal Allograft Rejection
ADULTS: **IV** Give a fixed dose of 15 mg/kg/day for 14 days, then every other day for 14 days, for a total of 21 doses in 28 days. Administer the first dose within 24 hr before or after the transplant.

Treatment of Allograft Rejection
ADULTS: **IV** The first dose can be delayed until the diagnosis of the first rejection episode. The recommended dose is 10 to 15 mg/kg/day for 14 days. Additional alternate-day therapy up to a total of 21 doses can be given.

Interactions
Immunosuppressants: Risk of infection may increase.

Lab Test Interferences None well documented.

Adverse Reactions Unless otherwise stated, the following adverse reactions occurred in less than 5% of patients.
CV: Chest pain; hypotension; hypertension; tachycardia; edema; CHF, vasculitis (postmarketing).
CNS: Fever; chills; headache; malaise; confusion, disorientation, dizziness, faintness, abnormal involuntary movements, paresthesia, rigidity, seizures, tremor (postmarketing).
DERM: Skin reactions common including rash, pruritus, wheal, flare, and urticaria; chemical phlebitis reported, along with pain, redness, or swelling at the injection site; rashes (27%), sweating (postmarketing).
EENT: Laryngospasm/edema, nosebleed (postmarketing).
GI: Stomatitis; diarrhea, nausea, vomiting (5% to 10%); abdominal, epigastric, and stomach pain, GI bleeding or perforation, sore mouth or throat (postmarketing).
GU: Renal failure; oliguria; elevated creatinine, BUN; abnormal renal function (5% to 10%); acute renal failure, enlarged or ruptured kidney, renal artery thrombosis (postmarketing).
HEMA: Thrombocytopenia (30%); leukopenia (14%); anemia, aplasia or pancytopenia, deep vein thrombosis, eosinophilia, hemolysis, hemolytic anemia, neutropenia or granulocytopenia, thrombophlebitis (postmarketing).
HEPA: Abnormal LFTs, viral hepatitis (postmarketing).
HYPERSEN: Anaphylactoid reactions. Symptoms may include respiratory distress, chest pain, flank pain, back pain, or hypotension. Anaphylaxis in fewer than 5% of patients; serum sickness common in patients with aplastic anemia or other hematological diseases.
METAB: Hyperglycemia (postmarketing).
MUSC: Arthralgia, back or flank pain (5% to 10%); leg pain, myalgia (postmarketing).
RESP: Apnea, dyspnea (5% to 10%); cough, pulmonary edema (postmarketing).
OTHER: Fever (51%); chills (16%); systemic infection (13%); serum sickness-like symptoms, chest pain (5% to 10%); lymphoproliferative disorders reported, including lymphomas (secondary malignancy); systemic infections; some studies have found an increased risk of cytomegalovirus infection; herpes simplex infection, pain, localized infection, lymphadenopathy (postmarketing).

> **WARNING:**
> Lymphocyte immune globulin should only be used by physicians experienced in immunosuppressive therapy in treatment of renal transplant or aplastic anemia. Patients should be treated in facilities equipped and staffed with adequate laboratory and supportive medical resources.

Precautions
Pregnancy: Category C.
Lactation: Undetermined.
Children: Experience with children has been limited. It has been administered safely to a small number of pediatric renal allograft recipients and pediatric aplastic anemia patients at dosage levels comparable to those in adults.
Hypersensitivity: Hypersensitivity may occur at any time during therapy.
Special risk patients: Because an immunosuppressive agent and antimetabolites are usually coadministered with this product, monitor patients carefully for signs of leukopenia, thrombocytopenia, or concurrent infection.
Antibodies: Human antilymphocyte immune globulin antibodies develop in 78% of patients

treated with lymphocyte immune globulin. It is unknown whether such antibodies alter the clinical efficacy of repeated courses of therapy.
Discontinuation: Discontinue treatment if symptoms of anaphylaxis or severe and unremitting thrombocytopenia or leukopenia occur in renal transplant patients.
Disease transmission: Because this product is made using equine and human blood components, there is a risk of transmitting infectious agents (eg, viruses) and theoretically, the Creutzfeld-Jacob disease.

PATIENT CARE CONSIDERATIONS
Administration/Storage

- Dose, frequency of administration, and duration of therapy are variable, depending on indication for use and patient response.
- For administration by IV infusion only. Not for intradermal, subcutaneous, IM, IV bolus, or intra-arterial administration.
- Before administering lymphocyte immune globulin, test patient with an intradermal injection of 0.1 mL of a freshly prepared 1:1,000 dilution of lymphocyte immune globulin in normal saline and a contralateral sodium chloride injection control.
- Do not shake diluted or undiluted solution. Shaking may cause foaming and/or denaturation of the protein.
- Dilute solution in an inverted bottle of compatible, sterile, saline-containing diluent so the undiluted lymphocyte immune globulin does not contact the air inside the bottle. Gently rotate or swirl the diluted solution to thoroughly mix. Final concentration should not exceed 4 mg of lymphocyte immune globulin/mL.
- Do not dilute with dextrose injection. Low salt concentrations may result in precipitation.
- Do not administer if solution is discolored, cloudy, turbid, or if particulate matter is noted.
- Allow solution to reach room temperature before infusion.
- Infuse prescribed dose through inline filter with pore size of 0.2 to 1 micron into vascular shunt, arterial venous fistula, or high-flow central vein catheter, over a period of no less than 4 hr.
- Store ampules in refrigerator (36° to 46°F). Protect from freezing. If not administered immediately, store diluted solution in refrigerator for up to 24 hr (including infusion time).

Dosage adjustment for hematologic toxicity: Consider dosage reduction in patients with profound bone marrow suppression; no specific guidelines available.
Extravasation: Local irritation or phlebitis may occur. Refer to your institution-specific protocol.
Hemolysis: Clinically significant hemolysis has been reported.
Serum sickness: Serum sickness reactions typically occur within 6 to 18 days of starting therapy, although reactions have been reported after drug discontinuation.

Assessment/Interventions

- Obtain patient history, including drug history and any known allergies. Note history of severe systemic reaction during prior administration of lymphocyte immune globulin or any other equine gamma globulin preparation.
- Ensure intradermal skin test has been considered before administering lymphocyte immune globulin and that patient and skin test site are evaluated every 15 to 20 minutes over the first hour following the intradermal injection. Document response to skin test.
- Ensure CBC and differential are determined at baseline and periodically during course of therapy.
- Implement infection control measures if WBC drops; implement bleeding precautions if platelet count drops. Discontinue therapy if severe and unremitting thrombocytopenia or leukopenia develops in renal transplant patient.
- Ensure resuscitation equipment is available at patient's bedside during intradermal skin test and while lymphocyte immune globulin is being infused.
- Monitor patient for signs of anaphylaxis or severe allergic reaction. Discontinue therapy and immediately notify health care provider if noted. Be prepared to treat appropriately.
- Closely monitor patient for development of previously masked reactions to lymphocyte immune globulin when dose of corticosteroids and other immunosuppressants is being reduced.
- Monitor patient for CV, GI, CNS, RESP, general body side effects, and infusion site reactions. Inform health care provider if noted and significant.

Patient/Family Education
- Explain name, actions, and potential side effects of the treatment regimen. Review the treatment regimen including dosing schedule, duration of treatment, and monitoring that will be required.
- Review benefits of therapy and risks, including potential to transmit disease and unknown infectious agents.
- Advise patient, family, or caregiver that medication will be prepared and administered by health care provider in a health care setting.
- Advise patient, family, or caregiver that medication will be used in combination with other agents to achieve max benefit possible.
- Advise patient, family, or caregiver that a skin test may be performed before the first dose is administered.
- Advise patient, family, or caregiver to immediately report any of the following to health care provider: rash; itching; hives; difficulty breathing; fever, chills, or other signs of infection; bleeding or unusual bruising; pain, redness, or swelling at injection site.
- Advise patient, family, or caregiver that after discharge frequent follow-up visits and laboratory tests will be required to monitor therapy and to keep appointments.

Magaldrate (Hydroxymagnesium Aluminate)

(MAG-al-drate)

Class Antacid

How Supplied
Iosopan Liquid 540 mg/5 mL ◆ *Riopan* Suspension 540 mg/5 mL

Action
PHARMACOLOGY: Neutralizes gastric acid, thereby increasing pH of stomach and duodenal bulb. Increases lower esophageal sphincter tone and inhibits smooth muscle contraction and gastric emptying.

Indications Symptomatic relief of upset stomach associated with hyperacidity, including heartburn, gastroesophageal reflux, acid indigestion and sour stomach; relief of hyperacidity associated with peptic ulcer, gastritis, peptic esophagitis, gastric hyperacidity and hiatal hernia.

Contraindications Severe renal dysfunction; hypophosphatemia; nausea; vomiting; severe abdominal pain; acute surgical abdomen; impaction; intestinal obstruction.

Route/Dosage
ADULTS: **PO** 480 to 1080 mg qid prn or to aid in peptic ulcer healing or chronic reflux, give 1 hr and 3 hr after meals and at bedtime (7 doses/day).
CHILDREN: **PO** 5 to 10 mg/dose q 3 to 6 hr or 1 hr and 3 hr after meals and at bedtime for peptic ulcer.

Interactions
Iron: Decreased pharmacologic effect of iron.
Ketoconazole: Decreased pharmacologic effect of ketoconazole.
Nitrofurantoin: Decreased effects of nitrofurantoin.
Penicillamine: Decreased pharmacologic effect of penicillamine.
Quinidine: Increased pharmacologic effect of quinidine.
Quinolones: Decreased pharmacologic effect of quinolones.
Salicylates: Decreased pharmacologic effect of salicylates.
Sodium polystyrene sulfonate: Concomitant use may cause metabolic alkalosis in patients with renal failure.
Tetracyclines: Decreased pharmacologic effect of tetracyclines.

Lab Test Interferences None well documented.

Adverse Reactions
CNS: Neurotoxicity; encephalopathy.
GI: Diarrhea; constipation; intestinal obstruction; rebound hyperacidity.
METAB: Hypophosphatemia; hypermagnesemia.
OTHER: Osteomalacia; bone pain; muscular weakness; malaise; decreased fluoride absorption; aluminum accumulation in serum, bone and CNS; milk-alkali syndrome.

Precautions
Pregnancy: Pregnancy category undetermined.
Lactation: Undetermined.
Renal function impairment: Use with caution in patients with renal impairment to avoid hypermagnesemia and toxicity.
GI hemorrhage: Use with care in patients with recent massive upper GI hemorrhage.

Overdosage: Signs and Symptoms
Nausea, vomiting, diarrhea, constipation, hypermagnesemia, hypophosphatemia.

PATIENT CARE CONSIDERATIONS

Administration/Storage
- Administer 1 hr and 3 hr after meals and at bedtime when ordered for treatment of ulcers or 4 times/day when ordered as necessary for relief of symptoms.
- If possible, administer antacid 1 to 2 hr before or after other medications.
- Shake suspension vigorously before pouring. Administer with sufficient water (approximately 4 oz) to ensure that drug reaches stomach.
- Chewable tablet should be chewed thoroughly before swallowing, followed by half a glass of water.
- Store at room temperature (59° to 86°F).

Assessment/Interventions
- Obtain patient history, including drug history and any allergies.
- Assess for heartburn and indigestion, noting location, duration, character and precipitating factors of GI pain.
- Monitor serum magnesium level in patients with renal impairment.
- Monitor level of relief obtained by patient following medication.

Patient/Family Education
- Instruct patient to take medication 1 and 3 hr after meals and at bedtime.
- Warn patient not to take other medications within 2 hr of antacid.

- Review proper use of suspension or tablet form.
- Advise patient to consult health care provider if problem recurs, if any symptoms that suggest bleeding occur (eg, black tarry stools) or if patient has taken antacids for more than 2 wk.

Magnesium Citrate

(mag-NEE-zee-uhm SIH-trate)
Class Laxative

How Supplied
Citrate of Magnesia ♦ *Citro-Nesia* ♣ *Citro-Mag*

Action
PHARMACOLOGY: Attracts and retains water in intestinal lumen, thereby increasing intraluminal pressure and inducing urge to defecate.

PHARMACOKINETICS/DYNAMICS:
Absorption: Up to 20% magnesium citrate is absorbed.

Excretion: Magnesium citrate is excreted by renal elimination

Onset: Onset is 0.5 to 5 hr.

Indications
Short-term treatment of constipation; evacuation of colon for rectal and bowel evaluations.

Contraindications
Hypersensitivity to any ingredient; nausea, vomiting or other symptoms of appendicitis; acute surgical abdomen; fecal impaction; intestinal obstruction; undiagnosed abdominal pain; intestinal bleeding; renal disease.

Route/Dosage
ADULTS: **PO** 1 glassful (approximately 240 mL) prn.
CHILDREN (6 TO 12 YR): **PO** 50 to 100 mL. Repeat if necessary.
CHILDREN (2 TO 6 YR): **PO** 4 to 12 mL.

Interactions
Nitrofurantoin: Reduced anti-infective action.
Penicillamine: Reduced action of penicillamine.
Tetracyclines: Impaired absorption of tetracyclines.

Lab Test Interferences None well documented.

Adverse Reactions
CV: Palpitations.
CNS: Dizziness; fainting.
GI: Excessive bowel activity (eg, cramping, diarrhea, nausea, vomiting); perianal irritation; bloating; flatulence; abdominal cramping.
OTHER: Sweating; weakness; fluid and electrolyte imbalance.

Precautions
Pregnancy: Pregnancy category undetermined.
Lactation: Undetermined.
Children: Exercise caution; consult health care provider. One 6-wk old infant developed magnesium poisoning after several doses for constipation.
Renal function impairment: Avoid in patients with renal dysfunction. Hypermagnesemia and toxicity may occur due to decreased clearance of magnesium ion.
Abuse/dependency: Chronic use of laxatives may lead to laxative dependency, which may result in fluid and electrolyte imbalances, steatorrhea, osteomalacia and vitamin and mineral deficiencies.
Fluid and electrolyte imbalance: Excessive laxative use may lead to significant fluid and electrolyte imbalance.
Rectal bleeding or failure to respond: May indicate serious condition requiring further attention.

Overdosage: Signs and Symptoms
Severe/protracted diarrhea, fluid and electrolyte disturbances, hypermagnesemia.

PATIENT CARE CONSIDERATIONS
Administration/Storage
- Chilling medication or giving with ice may improve palatability.
- Administer on empty stomach and give with full glass of water to increase effectiveness of medication.
- Store in tightly closed container in cool dry place.

Assessment/Interventions
- Obtain patient history, including drug history and any known allergies. Note symptoms of appendicitis, fecal impaction, renal disease or small bowel obstruction.
- Observe for distended abdomen and auscultate for presence of bowel sounds.
- Monitor for electrolyte imbalances and dehydration.
- If nausea, diarrhea, abdominal distention, increased abdominal pain or rectal bleeding occur, notify health care provider.

Patient/Family Education
- Explain that drug should not be used routinely for constipation; dependence can result.
- Instruct patient to report any of the following symptoms to health care provider: unrelieved constipation, vomiting, diarrhea, abdominal fullness, rectal bleeding, dizziness and muscle cramps.
- Review information on proper use and storage of medication.

Magnesium Oxide

(mag-NEE-zee-uhm OX-ide)

Class Antacid

How Supplied
Mag-Ox 400 Tablets 400 mg ♦ Maox 420 Tablets 420 mg ♦ Uro-Mag Capsules 140 mg

Action
PHARMACOLOGY: Neutralizes gastric acid, thereby increases pH of stomach and duodenal bulb; also increases lower esophageal sphincter tone.

PHARMACOKINETICS/DYNAMICS:
Excretion: Magnesium Oxide is eliminated renally and fecally.
Duration: Duration is 4 to 6 hr.

Indications Symptomatic relief of upset stomach associated with hyperacidity, including heartburn, gastroesophageal reflux, acid indigestion and sour stomach; relief of hyperacidity associated with peptic ulcer, gastritis, peptic esophagitis, gastric hyperacidity and hiatal hernia. Also used for treatment of hypomagnesemia, or magnesium depletion resulting from malnutrition, restricted diet, alcoholism or magnesium-depleting drugs.

Contraindications Standard considerations.

PATIENT CARE CONSIDERATIONS

Administration/Storage
- Administer caps or tabs with full glass of water or other liquid.
- Give 1 to 2 hr before or after other medications if possible.
- Store in airtight container in cool location unless otherwise specified by manufacturer.

Assessment/Interventions
- Obtain patient history, including drug history and any known allergies. Note renal disease.
- Monitor for symptoms of renal insufficiency (eg, elevated BUN and creatinine, decreased urine output).
- Encourage patient to increase fluid intake.
- Monitor serum magnesium levels in patients being treated for hypomagnesemia and in patients with impaired renal function.
- Assess for heartburn and indigestion. Note location, duration, character, and precipitating factors.

Patient/Family Education
- Advise patient that drug may be laxative and cause diarrhea.
- If being used for antacid effect, instruct patient to notify health care provider if symptoms are not relieved or if black, tarry stools or "coffee-ground" vomitus occurs. These symptoms can indicate bleeding.
- Explain that drug should not be used routinely for laxative effect. Advise patient to use other forms of bowel regulation such as increasing fluid intake, mobility and bulk in diet.
- Warn patient not to take other medications within 2 hr of antacids.

Route/Dosage
ADULTS: PO 140 mg (caps) 3 to 4 times/day or 400 to 840 mg/day (tabs).

Interactions
Iron: Decreased pharmacological effect of iron.
Nitrofurantoin: Decreased pharmacological effect of nitrofurantoin.
Penicillamine: Decreased pharmacological effect of penicillamine.
Tetracyclines: Decreased pharmacological effect of tetracyclines.

Lab Test Interferences None well documented.

Adverse Reactions
GI: Laxative effect (diarrhea); rebound hyperacidity.
METAB: Hypermagnesemia.
OTHER: Milk-alkali syndrome.

Precautions
Pregnancy: Category B.
Lactation: Undetermined.
Renal function impairment: Use caution in patients with renal impairment to avoid hypermagnesemia and toxicity.

Overdosage: Signs and Symptoms
Diarrhea, fluid and electrolyte abnormalities, hypermagnesemia.

Magnesium Sulfate

(mag-NEE-zee-uhm SULL-fate)

Class Anticonvulsant/Electrolyte/Laxative

How Supplied
Epsom Salt Granules see care instructions ♦ Magnesium sulfate Injection 4% (0.325 mEq/mL), Injection 8% (0.65 mEq/mL), Injection 12.5% (1 mEq/mL), Injection 50% (4 mEq/mL).

Action
PHARMACOLOGY: Magnesium has CNS depressant effect; prevents/controls seizures by blocking neuromuscular transmission and decreasing amount of acetylcholine liberated at end plate by motor nerve impulse. Orally it attracts/retains

water in intestinal lumen, thereby increasing intraluminal pressure and inducing urge to defecate.

Indications
Parenteral: Seizure prevention and control in severe preeclampsia or eclampsia without deleterious CNS depression in mother, fetus, or newborn; replacement therapy in magnesium deficiency, especially in acute hypomagnesemia accompanied by signs of tetany similar to those observed in hypocalcemia; corrects or prevents hypomagnesemia by addition to total parenteral nutrition admixture. **Unlabeled use(s):** Control of hypertension, encephalopathy, and convulsions in children with acute nephritis; inhibition of premature labor; treatment of life-threatening ventricular arrhythmias; prevention and treatment of nutritional magnesium deficiency; laxative (oral).

Contraindications
Toxemia of pregnancy during 2 hr preceding delivery; MI; myocardial damage; heartblock.

Route/Dosage
Eclampsia
IM/IV 10 to 14 g of magnesium sulfate (as a combination of IM and IV administration) appropriately diluted.

Hyperalimentation
ADULTS: **TPN** Maintenance dose ranges from 8 to 24 mEq (1 to 3 g) daily.
INFANTS: **TPN** Maintenance dose ranges from 2 to 10 mEq (0.25 to 1.25 g) daily.

Laxative
Usually 1-time dose.
ADULTS: **PO** 10 to 15 g.
CHILDREN: **PO** 5 to 10 g.

Magnesium Deficiency
Mild magnesium deficiency – **IM** Usual dose is 1 g, equivalent to 8.12 mEq magnesium (2 mL of 50% solution) injected q 6 hr for 4 doses, equivalent to a total of 32.5 mEq of magnesium per 24 hr.
Severe hypomagnesemia – As much as 250 mg (approximately 2 mEq) per kg (0.5 mL of the 50% solution) may be given within a period of 4 hr if necessary. Alternatively, 5 g (approximately 40 mEq) can be added to 1 L of 5% dextrose injection, or 0.9% sodium chloride injection, for slow IV infusion over a 3-hr period. Use caution so as not to exceed the renal excretion capacity.

Seizures Associated with Epilepsy, Glomerulonephritis, or Hypothyroidism
ADULTS: **IM/IV** 1 g.

PATIENT CARE CONSIDERATIONS
Administration/Storage
♦ Store granules and injection at ambient room temperature (59° to 86°F).

Interactions
Cardiac glycosides (eg, digoxin): Administer magnesium sulfate with extreme caution because of serious changes in cardiac conduction, which can result in heart block, may occur if administration of calcium is required to treat magnesium toxicity.
CNS depressants (eg, barbiturates, narcotics): Possible additive CNS depressant effects.
Neuromuscular blocking agents: Potentiation of neuromuscular blockade.
Nitrofurantoin: Decreased absorption of nitrofurantoin (oral magnesium).
Penicillamine: Reduced penicillamine effects (oral magnesium).
Tetracyclines: Decreased absorption of tetracyclines (oral magnesium).
INCOMPATIBILITIES: Alcohol (in high concentrations), alkali carbonates and bicarbonates, alkali hydroxides, arsenates, barium, calcium, clindamycin phosphate, heavy metals, hydrocortisone sodium succinate, phosphates, polymyxin B sulfate, procaine hydrochloride, salicylates, streptomycin, strontium, tartrates, tetracycline, tobramycin.

Lab Test Interferences
None well documented.

Adverse Reactions
CV: Cardiac depression; circulatory collapse; hypotension; cardiac arrest.
CNS: CNS depression; depressed reflexes; muscle weakness; flaccid paralysis.
METAB: Hypocalcemia.
RESP: Respiratory paralysis.
OTHER: Flushing; sweating; hypothermia.

Precautions
Pregnancy: Category A.
Lactation: Excreted in breast milk during parenteral use.
Renal function impairment: Use with caution; renal insufficiency may lead to magnesium intoxication.
Eclampsia: Use IV form only for immediate control of life-threatening convulsions.

Overdosage: Signs and Symptoms
Early signs: Sweating, flushing, thirst, decreased deep tendon reflexes, weakness.
Later signs: Sedation, loss of deep tendon reflexes, hypothermia, hypotension, heart block, respiratory paralysis.

Granules:
♦ Administer prescribed dose early in day on empty stomach.

- Mix granules in at least a half-glass of water before administering. Follow with full glass of water. May mix with ice chips or flavor with lemon or orange juice to make more palatable.

Injection:

- Dose is individualized depending on condition being treated.
- For IM or IV administration only. Not for intradermal, subcutaneous, or intra-arterial administration.
- Fifty percent solution may be administered undiluted to adults if given by deep IM injection. Rotate injection sites to reduce tissue irritation.
- Fifty percent solution must be diluted, with 0.9% sodium chloride injection or 5% dextrose injection, to a concentration of 20% or less before IV administration or IM administration in infants and children.
- When administering via IV route, use infusion pump. Deliver in separate line and do not mix with other IV drugs unless compatibility has been established.
- Do not administer if particulate matter, cloudiness, or discoloration noted.
- Discard any unused solution.

Assessment/Interventions

- Obtain patient history, including drug history and any known allergies. Note renal impairment. When using injection, note heart block, myocardial damage, or concurrent use of CNS depressants, digoxin, or neuromuscular blocking agents. When using granules, note nausea, vomiting, or other symptoms of appendicitis, fecal impaction, intestinal obstruction, and undiagnosed abdominal pain.

Granules:

- Assess bowel sounds, abdominal distention, and bowel patterns when using oral magnesium as a laxative. Document response to therapy.
- Ensure that proper dietary fiber intake and adequate hydration are being used to prevent constipation from recurring.
- Monitor patient for GI (eg, nausea, vomiting, bloating) and general body (eg, muscle cramps, weakness, dizziness) side effects. Inform health care provider if noted and significant.

Injection:

- Ensure that baseline ECG, calcium, phosphorous, magnesium, BUN, and creatinine levels have been obtained before beginning parenteral magnesium administration. Monitor regularly during therapy. Serum magnesium levels should be obtained as necessary based on condition being treated (eg, eclampsia, hypomagnesemia) or when toxicity is suspected.
- Obtain baseline vital signs, patellar reflex, and neurologic assessment. Continue to assess throughout parenteral magnesium administration.
- If magnesium is being administered to prevent preterm labor, assess fetal heart rate and uterine contractions prior to first dose and continuously during administration.
- Maintain strict, hourly I&O and keep patient well hydrated. Urine output should be at least 25 mL per hr while administering parenteral magnesium.
- Monitor patient for magnesium intoxication (eg, sweating, flushing, hypotension, loss of patellar reflex, respiratory depression, ECG changes including increased PR interval, increased QRS complex, prolonged QT interval, and heart block). Discontinue therapy and inform health care provider immediately if noted. Be prepared to treat appropriately (eg, respiratory assistance, IV calcium salts).
- Keep 10% calcium chloride at bedside for adult patient (calcium gluconate for newborns and pediatric patients).
- If magnesium is being given for preeclampsia or convulsions, maintain seizure precautions. Provide a quiet, nonstimulating environment.
- If magnesium was administered during labor, prepare for neonatal resuscitation. Monitor newborn for magnesium toxicity. Be prepared to treat appropriately (eg, respiratory assistance, IV calcium gluconate) if noted.

Patient/Family Education

- Explain name, action, and potential side effects of drug.

Injection:

- Advise patient that medication will be prepared and administered by a health care professional in a hospital setting.

Oral:

- Advise patient to mix granules in at least a half-glass of water before swallowing and to follow with full glass of water. Advise patient to mix with ice chips or flavor with lemon or orange juice to make more palatable.
- Educate patient regarding other measures that may help prevent constipation (eg, dietary fiber, adequate fluid intake, regular exercise).
- Caution patient that drug is for short-term laxative use only and that prolonged use can lead to dehydration and electrolyte imbalance.
- Advise patient to discontinue use and notify health care provider of the following: unrelieved constipation, rectal bleeding, symptoms of electrolyte imbalance (eg, muscle cramps or pain, weakness, dizziness)

Malathion

(mal-ah-THIGH-ahn)

Class Pediculicide

How Supplied
Ovide Lotion 0.5%

Action
PHARMACOLOGY: Inhibits cholinesterase activity.

Indications Treatment of head lice (*Pediculus humanus capitis*) and their ova of the scalp hair.

Contraindications Neonates and infants; hypersensitivity to any component of the product.

Route/Dosage
ADULTS AND CHILDREN 6 YR AND OLDER:
Topical Apply lotion on dry hair in amount just sufficient to thoroughly wet the hair and scalp, paying particular attention to back of head and neck. Wash hands after application. Allow hair to dry normally, without use of electric heat source, and allow hair to remain uncovered. Shampoo hair after 8 to 12 hr. Rinse and use a fine-toothed (nit) comb to remove dead lice and eggs. If lice are still present after 7 to 9 days, repeat with a second application.

Interactions None well documented.

Lab Test Interferences None well documented.

Adverse Reactions
DERM: Irritation to skin and scalp.
EENT: Conjunctivitis caused by accidental contact with eyes.

Precautions
Pregnancy: Category B..
Lactation: Undetermined; however, malathion is absorbed through the skin.
Children: Safety and efficacy not established in children under 6 yr.
External use: Avoid contact with eyes; if accidentally placed in eye, flush immediately with water.
Flammable: Because product contains alcohol, it should not be exposed to open flame or electric heat, including hair dryers and electric curlers; do not smoke while applying lotion or while hair is wet.

Overdosage: Signs and Symptoms
Severe respiratory distress.

PATIENT CARE CONSIDERATIONS

Administration/Storage
- For topical use only. Not for ophthalmic, oral, or intravaginal use.
- Lotion is flammable. Do not expose treated hair to open flames or electric heat sources (eg, hair dryer, electric curler) until hair is dry.
- Avoid contact with eyes. If eye contact occurs, flush immediately and thoroughly with water.
- Use gloves if applying to patient; apply lotion on dry hair in amount just sufficient to thoroughly wet hair and scalp; wash hands after applying lotion; allow hair to dry naturally; after 8 to 12 hr (eg, overnight) shampoo hair; rinse and use fine-toothed (nit) comb to remove dead lice and eggs.
- Treatment may be repeated once after 7 to 9 days if lice are still present.
- Store lotion at controlled room temperature (68° to 77°F). Keep bottle tightly capped and away from heat and open flame.

Assessment/Interventions
- Obtain patient history, including drug history and any known allergies.
- Monitor application site for evidence of irritation. If irritation is noted, wash scalp and hair immediately. If irritation clears, reapply lotion. If irritation reoccurs, wash scalp and hair again and notify health care provider.

Patient/Family Education
- Explain name, dose, action, and potential side effects of drug.
- Caution patient or caregiver that medication has potential for causing serious harm and not to exceed prescribed dose or apply more frequently than prescribed by health care provider. Advise patient or caregiver to not reapply unless specifically advised by health care provider.
- Caution patient or caregiver to avoid contact with eyes and that if accidental eye contact occurs to immediately flush the eyes with water to remove medication. Advise patient or caregiver to notify health care provider if eye irritation or sensitivity follows exposure to the eyes.
- Caution patient or caregiver that medication may be toxic if swallowed and to seek medical care immediately in case of accidental ingestion.
- Teach patient or caregiver proper technique for applying lotion: apply lotion on dry hair in amount just sufficient to thoroughly wet hair and scalp; wash hands after applying lotion; allow hair to dry naturally; after 8 to 12 hr (eg, overnight) shampoo hair; rinse and use fine-toothed (nit) comb to remove dead lice and eggs.
- Caution patient or caregiver that lotion is

flammable and not to smoke while applying lotion or expose treated hair to open flames or electric heat sources (eg, hair dryer, electric curler) until hair is dry.
- Advise patient or caregiver that slight stinging sensations may be noted following application but that this is expected and should not be bothersome.
- Advise patient or caregiver that if skin irritation occurs to wash scalp and hair immediately. If irritation clears, lotion may be reapplied. If irritation reoccurs, wash scalp and hair again and notify health care provider.
- Advise patient or caregiver that follow-up visits may be necessary and to keep appointments.

Maprotiline Hydrochloride

(ma-PRO-tih-leen HIGH-droe-KLOR-ide)

Class Tetracyclic antidepressant

How Supplied
Ludiomil Tablets 25 mg, Tablets 50 mg, Tablets 75 mg
🍁 *Novo-Maprotiline*

Action
PHARMACOLOGY: Inhibits norepinephrine (but not serotonin) reuptake.

PHARMACOKINETICS/DYNAMICS:
Absorption: Mean T_{max} is 12 hr.
Distribution: Maprotiline protein binding is 88% and apparent Vd is 13 to 24 L/kg.
Metabolism: Maprotiline is metabolized in the liver.
Excretion: Maprotiline is excreted in urine and feces. The mean t½ is 51 hr.

Indications Depression; anxiety associated with depression. **Unlabeled use(s):** Relief of chronic neurogenic pain.

Contraindications Hypersensitivity to tricyclic antidepressants; MI acute recovery period; seizure disorder; concomitant use with MAO inhibitors.

Route/Dosage
ADULTS:
Initial dose: **PO** 25 to 75 mg/day as single dose or divided doses. May be increased to 150 mg/day (outpatient) or 225 mg/day (inpatient).

Interactions
Alcohol, CNS depressants: Additive CNS effects possible.
MAO inhibitors: May precipitate hypertensive crisis and convulsions with possibly fatal results. Discontinue at least 14 days before starting maprotiline.

Lab Test Interferences None well documented.

Adverse Reactions
CV: Syncope; tachycardia; palpitations; orthostatic hypotension; hypertension; MI; arrhythmias; heart block.
CNS: Drowsiness; dizziness; hallucinations; disorientation; mania; exacerbation of psychosis; nervousness; fatigue; headache; anxiety; tremor; insomnia; agitation; seizures.
EENT: Blurred vision; mydriasis.
GI: Dry mouth; constipation; nausea; diarrhea.
GU: Impotence; urinary retention.
HEMA: Bone marrow depression, including agranulocytosis; eosinophilia; purpura; thrombocytopenia; leukopenia.
HEPA: Increased bilirubin and alkaline phosphatase.
METAB: Altered blood glucose levels.
OTHER: Hypersensitivity (eg, rash, itching, photosensitivity, petechiae, edema, drug fever).

Precautions
Pregnancy: Category B.
Lactation: Excreted in breast milk.
Children: Safety and efficacy not established.
Elderly: Use lower doses.
Special risk patients: Use with caution in patients with history of seizures, urinary retention, urethral or ureteral spasm, angle-closure glaucoma or increased IOP, CV disorders, hyperthyroid patients or those receiving thyroid medication, hepatic or renal impairment, schizophrenic or paranoid patients.
Severe depression: Do not allow patient to possess more than small quantities of drug.
Seizures: May occur in therapeutic dose or overdose.

Overdosage: Signs and Symptoms
Hypotension, tachycardia, ventricular arrhythmias, CNS depression, seizures, respiratory depression, coma.

PATIENT CARE CONSIDERATIONS

Administration/Storage
- Administer at bedtime to reduce side effects.
- Store in cool, dry place.

Assessment/Interventions
- Obtain patient history, including drug history and any known allergies. Note MI, seizure disorder, hypersensitivity to drug and concomitant use of MAO inhibitors.
- Ensure that CBC with differential is obtained prior to initial dose and monitored routinely throughout therapy.
- Take baseline vital signs with postural BP and pulse on initiation and reassess routinely.

- Monitor blood glucose closely in diabetic patients.
- Monitor patient's mood and affect closely. If mood changes or suicidal tendencies develop, notify health care provider and take suicide precautions.
- Assess patient's level of sedation. If patient becomes too lethargic or becomes restless and agitated, notify health care provider.
- Observe for signs of dizziness, palpitations, orthostatic hypotension, drowsiness, chest pain, tremors, or seizures. Notify health care provider if these symptoms occur.
- If constipation occurs, increase fiber and fluid intake and mobility.
- Observe for inability to urinate or bladder fullness. If these symptoms occur, notify health care provider.

Patient/Family Education
- Explain that full effectiveness of drug may not occur until after several doses.
- Instruct patient that if dose is missed, it should be taken as soon as possible unless close to time of next dose.
- Warn patient not to double up doses and to notify health care provider if more than one dose is missed.
- Explain that drug may cause dry mouth and constipation. Advise patient about measures to manage these side effects.
- Advise diabetic patient that drug may alter blood glucose level.
- Instruct patient not to take OTC medications without consulting health care provider.
- Instruct patient to avoid intake of alcoholic beverages or other CNS depressants.
- Instruct patient to report these symptoms to health care provider: difficult or infrequent voiding, dizziness, chest pain, palpitations, anxiety, depression, blurred vision, excessive dry mouth, mouth sores, severe constipation.
- Advise patient that drug may cause drowsiness and to use caution while driving or performing other tasks requiring mental alertness.

Masoproc

(mass-OH-prah-KOLE)

Class Topical/Antiproliferative

How Supplied
Actinex Cream 10%

Action
PHARMACOLOGY: Thought to have antiproliferative activity against keratinocytes.

Indications Topical treatment of actinic (solar) keratoses.

Contraindications Standard considerations.

Route/Dosage
ADULTS: **Topical** Massage evenly into area containing actinic keratoses each morning and evening for 28 days.

Interactions None well documented.

PATIENT CARE CONSIDERATIONS

Administration/Storage
- Before application, wash, rinse, and dry affected area.
- Apply each morning and evening for 28 days. Gently and evenly massage into affected area.
- Wash hands immediately after application.
- Avoid contact with eyes or mucous membranes. If contact occurs, promptly flush eye or mucous membranes with water.
- Do not cover with occlusive dressing.
- Store at room temperature (59° to 86°F).

Assessment/Interventions
- Obtain patient history, including drug history

Lab Test Interferences None well documented.

Adverse Reactions
DERM: Erythema; flaking; itching; dryness; edema; burning; soreness; bleeding; crusting; oozing; rash; skin irritation; stinging; tightness; tingling.
EENT: Eye irritation.

Precautions
Pregnancy: Category B.
Lactation: Undetermined.
Children: Safety and efficacy not established.
Sulfite sensitivity: Use caution in sulfite-sensitive individuals; preparation contains bisulfites.
Application: Occlusive dressings should not be used with this product.
External use: This product is for external use only. Avoid contact with eyes and mucous membranes.

and any known allergies.
- Assess number and severity of lesions before beginning therapy and throughout use of medication.
- Assess area after administration for local reactions such as redness, flaking, itching, dryness, swelling, continued burning, oozing, blistering or bleeding.
- If adverse reactions occur, notify health care provider immediately.

Patient/Family Education
- Explain proper method of administration. Tell patient that temporary stinging or burning

sensation is common but should disappear quickly.
- Warn patient that medication may stain clothing or other fabrics.
- Advise patient not to use makeup or other skin products without consulting health care provider.
- Caution patient to avoid excessive exposure to sun.
- Instruct patient to avoid taking any other medications unless prescribed by health care provider.

Measles, Mumps and Rubella Vaccine, Live

(MEE-zuhls, mumps and roo-BELL-uh vaccine, live)

Class Vaccine/Live virus

How Supplied
M-M-R-II Powder for Injection Mixture of 3 viruses: at least 1000 measles $TCID_{50}$ (tissue culture infectious doses), at least 20,000 mumps $TCID_{50}$ and at least 1000 rubella $TCID_{50}$ per 0.5 mL dose

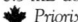 Priorix

Action
PHARMACOLOGY: Induces protective antibodies against measles, mumps, and rubella viruses.

Indications Vaccination of individuals known to be susceptible to measles, mumps, or rubella; prevention of occurrence of congenital rubella syndrome (CRS) among offspring of women who contract rubella during pregnancy. Preferred immunizing agent for most children and many adults.

Contraindications Pregnancy; moderate to severe hypersensitivity reaction to eggs; immunosuppressive therapy; blood dyscrasia, leukemia, lymphoma of any type or other malignant neoplasms affecting the bone marrow or lymphatic systems; primary or acquired immunodeficiency; active untreated tuberculosis; family history of congenital or hereditary immunodeficiency, until immune competence of potential vaccine recipient is demonstrated.
Exception: Vaccinate asymptomatic children with HIV infection.

Route/Dosage
ADULTS AND CHILDREN: SC 0.5 mL. Optimal schedule: Give first dose at 12 to 15 mo; revaccinate routinely at 5 to 6 yr or 11 to 12 yr.

Interactions
Human antibody products: To avoid inactivating vaccine, give MMR 2 to 4 wk before or 3 to 11 mo after AGIV, depending on dose. Susceptible postpartum women who received blood products or Rho(D) immune globulin may receive rubella vaccine prior to discharge, provided that rubella titer is measured 6 to 8 wk after vaccination to ensure seroconversion.
Immunosuppressants, interferon, meningococcal vaccine: May inhibit response to MMR vaccine.

Lab Test Interferences May cause delayed hypersensitivity skin tests (eg, tuberculin, histoplasmin) to appear falsely negative. Effect may persist for several weeks after vaccination. Methacoline inhalation challenge may be falsely positive for a few days.

Adverse Reactions
CNS: Fever; headache; encephalitis; dizziness; polyneuritis; arthralgia; arthritis (rarely chronic); convulsions or seizures.
DERM: Urticaria; rash; erythema multiforme.
EENT: Sore throat; optic neuritis.
GI: Nausea; vomiting; diarrhea.
HEMA: Thrombocytopenia; purpura.
OTHER: Local pain, induration, erythema or allergic reaction at injection site; mild regional lymphadenopathy; malaise.

Precautions
Pregnancy: Category C (contraindicated).
Lactation: Excreted in breast milk (vaccine-strain rubella).
Acute febrile illness: Defer immunization during course of any acute febrile illness.

PATIENT CARE CONSIDERATIONS

Administration/Storage
- If patient is febrile, delay administration if possible.
- Reconstitute using supplied diluent.
- With 25-gauge ⅝-inch needle, inject total volume of reconstituted vaccine SC, preferably into outer aspect of upper arm.
- Refrigerate before and after reconstitution and protect from light.
- Discard unused reconstituted vaccine if not used within 8 hr.

Assessment/Interventions
- Obtain patient history, including drug history and any known allergies. Note untreated tuberculosis, history of immunocompromised disease, immunosuppressive therapy, or hypersensitivity to eggs, egg products, or neomycin.
- Ensure that pregnancy test has been performed on sexually active women.

- Observe for local redness and warmth at injection site.
- Monitor for fever, dizziness, arthritis or rash. Notify health care provider if these symptoms occur.
- Record immunization in patient's record.

Patient/Family Education
- Advise patient that tenderness, redness, swelling, and warmth at site of injection may occur.
- Applying warm compress to site will decrease these symptoms.
- Instruct patient to notify health care provider if local symptoms persist.
- Caution sexually active women to avoid pregnancy for 3 mo after vaccination.

Mebendazole

(meh-BEND-uh-zole)

Class Antihelmintic

How Supplied
Vermox Tablets, chewable 100 mg

Action
PHARMACOLOGY: Kills parasitic worms by blocking glucose uptake, thus depleting stored glycogen. Without glycogen, parasite cannot reproduce or survive.

PHARMACOKINETICS/DYNAMICS:
Absorption: Mebendazole is poorly absorbed (approximately 5% to 10%). T_{max} is 0.5 to 7 hr and C_{max} is 0.03 mcg/mL. Food increases the absorption of mebendazole.

Distribution: Mebendazole is distributed to serum, cyst fluids, liver, omental fat, pelvic cysts, pulmonary cysts, hepatic cysts, and muscles. Mebendazole also crosses the placenta. Protein binding is 90% to 95%.

Metabolism: All metabolites are inactive. The major metabolite is 2-amino-5-benzoylbenzimidazole. Mebendazole is primarily metabolized hepatically.

Excretion: Mebandazole is excreted in the feces and a small amount in urine. The t½ is 2.5 to 9 hr.

Special Populations:
Hepatic Function Impairment – The t½ is prolonged to approximately 30 hr.

Indications Treatment of pinworm (*Enterobius vermicularis*), round worm (*Ascaris lumbricoides*), common hookworm (*Ancylostoma duodenale*), American hookworm (*Necator americanus*), and whipworm (*Trichuris trichiura*) in single or mixed parasitic infections.

Contraindications Standard considerations.

Route/Dosage
Trichuriasis, Ascariasis, and Hookworm Infection
ADULTS AND CHILDREN: PO 100 mg tablet AM and PM on 3 consecutive days.

Ascaris Infection
ADULTS AND CHILDREN:
Alternative dose: PO 500 mg as single dose.

Enterobiasis
ADULTS AND CHILDREN: PO 100 mg as single dose.

Interactions
Carbamazepine; hydantoins (eg, phenytoin): Pharmacological effects of mebendazole may be decreased.

Lab Test Interferences None well documented.

Adverse Reactions
GI: Transient abdominal pain and diarrhea.
OTHER: Fever.

Precautions
Pregnancy: Category C.
Lactation: Undetermined.
Children: Safety and efficacy in children younger than 2 yr not established.

Overdosage: Signs and Symptoms
GI complaints.

PATIENT CARE CONSIDERATIONS

Administration/Storage
- Give with food; crush or allow patient to chew tablets if patient has difficulty tolerating ingestion.
- Store in tightly closed container.

Assessment/Interventions
- Obtain patient history, including drug history and any known allergies.
- Monitor results of stool testing prior to and 3 wk after treatment is initiated.
- Obtain baseline vital signs and monitor throughout therapy.
- Notify health care provider of new-onset fever after initiation of therapy and diarrhea during expulsion of worms.
- Report to health care provider any signs of abdominal pain with diarrhea.
- Disinfect toilet facilities, towels, bed linens, and clothing daily.
- Avoid self-contamination. Practice thorough hand washing.
- Check for infection in other family members.

Patient/Family Education
- Advise patient to chew tablet or to crush tablet and mix with food.
- Instruct patient to wash clothing, bed linens, and towels daily and to disinfect bathroom facilities daily.
- Advise that infected person sleep alone.
- Caution patient not to put fingers in mouth.
- Emphasize importance of thorough hand washing, especially after toileting, to avoid reinfecting self.
- Explain that all family members should be treated to eradicate infestation.
- Tell patient that second treatment is sometimes necessary.
- Instruct family/patient to call health care provider if fever, abdominal pain, or diarrhea develops.

Mecamylamine Hydrochloride

(Mek-ah-MILL-oh-meen HIGH-dore-KLORide)

Class Antihypertensive/Antiadrenergic, peripherally acting

How Supplied
Inversine Tablets 2.5 mg

Action
PHARMACOLOGY: Potent ganglionic blocking agent.
PHARMACOKINETICS/DYNAMICS:
Absorption: Mecamylamine is almost completely absorbed.
Distribution: Mecamylamine crosses the placenta and blood-brain barrier.
Excretion: Slowly excreted in urine unchanged. Alkalinization of urine reduces, and acidification promotes renal excretion.
Onset: Onset is 0.5 to 2 hr.
Duration: Duration is 6 to 12 hr.

Indications Treatment of moderately severe to severe essential hypertension; uncomplicated malignant hypertension.

Contraindications Coronary insufficiency; recent MI; uremia; patients receiving antibiotics and sulfonamides; glaucoma; organic pyloric stenosis; mild, moderate, or labile hypertension; uncooperative patients; hypersensitivity to any component of product.

Route/Dosage
ADULTS:
Initial dose: **PO** 2.5 mg bid. Adjust dose in increments of 2.5 mg at intervals of at least 2 days until the desired BP response occurs.

Interactions
Alcohol, anesthetics, other antihypertensives: May potentiate the effects of mecamylamine.
Antibiotics, sulfonamides: Patients receiving these drugs generally should not be treated with ganglionic blocking agents.

Lab Test Interferences None well documented.

Adverse Reactions
CV: Orthostatic dizziness; syncope; postural hypotension.
CNS: Weakness; fatigue; sedation; paresthesia; tremor; choreiform movements; mental aberrations; convulsions.
EENT: Glossitis; dilated pupils; blurred vision.
GI: Anorexia; dry mouth; nausea; vomiting; constipation; ileus.
GU: Decreased libido; impotence; urinary retention.
RESP: Interstitial pulmonary edema; fibrosis.

Precautions
Pregnancy: Category C.
Lactation: Discontinue nursing or discontinue the drug.
Children: Safety and efficacy not established.
Renal function impairment: Give with caution, if at all, in patients with renal insufficiency manifested by a rising or elevated BUN.
CV function: Use with caution in patients with marked cerebral and coronary arteriosclerosis or after recent cerebral vascular accident.
Discontinuation of therapy: To prevent hypertension, fatal cerebral vascular accidents, or acute CHF, withdraw drug gradually, and substitute other antihypertensive therapy.
Paralytic ileus: Consider the possibility if frequent loose bowel movements with abdominal distention and decreased borborygmi occur.
Potentiation of effects: Mecamylamine's effects may be potentiated by excessive heat, fever, infection, hemorrhage, pregnancy, anesthesia, surgery, vigorous exercise, other antihypertensive agents, alcohol, salt depletion, vomiting, excessive sweating, or diuretics.
Urinary retention: Because urinary retention may occur, use with caution in patients with prostatic hypertrophy, bladder neck obstruction, and urethral stricture.

Overdosage: Signs and Symptoms
Hypotension, postural hypotension, nausea, vomiting, diarrhea, constipation, paralytic ileus, urinary retention, dizziness, anxiety, dry mouth, mydriasis, blurred vision, palpitations, increase in IOP.

PATIENT CARE CONSIDERATIONS

Administration/Storage
- Administer alone or in combination with other antihypertensives.
- Administer prescribed dose bid to qid times a day as ordered.
- Administer after meals or snacks to slow absorption of medication and provide smoother control of BP. Timing of doses in relation to meals should be consistent to minimize variation in BP control.
- Store tablets at controlled room temperature (59° to 86°F).

Assessment/Interventions
- Obtain patient history, including drug history and any known allergies. Note renal impairment, cerebral or coronary arteriosclerosis, prostatic hypertrophy, bladder neck obstruction, urethral stricture, or concurrent use of antibiotics or sulfonamides.
- Review patient's health history for any condition that could contraindicate mecamylamine therapy: recent MI; coronary insufficiency; uremia; glaucoma; pyloric stenosis; hypersensitivity to mecamylamine.
- Monitor and record BP and pulse with patient in erect position. If hypotension, dizziness, lightheadedness, or fainting result, hold medication and notify health care provider.
- Take safety precautions if orthostatic hypotension occurs.
- Ensure that therapy is periodically reviewed to determine if medication needs to be continued without change or if a dose change (eg, increase, decrease, discontinuation) is indicated.
- If treatment is to be discontinued, gradually taper the dose while other antihypertensive therapy is substituted to prevent rapid increase in BP.
- Monitor patient for GI, CV, CNS, PSYCH, and general body side effects. Inform health care provider if significant.

Patient/Family Education
- Explain name, dose, action, and potential side effects of drug.
- Advise patient that dose may be increased slowly until maximum benefit is obtained.
- Advise patient to take every day exactly as prescribed. Advise patient to take prescribed dose after meals or snacks to slow absorption of medication and provide smoother control of BP.
- Advise patient that timing of doses in relation to meals must be consistent.
- Caution patient not to change the dose or stop taking unless advised by health care provider.
- Inform patient that drug controls but does not cure hypertension and to continue taking drug as prescribed even when BP is not elevated.
- Instruct patient to continue taking other BP medications as prescribed by health care provider.
- Instruct patient in BP and pulse measurement skills.
- Advise patient to monitor and record BP and pulse at home in a standing position and to inform health care provider if abnormal measurements are noted. Also advise patient to take record of BP and pulse to each follow-up visit.
- Advise patient that dizziness, lightheadedness, or fainting can occur, especially when rising from a lying or sitting position. Inform patient that getting up slowly from a lying or sitting position will reduce the chance of this occurring.
- Caution patient that alcohol ingestion, fever, excessive heat, vigorous exercise, inadequate fluid intake, salt-depletion, and excessive perspiration, diarrhea, or vomiting can lead to excessive fall in BP resulting in dizziness, lightheadedness, or fainting.
- Instruct patient to lie or sit down if experiencing dizziness or lightheadedness when standing.
- Advise patient to stop taking the medication and immediately inform health care provider if any of the following occur: fainting; frequent loose bowel movements with stomach distention and "rumbling" sounds in the intestines; difficult urination; inability to urinate; mood changes or changes in thoughts; tremors or uncontrollable muscle movements.
- Emphasize to hypertensive patient importance of other modalities on BP: weight control, regular exercise, smoking cessation, moderate intake of alcohol and salt.
- Advise women to notify health care provider if pregnant, planning to become pregnant, or breastfeeding.
- Caution patient not to take any prescription or OTC medications, herbal preparations, or dietary supplements unless advised by health care provider.
- Advise patient that follow-up visits and lab tests may be required to monitor therapy and to keep appointments.

Mechlorethamine Hydrochloride

(meh-klor-ETH-ah-meen)
Class Alkylating agent/Nitrogen mustard

How Supplied
Mustargen Powder for injection 10 mg

Action
PHARMACOLOGY: An alkylating agent with cytotoxic, mutagenic, and radiomimetic actions that inhibit rapidly proliferating cells.

PHARMACOKINETICS/DYNAMICS:
Metabolism: Mechlorethamine is rapidly inactivated in body fluids or water within a few minutes.
Excretion: Apparently eliminated renally.
Onset: Onset happens within a few seconds or minutes.

Indications
Hodgkin disease (stage III and IV), lymphosarcoma, chronic myelocytic or lymphocytic leukemia, polycythemia vera, mycosis fungoides (topical), bronchogenic carcinoma; palliative treatment of malignant effusion (intrapleural, intraperitoneal, or intrapericardial use only).

Contraindications
Infectious disease; previous anaphylactic reactions to the drug.

Route/Dosage
ADULTS: **IV** Total dose of 0.4 mg/kg of body weight for each course (as single dose or divided doses of 0.1 to 0.2 mg/kg/day). Dose based on ideal dry body weight. May repeat courses as early as 3 wk after treatment.

Interactions
None well documented.

Lab Test Interferences
None well documented.

Adverse Reactions
DERM: Alopecia; erythema multiforme; herpes zoster; maculopapular eruptions.
EENT: Diminished hearing; tinnitus; vertigo.
GI: Anorexia; diarrhea; nausea; vomiting.
GU: Azoospermia; total germinal aplasia; impaired spermatogenesis; amenorrhea; delayed menses; oligomenorrhea; hyperuricemia.
HEMA: Agranulocytosis; granulocytopenia; hematopoietic depression; hyperheparinemia; lymphocytopenia; thrombocytopenia; hemolytic anemia; pancytopenia.
HEPA: Jaundice.
LOCAL: Extravasation; thrombosis; thrombophlebitis.
OTHER: Chromosomal abnormalities; anaphylaxis.

> **WARNING:**
> *Extravasation:* Mechlorethamine is a vesicant; extravasation can cause severe local necrosis.
> Follow procedures for proper handling and disposal of anticancer drugs. Wear gloves and avoid skin exposure and inhalation of fumes. Avoid exposure during pregnancy.

Precautions
Pregnancy: Category D.
Lactation: Undetermined.
Children: Safety and efficacy in children not established.
Hypersensitivity: Reactions, including anaphylaxis, have occurred.
Carcinogenesis: Therapy with nitrogen mustard may be associated with an increased incidence of second malignant tumor.
Fertility impairment: Impaired spermatogenesis, azoospermia, and total germinal aplasia have occurred in men.
Amyloidosis: Nitrogen mustard therapy may contribute to extensive and rapid development of amyloidosis; use only if foci or acute and chronic suppurative inflammation are absent.
Chronic lymphatic leukemia: Drug toxicity, especially sensitivity to bone marrow failure, appears to be more common in chronic lymphatic leukemia than in other conditions; administer with great caution in this condition, if at all.
GI: Nausea and vomiting usually begins 1 to 3 hr after use. Vomiting may persist for the first 8 hr, nausea for 24 hr.
Hematologic: The usual course of treatment produces lymphocytopenia within 24 hr after the first injection; significant granulocytopenia occurs within 6 to 8 days and lasts for 10 days to 3 wk. Severe thrombocytopenia may lead to bleeding from the gums and GI tract, petechiae, and small subcutaneous hemorrhages. Erythrocyte and hemoglobin levels may decline, but rarely significantly, during the first 2 wk after therapy. Depression of the hematopoietic system may occur up to 50 days or more after starting therapy.
Herpes zoster: Herpes zoster, common with lymphomas, may first appear after therapy is instituted and may be precipitated by treatment.
Hyperuricemia: Urate precipitation may develop during therapy, particularly in the treatment of lymphomas.
Intercavitary administration Pain occurs rarely with intrapleural use; it is common with intraperitoneal injection and is often associated with

nausea, vomiting, and diarrhea of 2 to 3 days duration. Transient cardiac irregularities may occur with intrapericardial injection.
Tumors: Tumors of bone and nervous tissue respond poorly to therapy.

PATIENT CARE CONSIDERATIONS
Administration/Storage

- For IV and intracavitary administration only. Not for intradermal, subcutaneous, IM, intra-arterial, or oral administration.
- Dose and frequency of administration vary with condition being treated and clinical situation. Medication may be given as a single dose or in 2 to 4 divided doses.
- Mechlorethamine is highly toxic. Handle and administer powder and solution with extreme care.
- Diligently follow institutional and National Institutes of Health (NIH) procedures for handling, administration, and disposal of anticancer drugs. Wear appropriate protective equipment when preparing and administering mechlorethamine. Avoid inhalation of dust or vapors and contact with skin, mucus membranes, and eyes.
- Examine vial before reconstitution. Do not use if droplets of water are visible.
- Reconstitute powder with 10 mL sterile water for injection or sodium chloride injection. Resulting solution contains 1 mg/mL of mechlorethamine.
- Do not administer if particulate matter, cloudiness, or discoloration noted.
- Premedicate patient with antiemetics and sedatives as ordered by health care provider.
- If possible, administer at night when sedation for side effects is required.
- To reduce risk of extravasation, inject prescribed dose into the rubber or plastic tubing of a freely flowing IV infusion set.
- To reduce loss of potency, administer prescribed dose immediately after reconstitution by IV infusion over a few minutes. Do not add to entire volume of infusion solution.
- Dispose of mechlorethamine vials and any remaining solution after neutralizing with an equal volume of 5% sodium thiosulfate and 5% sodium bicarbonate solution. Allow mixture to stand for 45 min.
- Decontaminate administration equipment (eg, rubber gloves, tubing, glassware) by soaking in solution containing equal volumes of 5% sodium thiosulfate and 5% sodium bicarbonate for 45 min.
- Store unopened vials at controlled room temperature (59° to 86°F). Protect from light and humidity. Administer solution immediately after reconstitution.

Overdosage: Signs and Symptoms
Severe leukopenia, anemia, thrombocytopenia, hemorrhagic diathesis, death.

Assessment/Interventions

- Obtain patient history, including drug history and any known allergies. Note acute or chronic suppurative inflammation, recent X-ray therapy, or evidence of active infection.
- Ensure women of childbearing potential are not pregnant when therapy is initiated and use effective contraception during treatment.
- Ensure X-ray therapy or other chemotherapy in alternating courses is not administered until bone marrow function has recovered following a course of mechlorethamine therapy.
- Ensure risk of developing hyperuricemia is evaluated before starting therapy and hypouricemic therapy, including adequate fluid intake and monitoring of uric acid, is initiated before starting treatment in patient determined to be at risk for developing hyperuricemia and urate precipitation.
- Ensure CBC with differential and platelet count, renal function, and liver enzymes are evaluated before starting therapy and then frequently during therapy.
- Implement infection control measures if WBC drops; implement bleeding precautions if platelet count drops.
- Ensure subsequent courses of mechlorethamine are not administered until hematologic recovery from a previous course of therapy has been documented.
- Monitor patient for signs of anaphylactic or serious allergic reactions. Discontinue therapy and immediately notify health care provider if noted. Be prepared to treat appropriately.
- Ensure 2% sodium thiosulfate solution is readily available in the event of accidental skin exposure to mechlorethamine.
- Should accidental skin contact occur, irrigate affected part immediately with copious amounts of water for at least 15 min while removing contaminated clothing, followed by irrigation with 2% thiosulfate solution. Notify health care provider immediately. Destroy contaminated clothing.
- If accidental eye contact occurs, immediately institute copious irrigation with water, normal saline, or a balanced salt ophthalmic irrigation solution. Notify health care provider immediately and be prepared to have patient

undergo a prompt ophthalmologic consultation.
- Ensure that 1/6 molar sterile isotonic sodium thiosulfate is readily available in the event extravasation occurs.
- Assess injection site frequently for signs or symptoms of extravasation (eg, burning, pain, induration). Discontinue infusion immediately if suspected and notify health care provider. Be prepared to infiltrate area with 1/6 molar sterile isotonic sodium thiosulfate and apply ice compresses for 6 to 12 hr to minimize local reaction.
- Ensure that patient who has received intracavitary mechlorethamine is repositioned every 5 to 10 min for an hour following the procedure.
- Monitor patient for GI, DERM, and general body side effects. Report to health care provider if noted and significant.
- Monitor patient for signs and symptoms of bacterial, viral, or fungal infection. Report to health care provider immediately if noted.

Patient/Family Education
- Explain name, action, and potential side effects of drug.
- Advise patient, family, or caregiver that medication will be prepared and administered by health care provider in a health care setting.
- Advise patient, family, or caregiver that medication may be used in combination with other agents, including antiemetics and sedatives, to achieve max benefit possible.
- Advise patient, family, or caregiver to immediately report any of the following to health care provider: rash; hives; difficulty breathing; fever, chills, or other signs of infection; unusual bleeding or bruising; pain, redness, or swelling at injection site.
- Advise patient, family, or caregiver to report any of the following to health care provider: persistent nausea, vomiting, diarrhea, or appetite loss; persistent or worsening general body weakness.
- Instruct patient not to take any prescription or OTC medications, herbal preparations, or dietary supplements unless advised by health care provider.
- Caution women of childbearing potential to avoid becoming pregnant during therapy.
- Advise women of childbearing potential to notify health care provider if pregnant, planning to become pregnant, or breastfeeding.
- Advise men that therapy may temporarily or permanently impair fertility.
- Advise patient, family, or caregiver that, following discharge, frequent follow-up visits and laboratory tests will be required to monitor therapy and to keep appointments.

Meclizine
(MEK-lih-zeen)

Class Antiemetic/Antivertigo/Anticholinergic

How Supplied
Antivert Tablets 12.5 mg, Tablets 25 mg, Tablets 50 mg ◆ *Antrizine* Tablets 12.5 mg ◆ *Dramamine Less Drowsy* Tablets 25 mg ◆ *Meni-D* Capsules 25 mg ◆ *Vergon* Capsules 25 mg
✤ *Bonamine*

Action
PHARMACOLOGY: Acts on CNS to decrease vestibular stimulation and depress labyrinthine activity.

PHARMACOKINETICS/DYNAMICS:
Excretion: The $t_{1/2}$ is 6 hr.
Onset: Onset is 30 min to 1 hr (oral).
Duration: Duration is 4 to 6 hr (25 mg) and 12 to 24 hr (30 mg).

Indications
Prevention and treatment of nausea, vomiting, and dizziness of motion sickness; possibly effective treatment for vertigo of vestibular dysfunction origin.

Contraindications
Hypersensitivity to cyclizine; asthma; glaucoma; emphysema; chronic pulmonary disease; shortness of breath; difficulty breathing; urinary retention caused by enlarged prostate.

Route/Dosage
Motion Sickness
ADULTS: **PO** 25 to 50 mg 1 hr before travel; may repeat q 24 hr during travel.

Vertigo
ADULTS: **PO** 25 to 100 mg/day in divided doses.

Interactions
Alcohol, CNS depressants: Additive CNS effects.

Lab Test Interferences
False-negative result in allergy skin testing.

Adverse Reactions
CV: Hypotension; tachycardia; palpitations.
CNS: Drowsiness; excitation; nervousness; restlessness; insomnia; euphoria; vertigo; hallucinations.
DERM: Rash; urticaria.
EENT: Dry nose and throat; visual disturbances; tinnitus.

GI: Nausea; vomiting; dry mouth; diarrhea; constipation; anorexia.
GU: Urinary frequency; urinary retention; difficulty urinating.

Precautions
Pregnancy: Category B.
Lactation: Undetermined.

Children: Safety and efficacy not established. Not recommended in children younger than 12 yr.

Overdosage: Signs and Symptoms
Hyperexcitability, drowsiness, hallucinations, convulsions.

PATIENT CARE CONSIDERATIONS

Administration/Storage
- Tablets may be chewed, swallowed whole or allowed to dissolve in water.
- Store at room temperature (59° to 86°F).

Assessment/Interventions
- Obtain patient history, including drug history and any known allergies. Note glaucoma and prostatic hypertrophy.
- Monitor for side effects, especially sedation, hypotension, tachycardia, and urinary retention.
- Implement safety precautions (eg, keep bed in low position and instruct patient to call for assistance when rising) if patient is experiencing sedation or vertigo.

Patient/Family Education
- When given for motion sickness, inform patient that first dose should be taken 1 hr before exposure to motion.
- Instruct patient to take sips of water frequently, suck on ice chips or sugarless hard candy or chew sugarless gum if dry mouth occurs.
- Explain that high-fiber diet and drinking plenty of fluids may help to prevent constipation, which is common side effect.
- Instruct patient to report the following symptoms to health care provider: sedation, dizziness, palpitations, difficulty urinating, or urinary retention.
- Instruct patient to notify health care provider if vomiting increases or becomes severe.
- Advise patient that drug may cause drowsiness and to use caution while driving or performing other tasks requiring mental alertness.
- Instruct patient to avoid intake of alcoholic beverages or other CNS depressants.
- Advise patient not to take OTC medications or other prescription medications without consulting health care provider.

Meclofenamate Sodium

(mek-loe-FEN-uh-mate SO-dee-uhm)

Class Analgesic/NSAID

How Supplied
Meclofenamate sodium Capsules 50 mg, Capsules 100 mg

Action
PHARMACOLOGY: Decreases inflammation, pain and fever, probably through inhibition of cyclooxygenase activity and prostaglandin synthesis.

PHARMACOKINETICS/DYNAMICS:
Absorption: T_{max} is 0.5 to 2 hr and the bioavailability is approximately 100%.
Distribution: Vd is 23 L and the protein binding is greater than 99%.
Excretion: Meclofenamate is excreted renally (70%) and fecally (30%). The $t_{½}$ is 1.3 hr and clearance is 206 mL/min.

Indications Treatment of rheumatoid and osteoarthritis; treatment of primary dysmenorrhea; relief of mild to moderate pain; idiopathic heavy menstrual blood loss. **Unlabeled use(s):** Relief of sunburn; pain; migraine (abort acute attacks).

Contraindications Patients in whom aspirin, iodides, or any NSAID has caused allergic-type reactions.

Route/Dosage
Osteoarthritis or Rheumatoid Arthritis; Mild to Moderate Pain
ADULTS: PO 200 to 400 mg/day in 3 to 4 equally divided doses.

Excessive Menstrual Blood Loss; Primary Dysmenorrhea
ADULTS: PO 100 mg tid for up to 6 days.

Interactions
Anticoagulants: Increased risk of gastric erosion and bleeding.
Cyclosporine: Nephrotoxicity of both agents may be increased.
Lithium: Serum lithium levels may be increased.
Methotrexate: Increased methotrexate levels.
Salicylates: Additive GI toxicity.

Lab Test Interferences May prolong bleeding time.

Adverse Reactions
CV: Edema.

CNS: Headache; vertigo; drowsiness; dizziness; tinnitus.
DERM: Rash; urticaria; fasciitis.
EENT: Tinnitus.
GI: Diarrhea; vomiting; nausea; abdominal pain; dyspepsia; peptic ulcer; GI bleeding; constipation; flatulence; anorexia; stomatitis; heartburn.
GU: Acute renal failure; nephrotic syndrome.
HEMA: Fall in hemoglobin; positive Coombs' test; bruising; prolonged bleeding time; thrombocytopenia purpura; anemia.
HEPA: Abnormal LFT results.
METAB: Porphyria; hyponatremia.
RESP: Breathing difficulties in aspirin-sensitive individuals.

Precautions

Pregnancy: Safety not established; avoid use, especially during first and last trimester.
Lactation: Undetermined.
Children: Not recommended for children younger than 14 yr.
Elderly: Increased risk of adverse reactions.
Hypersensitivity: May occur; use with caution in aspirin-sensitive individuals due to possible cross-sensitivity.
Renal function impairment: Acute renal insufficiency, interstitial nephritis, hyperkalemia, hyponatremia and renal papillary necrosis may occur. Lower doses may be necessary in patients with renal impairment.
Diarrhea: If diarrhea occurs, reduce dosage or temporarily discontinue.
GI toxicity: Bleeding, ulceration, or perforation can occur at any time, with or without warning symptoms.
Heavy menstrual flow: It is recommended that meclofenamate sodium treatment not be prescribed for heavy menstrual flow without establishing its idiopathic nature.

Overdosage: Signs and Symptoms

Sweating, disorientation, vomiting, convulsions, electrolyte imbalance, metabolic acidosis.

PATIENT CARE CONSIDERATIONS

Administration/Storage

- Administer with meals, followed by full glass of water or milk to reduce GI or esophageal irritation. May be given with antacids if stomach upset occurs.
- Store at room temperature (59° to 86°F) in tightly closed, light-resistant container.

Assessment/Interventions

- Obtain patient history, including drug history and any known allergies. Note chronic alcohol use, fluid retention, nasal polyps, bronchospastic disease, or hypersensitivity to aspirin or NSAIDs.
- Monitor carefully for hypersensitivity. Note any ecchymosis or rash.
- Notify health care provider if stomach pain develops or continues.
- Monitor renal and liver function and blood studies throughout treatment.
- Monitor for diarrhea or blood in stools. If diarrhea occurs, notify health care provider. Dosage may need to be reduced or drug temporarily withheld.
- Weigh patient daily if fluid retention is a concern.

Patient/Family Education

- Explain that therapeutic effects may take up to 1 mo to be noticed.
- Instruct patient to report the following symptoms to health care provider: rash, dark stools, persistent headache or stomach pain, unusual bruising or bleeding, decreased urinary output.
- Advise patient to avoid intake of alcoholic beverages.
- Caution patient to avoid exposure to sunlight and to use sunscreen or wear protective clothing to avoid photosensitivity reaction.
- Instruct patient that drug may cause dizziness and to use caution while driving or performing other activities requiring mental alertness until effects of drug are known.
- Tell patient to notify health care provider if diarrhea occurs. Review symptoms of dehydration. Explain that if diarrhea becomes severe or nausea and vomiting are severe, patient should stop taking medication and contact health care provider.
- Instruct patient to weigh self twice weekly and to notify health care provider if weight gain of more than 3 to 4 lb/wk occurs.
- Instruct patient not to take OTC medications, including aspirin and ibuprofen, or other prescription medications, without consulting health care provider.
- Warn patient about potential for bleeding and advise to notify other health care professionals that drug is being taken.
- Advise women who are taking meclofenamate sodium for heavy menstrual flow to consult their doctor if they have spotting or bleeding between cycles or worsening of their menstrual blood flow. These symptoms may be signs of the development of a more serious condition that is not appropriately treated with meclofenamate sodium.

Medroxyprogesterone Acetate

(meh-DROX-ee-pro-JESS-tuh-rone ASS-uh-TATE)

Class Progestin

How Supplied
Amen Tablets 10 mg ♦ *Curretab* Tablets 10 mg ♦ *Cycrin* Tablets 2.5 mg, Tablets 5 mg, Tablets 10 mg ♦ *Depo-Provera* Injection 150 mg/mL, Injection 400 mg/mL ♦ *Provera* Tablets 2.5 mg, Tablets 5 mg, Tablets 10 mg
🍁 *Gen-Medroxy* ♦ *Novo-Medrone* ♦ *ratio*-MPA

Action

PHARMACOLOGY: Inhibits secretion of pituitary gonadotropins, thereby preventing follicular maturation and ovulation (contraceptive effect); inhibits spontaneous uterine contraction; transforms proliferative endometrium into secretory endometrium; produces antineoplastic effect in advanced endometrial or renal carcinoma.

PHARMACOKINETICS/DYNAMICS:

Absorption: T_{max} is 2 to 4 hr. Food increases the bioavailability of medroxyprogesterone acetate.

Distribution: Medroxyprogesterone protein binding is approximately 90%.

Metabolism: Medroxyprogesterone is extensively metabolized in the liver by hydroxylation with subsequent conjugation. At least 16 metabolites have been identified.

Excretion: Most of the metabolites are excreted in urine. The t½ is approximately 12 hr.

Special Populations:
Hepatic Function Impairment – Metabolism and Cl are decreased in patients with hepatic impairment. Lower doses or less frequent administration is recommended in patients with mild or moderate hepatic impairment and is contraindicated in patients with severe hepatic impairment.

Indications

PO: Treatment of secondary amenorrhea and abnormal uterine bleeding caused by hormonal imbalance; reduction of incidence of endometrial hyperplasia in nonhysterectomized postmenopausal women receiving 0.625 mg conjugated estrogen.

Parenteral: Prevention of pregnancy; adjunctive and palliative treatment of inoperable, recurrent, and metastatic endometrial or renal carcinoma.

Contraindications

Hypersensitivity to progestins; current or history of thrombophlebitis, thromboembolic disorders, cerebrovascular disease, or cerebral hemorrhage; impaired liver function; breast or genital organ cancer; undiagnosed vaginal bleeding; missed abortion; diagnostic test for pregnancy; known or suspected pregnancy.

Route/Dosage

Abnormal Uterine Bleeding
ADULTS: **PO** 5 to 10 mg/day for 5 to 10 days beginning on 16th or 21st day of menstrual cycle.

Contraceptive
ADULTS: **IM** 150 mg q 3 mo.

Endometrial or Renal Carcinoma
ADULTS:
Initial: **IM** 400 to 1,000 mg/wk.
Maintenance: **IM** 400 mg/mo.

Reduction of Endometrial Hyperplasia
ADULTS: **PO** 5 to 10 mg daily for 12 to 14 consecutive days per month, beginning on the 1st or 16th day of cycle.

Secondary Amenorrhea
ADULTS: **PO** 5 to 10 mg/day for 5 to 10 days.

Interactions

Aminoglutethimide: May increase metabolism and decrease effect of medroxyprogesterone.

Lab Test Interferences Endocrine, coagulation (increased amounts of some clotting factors), thyroid, and LFT results may be affected by progestins; may decrease glucose tolerance; decreased plasma and urinary steroid levels; decreased gonadotropin levels; decreased sex-hormone-binding-globulin concentrations.

Adverse Reactions

CV: Thrombophlebitis; edema.
CNS: Depression; headache; nervousness; dizziness; insomnia; fatigue; somnolence.
DERM: Rash; acne; melasma; chloasma; alopecia; hirsutism; photosensitivity; pruritus; urticaria.
GI: Abdominal pain or discomfort; nausea.
GU: Breakthrough bleeding; spotting; change in menstrual flow; amenorrhea; decrease in libido; changes in cervical erosion and secretions.
HEPA: Cholestatic jaundice.
RESP: Pulmonary embolism.
OTHER: Breast tenderness; masculinization of female fetus; edema; weight changes, especially weight gain; anaphylactoid reactions; bone mineral density changes, increasing risk of osteoporosis; hyperglycemia; pyrexia; galactorrhea.

Precautions

Pregnancy: Category X.
Lactation: Excreted in breast milk.
Children: Safety and efficacy not established.
Conception: May prolong contraceptive effect, which may delay time to potential conception once therapy is discontinued.
Contraception: If period between injections is longer than 14 days, determine that patient is

not pregnant before administering drug.

Fluid retention: Use with careful observation when conditions that might be affected by this factor are present (eg, asthma, cardiac or renal dysfunction, epilepsy).

Mental depression: Carefully observe patients with history of depression.

Ophthalmic effects: Discontinue medication if there are any sudden changes in vision, sudden onset of proptosis, diplopia, migraine, papilledema, or retinal vascular lesions.

Prolonged use: Effect of prolonged use on pituitary, ovarian, adrenal, hepatic, and uterine function not known.

Thromboembolic: Discontinue if occurring or suspected.

Vaginal bleeding: With irregular vaginal bleeding, including breakthrough bleeding, nonfunctional causes should be considered and adequate diagnostic measures undertaken.

PATIENT CARE CONSIDERATIONS

Administration/Storage

- Store tablets and injection at controlled room temperature (68° to 77°F).

Tablets:

- Administer without regard to meals but administer with food if GI upset occurs.

Injection:

- For IM injection only. Not for intradermal, subcutaneous, or intra-arterial administration.
- Use povidone-iodine solution or similar product to cleanse vial top of multidose vial prior to withdrawing dose.
- Shake vial vigorously just before use to ensure that dose is being administered as a uniform suspension.
- Do not administer if particulate matter, cloudiness, or discoloration is noted.
- Administer by deep IM injection into gluteal or deltoid muscle. Rotate injection sites.
- When using as contraceptive, administer prescribed dose during first 5 days after the onset of a normal menstrual period, within 5 days postpartum if not breastfeeding, or if breastfeeding, at 6 wk postpartum.

Assessment/Interventions

- Obtain patient history, including drug history and any known allergies. Note renal or hepatic impairment, depression or history of depression, epilepsy, migraine headaches, asthma, or cardiac dysfunction.
- Review patient's health history for any condition that would contraindicate use of medroxyprogesterone: previous allergic reaction to progesterone; known or suspected pregnancy; known or suspected cancer of the breast or genital organs; undiagnosed vaginal bleeding; active or past history of thromboembolic disorders or stroke; severe liver dysfunction or disease; or missed abortion.
- Ensure that breast, abdominal and pelvic examination and Pap smear have been completed and documented before starting therapy.
- Monitor blood sugar in diabetic patient when therapy with estrogen and medroxyprogesterone therapy is started. Report significant changes to health care provider.
- Assess BP at beginning of therapy with estrogen and medroxyprogesterone and periodically during treatment.
- Assess patient for GI, CNS, PSYCH, GU, and general body side effects. Inform health care provider if noted and significant.
- Inform health care provider immediately if any of the following are noted: pain in groin or calves; sharp chest pain, coughing blood, or sudden shortness of breath; crushing chest pain or heaviness in chest; abnormal vaginal bleeding; breast lumps; sudden severe headache; dizziness or fainting tremors or seizures; vision or speech problems; weakness or numbness of arms or legs; abdominal swelling or severe pain; jaundice; symptoms of depression.

Injection:

- Document site of each injection.
- Assess injection sites for reaction. Inform health care provider if noted and significant.
- If period between injections for contraception is greater than 14 wk, ensure patient is not pregnant before administering dose.

Patient/Family Education

- Explain name, dose, action, and potential side effects of drug.
- Advise patient to read *Patient Information* leaflet before using the first time and with each refill.
- Instruct diabetic patient taking estrogen and medroxyprogesterone to monitor blood glucose more frequently when therapy is started and to inform health care provider of significant changes in readings
- Teach patient proper method of breast self-examination, and remind patient to perform monthly.
- Instruct patient to immediately report any of the following symptoms to health care provider: pain in groin or calves; sharp chest pain, coughing blood, or sudden shortness of breath; crushing chest pain or heaviness in chest; abnormal vaginal bleeding; breast lumps; sudden severe headache; dizziness or fainting; tremors or seizure; vision or speech problems; weakness or numbness of arms or legs; severe abdominal pain; depression; yel-

lowing of the skin or eyes; persistent pain, pus, or bleeding at injection site.
- Advise women to notify health care provider if pregnant, planning to become pregnant, or breastfeeding.
- Advise patient that follow-up visits and examinations, including Pap smear, at least once a year, will be required to monitor therapy and to keep appointments.

Tablets:
- Advise patient to take each dose without regard to meals but to take with food if stomach upset occurs.

Injection:
- Advise patient that injection will be prepared and administered by a health care provider in a medical setting.
- Advise patient that menstrual cycle may be disrupted (eg, irregular or unpredictable bleeding, or spotting) but that this usually decreases over several months to the point of no menstrual flow. Advise patient to notify health care provider if abnormal bleeding persists or is severe.
- Advise patient that contraceptive injection does not protect against HIV infection and other sexually transmitted diseases.

Medroxyprogesterone Acetate/Estradiol Cypionate

(Meh-DROX-ee-por-JESS-tuh-rone ASS-uh-TATE/ESS-truh-DIE-ole SIP-ee-oh-nate)

Class Progestin/Estrogen

How Supplied
Lunelle Injection 25 mg medroxyprogesterone acetate and 5 mg estradiol cypionate per 0.5 mL

Action
PHARMACOLOGY:
Medroxyprogesterone: Inhibits secretion of pituitary gonadotropins, thereby preventing follicular maturation and ovulation.
Estradiol: Inhibits ovulation.

Indications Prevention of pregnancy.

Contraindications Known or suspected pregnancy; thrombophlebitis or thromboembolic disorders; past history of deep-vein thrombophlebitis or thromboembolic disorders; cerebral vascular or coronary artery disease; undiagnosed abnormal genital bleeding; liver dysfunction or disease (such as history of hepatic adenoma or carcinoma); history of cholestatic jaundice or pregnancy; jaundice with prior hormonal contraceptive use (including severe pruritus of pregnancy); carcinoma of the endometrium, breast, or other known or suspected estrogen-dependent neoplasia; heavy smoking (at least 15 cigarettes/day) and over 35 yr; severe hypertension; diabetes with vascular involvement; headaches with focal neurological symptoms; valvular heart disease with complication; known hypersensitivity to any ingredient of product.

Route/Dosage
ADULTS (WOMEN AND POSTPUBERTAL ADOLESCENT FEMALES): **IM** 0.5 mL administered by IM injection into the deltoid, gluteus maximus, or anterior thigh. Give first injection within first 5 days of onset of normal menstrual period or within 5 days of complete first trimester abortion or no earlier than 4 wk postpartum if not breastfeeding (no earlier than 6 wk postpartum if breastfeeding). Give subsequent injections monthly (28 to 30 days) after previous injection, not to exceed 33 days.

Interactions
Acetaminophen, ascorbic acid: Estrogen plasma levels may be elevated, increasing the risk of side effects.
Antibiotics (eg, tetracycline), anticonvulsants (eg, carbamazepine, phenytoin), phenylbutazone, rifampin, St. John's wort: Contraceptive efficacy may be reduced.
Clofibric acid, morphine, salicylic acid, temazepam: Plasma levels of these agents may be reduced, decreasing their therapeutic effect.
Cyclosporine, prednisolone, theophylline: Plasma levels of these agents may be elevated, increasing the risk of side effects.

Lab Test Interferences Certain endocrine and LFTs and blood components may be affected by combined hormonal contraceptives. The following laboratory tests may be affected by progestins including *Lunelle* monthly contraceptive injection:

- Increased prothrombin and factors VII, VIII, IX, and X, decreased antithrombin 3, increased norepinephrine-induced platelet aggregability.
- Increased thyroid binding globulin (TBG) leading to increased circulating total thyroid hormone, as measured by protein-bound iodine (PBI). T4 by column or by radioimmunoassay. Free T3 resin uptake is decreased, reflecting the elevated TBG, free T4 concentration is unaltered.
- Other binding proteins may be elevated in serum.
- Sex-hormone-binding-globulins are increased and result in elevated levels of total circulating sex steroids and corticoids: however, free or biologically active levels remain unchanged.
- Triglycerides may be increased.

- Glucose tolerance may be decreased.
- Serum folate levels may be depressed by combined hormonal contraceptive therapy. This may be of clinical significance if a woman becomes pregnant shortly after discontinuing combined hormonal contraceptives.
- The pathologist should be advised of progestogen and estrogen therapy when relevant tissue specimens are submitted.
- Plasma and urinary steroid levels are decreased (eg, progesterone, estradiol, pregnanediol, testosterone, cortisol).
- Gonadotropin levels are decreased.
- Sex-hormone-binding-globulin concentrations are decreased.
- Sulfobromophthalein and other LFT values may be increased.

Adverse Reactions

CV: Arterial thromboembolism; cerebral hemorrhage; cerebral thrombosis; hypertension; MI; pulmonary embolism; thrombophlebitis; mesenteric thrombosis; retinal thrombosis.

CNS: Depression; headache; dizziness; nervousness; migraine; emotional lability; change in appetite.

DERM: Acne; alopecia; erythema multiforme; erythema nodosum; hirsutism.

EENT: Corneal curvature changes (eg, steepening); intolerance to contact lenses; cataract.

GI: Nausea; colitis.

GU: Amenorrhea; dysmenorrhea; menorrhagia; metrorrhagia; breast tenderness; breast pain; vaginal spotting; decreased libido; vaginal moniliasis; vulvovaginal disorder; breast changes (eg, enlargement, secretion); cervical changes; temporary infertility after treatment discontinuation; diminution in lactation when given immediately postpartum; changes in libido; premenstrual syndrome; vaginitis; cystitis-like syndrome; impaired renal function; gallbladder disease.

HEMA: Hemolytic uremic syndrome; porphyria; hemorrhagic eruption.

HEPA: Hepatic adenoma or benign liver tumor; cholestatic jaundice; Chiari syndrome.

METAB: Weight gain and decrease; reduced carbohydrate tolerance.

OTHER: Hypersensitivity (eg, anaphylactic reactions, rash); abdominal pain; asthenia; enlarged abdomen; edema; persistent melasma.

Precautions

Pregnancy: Category X.

Lactation: Undetermined.

Children: Use of this product before menarche is not indicated.

Special risk patients: Contraceptive use is associated with increased risks of MI, thromboembolism, stroke, hepatic neoplasm, and gallbladder disease.

Anaphylaxis and anaphylactoid reactions: This reaction may occur.

Bone mineral density changes: Use of injectable progestogen-only methods is among the risk factors for development of osteoporosis.

Cigarette smoking: May increase risk of serious cardiovascular side effects from contraceptives containing estrogen. These risks increase with age (women more than 35 yr) and with smoking more than 15 cigarettes/day.

Depression: Carefully observe patients with history of depression.

Elevated blood pressure: Increased BP during estrogen replacement has been attributed to idiosyncratic reactions.

Familial hyperlipoproteinemia: May be associated with massive elevations of plasma triglycerides.

Fluid retention: Use with careful observation when conditions that might be affected by fluid retention are present (eg, asthma, cardiac or renal dysfunction, epilepsy).

Headache: Development of headache or onset or exacerbation of migraine with a new pattern that is recurrent, persistent, or severe requires evaluation of the cause before further injection of product.

Hypercalcemia: In patients with breast cancer or bone metastases, severe hypercalcemia has occurred with estrogen therapy.

Induction of malignant neoplasm: May increase risk of endometrial or other carcinomas.

Lipid disorders: Because some progestogens may elevate LDL, monitor women who are being treated for hyperlipidemias closely.

Uterine bleeding: Certain patients may develop abnormal uterine bleeding.

Visual abnormalities: Retinal thrombosis has been associated with oral contraceptive use. Discontinue medication if there are any sudden changes in vision, sudden onset of proptosis, diplopia, migraine, papilledema, or retinal vascular lesions.

Overdosage: Signs and Symptoms

Nausea, vomiting, vaginal bleeding, menstrual irregularities.

PATIENT CARE CONSIDERATIONS

Administration/Storage

- For IM injection only. Not for intradermal, SC, or intra-arterial administration.
- Inject prescribed dose every 28 to 30 days.
- Inject first dose during first 5 days of normal menstrual cycle.
- Store at controlled room temperature (59° to 86°F).
- The aqueous suspension must be vigorously shaken just before use to ensure a uniform suspension of 25 mg medroxyprogesterone acetate and 5 mg estradiol cypionate.

Assessment/Interventions
- Obtain patient history, including drug history and any known allergies.
- Review patient's health history for any condition that would contraindicate use of conjugated estrogens/progesterone: previous allergic reaction to either drug; known or suspected pregnancy; known or suspected cancer of the breast; known or suspected estrogen-dependent cancer; undiagnosed abnormal uterine bleeding; active or past history of thromboembolic disorders or stroke; liver dysfunction or disease; heavy smoking and age greater than 35; severe hypertension; diabetes with vascular involvement; headaches with focal neurological symptoms; valvular heart disease with complications.
- Ensure that breast, abdominal, and pelvic examination and Pap smear have been completed and documented before starting therapy.
- Document time of last injection. If less than 28 days or more than 33 days, notify health care provider before administering.
- Monitor blood sugar in diabetic patient when therapy is started. Report significant changes to health care provider.
- Assess BP at beginning of therapy and periodically during treatment.
- Assess patient for GI, CNS, GU, and general body side effects. Inform health care provider if noted and significant.
- Notify health care provider immediately if any of the following are noted: pain in groin or calves; sharp chest pain, coughing blood, or sudden shortness of breath; crushing chest pain or heaviness in chest; abnormal vaginal bleeding; breast lumps; sudden severe headache; dizziness or fainting; vision or speech problems; weakness or numbness of arms or legs; severe abdominal pain; symptoms of depression; yellowing of skin or eyes.

Patient/Family Education
- Explain name, dose, action, and potential side effects of drug.
- Advise patient that medication will be prepared and administered by a health care provider in a medical setting.
- Advise patient that medication must be administered every 28 to 30 days, but no later than 33 days following the last injection.
- Instruct diabetic patient to monitor blood glucose more frequently when drug is started and to inform health care provider of significant changes in readings.
- Caution patient that this medication does not protect against HIV infection or other sexually transmitted diseases.
- Instruct patient to immediately report these symptoms to health care provider: pain in groin or calves; sharp chest pain, coughing blood, or sudden shortness of breath; crushing chest pain or heaviness in chest; abnormal vaginal bleeding; breast lumps; sudden severe headache; dizziness or fainting; vision or speech problems; weakness or numbness of arms or legs; severe abdominal pain; yellowing of skin or eyes; depression; persistent pain, pus, or bleeding at injection site.
- Instruct patient to notify health care provider if any of the following occur: missed menstrual period; persistent or bothersome altered menstrual bleeding; excessive weight gain; intolerance to contact lenses or change in vision while wearing contact lenses; swelling of fingers or ankles; other bothersome effects.
- Advise women to notify health care provider if pregnant, planning to become pregnant, or breastfeeding.
- Teach patient proper method of breast self-examination.
- Advise patient that follow-up visits and examinations, including Pap smear, at least once a year, will be required to monitor therapy and to keep appointments.

Mefenamic Acid

(MEH-fen-AM-ik acid)
Class Analgesic/NSAID

How Supplied
Ponstel Capsules 250 mg
❋ *Apo-Mefenamic* ♦ *Nu-Mefenamic* ♦ *PMS-Mefenamic Acid* ♦ *Ponstan*

Action
PHARMACOLOGY: Decreases inflammation, pain, and fever, probably through inhibition of cyclooxygenase activity and prostaglandin synthesis.

Indications Relief of moderate pain lasting less than 1 wk; treatment of primary dysmenorrhea. **Unlabeled use(s):** Treatment of sunburn, migraine (acute attack), PMS.

Contraindications Patients in whom aspirin, iodides, or any NSAID has caused allergic-type reactions; preexisting renal disease; active ulceration or chronic inflammation of GI tract.

Route/Dosage
Acute Pain
ADULTS AND CHILDREN (14 YR AND OLDER): PO 500 mg, followed by 250 mg q 6 hr prn. Usually not used more than 1 wk.

Primary Dysmenorrhea
ADULTS AND CHILDREN (14 YR AND OLDER):
PO 500 mg, followed by 250 mg q 6 hr starting with onset of bleeding and associated symptoms.

Interactions
Anticoagulants: Increased risk of gastric erosion and bleeding.
Cyclosporine: Nephrotoxicity of both agents may be increased.
Cytochrome P450: Exercise caution when coadministering mefenamic acid with drugs known to inhibit the isoenzyme 2C9.
Lithium: Serum lithium levels may be increased.
Methotrexate: Increased methotrexate levels.
Salicylates: Additive GI toxicity.

Lab Test Interferences
May cause prolonged bleeding time or false-positive reaction for urinary bile using diazo tablet test.

Adverse Reactions
CV: Edema; weight gain; CHF; altered BP; palpitations; chest pain; bradycardia; tachycardia.
CNS: Headache; vertigo; drowsiness; dizziness; insomnia.
DERM: Rash; urticaria; purpura.
EENT: Blurred vision; tinnitus; salivation; glossitis.
GI: Diarrhea; dry mouth; vomiting; abdominal pain; dyspepsia; GI bleeding; nausea; constipation; flatulence.
GU: Hematuria; proteinuria; dysuria; renal failure.
HEMA: Decreased hematocrit; bleeding; neutropenia; leukopenia; pancytopenia; eosinophilia; thrombocytopenia.
HEPA: Mild elevations in LFT results.
RESP: Bronchospasm; laryngeal edema; rhinitis; dyspnea; pharyngitis; hemoptysis; shortness of breath.
OTHER: Autoimmune hemolytic anemia may occur if used long term.

Precautions
Pregnancy: Category C.
Lactation: Undetermined.
Children: Not recommended for children younger than 14 yr.
Elderly: Increased risk of adverse reactions.
Hypersensitivity: May occur; use with caution in aspirin-sensitive individuals because of possible cross sensitivity.
Renal function impairment: Acute renal insufficiency, interstitial nephritis, hyperkalemia, hyponatremia, and renal papillary necrosis may occur. Lower doses may be necessary in patients with renal impairment.
Diarrhea: If diarrhea occurs, reduce dosage or temporarily discontinue.
GI toxicity: Bleeding, ulceration, or perforation can occur at any time, with or without warning symptoms.
Rash: Promptly discontinue if rash develops.

Overdosage: Signs and Symptoms
Acute renal failure, coma, grand mal seizures, muscle twitching, status epilepticus.

PATIENT CARE CONSIDERATIONS
Administration/Storage
- Administer with meals, followed by full glass of water or milk to avoid GI and esophageal irritation. May be given with antacids if stomach upset occurs.
- Exercise caution when initiating treatment in patients with considerable dehydration. Rehydrate patients first and then start therapy with mefenamic acid.
- Store at room temperature (59° to 86°F) in tightly closed, light-resistant container.

Assessment/Interventions
- Obtain patient history, including drug history and any known allergies. Note chronic alcohol use, fluid retention, nasal polyps, bronchospastic disease or hypersensitivity to aspirin or NSAIDs.
- Weigh patient daily if fluid retention is a concern.
- Monitor carefully for hypersensitivity. Note any ecchymosis or rash.
- Monitor renal and liver function and blood studies throughout treatment.
- Monitor for diarrhea or blood in stools. If diarrhea occurs, notify health care provider. Dosage may need to be reduced or drug temporarily withheld.
- Notify health care provider if stomach pain develops or continues.

Patient/Family Education
- Inform patient not to use drug for longer than 1 wk. If given for dysmenorrhea, instruct patient to begin taking drug with onset of bleeding and associated symptoms.
- Warn patient about potential for bleeding, and advise patient to notify other health care professionals that drug is being taken.
- Advise patient to discontinue medication if rash develops and to contact health care provider.
- Instruct patient to report the following symptoms to health care provider: rash, visual problems, dark stools, decreased urinary output, persistent headache or stomach pain and unusual bruising or bleeding.
- Advise patient to avoid intake of alcoholic beverages.
- Instruct patient that drug may cause drowsi-

ness and to use caution while driving or performing other activities requiring mental alertness.
- Caution patient to avoid prolonged exposure to sunlight and to use sunscreen or wear protective clothing to avoid photosensitivity reaction.
- Instruct patient not to take OTC medications, including aspirin and ibuprofen or other prescription drugs, without consulting health care provider.

Mefloquine Hydrochloride

(MEH-flow-kwin)

Class Antimalarial

How Supplied
Mefloquine Hydrochloride Tablets 250 mg ♦
Lariam Tablets 250 mg

Action
PHARMACOLOGY: Antimalarial agent that acts as a blood schizonticide. Mechanism of action is unknown.

PHARMACOKINETICS/DYNAMICS:
Distribution: Mefloquine Vd is approximately 20 L/kg and the protein binding is 98%.
Metabolism: At least 1 metabolite has been identified.
Excretion: Metabolism of mefloquine is primarily hepatic. The total clearance is 30 mL/min and the $t_{1/2}$ is 13 to 24 days (mean, approximately 3 wk).

Indications Treatment of mild to moderate malaria caused by mefloquine-susceptible strains of *Plasmodium falciparum* or *P. vivax*. Prevention of malaria caused by *P. falciparum* or *P. vivax*. Patients with acute *P. vivax* need subsequent treatment with 8-aminoquinolone to prevent relapse.

Contraindications Acute depression; history of psychosis or convulsions; hypersensitivity to the drug or related compounds (eg, quinine, quinidine).

Route/Dosage
Treatment of Malaria
ADULTS: **PO** 5 tablets (1250 mg) as a single dose with food and at least 240 mL of water.
CHILDREN: **PO** 20 to 25 mg/kg as a single dose or split into 2 doses 6 to 8 hr apart with food and at least 240 mL of water.

Prevention of Malaria
ADULTS: **PO** 250 mg once weekly starting 1 wk before exposure and continuing 4 wk after with food and at least 240 mL of water.
CHILDREN: **PO** 3 to 5 mg/kg once weekly starting with 1 wk before exposure and continuing 4 wk after. Take with food and at least 240 mL of water.
Weight up to 19 kg: **PO** ¼ tablet.
Weight 20 to 30 kg: **PO** ½ tablet.
Weight 31 to 45 kg: **PO** ¾ tablet.
Weight more than 45 kg: **PO** 1 tablet.

Interactions
Anticonvulsants: Reduced seizure control.
Drugs known to alter cardiac conduction (eg, antiarrhythmic, beta-adrenergic blockers, CCB, antihistamines, H_2 blockers, tricyclic antidepressants, phenothiazines): Potential for QTc interval prolongation.
Halofantrine: Concurrent use can cause potentially fatal QTc interval prolongation.
Related compounds (eg, quinine, quinidine, chloroquine): Increased risk of seizures and ECG abnormalities.
Typhoid vaccines, live: Reduced effectiveness.

Lab Test Interferences Hematocrit, decrease; leukocytosis (during prophylactic treatment); leukopenia; thrombocytopenia; transaminase, transient increase.

Adverse Reactions
CNS: Dizziness; headache; somnolence.
GI: Nausea; vomiting; diarrhea; abdominal pain; loss of appetite.
OTHER: Myalgia; fever; chills; rash; fatigue; tinnitus.

Precautions
Pregnancy: Category C.
Lactation: Eliminated in breast milk.
Children: Safety and efficacy in children younger than 6 mo not established.
Hepatic function impairment: Impaired elimination of mefloquine.
Special risk patients: Use caution in patients with acute depression or history of psychosis or convulsions.
CV: Risk of ECG alterations, sinus bradycardia, sinus arrhythmia, first degree AV block, prolonged QTc interval, and abnormal T waves.
Epileptic patients: Increased risk of seizures.

PATIENT CARE CONSIDERATIONS
Administration/Storage
Adults:
- Administer prescribed dose with at least 8 oz of water. Do not administer on an empty stomach.

Children:
- Administer prescribed dose with ample water. Do not administer on an empty stomach.
- Splitting total malaria treatment dose into 2 doses given 6 to 8 hr apart may decrease occurrence or severity of side effects.
- Tablets may be crushed, mixed with water or sugar water, and administered via an oral syringe to children who cannot swallow tablet.
- Repeat dose if vomiting occurs within 30 min of taking tablet(s).
- Administer additional half dose if vomiting occurs within 30 to 60 min of taking tablet(s).
- Store tablets at controlled room temperature (59° to 86°F).

Assessment/Interventions
- Obtain patient history, including drug history and any known allergies. Note presence of active depression or concurrent use of quinine, quinidine, chloroquine or halofantrine. Note history of liver disease, heart disease, depression, convulsions, generalized anxiety disorder, psychosis, schizophrenia, or other major psychiatric disorders.
- Monitor patient for development of psychiatric symptoms (eg, depression, anxiety, confusion). Inform health care provider if noted.
- Monitor patient for GI, CNS, and musculoskeletal side effects. Inform health care provider if noted and significant.
- If oral live typhoid vaccine is to be administered, ensure that last dose of typhoid vaccine is taken at least 3 days before the first dose of mefloquine.

Patient/Family Education
- Explain name, dose, action, and potential side effects of drug.
- Advise patient to take each prophylactic dose at the same time each day with food and at least 8 oz of water.
- Instruct patient taking mefloquine for prophylaxis that first dose should be taken 1 wk prior to arrival in malaria-infected area and that subsequent doses should be taken on the same day of the week while in the malaria-infected area and for 4 wk after leaving the malaria-infected area.
- Advise patient that protective clothing, insect repellants, and bednets are important components of malaria prophylaxis.
- Instruct patient taking prophylactic doses to discontinue drug and notify health care provider immediately if any of the following develop: acute anxiety, depression, restlessness, confusion, paranoia, hallucinations, or change in behavior. Alternative therapy will be necessary if mefloquine is discontinued.
- Advise patient to notify health care provider if severe or persistent vomiting or diarrhea develop, vomiting within 1 hr of taking dose occurs often, other bothersome side effects, or if therapy is prematurely discontinued for any reason.
- Advise patient that drug may cause dizziness or other nervous system disorders and to use caution while driving or performing other tasks requiring mental alertness until tolerance is determined.
- Advise women of childbearing potential to use effective contraception while taking mefloquine for malaria prophylaxis.
- Advise patient that if a febrile illness develops during or after return from a malaria-endemic area, seek health care and inform the doctor of possible malaria exposure.

Megestrol Acetate

(meh-JESS-trole ASS-uh-TATE)

Class Progestin

How Supplied
Megace Suspension 40 mg/mL, Tablets 40 mg
✤ *Apo-Megestrol* ◆ *Linmegestrol* ◆ *Megace OS* ◆ *Nu-Megestrol*

Action
PHARMACOLOGY: Inhibits secretion of pituitary gonadotropins, thereby preventing follicular maturation and ovulation (contraceptive effect); inhibits spontaneous uterine contraction; transforms proliferative endometrium into secretory endometrium.

PHARMACOKINETICS/DYNAMICS:
Absorption: C_{max} is 10 to 56 ng/mL and T_{max} is 1 to 3 hr for tablets. C_{max} is approximately 752 ng/mL and T_{max} is approximately 5 hr for suspension at steady state.

Metabolism: The megestrol acetate metabolites are negligible.

Excretion: The major route for elimination is urine; minor routes are feces and respiratory, as CO_2. The t½ is 13 to 104.9 hr (mean, 34.2 hr).

Indications Palliative treatment of advanced

inoperable, recurrent, or metastatic carcinoma of breast or endometrium. **Unlabeled use(s):** Appetite stimulation in HIV-related cachexia.

Contraindications Hypersensitivity to progestins; as diagnostic test for pregnancy.

Route/Dosage
Breast Cancer
ADULTS: PO 40 mg qid.

Endometrial Cancer
ADULTS: PO 40 to 320 mg/day in divided doses.

Interactions None well documented.

Lab Test Interferences Endocrine, coagulation (increased amounts of coagulation factors), thyroid and LFT results may be affected by progestins; may alter metyrapone test results; may decrease glucose tolerance.

Adverse Reactions
CV: Hypertension; thromboembolic phenomena, including thrombophlebitis and pulmonary embolism.
CNS: Insomnia; fatigue.
DERM: Rash; alopecia; mild acne.
GI: Abdominal pain or discomfort; nausea; vomiting.
GU: Breakthrough bleeding; change in menstrual flow; changes in cervical erosion and secretions; impotence.
HEPA: Cholestatic jaundice.
RESP: Dyspnea.
OTHER: Breast tenderness; masculinization of female fetus; edema; weight changes; decreased libido; tumor flare; carpal tunnel syndrome; increased appetite.

Precautions
Pregnancy: Category D.
Lactation: Excreted in breast milk.
Children: Safety and efficacy not established.
Hepatic function impairment: Use with caution and with close monitoring in patients with liver dysfunction.
Fluid retention: Use with careful observation when conditions that might be affected by this factor are present (eg, asthma, cardiac or renal dysfunction, epilepsy).
Mental depression: Carefully observe patients with history of depression.
Ophthalmic effects: Discontinue if there are any sudden changes in vision, sudden onset of proptosis, diplopia, migraine, papilledema, or retinal vascular lesions.
Thromboembolic disease: Use with caution in patients with history of thromboembolic disease.

PATIENT CARE CONSIDERATIONS

Administration/Storage
♦ Store in dry, cool place at room temperature (59° to 86°F).

Assessment/Interventions
♦ Obtain complete patient history, including drug history and any known allergies. Note history of thromboembolic disease.
♦ Assess results of baseline liver, thyroid, and coagulation tests prior to initiation of therapy and routinely during therapy.
♦ Monitor blood glucose in patients with diabetes.
♦ Monitor patient's mental status: affect, mood, depression, behavioral changes.
♦ Notify health care provider if any of these symptoms occur: pain in calves accompanied by swelling, warmth and redness; severe sudden headache; visual disturbances; numbness in extremities; signs of depression; signs of liver dysfunction (eg, dark urine, jaundice); breakthrough bleeding.

Patient/Family Education
♦ Caution patient that this medication must not be taken during pregnancy or when pregnancy is possible. Advise patient to use reliable form of birth control while taking this drug.
♦ Explain potential significance of breakthrough bleeding, irregular menstrual cycles, and possible lack of menstrual cycle. Tell patient to notify health care provider of heavy or continuous menstrual flow.
♦ Encourage patients with diabetes to monitor blood glucose more frequently until effect on diabetes control has been determined.
♦ Instruct patient to report these symptoms to health care provider: pain in calves of legs with redness, warmth and swelling; sudden severe headache; visual disturbances; numbness in extremities; dyspnea; chest pain; edema; jaundice; dark urine; clay-colored stools.
♦ Caution patient to avoid exposure to sunlight and other sources of ultraviolet light and to use sunscreen or wear protective clothing to avoid photosensitivity reaction.

Meloxicam

(mell-ox-ih-kam)

Class Analgesic/NSAID

How Supplied
Mobic Tablets 7.5 mg, Tablets 15 mg, Oral suspension 7.5 mg per 5 mL
✤ Mobicox

Action
PHARMACOLOGY: Decreases inflammation, pain, and fever, probably through inhibition of cyclooxygenase activity and prostaglandin synthesis.

PHARMACOKINETICS/DYNAMICS:
Absorption: Bioavailability is 89%; T_{max} is 4 to 5 hr.
Distribution: Mean Vd is approximately 10 L; protein binding is approximately 99.4%.
Metabolism: Meloxicam is almost completely metabolized to 4 inactive metabolites. Cytochromes P450 2C9 and 3A4 are also involved in metabolism.
Excretion: Meloxicam is equally excreted in the urine and feces, mainly in the form of metabolites. Mean $t_{½}$ is 15 to 20 hr; Cl is 7 to 9 mL/min. Meloxicam is not eliminated through hemodialysis.

Special Populations:
Renal Function Impairment – Meloxicam plasma concentration is decreased and Cl is increased in patients with renal impairment. There is no need for dose adjustment for mild to moderate renal failure (Ccr more than 15 mL/min). Meloxicam is not recommended for severe renal failure.

Indications Relief of signs and symptoms of osteoarthritis and rheumatoid arthritis.

Contraindications Patients who have experienced asthma, urticaria, or allergic-type reactions after taking aspirin or other NSAIDs; hypersensitivity to any component of product.

Route/Dosage
7.5 to 15 mg once daily (max, 15 mg/day).

Interactions
ACE inhibitors (eg, captopril): Antihypertensive effects may be decreased.
Aspirin: Additive GI toxicity.
Cholestyramine: Plasma levels of meloxicam may be reduced.
Lithium: May increase lithium levels.
Loop diuretics (eg, furosemide), thiazide diuretics (eg, chlorothiazide): Diuretic effects may be decreased.
Warfarin: May increase risk of gastric erosion and bleeding.

Lab Test Interferences None well documented.

Adverse Reactions
CV: Angina pectoris, cardiac failure, hypertension, hypotension, MI, vasculitis, arrhythmia, palpitation tachycardia (less than 2%).
CNS: Dizziness, headache, insomnia (4%); fatigue, convulsions, paresthesia, tremor, vertigo, abnormal dreaming, anxiety, increased appetite, confusion, depression, nervousness, somnolence (less than 2%).
DERM: Rash (3%); pruritus (2%); alopecia, angioedema, bullous eruption, photosensitivity reaction, increased sweating, urticaria (less than 2%); erythema multiforme, Stevens-Johnson syndrome, toxic epidermal necrolysis (postmarketing).
EENT: Pharyngitis (3%); abnormal vision, conjunctivitis, taste perversion, tinnitus (less than 2%).
GI: Diarrhea (8%); nausea (7%); dyspeptic signs and symptoms (6%); abdominal pain (5%); constipation, flatulence, vomiting (3%); colitis, dry mouth, duodenal ulcer, eructation, esophagitis, gastric ulcer, gastritis, gastroesophageal reflux, GI hemorrhage, hematemesis, hemorrhagic duodenal ulcer, hemorrhagic gastric ulcer, intestinal perforation, melena, pancreatitis, perforated duodenal ulcer, perforated gastric ulcer, ulcerative stomatitis (less than 2%).
GU: UTI (7%); micturition frequency (2%); albuminuria, increased BUN and creatinine, hematuria, renal failure (less than 2%); interstitial nephritis (postmarketing).
HEMA/LYMPH: Anemia (4%); leukopenia, purpura, thrombocytopenia (less than 2%); agranulocytosis (postmarketing).
HEPA: Increased ALT and AST, bilirubinemia, hepatitis, increased gamma-glutamyl-transferase (less than 2%); jaundice, liver failure (postmarketing).
M/N: Weight decrease or increase, dehydration (less than 2%).
MUSC: Arthralgia (5%); back pain (3%); joint related signs and symptoms (2%).
RESP: Upper respiratory tract infection (8%); coughing (2%); asthma, bronchospasm, dyspnea (less than 2%).
OTHER: Influenza-like symptoms (6%); household accidents, edema, pain (5%); fall (3%); allergic reaction, face edema, fever, hot flushes, malaise, syncope (less than 2%); anaphylactic reactions including shock (postmarketing).

Precautions
Pregnancy: Category C.
Lactation: Undetermined.
Children: Safety and efficacy not established.

Elderly: Use with caution.
Renal function impairment: Assess function before and during therapy because NSAID metabolites are eliminated by the kidney.
Hepatic function impairment: Assess liver function while on therapy.
CV disease: Because fluid retention and edema can occur, use with caution in patients with fluid retention, hypertension, or heart failure.
GI effects: Serious GI toxicity (eg, bleeding, ulceration, perforation) can occur at any time, with or without warning signs.

Pre-existing asthma: Patients with asthma may have aspirin sensitive asthma, which has been associated with severe, sometimes fatal bronchospasm.

Overdosage: Signs and Symptoms
Lethargy, drowsiness, nausea, vomiting, epigastric pain, GI bleeding, hypertension, acute renal failure, hepatic dysfunction, respiratory depression, coma, convulsions, CV collapse, cardiac arrest.

PATIENT CARE CONSIDERATIONS

Administration/Storage
- Administer prescribed dose once daily without regard to meals. Administer with food if GI upset occurs.
- Shake suspension well before measuring dose. Measure and administer prescribed dose using dosing spoon, syringe, or cup.
- Store tablets and suspension at controlled room temperature (59° to 86°F). Protect tablets from moisture. Keep suspension tightly closed.

Assessment/Interventions
- Obtain patient history, including drug history and any known allergies. Note history of GI bleeding or ulcers, allergic reaction to aspirin or other NSAIDs, dehydration, hypertension, heart failure, asthma, or renal or hepatic impairment.
- Obtain baseline assessments of pain and ability to perform activities of daily living.
- Frequently assess patient for response to treatment. Notify health care provider if condition does not appear to be improving or worsens.
- Ensure that therapy is periodically reviewed to determine if it needs to be continued without change or if a dose change (eg, increase, decrease, discontinuation) is indicated.
- Monitor patient for signs and symptoms of liver dysfunction (eg, flu-like symptoms, persistent nausea, fatigue, right upper quadrant abdominal pain, yellowing of skin or eyes, dark urine). If noted, discontinue therapy immediately and inform health care provider.
- Ensure that renal function has been assessed prior to initiating therapy and periodically during therapy in patient with renal impairment.
- Notify health care provider if indigestion, epigastric pain, dark tarry stools, or bleeding or unusual bruising occur.
- Monitor patient for GI, CNS, and general body side effects. Report to health care provider if noted and significant.

Patient/Family Education
- Explain name, dose, action, and potential side effects of drug.
- Advise patient that dose is individualized based upon severity of symptoms and response to therapy.
- Instruct patient to take prescribed dose once daily without regard to meals. Advise patient to take with food if stomach upset occurs.
- Advise patient using suspension to shake suspension well before measuring dose and to use dosing spoon, syringe, or cup to measure and take dose.
- Caution patient not to change the dose or stop taking unless advised by health care provider. Advise patient to notify health care provider if medication does not adequately control arthritis symptoms.
- Caution patient to avoid smoking, alcohol, and self administration of aspirin-containing medications while taking meloxicam.
- Advise patient that if a dose is missed, take it as soon as possible, but if close to the next to skip that dose and take the next dose at the regularly scheduled time. Caution patient not to double the dose to catch up.
- Advise patient to discontinue drug and notify health care provider if any of the following occur: persistent or recurrent GI upset, skin rash, itching, visual disturbances, black stools, rapid weight gain or swelling, changes in urine patterns, joint pain, fever, bleeding or unusual bruising, persistent nausea, fatigue, yellowing of the skin or eyes.
- Advise women to notify health care provider if pregnant, planning to become pregnant, or breastfeeding.
- Instruct patient not to take any prescription or OTC medications, herbal preparations, or dietary supplements unless advised by health care provider.
- Advise patient that follow-up examinations and lab tests may be required to monitor therapy and to keep appointments.

Melphalan

(MELL-fuh-lan)

Class Alkylating agent/Nitrogen mustard

How Supplied
Alkeran Tablets 2 mg, Powder for injection 50 mg

Action
PHARMACOLOGY: Melphalan is a bifunctional, alkylating agent of the bischloroethylamine type. Its cytotoxicity appears to be related to the extent of its interstrand cross-linking with DNA. Like other bifunctional alkylating agents, it is active against resting and rapidly dividing tumor cells.

PHARMACOKINETICS/DYNAMICS:
Absorption: C_{max} is 0.166 to 3741 mcg/mL; may vary depending on absorption or metabolism.

Distribution: Vdss is 0.54 kg; protein binding is 60% to 90% (approximately 30% irreversibly bound). CSF penetration is low.

Metabolism: Melphalan undergoes hydrolysis to form monohydroxy and dihydroxy melphalan.

Excretion: The t½ is approximately 75 min for IV and approximately 90 min for oral.

Indications Palliative therapy of multiple myeloma (oral and IV) and non-resectable epithelial carcinoma of the ovary (oral).

Unlabeled use(s): Breast carcinoma, testicular carcinoma, bone marrow transplantation.

Contraindications Standard considerations.

Route/Dosage

Multiple Myeloma
ADULTS: PO 6 mg/day for 2 to 3 wk as a single daily dose. Resume therapy with 2 mg/day after a rest period at no more than 4 wk and increase dose as necessary.
Alternate regimens: PO 0.25 mg/kg/day for 4 to 7 days or 0.15 mg/kg/day for 7 days. Either regimen can be repeated at 4- to 6-wk intervals after toxicity has resolved. Continuous daily dosing may increase the risk of severe bone marrow depression and secondary malignancy.
ADULTS: IV 16 mg/m² q 2 wk for 4 doses, then as tolerated q 4 wk. The dose should be decreased 50% in patients with BUN at least 30 mg/dL (or serum creatinine at least 1.5 mg/dL).

Epithelial Ovarian Cancer
ADULTS: PO 0.2 mg/kg/day for 5 days q 4 to 5 wk.

Dosage Adjustments
ADULTS: PO/IV All doses should be adjusted based on hematological parameters at nadir. If WBC is at least 4000 cells/mm³ and platelet count is at least 100,000 cells/mm³, administer 100% of prior dose. If WBC is at least 3000 cells/mm³ and platelet count is at least 75,000 cells/mm³, administer 75% of prior dose. If WBC is at least 2000 cells/mm³ and platelet count is at least 50,000 cells/mm³, administer 50% of prior dose. If WBC is less than 2000 cells/mm³ and platelet count is at least 50,000 cells/mm³, no prior dose is to be given. The manufacturer recommends discontinuing drug for leukocyte count is less than 3000/mm³ or platelet count is less than 100,000/mm³.

Interactions
Carmustine: Melphalan may increase the likelihood of carmustine pulmonary toxicity.
Cimetidine and interferon alfa: May decrease serum concentrations of melphalan.
Cisplatin: May alter melphalan clearance, resulting in renal dysfunction.
Cyclosporine: Bone marrow transplant patients receiving melphalan followed by cyclosporine had a high frequency of severe renal dysfunction in 1 study.

Lab Test Interferences None well documented.

Adverse Reactions
DERM: Alopecia.
ENDO: Syndrome of inappropriate antidiuretic hormone secretion with high IV doses.
GI: Very low potential for nausea and vomiting with oral use; moderate potential for nausea and vomiting when used IV in bone marrow transplantation; diarrhea, mucositis; hepatic veno-occlusive disease after bone marrow transplantation.
GU: Ovarian and testicular suppression.
HEMA: Bone marrow suppression, nadir at 2 to 3 wk.
HYPERSEN: Anaphylactoid reaction (2.4% frequency) after IV administration may require stopping the infusion and giving fluids, corticosteroids, antihistamines, or pressors.
RESP: Pulmonary fibrosis, interstitial pneumonitis.
OTHER: Increased risk of acute leukemia or myeloproliferative syndrome with high cumulative doses and long duration of therapy.

> **WARNING:**
> Hypersensitivity reactions including anaphylaxis have occurred with both oral and injection (2% with IV use). Whether routine dosage reductions are needed in impaired Ccr is unknown for oral administration.
>
> *Bone marrow suppression:* Excessive dosage will produce marked bone marrow suppression, which is the most significant toxicity associated with IV melphalan in most patients.
>
> *Carcinogenesis/mutagenesis:* Secondary malignancies, including acute nonlymphocytic leukemia, myeloproliferative syndrome, and carcinoma have occurred in cancer patients following therapy with alkylating agents. Melphalan causes chromatid or chromosome damage and has mutagenic potential in humans.

Precautions
Pregnancy: Category D.
Lactation: Undetermined.
Children: Safety and efficacy in children have not been established.
Renal function impairment: Consider dose reduction in patients with renal insufficiency receiving IV melphalan.
Fertility impairment: Suppression of ovarian function may occur in premenopausal women, resulting in amenorrhea.
Extravasation: IV melphalan is a vesicant; extravasation can cause severe local necrosis.
Prior radiation and chemotherapy: Use with extreme caution in patients whose bone marrow reserve may have been compromised by prior irradiation or chemotherapy or whose marrow function is recovering from previous cytotoxic therapy.

Overdosage: Signs and Symptoms
Severe nausea; vomiting; decreased consciousness; convulsions; muscular paralysis; cholinomimetic effects; severe mucositis; stomatitis; colitis; diarrhea; hemorrhage of the GI tract.

PATIENT CARE CONSIDERATIONS
Administration/Storage
- Store at room temperature (59° to 86°F) and protect from light. Store tablets in glass containers.
- Reconstitute by rapidly injecting 10 mL of supplied diluent into the vial and shaking vigorously until the solution is clear (final concentration is 5 mg/mL). The dose can be diluted with 0.9% Sodium Chloride to a concentration of no more than 0.45 mg/mL. It can also be given undiluted through a central venous catheter.
- Melphalan injection is rapidly hydrolyzed. The undiluted solution is stable for 90 min. With further dilution immediately after reconstitution, it is stable for 60 min.
- Administer PO or IV.
- Give oral melphalan on an empty stomach. Food markedly reduces bioavailability.
- IV melphalan degrades rapidly; give as soon as possible after reconstitution. Give over 15 to 20 min by IV push injection or IV side arm into a running IV infusion. Protection from light during infusion is not necessary. Bolus doses of undiluted solution are also tolerated via a central venous catheter.
- Follow procedures for proper handling and disposal of anticancer drugs. Wear gloves and avoid skin exposure and inhalation of fumes.

Assessment/Interventions
- For patients receiving melphalan for bone marrow ablation, hydration with IV fluids may begin 12 hr before the dose and continue for 24 hr after the dose. Furosemide may also be given to induce diuresis.
- Hyperuricemia may occur because of rapid cell lysis; monitor serum uric acid. Minimize effects of hyperuricemia with hydration, urinary alkalinization, and allopurinol.
- Perform the following tests at the start of therapy and prior to each subsequent dose: Platelet count, hemoglobin, WBC count, and differential. Thrombocytopenia or leukopenia are indications to withhold further therapy until the blood counts have sufficiently recovered. Discontinue the drug or decrease the dosage upon evidence of bone marrow suppression. Consider dose adjustment on the basis of blood counts at the nadir and day of treatments. If leukocyte count falls to less than 3000/mm^3 or platelet count to less than 100,000/mm^3, discontinue drug until peripheral blood cell counts have recovered.

Patient/Family Education
- Inform patients that the major toxicities are related to myelosuppression, hypersensitivity, GI toxicity, pulmonary toxicity, infertility, and non-lymphocytic leukemia. Do not take without close medical supervision.

- Notify health care provider of unusual bleeding or bruising, fever, chills, sore throat, shortness of breath, yellow discoloration of skin or eyes, persistent cough, flank or stomach pain, joint pain, mouth sores, black tarry stools, skin rash, vasculitis, amenorrhea, nausea, vomiting, weight loss, or unusual lumps or masses.
- Contraceptive measures are recommended during therapy.

Memantine Hydrochloride

(meh-MAN-teen HIGH-droe-KLOR-ide)
Class NMDA receptor antagonist
How Supplied
Namenda Tablets 5 mg, Tablets 10 mg
Action
PHARMACOLOGY: It is postulated that memantine exerts its therapeutic effect as a low to moderate affinity, uncompetitive nervous system N-methyl-D-aspartate (NMDA) receptor antagonist by binding preferentially to the NMDA receptor-operated cation channels.

PHARMACOKINETICS/DYNAMICS:
Absorption: Well absorbed from the GI tract, reaching C_{max} in about 3 to 7 hr.
Distribution: Vd is 9 to 11 L/kg. Plasma protein binding is 45%.
Metabolism: Little metabolism with 57% to 82% excreted unchanged in the urine and remainder eliminated as 3 polar metabolites that possess minimal activity.
Excretion: Terminal elimination t½ is about 60 to 80 hr. Renal elimination involves active tubular secretion moderated by pH dependent tubular reabsorption.

Special Populations:
Gender – Women had about 45% greater exposure than men; however, there was no difference in exposure when body weight was taken into account.

Indications Treatment of moderate to severe dementia of the Alzheimer type. **Unlabeled use(s):** Treatment of vascular dementia.

Contraindications Standard considerations.

Route/Dosage
ADULTS: **PO** Start with 5 mg qd. The dose should be increased in 5 mg increments to 5 mg bid, 15 mg/day (5 and 10 mg as separate doses), and 10 mg bid. The minimum recommended interval between dose increases is 1 wk.

Interactions
Drugs eliminated via renal mechanisms (eg, cimetidine, hydrochlorothiazide, nicotine, quinidine, ranitidine, triamterene) Plasma concentrations of both drugs may be altered.
Urinary alkalinizers (eg, carbonic anhydrase inhibitors, sodium bicarbonate): Renal Cl of memantine is reduced about 80% under alkaline urine conditions at pH 8.

Lab Test Interferences None well documented.

Adverse Reactions
CV: Hypertension (4%); cardiac failure (at least 1%).
CNS: Dizziness (7%); headache, confusion (6%); somnolence, hallucination (3%); transient ischemic attack, cerebrovascular accident, vertigo, ataxia, hypokinesia, aggressive reaction (at least 1%).
DERM: Rash (at least 1%).
EENT: Cataract, conjunctivitis (at least 1%).
GI: Constipation (5%); vomiting (3%).
GU: Frequent micturition (at least 1%).
HEMA: Anemia (at least 1%).
M/N: Increased alkaline phosphatase, decreased weight (at least 1%).
MUSC: Back pain (3%).
RESP: Coughing (4%); dyspnea (2%); pneumonia (at least 1%).
OTHER: Pain (3%); fatigue (2%); syncope (at least 1%).

Precautions
Pregnancy: Category B.
Lactation: Undetermined.
Children: Safety and efficacy not established.
Renal function impairment: It is likely that memantine exposure will be increased in patients with moderate renal impairment. Consider dose reduction. Administration of memantine is not recommended in severe renal impairment.
GU conditions: Conditions that raise urine pH may decrease urinary elimination of memantine, resulting in increased plasma levels.

Overdosage: Signs and Symptoms
Restlessness, psychosis, visual hallucinations, somnolence, stupor, loss of consciousness.

PATIENT CARE CONSIDERATIONS

Administration/Storage
- Administer prescribed dose without regard to meals. Administer with food if GI upset occurs.
- Dose is gradually increased at 1-wk intervals.
- May be administered alone or in combination with other medications for dementia.

- Store tablets at controlled room temperature (59° to 86°F).

Assessment/Interventions
- Obtain patient history, including drug history and any known allergies. Note renal impairment or conditions (eg, renal tubular acidosis) or therapy (eg, carbonic anhydrase inhibitor) that raise urine pH.
- Consider dose reduction in patient with moderate renal impairment.
- Evaluate patient's mental status and function prior to initiation of therapy.
- Monitor patient for signs of improvement after therapy is started.
- Assess patient for CNS, GI, GU, CV, respiratory, and general body side effects. Report to health care provider if noted and significant.

Patient/Family Education
- Explain name, dose, action, and potential side effects of drug.
- Advise patient or caregiver that this drug does not alter the Alzheimer process, and the effectiveness of the medication may lessen over time.
- Instruct patient or caregiver to continue using other medications for dementia as prescribed by health care provider.
- Advise patient or caregiver that medication is started at a low dose and gradually increased (no more often than q 1 wk) as tolerated.
- Advise patient or caregiver that doses greater than 5 mg are taken bid without regard to meals, but to take with food if GI upset occurs.
- Advise patient or caregiver not to discontinue the drug or change the dose unless advised by health care provider.
- Advise women to notify health care provider if pregnant, planning to become pregnant, or breastfeeding.
- Instruct patient or caregiver not to use any prescription or OTC medications or dietary supplements unless advised by health care provider.
- Advise patient or caregiver that follow-up visits may be required to monitor therapy and to keep appointments.

Menotropins

(MEN-oh-trope-inz)

Class Sex hormones/Ovulation stimulant

How Supplied
Pergonal Powder or pellet for injection, lyophilized 75 IU FSH activity, 75 IU LH activity ♦
Repronex Powder or pellet for injection, lyophilized 150 IU FSH activity, 150 IU LH activity

Action
PHARMACOLOGY: Stimulates ovarian follicular growth in women who do not have primary ovarian failure.

PHARMACOKINETICS/DYNAMICS:
Absorption: Mean FSH C_{max} is 5.62 mIU/mL (SC) and 4.15 mIU/mL (IM); mean FSH AUC is 385.2 mIU•hr/mL (SC) and 320.1 mIU•hr/mL (IM); median FSH T_{max} is 12 hr (SC) and 18 hr (IM).

Excretion: Mean FSH t½ is 53.7 hr (SC) and 59.2 hr (IM).

Indications
Women: In conjunction with human chorionic gonadotropin (hCG), for multiple follicular development and ovulation induction in patients who have previously received pituitary suppression.
Men: In conjunction with hCG for stimulation of spermatogenesis in primary or secondary hypogonadotropic hypogonadism caused by a congenital factor or prepubertal hypophysectomy and in secondary hypogonadotropic hypogonadism caused by hypophysectomy, craniopharyngioma, cerebral aneurysm, or chromophobe adenoma.

Contraindications Women who have high follicle stimulating hormone (FSH) level indicating primary ovarian failure; uncontrolled thyroid and adrenal dysfunction; organic intracranial lesion (eg, pituitary tumor); presence of any cause of infertility other than anovulation unless patient is candidate for in vitro fertilization; abnormal bleeding of undetermined origin; ovarian cysts or enlargement not caused by polycystic ovary syndrome; pregnancy; prior hypersensitivity to menotropins. Men (*Pergonal*) who have normal gonadotropin levels indicating normal pituitary function; elevated gonadotropin levels indicating primary testicular failure; infertility disorders other than hypogonadotropic hypogonadism.

Route/Dosage
Follicular Development and Ovulation Induction
ADULT (WOMEN): *Repronex:* **SC/IM** Start with 150 IU for 5 days, then based on patient response, adjust dose. Do not make adjustments more frequently than once q 2 days and do not exceed 75 to 150 IU per adjustment (max, 450 IU/day). Do not dose beyond 12 days. If response is appropriate, give hCG 5000 to 10,000 U 1 day following the last dose of menotropins. Withhold hCG if serum estradiol is greater than 2000 pg/mL.
PERGONAL: **IM** Start with 75 IU FSH/75 IU

luteinizing hormone (LH) daily for 7 to 12 days, followed by 5000 to 10,000 U hCG 1 day after the last dose of menotropins. Do not exceed 12 days of menotropins administration.

Repeat dose: **IM** If there is evidence of ovulation, but no pregnancy, repeat the regimen for at least 2 more courses before increasing the dose to 150 IU FSH/150 IU LH/day for 7 to 12 days, followed by 5000 to 10,000 U hCG 1 day after the last dose of menotropins. If there is evidence of ovulation, but no pregnancy, repeat the same dose for 2 more courses.

Stimulation of Spermatogenesis

ADULTS (MEN): **IM** Pretreat with hCG alone (5000 U 3 times/wk). Continue hCG for a period sufficient to achieve serum testosterone levels within normal range and masculinization (ie, appearance of secondary sex characteristics), which may take 4 to 6 mo.

ADULTS (MEN): *Pergonal*: **IM** 75 IU FSH/75 IU LH 3 times/wk and hCG 2000 U twice weekly for at least 4 mo to ensure spermatozoa in ejaculate. If patient has not responded with increased spermatogenesis at the end of 4 mo continue treatment with 75 IU FSH/75 IU LH 3 times/wk or increase the dose to 150 IU FSH/150 IU LH 3 times/wk, with the hCG dose unchanged.

Interactions None well documented.

Lab Test Interferences None well documented.

Adverse Reactions

CV: Vascular complications (eg, stroke); tachycardia.
CNS: Dizziness; headache.
DERM: Rash; swelling and irritation at injection site; body rashes.
GI: Nausea; vomiting; diarrhea; abdominal cramps; bloating; enlarged abdomen.
GU: Mild to moderate ovarian enlargement; ovarian cysts; ectopic pregnancy; congenital abnormalities; ovarian hyperstimulation syndrome; vaginal hemorrhage; ovarian disease; pelvic pain; breast tenderness; gynecomastia (men).
RESP: Pulmonary complications (eg, thrombolic events); dyspnea; tachypnea.
OTHER: Hemoperitoneum; adnexal torsion; abdominal pain; hypersensitivity; flu-like symptoms; pain; injection site edema; infection.

Precautions

Pregnancy: Category X.
Lactation: Undetermined.
Children: Safety and efficacy not established.
Elderly: Safety and efficacy not established.
Health care professional use: Menotropins should be used only by health care professionals thoroughly familiar with infertility problems and their management.
Multiple births: Multiple pregnancies have occurred.
Ovarian enlargement: Mild to moderate uncomplicated ovarian enlargement may occur in approximately 20% treated and generally regresses without treatment with 2 to 3 wk.
Ovarian hyperstimulation syndrome: Warning signs include pelvic pain, nausea, vomiting, distention, and weight gain. May progress within 24 hr to several days to become a serious medical event.
Pulmonary and vascular complications: May occur, resulting in intravascular thrombosis and embolism, which reduce blood flow to critical organs (may result in pulmonary infarct) or extremities (which may cause loss of limbs).

Overdosage: Signs and Symptoms

Ovarian hyperstimulation.

PATIENT CARE CONSIDERATIONS

Administration/Storage

- Follow manufacturer's instructions for reconstituting the Powder or Pellet for Injection. Administer prescribed dose immediately after reconstitution.
- Reconstitute by dissolving contents of 1 or more ampules in 0.5 to 1 mL of Sterile Water for Injection. Administer prescribed dose immediately after reconstitution.
- Do not administer if particulate matter or discoloration noted.
- Administer *Repronex* only by SC or IM injection. Not for intradermal or IV administration.
- Administer *Pergonal* only by IM injection. Not for intradermal, SC, or IV administration.
- With patient lying down or sitting, administer drug by SC or IM injection. Rotate injection sites.
- To minimize bleeding do not rub site after injection.
- Discard any unused reconstituted material.
- Store ampules and vials in refrigerator or at controlled room temperature 3° to 25°C (37° to 77°F). Protect from light.

Assessment/Interventions

- Obtain patient history, including drug history and any known allergies.
- Review patient's health history for any condition that could contraindicate menotropins (eg, previous allergic reaction to menotropins, high levels of FSH, uncontrolled thyroid or adrenal dysfunction, intracranial lesion, sex hormone dependent tumors, and in women,

abnormal uterine bleeding of undetermined origin, ovarian cyst or enlargement of undetermined origin, pregnancy).
- Ensure that women have had a thorough gynecological and endocrinological evaluation before starting therapy.
- Ensure that men have had a thorough medical and endocrinological evaluation before starting therapy.
- Monitor women for signs of overstimulation of the ovary (eg, difficulty breathing, severe pelvic pain, nausea, vomiting, weight gain, stomach pain or bloating, diarrhea, infrequent urination) and report to health care provider immediately if noted.

Patient/Family Education
- Explain name, dose, action, and potential side effects of drug. Review the treatment regimen including duration and monitoring that will be required.
- If patient will be administering at home, teach patient how to store, prepare, and administer the dose, and dispose of used equipment and supplies.
- Remind women that drug is administered to promote follicular growth and egg production, and that hCG will need to be administered to induce ovulation.
- Encourage patient receiving drug for infertility to have intercourse daily, beginning on the day prior to administration of hCG until ovulation has become apparent.
- Warn women that close monitoring for overstimulation of the ovary is required and to report any of the following immediately to health care provider: difficulty breathing, severe pelvic pain, nausea, vomiting, weight gain, stomach pain or bloating, diarrhea, infrequent urination.
- Remind men that drug is administered to promote sperm development and that hCG also will need to be administered to normalize testosterone levels.
- Advise patient that follow-up visits and laboratory tests will be required to monitor therapy and to keep appointments.

Mepenzolate Bromide

(meh-PEN-zoe-late BROE-mide)
Class Anticholinergic/Antispasmodic

How Supplied
Cantil Tablets 25 mg

Action
PHARMACOLOGY: Diminishes gastric acid and pepsin secretion; suppresses spontaneous contractions of the colon. It is a post-ganglionic parasympathetic inhibitor.

PHARMACOKINETICS/DYNAMICS:
Absorption: Oral absorption is low.
Excretion: Over a 5-day period, 3% to 22% is excreted in the urine, with the majority appearing on day 1. The remainder appears in the feces and is presumed not to have been absorbed.

Indications Adjunctive therapy in the treatment of peptic ulcer.

Contraindications Glaucoma; obstructive uropathy (eg, bladder neck obstruction caused by prostatic hypertrophy); obstructive GI tract disease (eg, pyloric duodenal stenosis); paralytic ileus; intestinal atony of the elderly or debilitated patient; unstable CV status in acute GI hemorrhage; toxic megacolon complicating ulcerative colitis; myasthenia gravis; allergic or idiosyncratic reactions to any component of the product or related compounds.

Route/Dosage
ADULTS: **PO** 25 or 50 mg qid, preferably with meals and at bedtime.

Interactions
Agents used to treat achlorhydria: May antagonize the effect of mepenzolate.
Amantadine, antiarrhythmic agents of class I (eg, quinidine), antihistamines, antipsychotic agents (eg, phenothiazines), benzodiazepines, MAO inhibitors, narcotic analgesics (eg, meperidine), nitrates, nitrites, sympathomimetic agents, tricyclic antidepressants, other drugs with anticholinergic activity: These agents may increase certain actions or side effects of anticholinergic drugs.
Antacids: May interfere with mepenzolate absorption; avoid simultaneous administration.
Antiglaucoma agents: Action may be antagonized by mepenzolate.
Digoxin: Serum digoxin levels may be increased in patients taking slow-dissolving dosage forms.
Drugs that alter GI motility (eg, metoclopramide): Action may be antagonized by mepenzolate.

Lab Test Interferences None well documented.

Adverse Reactions
CV: Tachycardia; palpitations.
CNS: Mental confusion; dizziness; weakness; drowsiness; headache; nervousness; insomnia; psychosis (including signs and symptoms of confusion, disorientation, short-term memory loss, hallucinations, dysarthria, ataxia, coma, euphoria, decreased anxiety, fatigue, insomnia, agitation, inappropriate affect).
DERM: Urticaria.
EENT: Increased ocular tension; cycloplegia; blurred vision; dilated pupil.
GI: Vomiting; nausea; constipation; loss of taste; bloated feeling; dry mouth.

GU: Urinary retention; urinary hesitancy; suppression of lactation; impotence.
OTHER: Anaphylaxis; decreased sweating.

Precautions
Pregnancy: Category B.
Lactation: Undetermined.
Children: Safety and efficacy not established.
Special risk patients: Use with caution in the elderly and in patients with autonomic neuropathy, hepatic or renal disease, ulcerative colitis, coronary heart disease, CHF, cardiac arrhythmia, tachycardia, hypertension, prostatic hypertrophy, or hyperthyroidism.
Diarrhea: May be symptom of incomplete intestinal obstruction, especially in patients with ileostomy or colostomy. Treatment of diarrhea with drug is inappropriate and possibly harmful.
Heat prostration: Can occur in presence of high environmental temperature.

Overdosage: Signs and Symptoms
Headache, nausea, vomiting, blurred vision, dilated pupils, hot, dry skin, dizziness, dryness of the mouth, difficulty swallowing, CNS stimulation, curare-like action (neuromuscular blockade).

PATIENT CARE CONSIDERATIONS
Administration/Storage
- Administer prescribed dose with meals and at bedtime.
- Store at controlled room temperature (59° to 86°F). Protect from excessive heat.

Assessment/Interventions
- Obtain patient history, including drug history and any known allergies. Note tartrazine sensitivity, kidney or liver disease, obstructive uropathy (eg, prostatic hypertrophy), hiatal hernia with reflux esophagitis, glaucoma, myocardial ischemia, obstructive GI disease (eg, achalasia, pyloroduodenal stenosis), paralytic ileus, intestinal atony, ulcerative colitis, myasthenia gravis, autonomic neuropathy, hyperthyroidism, hypertension, heart failure, rapid heart rate, arrhythmia.
- Assess symptoms before starting therapy and periodically during treatment. Inform health care provider if symptoms do not improve or appear to be getting worse.
- Ensure that progress of the peptic ulcer under treatment is being followed appropriately (eg, contrast radiology, endoscopy) and that tests for occult blood in the stool, hemoglobin and hematocrit are being periodically evaluated to rule out bleeding from the ulcer.
- Monitor patient for CV, CNS, GI, GU, and general body side effects. Inform health care provider if noted and significant.
- Discontinue therapy and notify health care provider immediately if any of the following occur: rash, eye pain, urinary retention.

Patient/Family Education
- Explain name, dose, action, and potential side effects of drug.
- Advise patient to take prescribed dose with meals and at bedtime.
- Advise patient that dose may be changed periodically to achieve max benefit.
- Advise patient to avoid strenuous activity during periods of high temperature or humidity.
- Advise patient to take sips of water, suck on ice chips or sugarless hard candy, or chew sugarless gum if dry mouth occurs.
- Advise patient that drug may cause drowsiness or blurred vision and to use caution while driving or performing other tasks requiring mental alertness until tolerance is determined.
- Advise patient to notify health care provider if symptoms do not improve or appear to be getting worse.
- Advise patient to stop taking the drug and notify health care provider immediately if any of the following occur: rash, flushing, eye pain, inability to urinate.
- Advise patient that medication may cause dry mouth, urination difficulties, or constipation and to notify health care provider if they occur and are bothersome.
- Advise women to notify health care provider if pregnant, planning to become pregnant, or breastfeeding.
- Warn patient not to take any prescription or OTC drugs or dietary supplements without consulting health care provider.
- Advise patient that follow-up visits may be necessary to monitor therapy and to keep appointments.

Meperidine Hydrochloride

(meh-PEHR-ih-deen HIGH-droe-KLOR-ide)

Class Narcotic analgesic

How Supplied
Demerol Hydrochloride Tablets 50 mg, Tablets 100 mg, Syrup 50 mg/5 mL

Action
PHARMACOLOGY: Relieves pain by stimulating opiate receptors in CNS; also causes respiratory depression, peripheral vasodilation, inhibition of intestinal peristalsis, sphincter of Oddi spasm, stimulation of chemoreceptors that cause vomiting and increased bladder tone.

PHARMACOKINETICS/DYNAMICS:

Distribution: Meperidine protein binding is high.

Excretion: The primary route for excretion is renal. The t½ is 3 to 4 hr.

Onset: Onset is 10 to 45 min.

Peak: The times to peak effect are 3 to 50 min (IM/SC), 60 to 90 min (oral), and 5 to 7 min (IV).

Duration: Duration is 2 to 4 hr.

Indications
Oral and parenteral: Relief of moderate to severe pain.

Parenteral: Preoperative sedation; support of anesthesia; obstetrical analgesia.

Contraindications Upper airway obstruction; acute asthma; diarrhea due to poisoning or toxins; patients who are receiving or have received MAO inhibitor within last 14 days.

Route/Dosage

Pain
ADULTS: **IM/SC/PO** 50 to 150 mg q 3 to 4 hr prn. If IV administration is required, reduce dose and administer slowly.
CHILDREN: **IM/SC/PO** 1 to 1.8 mg/kg (up to adult dose) q 3 to 4 hr prn.

Preoperative Sedation
ADULTS: **IM/SC** 50 to 100 mg 30 to 90 min before anesthetic.
CHILDREN: **IM/SC** 1 to 2 mg/kg (0.5 to 1 mg/lb), up to adult dose, 30 to 90 min before beginning anesthesia.

Support of Anesthesia
ADULTS: **IV** Repeated doses diluted to 10 mg/mL by slow injection or by continuous infusion diluted to 1 mg/mL.

Obstetrical Analgesia
ADULTS: **IM/SC** 50 to 100 mg q 1 to 3 hr prn when pains become regular.

Interactions
CNS depressants (eg, tranquilizers, sedatives, alcohol): Additive CNS depression.
Cimetidine: Monitor for increased respiratory and CNS depression.
Hydantoins: Hydantoins may decrease the pharmacologic effects of meperidine, possibly because of increased hepatic metabolism of the narcotic.
MAO inhibitors, furazolidone: Potentially fatal reactions can occur if meperidine is used in patients within 14 days of receiving MAO inhibitor or furazolidone.
Phenothiazines: Excessive sedation and hypotension.
INCOMPATIBILITIES: Do not co-infuse with solutions of soluble barbiturates, aminophylline, heparin, morphine, methicillin, phenytoin, sodium bicarbonate, iodine, sulfadiazine and sulfisoxazole.

Lab Test Interferences Increased amylase and lipase may occur up to 24 hr after dose.

Adverse Reactions
CV: Hypotension; orthostatic hypotension; bradycardia; tachycardia.
CNS: Lightheadedness; dizziness; sedation; disorientation; incoordination; seizures.
DERM: Sweating; pruritus; urticaria.
GI: Nausea; vomiting; constipation; abdominal pain.
GU: Urinary retention or hesitancy.
RESP: Respiratory depression; laryngospasm; depression of cough reflex.

Precautions
Pregnancy: Pregnancy category undetermined. Safety not established.
Lactation: Excreted in breast milk.
Renal function impairment: Dosage reduction may be necessary in patients with renal impairment.
Hepatic function impairment: Dosage reduction may be necessary in patients with hepatic impairment.
Special risk patients: Use with caution in patients with myxedema, acute alcoholism, acute abdominal conditions, ulcerative colitis, decreased respiratory reserve, head injury or increased intracranial pressure, hypoxia, supraventricular tachycardia, depleted blood volume, circulatory shock or renal dysfunction.
Sulfite sensitivity: Some parenteral products contain sulfites; may cause allergic-type reactions in susceptible individuals.
Drug dependence: Tolerance and psychological and physical dependence may occur with chronic use.

Neurotoxicity: Can cause dysphoria, hallucinations and seizures in patients with renal impairment or with chronic high-dose therapy.

PATIENT CARE CONSIDERATIONS
Administration/Storage
- Administer as soon as pain occurs or prophylactically 30 min before painful procedures. Effect is reduced as pain severity increases.
- Administer meperidine syrup with half glass of water to avoid anesthetizing oral mucous membranes.
- Give oral preparations with food if stomach upset occurs.
- IM administration is preferred for repeated doses.
- Prepare IV injection or solution by diluting in 5% Dextrose and Lactated Ringer's; Dextrose-Saline combinations; 2.5%, 5%, or 10% Dextrose in Water; Lactated Ringer's or Ringer's; 0.45% or 0.9% Sodium Chloride; or ⅙ Molar Sodium Lactate.
- Administer direct IV over at least 3 min.
- Place patient in reclining position and institute safety measures before administering parenteral medication.
- Do not administer if solution is cloudy or if precipitate is present.
- Do not administer IV solution if antidote is not readily available.
- Store at room temperature (59° to 86°F) in tightly closed, light-resistant container.

Assessment/Interventions
- Obtain patient history, including drug history and any known allergies.
- Reduce environmental stimuli and provide maximum comfort measures before administration.
- Obtain vital signs before administration. If

Overdosage: Signs and Symptoms
Miosis, respiratory and CNS depression, circulatory collapse, seizures, cardiopulmonary arrest, death.

respirations are diminished (or 12 breaths/min), withhold medication and notify health care provider.
- Reassess vital signs 30 min after administration (5 to 10 min after direct IV administration).
- Assess bowel and bladder function regularly in patients receiving repeated dosages.
- Encourage coughing and deep breathing exercises q 2 hr while awake.

Patient/Family Education
- Instruct patient that if dose is missed, it should be taken as soon as possible unless close to time of next dose. Do not double up doses.
- If medication is given long term, explain that dosage will be tapered gradually before stopping to prevent withdrawal symptoms.
- Instruct patient not to wait until pain level is high to self-medicate because drug will not be as effective.
- Encourage increased fluid intake and moderate exercise to prevent constipation. Stool softeners or fiber laxative may also be used.
- Advise patient to use humidifier to liquefy secretions. Teach deep breathing exercises.
- Instruct patient to avoid sudden position changes to avoid orthostatic hypotension.
- Tell patient to avoid intake of alcoholic beverages or other CNS depressants (eg, sleeping pills, antihistamines).
- Advise patient that drug may cause drowsiness and to use caution while driving or performing other tasks requiring mental alertness.

Mephentermine Sulfate
(meh-FEN-ter-meen SULL-fate)

Class Vasopressor

How Supplied
Wyamine Sulfate Injection 15 mg/mL, Injection 30 mg/mL

Action
PHARMACOLOGY: Acts directly and indirectly (via release of norepinephrine) on beta and alpha receptors, causing increase in cardiac contraction and, to lesser degree, increase in peripheral vasoconstriction.

PHARMACOKINETICS/DYNAMICS:
Metabolism: Mephentermine sulfate metabolism is hepatic via N-demethylation with subsequent p-hydroxylation.

Excretion: Mephentermine sulfate is excreted renally. The t½ is 17 to 18 hr.

Onset: Onset is 5 to 15 min for IM and almost immediately for IV.

Duration: Duration is 1 to 2 hr for IM and 15 to 30 min for IV.

Indications Treatment of hypotension secondary to ganglionic blockade and to spinal anesthesia; maintenance of blood pressure until blood or blood substitutes may be administered during hypovolemic shock.

Contraindications Hypotension induced by chlorpromazine; use of MAO inhibitors.

Route/Dosage
Shock and Hypotension
ADULTS: IM 0.5 mg/kg undiluted.
ADULTS: IV 1 mg/mL solution in D5W titrated to clinical response.

Hypotension Following Spinal Anesthesia
ADULTS: IV 30 to 45 mg; repeat doses of 30 mg prn; or give as 1 mg/mL infusion in D5W titrated to clinical response.

Prevention of Hypotension Following Spinal Anesthesia
ADULTS: IM 30 to 45 mg 10 to 20 min prior to anesthesia, operation, or termination of operative procedure.

Hypotension Secondary to Spinal Anesthesia During Cesarean Section
ADULTS: IV 15 mg; repeat prn.

Hemorrhagic Shock
ADULTS: IV Continuous infusion of 1 mg/mL solution in D5W until whole blood replacement can be accomplished.

Interactions
Guanethidine: Antihypertensive effects of guanethidine may be negated.
Halogenated hydrocarbon anesthetics: May sensitize myocardium to arrhythmogenic effects of catecholamines.
MAO inhibitors, furazolidone, rauwolfia alkaloids, methyldopa: May significantly increase pressor response, possibly resulting in hypertensive crisis and intracranial hemorrhage.
Oxytoxic drugs: Synergistic or additive vasoconstrictive effects may occur, resulting in hypertension and possible gangrene in the extremities.
Tricyclic antidepressants: May decrease pressor response.

Lab Test Interferences
None well documented.

Adverse Reactions
CV: Cardiac arrhythmias; excessive hypertension, especially in patients with heart disease.
CNS: Anxiety; seizures.

Precautions
Pregnancy: Category C.
Lactation: Undetermined.
CV effects: May be profound. Use with caution in chronically ill patients and patients with known CV disease or hyperthyroidism.
Hypovolemia: Avoid in patients with uncorrected hypovolemia. Persistent hypotension may indicate hypovolemia.

Overdosage: Signs and Symptoms
Hypertension, cardiac arrhythmias, seizures.

PATIENT CARE CONSIDERATIONS
Administration/Storage
- If solution is discolored, do not use; discard.
- IV solution can be prepared by adding 10 or 20 mL of 30 mg/mL mephentermine to 250 mL or 500 mL of D5W, respectively.
- Store reconstituted solution no longer than 24 hr.

Assessment/Interventions
- Obtain patient history, including drug history and any known allergies.
- Use electronic infusion device for IV administration.
- Monitor I&O. If urinary output is less than 30 mL/hr, notify health care provider.
- Monitor BP during IV administration and q 5 min after IM administration.

Patient/Family Education
- Instruct patient and family to notify health care provider if any OTC cold or allergy preparation has been used within 3 days of surgery.
- Inform health care provider of use of MAO inhibitors or tricyclic antidepressants within 1 mo of surgery.

Mephobarbital

(meh-foe-BAR-bih-tahl)

Class Sedative and hypnotic/Barbiturate/Anticonvulsant

How Supplied
Mebaral Tablets 32 mg, Tablets 50 mg, Tablets 100 mg

Action
PHARMACOLOGY: Depresses sensory cortex, decreases motor activity, alters cerebellar function, and produces drowsiness, sedation, and hypnosis.

PHARMACOKINETICS/DYNAMICS:
Absorption: Approximately 50% of an oral dose is absorbed from the GI tract.
Metabolism: Metabolized in the liver to phenobarbital. About 75% of the oral dose is converted to phenobarbital in 24 hr.
Excretion: The metabolite, phenobarbital, may be excreted unchanged in the urine or further metabolized and excreted in the urine as glucuronide or sulfate conjugates.
Onset: 30 to 60 min after an oral dose.
Duration: 10 to 16 hr.

Indications As a sedative for relief of anxiety, tension, and apprehension; as an anticonvulsant for the treatment of grand mal and petit mal epilepsy.

Contraindications Manifest or latent porphyria; hypersensitivity to any barbiturate.

Route/Dosage
Epilepsy
ADULTS: **PO** 400 to 600 mg/day.
CHILDREN OVER 5 YR: **PO** 32 to 64 mg tid or qid.
CHILDREN UNDER 5 YR: **PO** 16 to 32 mg tid or qid.

Interactions
Alcohol, CNS depressants: May enhance CNS depressant effects.
Anticoagulants (eg, warfarin), beta-blockers (eg, metoprolol), doxycycline, felodipine, griseofulvin, methadone, metronidazole, nifedipine, quinidine, theophyllines, verapamil: Activity of these drugs may be reduced by mephobarbital.
Anticonvulsants: Serum levels of carbamazepine, valproic acid, and succinimides may be reduced. Valproic acid may increase mephobarbital levels.
Estrogens, estrogen-containing oral contraceptives: May reduce contraceptive effectiveness.
MAO inhibitors: The effects of mephobarbital may be prolonged.
Methoxyflurane: Risk of renal toxicity may be increased.
Phenytoin: May increase mephobarbital levels while phenytoin levels may increase or decrease.

Lab Test Interferences Decreased serum bilirubin; false-positive phentolamine test results; decreased response to metyrapone.

Adverse Reactions
CV: Bradycardia; hypotension; syncope.
CNS: Agitation; confusion; hyperkinesia; ataxia; CNS depression; nightmares; nervousness; psychiatric disturbance; hallucinations; insomnia; anxiety; dizziness; thinking abnormality; headache.
GI: Nausea; vomiting; constipation.
HEMA: Megaloblastic anemia.
HEPA: Liver damage.
RESP: Hypoventilation; apnea.
OTHER: Hypersensitivity reactions including angioedema, skin rashes, exfoliative dermatitis; fever.

Precautions
Pregnancy: Category D.
Lactation: Excreted in breast milk.
Children: See Route/Dosage section.
Elderly: More sensitive to drug effects; dosage should be reduced.
Renal function impairment: Use with caution and in reduced dosage.
Hepatic function impairment: Use with caution and in reduced dosage.
Special risk patients: Use with caution in patients with a history of drug abuse who are mentally depressed or have suicidal tendencies, and those with myasthenia gravis, myxedema, or impaired cardiac or respiratory function.
Abrupt discontinuation: Status epilepticus may result from the abrupt discontinuation of mephobarbital, even when administered in small daily doses in the treatment of epilepsy.
Acute or chronic pain: Because paradoxical excitement may be induced, use with caution.
Debilitated patients: Increased sensitivity to drug effects; dosage should be reduced.
Dependence: May be habit forming; tolerance or psychological and physical dependence may occur with continued use.
Vitamin D deficiency: Mephobarbital may increase vitamin D requirements. Rarely, rickets and osteomalacia have been reported following prolonged use.
Vitamin K: Bleeding in the early neonatal period caused by coagulation defects may follow exposure to anticonvulsant drugs in utero; therefore, vitamin K should be given to the mother before delivery or to the child at birth.

Overdosage: Signs and Symptoms
CNS and respiratory depression, Cheyne-Stokes respiration, areflexia, constriction of pupils, oliguria, tachycardia, hypotension, lowered body temperature, coma, shock syndrome (including apnea, circulatory collapse, respiratory arrest, and death).

PATIENT CARE CONSIDERATIONS
Administration/Storage
- Administer alone or in combination with other anticonvulsant medications.
- Administer prescribed dose without regard to meals but administer with food if GI upset occurs.
- Administer at night if seizures occur during the night and during the day if seizures are diurnal.
- Store tablets at controlled room temperature (less than 77°F).

Assessment/Interventions
- Obtain patient history, including drug history and any known allergies. Note hepatic or renal impairment, porphyria, depression, suicidal tendency, CV disease, respiratory disease, myasthenia gravis, myxedema, acute or chronic pain, history of drug abuse, or sensitivity to barbiturates.

- Ensure that reduced initial dose and slower dose escalation is used in elderly or debilitated patient, or patient with renal or hepatic impairment.
- Ensure that CBC with differential, renal function, and hepatic function are evaluated before starting therapy and periodically during prolonged treatment.
- Frequently assess patient for response to treatment. Notify health care provider if condition does not appear to be improving or is worsening.
- Ensure that therapy is periodically reviewed to determine if it needs to be continued without change or if a dose change (eg, increase, decrease, discontinuation) is indicated.
- Monitor patient for CNS, RESP, CV, GI, and general body side effects. Report to health care provider if noted and significant. Implement safety precautions if excessive drowsiness or dizziness occurs.
- If treatment needs to be discontinued, attempt to gradually taper the dose over at least a 2-wk interval in patient who has been on prolonged therapy. Monitor patient for withdrawal symptoms (eg, increased anxiety, tremor, muscle or abdominal cramps, sweating). If significant withdrawal symptoms develop, reinstitute previous dosing schedule and attempt a less rapid tapering regimen after patient has stabilized.

Patient/Family Education

- Explain name, dose, action, and potential side effects of drug.
- Advise patient or caregiver to read the *Patient Information* leaflet before starting therapy and with each refill.
- Instruct patient with seizures to continue to take other medications for the condition unless advised otherwise by health care provider.
- Advise patient with anxiety to take as needed and to seek alternative methods for controlling or preventing anxiety (eg, stress reduction, counseling).
- Advise patient that medication is usually started at a low dose and then gradually increased as tolerated until maximum benefit is obtained.
- Advise patient that medication may be habit forming, to take as prescribed, and not to stop taking or change the dose unless advised by health care provider.
- Advise patient to take each dose without regard to meals but to take with food if stomach upset occurs.
- Advise patient that if a dose is missed to skip that dose and take the next dose at the regularly scheduled time. Caution patient to never take 2 doses at the same time.
- Advise patient that if medication needs to be discontinued, it will usually be slowly withdrawn over 2 wk or more unless safety concerns (eg, rash) require a more rapid withdrawal.
- Instruct patient to avoid alcoholic beverages and other depressants while taking this medication.
- Instruct patient with seizures to contact health care provider if seizures get worse, new types of seizures occur, or bothersome side effects (eg, drowsiness, indigestion) occur.
- Advise patient that drug may impair judgment, thinking, or motor skills, or cause drowsiness and to use caution while driving or performing other tasks requiring mental alertness until tolerance is determined.
- Advise women to notify health care provider if pregnant, planning to become pregnant, or breastfeeding.
- Caution patient not to take any prescription or OTC drugs or dietary supplements without consulting health care provider.
- Advise patient that follow-up visits and lab tests may be necessary to monitor therapy and to keep appointments.

Meprobamate

(meh-pro-BAM-ate)

Class Antianxiety

How Supplied
Equanil, Tablets 200 mg, Tablets 400 mg ◆
Miltown, Tablets 200 mg, Tablets 400 mg, Tablets 600 mg
✽ *Apo-Meprobamate*

Action
PHARMACOLOGY: Produces CNS depressant action at multiple sites, including thalamic and limbic systems.

PHARMACOKINETICS/DYNAMICS:
Absorption: Meprobamate is well absorbed. T_{max} is 1 to 3 hr.

Distribution: Meprobamate protein binding is approximately 15%.

Metabolism: 80% to 92% is metabolized in the liver.

Excretion: 90% is excreted renally and approximately 10% in feces. Plasma t½ is 6 to 14 hr for a single dose and 24 to 48 hr for chronic dosing.

Indications Management of anxiety.

Contraindications Hypersensitivity to

meprobamate or related compounds, such as carisoprodol; acute intermittent porphyria.

Route/Dosage
ADULTS: **PO** 1.2 to 1.6 g/day in 3 to 4 divided doses (max, 2.4 g/day).
CHILDREN (6 TO 12 YR): **PO** 100 to 200 mg bid to tid.

Interactions
Alcohol, CNS depressants: May produce additive CNS depression.

Lab Test Interferences
None well documented.

Adverse Reactions
CV: Palpitations; tachycardia; syncope; hypertension; hypotensive crisis; arrhythmias.
CNS: Drowsiness; ataxia; euphoria; slurred speech; dizziness; headache; paradoxical excitement.
GI: Nausea; vomiting; diarrhea.
HEMA: Leukopenia; thrombocytopenia; agranulocytosis; aplastic anemia.
OTHER: Hypersensitivity (eg, rash, itching, fever, chills, edema, bronchospasm, anaphylaxis, erythema multiforme, exfoliative dermatitis, Stevens-Johnson syndrome, bullous dermatitis); exacerbation of porphyria symptoms.

Precautions
Pregnancy: Category D. Use with extreme caution, if at all.
Lactation: Excreted in breast milk.
Children: Do not give to children younger than 6 yr; safety and efficacy not established. Do not give 600 mg tablet to children.
Elderly: Use lowest effective dose to avoid oversedation.
Hypersensitivity: Usually seen between first and fourth dose in patients without previous exposure.
Renal function impairment: Use drug with caution to avoid accumulation in patients with renal impairment.
Hepatic function impairment. Use drug with caution to avoid accumulation in patients with hepatic impairment.
Dependence: Physical and psychological dependence and abuse may occur. Avoid prolonged use, especially in patients prone to addiction. Abrupt discontinuation after prolonged or excessive use may precipitate withdrawal symptoms with risk of seizures.
Debilitated patients: Use lowest effective dose to avoid oversedation.

Overdosage: Signs and Symptoms
Drowsiness, lethargy, stupor, ataxia, coma, shock, vasomotor and respiratory collapse, death.

PATIENT CARE CONSIDERATIONS
Administration/Storage
- Do not alter medication form prior to administration.
- Store in dry, cool place.

Assessment/Interventions
- Obtain patient history, including drug history and any known allergies.
- Monitor results of liver and renal function tests throughout therapy.
- Watch patient take medication to ensure that it is swallowed.
- Notify health care provider if tachycardia, syncope, or palpitations occur.
- Monitor blood studies and CBC during long-term therapy.
- Notify health care provider if patient experiences signs of hypersensitivity, and withhold drug.
- Assess for signs of drowsiness, ataxia, lethargy, itching, rash, or stupor and report findings to health care provider.
- Assist patient with ambulation during beginning of therapy.
- Institute safety measures (eg, siderails).
- Monitor mental status: mood, sensorium, affect, sleeping patterns.
- Monitor pulse and lying and standing BP; if BP is less than 20 mm Hg, withhold drug and notify health care provider.

Patient/Family Education
- Instruct patient not to crush or chew tablets or capsules.
- Advise patient that drug may cause drowsiness and to use caution while driving or performing other tasks requiring mental alertness.
- Instruct patient to avoid intake of alcoholic beverages or other CNS depressants.
- Explain potential side effects, and encourage patient to notify healthcare provider if signs of itching, rash, fever, drowsiness, dizziness, difficulty walking, nausea, vomiting, diarrhea, palpitations, shortness of breath, or sore throat occur.
- Caution patient to change position slowly to minimize orthostatic hypotension.
- Caution patient not to discontinue taking drug abruptly because doing so may precipitate preexisting symptoms or withdrawal reactions.
- Advise women that if they become pregnant or intend to become pregnant to consult their health care provider about continued use of this drug.

Mercaptopurine

(mer-cap-toe-PURE-een)
Class Purine antimetabolite
How Supplied
Purinethol Tablets 50 mg
Action
PHARMACOLOGY: Mercaptopurine competes with hypoxanthine and guanine for the enzyme hypoxanthine-guanine phosphoribosyltransferase and is converted to thioinosinic acid (TIMP). This intracellular nucleotide inhibits several reactions involving inosinic acid (IMP). In addition, 6-methylthioinosinate (MTIMP) is formed by the methylation of TIMP. Both TIMP and MTIMP inhibit de novo purine ribonucleotide synthesis.

PHARMACOKINETICS/DYNAMICS:
Absorption: Mercaptopurine absorption is incomplete and variable; averaging 50%.

Distribution: Protein binding is approximately 19% (over concentration of 10 to 50 mcg/mL). Entry into CSF is negligible.

Metabolism: The major pathways for metabolism are hepatic via methylation and oxidation.

Excretion: Approximately 50% is excreted in urine within 24 hr as parent drug and metabolites. Plasma t½ is 47 minutes in adults.

Special Populations:
Pediatrics – Plasma t½ is 21 minutes.

Indications For maintenance therapy of acute lymphatic (lymphocytic, lymphoblastic) leukemia.

Contraindications Prior resistance to this drug; hypersensitivity to the drug or any component of this formulation.

Route/Dosage
Acute Lymphatic Leukemia, Maintenance
ADULTS: **PO** Usual range is 1.5 to 2.5 mg/kg/day as a single dose.
PEDIATRIC: **PO** Superior results have been obtained when mercaptopurine has been combined with other agents, most frequently methotrexate, for remission maintenance. Mercaptopurine should rarely be relied upon as a single agent for maintenance of remissions induced in acute leukemia.

DOSAGE WITH CONCOMITANT ALLOPURINOL
When allopurinol and mercaptopurine are administered concomitantly, the dose of mercaptopurine must be reduced to ⅓ to ¼ of the usual dose.

Interactions
Allopurinol: Inhibition of mercaptopurine metabolism; coadministration may cause increased toxicity. Reduce dose of mercaptopurine to ⅓ to ¼ of the usual dose.
Cotrimoxazole: Potentiates bone marrow suppression associated with mercaptopurine.
Methotrexate: May increase oral bioavailability of mercaptopurine.
Warfarin: Mercaptopurine may decrease the hypoprothrombinemic effect of warfarin; monitor and adjust warfarin therapy as necessary.

Lab Test Interferences None well documented.

Adverse Reactions
DERM: Alopecia; hyperpigmentation; rash.
GI: Anorexia; intestinal ulceration; mild diarrhea; nausea; oral lesions resembling thrush; sprue-like symptoms; vomiting.
GU: Hyperuricemia; hyperuricosuria; oligospermia.
HEMA: Bone marrow suppression; bone marrow toxicity; marrow hypoplasias.

Precautions
Pregnancy: Category D.
Lactation: Undetermined.
Elderly: Use with caution because of the greater frequency of decreased hepatic, renal, or cardiac function, and concomitant diseases or other drug therapy. Start at the low end of the dosing range.
Renal function impairment: Start with smaller doses because of the possibility of slower drug elimination and a greater cumulative effect in patients with renal impairment.
Hepatic function impairment: Start with smaller doses because of the possibility of slower drug elimination and a greater cumulative effect in patients with hepatic impairment.
Bone marrow toxicity: Most consistent dose-related toxicity is bone marrow suppression manifested by anemia, leukopenia, or thrombocytopenia.
Enzyme deficiency: There are patients with inherent deficiency of the enzyme thiopurine methyltransferase who may be unusually sensitive to the myelosuppressive effects of mercaptopurine and prone to developing rapid bone marrow suppression.
Hepatotoxicity: Hepatotoxicity occurs with greatest frequency when doses of 2.5 mg/kg/day are exceeded. Deaths have occurred from hepatic necrosis.
Immunosuppression: Induction of immunity to infectious agents or vaccines will be subnormal in patients receiving mercaptopurine. Carefully consider effect with regard to intercurrent infections and risk of subsequent neoplasm.

Overdosage: Signs and Symptoms
Anorexia, nausea, vomiting, diarrhea, myelosuppression, liver dysfunction, gastroenteritis.

PATIENT CARE CONSIDERATIONS

Administration/Storage
- Follow institutional and NIH procedures for handling, administration, and disposal of anticancer drugs.
- Administer as single daily dose.
- Store tablets at controlled room temperature (59° to 77°F). Protect from moisture.

Assessment/Interventions
- Obtain patient history, including drug history and any known allergies. Note prior resistance to drug, renal impairment, liver disease, bone marrow impairment, or concurrent treatment with allopurinol or medications that inhibit thiopurine-S-methyltransferase (eg, olsalazine, mesalazine).
- Ensure that reduced initial dose has been considered for patient with renal or hepatic impairment.
- Ensure that women of childbearing potential are not pregnant when therapy is initiated and use effective contraception during treatment.
- Ensure that risk of developing hyperuricemia is evaluated before starting therapy and that hypouricemic therapy (including adequate fluid intake) and monitoring of uric acid is initiated before starting treatment in patient determined to be at risk for developing hyperuricemia and urate precipitation.
- Ensure that CBC with differential and quantitative platelet count is evaluated before starting therapy and then weekly (or more often if clinically indicated) during therapy.
- Implement infection control measures if WBC drops; implement bleeding precautions if platelet count drops. Be prepared to administer platelet transfusions for bleeding, and antibiotics and granulocytes transfusions for sepsis.
- Ensure that mercaptopurine is temporarily withdrawn at the first sign of an unexpected abnormally large fall in any of the formed elements of the blood, if not attributable to another drug or disease process.
- Ensure that TPMT (thiopurine-S-methyltransferase) testing is considered for patient who exhibits clinical or laboratory evidence of severe toxicity, particularly myelosuppression.
- Ensure that serum transaminase levels, alkaline phosphatase, and bilirubin levels are monitored weekly when therapy is initiated and then monthly thereafter during prolonged treatment. Consider more frequent monitoring in patients with preexisting liver disease or those concurrently taking potentially hepatotoxic drugs. Inform health care provider if abnormalities are noted or if symptoms of hepatic injury (eg, jaundice, hepatomegaly, anorexia with tenderness in right upper quadrant) are documented. Be prepared to discontinue therapy.
- Monitor patient for signs of anaphylactic or serious allergic reactions. Discontinue therapy and immediately notify health care provider if noted. Be prepared to treat appropriately.
- Monitor patient for HEMA, GI, DERM, and general body side effects. Report to health care provider if noted and significant.
- Monitor patient for signs and symptoms of bacterial, viral, or fungal infection. Report to health care provider immediately if noted.

Patient/Family Education
- Explain name, action, and potential side effects of the treatment regimen. Review the treatment regimen including dosing schedule, duration of treatment, and monitoring that will be required.
- Advise patient, family, or caregiver that medication may be used in combination with other agents to achieve maximum benefit possible.
- Advise patient to take as a single daily dose.
- Advise patient, family, or caregiver to immediately report any of the following to health care provider: rash; hives; difficulty breathing; fever, chills, or other signs of infection; bleeding or unusual bruising; sores in mouth; dark urine; yellowing of skin or eyes.
- Advise patient, family, or caregiver to report any of the following to health care provider: persistent nausea, vomiting, diarrhea, or appetite loss; persistent or worsening general body weakness.
- Instruct patient not to take any prescription or OTC medications, herbal preparations, or dietary supplements unless advised by health care provider.
- Advise women of childbearing potential to avoid becoming pregnant during therapy.
- Advise women to notify health care provider if pregnant, planning to become pregnant, or breastfeeding.
- Advise patient, family, or caregiver that frequent follow-up visits and laboratory tests will be required to monitor therapy and to keep appointments.

Meropenem

(mare-oh-PEN-em)

Class Anti-infective/Carbapenem

How Supplied
Merrem Powder for Injection 500 mg, Powder for Injection 1 g

Action
PHARMACOLOGY: Inhibits cell wall synthesis.

PHARMACOKINETICS/DYNAMICS:
Absorption: The T_{max} is approximately 1 hr after start of infusion. The mean C_{max} for a 30-min infusion is 23 mcg/mL (500 mg) and 49 mcg/mL (1 g) and the mean C_{max} for a 5-min injection is 45 mcg/mL (500 mg) and 112 mcg/mL (1 g).

Distribution: Meropenem protein binding is approximately 2% and penetrates well into most body fluids and tissues, including CSF.

Metabolism: There is 1 metabolite that is inactive.

Excretion: Approximately 70% is excreted in urine as unchanged over 12 hr. The elimination t½ is approximately 1 hr.

Special Populations:
Renal Function Impairment – Clearance correlates with Ccr in patients with renal impairment. Dosage adjustments may be necessary.
Children – The t½ in children 3 mo to 2 yr is approximately 1.5 hr.

Indications Treatment of intra-abdominal infections in adults and children at least 3 mo and meningitis in children at least 3 mo when caused by susceptible microorganisms.

Contraindications Hypersensitivity to any component of this product or to other drugs in the same class or in patients who have demonstrated anaphylactic reactions to B-lactams.

Route/Dosage
Intra-Abdominal Infections
ADULTS: **IV** 1 g IV q 8 hr.
CHILDREN (AT LEAST 3 MO): **IV** 20 mg/kg q 8 hr.
Max dose: 2 g q 8 hr.

Meningitis
CHILDREN (AT LEAST 3 MO): **IV** 40 mg/kg q 8 hr.
Max dose: 2 g q 8 hr.

Interactions
Probenecid: Inhibits renal excretion of meropenem. Coadministration is not recommended.
INCOMPATIBILITIES: Do not physically mix with solutions containing other drugs.

Lab Test Interferences None well documented.

Adverse Reactions
RESP: Apnea.
CNS: Headache.
DERM: Rash; pruritus.
EENT: Stomatitis.
GI: Diarrhea; nausea; vomiting; constipation.
GU: Vaginitis.
OTHER: Injection site reactions (eg, pain, edema, inflammation).

Precautions
Pregnancy: Category B.
Lactation: Undetermined.
Children: Safety and efficacy in children younger than 3 mo not established.
Hypersensitivity: Administer drug with caution to penicillin-sensitive patients because of possible cross-reactivity.
Renal function impairment: Reduced clearance may occur in patients with renal impairment. Adjust dose downward accordingly in patients with Ccr less than 50 mL/min. Refer to manufacturer's package insert for dose calculations. Thrombocytopenia, without bleeding, has been observed.
Superinfection: May result in bacterial or fungal overgrowth of nonsusceptible organisms.
CNS: Seizures and other CNS adverse events have occurred. Use with caution in patients with CNS disorders, meningitis or renal dysfunction.
Pseudomembranous colitis: Consider possibility in patients with diarrhea.

Overdosage: Signs and Symptoms
Seizures.

PATIENT CARE CONSIDERATIONS

Administration/Storage
- For IV administration only. Do not use solution if discolored or if particulate matter is seen.
- For IV bolus administration, reconstitute with sterile water for injection. Shake to dissolve and let stand until clear. May administer over 3 to 5 min.
- For IV infusion, reconstitute infusion vial with compatible infusion fluid or use ADD-Vantage flexible diluent container for ADD-Vantage vial following instructions. Can administer over 15 to 30 min.
- Store dry powder for reconstitution at controlled room temperature (59° to 86°F).
- Stability of reconstituted meropenem is dependent on diluent and container (eg, syringe, infusion vial, minibag, ADD-Vantage diluent bag). Refer to manufacturer's package insert for guidelines.

Assessment/Interventions
- Obtain complete patient history, including drug history and any known allergies, especially to penicillin and B-lactam antibiotics.
- Notify health care provider if signs of superinfection (eg, vaginitis, stomatitis) or pseudomembranous colitis (eg, diarrhea with blood or pus) occurs.
- Assess for signs and symptoms of anaphylaxis (shortness of breath, wheezing, laryngeal edema). Have resuscitation equipment available.
- If seizures occur, withhold drug, institute safety measures and notify health care provider.
- If culture and sensitivity is ordered, obtain specimen(s) prior to first dose.
- Withhold drug and notify health care provider if any of the following occur: fever, rash, hives.
- Monitor vital signs, sputum, urine, stool and WBC at beginning of and throughout therapy.

Patient/Family Education
- Instruct patient to report itching, rash, hives, difficulty breathing, diarrhea, black "furry" tongue, loose, foul-smelling stool, or vaginal itching or discharge to health care provider.

Mesalamine (5-aminosalicylic acid, 5-ASA)

(me-SAL-uh-MEEN)

Class Intestinal anti-inflammatory/ Aminosalicylic acid derivative

How Supplied
Asacol Tablets, delayed release 400 mg ♦ *Pentasa* Capsules, controlled release 250 mg ♦ *Rowasa* Suppositories 500 mg, Rectal Suspension 4 g/60 mL
✤ *Mesacal* ♦ *Novo-5 ASA* ♦ *Salofalk*

Action
PHARMACOLOGY: Reduces inflammation of colon topically by preventing production of substances involved in inflammatory process such as arachidonic acid.

PHARMACOKINETICS/DYNAMICS:
Absorption: Approximately 20% to 30% of mesalamine is absorbed. The T_{max} is approximately 3 hr (N-acetylmesalamine) and the C_{max} is 1.8 mcg/mL (N-acetylmesalamine).

Metabolism: Mesalamine is rapidly acetylated in the gut mucosal wall and liver. The major metabolite is N-acetylmesalamine.

Excretion: Unabsorbed amount of mesalamine is excreted in feces; absorbed amount excreted mainly in the kidney as N-acetyl-5-aminosalicylic acid. Mean t½ is 42 min (IV, mesalamine).

Indications Treatment of active, mild to moderate distal ulcerative colitis, proctosigmoiditis, or proctitis. **Unlabeled use(s):** Treatment of Crohn disease.

Contraindications Hypersensitivity to salicylates.

Route/Dosage
CONTROLLED-RELEASE TABLETS OR CAPSULES
ADULTS: PO 800 mg tid for total of 2.4 g/day for 6 wk.

SUPPOSITORIES
ADULTS: PR 500 mg suppository bid for up to 6 wk. Retain suppository in rectum for at least 1 to 3 hr to achieve max benefit.

SUSPENSION ENEMA
ADULTS: PR 4 g in 60 mL as rectal instillation q day for up to 6 wk, preferably at bedtime, retained for 8 hr.

Interactions None well documented.

Lab Test Interferences May cause transient asymptomatic elevations in LFT results (eg, AST, ALT, alkaline phosphatase) and serum creatinine. Hepatitis is rare.

Adverse Reactions
CV: Chest pain.
CNS: Headache; asthenia; chills; dizziness; fever; sweating; malaise.
DERM: Acne; itching; rash.
EENT: Rhinitis; sore throat; pharyngitis.
GI: Abdominal pain; cramps; discomfort; colitis exacerbation; constipation; diarrhea; dyspepsia; vomiting; flatulence; nausea; eructation; rectal pain; soreness; burning.
RESP: Cough.
OTHER: Arthralgia; back pain; hypertonia; myalgia; dysmenorrhea; edema; flu syndrome; pain.

Precautions
Pregnancy: Category B.
Lactation: Excreted in breast milk.
Children: Safety and efficacy not established.

Renal function impairment: Patients with history of renal disease or dysfunction may have worsening of renal function.

Sulfite sensitivity: Some products may contain sulfites, which may cause allergic reactions in susceptible individuals.

Intolerance and colitis exacerbation: Some patients develop acute intolerance syndrome or exacerbation of colitis characterized by cramping, acute abdominal pain and bloody diarrhea, and occasionally fever, headache, malaise, pruritus, conjunctivitis and rash. Symptoms generally abate when mesalamine is discontinued.

Pericarditis: Rarely, pericarditis has been reported. Observe for chest pain or dyspnea.

Pyloric stenosis: Gastric retention of oral mesalamine may occur in patients with pyloric stenosis.

PATIENT CARE CONSIDERATIONS
Administration/Storage
- Instruct patient to swallow tablets or capsules whole.
- Do not alter form of medication prior to administration.
- Shake suspension well and position patient in knee-chest position or on left side with lower leg extended and upper right leg flexed for administration.
- Be certain that suppositories are retained for 1 to 3 hr and enemas retained for about 8 hr (preferably at bedtime) to achieve maximum effectiveness.
- Full course of therapy may last up to 6 wk and patient response may occur within 3 to 12 days.
- Store at room temperature (59° to 86°F).

Assessment/Interventions
- Obtain patient history, including drug history and any known allergies.
- Monitor results of renal function tests throughout therapy.
- Assess for increased abdominal pain, nausea, diarrhea, and vomiting, and notify health care provider of any problems.
- Document character and frequency of stools.

Patient/Family Education
- Tell patient to swallow capsules or tablets whole. Explain that outer coating must be intact to pass through stomach and travel to sigmoid colon.
- Tell patient to notify health care provider if any remnant of capsule or tablet is seen in stool.
- Tell patient to retain suppository 1 to 3 hr or to retain enema for 8 hr.
- Teach patient proper positioning and technique for self-administering enema. Include knee-chest and left side positions to promote medication advancement to sigmoid colon.
- Tell patient to report the following symptoms to health care provider: increase in abdominal pain, diarrhea or vomiting.
- Instruct patient to notify health care provider of hives, itching, wheezing, rash, or fever.

Mesna
(MESS-nah)

Class Uroprotectant

How Supplied
Mesnex Tablets 400 mg, Injection 100 mg/mL
✤ Uromitexan

Action
PHARMACOLOGY: Mesna is used to reduce the incidence of ifosfamide-induced hemorrhagic cystitis. Mesna disulfide is reduced to the free thiol compound, mesna, which reacts chemically with the urotoxic ifosfamide metabolites, resulting in their detoxification.

PHARMACOKINETICS/DYNAMICS:
Absorption: Urinary bioavailability of oral mesna is 45% to 79%.

Distribution: Protein binding is 69% to 75%; Vd is 0.652 L/kg.

Metabolism: The major metabolite is dimesna.

Excretion: Approximately 32% is excreted in urine within 24 hr. The $t_½$ is 1.2 to 8.3 hr (after IV plus oral dose); the plasma Cl is 1.23 L/kg/hr. The mesna disulfide is reduced to the free thiol compound that reacts chemically with the urotoxic ifosfamide metabolites, resulting in their detoxification. At doses of 2 to 4 g, the terminal elimination $t_½$ is approximately 4 to 8 hr. It is rapidly eliminated by the kidneys.

Indications Prevention of ifosfamide-induced hemorrhagic cystitis. **Unlabeled use(s):** Prevention of cyclophosphamide-induced hemorrhagic cystitis.

Contraindications Standard considerations.

Route/Dosage
Prevention of Ifosfamide-Induced Hemorrhagic Cystitis
ADULTS: IV Mesna dose is given as bolus injections in a dosage equal to 20% of ifosfamide dose at time of administration, 4 hr after, and 8 hr after each ifosfamide dose (eg, for ifosfamide 1,200 mg/m^2, give mesna 240 mg/m^2 at 0, 4, and 8 hr after each ifosfamide dose). The total daily dose of mesna is 60% of the ifosfamide dose. Repeat this dosing schedule on each

day that ifosfamide is administered. When the dosage of ifosfamide is adjusted, modify the dose of mesna accordingly.

ADULTS: **PO** Following the initial IV mesna dose (20% of ifosfamide dose), the oral mesna dose is 40% of ifosfamide dose 2 and 6 hr after each ifosfamide dose.

Interactions None well documented.

Lab Test Interferences A false-positive test for urinary ketones may arise in patients treated with mesna.

Adverse Reactions Because mesna is used in combination with ifosfamide or ifosfamide-containing regimens, it is difficult to distinguish the adverse reactions that may be caused by mesna from those caused by coadministered cytotoxic agents. The following adverse reactions are reasonably associated with mesna administration in patients also receiving ifosfamide or ifosfamide-containing regimens.
CV: Tachycardia (6%); hypotension (5%); ST-segment elevation (postmarketing).
CNS: Fatigue (20%); anorexia (18%); headache (11%); somnolence (10%); insomnia (9%); dizziness (8%); anxiety, confusion (6%).
DERM: Alopecia (11%); flushing (5%); injection site reaction including pain and erythema (postmarketing).
GI: Nausea (54%); vomiting (38%); constipation (24%); diarrhea (14%); dyspepsia (5%).
GU: Hematuria (7%).
HEPA: Increased liver enzymes (postmarketing).
HEMA/LYMPH: Leukopenia (21%); thrombocytopenia, anemia (18%); granulocytopenia (13%).
M/N: Hypokalemia (9%); dehydration (6%).
MUSC: Myalgia (postmarketing).
RESP: Dyspnea (9%); coughing (8%); pneumonia (7%); tachypnea (postmarketing).
OTHER: Fever (20%); asthenia (18%); abdominal pain (15%); chest pain, pain, increased sweating, injection site reaction (8%); back pain(7%); edema (8%) peripheral edema (7%); face edema, pallor (5%); allergic reactions, limb pain, malaise (postmarketing).

Precautions
Pregnancy: Category B.
Lactation: Undetermined.
Children: Safety and efficacy not established.
Hypersensitivity: Allergic reactions were reported ranging from mild hypersensitivity to systemic anaphylactic reactions.
Benzyl alcohol: Benzyl alcohol, contained in this product as a preservative, has been associated with a fatal "gasping syndrome" in premature infants.
Hematuria: Mesna does not prevent hemorrhagic cystitis in all patients Up to 6% treated have developed hematuria (more than 50 rbc/hpf or WHO grade 2 and above).
Ifosfamide toxicities: Mesna prevents ifosfamide-induced hemorrhagic cystitis. It will not prevent or alleviate other adverse reactions or toxicities associated with ifosfamide therapy.

PATIENT CARE CONSIDERATIONS
Administration/Storage
♦ Injection may be used alone. Tablets are administered in sequence with parenteral therapy.
Tablets:
♦ Administer prescribed dose without regard to meals but administer with food if GI upset occurs.
♦ Repeat the oral dose or administer IV bolus dose if patient vomits within 2 hr of administration.
♦ Store tablets at controlled room temperature (68° to 77°F).
Injection:
♦ For IV bolus administration only. Not for intradermal, subcutaneous, IM, or intra-arterial administration.
♦ Dilute IV concentrate to final concentration of 20 mg/mL with a compatible IV fluid following manufacturer's recommendations.
♦ Do not administer if cloudiness or particulate matter is noted.

♦ Administer first dose as IV bolus at the same time as ifosfamide administration.
♦ Store vials at controlled room temperature (68° to 77°F). Multidose vial can be used for up to 8 days following initial opening. Diluted solutions are stable for up to 24 hr if stored at temperature less than 77°F. Discard any unused solution after 24 hr.

Assessment/Interventions
♦ Obtain patient history, including drug history and any known allergies. Note autoimmune disorder or hypersensitivity to thiol (sulfur containing) compounds.
♦ Ensure that patient maintains good hydration (at least 32 oz of liquid daily) during therapy.
♦ Ensure that urinalysis is performed each morning before ifosfamide therapy. If hematuria develops, consider reducing the chemotherapy dose or discontinuing chemotherapy.
♦ Monitor patient for signs of allergic reaction. Discontinue therapy and immediately notify health care provider if noted. Be prepared to treat appropriately.

- Assess patient for GI, CNS, DERM, HEMA, and general body side effects. Report to health care provider if noted and significant.

Patient/Family Education
- Explain name, action, and potential side effects of drug.
- Advise patient, family, or caregiver to review the *Patient Information* sheet before using the first time and with each course of therapy.
- Advise patient, family, or caregiver that injectable medication will be prepared and administered by a health care provider in a health care setting.
- Review dosing schedule with patient, family, or caregiver.
- Instruct patient to take tablets at the exact times given to them by health care provider.
- Advise patient that if a dose is missed, to take it as soon as remembered and then contact health care provider for further instructions. Caution patient not to double the dose.
- Advise patient taking tablets to contact health care provider immediately if vomiting occurs within 2 hr of taking the dose.
- Advise patient to drink at least 4 cups (1 quart) of liquid each day that mesna is being used.
- Advise patient, family, or caregiver to immediately report any of the following to health care provider: red or pink-colored urine; rash; itching; hives.
- Advise patient, family, or caregiver to report any of the following to health care provider: persistent nausea, vomiting, diarrhea, appetite loss.
- Caution patient not to take any prescription or OTC medications, dietary supplements, or herbal preparations unless advised by health care provider.
- Advise women to notify health care provider if pregnant, planning to become pregnant, or breastfeeding.
- Advise patient that follow-up visits and laboratory tests will be required to monitor therapy and to keep appointments.

Mesoridazine

(Mez-oh-RID-uh-zeen)

Class Antipsychotic/Phenothiazine

How Supplied
Serentil Tablets 10 mg, Tablets 25 mg, Tablets 50 mg, Oral concentrate 25 mg/mL

Action
PHARMACOLOGY: Blocks dopamine receptor in CNS.

PHARMACOKINETICS/DYNAMICS:
Absorption: Mesoridazine besylate is well absorbed from the GI tract.

Distribution: Mesoridazine besylate crosses the placenta and is present in breast milk. Protein binding is more than 90% and Vd is large.

Metabolism: Mesoridazine besylate is metabolized hepatically.

Excretion: Mesoridazine besylate is eliminated through urinary and biliary excretion. The t½ is 24 to 48 hr.

Indications Management of schizophrenia in patients who fail to respond adequately to treatment with other antipsychotic agents.

Contraindications Congenital QT interval prolongation; concurrent drugs that prolong the QT interval; history of cardiac arrhythmias; severe CNS depression or comatose states (including drug-induced CNS depression); hypersensitivity to mesoridazine.

Route/Dosage
Because of potentially serious side effects, use the minimal effective dose.
ADULTS: **PO** Start with 50 mg tid (optimal dose range, 100 to 400 mg/day).

Interactions
Alcohol and other CNS depressants: May result in increased CNS depression and may precipitate extrapyramidal reaction.
Anticholinergics: May reduce therapeutic effects of mesoridazine and worsen anticholinergic effects of mesoridazine. May lead to tardive dyskinesia.
Drugs that prolong the QT interval: May increase the risk of life-threatening cardiac arrhythmias (including torsades de pointes). Coadministration of these agents is contraindicated.
Guanethidine: The hypotensive effect of guanethidine may be inhibited.

Paroxetine: Plasma levels of mesoridazine may be elevated, increasing the risk of side effects.

Lab Test Interferences None well documented.

Adverse Reactions
CV: Hypotension; prolongation of QTc interval, which is associated with life-threatening cardiac arrhythmias; ventricular arrhythmias; changes in terminal portion of ECG.
CNS: Drowsiness; tremor; muscular rigidity; Parkinson syndrome; dizziness; weakness; restlessness; ataxia; slurring; akathisia; fainting; agitation; motor restlessness; dystonic reactions; trismus; torticollis; opisthotonos; oculogyric crises; tardive dyskinesia; bizarre dreams; aggravation of psychoses; toxic confessional state.
DERM: Itching; rash; hypertrophic papilla of tongue; erythema; exfoliative dermatitis; contact dermatitis.
EENT: Stuffy nose; photophobia; blurred vision; miosis; discoloration of sclera and cornea; opacities of the anterior lens and cornea.
GI: Dry mouth; nausea; vomiting; constipation; anorexia; paralytic ileus; obstipation.
GU: Inhibition of ejaculation; impotence; enuresis; incontinence; priapism; menstrual irregularities; altered libido; gynecomastia; lactation; urinary retention.
HEMA: Agranulocytosis; leukopenia; eosinophilia; thrombocytopenia; anemia; aplastic anemia; pancytopenia.
HEPA: Jaundice; biliary stasis.
METAB: Weight gain.
OTHER: Fever; laryngeal edema; angioneurotic edema; asthma; edema; hyperpyrexia; systemic lupus erythematosus-like syndrome; elevated prolactin levels.

> **WARNING:**
> QTc prolongation is dose related. Torsades de pointes type arrhythmias and sudden death have occurred. This drug is reserved for use only in refractory schizophrenia in patients who have failed to show an acceptable response to adequate course therapy or other antipsychotics.

Precautions
Pregnancy: Safety and efficacy not established.
Lactation: Undetermined.
Children: Safety and efficacy not established.
Neuroleptic malignant syndrome (NMS): Has occurred with this class of agents; potentially life-threatening. Signs and symptoms include hyperpyrexia, muscle rigidity altered mental status, irregular pulse and BP, tachycardia, and diaphoresis.
Tardive dyskinesia: May occur with this class of agents and may become irreversible, depending on the duration of treatment and total cumulative dose. The syndrome consists of involuntary, dyskinetic movements.

Overdosage: Signs and Symptoms
Drowsiness, confusion, disorientation, agitation, dry mouth, edema of glottis, laryngeal spasms, nasal congestion, blurred vision, vomiting, hyperpyrexia, dilated pupils, muscle rigidity, hyperactive reflexes, areflexia, stupor, CNS depression or stimulation with convulsions followed by respiratory depression, cardiac abnormalities (including QRS changes), tachycardia, hypotension, bilateral bundle branch block, ventricular fibrillation, shock, cardiac arrest, congenital heart failure, coma, death.

PATIENT CARE CONSIDERATIONS
Administration/Storage
- Administer tablets or oral concentrate in divided doses tid.
- Measure prescribed dose of oral concentrate using measuring dropper supplied with bottle.
- Oral concentrate may be diluted with distilled water, orange juice, or grape juice just prior to administration. Do not prepare dilutions ahead of time and store.
- Store tablets at controlled room temperature (59° to 86°F). Store oral concentrate below 77°F. Protect oral concentrate from light.

Assessment/Interventions
- Obtain patient history, including drug history and any known allergies. Note history of the following: allergy to mesoridazine or other phenothiazines, cardiac arrhythmias, bradycardia, hypokalemia, congenital QT interval prolongation, concomitant use of other drugs that prolong the QT interval, or previous episodes of NMS.
- Ensure that baseline ECG is performed and serum potassium level is determined before starting therapy and periodically during treatment.
- Do not administer to patient with QTc interval greater than 450 msec at baseline. Discontinue therapy if QTc interval prolongs to greater than 500 msec during therapy.
- Ensure that medication is discontinued at least 48 hr before myelography and not resumed until at least 24 hr after procedure to reduce chance of seizures occurring.
- Frequently assess patient for response to treatment. Notify health care provider if condition being treated is not improving or is worsening.
- Ensure that therapy is periodically reviewed to determine if therapy needs to be continued

without change or if a dose change (eg, increase, decrease, discontinuation) is indicated.
- Avoid sudden discontinuation of therapy if possible. Attempt to gradually reduce dose if decision to discontinue medication is made.
- Inform health care provider immediately if hyperpyrexia, muscle rigidity, altered mental status, irregular pulse and BP, tachycardia, and diaphoresis develop.
- Notify health care provider immediately if palpitations or syncope occur.
- Assess neurologic status before and during treatment. Observe for involuntary body and facial movements, excessive drowsiness, agitation, tremor, or anxiety. Inform health care provider if noted.
- Monitor patient for CNS, CV, GI, GU, psychiatric, musculoskeletal, and general body side effects. Inform health care provider if noted and significant.
- Assess medication compliance.

Patient/Family Education
- Explain name, dose, action, and potential side effects of drug.
- Instruct patient, family, or caregiver to measure prescribed dose of oral concentrate using measuring dropper supplied with bottle.
- Advise patient, family, or caregiver that oral concentrate may be diluted with distilled water, orange juice, or grape juice prior to administration. Caution not to prepare dilutions ahead of time and store.
- Instruct patient not to stop taking mesoridazine when feeling better.
- Instruct patient, family, or caregiver to immediately report fainting or loss of consciousness, palpitations, dizziness, high fever, muscle rigidity, altered mental status, irregular pulse, or unexplained sweating to health care provider.
- Advise patient to avoid strenuous activity during periods of high temperature or humidity.
- Instruct patient to avoid alcoholic beverages and other depressants while taking this medication.
- Instruct patient to get up slowly from lying or sitting position and to avoid sudden position changes to prevent postural hypotension. Advise patient to report dizziness with position changes to health care provider. Caution patient that hot tubs and hot showers or baths may make dizziness worse.
- Advise patient to take sips of water, suck on ice chips or sugarless hard candy, or chew sugarless gum if dry mouth occurs.
- Advise patient that drug may cause drowsiness and impaired judgment or thinking skills and to use caution when driving or performing other tasks requiring mental alertness until tolerance is determined.
- Caution patient that medication may cause sensitivity to sunlight and to avoid unnecessary exposure to UV light (eg, sunlight, tanning booths) and to use sunscreen and wear protective clothing when exposed to UV light until tolerance is determined.
- Advise women to notify health care provider if pregnant, planning to become pregnant, or breastfeeding.
- Advise patient, family, or caregiver to notify health care provider of the following: excessive drowsiness, increased agitation or anxiety, or involuntary body or facial movements.
- Instruct patient not to take any prescription or OTC medications or dietary supplements unless advised by health care provider.
- Advise patient that follow-up visits may be required to monitor therapy and to keep appointments.

Metaproterenol Sulfate

(MEH-tuh-pro-TEHR-uh-nahl SULL-fate)
Class Bronchodilator/Sympathomimetic

How Supplied
Alupent Syrup 10 mg/5 mL, Aerosol 75 mg as micronized powder in inert propellant (100 inhalations). Each dose delivers 0.65 mg, Aerosol 150 mg as micronized powder in inert propellant (200 inhalations). Each dose delivers 0.65 mg, Solution for inhalation 0.4%, Solution for inhalation 0.6%, Solution for inhalation 5%

Action
PHARMACOLOGY: Relaxes bronchial smooth muscle through beta-2 receptor stimulation.

PHARMACOKINETICS/DYNAMICS:
Absorption: Less than 10% is absorbed intact.
Metabolism: Metaproterenol sulfate is metabolized through sulfate conjugation in the GI tract. The major metabolite is metaproterenol-o-sulfate.
Excretion: Metaproterenol sulfate is excreted fecally.
Onset: Onset is approximately 30 min (oral) and 5 to 30 min (inhalation).
Peak: Time to peak effect is 30 to 90 min.
Duration: Duration is 3 to 6 hr.

Indications Treatment of bronchial asthma and reversible bronchospasm associated with bronchitis and emphysema; control of acute asthma attacks in children at least 6 yr (inhalation solution only).

Contraindications Cardiac arrhythmias associated with tachycardia.

Route/Dosage

AEROSOL
ADULTS AND CHILDREN (AT LEAST 12 YR): Inhalation 2 to 3 inhalations q 3 to 4 hr, not to exceed 12 inhalations/day.

HAND NEBULIZER
ADULTS AND CHILDREN (AT LEAST 12 YR): Inhalation 5 to 15 inhalations q 4 hr prn.

INTERMITTENT POSITIVE PRESSURE BREATHING APPARATUS
ADULTS AND CHILDREN (AT LEAST 12 YR): Inhalation 0.2 to 0.3 mL of 5% solution in 2.5 mL of diluent q 4 hr prn.

NEBULIZER
ADULTS AND CHILDREN (AT LEAST 12 YR): Inhalation 0.1 to 0.2 mL in saline to a total volume of 3 mL.

Interactions
MAO inhibitors, tricyclic antidepressants: Pressor effects may be potentiated.

Lab Test Interferences
None well documented.

Adverse Reactions
CV: Palpitations; hypertension; tachycardia; cardiac arrest; palpitations; tachycardia; blood pressure changes/hypertension.
CNS: Tremor; dizziness; nervousness; weakness; headache; shakiness/nervousness/tension; drowsiness; insomnia.
DERM: Rash.
EENT: Throat irritation; bad taste; taste/smell change.
GI: GI distress; nausea; vomiting; dry mouth.
RESP: Cough; asthma exacerbation; throat dryness/irritation; pharyngitis; asthma exacerbation; hoarseness; nasal congestion.
OTHER: Fatigue; skin reaction.

Precautions
Pregnancy: Category C.
Lactation: Undetermined.
Children: May be used in children at least 6 yr.
Elderly: Lower doses may be required.
Labor and delivery: May inhibit uterine contractions and delay preterm labor.
Hypersensitivity: Hypersensitivity (allergic) reactions can occur after administration.
CNS effects: CNS stimulation may occur; use drug with caution in patients with history of seizures or hypothyroidism.
CV disorders: Toxic symptoms may occur.
Diabetes mellitus: Dosage adjustment of insulin or oral hypoglycemic agent may be required.
Excessive use: Paradoxical bronchospasm and cardiac arrest have been associated with excessive inhalant use.
Tolerance: May occur.

Overdosage: Signs and Symptoms
Tremor, palpitations, angina, arrhythmias, tachycardia, elevated or decreased BP, seizures, nervousness, headache, dry mouth, nausea, dizziness, fatigue, malaise, insomnia.

PATIENT CARE CONSIDERATIONS

Administration/Storage
- Oral form may be given with food to minimize GI upset.
- Instruct patient to exhale through nose as completely as possible; tilt head back, and put inhaler mouthpiece between lips or 2 inches from open mouth. Tell patient to inhale slowly, press down on canister, hold breath at least 10 sec or as long as comfortable, then exhale slowly.
- Administer pressurized inhalation during second half of inspiration to achieve better distribution of medication. Instruct patient to wait at least 2 full min between inhalations.
- Store metered-dose inhaler in pressurized container at room temperature (59° to 86°F); do not freeze. Keep away from extreme heat. Do not use near open flame or discard in incinerator.
- Refrigerate unit dose nebulizer vials at 35° to 46°F. Protect from excessive heat and light.

Assessment/Interventions
- Obtain patient history, including drug history and any known allergies.
- Review baseline ECG for cardiac dysrhythmias associated with tachycardia.
- Obtain baseline blood values and monitor during therapy. Notify health care provider of abnormal results.
- Take vital signs before, during, and after treatment, noting elevations in BP and pulse. If tachycardia, cardiac arrhythmia or chest pain are present, withhold medication and notify health care provider immediately.
- Assess baseline respiratory function, vital capacity and forced expiratory volume.
- Auscultate lung sounds before and after treat-

ment. If increase in extra sounds, notify health care provider.
- Observe for signs of tremors and anxiety. If present, discontinue therapy and notify health care provider.
- Have epinephrine 1:1000 available for immediate or delayed hypersensitivity reaction.

Patient/Family Education
- Ask patient to demonstrate correct use of inhaler. It may be necessary to repeat instructions and demonstrations more than once.
- Instruct patient that if more than 1 inhalation is necessary, to wait at least 2 min between doses.
- Instruct patient to wash and dry inhaler every day in warm water.
- Explain that tolerance may occur with prolonged use, but temporary cessation of drug usually restores its original effectiveness.
- Instruct patient to notify health care provider if medication is ineffective.
- Warn patient to avoid excessive use (no more than q 4 hr), which can lead to side effects or loss of effectiveness.
- Advise patient to increase fluid intake to liquefy secretions.
- Instruct patient to report the following symptoms to health care provider: palpitations, nervousness, dizziness, shortness of breath, rash, asthma exacerbation.
- Caution patient to avoid getting aerosol medication in eyes.
- Advise patient to avoid smoke-filled rooms and smoking.
- Instruct patient not to take OTC medications without consulting health care provider.
- Instruct patient to rinse mouth with water after each use.

Metaraminol

(met-uh-RAM-in-ole)

Class Vasopressor

How Supplied
Aramine Injection 10 mg/mL (1%, as bitartrate)

Action
PHARMACOLOGY: Acts directly on alpha receptors, causing peripheral vasoconstriction. Increase in systolic, diastolic blood and pulmonary pressure results, as does increase in cardiac output.

PHARMACOKINETICS/DYNAMICS:
Metabolism: Metaramine is metabolized hepatically.

Onset: Onsets of action are 1 to 2 min (IV), approximately 10 min (IM), and 5 to 20 min (SC).

Duration: Duration is 20 min to 1 hr.

Indications Prevention and treatment of acute hypotensive state occurring with spinal anesthesia; adjunctive treatment of hypotension due to hemorrhage, reactions to medications, surgical complications and shock associated with brain damage due to trauma or tumor. Probably effective as adjunct in hypotension due to cardiogenic shock or septicemia.

Contraindications Use with cyclopropane or halothane anesthesia unless essential.

Route/Dosage
Prevention of Hypotension
ADULTS: **SC/IM** 2 to 10 mg; wait at least 10 min before readministering.
CHILDREN: **SC/IM** 0.1 mg/kg.

Treatment of Hypotension
ADULTS: **IV** 15 to 100 mg in 250 to 500 mL of normal saline or D5W; adjust rate to response; may concentrate further in fluid-restricted states.
CHILDREN: **SC/IM** 0.1 mg/kg.

Treatment of Severe Shock
ADULTS: **IV** Push 0.5 to 5 mg followed by infusion of 15 to 100 mg in 500 mL of normal saline or D5W.
CHILDREN: **IV** 0.01 mg/kg as single dose or via infusion of 1 mg/25 mL in normal saline or D5W.

Interactions
Guanethidine: Antihypertensive effects of guanethidine may be negated.
MAO inhibitors, furazolidone, rauwolfia alkaloids, methyldopa: May significantly increase pressor response, possibly resulting in hypertensive crisis and intracranial hemorrhage.
Tricyclic antidepressants: May decrease pressor response.
INCOMPATIBILITIES: Metaraminol is incompatible with many drugs; consult reference prior to admixture.

Lab Test Interferences None well documented.

Adverse Reactions
CV: Sinus or ventricular tachycardia or other arrhythmias, especially in predisposed patients; hypertension or hypotension following cessation of drug; cardiac arrest; palpitations; flushing.
CNS: Headaches; dizziness; apprehension.
GI: Nausea.
OTHER: Sweating; abscess formation; tissue necrosis; sloughing at injection site.

Precautions
Pregnancy: Category C.
Lactation: Undetermined.
Sulfite sensitivity: Use caution in sulfite-sensitive individuals; some preparations contain sodium bisulfite.
Extravasation: Avoid by infusing into large vein and monitoring carefully.

PATIENT CARE CONSIDERATIONS
Administration/Storage
- Dilute in normal saline or D5W. Use large veins to decrease irritation or tissue necrosis at parenteral administration sites. If given directly IV, follow with infusion to decrease possibility of necrosis.
- After administration, observe patient for effects before repeating dose. Pressor effects occur 1 to 2 min after IV dose, 10 min after IM dose, and 5 to 20 min after SC dose.
- Avoid IM injection to prevent tissue sloughing at injection site.
- Use infusion solutions within 24 hr of mixing.
- Avoid exposing drug to excessive heat. Protect from light.

Assessment/Interventions
- Obtain patient history, including drug history and any known allergies.
- Monitor cardiac status, BP, pulse, and respiration rate frequently, especially with IV administration. Fall in BP may occur with repeated use of metaraminol. Check BP q 5 min until stabilized and then check q 5 min throughout therapy.
- Notify health care provider if significant changes or arrhythmias occur.

Overdosage: Signs and Symptoms
Convulsions, severe hypertension, cerebral hemorrhage, cardiac arrhythmias, headache, constricting sensation in chest, nausea, vomiting, euphoria, sweating, pulmonary edema, MI, cardiac arrest, convulsions.

- Monitor I&O.
- Monitor patient for the following sympathomimetic side effects: dizziness, headaches, restlessness, faintness, anxiety flushing and apprehension.
- Monitor for hypertensive crisis and intracranial hemorrhage if given with MAO inhibitors, furazolidone, rauwolfia alkaloids and methyldopa.
- Observe for metabolic acidosis with prolonged use.
- When infusion is to be discontinued, gradually reduce flow rate.
- Document any side effects or adverse reactions, including arrhythmias, hypertension or hypotension after stopping drug, cardiac arrest and nausea.

Patient/Family Education
- Alert patient to the possible problems of extravasation. Instruct patient to report symptoms such as paresthesia, respiratory distress, chest pain, palpitations or irritation or pain at injection site.
- Educate patient and family regarding sympathomimetic side effects.

Metaxalone

(me-TAX-a-lone)
Class Skeletal muscle relaxant
How Supplied
Skelaxin Tablets 400 mg
Action
PHARMACOLOGY: Mechanism of action not established, but may be caused by general CNS depression. No direct action on the contractile mechanism of striated muscle, the motor endplate, or the nerve fiber. Does not directly relax tense skeletal muscles.

PHARMACOKINETICS/DYNAMICS: Under fasting conditions, C_{max} is 1653 ng/mL, T_{max} is approximately 3 hr and mean t½ is 8 hr. Under fed conditions, C_{max} increased by 194%, T_{max} is approximately 4.9 hr and mean t½ is 4.2 hr (single 800 mg dose).

Indications As an adjunct to rest, physical therapy, and other measures for the relief of discomfort associated with acute, painful, musculoskeletal conditions.

Contraindications Standard considerations; known tendency to drug-induced hemolytic or other anemias; significantly impaired renal or hepatic function.

Route/Dosage
ADULTS AND CHILDREN OVER 12 YR: PO 800 mg tid to qid.

Interactions
Alcohol, barbiturates, CNS depressants: Effects may be enhanced by metaxalone.

Lab Test Interferences False-positive Benedict tests, caused by an unknown reducing substance, have been noted. A glucose-specific test will differentiate findings.

Adverse Reactions

CNS: Drowsiness; dizziness; headache; nervousness; irritability.
GI: Nausea; vomiting; GI upset.
OTHER: Hypersensitivity reaction (light rash with or without pruritus); leukopenia; hemolytic anemia; jaundice; anaphylactoid reactions (rare).

Precautions

Pregnancy: Do not use during pregnancy, especially during early pregnancy, or in women who may become pregnant, unless the potential benefits outweigh the potential hazards to the fetus.
Lactation: Undetermined.
Children: Safety and efficacy not determined in children younger than 12 yr.
Hepatic function impairment: Administer with great care to patients with preexisting liver damage and perform serial liver function studies as required.

PATIENT CARE CONSIDERATIONS

Administration/Storage

- Administer prescribed dose without regard to meals but administer with food if GI upset occurs.
- Store tablets at controlled room temperature (59° to 86°F).

Assessment/Interventions

- Obtain patient history, including drug history and any known allergies. Note hepatic or renal impairment, anemia, and history of drug-induced or hemolytic anemia.
- Ensure that reduced dose and slower dose escalation is used in patient with hepatic impairment and that liver function is periodically evaluated during prolonged treatment.
- Ensure that adjunctive therapy (eg, rest, physical therapy) is being used in conjunction with metaxalone.
- Frequently assess patient for response to treatment. Notify health care provider if condition does not appear to be improving or is worsening.
- Ensure that therapy is periodically reviewed to determine if it needs to be continued without change or if a dose change (eg, increase, decrease, discontinuation) is indicated.
- Monitor patient for CNS, GI, general body side effects. Report to health care provider if noted and significant. Implement safety precautions if excessive drowsiness or dizziness occurs.

Patient/Family Education

- Explain name, dose, action, and potential side effects of drug.
- Advise patient or caregiver to read the *Patient Information* leaflet before starting therapy and with each refill.
- Advise patient that medication is usually started at a low dose and then gradually increased until max benefit is obtained.
- Caution patient to take as prescribed and not to stop taking or change the dose unless advised by health care provider.
- Advise patient to take each dose without regard to meals but to take with food if stomach upset occurs.
- Advise patient that if a dose is missed to skip that dose and take the next dose at the regularly scheduled time. Caution patient to never take 2 doses at the same time.
- Instruct patient to avoid alcoholic beverages and other depressants while taking this medication.
- Emphasize importance of other adjunctive measures (eg, rest, physical therapy) as part of the management of musculoskeletal conditions.
- Instruct patient to contact health care provider if symptoms do not appear to be getting better, are getting worse, or if skin rash, yellowish discoloration of the skin or eyes, or bothersome side effects (eg, drowsiness, dizziness, nausea) occur.
- Advise patient that drug may cause drowsiness or dizziness and to use caution while driving or performing other tasks requiring mental alertness until tolerance is determined.
- Advise women to notify health care provider if pregnant, planning to become pregnant, or breastfeeding.
- Advise patient not to take any prescription or OTC drugs or dietary supplements without consulting health care provider.
- Advise patient that follow-up visits and lab tests may be necessary to monitor therapy and to keep appointments.

Metformin Hydrochloride

(met-FORE-min HIGH-droe-KLOR-ide)

Class Antidiabetic/Biguanide

How Supplied
Glucophage Tablets 500 mg, Tablets 850 mg ♦ Glucophage XR Tablets, extended-release 500 mg, Tablets, extended-release 750 mg
🍁 Apo-Metformin ♦ Gen-Metformin ♦ Novo-Metformin ♦ Nu-Metformin ♦ PMS-Metformin ♦ ratio-Metformin ♦ Rhoxal-metformin ♦ Rhoxal-metformin FC

Action
PHARMACOLOGY: Decreases blood glucose by decreasing hepatic glucose production. May also decrease intestinal absorption of glucose and increase response to insulin.

PHARMACOKINETICS/DYNAMICS:

Absorption: Absolute bioavailability is approximately 50% to 60%. T_{max} is 4 to 8 hr and C_{max} is approximately 0.6 to 1.8 mcg/mL (extended-release). Food decreases the extent of absorbtion and increases the T_{max} (immediate-release).

Distribution: The apparent Vd is approximately 654 L and the protein binding is negligible.

Excretion: The major route for excretion is renal via tubular secretion as unchanged. The plasma t½ is 6.2 hr; t½ in blood is 17.6 hr.

Indications Adjunct to diet to lower blood glucose in patients with type 2 diabetes mellitus whose hyperglycemia cannot be controlled by diet alone.

Contraindications Renal disease or dysfunction as suggested by serum creatinine above 1.5 mg/dL in men or above 1.4 mg/dL in females or abnormal Ccr; conditions which predispose to renal dysfunction (eg, CV collapse, acute MI, septicemia); in patients undergoing radiologic studies involving parenteral administration of iodinated contrast material (potential to acutely alter renal function); acute or chronic metabolic acidosis, including diabetic ketoacidosis.

Route/Dosage
ADULTS:
Initial dose: **PO** 500 mg bid, increase by 500 mg q wk (max, 2500 mg/day in divided doses).
ADULTS:
Initial dose: **PO** 850 mg qd, increase by 850 mg q 2 wk (max, 2550 mg/day in divided doses).

GLUCOPHAGE XR
ADULTS:
Initial dose: **PO** 500 mg qd with evening meal, increase by 500 mg q wk (max, 2000 mg once daily). If higher doses of metformin are required, administer at total daily dose up to 2500 mg in divided daily doses as described above.

Interactions
Alcohol: Potentiates effect of metformin on lactate metabolism.
Cationic drugs (eg, amiloride, digoxin, quinidine): May increase metformin serum concentration by competing for tubular secretion.
Cimetidine: Increases metformin serum concentration.
Furosemide: May increase metformin serum concentration; metformin may reduce furosemide serum concentration.
Iodinated contrast material: May cause acute renal failure and has been associated with lactic acidosis in patients receiving metformin.
Nifedipine: Increases metformin serum concentration.

Lab Test Interferences None well documented.

Adverse Reactions
EENT: Unpleasant/metallic taste.
GI: Diarrhea; nausea; vomiting; abdominal bloating; flatulence; anorexia.
METAB: Lactic acidosis.
OTHER: Subnormal vitamin B_{12} levels.

Precautions
Pregnancy: Category B. Insulin is recommended to maintain blood glucose levels during pregnancy.
Lactation: Undetermined.
Children: Safety and efficacy not established.
Elderly: Use with caution. Maximum doses are generally not used because of age-related decreases in renal function.
Renal function impairment: Decreased renal function results in decreased renal clearance and prolongation of the metformin t½ in patients with renal impairment. Comedications that affect renal function, result in significant hemodynamic changes or interfere with disposition of metformin (eg, cationic drugs eliminated by renal tubular secretion) should be used with caution.
Hepatic function impairment: Avoid metformin in patients with clinical or laboratory evidence of hepatic disease.
GI symptoms: GI symptoms occurring after a patient is stabilized on metformin are unlikely to be drug related but could be because of lactic acidosis or other serious disease.
Iodinated contrast material: Withhold metformin for at least 48 hr before parenteral contrast studies with iodinated materials. Reinstitute therapy 48 hr after the study and after renal function has been determined to be normal.
Lactic acidosis: Can occur and be fatal in approximately 50% of cases, as a result of

metformin accumulation (eg, renal impairment) or with pathophysiologic conditions associated with tissue hypoperfusion and hypoxia. The risk of lactic acidosis increases with the degree of renal dysfunction and the patient's age.

PATIENT CARE CONSIDERATIONS
Administration/Storage
- Administer in divided doses with meals starting with a low dose with gradual escalation of dose.
- Dosage of metformin should be individualized on basis of effectiveness and tolerance.
- Ensure determination of fasting plasma level prior to initial dose to ascertain therapeutic response to metformin.
- Metformin can be administered alone or in combination with a sulfonylurea.
- Monitor for possible hypoglycemic effects.
- A reduced dose may be needed in elderly and debilitated or malnourished patients.
- Monitor blood glucose as indicated to ensure blood sugar control; measure glycosylated hemoglobin at intervals of approximately 3 mo.
- Do not administer during pregnancy; insulin is usually given.

Assessment/Interventions
- Obtain patient history.
- Monitor patient for signs and symptoms of hypoglycemia.
- Assess for potential drug-drug interactions. A patient receiving hyperglycemic agents should be closely monitored to maintain adequate glycemic control.
- Assess patient for high risk factors for lactic acidosis.
- Do not use metformin if patient is to have an x-ray procedure with contrast dyes or surgery.
- Should the patient become ill, review laboratory studies as indicated for abnormalities in serum electrolytes, CBC, and blood glucose levels for signs of acidosis and dehydration.
- Assess for GI symptoms, especially with higher doses.
- When transferring from standard oral hypoglycemic agents, other than chlorpropamide, no transition period is usually necessary; however, when transferring from chlorpropamide, care should be exercised during the first 2 wk because of the long retention of chlorpropamide in the body, leading to overlapping drug effects and possible hypoglycemia.
- Determine possible pregnancy or lactation, as safety for these conditions has not been established.
- Administer with caution to elderly patients.

Overdosage: Signs and Symptoms
Lactic acidosis: Malaise, myalgia, respiratory distress, increased somnolence, abdominal distress.

- Store in a tightly closed container at room temperature (59° to 86°F).

Patient/Family Education
- Emphasize the importance of taking this medication exactly as prescribed and not double dosing.
- Caution patient to inform health care provider of OTC or other prescription drug use.
- Evaluate patient's knowledge of type 2 diabetes mellitus and its relationship to metformin therapy.
- Explain the difference between metformin and other glucose-control medications.
- Inform patient of the importance of following dietary instructions, of a regular exercise program, and of regular testing of blood glucose, glycosylated hemoglobin, renal function, and hematologic parameters.
- Instruct patient to take the medication as prescribed at the same time each day.
- Instruct patient in the proper techniques of glucose monitoring.
- Explain that metallic or unpleasant taste is sometimes present at the start of therapy and should be temporary.
- Caution patient to inform health care provider immediately if GI discomfort is severe. If symptoms do not go away within the first few weeks, or if symptoms come back after or start later on during the therapy, patient should inform health care provider so that the dosage can be adjusted.
- Caution patient to be aware of signs and symptoms of hypoglycemia.
- Caution patient to be aware of the signs and symptoms of lactic acidosis.
- Caution patient to not take metformin if having chronic liver or kidney problems; drinking alcohol excessively; severely dehydrated; having a diagnostic procedure with contrast agents; having surgery; or developing a serious condition such as MI, severe infection, or stroke.
- Caution patient to inform health care provider if having an illness that results in severe vomiting, diarrhea, or fever.
- Instruct female patients to inform health care provider if they are or plan to become pregnant, as metformin should not be taken during pregnancy.

Methadone Hydrochloride

(METH-uh-dohn HIGH-droe-KLOR-ide)

Class Narcotic analgesic

How Supplied
Dolophine Hydrochloride Tablets 5 mg, Tablets 10 mg, Injection 10 mg/mL ◆ *Methadose* Tablets 5 mg, Tablets 10 mg, Tablets, dispersible 40 mg, Concentrate, oral 10 mg/mL
🍁 *Metadol*

Action
PHARMACOLOGY: Relieves pain by stimulating opiate receptors in CNS; also causes respiratory depression, peripheral vasodilation, inhibition of intestinal peristalsis, sphincter of Oddi spasm, stimulation of chemoreceptors that cause vomiting and increased bladder tone.

PHARMACOKINETICS/DYNAMICS:
Distribution: Protein binding is high.

Metabolism: Methadone is metabolized hepatically and in intestinal mucosa.

Excretion: The primary route for elimination is renal; minor route is biliary. The t½ is 15 to 30 hr (repeated dosing).

Onset: Onsets of action are 30 to 60 min (oral) and 10 to 20 min (IM).

Peak: Times to peak effect are 90 to 120 min (oral), 60 to 120 min (IM), and 15 to 30 min (IV).

Duration: Durations are 4 to 6 hr (repeated oral dosing), 4 to 5 hr (IM), and 3 to 4 hr (IV).

Indications Management of severe pain; detoxification and temporary maintenance treatment of narcotic addiction.

Contraindications Standard considerations.

Route/Dosage
Pain
ADULTS: **IM/SC/PO** 2.5 to 10 mg q 3 to 4 hr prn. May need higher doses in patients with severe pain or tolerance.

Detoxification
ADULTS: **PO** 15 to 20 mg initially to suppress withdrawal symptoms. Additional doses may be needed.

PATIENTS PHYSICALLY DEPENDENT ON HIGH DOSES OF NARCOTICS: **PO** 40 mg/day may be given for 2 to 3 days; decrease dose q 1 to 2 days.

MAINTENANCE: **PO** 20 to 40 mg initially to suppress withdrawal symptoms in patients who are heavy heroin users. Additional 10 mg doses can be given prn. Adjust dose as tolerated and required, up to 120 mg/day.

Interactions
Barbiturate anesthetics: Drug actions may be additive.
Cimetidine, protease inhibitors: Monitor for increased respiratory and CNS depression.
CNS depressants (eg, tranquilizers, sedatives, alcohol): Additive CNS depression.
Fluvoxamine: Monitor for increased CNS depression when taken with methadone. Monitor for signs and symptoms of withdrawal when fluvoxamine is discontinued.
Hydantoins, rifampin, barbiturates: May decrease effectiveness of methadone.
Urinary acidifiers: May increase renal clearance of methadone.

Lab Test Interferences Increased amylase and lipase may occur up to 24 hr after dose.

Adverse Reactions
CV: Hypotension; palpitations; bradycardia; tachycardia.
CNS: Lightheadedness; euphoria; dysphoria; headache; insomnia; dizziness; sedation; disorientation; incoordination.
DERM: Sweating; pruritus; urticaria.
GI: Nausea; vomiting; constipation; abdominal pain; dry mouth.
GU: Urinary retention or hesitancy.
HEMA: Thrombocytopenia.
RESP: Laryngospasm; depression of cough reflex.
OTHER: Tolerance; psychological and physical dependence with chronic use.

> **WARNING:**
> Use in withdrawal syndromes must be dispensed by approved pharmacy/maintenance programs. Avoid use of narcotic antagonist as it may precipitate an acute withdrawal syndrome.

Precautions
Pregnancy: Pregnancy category undetermined. Methadone use has been associated with low infant birthweight.
Lactation: Excreted in breast milk.
Children: Not recommended for children; dosage is not well defined.
Renal function impairment: May need to decrease dose in patients with renal impairment.
Hepatic function impairment: May need to decrease dose in patients with hepatic impairment.
Special risk patients: Use drug with caution in patients with myxedema, acute alcoholism, acute abdominal conditions, ulcerative colitis, decreased respiratory reserve head injury or increased intracranial pressure, hypoxia, supra-

ventricular tachycardia, depleted blood volume or circulatory shock.

Drug dependence: Methadone has abuse potential.

Obstetrical analgesia: Do not use methadone for obstetrical analgesia. Its long duration of action increases the probability of neonatal respiratory depression.

Treatment of drug addiction: Methadone for detoxification should not be given for more than 21 days and treatment should not be repeated within 4 wk. More than 3 wk in methadone treatment of narcotic dependence is considered maintenance therapy; only approved programs can provide this therapy.

Overdosage: Signs and Symptoms

Miosis, respiratory and CNS depression, cool/clammy skin, skeletal muscle flaccidity, circulatory collapse, seizures, cardiopulmonary arrest, apnea, hypotension, coma, death.

PATIENT CARE CONSIDERATIONS

Administration/Storage

- If GI upset occurs, give with food.
- Adjust dose as tolerated and required (up to 120 mg/day) for adequate pain relief. When withdrawing methadone, decrease by 10% q 1 to 2 days.
- Use reduced dose in elderly or debilitated patients.
- IM administration is preferred over SC injection, which can cause local irritation.
- Rotate injection sites.
- Store at room temperature (59° to 86°F) in light-resistant container.

Assessment/Interventions

- Obtain patient history, including drug history and any known allergies.
- Monitor vital signs, especially respirations.
- Monitor bowel function and treat constipation as indicated.
- Monitor I&O. Observe for urinary retention.
- Assess for pain relief.
- Have patient turn, cough and deep breathe q 2 hr.
- Watch for additive CNS effects when used with other CNS depressants.
- Carefully monitor patients with acute abdominal problems, acute alcoholism, myxedema, respiratory disease, supraventricular tachycardia or shock.
- Document and notify health care provider of any side effects, including hypotension, bradycardia, tachycardia, laryngospasm, decreased cough reflex, dizziness, disorientation, nausea and vomiting, constipation, urinary retention, sweating, pruritus, physical and psychological dependence with long-term use.

Patient/Family Education

- Tell patient to take methadone regularly, as prescribed. If dose is missed, tell patient to take as soon as possible. If close to next dose, wait and take next regularly scheduled dose.
- Advise patient that drug may cause dizziness, drowsiness, or blurred vision and to use caution while driving or performing other hazardous tasks.
- Caution patient to avoid intake of alcoholic beverages or other CNS depressants.
- If constipation occurs, tell patient to increase fluids and fiber or to use fiber laxative.
- Explain that use of methadone before pain becomes acute will allow it to alleviate pain better.
- Caution patient to avoid sudden position changes to prevent orthostatic hypotension.
- Explain types and potential significance of sympathomimetic side effects.

Methamphetamine Hydrochloride (Desoxyephedrine Hydrochloride)

(meth-am-FET-uh-meen HIGH-droe-KLOR-ide)

Class CNS stimulant/Amphetamine

How Supplied
Desoxyn Tablets 5 mg

Action

PHARMACOLOGY: Activates noradrenergic neurons causing CNS and respiratory stimulation; stimulates the satiety center in the brain, causing appetite suppression.

PHARMACOKINETICS/DYNAMICS:

Absorption: Methamphetamine is rapidly absorbed from the GI tract.

Metabolism: Primary site for metabolism is the liver, by aromatic hydroxylation, N-dealkylation, and deamination. There are at least 7 metabolites.

Excretion: Primary route for excretion is urine (dependent on pH) and the t½ is 4 to 5 hr.

Indications Treatment of attention deficit disorder in children; short-term exogenous obesity adjunct.

Contraindications Advanced arteriosclerosis; symptomatic CV disease; moderate to severe hypertension; hyperthyroidism; hypersensitivity to sympathomimetic amines; glaucoma; agitated states; history of drug abuse. Drug should not be used concomitantly with or within 14 days of MAO inhibitor use.

Route/Dosage
Attention Deficit Disorder
CHILDREN: PO 5 mg 1 to 2 times/day; may be increased weekly by 5 mg to max of 20 to 25 mg/day in divided doses.

Exogenous Obesity
ADULTS AND CHILDREN (OLDER THAN 12 YR): PO 5 mg 1 to 3 times/day 30 min before meals. Not to be used beyond a few weeks.

Interactions
Guanethidine: Amphetamines may decrease effectiveness.
MAO inhibitors, furazolidone: Hypertensive crisis and intracranial hemorrhage may occur.
Tricyclic Antidepressants: Decreased amphetamine effect.
Urinary acidifiers: Decreased amphetamine levels.
Urinary alkalinizers: Increased amphetamine levels.

Lab Test Interferences Plasma and urinary steroid levels may be altered.

PATIENT CARE CONSIDERATIONS
Administration/Storage
- Administer last dose several hours before bedtime.
- Store in tightly closed container at room temperature (59° to 86°F).

Assessment/Interventions
- Obtain patient history, including drug history and any known allergies. Note CV disease, hyperthyroidism, glaucoma, or sensitivity to sympathomimetic drugs.
- Take vital signs and auscultate heart and lungs before administration; monitor closely during treatment.
- Assess the following mental states: mood, sensorium, affect, stimulation, insomnia, aggressiveness. Depressed patients are more likely to misuse drug to induce euphoria and mood elevation.
- Monitor renal function.
- Monitor blood glucose level closely in diabetic patient. Changes in appetite and food intake will occur.
- Monitor for weight loss (may be desired effect).

Adverse Reactions
CV: Palpitations; tachycardia; hypertension; arrhythmias.
CNS: Hyperactivity; dizziness; insomnia; euphoria; restlessness; tremors; headache.
DERM: Urticaria.
GI: Dry mouth; unpleasant taste; diarrhea; constipation; anorexia.
GU: Impotence.

> **WARNING:**
> High abuse/diversion potential. Drug dependence may develop with chronic use. Avoid long periods of use. Prescribe and dispense sparingly because of high diversion potential.

Precautions
Pregnancy: Category C.
Lactation: Excreted in breast milk.
Children: Not recommended as anorectic agent in children less than 12 yr.
Tartrazine sensitivity: Some products contain tartrazine, which may cause allergic reactions in susceptible individuals.
Tolerance: Tolerance may occur; do not exceed recommended dose.

Overdosage: Signs and Symptoms
Restlessness, tremor, hyperreflexia, rapid respiration, confusion, assaultiveness, hallucinations, panic attack, hyperpyrexia.

- If hypertension, dysrhythmias, marked agitation, restlessness, or confusion occur, withhold medication and notify health care provider.

Patient/Family Education
- Instruct patient to take medication exactly as prescribed and not to increase dosage unless advised by health care provider.
- Advise patient to take sips of water frequently, suck on ice chips or sugarless hard candy, or chew sugarless gum if dry mouth occurs.
- Instruct patient to report excessive dryness of mouth, constipation, or prolonged insomnia as dosage may need to be adjusted.
- Tell patient to avoid caffeine, which increases drug effect.
- Advise patient that drug may cause dizziness and to use caution while driving or performing other tasks requiring mental alertness or coordination.
- Instruct patient not to take OTC medications without consulting health care provider.
- Tell parents to report decreased appetite to pediatrician.

Methazolamide

(meth-ah-ZOLE-ah-mide)

Class Carbonic anhydrase inhibitor

How Supplied
Methazolamide Tablets 25 mg, Tablets 50 mg

Action
PHARMACOLOGY: Inhibits carbonic anhydrase enzyme, reducing rate of aqueous humor secretion and, thus, lowering IOP.

PHARMACOKINETICS/DYNAMICS:
Absorption: Well absorbed from the GI tract, reaching peak plasma levels in 1 to 2 hr. The C_{max} for the 25, 50, and 100 mg bid dosing regiments are 2.5, 5.1, and 10.7 mcg/mL, respectively. The AUCs are 1130, 2571, and 5418 mcg•min/mL, respectively.

Distribution: Methazolamide is distributed throughout the body including plasma, cerebrospinal fluid, aqueous humor, RBC, bile, and extracellular fluid. The Vd ranges from 17 to 23 L. Approximately 55% is bound to plasma proteins.

Excretion: Mean steady-state plasma elimination t½ is about 14 hr. Approximately 25% is recovered unchanged in the urine over the dosing interval and renal Cl accounts for 20% to 25% of the total Cl.

Onset: Decrease in IOP usually occurs in 2 to 4 hr.

Peak: About 6 to 8 hr.

Duration: About 10 to 18 hr.

Indications Treatment of ocular conditions where lowering IOP is likely to be of therapeutic benefit (eg, chronic open-angle glaucoma, secondary glaucoma, preoperatively in acute angle-closure glaucoma).

Contraindications Situations in which sodium and/or potassium serum levels are depressed; in cases of marked kidney or liver disease or dysfunction, in adrenal gland failure, and in hyperchloremic acidosis; in patients with cirrhosis (may precipitate hepatic encephalopathy); long-term administration in patients with angle-closure glaucoma.

Route/Dosage
ADULTS: PO 50 to 100 mg bid or tid.

Interactions
Aspirin (high-dose): Anorexia, tachypnea, lethargy, coma, and death have been reported.
Steroids: Use with caution because of risk of developing hypokalemia.

Lab Test Interferences None well documented.

Adverse Reactions
CNS: Paresthesias; malaise; drowsiness; confusion; loss of appetite; convulsions.
DERM: Urticaria; Stevens-Johnson syndrome; toxic epidermal necrolysis.
EENT: Hearing dysfunction; tinnitus; transient myopia.
ELECDIST: Electrolyte imbalance.
GI: Taste alteration; GI disturbance (including nausea, vomiting, diarrhea); melena.
GU: Polyuria; hematuria; glucosuria; crystalluria; renal calculi.
HEMA: Agranulocytosis; aplastic anemia; other blood dyscrasias.
HEPA: Hepatic insufficiency; fulminant hepatic necrosis.
METAB: Metabolic acidosis.
MUSC: Flaccid paralysis.
OTHER: Photosensitivity.

Precautions
Pregnancy: Category C.
Lactation: Undetermined.
Children: Safety and efficacy not established.
Hypersensitivity: Patients with known sulfonamide sensitivity may show allergic reactions to methazolamide.
Hepatic function impairment: Use could precipitate hepatic coma.
Pulmonary conditions: Use in pulmonary obstruction and emphysema may aggravate or precipitate acidosis.

Methenamine and Methenamine Salts

(meh-THEN-uh-meen and meh-THEN-uh-meen salts)

Class Urinary anti-infective

How Supplied
Methenamine Hippurate
Hiprex Tablets 1 g ♦ Urex Tablets 1 g

Methenamine Mandelate
Mandameth Tablets 0.5 mg, Tablets, enteric-coated 1 g ♦ Mandelamine Tablets 0.5 g, Tablets 1 g

Action
PHARMACOLOGY: In acidic urine, methenamine is hydrolyzed to ammonia and formaldehyde, which is bactericidal to certain bacteria in urine. Acid salts (methenamine mandelate and hippurate) have some nonspecific bacteriostatic activity and help to maintain low urine pH.

Pharmacokinetics/Dynamics:

Absorption: Methenamine absorbtion is rapid (30% to 60% hydrolized by gastric acid if not enteric-coated). T_{max} of urinary formaldehyde concentrations are 0.5 to 1.5 hr for methenamine, 2 hr for methenamine hippurate, and 3 to 8 hr for methenamine mandalate.

Distribution: Methenamine is freely distributed to body tissues and fluids. Vd is approximately 0.56 L/kg.

Metabolism: Methenamine is metabolized in the liver (approximately 10 to 25%) and through hydroysis in acidic urine (pH at least 5.5) to ammonia and formaldehyde.

Excretion: Methenamine is eliminated renally via glomerular filtration and tubular secretion. The t½ is 3 to 6 hr.

Indications Suppression or elimination of bacteriuria associated with pyelonephritis, cystitis and other chronic UITs; treatment of infected residual urine, sometimes accompanying neurologic disease or diabetes.

Contraindications Renal insufficiency; severe dehydration; severe hepatic insufficiency with hyperammonemia; acute UTIs involving renal parenchyma.

Route/Dosage

Methenamine Hippurate
ADULTS AND CHILDREN (OLDER THAN 12 YR): PO 1 g bid.
CHILDREN (6 TO 12 YR): PO 500 mg to 1 g bid.

Methenamine Mandelate
ADULTS: PO 1 g qid after meals and at bedtime.
CHILDREN (6 TO 12 YR): PO 500 mg qid.
CHILDREN (YOUNGER THAN 6 YR): PO 250 mg for q 30 lb body weight qid (18.4 mg/kg qid).

Interactions

Sulfonamides: May increase chance of crystalluria.

Urine alkalizers (acetazolamide, sodium bicarbonate, carbonate): Prevents hydrolysis of methenamine to formaldehyde with possible decrease in antimicrobial action.

Lab Test Interferences Methenamine may interfere with laboratory urine determinations of 17-hydroxycorticosteroids, catecholamines and vanillylmandelic acid (false increases) and 5-hydroxyindoleacetic acid (false decrease). Taken during pregnancy, can interfere with laboratory tests for urine estriol (false decrease) when acid hydrolysis procedure is used; use enzymatic hydrolysis procedure.

Adverse Reactions

CNS: Headache.
DERM: Pruritus; urticaria; erythematous eruptions; rash.
GI: Nausea; vomiting; cramps; diarrhea; stomatitis; anorexia.
GU: Bladder irritation; dysuria; proteinuria; hematuria; frequency; urgency; crystalluria.
HEMA: Serum transaminase elevation.
RESP: Dyspnea.
OTHER: Generalized edema.

Precautions

Pregnancy: Category C.
Lactation: Undetermined.
Special risk patients: Use with caution to avoid inducing lipoid pneumonia in debilitated patients and patients with swallowing difficulty.
Tartrazine sensitivity: Some products contain tartrazine, which may cause rash or bronchial asthma in susceptible patients.
Acid urine: If acidification of urine cannot be obtained or is contraindicated, drug is not recommended.
Gout: May cause precipitation of urate crystals in urine.
Lipoid pneumonia: Methenamine mandelate oral suspension is vegetable oil-based; aspiration could result in lipoid pneumonitis.

PATIENT CARE CONSIDERATIONS

Administration/Storage

- Administer after meals and at bedtime to minimize GI distress.
- Reconstitute granules by dissolving 1 packet (500 mg to 1 g) in 60 to 120 mL of water immediately before use. Solution may be cloudy.
- Urinary acidification using ascorbic acid to maintain low pH may be necessary.
- Store at room temperature (59° to 86°F) in tightly closed container. Protect from excessive heat.

Assessment/Interventions

- Obtain patient history, including drug history and any known allergies.
- Obtain clean-catch urine specimen for culture and sensitivity before beginning therapy.
- Monitor I&O, and watch for bladder irritation (eg, painful/frequent urination, proteinuria, hematuria); dose may need to be decreased if these symptoms occur. Fluid intake should be maintained at 1500 to 2000 mL/day (if medically acceptable).
- Monitor LFT results for transient increase in enzymes.
- Avoid concurrent use of sulfonamides (may cause precipitates), or any drugs that will alkalize urine.

Patient/Family Education

- Explain significance of adequate hydration.
- Tell patient to report the following symptoms to health care provider: painful urination,

skin rash, headache, swelling or severe stomach upset.
- Instruct patient to avoid use of milk products and antacids while taking drug to help keep urine acidic and allow drug to work better. Instruct patient to take vitamin C and drink cranberry or prune juice to acidify urine.
- Caution patient not to self-medicate with OTC medications containing sodium bicarbonate or sodium carbonate.
- Teach patient how to read dipstick tests for urine pH and specific gravity and to report to health care provider if required values are not attained.

Methimazole

(meth-IMM-uh-zole)
Class Antithyroid
How Supplied
Tapazole Tablets 5 mg, Tablets 10 mg
Action
PHARMACOLOGY: Inhibits synthesis of thyroid hormones.

PHARMACOKINETICS/DYNAMICS:
Absorption: Methimazole bioavailability is 80% to 95%.

Distribution: A high amount of methimazole is excreted in breast milk, has high transplacental passage, and is 0% protein bound.

Metabolism: Methimazole is rapidly metabolized.

Excretion: Less than 10% is excreted in urine. The t½ is 6 to 13 hr.

Indications Long-term therapy of hyperthyroidism; amelioration of hyperthyroidism in preparation for subtotal thyroidectomy or radioactive iodine therapy.

Contraindications Use in nursing women.

Route/Dosage
ADULTS:
Initial dose: **PO** 15 to 60 mg/day in 3 equal doses at approximately 8-hr intervals.
Maintenance: **PO** 5 to 15 mg/day.
CHILDREN:
Initial dose: **PO** 0.4 mg/kg/day.
Maintenance: **PO** Approximately ½ initial dose. Alternately, children may be given 0.5 to 0.7 mg/kg/day in 3 divided doses as initial therapy and ⅓ to ⅔ of initial dose for maintenance.

Interactions
Anticoagulants: May decrease or increase anticoagulant action.
Beta blockers: May increase effects of beta blockers, resulting in toxicity.
Digoxin: May cause increase in effects of digitalis glycosides, including toxicity.
Theophyllines: May alter theophylline clearance in hyperthyroid or hypothyroid patients.

Lab Test Interferences None well documented.

Adverse Reactions
CNS: Paresthesias; neuritis; headache; vertigo; drowsiness; neuropathies; CNS stimulation; depression.
DERM: Rash; urticaria; pruritus; erythema nodosum; skin pigmentation; exfoliative dermatitis; lupus-like syndrome including splenomegaly, hepatitis, periarteritis, hypoprothrombinemia and bleeding.
EENT: Loss of taste; sialadenopathy.
GI: Nausea; vomiting; epigastric distress.
GU: Nephritis.
HEPA: Jaundice; hepatitis.
HEMA: Inhibition of myelopoiesis (eg, agranulocytosis, granulocytopenia, thrombocytopenia); aplastic anemia; hypoprothrombinemia; periarteritis.
OTHER: Abnormal hair loss; arthralgia; myalgia; edema; lymphadenopathy; drug fever; interstitial pneumonitis; insulin autoimmune syndrome.

Precautions
Pregnancy: Category D.
Lactation: Avoid nursing.
Agranulocytosis: Potentially most serious side effect. Discontinue drug in presence of agranulocytosis, aplastic anemia, hepatitis, fever or exfoliative dermatitis.
Hemorrhage: May cause hypoprothrombinemia and bleeding. Monitor PT.

Overdosage: Signs and Symptoms
Nausea, vomiting, epigastric distress, headache, fever, arthralgia, pruritus, edema, pancytopenia, agranulocytosis, exfoliative dermatitis, hepatitis, neuropathies, CNS stimulation or depression.

PATIENT CARE CONSIDERATIONS

Administration/Storage
- Administer around clock in 3 equal doses (ie, q 8 hr).
- Administer each dose with same amount of food to facilitate uniform absorption.
- Store in light-resistant container at room temperature (59° to 86°F).

Assessment/Interventions
- Obtain patient history, including drug history and any known allergies.

- Assess for history of liver disease.
- Assess symptoms of hyperthyroidism that patient is experiencing.
- Obtain baseline vital signs and monitor during treatment.
- Obtain baseline hepatic blood work including bilirubin and liver enzymes.
- Obtain baseline CBC and monitor carefully during first 2 mo of treatment.
- Obtain baseline thyroid levels and monitor monthly initially and q 2 to 3 mo for long-term therapy.
- Monitor drug's effects on hyperthyroid symptoms.
- Monitor PT, especially before surgery, to assess increased risk of bleeding.
- Observe for potential adverse reactions including rash or fever, and notify health care provider if any occur.

Patient/Family Education
- Instruct patient in importance of taking proper dose exactly as scheduled.
- Advise patient not to stop, start or adjust dose of any medications, including OTC, without discussing with health care provider.
- Explain to patient the importance of complying with follow-up appointments and lab work.
- Instruct patient to check pulse daily.
- Advise patient that iodine-restrictive diet may be necessary.
- Inform patient that response to therapy may take months.
- Instruct patient to report the following symptoms to health care provider: rash, fever, sore throat, bruising or signs of infection or jaundice.
- Advise patient that drug may cause drowsiness and to use caution while driving or performing other tasks requiring mental alertness.

Methocarbamol

(meth-oh-CAR-buh-mahl)

Class Skeletal muscle relaxant, centrally acting

How Supplied
Robaxin Tablets 500 mg, Injection 100 mg/mL ♦ *Robaxin-750* Tablets 750 mg

Action
PHARMACOLOGY: May cause relaxation of skeletal muscle via general CNS depression. Does not directly relax tense skeletal muscles.
PHARMACOKINETICS/DYNAMICS:
Absorption: T_{max} is 2 hr.
Distribution: Methocarbamol protein binding is 46% to 50%.
Excretion: Inactive metabolites are excreted in urine and small amounts in feces. The t½ is 1 to 2 hr.
Onset: Onset is 30 min.
Special Populations:
Renal Function Impairment – Cl is decreased approximately 40% in patients with severe renal impairment.
Hepatic Function Impairment – Cl is decreased approximately 70%; t½ is prolonged to approximately 3.4 hr in cirrhosis patients.
Children – Safety and efficacy in children younger than 16 yr of age not established, except in tetanus.

Indications Adjunctive therapy for relief of painful, acute musculoskeletal conditions; control of neuromuscular manifestations of tetanus.

Contraindications Renal pathologic disorders (parenteral form); standard considerations.

Route/Dosage
Skeletal Muscle Relaxation
ADULTS:
Initial dose: **IV/IM** 3 g over no more than 3 consecutive days. Repeat course after 48-hr lapse if condition persists. **PO** 1.5 g qid.
Maintenance: **PO** 1 g qid, 750 mg q 4 hr, or 1.5 g tid. For first 48 to 72 hr, 6 to 8 g/day is recommended; then reduce to 4 g/day.

Tetanus
ADULTS: **IV** 1 to 2 g; additional 1 to 2 g may be added to infusion up to 3 g total. Repeat q 6 hr until oral form may be administered.
CHILDREN: **IV/IV infusion** 15 mg/kg initially; then 15 mg/kg q 6 hr.

Interactions
Alcohol, CNS depressants: CNS depressant effects may be additive.
Anticholinesterase agents (eg, pyridostigmine): Because effects may be inhibited by methocarbamol, use with caution in patients with myasthenia gravis who are receiving anticholinergic agents.

Lab Test Interferences
Screening tests for 5-hydroxy-indoleacetic acid or vanillylmandelic acid: Drug may cause color interference.

Adverse Reactions
CV: Bradycardia; hypotension; syncope; thrombophlebitis.
CNS: Headache; amnesia; confusion; dizziness/lightheadedness; drowsiness; insomnia; mild muscular incoordination; sedation; seizures (including grand mal); vertigo.
DERM: Flushing; pruritus; rash; urticaria.

EENT: Diplopia; nystagmus; blurred vision; conjunctivitis; nasal congestion.
GI: Dyspepsia; nausea; vomiting; metallic taste.
HEMA: Leukopenia.
HEPA: Jaundice (including cholestatic jaundice).
OTHER: Hypersensitivity reactions, anaphylactic reactions; angioneurotic edema; fever.

Precautions
Pregnancy: Category C.
Lactation: Undetermined.
Children: Safety and efficacy in children younger than 16 yr of age not established, except for management of tetanus.

Overdosage: Signs and Symptoms
Frequently occurs in conjunction with alcohol or other CNS depressants and includes nausea, drowsiness, blurred vision, hypotension, seizures, and coma.

PATIENT CARE CONSIDERATIONS

Administration/Storage
Tablets:
- Administer prescribed dose without regard to meals but administer with food if GI upset occurs.
- Tablets may be crushed and suspended in water or saline for administration through nasogastric tube.
- Store tablets at controlled room temperature (68° to 77°F).

Injection:
- For IV or IM administration only. Not for intradermal, subcutaneous, or intra-arterial administration.
- Administer direct IV injection of undiluted methocarbamol at max rate of 3 mL/min.
- For IV infusion dilute prescribed dose in no more than 250 mL of sodium chloride injection or 5% dextrose injection.
- Use diluted solution as soon as possible. Do not refrigerate diluted solution for IV administration.
- Administer prescribed IM dose by deep, slow injection into gluteal region. Do not inject more than 5 mL at 1 site. Rotate injection sites.
- Do not administer injection if particulate matter, cloudiness, or discoloration noted.
- Store vials for injection at controlled room temperature (68° to 77°F).

Assessment/Interventions
- Obtain patient history, including drug history and any known allergies. Note hepatic or renal impairment or seizure disorder (injection only).
- Assess MUSC symptoms before starting therapy and periodically during treatment. Notify health care provider if condition does not appear to be improving or is worsening.
- Ensure that therapy is periodically reviewed to determine if it needs to be continued without change or if a dose change (eg, increase, decrease, discontinuation) is indicated.
- Monitor patient for CNS, GI, and general body side effects and injection site reaction. Report to health care provider if noted and significant.

Injection:
- Ensure that injectable methocarbamol is not administered to patient with known or suspected renal pathology.
- Ensure that patient is in recumbent position during and for 10 to 15 min following IV injection.
- Ensure that total dose does not exceed 3 g for more than 3 days, except in patient being treated for tetanus. The course of therapy can be repeated, if needed, after a lapse of 48 hr.
- Ensure that patient is converted to oral methocarbamol as soon as possible.

Patient/Family Education
- Explain name, dose, action, and potential side effects of drug.
- Advise patient or caregiver that injectable medication will be prepared and administered by a health care provider in a medical setting.
- Advise patient that medication will be most effective when combined with rest and prescribed physical therapy.
- Advise patient that dose may be adjusted periodically in order to achieve max benefit.
- Advise patient to take prescribed dose as needed for muscle spasm or limited mobility.
- Advise patient to take without regard to meals but to take with food if stomach upset occurs.
- Instruct patient to avoid alcoholic beverages and sedatives (eg, diazepam) while taking methocarbamol.
- Advise patient that medication may cause urine to turn a dark brown, black, or green and not to be concerned; this is expected and not harmful.
- Advise patient that drug may cause drowsiness or dizziness and to use caution while driving or performing other tasks requiring mental alertness until tolerance is determined.
- Advise patient to stop taking and notify health care provider if any of the following occur: allergic reaction, persistent dizziness, excessive sedation.

- Advise women to notify health care provider if pregnant, planning to become pregnant, or breastfeeding.
- Instruct patient not to take any prescription or OTC drugs, dietary supplements, or herbal preparations unless advised by health care provider.
- Advise patient that follow-up visits may be necessary to monitor therapy and to keep appointments.

Methocarbamol/Aspirin

(Meth-oh-CAR-buh-mahl/ASS-pihr-in)
Class Skeletal muscle relaxant/Analgesic

How Supplied
Robaxisal Tablets 400 mg methocarbamol and 325 mg aspirin

Action
PHARMACOLOGY: May cause relaxation of skeletal muscle via general CNS depression. Aspirin: Inhibits prostaglandin synthesis, resulting in analgesia, anti-inflammatory activity, and inhibition of platelet aggregation.

Indications Adjunct to rest, physical therapy, and other measures for the relief of discomfort associated with acute, painful, musculoskeletal conditions.

Contraindications Hypersensitivity to methocarbamol, aspirin, related compounds, or any component of the product.

Route/Dosage
ADULTS: PO 2 tablets qid, or 3 tablets qid in severe conditions for 1 to 3 days.

Interactions
Alcohol, CNS drugs: Effects may be additive, increasing the amount of CNS depression.
Anticoagulants (eg, warfarin), antidiabetic agents, mercaptopurine, methotrexate, NSAIDs: The pharmacologic or adverse effects of these agents may be increased by aspirin.
Corticosteroids: May increase the renal Cl of aspirin; be prepared for possible increased levels of aspirin if corticosteroid therapy is stopped.
Pyridostigmine: Therapeutic effects may be inhibited by methocarbamol.
Uricosuric agents (eg, probenecid, sulfinpyrazone): The effects may be decreased by aspirin.

Lab Test Interferences Methocarbamol may cause a color interference in certain screening tests for 5-hydroxyindoleacetic acid using nitroso naphthol reagent and in screening tests for urinary vanillylmandelic acid using the Gitlow method. Aspirin may interfere with the following laboratory determinations in blood: serum amylase, fasting blood glucose, cholesterol, protein, serum glutamic-oxaloacetic transaminase, uric acid, prothrombin time, and bleeding time. Aspirin may interfere with the following laboratory determinations in urine: glucose, 5 hydroxyindoloacetic acid, Gerhardt ketone, vanillylmandelic acid, uric acid, diacetic acid and spectrophotometric detection of barbiturates.

Adverse Reactions
CV:
Methocarbamol – Bradycardia; flushing; hypotension; syncope.
CNS:
Methocarbamol – Headache; amnesia; confusion; diplopia; dizziness; lightheadedness; drowsiness; insomnia; mild muscular incoordination; seizures (including grand mal); vertigo.
DERM: Pruritus; urticaria; rash.
EENT:
Methocarbamol – Nystagmus; blurred vision; conjunctivitis with nasal congestion; metallic taste.
GI:
Methocarbamol – Dyspepsia; nausea; vomiting.
Aspirin – Nausea; GI discomfort; gastritis; gastric erosion; vomiting; constipation; diarrhea.
HEMA:
Methocarbamol – Leukopenia.
HEPA:
Methocarbamol – Jaundice (including cholestatic jaundice).
RESP:
Aspirin – Asthma.
OTHER:
Methocarbamol – Anaphylactic reaction; fever.
Aspirin – Angioedema; anaphylactic shock and other severe allergic reactions.

Precautions
Pregnancy: Category C.
Lactation: Undetermined.
Children: Safety and efficacy not established. Reye syndrome has been associated with aspirin administration in children (including teenagers) with acute febrile illness.
Special risk patients: Administer with caution to patients with gastritis, peptic ulceration, asthma, coagulation abnormalities, hypoprothrombinemia, vitamin K deficiency, or those who are receiving anticoagulant therapy.
CNS depressant effects: Caution about combined effects with alcohol or other CNS depressants.

Overdosage: Signs and Symptoms
Methocarbamol: Coma, CNS depression, nausea, drowsiness, blurred vision, hypotension, seizures.
Aspirin: CV and respiratory insufficiency, hyperthermia, dehydration, respiratory alkalosis, metabolic acidosis, death.

PATIENT CARE CONSIDERATIONS

Administration/Storage
- Administer 2 tablets as prescribed, up to qid if needed.
- Administer without regard to meals but administer with food if GI upset occurs.
- Store at controlled room temperature (68° to 77°F).

Assessment/Interventions
- Obtain patient history, including drug history and any known allergies. Note history of bleeding or coagulation disorders, hepatic or renal impairment, peptic ulcer or other serious GI lesions, or the syndrome of nasal polyps, rhinitis, and bronchospastic reactivity to aspirin or other NSAIDs.
- Assess musculoskeletal symptoms before starting therapy and periodically during treatment.
- Monitor patient for CNS, GI, and general body side effects. Report to health care provider if noted and significant.
- Discontinue therapy and notify health care provider immediately if any of the following occur: allergic reaction, unusual bleeding or bruising, shortness of breath, black or tarry stools, vomiting of blood or coffee ground-like material.

Patient/Family Education
- Explain name, dose, action, and potential side effects of drug.
- Advise patient to take 2 tablets as prescribed, up to qid if needed for muscle pain, muscle spasm, or limited mobility.
- Advise patient to take without regard to meals but to take with food if GI upset occurs.
- Instruct patient to avoid alcoholic beverages and other depressants while taking this medication.
- Advise patient that drug may cause drowsiness or dizziness and to use caution while driving or performing other tasks requiring mental alertness until tolerance is determined.
- Advise patient to stop taking the drug and notify health care provider if any of the following occur: allergic reaction, unusual bleeding or bruising, shortness of breath, black or tarry stools, vomiting of blood or coffee ground-like material, or excessive sedation.
- Advise women to notify health care provider if pregnant, planning to become pregnant, or breastfeeding.
- Warn patient not to take any prescription or OTC drugs or dietary supplements without consulting health care provider.
- Advise patient that follow-up visits may be necessary to monitor therapy and to keep appointments.

Methotrexate (MTX)

(meth-oh-TREK-sate)

Class Antineoplastic/Antimetabolite/Antipsoriatic/Antiarthritic

How Supplied
Methotrexate LPF *Sodium* Injection 25 mg/mL ◆ Methotrexate *Sodium* Injection 25 mg/mL ◆ Methotrexate *Sodium* Powder for injection 20 mg, Powder for injection 1 g ◆ *Rheumatrex Dose Pack* Tablets 2.5 mg ◆ *Trexall* Tablets 5 mg, Tablets 7.5 mg, Tablets 10 mg, Tablets 15 mg
✤ ratio-Methotrexate

Action
PHARMACOLOGY: Competitively inhibits dihydrofolic acid reductase and thereby inhibits DNA synthesis and cellular replication. In rheumatoid arthritis, believed to reduce immune function.

PHARMACOKINETICS/DYNAMICS:

Absorption: Oral absorption is dose dependent. T_{max} is 1 to 2 hr (oral) and 30 to 60 min (IM). The mean bioavailability is 60%. Absorption of doses more than 80 mg/m^2 is significantly less, possibly because of a saturation effect. Food delays absorption and reduces peak concentration.

Distribution: Initial Vd is 0.18 L/kg (18% of body weight); steady state Vd is approximately 0.4 to 0.8 L/kg (40% to 80% of body weight). Approximately 50% is protein bound. Methotrexate does not penetrate the blood-cerebrospinal fluid barrier in therapeutic amounts when given orally or parenterally, but it has been detected in breast milk.

Metabolism: Methotrexate undergoes hepatic and intracellular metabolism to active polyglutamated forms and is partially metabolized by intestinal flora after oral administration. Major metabolite is 7-hydroxymethotrexate.

Excretion: Renal excretion is the primary route of elimination and is dependent upon dosage and route of administration. With IV administration, 80% to 90% is excreted unchanged in urine within 24 hr and less than 10% through biliary excretion. The t½ for doses less than 30 mg/m^2 is approximately 3 to 10 hr; 8 to 15 hr for high doses.

Special Populations:
Renal Function Impairment – An increase in serum levels occurs because of decreased elimination in patients with renal impairment.

Indications Antineoplastic chemotherapy for treatment of gestational choriocarcinoma, chorioadenoma destruens, hydatidiform mole; treatment and prophylaxis of acute (meningeal) lymphocytic leukemia; treatment of breast cancer, epidermoid cancers of head and neck, advanced mycosis fungoides, and lung cancer; in combination therapy with advanced-stage non-Hodgkin lymphoma; as adjunct in high doses followed by leucovorin rescue in nonmetastatic osteosarcoma (postsurgically); symptomatic control of severe psoriasis and severe rheumatoid arthritis; polyarticular-course juvenile rheumatoid arthritis (JRA).

Contraindications Use in nursing mothers. In patients with psoriasis or rheumatoid arthritis, methotrexate is contraindicated in pregnancy, alcoholism, alcoholic liver disease, chronic liver disease, overt or laboratory evidence of immunodeficiency syndrome, and preexisting blood dyscrasias (eg, leukopenia, thrombocytopenia); hypersensitivity to the drug.

Route/Dosage

Choriocarcinoma and Thromboplastic Diseases
ADULTS: **PO/IM** 15 to 30 mg for 5 days. Repeat courses 3 to 5 times as required, with rest periods of more than 1 wk between courses.

Leukemia
ADULTS AND CHILDREN:
Induction: **PO/IM** 3.3 mg/m^2/day in combination with prednisone 60 mg/m^2/day usually for 4 to 6 wk.
Postremission maintenance therapy (usually in combination with other drugs): **PO/IM** 2 times/wk in total weekly doses of 30 mg/m^2 or **IV** 2.5 mg/kg q 14 days.

Lymphoma (Burkitt Lymphoma, Stages 1 and 2)
ADULTS: **PO** 10 to 25 mg/day for 4 to 8 days. Provide 7- to 10-day rest period between courses.

Meningeal Leukemia
ADULTS: **Intrathecal** 12 mg/m^2 (max, 15 mg). Administer q 2 to 5 days until cell count of CSF returns to normal, then give 1 additional dose.

Dose reduction may be required in elderly patients because of differences in CSF volume.
CHILDREN AT LEAST 3 YR OF AGE: **Intrathecal** 12 mg. Administer q 2 to 5 days until CSF cell count returns to normal.
CHILDREN 2 YR OF AGE: **Intrathecal** 10 mg.
CHILDREN 1 YR OF AGE: **Intrathecal** 8 mg.
CHILDREN YOUNGER THAN 1 YR OF AGE: **Intrathecal** 6 mg.

Mycosis Fungoides
ADULTS: Dosage in early stages is usually 5 to 50 mg/wk. In patients responding poorly to weekly therapy, methotrexate has also been administered as 15 to 37.5 mg twice weekly. Combination chemotherapy regimens that include IV methotrexate at higher doses (with leucovorin rescue) have been used in advanced stages of the disease.

Osteosarcoma
Complex high dose with leucovorin rescue and other chemotherapeutic agents. Starting dose for high-dose methotrexate is 12 g/m^2.

Polyarticular-Course JRA
PO start with 10 mg/m^2/wk.

Psoriasis
Individualize dosage. Administer 5 to 10 mg parenteral test dose 1 wk prior to therapy.
ADULTS: **IM/IV/PO** 10 to 25 mg/wk (max, 30 mg/wk).
ADULTS: **PO** 2.5 mg q 12 hr for 3 doses every wk (max, 30 mg/wk).

Rheumatoid Arthritis
ADULTS:
Initial therapy: **PO** 7.5 mg/wk in single dose or 2.5 mg q 12 hr for 3 doses each wk. Gradually adjust dosage to max response; do not exceed 20 mg/wk.

Stage 3 Lymphosarcoma As Part of Combination Therapy
ADULTS: **PO** 0.625 to 2.5 mg/kg/day.

Interactions
Acitretin, etretinate, NSAIDs, penicillins, probenecid, salicylates, sulfonamides, tetracyclines: May increase methotrexate blood levels and toxicity.
Antibiotics (oral) such as chloramphenicol, nonabsorbable broad spectrum antibiotics (eg, neomycin), and tetracycline: May decrease intestinal absorption of methotrexate or interfere with enterohepatic circulation.

Charcoal: May reduce methotrexate efficacy.
Digoxin: May reduce serum digoxin levels and actions.
Folic acid: May decrease responses to systemically administered methotrexate.
Hydantoins: May reduce plasma levels.
Mercaptopurine: Plasma concentrations may be increased by methotrexate.
Theophylline: Methotrexate decreases Cl of theophylline.
Trimethoprim: May increase risk of methotrexate-induced bone marrow suppression and megaloblastic anemia.

Lab Test Interferences None well documented.

Adverse Reactions

CNS: Dizziness (1% to 3%); fatigue; headache; aphasia; hemiparesis; paresis; convulsions; leukoencephalopathy (IV after craniospinal irradiation); chemical arachnoiditis; transient paresis; neurotoxicity.

DERM: Erythematous rashes, pruritus, alopecia (1% to 3%); urticaria; photosensitivity; pigmentary changes; ecchymosis; telangiectasia; acne; furunculosis; aggravation of psoriasis by ultraviolet light; Stevens-Johnson syndrome.

EENT: Blurred vision; ulcerative stomatitis; gingivitis; pharyngitis.

GI: Nausea, vomiting (10%); enteritis, stomatitis (3% to 10%); diarrhea (1% to 3%); abdominal distress (common); anorexia; hematemesis; melena; GI ulceration and bleeding.

GU: Renal failure; azotemia; cystitis; hematuria; severe nephropathy; reproductive disorders; infertility; abortion; fetal defects.

HEMA: Thrombocytopenia (3% to 10%); leukopenia, pancytopenia (1% to 3%); bone marrow depression; anemia; hypogammaglobulinemia; hemorrhage; septicemia.

HEPA: Elevated LFTs (15%); hepatotoxicity; hepatic cirrhosis and fibrosis.

RESP: Deaths from interstitial pneumonitis; chronic interstitial obstructive pulmonary disease.

OTHER: Malaise; chills; fever; lower resistance to infections; arthralgia; myalgia; diabetes; osteoporosis; anaphylactoid reaction; sudden death.

> **WARNING:**
> *Deaths:* Deaths have occurred.
> *Rheumatoid arthritis treatment:* Restrict use to patients with severe, recalcitrant, disabling disease not adequately responsive to other forms of therapy.
> *Pregnancy:* Fetal death or congenital anomalies have occurred.
> *Periodic monitoring:* Periodically monitor for toxicity, including CBC with differential and platelet counts and liver and renal function.
> *Liver:* Methotrexate may cause hepatotoxicity, fibrosis, and cirrhosis.
> *Lung disease:* Lung disease, a potentially dangerous lesion, may occur any time during therapy.
> *Severe reactions:* Unexpectedly severe and sometimes fatal marrow suppression, aplastic anemia, and GI toxicity have been reported with coadministration of NSAIDs.
> *Renal impairment:* Use with caution because methotrexate elimination will be prolonged.
> *Skin reactions:* Severe and occasionally fatal skin reactions have been reported.
> *Opportunistic infections:* Potentially fatal opportunistic infections may occur.
> *Radiotherapy:* The risk of soft tissue necrosis and osteonecrosis may be increased by concurrent radiotherapy.
> *GI:* Death from intestinal perforation may occur. Diarrhea and ulcerative stomatitis require interruption of therapy.
> *Diluents:* Do not use methotrexate formulations and diluents containing preservatives for intrathecal or experimental high-dose methotrexate therapy.
> *Malignant lymphomas:* Malignant lymphomas, which may regress following discontinuation of methotrexate, may occur.
> *Tumor lysis syndrome:* May occur in patients with rapidly growing tumors.

Precautions
Pregnancy: Category X (for rheumatoid arthritis and psoriasis); Category D (other uses).
Lactation: Contraindicated in nursing mothers.
Children: Safety and efficacy not established other than for cancer treatment and polyarticular-course JRA.
Elderly: Use with caution because of the greater frequency of decreased hepatic, renal, or cardiac function, and concomitant diseases or other drug therapy.
Renal function impairment: Determine renal status before and during therapy.
Infection: Severe reactions may occur if live vaccines are administered.
Intrathecal therapy: Large doses may cause convulsions and systemic toxicity. Dosage regimens based on age may be more effective and associated with fewer neurotoxic side effects.
GI toxicity: Use with caution in presence of peptic ulcer disease or ulcerative colitis. Vomiting, diarrhea, or stomatitis may lead to dehydration.

Hematologic toxicity: Suppression of hematopoiesis, which may cause anemia, aplastic anemia, pancytopenia, leukopenia, neutropenia, and thrombocytopenia, may occur.
Hepatic toxicity: Acute and chronic hepatotoxicity, which may be fatal, may occur.
Pulmonary symptoms: Pulmonary symptoms (eg, dry nonproductive cough) or a nonspecific pneumonitis may be indicative of a potentially dangerous lesion, requiring interruption of treatment.
Renal damage: Renal damage, leading to acute renal failure, may occur.
Severe effects: Potential toxicities include bone marrow depression, hepatotoxicity, lung disease (suggested by symptoms of dry, nonproductive cough), nephrotoxicity, and GI toxicity.

Overdosage: Signs and Symptoms
Hepatotoxicity, nephrotoxicity, GI toxicity, bone marrow toxicity, pulmonary toxicity.
Intrathecal: Headache, nausea, vomiting, seizure or convulsion, acute toxic encephalopathy.

PATIENT CARE CONSIDERATIONS
Administration/Storage
- Dose, route, and duration of therapy are dependent on condition being treated.
- Use alone or in combination with other medications for condition being treated.
- Store tablets, injection, and powder for injection at controlled room temperature (59° to 86°F). Protect from light.

Oral:
- Administer prescribed dose without regard to meals. Administer with food if GI upset occurs.

Injection:
- Follow institutional procedures for proper handling and disposal of anticancer drugs. Wear gloves and avoid skin exposure and inhalation of fumes.
- Ensure that leucovorin is available before beginning high-dose methotrexate therapy.
- Preservative-free methotrexate may be administered IM, IV, intra-arterially, or intrathecally.
- Do not administer preserved formulation in high-dose therapy or intrathecally.
- Reconstitute immediately prior to use.
- For intrathecal use, reconstitute immediately prior to administration using preservative-free diluent (eg, 0.9% sodium chloride injection).
- Follow manufacturer's guidelines for reconstitution and dilution of powder for injection and dilution of isotonic injection.
- Do not administer if solution is discolored or cloudy, or if particulate matter is noted.

Assessment/Interventions
- Obtain patient history, including drug history and any known allergies. Note impaired renal function, pleural effusion, ascites, active infection, or immunodeficiency syndrome. Note history of peptic ulcer disease or ulcerative colitis.
- Review patient's health history for any condition that could contraindicate methotrexate therapy (eg, pregnancy, breastfeeding, alcoholism, alcoholic liver disease or other chronic liver disease, immunodeficiency syndrome, preexisting blood dyscrasia).
- Ensure that CBC with differential and platelet count, kidney and liver function, and chest X-ray are evaluated prior to starting and periodically during therapy. Frequency is determined by condition being treated and individual patient characteristics.
- Determine need for baseline and follow-up pulmonary function tests and liver biopsies.
- When administering methotrexate therapy with leucovorin rescue, carefully follow manufacturer's guidelines regarding laboratory monitoring, evaluation of renal function, hydration, urinary alkalization, and leucovorin dosing.
- Ensure that women of childbearing potential are not pregnant when therapy is started and use effective contraception during and for at least 1 ovulatory cycle after therapy is completed.

- Ensure that female partner of male patient is not pregnant when therapy is started and uses effective contraception during and for at least 3 mo after therapy has been completed by her partner.
- Be prepared to discontinue therapy and implement infection control measures if WBC drops.
- Be prepared to discontinue therapy and implement bleeding precautions if platelet count drops.
- Be prepared to discontinue therapy if severe vomiting, diarrhea, or stomatitis develops.
- Monitor patient for CNS, GI, and general body side effects. Report to health care provider if noted and significant. Immediately report any of the following: dry, nonproductive cough, or difficulty breathing; diarrhea; sores in mouth; fever; sore throat; or other signs of infection; rash or other skin reaction; bleeding or unusual bruising; jaundice; edema.
- Do not administer live virus vaccines while patient is on therapy.

Patient/Family Education

- Explain name, action, and potential side effects of drug.
- Advise patient, family, or caregiver of patient receiving parenteral or intrathecal methotrexate that medication will be prepared and administered by a health care provider in a medical setting.
- Review dose and appropriate dosing schedule, depending on condition being treated (eg, rheumatoid arthritis, psoriasis, neoplastic disease). Instruct patient to take medication exactly as prescribed and not to stop taking or change the dose unless advised by health care provider.
- Reinforce to patient taking methotrexate for rheumatoid arthritis or psoriasis that prescribed dose is taken once weekly, on the same day each week, and that taking more frequently can cause serious toxicity.
- Advise patient that medication can be taken without regard to meals but to take with food if stomach upset occurs.
- Caution patient to avoid using alcohol while taking methotrexate.
- Caution patient to avoid taking aspirin and other NSAIDs (eg, ibuprofen) while taking methotrexate unless advised by health care provider.
- Caution patient to avoid unnecessary exposure to UV light (sunlight, tanning booths) and to use sunscreen and wear protective clothing to avoid photosensitivity reaction.
- Advise patient that drug may cause drowsiness or dizziness and to use caution while driving or performing other tasks requiring mental alertness or coordination until tolerance is determined.
- Advise patient with rheumatoid arthritis that dose of medication may be changed based on tolerance and response and that therapy for up to at least 12 wk may be required before max benefit is noted.
- Advise patient with rheumatoid arthritis or psoriasis to continue to take other arthritis or psoriasis medications as prescribed by health care provider.
- Instruct patient to immediately report any of the following to health care provider: cough; difficulty breathing; diarrhea; stomach pain; sores in or around the mouth; fever, sore throat, or other signs of infection; rash or other skin reaction; bleeding or unusual bruising; yellow discoloration of skin or eyes; swelling of legs or feet.
- Advise patient to contact health care provider if medication does not control lesions and/or symptoms or if intolerable side effects develop.
- Advise women of childbearing potential to use effective contraception during and for at least 1 ovulatory cycle after therapy is completed.
- Advise women to notify health care provider if pregnant, planning to become pregnant, or breastfeeding.
- Advise female partner of male patient to use effective contraception during and for at least 3 mo after therapy has been completed by her partner.
- Instruct patient not to take any prescription or OTC medications, herbal preparations, or dietary supplements unless advised by health care provider. Folic acid, an ingredient in some OTC products, can reduce methotrexate efficacy.
- Advise patient that follow-up visits and lab tests will be necessary to monitor therapy and to keep appointments.

Methoxsalen

(meth-OX-ah-len)

Class Psoralen

How Supplied
8-MOP Capsules 10 mg ♦ Oxsoralen-Ultra Capsules, soft gelatin 10 mg ♦ Oxsoralen Lotion 1% (10 mg/mL) ♦ Uvadex Solution 20 mcg/mL

Action

PHARMACOLOGY: Exact mechanism not known; however, methoxsalen acts as a photosensitizer.

PHARMACOKINETICS/DYNAMICS:
Absorption:
8-MOP – Max bioavailability is reached 1.5 to 3 hr after oral administration and lasts up to 8 hr.
Oxsoralen-Ultra – Reaches peak blood drug levels in 0.5 to 4 hr, and detectable levels are observed up to 12 hr.
Distribution: Methoxsalen is reversibly bound to serum albumin and preferentially taken up by epidermal cells.
Metabolism: Methoxsalen is rapidly metabolized.
Excretion: Approximately 95% is excreted as a series of metabolites in the urine within 24 hr.
Oxsoralen-Ultra – The t½ is approximately 2 hr.
Duration:
Oxsoralen-Ultra – Time of peak photosensitivity is 1.5 to 2.1 hr.

Indications Symptomatic control of severe, recalcitrant, disabling psoriasis not responsive to other forms of therapy and when diagnosis supported by biopsy (*Oxsoralen-Ultra*, 8-MOP capsule); use in conjunction with long wave UV radiation for repigmentation of idiopathic vitiligo (8-MOP capsule, *Oxsoralen* lotion); with long wave UV radiation of white blood cells (photopheresis) with the UVAR Photopheresis System in the palliative treatment of skin manifestations of cutaneous T-cell lymphoma in people not responsive to other forms of treatment (8-MOP capsule, *Oxsoralen* lotion); extracorporeal administration with UVAR Photopheresis System in the palliative treatment of skin manifestation of cutaneous T-cell lymphoma that is unresponsive to other forms of treatment (*Uvadex* solution).

Contraindications Patients exhibiting idiosyncratic reactions to psoralen compounds; specific history of light-sensitive disease states should not initiate methoxsalen therapy (eg, lupus erythematosus, porphyria cutanea tarda, erythropoietic protoporphyria, variegate porphyria, xeroderma pigmentosum, albinism); patients exhibiting melanoma or possessing a history of melanoma; patients exhibiting invasive squamous cell carcinomas; patients with aphakia, because of increased risk of retinal damage caused by absence of lenses.

Route/Dosage
Vitiligo
ADULTS:
8-MOP: PO Take 20 mg daily in 1 dose with milk or food 2 to 4 hr prior to UV exposure. Take on alternate days and never on 2 consecutive days. Sun exposure is based on basic skin color. Initial sun exposure should be 15 min for light skin, 20 min for medium-colored skin, and 25 min for dark skin. The second, third, and fourth exposures may be increased by 5 min/each exposure (if basic skin color is light, the second exposure can be increased to 20 min, the third exposure to 25 min, and the fourth exposure to 30 min). Subsequent exposures may gradually be increased based on erythema and tenderness of amelanotic skin (max, 0.6 mg/kg). Oxsoralen lotion: Apply lotion to a small, well-defined, vitiliginous lesion, then expose this area to UVA light. Initial exposure time must not exceed one half the minimal erythema dose. Regulate treatment intervals by erythema response (once weekly or less, depending on the results). Pigmentation may begin after a few weeks; significant repigmentation may take up to 6 to 9 mo. Periodic treatment may be needed to retain the new pigmentation.

Psoriasis
ADULTS: *Oxsoralen-Ultra*: PO Take with food or milk 1.5 to 2 hr prior to UVA exposure.
8-MOP: PO Take with food or milk 2 hr prior to UVA exposure. Take according to the following recommendations: Generally, elderly patients should be started at the low end of the dose recommended according to body weight and closely monitored during PUVA therapy. No treatments should be given more often than once every other day because the full extent of phototoxic reactions may not be evident until 48 hr after each exposure. Dosage may be increased by 10 mg after the fifteenth treatment. Patients weighing:

- Less than 30 kg take 10 mg
- 30 to 50 kg take 20 mg
- 51 to 65 kg take 30 mg
- 66 to 80 kg take 40 mg
- 81 to 90 kg take 50 mg
- 91 to 115 kg take 60 mg
- Greater than 115 kg take 70 mg

Cutaneous T-Cell Lymphoma
ADULTS: *Uvadex*: **Extracorporeal with the UVAR Photopheresis System only. (Not for parenteral administration.)** Normal treatment schedule: Treatment is given on 2 consecutive days q 4 wk for a minimum of 7 treatment cycles (6 mo). Accelerated treatment schedule: If assessment of the patient during the fourth treatment cycle (approximately 3 mo) reveals an increased skin score from the baseline score, the frequency of treatment may be increased to 2 consecutive treatments q 2 wk. If a 25% improvement in the skin score is attained after 4 consecutive wk, the regular treatment schedule may be resumed (max, 20 cycles). Consult UVAR Photopheresis System Operator's Manual before using this product. Treatment involves collection of leukocytes, photoactivation, and reinfusion of photoactivated cells. During each photopheresis treatment, 200 mcg (10 mL) of *Uvadex* is injected directly into photoactivation bag during the first buffy coat collection cycle. At the end of 6 cycles, a total of 740 mL (240 mL of buffy coat, 300 mL of plasma, and 200 mL of normal saline priming fluid) is collected and mixed with the 200 mcg of *Uvadex* present in the photoactivation bag. After photoactivation, the cells are reinfused.

Interactions
Known photosensitizers *(eg, anthralin, coal tar, coal tar derivatives, fluoroquinolone antibiotics, griseofulvin, halogenated salicylanilides, nalidixic acid, organic staining dyes [eg, methylene blue, methyl orange, rose bengal, toluidine blue], phenothiazines, sulfonamides, tetracyclines, thiazide diuretics)*: Exercise care when using these agents and methoxsalen concurrently.

Lab Test Interferences
None well documented.

Adverse Reactions
CV:
8-MOP, *Oxsoralen-Ultra* – Hypotension.
Uvadex – Hypotension (secondary to extracorporeal volume [greater than 1%]).
CNS:
8-MOP, *Oxsoralen-Ultra* – Dizziness; headache, malaise, depression.
DERM:
8-MOP, *Oxsoralen-Ultra* – Pruritus (10%); erythema; hypopigmentation; vesiculation and bullae formation; nonspecific rash; urticaria; folliculitis; cutaneous tenderness; extension of psoriasis.
GI:
8-MOP, *Oxsoralen-Ultra* – Nausea (10%); GI disturbances.
OTHER:
8-MOP, *Oxsoralen-Ultra* – Edema; herpes simplex; miliaria; leg cramps.
Uvadex – Infection.

> **WARNING:**
> Methoxsalen should only be used by physicians who have special competence in the diagnosis and treatment of psoriasis and vitiligo (8-MOP, *Oxsoralen-Ultra*) or cutaneous T-cell lymphoma (*Uvadex*) and who have special training and experience in photochemotherapy. 8-MOP may not be interchanged with *Oxsoralen-Ultra* capsules without retitration of the patient. *Oxsoralen-Ultra* has greater bioavailability and earlier photosensitization onset time than previous forms. Fully inform patient the possibilities of ocular damage, aging of the skin, and skin cancer.

Precautions
Pregnancy: Category C (8-MOP, *Oxsoralen-Ultra*).Category D (*Uvadex*).
Lactation: Undetermined.
Children: Safety and efficacy not established.
Elderly: Use with caution, start at low end of dosing range.
Hepatic function impairment: Because hepatic biotransformation is necessary for drug urinary excretion, use with caution.
Carcinogenesis: Risk of squamous cell carcinoma among PUVA-treated patients is increased (especially in patients who are fair-skinned or have had pre-PUVA exposure to prolonged tar and UVB treatment) ionizing radiation, or arsenic. Risk of basal cell carcinoma may also be increased.
Special risk patients: Diligently observe and treat patients with basal cell carcinoma or a history of basal cell carcinoma; diligently observe patients with a history of previous x-ray therapy, grenz ray therapy, or arsenic therapy for signs of carcinoma; patients with cardiac disease or others who may be unable to tolerate prolonged standing or exposure to heat stress should not be treated in a vertical UVA chamber.
Actinic degeneration: Exposure to sunlight and/or UV radiation may result in premature aging of the skin.
Cataract: Because the concentration of methoxsalen in the lens is proportional to the serum level, if the lens is exposed to UVA while methoxsalen is present, photochemical action may lead to irreversible binding of the methoxsalen to proteins and DNA components of the lens.
Sunbathing: The presence of sunburn may prevent the accurate evaluation of the patient's response to photochemotherapy.
Total dosage: Total cumulative dose of UVA that can be given safely over long periods of time has not been established.

PATIENT CARE CONSIDERATIONS
Administration/Storage
Capsules:
- 8-MOP capsules are not interchangeable with *Oxsoralen-Ultra* capsules unless the UVA-treatment dose is retitrated.
- Administer prescribed dose with food or milk. If nausea occurs, divide the dose into 2 portions and administer 30 min apart with food or milk.
- Administer methoxsalen dose 2 to 4 hr before UVA-treatment for vitiligo.
- Administer methoxsalen dose 2 hr before UVA-treatment for psoriasis.
- Store capsules at controlled room temperature (59° to 86°F).

Lotion:
- Use gloves or finger cots to apply lotion to patient. Contact of lotion with skin can cause photosensitization and possible burns.
- Apply small amount of lotion to well-defined, vitiliginous lesion before exposure to UVA-treatment.
- Store lotion at controlled room temperature (59° to 86°F).

Solution:
- For extracorporal use with the UVAR Photopheresis System only. Not for parenteral administration into patient.
- Store vials at controlled room temperature (59° to 86°F).

Assessment/Interventions
- Obtain patient history, including drug history and any known allergies. Note previous reaction to psoralens therapy, cataracts, basal cell carcinoma or history of basal cell carcinoma, previous x-ray or grenz ray therapy, previous arsenic therapy, liver disease, CV disease, or concurrent therapy with known photosensitizing agents (eg, anthralin, coal tar, phenothiazines).
- Review patient's health history for any condition that could contraindicate psoralens therapy: lupus erythematosus, porphyria cutanea tarda, erythropoietic protoporphyria, variegate porphyria, xeroderma pigmentosum, albinism, melanoma or history of melanoma, invasive squamous cell carcinoma, aphakia (absence of lens of eye).

Capsules:
- Carefully follow the manufacturer's methoxsalen and UVA-treatment dosing schedules for initial treatment and maintenance treatment.
- Ensure that UVA-absorbing/blocking goggles are worn by patient during UVA treatment.
- Ensure that an ophthalmologic exam is performed prior to therapy and yearly thereafter.
- Ensure that CBC, anti-nuclear antibodies, liver enzymes, and renal function are evaluated prior to starting therapy and then q 6 to 12 mo thereafter.
- Ensure that abdominal skin, breasts, genitalia, and other sensitive areas are protected for approximately 1/3 of the initial UVA exposure time until tanning occurs.
- Assess and document skin condition and reaction to UVA-treatment. Identify areas with pruritus, erythema, or blistering. Ensure that areas with pruritus or moderate or worse erythema are shielded during subsequent UVA-treatments until the pruritus or erythema resolve. Notify health care provider if pruritus, erythema, or blistering does not resolve within 48 hr.

Patient/Family Education
- Explain name, dose, action, and potential side effects of drug.
- Advise patient that response to therapy is not rapid and that it may take weeks to months to achieve max benefit.
- Advise women to notify health care provider if pregnant, planning to become pregnant, or breastfeeding.
- Instruct patient not to take any prescription or OTC medications, herbal preparations, or dietary supplements unless advised by health care provider.
- Advise patient that ingesting limes, figs, parsley, parsnips, mustard, carrots, or celery might cause an exaggerated response to the UVA treatments or the sun and to ingest carefully until tolerance is determined.
- Advise patient that follow-up visits will be required to monitor therapy and to keep appointments.

Capsules:
- Advise patient to read the *Patient Package Insert* before starting therapy and with each refill.
- Advise patient that nausea is a common side effect and to take each dose with food or milk to minimize this problem. If nausea still occurs advise patient to divide the dose into 2 portions taken approximately 30 min apart with food or milk.
- Caution patient to take the dose exactly as prescribed and to carefully follow the timing recommendations between taking the dose and starting the UVA treatment. Advise patient that serious burns can result if drug dosing schedules and/or UVA exposure schedules are not followed.
- Instruct patient to wear UVA-absorbing, wraparound sunglasses for the 24-hr period

following ingestion of methoxsalen, whether exposed to direct or indirect sunlight outside or through a glass window.
- Caution patient not to sunbathe during the 24 hr prior to and 48 hr after taking methoxsalen and UVA treatment.
- Caution patient to avoid exposure to sunlamps and the sun, even through windows or cloud cover, for at least 8 hr after taking methoxsalen. If sun exposure cannot be avoided, instruct patient to wear protective devices (eg, hat, gloves), and/or apply sunscreen that filters out UVA radiation ("UVA protection") with a sun protective factor (SPF) of 15 or greater. Instruct patient to apply sunscreen to all areas that might be exposed to the sun, including lips, but not to apply until after the UVA treatment.
- Advise patient that if itching occurs in UVA-treated areas to frequently apply a bland emollient. If itching persists or worsens, advise patient to notify health care provider.
- Advise patient to frequently examine their skin for small growths or sores that do not heal. Instruct patient to inform health care immediately if noted.
- Advise patient to notify health care provider if nausea, itching, redness, tenderness, or blistering of skin occurs and lasts more than 24 to 48 hr.

Lotion:
- Advise patient that lotion will be applied by a health care provider in a health care setting before undergoing UVA treatment.
- Instruct patient to keep the treated areas protected from sunlight by wearing protective clothing or applying a sunscreen with UVA protection and a sun protection factor (SPF) of 15 or greater. Advise patient that the area of application may be highly sensitive to sunlight or sunlamps for several days after application.

Solution:
- Advise that blood will be drawn and sent to the lab where this medication will be used to treat the patient's white blood cells. Once the treatment has been completed, the treated white blood cells will be returned to their body.
- Instruct patient to wear UVA-absorbing, wraparound sunglasses and cover exposed skin or use a sunblock with UVA protection and an SPF of 15 or greater for the 24-hr period following treatment of blood cells.

Methscopolamine Bromide

(meth-skoe-PAHL-uh-meen BRO-mide)
Class Antispasmodic/Anticholinergic

How Supplied
Pamine Tablets 2.5 mg ◆ *Pamine Forte* Tablets 5 mg

Action
PHARMACOLOGY: Competitively inhibits action of acetylcholine at muscarinic receptor.

PHARMACOKINETICS/DYNAMICS:
Absorption: Poorly and unreliably absorbed (10% to 25%).
Excretion: Primarily in urine and bile as well as unabsorbed drug in the feces.
Onset: 1 hr.
Duration: 4 to 6 hr.

Indications Adjunctive treatment of peptic ulcer.

Contraindications Glaucoma; obstructive uropathy (eg, bladder neck obstruction); obstructive disease of the GI tract (eg, pyloroduodenal stenosis); paralytic ileus; intestinal atony of the elderly or debilitated patient; unstable CV status in acute hemorrhage; severe ulcerative colitis; toxic megacolon complicating ulcerative colitis; myasthenia gravis; hypersensitivity to any component of the drug.

Route/Dosage
ADULTS: PO 2.5 mg one-half hr before meals and 2.5 to 5 mg at bedtime. A starting dose of 12.5 mg qd will be clinically effective in most patients. In patients experiencing severe abdominal pain or cramping or symptoms that demand prompt relief, methscopolamine may be started at 20 mg qd, administered in doses of 5 mg one-half hr before meals and at bedtime.

Interactions
Antacids: May interfere with the absorption of methscopolamine.
Antipsychotics, tricyclic antidepressants, drugs with anticholinergic effects: Additive anticholinergic effects may occur.

Lab Test Interferences None well documented.

Adverse Reactions
CV: Tachycardia; palpitation.
CNS: Headache; nervousness; mental confusion; drowsiness; dizziness; weakness; insomnia.
DERM: Decreased sweating; urticaria; other dermal manifestations.
EENT: Blurred vision; dilation of pupil; cycloplegia; increased ocular tension; loss of taste.
GI: Nausea; vomiting; constipation; bloated feeling.
GU: Impotence; suppression of lactation; urinary hesitancy and retention.

OTHER: Severe allergic reaction; drug idiosyncrasies including anaphylaxis; xerostomia.

Precautions

Pregnancy: Category C.
Lactation: Undetermined.
Children: Safety and efficacy not established.
Special risk patients: Use with caution in the elderly and in all patients with autonomic neuropathy, hepatic or renal disease, ulcerative colitis (large doses may produce paralytic ileus, precipitating or aggravating toxic megacolon), hyperthyroidism, coronary heart disease, CHF, tachyrhythmia, tachycardia, hypertension, or prostatic hypertrophy.
Diarrhea: May be a symptom of incomplete intestinal obstruction, especially in patients with ileostomy or colostomy. Treatment of diarrhea with drug is inappropriate and possibly harmful.
Heat prostration: Can occur in presence of high environmental temperature.

Overdosage: Signs and Symptoms

CNS disturbances (from restlessness and excitement to psychotic behavior), circulatory changes (flushing, fall in BP, circulatory failure), respiratory failure, paralysis, coma.

PATIENT CARE CONSIDERATIONS

Administration/Storage

- Administer prescribed dose 30 min before meals and at bedtime.
- Store at controlled room temperature (59° to 86°F).

Assessment/Interventions

- Obtain patient history, including drug history and any known allergies. Note kidney or liver disease, obstructive uropathy (eg, prostatic hypertrophy), hiatal hernia with reflux esophagitis, glaucoma, myocardial ischemia, obstructive GI disease (eg, achalasia, pyloroduodenal stenosis), paralytic ileus, intestinal atony, ulcerative colitis, myasthenia gravis, autonomic neuropathy, hyperthyroidism, hypertension, heart failure, rapid heart rate, or arrhythmia.
- Assess symptoms before starting therapy and periodically during treatment. Inform health care provider if symptoms do not improve or appear to be getting worse.
- Ensure that progress of the peptic ulcer under treatment is being followed appropriately (eg, contrast radiology, endoscopy) and that tests for occult blood in the stool, hemoglobin, and hematocrit are being periodically evaluated to rule out bleeding from the ulcer.
- Monitor patient for CV, CNS, GI, GU, and general body side effects. Inform health care provider if noted and significant.
- Discontinue therapy and notify health care provider immediately if any of the following occur: rash, eye pain, urinary retention.

Patient/Family Education

- Explain name, dose, action, and potential side effects of drug.
- Advise patient to take prescribed dose 30 min before meals and at bedtime.
- Advise patient that dose may be changed periodically to achieve max benefit.
- Advise patient to avoid strenuous activity during periods of high temperature or humidity.
- Advise patient to take sips of water, suck on ice chips or sugarless hard candy, or chew sugarless gum if dry mouth occurs.
- Advise patient that drug may cause drowsiness or blurred vision and to use caution while driving or performing other tasks requiring mental alertness until tolerance is determined.
- Advise patient to notify health care provider if symptoms do not improve or appear to be getting worse.
- Advise patient to stop taking the drug and notify health care provider immediately if any of the following occur: rash, flushing, eye pain, inability to urinate.
- Advise patient that medication may cause dry mouth, urination difficulties, or constipation and to notify health care provider if they occur and are bothersome.
- Advise women to notify health care provider if pregnant, planning to become pregnant, or breastfeeding.
- Warn patient not to take any prescription or OTC drugs or dietary supplements without consulting health care provider.
- Advise patient that follow-up visits may be necessary to monitor therapy and to keep appointments.

Methsuximide

(Meth-SUCK-sih-mide)
Class Anticonvulsant/Succinimide

How Supplied
Celontin Capsules 150 mg, Capsules 300 mg

Action
PHARMACOLOGY: Elevates seizure threshold and suppresses paroxysmal spike wave activity associated with lapses of consciousness common in absence (petit mal) seizures.

PHARMACOKINETICS/DYNAMICS:
Absorption: T_{max} is 1 to 4 hr and is readily absorbed.
Excretion: The t½ is 2.6 to 4 hr. Less than 1% recovered unchanged in urine.

Indications Control of absence (petit mal) seizures that are refractory to other drugs.

Contraindications Hypersensitivity to succinimides.

Route/Dosage
ADULTS AND CHILDREN:
Initial dose: PO 300 mg/day for the first week. Dosage may be increased at weekly intervals by 300 mg/day (max, 1200 mg/day).

Interactions
Hydantoins (eg, phenytoin), phenobarbital: Plasma concentrations may be elevated by methsuximide, increasing the risk of side effects.
Lamotrigine: Plasma concentrations may be reduced by methsuximide, decreasing the therapeutic effects.

Lab Test Interferences None well documented.

Adverse Reactions
CV: Hyperemia.
CNS: Drowsiness; ataxia; dizziness; irritability; nervousness; headache; insomnia; confusion; instability; mental slowness; depression; hypochondriacal behavior; auditory hallucinations; aggressiveness.
DERM: Urticaria; Stevens-Johnson syndrome; pruritic erythematous rash.
EENT: Periorbital edema; blurred vision.
GI: Nausea; vomiting; anorexia; diarrhea; weight loss; epigastric and abdominal pain; constipation; hiccups.
GU: Proteinuria; microscopic hematuria.
HEMA: Eosinophilia; leukopenia; monocytosis; pancytopenia (with and without bone marrow suppression).
OTHER: Photophobia.

Precautions
Pregnancy: Category C. Anticonvulsant drugs have been associated with an increase in the incidence of birth defects.
Lactation: Undetermined.
Renal function impairment: Use with caution.
Hepatic function impairment: Use with caution.
Dosage adjustment: Proceed slowly when increasing or decreasing the dose; do not withdraw drug abruptly as this may precipitate absence (petit mal) seizures.
Hematologic: Blood dyscrasias, including fatal cases, have occurred.
Systemic lupus: Systemic lupus has occurred.

Overdosage: Signs and Symptoms
Nausea, vomiting, CNS depression (including coma with respiratory depression).

PATIENT CARE CONSIDERATIONS

Administration/Storage
- May be used alone or in combination with other anticonvulsants.
- Administer qd or bid.
- May be administered without regard to meals. Administer with food if GI upset occurs.
- Administer capsules whole. Do not chew or break the capsule.
- Dose is gradually increased at 1-wk intervals.
- Store capsules at controlled room temperature (59° to 86°F). Protect from moisture and light.

Assessment/Interventions
- Obtain patient history, including drug history and any known allergies. Note history of renal or hepatic impairment.
- Ensure that periodic blood counts are performed during therapy.
- Monitor patient for seizure activity. Report seizure activity to health care provider.
- Monitor patient for GI, CNS, psychiatric, and general body side effects. Report to health care provider if noted and significant.
- Implement safety precautions for patients who experience dizziness or ataxia.
- Ensure that urinalysis and liver enzymes are evaluated before starting therapy and periodically thereafter.
- Frequently assess patient for response to treatment. Notify health care provider if seizures do not improve or appear to worsen.
- Ensure that therapy is periodically reviewed to determine if it needs to be continued without change or if a dose change (eg, increase, decrease, discontinuation) is indicated.
- Avoid sudden discontinuation of therapy if possible. Attempt to gradually reduce dose

over a period of several weeks if decision to discontinue medication is made.

Patient/Family Education
- Explain name, dose, action, and potential side effects of drug.
- Instruct patient to take exactly as prescribed and to not change the dose or stop taking unless advised by health care provider.
- Advise patient that dose may be gradually increased no more often than every week until max benefit is achieved.
- Advise patient to swallow capsule whole and to not chew or break the capsule.
- Advise patient that each dose may be taken without regard to meals but to take with food if GI upset occurs.
- Advise patient that if a dose is missed to take it as soon as possible. Caution patient that if several hours have passed or it is nearing time for the next dose not to double the dose in an effort to catch up and to take the next dose as scheduled.
- Advise patient that if medication needs to be discontinued it will be slowly withdrawn over a period of several weeks unless safety concerns (eg, rash) require a more rapid withdrawal.
- Caution patient that drug may cause drowsiness, dizziness, or blurred vision and to use caution while driving or performing other tasks requiring mental alertness until tolerance is determined.
- Advise women to notify health care provider if pregnant, planning to become pregnant, or breastfeeding.
- Instruct patient to contact health care provider immediately if any of the following occur: rash; joint pain; fever, sore throat, or other signs of infection; unusual bruising or bleeding; depression; aggressive behavior or other behavioral changes.
- Instruct patient to inform health care provider if seizures get worse of if new types of seizures occur.
- Advise patient not to take any prescription or OTC medications or dietary supplements unless advised by health care provider.
- Advise patient that laboratory tests and follow-up visits will be required to monitor therapy and to keep appointments.

Methyclothiazide/ Deserpidine

(meth-EE-kloe-THIGH-uh-zide/deh-SIHR pih-deen)

Class Antihypertensive combination

How Supplied
Enduronyl Tablets 5 mg methyclothiazide and 0.25 mg deserpidine

Action
PHARMACOLOGY:
Methyclothiazide: Inhibits renal tubular reabsorption of electrolytes.
Deserpidine: Depletes tissue stores of catecholamines (epinephrine and norepinephrine) from peripheral sites.

Indications Treatment of mild to moderately severe hypertension.

Contraindications Anuria, history of mental depression (especially suicidal tendencies); active peptic ulcer; ulcerative colitis; known hypersensitivity to sulfonamide-derived drug or any component of the product; patients receiving electroconvulsive therapy.

Route/Dosage
ADULTS: PO Once daily. Dosage should be determined by individual titration of the ingredients. Since at least 10 days to 2 wk may elapse before the full effects of the drugs become manifest, the dosage of the drugs should not be adjusted more frequently.

Interactions
Deserpidine:
Alcohol, CNS depressants – CNS depression may occur.
Antihypertensive agents, diuretics, phenothiazines – Hypotensive effects may potentiated by these drugs.
Digitalis, quinidine – Use with caution because cardiac arrhythmias may occur.
MAO inhibitors (eg, isocarboxazid) – Avoid or use with caution.
Methyclothiazide:
ACTH, steroids – May increase the risk of hypokalemia.
Antihypertensive agent – Additive or potentiation of effects.
Digitalis – Hypokalemia can sensitize or exaggerate the response to digitalis.
Insulin – Insulin requirements may be altered in diabetic patients.
Lithium – Renal Cl may be reduced, increasing the risk of lithium toxicity.
Norepinephrine – Arterial responsiveness to norepinephrine may be decreased.
NSAIDs (eg, ibuprofen) – The diuretic, natriuretic, and antihypertensive effects may be reduced by NSAIDs.
Tubocurarine – The responsiveness to tubocurarine may be increased.

Lab Test Interferences Methyclothiazide may decrease serum protein-bound iodine levels without signs of thyroid disturbances. Deserpidine may interfere with assay procedures for determination of 17-hydroxycorticosteroids and 17-ketosteroids.

Adverse Reactions
CV:
Deserpidine – Arrhythmias; syncope; angina-like symptoms; bradycardia; fluid retention.
Methyclothiazide – Orthostatic hypotension.
CNS:
Deserpidine – Headache; parkinsonian syndrome; extrapyramidal tract symptoms; dizziness; paradoxical anxiety; depression; nervousness; nightmares; dull sensorium; drowsiness; decreased libido.
Methyclothiazide – Headache; weakness; vertigo; dizziness; paresthesia; restlessness.
DERM:
Deserpidine – Rash; pruritus; flushing of the skin.
Methyclothiazide – Purpura; urticaria; rash.
EENT:
Deserpidine – Nasal congestion; deafness; optic atrophy; glaucoma; uveitis; conjunctival injection.
Methyclothiazide – Transient blurred vision; xanthopsia.
GI:
Deserpidine – Vomiting; diarrhea; nausea; anorexia; dryness of mouth; hypersecretion; increased motility; increased salivation.
Methyclothiazide – Pancreatitis; sialadenitis; vomiting; diarrhea; nausea; gastric irritation; constipation; anorexia.
GU:
Deserpidine – Nonpuerperal lactation; impotence; dysuria; gynecomastia; breast engorgement.
Methyclothiazide – Glycosuria.
HEMA:
Deserpidine – Thrombocytopenic purpura.
Methyclothiazide – Aplastic anemia; hemolytic anemia; agranulocytosis; leukopenia; thrombocytopenia.
HEPA:
Methyclothiazide – Jaundice (intrahepatic cholestatic).
METAB:
Deserpidine – Weight gain; methyclothiazide: hypokalemia; hypomagnesemia; hyperglycemia; hyperuricemia; electrolyte imbalance; hypercalcemia.
Methyclothiazide – Hyperglycemia; hyperuricemia; electrolyte imbalance; hypercalcemia.
RESP:
Deserpidine – Asthma; dyspnea; epistaxis.

PATIENT CARE CONSIDERATIONS
Administration/Storage
- Administer prescribed dose qd without regard to meals. Administer with food if GI upset occurs.

Methyclothiazide – Respiratory distress (including pneumonitis and pulmonary edema).
OTHER:
Deserpidine – Muscle aches.
Methyclothiazide – Cramping; hypersensitivity; anaphylactic reactions; necrotizing angiitis (vasculitis, cutaneous vasculitis); Stevens-Johnson syndrome; fever; photosensitivity; muscle spasms.

> **WARNING:**
> This fixed combination drug is not intended for initial therapy of hypertension. Hypertension requires therapy titrated to the individual patient. If the fixed combination represents the dosage determined, its use may be more convenient in patient management. The treatment of hypertension is not static, but must be reevaluated as conditions in each patient warrant.

Precautions
Pregnancy: Category C.
Lactation: Methyclothiazide and deserpidine are excreted in human milk.
Children: Safety and efficacy not established.
Special risk patients: Administer with caution to patients with a history of peptic ulcer, ulcerative colitis, or gallstones where biliary colic may be precipitated.
Depression: May occur.
Diabetes: Latent diabetes mellitus may become manifest.
Electrolyte imbalance: May occur; observe for signs and symptoms.
Hepatic impairment/renal disease: Use with caution.
Hyperlipidemia: Thiazides may cause increased concentrations of total serum cholesterol, total triglycerides, and low density lipoproteins.
Hyperuricemia/Gout: May be precipitated.
Postsympathectomy patients: Drug may enhance antihypertensive effects.
Systemic lupus erythematosus: Exacerbation or activation may occur.

Overdosage: Signs and Symptoms
Deserpidine: Flushing of skin, conjunctival injection, pupillary constriction, sedation, coma, hypotension, hypothermia, central respiratory depression, bradycardia.
Methyclothiazide: Electrolyte imbalance, signs of potassium deficiency (eg, confusion, dizziness, muscular weakness, GI disturbances.

- Administer alone or in combination with other antihypertensives.
- Store tablets at controlled room temperature (59° to 86°F).

Assessment/Interventions

- Obtain patient history, including drug history and any known allergies. Note history of depression, diabetes, lupus erythematosus, hyperkalemia, anuria, kidney disease, liver disease, peptic ulcer disease, ulcerative colitis, gallstones, electroconvulsive therapy, asthma, gout, or allergy to sulfonamides.
- Ensure that serum electrolytes, BUN, creatinine, and complete blood counts are monitored before and periodically during therapy.
- Monitor and record BP and pulse. Should hypotension result, hold medication and notify health care provider.
- Take safety precautions if orthostatic hypotension occurs.
- Monitor blood sugar in diabetic patient when drug is started or dose is changed. Report significant changes to health care provider.
- Monitor patient for GI, CV, and general body side effects. Inform health care provider if muscle cramps, depression, weakness, fatigue, or other significant effects are noted.

Patient/Family Education

- Explain name, dose, action, and potential side effects of drug.
- Advise patient to take qd as prescribed, without regard to meals but to take with food if GI upset occurs.
- Inform patient that drug controls, but does not cure, hypertension and to continue taking medication as prescribed even when BP is not elevated.
- Caution patient not to change the dose or stop taking unless advised by health care provider.
- Instruct patient to continue taking other BP medications as prescribed by health care provider.
- Instruct patient in BP and pulse measurement skills.
- Advise patient to monitor and record BP and pulse at home and to inform health care provider should abnormal measurements be noted. Also advise patient to take record of BP and pulse to each follow-up visit.
- Instruct patient to lie or sit down if experiencing dizziness or lightheadedness when standing.
- Caution patient that inadequate fluid intake, excessive perspiration, diarrhea, or vomiting can lead to excessive fall in BP resulting in lightheadedness or fainting.
- Instruct diabetic patient to monitor blood glucose more frequently when drug is started or dose is changed and to inform health care provider of significant changes in readings.
- Advise patient that drug may cause drowsiness or dizziness and to use caution while driving or performing other tasks requiring mental alertness until tolerance is determined.
- Instruct patient to avoid alcoholic beverages and other depressants while taking this medication.
- Caution patient to avoid unnecessary exposure to UV light (eg, sunlight, tanning booths) and to use sunscreen and wear protective clothing when exposed to UV light to avoid photosensitivity reaction.
- Emphasize to hypertensive patient importance of other modalities on BP: weight control, regular exercise, smoking cessation, moderate intake of alcohol and salt.
- Advise women to notify health care provider if pregnant, planning to become pregnant, or breastfeeding.
- Caution patient not to take any prescription or OTC medications or dietary supplements unless advised by health care provider.
- Instruct patient to immediately report any of the following symptoms to health care provider: depression, drowsiness, weakness, dry mouth, restlessness, muscle pain or cramps, nausea or vomiting, decreased urination, rapid heart rate.
- Advise patient that follow-up visits and lab tests may be required to monitor therapy and to keep appointments.

Methyldopa and Methyldopate Hydrochloride

(meth-ill-DOE-puh and meth-ill-DOE-pate HIGH-droe-KLOR-ide)

Class Antihypertensive/Antiadrenergic, centrally acting

How Supplied
Aldomet Tablets 125 mg methyldopa, Tablets 250 mg methyldopa, Tablets 500 mg methyldopa, Oral Suspension 50 mg methyldopa/mL, Injection 50 mg methyldopa hydrochloride/mL

🍁 *Apo-Methyldopa* ♦ *Nu-Medopa*

Action
PHARMACOLOGY: Causes central alpha-adrenergic stimulation, which inhibits sympathetic cardioaccelerator and vasoconstrictor centers; reduces plasma renin activity; reduces standing and supine BP.

PHARMACOKINETICS/DYNAMICS:
Absorption: Absorption is variable and incompletely absorbed. Mean bioavailability is approximately 50%.

Distribution: Methyldopa and Methyldopate

crosses the blood-brain and placental barriers, appears in cord blood and breast milk, and is approximately 8% protein bound.

Metabolism: Methyldopa and methyldopate are extensively metabolized. Approximately 17% appears in plasma as free methyldopa; active metabolite is alpha-methylnorepinephrine.

Excretion: Approximately 70% (oral) and approximately 49% (IV) is excreted in urine as methyldopa Mono-0-sulfate conjugate; excretion is complete in 36 hr after oral dose. The $t_{½}$ is 1.8 hr and the renal clearance is approximately 130 mL/min (oral) and 156 mL/min (IV).

Onset: Onset is 4 to 6 hr.

Peak: Time to peak effect is 12 to 24 hr.

Duration: Duration for methyldopa is 24 to 48 hr and 10 to 16 hr for methyldopate.

Special Populations:
Renal Function Impairment – Methyldopa is largely excreted by the kidneys. Patients with renal impairment may respond to smaller doses.

Indications Treatment of hypertension.

Contraindications Active hepatic disease or previous hepatic disease associated with methyldopa therapy; coadministration with MAO inhibitors.

Route/Dosage
ADULTS: **PO** 250 mg bid to tid in the first 48 hr initially, then 500 mg to 2 g/day in 2 to 4 divided doses. Adjust doses at intervals of not less than 2 days until adequate response is achieved.
IV 250 to 500 mg q 6 hr prn (max, 1 g q 6 hr).
CHILDREN: **PO** 10 mg/kg/day in 2 to 4 doses (max, 65 mg/kg/day or 3 g/day, whichever is less).
IV 20 to 40 mg/kg/day in divided doses every 6 hr (max, 65 mg/kg/day or 3 g/day, whichever is less).

Interactions
Anesthetics: May require reduced doses of anesthetics.
Barbiturates: Actions of methyldopa may be reduced.
Beta blockers: May cause paradoxical hypertension (rare).
Ferrous sulfate or gluconate: May decrease methyldopa absorption.
Haloperidol: May result in dementia or sedation.
Levodopa: BP lowering effects of methyldopa may be potentiated. Central effects of levodopa in Parkinson disease may be potentiated.
Lithium: May precipitate lithium toxicity.
MAO inhibitors: May lead to excessive sympathetic stimulation.
Phenothiazines: Serious elevations in BP may occur.

Sympathomimetics: May potentiate pressor effects of sympathomimetics and lead to hypertension.
Tolbutamide: Enhanced hypoglycemic effects may occur.
Tricyclic antidepressants: Reversal or attenuation of the hypotensive effects of methyldopa.

Lab Test Interferences May interfere with tests for urinary uric acid, serum creatinine, AST; may give falsely high levels of urinary catecholamines, abnormal LFT results, positive *Coombs'* test, or rise in BUN.

Adverse Reactions
CV: Bradycardia; prolonged carotid sinus hyperactivity; aggravation of angina pectoris; CHF; paradoxical pressor response with IV use; pericarditis; myocarditis; orthostatic hypotension; edema.
CNS: Dizziness; sedation; nightmares; headache; asthenia or weakness; paresthesias; lightheadedness; symptoms of cerebrovascular insufficiency; parkinsonism; Bell's palsy; decreased mental acuity; involuntary choreoathetotic movements.
DERM: Rash; toxic epidermal necrolysis.
EENT: Sore or "black" tongue; nasal stuffiness.
GI: Constipation; dry mouth; nausea; vomiting; distention; flatus; diarrhea; sialadentis.
GU: Impotence; decreased libido; rise in BUN.
HEPA: Abnormal LFTs; jaundice; hepatitis or liver disorders.
HEMA: Hemolytic anemia; bone marrow depression; leukopenia; granulocytopenia; thrombocytopenia; reduced WBC count; positive tests for anti-nuclear antibody, lupus erythematosus cells and rheumatoid factor.
METAB: Breast enlargement; gynecomastia; lactation; amenorrhea.
OTHER: Fever; lupus-like syndrome; mild arthralgia or myalgia.

Precautions
Pregnancy: Category B (methyldopa); Category C (methyldopate hydrochloride).
Lactation: Excreted in breast milk.
Children: Individualize dosage.
Elderly: Syncope in older patients may be related to an increased sensitivity and advanced arteriosclerotic vascular disease. May be avoided by lower doses.
Renal function impairment: Use with caution in patients with hepatic or renal dysfunction.
Hepatic function impairment: Use with caution in patients with hepatic or renal dysfunction.
IV use: Paradoxical pressor response has been reported.
Liver disorders: Jaundice, with or without fever, may occur. Fatal hepatic necrosis has been reported rarely. If symptoms or tests indicate

liver effects, the drugs may need to be discontinued.
Positive Coombs' test, hemolytic anemia, and liver disorders: May occur; monitor patient closely because of potentially fatal complications. *Blood transfusions:* Perform both a direct and an indirect *Coomb's* test. A positive direct *Coomb's* test alone will not interfere with typing or cross matching. If the indirect *Coomb's* test is also positive, problems may arise in the major crossmatch and assistance from a hematologist or transfusion expert will be needed.

Overdosage: Signs and Symptoms
Sedation, coma, acute hypotension, weakness, bradycardia, dizziness, lightheadedness, constipation, distention, flatus, diarrhea, nausea, vomiting, impaired atrioventricular conduction.

PATIENT CARE CONSIDERATIONS
Administration/Storage
- Add 100 mL of D5W to dose and infuse IV medication slowly over 30 to 60 min.
- Shake oral suspension well prior to administration.
- Make dosage increases with evening dose to avoid daytime drowsiness.

Methyldopa:
- Protect oral suspension from light. Avoid freezing.

Methyldopate Hydrochloride:
- Refrigerate. Do not freeze.

Assessment/Interventions
- Obtain patient history, including drug history and any known allergies. Determine whether patient has active hepatic or renal disease.
- Prior to therapy, perform baseline blood counts (hematocrit and hemoglobin or RBC count) and BP readings.
- During therapy monitor carefully for hemolytic anemia and liver disorders (eg, fever, jaundice).
- Monitor for paradoxical pressor response after IV administration of methyldopa or methyldopate hydrochloride.
- Monitor I&O and weight.
- Monitor renal studies for BUN, creatinine, protein.
- If *Coombs'* test-positive hemolytic anemia occurs, discontinue methyldopa and notify health care provider.

Patient/Family Education
- Encourage patient's compliance with health care provider recommendations of weight reduction, sodium and alcohol restriction, cessation of smoking, regular exercise, stress reduction, and other methods of BP control.
- Teach patient or family proper technique for BP monitoring at home.
- Prepare schedule for return visits to health care provider for additional monitoring of BP and hepatic function. Emphasize importance of return visits.
- Caution patient not to stop taking drug abruptly.
- Warn patient that dizziness may occur and that hot baths or showers may aggravate dizziness.
- Inform patient that nausea, vomiting, or diarrhea may cause increase in hypotensive effect because of dehydration. If this occurs, the patient should contact health care provider for dosage adjustment.
- Advise patient that urine may darken when exposed to air after voiding and assure patient that this is not a problem.
- Instruct patient to report the following symptoms to health care provider: fever, muscle aches, jaundice, flu-like symptoms.
- Advise patient to take sips of water frequently, suck on ice chips or sugarless hard candy, or chew sugarless gum if dry mouth occurs. Dry mouth usually does not continue for more than 2 wk; if it does, patient should report to health care provider.
- Caution patient to avoid sudden position changes to avoid orthostatic hypotension.
- Instruct patient to avoid intake of alcoholic beverages.
- Advise patient that drug may cause drowsiness, especially during first days of therapy or when dose is increased, and to use care while driving or performing other activities requiring mental alertness.
- Caution patient to avoid exposure to sunlight and to use sunscreen or wear protective clothing to avoid photosensitivity reaction.
- Instruct patient not to take OTC medications without consulting health care provider.

Methylergonovine Maleate

(METH-ill-err-go-NO-veen MAL-ee-ate)

Class Oxytocic

How Supplied
Methergine Tablets 0.2 mg, Injection 0.2 mg/mL

Action

PHARMACOLOGY: Acts directly on smooth muscle of the uterus and increases tone, rate, and amplitude of rhythmic contractions, thereby inducing a rapid and sustained tetanic uterotonic effect that shortens the third stage of labor and reduces blood loss.

PHARMACOKINETICS/DYNAMICS:
Absorption:
Oral – Bioavailability is about 60% with no accumulation after repeated doses. C_{max} is 3,243 pg/mL within 1.12 hr.
IM – Bioavailability is about 78%. C_{max} is 5,918 pg/mL observed at 0.41 hr. Decreased bioavailability following oral administration is probably caused by first-pass metabolism in liver.

Distribution: Vd about 56.1 L.
IV – Rapidly distributed to peripheral tissues within 3 min or less.

Metabolism: Plasma Cl about 14.4 L/hr. Hepatic metabolism.

Excretion: Hepatic excretion. The decline in plasma concentration is biphasic with a mean elimination t½ of 3.39 hr.

Indications Management after delivery of placenta; postpartum atony and hemorrhage; subinvolution; under full obstetric supervision, may be given in second stage of labor following delivery of the anterior shoulder.

Contraindications Because of the risk of vasospasm leading to cerebral ischemia and ischemia of the extremities, do not use potent CYP3A4 inhibitors (eg, azole antifungal agents, macrolide antibiotics, protease inhibitors) concurrently; hypertension; toxemia; pregnancy; hypersensitivity to any component of product.

Route/Dosage

ADULTS: **IM/IV** 0.2 mg after delivery of anterior shoulder, after delivery of placenta, or during puerperium. May repeat as required at intervals of 2 to 4 hr. IV route should not be used routinely (see Precautions).

PO 0.2 mg tid or qid in puerperium for a max of 1 wk.

Interactions

Less potent CYP3A4 inhibitors (eg, clotrimazole, fluconazole, fluoxetine, fluvoxamine, grapefruit juice, nefazodone, saquinavir, zileuton): Because of the increased risk of side effects, including vasospasm, use these agents with caution when administering with methylergonovine.

Potent CYP3A4 inhibitors (eg, azole antifungal agents [eg, itraconazole, ketoconazole, voriconazole], macrolide antibiotics [eg, clarithromycin, erythromycin, troleandomycin], protease inhibitors [eg, delavirdine, indinavir, nelfinavir, ritonavir]): Because of the risk of vasospasm, leading to cerebral ischemia and ischemia of the extremities, use of these agents is contraindicated with methylergonovine.

Lab Test Interferences None well documented.

Adverse Reactions

CV: Hypertension; hypotension; acute MI; transient chest pains; palpitation.
CNS: Headache; seizure; hallucinations; dizziness.
DERM: Diaphoresis.
EENT: Tinnitus; nasal congestion.
GI: Nausea; vomiting; diarrhea; foul taste.
GU: Hematuria.
HYPERSEN: Anaphylaxis.
METAB: Water intoxication.
MUSC: Leg cramps.
RESP: Dyspnea.
OTHER: Thrombophlebitis.

Precautions

Pregnancy: Category C.
Lactation: Small quantity excreted in breast milk.
Children: Safety and efficacy not established.
Elderly: Use with caution because of the greater frequency of decreased hepatic, renal, or cardiac function, and concomitant diseases or other drug therapy.
Retained placenta: Manual removal of retained placenta should occur only rarely with proper technique and adequate allowance of time for spontaneous separation.
Special risk patients: Use with caution in patients with sepsis, obliterative vascular disease, hepatic or renal involvement, or in second stage of labor.
IV use: Because of possibility of inducing sudden hypertensive and cerebrovascular accidents, do not use IV administration for routine use. Consider administration as a lifesaving measure and give slowly over a period of no less than 60 sec with careful monitoring of BP.

Overdosage: Signs and Symptoms

Nausea, vomiting, abdominal pain, numbness, tingling of extremities, rise in BP, hypotension, respiratory depression, hypothermia, convulsions, coma.

PATIENT CARE CONSIDERATIONS
Administration/Storage
Tablets:
- Administer prescribed dose tid or qid for max of 1 wk.
- Administer without regard to meals but administer with food if GI upset occurs.
- Store tablets below 77°F.

Injection:
- For IM or IV administration only. Not for intradermal, subcutaneous, or intra-arterial administration.
- Do not administer if solution is discolored or cloudy or if particulate matter is noted.
- Administer prescribed dose q 2 to 4 hr as ordered.
- Administer IV dose slowly over a period of no less than 60 sec with careful monitoring of BP.
- Store ampules in refrigerator (36° to 46°F). Protect from light.

Assessment/Interventions
- Obtain patient history, including drug history and any known allergies. Note stage of labor, toxemia, hepatic or renal impairment, hypertension, peripheral vascular disease, ischemic or vasospastic coronary artery disease, hypertension, concurrent use of other vasoconstrictors or ergot alkaloids, concurrent use of potent CYP3A4 inhibitor (eg, azole antifungals, protease inhibitors, macrolide antibiotics), or nursing.
- Obtain baseline vital signs, with special attention to pulse and BP. Closely monitor BP during treatment, particularly during and after IV administration. Notify health care provider immediately if BP becomes elevated. Be prepared to discontinue therapy and treat appropriately.
- Monitor and document uterine response during and after parenteral administration. Notify health care provider if uterine contractions are not maintained.
- Monitor patient for CV, GI, and general body side effects. Report to health care provider if noted and significant.

Patient/Family Education
- Explain name, dose, action, and potential side effects of drug.
- Advise patient that injection will be prepared and administered by a health care provider in a medical setting.
- Advise patient taking tablets to take each dose without regard to meals but to take with food if stomach upset occurs.
- Advise patient to stop taking the medication and notify health care provider if any of the following occur: numbness, tingling, coldness, or paleness in the fingers or toes; muscle pain in arms or legs; weakness in the legs; chest pain, tightness, or pressure; changes in heart rate.
- Warn patient not to take any prescription or OTC drugs, herbal preparations, or dietary supplements without consulting health care provider.
- Advise patient that follow-up visits will be necessary to monitor therapy and to keep appointments.

Methylphenidate Hydrochloride

(meth-ill-FEN-ih-date HIGH-droe-KLOR-ide)

Class Psychotherapeutic/CNS stimulant

How Supplied
Ritalin Tablets 5 mg, Tablets 10 mg, Tablets 20 mg ◆ *Metadate ER* Tablets, extended-release 10 mg, Tablets, extended-release 20 mg ◆ *Methylin* Tablets 5 mg, Tablets 10 mg, Tablets 20 mg, Tablets, chewable 2.5 mg, Tablets, chewable 5 mg, Tablets, chewable 10 mg ◆ *Methylin ER* Tablets, extended-release 10 mg, Tablets, extended-release 20 mg ◆ *Concerta* Tablets, extended-release 18 mg, Tablets, extended-release 27 mg, Tablets, extended-release 36 mg, Tablets, extended-release 54 mg ◆ *Ritalin-SR* Tablets, sustained-release 20 mg ◆ *Metadate CD* Capsules, extended-release 10 mg, Capsules, extended-release 20 mg, Capsules, extended-release 30 mg ◆ *Ritalin LA* Capsules, extended-release 10 mg, Capsules, extended-release 20 mg, Capsules, extended-release 30 mg, Capsules, extended-release 40 mg

🍁 *PMS-Methylphenidate* ◆ *ratio-Methylphenidate*

Action
PHARMACOLOGY: Acts as mild cortical stimulant with CNS action; exact mechanism of action unknown.

PHARMACOKINETICS/DYNAMICS:
Absorption: The extended-release and sustained-release tablets are absorbed more slowly but as extensively as the immediate-release. In children, the T_{max} is 4.7 hr (1.3 to 8.2 hr) for sustained-release and 1.9 hr (0.3 to 4.4 hr) for immediate-release. The relative bioavailabilities of SR tablets compared with regular tablets are 105% in children and 101% in adults. Chewable tablets are readily absorbed; T_{max} is 1 to 2 hr.

Metabolism: Methylphenidate is metabolized

primarily through de-esterification to alpha-phenyl-piperidine acetic acid (metabolite). 80% of dose is metabolized to ritalinic acid.

Excretion: 80% is excreted in urine. The t½ is 2.8 and 3 hr for the immediate-release and chewable tablets, respectively.

Indications Treatment of attention-deficit hyperactivity disorder (ADHD); treatment of narcolepsy (*Ritalin, Ritalin SR, Metadate ER, Methylin*).

Contraindications Marked anxiety, agitation, and tension; glaucoma; motor tics; family history or diagnosis of Tourette syndrome; concurrent treatment with MAO inhibitors and within a minimum of 14 days following discontinuation of a MAO inhibitor.

Route/Dosage

ADULTS: **PO** 10 to 60 mg/day in 2 to 3 divided doses.

CHILDREN (6 YR AND OLDER): **PO** 5 mg before breakfast and lunch initially; increase by increments of 5 to 10 mg/wk up to 60 mg/day. Give sustained-release (SR) tablets at 8-hr intervals.

CONCERTA

ADULTS AND CHILDREN (6 YR AND OLDER): **PO** In patients new to methylphenidate, start with 18 mg qd in the morning, then adjust dose in 18 mg increments at weekly intervals (max, 54 mg qd in the morning). In patients being converted from methylphenidate regimens to *Concerta*, start with 18 mg of *Concerta* every morning in patients receiving methylphenidate 5 mg bid or tid or 20 mg SR; start with 36 mg of *Concerta* every morning in patients receiving methylphenidate 10 mg bid or tid or 40 mg SR; start with 54 mg of *Concerta* every morning for patients receiving methylphenidate 15 mg bid or tid or 60 mg SR. The dose of *Concerta* may be adjusted in 18 mg increments at weekly intervals (max, 54 mg qd in the morning).

METADATE CD

ADULTS AND CHILDREN (6 YR AND OLDER): **PO** Start with 20 mg once daily in the morning before breakfast, then adjust dose in 20 mg increments at weekly intervals (max, 60 mg qd in the morning).

RITALIN LA

ADULTS AND CHILDREN (6 YR AND OLDER): **PO** In patients new to methylphenidate, start with 20 mg qd in the morning, then adjust dose in 10 mg increments at weekly intervals (max, 60 mg qd in the morning). In patients currently using methylphenidate immediate-release or sustained-released, start with 20 mg of *Ritalin LA* qd in patients receiving 10 mg bid or 20 mg SR; start with 30 mg of *Ritalin LA* qd in patients receiving 15 mg bid; start with 40 mg of *Ritalin LA* qd in patients receiving 20 mg bid or 40 mg SR; start with 60 mg of *Ritalin LA* qd in patients receiving 30 mg bid or 60 mg SR.

Interactions

Anticonvulsants (eg, phenobarbital, phenytoin, primidone), selective serotonin reuptake inhibitors (eg, fluoxetine), tricyclic antidepressants (eg, imipramine), coumarin anticoagulants: Plasma levels of these agents may be increased by methylphenidate, increasing the risk of side effects.

Guanethidine: The antihypertensive effects of guanethidine may be decreased.

MAO inhibitors (eg, phenelzine): Because of the risk of hypertensive crisis, methylphenidate is contraindicated in patients receiving MAO inhibitors and for a minimum of 14 days after discontinuation of a MAO inhibitor.

Lab Test Interferences None well documented.

Adverse Reactions

CV: Changes in pulse and BP; tachycardia; angina; cardiac arrhythmias; palpitations.
CNS: Nervousness; insomnia; dizziness; headache; dyskinesias; drowsiness; convulsions; toxic psychosis; motor tics.
EENT: Blurred vision.
GI: Anorexia; nausea; abdominal pain; weight loss during prolonged therapy.
HEMA: Leukopenia; anemia.
RESP: Upper respiratory tract infection; cough; pharyngitis; sinusitis.
OTHER: Tourette syndrome; hypersensitivity reactions (eg, rash, itching, fever, joint pain, exfoliative dermatitis, erythema multiforme, thrombocytopenia, purpura).

> **WARNING:**
> Tolerance/psychological dependence may result from chronic abusive use. Psychotic episodes have been reported, especially with parenteral abuse. Monitor during drug withdrawal for severe depression and effects of chronic overactivity. Long-term follow-up is needed. Use with caution in emotionally unstable patients or patients with a history of drug dependence or alcoholism as these patients may increase doses at own initiative.

Precautions

Pregnancy: Category C.
Lactation: Undetermined.
Children: Do not give to children less than 6 yr because safety and efficacy not established. Carefully monitor children on long-term therapy, especially for growth in height and weight gain.

Depression/Fatigue: Do not use to treat severe depression or normal fatigue.

GI obstruction: Because the Concerta tablet is nondeformable and does not change shape in the GI tract, do not administer to patients with preexisting, severe GI narrowing.

Hypertension: Use drug with caution; monitor BP.

Seizure disorders: Drug may lower seizure threshold in susceptible patients. Safe concomitant use with anticonvulsants is not established. If seizures occur, notify health care provider and consider withholding drug.

Overdosage: Signs and Symptoms

Vomiting, agitation, tremors, hyperreflexia, muscle twitching, convulsions, euphoria, confusion, hallucinations, delirium, sweating, flushing, headache, hyperpyrexia, tachycardia, palpitations, cardiac arrhythmias, hypertension, mydriasis, dry mucous membranes.

PATIENT CARE CONSIDERATIONS

Administration/Storage

- Discontinue MAO inhibitors at least 14 days before initiating therapy.
- Administer prescribed dose 30 to 45 min before meals. Administer with food if GI upset occurs.
- Administer last dose before 6 PM to patient who is unable to sleep if medication is taken late in the day.
- Dosage adjustments may be made at weekly intervals.
- Store at controlled room temperature (59° to 86°F). Protect from moisture and light.

Extended-Release Tablets and Capsules:

- Have patient swallow whole with aid of liquid. Do not crush, chew, or divide.
- Metadate CD capsules may be opened and the entire contents sprinkled onto a small amount of soft food (eg, applesauce). Administer dose immediately after sprinkling, without chewing, then provide a liquid (eg, water) to help wash the applesauce down.

Chewable Tablet:

- Do not administer chewable tablet to patient with phenylketonuria without first discussing with health care provider.
- Administer with at least 8 oz (full glass) of water to help prevent choking.

Assessment/Interventions

- Obtain patient history, including drug history and any known allergies. Note marked anxiety, tension, and agitation; glaucoma; motor tics; Tourette syndrome; family history of Tourette syndrome; seizures; hypertension; heart failure; hyperthyroidism; recent MI; behavior disturbance or thought disorder; history of drug dependence or alcoholism; or concurrent or recent (within 14 days) use of MAO inhibitor.
- Note any condition that would contraindicate use of Concerta extended-release tablet: preexisting GI narrowing, esophageal motility disorder, small bowel inflammatory disease, short-bowel syndrome, cystic fibrosis, chronic intestinal pseudo-obstruction, Meckel diverticulum, or history of pancreatitis.
- Ensure that medication is used as part of a total treatment program for ADHD that may include psychological, educational, and social interventions.
- Monitor BP frequently when medication is started and following changes in dose. Inform health care provider if elevated BP readings are noted.
- Monitor patient for response to therapy. With parental permission, consult with school personnel regarding medication's effectiveness.
- Monitor height and weight in children before starting therapy and periodically during therapy.
- Ensure that CBC, differential, and platelet count are periodically evaluated during long-term treatment.
- Monitor patient for CNS, CV, GI, and general body side effects. Report to health care provider if noted and significant.
- Discontinue medication periodically to assess behavior and determine need to continue therapy.

Patient/Family Education

- Explain name, dose, action, and potential side effects of drug.
- Advise patient, family, or caregiver to read *Patient Information* sheet provided with medication when available.
- Advise patient, family, or caregiver that this drug is part of a total treatment program for ADHD that should also include psychological, educational, and social interventions.
- Advise family or caregiver to notify school or day care personnel about medication use and administration.
- Advise patient or caregiver that last dose should be taken before 6 PM (or take the qd extended-release form in the morning) to avoid sleeplessness.
- Advise patient, family, or caregiver that health care provider may periodically change the dose to obtain max benefit, to take as prescribed, and not to stop taking or change the dose unless advised by health care provider.

- Advise patient, family, or caregiver that health care provider may discontinue medication periodically to assess behavior and determine need to continue therapy.
- Caution patient that drug may cause dizziness or drowsiness and to use caution while driving or performing other tasks requiring mental alertness until tolerance is determined.
- Advise patient, family, or caregiver to notify health care provider if appetite loss, nervousness, or difficulty sleeping occur and are bothersome.
- Advise patient or caregiver to notify health care provider if any unusual or unexplained symptoms are noted.
- Advise women to notify health care provider if pregnant, planning to become pregnant, or breastfeeding.
- Warn patient, family, or caregiver not to take/give any prescription or OTC drugs or dietary supplements without consulting health care provider.
- Advise patient, family, or caregiver that follow-up visits and lab tests may be necessary to monitor therapy and to keep appointments.

Extended-Release Tablets:

- Advise patient to swallow whole with the aid of liquids and not to crush, chew, or divide.
- Advise patient that the tablet shell passes through the intestine, is not absorbed, and may appear in the stool. Advise patient that this is normal.

Extended-Release Capsules:

- Advise patient to swallow capsule whole with the aid of liquids.
- Advise patient, family, or caregiver that *Metadate CD* capsules may be opened and the entire contents sprinkled onto a small amount of soft food (eg, applesauce) and consumed immediately without chewing. Advise patient, family, or caregiver that fluids (eg, water) should be given to help wash the applesauce down. Caution patient, family, or caregiver not to prepare ahead of time and store for future use.

Chewable Tablet:

- Instruct patient to take each dose 30 to 45 min before a meal with a full glass (8 oz) of water to help prevent choking. Instruct patient to immediately seek medical attention if experiencing any of the following after taking the chewable tablet: chest pain, vomiting, difficulty swallowing or breathing.
- Advise patient with phenylketonuria that the chewable tablet contains phenylalanine.

Methylprednisolone

(METH-ill-pred-NIH-suh-lone)

Class Corticosteroid

How Supplied

Medrol Tablets 2 mg, Tablets 4 mg, Tablets 8 mg, Tablets 16 mg, Tablets 24 mg, Tablets 32 mg ✤ *Depo-Medrol*

Methylprednisolone Sodium Succinate

A-Methapred Powder for injection 125 mg per vial, Powder for injection 500 mg per vial, Powder for injection 1 g per vial ♦ *Solu-Medrol* Powder for injection 125 mg per vial, Powder for injection 500 mg per vial, Powder for injection 1 g per vial, Powder for injection 2 g per vial

Methylprednisolone Acetate

depMedalone 40 Injection 40 mg/mL suspension ♦ *depMedalone 80* Injection 80 mg/mL suspension ♦ *Depo-Medrol* Injection 20 mg/mL suspension, Injection 40 mg/mL suspension, Injection 80 mg/mL suspension ♦ *Depopred-40* Injection 40 mg/mL suspension ♦ *Depopred-80* Injection 80 mg/mL suspension ♦ *Duralone-40* Injection 40 mg/mL suspension ♦ *Duralone-80* Injection 80 mg/mL suspension ♦ *Medralone 40* Injection 40 mg/mL suspension ♦ *Medralone 80* Injection 80 mg/mL suspension

Action

PHARMACOLOGY: Depresses formation, release and activity of endogenous mediators of inflammation including prostaglandins, kinins, histamine, liposomal enzymes and complement system. Modifies body's immune response.

PHARMACOKINETICS/DYNAMICS:

Excretion: Plasma t½ is longer than 3.5 hr.

Onset: Onset is 6 to 48 hr (IM).

Peak: Times to peak effect are 4 to 8 days (IM) and 1 to 2 hr (oral).

Duration: Durations are 1.25 to 1.5 days (oral) and 1 to 4 wk (IM).

Indications Replacement therapy in primary or secondary adrenal cortex insufficiency; adjunctive therapy for short-term administration in rheumatic disorders; exacerbation or maintenance therapy in collagen diseases; treatment of dermatologic diseases; control of allergic states or allergic and inflammatory ophthalmic processes; management of respiratory diseases; treatment of hematologic disorders; palliative management of neo-plastic diseases; management of cerebral edema associated with primary or metastatic brain tumor, craniotomy or head injury; induction of diuresis in edematous states (from nephrotic syndrome); management of critical exacerbations of GI diseases; management of acute exacerbations of multiple sclerosis; treatment of tuberculous meningitis; management of trichinosis with neurologic or myocardial involvement.

Intra-articular or soft tissue administration: Adjunctive therapy for short-term administration in synovitis of osteoarthritis, rheumatoid arthritis, bursitis, acute gouty arthritis, epicondylitis, acute nonspecific tenosynovitis and posttraumatic osteoarthritis.

Intralesional administration: Management of keloids; treatment of localized hypertrophic, infiltrated, inflammatory lesions of lichen planus, psoriatic plaques, granuloma annulare, lichen simplex chronicus; treatment of discoid lupus erythematosus, necrobiosis lipoidica diabeticorum, alopecia areata and cystic tumors of aponeurosis or tendon.

Topical administration: Treatment of inflammatory and pruritic manifestations of corticosteroid-responsive dermatoses. **Unlabeled use(s):** Reduction of mortality in severe alcoholic hepatitis; prevention of respiratory distress syndrome; treatment of septic shock; improvement of neurologic function in acute spinal cord injury.

Contraindications Systemic fungal infections; idiopathic thrombocytopenic purpura (IM administration); administration of live virus vaccines; topical monotherapy in primary bacterial infections; topical use on face, groin or axilla; use in premature infants (sodium succinate salt).

Route/Dosage

METHYLPREDNISOLONE
ADULTS: **PO** 4 to 48 mg/day.

METHYLPREDNISOLONE SODIUM SUCCINATE
ADULTS: **IV/IM** 10 to 40 mg administered over 1 to several min. In severe condition, 30 mg/kg infused over 30 min; may repeat q 4 to 6 hr for 48 to 72 hr.

INFANTS AND CHILDREN: **IV/IM** Not less than 0.5 mg/kg/24 hr.

METHYLPREDNISOLONE ACETATE
ADULTS: **IM** 40 to 120 mg q wk for 1 to 4 wk. **Intra-articular/intralesional** 4 to 80 mg into joints or lesions. **Topical** Apply sparingly to affected areas bid to qid.

Interactions

Anticholinesterases: May antagonize anticholinesterase effects in myasthenia gravis.
Barbiturates: May decrease pharmacologic effect of methylprednisolone.
Hydantoins, rifampin: May increase clearance and decrease efficacy of methylprednisolone.
Ketoconazole: May decrease clearance of methylprednisolone.
Macrolide antibiotics: Significantly decreases methylprednisolone clearance; may need to decrease dose.
Salicylates: May reduce serum levels and efficacy of salicylates.

Lab Test Interferences Drug may cause increased levels of urine glucose and serum cholesterol, decreased serum levels of potassium, T_3 and T_4, decreased uptake of thyroid I^{131}, false-negative result in nitroblue-tetrazolium test for systemic bacterial infection and suppression of skin-test reactions.

Adverse Reactions

CV: Thromboembolism or fat embolism; thrombophlebitis; necrotizing angiitis; cardiac arrhythmias or ECG changes syncopal episodes; hypertension; myocardial rupture; fatal arrest; circulatory collapse; CHF.
CNS: Convulsions; pseudotumor cerebri (increased intracranial pressure with papilledema); vertigo; headache; neuritis; paresthesias; psychosis.
DERM: Impaired wound healing; thin, fragile skin; petechiae and ecchymoses; erythema; lupus erythematosus-like lesions; subcutaneous fat atrophy; striae; hirsutism; acneiform eruptions; allergic dermatitis; urticaria; angioneurotic edema; perineal irritation; hyperpigmentation or hypopigmentation; burning, itching, irritation, dryness, folliculitis, hypertrichosis, pruritus, perioral dermatitis, allergic contact dermatitis, stinging, cracking and tightening of skin, secondary infections, skin atrophy, miliaria, telangiectasia (topical).
EENT: Posterior subcapsular cataracts; increased intraocular pressure; glaucoma; exophthalmos.
GI: Pancreatitis; abdominal distention; ulcerative esophagitis; nausea; vomiting; increased appetite and weight gain; peptic ulcer with perforation and hemorrhage; bowel perforation.
GU: Increased or decreased motility and number of spermatozoa.
HEMA: Leukocytosis.
METAB: Sodium and fluid retention; hypokalemia; hypokalemic alkalosis; metabolic alkalosis; hypocalcemia.
OTHER: Musculoskeletal effects (eg, weakness, myopathy, muscle mass loss, osteoporosis, spontaneous fractures); endocrine abnormalities (eg, menstrual irregularities, cushingoid state, growth suppression in children, sweating, decreased carbohydrate tolerance, hyperglycemia, glycosuria, increased insulin or sulfonylurea requirements in diabetic patients, hirsutism); anaphylactoid or hypersensitivity reactions; aggravation or masking of infections; fatigue; insomnia; osteonecrosis, tendon rupture, infection, skin atrophy, postinjection flare, hypersensitivity, facial flushing (intra-articular administration). Topical

application may produce adverse reactions seen with systemic use because of absorption.

Precautions
Pregnancy: Pregnancy category undetermined (systemic use); Category C (topical use).
Lactation: Excreted in breast milk.
Children: May be more susceptible to adverse effects from topical use. Benzyl alcohol/gasping syndrome may occur with use of methylprednisolone sodium succinate.
Elderly: May require lower doses.
Hypersensitivity: Reactions, including anaphylaxis, may occur rarely.
Tartrazine sensitivity: May contain tartrazine, which may cause allergic-type reactions in susceptible individuals.
Adrenal suppression: Prolonged therapy may lead to hypothalamic-pituitary-adrenal suppression.
Hepatitis: Drug may be harmful in chronic active hepatitis positive for hepatitis B surface antigen.
Immunosuppression: Because drug causes immunosuppressed state, do not administer live virus vaccines during treatment.
Infections: May mask signs of infection. May decrease host-defense mechanisms to prevent dissemination of infection.
Ocular effects: Use drug systemically with caution in ocular herpes simplex because of risk of possible corneal perforation.
Peptic ulcer: Drug may contribute to peptic ulceration, especially in large doses.
Repository injections: Do not inject subcutaneously. Avoid injection into deltoid muscle and repeated intramuscular injection into same site.
Stress: Increased dosage of rapidly acting corticosteroid may be needed before, during and after stressful situations.

Overdosage: Signs and Symptoms
Cushingoid changes, moonface, central obesity, striae, hirsutism, acne, ecchymoses, hypertension, osteoporosis, myopathy, sexual dysfunction, diabetes mellitus, hyperlipidemia, peptic ulcer, increased susceptibility to infection, electrolyte and fluid imbalance.

PATIENT CARE CONSIDERATIONS

Administration/Storage
- When initiating or discontinuing drug therapy, taper dose.
- With oral administration, give with food. Tablets can be crushed and given with fluid.
- Administer once-daily dose or alternate-day dosing in morning before 9 am.
- Administer multiple doses at evenly spaced intervals throughout day. When large doses are given, administer antacids between meals to help to prevent peptic ulcers. For long-term use, alternate-day regimen may be used.
- With intra-articular injection, inject into synovial space. Do not inject unstable joints.
- When treating conditions such as tendonitis or tenosynovitis, inject into tendon sheath rather than into substance of tendon.
- When treating conditions such as epicondylitis, outline area of greatest tenderness and infiltrate drug into area.
- When treating ganglia of tendon sheaths, inject drug directly into cyst.
- When treating dermatologic conditions, avoid injection of sufficient material to cause blanching, which may cause small slough.
- Do not inject into deltoid muscle. Administer IM injection deeply into gluteal muscle.
- If giving as injection, rotate sites.
- Although methylprednisolone sodium succinate can be given both IM and IV, methylprednisolone acetate can only be administered IM; it cannot be administered IV.
- With topical application, once ointment is applied, plastic wrap can be used over area to increase absorption. To avoid skin irritation, do not leave plastic wrap in place longer than 12 hr. Wash hands before and after application.
- Do not use topically on face, groin, or axilla.
- Use solution within 48 hr of mixing.
- Store at room temperature (59° to 86°F).

Assessment/Interventions
- Obtain patient history, including drug history and any known allergies. Note renal and liver function; state of mental health; hemologic, cardiac, vision, and skin problems; history of frequent fungal infections.
- Assess baseline renal function (ie, creatinine, electrolytes, frequency, 24-hr urine output).
- Check for history of hepatitis B.
- Assess for signs of adrenal insufficiency: low blood glucose, nausea, anorexia, weakness, dizziness, weight loss, diarrhea.
- Obtain baseline vital signs, weight and lab test results (ie, electrolytes, CBC, T_3, T_4, cholesterol, urine glucose).
- Observe growth and development of infants and children on prolonged therapy.
- Monitor renal function, especially in patients with renal impairment.
- If skin irritation occurs, withhold medication and notify health care provider.
- If signs of infection, renal or liver dysfunction, bleeding, circulatory problems, edema, weight

gain, or respiratory changes occur, notify health care provider.
- If difficulties with GI tract or vision changes occur, notify health care provider.
- If patient is having difficulty with weight control, obtain dietary counseling.
- If patient is diabetic, monitor closely for possible increased requirements for insulin or sulfonylurea.

Patient/Family Education
- Instruct patient to take medication at same time each day and with food if taking orally.
- With cream or ointment application, instruct patient to soak area of skin before gently applying light film of medication, to increase absorption. Caution patient to wash hands before and after application.
- Encourage patient to eat low-sodium, low-fat foods.
- Advise patient to practice frequent, thorough handwashing to help to prevent infections.
- Advise patient on chronic steroid therapy to wear or carry identification (eg, *Medi-Alert*) indicating condition and medication regimen.
- Inform patient of potential for mood swings.
- Warn patient regarding increasing appetite and consequent weight gain. Instruct patient to weigh self daily.
- Inform patient of moonface, which often occurs with this medication.
- Advise patient of acne and skin flushing, which are often associated with this medication. Instruct patient in proper skin care practices to help to prevent irritation and/or acne.
- Instruct patient to report the following symptoms to health care provider: swelling in feet and ankles, signs of infection (eg, fever, overgrowth in mouth, vaginal yeast, wound not healing or with drainage), diarrhea, nausea, vomiting, weight loss, discolored or painful urine, vision changes, menstrual irregularity and fatigue.

Methyltestosterone

(METH-ill-tess-TAHS-ter-ohn)

Class Androgen

How Supplied
Android Capsules 10 mg ◆ *Methitest* Tablets 10 mg, Tablets 25 mg ◆ *Methyltestosterone* Tablets, buccal 10 mg ◆ *Testred* Capsules 10 mg ◆ *Virilon* Capsules 10 mg ◆ *Virilon IM* Injection 200 mg/mL

Action
PHARMACOLOGY: Promotes growth and development of male reproductive organs, maintains secondary sex characteristics, increases protein anabolism, and decreases protein catabolism.

PHARMACOKINETICS/DYNAMICS:
Metabolism: Because methyltestosterone is less extensively metabolized by the liver and has a longer t½ than testosterone, methyltestosterone is more suitable than testosterone for oral administration.

Indications Replacement therapy in the following conditions associated with a deficiency or absence of endogenous testosterone: primary hypogonadism (congenital or acquired); hypogonadotropic hypogonadism (congenital or acquired); delayed puberty (males); used secondarily in advancing inoperable metastatic (skeletal) mammary cancer (females).

Contraindications Men with carcinoma of the breast; men with known or suspected carcinoma of the prostate gland; women known or suspected to be pregnant; hypersensitivity to any component of the product.

Route/Dosage
Congenital or Acquired Primary Hypogonadism, Hypogonadotropic Hypogonadism
ADULTS (MEN): **PO** 10 to 50 mg/day. **IM** 50 to 400 mg injected deeply into gluteal muscle q 2 to 4 wk.

Delayed Puberty
ADULTS (MEN): **PO/IM** Doses are generally in the lower range of the above doses for hypogonadism and for a limited duration (eg, 4 to 6 mo).

Metastatic Breast Carcinoma
ADULTS (WOMEN): **PO** 50 to 200 mg/day. **IM** 200 to 400 mg injected deeply into gluteal muscle q 2 to 4 wk.

Interactions
Insulin: Blood glucose levels may be reduced by methyltestosterone, decreasing insulin requirements.
Oral anticoagulants (eg, warfarin): Effects of oral anticoagulant may be increased. Dosage reduction may be required.

Lab Test Interferences Thyroxine-binding globulin levels may be decreased; however, thyroid hormone levels remain unchanged and there is no clinical evidence of thyroid dysfunction.

Adverse Reactions
CNS: Increased and decreased libido; headache; anxiety; depression; generalized paresthesia.
DERM: Hirsutism; male pattern baldness; acne.
ELECDIST: Retention of sodium, chloride, water, potassium, calcium, and inorganic phosphates.

GI: Nausea.
GU: Amenorrhea, menstrual irregularities, inhibition of gonadotropin secretion, virilization (including deepening of voice and clitoral enlargement for women); gynecomastia; excessive frequency and duration of penile erection, oligospermia (men).
HEMA: Suppression of clotting factors II, V, VII, and X; bleeding in patients with polycythemia.
HEPA: Cholestatic jaundice; alterations in LFTs; hepatocellular neoplasms; peliosis hepatitis.
METAB: Increased serum cholesterol.
OTHER: Anaphylactoid reactions.

Precautions

Pregnancy: Category X.
Lactation: Undetermined.
Children: Use with caution and only by specialists aware of the adverse effects on bone maturation.
Elderly: Elderly men may be at increased risk of developing prostatic hypertrophy or carcinoma.

Athletic performance: Abuse of this agent to enhance athletic performance has potential risk of serious side effects.
Delayed puberty: Because bone maturation without producing compensatory linear growth can occur, use with caution in males with delayed puberty.
Edema: Use with caution in patients with conditions that might be affected by fluid retention (eg, renal, hepatic, cardiac disease).
Gynecomastia: May occur and persist in patients being treated for hypogonadism.
Hepatic effects: Cholestatic hepatitis and jaundice may occur. Prolonged use of high doses may result in hepatic adenomas, hepatocellular carcinoma, and peliosis hepatitis.
Hypercalcemia: May cause hypercalcemia when used in patients with breast cancer.
Oligospermia and reduced ejaculatory volume: May occur after prolonged use.
Priapism: May be indicative of excessive dosage.
Virilization: May occur in women using high-dose androgens.

PATIENT CARE CONSIDERATIONS

Administration/Storage

- Dose is variable, depending on the condition being treated and the age and sex of the patient.
- Store tablets, capsules, and injection at ambient room temperature (59° to 86°F). Protect from light, moisture, and heat.

Oral Tablets and Capsules:

- Administer prescribed dose without regard to meals. Administer with food if GI upset occurs.

Buccal Tablets:

- Place buccal tablet between the cheek and gum and advise patient to allow to dissolve. Caution patient not to swallow tablet and to avoid eating or drinking anything while the tablet is in the mouth.

Injection:

- For IM administration only. Not for intradermal, subcutaneous, or IV administration.
- Inspect solution visually before administration. Do not administer if solution is cloudy, discolored, or contains particulate matter. Crystals may form if solution is stored at low temperature but will dissolve readily by warming solution and shaking vial.
- Administer prescribed dose by deep IM injection into upper outer quadrant of gluteal muscle. Rotate injection sites.

Assessment/Interventions

- Obtain patient history, including drug history and any known allergies. Note renal, hepatic, or cardiac disease.
- Review patient's health history for any condition that could contraindicate methyltestosterone (eg, men with carcinoma of the breast or known or suspected carcinoma of the prostate, women who are or may become pregnant).
- Ensure that urine and serum calcium levels are evaluated frequently during treatment of women with metastatic breast cancer. Notify health care provider if hypercalcemia noted and be prepared to discontinue therapy.
- Ensure that women of childbearing potential are not pregnant when therapy is started and use effective contraception during therapy.
- Ensure that transaminases are evaluated before starting therapy and periodically thereafter during prolonged therapy. Immediately notify health care provider if transaminases become elevated or if patient develops jaundice.
- Monitor women for signs or symptoms of virilization (eg, deepening of voice, hirsutism, acne, clitoromegaly, menstrual irregularity). Inform health care provider if noted.
- In adolescent males being treated for delayed puberty, ensure that bone maturation is monitored by assessing bone age of the wrist and hand by x-ray evaluation q 6 mo during treatment.
- Ensure that hemoglobin and hematocrit are evaluated periodically for polycythemia in patient receiving high-dose therapy.

- Monitor blood sugar in diabetic patient when drug is started or dose is changed. Report significant changes to health care provider.
- Monitor patient for GI, GU, DERM, and general body side effects. Report frequent, persistent erections, nausea or vomiting, change in skin color, ankle swelling, or any other significant side effect to health care provider.
- Assess elderly men for evidence of prostatic hypertrophy (eg, difficult or painful urination, urinary hesitancy, inability to urinate). Inform health care provider if noted.

Buccal System:
- Inspect application site frequently. Report tenderness or irritation to health care provider.

Patient/Family Education
- Advise patient to review *Patient Information* leaflet before starting therapy and with each refill.
- Advise patient receiving IM injection that medication will be prepared and administered by a health care professional in a health care setting.
- Instruct patient to take as prescribed and not to change the dose or stop taking unless advised by health care provider.
- Advise patient taking tablets or capsules that medication can be taken without regard to meals, but to take with food if GI upset occurs.
- Advise patient using buccal tablets to place buccal tablet between the cheek and gum and allow to dissolve. Caution patient not to chew or swallow tablet and avoid eating or drinking anything while the tablet is in the mouth.
- Advise patient to regularly inspect gum region where buccal system is applied and to report any abnormality (including gum tenderness or irritation) to health care provider.
- Advise women to immediately report any of the following to health care provider: deepening of voice, unusual hair growth, acne, enlargement of clitoris, menstrual irregularity.
- Advise men to report any of the following to health care provider: frequent, persistent erections, difficult or painful urination, urinary hesitancy, inability to urinate.
- Advise patient to report any of the following to health care provider: persistent nausea or vomiting, yellowing of skin or eyes, ankle swelling, any other unusual symptom.
- Instruct diabetic patient to monitor blood glucose more frequently when drug is started or dose is changed and to inform health care provider of significant changes in readings.
- Caution patient that medication has not been shown to be safe or effective for the enhancement of athletic performance and not to use for this purpose.
- Advise women of childbearing potential to use effective contraception during therapy.
- Advise women to notify health care provider if pregnant, planning to become pregnant, or breastfeeding.
- Instruct patient not to take any prescription or OTC medications, dietary supplements, or herbal preparations unless advised by health care provider.
- Advise patient that follow-up examinations and lab tests may be required to monitor therapy and to keep appointments.

Methysergide Maleate

(METH-ih-SIR-jide MAL-ee-ate)

Class Analgesic/Migraine

How Supplied
Sansert Tablets 2 mg

Action
PHARMACOLOGY: Semisynthetic ergot derivative possessing no intrinsic vasoconstrictor activity; believed to work by antagonizing effects of serotonin in lowering pain threshold.

PHARMACOKINETICS/DYNAMICS:
Absorption: Absorption is rapid.
Metabolism: Metabolism is probably hepatic.
Onset: Onset is 1 to 2 days.
Duration: Duration is 1 to 2 days.

Indications Prevention or reduction of intensity of severe and frequent (once weekly or more) vascular headaches; prophylaxis of vascular headache. Not for management of acute attack.

Contraindications Pregnancy; peripheral vascular disease; severe arteriosclerosis; severe hypertension; coronary artery disease; phlebitis or cellulitis in lower limbs; pulmonary disease; collagen disease or fibrotic processes; impaired liver or renal function; valvular heart disease; debilitated states; serious infections.

Route/Dosage
ADULTS: **PO** 4 to 8 mg/day with meals. There must be drug-free interval of 3 to 4 wk after 6 mo of treatment.

Interactions
Beta blockers: May result in peripheral ischemia, manifested by cold extremities with possible peripheral gangrene.

Lab Test Interferences None well documented.

Adverse Reactions

CV: Encroachment of retroperitoneal fibrosis on aorta, inferior vena cava and common iliac branches may cause vascular insufficiency of lower limbs; fibrotic thickening of cardiac valves; murmurs; bruits; arterial vasoconstriction causing chest pain; coldness, numbness or pain in extremities; diminished or absent pulse; ischemic tissue damage; orthostatic hypotension; tachycardia; peripheral edema.
CNS: Insomnia; drowsiness; mild euphoria; dizziness; ataxia; weakness; lightheadedness; hyperesthesia; hallucinatory dissociation; parasthesias.
DERM: Facial flush; telangiectasia; rash; initial increased hair loss.
GI: Nausea; vomiting; diarrhea; heartburn; abdominal pain; constipation.
HEMA: Neutropenia; eosinophilia.
RESP: Pleuropulmonary fibrosis.
OTHER: Arthralgia; myalgia; weight loss.

PATIENT CARE CONSIDERATIONS

Administration/Storage
- Administer as supplied; do not crush.
- Give with meals.

Assessment/Interventions
- Obtain patient history, including drug history and any known allergies. Note tartrazine sensitivity.
- Obtain cardiac and renal function studies, blood count and sedimentation rate before administration and monitor throughout therapy.
- Palpate for diminished or absent peripheral pulses, changes in extremity color/temperature or peripheral edema throughout prolonged therapy.
- Implement appropriate safety precautions, as patient may be at risk for falls due to insomnia, lightheadedness, hyperesthesia or hallucinatory experiences.
- Notify health care provider of orthostatic hypotension or tachycardia, chest or flank pain, leg cramps or shortness of breath.

Patient/Family Education
- Caution patient that this medication must not be taken during pregnancy or when pregnancy is possible. Advise patient to use reliable form of birth control while taking this drug.
- Explain that medication can be taken with food or milk if GI upset occurs.
- Tell patient that medication may cause drowsiness and to use caution while driving or performing other tasks requiring mental alertness, coordination, dexterity.
- Instruct patient or family member to check regularly for cold or numb extremities.
- Advise patient to report these symptoms to health care provider immediately: leg cramps, chest pain, flank pain, shortness of breath or painful urination.
- Caution patient to avoid sudden position changes to prevent orthostatic hypotension.
- Tell patient to consult health care provider after 6 mo of therapy regarding tapering of regimen.
- Explain that medication should not be discontinued abruptly; which may cause rebound headache.
- Educate patient to report rapid weight gain and to check for peripheral edema. Explain benefits of low salt, reduced calorie diet if necessary.

Precautions
Pregnancy: Contraindicated in pregnancy because of oxytocic properties.
Lactation: Excreted in breast milk.
Children: Not recommended for children.
Tartrazine sensitivity: Contains tartrazine, which may cause allergic reactions in susceptible people.
Fibrosis: Long-term methylsergide therapy may cause retroperitoneal fibrosis, pleuropulmonary fibrosis and fibrotic complications within CV system. These may be reversible. This drug should be reserved for prophylaxis of frequent, severe or uncontrollable vascular headaches under close supervision. To reduce fibrotic risks, continuous use should not exceed 6 mo. Reduce dosage gradually over 2 to 3 wk to avoid "rebound headache." Provide 3 to 4 wk drug-free interval between each 6-mo course of therapy.

Overdosage: Signs and Symptoms
Peripheral vasospasm, cyanotic extremities, coldness of extremities.

Metipranolol

(meh-tih-PRAN-oh-lahl)
Class Beta-adrenergic blocker

How Supplied
OptiPranolol Ophthalmic solution 0.3%

Action
PHARMACOLOGY: Reduces IOP, probably by reducing aqueous humor production and to a minor extent by slightly increasing outflow.

PHARMACOKINETICS/DYNAMICS:
Onset: 30 min after a single administration.

Peak: Max effect occurs at about 2 hr.
Duration: Reduced IOP can be demonstrated 24 hr after a single application.

Indications Treatment of elevated IOP in patients with ocular hypertension or glaucoma.

Contraindications Patients with bronchial asthma, history of bronchial asthma, or severe COPD; symptoms of sinus bradycardia; greater than first degree AV block; cardiogenic shock; overt cardiac failure; hypersensitivity to any component.

Route/Dosage
ADULTS: **Ophthalmic** 1 gtt in affected eye(s) bid.

Interactions
Adrenergic psychotropic drugs: Use with caution.
Calcium channel antagonists, digoxin: May prolong AV conduction time.
Calcium channel antagonists (eg, diltiazem): May precipitate left ventricular failure and hypotension.
Catecholamine-depleting drugs (eg, reserpine): Possible additive effects and the production of hypotension and/or bradycardia.
Oral beta-adrenergic blockers (eg, propranolol): Possible additive effects.

Lab Test Interferences None well documented.

Adverse Reactions
CV: Angina; atrial fibrillation; bradycardia; hypertension; MI; palpitation.
CNS: Headache; anxiety; depression; dizziness; nervousness; somnolence.
DERM: Rash.
EENT: Transient discomfort; abnormal vision; blepharitis; blurred vision; brow ache; conjunctivitis; edema; eyelid dermatitis; photophobia; tearing; uveitis; epistaxis; rhinitis.
GI: Nausea.
MUSC: Arthritis; asthenia; myalgia.
RESP: Bronchitis; coughing; dyspnea.
OTHER: Allergy.

Precautions
Pregnancy: Category C.
Lactation: Undetermined.
Children: Safety and efficacy not established.
Special risk patients: Use with caution in patients with history of cardiac failure, cerebrovascular insufficiency, diabetes, or COPD.
Anaphylaxis: Patients with a history of severe anaphylactic reaction to a variety of allergens may be more reactive to repeated challenge, either accidental, diagnostic, or therapeutic. Such patients are unresponsive to the usual doses of epinephrine used to treat allergic reactions.
Angle-closure glaucoma: To effectively reduce elevated IOP in angle-closure glaucoma, use with miotic agent.
Surgery: Some authorities recommend gradual withdrawal of beta-adrenergic receptor blocking agents in patient undergoing elective surgery.
Systemic absorption: Ophthalmic solution may produce same adverse reactions seen with systemic use because of absorption.
Thyrotoxicosis: May mask signs of developing or continuing hyperthyroidism. Abrupt withdrawal may exacerbate symptoms of hyperthyroidism, including thyroid storm.

Overdosage: Signs and Symptoms
Bradycardia, hypotension, acute cardiac failure.

PATIENT CARE CONSIDERATIONS

Administration/Storage
- Instill 1 gtt into affected eye(s) bid.
- If using other topical ophthalmic drugs, separate each medication by at least 10 min.
- Store at room temperature (59° to 86°F). Keep dropper bottle tightly closed.

Assessment/Interventions
- Obtain patient history, including drug history and any known allergies. Note renal or hepatic impairment, asthma, severe COPD, bradycardia, AV block, heart failure, diabetes, cerebrovascular insufficiency, myasthenia gravis, or hyperthyroidism.
- Ensure that IOPs have been measured and documented in the patient's record before starting therapy and periodically thereafter.
- Monitor patient for ocular and systemic reactions. Inform health care provider immediately if noted.

Patient/Family Education
- Explain name, dose, action, and potential side effects of drug.
- Advise patient that usual dose is 1 gtt instilled into the affected eye(s) bid.
- Teach patient proper technique for instilling eye gtt: wash hands; do not allow dropper tip to touch eye. Tilt head back; look up; pull lower eyelid down; instill prescribed number of gtt. Close eye for 1 to 2 min and apply gentle pressure to bridge of nose for 3 to 5 min. Do not rub eye.
- Advise patient that if more than 1 topical ophthalmic drug is being used, to administer the drugs at least 10 min apart.
- Advise patient who wears contact lenses to remove lenses before instilling this medicine and to wait at least 15 min after instilling eye gtt before reinserting lenses.

- Inform patient that temporary stinging or eye discomfort are the most common side effects and to contact health care provider if they occur and are bothersome.
- Advise patient that medication may cause temporary blurring of vision and to use caution driving or performing other tasks requiring good vision until tolerance is determined.
- Advise patient to discontinue therapy and immediately notify health care provider if serious or unusual reactions occur in the eye (eg, eye or eyelid inflammation).
- Advise patient to contact eye doctor if eye is injured or if having eye surgery.
- Advise women to notify health care provider if pregnant, planning to become pregnant, or breastfeeding.
- Instruct patient not to take any prescription or OTC medications or dietary supplements unless advised by health care provider.
- Remind patient that eye examinations and measurement of IOP will be necessary while using this medication and to keep appointments.

Metoclopramide

(MET-oh-kloe-PRA-mide)

Class Dopamine antagonist antiemetic agent

How Supplied

Maxolon Tablets 10 mg (as monohydrochloride monohydrate) ◆ *Octamide* Tablets 10 mg (as monohydrochloride monohydrate) ◆ *Octamide PFS* Injection 5 mg/mL (as monohydrochloride monohydrate) ◆ *Reglan* Tablets 5 mg (as monohydrochloride monohydrate), Tablets 10 mg (as monohydrochloride monohydrate), Syrup 5 mg/5 mL (as monohydrochloride monohydrate), Injection 5 mg/5 mL (as monohydrochloride monohydrate)
✤ APO-Metoclop ◆ Maxeran ◆ Metoclopramide Omega ◆ Nu-Metoclopramide

Action

PHARMACOLOGY: Stimulates upper GI tract motility, resulting in accelerated gastric emptying and intestinal transit and increased resting tone of lower esophageal sphincter. Exerts antiemetic properties through antagonism of central and peripheral dopamine receptors.

PHARMACOKINETICS/DYNAMICS:

Absorption: Absolute oral bioavailability is approximately 80%; T_{max} is 1 to 2 hr.

Distribution: Approximately 30% is protein bound; Vd is approximately 3.5 L/kg.

Excretion: Approximately 85% of dose appears in urine within 72 hr (50% of the 85% is present as free n conjugated metoclopramide). The $t_½$ is 5 to 6 hr.

Onset: Onsets are 1 to 3 hr (IV), 10 to 15 min (IM), and 30 to 60 min (oral).

Duration: Duration is 1 to 2 hr.

Special Populations:
Renal Function Impairment – The reduction in clearance suggests that adjustment downward of maintenance dosage should be done to avoid drug accumulation.

Indications

PO: Relief of symptoms associated with acute and recurrent diabetic gastroparesis; short-term therapy of symptomatic, documented gastroesophageal reflux disease in adults who fail to respond to conventional therapy.
Parenteral: Prevention of nausea and vomiting associated with emetogenic cancer chemotherapy; prophylaxis of postoperative nausea and vomiting when nasogastric suction is undesirable; facilitation of small bowel intubation when tube does not pass pylorus with conventional maneuvers. **Unlabeled use(s):** Treatment of hiccoughs, migraines, postoperative gastric bezoars, improvement in lactation, radiation-induced emesis.

Contraindications

Patients in whom increase in GI motility could be harmful (eg, in presence of GI hemorrhage, mechanical obstruction, perforation); pheochromocytoma; epilepsy; patients receiving drugs likely to cause extrapyramidal reactions.

Route/Dosage

Nausea and Vomiting Caused by Highly Emetogenic Chemotherapy

ADULTS: **IV** 2 mg/kg by infusion for 2 doses; give the first dose 30 min before chemotherapy, the second dose 2 hr later. If vomiting persists, 3 additional doses of 2 mg/kg may be given q 3 hr. If vomiting is controlled, 3 additional doses of 1 mg/kg may be given q 3 hr. **PO** 2 mg/kg 1 hr before chemotherapy, followed by 3 more doses at 2-hr intervals. If vomiting persists, 2 additional doses may be given q 3 hr (total daily dose of 12 mg/kg).

Nausea and Vomiting with Less Emetogenic Chemotherapy

ADULTS: **IV** 1 mg/kg by infusion 30 min before chemotherapy, repeated q 2 hr for 3 doses.

Prevention of Delayed Nausea and Vomiting Caused by Chemotherapy

ADULTS: **PO** 0.5 mg/kg qid for 4 days beginning 16 to 24 hr after chemotherapy given, in combination with dexamethasone. May be given IV in patients unable to take PO.

Adjustment in Renal Insufficiency

Reduce initial dose 50% in patients with Ccr less than 40 mL/min. Titrate subsequent doses based on patient response.

Interactions

Acetaminophen, cyclosporine, ethanol, levodopa, tetracycline: Metoclopramide may increase oral bioavailability or absorption of these drugs.
Anticholinergic, opioid analgesics, levodopa: May decrease effect of metoclopramide on gastric emptying.
Cefprozil, cimetidine, digoxin: Metoclopramide may decrease oral absorption of these drugs.
CNS depressants (eg, alcohol, anesthetics, barbiturates, opiates): May potentiate CNS depressant effects of metoclopramide.
Succinylcholine and possibly mivacurium: By inhibiting plasma cholinesterase metoclopramide may prolong neuromuscular blocking effects such as respiratory depression and paralysis.
INCOMPATIBILITIES: Cephalothin, chloramphenicol, sodium bicarbonate.

Lab Test Interferences None well documented.

Adverse Reactions

CNS: Dizziness; drowsiness; depression; hallucinations; extrapyridal symptoms which respond rapidly to treatment with anticholinergic agents (eg, diphenhydramine IV); exacerbation of Parkinson disease; tardive dyskinesia; akathisia.
DERM: Transient flushing of face or upper body with high IV doses.
ENDO: Hyperprolactinemia; galactorrhea; gynecomastia (in men).
GI: Diarrhea.
GU: Urinary frequency; incontinence; amenorrhea.
HYPERSEN: Injectable solutions may contain sodium metabisulfite, a sulfite. Sensitive individuals may experience allergic reactions (eg, anaphylaxis, bronchospasm, angioedema).

Precautions

Pregnancy: Category B.
Lactation: Excreted in breast milk.
Children: Some efficacy has been demonstrated. However, methemoglobinemia has occurred in newborns.
Carcinogenesis: Because the drug elevates serum prolactin concentration, use caution if administration of metoclopramide is considered in patient with previously detected breast cancer.
Anastomosis or closure of gut: Drug could theoretically put increased pressure on suture lines after gut anastomosis or closure.
Depression: Depression has occurred with or without history of depression. Symptoms have ranged from mild to severe and have included suicidal ideation and suicide.
Extrapyramidal symptoms: Manifest primarily as acute dystonic reactions, occurring usually during first 24 to 48 hr and more frequently in children and young adults or at higher doses.
Hypertension: Use with caution.
Parkinson-like symptoms: Occur more commonly within first 6 mo of treatment but also can occur after longer periods. Symptoms generally subside within 2 to 3 mo after drug discontinuation. Give drug cautiously, if at all, to patients with preexisting Parkinson disease.
Tardive dyskinesia: Tardive dyskinesia may develop, especially in the elderly. Risk of development and likelihood of irreversibility increases with treatment duration and total cumulative dose.

Overdosage: Signs and Symptoms

Drowsiness, disorientation, extrapyramidal reactions, muscle hypertonia, irritability, agitation.

PATIENT CARE CONSIDERATIONS

Administration/Storage

- Administer oral form 30 min before meals and at bedtime.
- For IV admixture, when diluted in parenteral solution, administer slowly over at least 15 min.
- For IM and IV bolus, inject slowly over 1 to 2 min.
- For parenteral doses more than 10 mg, dilute in 50 mL Sodium Chloride Injection.
- Store all dosage forms at room temperature (59° to 86°F) in tight, light-resistant containers.
- Administer PO, IM injection, direct IV injection, or intermittent IV infusion (doses more than 10 mg).
- Dilute the oral concentration (10 mg/mL) with liquid (eg, water, juice, soda) or mix with semisolid food (eg, applesauce, pudding) immediately before giving.

Assessment/Interventions

- Obtain patient history, including drug history and any known allergies. Note history of epilepsy, seizures, hypertension, Parkinson disease, GI bleeding, or bowel obstruction.
- Take safety precautions because of high risk for falls caused by drowsiness and decreased dexterity.
- Notify health care provider of acute CNS reactions, arrhythmias, hypotension, hypertension, and suicidal ideations.

Patient/Family Education
- Instruct patient to take medication 30 min before meals.
- Instruct patient to report the following symptoms to the health care provider: involuntary movement of eyes, face, or limbs.
- Caution patient to avoid intake of alcoholic beverages.
- Advise patient that drug may cause drowsiness and to use caution while driving or performing other tasks requiring mental alertness.

Metolazone

(meh-TOLE-uh-ZONE)

Class Thiazide-like diuretic

How Supplied
Zaroxolyn Tablets 2.5 mg, Tablets 5 mg, Tablets 10 mg ◆ Mykrox Tablets 0.5 mg

Action
PHARMACOLOGY: Increases urinary excretion of sodium and chloride by inhibiting reabsorption in ascending limb of loop of Henle and early distal tubules.

PHARMACOKINETICS/DYNAMICS:

Absorption: Steady states are usually reached in 4 to 5 days with 65% absorbed. T_{max} is approximately 8 hr (2 to 4 hr for Mykrox); C_{max} is 0.5 to 2 mg (dose dependent for Mykrox).

Metabolism: A small fraction of metolazone is metabolized.

Excretion: Most is excreted in the unconcentrated form in urine. The t½ is approximately 14 hr.

Onset: Onset is 1 hr.

Peak: Time to peak is 2 hr.

Duration: Duration is 12 to 24 hr.

Indications
Treatment of edema and hypertension. **Unlabeled use(s):** Prevention of calcium nephrolithiasis; reduction of postmenopausal osteoporosis; reduction of urine volume in diabetes insipidus.

Contraindications
Anuria; renal decompensation; hepatic coma or precoma.

Route/Dosage
ADULTS: **PO** 0.5 to 1 mg/day (Mykrox) or 2.5- to 20 mg/day (Zaroxolyn). Do not interchange Mykrox with Zaroxolyn. Mykrox is absorbed more rapidly and completely than Zaroxolyn.

Interactions
Cholestyramine, colestipol: May decrease effects of metolazone by decreasing absorption.
Diazoxide: Concurrent use may produce severe hyperglycemia.
Digitalis glycosides (eg, digoxin): Urinary loss of potassium and magnesium may predispose patient to digitalis-induced arrhythmia.
Lithium: Metolazone may decrease renal elimination of lithium, resulting in toxicity.
Loop diuretics (eg, furosemide): Concurrent use may produce profound diuresis and electrolyte abnormalities.
Sulfonylureas (eg, tolbutamide): Metolazone may decrease hypoglycemic effect of sulfonylureas by increasing blood glucose.

Lab Test Interferences
None well documented.

Adverse Reactions
CV: Rapid-acting formulation: Orthostatic hypotension; palpitations; chest pain; cold extremities; edema. Slow-acting formulation: Venous thrombosis, palpitations; chest pain; excessive volume depletion; hemoconcentration.
CNS: Rapid-acting formulation: Dizziness; headache; weakness; "weird" feeling; neuropathy; fatigue; lethargy; lassitude; depression. Slow-acting formulation: Dizziness; syncope; neuropathy; vertigo; headache; weakness; fatigue; lethargy; lassitude; anxiety; depression; nervousness.
DERM: Rapid-acting formulation: Necrotizing angiitis; vasculitis; cutaneous vasculitis; dry skin. Slow-acting formulation: Photosensitivity; necrotizing angiitis; vasculitis; cutaneous vasculitis.
EENT: Bitter taste.
GI: Rapid-acting formulation: Nausea. Slow-acting formulation: Nausea; anorexia; pancreatitis.
GU: Slow-acting formulation: Impotence.
HEMA: Slow-acting formulation: Leukopenia; agranulocytosis; aplastic anemia.
HEPA: Slow-acting formulation: Jaundice; hepatitis.
METAB: Hypokalemia; hyperuricemia; hyponatremia; hypochloremia; hypochloremic alkalosis.
RESP: Rapid-acting formulation: Cough; epistaxis; sinus congestion; sore throat.
OTHER: Rapid-acting formulation: Impotence; joint pain; back pain; itching eyes; tinnitus; muscle cramps and spasms. Slow-acting formulation: Swelling; chills; acute gouty attack; hyperglycemia; glucosuria; muscle cramps and spasms.

Precautions
Pregnancy: Category B.
Lactation: Undetermined.
Children: Not recommended for children.
Hypersensitivity: May occur; cross-sensitivity to sulfonamides or thiazides possible.
Renal function impairment: May precipitate azotemia; use drug with caution.
Hepatic function impairment: May precipitate hepatic coma; use drug with caution.

Tartrazine sensitivity: Some products contain tartrazine, which may cause allergic-type reactions (eg, bronchial asthma).
Fluid and electrolytes: May be altered; periodic determinations of serum electrolytes, BUN, uric acid and glucose are indicated.
Hyperuricemia: May increase serum uric acid and precipitate gout.
Lipids: May cause increases in total serum cholesterol, triglycerides and LDL.

Lupus erythematosus: May be activated or exacerbated.
Postsympathectomy patients: Antihypertensive effects may be increased.

Overdosage: Signs and Symptoms
Orthostatic hypotension, syncope, lethargy, GI hypermotility, dizziness, electrolyte abnormalities, CNS depression, drowsiness, hemoconcentration, GI irritation.

PATIENT CARE CONSIDERATIONS
Administration/Storage
- For treatment of edema, establish schedule for intermittent therapy every other day or 3 to 5 days/wk schedule to reduce potential for electrolyte imbalance.
- For treatment of hypertension, check orders for dosage adjustments of other agents to prevent hypotension.
- Do not interchange product with other brand or generic forms because some formulations are more rapidly bioavailable and not therapeutically equivalent at same doses of other thiazides.
- Administer medication in morning to prevent nocturia.
- Store at room temperature (59° to 86°F) in tight, light-resistant container.

Assessment/Interventions
- Obtain patient history, including drug history and any known allergies.
- Assess for signs of fluid or electrolyte imbalance (dry mouth, thirst, confusion, muscle fatigue, hypotension, tachycardia).
- Maintain accurate I&O records.
- Monitor blood sugar closely for diabetic patients.
- Monitor serum uric acid levels periodically.
- Assess initial and periodic determinations of serum electrolytes and uric acid levels.
- For treatment of diabetic patients, monitor output. If output increases dosage may need to be increased.

Patient/Family Education
- Advise patient to take early in day to avoid sleep disruption.
- Tell patient to take with food if stomach upset occurs.
- Explain significance of potential potassium loss, and identify appropriate supplemental food sources (eg, bananas, orange juice, dates, citrus fruits, apricots). Teach patient signs and symptoms of hypokalemia (muscle weakness, cramping).
- Explain that dizziness or lightheadedness may occur if patient stands up too fast.
- Tell patient to avoid exposure to sunlight and to use sunscreen or wear protective clothing until tolerance to sunlight can be established.
- Explain that BP should be checked periodically by patient or family member.
- Review signs and symptoms of fluid imbalance.

Metoprolol
(meh-TOE-pro-lahl)
Class Beta-adrenergic blocker

How Supplied
Lopressor Tablets 50 mg, Tablets 100 mg, Injection 1 mg/mL ◆ *Toprol XL* Tablets, extended release 25 mg (23.75 mg metoprolol succinate equivalent to 25 mg metoprolol tartrate), Tablets, extended release 50 mg (47.5 mg metoprolol succinate equivalent to 50 mg metoprolol tartrate), Tablets, extended release 100 mg (95 mg metoprolol succinate equivalent to 100 mg metoprolol tartrate), Tablets, extended release 200 mg (190 mg metoprolol succinate equivalent to 200 mg metoprolol tartrate)
✤ *Apo-Metoprolol* ◆ *Apo-Metoprolol (Type L)* ◆ *Betaloc* ◆ *Betaloc Durules* ◆ *Gen-Metoprolol* ◆ *Novo-Metoprol* ◆ *Nu-Metop* ◆ *PMS-Metoprolol-B*
◆ *PMS-Metoprolol-L*

Action
PHARMACOLOGY: Blocks beta receptors, primarily affecting CV system (decreases heart rate, decreases contractility, decreases BP) and lungs (promotes bronchospasm).

PHARMACOKINETICS/DYNAMICS:
Absorption: 95% is absorbed; oral bioavailability is 40% to 50%.

Distribution: 12% is protein bound, rapidly enters the CNS, and has moderate lipid solubility.

Metabolism: Metabolized hepatically (primarily by CYP2D6).

Excretion: Elimination is mainly by biotransformation in the liver. Approximately 95% excreted renally and less than 5% unchanged in urine. The t½ is 3 to 7 hr.

Peak: Times to peak are 1 to 2 hr (oral, regular), 6 to 12 hr (oral, long-acting), and 20 min (IV).

Indications Used alone or in combination with other antihypertensive agents, for management of hypertension, long-term management of angina pectoris, MI (immediate-release tablets and injection), treatment of stable, symptomatic (NYHA class II or III) heart failure of ischemic, hypertensive, or cardiomyopathic origin (*Toprol-XL* 25 mg only).

Contraindications Greater than first-degree heart block; CHF unless secondary to tachyarrhythmia treatable with beta-blockers; overt or moderate to severe cardiac failure; sinus bradycardia; cardiogenic shock; hypersensitivity to beta-blockers; systolic BP below 100 mm Hg; MI in patients with heart rate less than 45 bpm.

Route/Dosage

Hypertension
ADULTS: Initial: **PO** 100 mg/day in single or divided doses. Give 50 to 100 mg/day in a single dose, extended-release tablet.
Maintenance: **PO** 100 to 450 mg/day.

Angina
ADULTS: Initial: **PO** 100 mg/day in 2 divided doses. 100 mg/day in a single dose, extended-release tablet.
Maintenance: **PO** 100 to 400 mg/day.

MI
ADULTS: **IV bolus injection** 5 mg slowly; may repeat q 2 min up to 15 mg. If tolerated, give **PO** 50 mg q 6 hr beginning 15 min after last IV dose; continue for 48 hr followed by **PO** 100 mg bid for 1 to 3 yr. If patient is intolerant of full IV dose, give **PO** 25 to 50 mg q 6 hr starting 15 min after last IV dose.

CHF
ADULTS: Extended-release tablet: **PO** Start with 25 mg qd for 2 wk in patients with NYHA class II heart failure and 12.5 mg qd in patients with more severe heart failure; then double the dose q 2 wk to highest dosage tolerated by patient (max, 200 mg).

Interactions
Barbiturates: Bioavailability of metoprolol may decrease.
Cimetidine: May increase metoprolol levels.
Clonidine: May enhance or reverse antihypertensive effect; potentially life-threatening situations may occur, especially on abrupt withdrawal of clonidine.
Hydralazine: Serum levels of both drugs may increase.
Lidocaine: Lidocaine levels may increase, leading to toxicity.
NSAIDs: Some agents may impair antihypertensive effect.
Prazosin: Orthostatic hypotension may increase.
Methimazole, propafenone, propylthiouracil, quinidine: Effects of metoprolol may increase.
Rifampin: May decrease effects of metoprolol.
Verapamil: Effects of both drugs may be increased.

Lab Test Interferences Antinuclear antibodies may develop but are usually reversible on discontinuation.

Adverse Reactions
CV: Hypotension; edema; flushing; bradycardia (3%); palpitations; CHF; arterial insufficiency; peripheral edema.
CNS: Headache; fatigue; dizziness (10%); depression (5%); lethargy; drowsiness; forgetfulness; sleepiness (10%); vertigo; paresthesias.
DERM: Rash (5%); facial erythema; alopecia; urticaria; pruritus (5%).
EENT: Dry eyes; visual disturbances.
GI: Nausea; vomiting; diarrhea (5%); dry mouth; gastric pain; constipation; heartburn; flatulence.
GU: Impotence; urinary retention; difficulty with urination.
RESP: Shortness of breath (3%); bronchospasm; dyspnea; wheezing.
OTHER: Increased hypoglycemic response to insulin; may mask hypoglycemic signs; muscle cramps; asthenia; systemic lupus erythematosus; cold extremities.

> **WARNING:**
>
> *Abrupt withdrawal:* In patients with angina pectoris or coronary artery disease (CAD), metoprolol may cause exacerbation of angina, occurrence of MI, and ventricular arrhythmias. Monitor patients closely. Because CAD is common and often unrecognized, it may be prudent not to discontinue beta-blocker therapy abruptly in patients being treated for hypertension.

Precautions
Pregnancy: Category C.
Lactation: Excreted in breast milk.
Children: Safety and efficacy not established.
Hepatic function impairment: Reduced daily dose advised.
Anaphylaxis: Deaths have occurred; aggressive therapy may be required.
AV block: Slows AV conduction and may cause heart block.
Bradycardia: Metoprolol decreases heart rate in most patients.
Bronchospastic disease: Use with caution. Administer in smaller divided doses.

CHF: Administer cautiously in CHF patients controlled by digitalis and diuretics. Notify health care provider at first sign or symptom of CHF or of unexplained respiratory symptoms in any patient.
Diabetes: May mask tachycardia associated with hypoglycemia.
Hypokalemia: Usually transient decreases in serum potassium levels may occur caused by intracellular shunting, which can produce adverse cardiovascular effects.

PATIENT CARE CONSIDERATIONS
Administration/Storage
- When switching from immediate-release tablets, give same total daily dose.
- Give drug at same time consistently with or without meals. Food slightly enhances drug's bioavailability.
- Store at room temperature (59° to 86°F) and protect from light.

Tablets (immediate release) and injection:
- Give at same time every day.

Assessment/Interventions
- Obtain patient history, including drug history and any known allergies.
- Implement periodic ECG or telemetry monitoring, as ordered, if bradyarrhythmia occurs.
- Check BP and pulse q 8 hr.
- Monitor levels of BUN, LDH, and uric acid and glucose tolerance.
- In diabetic patients, monitor blood sugar closely.
- Notify health care provider of CNS changes, unstable diabetes, rash, pruritus, visual disturbance or eye irritation, dyspnea, bronchospasm, asthma, arthralgia, and muscle cramps.
- Avoid abrupt withdrawal of therapy, which may precipitate ventricular arrhythmia, angina, MI, or death.
- Assess peripheral pulses for evidence of arterial occlusion.

Patient/Family Education
- Teach patient how to check pulse and BP.
- Advise patient to contact health care provider if pulse is less than 50 bpm.
- Explain why medication should not be discontinued abruptly.
- Tell diabetic patient to check blood sugar regularly and consult health care provider if levels are unstable.
- Explain that adverse effects are usually mild and transient and will generally subside with continued therapy.
- Instruct patient to report the following symptoms to health care provider: difficulty breathing, night cough, edema.
- Advise patient that drug may cause drowsiness and to use caution while driving or performing tasks requiring mental alertness.
- Instruct patient not to take OTC cold preparations without consulting health care provider.

Peripheral vascular disease: May precipitate or aggravate symptoms of atrial insufficiency.
Thyrotoxicosis: May mask clinical signs (eg, tachycardia) of developing or continuing hyperthyroidism. Abrupt withdrawal may exacerbate symptoms of hyperthyroidism, including thyroid storm.

Overdosage: Signs and Symptoms
Bradycardia, hypotension, bronchospasm, cardiac failure.

Metronidazole
(meh-troe-NID-uh-zole)
Class Anti-infective

How Supplied
Flagyl Tablets 250 mg, Tablets 500 mg ♦ *Flagyl ER* Tablets, extended-release 750 mg ♦ *Flagyl 375* Capsules 375 mg ♦ *Flagyl I.V.* Powder for Injection, lyophilized 500 mg ♦ *Flagyl I.V. RTU* Injection 5 mg/mL ♦ *Metric 21* Tablets 250 mg ♦ *MetroCream* Cream 0.75% ♦ *MetroGel* Gel 0.75% ♦ *MetroGel-Vaginal* Gel 0.75% ♦ *MetroLotion* Lotion 0.75% ♦ *Noritate* Cream 1% ♦ *Protostat* Tablets 250 mg, Tablets 500 mg
✽ *Apo-Metronidazole* ♦ *Florazole ER* ♦ *Nida Gel* ♦ *Novo-Nidazol*

Action
PHARMACOLOGY: Enters bacterial or protozoal cell and impairs synthesis of DNA, resulting in cell death.

PHARMACOKINETICS/DYNAMICS:
Absorption: Oral metronidazole is well absorbed; topical application is less complete and more prolonged. Following administration, T_{max} is 1 to 2 hr, and C_{max} is 25 mg/mL. Oral bioavailability is not affected by food, but peak serum levels will be delayed to 2 hr.

Distribution: Metronidazole appears in cerebrospinal fluid, saliva, and breast milk in concentrations similar to those found in plasma. Less than 20% is protein bound.

Metabolism: Metabolites are 2–hydroxymethyl and acidic metabolite.

Excretion: Routes of elimination are via urine (60% to 80%) and feces (6% to 15%). Renal Cl is approximately 10 mL/min per 1.73 m^2. The t½ is 8 hr in healthy adults, and the hydroxy-metabolite t½ is 15 hr.

Special Populations:
Hepatic Function Impairment – Patients with hepatic dysfunction metabolized metronidazole slower; accumulation of drug may occur. Cautiously administer doses below the usual recommended dose.

Elderly – Because the pharmacokinetics of metronidazole may be altered in the elderly, monitoring of serum levels may be necessary to adjust the dosage accordingly.

Indications Treatment of serious infections caused by susceptible anaerobic bacteria; prophylaxis of postoperative infection in patients undergoing colorectal surgery; treatment of amebiasis; treatment of trichomoniasis and asymptomatic partners of infected patients; bacterial vaginosis (*Flagyl ER* only).

Topical: Treatment of inflammatory papules, pustules, and erythema of acne rosacea.
Vaginal: Treatment of bacterial vaginosis.

Unlabeled use(s): Treatment of hepatic encephalopathy, Crohn disease, antibiotic-associated pseudomembranous colitis, *Helicobacter pylori* infections.

Contraindications Hypersensitivity to nitroimidazole derivatives or any component of the products; first trimester of pregnancy in patients with trichomoniasis.

Route/Dosage
Amebiasis
ADULTS: **PO**
Flagyl 375 capsules: Acute amebic dysentery and amebic liver abscess: 750 mg tid for 5 to 10 days.
Flagyl 250 mg tablets: Acute amebic dysentery: 750 mg tid for 5 to 10 days. Amebic liver abscess: 500 or 750 mg tid for 5 to 10 days.
CHILDREN: **PO**
Flagyl 375, Flagyl 250 mg tablets: 35 to 50 mg/kg per 24 hr divided into 3 daily doses for 10 days.

Anaerobic Bacterial Infections
Give IV initially when treating most serious anaerobic infections.
ADULTS: **IV** 15 mg/kg loading dose infused over 1 hr (approximately 1 g for a 70 kg adult); then a maintenance dose of 7.5 mg/kg infused over 1 hr q 6 hr (approximately 500 mg for a 70 kg adult). The first maintenance dose should be given 6 hr following initiation of loading dose. Do not exceed 4 g in 24 hr. May follow with similar oral dose. For prophylaxis, loading dose is to be completed 1 hr before surgery, followed by maintenance dose 6 and 12 hr later.
Duration: The usual duration is 7 to 10 days; however, infections of the bone, joint, lower respiratory tract, and endocardium may require longer treatment.
ADULTS: **PO**
Flagyl 375, Flagyl 250 mg tablets: Usual dosage is 7.5 mg/kg (approximately 500 mg for a 70 kg adult) q 6 hr (max, 4 g per 24 hr) for 7 to 10 days; however, infections of the bone, joint, lower respiratory tract, and endocardium may require longer treatment.

Bacterial Vaginosis
ADULTS: **PO** 750 mg (*Flagyl ER*) daily for 7 consecutive days. **Vaginal** 1 applicator-full (approximately 37.5 mg metronidazole) intravaginally once or twice a day for 5 days; for daily dosing, administer at bedtime

Inflammatory Papules, Pustules of Rosacea
ADULTS: **Topical** Apply thin layer once daily (1% cream) or bid to entire affected areas after washing. Use morning and evening or as directed by health care provider. Avoid application close to eyes.

Trichomoniasis
Individualize treatment for women and men.
ADULTS: **PO**
Flagyl 375 capsules: Women: 375 mg bid for 7 consecutive days. When a repeat course is required, a lapse of 4 to 6 wk between courses is recommended.
Flagyl 250 mg tablets: 250 mg tid for 7 consecutive days.
One-day treatment: 2 g as a single dose or in 2 divided doses of 1 g each given on the same day.
CHILDREN: **PO** 5 mg/kg/dose tid for 7 days.

Interactions
Anticoagulants: Anticoagulant effect may be increased.
Barbiturates, phenytoin: Therapeutic failure of metronidazole may occur.
Cimetidine: May prolong the t½ and decrease plasma Cl of metronidazole.
Disulfiram: Concurrent use may result in acute psychosis or confusional state. Do not give metronidazole to patients who have taken disulfiram within last 2 wk.
Ethanol: Disulfiram-like reaction including flushing, palpitations, tachycardia, nausea, and vomiting may occur with concurrent use.
Lithium: Plasma levels may be elevated by metronidazole, increasing the risk of lithium toxicity.
INCOMPATIBILITIES: Do not use aluminum-containing equipment with metronidazole because solution will turn orange/rust color.

Lab Test Interferences May interfere with chemical analyses for AST, ALT, LDH, triglycerides, and hexokinase glucose; zero values may occur.

Adverse Reactions When known, dose form and percentage are stated.
CV: Flattening of T-wave.
CNS: Seizures; peripheral neuropathy; dizziness; vertigo; incoordination; ataxia; confusion; depression; insomnia; syncope; irritability; weakness. *Flagyl ER*: Headache (18%); dizziness (4%). *MetroGel Vaginal*: Headache (5%); dizziness (2%).
DERM: Thrombophlebitis; urticaria; erythematous rash; flushing. *MetroGel Vaginal*: Generalized itching or rash, skin irritation, transient skin erythema, mild skin dryness and burning (2%). *MetroLotion/Cream/Gel Topical*: erythema, local allergic reaction, contact dermatitis, pruritus, skin discomfort (burning, stinging), worsening of rosacea, dry skin, transient redness.
EENT: Metallic taste; glossitis; stomatitis. *Flagyl ER*: Rhinitis (4%); sinusitis, pharyngitis (3%).
GI: Nausea; anorexia; vomiting; diarrhea; constipation; epigastric distress; cramps; pseudomembranous colitis; furry tongue; glossitis; stomatitis. *Flagyl ER*: Nausea (10%); metallic taste (9%); abdominal pain, diarrhea (4%); dry mouth (2%). *MetroGel Vaginal*: GI discomfort (7%); nausea, vomiting (4%); unusual taste (2%); diarrhea, loose stools, decreased appetite (1%).
GU: Darkening of urine; dysuria; cystitis; sense of pelvic pressure; polyuria; incontinence; vaginal *Candida* proliferation; decreased libido; proctitis. *Flagyl ER*: Vaginitis (15%); genital pruritus (5%); abnormal urine, dysmenorrhea (3%); UTI (2%). *MetroGel Vaginal*: Vaginal discharge (12%); symptomatic *Candida* cervicitis/vaginitis (10%); vulva/vaginal irritative symptoms (9%); pelvic discomfort (3%).
HEMA: Mild leukopenia; reversible thrombocytopenia.

RESP: *Flagyl ER*: Upper respiratory tract infection (4%).
OTHER: Hypersensitivity reactions including dermatologic reactions, nasal congestion, dry mouth or vagina, and fever; fleeting joint pain; pancreatitis. Topical or vaginal use may cause similar adverse effects. After prolonged IV use, thrombophlebitis may occur. *Flagyl ER*: Bacterial infection (7%); influenza-like symptoms (6%); moniliasis (3%). *MetroGel Vaginal*: Unspecified cramping (1%).

> **WARNING:**
> Oral and IV metronidazole have been carcinogenic in mice and rats. Avoid unnecessary use.

Precautions
Pregnancy: Category B.
Lactation: Excreted in breast milk.
Children: Safety and efficacy not established, except for amebiasis.
Elderly: Monitoring serum levels may be necessary for proper dosing.
Hepatic function impairment: Patients with severe hepatic disease metabolize drug slowly; use caution and lower dose.
Candidiasis: Known or previously unrecognized candidiasis may present more prominent symptoms during therapy.
Hematologic effects: Use with caution in patients with a history of blood dyscrasia.
Neurologic effects: Seizures and peripheral neuropathy have occurred. Use extra caution with prolonged use, high doses, or history of CNS disease.

Overdosage: Signs and Symptoms
Nausea, vomiting, ataxia, seizures, peripheral neuropathy.

PATIENT CARE CONSIDERATIONS
Administration/Storage
- Dose and dosing frequency are variable, depending on condition being treated.
- Store extended-release tablets, vaginal gel, topical cream, and topical gel at controlled room temperature (59° to 86°F). Store tablets, capsules, topical lotion, and injection below 77°F. Protect injection from light until use.

Tablets and capsules:
- Administer prescribed dose without regard to meals. Administer with food if GI upset occurs.

Extended-release tablets:
- Administer prescribed dose daily, 1 hr before or 2 hr after a meal.

- Have patient swallow extended-release tablet whole. Do not crush, chew, or divide.

Vaginal gel:
- For intravaginal use only. Not for ophthalmic, dermal, or oral administration.
- Administer gel using disposable applicator provided with medication.
- If accidental contact of vaginal gel with the eye(s) occurs, rinse the eye(s) with copious amounts of cool tap water.

Topical:
- For topical use only. Not for ophthalmic, vaginal, or oral administration.

♦ Cleanse areas to be treated before applying medication. Apply and rub in a thin film of medication bid to entire affected areas. Avoid contact with the eyes.

Injection:
♦ Administer by IV infusion only. Not for intradermal, subcutaneous, or IM administration.
♦ Solution is administered directly from original IV container. No further dilution is required.
♦ Do not administer using equipment containing aluminum (eg, needles, cannulae) that may come in or make contact with the drug solution.
♦ Administer prescribed dose over 30 to 60 min.
♦ Do not administer if particulate matter, cloudiness, or discoloration are noted or if the seals are not intact.
♦ Do not add other drugs to the metronidazole infusion bag.
♦ If other drugs are being administered through the same IV line, flush it before and after infusion of metronidazole. If being used with a primary IV fluid system, discontinue the primary solution during metronidazole infusion.
♦ Reconstituted *Flagyl IV* is stable for 96 hr when stored above 86°F. Use diluted and neutralized IV solutions within 24 hr.
♦ For proper reconstitution, dilution, and neutralization of IV solutions, see manufacturer's guidelines.

Assessment/Interventions

♦ Obtain patient history, including drug history and any known allergies. Note renal impairment, severe hepatic impairment, CNS disease, blood dyscrasia, history of blood dyscrasia, or current or recent (within 2 wk) use of disulfiram.
♦ Review results of culture and sensitivity testing as available.
♦ Ensure that CBC with differential is obtained before starting therapy and after therapy has been completed.
♦ Monitor for signs of infection, especially fever, and for positive response to antibiotic therapy.
♦ Monitor patient for GI, CNS, musculoskeletal, and general body side effects. Report to health care provider if noted and significant. Immediately report any abnormal neurologic signs or symptoms (eg, seizures, extremity numbness, abnormal skin sensations).

Patient/Family Education

♦ Explain name, dose, action, and potential side effects of drug.
♦ Instruct patient to take exactly as prescribed and not to change the dose or discontinue therapy unless advised by health care provider.
♦ Instruct patient to notify health care provider if infection does not appear to be improving or appears to be getting worse.
♦ Caution patient to avoid alcoholic beverages while taking metronidazole and for at least 3 days following completion of therapy.
♦ Advise patient that metallic taste is a common side effect of therapy but that this will resolve when therapy has been discontinued.
♦ Advise patient to report any other bothersome side effects to health care provider and to immediately report any abnormal neurologic signs or symptoms (eg, seizures, extremity numbness, abnormal skin sensations).
♦ Advise women to notify health care provider if pregnant, planning to become pregnant, or breastfeeding.
♦ Instruct patient not to take any prescription or OTC medications, dietary supplements, or herbal preparations unless advised by health care provider.
♦ Advise patient that follow-up examinations and lab tests may be required to monitor therapy and to keep appointments.

Tablets and capsules:
♦ Advise patient to take prescribed dose without regard to meals but to take with food if GI upset occurs.

Extended-release tablets:
♦ Advise patient to take prescribed dose daily, 1 hr before or 2 hr after a meal.
♦ Caution patient to swallow extended-release tablet whole and not to crush, chew, or divide.

Vaginal gel:
♦ Review instructions for filling applicator, administering medication, and care of applicator.
♦ Advise patient that if accidental contact of the gel with the eye(s) occurs, to rinse the eye(s) with copious amounts of cool tap water. Advise patient to notify health care provider if eye irritation persists after rinsing.
♦ Advise patient to avoid vaginal intercourse during treatment.
♦ Advise patient to discontinue use and notify health care provider if vaginal irritation develops while using the medication.

Topical:
♦ Advise patient to cleanse areas to be treated before applying medication, then apply and rub in a thin film bid to entire affected areas.
♦ Advise patient that cosmetics may be applied after application of medication but if using lotion, to allow it to dry first.
♦ Advise patient that if local irritation occurs to apply the medication less frequently. If

irritation persists, advise patient to discontinue use and notify health care provider.
Injection:
• Advise patient, family, or caregiver that medication will be prepared and administered by a health care provider in a health care setting.
• Advise patient to report injection site pain or redness.

Mexiletine Hydrochloride

(MEX-ih-leh-teen HIGH-droe-KLOR-ide)
Class Antiarrhythmic
How Supplied
Mexitil Capsules 150 mg, Capsules 200 mg, Capsules 250 mg
✤ *Novo-Mexiletine*

Action
PHARMACOLOGY: Reduces rate of rise of action potential; decreases effective refractory period in Purkinje fibers; has local anesthetic actions.

PHARMACOKINETICS/DYNAMICS:
Absorption: Mexiletine is well absorbed with approximately 90% from the GI tract. T_{max} is 2 to 3 hr, and the therapeutic range is 0.5 to 2 mcg/mL.

Distribution: Approximately 50% to 60% is protein bound. Vd is 5 to 7 L/kg.

Metabolism: First-pass metabolism occurs in the liver. N-methylmexiletine metabolite is the most active, but less than 20% as potent as mexiletine.

Excretion: 10% is excreted unchanged by the kidney, and less than 0.5% of N-methylmexiletine is excreted in urine. The plasma t½ is 10 to 12 hr. Urinary acidification accelerates excretion.

Special Populations:
Renal Function Impairment – Patients with severe renal impairment may require lower doses. Monitor closely. Mean t½ is 15.7 hr with Ccr less than 10 mL/min.
Hepatic Function Impairment – Prolonged elimination t½; mean t½ is approximately 25 hr.

Indications
Treatment of documented life-threatening ventricular arrhythmias such as sustained ventricular tachycardia (VT).

Contraindications
Preexisting second- or third-degree AV block (if pacemaker is not present); cardiogenic shock.

Route/Dosage
Ventricular Arrhythmias
ADULTS: PO 200 mg q 8 hr initially, increasing up to 400 mg q 8 hr if necessary (max, 1,200 mg/day). Adjust dose by 50 to 100 mg increments q 2 to 3 days. For rapid control of ventricular arrhythmias, give loading dose of 400 mg followed by 200 mg in 8 hr. When adequate suppression is achieved on a dose of 300 mg or less given q 8 hr, the same total daily dose may be given in divided doses q 12 hr (max, 450 mg q 12 hr).

Interactions
Aluminum-magnesium hydroxide, atropine, narcotics: May slow absorption.
Caffeine: Cl may be decreased by 50%.
Cimetidine: May increase or decrease mexiletine plasma levels.
Fluvoxamine: Cl of mexiletine may be decreased.
Hydantoins, rifampin, phenobarbital: May increase mexiletine Cl.
Metoclopramide: May accelerate absorption of mexiletine.
Propafenone: May inhibit mexiletine metabolism, which may elevate mexiletine plasma levels in extensive metabolizers and increase the risk of side effect.
Theophylline: May increase serum theophylline levels.

Lab Test Interferences
May result in abnormal LFTs, positive ANA titer, or thrombocytopenia.

Adverse Reactions
CV: Palpitations, chest pain (8%); increased ventricular arrhythmias/PVCs, angina or angina-like pain (2%); exacerbation of CHF (postmarketing).
CNS: Dizziness, lightheadedness (26%); tremor (13%); nervousness (11%); coordination difficulties (10%); headache (8%); changes in sleep habits (7%); weakness (5%); paresthesias, numbness, fatigue (4%); speech difficulties, confusion, clouded sensorium (3%); depression (2%); drowsiness, ataxia (postmarketing).
DERM: Rash (4%).
EENT: Blurred vision, visual disturbances (8%); tinnitus (2%); nystagmus (postmarketing).
GI: Nausea, vomiting, heartburn (40%); diarrhea (5%); constipation (4%); changes in appetite, dry mouth (3%); abdominal pain, cramps or discomfort (1%); dyspepsia (postmarketing).
HEMA/LYMPH: Blood dyscrasias.
MUSC: Arthralgia (1.7%); myelofibrosis.
RESP: Dyspnea (6%).
OTHER: Non-specific edema (4%); fever (1%); hypersensitivity (postmarketing).

> **WARNING:**
> Mortality risks noted for flecainide and/or encainide (type 1C antiarrhythmics). Reserved for use in patients with life-threatening ventricular arrhythmias.

Precautions
Pregnancy: Category C.
Lactation: Excreted in breast milk.
Children: Safety and efficacy not established.
Hepatic function impairment: Use drug with caution in patients with hepatic impairment. Reduce dosage in patients with severe liver disease.

PATIENT CARE CONSIDERATIONS
Administration/Storage
- May be used alone or in combination with other antiarrhythmic medications.
- Initiate therapy for life-threatening arrhythmias in-hospital with close monitoring of cardiac rhythm.
- Administer dose q 8 or 12 hr as prescribed.
- Administer with food or antacid to reduce GI upset
- Do not increase dose more often than q 2 days during dosage titration as optimal effect may not be achieved during the first 2 days following initiation of therapy or dose change.
- When converting from lidocaine infusion to mexiletine, discontinue lidocaine infusion when first dose of mexiletine is administered.
- Store capsules at controlled room temperature (59° to 86°F).

Assessment/Interventions
- Obtain patient history, including drug history and any known allergies. Note hepatic impairment, sinus node dysfunction, intraventricular conduction abnormalities, hypotension, CHF, seizure disorder, or concurrent use of propafenone.
- Review patient's health history and current situation for any condition that would contraindicate mexiletine therapy: hypersensitivity to mexiletine; pre-existing second- or third-degree AV block unless pacemaker is present; cardiogenic shock.
- Ensure liver enzymes are evaluated before initiating therapy and periodically thereafter during long-term treatment. Monitor liver enzymes more frequently in patient with pre-existing liver disease or if signs or symptoms suggesting liver dysfunction develop. Be prepared to discontinue therapy if persistent or worsening elevation of hepatic enzymes is noted.

CV effects: Has proarrhythmic effect; initiate therapy in hospital.
Convulsions: Have occurred; use drug with caution in patients with known seizure disorder.
Special risk patients: Use with caution in patients with CHF or hypotension.
Urinary pH: Marked alterations in urinary pH may alter mexiletine elimination; avoid drugs or diets that alter pH.

Overdosage: Signs and Symptoms
Coma, respiratory arrest, dizziness, drowsiness, nausea, hypotension, sinus bradycardia, paresthesia, seizures, confusion, bundle branch block, AV heart block, asystole, ventricular tachyarrhythmias including ventricular fibrillation.

- Review baseline ECG. Monitor cardiac rhythm while initiating therapy or when adjusting dose. Notify health care provider immediately of increase in ventricular rate, new or worsening premature ventricular contractions, VT, or ventricular fibrillation. Be prepared to treat appropriately.
- Monitor and record BP and pulse frequently during treatment. Notify health care provider of any significant changes.
- Ensure mexiletine plasma levels are periodically evaluated during prolonged therapy. Monitor plasma levels more frequently if toxic or subtherapeutic dosage regimens are suspected.
- Monitor patient for GI, CNS, CV, and general body side effects. Inform health care provider if noted and significant.

Patient/Family Education
- Explain name, dose, action, and potential side effects of drug.
- Advise patient that dose of medication may be changed periodically to obtain max benefit.
- Caution patient to take prescribed dose q 8 or 12 hr exactly as ordered. Advise patient that serious heart disturbances can result from missing doses.
- Advise patient to take each dose with food or antacid to prevent stomach upset.
- Caution patient not to change the dose or stop taking unless advised by health care provider. Advise patient that serious side effects can result from increasing or decreasing the dose without medical supervision.
- Inform patient that drug controls, but does not cure, abnormal heart rhythm and to continue taking as prescribed once the heart rhythm has been controlled.

- Instruct patient to continue taking other heart medications as prescribed by health care provider.
- Instruct patient in BP and pulse measurement skills.
- Advise patient to monitor and record BP and pulse at home and to inform health care provider if abnormal measurements are noted. Also advise patient to take record of BP and pulse to each follow-up visit.
- Instruct patient to lie or sit down if experiencing dizziness or lightheadedness when standing.
- Advise patient to notify health care provider if any of the following occur: frequent episodes of dizziness or lightheadedness, persistent nausea, tremor, any other unusual or unexplained symptom or sign.
- Instruct patient to immediately report fainting, pounding in chest, change in pulse or heart rhythm, yellowing of skin or eyes, unexplained fever, sore throat, bleeding, or unusual bruising to health care provider.
- Caution patient that drug may cause dizziness, lightheadedness, or coordination difficulties, and to use caution while driving or performing other tasks requiring mental alertness or coordination until tolerance is determined.
- Advise women to notify health care provider if pregnant, planning to become pregnant, or breastfeeding.
- Advise patient to carry medical identification (eg, *Medi-Alert*) describing cardiac condition and medication regimen.
- Caution patient not to take any prescription, herbal preparations, or OTC medications or dietary supplements unless advised by health care provider.
- Offer family instruction in basic life support.
- Advise patient that follow-up visits and lab tests will be required to monitor therapy and to keep appointments.

Mezlocillin Sodium

(MEZZ-low-SILL-in SO-dee-uhm)

Class Antibiotic/Penicillin

How Supplied
Mezlin Powder for injection 1 g (as sodium; contains 1.85 mEq sodium/g), Powder for injection 2 g (as sodium), Powder for injection 3 g (as sodium), Powder for injection 4 g (as sodium), Powder for injection 20 g (as sodium)

Action
PHARMACOLOGY: Inhibits biosynthesis of bacterial cell wall mucopeptide.

PHARMACOKINETICS/DYNAMICS:
Absorption: T_{max} is 0.5 to 1 hr (IM); C_{max} is 35 to 45 mcg/mL (1g IM) and 254 mcg/mL (4 g IV).

Distribution: Protein binding is 16% to 42% and Vd is 0.23 L/kg.

Metabolism: Metabolism is 20% to 30% hepatic.

Excretion: 55% to 60% is excreted renally as unchanged. The t½ is 0.8 to 1.1 hr. Mezlocillin is removed by hemodialysis.

Special Populations:
Renal Function Impairment – The t½ for Ccr 10 to 30 mL/min is 2 hr and 2.6 hr for Ccr less than 10 mL/min.

Indications Treatment of infections of lower respiratory tract, urinary tract, skin or skin structure; intra-abdominal infections; uncomplicated gonorrhea; gynecological infections; septicemia; streptococcal infections; severe infections; and *Pseudomonas* infections caused by susceptible strains of specific microorganisms and prophylaxis.

Contraindications Hypersensitivity to penicillins.

Route/Dosage
ADULTS: **IM/IV** 200 to 300 mg/kg/day in 4 to 6 divided doses. Usual doses are 3 g q 4 hr or 4 g q 6 hr. **IM** Doses should not exceed 2 g/injection.
CHILDREN (OLDER THAN 1 MO TO YOUNGER THAN 12 YR): **IM/IV** 50 mg/kg q 4 hr.
NEWBORNS: **IV** 75 mg/kg q 6 to 12 hr.

Interactions
Contraceptives, oral: May reduce efficacy of oral contraceptives.
Tetracyclines: May impair bactericidal effects of mezlocillin.
INCOMPATIBILITIES: Parenteral aminoglycosides may inactivate aminoglycosides in vitro; do not mix in same IV solution.

Lab Test Interferences
Antiglobulin (Coombs) test: Drug may cause false-positive results in certain patient groups.
Urine glucose test: Drug may cause false-positive results with copper sulfate tests (eg, *Benedict* test, *Fehling* test, or *Clinitest* tablets); enzyme-based tests (eg, *Clinistix, Tes-tape*) are not affected.
Urine protein determinations: Drug may cause false-positives with sulfosalicylic acid and boiling test, acetic acid test, biuret reaction and nitric acid test; bromphenol blue test (*Multi-Stix*) not affected.

Adverse Reactions
CNS: Neurotoxicity (eg, lethargy, neuromuscular irritability, hallucinations, convulsions, seizures); dizziness; fatigue; insomnia; reversible hyperactivity; prolonged muscle relaxation.
DERM: Ecchymosis.
EENT: Itchy eyes.
GI: Nausea; vomiting; abdominal pain or cramp; diarrhea or bloody diarrhea; rectal bleeding; flatulence; enterocolitis; pseudomembranous colitis; anorexia.
GU: Interstitial nephritis (oliguria, proteinuria, hematuria, hyaline casts, pyuria); nephropathy; elevated creatinine or BUN.
HEPA: Transient hepatitis; cholestatic jaundice.
HEMA: Anemias; thrombocytopenia; eosinophilia; leukopenia; granulocytopenia; neutropenia; bone marrow depression; agranulocytosis; reduced hemoglobin or hematocrit; prolongation of bleeding time and PT; altered blood cell counts.
METAB: Elevated serum alkaline phosphatase; hypernatremia; reduced serum potassium, albumin, total proteins, and uric acid.
OTHER: Hypersensitivity reactions that may lead to death; vaginitis; hyperthermia; pain at site of injection; deep vein thrombosis; hematomas; vein irritation; phlebitis; sciatic neuritis.

Precautions
Pregnancy: Category B.
Lactation: Excreted in breast milk.
Hypersensitivity: Reactions range from mild to life threatening. Administer cautiously to cephalosporin-sensitive patients because of possible cross reactivity.
Superinfection: May result in bacterial or fungal overgrowth of nonsusceptible organisms.
Bleeding abnormalities: Hemorrhagic manifestations associated with abnormalities of coagulation tests (bleeding time, PT, platelet aggregation) may occur. Abnormalities should revert to normal when drug is discontinued.
Pseudomembranous colitis: Consider in patients with diarrhea.
Sodium content: 1.85 mEq sodium/g.

Overdosage: Signs and Symptoms
Neuromuscular hyperexcitability, seizures, convulsive seizures, agitation, confusion, asterixis, hallucinations, stupor, coma, multifocal myoclonus, encephalopathy, hyperkalemia.

PATIENT CARE CONSIDERATIONS
Administration/Storage
- For IV administration reconstitute each gram of mezlocillin sodium with 9 to 10 mL of sterile water, D5W, or 0.9% Sodium Chloride Injection; shake vigorously.
- Temporarily discontinue administration of any other solution during infusion.
- May inject reconstituted solution at least 10% into vein or IV tubing; infuse slowly over 3 to 5 min.
- For IM administration reconstitute each gram of mezlocillin sodium with 3 to 4 mL of 0.5% to 1% lidocaine hydrochloride without epinephrine. Inject into large muscle slowly (12 to 15 sec) to minimize discomfort.
- Store unreconstituted mezlocillin at room temperature.

Assessment/Interventions
- Obtain patient history, including drug history and any allergies.
- Monitor I&O throughout therapy.
- Monitor liver function, hematology (eg, WBC, RBC, hgb, hct, bleeding time), and renal function.
- Assess bowel function.
- Assess respiratory status.
- Observe IV site for thrombophlebitis.
- Notify health care provider of hemorrhagic manifestations associated with abnormalities in coagulation time.

Patient/Family Education
- Instruct patient to report the following symptoms to health care provider: Skin rash, itching, hives, severe diarrhea, shortness of breath, wheezing, black tongue, sore throat, nausea, vomiting, fever, swollen joints, or any unusual bleeding or bruising.

Miconazole

(my-KAHN-uh-zole)

Class Anti-infective/Antifungal

How Supplied
Absorbine Antifungal Foot Powder Powder 2% ♦ *Breezee Mist Antifungal* Powder 2% ♦ *Femizol-M* Vaginal Cream 2% ♦ *Fungoid Cream* Cream 2% ♦ *Fungoid Tincture* Solution 2% ♦ *Lotrimin AF* Spray Liquid 2%, Spray Powder 2%, Powder 2% ♦ *M-Zole 3 Combination Pack* Vaginal Suppositories 200 mg, Topical Cream 2% ♦ *M-Zole 7 Dual Pack* Vaginal Suppositories 100 mg, Topical Cream 2% ♦ *Maximum Strength Desenex Antifungal Cream* 2% ♦ *Micatin* Cream 2%, Spray Liquid 2%, Spray Powder 2%, Powder 2% ♦ *Monistat 3* Vaginal Suppositories 200 mg ♦ *Monistat 7* Vaginal Suppositories 100 mg, Vaginal Cream 2% ♦ *Monistat 7 Combination Pack* Vaginal Suppositories 100 mg, Topical Cream 2% ♦ *Monistat-Derm* Topical Cream 2% ♦

MICONAZOLE

Monistat Dual-Pak Vaginal Suppositories 200 mg, Topical Cream 2% ♦ Only-Clear Spray 2% ♦ Prescription Strength Desenex Spray powder 2%, Spray liquid 2% ♦ Tetterine Ointment 2% ♦ Zeasorb-AF Powder 2%

🍁 Micozole ♦ Monistat 1 Combination Pack ♦ Monistat 1 Vaginal Ovule ♦ Monistat 3 Vaginal Ovules ♦ Monistat Derm Cream

Action
PHARMACOLOGY: Alters permeability of fungal cell membrane, leading to cell death.

Indications
Parenteral form: Treatment of severe systemic fungal infections.
Vaginal form: Local treatment of vulvovaginal candidiasis (moniliasis).
Topical form: Treatment of topical fungal infections, including tinea infections and candidiasis.

Contraindications
Hypersensitivity to imidazoles.

Route/Dosage
Systemic Infections
ADULTS: **IV** 200 to 3600 mg/day. May divide into 3 doses. Treatment of meningitis is supplemented by intrathecal injections of 20 mg/dose. Treatment of bladder infections is supplemented by bladder instillations of 200 mg per dose.
CHILDREN (1 TO 12 YR): **IV** 20 to 40 mg/kg/day (max, 15 mg/kg/dose).
CHILDREN (YOUNGER THAN 1 YR): **IV** 15 to 30 mg/kg/day (max, 15 mg/kg/dose).

Vaginal Infections
ADULTS: **Intravaginal** 1 suppository (200 mg) at bedtime for 3 days or 1 suppository (100 mg) for 7 days or 1 applicatorful at bedtime for 7 days.

Topical Infections
ADULTS: **Topical** Apply to infected area bid.

Interactions
Anticoagulants, oral: May cause increased anticoagulant effect.
Antihistamines, nonsedating type (eg, astemizole, terfenadine): Cardiotoxicity, including arrhythmias and death, has occurred when agents of this type were used together with azole-type antifungals.

Lab Test Interferences
None well documented.

Adverse Reactions
CV: Tachycardia; arrhythmia; cardiorespiratory arrest.
DERM: Phlebitis at infusion site; pruritus; rash; skin irritation, sensitization and burning from topical preparations.
GI: Nausea; vomiting; diarrhea; anorexia.
HEMA: Transient decreases in hematocrit; thrombocytopenia.
METAB: Hyperlipemia possibly caused by vehicle.
OTHER: Anaphylaxis; fever; chills. Topical or vaginal forms may cause similar reactions.

Precautions
Pregnancy: Category C.
Lactation: Undetermined.
Children: Safety and efficacy in children younger than 1 yr not studied sufficiently.
Cardiac effects: Have occurred, possibly because of too-rapid administration.
Cremophor-type vehicle: Present in IV formulation; may cause electrophoretic abnormalities of lipoprotein; usually reversible.

PATIENT CARE CONSIDERATIONS

Administration/Storage
- Dilute IV admixture in 200 mL of 0.9% Sodium Chloride Injection or D5W. Infuse at rate of 2 hr/amp.
- Continue treatment until clinical and lab tests indicate absence of fungal infection.
- Topical lotion is preferred in intertriginous areas. If cream is used, use sparingly to avoid maceration effects.
- Spray or sprinkle powder liberally over affected area bid.

Assessment/Interventions
- Obtain patient history, including drug history and any known allergies. Note history of blood dyscrasias and hyperlipidemia.
- Monitor hemoglobin, hematocrit, electrolytes and lipids.
- Avoid having topical products come into contact with eyes.
- Refrigerate suppositories.

Patient/Family Education
- With topical therapy, instruct patient to use for full treatment time, even if symptoms improve. Advise patient to notify health care provider if there is no improvement in 2 wk.
- With topical therapy, if condition worsens or if burning, itching or redness occurs, instruct patient to discontinue use and notify health care provider.
- With vaginal therapy, instruct patient to refrain from sexual intercourse or to have partner use condom for protection and to prevent reinfection. Advise patient to apply medication at bedtime.
- Suggest patient use sanitary pad to prevent staining of clothing.
- With vaginal therapy, instruct patient not to discontinue use during menstruation.

Midazolam hydrochloride

(meh-DAZE-oh-lam HIGH-droe-KLOR-ide)
Class General anesthetic/Benzodiazepine

How Supplied
Versed Syrup 2 mg/mL, Injection 1 mg (as hydrochloride)/mL, Injection 5 mg (as hydrochloride)/mL
🍁 *Apo-Midazolam*

Action
PHARMACOLOGY: Depresses all levels of CNS, including limbic and reticular formation, probably through increased action of GABA, which is major inhibitory neurotransmitter in brain.

PHARMACOKINETICS/DYNAMICS:
Absorption: Midazolam is rapidly absorbed. The oral AUC ratio of metabolite to midazolam is higher than IV. Mean T_{max} is 0.17 to 2.65 hr and the absolute bioavailability is 36%.

Distribution: Midazolam exhibits linear pharmacokinetics (dose 0.25 to 1 mg/kg). Approximately 97% is protein bound (mainly to albumin). The mean steady-state Vd is 1.24 to 2.02 L/kg in children 6 mo to less than 16 yr receiving 0.15 mg/kg IV.

Metabolism: Midazolam is subject to substantial intestinal and hepatic first-pass metabolism by cytochrome P450 3A4. Active metabolite is alpha-hydroxymidazolam.

Onset: Onset is 10 to 20 min.

Special Populations:
Hepatic Function Impairment – Following oral administration (15 mg), C_{max} and bioavailability were 43% and 100% higher, respectively. The clearance was reduced 40% and t½ increased 90%. Doses should be titrated.
CHF – Following oral administration (7.5 mg), t½ increased 43%.

Indications Preoperative sedative; conscious sedation prior to diagnostic, therapeutic or endoscopic procedures; induction of general anesthesia; supplement to nitrous oxide and oxygen for short surgical procedures; infusion for sedation of intubated and mechanically ventilated patients as a component of anesthesia or during treatment in critical care setting.

Unlabeled use(s): Treatment of epileptic seizures; alternative for the termination of refractory status epilepticus.

Contraindications Hypersensitivity to benzodiazepines; uncontrolled pain; existing CNS depression; shock; acute narrow-angle glaucoma; acute alcohol intoxication; coma.

Route/Dosage
Preoperative Sedative
ADULTS: **IM** 0.07 to 0.08 mg/kg approximately 1 hr before surgery.

Conscious Sedation
ADULTS: **IV** 1 to 2.5 mg as 1 mg/mL dilution over 2 min. Increase by small increments to total dose of no more than 5 mg in at least 2 min intervals; use less if patient is premedicated with other CNS depressants.
CHILDREN: **IM** 0.1 to 0.15mg/kg. Doses up to 0.5 mg/kg have been used for more anxious patients. Total dose usually does not exceed 10 mg.
CHILDREN (YOUNGER THAN 6 MO): **IV** Titrate in small increments to clinical effect and monitor carefully.
CHILDREN (6 MO TO 5 YR): **IV** 0.05 to 0.1 mg/kg. Total dose up to 0.6 mg/kg may be necessary. Do not exceed 6 mg.
CHILDREN (6 TO 12 YR): **IV** 0.025 to 0.05 mg/kg. Total dose up to 0.4 mg/kg. Do not exceed 10 mg.
CHILDREN (12 TO 16 YR): **IV** Dose as adults.

Induction of General Anesthesia
UNPREMEDICATED ADULTS: **IV** 0.3 to 0.35 mg/kg as 1 mg/mL dilution over 20 to 30 sec, allowing 2 min for effect; may use increments of approximately 25% of initial dose.
PREMEDICATED ADULTS: **IV** 0.15 to 0.35 mg/kg over 20 to 30 sec.

Continuous Infusion
ADULTS:
Loading dose: 0.01 to 0.05 mg/kg given slowly over several minutes. May be repeated at 10- to 15-min intervals until adequate sedation is achieved.
Maintenance: 0.02 to 0.1 mg/kg/hr (1 to 7 mg/hr).
PEDIATRIC (NON-NEONATAL): **IV** 0.05 to 0.2 mg/kg over at least 2 to 3 min in patients whose trachea is intubated. Loading dose may be followed by continuous IV infusion at 0.06 to 0.12 mg/kg/hr (1 to 2 mcg/kg/min). Increase or decrease approximately 25% of the initial infusion rate or subsequent infusion rate.
INTUBATED PRETERM AND TERM NEWBORNS (YOUNGER THAN 32 WK): 0.03 mg/kg/hr (0.5 mcg/kg/min).
INTUBATED PRETERM AND TERM NEWBORNS (YOUNGER THAN 32 WK): 0.06 mg/kg/hr (1 mcg/kg/min).

Maintenance Of Anesthesia
IV Increments of approximately 25% of induction dose in response to signs of lightening of anesthesia and repeat as necessary.

Interactions
Anesthetics, inhalation: Inhalation anesthetics may need to be reduced if midazolam is used as

an induction agent. IV administration decreases minimum alveolar concentration of halothane required for general anesthesia.

Azole antifungal agents: Serum concentration of certain benzodiazepines may be increased and prolonged, producing enhanced CNS depression and prolonged effects.

Barbiturates, alcohol, other CNS depressants: May prolong effect and increase risk of underventilation or apnea.

Cimetidine: May increase midazolam levels.

Contraceptives, oral: Coadministration may result in prolongation of benzodiazepine t½.

Droperidol, narcotics, secobarbital: May accentuate hypnotic effect of midazolam.

Ethanol: Increased CNS effects with acute ethanol ingestion.

Fluvoxamine: Reduced clearance, prolonged t½ and increased serum concentrations of certain benzodiazepines may occur. Sedation or ataxia may be increased.

Indinavir: Possibly severe sedation and respiratory depression.

Propofol: Pharmacologic effects of propofol may be increased.

Rifamycins: Pharmacokinetic parameters of benzodiazepines may be altered.

Ritonavir: Possibly severe sedation and respiratory depression.

Theophyllines: Sedative effects of benzodiazepines may be antagonized.

Thiopental: Moderate reduction in induction dosage requirements has been noted following use of IM midazolam for premedication.

Valproic acid: Pharmacokinetic parameters of benzodiazepines may be increased. Liver metabolism may be decreased.

Verapamil: Effects of certain benzodiazepines may be increased, producing increased CNS depression and prolonged effects.

INCOMPATIBILITIES: Dimenhydrinate, pentobarbital, perphenazine, prochlorperazine, ranitidine.

Lab Test Interferences None well documented.

Adverse Reactions

CV: Bigeminy; hypotension; PVCs; tachycardia; cardiac arrest; vasovagal episode; bradycardia; nodal rhythm.

CNS: Headache; oversedation; retrograde amnesia; euphoria or dysphoria; confusion; argumentativeness; anxiety; emergence delirium and dreaming; nightmares; tonic/clonic movements; tremor; athetoid movements; ataxia; dizziness; slurred speech; paresthesia; weakness; loss of balance; drowsiness; nervousness; agitation; restlessness; prolonged emergence from anesthesia; insomnia; dysphonia.

DERM: Hives; hive-like elevation at injection site; swelling or feeling of burning; warmth or coldness at injection site; rash; pruritus.

EENT: Vision disturbances; nystagmus; pinpoint pupils; cyclic eyelid movements; blocked ears; blurred vision; diplopia; difficulty focusing; loss of balance.

GI: Nausea; vomiting; acid taste; excessive salivation; retching.

RESP: Respiratory depression or arrest; decreased tidal volume, decreased respiratory rate; apnea, coughing; laryngospasm; bronchospasm; dyspnea; hyperventilation; wheezing; shallow respirations; airway obstruction; tachypnea.

OTHER: Pain, tenderness and induration at injection site; yawning; chills; lethargy; weakness; toothache; faint feeling; hematoma; desaturation, apnea, hypotension, paradoxical reactions, hiccough, seizure-like activity, nystagmus (children).

> **WARNING:**
> Respiratory depression/arrest has been reported with use for sedation in noncritical care settings and occurs most often with concurrent CNS depressants. Midazolam should only be used in settings that can provide continuous monitoring for respiratory and cardiac function. Severe hypotension and seizures have been reported in neonates after rapid IV injection, particularly with concurrent fentanyl. Do not administer via rapid injection in this population.

Precautions

Pregnancy: Category D.

Lactation: Midazolam is excreted in breast milk. Exercise caution when administering to a nursing mother.

Children: As a group, pediatric patients generally require higher dosages of midazolam (mg/kg) than do adults. Pediatric patients (younger than 6 yr) may require higher dosages (mg/kg) than older pediatric patients and may require closer monitoring. In obese pediatric patients, calculate the dose based on ideal body weight.

Elderly: May need to decrease dosage. Titration should be more gradual.

Labor and delivery: Drug not recommended because of transplacental transfer.

Renal function impairment: Patients with renal impairment may have longer t½ for midazolam, which may result in slower recovery.

Special risk patients: High-risk surgical patients require lower doses. Patients with COPD are unusually sensitive to respiratory depressant effects. In renal or heart failure patients, give less frequently. Exercise care when administering to patients with uncompensated acute illness (eg, severe fluid or electrolyte disturbances).

Hazardous tasks: No patient should operate hazardous machinery or a motor vehicle until the side effects of the drug have subsided or until the day after anesthesia and surgery, whichever is longer.

Abrupt withdrawal: Withdrawal symptoms (convulsions, hallucinations, tremor, abdominal and muscle cramps, vomiting, and sweating) may occur following abrupt discontinuation.

Benzyl alcohol: The midazolam injection contains benzyl alcohol, which has been associated with a fatal "gasping syndrome" in premature infants.

Debilitated patients: May need to decrease dosage. Titration should be more gradual.

Serious cardiorespiratory events: Have occurred, including respiratory depression, airway obstruction, desaturation, permanent neurologic injury, apnea, respiratory arrest or cardiac arrest, sometimes resulting in death.

Improper dosing: Reactions such as agitation, involuntary movements, hyperactivity and combativeness have been reported.

Ophthalmic: Moderate lowering of IOP following induction with midazolam.

Intra-arterial injection: Unknown.

Intracranial pressure/circulatory side effects: Does not protect against the increase in intracranial pressure or circulatory effects associated with endotracheal intubation under light general anesthesia.

Overdosage: Signs and Symptoms

Sedation, impaired coordination and reflexes, hypotension, hypoventilation, somnolence, coma, confusion.

PATIENT CARE CONSIDERATIONS

Administration/Storage

- For IM administration, inject deeply in large muscle mass.
- Prior to IV administration, ensure availability of resuscitative equipment.
- For IV administration, titrate slowly to achieve desired effect (initiation of slurred speech).
- Do not use IV loading dose in newborns; the infusion may be run more rapidly for the first several hours to establish therapeutic plasma levels.
- Frequently reassess the rate of infusion, particularly after the first 24 hr, so as to administer the lowest dose and reduce the potential for drug accumulation.
- Give no more than 2.5 mg over at least 2 min; wait additional 2 min to fully evaluate the sedative effect.
- Continuously monitor patients for hypoventilation or apnea.
- Do not administer IV medication as rapid or bolus dose. Excessive or rapid IV dosing may result in respiratory arrest.
- Avoid intra-arterial injection.
- Avoid extravasation.
- May mix midazolam in same syringe as morphine, meperidine, atropine or scopolamine.
- Midazolam is compatible with Sodium Chloride for Injection, D5W, Ringer's Lactate Solution for 24 hr.
- Store at room temperature (59° to 86°F).

Assessment/Interventions

- Obtain patient history, including drug history and any known allergies. Note history of glaucoma, hypersensitivity to benzodiazepines and existing CNS depression.
- Continuously monitor patient for hypoventilation or apnea.
- Assist with ambulation after procedure until drowsiness resolves.
- Because serious life-threatening cardiorespiratory events have been reported, make provision for monitoring, detection and correction of these reactions for every patient regardless of health status.

Patient/Family Education

- Inform patient and family pre-operatively about possibility of temporary postoperative amnesia.
- Advise patient that drug may cause drowsiness and to use caution while driving or performing other tasks requiring mental alertness until drowsiness has subsided or until day after administration, whichever is longer.
- Advise patient to avoid alcohol and other CNS depressants for 24 hr following administration.
- The patient should inform her health care provider if she is pregnant, planning to become pregnant or is breastfeeding.
- Patients receiving continuous infusion in critical care settings over an extended period of time may experience symptoms of withdrawal following abrupt discontinuation.

Midodrine Hydrochloride

(mid-OH-drean HIGH-droe-KLOR-ide)

Class Vasopressor/Antihypotensive

How Supplied
ProAmatine Tablets 2.5 mg, Tablets 5 mg, Tablets 10 mg

Action

PHARMACOLOGY: Activates arteriolar and venous α-adrenergic receptors, resulting in an increase in vascular tone and elevation of BP.

PHARMACOKINETICS/DYNAMICS:

Absorption: Midodrine is rapidly absorbed. Absolute bioavailability is 93%, prodrug T_{max} is 30 min, and metabolite T_{max} is 1 to 2 hr.

Distribution: Neither prodrug nor metabolite is bound to plasma proteins to any significant extent.

Metabolism: Major active metabolite is desglymidodrine. Declycination of midodrine to desglymidodrine takes place in many tissues. Both compounds are metabolized in part by the liver.

Excretion: Renal Cl of desglymidodrine is 385 mL/min (approximately 80% by active renal secretion). The t½ is 25 min (midodrine) and 3 to 4 hr (desglymidodrine).

Peak: Time to peak is 1 hr.

Duration: Duration is 2 to 3 hr.

Special Populations:

Renal Function Impairment – Use cautiously in patients with urinary retention problems. A lower starting dose (2.5 mg) may be necessary. Assess renal function prior to initial use.

Hepatic Function Impairment – Use with caution, as the liver has a role in the metabolism.

Indications Treatment of symptomatic orthostatic hypotension in patients whose lives are considerably impaired despite standard clinical care, including support stockings, fluid expansion, and lifestyle changes. **Unlabeled use(s):** Management of urinary incontinence.

Contraindications Severe organic heart disease, acute renal failure, urinary retention, phenochromocytoma, thyrotoxicosis, or in patients with persistent and excessive supine hypertension.

Route/Dosage
ADULTS: PO 10 mg tid during daytime hours.

Renal Function Impairment
ADULTS: PO Start with 2.5 mg/dose.

Interactions

Alpha-blocking agents (eg, prazosin, terazosin, doxazosin): May antagonize pressor effects of midodrine.

Cardiac glycosides (ie, digitalis), beta-blockers: May precipitate bradycardia, AV block, or arrhythmia.

Fludrocortisone: May exacerbate supine hypertension.

Vasoconstrictors (eg, dihydroergotamine, ephedrine, phenylephrine, phenylpropanolamine, pseudoephedrine): May enhance pressor effects of midodrine.

Lab Test Interferences None well documented.

Adverse Reactions

CV: Supine and sitting hypertension (7%); bradycardia.

CNS: Paresthesia (18%); headache; confusion; nervousness; anxiety; confusion; abnormal thinking.

DERM: Piloerection (13%); scalp pruritus (12%); rash (2%).

GI: Abdominal pain; dry mouth.

GU: Dysuria (frequency, impaired micturition, urinary retention, urinary urgency) (13%).

OTHER: Pain, chills (5%); facial flushing; feeling of fullness/pressure in head.

> **WARNING:**
>
> Hypertension: Because the drug can cause significant hypertension, use only in patients whose lives are considerably impaired despite critical care. Clinical benefits have not been verified.

Precautions

Pregnancy: Category C.

Lactation: Undetermined.

Children: Safety and efficacy not established.

Renal function impairment: Use with caution. Initiate therapy with smaller doses.

Hepatic function impairment: Use with caution.

Bradycardia: May occur because of vagal reflex. Use caution when coadministering other agents that can reduce heart rate (eg, cardiac glycosides, beta-blockers, psychopharmacologic agents).

Diabetes: Use with caution.

Supine hypertension: Potentially most serious adverse reaction. Most common in patients with elevated pretreatment supine systolic BP (mean 170 mm Hg). Use is not recommended in patients with pretreatment supine systolic BP above 180 mm Hg. Monitor supine and sitting BPs.

Urinary retention: Use with caution because of effect on α-adrenergic receptors of bladder neck.

Overdosage: Signs and Symptoms

Hypertension, piloerection sensation of coldness, urinary retention.

PATIENT CARE CONSIDERATIONS
Administration/Storage
- Administer prescribed dose without regard to meals but administer with food if GI upset occurs.
- Medication is taken during daytime hours when patient is upright, at roughly 4-hr intervals, with first dose given before or upon rising in the morning. Medication may be given at 3-hr intervals if necessary to control symptoms of orthostatic hypotension.
- Do not administer after evening meal or less than 4 hr before bedtime to reduce risk of supine hypertension.
- Store tablets at controlled room temperature (59° to 86°F).

Assessment/Interventions
- Obtain patient history, including drug history and any known allergies. Note renal or hepatic impairment, heart disease, urinary retention, pheochromocytoma, thyrotoxicosis, excessive supine hypertension (eg, systolic BP greater than 170 mm Hg), or concurrent use of fludrocortisone or vasoconstrictors.
- Ensure that reduced initial dose and slower dose escalation is used in patient with renal impairment.
- Ensure that renal and hepatic function are evaluated before starting therapy and periodically during prolonged treatment.
- Monitor supine, sitting, and standing BP and pulse frequently during initiation of therapy.
- If supine hypertension noted, have patient sleep with head of bed elevated.
- Frequently assess patient for response to treatment. Discontinue medication and notify health care provider if supine hypertension (systolic BP greater than 180 mm Hg) persists or occurs or if patient develops symptomatic bradycardia.
- Ensure that therapy is periodically reviewed to determine if therapy needs to be continued without change or if a dose change (eg, increase, decrease, discontinuation) is indicated.
- Monitor patient for CNS, GU, DERM, and general body side effects. Report to health care provider if noted and significant.

Patient/Family Education
- Explain name, dose, action, and potential side effects of drug.
- Advise patient to read the *Patient Information* leaflet before starting therapy and with each refill.
- Ensure that patient understands dosing schedule and importance of taking last dose more than 4 hr before bedtime to minimize supine hypertension.
- Advise patient to take as prescribed and not to stop taking or change the dose unless advised by health care provider.
- Advise patient to take each dose without regard to meals but to take with food if stomach upset occurs.
- Advise patient to skip dose before lying down for any length of time (eg, nap).
- Ensure that patient has, and can use, a home BP monitoring device. Advise patient to monitor and record BP and pulse at regular intervals and in lying, sitting, and standing positions. Advise patient to inform health care provider if persistent hypertension noted or if heart rate is persistently slow.
- Advise patient to sleep with head of bed elevated if supine hypertension noted.
- Advise patient to discontinue therapy and notify health care provider immediately if any of the following occur: cardiac awareness, pounding in the ears, headache, blurred vision, slowing of heart rate, dizziness, fainting.
- Advise patient that abnormal skin sensations, goosebumps, itching, and painful or difficult urination are most common side effects and to inform health care provider if these or any other unexplained sensation or feeling occur and are bothersome.
- Advise patient to inform health care provider of any unexplained feeling or sensation.
- Advise women to notify health care provider if pregnant, planning to become pregnant, or breastfeeding.
- Caution patient not to take any prescription or OTC drugs or dietary supplements without consulting health care provider.
- Advise patient that follow-up visits and lab tests may be necessary to monitor therapy and to keep appointments.

Mifepristone
(mi-FE-pri-stone)
Class Abortifacient
How Supplied
Mifeprex Tablets 200 mg
Action
PHARMACOLOGY: Competes with progesterone at progesterone-receptor sites.

PHARMACOKINETICS/DYNAMICS:
Absorption: T_{max} is approximately 90 min, C_{max} is 1.98 mg/L, and absolute bioavailability (20 mg oral) is 69%.

Distribution: Mifepristone is 98% protein bound and displays nonlinear kinetics.

Metabolism: Metabolized via pathways involving N-demethylation and terminal hydroxylation of the 17–propynyl chain. In vitro, CYP450 3A4 is primarily responsible for metabolism. Major metabolite is N-monodemethyated metabolite.

Excretion: 83% is excreted in feces and 9% in urine. Elimination is slow at first (50% eliminated in 12 to 72 hr) and then becomes more rapid with t½ at 18 hr.

Indications Termination of pregnancy through day 49 of pregnancy. **Unlabeled use(s):** Postcoital contraception; intrauterine fetal death/nonviable early pregnancy; unresectable meningioma; endometriosis; Cushing syndrome.

Contraindications Confirmed or suspected ectopic pregnancy or undiagnosed adnexal mass; IUD in place; chronic adrenal failure; concurrent long-term corticosteroid therapy; history of allergy to mifepristone, misoprostol, or other prostaglandin; hemorrhagic disorders or concurrent anticoagulant therapy; inherited porphyrias.

Route/Dosage
ADULT:
Day 1: **PO** Patient takes 600 mg mifepristone in a single dose.
Day 3: **PO** Unless a confirmed abortion has occurred, patient takes 400 mcg misoprostol.
Day 14: **PO** Follow-up visit to confirm by clinical examination or ultrasonographic scan that a complete termination of pregnancy has occurred.

Interactions
Erythromycin, grapefruit juice, itraconazole, ketoconazole: May increase mifepristone plasma levels.
Carbamazepine, dexamethasone, phenobarbital, phenytoin, rifampin, St. John's wort: May decrease mifepristone plasma levels.

Lab Test Interferences None well documented.

Adverse Reactions
CNS: Headache; dizziness; insomnia; anxiety; syncope; fainting.
EENT: Sinusitis.
GI: Abdominal pain and cramping; nausea; vomiting; diarrhea; dyspepsia.
GU: Uterine cramping and hemorrhage; vaginitis; pelvic pain.
HEMA: Anemia; decreased hemoglobin.
OTHER: Fatigue; back pain; fever; viral infections; rigors; chills; shaking; asthenia; leg pain; leukorrhea.

> WARNING:
> Incomplete abortion may occur and require surgical intervention. Prior to prescribing, determine a surgical site and provider in the event of an emergency. Review patient agreement prior to initiation of therapy.

Precautions
Pregnancy: Indicated for termination of pregnancy.
Lactation: Undetermined.
Children: Safety and efficacy not established.
Elderly: Safety and efficacy not established.
Monitoring: Qualified health care provider must supervise administration.
Availability: Available only through selected health care provider offices.
Surgical intervention: Facilities for transfusions and resuscitation may be necessary in incomplete abortion.
Vaginal bleeding: Occurs in almost all patients.

Overdosage: Signs and Symptoms
Adrenal failure.

PATIENT CARE CONSIDERATIONS
Administration/Storage
- This medication can only be administered in a clinic, medical office, or hospital, by or under the supervision of a physician able to assess how far the pregnancy has progressed and to diagnose ectopic pregnancies.
- Do not administer until the patient has read the Medication Guide and read and signed the Patient Agreement.
- The dose of mifepristone is three 200 mg tablets (600 mg) taken as a single oral dose.
- Store at controlled room temperature (59° to 86°F).

Assessment/Interventions
- Obtain patient history, including drug history and any known allergies. Ensure that duration of pregnancy has been determined and documented and does not exceed 49 days.
- Review patient's health history for any condition that could contraindicate mifepristone therapy (eg, confirmed or suspected ectopic pregnancy or undiagnosed adnexal mass, IUD in place, chronic adrenal failure, concurrent long-term corticosteroid therapy, hemorrhagic disorders or concurrent anticoagulant therapy, inherited porphyries, or allergy to mifepristone, misoprostol or other prostaglandin).
- Ensure that patient understands the effects of the treatment procedure and the complete regimen that must be followed.
- Ensure that patient has clear instructions on whom to call and what to do in the event of an emergency following administration of mifepristone.

Patient/Family Education
- Explain name, dose, action, and potential side effects of drug. Advise patient that vaginal bleeding and uterine cramping probably will occur.
- Give patient a copy of the Medication Guide and review its contents with patient.
- Provide instructions on whom to call and what to do in the event of an emergency following administration.
- Warn patient of the necessity of completing the treatment schedule including the follow-up visits 2 days (to receive misoprostol if abortion has not occurred) and 14 days (to confirm that complete termination of pregnancy has occurred) after taking mifepristone.

Miglitol

(mig-LIH-tall)

Class Antidiabetic/Alpha-glucosidase inhibitor

How Supplied
Glyset Tablets 25 mg, Tablets 50 mg, Tablets 100 mg

Action
PHARMACOLOGY: Inhibits intestinal enzymes that digest carbohydrates, thereby reducing carbohydrate digestion after meals, which lowers postprandial glucose elevation in diabetics.

PHARMACOKINETICS/DYNAMICS:
Absorption: Absorption is saturable at high doses (ie, 25 mg dose is completely absorbed vs 100 mg dose is only 50% to 70% absorbed). T_{max} is 2 to 3 hr.

Distribution: Distributes primarily into the extracellular fluid. Less than 4% is protein bound and Vd is 0.18 L/kg.

Metabolism: Miglitol is not metabolized.

Excretion: Eliminated by renal excretion as unchanged. More than 95% is recovered in the urine within 24 hr. Plasma t½ is approximately 2 hr.

Special Populations:
Renal Function Impairment – Because miglitol is excreted primarily by the kidneys, accumulation is expected. However, dosage adjustment to correct the increased plasma concentrations is not feasible because miglitol acts locally.

Indications
Patients with NIDDM who have failed dietary therapy. May be used alone or in combination with sulfonylureas.

Contraindications
Diabetic ketoacidosis; inflammatory bowel disease; colonic ulceration; intestinal disorders of digestion or absorption; partial or predisposition to intestinal obstruction; conditions that may deteriorate as a result of increased intestinal gas production.

Route/Dosage
ADULTS: PO 25 mg tid at the start of each meal. After 4 to 8 wk can increase to 50 mg/dose for 3 mo. If glycosylated hemoglobin level not acceptable after 3 mo can increase at 100 mg tid (max dose).

Interactions
Intestinal absorbents (eg, charcoal), digestive enzymes: May lower efficacy of miglitol.
Drugs that produce hyperglycemia (eg, corticosteroids, diuretics, thyroid preparations): May lead to loss of glucose control.
Ranitidine: Reduced ranitidine bioavailability.
Propranolol: Reduced propranolol bioavailability.

Lab Test Interferences
Transient decreases in serum iron that are not associated with hemoglobin reduction or other changes in hematologic indices.

Adverse Reactions
DERM: Rash.
GI: Abdominal pain; diarrhea; flatulence.

Precautions
Pregnancy: Category B.
Lactation: Excreted in breast milk.
Children: Safety and efficacy not established.
Renal function impairment: Miglitol not recommended if serum creatinine is more than 2 mg/dL.
Hypoglycemia: Miglitol does not produce hypoglycemia; however, hypoglycemia may develop if used together with sulfonylureas. Use glucose (dextrose) and not cane sugar (table sugar) or fruits/fruit juices to treat hypoglycemia.

Loss of blood glucose control: Certain medical conditions (eg, surgery, fever, infection, or trauma) and drugs (eg, diuretics, corticosteroids, oral contraceptives) affect glucose control. In these situations, it may be necessary to adjust the dose of miglitol and other antidiabetic drugs.

Overdosage: Signs and Symptoms
Increased flatulence, diarrhea, abdominal discomfort.

PATIENT CARE CONSIDERATIONS

Administration/Storage
- The medication should be taken with the first bite of each meal.
- Store at room temperature (59° to 86°F) in a tightly closed container, protected from moisture.

Assessment/Interventions
- Therapy is monitored by 1-hr postprandial blood glucose tests and periodic glycosylated hemoglobin determinations.
- If hypoglycemia develops, use oral or parenteral glucose (dextrose) to increase blood glucose instead of sucrose (cane or table sugar) or fruits/fruit juice, since the metabolism of sucrose is inhibited by miglitol.
- Renal function should be assessed prior to starting medication.
- Monitor patient for GI side effects. Notify health care provider if intolerable.
- Monitor patient for hypoglycemia if this medication is combined with sulfonylurea.

Patient/Family Education
- Advise patient to take the drug with the first bite of each meal. If necessary, it may be taken during the meal if not taken with the first bite. Do not take after the meal is complete or if skipping a meal
- Advise patient not to change the dose or dosing interval or discontinue the drug without consulting with health care provider.
- Encourage patient to continue to adhere to a regular exercise program and follow their diabetic meal plan.
- Counsel patient on proper monitoring of blood glucose.
- Advise women of childbearing age that this medication should not be used during pregnancy. Insulin is the preferred agent to control blood glucose.
- Advise patient family that "cane sugar" (sucrose or table sugar) or fruits or fruit juices should not be used to treat hypoglycemic reactions. Glucose (dextrose) or glucagon are necessary to increase blood sugar.
- Advise patient that GI side effects (eg, gas, diarrhea, or abdominal discomfort) usually occur during the first few weeks of therapy but generally go away. Advise patient to inform healthcare provider if these effects persist or become intolerable.

Miglustat

(MIG-loo-stat)

Class Enzyme inhibitor

How Supplied
Zavesca Capsule 100 mg

Action
PHARMACOLOGY: Competitive and reversible inhibitor of the enzyme glucosylceramide synthase.

PHARMACOKINETICS/DYNAMICS:
Absorption: Bioavailability is about 97%. C_{max} observed in 2 to 2.5 hr. Effective t½ is about 6 to 7 hr, predicting a steady-state in 1.5 to 2 days.
Distribution: Vd is 83 to 105 L. No protein binding.
Excretion: Excreted unchanged in the urine.
Special Populations:
Renal insufficiency – Based on Ccr levels, dosage adjustment in mild and moderate renal impairment is justified.

Indications Treatment of adult patients with mild to moderate type 1 Gaucher disease for whom enzyme replacement therapy is not an option (eg, hypersensitivity).

Contraindications Pregnancy; standard considerations.

Route/Dosage
ADULTS: PO 100 mg tid at regular intervals. It may be necessary to reduce the dose to 100 mg qd or bid in patients experiencing adverse effects (eg, diarrhea, tremor).

Renal insufficiency
ADULTS: PO Ccr 50 to 70 mL/min, start with 100 mg bid; Ccr 30 to 50 mL/min, start with 100 mg qd. Administration to patient with severe renal impairment (Ccr less than 30 mL/min) is not recommended.

Interactions None well documented.

Lab Test Interferences None well documented.

Adverse Reactions
CNS: Headache (22%); tremor, dizziness, leg cramps (11%); unsteady gait, memory loss (8%); paresthesia (7%); migraine (6%).
EENT: Visual disturbance (17%).

GI: Diarrhea (85%); abdominal pain (50%); flatulence (44%); nausea (22%); vomiting (11%); constipation, dry mouth (8%); anorexia, dyspepsia (7%); bloating, epigastric pain (6%).
GU: Menstrual disorder (6%).
HEMA: Thrombocytopenia (7%).
METAB: Weight loss (65%).
MUSC: Cramps (11%)
OTHER: Generalized weakness (17%); abdominal distension and gaseous abdominal distension, back pain, heaviness in limbs (8%).

PATIENT CARE CONSIDERATIONS
Administration/Storage
* Do not administer to patient with severe renal impairment (Ccr less than 30 mL/min) or to women who are pregnant.
* Administer prescribed dose tid without regard to meals. Administer with food if GI upset occurs. Have patient swallow capsule whole with a glass of water.
* Store capsules at controlled room temperature (68° to 77°F).

Assessment/Interventions
* Obtain patient history, including drug history and any known allergies. Note renal impairment or current use of imiglucerase.
* Ensure that patient has neurologic exam before starting therapy and q 6 mo during treatment. Notify health care provider if tremor develops or worsens or if symptoms of peripheral neuropathy (eg, numbness, tingling, burning, pain) are noted during treatment. Be prepared to reduce the dose or discontinue medication after patient has been evaluated by health care provider.
* Administer reduced dose to patient with renal impairment (following manufacturer's guidelines) or significant side effects (eg, severe diarrhea, weight loss, tremor).
* Ensure that women of childbearing potential are using effective contraception before starting treatment and during therapy.
* Ensure that sexually-active men use reliable contraceptive methods during and for 3 mo after therapy has been discontinued.
* Assess patient for GI, CNS, musculoskeletal, and general body side effects. Inform health care provider if noted and significant. If diarrhea develops, facilitate change in diet to reduce carbohydrate intake and administer OTC antidiarrheals (eg, loperamide) as ordered.

Precautions
Pregnancy: Category X.
Lactation: Undetermined.
Children: Safety and efficacy not established.
Elderly: Use with caution and start at the lower end of the dose range because of the greater frequency of decreased hepatic, renal, or cardiac function, and concomitant diseases or other drug therapy.
Renal function impairment: Dosage adjustment is recommended.
Peripheral neuropathy: Has been reported.

Patient/Family Education
* Advise patient to read the patient information leaflet before starting therapy and with each refill.
* Explain name, dose, action, and potential side effects of drug.
* Advise patient to take prescribed dose without regard to meals but to take with food if stomach upset occurs. Advise patient to swallow each capsule whole with a glass of water.
* Advise patient that diarrhea is most common side effect and that reducing carbohydrate intake may be helpful. If diarrhea develops, advise patient to discuss use of OTC antidiarrheals (eg, loperamide) with health care provider.
* Advise patient that if a dose is missed to skip that dose and take the next dose at the regularly scheduled time.
* Instruct women of childbearing potential to use effective contraception during treatment.
* Advise women of childbearing potential to notify health care provider if pregnant, planning to become pregnant, or breastfeeding.
* Instruct sexually active men to use reliable contraceptive methods during treatment and for 3 mo after therapy has been discontinued.
* Instruct patient to immediately report the following symptoms to health care provider: numbness, pain, burning, or tingling in hands or feet; tremor; worsening of existing tremor.
* Advise patient to inform health care provider if persistent diarrhea does not respond to OTC antidiarrheals or unexplained weight loss occurs.
* Instruct patient not to take any prescription or OTC medications or dietary supplements unless advised by health care provider.
* Advise patient that follow-up examinations and laboratory tests will be required to monitor therapy and to keep appointments.

Milrinone Lactate

(MILL-rih-nohn LAK-tate)

Class Cardiovascular

How Supplied
Primacor Injection 1 mg/mL, Injection, premixed 200 mcg/mL in 5% Dextrose Injection

Action
PHARMACOLOGY: Has direct arterial vasodilator activity and positive inotropic effect; increases myocardial contractility.

PHARMACOKINETICS/DYNAMICS:
Absorption: Steady state is reached after approximately 6 to 12 hr of infusion of 0.5 mcg/kg/min. Therapeutic range is 100 to 300 ng/mL.
Distribution: Approximately 70% is protein bound and Vd is 0.38 L/kg.
Metabolism: Metabolite is 0-glucuronide.
Excretion: Primary route of excretion is via urine. Major urinary excretions of orally administered milrinone is 83% and 12% for 0-glucuronide metabolite. Mean t½ is 2.3 hr and clearance is 0.13 L/kg/hr.
Duration: Duration depends on patient's responsiveness (approximately 5 days).

Indications Short-term treatment of CHF.

Contraindications Standard considerations.

Route/Dosage
ADULTS:
Loading dose: **IV** 50 mcg/kg over 10 min; adjust infusion rate according to hemodynamic and clinical response.

Interactions None well documented.
INCOMPATIBILITIES: Precipitate forms if furosemide is injected into same IV line as milrinone; do not administer both in same IV line.

Lab Test Interferences None well documented.

Adverse Reactions
CV: Ventricular arrhythmia (eg, ventricular ectopic activity, nonsustained ventricular tachycardia, sustained ventricular tachycardia, ventricular fibrillation); supraventricular arrhythmia; hypotension; angina.
CNS: Headaches; tremor.
HEMA: Thrombocytopenia.
OTHER: Hypokalemia.

Precautions
Pregnancy: Category C.
Lactation: Undetermined.
Children: Safety and efficacy not established.
Renal function impairment: Use drug with caution; monitor renal function. Dosage reduction, based on Ccr, may be needed.
CV effects: Do not use in patients with severe obstructive aortic or pulmonic valvular disease; may exacerbate hypertrophic subaortic stenosis; may cause supraventricular and ventricular arrhythmias; may shorten atrioventricular node conduction.

Overdosage: Signs and Symptoms
Hypotension.

PATIENT CARE CONSIDERATIONS

Administration/Storage
- For short-term (up to 5 days) IV use only.
- Prepare drug for IV infusion by diluting with 0.45% or 0.9% Sodium Chloride Injection D5W.
- Use infusion pump for administration.
- Adjust maintenance infusion rate on the basis of hemodynamic and clinical response (max rate is 0.75 mcg/kg/min or 1.13 mg/kg/day).
- Store at room temperature (59° to 86°F) and protect from light.

Assessment/Interventions
- Obtain patient history, including drug history and any known allergies.
- Evaluate renal function and identify whether patient has severe obstructive aortic or pulmonic valvular disease.
- Provide close cardiac and BP monitoring.
- Be especially observant for supraventricular and ventricular arrhythmias and excessive decreases in BP and report to health care provider.
- Carefully monitor fluid and electrolyte changes as well as renal function during therapy.
- Observe IV site for signs of irritation. Rotate injection site q 48 hr.
- Correct hypokalemia by potassium supplementation prior to and during use of drug.
- Observe for other common side effects (eg, headaches, hypokalemia, tremor and thrombocytopenia) and report to health care provider.

Patient/Family Education
- Explain what medication does.
- Inform patient that treatment with this drug usually does not exceed 5 days.
- Instruct patient to report the following symptoms to health care provider: headache or tremors.

Minocycline

(min-oh-SIGH-kleen)

Class Antibiotic/Tetracycline

How Supplied

Arestin Microspheres, sustained-release 1 mg (as hydrochloride) ♦ *Dynacin* Tablets 50 mg (as hydrochloride), Tablets 75 mg (as hydrochloride), Tablets 100 mg (as hydrochloride), Capsules 50 mg (as hydrochloride), Capsules 100 mg (as hydrochloride) ♦ *Minocin* Capsules, pellet-filled 50 mg (as hydrochloride), Capsules, pellet-filled 100 mg (as hydrochloride), Powder for injection, cryodesiccated 100 mg

✤ Apo-Minocycline ♦ Gen-Minocycline ♦ Novo-Minocycline ♦ PMS-Minocycline ♦ ratio-Minocycline ♦ Rhoxal-minocycline

Action

PHARMACOLOGY: Inhibits bacterial protein synthesis.

PHARMACOKINETICS/DYNAMICS:

Absorption: T_{max} is 1 to 4 hr after a single dose. Food does not affect extent of absorption, but C_{max} is slightly decreased and delayed by 1 hr.

Distribution: Minocycline has a very high lipid solubility, readily penetrates the CSF, and displays a good penetration of saliva, brain, eye, and prostate. 70% to 80% is protein bound.

Metabolism: Metabolism is concentrated by the liver in the bile.

Excretion: 1% to 12% is excreted unchanged in urine. Serum t½ is approximately 11 to 23 hr in healthy volunteers. Hemodialysis and peritoneal dialysis have little effect.

Special Populations:
Renal Function Impairment – Serum t½ is 18 to 69 hr.
Hepatic Function Impairment – Serum t½ is 11 to 16 hr.

Indications Treatment of periodontitis as an adjunct to scaling and root planing. Treatment of infections caused by susceptible strains of gram-positive and gram-negative bacteria, *Rickettsia* and *Mycoplasma* pneumonia, and trachoma; treatment for susceptible infections when penicillins are contraindicated; adjunctive treatment of acute intestinal amebiasis; treatment of asymptomatic carriers of *Neisseria meningitidis* to eliminate meningococci from nasopharynx, chlamydia, inflammatory acne, syphilis, gonorrhea.

Contraindications Standard considerations.

Route/Dosage

Inflammatory Acne
ADULTS: **PO** 50 mg 1 to 3 times per day.

Meningococcal Carrier State
ADULTS: **PO** 100 mg q 12 hr for 5 days.

Mycobacterium Marinum Infections
ADULTS: **PO** 100 mg q 12 hr for 6 to 8 wk, although optimal doses have not been established.

Periodontitis
ADULTS: **Subgingival** 1 mg microspheres are to be inserted by an oral health care professional.

Primary/Secondary Syphilis
ADULTS: **PO** 200 mg initially then 100 mg q 12 hr for 10 to 15 days.

Renal Impairment
Do not exceed 200 mg per 24 hr.

Susceptible Infections
ADULTS: **PO/IV** 200 mg initially, then **PO/IV** 100 mg q 12 hr or **PO** 50 mg qid (max, parenteral 400 mg per 24 hr).
CHILDREN OLDER THAN 8 YR OF AGE: **PO/IV** 4 mg/kg initially, then 2 mg/kg q 12 hr (max, usual adult dose).

Uncomplicated Gonococcal Infections Except Urethritis and Anorectal Infections in Men
ADULTS: **PO** 200 mg initially followed with 100 mg q 12 hr for at least 4 days, with posttherapy cultures within 2 to 3 days.

Uncomplicated Gonococcal Urethritis in Men
ADULTS: **PO** 100 mg q 12 hr for 5 days.

Uncomplicated Urethral, Endocervical, or Rectal Infections in Adults Caused by C. Trachomatis or Ureaplasma Urealyticum
ADULTS: **PO** 100 mg q 12 hr for at least 7 days.

Interactions

Antacids (containing aluminum, calcium, magnesium, zinc), bismuth salts, divalent or trivalent cations: May decrease oral absorption of minocycline.
Anticoagulants, oral: Increased anticoagulant activity.
Contraceptives, oral: May reduce effect of oral contraceptives.
Digoxin: May increase digoxin serum levels.
Insulin: Increases hypoglycemic potential.
Iron salts: May decrease absorption of minocycline.
Isotretinoin: Because the risk of pseudotumor cerebri may be increased, avoid isotretinoin administration shortly before, during, or after minocycline therapy.
Methoxyflurane: Increased potential for nephrotoxicity exists; do not coadminister.
Milk and dairy products: Although the effects of milk and dairy products on minocycline absorption are less than observed with other tetracycline derivatives, it would be prudent to avoid the administration of milk or dairy products with all tetracycline derivatives.

Penicillins: May interfere with bactericidal action of penicillins.
Urinary alkalinizers, zinc salts: May decrease serum minocycline levels.
INCOMPATIBILITIES: Do not mix before or during administration with adrenocorticotropic hormone, aminophylline, amobarbital sodium, amphotericin B, bicarbonate infusion mixtures, calcium gluconate or chloride, carbenicillin, cephalothin sodium, cefazolin sodium, chloramphenicol succinate, colistin sulfate, heparin sodium, hydrocortisone sodium succinate, iodine sodium, methicillin sodium, novobiocin, penicillin, pentobarbital, phenytoin sodium, polymyxins, prochlorperazine, sodium ascorbate, sulfadiazine, sulfisoxazole, thiopental sodium, vitamin K (sodium bisulfate or sodium salt), whole blood.

Lab Test Interferences False increase in urinary catecholamines with fluorometric method.

Adverse Reactions
CNS: Convulsions; dizziness; hypoesthesia; paresthesia; sedation; vertigo; bulging fontanels in infants; benign intracranial hypertension (pseudotumor cerebri) in adults; headache.
DERM: Alopecia; erythema nodosum; hyperpigmentation of nails; pruritus; toxic epidermal necrolysis; vasculitis; maculopapular and erythematous rashes; exfoliative dermatitis; fixed drug eruptions; balanitis due to lesions on the penis; erythema multiforme; Stevens-Johnson syndrome; photosensitivity.
EENT: Tinnitus; decreased hearing.
GI: Anorexia; nausea; vomiting; diarrhea; dyspepsia; stomatitis; glossitis; dysphagia; enamel hypoplasia; enterocolitis; pseudomembranous colitis; pancreatitis; inflammatory lesions (with monilial overgrowth) in oral and anogenital regions; esophagitis; esophageal ulceration; tooth discoloration; oral cavity discoloration (including tongue, lips, and gums).
GU: Vulvovaginitis.
HEPA: Hyperbilirubinemia; hepatic cholestasis; increased liver enzymes, fatal hepatic failure; jaundice; hepatitis (including autoimmune hepatitis); liver failure.
HEMA/LYMPH: Agranulocytosis; hemolytic anemia; thrombocytopenia; leukopenia; neutropenia; pancytopenia; eosinophilia.
HYPERSEN: Urticaria; angioneurotic edema; polyarthralgia; anaphylaxis/anaphylactoid reaction (including shock and death); anaphylactoid purpura; myocarditis; pericarditis; exacerbation of SLE; pulmonary infiltrates with eosinophilia; transient lupus-like syndrome; serum sickness-like reactions; hypersensitivity syndrome (including rash, exfoliative dermatitis, eosinophilia, fever, lymphadenopathy and one or more of the following hepatitis, pneumonitis, nephritis, myocarditis, pericarditis).
MUSC: Arthralgia; arthritis bone discoloration; myalgia; joint stiffness; joint swelling.
RENAL: Interstitial nephritis; elevations in BUN; reversible renal failure.
RESP: Cough; dyspnea; bronchospasm; exacerbation of asthma; pneumonitis.
OTHER: Fever, discoloration of secretions; brown-black microscopic discoloration of the thyroid gland.

Precautions
Pregnancy: Category D.
Lactation: Excreted in breast milk. Advise against nursing.
Children: Avoid in children younger than 8 yr of age unless other appropriate drugs are ineffective or contraindicated because abnormal bone formation and discoloration of teeth may occur.
Renal function impairment: May increase BUN, may lead to azotemia, hyperphosphatemia, and acidosis.
Superinfection: Prolonged use may result in bacterial or fungal overgrowth.
Photosensitivity: May cause exaggerated sunburn reactions.
Expiration: Do not use outdated product; degraded product is highly nephrotoxic.
Hepatotoxicity: Has been reported. Use with caution in patients with hepatic dysfunction and in conjunction with hepatotoxic drugs.
Parenteral therapy: Prolonged periods of parenteral use may result in thrombophlebitis.
Pseudotumor cerebri (benign intracranial hypertension): Has been reported in adults. Usual manifestations are headache and blurred vision.
Tooth discoloration: May cause permanent discoloration of the teeth.

Overdosage: Signs and Symptoms
Dizziness, nausea, vomiting.

PATIENT CARE CONSIDERATIONS
Administration/Storage
♦ Route of administration, dose, and dosing frequency are variable, depending on condition being treated.

Oral:
♦ Administer prescribed dose without regard to meals but administer with food if GI upset occurs.

- Administer capsules with a full glass of water.
- Administer oral minocycline 1 hr before or 2 hr after antacids containing aluminum, calcium, or magnesium, or preparations containing iron or zinc.
- Store capsules at controlled room temperature (68° to 77°F). Protect from light, moisture, and excessive heat.

Injection:
- For IV infusion only. Not for intradermal, subcutaneous, IM, intra-arterial, or IV bolus administration.
- Because of the risk of thrombophlebitis, use parenteral therapy only when oral therapy is not indicated. Institute oral therapy as soon as possible.
- Follow manufacturer's guidelines for reconstituting and further diluting the powder for injection.
- Do not administer if particulate matter, cloudiness, or discoloration is noted.
- Diluted solution should be administered immediately, but can be stored at room temperature (68° to 77°F) for up to 24 hr. Discard any unused solution after 24 hr.
- Store powder for injection at controlled room temperature (68° to 77°F). Protect from light moisture and excessive heat.

Subgingival Microspheres:
- *Arestin* is for instillation into periodontal pockets. Not for oral, intradermal, subcutaneous, IM, IV, or intra-arterial administration.
- Medication will be instilled by a dental professional.
- Store at controlled room temperature (59° to 86°F). Avoid exposure to excessive heat.

Assessment/Interventions
- Obtain patient history, including drug history and any known allergies. Note renal or hepatic impairment, or history of allergy or intolerance to other tetracycline antibiotics.
- Ensure that expiration date has not been exceeded.
- Review results of culture and sensitivity testing as appropriate.
- Ensure that women are not pregnant or breastfeeding.
- Ensure that CBC, liver enzymes, and renal function are periodically evaluated during prolonged therapy.
- Monitor patient's response to therapy. Notify health care provider if infection does not appear to be improving or is worsening.
- Monitor patient for signs of allergic reaction. Discontinue therapy and immediately notify health care provider if noted. Be prepared to treat appropriately.
- Monitor patient for GI, CNS, DERM, general body side effects, and signs of superinfection. Report to health care provider if noted and significant. Immediately report severe diarrhea, diarrhea containing blood or pus, or severe abdominal cramping.
- In venereal disease when coexistent syphilis is suspected, a dark field examination should be done before treatment is started and blood serology repeated monthly for at least 4 months.

Patient/Family Education
- Explain name, dose, action, and potential side effects of drug.
- Review dosing schedule and prescribed length of therapy with patient. Advise patient that dose and duration of therapy are dependent on site and cause of infection.
- Instruct patient using capsules to take prescribed dose with a full glass of water.
- Instruct patient or caregiver using oral suspension to measure and administer prescribed dose using dosing spoon, dosing syringe, or medicine cup.
- Advise patient to take without regard to meals, but to take with food if GI upset occurs.
- Advise patient to take 1 hr before or 2 hr after antacids containing aluminum, calcium, or magnesium, or preparations containing iron or zinc.
- Instruct patient to complete entire course of therapy, even if symptoms of infection have disappeared.
- Advise patient to discontinue therapy and contact health care provider immediately if skin rash, hives, itching, shortness of breath, headache, or blurred vision occur.
- Advise patient that medication may cause photosensitivity (sensitivity to sunlight) and to avoid unnecessary exposure to sunlight or tanning lamps and to use sunscreens and wear protective clothing to avoid photosensitivity reactions.
- Caution women taking oral contraceptives that minocycline may make birth control pills less effective and to use nonhormonal forms of contraception during treatment.
- Advise women to notify health care provider if pregnant, planning to become pregnant, or breastfeeding.
- Caution patient that drug may cause dizziness, light-headedness, or blurred vision and to use caution while driving or performing other hazardous tasks until tolerance is determined.
- Advise patient to report signs of superinfection to health care provider: black furry

tongue, white patches in mouth, foul-smelling stools, vaginal itching, or discharge.
* Warn patient that diarrhea containing blood or pus may be a sign of a serious disorder and to seek medical care if noted and not treat at home.
* Caution patient not to take any prescription or OTC medications, dietary supplements, or herbal preparations unless advised by health care provider.
* Advise patient to discard any unused minocycline by the expiration date noted on the label.
* Advise patient that follow-up examinations and lab tests may be required to monitor therapy and to keep appointments.

Subgingival Microspheres:
* Caution patient to avoid touching treated areas and to avoid brushing for 12 hr following treatment. Advise patient to avoid eating hard, crunchy, or sticky foods for 1 wk following treatment and postpone use of interproximal cleaning devices for 10 days.
* Advise patient that mild to moderate sensitivity is expected after treatment, but to notify dental professional immediately if pain, swelling, or other problems occur.

Minoxidil

(min-OX-ih-dill)

Class Antihypertensive/Topical hair growth

How Supplied
Loniten Tablets 2.5 mg, Tablets 10 mg ♦ *Monoxidil* Tablets 2.5 mg, Tablets 10 mg ♦ *Minoxidil for Men* Topical Solution 2% ♦ *Rogaine* Solution 2%
♣ *APO-Gain Topical Solution*

Action
PHARMACOLOGY: Directly dilates vascular smooth muscle by mechanism possibly related to blockade of calcium uptake or stimulation of catecholamine release; reduces elevated systolic and diastolic BP by decreasing peripheral arteriolar resistance; triggers sympathetic, vagal inhibitory and renal homeostatic mechanisms including increased renin release, which results in increased cardiac rate and output and fluid retention; stimulates hair growth by unknown mechanism but likely is related to its arterial vasodilating action.

PHARMACOKINETICS/DYNAMICS:
Absorption: At least 90% is absorbed. T_{max} is 1 hr.

Distribution: 0% is protein bound.

Metabolism: Approximately 90% is primarily metabolized by glucuronic acid conjugation.

Excretion: Primary route of excretion is urine. Mean t½ is 4.2 hr. Hemodialysis does not remove minoxidil or its metabolites.

Onset: Onset is 30 min.

Peak: Time to peak is 2 to 3 hr.

Duration: Duration is approximately 75 hr.

Indications
Oral form: Management of severe hypertension associated with target organ damage in patients who have failed to respond to max doses of a diuretic plus 2 other antihypertensive drugs.
Topical form: Treatment of androgenic alopecia.

Unlabeled use(s): Treatment of alopecia areata (topical).

Contraindications Pheochromocytoma; standard considerations.

Route/Dosage
ADULTS AND CHILDREN (OLDER THAN 12 YR): PO 5 mg/day initially. If necessary, can increase to 10, 20, and then 40 mg/day in single or divided doses (max, 100 mg/day).

CHILDREN (YOUNGER THAN 12 YR): PO 0.2 mg/kg/day as single dose initially. May increase in 50% to 100% increments until optimal BP control is achieved (usually 0.25 to 1 mg/kg/day; max, 50 mg/day).

ADULTS: **Topical** Apply 1 mL to affected scalp areas morning and evening (max, 2 mL/day).

Interactions
Guanethidine: May result in profound orthostatic hypotensive effects; discontinue guanethidine before minoxidil therapy.
Topical corticosteroids or retinoids, petrolatum: May enhance cutaneous drug absorption of topically applied minoxidil.

Lab Test Interferences None well documented.

Adverse Reactions
CV: Changes in T-waves (60%); pericardial effusion leading to tamponade (3%); edema, chest pain, BP changes, palpitations, heart rate changes (topical); tachycardia, edema, angina, rebound hypertension following withdrawal (systemic).
CNS: Headache; dizziness, faintness (topical); fatigue (systemic).
DERM: Hypertrichosis (80%); irritant or allergic dermatitis, eczema, local erythema, pruritus, dry scalp, exacerbation of hair loss, alopecia (topical).
GI: Diarrhea; nausea; vomiting.
HEMA: Hct, Hgb, and RBC counts may fall but return to normal (7%, systemic); thrombocytopenia, leukopenia (rare).

OTHER: Temporary edema (7%); breast tenderness (less than 1%); darkening of skin (systemic).

> **WARNING:**
> Serious side effects may occur including pericardial effusion, occasionally progressing to tamponade, which can exacerbate angina pectoris. When first administering minoxidil, hospitalize and monitor patients with malignant hypertension and those patients already receiving guanethidine to avoid too rapid or large orthostatic decreases in BP.

Precautions
Pregnancy: Category C.
Lactation: Excreted in breast milk. In general, nursing should not be undertaken.
Children: Safety and efficacy not established.
Elderly: Use with caution because of the greater frequency of decreased hepatic, renal, or cardiac function, and concomitant diseases or other drug therapy.
Hypersensitivity: Can occur and is manifested by rash, bullous eruptions, and Stevens-Johnson syndrome.

PATIENT CARE CONSIDERATIONS
Administration/Storage
- Dry hair and scalp before topical administration.
- Wear gloves to apply topical form.
- Wash hands after topical administration.
- Administer oral form with diuretic to counteract fluid retention and with beta-blocker to counteract tachycardia.
- Give oral medication with meals to minimize GI symptoms.
- Store tablets at room temperature (59° to 86°F) in tightly closed container.
- Store topical solution at room temperature.

Assessment/Interventions
- Obtain patient history, including drug history and any known allergies. Note renal insufficiency or cardiac disease.
- Perform urinalysis, renal function tests, ECG, chest x-ray and echocardiogram at initiation of therapy. Repeat any tests with abnormal results q 1 to 3 mo. After stabilization occurs, repeat tests at 6- to 12-mo intervals.
- Monitor fluid and electrolyte balance and body weight.
- Avoid too rapid control of very severe high BP; syncope, cerebrovascular accidents, MI and ischemia of special sense organs, decreasing hearing and vision, may result.
- Closely supervise patients with renal impairment to prevent cardiac failure or exacerbation of renal failure.

Renal failure or dialysis: Patients may require smaller doses and should have close medical supervision to prevent exacerbation of renal failure or precipitation of cardiac failure.
Abnormal scalp: Use of topical form of drug may result in increased absorption and systemic effects; avoid use on scalps with decreased integrity.
ECG changes: T-wave changes may occur; significance unknown.
Fluid/electrolytes imbalance: Sodium and water retention occur, leading to edema and possible CHF.
Heart disease: Patients may be predisposed to CV side effects.
Pericardial effusion: Has occurred rarely, sometimes with tamponade.
Severe hypertension: Too rapid BP correction can precipitate syncope, cerebrovascular accidents, MI, and ischemia of special sense organs with resulting loss of vision or hearing. Patients should be hospitalized to monitor carefully.
Tachycardia: Can be prevented by concomitant use of beta-blocker or other agent.

Overdosage: Signs and Symptoms
Exaggerated hypotension, fluid retention, tachycardia.

- Observe for tachycardia or angina and report to health care provider.
- Report patient complaints of nausea, vomiting, diarrhea, dizziness, lightheadedness, rash or skin irritation to health care provider.
- Observe patients, especially those with renal impairment, closely for signs of pericardial effusion. If condition is suspected, notify health care provider; ECG must be performed.
- Monitor patients receiving topical therapy for possible systemic effects after 1 mo of therapy and q 6 mo thereafter.
- If systemic effects appear in patients using drug topically, discontinue drug and notify health care provider.

Patient/Family Education
- Advise patient not to change dose without health care provider direction.
- Tell patient that diuretic and beta-blocker are necessary to enhance effectiveness and to decrease side effects of minoxidil.
- Instruct patient to notify health care provider of heart rate at least 20 beats/min over normal, rapid weight gain of more than 5 lb, unusual swelling, breathing difficulty, angina symptoms, dizziness, or lightheadedness.

- Tell patient to report the following symptoms to health care provider: skin irritation, diarrhea, vomiting, rash, or other bothersome physical complaints.
- Warn patient taking oral form that enhanced growth and darkening of fine body hair may occur. It may take 1 to 6 mo to return to pretreatment appearance.
- Inform patient using topical form that 4 mo of continuous use is required before hair growth is seen and that stopping treatment will lead to hair loss within a few mo.
- Advise patient using topical form that more frequent applications or use of larger doses will not enhance hair growth and may lead to side effects.
- Inform patient using topical form to expect initial hair growth to be soft, downy, colorless, and barely visible and that after further treatment new hair should match other scalp hair.
- Tell patient using topical form not to use it in conjunction with other topical scalp medications, to apply drug only to healthy areas of scalp, not to use if scalp becomes irritated or sunburned, and not to use it on other parts of body.
- For topical application; instruct patient to dry head and scalp before application and to wash hands after application.
- Explain that product contains significant amount of alcohol as base. Caution patient to avoid having topical form coming into contact with eyes, mucous membranes or sensitive skin areas. If accidental contact occurs, instruct patient to rinse area with large amounts of cool tap water and to notify health care provider.

Mirtazapine

(mer-TAZ-ah-peen)

Class Tetracyclic antidepressant

How Supplied
Remeron Tablets 15 mg, Tablets 30 mg, Tablets 45 mg

Action
PHARMACOLOGY: Unknown. May enhance central nonadrenergic and serotonergic activity.

PHARMACOKINETICS/DYNAMICS:
Absorption: Tablets are rapidly and completely absorbed following oral administration. Steady-state plasma levels are attained within 5 days, with about 50% accumulation. T_{max} is approximately 2 hr.

Distribution: Plasma levels are linearly related to dose (15 to 80 mg) and approximately 85% is protein bound.

Metabolism: Mirtazapine is extensively metabolized with 8–hydroxy, N-desmethyl, and N-oxide as the metabolites. Major pathways are demethylation and hydroxylation followed by glucuronide conjugation. In vitro, cytochrome 2D6 and 1A2 are involved in the formation of the 8–hydroxymetabolite. Cytochrome 3A4 is responsible for the formation of the N-desmethyl and N-oxide metabolites.

Excretion: Primary route of excretion is urine (75%) and feces (15%). Mean t½ is approximately 20 to 40 hr with women exhibiting a longer t½. The (-) enantiomer t½ is twice as long as (+) enantiomer.

Special Populations:
Renal Function Impairment – Caution is indicated in administration because of decreased clearance.

Hepatic Function Impairment – Caution is indicated in administration because of decreased clearance.

Elderly – Caution is indicated in administration because of decreased clearance.

Indications Treatment of depression.

Contraindications Hypersensitivity to maprotiline or mirtazapine; concomitant use with MAO inhibitors.

Route/Dosage
ADULTS:
Initial dose: **PO** 15 mg/day as single dose. May be increased to 45 mg/day. For acute episodes, continue therapy of depression for at least 6 mo.

Interactions
Alcohol, CNS depressants: Additive CNS effects.
MAO inhibitors: May precipitate hypertensive crisis and convulsions with possible fatal results. Do not use mirtazapine in combination with an MAO inhibitors, or within 14 days of starting or stopping therapy with an MAO inhibitors.

Lab Test Interferences None well documented.

Adverse Reactions
CV: Hypotension; vasodilation; hypertension.
CNS: Somnolence; asthenia; dizziness; abnormal dreams; abnormal thinking; tremor; confusion; hypesthesia; apathy; depression; hypokinesis; twitching; agitation; anxiety; amnesia; hyperkinesia; paresthesia.
DERM: Pruritus; rash.
GI: Nausea; dry mouth; constipation; vomiting; appetite changes; abdominal pain.
GU: Urinary frequency.
HEMA: Agranulocytosis; leukopenia; thrombocytopenia; anemia.

METAB: Weight gain.
EENT: Sinusitis.
RESP: Cough; dyspnea.
OTHER: "Flu-like" syndrome; back pain; myasthenia; myalgia; arthralgia; peripheral edema; thirst.

Precautions
Pregnancy: Category C.
Lactation: Undetermined.
Children: Safety and efficacy not established.
Elderly: Use with caution.
Renal function impairment: Use with caution.
Hepatic function impairment: Use with caution. Transaminase elevations may occur without symptoms of compromised liver function.
Special risk patients: Use with caution in patients with known CV or cerebrovascular disease that could be exacerbated by hypotension (eg, history of MI, angina, ischemic stroke) and conditions that would predispose patients to hypotension (eg, dehydration, hypovolemia, treatment with antihypertensive agents).
Agranulocytosis: Has occurred. Warn patients about risk and symptoms of agranulocytosis.
Cholesterol/Triglycerides: Increases have been reported.
Increased appetite/weight gain: Increases in appetite and weight gain have been reported.
Severe depression: Closely supervise during initial drug therapy. Do not allow patient to possess more than small quantities of drug.

Overdosage: Signs and Symptoms
Disorientation, drowsiness, impaired memory, tachycardia.

PATIENT CARE CONSIDERATIONS

Administration/Storage
- Administer as a single daily dose, preferably in the evening prior to sleep.
- May be administered without regard to food.
- Dosage changes should be made in more than 1- to 2-wk intervals.
- Store at room temperature (59° to 86°F). Protect from light and moisture.
- Do not attempt to split oral disintegrating tablet.
- Use oral disintegrating tablet immediately after removal from blister; do not store.
- Water is not needed with disintegrating tablet.

Assessment/Interventions
- Obtain patient history, including drug history and any known allergies. Note history of sensitivity to drug or maprotiline, MI, angina, and concomitant or recent use of MAO inhibitors.
- Monitor patient's mood and affect closely. If mood changes or suicidal tendencies develop, notify health care provider and institute suicide precautions.
- Assess patient for side effects. Notify health care provider if present.
- If constipation occurs, increase fiber and fluid intake and mobility.

Patient/Family Education
- Explain that full effectiveness of the drug may take several weeks to develop.
- Advise patient to take as a single dose in the evening prior to sleep.
- Instruct patient that if a dose is missed, to take it as soon as possible unless close to time of next dose.
- Warn patient not to double up doses and to notify health care provider if more than 1 dose is missed.
- Advise patient not to change the dose or discontinue the medication without consulting with health care provider.
- Warn patient that drug may impair judgment, thinking and particularly, motor skills, because of prominent sedative effect and that this may impair ability to drive, use machines or perform tasks that require alertness, coordination, or physical dexterity.
- Caution patient about engaging in hazardous activities until reasonably certain that the drug does not affect the patient's ability to engage in such activities.
- Advise patient to avoid alcohol and other CNS depressants because of additive impairment of cognitive and motor skills.
- Advise patient to inform their health care provider if they are taking, or intend to take any prescription or OTC drugs because of the potential for interactions with mirtazapine.
- Advise women to notify health care provider if becoming pregnant, intending to become pregnant, or if breastfeeding while taking this drug.
- Warn patient about the risk of developing agranulocytosis and to contact the health care provider health care provider if experiencing any indication of infection (eg, "flu-like" symptoms, fever, chills, sore throat, mucous membrane ulceration).
- Explain that drug may cause dry mouth and constipation. Advise patient about measures to manage these side effects.
- Advise patient to report the following symptoms to health care provider: excessive sedation; dizziness; abnormal dreams or thinking; tremors; confusion; anxiety; agitation; rash; itching; excessive dry mouth; severe constipation.

- Advise patient not to split disintegrating tablet.
- Instruct patient to take disintegrating tablet immediately after removal from blister pack and not to store tablet after removal from blister pack.
- Explain that disintegrating tablet disintegrates rapidly on the tongue and can be swallowed with saliva; water is not needed.

Misoprostol

(MY-so-PRAHST-ole)
Class Prostaglandin

How Supplied
Cytotec Tablets 100 mcg, Tablets 200 mcg
♣ *Apo-Misoprostol* ♦ *Novo-Misoprostol*

Action
PHARMACOLOGY: Synthetic prostaglandin E_1 analog that inhibits gastric acid secretion and exerts mucosal-protective properties.

PHARMACOKINETICS/DYNAMICS:
Absorption: Misoprostol is extensively absorbed. T_{max} is approximately 12 min. Food decreases C_{max} and total availability of misoprostol acid is reduced by the use of concomitant antacid.

Distribution: Less than 90% is protein bound and displays linear kinetics.

Metabolism: Misoprostol undergoes rapid de-esterification to its free acid, which is responsible for its clinical activity. It does not affect the hepatic mixed function oxidase cytochrome P450 enzyme system.

Excretion: Approximately 80% is detected in urine and the t½ is 20 to 40 min.

Special Populations:
Renal Function Impairment – C_{max}, AUC, and t½ are almost doubled, but no clear correlation between degree of impairment and AUC is shown. No dosage adjustment is recommended. However, dose reduction my be needed if patient does not tolerate.

Elderly – AUC is increased in patients older than 64 yr. However, no dose adjustment is needed.

Indications
Prevention of gastric ulcers in high-risk patients who are taking NSAIDs.

Contraindications
History of allergy to prostaglandins; pregnancy.

Route/Dosage
ADULTS: **PO** 100 to 200 mcg qid, in conjunction with NSAID therapy.

Interactions
None well documented.

Lab Test Interferences
None well documented.

Adverse Reactions
CNS: Headache (2%).
GI: Diarrhea (14% to 40% [dose-related]); abdominal pain (13% to 20%); nausea, flatulence (3%); dyspepsia (2%); vomiting, constipation (1%).

> **WARNING:**
> Abortion, premature birth, birth defects, and uterine rupture have been reported when misoprostol is administered in pregnant women to induce labor or abortion beyond week 3 of pregnancy. Misoprostol should not be taken by pregnant women for risk reduction of NSAID ulcers. Counsel patients on abortifacient properties.
> *Monitoring recommendations:* Prescribe for NSAID ulcer reduction in women only if serum pregnancy test is negative when administered within 2 wk prior to therapy and patient is capable of contraception compliance. Written and oral patient counseling is required. Begin therapy only on second or third day of the next menstrual period.

Precautions
Pregnancy: Category X.
Lactation: Undetermined.
Children: Safety and efficacy not established in children younger than 18 yr
Elderly: Reduce dosage if usual dose is not tolerated.
Renal function impairment: May reduce drug Cl; routine dosage adjustment is not recommended unless usual dose is not tolerated.
Fertility impairment: May adversely affect fertility.
Diarrhea: Dose related (13% to 40%); usually develops early in course of therapy (after 13 days) and is usually self-limiting (resolving after 8 days).
Duodenal ulcers: Not for prevention of duodenal ulcers in patients on NSAIDs.

Overdosage: Signs and Symptoms
Sedation, tremor, seizure, dyspnea, abdominal pain, diarrhea, fever, palpitations, hypotension, bradycardia.

PATIENT CARE CONSIDERATIONS

Administration/Storage
* Administer prescribed dose with or after meals to minimize diarrhea.
* Take the last dose of the day at bedtime.
* Antacids can be administered as needed. Avoid magnesium-containing antacids because of association with misoprostol-induced diarrhea.
* Store tablets below 77° F. Protect from moisture.

Assessment/Interventions
* Obtain patient history, including drug history and any known allergies. Note pregnancy, CV disease, duodenal ulcers(s), inflammatory bowel disease, or history of sensitivity to prostaglandins.
* Ensure that women of childbearing potential are not pregnant when therapy is initiated and are using an effective method of contraception.
* Assess patient for symptoms of gastric ulceration (eg, indigestion, abdominal pain) before starting therapy and periodically during treatment. Inform health care provider if symptoms of gastric ulceration develop.
* Monitor patient for GI, GU, CNS, and general body side effects. Inform health care provider if noted and significant.

Patient/Family Education
* Explain name, dose, action, and potential side effects of drug.
* Advise patient to read *Patient Information* leaflet before starting therapy and with each refill.
* Advise patient that medication is not used to treat stomach ulcers but is being used to prevent the NSAID from causing stomach ulcers and that the medication must be taken regularly, as prescribed, for this beneficial effect to occur.
* Advise patient to take prescribed dose with or after a meal to reduce risk of diarrhea.
* Advise patient to take the last dose of the day just before bedtime.
* Caution patient not to change the dose or stop taking unless advised by health care provider.
* Advise patient that diarrhea is the most common side effect of misoprostol and that taking each dose with or after meals and avoiding magnesium-containing antacids may minimize this problem.
* Advise patient to notify health care provider if symptoms of stomach ulcer develop (eg, indigestion, stomach pain), or if intolerable side effects (eg, diarrhea, cramping) develop.
* Caution women of childbearing potential to use an effective method of contraception while taking this medication and for 1 mo or for 1 menstrual cycle after misoprostol has been discontinued.
* Advise women to notify health care provider if pregnant, planning to become pregnant, or breastfeeding.
* Advise patient not to take any prescription or OTC drugs or dietary supplements without consulting health care provider.
* Advise patient that follow-up visits may be necessary to monitor therapy and to keep appointments.

Mitomycin

(MY-toe-MY-sin)

Class Antineoplastic antibiotic

How Supplied
Mutamycin Powder for injection 5 mg (10 mg mannitol) vials, Powder for injection 20 mg (40 mg mannitol) vials, Powder for injection 40 mg (80 mg mannitol) vials

Action
PHARMACOLOGY: An antibiotic that inhibits the synthesis of DNA.

PHARMACOKINETICS/DYNAMICS:

Absorption: Mitomycin is rapidly cleared from the serum. C_{max} is 2.4 mch/mL (after 30 mg IV injection), 1.7 mcg/mL (after 20 mg IV), and 0.5 mcg/mL (after 10 mg IV).

Metabolism: Metabolism is primarily hepatic and has saturable metabolic pathways.

Excretion: Approximately 10% is excreted in urine (increases as dose increases) and clearance is affected primarily by hepatic metabolism. Serum t½ is 17 min after 30 mg bolus.

Special Populations:
Renal Function Impairment – Observe patients for evidence of renal toxicity. Do not give to patients with a serum creatinine more than 1.7 mg/dL.

Indications Palliative treatment of disseminated adenocarcinoma of stomach or pancreas. **Unlabeled use(s):** Bladder, colorectal, or breast cancer; squamous cell carcinoma of head and neck, lungs, or cervix; pterygium.

Contraindications Primary therapy as a single agent; to replace surgery or radiotherapy; hypersensitivity or idiosyncratic reaction to mitomycin; thrombocytopenia; coagulation disorder; increase in bleeding tendency caused by other causes.

Route/Dosage
Mitomycin 0.02% Eye Drops for Pterygium
ADULTS: Reconstitute 5 mg vial of mitomycin with 10 mL sterile water for injection to a concentration of 0.5 mg/mL. Transfer 6 mL (3 mg) to a sterile 15 mL eye dropper bottle. Add 9 mL of sterile water for injection for a final concentration of 0.2 mg/mL (0.02% solution). This solution is stable for 1 wk at room temperature (59° to 86°F) and 2 wk refrigerated.

Mitomycin 0.2 mg/mL Ophthalmic Solution for Intraoperative Use
ADULTS: Reconstitute 5 mg vial of mitomycin with 10 mL sterile water for injection. Transfer the contents of the vial to a 30 mL sterile vial. Add 15 mL of sterile water for injection for a final volume of 25 mL (0.2 mg/mL). This solution is stable for 52 wk frozen, 2 wk under refrigeration, and 24 hr at room temperature (59° to 86°F).

Palliative Treatment of Disseminated Adenocarcinoma of Stomach or Pancreas
ADULTS AND PEDIATRICS:
Initial dose: 10 to 20 mg/m^2, q 6 to 8 wk. Fully reevaluate patients after each course of therapy. Do not exceed 20 mg/m^2. Give an additional course of therapy only after the leukocyte and platelet counts have recovered. Subsequent doses of mitomycin may be adjusted according to the following schedule.

For dosage adjustments of mitomycin, nadir after prior dose (cells/mm^3): 100% of prior dose to be given to more than 3000 leukocytes and more than 75,000 platelets; 70% of prior dose to be given to 2000 to 2999 leukocytes and 25,000 to 74,999 platelets; 50% of prior dose to be given to less than 2000 leukocytes and less than 25,000 platelets.

If disease progression continues after 2 courses, discontinue therapy.

Interactions Use of vinca alkaloids in patients who have previously or simultaneously received mitomycin has resulted in acute shortness of breath and severe bronchospasm.

Lab Test Interferences None well documented.

Adverse Reactions
DERM: Alopecia; desquamation; pruritus.
GI: Moderate to low potential for nausea and vomiting; anorexia; mucositis; hepatic artery thrombosis (intra-arterial administration only).
GU: Amenorrhea.
HEMA: Bone marrow suppression; thrombocytopenia nadir at 4 to 6 wk; leukopenia nadir at 6 wk (can be delayed 8 wk or less).
RENAL: Increased serum creatinine and BUN; glomerular sclerosis; hemolytic uremic syndrome may result in irreversible renal failure.
RESP: Interstitial pneumonitis; pulmonary fibrosis.
OTHER:
Hemolytic uremic syndrome – Usually occurs after 6 mo of therapy. Course may be chronic or fulminant. Plasmapheresis may be indicated for treatment. Fever.

> **WARNING:**
> *Bone marrow suppression:* Thrombocytopenia and leukopenia may occur any time within 8 wk (average, 4 wk) of therapy; recovery after therapy is within 10 wk. They may contribute to overwhelming infection in an already compromised patient.
>
> *Hemolytic uremic syndrome:* Hemolytic uremic syndrome has been reported and may occur with monotherapy or combination therapy. Usually occurs with doses of at least 60 mg. Blood product transfusion may exacerbate symptoms.

Precautions
Pregnancy: Safety for use during pregnancy has not been established. Teratological changes have been noted in animal studies.
Renal function impairment:
Dosage adjustment for renal insufficiency – Do not give to patients with a serum creatinine more than 1.7 mg/dL.

Mitomycin Dosage Adjustment Based on Renal Function	
Ccr	Percent of Usual Dose
> 60 mL/min	100
30 to 60 mL/min	75
10 to 29 mL/min	75
< 10 mL/min	50

Adult respiratory distress syndrome: Exercise caution to use only enough oxygen to provide adequate arterial saturation since oxygen itself is toxic to the lungs. Pay careful attention to fluid balance; avoid overhydration.
Extravasation risk: Local irritation or phlebitis may occur. Refer to your institution specific protocol.

PATIENT CARE CONSIDERATIONS
Administration/Storage
- Protect powder for injection from light and store at room temperature (59° to 86°F).
- Dilute with sterile water for injection. Shake the vial; allow to stand at room temperature for complete dissolution. Maximum concentration is 0.5 mg/mL; more concentrated solutions crystallize easily.
- Reconstituted mitomycin contains no preservative and should be used within 24 hr.
- Diluted in various IV fluids at room temperature to a concentration of 20 to 40 mcg/mL, stability is as follows: 5% Dextrose Injection, 3 hr; 0.9% NaCl Injection, 12 hr; Sodium Lactate Injection, 24 hr.
- The combination of mitomycin (5 to 15 mg) and heparin (1000 to 10,000 units) in 30 mL of 0.9% NaCl Injection is stable for 48 hr at room temperature.
- Administer IV, intra-arterial, or intravesical.
- Administer by IV push injection or IV side arm into a running infusion.

Assessment/Interventions
- Monitor for evidence of renal or pulmonary toxicity.
- Perform hematologic studies (eg, platelet count, WBC, differential, hemoglobin) during therapy and for at least 8 wk following discontinuation of the drug.
- Avoid use in patients with thrombocytopenia, coagulation disorders, or an increased bleeding tendency, and patients with a serum creatinine more than 1.7 mg/dL.
- Advise patients of potential bone marrow suppression.
- Monitor patients receiving at least 60 mg for unexplained anemia with fragmented cells on peripheral blood smear, thrombocytopenia, and decreased renal function.

Patient/Family Education
- Explain name, action, and potential side effects of drug.
- Advise patient, family, or caregiver that medication will be prepared and administered by health care provider in a health care setting.
- Advise patient, family, or caregiver that medication will be used in combination with other agents to achieve maximum benefit possible.
- Review dosing schedule with patient, family, or caregiver.
- Advise patient, family, or caregiver to immediately report any of the following to health care provider: rash; hives; shortness of breath or difficulty breathing; fever, chills or other signs of infection; sores in mouth; unusual bleeding or bruising; pain, redness or swelling at injection site.
- Advise patient, family, or caregiver to report any of the following to health care provider: persistent nausea, vomiting, diarrhea or appetite loss; persistent or worsening general body weakness.
- Instruct patient to not take any prescription or OTC medications or dietary supplements unless advised to do so by health care provider.
- Caution women of childbearing potential to avoid becoming pregnant during therapy.
- Advise women to notify health care provider if pregnant, planning to become pregnant, or breastfeeding.
- Advise patient, family, or caregiver that following discharge frequent follow-up visits and laboratory tests will be required to monitor therapy and to be sure to keep appointments.

Mitotane
(MY-toe-TANE)

Class Adrenal cortex suppressant

How Supplied
Lysodren Tablets 500 mg

Action
PHARMACOLOGY: The primary action is on the adrenal cortex. The production of adrenal steroids is reduced. The biochemical mechanism of action is unknown. Data suggest that the drug modifies the peripheral metabolism of steroids and directly suppresses the adrenal cortex. Use of mitotane alters the peripheral metabolism of cortisol, even though plasma levels of corticosteroids do not fall. The drug causes increased formation of 6-beta-hydroxycortisol.

PHARMACOKINETICS/DYNAMICS:
Absorption: Approximately 40% of oral dose is absorbed.

Distribution: Mitotane is found in most tissues, but mainly in fat tissues.

Metabolism: Primary metabolites are oxidation products.

Excretion: Approximately 10% is recovered in the urine as a water-soluble metabolite. No unchanged metabolites are found in urine or bile. Up to 60% is excreted unchanged in feces; 1% to 17% of metabolite is excreted in bile with the rest stored in the tissues. The $t_{½}$ is 18 to 159 days.

Special Populations:
Hepatic Function Impairment – Administer with care in patients with liver disease other than

metastatic lesions of the adrenal cortex. Interference with metabolism may occur, causing drug accumulation.

Indications Inoperable adrenal cortical carcinoma.

Contraindications Standard considerations.

Route/Dosage
Inoperable Adrenal Cortical Carcinoma
ADULTS: PO Initially 2 to 6 g/day in divided doses, tid or qid. Titrate at least 9 to 10 g/day until adverse effects occur. The max tolerated dose ranges from 2 to 16 g/day. Doses as high as 18 to 19 g/day have been used.

Interactions
CNS depressants (eg, narcotics, analgesics, alcohol, antiemetics, benzodiazepines, sedatives, tranquilizers): Potentiation of CNS effects with mitotane.
Corticosteroids: May increase corticosteroid metabolism, requiring higher corticosteroid doses with long-term mitotane therapy.
Spironolactone: May block the adrenolytic effects of mitotane.
Warfarin: Increases warfarin metabolism; increased warfarin doses may be required.

Lab Test Interferences Protein-bound iodine levels and urinary 17-hydroxycorticosteroids may be decreased by mitotane.

Adverse Reactions
CV: Hypertension, orthostatic hypotension, flushing (infrequent).
CNS: Lethargy, somnolence (25%); dizziness, vertigo (15%).
DERM: Skin toxicity (primarily rash [15%]).
EENT: Toxic retinopathy, visual blurring, diplopia, lens opacity (infrequent).
GI: Anorexia, nausea, vomiting, diarrhea (80%).
GU: Hematuria, hemorrhagic cystitis, albuminuria (infrequent).
OTHER: Generalized aching, hyperpyrexia (infrequent).

> **WARNING:**
> Temporarily stop therapy after shock or severe trauma as drug's prime action is adrenal suppression. Administer exogenous steroids in such cases as depressed adrenal function may not immediately return.

Precautions
Pregnancy: Category C.
Lactation: Undetermined.
Children: Safety and efficacy not established.
Hepatic function impairment: Administer with care to patients with liver disease other than metastatic lesions of the adrenal cortex. Patients with hepatic insufficiency may require a decrease in mitotane dosage; however, specific recommendations are not established.
Adrenal insufficiency: Adrenal insufficiency may develop; consider adrenal steroid replacement in these patients.
Long-term therapy: Continuous administration of high doses may lead to brain damage and impairment of function.
Tumor tissue: Surgically remove all possible tumor tissue from large metastatic masses before administration to minimize the possibility of infarction and hemorrhage in the tumor caused by a rapid, cytotoxic effect of the drug.

PATIENT CARE CONSIDERATIONS

Administration/Storage
- Follow institutional procedures for handling, administration, and disposal of anticancer drugs.
- Administer prescribed dose without regard to meals. Administer with food if GI upset occurs.
- Store tablets at controlled room temperature (59° to 86°F).

Assessment/Interventions
- Obtain patient history, including drug history and any known allergies. Note hepatic impairment.
- Ensure that treatment is temporarily discontinued and exogenous corticosteroid therapy is initiated in any situation that could cause acute adrenal insufficiency (eg, shock, trauma, infection).
- Ensure that behavioral and neurological assessments are made before initiating therapy and periodically thereafter when continuous treatment with mitotane exceeds 2 yr.
- Carefully assess patient for signs of adrenal insufficiency during treatment (eg, hypotension, malaise, weakness, fever). Notify health care provider if suspected and be prepared to administer exogenous corticosteroids.
- Frequently assess patient for response to treatment (eg, reduction in tumor mass, pain, weakness, anorexia, symptoms or signs of excessive steroid production). Notify health care provider if symptoms do not appear to be improving or are worsening.
- Ensure that therapy is periodically reviewed to determine if it needs to be continued without change or if a dose change (eg, increase, decrease, discontinuation) is indicated.
- Monitor patient for GI, CNS, DERM, and general body side effects. Report to health care provider if noted and significant.

- Implement safety precautions for patients who experience dizziness or ataxia.

Patient/Family Education
- Explain name, dose, action, and potential side effects of drug.
- Advise patient to read the *Patient Information* leaflet before starting therapy and with each refill.
- Advise patient that medication is usually started in the hospital while the dose is being adjusted and stabilized.
- Instruct patient to take exactly as prescribed and not to change the dose or discontinue unless advised by health care provider.
- Advise patient that dose is started low and increased as tolerated until max has been obtained.
- Advise patient that each dose may be taken without regard to meals but to take with food if stomach upset occurs.
- Advise patient that if a dose is missed to take it as soon as remembered, but if several hours have passed or it is nearing the time for the next scheduled dose, to skip that dose and take the next dose at the regularly scheduled time. Caution patient to never double the dose to catch up.
- Instruct patient to inform health care provider if any of the following occur: excessive drowsiness or dizziness; persistent nausea, vomiting, diarrhea; fever; low BP or dizziness when arising from a sitting or lying position; skin rash; recurrence or worsening of symptoms of tumors.
- Caution patient that drug may cause drowsiness and dizziness and to use caution while driving or performing other tasks requiring mental alertness until tolerance is determined.
- Advise women of childbearing potential to use effective contraception during treatment and for 3 mo following discontinuation of mitotane.
- Advise women to notify health care provider if pregnant, planning to become pregnant, or breastfeeding.
- Advise patient not to take any prescription or OTC medications or dietary supplements unless advised by health care provider.
- Advise patient that laboratory tests and follow-up visits will be required to monitor therapy and to keep appointments.

Mitoxantrone

(MY-toe-ZAN-trone)

Class Antineoplastic antibiotic

How Supplied
Novantrone Sterile solution for injection 2 mg/mL

Action
PHARMACOLOGY: It has a cytocidal effect on proliferating and nonproliferating cultured human cells, suggesting lack of cell cycle phase specificity.

PHARMACOKINETICS/DYNAMICS:
Distribution: Distribution to tissues is extensive and is 78% protein bound over a 26 to 455 ng/mL concentration range. Vd exceeds 1,000 L/m^2.

Excretion: Elimination is slow via renal and hepatobiliary systems. Only 11% is recovered in urine within 5 days (65% unchanged, 35% as metabolite); hepatobiliary is more significant with 25% recovered in feces within 5 days. The elimination t½ is 23 to 215 hr (median is approximately 75 hr).

Special Populations:
Hepatic Function Impairment – Patients with multiple sclerosis (MS) who have hepatic impairment should not ordinarily be treated with mitoxantrone. Dosage adjustment may be required for other patients with hepatic impairment.

Indications Adult acute nonlymphocytic leukemia (ANLL) as adjunctive therapy; advanced hormone-refractory prostate cancer (in combination with corticosteroids); secondary (chronic) progressive, progressive-relapsing, or worsening relapsing-remitting MS.

Contraindications Standard considerations.

Route/Dosage
Combination Initial Therapy for ANLL
ADULTS: **IV** For induction, give 12 mg/m^2 per day on days 1 to 3, and give 100 mg/m^2 of cytarabine for 7 days as a continuous 24-hr infusion on days 1 to 7. A second induction course may be given. Give mitoxantrone for 2 days and cytarabine for 5 days using the same daily dosage levels.

MS
ADULTS: **IV** The recommended dosage of mitoxantrone is 12 mg/m^2 given as a short

(approximately 5 to 15 min) IV infusion q 3 mo. Do not administer to MS patients who have received a cumulative lifetime dose of 140 mg/m^2 or more, or those with either left ventricular ejection fraction (LVEF) of less than 50% or a clinically significant reduction in LVEF.

Prostate Cancer
ADULTS: **IV** Recommended dosage of mitoxantrone is 12 to 14 mg/m^2 given as a short IV infusion q 21 days.

Interactions
Quinolone antibiotics: Mitoxantrone may decrease oral absorption of quinolone antibiotics.

Lab Test Interferences None well documented.

Adverse Reactions
CV: Arrhythmia (18%); abnormal ECG (11%).
CNS: Headache (6%).
DERM: Alopecia (61%).
EENT: Sinusitis (6%).
GI: Nausea (76%); diarrhea (25%); stomatitis (19%); constipation (14%).
GU: Menstrual disorder (61%); amenorrhea (43%); UTI (32%); abnormal urine (11%).
HEMA: Leukopenia (19%); granulocytopenia, anemia (6%).
METAB: Increased gamma-GT (15%); increased AST (9%); increased ALT (6%).
RESP: Upper respiratory tract infection (53%).
OTHER: Back pain (8%).

> **WARNING:**
> *Administration:* Administer mitoxantrone under the supervision of a physician experienced in the use of cytotoxic chemotherapy. Administer into a free-flowing IV infusion.

Extravasation risk: Local irritation or phlebitis may occur. Refer to institution-specific protocol.
Intrathecal: Not for intrathecal use.
Leukemia: Secondary acute myelogenous leukemia has been reported in cancer patients treated with agents related to mitoxantrone.
Myocardial toxicity: Myocardial toxicity, including fatal CHF, may occur during and for years after stopping mitoxantrone therapy.
Neutropenia: Except for the treatment of ANLL, do not administer to patients with baseline neutrophil counts less than 1,500 cells/mm^3.

Precautions
Pregnancy: Category D.
Lactation: Excreted in breast milk. Discontinue breastfeeding upon starting treatment.
Children: Safety and efficacy for use in children not established.
Hepatic function impairment: There is no laboratory measurement that allows for dose adjustment recommendations. Patients with MS who have hepatic impairment should ordinarily not be treated with mitoxantrone. A dosage adjustment may be required for other patients with hepatic impairment.
Cardiac: Functional cardiac changes, including irreversible CHF and decreased LVEF, can occur.
Myelosuppression: Mitoxantrone administered at any dose can cause myelosuppression. Patients with preexisting myelosuppression as the result of prior drug therapy should not receive mitoxantrone.

PATIENT CARE CONSIDERATIONS
Administration/Storage
- Do not administer to patient with neutrophil count less than 1,500 cells/mm^3 unless patient has ANLL.
- Dose, frequency, and duration of therapy are dependent on condition being treated.
- May be used alone or in combination with other agents.
- For IV administration only. Not for intradermal, subcutaneous, IM, intra-arterial, or intrathecal administration.
- Concentrate must be diluted following manufacturer's recommendations before administration. Administer immediately after dilution.
- Do not administer if particulate matter or discoloration noted.
- Administer prescribed dose slowly (over period of not less than 3 min) into free-flowing IV infusion.
- Do not mix with other medications.
- Discard any unused infusion solution.
- Follow procedures for proper handling and disposal of anticancer drugs. Wear goggles, gloves, and protective gowns during preparation and administration.
- Store unopened vials at controlled room temperature (59° to 77°F). Do not freeze. After penetration of multidose vial stopper, the remaining undiluted concentrate can be stored for up to 7 days at room temperature (59° to 77°F) or for up to 14 days refrigerated (36° to 46°F). Do not freeze.

Assessment/Interventions

- Obtain patient history, including drug history and any known allergies. Note impaired liver function, cardiac disease, decreased left ventricular function, myelosuppression from previous drug therapy, previous or concurrent treatment with radiotherapy to mediastinum/pericardial area, previous treatment with anthracyclines or anthracenediones, or concomitant use of other cardiotoxic drugs.
- Note cumulative dose (mg/m^2) before each course of therapy or cycle.
- Ensure that left ventricular function (eg, echocardiogram, multiple-gated acquisition scan) is evaluated in patient with MS before starting therapy, before all subsequent doses if signs or symptoms of heart failure develop, or in patient who has received a cumulative dose greater than 100 mg/m^2.
- Ensure that CBC with differential and platelet count are evaluated before each course of therapy and in the event signs or symptoms of an infection develop. Ensure that liver enzymes are evaluated before each course of therapy.
- Ensure that hypouricemic therapy is initiated before starting treatment for leukemia and that uric acid levels are monitored frequently during treatment.
- Ensure women being treated for MS have a negative pregnancy test before starting therapy and before each subsequent dose.
- Ensure women of childbearing potential are not pregnant when therapy is started and use effective contraception during therapy.
- Take steps to avoid extravasation at the infusion site and to avoid contact of medication with skin, mucus membranes, or eyes. If skin contact occurs, wash area copiously with warm water. If eye contact occurs, irrigate copiously.
- Assess injection site frequently for signs or symptoms of extravasation (eg, burning, pain, pruritus, erythema, swelling, blue discoloration, ulceration). If noted, discontinue infusion immediately and restart in another vein. Elevate affected extremity and place ice packs intermittently over area of extravasation.
- Implement infection control measures if WBC drops; implement bleeding precautions if platelet count drops.
- Monitor patient for CNS, GI, GU, and general body side effects. Report to health care provider if noted and significant. Immediately report any of the following: cough, shortness of breath on exertion, edema, or other signs of heart failure; sores in mouth; fever, sore throat, or other signs of infection; bleeding or unusual bruising.

Patient/Family Education

- Advise patient to read patient package insert before starting therapy and prior to each treatment.
- Explain name, action, and potential side effects of drug.
- Advise patient, family, or caregiver that medication will be prepared and administered by a health care provider in a medical setting.
- Review dose and dosing schedule, depending on condition being treated.
- Advise patient, family, or caregiver urine may have a blue-green color for 24 hr after administration and bluish discoloration of the sclera may occur but these are expected and are of no concern.
- Instruct patient to immediately report any of the following to health care provider: infusion site reaction or pain; cough or difficulty breathing on exertion; swelling of legs or feet; sores in or around the mouth; fever, sore throat, or other signs of infection; bleeding or unusual bruising.
- Advise women of childbearing potential to use effective contraception during therapy.
- Advise women to notify health care provider if pregnant, planning to become pregnant, or breastfeeding.
- Instruct patient not to take any prescription or OTC medications, herbal preparations, or dietary supplements unless advised by health care provider.
- Advise patient that follow-up visits and lab tests will be necessary to monitor therapy and to keep appointments.

Mivacurium Chloride

(mih-vuh-CURE-ee-uhm KLOR-ide)

Class Muscle relaxant/Nondepolarizing neuromuscular blocker

How Supplied
Mivacron Injection 0.5 mg/mL, Injection 2 mg/mL

Action

PHARMACOLOGY: Binds competitively to cholinergic receptors on motor end-plate to antagonize action of acetylcholine, resulting in block of neuromuscular transmission.

PHARMACOKINETICS/DYNAMICS:
Distribution: Mean Vd's are 0.15 (trans-trans isomer), 0.27 (cis-trans isomer), and 0.31 min (cis-cis isomer).

Metabolism: Rapid hydrolysis by plasma cholinesterase.

Excretion: Mean t½ is 2.3 min (trans-trans isomer), 2.1 min (cis-trans isomer), and 55 min (cis-cis isomer). Mean plasma clearance is 53 (trans-trans isomer), 99 (cis-trans isomer), and 4.2 mL/nim/kg (cis-cis isomer).

Peak: Time to peak effect is 2.3 to 4.9 min (dose dependent).

Duration: 95% recovery; 21 to 34 min (dose dependent).

Special Populations:
Renal Function Impairment – Increased duration of action and decreased clearance.
Hepatic Function Impairment – Increased duration of action and decreased clearance.
Elderly – Increased duration of action and decreased clearance.

Indications Adjunct to general anesthesia; facilitation of tracheal intubation.

Contraindications Hypersensitivity to mivacurium or similar agents; use of multidose vials in benzyl alcohol-sensitive patients.

Route/Dosage
ADULTS:
Initial dose: **IV** 0.15 mg/kg over 5 to 15 sec.
Maintenance: **IV** 0.1 mg/kg q 15 min prn or 9 to 10 mcg/kg/min infusion initially followed by titration (range 1 to 15 mg/kg/min).
CHILDREN (2 TO 12 YR):
Initial dose: **IV** 0.2 mg/kg over 5 to 15 sec.
Maintenance: **IV** 14 mcg/kg/min infusion initially followed by titration (range 5 to 31 mcg/kg/min).

Interactions
Aminoglycosides, clindamycin, inhalation anesthetics ketamine, parenteral magnesium salts, polypeptide antibiotics, quinidine, quinine, trimethaphan, verapamil: Action of mivacurium potentiated.
Azathioprine: Action of mivacurium may be decreased or reversed.
Carbamazepine: Shortened action of mivacurium and decreased effectiveness.
Theophyllines: Dose-dependent reversal of neuromuscular blockade.
Trimethaphan: Prolonged apnea.
Verapamil: Enhanced action of mivacurium (eg, respiratory depression).
INCOMPATIBILITIES: Alkaline solutions (pH more than 8.5).

Lab Test Interferences None well documented.

Adverse Reactions
CV: Flushing; hypotension; tachycardia; bradycardia; arrhythmia; phlebitis.
DERM: Rash; urticaria; erythema; injection site reaction.
RESP: Bronchospasm; wheezing; hypoxemia.
OTHER: Dizziness; muscle spasms.

Precautions
Pregnancy: Category C.
Lactation: Undetermined.
Children: Safety and efficacy in children younger than 2 yr not established.
Elderly: Neuromuscular blockade may be longer.
Renal function impairment: Duration of action is longer; use lower maintenance doses.
Hepatic function impairment: Duration of action is longer; use lower maintenance doses.
Cachectic or debilitated patients, patients with neuromuscular disease, burns: Use test dose of no more than 0.015 to 0.02 mg/kg.
CV disease or allergy/sensitivity (eg, asthma): Administer initial dose of no more than 0.15 mg/kg over 60 sec.
Obese patients: Use ideal body weight to determine initial dose.
Reduced plasma cholinesterase activity: Use drug with great caution, if at all.

Overdosage: Signs and Symptoms
Flaccid paralysis, apnea, hypotension.

PATIENT CARE CONSIDERATIONS

Administration/Storage
- Administer via IV route only.
- Administer only under supervision of health care provider familiar with drug actions and possible complications.
- Ensure that personnel and facilities for resuscitation and life support (tracheal intubation, artificial ventilation, oxygen therapy) are available and have antagonist of drug (anticholinesterase) immediately available.
- Administer to unconscious patients only.
- Prepared drug dilutions in compatible solutions may be stored at room temperature (59° to 86°F) for up to 24 hr when protected from ultraviolet light and from temperature extremes.
- Do not introduce additives into infusion solution.
- Discard unused portion of diluted drug after each use.

Assessment/Interventions
- Obtain patient history, including drug history and any known allergies. Note CV disease, asthma or other conditions resulting in sensitivity to release of histamine or related mediators; neuromuscular disease; carcinomatosis; renal or hepatic impairment; history of reduced plasma cholinesterase activity.

- Observe for flushing, hypotension, increases or decreases in heart rate, dizziness or muscle spasms and report to health care provider.
- Use nerve stimulator to assess neuromuscular blockade.
- Maintain adequate hydration and monitor hemodynamic status in patients with clinically significant CV disease and with asthma or other conditions resulting in sensitivity to release of histamine or related mediators.
- Perform eye care (eg, artificial tears, covering eye) frequently to prevent corneal drying.

Patient/Family Education
- Explain that drug will be administered while patient is unconscious.
- Advise patient that dizziness or muscle spasms sometimes occur during recovery.

Modafinil

(moe-DAFF-ih-nill)
Class CNS stimulant/Analeptic

How Supplied
Provigil Tablets 100 mg, Tablets 200 mg
 Alertec

Action
PHARMACOLOGY: Wakefulness-promoting agent; however, precise mechanism(s) unknown.

PHARMACOKINETICS/DYNAMICS:
Absorption: T_{max} is 2 to 4 hr. Food delays T_{max} approximately 1 hr.
Distribution: Apparent Vd is 0.9 L/kg and protein binding is approximately 60%.
Metabolism: Primary site is hepatic via hydrolytic deamination, S-oxidation, aromatic ring hyroxylation, and glucuronide conjugation. Major inactive metabolites are modafinil acid and modafinil sulfone. Modafinil induces it own metabolism via cytochrome P450 3A4 after chronic administration.
Excretion: Approximately 80% (urine) and 1% (feces) are excreted in 11 days. The t½ is approximately 15 hr.

Special Populations:
Hepatic Function Impairment – In severe hepatic impairment, Cl is decreased approximately 60%, and steady-state concentrations are doubled. Dose reduction is recommended.

Indications Improve wakefulness in patients with excessive daytime sleepiness associated with narcolepsy, obstructive sleep apnea/hypopnea syndrome (OSAHS), and shift work sleep disorder (SWSD). **Unlabeled use(s):** Treatment of fatigue associated with multiple sclerosis.

Contraindications Standard considerations.

Route/Dosage
ADULTS AND CHILDREN (16 YR OF AGE AND OLDER): **PO** 200 mg/day as a single dose. Patients with narcolepsy or OSAHS should take dose in the morning, while patients with SWSD should take dose 1 hr prior to start of work shift. Dosage adjustment should be considered for concomitant medications that are substrates for CYP3A4, such as triazolam and cyclosporine.
ELDERLY: Consider using a lower dose in this population.
Hepatic impairment – A dose reduction of 50% is recommended.

Interactions
Certain tricyclic antidepressants (eg, clomipramine, desipramine): Plasma levels of certain tricyclic antidepressants may be increased.
Clomipramine: Plasma levels may be increased by modafinil.
Contraceptives, oral: Efficacy may be decreased by modafinil, increasing the risk of unintended pregnancy.
Cyclosporine: Blood levels may be decreased by modafinil.
MAO inhibitors (eg, isocarboxazid): Use with caution.
Methylphenidate: May delay the absorption of modafinil.
Phenytoin: Increased risk of phenytoin toxicity.
Triazolam: Triazolam concentration may be decreased, reducing the clinical effect.
Warfarin: Monitor PT.

Lab Test Interferences None well documented.

Adverse Reactions
CV: Hypertension (3%); palpitation, tachycardia, vasodilatation (2%).
CNS: Headache (34%); nervousness (7%); anxiety, dizziness, insomnia (5%); depression, emotional lability, paresthesia, somnolence (2%); anxiety, confusion, dyskinesia, hyperkinesias, hypertonia, tremor, vertigo (1%); symptoms of mania or psychosis (postmarketing).
DERM: Sweating, herpes simplex (1%).
EENT: Rhinitis (7%); pharyngitis (4%); abnormal vision, amblyopia, epistaxis, eye pain (1%).
GI: Nausea (11%); diarrhea (6%); dyspepsia (5%); anorexia, dry mouth (4%); constipation (2%); flatulence, mouth ulceration, thirst, (1%); taste perversion (1%).
GU: Hematuria, pyuria, urine abnormality (1%).
HEMA/LYMPH: Eosinophilia (1%); agranulocytosis (postmarketing).
HEPA: Abnormal liver function (2%).

LABTESTABS: Increased gamma glutamyltransferase and alkaline phosphatase.
M/N: Edema (1%).
MUSC: Back pain (6%); neck pain (1%).
RESP: Lung disorder (2%); asthma (1%).
OTHER: Flu-like syndrome (4%); chest pain (3%); chills (1%).

Precautions

Pregnancy: Category C.
Lactation: Undetermined.
Children: Safety and efficacy in children younger than 16 yr of age not established.
Hepatic function impairment: Dosage reduction is recommended in patients with severe hepatic impairment.
CNS: Psychotic episodes have been reported.
CV system: Not recommended for use in patients with history of left ventricular hypertrophy or mitral valve prolapse who have experienced mitral valve prolapse syndrome when receiving CNS stimulants.
Drug dependence: Because of psychoactive and euphoric effects, modafinil has potential for abuse.
MI/Unstable angina: Use with caution.
Wakefulness: May not return to normal in patients taking modafinil.

Overdosage: Signs and Symptoms

Excitation, agitation, insomnia, slight to moderate elevations in hemodynamic parameters, anxiety, irritability, aggressiveness, confusion, nervousness, tremor, palpitations, sleep disturbances, nausea, diarrhea, decreased PT.

PATIENT CARE CONSIDERATIONS

Administration/Storage

- Administer prescribed dose once daily.
- Administer prescribed dose in morning to minimize sleep disturbances when improving wakefulness in patient with narcolepsy or OSAHS.
- Administer prescribed dose 1 hr prior to start of shift work when using medication to improve wakefulness in SWSD.
- Administer without regard to food but administer with meals if GI upset occurs.
- Store tablets at controlled room temperature (68° to 77°F).

Assessment/Interventions

- Obtain patient history, including drug history and any known allergies. Note hepatic impairment, left ventricular hypertrophy, recent MI, unstable angina, history of psychosis, history of drug and/or stimulant abuse, history of significant manifestations of mitral valve prolapse (chest pain, palpitations, dyspnea, ischemic ECG changes) with previous CNS stimulant use, or concurrent use of CYP3A4 or CYP2C19 substrates.
- Ensure that medication is used only in patient who has had a complete evaluation of excessive sleepiness, and in whom a diagnosis of narcolepsy, OSAHS, and/or SWSD has been made in accordance with International Classification of Sleep Disorders (ICSD) or DSM diagnostic criteria.
- Ensure that modafinil dose has been reduced 50% in patient with severe hepatic impairment.
- Ensure that use of lower dose has been considered for elderly patient.
- Monitor BP before starting therapy and periodically thereafter in patient with history of hypertension. Notify health care provider of any significant changes.
- Frequently assess patient for response to treatment. Notify health care provider if modafinil does not appear to be improving wakefulness.
- Follow patient closely, especially patient with history of drug and/or stimulant abuse, for signs of drug misuse or abuse (eg, incrementation of doses, drug seeking behavior). Notify health care provider if drug misuse or abuse is suspected.
- Monitor patient for CNS, CV, GI, and general body side effects. Report to health care provider if noted and significant.

Patient/Family Education

- Explain name, dose, action, and potential side effects of drug. Advise patient that medication will not cure sleep disorder and is not a replacement for sleep.
- Advise patient to read *Patient Information Leaflet* before beginning therapy and to reread it each time medication is renewed.
- Advise patient that medication is taken only once a day.
- Advise patient using modafinil for narcolepsy or OSAHS to take prescribed dose in the morning to minimize sleep disturbances.
- Advise patient using modafinil for SWSD to take prescribed dose 1 hr prior to start of shift work.
- Advise patient to take each dose without regard to meals but to take with food if stomach upset occurs.
- Advise patient to continue to take previously prescribed treatments (eg, CPAP for patient with OSAHS) as instructed by health care provider.
- Caution patients not to alter previous behavior with regard to potentially dangerous activities (eg, driving, operating machinery) or other activities requiring appropriate levels of wakefulness until, and unless, treatment

with modafinil has been shown to produce levels of wakefulness that permit such activities.
- Advise patient to take medication as prescribed and to not stop taking or change the dose unless advised by health care provider.
- Caution patient that drug may alter judgment, thinking, or motor skills and to use caution while driving or performing other tasks requiring mental alertness and coordination until tolerance is determined.
- Caution patient that the use of modafinil in combination with alcohol has not been studied, and it is prudent to avoid alcohol while taking modafinil.
- Advise patient to notify health care provider if appetite loss, nervousness, difficulty sleeping, or other bothersome side effects occur.
- Advise patient to stop taking modafinil and immediately notify health care provider if chest pain, mental problems, or rash, hives, or other symptoms of an allergic reaction occur.
- Advise women using hormonal contraception (oral, depot, or implantable) to use alternative or concomitant methods of contraception with, and for 1 mo following discontinuation of, therapy.
- Advise women to notify health care provider if pregnant, planning to become pregnant, or breastfeeding.
- Warn patient not to take any prescription, OTC drugs, herbal preparations, or dietary supplements without consulting health care provider.
- Advise patient or caregiver that follow-up visits and lab tests may be necessary to monitor therapy and to keep appointments.

Moexipril Hydrochloride

(moe-EX-ah-pril HIGH-droe-KLOR-ide)

Class Antihypertensive/ACE inhibitor

How Supplied
Univasc Tablets 7.5 mg, Tablets 15 mg

Action
PHARMACOLOGY: Competitively inhibits angiotensin I-converting enzyme, preventing conversion of angiotensin I to angiotensin II, which is a potent vasoconstrictor and also stimulates aldosterone secretion from the adrenal cortex. This results in decrease in sodium and fluid retention, decrease in BP, and increase in diuresis.

PHARMACOKINETICS/DYNAMICS:

Absorption: Moexipril is incompletely absorbed and the bioavailability is approximately 13%. Food markedly reduces absorption.

Distribution: Approximately 50% is protein bound and Vd is approximately 183 L.

Metabolism: Active metabolite is moexiprilat.

Excretion: Moexipril is excreted in urine (13%, 1% unchanged) and feces (53%, 1% unchanged). The $t_{½}$ is 2 to 9 hr, and the clearances are 441 mL/min (moexipril) and 232 mL/min (moexiprilat).

Onset: 1 hr.

Peak: 3 to 6 hr.

Duration: 24 hr.

Special Populations:
Renal Function Impairment – Effective elimination $t_{½}$ and AUC of moexipril and moexiprilat are increased with decreasing renal function.

Indications Treatment of hypertension.

Contraindications Hypersensitivity to ACE inhibitors; history of angioedema related to previous treatment with an ACE inhibitor.

Route/Dosage
ADULTS:
Initial dose: **PO** 7.5 mg qd.
Maintenance: **PO** 7.5 to 30 mg/day in 1 or 2 divided doses; may add diuretic if needed and decrease dose.
Renal function impairment – Cautiously use 3.75 mg qd in patients with Ccr no more than 40 mL/min/1.73 m^2. Dosage may be titrated up to a max of 15 mg/day.

Interactions
Capsaicin: Cough may be exacerbated.
Digoxin: May increase or decrease plasma digoxin levels.
Diuretics: Excessive reductions in BP may occur.
Indomethacin, salicylates (eg, aspirin): Reduced hypotensive effects, especially in low-renin or volume-dependent hypertensive patients.
Lithium: Increased lithium levels and symptoms of lithium toxicity.
Phenothiazines: May increase the pharmacologic effect of moexipril.
Potassium-sparing diuretics, potassium preparations: May increase serum potassium levels.

Lab Test Interferences False elevation of liver enzymes and uric acid may occur.

Adverse Reactions
CNS: Dizziness (4%); fatigue (2%).
DERM: Rash (2%).
EENT: Pharyngitis (2%).
GI: Diarrhea (3%).
HEMA/LYMPH: Neutropenia; agranulocytosis.
METAB: Hyperkalemia.
MUSC: Myalgia (1%).

RESP: Cough (6%).
OTHER: Flu syndrome (3%); flushing (2%); anaphylactoid reactions.

> **WARNING:**
> *Pregnancy:* Use in second and third trimesters may cause injury and death to fetus.

Precautions
Pregnancy: Category D (second and third trimester); Category C (first trimester).
Lactation: Undetermined.
Children: Safety and efficacy not established.
Elderly: Use with caution, usually starting at the low end of the dose range, because of the greater frequency of decreased hepatic, renal, or cardiac function, and concomitant diseases or other drug therapy.
Renal function impairment: In renal insufficiency, increased serum creatinine may occur due to inadequate renal perfusion; monitor renal function during first few weeks of therapy and adjust dosage carefully; for patients with Ccr less than 40 mL/1.73 m^2, give an initial dose of 3.75 mg. Doses may be carefully titrated to max of 15 mg/day.

Hepatic function impairment: Hepatic failure has been associated with other ACE inhibitors. Patients who develop jaundice or marked elevations of liver enzymes should discontinue drug and receive medical follow-up.
Angioedema: Use with extreme caution in patients with hereditary angioedema.
Hepatic failure: Rarely, ACE inhibitors have been associated with a syndrome that starts with cholestatic jaundice and progresses to fulminant hepatic necrosis and sometimes death.
Hypotension/first dose effect: Significant decreases in BP may occur after the first dose, especially in severely salt- or volume-depleted patients or in those with heart failure. Minimize risk by discontinuing diuretics, decreasing dose, or increasing salt intake approximately 2 to 3 days prior to initiating drug.
Neutropenia/agranulocytosis: Has been reported with other ACE inhibitors. Risk appears greater in patients with renal dysfunction, heart failure, or immunosuppression.

Overdosage: Signs and Symptoms
Hypotension.

PATIENT CARE CONSIDERATIONS

Administration/Storage
- Administer alone or in combination with other antihypertensives.
- Give qd or bid as prescribed, 1 hr before or 2 hr after meals.
- Do not administer to pregnant women during second and third trimesters as fetal and neonatal morbidity and death can occur.
- Store tablets at controlled room temperature (68° to 77°F). Protect from moisture.

Assessment/Interventions
- Obtain patient history, including drug history and any known allergies. Note renal or hepatic impairment, conditions predisposing to volume depletion (eg, prolonged diuretic therapy), diabetes, heart failure, anuria, hereditary or idiopathic angioedema, lupus erythematosus, left ventricular outflow obstruction, allergy to any other ACE inhibitor, and concurrent use of potassium-containing salt substitutes, potassium supplements, or potassium-sparing diuretics.
- Ensure that reduced dose is administered to patient with severe renal impairment (Ccr less than 40 mL/min).
- Ensure that volume and/or salt depletion have been corrected before initiating therapy.
- Ensure that serum electrolytes and renal function are monitored periodically.
- Ensure that CBC with differential are evaluated prior to starting therapy, at 2 wk intervals for 3 mo, and periodically thereafter in patient with renal impairment.
- Monitor and record BP and pulse. Should symptomatic hypotension occur, hold medication and notify health care provider.
- Take safety precautions if orthostatic hypotension occurs.
- Monitor for signs of hypersensitivity including angioedema involving swelling of the face, lips, eyelids, and tongue. Discontinue medication and notify health care provider immediately if noted. Be prepared to treat appropriately.
- Assess patient for GI, CNS, and general body side effects. Inform health care provider if noted and significant.

Patient/Family Education
- Explain name, dose, action, and potential side effects of drug.
- Advise patient to take qd or bid as prescribed.
- Advise patient to take medication 1 hr before or 2 hr after meals because food can reduce absorption and benefits of medication.
- Advise patient to try to take each dose at about the same time each day.
- Inform patient that drug controls, but does not cure, hypertension and to continue taking drug as prescribed even when BP is not elevated.

- Caution patient not to change the dose or stop taking unless advised by health care provider.
- Instruct patient to continue taking other BP medications as prescribed by health care provider.
- Instruct patient in BP and pulse measurement skills.
- Advise patient to monitor and record BP and pulse at home and to inform health care provider if abnormal measurements are noted. Also advise patient to take record of BP and pulse to each follow-up visit.
- Caution patient to avoid sudden position changes to prevent orthostatic hypotension.
- Instruct patient to lie or sit down if experiencing dizziness or lightheadedness when standing.
- Emphasize importance of other modalities on BP control: weight control, regular exercise, smoking cessation, and moderate intake of alcohol and salt.
- Caution patient that inadequate fluid intake, excessive perspiration, diarrhea, or vomiting can lead to excessive fall in BP, resulting in lightheadedness or fainting.
- Advise patient that medication may cause dizziness or lightheadedness and to use caution while driving or performing other tasks requiring mental alertness until tolerance is determined.
- Caution patient to avoid unnecessary exposure to UV light (sunlight, tanning booths) and to use sunscreen and wear protective clothing when exposed to UV light to avoid photosensitivity reaction.
- Instruct women to inform health care provider if pregnant, planning to become pregnant, or breastfeeding.
- Instruct patient to stop taking drug and immediately report any of the following symptoms to health care provider: sore throat, fever, swelling of the hands or feet, irregular heartbeat, chest pains, fainting, swelling of the face, lips, eyelids, or tongue, difficulty breathing.
- Instruct patient to inform health care provider if a persistent cough develops while taking this medication.
- Caution patient to not take any prescription or OTC medications, potassium-containing salt substitutes, potassium supplements, or dietary supplements unless advised by health care provider.
- Advise patient that follow-up visits and lab tests will be required to monitor therapy and to keep appointments.

Molindone Hydrochloride

(moe-LIN-dohn HIGH-droe-KLOR-ide)

Class Antipsychotic

How Supplied
Moban Tablets 5 mg, Tablets 10 mg, Tablets 25 mg, Tablets 50 mg

Action
PHARMACOLOGY: Unknown. Exerts its effect on ascending reticular activating system.

PHARMACOKINETICS/DYNAMICS:
Absorption: Molindone is rapidly absorbed.
Metabolism: Metabolism is rapid.
Excretion: Thirty-six metabolites are recognized with less than 2% to 3% unmetabolized molindone excreted in urine and feces.
Peak: Time to peak is 1.5 hr.
Duration: Duration is 24 to 36 hr.

Indications Management of schizophrenia.

Contraindications Comatose or severe drug-induced depressed states (eg, barbiturates); hypersensitivity to the drug.

Route/Dosage
ADULTS AND CHILDREN 12 YR AND OLDER:
Initial dose: PO 50 to 75 mg/day, increasing dose to 100 mg/day in 3 or 4 days. Patients with severe symptoms may require 225 mg/day. Start elderly and debilitated patients on lower dosage.
Maintenance dose:
Mild symptoms: PO 5 to 15 mg tid or qid.
Moderate symptoms: PO 10 to 25 mg tid or qid.
Severe symptoms: PO 225 mg/day may be required.

Interactions None well documented.

Lab Test Interferences None well documented.

Adverse Reactions
CV: Tachycardia; transient, nonspecific T-wave changes; hypotension.
CNS: Drowsiness; depression; hyperactivity; euphoria; extrapyramidal reactions; akathisia; Parkinson syndrome; dystonic syndrome; tardive dyskinesia; increased libido; seizures.
DERM: Skin rash.
EENT: Blurred vision.
GI: Dry mouth; salivation; constipation; nausea.
GU: Urinary retention; priapism; amenorrhea; gynecomastia; heavy menses (initially).
HEPA: Altered liver function.
METAB: Galactorrhea.

Precautions
Pregnancy: Category C.
Lactation: Undetermined.

Children: Safety and efficacy not established in children younger than 12 yr.
Elderly: Start therapy with a reduced dosage.
Debilitated patients: Start therapy with a reduced dosage.
Neuroleptic malignant syndrome (NMS): This potentially fatal condition has been reported in association with antipsychotic agents. Signs and symptoms include hyperpyrexia, muscle rigidity, altered mental status, irregular pulse or BP, tachycardia, diaphoresis, cardiac arrhythmias.

Prolactin levels: Antipsychotic drugs elevate prolactin levels; elevation persists during chronic administration.
Seizures: Convulsive seizures have been reported.
Tardive dyskinesia: This syndrome of potentially irreversible, involuntary dyskinetic movements has occurred with other antipsychotic agents. Incidence appears to be highest among the elderly, especially elderly women.

PATIENT CARE CONSIDERATIONS

Administration/Storage
- Administer prescribed dose tid to qid.
- Store at controlled room temperature (59° to 86°F). Protect from light.

Assessment/Interventions
- Obtain patient history, including drug history, any known allergies, and previous episodes of NMS.
- Inform health care provider immediately if hyperpyrexia, muscle rigidity, altered mental status, irregular pulse and BP, tachycardia, or diaphoresis develop.
- Assess baseline neurological status and during treatment observe for involuntary body and facial movements and excessive drowsiness. Inform health care provider if noted.
- Assess and document effect of medication on psychotic symptoms.
- Assess medication compliance.
- Ensure that therapy is periodically reviewed to determine if therapy needs to be continued without change or if a dose change (eg, increase, decrease, discontinuation) is indicated.
- Avoid sudden discontinuation of therapy if possible. Attempt to gradually reduce dose if decision to discontinue medication is made.
- Monitor patient for CNS and general body side effects. Inform health care provider if noted and significant.

Patient/Family Education
- Explain name, dose, action, and potential side effects of drug.
- Advise patient that dose may be slowly increased until max benefit is achieved and not to take more than prescribed or increase the dose more rapidly than advised.
- Instruct patient not to stop taking molindone when symptoms have improved.
- Tell patient to immediately report high fever, muscle rigidity, involuntary body or facial movements, altered mental status, irregular pulse, or sweating to health care provider.
- Advise patient to avoid strenuous activity during periods of high temperature or humidity.
- Advise patient that drug may cause drowsiness and to use caution while driving or performing other tasks requiring mental alertness.
- Advise women to notify health care provider if pregnant, planning to become pregnant, or breastfeeding.
- Advise patient to notify health care provider if excessive drowsiness occurs.
- Instruct patient not to take any prescription or OTC medications or dietary supplements unless advised by the health care provider.
- Advise patient that follow-up visits will be required to monitor therapy and to keep appointments.
- Advise patient, family, or caregiver not to change the dose or stop taking molindone unless advised by health care provider.
- Instruct patient to avoid alcoholic beverages and other depressants while taking this medication.

Mometasone

(moe-MET-a-sone)
Class Corticosteroid
How Supplied
Nasonex Spray 50 mcg
Action
PHARMACOLOGY: Has potent anti-inflammatory effects on the nasal passages.

PHARMACOKINETICS/DYNAMICS:
Distribution: Approximately 98% to 99% is protein bound in vitro. Mometasone furoate and its major metabolites are undetectable in plasma.

Metabolism: Portion of dose which is swallowed and absorbed undergoes extensive metabolism to multiple metabolites. Formation of metabolite is regulated by cytochrome P450 3A4.

Excretion: Any absorbed drug is excreted as metabolites mostly via bile and urine, to a limited extent. Plasma t½ is 5.8 hr.

Indications Prophylaxis and treatment of seasonal allergic rhinitis symptoms; treatment of perennial allergic rhinitis symptoms; prophylaxis in patients with a known seasonal allergen that precipitates nasal symptoms of seasonal allergic rhinitis.

Contraindications Standard considerations

Route/Dosage

Prophylaxis and treatment of seasonal allergic rhinitis/Treatment of perennial allergic rhinitis
ADULTS AND CHILDREN (AT LEAST 12 YR): Nasal Inhalation 2 sprays in each nostril once daily.
CHILDREN (3 TO 11 YR): Nasal Inhalation 1 spray in each nostril once daily.

Prophylaxis for seasonal allergic rhinitis
ADULTS & CHILDREN (AT LEAST 12 YR): Nasal Inhalation 2 sprays in each nostril once daily beginning 2 to 4 wk prior to the anticipated start of the pollen season.

Interactions None well documented

Lab Test Interferences None well documented

PATIENT CARE CONSIDERATIONS

Administration/Storage
- For nasal use only.
- Usual dose is 1 to 2 sprays once daily.
- Prime unit with 10 actuations before first use or with 2 actuations if spray has not been used for more than 7 days.
- Have patient prepare nostrils before use by gently blowing nose and pretreating with topical decongestant and saline lavage if indicated.
- Instruct patient in proper administration technique and monitor for proper use.
- Store at controlled room temperature (59° to 86°F) protected from prolonged exposure to direct light.

Assessment/Interventions
- Obtain patient history, including drug history and any known allergies.
- Note history of recent nasal trauma or surgery or nasal septum ulcers.
- If change is made from systemic (oral) to intranasal corticosteroid, observe patient carefully for signs of steroid withdrawal (eg, nausea, fatigue, dizziness, hypotension, depression, joint and muscle pain). Notify health care provider if these signs occur.
- Monitor patient for improvement in nasal symptoms.

Adverse Reactions
CNS: Headache.
CV: Chest pain.
RESP: Coughing; upper respiratory tract infection; asthma; bronchitis; wheezing.
GI: Vomiting; diarrhea; dyspepsia; nausea.
EENT: Earache; conjunctivitis; otitis media; pharyngitis; epistaxis/blood tinged mucus; rhinitis; sinusitis; nasal irritation.
OTHER: Viral Infection; dysmenorrhea; musculoskeletal pain; arthralgia; flu-like symptoms; myalgia.

Precautions
Pregnancy: Category C.
Lactation: Undetermined. Because other corticosteroids are excreted in human milk, use caution.
Children: Safety and efficacy in children younger than 3 yr not established. Oral corticosteroids may suppress growth in children and adolescents, particularly with higher doses over extended periods.
Immunology: Patients receiving immunosuppressant agents are more susceptible to infections than healthy adults. If a patient is exposed to measles or chickenpox, appropriate prophylaxis and treatment may be indicated.

Patient/Family Education
- Explain name, dose, action, and potential side effects of drug.
- Advise patient to read and follow the Patient's Instructions for Use carefully.
- Advise patient that medication is used once daily to prevent or control nasal symptoms and is not intended to be used on an "as needed" basis.
- Instruct patient that pump must be primed before using for the first time by actuating 10 times or until a fine mist appears. Remind patient that further priming is not necessary unless medication has not been used for more than 1 wk, in which case repriming with 2 actuations or until fine mist appears is advised.
- Instruct patient to shake medication well before each use.
- Instruct patient on proper administration technique: blow nose gently to clear nasal passages; if congested, use a topical nasal decongestant 5 to 10 min before medication administration; use saline lavage if necessary to remove secretions; clean outer portion of nose with damp tissue; insert nozzle into nostril; while using finger to keep other nostril closed, inhale while activating the pump; repeat with other nostril.

- Caution patient to not spray directly into the eyes or onto the nasal septum.
- Inform patient that symptoms should begin to improve within 2 days of starting therapy but may take up to 2 wk before max benefit is noted.
- Warn patient that increasing the number of sprays or frequency of use does not increase the effectiveness of the drug but may increase the incidence and severity of side effects.
- Advise patient to contact health care provider if symptoms do not improve or become worse while using this medication.
- If patient is being converted from oral steroids to nasal steroids, review signs and symptoms of adrenal insufficiency that may occur days or weeks after conversion is complete.
- Warn patients who are also taking immunosuppressant doses of corticosteroids to avoid exposure to measles or chickenpox and, if exposed, to seek medical advice without delay.

Mometasone Furoate

(moe-MET-uh-SONE FYU-roh-ate)

Class Topical corticosteroid

How Supplied
Elocon Ointment 0.1%, Cream 0.1%, Lotion 0.1%

 Elocon

Action
PHARMACOLOGY: Medium-potency topical corticosteroid that depresses formation, release, and activity of endogenous mediators of inflammation including prostaglandins, kinins, histamine, liposomal enzymes, and complement system; modifies body's immune response.

Indications
Topical: Relief of inflammatory and pruritic manifestations of corticosteroid-responsive dermatoses.
Intranasal: Treatment and prophylaxis of nasal symptoms of seasonal allergic and perennial allergic rhinitis.

Contraindications Hypersensitivity to other corticosteroids; monotherapy in primary bacterial infections; ophthalmic use.

Route/Dosage
ADULTS: **Topical** Apply sparingly to affected areas once daily.
ADULTS AND CHILDREN (AT LEAST 12 YR): **Intranasal** 2 sprays (50 mcg/spray) in each nostril once daily (total daily dose, 200 mcg). Prophylaxis with 200 mcg/day is recommended 2 to 4 wk prior to the anticipated start of pollen season for patients with a known seasonal allergen that precipitates nasal symptoms.
CHILDREN (3 TO 11 YR): **Intranasal** 1 spray (50 mcg/spray) in each nostril once daily (total daily dose, 100 mcg).

Interactions None well documented.

Lab Test Interferences None well documented.

Adverse Reactions
DERM: Burning; itching; irritation; erythema; dryness; folliculitis; hypertrichosis; acneiform eruptions; hypopigmentation; perioral dermatitis; allergic contract dermatitis; numbness of fingers; stinging; cracking and tightening of skin; skin maceration; secondary infection; skin atrophy; striae; miliaria; telangiectasis.
EENT: Cataracts; glaucoma.
OTHER: Systemic absorption may produce reversible hypothalamic pituitary adrenal (HPA) axis suppression, manifestations of Cushing syndrome, hyperglycemia, and glycosuria.

Precautions
Pregnancy: Category C.
Lactation: May be excreted in breast milk.
Children: May be more susceptible to topical corticosteroid-induced HPA axis suppression and Cushing syndrome.
Occlusive therapy: Do not use with mometasone treatment regimens.

Overdosage: Signs and Symptoms
Hypothalamic-pituitary-adrenal suppression, Cushing syndrome.

PATIENT CARE CONSIDERATIONS

Administration/Storage
- For topical use only.
- Apply as thin film, rubbing in lightly. Washing or soaking area before application may enhance drug penetration.
- Avoid prolonged use near eyes, on face, on genital and rectal areas, and in skinfolds.
- Do not use with occlusive dressings.
- When applied in diaper area, avoid using tight-fitting diapers or plastic pants.
- Store at room temperature (59° to 86°F).

Assessment/Interventions
- Obtain patient history, including drug history and any known allergies. Note liver failure, diabetes, Cushing disease, or HPA axis suppression.
- Observe for local irritation. If redness, itching, or other skin changes occur, notify health care provider.

- Observe for signs of systemic absorption (eg, HPA axis suppression, manifestations of Cushing syndrome, hyperglycemia, glycosuria), particularly in children, in patients with liver failure and in those receiving high doses of drug.
- If systemic absorption is suspected, ensure that appropriate tests (eg, morning plasma cortisol, urinary free cortisol, ACTH stimulation) are performed.

Patient/Family Education
- Explain that product is for topical use only.
- Tell patient to not put other skin products, cosmetics, bandages, or dressings over affected area.
- Remind patient to wash hands before and after application of drug.
- Warn patient to avoid contact with eyes and prolonged use around eyes.
- Instruct patient in proper application (eg, apply sparingly once daily; washing or soaking area before application will increase effectiveness).
- Instruct patient to notify health care provider if condition worsens or if local irritation occurs.

Monoctanoin

(MAHN-ahk-tuh-NO-in)

Class Gallstone solubilizer

How Supplied
Moctanin Infusion Glyceryl-l-mono-octanoate (80% to 85%), glyceryl-l-mono-decanoate (10% to 15%), glyceryl-l-2-di-octanoate (10% to 15%), free glycerol (2.5% max)

Action
PHARMACOLOGY: Dissolves cholesterol gallstones via perfusion of common bile duct.

PHARMACOKINETICS/DYNAMICS:
Absorption: Hydrolysis products are readily absorbed from the portal vein.

Metabolism: Monoctanoin is rapidly hydrolyzed by pancreatic and other lipases to fatty acids and glycerol. Octanoic acid is metabolized to CO_2 in the liver.

Indications Solubilizing agent for cholesterol (radiolucent) gallstones retained in biliary tract after cholecystectomy, via perfusion of common bile duct, when other means of removing them have failed or cannot be undertaken.

Contraindications Impaired hepatic function, significant biliary tract infection or history of recent duodenal ulcer or jejunitis; portosystemic shunting, so that there is saturation of hepatic uptake and metabolism of material absorbed from gut lumen; acute pancreatitis; any active life-threatening problems that would be complicated by perfusion into biliary tract.

Route/Dosage
ADULTS: **Biliary/nasobiliary** 3 to 5 mL/hr continuous perfusion for 2 to 10 days.

Interactions None well documented.

Lab Test Interferences None well documented.

Adverse Reactions
CNS: Fatigue; lethargy; depression; headache.
DERM: Pruritus.
GI: Abdominal pain or discomfort; nausea; vomiting; diarrhea; loose stools; anorexia; indigestion; burning; increased fistula drainage; irritation of duodenal mucosa.
HEMA: Leukopenia.
HEPA: Increased serum amylase; bile shock.
METAB: Hypokalemia.
OTHER: Fever; chills; diaphoresis; allergic reaction.

Precautions
Pregnancy: Category C.
Lactation: Undetermined.
Children: Safety and efficacy not established.
Hepatic function impairment: Patients with impaired hepatic function may experience metabolic acidosis during drug perfusion.

Overdosage: Signs and Symptoms
Abdominal pain.

PATIENT CARE CONSIDERATIONS

Administration/Storage
- Use caution in patients with obstructive jaundice due to stones.
- Not for parenteral (IM/IV) use.
- Prepare vials by adding 13 mL of Sterile Water for Injection.
- Continuously perfuse on a 24-hr basis at a rate of 3 to 5 mL/hr. Continuous perfusion usually requires 2 to 10 days for elimination or size reduction of stones. If, after 10 days, cholangiography shows neither elimination nor reduction in size or density of stones, an endoscopy should be performed to determine advisability of additional perfusion based on friability, softness or reduction of stone density.
- Maximize benefits of therapy by administering drug at 37°C (98.6°F).
- Perfuse into biliary tract either directly via catheter inserted through T-tube or via catheter inserted through mature sinus tract through nasobiliary tube placed endoscopically.
- Place tip of catheter as close to stone as possible. Drug is effective only when in direct contact with stone.

- Store at room temperature (59° to 86°F). If stored below 59°F (15°C), drug may form semisolid, which will reliquefy on rewarming.

Assessment/Interventions
- Obtain patient history, including drug history and any known allergies. Note impaired hepatic function, significant biliary tract infection, acute pancreatitis, recent duodenal ulcer, recent jejunitis, portosystemic shunting or active life-threatening problems that would be complicated by perfusion into biliary tract.
- Ensure that LFTs are performed routinely in patients with impaired liver function.
- Monitor flow rate and pressure carefully. Irritation to GI and biliary tracts is related to perfusion pressure and rate of administration.
- Monitor for intolerable abdominal pain, nausea, diarrhea or emesis. If symptoms occur, stop perfusion for 1 hr, aspirate duct, then restart. If symptoms persist, stop perfusion for 1 hr, aspirate duct, then restart at reduced rate of 3 mL/hr. If symptoms still persist, temporarily discontinue perfusion during mealtimes.
- Observe for fever, anorexia, chills, severe right upper quadrant abdominal pain or jaundice. If the following symptoms occur, discontinue drug and notify health care provider.

Patient/Family Education
- Instruct patient to report these symptoms to health care provider: fever, chills, anorexia, severe right upper quadrant abdominal pain, jaundice, fatigue, lethargy abdominal pain or discomfort, nausea, vomiting, diarrhea, anorexia, depression or any other problem.

Montelukast Sodium
(mahn-teh-LOO-kast)

Class Leukotriene receptor antagonist

How Supplied
Singulair Tablets 10 mg, Tablets, chewable 4 mg, Tablets, chewable 5 mg

Action
PHARMACOLOGY: Blocks the effects of specific leukotrienes in the respiratory airways, thereby reducing bronchoconstriction, edema, and inflammation.

PHARMACOKINETICS/DYNAMICS:
Absorption: T_{max} is 3 to 4 hr and bioavailability is 64% for 10-mg dose. T_{max} is 2 to 2.5 hr and bioavailability is 73% for 5-mg chewable dose (63% if taken with food).

Distribution: More than 99% is protein bound and Vd is 8 to 11 L/kg. There is minimal distribution across the blood-brain barrier and displays linear kinetics (up to 50 mg).

Metabolism: Montelukast is extensively metabolized and plasma concentrations of metabolites are undetectable at steady state. Cytochrome P450 3A4 and 2C9 are involved in metabolism.

Excretion: Montelukast was recovered in feces (86%) and urine (less than 0.2%) within 5 days. Plasma clearance is approximately 45 mL/min and the mean plasma t½ is 2.7 to 5.5 hr.

Special Populations:
Hepatic Function Impairment – No dosage adjustment required. However, AUC is approximately 41% higher and t½ is prolonged to 7.4 hr.
Elderly – Plasma t½ is slightly longer. No dosage adjustment is required.

Indications Prophylaxis and chronic treatment of asthma in patients 12 mo and older; relief of symptoms of seasonal allergic rhinitis in patients 2 yr and older.

Contraindications Standard considerations.

Route/Dosage
ADULTS AND CHILDREN (AT LEAST 15 YR): PO 10 mg once daily in the evening.
CHILDREN (6 TO 14 YR): PO 5 mg chewable tablet once daily in the evening.
CHILDREN (2 TO 5 YR): PO 4 mg chewable tablet once daily in the evening.
CHILDREN (12 TO 23 MO): PO 1 packet of 4 mg granules daily in the evening.

Interactions
Phenobarbital, rifampin: Decreased montelukast levels.

Lab Test Interferences None well documented.

Adverse Reactions
CNS: Dizziness; headache.
DERM: Rash; urticaria.
EENT: Dental pain; pharyngitis; laryngitis; nasal congestion; sinusitis; otitis; cough; ear pain; sneezing.
GI: Dyspepsia; gastroenteritis; nausea; diarrhea; abdominal pain.
HEPA: Increased AST and ALT.
RESP: Bronchitis.
OTHER: Asthenia; fatigue; viral infection; influenza; pyuria; fever; leg pain; thirst.

Precautions
Pregnancy: Category B.
Lactation: Undetermined.
Children: Safety and efficacy in children less than 12 mo not established.
Acute asthma attacks: Do not use for the reversal of bronchospasm in acute asthma attacks, including status asthmaticus.

PATIENT CARE CONSIDERATIONS
Administration/Storage
- Administer in the evening.
- Store tablets at room temperature (59° to 86°F). Protect from light and moisture.

Assessment/Interventions
- Review patient history, including drug history.
- If potent cytochrome P450 enzyme inducers, such as phenobarbital, are prescribed, employ appropriate clinical monitoring.
- Review history and laboratory tests for signs of decreased severe hepatic function.
- Do not administer alone for acute attacks. This drug is for prophylaxis only. Have short-acting inhaled beta-agonists available for respiratory emergencies.
- Monitor patient appropriately.
- Monitor patient for effective prophylaxis and lessening of asthma symptoms.

Patient/Family Education
- Provide patient information pamphlet.
- Advise patient to take montelukast daily in the evening as prescribed, even when asymptomatic, as well as during periods of worsening asthma.
- Advise patient that oral montelukast tablets are not for treatment of acute asthma attack but for prophylaxis purposes.
- Advise patient to have short-acting inhaled beta-agonists available for respiratory emergencies to treat asthma exacerbations.
- Instruct patient to seek medical attention if short-acting inhaled bronchodilators are needed more often than usual or respiratory difficulties are present.
- Inform patient with phenylketonuria that the 4- and 5-mg chewable tablets contain phenylalanine.
- Instruct patient who has exacerbations of asthma after exercise to use the usual treatment of inhaled beta-agonists for prophylaxis as prescribed.
- Caution patient with known aspirin sensitivity to avoid aspirin or NSAIDs while taking montelukast.
- Instruct patient not to decrease the dose or stop taking any other anti-asthma medication unless instructed by a health care provider.

Moricizine Hydrochloride
(MAHR-IH-sizz-een HIGH-droe-KLOR-ide)

Class Antiarrhythmic agent

How Supplied
Ethmozine Tablets 200 mg, Tablets 250 mg, Tablets 300 mg

Action
PHARMACOLOGY: Moricizine is a class 1 antiarrhythmic agent with potent local anesthetic activity and myocardial membrane stabilizing effects. Moricizine reduces the fast inward current carried by sodium ions.

PHARMACOKINETICS/DYNAMICS:

Absorption: Bioavailability approximately 38% caused by first-pass metabolism. C_{max} usually reached in 0.5 to 2 hr.

Distribution: Vd is 300 L or more. Protein binding approximately 95%.

Metabolism: Moricizine induces its own metabolism. Undergoes extensive first-pass metabolism. Extensive biotransformation to at least 26 metabolites. In an animal model, 2 metabolites are active, moricizine sulfate and phenothiazine-2carbamic acid ethyl ester sulfoxide.

Excretion: Less than 1% excreted unchanged in urine. Plasma t½ is 1.5 to 3.5 hr. Approximately 56% excreted in feces and 39% in urine. Some enterohepatic recirculation occurs.

Indications
Treatment of documented life-threatening ventricular arrhythmias (eg, sustained ventricular tachycardia).

Contraindications
Preexisting second- or third-degree AV block; right bundle branch block associated with left hemiblock (bifascicular) unless a pacemaker is present; cardiogenic shock; hypersensitivity to any component of product.

Route/Dosage
ADULTS: **PO** Between 600 and 900 mg/day, given q 8 hr in 3 equally divided doses. Within this range, adjust dose in increments of 150 mg/day at 3-day intervals, until desired effect obtained. Patients exhibiting beneficial response as judged objectively (eg, Holter monitoring) can be maintained on chronic moricizine therapy. Because the antiarrhythmic effect persists for longer than 12 hr, some patients, whose arrhythmias are well controlled on an q 8 hr regimen, may be given the same total daily dose on a 12 hr regimen to increase convenience and compliance.

Hepatic/Renal Function Impairment
ADULTS: **PO** Start with 600 mg/day or less and monitor closely, including ECG interval measurements, before dosage adjustment.

Interactions
Cimetidine, diltiazem: Plasma levels of moricizine may be elevated, increasing the pharmacologic and adverse effects.

Digoxin, propranolol: Additive prolongation of PR interval.
Diltiazem, theophylline: Levels may be reduced by moricizine, decreasing the pharmacologic effects.
Warfarin: Anticoagulant effect may be increased.

Lab Test Interferences None well documented.

Adverse Reactions
CV: Palpitations (6%); cardiac chest pain, cardiac death, CHF, sustained ventricular tachycardia (2% to less than 5%); bradycardia, cardiac arrest, cerebrovascular events, hypertension, hypotension, MI, pulmonary embolism, superventricular arrhythmias, syncope, thrombophlebitis, vasodilation (less than 2%).
CNS: Headache (8%); fatigue (6%); asthenia, hypesthesia, nervousness, paresthesia, sleep disorder (2% to less than 5%); abnormal coordination and gait, agitation, akathisia, anxiety, ataxia, coma, confusion, decreased libido, depression, diplopia, dyskinesia, euphoria, hallucination, memory loss, nystagmus, seizure, somnolence, speech disorder, tremor, vertigo (less than 2%).
DERM: Sweating (2% to less than 5%); dry skin, rash, pruritus, urticaria (less than 2%).
EENT: Blurred vision, eye pain, pharyngitis, tinnitus (less than 2%).
GI: Nausea (10%); abdominal pain, diarrhea, dry mouth, dyspepsia, vomiting (2% to less than 5%); anorexia, bitter taste, dysphagia, flatulence, ileus (less than 2%).
GU: Dysuria, impotence, kidney pain, urinary incontinence, urinary retention or frequency (less than 2%).
HEMA/LYMPH: Thrombocytopenia.
HEPA: Elevated LFTs, jaundice (rare).

MUSC: Musculoskeletal pain (2% to less than 5%).
RESP: Dyspnea (6%); apnea, asthma, cough, hyperventilation, sinusitis (less than 2%).
OTHER: Drug fever, hypothermia, periorbital edema, swelling of lips and tongue, temperature intolerance (less than 2%).

> **WARNING:**
> Because of the known proarrhythmic properties of moricizine and the lack of evidence of improved survival for any antiarrhythmic agent in patients without life-threatening arrhythmias, it is prudent to reserve the use of moricizine for patients with life-threatening ventricular arrhythmias.

Precautions
Pregnancy: Category B.
Lactation: Excreted in breast milk.
Children: Safety and efficacy not established.
Electrolyte disturbances: Because may alter the effects of class 1 antiarrhythmic agents, correct electrolyte imbalance before administration.
Hepatic/Renal impairment: Use with caution and start with lower doses.
Proarrhythmic effect: Can provoke new rhythm disturbances or make existing arrhythmias worse.
Sick sinus syndrome: Because moricizine may cause sinus bradycardia, sinus pause, or sinus arrest, use with caution.
Survival: Has not been proven to favorably affect survival or incidence of sudden death.

Overdosage: Signs and Symptoms
Emesis, lethargy, coma, syncope, hypotension, conduction disturbances, exacerbation of CHF, MI, sinus arrest, arrhythmias, respiratory failure, death.

PATIENT CARE CONSIDERATIONS
Administration/Storage
- May be used alone or in combination with other antiarrhythmic medications.
- Therapy for life-threatening arrhythmias should be initiated in-hospital with close monitoring of cardiac rhythm.
- Administer dose q 8 or 12 hr as prescribed.
- Administer without regard to meals but administer with food if GI upset occurs.
- Do not increase dose by more than 150 mg/day q 3 days during dosage titration.
- When converting from other antiarrhythmic agents to moricizine, withdraw previous antiarrhythmic therapy for 1 to 2 plasma half-lives before starting moricizine.
- Store tablets at controlled room temperature (59° to 86°F). Protect from light.

Assessment/Interventions
- Obtain patient history, including drug history and any known allergies. Note renal or hepatic impairment, sick sinus syndrome, sinus node dysfunction, intraventricular conduction abnormalities, hypotension, or CHF.
- Review patient's health history and current situation for any condition that would contraindicate moricizine therapy: hypersensitivity to moricizine; preexisting second- or third-degree AV block unless pacemaker is present; cardiogenic shock.
- Ensure that lower starting dose and close monitoring, including measurement of ECG intervals before dosage adjustment, are used in patient with renal or hepatic impairment.
- Ensure that preexisting electrolyte disorders have been corrected before initiating therapy.

- Review baseline ECG. Monitor cardiac rhythm while initiating therapy or when adjusting dose. Notify health care provider immediately of any significant changes.
- Monitor and record BP and pulse frequently during treatment. Notify health care provider of any significant changes.
- Ensure that pacing threshold is determined before starting therapy, and periodically thereafter, in patient with pacemaker.
- Carefully monitor patient with preexisting heart failure for worsening heart failure when therapy with moricizine is initiated. Notify health care provider if symptoms or signs of worsening heart failure are noted or suspected.
- Monitor patient for GI, CNS, CV, and general body side effects. Inform health care provider if noted and significant.

Patient/Family Education

- Explain name, dose, action, and potential side effects of drug.
- Advise patient that dose of medication may be changed periodically to obtain maximum benefit.
- Caution patient to take prescribed dose q 8 or 12 hr exactly as ordered. Advise patient that serious heart disturbances can result from missing doses or taking more often than prescribed.
- Advise patient to take each dose without regard to meals but to take with food if stomach upset occurs.
- Caution patient not to change the dose or stop taking unless advised by health care provider. Advise patient that serious side effects can result from increasing or decreasing the dose without medical supervision
- Inform patient that drug controls, but does not cure, abnormal heart rhythm and to continue taking as prescribed once the heart rhythm has been controlled.
- Instruct patient to continue taking other heart medications as prescribed by health care provider.
- Instruct patient in BP and pulse measurement skills.
- Advise patient to monitor and record BP and pulse at home and to inform health care provider if abnormal measurements are noted. Also advise patient to take record of BP and pulse to each follow-up visit.
- Instruct patient to lie or sit down if experiencing dizziness or lightheadedness when standing.
- Advise patient to notify health care provider if any of the following occur: frequent episodes of dizziness or lightheadedness, persistent nausea, any other unusual or unexplained symptom.
- Instruct patient to immediately report fainting, pounding in chest, change in pulse or heart rhythm, or unexplained fever to health care provider.
- Caution patient that drug may cause dizziness or lightheadedness and to use caution while driving or performing other tasks requiring mental alertness or coordination until tolerance is determined.
- Advise women to notify health care provider if pregnant, planning to become pregnant, or breastfeeding.
- Advise patient to carry medical identification (eg, *Medi-Alert*) describing cardiac condition and medication regimen.
- Caution patient not to take any prescription or OTC medications, herbal preparations, or dietary supplements unless advised by health care provider.
- Offer family instruction in basic life support.
- Advise patient that follow-up visits and lab tests will be required to monitor therapy and to keep appointments.

Morphine Sulfate

(moRE-feen SULL-fate)

Class Narcotic analgesic

How Supplied

Astramorph PF Injection 0.5 mg/mL, Injection 1 mg/mL ♦ *Duramorph* Injection 0.5 mg/mL, Injection 1 mg/mL ♦ *Infumorph* Injection 10 mg/mL, Injection 25 mg/mL ♦ *Kadian* Capsules, sustained-release 20 mg, Capsules, sustained-release 50 mg, Capsules, sustained-release 100 mg ♦ *MS Contin* Tablets, controlled-release 15 mg, Tablets, controlled-release 30 mg, Tablets, controlled-release 60 mg, Tablets, controlled-release 100 mg, Tablets, controlled-release 200 mg ♦ *MSIR* Tablets 15 mg, Tablets 30 mg, Capsules 15 mg, Capsules 30 mg, Solution 10 mg/5 mL, Solution 20 mg/5 mL, Solution 20 mg/mL ♦ *Oramorph SR* Tablets, controlled-release 15 mg, Tablets, controlled-release 30 mg, Tablets, controlled-release 60 mg, Tablets, controlled-release 100 mg ♦ *OMS Concentrate* Solution 20 mg/mL ♦ *RMS* Rectal Suppositories 5 mg, Rectal Suppositories 10 mg, Rectal Suppositories 20 mg, Rectal Suppositories 30 mg ♦ *Roxanol* Solution 20 mg/mL ♦ *Roxanol Rescudose* Solution 10 mg/2.5 mL ♦ *Roxanol 100* Solution 100 mg/5 mL ♦ *Roxanol T* Solution 20 mg/mL ♦ *Roxanol UD* Solution 10 mg/ 2.5 mL, Solution 20 mg/ 5 mL, Solution 30 mg/ 1.5 mL

♦ M-Eslon ♦ Morphine HP ♦ M.O.S.-Sulfate ♦ ratio-Morphine SR ♦ Statex

Action

PHARMACOLOGY: Relieves pain by stimulating opiate receptors in CNS; also causes respiratory depression, peripheral vasodilation, inhibition of intestinal peristalsis, sphincter of Oddi spasm, stimulation of chemoreceptors that cause vomiting and increased bladder tone.

PHARMACOKINETICS/DYNAMICS:
Absorption: Mean T_{max} is 3.7 hr and mean C_{max} is 9.9 to 27.4 ng/mL (dose dependent) for sustained-release form. Bioavailability is approximately 40%.

Distribution: Morphine distributes to skeletal muscle, kidneys, liver, intestinal tract, lungs, spleen, and brain; crosses the placental membrane and is found in breast milk.

Metabolism: Virtually all converted into glucuronide metabolites; small fraction is demethylated in the liver. Major metabolite is morphine-3–glucuronide (55% to 75%).

Excretion: The t½ is approximately 2 to 4 hr.

Onset: Onset is 15 to 60 min (intrathecal/epidural).

Duration: Duration is 3 to 7 hr.

Indications Relief of moderate to severe acute and chronic pain; relief of pain in patients who require opioid analgesics for more than a few days (sustained-release only); management of pain not responsive to nonnarcotic analgesics; dyspnea associated with acute left ventricular failure and pulmonary edema; preoperative sedation; adjunct to anesthesia; analgesia during labor.

Contraindications Hypersensitivity to opiates; upper airway obstruction; acute asthma; diarrhea caused by poisoning or toxins.
Injection: Heart failure secondary to chronic lung disease; cardiac arrhythmias; brain tumor; acute alcoholism; delirium tremens; idiosyncrasy to the drug; convulsive states (eg, status epilepticus, tetanus, strychnine poisoning).
Immediate-release oral solution: Respiratory insufficiency; severe CNS depression; heart failure secondary to chronic lung disease; cardiac arrhythmias; increased intracranial or cerebrospinal pressure; head injuries; brain tumor; acute alcoholism; delirium tremens; convulsive disorders; after biliary tract surgery; suspected surgical abdomen; surgical anastomosis; idiosyncrasy to the drug; concomitantly with MAO inhibitors or within 14 days of such treatment.
Intrathecal/epidural: Infection at injection site; anticoagulation; bleeding condition; parenteral corticosteroids within past 2 wk; any other drug or condition that would contraindicate intrathecal/epidural therapy.

Route/Dosage

ADULTS: **PO** 10 to 30 mg q 4 hr prn. **SC/IM** 5 to 20 mg/70 kg q 4 hr prn. **IV** 2.5 to 15 mg/70 kg in 4 to 5 mL Water for Injection over 5 min prn. **IV (open-heart surgery)** 0.5 to 3 mg/kg. **IV (MI pain)** 8 to 15 mg; for very severe pain, additional smaller doses may be given q 3 to 4 hr. **PR** 10 to 20 mg q 4 hr prn. **Epidural** Initial injection of 5 mg may provide pain relief for up to 24 hr; if pain is not controlled within 1 hr, give incremental doses of 1 to 2 mg. Do not exceed 10 mg/24 hr. **Intrathecal** Usual dose is 10% of epidural dose. Single injection of 0.2 to 1 mg may provide pain relief for 24 hr. Do not inject more than 2 mL of 5 mg/10 mL ampul or 1 mL of 10 mg/10 mL ampul. Repeat injections not recommended.
CHILDREN: **SC/IM** 0.1 to 0.2 mg/kg q 4 hr. Max dose: 15 mg.

Interactions

Acyclovir, barbiturates, furosemides, heparin, sargramostim, sodium bicarbonate: Precipitation of IV solutions.
Antihistamines, chloral hydrate, glutethimide, methocarbamol: Depressant effects of morphine may be enhanced.
Cimetidine: Monitor for increased respiratory and CNS depression. Concomitant administration of cimetidine and morphine has been reported to precipitate apnea, confusion, and muscle twitching in an isolated report.
Clomipramine, nortriptyline, amitriptyline: Monitor for increased CNS and respiratory depression when administered with morphine.
CNS depressants (eg, alcohol, sedatives, tranquilizers): Additive CNS depression.

Lab Test Interferences Increased amylase and lipase may occur up to 24 hr after dose.

Adverse Reactions

CV: Hypotension; orthostatic hypotension; bradycardia; tachycardia; palpitations.
CNS: Lightheadedness; dizziness; drowsiness; sedation; euphoria; dysphoria; delirium; disorientation; incoordination.
DERM: Sweating; pruritus; urticaria.
EENT: Blurred vision; miosis.
GI: Nausea; vomiting; constipation; abdominal pain.
GU: Urinary retention or hesitancy.
RESP: Respiratory depression; apnea; respiratory arrest; laryngospasm; depression of cough reflex.
OTHER: Tolerance; psychological and physical dependence with chronic use; pain at injection site; local irritation and induration following SC use.

> **WARNING:**
> Monitor patient for at least 24 hr after initial dose because of reports of severe adverse reactions with epidural/intrathecal use. Improper substitution of *Infumorph* for regular *Duramorph* may result in serious overdose.

Precautions

Pregnancy: Category C.
Lactation: Excreted in breast milk.
Children: Safety not established in children.
Elderly: Dosage reduction may be necessary.
Labor and delivery: Therapeutic morphine doses have increased duration of labor.
Renal function impairment: May need to reduce dose.
Hepatic function impairment: May need to reduce dose.
Special risk patients: Use drug with caution in patients with myxedema, acute alcoholism, acute abdominal conditions, ulcerative colitis, decreased respiratory reserve, head injury or increased intracranial pressure, hypoxia, supraventricular tachycardia, depleted blood volume or circulatory shock.
Asthma and other respiratory conditions: Bisulfites and morphine may potentiate each other, preventing use by cause severe adverse reactions.
Drug dependence: Has abuse potential.

Overdosage: Signs and Symptoms

Miosis, respiratory and CNS depression, circulatory collapse, seizures, cardiopulmonary arrest, death.

PATIENT CARE CONSIDERATIONS

Administration/Storage

- Administer medication as soon as pain occurs. Effect is reduced as pain increases.
- Give oral form with food to decrease GI upset.
- Administer antiemetic for nausea and vomiting, if ordered.
- Controlled-release tablets should not be chewed or crushed.
- Prepare IV solution by diluting in 4 to 5 mL of Water for Injection. Administer over 4 to 5 min.
- For continuous IV infusion, add drug to prepare solution of 0.1 to 1 mg/mL in D5W. Control infusion with electronic infusion device.
- Do not administer IV solution if cloudy, precipitate is present or antidote is not readily available.
- Intrathecal and epidural injection should be administered only in lumbar region.
- To reduce chance of adverse effects with intrathecal administration, constant IV infusion of naloxone (0.6 mg/hr for 24 hr after intrathecal injection) is recommended.
- Subcutaneous injection can irritate tissues; use IM injection for repeated doses.
- Store at room temperature (59° to 86°F).

Assessment/Interventions

- Obtain patient history, including drug history and any known allergies.
- Assess type, location and intensity of pain before and 30 to 60 min after administration.
- Assess vital signs before and periodically during therapy.
- Assess bowel and bladder function regularly in patients receiving repeated doses.
- Assist patient with ambulation. Keep siderails up and call bell within reach.
- Evaluate therapeutic response. Prolonged use may lead to physical dependence and tolerance. Progressively higher doses may be necessary to control pain in patients receiving long-term therapy.
- With continuous infusion, titrate dose to ensure adequate pain relief without excessive sedation, respiratory depression or hypotension.
- Monitor for CNS changes: dizziness, drowsiness, hallucinations, euphoria, level of consciousness, pupil reaction.

Patient/Family Education

- Instruct patient to take oral preparations with food or juice if GI upset occurs.
- Tell patient not to crush or chew controlled-release tablets.
- Explain that full effectiveness of drug may not occur for 30 to 60 min after administration. Emphasize that drug is more effective if taken regularly to prevent pain rather than to treat pain after it occurs.
- If patient is to receive patient-controlled analgesia (PCA), instruct on use of PCA pump.
- Explain that physical dependency may occur with long-term therapy and that dosage will be tapered slowly before stopping to prevent withdrawal symptoms (nausea, vomiting, cramps, fever, faintness, anorexia).
- Encourage patient to turn, cough and breathe deeply q 2 hr to prevent atelectasis.
- Advise patient to consult with health care provider if excessive sedation occurs or if pain relief is inadequate.

- Inform patient that drug may cause constipation. Stool softener, fiber laxative, increased fluid intake and bulk in diet may help alleviate problem.
- Caution patient to avoid sudden position changes to prevent orthostatic hypotension.
- Instruct patient to avoid intake of alcoholic beverages and other CNS depressants.
- Advise patient that drug may cause drowsiness, dizziness or blurred vision and to use caution while driving or performing other tasks requiring mental alertness.
- Instruct patient not to take OTC medications without consulting health care provider.

Moxifloxacin Hydrochloride

(mox-ih-FLOX-ah-sin HIGH-droe-KLOR-ide)

Class Antibiotic/Fluoroquinolone

How Supplied
Avelox Tablets 400 mg ♦ Avelox IV Injection (premix) 400 mg ♦ Vigamox Solution, ophthalmic 0.5% (5 mg/mL)

Action
PHARMACOLOGY: Interferes with microbial DNA synthesis.

PHARMACOKINETICS/DYNAMICS:

Absorption: Bioavailability is approximately 90%; AUC is approximately 48 mcg•hr/mL, mean C_{max} is 4.5 mcg/mL (multiple 400 mg oral dose).

Distribution: Protein binding is approximately 50%; Vd is 1.7 to 2.7 L/kg.

Metabolism: Metabolized via glucuronide (approximately 14%) and sulfate (approximately 38%) conjugation in the liver.

Excretion: Moxifloxacin is eliminated in urine (approximately 20% unchanged) and feces (approximately 25%); sulfate conjugate is excreted in feces and glucuronide conjugate is excreted in urine. The t½ is approximately 12 hr; mean apparent total Cl is approximately 12 L/hr; renal Cl is approximately 2.6 L/hr.

Indications Treatment of acute bacterial sinusitis, acute bacterial exacerbation of chronic bronchitis, community-acquired pneumonia, uncomplicated skin and skin structure infections, and conjunctivitis caused by susceptible organisms.

Contraindications Standard considerations.

Route/Dosage

Acute Bacterial Exacerbation of Chronic Bronchitis
ADULTS: IV/PO 400 mg/day for 5 days.

Acute Bacterial Sinusitis
ADULTS: IV/PO 400 mg/day for 10 days.

Community-Acquired Pneumonia
ADULTS: IV/PO 400 mg/day for 7 to 14 days.

Conjunctivitis
ADULTS AND CHILDREN AT LEAST 1 YR: **Ophthalmic** Instill 1 drop in affected eye(s) tid for 7 days.

Uncomplicated Skin and Skin Structure Infections
ADULTS: IV/PO 400 mg/day for 7 days.

Interactions
Antacids containing aluminum, calcium, or magnesium; drug formulations containing divalent or trivalent cations (eg, some didanosine formulations); metal cations (eg, iron); multivitamins containing iron or zinc; sucralfate: May decrease the absorption of moxifloxacin.

Cisapride; class IA antiarrhythmic agents (eg, procainamide, quinidine); class III antiarrhythmic agents (eg, amiodarone, sotalol); erythromycin; pentamidine; phenothiazines; tricyclic antidepressants; any other drug known to prolong the QTc interval: Increased risk of torsades de pointes or other ventricular arrhythmias.

Lab Test Interferences None well documented.

Adverse Reactions
CV: Palpitation, tachycardia, hypertension, peripheral edema, QT interval prolongation (less than 3%); ventricular tachyarrhythmias (postmarketing).
CNS: Dizziness (3%); headache, insomnia, nervousness, anxiety, confusion, somnolence, tremor, vertigo, paresthesia (less than 3%); psychotic reaction (postmarketing).
DERM: Injection-site reaction, rash (maculopapular, purpuric, pustular), pruritus, sweating (less than 3%); Stevens-Johnson syndrome (postmarketing).
GI: Nausea (7%); diarrhea (6%); vomiting, abnormal LFT, dyspepsia, dry mouth, constipation, oral moniliasis, anorexia, stomatitis, glossitis, flatulence, GI disorder, taste perversion (less than 3%); pseudomembranous colitis (postmarketing).
GU: Vaginal moniliasis, vaginitis (less than 3%).
HEPA: Hepatitis (postmarketing).
HEMA/LYMPH: Prothrombin decrease (PT/INR increased), thrombocythemia, thrombocytopenia, eosinophilia, leukopenia (less than 3%).
M/N: Amylase increased, lactic acid dehydrogenase increased (less than 3%).
MUSC: Arthralgia, myalgia (less than 3%); tendon rupture (postmarketing).
RESP: Dyspnea (less than 3%); syncope (postmarketing).

OTHER: Abdominal pain, asthenia, moniliasis, pain, malaise, allergic reaction, leg pain, back pain, chest pain (less than 3%); angioedema (including laryngeal edema), anaphylactic reaction, anaphylactic shock (postmarketing).

Precautions

Pregnancy: Category C.
Lactation: Undetermined; however, other fluoroquinolones have been shown to be excreted in breast milk.
Children:
PO/IV – Safety and efficacy not established.
Ophthalmic – Safety and efficacy in children under 1 yr not established.
Hypersensitivity: Acute anaphylactic reactions and serious dermatological hypersensitivity reactions reported.
Superinfection: Use of antibiotics may result in bacterial or fungal overgrowth.

Convulsions and toxic psychosis: CNS stimulation, lowering of the seizure threshold, and psychotic reactions have been reported with similar agents. Use with caution in patients with seizures or other CNS disorders.
Pseudomembranous colitis: Consider possibility in patients with diarrhea.
QT interval: QT interval may be prolonged in some patients; avoid use in patients with known prolongation of QT interval or uncorrected hypokalemia and patients receiving class IA or III antiarrhythmics.
Tendonitis: Inflammation and rupture of tendons may occur. The risk may be increased in patients receiving corticosteroids, especially in the elderly.

Overdosage: Signs and Symptoms

Possible QTc prolongation, somnolence, tremor, convulsions.

PATIENT CARE CONSIDERATIONS

Administration/Storage

- No dosage adjustment is necessary when switching from IV to oral therapy.

Tablets:

- Administer tablets with a full glass of water without regard to meals. Administer with food if GI upset occurs.
- Administer moxifloxacin 4 hr before or 8 hr after sucralfate, antacids containing magnesium or aluminum, didanosine-buffered tablets or pediatric powder, or other products containing iron or zinc.
- Store tablets at controlled room temperature (59° to 86°F). Avoid high humidity.

Ophthalmic Solution:

- Instill 1 drop tid.
- If using other topical ophthalmic drugs, separate each medication by at least 5 min.
- Store in refrigerator (36° to 46°F) or at controlled room temperature (47° to 77°F). Keep container tightly closed.

Injection:

- For IV infusion only. Not for intradermal, intrathecal, intraperitoneal, SC, or IM administration.
- Inspect solution visually before administration. Do not administer if solution is cloudy, discolored, or contains particulate matter.
- Infuse prescribed dose over 60 min by direct infusion or through a Y-type infusion set. Avoid rapid or bolus administration because of risk of prolonging QT interval.
- Do not add other medications or additives to moxifloxacin injection bag.
- If other drugs are being administered through the same IV line, administer each medication separately and flush IV line with compatible solution before and after infusion of moxifloxacin.
- Premixed flexible containers are for single use only; discard any unused solution.
- Store flexible injection bags at controlled room temperature (59° to 86°F). Do not refrigerate.

Assessment/Interventions

- Obtain patient history, including drug history and any known allergies. Note prolongation of QT interval, hypokalemia, bradycardia, ischemic heart disease, epilepsy, predisposition to convulsions, cerebral arteriosclerosis, allergy to quinolone antibiotics, or concurrent use of class IA antiarrhythmics (eg, quinidine), class III antiarrhythmics (eg, amiodarone), or other medications known to cause QT prolongation (eg, erythromycin).
- Review results of culture and sensitivity testing as available.
- Monitor for signs of infection, especially fever, and for positive response to antibiotic therapy.
- Monitor patient for signs of allergic reaction. Discontinue therapy and immediately notify health care provider if noted. Be prepared to treat appropriately.
- Monitor patient for evidence of CNS stimulation or psychiatric changes (eg, dizziness, tremors, depression, restlessness, lightheadedness, confusion, hallucinations, agitation, anxiety, sleep disturbance). Inform health care provider if noted and be prepared to discontinue therapy.
- Monitor patient for GI, CV, DERM, and general body side effects. Report to health care provider if noted and significant.

Ophthalmic Solution:
* Monitor patient's response to therapy. Notify health care provider if eye or eyelid inflammation is noted or if symptoms do not improve or worsen.

Patient/Family Education
* Explain name, dose, action, and potential side effects of drug.
* Advise patient to read *Patient Information* leaflet before starting therapy and with each refill.
* Review dosing schedule and prescribed length of therapy with patient.

Tablets:
* Advise patient that medication can be taken with a full glass of water without regard to meals but to take with food if GI upset occurs.
* Advise patient that if a dose is missed to take as soon as remembered. However, if it is nearing the time for the next dose, to skip the dose and take the next dose at the regularly scheduled time.
* Advise patient to take moxifloxacin 4 hr before or 8 hr after sucralfate, antacids containing magnesium or aluminum, didanosine-buffered tablets or pediatric powder, or other products containing iron or zinc.
* Remind patient to complete entire course of therapy, even if symptoms of infection have disappeared.
* Advise patient to inform health care provider if infection does improve or worsens.
* Advise patient to discontinue therapy and contact health care provider immediately if skin rash, hives, itching, shortness of breath, palpitations, fainting, pain, tenderness, or rupture of tendon occur.
* Advise patient to report the following signs of superinfection to health care provider: black furry tongue, white patches in mouth, foul-smelling stools, vaginal itching or discharge.
* Warn patient that diarrhea containing blood or pus may be a sign of a serious disorder and to seek medical care if noted and not to treat at home.
* Caution patient that drug may cause dizziness and lightheadedness and to use caution while driving or performing other tasks requiring mental alertness until tolerance is determined.
* Advise patient to avoid unnecessary exposure to direct and indirect sunlight or tanning lamps and to use sunscreen and wear protective clothing to avoid photosensitivity reactions during therapy. Advise patient to discontinue therapy and notify health care provider if any of the following occur after exposure to sunlight or artificial UV light (eg, sunlamp): sensation of skin burning, redness, swelling, blistering, rash or itching.
* Advise women to notify health care provider if pregnant, planning to become pregnant, or breastfeeding.
* Instruct patient not to take any prescription or OTC medications or dietary supplements unless advised by health care provider.
* Advise patient that follow-up examinations may be required to monitor therapy and to keep appointments.

Ophthalmic Solution:
* Review prescribed dosing schedule with patient.
* Teach patient proper technique for instilling eye drops: wash hands; do not allow dropper to touch eye. Tilt head back, look up; pull lower eyelid down; instill prescribed number of drops. Close eye for 1 to 2 min and apply gentle pressure to bridge of nose for 3 to 5 min. Do not rub eye.
* Advise patient that if more than 1 topical ophthalmic drug is being used, administer the drugs at least 5 min apart.
* Inform patient that temporary blurred vision, eye itching, eye pain, or discomfort are the most common side effects and to contact health care provider if they occur and are bothersome.
* Advise patient to contact eye doctor if eye or eyelid inflammation is noted or if eye symptoms do not improve or worsen.
* Advise patient that the entire course of therapy must be completed to ensure maximal benefit and to complete full course of therapy even if symptoms have resolved.
* Instruct patient not to wear contact lenses during treatment.

Injection:
* Advise patient that medication will be prepared and administered by a health care professional in a health care setting when oral therapy is not feasible but that the patient will be switched to oral therapy when health care provider believes it is appropriate.

Mupirocin (Pseudomonic Acid A)

(myoo-PIHR-oh-sin)
Class Topical/Anti-infective

How Supplied
Bactroban Ointment 2%, Cream 2% ♦ Bactroban Nasal Ointment 2%

Action
PHARMACOLOGY: Inhibits bacterial protein synthesis.

PHARMACOKINETICS/DYNAMICS:
Absorption:
Cream – Systemic absorption of mupirocin through human intact skin is minimal by detection of the metabolite, monic acid, in urine. More frequent occurrence of percutaneous absorption in children (90%) was found compared with adults (44%). Mupirocin is highly protein bound (more than 97%).
Ointment – Measurable systemic absorption.
Nasal – No evidence of systemic absorption.

Metabolism: Any mupirocin reaching the systemic circulation is rapidly metabolized, predominantly to inactive monic acid, which is eliminated by renal excretion. The elimination t½ after IV administration was 20 to 40 min for mupirocin and 30 to 80 min for monic acid.

Indications Treatment of impetigo caused by *Staphylococcus aureus* and *Streptococcus pyogenes* (topical ointment); treatment of secondarily infected traumatic skin lesions (up to 10 cm in length or 100 cm² in area) caused by susceptible strains of *S. aureus* and *S. pyogenes* (topical cream); eradication of nasal colonization with methicillin-resistant *S. aureus* in adult patients and health care workers (nasal).

Contraindications Standard considerations.

Route/Dosage
ADULTS AND CHILDREN: **Topical ointment** Apply small amount to affected area tid. Reevaluate lesions not showing a response in 3 to 5 days. **Topical cream** Apply small amount to affected area tid for 10 days. Reevaluate lesions not showing a response in 3 to 5 days.

ADULTS AND CHILDREN 12 YR AND OLDER:
Nasal Divide approximately one-half of the ointment from a single-use tube between the nostrils and apply morning and evening for 5 days.

Interactions None well documented.

Lab Test Interferences None well documented.

Adverse Reactions
CNS:
Topical – Headache (2%).
Nasal – Headache (9%).
DERM:
Topical – Burning, stinging, pain, pruritus (2%); itching (1%); secondarily infected eczema.
Nasal – Burning, stinging (2%); pruritus (1%).
EENT:
Nasal – Rhinitis (6%); pharyngitis (4%); taste perversion (3%); burning, stinging cough (2%).
GI:
Topical – Nausea (5%) (secondary infected eczema).
RESP:
Nasal – Respiratory disorder (5%); cough (2%).

Precautions
Pregnancy: Category B.
Lactation: Undetermined.
Children:
Ointment and cream – Safety and efficacy have been established in children 2 mo to 16 yr (ointment) and in children 3 mo to 16 yr (cream).
Nasal – Safety and efficacy not established in children under 12 yr.
Hypersensitivity: Chemical irritation may occur.
Superinfection: Prolonged use of antibiotics may result in overgrowth of nonsusceptible organisms, including fungi.
Open wounds (ointment only): Because polyethylene glycol can be absorbed from open wounds and damaged skin and is excreted by the kidneys, do not use if absorption of large quantities is possible, especially if evidence of moderate or severe renal impairment.
Prophylaxis: Insufficient data to recommend use of mupirocin nasal for general prophylaxis of any infection.

PATIENT CARE CONSIDERATIONS

Administration/Storage
- Apply topically only; avoid contact with eyes and mucous membranes. Treated area may be covered with gauze dressing.
- Wash hands before and after application.

Assessment/Interventions
- Obtain patient history, including drug history and any known allergies.
- Assess for signs of superinfection (bacterial or fungal overgrowth of nonsusceptible organisms).
- Assess for therapeutic response (decrease in size and number of lesions).
- If a skin reaction develops, discontinue therapy, wash affected area, and notify health care provider.

Patient/Family Education
- Warn the patient to avoid contact of drug with eyes and mucous membranes.
- Instruct patient to wash hands before and after application.
- Tell patient to inform health care provider if no improvement is seen within 3 to 5 days or if condition worsens.
- Advise patient to keep fingernails well trimmed to prevent scratching.
- Review with patient and family appropriate hygiene measures to prevent spread of impetigo.
- Instruct patient to report the following symptoms to health care provider: burning, stinging, pain, nausea, tenderness, swelling, rash, dry skin, increased exudate.

Muromonab-CD3
(MYOO-row-MOE-nab-CD3)

Class Murine monoclonal antibody

How Supplied
Orthoclone OKT3 Injection 5 mg per 5 mL

Action
PHARMACOLOGY: Blocks T-cell function, which plays major role in graft rejection, by reacting with and blocking T3 (CD3) molecule on membrane of human T cells associated with antigen recognition. Serum levels are measured with an enzyme-linked immunosorbent assay (ELISA).

PHARMACOKINETICS/DYNAMICS:

Absorption: Time to steady-state trough levels is 3 days and C_{min} is 0.9 mcg/mL with 5 mg/day (steady-state).

Onset: Onset within minutes.

Duration: Duration is approximately 1 wk.

Indications
Treatment of renal, steroid resistant cardiac, or hepatic allograft rejection.

Contraindications
Hypersensitivity to any product of murine origin; anti-mouse antibody titers at least 1:1,000; fluid overload or uncompensated heart failure; seizures or predisposition to seizures; pregnancy; breastfeeding; uncontrolled hypertension.

Route/Dosage
ADULTS: **IV** 5 mg/day as bolus given over less than 1 min for 10 to 14 days.

PEDIATRIC: **IV** 2.5 mg/day in patients weighing 30 kg or less, and 5 mg/day in patients over 30 kg. As a single bolus given over less than 1 min for 10 to 14 days. Daily increases in doses (ie, 2.5 mg increments) may be required.

Interactions
Immunosuppressants (eg, azathioprine, corticosteroids, cyclosporine): Psychosis, infections, malignancies, seizures, encephalopathy, and thrombotic events have occurred with immunosuppressants alone and in conjunction with muromonab-CD3.

Indomethacin: May increase risk of encephalopathy and other CNS effects.

Lab Test Interferences None well documented.

Adverse Reactions
CV: CV collapse; angina; MI; chest pain/tightness; bradycardia; tachycardia; hypertension; profound hypotension including shock, heart failure, pulmonary edema, arrhythmias; intravascular thrombosis; cerebrovascular accidents; transient ischemic attacks; hemodynamic instability, left ventricular dysfunction (postmarketing).

CNS: Headache; tremor; dizziness; confusion; agitation; auditory and visual hallucinations; obtundation; mood changes; hypotonus; encephalopathy; cerebral edema; aseptic meningitis; encephalitis; aphasia; quadri- or paraparesis; hemiparesis; subarachnoid hemorrhage; vertigo; sixth cranial nerve palsy; hyperreflexia; myoclonus; hypotonus; asterixis; involuntary movements; tremor; cerebritis, cerebral herniation, cerebrovascular accident, CNS infection, CNS malignancy, intracranial hemorrhage, impaired cognition, status epilepticus, stupor, transient ischemic attack (postmarketing).

DERM: Rash; urticaria; pruritus; erythema; flushing; diaphoresis; Stevens-Johnson syndrome (postmarketing).

GI: Anorexia; bowel infarction; elevated LFTs; hepatomegaly; splenomegaly or hepatitis.

GU: Anuria; oliguria; delayed renal graft function; transient and reversible increases in blood urea nitrogen and serum creatinine; abnormal urinary cytology (eg, exfoliation of damaged lymphocytes and cellular casts); azotemia (postmarketing).

HEMA: Pancytopenia; aplastic anemia; neutropenia; leukopenia; thrombocytopenia; lymphopenia; leukocytosis; lymphadenopathy; disturbances of coagulation; arterial venous and capillary thrombosis of allografts and other vascular beds (eg, bowel, brain, heart, lung); disseminated intravascular coagulation, microangiopathic changes (eg, platelet microthrombi), microangiopathic hemolytic anemia (postmarketing).

HYPERSEN: Anaphylactic reaction, usually occurring with 10 min of administration; angioedema; reduced efficacy of treatment; serum sickness; arthritis; allergic interstitial nephritis; immune complex deposition resulting in glomerulonephritis, vasculitis (including temporal and retinal) and eosinophilia.

MUSC: Arthralgia; arthritis; myalgia; stiffness.

RESP: Dyspnea; shortness of breath; tachypnea; bronchospasm; respiratory arrest; adult respiratory distress syndrome; hypoxemia; apnea can occur during Cytokine Release Syndrome (CRS); nasal stuffiness.

SPEC SENSE: Blindness; blurred vision; diplopia; photophobia; conjunctivitis; hearing loss; otitis media; tinnitus; ear stuffiness.

OTHER: Lymphoproliferative disorders including lymphomas; patients who receive more than 1 course may have an increased risk of malignancy; infections; immunosuppression; fever, chills, rigors, headache, tremor, nausea, vomiting, diarrhea, abdominal pain, malaise, muscle aches, joint aches, generalized weakness, most frequently develops within 30 to 60 min of administering the first 2 to 3 doses (CRS); flu-like syndrome (postmarketing).

> **WARNING:**
> Anaphylactic and anaphylactoid reactions may occur following administration of any dose or course. CRS has been reported.
>
> *Cardiotoxicity, CNS and systemic reactions:* Potentially life-threatening reactions including pulmonary edema, shock, CV collapse, cardiac/respiratory arrest, seizures, coma, cerebral edema, cerebral herniation, blindness, and paralysis have been reported.
>
> *Monitoring recommendations:* Carefully monitor fluid status at baseline and during therapy. Consider pretreatment with methylprednisolone to minimize CRS.

Precautions

Pregnancy: Category C.

Lactation: Undetermined.

Children: Safety and effectiveness have been established in infants (1 mo to 2 yr of age); children (2 yr to 12 yr of age); and adolescents (12 yr to 16 yr of age).

Aseptic meningitis syndrome: The incidence of aseptic meningitis syndrome was 6%. Fever (89%), headache (44%), meningismus (14%), and photophobia (10%) were the most common symptoms. Approximately ⅓ with this diagnosis had coexisting signs and symptoms of encephalopathy.

Cerebral edema: Signs of increased vascular permeability (eg, otitis media, nasal and ear stuffiness).

CRS: Temporally associated with administration of first few doses of drug and linked to release of cytokines. Reactions range from mild flu-like illness to more rare and serious shock-like CV and CNS manifestations. Common reactions include high, spiking fever; chills; rigors; headache; tremor; nausea; vomiting; diarrhea; abdominal pain; malaise; muscle and joint aches; weakness. Cardiorespiratory findings include dyspnea; shortness of breath; bronchospasm; tachypnea; respiratory arrest; CV collapse; cardiac arrest; angina; MI; chest pain; tachycardia; hypertension; hemodynamic instability; hypotension; adult respiratory distress syndrome; pulmonary edema; hypoxemia; apnea; arrhythmias. Decreased urine output may occur.

Encephalopathy: May include impaired cognition, confusion, altered mental status, psychosis, mood changes, hyperreflexia, monoclonus, tremor, asterixis, major motor seizures, lethargy, auditory/visual hallucinations.

Fluid status: Assess patient's fluid status prior to administration. No clinical evidence of volume overload or uncompensated heart failure, including a clear chest x-ray and weight restriction of 3% or less above the patient's minimum weight during the week prior to injection.

Headache: Headache is frequently seen after first few doses.

Immunosuppression: Increases risk, severity, and morbidity from infectious complications.

Intravascular thrombosis: Arterial or venous thromboses of allografts and other vascular beds have been reported.

Neoplasia: Immunosuppression can increase risk of malignancies developing.

Neuropsychiatric events: Have occurred even after first dose and include seizures, encephalopathy, cerebral edema, aseptic meningitis syndrome, headache.

Seizures: Seizures, some with loss of consciousness, cardiorespiratory arrest, or death, have occurred.

Serum creatinine: During the first 1 to 3 days of therapy, some patients have experienced an acute and transient decline in glomerular filtration rate and diminished urine output with an increase in serum creatinine.

Overdosage: Signs and Symptoms

Hyperthermia; severe chills; myalgia; vomiting; diarrhea; edema; oliguria; pulmonary edema; acute renal failure; microangiopathic hemolytic anemia syndrome.

PATIENT CARE CONSIDERATIONS
Administration/Storage
- For IV bolus only. Not for IV infusion, intradermal, subcutaneous, IM, or intra-arterial administration.
- Do not administer if solution is discolored or cloudy. Fine translucent particles may be noted, but this does not affect potency.
- Once ampule has been opened, use immediately and discard any unused solution. Do not save unused solution for later use.
- Prepare injection by drawing solution into syringe though low protein-binding 0.2 or 0.22 micrometer (mcm) filter. Detach filter and attach new needle for the IV bolus injection.
- Do not mix with other IV substances or additives or infuse simultaneously through the same IV line. If the same IV line is used for sequential infusion of different medications, flush line with saline solution before and after injection of muromonab-CD3.
- Administer prescribed dose by IV bolus (less than 1 min).
- Store unopened vials in refrigerator (36° to 46° F). Do not freeze or shake.

Assessment/Interventions
- Obtain patient history, including drug history and any known allergies. Note volume depletion, uncontrolled hypertension, unstable angina, recent MI, pulmonary edema, symptomatic ischemic heart, heart failure, history of seizures, COPD, cerebrovascular disease, vascular disease, history of thrombosis, neuropathy, or septic shock.
- Review patient's health history and current status for any condition that would contraindicate muromobab-CD3 therapy: previous allergic reaction to muromonab-CD3, hypersensitivity to any product of murine origin, anti-mouse antibody titers greater than 1:1,000, fluid overload, uncompensated heart failure as evidenced by chest x-ray or greater than 3% weight gain within week prior to treatment, history of seizures or predisposition to seizures, pregnancy, or breastfeeding.
- Ensure that BUN, serum creatinine, transaminases, alkaline phosphatase, bilirubin, and CBC with differential and platelet count are evaluated prior to and during muromonab-CD3 therapy. Inform health care provider if abnormalities noted.
- Ensure that muromonab-CD3 levels or T-cell Cl are periodically monitored during therapy. Notify health care provider if muromonab-CD3 level is less than 800 ng/mL or if CD3 positive T cells are greater than 25 cells/mm^3.
- Ensure that muromonab-CD3 levels and T-cell Cl are monitored daily during therapy in pediatric patient. Notify health care provider if muromonab-CD3 levels are less than 800 ng/mL or if CD3 positive T cells are greater than 25 cells/mm^3.
- Ensure that human anti-mouse antibodies are measured before administering repeat course of therapy or if patient has received other murine-derived products.
- Ensure that there is no evidence of volume overload, uncontrolled hypertension, or uncompensated heart failure prior to administering muromonab-CD3.
- Weigh patient daily. Patient should not weigh more than 3% above their minimum weight during the week prior to starting therapy.
- Ensure that need for anti-infective prophylaxis is evaluated in pediatric and other high risk patients.
- Ensure that fluid status is carefully monitored prior to and during medication administration.
- Ensure that antipyretics are administered before monomurab-CD3 in patient with temperature greater than 100°F.
- Ensure that consideration has been given to using an antihistamine and acetaminophen concomitantly with muromonab-CD3 in effort to reduce early systemic reactions.
- Ensure that consideration has been given to pretreatment with systemic corticosteroid (eg, methylprednisolone) 1 to 4 hr before initial dose to minimize symptoms of CRS.
- Monitor patient for signs and symptoms of CRS (eg, flu-like symptoms, high fever, chills, rigors, headache, tremor, nausea, vomiting, diarrhea, abdominal pain, dyspnea, shortness of breath, bronchospasm, hemodynamic instability, hypertension, pulmonary edema, hypoxia, arrhythmias). Inform health care provider immediately if noted. Be prepared to treat serious presentations of the syndrome.
- Monitor patient closely for neurologic symptoms during the first 24 hr following each of the first few doses of muromonab-CD3. Inform health care provider immediately if any neurologic symptoms develop. Ensure that the possibility of infection is evaluated in patient developing clinical signs of meningitis.
- Monitor patient for signs of allergic reaction. Discontinue therapy and immediately notify health care provider if noted. Be prepared to treat serious allergic events appropriately.
- Ensure that doses of other immunosuppressive agents are reduced to lowest level compatible

with an effective therapeutic response during treatment with muromonab-CD3 and are returned to maintenance levels about 3 days prior to cessation of muromonab-CD3 treatment.
- Ensure that following initiation of monomurab-CD3 therapy that patient is continuously monitored for evidence of lymphoproliferative disorders.
- Monitor patient for GI, CNS, CV, RESP, HEMA, and general body side effects. Report to health care provider if noted and significant.

Patient/Family Education
- Explain name, action, and potential side effects of drug.
- Advise patient, family, or caregiver that it will be necessary to resume lifelong therapy with other immunosuppressive medications after completing therapy with muromonab-CD3.
- Advise patient, family, or caregiver that medication will be prepared and administered by health care provider in a health care setting with close monitoring.
- Review dosing schedule with patient, family, or caregiver.
- Review signs and symptoms associated with the CRS and the potentially serious nature of this syndrome.
- Instruct patient to seek medical attention if any of the following occur: skin rash, hives, rapid heart beat, difficulty breathing or unexplained shortness of breath, difficult or painful swallowing, any swelling suggesting an allergic reaction.
- Caution patient that medication may impair mental alertness and coordination and to use caution when driving or performing other tasks that require mental alertness or coordination until tolerance is determined.
- Caution patient not to take any prescription or OTC medications, herbal preparations, or dietary supplements unless advised by health care provider.
- Advise patient, family, or caregiver that frequent follow-up visits and laboratory tests will be required to monitor therapy and to keep appointments.

Mycophenolate Mofetil

(my-koe-FEN-oh-late moE-feh-till)
Class Immunosuppressive

How Supplied
CellCept Capsules 250 mg, Tablets 500 mg, Powder for Injection 500 mg as hydrochloride
✣ *CellCept* I.V.

Action
PHARMACOLOGY: Inhibits immune-mediated inflammatory responses, but exact mechanism not known.

PHARMACOKINETICS/DYNAMICS:
Absorption: Mean absolute bioavailability is 94%. Food decreases MPA C_{max} 40%.

Distribution: Protein binding is 97% (MPA) and 82% (MPAG). Mean apparent Vd is 3.6 L/kg (IV) and 4 L/kg (oral).

Metabolism: Metabolism is rapid and complete to MPA. MPA (active metabolite) is metabolized to MPAG (inactive metabolite) by glucuronyl transferase. MPAG undergoes enterohepatic recycling where it is converted to MPA.

Excretion: Mycophenolate is excreted in urine (93%, mostly as MPAG) and feces (6%). Mean apparent $t_{½}$ is approximately 18 hr and mean plasma clearance is approximately 193 mL/min (oral).

Indications In combination with cyclosporine and corticosteroids for prophylaxis of organ rejection in patients receiving allogenic renal or cardiac transplants.

Contraindications Hypersensitivity to the drug, mycophenolic acid, or any component of the drug product; persons with a sensitivity to polysorbate 80 (Tween) (IV only).

Route/Dosage
Renal Transplantation
ADULTS: PO/IV 1 g administered over at least 2 hr bid (daily dose of 2 g).

Cardiac Transplantation
ADULTS: PO/IV 1.5 g administered over at least 2 hr bid (daily dose of 3 g).

Interactions
Acyclovir: Possible increased plasma concentrations of both drugs.
Antacids containing magnesium and aluminum hydroxides: Decreased absorption of mycophenolate; do not administer simultaneously.
Azathioprine: Avoid use due to lack of clinical studies.
Cholestyramine: Decreased mycophenolate plasma concentrations; do not give mycophenolate with cholestyramine or other agents that may interfere with enterohepatic recirculation.
Ganciclovir: Possible increased plasma concentrations of both drugs.
Phenytoin: MPA decreased protein binding of phenytoin and may, therefore, increase free phenytoin levels.
Probenecid: May increase plasma concentrations of mycophenolate.

Salicylates: Coadministration increased the free fraction of MPA.
Theophylline: MPA decreased protein binding of theophylline and may, therefore, increase free theophylline levels.

Lab Test Interferences None well documented.

Adverse Reactions

CV: Hypertension; hypotension; orthostatic hypotension; peripheral edema; tachycardia; chest pain; palpitations; ventricular extrastystole; CHF; supraventricular tachycardia; ventricular tachycardia; atrial flutter; pulmonary hypertension; heart arrest; venous pressure increase; syncope; supraventricular extrasystoles; extrastystoles; pallor; vasospasm.
CNS: Headache; tremor; insomnia; dizziness; anxiety; depression; somnolence; paresthesia; emotional lability; neuropathy; convulsion; hallucinations; abnormal thinking; vertigo.
DERM: Acne; rash; alopecia; pruritus; sweating; hemorrhage; skin carcinoma.
EENT: Amblyopia; cataracts; conjunctivitis; rhinitis; sinusitis; pharyngitis; ear pain; deafness; ear disorder; tinnitus; abnormal vision; lacrimation disorder; eye hemorrhage.
GI: Diarrhea; constipation; nausea; abdominal pain; dyspepsia; vomiting; oral moniliasis; anorexia; esophagitis; flatulence; gastritis; GI hemorrhage; gingivitis; gingival hyperplasia; ileus; GI disorder; liver damage; dysphagia; jaundice; stomatitis; thirst.
GU: UTI or disorder; hematuria; kidney tubular necrosis; dysuria; impotence; pyelonephritis; urinary frequency; nocturia; kidney failure; urine abnormality; hematuria; urinary incontinence; prostatic disorder; urinary retention.
HEMA: Anemia; hypochromic anemia; leukopenia; thrombocytopenia; leukocytosis.
HEPA: Elevated LFTs.
METAB: Hypercholesterolemia; hypophosphatemia; hypokalemia; hyperkalemia; hyperglycemia; edema.
RESP: Infection; dyspnea; cough; bronchitis; asthma; pulmonary edema; pleural effusion; pneumonia; meningitis; infectious endocarditis; tuberculosis; atypical mycobaterial infection; atelectasis; hiccup; pneumothorax; increased sputum; epistaxis; apnea; voice alteration; pain; hemoptysis; neoplasm; respiratory acidosis.
OTHER: Body/back pain; fever; chills; infection; sepsis; asthenia; arthralgia; myalgia; leg cramps; myasthenia; lymphoma/lymphoproliferative disease; nonmelanoma skin carcinoma; Cushing's syndrome; hypothyroidism; neck pain; cellulitis; increased prothrombin; decreased thromboplastin; petechia; phlebitis; thrombosis; weight gain/loss; abnormal healing; dehydration.

> **WARNING:**
> Should be administered under the supervision of a physician experienced in immunosuppressive therapy and management of organ transplantation, and in an equipped facility. Increased risk of lymphoma and increased susceptibility to infection may be related to immunosuppression.

Precautions
Pregnancy: Category C.
Lactation: Undetermined.
Children: Safety and efficacy not established.
Renal function impairment: Do not exceed 2 g per day doses in patients with GFR less than 25 mL/min/1.73 m^2; carefully monitor these patients.
Monitoring: Complete blood counts should be performed weekly during the first month, twice monthly during the second and third months, then monthly through the first year.
GI hemorrhage: GI tract hemorrhage has been observed; administer with caution to patients with active serious digestive system disease.
Lymphomas/Malignancies: Patients receiving immunosuppressive regimens involving combinations of drugs are at increased risk of developing lymphomas and other malignancies, particularly of the skin. Risk appears to be related to intensity and duration of immunosuppression rather than to any specific agent.
Neutropenia: Monitor patients for neutropenia; dosage changes may be indicated.
Women of childbearing potential: Have a negative serum or urine pregnancy test within 1 wk of beginning therapy; effective contraception (abstinence or two reliable methods) must be used before, during and for 6 wk following discontinuation of therapy.

Overdosage: Signs and Symptoms
Nausea, vomiting, diarrhea, neutropenia.

PATIENT CARE CONSIDERATIONS

Administration/Storage

- Initial oral dose as soon as possible following transplantation.
- Oral medication is most effective on an empty stomach.
- Medication should be used concurrently with cyclosporine and corticosteroids.
- Do not open or crush capsules. Avoid inhalation or direct contact with skin or mucous membranes of the capsule powder. If contact occurs, wash thoroughly with soap and water; rinse eyes with plain water.

- Store at room temperature (59° to 86°F).

Assessment/Interventions
- Obtain patient history.
- Obtain baseline laboratory tests, including BUN, creatinine, lipid levels, potassium, WBC with diff and CBC. Perform and evaluate these tests periodically during treatment.
- Assess for any signs of infection, bleeding or bruising.
- Maintain medical asepsis and eliminate any potential sources of environmental contamination.
- Monitor for signs and symptoms of organ rejection.

Patient/Family Education
- Instruct patient not to change dose or discontinue medication without consulting health care provider.
- Instruct patient to check with healthcare provider before taking any OTC or prescription medications, and vaccinations.
- Instruct patient to report any serious side effects to health care provider, including: tremors, headaches, diarrhea, hypertension, nausea and low urine output.
- Inform patient of need for frequent laboratory tests while taking this medication. Be sure to keep appointments.
- Instruct patient to avoid contact with others who may have infections.
- Instruct patient to use a soft toothbrush and to practice frequent oral hygiene.
- Instruct patient to take medication 30 min before or 2 hr after meals. If medication causes GI upset, take with a full glass of water. May be taken with food, but is less effective.
- Instruct women of childbearing potential to use effective contraception before beginning therapy, during therapy and for 6 wk after stopping therapy.
- Instruct patients with increased risk for skin cancer to limit exposure to sunlight and UV light by wearing protective clothing and using a strong sunscreen.

Nabumetone

(nab-YOU-meh-TONE)

Class Analgesic/NSAID

How Supplied
Relafen Tablets 500 mg, Tablets 750 mg
✤ *Apo-Nabumetone* ♦ *Gen-Nabumetone* ♦ *Rhoxal-nabumetone*

Action

PHARMACOLOGY: Decreases inflammation, pain and fever, probably through inhibition of cyclooxygenase activity and prostaglandin synthesis.

PHARMACOKINETICS/DYNAMICS:

Absorption: Nabumetone is well absorbed from the GI tract. Food increases the rate of absorption and plasma concentration of 6-methoxy-2-naphthylacetic acid (6 MNA). Bioavailability is greater than 80%.

Distribution: Protein binding is more than 99% (active metabolite) and the Vd is at 0.1 to 0.2 L/kg.

Metabolism: Undergoes rapid biotransformation to main active metabolite 6 MNA approximately 35% and the remaining unidentified metabolites approximately 50%. 6 MNA is metabolized in the liver to inactive metabolites.

Excretion: 80% recovered in urine, 9% in feces. The t½ of major metabolite is 22.5 to 24 hr and plasma clearance is 20 to 30 mL/min.

Special Populations:
Renal Function Impairment – Terminal half-life of 6 MNA was increased.
Elderly – Steady state concentrations are generally higher.

Indications Relief of symptoms of chronic and acute rheumatoid arthritis and osteoarthritis.

Contraindications Hypersensitivity to aspirin, iodides, or any NSAID.

Route/Dosage

Osteoarthritis/Rheumatoid Arthritis
ADULTS: PO 1000 mg initially; may increase to 1500 to 2000 mg daily in 1 to 2 divided doses.

Interactions
Anticoagulants: May increase effect of anticoagulants. May increase risk of gastric erosion and bleeding.
Cyclosporine: Neurotoxicity of both agents may be increased.
Lithium: May increase lithium levels.

PATIENT CARE CONSIDERATIONS

Administration/Storage
♦ Give medication with full glass of water, either with or without food.

Methotrexate: Increased risk of methotrexate toxicity.
Salicylates: Additive GI toxicity.

Lab Test Interferences May prolong bleeding time.

Adverse Reactions

CV: Edema; weight gain; congestive heart failure; alterations in BP; vasodilation; palpitations; tachycardia; chest pain; bradycardia.
CNS: Dizziness; lightheadedness; drowsiness; confusion; increased sweating; vertigo; headaches; nervousness; migraine; anxiety; aggravated Parkinson or epilepsy; paresthesia; peripheral neuropathy; myalgia; tremors; fatigue.
DERM: Rash; urticaria; purpura.
EENT: Blurred vision; tinnitus; rhinitis; salivation; glossitis; pharyngitis.
GI: Diarrhea; ulceration; dry mouth; heartburn; dyspepsia; nausea; vomiting; anorexia; diarrhea; constipation; flatulence; indigestion; appetite changes; abdominal cramps; epigastric pain; hematemesis; peptic ulcer; stomatitis.
GU: Acute renal insufficiency; interstitial nephritis; hyperkalemia; hyponatremia; papillary necrosis; melena; menometrorrhagia; impotence; menstrual disorders; hematuria; cystitis; nocturia; proteinuria.
HEPA: Hepatitis.
HEMA: Increased prothrombin time; bleeding; anemia; neutropenia; leukopenia; pancytopenia; eosinophilia; thrombocytopenia.
RESP: Bronchospasm; laryngeal edema; dyspnea; hemoptysis; shortness of breath.
OTHER: Photosensitivity.

Precautions

Pregnancy: Category C.
Lactation: Undetermined.
Children: Safety and efficacy not established.
Elderly: Increased risk of adverse reactions.
Hypersensitivity: May occur; use drug with caution in aspirin-sensitive patients because of possible cross-sensitivity.
Renal function impairment: Lower doses may be necessary in patients with renal impairment.
GI effects: Serious GI toxicity (eg, bleeding, ulceration, perforation) can occur at any time, with or without warning symptoms.

Overdosage: Signs and Symptoms

Drowsiness, dizziness, confusion, disorientation, lethargy, numbness, vomiting, gastric irritation, nausea, abdominal pain, headache, tinnitus, sweating, convulsions, blurred vision, renal failure, coma.

♦ Store in tightly closed, light-resistant container at room temperature (59° to 86°F).

Assessment/Interventions
- Obtain patient history, including drug history and any known allergies. Note fluid retention, nasal polyps, bronchospastic disease, and hypersensitivity to aspirin or other NSAIDs.
- Obtain baseline assessments of pain and ability to perform activities of daily living.
- For patients undergoing long-term therapy or with history of GI or renal disease, monitor for abnormalities/trends in liver/kidney function test results, hematocrit, hemoglobin, and platelets.
- Use caution if patient is receiving anticoagulants or thrombolytics.
- Monitor for signs and symptoms of GI distress or bleeding.

Patient/Family Education
- Remind patient to take medication with full glass of water, either with or without food.
- Explain that therapeutic effects may take up to 1 mo to be noted.
- Instruct patient to report the following symptoms to health care provider: rash, visual disturbance, ringing in ears, dark stools, persistent headache or abdominal pain, unusual bleeding or bruising, decreased urinary output, weight gain, edema.
- Caution patient to avoid intake of alcoholic beverages and to avoid smoking.
- Advise patient that drug may cause drowsiness and to use caution while driving or performing other tasks requiring mental alertness.
- Caution patient to avoid exposure to sunlight and to use sunscreen or wear protective clothing to avoid photosensitivity reaction.

Nadolol

(nay-DOE-lahl)

Class Beta-adrenergic blocker

How Supplied
Corgard Tablets 20 mg, Tablets 40 mg, Tablets 80 mg, Tablets 120 mg, Tablets 160 mg
❋ *Apo-Nadol* ♦ *Novo-Nadolol* ♦ *ratio-Nadolol*

Action
PHARMACOLOGY: Blocks beta-receptors, which primarily affect cardiovascular system (decreases heart rate, contractility, and BP) and lungs (promotes bronchospasm).

PHARMACOKINETICS/DYNAMICS:

Absorption: Oral absorption is approximately 30%. T_{max} is 3 to 4 hr and steady state is 6 to 9 days.

Distribution: Widely distributed into body tissues and into milk. Protein binding is approximately 30%.

Metabolism: Not metabolized.

Excretion: Nadolol is eliminated unchanged primarily through kidneys. Plasma t½ is 20 to 24 hr; increases in renal failure.

Special Populations:
Renal Function Impairment – Half-life increases.

Indications Management of hypertension and angina pectoris.

Contraindications Hypersensitivity to beta-blockers; greater than first-degree heart block; CHF unless secondary to tachyarrhythmia treatable with beta-blockers or untreated hypotension; overt cardiac failure; sinus bradycardia; cardiogenic shock; bronchial asthma or bronchospasm, including severe COPD.

Route/Dosage
Hypertension
ADULTS: **PO** Initiate with 40 mg/day; titrate in 40 to 80 mg increments to desired response.
Maintenance: **PO** 40 to 320 mg/day.

Angina
ADULTS: **PO** Initiate with 40 mg/day; titrate in 40 to 80 mg increments at 3- to 7-day intervals to desired response.
Maintenance: **PO** 40 to 240 mg/day. Dosage intervals may need to be altered in patients with decreased renal function.

Interactions
Clonidine: May enhance or reverse antihypertensive effect; potentially life-threatening situations may occur, especially on withdrawal.
Epinephrine: Initial hypertensive episode followed by bradycardia may occur.
Ergot derivatives: Peripheral ischemia, manifested by cold extremities and possible gangrene, may occur.
Insulin: Prolonged hypoglycemia with masking of symptoms may occur.
Lidocaine: Lidocaine levels may increase, leading to toxicity.
NSAIDs: Some agents may impair antihypertensive effect.

Prazosin: Orthostatic hypotension may be increased.
Verapamil: Effects of both drugs may be increased.

Lab Test Interferences Serum glucose may decrease; may interfere with glucose or insulin intolerance tests.

Adverse Reactions
CV: Bradycardia; hypotension; CHF; cold extremities; heart block; worsening angina; edema.
CNS: Depression; fatigue; lethargy; drowsiness; short-term memory loss; headache; dizziness.
DERM: Alopecia; rash.
EENT: Dry eyes; visual disturbances.
GI: Nausea; vomiting; diarrhea.
GU: Impotence; urinary retention; difficulty with urination.
HEMA: Agranulocytosis.
METAB: May increase or decrease blood glucose; elevated triglycerides and total cholesterol; decreased HDL cholesterol.
RESP: Wheezing; bronchospasm; difficulty breathing.
OTHER: Increased sensitivity to cold.

> **WARNING:**
>
> *Abrupt withdrawal:* In patients with angina pectoris or coronary artery disease (CAD), abrupt withdrawal may cause exacerbation of angina, occurrence of MI and ventricular arrhythmias. Monitor patients closely. Because CAD is common and unrecognized, it may be prudent not to discontinue beta-blocker therapy abruptly in patients treated only for hypertension.

Precautions
Pregnancy: Category C.
Lactation: Excreted in breast milk.
Children: Safety and efficacy not established.
Renal function impairment: Reduced dosage advised in patients with renal impairment.
Hepatic function impairment Reduced dosage advised in patients with hepatic impairment.
Abrupt withdrawal: Beta-blocker withdrawal syndrome (eg, hypertension, tachycardia, anxiety, angina, MI) may occur 1 to 2 wk following sudden discontinuation of systemic beta-blocker therapy. Withdraw treatment gradually over 1 to 2 wk.
Anaphylaxis: Deaths have occurred; aggressive therapy may be required.
CHF: Administer cautiously in CHF patients controlled by digitalis and diuretics. Notify health care provider at first sign or symptom of CHF or unexplained respiratory symptoms in any patient.
Diabetics: May mask signs and symptoms of hypoglycemia (eg, tachycardia, BP changes). May potentiate insulin-induced hypoglycemia.
Nonallergic bronchospasm: Give drug with caution in patients with bronchospastic disease.
Peripheral vascular disease: May precipitate or aggravate symptoms of arterial insufficiency.
Thyrotoxicosis: May mask clinical signs (eg, tachycardia) of developing or continuing hyperthyroidism. Abrupt withdrawal may exacerbate symptoms of hyperthyroidism, including thyroid storm.

Overdosage: Signs and Symptoms
Bradycardia, cardiogenic shock, intraventricular conduction disturbances, hypotension, AV block, depressed consciousness, CHF, asystole, coma.

PATIENT CARE CONSIDERATIONS

Administration/Storage
- Assess heart rate and BP before administering medication.
- Administer on regular schedule.
- Give medication with full glass water, either with or without food.
- Discontinue drug gradually over 1 to 2 wk.
- Store in tightly closed, light-resistant container at room temperature (59° to 86°F).

Assessment/Interventions
- Obtain patient history, including drug history and any known allergies. Note CHF, asthma, diabetes mellitus, or hyperthyroidism.
- Obtain baseline cardiac assessment including heart rate, BP, capillary refill, pulse rhythm, and presence of angina. Monitor BP and pulse frequently during initial phase of therapy and when changing dosage.
- If patient is scheduled for surgery, confer with health care provider regarding use of medication prior to surgery.
- For postoperative patients, monitor for trends in heart rate and BP.
- Monitor I&O and weigh patient daily.
- Withhold medication and notify health care provider if heart rate is less than 60 bpm or systolic BP is less than 90 mm Hg. Atropine may be needed for treatment of persistent bradycardia.
- For diabetic patients receiving hypoglycemic agents, monitor blood glucose test results. Signs and symptoms of hypoglycemia may be masked with nadolol.
- For patients discontinuing medication, moni-

tor for signs or symptoms of thyroid storm. Abrupt withdrawal may precipitate thyrotoxicosis.
- Observe for signs of beta-blocker withdrawal syndrome (eg, hypotension, tachycardia, anxiety, angina, MI) if medication is discontinued suddenly.
- Use caution in patients with CHF, COPD, or asthma. Monitor cardiovascular and respiratory status carefully and frequently.

Patient/Family Education
- Teach patient how to measure pulse rate before taking medication. Explain that if pulse rate is less than 50 bpm, patient needs to discontinue taking medication immediately and notify health care provider.
- Ensure that patient has independently demonstrated how to measure pulse rate.
- Show patient how to monitor blood sugar levels, and explain that signs and symptoms of low blood sugar levels may be masked.
- Caution patient not to stop taking medication abruptly but to consult health care provider for instructions on safest way to discontinue medication.
- Instruct patient to report the following symptoms to health care provider: bradycardia, palpitations, dizziness, fatigue, insomnia or sleep disturbances, altered sensorium, GI symptoms, and changes in blood sugar levels.
- Advise patient that drug may cause drowsiness and to use caution while driving or performing other tasks requiring mental alertness.
- Instruct patient not to take OTC medications without consulting health care provider.

Nafarelin Acetate

(NAFF-uh-RELL-in ASS-uh-TATE)

Class Gonadotropin-releasing hormone

How Supplied
Synarel Nasal solution 2 mg/mL (as nafarelin base)

Action
PHARMACOLOGY: Initially causes synthesis and release of luteinizing hormone (LH) and follicle-stimulating hormone (FSH). With continued use (more than 4 wk) suppresses secretion of LH and FSH.

PHARMACOKINETICS/DYNAMICS:
Absorption: Nafarelin acetate is rapidly absorbed into system circulation after intranasal administration. T_{max} is 10 to 40 min, C_{max} is 0.6 to 1.8 ng/mL, and serum bioavailability is 2.8%.
Distribution: Plasma protein binding is 80%.
Excretion: Nafarelin acetate is eliminated in urine (3% as unchanged) and feces. Serum t½ is about 3 hr (adults), 2.5 hr (children), and 85.5 hr (metabolites).

Indications Treatment of endometriosis, central precocious puberty in children of both sexes.

Contraindications Hypersensitivity to gonadotropin-releasing hormone (GnRH); or GnRH-agonist analogs; undiagnosed abnormal vaginal bleeding; pregnancy; lactation.

Route/Dosage
Endometriosis
ADULTS: **Intranasal** 400 mcg/day (200 mcg [1 spray] in 1 nostril in morning and 200 mcg [1 spray] in other nostril in evening. For long-term suppression, 800 mcg/day (1 spray in each nostril bid) may be necessary.

Central Precocious Puberty
CHILDREN: **Intranasal** 1600 mcg/day (400 mcg [2 sprays] in each nostril in morning and 400 mcg [2 sprays] in each nostril in evening). In some patients 1800 mcg/day (3 sprays in alternating nostrils tid) may be necessary.

Interactions None well documented.

Lab Test Interferences Diagnostic tests of pituitary gonadotropic and gonadal function during treatment and 4 to 8 wk after discontinuation of treatment may be misleading.

Adverse Reactions
CNS: Headaches; insomnia; depression.
DERM: Acne; seborrhea.
EENT: Nasal irritation.
GU: Vaginal dryness.
OTHER: Hot flushes; decreased libido; emotional lability; myalgia; reduced breast size; edema; weight gain; hirsutism; decreased bone density.

Precautions
Pregnancy: Category X.
Lactation: Do not use in lactating women.
Bone density loss: May be small loss in bone density during therapy, some of which may not be reversible. Risk is greater in patients who smoke or have osteoporosis and in alcoholics.
Intercurrent rhinitis: If patient must use topical nasal decongestant during nafarelin therapy, should be used at least 2 hr after nafarelin dosing to decrease possibility of reduced absorption.
Menstruation: Should stop with effective doses.
Noncompliance: Irregular or incomplete doses may result in stimulation of pituitary-gonadal axis.
Ovarian cysts: Have occurred in first 2 mo of therapy.

PATIENT CARE CONSIDERATIONS
Administration/Storage
- When treating endometriosis, begin treatment between days 2 and 4 of menstrual cycle.
- Administer intranasally with metered-spray pump. Patient's head should be tilted back slightly.
- If administering more than 1 spray per nostril, wait 30 sec between sprays.
- Store container upright at room temperature (59° to 86°F).
- Protect from light.

Assessment/Interventions
- Obtain patient history, including drug history and any known allergies.
- Obtain baseline assessments of last menstrual period, pregnancy status in patients with endometriosis, and height and weight in patients with central precocious puberty.
- Monitor menstrual cycles.
- Monitor for drug-related hypoestrogenism. Note patient complaints of hot flushes, libido decrease, vaginal dryness, headaches, and emotional lability.
- Monitor for signs of androgenism, including acne, myalgia, breast size reduction, edema, and weight gain.

Patient/Family Education
- Caution patient that this medication must not be taken during pregnancy or when pregnancy is possible. Advise patient to use nonhormonal form of birth control while taking this drug.
- Advise patient regarding proper administration techniques and storage information.
- Tell patient to begin treatment between days 2 and 4 of menstrual cycle if being treated for endometriosis.
- Instruct patient not to blow nose, and to avoid sneezing immediately after administration.
- Tell patient using topical nasal decongestant to use 2 hr after nafarelin has been administered.
- Advise patient that each bottle contains about 60 sprays and plan refills accordingly.
- Explain side effects of medication and instruct patient to report the following symptoms to health care provider: bleeding/menses continues, breakthrough bleeding or adverse/side effects.

Nafcillin Sodium

(naff-SILL-in SO-dee-uhm)

Class Penicillinase-resistant penicillin

How Supplied
Nafcillin Sodium Injection 1 g (as base), Injection 2 g (as base)

Action
PHARMACOLOGY: Inhibits bacterial cell wall mucopeptide synthesis.

PHARMACOKINETICS/DYNAMICS:
Absorption: T_{max} is 0.5 to 1 hr.

Distribution: Nafcillin is widely distributed in various body fluids (eg, bile, pleural, amniotic, synovial) and has high CSF penetration in presence of inflamed meninges. Protein binding is 89.9%, mainly albumin.

Metabolism: Nafcillin is metabolized mainly in the liver.

Excretion: Nafcillin is excreted in urine (30% as unchanged), and primarily eliminated in bile. Serum t½ is 33 to 61 min (IV).

Special Populations:
Biliary obstruction and cirrhosis – Plasma clearance is significantly decreased and excretion in urine was significantly increased from approximately 30% to 50%.

Indications Treatment of infections caused by penicillinase-producing staphylococci.

Contraindications Standard considerations.

Route/Dosage
ADULTS: **IV** Usual, 500 mg q 4 hr. Severe infections, 1 g q 4 hr. Infuse over at least 30 to 60 min.

Interactions
Cyclosporine: May reduce blood levels of cyclosporine.
Disulfiram: May increase nafcillin levels.
Probenecid: May increase nafcillin levels.
Tetracycline: May reduce effectiveness of nafcillin.
Warfarin: May increase warfarin effects.

Lab Test Interferences May cause false-positive urine reaction for protein when the sulfosalicylic acid test is used.

Adverse Reactions
GI: Pseudomembranous colitis.
GU: Renal tubular damage; interstitial nephritis.
HYPERSEN: Immediate hypersensitivity reactions including urticaria; pruritus; angioneurotic edema; laryngospasm; bronchospasm; hypotension; vascular collapse. Delayed reactions including fever, malaise, urticaria, myalgia, arthralgia, abdominal pain, and rashes
METAB: Agranulocytosis; neutropenia; bone marrow depression.

OTHER: Local reactions include pain, swelling, phlebitis, thrombophlebitis, inflammation at the injection site.

Precautions
Pregnancy: Category B.
Lactation: Secreted into breast milk.
Children: Excretion may be impaired in newborns. Not approved for IV use in neonates or children.

Hypersensitivity: Use with caution in patients with histories of significant allergies to penicillins or asthma.
Renal function impairment: May reduce nafcillin elimination.
Hepatic function impairment: May reduce nafcillin elimination.
Superinfection: May result in overgrowth of nonsusceptible organisms.

PATIENT CARE CONSIDERATIONS

Administration/Storage
- For IV administration only. Do not administer intradermal, SC, or IM.
- Infuse prescribed dose q 4 hr.
- Infuse over 30 to 60 min to reduce risk of vein irritation and extravasation.
- Thaw frozen container at room temperature (77°F) or under refrigeration (41°F). Do not force thawing by immersion in water or by microwave irradiation.
- Check thawed IV container for minute leaks by squeezing bag firmly. If leaks are detected discard solution because sterility may be impaired.
- Agitate thawed IV container and inspect visually. Do not administer if thawed solution is cloudy, discolored, or contains particulate matter or if any seal or outlet port is not intact.
- Do not add other medications to IV container.
- Follow manufacturer's instructions for preparing the IV container for administration.
- Do not use plastic nafcillin containers in series to reduce risk of air embolism.
- Store IV bag in freezer at -4°F. Thawed solutions are stable for 21 days under refrigeration (41°F) or for 72 hr at room temperature (77°F). Do not refreeze thawed solutions.

Assessment/Interventions
- Obtain patient history, including drug history and any known allergies, especially to penicillin and beta-lactam antibiotics. Note history of asthma, multiple allergies, or concomitant liver and renal impairment.
- Ensure that culture and susceptibility test results indicate sensitivity to nafcillin.
- Ensure that nafcillin is discontinued and another antimicrobial agent is started if culture and sensitivity tests indicate that the infection is caused by an organism other than a pencillinase-producing staphylococci.
- Ensure that WBC and differential are determined prior to starting therapy and periodically during therapy.
- Ensure that periodic urinalysis, liver enzymes, and renal function are determined periodically during prolonged therapy.
- Ensure that nafcillin serum levels are determined periodically in patients with concomitant renal and hepatic dysfunction and that the nafcillin dose is changed appropriately.
- Monitor for signs of infection, especially fever, and for positive response to antibiotic therapy.
- Monitor patient for signs of anaphylaxis or severe allergic reaction. If noted discontinue therapy and immediately notify health care provider. Be prepared to treat appropriately.
- Monitor administration site for pain, inflammation, swelling, or phlebitis. Change administration site and treat injection site reaction appropriately if noted.
- Monitor patient for GI, CNS, and general body side effects. Report to health care provider if noted and significant.
- If seizure occurs, withhold drug, institute safety measures, and notify health care provider.
- Withhold drug and notify health care provider if any of the following occurs: severe diarrhea; loose, foul-smelling stools; vaginal itching or discharge.

Patient/Family Education
- Explain name, dose, action, and potential side effects of drug.
- Explain to patient or caregiver that medication is usually prepared and administered by a health care provider in a health care setting but may be used at home in some situations if ordered by the patient's health care provider.
- If patient or caregiver is administering at home ensure that the patient or caregiver understands how to store, prepare and administer the dose, and dispose of used equipment and supplies. The first injection should be performed under the supervision of a qualified health professional.
- Review dosing schedule and prescribed length of therapy with patient. Advise patient that dose and duration of therapy are dependent on site and cause of infection and response to therapy.
- Instruct patient to report the following to health care provider: itching; rash; hives; diffi-

culty breathing; diarrhea; loose, foul-smelling stools; injection site reaction.
• Advise patient that follow-up visits and lab tests may be needed to monitor therapy and to keep appointments.

Nalbuphine Hydrochloride
(NAL-byoo-FEEN HIGH-droe-KLOR-ide)
Class Narcotic agonist-antagonist analgesic
How Supplied
Nubain Injection 10 mg/mL, Injection 20 mg/mL
❧ *Nubain*

Action
PHARMACOLOGY: An opiate analgesic with both narcotic agonist and antagonist actions. Analgesic potency is about equal to that of morphine, and antagonist potency is about ½₅ that of naloxone. May cause sphincter of Oddi spasm. Does not increase pulmonary artery pressure, systemic vascular resistance or myocardial work load.

PHARMACOKINETICS/DYNAMICS:
Absorption: When nalbuphine is taken orally, it is not effective for pain relief as when given IM, mainly because of first-pass metabolism in GI and liver. T_{max} is 30 min (IM).
Distribution: Nalbuphine is not bound to plasma proteins. Nalbuphine crosses the placenta.
Metabolism: Metabolized in the liver.
Excretion: Approximately 7% eliminated in urine unchanged, and in feces. Plasma t½ is 5 hr and t½ is 2.4 hr.
Onset: Onset of IV nalbuphine is 2 to 3 min. Onset of SC and IM nalbuphine is less than 15 min.
Duration: Duration of analgesic activity is 3 to 6 hr.

Indications Management of moderate-to-severe pain; preoperative and postoperative analgesia; supplement to balanced anesthesia; obstetrical analgesia during labor and delivery.
Contraindications Standard considerations.
Route/Dosage
ADULTS: SC/IM/IV 10 mg/70 kg q 3 to 6 hr prn. Individualize dosage. In nontolerant patients, do not exceed 20 mg/dose or 160 mg/day.

Interactions
CNS depressants, including barbiturate anesthetics: Increased respiratory and CNS depression.
INCOMPATIBILITIES: Diazepam, pentobarbital, promethazine.

Lab Test Interferences None well documented.
Adverse Reactions
CV: Hypertension; hypotension; bradycardia; tachycardia; pulmonary edema.
CNS: Sedation; dizziness; vertigo; headache.
DERM: Urticaria.
EENT: Miosis.
GI: Nausea; vomiting; constipation; dry mouth.
RESP: Respiratory depression.
OTHER: Sweaty or clammy feeling.

Precautions
Pregnancy: Pregnancy category undetermined. Safety (except during labor) is unknown. May cause respiratory depression in newborn; use drug with caution in women delivered of premature infants.
Lactation: Undetermined.
Children: Not recommended in patients younger than 18 yr.
Renal function impairment: Duration of action may be prolonged in patients with renal impairment; may need to reduce dose.
Hepatic function impairment: Duration of action may be prolonged in patients with hepatic impairment; may need to reduce dose.
Special risk patients: Use drug with caution in patients with impaired respiration, head injury, increased intracranial pressure, or MI with nausea or vomiting and in patients about to undergo biliary tract surgery
Sulfite sensitivity: Contains sodium metabisulfite, which may cause allergic-type reactions including anaphylactic symptoms and life-threatening asthma.
Dependence: Low abuse potential; however, withdrawal symptoms can occur after long-term use. Use drug with caution in patients who are emotionally unstable or have history of narcotic abuse.
Opiate-dependent patients: Nalbuphine can precipitate withdrawal; small doses of morphine can be given to relieve discomfort. If patient has received morphine, meperidine, codeine or other opiate of similar duration, give 25% of normal nalbuphine dose first. Observe for signs of withdrawal and increase nalbuphine dose slowly.

Overdosage: Signs and Symptoms
Respiratory depression, hypoxemia, sedation.

PATIENT CARE CONSIDERATIONS

Administration/Storage
- Administer via parenteral route only.
- Store in light-resistant container at room temperature (59° to 86°F).

Assessment/Interventions
- Obtain patient history, including drug history and any known allergies.
- Obtain baseline assessments of pain, respiratory rate and level of consciousness. Withhold medication and notify health care provider if respiratory rate is less than 10/min.
- For patients receiving opiate agonists (eg, morphine, codeine), assess for signs and symptoms of withdrawal, which may include restlessness, abdominal cramps, nausea, vomiting, lacrimation, piloerection, increased temperature. Check health care provider's orders for notes on use of morphine sulfate to relieve withdrawal symptoms.
- Monitor effectiveness of medication by evaluating patient's pain perception.
- Monitor for sedation. May need to take precautions against falling to ensure patient safety.
- Carefully monitor patients with neurologic injury.
- Monitor for constipation and urinary retention.

Patient/Family Education
- Explain importance of communicating effectiveness of pain relief.
- Tell patient to inform health care provider if difficulty breathing, dizziness, drowsiness, or lethargy occurs.
- Explain importance of fall precautions and of asking for assistance with ambulation.
- Emphasize importance of informing caregivers of potential problems, including sedation, dizziness, headache, vertigo, nausea, vomiting, dry mouth, itching, shortness of breath, blurred vision, flushing.
- Instruct patient to avoid intake of alcoholic beverages or other CNS depressants.
- Advise patient that drug may cause drowsiness and to use caution while driving or performing other tasks requiring mental alertness.

Nalidixic Acid

(nal-ih-DIK-sik acid)

Class Urinary anti-infective

How Supplied
NegGram Caplets 250 mg, Caplets 500 mg, Caplets 1 g, Suspension 250 mg/5 mL

Action

PHARMACOLOGY: Interferes with DNA formation of certain bacteria.

PHARMACOKINETICS/DYNAMICS:

Absorption: Nalidixic acid is rapidly absorbed from GI tract. C_{max} is 20 to 40 mcg/mL and T_{max} is 1 to 2 hr.

Distribution: Nalidixic acid protein binding is 93% to 97% (parent) and 63% (hydroxynalidixic acid), and concentrates in renal tissue and seminal fluid.

Metabolism: Nalidixic acid is partially metabolized in liver to hydroxynalidixic acid (activity similar to nalidixic acid) and inactive conjugates.

Excretion: Nalidixic acid is excreted in urine as unchanged drug and 85% as active metabolites; 4% in feces. The t½ is approximately 6 hr in urine.

Special Populations:
Renal Function Impairment – Significantly affects renal clearance, increases serum concentrations, and decreases urine levels of parent and metabolites.

Indications Treatment of UTIs caused by susceptible gram-negative bacteria, including most Proteus strains, *Klebsiella* and *Enterobacter* species and *E. coli.*

Contraindications History of seizures.

Route/Dosage

ADULTS:
Initial therapy: **PO** 1 g qid for 1 or 2 wk.
Prolonged therapy: **PO** 1 g bid after initial therapy.

CHILDREN (3 MO TO 2 YR):
Initial therapy: **PO** 55 mg/kg/day divided into 4 equal doses.
Prolonged therapy: **PO** 33 mg/kg/day in 4 divided doses after initial therapy.

Interactions
Oral anticoagulants: May enhance anticoagulant effect.

Lab Test Interferences False-positive urinary glucose results with *Benedict's* or *Fehling's* solutions or *Clinitest* reagent tablets; use *Clinistix* or *Tes-tape*. Urinary 17-keto and ketogenic steroids may be falsely elevated; Porter-Silber method should be used.

Adverse Reactions
CNS: Drowsiness; weakness; headache; dizziness; vertigo; seizures; intracranial hypertension;

increased intracranial pressure; sixth cranial nerve palsy in children and infants.
DERM: Rash; pruritus; urticaria; angioedema; photosensitivity.
EENT: Visual disturbances.
GI: Abdominal pain; nausea; vomiting; diarrhea.
HEMA: Thrombocytopenia; leukopenia, eosinophilia or hemolytic anemia (associated with G-6-PD deficiency or acute immune reaction).
HEPA: Cholestatic jaundice; cholestasis.
METAB: Metabolic acidosis.

Precautions
Pregnancy: Pregnancy category undetermined. Do not use during first trimester.
Lactation: Excreted in breast milk.
Children: Use drug with caution in prepubertal children; may affect cartilage and joints.
Renal function impairment: Patients with compromised renal function may fail to accumulate nalidixic acid, decreasing its effectiveness.
CNS effects: Convulsions, increased intracranial pressure and toxic psychosis may occur with overdose or predisposing factors (eg, epilepsy, cerebral arteriosclerosis).
Hematologic: Can produce clinically significant hemolysis in patients with G-6-PD deficiency.

Overdosage: Signs and Symptoms
Increased intracranial pressure, metabolic acidosis, lethargy, psychosis, nausea, hyperglycemia, convulsions, vomiting.

PATIENT CARE CONSIDERATIONS

Administration/Storage
- Give medication at least 1 hr before meals.
- Shake suspension well before use.
- Store in tightly closed container at room temperature (59° to 86°F). Do not freeze.

Assessment/Interventions
- Obtain patient history, including drug history and any known allergies.
- Obtain baseline assessments of burning/pain with urination, urinary urgency or frequency, level of consciousness.
- Assess for adverse reactions, primarily with CNS and GI systems.
- Obtain urine specimens as needed for culture and sensitivity.
- Monitor blood counts, liver, and renal function test values if treatment is continued longer than 2 wk.
- Re-evaluate patient for improvement of symptoms.

Patient/Family Education
- Tell patient to take with food or milk.
- Explain importance of adequate hydration and encourage intake of 1500 to 3000 mL fluids/day, unless otherwise specified by health care provider.
- Instruct patient to report the following symptoms to health care provider: if no improvement of UTI discomfort, signs or symptoms 48 hr after initiation of treatment and if adverse effects occur.
- Advise patient that drug may cause drowsiness or dizziness and to use caution while driving or performing other tasks requiring mental alertness.
- Caution patient to avoid exposure to ultraviolet light and sunlight and to use sunscreen or wear protective clothing and to use sunglasses when outdoors. Explain that photosensitivity may last up to 3 mo after last dose.

Naloxone Hydrochloride
(NAL-ox-ohn HIGH-droe-KLOR-ide)

Class Narcotic antagonist

How Supplied
Naloxone Hydrochloride Neonatal injection 0.02 mg/mL ♦ *Narcan* Injection 0.4 mg/mL, Injection 1 mg/mL

Action
PHARMACOLOGY: Evidence suggests that naloxone antagonizes opioid effects by competing for opiate receptor sites in the CNS.

PHARMACOKINETICS/DYNAMICS:
Distribution: Rapidly distributed in the body and readily crosses the placenta. Plasma protein binding is relatively weak.
Metabolism: Metabolized in the liver primarily by glucuronidation (major metabolite naloxone-3-glucuronide).
Excretion: In adults the t½ ranges from 30 to 81 min, while in neonates the t½ is about 3 hr. Approximately 25% to 40% is excreted as metabolites in the urine within 6 hr, about 50% in 24 hr, and 60% to 70% in 72 hr.
Onset: Following IV administration, the onset of action is usually apparent within 2 min.
Duration: Duration of effect is more prolonged after IM injection compared with IV administration.

Indications Complete or partial reversal of opioid depression, including respiratory depression, induced by natural and synthetic opioids, including propoxyphene; diagnosis of suspected or known opioid overdosage; adjunctive agent to increase BP in management of septic shock.

Contraindications Standard considerations.

Route/Dosage

Opioid-induced Depression
NEONATES: **IV/IM/SC** 0.01 mg/kg. Dose may be repeated in accordance with adult administration guidelines for postoperative opioid depression.

Opioid Overdosage
ADULTS: **IV** (**IM/SC** if **IV** route is not available) 0.4 to 2 mg; dose may be repeated at 2 to 3 min intervals if desired degree of counteraction and improvement in respiratory function are not obtained. If no response is observed after administration of 10 mg of naloxone, question the diagnosis.
CHILDREN: **IV** (**IM/SC** if **IV** route is not available) Initial dose is 0.01 mg/kg; may give a subsequent dose of 0.1 mg/kg.

Postoperative Opioid Depression
ADULTS: **IV** Small doses are usually sufficient. Titrate dose in increments of 0.1 to 0.2 mg IV at 2- to 3-min intervals to the desired degree of reversal (eg, adequate ventilation without significant pain). Repeat doses may be required at 1- or 2-hr intervals, depending on amount, type, and time interval since last administration of an opiate.
CHILDREN: **IV** Inject in increments of 0.005 to 0.01 mg at 2- to 3-min intervals to the desired degree of reversal of respiratory depression. Follow recommendation and cautions for adults.

Septic Shock
ADULTS: Optimal dose and duration of treatment of hypotension in septic shock have not been established.

Interactions None well documented.

Lab Test Interferences None well documented.

Adverse Reactions

CV: Hypotension; hypertension; ventricular tachycardia and fibrillation; pulmonary edema; cardiac arrest; death.
CNS: Agitation; seizures; convulsions; paresthesia; hallucinations; tremulousness.
DERM: Sweating; injection site reactions; flushing.
GI: Nausea; vomiting.
RESP: Dyspnea; respiratory depression; hypoxia.
OTHER: Coma; encephalopathy; withdrawal.

Precautions

Pregnancy: Category B.
Lactation: Undetermined.
Children: May be given IV/IM/SC in children and neonates to reverse the effects of opiates. IM/SC route for opiate intoxication is not endorsed by the American Academy of Pediatrics because absorption may be erratic or delayed. Safety and efficacy in septic shock not established. It is preferable to administer directly to the neonate if needed after delivery.
Elderly: Use with caution because of the greater frequency of decreased hepatic, renal, or cardiac function, and concomitant diseases or other drug therapy.
Renal function impairment: Use with caution.
Hepatic function impairment: Use with caution.
Opiate duration: Because duration of action of some opiates may exceed that of naloxone, keep patients under continuous surveillance.
Postoperative: Abrupt postoperative reversal of opioid depression may result in nausea, vomiting, sweating, tremulousness, tachycardia, increased BP, seizures, ventricular tachycardia and fibrillation, pulmonary edema, and cardiac arrest, which may result in death.
Withdrawal: Use with caution in patients, including neonates of mothers suspected to be physically dependent on opioids because an acute withdrawal syndrome may be precipitated.

Overdosage: Signs and Symptoms

Seizures, severe hypertension, bradycardia, cognitive impairment, behavioral symptoms (including irritability, anxiety, tension, suspiciousness, sadness, difficulty concentrating, lack of appetite), somatic symptoms (including dizziness, heaviness, sweating, nausea, stomachaches).

PATIENT CARE CONSIDERATIONS

Administration/Storage

- For IV, IM, or SC injection.
- Administer prescribed dose via IV route for most rapid onset of action.
- Initial doses may be repeated at 2- to 3-min intervals until desired degree of narcotic reversal is achieved.
- Dilute prescribed dose in normal saline or 5% dextrose solution for IV infusion.
- Do not administer if particulate matter, cloudiness, or discoloration noted.
- Discard any unused solution in single-dose ampule. Do not save for future use.
- Store vials and ampules at controlled room temperature (59°F to 86°F). Protect from light. Use diluted solution for infusion within 24 hr. Discard any unused infusion solution after 24 hr.

Assessment/Interventions

- Obtain patient history, including drug history and any known allergies. Note physical dependence on opioids, renal or hepatic

impairment, cardiac disease, or concurrent use of cardiotoxic medications.
- Ensure that oxygen, resuscitation, and intubation equipment are available for use if needed.
- Continuously assess patient for need of repeat doses.
- Frequently assess opioid-dependent patient for evidence of narcotic withdrawal symptoms (eg, body aches, diarrhea, runny nose, sneezing, piloerection, sweating, yawning). Inform health care provider if noted and significant.
- Frequently assess postoperative patient for evidence of excessive narcotic reversal (eg, loss of pain control, tachycardia, nausea). Inform health care provider immediately if noted and significant.
- Monitor patient for CV, respiratory, and CNS side effects. Report to health care provider if noted and significant.

Patient/Family Education
- Explain name, action, and potential side effects of drug.
- Advise patient or caregiver that medication will be prepared and administered by a health care professional in a medical setting.

Naltrexone Hydrochloride

(nal-TREX-ohn HIGH-droe-KLOR-ide)

Class Narcotic antagonist

How Supplied
ReVia Tablets 50 mg

Action
PHARMACOLOGY: Opioid receptor antagonist, markedly attenuating or completely blocking, reversibly, the subjective effects of IV administered opioids.

PHARMACOKINETICS/DYNAMICS:
Absorption: Rapidly and nearly completely absorbed (96%) from the GI tract.
Distribution: Vd estimated to be 1,350 L. Plasma protein binding 21%.
Metabolism: Over 98% metabolized and extrahepatic sites may exist. The major metabolite is 6-β-naltrexol, which accounts for 43% of an oral dose. There are 2 minor metabolites.
Excretion: Renal Cl of naltrexone ranges from 30 to 127 mL/min, suggesting that renal elimination is primarily glomerular filtration. Urinary excretion of unchanged naltrexone is less than 2%, while urinary excretion of unchanged and conjugated 6-β-naltrexol accounts for 43%. Naltrexone and its metabolites may undergo enterohepatic recirculation.

Indications Treatment of alcohol dependence; blockade of exogenously administered opioids. **Unlabeled use(s):** Eating disorders; postconcussional syndrome unresponsive to other treatments.

Contraindications Patients receiving opioid analgesics; patients currently dependent on opioids, including those maintained on opiate agonists (eg, methadone); patients in acute opioid withdrawal; any individual who has failed the naloxone challenge test or who has positive urine screen for opioids; any individual with acute hepatitis or liver failure; any individual with a history or sensitivity to naloxone or the phenanthrene-containing opioids.

Route/Dosage
Treatment of Alcoholism
ADULTS: **PO** 50 mg once daily for up to 12 wk is sufficient for most patients.

Treatment of Opioid Dependence
ADULTS: **PO** Start with 25 mg; if no withdrawal signs occur, patient may be started on 50 mg daily thereafter. Do not attempt treatment if patient has not remained opioid-free for at least 7 to 10 days or if signs of opioid withdrawal are observed following naloxone challenge.

Interactions
Disulfiram: May increase the risk of hepatotoxicity.
Opioid-containing medication: Because of antagonistic effects of naltrexone, patients may not benefit from opioid medication.
Thioridazine: Lethargy and somnolence have been reported with coadministration of naltrexone.

Lab Test Interferences None well documented.

Adverse Reactions
CNS: Headache (7%); dizziness, fatigue (4%); insomnia (3%); anxiety, somnolence (2%); nervousness, low energy (more than 10%); increased energy, feeling down, irritability, loss of appetite (less than 10%); depression (0% to 15%); suicidal attempt/ideation (0% to 1%).
DERM: Skin rash (less than 10%).
GI: Abdominal cramps (more than 10%); nausea (10%); diarrhea, constipation, vomiting (3%); increased thirst (less than 10%).
GU: Delayed ejaculation, decreased potency (less than 10%).
HEPA: Hepatocellular injury.
MUSC: Joint and muscle pain (more than 10%).

> **WARNING:**
> *Hepatotoxicity:* Naltrexone has capacity to cause hepatocellular injury when given in excessive doses.

Precautions

Pregnancy: Category C.
Lactation: Undetermined.
Children: Safety and efficacy not established.
Abstinence syndrome: To prevent occurrence of an acute abstinence syndrome, patient must be opioid-free for a minimum of 7 to 10 days.
Accidental precipitation of withdrawal: Severe opioid withdrawal syndromes precipitated by accidental ingestion of naltrexone may occur in opioid-dependent individuals. Withdrawal symptoms may appear within 5 min and last 48 hr.
Naloxone challenge: Should not be performed in patients showing clinical signs or symptoms of opioid withdrawal or in patients whose urine contains opioids.
Overcoming blockade: Overcoming the antagonism by taking opioids is dangerous and may lead to fatal overdose.
Rapid opioid withdrawal: Safe use has not been established.
Special risk patients: Use with caution in patients with renal or hepatic impairment.
Suicide: Risk is not abated by naltrexone treatment.

PATIENT CARE CONSIDERATIONS

Administration/Storage

- Dose and frequency of administration are dependent on condition being treated (eg, alcohol dependence, narcotic addiction) and specific patient factors (eg, side effects, compliance issues).
- Administer prescribed dose without regard to meals but administer with food if GI upset occurs.
- Store tablets at controlled room temperature (59° to 86°F).

Assessment/Interventions

- Obtain patient history, including drug history and any known allergies. Note renal impairment, active liver disease, acute hepatitis, liver failure, current dependence on opioids (including opiate maintenance medications such as methadone), acute opioid withdrawal, positive urine screen for opioids, or concurrent use of opioid analgesics.
- Assess patient for occult opioid dependence. If in doubt, perform naloxone challenge test. Do not administer naltrexone until naloxone challenge test is negative.
- Before initiating treatment in patient with narcotic addiction, ensure patient has remained opioid-free for 7 to 10 days, has a negative naloxone challenge test, and is not manifesting signs of, nor reporting symptoms of, narcotic withdrawal.
- To enhance potential success of treatment, ensure the following: good medication compliance is maintained; the patient is involved in a community-based support group; comorbid conditions are appropriately managed.
- Ensure liver function (eg, transaminases, bilirubin, alkaline phosphatase) is evaluated before starting therapy and periodically thereafter based on clinical situation, and dose of naltrexone, for duration of therapy
- Ensure therapy is periodically reviewed to determine if it needs to be continued without change or if a dose change (eg, increase, decrease, discontinuation) is indicated.
- Monitor patient for GI, CNS, PSYCH, MUSC, and general body side effects. Report to health care provider if noted and significant. Immediately report any symptoms or signs suggestive of hepatitis.

Patient/Family Education

- Explain name, dose, action, and potential side effects of drug.
- Advise patient that medication will be most effective when taken exactly as prescribed and combined with participation in a community-based support group.
- Advise patient that dose may be adjusted periodically in order to achieve max benefit.
- Advise patient to take without regard to meals but to take with food if stomach upset occurs.
- Advise patient to carry or wear medical identification (eg, *Medi-Alert*) indicating naltrexone use.
- Advise patient that self-administration of small doses of heroin or any other opiate will not produce noticeable effects. Caution patient that self-administration of large doses of heroin or any other opiate may overcome the naltrexone blockade and can cause coma or death.
- Advise patient that drug may cause dizziness and to use caution while driving or performing other tasks requiring mental alertness and coordination until tolerance is determined.
- Advise patient to stop taking and notify health care provider of any of the following: allergic reaction; stomach pain lasting more that a few days; white bowel movements; dark urine; yellowing of the eyes.

- Advise women to inform health care provider if pregnant, planning to become pregnant, or breastfeeding.
- Instruct patient not to take any prescription or OTC drugs, herbal preparations, or dietary supplements unless advised by health care provider.
- Advise patient that follow-up visits and lab tests may be necessary to monitor therapy and to keep appointments.

Naproxen

(nay-PROX-ehn)
Class Analgesic/NSAID

How Supplied
EC *Naprosyn* Tablets, delayed-release 375 mg, Tablets, delayed-release 500 mg ♦ *Naprosyn* Tablets 250 mg, Tablets 375 mg, Tablets 500 mg, Suspension 125 mg/5 mL
❋ *Apo-Naproxen* ♦ *Apo-Naproxen SR* ♦ *Gen-Naproxen EC* ♦ *Naxen* ♦ *Novo-Naprox* ♦ *Novo-Naprox EC* ♦ *Nu-Naprox* ♦ *ratio-Naproxen*

Naproxen Sodium
Aleve Tablets 200 mg (220 mg naproxen sodium) ♦ *Anaprox* Tablets 250 mg (275 mg naproxen sodium) ♦ *Anaprox DS* Tablets 500 mg (550 mg naproxen sodium) ♦ *Naprelan* Tablets, controlled-release 375 mg (412.5 mg naproxen sodium), Tablets, controlled-release 500 mg (550 mg naproxen sodium)
❋ *Apo-Napro-Na* ♦ *Apo-Napro-Na DS* ♦ *Novo-Naprox Sodium* ♦ *Novo-Naprox SR* ♦ *Novo-Naprox Sodium DS*

Action
PHARMACOLOGY: Decreases inflammation, pain and fever, probably through inhibition of cyclooxygenase activity and prostaglandin synthesis.

PHARMACOKINETICS/DYNAMICS:
Absorption: Naproxen is completely absorbed from the GI tract. Tablet T_{max} is 2 to 4 hr (immediate-release); suspension T_{max} is 1 to 4 hr; fasted patients' T_{max} is 4 to 6 hr (delayed-release); bioavailability is 95%; steady state is reached in 4 to 5 days.
Distribution: Vd is 0.16 L/kg and protein binding is 99% albumin-bound.
Excretion: Naproxen is eliminated in urine (95%), primarily as naproxen less than 1%, 6-0-desmethylnaproxen less than 1%, or their conjugates (66% to 92%). Naproxen t½ is 12 to 17 hr; clearance is 0.13 mL/min/kg; t½ of metabolites and conjugates is less than 12 hr.
Special Populations:
Renal Function Impairment – Metabolites and conjugates may accumulate.

Indications
Rx: Management of mild to moderate pain, symptoms of rheumatoid or osteoarthritis, bursitis, tendonitis, ankylosing spondylitis, primary dysmenorrhea, acute gout. Naproxen (not naproxen sodium) also indicated for treatment of juvenile rheumatoid arthritis. Delayed-release naproxen is not recommended for initial treatment of acute pain because absorption is delayed compared to other naproxen formulations.
OTC: Temporary relief of minor aches and pains associated with the common cold, headache, toothache, muscular aches, backache, minor arthritis pain, pain of menstrual cramps, and reduction of fever. **Unlabeled use(s):** Sunburn, migraine, PMS.

Contraindications
Allergy to aspirin, iodides or any NSAID; patients in whom aspirin or other NSAIDs induce symptoms of asthma, rhinitis or nasal polyps.

Route/Dosage
NAPROXEN
Rheumatoid Arthritis, Osteoarthritis, Ankylosing Spondylitis
ADULTS: PO 250 to 500 mg bid; max dose of 1.5 g/day should be used short term only. Delayed-release: PO 375 to 500 mg bid. Controlled release: PO 750 to 1000 mg qd. Individualize dosage. Do not exceed 1500 mg/day. Suspension: PO 250 mg (10 mL), 375 mg (15 mL), or 500 mg (20 mL) bid.

Pain, Dysmenorrhea, Bursitis, Tendinitis
ADULTS: PO 500 mg initially, then 250 mg q 6 to 8 hr. Do not exceed 1250 mg/day.

Juvenile Rheumatoid Arthritis
CHILDREN: PO 10 mg/kg/day in 2 divided doses. For children requiring suspension, 2.5 mL bid can be given for weights of at least 13 kg; 5 mL bid for weights of at least 25 kg, or 7.5 mL bid for weights of at least 38 kg.

Acute Gout
ADULTS: PO 750 mg, followed by 250 mg q 8 hr until the attack subsides.

NAPROXEN SODIUM
Rheumatoid Arthritis, Osteoarthritis, Ankylosing Spondylitis
ADULTS: PO 275 to 550 mg bid. May increase to 1.65 g for limited periods.

Acute Gout
ADULTS: PO 825 mg initially, then 275 mg q 8 hr prn.
Controlled-release: PO 1000 to 1500 mg once daily on the first day, then 1000 mg once daily until attack has subsided.

Pain, Dysmenorrhea, Tendinitis, Bursitis
ADULTS: PO 500 mg initially, then 275 mg q 6 to 8 hr prn. Do not exceed 1375 mg/day.

Controlled release: **PO** 750 to 1000 mg once daily. Individualize dosage. Do not exceed 1500 mg/day.

Interactions

Anticoagulants: May increase effect of anticoagulants because of decreased plasma protein binding. May increase risk of gastric erosion and bleeding.
Lithium: May decrease lithium clearance.
Methotrexate: May increase methotrexate levels.

Lab Test Interferences

May falsely increase urinary 17-ketosteroid values; may interfere with urinary assays for 5-hydroxy-indoleacetic acid.

Adverse Reactions

CV: Edema; weight gain; CHF; alterations in BP; vasodilation; palpitations; tachycardia; chest pain; bradycardia.
CNS: Headache; dizziness; drowsiness; vertigo; lightheadedness; mental depression; nervousness; irritability; fatigue; malaise; insomnia; sleep disorders; dream abnormalities; aseptic meningitis.
DERM: Rash; urticaria; purpura; skin eruptions.
EENT: Visual changes; tinnitus; rhinitis; pharyngitis; stomatitis.
GI: Constipation; heartburn; abdominal pain; peptic ulceration and bleeding; nausea; dyspepsia; diarrhea; vomiting; anorexia; colitis; flatulence.
GU: Glomerulonephritis; interstitial nephritis; nephrotic syndrome; acute renal insufficiency and renal failure; dysuria; hyperkalemia; hyponatremia; renal papillary necrosis.
HEPA: Increased LFT results.
HEMA: Increased bleeding time; leukopenia; thrombocytopenia; granulocytopenia; eosinophilia; ecchymosis.
RESP: Bronchospasm; laryngeal edema; dyspnea; shortness of breath.

Precautions

Pregnancy: Category B.
Lactation: Excreted in breast milk.
Children: Safety and efficacy in children younger than 2 yr not established (Rx); do not give to children younger than 12 yr except under the advice and supervision of a health care provider (OTC).
Elderly: Increased risk of adverse reactions.
Renal function impairment: Assess function before and during therapy in patients with renal impairment because NSAID metabolites are eliminated renally.
Hepatic function impairment: May need to reduce dose in patients with hepatic failure.
Cardiovascular disease: Drug may worsen CHF and may decrease hypertension control.
Concomitant therapy: Do not use naproxen sodium and naproxen concomitantly; both drugs circulate as naproxen anion.
GI effects: Serious GI toxicity (eg, bleeding, ulceration, perforation) can occur at any time, with or without warning symptoms.

Overdosage: Signs and Symptoms

Drowsiness, nausea, heartburn, vomiting, indigestion, seizures.

PATIENT CARE CONSIDERATIONS

Administration/Storage

- Give with meals, milk, or antacids.
- To facilitate dosing accuracy, for juvenile rheumatoid arthritis use suspension only.
- Store in tightly closed, light-resistant container at room temperature (59° to 86°F).

Assessment/Interventions

- Obtain patient history, including drug history and any known allergies.
- Obtain baseline assessments of pain and ability to perform activities of daily living.
- Review baseline CBC, renal, and hepatic studies, and coagulation studies.
- For patients on long-term therapy, history of GI or renal disease, monitor LFT results, serum creatinine, hematocrit, hemoglobin, and platelets.
- Carefully monitor patients also receiving anticoagulants or thrombolytics. Be alert for GI bleeding.

Patient/Family Education

- Tell patient to take with milk, meals or antacids; follow with ½ to 1 glass of water to reduce GI upset.
- Advise patient to shake oral suspension before measuring.
- Explain that it may take 2 to 4 wk with naproxen and 1 to 2 days with naproxen sodium for anti-inflammatory effects to occur. Peak analgesic effect may occur in 1 to 2 hr.
- Caution patient that use with aspirin, alcohol, steroids and other GI irritants may cause increased GI upset.
- Instruct patient to report the following symptoms to health care provider: visual problems, abdominal pain, symptoms of gastric bleeding.
- Caution patient to avoid intake of alcoholic beverages and smoking.
- Advise patient to use caution while driving or performing other activities that require coordinated motor movements and mental alertness.

Naratriptan

(NAHR-ah-trip-tan)
Class Analgesic/Migraine

How Supplied
Amerge Tablets 1 mg (as hydrochloride), Tablets 2.5 mg (as hydrochloride)

Action
PHARMACOLOGY: Binds to serotonin (5-HT) 1_B and 1_D receptors in intracranial arteries leading to vasoconstriction and subsequent relief of migraine headache.

PHARMACOKINETICS/DYNAMICS:
Absorption: Bioavailability of naratriptan is 70%, AUC is 98 mcg/L•hr, T_{max} is 2 to 3 hr, T_{max} during migraine attack is 3 to 4 hr, and C_{max} is 12.6 mcg/L.
Distribution: Naratriptan Vd is 170 L and protein binding is 28% to 31%.
Metabolism: Naratriptan is metabolized in the liver by CYP450 enzymes to inactive metabolites.
Excretion: Naratriptan is eliminated in urine, 50% unchanged and 30% as metabolites (inactive). The t½ is 6 hr, systemic Cl is 6.6 mL/min/kg, and renal Cl is 220 mL/min.

Special Populations:
Renal Function Impairment – Naratriptan Cl is reduced 50% with moderate impairment (Ccr 18 to 39 mL/min). This resulted in an increase of t½ from 6 to 11 hr, and mean C_{max} was increased about 40%.
Hepatic Function Impairment – Naratriptan Cl is decreased 30%, which resulted in about a 40% increase in the t½ from 8 to 16 hr.
Gender – C_{max} is 50% higher in women.

Indications
Treatment of acute migraine attacks with or without aura.

Contraindications
Patients with history, signs, or symptoms of ischemic heart disease (eg, angina, including Prinzmetal variant, MI, silent myocardial ischemia), cerebrovascular or peripheral vascular syndromes, uncontrolled hypertension, severe renal or hepatic insufficiency, patients with hemiplegic or basilar migraine, or hypersensitivity to any component of the product. Naratriptan is contraindicated within 24 hr of use with other serotonin agonists, ergotamine compounds, or methysergide.

Route/Dosage
ADULTS: PO 1 or 2.5 mg with onset of migraine headache. Dose is individualized based on response and side effects. The dose may be repeated once after 4 hr if partial response or if the headache returns. The max daily dose is 5 mg in 24 hr.

Interactions
5-HT_1 agonists (eg, sumatriptan): Increased risk of vasospastic reactions; therefore, coadministration of two 5-HT_1 agonists within 24 hr of each other is contraindicated.
Ergot-containing drugs: May cause additive, prolonged vasospasm.
Selective serotonin reuptake inhibitors (eg, citalopram, fluoxetine, fluvoxamine, paroxetine, sertraline): Weakness, hyperreflexia, and incoordination have been rarely reported.
Sibutramine: Serotonin syndrome, including CNS irritability, motor weakness, shivering, myoclonus, and altered consciousness may occur.

Lab Test Interferences
None well documented.

Adverse Reactions
CV: Angina, MI (postmarketing).
CNS: Dizziness, drowsiness, malaise/fatigue, paresthesia (2%); vertigo (at least 1%); cerebral vascular accident, including transient ischemic attack, subarachnoid hemorrhage, and cerebral infarction (postmarketing).
EENT: Ear, nose, and throat infections, photophobia (at least 1%).
GI: Nausea (5%); hyposalivation, vomiting (at least 1%); colonic ischemia (postmarketing).
HYPERSEN: Hypersensitivity, including anaphylaxis/anaphylactoid reactions (postmarketing).
RESP: Dyspnea (postmarketing).
OTHER: Atypical sensation (4%); pain and pressure in neck and throat (2%); warm/cold temperature sensation, sensations of pressure, tightness, and heaviness (at least 1%).

Precautions
Pregnancy: Category C.
Lactation: Undetermined.
Children: Safety and efficacy not established.
Elderly: Not recommended.
Hypersensitivity: Hypersensitivity reactions (including anaphylaxis and anaphylactoid reactions) may occur.
Cardiac: May cause coronary vasospasm in patients with coronary artery disease (CAD).
Cerebrovascular events: Cerebral hemorrhage, subarachnoid hemorrhage, stroke, and other cerebrovascular events have been reported with 5-HT_1 agonists.
Hypertensive crisis: Elevation in BP, including hypertensive crisis, have been reported with administration of 5-HT_1 agonists.

Overdosage: Signs and Symptoms
Hypertension, cardiac ischemia, lightheadedness, neck tension, loss of coordination.

PATIENT CARE CONSIDERATIONS

Administration/Storage
- Administer prescribed dose at onset of migraine symptoms.
- Administer without regard to meals.
- Do not administer within 24-hr of treatment with another 5-HT$_1$ agonist or ergot-containing drug.
- If headache recurs after initial relief or if there was only a partial response, a second tablet may be administered, providing there is an interval of at least 4 hr between doses.
- If first dose is ineffective, do not administer a second dose unless prescribed by health care provider.
- Do not administer more than 5 mg per 24-hr period in patient with normal renal function or more than 2.5 mg per 24-hr period in patient with mild to moderate renal impairment or mild to moderate hepatic impairment.
- Store tablets at controlled room temperature (68° to 77°F).

Assessment/Interventions
- Obtain patient history, including drug history and any known allergies. Note renal or hepatic impairment, ischemic or vasospastic CAD, uncontrolled hypertension, peripheral vascular disease, ischemic bowel disease, stroke, transient ischemic attacks, or hemiplegic or basilar migraine.
- Ensure that medication is not administered to patient with severe renal impairment (Ccr less than 15 mL/min) or severe hepatic impairment (Child-Pugh grade C).
- Note recent (within 24 hr) use of other 5-HT$_1$ agonists or ergotamine-containing or ergot-type drugs.
- Assess pain location, intensity, duration, and associated symptoms of migraine attack and response to treatment.
- Provide quiet, calm environment. Decrease stimuli, noise, and light.
- Ensure patients with potential for CAD, including postmenopausal women, men over 40 yr of age, and patients with risk factors for CAD (eg, hypertension, hypercholesterolemia, obesity, diabetes, smokers, family history), undergo a CV evaluation before initiating therapy.
- Administer first dose in physician's office or other adequately staffed medical facility to patient with potential for CAD whose CV evaluation provided clinical evidence that patient is reasonably free of coronary artery and ischemic myocardial disease or other significant underlying CV disease. Consider obtaining an ECG during the interval immediately following administration of the first dose of medication to patient with potential for CAD.
- Monitor patient for signs of allergic reaction. Discontinue therapy and immediately notify health care provider if noted. Be prepared to treat appropriately.
- Ensure that patient who is a long-term user of triptans, such as naratriptan, undergoes periodic CV evaluation.
- Monitor patient for CNS, CV, GI, and general body side effects. Report to health care provider if noted and significant.

Patient/Family Education
- Explain name, dose, action, and potential side effects of drug.
- Advise patient to read the *Patient Information* leaflet before starting therapy and again with each refill.
- Explain that drug is to be used only during migraine and does not prevent or reduce the number of attacks. Emphasize that drug is used only to treat actual migraine attack and should not be used to prevent migraine headaches or treat headaches caused by other conditions.
- Advise patient that drug is to be taken as soon as symptoms of migraine appear. A second dose may be taken if symptoms return, but no sooner than 4 hr following the first dose. For a given attack, if there is no response to the first tablet, do not take a second tablet without first consulting with health care provider. Caution patient not to take more than 2 doses in any 24-hr period.
- Advise patient that safety of treating more than 4 headaches in a 30-day period has not been established and to inform health care provider if headaches are occurring more frequently.
- Advise patient to immediately notify health care provider if any of the following occur after taking a dose of naratriptan: severe chest pain or chest pain that does not go away; sudden and/or severe stomach pain; shortness of breath; wheezing; swelling of eyelids, face, or lips.
- Advise patient that if tightness, pain, pressure, or heaviness in chest, throat, neck, or jaw occur when using sumatriptan, to discuss these symptoms with health care provider before using again.
- Advise patient to notify health care provider if feelings of tingling, heat, flushing, tiredness, dizziness, heaviness, or pressure occur after treatment.

- Advise patient that drug may cause fatigue or dizziness and to use caution while driving or performing other activities requiring mental alertness.
- Advise patient to avoid unnecessary exposure to sunlight or tanning lamps and to use sunscreen and wear protective clothing to avoid photosensitivity reactions.
- Instruct patient to continue taking prescribed migraine prophylactic medications daily as directed.
- Advise patient not currently taking migraine prophylactic drugs to discuss the use of such drugs with health care provider.
- Advise women to notify health care provider if pregnant, planning to become pregnant, or breastfeeding.
- Warn patient not to take any prescription or OTC drugs, dietary supplements, and herbal preparations without consulting health care provider.
- Advise patient that follow-up visits may be necessary to monitor therapy and to keep appointments.

Natamycin

(NAT-uh-MY-sin)
Class Ophthalmic/Anti-infective

How Supplied
Natacyn Suspension 5%

Action
PHARMACOLOGY: Binds to fungal cell membrane, altering membrane permeability and depleting essential cellular constituents.

Indications Treatment of fungal blepharitis, conjunctivitis and keratitis caused by susceptible organisms.

Contraindications Standard considerations.

Route/Dosage
ADULTS: **Ophthalmic** 1 gtt in conjunctival sac q 1 to 2 hr initially; after 3 to 4 days, frequency of instillation usually reduced to 1 gtt 6 to 8 times/day. Continue for 14 to 21 days or until there is resolution of active fungal keratitis.

Interactions None well documented.

Lab Test Interferences None well documented.

Adverse Reactions
EENT: Conjunctival chemosis; hyperemia.

Precautions
Pregnancy: Category C.
Lactation: Undetermined.
Children: Safety and efficacy not established.
Keratitis: Continue medication for 14 to 21 days or until active fungal keratitis has resolved, to avoid recurrence.

PATIENT CARE CONSIDERATIONS

Administration/Storage
- Administer as topical ophthalmic suspension.
- Shake well before administering medication.
- To administer, wash hands thoroughly. Have patient tilt head back. Pull lower eyelid down to create pocket. Place prescribed number of drops in pocket, taking care not to touch eye or allow dropper to touch eye, eyelid or other surfaces. Wash hands again after instillation.
- Store at room temperature (59° to 86°F) or refrigerate. Do not freeze. Protect from light and excessive heat.

Assessment/Interventions
- Obtain patient history, including drug history and any known allergies.
- Obtain the following baseline ophthalmic assessment: presence of pain, visual changes, signs and symptoms that prompted patient to seek treatment.
- Assess for ocular inflammation or irritation. Note presence of discharge, including amount and characteristics.
- Re-evaluate patient regularly for effectiveness of therapy.

Patient/Family Education
- Review proper method of instillation of medication. Instruct patient to clean excessive exudate before instilling drops and to apply light pressure to lacrimal sac for 1 min after drops are instilled.
- Emphasize importance of thorough handwashing before and after instillation and the need to avoid touching of the eye or allowing dropper to touch eye, lids, or other surfaces, to prevent spread of infection to unaffected eye or others.
- Warn patient to avoid scratching, rubbing, or touching eyes.
- Instruct patient to consult health care provider before applying medication while wearing contact lenses.
- Advise patient to notify health care provider if there is no improvement in 7 to 10 days.
- Instruct patient to report conjunctivitis (ie, pain, itching, changes in vision and sense of foreign body in eye) to the health care provider.

Nateglinide

(nah-TEG-lih-nide)
Class Antidiabetic/Meglitinide

How Supplied
Starlix Tablets 60 mg, Tablets 120 mg

Action

PHARMACOLOGY: Lowers blood glucose levels by stimulating insulin secretion from the pancreas.

PHARMACOKINETICS/DYNAMICS:
Absorption: Rapidly absorbed immediately prior to a meal. Oral T_{max} is 1 hr (prior to a meal); bioavailability is approximately 73%. Food delays T_{max} and C_{max}.

Distribution: Nateglinide protein binding is 98% (primarily albumin, lesser extent to alpha$_1$-acid glycoprotein). Vd is 10 L (IV).

Metabolism: Hydroxylation followed by glucuronide conjugation via CYP2C9 (70%) and CYP3A4 (30%).

Excretion: Nateglinide is eliminated in urine (83% as metabolites, 16% as parent compound) and feces (10%). The t½ is 1.5 hr.

Special Populations:
Hepatic Function Impairment – The peak and total exposure of nateglinide were increased 30% (mild hepatic insufficiency). Use with caution (chronic hepatic insufficiency).

Indications
As monotherapy to lower blood glucose in patients with type 2 diabetes mellitus (non-insulin-dependent diabetes mellitus) whose hyperglycemia cannot be adequately controlled by diet and exercise and who have not been chronically treated with other antidiabetic agents; in combination with metformin or a thiazolidinedione, in patients whose hyperglycemia is inadequately controlled with metformin, or after a therapeutic response to a thiazolidinedione. Do not use as a substitute for those drugs.

Contraindications
Type 1 diabetes; diabetic ketoacidosis; hypersensitivity to nateglinide or its ingredients.

Route/Dosage
ADULTS: **PO** 120 mg tid, 1 to 30 min before meals, alone or in combination with metformin or a thiazolidinedione. The 60 mg dose of nateglinide may be used, alone or in combination with metformin or a thiazolidinedione, in patients whose glycosylated hemoglobin (HbA$_{1c}$) is near goal levels when treatment is initiated.

Interactions
Corticosteroids, rifamycins, sympathomimetics, thiazide diuretics, thyroid products: May reduce the hypoglycemic effects of nateglinide.
Fluconazole, MAO inhibitors, nonselective beta-adrenergic blocking agents, NSAIDs, salicylates: May potentiate the hypoglycemic effects of nateglinide.

Lab Test Interferences
Uric acid levels may be increased.

Adverse Reactions
CNS: Dizziness (4%).
GI: Diarrhea (3%).
HYPERSEN: Rash, itching, urticaria (postmarketing).
M/N: Hypoglycemia (2%).
RESP: Upper respiratory tract infection (11%); bronchitis (3%); coughing (2%).
OTHER: Back pain, flu-like symptoms (4%); arthropathy, accidental trauma (3%).

Precautions
Pregnancy: Category C. Insulin is recommended to maintain blood glucose levels during pregnancy.
Lactation: Undetermined.
Children: Safety and efficacy not established.
Hepatic function impairment: Use with caution in patients with moderate to severe or chronic liver disease.
Special risk patients: Patients with type 2 diabetes and renal failure on dialysis may exhibit reduced overall drug exposure.
Secondary failure: Transient loss of glycemic control may occur in patients with fever, infection, trauma, or surgery. At such times, it may be necessary to discontinue nateglinide and administer insulin.

Overdosage: Signs and Symptoms
Exaggerated glucose lowering with hypoglycemic symptoms, coma, seizure, neurological symptoms.

PATIENT CARE CONSIDERATIONS

Administration/Storage
- May be used alone or in combination with metformin or a thiazolidinedione. Not to be used in combination with sulfonylureas or other secretogogues or for the treatment of type 1 diabetes.
- Administer prescribed dose immediately before or up to 30 min before each meal.
- If a meal is skipped, the dose should be skipped to reduce the risk of hypoglycemia.
- Store tablets at controlled room temperature (59° to 86°F). Keep tightly closed.

Assessment/Interventions
- Obtain patient history, including drug history and any known allergies. Note liver disease

and the nature of the patient's diabetes (type 1 vs type 2).
- Check blood sugars frequently and observe for signs of hypoglycemia and hyperglycemia. Inform health care provider if blood sugar readings are outside target range or if hypoglycemic events are noted. Be prepared to treat hypoglycemic reactions.
- Ensure therapy is periodically reviewed to determine if it needs to be continued without change or if a dose change (eg, increase, decrease, discontinuation) is indicated.

Patient/Family Education
- Explain name, dose, action, and potential side effects of drug.
- Advise patient or caregiver to read *Patient Information* leaflet before using the first time and with each refill.
- Instruct patient to take prescribed dose immediately before or up to 30 min before each meal.
- Instruct patient if meal is missed, to skip the dose for that meal to reduce risk of hypoglycemia.
- Educate patient or caregiver regarding diabetes and its management, including target ranges for blood sugar control. Instruct patient or caregiver that this medication is not a substitute for diet and exercise and to continue to follow prescribed regimens.
- Educate patient or caregiver regarding potential long-term complications of diabetes and need for regular general physical and eye examinations.
- Ensure patient or caregiver understands how to use home glucose monitor and has a plan for monitoring and recording blood sugar measurements (eg, log). Advise patient to take log to each visit with health care provider.
- Educate patient regarding value of periodic A_{1c} testing to confirm level of glucose control.
- Review symptoms of hypoglycemia (eg, low blood sugar) and hyperglycemia (eg, high blood sugar), and action plans to undertake in the event either occur.
- Advise patient to discuss with health care provider a plan for managing each of the following situations: medication dosing during intercurrent conditions (eg, vomiting, infection, trauma, stress, sick days); accidental ingestion of too little or too much medication; missed dose of medication; inadequate food intake or a skipped meal; travel across time zones; change in physical activity.
- Instruct patient to notify health care provider if experiencing severe, continuous, or frequent hypoglycemic episodes; hypoglycemic episodes with few or no warning symptoms; or continuous or severe hyperglycemia.
- Advise patient to carry medical identification of diabetes (eg, *Medi-Alert*).
- Advise women to notify health care provider if pregnant, planning to become pregnant, or breastfeeding.
- Instruct patient not to take prescription or OTC drugs, dietary supplements, or herbal preparations without consulting health care provider.
- Advise patient that follow-up visits and lab tests will be required to monitor therapy and to keep appointments.

Nedocromil Sodium

(NEH-doe-KROE-mill SO-dee-uhm)
Class Respiratory inhalant

How Supplied
Alocril Solution, ophthalmic 2% (20 mg/mL) ♦ *Tilade* Aerosol 1.75 mg/actuation

Action
PHARMACOLOGY: Inhibits release of mediators from inflammatory cell types associated with asthma, including histamine from mast cells and betaglucuronidase from macrophages. May also suppress local production of leukotrienes and prostaglandins. Inhibits development of bronchoconstriction responses to inhaled antigen and other challenges such as cold air.

PHARMACOKINETICS/DYNAMICS:
Absorption: Nedocromil sodium bioavailability is 8% to 17%, C_{max} is 1.6 to 2.8 ng/mL, and T_{max} is 5 to 90 min.

Distribution: Plasma protein binding is approximately 89%.

Metabolism: Nedocromil sodium is not metabolized.

Excretion: Nedocromil is eliminated unchanged in urine 64% and feces 36%. The t½ is 1.5 to 3.3 hr.

Indications Maintenance of mild to moderate bronchial asthma; treatment of itching caused by allergic conjunctivitis.

Contraindications Standard considerations.

Route/Dosage
SYMPTOMATIC ADULTS AND CHILDREN (OLDER THAN 12 YR): **Aerosol inhalation** 2 inhalations qid at regular intervals to provide 14 mg/day. May attempt lower frequency of doses in well-controlled patients.

Interactions None well documented.

Lab Test Interferences None well documented.

Adverse Reactions
CNS: Headache.
EENT: Ocular burning; irritation and stinging; unpleasant taste; nasal congestion; conjunctivitis; eye redness; photophobia.
GI: Nausea; vomiting; dyspepsia; abdominal pain.
RESP: Rhinitis; upper respiratory tract infection; asthma.
OTHER: Unpleasant taste.

Precautions
Pregnancy: Category B.

Lactation: Undetermined.
Children: Safety and efficacy in children younger than 6 yr not established (aerosol inhalation). Safety and efficacy in children younger than 3 yr not established (ophthalmic).
Acute bronchospasm: Do not use for reversal of acute bronchospasm, particularly status asthmaticus. However, continue to administer during acute exacerbations, unless patient becomes intolerant to inhaled dosage forms.
Cough/Bronchospasm: If cough or bronchospasm follow inhalation, may need to discontinue.
Dosing interval: Optimal effect depends on administration at regular intervals, even during symptom-free periods.

PATIENT CARE CONSIDERATIONS

Administration/Storage
- Shake container well and invert before activation.
- Clean inhaler at least 2 times/wk.
- Store in light-resistant container at room temperature (59° to 86°F).
- Protect from heat and moisture.

Assessment/Interventions
- Obtain patient history, including drug history and any known allergies.
- Obtain baseline respiratory assessment, carefully documenting any shortness of breath, presence of mucus and breath sounds.

Patient/Family Education
- Ensure appropriate demonstration of how to connect medication and inhalant cartridge. Supply adequate information for home use.
- Provide appropriate demonstration of how to administer inhalant dose.
- Advise patient to increase fluid intake (if not contraindicated) to promote flow of nasal secretions.
- Caution patient to avoid exhaling into mouthpiece to avoid moisture accumulation.
- Tell patient to notify health care provider if coughing and bronchospasm occur with inhalation therapy. Alternative therapy may be needed.
- Explain that therapeutic effect may take about 2 wk.
- Tell patient that nedocromil sodium cannot be substituted for bronchodilator (for acute attacks) or steroids.
- If patient is being tapered from steroids, explain that increased asthmatic symptoms may occur and to notify health care provider if this occurs.
- Demonstrate proper method of cleaning inhaler and remind patient to clean inhaler at least 2 times/wk.
- Tell patient to report any adverse effects.

Nefazodone Hydrochloride

(neff-AZE-oh-dohn HIGH-droe-KLOR-ide)http://www.fda.gov/medwatch/SAFETY/2004/safety04.htm#antidepressants

Class Antidepressant

How Supplied
Serzone Tablets 50 mg, Tablets 100 mg, Tablets 150 mg, Tablets 200 mg, Tablets 250 mg
✽ Apo-Nefazodone ◆ Lin-Nefazodone ◆ Serzone-5HT2

Action
PHARMACOLOGY: Undetermined; inhibits neuronal uptake of serotonin and norepinephrine; antagonizes alpha$_1$-adrenergic receptors.

PHARMACOKINETICS/DYNAMICS:
Absorption: Absorbtion is rapid and complete. Absolute bioavailability is approximately 20%, T_{max} is about 1 hr, and steady state is 4 to 5 days (parent and metabolite). Food delays absorption and decreases bioavailability.

Distribution: Nefazodone is widely distributed in body tissues, including CNS, and exhibits nonlinear kinetics for dose and time. Nefazodone Vd is 0.22 to 0.87 L/kg and plasma protein binding is more than 99%.

Metabolism: Nefazodone is extensively metabolized in the liver by n-dealkylation and aliphatic and aromatic hydroxylation. Three active metabolites are hydroxynefazodone (HO-NEF), meta-chlorophenylpiperazine (mCPP), and triazole-dione.

Excretion: Nefazodone is eliminated in urine (less than 1% excreted as unchanged) and feces. The t½ is 2 to 4 hr (parent compound), 1.5 to 4 hr (HO-NEF), 4 to 8 hr (mCPP), and 18 hr (triazole-dione).

Special Populations:
Elderly – C_{max} and AUC for nefazodone and HO-NEF were twice as high. Initiate at half the dose, especially in elderly women.

Gender – Nefazodone has a higher C_{max} and AUC in women in single dose, but no difference after multiple doses.

Liver Cirrhosis – AUC for nefazodone and HO-NEF at steady state were approximately 25% greater.

Indications Treatment of depression.

Contraindications Coadministration with carbamazepine, cisapride, or pimozide; hypersensitivity to nefazodone or other phenylpiperazine antidepressants (eg, trazodone).

Route/Dosage
ADULTS: PO 100 mg bid initially; increase by 100 to 200 mg increments q wk (max, 600 mg/day).

ELDERLY AND DEBILITATED PATIENTS: PO 50 mg bid initially; increase by 100 mg increments q wk (max, 600 mg/day).

Interactions
Benzodiazepines: Increased plasma concentrations and effects of alprazolam and triazolam.

Buspirone: Elevated buspirone concentrations and decreased buspirone metabolite plasma concentrations.

Carbamazepine: Elevated serum carbamazepine concentrations with possible increase in side effects may occur.

Cisapride: Increased cisapride plasma concentrations with cardiotoxicity may occur.

Digoxin: Increased plasma levels of digoxin.

Haloperidol: Decreased haloperidol clearance; may need to adjust haloperidol dose.

HMG-CoA reductase inhibitors (eg, simvastatin): The risk of rhabdomyolysis occurrence may be increased.

MAO inhibitors: Do not use nefazodone concurrently or within 14 days of discontinuing a MAO inhibitors; do not start MAO inhibitors within 1 wk of stopping nefazodone.

Pimozide: Increased plasma concentrations of pimozide may occur associated with QT prolongation and rare cases of serious cardiovascular adverse events, including death, principally caused by ventricular tachycardia of the torsades de pointes type.

Propranolol: Nefazodone may decrease propranolol serum concentration; propranolol may interfere with nefazodone metabolism.

St. John's wort: Increased sedative-hypnotic effects may occur.

Sibutramine, sumatriptan, trazodone: Serotonin syndrome, including irritability, increased muscle tone, shivering, myoclonus, and altered consciousness may occur.

Lab Test Interferences None well documented.

Adverse Reactions
CV: Postural hypotension, vasodilation (4%); hypotension (2%); sinus bradycardia (1.5%).
CNS: Headache (36%); somnolence (28%); dizziness (22%); asthenia, insomnia (11%); lightheadedness (10%); confusion (8%); memory impairment, paresthesia (4%); abnormal dreams, decreased concentration (3%); ataxia, incoordination, psychomotor retardation, tremor (2%); hypertonia, decreased libido (1%); convulsions (postmarketing).
DERM: Pruritus, rash (2%); Stevens-Johnson syndrome (postmarketing).
EENT: Abnormal vision (10%); blurred vision (9%); pharyngitis (6%); tinnitus (3%); taste perversion, visual field defect (2%).
GI: Dry mouth (25%); nausea (23%); constipation (17%); dyspepsia (9%); diarrhea (8%); increased appetite (5%); nausea and vomiting (2%); gastroenteritis (at least 1%).
GU: Urinary frequency, UTI, urinary retention, vaginitis (2%); breast pain (1%); impotence (at least 1%); gynecomastia (male), priapism (postmarketing).
HEMA: Thrombocytopenia (postmarketing).
HEPA: Liver necrosis, liver failure (postmarketing).
LABTESTABS: Decreased hematocrit (3%).
METAB: Peripheral edema (3%); thirst (1%); galactorrhea, hyponatremia increased prolactin (postmarketing).
MUSC: Arthralgia (1%).
RESP: Increased cough (3%); dyspnea, bronchitis (at least 1%).
OTHER: Infection (8%); flu-like syndrome (3%); chills, fever (2%); neck rigidity (1%); anaphylactic reactions, angioedema, serotonin syndrome (postmarketing).

> **WARNING:**
> Life-threatening cases of hepatic failure have been reported. Counsel patient about and immediately report signs of liver dysfunction. Do not initiate therapy in patients with active liver disease or elevated baseline serum transaminases. There is no evidence that preexisting liver disease increases risk of liver failure, but it can complicate patient monitoring. Withdraw therapy and do not consider retreatment if serum AST or ALT is 3 times the upper limit of normal or more.

Precautions

Pregnancy: Category C.
Lactation: Undetermined.
Children: Safety and efficacy not established.
Elderly: Initiate treatment at half the usual dose. Dosage range same as younger patients.
Bradycardia: Sinus bradycardia reported in 1.5% of patients; use with caution in patients with recent MI or unstable heart disease.

Mania/Hypomania: May activate mania/hypomania; use with caution in patients with history of mania.
Postural hypotension: Use with caution in patients with known cardiovascular or cerebrovascular disease that could be exacerbated by hypotension (eg, history of MI, angina, ischemic stroke) and conditions that would predispose to hypotension (eg, dehydration, hypovolemia, treatment with antihypertensive medications).
Priapism: Priapism (eg, prolonged, painful, inappropriate penile erection) has been reported with closely related antidepressants. Discontinuation of therapy is necessary.
Seizures: Rare cases of petit mal and grand mal seizures reported.
Suicide: Closely monitor patients at risk, and do not give them access to excessive quantities.
Visual disturbances: Visual disturbances, including blurred vision, scotoma, and visual trails reported.

Overdosage: Signs and Symptoms

Nausea, vomiting, somnolence.

PATIENT CARE CONSIDERATIONS

Administration/Storage

- Do not administer with, or within 14 days of MAO inhibitor administration.
- Do not administer to patients with clinical evidence of active liver disease or elevated liver enzymes (ALT more than 3 times upper limit of normal).
- Administer prescribed dose bid without regard to meals. Administer with food if GI upset occurs.
- Store tablets at controlled room temperature (59° to 86°F).

Assessment/Interventions

- Obtain patient history, including drug history and any known allergies. Determine whether any MAO inhibitors have been used in the past 14 days. Note liver disease, cardiovascular disease, cerebrovascular disease, recent MI, or current use of cisapride, pimozide, carbamazepine, triazolam, or antihypertensive therapy.
- Ensure that elderly patient receives a reduced initial dose.
- Ensure that liver enzymes are determined before starting therapy and periodically during therapy.
- Ensure that increases in dose are made no more frequently than q 7 days.
- Continue suicide monitoring of high-risk patients.
- Observe for signs of mood change and report to physician.
- Assess patient for evidence of liver dysfunction (nausea, vomiting, abdominal pain, fatigue, anorexia, dark urine, and/or or yellowing of the skin or eyes) and notify health care provider immediately if noted.
- Monitor and record BP and pulse periodically during treatment. If symptomatic hypotension (eg, postural hypotension) develops, notify health care provider.
- Assess patient for CNS, GI, psychiatric, musculoskeletal, GU, and general body side effects. Report to health care provider if noted and significant.

Patient/Family Education

- Explain name, dose, action, and potential side effects of drug.
- Advise patient to read Patient Information leaflet before starting therapy and with each refill.
- Advise patient that medication will be started at a low dose and then gradually increased as tolerated until max benefit is obtained.
- Advise patient to take prescribed dose bid without regard to meals but to take with food if stomach upset occurs.
- Advise patient that if a dose is missed to skip that dose and take the next dose at the regularly scheduled time. Caution patient to never take 2 doses at the same time.
- Advise patient not to change the dose or stop taking unless advised by health care provider.
- Inform patient that it may take 1 to 4 wk to note improvement in symptoms and to con-

tinue with the prescribed therapy once improvement has been noted.
- Advise patient to take frequent sips of water, suck on ice chips or sugarless hard candy, or chew sugarless gum if dry mouth occurs.
- Advise patient to avoid alcoholic beverages.
- Advise patient that drug may cause drowsiness or impair judgment, thinking, or reflexes and to use caution while driving or performing other tasks requiring mental alertness until tolerance is determined.
- Advise patient to immediately report any of the following to health care provider: nausea, vomiting, abdominal pain, fatigue, anorexia, dark urine, yellowing of the skin or eyes, seizure, or fainting.
- Advise patient to contact health care provider if rash, hives, or other symptoms of an allergic reaction develop, if a painful or prolonged erection occurs, or if experiencing bothersome side effects such as visual disturbances, headache, insomnia, or drowsiness.
- Instruct patient not to take prescription or OTC drugs or dietary supplements unless advised by health care provider.
- Advise women to notify health care provider if pregnant, planning to become pregnant, or breastfeeding.
- Advise patient that follow-up visits will be necessary to monitor therapy and to keep appointments.

Nelfinavir Mesylate

(nell-FIN-ah-veer)
Class Antiretroviral/Protease inhibitor

How Supplied
Viracept Tablets 250 mg, Powder 50 mg/g

Action
PHARMACOLOGY: Inhibits human immunodeficiency virus (HIV) protease, the enzyme required to form functional proteins in HIV-infected cells.

PHARMACOKINETICS/DYNAMICS:
Absorption: Food increased maximum plasma concentration and AUC by 2- to 3-fold. T_{max} was 2 to 4 hr and C_{max} was 3 to 4 hr.
Distribution: Nelfinavir's Vd is 2 to 7 L/kg and protein binding is greater than 98%.
Metabolism: Nelfinavir is metabolized by multiple cytochrome P450 isoforms, including CYP3A. Major metabolite has activity comparable to parent drug.
Excretion: The t½ is 3.5 to 5 hr; 87% excreted in feces (78% metabolites, 22% unchanged) and 1% to 2% in urine (unchanged).

Indications
Treatment of HIV infection in combination with other antiretroviral agents.

Contraindications
Hypersensitivity to nelfinavir or any component of the product. Concomitant therapy with amiodarone, ergot derivatives, quinidine, lovastatin, midazolam, pimozide, simvastatin, and triazolam.

Route/Dosage
ADULTS AND CHILDREN (OLDER THAN 13 YR): PO 1250 mg bid or 750 mg tid in combination with nucleoside analogs.
CHILDREN (2 TO 13 YR): PO 20 to 30 mg/kg/dose tid.

Interactions
Alprazolam, clorazepate, diazepam, estazolam, flurazepam, midazolam, triazolam, zolpidem: Nelfinavir may increase blood levels of these drugs, which may produce extreme sedation and respiratory depression. Do not coadminister.
Amiodarone, cisapride, cyclosporine, lovastatin, pimozide, quinidine, rifabutin, sildenafil, simvastatin, sirolimus, tacrolimus: Nelfinavir may elevate blood levels of these drugs, which may increase the risk of arrhythmias or other potential serious adverse effects.
Carbamazepine, phenobarbital, St. John's wort: May decrease nelfinavir plasma concentrations.
Indinavir: Nelfinavir may increase indinavir blood levels.
Indinavir, ritonavir: May increase nelfinavir plasma concentrations.
Methadone: May decrease methadone concentration.
Oral contraceptives: Concentrations of ethinyl estradiol, a component of oral contraceptives, may be reduced.
Phenytoin: Nelfinavir may decrease blood levels of phenytoin.
Rifabutin: May increase rifabutin concentration and decrease nelfinavir concentration.
Rifampin: May decrease plasma concentrations of nelfinavir.

Lab Test Interferences
None well documented.

Adverse Reactions
CNS: Headache; paresthesia; dizziness; insomnia; somnolence; anxiety; depression; seizures; emotional lability; hyperkinesia; migraine; sleep disorder.
DERM: Rash (2%); pruritus; sweating; urticaria; dermatitis folliculitis.
EENT: Pharyngitis; rhinitis; sinusitis; acute iritis; eye disorder.

GI: Anorexia; diarrhea (20%); dyspepsia; flatulence; nausea (3%); vomiting; abdominal pain; pancreatitis; bleeding; mouth ulcerations.
GU: Sexual dysfunction; kidney calculus; urine abnormality.
HEMA: Anemia; leukopenia; thrombocytopenia.
HEPA: Hepatitis.
METAB: Increased alkaline phosphatase; LFTs; creatine phosphokinase; hyperlipidemia; amylase; lactic dehydrogenase; hyperuricemia; hyperglycemia; hypoglycemia; dehydration; gamma glutamyl transpeptidase.
RESP: Dyspnea.
OTHER: Asthenia; fever; myalgia; back pain; malaise; arthralgia; myasthenia; myopathy; accidental injury; allergic reaction; arthralgia; cramps.

Precautions
Pregnancy: Category B.

PATIENT CARE CONSIDERATIONS
Administration/Storage
- Administer with food.
- The oral powder may be mixed with a small amount of water, milk, formula, soy formula, soy milk, or dietary supplement (eg, *Ensure*). Once mixed, consume the entire contents to obtain full dose. If mixture is not consumed immediately, it must be stored under refrigeration and used within 6 hr of mixing.
- Do not mix oral powder with acidic food or juice (eg, orange juice, apple juice, apple sauce) because of bitter taste.
- Store tablets and powder at room temperature (59° to 86°F).

Assessment/Interventions
- Obtain patient history, including drug history and any known allergies. Note hepatic function impairment, phenylketonuria, or diabetes.
- Obtain baseline triglycerides, ALT, AST, GGT, CPK, blood sugar, and uric acid. Monitor periodically during treatment.
- Monitor HCT, HGB, WBC, and differential. Note any significant change.
- Monitor patient for diarrhea, the most frequent side effect. This may be treated with OTC antidiarrheals such as loperamide.

Patient/Family Education
- Advise patient to take medication exactly as prescribed, including taking each dose with food to increase absorption.
- Warn patient not to alter dose or discontinue the medication without consulting health care provider.

Lactation: Undetermined. HIV-infected mothers should not breastfeed their infants.
Children: Safety and efficacy not established for children younger than 2 yr.
Hepatic function impairment: Use caution in patients with hepatic impairment; decreased nelfinavir clearance may occur.
Diabetes: New onset diabetes and exacerbation of pre-existing diabetes mellitus has been reported in postmarking surveillance.
Fat redistribution: Redistribution/accumulation of body fat has been observed in patients receiving antiretroviral therapy.
Hemophilia: There have been reports of increased bleeding, including skin hematomas and hemarthrosis in patients with hemophilia type A and B treated with protease inhibitors. A causal relationship not established.
Phenylketonuria: Nelfinavir powder contains 11.2 mg phenylalanine/g of powder.

- Advise patient that if a dose is missed, to take it as soon as possible and then return to normal dose. However, if a dose is skipped, the patient should not double the next dose.
- Instruct patient not to take any other medications, including OTC medications, without checking with health care provider. This medication interacts with a wide range of all types of medications.
- Explain that the patient will be required to have frequent follow-up blood and urine tests during the course of treatment and to keep appointments.
- Inform patient that this medication is not a cure for HIV infection and that the patient may continue to acquire secondary illnesses associated with the disease.
- Emphasize to patient, family, and significant others that this medication does not reduce the risk of transmitting HIV to others through sexual contact or blood contamination.
- Inform patient that diarrhea is the most common adverse effect and that it can usually be controlled by OTC antidiarrheals such as loperamide.
- Inform patient to report serious or bothersome side effects to the health care provider.
- Explain that the long-term effects of this medication are not known at this time.
- Inform patients taking oral contraceptives that alternate or additional contraceptive measures should be used during therapy with nelfinavir.

Neomycin Sulfate

(NEE-oh-MY-sin SULL-fate)
Class Anti-infective/Aminoglycoside

How Supplied
Neomycin Sulfate Tablets 500 mg ♦ *Neo-fradin* Oral solution 125 mg per 5 mL

Action
PHARMACOLOGY: Inhibits production of protein in bacteria, causing bacterial cell death.

PHARMACOKINETICS/DYNAMICS:
Absorption: Poorly absorbed from the GI tract (3%).

Distribution: Small amount absorbed is rapidly distributed to the tissues. Removed by dialysis.

Excretion: Small fraction absorbed is eliminated by the kidney. The unabsorbed portion (97%) is eliminated unchanged in the feces.

Indications
As adjunctive treatment for suppression of normal bacterial flora of the bowel (tablet); as adjunctive therapy in hepatic coma to reduce ammonia-forming bacteria in the intestinal tract (tablet and solution).

Contraindications
Patients with intestinal obstruction; inflammatory or ulcerative GI disease; history of sensitivity to aminoglycosides or any component of the product.

Route/Dosage
Hepatic Coma
ADULTS: PO 4 to 12 g/day in divided doses. Treatment should be continued over a period of 5 to 6 days.

Preoperative Prophylaxis
ADULTS: PO As part of a bowel preparation regimen, 1 g of neomycin and 1 g of erythromycin are given orally on pre-op day 1 at 1 PM, 2 PM, and 11 PM.

Interactions
Aminoglycosides, polymyxins, neurotoxic or nephrotoxic agents: Neomycin ototoxicity or nephrotoxicity may be enhanced.
Anticoagulants (eg, warfarin): May increase the anticoagulant effects by decreasing vitamin K availability.
Digoxin, fluorouracil, methotrexate, penicillin V, vitamin B-12: Intestinal absorption of these agents may be inhibited by neomycin.

Potent diuretics (eg, ethacrynic acid, furosemide): When administered IV, diuretics may enhance neomycin toxicity by altering the concentration in serum and tissue.

Lab Test Interferences
None well documented.

Adverse Reactions
EENT: Ototoxicity.
GI: Nausea; vomiting; diarrhea.
GU: Nephrotoxicity.
METAB: Malabsorption syndrome.
MUSC: Neuromuscular blockade.

> **WARNING:**
> Systemic absorption of neomycin occurs after oral administration, and toxic reactions may occur (eg, ototoxicity, nephrotoxicity). Neuromuscular blockade and respiratory paralysis have been reported. The risk of toxicity may be increased by dehydration or advanced age.

Precautions
Pregnancy: Category D.
Lactation: Undetermined.
Children: Safety and efficacy not established.
Renal function impairment: If renal insufficiency develops during oral therapy, consider reducing the neomycin dose or discontinuing therapy.
Special risk patients: Use with caution in patients with muscular disorders (eg, myasthenia gravis, parkinsonism) because neomycin may aggravate muscle weakness.
Superinfection: Prolonged or repeated use may result in bacterial or fungal overgrowth of nonsusceptible organisms and secondary infections.
Bile acid: Bile acid fecal excretion may be increased.
Hearing loss: Risk may continue after drug withdrawal.
Lactase: Intestinal lactase activity may be reduced.
Malabsorption syndrome: Oral neomycin (12 g/day) produces malabsorption of a variety of substances including fat, nitrogen, cholesterol, carotene, glucose, xylose, lactose, sodium, calcium, cyanocobalamin, and iron.

Overdosage: Signs and Symptoms
Neurotoxicity, ototoxicity, nephrotoxicity.

PATIENT CARE CONSIDERATIONS
Administration/Storage
- Administer prescribed dose without regard to meals. Administer with food if GI upset occurs.
- Store tablets at controlled room temperature (68° to 77°F). Store oral solution at ambient room temperature (59° to 86°F).

Oral Solution:
- For oral use only. Not for injection or topical use.

Assessment/Interventions
- Obtain patient history, including drug history and any known allergies. Note hepatic or renal impairment, dehydration, intestinal

obstruction, inflammatory or ulcerative GI disease, muscular disorder (eg, myasthenia gravis, Parkinson disease), history of hypersensitivity or serious toxic reaction to other aminoglycoside antibiotics, or concurrent use of loop diuretics or drugs with nephrotoxic or neurotoxic potential.
- Ensure that erythromycin is administered concurrently when using neomycin tablets for preoperative preparation of bowel.
- Ensure that urinalysis, renal function tests, and audiometric and vestibular testing are performed prior to and periodically during prolong therapy.
- Document baseline neurologic function in patient with hepatic coma. Reassess periodically to document response to therapy.
- Monitor patient for neuromuscular blockage and respiratory paralysis. Inform health care provider immediately if noted and be prepared to treat appropriately (eg, respiratory assistance, IV calcium salts).
- Monitor patient for GI and general body side effects. Inform health care provider if noted and significant. Immediately report ringing in the ears, hearing loss, vestibular symptoms (eg, vertigo, ataxia), severe diarrhea, muscle twitching, numbness, skin tingling, or loose, foul-smelling stools.

Patient/Family Education
- Explain name, dose, action, and potential side effects of drug.
- Review dosing schedule and prescribed length of therapy with patient.
- Advise patient to take each dose without regard to meals but to take with food if stomach upset occurs.
- Remind patient to complete entire course of therapy.
- Caution patient not to change the dose or discontinue therapy unless advised by health care provider.
- Warn patient that diarrhea containing blood or pus may be a sign of a serious disorder and to seek medical care if noted and not treat at home.
- Advise patient to contact health care provider immediately if experiencing ringing in the ears, hearing loss, vestibular symptoms (eg, dizziness, incoordination), severe diarrhea, muscle twitching, numbness, skin tingling, or loose, foul-smelling stools.
- Advise women to notify health care provider if pregnant, planning to become pregnant, or breastfeeding.
- Instruct patient not to take any prescription or OTC medications, dietary supplements, or herbal preparations unless advised by health care provider.
- Advise patient that follow-up examinations and lab tests will be required to monitor therapy and to keep appointments.

Neomycin/Polymyxin B Sulfates/Bacitracin Zinc

(NEE-oh-MY-sin/pal-ee-MIX-in BEE SULL-fates/Bass-ih-TRAY-sin zingk)

Class Antibiotic

How Supplied
Neosporin Ophthalmic Ointment 10,000 units/g polymixin B sulfate, 3.5 mg/g neomycin, and 400 units/g bacitracin zinc
🌺 Neosporin Ointment

Action
PHARMACOLOGY:
Prednisolone: Depresses formation, release, and activity of endogenous mediators of inflammation including prostaglandins, kinins, histamine, liposomal enzymes, and complement system.
Neomycin: Inhibits protein synthesis by binding to ribosomal RNA, causing bacterial genetic code misreading.
Polymyxin B: Interacts with phospholipid components of bacterial cell membrane, increasing cell wall permeability.

Indications Treatment of steroid-responsive inflammatory ocular conditions for which a corticosteroid is indicated and where bacterial infection or a risk of bacterial ocular infection exists; inflammatory conditions of the palpebral and bulbar conjunctiva, cornea, and anterior segment of the globe where the inherent risk of steroid use in certain infective conjunctivitis is accepted to obtain a diminution in edema and inflammation; chronic anterior uveitis and corneal injury from chemical, radiation, or thermal burns or penetration of foreign bodies; when risk of infection is high or where there is expectation that potentially dangerous numbers of bacteria will be present in the eye.

Contraindications Epithelial herpes simplex keratitis (dendritic keratitis), vaccinia, varicella, and many other viral diseases of the corneal and conjunctiva; mycobacterial eye infections; fungal diseases of the ocular structures; uncomplicated removal of a corneal foreign body; hypersensitivity to any component of the product.

Route/Dosage
Eye: OPHTHALMIC Instill 1 or 2 gtt in the

eye q 3 or 4 hr or more frequently as required. Acute infections may require administration every 30 min, with decreasing frequency as the infection is brought under control.
Lids: **OPHTHALMIC** Instill 1 or 2 gtt in the eye q 3 to 4 hr, close the eye, and rub the excess on the lids and lid margins.

Interactions None well documented.

Lab Test Interferences None well documented.

Adverse Reactions
EENT: Elevated IOP with possible development of glaucoma; optic nerve damage; posterior subcapsular cataract formation; delayed wound healing; secondary infection; fungal infection; acute anterior uveitis and perforation of the globe.
OTHER: Allergic sensitivity.

Precautions
Pregnancy: Category C.
Lactation: Excreted in breast milk.
Children: Safety and efficacy have not been established.
Superinfection: Prolonged use may result in bacterial or fungal overgrowth of nonsusceptible microorganisms.
Cross-sensitivity: Allergic cross-sensitivity to kanamycin, paromomycin, streptomycin, and, possibly, gentamicin may occur.
Glaucoma: Prolonged use may result in glaucoma with damage to the optic nerve, defects in visual acuity and fields of vision, and posterior subcapsular cataract formation.
Secondary infection: Secondary bacterial ocular infection following suppression of host responses may occur.

PATIENT CARE CONSIDERATIONS
Administration/Storage
- For ophthalmic use only. Not for use in the ears or on the skin.
- Shake well before instilling gtt.
- Instill 1 to 2 gtt into conjunctival sac(s) as prescribed.
- Do not allow tip of dropper bottle to touch eye, eyelid, fingers, or any other surface.
- If using other topical ophthalmic medications, instill drops first, wait at least 5 min, and instill ointment last.
- Store at controlled room temperature (less than 77°F). Keep bottle tightly capped and protect from freezing.

Assessment/Interventions
- Obtain patient history, including drug history and any known allergies. Note history of viral, mycobacterial, or fungal infection of the eye(s).
- Monitor patient's response to therapy. Notify health care provider if eye or eyelid inflammation is noted or if symptoms do not improve or worsen.
- Ensure that intraocular pressure is measured if therapy is continued beyond 10 days.

Patient/Family Education
- Explain name, dose, action, and potential side effects of drug.
- Review prescribed dosing schedule with patient, family, or caregiver.
- Remind patient, family, or caregiver that suspension is for use in the eye only.
- Teach patient, family, or caregiver proper technique for instilling suspension: wash hands; do not allow tip of dropper bottle to touch eye, eyelid, fingers, or any other surface. Tilt head back, look up; pull lower eyelid down to form pocket; place prescribed number of drops in the pocket. Look downward before closing eye. Do not rub eye.
- Advise patient, family, or caregiver that if more than 1 topical ophthalmic drug is being used, instill eye drops first, wait at least 5 min and then instill ointment last.
- Inform patient that temporary blurred vision and stinging of the eye are the most common side effects and to contact health care provider if these symptoms occur and are bothersome.
- Advise patient to contact eye doctor if eye or eyelid inflammation is noted or if eye symptoms do not improve or worsen.
- Advise patient that the entire course of therapy must be completed to ensure maximal benefit and to complete full course of therapy even if symptoms have resolved.
- Instruct patient not to wear contact lenses during treatment.
- Remind patient, family, or caregiver that follow-up eye examinations may be necessary while using this medication and to keep appointments.

Neomycin Sulfate/Polymyxin B Sulfate/Dexamethasone

(NEE-oh-MY-sin SULL-fate/pahl-ee-MIX-in BEE SULL-fate/DEX-uh-METH-uh-sone)

Class Antibacterial/Corticosteroid

How Supplied
AK-Trol Ointment 0.1% dexamethasone, neomycin sulfate equivalent to 0.35% neomycin base, and 10,000 units polymyxin B sulfate, Ophthalmic Suspension 0.1% dexamethasone, neomycin sulfate equivalent to 0.35% neomycin base, and 10,000 units/mL polymyxin B sulfate
◆ Dexacine Ointment 0.1% dexamethasone, neomycin sulfate equivalent to 0.35% neomycin base, and 10,000 units polymyxin B sulfate ◆
Maxitrol Ophthalmic Suspension 0.1% dexamethasone, neomycin sulfate equivalent to 0.35% neomycin base, and 10,000 units/mL polymyxin B sulfate

Action
PHARMACOLOGY:
Neomycin: Inhibits protein synthesis by binding to ribosomal RNA, causing bacterial genetic code misreading.
Polymyxin B: Interacts with phospholipid components of bacterial cell membranes, increasing cell wall permeability.
Dexamethasone: Depresses formation, release, and activity of endogenous mediators of inflammation including prostaglandins, kinins, histamine, liposomal enzymes, and complement systems.

Indications Treatment of steroid-responsive inflammatory ocular conditions for which a corticosteroid is indicated and where bacterial infection or a risk of bacterial ocular infection exists; inflammatory conditions of the palpebral and bulbar conjunctiva, cornea, and anterior segment of the globe where the inherent risk of steroid use in certain infective conjunctivitis is accepted to obtain a diminution in edema and inflammation; chronic anterior uveitis and corneal injury from chemical, radiation, or thermal burns or penetration of foreign bodies; when risk of infection is high or where there is expectation that potentially dangerous numbers of bacteria will be present in the eye.

Contraindications Epithelial herpes simplex keratitis (dendritic keratitis), vaccine, vericella, and many other viral diseases of the corneal and conjunctiva; mycobacterial eye infections; fungal diseases of the ocular structures; uncomplicated removal of a corneal foreign body; hypersensitivity to any component of the product.

Route/Dosage
OPHTHALMIC Suspension Instill 1 or 2 drops into the conjunctival sac(s) up to 4 to 6 times/day in mild disease. In severe disease, drops may be used hourly, tapering to discontinuation as the inflammation subsides.
OPHTHALMIC Ointment Apply a small amount (eg, ½ inch) into the conjunctival sac(s) up to tid or qid.

Interactions None well documented.

Lab Test Interferences None well documented.

Adverse Reactions
EENT: Elevated intraocular pressure (IOP) with possible development of glaucoma; optic nerve damage; posterior subcapsular cataract formation; delayed wound healing; secondary infection; fungal infection.
OTHER: Allergic hypersensitivity.

Precautions
Pregnancy: Category C.
Lactation: Undetermined.
Children: Safety and efficacy have not been established.
Superinfection: Prolonged use may result in bacterial or fungal overgrowth of nonsusceptible microorganisms.
Glaucoma: Prolonged use may result in glaucoma with damage to the optic nerve, defects in visual acuity and fields of vision, and in posterior subcapsular cataract formation.
Secondary infection: Secondary bacterial ocular infection following suppression of host responses may occur.

PATIENT CARE CONSIDERATIONS

Administration/Storage
- For ophthalmic use only. Not for use in the ears or on the skin.
- Shake well before instilling drops.
- Instill 1 to 2 drops into conjunctival sac(s) as prescribed.
- Instill prescribed amount of ointment as ordered.
- Do not allow tip of dropper bottle or tube to touch eye, eyelid, fingers, or any other surface.
- If using other topical ophthalmic medications, instill drops first, wait at least 5 min, and instill ointment last.
- Store at controlled room temperature (59° to 86°F). Keep bottle or tube tightly capped.

Assessment/Interventions
- Obtain patient history, including drug history and any known allergies. Note history of

viral, mycobacterial, or fungal infection of the eye(s).
- Monitor patient's response to therapy. Notify health care provider if eye or eyelid inflammation is noted or if symptoms do not improve or worsen.
- Ensure that IOP is measured if therapy is continued beyond 10 days.

Patient/Family Education
- Explain name, dose, action, and potential side effects of drug.
- Review prescribed dosing schedule with patient, family, or caregiver.
- Remind patient, family, or caregiver that suspension and ointment are for use in the eye only.
- Teach patient, family, or caregiver proper technique for instilling suspension: wash hands; do not allow tip of dropper bottle to touch eye, eyelid, fingers, or any other surface. Tilt head back and look up; pull lower eyelid down to form pocket; place prescribed number of drops in the pocket. Look downward before closing eye. Do not rub eye.
- Teach patient or caregiver proper technique for instilling ointment: wash hands; do not allow tip of tube to touch eye, eyelid, fingers, or any other surface. Tilt head back and look up; pull lower eyelid down to form pocket; place prescribed amount of ointment in the pocket. Look downward before closing eye. Do not rub eye.
- Advise patient, family, or caregiver that if more than 1 topical ophthalmic drug is being used, instill eye drops first, wait at least 5 min, and then instill ointment last.
- Inform patient that temporary blurred vision and stinging of the eye are the most common side effects and to contact health care provider if occurring and bothersome.
- Advise patient to contact eye doctor if eye or eyelid inflammation is noted or if eye symptoms do not improve or worsen.
- Advise patient that the entire course of therapy must be completed to ensure maximal benefit and to complete full course of therapy even if symptoms have resolved.
- Instruct patient not to wear contact lenses during treatment.
- Remind patient, family, or caregiver that follow-up eye examinations may be necessary while using this medication and to keep appointments.

Neomycin Sulfate/Polymyxin B Sulfate/Gramicidin

(NEE-oh-MY-sin SULL-fate/pahl-ee-MIX-in BEE SULL-fate/gram-ih-SIGH-din)

Class Antibacterial

How Supplied
Neosporin Ophthalmic Solution 10,000 units/mL polymyxin B sulfate, 1.75 mg/mL neomycin, and 0.025 mg/mL gramicidin

✤ *Neosporin Eye and Ear Solution* ◆ *Optimyxin Plus Solution*

Action
PHARMACOLOGY:
Neomycin: Inhibits protein synthesis by binding to ribosomal RNA, causing bacterial genetic code misreading.
Polymyxin B: Interacts with phospholipid components of bacterial cell membranes, increasing cell wall permeability.
Gramicidin: Increases the permeability of the bacterial cell wall to inorganic cations by forming a network of channels through the normal lipid bilayer of the membrane.

Indications Topical treatment of superficial infections of the external eye and its adnexa caused by susceptible bacteria.

Contraindications Hypersensitivity to any component of the product.

Route/Dosage
ADULTS: OPHTHALMIC Instill 1 or 2 drops into the affected eye q 4 hr for 7 to 10 days. In severe infections, the dosage may be increased to as many as 2 drops q hr.

Interactions None well documented.

Lab Test Interferences None well documented.

Adverse Reactions
EENT: Hypersensitivity, including itching, swelling, and conjunctival erythema; local irritation.
OTHER: Allergic hypersensitivity, including anaphylaxis.

Precautions
Pregnancy: Category C.
Lactation: Undetermined.
Children: Safety and efficacy not established.
Superinfection: Prolonged use may result in bacterial or fungal overgrowth of nonsusceptible microorganisms.
Bacterial keratitis: Has been reported with use of topical ophthalmic products in multiple-dose containers that have been inadvertently contaminated by patients who frequently had concurrent corneal disease or a disruption of the ocular epithelial surface.
Bacterial resistance: May develop.
Cross-sensitivity: Allergic cross-sensitivity to kanamycin, paromomycin, streptomycin, and possible gentamicin may occur.

PATIENT CARE CONSIDERATIONS
Administration/Storage
- For ophthalmic use only. Not for use in the ears or on the skin.
- Instill 1 to 2 drops into conjunctival sac(s) q 4 hr or as prescribed.
- Do not allow tip of dropper bottle to touch eye, eyelid, fingers, or any other surface.
- If using other topical ophthalmic medications, instill drops first, wait at least 5 min, and instill ointment last.
- Store at controlled room temperature (59° to 86°F). Keep bottle tightly capped and protect from light.

Assessment/Interventions
- Obtain patient history, including drug history and any known allergies.
- Monitor patient's response to therapy. Notify health care provider if eye or eyelid inflammation is noted or if symptoms do not improve or worsen.

Patient/Family Education
- Explain name, dose, action, and potential side effects of drug.
- Review prescribed dosing schedule with patient, family, or caregiver.
- Remind patient, family, or caregiver that solution is for use in the eye only.
- Teach patient, family, or caregiver proper technique for instilling solution: wash hands; do not allow tip of dropper bottle to touch eye, eyelid, fingers, or any other surface. Tilt head back and look up; pull lower eyelid down to form pocket; place prescribed number of drops in the pocket. Look downward before closing eye. Do not rub eye.
- Advise patient, family, or caregiver that if more than 1 topical ophthalmic drug is being used, instill eye drops first, wait at least 5 min, and then instill ointment last.
- Inform patient that temporary blurred vision and stinging of the eye are the most common side effects and to contact health care provider if they occur and are bothersome.
- Advise patient to contact eye doctor if eye or eyelid inflammation is noted or if eye symptoms do not improve or worsen.
- Advise patient that the entire course of therapy must be completed to ensure maximal benefit and to complete full course of therapy even if symptoms have resolved.
- Instruct patient not to wear contact lenses during treatment.
- Remind patient, family, or caregiver that follow-up eye examinations may be necessary while using this medication and to keep appointments.

Neostigmine

(nee-oh-STIGG-meen)

Class Cholinergic muscle stimulant/Anticholinesterase

How Supplied
Prostigmin Tablets 15 mg, Injection 1:1,000, Injection 1:2,000, Injection 1:4,000

Action
PHARMACOLOGY: Facilitates myoneural junction impulse transmission by inhibiting acetylcholine destruction by cholinesterase.

PHARMACOKINETICS/DYNAMICS:

Absorption: Rapid absorption of neostigmine methylsulfate. T_{max} is 30 min.

Distribution: Neostigmine protein binding is 15% to 25% serum albumin.

Metabolism: Neostigmine is metabolized in the liver by microsomal enzymes.

Excretion: Neostigmine is eliminated in urine (50% as unchanged), t½ is 51 to 90 min, and plasma t½ is 47 to 60 min.

Onset: Onset of IM neostigmine is 20 to 30 min.

Duration: Duration of IM neostigmine is 2.5 to 4 hr.

Indications
Neostigmine bromide (oral) and methylsulfate (injection): Symptomatic control of myasthenia gravis; antidote for nondepolarizing neuromuscular blocking agents after surgery.
Neostigmine methylsulfate: Prevention and treatment of postoperative distention and urinary retention.

Contraindications
Hypersensitivity to anticholinesterases and bromides; mechanical intestinal or urinary obstruction; peritonitis.

Route/Dosage
Antidote
ADULTS: **IV** 0.5 to 2 mg by slow infusion repeated as needed, preceded by 0.6 to 1.2 mg of atropine sulfate. May be repeated prn up to total dose of 5 mg.

Control of Myasthenia Gravis
ADULTS: **PO** 15 to 375 mg/day; **SC/IM** 1 mL of 1:2,000 solution (0.5 mg); individualize subsequent doses.

Prevention of Postoperative Urinary Distention and Retention
ADULTS: SC/IM 1 mL of 1:4,000 solution (0.25 mg) after surgery; repeat q 4 to 6 hr for 2 or 3 days.

Treatment of Postoperative Distention
ADULTS: SC/IM 1 mL of 1:2,000 solution (0.5 mg), as required.

Treatment of Urinary Retention
ADULTS: SC/IM 1 mL of 1:2,000 solution (0.5 mg) after bladder is emptied; continue 0.5 mg injection q 3 hr for at least 5 injections.

Interactions
Corticosteroids: May antagonize anticholinesterases in myasthenia gravis, producing profound muscular depression.
Local/general anesthetics, antiarrhythmic agents: Use with caution, may interfere with neuromuscular transmission.
Streptomycin, kanamycin: May accentuate neuromuscular block.
Succinylcholine: Neuromuscular blockade produced by succinylcholine may be prolonged.

Lab Test Interferences
None well documented.

Adverse Reactions
CV: Arrhythmia (bradycardia, tachycardia, AV block, nodal rhythm); nonspecific ECG changes; cardiac arrest; hypotension; syncope.
CNS: Convulsions; dysarthria; dysphonia; dizziness; loss of consciousness; drowsiness; headache.
DERM: Rash; urticaria; flushing.
EENT: Miosis.
GI: Vomiting; increased peristalsis; flatulence.
GU: Urinary frequency.
RESP: Increased oral, pharyngeal, and bronchial secretions, dyspnea; respiratory depression, respiratory arrest, and bronchospasm (injectable form).
OTHER: Allergy and anaphylaxis; weakness; fasciculations; muscle cramps and spasms; arthralgia; diaphoresis.

Precautions
Pregnancy: Category C.
Lactation: Undetermined.
Children: Safety and efficacy not established.
Hypersensitivity: Anaphylaxis may occur. Have atropine and antishock medications available.
Special risk patients: Use with caution in patients with epilepsy, bronchial asthma, bradycardia, recent coronary occlusion, vagotonia, hyperthyroidism, cardiac arrhythmias, or peptic ulcer.
Anticholinesterase insensitivity: May develop.

Overdosage: Signs and Symptoms
Abdominal cramps, miosis, diarrhea, sweating, excessive salivation, panic attacks, progressive muscle weakness leading to paralysis and death, urinary urgency, anxiety.

PATIENT CARE CONSIDERATIONS
Administration/Storage
♦ Store tablets and injection at controlled room temperature (59° to 86°F). Keep injection in carton until ready to use and protect from light.

Tablets:
♦ Administer as prescribed. Size of dose (eg, number of tablets) and frequency of administration will be adjusted to provide max relief of myasthenia gravis symptoms.
♦ Administer without regard to meals. Administer with food if GI upset occurs.

Injection:
♦ For IV, subcutaneous, or IM administration. Not for intradermal or intra-arterial administration.
♦ Administer as prescribed. Dose and route of administration depend on patient and indication for use.
♦ Do not administer if particulate matter or discoloration noted.

Assessment/Interventions
♦ Obtain patient history, including drug history and any known allergies. Note peritonitis, mechanical obstruction of the intestinal or urinary tract, epilepsy, asthma, bradycardia, recent myocardial occlusion, vagotonia, hyperthyroidism, cardiac arrhythmias, or peptic ulcer.
♦ Assess pulse, BP, and respiratory rate before starting therapy and periodically during treatment. Notify health care provider immediately of any significant changes.
♦ Ensure that emergency airway and resuscitation equipment are available.
♦ Ensure that parenteral atropine is available for emergency treatment of cholinergic crisis.
♦ Frequently assess muscle strength and function in patient with myasthenia gravis or patient recovering from nondepolarizing neuromuscular blocking agent. Notify health care provider immediately of increasing muscle weakness and/or respiratory distress.
♦ If used for urinary retention, assess patients response to therapy. Notify health care provider if urination does not occur within 1 hr of administration and be prepared to catheterize the patient.
♦ Monitor patient for signs and symptoms of anaphylactic or serious allergic reactions. Be

prepared to discontinue therapy and treat appropriately.
- Assess patient for GI, RESP, CNS, CV, MUSC, and general body side effects. Inform health care provider if noted and significant.

Patient/Family Education
- Explain name, dose, action, and potential side effects of drug.
- Advise patient or caregiver that injection will be prepared and administered by a health care provider in a medical setting.
- Advise patient that dose and frequency of administration may be adjusted to achieve max benefit.
- Advise patient to take exactly as prescribed and not to change the dose or stop taking unless advised by health care provider.
- Advise patient to take prescribed dose without regard to meals but to take with food if stomach upset occurs.
- Advise patient with myasthenia gravis to keep a diary of medication administration times and times when muscle weakness or other symptoms occur. This log will help the health care provider adjust the dose and dosing interval to establish the most effective dose and times of administration.
- Instruct patient to contact health care provider immediately if any of the following occur: worsening muscle weakness, difficulty breathing, slow or irregular heart rate, dizziness, fainting, vomiting, severe abdominal pain.
- Advise patient that diarrhea, increased salivation, sweating, and nausea are common side effects and to notify health care provider if any occur and are bothersome.
- Advise women to notify health care provider if pregnant, planning to become pregnant, or breastfeeding.
- Instruct patient to not take any prescription or OTC medications, dietary supplements, or herbal preparations unless advised by health care provider.
- Advise patient that follow-up visits will be required to monitor therapy and to keep appointments.

Nesiritide

(nih-SIR-ih-tide)

Class Vasodilator

How Supplied
Natrecor Powder for injection, lyophilized 1.58 mg

Action
PHARMACOLOGY: Binds to the particulate guanylate cyclase receptor of vascular smooth muscle and endothelial cells, leading to dose-dependent reductions in pulmonary capillary wedge pressure and systemic arterial pressure in patients with heart failure.

PHARMACOKINETICS/DYNAMICS:
Distribution: The mean Vd of the central compartment is estimated to be 0.073 L/kg and the mean Cl is approximately 9.2 mL/min/kg. Following IV administration to patients with CHF, disposition from the plasma is biphasic.

Excretion: The mean terminal elimination $t_{½}$ is approximately 18 min and is associated with approximately 2/3 of the AUC. The mean initial elimination phase is about 2 min.

Onset: With administration of the recommended dosing regimen of 2 mcg/kg IV bolus followed by 0.01 mcg/kg/min, 60% of the 3-hr effect on pulmonary capillary wedge pressure reduction is achieved within 15 min after the bolus. Approximately 70% of the 3-hr effect on standing BP reduction is reached within 15 min.

Peak: 95% of the 3-hr effect is achieved within 1 hr.

Duration: The pharmacodynamic $t_{½}$ of the onset and offset of the hemodynamic effect is longer than predicted by the pharmacokinetic $t_{½}$.

Indications Treatment of patients with acutely decompensated CHF who have dyspnea at rest or with minimal activity.

Contraindications Primary treatment for patients with cardiogenic shock; systolic BP less than 90 mm Hg; hypersensitivity to any component of the product.

Route/Dosage
ADULTS: **IV** Recommended dose is 2 mcg/kg IV bolus followed by continuous infusion at a dose of 0.01 mcg/kg/min. If hypotension occurs during administration, reduce or discontinue the dose and start other measures to support BP.

Interactions
ACE inhibitors (eg, captopril): Coadministration may cause an increase in symptomatic hypotension.
INCOMPATIBILITIES: Physically and chemically incompatible with injectable formulations of bumetanide, enalaprilat, ethacrynate sodium, furosemide, hydralazine, heparin, and insulin. These agents should not be administered as infusions with nesiritide through the same IV catheter. Sodium metabisulfite preservative is incompatible with nesiritide. Since nesiritide

binds with heparin, do not administer through a central heparin-coated catheter.

Lab Test Interferences None well documented.

Adverse Reactions

CV: Hypotension (symptomatic and asymptomatic) (11%); ventricular tachycardia (3%); nonsustained ventricular tachycardia (3%); ventricular extrasystoles (3%); angina pectoris; bradycardia; tachycardia; atrial fibrillation; AV node conduction abnormalities.
CNS: Headache (8%); insomnia; dizziness (3%); anxiety (3%); confusion; paresthesia; somnolence; tremor.
DERM: Sweating; pruritus; rash.
EENT: Amblyopia.
GI: Nausea (4%); vomiting.
HEMA: Anemia.
RESP: Increased cough; hemoptysis; apnea.
OTHER: Abdominal pain; back pain; catheter pain; fever; injection site reaction; increased creatinine; leg cramps.

Precautions

Pregnancy: Category C.
Lactation: Undetermined.
Children: Safety and efficacy not established.
Renal function impairment: Renal function may be affected in susceptible patients; azotemia may occur in patients with severe heart failure whose renal function may depend on the activity of the renin-angiotensin-aldosterone system.
Cardiac: Avoid administration in patients suspected of having or known to have low cardiac filling pressures. Not recommended for use in patients for whom vasodilating agents are not approved (eg, significant valvular stenosis; restrictive or obstructive cardiomyopathy).
Hypotension: May occur at recommended or adjustable doses.

Overdosage: Signs and Symptoms
Hypotension.

PATIENT CARE CONSIDERATIONS

Administration/Storage

- For IV administration only. Do not administer intradermally, IM, or SC.
- Follow manufacturer's instructions for reconstitution of powder and final dilution for infusion solution.
- Do not shake or agitate vials during reconstitution or dilution. Do not use filter needles during preparation of infusion.
- Inspect solution visually before administration. Do not administer if solution is cloudy, discolored, or contains particulate matter.
- Prime IV tubing with infusion solution prior to connecting to patient's vascular access port and prior to administering bolus dose and starting infusion.
- Administer prescribed bolus dose over 60 sec through IV port on tubing. Immediately following bolus dose begin infusion at prescribed rate.
- Infusion rate may be increased by 0.005 mcg/kg/min, no more often than q 3 hr up to a max of 0.03 mcg/kg/min. Increases in infusion rate should be preceded by a bolus dose of 1 mcg/kg.
- Do not administer through a central heparin-coated catheter.
- Flush catheter between administration of nesiritide and any incompatible injectable medication.
- Store vials at controlled room temperature (68° to 77°F) in original carton. Reconstituted solution should be used immediately. If immediate use is not possible, the reconstituted solution may be stored for up to 24 hr in refrigerator (36° to 46°F) or at controlled room temperature.

Assessment/Interventions

- Obtain patient history, including drug history and any known allergies. Note presence of significant valvular stenosis, restrictive or obstructive cardiomyopathy, constrictive pericarditis, pericardial tamponade, low cardiac filling pressures, systolic BP less than 100 mm Hg, and concurrent use of medications that may cause hypotension.
- Use, as appropriate, central hemodynamic monitoring to assess patient's hemodynamic status and response to therapy.
- Monitor BP closely during infusion. Be prepared to reduce the infusion rate or even discontinue the infusion if hypotension occurs. Be prepared to support BP (eg, IV fluids, change in body position) if necessary.
- Administer reduced dose and no bolus to patient who has previously developed hypotension with nesiritide.
- Monitor ECG closely during infusion. Inform health care provider if arrhythmias or significant changes in heart rate are noted.
- Assess patient for CNS, GI, and general body side effects. Inform health care provider if noted and significant.

Patient/Family Education

- Explain name, action, dosing regimen, and potential side effects of drug.
- Advise patient, family, or caregiver that medication will be prepared and administered by highly trained health care providers in an intensive care setting.

Nevirapine

(nuh-VEER-uh-peen)

Class Antiretroviral/Non-nucleoside reverse transcriptase inhibitor

How Supplied
Viramune Tablets 200 mg, Oral solution 50 mg/mL (as hemihydrate)

Action

PHARMACOLOGY: Inhibits replication of retroviruses, including HIV.

PHARMACOKINETICS/DYNAMICS:

Absorption: Nevirapine oral absorption is more than 90%, bioavailability is 93% (tablets) and 91% (oral solution), T_{max} is 4 hr, and C_{max} is approximately 2 mcg/mL.

Distribution: Nevirapine crosses the placenta and is found in breast milk. Protein binding is approximately 60% and is highly lipophilic and widely distributed. Nevirapine Vd is 1.21 L/kg (IV), and cerebrospinal fluid approximates 45% of concentration in plasma.

Metabolism: Nevirapine is eliminated in urine (81.3%) and feces (10.1%). Less than 3% of the parent compound is excreted in urine. Autoinduction results in a decrease of the $t_½$ from 45 hr (single dose) to approximately 25 to 30 hr (multiple dose).

Indications In combination with other antiretroviral agents for treatment of HIV-1 infection.

Contraindications Standard considerations.

Route/Dosage

ADULTS:
Initial therapy: **PO** 200 mg daily for 14 days. Total daily dose not to exceed 400 mg.
Maintenance therapy: **PO** 200 mg bid in combination with other antiretroviral agents.
CHILDREN (2 MO TO 8 YR OF AGE): **PO** 4 mg/kg daily for 14 days followed by 7 mg/kg bid. Total daily dose not to exceed 400 mg.
CHILDREN (AT LEAST 8 YR OF AGE): **PO** 4 mg/kg daily for 14 days followed by 4 mg/kg bid. Total daily dose not to exceed 400 mg.

Interactions

Clarithromycin: Clarithromycin concentrations may be reduced, while concentrations of the active metabolite of clarithromycin may be increased.
Contraceptives, oral: Lower hormone levels and potential contraceptive failure.
Efavirenz, methadone: Concentrations of these agents may be decreased by nevirapine.
Fluconazole: Nevirapine concentrations may be increased.
Ketoconazole: Coadministration resulted in significant reduction in ketoconazole plasma concentrations. Do not coadminister ketoconazole and nevirapine.
Protease inhibitors: Lower protease inhibitor plasma levels.
Rifabutin: Rifabutin concentrations may be increased.
Rifampin, rifabutin: Lower nevirapine plasma levels.
St. John's wort: May reduce nevirapine concentrations, resulting in loss of virologic response and possible resistance to nevirapine and the class of non-nucleoside reverse transcriptase inhibitors.
Warfarin: Plasma concentrations of warfarin may be altered, resulting in potential increases in coagulation time.

Lab Test Interferences None well documented.

Adverse Reactions

CNS: Fatigue (5%); headache (4%); somnolence, paresthesia, malaise (postmarketing).
DERM: Rash (all grades 24% [life-threatening 2%]); Stevens-Johnson syndrome; toxic epidermal necrolysis; angioedema, bullous eruptions, urticaria, blistering (postmarketing); facial edema.
EENT: Conjunctivitis (postmarketing).
GI: Nausea (9%); abdominal pain, diarrhea (2%); vomiting, ulcerative stomatitis, oral lesions (postmarketing).
HEPA: Hepatitis (including fatal fulminant hepatitis); hepatic failure; jaundice, cholestatic hepatitis, hepatic necrosis (postmarketing).
HEMA/LYMPH: Eosinophilia; granulocytopenia; lymphadenopathy; anemia, neutropenia (postmarketing).
HYPERSEN: Hypersensitivity, including severe rash or rash accompanied by fever, general malaise, fatigue, muscle or joint aches, blisters, oral lesions, conjunctivitis, facial edema; anaphylaxis (postmarketing).
LABTESTABS: Abnormal LFTs (7%).
METAB: Redistribution and accumulation of body fat (postmarketing).
MUSC: Arthralgia, muscle and joint pain (postmarketing).
RENAL: Renal dysfunction.
OTHER: Fever (postmarketing).

> **WARNING:**
> *Dermal reactions:* Severe, life-threatening skin reactions (sometimes fatal) occurred during therapy. Cases include Stevens-Johnson syndrome, toxic epidermal necrolysis, and hypersensitivity reactions.
> *Dosing:* A 14-day initiation period (200 mg/day) must be strictly followed.
> *Hepatotoxicity:* Severe, life-threatening, and in some cases fatal, including fulminant and cholestatic hepatitis, necrosis, and failure.
> *Patient monitoring:* Closely monitor for first 18 wk to detect signs and symptoms of skin/hepatic reactions.

Precautions

Pregnancy: Category C.
Lactation: Excreted in breast milk. HIV-infected mothers should not breastfeed their infants.
Children: For use in pediatric patients at least 2 mo of age. Nevirapine Cl at least 2-fold greater in children younger than 8 yr of age.
Renal function impairment: Use with caution in patients with renal impairment.
Hepatic function impairment: Use with caution in patients with moderate hepatic impairment. Do not administer to patients with severe hepatic impairment.

Monitoring: Perform clinical chemistry tests, including LFTs, prior to initiating therapy and at regular intervals during therapy.
Fat redistribution: Redistribution or accumulation of body fat, including central obesity, dorsocervical fat enlargement, peripheral wasting, facial wasting, breast enlargement, and cushingoid appearance may occur.
Hepatotoxicity: Permanently discontinue therapy if hepatotoxicity occurs.
Missed doses: Patients who interrupt maintenance dosing for more than 7 days should restart the recommended dosing (1 daily for 14 days followed by 1 bid).
Resistance: When used as monotherapy, resistant virus emerges rapidly and uniformly.
Skin reactions: Discontinue drug if skin rash accompanied by constitutional symptoms (eg, fever, blistering, oral lesions, conjunctivitis, swelling, muscle or joint aches, general malaise) occurs. If rash is mild to moderate in severity and not accompanied by constitutional symptoms, the drug can be continued with close monitoring. If rash develops during first 14 days of therapy, do not increase dose beyond 200 mg daily until rash resolves.

Overdosage: Signs and Symptoms

Edema, erythema nodosum, fatigue, fever, headache, insomnia, nausea, pulmonary infiltrates, rash, vertigo, vomiting, weight decrease.

PATIENT CARE CONSIDERATIONS

Administration/Storage

- Tablets and oral suspension are interchangeable on a mg-to-mg basis at doses up to 200 mg.
- Administer prescribed dose without regard to meals. Administer with food if GI upset occurs.
- Shake suspension before measuring dose. Administer prescribed dose using oral dosing syringe or dosing cup. If using dosing cup, thoroughly rinse dosing cup with water and administer rinse water to patient.
- Store tablets and oral suspension at ambient room temperature (59° to 86°F).

Assessment/Interventions

- Obtain patient history, including drug history and any known allergies. Note hepatic or renal impairment, history of previous hepatic, skin or hypersensitivity reaction to nevirapine, or co-infection with hepatitis B or C.
- Ensure that medication is used in combination with other antiretroviral agents.
- Ensure that medication is not administered to patient with severe hepatic impairment.
- Ensure that medication is not restarted in patient who has previously experienced a severe hepatic, skin, or hypersensitivity reaction to nevirapine.
- Ensure that 14-day lead-in period (200 mg/day for adults, or 4 mg/kg/day for children) is followed to reduce frequency of skin rash when initiating or restarting therapy following interruption of therapy for more than 7 days.
- Ensure that patient is intensively monitored for clinical and laboratory evidence of life-threatening hepatic events or skin reactions during the first 18 wk of therapy and then frequently thereafter. Ensure that liver enzymes are determined before starting therapy, before dose escalation, and at 2 wk following dose escalation.
- Closely monitor patient for signs or symptoms of liver disease, skin reactions, or hypersensitivity reactions. Discontinue use and notify health care provider immediately if any of the following are noted: severe skin rash or rash accompanied by fever, general body discomfort, nausea, appetite loss fatigue, muscle or joint aches, blisters, mouth sores, conjunctivi-

tis, facial swelling, swollen lymph nodes, decreased urination, dark urine, pale stools, yellowing of skin or eyes. Ensure that liver enzymes are evaluated in patient suspected of experiencing nevirapine-associated rash.
* Monitor patient for evidence of redistribution or accumulation of body fat and CNS, GI, and general body side effects. Inform health care provider if noted and significant.

Patient/Family Education
* Explain name, dose, action, and potential side effects of drug.
* Warn patient that this drug is not to be used by itself but is combined with other antiretroviral agents and not to change the dose or stop taking any of the antiretroviral agents unless advised by health care provider.
* Advise patient to review *Patient Information* leaflet before starting therapy and with each refill of the medication.
* Advise patient to take prescribed dose without regard to meals but to take with food if stomach upset occurs.
* Advise patient or caregiver using suspension to shake suspension before measuring dose and to administer prescribed dose using oral dosing syringe or dosing cup. If using dosing cup, advise patient or caregiver to thoroughly rinse the dosing cup with water and administer rinse water to patient.
* Advise patient that a 14-day lead-in period (lower dose) is used to reduce frequency of rash and not to exceed the prescribed dose during this period.
* Advise patient that if a dose is missed, to take the dose as soon as possible and then return to the normal schedule. However, if it is almost time for the next dose, advise patient to skip the dose and take the next dose at the regular time. Caution patient not to double the dose to catch up.
* Instruct patient that if therapy is stopped for longer than 7 days for any reason, not to restart therapy without discussing how to restart nevirapine with health care provider. Advise patient that therapy may have to be restarted using the 14-day lead-in dose again.
* Instruct patient to discontinue use and notify health care provider immediately if any of the following are noted: severe skin rash or rash accompanied by fever, general body discomfort, nausea, appetite loss, fatigue, muscle or joint aches, blisters, mouth sores, red or inflamed eyelids, facial swelling, swollen lymph nodes, decreased urination, dark urine, pale stools, tenderness on right side below ribs, or yellowing of skin or eyes.
* Advise patient that changes in body fat (increased fat in upper back and neck, breast, or around the trunk and loss of fat from legs, arms, or face) may occur but that the cause and long-term health effects of these changes are not known at this time. Advise patient to discuss with health care provider if noted and significant.
* Inform patient that drug does not completely eliminate HIV virus and, therefore, does not reduce risk of transmitting HIV. Appropriate precautions must still be followed.
* Advise patient that drug is not a cure for HIV infection and that illnesses associated with HIV infection, including opportunistic infections, may still be acquired. Patient should remain under a physician's care.
* Instruct patient not to take any prescription or OTC medications, dietary supplements, or herbal preparations (including St. John's wort) unless advised by health care provider.
* Advise women using combination oral contraceptives to use an additional nonhormonal form of contraception because nevirapine can reduce the effectiveness of combination oral contraceptives.
* Advise women to notify health care provider if pregnant, planning to become pregnant, or breastfeeding. Caution HIV-infected mother that breastfeeding a baby could cause HIV infection in the baby.
* Remind patient that examinations and laboratory tests will be required to monitor therapy and to keep appointments.

Niacin (B$_3$; nicotinic acid)

(NYE-uh-sin)
Class Vitamin/Antihyperlipidemic
How Supplied
Slo-Niacin Tablets, controlled-release 250 mg, Tablets, controlled-release 500 mg, Tablets, controlled-release 750 mg ◆ *Niaspan* Tablets, extended-release 500 mg, Tablets, extended-release 750 mg, Tablets, extended-release 1000 mg

Action
PHARMACOLOGY: Necessary for lipid metabolism, tissue respiration and glycogenolysis. At pharmacologic doses, it reduces total cholesterol, LDL cholesterol, and triglycerides while increasing HDL cholesterol. Also causes peripheral vasodilation, especially cutaneous vessels.

PHARMACOKINETICS/DYNAMICS:
Absorption: Niacin is rapidly and extensively absorbed from GI tract. T_{max} is 30 to 60 min and C_{max} is 15 to 30 mcg/mL.

Metabolism: Rapid and extensive first-pass metabolism of niacin in liver.

Excretion: Niacin is eliminated in urine (approximately 88% as unchanged and nicotinuric acid). Plasma t½ is 20 to 45 min.

Special Populations:
Gender – Steady state plasma concentrations and metabolites are generally higher in women.
Liver disease – Extended-release tablets are contraindicated in patients with active liver disease.

Indications Prevention and treatment of niacin deficiency or pellagra; treatment of hyperlipidemia (types IV and V); adjunct to diet for the reduction of elevated total and LDL levels in patients with primary hypercholesterolemia when the response to diet and other nonpharmacologic measures alone has been inadequate.

Contraindications Significant liver disease; active peptic ulcer; severe hypotension; arterial hemorrhaging.

Route/Dosage
Pellagra
ADULTS: PO Up to 500 mg/day in divided doses.

ADULTS: **Slow IV/SC/IM** When oral route is not possible.

Dietary Supplementation
ADULTS: PO RDA is 15 to 20 mg/day for adult men and 13 to 15 mg/day for adult women. Increase niacin to 17 to 20 mg/day during pregnancy and lactation.
CHILDREN: PO RDA is 5 to 20 mg/day.

Hyperlipidemia
ADULTS:
Extended release: **PO** 500 mg at bedtime for 1 to 4 wk, then 1000 mg at bedtime during wk 5 to 8. If response is inadequate and patient tolerates dose, the dose may be increased by no more than 500 mg in a 4-wk period (max, 2000 mg/day).
Immediate release: **PO** Initiate therapy at 250 mg with evening meal. The frequency of dose and total daily dose can be increased q 4 to 7 days until a dose of 1.5 to 2 g/day (in divided doses) is reached. If hyperlipidemia is not adequately controlled after 2 mo, increase dosage at 2- to 4-wk intervals to 1 g tid (max, 6 g/day).

Interactions
Adrenergic-blocking agent: May potentiate hypotensive effect.

HMG-CoA reductase inhibitors: Increased risk of myopathy and rhabdomyolysis.

Lab Test Interferences May produce fluorescent substances, which may cause false elevation in some fluorometric measurements of urinary catecholamines. May produce false-positive reaction with cupric sulfate solution used for urinary glucose determination.

Adverse Reactions
CV: Hypotension; tachycardia.
CNS: Dizziness; syncope; headache.
DERM: Flushing; pruritus; burning or tingling sensation; rash; hyperpigmentation (acanthosis nigricans); dry skin.
EENT: Blurred vision; xerostomia.
GI: Nausea; bloating; flatulence; hunger; vomiting; heartburn; diarrhea; activation of peptic ulcer; abdominal pain; dyspepsia.
HEPA: Jaundice; liver damage; abnormal LFT results.
OTHER: Hyperuricemia; hyperglycemia; decreased glucose tolerance test results; toxic amblyopia; atrial fibrillation and other cardiac arrhythmias; cystoid macular edema; orthostasis.

Precautions
Pregnancy: Category A. (Category C if used in doses above RDA.)
Lactation: Actively excreted in breast milk.
Children: Safety and efficacy not established for doses exceeding nutritional requirements. Extended-release preparations not recommended for children.
Special risk patients: Use drug with caution when administering to patients with gallbladder disease, history of jaundice, diabetes mellitus, gout, peptic ulcer, or allergy. Also, patients allergic to aspirin may be allergic to this product.
Tartrazine sensitivity: Products containing FD&C yellow #5 may cause asthma in susceptible patients.
Flushing: Commonly appears with oral therapy. Aspirin (325 mg) 30 min to 1 hr before niacin may decrease flushing.
Long-acting dosage form: Increases risk of jaundice and hepatitis. Avoid use if possible.
Heart disease: People who have recurrent chest pain (angina) or who recently suffered a heart attack should take niacin only under the supervision of a health care provider.

Overdosage: Signs and Symptoms
Nausea, dizziness, pruritus, vomiting, tachycardia, GI distress, hypotension, flushing.

PATIENT CARE CONSIDERATIONS
Administration/Storage
- When giving orally, start with small doses, then increase gradually.
- Administer with food.
- Do not crush or break oral medication.

Assessment/Interventions
- Obtain patient history, including drug history and any known allergies.
- If giving for hyperlipidemia, check baseline and monitor cholesterol level.

- Check blood glucose, LFTs, and uric acid level as ordered.
- Monitor vital signs.
- Assess for signs of jaundice, light-colored stools, dizziness, or faint feeling.
- Notify health care provider of changes from baseline assessment.

Patient/Family Education
- Tell patient not to break up medication if taking orally.
- Explain that flushing may appear after taking medication but should dissipate with continued therapy.
- Tell patient to take medication with food.
- Identify specific elements of well-balanced, low-fat diet.
- Instruct patient to report the following symptoms to health care provider: jaundice, light-colored stools, excessive thirst, urinary frequency, dizziness, or faint feeling.
- Caution patient to avoid sudden position changes, especially lying to sitting, to prevent dizziness.
- Advise patient to avoid intake of alcoholic beverages or hot drinks and large doses of medication (more than 500 mg) at one time to minimize flushing and warmth sensation.
- Advise diabetic patients to notify health care provider if a change in blood glucose occurs.
- Instruct patient to inform health care provider if taking vitamins or other nutritional supplements containing niacin or a related compound such as nicotinamide.

Niacin/Lovastatin

(NYE-uh-sin/LOW-vuh-STAT-in)

Class Antihyperlipidemic combination

How Supplied
Advicor Tablets 500/20 mg, Tablets 1,000/20 mg

Action

PHARMACOLOGY:

Niacin: Necessary for lipid metabolism, tissue respiration, and glycogenolysis; reduces total cholesterol, LDL cholesterol, and triglycerides (TG) while increasing HDL cholesterol.
Lovastatin: Increases rate at which body removes cholesterol from blood and reduces production of cholesterol in body by inhibiting enzyme that catalyses early rate-limiting step in cholesterol synthesis; increases HDL; reduces LDL, VLDL, and TG.

PHARMACOKINETICS/DYNAMICS:

Absorption: C_{max} of niacin averaged about 18 mcg/mL about 5 hr after dosing; lovastatin C_{max} averaged about 11 ng/mL about 2 hr after dosing. The extent of niacin and lovastatin absorption was increased by administration with food.

Distribution: Niacin is less than 20% bound to human serum proteins and distributes into milk. Niacin and its metabolites concentrate in the liver, kidney, and adipose tissue. Both lovastatin and its beta-hydroxyacid metabolite are highly bound (more than 95%) to human plasma proteins. Lovastatin is concentrated in the liver and crosses the blood-brain and placental barriers.

Metabolism: Niacin undergoes rapid and extensive first-pass metabolism forming nicotinuric acid and nicotinamide. Lovastatin undergoes extensive first-pass extraction and metabolism by cytochrome P450 3A4 in the liver. The major active metabolites are the beta-hydroxyacid of lovastatin (lovastatin acid), its 6'-hydroxy derivative.

Excretion: Niacin is primarily excreted in urine mainly as metabolites. The plasma $t_{½}$ was about 4.5 hours for lovastatin and about 20 to 48 minutes for niacin.

Indications Treatment of primary hypercholesterolemia (heterozygous familial and nonfamilial) and mixed dyslipidemia (Frederickson Types IIa and IIb) in patients treated with lovastatin who require further TG-lowering or HDL-raising who may benefit from having niacin added to their regimen; patients treated with niacin who require further LDL-lowering who may benefit from having lovastatin added to their regimen.

Contraindications Pregnancy, lactation, active liver disease, unexplained persistent elevations in serum transaminases, active peptic ulcer disease, arterial bleeding, hypersensitivity to any component of product.

Route/Dosage

ADULTS: **PO** Patients receiving a stable dose of *Niaspan* (niacin extended-release tablets) may be switched directly to a niacin-equivalent dose of *Advicor*. Patients receiving a stable dose of lovastatin may receive concomitant dosage titration with *Niaspan* and switch to *Advicor* once a stable dose of *Niaspan* has been reached. *Advicor* should be taken at bedtime.

Interactions

Antihypertensive therapy (eg, ganglionic agents, vasoactive agents): Niacin may potentiate effects resulting in postural hypotension.
Aspirin: Metabolic Cl of niacin may be decreased.
Bile acid sequestrants: Because of possible binding of niacin to these agents, allow 4 to 6 hr (or as long an interval as possible) to elapse

between the ingestion of bile acid-binding resins and administration of *Advicor*.

Clarithromycin, cyclosporine, erythromycin, gemfibrozil, HIV protease inhibitors (eg, ritonavir), itraconazole, ketoconazole, nefazodone, niacin: May increase the risk of skeletal muscle disorders (eg, rhabdomyolysis).

Coumarin anticoagulants (eg, warfarin): Bleeding and increased PT may occur. Monitor anticoagulant parameters when starting, stopping, or changing the *Advicor* dose.

Hot beverages or alcohol: May increase the side effects of flushing and pruritus with niacin and should be avoided.

Lab Test Interferences Niacin may produce false elevations in some fluorometric determinations of plasma or urinary catecholamines; niacin may give false-positive reactions with cupric sulfate solution (*Benedicts* reagent) in urine glucose tests.

Adverse Reactions The incidence stated for the following adverse reactions were reported with *Advicor* (niacin/lovastatin) administration. Adverse reactions occurring with administration of either niacin or lovastatin listed in their respective monographs.

CNS: Headache (9%); asthenia (5%).
DERM: Flushing (71%); pruritus (7%); rash (5%).
GI: Nausea (7%); diarrhea (6%); abdominal pain (4%); dyspepsia, vomiting (3%).
M/N: Hyperglycemia (4%).
MUSC: Back pain (5%); myalgia (3%).
OTHER: Infection (20%); pain (8%); flu syndrome (6%).

Precautions
Pregnancy: Category X.

Lactation:
Niacin – Excreted in breast milk.
Lovastatin – Undetermined.
Children: Safety and efficacy not established.
Special risk patients: Use with caution in patients with unstable angina or in the acute phase of MI, or in patients predisposed to gout; use with caution in patients with a history of jaundice or hepatobiliary disease; administer with caution in patients with peptic ulcers and in patients who consume substantial quantities of alcohol and/or who have a history of liver disease

Dose equivalence: Equivalent doses of *Advicor* may be substituted for equivalent doses of *Niaspan* but should not be substituted for other modified-release niacin preparations or immediate-release niacin preparations.

Fasting blood sugar: A dose related rise may be experienced in diabetic patients.

Liver dysfunction: Severe hepatic toxicity, including fulminant hepatic necrosis, has occurred in patients substituting sustained-release niacin for immediate-release niacin in equivalent doses.

Myopathy/Rhabdomyolysis: Have been reported when lovastatin is used in combination with lipid altering doses (at least 1 g/day) of niacin.

Transaminase levels: Because lovastatin may increase creatine phosphokinase and transaminase levels, this should be considered in differential diagnosis of chest pain.

Overdosage: Signs and Symptoms
Niacin: Severe flushing, nausea, vomiting, diarrhea, dyspepsia, dizziness, syncope, hypotension, possible cardiac arrhythmias, clinical laboratory abnormalities.

PATIENT CARE CONSIDERATIONS

Administration/Storage

- May be used alone or in combination with other cholesterol-lowering medications.
- Do not substitute for equivalent doses of sustained-release, time-release, or immediate-release niacin.
- Administer prescribed dose at bedtime with a low-fat snack.
- Do not increase dose by more than 500 mg daily (based on extended-release niacin component) q 4 wk.
- Administer niacin/lovastatin at least 2 hr before or 4 hr or more after administration of a bile acid sequestrant (eg, cholestyramine).
- Store tablets at controlled room temperature (68° to 77°F).

Assessment/Interventions

- Obtain patient history, including drug history and any known allergies. Note renal disease, active liver disease or past history of liver disease, unexplained elevations of serum transaminases, active peptic ulcer disease, arterial bleeding, pregnancy, breastfeeding, alcohol consumption, unstable angina, gout, concurrent use of potent inhibitors of CYP3A4 (eg, cyclosporine, ketoconazole), and concurrent therapy with medications known to increase the risk of myopathy (eg, fibrates).
- Ensure secondary causes of hypercholesterolemia (eg, poorly controlled diabetes, hypothyroidism, drugs that increase LDL-C and decrease HDL-C) are excluded, or if appropriate, treated, before starting therapy.
- Ensure patient is on a cholesterol-lowering diet before starting therapy and diet is continued during treatment.
- Ensure dose does not exceed 1,000/20 mg/day in patient taking cyclosporine or a fibrate.

- Monitor blood sugar in diabetic patient when drug is started or dose is changed. Report significant changes to health care provider.
- Ensure fasting blood glucose is evaluated before starting therapy and periodically thereafter during therapy in patient with risk factors for diabetes mellitus (eg, obesity, family history of diabetes).
- Ensure phosphorous levels are monitored periodically in patient at risk for hypophosphatemia (eg, malabsorption syndrome, small bowel bypass).
- Ensure preoperative INR and platelet count are evaluated in patient undergoing surgery.
- Ensure lipid levels are determined at intervals of no less than 4 wk and dosage is adjusted according to patient's response to therapy.
- Ensure therapy is temporarily withheld before elective major surgery and when any major acute medical or surgical condition supervenes.
- Ensure consideration is given to temporarily discontinuing therapy during a course of therapy with a systemic antifungal azole or macrolide antibiotic.
- Ensure serum transaminases are determined before starting therapy, q 6 to 12 wk for the first 6 mo of therapy, and periodically (eg, q 6 mo) thereafter as clinically indicated.
- If elevated serum transaminase levels develop during treatment, repeat levels more frequently. If transaminase levels rise to 3 times upper limit of normal or greater and persist, or if they are associated with symptoms of nausea, fever, and/or malaise, notify health care provider. Be prepared to discontinue therapy.
- Monitor patient for symptoms of myopathy (eg, muscle pain, tenderness, weakness) when medication is started and when dose is increased. Discontinue therapy and immediately notify health care provider if myopathy is suspected.
- Assess patient for CV, GI, and general body side effects. Inform health care provider if noted and significant.

Patient/Family Education

- Explain name, dose, action, potential side effects of medication, and LDL-C and TG goals.
- Advise patient that dose of medication may change, based on results of cholesterol and TG blood tests, in an effort to reach LDL-C and TG goals.
- Review other substances (eg, grapefruit juice) and medications (eg, potent CYP3A4 inhibitors, nutritional supplements containing niacin or nicotinamide) that should not be taken with this medication.
- Advise patient to take prescribed dose once daily at bedtime with a low-fat snack.
- Instruct patient to swallow tablets whole and not to crush, chew, or break the tablets.
- Caution patient that taking this medication on an empty stomach increases the risk of experiencing flushing, itching, and stomach distress.
- Caution patient that drinking alcohol or hot drinks around the time of medication administration will increase the risk of flushing.
- Caution patient not to change the dose or stop taking unless advised by health care provider.
- Caution patient that if medication is not taken for an extended length of time (eg, more than 7 days) to contact health care provider before restarting the medication. Advise patient that retitration of the dose of medication may be required.
- Emphasize to patient importance of other modalities on cholesterol control: dietary changes (reduced saturated fat intake, increase soluble fiber intake), weight control, regular exercise, smoking cessation.
- Advise patient that drug helps control, but not does cure, cholesterol abnormality and to continue taking drug as prescribed when LDL-C and TG goals have been met.
- Instruct patient to continue taking other cholesterol-lowering medications as prescribed by health care provider.
- Advise patient that flushing, which may last for several hours after dosing, is a common side effect of therapy but that it usually goes away after several weeks of consistent use.
- Caution patient that if flushing awakens them during the night to rise slowly to reduce the chances of dizziness or fainting.
- Advise patient that if flushing occurs and is bothersome, that taking aspirin or another NSAID (eg, ibuprofen) 30 minute before taking niacin/lovastatin may minimize flushing.
- Advise patient who also is taking a bile acid sequestrant (eg, cholestyramine) to take the niacin/lovastatin at least 2 hr before or 4 hr or more after the sequestrant.
- Instruct patient to immediately notify health care provider if experiencing any unexplained muscle pain, tenderness and/or weakness, unquenchable thirst, frequent urination, frequent episodes of dizziness, fainting, or if any other unusual or unexplained feelings are noted.
- Instruct diabetic patient to monitor blood glucose more frequently when drug is started or dose is changed and to inform health care provider of significant changes in readings.

- Advise women of childbearing potential to use effective contraception during treatment with niacin/lovastatin.
- Advise women to notify health care provider if pregnant, planning to become pregnant, or breastfeeding.
- Caution patient not to take any prescription or OTC medications, herbal preparations, dietary supplements, other forms of niacin, or nicotinamide unless advised by health care provider.
- Advise patient that follow-up visits and lab tests will be required to monitor therapy and to keep appointments.

Nicardipine Hydrochloride

(NYE-CAR-dih-peen HIGH-droe-KLOR-ide)

Class Calcium channel blocker

How Supplied
Cardene Capsules 20 mg, Capsules 30 mg ♦ *Cardene I.V.* Injection 2.5 mg/mL ♦ *Cardene SR* Capsules, sustained-release 30 mg, Capsules, sustained-release 45 mg, Capsules, sustained-release 60 mg

Action
PHARMACOLOGY: Inhibits movement of calcium ions across cell membrane in systemic and coronary vascular smooth muscle and myocardium.

PHARMACOKINETICS/DYNAMICS:

Absorption: Nicardipine is absorbed approximately 100% following oral administration. C_{max} is 28 to 50 mg/mL; steady state is 24 to 48 hr (IV), 2 to 30 hr (oral); T_{max} is 0.5 to 2 hr (oral); absolute bioavailability is 35% (less for oral administration because of first pass metabolism). Food is administered 3 hr after high-fat meal. C_{max} is less than 20% and AUC is less than 30%.

Distribution: Rapid early distribution phase, intermediate phase, and a slow terminal phase. Vd: 8.3 L/kg; protein binding is approximately 95%.

Excretion: Eliminated by urine (less than 1% unchanged, 49% of dose recovered) and feces (43%). Plasma clearance is 0.4 L/hr/kg; plasma t½ is 8.6 hr (oral); t½ is 2 to 4 hr (oral); alpha t½ is 2.7 min (IV); beta t½ is 44.8 min (IV); gamma t½ is 14.4 hr (IV).

Onset: Approximately 20 min (oral).

Special Populations:
Renal Function Impairment – Significant reduction in glomerular filtration rate (GFR), significant systemic clearance, and higher AUC.
Severe Liver Insufficiency – Plasma concentrations increased and half-life was prolonged to 19 hr.

Indications
Treatment of chronic stable (effort-associated) angina (immediate-release capsules); management of hypertension (immediate- and sustained-release capsules); IV when oral therapy not feasible or desirable).

Contraindications Sick sinus syndrome; second- or third-degree atrioventricular (AV) block except with functioning pacemaker; advanced aortic stenosis.

Route/Dosage
Angina (Immediate-Release Only)
ADULTS: PO Usual initial dose 20 mg tid (range, 20 to 40 mg tid).

Hypertension
ADULTS:
Immediate-release: PO Usual dose 20 mg tid (range, 20 to 40 mg tid).
Sustained-release: PO Start with 30 mg bid (range, 30 to 60 mg bid). IV Individualize dosage based on severity of hypertension and response of patient during dosing.

Interactions
Cyclosporine: May cause increased cyclosporine levels with possible toxicity.
Other hypertensive agents: May have additive effects.

Lab Test Interferences None well documented.

Adverse Reactions
CV: Peripheral edema; palpitations; AV block; MI; angina; tachycardia; abnormal ECG.
CNS: Dizziness; lightheadedness; asthenia; psychiatric disturbances; headache; paresthesia; somnolence; weakness.
DERM: Rash.
GI: Nausea; abdominal discomfort; cramps; dyspepsia; dry mouth; thirst.
OTHER: Flushing; allergic reaction; myalgia.

Precautions
Pregnancy: Category C.
Lactation: Undetermined.
Children: Safety and efficacy not established.
Renal function impairment: Adjust dose in patients with renal dysfunction.
Hepatic function impairment: Adjust dosage and use drug with caution in patients with impaired hepatic function or reduced hepatic blood flow.
Antiplatelet effects: Calcium channel blockers may inhibit platelet function.
Beta-blocker withdrawal: Patients withdrawn from beta-blockers while taking nicardipine may experience increased angina. Gradually taper beta-blocker dose.
CHF: Use drug with caution in patients with CHF.

Increased angina: Occasionally patients have increased frequency, duration, or severity of angina on starting or increasing dose.
Withdrawal: Abrupt withdrawal may cause increased frequency and duration of angina.

PATIENT CARE CONSIDERATIONS
Administration/Storage
- Administer without regard to meals. Avoid giving with high-fat meals.
- If patient is taking sustained-released capsules, instruct patient to swallow capsule whole and not to chew, divide, or crush.
- If stopping medication, taper dose slowly. Stopping drug quickly could result in immediate angina.
- If patient has history of liver or renal disease, start with low doses and titrate.
- Do not increase dose for minimum of 3 days after starting medication or dose changes.
- When converting from immediate-release form to sustained-release form, note that dosage may differ.
- Store at controlled room temperature (56° to 86°F) in tight, light-resistant container.

Assessment/Interventions
- Obtain patient history, including drug history and any known allergies.
- Evaluate cardiac, hepatic, renal, and thyroid function.
- Obtain baseline vital signs and monitor 1 to 2 hr and 8 hr after administration of immediate-release product and 2 to 4 hr and at end of dosing interval if sustained-release product is used.
- Obtain baseline ECG and any follow-up ECGs as ordered by health care provider.

Overdosage: Signs and Symptoms
Nausea, weakness, dizziness, drowsiness, confusion, slurred speech, marked and prolonged hypotension, bradycardia, functional rhythms, second- or third-degree AV block, palpitations, flushing, nervousness, vomiting.

- Assess for edema, dizziness, headache, sore throat, renal changes, palpitations, liver dysfunction, or flushing.
- If patient has history of liver, renal, or cardiac dysfunction, monitor patient closely for changes from baseline.
- If there are any changes from baseline assessment, notify health care provider.
- If used to treat angina, monitor frequency of anginal episodes and consumption of sublingual nitroglycerin.

Patient/Family Education
- Instruct patient to swallow sustained-release capsules whole and not to crush or chew.
- Caution patient that increased angina may occur initially when starting, changing dose, or stopping medication.
- Advise patient not to stop taking drug abruptly.
- Instruct patient to report the following symptoms to health care provider: any unusual bleeding, bruising, rash, palpitations, irregular heartbeat, shortness of breath, nausea, change in angina, constipation, changes in gums, dizziness, or swelling in hands or feet.
- Advise patient that drug may cause dizziness or drowsiness and to use caution while driving or performing other tasks requiring mental alertness.

Nicotine

(NIK-oh-TEEN)

Class Smoking deterrent

How Supplied
Commit Lozenges 2 mg, Lozenges 4 mg ♦ *Habitrol* Transdermal system 17.5 mg, Transdermal system 35 mg, Transdermal system 52.5 mg ♦ *Nicoderm* Transdermal system 36 mg, Transdermal system 78 mg, Transdermal system 114 mg ♦ *Nicorette* Chewing gum 2 mg/square ♦ *Nicorette DS* Chewing gum 4 mg/square ♦ *Nicotrol* Transdermal system 8.3 mg, Transdermal system 16.6 mg, Transdermal system 24.9 mg ♦ *Nicotrol NS* Spray pump 0.5 mg nicotine/actuation ♦ *Nicotrol Inhaler* Inhaler 4 mg delivered (10 mg/cartridge) ♦ *ProStep* Transdermal system 15 mg, Transdermal system 30 mg
🍁 *Nicorette Plus*

Action
PHARMACOLOGY: Reduces nicotine withdrawal symptoms by providing nicotine levels lower than those associated with smoking.

Indications Aid to smoking cessation. Part of comprehensive behavioral smoking-cessation program.

Contraindications Nonsmokers; during immediate post-MI period; life-threatening arrhythmias; severe or worsening angina pectoris; active temporomandibular joint disease (nicotine polacrilex gum).

Route/Dosage
Advise patient to stop smoking completely when beginning to use smoking cessation therapy.

Nicotine Gum
ADULTS: **PO** If patient smokes less than 25 cigarettes/day, chew 2 mg gum (max, 24 pieces/day) for up to 12 wk. If patient smokes at least 25 cigarettes/day, chew 4 mg gum (max, 24 pieces/day) for up to 12 wk.

Nicotine Lozenges
ADULTS: **PO** If patient smokes first cigarette more than 30 min after waking up, start with the 2 mg lozenge. If patient smokes first cigarette within 30 min after waking up, start with the 4 mg lozenge. Week 1 to 6, slowly dissolve 1 lozenge in the mouth q 1 to 2 hr; week 7 to 9, slowly dissolve 1 lozenge in the mouth q 2 to 4 hr; week 10 to 12, slowly dissolve 1 lozenge in the mouth q 4 to 8 hr.

Nicotine Inhaler
ADULTS: **Inhaler** 6 to 16 cartridges/day for up to 6 mo.

Nicotine Transdermal Patches
ADULTS:
Habitrol: **Topical** If patient smokes at least 10 cigarettes/day, start with 21 mg/day for first 4 wk, then decrease dose to 14 mg/day for next 2 wk, then decrease dose to 7 mg/day for last 2 wk. If patient smokes less than 10 cigarettes/day, start with 14 mg/day for 6 wk then decrease dose to 7 mg/day for last 2 wk.
Nicoderm: **Topical** If patient smokes at least 10 cigarettes/day, start with 21 mg/day for first 6 wk then decrease dose to 14 mg/day for next 2 wk, then decrease dose to 7 mg/day for last 2 wk. If patient smokes less than 10 cigarettes/day, start with 14 mg/day for 6 wk then decrease dose to 7 mg/day for last 2 wk.
Nicotrol: **Topical** Use 15 mg/16 hr for 6 wk.

Nicotine Nasal Spray
ADULTS: **Spray** (Each actuation delivers 50 mcL spray containing 0.5 mg nicotine.) 8 to 40 doses/day for 3 to 6 mo.

Interactions
Acetaminophen, caffeine, imipramine, oxazepam, pentazocine, propanolol, theophylline: Smoking tends to increase metabolism and may lower blood levels of these drugs or others. Smoking cessation, with or without nicotine medication, may reverse these effects.
Food: Effective absorption of nicotine gum depends on mildly alkaline saliva. Coffee, cola, and other drinks or food may reduce salivary pH and should probably be avoided 15 min before and during chewing of gum.

Lab Test Interferences
None well documented.

Adverse Reactions
CV: Edema; flushing; hypertension; palpitations; tachyarrhythmias; tachycardia; MI; CHF; cardiac arrest; cerebrovascular accident.
CNS: Insomnia; dizziness; lightheadedness; irritability; headache; impaired concentration; confusion; convulsions; depression; paresthesia; abnormal dreams.
DERM: Erythema; rash; itching; urticaria.
EENT: Buccal cavity irritation; mouth or throat soreness or dryness. With gum chewing: traumatic injury to oral mucosa or teeth; jaw ache; changes in taste perception.
GI: GI distress; belching; indigestion; nausea; vomiting; excess salivation; hiccoughs; anorexia; constipation; diarrhea.
HEPA: Alterations of LFTs.
RESP: Increased cough; pharyngitis; sinusitis; difficulty breathing; hoarseness; sneezing.
OTHER: Pain; myalgia; arthralgia; dysmenorrhea.

Precautions
Pregnancy: Category C (nicotine polacrilex gum); Category D (inhaler, spray, transdermal nicotine).
Lactation: Excreted in breast milk.
Children: Safety and efficacy not established.
Elderly: May be more susceptible to adverse effects.
Hepatic function impairment: Hepatic impairment may reduce nicotine clearance.
Abuse/Dependence: Transference of nicotine dependence from smoking to deterrent product exists. If patient continues to smoke while on nicotine therapy, severe effects caused by higher nicotine levels may be experienced.
Cardiovascular effects: Patients with coronary heart disease, serious cardiac arrhythmias, systemic hypertension, or vasospastic disease need to be carefully evaluated and monitored closely because of cardiac effects.
Debilitated patients: May be more susceptible to adverse effects.
Dental problems: Might be exacerbated by chewing nicotine gum.
Endocrine effects: Use with caution in patients with hyperthyroidism, pheochromocytoma, or insulin-dependent diabetes because of action of nicotine on adrenal medulla.
GI effects: May delay healing in patients with peptic ulcer disease.

Overdosage: Signs and Symptoms
Nausea, salivation, abdominal pain, vomiting, diarrhea, cold sweat, headache, dizziness, disturbed hearing and vision, mental confusion, marked weakness, faintness, prostration, hypotension, difficult breathing, rapid, weak, irregular pulse, respiratory collapse.

PATIENT CARE CONSIDERATIONS
Administration/Storage
Transdermal system:
- Apply patch promptly on removal from pouch.
- Apply patch once daily to nonhairy, clean, dry skin site on upper body or upper outer arm.
- After patch has been on for 24 hr, remove and apply new patch to alternate skin site. Do not reuse skin sites for at least 1 wk (exception is *Nicotrol*, which is applied on awakening and removed at bedtime).
- After handling active patch, wash hands with water alone, because soap may increase nicotine absorption. Do not touch eyes.
- After removing used patch from skin, fold over, place in protective pouch, and immediately dispose of it so that it is inaccessible to children and pets.
- Store in cool location. Do not store out of pouch.

Nicotine chewing gum:
- Instruct patient to chew gum 1 piece at a time.
- Tell patient to chew intermittently for about 30 min. Proper chewing technique is slow-paced chewing and intermittent "parking."
- If gum is chewed fast, increased side effects will result.
- Do not allow patient to eat or drink for 15 min before chewing and during chewing.

Nasal spray:
- Administer with the head tilted back slightly.
- Should even a small amount of the spray come in contact with the skin, lips, mouth, eye or eyes, wash the area immediately with water only.
- Store at room temperature (59° to 86°F).

Assessment/Interventions
- Obtain patient history, including drug history and any known allergies.
- Assess for edema, cardiac irregularities or changes, headache, dizziness, inability to sleep, GI distress, or signs of liver dysfunction.
- Assess for history or signs of depression. If present, notify health care provider.
- If patient is diabetic, monitor blood sugar closely.
- Monitor oral mucosa and teeth for traumatic injury related to medicated gum.
- Report cardiac, hepatic, or CNS changes from baseline assessment to health care provider.

Patient/Family Education
- Review package insert information with patient.
- Inform patient of serious effects if continuing to smoke while chewing gum or using patch. Instruct patient to stop smoking. Encourage patient to participate in comprehensive smoking cessation program.
- Warn patient of possible dependence of medication.
- Tell patient that gum or patch is not for long-term use and that dose will be gradually tapered off over course of a few weeks to a month.
- Inform patient it will take a few days to adjust to taste of gum.
- Instruct patient to avoid drinking or eating 15 min before and during chewing of gum.
- Advise patient to chew gum slowly 1 piece at a time when urge to start smoking is felt.
- Instruct patient regarding proper use of gum (intermittent technique of slow-paced chewing and "parking").
- Advise patient not to exceed 30 pieces of gum/day (2 mg size) or 20 pieces/day (4 mg size) and to decrease this number gradually over first month.
- Tell patient to inspect mouth daily (if chewing gum) for signs of irritation.
- Instruct patient in proper use and disposal of patch. Tell patient to always remove old patch before applying new one, and to wash hands after applying patch.
- Advise patient regarding proper storage of patch (eg, heat sensitive, rapid evaporation once opened).
- Instruct patient to report the following symptoms to health care provider: GI distress (ie, constipation, diarrhea, nausea), headache, depression, dizziness, hiccoughs, sore throat or pain, or mouth discomfort.

Nasal spray:
- Encourage patient to participate in a smoking cessation program.
- If the patient has not stopped smoking by the fourth week of therapy, discontinue treatment.

Nifedipine

(nye-FED-ih-peen)
Class Calcium channel blocker

How Supplied
Adalat Capsules 10 mg, Capsules 20 mg ♦ *Adalat CC* Tablets, extended-release 30 mg, Tablets, extended-release 60 mg, Tablets, extended-release 90 mg ♦ *Afeditab CR* Tablets, extended-release 30 mg, ♦ *Nifedical XL* Tablets, extended-release 30 mg, Tablets, extended-release 60 mg ♦ *Procardia* Capsules 10 mg ♦ *Procardia XL* Tablets, extended-release 30 mg, Tablets, extended-release 60 mg, Tablets, extended-release 90 mg
✸ *Adalat XL* ♦ *Apo-Nifed* ♦ *Apo-Nifed PA* ♦ *Novo-Nifedin* ♦ *Nu-Nifed* ♦ *Nu-Nifedipine*

Action
PHARMACOLOGY: Inhibits movement of calcium ions across cell membrane in systemic and coronary vascular smooth muscle and myocardium. Increases CO and decreases peripheral vascular resistance. Minimal effect on sinoatrial and AV nodal conduction. Reduces myocardial oxygen demand; relaxes and prevents coronary artery spasm.

PHARMACOKINETICS/DYNAMICS:
Absorption: Nifedipine is rapidly and fully absorbed (100%). T_{max} is about 30 min (immediate-release) and 2.5 to 5 hr (extended-release). Bioavailability is 84% to 89% (extended-release) and 45% to 75% (immediate-release).
Distribution: Nifedipine protein binding is 92% to 98%.
Metabolism: Nifedipine is metabolized extensively in the liver to inactive metabolites.
Excretion: Nifedipine is eliminated in urine (0.1% unchanged) and in small amounts in feces. The t½ is about 7 hr (extended-release) and 2 hr (immediate-release). Plasma t½ is approximately 2 hr; 60% to 80% excreted in urine and the remainder in feces in metabolized form.

Special Populations:
Renal Function Impairment – Absorption of nifedipine from extended-released form could be modified by renal disease. Use with caution.
Elderly – Mean C_{max} is 36% higher and plasma concentration is 70% greater in elderly patients.
Liver Cirrhosis – Longer t½, higher bioavailability, and reduced protein binding may occur.

Indications
Treatment of vasospastic (Prinzmetal's or variant) angina, chronic stable angina, hypertension (sustained-release tablets only).

Contraindications
Sick sinus syndrome; second- or third-degree AV block, except with functioning pacemaker.

Route/Dosage
Capsules
ADULTS: PO 10 mg tid (usual dose range, 10 to 20 mg tid); swallow whole. Some patients (eg, coronary artery spasm) respond only to higher doses administered more frequently (eg, 20 to 30 mg tid to qid; max, 180 mg/day). In hospitalized patients, under close observation, dose may be increased in 10 mg increments throughout 4- to 6-hr periods as required to control pain and arrhythmias caused by ischemia. A single dose rarely exceeds 30 mg.

Extended-release tablets
ADULTS:
Procardia XL and *Nifedical XL*: PO 30 or 60 mg once daily, titrated over 7- to 14-day period (max, 120 mg/day).
Adalat CC (hypertension): PO Start with 30 mg/day and titrate dose over 7- to 14-day period (max, 90 mg/day).

Interactions
Barbiturates, rifampin: May reduce nifedipine levels, decreasing the therapeutic effect.
Cimetidine: May increase bioavailability of nifedipine.
Cisapride, diltiazem: May elevate nifedipine levels, increasing the risk of side effects.
Fentanyl, parenteral magnesium: Hypotension may occur.
Melatonin: May interfere with the antihypertensive effects of nifedipine.
Tacrolimus: Tacrolimus trough concentrations may be elevated, increasing the risk of toxicity.
Other hypertensive agents: May have additive effects.

Lab Test Interferences
None well documented.

Adverse Reactions
CV: Peripheral edema; hypotension; palpitations; syncope; CHF; MI; arrhythmia; pulmonary edema; angina; tachycardia.
CNS: Dizziness; lightheadedness; giddiness; nervousness; headache; sleep disturbances; insomnia; abnormal dreams; blurred vision; equilibrium disturbances; weakness; jitteriness; paresthesia; somnolence; malaise; anxiety.
DERM: Dermatitis; rash; pruritus; urticaria; Stevens-Johnson syndrome.
EENT: Tinnitus; sinusitis; rhinitis.
GI: Nausea; diarrhea; constipation; abdominal discomfort; cramps; dyspepsia; dry mouth; flatulence.
GU: Micturition disorders; sexual difficulties.

HEPA: Hepatitis; hepatotoxicity; elevations of LFT enzymes.
HEMA: Anemia; leukopenia; thrombocytopenia; bruising; positive *Coombs'* test with or without hemolytic anemia.
RESP: Nasal or chest congestion; shortness of breath; wheezing; cough; respiratory infection.
OTHER: Flushing; gingival hyperplasia; sweating; muscle cramps, pain and inflammation; joint stiffness, pain, or arthritis; chills; fever; thirst.

Precautions
Pregnancy: Category C.
Lactation: Excreted in breast milk in small amounts.
Children: Safety and efficacy not established.
Elderly: May experience greater hypotensive effects.
Hepatic function impairment: Use drug with caution in patients with impaired hepatic function, reduced hepatic blood flow, or hepatic cirrhosis.
Acute hepatic injury: In rare instances, nifedipine has been associated with significant elevations in liver enzymes, symptoms consistent with acute hepatic injury, cholestasis with or without jaundice and allergic hepatitis.
Antiplatelet effects: Nifedipine decreases platelet aggregation and can increase bleeding time in some patients.
Beta-blocker withdrawal: Patients withdrawn from beta-blockers while taking nifedipine may experience increased angina.
CHF: Use drug with caution in patients with CHF.
Edema: Nifedipine has been associated with edema in some cases and should be distinguished from fluid retention secondary to heart failure.
Increased angina: Occasional patients may have increased frequency, duration, or severity of angina at start of therapy or when dose is increased.
Withdrawal: Abrupt withdrawal may cause increased frequency and duration of angina.

Overdosage: Signs and Symptoms
Hypotension, nausea, weakness, dizziness, drowsiness, confusion, slurred speech, second- or third-degree AV block, marked and prolonged hypotension and bradycardia, decreased cardiac output, functional rhythms.

PATIENT CARE CONSIDERATIONS

Administration/Storage
* Taper initiation and discontinuation of drug over 7 to 14 days.
* May be administered without regard to meals.
* Have patient swallow sustained-release tablets whole; do not allow patient to chew, divide, or crush.
* *Procardia XL* and *Adalat CC* are not rated as generic equivalents; do not be interchanged without health care provider's authorization.
* If beta-blockers are being withdrawn while patient is taking nifedipine, gradually taper beta-blocker dose.
* Start patients with impaired hepatic function with low doses.
* When using immediate-release capsules for treatment of hypertensive emergencies, puncture capsules, and squeeze liquid contents under tongue, or puncture capsule several times and have patient chew.
* Store capsules at room temperature (59° to 86°F) and protect from light and moisture.

Assessment/Interventions
* Obtain history, including drug history and any known allergies. Evaluate cardiac, endocrine, respiratory, hepatic, CNS, renal, and GI systems.
* Obtain baseline and follow-up vital signs; assess for chest pain.
* If drug is used as antihypertensive, routinely monitor BP and note any orthostatic hypotension.
* Inspect skin for rashes.
* Assess for any unusual bruising or bleeding.
* Check BP at least once daily when patient is taking both nifedipine and cimetidine. If possible, another H_2 antagonist may be prescribed instead of cimetidine.
* Administer sublingual nitroglycerin if breakthrough chest pain occurs. Record frequency and duration of anginal attacks and use of sublingual nitroglycerin.
* If any changes from baseline vital signs occur, notify health care provider.

Patient/Family Education
* Remind patient that sustained-release capsules must be swallowed whole, not chewed, divided, or crushed.
* Teach patient the importance of good dental care, and advise that patient visit dentist on routine basis because gum swelling may occur.
* Instruct patient to maintain increased fluid intake (if not contraindicated) to avoid constipation.
* Instruct patient that medication must be used chronically to obtain benefit and to notify health care provider if at least 2 doses are missed.
* Teach patient/family to notify health care provider of any changes from baseline evalua-

tion (ie, chest pain, shortness of breath).
- Inform patient that there may be increased chest pain at start of medication and with dose changes, but that this effect is transient. If it persists, notify health care provider.
- If health care provider prescribes coadministration of sublingual nitroglycerin, teach patient how to take nitroglycerin sublingually.
- Explain that when sustained-release form is used, partially undigested tablet may appear in feces but that this effect is no cause for concern.
- Instruct patient to report the following symptoms to the health care provider: ringing in ears, swollen gums, respiratory changes, inability to sleep, fever, or chills.
- Advise patient that drug may cause dizziness, lightheadedness, and blurred vision, and to use caution while driving or performing other tasks requiring mental alertness.

Nilutamide

(nye-LOO-tah-mide)
Class Antiandrogen

How Supplied
Nilandron Tablets 50 mg
✤ *Anandron*

Action
PHARMACOLOGY: Nonsteroidal with antiandrogen activity. It blocks the effects of testosterone at the androgen receptor level. The drug is rapidly and completely absorbed. There is moderate binding of the drug to plasma proteins. It is extensively metabolized. The majority is eliminated in the urine. Fecal elimination is negligible. The mean t½ ranged from 38 to 59.1 hr. Metabolic enzyme inhibition may occur for this drug.

PHARMACOKINETICS/DYNAMICS:
Absorption: Nilutamide is rapidly and completely absorbed. Steady state is 2 to 4 weeks (multiple dosing).
Distribution: Nilutamide is moderately binding to plasma proteins and low binding to erythrocytes.
Metabolism: Nilutamide is extensively metabolized. Five metabolites have been isolated with several active.
Excretion: Nilutamide is excreted in urine 62% (2% as unchanged) and feces 1.4% to 7%. The t½ is 38 to 59.1 hr.

Indications Metastatic prostate cancer in combination with surgical castration.

Contraindications Severe hepatic impairment; severe respiratory insufficiency; hypersensitivity to nilutamide or any component of this preparation.

Route/Dosage
Prostate Cancer
ADULTS:
Initial dose: **PO** 300 mg (6 tablets) once daily for 30 days.
Maintenance dose: **PO** 150 mg (3 tablets) once daily.

Interactions Inhibits hepatic cytochrome P450 enzymes. May alter the elimination of other agents metabolized by the cytochrome P450 system. Monitor patients for increased serum levels and toxicity during concomitant therapy with warfarin, phenytoin, or theophylline.

Lab Test Interferences Increased ALT and AST.

Adverse Reactions
CV: Peripheral edema, hypertension, chest pain; heart failure.
CNS: Insomnia; headache; dizziness; depression; hypesthesia; asthenia; paresthesia.
DERM: Sweating; loss of body hair; dry skin.
ENDO: Hot flashes.
GI: Low potential for nausea and vomiting; constipation; anorexia; abdominal pain; hemorrhage or melena (2%).
GU: Testicular atrophy; UTI.
HEMA: Anemia.
METAB: Alcohol intolerance.
MUSC: Pain; bone pain.
RESP: Dyspnea; pneumonia; intestinal pneumonitis.
SPEC SENSE: Delayed adjustment to dark or light; abnormal vision; cataract.
OTHER: Flu-like syndrome.

> **WARNING:**
> *Interstitial pneumonitis:* Interstitial pneumonitis has been reported in 2% of patients in clinical trials. Reports of interstitial changes including pulmonary fibrosis leading to hospitalization and death rarely reported in postmarketing surveillance. Most cases were reversible with discontinuation and occurred within the first 3 mo of therapy.

Precautions
Pregnancy: Category C.
Children: Safety and efficacy in pediatric patients have not been established.
Delay in adaptation to the dark: When passing from a lighted area to a dark area.

Hepatitis: Severe liver injury has been reported. Hepatotoxicity in these reports generally occurred within the first 3 to 4 mo of treatment. *Women:* Nilutamide has no indication for women.

PATIENT CARE CONSIDERATIONS
Administration/Storage
- Store at room temperature (59° to 86°F); protect from light.
- Initiate therapy on day of surgical castration or the day after surgery. Nilutamide may be taken without regard to meals.

Assessment/Interventions
- Monitor LFTs at baseline and at 3-mo intervals during therapy.
- Measure serum transaminase levels prior to starting treatment and at regular intervals for the first 4 mo of treatment and periodically thereafter. Obtain LFTs at the first sign or symptoms suggestive of liver dysfunction (eg, nausea, vomiting, abdominal pain, fatigue, anorexia, flu-like symptoms, dark urine, jaundice, right upper quadrant tenderness).
- Perform a routine chest x-ray prior to initiating treatment. Baseline pulmonary function tests may be considered.
- If at any time, a patient has jaundice or their ALT rises above 2 times the upper limit of normal, discontinue nilutamide with close follow up of LFTs until resolution.

Patient/Family Education
- Start nilutamide tablets on the day of, or the day after, surgical castration. Patients should not interrupt their dosing of nilutamide or stop taking the medication without consulting their health care provider.
- Delays of visual adaptation from light to dark may occur. Advise patients to use caution when driving at night or through tunnels. Patients can use tinted glasses to help decrease the problem.
- Nilutamide may cause alcohol-intolerance. Avoid alcohol if facial flushing, malaise, or hypotension occurs after consuming alcoholic beverages.
- Notify your doctor at the first sign or symptoms suggestive of liver dysfunction (eg, nausea, vomiting, abdominal pain, fatigue, anorexia, flu-like symptoms, dark urine, jaundice, right upper quadrant tenderness).
- Tell health care provider immediately of any dyspnea or aggravation of preexisting dyspnea.
- Instruct patients to report any new or worsening shortness of breath that they experience while on nilutamide. If symptoms occur, discontinue nilutamide immediately until it can be determined if the symptoms are drug-related.

Overdosage: Signs and Symptoms
GI disorders, including nausea and vomiting, malaise, headache, dizziness (600 and 900 mg/day).

Nimodipine
(NYE-moE-dih-peen)
Class Calcium channel blocker
How Supplied
Nimotop Capsules, liquid 30 mg
Action
PHARMACOLOGY: Inhibits movement of calcium ions across cell membrane in systemic and coronary vascular smooth muscle and myocardium. Has greater effect on cerebral arteries than on other arteries.

PHARMACOKINETICS/DYNAMICS:

Absorption: Nimodipine is rapidly absorbed after oral administration. Bioavailability is 13% and, T_{max} is approximately 1 hr. Food decreases peak plasma concentration 68% and bioavailability 38%.

Distribution: Nimodipine protein binding is over 95%.

Metabolism: Extensive first-pass metabolism in the liver.

Excretion: Nimodipine is eliminated in urine (less than 1% unchanged), and elimination of metabolites are considerably less active than parent compound. Terminal $t_{½}$ is 8 to 9 hr, and initial $t_{½}$ is 1 to 2 hr.

Special Populations:
Elderly – AUC and C_{max} was approximately 2–fold higher, and is not considered significant. Liver Cirrhosis – Nimodipine bioavailability is significantly increased, C_{max} almost doubles, and dosage adjustment is necessary.

Indications Improvement of neurologic deficits caused by vasospasm after subarachnoid hemorrhage from ruptured congenital intracranial aneurysms. **Unlabeled use(s):** Treatment of common and classic migraine and chronic cluster headache.

Contraindications Standard considerations.

Route/Dosage
Subarachnoid Hemorrhage
ADULTS: PO/Nasogastric 60 mg q 4 hr for 21 consecutive days. Initiate therapy within 96 hr of subarachnoid hemorrhage.

Headaches
ADULTS: PO 30 mg tid.

Interactions
Beta-blockers: May cause increased adverse effects because of myocardial contractility or atrioventricular (AV) conduction depression.
Fentanyl: May cause severe hypotension or increased fluid requirements.
Other hypertensive agents: May have additive effects.

Lab Test Interferences None well documented.

Adverse Reactions
CV: Peripheral edema; hypotension; hypertension; bradycardia; CHF; tachycardia; abnormal ECG.
CNS: Rebound vasospasm; headache; dizziness; psychiatric disturbances.
DERM: Rash; acne.
GI: Nausea; diarrhea; abdominal discomfort; cramps; dyspepsia; GI hemorrhage.
HEMA: Disseminated intravascular coagulation; thrombocytopenia; deep vein thrombosis.
HEPA: Hepatitis; hepatotoxicity; elevated LDH, alkaline phosphatase and ALT levels.
RESP: Shortness of breath; wheezing.
OTHER: Flushing; muscle cramps, pain, and inflammation.

Precautions
Pregnancy: Category C.
Lactation: Undetermined.
Children: Safety and efficacy not established.
Hepatic function impairment Use drug with caution in patients with impaired hepatic function or reduced hepatic blood flow.
Antiplatelet effects: Calcium channel blockers may inhibit platelet function.

Overdosage: Signs and Symptoms
Nausea, weakness, dizziness, drowsiness, confusion, slurred speech, marked and prolonged hypotension, bradycardia, decreased cardiac output, junctional rhythms, second-or third-degree AV block, palpitations, flushing, nervousness, loss of consciousness, vomiting, generalized edema.

PATIENT CARE CONSIDERATIONS
Administration/Storage
- If capsule cannot be swallowed, make hole in both ends of capsule with 18-gauge needle and extract contents into syringe. Empty contents into patient's nasogastric tube and wash down tube with 30 mL of normal saline solution.
- Patient may require decreased dose if liver dysfunction is present.
- Administer drug around the clock.
- Do not abruptly withdraw drug; dosage must be tapered.
- Store at room temperature (59° to 86°F) in original foil packaging.

Assessment/Interventions
- Obtain patient history, including drug history and any known allergies. Note liver dysfunction, respiratory difficulties, unusual bruising or bleeding, GI problems, rashes, acne, joint pain, deep vein thrombosis or muscle cramping.
- Obtain baseline vital signs.
- Assess patient's neurological status and document any deficits.
- If patient has history of liver, renal, or cardiac dysfunction, monitor closely for change from baseline.
- If patient is hypotensive or bradycardic or has respiratory difficulties, notify health care provider.
- If nausea, vomiting, diarrhea, abdominal cramping, or increased bruising or bleeding occurs, notify health care provider.

Patient/Family Education
- Explain that medication needs to be taken around the clock for 21 days.
- Instruct patient to report the following symptoms to health care provider: Shortness of breath, nausea, abdominal cramping, diarrhea, unusual bruising or bleeding, palpitations, dizziness, faint feeling, or swelling of hands or feet.

Nisoldipine
(nye-SOLD-ih-peen)
Class Calcium channel blocker

How Supplied
Sular Tablets, extended-release 10 mg, Tablets, extended-release 20 mg, Tablets, extended-release 30 mg, Tablets, extended-release 40 mg

Action
PHARMACOLOGY: Inhibits movement of calcium ions across cell membrane in systemic and coronary vascular smooth muscle and myocardium.

PHARMACOKINETICS/DYNAMICS:
Absorption: Nisoldipine is well absorbed. Absolute bioavailability is 5% and T_{max} is 6 to 12 hr. High fat food significantly affects release of drug from coat-core formulation, resulting in significant increase in peak concentration.

Metabolism: Presystemic metabolism of nisoldipine in gut wall and liver by CYP450 enzymes.

Excretion: Nisoldipine is eliminated 60% to 80% in urine (traces unchanged), 5 urinary metabolites and only 1 active. The t½ is 7 to 12 hr.

Special Populations:
Elderly – Higher nisoldipine plasma concentrations (C_{max} and AUC) have been found in elderly.

Liver Cirrhosis – Increased plasma concentrations. Use lower starting and maintenance doses.

Indications Treatment of hypertension, alone or in combination with other antihypertensive agents.

Contraindications Sensitivity to dihydropyridine calcium channel blockers.

Route/Dosage
ADULTS: **PO** Initiate therapy with 20 mg once daily, then increase by 10 mg/wk, or at longer intervals, to attain adequate BP control. Doses greater than 60 mg once daily are not recommended.

Interactions
Azole antifungal agents (eg, ketoconazole), cimetidine, grapefruit juice: May increase nisoldipine concentrations and effects.
Hydantoins (eg, phenytoin): May decrease nisoldipine levels and effects.

Lab Test Interferences None well documented.

Adverse Reactions
CV: Vasodilation; palpitation; chest pain.
CNS: Headache; dizziness.
DERM: Rash.
EENT: Sinusitis; pharyngitis.
GI: Nausea.
OTHER: Peripheral edema.

Precautions
Pregnancy: Category C.
Lactation: Undetermined.
Children: Safety and efficacy not established.
Elderly: Start with doses no greater than 10 mg in patients over 65 yr.
Hepatic function impairment: Use drug with caution in patients with severe hepatic dysfunction. Start with doses no greater than 10 mg/day.
CHF: Use drug with caution in patients with CHF.
Increased angina, MI: Occasional patients, particularly those with severe obstructive coronary artery disease, may have increased frequency, duration, or severity of angina or acute MI at start of therapy or when dose is increased.

Overdosage: Signs and Symptoms
Pronounced hypotension.

PATIENT CARE CONSIDERATIONS

Administration/Storage
- Available in extended-release tablets only.
- Have patient swallow tablets whole. Do not allow patient to crush, chew, or divide.
- Administer once daily. Do not administer with a high fat meal. Avoid grapefruit products before and after dosing.
- Start elderly patients over 65 yr and patients with impaired hepatic function with doses no greater than 10 mg/day.
- Store at room temperature (59° to 86°F) protected from light and moisture.

Assessment/Interventions
- Obtain patient history, including drug history, and any known allergies.
- Evaluate hepatic function tests prior to therapy.
- Monitor BP and pulse prior to therapy, during titration, and periodically during therapy.
- Administer SL nitroglycerin for chest pain. Record frequency and duration of anginal attacks and use of SL nitroglycerin.
- Monitor patient for development of peripheral edema, headaches, palpitations, increasing angina. Notify health care provider if present.

Patient/Family Education
- Instruct patient not to chew, crush, or divide extended-release tablets.
- Advise patient not to take with a high-fat meal and to avoid grapefruit products before and after dosing.
- Advise patient to take the medication once daily as directed even if they have no symptoms.
- Teach patient correct technique for monitoring BP and pulse daily.
- Advise patient not to stop or change the dose unless advised by the health care provider.
- Advise patient that drug may cause dizziness and to use caution while driving or performing other tasks requiring mental alertness.
- Instruct patient to report the following symptoms to health care provider: palpitations; increasing chest pain; swelling of ankles, feet or hands; headache; dizziness.
- Stress the need to comply with the other components of the hypertensive regimen, such as dietary changes, weight loss, and exercise.
- Instruct patient never to stop taking the medication suddenly.

Nitrofurantoin

(nye-troe-FYOOR-an-toyn)

Class Urinary anti-infective

How Supplied
Furadantin Oral suspension 25 mg/5 mL ♦ *Macrobid* Capsules 100 mg (as 25 mg macrocrystals, 75 mg monohydrate) ♦ *Macrodantin* Capsules 25 mg, Capsules 50 mg, Capsules 100 mg ❋ *Apo-Nitrofurantoin* ♦ *Novo-Furantoin*

Action
PHARMACOLOGY: May interfere with bacterial cell wall formation and bacterial duplication. Inhibits bacterial carbohydrate metabolism. Bacteriostatic in low concentrations; bactericidal at higher concentrations.

PHARMACOKINETICS/DYNAMICS:

Absorption: Nitrofurantoin is well absorbed from the GI tract, macrocrystalline form is absorbed more slowly, and food increases bioavailability.

Distribution: Nitrofurantoin protein binding is approximately 60%.

Metabolism: Approximately 50% to 70% of nitrofurantoin is rapidly metabolized by body tissues.

Excretion: Nitrofurantion is eliminated in urine (30% to 50% unchanged). The t½ in healthy patients is 20 min and the t½ in anephric patients is 60 min.

Special Populations:
Renal Function Impairment – Nitrofurantoin accumulates in serum.

Indications
Treatment of urinary tract infections caused by susceptible strains of *E. coli*, enterococci, *Staphylococcus aureus*, certain strains of *Klebsiella*, *Enterobacter*, and *Proteus* species.

Contraindications
Renal impairment (Ccr less than 40 mL/min); anuria or oliguria; pregnant women at term; infants younger than 1 mo.

Route/Dosage

ADULTS AND CHILDREN (OLDER THAN 12 YR): **PO** 50 to 100 mg qid with meals for 7 days min and for at least 3 days after sterile urine is obtained.

CHILDREN (OLDER THAN 1 MO): **PO** 5 to 7 mg/kg/24 hr in 4 divided doses with meals and at bedtime for min of 7 days and for at least 3 days after sterile urine is obtained.

Long-Term Suppressive Therapy
ADULTS: **PO** 50 to 100 mg at bedtime.
CHILDREN: **PO** 1 mg/kg/24 hr as single or 2 divided doses.

Interactions
Anticholinergic drugs and food: Increased absorption of nitrofurantoin.
Magnesium salts: May reduce anti-infective action by decreasing absorption.
Probenecid: May increase nitrofurantoin serum levels by reducing renal elimination.

Lab Test Interferences
Urinary creatinine elevation and false-positive urine glucose determination with *Benedict's* reagent (copper sulfate solution) may occur.

Adverse Reactions
CNS: Peripheral neuropathy; headache; dizziness; nystagmus; drowsiness.
DERM: Exfoliative dermatitis; erythema multiforme; maculopapular, erythematous or eczematous eruption; pruritus; urticaria; angioedema; alopecia; photosensitivity.
GI: Anorexia; nausea; emesis; abdominal pain; diarrhea; parotiditis; pancreatitis.
GU: Superinfection.
HEPA: Hepatitis; hepatotoxicity; jaundice; increased bilirubin and alkaline phosphatase; permanent liver dysfunction.
HEMA: Hemolytic anemia from G-6-PD deficiency; granulocytopenia; agranulocytosis; leukopenia; thrombocytopenia; eosinophilia; megaloblastic anemia; aplastic anemia.
RESP: Acute, subacute or chronic pulmonary reaction (eg, shortness of breath, chest pain, cough, fever, chills); permanent pulmonary impairment.
OTHER: Anaphylaxis; asthmatic attack in patient with history of asthma; drug fever; arthralgia; sialadenitis; muscular aches.

Precautions
Pregnancy: Category B. Contraindicated in women at term. Do not give to pregnant patient with G-6-PD deficiency.
Lactation: Excreted in breast milk.
Children: Contraindicated in infants less than 1 mo.
Superinfection: Prolonged or repeated therapy with antibiotics may result in overgrowth of nonsusceptible bacteria or fungi.
Hemolysis: Hemolytic anemia has occurred, apparently linked to G-6-PD deficiencies. Discontinue at any sign of hemolysis.
Peripheral neuropathy: May become severe or irreversible; fatalities have been reported. Predisposing conditions such as renal impairment, anemia, diabetes, electrolyte imbalance, vitamin B deficiency and debilitating diseases may increase risk.
Pulmonary reactions: Acute and chronic reactions, including interstitial pneumonia, respiratory failure and death, have occurred. Do not

give to any patient who has had pulmonary reaction to drug.

PATIENT CARE CONSIDERATIONS

Administration/Storage

- Administer with food or milk.
- Oral suspension can be mixed with water, juice, or formula.
- Have patient rinse mouth after administration to avoid staining teeth.
- Have patient swallow tablets or capsules whole. Instruct patient not to open capsule or crush tablets.
- Nitrofurantoin and nitrofurantoin macrocrystalline are not interchangeable because of differences in absorption. *Macrobid* brand is formulated for q 12-hr administration.
- Store at room temperature (59° to 86°F) in tightly closed container. Protect from light.

Assessment/Interventions

- Obtain patient history, including drug history and any known allergies.
- Obtain urine for culture and sensitivity prior to starting drug.
- Obtain results of CBC and other lab tests ordered by health care provider (ie, creatinine, electrolytes, alkaline phosphatase, bilirubin).
- Obtain vital signs. Monitor weight and I&O.
- Evaluate for signs of infection (ie, fever, chills, drainage, burning, frequency or hesitancy).

Overdosage: Signs and Symptoms
Nausea, anorexia, vomiting, diarrhea.

- Evaluate for dizziness, headaches, GI upset, skin changes, hearing, or vision changes.
- If patient exhibits shortness of breath, chest pain, continued fever, numbness, tingling, headache, dizziness, drowsiness, nystagmus, blood in urine, or signs of hemolysis, notify health care provider.

Patient/Family Education

- Remind patient to shake nitrofurantoin suspension before measuring dose.
- Instruct patient to take medication with food or milk.
- Inform patient to expect urine to be orange or brown in color while taking medication.
- Teach patient importance of completing full course of antibiotic to avoid recurrent infection.
- Instruct patient to report the following symptoms to health care provider: shortness of breath, difficulty breathing, changes in urination (other than orange discoloration), nausea, vomiting, diarrhea, cramping, skin changes, chest pain, cough, fever, headache, dizziness, vision changes, unusual bleeding (ie, red or black urine or stool), yellowing of skin, light-colored stools or edema.
- Caution patient to avoid exposure to sunlight and to use sunscreen or wear protective clothing to avoid photosensitivity reaction.

Nitroglycerin

(nye-troe-GLIH-suh-rin)

Class Antianginal

How Supplied

Deponit Transdermal systems 16 mg, Transdermal systems 32 mg ♦ *Minitran* Transdermal systems 9 mg, Transdermal systems 18 mg, Transdermal systems 36 mg, Transdermal systems 54 mg ♦ *Nitrek* Transdermal systems 22.4 mg, Transdermal systems 44.8 mg, Transdermal systems 67.2 mg ♦ *Nitro-Bid* Ointment, topical 2% in a lanolin-petrolatum base ♦ *Nitro-Bid IV* Injection, IV 5 mg/mL ♦ *Nitro-Dur* Transdermal systems 20 mg, Transdermal systems 40 mg, Transdermal systems 60 mg, Transdermal systems 80 mg, Transdermal systems 100 mg, Transdermal systems 120 mg, Transdermal systems 160 mg ♦ *Nitro-Time* Capsules, sustained-release 2.5 mg, Capsules, sustained-release 6.5 mg, Capsules, sustained-release 9 mg ♦ *Nitrodisc* Transdermal systems 16 mg, Transdermal systems 24 mg, Transdermal systems 32 mg ♦ *Nitrogard* Tablets, buccal, controlled-release (transmucosal) 2 mg, Tablets, buccal, controlled-release (transmucosal) 3 mg ♦ *Nitrol* Ointment, topical 2% in a lanolin-petrolatum base ♦ *Nitrolingual* Aerosol spray, translingual 0.4 mg/metered dose ♦ *NitroQuick* Tablets, sublingual 0.3 mg, Tablets, sublingual 0.4 mg, Tablets, sublingual 0.6 mg ♦ *Nitrostat* Tablets, sublingual 0.3 mg, Tablets, sublingual 0.4 mg, Tablets, sublingual 0.6 mg ♦ *Transderm-Nitro* Transdermal systems 12.5 mg, Transdermal systems 25 mg, Transdermal systems 50 mg, Transdermal systems 75 mg
✤ *Gen-Nitro* ♦ *Nitrolingual Pumpspray*

Action

PHARMACOLOGY: Relaxation of smooth muscle of venous and arterial vasculature.

PHARMACOKINETICS/DYNAMICS:
Absorption: Rapid.

Distribution: Vd: 3 L/kg. Plasma protein binding is approximately 60% (parent); 1,2 dinitroglycerin 60%; 1,3 dinitroglycerin 30%.

Metabolism: Extensive in liver by nitrate reductase; known sites of extrahepatic metabolism include red blood cells and vascular walls.

Metabolized to inorganic nitrate and the active 1,2 and 1,3 dinitroglycerols which are less effective vasodilators but have longer plasma half-lives than parent compound.

Excretion: Eliminated by urine as inactive metabolites. Serum t½ is 3 min (IV) and 1 to 4 min (sublingual). Clearance is 1 L/kg/min.

Onset: 1 to 2 min (IV) and 1 to 3 min (sublingual).

Duration: 3 to 5 min (IV), 30 to 60 min (sublingual), and 3 to 5 hr (buccal).

Indications Treatment of acute angina (SL, translingual, IV, transmucosal); prophylaxis of angina (SL, transmucosal, translingual, sustained release, transdermal, topical); control of BP in perioperative or intraoperative hypertension (IV); CHF associated with MI (IV). **Unlabeled use(s):** Reduce cardiac workload in patients with MI and in refractory CHF (SL, topical, oral, IV); adjunctive treatment of Raynaud disease (topical); treatment of hypertensive crisis (IV).

Contraindications Hypersensitivity to nitrates; severe anemia; closed-angle glaucoma; orthostatic hypotension; early MI; pericarditis or pericardial tamponade; head trauma or cerebral hemorrhage; allergy to adhesives (transdermal); hypotension or uncorrected hypovolemia (IV); increased intracranial pressure or decreased cerebral perfusion (IV).

Route/Dosage

Perioperative Hypertension
ADULTS: **IV** 5 mcg/min using nonperipheral vein catheter (PVCP) IV administration set initially; titrate to response.

Angina
ADULTS: **PO** 2.5 or 2.6 mg (sustained-release form) tid to qid initially; titrate to response. **SL** 0.15 to 0.6 mg dissolved under tongue or in buccal pouch at first sign of acute angina attack; repeat q 5 min (do not exceed 3 tablets in 15 min). **Topical** 1 to 2 inches q 8 hr up to 4 to 5 inches spread over 3 × 4 inch area and cover with plastic wrap to prevent staining of clothes or application q 4 hr prn. Allow a nitrate-free period of 10 to 12 hr/day. **Transdermal** 0.2 to 0.4 mg/hr patch initially applied once daily; titrate dose to response. **Translingual** 1 to 2 sprays onto or under tongue at first onset of attack. **Transmucosal** 1 mg q 3 to 5 hr during waking hours; tablet placed between lip or cheek and gum.

Refractory Angina, CHF Secondary to Acute MI
ADULTS: **IV** 5 mcg/min initially; titrate according to hemodynamic readings (eg, BP, heart rate, pulmonary capillary wedge pressure).

Interactions
Alcohol: Severe hypotension and cardiovascular collapse may occur.
Calcium channel blockers: Symptomatic orthostatic hypotension may occur.
Dihydroergotamine: May increase systolic BP and decrease antianginal effects.
Heparin: May decrease anticoagulation effect when used in conjunction with IV nitroglycerin.

Lab Test Interferences May cause false report of reduced serum cholesterol with Zlatkis-Zak color reaction. May cause false-positive result in urinary catecholamines and VMA determinations.

Adverse Reactions
CV: Tachycardia; palpitations; hypotension; syncope; arrhythmias.
CNS: Headache; apprehension; weakness; vertigo; dizziness; agitation; insomnia.
DERM: Cutaneous vasodilation with flushing; contact dermatitis (transdermal); topical allergic reactions (ointment); local burning or tingling sensation in oral cavity (sublingual).
EENT: Blurred vision.
GI: Nausea; vomiting; diarrhea; dyspepsia.
GU: Dysuria; urinary frequency; impotence.
HEMA: Methemoglobinemia; hemolytic anemia.
RESP: Bronchitis; pneumonia.
OTHER: Arthralgia; perspiration; pallor; cold sweat; edema.

Precautions
Pregnancy: Category C.
Lactation: Undetermined.
Children: Safety and efficacy not established.
Renal function impairment: Use IV product with caution in patients with renal impairment.
Hepatic function impairment: Use IV product with caution in patients with hepatic impairment.
Alcohol intoxication: Has occurred in patients receiving high doses of IV nitroglycerin.
Angina: May aggravate angina caused by hypertrophic cardiomyopathy
Defibrillator: Do not discharge cardioverter/defibrillator through paddle electrode overlying transdermal system. Arcing may occur and burn patient.
Glaucoma: May increase intraocular pressure; administer with caution in patients with glaucoma.
Hypotension: Avoid excessive, prolonged hypotension with IV product because of possible harmful effects on brain, heart, liver and kidneys.
MI: Safety of oral or sublingual products in acute MI not established; use only with close observation and monitoring. However, IV nitro-

glycerin is drug of choice in acute MI.
Orthostatic Hypotension: May occur even with small doses; alcohol accentuates this reaction.
Sublingual administration: Absorption is dependent on salivary secretion; dry mouth decreases absorption.
Transdermal nitroglycerin: Not for immediate relief of anginal attacks.

PATIENT CARE CONSIDERATIONS
Administration/Storage
IV:
- Dilute in D5W or 0.9% Sodium Chloride injection prior to infusion. Do not mix with any other infusions. Use glass bottles only and non-PVC tubing provided. Use with infusion pump. Do not use IV filter. Store premixed IV solution in dark. Do not freeze.

Topical:
- Apply uniform layer with applicator or on dose-measuring paper. Apply in thin, uniform layer on nonhairy area on upper arm or upper torso. After spreading measured dose, cover skin with plastic wrap to prevent staining of clothes. Wash hands after application. Store in original tube. Do not freeze.

Sublingual:
- Give while patient is lying or sitting. Place in buccal pouch to decrease stinging. Do not swallow. Store at room temperature (59° to 86°F) in original, brown glass container. If cotton is in bottle, remove and discard after opening. Do not place cotton or other materials within bottle because they may absorb nitroglycerin. Protect from moisture. Discard unused amounts after 6 mo.

PO (sustained-release):
- Tell patients not to chew or dissolve capsule in mouth. Store at room temperature (59° to 86°F).

Transdermal:
- Apply patch to nonhairy area on upper arm or torso. Do not apply over cuts or abrasions. Remove old patch prior to applying new patch. Store at room temperature (59° to 86°F). Do not open until ready to use.

Translingual:
- Do not shake canister prior to using. Patient should release spray under tongue. Do not inhale spray.

Assessment/Interventions
- Obtain patient history, including drug history and any known allergies.
- Assess baseline vital signs, ECG, lung, and heart sounds.
- All other forms: Monitor vital signs, I&O. Assess for tolerance of drug effects.
- Monitor for nausea, diarrhea, incontinence,

Overdosage: Signs and Symptoms
Hypotension, tachycardia, flushing, excessive sweating, headache, vertigo, palpitations, visual disturbances, nausea, vomiting, confusion and dyspnea may occur as a result of vasodilation and methemoglobinemia.

---

abdominal pain, chest pain, bradycardia, flushing, pruritus, rash, or contact dermatitis.
- Notify health care provider of any muscle twitching, diaphoresis, pallor, edema, blurred vision, wheezing, hypotension, or chest pain.

IV:
- Assess lung and heart sounds regularly during IV therapy.
- Monitor vital signs frequently while patient is receiving infusion and titrate dosage to systolic BP or pain relief as prescribed.
- Monitor LOC. Notify health care provider of any significant hypotension, bradycardia, headache, or no reduction of anginal pain. Keep patient on bedrest.
- Monitor pulmonary capillary wedge pressure and I&O.

Patient/Family Education
- Review with patient and family the following signs of angina: Pressure-like chest pain of acute onset, often associated with physical activity, that may radiate down to left arm or up to neck and jaw.

Sublingual:
- Advise patient to dissolve tablet under tongue and not to swallow. If pain remains, the dose may be repeated q 5 min until 3 tablets are taken. If pain still persists or becomes more intense, patient should be taught to call 911 or appropriate local number to obtain emergency services.
- Tell patient to place tablet between gum and cheek if stinging sensation occurs.
- Caution patient to sit or lie down while taking and for 20 minutes after initial dose. If dizziness occurs, instruct patient to lie down.
- Teach patient storage instructions (per Administration/Storage information).
- Advise patient to discard 6 mo after opening package.
- Instruct patient to report these symptoms to health care provider: Severe headache, blurred vision, dry mouth, dizziness or flushing.

Ointment, Spray, Sustained-Release, Transdermal:
- Advise patient to wear gloves or use dose-

determining applicator when applying ointment.
- Teach patient to leave a 10 to 12 hr nitrate-free period at night to decrease likelihood of developing tolerance.
- For transdermal form, tell patient to change site of application to avoid skin sensitization.
- Explain that swimming or bathing does not affect effectiveness of drug
- Advise patient to notify health care provider of any decrease in effectiveness of medication.
- Caution patient to avoid sudden position changes to prevent orthostatic hypotension.
- Instruct patient to avoid intake of alcoholic beverages.

Nitroprusside Sodium

(nye-troe-PRUSS-ide SO-dee-uhm)

Class Agent for hypertensive emergencies

How Supplied
Nitropress Powder for injection 50 mg/vial

Action
PHARMACOLOGY: Relaxes vascular smooth muscle and dilates peripheral veins and arteries.

Indications Immediate reduction of BP in hypertensive crisis; production of controlled hypotension to reduce bleeding during surgery; for acute congestive heart failure. **Unlabeled use(s):** Has been used alone or with dopamine in acute MI.

Contraindications Treatment of compensatory hypertension, in which primary hemodynamic lesion is aortic coarctation or arteriovenous shunting; to produce hypotension during surgery in patients with known inadequate cerebral circulation or in moribund patients (A.S.A. Class 5E) coming to emergency surgery; patients with congenital (Leber's) optic atrophy or with tobacco amblyopia; acute CHF associated with reduced peripheral vascular resistance.

Route/Dosage
Give by IV infusion using infusion pump, preferably volmetric pump.
ADULTS AND CHILDREN: **IV** 0.3 mcg/kg/min initially; titrate upward gradually every few minutes to desired effect. Do not exceed 10 mcg/kg/min. Do not use maximum rate for more than 10 min. Average rate of infusion is 3 mcg/kg/min; some patients require much lower doses, especially if other hypotensive agents are used.

Interactions
Antihypertensives, ganglionic blocking agents, volatile anesthetics (eg, enflurane, halothane): Additive hypotensive effects.

Lab Test Interferences None well documented.

Adverse Reactions
CV: Evidence of rapid BP reduction (eg, abdominal pain; apprehension; diaphoresis; dizziness; headache; muscle twitching; nausea; palpitations; restlessness; retching; retrosternal discomfort); bradycardia; ECG changes; tachycardia.
GI: Ileus.
HEMA: Methemoglobinemia; decreased platelet aggregation.
DERM: Flushing; venous streaking; irritation at infusion site; rash.
METAB: Hypothyroidism.
OTHER: Thiocyanate toxicity; cyanide toxicity; increased intracranial pressure.

> **WARNING:**
> *Administration:* Administration is not suitable for direct injection and requires dilution prior to infusion.
> *Cyanide toxicity:* Accumulation of cyanide ion may occur.
> *Hypotension:* Hypotension can cause significant drops in BP leading to irreversible ischemic injury or death. Requires appropriate monitoring equipment and experienced personnel.

Precautions
Pregnancy: Category C.
Lactation: Undetermined.
Elderly: May be more sensitive to hypotensive effects.
Hepatic function impairment: Cyanide may accumulate in patients with hepatic impairment.
Anesthesia: Patient's ability to compensate for anemia and hypovolemia may be diminished during anesthesia.
Cyanide toxicity: Infusions faster than 2 mcg/kg/min generate cyanide faster than body can dispose of it. Symptoms of cyanide toxicity include venous hyperoxemia with bright red venous blood, metabolic (lactic) acidosis, air hunger, confusion and death.
Intracranial pressure: Use with extreme caution in patients with elevated intracranial pressure; nitroprusside can increase intracranial pressure.
Methemoglobinemia: Clinically significant methemoglobinemia is seen rarely, but suspect condition in patients who have received more than 10 mg/kg of nitroprusside and who have signs of impaired oxygen delivery despite adequate cardiac output and arterial Po_2. Blood may be chocolate brown.
Severe renal disease, anuria: Thiocyanate may accumulate.
Thiocyanate toxicity: Cyanide is eliminated in form of thiocyanate. When cyanide elimination

is accelerated by infusion of thiosulfate or when prolonged infusions are used, thiocyanate levels may increase. Thiocyanate is neurotoxic (tinnitus, miosis, hyperreflexia) and toxicity may be life threatening.

PATIENT CARE CONSIDERATIONS
Administration/Storage
* Dilute 50 mg in 2 mL D5W. Add to 250 to 500 mL D5W. Resulting solution is 200 mcg/mL or 100 mcg/mL. Use only D5W; no other diluent should be used. No other medication should be infused with nitroprusside medication. Protect solution from light, usually by wrapping with aluminum foil. However, it is not necessary to protect drip chamber or tubing.
* Do not use if solution is discolored or if particulate matter is seen.
* Store diluted solution at room temperature (59° to 86°F) for no longer than 24 hr and protect from light.
* Do not give by bolus infusion; infuse slowly using pump or controller to regulate rate.

Avoidance of excessive hypotension:
* While the average effective rate in adults and children is about 3 mcg/kg/min, some patients will become dangerously hypotensive when they receive nitroprusside at this rate. Start at a very low rate (0.3 mcg/kg/min), with gradual upward titration every few minutes until the desired effect is reached or the max recommended infusion rate (10 mcg/kg/min) has been reached.

CHF:
* Nitroprusside can be titrated by increasing the infusion rate until measured cardiac output is no longer increasing, systemic BP cannot be further reduced without compromising the perfusion of vital organs or the maximum recommended infusion rate has been reached, whichever comes earliest.

Overdosage: Signs and Symptoms
Severe hypotension, dyspnea, loss of consciousness, metabolic acidosis, headache, death.

Assessment/Interventions
* Obtain patient history, including drug history and any known allergies.
* Assess baseline vital signs, ECG, heart sounds, and lung sounds.
* Assess baseline neurological status.
* Place patient in Trendelenburg position to increase venous return.
* Perform continuous ECG monitoring.
* Monitor vital signs q 15 min while on drip and q 5 min while infusion is being titrated.
* Monitor I&O throughout therapy.
* Monitor plasma cyanogen level if used for more than 48 hr or with hepatic impairment.
* Monitor thiocyanate level (less than 10 mg/dL) if used for more then 48 hr or in severe renal dysfunction.
* Monitor for chest pain or flushing.
* Notify health care provider of severe hypotension, abdominal pain, apprehension, dizziness, headache, vomiting, bradycardia or tachycardia, ECG changes, or syncope.
* Notify health care provider of signs of cyanide toxicity such as bright red venous blood, metabolic acidosis, air hunger, and mental confusion.
* Monitor for and notify health care provider of signs of thiocyanate toxicity (ie, tinnitus, miosis, hyperreflexia).

Patient/Family Education
* Instruct patient to report the following symptoms to health care provider: dizziness; retching, nausea, abdominal pain, chest pain, palpitations, tinnitus, or flushing.
* Caution patient to avoid sudden position changes to prevent orthostatic hypotension.

Nizatidine

(nye-ZAT-ih-deen)

Class Histamine H_2 antagonist

How Supplied
Axid AR Tablets 75 mg ◆ *Axid Pulvules* Capsules 150 mg, Capsules 300 mg
🍁 *Apo-Nizatidine* ◆ *Novo-Nizatidine* ◆ *PMS-Nizatidine*

Action
PHARMACOLOGY: Reversibly and competitively blocks histamine at H_2 receptors, particularly those in gastric parietal cells, leading to inhibition of gastric acid secretion.

PHARMACOKINETICS/DYNAMICS:

Absorption: Absolute bioavailability is more than 70%, C_{max} is 700 to 1800 mcg/L (150 mg dose) and 1400 to 3600 mcg/L (300 mg dose), and T_{max} is 0.5 to 3 hr. Food increases nizatidine AUC and C_{max} by approximately 10%.

Distribution: Vd is 0.8 to 1.5 L/kg and the plasma protein binding is about 35%, mainly to alpha$_1$–acid glycoprotein.

Metabolism: Less than 7% of nizatidine is metabolized as N2–monodes-methylnizatidine (main metabolite). Other metabolites include N2–oxide (less than 5%) and S-oxide (less than 6%).

Excretion: Nizatidine is eliminated in urine (90% excreted; 60% as unchanged) and feces (less than 6%). The $t_{½}$ is 1 to 2 hr, plasma clearance is 40 to 60 L/hr, and renal clearance is 500 mL/min.

Special Populations:
Renal Function Impairment – Moderate to severe renal insufficiency prolongs nizatidine half-life and decreased clearance. Reduce amount and frequency of dose according to severity.

Indications Treatment and maintenance of duodenal ulcer, gastroesophageal reflux disease (GERD, including erosive or ulcerative disease) and benign gastric ulcer. Prevention of heartburn, acid indigestion and sour stomach brought on by consuming food and beverages.

Contraindications Hypersensitivity to H_2 antagonists.

Route/Dosage
Duodenal Ulcer (Active)
ADULTS: **PO** 300 mg at bedtime or 150 mg bid for up to 8 wk.
Maintenance: **PO** 150 mg at bedtime.

Benign Gastric Ulcer (Acute)
ADULTS: **PO** 300 mg at bedtime or 150 mg bid.

GERD
ADULTS: **PO** 150 mg bid.

Moderate to Severe Renal Insufficiency
Dosage adjustment recommended.

Acid Reduction
ADULTS: **PO** 75 mg with water 30 min to 1 hr before consuming food and beverages that may cause symptoms.

Interactions
Aspirin: Increased salicylate levels in patients taking very high doses of aspirin (3.9 g/day).
Ketoconazole: Effects of ketoconazole may be reduced.

Lab Test Interferences False-positive tests for urobilinogen with *Multistix* may occur.

Adverse Reactions
CV: Cardiac arrhythmias.
CNS: Headache; somnolence; fatigue; dizziness.
DERM: Exfoliative dermatitis; erythroderma; rash; pruritus; urticaria.
GI: Diarrhea; constipation; nausea; vomiting; abdominal discomfort; anorexia; cholestatic or hepatocellular effects.
GU: Hyperuricemia unassociated with gout or nephrolithiasis.
HEMA: Thrombocytopenia; eosinophilia.
HEPA: Hepatocellular injury; elevated AST, ALT, and alkaline phosphatase concentrations.
OTHER: Gynecomastia; sweating; fever.

Precautions
Pregnancy: Category B.
Lactation: Excreted in breast milk.
Children: Safety and efficacy not established.
Elderly: May have reduced renal function; decreased clearance may be more common.
Renal function impairment: Decreased clearance may occur in patients with renal impairment; reduced dosage may be needed.
Hepatic function impairment: Use drug with caution in patients with hepatic impairment; decreased clearance may occur. In patients with normal renal function and uncomplicated hepatic dysfunction, nizatidine disposition is generally normal.
Hepatocellular injury: Abnormalities appear to be reversible after discontinuation of drug.

PATIENT CARE CONSIDERATIONS

Administration/Storage
- Give twice daily after breakfast and at bedtime, or if once daily, give at bedtime.
- Do not administer within 1 hr of antacids.
- Store at room temperature (59° to 86°F).

Assessment/Interventions
- Obtain patient history, including drug history and any known allergies.
- Assess baseline AST, ALT, and alkaline phosphatase levels.
- Monitor LFT results, CBC, BUN, and creatinine levels.
- Assess for constipation and encourage increased fluid intake.
- Assess for fatigue, somnolence, skin rashes, and diaphoresis.

Patient/Family Education
- Advise patient to take medication after breakfast and at bedtime if prescribed for twice-daily regimen or at bedtime if prescribed for once-daily dosage.
- Caution patient to stay active and to increase fluid and roughage in diet to prevent constipation.
- Instruct patient to take missed dose as soon as possible, and caution not to double doses.
- Advise patient to avoid cigarette smoking, which increases gastric acid secretions and therefore decreases effectiveness of nizatidine therapy.
- Instruct patient to report the following symptoms to health care provider: abdominal pain, coffee-ground emesis, tarry stools, extreme fatigue, or weakness.

Norepinephrine (Levarterenol)

(NOR-eh-pih-NEFF-reen)
Class Vasopressor
How Supplied
Levophed Injection 1 mg (as bitartrate)/mL
Action
PHARMACOLOGY: Stimulates alpha-receptors in arterial and venous beds and beta$_1$ receptors of heart, resulting in peripheral vasoconstriction and stimulation of heart rate and contractility. Coronary vasodilation occurs secondary to enhanced myocardial contractility.

PHARMACOKINETICS/DYNAMICS:
Absorption: Norepinephrine is ineffective orally, SC absorption is poor, and IV absorption is immediate.

Distribution: Norepinephrine is localized mainly in sympathetic nervous tissue and crosses the placenta.

Excretion: Norepinephrine is excreted in urine (small amount eliminated as unchanged).

Onset: Onset of IV norepinephrine is rapid.

Duration: Duration of norepinephrine is 1 to 2 min (discontinuation of IV).

Indications Restoration of BP in certain acute hypotensive states; adjunct in treatment of cardiac arrest and profound hypotension.

Contraindications Hypovolemic states, except temporarily until blood volume replacement is accomplished; mesenteric or peripheral vascular thrombosis, unless essential; generally contraindicated during cyclopropane and halothane anesthesia; profound hypoxia or hypercarbia.

Route/Dosage
Acute Hypotensive States
ADULTS: IV 2 to 3 mL/min of 4 mcg base/mL solution (8 to 12 mcg/min); adjust to response. Higher concentration (up to 16 mcg/mL) may be used in fluid-restricted patients. Usual maintenance dose is 2 to 4 mcg/min, but higher doses and prolonged therapy may be needed.

Interactions
Blood or plasma: Chemically incompatible with norepinephrine.
Furazolidone, guanethidine, MAO inhibitors, methyldopa, rauwolfia alkaloids: May increase pressor response, resulting in severe hypertension.
Normal saline: Norepinephrine may lose potency in normal saline solution.
Oxytocic drugs: May cause severe, persistent hypertension.
Phenothiazines (eg, chlorpromazine): May decrease pressor effect.
Tricyclic antidepressants: May increase pressor response.

Lab Test Interferences None well documented.

Adverse Reactions
CV: Hypotension; increased peripheral vascular resistance; decreased carbon monoxide; precordial pain; ventricular arrhythmias; reflex bradycardia.
CNS: Headache; dizziness; tremor; insomnia; anxiety.
METAB: Metabolic acidosis; hyperglycemia.
RESP: Respiratory difficulties.
OTHER: Gangrene (when infused into small vein); thyroid enlargement; irritation from extravasation; decreased urinary output.

Precautions
Pregnancy: Category D.
Lactation: Undetermined.
Children: Safety and efficacy not established.
Sulfite sensitivity: Use caution in sulfite-sensitive individuals; some preparations contain sodium bisulfite.
Extravasation: Avoid by infusion into large vein and monitoring carefully.

Overdosage: Signs and Symptoms
Severe hypertension, reflex bradycardia, decreased cardiac output, increased peripheral vascular resistance, ventricular arrhythmias, tissue hypoxia and ischemic injury.

PATIENT CARE CONSIDERATIONS

Administration/Storage
- Administer in D5W or 5% Dextrose in saline. Do not prepare infusion with normal saline alone because doing so may cause degradation.
- Use infusion pump and plastic catheter. Enter antecubital or other large vein.
- Do not discontinue therapy abruptly.
- Discard solution after 24 hr.
- Store undiluted solution at room temperature (59° to 86°F). Protect from light.

Assessment/Interventions
- Obtain patient history, including drug history and any known allergies.
- Obtain baseline vital signs, neurological assessment, urinary output, and ECG.
- Monitor vital signs, ECG, I&O, and neurological status regularly during therapy.
- Monitor for cyanosis (eg, bluish skin color and cold extremities).
- Assess for signs of extravasation (eg, blanching and coolness of skin over vein) at infu-

sion site. If this occurs, notify health care provider immediately and change infusion site as soon as possible. Have phentolamine readily available for local infiltration in case extravasation occurs.

Patient/Family Education
- Advise patient to notify nurse if IV site feels cool or painful.
- Instruct patient to report the following symptoms to health care provider: dizziness, nausea, syncope, abdominal pain, chest pain or confusion.
- Caution patient to avoid sudden position changes to prevent orthostatic hypotension.

Norethindrone Acetate

(nor-eth-IN-drone ASS-uh-TATE)

Class Progestin

How Supplied
Aygestin Tablets 5 mg
✣ *Norlutate*

Action
PHARMACOLOGY: Inhibits secretion of pituitary gonadotropins, thereby preventing follicular maturation and ovulation.

PHARMACOKINETICS/DYNAMICS:
Absorption: Norethindrone acetate is rapidly absorbed from GI tract. T_{max} is approximately 2 hr.

Distribution: Rapid distribution of dorethindrone acetate.

Metabolism: Norethindrone is metabolized in the liver.

Excretion: Norethindrone elimination is rapid, primarily in feces.

Indications
Treatment of secondary amenorrhea; endometriosis; abnormal uterine bleeding caused by hormonal imbalance in the absence of organic pathology (eg, uterine cancer).

Contraindications
Thrombophlebitis, thrombolic disorders, cerebral apoplexy, or a history of these conditions; markedly impaired liver function or liver disease; known or suspected carcinoma of the breast; undiagnosed vaginal bleeding; missed abortion; as a diagnostic test for pregnancy.

Route/Dosage
Secondary Amenorrhea, Abnormal Uterine Bleeding
ADULTS: PO 2.5 to 10 mg/day for 5 to 10 days during second half of the theoretical menstrual cycle.

Endometriosis
ADULTS: PO 5 mg/day initially for 2 wk, then increase in increments of 2.5 mg/day q 2 wk until 15 mg/day is achieved. Therapy may be continued at this level for 6 to 9 mo or until breakthrough bleeding demands temporary termination.

Interactions
Rifampin: Elimination of norethindrone may be increased, decreasing the therapeutic effect.

Lab Test Interferences Pregnanediol determinations may be altered; thyroid and LFT results may be affected; increased amounts of coagulation factors; reduced response to metyrapone test.

Adverse Reactions
CV: Thrombophlebitis; cerebral thrombosis and embolism; hypertension; edema.
CNS: Depression; changes in libido; changes in appetite; headache; nervousness; dizziness; fatigue.
DERM: Allergic rash; melasma; chloasma; hirsutism; alopecia; erythema multiforme; erythema nodosum; hemorrhagic eruption; itching.
EENT: Neuro-ocular lesions (eg, retinal thrombosis, optic neuritis).
GU: Breakthrough bleeding; spotting; amenorrhea; increased cervical erosion and secretion; cystitis.
HEPA: Cholestatic jaundice.
METAB: Weight gain and loss.
RESP: Pulmonary embolism.
OTHER: Premenstrual syndrome; backache.

Precautions
Pregnancy: Category X.
Lactation: Excreted in breast milk.
Children: Safety and efficacy not established.
Fluid retention: Use with careful observation when conditions that might be affected by fluid retention are present (eg, asthma, cardiac or renal dysfunction, epilepsy).
Mental depression: Carefully observe patients with history of depression.
Ophthalmic effects: Discontinue therapy if there are any sudden changes in vision or onset of proptosis, diplopia, migraine papilledema, or retinal vascular lesions.

PATIENT CARE CONSIDERATIONS
Administration/Storage
- Administer prescribed dose once daily, without regard to meals. Administer with food if GI upset occurs.

- Store at controlled room temperature (59° to 86°F).

Assessment/Interventions
- Obtain patient history, including drug history and any known allergies.
- Review patient's health history for any condition that would contraindicate norethindrone (eg, previous allergic reaction, known or suspected pregnancy, missed abortion, known or suspected cancer of the breast, undiagnosed vaginal bleeding, active or past history of thromboembolic disorders or stroke, liver dysfunction or disease).
- Ensure that breast and pelvic examination and Pap smear have been completed and documented before starting therapy.
- Monitor blood sugar in diabetic patient more frequently when drug is started or dose is changed. Report significant changes in blood sugar to health care provider.
- Monitor patient for CNS, RESP, CV, and general body side effects. Report to health care provider if noted and significant.
- Notify health care provider of the following symptoms: pain, swelling, redness or warmth in calves; sharp chest pain or sudden shortness of breath; sudden severe headache or migraine headache; visual disturbances; signs of liver dysfunction (eg, dark urine, jaundice); signs of depression.

Patient/Family Education
- Explain name, dose, action and potential side effects of drug.
- Instruct patient to take once daily as prescribed.
- Advise patient that medication can be taken without regard to meals, but to take with food if GI upset occurs.
- Warn women of childbearing potential of significant risks associated with taking this medication and becoming pregnant.
- Instruct diabetic patient to monitor blood glucose more frequently when drug is started or dose is changed and to inform health care provider of significant changes in readings.
- Instruct patient to report the following symptoms to health care provider: pain in groin or calves; sharp chest pain or sudden shortness of breath; abnormal vaginal bleeding; sudden severe headache or migraine headache; vision problems; yellowing of skin or eyes; or depression.
- Instruct women to notify health care provider if becoming pregnant, planning to become pregnant, or are breastfeeding.
- Instruct patient to not take any prescription or OTC medications or dietary supplements unless advised to do so by the health care provider.
- Advise patient that follow-up visits and examinations may be required to monitor therapy and to be sure to keep appointments.

Norfloxacin

(nor-FLOX-uh-SIN)

Class Antibiotic/Fluoroquinolone

How Supplied
Chibroxin Solution 3 mg/mL ♦ *Noroxin* Tablets 400 mg
✤ *Apo-Norflox* ♦ *Novo-Norfloxacin*

Action

PHARMACOLOGY: Interferes with microbial DNA synthesis.

PHARMACOKINETICS/DYNAMICS:

Absorption: Norfloxacin is rapidly absorbed; 30% to 40% absorbed in fasting patients. Food and dairy products decrease absorption. Steady state is 2 days, C_{max} is 0.8 to 2.4 mcg/mL, and T_{max} is approximately 1 hr after dosing.

Distribution: Protein binding is 10% to 15% and crosses the placenta.

Metabolism: Suggested as first-pass metabolism; however, further study is needed.

Excretion: Norfloxacin is eliminated in urine (26% to 32% as norfloxacin, 5% to 8% as active metabolites) and feces (30%).

Special Populations:
Renal Function Impairment – Renal insufficiency increases half-life. Alteration of dose is necessary.

Indications Oral treatment of urinary tract infections (UTIs) caused by susceptible organisms; treatment of STDs caused by *Neisseria gonorrhoeae*; ocular solution for treatment of superficial ocular infections due to strains of susceptible organisms; prostatitis caused by *E. coli*.

Contraindications Hypersensitivity to fluoroquinolones, quinolones, or any component; tendonitis or tendon rupture associated with quinolone use.
Ophthalmic use: Epithelial herpes simplex keratitis; fungal disease of ocular structure; mycobacterial infections of eye; vaccinia; varicella.

Route/Dosage
UTIs
ADULTS: **PO** 400 mg q 12 hr for 3 to 21 days.
STDs
ADULTS: **PO** 800 mg as single dose.

Ocular Infections
ADULTS AND CHILDREN:
Acute infection: **Topical** 1 to 2 gtt q 15 to 30 min
Moderate infection: **Topical** 1 to 2 gtt 4 to 6 times/day.

Prostatitis Caused By E. coli
ADULTS: **PO** 400 mg q 12 h for 28 days.

Interactions
Antacids, iron salts, zinc salts, sucralfate, didanosine: May decrease oral absorption of norfloxacin.
Antineoplastic agents: Serum norfloxacin levels may be decreased.
Cyclosporine: Elevated serum cyclosporine levels.
Theophylline: Decreased clearance and increased plasma levels of theophylline may result in toxicity.

Lab Test Interferences
None well documented.

Adverse Reactions
CNS: Headache; dizziness; fatigue; drowsiness.
DERM: Rash.
EENT: Conjunctival hyperemia, chemosis, photophobia, transient burning, itching, or stinging.
GI: Diarrhea; nausea; vomiting; abdominal pain/discomfort.
GU: Increased serum creatinine and BUN.
HEMA: Eosinophilia; leukopenia; neutropenia.
HEPA: Increased ALT, AST, LDH.

Precautions
Pregnancy: Category C.
Lactation: Undetermined.
Children: Safety and efficacy not established (oral form).
Renal function impairment: Reduced clearance may occur in patients with renal impairment; adjust dose accordingly.
Superinfection: Use of antibiotics may result in bacterial or fungal overgrowth.
Photosensitivity: Moderate to severe reactions have occurred; avoid excessive sunlight and ultraviolet light.
Convulsions: CNS stimulation can occur; use drug with caution in patients with known or suspected CNS disorders.
Pseudomembranous colitis: Consider possibility in patients who develop diarrhea.

Overdosage: Signs and Symptoms
Nausea, headache, dizziness, crystalluria, vomiting, drowsiness, seizures.

PATIENT CARE CONSIDERATIONS
Administration/Storage
Ophthalmic:
- Store at room temperature (59° to 86°F) in original container.

Tablets:
- Store at room temperature (59° to 86°F).
- Give 1 hr before or 2 hr after meals with full glass of water.
- Do not administer antacids within 2 hr of dose.

Assessment/Interventions
- Obtain patient history, including drug history and any known allergies.
- Assess baseline CBC, taste alterations, conjunctivitis, or mycobacterial infections.
- Review baseline BUN, creatinine, ALT, AST, and LDH.
- Monitor vital signs, elimination patterns, food intolerance, sedation, and sleep patterns.
- Monitor conjunctival color and edema if using eyedrop preparation.
- Encourage fluid intake; take full glass with each dose and full glass between each dose if not medically contraindicated.
- Notify health care provider of any nausea, rashes, diarrhea, shortness of breath, dizziness, extreme headache, or lethargy.

Patient/Family Education
- For ophthalmic use, demonstrate and observe return demonstration of correct technique for instillation of drops.
- Advise patient to take medication on empty stomach with full glass of water.
- Caution patient to avoid exposure to sunlight and to use sunscreen or wear protective clothing to avoid photosensitivity reaction.
- Advise patient not to double dose if one dose is missed and to notify health care provider if more than 1 dose is missed.
- Advise patient to notify health care provider of any nausea, rashes, diarrhea, shortness of breath, dizziness, unusual headache, or lethargy.
- Instruct patient to maintain increased fluid intake (if not contraindicated) while taking this medication.
- Advise patient to use caution when driving or performing tasks that require mental alertness until effects of medication are determined.

- Remind patient to complete full course of therapy, even if symptoms of urinary tract or eye infection have resolved.
- Instruct patient to stop treatment and inform health care provider if experiencing pain, inflammation, or rupture of tendon, and to rest or refrain from exercise until diagnosis of tendonitis or tendon rupture is excluded.

Nortriptyline Hydrochloride

(nor-TRIP-tih-leen HIGH-droe-KLOR-ide)

Class Tricyclic antidepressant

How Supplied
Aventyl Hydrochloride Solution 10 mg base/5 mL
- Aventyl Hydrochloride Pulvules Capsules 10 mg, Capsules 25 mg ♦ Pamelor Capsules 10 mg, Capsules 25 mg, Capsules 50 mg, Capsules 75 mg, Solution 10 mg base/5 mL

❀ Apo-Nortriptyline ♦ Gen-Nortriptyline ♦ Novo-Nortriptyline ♦ Nu-Nortriptyline ♦ PMS-Nortriptyline ♦ ratio-Nortriptyline

Action
PHARMACOLOGY: Inhibits reuptake of norepinephrine and serotonin in CNS.

Indications Relief of symptoms of depression.

Unlabeled use(s): Treatment of panic disorder, premenstrual depression, dermatologic disorders (eg, chronic urticaria, angioedema, nocturnal pruritus in atopic eczema).

Contraindications
Hypersensitivity to any tricyclic antidepressant. Generally, not to be given in combination with or within 14 days of treatment with MAO inhibitors or during acute recovery phases of MI.

Route/Dosage
ADULTS: PO 25 mg tid to qid. Doses more than 150 mg/day are not recommended.

ELDERLY AND ADOLESCENTS: PO 30 to 50 mg/day in divided doses.

Interactions
Anticoagulants: Dicumaral actions may increase.
Carbamazepine: Carbamazepine levels may increase; nortriptyline levels may decrease.
Cimetidine, fluoxetine: Coadministration may increase nortriptyline blood levels and effects.
CNS depressants: Depressant effects may be additive.
Clonidine: May result in hypertensive crisis.
Guanethidine: Hypotensive action may be inhibited.
MAO Inhibitors: Hyperpyretic crisis, convulsions and death may occur.
Sympathomimetics: Pressor response may decrease.

Lab Test Interferences None well documented.

Adverse Reactions
CV: Orthostatic hypotension; hypertension; tachycardia; palpitations; arrhythmias; ECG changes; stroke; heart block; CHF.
CNS: Confusion; hallucinations; delusions; nervousness; restlessness; agitation; panic; insomnia; nightmares; mania; exacerbation of psychosis; drowsiness; dizziness; weakness; fatigue; emotional lability; seizures; tremors; extrapyramidal symptoms (eg, pseudoparkinsonism, movement disorders, akathisia).
DERM: Rash; pruritus; photosensitivity reaction; dry skin; acne.
EENT: Nasal congestion; tinnitus; conjunctivitis; mydriasis; blurred vision; increased IOP; peculiar taste in mouth.
GI: Nausea; vomiting; anorexia; GI distress; diarrhea; flatulence; dry mouth; constipation.
GU: Impotence; sexual dysfunction; nocturia; urinary frequency; urinary tract infection; vaginitis; cystitis; dysmenorrhea; amenorrhea; urinary retention and hesitancy.
HEMA: Bone marrow depression including agranulocytosis; eosinophilia; purpura; thrombocytopenia; leukopenia.
HEPA: Hepatitis; jaundice.
METAB: Elevation or depression of blood sugar.
RESP: Pharyngitis; rhinitis; sinusitis; laryngitis; coughing.
OTHER: Numbness; breast enlargement.

Precautions
Pregnancy: Category D. Safety not established. Limb reduction anomalies have been reported with nortriptyline.
Lactation: Excreted in breast milk.
Children: Safety and efficacy not established.
Special risk patients: Use drug with caution in patients with history of seizures, urinary retention, urethral or ureteral spasm, angle-closure glaucoma or increased IOP, CV disorders, hyperthyroid patients or those receiving thyroid medication, patients with hepatic or renal impairment, schizophrenia, or paranoia.

Overdosage: Signs and Symptoms
Confusion, vomiting, muscle rigidity, ECG abnormalities, seizures, agitation, fever, hyperactive reflexes, CHF, coma, respiratory depression, death.

PATIENT CARE CONSIDERATIONS
Administration/Storage
- Give with food or milk.
- Store at room temperature (59° to 86°F) in tight container.
- If prescribed as single daily dose, give at bedtime to reduce side effects.

Assessment/Interventions
- Obtain patient history, including drug history and any known allergies.
- Obtain baseline renal function tests, LFTs, CBC, and ECG, and monitor throughout therapy.
- Drug levels may be obtained to determine if patient is in optimal range (50 to 150 ng/mL).
- Assess emotional status (eg, appearance, speech patterns, mood, level of interest), and monitor level of consciousness and suicidal ideation.
- Monitor daily elimination pattern, BP, and pulse, and notify health care provider of potential problems.
- Assess for bladder distention and constipation.

Patient/Family Education
- Advise patient to avoid sudden position changes to prevent orthostatic hypotension.
- Explain that it may take up to 2 wk for therapeutic effects to become evident.
- Caution patient to avoid exposure to sunlight and to use sunscreen or wear protective clothing to avoid photosensitivity reaction.
- Instruct patient to notify health care provider of visual disturbances.
- Advise patient to take sips of water frequently, suck on ice chips or sugarless hard candy or chew sugarless gum if dry mouth occurs.
- Caution patient that drug may cause drowsiness and to use caution while driving or performing other tasks requiring mental alertness.
- Instruct patient not to double dose if one is missed and to notify health care provider if more than 1 dose is missed.
- Advise that side effects will be decreased if taken at bedtime if prescribed as once-daily dose.

Nystatin
(nye-STAT-in)

Class Anti-infective/Antifungal

How Supplied
Mycostatin Vaginal tablets 100,000 units, Ointment 100,000 units/g, Powder 100,000 units/g ♦ *Mycostatin Pastilles* Troches 200,000 units ♦ *Nilstat* Oral suspension 100,000 units, Bulk powder 150 million units, Bulk powder 1 billion units, Bulk powder 2 billion units, Cream 100,000 units, Ointment 100,000 units ♦ *Pedi-Dri* Powder 100,000 units/g

✽ *Candistatin* ♦ *Nyaderm* ♦ *PMS-Nystatin* ♦ *ratio-Nystatin*

Action
PHARMACOLOGY: Binds to fungal cell membrane, changing membrane permeability and allowing leakage of intracellular components.

Indications Treatment of intestinal, oral, vulvovaginal, cutaneous, or mucocutaneous candidiasis.

Contraindications Standard considerations.

Route/Dosage
Intestinal Candidiasis
ADULTS AND CHILDREN: **PO** 500,000 to 1,000,000 U tid. Continue treatment for at least 48 hr after clinical cure.

Oral or Mucocutaneous Candidiasis
ADULTS AND CHILDREN: **PO** (suspension) 200,000 to 600,000 U qid; swish and swallow, or (oral pastilles) 1 to 2 pastilles (200,000 to 400,000 U) dissolved in mouth 4 to 5 times/day.
INFANTS: **PO** 200,000 U qid.

Vaginal Candidiasis
ADULTS: **Intravaginal** 100,000 U qd for 2 wk.

Cutaneous Candidiasis
ADULTS AND CHILDREN: **Topical** Apply to affected areas bid to tid.

Interactions None well documented.

Lab Test Interferences None well documented.

Adverse Reactions
GI: Diarrhea; GI distress; nausea; vomiting (with large oral doses).
DERM: Irritation (with topical use).

Precautions
Pregnancy: Category C (oral); Category A (vaginal).
Lactation: Undetermined.
Effectiveness: Has no activity against bacteria or trichomonads. Not indicated for systemic mycoses.
Topical preparations: Not for ophthalmic use.

Overdosage: Signs and Symptoms
Nausea, diarrhea, vomiting.

PATIENT CARE CONSIDERATIONS
Administration/Storage
- For troche/pastilles administration, have patient dissolve troche in mouth. Instruct patient not to chew or swallow troche whole. Have patient retain troche in mouth as long as possible before swallowing.
- For administration of oral suspension, place half of dose in each side of mouth. Have patient swish thoroughly around in mouth and retain in mouth as long as possible before swallowing. Shake suspension well. Use calibrated dropper provided.
- Do not mix oral suspension in foods.
- To use powder for extemporaneous compounding, reconstitute ⅛ tsp (500,000 U) in half glass of water and stir well. Use immediately; do not store. Can be administered in form of flavored frozen popsicle.
- Cream or ointment is preferred for affected intertriginous areas. Wash and dry affected area before application. Use gloves or swabs to apply enough medication to cover lesion completely.
- To use powder, clean and dry affected area before application. Dust powder on feet and in socks and shoes for infection of feet. Very moist lesions are best treated with powder.
- For vaginal use, insert 1 tablet high into vagina with applicator.
- Refrigerate vaginal tablets.
- Avoid contact with eyes.
- Store oral suspension in refrigerator. Protect from heat, light, moisture, and air.

Assessment/Interventions
- Obtain patient history, including drug history and any known allergies.
- Although allergic reactions are rare, assess for rash, urticaria, burning, stinging, redness, and swelling.
- Assess for factors predisposing to infection: pregnancy, antibiotic therapy, diabetes, infected sexual partners (vaginal infections). However, vaginal yeast infections are common and may not be associated with any of these factors.
- Inspect mucous membranes before and frequently throughout course of therapy.

Patient/Family Education
- Instruct patient that long-term therapy may be needed to clear infection and that patient should complete entire course of medication. Take drug for 2 days after symptoms have disappeared or as directed.
- Advise patient using vaginal preparations to wear light-day pad; drug may stain clothing and linens.
- Advise patient to notify health care provider if irritation occurs.
- Assure patient that relief from itching may occur after 24 to 72 hr.
- Instruct patient to practice good hand washing before and after each application of topical or vaginal medication. Remind patient to wash applicator after each use.
- Advise patient with oral candidiasis not to use mouthwash, which may alter normal flora and promote infections.
- Teach patient to continue using vaginal tablets even when menstruating because treatment should be continued for 2 wk. Instruct patient to avoid using tampons.
- Explain to patient that during pregnancy, use of vaginal applicator may be contraindicated, and manual insertion of vaginal tablets may be preferred.
- Advise patient to prevent reinfection (ie, avoid intercourse during therapy or use condoms).
- Instruct patient to discontinue drug and notify health care provider if vaginal tablets cause irritation, redness, or swelling.

Nystatin/Triamcinolone Acetonide

(nye-STAT-in/TRY-am-SIN-oh-lone ah-SEE-toe-nide)

Class Corticosteroid/Antifungal combination

How Supplied
Mycogen II Cream 100,000 units/g nystatin, 0.1% triamcinolone, Ointment 100,000 units/g nystatin, 0.1% triamcinolone ◆ *Mycolog II* Cream 100,000 units/g nystatin, 0.1% triamcinolone, Ointment 100,000 units/g nystatin, 0.1% triamcinolone ◆ *Mytrex* Cream 100,000 units/g nystatin, 0.1% triamcinolone, Ointment 100,000 units/g nystatin, 0.1% triamcinolone

Action
PHARMACOLOGY: The antifungal binds to fungal cell membrane, changing membrane permeability and allowing leakage of intracellular components; the corticosteroid adds anti-inflammatory, antipruritic, and vasoconstrictive action.

Indications Cutaneous candidiasis.

Contraindications Standard considerations.

Route/Dosage
ADULT AND CHILDREN: **Topical** Apply as a thin film to affected area(s) bid.

Interactions None well documented.

Lab Test Interferences None well documented.

Adverse Reactions
DERM: Acneiform eruptions; burning; itching; irritation; dryness; folliculitis; hypertrichosis; hypopigmentation; perioral dermatitis; allergic contact dermatitis; maceration; secondary infection; skin atrophy; striae; miliaria.

PATIENT CARE CONSIDERATIONS
Administration/Storage
- For topical use only. Not for ophthalmic or otic use.
- Apply a thin film to affected area(s) bid. Use gloves or applicator as applicable.
- Store at controlled room temperature (59° to 86°F). Keep tube tightly closed.

Assessment/Interventions
- Obtain patient history, including drug history and any known allergies.
- Limit use to 25 days.
- Monitor patient's response to therapy. Notify health care provider if skin inflammation, irritation, or sensitization are noted, or if symptoms do not improve or worsen.

Patient/Family Education
- Explain name, dose, action, and potential side effects of medication.

Precautions
Pregnancy: Category C.
Lactation: Undetermined.
Children: Greater risk of HPA axis suppression, Cushing syndrome, intracranial hypertension.
Risk of HPA axis suppression, Cushing syndrome, hyperglycemia, glycosuria: Conditions that augment cutaneous absorption include use of large body surface area, prolonged use, and occlusive dressings.

- Review prescribed dosing schedule with patient or caregiver.
- Remind patient or caregiver that medicine is not to be used in the eye or ear.
- Teach patient or caregiver proper technique for applying medicine: wash hands; apply thin film to affected area(s) using fingers or applicator. Wash hands after application.
- Caution patient or caregiver not to occlude treated skin area with bandage, cover, or wrap.
- Advise patient or caregiver to contact health care provider if local redness or swelling develops, or if skin lesions do not improve or worsen.
- Remind patient or caregiver that follow-up examinations may be necessary while using this medication and to keep appointments.

Octreotide Acetate
(ock-TREE-oh-tide ASS-uh-TATE)
Class Hormone

How Supplied
Sandostatin Injection 0.05 mg/mL, Injection 0.1 mg/mL, Injection 0.2 mg/mL, Injection 0.5 mg/mL, Injection 1 mg/mL ♦ *Sandostatin LAR Depot* Injection 10 mg/5 mL, Injection 20 mg/5 mL, Injection 30 mg/5 mL

Action
PHARMACOLOGY: Actions mimic those of natural hormone somatostatin. Suppresses secretion of serotonin and gastroenteropancreatic peptides (eg, gastrin, insulin, glucagon, secretin, motilin). Also suppresses growth hormone.

PHARMACOKINETICS/DYNAMICS:
Absorption: Octreotide is rapidly and completely absorbed (SC).
The bioavailability is 100% (SC). C_{max} is 5.2 ng/mL.
Distribution: Vd is 13.6 L. Protein binding is 65% and is bound mainly to lipoprotein, and, to a lesser extent, albumin.
Excretion: The $t_{1/2}$ is 1.7 hr. 32% is eliminated unchanged through the urine. Cl is 10 L/hr.
Duration: May extend up to 12 hr.
Special Populations:
Elderly – There is a 46% increase in the half-life of the drug, and a 26% decrease in clearance. Dosage adjustment may be necessary.
Severe Renal Insufficiency – Clearance may be reduced by about 50%.

Indications
Symptomatic treatment of diarrhea associated with carcinoid tumors; treatment of profuse watery diarrhea associated with vasoactive intestinal peptide tumors (VIPoma); to reduce blood levels of growth hormone and IGF-1 in acromegaly patients who have had inadequate response to or cannot be treated with resection, pituitary irradiation and bromocriptine at maximally tolerated doses.

Unlabeled use(s):
To reduce output from GI fistulas; for variceal bleeding; for relief of diarrhea associated with a variety of conditions; to reduce output from pancreatic fistulas; to treat irritable bowel syndrome; to treat dumping syndrome; to treat the following conditions: Enteric fistula; pancreatitis; pancreatic surgery; glucagonoma; insulinoma; gastrinoma (Zollinger-Ellison syndrome); intestinal obstruction; local radiotherapy; chronic pain management; antineoplastic therapy; decrease insulin requirements in diabetes mellitus; thyrotropin- and TSH-secreting tumors.

Contraindications
Standard considerations.

Route/Dosage
Carcinoid Tumors
ADULTS: SC 100 to 600 mcg/day in 2 to 4 divided doses, adjusting to response.
VIPoma
ADULTS: SC 200 to 300 mcg/day in 2 to 4 divided doses, adjusting to response.
Acromegaly
ADULTS: SC 50 mcg to 500 mcg/tid. Most common dose is 100 mcg/tid; doses more than 300 mcg/day seldom result in additional benefit.

Interactions
Cyclosporine: May decrease plasma levels of cyclosporine.
INCOMPATIBILITIES: Parenteral nutrition solutions.

Lab Test Interferences
None well documented.

Adverse Reactions
CNS: Headache; dizziness; lightheadedness; fatigue; sinus bradycardia; conduction abnormalities; arrhythmias.
GI: Nausea; constipation; flatulence; diarrhea; abdominal pain or discomfort; loose stools; vomiting; fat malabsorption.
HEPA: Increased liver transaminase.
METAB: Hyperglycemia; hypoglycemia.
OTHER: Injection site pain; flushing; asthenia; weakness.

Precautions
Pregnancy: Category B.
Lactation: Undetermined.
Children: Has been used in children as young as 1 mo.
Elderly: Dose adjustments may be necessary due to significant increases in half-life and significant decrease in the clearance of octreotide.
Renal function impairment: Dosage reduction may be necessary.
Cardiac effects: In acromegalics, bradycardia, conduction abnormalities and arrhythmias have occurred. Other ECG changes observed include QT prolongation, axis shifts, early repolarization, low voltage, R/S transition and early wave progression. Dose adjustments in drugs such as beta blockers that have bradycardia effects may be necessary.
Pancreatitis: Several cases have occurred in patients receiving octreotide.
Cholelithiasis: Cholelithiasis may occur; periodically monitor gallbladder function.
Hypoglycemia or hyperglycemia: Serum glucose control may be altered; carefully monitor patient and adjust insulin requirements accordingly.

Overdosage: Signs and Symptoms
Possible hyperglycemia and hypoglycemia.

PATIENT CARE CONSIDERATIONS
Administration/Storage
- Do not administer if particulate matter or discoloration is observed.
- Rotate sites for SC injection.
- Store ampules at room temperature for day of use.
- Refrigerate for prolonged storage.

Assessment/Interventions
- Obtain patient history, including drug history and any known allergies.
- Monitor glucose, CBC, T_3, T_4, TSH, renal function tests, BUN, creatinine, and electrolytes, and obtain baseline weight and BP.
- Assess for nausea, headache, shortness of breath, hyperglycemia/hypoglycemia, or abdominal pain.
- Monitor I&O and daily weight.
- Monitor BP, pulse, and respiration weekly during treatment.
- Assess frequency and consistency of stools.
- Assess lung sounds, and report any edema or decrease in urine output.
- Dietary fat absorption may be altered in some patients. Perform periodic quantitative 72-hr fecal fat and serum carotene determination to aid in assessment of possible drug-induced aggravation of fat malabsorption.

Patient/Family Education
- Instruct and observe return demonstration of correct technique for SC injection. Explain that preferred sites for injection are abdomen, thigh, and hip.
- Advise patient of importance of regular follow-up with health care provider.
- Caution patient to report the following symptoms to health care provider: icterus, jaundice, dark urine, or clay-colored stools.
- Advise patient to notify health care provider of abdominal pain, edema, chest pain, fainting, dry mouth, or shortness of breath.
- Advise patient that various laboratory tests may be required during therapy.

Ofloxacin

(oh-FLOX-uh-SIN)

Class Antibiotic/Fluoroquinolone

How Supplied
Floxin Tablets 200 mg, Tablets 300 mg, Tablets 400 mg, Injection 200 mg, Injection 400 mg ♦ *Ocuflox* Ophthalmic Solution 3 mg/mL
❦ *Apo-Oflox*

Action
PHARMACOLOGY: Interferes with microbial DNA synthesis.

PHARMACOKINETICS/DYNAMICS:

Absorption: C_{max} is 2.7 to 4 mcg/mL. T_{max} is 1 to 2 hr (oral).

Distribution: Widely distributed to body tissues and fluids. 32% protein bound. Bioavailability is 98%.

Metabolism: Pyridobenzoxazine ring appears to decrease the extent of parent compound metabolism.

Excretion: The t½ is 6 hr (IV) and 4 to 5 hr (oral). Less than 5% is eliminated by the kidneys as desmethyl or N-oxide metabolites; 4% to 8% by feces.

Special Populations:
Renal Function Impairment – Less than 50 mL/min; Cl is reduced. Dosage adjustment is necessary.

Elderly – Longer plasma t½ is approximately 6.4 to 7.4 hr.

Indications
Treatment of acute bacterial exacerbations of chronic bronchitis, community acquired pneumonia, uncomplicated skin and skin structure infections, acute uncomplicated urethral and cervical gonorrhea, nongonococcal urethritis, cervicitis, acute pelvic inflammatory disease, uncomplicated cystitis, complicated UTI, prostatitis caused by *Escherichia coli*.
Ophthalmic: Treatment of conjunctivitis and corneal ulcer infections caused by susceptible organisms.
Otic: Treatment of otitis externa, chronic suppurative otitis media in patients with perforated tympanic membranes, and acute otitis media in pediatric patients with tympanostomy tubes.

Contraindications
Standard considerations.
Ophthalmic: Epithelial herpes simplex keratitis; vaccinia; varicella; fungal disease of ocular structure; mycobacterial infections of the eye.

Route/Dosage
Acute Otitis Media in Pediatric Patients with Tympanostomy Tubes
CHILDREN 1 TO 12 YR: **OTIC** 5 gtt (0.25 mL, 0.75 mg ofloxacin) instilled into affected ear bid for 10 days.

Acute Pelvic Inflammatory Disease
ADULTS: **PO/IV** 400 mg q 12 hr for 10 to 14 days.

Acute Uncomplicated Urethral and Cervical Gonorrhea
ADULTS: PO/IV 400 mg as single dose.

Bacterial Conjunctivitis
ADULTS AND CHILDREN 1 YR OR OLDER: **Ophthalmic** Days 1 and 2 instill 1 to 2 gtt q 2 to 4 hr in affected eye(s). Days 3 through 7 instill 1 to 2 gtt qid.

Bacterial Corneal Ulcer
ADULTS AND CHILDREN 1 YR OR OLDER: **Ophthalmic** Days 1 and 2 instill 1 to 2 gtt into affected eye q 30 min while awake, awaken at approximately 4 to 6 hr after retiring and instill 1 to 2 gtt; days 3 through 7 to 9 instill 1 to 2 gtt q hr while awake; days 7 to 9 instill 1 to 2 gtt qid.

Cervicitis/Urethritis
ADULTS: PO/IV 300 mg q 12 hr for 7 days.

Chronic Bronchitis, Community-Acquired Pneumonia, Uncomplicated Skin and Skin Structure Infections
ADULTS: PO/IV 400 mg q 12 hr for 10 days.

Chronic Suppurative Otitis Media with Perforated Tympanic Membranes
ADULTS AND CHILDREN 12 YR AND OLDER: **OTIC** 10 gtt (0.5 mL, 1.5 mg ofloxacin) instilled into affected ear bid for 10 days.

Complicated UTI
ADULTS: PO/IV 200 mg q 12 hr for 10 days.

Epididymitis
ADULTS: PO 300 mg bid for 10 days.

Otitis Externa
ADULTS AND CHILDREN 12 YR AND OLDER: **OTIC** 10 gtt (0.5 mL, 1.5 mg ofloxacin) instilled into affected ear bid for 10 days.
CHILDREN 1 TO 12 YR: **OTIC** 5 gtt (0.25 mL, 0.75 mg ofloxacin) instilled into affected ear bid for 10 days.

Prostatitis
ADULTS: PO/IV 300 mg q 12 hr for 6 wk.

Uncomplicated Cystitis Caused by E. Coli or Klebsiella Pneumoniae
ADULTS: PO/IV 200 mg q 12 hr for 3 days.

Uncomplicated Cystitis Caused by Other Pathogens
ADULTS: PO/IV 200 mg q 12 hr for 7 days.

Interactions
Antacids, didanosine, iron salts, sucralfate, zinc salts: May decrease oral absorption of ofloxacin.
Antineoplastic agents: Serum ofloxacin levels may be decreased.
NSAIDs: Coadministration with ofloxacin may increase risk of CNS stimulation and seizures.
Procainamide: Plasma levels of procainamide may be elevated, increasing the risk of toxicity.
Theophylline: Decreased Cl and increased plasma levels of theophylline may result in toxicity.

Lab Test Interferences
None well documented.

Adverse Reactions
CV: Chest pain.
CNS: Dizziness, vertigo (1%, otic); headache; dizziness; fatigue; lethargy; drowsiness; insomnia; nervousness.
DERM: Pruritus, rash (4%, otic); rash, pruritus.
EENT: Tearing, dryness, eye pain, visual disturbances, transient burning, itching, stinging, inflammation, facial edema (ophthalmic use); earache (otic).
GI: Taste perversion (7%, otic); diarrhea; nausea; vomiting; abdominal pain or discomfort; dry or painful mouth; flatulence; dysgeusia.
GU: Vaginal discharge; genital pruritus.
HEMA: Eosinophilia; lymphocytopenia.
HEPA: Increased ALT, AST.
OTHER: Application site reaction (3%), paresthesia (otic); vaginitis; fever; decreased appetite. Ophthalmic use may possibly cause same adverse reactions seen with systemic use because of absorption.

Precautions
Pregnancy: Category C.
Lactation: Excreted in breast milk.
Children: Safety and efficacy not established in children under 18 yr. **Otic** Safety and efficacy not established in children under 1 yr.
Hypersensitivity: Serious and occasionally fatal reactions (eg, anaphylactic) have occurred, some after the first dose.
Renal function impairment: Reduced Ccr may occur; decrease dose accordingly.
Superinfection: May result in bacterial or fungal overgrowth of nonsusceptible microorganisms.
Photosensitivity: Moderate to severe reactions may occur; avoid excessive sunlight and ultraviolet light.
Convulsions/Toxic psychosis: CNS stimulation can occur; use drug with caution in patients with known or suspected CNS disorders.
Pseudomembranous colitis: Consider possibility in patients who develop diarrhea.
Syphilis: Not effective for treating syphilis.
Tendonitis: Inflammation and rupture of tendons have been associated with the use of fluoroquinolone antibiotics.

Overdosage: Signs and Symptoms
Nausea, dizziness, crystalluria, facial swelling and numbness, vomiting, drowsiness, hot and cold flushes.

PATIENT CARE CONSIDERATIONS
Administration/Storage
IV:
- Store at room temperature (59° to 86°F).
- IV solution is stable after dilution for 72 hr at room temperature and 2 wk if refrigerated.
- Discard unused portion of IV preparation.
- Do not give as IV push or bolus. To reduce likelihood of hypotension, infuse over 60 min.
- Dilute to concentration of 4 mg/mL.
- Do not infuse in IV line with any other drug.

Oral:
- Store at room temperature.
- Do not coadminister with antacids.
- Administer with full glass of water.

Assessment/Interventions
- Obtain patient history, including drug history and any known allergies.
- Obtain baseline CBC, renal and LFTs, and electrolytes.
- Assess for any rashes. Notify health care provider if rash occurs.
- Monitor for convulsions, dizziness, confusion, tremors, hallucinations, depression, or suicidal thoughts; if occurring, discontinue medication and refer for appropriate treatment.
- Monitor for signs of arthropathy, pain, inflammation, or rupture of tendon; if present, discontinue medication.
- Obtain baseline vital signs. Monitor vital signs at least bid while administering medication.
- Monitor patterns of elimination and stool consistency.
- Monitor for signs of superinfection (eg, vaginitis, stomatitis, diarrhea).
- Encourage fluid intake.
- Notify health care provider if vomiting, fatigue, lymphocytopenia, increased LFTs, seizures, or visual disturbances occur.
- Notify health care provider if extreme burning, angioneurotic edema, or dermatitis occurs with ophthalmic use.

Patient/Family Education
- Instruct patient to avoid taking antacids, sucralfate, vitamins with iron or minerals within 2 hr before or 2 hr after dose.
- Advise diabetic patient to discontinue if a hypoglycemic reaction occurs and notify health care provider.
- Encourage patient to drink fluids liberally.
- Caution patient to avoid exposure to sunlight, and to use sunscreen or wear protective clothing to avoid photosensitivity reaction.
- Advise patient to notify health care provider of signs of superinfection.
- Caution patient to report the following symptoms to health care provider: seizures, nausea, rash, itching, diarrhea, shortness of breath, dizziness, headache.
- Instruct patient to complete full course of therapy, even if symptoms have resolved.
- Instruct patient to stop treatment and inform health care provider if experiencing pain, inflammation, or rupture of tendon, and to rest or refrain from exercise until diagnosis of tendonitis or tendon rupture is excluded.

Ophthalmic:
- Demonstrate and observe correct technique for instillation of ophthalmic drops.
- Advise patient using ophthalmic solution to discontinue medication and notify health care provider of rash or allergic reaction.

Otic:
- Caution patient to avoid contaminating the applicator tip with material from fingers or other sources.
- Instruct patient to warm the solution by holding the bottle in the hand for 1 or 2 min to avoid dizziness, which may result from the instillation of cold solution.

Olanzapine

(oh-LAN-zah-peen)

Class Atypical antipsychotic

How Supplied
Zyprexa Tablets 2.5 mg, Tablets 5 mg, Tablets 7.5 mg, Tablets 10 mg, Tablets 15 mg, Tablets 20 mg ♦ *Zyprexa Zydis* Tablets, orally disintegrating 5 mg, Tablets, orally disintegrating 10 mg, Tablets, orally disintegrating 15 mg, Tablets, orally disintegrating 20 mg ♦ *Zyprexa IntraMuscular* Powder for injection 10 mg

Action
PHARMACOLOGY: Unknown. May control psychotic symptoms through antagonism of selected dopamine and serotonin receptors in the CNS.

PHARMACOKINETICS/DYNAMICS:
Absorption: Readily absorbed orally and intramuscularly. C_{max} is approximately 6 hr (oral) and 15 to 45 min (IM). Steady state is approximately 1 wk.

Distribution: Extensively distributed throughout the body. Vd is approximately 1,000 L; 93% is protein bound.

Metabolism: In liver by glucuronidation and CYP450-mediated oxidation; major circulating metabolites are inactive.

Excretion: Elimination is 57% in urine (7% unchanged); 30% eliminated in feces. The t½ is 21 to 54 hr. Plasma Cl is 12 to 47 L/hr.

Special Populations:
Elderly – The t½ increases 1.5 times. Use caution when dosing.
Gender – Cl is 30% lower in women.
Smoking – Cl is approximately 40% higher in smokers.

Indications Treatment of schizophrenia; short-term treatment of acute mixed or manic episodes with bipolar I disorder.

Contraindications Standard considerations.

Route/Dosage

Bipolar Mania
ADULTS: **PO** Start with 10 to 15 mg/day and adjust at 5 mg increments or decrements in intervals no less than 24 hr (safety of doses more than 20 mg/day not evaluated). When administered in combination with lithium or valproate, oral olanzapine dosing should generally begin with 10 mg daily without regard to meals.
IM Recommended dose is 10 mg; a lower dose of 5 to 7.5 mg may be considered. If agitation persists, subsequent doses up to 10 mg may be given. Safety of total daily doses greater than 30 mg, or 10 mg given more than 2 hr after initial dose and 4 hr after second dose, have not been evaluated.

Schizophrenia
ADULTS: **PO** Start with 5 to 10 mg/day and adjust dosage at 5 mg increments or decrements in intervals of no less than 1 wk (safety of doses above 20 mg/day not evaluated). **IM** Recommended dose is 10 mg; a lower dose of 5 to 7.5 mg may be considered. If agitation persists, subsequent doses up to 10 mg may be given. Safety of total daily doses greater than 30 mg, or 10 mg given more than 2 hr after initial dose and 4 hr after second dose, have not been evaluated.

Special Populations
ADULTS (EG, DEBILITATED, PREDISPOSED TO HYPOTENSION, ELDERLY): **PO** Start with 5 mg/day. **IM** 5 mg (elderly); a lower dose of 2.5 mg for debilitated patients who are predisposed to hypotension.

Interactions
Antihypertensive drugs: Olanzapine may enhance hypotensive effects.
Carbamazepine: Olanzapine Cl increases 50%, resulting in lower plasma levels.
Fluvoxamine: May elevate olanzapine plasma levels.
Levodopa and other dopamine agonists: Olanzapine may antagonize effects by inhibiting dopamine receptors.
Sedating drugs and alcohol: Additive CNS depression; motor and cognitive impairment.

Lab Test Interferences None well documented.

Adverse Reactions
CV: Postural hypotension (5%); tachycardia (3%); hypertension (2%); hypotension (at least 1%).
CNS: Somnolence (35%); dizziness (18%); parkinsonism (14%); insomnia (12%); personality disorder (8%); tremor, abnormal gait, increased appetite (6%); akathisia (5%); hypertonia, dystonia (3%); articulation impairment (2%); abnormal dreams, emotional lability, euphoria, decreased libido, paresthesia, schizophrenic reaction (at least 1%).
DERM: Ecchymosis (5%); sweating (at least 1%).
EENT: Rhinitis (7%); pharyngitis (4%); amblyopia (3%); conjunctivitis (at least 1%).
GI: Dry mouth (22%); constipation, dyspepsia (11%); nausea (9%); increased appetite (6%); vomiting (4%); increased salivation and thirst (at least 1%).
GU: Urinary incontinence, UTI (2%); amenorrhea, hematuria, metrorrhagia, vaginitis, priapism (postmarketing).
HEMA: Leukopenia (at least 1%).
METAB: Weight gain (6%); peripheral edema (3%); diabetic coma (postmarketing).
RESP: Increased cough (6%); dyspnea (at least 1%).
OTHER: Asthenia (15%); accidental injury (12%); fever (6%); back pain, extremity pain, joint pain (5%); chest pain (3%); dental pain, flu-like syndrome, suicide attempt, intentional injury, joint stiffness and twitching (at least 1%); allergic reactions (eg, anaphylactoid reaction, angioedema, pruritus, urticaria), pancreatitis (postmarketing).

Precautions
Pregnancy: Category C.
Lactation: Undetermined.
Children: Safety and efficacy not established.
Hepatic function impairment: Use with caution.
Body temperature regulation: Antipsychotics disrupt the ability to reduce core body temperature. Use with caution in patients who will experience conditions that may contribute to an elevation in core body temperature (eg, strenuous exercise, exposure to extreme heat, concomitant anticholinergic therapy, subject to dehydration).
Cerebrovascular adverse events (CVAE): CVAE (eg, stroke, transient ischemic attack), including fatalities, may occur.

Cognitive and motor impairment: Caution patients about operating potentially hazardous machinery (eg, driving) until they know whether the drug impairs their ability. Avoid use of alcohol.
Dysphagia: Use with caution in patients at risk for aspiration pneumonia.
Hyperglycemia: Hyperglycemia, in some cases extreme and associated with ketoacidosis or hyperosmolar coma or death, may occur.
Hyperprolactinemia: Olanzapine-treated patients often have elevation in prolactin levels; however, there is no evidence of increased breast tumor risk.
Liver disease: Monitor LFTs in patients with significant hepatic disease.
Neuroleptic malignant syndrome (NMS): NMS has occurred and is potentially fatal. Signs and symptoms are hyperpyrexia, muscle rigidity, altered mental status, irregular pulse, irregular BP, tachycardia, and diaphoresis.
Orthostatic hypotension: May occur with associated symptoms of dizziness, tachycardia, and syncope. Most common during titration period and in patients with CV disease, cerebrovascular disease, and conditions that predispose to hypotension (eg, dehydration, hypovolemia, treatment with antihypertensive agents). Reduce risk by initiating therapy with 5 mg daily.
Seizures: Use with caution in patients with a history of seizures or with conditions that lower the seizure threshold (eg, Alzheimer disease, dementia).
Suicide: Possible suicide attempts are inherent in schizophrenia and in bipolar disorder. Closely supervise high-risk patients. Write prescriptions for the smallest quantity consistent with good patient management.
Tardive dyskinesia: Syndrome of potentially irreversible, involuntary dyskinetic movements may develop. Prevalence is highest in elderly, especially women. Use smallest effective dose for shortest period of time needed.

Overdosage: Signs and Symptoms

Drowsiness, slurred speech, agitation/aggressiveness, dysarthria, tachycardia, various extrapyramidal symptoms, reduced level of consciousness, sedation to coma, aspiration, cardiopulmonary arrest, cardiac arrhythmias (such as supraventricular tachycardia), sinus pause, delirium, possible neuroleptic malignant syndrome, respiratory depression/arrest, convulsion, hypertension, hypotension, death.

PATIENT CARE CONSIDERATIONS

Administration/Storage

- Administer prescribed dose daily without regard to meals.
- Administer with food if GI upset occurs.
- Administer disintegrating tablet by peeling back foil on blister pack (do not push tablet through foil) and, using dry hands, remove tablet from foil and place in patient's mouth; tablet will disintegrate with or without liquid.
- Do not administer orally disintegrating tablet to patient with phenylketonuria without first discussing it with health care provider.
- Store at controlled room temperature (59° to 86°F). Protect from light and moisture.

Injection:

- For IM administration only. Not for intradermal, subcutaneous, IV, or intra-arterial administration.
- Reconstitute powder for injection using 2.1 mL sterile water for injection. Resulting solution contains approximately 5 mg/mL.
- Do not mix with other medications or use other diluents.
- Do not administer if particulate matter or cloudiness are noted. Solution should be clear and yellow.
- Administer within 1 hr of reconstitution.
- Administer by slow, deep injection into muscle mass.
- Discard any unused solution. Do not save unused solution for later administration.
- Store powder for injection at controlled room temperature (68° to 77°F). Protect from light and freezing. Following reconstitution, the injection can be stored for up to 1 hr at controlled room temperature if necessary.

Assessment/Interventions

- Obtain patient history, including drug history and any known allergies. Note history of liver disease, CV disease, cerebrovascular disease, cardiac arrhythmias, previous episodes of NMS, seizures or conditions that predispose to seizures (eg, Alzheimer disease), or conditions that would predispose to hypotension (eg, dehydration, hypovolemia, treatment with antihypertensive medications).
- Monitor patient for CNS, GI, CV, PSYCH, and general body side effects. Inform health care provider if noted and significant.
- Ensure that liver enzymes are assessed prior to and periodically during therapy in patient with liver disease.
- Monitor blood sugar in diabetic patient when drug is started or dose is changed. Report significant changes to health care provider.
- Ensure that fasting blood glucose is evaluated before starting therapy and periodically thereafter during therapy in patient with risk fac-

tors for diabetes mellitus (eg, obesity, family history of diabetes).
- Monitor cardiac patients during initiation of drug for orthostatic hypotension; notify health care provider if noted.
- Take safety precautions if orthostatic hypotension occurs.
- Inform health care provider immediately if symptoms of NMS (eg, hyperpyrexia, muscle rigidity, altered mental status, irregular pulse and BP, tachycardia, diaphoresis) develop.
- Notify health care provider if any of the following symptoms develop: hypotension; tachycardia; excessive drowsiness; constipation; symptoms of hyperglycemia (eg, polyuria, polydipsia, polyphagia); persistent nausea, vomiting, or indigestion.
- Assess baseline neurologic status and, during treatment, observe for involuntary body and facial movements, drowsiness, agitation, anxiety, aggressive reaction, or seizure activity.
- Frequently assess patient for response to treatment. Notify health care provider if condition does not appear to be improving or is worsening.
- Ensure that therapy is periodically reviewed to determine if it needs to be continued without change or if a dose change (eg, increase, decrease, discontinuation) is indicated.
- Monitor patient for suicidal tendencies often associated with schizophrenia.
- Assess medication compliance.
- Assess for orthostatic hypotension prior to the administration of any subsequent IM doses.

Patient/Family Education

- Explain name, dose, action, and potential side effects of drug.
- Instruct patient to take prescribed dose daily without regard to meals but to take with food if GI upset occurs.
- Caution patient using disintegrating tablet not to open the blister until ready to take the dose.
- Advise patient that if a dose is missed to take it as soon as possible and then return to the normal schedule. Instruct patient that if a dose is skipped not to double the dose to catch up.
- Advise patient that dose will be started low and then increased until max benefit is obtained.
- Instruct patient not to change the dose or stop taking unless advised by health care provider.
- Instruct patient not to stop taking olanzapine when feeling better.
- Advise patient to take frequent sips of water, suck on ice chips or sugarless hard candy, or chew sugarless gum if dry mouth occurs.
- Instruct diabetic patient to monitor blood glucose more frequently when drug is started or dose is changed and to inform health care provider of significant changes in readings.
- Tell patient to immediately report high fever, muscle rigidity, altered mental status, irregular pulse, sweating, seizures, racing thoughts, mood swings, irritability, unquenchable thirst, frequent urination, unusual hunger, rash, or hives to health care provider.
- Advise patient to notify health care provider of the following: excessive drowsiness, swelling in the feet or ankles, weight gain, involuntary body or facial movements, rapid pulse, change in personality or mood.
- Advise patient to avoid strenuous activity during periods of high temperature or humidity.
- Instruct patient to avoid alcoholic beverages and sedatives (eg, diazepam) while taking olanzapine.
- Instruct patient to get up slowly from lying or sitting position and to avoid sudden position changes to prevent postural hypotension. Advise patient to report dizziness with position changes to health care provider. Caution patient that hot tubs and hot showers or baths may make dizziness worse.
- Advise patient taking antihypertensives to monitor BP at regular intervals.
- Advise patient that drug may impair judgment, thinking, or motor skills or cause drowsiness and to use caution while driving or performing other tasks requiring mental alertness until tolerance is determined.
- Advise women to notify health care provider if pregnant, planning to become pregnant, or breastfeeding.
- Instruct patient not to take any prescription or OTC medications, dietary supplements, or herbal preparations unless advised by health care provider.
- Advise patient that follow-up visits will be required to monitor therapy and to keep appointments.

Olanzapine/Fluoxetine Hydrochloride

(oh-LAN-zah-peen/flew-OX-uh-tee HIGH-droe-KLOR-ide)

Class Antidepressant

How Supplied

Symbyax Capsules 6 mg olanzapine/25 mg fluoxetine hydrochloride, Capsules 6 mg olanzapine/50 mg fluoxetine hydrochloride, Capsules 12 mg olanzapine/25 mg fluoxetine hydrochloride, Capsules 12 mg olanzapine/50 mg fluoxetine hydrochloride

Action

PHARMACOLOGY: Unknown; however, it is suspected that activation of 3 monoaminergic neural systems (serotonin, norepinephrine, and dopamine) is responsible for an enhancement of the antidepressant effect.

Indications Treatment of depressive episodes associated with bipolar disorder.

Contraindications Coadministration with thioridazine (or within at least 5 wk of stopping olanzapine/fluoxetine) or an MAO inhibitor (or within 14 days of discontinuing an MAO inhibitor and at least 5 wk after stopping olanzapine/fluoxetine); hypersensitivity to any component of the product.

Route/Dosage

ADULTS: **PO** Start with 6 mg olanzapine/25 mg fluoxetine qd in the evening. If indicated, dosage adjustments can be made based on efficacy and tolerability. Antidepressant efficacy has been demonstrated up to 12 mg olanzapine/50 mg fluoxetine. Safety of doses above 18 mg olanzapine/75 mg fluoxetine have not been evaluated.

Interactions

Antihypertensives: Antihypertensive effects may be enhanced by olanzapine.

Anti-Parkinsonian agents (eg, levodopa, dopamine antagonists): Effects may be antagonized by olanzapine.

Benzodiazepines (eg, alprazolam, diazepam): The orthostatic hypotensive effects of olanzapine may be potentiated by diazepam; the t½ of diazepam may be prolonged by fluoxetine; plasma concentrations of alprazolam may be increased.

Carbamazepine: Plasma concentrations of olanzapine may be decreased by carbamazepine, and plasma levels of carbamazepine may be increased by fluoxetine.

Clozapine, haloperidol, phenytoin, tricyclic antidepressants (eg, desipramine, imipramine): Blood levels of these agents may be increased by fluoxetine.

Digoxin, warfarin: May be displaced from protein binding site by fluoxetine, increasing the risk of adverse effects.

Ethanol: May potentiate sedation and orthostatic hypotension of olanzapine/fluoxetine combination.

Fluvoxamine: May inhibit the metabolism of olanzapine, elevating olanzapine plasma levels and increasing the risk of side effects.

Lithium: Fluoxetine may increase or decrease lithium levels. Lithium toxicity and increased serotonergic effects have been reported.

MAO inhibitors (eg, isocarboxazid): Administration with olanzapine/fluoxetine (or administration within 14 days of discontinuing an MAO inhibitor and at least 5 wk after stopping olanzapine/fluoxetine) is contraindicated; death has been reported with coadministration of MAO inhibitors and fluoxetine.

Omeprazole, rifampin: May decrease olanzapine concentrations.

Pimozide: Bradycardia has been reported during coadministration with fluoxetine.

Sumatriptan: Weakness, hyperreflexia, and incoordination have been reported with coadministration of sumatriptan and an SSRI (eg, fluoxetine).

Thioridazine: Administration with olanzapine/fluoxetine or within a minimum of 5 wk after discontinuing olanzapine/fluoxetine is contraindicated.

Lab Test Interferences None well documented.

Adverse Reactions

CV: Hypertension, tachycardia (at least 2%); increase in QTc interval, bradycardia, orthostatic hypotension, migraine, vasodilation (postmarketing).

CNS: Somnolence, abnormal thinking, tremor (at least 5%); decreased libido, hyperkinesias, personality disorder, sleep disorder, amnesia (at least 2%).

EENT: Pharyngitis (at least 5%); amblyopia, ear pain, otitis media (at least 2%); abnormal vision, taste perversion, tinnitus (postmarketing).

GI: Increased appetite (at least 5%); diarrhea, dry mouth, tooth disorder (at least 2%); increased salivation, thirst (postmarketing).

GU: Abnormal ejaculation, impotence, anorgasmia (at least 2%); priapism, breast pain, menorrhagia, urinary frequency, urinary incontinence, UTI (postmarketing).

LABTESTABS: Increases in alkaline phosphatase, cholesterol, glucose tolerance test, uric acid, serum prolactin decrease in hemoglobin (postmarketing); abnormal ejaculation.

M/N: Edema, peripheral edema, weight gain (at least 5%); weight loss, generalized edema (postmarketing).
MUSC: Joint disorder, twitching, arthralgia (at least 2%).
RESP: Dyspnea (at least 2%); lung disorder (postmarketing); bronchitis.
OTHER: Asthenia (at least 5%); accidental injury, fever, speech disorder (at least 2%); chest pain (at least 1%); chills, infection, neck pain and rigidity, photosensitivity reaction (postmarketing).

Precautions

Pregnancy: Category C.
Lactation: Undetermined; however, fluoxetine is excreted in breast milk.
Children: Safety and efficacy not established.
Elderly: Use with caution because of the greater frequency of decreased hepatic, renal, or cardiac function and concomitant diseases or other drug therapy.
Body temperature regulation: Antipsychotics disrupt the ability to reduce core body temperature. Use with caution in patients who will experience conditions that may contribute to an elevation in core body temperature (eg, strenuous exercise, exposure to extreme heat, concomitant anticholinergic therapy, subject to dehydration).
Cerebrovascular adverse events (CVAE): CVAE (eg, stroke, transient ischemic attack), including fatalities, may occur.
Cognitive and motor impairment: Caution patients about operating potentially hazardous machinery (eg, driving) until it is known if the drug impairs ability. Avoid use of alcohol.
Dose changes: Because of the long elimination t½ of fluoxetine, changes in dose will not be fully reflected in plasma for several weeks, affecting titration to final dose and withdrawal from treatment.
Dysphagia: Use with caution in patients at risk of aspiration pneumonia.

Hyperglycemia: Hyperglycemia, in some cases extreme and associated with ketoacidosis, hyperosmolar coma, or death, may occur.
Hyperprolactinemia: Olanzapine-treated patients often have elevation in prolactin levels; however, there is no evidence of increased breast tumor risk.
Mania/Hypomania: May be precipitated by fluoxetine in susceptible patients.
Neuroleptic malignant syndrome (NMS): Has occurred and is potentially fatal. Signs and symptoms include hyperpyrexia, muscle rigidity, altered mental status, irregular pulse, irregular BP, tachycardia, and diaphoresis.
Orthostatic hypotension: Orthostatic hypotension, associated with dizziness, tachycardia, bradycardia, and syncope may occur.
Seizures: May occur; use with caution in patients with a history of seizures.
Suicide: Supervise depressed patients at risk during initial therapy. Prescribe the smallest quantity consistent with good patient management in order to reduce the risk of overdose.
Tardive dyskinesia: Syndrome of potentially irreversible, involuntary dyskinetic movements may develop. Prevalence is higher in elderly, especially women. Use smallest effective dose for shortest period of time needed.

Overdosage: Signs and Symptoms

Olanzapine: Agitation, aggressiveness, dysarthria, tachycardia, various extrapyramidal symptoms, reduced level of consciousness (from sedation to coma), aspiration, cardiopulmonary arrest, cardiac arrhythmias (eg, supraventricular tachycardia), delirium, possible NMS, respiratory arrest, convulsion, hypertension, hypotension.
Fluoxetine: Abnormal accommodation, abnormal gait, confusion, unresponsiveness, nervousness, pulmonary dysfunction, vertigo, tremor, elevated BP, impotence, movement disorder, hypomania, seizures, somnolence, nausea, tachycardia, vomiting, death.

PATIENT CARE CONSIDERATIONS

Administration/Storage

- Do not administer with, or within 14 days of MAO inhibitor administration. Do not administer MAO inhibitors within at least 5 wk of olanzapine/fluoxetine discontinuation.
- Do not administer with thioridazine. Do not administer thioridazine within at least 5 wk of olanzapine/fluoxetine discontinuation.
- Administer prescribed dose qd in the evening without regard to meals. Administer with food if GI upset occurs.
- Store capsules at controlled room temperature (59° to 86°F). Protect from moisture.

Assessment/Interventions

- Obtain patient history, including drug history and any known allergies. Note hepatic impairment, pregnancy, breastfeeding, diabetes, CV disease, cerebrovascular disease, dementia-related psychosis, difficulty swallowing, cardiac arrhythmias, previous episodes of NMS, seizures, or conditions that predispose to seizures (eg, Alzheimer disease), conditions that would predispose to hypotension (eg, dehydration, hypovolemia, treatment with antihypertensive medications), prostatic hypertrophy, narrow angle glaucoma, history

of paralytic ileus, previous hypersensitivity reaction to SSRI, concurrent or recent (eg, within 14 days) use of MAO inhibitor, concurrent or recent use of thioridazine, fluoxetine-containing (eg, *Sarafem*) or olanzapine-containing (eg, *Zyprexa*) medications, potentially hepatotoxic drug (eg, pioglitazone), aspirin, NSAIDs, or other medications that can affect coagulation.
- Ensure that lowest starting dose and slower dose escalation are used in patient with hepatic impairment, predisposition to hypotensive reactions, or combination of factors that may slow metabolism of medication (eg, nonsmokers, elderly, women).
- Ensure that liver enzymes are assessed prior to and periodically during therapy in patient with liver disease. Inform health care provider if elevated transaminases are noted.
- Monitor blood sugar in diabetic patient when drug is started or dose is changed. Report significant changes to health care provider.
- Ensure that fasting blood glucose is evaluated before starting therapy and periodically thereafter during therapy in patient with risk factors for diabetes mellitus (eg, obesity, family history of diabetes).
- Monitor cardiac patients during initiation of drug for orthostatic hypotension; notify health care provider if noted and implement safety precautions.
- Inform health care provider immediately if symptoms of NMS (hyperpyrexia, muscle rigidity, altered mental status, irregular pulse and BP, tachycardia, diaphoresis) develop.
- Assess baseline neurologic status and, during treatment, observe for involuntary body and facial movements, excessive drowsiness, agitation, anxiety, aggressive reaction, or seizure activity.
- Monitor patient for suicidal tendencies often associated with bipolar disorder.
- Frequently assess patient for response to treatment. Notify health care provider if condition does not appear to be improving or is worsening.
- Ensure that therapy is periodically reviewed to determine if it needs to be continued without change or if a dose change (eg, increase, decrease, discontinuation) is indicated.
- Monitor patient for development of skin rash, symptoms of hyperglycemia (eg, polydipsia, polyuria, polyphagia, weakness). Inform health care provider if noted.
- Monitor patient for CNS, GI, PSYCH, MUSC, GU, and general body side effects. Report to health care provider if noted and significant.
- Assess medication compliance.

Patient/Family Education
- Explain name, dose, action, and potential side effects of drug.
- Advise patient to read *Patient Information* leaflet before starting therapy and with each refill.
- Advise patient that dose will be started low and then increased until max benefit is obtained.
- Instruct patient to take prescribed dose qd in the evening without regard to meals but to take with food if GI upset occurs.
- Advise patient that if a dose is missed to take it as soon as possible and then return to the normal schedule. However, if it is almost time for the next dose, to skip the missed dose and take the next dose at the regularly scheduled time. Instruct patient that if a dose is skipped, not to double the dose to catch up.
- Instruct patient not to change the dose or stop taking unless advised by health care provider.
- Instruct patient not to stop taking the medication when feeling better.
- Caution patient not to take aspirin or aspirin-containing products, NSAIDS, Ginkgo biloba, or any other medication or herb that can affect coagulation because of increased risk of serious bleeding.
- Instruct patient to contact health care provider if symptoms do not appear to be getting better, are getting worse, or if bothersome side effects (eg, excessive drowsiness, diarrhea, tremors, nausea, nervousness, changes in sexual function) occur.
- Advise patient to take frequent sips of water, suck on ice chips or sugarless hard candy, or chew sugarless gum if dry mouth occurs.
- Instruct diabetic patient to monitor blood glucose more frequently when drug is started or dose is changed and to inform health care provider of significant changes in readings.
- Tell patient to immediately report high fever, muscle rigidity, altered mental status, irregular pulse, sweating, seizures, racing thoughts, mood swings, irritability, unquenchable thirst, frequent urination, unusual hunger, or rash or hives to health care provider.

- Advise patient to notify health care provider if excessive drowsiness, swelling in the feet or ankles, weight gain, involuntary body or facial movements, rapid pulse, or change in personality or mood occurs.
- Advise patient to avoid strenuous activity during periods of high temperature or humidity.
- Instruct patient to avoid alcoholic beverages and sedatives or depressants (eg, diazepam) while taking medication.
- Instruct patient to get up slowly from lying or sitting position and to avoid sudden position changes to prevent postural hypotension. Advise patient to report dizziness with position changes to health care provider. Caution patient that hot tubs and hot showers or baths may make dizziness worse.
- Advise patient taking antihypertensives to monitor BP at regular intervals.
- Advise patient that drug may impair judgment, thinking, or motor skills or cause drowsiness and to use caution while driving or performing other tasks requiring mental alertness until tolerance is determined.
- Advise women to notify health care provider if pregnant, planning to become pregnant, or breastfeeding.
- Instruct patient not to take any prescription or OTC medications or dietary supplements unless advised by health care provider.
- Advise patient that follow-up visits will be required to monitor therapy and to keep appointments.

Olmesartan Medoxomil

(ole-mih-SAR-tan meh-DOX-oh-mill)

Class Antihypertensive/Angiotensin II antagonist

How Supplied
Benicar Tablets 5 mg, Tablets 20 mg, Tablets 40 mg

Action
PHARMACOLOGY: Blocks vasoconstrictor effects of angiotensin II by selectively blocking the binding of angiotensin II to the AT_1 receptor in vascular smooth muscle.

PHARMACOKINETICS/DYNAMICS:

Absorption: Rapidly and completely absorbed from the GI tract. The steady state is 3 to 5 days. The bioavailability is approximately 26%. The T_{max} is 1 to 2 hr.

Distribution: The Vd is 17 L. 99% is protein bound.

Excretion: About 35% to 50% is eliminated through urine. The remainder is eliminated in feces via bile (50% to 65% recovered).

The total plasma clearance is 1.3 L/hr. Renal clearance is 0.6 L/hr. The $t_{1/2}$ is approximately 13 hr.

Special Populations:
Renal Function Impairment – Ccr is less than 20 mL/min. AUC is approximately tripled.
Hepatic Function Impairment – AUC increased by approximately 60%. C_{max} increased.
Elderly – AUC increased by 33%, and there is a 30% reduction in renal clearance.
Gender – AUC increased 10% and C_{max} increased by 15% in women. Minor differences.

Indications Treatment of hypertension.

Contraindications Standard considerations.

Route/Dosage
ADULTS: **PO** Start with 20 mg once daily; after 2 wk, dosage may be increased to 40 mg/day if further reduction in BP is needed.

Interactions None well documented.

Lab Test Interferences
Lithium: Plasma concentrations may be increased by olmesartan, resulting in an increase in the pharmacologic and adverse effects of lithium.

Adverse Reactions
CV: Tachycardia.
CNS: Dizziness; fatigue; vertigo; insomnia.
DERM: Rash.
GI: Abdominal pain; dyspepsia; gastroenteritis; nausea.
GU: UTI.
METAB: Hypercholesterolemia; hyperlipemia; hyperuricemia.
OTHER: Chest pain; pain; peripheral edema; arthritis; myalgia; skeletal pain.

Precautions
Pregnancy: Category C (first trimester); Category D (second and third trimester). Can cause injury or death to the fetus if used during second or third trimester.
Lactation: Undetermined.
Children: Safety and efficacy not established.
Renal function impairment: In patients whose renal function may depend on activity of the renin-angiotensin-converting enzyme system (eg, patients with severe CHF), treatment with olmesartan may be associated with oliguria and progressive azotemia, rarely resulting in acute renal failure or death.

Overdosage: Signs and Symptoms
Hypotension, tachycardia, bradycardia.

PATIENT CARE CONSIDERATIONS

Administration/Storage
- Give prescribed dose once daily, with or without food.
- Administer with food if GI upset occurs.
- Store tablets at controlled room temperature (68° to 77°F).

Assessment/Interventions
- Obtain patient history, including drug history and any known allergies. Note history of impaired renal function, severe CHF, renal artery stenosis, volume depletion or dehydration, or allergy to olmesartan or other angiotensin II receptor antagonists.
- Ensure that serum electrolytes are monitored periodically.
- Monitor and record BP and pulse. Should hypotension result, withhold medication and notify health care provider.
- Take safety precautions if orthostatic hypotension occurs.
- Monitor for signs of hypersensitivity, including angioedema involving swelling of the face, lips, eyelids, and tongue. Discontinue medication and contact health care provider immediately if noted.

Patient/Family Education
- Explain name, dose, action, and potential side effects of drug.
- Advise patient to take once daily as prescribed, without regard to meals, but to take with food if GI upset occurs.
- Advise patient to take each dose at about the same time each day.
- Inform patient that the drug controls, but not does cure, hypertension and to continue taking the drug as prescribed, even when BP is not elevated.
- Caution patient not to change the dose or stop taking unless advised by health care provider.
- Instruct patient to continue taking other BP medications as prescribed by health care provider.
- Instruct patient in BP and pulse measurement skills.
- Advise patient to monitor and record BP and pulse at home and to inform health care provider should abnormal measurements be noted. Advise patient to take record of BP and pulse to each follow-up visit.
- Instruct patient to lie or sit down if experiencing dizziness or lightheadedness when standing.
- Caution patient that inadequate fluid intake, excessive perspiration, diarrhea, or vomiting can lead to an excessive fall in BP resulting in lightheadedness or fainting.
- Emphasize to hypertensive patient the importance of the following other modalities on BP: weight control, regular exercise, smoking cessation, moderate intake of alcohol and salt.
- Instruct women to notify health care provider if pregnant, plan on becoming pregnant, or breastfeeding.
- Instruct patient to stop taking drug and immediately report any of the following symptoms to health care provider: fainting; swelling of the face, lips, eyelids, or tongue.
- Caution patient to not take any prescription or OTC medications, salt substitutes, or dietary supplements unless advised by health care provider.
- Advise patient that follow-up visits and lab tests may be required to monitor therapy and to keep appointments.

Olopatadine Hydrochloride

(oh-low-pat-AD-een HIGH-droe-KLOR-ide)

Class Ophthalmic Antihistaminic Agent

How Supplied
Patanol Solution 0.1%

Action
PHARMACOLOGY: Inhibits release of histamine from mast cells and relatively selective histamine H1 antagonist. Inhibits type 1 immediate hypersensitivity reactions.

Indications Temporary relief of itching caused by allergic conjunctivitis.

Contraindications Standard considerations.

Route/Dosage
ADULTS AND CHILDREN: 1 to 2 drops in affected eye(s) twice daily, 6 to 8 hrs apart.

Interactions None well documented.

Lab Test Interferences None well documented.

Adverse Reactions
OPHTH: Burning, dry eye, foreign body sensation, hyperemia, keratitis, lid edema, pruritus, stinging.
OTHER: Asthenia, cold syndrome, dysgeusia, headache, pharyngitis, rhinitis, sinusitis.

Precautions
Pregnancy: Category C.

Lactation: Secreted into animal breast milk.
Children: Safety and effectiveness younger than 3 yr of age are not established.
Do not instill while wearing contact lenses.

PATIENT CARE CONSIDERATIONS

Administration/Storage
- For topical use in the eye only.
- Instill 1 drop in affected eye(s) bid, 6 to 8 hr apart.
- If using other topical ophthalmic drugs, separate each medication by 5 min or more.
- Store at controlled room temperature. Keep bottle tightly closed.

Assessment/Interventions
- Obtain patient history, including drug history and any known allergies.
- Monitor patient for clinical response as well as side effects. Report side effects to health care provider.

Patient/Family Education
- Explain name, dose, action, and potential side effects of drug.
- Advise patient that usual dose is 1 drop in affected eye(s) bid at an interval of 6 to 8 hr.
- Teach patient proper technique for instilling eye drops: Wash hands; do not allow dropper to touch eye; tilt head back, look up; pull lower eyelid down; instill prescribed number of drops; close eye for 1 to 2 min and apply gentle pressure to bridge of nose; do not rub eye.
- Advise patients who wear contact lenses to remove their lenses before instilling this medicine and to wait at least 10 min after instilling eye drop before inserting their lenses. Also, caution these patients to not wear their lenses if the eye is red.
- Advise patient that if more than 1 topical ophthalmic drug is being used, administer the drugs at least 5 min apart.
- Advise patient to inform health care provider if experiencing side effects or if eye symptoms do not improve or worsen.

Olsalazine Sodium

(OLE-SAL-uh-zeen SO-dee-uhm)

Class Intestinal anti-inflammatory/Aminosalicylic acid derivative

How Supplied
Dipentum Capsules 250 mg

Action
PHARMACOLOGY: Bioconverted to 5-aminosalicylic acid (mesalamine) in colon. Although mechanism of action is unknown, it probably reduces inflammation of colon topically by preventing production of substances involved in inflammatory process such as arachidonic acid.

PHARMACOKINETICS/DYNAMICS:
Absorption: Little is systematically absorbed. T_{max} is approximately 1 hr. Steady state is 2 to 3 wk (metabolite olsalazine-s).

Distribution: Once the drug metabolized to 5-aminosalicylic (5-ASA), the drug is slowly absorbed from the colon resulting in high concentration levels. More than 99% of olsalazine and olsalazine-s is protein bound. 74% of 5-ASA is protein bound.

Metabolism: 0.1% of dose is metabolized in liver to olsalazine-o-sulfate metabolite. The remainder reaches the colon and is rapidly converted to 5–ASA by colonic bacteria.

Excretion: Less than 1% is recovered in the urine. A small amount is recovered in the feces. The $t_{1/2}$ (serum) is 0.9 hr for olsalazine and 7 days for olsalazine-s.

Indications
Maintenance of remission of ulcerative colitis in patients intolerant of sulfasalazine.

Contraindications
Hypersensitivity to salicylates or any product component.

Route/Dosage
ADULTS: PO 500 mg bid (2 capsules) (total of 1 g/day).

Interactions
None well documented.

Lab Test Interferences
None well documented.

Adverse Reactions
CNS: Headache; fatigue; drowsiness; lethargy; depression.
DERM: Rash; itching.
GI: Diarrhea; abdominal pain; cramps; nausea; dyspepsia; bloating; anorexia.
OTHER: Arthralgia; upper respiratory infection.

Precautions
Pregnancy: Category C.
Lactation: Undetermined.
Children: Safety and efficacy not established.
Renal function impairment: Patients with history of renal disease or dysfunction may have worsening of renal function.

PATIENT CARE CONSIDERATIONS
Administration/Storage
- Administer with meals.
- Store at room temperature.

Assessment/Interventions
- Obtain patient history, including drug history and any known allergies.
- Assess baseline vital signs, weight, BUN, creatinine, ALT, and AST.
- Monitor elimination patterns, color, and consistency of stools.
- Assess for rashes, respiratory difficulty, abdominal pain, vomiting, diarrhea, abdominal distention, or lethargy, and notify health care provider of any problems.

Patient/Family Education
- Caution patient to notify health care provider of rashes, respiratory difficulty, lethargy, muscle weakness, vomiting, diarrhea or abdominal distention, or worsening of abdominal pain.
- Advise patient not to take double doses if one is missed. If more than 1 dose is missed, tell patient to notify health care provider.

Omalizumab
(oh-mah-lie-ZOO-mab)

Class Monoclonal antibody

How Supplied
Xolair Powder for Injection, lyophilized 202.5 mg (150 mg/1.2 mL after reconstitution)

Action
PHARMACOLOGY: Selectively binds to human IgE, inhibiting the binding of IgE to the high-affinity IgE receptor on the surface of mast cells and basophils and limiting the degree of release of mediators of the allergic response.

PHARMACOKINETICS/DYNAMICS:

Absorption: Average absolute bioavailability after SC administration is 62%. C_{max} reached in about 7 to 8 days. AUC from day 0 to 14 at steady state is up to 6-fold higher than those after the first dose.

Distribution: Vd 78 mL/kg.

Metabolism: Degraded by the liver.

Excretion: Average serum elimination t½ 26 days.

Indications
Treatment of moderate to severe persistent asthma in patients who have a positive skin test or in vitro reactivity to a perennial aero-allergen and whose symptoms are inadequately controlled with inhaled corticosteroids.

Unlabeled use(s): Seasonal allergic rhinitis.

Contraindications
Standard considerations.

Route/Dosage
ADULTS AND CHILDREN 12 YR AND OLDER: SC 150 to 375 mg q 2 or 4 wk. Doses (mg) and dosing frequency are determined by serum total immunoglobulin E (IgE) level (U/mL), measured before the start of treatment, and body weight (kg). Doses greater than 150 mg are divided among more than 1 injection site in order to limit injections to not more than 150 mg/site.

DOSAGE ADJUSTMENTS: Because total IgE levels are elevated during treatment and remain elevated for up to 1 yr after discontinuation of treatment, retesting of IgE levels during omalizumab treatment cannot be used as a guide for dose determination. Base dose determination after treatment interruptions lasting less than 1 yr on serum IgE levels obtained at the initial dose determination. If treatment is interrupted for 1 yr or more, IgE levels may be retested for dose determination. Adjust doses for significant changes in body weight.

Interactions
None well documented.

Lab Test Interferences
Elevated serum total IgE levels may persist for up to 1 yr after discontinuation of omalizumab; therefore, serum total IgE levels obtained during this time may not reflect steady state free IgE levels and should not be used to reassess the dosing regimen.

Adverse Reactions
CNS: Headache (15%); fatigue, dizziness (3%).
DERM: Pruritus, dermatitis (2%).
EENT: Sinusitis (16%); pharyngitis (11%); earache (2%).
RESP: Upper respiratory tract infections (20%).
OTHER: Injection site reactions (including bruising, redness, warmth, burning, stinging, itching, hive formation, pain, indurations, mass, inflammation [45%]); viral infections (23%); arthralgia (8%); pain (7%); leg pain (4%); fracture, arm pain (2%); malignancy (0.5%); hypersensitivity (including urticaria, dermatitis, pruritus, anaphylaxis).

Precautions
Pregnancy: Category B.
Lactation: Undetermined.
Children: Safety and efficacy not established in children under 12 yr.
Hypersensitivity: Anaphylaxis has occurred within 2 hr of the first or subsequent administration of omalizumab.

Asthma: Should not be used to treat acute bronchospasm or status asthmaticus.
Corticosteroid reduction: Do not abruptly discontinue corticosteroids upon initiation of omalizumab therapy.

PATIENT CARE CONSIDERATIONS
Administration/Storage
- For SC administration only. Not for intradermal, IM, or IV administration.
- Prescribed dose is usually administered q 2 or 4 wk.
- Follow manufacturer's instructions for reconstituting the lyophilized powder.
- Swirl vial during reconstitution. Do not shake. Reconstitution may take up to 40 min. Do not use if contents of vial do not dissolve completely by 40 min.
- Do not administer if particulate matter is noted.
- Reconstituted solution is slightly viscous and may take 5 to 10 sec to inject.
- Rotate injection sites (thigh, abdomen, upper arm). Give new injections at least 1 inch from old site and never into areas where the skin is tender, bruised, red, or hard.
- Discard any unused solution. Do not save unused solution for later administration.
- Store vials in refrigerator (36° to 46°F). After reconstitution the solution should be used within 8 hr if stored in refrigerator or within 4 hr if stored at room temperature. Protect reconstituted solution from direct sunlight.

Assessment/Interventions
- Obtain patient history, including drug history and any known allergies.
- Ensure that serum total IgE level and body weight are determined before initiating therapy and are used to calculate the appropriate dose and frequency of administration using the manufacturer's Dose Determination chart.
- Ensure that doses greater than 150 mg are divided among more than 1 injection site so that no more than 150 mg is administered into 1 site.
- Ensure that medication is not used to treat an acute exacerbation of asthma or status asthmaticus.

Malignancy: Malignant neoplasms were observed; variety of types with breast, non-melanoma skin, prostate, melanoma, and parotid.

- Ensure that patient is continued on maintenance controller and bronchodilator therapy during initiation of therapy.
- Monitor patient for signs and symptoms of anaphylactic or serious allergic reactions. Be prepared to treat appropriately.
- Monitor patient for CNS, musculoskeletal, and general body side effects, and injection site reactions. Report to health care provider if noted and significant.

Patient/Family Education
- Explain name, dose, action, and potential side effects of drug.
- Advise patient that medication will be prepared and administered by a health care provider in a medical setting.
- Instruct patient to continue taking other asthma medications as prescribed by health care provider and to not change the dose or stop taking unless advised by health care provider.
- Advise patient that therapy will not immediately improve asthma symptoms but that improvement should be noted as therapy is continued.
- Advise patient that injection site reactions are common but that these should become less of a problem as therapy continues.
- Advise patient to report any of the following to health care provider: intolerable injection site reactions or any unexplained symptoms.
- Advise women to notify health care provider if pregnant, planning to become pregnant, or breastfeeding.
- Instruct patient not to take any prescription or OTC medications or dietary supplements unless advised by health care provider.
- Remind patient that office visits will be required to monitor therapy and to keep appointments.

Omeprazole

(oh-MEH-pray-ZAHL)

Class GI

How Supplied
Prilosec Capsules, delayed-release 10 mg, Capsules, delayed-release 20 mg, Capsules, delayed-release 40 mg
✤ *Losec*

Action
PHARMACOLOGY: Suppresses gastric acid secretion by blocking "acid (proton) pump" within gastric parietal cell.

PHARMACOKINETICS/DYNAMICS:
Absorption: Absorption is rapid. T_{max} is 0.5 to 3.5 hr. Bioavailability is 30% to 40% and increases upon repeat administration.

Distribution: 95% is protein bound.

Metabolism: Extensive in the liver.

Excretion: Little is unchanged in the urine. Approximately 77% is eliminated as 6 metabolites; the remainder is eliminated in the feces. The $t_{1/2}$ is 0.5 to 1 hr. Total body clearance is 500 to 600 mL/min.

Duration: 72 hours or more.

Special Populations:
Elderly – The elimination rate is decreased. Bioavailibility is increased. No dosage adjustment is necessary
Race – The increase in AUC is approximately 4-fold in Asians. Consider dose adjustment.
Chronic hepatic insufficiency – Bioavailability is increased. Plasma half-life is increased to 3 hr. Plasma clearance is decreased. However, no dosage adjustment is necessary.
Chronic renal insufficiency – There is slight increase in bioavailability. No dose adjustment necessary.

Indications
Short-term treatment of active duodenal ulcer, gastroesophageal reflux disease (GERD), including erosive esophagitis and symptomatic GERD; long-term treatment of pathologic hypersecretory conditions (eg, Zollinger-Ellison syndrome, multiple endocrine adenomas, systemic mastocytosis); to maintain healing of erosive esophagitis; in combination with clarithromycin to eradicate *H. pylori*, use clarithromycin and amoxicillin in combination with omeprazole in patients with a 1-yr history of duodenal ulcers or active duodenal ulcers to eradicate *H. pylori*; short-term treatment of active benign gastric ulcer. **Unlabeled use(s):** Posterior laryngitis; enhanced efficacy of pancreatin for treatment of steatorrhea in cystic fibrosis.

Contraindications
Standard considerations.

Route/Dosage
Active Duodenal Ulcer
ADULTS: **PO** 20 mg/day for 4 to 8 wk.

Erosive Esophagitis
ADULTS: **PO** 20 mg/day for 4 to 8 wk. For maintenance treatment, give 20 mg/day.

Pathologic Hypersecretory Conditions
ADULTS: **PO** For initial dose, give 60 mg/day. Doses up to 120 mg tid have been given. Divide daily doses more then 80 mg.

H. pylori
ADULTS (TRIPLE THERAPY): **PO** 20 mg omeprazole plus clarithromycin 500 mg plus amoxicillin 1000 mg each given bid for 10 days; continue omeprazole 20 mg/day for an additional 18 days if an ulcer is present at start of therapy.

ADULTS (DUAL THERAPY): **PO** 40 mg omeprazole once daily plus clarithromycin 500 mg tid for 14 days; continue omeprazole 20 mg/day for an additional 14 days if an ulcer is present at start of therapy.

Gastric ulcer
ADULTS: **PO** 40 mg once daily for 4 to 8 wk.

GERD
ADULTS (WITHOUT ESOPHAGEAL LESIONS): **PO** 20 mg/day for 4 wk.
ADULTS (WITH EROSIVE ESOPHAGITIS): **PO** 20 mg/day for 4 to 8 wk.

Interactions
Benzodiazepines: Clearance of benzodiazepines may be decreased.
Cilostazol: Plasma levels may be increased by omeprazole, increasing the therapeutic and adverse effects.
Clarithromycin: Serum concentrations of clarithromycin and omeprazole may be increased.
Drugs depending on gastric pH for bioavailability (eg, ketoconazole, iron salts, ampicillin): Absorption of these drugs may be affected.
Phenytoin: Decreased plasma clearance and increased phenytoin half-life.
Warfarin: Prolonged warfarin elimination.

Lab Test Interferences
None well documented.

Adverse Reactions
CV: Angina; tachycardia; bradycardia; palpitation.
CNS: Headache; dizziness.
DERM: Rash.
GI: Diarrhea; abdominal pain; acid regurgitation; nausea; vomiting; constipation; flatulence.
RESP: Cough; upper respiratory tract infection.
OTHER: Asthenia; back pain.

Precautions
Pregnancy: Category C.
Lactation: Undetermined.
Children: Safety and efficacy in children not established.

PATIENT CARE CONSIDERATIONS
Administration/Storage
- Do not open, chew, or crush capsule. Instruct patient to swallow capsule whole.
- Divide daily doses greater than 80 mg.
- Give before meals or as one-time daily dose. If medication is administered once daily, give before dinner.
- Store at room temperature in original container tightly closed and protected from light.

Assessment/Interventions
- Obtain patient history, including drug history and any known allergies.
- Review baseline CBC and LFT results, and monitor as indicated.
- Assess for coffee ground emesis, tarry stools, or constipation.
- Assess for any symptoms of hyperacidity (eg, dyspepsia, nausea, vomiting).

Overdosage: Signs and Symptoms
Confusion, drowsiness, blurred vision, tachycardia, nausea, diaphoresis, flushing, headache, dry mouth.

- Monitor elimination patterns and document any problems such as constipation.
- Assess skin for rashes or hives.
- Encourage adequate fluid intake and roughage in diet.

Patient/Family Education
- Advise patient not to chew or crush medication, and to swallow medication whole.
- Remind patient to take medication before meals.
- Inform patient that antacids may be taken concurrently with omeprazole.
- Advise patient to avoid tasks requiring alertness until response to medication is established.
- Caution patient to report the following symptoms to health care provider: cramping, diarrhea, rash, hives.

Ondansetron Hydrochloride
(ahn-DAN-SEH-trahn HIGH-droe-KLOR-ide)

Class Antiemetic/Antivertigo

How Supplied
Zofran Tablets 4 mg (as hydrochloride dihydrate), Tablets 8 mg (as hydrochloride dihydrate), Tablets 24 mg (as hydrochloride dihydrate), Solution, oral 4 mg/5 mL (5 mg as hydrochloride dihydrate), Injection 2 mg/mL (as hydrochloride dihydrate), Injection 32 mg/50 mL (as hydrochloride dihydrate) ♦ *Zofran ODT* Tablets, orally-disintegrating 4 mg (as base), Tablets, orally-disintegrating 8 mg (as base)

Action
PHARMACOLOGY: Selective serotonin (5-HT$_3$) receptor antagonist that inhibits serotonin receptors in GI tract or chemoreceptor trigger zone.

PHARMACOKINETICS/DYNAMICS:
Absorption: Passively and completely absorbed from GI tract. Bioavailability is 48% to 75% and is slightly enhanced with food.

C_{max} for males is 24.1 to 37 ng/mL (8 mg oral dose). C_{max} for females is 42.7 to 52.4 ng/mL (8 mg oral dose). C_{max} for injection is 102 to 170 ng/mL. T_{max} for males is 2 to 4.1 hr (8 mg dose). T_{max} for females is 1.7 to 4.9 hr (8 mg dose).

Distribution: Plasma protein binding is 70% to 76%.

Metabolism: Extensively metabolized in the liver by hydroxylation, followed by glucuronide or sulfate conjugation; CYP1A2, CYP2D6, CYP3A4 are the main hepatic enzymes.

Excretion: Approximately 5% is eliminated as parent compound in urine. The $t_{1/2}$ for males is 2.1 to 4.5 hr (8 mg oral dose). The $t_{1/2}$ for females is 1.9 to 6.2 hr (8 mg dose). The $t_{1/2}$ for injection is 3.5 to 5.5 hr. Plasma clearance is 0.262 to 0.381 L/hr/kg.

Special Populations:
Elderly – In elderly over 75 yr, there is a reduction in clearance and an increase in elimination half-life. No dosage adjustment is necessary.
Gender – The extent and rate of absorption is greater in women than in men. There is slower clearance, a smaller volume of distribution, and higher bioavailability in women.
Severe hepatic insufficiency – Clearance is reduced 2- to 3-fold. The volume of distribution is increased. The half-life is increased to 20 hr. Bioavailability approaches 100%. A total daily dose of 8 mg should not be exceeded.
Severe renal insufficiency – There is a reduction in clearance. Oral plasma clearance was reduced by 50%. No dosage adjustment is necessary.

Indications
Parenteral and oral: Prevention of nausea and vomiting with initial and repeat courses of emetogenic cancer chemotherapy, including high-dose cisplatin; prevention of postoperative nausea or vomiting.

Oral: Prevention of nausea and vomiting associated with radiotherapy in patients receiving either total body irradiation, single high-dose fraction to the abdomen, or daily fractions to the abdomen; prevention of nausea and vomiting associated with highly emetogenic cancer chemotherapy, including cisplatin 50 mg/m^2 or more. **Unlabeled use(s):** Treatment of nausea and vomiting associated with acetaminophen poisoning or prostacyclin therapy; treatment of acute levodopa-induced psychosis (visual hallucinations); reduction in bulimic episodes due to bulimia nervosa; treatment of spinal or epidural morphine-induced pruritus; management of social anxiety disorder.

Contraindications Standard considerations.

Route/Dosage

Prevention of Chemotherapy-Induced Nausea and Vomiting
ADULTS: **IV** 0.15 mg/kg infused over 15 min beginning 30 min before emetogenic chemotherapy with 2 additional 0.15 mg/kg doses 4 and 8 hr after the first dose. Alternatively, infuse 32 mg over 15 min, starting 30 min prior to emetogenic chemotherapy.

ADULTS AND CHILDREN 12 YR AND OLDER: **PO** (moderately emetogenic cancer chemotherapy) 8 mg bid, administering the first dose 30 min prior to starting emetogenic chemotherapy and the second dose 8 hr after the first dose; subsequent 8 mg doses may be given q 12 hr for 1 to 2 days after completion of chemotherapy.

CHILDREN 4 TO 11 YR: **PO** 4 mg tid, starting 30 min prior to chemotherapy, with subsequent doses 4 and 8 hr after the first dose; give 4 mg q 8 hr for 1 to 2 days after completion of chemotherapy.

Prevention of Radiotherapy-Induced Nausea and Vomiting
ADULTS: **PO** 8 mg tid.

Total Body Irradiation
ADULTS: **PO** 8 mg 1 to 2 hr prior to each fraction of radiotherapy administered each day.

Single High-Dose Fraction Radiotherapy to the Abdomen
ADULTS: **PO** 8 mg 1 to 2 hr prior to radiotherapy, with subsequent doses q 8 hr after the first dose for 1 to 2 days after completion of radiotherapy.

Daily Fractionated Radiotherapy to the Abdomen
ADULTS: **PO** 8 mg 1 to 2 hr prior to radiotherapy, with subsequent doses q 8 hr after the first dose for each day radiotherapy is given.

Prevention of Postoperative Nausea and Vomiting
ADULTS: **IV** 4 mg (undiluted) over 30 sec (preferably over 2 to 5 min) or **IM** 4 mg (undiluted) as a single injection. **PO** 16 mg as a single dose 1 hr prior to induction of anesthesia.
CHILDREN (2 TO 12 YR WEIGHING 40 KG OR LESS): **IV** 0.1 mg/kg
CHILDREN (MORE THAN 40 KG): **IV** 4 mg single dose. Administer over 30 sec or longer, preferably over 2 to 5 min.

Prevention of Nausea and Vomiting due to Highly Emetogenic Cancer Chemotherapy
ADULTS: **PO** 24 mg given 30 min prior to start of single-day highly emetogenic chemotherapy, including 50 mg/m^2 or more cisplatin.

Interactions
Rifamycins (eg, rifampin): Plasma levels of ondansetron may be reduced, decreasing the antiemetic effect.
INCOMPATIBILITIES: Alkaline solutions.

Lab Test Interferences None well documented.

Adverse Reactions
CV: Chest pain; tachycardia.
CNS: Headache; seizures.
DERM: Rash.
GI: Dry mouth; constipation; abdominal pain.
METAB: Hypokalemia.
RESP: Bronchospasm.
OTHER: Fever; anaphylaxis; weakness.

Precautions
Pregnancy: Category B.
Lactation: Undetermined.
Children: Dosing in children younger than 4 yr is not well defined.
Hepatic function impairment: In patients with severe hepatic impairment, do not exceed 8 mg/day oral dose. For IV use, give single 8 mg/day dose over 15 min beginning 30 min before chemotherapy.
Peristalsis: Ondansetron does not stimulate gastric or intestinal peristalsis; may mask progressive ileus or gastric distention.

Overdosage: Signs and Symptoms
Hypotension, constipation.

PATIENT CARE CONSIDERATIONS
Administration/Storage
- Dilute solution in 50 mL of 5% Dextrose in Water or 0.9% Sodium Chloride for Injection.
- Do not mix with solutions for which compatibility has not been established.
- Preparation is stable for 48 hr at room temperature following dilution.
- Rectal suppositories and oral solutions may be extemporaneously compounded.

Assessment/Interventions
- Obtain patient history, including drug history and any known allergies. Note hepatic impairment.
- Ensure that baseline hepatic studies have been performed before beginning therapy.
- Assess patient for nausea, vomiting, and bowel sounds.
- Monitor I&O carefully.
- Be prepared to give additional IV fluids to patient who is vomiting, but do not overhydrate.
- Discontinue IV infusion if signs of hypersensitivity develop.

Patient/Family Education
- Advise patient that headache is a common side effect.
- Advise patient that medication will greatly reduce likelihood of nausea and vomiting, but that these are still possible.

Oprelvekin

(oh-PRELL-veh-kin)

Class Thrombopoietic factor

How Supplied
Neumega Powder for injection 5 mg

Action
PHARMACOLOGY: Interleukin 11 (IL-11) is a thrombopoietic growth factor that directly stimulates the proliferation of hematopoietic stem cells and megakaryocyte progenitor cells and induces megakaryocyte maturation, resulting in increased platelet production.

PHARMACOKINETICS/DYNAMICS:
Absorption: C_{max} is 17.4 ng/mL. T_{max} is 3.2 hr.
Distribution: The bioavailability is more than 80%.
Excretion: Renal. The $t_{1/2}$ (terminal) is 6.9 hrs.
Special Populations:
Renal Function Impairment – C_{max} was 2.2-fold higher. AUC was 2.6-fold higher. Clearance was approximately 40% of the value seen in normal renal patients.
Elderly – Clearance decreases with age.
Children – Clearance increases approximately 1.2- to 1.6-fold in infants and children.

Indications
Prevent severe thrombocytopenia and reduce the need for platelet transfusions following myelosuppressive chemotherapy in patients with nonmyeloid malignancies.

Contraindications
Standard considerations.

Route/Dosage
Prevent Severe Thrombocytopenia and Reduce the Need for Platelet Transfusions Following Myelosuppressive Chemotherapy in Patients with Nonmyeloid Malignancies
ADULTS: SC 50 mcg/kg once daily, starting 6 to 24 hr after completing chemotherapy. Continue therapy until the postnadir platelet count is at least 50,000/mm³ or for a maximum of 21 days. Discontinue oprelvekin at least 2 days before starting the next chemotherapy cycle.

Interactions
None well documented.

Lab Test Interferences
None well documented.

Adverse Reactions
CV: Plasma volume expansion; symptomatic atrial arrhythmias, syncope, tachycardia, peripheral edema.
CNS: Headache, fatigue, dizziness.
DERM: Transient rash at injection site.
EENT: Transient visual blurring, papilledema.
GI: Nausea; vomiting; mucositis; diarrhea; oral moniliasis.
HEMA: Dilutional anemia.
METAB: Weight gain.
RESP: Dyspnea, rhinitis; increased cough; pharyngitis; pleural effusion.
OTHER: Edema; neutropenic fever; fever.

Precautions
Pregnancy: Category C.
Lactation: Undetermined.
Children: Safety and efficacy not established.
Fluid retention: Oprelvekin is known to cause fluid retention; use with caution in patients with clinically evident CHF, patients who may be susceptible to developing CHF, and patients with a history of heart failure. Patients have commonly experienced mild to moderate fluid retention as indicated by peripheral edema or dyspnea on exertion. Monitor preexisting fluid collections, including pericardial effusions or ascites. Sudden deaths have occurred in oprelvekin-treated patients receiving chronic diuretic therapy and ifosfamide who developed severe hypokalemia.
Cardiovascular events: Use with caution in patients with a history of atrial arrhythmia. Transient atrial arrhythmias (atrial fibrillation or flutter) have occurred in approximately 10% of patients following treatment with oprelvekin.
Ophthalmologic events: Transient, mild visual blurring has occasionally been reported.
Antibody formation/allergic reactions: A small proportion (1%) of patients developed antibodies to oprelvekin and transient rashes were occasionally observed at the injection site.

Chronic administration: Oprelvekin has been administered safely using the recommended dosing schedule for no more than 6 cycles following chemotherapy. Continuous dosing (2 to 13 wk) in primates produced joint capsule, tendon fibrosis, and periosteal hyperostosis.

Chemotherapy: The safety and efficacy of administering oprelvekin before or concurrently with chemotherapy has not been evaluated.

Overdosage: Signs and Symptoms
Doses of oprelvekin more than 50 mcg/kg may be associated with an increased incidence of cardiovascular events in adult patients.

PATIENT CARE CONSIDERATIONS

Administration/Storage
- Refrigerate sterile powder; do not freeze. Unreconstituted vials are stable at room temperature for no more than 3 days.
- Reconstitute vial with 1 mL of sterile water for injection, for a final concentration of 5 mg/mL. Direct sterile water at side of vial and swirl contents gently. Do not shake vial or excessive foaming will occur.
- The diluent vial supplied contains 1 mL of sterile water for injection. Use only 1 mL of sterile water to reconstitute oprelvekin powder.
- After reconstitution, oprelvekin is stable for no more than 3 hr refrigerated or at room temperature.
- Administer by SC injection.

Assessment/Interventions
- During dosing with oprelvekin, monitor fluid balance. If a diuretic is used, carefully monitor fluid and electrolyte balance.
- Obtain a complete blood count prior to chemotherapy and at regular intervals during oprelvekin therapy. Monitor platelet counts during the time of the expected nadir and until adequate recovery has occurred (postnadir counts at least 50,000).
- Begin dosing with oprelvekin 6 to 24 hr following the completion of chemotherapy dosing.

- Oprelvekin has not been evaluated in patients receiving chemotherapy regimens of more than 5 days duration or regimens associated with delayed myelosuppression (eg, nitrosoureas, mitomycin-C).

Patient/Family Education
- Instruct people who will be administering oprelvekin as to the proper dose and the method for reconstituting and administering oprelvekin. Instruct patients in the importance of proper disposal and caution against the reuse of needles, syringes, drug product, and diluent.
- Inform patients of the most common adverse reactions associated with oprelvekin administration, including those symptoms related to fluid retention. Mild to moderate peripheral edema and shortness of breath on exertion can occur within the first week of treatment and may continue for the duration of administration. Advise patients who have preexisting pleural or other effusions or a history of CHF to contact their health care provider if dyspnea worsens.
- Most patients who receive oprelvekin develop some anemia.
- Contact health care provider if symptoms attributable to atrial arrhythmia develop and are not transient.
- Advise women of childbearing potential of the possible risks of oprelvekin to the fetus.

Orlistat
(ORE-lih-stat)

Class Gastrointestinal Lipase Inhibitor

How Supplied
Xenical Capsules 120 mg

Action
PHARMACOLOGY: Reversible lipase inhibitor for obesity management that acts by inhibiting absorption of dietary fats.

PHARMACOKINETICS/DYNAMICS:
Absorption: Systemic absorption is minimal. T_{max} is approximately 8 hr.
Distribution: More than 99% is protein bound to plasma, mainly albumin and lipoprotein.

Metabolism: Occurs mainly in the GI wall. Two metabolites are M1 (4-member lactone ring hydrolyzed) and M3 (M1 with N-formyl leucine moiety cleaved); considered pharmacologically inconsequential.

Excretion: Eliminated by fecal excretion (major route); biliary excretion for metabolites. 97% eliminated through feces, 83% as unchanged drug, and less than 2% through urine.

The $t_{1/2}$ for M1 metabolite is approximately 3 hr. The $t_{1/2}$ for M3 metabolite is approximately 13.5 hr. The $t_{1/2}$ is 1 to 2 hr.

Indications
Obesity management including weight loss and weight maintenance when used in combination with a reduced-calorie diet; reduce the risk for weight regain after prior weight loss.

Contraindications Chronic malabsorption syndrome or cholestasis, and standard considerations.

Route/Dosage
PO 1 capsule tid with each main meal containing fat (during or up to 1 hr after the meal).

Interactions
Cyclosporine: Because changes in cyclosporine absorption have been reported with variations in dietary intake, use caution with orlistat plus diet in patients receiving orlistat.
Fat-soluble vitamins: Thirty percent reduction in beta-carotene supplement absorption was shown when administered with orlistat. Orlistat inhibited absorption of a vitamin E acetate supplement approximately 60%. The effect on the absorption of supplemental vitamin D, vitamin A, and nutritionally derived vitamin K is unknown.
Pravastatin: In 24 healthy-weight, mildly hypercholesterolemic subjects receiving orlistat 120 mg 3 times a day for 10 days, the effect was additive to the lipid-lowering effect of pravastatin. Modest increases (approximately 30%) in pravastatin plasma concentrations were observed during coadministration with orlistat.
Warfarin: Vitamin K levels tended to decline in subjects taking orlistat. Therefore, as vitamin K absorption may be decreased with orlistat, monitor patients on chronic stable doses of warfarin who are prescribed orlistat closely for changes in coagulation parameters.

Lab Test Interferences None well documented.

PATIENT CARE CONSIDERATIONS
Administration/Storage
- Administer each dose during or up to 1 hr after each main meal containing fat.
- Store at controlled room temperature. Keep bottle tightly closed.

Assessment/Interventions
- Obtain patient history, including drug history and any known allergies. Note history of chronic malabsorption, cholestasis, anorexia nervosa, bulimia, hyperoxaluria, or calcium oxalate nephrolithiasis.
- Ensure that patient is on a nutritionally balance, reduced-calorie diet containing no more than 30% of calories from fat.
- Ensure that patient is taking a multivitamin containing fat-soluble vitamins qd.
- Monitor patient for GI and general body side effects. Report to health care provider if noted and significant.

Adverse Reactions
CNS: Anxiety; depression; dizziness; headache
DERM: Dry skin; rash
GI: Abdominal pain/discomfort; oily spotting; flatus with discharge; fecal urgency; fatty/oily stool; oily evacuation; increased defecation; fecal incontinence; infectious diarrhea; nausea; rectal pain/discomfort; vomiting.
GU: Menstrual irregularity; vaginitis.
MUSC: Arthritis; back pain; joint disorder; myalgia; lower extremity pain; tendonitis.
RESP: Ear, nose, and throat symptoms; influenza; lower respiratory tract infections; upper respiratory tract infections.
OTHER: Fatigue; pedal edema; sleep disorder; urinary tract infection.

Precautions
Pregnancy: Category B.
Lactation: Not known if orlistat excreted in human milk.
Children: Safety and efficacy data in children not established.
Special risk patients: Patients with anorexia nervosa or bulimia should not take orlistat because of the potential for misuse. Exercise caution when prescribing orlistat to patients with a history of hyperoxaluria or calcium oxalate nephrolithiasis because of the risk of development of increased levels of urinary oxalate following treatment with orlistat.
Diabetic patients – Weight-loss induction by orlistat may be accompanied by improved metabolic control in diabetic patients, which might require a reduction in dose of oral hypoglycemic medication or insulin.

Patient/Family Education
- Explain name, dose, action, and potential side effects of drug.
- Remind patient to read the Patient Information sheet before starting treatment and with each refill.
- Advise patient to take prescribed dose tid with each main meal containing fat.
- Dose should be taken during or up to 1 hr after the meal.
- Advise patient that drug may be omitted if a meal is missed or the meal contains no fat.
- Warn patient that drug must be used in conjunction with a nutritionally balanced, reduced-calorie diet.
- Advise patient that taking more drug than prescribed does not increase weight loss.
- Instruct patient to take a multivitamin supplement containing fat-soluble vitamins qd

at least 2 hr before or after taking drug, such as at bedtime.
- Warn patient that daily intake of fat must be less than 30% and that ingesting larger quantities of fat in the diet will result in GI side effects.
- Advise female patient to inform health care provider if pregnant, planning on becoming pregnant, or breastfeeding.
- Advise patient to report bothersome side effects to health care provider.

Orphenadrine Citrate

(ore-FEN-uh-dreen SIH-trate)
Class Skeletal muscle relaxant/Centrally acting

How Supplied
Banflex Injection 30 mg/mL • *Flexoject* Injection 30 mg/mL • *Flexon* Injection 30 mg/mL • *Norflex* Tablets, sustained-release 100 mg, Injection 30 mg/mL
❦ *Orfenace* • *Rhoxal-orphenadrine*

Action
PHARMACOLOGY: Unknown; may be related to analgesic properties since drug acts on brain stem and does not act directly on muscles; possesses anticholinergic actions.

PHARMACOKINETICS/DYNAMICS:
Absorption: Readily absorbed from the GI tract. T_{max} is 2 hr.
Distribution: Not fully characterized.
Metabolism: Degraded to 8 known metabolites.
Excretion: Eliminated through urine (as metabolites, small amount as unchanged) and feces. The $t_{1/2}$ is approximately 14 hr (parent drug). The $t_{1/2}$ is 2 to 25 hr (metabolites).
Duration: 4 to 6 hr.

Indications Adjunctive treatment for acute, painful musculoskeletal conditions. **Unlabeled use(s):** Treatment of quinine-resistant leg cramps.

Contraindications Glaucoma; pyloric or duodenal obstruction; stenosing peptic ulcers; prostatic hypertrophy; obstruction of bladder neck; esophageal achalasia; myasthenia gravis.

Route/Dosage
ADULTS: **IV/IM** 60 mg q 12 hr prn.
ADULTS: **PO** 100 mg bid.

Interactions
Alcohol, other CNS depressants: Increased CNS depression.

Haloperidol: Worsening schizophrenic symptoms, decreased haloperidol levels, tardive dyskinesia.
Phenothiazines: Decreased effects of phenothiazines.

Lab Test Interferences None well documented.

Adverse Reactions
CV: Tachycardia; palpitations; transient syncope.
CNS: Weakness; headache; dizziness; lightheadedness; confusion (especially in elderly); hallucinations; agitation; tremor; drowsiness.
DERM: Hypersensitivity reactions (eg, rashes).
EENT: Blurred vision; pupil dilation; increased ocular tension.
GI: Dry mouth; vomiting; nausea; constipation; gastric irritation.
GU: Urinary hesitancy and retention.

Precautions
Pregnancy: Category C.
Lactation: Undetermined.
Children: Safety and efficacy not established.
Elderly: May be more sensitive to anticholinergic effects.
Hypersensitivity: May occur.
Sulfite sensitivity: Some products contain bisulfites, which may cause allergic-type reactions in certain persons.
Cardiac disease: Use drug with caution in patients with cardiac decompensation, coronary insufficiency, cardiac arrhythmias or tachycardia.
Heat prostration: Can occur in presence of high environmental temperature.

Overdosage: Signs and Symptoms
Cardiac arrhythmias, seizures, coma, shock.

PATIENT CARE CONSIDERATIONS

Administration/Storage
- Do not crush or have patient chew sustained-release preparations.
- Give IV solution over 5 min with patient in supine position. Administer carefully; intoxication is very rapid and can be lethal.
- Store at room temperature.

Assessment/Interventions
- Obtain patient history, including drug history and any known allergies.
- Monitor patient's vital signs.
- Monitor blood, urine, and liver function values during long-term therapy.
- Assess degree of pain relief obtained.

- Implement safety precautions if patient becomes drowsy or dizzy.
- Notify health care provider if rapid heart rate, palpitations, or mental confusion occurs.
- Carefully document voiding.

Patient/Family Education
- Tell patient not to increase dosage of medication. Even slight overdose may be highly toxic.
- Instruct patient to take sips of water frequently, suck on ice chips or sugarless hard candy, or chew sugarless gum if dry mouth occurs.
- Advise patient that drug may cause drowsiness or dizziness, and to use caution while driving or performing other tasks requiring mental alertness.
- Instruct patient to report the following symptoms to health care provider: urinary retention, constipation, palpitations, or tremors.
- Instruct patient to avoid alcohol or other CNS depressants.

Orphenadrine Citrate/Aspirin/Caffeine

(Ore-FEN-uh-dreen SIH-trate/ASS-pihr-in/kaff-EEN)

Class Skeletal muscle relaxant/Analgesic

How Supplied
Norgesic Tablets 25 mg orphenadrine citrate/385 mg aspirin/30 mg caffeine ♦ *Norgesic Forte* Tablets 50 mg orphenadrine citrate/770 mg aspirin/60 mg caffeine

Action

PHARMACOLOGY:

Orphenadrine: May be related to analgesic properties.

Aspirin: Inhibits prostaglandin synthesis, resulting in analgesia, anti-inflammatory activity, and inhibition of platelet aggregation.

Caffeine: Is thought to produce constriction of cerebral blood vessels.

Indications Symptomatic relief of mild to moderate pain of acute musculoskeletal disorders; adjunct to rest, physical therapy, and other measures for the relief of discomfort with acute painful musculoskeletal conditions.

Contraindications Patients with glaucoma, pyloric or duodenal obstruction, achalasia (eg, failure of visceral openings or sphincter muscle to relax), prostatic hypertrophy or obstructions at the bladder neck, myasthenia gravis; hypersensitivity to any component of the product.

Route/Dosage
ADULTS: **PO** *Norgesic* 1 to 2 tablets tid to qid; *Norgesic Forte* ½ to 1 tablet tid to qid.

Interactions
Anticoagulants (eg, warfarin): Effects of anticoagulants may be enhanced by aspirin, increasing the risk of bleeding.
Uricosuric agents (probenecid): Effects may be inhibited by aspirin.

Adverse Reactions
CV: Tachycardia; palpitation.
CNS: Weakness; confusion; excitation; hallucinations; headache; lightheadedness; dizziness; syncope.
DERM: Urticaria and other dermatoses.
EENT: Blurred vision; dilation of the pupil; increased intraocular tension; drowsiness.
GI: Dry mouth; nausea; vomiting; hemorrhage.
GU: Urinary hesitancy or retention; constipation.

Precautions
Pregnancy: Safety and efficacy not established.
Lactation: Undetermined.
Children: Safety and efficacy not established.
Reye syndrome – Has been associated with aspirin administration to children (including teenagers) with acute febrile illness.
Peptic ulcers: Use with extreme caution.

PATIENT CARE CONSIDERATIONS

Administration/Storage
- Administer prescribed dose tid to qid if needed.
- Administer without regard to meals but administer with food if GI upset occurs.
- Store below 86°F. Protect from moisture.

Assessment/Interventions
- Obtain patient history, including drug history and any known allergies. Note history of hemorrhagic diathesis or coagulation disorders, severe hepatic or renal impairment, peptic ulcer or other serious GI lesions, glaucoma, pyloric or duodenal obstruction, achalasia, prostatic hypertrophy, bladder neck obstruction, myasthenia gravis, the syndrome of nasal polyps, angioedema, and bronchospastic reactivity to aspirin or other NSAIDs.
- Assess musculoskeletal symptoms before starting therapy and periodically during treatment.
- Monitor patient for CNS, GI, and general body side effects. Report to health care provider if noted and significant.

- Discontinue therapy and notify health care provider immediately if any of the following occur: allergic reaction, unusual bleeding or bruising, shortness of breath, black or tarry stools, vomiting of blood or coffee ground-like material.

Patient/Family Education
- Explain name, dose, action, and potential side effects of drug.
- Advise patient to take prescribed dose tid to qid if needed for muscle pain, muscle spasm, or limited mobility.
- Advise patient to take without regard to meals but to take with food if GI upset occurs.
- Instruct patient to avoid alcoholic beverages and other depressants while taking this medication.
- Advise patient that drug may cause drowsiness, dizziness, or blurred vision and to use caution while driving or performing other tasks requiring mental alertness until tolerance is determined.
- Advise patient to stop taking the drug and notify health care provider if any of the following occur: allergic reaction, unusual bleeding or bruising, shortness of breath, black or tarry stools, vomiting of blood or coffee ground-like material.
- Advise women to notify health care provider if pregnant, planning to become pregnant, or breastfeeding.
- Warn patient not to take any prescription or OTC drugs or dietary supplements without consulting health care provider.
- Advise patient that follow-up visits may be necessary to monitor therapy and to keep appointments.

Oseltamivir Phosphate

(oh-sell-TAM-ih-veer FOSS-fate)

Class Anti-infective/Antiviral

How Supplied
Tamiflu Capsules 75 mg, Powder for oral suspension 12 mg/mL

Action
PHARMACOLOGY: Inhibition of influenza virus neuraminidase with possible alteration of virus particle aggregation and release.

PHARMACOKINETICS/DYNAMICS:
Absorption: Readily absorbed from GI tract. C_{max} for oseltamivir is 65.2 ng/mL. C_{max} for metabolite is 348 ng/mL. AUC $_{(0-12\ hr)}$ for oseltamivir is 112 ng•hr/mL. AUC $_{(0-12\ hr)}$ for metabolite is 2719 ng•hr/mL.

Distribution: At least 75% of the dose reaches systemic circulation as oseltamivir carboxylate (bioavailability). The Vd is 23 to 26 L (metabolite). 3% is protein bound (metabolite); 42% is protein bound (parent drug).

Metabolism: Converted to active oseltamivir carboxylate by esterases located predominantly in the liver.

Excretion: The t½ is 6 to 10 hr for the metabolite. The t½ for the parent drug is 1 to 3 hr. More than 90% of oseltamivir is metabolized to oseltamivir carboxylate, which is entirely (more than 99%) eliminated by renal excretion. Less than 20% of the oral dose is eliminated through feces.

Special Populations:
Children – Children 12 yr and younger clear the prodrug and active metabolite faster, resulting in a lower exposure mg/kg/dose.

Indications Treatment of uncomplicated acute illness caused by influenza infection in patients older than 1 yr who have been symptomatic for 2 days or less; prophylaxis of influenza in patients 13 yr and older.

Contraindications Standard considerations.

Route/Dosage
Influenza Prophylaxis
ADULTS AND ADOLESCENTS 13 YR AND OLDER: PO 75 mg qd for 7 days or more, starting within 2 days of exposure.
RENAL IMPAIRMENT (CCR 10 TO 30 ML/MIN): PO 75 mg qod or 30 mg of oral suspension qd.

Treatment of Influenza
ADULTS AND ADOLESCENTS 13 YR AND OLDER: PO 75 mg bid for 5 days, starting within 2 days of onset of symptoms.
RENAL IMPAIRMENT (CCR 10 TO 30 ML/MIN): PO 75 mg qd for 5 days.
ADULTS AND CHILDREN 1 YR AND OLDER (WHO CANNOT SWALLOW CAPSULES): **Suspension PO** 15 kg or less (33 lbs or less) administer 30 mg (2.5 mL) bid; 16 to 23 kg (34 to 51 lbs) administer 45 mg (3.8 mL) bid; 24 to 40 kg (52 to 88 lbs) administer 60 mg (5 mL) bid; more than 40 kg (more than 88 lbs) administer 75 mg (6.2 mL) bid.

Interactions None well documented.

Lab Test Interferences None well documented.

Adverse Reactions
CNS: Insomnia, vertigo (1%); seizure, confusion (postmarketing).
DERM: Rash, swelling of face (postmarketing).
GI: Nausea (10%); vomiting (9%); swelling of tongue (postmarketing).

METAB: Aggravation of diabetes (postmarketing).
RESP: Bronchitis (2%).

Precautions
Pregnancy: Category C.
Lactation: Undetermined.
Children:
Influenza treatment – Safety and efficacy not established in children younger than 1 yr.
Influenza prophylaxis – Safety and efficacy not established in children younger than 13 yr.
Renal function impairment: Administer with caution.
Repeated courses: Safety and efficacy not established.

Overdosage: Signs and Symptoms
Nausea, vomiting.

PATIENT CARE CONSIDERATIONS

Administration/Storage
- Initiate therapy within 40 hr of onset of influenza symptoms or exposure to influenza-infected individual.
- Administer prescribed dose without regard to meals but administer with food if GI upset occurs.
- Shake suspension well before measuring dose. Measure and administer dose using supplied dosing dispenser.
- Store capsules and dry powder for suspension at controlled room temperature (59° to 86°F). Store reconstituted suspension in refrigerator (36° to 46°F) or at controlled room temperature. Do not freeze. Discard any unused suspension after 10 days.

Assessment/Interventions
- Obtain patient history, including drug history and any known allergies. Note renal or hepatic impairment, asthma, COPD, or cardiac disease.
- Ensure that reduced dose is administered to patient with renal impairment (Ccr less than 30 mL/min) following manufacturer's recommendations.
- Monitor patient's response to therapy. Inform health care provider if influenza symptoms are not improving, are getting worse, or if new symptoms develop during treatment.
- Monitor patient for signs of allergic reaction. Discontinue therapy and immediately notify health care provider if noted. Be prepared to treat appropriately.
- Monitor patient for GI, RESP, CNS, and general body side effects. Report to health care provider if noted and significant.

Patient/Family Education
- Explain name, dose, action, and potential side effects of drug.
- Advise patient to read patient information leaflet before starting therapy.
- Review dosing schedule and prescribed length of therapy with patient. Caution patient that medication must be started within 40 hr of onset of influenza symptoms or exposure to influenza-infected individual in order to be effective.
- Advise patient to take prescribed dose without regard to meals but administer with food if GI upset occurs.
- Advise patient or caregiver using suspension to shake well before measuring dose and to measure and administer dose using supplied dosing dispenser.
- Advise patient that if a dose is missed to take as soon as remembered. However, if it is within 2 hr of the time for the next dose, to skip the dose and take the next dose at the regularly scheduled time. Caution patient not to take 2 doses at the same time to catch up.
- Review other modalities for alleviating influenza symptoms (eg, rest, hydration, OTC antipyretics and analgesics).
- Remind patient to complete entire course of therapy, even if feeling better.
- Advise patient that oseltamivir is not a substitute for flu vaccination and to continue to obtain an annual flu vaccination.
- Advise patient to inform health care provider if flu symptoms do not appear to be improving, are getting worse, or if new symptoms develop during or after treatment.
- Instruct patient to discontinue therapy and contact health care provider immediately if experiencing signs or symptoms of an allergic reaction (eg, rash, hives, swelling of throat).
- Advise women to notify health care provider if pregnant, planning to become pregnant, or breastfeeding.
- Instruct patient not to take any prescription or OTC medications or dietary supplements unless advised by health care provider.
- Advise patient that follow-up examinations and lab tests may be required to monitor therapy and to keep appointments.

Oxacillin Sodium

(ox-uh-SILL-in SO-dee-uhm)

Class Antibiotic/Penicillin

How Supplied
Oxacillin Sodium Powder for oral solution 250 mg/5 mL, Powder for injection 500 mg, Powder for injection 1 g, Powder for injection 2 g, Powder for injection 10 g

Action
PHARMACOLOGY: Inhibits mucopeptide synthesis in bacterial cell wall.

PHARMACOKINETICS/DYNAMICS:
Absorption: 30% to 35% of the oral dose is absorbed from the GI tract. The T_{max} is 5 min (IV), 30 min (IM), and 30 min to 2 hr (oral). The C_{max} is 43 mcg/mL (IV), 2.6 to 3.9 mcg (oral), and 5.3 to 10.9 mcg/mL (IM). Food decreases the rate and extent of absorption.

Distribution: Varies. Concentrations are found in CSF and aqueous humor, pleural, bile, and amniotic fluids. Protein binding is approximately 94.2%, mainly albumin. Crosses the placenta and distributes into milk.

Metabolism: Metabolized to active and inactive metabolites.

Excretion: Rapidly excreted primarily as unchanged drug in urine. The $t_{1/2}$ for elimination is 30 min. The $t_{1/2}$ for serum is 20 to 30 min.

Indications
Treatment of infections caused by penicillinase-producing staphylococci; initial therapy of suspected staphylococcal infection.

Contraindications
Hypersensitivity to penicillins. Do not treat severe pneumonia, empyema, bacteremia, pericarditis, meningitis and purulent or septic arthritis with oral oxacillin during acute state.

Route/Dosage
ADULTS: **PO/IV/IM** 250 mg to 1 g q 4 to 6 hr.
CHILDREN (LESS THAN 40 KG): **PO/IV/IM** 50 to 100 mg/kg/day in divided doses q 4 to 6 hr.
PREMATURE/NEONATES: **IV/IM** 25 mg/kg/day.

Interactions
Contraceptives, oral: Reduced efficacy of oral contraceptives.
Probenecid: Increased oxacillin levels.
Tetracyclines: Impaired bactericidal effects of oxacillin.
INCOMPATIBILITIES: Aminoglycosides.

Lab Test Interferences
Antiglobulin (Coombs') test: Drug may cause false-positive results.
Urine and serum protein determinations: Drug may cause false-positive reactions with sulfosalicylic acid and boiling test, acetic acid test, biuret reaction, and nitric acid test but not with bromphenol blue test (*Multi-Stix*).
Urine glucose test: May cause false-positive urine glucose test result with *Benedict* solution, *Fehling* solution, or *Clinitest* tablets but not with enzyme-based tests (eg, *Clinistix*, *Tes-tape*).

Adverse Reactions
CNS: Neurotoxicity (eg, lethargy, neuromuscular irritability, hallucinations, convulsions and seizures); dizziness; fatigue; insomnia; reversible hyperactivity; prolonged muscle relaxation.
DERM: Ecchymosis.
EENT: Itchy eyes; abnormal taste perception.
GI: Glossitis; stomatitis; gastritis; sore mouth or tongue; dry mouth; furry tongue; black "hairy" tongue; nausea; anorexia; vomiting; abdominal pain or cramp; diarrhea or bloody diarrhea; rectal bleeding; flatulence; enterocolitis; pseudomembranous colitis; anorexia.
GU: Interstitial nephritis (eg, oliguria, proteinuria, hematuria, hyaline casts, pyuria); nephropathy; increased creatinine and BUN; vaginitis.
HEMA: Deep vein thrombosis; hematomas; phlebitis; anemias; thrombocytopenia; eosinophilia; leukopenia; granulocytopenia; neutropenia; bone marrow depression; agranulocytosis; reduced Hgb or Hct; prolongation of bleeding and prothrombin time.
HEPA: Transient hepatitis; cholestatic jaundice; increased LFT results.
METAB: Elevated serum alkaline phosphatase, AST, ALT, bilirubin, and LDH; hypernatremia; hypokalemia; reduced albumin, total proteins, and uric acid.
OTHER: Hypersensitivity reactions that may lead to death; hyperthermia; pain at site of injection; hyperthermia; sciatic neuritis.

Precautions
Pregnancy: Category B.
Lactation: Excreted in breast milk.
Hypersensitivity: Reactions range from mild to life-threatening. Administer cautiously to cephalosporin-sensitive or imipenem-sensitive patients because of possible crossreactivity.
Superinfection: May result in bacterial or fungal overgrowth of nonsusceptible organisms.
Pseudomembranous colitis: Consider pseudomembranous colitis in patients who develop diarrhea.
Sodium content: Contains 2.5 to 3.1 mEq sodium/g.

Overdosage: Signs and Symptoms
Neuromuscular hyperexcitability, stupor, agitation, confusion, asterixis, hallucinations, coma, multifocal myoclonus, seizures, encephalopathy.

PATIENT CARE CONSIDERATIONS

Administration/Storage
- Administer at regular intervals around the clock.
- Administer oral doses on empty stomach at least 1 hr before or 2 hr after meals.
- Reconstitute IM preparation to dilution of 250 mg/1.5 mL. Use deep, slow injection. Rotate sites to prevent tissue irritation.
- Reconstitute IV preparation with Sterile Water for Injection or Sodium Chloride for Injection. Administer slowly over approximately 10 min to prevent vein irritation.
- IM solution is stable for up to 3 days at room temperature or 7 days under refrigeration.
- IV solutions are stable for at least 6 hr at room temperature.
- Reconstituted oral solution is stable for 14 days if refrigerated.

Assessment/Interventions
- Obtain patient history, including drug history and any known allergies.
- Ensure that specimens for culture and sensitivity have been obtained before starting therapy.
- Assess for infection at beginning and throughout course of therapy (eg, fever, appearance of wound, increased WBC).
- Observe patient for signs and symptoms of anaphylaxis (eg, rash, pruritus, laryngeal edema, wheezing). Discontinue drug if these symptoms occur.
- Keep resuscitation equipment, adrenaline, and antihistamines available.
- Notify health care provider if unusual bleeding or bruising occurs.

Patient/Family Education
- Advise patient to complete full course of therapy, even if symptoms abate, to prevent reoccurrence of infection.
- Instruct patient to discard any liquid forms of medication after 7 days if stored at room temperature; after 14 days if refrigerated.
- Instruct patient to notify health care provider if symptoms of infection do not improve.
- Advise patient to report pruritus and rash immediately.
- Instruct patient to report the following signs of superinfection: black, "furry" tongue, loose or foul-smelling stools, vaginal itching, discharge.

Oxaprozin

(ox-uh-PRO-zin)

Class Analgesic/NSAID

How Supplied
Daypro Caplets 600 mg
✤ *Apo-Oxaprozin* ◆ *Rhoxal-oxaprozin*

Action
PHARMACOLOGY: Decreases inflammation, pain and fever, probably through inhibition of cyclooxygenase activity and prostaglandin synthesis.

PHARMACOKINETICS/DYNAMICS:
Absorption: Bioavailability is 95%. T_{max} is 3 to 5 hr.

Distribution: 99% is protein bound (plasma). Vd is 10 to 12.5 L.

Metabolism: Metabolized in the liver by microsomal oxidation (65%) and glucuronic acid conjugation (35%). 5% of active phenolic metabolites.

Excretion: 65% glucuronide metabolites are eliminated in the urine and 35% in the feces. The $t_{1/2}$ is 42 to 50 hr. Clearance is 0.25 to 0.34 L/hr.

Special Populations:
Renal Function Impairment – Alters binding and reduces unbound clearance and unbound volume of distribution. Dosage reduction is recommended.

Indications Relief of symptoms of rheumatoid arthritis and osteoarthritis.

Contraindications Hypersensitivity to aspirin, iodides, or any other NSAID.

Route/Dosage
ADULTS: PO 1200 mg once a day (max, 1800 mg/day or 26 mg/kg, whichever is lower).

Interactions
Beta-blockers: Antihypertensive effects may be decreased.
Lithium: May increase lithium levels.
Loop diuretics: Diuretic effects may be decreased.
Methotrexate: May increase methotrexate levels.
Warfarin: May increase risk of gastric erosion and bleeding.

Lab Test Interferences False-positive urine immunoassay screening tests for benzodiazepines have been reported in patients taking oxaprozin.

Adverse Reactions
CV: Edema; blood pressure changes; worsening or precipitation of CHF.
CNS: Depression; sedation; somnolence; confusion; disturbed sleep.
DERM: Rash; pruritus; erythema; photosensitivity; ecchymosis.

EENT: Visual disturbances; tinnitus.
GI: Gastric distress; peptic ulcers; occult blood loss; diarrhea; constipation; vomiting; nausea; dyspepsia; flatulence; anorexia; abdominal distress/cramps/pain; stomatitis.
GU: Difficult or painful urination; urinary frequency; decreased menstrual flow.
HEMA: Anemia; neutropenia; thrombocytopenia; leukopenia.
HEPA: Hepatitis.

Precautions
Pregnancy: Category C.
Lactation: Undetermined.
Children: Safety and efficacy not established.
Elderly: Increased risk of adverse reactions.

PATIENT CARE CONSIDERATIONS
Administration/Storage
- Food may reduce the rate of absorption but not the extent. Antacids have no effect on rate or extent of absorption.
- Not recommended for patients with renal or hepatic disease, low body weight, advanced age, a known ulcer susceptibility or known sensitivity to other NSAIDs.
- Store less than 86°F in a tight, light-resistant container.

Assessment/Interventions
- Obtain patient history.
- Closely monitor patients at risk for peptic ulcer disease such as those with a history of serious GI problems, alcoholism, smoking or other ulcer-associated factors.
- Determine if patient is taking aspirin, oral anticoagulants, H_2-receptor antagonists, beta-blockers, iodides, or other NSAIDs as drug interactions can occur and discontinuation or adjustment in therapy would be indicated.
- Assess for adverse reactions. Notify health care provider if the following adverse reactions occur: abdominal pain, anorexia, dyspepsia, flatulence, nausea, vomiting, depression, sedation, somnolence, confusion, sleep disturbances, rash, tinnitus and dysuria, frequency of urination.
- Ensure dosage is individualized to the lowest effective dose to minimize adverse effects.
- Anticipate a greater risk of reactions from patients on higher dosages or elderly patients.
- Monitor renal function tests (eg, creatinine, BUN).
- Monitor CBC, especially hemoglobin, hematocrit and platelets.
- If patient is taking beta-blockers, monitor blood pressure when starting therapy for increases in sitting and standing blood pressure.

Renal function impairment: May need to reduce dose.
Hepatic function impairment: Exercise caution when administering to patients with impaired hepatic function or history of liver disease.
GI effects: Serious GI toxicity (eg, bleeding, ulceration, perforation) can occur at any time, with or without warning symptoms.
Platelet aggregation: Can inhibit platelet aggregation; use with caution in patients with intrinsic coagulation defects or those on anticoagulant therapy.

Overdosage: Signs and Symptoms
Drowsiness, nausea, heartburn, vomiting, indigestion, seizures.

Patient/Family Education
- Instruct patient to take medication as prescribed and not to make up missed doses.
- Inform patient that analgesic effects are usually achieved after a single dose, but that it requires several days of dosing to reach the maximum effect.
- Inform patient concerning the expected therapeutic effects of the medication, which include analgesic, antipyretic and anti-inflammatory benefits.
- Instruct patient to inform the health care provider of symptom relief so that the dosage is individualized to the lowest effective dose to minimize adverse effects.
- Instruct patient to take the dose exactly as prescribed about the same time each day with a full glass of water.
- Caution patient to avoid taking other NSAIDs, aspirin, alcohol, or other *otc* medications unless advised to do so by the health care provider.
- Instruct patient concerning drug/drug interactions as applicable to their situation.
- Advise patient to discontinue drug and notify health care provider if any of the following occurs: persistent GI upset or headache, skin rash, itching, visual disturbances, black stools, weight gain or edema, changes in urine pattern, joint pain, fever, or blood in urine.
- Caution patient regarding the serious GI, renal, hepatic, hematologic and dermatologic adverse effects that can occur at any time, with or without warning symptoms.
- Advise patient on long-term therapy that lab tests may be required and to keep appointments.
- Caution patient to inform dentist or surgeon oxaprozin use prior to any procedure.

- Advise elderly or debilitated patients regarding their increased risk of adverse reactions.
- Caution patient regarding possibility of photosensitivity and to use protective measures until tolerance is determined.
- Advise patient that medication may cause drowsiness, and to use caution while driving or performing other tasks requiring mental alertness.

Oxazepam

(ox-AZE-uh-pam)
Class Antianxiety/Benzodiazepine

How Supplied
Serax Tablets 15 mg, Capsules 10 mg, Capsules 15 mg, Capsules 30 mg
✤ *Apo-Oxazepam*

Action
PHARMACOLOGY: Potentiates action of GABA, an inhibitory neurotransmitter, resulting in increased neuronal inhibition and CNS depression, especially in limbic system and reticular formation.

PHARMACOKINETICS/DYNAMICS:
Absorption: Readily absorbed orally. T_{max} is 2 to 4 hr; C_{max} is approximately 450 mg/mL.
Distribution: Protein bound approximately 87%.
Metabolism: In liver to inactive compounds (glucuronide conjugates).
Excretion: Excreted in the urine. The t½ is 8.2 hr.
Onset: Slow.

Indications
Control of anxiety, anxiety associated with depression; control of anxiety, tension, agitation, and irritability in elderly; treatment of alcoholic patients with acute tremulousness, inebriation, or anxiety associated with alcohol withdrawal.

Contraindications
Hypersensitivity to benzodiazepines; psychoses.

Route/Dosage
Mild to Moderate Anxiety with Associated Tension, Irritability, and Agitation
ADULTS: PO 10 to 15 mg tid to qid.

Severe Anxiety Syndromes, Agitation or Anxiety Associated with Depression, Alcoholics with Acute Inebriation and Tremulousness, or Anxiety on Withdrawal
ADULTS: PO 15 to 30 mg tid to qid.
ELDERLY: PO 10 mg tid; increase cautiously up to 15 tid to qid.

Interactions
Alcohol, CNS depressants: Additive CNS depressant effects.
Digoxin: Increased serum digoxin concentrations.
Theophyllines: May antagonize sedative effects of oxazepam.

Lab Test Interferences None well documented.

Adverse Reactions
CV: Changes in ECG pattern; hypotension; syncope.
CNS: Drowsiness; dizziness; lethargy; vertigo; tremor; fatigue; memory impairment; disorientation; anterograde amnesia; ataxia; hallucinations; restlessness; headache; slurred speech; stupor; euphoria; paradoxical reactions (eg, anger, hostility, mania, insomnia).
DERM: Rashes (morbilliform, urticaria, maculopapular).
EENT: Blurred vision; diplopia.
GI: Nausea.
HEMA: Blood dyscrasias including agranulocytosis; leukopenia.
HEPA: Hepatic dysfunction and jaundice.
OTHER: Dependence/withdrawal syndrome (eg, confusion, abnormal perception of movement, depersonalization, muscle twitching, psychosis, paranoid delusions, seizures); edema; altered libido; incontinence; fever; menstrual irregularities.

Precautions
Pregnancy: Category D.
Lactation: Undetermined.
Children: Dosage and efficacy not established in children under 6 yr; absolute dosage not established for patients 6 to 12 yr.
Elderly: For elderly and debilitated patients, initial dose should be small; increase gradually.
Dependence: Prolonged use may lead to dependence. Withdrawal syndrome has occurred within 4 to 6 wk of treatment with therapeutic doses, especially if abruptly discontinued. Use caution and taper dosage.
Long-term use (more than 4 mo): Effectiveness has not been assessed.
Psychiatric disorders: Not intended for use in patients with primary depressive disorder, psychoses, or disorders in which anxiety is not prominent.
Suicide: Use drug with caution in patients with suicidal tendencies; do not allow access to large quantities of drug.

Overdosage: Signs and Symptoms
Drowsiness, mental confusion, lethargy, ataxia, hypotonia, hypotension, hypnotic state, coma, death.

PATIENT CARE CONSIDERATIONS
Administration/Storage
- Administer prescribed dose without regard to meals but administer with food if GI upset occurs.
- Store capsules at controlled room temperature (59° to 86°F).

Assessment/Interventions
- Obtain patient history, including drug history and any known allergies. Note hepatic or renal impairment, pulmonary disease, acute narrow-angle glaucoma, depression, suicidal tendency, seizure disorder, history of drug abuse, sensitivity to other benzodiazepines, or concurrent use of other psychotropic medications or CNS depressants.
- Ensure that reduced dose and slower dose escalation is used in elderly patient or patient with debilitating disease.
- Ensure that women of childbearing potential are not pregnant when therapy is initiated.
- Ensure that CBC with differential and liver enzymes are evaluated periodically in patient on prolonged therapy.
- Frequently assess patient for response to treatment. Notify health care provider if condition does not appear to be improving or is worsening.
- Ensure that therapy is periodically reviewed to determine if it needs to be continued without change or if a dose change (eg, increase, decrease, discontinuation) is indicated.
- If treatment is to be discontinued or the dose reduced, gradually taper the dose. Monitor patient for withdrawal symptoms (eg, increased anxiety, tremor, muscle or abdominal cramps, sweating). If significant withdrawal symptoms develop, reinstitute previous dosing schedule and attempt a less rapid tapering regimen after patient has stabilized.
- Monitor patient for CNS, GI, PSYCH, and general body side effects. Report to health care provider if noted and significant. Implement safety precautions if excessive drowsiness or dizziness occurs.

Patient/Family Education
- Explain name, dose, action, and potential side effects of drug.
- Advise patient or caregiver to read the *Patient Information* leaflet before starting therapy and with each refill.
- Advise patient that medication is usually started at a low dose and then gradually increased until max benefit is obtained.
- Caution patient that medication may be habit forming, to take as prescribed, and not to stop taking or change the dose unless advised by health care provider.
- Advise patient to take each dose without regard to meals but to take with food if stomach upset occurs.
- Advise patient that if a dose is missed to skip that dose and take the next dose at the regularly scheduled time. Caution patient to never take 2 doses at the same time.
- Advise patient that if medication needs to be discontinued it will be slowly withdrawn unless safety concerns (eg, rash) require a more rapid withdrawal.
- Instruct patient to avoid alcoholic beverages and other depressants while taking this medication.
- Advise patient with anxiety to take as needed and to seek alternative methods for controlling or preventing anxiety (eg, stress reduction, counseling).
- Instruct patient to contact health care provider if symptoms do not appear to be getting better, are getting worse, or if bothersome side effects (eg, drowsiness, memory impairment) occur.
- Advise patient that drug may cause drowsiness or impair judgment, thinking, or reflexes and to use caution while driving or performing other tasks requiring mental alertness until tolerance is determined.
- Advise women to notify health care provider if pregnant, planning to become pregnant, or breastfeeding.
- Warn patient not to take any prescription or OTC drugs or dietary supplements without consulting health care provider.
- Advise patient that follow-up visits may be necessary to monitor therapy and to keep appointments.

Oxcarbazepine
(ox-kar-BAZE-uh-peen)
Class Antiepileptic
How Supplied
Trileptal Tablets 150 mg, Tablets 300 mg, Tablets 600 mg, Suspension 300 mg/5 mL

Action
PHARMACOLOGY: The pharmacologic activity is primarily through the 10-monohydroxy metabolite (MHD) of oxcarbazepine, but the exact mechanism is unknown. It may block voltage-sensitive sodium channels resulting in stabilization of hyperexcited neural membranes,

inhibition of repetitive neuronal firing, and diminution of propagation of synaptic impulses.

PHARMACOKINETICS/DYNAMICS:
Absorption: Completely absorbed and extensively metabolized to active 10-monohydroxy metabolite (MHD). In the steady state, MHD is reached in 2 to 3 days. For tablet form, the T_{max} is 4.5 hr. For the oral suspension form, the T_{max} is 6 hr.

Distribution: The Vd for MHD is 49 L. 40% of serum is protein bound for the MHD; predominantly albumin.

Metabolism: Rapidly reduced by cytosolic enzymes in the liver to 10-MHD metabolite primarily responsible for pharmacologic effect. MHD metabolized further by conjugation with glucuronic acid. Four percent oxidized to inactive 10, 11-dihydroxy metabolite (DHD).

Excretion: Less than 1% eliminated unchanged through the kidneys. Eighty percent excreted as glucuronides of MHD (49%) or as unchanged MHD (27%). Inactive DHD accounts for 3%; conjugates of MHD and oxcarbazepine account for 13%. The t½ for the parent drug is approximately 2 hr. The t½ for MHD is approximately 9 hr.

Special Populations:
Renal Function Impairment – If less than 30 mL/min, elimination t½ of MHD is prolonged to 19 hr; 2-fold increase in AUC. Dose adjustment recommended.

Elderly – Max plasma concentration and AUC values of MHD were 30% and 60% higher.

Indications As monotherapy or adjunctive therapy in the treatment of partial seizures in patients with epilepsy.

Contraindications Standard considerations.

Route/Dosage
Adjunctive Therapy
ADULTS: **PO** Initial dose of 300 mg bid; may be increased by a max of 600 mg/day at weekly intervals; recommended daily dose is 1200 mg/day.

CHILDREN 4 TO 16 YR: **PO** Initial dose of 8 to 10 mg/kg generally not to exceed 600 mg/day, given bid; target maintenance dose should be achieved over 2 wk and is dependent upon patient's weight (900 mg/day for 20 to 29 kg; 1200 mg/day for 29.1 to 39 kg; 1800 mg/day for over 39 kg).

Conversion to Monotherapy
ADULTS: **PO** Initial dose of 300 mg bid while simultaneously initiating the reduction of the dose of the concomitant antiepileptic drugs (AEDs). These should be completely withdrawn over 3 to 6 wk while the max dose of the oxcarbazepine should be reached in 2 to 4 wk. Oxcarbazepine may be increased 600 mg/day at weekly intervals; recommended daily dose is 2400 mg/day.

CHILDREN 4 TO 16 YR: **PO** Initial dose of 8 to 10 mg/kg/day given in 2 divided doses while simultaneously reducing the dose of concomitant AEDs. The AEDs can be completely withdrawn over 3 to 6 wk while oxcarbazine may be increased by a max increment of 10 mg/kg/day at weekly intervals.

Initiation of Monotherapy
ADULTS: **PO** Initial dose of 300 mg bid; increase dose q 3 days by 300 mg/day to a dose of 1200 mg/day.

CHILDREN 4 TO 16 YR: **PO** Initial dose of 8 to 10 mg/kg/day given in 2 divided doses. The dose may be increased by 5 mg/kg/day q 3 days to the maintenance dose based on the following body weights.

- Weight 20 kg: daily dose 600 to 900 mg/day.
- Weight 25 to 30 kg: daily dose 900 to 1200 mg/day.
- Weight 35 to 40 kg: daily dose 900 to 1500 mg/day.
- Weight 45 kg: daily dose 1200 to 1500 mg/day.
- Weight 50 to 55 kg: daily dose 1200 to 1800 mg/day.
- Weight 60 to 65 kg: daily dose 1200 to 2100 mg/day.
- Weight 70 kg: daily dose 1500 to 2100 mg/day.

Renal function impairment – (Ccr less than 30 mL/min): Initiate therapy at 50% of the starting dose; titrate more slowly until the desired response is achieved.

Interactions May inhibit CYP2C19 and induce CYP3A4/5.
Carbamazepine: May decrease oxcarbazepine's active metabolite (MHD).
Contraceptives, oral: May decrease ethinyl estradiol and levonorgestrel AUC.
Felodipine: May decrease felodipine AUC.
Lamotrigine: Levels may be reduced by oxcarbazine.
Phenobarbital: May decrease MHD and may increase phenobarbital AUC.
Phenytoin: May decrease MHD and may increase phenytoin AUC.
Valproic acid: May decrease oxcarbazepine AUC.
Verapamil: May decrease MHD.

Lab Test Interferences None well documented.

Adverse Reactions
CV: Hypotension.
CNS: Ataxia; abnormal coordination; fatigue; asthenia; headache; dizziness; somnolence; anxiety; abnormal gait; insomnia; tremor; amnesia;

nervousness; agitation; confusion; speech disorder; aggravated convulsions.
DERM: Acne; hot flashes; purpura; rash; Stevens-Johnson syndrome (postmarketing).
EENT: Nystagmus; diplopia; vertigo; taste perversion; earache; ear infection; abnormal vision.
GI: Nausea; vomiting; abdominal pain; anorexia; dry mouth; diarrhea; dyspepsia; constipation; gastritis; rectum hemorrhage; toothache.
GU: UTI; micturition frequency; vaginitis.
METAB: Hyponatremia; thirst; generalized edema; leg edema.
RESP: Rhinitis; upper respiratory tract infection; cough; bronchitis; pharyngitis; epistaxis; sinusitis.
OTHER: Muscle weakness; back pain; sprains/strains; fever; allergy; chest pain; weight increase; infection; lymphadenopathy (postmarketing).

Precautions
Pregnancy: Category C.
Lactation: Oxcarbazepine and MHD are excreted in the breast milk. Effects on the infant are undetermined.
Children: Safety and efficacy have not been determined in patients less than 4 yr.
Elderly: Because of age-related reductions in Ccr, the C_{max} and AUC may be elevated.
Hypersensitivity: Approximately 25% to 30% of patients who have a hypersensitivity to carbamazepine will experience a hypersensitivity reaction to oxcarbazepine.
Renal function impairment: Use with caution; dosage adjustment may be required (see Route/Dosage).
CNS effects: Oxcarbazine has been associated with symptoms including psychomotor slowing; difficulty with concentration speech, or language; somnolence or fatigue; and coordination abnormalities, including ataxia and gait disturbances.
Hyponatremia: May occur.
Withdrawal: Withdraw therapy gradually to minimize potential of increased seizure frequency.

PATIENT CARE CONSIDERATIONS

Administration/Storage
- May be used alone or in combination with other AEDs.
- Administer prescribed dose bid without regard to meals. Administer with food if GI upset occurs.
- Shake suspension well before measuring dose. Measure dose using dosing cup, spoon, or syringe.
- Store tablets and suspension at controlled room temperature (59° to 86°F). Discard any unused suspension 7 wk after first opening.

Assessment/Interventions
- Obtain patient history, including drug history and any known allergies. Note renal impairment or history of sensitivity to carbamazepine.
- Ensure that initial dose is reduced and slower dose escalation is used in patient with Ccr less than 30 mL/min.
- Ensure that serum sodium is evaluated periodically during prolonged therapy, especially in patient receiving other medications known to decrease serum sodium (eg, medications for SIADH).
- Evaluate serum sodium if symptoms possibly indicating hyponatremia develop (eg, nausea, malaise, headache, lethargy, confusion, obtundation, increase in seizure frequency or severity).
- Closely observe patient and monitor plasma levels of other coadministered antiepileptic drugs when adding, increasing, or decreasing the dose of oxcarbazepine.
- Frequently assess patient for response to treatment. Notify health care provider if seizures do not improve or appear to worsen.
- Ensure that therapy is periodically reviewed to determine if it needs to be continued without change or if a dose change (eg, increase, decrease, discontinuation) is indicated.
- Avoid sudden discontinuation of therapy if possible. Attempt to gradually reduce dose over a period of several weeks if decision to discontinue medication is made.
- Monitor patient for GI, CNS, PSYCH, and general body side effects. Report to health care provider if noted and significant.
- Implement safety precautions for patients who experience dizziness or ataxia.

Patient/Family Education
- Explain name, dose, action, and potential side effects of drug.
- Instruct patient to continue to take other antiepileptic medications as prescribed by health care provider.
- Advise patient to read the *Patient Information* leaflet before starting therapy and with each refill.
- Instruct patient to take exactly as prescribed and not to change the dose or discontinue unless advised by health care provider.
- Advise patient that dose is gradually increased as tolerated until max benefit has been obtained.
- Advise patient or caregiver to shake suspension well before measuring dose and to mea-

sure prescribed dose using dosing cup, spoon, or syringe.
- Advise patient that each dose may be taken without regard to meals but to take with food if stomach upset occurs.
- Advise patient that if a dose is missed to take it as soon as remembered; however, if several hours have passed or it is nearing the time for the next scheduled dose, the missed dose should be skipped and the next dose taken at the regularly scheduled time. Caution patient to never double the dose to catch up.
- Advise patient that if medication needs to be discontinued it will be slowly withdrawn over a period of several weeks unless safety concerns (eg, rash) require a more rapid withdrawal.
- Advise patient to avoid alcoholic beverages and other depressants while taking this medication.
- Instruct patient or caregiver to immediately notify health care provider if any of the following occur: confusion, unresponsiveness to stimulation, general body discomfort, persistent nausea or headache.
- Instruct patient to contact health care provider if developing difficulty with concentration, speech or language problems, excessive drowsiness or fatigue, or coordination problems.
- Instruct patient to inform health care provider if seizures get worse, if new types of seizures develop, or if bothersome side effects occur.
- Caution patient that drug may cause drowsiness and dizziness and to use caution while driving or performing other tasks requiring mental alertness until tolerance is determined.
- Advise women using combination oral contraceptive to use additional nonhormonal form of contraception because oxcarbazepine causes a reduction in effectiveness of combination oral contraceptives.
- Advise women to notify health care provider if pregnant, planning to become pregnant, or breastfeeding.
- Advise patient not to take any prescription or OTC medications or dietary supplements unless advised by health care provider.
- Advise patient that laboratory tests and follow-up visits will be required to monitor therapy and to keep appointments.

Oxybutynin Chloride

(OX-ee-BYOO-tih-nin KLOR-ide)

Class Urinary tract product/Antispasmodic

How Supplied
Ditropan Tablets 5 mg, Syrup 5 mg/5 mL ♦ *Ditropan XL* Tablets, extended-release 5 mg, Tablets, extended-release 10 mg, Tablets, extended-release 15 mg ♦ *Oxytrol* Transdermal system 36 mg of oxybutinin delivering 3.9 mg of oxubutinin/day.

❀ *Apo-Oxybutynin* ♦ *Gen-Oxybutynin* ♦ *Novo-Oxybutynin* ♦ *Nu-Oxybutynin* ♦ *PMS-Oxybutynin*

Action
PHARMACOLOGY: Increases bladder capacity, diminishes frequency of uninhibited contractions of detrusor muscle and delays initial desire to void.

PHARMACOKINETICS/DYNAMICS:
Absorption:
Extended-release – Following oral administration of the oxybutynin extended-release (ER) tablet, plasma levels rise for 4 to 6 hr; thereafter, steady levels are maintained for up to 24 hr. Steady-state levels are achieved by day 3 of repeated ER dosing.
Transdermal system – Following application of the first 3.9 mg/day system, plasma levels increase for approximately 24 to 48 hr; reaching C_{max} of 3 to 4 ng/mL.

Distribution:
Extended-release – Plasma concentrations of oxybutynin decline biexponentially following IV or oral administration. The Vd is 193 L after IV administration of 5 mg oxybutynin chloride.
Transdermal system – Widely distributed to body tissues. The Vd was estimated to be 193 L after IV administration of 5 mg oxybutynin chloride.

Metabolism: Extensively metabolized by the liver. Primarily by the CYP3A4 isozyme in the liver and gut wall. Transdermal administration bypasses the first-pass GI and hepatic metabolism.

Excretion: Less than 0.1% excreted unchanged in the urine.

Indications Treatment of symptoms of bladder instability associated with voiding in patients with uninhibited and reflex neurogenic bladder (eg, urinary leakage, dysuria). Treatment of overactive bladder with symptoms of urge urinary incontinence, urgency, and frequency (ER tablet).

Contraindications Untreated angle-closure glaucoma; untreated narrow anterior chamber angles; GI obstruction; paralytic ileus; intestinal atony of elderly or debilitated patients; toxic megacolon complicating ulcerative colitis; severe colitis; obstructive uropathy; myasthenia gravis; unstable cardiovascular status in acute hemorrhage.

Route/Dosage

ADULTS (IMMEDIATE-RELEASE TABLET OR SYRUP): **PO** 5 mg bid to tid (max, 5 mg qid).
CHILDREN OVER 5 YR: **PO** 5 mg bid (max, 5 mg tid).
ADULTS (ER TABLET): **PO** 5 mg qd adjusted in 5 mg increments at weekly intervals (max, 30 mg/day).

TRANSDERMAL SYSTEM

ADULTS: **Transdermal** 3.9 mg/day applied twice/wk (q 3 or 4 days) to dry, intact skin on abdomen, hip, or buttock, selecting a new application site with each system and avoiding using the same site within 7 days.

Interactions

Anticholinergic drugs (eg, amantadine): Increased risk of anticholinergic side effects.
Beta-blockers (eg, atenolol): Atenolol plasma levels may be elevated, increasing the risk of side effects.
Digoxin: Increased plasma levels of slow-dissolution oral tablets may be increased.
Haloperidol: Worsening of schizophrenic symptoms; tardive dyskinesia; decreased serum haloperidol concentrations, reducing therapeutic effect.
Phenothiazines: Decreased therapeutic effects of phenothiazines; increased incidence of anticholinergic side effects.

Lab Test Interferences None well documented.

Adverse Reactions

CV:
ER tablets – Tachycardia, palpitations, vasodilatation, hypertension, palpitation, vasodilation (2% to less than 5%).
Immediate-release tablets and syrup – Palpitations; tachycardia; vasodilation.
CNS:
ER tablets – Somnolence (11.9%); headache (9.8%); dizziness (6.3%); drowsiness, hallucinations, restlessness, insomnia, nervousness, confusion (2% to less than 5%).
Immediate-release tablets and syrup – Dizziness; drowsiness; hallucinations; insomnia; restlessness.
Transdermal system – Fatigue; somnolence; headache (more than 1%).
DERM:
ER tablets – Rash, dry skin (2% to less than 5%).
Immediate-release tablets and syrup – Decreased sweating; rash.
Transdermal system – Application site pruritus, erythema, vesicles, rash and macules (2% or more).
EENT:
ER tablets – Blurred vision (7.7%); dry eyes (6.1%); decreased lacrimation; mydriasis; amblyopia; cycloplegia; rhinitis; sinusitis; dry nasal and sinus mucous membranes; pharyngitis.
Immediate-release tablets and syrup – Amblyopia; cycloplegia; decreased lacrimation; mydriasis.
Transdermal system – Abnormal vision (2% or more).
GI:
ER tablets – Dry mouth (60.8%); constipation (13.1%); diarrhea (9.1%); nausea (8.9%); dyspepsia (6.8%); vomiting, decreased GI motility, flatulence, gastroesophageal reflux (2% to less than 5%).
Immediate-release tablets and syrup – Constipation; decreased GI motility; dry mouth; nausea.
Transdermal system – Dry mouth, diarrhea, constipation (2% or more); abdominal pain, nausea, flatulence (more than 1%).
GU:
ER tablets – Impotence, urinary tract infection, increased postvoid residual volume, cystitis (2% to less than 5%).
Immediate-release tablets and syrup – Urinary retention and hesitancy.
Transdermal system – Dysuria (2% or more).
RESP:
ER tablets – Upper respiratory tract infection, cough, bronchitis (2% to less than 5%).
OTHER:
ER tablets – Asthenia, pain (6.8%); rhinitis (5.6%); UTI (5.1%); decreased sweating, suppression of lactation, abdominal pain, accidental injury, back pain, flu-like syndrome, arthritis (2% to less than 5%).
Immediate-release tablets and syrup – Asthenia; impotence; suppression of lactation.
Transdermal system – Flushing, back pain, application site burning (more than 1%).

Precautions

Pregnancy: Category B.
Lactation: Undetermined.
Children: Safety and efficacy in children younger than 5 yr not established.
Special risk patients: Use with caution in the elderly and in patients with renal or hepatic function impairment or autonomic neuropathy.
Anticholinergic effects: Use cautiously with phenothiazines or other drugs with anticholinergic properties because side effects will be additive.
Cardiac and other effects: May aggravate symptoms of hyperthyroidism, coronary heart disease, CHF, cardiac arrhythmias, tachycardia, hypertension, hiatal hernia, and prostatic hypertrophy.
Diarrhea: Diarrhea may be an early symptom of intestinal obstruction in which oxybutynin is contraindicated.
GI disorders: Administration to patients with ulcerative colitis may suppress GI motility and produce paralytic ileus, precipitating or aggravating toxic megacolon.

Heat prostration: Heat prostration may occur when exposed to high environmental temperature.

Urinary retention: Because risk may be increased, use with caution.

PATIENT CARE CONSIDERATIONS

Administration/Storage

- If patient experiences nausea, administer with food.
- Store in tightly closed container at room temperature.
- Oxybutynin ER tablet should be taken whole with liquid and not chewed, divided, or crushed.

Transdermal system:

- Patch is applied twice/wk (eg, q 3 to 4 days).
- Remove patch from foil pouch, remove plastic strips covering adhesive layer, and immediately apply to dry, intact skin on the abdomen, buttock, or hip.
- Rotate application sites to avoid reapplication to same site within 7 days.
- To discard used patch, fold used patch, place in foil pouch from new patch, and discard in trash.
- Store patches in foil pouch at controlled room temperature (59° to 86°F). Protect from moisture and humidity. Do not store patches outside foil pouch.

Assessment/Interventions

- Obtain patient history, including drug history and any known allergies. Note presence of hepatic or renal impairment, autonomic neuropathy, bladder outflow obstruction, GI obstructive disorder, ulcerative colitis, intestinal atony, myasthenia gravis, gastroesophageal reflux, or concurrent therapy with drugs that can cause or exacerbate esophagitis (eg, bisphosphonates).
- Note conditions which would contraindicate use of oxybutynin, including presence or risk of urinary retention, gastric retention, or uncontrolled narrow-angle glaucoma.
- Assess patient for urinary retention before administering drug and periodically during treatment. If symptoms of urinary retention (eg, suprapubic pain in conjunction with urgency and frequency with voiding of small amounts) occur, notify health care provider.
- If signs of heat stroke develop (eg, elevation in body temperature, dehydration, mental changes), move patient to a cooler area; cover torso with wet towels, and/or use fans or air conditioners. Give extra fluids.
- If patient has difficulty voiding, use bladder massage.

Overdosage: Signs and Symptoms

CNS excitation, flushing, fever, tachycardia, nausea, respiratory depression, coma.

- If passing urinary catheter becomes difficult, use extra lubricant and inflexible catheter, and allow time for spasms to diminish.
- If diarrhea occurs, discontinue use and notify health care provider.

Transdermal system:

- Assess application site for redness, itching, or other signs of reaction. Inform health care provider if reactions are bothersome or appear to occur with each application.
- If patch comes off before scheduled replacement, discard and apply new patch to new application site and establish new reapplication schedule.

Patient/Family Education

- Instruct patient to take sips of water frequently, suck on ice chips or sugarless hard candy, or chew sugarless gum if dry mouth occurs.
- Teach patient to use bladder massage to empty bladder.
- Advise patient to use caution in hot weather to reduce risk of heat stroke.
- Advise patient that drug may cause drowsiness or dizziness, and to use caution while driving or performing other tasks requiring mental alertness.
- Advise patient to take oxybutynin ER tablet whole with liquids and not to chew, divide, or crush.
- Inform patient not to be concerned if noticing a tablet in the stool; the tablet shell is eliminated from the body but the drug is released from the tablet at a controlled rate.
- Advise women to notify health care provider if pregnant, planning to become pregnant, or breastfeeding.
- Instruct patient not to take any prescription or OTC medications or dietary supplements unless advised by health care provider.
- Advise patient that follow-up visits may be required to monitor therapy and to keep appointments.

Transdermal system:

- Advise patient to review "Patient Information" leaflet that comes with each prescription before using the first time and with each refill.
- Ensure that patient understands how to store, apply, and discard patches.

- Advise patient that new patch is applied twice/wk (eg, q 3 to 4 days) and to rotate application sites to avoid reapplication to the same site within 7 days.
- Advise patient that if patch comes off before scheduled replacement, to discard and apply new patch to new application site and establish new reapplication schedule.
- Advise patient to notify health care provider if application site reactions occur and are bothersome or occur with each application.

Oxycodone Hydrochloride

(OX-ee-KOE-dohn HIGH-droe-KLOR-ide)

Class Narcotic analgesic

How Supplied

M-oxy Tablets 5 mg ◆ Endocodone Tablets 5 mg ◆ OxyIR Capsules, immediate-release 5 mg ◆ OxyContin Tablets, controlled-release 10 mg, Tablets, controlled-release 20 mg, Tablets, controlled-release 40 mg, Tablets, controlled-release 80 mg, Tablets, controlled-release 160 mg ◆ Oxydose Solution, concentrate 20 mg/mL ◆ OxyFAST Solution, concentrate 20 mg/mL ◆ Percolone Tablets 5 mg ◆ Roxicodone Tablets 5 mg, Solution, oral 5 mg/5 mL ◆ Roxicodone Intensol Solution, concentrate 20 mg/mL
♣ Supeudol

Action

PHARMACOLOGY: Relieves pain by stimulating opiate receptors in CNS; may cause respiratory depression, peripheral vasodilation, inhibition of intestinal peristalsis, sphincter of Oddi spasm, stimulation of chemoreceptors that cause vomiting and increased bladder tone.

PHARMACOKINETICS/DYNAMICS:

Absorption: High oral availability due to low presystemic or first-pass metabolism. Exhibits a biphasic absorption pattern. The immediate-release oral bioavailability is 100%. The oral bioavailability is 60% and 87%. Peak plasma concentration increased by 25% with a high fat meal. Once absorbed it is distributed to skeletal muscle, liver, intestinal tract, lungs, spleen, and brain.

Distribution: The Vd is 2.6 L/kg (IV). It is found in breast milk.

Metabolism: Extensively metabolized in the liver to noroxycodone (a major metabolite), oxymorphone, and their glucuronides.

Excretion: Excreted through the urine, with less than 19% as free oxycodone, less than 50% as conjugated oxycodone, and less than 14% as conjugated oxymorphone. The $t_{1/2}$ for immediate release is 0.4 hr. Clearance is 0.8 L/min. Elimination on $t_{1/2}$ is 3.2 hr (immediate release).

Onset: 15 to 30 min.

Peak: 1 hr.

Duration: 4 to 6 hr.

Special Populations:
Severe Renal Insufficiency – For less than 60 mL/min, higher peak plasma oxycodone (50%), and noroxycodone (20%), higher AUC for oxycodone (60%), noroxycodone (50%), oxymorphone (40%). There is an increased $t_{1/2}$ of oxycodone elimination of only 1 hr.
Mild to Moderate Hepatic Insufficiency – Peak plasma oxycodone and noroxycodone concentrations 50% and 20% higher; AUC values are 95% and 65% higher, respectively. Oxymorphone peak plasma concentration and AUC values are lower by 30% and 40%. The $t_{1/2}$ elimination for oxycodone is increased by 2.3 hr.

Indications Relief of moderate to moderately severe pain.

Contraindications Hypersensitivity to opiates; upper airway obstruction; acute asthma; diarrhea due to poisoning or toxins.

Route/Dosage

Individualize dosing regimen for each patient.

Immediate-Release

ADULTS: **PO** 10 to 30 mg q 4 hr (5 mg q 6 hr for OxyIR, oxycodone immediate-release capsules, Oxydose, and OxyFAST) prn.

Controlled-Release

ADULTS: **PO** 10 to 160 mg bid (80 and 160 mg controlled-release tablets are for use in opioid-tolerant patients only).

Interactions

CNS depressants (eg, alcohol, barbiturate anesthetics, phenothiazines, sedatives, tricyclic antidepressants, other narcotics): Additive CNS depression.

Lab Test Interferences Increased amylase and lipase may occur up to 24 hr after administration.

Adverse Reactions

CV: Hypotension; orthostatic hypotension; bradycardia; tachycardia.
CNS: Lightheadedness; dizziness; sedation; disorientation; incoordination.
DERM: Sweating; pruritus; urticaria.
GI: Nausea; vomiting; constipation; abdominal pain.
GU: Urinary retention or hesitancy.
RESP: Respiratory depression; laryngospasm; depression of cough reflex.
OTHER: Tolerance; psychological and physical dependence with chronic use.

> **WARNING:**
> *Controlled release:* Controlled release is for management of moderate to severe pain with around-the-clock dosing. Not intended for prn use. Use 80 and 160 mg tablets in opioid tolerant patients only. Respiratory depression reported when used in opioid-naive patients. Swallow tablets whole. Do not crush, chew, or break; may result in potential fatal dose of oxycodone.

Precautions
Pregnancy: Category C.
Lactation: Excreted in breast milk.
Children: Not recommended for children.

PATIENT CARE CONSIDERATIONS
Administration/Storage
- Administer with food or milk to minimize GI irritation.
- Store at room temperature in tightly closed container; protect from light.

Assessment/Interventions
- Obtain patient history, including drug history and any known allergies.
- Assess type, location, and intensity of pain before administration and frequently during treatment.
- Assess vital signs before administration and periodically during treatment.
- Assess for signs of narcotic dependence.
- Assess bowel function routinely. If constipation develops, provide additional fluids, high-fiber foods, or stool softeners. Administer laxative if indicated.
- If respiratory depression develops, notify health care provider immediately and prepare emergency equipment.
- If sedation or confusion develops, take safety precautions (eg, keep side rails up, assist with ambulation).

Renal function impairment: Dosage reduction may be necessary.
Hepatic function impairment: Dosage reduction may be necessary.
Special risk patients: Use with caution in elderly and debilitated patients and patients with myxedema, acute alcoholism, acute abdominal conditions, ulcerative colitis, decreased respiratory reserve, head injury or increased intracranial pressure, hypoxia, supraventricular tachycardia, depleted blood volume, or circulatory shock.
Drug dependence: Has abuse potential.

Overdosage: Signs and Symptoms
Miosis, respiratory depression, CNS depression (somnolence progressing to stupor or coma), circulatory collapse, seizures, cardiopulmonary arrest, death.

- Evaluate patient's continuing need for therapy since psychological and physical dependence and tolerance may develop.

Patient/Family Education
- Instruct patient to take medication before pain becomes severe for greatest effectiveness.
- Instruct patient on methods of preventing constipation.
- Instruct patient to make position changes slowly if lightheadedness or sedation occur.
- Advise patient to avoid intake of alcoholic beverages or products containing alcohol while using this medication.
- Advise patient that drug may cause drowsiness, and to use caution while driving or performing other tasks requiring mental alertness.
- Instruct patient not to take any OTC medications without consulting health care provider.
- Explain that physical dependency may occur and that withdrawal symptoms may be noted on discontinuation after long-term therapy.
- Instruct and alert patient to swallow the controlled-release tablets whole and not to break, chew, or crush them before ingestion.

Oxycodone/Acetaminophen

(OX-ee-KOE-dohn/ass-cet-ah-MEE-noe-fen)

Class Narcotic analgesic combination

How Supplied
Percocet Tablets 5 mg oxycodone hydrochloride/325 mg acetaminophen, Tablets 7.5 mg oxycodone hydrochloride/500 mg acetaminophen, Tablets 10 mg oxycodone hydrochloride/650 mg acetaminophen ◆ *Roxicet* Tablets 5 mg oxycodone hydrochloride/325 mg acetaminophen, Solution, oral 5 mg oxycodone hydrochloride/325 mg acetaminophen ◆ *Roxicet 5/500* Caplets 5 mg oxycodone/500 mg acetaminophen ◆ *Roxilox* Capsules 5 mg oxycodone hydrochloride/500 mg acetaminophen ◆ *Tylox* Capsules 5 mg oxycodone hydrochloride/500 mg acetaminophen ❋ *Percocet-Demi* ◆ *ratio-Oxycocet*

Action
PHARMACOLOGY: Acetaminophen inhibits synthesis of prostaglandins and peripherally blocks pain impulse generation, whereas, oxycodone binds to opiate receptors in CNS. Combination has synergistic effect on alleviating pain.

Indications Relief of moderate to moderately severe pain.

Contraindications Hypersensitivity to acetaminophen, oxycodone, or similar compounds.

Route/Dosage
ADULTS: **PO** 5 mg (1 tablet, caplet, or teaspoonful) q 6 hr prn.

Interactions
Anesthetics: Additive CNS depression.
Carbamazepine, hydantoins, sulfinpyrazone: Increased risk of hepatotoxicity.
CNS depressants (eg, barbiturates, tricyclic antidepressants, phenothiazines, sedatives, hypnotics, alcohol, other narcotics): Additive CNS depression.

Lab Test Interferences With *Chemstrip bG*, *Dextrostix*, and *Visidex II* home blood glucose systems, may cause false decrease in mean glucose values.

Adverse Reactions
CV: Hypotension; bradycardia; tachycardia.
CNS: Lightheadedness; dizziness; weakness; fatigue; sedation; euphoria; dysphoria; nervousness; headache; confusion.
DERM: Pruritus; rash.
GI: Nausea; vomiting; constipation; abdominal pain; anorexia; biliary spasm; dry mouth.
GU: Urinary retention or hesitancy.
RESP: Dyspnea; respiratory depression.
OTHER: Malaise; tolerance; psychological and physical dependence with chronic use.

Precautions
Pregnancy: Category C.
Lactation: Undetermined.
Children: Safety and efficacy not established.
Hepatic function impairment: Chronic alcoholics should limit acetaminophen intake to less than 2 g/day.
Special risk patients: Use with caution in elderly, debilitated patients and those with hepatic or kidney failure or conditions accompanied by hypoxia or hypercapnia; monitor carefully to avoid decrease in pulmonary ventilation. Also use cautiously in patients sensitive to CNS depressants, postoperatively and in patients with pulmonary disease.
Sulfite sensitivity: Use with caution in patients known to be sensitive, as some products contain bisulfites.
Acute abdominal conditions: Diagnosis may be obscured; use with caution.
Dependence: Can produce drug dependence; has abuse potential.
Head injury: Respiratory depression and elevation of CSF pressure may be exacerbated.

Overdosage: Signs and Symptoms
Miosis, respiratory depression, CNS depression (somnolence progressing to stupor or coma), hepatic damage, circulatory collapse, cardiopulmonary arrest, death.

PATIENT CARE CONSIDERATIONS
Administration/Storage
- Administer with food or milk to minimize GI irritation.
- Store at room temperature in tightly-closed container.

Assessment/Interventions
- Obtain patient history, including drug history and any known allergies.
- Assess type, location, and intensity of pain before administration and frequently during treatment.
- Assess vital signs before administration and periodically during treatment.
- Assess for signs of narcotic dependence.
- Assess bowel function routinely. If constipation develops, provide additional fluids, high-fiber foods, or stool softeners.
- If respiratory depression develops, notify health care provider immediately and prepare emergency equipment.
- If sedation or confusion develops, take safety precautions (eg, keep side rails up, assist with ambulation).
- Evaluate patient's continuing need for therapy since psychological and physical dependence and tolerance may develop.

Patient/Family Education
- Instruct patient to take medication before pain becomes severe for greatest effectiveness.
- Teach patient methods to prevent constipation.
- Instruct patient to make position changes slowly if lightheadedness or sedation occurs.
- Advise patient to avoid intake of alcoholic beverages or products containing alcohol while using this medication.
- Advise patient that drug may cause drowsiness, and to use caution while driving or performing other tasks requiring mental alertness.
- Caution patient that physical dependency and withdrawal symptoms may occur following discontinuation of long-term therapy.
- Instruct patient not to take any *otc* medications without consulting health care provider.

Oxycodone Hydrochloride/ Aspirin

(OX-ee-KOE-dohn HIGH-droe-KLOR-ide/ ASS-pihr-in)

Class Narcotic analgesic/Analgesic

How Supplied
Percodan Tablets 4.5 mg oxycodone hydrochloride/ 0.38 mg oxycodone terephthalate/325 mg aspirin
♣ *ratio-Oxycodan*

Action
PHARMACOLOGY:
Oxycodone: Relieves pain by stimulating opiate receptors in CNS
Aspirin: Inhibits prostaglandin synthesis, resulting in analgesia, anti-inflammatory activity, and inhibition of platelet aggregation.

Indications For the relief of moderate to moderately severe pain.

Contraindications Hypersensitivity to any component of the product.

Route/Dosage
ADULTS: **PO** Usual dose is 1 tablet q 6 hr prn for pain (max, 12 tablets [4 g aspirin] q 24 hr).

Interactions
Anticoagulants (eg, warfarin): Effects of anticoagulants may be enhanced by aspirin, increasing the risk of bleeding.
CNS depressants (eg, alcohol, phenobarbital), general anesthetics, opioid analgesics, phenothiazines, sedative-hypnotics, tranquilizers: Effects may be additive.
Uricosuric agents (eg, probenecid): Effects may be inhibited by aspirin.

Lab Test Interferences None well documented.

Adverse Reactions
CNS: Lightheadedness; dizziness; sedation; euphoria; dysphoria.
DERM: Pruritus.
GI: Nausea; vomiting; constipation.

Precautions
Pregnancy: Safety of use has not been established.
Children: Safety and efficacy not established. Reye syndrome has been associated with aspirin administration to children (including teenagers) with acute febrile illness.
Special risk patients: Use with caution in the elderly or debilitated and patients with severe impairment of hepatic or renal function, peptic ulcers, hypothyroidism, Addison disease, and prostatic hypertrophy or urethral stricture.
Acute abdominal conditions: Diagnosis or clinical course may be obscured.
Ambulatory patients: Mental and physical abilities may be impaired.
Dependency: Oxycodone has abuse potential.
Head injury and increased intracranial pressure: Cerebrospinal fluid pressure may be markedly exaggerated in the presence of head injury.
Peptic ulcers: Use with caution in the presence of peptic ulcer.

Overdosage: Signs and Symptoms
Respiratory depression, extreme somnolence progressing to stupor or coma, skeletal muscle flaccidity, cold and clammy skin, bradycardia, hypotension, apnea, circulatory collapse, cardiac arrest, death.

PATIENT CARE CONSIDERATIONS

Administration/Storage
- Administer 1 to 2 tablets as prescribed q 6 hr if needed.
- Do not exceed 12 tablets in 24 hr.
- Administer without regard to meals but administer with food if GI upset occurs.
- Store at controlled room temperature (59° to 86°F).

Assessment/Interventions
- Obtain patient history, including drug history and any known allergies. Note history of addiction, bleeding or coagulation disorders, hepatic or renal impairment, peptic ulcer or other serious GI lesions, head injury, increased intracranial pressure, acute abdominal conditions, hypothyroidism, prostatic hypertrophy, urethral stricture, or the syndrome of nasal polyps, rhinitis, and bronchospastic reactivity to aspirin or other NSAIDs.
- Assess pain before starting therapy and periodically during treatment.
- Monitor patient for CNS, GI, and general body side effects. Report to health care provider if noted and significant.
- Discontinue therapy and notify health care provider immediately if any of the following occur: allergic reaction, unusual bleeding or bruising, shortness of breath, black or tarry stools, vomiting of blood or coffee ground-like material.

Patient/Family Education
- Explain name, dose, action, and potential side effects of drug.
- Advise patient to take 1 tablet q 6 hr or as prescribed if needed for pain but to not take more than 12 tablets in 24 hr.
- Advise patient to take without regard to meals but to take with food if GI upset occurs.

- Instruct patient to avoid alcoholic beverages and other depressants while taking this medication.
- Advise patient that drug may impair judgment, thinking, or motor skills or cause drowsiness and to use caution while driving or performing other tasks requiring mental alertness until tolerance is determined.
- Advise patient to stop taking the drug and notify health care provider if any of the following occur: allergic reaction, unusual bleeding or bruising, shortness of breath, black or tarry stools, vomiting of blood or coffee ground-like material, excessive sedation.
- Advise women to notify health care provider if pregnant, planning to become pregnant, or breastfeeding.
- Warn patient not to take any prescription or OTC drugs or dietary supplements without consulting health care provider.
- Advise patient that follow-up visits may be necessary to monitor therapy and to keep appointments.

Oxymorphone Hydrochloride

(ox-ee-MORE-fone HIGH-droe-KLOR-ide)

Class Narcotic analgesic

How Supplied
Numorphan Injection 1 mg/mL, Injection 1.5 mg/mL, Suppositories 5 mg

Action
PHARMACOLOGY: Relieves pain by stimulating opiate receptors in the CNS.

PHARMACOKINETICS/DYNAMICS:
Distribution: Vd is 3.08 L/kg.
Metabolism: Undergoes extensive hepatic metabolism.
Excretion: Mean terminal t½ is 1.3 hr. Following a 10 mg oral dose, 49% is excreted in the urine over a 5-day period.
Onset: After parenteral administration, effects are seen within 5 to 10 min.
Duration: Duration of effect is 3 to 6 hr.

Indications
Relief of moderate to severe pain.

Contraindications
Hypersensitivity to morphine analogs; hypersensitivity to any component of the product.

Route/Dosage
ADULTS: **IM/SC** Initially, 1 to 1.5 mg, repeated q 4 to 6 hr prn.
IV Initially, 0.5 mg. In nondebilitated patients, the dose may be cautiously increased until satisfactory pain relief is achieved.
PR 1 suppository (5 mg), q 4 to 6 hr. In nondebilitated patients, the dose may be cautiously increased until satisfactory pain relief is achieved.

Labor
ADULTS: **IM** 0.5 to 1 mg is recommended.

Interactions
Anticholinergics or drugs with anticholinergic activity: Increased risk of urinary retention and severe constipation, possibly leading to paralytic ileus.
CNS depressants (eg, alcohol, hypnotics, sedatives, tranquilizers): Additive CNS depressant effects. Respiratory depression, hypotension, profound sedation, or coma may occur.
Propofol: Increased risk of bradycardia.

Lab Test Interferences
None well documented.

Adverse Reactions
CV: Hypotension; orthostatic hypotension; tachycardia; bradycardia; palpitations; flushing.
CNS: Drowsiness; lightheadedness; unusual tiredness or weakness; headache; dysphoria; euphoria; nervousness; restlessness; confusion; mental clouding; trouble sleeping; paradoxical CNS stimulation; hallucinations; mental depression.
DERM: Itching; sweating; injection site reaction; allergic reaction (eg, skin rash, hives, swelling of the face).
EENT: Miosis; diplopia; blurred vision.
GI: Nausea; vomiting; dry mouth; constipation; biliary tract spasm; cramps or pain; loss of appetite; paralytic ileus or toxic megacolon in patients with inflammatory bowel disease.
GU: Ureteral spasm; urinary hesitancy or retention; antidiuretic effect.
RESP: Respiratory depression; atelectasis; allergic bronchospastic reaction; allergic laryngeal edema; allergic laryngospasm.

Precautions
Pregnancy: Category C.
Lactation: Undetermined.
Children: Safety and efficacy not established in patients younger than 18 yr
Special risk patients: Use with caution in elderly and debilitated patients and in patients known to be sensitive to CNS depressants (eg, CV, pulmonary, renal, or hepatic disease); use with caution in patients with hypothyroidism, acute alcoholism, delirium tremens, convulsive disorders, Addison disease, gallbladder disease or gallstones, prostatic hypertrophy, or urethral stricture; recent GI or GU tract surgery, inflammatory bowel disease. diarrhea secondary to poisoning until toxin is eliminated.

Acute abdominal conditions: Diagnosis or clinical course of patient may be obscured.
Drug dependence: Has abuse potential.
Head injury: Respiratory depressant effects may be markedly exaggerated in the presence of head injury, intracranial lesions, or preexisting increased intracranial pressure.
Hypotension: May cause severe hypotension in postoperative patients or in individuals whose ability to maintain BP is compromised (eg, volume depletion). May cause orthostatic hypotension in ambulatory patients.
Respiratory depression: May cause serious or potentially fatal respiratory depression if given in excessive dose, too frequently, or in full dosage to compromised patients. Use with caution in patients with impaired respiratory reserve or respiratory depression.

Overdosage: Signs and Symptoms
Respiratory depression, CNS depression, extreme somnolence progressing to stupor or coma, skeletal muscle flaccidity, cold and clammy skin, constricted pupils, bradycardia, hypotension, apnea, circulatory collapse, cardiac arrest, death.

PATIENT CARE CONSIDERATIONS

Administration/Storage
Injection:
- For SC, IM, or IV administration. Not for intradermal or intra-arterial administration.
- Do not administer if particulate matter or discoloration noted.
- Discard any unused medication per institutional policy and procedure for schedule II controlled substances.
- Store injection at controlled room temperature (59° to 86°F). Protect from light.

Suppository:
- Remove foil over-wrap just prior to use.
- Multiple suppositories can be used for total doses greater than 5 mg.
- Store suppositories in refrigerator (36° to 46°F).

Assessment/Interventions
- Obtain patient history, including drug history and any known allergies. Note renal or hepatic impairment, CV disease, pulmonary disease, severe respiratory depression, upper airway obstruction, paralytic ileus, acute abdominal condition, head injury, brain tumor, seizures, hypothyroidism, Addison disease, prostatic hypertrophy or urethral stricture, recent GI surgery, elevated IOP, inflammatory bowel disease, concurrent use of CNS depressant medications, or history of allergy or intolerance to morphine or analogs of morphine.
- Ensure that reduced dose and slower dose escalation are used in elderly or debilitated patient or patient with hepatic impairment.
- Assess pain type and intensity prior to administration; assess effectiveness of pain relief after medication administration. Notify health care provider if optimal pain control is not achieved.
- Ensure that therapy is periodically reviewed to determine if it needs to be continued without change or if a dose change (eg, increase, decrease, discontinuation) is indicated.
- Monitor cardiac patients during initiation of drug for orthostatic hypotension; notify health care provider if noted and implement safety precautions.
- Monitor patient for CNS, GI, CV, RESP, and general body side effects. Report to health care provider if noted and significant.
- If treatment is to be discontinued or the dose reduced, gradually taper the dose and monitor patient for withdrawal symptoms. If significant withdrawal symptoms (eg, sweating, muscle cramps, abdominal pain, piloerection) develop notify health care provider. Be prepared to reinstitute previous dosing schedule and attempt a less rapid tapering regimen after patient has stabilized.

Injection:
- Ensure that an opioid antagonist, oxygen, and resuscitation and intubation equipment are available for use if needed.
- Frequently monitor patient and vital signs. Report significant changes to health care provider. Be prepared to appropriately treat respiratory depression, apnea, or any other potentially life-threatening event.

Patient/Family Education
- Explain name, action, and potential side effects of drug.

Suppository:
- Instruct patient or caregiver that medication may be habit forming and to use exactly as prescribed and not to change the dose or discontinue therapy unless advised by health care provider. Advise patient or caregiver to notify health care provider if medication does not adequately control pain.
- Advise patient, family, or caregiver that if medication needs to be discontinued after prolonged use that it will usually be slowly withdrawn unless safety concerns (eg, rash) require a more rapid withdrawal.
- Advise patient or caregiver to notify health care provider if any of the following occur: excessive sedation or drowsiness; slow or shal-

low breathing; low BP; slow heart rate; severe constipation.
- Instruct patient to get up slowly from lying or sitting position and to avoid sudden position changes to prevent postural hypotension. Advise patient to report dizziness with position changes to health care provider. Caution patient that hot tubs and hot showers or baths may make dizziness worse.
- Caution patient that drug may cause dizziness or drowsiness and to use caution while driving or performing other tasks requiring mental alertness or coordination until tolerance is determined.
- Advise women to notify health care provider if pregnant, planning to become pregnant, or breastfeeding.
- Caution patient to avoid alcohol and other CNS depressant medications while using this medication.
- Advise patient, family, or caregiver not to take (give) any prescription or OTC medications or dietary supplements unless advised by health care provider.

Injection:
- Advise patient or caregiver that medication will be prepared and administered by a health care professional in a health care setting.

Oxytocin

(ox-ih-TOE-sin)
Class Oxytocic hormone
How Supplied
Pitocin Injection 10 units/mL

Action
PHARMACOLOGY: Endogenous hormone with uterine stimulant properties and vasopressive and antidiuretic effects.

PHARMACOKINETICS/DYNAMICS:
Distribution: Distributed throughout the extracellular fluid. Small amounts may reach fetal circulation.

Excretion: Small amounts are unchanged in the urine. The t½ of plasma is 1 to 6 min.

Onset: Onset of uterine contraction occurs almost immediately in the IV form. In the IM form, it occurs between 3 to 5 min.

Duration: IM is 2 to 3 hr. IV is 1 hr.

Indications Initiation or improvement of uterine contractions to achieve early vaginal delivery for maternal or fetal reasons (IV); as adjunctive therapy in the management of inevitable or incomplete abortion (IV); stimulation of uterine contractions during third stage of labor (IV); stimulation reinforcement of labor, as in selected cases of uterine inertia (IV); control of postpartum bleeding or hemorrhage (IV, IM); induction of labor in patients with a medical indication for the initiation of labor (eg, Rh problems, maternal diabetes, preeclampsia at or near term) when in the best interest of mother and fetus or when membranes are prematurely ruptured and delivery is indicated (IV).

Contraindications Hypersensitivity to the drug; significant cephalopelvic disproportion; inadequate, undeliverable fetal position; obstetric emergencies in which surgical intervention is preferred; cases of fetal distress in which delivery is not imminent; prolonged use in uterine inertia or severe toxemia; hypertonic or hyperactive uterine patterns; when adequate uterine activity fails to achieve satisfactory response; when vaginal delivery is contraindicated (eg, invasive cervical carcinoma, active herpes genitalis, total placenta previa, vasa previa, prolapse of the cord).

Route/Dosage
Induction or Stimulation of Labor
ADULTS: **IV infusion (drip method) or IV** 0.5 to 2 milliunits/min; adjust by no more than 1 to 2 milliunits/min at 30- to 60-min intervals until contraction pattern similar to normal labor is obtained. Once the desired frequency of contractions has been reached, the dose may be reduced by similar increments.

Treatment of Incomplete, Inevitable, or Elective Abortion
IV infusion 10 to 20 milliunits/min (max, 30 units in 12 hr).

Control of Postpartum Uterine Bleeding
IV infusion (drip method) 10 to 40 units in 1,000 mL diluent to run as infusion at rate necessary to control uterine atony. **IM** 10 units (1 mL) after delivery of placenta.

Interactions
Cyclopropane anesthesia: May cause maternal hypotension, bradycardia, and abnormal AV rhythms.
Vasoconstrictors/Caudal block anesthesia: Severe hypertension occurred when oxytocin was given 3 to 4 hr following prophylactic administration of a vasoconstrictor in conjunction with caudal block anesthesia.
INCOMPATIBILITIES: Sodium bicarbonate. Oxytocin is rapidly decomposed in the presence of sodium bisulfite.

Lab Test Interferences None well documented.

Adverse Reactions
CV: Maternal reactions include cardiac arrhythmias, premature ventricular contractions, hypertensive episodes; fetal or neonatal reactions include bradycardia, premature ventricular contractions, other arrhythmias.

CNS: Fetal or neonatal reactions include permanent CNS or brain damage and seizures.
EENT: Fetal or neonatal reactions include retinal hemorrhage.
GI: Maternal reactions include nausea and vomiting.
GU: Maternal reactions include rupture of uterus, uterine hypertonicity.
HEPA: Fetal or neonatal reactions include jaundice.
M/N: Maternal reactions include severe water intoxication with convulsion, coma, and death.
OTHER: Maternal reactions include anaphylactic reaction, fatal absence of fibrinogen in the plasma, pelvic hematoma, postpartum hemorrhage, subarachnoid hemorrhage; fetal and neonatal reactions include death, low Apgar scores at 5 min.

> **WARNING:**
> Oxytocin is not indicated for elective induction of labor.

Precautions
Pregnancy: No indication for use in first trimester unless related to spontaneous or induced abortion.
Lactation: Undetermined.

Special risk patients: Not recommended in prematurity, borderline cephalopelvic disproportion, previous major surgery on cervix or uterus (including cesarean section), uterine overdistention, grand multiparity, history of uterine sepsis, traumatic delivery, fetal distress, hydramnios, partial placenta previa, or invasive cervical carcinoma, except in unusual circumstances.
Mortality: Hypertensive episodes, subarachnoid hemorrhage, and rupture of uterus have resulted in maternal deaths. Fetal deaths and infant brain damage have been reported with IV use during first and second stages of labor.
Overstimulation of uterus: Overstimulation of uterus can occur and can be hazardous to mother and fetus.
Water intoxication: Consider possibility when patient is receiving oxytocin by IV infusion and fluids by mouth.

Overdosage: Signs and Symptoms
Uterine hyperactivity (hyperstimulation with hypertonic or tetanic contractions), uterine rupture, cervical and vaginal lacerations, postpartum hemorrhage, uteroplacental hypoperfusion, variable deceleration of fetal heart, fetal hypoxia, hypercapnia, perinatal hepatic necrosis, death, water intoxication with seizures.

PATIENT CARE CONSIDERATIONS
Administration/Storage
- Dosage is individualized and determined by uterine response.
- Do not administer if solution is discolored or cloudy, or if particulate matter is noted.
- Store ampuls, disposable syringes, and vials in refrigerator (36° to 46°F). May store at controlled room temperature (59° to 77°F) for up to 30 days. Discard after 30 days if stored at room temperature.
- Store oxytocin vials at controlled room temperature (59° to 86°F).

Induction or Stimulation of Labor:
- Administer by IV infusion only. Not for intradermal, subcutaneous, IM, IV bolus, or intra-arterial administration in this situation.
- For IV infusion add 1 mL (10 units) of oxytocin to 1,000 mL 0.9% sodium chloride injection or Ringer's lactate to produce solution containing 10 milliunits/mL (0.01 units/mL). Rotate infusion bottle to ensure thorough mixing. Administer via constant infusion pump to accurately control rate of infusion.
- Piggy-back oxytocin infusion on a physiologic electrolyte solution (eg, 0.9% sodium chloride injection).

Control of Postpartum Uterine Bleeding:
- Administer by IM injection or IV infusion only. Not for intradermal, subcutaneous, IV bolus, or intra-arterial administration in this situation.
- For IV infusion add 10 to 40 units (1 to 4 mL) of oxytocin to patient's IV infusion solution as ordered (do not exceed 40 units in 1,000 mL). Adjust infusion rate to sustain uterine contraction and control uterine atony.
- For IM administration, inject 10 units (1 mL) after delivery of placenta as ordered.

Treatment of Incomplete, Inevitable, or Elective Abortion:
- Administer by IV infusion only. Not for intradermal, subcutaneous, IM, IV bolus, or intra-arterial administration in this situation.
- For IV infusion add 10 units (1 mL) of oxytocin to 500 mL of physiologic saline solution or 5% dextrose-in-water solution.

Assessment/Interventions
- Obtain patient history, including drug history and any known allergies. Note fetal distress, hydramnios, partial placenta previa, prematurity, borderline cephalopelvic disproportion, any condition predisposing to uterine rupture

(eg, previous major surgery on cervix or uterus), concurrent or recent use of vasoconstrictor, or concurrent use of cyclopropane anesthesia.
- Review patient's health history for any of the following conditions that could contraindicate oxytocin therapy: hypersensitivity to oxytocin; significant cephalopelvic disproportion; unfavorable fetal position or presentation that is undeliverable without conversion prior to therapy; obstetrical emergency where benefit-to-risk ratio for the fetus or mother favors surgical intervention; fetal distress and delivery is not imminent; adequate uterine activity has failed to achieve satisfactory progress; uterus is already hyperactive or hypertonic; situation in which vaginal delivery is contraindicated (eg, active herpes genitalis, total placenta previa).
- Ensure that emergency resuscitation equipment is readily available.
- Obtain baseline vital signs, with special attention to pulse and BP. Closely monitor BP during treatment. Notify health care provider immediately if BP becomes elevated. Be prepared to discontinue therapy and treat appropriately.
- Ensure the uterine activity and fetal heart rate are electronically monitored throughout the infusion of oxytocin. Document fetal heart rate, resting uterine tone, and frequency, duration, and force of uterine contractions. Immediately discontinue infusion and notify health care provider in the event of uterine hyperactivity and/or fetal distress. Be prepared to treat appropriately (eg, place mother in a lateral position, administer oxygen).
- Monitor patient for signs of water intoxication during prolonged infusion, particularly when the patient is receiving fluids by mouth. If signs of water intoxication are noted or suspected (eg, drowsiness, listlessness, confusion, headache, anuria) immediately discontinue the infusion and notify health care provider.

Patient/Family Education
- Explain name, action, and potential side effects of drug to patient and family.
- Advise patient and family that medication will be prepared and administered by a health care provider in a medical setting with very close monitoring of the effects of the medication.

Oxytetracycline Hydrochloride/Polymyxin B Sulfate

(ox-ee-the-tra-SIGH-kleen HIGH-droe-KLOR-ide/pahl-ee-MIX-in BEE SULL-fate)

Class Ophthalmic Antibiotic

How Supplied
Terak with Polymyxin B Sulfate Ophthalmic Ointment 10,000 units/g polymyxin B sulfate and 5 mg/g oxytetracycline hydrochloride ♦
Terramycin with Polymyxin B Sulfate Ophthalmic Ointment 10,000 units/g polymyxin B sulfate and 5 mg/g oxytetracycline hydrochloride

Action
PHARMACOLOGY:
Oxytetracycline: Inhibits bacterial protein synthesis
Polymyxin B: Interacts with phospholipid components of bacterial cell membrane, increasing cell wall permeability.

Indications Treatment of superficial ocular infections involving the conjunctiva and/or cornea caused by susceptible organisms.

Contraindications Standard considerations.

Route/Dosage
Ophthalmic Approximately ½ inch of ointment squeezed from the tube onto the lower lid of the infected eye bid to qid.

Interactions None well documented.

Lab Test Interferences None well documented.

Adverse Reactions
SPEC SENSE: Blurred vision; stinging of the eye.
OTHER: Allergic hypersensitivity.

Precautions
Superinfection: Prolonged use may result in bacterial or fungal overgrowth of nonsusceptible microorganisms.

PATIENT CARE CONSIDERATIONS
Administration/Storage
- For ophthalmic use only. Not for use on the skin.
- Instill prescribed amount of ointment bid to qid.
- Do not allow tip of tube to touch eye, eyelid, fingers, or any other surface.
- If using other topical ophthalmic medications, instill drops first, wait at least 5 min, and instill ointment last.
- Store at controlled room temperature (59° to 77°F). Keep tube tightly closed.

Assessment/Interventions
- Obtain patient history, including drug history and any known allergies.
- Monitor patient's response to therapy. Notify health care provider if eye or eyelid inflammation is noted or if symptoms worsen or do not improve.

Patient/Family Education
- Explain name, dose, action, and potential side effects of drug.
- Review prescribed dosing schedule with patient, family, or caregiver.
- Remind patient, family, or caregiver that ointment is for use in the eye only.
- Teach patient, family, or caregiver proper technique for instilling ointment: wash hands; do not allow tip of tube to touch eye, eyelid, fingers, or any other surface. Tilt head back, look up; pull lower eyelid down to form pocket; place prescribed amount of ointment in the pocket. Look downward before closing eye. Do not rub eye.
- Advise patient, family, or caregiver that if more than 1 topical ophthalmic drug is being used, instill eye drops first, wait at least 5 min, and then instill ointment last.
- Inform patient that temporary blurred vision and stinging of the eye are the most common side effects and to contact health care provider if these symptoms occur and are bothersome.
- Advise patient to contact eye doctor if eye or eyelid inflammation is noted or if eye symptoms worsen or do not improve.
- Advise patient that the entire course of therapy must be completed to ensure maximal benefit and to complete full course of therapy even if symptoms have resolved.
- Instruct patient not to wear contact lenses during treatment.
- Remind patient, family, or caregiver that follow-up eye examinations may be necessary while using this medication and to keep appointments.

Paclitaxel

(pak-lih-TAX-uhl)

Class Mitotic inhibitor

How Supplied
Taxol Solution for injection 6 mg/mL

Action
PHARMACOLOGY: Paclitaxel is a novel antimicrotubule agent that promotes the assembly of microtubules from tubulin dimers and stabilizes microtubules. This stability inhibits the normal dynamic reorganization of the microtubule network that is essential for vital interphase and mitotic cellular functions. In addition, paclitaxel induces abnormal arrays or "bundles" of microtubules throughout the cell cycle and multiple esters of microtubules during mitosis, further disrupting cell function.

PHARMACOKINETICS/DYNAMICS:

Absorption: Following IV, the drug exhibits biphasic decline in plasma concentration.

Distribution: Initial rapid decline represents distribution to the peripheral compartment and elimination of the drug. Extensive extravascular distribution or tissue binding Vd is 227 to 688 L/m^2 over 24 hr infusion. The drug is 89% to 98% plasma protein bound. Major plasma proteins involved are α_1-acid glycoprotein, albumin, and lipoproteins.

Metabolism: Paclitaxel is metabolized primarily to 6α-hydroxypaclitaxel by isoenzyme CYP2C8 and to 2 minor metabolites, 3'-p-hydroxypaclitaxel and 6α_1 3'-p-dihydroxypaclitaxel, by CYP3A4.

Excretion: Following IV, the drug exhibits biphasic decline in plasma concentrations. 14% is excreted in the urine, 71% in the feces. Following 3 and 24 hr infusions, the elimination t½ is 13.1 to 52.7 hr and total body clearance is 12.2 to 23.8 L/hr/m^2.

Indications
Advanced ovarian carcinoma, breast cancer, AIDS-related Kaposi's sarcoma, non-small lung cancer. **Unlabeled use(s):** Squamous cell head and neck cancer, small-cell lung cancer, bladder cancer.

Contraindications
Hypersensitivity reactions to paclitaxel or other drugs formulated in *Cremophor EL* (polyoxyethylated castor oil) or polyoxyl 35 castor oil; patients with solid tumors who have baseline neutrophil count of fewer than 1500 cells/mm^3 or in patients with AIDS-related Kaposi's sarcoma with baseline neutrophil counts of less than 1000 cells/mm^3.

Route/Dosage
Usual Dose
ADULTS: **IV** Usual dose ranges from 135 mg/m^2 to 250 mg/m^2 per course of therapy.

Repeat Doses
ADULTS: **IV** After the initial course, hold further courses of therapy until neutrophil count is at least 1500/mm^3 and platelet count is no less than 100,000/mm^3. Reduce dose 20% for subsequent courses in patients who develop severe neutropenia or severe neuropathy. Hold therapy until neutrophil count is at least 1000/mm^3 in AIDS patients.

Ovarian Carcinoma
ADULTS: **IV infusion** For single agents, use 135 to 175 mg/m^2 over 3 hr q 3 wk. When combined with other agents, use 135 mg/m^2 by IV infusion over 24 hr q 3 wk.

Breast Cancer
ADULTS: **IV infusion** 175 mg/m^2 over 3 hr q 3 wk.

Non-Small Cell Lung Cancer
ADULTS: **IV infusion** When combined with other agents, use 135 mg/m^2 over 24 hr q 3 wk.

Kaposi's Sarcoma
ADULTS: **IV infusion** 135 mg/m^2 over 3 hr q 3 wk. As an alternate regiment, use 100 mg/m^2 by IV infusion over 3 hr q 2 wk.

Pretreatment Regimen
ADULTS: **PO** or **IV** Reduce incidence of hypersensitivity reactions. Premedicate with each of the following:
Corticosteroid: Dexamethasone 20 mg **PO** or **IV** 12 and 6 hr before paclitaxel administration. Reduce each dexamethasone dose to 10 mg in AIDS patients. Some clinicians give a third dexamethasone dose immediately prior to paclitaxel.
Diphenhydramine: 50 mg **IV** 30 to 60 min before paclitaxel.
Histamine H$_2$ antagonist: Cimetidine 300 mg, ranitidine 50 mg, or famotidine 20 mg **IV** 30 to 60 min before paclitaxel administration.

Interactions
Cisplatin: Paclitaxel clearance may decrease when given after cisplatin, resulting in increased hematologic toxicity.
CYP450 inducers: May induce the metabolism of paclitaxel.
CYP450 inhibitors: May decrease the metabolism of paclitaxel.
Doxorubicin: Paclitaxel may increase plasma concentrations of doxorubicin and its active metabolite, doxorubicinol.

Ketoconazole: Ketoconazole may inhibit paclitaxel metabolism.

Lab Test Interferences None well documented.

Adverse Reactions
CV: Hypotension, bradycardia.
CNS: Peripheral neuropathy.
DERM: Alopecia, radiation recall.
GI: Nausea, vomiting, diarrhea, mucositis, elevated LFTs.
HEMA: Bone marrow suppression, neutrophil nadir at 11 days, platelet nadir at 8 to 9 days.
HYPERSEN: Acute anaphylactic reactions with symptoms of dyspnea, hypotension, angioedema, and generalized urticaria.
MUSC: Arthralgias and myalgias.

> **WARNING:**
> Anaphylaxis and severe hypersensitivity reactions have occurred in 2% to 4% of patients. Fatal reactions have occurred despite premedication. Pretreat patients receiving paclitaxel with corticosteroids, diphenhydramine, and H_2 antagonists to prevent these reactions. Do not rechallenge patients who experience severe hypersensitivity reactions to paclitaxel with the drug. Contraindicated in solid tumor patients with baseline neutrophil counts less than 1500 cells/mm^3 and in AIDS-related Kaposi sarcoma patients with baseline neutrophil counts less than 1000 cells/mm^3.

Precautions
Pregnancy: Category D.
Lactation: Undetermined.
Children: Safety and efficacy not established.
Hypersensitivity: Do not use in patients with a history of severe hypersensitivity reactions to products containing *Cremophor EL* (polyoxyethylated castor oil). Pretreat patients with corticosteroids, diphenhydramine, and H_2 antagonists. Patients with a history of allergic reactions to bee stings may have an increased risk for a hypersensitivity reaction with paclitaxel.
Hepatic function impairment: May require dosage reduction. Exercise caution when administering to patients with moderate to severe hepatic impairment and consider dose adjustments.
Extravasation: Can cause local irritation or phlebitis.
Bone marrow suppression: Bone marrow suppression (primarily neutropenia) is dose-dependent and is the major dose-limiting toxicity. Do not administer to patients with baseline neutrophil counts of less than 1500 cells/mm^3.
Cardiac effects: Severe conduction abnormalities have been documented in fewer than 1% of patients during therapy, sometimes requiring a pacemaker. Hypotension, hypertension, and bradycardia also observed.
CNS: Peripheral neuropathy (glove-and-stocking distribution) occurs frequently.

Overdosage: Signs and Symptoms
Bone marrow suppression, peripheral neurotoxicity, mucositis.

PATIENT CARE CONSIDERATIONS

Administration/Storage
- Store at room temperature and protect from light. Diluted 0.3 to 1.2 mg/mL solutions are stable for no more than 27 hr at room temperature under normal room lighting.
- Dilute to a final concentration of 0.3 to 1.2 mg/mL with any of the following solutions: 0.9% Sodium Chloride, 5% Dextrose, or 0.9% Sodium Chloride with 5% Dextrose.
- Solution may appear hazy.
- May leach DEHP from PVC infusion sets or bags. Use glass, polypropylene, or polyolefin containers.
- IV infusion over 1 to 24 hr via non-PVC-containing administration sets.
- Administer through an in-line 0.22 micron filter.

Assessment/Interventions
- Monitor WBC and platelet counts at baseline and throughout therapy. For WBC less than 1500/mm^3 or platelet count less than 100,000/mm^3, withhold therapy.
- Avoid use in patients with previous hypersensitivity reactions to *Cremophor EL* (eg, cyclosporine injection, teniposide injection).
- Frequently monitor vital signs, particularly during the first hour of infusion.

Patient/Family Education
- Explain name, action, and potential side effects of drug.
- Advise patient, family, or caregiver that medication will be prepared and administered by health care provider in a health care setting.
- Advise patient, family, or caregiver that medication may be used in combination with other agents to achieve maximum benefit possible.
- Review dosing schedule with patient, family, or caregiver.
- Advise patient, family or caregiver that additional medications will be given before

paclitaxel administration to reduce side effects of paclitaxel.
- Advise patient, family, or caregiver to immediately report any of the following to health care provider: rash; hives; shortness of breath or difficulty breathing; fever, chills or other signs of infection; sores in mouth; unusual bleeding or bruising; pain, redness or swelling at injection site.
- Advise patient, family, or caregiver to report any of the following to health care provider: persistent nausea, vomiting, diarrhea or appetite loss; numbness, tingling or burning in arms or legs; persistent muscle or joint pain.
- Advise patient, family, or caregiver that medication may cause hair loss but that this is reversible when therapy is stopped.
- Instruct patient to not take any prescription or OTC medications or dietary supplements unless advised by health care provider.
- Caution women of childbearing potential to avoid becoming pregnant while being treated.
- Instruct women of childbearing potential to notify health care provider if they become pregnant, plan on becoming pregnant, or are breastfeeding.
- Advise patient that after discharge follow-up visits and laboratory tests will be required to monitor therapy and to be sure to keep appointments.

Palivizumab

(pal-eh-VIZ-u-mab)
Class Monoclonal antibody
How Supplied
Synagis Powder for injection, lyophilized 50 mg, Powder for injection, lyophilized 100 mg
Action
PHARMACOLOGY: Neutralizing and fusion-inhibitory activity against respiratory syncytial virus (RSV), inhibiting RSV replication.
PHARMACOKINETICS/DYNAMICS:
Excretion: The t½ is 20 days in children younger than 24 mo.
Indications Prevention of serious lower respiratory tract disease caused by RSV in pediatric patients at high risk of RSV disease.
Contraindications Standard considerations.
Route/Dosage
PEDIATRICS: **IM** 15 mg/kg monthly, preferably in anterolateral aspect of thigh. Give doses greater than 1 mL in divided doses.
Interactions None well documented.
Lab Test Interferences None well documented.
Adverse Reactions
DERM: Rash.
EENT: Otitis media, rhinitis (at least 1%).
GI: Diarrhea; vomiting; gastroenteritis.
HEPA: Increased AST (at least 1%).
RESP: Upper respiratory tract infection (at least 1%); cough; wheezing.
OTHER: Fever (at least 1%); hypersensitivity including dyspnea, cyanosis, respiratory failure, urticaria, pruritus, angioedema, hypotonia, and unresponsiveness (postmarketing).
Precautions
Pregnancy: Category C.
Hypersensitivity: Rare cases of anaphylaxis have been reported following re-exposure; rare severe cases of acute hypersensitivity reactions have been reported on initial or re-exposure.
Adults: Not indicated for adult use.

PATIENT CARE CONSIDERATIONS

Administration/Storage
- For IM administration only. Not for intradermal, SC, or IV administration.
- Dose is usually administered once every month during RSV season. Administer the first dose prior to the beginning of RSV season.
- Reconstitute powder for injection following manufacturer's guidelines using sterile water for injection.
- Do not shake the vial during reconstitution. Allow vial to stand, undisturbed, for a minimum of 20 min at room temperature until solution clarifies.
- Administer reconstituted solution immediately; store, if necessary, for up to 6 hr at room temperature (59° to 86°F).
- Do not administer if particulate matter or discoloration is noted.
- Administer prescribed dose by IM injection, preferably in the anterolateral aspect of the thigh. Do not use gluteal muscle routinely as injection site because of risk of damage to sciatic nerve.
- Give injection volumes greater than 1 mL as a divided dose.
- Discard any unused solution. Do not save for future administration.
- Store powder for injection in refrigerator (36° to 46°F). Do not freeze.

Assessment/Interventions
- Obtain patient history, including drug history and any known allergies. Note thrombocyto-

penia, coagulation disorder, or history of previous reaction to palivizumab.
* Ensure that dose is administered as soon as possible to a patient who has undergone cardiopulmonary bypass procedure, even if it has not been 1 mo since the previous dose. Ensure further doses are administered monthly thereafter.
* Monitor patient for signs and symptoms of anaphylactic or serious allergic reaction. Notify health care provider immediately and be prepared to treat appropriately.
* Monitor patient for RESP, GI, general body side effects, and injection site reactions. Report to health care provider if noted and significant.

Patient/Family Education
* Explain name, dose, action, and potential side effects of drug.
* Advise family or caregiver that medication will be prepared and administered by a health care professional in a health care setting.
* Educate family or caregiver of importance of monthly injection in helping to prevent RSV infection during the RSV season.
* Advise family or caregiver to report any of the following to health care provider: injection site reactions; fever or other signs of infection; sore throat; rash; itching; hives; swelling of the face, lips, eyes, or tongue; diarrhea; wheezing; shortness of breath; difficulty breathing.
* Instruct family or caregiver not to administer any prescription or OTC medications or dietary supplements unless advised by health care provider.
* Advise family or caregiver that follow-up office visits will be required to administer and monitor therapy and to keep appointments.

Palonosetron

(pal-oh-NO-seh-trahn)
Class Antiemetic
How Supplied
Aloxi Injection 0.25 mg
Action
PHARMACOLOGY: Selective antagonist for the 5-HT$_3$ receptor with a strong binding affinity for this receptor.

PHARMACOKINETICS/DYNAMICS:
Absorption: Following IV administration, the C$_{max}$ and AUC are generally dose-proportional. After a single IV dose at 3 mcg/kg, the mean C$_{max}$ was approximately 5.6 ng/mL and the AUC was 35.8 ng•hr/mL.

Distribution: Vd is approximately 8.3 L/kg and protein binding is about 62%.

Metabolism: Approximately 50% is metabolized to 2 metabolites that have less than 1% of the activity of palonosetron. The major isozyme responsible for metabolism appears to be CYP2D6 and, to a lesser degree, CYP1A2 and CYP3A are involved.

Excretion: Approximately 80% of the dose is recovered in the urine. The terminal t½ is approximately 40 hr.

Indications Prevention of acute nausea and vomiting associated with moderately and highly emetogenic cancer chemotherapy; prevention of delayed nausea and vomiting associated with moderately emetogenic cancer chemotherapy.

Contraindications Standard considerations.

Route/Dosage
ADULTS: **IV** 0.25 mg as a single dose approximately 30 min before the start of chemotherapy. Repeated dosing within a 7 day interval is not recommended.

Interactions None well documented.
Incompatibilities: Do not mix with other drugs.

Lab Test Interferences None well documented.

Adverse Reactions
CV: Nonsustained tachycardia, bradycardia, hypotension (1%).
CNS: Headache (9%); dizziness, anxiety (1%).
GI: Constipation (5%); diarrhea (1%).
METAB: Hyperkalemia (1%).
OTHER: Weakness (1%).

Precautions
Pregnancy: Category B.
Lactation: Undetermined.
Children: Safety and efficacy not established.
Hypersensitivity: May occur in patients who have exhibited hypersensitivity to other selective 5-HT$_3$ receptor antagonists.
CV effects: Although palonosetron has been safely administered to patients with pre-existing cardiac impairment, administer with caution in patients who have or may develop prolongation of cardiac conduction intervals, particularly QTc.

PATIENT CARE CONSIDERATIONS
Administration/Storage
* For IV administration only. Not for intradermal, SC, or IM administration.
* Do not administer if particulate matter, cloudiness, or discoloration noted.
* Administer prescribed dose via 30 sec IV infusion 30 min before start of chemotherapy.

- Discard any unused solution. Do not save unused solution for later administration.
- Do not repeat dose within 7 days.
- Do not mix with other medications.
- Store vials at controlled room temperature (59° to 86°F). Protect from light and freezing.

Assessment/Interventions
- Obtain patient history, including drug history and any known allergies. Note hypokalemia, hypomagnesemia, cumulative high dose anthracycline therapy, or concurrent use of diuretics or other medications that can prolong the QT interval. Note history of congenital QT syndrome and prior use and effectiveness of antiemetic therapy.
- Monitor patient for antiemetic efficacy. Notify health care provider if nausea or vomiting are not prevented.
- Assess patient for CNS, GI, and general body side effects. Inform health care provider if noted and significant.

Patient/Family Education
- Explain name, action, and potential side effects of drug.
- Advise patient, family, or caregiver that medication will be prepared and administered by health care professional in a medical facility.
- Advise patient, family, or caregiver that medication will greatly reduce likelihood of nausea or vomiting but these are still possible.
- Instruct patient to inform health care provider if medication does not prevent nausea or vomiting.
- Advise patient to report any of the following to health care provider: intolerable headache; persistent or intolerable constipation or diarrhea.

Pamidronate Disodium

(pam-IH-DROE-nate die-SO-dee-uhm)

Class Bisphosphonate

How Supplied
Aredia Powder for injection, lyophilized 30 mg, Powder for injection, lyophilized 90 mg ♦ *Pamidronate Disodium* Injection 3 mg/mL, Injection 6 mg/mL, Injection 9 mg/mL

Action
PHARMACOLOGY: Inhibits normal and abnormal bone resorption.

PHARMACOKINETICS/DYNAMICS:
Distribution: Adsorbed to bone in areas of high turnover.
Metabolism: Not metabolized.
Excretion: Renal excretion (46% unchanged). The t½ is 28 hr. Renal Cl is 49 mL/min.

Indications Treatment of moderate to severe hypercalcemia associated with malignancy with or without bone metastases; treatment of moderate to severe Paget disease of bone; treatment of osteolytic bone lesions of multiple myeloma and bone metastases of breast cancer in conjunction with standard chemotherapy. **Unlabeled use(s):** Treatment of postmenopausal osteoporosis; treatment of hyperparathyroidism; prevention of glucocorticoid-induced osteoporosis; management of immobilization-related hypercalcemia; reduction of bone pain in prostatic carcinoma.

Contraindications Hypersensitivity to bisphosphonates.

Route/Dosage
Moderate to Severe Hypercalcemia of Malignancy
ADULTS: IV For moderate, give 60 to 90 mg as an initial single-dose infusion over 2 to 24 hr. For severe, give 90 mg as an initial single-dose infusion over 2 to 24 hr. For retreatment, same as initial therapy, at least 7 days after initial dose.

Paget Disease
ADULTS: IV 30 mg/day as a 4-hr infusion on 3 consecutive days for a total dose of 90 mg. For retreatment, same as initial therapy, when clinically indicated.

Osteolytic Bone Metastases of Breast Cancer
ADULTS: IV 90 mg as a 2-hr infusion q 3 to 4 wk.

Osteolytic Bone Lesions of Multiple Myeloma
ADULTS: IV 90 mg as a 4-hr infusion on a monthly basis.

Interactions None well documented.
INCOMPATIBILITIES: Calcium-containing infusion solutions (eg, Ringer's solution). Do not mix.

Lab Test Interferences None well documented.

Adverse Reactions
CV: Atrial fibrillation; atrial flutter; cardiac failure; hypertension; syncope; tachycardia.
CNS: Asthenia; anxiety; fatigue; headache; insomnia; paresthesia; psychosis; somnolence.
DERM: Sweating.
ENDO: Hypothyroidism.

GI: Abdominal pain; anorexia; constipation; diarrhea; dyspepsia; GI hemorrhage; nausea; stomatitis; vomiting.
GU: UTI; uremia; renal toxicity.
HEMA/LYMPH: Anemia; granulocytopenia; leukopenia; neutropenia; thrombocytopenia.
LAB TESTS ABS: Hypocalcemia; hypokalemia; hypomagnesemia; hypophosphatemia.
LOCAL: Infusion-site reaction.
MUSC: Arthralgia; arthrosis; back pain; bone pain; musculoskeletal pain; myalgia; osteonecrosis primarily of the jaws (postmarketing).
RESP: Coughing; dyspnea; pleural effusion; rales; rhinitis; sinusitis; upper respiratory infection.
OTHER: Edema; fever; metastases; moniliasis; pain; allergic manifestations (eg, hypotension, dyspnea, angioedema, anaphylactic shock) (postmarketing).

Precautions

Pregnancy: Category D.
Lactation: Undetermined.
Children: Safety and efficacy not established.
Hypocalcemia: Hypocalcemia has occurred.
GI disorders: Use with caution in patients with active upper GI problems such as dysphagia (eg, difficulty swallowing), symptomatic esophageal diseases, gastritis, duodenitis, or ulcers.
Osteonecrosis of the jaw: Has been reported in patients with cancer receiving treatment regimens that include bisphosphonates. Risk factors include cancer chemotherapy, corticosteroid administration, and poor oral hygiene.
Renal insufficiency: Because pamidronate is excreted primarily by the kidney, the risk of adverse reactions may be increased in patients with impaired renal function. In patients receiving pamidronate for bone metastases and who have evidence of renal function deterioration, the drug should be withheld until renal function returns to baseline. Pamidronate has not been tested in patients with class Dc renal impairment (creatinine above 5 mg/dL).

Overdosage: Signs and Symptoms

High fever, hypotension, hypocalcemia, transient taste perversion.

PATIENT CARE CONSIDERATIONS

Administration/Storage

- For IV administration only. Not for intradermal, subcutaneous, IM, intra-arterial, or oral administration.
- Concentrated injection solution must be further diluted before administration.
- Reconstitute lyophilized powder with 10 mL sterile water for injection. Allow drug to dissolve completely before withdrawing for further dilution.
- Do not mix pamidronate with calcium-containing IV solutions (eg, Ringer's solution) or other IV medications.
- Do not administer if particulate matter or discoloration noted.
- Administer diluted solution via separate IV line.
- Store unopened vials below 86°F. Powder reconstituted with sterile water for injection may be stored in refrigerator (36° to 46°F) for up to 24 hr. Diluted solution for infusion may be stored at room temperature for up to 24 hr.

Hypercalcemia of malignancy:

- Dilute the recommended dose in 1,000 mL 0.45% or 0.9% sodium chloride or 5% dextrose injection. Infuse prescribed dose over 2 to 24 hr as ordered. Do not retreat for at least 7 days.

Paget Disease:

- Dilute the recommended dose in 500 mL 0.45% or 0.9% sodium chloride or 5% dextrose injection. Infuse prescribed dose over 4 hr on 3 consecutive days.

Osteolytic bone lesions of multiple myeloma:

- Dilute the recommended dose in 500 mL 0.45% or 0.9% sodium chloride or 5% dextrose injection. Infuse prescribed dose over 4 hr q 4 wk as ordered.

Osteolytic bone metastases of breast cancer:

- Dilute the recommended dose in 500 mL 0.45% or 0.9% sodium chloride or 5% dextrose injection. Infuse prescribed dose over 2 hr q 3 to 4 wk as ordered.

Assessment/Interventions

- Obtain patient history, including drug history and any known allergies. Note renal impairment, hypersensitivity to bisphosphonates, or concurrent use of nephrotoxic drug.
- Record dates and response to any previous treatment with pamidronate or other bisphosphonates.
- To reduce risk of renal toxicity ensure that single dose does not exceed 90 mg.
- Ensure that women of childbearing potential are not pregnant when therapy begins and use effective contraception during treatment.
- Ensure that serum creatinine is assessed before each dose of pamidronate. Be prepared to withhold therapy in patient being treated for bone metastases if renal function is noted to have deteriorated (Scr increases 0.5 mg/dL in patient with normal baseline creatinine or Scr increases 1 mg/dL in patient with abnormal baseline creatinine).
- Ensure that serum calcium, phosphate, magnesium, and potassium are monitored and

recorded before and periodically during therapy. Notify health care provider if abnormalities noted. Be prepared to treat symptomatic hypocalcemia.
- Ensure that a dental examination is performed, and preventive dentistry is completed, before starting therapy in patient at risk for developing osteonecrosis of the jaw (eg, cancer, chemotherapy, corticosteroids, poor oral hygiene). While on treatment, avoid invasive dental procedures if possible.
- Ensure that CBC, differential, hemoglobin, and hematocrit are determined before therapy is initiated. Monitor these parameters closely for the first 2 wk of therapy if preexisting anemia, leukopenia, or thrombocytopenia is noted.
- Ensure that vigorous saline hydration is utilized in patient being treated for hypercalcemia of malignancy.
- Monitor patient for signs of fluid overload during saline hydration. Notify health care provider if noted or suspected and be prepared to administer diuretics if ordered.
- Monitor and record temperature before and during treatment.
- If infusion site reaction develops (eg, redness, swelling, induration, pain) discontinue infusion, elevate site, and apply ice pack for 15 to 20 min q 4 to 6 hr for 72 hr.
- Monitor patient for signs of allergic reaction during and shortly after infusion. Discontinue therapy and immediately notify health care provider if noted. Be prepared to treat appropriately.
- Assess patient for GI, CNS, MUSC, and general body side effects. Report to health care provider if noted and significant.

Patient/Family Education
- Explain name, dose, action, and potential side effects of drug.
- Advise patient that medication will be prepared and administered by a health care provider in a health care setting and that medication will not be administered at home.
- Advise patient that infusion-site reactions (eg, redness, swelling, hardness, pain) can be treated with local measures (eg, warm or cold packs) and oral OTC analgesics (eg, acetaminophen, ibuprofen). Advise patient to report infusion-site reactions that do not respond to symptomatic treatment to health care provider.
- Instruct patient to report the following symptoms to health care provider: tingling, numbness, muscle spasms, stomach pain, fever, fatigue, swelling, nausea, appetite loss, constipation, diarrhea, vomiting, inflammation of the mouth, difficulty breathing, muscle or bone pain.
- Advise women of childbearing potential to use effective contraception during treatment with pamidronate.
- Advise women to notify health care provider if pregnant, planning to become pregnant, or breastfeeding.
- Instruct patient not to take any prescription or OTC medications, herbal preparations, or dietary supplements unless advised by health care provider.
- Advise patient that follow-up visits and laboratory tests will be required to monitor therapy and to keep appointments.

Pancrelipase

(pan-KREE-lih-pace)

Class Digestive enzyme

How Supplied
Creon 5 Capsules, delayed-release 5000 U lipase/18,750 U protease/16,600 U amylase ♦ *Creon 10* Capsules, delayed-release 10,000 U lipase/37,500 U protease/33,200 U amylase ♦ *Creon 20* Capsules, delayed-release 20,000 U lipase/75,000 U protease/66,400 U amylase ♦ *Kutrase* Capsules 2400 U lipase/30,000 U protease/30,000 U amylase ♦ *Ku-Zyme* Capsules 1200 U lipase/15,000 U protease/15,000 U amylase ♦ *Ku-Zyme HP* Capsules 8000 U lipase/30,000 U protease/30,000 U amylase/lactose ♦ *Lipram* 4500 Capsules, delayed-release 4500 U lipase/25,000 U protease/20,000 U amylase ♦ *Lipram-CR5* Capsules, delayed-release 5000 U lipase/18,750 U protease/16,600 U amylase ♦ *Lipram-CR10* Capsules, delayed-release 10,000 U lipase/37,500 U protease/33,200 U amylase ♦ *Lipram-CR20* Capsules, delayed-release 20,000 U lipase/75,000 U protease/66,400 U amylase ♦ *Lipram-PN10* Capsules, delayed-release 10,000 U lipase/30,000 U protease/30,000 U amylase ♦ *Lipram-PN16* Capsules, delayed-release 16,000 U lipase/48,000 U protease/48,000 U amylase ♦ *Lipram-PN20* Capsules, delayed-release 20,000 U lipase/44,000 U protease/56,000 U amylase ♦ *Lipram-UL12* Capsules, delayed-release 12,000 U lipase/39,000 U protease/39,000 U amylase ♦ *Lipram-UL18* Capsules, delayed-release 18,000 U lipase/58,500 U protease/58,500 U protease ♦ *Lipram-UL20* Capsules, delayed-release 20,000 U lipase/65,000 U protease/65,000 U protease ♦ *Pancrease* Capsules 4500 U lipase/25,000 U protease/20,000 U amylase ♦ *Pancrease MT 4* Capsules 4000 U lipase/12,000 U protease/12,000 U amylase ♦ *Pancrease MT 10* Capsules 10,000 U lipase/30,000 U

protease/30,000 U amylase ♦ *Pancrease MT 16 Capsules* 16,000 U lipase/48,000 U protease/48,000 U amylase ♦ *Pancrease MT 20 Capsules* 20,000 U lipase/44,000 U protease/56,000 U amylase ♦ *Pancrecarb MS-4 Capsules*, delayed-release 4000 U lipase/25,000 U protease/25,000 U amylase ♦ *Pancrecarb MS-8 Capsules*, delayed-release 8000 U lipase/45,000 U protease/40,000 U amylase ♦ *Pancrelipase Capsules* 4500 U lipase/25,000 U protease/20,000 U amylase, Tablets 8000 U lipase/30,000 U protease/30,000 U amylase, Capsules 16,000 U lipase/48,000 U protease/48,000 U amylase, Tablets 16,000 U lipase/60,000 U protease/60,000 U amylase ♦ *Panokase* Tablets 8000 U lipase/30,000 U protease/30,000 U amylase ♦ *Plaretase* 8000 Tablets 8000 U lipase/30,000 U protease/30,000 U amylase ♦ *Ultrase* Capsules 4500 U lipase/25,000 U protease/20,000 U amylase ♦ *Ultrase MT 12* Capsules 12,000 U lipase/39,000 U protease/39,000 U amylase ♦ *Ultrase MT 18* Capsules 18,000 U lipase/58,500 U protease/58,500 U protease ♦ *Ultrase MT 20* Capsules 20,000 U lipase/65,000 U protease/65,000 U protease ♦ *Viokase* Powder 16,000 U lipase/60,000 U protease/60,000 U amylase ♦ *Viokase 8* Tablets 8000 U lipase/30,000 U protease/30,000 U amylase ♦ *Viokase 16* Tablets 16,000 U lipase/60,000 U protease/60,000 U amylase

🍁 *Creon 5* ♦ *Creon 10* ♦ *Creon 20* ♦ *Pancrease MT*

Action

PHARMACOLOGY: Helps to digest and absorb fats, proteins, and carbohydrates from food.

Indications Enzyme replacement therapy in patients who do not produce enough pancreatic enzymes because of cystic fibrosis, chronic pancreatitis, postpancreatectomy, ductal obstructions caused by cancer of pancreas or common bile duct, pancreatic insufficiency; treatment of steatorrhea of malabsorption syndrome; postgastrectomy or after GI surgery; pancreatic function testing.

Contraindications Hypersensitivity to pork protein or enzymes; acute pancreatitis; acute exacerbations of chronic pancreatic disease.

Route/Dosage

Dosage is adjusted based on severity of the exocrine pancreatic enzyme deficiency. Dosage recommendation varies with the brand and formulation. Take capsules or tablets with meals or snacks.

KU-ZYME, PANCRECARB, ULTRASE, ULTRASE MT

ADULTS: **PO** Start with 1 or 2 capsules with each meal or snack.

KUTRASE

ADULTS: **PO** Take 1 capsule with each meal or snack.

KU-ZYME HP

ADULTS: **PO** Take 1 to 3 capsules with each meal or snack. In severe deficiencies, increase the dose to 8 capsules with meals or increase the frequency to hourly intervals if nausea, cramps, or diarrhea do not occur.

PANCREASE, PANCREASE MT 4

CHILDREN (OVER 4 YR): **PO** Start with 400 lipase U/kg/meal up to a max of 2500 lipase U/kg/meal.

CHILDREN (UNDER 4 YR): **PO** Start with 1000 lipase U/kg with each meal up to a max of 2500 lipase U with each meal.

CHILDREN (UP TO 12 MO): **PO** 2000 to 4000 lipase U/120 mL of formula or breast milk.

PANCRELIPASE, LIPRAM

ADULTS: **PO** 4000 to 20,000 lipase U with each meal and with snacks.

CHILDREN (7 TO 12 YR): **PO** 4000 to 12,000 lipase U with each meal and with snacks.

CHILDREN (1 TO 6 YR): **PO** 4000 to 8000 lipase U with each meal and 4000 U with each snack.

CHILDREN (6 MO TO UNDER 1 YR): **PO** 2000 lipase U with each meal.

CREON 5

ADULTS AND CHILDREN (OVER 6 YR): **PO** Usual starting dose is 2 to 4 capsules with each meal or snack.

CHILDREN (UNDER 6 YR): **PO** Start with 1 to 2 capsules with each meal or snack. Select exact dose based on clinical experience with this age group.

Cystic Fibrosis Patients
PO Usual doses are 1500 to 3000 lipase U/kg with each meal (max, 6000 lipase U/kg/meal).

CREON 10

ADULTS AND CHILDREN (OVER 6 YR): **PO** Usual starting dose is 1 to 2 capsules with each meal or snack.

CHILDREN (UNDER 6 YR): **PO** Usual starting dose is up to 1 capsule with each meal or snack.

Cystic Fibrosis Patients
PO Usual doses are 1500 to 3000 lipase U/kg with each meal (max, 6000 lipase U/kg/meal).

CREON 20

ADULTS AND CHILDREN (OVER 6 YR): **PO** Start with 1 capsule with each meal or snack.

CHILDREN (UNDER 6 YR): **PO** Select exact dose based on clinical experience with this age group.

Cystic Fibrosis Patients
PO Usual starting doses are 1500 to 3000 lipase U/kg with each meal (max, 6000 lipase U/kg/meal).

PANOKASE, PLARETASE, VIOKASE (TABLETS)
Cystic Fibrosis and Chronic Pancreatitis Patients
PO Dose ranges from 8000 to 32,000 lipase U (1 to 4 tablets [Plaretase, Panokase, Viokase 8] or 1 to 2 tablets [Viokase 16]) with each meal.

Pancreatectomy or Obstruction of Pancreatic Ducts
PO 1 to 2 tablets (Plaretase, Panokase, Viokase 8) or 1 tablet (Viokase 16) q 2 hr.

VIOKASE (POWDER)
Cystic Fibrosis
PO 0.7 g (1/4 tsp) with each meal.

Interactions
Antacids: Calcium carbonate or magnesium hydroxide may negate beneficial effect of enzymes.
Iron: Serum iron response to oral iron may be decreased with concomitant pancreatic enzyme administration.

Lab Test Interferences None well documented.

PATIENT CARE CONSIDERATIONS
Administration/Storage
- Do not crush or allow patient to chew enteric-coated formulations.
- Give with or before meals.
- If powder spills on hands, wash with soap and water immediately.
- If patient has difficulty swallowing capsule, open capsule and shake onto small quantity of soft, non-hot food (eg, applesauce, gelatin) that does not require chewing. Have patient swallow immediately without chewing to avoid irritating GI mucosa. Follow with glass of juice or water.
- Be careful not to inhale powder, which can irritate mucosal surfaces and cause asthma attack.
- Store at room temperature in tightly closed container. Protect from moisture.

Assessment/Interventions
- Obtain patient history, including drug history and any known allergies.
- Assess bowel status before and during treatment.

Adverse Reactions
DERM: Perianal irritation.
GI: Colonic strictures; diarrhea; abdominal pain; intestinal obstruction; vomiting; intestinal stenosis; constipation; flatulence; nausea; bloating; cramping.
OTHER: Hypersensitivity reaction.

Precautions
Pregnancy: Category B (Pancrease, Pancrease MT); Category C (Creon, Ku-Zyme, Ku-Zyme HP, Kutrase, Lipram, Pancrelipase, Panokase, Plaretase, Ultrase, Ultrase MT, Viokase).
Lactation: Undetermined.
Asthma: Inhalation of airborne pancrelipase powder can precipitate asthma attack.
Colonic strictures: Colonic strictures reported primarily in cystic fibrosis patients often at dosages above the recommended range.
Skin irritation: Contact of pancrelipase with skin can cause irritation.

Overdosage: Signs and Symptoms
Nausea, vomiting, abdominal cramps, diarrhea, hyperuricosuria, hyperuricemia.

- Maintain growth chart on children.
- Assess for steatorrhea.
- If symptoms of sensitivity occur, discontinue drug and initiate symptomatic and supportive therapy.
- If nausea, abdominal cramps, or diarrhea develop, notify health care provider.

Patient/Family Education
- Tell patient not to change brands without notifying health care provider. Products are not bioequivalent.
- Advise patient not to take pancrelipase with antacid containing calcium carbonate or magnesium hydroxide.
- Stress to patient the importance of taking drug before or with meals to enhance effectiveness of drug.
- Instruct patient to avoid inhaling powder to reduce chance of irritating mucous membranes or precipitating asthma attack.
- Advise patient to follow any special dietary recommendations from health care provider or dietitian.

Pancuronium Bromide

(PAN-cue-ROW-nee-uhm BROE-mide)

Class Nondepolarizing neuromuscular blocker

How Supplied
Pancuronium Bromide Injection 1 mg/mL, Injection 2 mg/mL

Action
PHARMACOLOGY: Binds competitively to cholinergic receptors on motor end-plate to antagonize action of acetylcholine, resulting in block of neuromuscular transmission.

PHARMACOKINETICS/DYNAMICS:
Distribution: Vd is 241 to 280 mL/kg. Plasma protein binding is 87%; strong binding to gamma globulin and moderate to albumin.

Metabolism: Hepatic to active 3-hydroxy metabolite, which is half as potent a blocking agent as pancuronium. Other less potent metabolites include 17-hydroxy metabolite and 3,17-dihydroxy metabolite.

Excretion: Urine (40% as unchanged), bile (11% as metabolites). The $t_{½}$ is 89 to 161 min. Plasma Cl is approximately 1.1 to 1.9 mL/min/kg.

Special Populations:
Renal Function Impairment – Elimination $t_{½}$ doubles, plasma Cl reduces 60%, and Vd may be elevated and variable.
Hepatic Function Impairment – In patients with cirrhosis, the Vd increases approximately 50%, plasma Cl decreases 22%, and elimination $t_{½}$ doubles.
Biliary obstruction – Plasma Cl decreases 50%, Vd increases approximately 50%, and elimination $t_{½}$ doubles.

Indications
Adjunct to general anesthesia for induction of skeletal muscle relaxation; facilitation of management of patients undergoing mechanical ventilation; facilitation of tracheal intubation.

Contraindications
Standard considerations.

Route/Dosage
Individualize dose to each case.
Endotracheal Intubation
ADULTS AND CHILDREN OLDER THAN 1 MO OF AGE: **IV** bolus 0.06 to 0.1 mg/kg. Skeletal muscle relaxation usually occurs in 2 to 3 min.
NEWBORNS YOUNGER THAN 1 MO OF AGE: **IV** For test dose, use 0.02 mg/kg.

Surgical Procedures
ADULTS AND CHILDREN OLDER THAN 1 MO OF AGE: **IV** 0.04 to 0.1 mg/kg initially. For maintenance therapy, use incremental doses q 25 to 60 min beginning with 0.01 mg/kg.
NEWBORNS YOUNGER THAN 1 MO OF AGE: **IV** For test dose, use 0.02 mg/kg.

Interactions
Aminoglycosides, bacitracin, clindamycin, colymycin, inhalational anesthetics, ketamine, lincomycin, magnesium salts, polymyxin B, quinidine, quinine, succinylcholine, tetracyclines, vancomycin: May augment action of pancuronium.
Azathioprine, mercaptopurine: May cause reversal of neuromuscular blocking effects of pancuronium.
Carbamazepine, hydantoins: May decrease duration and effect of pancuronium.
Halothane/tricyclic antidepressants: Patients receiving chronic TCA therapy who are anesthetized with halothane should use pancuronium with caution; severe ventricular arrhythmias may result.
Theophyllines: May cause possible resistance to, or reversal of, effects of pancuronium; cardiac arrhythmias may occur.
Trimethaphan: May cause prolonged apnea.

Lab Test Interferences
None well documented.

Adverse Reactions
CV: Rise in arterial pressure, cardiac output, and heart rate. Decrease in central venous pressure.
DERM: Transient rash.
GI: Salivation.
RESP: Respiratory insufficiency; apnea.
OTHER: Skeletal muscle weakness to complete relaxation; hypersensitivity reactions (eg, bronchospasm, flushing, redness, hypotension, tachycardia).

> **WARNING:**
> Administer via trained personnel. Have equipped facility available to monitor, assist, and control respiration.

Precautions
Pregnancy: Category C; do not use in early pregnancy.
Children: Prolonged use in newborns undergoing mechanical ventilation has been associated with severe skeletal muscle weakness and methemoglobinemia. Contains benzyl alcohol, which is related to a fatal gasping syndrome in premature infants.
Labor and delivery: Reduce dosage in cesarean section if patient is receiving magnesium sulfate.
Renal function impairment: Renally excreted; may require lower doses or less frequent maintenance doses.
Altered circulation time (eg, elderly patients, patients with CV disease or edema): Delay in onset of action.
Electrolyte imbalance: Neuromuscular blockade

may be altered depending on nature of imbalance.
Hepatic or biliary tract disease: Results in slower onset and prolonged duration.
Myasthenia gravis: Small doses may have profound effects.
Obesity/Neuromuscular disease: Require special attention to airway maintenance and ventilatory support.

PATIENT CARE CONSIDERATIONS
Administration/Storage
- For IV administration only. Not for intradermal, subcutaneous, IM, or intra-arterial administration.
- May be diluted with 0.9% sodium chloride injection, 5% dextrose injection, 5% dextrose and sodium chloride injection, or lactated Ringer's injection.
- Inspect solution visually before administration. Do not administer if solution is cloudy, discolored, or contains particulate matter.
- Store undiluted product in refrigerator (36° to 46°F) to maintain potency for 24 mo, or at controlled room temperature (65° to 72°F) to maintain potency for 6 mo. Diluted solution is stable for 48 hr at controlled room temperature.

Assessment/Interventions
- Obtain patient history, including drug history and any known allergies. Note liver, biliary tract, kidney, CV, or lung disease, edematous state, myasthenia gravis or myasthenic syndrome, neuromuscular disease, severe obesity, electrolyte imbalance, coadministration of antibiotics or magnesium salts, or acid-base abnormality.
- Ensure that resuscitative and tracheal intubation equipment, oxygen, and an antagonist (eg, neostigmine) are available at all times.
- Ensure that peripheral nerve stimulator is used to monitor neuromuscular function during administration in order to monitor effectiveness of dosing, need for additional doses, and confirm recovery from neuromuscular blockade.

Pain/Anxiety: Pancuronium does not have analgesic or antianxiety effects. Paralyzed patient will still need analgesic or sedative agents if indicated.

Overdosage: Signs and Symptoms
Skeletal muscle relaxation, decreased respiratory reserve, low tidal volume, apnea, prolonged neuromuscular blockade.

- Ensure that patient has adequate anesthesia or sedation before administering pancuronium because drug has no known effect on consciousness, pain threshold, or cerebration.
- Administer reduced dose to patient with neuromuscular disease (eg, myasthenia gravis).
- To avoid inaccurate dosing in patient with hemiparesis or paraparesis, monitor neuromuscular function on a nonparetic limb.
- Provide total care for immobilized patient.
- Check mechanical ventilator settings frequently.
- Assess respiratory status frequently. Inform health care provider immediately if deterioration in respiratory status or blood gases are noted.
- Monitor vital signs frequently. Inform health care provider immediately if CV instability is noted.
- Assess injection site frequently. If extravasation occurs, discontinue injection immediately and restart in another vein.

Patient/Family Education
- Explain name, action, and potential side effects of drug.
- Advise patient, family, or caregiver that medication will be prepared and administered by a health care provider in a health care setting.
- Reassure patient, family, or caregiver that breathing will be closely monitored and supported while medication is administered and that breathing and muscle function will return to normal after medication is discontinued.

Pantoprazole Sodium
(pahn-TOE-prazz-ole)
Class GI

How Supplied
Protonix Tablets, delayed-release 40 mg ♦ *Protonix IV* Powder for Injection 40 mg/vial
✤ *Panto IV* ♦ *Pantoloc*

Action
PHARMACOLOGY: Suppresses gastric acid secretion by blocking "acid (proton) pump" within gastric parietal cells.

PHARMACOKINETICS/DYNAMICS:
Absorption: Rapid. C_{max} is 2.5 mcg/mL (oral) and 5.52 mcg/mL (IV); bioavailability is approximately 77% (oral). T_{max} is 2.4 hr. Oral

administration with food may delay absorption up to 2 hr or longer.

Distribution: Pantoprazole distributes mainly in extracellular fluid. Vd is 11 to 23.6 L. Protein binding is approximately 98%, mainly albumin.

Metabolism: Pantoprazole is extensively metabolized in the liver through CYP450. The main metabolic pathway is demethylation by CYP2C19 and oxidation by CYP3A4. No evidence of metabolites with pharmacologic activity. CYP2C19 displays genetic polymorphism due to deficiency in some populations (3% white, 17% black, 23% Asian); these patients are known to be slow metabolizers of pantoprazole.

Excretion: Urine (71%), feces (18%); no renal excretion of unchanged drug. The t½ is 1 hr, and 3.5 to 10 hr in slow metabolizers. Total clearance is 7.6 to 14 L/hr.

Duration: More than 24 hr.

Special Populations:
Hepatic Function Impairment – With oral administration, there is an increase in serum elimination half-life from 7 to 9 hr; AUC increases by 5- to 7-fold. No dosage adjustment is necessary.
Elderly – Moderate increase in AUC (43%) and C_{max} (26%). No dosage adjustment is recommended.
Gender – Oral administration produces a modest increase in AUC and C_{max} in women. No dosage adjustment is recommended.

Indications
Oral: Short-term (no more than 8 wk) treatment in the healing and symptomatic relief of erosive esophagitis associated with gastroesophageal reflux disease (GERD); long-term treatment of pathological hypersecretory conditions, including Zollinger-Ellison syndrome; maintenance of healing of erosive esophagitis.
IV: Short-term (7- to 10-day) treatment of GERD, as an alternative to oral therapy in patients unable to continue oral pantoprazole; hypersecretory conditions associated with Zollinger-Ellison syndrome or other neoplastic conditions.

Contraindications
Standard considerations.

Route/Dosage
Maintenance of Healing of Erosive Esophagitis
ADULTS: **PO** 40 mg/day.

Treatment of Erosive Esophagitis
ADULTS: **PO** 40 mg/day for up to 8 wk; an additional 8-wk course of treatment may be considered in patients who have not healed after 8 wk.
ADULTS: **IV** 40 mg/day for 7 to 10 days.

Pathological Hypersecretion Associated with Zollinger-Ellison Syndrome
ADULTS: **IV** 80 mg q 12 hr; based upon individual patient needs, the dose may be increased to 80 mg q 8 hr.

Interactions
None well documented.

Lab Test Interferences
None well documented.

Adverse Reactions
CV: Angina; arrhythmia; MI; palpitation; chest pain.
CNS: Headache; migraine; anxiety; dizziness.
DERM: Rash; erythema multiforme; Stevens-Johnson syndrome; toxic epidermal necrolysis.
EENT: Pharyngitis; rhinitis; sinusitis.
GI: Diarrhea; flatulence; abdominal pain; constipation; dyspepsia; gastroenteritis; nausea; vomiting.
GU: Urinary frequency; UTI.
HEPA: Abnormal LFTs; increased ALT.
RESP: Bronchitis; increased cough; dyspnea; upper respiratory tract infection.
OTHER: Asthenia; back pain; neck pain; flu syndrome; pain; arthralgia; hypertonia.

Precautions
Pregnancy: Category B.
Lactation: Undetermined.
Children: Safety and efficacy not established.

PATIENT CARE CONSIDERATIONS
Administration/Storage
- Give oral preparation once daily without regard to meals.
- Do not split, chew, or crush. Instruct patient to swallow tablet whole.
- IV preparation is only used when patient cannot take tablets and for no more than 10 days.
- Reconstitute IV preparation with 10 mL of 0.9% Sodium Chloride Injection, then further dilute by mixing with 100 mL of 0.9% Sodium Chloride Injection, 5% Dextrose Injection, or Lactated Ringer's Injection.
- Administer IV preparation once daily by infusing over a period of about 15 min through a dedicated line using the inline filter provided. If administered through a Y-site, the in-line filter must be positioned below the Y-site that is closest to the patient.
- The inline filter removes precipitates that may form when the reconstituted drug product is mixed with recommended IV solutions but does not reduce the total amount of drug administered.
- Flush IV line before and after administration with 5% Dextrose Injection, 0.9% Sodium

Chloride Injection, or Lactated Ringer's Injection.
- Do not simultaneously administer IV pantoprazole through the same line with other IV solutions.
- Store tablets at controlled room temperature. Store powder for injection in refrigerator, protected from light. Reconstituted solution may be stored for up to 2 hr at room temperature before further dilution. The diluted solution may be stored for up to 12 hr at room temperature before infusion. Reconstituted and diluted solutions do not need to be protected from light. Store inline filters at room temperature.

Assessment/Interventions
- Obtain patient history, including drug history and any known allergies. Note history of liver disease.
- Assess for bloody or coffee ground emesis and black tarry stools.
- Assess for symptoms of esophageal reflux (eg, heart burn, acid regurgitation) or peptic ulcer activity (eg, indigestion, abdominal pain, nausea).

Patient/Family Education
- Explain name, dose, action, and potential side effects of drug.
- Advise patient to not split, crush, or chew medication and to swallow the tablet whole.
- Remind patient to take dose once daily without regard to meals.
- Inform patient that antacids may be taken concurrently with pantoprazole.
- Remind patient that pantoprazole is to be taken every day and not "as needed" or only when symptoms are present.
- Instruct women to notify health care provider if pregnant, planning to become pregnant, or breastfeeding.
- Advise patient to report any of the following to the health care provider: bloody or coffee ground emesis; black tarry stools; recurrent heart burn; recurrent indigestion or abdominal pain; increasing need for antacid use.

Papaverine Hydrochloride
(pap-PAV-uhr-een HIGH-droe-KLOR-ide)
Class Peripheral vasodilator

How Supplied
Pavabid Plateau Caps Capsules, timed-release 150 mg ♦ *Pavagen TD* Capsules, timed-release 150 mg

Action
PHARMACOLOGY: Directly relaxes tone of all smooth muscle, especially when spasmodically contracted. Causes vasodilatation of blood vessels of the coronary, cerebral, pulmonary and peripheral arteries; relaxes musculature of bronchi, GI tract, ureters and biliary system.

PHARMACOKINETICS/DYNAMICS:
Absorption: Readily absorbed from GI tract. Oral bioavailability is approximately 54%. T_{max} is 1 to 2 hr after a dose.

Distribution: Drug localizes in fat depots and in the liver; remainder is distributed throughout the body. Protein binding is 90%.

Metabolism: Liver.

Excretion: Urine (inactive form). $T_{½}$ is 0.5 to 2 hr. $T_{½}$ varies widely; constant levels can be maintained by giving drug at 6-hr intervals.

Indications
Oral form: Relief of cerebral and peripheral ischemia associated with arterial spasm and myocardial ischemia complicated by arrhythmias.

Parenteral form: Vascular spasm associated with acute MI (coronary occlusion), angina pectoris, peripheral and pulmonary embolism, peripheral vascular disease in which there is a vasospastic element, certain cerebral angiospastic states, visceral spasm (eg, ureteral, biliary, and GI colic). **Unlabeled use(s):** Intracavernous injection for impotence.

Contraindications Complete atrioventricular (AV) heart block; intracorporeal injection for impotence.

Route/Dosage
Ischemia
ADULTS: **PO** 100 to 300 mg 3 to 5 times daily (immediate-release tablets) or 150 mg q 8 to 12 hr or 300 mg q 12 hr (sustained-release capsules).

Vascular Occlusion
ADULTS: **IV/IM** Initial dose is 30 mg. Repeat doses are 30 to 120 mg q 3 hr prn.

Impotence
ADULTS: **IV** 2.5 to 60 mg as intracavernous injection (usually combined with phentolamine mesylate).

Interactions
CNS depressants: Effects may be additive.
Levodopa: May reduce effectiveness of levodopa.
INCOMPATIBILITIES: Lactated Ringer's solution incompatible with parenteral formulation; do not mix.

Lab Test Interferences None well documented.

Adverse Reactions

CV: Increase in heart rate; slight increase in BP.
CNS: Depression; dizziness; vertigo; headache; drowsiness; sedation; lassitude; malaise; lethargy.
DERM: Flushing of face; sweating; pruritus.
GI: Constipation; nausea; diarrhea; abdominal distress; dry mouth; anorexia.
HEMA: Eosinophilia.
HEPA: Jaundice; hepatitis.
RESP: Increased depth of respiration.

Precautions

Pregnancy: Category C.
Lactation: Unknown.
Children: Safety and efficacy not established.
Glaucoma: Use drug with caution.
Hepatic hypersensitivity: Hepatic hypersensitivity reported.

Overdosage: Signs and Symptoms

Drowsiness, weakness, diplopia, lassitude, depression, nystagmus, incoordination, coma, cyanosis, respiratory depression, anxiety, ataxia, headache, pruritic skin rashes, nausea, CNS depression, blurred vision, GI upset, vomiting, diaphoresis, sinus tachycardia, metabolic acidosis, hyperventilation, hyperglycemia, hypokalemia.

PATIENT CARE CONSIDERATIONS

Administration/Storage

- Give at evenly spaced intervals throughout day.
- Do not crush or allow patient to chew sustained-release capsules.
- Do not administer in Lactated Ringer's solution because precipitate will develop.
- Administer parenteral form slowly over 1 to 2 min to minimize adverse effects.
- Store at room temperature.

Assessment/Interventions

- Obtain patient history, including drug history and any known allergies.
- Assess mental status before and during therapy (eg, lassitude, sedation, malaise, headache, depression).
- Assess bowel status and bowel sounds before administering drug and periodically during treatment.
- Monitor patient's BP, both lying and standing.
- Monitor LFTs.
- Monitor ECG. If cardiac changes occur on ECG, notify health care provider immediately.
- If AV block, flushing, headache, jaundice, abdominal distress, constipation, or diarrhea develop, notify health care provider.

Patient/Family Education

- Instruct patient to take medication at evenly spaced intervals throughout day.
- Advise patient with glaucoma to undergo regular eye examinations.
- Instruct patient to report the following symptoms to health care provider: flushing, sweating, headache, tiredness, jaundice, skin rash, nausea, anorexia, abdominal distress, constipation, or diarrhea.
- Advise patient to avoid smoking and intake of alcoholic beverages or other CNS depressants.
- Caution patient to avoid sudden position changes to prevent orthostatic hypotension.
- Advise patient that drug may cause dizziness, vertigo, and drowsiness, and to use caution while driving or performing other tasks requiring mental alertness.

Paromomycin Sulfate

(par-oh-moe-MY-sin SULL-fate)
Class Anti-infective/Amebicide/Aminoglycoside

How Supplied
Humatin Capsules 250 mg

Action
PHARMACOLOGY: Inhibits production of protein in bacteria, causing bacterial cell death.
PHARMACOKINETICS/DYNAMICS:
Absorption: Poorly absorbed orally.
Excretion: Feces (100% unchanged).

Indications Treatment of acute and chronic intestinal amebiasis. Adjunctive therapy in management of hepatic coma. **Unlabeled use(s):** Treatment of other parasitic infections.

Contraindications Intestinal obstruction; extraintestinal amebiasis; hypersensitivity to aminoglycosides.

Route/Dosage
Intestinal Amebiasis
ADULTS AND CHILDREN: **PO** 25 to 35 mg/kg/day in 3 divided doses with meals for 5 to 10 days.

Hepatic Coma
ADULTS: **PO** 4 g/day in divided doses at regular intervals for 5 to 6 days.

Interactions
Digoxin: May reduce rate and extent of digoxin absorption; this may be offset by decreased digoxin metabolism.
Methotrexate: Decreased absorption of methotrexate.
Neuromuscular blockers: Increased action of both depolarizing and nondepolarizing neuromuscular blocking agents, may prolong need for respiratory support.
Neurotoxic, nephrotoxic, or ototoxic medications (eg, polypeptide antibiotics): Additive adverse effects may occur with concurrent or sequential administration of medications with similar toxic profiles.

Lab Test Interferences None well documented.

Adverse Reactions
GI: Nausea; vomiting; abdominal cramps; anorexia; epigastric burning; pruritus ani; diarrhea.
OTHER: Malabsorption syndrome.

> **WARNING:**
> *Neurotoxicity:* Manifests as both auditory and vestibular ototoxicity, and primarily occurs in patients with pre-existing renal damage or with prolonged therapy. Partial or total irreversible deafness may continue to develop after drug is stopped. Other features of neurotoxicity include paresthesias, twitching, and seizures.
> *Nephrotoxicity:* Usually reversible.
> Paromomycin is teratogenic in pregnancy. Closely monitor renal and eighth nerve function in patients with suspected renal dysfunction. Monitor peak and trough concentrations. Renal impairment requires dosage adjustments.

Precautions
Pregnancy: Category D.
Lactation: Excreted in breast milk.
Superinfection: Prolonged or repeated therapy may result in bacterial or fungal overgrowth of nonsusceptible organisms and secondary infections.
Muscular disorders: Patients with muscular disorders such as myasthenia gravis or parkinsonism may have worsening of their disease because of potential effect of aminoglycosides on neuromuscular junction.

Overdosage: Signs and Symptoms
Neurotoxicity, nephrotoxicity, ototoxicity.

PATIENT CARE CONSIDERATIONS

Administration/Storage
- Administer medication with meals.
- Store at room temperature in a tight container.

Assessment/Interventions
- Obtain patient history, including drug history and any known allergies.
- Assess patient for adverse reactions to paromomycin (eg, altered auditory sensory perception, GI dysfunction, nephrotoxicity, neuromuscular blockage).
- Observe for signs of superinfection.
- If nausea, vomiting or diarrhea occur, give antiemetic or antidiarrheal medication as prescribed.
- If hearing loss occurs or if audiometric testing becomes abnormal or if casts or protein appear in urinalysis, notify health care provider.

Patient/Family Education
- Stress to patient the importance of taking full course of therapy.
- Emphasize to patient the importance of personal hygiene, especially handwashing.

- Explain to patient the symptoms of superinfection and ask patient to watch for symptoms if on prolonged therapy.
- Instruct patient to report the following symptoms to health care provider: ringing in ears, hearing impairment, or dizziness.

Paroxetine

(puh-ROKS-uh-teen)

Class Antidepressant

How Supplied

Paroxetine Hydrochloride
Paxil Tablets 10 mg, Tablets 20 mg, Tablets 30 mg, Tablets 40 mg, Oral suspension 10 mg/ 5 mL ♦ Paxil CR Tablets, controlled-release 12.5 mg, Tablets, controlled-release 25 mg, Tablets, controlled-release 37.5 mg

Paroxetine Mesylate
Pexeva Tablets 10 mg, Tablets 20 mg, Tablets 30 mg, Tablets 40 mg

Action

PHARMACOLOGY: Blocks reuptake of serotonin, enhancing serotonergic function.

PHARMACOKINETICS/DYNAMICS:

Absorption: Completely absorbed. Steady state is 10 days (hydrochloride; immediate release), 13 days (mesylate), 2 wk (controlled release). C_{max} is 61.7 ng/mL (hydrochloride; immediate release), 81.3 ng/mL (mesylate), 30 ng/mL (controlled release). T_{max} is 5.2 hr (hydrochloride; immediate release), 8.1 hr (mesylate), 6 to 10 hr postdose (controlled release). Food increases AUC 6%, C_{max} 29%. Time to reach peak plasma concentration decreased from 6.4 hr postdosing to 4.9 hr.

Distribution: Distributes throughout the body, including CNS; only 1% remains in plasma. Protein binding is 93% to 95%. Distributes into breast milk.

Metabolism: Extensive first-pass metabolism in liver by CYP450 2D6. Principal metabolites are polar and conjugated products of oxidation and methylation.

Excretion: Urine (64% dose excreted in urine, 2% as parent compound, 62% as metabolites); feces (36% excreted mostly as metabolites). The $t_{½}$ is 21 hr (hydrochloride; immediate release), 33.2 hr (mesylate), 15 to 20 hr (controlled release).

Onset: 1 to 4 wk (antidepressant effects).

Special Populations:
Renal Function Impairment – Mean plasma concentrations increased approximately 4 times (Ccr below 30 mL/min). Plasma concentrations increased 2-fold (Ccr 30 to 60 mL/min). Dose reduction should take place in these patients.
Hepatic Function Impairment – 2-fold increase in plasma concentrations; dose reduction may be necessary.
Elderly – Minimum concentrations were 70% to 80% greater. Reduce initial dosage.

Indications Panic disorder or social anxiety disorder (except *Pexeva*), as defined in the DSM-IV; major depressive disorder, as defined in DSM-III (immediate release) or DSM-IV (controlled release).
Immediate release only: Obsessive-compulsive disorder (OCD); generalized anxiety disorder (GAD) (except *Pexeva*); posttraumatic stress disorder (PTSD), as defined in the DSM-IV (except *Pexeva*).
Controlled release only: Premenstrual dysphoric disorder (PMDD), as defined in the DSM-IV.

Contraindications Standard considerations. Concomitant use in patients taking MAO inhibitors or thioridazine.

Route/Dosage

Depression
ADULTS: PO
Immediate release: 20 mg/day initially; may increase by 10 mg/day at intervals of at least 7 days (max, 50 mg/day). Administer as single daily dose, usually in morning.
Controlled release: 25 mg/day as a single dose, usually in the morning (usual dose range, 25 to 62.5 mg/day). The dose may be increased in increments of 12.5 mg/day at intervals of at least 1 wk (max, 62.5 mg/day).

Elderly, Debilitated, or Patients with Severe Renal or Hepatic Impairment
PO
Immediate release – 10 mg/day initially; do not exceed 40 mg/day.
Controlled release – 12.5 mg/day initially; do not exceed 50 mg/day.

GAD/PTSD
ADULTS: PO
Immediate release: 20 mg/day administered as a single dose with or without food, usually in the morning. May increase dose by 10 mg/day at intervals of 1 wk. Usual range, 20 to 50 mg/day.

OCD
ADULTS: PO
Immediate release: 20 mg/day initially; recommended dose is 40 mg/day. May increase dose by 10 mg/day at intervals of at least 7 days (max, 60 mg/day). Administer as single daily dose, usually in morning.

Panic Disorder
ADULTS: PO
Immediate release: 10 mg/day initially; recommended dose is 40 mg/day. May increase dose by 10 mg/day at intervals of at least 7 days (max,

60 mg/day). Administer as single daily dose, usually in morning.
Controlled release: 12.5 mg/day as a single dose, usually in the morning. The dose may be increased in increments of 12.5 mg/day at intervals of at least 1 wk (max, 75 mg/day).

PMDD
ADULTS: PO
Controlled release: 12.5 mg/day initially, usually in the morning; change doses at intervals of at least 1 wk; usual range is 12.5 to 25 mg/day. May be administered either daily throughout the menstrual cycle or limited to the luteal phase of the menstrual cycle.

Social Anxiety Disorder
ADULTS: **PO**
Immediate release: 20 mg/day administered as a single daily dose with or without food, usually in the morning. Usual range is 20 to 60 mg/day.
Controlled release: 12.5 mg initially, usually in the morning. Usual range is 12.5 to 37.5 mg/day. The dose may be increased in increments of 12.5 mg/day at intervals of at least 1 wk (max, 37.5 mg/day).

Interactions
5-HT$_1$ agonists (eg, naratriptan, sumatriptan, zolmitriptan): Weakness, hyperreflexia, and incoordination reported rarely.
Alcohol: Causes additive CNS effects; concurrent use is not recommended.
Cimetidine: May increase paroxetine concentrations.
Cyclosporine: Concentrations of cyclosporine may be elevated, increasing the risk of toxicity.
Cyproheptadine: Pharmacologic effects of paroxetine may be decreased or reversed.
CYP2D6 system: Approach coadministration with other drugs metabolized by cytochrome P450 2D6 (eg, certain antidepressants, phenothiazines, type IC antiarrhythmics) or drugs that inhibit this enzyme (eg, quinidine) with caution.
Digoxin: May decrease digoxin levels.
Hemostatic agents (eg, aspirin, NSAIDs, warfarin): Risk of bleeding (eg, GI bleeding) may be increased.
MAO inhibitors: Can cause serious, sometimes fatal reactions. Do not use concomitantly or within 14 days of each other.
Phenobarbital, phenytoin: May decrease paroxetine concentration; may reduce phenytoin concentration.
Procyclidine: Reduction of procyclidine dose may be necessary if anticholinergic effects (eg, dry mouth, blurred vision, urinary retention) occur.
Protein bound agents: Highly protein bound agents may be displaced by paroxetine or paroxetine may be displaced, increasing plasma levels and the risk of adverse effects.
Sibutramine: The risk of occurrence of serotonin syndrome may be increased.
St. John's wort: Sedative-hypnotic effects may be increased.
Sympathomimetics (eg, amphetamine): Sensitivity of sympathomimetics and risk of serotonin syndrome may be increased.
Theophylline: Elevated theophylline levels have occurred with paroxetine. Monitor theophylline levels when coadministered.
Thioridazine: May increase thioridazine levels, leading to an increased risk of QTc prolongation, ventricular arrhythmias, and death. Concomitant use is contraindicated.
Tricyclic antidepressants (eg, amitriptyline): Metabolism may be inhibited by paroxetine, increasing plasma levels, and adverse effects.
Tryptophan: May cause headache, nausea, sweating, and dizziness.
Warfarin: Increased risk of bleeding.
Zolpidem: The effect of zolpidem may be increased.

Lab Test Interferences None well documented.

Adverse Reactions Incidences of adverse reactions are stated in broad ranges because those reported varied depending on the dose or indication.
CV: Palpitation, vasodilation, hypertension, syncope, tachycardia (1% to 4%); ventricular fibrillation, ventricular tachycardia (including torsades de pointes) (postmarketing).
CNS: Headache, somnolence, dizziness, insomnia, tremor, nervousness, anxiety, decreased libido (5% or greater); paresthesia, drugged feeling, confusion, agitation, abnormal dreams, migraine, impaired concentration, depersonalization, myoclonus, amnesia, stimulation, depression, emotional lability, vertigo (1% to 4%); neuroleptic malignant syndrome, extrapyramidal symptoms, status epilepticus, eclampsia (postmarketing).
DERM: Sweating (5% or greater); rash, pruritus (1% to 4%); vasculitic syndrome, toxic epidermal necrolysis (postmarketing).
EENT: Blurred vision, taste perversion, rhinitis, pharyngitis, sinusitis, abnormal vision (1% to 4%); laryngismus, optic neuritis (postmarketing).
GI: Nausea, dry mouth, constipation, diarrhea, abdominal pain, decreased appetite (5% or greater); flatulence, oropharynx disorder, dyspepsia, increased appetite, vomiting (1% to 4%).
GU: Ejaculatory disturbances and other male genital disorders, impotence (5% or greater); urinary frequency, urinary disorder, female genital disorders, vaginitis, dysmenorrhea, impaired

urination, UTI (1% to 4%); priapism (postmarketing).
HEMA: Thrombocytopenia, impaired hematopoiesis (including aplastic anemia, pancytopenia, bone marrow aplasia, agranulocytosis), hemolytic anemia (postmarketing).
HEPA: Liver necrosis, grossly elevated transaminases levels, severe liver dysfunction (postmarketing).
M/N: Weight gain or loss (1% to 4%); SIADH (postmarketing).
MUSC: Myopathy, hypertonia, myalgia, myasthenia, arthralgia (1% to 4%).
RESP: Yawn, increased cough (1% to 4%); pulmonary hypertension, allergic alveolitis (postmarketing).
OTHER: Asthenia (5% or greater); chest pain, back pain, chills, trauma, allergic reaction, photosensitivity, malaise (1% to 4%); Guillain-Barré syndrome, prolactinemia, galactorrhea, serotonin syndrome, anaphylaxis (postmarketing).

Precautions
Pregnancy: Category C.
Lactation: Secreted in breast milk. Use with caution.
Children: Safety and efficacy not established.
Renal function impairment: May increase plasma concentrations of paroxetine; adjust dosage.
Hepatic function impairment: May increase plasma concentrations of paroxetine; adjust dosage.

Special risk patients: Use with caution in patients with history of seizure, mania, hypomania, suicidal tendencies, concomitant illness, narrow-angle glaucoma, drug abuse, or dependence.
Altered platelet function: Altered platelet function or abnormal results from lab studies have occurred.
Depression/Suicide: Patients with major depressive disorder may experience worsening of depression and/or emergence of suicidal ideation and behavior, whether or not they are taking antidepressant medication, and risk may persist until significant remission occurs. Monitor patients closely for clinical worsening of depression and suicidal ideation.
Discontinuation: Avoid abrupt cessation. Gradually reduce dose.
Hyponatremia: Hyponatremia has occurred. Use drug with caution in elderly, patients taking diuretics, and volume-depleted patients.
Mania/Hypomania: Paroxetine may activate hypomania or mania. Use cautiously in patients with history of mania.

Overdosage: Signs and Symptoms
Nausea, vomiting, drowsiness, sinus tachycardia, dilated pupils, dizziness, sweating, tremor, confusion, somnolence, coma.

PATIENT CARE CONSIDERATIONS
Administration/Storage
- Do not administer with or within 14 days of MAO inhibitor administration.
- Administer prescribed dose daily, preferably in the morning. Administer without regard to meals but administer with food if GI upset occurs.
- Have patient swallow controlled-release tablet whole. Do not crush, chew, divide, or break tablet.
- Shake suspension well before measuring dose. Use dosing cup or spoon to measure and administer dose.
- Increase dose no more often than q 7 days.
- Store immediate-release tablets at controlled room temperature (59° to 86°F). Store controlled-release tablets and suspension below 77°F.

Assessment/Interventions
- Obtain patient history, including drug history and any known allergies. Note renal or hepatic impairment, mania, seizure disorder, history of seizure, narrow angle glaucoma, concurrent or recent (eg, within 14 days) use of MAO inhibitor, concurrent use of thioridazine, or concurrent use of aspirin, NSAIDs or other medications that can affect coagulation.
- Ensure reduced initial dose and slower dose escalation are used in elderly patient, debilitated patient, or patient with severe renal or hepatic impairment.
- Ensure serum electrolytes, BUN, and creatinine are regularly evaluated in patient with SIADH, edema, adrenal disease, or condition associated with fluid loss.
- Continue suicide monitoring of high-risk patients.
- Frequently assess patient for response to treatment. Notify health care provider if condition does not appear to be improving or is worsening.
- Ensure therapy is periodically reviewed to determine if it needs to be continued without change or if a dose change (eg, increase, decrease, discontinuation) is indicated.
- Observe for signs of mood change and report to health care provider.
- If treatment is to be discontinued, or the dose reduced, gradually taper the dose and monitor patient for withdrawal symptoms (eg, dizziness, abnormal skin sensations, agitation, anxiety, nausea, sweating). If significant with-

drawal symptoms develop, reinstitute previous dosing schedule and attempt a less rapid tapering regimen after patient has stabilized.
• Monitor patient for CNS, GI, PSYCH, MUSC, GU, and general body side effects. Report to health care provider if noted and significant.

Patient/Family Education
• Explain name, dose, action, and potential side effects of drug.
• Advise patient to read *Patient Information Leaflet* before starting therapy and with each refill.
• Advise patient that medication is usually started at a low dose and then gradually increased until max benefit is obtained.
• Advise patient that medication is usually administered as a single daily dose, preferably in the morning.
• Instruct patient taking controlled-release tablet to swallow tablet whole and not crush, chew, divide, or break tablet.
• Advise patient using suspension to shake well before measuring dose and use a dosing cup or spoon to measure prescribed dose.
• Advise patient to take prescribed dose without regard to meals, but to take with food if stomach upset occurs.
• Advise patient not to change the dose or stop taking unless advised by health care provider.
• Inform patient that it may take 1 to 4 wk to note improvement in symptoms and to continue with the prescribed therapy once improvement has been noted.
• Instruct patient to contact health care provider if symptoms do not appear to be getting better, are getting worse, or if bothersome side effects (eg, unusual sweating, headache, drowsiness, insomnia, nausea, diarrhea, nervousness, changes in sexual function) occur.
• Advise patient that if medication needs to be discontinued, it will be slowly withdrawn unless safety concerns (eg, rash) require a more rapid withdrawal.
• Advise patient to take frequent sips of water, suck on ice chips or sugarless hard candy, or chew sugarless gum if dry mouth occurs.
• Instruct patient to avoid alcoholic beverages and other depressants while taking this medication.
• Advise patient that drug may impair judgment, thinking, or reflexes and to use caution while driving or performing other tasks requiring mental alertness until tolerance is determined.
• Instruct patient not to take prescription or OTC drugs, herbal preparations, or dietary supplements without consulting with health care provider.
• Advise women to notify health care provider if pregnant, planning to become pregnant, or breastfeeding.
• Advise patient that follow-up visits may be necessary to monitor therapy and to keep appointments.

Pegaspargase

(peh-ASS-par-jase)
Class Modified enzyme
How Supplied
Oncaspar Injection 750 IU/mL

Action
PHARMACOLOGY: Leukemic cells are unable to synthesize asparagine because of a lack of asparagine synthetase and are dependent on an exogenous source of asparagine for survival. Rapid depletion of asparagine, which results from treatment with the enzyme L-asparaginase, kills the leukemic cells.

PHARMACOKINETICS/DYNAMICS:
Absorption: Levels are detectable for at least 15 days after IV.
Distribution: Found in lymph at 20% of the concentration in plasma.
Metabolism: Unknown.
Excretion: Unknown. $T_{½}$ is 5.73 days (children), 3.24 days (previously hypersensitive adults), and 5.69 days (nonhypersensitive adults).

Indications
Adults and pediatrics: Combination therapy of acute lymphocytic leukemia in patients who are hypersensitive to the native form of L-asparaginase; may be used for single agent therapy in these patients when combination therapy is inappropriate.

Contraindications Pancreatitis or history of pancreatitis; significant hemorrhagic events associated with prior L-asparaginase therapy; previous serious allergic reactions.

Route/Dosage
Combination or Single Agent Therapy of Acute Lymphocytic Leukemia
ADULTS: **IM** or **IV** 2500 IU/m^2 q 14 days.
PEDIATRIC: **IM** or **IV** Dose may be determined by body surface area or body weight. Administer

dose every 14 days. The recommended dose for children with a body surface area of at least 0.6 m^2 is 2500 IU/m^2. The recommended dose for children with a body surface area less than 0.6 m^2 is 82.5 IU/kg.

Interactions

Methotrexate: Pegaspargase may interfere with drugs such as methotrexate which require cell replication for their lethal effects.

Protein-bound drugs: Depletion of serum proteins by pegaspargase may increase the toxicity of other drugs which are protein bound.

Warfarin, heparin, dipyridamole, aspirin, or nonsteroidal anti-inflammatory agents: Pegaspargase may increase or decrease the anticoagulant effects of warfarin, heparin, dipyridamole, aspirin, or nonsteroidal anti-inflammatory agents. Patients may be at increased risk for bleeding or thrombosis.

Lab Test Interferences
None well documented.

Adverse Reactions

CV: Superficial, deep vein, catheter or atrial thrombosis.

CNS: Malaise, headache, seizures, paresthesias, confusion, emotional lability, Parkinson-like syndrome.

DERM: Rashes, urticaria.

ENDO: Hyperglycemia, hypoglycemia, hyperuricemia.

GI: Nausea and vomiting, abdominal pain, diarrhea, anorexia, jaundice, elevation of LFTs, fatty changes in the liver, fatal hemorrhagic pancreatitis (rare).

HEMA: Hypofibrinogenemia, leukopenia, thrombocytopenia, hemolytic anemia, disseminated intravascular coagulation, prolonged prothrombin time and partial thromboplastin time.

HYPERSEN: Acute anaphylactoid reactions are common, discontinuation of therapy and administration of fluids, corticosteroids, antihistamines, or pressors may be required.

MUSC: Arthralgia, myalgia.

RENAL: Prerenal azotemia, transient proteinuria.

OTHER: Fever, chills, night sweats.

Precautions

Pregnancy: Category C.

Lactation: Undetermined.

Bleeding: Patients taking pegaspargase are at higher than usual risk for bleeding problems, especially with simultaneous use of other drugs that have anticoagulant properties, such as aspirin and NSAIDs.

Infection: Pegaspargase may have immunosuppressive activity. Therefore, it is possible that use of the drug may predispose patients to infection.

Hepatic/CNS toxicity: Severe hepatic and CNS toxicity following multi-agent chemotherapy that includes pegaspargase may occur. Caution appears warranted when treating patients with pegaspargase in combination with hepatotoxic agents, particularly when liver dysfunction is present.

Overdosage: Signs and Symptoms
Slight increase in liver enzymes; rash.

PATIENT CARE CONSIDERATIONS

Administration/Storage

- Refrigerate solution for injection, but do not freeze. Do not administer if there is any indication that the drug has been frozen. Freezing destroys activity of product. Do not use solution stored at room temperature for greater than 48 hr or if it has been frozen.
- Avoid excessive agitation; do not shake.
- Discard single-dose vials after a single use. Use solution only if clear.
- Use only 1 dose per vial; do not re-enter the vial. Do not save unused drug for alter administration.
- Administer by IV infusion or IM injection.
- IV administration is associated with a higher incidence of adverse effects than IM administration.
- This drug may be a contact irritant. Gloves are recommended. Inhalation of vapors and contact with skin or mucous membranes must be avoided. In case of contact, wash with copious amounts of water for at least 15 min.

IV:
- Dilute dose in 100 mL of 0.9% Sodium Chloride or 5% Dextrose.
- Infuse diluted solution through a running IV line over 1 to 2 hr.

IM:
- Use solution for injection as commercially prepared. Syringes prepared for IM administration should contain less than or equal to 2 mL; prepare multiple syringes for larger doses.
- The volume of a single IM injection should not exceed 2 mL.

Assessment/Interventions

- Hypersensitivity reactions to pegaspargase, including life-threatening anaphylaxis, may occur during therapy. As a routine precaution, keep patient under observation for 1 hr with resuscitation equipment and other agents necessary to treat anaphylaxis.
- Monitor peripheral blood count and bone marrow, serum amylase determinations to detect early evidence of pancreatitis, glucose

because hyperglycemia may occur, LFTs, and ammonia. Blood ammonia may increase during therapy. Monitoring of fibrinogen, PT, and PTT may be indicated.

Patient/Family Education
- Inform patients of the possibility of hypersensitivity reactions.
- Instruct patients that the simultaneous use of pegaspargase with other drugs that may increase the risk of bleeding should be avoided.
- May predispose the patient to infection. Patients should notify the health care provider of any adverse reactions that occur.

Pegfilgrastim
(peg-fill-GRAH-stim)

Class Colony-stimulating factor

How Supplied
Neulasta Solution for injection 10 mg/mL

Action
PHARMACOLOGY: Stimulates neutrophil production within bone marrow.

PHARMACOKINETICS/DYNAMICS:
Excretion: T½ is 15 to 80 hr (SC injection). Serum clearance is directly related to the number of neutrophils.

Indications Decrease incidence of infection, manifested by febrile neutropenia, in patients with nonmyeloid malignancies receiving myelosuppressive anticancer drugs associated with febrile neutropenia.

Contraindications Hypersensitivity to *Escherichia coli*-derived proteins, filgrastim, pegfilgrastim, or any component of the product.

Route/Dosage
ADULTS: SC 6 mg once per chemotherapy cycle. Do not administer in period between 14 days before and 24 hr after administration of cytotoxic chemotherapy. Do not administer the 6 mg fixed-dose formulation in infants, children, and smaller adolescents weighing less than 45 kg.

Interactions
Drugs potentiating the release of neutrophils (eg, lithium): Use drugs that potentiate the release of neutrophils with caution.

Lab Test Interferences None well documented.

Adverse Reactions
CNS: Fatigue; headache; insomnia; dizziness.
DERM: Alopecia.
GI: Nausea; diarrhea; vomiting; constipation; anorexia; taste perversion; dyspepsia; abdominal pain; stomatitis.
HEMA: Granulocytopenia; leukocytosis.
MUSC: Skeletal pain; myalgia; arthralgia; medullary bone pain.
OTHER: Fever; generalized weakness; peripheral edema; mucositis; neutropenic fever.

Precautions
Pregnancy: Category C.
Lactation: Undetermined.
Children: Safety and efficacy not established. Do not administer 6 mg fixed-dose formulation in infants, children, and smaller adolescents weighing less than 45 kg.
Hypersensitivity: Allergic-type reactions, including anaphylaxis, skin rash, and urticaria may occur.
Adult respiratory distress syndrome: Adult respiratory distress syndrome may occur.
Sickle cell disease: Use with caution because severe sickle cell crisis may occur in patients with sickle cell disease.
Splenic rupture: Because splenic rupture may occur, do not use pegfilgrastim for peripheral blood progenitor cell mobilization.

PATIENT CARE CONSIDERATIONS
Administration/Storage
- Administer via SC route only. Not for IM or IV administration.
- Avoid shaking syringe.
- Dose is administered once per chemotherapy cycle but not in the time period from 14 days before to 24 hr after administration of cytotoxic chemotherapy.
- Do not administer if particulate matter, cloudiness, or discoloration noted.
- Store prefilled syringes in original carton in refrigerator (36° to 46°F). Do not freeze. If accidentally frozen, allow to thaw in refrigerator before using. Discard syringe if frozen a second time. May allow syringe to reach room temperature before administering. If removed from refrigerator, keep syringe in original carton to protect from light and use within 48 hr. Discard syringe if left at room temperature for greater than 48 hr.

Assessment/Interventions
- Obtain patient history, including drug history and any known allergies. Note history of the following: allergy to *E. coli*-derived proteins or filgrastim; sickle cell disease.
- Ensure that CBC and platelet count are obtained before therapy and periodically during treatment.
- Monitor patient for signs and symptoms of splenic enlargement (eg, left upper abdominal pain, shoulder tip pain). Inform health care provider immediately if noted.

- Monitor patient for signs and symptoms of adult respiratory distress syndrome (eg, fever, respiratory distress). Inform health care provider immediately if noted.
- Monitor patient with sickle cell disease for signs and symptoms of sickle cell crisis. Notify health care provider immediately if noted and be prepared to treat appropriately.
- Monitor patient for signs and symptoms of anaphylactic or serious allergic reactions. Be prepared to treat appropriately.
- Monitor patient for CNS, GI, and general body side effects. Report to health care provider if noted and significant.

Patient/Family Education
- Explain name, dose, action and potential side effects of drug. If patient or caregiver will be administering at home, review "Information for Patients and Caregivers" insert with the patient or caregiver. Ensure that the patient or caregiver understands how to store, prepare, and administer the dose, and dispose of used equipment and supplies. The first injection should be performed under the supervision of a qualified health professional.
- Caution patient or caregiver that medication is not to be administered during the time interval beginning 14 days before to 24 hr after administration of chemotherapy.
- Advise patient or caregiver to immediately report any of the following to their health care provider: fever or other signs of infection; sore throat; left upper stomach pain; shoulder tip pain; difficulty breathing; rash or hives.
- Advise patient or caregiver to report intolerable injection site reactions or unusual symptoms to their health care provider.
- Instruct women to notify health care provider if becoming pregnant, planning on becoming pregnant, or breastfeeding.
- Instruct patient not to take any prescription or OTC medications or dietary supplements unless advised by health care provider.
- Remind patient or caregiver that office visits and laboratory tests will be required to monitor therapy and to be sure to keep appointments.

Peginterferon Alfa-2a

(peg-IN-ter-FEER-ahn AL-fuh-2a)
Class Interferon/Immunomodulator
How Supplied
PEGASYS Injection 180 mcg/mL
Action
PHARMACOLOGY: Binds to specific receptors on cell surface and initiates a complex sequence of intracellular events (eg, inhibition of viral replication and inhibition of cell proliferation).
PHARMACOKINETICS/DYNAMICS:
Absorption: T_{max} is 72 to 96 hr. Steady-state is reached within 5 to 8 wk.
Excretion: Cl is approximately 94 mL/hr; t½ is approximately 80 hr.
Special Populations:
Renal Function Impairment – Cl decreased 25% to 45% in those with end-stage renal disease undergoing hemodialysis.
Elderly – AUC increased, but C_{max} did not.

Indications Treatment of chronic hepatitis C in patients with compensated liver disease and not treated previously with interferon alfa.

Contraindications Autoimmune hepatitis; decompensated hepatic disease prior to or during treatment with interferon alfa-2a; hypersensitivity to any component of the product.

Route/Dosage
ADULTS: **SC** 180 mcg (1 mL) once weekly for 48 wk.

Dose reduction
Adverse reactions – When dose reduction is required for moderate to severe adverse reactions, initial dose reduction to 135 mcg is generally adequate; however, in some cases, a dose reduction to 90 mcg may be needed. The dose may be re-escalated following improvement of the adverse reaction.
Hematologic toxicity – Dose reduction to 135 mcg of peginterferon alfa-2a is recommended if the neutrophil count is less than 750 cells/mm^3. Suspend treatment in patients with an absolute neutrophil count below 500 cells/mm^3 until the count returns to more than 1000 cells/mm^3. Reinstitute therapy at 90 mcg of peginterferon alfa-2a and monitor the neutrophil count. A dose reduction to 90 mcg of peginterferon alfa-2a is recommended if the platelet count is less than 50,000 cells/mm^3. Cessation of therapy is recommended when the platelet count is below 25,000 cells/mm^3.
Renal function impairment – A dose reduction to 135 mcg of peginterferon alfa-2a is recommended in patients with end-stage renal disease requiring hemodialysis.
Hepatic function impairment – A dose reduction to 90 mcg of peginterferon alfa-2a is recommended in patients with progressive ALT increases above baseline values. Discontinue peginterferon alfa-2a immediately if ALT increases are progressive despite dose reduction or accompanied by increased bilirubin or evidence of hepatic decompensation.

Interactions

Theophylline: Plasma concentrations of theophylline may be elevated, increasing the risk of side effects.

Lab Test Interferences
None well documented.

Adverse Reactions

CV: Arrhythmia; endocarditis.
CNS: Depression; irritability; anxiety; headache; insomnia; dizziness; concentration impairment; memory impairment; suicidal ideation.
DERM: Alopecia; pruritus; sweating; dermatitis; rash.
EENT: Corneal ulcer.
GI: Nausea; anorexia; diarrhea; abdominal pain; dry mouth; vomiting; peptic ulcer; GI bleeding; pancreatitis; colitis.
HEMA: Neutropenia; thrombocytopenia.
HEPA: Hepatic dysfunction; fatty liver; cholangitis.
METAB: Diabetes mellitus.
RESP: Pneumonia; interstitial pneumonitis; pulmonary embolism.
OTHER: Flu-like symptoms; myalgia; arthralgia; back pain; fatigue; pyrexia; rigors; injection-site reaction; pain; asthenia; suicide; autoimmune phenomena; peripheral neuropathy; coma; myositis; cerebral hemorrhage.

> **WARNING:**
>
> *Neuropsychiatric, autoimmune, ischemic, and infectious disorders:* Interferons may cause or aggravate fatal or life-threatening disorders of this nature. Persistent, severe, or worsening signs or symptoms may necessitate discontinuation of therapy. Closely monitor patients with periodic clinical and laboratory evaluations.
>
> *Use with ribavirin:* May cause birth defects and/or death of the fetus. Extreme care must be taken to avoid pregnancy in female patients and in female partners of male patients. Ribavirin causes hemolytic anemia, which may result in a worsening of cardiac disease. Ribavirin is genotoxic and mutagenic and should be considered a potential carcinogen.

Precautions

Pregnancy: Category C.
Lactation: Undetermined.
Children: Safety and efficacy not established.
Elderly: Use with caution because of increased likelihood of decreased renal function.
Renal function impairment: Use with caution and adjust dose accordingly.
Autoimmune disorders: Use with caution.
Bone marrow toxicity: Bone marrow function may be suppressed.
Cardiovascular disorders: Use with caution in patients with preexisting cardiac disease, including hypertension, supraventricular arrhythmias, chest pain, and MI.
Colitis: Fatal and nonfatal ischemic and hemorrhagic colitis have been observed. Discontinue use immediately in patients who develop symptoms.
Endocrine disorders: May cause or aggravate hypothyroidism and hyperthyroidism. Hyperglycemia, hypoglycemia, and diabetes mellitus have occurred during treatment with peginterferon alfa-2a; therefore, do not begin peginterferon alfa-2a therapy in patients with these conditions at baseline who cannot be effectively treated by medication. Patients who develop these conditions during treatment and cannot be controlled by medication may require discontinuation of peginterferon alfa-2a therapy.
Ophthalmologic disorders: Decreased or loss of vision, retinopathy including macular edema, retinal hemorrhage, cotton wool spots, and retinal artery or vein obstruction have been observed.
Pancreatitis: Fatal and nonfatal pancreatitis has been observed. Discontinue use in patients who develop symptoms.
Pulmonary disorders: Dyspnea, pulmonary infiltrates, pneumonia, bronchiolitis obliterans, interstitial pneumonitis, and sarcoidosis have been associated with use.

Overdosage: Signs and Symptoms

Fatigue, elevated liver enzymes, neutropenia, thrombocytopenia.

PATIENT CARE CONSIDERATIONS
Administration/Storage
- For SC administration only. Not for intradermal, IM, or IV administration.
- Do not administer if particulate matter or discoloration noted.
- If severe adverse reactions develop, dosage adjustment or discontinuation of therapy may be appropriate.
- Use only 1 dose/vial. Do not re-enter vial. Discard any unused portions. Do not save unused solution for later administration.
- Store unused vials in refrigerator (36° to 46°F). Do not freeze or shake. Protect from light.

Assessment/Interventions
- Obtain patient history, including drug history and any known allergies. Note evidence of decompensated liver disease or diagnosis of autoimmune hepatitis. Note history of psychiatric disorders, autoimmune disorders, cardiac disease, thyroid disease, diabetes, or previous treatment with alpha interferon.
- Ensure that the following laboratory tests are performed and reviewed prior to beginning therapy and periodically thereafter during the 48 wk of therapy: platelet count; hemoglobin; absolute neutrophil count; liver enzymes and bilirubin; serum creatinine or creatinine clearance; TSH.
- Ensure that all patients have an ophthalmic examination prior to beginning therapy and that patients with preexisting ophthalmic disorders (eg, diabetic or hypertensive retinopathy) receive periodic ophthalmic examinations during therapy.
- Monitor patient for life-threatening neuropsychiatric reactions (eg, depression, suicidal ideation, suicidal attempt). If noted, inform health care provider immediately.
- Assess patient for GI, CV, HEMA, respiratory, and DERM side effects. If noted and significant inform health care provider.
- If patient experiences adverse CNS symptoms, implement safety precautions such as lowering bed, putting side rails up, and supervising ambulation.
- Assess for flu-like symptoms (eg, fever, rigors, headache, fatigue, arthralgia, myalgia, chills, sweating). If such symptoms occur, administer drug in the evening and give nonnarcotic analgesics as prescribed.
- Implement infection control measures if WBC drops; implement bleeding precautions if platelet count drops.
- Reduce dose 25% if absolute neutrophil count is less than 750/mm^3.
- Reduce dose 50% if platelet count is less than 50,000/mm^3.
- Suspend therapy if absolute neutrophil count is less than 500/mm^3 or if platelet count is less than 25,000/mm^3.
- Reduce dose 25% in patient with end-stage renal disease on hemodialysis.
- Reduce dose 50% in patient with progressive ALT increases above baseline values. Discontinue therapy if ALT increases progress in spite of dose reduction or if hepatic decompensation or increased bilirubin are noted.
- Reduce dose 25% if moderate to severe adverse reactions occur. Further reduce dose to 50% if adverse reactions persist. Discontinue therapy if the reaction does not become tolerable at the reduced dose.
- Ensure that women of child bearing potential is using effective contraception during therapy.

Patient/Family Education
- Explain name, dose, action, and potential side effects of drug. If patient will be administering at home, review "Medication Guide" with the patient. Ensure that the patient understands how to store, prepare, and administer the dose, and dispose of used equipment and supplies.
- Teach patient infection control and bleeding precautions.
- Advise patient that drug may cause confusion, drowsiness, or dizziness and to use caution while driving or performing other activities requiring mental alertness.
- Advise women of childbearing potential to use effective contraception during treatment.
- Instruct women to contact health care provider if pregnant, planning to become pregnant, or breastfeeding.
- Advise patient that it is not known if this drug will prevent transmission of hepatitis C to others nor is it known if it can prevent cirrhosis, liver failure, or liver cancer that may develop as a result of hepatitis C infection.
- Advise patient to report any of the following: signs or feelings of depression; persistent fever; sore throat; unusual bleeding or bruising; stomach pain; bloody diarrhea; rapid or irregular pulse; difficulty breathing.
- Instruct patient to not take any prescription or OTC medications or dietary supplements unless advised by the health care provider.
- Advise patient that follow-up visits and lab tests will be required to monitor therapy; keep appointments.

Peginterferon Alfa-2b

(peg-IN-ter-FEER-ahn AL-fuh-2b)
Class Interferon/Immunomodulator

How Supplied
PEG-Intron Powder for injection, lyophilized 100 mcg/mL (reconstituted), Powder for injection, lyophilized 160 mcg/mL (reconstituted), Powder for injection, lyophilized 240 mcg/mL (reconstituted), Powder for injection, lyophilized 300 mcg/mL (reconstituted)

Action
PHARMACOLOGY: Binds to specific membrane receptors on cell surface and initiates a complex sequence of intracellular events (eg, suppression of cell proliferation, enhancement of phagocytic activity of macrophages).

PHARMACOKINETICS/DYNAMICS:
Absorption: T_{max} is 15 to 44 hr (postdose). Bioavailability increases with multiple dosing. Both AUC and C_{max} increased 70% when administered with a high-fat meal.
Excretion: Renal excretion is 30%. The $t_½$ absorption is 4.6 hr (subcutaneous) and elimination is approximately 40 hr. Apparent Cl is 22 mL/hr•kg.
Duration: Duration is 48 to 72 hr.
Special Populations:
Renal Function Impairment – Cl decreases 50% when Ccr is less than 50 mL/min.

Indications For use alone or in combination with ribavirin for the treatment of chronic hepatitis C in patients not previously treated with interferon alfa who have compensated liver disease. **Unlabeled use(s):** Renal carcinoma.

Contraindications Autoimmune hepatitis; decompensated liver disease; hypersensitivity to the drug.

Route/Dosage
Once Weekly (on Same Day of Week) for 1 yr; Initial Dose Based on Weight
ADULTS: **Subcutaneous** For patients weighing 45 kg or less, administer 40 mcg; 46 to 56 kg, administer 50 mcg; 57 to 72 kg, administer 64 mcg; 73 to 88 kg, administer 80 mcg; 89 to 106 kg, administer 96 mcg; 107 to 136 kg, administer 120 mcg; 137 to 160 kg, administer 150 mcg.

Peginterferon Alfa-2b Dose in Combination Therapy with Ribavirin
ADULTS: **Subcutaneous** For patients weighing less than 40 kg, administer 50 mcg; 40 to 50 kg, administer 64 mcg; 51 to 60 kg, administer 80 mcg; 61 to 75 kg, administer 96 mcg; 76 to 85 kg, administer 120 mcg; greater than 85 kg, administer 150 mcg.

Dose Reduction
If a serious adverse reaction develops during treatment, discontinue or modify dosage to 50% of the starting dose until reaction abates or decreases in severity.

Interactions None well documented.

Lab Test Interferences None well documented.

Adverse Reactions
CV: Cardiac ischemia (postmarketing).
CNS: Fatigue/asthenia (66%); headache (62%); anxiety, emotional lability, irritability (47%); insomnia (40%); depression (31%); dizziness (21%); impaired concentration (17%); agitation, nervousness (8%); peripheral neuropathy, seizures, vertigo (postmarketing).
DERM: Alopecia (36%); pruritus (29%); rash, dry skin (24%); increased sweating (11%); flushing (6%); erythema multiforme, Stevens-Johnson syndrome, toxic epidermal necrolysis (postmarketing).
EENT: Pharyngitis (12%); rhinitis (8%); blurred vision (5%); conjunctivitis (4%); hearing impairment or loss (postmarketing).
ENDO: Hypothyroidism (5%).
GI: Nausea (43%); anorexia (32%); diarrhea (22%); abdominal pain (15%); vomiting (14%); dry mouth (12%); dyspepsia, taste perversion (9%); constipation (5%); stomatitis (postmarketing).
GU: Menstrual disorder (7%); renal failure, renal insufficiency (postmarketing).
HEMA/LYMPH: Neutropenia (26%); anemia (12%); leukopenia (6%); thrombocytopenia (5%).
HEPA: Hepatomegaly (6%).
LABTESTABS: Decreased neutrophils (70%); decreased platelets (20%); hypothyroidism (5%); hyperthyroidism (3%).
LOCAL: Injection site inflammation/reaction (75%).
M/N: Decreased weight (29%).
MUSC: Myalgia (56%); rigors (48%); arthralgia (34%); MUSC pain (28%); rhabdomyolysis (postmarketing).
RESP: Dyspnea (26%); coughing (23%); sinusitis (6%).
OTHER: Right upper quadrant pain (48%); fever (46%); viral infection (12%); chest pain (8%); malaise (7%); fungal infection (6%).

> **WARNING:**
> *Neuropsychiatric, autoimmune, ischemic, and infectious disorders:* Interferons may cause or aggravate fatal or life-threatening disorders of this nature. Persistent, severe, or worsening signs or symptoms may necessitate discontinuation of therapy. Closely monitor patients with periodic clinical and laboratory evaluations.

Precautions
Pregnancy: Category C.
Lactation: Undetermined.
Children: Safety and efficacy not established.
Elderly: Use with caution.
Renal function impairment: Use with caution and monitor for signs and symptoms of interferon toxicity.
Autoimmune disorders: Because interferon alfa may cause or exacerbate autoimmune disorders (eg, thyroiditis, SLE), use with caution in patients with history of autoimmune disorders. Discontinue use in patients with persistently severe or worsening signs or symptoms.
Bone marrow toxicity: Bone marrow function may be suppressed.
CV events: Use with caution in patients with CV disease, including hypotension, arrhythmia, tachycardia, cardiomyopathy, and MI.
Colitis: Fatal and nonfatal ulcerative and hemorrhagic colitis have been observed. Discontinue use immediately in patients who develop symptoms.
Endocrine disorders: Hypo- and hyperthyroidism may occur or be aggravated. Diabetes mellitus has been observed in treated patients.
Hypersensitivity: Serious, acute hypersensitivity reactions (eg, angioedema, anaphylaxis) may occur with alfa interferon therapy.
Infectious disorders: Because life-threatening infectious disorders may occur, use with caution and monitor with periodic clinical and laboratory evaluations. Discontinue use in patients with persistently severe or worsening signs or symptoms.
Neuropsychiatric events: Because life-threatening or fatal neuropsychiatric events, including suicide, suicidal and homicidal ideation, depression, relapse of drug addiction, and aggressive behavior have occurred, use with caution, especially in patients with history of psychiatric disorder. Discontinue use in patients with persistently severe or worsening signs or symptoms.
Ophthalmic disorders: Decrease or loss of vision, retinal hemorrhages, cotton wool spots, and retinal artery or vein obstruction have been observed.
Pancreatitis: Fatal and nonfatal pancreatitis has been observed. Discontinue use in patients who develop symptoms.
Pulmonary disorders: Dyspnea, pulmonary infiltrates, pneumonia, pneumonitis and sarcoidosis, some resulting in respiratory failure and/or patient deaths have been associated with use.
Triglycerides: Elevated triglyceride levels may occur.

PATIENT CARE CONSIDERATIONS
Administration/Storage
- For use alone or in combination with ribavirin.
- For subcutaneous administration only. Not for intradermal, IM, IV, or intra-arterial administration.
- Administer prescribed dose at bedtime to minimize flu-like symptoms.
- Administer antipyretics as ordered as pretreatment to minimize flu-like symptoms.
- Reconstitute powder for injection in vials or *Redipen* following manufacturer's instructions.
- Do not reconstitute with any solution other than that provided with the powder for injection nor add any other medications to reconstituted solution.
- Do not shake solution during reconstitution process. Gently invert *Redipen* or gently swirl contents in vial to obtain a clear, colorless solution.
- Do not administer if solution is discolored or cloudy, or if particulate matter is noted.
- Use only 1 dose/vial or pen. Do not re-enter vial. Discard any unused portions. Do not save unused solution for later administration.
- Store unopened vials at controlled room temperature (59° to 86°F). Store *Redipen* in refrigerator (36° to 46°F). Administer reconstituted solution immediately or store for up to 24 hr in refrigerator. Do not freeze.

Assessment/Interventions
- Obtain patient history, including drug history and any known allergies. Note evidence of decompensated liver disease, diagnosis of autoimmune hepatitis, or renal impairment. Note history of cardiac disease, psychiatric disorder, thyroid disease, diabetes, lung disease, autoimmune disorder (eg, lupus erythematosus, rheumatoid arthritis), or previous treatment with alfa interferon.
- Ensure that hepatitis C virus levels are determined before starting therapy and after 6 mo of therapy. Be prepared to discontinue therapy if viral levels remain high after 6 mo of therapy.

- Ensure the following laboratory tests are performed and reviewed prior to beginning therapy and periodically thereafter during the 52 wk of therapy: CBC with differential and platelet count; liver enzymes and bilirubin; serum creatinine or Ccr; TSH.
- Be prepared to either reduce the dose or discontinue therapy following manufacturer's guidelines if moderate to severe depression is noted, or if significant hematologic abnormalities (eg, HGB less than 8.5 g/dL; WBC count less than $1,500/mm^3$ or neutrophil count less than $750/mm^3$; or platelet count less than $80,000/mm^3$) develop.
- Ensure that all patients have an ophthalmic examination prior to beginning therapy and that patients with preexisting ophthalmic disorders (eg, diabetic, hypertensive retinopathy) receive periodic ophthalmic examinations during therapy.
- Ensure that patient with preexisting cardiac abnormality has an ECG evaluated prior to initiating therapy.
- Ensure that women of child-bearing potential are not pregnant when therapy is started and use effective contraception during therapy.
- Assess patient for CNS, GI, PSYCH, CV, HEMA, RESP, DERM, and MUSC side effects, and injection site reactions. Inform health care provider if noted and significant.
- Assess for flu-like symptoms (eg, fever, rigors, headache, fatigue, arthralgia, myalgia, chills, sweating). If symptoms occur, administer drug in the evening and give nonhepatnarcotic analgesics as prescribed.
- If patient experiences adverse CNS symptoms, implement safety precautions such as lowering bed, putting side rails up, and supervising ambulation.
- Implement infection control measures if WBC drops; implement bleeding precautions if platelet count drops.

Patient/Family Education
- Explain name, dose, action, and potential side effects of drug.
- If patient will be self-administering at home, review *Medication Guide* with the patient. Ensure that the patient understands how to store, prepare, and administer the dose, and dispose of used equipment and supplies.
- Remind patient that prescribed dose is administered once weekly and should be administered on the same day of the week.
- Caution patient not to change the dose or stop taking unless advised by health care provider.
- Advise patient that dose may be reduced or the medication stopped if it causes depression or significant changes in blood cell counts.
- Teach patient infection control and bleeding precautions.
- Advise patient that it is not known if this drug will prevent transmission of hepatitis C to others, nor is it known if it can prevent cirrhosis, liver failure, or liver cancer that may develop as a result of hepatitis C infection.
- Instruct patient to immediately report any of the following to health care provider: signs or feelings of depression and/or suicidal ideation; fever; sore throat; unusual bleeding or bruising; stomach pain; bloody diarrhea; rapid or irregular pulse; difficulty breathing or unexplained shortness of breath.
- Advise women of childbearing potential to use effective contraception during treatment.
- Advise women to notify health care provider if pregnant, planning to become pregnant, or breastfeeding.
- Caution patient not to take any prescription or OTC medications, herbal preparations, or dietary supplements unless advised by health care provider.
- Advise patient that follow-up visits and frequent lab tests will be required to monitor therapy and keep appointments.

Pegvisomant

(peg-VIE-so-mant)
Class Pegvisomant
How Supplied
Somavert Injection 10 mg, Injection 15 mg, Injection 20 mg

Action
PHARMACOLOGY: Selectively binds to growth hormone receptors on cell surfaces, where it blocks the binding of endogenous growth hormone, interfering with growth hormone transduction.

PHARMACOKINETICS/DYNAMICS:
Absorption: Following SC administration, C_{max} is generally not attained until 33 to 77 hr.
Distribution: Mean apparent Vd is 7 L.
Excretion: After multiple dosing, the mean total body clearance is estimated to range between 36 to 28 mL/hr for SC doses ranging from 10 to 20 mg/day, respectively. Following either single or multiple doses, the mean elimination t½ is approximately 6 days.

Indications Treatment of acromegaly in patients who have had an inadequate response to surgery or radiation therapy or other medical therapies.

Contraindications Standard considerations.

Route/Dosage

ADULTS: **SC** 40 mg loading dose under health care provider supervision; then instruct patient to begin daily injections of 10 mg. Measure serum insulin-like growth factor-I (IGF-I) levels every 4 to 6 wk, at which time, increase the dose in 5 mg increments if IGF-I levels are still elevated or decrease the dose in 5-mg decrements if IGF-I levels have decreased below the normal range.

Interactions

Insulin, oral hypoglycemic agents: Dose may need to be reduced after starting pegvisomant.
Opioids: May need higher pegvisomant serum levels to achieve appropriate IGF-I suppression.

Lab Test Interferences Because of structural similarities, pegvisomant may cross-react in commercially available growth hormone assays.

Adverse Reactions

CV: Hypertension.
CNS: Dizziness.
DERM: Injection site reaction.
EENT: Sinusitis.
GI: Diarrhea; nausea.
HEMA: Elevated ALT and AST.
OTHER: Infection; accidental injury; back pain; pain; peripheral edema; chest pain; flu-like syndrome; paresthesia.

Precautions

Pregnancy: Category B.
Lactation: Undetermined.
Children: Safety and efficacy not established.
Elderly: Select dose with caution, reflecting greater frequency of decreased hepatic, renal, or cardiac function, and comorbidity.
Glucose metabolism: Because growth hormone opposes the effects of insulin on carbohydrate metabolism by decreasing insulin sensitivity, glucose tolerance may increase in some patients.
Growth hormone deficiency: A state of functional growth hormone deficiency may occur.
LFTs: Elevations of serum concentrations of ALT and AST greater than 10 times the upper limit of normal have been reported.
Tumor growth: Tumors that secrete growth hormone may expand and cause serious complications.

Overdosage: Signs and Symptoms
Fatigue.

PATIENT CARE CONSIDERATIONS

Administration/Storage

- For SC administration only. Not for intradermal, IM, or IV administration.
- Follow manufacturer's instructions for reconstitution of powder for injection.
- Do not shake vial during reconstitution process.
- Do not administer if particulate matter, cloudiness, or discoloration noted.
- Rotate injection sites (eg, thigh, abdomen, upper arm). Give new injections at least 1 inch from old site and never into areas where the skin is tender, bruised, red, or hard.
- Discard any unused solution. Do not save unused solution for later administration.
- Store unopened vials in refrigerator (36° to 46°F). Do not freeze. Use reconstituted solution within 6 hr.

Assessment/Interventions

- Obtain patient history, including drug history and any known allergies. Note history of latex sensitivity.
- Ensure that liver enzymes are determined prior to starting therapy. Do not start therapy if liver enzymes are greater than 3 times upper limit of normal. Monitor liver enzymes monthly for 1 yr and then biannually for 1 yr if liver enzymes are elevated but are less than 3 times upper limit of normal.
- Monitor blood sugar in diabetic patient when drug is started or dose is changed. Report significant changes to health care provider. Be prepared to reduce the dose of insulin or oral hypoglycemic agents.
- Monitor patient for CNS, GI, respiratory, and general body side effects, and injection site reactions. Report to health care provider if noted and significant.
- Discontinue therapy and immediately inform health care provider if any signs or symptoms of liver injury (eg, jaundice, nausea or vomiting, right upper quadrant pain, ascites, edema, easy bruising) are noted.

Patient/Family Education

- Explain name, dose, action, and potential side effects of drug.
- Advise patient or caregiver that dose will be carefully adjusted based on results of lab tests that are done periodically.
- If patient or caregiver will be administering at home, review "Patient Information" insert with the patient or caregiver. Ensure that the patient or caregiver understands how to store, prepare, and administer the dose, and dispose of used equipment and supplies. The first injection should be performed under the supervision of a qualified health professional.
- Advise patient that if a dose is missed, to inject the missed dose as soon as remembered

and then inject the next dose at the regularly scheduled time.
- Advise patient to report any of the following to health care provider: intolerable injection site reactions, fatigue, persistent nausea or vomiting, unexplained bruising, bloating, stomach pain, or swelling.
- Instruct patient to stop taking and immediately inform health care provider if yellowing of skin or eyes is noted.
- Instruct diabetic patient to monitor blood glucose more frequently when drug is started or dose is changed and to inform health care provider of significant changes in readings.
- Advise women to notify health care provider if pregnant, planning to become pregnant, or breastfeeding.
- Instruct patient to not take any prescription or OTC medications or dietary supplements unless advised by health care provider.
- Remind patient that office visits and laboratory tests will be required to monitor therapy and to keep appointments.

Pemetrexed
(pem-eh-TREX-ehd)
Class Antineoplastic
How Supplied
Alimta Injection 500 mg
Action
PHARMACOLOGY: Disrupts folate-dependent metabolic processes essential for cell replication.
PHARMACOKINETICS/DYNAMICS:
Distribution: Vd is about 16.1 L. Protein binding approximately 81%.
Metabolism: Not appreciably metabolized.
Excretion: Primarily eliminated in the urine. Elimination t½ is 3.5 hr.
Indications In combination with cisplatin for the treatment of malignant pleural mesothelioma in patients whose disease is unresectable or who are otherwise not candidates for curative surgery.
Contraindications Standard considerations.
Route/Dosage
ADULTS: **IV** Recommended dose is 500 mg/m^2 infused over 10 min on day 1 of each 21-day cycle.
Dosage Modification
ADULTS: **IV** Reduce the dose of pemetrexed to 75% of previous dose in patients with nadir absolute neutrophil count (ANC) below 500/mm^3 and nadir platelets at least 50,000/mm^3, any grade 3 or 4 toxicities (except mucositis), any diarrhea requiring hospitalization. Reduce the dose to 50% of previous dose in patients with nadir platelets below 50,000/mm^3 regardless of nadir ANC, grade 3 or 4 mucositis. Discontinue immediately if grade 3 or 4 neurotoxicity occurs or if a patient experiences any hematologic or nonhematologic grade 3 or 4 toxicity after 2 dose reductions.
Interactions
Nephrotoxic drugs or drugs secreted by the renal tubules (eg, probenecid): May delay Cl of pemetrexed.
NSAIDs with longer half-lives (or NSAIDs with short elimination half-lives in patients with mild to moderate renal insufficiency): Patients should interrupt NSAID dosing for at least 5 days before (2 days for NSAIDs with short elimination half-lives in patients with mild to moderate renal insufficiency), the day of, and 2 days following pemetrexed administration.
Incompatibilities: Calcium (including lactated Ringer's injection and Ringer's injection).
Lab Test Interferences None well documented.
Adverse Reactions Percentages of adverse reactions reported are for all grades of toxicity with patients receiving pemetrexed plus cisplatin.
CV: Thrombosis/embolism (7%).
CNS: Fatigue (80%); neuropathy (17%); mood alteration, depression (14%).
DERM: Rash/desquamation (22%).
EENT: Pharyngitis (28%).
GI: Nausea (84%); vomiting (58%); constipation (44%); anorexia (35%); stomatitis (28%); diarrhea (26%); esophagitis (6%).
HEMA/LYMPH: Neutropenia (58%); leukopenia (55%); anemia (33%); thrombocytopenia (27%).
HYPERSEN: Allergic reaction/hypersensitivity (2%).
M/N: Dehydration (7%).
RENAL: Creatinine elevation (16%); renal failure (2%).
RESP: Dyspnea (66%).
OTHER: Chest pain (40%); fever (17%); infection without neutropenia (11%); dysphagia, odynophagia, infection with grade 3 or 4 neutropenia (6%); febrile neutropenia (1%).
Precautions
Pregnancy: Category D.
Lactation: Undetermined.
Children: Safety and efficacy not established.
Renal function impairment: Decreased renal function will result in reduced Cl and greater exposure to pemetrexed. Do not administer to patients with Ccr less than 45 mL/min.

Bone marrow suppression: Suppression of bone marrow function, manifested in neutropenia, thrombocytopenia, and anemia may occur.
Hematologic and GI toxicity: Folic acid and vitamin B_{12} supplementation should be taken to reduce treatment-related hematologic and GI toxicity.

Overdosage: Signs and Symptoms
Neutropenia, anemia, thrombocytopenia, mucositis, rash, infection (with or without fever), diarrhea.

PATIENT CARE CONSIDERATIONS
Administration/Storage
- Administer in combination with cisplatin.
- For IV infusion only. Not for IV bolus, intradermal, subcutaneous, IM, or intra-arterial administration.
- Follow institutional procedures for handling, administration, and disposal of anticancer drugs.
- Reconstitute powder for injection with 20 mL preservative-free 0.9% sodium chloride injection following manufacturer's guidelines. Gently swirl to mix. Reconstituted solution contains 25 mg/mL of pemetrexed. Further dilute prescribed amount of reconstituted solution to 100 mL with preservative-free 0.9% sodium chloride injection.
- Do not mix with any other medications or diluents.
- Do not administer if particulate matter or cloudiness is noted. A slight yellow or green-yellow coloration is normal and of no concern.
- Administer prescribed dose by IV infusion over 10 min.
- If pemetrexed solution contacts the skin, wash the skin immediately and thoroughly with soap and water. If pemetrexed contacts mucous membranes, flush thoroughly with water.
- Discard unused portions of vial. Do not save any unused portions for future use.
- Store unopened vials at controlled room temperature (59° to 86°F). Reconstituted solution should be used immediately or used within 24 hr if stored in refrigerator (36° to 46°F) or at controlled room temperature and lighting conditions. Discard solution if not used within 24 hr.

Assessment/Interventions
- Obtain patient history, including drug history and any known allergies. Note renal or hepatic impairment.
- Ensure that CBC with differential and platelet count is evaluated before starting therapy, on days 8 and 15 of each cycle, and before starting new cycle.
- Do not begin a cycle unless absolute neutrophil count is 1,500/mm^3 or higher, platelet count is 100,000/mm^3 or higher, and Ccr is 45 mL/min or more.
- Ensure that renal and hepatic function are evaluated before starting therapy and periodically during therapy.
- Ensure that medication is not administered to patient with renal impairment (Ccr less than 45 mL/min).
- Ensure that dose adjustments for subsequent cycle are made for hematologic and nonhematologic (eg, neurologic, GI) toxicity from preceding cycle per manufacturer's guidelines.
- Ensure that premedication regimen consisting of corticosteroid (to reduce incidence and severity of cutaneous reactions), folic acid, and injectable vitamin B_{12} (to reduce hematologic and GI toxicity) has been ordered.
- Ensure that women of childbearing potential are not pregnant and are using effective contraception during treatment.
- Because of potential risk of increased toxicity, do not administer short-acting NSAIDs (eg, ibuprofen) for a period of 2 days before, the day of, and for 2 days following administration of pemetrexed. If coadministration cannot be avoided, closely monitor patient for myelosuppression, and renal and GI toxicity.
- Because of potential risk of increased toxicity, do not administer long-acting NSAIDs (eg, piroxicam) for a period of 5 days before, the day of, and for 2 days following administration of pemetrexed in patient with mild renal insufficiency (Ccr from 45 to 79 mL/min). If coadministration cannot be avoided, closely monitor patient for myelosuppression, and renal and GI toxicity.
- Monitor patient for signs or symptoms of infection or bleeding. Inform health care provider immediately if noted and be prepared to treat appropriately.
- Implement infection control measures if WBC drops; implement bleeding control measures if platelet count drops.

- Assess patient for GI, CNS, RESP, DERM, HEMA, and general body side effects. Report to health care provider if noted and significant.

Patient/Family Education
- Explain name, action, and potential side effects of drug.
- Advise patient, family, or caregiver that medication will be prepared and administered by health care provider in a health care setting.
- Review dosing schedule with patient, family, or caregiver.
- Instruct patient to carefully follow premedication orders for folic acid, vitamin B_{12} supplementation, and corticosteroid as ordered to reduce toxic effects of chemotherapy.
- Caution patient with mild renal insufficiency (Ccr from 45 to 79 mL/min) to avoid taking short-acting NSAIDs (eg, ibuprofen) for a period of 2 days before, the day of, and for 2 days following administration of pemetrexed.
- Caution patient to avoid taking long-acting NSAIDs (eg, piroxicam) for a period of 5 days before, the day of, and for 2 days following administration of pemetrexed.
- Advise patient, family, or caregiver to immediately report any of the following to health care provider: fever, chills, or other signs of infection; unusual bleeding or bruising; pain, redness, or swelling at injection site.
- Advise patient, family, or caregiver to report any of the following to health care provider: persistent nausea, vomiting, diarrhea, or appetite loss; sores in mouth; persistent or worsening general body weakness or fatigue.
- Caution women of childbearing potential to avoid becoming pregnant during therapy.
- Advise women to notify health care provider if pregnant, planning to become pregnant, or breastfeeding.
- Instruct patient not to take any prescription or OTC medications, herbal preparations, or dietary supplements unless advised by health care provider.
- Advise patient, family, or caregiver that frequent follow-up visits and laboratory tests will be required to monitor therapy and to keep appointments.

Pemoline

(PEM-oh-leen)
Class Psychotherapeutic

How Supplied
Cylert Tablets 18.75 mg, Tablets 37.5 mg, Tablets 75 mg, Tablets, chewable 37.5 mg

Action
PHARMACOLOGY: Acts as a CNS stimulant but with minimal sympathomimetic effects; exact mechanism of action unknown.

PHARMACOKINETICS/DYNAMICS:
Absorption: Pemoline is rapidly absorbed from GI tract. T_{max} is 2 to 4 hr. Steady state is 2 to 3 days.

Distribution: Widely distributed throughout tissues, including the brain. Protein binding is approximately 50%.

Metabolism: Metabolized in the liver to metabolites including pemoline conjugate, pemoline dione, mandelic acid, and unidentified polar compounds.

Excretion: Pemoline is excreted 50% unchanged through the kidneys. Serum t½ is approximately 12 hr.

Peak: 3 to 4 wk.

Indications Treatment of attention-deficit hyperactivity disorder (ADHD). **Unlabeled use(s):** Treatment of narcolepsy and excessive daytime sedation.

Contraindications Hepatic insufficiency.

Route/Dosage
ADULTS AND CHILDREN 6 YR AND OLDER: **PO** 37.5 mg/day as a single dose in the morning initially; increase by increments of 18.75 mg weekly until desired response is obtained (max daily dose, 112.5 mg/day).

Interactions None well documented.

Lab Test Interferences None well documented.

Adverse Reactions
CNS: Insomnia; Tourette syndrome; hallucinations; dyskinetic movements of tongue, lips, face, and extremities; abnormal oculomotor function (eg, nystagmus, oculogyric crisis); depression; dizziness; irritability; headache; drowsiness; seizures.
DERM: Rash.
GI: Anorexia; transient weight loss; stomach ache; nausea.
HEPA: Elevated liver enzymes; hepatitis; jaundice.
OTHER: Growth suppression.

> **WARNING:**
> Life-threatening hepatotoxicity limits use as first-line agent in ADHD; may have long latency period. Obtain written informed consent from patient prior to initiation.

Precautions
Pregnancy: Category B.
Lactation: Undetermined.
Children: Safety and efficacy in children younger than 6 yr not established.
Renal function impairment: Use with caution in patients with significantly impaired renal function.
Hepatic function impairment: Pemoline is not usually considered first-line therapy.
Drug abuse and dependence: Can occur; use with caution in emotionally unstable patients who may increase the dosage on their own initiative.

Overdosage: Signs and Symptoms
Vomiting, agitation, tremors, hyperreflexia, muscle twitching, convulsions (followed by coma), euphoria, confusion, hallucinations, delirium, sweating, flushing, headache, high fever, tachycardia, hypertension, dilated pupils.

PATIENT CARE CONSIDERATIONS
Administration/Storage
- Do not administer if LFTs are abnormal.
- Administer as a single dose each morning and ensure that chewable tablets are completely chewed and swallowed.
- Administer with caution to emotionally unstable patients. Administration may intensify symptoms of behavior disturbance and thought disorder.
- Administer with caution to patients with impaired renal function.
- Store at controlled room temperature (56° to 86°F) in a tight, dry container.

Assessment/Interventions
- Obtain patient history.
- Clinically assess for tics and Tourette syndrome in children and their families before use of this drug.
- Monitor growth of children during treatment, as long-term administration is associated with growth inhibition.
- Ensure LFTs are performed prior to and periodically during therapy.
- Assess therapeutic effects of medication. Medication is often interrupted at intervals to determine therapeutic effects and to ascertain if there are sufficient behavioral symptoms present to require continued therapy.
- Ensure that dosage is decreased gradually following long-term therapy to prevent withdrawal symptoms.

Patient/Family Education
- Advise patient that clinical improvement is gradual and benefits may not occur until week 3 or 4 of administration.
- Instruct patient to take pemoline as prescribed and not to make up missed doses.
- Caution patient to avoid taking large doses of caffeine or using other stimulants that could adversely potentiate the effects of pemoline.
- Instruct patient to take medication in the morning to avoid sleep disturbance. Notify health care provider if problems with sleeping occur.
- Instruct patient to notify health care provider of adverse reactions; the dosage may need to be reduced or the drug discontinued.
- Advise patient that medication can cause dizziness or drowsiness and to avoid driving and other tasks requiring mental alertness.
- Instruct patient not to increase the dose amount or take the medication more frequently because of a high dependence and abuse potential. In addition, psychotic symptoms could occur following long-term misuse of excessive oral doses.
- Instruct caregiver, patient, or family to be aware of the symptoms of overdose and take immediate and appropriate action, such as notifying a poison control center.
- Instruct patient to take daily dose in the morning.
- Advise patient to follow health care provider instructions for LFTs.
- Advise patient to be alert for signs and symptoms of liver dysfunction (eg, jaundice, anorexia, malaise, GI complaints) and to report them immediately to the health care provider.

Penbutolol Sulfate
(pen-BYOO-toe-lole SULL-fate)
Class Beta-adrenergic blocker
How Supplied
Levatol Tablets 20 mg
Action
PHARMACOLOGY: Nonselectively blocks beta-adrenergic receptors, primarily affecting the cardiovascular system (eg, decreased heart rate, decreased cardiac contractility, decreased BP) and lungs (promotes bronchospasm).

PHARMACOKINETICS/DYNAMICS:
Absorption: Absorption is rapid and complete (100%). The t_{max} is 2 to 3 hr.
Distribution: Protein binding is 80% to 98%.

Penbutolol crosses the placenta.

Metabolism: Hepatic metabolism is by conjugation and oxidation.

Excretion: Urine (90% excreted in urine, ⅙ as penbutolol conjugate). Penbutolol plasma t½ is approximately 5 hr; conjugated penbutolol is approximately 20 hr, 25 hr in the elderly, and approximately 100 hr in patients on renal dialysis.

Special Populations:
Renal Function Impairment – Accumulation of penbutolol conjugates may be expected.

Indications Management of mild to moderate hypertension.

Contraindications Greater than first-degree heart block; CHF unless secondary to tachyarrhythmia or untreated hypertension treatable with beta-blockers; overt cardiac failure; sinus bradycardia; cardiogenic shock; hypersensitivity to beta-blockers; untreated bronchial asthma or bronchospasm, including severe COPD.

Route/Dosage
ADULTS: **PO** 20 mg qd.

Interactions
Clonidine: May attenuate or reverse antihypertensive effect; potentially life-threatening increases in BP, especially on withdrawal.
Epinephrine: Initial hypertensive episodes followed by bradycardia may occur.
Ergot derivatives: Peripheral ischemia, manifested by cold extremities and possible gangrene.
Insulin: Prolonged hypoglycemia with masking of symptoms.
Lidocaine: Increased lidocaine levels, leading to toxicity.
Nonsteroidal anti-inflammatory agents: Some agents may impair antihypertensive effects.
Theophylline: Elimination of theophylline may be reduced; effects of both drugs may be reduced by pharmacologic antagonism.
Verapamil: Effects of both drugs may be increased.

Lab Test Interferences None well documented.

Adverse Reactions
CV: Bradycardia; hypotension; CHF; edema; worsening angina, atrioventricular (AV) block.
CNS: Dizziness; tiredness; fatigue; headache; insomnia; depression; short-term memory loss; emotional lability.
DERM: Sweating.
EENT: Dry eyes; visual disturbances.
GI: Diarrhea; nausea; dyspepsia.
GU: Impotence.
HEMA: Agranulocytosis; nonthrombocytopenic and thrombocytopenic purpura.
METAB: May increase or decrease blood sugar.
RESP: Cough; dyspnea; bronchospasm.

Precautions
Pregnancy: Category C.
Lactation: Undetermined.
Children: Safety and efficacy not established.
CHF: Administer cautiously in CHF patients controlled with digitalis and diuretics.
Diabetics: May mask signs and symptoms of hypoglycemia (eg, tachycardia, BP changes). May potentiate insulin-induced hypoglycemia.
Nonallergic bronchospasm: Give drug with caution to patients with bronchospastic disease.
Thyrotoxicosis: May mask clinical signs of developing or continuing hyperthyroidism (eg, tachycardia). Abrupt withdrawal may exacerbate symptoms of hyperthyroidism, including thyroid storm.
Abrupt withdrawal: A beta-blocker withdrawal syndrome (eg, hypertension, tachycardia, anxiety, angina, MI) may occur 1 to 2 wk after sudden discontinuation of systemic beta-blockers. If possible, gradually withdraw therapy over 1 to 2 wk.
Anaphylaxis: May be unresponsive to usual doses of epinephrine; aggressive therapy may be required.
Peripheral vascular disease: May precipitate or aggravate symptoms of arterial insufficiency.

Overdosage: Signs and Symptoms
Bradycardia, hypotension, CHF, AV block, intraventricular conduction defects, asystole, coma.

PATIENT CARE CONSIDERATIONS

Administration/Storage
- May be taken with or without food.
- Store tablets at room temperature in a tightly closed, light-resistant container.

Assessment/Interventions
- Obtain patient history.
- Evaluate current ECG for signs of bradycardia or heart block.
- Monitor for bradycardia, hypotension, respiratory difficulty, and heart block that may indicate need for reduced dosage.
- Avoid use in patients with asthma, chronic bronchitis, and other chronic respiratory diseases.
- Monitor I&O and daily weight during therapy for signs of fluid retention. If sudden, severe dyspnea or edema of hands and feet develop, withhold medication and notify health care provider.
- Notify health care provider at first sign or symptom of CHF or unexplained respiratory symptoms in any patient.

Patient/Family Education
- Warn patient to never stop taking this medication suddenly. Rebound effects can produce angina, and even MI. Explain that medication will be tapered slowly before discontinuation.
- Instruct patient to take medication at the same time every day.
- Advise patient not to take any *otc* medications such as nasal decongestants, diet aids, cold preparations, or antihistamines without consulting the health care provider first.
- Teach patient and family how to take pulse. Instruct them to check it before taking the medication. If the pulse is irregular or has a rate less than 60 bpm, notify health care provider before taking the medication.
- Instruct patient and family on how to take BP. If BP is markedly lower than normal, notify health care provider.
- Warn patient that sudden position changes may cause dizziness caused by postural hypotension.
- Instruct patient to notify health care provider if any of the following occur: confusion, depression, memory loss, rash, shortness of breath, slowed pulse rate, or unusual bruising or bleeding.

Penciclovir

(pen-SICK-low-vihr)

Class Topical anti-infective/Antiviral

How Supplied
Denavir Cream 10 mg/g

Action
PHARMACOLOGY: Selectively inhibits herpes viral DNA synthesis and replication.

Indications Treatment of recurrent herpes labialis (cold sores) in adults.

Contraindications Standard considerations.

Route/Dosage
ADULTS: **Topical** Apply to lesions q 2 hr while awake for 4 days. Start treatment as early as possible, during the prodrome or when lesions first appear.

Interactions None well documented.

Lab Test Interferences None well documented.

Adverse Reactions
DERM: Application site reaction.

Precautions
Pregnancy: Category B.
Lactation: Undetermined.
Children: Safety and efficacy not established.
Elderly: Side effect profile similar to younger patients.

PATIENT CARE CONSIDERATIONS

Administration/Storage
- Available as a topical cream.
- Wash hands before and after application.
- Apply small amount using finger cot or glove every 2 hr directly on lesion. Avoid application in or near eyes or mucous membranes.
- Store at room temperature (59° to 86°F). Do not freeze.

Assessment/Interventions
- Assess lesions prior to and daily during therapy.
- Report any local reaction to health care provider.

Patient/Family Education
- Obtain patient history, including drug history and any known allergies.
- Instruct patient to begin treatment as soon as possible, during the prodrome, or as soon as lesions appear.
- Advise patient to apply the medication exactly as directed and to only apply to lesions on the face and lips.
- Advise patient to avoid applying cream to mucous membranes, within or near eyes.
- Advise patient to wash hands before and after applying cream.
- Advise patient to discontinue use and notify health care provider if local irritation develops.
- Advise the patient that the use of additional OTC creams or ointments may delay the healing process or even spread the disease.
- Instruct the patient to notify the health care provider if the symptoms do not improve in 7 days of topical therapy.
- Instruct the patient to apply sufficient ointment to cover all lesions q 2 hr while awake.
- Advise the patient to use a finger cot or glove when applying the ointment to prevent the spread of virus.

Penicillamine

(PEN-ih-SILL-ah-meen)

Class Cystine-depleting agents

How Supplied
Cuprimine Capsules 125 mg, Capsules 250 mg ♦
Depen Tablets, titratable 250 mg

Action
PHARMACOLOGY: Unknown; however, appears to suppress disease activity.

Indications Treatment of Wilson disease; cystinuria; and severe, active rheumatoid arthritis.

Contraindications Pregnancy (except in treatment of Wilson disease or certain cases of cystinuria); penicillamine-related aplastic anemia or agranulocytosis; rheumatoid arthritis patients with a history of renal insufficiency; breastfeeding.

Route/Dosage

Cystinuria
ADULTS: PO Initially, 250 mg/day, and increasing gradually to the requisite amount. Range 1 to 4 g/day. Daily dose should be divided into 4 doses.
CHILDREN: PO 30 mg/kg/day divided into 4 doses. If 4 equal doses are not feasible, give the larger portion at bedtime.

Rheumatoid Arthritis
ADULTS: PO Start with a single daily dose of 125 or 250 mg/day. The dose may be increased at 1- to 3-mo intervals by 125 or 250 mg/day, as patient response and tolerance indicate. Continue dosage associated with satisfactory remission. If there is no improvement or no signs of potentially serious toxicity after 2 to 3 mo of treatment with 500 to 750 mg/day, increases of 250 mg/day at 2- to 3-mo intervals may be continued until satisfactory remission or signs of toxicity develop. If there is no discernible improvement after 3 or 4 mo of treatment with 1000 to 1500 mg/day, penicillamine should be discontinued.
Maintenance therapy: Many patients respond satisfactorily to dosage within the 500 to 750 mg/day range.
Duration: If a patient has been in remission for 6 mo or more, a gradual, stepwise dosage reduction in decrements of 125 or 250 mg at about 3-mo intervals may be attempted.

Wilson Disease
ADULTS: PO 0.25 mg to 2 g/day. Optimal dosage can be determined by measurement of urinary copper excretion and determination of free copper in the serum.

Interactions
Aluminum salts (eg, aluminum carbonate, sucralfate): GI absorption of penicillamine may be reduced.

Lab Test Interferences None well documented.

Adverse Reactions
CNS: Peripheral sensory and motor neuropathies (including Guillain-Barré syndrome); psychic disturbances; mental disorders; agitation; anxiety.
DERM: Urticaria; exfoliative dermatitis; alopecia; failing hair; lichen planus; toxic epidermal necrolysis; cutaneous macular atrophy; increased skin friability; excessive wrinkling; development of small white papules at venipuncture and surgical sites; yellow nail syndrome.
EENT: Tinnitus; optic neuritis; visual disturbances.
GI: Anorexia, epigastric pain, nausea, vomiting, diarrhea (17%); diminished taste perception (12%); peptic ulcers; pancreatitis; oral ulcers.
ENDO: Thyroiditis.
HEMA: Thrombocytopenia (4%); leukopenia (2%); agranulocytosis; aplastic anemia; sideroblastic anemia; hemolytic anemia; thrombotic thrombocytopenic purpura; red cell aplasia; monocytosis; leukocytosis; eosinophilia; thrombocytosis.
HEPA: Intrahepatic cholestasis; toxic hepatitis.
MUSC: Migratory polyarthralgia; myasthenia gravis; dystonia.
RENAL: Proteinuria (6%); hematuria; nephrotic syndrome; renal failure.
RESP: Allergic alveolitis, obliterative bronchiolitis; interstitial pneumonitis; pulmonary fibrosis; bronchial asthma.
OTHER: Allergy, including generalized pruritus with early and late rashes (5%); pemphigus; drug eruptions (accompanied by fever, arthralgia, lymphadenopathy); lupus erythematosus-like syndrome; thrombophlebitis; hyperpyrexia; polymyositis; dermatomyositis; mammary hyperplasia; elastosis perforans serpiginosa; Goodpasture syndrome; vasculitis (including fatal renal vasculitis).

> **WARNING:**
> Physicians should be thoroughly familiar with penicillamine toxicity, special dosage considerations, and therapeutic benefits. Patients should promptly report any symptoms of toxicity.

Precautions
Pregnancy: Contraindicated in pregnancy.
Lactation: Breastfeeding is contraindicated.

Children: Safety and efficacy not established in pediatric patients with juvenile rheumatoid arthritis.
Allergy: Skin and mucous membranes should be observed for allergic reactions.
Pemphigus: Pemphigus vulgaris or pemphigus foliaceus may be late complications of therapy.

Severe reactions: Penicillamine therapy has a high incidence of adverse reactions, some of which are potentially fatal. Treatment has been associated with aplastic anemia, agranulocytosis, thrombocytopenia, Goodpasture syndrome, myasthenia gravis, proteinuria, hematuria, and obliterative bronchiolitis.

Penicillin G

(pen-ih-SILL-in G)
Class Antibiotic/Penicillin

How Supplied

Penicillin G Potassium
Pfizerpen Powder for injection 1,000,000 units, Powder for injection 5,000,000 units, Powder for injection 20,000,000 units

Penicillin G Procaine
Wycillin Injection, IM 600,000 units, Injection, IM 1,200,000 units, Injection, IM 2,400,000 units

Penicillin G Sodium
Penicillin G Sodium Powder for injection 5,000,000
♣ *Crystapen*

Penicillin G Benzathine
Bicillin L-A Injection, IM 300,000 units/mL, Injection, IM 600,000 units/dose, Injection, IM 1,200,000 units/dose, Injection, IM 2,400,000 units/dose ♦ *Permapen* Injection 1,200,000 units/dose

Action

PHARMACOLOGY: Inhibits mucopeptide synthesis of bacterial cell wall.

PHARMACOKINETICS/DYNAMICS:
Absorption: Varies considerably, 15% to 30% (oral) and slow absorption (IM). T_{max} is 1 to 2 hr (oral), and 24 hr (benzathine IM), 4 hr (procaine IM). C_{max} is 2.2 to 17 mcg/mL (IV), 0.03 to 0.05 mcg/mL (benzathine IM).

Distribution: Distributed throughout body tissues; highest levels found in kidneys with lesser amount in liver, skin, and intestines. Also, penetrates CSF; however, concentrations are low with noninflammed meninges, as is penetration in purulent bronchial secretions. Protein binding is 60% (oral), primarily albumin. Vd is 0.5 to 0.7 L/kg (oral). Crosses the placenta; distributes into breast milk.

Metabolism: Hepatic metabolism accounts for less than 30% of the biotransformation.

Excretion: Renal (largely unchanged); hepatic inactivation and excretion in bile; t½ 1.4 hr or less.

Duration: Sustaining levels for up to 4 wk (benzathine).

Special Populations:
Renal Function Impairment – Neonates and young infants with impaired renal function have delayed excretion.

Indications
Penicillin G: Treatment of infections caused by susceptible microorganisms.
Penicillin G Procaine: Treatment of moderately severe infections caused by penicillin-G-sensitive microorganisms that are sensitive to low and persistent serum levels achieved with this dose form.
Penicillin G Benzathine: Mild to moderate upper respiratory tract infections, venereal diseases, and prophylaxis of rheumatic fever or chorea caused by penicillin-G-sensitive microorganisms that are susceptible to the low and very prolonged serum levels common to this dosage form.

Contraindications
Hypersensitivity to penicillins. Do not treat severe pneumonia, empyema, bacteremia, pericarditis, meningitis, and purulent or septic arthritis with oral penicillin G during acute stage.

Route/Dosage

Dosage may vary with site of infection and organism being treated.

PENICILLIN G (AQUEOUS POTASSIUM OR SODIUM)
ADULTS: **IV/IM** 1 to 24 million U/day in divided doses q 4 to 6 hr.
CHILDREN: **IV/IM** 100,000 to 250,000 U/kg/day in divided doses q 4 hr.
INFANTS (OVER 7 DAYS AND MORE THAN 2000 G): **IV/IM** 100,000 U/kg/day in divided doses q 6 hr (meningitis: 200,000 U/kg/day in divided doses q 6 hr).
INFANTS (UNDER 7 DAYS AND MORE THAN 2000 G): **IV/IM** 50,000 U/kg/day in divided doses q 8 hr (meningitis: 150,000 U/kg/day in divided doses q 8 hr).
INFANTS (UNDER 7 DAYS AND LESS THAN 2000 G): **IV/IM** 50,000 U/kg/day in divided doses q 12 hr (meningitis: 100,000 U/kg/day in divided doses q 12 hr).

PENICILLIN G POTASSIUM
ADULTS AND CHILDREN OLDER THAN 12 YR: **PO** 200,000 to 500,000 U q 6 to 8 hr.

INFANTS AND CHILDREN YOUNGER THAN 12 YR: PO 25,000 to 90,000 U/kg/day in 3 to 6 divided doses.

PENICILLIN G PROCAINE (AQUEOUS)
ADULTS AND CHILDREN (AT LEAST 27 KG): IM 600,000 to 1.2 million U/day in 1 to 2 doses.
CHILDREN (UNDER 27 KG): IM 300,000 U/day.

Congenital Syphilis
CHILDREN (UNDER 32 KG): IM 50,000 U/kg/day as a single dose for 10 to 14 days.

Neurosyphilis
ADULTS: IM 2.4 million U/day plus probenecid 500 mg PO qid, both for 10 to 14 days.

PENICILLIN G BENZATHINE
ADULTS: IM 1.2 to 2.4 million U in 1 dose.
CHILDREN MORE THAN 27 KG: IM 900,000 to 1.2 million U in 1 dose.
CHILDREN AND INFANTS LESS THAN 27 KG: IM 300,000 to 1.2 million U in 1 dose.
NEWBORNS: IM 50,000 U/kg in 1 dose.

PENICILLIN G BENZATHINE AND PROCAINE COMBINED
ADULTS AND CHILDREN MORE THAN 27 KG: IM 2.4 million U in 1 dose.
CHILDREN 14 TO 27 KG: IM 900,000 to 1.2 million U in 1 dose.
CHILDREN AND INFANTS LESS THAN 14 KG: IM 600,000 U in 1 dose.

Interactions
Anticoagulants (oral and heparin): May increase bleeding risks of anticoagulant by prolonging bleeding time.
Beta-blockers: May potentiate anaphylactic reactions of penicillin.
Chloramphenicol: May cause synergism or antagonism to develop.
Contraceptives, oral: May reduce efficacy of oral contraceptives.
Erythromycin: May cause synergism or antagonism to develop.
Probenecid: Increases penicillin serum concentration.
Tetracyclines: May impair bactericidal effects of penicillin G.
INCOMPATIBILITIES:
Aminoglycosides, parenteral: Penicillin may inactivate aminoglycosides in vitro; do not mix in same IV solution. May be used in combination for synergy if administered separately.
Carbohydrate solutions at alkaline pH: Penicillin solutions are rapidly inactivated.

Lab Test Interferences
Antiglobulin (*Coombs'* test): Drug may cause false-positive results. Urine glucose test: Drug may cause false-positive results with copper sulfate tests (*Benedict's* test, *Fehling's* test, or *Clinitest* tablets); enzyme-based tests (eg, *Clinistix*, *Tes-tape*) are not affected. Urine protein determinations: Drug may cause false-positive reactions with sulfosalicylic acid and boiling test, acetic acid test, biuret reaction, and nitric acid test; bromphenol blue test (*Multi-Stix*) is not affected.

Adverse Reactions
CNS: Dizziness; fatigue; insomnia; reversible hyperactivity; neurotoxicity (eg, lethargy, neuromuscular irritability, hallucinations, convulsions, seizures).
EENT: Itchy eyes; stomatitis; gastritis; sore mouth or tongue; furry tongue; black "hairy" tongue; abnormal taste perception.
GI: Glossitis; dry mouth; nausea; anorexia; vomiting; abdominal pain or cramp; epigastric distress; diarrhea or bloody diarrhea; rectal bleeding; flatulence; enterocolitis; pseudomembranous colitis.
GU: Interstitial nephritis (eg, oliguria, proteinuria, hematuria, hyaline casts, pyuria); nephropathy; increased BUN and creatinine.
HEMA: Decreased hemoglobin, hematocrit, RBC, WBC, neutrophils, lymphocytes, platelets; increased lymphocytes, monocytes, basophils, eosinophils and platelets; abnormal coagulation tests.
METAB: Elevated serum alkaline phosphatase, hypernatremia; hypokalemia; hyperkalemia.
OTHER: Hypersensitivity reactions (eg, urticaria, angioneurotic edema, laryngospasm, laryngeal edema, bronchospasm, hypotension, vascular collapse, death, maculopapular to exfoliative dermatitis, vesicular eruptions, erythema multiforme, serum sickness, skin rashes); vaginitis; hyperthermia.

Precautions
Pregnancy: Category B.
Lactation: Small amount excreted in breast milk. May cause diarrhea, candidiasis, or allergic response in nursing infant.
Hypersensitivity: Reactions range from mild to life threatening. Administer drug with caution to cephalosporin-sensitive patients because of possible crossreactivity.
Renal function impairment: Use drug with caution; may require dosage adjustment.
Superinfection: May result in bacterial or fungal overgrowth of nonsusceptible organisms.
Tartrazine sensitivity: Some products contain tartrazine, which may cause allergic-type reactions in susceptible individuals.
Electrolyte content: Penicillin G aqueous sodium contains 2 mEq sodium/1 million U. Penicillin G aqueous potassium contains 1.7 mEq potassium and 0.3 mEq sodium/1 million U. Beware of iatrogenic electrolyte abnormalities and fluid overload.
Procaine sensitivity: If sensitivity to procaine in penicillin G procaine is suspected, inject 0.1 mL

of 1% to 2% procaine solution intradermally. If erythema, wheal, flare, or eruption develops, do not use procaine penicillin preparations.
Pseudomembranous colitis: May occur because of overgrowth of clostridia.

PATIENT CARE CONSIDERATIONS
Administration/Storage
- Depending on route of administration, prepare solution using Sterile Water for Injection, Isotonic Sodium Chloride Injection, or Dextrose Injection.
- Administer at regular intervals around clock.
- Give oral form on empty stomach with full glass of water at least 1 hr before or 2 hr after meals.
- Do not administer with acidic juices or carbonated beverages, which may decrease absorption of penicillin G.
- For IM administration, inject deeply into upper outer quadrant of buttock in adults. In infants and small children, inject in midlateral aspect of thigh. With repeated doses, rotate injection sites.
- For IV administration, administer continuously or intermittently. For intermittent infusion, infuse each dose over 1 to 2 hr (adults) or 15 to 30 min (newborns and children).
- Solutions prepared for IV infusion are stable at room temperature for at least 24 hr.
- Dry powder is stable and does not require refrigeration.
- Sterile solutions may be kept in refrigerator for 1 wk.

Assessment/Interventions
- Obtain patient history, including drug history and any known allergies.
- Assess patient for infection at beginning and throughout therapy (eg, fever, WBC, appearance of wound).
- Obtain specimens for culture and sensitivity before beginning therapy.
- Have emergency medication (eg, epinephrine, antihistamine) and equipment readily available in case of anaphylaxis.
- Observe for anaphylaxis. People with no history of hypersensitivity may have allergic response.

Overdosage: Signs and Symptoms
Neuromuscular hyperexcitability, convulsions, agitation, confusion, asterixis, hallucinations, stupor, coma, multifocal myoclonus, seizures, encephalopathy, hyperkalemia.

- Assess for signs of superinfection (eg, bacterial or fungal overgrowth of nonsusceptible organisms).
- Monitor newborns closely for signs of toxicity or adverse effects.
- Monitor renal function, especially in patients with renal impairment. Monitor I&O strictly. If urinary output is decreased, notify health care provider.
- If patient develops rash, pruritus, laryngeal edema, evidence of hemolysis, wheezing, or other signs of allergic reaction, discontinue drug and notify health care provider.
- If sudden elevation in temperature develops, notify health care provider; it may be drug fever.
- Discontinue penicillin G if signs of hemolytic anemia develop (positive *Coomb* test).

Patient/Family Education
- Instruct patient to finish course of therapy even if feeling better.
- Advise patient to take oral penicillin at intervals around clock on empty stomach 1 hr before or 2 hr after meal with full glass of water, not fruit juice or carbonated beverage.
- Instruct penicillin allergic patient to carry *Medi-Alert* necklace or bracelet.
- Advise patient to use nonhormonal form of contraceptive while taking penicillin.
- Inform patient of signs of hypersensitivity (eg, skin rash, itching, hives, shortness of breath, wheezing) and other side effects, such as black tongue, sore throat, nausea, vomiting, severe diarrhea, fever, swollen joints, and instruct patient to notify health care provider should they occur.
- Instruct patient to notify health care provider if there is no improvement in symptoms of infection.
- Advise patient to notify health care provider of signs of superinfection (eg, vaginitis, black "hairy" tongue).

Penicillin G Benzathine/ Penicillin G Procaine

(pen-ih-SILL-in G BENZ-ah-theen/pen-ih-SILL-in G PRO-cane)

Class Antibiotic/Penicillin

How Supplied
Bicillin C-R Injection 600,000 units/dose (300,000 units each penicillin G benzathine and penicillin G procaine), Injection 1,200,000 units/dose (600,000 units each penicillin G benzathine and penicillin G procaine), Injection 2,400,000 units/dose (1,200,000 units each penicillin G benzathine and penicillin G procaine) ♦ *Bicillin C-R 900/300* Injection 1,200,000 units/dose (900,000 units penicillin G benzathine and 300,000 units penicillin G procaine)

Action
PHARMACOLOGY: Inhibits mucopeptide synthesis of bacterial cell wall.

Indications Treatment of moderately severe infections caused by penicillin-G susceptible microorganisms that are susceptible to serum levels common to this particular dosage form; moderately severe to severe infections of the upper respiratory tract, scarlet fever, erysipelas, and skin and soft-tissue infections caused by susceptible streptococci; moderately severe pneumonia and otitis media caused by susceptible organisms. Severe pneumonia, empyema, bacteremia, pericarditis, meningitis, peritonitis, and arthritis of pneumococcal etiology are better treated with penicillin G sodium or potassium during the acute stage. When high, sustained serum levels are required, penicillin G sodium or potassium, either IM or IV, should be used. This drug should not be used in the treatment of venereal diseases, including syphilis, gonorrhea, yaws, bejel, and pinta.

Contraindications Hypersensitivity to any penicillin or to procaine.

Route/Dosage
Streptococcal Infections Group A (upper-respiratory tract, skin and soft-tissue infections, scarlet fever, and erysipelas)
ADULTS AND CHILDREN OVER 60 LBS: **IM** 2,400,000 units.
CHILDREN 30 TO 60 LBS: **IM** 900,000 to 1,200,000 units.
CHILDREN UNDER 30 LBS: **IM** 600,000 units.

Pneumococcal Infections (except pneumococcal meningitis)
ADULTS: **IM** 1,200,000 units repeated q 2 or 3 days until temperature is normal for 48 hr.
CHILDREN: **IM** 600,000 units repeated q 2 or 3 days until temperature is normal for 48 hr.

Interactions
Probenecid: Increases and prolongs serum penicillin levels.
Tetracycline: May antagonize the bactericidal effect of penicillin.

Adverse Reactions
CV: Cardiac arrest; hypotension; tachycardia; palpitations; pulmonary hypertension; pulmonary embolism; vasodilation; vasovagal reaction; cerebrovascular accident; syncope.
CNS: Neuropathy; headache; fatigue; asthenia; nervousness; tremors; dizziness; somnolence; confusion; anxiety; euphoria; transverse myelitis; seizures; coma; a CNS syndrome with symptoms of severe agitation, convulsion, visual and auditory hallucinations and fear of impending death, psychosis, seizures, dizziness, tinnitus, cyanosis, palpitations, tachycardia, and abnormal taste perception.
DERM: Diaphoresis.
EENT: Blurred vision; blindness.
GI: Pseudomembranous colitis; nausea; vomiting; blood in stool; intestinal necrosis.
GU: Nephropathy; neurogenic bladder, hematuria, proteinuria, renal failure, impotence; priapism.
HEMA: Hemolytic anemia; leukopenia; thrombocytopenia; lymphadenopathy.
METAB: Elevated BUN, creatinine, and AST.
RESP: Hypoxia; apnea; dyspnea.
OTHER: Allergic hypersensitivity (including skin eruptions [maculopapular to exfoliative dermatitis], urticaria, laryngeal edema, fever, eosinophilia); serum sickness-like reactions (including chills, fever, edema, arthralgia, prostration); anaphylaxis (including shock and death); injection site reactions (including pain, inflammation, lump, abscess, necrosis, edema, hemorrhage, cellulitis, hypersensitivity, atrophy, ecchymosis, skin ulcer); neurovascular reactions (including warmth, vasospasm, pallor, mottling, gangrene, numbness and cyanosis of the extremities, neurovascular damage); joint disorder; periostitis; exacerbation of arthritis; myoglobinuria; rhabdomyolysis.

Precautions
Pregnancy: Category B.
Lactation: Excreted in breast milk.
Hypersensitivity: Serious and sometimes fatal hypersensitivity reactions have occurred.
Superinfection: Prolonged use of antibiotics may result in bacterial or fungal overgrowth of nonsusceptible microorganisms.
Administration: Do not inject into or near an artery or nerve because such injections may produce neurovascular damage.
Pseudomembranous colitis: May occur because of overgrowth of clostridia; consider the possibility in patients in whom diarrhea develop.

PATIENT CARE CONSIDERATIONS

Administration/Storage
- For deep IM administration only. Do not administer intradermally, SC, or IV.
- Do not inject into or near an artery or nerve.
- To avoid intravascular administration, aspirate injection site before anesthetic solution is injected.
- Multiple concentrations are available. Ensure that the proper concentration is being used.
- Inject prescribed dose into the upper outer quadrant of the buttock in adults or midlateral aspect of thigh in neonates, infants, or small children.
- Administer injection at a slow, steady rate to prevent blocking the needle.
- Multiple IM sites may be used to administer total dose in 1 session. An alternate regimen involves administering ½ the dose on day 1 and ½ the dose on day 3.
- Discontinue the injection if the patient complains of, or gives any indication of, severe immediate pain at the injection site.
- Vary injection site if multiple doses are administered.
- Do not admix with IV solutions.
- Store in refrigerator 36° to 46°F. Protect from freezing.

Assessment/Interventions
- Obtain patient history, including drug history and any known allergies, especially to penicillin and β-lactam antibiotics. Note history of asthma or multiple allergies.
- Ensure that culture and susceptibility test results indicate sensitivity to penicillin G.
- Ensure that penicillin G is discontinued and another antimicrobial agent is started if culture and sensitivity tests indicate that the infection is resistant to penicillin G.
- Ensure that WBC and differential are determined prior to starting therapy and periodically during therapy.
- Monitor for signs of infection, especially fever, and for positive response to antibiotic therapy.
- Monitor patient for signs of anaphylaxis or severe allergic reaction. If noted, discontinue therapy and immediately notify health care provider. Be prepared to treat appropriately.
- Notify health care provider if any of the following occurs: severe diarrhea or loose, foul-smelling stools.

Patient/Family Education
- Explain name, dose, action, and potential side effects of drug.
- Explain to patient or caregiver that medication will be prepared and administered by a health care provider in a health care setting.
- Review dosing schedule and prescribed length of therapy with patient. Advise patient dose and duration of therapy are dependent on site, cause of infection, and response to therapy.
- Instruct patient to report the following to health care provider: itching, rash, hives, difficulty breathing, diarrhea, loose, foul-smelling stools, injection site reaction.
- Advise patient that follow-up visits and lab tests may be needed to monitor therapy and to keep appointments.

Penicillin V (Phenoxymethyl Penicillin, Penicillin V Potassium)

(pen-ih-SILL-in V)

Class Antibiotic/Penicillin

How Supplied
Beepen-VK Tablets 250 mg, Tablets 500 mg, Powder for oral solution 125 mg/5 mL, Powder for oral solution 250 mg/5 mL ♦ Pen-Vee K Tablets 250 mg, Tablets 500 mg, Powder for oral solution 125 mg/5 mL, Powder for oral solution 250 mg/5 mL ♦ Penicillin VK Tablets 250 mg, Tablets 500 mg, Powder for oral solution 125 mg/5 mL, Powder for oral solution 250 mg/5 mL ♦ Veetids Tablets 250 mg, Tablets 500 mg, Powder for oral solution 125 mg/5 mL ♦ Veetids '250' Powder for oral solution 250 mg/5 mL
🍁 APO-Pen VK ♦ Nadopen-V ♦ Novo-Pen-VK ♦ Nu-Pen-VK ♦ Pen-Vee ♦ PVF K

Action
PHARMACOLOGY: Inhibits mucopeptide synthesis of bacterial cell wall.

PHARMACOKINETICS/DYNAMICS:

Absorption: Oral absorption is 60% to 73%. T_{max} is 0.5 to 1 hr. C_{max} is 2 to 3 mcg/mL.

Distribution: Widely distributed to most tissues and body fluids; distribution into CSF is low with noninflamed meninges. Protein binding is 80%. Vd is 0.5 L/kg. Crosses the placenta and distributes into breast milk.

Metabolism: Hepatic biotransformation is 55%.

Excretion: Mainly renal (20% to 40% as unchanged). $T_{1/2}$ is 0.5 to 1 hr.

Special Populations:
Renal Function Impairment – For Ccr less than 10 mL/min, $t_{1/2}$ increased to 4.1 hr.

Indications
Treatment of upper respiratory tract infections; treatment of pneumococcal, streptococci, and staphylococcal infections and

fusospirochetosis (Vincent's infection) of oropharynx caused by susceptible microorganisms.
Unlabeled use(s): Prophylactic treatment of sickle cell anemia in children; treatment of anaerobic infections; treatment of Lyme disease (*Borrelia burgdorferi*).

Contraindications Hypersensitivity to penicillins. Do not treat severe pneumonia, empyema, bacteremia, pericarditis, meningitis, and purulent or septic arthritis with oral penicillin V during acute stage.

Route/Dosage
ADULTS AND CHILDREN OVER 12 YR: **PO** 125 to 500 mg qid.

Interactions
Beta-blockers: May potentiate anaphylactic reactions of penicillin.
Contraceptives, oral: May reduce efficacy of oral contraceptives.
Erythromycin: May cause synergism or antagonism to develop.
Tetracyclines: May impair bactericidal effects of penicillin V.

Lab Test Interferences
Antiglobulin (Coombs') test: Drug may cause false-positive results.
Urine glucose test: Drug may cause false-positive results with copper sulfate tests (*Benedict's* test, *Fehling's* test or *Clinitest* tablets); enzyme-based tests (eg, *Clinistix*, *Tes-tape*) are not affected.
Urine protein determinations: Drug may cause false-positive reactions with sulfosalicylic acid and boiling test, acetic acid test, biuret reaction and nitric acid test; bromphenol blue test (*Multi-Stix*) is not affected.

Adverse Reactions
CNS: Dizziness; fatigue; insomnia; reversible hyperactivity; neurotoxicity (eg, lethargy, neuromuscular irritability, hallucinations, convulsions, seizures).
EENT: Itchy eyes; furry tongue; black "hairy" tongue; stomatitis; sore mouth or tongue.
GI: Glossitis; gastritis; dry mouth; nausea; vomiting; abdominal pain or cramp; epigastric distress; diarrhea or bloody diarrhea; rectal bleeding; flatulence; enterocolitis; pseudomembranous colitis.
GU: Interstitial nephritis (eg, oliguria, proteinuria, hematuria, hyaline casts, pyuria); nephropathy; increased BUN and creatinine.
HEMA: Decreased hemoglobin, hematocrit, RBC, WBC, neutrophils, lymphocytes, platelets; increased lymphocytes, monocytes, basophils, eosinophils, and platelets.
METAB: Elevated serum alkaline phosphatase; hypernatremia; hypokalemia; albumin, total proteins and uric acid.
OTHER: Hypersensitivity reactions (eg, urticaria, angioneurotic edema, laryngospasm, laryngeal edema, bronchospasm, hypotension, vascular collapse, death, maculopapular to exfoliative dermatitis, vesicular eruptions, erythema multiforme, serum sickness, skin rashes, prostration); vaginitis; hyperthermia.

Precautions
Pregnancy: Category B.
Lactation: Small amount excreted in breast milk. May cause diarrhea, candidiasis, or allergic response in nursing infant.
Hypersensitivity: Reactions range from mild to life threatening. Administer drug with caution to cephalosporin-sensitive patients because of possible crossreactivity.
Renal function impairment: Use drug with caution; dosage adjustment may be necessary.
Superinfection: May result in bacterial or fungal overgrowth of nonsusceptible organisms.
Pseudomembranous colitis: May occur because of overgrowth of clostridia.
Streptococcal infections: Therapy must be minimum of 10 days.

Overdosage: Signs and Symptoms
Neuromuscular hyperexcitability, agitation, confusion, asterixis, hallucinations, stupor, coma, multifocal myoclonus, encephalopathy, hyperkalemia.

PATIENT CARE CONSIDERATIONS

Administration/Storage
- Administer without regard to food.
- Administer at regular intervals around the clock.
- Reconstituted oral suspension is stable for 14 days when refrigerated. Shake well before using.

Assessment/Interventions
- Obtain patient history, including drug history and any known allergies.
- Assess patient for infection at beginning and throughout therapy (eg, fever, WBC, appearance of wound).
- Obtain specimens for culture and sensitivity before beginning therapy.
- Observe for anaphylaxis. People with no history of hypersensitivity may develop allergic response.
- Assess for signs of superinfection (eg, bacterial or fungal overgrowth of nonsusceptible organisms).
- Monitor renal function, especially in patients with renal impairment.
- If patient develops rash, pruritus, laryngeal edema, wheezing or evidence of hemolytic anemia (positive *Coomb's* test), or other signs

of an allergic reaction, discontinue drug and notify health care provider.
- If sudden elevation in temperature develops, notify health care provider; it may be drug fever.
- Discontinue use of penicillin V if signs of hemolytic anemia develop (positive *Coomb's* test).

Patient/Family Education
- Instruct patient to complete entire course of therapy even if feeling better.
- Advise patient to use calibrated measuring device for liquid preparation.
- Instruct penicillin allergic patient to carry *Medi-Alert* necklace or bracelet.
- Advise patient to use nonhormonal form of contraceptive during penicillin V therapy.
- Inform patient of the signs of hypersensitivity (eg, skin rash, itching, hives, shortness of breath, wheezing) and other side effects, such as black tongue, sore throat, nausea, vomiting, severe diarrhea, fever, swollen joints. Instruct patient to notify health care provider if these symptoms occur.
- Instruct patient to notify health care provider if there is no improvement in symptoms of infection.
- Instruct patient to notify health care provider of signs of superinfection (eg, vaginitis, black "hairy" tongue).

Pentamidine Isethionate

(pen-TAM-ih-deen ice-uh-THIGH-uh-nate)
Class Anti-infective/Antiprotozoal

How Supplied
NebuPent Aerosol 300 mg ◆ *Pentacarinat* Injection 300 mg ◆ *Pentam 300* Injection 300 mg

Action
PHARMACOLOGY: Mechanism of action not fully understood. Interferes with synthesis of DNA, RNA, phospholipids, and proteins.

PHARMACOKINETICS/DYNAMICS:
Absorption: Well absorbed after IM administration and detectable in the blood briefly due to extensive tissue binding.
C_{max} is 612 ng/mL (single 2-hr IV infusion).
T_{max} is 0.5 to 1 hr (IM), 1 to 2 hr (IV).
Distribution: Rapidly distributed with highest concentrations in liver, kidneys, adrenal glands, and spleen; smaller amount in lungs, and slow uptake into CNS and brain tissue.
Vd is 3 to 32 L/kg (at steady state).
Metabolism: Unknown in humans.
Excretion: Urine (12% as unchanged).
$T_{1/2}$ is 6.4 hr (IV), 9.1 to 13.2 hr (IM).
Clearance is 248 L/hr (IV).
Terminal $t_{1/2}$ is 2 to 4 wk.
Special Populations:
Renal Function Impairment – Pentamidine may accumulate in renal failure.

Indications
Parenteral form: Treatment of *Pneumocystis carinii* pneumonia (PCP).
Inhalation: Prevention of PCP in high risk HIV-infected patients. **Unlabeled use(s):** Treatment of trypanosomiasis and visceral leishmaniasis.

Contraindications
Parenteral form: Once diagnosis of PCP is made, there are no absolute contraindications. *Inhalation:* History of anaphylactic reaction to pentamidine.

Route/Dosage
ADULTS AND CHILDREN: **IM/IV** 4 mg/kg qd for 14 days.
ADULTS: **Inhalation** 300 mg once q 4 wk administered via *Respirgard II* nebulizer.

Interactions
INCOMPATIBILITIES: Do not reconstitute with saline solutions. Do not mix with other drugs.

Lab Test Interferences None well documented.

Adverse Reactions
CV: Hypotension; ventricular tachycardia; cardiac arrhythmias; chest pain; edema; phlebitis.
CNS: Confusion; hallucinations; dizziness; fatigue; headache.
DERM: Stevens-Johnson syndrome; sterile abscess, pain or induration at IM injection site; rash.
EENT: Bad or metallic taste.
GI: Nausea; anorexia; vomiting; diarrhea; abdominal pain.
GU: Acute renal failure; elevated serum creatinine.
HEMA: Leukopenia; thrombocytopenia; anemia; pancytopenia.
HEPA: Elevated LFT results.
METAB: Hypoglycemia; hypocalcemia; hyperkalemia.
RESP: Shortness of breath; cough; pharyngitis; chest congestion; bronchospasm; pneumothorax (generally associated with inhalation).
OTHER: Neuralgia; myalgia; night sweats; chills.

Precautions

Pregnancy: Category C.
Lactation: Undetermined.
Children: Safety and efficacy of inhalation solution not established.
Renal function impairment: Reduction of dosage, longer infusion time, or extension of dosing interval may be required.
Special risk patients: Use drug with caution in patients with hypertension, hypotension, hypoglycemia, hyperglycemia, hypocalcemia, leukopenia, thrombocytopenia, anemia, hepatic or renal dysfunction, ventricular tachycardia, pancreatitis, Stevens-Johnson syndrome.
Development of acute PCP: Acute PCP may develop despite pentamidine prophylaxis.
Fatalities: Fatalities from severe hypotension (even after one dose), hypoglycemia and cardiac arrhythmias have been reported with IM and IV routes.

PATIENT CARE CONSIDERATIONS

Administration/Storage

- For parenteral use, dissolve contents of vial in Sterile Water for Injection or D5W as directed.
- For IV infusion, solution may be diluted further in D5W.
- Infuse pentamidine IV over 1 hr with patient supine to minimize severe hypotension and arrhythmias.
- Monitor BP continuously throughout infusion, every 30 min for 2 hr thereafter and then q 4 hr until BP stabilizes.
- For IM administration, inject deeply and rotate sites.
- Reconstitute medication for inhalation in Sterile Water for Injection. Do not mix with any other drugs.
- Deliver aerosol dose until nebulizer chamber is empty (approximately 30 to 45 min).
- Reconstituted aerosol preparation is stable up to 48 hr at room temperature, if protected from light source. Discard unused portion.
- IV solutions prepared with D5W are stable at room temperature for up to 48 hr. Discard unused portion.
- Store unopened vial at room temperature. Protect from light.

Assessment/Interventions

- Obtain patient history, including drug history and any known allergies.
- Assess for adverse reactions throughout course of therapy (eg, hypotension, chest pain, neuralgia, phlebitis, edema, headache, nausea, night sweats, chills).
- If patient is coughing, provide physical support to patient's chest. Institute measures to reduce nonproductive coughing to decrease expenditure and chest pain.
- Protect immunocompromised patient from additional infections and stress.
- Consult with nutritionist to maintain optimal diet for patient.
- Inspect injection sites periodically for signs of induration or sterile abscess.
- Obtain prescription for antiemetic agent if needed.
- Keep emergency resuscitation equipment available.
- Monitor lab studies for leukopenia, thrombocytopenia, elevated serum creatinine, elevated liver function studies, hypoglycemia, hypocalcemia, or hyperkalemia.
- Monitor vital signs greater than or equal to q 4 hr during therapy.
- Monitor BP before, during, and after pentamidine administration.
- Monitor I&O throughout therapy. If urinary output is decreased, notify health care provider immediately.
- If patient experiences anorexia, nausea, and vomiting, increased hydration will be necessary.
- If vertigo, emotional changes, or seizures occur, take safety precautions.
- Notify health care provider if GI reactions persist or worsen.

Patient/Family Education

- Inform the patient that there may be pain at the injection site with IM administration.
- Caution patient to avoid crowds and persons with known infections.
- Instruct patient to report the following symptoms to health care provider: nausea, vomiting, anorexia, diarrhea, oliguria, dizziness, chest pain, or edema.
- Advise patient that drug may cause dizziness, and to use caution while driving or performing other tasks requiring mental alertness.

Pentazocine

(pen-TAZ-oh-seen)

Class Narcotic agonist-antagonist analgesic

How Supplied
Talacen Tablets 25 mg pentazocine (as hydrochloride)/650 mg acetaminophen ♦ *Talwin* Injection 30 mg/mL (as lactate) ♦ *Talwin Compound* Tablets 12.5 mg pentazocine (as hydrochloride)/325 mg aspirin ♦ *Talwin NX* Tablets 50 mg pentazocine (as hydrochloride)/0.5 naloxone

Action
PHARMACOLOGY: Produces analgesia by an agonistic effect at the kappa opioid receptor. Weakly antagonizes effects of opiates at mu opioid receptor; does not appear to increase biliary tract pressure.

PHARMACOKINETICS/DYNAMICS:
Absorption: Well absorbed from GI tract and from SC and IM sites. Bioavailability is less than 20% (oral).

Distribution: Moderate protein binding. Passes into fetal circulation.

Metabolism: Hepatic, extensive first-pass; also in intestinal mucosa.

Excretion: Primarily kidney (less than 5% unchanged), small amount biliary. T½ is 2 to 3 hr.

Onset: IM/SC is 15 to 20 min; IV is 2 to 3 min; oral is 15 to 30 min.

Peak: For analgesic effect, IM/SC is 30 to 60 min; IV is 15 to 30 min; oral is 60 to 90 min.

Duration: IM is 2 to 3 hr; SC is 2 to 3 hr; IV is 2 to 3 hr; oral is 3 hr.

Special Populations:
Hepatic Function Impairment – Oral bioavailability is increased by 3-fold in cirrhotic patients.

Indications
Oral and parenteral forms: Management of moderate to severe pain.
Parenteral form: Preoperative or preanesthetic medication; supplement to surgical anesthesia.

Contraindications
Hypersensitivity to naloxone (in *Talwin NX*) or sulfites.

Route/Dosage
Labor
ADULTS: **IM** 30 mg as single dose; alternatively, when contractions are regular, **IV** 20 mg for 2 to 3 doses given q 2 to 3 hr.

PENTAZOCINE
Moderate to Severe Pain
ADULTS: **IM/SC/IV** 30 mg q 3 to 4 hr prn (max, 360 mg/day). Doses greater than 30 mg **IV** or 60 mg **SC/IM** are not recommended.
ADULTS: **PO** 50 mg q 3 to 4 hr; increase to 100 mg if necessary (max, 600 mg/day).

PENTAZOCINE 12.5 MG WITH ASPIRIN 325 MG (TALWIN COMPOUND)
Moderate to Severe Pain
ADULTS: **PO** 2 tablets tid to qid.

PENTAZOCINE 25 MG WITH ACETAMINOPHEN 650 MG (TALACEN)
Moderate to Severe Pain
ADULTS: **PO** 1 tablet q 4 hr (max, 6 tablets/day).

Interactions
Alcohol: Causes additive CNS depression.
Barbiturate anesthetics and any other CNS depressants (eg, benzodiazepines, antidepressants): Causes increased CNS and respiratory depression.
INCOMPATIBILITIES:
Barbiturates: Do not mix in the same syringe with pentazocine; precipitation will occur.

Lab Test Interferences None well documented.

Adverse Reactions
CV: Hypotension; hypertension; tachycardia; circulatory depression; shock.
CNS: Lightheadedness; dizziness; euphoria; hallucinations; disorientation; confusion; seizures.
DERM: Nodules, soft tissue induration, depressions, sclerosis and ulceration at injection sites.
EENT: Visual disturbances.
GI: Nausea.
GU: Urinary retention.
HEMA: Granulocytopenia.
RESP: Respiratory depression; transient apnea in newborns whose mothers received parenteral pentazocine during labor.
OTHER: Anaphylaxis; tolerance; psychological and physical dependence in long-term use.

Precautions
Pregnancy: Category C. Neonatal abstinence syndrome may develop.
Children: Not recommended for children less than 12 yr.
Labor and delivery: Pentazocine rapidly crosses placenta with cord blood levels 40% to 70% of maternal serum levels. Use drug with caution in women delivering premature infants.
Special risk patients: Use with caution in patients with MI, decreased respiratory reserve, asthma, respiratory depression, head injury or increased intracranial pressure.
Sulfite sensitivity: Drug may cause allergic-type reactions (eg, hives, itching, wheezing, anaphylaxis) in susceptible persons.
Abuse/Dependence/Withdrawal: Abuse potential exists. Abrupt discontinuation after long-term use may cause withdrawal symptoms. Do not substitute other opiates in pentazocine withdrawal syndrome. Pentazocine may induce with-

drawal symptoms in narcotic-dependent patients.

Acute CNS manifestations: Hallucinations, disorientation, confusion, and seizures.

Renal or hepatic impairment: Duration of action may be prolonged; dosage reduction may be required.

"Ts and Blues": Refers to drug abuse by IV injection of oral pentazocine and tripelennamine (antihistamine) as substitute for heroin. Complications of injecting oral pentazocine include pulmonary emboli, vascular occlusion, ulceration, seizures, strokes, and CNS infections. Addition of naloxone to pentazocine tablets (*Talwin NX*) prevents this drug abuse; it may cause withdrawal in narcotic-dependent individuals.

Tissue damage: Severe sclerosis of skin, SC tissues, and underlying muscle have occurred at injection sites.

Overdosage: Signs and Symptoms

Respiratory depression, hypertension, tachycardia.

PATIENT CARE CONSIDERATIONS

Administration/Storage

- Pentazocine is a schedule IV drug; keep it locked according to hospital policy.
- When anti-inflammatory or antipyretic effects are desired in addition to analgesia, aspirin or acetaminophen can be administered concomitantly with oral form of pentazocine.
- Do not mix barbiturate in same syringe with pentazocine; precipitation will occur.
- If frequent injections are needed, rotate sites.
- For IM administration; inject deep into well-developed tissue.
- For IV administration; inject undiluted by slow bolus. Do not exceed a 30 mg dose.
- Administer SC only when necessary; severe tissue damage is possible at injection sites.
- Store in tightly closed, light-resistant containers.

Assessment/Interventions

- Obtain patient history, including drug history and any known allergies.
- Assess for signs of physical and psychological dependence throughout course of therapy.
- Assess respiratory rate and quality, BP, and pulse before administering drug and periodically during therapy.
- Assess for adverse reactions (eg, hypotension, shock, dizziness, hallucinations, seizures, urinary retention, tissue changes from injections).
- Assess newborns whose mothers received parenteral pentazocine for apnea.
- Rate patient's pain before and after each dose. Determine and record onset, durations, location, intensity, and quality of pain.
- Notify health care provider if medication does not relieve patient's pain.
- If anaphylaxis occurs, prepare to institute emergency oxygen, mechanical ventilation, IV fluids, and vasopressors.
- If constipation occurs, give stool softeners or laxative, teach high-fiber diet and increase fluid consumption to 2 to 3 L/day if tolerated.

Patient/Family Education

- For maximum effectiveness, instruct patient to take medication before intolerable pain develops.
- Tell patient to take medication exactly as prescribed, to minimize dependence.
- Teach patient to consume 2 to 3 L of fluids each day, if tolerated, to prevent constipation.
- Inform patient that aspirin or acetaminophen may be taken concurrently for additive analgesia as well as its anti-inflammatory and antipyretic effects.
- Explain therapeutic value of pentazocine prior to administration to enhance the analgesic effect.
- Caution patient not to stop taking drug abruptly without consulting health care provider.
- Advise patient to avoid sudden position changes to prevent orthostatic hypotension.
- Instruct patient to avoid intake of alcoholic beverages or other CNS depressants.
- Advise patient that drug may cause dizziness and to use caution while driving or performing other tasks requiring mental alertness.

Pentobarbital Sodium

(pen-toe-BAR-bih-tahl SO-dee-uhm)

Class Sedative and hypnotic/Barbiturate, Short-acting/Anticonvulsant

How Supplied

Nembutal Sodium Capsules 50 mg, Capsules 100 mg, Suppositories 30 mg, Suppositories 60 mg, Suppositories 120 mg, Suppositories 200 mg, Elixir Equivalent to 20 mg/5 mL, Injection 50 mg/mL

Action

PHARMACOLOGY: Depresses sensory cortex, decreases motor activity, alters cerebellar function and produces drowsiness, sedation and hypnosis.

PHARMACOKINETICS/DYNAMICS:

Absorption: Pentobarbital sodium is absorbed in varying degrees. T_{max} is 15 min (IV), maximal CNS depression.

Distribution: Rapidly distributed to all tissues and fluids with high concentration in brain, liver, and kidneys due to lipid solubility. Protein binding is 60% to 70%. Pentobarbital sodium distributes into breast milk.

Metabolism: Metabolized by hepatic microsomal enzyme system.

Excretion: Urine (very little unchanged); in the feces is less common. The t½ is 15 to 50 hr.

Onset: Immediate following IV administration.

Duration: 3 to 4 hr.

Indications Sedation; short-term treatment of insomnia; preanesthesia; emergency control of convulsions (parenteral form).

Contraindications Hypersensitivity to barbiturates; manifest or latent porphyria.

Route/Dosage

Insomnia
ADULTS: **PO/IV** 100 mg (max IV rate, 50 mg/min). **IM/PR** 120 to 200 mg (max IM dose, 500 mg or 5 mL volume regardless of concentration).

Sedation
ADULTS: **PO/PR** 20 to 30 mg bid to qid.
CHILDREN: **PO/IM** 2 to 6 mg/kg (max, 100 mg). **IV** 50 mg.

Convulsions
ADULTS: **IV** Use minimum dose to avoid compounding depression. Administer slowly to allow time for drug to penetrate the blood-brain barrier. Do not exceed 50 mg/min.

Pediatric Patients Unable to Take Orally or by Injection
CHILDREN 12 TO 14 YR (36.4 TO 50 KG): **PR** 60 or 120 mg.
CHILDREN 5 TO 12 YR (18.2 TO 36.4 KG): **PR** 60 mg.
CHILDREN 1 TO 4 YR (9 TO 18.2 KG): **PR** 30 or 60 mg.
CHILDREN 2 MO TO 1 YR (4.5 TO 9 KG): **PR** 30 mg.

Interactions
Alcohol, CNS depressants: May produce additive depressant effects.
Anticoagulants, beta-blockers, calcium-channel blockers (eg, nifedipine, verapamil), theophylline: Activity of these drugs may be reduced.
Anticonvulsants: Serum concentrations of carbamazepine, valproic acid and succinimides may be reduced. Valproic acid may increase barbiturate serum levels.
Corticosteroids: Effectiveness may be reduced.
Estrogen, estrogen-containing oral contraceptives: May cause decreased contraceptive and estrogen effect.
Griseofulvin: Decreased griseofulvin levels.

Lab Test Interferences Decreased serum bilirubin concentrations, false-positive phentolamine test, decreased response to metyrapone and impaired absorption of radioactive cyanocobalamin.

Adverse Reactions
CV: Bradycardia; hypotension; syncope.
CNS: Drowsiness; agitation; confusion; headache; hyperkinesia; ataxia; CNS depression; paradoxical excitement; nightmares; psychiatric disturbances; hallucinations; insomnia; dizziness.
GI: Nausea; vomiting; constipation.
HEPA: Liver damage.
HEMA: Blood dyscrasias (eg, agranulocytosis, thrombocytopenia).
RESP: Hypoventilation; apnea; laryngospasm; bronchospasm.
OTHER: Hypersensitivity reactions (eg, angioedema, rashes, exfoliative dermatitis); fever; injection site reactions (eg, local pain, thrombophlebitis).

Precautions
Pregnancy: Category D.
Lactation: Excreted in breast milk.
Children: May respond with excitement rather than depression.
Elderly: More sensitive to drug effects; dosage reduction is required.
Renal function impairment: Use drug with caution; dosage reduction may be required.
Hepatic function impairment: Use drug with caution; dosage reduction may be required.
Dependence: Tolerance or psychological and physical dependence may occur with continued use.
IV administration: Do not exceed max IV rate; respiratory depression, apnea and hypotension may result. Parenteral solutions are highly alkaline; extravasation may cause tissue damage and necrosis. Inadvertent intra-arterial injection may lead to arterial spasm, thrombosis, and gangrene.
Seizure disorders: Status epilepticus may result from abrupt discontinuation.

Overdosage: Signs and Symptoms
CNS and respiratory depression, Cheyne-Stokes respiration, areflexia, constriction of pupils, oliguria, tachycardia, hypotension, lowered body temperature, coma, apnea, circulatory collapse, respiratory arrest, death.

PATIENT CARE CONSIDERATIONS
Administration/Storage
- Give IM injections deeply into large muscle. Do not exceed max IM dose of 500 mg or 5 mL of volume (regardless of concentration).
- For IV administration, inject into large vein; do not exceed max IV rate of 50 mg/min, do not administer into artery and do not allow perivascular extravasation.
- Administer with caution to patients with history of substance abuse.
- Do not use as sleep aid for greater than 2 wk.
- Store parenteral form at room temperature. Do not use if discolored or if precipitate forms.
- Store suppositories in refrigerator. Do not divide.

Assessment/Interventions
- Obtain patient history, including drug history and any known allergies. Note presence of liver disease, respiratory disease, and porphyria.
- Observe for common side effects such as sedation or dizziness and report to health care provider.
- With prolonged therapy monitor lab test results for liver, renal, and hematopoietic functions.
- Monitor patient carefully during IV use for potential respiratory depression.
- Assess infants of lactating mothers and report drowsiness to health care provider.
- In children, monitor for possible paradoxical response of increased agitation and report to health care provider.
- Notify health care provider of the following signs of barbiturate intoxication: unsteady gait, slurred speech, confusion or irritability.
- Watch for behavior indicative of drug dependency such as inordinate requests for more medication or need to refill prescription early.

Patient/Family Education
- Warn patient that medication may be habit forming and for this reason it is important to take medicine as directed. Taking too little or too much can have serious complications.
- Instruct patient to report the following symptoms to health care provider: nausea, vomiting, drowsiness, dizziness, fever, sore throat, mouth sores, easy bleeding bruising, skin irritation, or exaggerated sunburn.
- Caution patient to avoid intake of alcoholic beverages or other CNS depressants.
- Advise patient that drug may cause drowsiness, and to use caution while driving or performing other tasks requiring mental alertness.

Pentosan Polysulfate Sodium
(PEN-toe-san)

Class Urinary Analgesic

How Supplied
Elmiron Capsules 100 mg

Action
PHARMACOLOGY: Unknown. Adheres to and may protect the mucosal membrane of the bladder.

PHARMACOKINETICS/DYNAMICS:
Absorption: Absorption is approximately 3% of dose.
Distribution: Distributed to the uroepithelium of the GU tract with lesser amounts in liver, spleen, lung, skin, periosteum, and bone marrow. Erythrocyte penetration is low.
Metabolism: 68% of dose undergoes desulfation in liver and spleen 1 hr after IV administration; partial depolymerization occurs in the kidney.
Excretion: Renal excretion is 3% as unchanged drug. The t½ is 24 hr (IV) and 4.8 hr (oral).

Indications For relief of bladder pain or discomfort associated with interstitial cystitis.

Contraindications Standard considerations.

Route/Dosage
ADULTS: PO 100 mg tid.

Interactions
Anticoagulants, antiplatelet agents, thrombolytics: Pentosan has weak anticoagulant properties and may potentiate the pharmacological action of other anticoagulants, antiplatelet, or thrombolytic drugs.

Lab Test Interferences None reported.

Adverse Reactions
CNS: Headache; emotional lability; depression; dizziness.
DERM: Alopecia; rash.
GI: Nausea; abdominal pain; diarrhea; dyspepsia.
HEPA: Liver function abnormalities.

Precautions
Pregnancy: Category B.
Lactation: Unknown.
Children: Safety and efficacy not established.
Anticoagulant effects: Since drug has weak anticoagulant effects, carefully evaluate patients with diseases such as aneurysms, thrombocytopenia, hemophilia, GI ulcerations, polyps or diverticula before initiating therapy.

Hepatic/Splenic function impairment: Use with caution.
Thrombocytopenia: Use with caution in patients with a history of heparin-induced thrombocytopenia.

PATIENT CARE CONSIDERATIONS
Administration/Storage
- Administer with water greater than or equal to 1 hr before or 2 hr after meals.
- Store at room temperature (68° to 77°F) in tightly closed container.

Assessment/Interventions
- Obtain patient history including drug history and any known allergies. Note presence of hepatic or splenic disease or disease which may predispose to bleeding (eg, hemophilia) and history of heparin-induced thrombocytopenia.
- Monitor patients for signs of bleeding, especially those on anticoagulant or antiplatelet therapy.
- Assess for pain relief or improvement to help determine effectiveness of treatment.
- Monitor for adverse reactions and report to health care provider any notable findings.

Patient/Family Education
- Instruct patient to take as prescribed and not more frequently than directed.
- Instruct patient to take pentosan polysulfate sodium greater than or equal to 1 hr before or 2 hr after meals with a full glass of water.
- Inform patient of possible adverse reactions with other drugs or foods they may be taking.
- Advise patient to consult with health care provider before taking any other medications including OTCs.
- Instruct patient to assess pain relief or improvement and report to the primary care provider greater than or equal to q 3 mo to determine effectiveness of treatment.
- Instruct patient to be aware of adverse effects such as bleeding complications (eg, ecchymosis, epistaxis, gum hemorrhage) and alopecia areata. Inform health care provider if noted.
- Instruct patient to inform health care provider if needing invasive dental work, surgery, or other procedures that might expose patient to increased risk for bleeding.
- Advise the patient to notify primary caregiver if experiencing jaundice or other signs of liver disease.
- Instruct female patients to notify primary care provider if pregnant, planning to become pregnant, or planning to breastfeed.

Overdosage: Signs and Symptoms
Unknown. Based on its pharmacology, overdose is likely to manifest as an increased risk of anticoagulation, thrombocytopenia, gastric pain, and liver function abnormalities.

Pentostatin
(PEN-toe-STAT-in)

Class Purine antimetabolite

How Supplied
Nipent Powder for injection 10 mg/vial

Action
PHARMACOLOGY: Pentostatin is a potent transition state inhibitor of the enzyme adenosine deaminase (ADA) that leads to cytotoxicity because of elevated intracellular levels of dATP that can block DNA synthesis through inhibition of ribonucleotide reductase. Pentostatin can also inhibit RNA synthesis as well as cause increased DNA damage.

PHARMACOKINETICS/DYNAMICS:
Distribution: Concentrations are highest in the kidneys with little CNS penetration. Protein binding is approximately 4%. The distribution $t_{1/2}$ half-life is 11 minutes. Pentostatin crosses the blood brain barrier. CSF concentrations are 10% to 12.5% of serum concentrations within 24 hr after a single dose.
Metabolism: Hepatic; only small amounts are metabolized.
Excretion: Urine (90% as unchanged or metabolites). Distribution $t_{1/2}$ is 11 minutes and terminal $t_{1/2}$ is 5.7 hr (single dose) and increases to 18 hr with renal impairment. Plasma Cl is 68 mL/min/m².

Onset: Time to achieve response is approximately 4.7 mo.
Duration: More than 1 wk after a single dose.
Special Populations:
Renal Function Impairment – The $t_{1/2}$ increased to 18 hr (Ccr less than 50 mL/min).

Indications Treatment for both untreated and alpha-interferon refractory hairy cell leukemia.
Unlabeled use(s): Palliative therapy of chronic lymphocytic leukemia, prolymphocytic leukemia, cutaneous T-cell lymphoma.

Contraindications Standard considerations.

Route/Dosage
Refractory Hairy Cell Leukemia
ADULTS: IV For patients with a Ccr at least 60 mL/min, give 4 mg/m² every other wk until complete response is achieved, then give 2 additional doses. Administer by IV bolus injection or diluted in a larger volume and give over 20 to 30 minutes. Assess patient response after

6 mo of therapy. If no response occurs, discontinue therapy. If a partial response occurs, continue therapy for no more than 6 mo then discontinue. Give 2 additional doses after achieving a complete response. Delay further therapy in patients whose absolute neutrophil count falls less than 200 cells/mm^3 from a baseline value greater than 500 cells/mm^3 and in patients with active infections, severe rash, or nervous system toxicity. Therapy may be resumed when infection is controlled.

Hydration
It is recommended that patients receive hydration with 500 to 1,000 mL of 5% dextrose in 0.5 mL normal saline before pentostatin administration. An additional 500 mL of 5% dextrose or equivalent should be administered after pentostatin is given.

Renal function impairment (Ccr greater than 60 mL/min)
Patients who have elevated serum creatinine should have their dose withheld and a Ccr determined.

Interactions
Allopurinol: May enhance toxicity of pentostatin.
Carmustine, cyclophosphamide, etoposide: Acute pulmonary edema, hypotension, and death have been reported when coadministered with pentostatin.
Fludarabine: Coadministration can result in severe pulmonary toxicity; coadministration is not recommended.
Vidarabine: Pentostatin may increase toxicity of vidarabine.

Lab Test Interferences None well documented.

Adverse Reactions
CV: Hemorrhage, hypotension (3% to 10%); angina pectoris, arrhythmia, AV block, bradycardia, ventricular extrasystoles; heart arrest, heart failure, hypertension, pericardial effusion, phlebitis, pulmonary embolus, sinus arrest, tachycardia, thrombophlebitis, vasculitis (less than 3%).
CNS: Fatigue (42%); headache (17%); neurologic disorder, asthenia (12%); anxiety, confusion, depression, dizziness, insomnia, nervousness, paresthesia, somnolence (3% to 10%); abnormal thinking and dreaming, amnesia, ataxia, convulsions, dysarthria, emotional lability, encephalitis, hallucination, hostility, hyperkinesias, meningism, neuralgia, neuritis, neuropathy, neurosis, paralysis, syncope, twitching, vertigo (less than 3%); CNS toxicity (1%).
DERM: Rash (43%); pruritus (21%); sweating (8%); skin disorder (4%); dry skin, urticaria (3% to 10%); acne alopecia, eczema, petechial rash, photosensitivity (less than 3%).
EENT: Abnormal vision, amblyopia, deafness, dry eyes, earache, labyrinthitis, lacrimation disorder, nonreactive eye, photophobia, retinopathy, tinnitus, watery eyes (less than 3%).
GI: Nausea/vomiting (63%); diarrhea (17%); abdominal pain (16%); anorexia (13%); stomatitis (12%); dental abnormalities, dyspepsia, flatulence, gingivitis (3% to 10%); constipation, dysphagia, glossitis, ileus, unusual taste (less than 3%).
GU: Abnormal kidney function, amenorrhea, breast lump, decreased libido, gout, impotence, nephropathy, renal failure, renal insufficiency, renal stone (less than 3%).
HEMA/LYMPH: Leukopenia (22%); anemia (8%); thrombocytopenia (6%); agranulocytosis (3% to 10%); acute leukemia, aplastic anemia, hemolytic anemia (less than 3%).
HEPA: Hepatic disorder/elevated LFTs (2%).
HYPERSEN: Allergic reaction (2%).
LABTESTABS: Elevated creatinine (3% to 10%); hypercalcemia, hyponatremia (less than 3%).
MUSC: Myalgia (19%); arthralgia (6%); arthritis (less than 3%).
RESP: Coughing/increased cough (20%); upper respiratory tract infection (13%); dyspnea, rhinitis, pharyngitis (11%); asthma (3% to 10%); bronchospasm, laryngeal edema (less than 3%).
OTHER: Fever (46%); chills (19%); pain, viral infection (8%); infection (7%); chest pain, death, face edema, peripheral edema (3% to 10%); flu-like symptoms, hangover effect, neoplasm (less than 3%).

> **WARNING:**
> Do not exceed recommended doses. Nephrotoxicity, hepatotoxicity, CNS, and pulmonary toxicity occurred in phase 1 studies that used higher doses than recommended.

Precautions
Pregnancy: Category D.
Lactation: Undetermined.
Children: Safety and efficacy not established.
Renal function impairment: Dosage reduction may be required in patients with impaired renal failure (Ccr less than 60 mL/min).
CNS toxicity: Withhold or discontinue therapy in those with evidence of CNS toxicity.
Myelosuppression: Patients may experience myelosuppression, primarily during the first few courses of treatment.
Neutropenia: Worsening of neutropenia may occur.
Rashes: Rashes, occasionally severe, were commonly reported and may worsen with continued treatment. Withholding of treatment may be required.

Renal toxicity: In patients treated at the recommended dose, elevations in serum creatinine were usually minor and reversible. Some patients who began treatment with normal renal function had evidence of mild to moderate toxicity at a final assessment.

Overdosage: Signs and Symptoms
Severe renal, hepatic, pulmonary, and CNS toxicity.

PATIENT CARE CONSIDERATIONS
Administration/Storage
- Do not administer to patient with renal impairment (Ccr less than 60 mL/min) or in combination with fludarabine.
- For IV bolus or infusion only. Not for intradermal, subcutaneous, IM, intra-arterial, or oral administration.
- Diligently follow institutional and NIH procedures for handling, administration, and disposal of anticancer drugs. Wear appropriate protective equipment when preparing and administering pentostatin. Avoid exposure by inhalation or by direct contact of the skin, mucous membranes, and eyes. Treat spills and wastes with a 5% sodium hypochlorite solution prior to disposal.
- If accidental skin or mucus membrane contact occurs, wash thoroughly with soap and water. If accidental eye contact occurs, immediately institute copious irrigation with plain water.
- Ensure that patient is hydrated with 500 to 1,000 mL 5% dextrose in 0.45% normal saline (or equivalent solution) before administering pentostatin and receives an additional 500 mL 5% dextrose (or equivalent solution) following administration of pentostatin.
- Reconstitute powder for injection with 5 mL sterile water for injection. Mix thoroughly to obtain complete dissolution. Resulting solution contains 2 mg/mL of pentostatin.
- Do not administer if particulate matter, cloudiness, or discoloration is noted.
- May administer reconstituted solution as bolus injection or may further dilute reconstituted solution with 25 to 50 mL of 5% dextrose in water or 0.9% sodium chloride injection for IV infusion over 20 to 30 minutes.
- Store unopened vials in refrigerator (36° to 46°F). Reconstituted solution or reconstituted solution further diluted contains no preservatives and may be stored at room temperature and ambient light but should be used within 8 hr of reconstitution.

Assessment/Interventions
- Obtain patient history, including drug history and any known allergies. Note active infection, renal impairment, concurrent treatment with fludarabine.
- Ensure that active infection has been controlled before initiating or resuming therapy with pentostatin.
- Ensure that periodic monitoring of the peripheral blood for hairy cells is performed to assess response to treatment. Discontinue therapy if patient has not achieved a complete or partial response after 6 mo of therapy. If partial response noted, therapy can be continued for an additional 6 mo. If complete response has not been achieved within this time period, discontinue treatment with pentostatin.
- Ensure that women of childbearing potential are not pregnant when therapy is initiated and use effective contraception during treatment.
- Ensure that risk of developing hyperuricemia is evaluated before starting therapy and that hypouricemic therapy (including adequate fluid intake) and monitoring of uric acid is initiated before starting treatment in patient determined to be at risk for developing hyperuricemia and urate precipitation.
- Ensure that CBC with differential and platelet count and renal function are evaluated before each dose of pentostatin and at other intervals as clinically indicted.
- Monitor patient for signs or symptoms of infection or bleeding. Inform health care provider immediately if noted and be prepared to treat appropriately (eg, IV antibiotics, colony stimulating factors, transfusions).
- Ensure that pentostatin is withheld in patient exhibiting severe hematologic (eg, absolute neutrophil count less than 200 cells/mm^3 in patient with initial neutrophil count greater than 500 cells/mm^3) or severe nonhematologic toxicity (eg, severe rash, neurotoxicity) in patient with active infection, or in patient with elevated serum creatinine until Ccr is determined.
- Monitor patient for signs of anaphylactic or serious allergic reactions. Discontinue therapy and immediately notify health care provider if noted. Be prepared to treat appropriately.

- Monitor patient for HEMA, GI, CNS, DERM, and general body side effects. Report to health care provider if noted and significant.
- Monitor patient for signs and symptoms of bacterial, viral, or fungal infection. Report to health care provider immediately if noted.

Patient/Family Education
- Explain name, action, and potential side effects of the treatment regimen. Review the treatment regimen including dosing schedule, duration of treatment, and monitoring that will be required.
- Advise patient, family, or caregiver that medication will be prepared and administered by health care providers in a health care setting.
- Advise patient, family, or caregiver that medication may be used in combination with other agents to achieve maximum benefit possible.
- Advise patient, family, or caregiver to immediately report any of the following to health care provider: rash; hives; difficulty breathing; fever, chills, or other signs of infection; bleeding or unusual bruising; sores in mouth; dark urine; yellowing of skin or eyes; pain, redness, or swelling at injection site.
- Advise patient, family, or caregiver to report any of the following to health care provider: persistent nausea, vomiting, diarrhea, or appetite loss; persistent or worsening general body weakness.
- Instruct patient not to take any prescription or OTC medications, herbal preparations, or dietary supplements unless advised by health care provider.
- Advise women of childbearing potential to avoid becoming pregnant during therapy.
- Advise women to notify health care provider if pregnant, planning to become pregnant, or breastfeeding.
- Advise patient, family, or caregiver that frequent follow-up visits and laboratory tests will be required to monitor therapy and to keep appointments.

Pentoxifylline

(pen-TOX-IH-fill-in)

Class Hemorheologic

How Supplied
Trental Tablets, controlled-release 400 mg
✤ *Nu-Pentoxifylline* ◆ *Pentoxifylline*

Action
PHARMACOLOGY: Improves blood flow by decreasing blood viscosity.

PHARMACOKINETICS/DYNAMICS:
Absorption: Pentoxifylline is almost completely absorbed. Food delays absorption and increases C_{max} by 28% and AUC by 13%. T_{max} is 1 hr (parent drug and metabolites) and 2 to 4 hr (controlled–release).

Distribution: Extensive first-pass metabolism. Protein binding to erythrocyte membrane. Both parent drug and metabolites distribute into breast milk.

Metabolism: Undergoes first-pass effect and, in the liver, some metabolites are active with 5 to 8 times the plasma levels of the parent drug.

Excretion: Urine (as metabolites), fecal (less than 4%). The plasma t½ is 0.4 to 0.8 hr (parent drug) and 1 to 1.6 hr (metabolites).

Onset: 2 to 4 wk (multiple doses).

Special Populations:
Elderly – Increases AUC and decreases elimination rate (60 to 68 yr).

Indications Intermittent claudication on basis of chronic occlusive arterial disease of limbs.

Unlabeled use(s): Treatment of psychopathological symptoms in patients with cerebrovascular insufficiency; treatment of diabetic angiopathies; reduction of incidence of stroke in patients with recurrent TIAs.

Contraindications Intolerance to methylxanthines (ie, caffeine, theophylline); recent cerebral or retinal hemorrhage.

Route/Dosage
ADULTS: **PO** 400 mg tid with meals for greater than or equal to 8 wk. If GI and CNS side effects occur, decrease to 400 mg bid. If side effects persist, discontinue.

Interactions
Antihypertensives: Small decreases in blood pressure possible with patients receiving pentoxifylline while using antihypertensive drugs. Monitor blood pressure. If indicated, reduce dosage of the antihypertensive.
Cimetidine: Effects of pentoxifylline may be increased.
Theophylline: Concomitant administration with pentoxifylline leads to increased theophylline levels and possible toxicity in some patients. Monitor and adjust closely.
Warfarin: Bleeding and prolonged prothrombin time possible in patients.

Lab Test Interferences None well documented.

Adverse Reactions
CV: Angina; edema; hypotension; dyspnea; arrhythmia; tachycardia.
CNS: Dizziness; insomnia; headache; tremor; anxiety; confusion.

DERM: Brittle fingernails; pruritus; rash; flushing; urticaria.
EENT: Blurred vision; conjunctivitis; nosebleed; bad taste; excessive salivation; sore throat.
GI: Dyspepsia; nausea; vomiting; belching; flatus; bloating; dry mouth.
HEPA: Hepatitis; jaundice.
HEMA: Leukopenia; pancytopenia; purpura; thrombocytopenia; decreased serum fibrinogen.
RESP: Flu-like symptoms; laryngitis.

Precautions
Pregnancy: Category C.
Lactation: Excreted in breast milk.
Children: Safety and efficacy for children less than 18 yr not established.

PATIENT CARE CONSIDERATIONS
Administration/Storage
- Give medication with meals.
- Reduced dosage may be needed if adverse GI or CNS effects develop.
- Store at room temperature in a tightly closed, light-resistant container.

Assessment/Interventions
- Obtain patient history, including drug history and any known allergies.
- Carefully assess for risk of hemorrhage (ie, recent surgery or peptic ulcer), and monitor PT/PTT and Hgb/Hct for indications of bleeding.
- Assess baseline BUN and creatinine, and monitor throughout therapy.
- Monitor patients taking pentoxifylline and anticoagulants for bleeding or changes in PT.

Patient/Family Education
- Explain that improvement in symptoms may take 2 to 4 wk to notice and up to 8 wk for max relief.

Renal function impairment: Drug may accumulate, producing toxicity; lower dose may be necessary.
Hemorrhage: Periodically examine patients with risk of hemorrhage for bleeding.

Overdosage: Signs and Symptoms
Symptoms appear to be dose related. They usually occur 4 to 5 hr after ingestion and last approximately 12 hr. Symptoms include flushing, hypotension, nervousness, agitation, tremors, convulsions, somnolence, loss of consciousness, fever, and agitation. Transient (less than 24 hr) bradycardia with first- or second-degree atrioventricular block may be seen.

- Explain importance of follow-up lab work for patients with high risk of bleeding or taking anticoagulant.
- In patients with occlusive peripheral vasospastic disorders, emphasize use of self-help measures to augment drug therapy (eg, exercise, weight control, no smoking).
- Review specifics of good foot care, including bathing of feet daily in lukewarm water and drying thoroughly, applying lanolin to feet after bathing, use of lambs wool between toes and feet, avoidance of extremes in temperature, wearing of clean cotton socks daily.
- Instruct patient to report the following symptoms to health care provider: dizziness, chest pain, fainting, excessive bruising, abnormal bleeding.
- Advise patient that drug may cause dizziness, and to use caution while driving or performing other tasks requiring mental alertness.

Pergolide Mesylate
(PURR-go-lide MEH-sih-LATE)

Class Antiparkinson

How Supplied
Permax Tablets 0.05 mg, Tablets 0.25 mg, Tablets 1 mg

Action
PHARMACOLOGY: Directly stimulates postsynaptic dopamine receptors in nigrostriatal system.

PHARMACOKINETICS/DYNAMICS:
Absorption: Oral bioavailability is unknown.
Distribution: Plasma protein binding is approximately 90%.
Metabolism: 10 metabolites have been detected, some active.
Excretion: Kidney (55%), 5% as expired carbon dioxide.

Indications Adjunctive treatment to levodopa-carbidopa in management of Parkinson disease.

Contraindications Hypersensitivity to ergot derivatives or any component of the product.

Route/Dosage
Administer in divided doses tid.
ADULTS: **PO** 0.05 mg/day first 2 days. Gradually increase dose by 0.1 to 0.15 mg/day q 3 days over next 12 days. Dose may then be increased by 0.25 mg/day q 3 days until optimum therapeutic dosage is achieved (mean therapeutic dose is 3 mg/day; max, 5 mg/day). During titration cautiously decrease levodopa-carbidopa (average daily concurrent dose is 650 mg/day of levodopa).

Interactions

Dopamine antagonists (eg, butyrophenones, metoclopramide, neuroleptics, phenothiazines, thioxanthenes): May diminish effectiveness of pergolide.

Lab Test Interferences None well documented.

Adverse Reactions

CV: Orthostatic hypotension (9%); vasodilation (3.2%); palpitations; hypotension; syncope; hypertension; arrhythmia; MI.
CNS: Dyskinesia (62.4%); dizziness (19.1%); hallucinations (13.8%); dystonia (11.6%); confusion (11.1%); somnolence (10.1%); insomnia (7.9%); anxiety (6.4%); personality disorder; psychosis; extrapyramidal syndrome; incoordination; akinesia; hypertonia; neuralgia; akathesia.
DERM: Rash; sweating.
EENT: Abnormal vision (5.8%); diplopia (2.1%); glaucoma; eye hemorrhage; photophobia; visual field defect; taste perversion; eye disorder.
GI: Nausea (24.3%); constipation (10.6%); diarrhea (6.4%); dyspepsia (6.4%); anorexia (4.8%); dry mouth (3.7%); vomiting (2.7%); abdominal pain (5.8%).
GU: Hematuria.
RESP: Rhinitis (12.2%); dyspnea (4.8%); epistaxis; hiccoughs.
OTHER: Pain (7%); accidental injury; flu syndrome; chills; peripheral edema (7.4%); facial edema; edema; weight gain; anemia; bursitis; myalgia; twitching; chest pain; infection.

Precautions

Pregnancy: Category B.
Lactation: Unknown.
Children: Safety and efficacy not established.
Elderly: Because elderly patients are more likely to have decreased renal function, monitor renal function and select dose with caution.
Carcinogenesis: Uterine neoplasia and endometrial sarcomas observed with high doses of pergolide in animal models and was probably a result of prolactin inhibition.
Cardiac arrhythmias: Exercise caution in patients with arrhythmias because of possible atrial premature contractions and sinus tachycardia.
Discontinuation: Abrupt discontinuation in patients receiving chronic pergolide as an adjunct to levodopa may precipitate hallucinations and confusion.
Hallucinosis: Hallucinations may occur in some patients.
Neuroleptic malignant syndrome (NMS): Symptoms resembling NMS (eg, elevated temperature, muscular rigidity, altered consciousness, autonomic instability) associated with rapid dose reduction, withdrawal, or changes in pergolide therapy.
Symptomatic hypotension: Either symptomatic or orthostatic hypotension may occur, especially during initial treatment. With gradual titration, tolerance to hypotension usually develops.

Overdosage: Signs and Symptoms

Vomiting, hypotension, agitation, hallucinations, involuntary movements and tingling of extremities, palpitations, ventricular extrasystoles.

PATIENT CARE CONSIDERATIONS

Administration/Storage

- Administer in divided doses 3 times/day.
- Store at room temperature (59° to 86°F).

Assessment/Interventions

- Obtain patient history, including drug history and any known allergies. Note reports of syncope, irregular heart beats, or palpitations.
- If symptomatic orthostatic or sustained hypotension occurs, take safety precautions. As dosage is gradually titrated, tolerance to hypotension usually develops.
- Provide regular ophthalmic exams.

Patient/Family Education

- Inform patient of risk of hypotension and teach safety measures to prevent falls from orthostatic hypotension (eg, dangling legs before getting out of bed. gradually rising from chairs).
- Instruct patient to report the following symptoms to health care provider: symptomatic orthostatic or sustained hypotension, hallucinations, dyskinesia, somnolence, insomnia, nausea, constipation, diarrhea, dyspepsia, and rhinitis.
- Tell patient to take sips of water frequently, suck on ice chips or sugarless hard candy, or chew sugarless gum if dry mouth occurs.
- Advise patient that drug may cause drowsiness, and to use caution while driving or performing other tasks requiring mental alertness.

Perindopril Erbumine

(per-IN-doe prill ehr-BYOO-meen)

Class Antihypertensive/Angiotensin-converting enzyme (ACE) inhibitor

How Supplied
Aceon Tablets 2 mg, Tablets 4 mg, Tablets 8 mg
✣ Coversyl

Action

PHARMACOLOGY: Competitively inhibits angiotensin I-converting enzyme, resulting in prevention of angiotensin I conversion to angiotensin II, a potent vasoconstrictor that also stimulates aldosterone release. Clinical consequences are a decrease in BP, reduced sodium resorption, and potassium retention.

PHARMACOKINETICS/DYNAMICS:

Absorption: Rapid absorption. Bioavailability is approximately 75% (perindopril) and approximately 25% (active metabolite perindoprilat). Food reduces bioavailability 35%. Steady state is 3 to 6 days. T_{max} is approximately 1 hr (perindopril) and 3 to 7 hr (active metabolite perindoprilat).

Distribution: Protein binding is 60% (perindopril) and 10% to 20% (active metabolite perindoprilat).

Metabolism: Extensively metabolized in liver to active metabolite perindoprilat and other metabolites by glucuronidation and cyclization via dehydration.

Excretion: Urine (4% to 12% unchanged, 4.5% to 22% as metabolites). Mean total body Cl is 219 to 362 mL/min and mean renal Cl is 23.3 to 28.6 mL/min (perindopril). The $t_{½}$ is 0.8 to 1 hr (perindopril). Apparent mean $t_{½}$ is 30 to 120 hr (metabolite perindoprilat).

Special Populations:

Renal Function Impairment – Ccr is 30 to 80 mL/min; metabolite AUC is approximately doubled.

Hepatic Function Impairment – Bioavailability of metabolite is increased and plasma concentrations are approximately 50% higher.

Elderly – Plasma concentrations of both perindopril and metabolite are approximately twice those observed in younger patients; renal excretion of metabolite decreases (70 yr and older).

Heart failure patients – Metabolite Cl is reduced in CHF, resulting in 40% higher dose interval AUC.

Indications Treatment of essential hypertension.

Contraindications Hypersensitivity or history of angioedema related to ACE inhibitor treatment.

Route/Dosage

Impaired Renal Function
ADULTS (CCR ABOVE 30 ML/MIN): **PO** Initial dose is 2 mg/day (max, 8 mg/day).

Uncomplicated Hypertension
ADULTS: **PO** Initial dose 4 mg qd; then titrate upward until BP, measured just before the next dose, is controlled (max, 16 mg/day). Usual maintenance dose is 4 to 8 mg/day.

PATIENTS OLDER THAN 65 YR: **PO** Initial dose 4 mg/day in 1 or 2 divided doses; then titrate upward until BP, measured just before the next dose, is controlled (max, 8 mg/day).

Use with Concomitant Diuretics
ADULTS: **PO** If BP is not adequately controlled with perindopril alone, a diuretic may be added. In patients being treated with a diuretic, to reduce the likelihood of the occurrence of symptomatic hypotension, discontinue the diuretic 2 to 3 days prior to beginning perindopril. If the diuretic cannot be discontinued, use an initial dose of 2 to 4 mg/day of perindopril and titrate the dose as above.

Interactions

Capsaicin: May increase cough.

Digoxin: May cause increased or decreased digoxin levels.

Diuretics: Increased risk of excessive reduction in BP.

Indomethacin, salicylates (eg, aspirin): May reduce hypotensive effects, especially in low renin or volume-dependent hypertensive patients.

Lithium: Increased risk of lithium toxicity.

Loop diuretics: Effects of loop diuretics may be decreased.

Phenothiazines: Enhanced hypotensive effects.

Potassium supplements, potassium-sparing diuretics (eg, spironolactone), drugs capable of increasing serum potassium (eg, cyclosporine, heparin, indomethacin): Increased risk of hyperkalemia.

Lab Test Interferences None well documented.

Adverse Reactions

CV: Palpitation (1%).

CNS: Dizziness (8%); cerebrovascular accident (0.2%).

EENT: Sinusitis (5%); ear infection (3%).

GI: Dyspepsia (2%).

GU: Proteinuria (2%).

HEMA: Neutropenia; agranulocytosis.

METAB: Hyperkalemia.

RESP: Cough (12%); pulmonary fibrosis (less than 0.1%).
OTHER: Back pain (6%); viral infection, upper extremity pain, hypertonia (3%); fever (2%); angioedema (0.1%); anaphylactoid reactions.

> **WARNING:**
> *Pregnancy:* Use in second and third trimesters may cause injury and death to fetus.

Precautions
Pregnancy: Category C (first trimester); category D (second and third trimesters).
Lactation: Undetermined.
Children: Safety and efficacy not established.
Elderly: Perindopril plasma concentrations may be increased.

Renal function impairment: Changes in renal function may occur in susceptible individuals.
Angioedema: May occur and is potentially fatal if laryngeal edema occurs. Use drug with extreme caution in patients with history of angioedema.
Cough: Chronic nonproductive cough may occur.
Hepatic failure: Hepatic failure has occurred rarely with other ACE inhibitors.
Hypotension: Symptomatic hypotension may occur.
Neutropenia and agranulocytosis: Has occurred rarely with other ACE inhibitors; risk appears greater with renal dysfunction, heart failure, or immunosuppression.

Overdosage: Signs and Symptoms
Hypotension, hypothermia, circulatory arrest, death.

PATIENT CARE CONSIDERATIONS
Administration/Storage
- Administer alone or in combination with other antihypertensives.
- Give without regard to meals.
- Do not administer to pregnant women during second and third trimesters as fetal and neonatal morbidity and death can occur.
- Store tablets at controlled room temperature (68° to 77°F). Protect from moisture.

Assessment/Interventions
- Obtain patient history, including drug history and any known allergies. Note renal or hepatic impairment, conditions predisposing to volume depletion (eg, prolonged diuretic therapy), diabetes, heart failure, anuria, hereditary or idiopathic angioedema, lupus erythematosus, left ventricular outflow obstruction, allergy to any other ACE inhibitor, and concurrent use of potassium-containing salt substitutes, potassium supplements, or potassium-sparing diuretics.
- Ensure that reduced dose is administered to patient with renal impairment or on current diuretic therapy.
- Ensure that volume and/or salt depletion have been corrected before initiating therapy.
- Ensure that serum electrolytes and renal function are monitored periodically.
- Ensure that CBC with differential is evaluated prior to starting therapy, at 2 wk intervals for 3 mo and then periodically thereafter in patient with renal impairment.
- Monitor and record BP and pulse. Should symptomatic hypotension occur, hold medication and notify health care provider.
- Take safety precautions if orthostatic hypotension occurs.
- Monitor for signs of hypersensitivity including angioedema involving swelling of the face, lips, eyelids, and tongue. Discontinue medication and notify health care provider immediately if noted. Be prepared to treat appropriately
- Assess patient for GI, CNS, and general body side effects. Inform health care provider if noted and significant.

Patient/Family Education
- Explain name, dose, action, and potential side effects of drug.
- Advise patient to take qd or bid as prescribed, without regard to meals, but to take with food if stomach upset occurs.
- Advise patient to try to take each dose at about the same time each day.
- Inform patient that drug controls, but does not cure, hypertension and to continue taking drug as prescribed even when BP is not elevated.
- Caution patient not to change the dose or stop taking unless advised by health care provider.
- Instruct patient to continue taking other BP medications as prescribed by health care provider.
- Instruct patient in BP and pulse measurement skills.
- Advise patient to monitor and record BP and pulse at home and to inform health care provider should abnormal measurements be noted. Also advise patient to take record of BP and pulse to each follow-up visit.
- Caution patient to avoid sudden position changes to prevent orthostatic hypotension.

- Instruct patient to lie or sit down if experiencing dizziness or lightheadedness when standing.
- Emphasize importance of the following: other modalities on BP control: weight control, regular exercise, smoking cessation, and moderate intake of alcohol and salt.
- Caution patient that inadequate fluid intake, excessive perspiration, diarrhea, or vomiting can lead to excessive fall in BP resulting in lightheadedness or fainting.
- Advise patient that medication may cause dizziness or lightheadedness and to use caution while driving or performing other tasks requiring mental alertness until tolerance is determined.
- Caution patient to avoid unnecessary exposure to UV light (sunlight, tanning booths) and to use sunscreen and wear protective clothing when exposed to UV light to avoid photosensitivity reaction.
- Advise women to notify health care provider if pregnant, planning to become pregnant, or breastfeeding.
- Instruct patient to stop taking drug and immediately report any of the following symptoms to health care provider: sore throat, fever, swelling of the hands or feet, irregular heartbeat, chest pains, fainting, swelling of the face, lips, eyelids, or tongue, difficulty breathing.
- Instruct patient to inform health care provider if a persistent cough develops while taking this medication.
- Caution patient not to take any prescription or OTC medications, potassium-containing salt substitutes, potassium supplements, or dietary supplements unless advised by health care provider.
- Advise patient that follow-up visits and lab tests will be required to monitor therapy and to keep appointments.

Permethrin

(per-METH-rin)

Class Scabicides/Pediculicides

How Supplied
Acticin Cream 5% ♦ *Elimite* Cream 5% ♦ *Permethrin* Lotion 1% ♦ *Nix Cream Rinse* Liquid 1% ❋ *Nix Creme Rinse* ♦ *Nix Dermal Cream*

Action
PHARMACOLOGY: Acts on the nerve cell membrane to disrupt the sodium channel current by which the polarization of the membrane is regulated. Delayed repolarization and paralysis of the pests is the outcome.

PHARMACOKINETICS/DYNAMICS:

Metabolism: Rapidly metabolized by ester hydrolysis to inactive metabolites.

Excretion: Excreted primarily in the urine.

Indications
Cream: Treatment of scabies (*Sarcoptes scabiei*) infestation.

Lotion/Cream rinse: Treatment of infestation with head lice (*Pediculus humanus capitis*) and its nits (eggs).

Liquid: Treatment of infestation with *Pediculus humanus* var. *capitis* (head louse) and its nits (eggs).

Contraindications Standard considerations.

Route/Dosage

Scabies

Cream Massage 30 g into the skin from head to soles of feet. Massage into hairline, neck, temple, and forehead of infants and geriatric patients. Remove cream by shower or bath after 8 to 14 hr. One application is generally curative.

Head Lice

Lotion/Cream rinse Apply to hair after washing with shampoo; rinse with water and towel dry. Apply a sufficient amount to saturate hair and scalp, especially behind the ears and nape of neck. Leave on hair for no longer than 10 min, then rinse with water. If lice are observed within 7 days after application, apply a second treatment. Remove remaining nits with nit comb provided.

Interactions None well documented.

Lab Test Interferences None well documented.

Adverse Reactions
CNS:
Cream – Dizziness (5%), headache, seizure (rare) (postmarketing).
DERM:
Cream – Mild transient burning/stinging (10%); itching (7%); tingling, numbness, erythema, rash (2% or less).
Lotion/Cream rinse – Itching, redness, swelling of scalp.
GI:
Cream – Abdominal pain, diarrhea, nausea, vomiting (5% [postmarketing]).
OTHER:
Cream – Fever (5% [postmarketing]).

Precautions
Pregnancy: Category B.
Lactation: Undetermined.
Children: Safety and efficacy established in patients greater than or equal to 2 mo.
Asthmatics: May cause breathing difficulties or exacerbate asthmatic episodes.
Dermatological effects: Elimite may temporarily exacerbate pruritus, edema, and erythema and is rarely a sign of treatment failure.

PATIENT CARE CONSIDERATIONS

Administration/Storage
- For topical use only. Not for ophthalmic, oral, or intravaginal use.
- Avoid contact with eyes. If eye contact occurs, flush immediately and thoroughly with water.
- Use glove if applying cream to patient; thoroughly massage cream into skin from the head to the soles of the feet; remove cream 8 to 14 hr after application by showering or bathing.
- Store cream at controlled room temperature (59° to 77°F). Keep tube tightly capped.

Assessment/Interventions
- Obtain patient history, including drug history and any known allergies. Note history of allergy to pyrethroid or pyrethrin.
- Assess and document skin condition before initial application and periodically throughout treatment.

Patient/Family Education
- Explain name, dose, action, and potential side effects of drug.
- Caution patient or caregiver to avoid contact with eyes and if accidental eye contact occurs, immediately flush the eyes with water to remove medication. Advise patient or caregiver to notify health care provider if eye irritation or sensitivity follows exposure to the eyes.
- Teach patient or caregiver proper technique for applying cream: wash hands; use gloves if applying to another person; thoroughly massage cream into skin from the head to the soles of the feet; 8 to 14 hr after application, remove cream by washing (shower or bath).
- Advise patient or caregiver that itching, mild burning, and/or stinging may occur after application of cream but that this should go away in 2 to 4 wk. If irritation persists, advise patient to notify health care provider.
- For proper nit removal, wash all personal articles and clothing (eg, coats, linen, combs, headgear) in hot water or seal in a plastic bag for approximately 2 wk. Thorough vacuuming of rooms is recommended.
- Advise patient to discontinue use and consult health care provider if irritation persists or infection is present or develops.
- Consult health care provider if infestation of eyebrows or eyelashes occur.
- Advise patient or caregiver that follow-up visits may be necessary and to keep appointments.

Perphenazine

(per-FEN-uh-zeen)

Class Antipsychotic/Phenothiazine/Antiemetic

How Supplied
Perphenazine Tablets 2 mg, Tablets 4 mg, Tablets 8 mg, Tablets 16 mg, Oral concentrate 16 mg/5 mL

✽ *Apo-Perphenazine*

Action
PHARMACOLOGY: Effects apparently caused by postsynaptic dopamine receptor blockade in CNS.

PHARMACOKINETICS/DYNAMICS:

Absorption: T_{max} is approximately 1 to 3 hr (parent), 2 to 4 hr (metabolite). Steady state is 72 hr. C_{max} is 984 pg/mL (parent compound), 7-hydroxyperphenazine (509 pg/mL).

Distribution: Readily crosses placenta, distributes into breast milk. Protein binding is greater than 90%.

Metabolism: Extensively metabolized in liver to a number of metabolites mediated by CYP2D6 and is subject to genetic polymorphism (7% to 10% of white patients, low percentage of Asian patients); therefore, they are poor metabolizers of CYP2D6 and will then metabolize the drug more slowly.

Excretion: Renal and biliary, some enterohepatic recycling. Terminal $t_{½}$ is 9.9 to 18.8 hr (metabolite). Plasma $t_{½}$ is 9 to 12 hr (perphenazine).

Onset: Gradual, up to several weeks, varies.

Indications Management of psychotic disorders; control of severe nausea/vomiting in adults.

Contraindications Comatose or severely depressed states; allergy to any phenothiazine; presence of large amounts of other CNS depressants; bone marrow depression or blood dyscrasias; liver damage; subcortical brain damage.

Route/Dosage
Psychiatric
ADULTS:
Nonhospitalized patients: **PO** 4 to 8 mg tid, reduce as soon as possible to minimum effective dosage.
Hospitalized patients: **PO** 8 to 16 mg bid to qid; avoid dosages greater than 64 mg/day.

Nausea/Vomiting
ADULTS: **PO** 8 to 16 mg/day in divided doses. Give elderly and debilitated patients lower doses and observe closely.

CHILDREN 12 YR AND OLDER: May be given lowest limit of adult dosage.

Interactions

Alcohol and other CNS depressants: May result in increased CNS depression and may precipitate extrapyramidal reaction.

Anticholinergics: May reduce therapeutic effects of perphenazine and worsen anticholinergic effects. Coadministration may worsen schizophrenic symptoms and lead to tardive dyskinesia (see Precautions).

Barbiturate anesthetics: Frequency and severity of neuromuscular excitation and hypotension may increase.

Cisapride, sparfloxacin: The risk of life-threatening cardiac arrhythmias, including torsades de pointes, may be increased.

Guanethidine: Hypotensive action of guanethidine may be inhibited.

Metrizamide: Possibility of seizure may be increased when subarachnoid metrizamide injection is used.

Paroxetine: Plasma levels of perphenazine may be elevated, increasing the risk of side effects.

Lab Test Interferences
May discolor urine pink to red-brown. False-positive pregnancy tests may occur but are less likely to occur with serum test. Increases in protein-bound iodine have been reported.

Adverse Reactions

CV: Orthostatic hypotension; hypertension; tachycardia; bradycardia; syncope; cardiac arrest; circulatory collapse; ECG changes.
CNS: Lightheadedness; faintness; dizziness; pseudoparkinsonism; dystonia; dyskinesia, motor restlessness; oculogyric crisis; dystonias; hyperreflexia; tardive dyskinesia; drowsiness; headache; fatigue; abnormalities of the cerebrospinal fluid proteins; paradoxical excitement or exacerbation of psychotic symptoms; catatonic-like states; weakness; tremor; paranoid reactions; lethargy; seizures; hyperactivity; nocturnal confusion; bizarre dreams; vertigo; insomnia.
DERM: Photosensitivity; skin pigmentation; dry skin; exfoliative dermatitis; urticarial rash; maculopapular hypersensitivity reaction; seborrhea; eczema; pruritus.
EENT: Pigmentary retinopathy; glaucoma; photophobia; blurred vision; mydriasis; increased IOP; dry mouth or throat; nasal congestion.
GI: Dyspepsia; adynamic ileus (may result in death); nausea; vomiting; constipation.
GU: Breast enlargement; galactorrhea; urinary hesitancy or retention; impotence; sexual dysfunction; menstrual irregularities.
HEMA: Agranulocytosis; eosinophilia; leukopenia; hemolytic anemia; thrombocytopenic purpura; pancytopenia.
HEPA: Jaundice.
METAB: Hyperglycemia; hypoglycemia; decreased cholesterol.
RESP: Laryngospasm; bronchospasm; dyspnea.
OTHER: Increases in appetite and weight; polydipsia; increased prolactin levels.

Precautions

Pregnancy: Pregnancy category undetermined.
Lactation: Undetermined.
Children: Not recommended in children younger than 12 yr.
Elderly: More susceptible to effects; consider lower dose.
Special risk patients: Use caution in patients with CV disease or mitral insufficiency, history of glaucoma, EEG abnormalities or seizure disorders, prior brain damage, hepatic or renal impairment, or those who will be exposed to extreme heat.
Antiemetic effects: Because of suppression of cough reflex, aspiration of vomitus possible.
CNS effects: May impair mental or physical abilities, especially during first few days of therapy.
Hepatic effects: Jaundice usually occurs between second and fourth weeks of treatment; considered hypersensitivity reaction. Usually reversible.
Neuroleptic malignant syndrome (NMS): Potentially fatal NMS has occurred with agents of this class. Signs and symptoms are hyperpyrexia, muscle rigidity, altered mental status, irregular pulse, irregular BP, tachycardia, and diaphoresis.
Pulmonary: Cases of bronchopneumonia, some fatal, have occurred.
Sudden death: Has been reported; predisposing factors may be seizures or previous brain damage. Flare-ups of psychotic behavior may precede death.
Suicide: Because of the possibility of suicide in depressed patients, avoid access to large quantities of this drug.
Tardive dyskinesia: Syndrome of potentially irreversible involuntary body and facial movements may develop. Prevalence highest in elderly, especially women. Use smallest effective doses for shortest possible time period.

Overdosage: Signs and Symptoms
CNS depression, hypotension, extrapyramidal symptoms, agitation, convulsions, fever, hypothermia, ECG changes, cardiac arrhythmias.

PATIENT CARE CONSIDERATIONS
Administration/Storage
- Dose and frequency of administration are variable, depending on condition being treated.
- Administer tablets as prescribed, without regard to meals. Administer with food if GI upset occurs.
- Shake oral concentrate well before measuring dose.
- Measure prescribed dose of oral concentrate using calibrated dropper supplied with medication.
- Dilute each 5 mL of oral concentrate with 2 oz of water, saline, 7-Up, homogenized milk, carbonated orange drink, or pineapple, apricot, prune, orange, V-8, tomato, or grapefruit juice just prior to administration. Do not prepare dilutions ahead of time and store.
- Do not dilute oral concentrate with beverages containing caffeine (eg, coffee), tannins (eg, tea), or pectins (eg, apple juice) because physical incompatibilities may occur.
- Store tablets at controlled room temperature (59° to 86°F). Store oral concentrate in refrigerator (36° to 46°F) or at controlled room temperature. Protect oral concentrate from light.

Assessment/Interventions
- Obtain patient history, including drug history and any known allergies. Note allergy to perphenazine or other phenothiazines, previous episode of jaundice with phenothiazine therapy, renal impairment, hepatic impairment, ischemic heart disease, heart failure, arrhythmias, cerebrovascular disease, asthma, emphysema, narrow angle glaucoma, epilepsy, mitral insufficiency, pheochromocytoma, prostatic hypertrophy, condition predisposing to hypotension (eg, dehydration, hypovolemia), concomitant use of antihypertensive drugs, or previous episodes of NMS.
- Ensure that medication is discontinued at least 48 hr before myelography and not resumed until at least 24 hr after procedure to reduce chance of seizures occurring.
- Frequently assess patient for response to treatment. Notify health care provider if condition being treated is not improving or is worsening.
- Ensure that therapy is periodically reviewed to determine if therapy needs to be continued without change or if a dose change (eg, increase, decrease, discontinuation) is indicated.
- Avoid sudden discontinuation of therapy if possible. Attempt to gradually reduce dose if decision to discontinue medication is made.
- Inform health care provider immediately if hyperpyrexia, muscle rigidity, altered mental status, irregular pulse, BP, tachycardia, or diaphoresis develop.
- Notify health care provider immediately if palpitations or syncope occur.
- Assess neurologic status before and during treatment. Observe for involuntary body and facial movements, excessive drowsiness, agitation, tremor, or anxiety. Inform health care provider if noted.
- Monitor patient for CNS, CV, GI, GU, psychiatric, musculoskeletal, and general body side effects. Inform health care provider if noted and significant.
- Assess medication compliance.

Patient/Family Education
- Explain name, dose, action, and potential side effects of drug.
- Advise patient, family, or caregiver that dose will be adjusted periodically until max benefit has been obtained.
- Advise patient, family, or caregiver not to change the dose or stop taking unless advised by health care provider.
- Instruct patient, family, or caregiver to measure prescribed dose of oral concentrate using calibrated dropper supplied with medication.
- Advise patient, family, or caregiver that each 5 mL of oral concentrate should be diluted with 2 oz of water, saline, 7-Up, homogenized milk, carbonated orange drink, or pineapple, apricot, prune, orange, V-8, tomato, or grapefruit juice just prior to administration. Caution patient, caregiver, or family not to prepare dilutions ahead of time and store.
- Caution patient, family, or caregiver not to dilute oral concentrate with beverages containing caffeine (eg, coffee), tannins (eg, tea) or pectins (eg, apple juice), because physical incompatibilities may occur.
- Instruct patient not to stop taking perphenazine when feeling better.
- Instruct patient, family, or caregiver to immediately report fainting or loss of consciousness, palpitations, dizziness, high fever, muscle rigidity, altered mental status, irregular pulse, sore throat, unusual bruising, or yellowing of the skin or eyes.
- Advise patient, family, or caregiver to notify health care provider of the following: excessive drowsiness, increased agitation or anxiety, involuntary body or facial movements.
- Advise patient to avoid strenuous activity during periods of high temperature or humidity.

- Instruct patient to avoid alcoholic beverages and other depressants while taking this medication.
- Instruct patient to get up slowly from lying or sitting position and to avoid sudden position changes to prevent postural hypotension. Advise patient to report dizziness with position changes to health care provider. Caution patient that hot tubs and hot showers or baths may worsen dizziness.
- Advise patient to take sips of water, suck on ice chips or sugarless hard candy, or chew sugarless gum if dry mouth occurs.
- Advise patient that drug may cause drowsiness or impaired judgment or thinking skills and to use caution while driving or performing other tasks requiring mental alertness until tolerance is determined.
- Caution patient that medication may cause sensitivity to sunlight and to avoid unnecessary exposure to UV light (sunlight, tanning booths) and to use sunscreen and wear protective clothing when exposed to UV light until tolerance is determined.
- Advise women to notify health care provider if pregnant, planning to become pregnant, or breastfeeding.
- Instruct patient not to take any prescription or OTC medications or dietary supplements unless advised by health care provider.
- Advise patient that follow-up visits may be required to monitor therapy and to keep appointments.

Perphenazine/Amitriptyline

(per-FEN-uh-zeen/am-ee-TRIP-tih-leen)

Class Psychotherapeutic combination

How Supplied
Etrafon 2-10 Tablets 2 mg perphenazine/10 mg amitriptyline ◆ *Etrafon* Tablets 2 mg perphenazine/25 mg amitriptyline ◆ *Etrafon-A* Tablets 4 mg perphenazine/10 mg amitriptyline ◆ *Etrafon-Forte* Tablets 4 mg perphenazine/25 mg amitriptyline

Action
PHARMACOLOGY: Amitriptyline blocks reuptake of serotonin and norepinephrine in CNS. Perphenazine appears to block postsynaptic dopamine receptors.

Indications
Treatment of moderate-to-severe anxiety or agitation and depressed mood; moderate to severe depression and anxiety associated with chronic physical disease; treatment of patients in whom depression and anxiety cannot be clearly differentiated; treatment of schizophrenia with associated depression.

Contraindications
Hypersensitivity to phenothiazines; depression of CNS due to drugs (eg, barbiturates, alcohol, narcotics, analgesics, antihistamines); bone marrow depression; hypersensitivity to tricyclic antidepressant. Should not be given concomitantly with MAO inhibitors, suspected or established subcortical brain damage. Not recommended for use during acute recovery phases of myocardial infarction.

Route/Dosage
ADULTS: **PO** Initially, usual dose is 2 to 4 mg perphenazine with 10 to 50 mg amitriptyline tid to qid.

Interactions
Alcohol: May result in increased CNS depression and may precipitate extrapyramidal reaction.
Amphetamines: May antagonize antipsychotic effects of perphenazine.
Anticholinergics: May reduce therapeutic effects of perphenazine and worsen anticholinergic effects. Concomitant administration may worsen schizophrenic symptoms and lead to tardive dyskinesia.
Barbiturate anesthetics: Frequency and severity of neuromuscular excitation and hypotension may increase.
Barbiturates, carbamazepine, charcoal: May cause decreased amitriptyline blood levels.
Cimetidine, fluoxetine, haloperidol, oral contraceptives: May cause increased amitriptyline blood levels.
Clonidine: May result in hypertensive crisis.
CNS depressants: Depressant effects may be addictive.
Guanethidine: Hypotensive action may be inhibited.
Lithium: Possible neurotoxicity with perphenazine and may increase effects of amitriptyline.
MAO inhibitors: Do NOT use this product with MAO inhibitors as hyperpyretic crisis, severe convulsions and death may result. When switching from MAO inhibitors, wait 14 days and initiate with low doses, increasing dosage gradually until desired response is achieved.
Metrizamide: Seizure risk may be increased.
Sympathomimetics: Increased pressor effects.

Lab Test Interferences
May discolor urine pink to red-brown. False positive pregnancy test results may occur, but are less likely to occur with serum test. Increases in protein bound iodine have been reported.

Adverse Reactions
CV: Orthostatic hypotension; hypertension; tachycardia; bradycardia; syncope; cardiac arrest; circulatory collapse; arrhythmias; lightheadedness; faintness; dizziness; EKG changes; palpitations.

CNS: Sedation; neurologic impairments; extrapyramidal symptoms (eg, pseudoparkinsonism); dystonia; dyskinesia; motor restlessness; oculogyric crisis; opisthotonos; hyperreflexia; tardive dyskinesia; drowsiness; headache; weakness; anxiety; agitation; mania; exacerbation of psychosis; dizziness; tremor; fatigue; slurring of speech; insomnia; vertigo; seizures; abnormalities of CSF proteins; paradoxical excitement or exacerbation of psychotic symptoms; catatonic-like states; paranoid reactions; lethargy; hyperactivity; nocturnal confusion; bizarre dreams.
DERM: Photosensitivity reaction; skin pigmentation; dry skin; exfoliative dermatitis; urticarial rash; maculopapular hypersensitivity reaction; seborrhea; eczema; acne; pruritus.
EENT: Pigmentary retinopathy; glaucoma; photophobia; rhinitis; pharyngitis; tinnitus; blurred vision; nasal congestion; mydriasis; increased IOP.
GI: Dyspepsia; adynamic ileus (may cause death); constipation; nausea; vomiting; anorexia; diarrhea; peculiar taste; dry mouth or throat.
GU: Urinary hesitancy or retention; impotence; sexual dysfunction; menstrual irregularities; nocturia.
HEMA: Agranulocytosis; eosinophilia; leukopenia; hemolytic anemia; thrombocytopenic purpura.
HEPA: Jaundice.
METAB: Hyperglycemia; hypoglycemia.
RESP: Laryngospasm; bronchospasm; dyspnea; cough.
OTHER: Increases in appetite and weight; polydipsia; breast enlargement; galactorrhea; increased prolactin levels.

Precautions
Pregnancy: Safety not established.
Lactation: Safety not established.
Elderly: More susceptible to adverse effects.
Special risk patients: Use caution in patients with cardiovascular disease or mitral insufficiency, history of glaucoma, EEG abnormalities or seizure disorders, prior brain damage, hepatic or renal impairment.
CNS effects: May impair mental or physical abilities, especially during first few days of therapy.
Neuroleptic malignant syndrome (NMS): Has occurred with agents of this class; is potentially fatal. Signs and symptoms are hyperpyrexia, muscle rigidity, altered mental status, irregular pulse, irregular blood pressure, tachycardia and diaphoresis.
Sudden death: Has been reported; predisposing factors may be seizures or previous brain damage. Flare-up of psychotic behavior may precede death.
Tardive dyskinesia: Syndrome of potentially irreversible involuntary body and facial movements may develop. Prevalence highest in elderly, especially women. Use smallest effective doses for shortest time possible.

Overdosage: Signs and Symptoms
Confusion, tachycardia, visual hallucinations, sedation, hypothermia, arrhythmias, congestive heart failure, dilated pupils, seizures, hypotension, coma, hyperpyrexia, muscle rigidity, hyperactive reflexes, death.

PATIENT CARE CONSIDERATIONS

Administration/Storage
- Administer oral medication with meals or with full glass of milk or water.
- Oral concentrate should be used in hospital setting only and diluted with water, milk, fruit juice, soup, saline, or lemon-lime carbonated soft drink.
- Store tablets in tightly covered, light-resistant container.

Assessment/Interventions
- Obtain patient history, including drug history and any known allergies.
- Monitor blood cell counts with differential, hepatic, and renal function studies, ECG, and ophthalmic status throughout therapy.
- Monitor for jaundice. If present, notify health care provider immediately.
- Monitor for potential signs of pseudoparkinsonism, dystonia, dyskinesia, or akathisia and report to health care provider.
- Monitor for evidence of tardive dyskinesia (eg, involuntary dyskinetic movements of tongue, lips, mouth, face or jaw) and report to health care provider.
- Assess for signs of orthostatic hypotension; take orthostatic blood pressures and report to health care provider.
- Report any significant unexplained temperature increase to health care provider.

Patient/Family Education
- Instruct patient to avoid intake of alcoholic beverages or other CNS depressants.
- Tell patient to use caution in driving or operating machinery.
- Advise patient that the medication may take days to weeks before having a full effect.
- Instruct patient to avoid becoming overheated.
- Caution patient to avoid exposure to sunlight and to use sunscreen or wear protective clothing to minimize photosensitivity reaction.
- Teach patient to change position slowly if dizziness occurs.

- Instruct patient to take sips of water frequently, suck on ice chips or sugarless hard candy, or chew sugarless gum if dry mouth occurs.
- Instruct patient to report the following symptoms to health care provider: dizziness, drooling, restlessness, tremors, stiffness, or muscle spasms.
- Instruct patient to report involuntary face, tongue, mouth, or lip movements to health care provider.
- Explain that urine may turn reddish-brown.

Phenazopyridine Hydrochloride

(fen-AZZ-oh-PIH-rih-deen HIGH-droe-KLOR-ide)

Class Urinary tract product/Analgesic

How Supplied
Azo-Standard Tablets 95 mg ♦ *Baridium* Tablets 100 mg ♦ *Geridium* Tablets 100 mg, Tablets 200 mg ♦ *Prodium* Tablets 95 mg ♦ *Pyridiate* Tablets 100 mg ♦ *Pyridium* Tablets 100 mg, Tablets 200 mg ♦ *Pyridium Plus* Tablets 150 mg ♦ *Urodine* Tablets 100 mg, Tablets 200 mg ♦ *Urogesic* Tablets 100 mg ♦ *UTI Relief* Tablets 97.2 mg
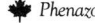 *Phenazo*

Action
PHARMACOLOGY: Exerts topical analgesic effect on urinary tract mucosa.

PHARMACOKINETICS/DYNAMICS:
Metabolism: Phenazopyridine hydrochloride metabolism is probably hepatic; also in other body tissues. One active metabolite is acetaminophen.
Excretion: Phenazopyridine hydrochloride is rapidly excreted by the kidneys, 65% as unchanged drug and metabolites.

Indications Symptomatic relief of pain, burning, urgency, frequency and other discomforts arising from irritation of lower urinary tract mucosa.

PATIENT CARE CONSIDERATIONS

Administration/Storage
- Administer after meals to avoid GI irritation.
- If patient has renal impairment, dosage reduction may be required.
- If being taken concomitantly with antibiotics for UTI, this medicine should be taken for only 2 days (6 doses).
- Do not crush tablets or make into a suspension.
- Store at room temperature in a tightly closed container.

Assessment/Interventions
- Obtain patient history, including drug history and any known allergies.
- Obtain BUN and creatinine to assess for renal dysfunction.

Contraindications Renal insufficiency.

Route/Dosage
ADULTS: **PO** 200 mg tid.
CHILDREN (6 TO 12 YR): **PO** 12 mg/kg/24 hr divided into 3 doses for 2 days.

Interactions None well documented.

Lab Test Interferences Possible interference with colorimetric lab test procedures and urinalysis based on spectrometry or color reactions.

Adverse Reactions
CNS: Headache.
DERM: Rash; pruritus.
GI: Occasional GI disturbances.
GU: Renal toxicity.
HEMA: Methemoglobinemia; hemolytic anemia.
HEPA: Hepatotoxicity.
OTHER: Anaphylactoid reaction.

Precautions
Pregnancy: Category B.
Lactation: Unknown.
Renal function impairment: May lead to accumulation, indicated by yellow tinge to skin and sclera.

Overdosage: Signs and Symptoms
Methemoglobinemia, hemolytic anemia, hemolysis, renal and hepatic impairment and failure.

Patient/Family Education
- Inform patient that this drug should not be taken long term for undiagnosed urinary tract pain.
- Advise patient to take drug after meals to avoid GI upset.
- Inform patient that urine may temporarily become reddish-orange in color and may stain fabric.
- Advise patient to wear glasses instead of contact lenses while taking this drug; contact lenses may become discolored.
- Inform patients with diabetes of possible interference with urine glucose test results.
- Instruct patient not to crush or chew tablets. Permanent teeth discoloration may occur.

Phendimetrazine Tartrate

(fen-dye-ME-tra-zeen TAR-trate)
Class CNS stimulant/Anorexiant

How Supplied
Bontril PDM Tablets 35 mg ♦ Bontril Slow-Release Tablets 35 mg ♦ Melfiat-105 Unicelles Tablets 35 mg ♦ Prelu-2 Capsules, sustained-release 105 mg

Action
PHARMACOLOGY: May stimulate satiety center in brain, causing appetite suppression.
PHARMACOKINETICS/DYNAMICS:
Absorption: Phendimetrazine is readily absorbed.
Metabolism: Phendimetrazine metabolism is hepatic. Some of the drug is metabolized to phenmetrazine and phendimetrazine-N-oxide.
Excretion: Excretion is via the kidneys and is increased by acidifying the urine. The t½ is 1.9 hr (immediate-release) and 9.8 hr (slow-release).
Duration: 4 hr.

Indications
Short-term (few weeks) adjunct to diet plan to reduce weight.

Contraindications
Hypersensitivity to sympathomimetic amines; pregnancy; advanced arteriosclerosis; symptomatic cardiovascular disease; moderate to severe hypertension; hyperthyroidism; glaucoma; agitated states; history of drug abuse; during or within 14 days following the administration of an MAOI.

Route/Dosage
ADULTS AND CHILDREN (GREATER THAN OR EQUAL TO 12 YR): PO Tablets or capsules 35 mg bid or tid before meals; sustained-release capsules 105 mg once daily in the morning before breakfast.

Interactions
Guanethidine: May decrease hypotensive effect of guanethidine.
MAOIs (eg, phenelzine); furazolidone: May cause hypertensive crisis and intracranial hemorrhage.
Selective serotonin reuptake inhibitors (eg, fluoxetine): Sympathomimetic effects of phendimetrazine and risk of "serotonin syndrome" may be increased.

Lab Test Interferences
None well documented.

Adverse Reactions
CV: Palpitation; tachycardia; hypertension.
CNS: Overstimulation; restlessness; dizziness; insomnia; euphoria; dysphoria; tremor; headache; psychosis.
DERM: Allergic urticaria.
GI: Dry mouth; unpleasant taste; diarrhea; constipation.
GU: Impotence; changes in libido.

Precautions
Pregnancy: Do not use in women who are pregnant or may become pregnant.
Lactation: Undetermined.
Children: Safety and efficacy not established in children less than 12 yr.
Special risk patients: Use with caution in patients with glaucoma, hypertension, diabetes mellitus.
Drug dependence: Psychological and physical dependence may occur with continued use; this class of drugs has been extensively abused.
Tolerance: Tolerance to the anorectic effect usually develops within a few weeks.

Overdosage: Signs and Symptoms
Restlessness, tremor, hyperreflexia, rapid respiration, confusion, assaultiveness, hallucinations, panic states, fatigue, depression, arrhythmias, hypertension, hypotension, circulatory collapse, nausea, vomiting, diarrhea, abdominal cramps, convulsions, coma, death.

PATIENT CARE CONSIDERATIONS

Administration/Storage
- Discontinue MAOIs greater than or equal to 14 days before initiating therapy.
- Administer sustained-release capsule once daily in the morning. Medication is slowly released over 12 hr.
- Swallow sustained-release capsule whole. Do not crush, chew, or open capsule.
- Administer immediate-release tablet bid to tid as prescribed, 1 hr before meals. Administer last dose several hours before bedtime.
- Store at controlled room temperature (59° to 86°F).

Assessment/Interventions
- Obtain patient history, including drug history and any known allergies. Note history of

advanced coronary artery disease, moderate to severe hypertension, hyperthyroidism, sensitivity to sympathomimetic amines, glaucoma, agitation, history of drug abuse, or concurrent or recent MAOI therapy.
* Ensure that patient receives dietary instructions regarding caloric restriction.
* Determine baseline weight. Weigh periodically during therapy to monitor response to therapy.
* Monitor blood sugar in diabetic patient more frequently when drug is started or dose is changed.
* Monitor patient for CNS, CV, GI, and general body side effects.

Patient/Family Education
* Explain name, dose, action, and potential side effects of drug.
* Advise patient using immediate-release tablet to take prescribed dose 1 hr before meals and to take last dose several hours before bedtime.
* Advise patient using sustained-release capsule that medication is slowly released over 12 hr and to take dose in the morning. Advise patient to swallow the capsule whole and to not crush or chew the capsule.
* Encourage patient to follow medically supervised weight reduction program. Emphasize that this medication will only work in conjunction with a caloric restricted diet and exercise program.
* Advise patient that medication should be taken as prescribed and to not stop taking or change the dose unless advised to do so by the health care provider.
* Explain that appetite suppressant effects are temporary and tolerance to medication and dependence can occur. Caution patient not to increase the dose in an effort to overcome the tolerance when it occurs.
* Remind diabetic patient to monitor blood sugar more frequently while implementing dietary restrictions and to notify health care provider if significant changes in blood sugar occur.
* Caution patient that drug may impair the ability to drive or perform other tasks requiring mental alertness.
* Advise patient to notify health care provider immediately if the following symptoms occur: chest pain, palpitations, nervousness, dizziness.
* Advise patient to notify health care provider if experiencing any unusual or unexplained symptoms.
* Advise women to inform the health care provider if becoming pregnant, planning on becoming pregnant, or breastfeeding.
* Warn patient not to take any prescription or *otc* drugs or dietary supplements without consulting the health care provider.
* Advise patient that follow-up visits may be necessary to monitor therapy and to be sure to keep appointments.

Phenelzine Sulfate

(FEN-uhl-zeen SULL-fate)
Class Antidepressant/MAO inhibitor
How Supplied
Nardil Tablets 15 mg (as sulfate)

Action
PHARMACOLOGY: Phenelzine blocks activity of enzyme MAO, thereby increasing monoamine (eg, epinephrine, norepinephrine, serotonin) concentrations in CNS.

PHARMACOKINETICS/DYNAMICS:
Absorption: Phenelzine is well absorbed. T_{max} is approximately 2 to 3 hr.
Metabolism: Phenelzine metabolism is hepatic. It is metabolized with the release of active metabolites. Inactivation is mainly by acetylation.
Excretion: Urine (mainly as metabolites).
Onset: As early as 7 to 10 days, may take up to 4 to 8 wk for full effect.
Duration: Up to 2 wk.

Indications Treatment of "atypical" ("nonendogenous" or "neurotic") depression; management of depression in patients unresponsive to other antidepressant drugs. **Unlabeled use(s):** Treatment of bulimia; treatment of cocaine addiction; control of panic disorder with agoraphobia.

Contraindications Hypersensitivity to MAO inhibitors; pheochromocytoma; CHF; abnormal liver function; history of liver disease; severe renal impairment; cerebrovascular defect; concurrent use of dextromethorphan or CNS depressants (eg, alcohol); sympathomimetic drugs (eg, amphetamine, dopamine, norepinephrine) or related drugs (eg, methyldopa); cardiovascular disease.

Route/Dosage
ADULTS: **PO** 15 mg tid initially; may titrate up to 90 mg/day. Elderly should receive no more than 60 mg/day. After max benefit is achieved, dose can be slowly decreased over several weeks to maintenance dose. Doses as low as 15 mg qod may be used for maintenance.

Interactions
Amine-containing foods: May cause severe hypertension or hemorrhagic strokes.
Anorexiants: May cause exaggerated pharmacologic effects (eg, severe headaches, hypertension, hyperpyrexia) of anorexiants (amphetamines and related compounds).
CNS depressants: May enhance CNS effects.
Dextromethorphan: Concurrent use has been associated with severe reactions (eg, hyperpyrexia, hypotension, death).
Fluoxetine, paroxetine, sertraline, trazodone: Although data are limited, interactions comparable to those of the tricycle antidepressants and phenelzine may occur.
Guanethidine: MAO inhibitors may antagonize the antihypertensive effect.
Insulin, sulfonylureas: May enhance hypoglycemic action.
Levodopa: May cause hypertensive reactions.
Meperidine: May lead to severe reactions, including hypotension, convulsions, respiratory depression, and vascular collapse.
Sympathomimetics: May cause severe headache, hypertensive crisis, and hyperpyrexia.
Tricyclic antidepressants, buspirone, cyclobenzaprine, carbamazepine, maprotiline, guanethidine, CNS stimulants, tyramine: May lead to potentially fatal reactions, including seizures and hypertensive crisis; mental status changes, hyperthermia.

Lab Test Interferences None well documented.

Adverse Reactions
CV: Orthostatic hypotension; edema; hypertensive crisis.
CNS: Dizziness; headache; sleep disturbances; tremors; hyperflexemia; manic symptoms; convulsions; toxic delirium; coma.
DERM: Rash; sweating; photosensitivity.
EENT: Blurred vision; glaucoma.
GI: Constipation; nausea; GI disturbances; anorexia.
GU: Sexual dysfunction; urinary retention; incontinence.
HEMA: Anemia; leukopenia; agranulocytosis; thrombocytopenia.
HEPA: Fatal progressive necrotizing hepatocellular damage; elevated serum transaminases; hepatitis.
METAB: Weight gain; hypermetabolic syndrome (eg, fever, tachycardia rapid breathing, rigidity, metabolism, acidosis, coma); hypernatremia.
OTHER: Transient respiratory and circulatory depression following electroconvulsive therapy.

Precautions
Pregnancy: Category C.
Lactation: Undetermined.
Children: Not recommended in patients less than 16 yr.
Elderly: Drug should be used cautiously in patients greater than 60 yr because of possibility of existing cerebral sclerosis with damaged vessels. If hypertension develops, the risk of stroke may be increased.
Depression associated with drug abuse/alcoholism: Use with caution; increased risk of serious drug interactions.
Epilepsy: May lower seizure threshold.
Diabetes: May alter glucose control.
Hypotension: Orthostatic hypotension is significant side effect and may lead to falling and changes in heart rate.
Pyridoxine: Phenelzine may cause pyridoxine deficiency, with symptoms of numbness, paresthesias and edema. Supplements may be required.
Suicidal patients: Strict supervision may be necessary in patients at risk.

Overdosage: Signs and Symptoms
Excitement, hypotension, dizziness, movement disorders, irritability, insomnia, weakness, severe headache, anxiety, restlessness, drowsiness, coma, convulsions, flushing, hypertension, sweating, tachypnea, acidosis, hyperpyrexia, tachycardia, cardiorespiratory arrest, incoherence, agitation, mental confusion, shock.

PATIENT CARE CONSIDERATIONS
Administration/Storage
- Tablets may be crushed if patient is unable to swallow them whole.
- Do not give greater than 60 mg/day to elderly.
- Do not administer several days before surgery. If possible, discontinue 7 to 14 days before elective surgery.
- Wait 14 days after discontinuing tricyclic antidepressants, other MAO inhibitors, carbamazepine, maprotiline, guanethidine, paroxetine, sertraline cyclobenzaprine or CNS stimulants to administer this medication. Wait 5 wk after discontinuing fluoxetine before starting phenelzine.
- Do not administer unless patient has been on tyramine-free diet for greater than or equal to 2 to 3 days. Continue on this diet for 2 wk after discontinuation of MAOI.
- Store in tightly-closed container and protect from heat and light.

Assessment/Interventions
- Obtain patient history, including drug history and any known allergies. Note CHF, cardiovascular disease, cerebrovascular disease,

hypertension, abnormal liver or renal function, pheochromocytoma, or severe headaches.
- Monitor patient's lying and standing BP before initiating therapy.
- Monitor liver function if jaundice or other signs of liver dysfunction occur, discontinue drug and notify health care provider.
- Obtain baseline CBC and LFTs.
- During initial therapy, monitor BP and pulse.
- Monitor I&O carefully until dosage is stabilized.
- Observe for onset of therapeutic effect (ie, improved mood, improved sleep patterns, socialization) in depressed patients in 7 to 14 days and full response in up to 6 wk.
- Continue to monitor potentially suicidal patients until they demonstrate definite significant, lasting improvement.
- Be alert for evidence of orthostatic hypotension, monitor orthostatic BP and report to health care provider.
- Monitor for signs of hypertensive crisis (eg, high BP, severe headache, palpitations, severe chest pain, sweating, nausea and vomiting, dilated pupils, photophobia). If signs occur, discontinue drug and notify health care provider. Have alpha-adrenergic blocking agent (eg, phentolamine) readily available to lower BP and external cooling mechanisms for hyperpyrexia.
- Monitor blood sugars of patients receiving insulin or other antidiabetic agents; coadministration may enhance hypoglycemic effect.

Patient/Family Education
- Inform patient that it may be 4 wk before improvement in mood is noticed.
- Instruct patient that antidepressant medications will not make him or her high or elevate mood; antidepressants restore depressed people to normal state.
- Instruct patient to avoid sudden position changes to prevent orthostatic hypotension.
- Instruct patient that it is important to consult health care provider before taking any medication and that it is especially important to avoid OTC cold, hay fever, or weight reduction preparations.
- Instruct patient to avoid tyramine- or tryptophan-containing foods while taking drug and for 2 wk after discontinuing medication. These are protein foods that are aged or fermented and include cheeses, pickled herring, liver, hard sausage (eg, Genoa salami or pepperoni), pods of broad beans, beer, red wine, yeast extract, yogurt, ginseng, soy sauce, bananas, raisins, and avocados. Advise patient to consult dietitian.
- Instruct patient to ingest caffeine and chocolate in moderation.
- Advise patient to weigh self 2 to 3 times/wk and report unusual gains.
- Instruct patient to stop taking phenelzine and to notify health care provider immediately if severe headache, severe chest pain, change in heart rate, photophobia, increased sweating, nausea and vomiting, or stiff or sore neck occurs.
- Advise patient not to use alcohol or any abuse drug.
- Advise patient that drug may cause drowsiness and to use caution while driving or performing other tasks requiring mental alertness.

Phenindamine Tartrate

(fen-IN-dah-meen TAR-trate)
Class Antihistamine
How Supplied
Nolahist Tablets 25 mg
Action
PHARMACOLOGY: Competitively antagonizes histamine at H_1 receptor sites.
PHARMACOKINETICS/DYNAMICS:
Excretion: Eliminated through the kidneys.
Duration: 4 to 6 hr.
Indications Temporary relief of runny nose, sneezing, itching of the nose or throat, and itchy, watery eyes caused by hay fever or other upper respiratory allergic rhinitis.
Contraindications Standard considerations.

Route/Dosage
ADULTS AND CHILDREN (AT LEAST 12 YR): PO 25 mg q 4 to 6 hr (max, 150 mg/24 hr).
CHILDREN (6 TO UNDER 12 YR): PO 12.5 mg q 4 to 6 hr (max, 75 mg/24 hr).

Interactions
Alcohol, sedatives, tranquilizers: Will potentiate the sedative effects of phenindamine.

Lab Test Interferences May interfere with diagnostic test results for skin tests using allergen extracts.

Adverse Reactions
CNS: Excitability (especially in children), drowsiness, nervousness, insomnia.
GI: Dry mouth, constipation.
GU: Urinary retention.

Precautions
Children: Safety and efficacy not established in children under 6 yr.

Special risk patients: Use with caution in patients with hypertension, heart disease, asthma, hyperthyroidism, increased IOP, diabetes mellitus, prostatic hypertrophy, bronchial asthma, difficulty in urination, breathing problems.

PATIENT CARE CONSIDERATIONS
Administration/Storage
- Give prescribed dose q 4 to 6 hr without regard to meals. Give with food if GI upset occurs.
- Store tablets at controlled room temperature (59° to 86°F). Protect from light.

Assessment/Interventions
- Obtain patient history, including drug history and any known allergies. Note history of narrow-angle glaucoma, stenosing peptic ulcer, pyloric obstruction, prostatic hypertrophy, bladder neck obstruction, asthma, chronic bronchitis, emphysema, and concurrent or recent use of MAO inhibitors.
- Assess for allergy symptoms (eg, rhinitis, nasal congestion, sneezing, itching, watery eyes) before and periodically throughout therapy.
- Monitor patient for dizziness and excessive drowsiness. If noted, hold therapy and notify health care provider.
- Monitor patient for CNS, CV, GI, respiratory, and general body side effects. Inform health care provider if noted and significant.

Patient/Family Education
- Explain name, dose, action, and potential side effects of drug.
- Advise patient to take as prescribed without regard to meals, but to take with food if GI upset occurs.
- Advise patient that if allergy symptoms are not controlled not to increase the dose of medication or frequency of use but to inform health care provider. Inform patient that larger or more frequent dosing does not increase effectiveness and may cause drowsiness or other unwanted effects.
- Advise patient that medication may cause drowsiness or dizziness and not to drive or perform other activities requiring mental alertness until tolerance is determined.
- Caution patient that alcohol and other CNS depressants (eg, sedatives) will have additional sedative effects if taken with phenindamine.
- Caution patient not to take any other OTC antihistamines while taking this medication unless advised by health care provider.
- Advise patient to take sips of water, suck on ice chips or sugarless hard candy, or chew sugarless gum if dry mouth occurs.
- If patient is to have allergy skin testing, advise to not take the medication for at least 7 days before the skin testing.
- Advise women to notify health care provider if pregnant, planning to become pregnant, or breastfeeding.
- Instruct patient to stop taking drug and immediately report any of the following symptoms to health care provider: dizziness, excessive drowsiness.
- Caution patient not to take any prescription or OTC medications or dietary supplements unless advised by health care provider.

Phenobarbital

(fee-no-BAR-bih-tahl)

Class Sedative and hypnotic/Barbiturate/Anticonvulsant

How Supplied
Phenobarbital
Bellatal Tablets 16.2 mg ◆ Solfoton Tablets 16 mg, Capsules 16 mg

Phenobarbital Sodium
Luminal Sodium Injection 130 mg/mL

Action
PHARMACOLOGY: Depresses sensory cortex, decreases motor activity, alters cerebellar function and produces drowsiness, sedation, and hypnosis.

PHARMACOKINETICS/DYNAMICS:
Absorption: The T_{max} is 8 to 12 hr (oral).

Distribution: Rapidly distributed to all tissues and fluids with high concentrations in the brain, liver, and kidneys. Lipid solubility plays a dominant factor in distribution. Protein binding is 20% to 45%.

Metabolism: Detoxified in liver by microsomal enzyme system.

Excretion: Eliminated in urine (25% to 50% as unchanged), and small amount in the feces. The $t_{½}$ plasma is 53 to 118 hr (adults), 60 to 180 hr (children).

Onset: Onset of action is 30 min.

Duration: Duration is 5 to 6 hr (oral).

Indications Short-term treatment of insomnia; long-term treatment of generalized tonic-clonic and cortical focal seizures; emergency control of acute convulsions; preanesthetic sedation. **Unlabeled use(s):** Treatment of febrile seizures in children; treatment and prevention of hyperbilirubinemia in newborns; management of chronic cholestasis.

Contraindications Hypersensitivity to barbiturates; history of addiction to sedative/hypnotic drugs; history of porphyria; severe liver impairment; respiratory disease with dyspnea; nephritic patients.

Route/Dosage

Insomnia
ADULTS: **PO/IM/IV** 100 to 320 mg.

Sedation
ADULTS: **PO** 30 to 120 mg/day in 2 to 3 divided doses.

Epilepsy
ADULTS: **PO** 60 to 250 mg/day.

Convulsions
ADULTS: **IV** 100 to 320 mg. Repeat if needed (max, 600 mg/24 hr).

Status Epilepticus
ADULTS: **IV** 10 to 20 mg/kg. Repeat if needed.
CHILDREN: **IV** 15 to 20 mg/kg over 10 to 15 min.

Preoperative Sedation
CHILDREN: **PO/IM/IV** 1 to 3 mg/kg.

Anticonvulsant
CHILDREN: **IM/IV** 4 to 6 mg/kg/day. For 10 days, then adjust to blood level. Alternatively, use **IM/IV** 10 to 15 mg/kg/day to reach therapeutic level more quickly. Max **IV** rate 60 mg/min. Max adult **IM** dose is 500 mg or 5 mL volume regardless of concentration.

Interactions

Alcohol, CNS depressants: May enhance CNS depressant effects.
Anticoagulants (eg, warfarin), beta-blockers (eg, metoprolol, propranolol), doxycycline, metronidazole, quinidine, theophyllines, verapamil: Activity of these drugs may be reduced.
Anticonvulsants: Serum concentrations of carbamazepine, valproic acid and succinimides may be reduced. Valproic acid may increase barbiturate serum levels.
Corticosteroids: May reduce effectiveness of corticosteroids.
Estrogens, estrogen-containing oral contraceptives: May reduce contraceptive effectiveness.
Phenytoin: May increase phenobarbital levels while phenytoin levels may increase or decrease.

Lab Test Interferences May cause decreased serum bilirubin concentrations; false-positive phentolamine test results; decreased response to metyrapone; impaired absorption of radioactive cyanocobalamin.

Adverse Reactions

CV: Bradycardia; hypotension; syncope.
CNS: Drowsiness; agitation; confusion; anxiety; headache; hyperkinesia; ataxia; CNS depression; paradoxical excitement; nightmares; psychiatric disturbances; hallucinations; insomnia; dizziness.
GI: Nausea; vomiting; constipation.
HEMA: Blood dyscrasias (eg, agranulocytosis, thrombocytopenia).
HEPA: Liver damage.
RESP: Hypoventilation; apnea; laryngospasm; bronchospasm.
OTHER: Hypersensitivity reactions (eg, angioedema, rashes, exfoliative dermatitis); fever; injection site reactions (eg, local pain, thrombophlebitis).

Precautions

Pregnancy: Category D.
Lactation: Excreted in breast milk.
Children: May respond with excitement rather than depression.
Elderly: More sensitive to drug effects; dosage reduction is required.
Renal function impairment: Use drug with caution; dosage reduction may be required.
Hepatic function impairment: Use drug with caution; dosage reduction may be required.
Abuse: Administer drug with caution to patients with history of drug abuse.
Debilitated patients: Use drug with extreme caution.
Dependence: Tolerance or psychologic and physical dependence may occur with continued use.
Seizure disorders: Status epilepticus may result from abrupt discontinuation.

Overdosage: Signs and Symptoms

CNS and respiratory depression, Cheyne-Stokes respiration, areflexia, constriction of pupils, oliguria, tachycardia, hypotension, lowered body temperature, coma, shock syndrome, pneumonia, pulmonary edema, cardiac arrhythmias, CHF, renal failure.

PATIENT CARE CONSIDERATIONS

Administration/Storage

- For oral administration, tablets may be crushed and mixed with fluid or food.
- For IM administration, inject deeply into large muscle. Do not exceed max IM dose of 500 mg or 5 mL of volume (regardless of concentration).
- For IV administration, inject into large vein. Do not exceed max IV rate of 60 mg/min; respiratory depression, apnea and hypotension may result.
- Do not base IV administration on response as there may be greater than 15-min delay in peak concentrations in brain.

- Avoid inadvertent intra-arterial injection; arterial spasm, thrombosis, and gangrene may result.
- Do not use as sleeping aid for greater than 2 wk.
- Store at room temperature. Protect from light.

Assessment/Interventions
- Obtain patient history, including drug history and any known allergies. Evaluate for history of substance abuse, liver disease, respiratory disease and porphyria.
- Monitor vital signs of patient undergoing IV administration at least every hour if indicated. Keep resuscitation equipment and drugs readily available.
- After IM administration (1 g dose), observe patient closely for greater than 30 min to ensure that necrosis is not excessive.
- Observe for common side effects such as sedation and dizziness and, if excessive, report to health care provider. Institute safety precautions for elderly patients to prevent accidental falls.
- In children, monitor for possible paradoxical response of increased agitation and notify health care provider.
- Be alert for evidence of barbiturate intoxication (eg, unsteady gait, slurred speech, confusion, irritability) and report to health care provider.
- Watch for behavior indicative of drug dependence such as inordinate requests for more medication or need to refill prescription early.
- With prolonged therapy monitor lab tests for liver, renal, and hematopoietic functions.

Patient/Family Education
- Advise patient to increase intake of vitamin D-fortified foods (eg, milk products) while taking this medication.
- Explain the following importances of maintaining adequate intake of folic acid: fresh vegetables, fruits, whole grains, liver.
- Instruct patient to report the following symptoms to health care provider: nausea, vomiting, drowsiness, dizziness, fever, sore throat, mouth sores or easy bleeding or bruising.
- Caution patient to avoid intake of alcoholic beverages or other CNS depressants.
- Warn patient that medication may be habit forming, and for that reason, it is important to take medicine as directed.
- Advise patient that drug may cause drowsiness, and to use caution while driving or performing other tasks requiring mental alertness.
- Instruct patient not to stop taking medication abruptly without consulting health care provider.

Phenoxybenzamine Hydrochloride

(fen-ox-ee-BEN-zuh-meen HIGH-droe-KLOR-ide)

Class Antihypertensive/Agent for pheochromocytoma

How Supplied
Dibenzyline Capsules 10 mg

Action
PHARMACOLOGY: Irreversibly blocks alpha-adrenergic receptors.

PHARMACOKINETICS/DYNAMICS:
Absorption: 20% to 30% of an oral dose is absorbed in the active form.

Metabolism: Phenoxybenzamine hydrochloride metabolism is hepatic.

Excretion: Phenoxybenzamine hydrochloride excretion is renal and biliary. The t½ is approximately 24 hr (IV); oral is unknown.

Duration: 3 to 4 days (IV).

Indications Control of episodes of hypertension and sweating in patients with pheochromocytoma. **Unlabeled use(s):** Treatment of micturition disorders resulting from neurogenic bladder; treatment of functional outlet obstruction and partial prostatic obstruction.

Contraindications Conditions in which fall in BP may be undesirable.

Route/Dosage
ADULTS: PO 10 mg bid initially. Usual dosage range is 20 to 40 mg bid to tid.
CHILDREN: PO 1 to 2 mg/kg/day in 3 to 4 divided doses.

Interactions
Epinephrine: Exaggerated hypotensive response and tachycardia may occur when epinephrine, or other agents that stimulate both alpha- and beta-receptors, are given concomitantly with phenoxybenzamine.

Lab Test Interferences None well documented.

Adverse Reactions
CV: Orthostatic hypotension; tachycardia.
CNS: Drowsiness; fatigue.
EENT: Miosis.
GI: Gastrointestinal irritation.

GU: Inhibition of ejaculation.
RESP: Nasal congestion.

Precautions
Pregnancy: Safety not established.
Lactation: Undetermined.
Special risk patients: Administer drug with caution to patients with marked cerebral or coronary arteriosclerosis or renal damage. Adrenergic blocking effects may aggravate respiratory infections.

Overdosage: Signs and Symptoms
Orthostatic hypotension, dizziness, fainting, tachycardia, vomiting, lethargy, shock.

PATIENT CARE CONSIDERATIONS

Administration/Storage
- Give drug with milk or in divided doses to reduce GI irritation.
- Store in airtight container and protect from light.

Assessment/Interventions
- Obtain patient history, including drug history and any known allergies.
- Instruct patient to change position slowly, especially from lying to sitting up or standing, and to dangle and move legs before standing.
- Assess for the following adverse reactions: orthostatic hypotension, tachycardia, nasal congestion.
- Assess for effectiveness (lowering of BP) periodically.
- Take safety precautions if patient develops lightheadedness.
- If shocklike state develops, place patient in Trendelenburg position. Notify health care provider and begin emergency interventions.
- During dosage adjustments, monitor BP and pulse (eg, quality, rate, rhythm) with patient in lying and standing position for 4 days.
- In patients with peripheral vasospastic problems, observe for improvement in skin color, temperature, and quality of peripheral pulses.

Patient/Family Education
- Advise patient to avoid alcoholic beverages.
- Stress to patient importance of weight reduction, sodium and alcohol restriction, discontinuation of smoking, regular exercise, and behavior modification.
- Instruct patient to avoid OTC cough, cold, or allergy medications containing sympathomimetics without consulting health care provider.
- Instruct patient to avoid sudden position changes to prevent orthostatic hypotension. Warn patient that taking a hot bath or shower may aggravate dizziness.
- Inform patient that drug may cause nasal congestion and constricted pupils.
- Advise patient that inhibition of ejaculation may occur, but reassure patient that this condition generally decreases with continued therapy.
- Advise patient that drug may cause drowsiness, and to use caution while driving or performing other tasks requiring mental alertness.

Phentermine Hydrochloride

(FEN-ter-meen)

Class CNS stimulant/Anorexiant

How Supplied
Phentermine Hydrochloride Tablets 8 mg (equiv. to 6.4 mg base), Tablets 30 mg (equiv. to 24 mg base), Tablets 37.5 mg (equiv. to 30 mg base), Capsules 15 mg (equiv. to 12 mg base), Capsules 18.75 mg (equiv. to 15 mg base), Capsules 37.5 mg (equiv. to 30 mg base) ◆ *Ionamin* Capsules 15 mg phentermine resin, Capsules 15 mg (as resin complex), Capsules 30 mg (as resin complex) ◆ *Adipex-P* Tablets 37.5 mg (equiv. to 30 mg base), Capsules 37.5 mg (equiv. to 30 mg base) ◆ *Obe-Nix 30* Capsules 37.5 mg (equiv. to 30 mg base) ◆ *Phentermine Resin* Capsules 15 mg (as resin complex), Capsules 30 mg (as resin complex)

Action
PHARMACOLOGY: May stimulate satiety center in brain, causing appetite suppression.

PHARMACOKINETICS/DYNAMICS:
Metabolism: Phentermine hydrochloride metabolism is hepatic; it is not significantly biotransformed.

Excretion: Phentermine hydrochloride excretion is primarily renal (70% to 80% excreted unchanged); excretion is increased by acidifying the urine. The t½ is 19 to 24 hr.

Indications Short-term (few weeks) adjunct to diet plan to reduce weight.

Contraindications Hypersensitivity to sympathomimetic amines; advanced arteriosclerosis; symptomatic cardiovascular disease; moderate to severe hypertension; hyperthyroidism; glaucoma; agitated states; history of drug abuse; during or within 14 days following the administration of an MAOI.

Route/Dosage
8 Mg Dose
ADULTS AND CHILDREN (GREATER THAN OR EQUAL TO 12 YR): **PO** 8 mg up to 3 times daily ½ hr before meals.

15 to 37.5 Mg Dose
ADULTS AND CHILDREN (GREATER THAN 16 YR): **PO** 15 to 37.5 mg as a single dose before breakfast or 2 hr after breakfast.

Interactions
Guanethidine: May decrease hypotensive effect of guanethidine.
MAOIs (eg, phenelzine); furazolidone: May cause hypertensive crisis and intracranial hemorrhage.
Selective serotonin reuptake inhibitors (eg, fluoxetine): Sympathomimetic effects of phentermine and risk of "serotonin syndrome" may be increased.

Lab Test Interferences
None well documented.

Adverse Reactions
CV: Regurgitant cardiac valvular disease; palpitation; tachycardia; hypertension.
CNS: Overstimulation; restlessness; dizziness; insomnia; euphoria; dysphoria; tremor; headache; psychotic episodes.
DERM: Allergic urticaria.
GI: Dry mouth; unpleasant taste; diarrhea; constipation.
GU: Impotence; changes in libido.
RESP: Primary pulmonary hypertension.

Precautions
Pregnancy: Category C.
Lactation: Undetermined.
Children:
8 mg dose – Safety and efficacy not established in children less than 12 yr.
16 mg dose – Safety and efficacy not established in children 16 yr or less.
Special risk patients: Use with caution in patients with glaucoma, hypertension, and diabetes mellitus.
Drug dependence: Psychological and physical dependence may occur with continued use; this class of drugs has been extensively abused.
Tolerance: Tolerance to the anorectic effect usually develops within a few weeks.
Primary pulmonary hypertension: Has been reported with concurrent use of phentermine and fenfluramine or dexfenfluramine.
Valvular heart disease: Serious regurgitant cardiac valvular disease has been reported with concurrent use of phentermine and fenfluramine or dexfenfluramine.

Overdosage: Signs and Symptoms
Restlessness, tremor, hyperreflexia, rapid respiration, confusion, assaultiveness, hallucinations, panic states, fatigue, depression, arrhythmias, hypertension, hypotension, circulatory collapse, nausea, vomiting, diarrhea, abdominal cramps, convulsions, coma, death.

PATIENT CARE CONSIDERATIONS
Administration/Storage
- Discontinue MAOIs greater than or equal to 14 days before initiating therapy.
- Administer 8 mg dose up to 3 times daily as prescribed, ½ hour before meals. Administer last dose several hours before bedtime.
- Administer 15 to 37.5 mg doses as a single daily dose before, or 2 hr after breakfast. Medication is slowly released over 10 to 14 hr. Swallow whole. Do not crush or chew 15 to 37.5 mg strength tablets or capsules.
- Store at controlled room temperature (59° to 86°F).

Assessment/Interventions
- Obtain patient history, including drug history and any known allergies. Note history of advanced coronary artery disease, moderate to severe hypertension, hyperthyroidism, sensitivity to sympathomimetic amines, glaucoma, agitation, history of drug abuse or concurrent or recent MAOI therapy.
- Ensure that patient receives dietary instructions regarding caloric restriction.
- Determine baseline weight. Weigh periodically to monitor response to therapy.
- Monitor blood sugar in patients with diabetes more frequently when drug is started or dose is changed.
- Monitor patient for CNS, RESP, CV, GI, and general body side effects.

Patient/Family Education
- Explain name, dose, action, and potential side effects of drug.
- Advise patient using 8 mg dose to take up to 3 times daily as prescribed, ½ hour before meals, and to take last dose several hours before bedtime.
- Advise patient using 15 to 37.5 mg dose as a single daily dose before, or 2 hr after, breakfast. Advise patient to swallow tablet or capsule whole and to not crush or chew the tablet or capsule.
- Encourage patient to follow medically supervised weight reduction program. Emphasize that this medication will only work in conjunction with a caloric-restricted diet and exercise program.
- Advise patient that medication should be taken as prescribed and to not stop taking or change the dose unless advised to do so by health care provider.

- Explain that appetite suppressant effects are temporary and tolerance to medication and dependence can occur. Caution patient not to increase the dose in an effort to overcome the tolerance when it occurs.
- Remind patients with diabetes to monitor blood sugar more frequently while implementing dietary restrictions and to notify health care provider if significant changes in blood sugar occur.
- Caution patient that drug may impair the ability to drive or perform other tasks requiring mental alertness.
- Advise patient to notify health care provider immediately if the following symptoms occur: decreased exercise tolerance, dyspnea, swelling of the feet or ankles, fainting, chest pain, palpitations, nervousness, or dizziness.
- Advise patient to notify health care provider if experiencing any unusual or unexplained symptoms.
- Advise women to inform health care provider if they become pregnant, plan on becoming pregnant, or are breastfeeding.
- Warn patient not to take any prescription or OTC drugs or dietary supplements without consulting health care provider.
- Advise patient that follow-up visits may be necessary to monitor therapy and to be sure to keep appointments.

Phentolamine

(fen-TOLE-uh-meen)

Class Antihypertensive/Agent for pheochromocytoma

How Supplied
Phentolamine Mesylate Powder for Injection 5 mg (as mesylate)/vial
✤ *Rogitine*

Action
PHARMACOLOGY: Decreases total peripheral resistance and venous return to heart by competitive blockade of presynaptic and postsynaptic alpha-adrenergic receptors.

PHARMACOKINETICS/DYNAMICS:
Absorption: Not determined.
Distribution: Not determined.
Metabolism: Not determined.
Excretion: Urine (13% as unchanged drug). $T_{1/2}$ is 19 min (IV).

Indications Prevention or control of hypertensive episodes in patients with pheochromocytoma; pharmacologic test for pheochromocytoma (not method of choice); prevention and treatment of dermal necrosis and sloughing following IV administration or extravasation of norepinephrine or dopamine. **Unlabeled use(s):** Control of hypertensive crises secondary to MAO inhibitor-sympathomimetic amine interactions or withdrawal of clonidine, propranolol or other antihypertensives; in conjunction with papaverine as intracavernous injection for impotence.

Contraindications Hypersensitivity to phentolamine or related compounds; MI, coronary insufficiency, angina, or other evidence suggestive of coronary artery disease.

Route/Dosage
Hypertensive Episodes in Pheochromocytoma
ADULTS: IM/IV 5 mg 1 to 2 hr before surgery. Repeat if necessary. During surgery, IV 5 mg as indicated.
CHILDREN: IM/IV 1 mg 1 to 2 hr before surgery. During surgery, IV 1 mg as indicated.

Prevention of Dermal Necrosis and Sloughing
ADULTS: IV Add 10 mg/1 L of solution containing norepinephrine.

Treatment of Dermal Necrosis or Sloughing After Norepinephrine Extravasation
ADULTS: 5 to 10 mg in 10 mL saline solution in area of extravasation within 12 hr.
CHILDREN: Infiltrate area 0.1 to 0.2 mg/kg (max, 10 mg).

Diagnosis of Pheochromocytoma
ADULTS: IM/IV 2.5 to 5 mg.
CHILDREN: IV 1 mg or IM 3 mg.

Interactions
Epinephrine, ephedrine: Vasoconstrictive and hypertensive effects of epinephrine and ephedrine are antagonized by phentolamine.

Lab Test Interferences None well documented.

Adverse Reactions
CV: Acute and prolonged hypotensive episodes; tachycardia; cardiac arrhythmias; orthostatic hypotension.
CNS: Weakness; dizziness.
EENT: Nasal stuffiness.
GI: Nausea; vomiting; diarrhea.
OTHER: Flushing.

Precautions
Pregnancy: Category C.
Lactation: Undetermined.
Cardiovascular effects: Marked hypotensive episodes and shocklike states may follow use of phentolamine and lead to MI, cerebrovascular spasm, or cerebrovascular occlusion.
Screening tests: Urinary assays of catecholamines or other biochemical assays have largely supplanted phentolamine and other pharmacologic

tests for pheochromocytoma. Phentolamine is usually used as confirmation. Follow specific guidelines for use of phentolamine.

PATIENT CARE CONSIDERATIONS

Administration/Storage
- Have patient remain supine during IV therapy.
- Dilute 5 mg in 1 mL Sterile Water for Injection. May dilute further with 5 to 10 mL Sterile Water for Injection.
- Use reconstituted solution immediately; do not store.
- Store unopened vial in light-resistant container at room temperature.
- When using phentolamine for managing hypertensive crisis or as a diagnostic test, inject drug by rapid IV bolus.

Assessment/Interventions
- Obtain patient history, including drug history and any known allergies.
- Obtain baseline lying and standing BP and pulse before starting therapy.
- Assess IV site for infiltration.

Overdosage: Signs and Symptoms
Severe hypotension, shock, tachycardia, flushing.

- Monitor BP q 2 min when beginning IV therapy until BP is stable.
- Notify health care provider immediately if symptoms of severe hypotension or shock develop.
- If chest pain develops during infusion, notify health care provider.
- If patient develops dizziness, take safety precautions (eg, bed in low position, supervise ambulation).

Patient/Family Education
- Instruct patient to avoid sudden position changes to prevent orthostatic hypotension.
- Instruct patient to notify health care provider if chest pain develops during infusion.
- Tell patient to report the following symptoms to health care provider: dizziness, fainting spells or weakness.

Phenylephrine Hydrochloride

(fen-ill-EFF-rin HIGH-droe-KLOR-ide)

Class Vasopressor/Decongestant

How Supplied
AH-chew D Tablets, chewable 10 mg ♦ AK-Dilate Solution 2.5%, Solution 10% ♦ Alconefrin Solution 0.5% ♦ Alconefrin 12 Solution 0.16% ♦ Alconefrin 25 Solution 0.25% ♦ Children's Nostril Solution 0.25% ♦ Mydfrin 2.5% Solution 2.5% ♦ Neo-Synephrine Solution 0.125%, Solution 0.25%, Solution 0.5%, Solution 1%, Solution 2.5%, Solution 10%, Injection 1% (10 mg/mL) ♦ Nostril Solution 0.5% ♦ Phenoptic Solution 2.5% ♦ Prefrin Liquifilm Solution 0.12% ♦ Relief Solution 0.12% ♦ Rhinall Solution 0.25% ♦ Sinex Solution 0.5%
✤ Minims Phenylephrine ♦ Novahistine Decongestant

Action
PHARMACOLOGY: Stimulates postsynaptic alpha-receptors, resulting in rise in intense arterial peripheral vasoconstriction. Causes marked increase in systolic, diastolic and pulmonary pressures as well as reflex bradycardia. Slightly decreases cardiac output and increases coronary blood flow.

PHARMACOKINETICS/DYNAMICS:
Absorption: Unknown.
Distribution: Unknown.
Metabolism: In liver and GI.
Excretion: Unknown.
Onset: Rapid (IV).
Duration: 20 min (IV); 50 min (SC).

Indications Treatment of vascular failure in shock, shock-like states, drug-induced hypotension or hypersensitivity; correction of paroxysmal supraventricular tachycardia; prolongation of spinal anesthesia; vasoconstriction in regional analgesia; maintenance of adequate level of BP during spinal and inhalation anesthesia; temporary relief of nasal congestion and of minor eye irritations; pupil dilation in uveitis; treatment of open-angle glaucoma; use in diagnostic procedures (funduscopy) and before surgery.

Contraindications Severe hypertension; ventricular tachycardia; pheochromocytoma; 10% ophthalmic solution contraindicated in infants and patients with aneurysms.

Route/Dosage

Mild or Moderate Hypotension
ADULTS: **SC/IM** 1 to 10 mg (usually 2 to 5 mg); do not exceed initial dose of 5 mg. **IV** 0.1 to 0.5 mg (usually 0.2 mg); do not exceed initial dose of 0.5 mg. Avoid repeat injections more often than q 10 to 15 min.

Severe Hypotension and Shock
ADULTS: **IV continuous infusion** For initial dose, give 100 to 180 mcg/min in of 1:25,000 or 1:50,000 solution (10 mg/250 to 500 mL D5W or Sodium Chloride); once BP has stabilized to low normal level, decrease to maintenance rate of 40 to 60 mcg/min. If prompt initial vasopres-

sor response is not obtained, increase dosage in increments greater than or equal to 10 mg and add to infusion; adjust rate until desired BP is obtained.

Hypotension of Spinal Anesthesia
ADULTS: SC/IM 2 to 3 mg 3 to 4 min before injection of anesthetic. For hypotensive emergencies during spinal anesthesia, inject 0.2 mg, increasing by no more than 0.1 to 0.2 mg/dose (max, 0.5 mg/dose).
CHILDREN: SC/IM 0.5 to 1 mg/25 lb (55 kg).

Prolongation of Spinal Anesthesia
ADULTS: 2 to 5 mg added to anesthetic solution increases duration of motor block by up to 50%.

Vasoconstriction for Regional Analgesia
ADULTS: At least 2 mg added to local anesthetic solution in concentration of 1:20,000 (1 mg/20 mL).

Paroxysmal Supraventricular Tachycardia
ADULTS: IV
Initial dose: 0.5 mg or less via rapid IV push (within 20 to 30 sec); subsequent doses should not exceed preceding dose by more than 0.1 to 0.2 mg (max, 1 mg/dose).

Nasal Congestion
ADULTS AND CHILDREN AT LEAST 12 YR: **Intranasal** 1 to 2 sprays or 3 gtt of 0.25%, 0.5% or 1% solution q 4 hr.
CHILDREN 6 TO 12 YR: **Intranasal** 2 to 3 sprays of 0.25% solution in each nostril q 3 to 4 hr.
CHILDREN 6 MO TO 6 YR: **Intranasal** 1 to 2 gtt of 0.16% solution in each nostril q 3 hr.

Vasoconstriction/Pupil Dilation
ADULTS: **Ophthalmic** Instill 1 gtt 2.5% or 10% on upper limbus. If necessary, repeat after 1 hr.

Uveitis/Prevention of Synechiae
ADULTS: **Ophthalmic** Instill 2.5% or 10% phenylephrine plus atropine.

To Free Recently Formed Posterior Synechiae
ADULTS: **Ophthalmic** Instill 1 gtt of 2.5% or 10% to upper surface of cornea.

Wide-Angle Glaucoma
ADULTS: **Ophthalmic** Instill 1 gtt of 10% on upper surface of cornea prn.

Open-Angle Glaucoma
ADULTS: **Ophthalmic** Instill 2.5% or 10% solution in conjunction with miotics.

Surgery
ADULTS: **Ophthalmic** Instill 2.5% or 10% solution 30 to 60 min before operation as short-acting mydriatic.

Refraction
ADULTS: **Ophthalmic** Instill 1 gtt 2.5% solution.
CHILDREN: **Ophthalmic** Instill 1 gtt 2.5% solution.

Ophthalmoscopic Examination
ADULTS: **Ophthalmic** Instill 1 gtt 2.5% solution in each eye.

Diagnostic Procedures/Provocative Test for Angle-block in Glaucoma
ADULTS: **Ophthalmic** Instill 2.5%.

Retinoscopy
ADULTS: **Ophthalmic** Instill 2.5% solution.

Blanching Test
ADULTS: **Ophthalmic** Instill 1 to 2 gtt of 2.5% solution.

Minor Eye Irritations
ADULTS: **Ophthalmic** Instill 1 to 2 gtt of 0.12% solution up to qid.

Interactions
Beta-blockers: Decrease phenylephrine's effect.
General anesthetics: Arrhythmias.
Guanethidine: May increase pressor response of phenylephrine; resulting in severe hypertension.
Halogenated hydrocarbon anesthetics: May sensitize myocardium to effects of catecholamines. Use extreme caution to avoid arrhythmias.
MAO inhibitors, furazolidone: May significantly increase pressor response resulting in hypertensive crisis and intracranial hemorrhage.
Oxytocic drugs: May cause severe persistent hypertension.
Tricyclic antidepressants: May decrease or increase response; use with caution.

Lab Test Interferences None well documented.

Adverse Reactions
CV: Reflex bradycardia; hypertension; angina; arrhythmias.
CNS: Headache; excitability; restlessness; tremor.
EENT: With ophthalmic and intranasal forms: Transitory stinging on initial instillation; blurring of vision; rebound congestion.

Precautions
Pregnancy: Category C.
Lactation: Undetermined.
Children: Ophthalmic use of phenylephrine 10% is contraindicated in infants.
Special risk patients: Administer drug with caution to patients with hyperthyroidism, bradycardia, partial heart block, myocardial disease, prostatic hypertrophy, diabetes mellitus, increased IOP or severe arteriosclerosis.
Sulfite sensitivity: Use drug with caution in sulfite-sensitive individuals; some commercial preparations contain sodium bisulfite.
Corneal effects: If corneal epithelium has been denuded or damaged, corneal clouding may occur if phenylephrine 10% is instilled.
Hypovolemia: Avoid use in uncorrected hypovolemic states unless used as temporary emergency

measure to maintain coronary and cerebral flow and in patients with tachyarrhythmias or ventricular fibrillation.

Narrow-angle glaucoma: Ordinarily any mydriatic is contraindicated in patients with glaucoma. However, when temporary dilation of pupil may free adhesions or when vasoconstriction of intrinsic vessels may lower intraocular tension, these advantages may temporarily outweigh danger from coincident dilation of pupil.

PATIENT CARE CONSIDERATIONS
Administration/Storage
- For vasopressor use, administer medication via continuous pump infusion. Administer IV through large vein, preferably central vein. Titrate carefully to avoid hypotension.
- With intranasal administration, do not share container. Instill spray into nose with head upright. Have patient sniff hard for a few minutes after administration. To instill drops, have patient recline on bed, hang head over edge and instill drops. Have patient remain in this position for several minutes after using and turn head from side to side. Do not allow tip of container to touch nasal passage. Discard after medication is no longer needed.
- To instill ophthalmic solution, tilt patient's head back, hold dropper over eye, drop medication inside lower lid, apply pressure to inside corner of eye for 1 min. Take care not to touch dropper to eye.
- Prolonged exposure of ophthalmic solution to air or strong light may cause oxidation and discoloration. Do not use if solution is discolored or cloudy or contains precipitate.
- Store parenteral and nasal solution at room temperature and protect from light.

Assessment/Interventions
- Obtain patient history, including drug history and any known allergies. Note history of cardiovascular disease such as hypertension and assess for MAO inhibitor use.
- For ocular or ophthalmic use, assess for intraocular lens implants due to possibility of dislodging lens. Also assess for history of damaged corneal epithelium.
- Check BP and pulse frequently.

Rebound congestion: May occur with extended use of intranasal or ophthalmic forms.

Overdosage: Signs and Symptoms
Severe hypertension, vomiting, ventricular extrasystoles, short paroxysms of ventricular tachycardia, sensation of fullness in head, tingling of extremities, somnolence, sedation, coma, profuse sweating, hypotension, shock.

- Monitor hemodynamic function.
- Observe IV site for extravasation and infiltration.

Patient/Family Education
Intranasal:
- Advise patient that intranasal form is for short-term use only and should not be used for more than 3 to 5 days.
- Inform patient that stinging, burning, or drying of the nose or an increase in nasal discharge may occur with intranasal form.
- Instruct patient to gradually stop taking intranasal form of this medicine rather than abruptly discontinuing it because rebound congestion can occur with sudden withdrawal. First stop using drug in one nostril and then in both nostrils.

Ophthalmic:
- Caution patient that ophthalmic form of drug can cause discoloration of contact lenses and advise patient to wear glasses during therapy.
- Instruct patient not to use ophthalmic form for greater than 72 hr without consulting health care provider.
- Advise patient to discontinue drug and notify health care provider if severe eye pain, headache, vision changes, floating spots, acute eye redness, pain with light exposure, insomnia, dizziness, weakness, tremor, or irregular heartbeat occurs.
- Advise patient that drug may cause temporary blurred or unstable vision and to use caution while driving or performing other tasks requiring mental alertness.

Phenylephrine Tannate/Chlorpheniramine Tannate

(Fen-ill-EFF-rin TAN-ate/klor-fen-AIR-uh-meen TAN-ate)

Class Vasopressor/Decongestant/Antihistamine

How Supplied
Rhinatate-NF Pediatric Suspension 5 mg phenylephrine tannate and 4.5 mg chlorpheniramine tannate ♦ *Nuhist* Suspension 5 mg phenylephrine tannate and 4.5 mg chlorpheniramine tannate ♦ *R-Tanna S* Pediatric Suspension 5 mg phenylephrine tannate and 4.5 mg chlorpheniramine tannate ♦ *Rynatan* Pediatric Suspension 5 mg phenylephrine tannate and 4.5 mg chlorpheniramine tannate

Action
PHARMACOLOGY:
Phenylephrine: Stimulates postsynaptic alpha-receptors, resulting in vasoconstriction, which reduces nasal congestion.
Chlorpheniramine: Competitively antagonizes histamine at H_1 receptor sites.

Indications Symptomatic relief of coryza and nasal congestion associated with common cold, sinusitis, allergic rhinitis, and other upper respiratory tract conditions.

Contraindications Newborns; nursing mothers; sensitivity to any component of product.

Route/Dosage
CHILDREN (OVER 6 YR): **PO** 5 to 10 mL (1 to 2 tsp) q 12 hr.
CHILDREN (2 TO 6 YR): **PO** 2.5 to 5 mL (½ to 1 tsp) q 12 hr.
CHILDREN (LESS THAN 2 YR): **PO** Titrate dose individually.

Interactions
MAO Inhibitors (eg, isocarboxazid): Avoid or use with caution in patients receiving MAO inhibitor therapy or within 14 days of stopping such treatment. May prolong and intensify the effects of chlorpheniramine and phenylephrine.

Lab Test Interferences May interfere with diagnostic test results for skin tests using allergen extracts.

Adverse Reactions
CNS: Drowsiness; sedation.
GI: GI effects.
OTHER: Dryness of mucous membranes.

Precautions
Pregnancy: Category C.
Lactation: Do not administer.
Elderly: Chlorpheniramine is more likely to cause dizziness, sedation, and hypotension in the elderly.
Special risk patients: Use with caution in patients with hypertension, heart disease, hyperthyroidism, narrow angle glaucoma, diabetes mellitus, or prostatic hypertrophy.
Excitation: Chlorpheniramine may cause excitation in pediatric patients; however, in combination with phenylephrine, it may cause mild stimulation or mild sedation.

Overdosage: Signs and Symptoms
CNS depression, CNS stimulation, convulsions, death, atropine-like signs and symptoms may be present.

PATIENT CARE CONSIDERATIONS
Administration/Storage
- Shake well before measuring dose.
- Give prescribed dose of suspension q 12 hr as needed.
- Give with food or milk if GI upset occurs.
- Use dosing spoon or syringe for pediatric doses.
- Store suspension at controlled room temperature (68° to 77°F). Keep tightly capped and protect from freezing.

Assessment/Interventions
- Obtain patient history, including drug history and any known allergies. Note history of peptic ulcer disease, diabetes, hypertension, hyperthyroidism, enlarged prostate, asthma, narrow angle glaucoma, urinary retention, severe hypertension, coronary artery disease, or concurrent use of or within 2 wk of stopping MAO inhibitor therapy.
- Assess for allergy symptoms (eg, rhinitis, nasal congestion, sneezing, itching, watery eyes) before and periodically throughout therapy.
- Monitor pulse and BP periodically during therapy.
- Monitor patient for nervousness, dizziness, and insomnia. If noted, hold therapy and notify health care provider.

Patient/Family Education
- Explain name, dose, action, and potential side effects of drug.
- Remind patient to shake well before measuring dose.
- Advise patient to take prescribed dose q 12 hr as needed.
- Advise caregiver to use dosing spoon or syringe when giving suspension to children.
- Advise patient to take with food or milk if GI upset occurs.
- Advise patient to take last dose late in the afternoon or early evening to reduce chance of drug causing sleeplessness.
- Advise patient that if a dose is missed to take as soon as remembered unless it is nearing time for the next dose. Caution patient to not double the dose to catch up.
- Advise patient that if allergy symptoms are not controlled, not to increase the dose of medication but to inform health care provider.
- Caution patient that drug may cause drowsiness and to use caution while driving or performing other tasks requiring mental alertness until tolerance is determined.

- Advise patient to avoid alcohol and other CNS depressants because of risk of excessive sedation.
- Caution patient not to take any OTC antihistamines or decongestants while taking this medication unless advised by health care provider.
- If patient is to have allergy skin testing, advise against taking the medication for at least 6 days before the skin testing.
- Advise women to notify health care provider if pregnant, planning to become pregnant, or breastfeeding.
- Instruct patient to stop taking drug and immediately report any of the following symptoms to health care provider: nervousness, dizziness, sleeplessness.
- Caution patient not to take any prescription or OTC medications or dietary supplements unless advised by health care provider.

Phenylephrine Tannate/ Chlorpheniramine Tannate/ Pyrilamine Tannate

(Fen-ill-EFF-rin TAN-ate/klor-fen-AIR-uh-meen TAN-ate/pie-RILL-ah-meen TAN-ate)

Class Vasopressor/Decongestant/Antihistamine

How Supplied
Triotann Pediatric Suspension 5 mg phenylephrine, 2 mg chlorpheniramine, 12.5 mg pyrilamine ♦ *Triotann-S Pediatric Suspension* 5 mg phenylephrine, 2 mg chlorpheniramine, 12.5 mg pyrilamine

Action
PHARMACOLOGY:
Phenylephrine: Stimulates postsynaptic alpha-receptors, resulting in vasoconstriction which reduces nasal congestion.
Chlorpheniramine and pyrilamine: Competitively antagonizes histamine at H_1 receptor sites.

Indications Symptomatic relief of coryza and nasal congestion associated with common cold, sinusitis, allergic rhinitis, and other upper respiratory tract conditions.

Contraindications Newborns; nursing mothers; sensitivity to any component of product.

Route/Dosage
CHILDREN OVER 6 YR: **PO** 5 to 10 mL (1 to 2 tsp) q 12 hr.
CHILDREN 2 TO 6 YR: **PO** 2.5 to 5 mL (½ to 1 tsp) q 12 hr.
CHILDREN LESS THAN 2 YR: **PO** Titrate dose individually.

PATIENT CARE CONSIDERATIONS
Administration/Storage
- Shake well before measuring dose.
- Give prescribed dose of suspension q 12 hr as needed.
- Give with food or milk if GI upset occurs.
- Use dosing spoon or syringe for pediatric doses.
- Store suspension at controlled room temperature (59° to 77°F). Keep tightly capped and protect from freezing.

Interactions
MAO Inhibitors (eg, isocarboxazid [certain drugs for depression, psychiatric or emotional condition, Parkinson disease]): Do not use in patients receiving MAO inhibitor therapy or within 14 days of stopping such treatment. May prolong and intensify the effects of chlorpheniramine, pyrilamine, and phenylephrine.

Lab Test Interferences May interfere with diagnostic test results for skin tests using allergen extracts.

Adverse Reactions
CNS: Drowsiness; sedation.
GI: GI effects.
OTHER: Dryness of mucous membranes.

Precautions
Pregnancy: Category C.
Lactation: Do not administer.
Elderly: Chlorpheniramine and pyrilamine are more likely to cause dizziness, sedation, and hypotension in the elderly.
Special risk patients: Use with caution in patients with hypertension, heart disease, hyperthyroidism, narrow angle glaucoma, diabetes mellitus, and prostatic hypertrophy.
Excitation: Chlorpheniramine and pyrilamine may cause excitation in pediatric patients; however, combination with phenylephrine may cause mild stimulation or mild sedation.

Overdosage: Signs and Symptoms
CNS depression, CNS stimulation, convulsions, death.

Assessment/Interventions
- Obtain patient history, including drug history and any known allergies. Note history of peptic ulcer disease, diabetes, hypertension, hyperthyroidism, enlarged prostate, asthma, narrow angle glaucoma, urinary retention, severe hypertension or coronary artery disease, or concurrent use of or within 2 wk of stopping MAO-inhibitor therapy.

- Assess for allergy symptoms (eg, rhinitis, nasal congestion, sneezing, itching, watery eyes) before and periodically throughout therapy.
- Monitor pulse and BP periodically during therapy.
- Monitor patient for nervousness, dizziness, and insomnia. If noted, hold therapy and notify health care provider.

Patient/Family Education
- Explain name, dose, action, and potential side effects of drug.
- Remind patient to shake well before measuring dose.
- Advise patient to take prescribed dose q 12 hr as needed.
- Advise caregiver to use dosing spoon or syringe when giving suspension to children.
- Advise patient to take with food or milk if GI upset occurs.
- Advise patient to take last dose late in the afternoon or early evening to reduce chance of drug causing sleeplessness.
- Advise patient that if a dose is missed to take as soon as remembered unless it is nearing time for the next dose. Caution patient to not double the dose to catch up.
- Advise patient that if allergy symptoms are not controlled, not to increase the dose of medication but to inform health care provider.
- Caution patient that drug may cause drowsiness and to use caution while driving or performing other tasks requiring mental alertness until tolerance is determined.
- Advise patient to avoid alcohol and other CNS depressants due to risk of excessive sedation.
- Caution patient not to take any OTC antihistamines or decongestants while taking this medication unless advised by health care provider.
- If patient is to have allergy skin testing, advise not to take the medication for at least 6 days before the skin testing.
- Advise women to notify health care provider if pregnant, planning to become pregnant, or breastfeeding.
- Instruct patient to stop taking drug and immediately report any of the following symptoms to health care provider: nervousness, dizziness, sleeplessness.
- Caution patient to not take any prescription or OTC medications or dietary supplements unless advised by health care provider.

Phenylephrine Hydrochloride/Guaifenesin

(Fen-ill-EFF-rin HIGH-droe-KLOR-ide /GWHY-fen-ah-sin)

Class Decongestant/Expectorant

How Supplied
Rescon-GG Liquid 5 mg phenylephrine hydrochloride and 100 mg guaifenesin ♦ *Entex* Liquid 7.5 mg phenylephrine hydrochloride and 100 mg guaifenesin ♦ *Guaifed-PD* Capsules 7.5 mg phenylephrine hydrochloride and 200 mg guaifenesin ♦ *Entex ER* Capsules 10 mg phenylephrine hydrochloride and 300 mg guaifenesin ♦ *Guaifed* Capsules 15 mg phenylephrine hydrochloride and 400 mg guaifenesin ♦ *SINUvent PE* Tablets 15 mg phenylephrine hydrochloride and 600 mg guaifenesin ♦ *Endal Nasal Decongestant* Tablets 20 mg phenylephrine hydrochloride and 300 mg guaifenesin ♦ *GFN 600/Phenylephrine 20* Tablets 20 mg phenylephrine hydrochloride and 600 mg guaifenesin ♦ *Liquibid-PD* Tablets 25 mg phenylephrine hydrochloride and 275 mg guaifenesin ♦ *Entex LA* Tablets 30 mg phenylephrine hydrochloride and 600 mg guaifenesin ♦ *Liquidbid-D* Tablets 40 mg phenylephrine hydrochloride and 600 mg guaifenesin ♦ *Liquibid-D 1200* Tablets 40 mg phenylephrine hydrochloride and 1200 mg guaifenesin

Action
PHARMACOLOGY:
Phenylephrine: Stimulates postsynaptic alpha-receptors, resulting in vasoconstriction, which reduces congestion.
Guaifenesin: May enhance output of respiratory tract fluid by reducing adhesiveness and surface tension, enhancing removal of viscous mucus and making nonproductive coughs more productive and less frequent.

Indications Temporary relief of symptoms of upper respiratory tract disorders such as sinusitis, vasomotor rhinitis, and hay fever; temporary relief of coughs associated with respiratory tract infections and related conditions such as sinusitis, pharyngitis, bronchitis, and asthma when tenacious mucus and/or mucus plugs and congestion complicate these conditions.

Contraindications Hypersensitivity to any component of product; hypersensitivity or idiosyncrasy to sympathomimetic amines, which may manifest by insomnia, dizziness, weakness, tremor, or arrhythmias. Phenylephrine is contraindicated in patients with hypertension or ventricular tachycardia and should be employed only with extreme caution in elderly patients or in patients with hyperthyroidism, bradycardia, partial heart block, myocardial disease, or severe arteriosclerosis. Phenylephrine is contraindicated in patents on monoamine oxidase (MAO) inhibitor therapy and for 14 days after stopping MAO therapy (see Interactions section).

Route/Dosage
ADULTS AND CHILDREN (12 YR AND OLDER):
Rescon-GG Liquid: **PO** 10 mL q 4 to 6 hr (up to 40 mL/day).
Entex Liquid: **PO** 5 to 10 mL q 4 to 6 hr (up to 40 mL/day).
Guaifed-PD Capsules: **PO** 1 to 2 q 12 hr.
Entex ER Capsules: **PO** 1 or 2 q 12 hr.
Guaifed Capsules: **PO** 1 q 12 hr.
SINUvent PE Tablets: **PO** 2 q 12 hr.
Endal Nasal Decongestant Tablets: **PO** 2 q 12 hr.
GFN 600/Phenylephrine 20 Tablets: **PO** 1 or 2 q 12 hr (up to 2/day).
Liquibid-PD Tablets: **PO** 1 or 2 q 12 hr (up to 4/day).
Liquibid-D Tablets: **PO** 1 q 12 hr.
Liquibid-D 1200 Tablets: **PO** 1 q 12 hr.
CHILDREN (6 TO 12 YR): **PO** ½ tablet q 12 hr (max, 1 tablets in 24 hr).

Interactions
Beta-adrenergic blockers, MAO inhibitors: May potentiate the pressor effect of phenylephrine.
Digitalis glycosides, other vasopressor drugs during halothane anesthesia: The risk of cardiac arrhythmias may be increased.
Guanethidine, mecamylamine, methyldopa, reserpine, veratrum alkaloids: Hypotensive effects of these agents may be reduced.
Tricyclic antidepressants: Effects of phenylephrine may be decreased.

Lab Test Interferences Guaifenesin may interfere with the interpretation of the test for urinary 5-hydroxyindoleacetic acid for the diagnosis of carcinoid syndrome; VMA test for catecholamines may be falsely elevated; guaifenesin may increase renal clearance for urate and thereby lower serum uric acid levels.

Adverse Reactions
CV: Tachycardia; palpitations; arrhythmias; cardiovascular collapse with hypotension.
CNS: Headache; dizziness; fear; anxiety; nervousness; restlessness; tremor; weakness; insomnia; hallucinations; convulsions; CNS depression.
GI: Nausea.
GU: Dysuria.
RESP: Respiratory difficulty.
OTHER: Pallor.

Precautions
Pregnancy: Category C.
Lactation: Small amounts of phenylephrine excreted in breast milk.
Children: Not recommended for use in children under 6 yr.
Elderly: Patients 60 yr or older are more likely to experience adverse sympathomimetic effects.
Special risk patients: Use with caution in patients with hypertension, heart disease, asthma, hyperthyroidism, increased intraocular pressure, diabetes mellitus, prostatic hypertrophy.
Drug abuse: Has abuse potential.

Overdosage: Signs and Symptoms
Cardiac arrhythmias, cerebral hemorrhage, pulmonary edema, palpitation, tremor, dizziness, vomiting, fear, labored breathing, headache, dryness of mouth, pallor, weakness, panic, anxiety, confusion, hallucinations, delirium.

PATIENT CARE CONSIDERATIONS

Administration/Storage
♦ Give dose as prescribed.
♦ Give with food if GI upset occurs.
♦ Tablets may be broken in half for ease of administration. Do not crush or chew tablets or half-tablets.
♦ Store tablets at controlled room temperature (59° to 86°F).
♦ Do not take MAO inhibitor while taking this medication.

Assessment/Interventions
♦ Obtain patient history, including drug history and any known allergies. Note history of diabetes, hypertension, hyperthyroidism, enlarged prostate, narrow angle glaucoma, urinary retention, severe coronary artery disease, ventricular arrhythmias, heart block pregnancy, or concurrent use of or within 2 wk of stopping MAO inhibitor therapy.

♦ Assess symptoms (eg, cough, sputum viscosity, color and volume, sinus congestion) before and periodically throughout therapy.
♦ Notify health care provider if any of the following occur: persistent or recurrent cough; cough associated with fever, rash, or persistent headache; bothersome side effects.
♦ Monitor patient for nervousness, dizziness, tachycardia, and palpitations. If noted, hold therapy and notify health care provider.

Patient/Family Education
♦ Explain name, dose, action, and potential side effects of drug.
♦ Advise patient how to properly take medication.
♦ Advise patient that tablets may be broken in half for ease of administration.
♦ Instruct patient to not chew or crush tablets or half-tablets and to swallow whole.

- Advise patient to take with food if GI upset occurs.
- Advise patient that if a dose is missed to take as soon as remembered unless it is nearing time for the next dose. Caution patient to not double the dose to catch up.
- Instruct patient to discontinue use and report any of the following symptoms to health care provider: nervousness, dizziness, sleeplessness; persistent or recurrent cough; cough associated with fever, rash, or persistent headache; bothersome side effects.
- Advise patient that if symptoms are not controlled, not to increase the dose of medication but to inform health care provider.
- Advise women to notify health care provider if pregnant, planning to become pregnant, or breastfeeding.
- Caution patient to not take any prescription or OTC medications, or dietary supplements unless advised by health care provider.
- Caution patient not to take MAO inhibitor while taking this medication.

Phenytoin

(FEN-ih-toe-in)

Class Anticonvulsant/Hydantoin

How Supplied

Phenytoin
Dilantin Infatab Tablets, chewable 50 mg ♦
Dilantin-125 Suspension, oral 125 mg/5 mL

Phenytoin Sodium
Dilantin Injection 50 mg/mL (46 mg phenytoin)
♦ *Dilantin Kapseals* Capsules 30 mg (27.6 mg phenytoin), Capsules 100 mg (92 mg phenytoin)
🍁 *Dilantin-30 Pediatric*

Action

PHARMACOLOGY: Appears to act at motor cortex in inhibiting spread of seizure activity. Possibly works by promoting sodium efflux from neurons, thereby stabilizing threshold against hyperexcitability. Also decreases posttetanic potentiation at synapse.

PHARMACOKINETICS/DYNAMICS:
Absorption: Slow and variable (oral); poor in neonates; rapid (IV); slow but complete (IM). Steady state is 7 to 10 days. T_{max} is 4 to 12 hr (*Kapseals*); 1.5 to 3 hr (*Infatabs, Dilantin-125* oral suspension).

Distribution: Distributes into CSF, saliva, semen, GI fluids, bile, breast milk, and crosses the placenta. Protein binding is high (more than 90%) but may be lower in neonates (84%).

Metabolism: Hydroxylated in the liver by an enzyme system, which is saturable at high plasma levels.

Excretion: Mostly excreted in bile as inactive metabolites, then reabsorbed from the intestinal tract and excreted in the urine (as metabolites). Plasma $t_{1/2}$ is 22 hr (oral phenytoin) and 14 hr (*Infatabs*). Excretion is enhanced by alkaline urine.

Indications Control of grand mal and psychomotor seizures; prevention and treatment of seizures occurring during or after neurosurgery; control of grand mal type of status epilepticus (parenteral administration). **Unlabeled use(s):** Control of arrhythmias, (particularly cardiac glycoside-induced arrhythmias); control of convulsions in severe preeclampsia; treatment of trigeminal neuralgia (tic douloureux), recessive dystrophic epidermolysis bullosa and junctional epidermolysis bullosa.

Contraindications Hypersensitivity to phenytoin or other hydantoins; sinoatrial block; sinus bradycardia; second- and third-degree atrioventricular block; Adams-Stokes syndrome.

Route/Dosage

Individualize dose within clinically effective therapeutic serum level of 10 to 20 mcg/mL.

Seizures
ADULTS: PO 100 mg (or 125 mg of suspension) tid initially.
Maintenance: 300 to 400 mg/day (max, 600 mg/day). Sometimes initial 1 g loading dose is divided into 3 doses (400, 300, and 300 mg) and is given at 2-hr intervals. Once seizure control is established, extended-release form (300 mg) may be administered for once-a-day dosing.
CHILDREN: PO 5 mg/kg/day in 2 to 3 divided doses initially.
Maintenance: 4 to 8 mg/kg/day (max, 300 mg/day).

Status Epilepticus
ADULTS: IV Loading dose of 10 to 15 mg/kg via slow IV. Then PO/IV 100 mg q 6 to 8 hr.
CHILDREN: IV Loading dose of 15 to 20 mg/kg at rate not exceeding 1 to 3 mg/kg/min.

Neurosurgery Prophylaxis
ADULTS: IM 100 to 200 mg at 4-hr intervals during surgery and postoperatively.

Interactions

Acetaminophen: May increase hepatotoxicity potential with chronic phenytoin use.
Amiodarone, chloramphenicol, disulfiram, estrogens, felbamate, fluconazole, isoniazid, cimetidine, trimethoprim, phenylbutazone, oxyphenbutazone, phenacemide, sulfonamides: May increase phenytoin serum levels.

Carbamazepine, sucralfate, antineoplastic agents, rifampin, rifabutin: May decrease phenytoin serum levels.

Corticosteroids, coumarin anticoagulants, doxycycline, estrogens, levodopa, felodipine, methadone, loop diuretics, oral contraceptives, quinidine, rifampin, rifabutin: May impair effects of these agents.

Cyclosporine: May reduce cyclosporine levels.

Disopyramide: May cause decreased disopyramide levels and bioavailability and may enhance anticholinergic actions.

Enteral nutritional therapy: May reduce phenytoin concentrations.

Folic acid: May cause folic acid deficiency.

Metyrapone: Phenytoin may cause subnormal response to metyrapone.

Mexiletine: May decrease mexiletine levels and effects.

Nondepolarizing muscle relaxants: May cause these agents to have shorter duration or decreased effects.

Phenobarbital, sodium valproate, valproic acid: May increase or decrease phenytoin levels. Phenytoin may increase phenobarbital and decrease valproic acid levels.

Primidone: May increase concentrations of primidone and metabolites.

Sympathomimetics (eg, dopamine): May cause profound hypotension and possibly cardiac arrest.

Theophyllines: Effects of either agent may be decreased.

INCOMPATIBILITIES: Do not mix with other drugs in syringe.

Lab Test Interferences Phenytoin may interfere with metapyrone and dexamethasone tests, causing inaccurate results because of increased metabolism of these agents. Drug may cause decreases in serum levels of protein-bound iodine. It may cause increased levels of glucose, alkaline phosphatase and gamma glutamyl transpeptidase.

Adverse Reactions

CV: CV collapse, hypotension, atrial and ventricular conduction depression, ventricular fibrillation (IV use).

CNS: Nystagmus; ataxia; dysarthria; slurred speech; mental confusion; dizziness; insomnia; transient nervousness; motor twitching; diplopia; fatigue; irritability; drowsiness; depression; numbness; tremor; headache; choreoathetosis (IV use).

DERM: Rashes, sometimes accompanied by fever; bullous, exfoliative or purpuric dermatitis; lupus erythematosus; Stevens-Johnson syndrome; toxic epidermal necrolysis; hirsutism; alopecia.

EENT: Conjunctivitis.

GI: Nausea; vomiting; diarrhea; constipation.

HEMA: Thrombocytopenia; leukopenia; granulocytopenia; agranulocytosis; pancytopenia; macrocytosis; megaloblastic anemia; eosinophilia; monocytosis; leukocytosis; simple anemia; hemolytic anemia; aplastic anemia.

HEPA: Toxic hepatitis and liver damage; hepatocellular degeneration and necrosis; hepatitis; jaundice; nephrosis.

OTHER: Gingival hyperplasia; coarsening of facial features; lip enlargement; Peyronie's disease; polyarthropathy; hyperglycemia; weight gain; chest pain; IgA depression; fever; photophobia; gynecomastia; periarteritis nodosa; pulmonary fibrosis; tissue injury at injection site; lymph node hyperplasia; hypothyroidism.

Precautions

Pregnancy: Pregnancy category undetermined. Consult health care provider. Possible risk of birth defects must be considered along with risk of seizures to fetus in untreated epileptic mothers.

Lactation: Excreted in breast milk.

Hypersensitivity: Rapid substitution of alternate therapy may be necessary.

Special risk patients: Use drug with caution with hepatic impairment, acute intermittent porphyria, alcohol abuse, hypotension, and severe myocardial insufficiency.

Bioavailability: Because products vary in bioavailability; brand interchange is not recommended.

Seizures: Drug should not be given to treat seizures due to hypoglycemia or other metabolic causes or petit mal (absence) epilepsy.

Withdrawal: Abrupt withdrawal may precipitate status epilepticus. Dosage must be reduced or other anticonvulsant medicine substituted gradually.

Overdosage: Signs and Symptoms

Nystagmus, ataxia, dysarthria, hypotension, diminished mental capacity, coma, unresponsive pupils, respiratory and cardiovascular depression.

PATIENT CARE CONSIDERATIONS

Administration/Storage

- Shake oral suspension well.
- Do not administer discolored capsules.
- Administer oral forms with food.
- Only extended-release capsules are recommended for once-a-day dosage.
- Do not crush or allow patient to chew extended-release capsules.
- Do not substitute one brand for another; bioequivalence problems exist.
- For parenteral administration, direct IV administration is recommended.

- Administer IV into large vein via large-gauge needle or cannula. Do not exceed rate of 50 mg/min for adults or 1 to 3 mg/kg/min in newborns. Immediately flush with normal saline solution. Avoid continuous infusion.
- Monitor BP for possible hypotension during IV infusion. Rate of infusion may need to be decreased.
- Avoid IM route when possible. If IM administration is needed for greater than 1 wk, consider alternatives such as gastric intubation.
- When patient is stabilized with oral phenytoin and switched from oral to IM route, dose must be increased by 50%. When patient returns to oral form after IM administration, ½ original oral dose should be given for 1 wk.
- Do not abruptly discontinue medication; withdrawal must be slowly tapered.
- Do not use parenteral solution if precipitates form that will not dissolve at room temperature.
- Do not use parenteral solution if it is hazy; faint, clear yellow color is acceptable for use.

Assessment/Interventions
- Obtain patient history, including drug history and any known allergies. Note hepatic impairment, cardiac disease and porphyria.
- Perform blood counts and urinalyses on initiation of therapy and at monthly intervals for several months.
- Observe for rash, which may signify hypersensitivity reaction that can lead to serious dermatological reactions. If rash occurs, withhold drug and notify health care provider.
- Monitor ECG and BP continuously.
- Monitor for elevated blood glucose values in diabetic patients and report to health care provider.
- Observe for side effects including nystagmus, ataxia, drowsiness, severe nausea or vomiting, gingival hyperplasia or jaundice, and report to health care provider.

Patient/Family Education
- Advise patient to take medication with food.
- Teach patient to shake oral suspension well.
- Instruct patient taking capsules not to use discolored ones.
- Tell patient to notify health care provider if skin rash develops.
- Instruct patient to report the following symptoms to health care provider: nystagmus, ataxia, drowsiness, severe nausea or vomiting, gingival hyperplasia, or jaundice.
- Caution patient to consult with health care provider before using alcohol or taking any other drug including OTC medications.
- Warn patient that stopping medication too quickly may precipitate seizures. Stress that dose should be changed only under health care provider's direction.
- Inform patient that it is important to maintain good oral hygiene and to inform dentist of phenytoin therapy.
- Instruct diabetic patient that changes may occur in blood sugars and to monitor and report any abnormal results to health care provider.
- Inform patient that urine may turn pink.
- Advise patient to carry identification such as *Medi-Alert* that identifies illness and medication.
- Warn patient to inform surgeon, health care provider, or dentist about this medication before any surgical, emergency, or dental procedure.
- Advise patient that drug may cause drowsiness, and to use caution while driving or performing other tasks requiring mental alertness.

Phytonadione (K_1; Phylloquinone; Methylphytyl Naphthoquinone)

(fye-toe-nuh-DIE-ohn)

Class Blood modifier/Vitamin K

How Supplied
AquaMEPHYTON Injection (aqueous colloidal solution) 2 mg/mL, Injection (aqueous dispersion) 10 mg/mL ♦ *Mephyton* Tablets 5 mg

Action
PHARMACOLOGY: Promotes hepatic synthesis of active prothrombin (factor II), proconvertin (factor VII), plasma thromboplastin component (factor IX) and Stuart factor (factor X).

PHARMACOKINETICS/DYNAMICS:

Absorption: GI tract via intestinal lymphatics in the presence of bile (oral); readily absorbed (SC).

Distribution: Concentrated in the liver initially, then concentration declines rapidly.

Metabolism: Rapidly metabolized in the liver; little tissue accumulation.

Excretion: Urine and bile.

Onset: 6 to 10 hr (oral) and 1 to 2 hr (parenteral); controls hemorrhage in approximately 3 to 6 hr.

Indications Management of coagulation disorders due to faulty formation of factors II, VII, IX and X when due to vitamin K deficiency or interference with vitamin K activity.

Oral/Parenteral: Treatment of anticoagulant-induced prothrombin deficiency; treatment of hypoprothrombinemia secondary to salicylates or antibacterial therapy or secondary to obstructive jaundice and biliary fistulas, provided bile salts are also given.

Parenteral: Treatment of hypoprothrombinemia secondary to conditions limiting absorption or synthesis of vitamin K prophylaxis and therapy of hemorrhagic disease of the newborn.

Contraindications Standard considerations.

Route/Dosage

ADULTS AND CHILDREN: **PO/SC/IM** 2.5 to 10 mg (in adults, up to 25 mg for serious bleeding; rarely, 50 mg), may repeat oral dose based on response in 6 to 8 hr or 12 to 48 hr; avoid oral route when disorder would prevent adequate absorption.

Hemorrhagic Disease (Prophylaxis)
NEWBORNS: **IM** Single dose 0.5 to 1 mg within 1 hr of birth.
INFANTS: **PO/SC/IM** 2 mg.

Hemorrhagic Disease (Treatment)
NEWBORNS: **SC/IM** 1 mg accompanied by laboratory evaluation.

Interactions

Oral anticoagulants: Effects are antagonized by vitamin K, particularly in patients with advanced liver disease.

Lab Test Interferences Paradoxical prolongation of prothrombin time (PT) after max doses of vitamin K.

Adverse Reactions

CV: Hypotension; cyanosis.
CNS: Headache; dizziness.
DERM: Pruritic erythematous plaques at IM injection site; rash; urticaria.
HEPA: Hyperbilirubinemia, including kernicterus, in newborns.
OTHER: Anaphylactoid reactions; pain, swelling and tenderness at injection site; death after IV injection.

> **WARNING:**
>
> *Phytonadione injection:* Severe reactions, including death, have occurred during and immediately after IV injection. Severe reactions have resembled hypersensitivity or anaphylaxis, including shock and cardiac and/or respiratory arrest. Events have occurred even when appropriate dilution was used to avoid rapid infusion. Some patients have exhibited symptoms on first administration of the drug. Thus, restrict IV use for situations where other routes are not feasible and benefit/risk ratio is assessed.

Precautions

Pregnancy: Category C.
Lactation: Vitamin K excreted in breast milk.
Hypersensitivity: Rash and urticaria; anaphylactoid reactions.
Hepatic function impairment: Giving vitamin K to correct hypoprothrombinemia associated with severe hepatitis or cirrhosis may further depress prothrombin concentration.
Anticoagulation: Patient may be refractory to oral anticoagulants, particularly large doses.
Bleeding: Giving vitamin K has no immediate coagulant effect. Management of bleeding involves standard measures (eg, transfusions).

Overdosage: Signs and Symptoms

Parenteral administration: Hypotension, asystole, chest pain, dyspnea, nausea, rash, pruritus.

PATIENT CARE CONSIDERATIONS

Administration/Storage

- After initial dose, determine subsequent doses by PT response or clinical condition. If in 6 to 8 hr after parenteral administration or 12 to 48 hr after oral administration, PT has not been shortened satisfactorily, repeat dose.
- Give SC or IM when possible. For adults and older children, inject IM in upper outer quadrant of buttocks. In infants and young children, anterolateral aspect of thigh or deltoid region is preferred.
- Protect from light at all times.
- Avoid IV route unless risk outweighs benefit. If IV administration is unavoidable, inject very slowly, not exceeding 1 mg/min.

Assessment/Interventions

- Obtain patient history, including drug history and any known allergies.
- When given for oral anticoagulant-induced hypoprothrombinemia, remember that phytonadione promotes synthesis of prothrombin by liver, but does not directly counteract effects of oral anticoagulants. Do not expect immediate coagulant effect; it takes minimum of 1 to 2 hr for measurable improvement in PT.
- Check PT prior to and after treatment with phytonadione.
- For prophylaxis or treatment of hemorrhagic disease of newborn, phytonadione (vitamin K_1) is safer than menadiol sodium diphosphate (vitamin K_4). A prompt response (shortening of the PT in 2 to 4 hr) is usually diagnostic of hemorrhagic disease of newborn; failure to respond indicates another diagnosis or coagulation disorder.

Patient/Family Education
- Explain that patient may experience temporary "flushing sensations" and "peculiar" sensations of taste. Rarely dizziness, rapid weak pulse, profuse sweating, or difficulty breathing may occur. Another rare occurrence is pain, swelling, or tenderness at injection site.
- Remind patients on anticoagulant and phytonadione therapy of importance of regular lab work to check PT. Anticoagulant effects are antagonized by vitamin K so temporary resistance to oral anticoagulants may result, especially when larger doses are used.
- Instruct patient to report any symptoms of bleeding.

Pilocarpine

(pie-low-CAR-peen)

Class Ophthalmic/Antiglaucoma/Mouth and throat product

How Supplied

Pilocarpine Hydrochloride

Adsorbocarpine Solution 1%, Solution 2%, Solution 4% ◆ *Akarpine* Solution 1%, Solution 2%, Solution 4% ◆ *Isopto-Carpine* Solution 0.35%, Solution 0.5%, Solution 1%, Solution 2%, Solution 3%, Solution 4%, Solution 5%, Solution 6%, Solution 8%, Solution 10% ◆ *Pilocar* Solution 0.5%, Solution 1%, Solution 2%, Solution 3%, Solution 4%, Solution 6% ◆ *Piloptic-1/2* Solution 0.5% ◆ *Piloptic-1* Solution 1% ◆ *Piloptic-2* Solution 2% ◆ *Piloptic-3* Solution 3% ◆ *Piloptic-4* Solution 4% ◆ *Piloptic-6* Solution 6% ◆ *Pilopine HS* Gel 4% ◆ *Pilostat* Solution 0.5%, Solution 1%, Solution 2%, Solution 3%, Solution 4%, Solution 6% ◆ *Salagen* Tablets 5 mg

Pilocarpine Ocular Therapeutic System

Ocusert Pilo-20 Ocular therapeutic system Releases 20 mcg/hr for 1 wk ◆ *Ocusert Pilo-40* Ocular therapeutic system Releases 40 mcg/hr for 1 wk

✤ *Minims-Pilocarpine*

Action

PHARMACOLOGY:

Ophthalmic: Decreases IOP by constricting pupil and stimulating ciliary muscles to open trabecular meshwork spaces and facilitate outflow of aqueous humor.

PO: Stimulates exocrine glands including mucous cells of respiratory tract and salivary glands in oral cavity.

PHARMACOKINETICS/DYNAMICS:

Absorption: T_{max} is 0.85 to 1.25 hr. C_{max} is 15 to 41 ng/mL. AUC is 33 to 108 hr•ng/mL. High-fat meals decreased the rate of absorption.

Metabolism: Limited information available; however, its thought to occur at neuronal synapses and probably in the plasma.

Excretion: Urine (as unchanged pilocarpine, minimal active/inactive degradation products). Half-life is 0.76 to 1.35 hr.

Onset: 20 min.

Peak: 1 hr.

Duration: 3 to 5 hr.

Special Populations:
Gender – Elderly females had C_{max} and AUC approximately twice that of elderly, young males.

Indications

Ophthalmic: Treatment of chronic simple glaucoma, chronic angle-closure glaucoma, acute angle-closure glaucoma, pre- and postoperative management of intraocular tension, treatment of mydriasis.

PO: Treatment of xerostomia in patients with malfunctioning salivary glands because of radiotherapy for cancer of head and neck, relieve dry mouth in patients with Sjogren syndrome.

Unlabeled use(s): Relief of dry mouth in patients with graft-vs-host disease (PO).

Contraindications Hypersensitivity; conditions in which cholinergic effects such as constriction are undesirable. Oral use also contraindicated in uncontrolled asthma, acute iritis, narrow-angle glaucoma, acute inflammatory disease of anterior segment of eye.

Route/Dosage

SOLUTION

ADULTS: Instill 1 to 2 drops of 1% or 2% solution in affected eye(s) 6 times or less/day. More concentrated solutions are sometimes used.

GEL

ADULTS: Apply 0.5-inch ribbon in lower conjunctival sac of affected eye(s) once daily at bedtime.

OCULAR THERAPEUTIC SYSTEM

ADULTS: Place system into conjunctival cul-de-sac of affected eye(s) at bedtime. Replace each unit q 7 days. **PO** 5 mg tid; may titrate 10 mg or less tid.

PO

ADULTS: **PO** Titrate dosage based on therapeutic response and tolerance. To reduce the incidence and severity of side effects, use the lowest effective dose. Do not exceed a maximum of 10 mg/dose.

Radiation-induced Xerostomia

ADULTS: **PO** 5 mg tid. If no response, increase dose to 10 mg tid. Continue uninterrupted for at least 12 wk before assessing for full therapeutic benefit.

Sjogren Syndrome
ADULTS: **PO** 5 mg qid. Continue uninterrupted for at least 6 wk before assessing for full therapeutic benefit.

Interactions
Anticholinergics: May antagonize action of pilocarpine (PO, ophthalmic).
Beta-blockers: Potential for cardiac conduction disturbances with oral pilocarpine.
Parasympathomimetics: Additive pharmacologic effects and increased toxicity possible.

Lab Test Interferences
None well documented.

Adverse Reactions
CV: Transient hypertension; tachycardia; edema; palpitations.
CNS: Chills; headache; dizziness; asthenia.
DERM: Excessive sweating; flushing.
EENT: Transient stinging and burning, tearing, ciliary spasm, conjunctival vascular congestion, temporal, peri-, or supraorbital headache, superficial keratitis-induced myopia, blurred vision, poor dark adaptation, conjunctival hyperemia, reduced visual acuity in poor illumination, lens opacity, subtle corneal granularity, conjunctival irritation, ciliary spasm, precipitation of angle closure, irritation, corneal abrasion, visual impairment (ophthalmic); rhinitis (PO).

GI: Excessive salivation; nausea; vomiting; diarrhea dyspepsia; abdominal pain.
GU: Urinary frequency (PO).
RESP: Bronchial spasm; pulmonary edema; rhinitis; sinusitis; pharyngitis; increased coughing; increases airway resistance; bronchial smooth muscle tone; bronchial secretions.
SPEC SENSE: Lacrimation; amblyopia; conjunctivitis; abnormal vision; excessive salivation.

Precautions
Pregnancy: Category C.
Lactation: Undetermined.
Children: Safety and efficacy not established.
Elderly: Elderly patients also may be at increased risk for certain adverse effects during therapy, including diarrhea, urinary frequency, and dizziness.
Special risk patients: Use oral pilocarpine with caution in acute cardiac failure, bronchial asthma, peptic ulcer, hypertension, hyperthyroidism, retinal disease, GI or biliary tract spasm or obstruction, urinary tract obstruction, Parkinson disease, angina pectoris, MI, chronic bronchitis, chronic obstructive pulmonary disease, underlying psychiatric disorders.

Overdosage: Signs and Symptoms
Salivation, lacrimation, nausea, vomiting, diarrhea, cramping, sweating, frequent urination, bradycardia, asystole, death (PO).

PATIENT CARE CONSIDERATIONS

Administration/Storage
PO:
- Administer PO.
- Administration with a high-fat meal reduces pilocarpine absorption.
- Store at room temperature.
- Give medication with food if GI distress occurs.

Optic:
- To avoid contamination, do not touch tip of container to any surface. Replace cap after administration. Gently apply pressure over nasolacrimal drainage system (bridge of nose) for 1 to 2 min.
- Keep bottle tightly closed when not in use.
- Wash hands before and after using.
- Keep out of reach of children.

Solution:
- Store at room temperature and protect from light.

Gel:
- Refrigerate until time of dispensation. Do not freeze.
- *Ocular Therapeutic System* is a small device that releases pilocarpine through a membrane when placed in the cul-de-sac of the eye.

- Wash hands with soap and water before touching or manipulating system.
- Read and follow directions on package insert.
- Check for presence of system at end and beginning of each shift.
- If displaced system contacts unclean surfaces, rinse with cool tap water before replacing. Discard contaminated systems and replace with fresh unit.
- Refrigerate; do not freeze.
- Place system into eye at bedtime. If keeping unit in eye is problem, move unit from lower to upper lid by gentle lid massage. If unit slips out during night, its effects continue for period of time similar to that following instillation of eyedrops.

Assessment/Interventions
- Obtain patient history, including drug history and any known allergies.
- During early treatment of adult glaucoma, perform hourly tonometric tests to monitor for transitory increase in IOP.
- Use health care provider- or manufacturer-recommended technique for patient application with contact lenses.
- Monitor for changes in vision, which could indicate potential retinal detachment.

PO:
- May cause increased sweating, resulting in dehydration.

Patient/Family Education
- For treatment of glaucoma, emphasize need to adhere to medical regimen to prevent blindness.
- Explain that long-term therapy may be required.
- Instruct patient to wash hands thoroughly before and after using ophthalmic preparation.
- Review proper procedure for administration of ophthalmic preparations.
- Explain that ophthalmic preparations may sting upon instillation, especially with first few doses.
- Tell patient to discard solution after expiration date.
- Explain that medication may cause headache or brow ache and that because of blurring, altered distance vision and night vision; patient should use caution while night driving or performing hazardous tasks.
- Explain that during acute phases, a miotic (agent that causes pupil to constrict) also must be instilled into unaffected eye to prevent occurrence of angle-closure glaucoma.
- Tell patients using *Ocular Therapeutic System* that signs of irritation, including mild redness with or without slight increase in mucus secretion may be noticed with first use but that these symptoms tend to lessen or disappear after first wk of therapy.
- Instruct patient to check for placement of system before retiring and on arising.

PO:
- Advise patients to drink additional water or noncaffeinated fluids during therapy.
- Tell patients using oral form to report the following symptoms to health care provider: sweating, nausea, nasal congestion, chills, flushing, frequent urination, dizziness, weakness, headache, indigestion, tearing, diarrhea, fluid retention.

Pimecrolimus

(pim-eh-CROW-lih-muss)

Class Topical Immunomodulator

How Supplied
Elidel Cream 1%

Action

PHARMACOLOGY: Mechanism in atopic dermatitis is not known; however, pimecrolimus inhibits T cell activation by blocking the transcription of early cytokines.

PHARMACOKINETICS/DYNAMICS:

Absorption: After topical application, blood levels are routinely at or below the limit of quantification.

Distribution: In vitro studies indicate that plasma protein binding is 74% to 87%.

Metabolism: No evidence of skin-mediated drug metabolism.

Indications Short-term and intermittent long-term treatment of mild to moderate atopic dermatitis in nonimmunocompromised patients.

Contraindications Standard considerations.

Route/Dosage

ADULTS AND CHILDREN 2 YR AND OLDER: **Topical** Apply a thin layer to the affected skin bid and rub in gently and completely. Re-evaluate patient if symptoms persist beyond 6 wk of treatment.

Interactions None well documented.

Lab Test Interferences None well documented.

Adverse Reactions

CNS: Headache.
DERM: Application site reactions (eg, burning sensation, irritation, erythema, pruritus); cutaneous infections; impetigo; urticaria; acne.
EENT: Nasopharyngitis; ear infection; otitis media; sinusitis; nasal congestion; rhinorrhea; rhinitis; sore throat; conjunctivitis.
GI: Gastroenteritis; upper abdominal pain; vomiting; diarrhea; nausea.
GU: Dysmenorrhea.
RESP: Upper respiratory tract infection; pneumonia; bronchitis; aggravated asthma; sinus congestion; asthma; cough.
OTHER: Bacterial infection; folliculitis; herpes simplex; chicken pox; pyrexia; flu-like symptoms; hypersensitivity; back pain; arthralgia.

Precautions

Pregnancy: Category C.
Lactation: Undetermined.
Children: Safety and efficacy not established in children less than 2 yr.
Lymphadenopathy: Investigate the etiology of lymphadenopathy occurring in patients receiving the topical ointment.
Viral infections: The topical ointment may be associated with increased risk of varicella zoster virus infection (chicken pox or shingles), herpes simplex virus infection, or eczema herpeticum.

PATIENT CARE CONSIDERATIONS

Administration/Storage
- For topical use only. Not for ophthalmic, oral, or intravaginal use.
- Avoid contact with eyes and areas of active cutaneous viral or bacterial infections.
- Cream is usually applied to affected areas bid.
- Apply a thin film of cream to cover the affected area(s).
- Store cream at controlled room temperature (59° to 86°F). Protect from freezing. Keep tube tightly capped.

Assessment/Interventions
- Obtain patient history, including drug history and any known allergies. Note Netherton syndrome, current viral or bacterial infection of affected skin, concurrent light therapy (eg, phototherapy), and concurrent use of other skin products.
- Ensure that clinical infections at treatment sites have been treated before starting therapy.
- Assess the skin and identify areas where medication is to be applied and areas that should be avoided (eg, infected site).
- Do not apply other topical products unless advised by health care provider.
- Assess and document skin condition before initial application and periodically throughout treatment. Inform health care provider if condition does not improve, worsens, or if application site reactions are bothersome.
- Monitor patient for development of lymphadenopathy. If noted inform health care provider.
- Assess patient for RESP, CNS, GI, general body side effects, and application site reactions. Inform health care provider if noted and significant.

Patient/Family Education
- Explain name, dose, action, and potential side effects of drug.
- Advise patient or caregiver to carefully read the "Patient Information" insert before using the first time and with each refill.
- Advise patient or caregiver that cream is applied topically to skin lesions bid.
- Teach patient or caregiver proper technique for applying cream: Wash hands. Apply a thin film of cream to cover skin areas with eczema. Wash hands after applying cream unless hands are also being treated.
- Advise patient to not bathe, shower, or swim after applying cream because this could wash the cream off.
- Advise patient not to stop using the cream until signs and symptoms of eczema have resolved. Advise patient to start applying the cream again and if symptoms return.
- Advise patient using moisturizers to apply them after applying pimecrolimus cream.
- Caution patient not to cover treated areas with bandages, dressings, or wraps.
- Warn patient to avoid contact with the eyes.
- Advise patient to wash eyes with large amounts of cool water if cream comes in contact with the eyes and to contact a health care provider if eye irritation persists.
- Advise patient that mild to moderate feelings of warmth and/or sensations of burning are the most common side effects and to notify health care provider if these side effects become severe or persist for more than 1 wk.
- Advise patient that if condition does not improve after 6 wk of treatment or if condition worsens to contact a health care provider.
- Advise patient to talk to a health care provider before using any other topical agents (eg, medicated soaps, astringents, cosmetics, other acne products) on treated skin.
- Warn patient to avoid unnecessary exposure to sun and sun lamps while using this medication. Advise patient to use sunscreens with minimum SPF of 15 and protective clothing over treated areas when exposure cannot be avoided.
- Advise women to notify health care provider if pregnant, planning to become pregnant, or breastfeeding.
- Warn patient not to take any prescription or OTC drugs or dietary supplements without consulting health care provider.
- Advise patient that follow-up visits to examine the skin lesions may be necessary and to keep appointments.

Pimozide

(Pih-moe-ZIDE)

Class Antipsychotic

How Supplied
Orap Tablets 1 mg, Tablets 2 mg

Action

PHARMACOLOGY: Blockage of dopaminergic receptors on neurons in the CNS.

PHARMACOKINETICS/DYNAMICS:
Absorption: More than 50% of oral dose absorbed. T_{max} is 6 to 8 hr.

Metabolism: Significant first-pass metabolism by N-dealkylation in the liver, catalyzed mainly by CYP3A enzymatic system and to a lesser extent by CYP1A2 producing 2 major metabolites of undetermined activity.

Excretion: Primarily in the kidney, small amount in feces. Serum t½ is approximately 55 hr.

Indications Suppression of motor and phonic tics in patients with Tourette syndrome who fail to respond satisfactorily to standard treatment.

Contraindications Treatment of simple tics or tics other than those associated with Tourette syndrome; drug-induced motor and phonic tics (eg, amphetamine, methylphenidate, pemoline) until it is determined whether the tics are caused by drugs or Tourette syndrome; patients with congenital long QT syndrome, history of cardiac arrhythmias; administration with other drugs that prolong the QT interval; patients receiving aprepitant or the azole antifungal agents itraconazole, ketoconazole, and voriconazole; patients receiving the macrolide antibiotics azithromycin, clarithromycin, dirithromycin, erythromycin, and troleandomycin; patients receiving protease inhibitors (eg, amprenavir, atazanavir, indinavir, nelfinavir, ritonavir, saquinavir); coadministration of nefazodone, sertraline, zileuton, or ziprasidone; severe toxic CNS depression or comatose states from any cause; hypersensitivity to pimozide.

Route/Dosage

ADULTS: **PO** For the initial dose, give 1 to 2 mg/day in divided doses, increasing the dose every other day. For the maintenance dose, give less than 0.2 mg/kg/day or 10 mg/day, whichever is less. Doses greater than 0.2 mg/kg/day or 10 mg/day are not recommended.

CHILDREN (AT LEAST 12 YR): **PO** For the initial dose, give 0.05 mg/kg/day (preferably at bedtime); increasing the dose every third day (max, 0.2 mg/kg, not to exceed 10 mg/day).

Interactions

CNS depressants (eg, analgesics, sedatives, anxiolytics): Pimozide may potentiate effects.
Drugs that may cause motor and phonic tics (eg, amphetamine, methylphenidate, pemoline): Coadministration of these agents with pimozide is contraindicated.
Drugs that prolong the QT interval (eg, aprepitant, azole antifungal agents [eg, ketoconazole], macrolide antibiotics [eg, erythromycin], nefazodone, phenothiazines [eg, thioridazine], protease inhibitors [eg, indinavir], sertraline, tricyclic antidepressants [eg, amitriptyline], voriconazole, zileuton, ziprasidone): Increased risk of life-threatening cardiac arrhythmias, including torsades de pointes. Coadministration of these agents with pimozide is contraindicated.

Grapefruit juice: May increase pimozide concentrations, increasing the pharmacologic and adverse effects. Avoid grapefruit juice.

Lab Test Interferences None well documented.

Adverse Reactions

CV: ECG changes, including prolongation of QT interval, flattening, notching, and inversion of T wave, and appearance of U waves; postural hypotension; hypotension; hypertension; tachycardia; palpitations.
CNS: Extrapyramidal reactions; motor restlessness; dystonia; akathisia; hyperpyrexia; opisthotonos; tardive dyskinesia; neuroleptic malignant syndrome (NMS); Parkinsonian syndrome; grand mal seizures; drowsiness; sedation; insomnia; rigidity; speech disorder; handwriting change; akinesia; depression; excitement; nervousness; adverse behavior; headache; abnormal dreaming; hyperkinesia; somnolence; torticollis; limb tremor; dizziness.
DERM: Rash; increased sweating; skin irritation.
EENT: Oculogyric crises; visual disturbances; taste change; sensitivity of eyes to light; decreased accommodation; spots before eyes; blurred vision; cataracts.
GI: Dry mouth; diarrhea; constipation; thirst; increased appetite; dysphagia; increased salivation; nausea; vomiting; anorexia; GI distress.
GU: Menstrual disorder; breast secretions; impotence; nocturia; urinary frequency; loss of libido.
OTHER: Sudden, unexpected death; hyperpyrexia; muscle cramps and tightness; stooped posture; asthenia; myalgia; chest pain; periorbital edema.

Precautions

Pregnancy: Category C.
Lactation: Undetermined.
Children: Limited information regarding use, efficacy, and safety in patients less than 12 yr.
Renal function impairment: Use with caution.
Hepatic function impairment: Use with caution.
Special risk patients: Use with caution in patients with conditions that may be aggravated by anticholinergic activity, patients receiving anticonvulsant medication, patients with history of seizures or EEG abnormalities.
NMS: This potentially fatal condition has been reported in association with antipsychotic agents. Signs and symptoms include hyperpyrexia, muscle rigidity, altered mental status, irregular pulse or BP, tachycardia, diaphoresis, cardiac arrhythmias.
Sudden death: Sudden, unexpected deaths have occurred in patients receiving dosages in the range of 1 mg/kg. Prolongation of the QT interval, predisposing patients to ventricular arrhyth-

mia, is one possible mechanism for the deaths.
Tardive dyskinesia: This syndrome of potentially irreversible, involuntary dyskinetic movements has occurred with other antipsychotic agents. Incidence appears to be highest among the elderly, especially women.

PATIENT CARE CONSIDERATIONS
Administration/Storage
- Administer prescribed dose bid to adults.
- Administer prescribed dose qd at bedtime to children.
- Store at controlled room temperature (59° to 86°F).

Assessment/Interventions
- Obtain patient history, including drug history and any known allergies. Note history of hypersensitivity to antipsychotic drugs, liver disease, kidney disease, congenital long QT syndrome, cardiac arrhythmias, previous episodes of NMS, seizures, or current use of anticonvulsants, pemoline, methylphenidate, amphetamines, macrolide antibiotics, protease inhibitors, azole antifungals, or drugs that prolong the QT interval.
- Ensure that baseline electrolytes are determined before starting therapy in patients taking diuretics.
- Ensure that ECG is performed before initiating therapy and periodically thereafter, especially during periods of dose adjustment. Ensure that hypokalemia is corrected before initiating therapy and normal potassium levels are maintained during therapy.
- Withhold therapy if QTc interval prolongs beyond 0.47 sec (children), 0.52 sec (adults), or more than 25% above baseline QTc.
- Inform health care provider immediately if hyperpyrexia, muscle rigidity, altered mental status, irregular pulse and BP, tachycardia, or diaphoresis develop.
- Notify health care provider immediately if palpitations or syncope occur.
- Assess baseline neurologic status and, during treatment, observe for involuntary body and facial movements, excessive drowsiness, behavior changes, and seizure activity. Inform health care and provider if noted.
- Assess and document effect of medication on motor and phonic tic activity.
- Assess medication compliance.

Overdosage: Signs and Symptoms
Severe extrapyramidal reactions, ECG abnormalities, hypotension, comatose state with respiratory depression.

Patient/Family Education
- Explain name, dose, action, and potential side effects of drug.
- Advise patient that dose may be increased slowly until max benefit is achieved and not to take more than prescribed or increase the dose more rapidly than advised.
- Instruct patient not to stop taking pimozide when symptoms improve.
- Tell patient to immediately report fainting or loss of consciousness, palpitations, high fever, muscle rigidity, involuntary body or facial movements, altered mental status, irregular pulse, sweating, or seizures to health care provider.
- Advise patient to avoid strenuous activity during periods of high temperature or humidity.
- Instruct patient to avoid alcoholic beverages, grapefruit juice, and grapefruit products.
- Advise patient to take sips of water, suck on ice chips or sugarless hard candy, or chew sugarless gum if dry mouth occurs.
- Advise patient that drug may impair mental or physical abilities and to use caution while driving or performing other tasks requiring mental alertness.
- Advise women to notify health care provider if pregnant, planning to become pregnant, or breastfeeding.
- Advise patient to notify health care provider of the following: excessive drowsiness, change in behavior, or rapid pulse.
- Instruct patient not to take any prescription or OTC medications or dietary supplements unless advised by health care provider.
- Advise patient that if a decision to withdraw therapy is made, not to stop the medication suddenly. Gradual withdrawal over several days to weeks may be necessary to prevent withdrawal symptoms.
- Advise patient that follow-up visits and lab tests, including ECGs, will be required to monitor therapy and to keep appointments.

Pindolol

(PIN-doe-lahl)
Class Beta-adrenergic blocker
How Supplied
Visken Tablets 5 mg, Tablets 10 mg
✤ Alti-Pindolol ♦ APO-Pindol ♦ Gen-Pindolol ♦ Novo-Pindol ♦ Nu-Pindol ♦ PMS-Pindolol

Action
PHARMACOLOGY: Nonselectively blocks beta receptors, which primarily affect heart (slows rate), vascular musculature (decreases blood pressure), and lungs (reduces function).
PHARMACOKINETICS/DYNAMICS:
Absorption: Rapidly and reproducibly absorbed (more than 95%). T_{max} is 1 hr. Bioavailability is approximately 100%.
Distribution: Protein binding is 40%. Evenly distributed between plasma red cells. Vd is 2 L/kg.
Metabolism: Metabolized in the liver (60% to 65%) as hydroxy metabolites.
Excretion: Urine (amount of dose excreted 60% to 65%; as unchanged 35% to 40%); feces (6% to 9%). $T_{1/2}$ is approximately 8 hr (polar metabolites). $T_{1/2}$ is 3 to 4 hr.
Special Populations:
Renal Function Impairment – 50% decreased in volume of distribution in uremic patients, generally excreted in less than 15% of dose as unchanged in the urine.
Hepatic Function Impairment – In cirrhosis patients, elimination was more variable in rate and slower, half-life ranged from 2.5 hr to more than 30 hr. Exercise caution; dosage adjustments may be necessary.
Elderly – In elderly hypertensive patients, the half-life is more variable, averaging 7 hr.

Indications Management of mild to moderate hypertension.

Contraindications Greater than first-degree heart block; CHF unless secondary to tachyarrhythmia treatable with beta-blockers; overt cardiac failure; sinus bradycardia; cardiogenic shock; hypersensitivity to beta-blockers; bronchial asthma or bronchospasm, including severe COPD.

Route/Dosage
ADULTS: PO 5 mg bid. May be increased by 10 mg q 3 to 4 wk until desired response; max dose is 60 mg/day.

Interactions
Clonidine: May enhance or reverse antihypertensive effect; potentially life-threatening situations may occur, especially on withdrawal.
Epinephrine: Initial hypertensive episode followed by bradycardia may occur.
Ergot derivatives: Peripheral ischemia, manifested by cold extremities and possible gangrene, may occur.
Insulin: Prolonged hypoglycemia with masking of symptoms may occur.
Lidocaine: Lidocaine levels may increase, leading to toxicity.
NSAIDs: Some agents may impair antihypertensive effect.
Prazosin: Orthostatic hypotension may be increased.
Theophyllines: Elimination of theophylline may be reduced. Also, effects of both drugs may be reduced by pharmacologic antagonism.
Verapamil: Effects of both drugs may be increased.

Lab Test Interferences None well documented.

Adverse Reactions
CV: Bradycardia; hypotension; CHF; edema; worsening angina.
CNS: Depression; visual disturbances; short-term memory loss; dizziness.
DERM: Skin rash; increased sensitivity to cold.
EENT: Dry eyes; visual disturbances.
GI: Nausea; vomiting; diarrhea.
GU: Impotence; urinary retention; difficulty with urination.
HEMA: Agranulocytosis.
HEPA: May increase AST or ALT; rarely increases LDH or alkaline phosphatase.
METAB: May increase or decrease blood glucose, uric acid.
RESP: Wheezing; bronchospasm; difficulty breathing (at higher doses).

Precautions
Pregnancy: Category B.
Lactation: Excreted in breast milk.
Children: Safety and efficacy not established.
Renal function impairment: Dosage may need to be reduced.
Hepatic function impairment: Dosage may need to be reduced.
Anaphylaxis: Deaths have occurred; aggressive therapy may be required.
CHF: Administer cautiously in CHF patients controlled with digitalis and diuretics. Notify health care provider at first sign or symptom of CHF or unexplained respiratory symptoms in any patient.
Diabetics: May mask signs and symptoms of hypoglycemia (eg, tachycardia, BP changes). May potentiate insulin-induced hypoglycemia.
Peripheral vascular disease: May precipitate or aggravate symptoms of arterial insufficiency.

Thyrotoxicosis: May mask clinical signs of developing or continuing hyperthyroidism (eg, tachycardia). Abrupt withdrawal may exacerbate symptoms of hyperthyroidism, including thyroid storm.

PATIENT CARE CONSIDERATIONS

Administration/Storage
- Give orally.
- Give medication at same time each day.
- May be taken without regard to meals.
- Store at room temperature and protect from moisture, light, and air.

Assessment/Interventions
- Obtain patient history, including drug history and any known allergies.
- Assess pulse and BP prior to initiation of therapy.
- Monitor BP, apical and radial pulses, I&O, daily weight, respiration, and circulation in extremities.
- Review baseline serum glucose level, results of hepatic and renal function studies, and monitor lab data throughout therapy.
- Monitor blood glucose closely for diabetic patients.
- Notify health care provider if symptoms of CHF occur (eg, difficulty breathing, cough, swelling in extremities).
- Report bothersome side effects to health care provider, especially new-onset depression.
- Reduce dose gradually upon discontinuation of therapy. Abrupt withdrawal is associated with adverse effects, including precipitation, or worsening of angina.

Patient/Family Education
- Teach patient and family technique for measuring BP and pulse rates and to keep written record.
- Instruct patient to notify health care provider if pulse rate is less than 50 bpm or systolic BP is less than 90 mm Hg.
- Warn patient not to engage in activities that require mental alertness until drug effects are apparent because it may cause blurred vision, drowsiness, and dizziness.
- Explain that decreased blood supply to extremities may cause patient to be more sensitive to cold temperatures.
- Encourage patients with diabetes to monitor blood glucose carefully.
- Advise patient to report the following symptoms to health care provider: any asthma-like symptoms, cough or nasal stuffiness, skin rash, fever, sore throat, unusual bleeding or bruising.
- Instruct patient not to take any OTC medications without consulting health care provider.
- Instruct patient to sit or lie down immediately if dizziness or faintness occurs.

Overdosage: Signs and Symptoms
Bradycardia, hypotension, seizures, respiratory depression.

Pioglitazone

(pye-oh-GLI-ta-zone)

Class Antidiabetic/Thiazolidinedione

How Supplied
Actos Tablet 15 mg, Tablet 30 mg, Tablet 45 mg

Action
PHARMACOLOGY: Increases insulin sensitivity in muscle, adipose tissue, and inhibits hepatic gluconeogenesis.

PHARMACOKINETICS/DYNAMICS:

Absorption: Rapid. T_{max} is 2 hr (3 to 4 hr if taken with food). Food slightly delays time to peak serum concentrations 3 to 4 hr. Steady state is 7 days.

Distribution: Vd is 0.63 L/kg (single dose). Protein binding is extensive (more than 99%); mainly albumin.

Metabolism: Extensively metabolized in the liver by hydroxylation and oxidation. The metabolites M-II (hydroxy derivative), M-IV (hydroxy derivative), and M-III (keto derivative) are active. The major isoforms involved include the CYP2C8, CYP3A4, and CYP1A1.

Excretion: Urine (15% to 30%, excreted primarily as metabolites). Bile (unchanged as metabolites) and then eliminated in the feces. Serum t½ is 3 to 7 hr (pioglitazone); 16 to 24 hr (pioglitazone and active metabolites). Apparent Cl is 5 to 7 L/hr.

Special Populations:

Hepatic Function Impairment – There is a 45% reduction in mean peak concentrations but no change in AUC values. Do not initiate therapy in these patients with active liver disease.

Elderly – AUC value is slightly higher; terminal t½ is slightly longer.

Gender – The mean C_{max} is increased 20% and the AUC increased 60% in women.

Indications Type 2 diabetes, as an adjunct to diet and exercise; also may be used in conjunction with a sulfonylurea, metformin, or insulin when diet, exercise, and a single agent alone does not result in adequate glycemic control in patients with type 2 diabetes mellitus.

Contraindications Standard considerations.

Route/Dosage
Monotherapy
PO Initially, 15 or 30 mg/day, up to 45 mg/day. If monotherapy is inadequate, consider combinations using same starting dose and adjust accordingly. May be given without regard to meals.

SULFONYLUREAS
Combination Therapy
ADULTS: PO In combination with sulfonylureas, the recommended dose of pioglitazone is 15 or 30 mg qd. If patient reports hypoglycemia, decrease the pioglitazone dose.

METFORMIN
Combination Therapy
ADULTS: PO In combination with metformin, pioglitazone may be initiated at 15 or 30 mg qd.

INSULIN
Combination Therapy
ADULTS: PO In combination with insulin, the recommended dose of pioglitazone is 15 or 30 mg qd. If the patient reports hypoglycemia or if plasma glucose concentrations decrease to less than 100 mg/dL, it is recommended that the insulin dose be decreased 10% to 25%. Individualize further adjustment based on glucose lowering response.

Interactions
Contraceptives, oral: Oral contraceptives may decrease both hormone components about 30%, potentially reducing contraceptive effectiveness.
P450 system: Cytochrome P450 isoform CYP3A4 is partially responsible for pioglitazone metabolism; therefore, other drugs affected by or affecting this system may interact.

Lab Test Interferences
Mean hemoglobin values may decline 2% to 4%, usually in first 4 to 12 wk of therapy, then stabilize; not associated with hematologic clinical effects.

Adverse Reactions
CV: CHF (postmarketing).
CNS: Headache (9%).
EENT: Pharyngitis (5%).
HEMA: Anemia (1%); decrease in hemoglobin and hematocrit.
METAB: Diabetes mellitus aggravated (8%).
RESP: Upper respiratory tract infection (13%); sinusitis (6%).
OTHER: Myalgia, edema (5%); tooth disorder, hypoglycemia (2%).

Precautions
Pregnancy: Category C.
Lactation: Undetermined.
Children: Safety and efficacy not established.
Hepatic function impairment: Related drugs have reported rare hepatotoxicity; monitor liver enzymes and symptoms.
Cardiac failure: Fluid retention may occur that may exacerbate or lead to heart failure.
Edema: Use caution, can cause fluid retention.
Ovulation: May result in ovulation in premenopausal anovulatory women; recommend contraception.
Weight gain: Dose-related weight gain has been seen alone and in combination with other hypoglycemic agents.

PATIENT CARE CONSIDERATIONS

Administration/Storage
- Do not administer to patients with clinical evidence of active liver disease or elevated liver enzymes (ALT above 2.5 × ULN) or to patients with type 1 diabetes mellitus.
- Administer dose qd, usually in the morning, with or without food.
- Store at controlled room temperature (59° to 86°F). Protect from moisture and humidity.

Assessment/Interventions
- Obtain patient history, including drug history and any known allergies. Note history of liver disease or CHF.
- Ensure that liver enzymes are determined before starting therapy and periodically during therapy (eg, q 2 mo for 1 yr, then periodically thereafter).
- Check blood sugar frequently and observe for signs of hypoglycemia and hyperglycemia; report to health care provider.

Patient/Family Education
- Explain name, dose, action, and potential side effects of drug.
- Advise patient to take qd without regard to meals.
- Educate patient, family, or caregiver regarding type 2 diabetes and its management.
- Instruct patient that this drug is not a substitute for diet and exercise and to follow prescribed regimens.
- Emphasize the importance of regular daily blood glucose monitoring and periodic glycosylated hemoglobin (HbA_{1c}) tests.
- Advise diabetic patient to carry medical identification (eg, *Medi-Alert*).
- Advise patient to report any of the following to health care provider immediately: nausea, vomiting, abdominal pain, fatigue, anorexia, dark urine, yellowing of skin or eyes.
- Review symptoms of hypoglycemia and hyperglycemia and action plans to undertake in the event either occur. Instruct patient to report hypoglycemic or hyperglycemic episodes to the health care provider.
- Advise patient that blood will be drawn to check liver function prior to starting therapy

and about q 2 mo for 1 yr and periodically thereafter. Remind patient to keep appointments.
- Caution women that drug can cause resumption of ovulation in premenopausal, anovulatory women with insulin resistance. Address adequate contraceptive measures for these women.
- Advise women to notify health care provider if pregnant, planning to become pregnant, or breastfeeding.
- Instruct patient not to take prescription or OTC drugs or dietary supplements without consulting health care provider.

Piperacillin Sodium

(PIH-per-uh-SILL-in SO-dee-uhm)

Class Antibiotic/Penicillin

How Supplied
Pipracil Powder for injection (contains 1.85 mEq [42.5 mg] sodium/g) 2 g, Powder for injection 3 g, Powder for injection 4 g, Powder for injection 40 g

Action
PHARMACOLOGY: Inhibits bacterial cell wall mucopeptide synthesis.

PHARMACOKINETICS/DYNAMICS:
Absorption: Not absorbed orally; rapidly absorbed IM. T_{max} is 30 min (IM) and immediately after completion (IV). C_{max} is 412 mcg/mL (IV).
Distribution: Widely distributed in human tissues and body fluids, including bone, prostate, and heart; reaches high concentrations in bile. Penetrates CSF in the presence of inflamed meninges. Protein binding is 16%. Vd is 0.23 L/kg. It crosses the placenta and distributes into breast milk.
Metabolism: Liver.
Excretion: Urine (60% to 80% unchanged), partially biliary. Serum t½ is 36 to 72 min; elimination t½ is 54 to 63 min.

Special Populations:
Renal Function Impairment – Elimination half-life is increased 2-fold in mild to moderate impairment, 5- to 6-fold in severe impairment.

Indications Treatment of intra-abdominal, urinary tract, gynecologic, lower respiratory tract infections, septicemia, skin and skin structure infections, bone and joint infections, and gonococcal urethritis; surgical prophylaxis; treatment of infection caused by susceptible microorganisms including infections caused by *Streptococcus* and *Pseudomonas* species.

Contraindications Hypersensitivity to penicillins or cephalosporins.

Route/Dosage
ADULTS: **IM/IV** 3 to 4 g q 4 to 6 hr (max, 24 g/day).
CHILDREN: **IM/IV** 200 to 500 mg/kg/day divided q 4 to 6 hr.
NEWBORNS: **IM/IV** 100 mg/kg/dose q 12 hr.

Interactions
Aminoglycosides, parenteral: May inactivate aminoglycosides in vitro; do not mix in same IV solution. May be used in combination for synergy.
Anticoagulants: May increase bleeding risks by prolonging bleeding time.
Chloramphenicol: Synergism or antagonism may develop.
Contraceptives, oral: May reduce efficacy of oral contraceptives. Use additional form of contraception during piperacillin therapy.
Erythromycin: Synergism or antagonism may develop.
Heparin: May increase bleeding risks of heparin by prolonging bleeding time.
Tetracyclines: May impair bactericidal effects of piperacillin.

Lab Test Interferences May cause false-positive urine glucose test results with *Benedict's* solution, *Fehling's* solution, or *Clinitest* tablets but not with enzyme-based tests (eg, *Clinistix*, *Tes-tape*); false-positive direct *Coombs'* test result in certain patient groups; positive direct antiglobulin tests; false-positive protein reactions with sulfosalicylic acid and boiling test, acetic acid test, biuret reaction and nitric acid test but not with the bromphenol blue test (*Multi-Stix*).

Adverse Reactions
CNS: Neurotoxicity (eg, lethargy, neuromuscular irritability, hallucinations, convulsions, seizures) especially with large dose or patient with renal failure; dizziness; fatigue; insomnia; reversible hyperactivity; prolonged muscle relaxation.
DERM: Ecchymosis.
EENT: Itchy eyes.
GI: Nausea; vomiting; abdominal pain or cramping; epigastric distress; diarrhea or bloody diarrhea; rectal bleeding; flatulence; enterocolitis; pseudomembranous colitis; anorexia.
GU: Interstitial nephritis (oliguria, proteinuria, hematuria, hyaline casts, pyuria); nephropathy; elevated creatinine or BUN; vaginitis; moniliasis.
HEMA: Anemia; hemolytic anemia; thrombocytopenia; thrombocytopenic purpura; eosinophilia; leukopenia; granulocytopenia; neutropenia; bone marrow depression; agranulocytosis;

reduced Hgb or Hct; prolongation of bleeding and prothrombin time; decrease in WBC and lymphocyte counts; increase in lymphocytes, monocytes, basophils, and platelets.
HEPA: Elevated AST or AST and bilirubin; transient hepatitis; cholestatic jaundice.
METAB: Elevated serum alkaline phosphatase; hypernatremia; hypokalemia, reduced albumin, total proteins, and uric acid.
OTHER: Hypersensitivity reactions (ie, urticaria, angioneurotic edema, laryngospasm, bronchospasm, hypotension, vascular collapse, death, maculopapular to exfoliative dermatitis, vesicular eruptions, erythema multiforme, serum sickness, laryngeal edema, skin rashes, prostration); vaginitis; hyperthermia; pain at site of injection; deep vein thrombosis; hematomas; vein irritation; phlebitis; hyperthermia; sciatic neuritis.

Precautions
Pregnancy: Category B.
Lactation: Excreted in breast milk.
Hypersensitivity: Reactions range from mild to life-threatening. Administer cautiously to cephalosporin-sensitive patients because of possible crossreactivity.
Renal function impairment: Dosage adjustment required.
Superinfection: May result in bacterial or fungal overgrowth of nonsusceptible organisms.
Bleeding abnormalities: Hemorrhagic manifestations associated with abnormalities of coagulation tests (bleeding time, prothrombin time, platelet aggregation) may occur. Abnormalities should revert to normal once drug is discontinued.
Cystic fibrosis patients: May experience higher incidence of side effects when treated with piperacillin.
Pseudomembranous colitis: May occur caused by overgrowth of clostridia.

Overdosage: Signs and Symptoms
Agitation, confusion, asterixis, hallucinations, stupor, coma, seizures, hyperexcitability.

PATIENT CARE CONSIDERATIONS

Administration/Storage
- Obtain culture and sensitivity before administering first dose.
- IM or IV route.
- For IM use, dilute to 1 g/2.5 mL. Lidocaine (0.5% to 1%) may be used to dilute (for IM use only).
- Do not give greater than 2 g IM at any one site.
- For IV injection, reconstitute each gram with greater than or equal to 5 mL compatible diluent.
- IV infusion is diluted further with 50 to 100 mL of D5W or normal saline and infused over 20 to 30 min.
- Time doses for even distribution throughout 24 hours.

Assessment/Interventions
- Obtain patient history, including drug history and any known allergies.
- Assess for drug reactions especially in patients with asthma, hay fever, urticaria, or allergy to cephalosporins.
- Assess baseline CBC and liver and renal function study results prior to initiating therapy and monitor throughout therapy.
- Monitor results of diagnostic cultures and sensitivity tests.
- Monitor patient for at least 20 min after administering penicillin to observe for signs or symptoms of anaphylaxis. Notify health care provider if skin rash, hives, wheezing, nausea, or vomiting occur.

Patient/Family Education
- Instruct patient to notify health care provider if symptoms of potential superinfection (eg, nausea/vomiting, diarrhea, black tongue, swollen joints, unusual bleeding or bruising) occur.
- Explain signs and symptoms of allergic reaction (eg, hives, wheezing, skin rash, itching) and importance of seeking medical supervision as soon as possible.
- Emphasize need for good hygiene to avoid superinfections.
- If patient develops allergy to piperacillin, advise patient to notify future caregivers of penicillin allergy and patient should wear *Medi-Alert* identification.

Piperacillin Sodium/Tazobactam Sodium

(PIH-per-uh-SILL-in SO-dee-uhm/TAZZ-oh-BACK-tam SO-dee-uhm Zosyn)

Class Extended spectrum penicillin

How Supplied
Zosyn Powder for Injection 2 g piperacillin, 0.25 g tazobactam, Powder for Injection 3 g piperacillin, 0.375 g tazobactam, Powder for Injection 4 g piperacillin, 0.5 g tazobactam, Powder for Injection 36 g piperacillin, 4.5 g tazobactam (bulk), Solution 2 g piperacillin, 0.25 g tazobactam, Solution 3 g piperacillin, 0.375 g tazobactam, Solution 4 g piperacillin, 0.5 g tazobactam

Action
PHARMACOLOGY: Inhibits bacterial cell wall mucopeptide synthesis.

Indications
Treatment of moderate to severe infections caused by piperacillin-resistant piperacillin/tazobactam-susceptible, β-lactamase producing strains of microorganisms in the following conditions: appendicitis (complicated by rupture or abscess); uncomplicated and complicated skin and skin structure infections; postpartum endometritis or pelvic inflammatory disease; community-acquired pneumonia (moderate severity only); nosocomial pneumonia (moderate to severe).

Contraindications
History of allergic reactions to penicillins, cephalosporins, or β-lactamase inhibitors; hypersensitivity to any component of the product.

Route/Dosage
Administer by IV infusion over 30 min.

Normal Renal Function (Ccr 90 mL/min or more)
ADULTS: **IV** 3.375 g q 6 hr totaling 13.5 g (12 g piperacillin/1.5 g tazobactam) for 7 to 10 days.

Nosocomial Pneumonia
ADULTS: **IV** Start with 4.5 g q 6 hr plus an aminoglycoside (administered separately) for 7 to 14 days.

Renal Insufficiency
ADULTS: **IV** Ccr greater than 40 mL/min: 3.375 g q 6 hr (all indications), and 4.5 g q 6 hr (nosocomial pneumonia). Cr 20 to 40 mL/min: 2.25 g q 6 hr (all indications), and 3.375 g q 6 hr (nosocomial pneumonia). Ccr 20 mL/min or less: 2.25 g q 8 hr (all indications), and 2.25 g q 6 hr (nosocomial pneumonia).

Hemodialysis
ADULTS: **IV** Max dose 2.25 g q 8 hr for nosocomial pneumonia and q 12 hr for other indications plus 1 additional dose of 0.75 g following each dialysis period.

Interactions
Aminoglycosides: May form microbiologically inactive complexes and should not be mixed in the same container.
Anticoagulants: Frequently monitor coagulation parameters.
Methotrexate: May reduce Cl.
Probenecid: Increases and prolongs half-life penicillin levels.
Vecuronium: Neuromuscular blockade may be prolonged.
INCOMPATIBILITIES: Lactated Ringers solution.

Lab Test Interferences
False-positive reaction for glucose in the urine using a copper-reduction method (eg, *Clinitest*).

Adverse Reactions
CV: Hypertension; chest pain; cardiac arrest; hypotension; supraventricular tachycardia; syncope; bradycardia; atrial and ventricular fibrillation; MI.
CNS: Headache; insomnia; agitation; dizziness; anxiety; confusion; convulsions.
DERM: Rash (including maculopapular, bullous, urticarial and eczematous); pruritus.
EENT: Rhinitis.
GI: Diarrhea; nausea; vomiting; constipation; dyspepsia; stool changes; abdominal pain; oral thrush; hiccough; duodenal ulcer; flatulence; pancreatitis; anorexia.
GU: Urinary incontinence, UTI.
HEMA: Thrombocytopenia; thrombocythemia.
METAB: Fluid overload; BUN increased; creatinine increased.
RESP: Pleural effusion; pneumothorax; pulmonary edema.
OTHER: Allergy; phlebitis; injection site reactions (including pain, inflammation, edema, thrombophlebitis); fever; moniliasis; diaphoresis; abnormal liver function tests.

Precautions
Pregnancy: Category B.
Lactation:
Piperacillin – Excreted in low concentrations in human milk.
Tazobactam – Undetermined.
Children: Safety and efficacy not established.
Hypersensitivity: Serious and sometimes fatal hypersensitivity reactions have occurred.
Renal function impairment: Adjust dose accordingly.
Superinfection: Prolonged use of antibiotics may result in bacterial or fungal overgrowth of nonsusceptible microorganisms.
Pseudomembranous colitis: May occur because of overgrowth of clostridium difficile; consider the possibility in patients in whom diarrhea develops.

Overdosage: Signs and Symptoms
Neuromuscular excitability, convulsions, nausea, vomiting, diarrhea.

PATIENT CARE CONSIDERATIONS

Administration/Storage

- For IV administration only. Do not administer intradermally, SC, or IM.
- Multiple concentrations are available. Ensure the proper concentration is being used.
- Reconstitute powder for injection following manufacturer's recommendations.
- Dilute reconstituted solution following manufacturer's recommendations before administration.
- Do not administer if solution is cloudy, discolored, or contains particulate matter.
- Administer prescribed dose by IV infusion over a period of at least 30 min.
- Do not mix with other IV medications.
- Use reconstituted solutions immediately. Discard any unused portion after 24 hr if stored at room temperature (68° to 77°F) or after 48 hr if stored in refrigerator (36° to 46°F).
- Store vials at controlled room temperature (68° to 77°F) prior to reconstitution.

Assessment/Interventions

- Obtain patient history, including drug history and any known allergies, especially to penicillins, cephalosporins, and β-lactamase inhibitors. Note history of renal impairment, asthma, or multiple allergies.
- Administer reduced dose to patient with renal impairment.
- Ensure that culture and susceptibility test results indicate sensitivity to medication.
- Ensure that medication is discontinued and another antimicrobial agent is started if culture and sensitivity tests indicate that the infection is resistant to piperacillin/tazobactam.
- Ensure that WBC and differential are determined prior to starting therapy and periodically during therapy.
- Monitor for signs of infection, especially fever, and for positive response to antibiotic therapy.
- Monitor patient for signs of anaphylaxis or severe allergic reaction. If noted discontinue therapy and immediately notify health care provider. Be prepared to treat appropriately.
- Notify health care provider if any of the following occurs: severe diarrhea, loose, foul-smelling stools.

Patient/Family Education

- Explain name, dose, action, and potential side effects of drug.
- Explain to patient or caregiver that medication will be prepared and administered by a health care provider in a health care setting.
- Review dosing schedule and prescribed length of therapy with patient. Advise patient that dose and duration of therapy are dependent on site and cause of infection and response to therapy.
- Instruct patient to report the following to health care provider: itching; rash; hives; difficulty breathing; diarrhea; loose, foul-smelling stools; injection site reaction.
- Advise patient that follow-up visits and lab tests may be needed to monitor therapy and to keep appointments.

Pirbuterol Acetate

(pihr-BYOO-tuh-role ASS-uh-TATE)

Class Bronchodilator/Sympathomimetic

How Supplied

Maxair Autohaler Aerosol 0.2 mg/actuation

Action

PHARMACOLOGY: Produces bronchodilation by relaxing bronchial smooth muscle through beta-2 receptor stimulation.

PHARMACOKINETICS/DYNAMICS:

Absorption: Rapidly absorbed following aerosol administration.

Excretion: 51% of the dose is excreted in the urine plus its sulfate conjugate. T½ and plasma is approximately 2 hr (oral).

Onset: 5 min (inhalation).

Duration: 5 hr (inhalation).

Indications

Prevention and treatment of reversible bronchospasm associated with asthma or other obstructive pulmonary diseases.

Contraindications

Hypersensitivity to drug components; cardiac arrhythmias associated with tachycardia.

Route/Dosage

ADULTS AND CHILDREN 12 YR AND OLDER:
Inhalation 1 to 2 inhalations q 4 to 6 hr; not to exceed 12 inhalations/day.

Interactions

MAO inhibitors, tricyclic antidepressants: May increase the effects of pirbuterol.

Lab Test Interferences

None well documented.

Adverse Reactions

CV: Palpitations; tachycardia; BP changes; chest tightness/pain/discomfort; angina; arrhythmias/skipped beats.
CNS: Tremor; anxiety; confusion; fatigue; dizziness; nervousness; headache; weakness; hyperactivity/hyperkinesia/excitement; insomnia.
EENT: Dry nose; throat irritation.

GI: GI distress; dry mouth; diarrhea; nausea/vomiting.
RESP: Cough; throat irritation.
OTHER: Flushing; anorexia/appetite loss; unusual/bad taste; taste/smell change.

Precautions
Pregnancy: Category C.
Lactation: Undetermined.
Children: Safety and efficacy in children 12 yr and younger not established.
Elderly: Lower doses may be required.
Labor and delivery: May inhibit uterine contractions and delay preterm labor.
Cardiovascular effects: Toxic symptoms in patients with cardiovascular disorders may occur.

CNS effects: CNS stimulation may occur; use cautiously in patients with history of seizure or hyperthyroidism.
Diabetes: Dosage adjustment of insulin or oral hypoglycemic agent may be required.
Excessive use: Paradoxical bronchospasm and cardiac arrest have been associated with excessive inhalant use.
Hypokalemia: Decreases in potassium levels have occurred.
Tolerance: If previously effective dose fails to provide relief therapy may need to be reassessed.

Overdosage: Signs and Symptoms
Tremor, palpitations, tachycardia, elevated blood pressure, anginal pain, hypokalemia, seizures.

PATIENT CARE CONSIDERATIONS
Administration/Storage
- Give pressurized inhalation during second half of breath intake.
- If more than 1 inhalation is needed, wait 1 to 2 min before administering second dose.
- Discard any discolored solutions of drug.
- Store at room temperature in light-resistant container.

Assessment/Interventions
- Obtain patient history, including drug history and any known allergies.
- Obtain baseline ABGs prior to initiation of therapy.
- Assess BP and pulse before and after each dose.
- Assess for CNS response, and adjust dose and frequency accordingly.
- To prevent respiratory depression, administer oxygen based on ABGs and symptoms.
- Assess vital capacity and forced expiratory volume.
- If 3 to 5 aerosol treatments have been given within 6 to 12 hr with minimal relief, notify health care provider and do not give further treatment.

Patient/Family Education
- Advise patient to take drug early in day to prevent insomnia.
- Explain that implementing therapy in morning and after meals may reduce fatigue and improve lung ventilation.
- Encourage patient to increase fluid intake to help liquify secretions.
- Tell patient to report the following symptoms to health care provider: Dizziness, chest pain, palpitations, muscle spasms, headache, difficult urination, dyspnea or nervous tremor.
- Explain that if no relief is obtained from normal daily dose, call health care provider instead of increasing dose. Also if more than 3 aerosol treatments are needed in 24 hr, notify health care provider.
- Tell patient to wait at least 1 to 2 min before administering second inhalation.
- Instruct patient that regular, consistent use of medication is required for maximum benefits.
- Explain benefits of and demonstrate technique for postural drainage and chest vibration.
- Instruct patient not to take any OTC medications without consulting health care provider.
- Emphasize that it is important to avoid getting aerosol medication in eyes.
- Tell patient to avoid smoking, smoke-filled rooms, and persons with respiratory infections.
- Explain how to use and care for inhalers and any other respiratory equipment.

Piroxicam

(pihr-OX-ih-kam)
Class Analgesic/NSAID

How Supplied
Feldene Capsules 10 mg, Capsules 20 mg
🍁 *Alti-Piroxicam* ♦ *Apo-Piroxicam* ♦ *Gen-Piroxicam* ♦ *Novo-Pirocam* ♦ *Nu-Pirox*

Action
PHARMACOLOGY: Decreases inflammation, pain, and fever, probably through inhibition of cyclooxygenase activity and prostaglandin synthesis.

PHARMACOKINETICS/DYNAMICS:
Absorption: Slight delay in the rate of absorption with food. Steady state is 7 to 12 days, up to 2 to 3 wk. T_{max} is 3 to 5 hr. Well absorbed. C_{max} is 3 to 8 mcg/mL (multiple doses), 1.5 to 2 mcg/mL (single doses).

Distribution: Vd is 0.14 L/kg. Protein binding is 99%. Excreted in breast milk.

Metabolism: In the liver by hydroxylation; no active metabolites.

Excretion: $T_{1/2}$ is approximately 50 hr. Eliminated primarily in the urine, small amount in feces; 5% excreted unchanged.

Peak: Therapeutic effect is 3 to 5 hr.

Special Populations:
Hepatic Function Impairment – Effect not established; however, the drug is extensively metabolized in the liver and may require reduced doses.

Indications Treatment of acute or long-term use of rheumatoid arthritis and osteoarthritis.

Unlabeled use(s): Symptomatic relief of primary dysmenorrhea, pain, sunburn, juvenile rheumatoid arthritis.

Contraindications Known allergy or hypersensitivity to aspirin, iodides, or any NSAID, including piroxicam.

Route/Dosage
Rheumatoid Arthritis, Osteoarthritis
ADULTS: **PO** Initiate and maintain at 20 mg/day in 1 to 2 divided doses.

Interactions
Alcohol: May augment risk of GI bleeding.
Anticoagulants: May increase effect of anticoagulants because of decreased plasma protein binding and inhibition of platelet aggregation. May increase risk of gastric erosion and bleeding.
Beta-blockers: Antihypertensive effect may be decreased.
Cholestyramine: Effects of piroxicam may be decreased.
Lithium: May decrease lithium clearance.
Methotrexate: May increase methotrexate levels and toxicity.
Ritonivir: May increase concentrations and possibly the toxicity of piroxicam by inhibiting its metabolism.

Lab Test Interferences May prolong bleeding time. May reversibly increase BUN and serum creatinine.

Adverse Reactions
CV: Edema; weight gain; CHF; alterations in BP; vasodilation; palpitations; tachycardia.
CNS: Headache; malaise; dizziness; somnolence; vertigo; depression; insomnia; nervousness.
DERM: Pruritus; rash; sweating; erythema; bruising; desquamation; erythema multiforme; toxic epidermal necrolysis.
EENT: Tinnitus; swollen eyes; blurred vision; eye irritation; rhinitis; pharyngitis.
GI: Epigastric distress; nausea; vomiting; anorexia; constipation; stomatitis; abdominal discomfort; diarrhea; flatulence; abdominal pain; indigestion; toxicity (bleeding, ulceration, perforation); heartburn; dyspepsia; anorexia.
GU: Hematuria; proteinuria; increased BUN and serum creatinine; acute renal insufficiency and failure; papillary necrosis; interstitial nephritis; nephrotic syndrome; hyperkalemia; hyponatremia.
HEMA: Increased bleeding time; decreased Hgb and Hct; anemia; leukopenia; eosinophilia, thrombocytopenia.
HEPA: Increased LFTs; elevated liver enzymes.
RESP: Bronchospasm; laryngeal edema; dyspnea; hemoptysis; shortness of breath.

Precautions
Pregnancy: Category C.
Lactation: Undetermined.
Children: Safety and efficacy not established.
Elderly: Increased risk of adverse reactions. May require decreased dosage.
Asthma: In certain patients (aspirin-allergic, nasal polyps) may precipitate asthma attacks.
Cardiovascular disease: May worsen CHF and hypertension.
Coagulation disorders: Increases risk of bleeding.
Dermatologic effects: Combination of dermatologic/allergic signs and symptoms (ie, arthralgias, pruritus, fever, fatigue, rash including vesiculobullous reactions, exfoliative dermatitis) suggestive of serum sickness have occurred.
GI effects: Serious GI toxicity can occur at any time, with or without warning symptoms.
Renal disease: Drug may accumulate, increasing the risk of toxicity. In cases of advanced kidney disease, treatment with piroxicam is not recommended.

Overdosage: Signs and Symptoms
Drowsiness, dizziness, mental confusion, disorientation, lethargy, paresthesia, numbness, vomiting, GI irritation, headache, tinnitus, seizure, increased BUN.

PATIENT CARE CONSIDERATIONS
Administration/Storage
- Give after meals to reduce GI effects.
- Store at room temperature.

Assessment/Interventions
- Obtain patient history, including drug history and any known allergies.
- Obtain baseline vital signs, weight, and lab results and monitor throughout therapy.
- Notify health care provider of any changes in creatinine and electrolyte values and of any signs of renal or liver dysfunction, bleeding, GI discomfort, or vision changes.

Patient/Family Education
- Explain that increased response may be seen after weeks of therapy.
- Caution patient to avoid exposure to sunlight, and to use sunscreen or wear protective clothing to avoid photosensitivity reaction.

- Identify signs and symptoms patient should report to health care provider, including changes in how food tastes, nausea, vomiting, constipation, diarrhea, cramping, black or red stool, discolored urine, changes in urination, fever, rash, unusual bruising or bleeding.
- Explain that taking medication with food will minimize GI distress.
- Inform patient to avoid aspirin and alcohol during therapy.
- Instruct patient not to take any OTC medications without consulting health care provider.
- Advise patient that drug may cause drowsiness and to use caution while driving or performing other tasks requiring mental alertness until the effects of the drug are known.
- Encourage patient to maintain adequate fluid intake.

Pneumococcal Vaccine, Polyvalent

(new-moe-KAH-kuhl vaccine)

Class Vaccine, inactivated bacteria

How Supplied
Pneumovax 23 Injection 25 mcg each of 23 polysaccharide isolates/0.5 mL dose ♦ *Pnu-Imune 23* Injection 25 mcg each of 23 polysaccharide isolates/0.5 mL dose

Action
PHARMACOLOGY: Induces antibodies against 23 capsular types of *Streptococcus pneumoniae*. Type-specific antibody facilitates bacterial destruction by complement-mediated lysis.

Indications Protection against pneumococcal pneumonia, pneumococcal bacteremia, and other pneumococcal infections.

Contraindications Patients with Hodgkin disease who have received extensive chemotherapy or nodal irradiation; patients with Hodgkin disease cannot have immunization less than 10 days before or during chemotherapy; children under 2 yr. Some packages contain thimerosal as preservative; use cautiously in mercury-sensitive patients or choose different brand.

Route/Dosage
ADULTS AND CHILDREN: **SC/IM** 0.5 mL. Booster dose: Revaccinate recipients of 14-valent pneumococcal vaccine (distributed from 1977 to 1983) who are also at highest risk of fatal pneumococcal infection (eg, asplenic patients), using 23-valent vaccine. Revaccinate adults who received 23-valent vaccine 6 or more yr earlier if they also are at highest risk or are likely to have rapid decline in antibody levels (eg, patients with asplenia, nephrotic syndrome, or renal failure; transplant recipients). Consider revaccination of children with nephrotic syndrome, asplenia or sickle-cell anemia after 3 to 5 yr, if these children would be under 10 yr at time of revaccination.

Interactions In patients anticipating immunosuppression, response to pneumococcal vaccine is best if administered 10 to 14 days prior to immunosuppressive chemotherapy or radiation. Pneumococcal and influenza vaccines and HIB, meningococcal and pneumococcal vaccines safely and effectively may be administered simultaneously at separate injection sites. As with other drugs administered by IM injection, give pneumococcal vaccine with caution to patients receiving anticoagulant therapy.

Lab Test Interferences None well documented.

Adverse Reactions
LOCAL: Erythema and soreness at injection site, usually less than 48 hr in duration. Local induration occurs less commonly.
SYST: Rash, arthralgia, adenitis, fever higher than 39°C (102°F), malaise myalgia, and asthenia occur rarely. Low-grade fever (under 38.3°C or 100.9°F) occurs occasionally and usually subsides within 24 hr. Patients with otherwise stabilized immune thrombocytopenic purpura may rarely experience relapse in thrombocytopenia, 2 to 14 days after vaccination lasting up to 2 wk. Anaphylactoid reactions rarely reported.

Precautions
Pregnancy: Category C. Vaccinate if risk of disease outweighs risk to patients.
Lactation: Undetermined.

PATIENT CARE CONSIDERATIONS

Administration/Storage
- Administer via SC or IM route only.
- Keep medication under refrigeration.

Assessment/Interventions
- Obtain patient history, including drug history and any known allergies. Note if patient is receiving immunosuppressive therapy or scheduled for surgery. Administer vaccine 2 or more wk prior to these procedures when possible.
- If needed, give 1 dose of acetaminophen to reduce pain at injection site and to prevent fever.

Patient/Family Education
- Instruct parents on risks and benefits of vaccination.
- Explain that tepid bath may reduce pain at injection site.
- Advise parents to complete all immunizations.
- Explain that low-grade fever is transient and should subside in 24 hr.
- Tell patient or parents to notify health care provider immediately if any serious adverse reactions occur (eg, shortness of breath, hives, wheezing).
- This vaccine is usually only needed once.

Pneumococcal 7-Valent Conjugate Vaccine

(new-moe-KAH-kuhl 7-valent conjugate vaccine)

Class Vaccine, bacterial

How Supplied
Prevnar Injection 2 mcg each of 6 polysaccharide isolates; 4 mcg of 1 polysaccharide isolate per 0.5 mL dose

Action
PHARMACOLOGY: Induces antibodies against (4, 6B, 9V, 14, 18C, 19F, and 23F) serotypes of *Streptococcus pneumoniae*, which are directly conjugated to the protein carrier CRM_{197} to form glycoconjugate.

Indications Active immunization of infants and toddlers against *Streptococcus pneumoniae*; active immunization of infants and toddlers against otitis media caused by serotypes included in the vaccine.

Contraindications Severe or moderate febrile illness; hypersensitivity to any component of the product.

Route/Dosage
Preferred sites of IM injection are the anterolateral aspect of the thigh in infants or deltoid muscle of the upper arm in toddlers and young children.

Vaccination schedule
CHILDREN AT LEAST 24 MO THROUGH 9 YR: **IM** 3 doses of 0.5 mL each, at approximately 2-mo intervals, followed by a fourth dose of 0.5 mL at 12 to 15 mo of age. Usually the first dose is at 2 mo of age; however, it can be given as young as 6 wk. The recommended dosing interval is 4 to 8 wk. Administer the fourth dose at least 2 mo after the third dose.

Previously Unvaccinated Older Infants and Children Beyond Age of Routine Infant Schedule
CHILDREN AT LEAST 24 MO THROUGH 9 YR: **IM** 1 dose of 0.5 mL.

CHILDREN 12 TO 23 MO: **IM** 2 doses of 0.5 mL at least 2 mo apart.
CHILDREN 7 TO 11 MO: **IM** 3 doses of 0.5 mL, administer 2 doses at least 4 wk apart and the third dose after the 1-yr birthday, separated from the second dose by at least 2 mo.

Interactions
Immunosuppressive agents (large amounts of corticosteroids, antimetabolites, alkylating agents, cytotoxic agents): Children may not respond optimally to active immunization.

Lab Test Interferences None well documented.

Adverse Reactions
CNS: Irritability; drowsiness; restless sleep.
DERM: Urticaria-like rash; erythema multiforme.
GI: Decreased appetite; vomiting; diarrhea.
OTHER: Fever; injection site reactions (including edema, pain or tenderness, redness, inflammation, skin discoloration, mass, local hypersensitivity reaction, dermatitis, urticaria, pruritus); hypersensitivity (including face edema, dyspnea, bronchospasm, anaphylactic or anaphylactoid reaction [including shock]); lymphadenopathy at region of injection site; angioneurotic edema.

Precautions
Pregnancy: Category C.
Lactation: Undetermined.
Children: Safety and efficacy not established in children under 6 wk of age or after the tenth birthday.
Elderly: Not recommended for use in adult population.
Efficacy: Will not protect against *S. pneumoniae* disease other than that caused by the 7 serotypes included in the vaccine.
Immunocompromised patients: Pneumococcal 7-valent conjugate vaccine does not replace the 23-valient pneumococcal polysaccharide vaccination in children at least 24 mo with sickle cell disease, asplenia, HIV infection, chronic illness or those who are immunocompromised.
Latex sensitivity: Use with caution because packaging contains dry natural rubber.

PATIENT CARE CONSIDERATIONS
Administration/Storage
- For IM injection only. Not for IV, SC, or intradermal administration.
- Do not administer to infants less than 6 wk or individuals 10 yr or older.
- Vaccination regimen consists of 3 doses, at approximately 2 mo intervals (4 to 8 wk), followed by a fourth dose at 12 to 15 mo of age (at least 2 mo after the third dose). First dose is usually administered at 2 mo of age but can be given as young as 6 wk.
- Follow manufacturer's recommendations for immunizing previously unvaccinated older infants and children.
- Can be administered simultaneously with DTP-HbOC or DtaP and HbOC, OPV or IPV, hepatitis B, MMR, and varicella vaccine.
- Use vaccine as supplied; no dilution or reconstitution is necessary.
- Shake vial vigorously immediately prior to use to obtain a uniform suspension.
- Examine vial after shaking. Suspension should be homogeneous and white. Do not use if particulate matter or discoloration are noted of if vaccine cannot be resuspended.
- Administer immediately after drawing vaccine into syringe.
- Administer IM into anterolateral thigh in infants or the deltoid muscle of the upper arm in toddlers and young children. Avoid injection into gluteal area or areas where there may be a major nerve trunk or blood vessel.
- Always record manufacturer's name and vaccine lot number in patient's permanent medical record file along with date of administration, and name and title of person administering vaccine.
- Store vials in refrigerator (36° to 46°F). Do not freeze.

Assessment/Interventions
- Obtain patient history, including drug history and any known allergies. Note history of the following: latex sensitivity anticoagulant therapy; bleeding disorder; thrombocytopenia.
- Check patient's immunization history to verify that administration regimen is being followed.
- Consider delaying immunization during course of moderate or severe acute febrile illness.
- Monitor patient for signs of anaphylaxis or severe allergic reaction. Discontinue therapy and immediately notify health care provider if noted. Be prepared to treat appropriately.

Patient/Family Education
- Explain name, action, and potential side effects of vaccine.
- Advise parent or guardian that vaccine provides protection against the 7 most common and serious bacterial infections in infants and toddlers but does not provide protection from other causes of bacterial infection.
- Review immunization schedule and advise parent or guardian that entire series must be completed to provide maximum benefit.
- Provide parent or guardian with immunization history record.
- Advise parent or guardian to use OTC analgesics (eg, acetaminophen or ibuprofen) for fever, pain, or discomfort at injection site.
- Advise parent or guardian to notify health care provider if bothersome side effects last more than 24 hr.

Poliovirus Vaccine, Live, Oral, Trivalent (OPV)

(POE-lee-oh-VYE-russ vaccine)

Class Vaccine, live virus

How Supplied
Orimune Suspension, oral Mixture of 3 viruses (Types 1, 2, and 3) propagated in monkey kidney tissue culture

Action
PHARMACOLOGY: Induces protective antibodies, reducing intestinal and pharyngeal excretion of poliovirus. OPV administration simulates natural infection, inducing active mucosal and systemic immunity against poliovirus types 1, 2, and 3.

Indications Prevention of poliomyelitis. Infants as young as 6 to 12 wk and all unimmunized children and adolescents up to 18 yr are usual candidates for routine OPV prophylaxis. OPV is also recommended for control of epidemic poliomyelitis. If less than 4 wk remain before protection is needed, single dose of OPV is recommended, with remaining vaccine doses given later if person remains at increased risk. Immunization with IPV may be indicated for unimmunized parents and those in other special situations in which protection may be needed. In household with immunocompromised member or other close contacts or in household with unimmunized adult, use only IPV for all those requiring poliovirus immunization.

Adults: Primary immunization with inactivated polio vaccine is recommended whenever feasible for unimmunized adults subject to increased risk of exposure, such as by travel to or contact with epidemic or endemic areas (eg, developing countries) and for those employed in medical and sanitation facilities.

Contraindications Do not administer OPV to any person with immunosuppression or to any household member of immunodeficient person. This includes combined immunodeficiency, hypogammaglobulinemia, agammaglobulinemia, thymic abnormalities, leukemia, lymphoma, generalized malignancy, and lowered resistance to infection from therapy with corticosteroids, alkylating drugs, antimetabolites, or radiation. Advise vaccine recipients to avoid contact with such persons for at least 6 to 8 wk. Do not give OPV to member of household in which there is family history of immunodeficiency until immune status of intended recipient and other children in family is determined to be normal. IPV is preferred for immunizing all persons in these circumstances.

Route/Dosage

OLDER CHILDREN, ADOLESCENTS AND ADULTS: PO 0.5 mL. Give 2 doses no less than 6 wk apart (or 8 wk apart or less) followed by third dose 6 to 12 mo later.

INFANTS: PO 0.5 mL. Administer at 2, 4, and 15 to 18 mo. A fourth dose is given when child begins school if third dose of primary series was administered before child's fourth birthday. OPV may be administered with any of following: distilled water, chlorinated tap water, simple syrup, milk, bread, sugar cube, cake.

Interactions Immune globulin (IG) does not interfere with immunity following OPV. However, do not administer OPV less than 7 days after IG administration unless unavoidable, such as unexpected travel to or contact with epidemic or endemic areas or persons. If OPV is given within 1 wk after IG, the OPV dose should probably be repeated 3 mo later, if immunity is still needed. Like all live viral vaccines, administration to patients or contacts of patients receiving immunosuppressant drugs, including steroids or radiation may predispose patients to disseminated infections or insufficient response to immunization. They may remain susceptible despite immunization. Several routine pediatric vaccines may safely and effectively be administered simultaneously at separate injection sites (eg, DTP, MMR, IPV, Hib, hepatitis B, influenza). National authorities recommend simultaneous immunization at separate sites as indicated by age or health risk. Live virus vaccines may cause delayed-hypersensitivity skin test results (eg, tuberculin, histoplasmin) to appear falsely negative. Effect may persist for several weeks after vaccination. Give tuberculin tests either prior to live-virus vaccination, simultaneously with it, or at least 6 wk after vaccination.

Lab Test Interferences None well documented.

Adverse Reactions

OTHER: Vaccine-associated paralysis occurs with frequency of 1 case per 2.6 million OPV vaccine doses distributed.

Precautions

Pregnancy: Category C. Use OPV in pregnancy if exposure is imminent and immediate protection is needed.

Lactation: Breastfeeding does not generally interfere with successful immunization of infants, despite IgA antibody secretion in breast milk.

Immunodeficient patients: Do not use OPV in immunodeficient people, including people with congenital or acquired immune deficiencies, whether because of genetics, disease, drug or radiation therapy. Contains live viruses. Avoid use in HIV-positive persons, regardless of whether symptomatic or asymptomatic. Poliovirus is shed for 6 to 8 wk in vaccinee's stool and by pharyngeal route.

PATIENT CARE CONSIDERATIONS

Administration/Storage

- Give medication orally.
- Administer directly or mix with distilled water, plain tap water, syrup, milk, or sugar cube. Changes in color of product are of no significance as long as product remains clear.
- Store in freezer. Drug may remain in liquid state to -14°C (7°F) because of sorbitol content.
- If frozen, vaccine must be thawed completely before use.
- Follow recommended schedule for immunization (2, 4, 15 or 18 mo and at 4 to 6 yr).
- Discard poliovirus pipettes in manner that will inactivate live virus (eg, autoclave, incinerator).
- Max of 10 freeze-thaw cycles are permitted provided that (1) temperature dose not exceed 8° C (46°F) and (2) vaccine remains thawed for no more than 24 hr total.

Assessment/Interventions

- Obtain patient history, including drug history and any known allergies.
- Note if patient has had hypersensitivity test within 48 hr. Live virus could cause false-negative result.
- Document manufacturer, lot number, date of administration, name, address, and title of person administering on patient's chart.
- Adhere to guidelines of Vaccine Adverse Event Reporting System for reporting adverse effects (800-822-7967).

Patient/Family Education
- Advise women to abstain from breastfeeding 2 to 3 hr before and after vaccination of infants to permit establishment of viruses in gut.
- Explain risks and benefits of vaccination. Point out to parents or patient that vaccine produces protective antibodies against poliomyelitis.
- Tell parents that child should receive dose at 2, 4, and 15 or 18 mo and at 4 to 6 yr to be fully immunized.
- Explain that attenuated live virus vaccine may be shed for a few weeks following vaccination. This virus is not harmful to normal individuals but may cause disease in immunocompromised patients. Therefore vaccine recipient must stay away from immunocompromised individuals.

Poliovirus Vaccine, Inactivated (IPV)

(POE-lee-oh-VYE-russ vaccine)

Class Vaccine, inactivated virus

How Supplied
IPOL Injection Suspension of 3 types of poliovirus (Types 1, 2, and 3) grown in monkey kidney cell cultures

Action
PHARMACOLOGY: Induces protective antipoliovirus antibodies, reducing pharyngeal excretion of poliovirus types 1, 2, and 3.

Indications Routine use in infants and children is not recommended; OPV is generally preferred. Prophylaxis for individuals traveling to regions where poliomyelitis is endemic or epidemic (eg, developing countries), who routinely are exposed to patients who may be excreting polioviruses or to laboratory specimens that may contain polioviruses, and for members of communities with disease caused by wild polioviruses. Offer IPV to individuals who decline OPV or in whom OPV is contraindicated. In household with immunocompromised member or close contacts, or in household with unimmunized adult, use only IPV for all those requiring poliovirus immunization. Previous clinical poliomyelitis (usually because of single poliovirus type) or incomplete immunization with OPV are not contraindications to completing primary series of immunization with IPV.

Contraindications History of hypersensitivity to any component of vaccine, including neomycin, streptomycin, and polymyxin B. Patients with acute febrile illness should not receive IPV until after recovery.

Route/Dosage
CHILDREN: **SC** 0.5 mL in deltoid region. In infants and small children, preferred site is anterolateral thigh muscle.

CHILDREN: Primary series consists of 3 doses of 0.5 mL. Separate first 2 doses by at least 4 wk, but preferably 8 wk; commonly given at 2 and 4 mo. Give third dose at least 6 mo, but preferably 12 mo, after second dose, commonly given at 15 to 18 mo. Give all children who received primary series of IPV or combination of IPV and OPV booster dose of OPV or IPV before entering school, unless third dose of primary series was administered on or after fourth birthday.

ADULTS: For unvaccinated adults at increased risk of exposure to poliovirus, give primary series of IPV: 2 doses at 1 to 2-mo interval, with third dose 6 to 12 mo later. If less than 3 mo, but older than 2 mo remain before protection is needed (eg, planned international travel), give 3 doses of IPV at least 1 mo apart. Likewise, if only 1 or 2 mo remain, give 2 doses of IPV 1 mo apart. If less than 4 wk remain, give single dose of either OPV or IPV. Give adults at increased risk of exposure who have had at least 1 dose of OPV, less than 3 doses of conventional IPV (available before 1988) or combination of conventional IPV and OPV totaling less than 3 doses, at least 1 dose of OPV or IPV. Give any additional doses needed to complete primary series if time permits. Give adults who have completed primary series with any poliovirus vaccine and who are at increased risk of exposure to poliovirus single dose of either OPV or IPV.

Interactions Several routine pediatric vaccines may safely and effectively be administered simultaneously at separate injection sites (eg, DTP, MMR, OPV, Hib, hepatitis B, influenza). National authorities recommend simultaneous immunization at separate sites as indicated by age or health risk.

Lab Test Interferences None well documented.

Adverse Reactions
LOCAL: IPV administration may result in erythema, induration and pain at injection site.
SYST: Temperatures 39°C (102°F) or higher reported in 38% of IPV vaccinees.

Precautions
Pregnancy: Category C. Vaccinate if risk of disease outweighs risk to patients.
Lactation: Undetermined.

PATIENT CARE CONSIDERATIONS
Administration/Storage
- Give 0.5 mL SC in deltoid for adults; preferred site for infants is vastus lateralis.
- If blood appears in syringe after aspiration, do not inject. Withdraw needle and discard syringe. Use new dose injected at different site.
- Document manufacturer and lot number of vaccine, date of administration, and name, address, and title of person administering vaccine in permanent record according to federal regulations.
- Store under refrigeration.

Assessment/Interventions
- Obtain patient history, including drug history and any known allergies.
- Advise adult patients to be vaccinated before traveling to developing country.
- Note if patient is immunocompromised or in household with unimmunized adult.
- If patient has acute febrile illness, notify health care provider and do not administer until after recovery.
- Assess patient for any adverse reactions and document properly in patient record. Report as required by Vaccine Adverse Event Reporting System (800-822-7967).

Patient/Family Education
- Advise patient to observe for fever, erythema, induration, or pain at injection site, and to report to health care provider immediately.
- Explain risks and benefits of vaccination.
- Advise patient and family about vaccine schedule. Explain that the series must be completed to offer full protection.

Poly-L-Lactic acid

(PAHL-ee EL LACK-tick AH-sid)

Class Physical adjunct

How Supplied
Sculptra Powder for Injection, freeze dried.

Action
PHARMACOLOGY: Injectable implant of microparticles of poly-L-lactic acid.

Indications Restoration and/or correction of signs of facial fat loss (lipoatrophy) in people with HIV.

Contraindications Standard considerations.

Route/Dosage
ADULTS: **Deep Dermal or Subcutaneous** Quantity and number of injection sessions vary by patient. Typical treatment course for severe facial fat loss involves 3 to 6 injection sessions separated by 2 or more wk. Full effects of treatment course are evident within weeks to months. Reevaluate patient no sooner than 2 wk after each injection session to determine need for additional correction.

Interactions None well documented.

Lab Test Interferences None well documented.

Adverse Reactions
CNS: Fatigue, malaise (postmarketing).
DERM: Bruising, erythema; application-site discharge, ectropion, hypertrophy of skin, injection-site abscess, atrophy, fat atrophy, granuloma, skin rash and roughness, telangiectasias, visible nodules with or without inflammation or dyspigmentation, brittle nails, hair breakage (postmarketing).
LOCAL: Discomfort; hematoma; inflammation; injection-site bleeding, induration, infection, lesion, and tenderness; injection-site subcutaneous papule.
MUSC: Aching joints (postmarketing).
OTHER: Fever; allergic reaction, angioedema, colitis, hypersensitivity, photosensitivity, Quincke edema (postmarketing).

Precautions
Pregnancy: Not established.
Lactation: Undetermined.
Children: Safety and efficacy not established.
Keloid formation/hypertrophic scarring/periorbital area: Safety not established for use in these conditions.
Long-term use: Safety and efficacy beyond 2 yr not established.
Skin inflammation/infection: Defer treatment until inflammation or infection process in or near treatment area has been controlled.
Special risk patients: Risk of hematoma or localized bleeding at injection site may be increased in patients taking anticoagulants.
Treatment effect: Do not overcorrect a contour deficiency because depression should gradually improve within several weeks as treatment effect occurs.

PATIENT CARE CONSIDERATIONS
Administration/Storage
- For mid to deep dermal or subcutaneous injection only. Not IM or IV administration.
- Reconstitute powder for injection with 3 to 5 mL sterile water for injection. Slowly add desired volume of sterile water for injection into vial and allow vial to stand, without agitation or shaking, for at least 2 hr to ensure complete hydration. After waiting at least 2 hr, and immediately before use, agitate vial (a single vial swirling agitator may be used) until a uniform suspension is obtained.
- Carefully follow manufacturer's guidelines for transferring suspension from vial to syringe used for injection, administration and injection technique, and posttreatment care (eg, ice pack to reduce swelling, thorough massage to evenly distribute product).
- Do not inject poly-L-lactic acid using needles with an internal diameter smaller than 26-gauge.
- Do not mix with other products prior to injection.
- Store unopened vials of powder for injection and reconstituted suspension at controlled room temperature (less than 86°F). Protect from freezing. Do not store reconstituted suspension in syringe. Administer suspension within 72 hr of reconstitution. Discard any material remaining after use or after 72 hr following reconstitution.

Assessment/Interventions
- Obtain patient history, including drug history and any known allergies. Note susceptibility to keloid formation or hypertrophic scaring, or concurrent use of anticoagulants or medications affecting platelet function (eg, aspirin).
- Assess injection site prior to administration. Avoid injecting into site with infection, skin disease, or active inflammatory process (eg, cysts, rash).
- Ensure posttreatment ice packs and massage of treatment area are implemented as ordered.
- Assess treatment area following injection session for procedure-related adverse events (eg, tenderness, bleeding, induration, infection). Inform health care provider if noted and significant.
- Ensure treatment area is evaluated no sooner than 2 wk following injection session to determine if additional correction is needed.

Patient/Family Education
- Explain name, dosing regimen, action, potential side effects, and expected response to treatment.
- Advise patient that treatment course may consist of 3 to 6 injection sessions separated by 2 or more wk. Explain importance of completing entire treatment course in order to obtain maximal benefit and advise patient that supplemental injection sessions may be required to maintain an optimal treatment effect.
- Advise patient that medication will be prepared and administered in a health care setting by a health care provider.
- Advise patient to review patient information sheet before starting therapy.
- Advise patient to apply an ice pack (avoiding direct contact of ice with skin) to treatment area for a few minutes at a time for the first 24 hr following injection session to reduce swelling.
- Advise patient to massage treatment area a few times each day for several days following injection session to promote a natural looking correction.
- Advise patient that mild to moderate treatment area reactions (eg, redness, swelling, bruising) are common and should resolve within hours to a week but to notify health care provider if treatment area reaction does not resolve or worsens.
- Advise patient that original skin depression may initially reappear, but the depression should gradually improve within several weeks as the beneficial effect of the medication occurs.
- Advise patient that small bumps may develop in the treatment area within 6 to 12 mo after the first treatment session. Advise patient that the bumps may not be visible and are only noted when pressing on the treatment area, or, they may become visible and eventually go away on their own. Advise patient to notify health care provider if visible bumps develop and are associated with redness or color change to treated area.
- Caution patient to minimize exposure of treatment area to excessive UV light (eg, sunlight, tanning lamps) until any initial redness and swelling have resolved.
- Advise patient that make-up may be applied a few hours after treatment session if no com-

plications (eg, open wound, bleeding, redness, swelling).
- Advise women to notify health care provider if pregnant, planning to become pregnant, or breastfeeding.
- Instruct patient not to take any prescription or OTC medications, herbal preparations, or dietary supplements unless advised by health care provider.
- Remind patient that office visits will be required to monitor therapy and to keep appointments.

Polyethylene Glycol (PEG)

(poli-eth-uh-leen gli-cawl)

Class Bowel evacuant

How Supplied
MiraLax Powder for Oral Solution 255 g PEG 3350, Powder for Oral Solution 527 g PEG 3350

Action
PHARMACOLOGY: Acts as an osmotic agent by causing water to be retained with the stool.

Indications Treatment of occasional constipation; use should be limited to 14 days or less.

Contraindications Known or suspected bowel obstruction; allergy to polyethylene glycol.

Route/Dosage
ADULTS: **PO** 17 g/day as directed by health care provider in 240 mL of water, juice, soda, coffee, or tea.

Interactions None well documented.

PATIENT CARE CONSIDERATIONS

Administration/Storage
- Usual dose is 17 g once daily.
- If using bulk powder, measure prescribed quantity using measuring cap supplied with product or use 1 heaping Tbsp. Dissolve powder in 8 oz of water, juice, soda, coffee, or tea before administering.
- If using individual packet, dissolve contents of 1 packet in 8 oz of water, juice, soda, coffee, or tea before administering.
- Store powder at controlled room temperature (59° to 86°F).

Assessment/Interventions
- Obtain patient history, including drug history and any known allergies. Note bowel obstruction or concurrent use of medications known to cause constipation.
- Ensure that patient with nausea, vomiting, abdominal pain, or distention is evaluated for possible bowel obstruction before initiating therapy.
- Assess and document bowel habits before and after initiating therapy. Notify health care provider if constipation does not improve, worsens, or if cramping, bloating, or diarrhea occur.

Lab Test Interferences None well documented.

Adverse Reactions
GI: Nausea; abdominal bloating; cramping; flatulence; diarrhea; excessive stool frequency.

Precautions
Pregnancy: Category C.
Children: Safety and efficacy not established.
Evaluation of constipation: Patients with complaints of constipation should have a thorough medical history and physical examination to detect associated metabolic, endocrine, and neurogenic conditions, and medications.
Symptoms of bowel obstruction: Patients with symptoms of bowel obstruction (eg, nausea, vomiting, abdominal pain or distention) should be evaluated to rule out this condition before starting therapy.

Overdosage: Signs and Symptoms
Diarrhea.

Patient/Family Education
- Explain name, dose, action, and potential side effects of drug.
- Educate patient regarding good defecatory and eating habits (eg, high fiber diet) and lifestyle changes (eg, adequate dietary fiber and fluid intake, regular exercise) that promote more regular bowel habits.
- Advise patient that PEG should be used for 2 wk or less unless specified otherwise by health care provider. Caution patient that prolonged, frequent, or excessive use may result in electrolyte imbalance and dependence on laxatives.
- Instruct patient to dissolve prescribed dose in 8 oz of water, juice, soda, coffee, or tea before taking.
- Advise patient that medication does not work immediately and that 2 to 4 days of therapy may be required to produce a bowel movement.
- Advise patient to notify health care provider if constipation does not improve, worsens, or if nausea, cramping, bloating, or diarrhea occur.

- Caution patient not to take any prescription or OTC drugs, dietary supplements, or herbal preparations unless advised by health care provider.
- Advise women to notify health care provider if pregnant, planning to become pregnant, or breastfeeding.
- Advise patient that follow-up visits may be necessary to monitor therapy and to keep appointments.

Polyethylene Glycol-Electrolyte Solution (PEG-ES)

(poli-eth-uh-leen gli-cawl)

Class Laxative

How Supplied

CoLyte Powder for oral solution 1 gal: 227.1 g PEG 3350, 21.5 g sodium sulfate, 6.36 g sodium bicarb, 5.53 g NaCl, 2,82 g KCl, Powder for oral solution 4L: 240 g PEG 3350, 22.72 g sodium sulfate, 6.72 g sodium bicab, 5.84 g NaCl, 2.98 g KCl ♦ *GoLYTELY* Powder for oral suspension 236 g PEG 3350, 22.74 g sodium sulfate, 6.74 g sodium bicarb, 5.86 g NaCl, 2.97 g KCl, Powder for oral suspension 227.1 g PEG 3350, 21.5 sodium sulfate, 6.36 g sodium bicarb, 5.53 g NaCl, 2.82 g KCl ♦ *NuLYTELY* Powder for reconstitution 420 g PEG 3350, 5.72 g sodium bicarb, 11.2 g NaCl, 1.48 g KCl ♦ *OCL* Oral solution 146 mg NaCl, 168 mg sodium bicarb, 1.29 g sodium sulfate decahydrate, 75 mg KCl, 6 g PEG 3350, 30 mg polysorbate 80/100 mL

Action

PHARMACOLOGY: Induces diarrhea, which rapidly cleanses bowel, usually within 4 hr.

PHARMACOKINETICS/DYNAMICS:
Absorption: Negligible.
Onset: 30 to 60 min.

Indications Bowel cleansing prior to GI examination. **Unlabeled use(s):** Management of acute iron overdose in children.

PATIENT CARE CONSIDERATIONS

Administration/Storage

- May be given via NG tube for patients unable or unwilling to drink solution.
- Reconstitute solution with tap water and shake container until powder is dissolved.
- Do not add flavorings or additional ingredients to solution before use. Chilling solution before administration improves palatability.
- Refrigerate reconstituted solution. Use within 48 hr.
- Administer minimum of 3 L of solution to achieve satisfactory bowel evacuation.

Assessment/Interventions

- Obtain patient history, including drug history and any allergies. Note history of ulcerative colitis.

Contraindications GI obstruction; gastric retention; bowel perforation; toxic colitis; toxic megacolon or ileus.

Route/Dosage

ADULTS: **PO/Nasogastric** 4 L prior to GI examination. Give orally as 240 mL q 10 min or via NG tube as 1.2 to 1.8 L/hr until 4 L are consumed or until rectal effluent is clear. Via nasogastric (NG) tube, use rate of 1.2 to 1.8 L/hr.

Interactions

Oral medication given within 1 hr of starting therapy: Medication may be flushed from GI tract and not absorbed.

Lab Test Interferences None well documented.

Adverse Reactions

DERM: Urticaria; dermatitis.
EENT: Rhinorrhea.
GI: Nausea; abdominal fullness; bloating; abdominal cramps; vomiting anal irritation.

Precautions

Pregnancy: Category C.
Children: Safety and efficacy not established.
Regurgitation/Aspiration: Use with caution in patients with impaired gag reflex.
Severe ulcerative colitis: Use with caution. If GI obstruction or perforation is suspected, rule out these contraindications before administration.

Overdosage: Signs and Symptoms

Diarrhea, bloating, abdominal pain.

- Do not administer if patient has, or is suspected to have, GI obstruction, gastric retention, bowel perforation, toxic colitis, toxic megacolon, or ileus.
- Observe patients with impaired gag reflex or patient who is otherwise prone to regurgitation or aspiration during administration, especially if solution is given via NG tube.
- Notify health care provider if patient is unable to tolerate solution or if rectal bleeding occurs.
- If patient complains of bloating, abdominal pain or distention, slow solution or discontinue until symptoms abate.

Patient/Family Education

- Explain that solution is given to cleanse bowel as preparation for GI examination.

- Explain that if discomfort becomes intolerable, patient should stop drinking solution temporarily or allow longer intervals between drink portions.
- Instruct patient not to eat or drink anything for 3 to 4 hr before ingestion and explain that only clear liquids are allowed after ingestion of solution.
- Tell patient to continue drinking solution until watery stool is clear and free of solid material.
- Instruct patient to report the following symptoms to health care provider: severe bloating, distention, or abdominal pain.

Porfimer Sodium

(PORE-fih-muhr SO-dee-uhm)

Class Photosensitizing agent

How Supplied
Photofrin Cake or Powder for Injection (freeze-dried) 75 mg

Action
PHARMACOLOGY: Porfimer is a photosensitizing agent used in the photodynamic therapy (PDT) of tumors. Cellular damage caused by porfimer PDT is a consequence of the propagation of radical reactions. Tumor death also occurs through ischemic necrosis secondary to vascular occlusion that appears to be partly mediated by thromboxane A_2 release. The laser treatment induces a photochemical, not a thermal, effect.

PHARMACOKINETICS/DYNAMICS:
Absorption: C_{max} is 15 mcg/mL.

Distribution: Vd is 0.49 L/kg. Protein binding is approximately 90%. Distributed through a variety of tissues and retained mostly in tumors, skin, liver, and spleen.

Excretion: The t½ is 250 hr. Total plasma Cl is 0.051 mL/min/kg.

Indications Esophageal cancer; endobronchial non-small cell lung cancer; Barrett esophagus.

Contraindications
PDT: Existing tracheoesophageal or bronchoesophageal fistula; tumors eroding into a major blood vessel.
Porfimer: Porphyria or in patients with known allergies to porphyrins.

Route/Dosage
Barrett Esophagus
ADULTS: **IV** 2 mg/kg as a single slow injection over 3 to 5 min. Patients may receive a second course of PDT a minimum of 90 days after the initial therapy; up to 3 courses of PDT, each separated by a minimum of 90 days can be given to previously treated segment that still show high-grade dysplasia.

Esophageal and Endobronchial Non-Small Cell Lung Cancer
ADULTS: **IV** 2 mg/kg as a single slow IV injection over 3 to 5 min. Patients may receive a second course of PDT a minimum of 30 days after the initial therapy; no more than 3 courses of PDT (each separated by a minimum of 30 days) can be given.

Interactions
Compounds that quench active oxygen species or scavenge radicals (eg, dimethyl sulfoxide, beta-carotene, ethanol, mannitol): Would be expected to decrease PDT activity.
Drugs that decrease clotting, vasoconstriction, or platelet aggregation (eg, thromboxane A_2 inhibitors): Could decrease the efficacy of PDT.
Glucocorticoid hormones: Given before or concomitantly with PDT, may decrease the efficacy of the treatment.
Photosensitizing agents: Concomitant use of other photosensitizing agents (eg, tetracyclines, sulfonamides, phenothiazines, hypoglycemic agents, thiazide diuretics, griseofulvin) could increase photosensitivity reaction.
Tissue ischemia, allopurinol, calcium channel blockers, and some prostaglandin synthesis inhibitors: Preclinical data also suggest that these could interfere with porfimer.

Lab Test Interferences None well documented.

Adverse Reactions Adverse reactions reported represent those occurring with porfimer with PDT as a 2-stage process. Adverse reactions listed were reported in at least 5% of patients treated with porfimer-PDT.
CV: Atrial fibrillation; cardiac failure; hypotension; tachycardia; hypertension.
CNS: Insomnia; confusion; anxiety; headache; fatigue; depression.
DERM: Photosensitivity; rash; pruritus; sunburn.
EENT: Sinusitis; bronchitis.
GI: Constipation; nausea; abdominal pain; vomiting; dysphagia; esophageal edema; tumor bleeding; hematemesis; dyspepsia; esophageal stricture; diarrhea; eructation; esophagitis; melena; esophageal narrowing; esophageal pain; hiccup; odynophagia.
M/N: Weight decrease; dehydration; anorexia.
RESP: Pleural effusion; dyspnea; pneumonia; pharyngitis; respiratory insufficiency; cough; tracheoesophageal fistula.
OTHER: Anemia; fever; chest pain; pain; back pain; moniliasis; UTI; peripheral edema; asthenia; substernal chest pain; generalized edema;

exudate; obstruction; stricture; ulceration; arthralgia.

Precautions

Pregnancy: Category C.

Lactation: Undetermined.

Children: Safety and efficacy in children have not been established.

Photosensitivity: All patients who receive porfimer sodium will be photosensitive and must observe precautions to avoid exposure of skin and eyes to direct sunlight or bright indoor light for at least 30 days. Exposure of the skin to ambient indoor light is beneficial because the remaining drug will be inactivated gradually and safely through a photobleaching reaction. Therefore, advise patients not to stay in a darkened room during this period and encourage them to expose their skin to ambient indoor light. Ultraviolet (UV) sunscreens are of no value in protecting against photosensitivity reactions.

Chest pain: Patients may complain of substernal chest pain because of inflammatory responses within the area of treatment.

Esophageal strictures: Esophageal strictures as a result of PDT of high-grade dysplasia in Barrett esophagus are common adverse events.

Esophageal varices: Treat patients with esophageal varices with extreme caution. Do not administer light directly to the variceal area because of a high risk of bleeding.

Extravasation risk: Local irritation or phlebitis may occur; in these cases, protect area from light. Refer to your institution-specific protocol.

Fistula: PDT is not recommended if the esophageal tumor is eroding into the trachea or bronchial tree and the likelihood of tracheoesophageal or bronchoesophageal fistula resulting from treatment is sufficiently high.

Ocular sensitivity: Ocular discomfort, commonly described as sensitivity to sun, bright lights, or car headlights has been reported. For 30 days, when outdoors, patients should wear dark sunglasses that have an average white light transmittance of less than 4%.

Respiratory distress: Closely monitor patients with endobronchial lesions between the laser light therapy and the mandatory debridement bronchoscopy for any evidence of respiratory distress.

Treatment-induced inflammation: Use PDT with extreme caution for endobronchial tumors in locations where treatment-induced inflammation could obstruct the main airway.

Use with radiotherapy: Allot sufficient time between the 2 therapies to ensure that the inflammatory response produced by the first treatment has subsided before commencing the second treatment. Allow 2 to 4 wk after PDT before commencing radiotherapy. Similarly, allow 4 wk after completing radiotherapy before giving PDT. Patients with obstructing lung cancer who have received prior radiation therapy have a higher incidence of fatal hemoptysis after PDT.

PATIENT CARE CONSIDERATIONS

Administration/Storage

- Photodynamic therapy with porfimer is a 2-stage process requiring administration of drug and laser light by trained practitioners. The first stage is the IV injection of porfimer, followed 40 to 50 hr later by illumination with laser lights constituting the second stage of therapy. A second laser light application may be given 96 to 120 hr after injection, preceded by gentle debridement of residual tumor
- For IV administration only. Not for intradermal, SC, IM, or intra-arterial administration.
- Avoid skin and eye contact during reconstitution. Use rubber gloves and eye protection. If accidental skin or eye exposure occurs, protect the exposed area from bright light.
- Reconstitute powder for injection following manufacturer's guidelines using D5W or 0.9% sodium chloride injection. Shake well until dissolved.
- Do not reconstitute with other diluents or mix with other medications in same vial.
- Protect reconstituted solution from light and administer immediately after reconstitution.
- Administer prescribed dose as a single slow IV injection over 3 to 5 min.
- Take precautions to prevent extravasation at injection site. If extravasation occurs protect the area from exposure to light.
- If injection solution is accidentally spilled, wipe up with damp cloth and dispose of in polyethylene bag following institutional guidelines.
- Store powder for injection at controlled room temperature (68° to 77°F).

Assessment/Interventions

- Obtain patient history, including drug history and any known allergies. Note porphyria, tracheoesophageal or bronchoesophageal fistula, tumor eroding into major blood vessel, esophageal or gastric varices, esophageal ulcer greater than 1 cm in diameter, previous radiotherapy to same region, or concurrent use of photosensitizing medications (eg, tetracyclines, sulfonylureas, thiazide diuretics), corticosteroids, or antioxidants.

- Ensure that women of childbearing potential are not pregnant when treatment is started and use effective contraception during therapy.
- Ensure that precautions are taken to avoid exposure of patient's skin and eyes to direct sunlight or bright indoor light (eg, examination lamps, operating room lamps, dental lamps, unshaded light bulbs at close range) following injection of porfimer. Inform health care provider if severe photosensitivity reaction (eg, severe sunburn) develops.
- For patient being treated for high-grade dysplasia in Barrett esophagus, ensure that endoscopic surveillance is conducted q 3 mo until 4 consecutive negative evaluations for high-grade dysplasia have been recorded, and then q 6 to 12 mo as indicated.
- Closely monitor patient with endobronchial lesions between laser light therapy and mandatory bronchoscopy for respiratory distress. Immediately inform health care provider if noted and be prepared for immediate bronchoscopy.
- Assess patient for GI, respiratory, CNS, CV, DERM, and general body side effects. Inform health care provider if noted and significant.

Patient/Family Education

- Explain name, dose, action, and potential side effects of drug.
- Advise patient, family, or caregiver that medication will be prepared and administered by health care provider in a health care setting and that laser light treatment will be administered 40 to 50 hr after porfimer administration has been completed.
- Advise patient, family, or caregiver that a second laser light treatment may be administered 96 to 120 hr after the porfimer has been administered.
- Caution patient that therapy will make them extremely sensitive to light (photosensitivity) for up to 30 days and to avoid exposure of skin and eyes to direct sunlight (including skylights and undraped windows) or bright indoor light (eg, examination lamps, dental lamps, unshaded light bulbs at close range).
- Advise patient to cover the skin as much as possible during daylight hours (eg, long-sleeved shirts, slacks, gloves, socks) even on cloudy days or when in a car.
- Advise patient to wear dark sunglasses when exposed to sunlight, bright lights, or car headlights to prevent eye discomfort. Advise patient that sunglasses should have an average white light transmittance of less than 4% and to check with an eye doctor if unsure.
- Caution patient that OTC sunscreens will not protect them against photosensitivity reactions.
- Advise patient not to stay in darkened room but to expose the skin to soft indoor light (eg, shaded lamps).
- Instruct patient how to check for residual photosensitivity after 30 days (eg, expose small area of skin other than face to sunlight for 10 min and note degree of redness, swelling, or blistering that occurs over the next 24 hr).
- Advise patient, family, or caregiver to immediately report any of the following to health care provider: shortness of breath or difficulty breathing; severe sunburn reaction.
- Advise patient, family, or caregiver to report persistent chest pain to health care provider.
- Instruct patient not to take any prescription or OTC medications or dietary supplements unless advised by health care provider.
- Advise women of childbearing potential to avoid becoming pregnant during therapy by using effective contraception.
- Advise women of childbearing potential to notify health care provider if pregnant, planning to become pregnant, or breastfeeding.
- Advise patient that follow-up visits will be required to monitor therapy and to keep appointments.

Potassium Products

(poe-TASS-ee-uhm)

Class Electrolyte

How Supplied

Cena-K Liquid 20 mEq/15 mL potassium and chloride (10% KCl), Liquid 40 mEq/15 mL potassium and chloride (20% KCl) ♦ *Effer-K* Tablets, effervescent 25 mEq potassium (as bicarbonate and citrate) ♦ *Gen-K* Powder 20 mEq potassium chloride/packet ♦ *K + 8* Tablets, extended-release 8 mEq potassium chloride ♦ *K + 10* Tablets, controlled-release 10 mEq (750 mg) potassium chloride in a wax matrix ♦ *K + Care* Powder 15 mEq potassium chloride/packet, Powder 20 mEq potassium chloride/packet, Powder 25 mEq potassium chloride/packet ♦ *K + Care ET* Tablets, effervescent 20 mEq potassium (from potassium bicarbonate), Tablets, effervescent 25 mEq potassium (from potassium bicarbonate) ♦ *K-Dur 10* Tablets, controlled-release 750 mg microencapsulated potassium chloride equiv. to 10 mEq ♦ *K-Dur 20* Tablets, controlled-release 1500 mg microencapsulated potassium chloride equiv. to 20 mEq ♦ *K-G Elixir* Liquid 20 mEq/15 mL potassium (as potassium gluconate) ♦ *K-Lor* Powder 20 mEq potassium chloride/packet ♦ *K•Lyte* Tablets, effervescent 25 mEq potassium (as bicarbonate and citrate) ♦ *K•Lyte DS* Tablets, effervescent 50 mEq potassium (from potassium bicarbonate and citrate and citric acid) ♦ *K•Lyte/Cl* Tablets, effervescent 25 mEq potassium (from potassium Cl and bicarbonate, I-lysine monohydrochloride, and citric acid), Powder 25 mEq potassium chloride/dose ♦ *K•Lyte/Cl 50* Tablets, effervescent 50 mEq potassium (from Cl and bicarbonate, I-lysine monohydrochloride, and citric acid) ♦ *K-Tab* Tablets, controlled-release 10 mEq (750 mg) potassium chloride in a wax matrix ♦ *K-vescent Potassium Chloride* Powder 20 mEq potassium and chloride from 1.5 g potassium chloride ♦ *Kaon* Liquid 20 mEq/15 mL potassium (as potassium gluconate) ♦ *Kaon-Cl* Tablets, controlled-release 6.7 mEq (500 mg) potassium chloride in a wax matrix ♦ *Kaon Cl-10* Tablets, controlled-release 10 mEq (750 mg) potassium chloride in a wax matrix ♦ *Kaon-Cl 20%* Liquid 40 mEq/15 mL potassium and chloride (20% KCl) ♦ *Kay Ciel* Liquid 20 mEq/15 mL potassium and chloride (10% KCl), Powder 20 mEq potassium chloride/packet ♦ *Kaylixir* Liquid 20 mEq/15 mL potassium (as potassium gluconate) ♦ *Klor-Con* Powder 20 mEq potassium chloride/packet ♦ *Klor-Con 8* Tablets, controlled-release 8 mEq (600 mg) potassium chloride in a wax matrix ♦ *Klor-Con 10* Tablets, controlled-release 10 mEq (750) mg potassium chloride in a wax matrix ♦ *Klor-Con/EF* Tablets, effervescent 25 mEq potassium (as bicarbonate and citrate) ♦ *Klor-Con/25* Powder 25 mEq potassium chloride/packet ♦ *Klor-Con M10* Tablets, extended-release 10 mEq potassium (from 750 mg potassium chloride) ♦ *Klor-Con M15* Tablets, extended-release 15 mEq potassium (from 1125 mg potassium chloride) ♦ *Klor-Con M20* Tablets, extended-release 20 mEq potassium (from 1500 mg potassium chloride) ♦ *Klorvess* Tablets, effervescent 20 mEq potassium (from potassium chloride and bicarbonate and lysine hydrochloride) ♦ *Klorvess* Liquid 20 mEq/15 mL potassium and chloride (10% KCl), Powder 20 mEq potassium and chloride (potassium chloride, bicarbonate, and citrate and lysine hydrochloride)/packet ♦ *Klotrix* Tablets, controlled-release 10 mEq (750 mg) potassium chloride in a wax matrix ♦ *Kolyum* Liquid 20 mEq potassium and 3.4 mEq potassium chloride/15 mL (from potassium gluconate and potassium chloride) ♦ *Micro-K Extencaps* Capsules, controlled-release 600 mg potassium chloride equiv. to 8 mEq potassium. Microencapsulated particles, Capsules, controlled-release 10 mEq (750 mg) potassium chloride. Microencapsulated particles ♦ *Micro-K LS* Powder 20 mEq potassium chloride/packet ♦ *Rum-K* Liquid 30 mEq/15 mL potassium and chloride (20% KCl) ♦ *Ter-K* Tablets, controlled-release 750 mg microencapsulated potassium chloride equiv. to 10 mEq ♦ *Tri-K* Liquid 45 mEq/15 mL potassium (from potassium acetate, potassium bicarbonate, and potassium citrate) ♦ *Twin-K* Liquid 20 mEq/15 mL potassium (as potassium gluconate and potassium citrate) ♦ *Potasalan* Liquid 20 mEq/15 mL potassium and chloride (10% KCl)

🍁 *Apo-Amoxi-Clav* ♦ *APO-K* ♦ *K-10 Solution* ♦ *Kaochlor-20 Concentrate* ♦ *K-Lor* ♦ *Kaoch*

Action
PHARMACOLOGY: Major intracellular cation, essential in maintaining acid base balance and isotonicity within cells. Functions in muscle contraction, nerve impulse transmission, gastric secretion, renal function and metabolism.

PHARMACOKINETICS/DYNAMICS:
Absorption: Absorbed from the GI tract.
Excretion: Renal (90%), fecal (10%), and a small extent in perspiration.

Indications
Treatment of hypokalemia; prevention of potassium depletion in certain conditions. Parenterally, as prophylaxis or treatment of moderate to severe potassium loss when oral therapy is not adequate or feasible. **Unlabeled use(s):** Treatment of thallium poisoning; with anticholinesterase agents in myasthenia gravis.

Contraindications
Severe renal impairment with concomitant azotemia or oliguria; hyperkalemia; diseases in which high potassium levels may be present include: renal failure and conditions in which potassium retention is present; anuria; trauma with muscle destruction; severe hemolytic reactions; adrenocortical insufficiency; heat cramps; acute dehydration; adynamica episodica hereditaria; early postoperative oliguria (except during GI drainage); use of potassium-sparing diuretics.

Route/Dosage
ADULTS: **PO** 20 to 100 mEq in divided doses. **IV** 10 to 40 mEq/hr.
INFANTS: **PO** 2 to 3 mEq/kg in divided doses.

Interactions
Digitalis: Cardiac arrhythmias may occur with potassium imbalance.
Potassium-sparing diuretics: Severe hyperkalemia may occur.

Lab Test Interferences None well documented.

Adverse Reactions
DERM: Rashes.
GI: Abdominal discomfort or distention; GI obstruction; bleeding; ulceration or perforation; nausea; vomiting; flatulence.
GU: Oliguria; anuria.

OTHER: Hyperkalemia (symptoms may include paresthesia of extremities; listlessness; confusion; weak or heavy limbs; flaccid paralysis; hypotension; arrhythmias; heart block; cardiac arrest; prolonged QT interval; wide QRS complex; peaked T waves; ST depression.

Precautions
Pregnancy: Category C.
Lactation: Undetermined.
Children: Safety and efficacy not established.
Special risk patients: Administer with caution to elderly patients or patients with decreased renal function. Use with caution in patients with cardiac disease.

GI lesions: May cause stenotic or ulcerative lesions of the small bowel and death. Discontinue immediately if bowel obstruction or perforation is suspected.
Hyperkalemia: May produce hyperkalemia or cardiac arrest in patients with impaired potassium excretion.

Overdosage: Signs and Symptoms
ECG changes, ventricular fibrillation, death, muscle weakness that may progress to paralysis of diaphragm.

PATIENT CARE CONSIDERATIONS

Administration/Storage
- Do not give tablets to patients who have physical conditions that may slow or stop tablet in GI track; use properly diluted concentrate form.
- Use whole tablets; do not crush or split tablets. Do not allow patient to chew or suck tablets.
- Administer tablets after meals or with food and full glass of water.
- Mix or dissolve completely oral liquids, soluble powders, or effervescent tablets in 3 to 8 oz of cold water, juice, or other beverage, and have patient drink slowly to minimize GI irritation.
- Do not give via IM route.
- Generally, do not begin IV administration until renal flow is established.
- Do not exceed IV administration rate of 20 mEq/hr and concentration of 40 mEq/L without performing cardiac monitoring. Rapid infusion may cause local pain; reduce rate to relieve irritation.
- Dilute parenteral concentrates before use. Direct injection may be instantly fatal.
- Maximum 24 hr dose should not exceed 200 mEq if serum potassium is more than 2.5 mEq/L; 400 mEq, if serum potassium is less than 2 mEq/L.

Assessment/Interventions
- Obtain patient history, including drug history and any known allergies. Note renal cardiac disease, untreated Addison disease, dehydration, or other conditions that may place patient at risk.
- Ensure that potassium level has been obtained before beginning therapy. Monitor potassium levels regularly during treatment. Cardiac monitoring is recommended when giving parenteral potassium at rates more than 20 mEq/hr.
- Monitor serum potassium levels closely in patients with renal impairment.
- Watch for ECG changes such as peaking of T waves, loss of P wave, depression of ST segment, prolongation of QT interval, lengthened P-R interval, or widened QRS complex during cardiac monitoring.
- Observe for the following overt signs of hyperkalemia: decreased BP, paresthesia, muscle weakness and flaccid paralysis of extremities, listlessness, mental confusion, shock, cardiac arrhythmias, or heart block. Notify health care provider immediately if these symptoms occur.
- Observe for phlebitis (IV) and for possible GI distress, including abdominal discomfort, nausea, vomiting, and diarrhea. Notify health care provider if these symptoms occur.
- Do not abruptly discontinue drug in patients who are also receiving digitalis; digitalis toxicity may occur.

Patient/Family Education
- Instruct patient to take oral medication after meals or with food and full glass of water.
- Advise patient to swallow tablets whole, without chewing, sucking, or crushing.
- Warn patient not to use salt substitutes and to avoid "salt-free" food unless approved by health care provider.
- Advise patients taking time-released drug that wax matrix may appear in stool. Emphasize that this is normal.
- Explain importance of avoiding ingestion of large amounts of potassium through excessive intake of foods such as avocados, bananas, broccoli, dried fruits, grapefruit, oranges, beans, nuts, spinach, tomatoes, and sunflower seeds.
- Instruct patient to promptly report the following symptoms to health care provider: Severe nausea or vomiting, abdominal pain, black stools, tingling of hands and feet, unusual fatigue or weakness, or feeling of heaviness in legs.

Potassium Citrate/Sodium Citrate/Citric Acid

(poe-TASS-ee-uhm SIH-trate/SO-dee-uhm SIH-trate/SIH-trik ASS-id)

Class Systemic alkalinizer/Urinary alkalinizer

How Supplied
Polycitra Syrup 550 mg potassium citrate, 500 mg sodium citrate, 334 mg citric acid/5 mL (1 mEq K, 1 mEq Na/mL; equiv. to 2 mEq bicarbonate)
♦ *Polycitra-LC* Solution 550 mg potassium citrate, 500 mg sodium citrate, 334 mg citric acid/5 mL (1 mEq K, 1 mEq Na/mL; equiv. to 2 mEq bicarbonate)

Action
PHARMACOLOGY: Potassium citrate and sodium citrate are metabolized to potassium bicarbonate and sodium bicarbonate, thus acting as systemic alkalizers.

Indications
Treatment of chronic metabolic acidosis, particularly when caused by renal tubular acidosis; conditions when long-term maintenance of an alkaline urine is desirable, in treatment of patients with uric acid and cystine calculi of the urinary tract and in conjunction with uricosurics in gout therapy to prevent uric acid nephropathy.

Contraindications
Severe renal impairment with oliguria; azotemia; untreated Addison disease; severe myocardial damage; certain situations when patients are on a sodium- or potassium-restricted diet.

Route/Dosage
ADULTS: **PO** 3 to 6 tsp (15 to 30 mL), diluted with water, qid after meals and at bedtime, or as directed by health care provider.

CHILDREN: **PO** 1 to 3 tsp (5 to 15 mL), diluted with water qid after meals and at bedtime, or as directed by health care provider.

Interactions
Potassium-containing medication, potassium-sparing diuretics (eg, spironolactone), ACE inhibitors (eg, captopril), or cardiac glycosides (eg, digoxin): Concurrent use may lead to toxicity.

Lab Test Interferences
None well documented.

Adverse Reactions
METAB: Alkalosis; hyperkalemia leading to listlessness, weakness, mental confusion, tingling of extremities, and other symptoms associated with high serum potassium concentrations (eg, ECG abnormalities).

Precautions
Pregnancy: Undetermined.
Lactation: Undetermined.
Special risk patients: Sodium salts should be used with caution in patients with cardiac failure, hypertension, impaired renal function, peripheral and pulmonary edema, and toxemia of pregnancy.
Low urinary output or reduced glomerular filtration rate: Because hyperkalemia or alkalosis can occur, use with caution.
GI effects: Dilute with water to minimize GI injury associated with oral ingestion of concentrated potassium salts.

Overdosage: Signs and Symptoms
Diarrhea, nausea, vomiting, hypernoia (excessive mental activity), convulsions, hyperkalemia, alkalosis.

PATIENT CARE CONSIDERATIONS

Administration/Storage
♦ Refrigerate solution prior to administration to enhance palatability.
♦ Dilute each dose with 1 to 3 oz of water and administer after meals to reduce saline laxative effect.
♦ Additional water may be given after the dose if desired by the patient.
♦ Store syrup at controlled room temperature (59° to 86°F). Keep tightly capped and protect from freezing or excessive heat.

Assessment/Interventions
♦ Obtain patient history, including drug history and any known allergies. Note history of sodium restricted diet, potassium-restricted diet, renal impairment, low urine output, heart failure, hypertension, edema states, toxemia of pregnancy, untreated Addison disease, or coadministration of aluminum-based antacids.
♦ Ensure that serum electrolytes and acid-base states are determined before and periodically throughout therapy.
♦ Notify health care provider if any of the following occur: edema, decreased urine output, persistent diarrhea.

Patient/Family Education
♦ Explain name, dose, action, and potential side effects of drug.
♦ Advise patient to take as prescribed and to not change the dose or stop taking unless advised by health care provider.
♦ Advise patient to dilute each dose with 1 to 3 oz of cold water and take after meals if possible to prevent laxative effect. Additional water may follow the dose if desired.
♦ Advise patient that if a dose is missed to take as soon as remembered unless it is nearing time for the next dose. Caution patient to not double the dose to catch up.

- Advise patient to inform health care provider if any of the following occur: edema, decreased urine production, persistent diarrhea, any other bothersome side effects.
- Advise women to notify health care provider if pregnant, planning to become pregnant, or breastfeeding.
- Caution patient to not take any prescription or OTC medications or dietary supplements unless advised by health care provider.
- Advise patient that follow-up visits and lab tests will be required to monitor therapy and to keep appointments.

Pramipexole Dihydrochloride

(pram-ih-PEX-ole)

Class Antiparkinson/Non-ergot dopamine receptor agonist

How Supplied
Mirapex Tablets 0.125 mg, Tablets 0.25 mg, Tablets 1 mg, Tablets 1.5 mg

Action
PHARMACOLOGY: Stimulates dopamine receptors in the corpus striatum, relieving parkinsonian symptoms.

PHARMACOKINETICS/DYNAMICS:

Absorption: Rapid absorption. T_{max} is approximately 2 hr; increased 1 hr if taken with food. Bioavailability is more than 90%. Steady state is 2 days.

Distribution: Extensively distributed, distributes into red blood cells, and indicated by an erythrocyte to plasma ratio of approximately 2. Vd is 500 L. Protein binding is 15%.

Excretion: Renal (90% mostly as unchanged in urine); nonrenal routes may contribute to a small extent. Renal Cl is 400 mL/min. The terminal $t_{1/2}$ is approximately 8 hr (adults) and approximately 12 hr (elderly).

Special Populations:

Renal Function Impairment – Cl is 75% lower in severe impairment (Ccr less than 20 mL/min) and about 60% lower with moderate impairment (Ccr less than 40 mL/min). Recommend lower starting and maintenance dose.

Elderly – At least 65 yr, half-life increases by approximately 40% and Cl decreases by approximately 30%, mostly because of reduced renal function with age.

Gender – Cl is approximately 30% lower in women.

Parkison disease – Clearance reduced by approximately 30%; appears to be related to reduced renal function in these patients.

Indications
Treatment of the signs and symptoms of idiopathic Parkinson disease. May be used in conjunction with L-dopa.

Contraindications
Standard considerations.

Route/Dosage
Individualize by careful titration.

ADULTS: **PO** Initial dose is 0.125 mg tid. For the maintenance dose, dosage may be increased q 5 to 7 days to max dose of 4.5 mg/day.

Interactions
Drugs eliminated via cationic renal secretion (eg, cimetidine, ranitidine, diltiazem, triamterene, verapamil, quinidine, quinine): May reduce oral clearance of pramipexole. Pramipexole dosage adjustment may be needed if therapy with any of these agents is started or stopped during treatment with pramipexole.

Dopamine antagonists (eg, butyrophenones, metoclopramide, phenothiazines, thioxanthenes): May reduce effectiveness of pramipexole.

Lab Test Interferences None well documented.

Adverse Reactions
CV: Orthostatic hypotension.
CNS: Dizziness; somnolence; headache; confusion; hallucinations; abnormal dreams; tremor; insomnia; aggravated Parkinson disease; dyskinesia; hypokinesia; hypesthesia; amnesia; extrapyramidal syndrome; abnormal thinking; hypertonia; akathisia; dystonia; delusions; paranoid reactions.
EENT: Abnormal vision; rhinitis.
GI: Nausea; dyspepsia; constipation; dry mouth; anorexia; dysphagia.
GU: Urinary tract infection; urinary frequency; urinary incontinence; impotence; decreased libido.
RESP: Dyspnea; pneumonia.
OTHER: Asthenia; edema; malaise; injury; fever; weight decrease; myoclonus.

Precautions
Pregnancy: Category C.
Lactation: Inhibits prolactin secretion. Do not give to nursing mothers.
Children: Safety and efficacy have not been established.
Elderly: Incidence of hallucinations appears to be increased with age.
Renal function impairment: Use with caution in presence of moderate to severe renal function impairment. Use lower initial and maintenance doses.
Abrupt withdrawal: Rapid withdrawal or dose reduction of antiparkinsonism drugs may produce symptoms resembling the neuroleptic malignant syndrome.
CNS effect: Use concomitant CNS depressants with caution because of additive sedative effects.

Concurrent L-dopa use: When pramipexole is used in combination with levodopa, the dose of levodopa may be reduced as tolerated.
Dyskinesia: Pramipexole may potentiate dopaminergic side effects of L-dopa and may cause or exacerbate pre-existing dyskinesias.
Hypotension: Postural hypotension may occur, especially during dose escalation.

Hallucinations: Can occur during pramipexole therapy. Frequency is greater when used in conjunction with L-dopa.
Retinal pathology: Pathological changes were observed in the retinas of albino rats receiving dopaminergic receptor agonists. The potential significance of this effect in humans has not been established but cannot be disregarded.

PATIENT CARE CONSIDERATIONS

Administration/Storage
- Administer tid without regard to food.
- If nausea occurs, administer each dose with food.
- Store at controlled room temperature protected from light.

Assessment/Interventions
- Obtain patient history, including drug history and any known allergies.
- Note renal function impairment.
- Complete baseline assessment of parkinsonian symptoms before instituting therapy.
- Assess for therapeutic effects, adverse reactions, and drug interactions throughout course of therapy.
- Assess for orthostatic hypotension, dizziness, and mental status changes during initial phase of therapy or following dose escalation.
- Assist patient with position changes and ambulation during initial therapy to prevent falling.
- Monitor blood pressure and pulse routinely during therapy.
- Do not administer if significant changes in BP, pulse, or mental status occur. Notify health care provider.

Patient/Family Education
- Instruct patient to take exactly as prescribed. Advise patient that dose may be taken without regard to meals but to take with food if nausea occurs.
- Inform patient that drug may cause drowsiness and to use caution while driving or performing other tasks requiring mental alertness.
- Instruct patient to avoid sudden position changes to prevent orthostatic hypotension.
- Instruct patient to report the following symptoms to health care provider: uncontrollable movements, dizziness, mood or mental changes, severe or persistent nausea, headache.
- Inform patient that hallucinations can occur and that elderly are more susceptible.
- Advise patient to use caution when taking other drugs with CNS depressant effects (eg, alcohol, sedatives).
- Advise patient not to take any other medications (including *otc*) without consulting health care provider.
- Advise patient to notify health care provider if becoming pregnant, planning to become pregnant, or breastfeeding while taking this medication.

Pravastatin Sodium

(PRUH-vuh-stuh-tin SO-dee-uhm)

Class Antihyperlipidemic/HMG-CoA reductase inhibitor

How Supplied
Pravachol Tablets 10 mg, Tablets 20 mg, Tablets 40 mg, Tablets 80 mg
❀ *Apo-Pravastatin* ♦ *Nu-Pravastatin*

Action
PHARMACOLOGY: Increases rate at which body removes cholesterol from blood and reduces production of cholesterol in body by inhibiting enzyme that catalyzes early rate-limiting step in cholesterol synthesis.

PHARMACOKINETICS/DYNAMICS:
Absorption: Rapidly absorbed (34%). T_{max} is 1 to 1.5 hr. Bioavailability is 17%. Food reduces systemic bioavailability.

Distribution: Protein binding is approximately 50%.

Metabolism: Extensive first-pass extraction in the liver. The major degradation product is 3-alpha-hydroxy isomeric metabolite.

Excretion: Urine (20% excreted); feces (70% excreted). The t½ is 77 hr.

Special Populations:
Elderly – Mean AUC was approximately 27% greater and mean cumulative urinary excretion was approximately 19% lower in elderly men. Mean AUC was approximately 46% higher and mean cumulative urinary excretion was approximately 18% lower in elderly women.

Indications As an adjunct to diet for reduction of elevated total and LDL cholesterol, apolipoprotein B, and triglyceride levels and to increase HDL cholesterol in patients with primary hypercholesterolemia and mixed dyslipidemia (Frederickson types IIa and IIb); as adjunctive therapy to diet for treatment of patients with elevated serum triglyceride levels (Frederickson type IV); treatment of primary dysbetalipoproteinemia (Frederickson type III) who do not respond adequately to diet; in hypercholesterolemic patients without clinically evident coronary heart disease (CHD) to reduce risk of MI or CV mortality with no increase in death from noncardiovascular causes; in patients with clinically evident CHD, to reduce risk of total mortality by reducing coronary death, MI, undergoing myocardial revascularization procedures, stroke, and stroke/transient ischemic attack and slow progression of coronary arteriosclerosis.

Contraindications Active liver disease or unexplained persistent elevations of LFTs; pregnancy; lactation.

Route/Dosage

ADULTS: **PO** 10 to 40 mg/day.
CHILDREN 8 TO 13 YR OF AGE: **PO** 20 mg once daily.
CHILDREN 14 TO 18 YR OF AGE: **PO** 40 mg once daily.

Interactions

Bile acid sequestrants: Large decrease in pravastatin bioavailability.
Cyclosporine, gemfibrozil: Severe myopathy or rhabdomyolysis; decreased urinary excretion and protein binding of pravastatin.
Protease inhibitors (eg, ritonavir): Pravastatin plasma levels may be reduced, decreasing the efficacy.

Lab Test Interferences None well documented.

Adverse Reactions

CV: Chest pain.
CNS: Headache; dizziness.
DERM: Rash; pruritus.
EENT: Dysfunction of certain cranial nerves (including alteration of taste, impairment of extraocular movement, facial paresis); lens opacities.
GI: Nausea; vomiting; diarrhea; abdominal pain; constipation; flatulence; heartburn; dyspepsia; pancreatitis.
GU: Urinary abnormality.
HEPA: Hepatitis; jaundice; fatty changes in liver; cirrhosis; fulminant hepatic necrosis; hepatoma; increased serum transaminases.
RESP: Common cold; rhinitis; cough; influenza.
OTHER: Localized pain; myalgia; myopathy; rhabdomyolysis; fatigue; paresthesia; peripheral neuropathy. An apparent hypersensitivity syndrome has been reported rarely that has included 1 or more of the following features: anaphylaxis; angioedema; lupus erythematous-like syndrome; polymyalgia rheumatica; vasculitis; purpura; thrombocytopenia; leukopenia; hemolytic anemia; positive antinuclear antibodies; increase in erythrocyte sedimentation rate; arthritis; arthralgia; urticaria; asthenia; photosensitivity; fever; chills; flushing; malaise; dyspnea; toxic epidermal necrolysis; erythema multiforme, including Stevens-Johnson syndrome.

Precautions

Pregnancy: Category X.
Lactation: Excreted in breast milk.
Children: Use in children not recommended.
Renal function impairment: Monitor patients closely.
Hepatic function impairment: Use with caution in patients who consume substantial quantities of alcohol or those with history of liver disease. Marked, persistent increases in serum transaminases have occurred.
Skeletal muscle effects: Rhabdomyolysis with renal dysfunction secondary to myoglobinuria has occurred.

PATIENT CARE CONSIDERATIONS

Administration/Storage

- May be used alone or in combination with other cholesterol-lowering medications.
- Administer prescribed dose once daily without regard to meals. Administer with food if GI upset occurs.
- Administer pravastatin at least 1 hr before or 4 hr after administration of a bile acid sequestrant (eg, cholestyramine).
- Store tablets at controlled room temperature (59° to 86°F). Protect from moisture and light

Assessment/Interventions

- Obtain patient history, including drug history and any known allergies. Note active liver disease, past history of liver disease, unexplained elevations of serum transaminases, renal insufficiency, pregnancy, breastfeeding, alcohol consumption, hypercholesterolemia caused by hyperalphalipoproteinemia, or concurrent therapy with medications known to increase the risk of myopathy (eg, fibrates, niacin, cyclosporine).
- Ensure that secondary causes of hypercholesterolemia (eg, poorly controlled diabetes, hypothyroidism, drugs that increase LDL-C and decrease HDL-C) are excluded or, if appropriate, treated before starting therapy.
- Ensure that patient is on a cholesterol-lowering diet before starting therapy and that diet is continued during treatment.
- Ensure that lower starting dose (eg, 10 mg) and cautious dose titration are used in patient

with history of significant renal or hepatic dysfunction or in patient taking immunosuppressive drugs such as cyclosporine.
♦ Ensure that lipid levels are measured before therapy is started, no less than 4 wk after starting pravastatin therapy or changing the dose, and then periodically thereafter.
♦ Ensure that therapy is temporarily withheld in patient with an acute, serious condition suggestive of myopathy or predisposing to the development of renal failure secondary to rhabdomyolysis (eg, sepsis, hypotension, major surgery).
♦ Ensure that serum transaminases are determined before starting therapy, before increasing the dose, and periodically thereafter as clinically indicated.
♦ If elevated serum transaminase levels develop during treatment, or if signs or symptoms of liver disease (flu-like symptoms, persistent nausea, fatigue, right upper quadrant abdominal pain, yellowing of skin or eyes, dark urine) are noted, repeat transaminase levels more frequently. If transaminase levels rise to 3 times upper limit of normal or greater and persist, notify health care provider. Be prepared to discontinue therapy.
♦ Monitor patient for symptoms of myopathy (muscle pain, tenderness, weakness) when medication is started and when dose is increased. Discontinue therapy and immediately notify health care provider if myopathy suspected.
♦ Assess patient for GI, CNS, and general body side effects. Inform health care provider if noted and significant.

Patient/Family Education
♦ Explain name, dose, action, potential side effects of medication, and LDL-C goal.
♦ Advise patient that dose of medication may change, based on results of cholesterol blood tests, in an effort to reach LDL-C goal.
♦ Advise patient to take prescribed dose once daily without regard to meals, but to take with food if stomach upset occurs.
♦ Advise patient to try to take each dose at about the same time each day.
♦ Advise patient that if a dose is missed to take as soon as remembered but to never take more than 1 dose of pravastatin a day.
♦ Caution patient not to change the dose or stop taking unless advised by health care provider.
♦ Advise patient that pravastatin helps control, but does not cure, cholesterol abnormality and to continue taking as prescribed when LDL-C goal has been reached.
♦ Instruct patient to continue taking other cholesterol-lowering medications as prescribed by health care provider.
♦ Advise patient who is also taking a bile acid sequestrant (eg, cholestyramine) to take the pravastatin at least 1 hr before or 4 hr after the sequestrant.
♦ Instruct patient to immediately notify health care provider if experiencing any unexplained muscle pain, tenderness, and/or weakness, or if they note any other unusual feelings.
♦ Emphasize to patient importance of other modalities on cholesterol control: dietary changes (reduced saturated fat intake, increase soluble fiber intake), weight control, regular exercise, and smoking cessation.
♦ Advise women of childbearing potential to use effective contraception during treatment with pravastatin.
♦ Advise women to notify health care provider if pregnant, planning to become pregnant, or breastfeeding.
♦ Caution patient not to take any prescription or OTC medications, herbal preparations, or dietary supplements unless advised by health care provider.
♦ Advise patient that follow-up visits and lab tests will be required to monitor therapy and to keep appointments.

Praziquantel

(pray-zih-KWAHN-tuhl)
Class Anti-infective/Antihelminthic
How Supplied
Biltricide Tablets 600 mg

Action
PHARMACOLOGY: Increases cell membrane permeability in susceptible worms, resulting in loss of intracellular calcium, massive contractions, and paralysis of their musculature. Phagocytes are thus able to attach to worms, causing their death.

PHARMACOKINETICS/DYNAMICS:
Absorption: Rapidly absorbed (80%). T_{max} is 1 to 3 hr.

Distribution: CSF levels are 14% to 20% of plasma concentration. Appears in breast milk. Protein binding is 80% to 85%.

Metabolism: Extensive first-pass metabolism, rapidly metabolized to inactive mono- and polyhydroxylated derivatives.

Excretion: Urine (as metabolites), small amounts in feces. Serum $t_{1/2}$ is 0.8 to 1.5 hr.

Special Populations:
Hepatic Function Impairment – Moderate to severe; plasma concentration were significantly elevated in one study.

Indications Infections caused by *Schistosoma mekongi, S. japonicum, S. mansoni, S. hematobium*, liver flukes, *Clonorchis sinensis,* and *Opisthorchis viverrini.* **Unlabeled use(s):** Treatment of neurocysticercosis, tissue flukes (opisthorchis, felineus, *Paragonimus westermani, Fasciola hepatica*), intestinal flukes (*Heterophyes heterophyes, Fasciolopsis buski*), and intestinal cestodes (*Diphyllobothrium latum, Taenia saginata, T. solium, Dipylidium caninum, Hymenolepsis nana*), and schistosomiasis (in concurrent use with oxamniquine).

Contraindications Ocular cysticercosis.

Route/Dosage
Schistosomiasis
ADULTS AND CHILDREN AT LEAST 4 YR: **PO** 60 mg/kg in 3 equally divided doses q 4 to 6 hr for 1 day.

Clonorchiasis and Opisthorchiasis
ADULTS: **PO** 75 mg/kg in 3 equally divided doses q 4 to 6 hr for 1 day.

Interactions
Cimetidine: Plasma levels of praziquantel may be elevated, increasing the pharmacologic and adverse effects.

Lab Test Interferences None well documented.

Adverse Reactions
CNS: Malaise; headache; fever; drowsiness; dizziness.
DERM: Urticaria.
GI: Abdominal discomfort, with or without nausea.
HEPA: Increased liver enzymes.

Precautions
Pregnancy: Category B.
Lactation: Excreted in breast milk. Lactating women should avoid breastfeeding on day of treatment and for subsequent 72 hr.
Children: Safety and efficacy not established in children under 4 yr.

PATIENT CARE CONSIDERATIONS
Administration/Storage
- Administer tablets during meals with liquids.
- Instruct patient not to chew tablets.
- Store at room temperature.

Assessment/Interventions
- Obtain patient history, including drug history and any known allergies. Note history of seizures.
- Monitor for side effects, especially malaise, headache, dizziness, abdominal pain, nausea, or fever.

Patient/Family Education
- Explain that treatment lasts only 1 day for most parasitic infections.
- Instruct patient to take drug with liquids during meals and not to chew tablets.
- Advise patient to have all family members examined for infestation.
- Emphasize need for follow-up examinations.
- Instruct patient to report the following symptoms to health care provider: malaise, headache, dizziness, abdominal pain, nausea, urticaria, or fever.
- Advise patient that drug may cause drowsiness and to use caution while driving or performing other tasks requiring mental alertness.

Prazosin
(PRAY-zoe-sin)

Class Antihypertensive/Antiadrenergic, peripherally acting

How Supplied
Minipress Capsules 1 mg, Capsules 2 mg, Capsules 5 mg
🍁 *Alti-Prazosi* ♦ *APO-Prazo* ♦ *Novo-Prazin* ♦ *Nu-Prazo*

Action
PHARMACOLOGY: Selectively blocks postsynaptic alpha-1 adrenergic receptors, resulting in dilation of arterioles and veins.

PHARMACOKINETICS/DYNAMICS:
Absorption: T_{max} is approximately 3 hr. Oral bioavailability is 48% to 68%.

Distribution: Protein binding is 92% to 97%.
Metabolism: Extensively metabolized by demethylation and conjugation in the liver.
Excretion: Urine (less than 10%); feces (less than 90%). Plasma $t_{1/2}$ is 2 to 3 hr.
Duration: Duration of antihypertensive effect is 10 hr.

Special Populations:
CHF – Elimination is slower.
Chronic renal failure – Elimination half-life prolonged, protein binding decreased, and peak plasma concentrations increased.

Indications Treatment of hypertension.

Contraindications Hypersensitivity to doxazosin, prazosin, or terazosin.

Route/Dosage
ADULTS:
Initial dose: **PO** 1 mg bid to tid.
Maintenance: **PO** 6 to 20 mg/day in divided doses (max, 40 mg/day).
CHILDREN: **PO** 0.5 to 7 mg tid has been suggested.

Interactions
Alcohol: Increased risk of hypotension.
Beta-blockers: Enhanced acute orthostatic hypotensive reaction after first dose of prazosin.
Verapamil: Increased serum prazosin levels and increased sensitivity to orthostatic hypotension.

Lab Test Interferences
May cause false elevation in vanillylmandelic acid.

Adverse Reactions
CV: Palpitations; orthostatic hypotension; hypotension; tachycardia.
CNS: Depression; dizziness; nervousness; paresthesia; asthenia; drowsiness; headache.
DERM: Pruritus; rash; sweating; alopecia; lichen planus.
EENT: Blurred vision; conjunctivitis; tinnitus; nasal congestion; epistaxis.
GI: Nausea; vomiting; dry mouth; diarrhea; constipation; abdominal discomfort or pain.
GU: Impotence; urinary frequency; incontinence; priapism.
RESP: Dyspnea.
OTHER: Arthralgia; edema; fever.

Precautions
Pregnancy: Category C.
Lactation: Excreted in breast milk.
Children: Safety and efficacy not established.
Concomitant therapy: When adding a diuretic or other antihypertensive agent, reduce dosage to 1 to 2 mg tid and then retitrate.
First-dose effect: May cause marked hypotension (especially orthostatic) and syncope at 30 min after first few doses, after reintroduction, with rapid increase (at least 2 mg) in dosing, or after addition of another antihypertensive. To avoid, initiate dosing with low dose (1 mg or up to 2 mg) and gradually increase after 2 wk.
Lipids: May decrease total cholesterol levels and LDLs and increase HDLs.

Overdosage: Signs and Symptoms
Drowsiness, depressed reflexes, hypotension.

PATIENT CARE CONSIDERATIONS
Administration/Storage
- Give initial dose at bedtime to avoid syncope.
- Dosage is increased slowly, usually q 2 wk, with increase given at bedtime dose.
- Give maintenance therapy in divided doses.
- Note that efficacy does not increase when dosage exceeds 20 mg/day.
- Store at room temperature in tightly-closed, light-resistant container.

Assessment/Interventions
- Obtain patient history, including drug history and any known allergies. Note current use of antihypertensives.
- Obtain baseline BP and pulse.
- Observe for possible retention of water and sodium.
- Monitor closely for first-dose effect. If syncope occurs, place patient in recumbent position and notify health care provider.
- Notify health care provider if patient complains of dizziness, palpitations, drowsiness, fatigue, tiredness, nausea, or headache.

Patient/Family Education
- Advise patient to take medication at same time each day.
- Warn patient about possibility of syncope or orthostasis.
- Instruct patient to report the following symptoms to health care provider: dizziness, palpitations, drowsiness, fatigue, nausea, headache.
- Caution patient to avoid sudden position changes to prevent orthostatic hypotension.
- Advise patient to avoid driving or performing other tasks requiring mental alertness for 12 to 24 hr after first dose, after dosage increase, and after resuming treatment after interruption. After the 12- to 24-hr period, advise patient to use caution.
- Instruct patient not to take OTC medications (eg, nonprescription weight loss products or cough, cold, or allergy medications) without consulting health care provider.

Prednisolone
(pred-NISS-oh-lone)
Class Corticosteroid

How Supplied
Prednisolone
Delta-Cortef Tablets 5 mg ♦ Prelone Syrup 5 mg/5 mL, Syrup 15 mg/5 mL
✤ Minims Prednisolone ♦ Novo-Prednisolone

Prednisolone Acetate
Econopred Suspension 0.125% ♦ Econopred Plus Suspension 1% ♦ Key-Pred 25 Injection 25 mg/mL suspension ♦ Key-Pred 50 Injection 50 mg/mL suspension ♦ Predcor-50 Injection 50 mg/mL suspension ♦ Predalone 50 Injection 50 mg/mL suspension ♦ Pred Forte Suspension 1% ♦ Pred Mild Suspension 0.12%

Prednisolone Sodium Phosphate
AK-Pred Solution 1% prednisolone sodium

phosphate, Solution 0.125% prednisolone sodium phosphate ♦ *Hydeltrasol* Injection 20 mg/mL prednisolone (as sodium phosphate) solution ♦ *Inflamase Forte* Solution 1% prednisolone sodium phosphate ♦ *Inflamase Mild* Solution 0.125% prednisolone sodium phosphate ♦ *Key-Pred-SP* Injection 20 mg/mL prednisolone (as sodium phosphate) solution ♦ *Pediapred* Oral liquid 5 mg prednisolone (as sodium phosphate)/5 mL

Prednisolone Tebutate
Prednisol TBA Injection 20 mg/mL suspension

Action
PHARMACOLOGY: Intermediate-acting glucocorticoid that depresses formation, release, and activity of endogenous mediators of inflammation including prostaglandins, kinins, histamine, liposomal enzymes, and complement system. Also modifies body's immune response.

PHARMACOKINETICS/DYNAMICS:
Absorption: Rapid and almost completely absorbed (oral, IV, IM). Slow, but completely absorbed (tebutate).

Distribution: Protein binding is high; crosses the placenta.

Metabolism: Primarily hepatic, also renal and tissue to mainly inactive metabolites.

Excretion: Renal (inactive metabolites). Plasma $t_{1/2}$ is 2.1 to 3.5 hr; biologic $t_{1/2}$ is 18 to 36 hr.

Onset: Slow, 1 to 2 days (tebutate).

Peak: 1 to 2 hr (oral); 1 hr (IV, IM).

Duration: 1.25 to 1.5 days (oral); up to 4 wk (IM). Duration of action for tebutate is 1 to 3 wk.

Indications
Oral/Parenteral administration: Endocrine disorders: rheumatic disorders; collagen diseases; dermatologic diseases; allergic and inflammatory ophthalmic processes; respiratory diseases; hematologic disorders; neoplastic diseases; edematous states caused by nephrotic syndrome; GI diseases; multiple sclerosis; tuberculous meningitis; trichinosis with neurologic or myocardial involvement.

Intra-articular or soft tissue administration: Short-term adjunctive therapy of synovitis of osteoarthritis, rheumatoid arthritis, bursitis, acute gouty arthritis, epicondylitis, acute nonspecific tenosynovitis, posttraumatic osteoarthritis.

Intralesional administration: Treatment of the following lesions: keloids; localized hypertrophic, infiltrated, inflammatory lesions of lichen planus, psoriatic plaques, granuloma annulare, lichen simplex chronicus; discoid lupus erythematosus; necrobiosis lipoidica diabeticorum; alopecia areata; cystic tumors of aponeurosis or tendon.

Ophthalmic administration: Treatment of steroid-responsive inflammatory conditions of palpebral and bulbar conjunctiva, lid, cornea and anterior segment of globe. **Unlabeled use(s):** Adjunctive therapy for tuberculous pleurisy.

Contraindications
Oral/Parenteral: Systemic fungal infections; administration of live virus vaccines.
IM: Idiopathic thrombocytopenic purpura; sulfite sensitivity.
Ophthalmic: Acute superficial herpes simplex keratitis; fungal diseases of ocular structures, vaccinia, varicella, and most other viral diseases of cornea and conjunctiva; ocular tuberculosis.

Route/Dosage
ADULTS: **PO** 5 to 60 mg/day (prednisolone, prednisolone sodium phosphate).
IM 4 to 60 mg/day (prednisolone acetate).
IV/IM 4 to 60 mg/day (prednisolone sodium phosphate).
Ophthalmic 1 to 2 gtt into conjunctival sac q hr during day and q 2 hr during night (prednisolone acetate, prednisolone sodium phosphate).

Intra-Articular, Intralesional, or Soft Tissue Administration
ADULTS: 4 to 100 mg (prednisolone acetate); 4 to 30 mg or lesions (prednisolone tebutate), or 2 to 30 mg prednisolone sodium phosphate.

Multiple Sclerosis
ADULTS: **PO** 200 mg/day for 1 wk, then 80 mg qod for 1 mo (prednisolone, prednisolone sodium phosphate). **IM** 200 mg/day for 1 wk, then 80 mg qod for 1 mo (prednisolone acetate).

Tuberculous Pleurisy
ADULTS: **PO** 0.75 mg/kg/day then taper as tolerated until patient is drug-free (prednisolone).

Interactions
Anticholinesterases: May antagonize anticholinesterase effects in myasthenia gravis.
Barbiturates: May decrease pharmacologic effect of prednisolone.
Contraceptives (oral), estrogens, ketoconazole: May decrease clearance of prednisolone.
Hydantoins, rifampin: May increase clearance and decrease efficacy of prednisolone.
Salicylate: May reduce serum levels and efficacy of salicylates.
Troleandomycin: May increase prednisolone effects.

Lab Test Interferences
May cause increased serum cholesterol; decreased serum levels of potassium, T_3 and T_4; decreased uptake of thyroid I^{131}; false-negative results of nitroblue-tetrazolium test for systemic bacterial infection; suppression of skin test reactions.

Adverse Reactions

CV: Thromboembolism or fat embolism; thrombophlebitis; necrotizing angiitis; cardiac arrhythmias or ECG changes; syncopal episodes; hypertension; myocardial rupture; CHF.

CNS: Convulsions; pseudotumor cerebri (increased intracranial pressure with papilledema); vertigo; headache; neuritis; paresthesias; psychosis.

DERM: Impaired wound healing; thin, fragile skin; petechiae and ecchymoses; erythema; lupus erythematosus-like lesions; SC fat atrophy; striae; hirsutism; acneiform eruptions; allergic dermatitis; urticaria; angioneurotic edema; perineal irritation; hyperpigmentation or hypopigmentation.

EENT: Posterior subcapsular cataracts; increased IOP; glaucoma; exophthalmos. With ophthalmic use: glaucoma with optic nerve damage; visual acuity and field defects; posterior subcapsular cataract formation; secondary ocular infections; transient stinging or burning; perforation of globe.

GI: Pancreatitis; abdominal distention; ulcerative esophagitis; nausea; vomiting; increased appetite and weight gain; peptic ulcer with perforation and hemorrhage; small and large bowel perforation.

GU: Increased or decreased motility and number of spermatozoa.

HEMA: Leukocytosis.

METAB: Sodium and fluid retention; hypokalemia; hypokalemic alkalosis; metabolic alkalosis; hypocalcemia; negative nitrogen balance.

OTHER: Musculoskeletal effects (eg, weakness, myopathy, muscle mass loss, tendon rupture, osteoporosis, aseptic necrosis of femoral and humoral heads, spontaneous fractures); endocrine abnormalities (eg, menstrual irregularities, cushingoid state, growth suppression in children, sweating, decreased carbohydrate tolerance, hyperglycemia, glycosuria, increased insulin or sulfonylurea requirements in diabetic patients, hirsutism); anaphylactoid or hypersensitivity reactions; aggravation or masking of infections; fatigue; insomnia. With intra-articular administration: osteonecrosis; tendon rupture; infection, skin atrophy; postinjection flare; hypersensitivity; facial flushing.

Precautions

Pregnancy: Category C (prednisolone sodium phosphate). Safety not established.
Lactation: Excreted in breast milk.
Children: Observe growth and development of infants and children on prolonged therapy.
Elderly: May require lower doses.
Hypersensitivity: Reactions may occur, including anaphylaxis.
Renal function impairment: Use drug with caution.
Adrenal suppression: Prolonged therapy may lead to HPA suppression.
Cardiovascular effects: Use drug with great caution in patient who has suffered recent MI.
Hepatitis: Drug may be harmful in patients with chronic active hepatitis positive for hepatitis B surface antigen.
Immunosuppression: Do not administer live virus vaccines during treatment.
Infections: Drug may mask signs of infection. May decrease host-defense mechanisms to prevent dissemination of infection.
Ocular effects: Use systemic drug with caution in ocular herpes simplex because of possible corneal perforation.
Ophthalmic use: Prolonged use may result in cataracts, glaucoma, or other complications.
Peptic ulcer: May contribute to peptic ulceration, especially in large doses.
Repository injections: Do not inject SC. Avoid injection into deltoid muscle and repeated IM injection to same site.
Stress: Increased dosage of rapidly acting corticosteroid may be needed before, during and after stressful situations.
Withdrawal: Abrupt discontinuation may result in adrenal insufficiency.

Overdosage: Signs and Symptoms

Cushingoid changes, moonfaced, striae, central obesity, hirsutism, acne, ecchymoses, hypertension, osteoporosis, myopathy, sexual dysfunction, diabetes mellitus, hyperlipidemia, peptic ulcer, GI bleeding, increased susceptibility to infection, electrolyte and fluid imbalance, psychosis.

PATIENT CARE CONSIDERATIONS

Administration/Storage

- Check drug name carefully to avoid confusion with prednisone.
- Administer oral medication with food.
- For long-term use, alternate-day regimen may be used.
- Do not inject SC or IM doses into deltoid muscle. Give IM injection in gluteal muscle. Rotate injection sites.
- Do not administer if patient has had live vaccine within last month.
- Discontinuation of drug must be done gradually.
- If giving ophthalmic solution, do not touch eye with dropper, place drops in lower lid and wait 5 min between drops. Apply pressure on lacrimal sac to prevent systemic effects. Wash hands before and after administering.
- Store dosage forms at room temperature and protect from light.

Assessment/Interventions
- Obtain patient history, including drug history and any known allergies. Note MI, diabetes, renal impairment, hepatitis, peptic ulcer disease, ocular herpes simplex, or current infections.
- If patient is at increased risk for herpes, chickenpox, or other viruses, notify health care provider.
- Ensure that baseline lab tests have been obtained before beginning therapy. Monitor for possible hyperglycemia, hypoglycemia, and hypocalcemia during treatment.
- Be aware that drug may mask signs of infection and that resistance to infection may be diminished.
- In patients with diabetes, monitor blood glucose carefully.
- Monitor renal function, especially in patients with renal impairment.
- Observe for possible delayed wound healing.
- If menstrual irregularities, muscle wasting or weakness, moon face, fluid retention, GI bleeding, or mental status changes occur, notify health care provider.
- Assess for signs of adrenal insufficiency (eg, fever, myalgia, arthralgia, malaise, anorexia, nausea, orthostatic hypotension, dizziness, fainting) and notify health care provider immediately if suspected.

Patient/Family Education
- Advise patient to take single daily or alternate-day doses in morning before 9 AM and to take multiple doses at evenly-spaced intervals throughout day.
- Instruct patient to take medication with meals or snacks to avoid GI irritation.
- Caution patient not to take drug with aspirin or other OTC medications containing salicylates unless directed by health care provider.
- Instruct patient to check weight at home daily at same time of day.
- Advise patient on chronic steroid therapy to wear *Medi-Alert* identification indicating condition and drug regimen.
- Remind patient to wash hands before and after instillation.
- Teach patient correct method for instilling eye drops.
- Instruct patient not to rub eyes or touch dropper into eye.
- Inform patient of increased appetite and counsel patient on appropriate diet management (ie, diet high in protein, calcium and potassium but low in sodium and carbohydrates).
- Advise family that medication may slow growth in children.
- Inform patient of the possible side effects of moonface, mood swings, and increased emotions.
- Teach patient to monitor for infection, eye burning, or increased bruising.
- Instruct patient not to drive soon after using eye drops because vision may be blurred initially.
- Inform patient that ophthalmic preparation may cause sensitivity to bright light and recommend use of sunglasses to minimize this effect.
- Instruct patient to report the following symptoms to health care provider: unusual weight gain, swelling of lower extremities, muscle weakness, black tarry stools, vomiting of blood, puffing of face, menstrual irregularities, prolonged sore throat, fever, cold, or infection.
- Tell patient to notify health care provider if the following symptoms occur after dosage reduction or withdrawal of therapy: fatigue, anorexia, nausea, vomiting, diarrhea, weight loss, weakness, dizziness or low blood sugar.

Prednisolone Acetate/ Gentamicin Sulfate

(pred-NISS-oh-lone ASS-uh-TATE/JEN-tuh-MY-sin SULL-fate Pred-G)

Class Corticosteroid/Antibiotic

How Supplied
Pred-G Ophthalmic Suspension 1% prednisolone acetate and gentamicin sulfate equiv. to 0.3% gentamicin base ♦ Pred-G S.O.P. Ophthalmic Ointment 0.6% prednisolone acetate and gentamicin sulfate equiv. to 0.3% gentamicin base

Action
PHARMACOLOGY:
Prednisolone: Depresses formation, release, and activity of endogenous mediators of inflammation as well as modifying body's immune response.
Gentamicin: Inhibits production of bacterial protein, causing bacterial cell death.

Indications Treatment of steroid-responsive inflammatory ocular conditions for which a corticosteroid is indicated and when superficial bacterial ocular infection or a risk of bacterial ocular infection exists; inflammatory conditions of the palpebral and bulbar conjunctiva, cornea, and anterior segment of the globe where the inherent risk of steroid use in certain infective conjunctivitides is accepted to obtain a diminution in edema and inflammation; chronic anterior uveitis; corneal injury from chemical, radiation, or thermal burns or penetration of foreign bodies; high risk of superficial ocular infection; expectation that potentially dangerous numbers of bacteria will be present.

Contraindications Epithelial herpes simplex keratitis (dendritic keratitis); vaccinia; varicella and many other viral diseases of the cornea and conjunctiva; mycobacterial eye infection; fungal diseases of the ocular structures; uncomplicated removal of a corneal foreign body; hypersensitivity to any component of the product.

Route/Dosage
ADULTS: **Topical Ointment** Apply small amount (½ inch ribbon) in the conjunctival sac 1 to 3 times/day. **Suspension** Instill 1 gtt into the conjunctival sac 2 to 4 times/day. During the initial 24 to 48 hr, the dosing frequency may be increased if necessary, up to 1 gtt q hr. If signs and symptoms fail to improve after 2 days, re-evaluate the patient.

PATIENT CARE CONSIDERATIONS

Administration/Storage
- For ophthalmic use only. Not for use in the ears or on the skin.
- Shake well before instilling gtt.
- Instill 1 to 2 gtt into conjunctival sac(s) as prescribed.
- Instill prescribed amount of ointment qd to tid as ordered.
- Do not allow tip of dropper bottle or tube to touch eye, eyelid, fingers, or any other surface.
- If using other topical ophthalmic medications, instill gtt first, wait at least 5 min, and instill ointment last.
- Store ointment at controlled room temperature (59° to 86°F). Keep tube capped.
- Store suspension at controlled room temperature (59° to 77°F). Keep bottle tightly capped and protect from freezing.

Assessment/Interventions
- Obtain patient history, including drug history and any known allergies. Note history of viral, mycobacterial, or fungal infection of the eye(s).
- Monitor patient's response to therapy. Notify health care provider if eye or eyelid inflammation is noted or if symptoms do not improve or worsen.
- Ensure that IOP is measured if therapy is continued beyond 10 days.

Interactions None well documented.
Lab Test Interferences None well documented.

Adverse Reactions
EENT: Ocular discomfort; irritation upon instillation; punctate keratitis; elevation of IOP with possible development of glaucoma; optic nerve damage; posterior subcapsular cataract formation; delayed wound healing; secondary infection; fungal infections of the cornea.
OTHER: Allergic sensitizations

Precautions
Pregnancy: Category C.
Lactation:
Prednisolone – Excreted in breast milk.
Children: Safety and efficacy not established.
Superinfection: Prolonged use may result in bacterial or fungal overgrowth of nonsusceptible microorganisms.
Bacterial Resistance: Bacterial resistance to components of the product may develop.
Ocular damage: Prolonged use may result in glaucoma, with damage to the optic nerve, defects in visual acuity and fields of vision, and in posterior subcapsular cataract formation.

Patient/Family Education
- Explain name, dose, action, and potential side effects of drug.
- Review prescribed dosing schedule with patient, family, or caregiver.
- Remind patient, family, or caregiver that suspension and ointment are for use in the eye only.
- Teach patient, family, or caregiver proper technique for instilling suspension: wash hands; do not allow tip of dropper bottle to touch eye, eyelid, fingers, or any other surface. Tilt head back and look up; pull lower eyelid down to form pocket; place prescribed number of gtt in the pocket. Look downward before closing eye. Do not rub eye.
- Teach patient or caregiver proper technique for instilling ointment: wash hands; do not allow tip of tube to touch eye, eyelid, fingers, or any other surface. Tilt head back and look up; pull lower eyelid down to form pocket; place prescribed amount of ointment in the pocket. Look downward before closing eye. Do not rub eye.
- Advise patient, family, or caregiver that if more than 1 topical ophthalmic drug is being used, instill eye gtt first, wait at least 5 min, and instill ointment last.
- Inform patient that temporary blurred vision and stinging of the eye are the most common

- side effects and to contact health care provider if these symptoms occur and are bothersome.
- Advise patient to contact eye doctor if eye or eyelid inflammation is noted or if eye symptoms do not improve or worsen.
- Advise patient that the entire course of therapy must be completed to ensure maximal benefit and to complete full course of therapy even if symptoms have resolved.
- Instruct patient not to wear contact lenses during treatment.
- Remind patient, family, or caregiver that follow-up eye examinations may be necessary while using this medication and to keep appointments.

Prednisolone Acetate/ Neomycin Sulfate/Polymyxin B Sulfate

(pred-NISS-oh-lone ASS-uh-TATE/NEE-oh-MY-sin SULL-fate/pahl-ee-MIX-in BEE SULL-fate)

Class Corticosteroid/Antibacterial

How Supplied
Poly-Pred Liquifilm Ophthalmic Suspension 0.5% prednisolone acetate/neomycin sulfate equiv. to 0.35% neomycin base/10,000 units/mL polymyxin B sulfate

Action

PHARMACOLOGY:
Prednisolone: Depresses formation, release, and activity of endogenous mediators of inflammation including prostaglandins, kinins, histamine, liposomal enzymes, and complement system.
Neomycin: Inhibits protein synthesis by binding to ribosomal RNA, causing bacterial genetic code misreading.
Polymyxin B: Interacts with phospholipid components of bacterial cell membrane, increasing cell wall permeability.

Indications Treatment of steroid-responsive inflammatory ocular conditions for which a corticosteroid is indicated and where bacterial infection or a risk of bacterial ocular infection exists; inflammatory conditions of the palpebral and bulbar conjunctiva, cornea, and anterior segment of the globe where the inherent risk of steroid use in certain infective conjunctivitis is accepted to obtain a diminution in edema and inflammation; chronic anterior uveitis and corneal injury from chemical, radiation, or thermal burns or penetration of foreign bodies; when risk of infection is high or where there is expectation that potentially dangerous numbers of bacteria will be present in the eye.

Contraindications Epithelial herpes simplex keratitis (dendritic keratitis), vaccinia, varicella, and many other viral diseases of the corneal and conjunctiva; mycobacterial eye infections; fungal diseases of the ocular structures; uncomplicated removal of a corneal foreign body; hypersensitivity to any component of the product.

Route/Dosage
Eye:
OPHTHALMIC Instill 1 or 2 gtt in the eye q 3 or 4 hr or more frequently as required. Acute infections may require administration every 30 min, with decreasing frequency as the infection is brought under control.
Lids:
OPHTHALMIC Instill 1 or 2 gtt in the eye q 3 to 4 hr, close the eye, and rub the excess on the lids and lid margins.

Interactions None well documented.

Lab Test Interferences None well documented.

Adverse Reactions
EENT: Elevated IOP with possible development of glaucoma; optic nerve damage; posterior subcapsular cataract formation; delayed wound healing; secondary infection; fungal infection; acute anterior uveitis and perforation of the globe.
OTHER: Allergic sensitivity.

Precautions
Pregnancy: Category C.
Lactation: Excreted in breast milk.
Children: Safety and efficacy have not been established.
Superinfection: Prolonged use may result in bacterial or fungal overgrowth of nonsusceptible microorganisms.
Cross-sensitivity: Allergic cross-sensitivity to kanamycin, paromomycin, streptomycin, and, possibly, gentamicin may occur.
Glaucoma: Prolonged use may result in glaucoma with damage to the optic nerve, defects in visual acuity and fields of vision, and posterior subcapsular cataract formation.
Secondary infection: Secondary bacterial ocular infection following suppression of host responses may occur.

PATIENT CARE CONSIDERATIONS
Administration/Storage
- For ophthalmic use only. Not for use in the ears or on the skin.
- Shake well before instilling gtt.
- Instill 1 to 2 gtt into conjunctival sac(s) as prescribed.

- Do not allow tip of dropper bottle to touch eye, eyelid, fingers, or any other surface.
- If using other topical ophthalmic medications, instill drops first, wait at least 5 min, and instill ointment last.
- Store at controlled room temperature (less than 77°F). Keep bottle tightly capped and protect from freezing.

Assessment/Interventions
- Obtain patient history, including drug history and any known allergies. Note history of viral, mycobacterial, or fungal infection of the eye(s).
- Monitor patient's response to therapy. Notify health care provider if eye or eyelid inflammation is noted or if symptoms do not improve or worsen.
- Ensure that intraocular pressure is measured if therapy is continued beyond 10 days.

Patient/Family Education
- Explain name, dose, action, and potential side effects of drug.
- Review prescribed dosing schedule with patient, family, or caregiver.
- Remind patient, family, or caregiver that suspension is for use in the eye only.
- Teach patient, family, or caregiver proper technique for instilling suspension: wash hands; do not allow tip of dropper bottle to touch eye, eyelid, fingers, or any other surface. Tilt head back, look up; pull lower eyelid down to form pocket; place prescribed number of drops in the pocket. Look downward before closing eye. Do not rub eye.
- Advise patient, family, or caregiver that if more than 1 topical ophthalmic drug is being used, instill eye drops first, wait at least 5 min and then instill ointment last.
- Inform patient that temporary blurred vision and stinging of the eye are the most common side effects and to contact health care provider if these symptoms occur and are bothersome.
- Advise patient to contact eye doctor if eye or eyelid inflammation is noted or if eye symptoms do not improve or worsen.
- Advise patient that the entire course of therapy must be completed to ensure maximal benefit and to complete full course of therapy even if symptoms have resolved.
- Instruct patient not to wear contact lenses during treatment.
- Remind patient, family, or caregiver that follow-up eye examinations may be necessary while using this medication and to keep appointments.

Prednisone
(PRED-nih-sone)

Class Corticosteroid

How Supplied
Deltasone Tablets 2.5 mg, Tablets 5 mg, Tablets 10 mg, Tablets 20 mg, Tablets 50 mg ♦ *Liquid Pred* Syrup 5 mg/5 mL ♦ *Meticorten* Tablets 1 mg ♦ *Orasone* Tablets 1 mg, Tablets 5 mg, Tablets 10 mg, Tablets 20 mg, Tablets 50 mg ♦ *Panasol-S* Tablets 1 mg ♦ *Prednicen-M* Tablets 5 mg ♦ *Prednisone Intensol Concentrate* Oral solution 5 mg/mL ♦ *Sterapred* Tablets 5 mg ♦ *Sterapred DS* Tablets 10 mg
✤ *Alti-Prednisone* ♦ *Apo-Prednisone* ♦ *Jaa Prednisone*

Action
PHARMACOLOGY: Intermediate-acting glucocorticoid that depresses formation, release, and activity of endogenous mediators of inflammation, including prostaglandins, kinins, histamine, liposomal enzymes, and complement system. Also modifies body's immune response.

PHARMACOKINETICS/DYNAMICS:
Absorption: Rapid, almost complete.
Distribution: Crosses placenta.
Metabolism: Mainly hepatic, also renal and in the tissue. Prednisone is inactive and rapidly metabolized to active prednisolone.
Excretion: Renal. Plasma $t_{1/2}$ is 3.4 to 3.8 hr.
Peak: 1 to 2 hr.
Duration: 1.25 to 1.5 days.

Indications Endocrine disorders; rheumatic disorders; collagen diseases; dermatologic diseases; allergic states; allergic and inflammatory ophthalmic processes; respiratory diseases; hematologic disorders; neoplastic diseases; edematous states (because of nephrotic syndrome); GI diseases; multiple sclerosis; tuberculous meningitis; trichinosis with neurologic or myocardial involvement. **Unlabeled use(s):** COPD; Duchenne muscular dystrophy; Graves ophthalmopathy.

Contraindications Systemic fungal infections; administration of live virus vaccines.

Route/Dosage
ADULTS: **PO** 5 to 60 mg/day.

COPD
ADULTS: **PO** 30 to 60 mg/day for 1 to 2 wk, then taper.

Duchenne Muscular Dystrophy
ADULTS: PO 0.75 to 1.5 mg/kg/day.

Graves Ophthalmopathy
ADULTS: PO 60 mg/day; taper to 20 mg/day.

Interactions
Anticholinesterases: Antagonizes anticholinesterase effects in myasthenia gravis.
Anticoagulants, oral: Alters anticoagulant dose requirements.
Barbiturates, hydantoins (eg, phenytoin), rifampin: Decreased pharmacologic effect of prednisone.
Cyclosporine: Enhanced cyclosporine toxicity.
Estrogens, ketoconazole, oral contraceptives: Decreased clearance of prednisone.
Nondepolarizing muscle relaxants: May potentiate, counteract, or have no effect on neuromuscular blocking action.
Salicylates: Reduced serum levels and efficacy of salicylates.
Somatrem: Inhibition of growth-promoting effects of somatrem.
Theophylline: Alterations in pharmacologic activity of either agent.

Lab Test Interferences May increase serum cholesterol; decrease serum levels of T_3 and T_4; decrease uptake of thyroid I^{131}; and cause false-negative result on nitroblue-tetrazolium test for systemic bacterial infection and suppression of skin test reactions.

Adverse Reactions
CV: Thromboembolism or fat embolism; thrombophlebitis; necrotizing angiitis; cardiac arrhythmias or ECG changes; syncopal episodes; hypertension; myocardial rupture; CHF.
CNS: Convulsions; pseudotumor cerebri (increased intracranial pressure with papilledema); vertigo; headache; neuritis/paresthesias; psychosis.
DERM: Impaired wound healing; thin fragile skin; petechiae and ecchymoses; erythema; lupus erythematosus-like lesions; SC fat atrophy; purpura; striae; hirsutism; acneiform eruptions; allergic dermatitis; urticaria; angioneurotic edema; perineal irritation.
EENT: Posterior subcapsular cataracts; increased IOP; glaucoma; exophthalmos.
GI: Pancreatitis; abdominal distention; ulcerative esophagitis; nausea; vomiting; increased appetite and weight gain; peptic ulcer with perforation and hemorrhage; small and large bowel perforation.
GU: Increased or decreased motility and number of spermatozoa.
HEMA: Leukocytosis.
METAB: Sodium and fluid retention; hypokalemia; hypokalemic alkalosis; metabolic alkalosis; hypocalcemia.
OTHER: Musculoskeletal effects (muscle weakness, steroid myopathy, muscle mass loss, tendon rupture, osteoporosis, aseptic necrosis of femoral and humeral heads, spontaneous fractures, including vertebral compression fractures and pathologic fracture of long bones); endocrine abnormalities (menstrual irregularities, cushingoid state, growth suppression in children secondary to adrenocortical and pituitary unresponsiveness, increased sweating, decreased carbohydrate tolerance, hyperglycemia, glycosuria, increased insulin or sulfonylurea requirements in diabetics, negative nitrogen balance because of protein catabolism, hirsutism); anaphylactoid/hypersensitivity reactions; aggravation or masking of infections; malaise; fatigue; insomnia.

Precautions
Pregnancy: Category C.
Lactation: Excreted in breast milk.
Children: Observe growth and development of infants and children on prolonged therapy.
Elderly: May require lower doses.
Hypersensitivity: May occur, including anaphylaxis.
Renal function impairment: Use with caution; monitor renal function.
Adrenal suppression: Prolonged therapy may lead to HPA suppression.
Cardiovascular effects: Use drug with great caution in patients who have suffered recent MI.
Hepatitis: Drug may be harmful in patients with chronic active hepatitis positive for hepatitis B surface antigen.
Immunosuppression: Do not administer live virus vaccines during treatment.
Infections: May mask signs of infection. May decrease host-defense mechanisms to prevent dissemination of infection.
Ocular effects: Use systemic drug cautiously in ocular herpes simplex because of possible corneal perforation.
Ophthalmic use: Prolonged use may result in glaucoma, cataracts, or other complications.
Peptic ulcer: May contribute to peptic ulceration, especially with large doses.
Stress: Increased dosage of rapidly acting corticosteroid may be needed before, during and after stressful situations.
Withdrawal: Abrupt discontinuation may result in adrenal insufficiency.

Overdosage: Signs and Symptoms
Cushingoid changes, moonfaced, striae, central obesity, hirsutism, acne, ecchymoses, hypertension, osteoporosis, myopathy, sexual dysfunction, diabetes mellitus, hyperlipidemia, peptic ulcer, GI bleeding, increased susceptibility to infection, electrolyte and fluid imbalance, psychosis.

PATIENT CARE CONSIDERATIONS
Administration/Storage
- Administer with meal or snack.
- Give single daily dose before 9 AM; space multiple doses evenly throughout day.
- Do not administer to patients who have received live virus vaccine within last month.

Assessment/Interventions
- Obtain patient history, including drug history and any known allergies. Note MI, diabetes, renal impairment, hepatitis, tuberculosis, peptic ulcer disease, ocular herpes simplex, or current infections.
- Ensure that baseline laboratory tests have been obtained before beginning therapy, and monitor for possible hyperglycemia, hypokalemia, and hypocalcemia during treatment.
- Be aware that drug may mask signs of infection and that resistance to infection may be diminished.
- Observe for possible delayed wound healing.
- Monitor blood glucose of diabetic patient carefully.
- If menstrual irregularities, muscle wasting or weakness, rounded moon facies, fluid retention, GI bleeding, or mental status changes occur, notify health care provider.
- Assess for signs of adrenal insufficiency (eg, fever, myalgia, arthralgia, malaise, anorexia, nausea, orthostatic hypotension, dizziness, fainting). Notify health care provider immediately if this condition is suspected.

Patient/Family Education
- Advise patient to take single daily doses or alternate day doses in morning (before 9 AM) and to take multiple doses at evenly spaced intervals throughout day.
- Instruct patient to take medication with meals or snack to avoid GI irritation.
- Caution patient not to discontinue drug suddenly, to avoid withdrawal syndrome. Explain that dosage will be tapered slowly (until 5 mg/day or less) before stopping.
- Warn patient to avoid people with known viral infections, particularly chickenpox or measles, and to inform health care provider if exposure occurs.
- Explain that patient should not receive live virus vaccinations.
- Instruct diabetic patients to monitor blood glucose closely.
- Advise patient to notify health care providers of drug regimen before any surgical procedure, emergency treatment, immunization, or skin test.
- Tell patient to carry medical identification card at all times describing medication being taken.
- Tell patient about symptoms of adrenal insufficiency (eg, fever, myalgia, malaise, anorexia, nausea, orthostatic hypotension, dizziness, fainting) and need to report these symptoms to health care provider immediately.
- Instruct patient to report the following symptoms to health care provider: black tarry stools, vomiting of blood, menstrual irregularities, unusual weight gain, swelling of lower extremities, puffy face, muscle weakness, prolonged sore throat, fever, or cold.

Primaquine Phosphate
(PRIM-uh-kween FOSS-fate)

Class Anti-infective/Antimalarial

How Supplied
Available as generic only Tablets 26.3 mg (equiv. to 15 mg base), Powder no strength

Action
PHARMACOLOGY: Disrupts metabolic processes of parasitic organism, eliminating tissue (exo-erythrocytic) infection and preventing development of blood (erythrocytic) forms of parasite responsible for relapses of vivax malaria.

PHARMACOKINETICS/DYNAMICS:

Absorption: Rapid. Bioavailability is approximately 96%. T_{max} is approximately 2 to 3 hr (primaquine), approximately 7 hr (metabolite carboxyprimaquine). C_{max} is 50 to 66 ng/mL (15 mg); 104 ng/mL (30 mg).

Distribution: Extensively distributed. Vd is 248 L. C_{max} is 291 to 736 ng/mL (metabolite) and 432 to 1240 ng/mL (metabolite).

Metabolism: Rapidly converted to carboxyprimaquine. Undetermined if the main plasma metabolite has activity.

Excretion: Urine (less than 2% of dose). $T_{1/2}$ is 5.8 hr (primaquine); 22 to 30 hr (metabolite carboxyprimaquine).

Indications Radical cure or prevention of relapse in vivax malaria; after termination of chloroquine phosphate suppressive therapy in areas where vivax malaria is endemic.

Unlabeled use(s): With clindamycin, treatment of *Pneumocystis carinii* pneumonia associated with AIDS.

Contraindications Concomitant administration of quinacrine and primaquine; acutely ill patient with systemic disease manifested by granulocytopenia (eg, rheumatoid arthritis, lupus erythematosus); concurrent administration of other potentially hemolytic or bone marrow depressant medications.

Route/Dosage
Begin therapy during last 2 wk of or after course of suppression with chloroquine or comparable drug.
ADULTS: PO 26.3 mg (15 mg base) for 14 days.
CHILDREN: PO 0.5 mg/kg/day (0.3 mg/kg/day of base) for 14 days (max, 15 mg/day of base).

Interactions
Quinacrine: May potentiate toxicity of antimalarial compounds that are structurally related to primaquine.

Lab Test Interferences
None well documented.

Adverse Reactions
GI: Nausea; vomiting; epigastric distress; abdominal cramps.
HEMA: Leukopenia; hemolytic anemia in G-6-PD deficiency; methemoglobinemia in NADH methemoglobin reductase deficiency.

Precautions
Pregnancy: Pregnancy category undetermined.
Lactation: Undetermined. To avoid adverse effects in the infant, do not give to lactating women.
Hemolytic anemia: May occur in patients with following conditions: G-6-PD deficiency, NADH methemoglobin reductase deficiency; idiosyncratic reactions (leukopenia, methemoglobinemia; hemolytic anemia). Discontinue drug if marked darkening of urine or sudden decrease in hemoglobin or leukocyte count occurs.
Max dose: Hemolytic reactions may occur with doses of drug exceeding recommended dose.

Overdosage: Signs and Symptoms
Anemia, methemoglobinemia, leukopenia, acute abdominal cramps, vomiting, epigastric distress, CNS and cardiovascular disturbances, granulocytopenia, hemolytic anemia.

PATIENT CARE CONSIDERATIONS

Administration/Storage
- Do not begin administration unless patient has completed or is within 2 wk of completing course of suppression with chloroquine or comparable drug.
- Do not administer to patient who is taking or has recently received quinacrine within past 3 mo.
- Administer with food if medicine causes GI upset.
- Store at room temperature in tightly closed, light-resistant container.

Assessment/Interventions
- Obtain patient history, including drug history and any known allergies. Note recent use of quinacrine and other antimalarial agents.
- Ensure that CBC with differentials have been obtained before beginning therapy and are performed routinely during therapy.
- Monitor for hemolytic reactions (eg, marked darkening of urine or sudden decrease in hemoglobin concentration or leukocyte or erythrocyte count); notify health care provider if these reactions occur.

Patient/Family Education
- Tell patient that medicine may be taken with food if stomach upset (eg, nausea, vomiting, abdominal cramps) occurs, and advise patient to contact health care provider if upset persists.
- Emphasize importance of compliance with drug regimen.
- Advise patient to report marked darkening of urine to health care provider.

Primidone

(PRIM-ih-dohn)

Class Anticonvulsant

How Supplied
Mysoline Tablets 50 mg, Tablets 250 mg
❋ *Apo-Primidone* ◆ *Sertan*

Action
PHARMACOLOGY: Primidone and its metabolites (phenobarbital and phenylethylmalonamide) have anticonvulsant activity, raising seizure threshold and altering seizure patterns.

PHARMACOKINETICS/DYNAMICS:
Absorption: Readily absorbed from the GI tract. T_{max} is 3 hr (primidone) and 7 to 8 hr (phenobarbital and phenylethylmalonamide [PEMA] metabolites). Bioavailability is 90% to 100%.

Distribution: Protein binding is negligible for primidone and PEMA; approximately 50% (phenobarbital). Distributes into breast milk. Vd is 0.64 to 0.86 L/kg.

Metabolism: Hepatic, 2 active metabolites: phenobarbital (15% to 25%) and PEMA. PEMA is the major metabolite and is less active than phenobarbital.

Excretion: Excreted in the urine (40% as unchanged and remainder excreted as metabolites). Plasma t½ is 5 to 15 hr (primidone), 10 to 18 hr (PEMA), and 53 to 140 hr (phenobarbital).

Indications Control of grand mal, psychomotor, or focal epileptic seizures; may control grand mal seizures refractory to other anticonvulsants.
Unlabeled use(s): Treatment of benign familial tremor (essential tremor).

Contraindications Hypersensitivity to barbiturates; porphyria.

Route/Dosage

ADULTS AND CHILDREN OVER 8 YR OF AGE: If no previous treatment, initiate as follows: **PO** For days 1 to 3, give 100 to 125 mg at bedtime; days 4 to 6, give 100 to 125 mg bid; days 7 to 9, give 100 to 125 mg tid; and day 10 through maintenance dose, give 250 mg tid or qid. May increase to 250 mg 5 to 6 times/day, but do not exceed 500 mg qid (2 g/day).

CHILDREN UNDER 8 YR OF AGE: **PO** For days 1 to 3, give 50 mg at bedtime; days 4 to 6, give 50 mg bid; days 7 to 9, give 100 mg bid; and day 10 through maintenance dose, give 125 to 250 mg tid or 10 to 25 mg/kg/day in divided doses.

Patients Already Taking Anticonvulsants
Initiate at 100 to 125 mg at bedtime, gradually increasing dose to maintenance level as other drug is gradually decreased. Complete switch to primidone should occur over more than 2 wk.

Interactions

Anticoagulants: Decreased anticoagulant effects.
Beta-blockers: Effects of beta-blockers may be reduced.
Carbamazepine: Decreased primidone levels; increased concentrations of carbamazepine.
Corticosteroids: Decreased effect of corticosteroids.
Doxycycline: Decreased doxycycline serum levels.
Estrogens, oral contraceptives: Contraceptive failure has been reported.
Ethanol: Additive CNS suppression.
Felodipine: Decreased effect of felodipine.
Griseofulvin: Decreased serum griseofulvin levels.
Hydantoins, valproic acid: Increased primidone serum levels.
Methadone: Plasma concentrations may be reduced by primidone, leading to opiate withdrawal.
Methoxyflurane: Enhanced renal toxicity may occur.
Metronidazole: Therapeutic failure of metronidazole.
Nifedipine: Decreased nifedipine levels.
Quinidine: Decreased quinidine serum levels.
Succinimides: Decreased primidone levels.
Theophyllines: Decreased theophylline levels.

Lab Test Interferences None well documented.

Adverse Reactions

CNS: Ataxia; vertigo; fatigue; hyperirritability; emotional disturbances; drowsiness; personality deterioration; mood changes; paranoia.
DERM: Morbilliform or maculopapular skin eruptions.
EENT: Diplopia; nystagmus.
GI: Nausea; anorexia; vomiting.
GU: Impotence; crystalluria.
HEMA: Megaloblastic anemia; granulocytopenia, agranulocytosis, red-cell hypoplasia, aplasia (rarely).

Precautions

Pregnancy: Category D. Consult health care provider regarding anticonvulsant use during pregnancy.
Lactation: Excreted in breast milk.
Status epilepticus: May be precipitated by abrupt withdrawal.

PATIENT CARE CONSIDERATIONS

Administration/Storage

- May be used alone or in combination with other antiepileptic drugs.
- Administer prescribed dose without regard to meals. Administer with food if GI upset occurs.
- Store tablets at controlled room temperature (59° to 86°F).

Assessment/Interventions

- Obtain patient history, including drug history and any known allergies. Note renal impairment, porphyria, or sensitivity to phenobarbital.
- Ensure that complete blood count and sequential multiple analysis-12 panel are evaluated before starting therapy and periodically (eg, q 6 mo) during prolonged therapy.
- Frequently assess patient for response to treatment, including periodic measurements of primidone blood levels. Notify health care provider if seizures do not improve or appear to worsen, or if primidone blood levels are above or below the therapeutic range of 5 to 12 mcg/mL.
- Ensure that therapy is periodically reviewed to determine if therapy needs to be continued without change or if a dose change (eg, increase, decrease, discontinuation) is indicated.
- Avoid sudden discontinuation of therapy to minimize potential of increased seizure frequency. Attempt to gradually reduce dose over a period of several weeks if decision to discontinue medication is made.

- Monitor patient for GI, CNS, and general body side effects. Report to health care provider if noted and significant.
- Implement safety precautions for patients who experience dizziness or ataxia.

Patient/Family Education
- Explain name, dose, action, and potential side effects of drug.
- Advise patient to read the *Patient Information* leaflet before starting therapy and with each refill.
- Instruct patient, family, or caregiver to continue to take other medications for seizures unless advised by health care provider.
- Instruct patient to take exactly as prescribed and to not change the dose or discontinue unless advised by health care provider.
- Advise patient that medication will be started at a low dose and then gradually increased until max benefit has been obtained.
- Advise patient that each dose may be taken without regard to meals but to take with food if stomach upset occurs.
- Advise patient that the most common side effects of therapy are dizziness, drowsiness, feeling of whirling motion, and incoordination and that they generally occur early in therapy or after a dose increase and tend to disappear with continued therapy.
- Advise patient that if medication needs to be discontinued it will be slowly withdrawn over a period of several weeks unless safety concerns (eg, rash) require a more rapid withdrawal.
- Caution patient that drug may cause dizziness, drowsiness, or coordination problems and to use caution while driving or performing other tasks requiring mental alertness or coordination until tolerance is determined.
- Advise women to notify health care provider if pregnant, planning to become pregnant, or breastfeeding.
- Instruct patient to contact health care provider immediately if rash or fever occur.
- Instruct patient to inform health care provider if seizures get worse of if new types of seizures occur.
- Advise patient to avoid alcoholic beverages and other depressants while taking this medication.
- Advise patient to carry identification (eg, *Medic Alert*) indicating medication usage and epilepsy.
- Advise patient not to take any prescription or OTC medications, dietary supplements, or herbal preparations unless advised by health care provider.

Probenecid

(pro-BEN-uh-sid)

Class Analgesic/Gout/Uricosuric

How Supplied
Probenecid Tablets 0.5 g
✤ Benuryl

Action
PHARMACOLOGY: Inhibits tubular reabsorption of urate, thus increasing urinary excretion of uric acid. Inhibits tubular secretion of most penicillin and cephalosporin antibiotics.

PHARMACOKINETICS/DYNAMICS:
Absorption: Well absorbed. T_{max} is 2 to 4 hr. C_{max} for a single 1 g dose is more than 30 mcg/mL. C_{max} for a single 2 g dose is 150 to 200 mcg/mL.
Distribution: Protein binding is 85% to 95%, albumin. Distributes into CSF, crosses the placenta, and appears in cord blood.
Metabolism: Rapid and extensive; hydroxylated to active metabolites and probenecid monoacylglucuronide in the liver.
Excretion: Excreted in the urine (mainly in metabolite form) 5% to 10% unchanged. $T_{1/2}$ is dose dependent and varies from less than 5 to greater than 8 hr.
Peak: Uricosuric is 30 min.
Duration: Approximately 8 hr.

Indications Treatment of hyperuricemia associated with gout and gouty arthritis; adjunctive therapy with penicillins or cephalosporins to elevate and prolong serum levels.

Contraindications Children less than 2 yr; blood dyscrasias or uric acid kidney stones. Do not start therapy until acute gout attack subsides.

Route/Dosage
Gout
ADULTS AND CHILDREN OVER 110 LB: **PO** 250 mg bid initially (for 1 wk), followed by 500 mg bid. For maintenance therapy, may reduce by 500 mg q 6 mo until serum uric acid increases.

In Conjunction with Antibiotic Therapy
PO 2 g/day in divided doses.
CHILDREN 2 TO 14 YR (UNDER 110 LB): **PO** 25 mg/kg or 0.7 g/m² initially. Maintenance dose is 40 mg/kg/day or 1.2 g/m², divided into 4 doses.

Interactions Interacts with many other drugs by altering their clearance and elimination.
Barbiturate anesthetics, dyphylline, methotrexate, oral hypoglycemic agents, zidovudine: Increased serum levels and effects of these drugs.
Salicylates: Inhibition of uricosuric effect of either drug.

Lab Test Interferences May produce false-positive results for glycosuria in some urine glucose tests and falsely high assays for theophylline with Schack and Waxler technique. May inhibit renal excretion of phenolsulfonphthalein, 17-ketosteroid, and sulfobromophthalein.

Adverse Reactions
CNS: Headaches; dizziness.
DERM: Dermatitis; pruritus.
GI: Anorexia; nausea; GI distress; vomiting; sore gums.
GU: Urinary frequency; hematuria; renal colic; nephrotic syndrome.
HEMA: Anemia; hemolytic anemia (possibly related to G-6-PD deficiency); aplastic anemia.
HEPA: Hepatic necrosis.
OTHER: Hypersensitivity reactions; anaphylaxis; fever; flushing; exacerbation of gout; uric acid stones; costovertebral pain.

PATIENT CARE CONSIDERATIONS

Administration/Storage
- Do not start therapy during acute gout attack; wait until attack subsides.
- Give with food or antacid to reduce GI upset.
- Colchicine is sometimes prescribed concurrently for first 3 to 6 mo of therapy because probenecid alone may aggravate gout.

Assessment/Interventions
- Obtain patient history, including drug history and any known allergies. Note renal impairment, blood dyscrasias, peptic ulcers, or uric acid kidney stones.
- Encourage liberal fluid intake and give sodium bicarbonate or potassium citrate to prevent urate crystallization in kidney.
- Monitor BUN and renal function test results.
- Monitor for GI tolerance. If nausea, vomiting, or diarrhea becomes a problem, notify health care provider.
- Observe for possible exacerbation of gout. If symptoms of exacerbation occur, notify health care provider; adjunctive therapy may be needed.
- Observe for possible allergic reaction. If reaction occurs, withhold drug and notify health care provider.

Precautions
Pregnancy: Pregnancy category undetermined. Probenecid crosses placenta and appears in cord blood.
Children: Not recommended for children under 2 yr.
Hypersensitivity: Severe allergic reactions and anaphylaxis, although rare, have occurred. These have usually been associated with prior probenecid use.
Renal function impairment: May require increased doses for gout (not to exceed 2 g/day). Probenecid may be ineffective in chronic renal insufficiency (ie, glomerular filtration rate of less than 30 mL/min). Drug is not recommended for use with penicillin in cases of known renal impairment.
Alkalinization of urine: May be needed to prevent hematuria, renal colic, costovertebral pain, formation of uric acid stones.
Exacerbation of gout: May occur; appropriate drug therapy (eg, colchicine or other appropriate therapy) is advisable.
History of peptic ulcer: Use with caution.

Overdosage: Signs and Symptoms
Nausea, vomiting, diarrhea, seizure.

Patient/Family Education
- Instruct patient to take drug with food or antacids if GI upset occurs.
- Advise patient that drinking 6 to 8 full glasses of water daily may help prevent formation of kidney stones.
- If health care provider has recommended restriction of intake of foods high in purine, review foods to be avoided (eg, organ meats, meat gravy, anchovies, sardines). Explain that moderate amounts of purine are found in other meats, fish and other seafood, asparagus, spinach, peas, dried legumes, and wild game.
- Inform patient to notify health care provider if GI upset, anorexia, or headaches become bothersome.
- Instruct patient to report the following symptoms to health care provider: painful urination, bloody urine, severe lower back pain, difficulty breathing, or rash.
- Advise patient to avoid intake of alcoholic beverages.
- Instruct patient not to take OTC medications (including aspirin) without consulting health care provider.
- Caution patient not to discontinue drug without consulting health care provider.

Probenecid/Colchicine

(pro-BEN-uh-sid/KOHL-chih-seen)

Class Analgesic/Uricosuric

How Supplied
Probenecid and Colchicine Tablets 500 mg probenecid and 0.5 mg colchicine

Action
PHARMACOLOGY:
Probenecid: Inhibits tubular reabsorption of urate, thus increasing urinary excretion of uric acid.
Colchicine: Inhibits inflammation and reduces pain and swelling associated with gouty arthritis.

Indications Treatment of chronic gouty arthritis when complicated by frequent, recurrent, acute attacks of gout.

Contraindications Hypersensitivity to any component of product; children under 2 yr; known blood dyscrasias; uric acid kidney stones; current acute gouty attack.

Route/Dosage
ADULTS: PO 1 tablet/day for 7 days, then 1 tablet bid thereafter. If necessary, the daily dosage may be increased by 1 tablet at 4-wk intervals as tolerated (usually not more than 4 tablets/day).

Interactions
Acetaminophen, indomethacin, ketoprofen, lorazepam, meclofenamate, naproxen, rifampin: Plasma levels of these agents may be increased.
Beta-lactam antibiotics, penicillins: Psychic disturbances may occur.
Induction anesthesia (eg, thiopental): Less anesthetic may be required.
Methotrexate: Probenecid increases plasma levels; methotrexate dose may need to be reduced.
Pyrazinamide, salicylates: Uricosuric action of probenecid may be antagonized.
Sulfonamides: Total sulfonamide (drug plus metabolite) levels may be increased.
Sulfonylureas: Risk of hypoglycemia may be increased.

Lab Test Interferences Falsely high reading for theophylline may occur when measured by the Schack and Waxler technique.

PATIENT CARE CONSIDERATIONS

Administration/Storage
- Administer prescribed dose as ordered.
- Administer without regard to meals but administer with food if GI upset occurs.
- Store tablets at controlled room temperature (59° to 86°F).

Adverse Reactions
CNS:
Probenecid – Headache; dizziness.
Colchicine – Peripheral neuritis.
DERM:
Probenecid – Urticaria; pruritus; dermatitis; alopecia; flushing.
Colchicine – Urticaria; purpura; alopecia; dermatitis.
GI:
Probenecid – Vomiting; nausea; anorexia; sore gums.
Colchicine – Nausea; vomiting; abdominal pain; diarrhea.
GU:
Probenecid – Nephrotic syndrome; uric acid stones with or without hematuria; renal colic; costovertebral pain; urinary frequency.
HEMA:
Probenecid – Aplastic anemia; leukopenia; hemolytic anemia.
Colchicine – Aplastic anemia; agranulocytosis.
HEPA:
Probenecid – Hepatic necrosis.
METAB:
Probenecid – Precipitation of acute gouty arthritis.
OTHER:
Probenecid – Anaphylaxis; fever.
Colchicine – Muscular weakness.

Precautions
Pregnancy: Category C.
Lactation: Undetermined.
Children: Safety and efficacy not established; contraindicated in children under 2 yr.
Renal function impairment: May not be effective in patients with chronic renal insufficiency (30 mL/min or less); dose may need to be increased.
Alkalinization of urine: May be needed to prevent hematuria, renal colic, costovertebral pain, formation of uric acid stones.
Exacerbation of gout: May occur.
Peptic ulcer: Use with caution in patients with history of peptic ulcer disease.

Overdosage: Signs and Symptoms
Diarrhea, generalized vascular damage, renal damage, hematuria, oliguria.

Assessment/Interventions
- Obtain patient history, including drug history and any known allergies. Note history of blood dyscrasias, uric acid kidney stones, renal impairment, pregnancy, or peptic ulcer disease.
- Ensure that acute gouty attack has subsided before starting therapy.

- Ensure that adequate fluids are given to maintain good hydration.
- Administer urinary alkalinizing agents as ordered by health care provider.
- Ensure that women of child bearing potential use adequate contraception during therapy.
- Monitor patient for CNS, GI, and general body side effects. Report to health care provider if noted and significant.
- Discontinue therapy and notify health care provider if persistent diarrhea or other GI side effects are noted, or if rash or other signs of hypersensitivity occur.

Patient/Family Education
- Explain name, dose, action, and potential side effects of drug.
- Advise patient to take tablets as prescribed by health care provider.
- Advise patient to take without regard to meals but to take with food if GI upset occurs.
- Inform patient that dose will be slowly increased until maximum benefit is obtained.
- Advise patient to maintain adequate fluid intake (at least eight 8 oz glasses of water/day) and to carefully follow any instructions regarding alkalinizing the urine that were provided by health care provider.
- Caution patient to not increase the dose of this medication if gout symptoms should recur. Instruct patient to discuss other treatments for acute gout while continuing this medication.
- Caution patient to avoid concurrent use of aspirin or aspirin-containing products. Advise patient to use acetaminophen for management of mild to moderate pain.
- Advise patient to stop taking the drug and notify health care provider if persistent diarrhea or other GI symptoms occur or if a rash or other signs of an allergic reaction develop.
- Advise women to notify health care provider if pregnant, planning to become pregnant, or breastfeeding.
- Warn patient not to take any prescription or OTC drugs or dietary supplements without consulting health care provider.
- Advise patient that follow-up visits and lab tests may be necessary to monitor therapy and to keep appointments.

Procainamide Hydrochloride

(pro-CANE-uh-mide HIGH-droe-KLOR-ide)

Class Antiarrhythmic

How Supplied
Procanbid Tablets, sustained-release 500 mg, Tablets, extended-release 1000 mg ♦ *Pronestyl* Tablets 250 mg, Tablets 375 mg, Tablets 500 mg, Capsules 250 mg, Capsules 375 mg, Capsules 500 mg, Injection 100 mg/mL, Injection 500 mg/mL ♦ *Pronestyl-SR* Tablets, sustained-release 500 mg

✦ *Apo-Procainamide* ♦ *Procan SR*

Action
PHARMACOLOGY: Increases effective refractory period of atria and bundle of His-Purkinje system; reduces impulse conduction velocity and myocardial excitability in atria, Purkinje fibers, and ventricles.

PHARMACOKINETICS/DYNAMICS:

Absorption: Rapid absorption (IM), immediate absorption (IV). Well absorbed from entire small intestinal surface (oral).

Distribution: Protein binding is 15% to 20%, also bound to tissues of the heart, liver, lung, and kidney. Vd is 2 L/kg. The drug distributes into breast milk (procainamide and N-acetylprocainamide [NAPA]).

Metabolism: Metabolized in liver to NAPA, an active metabolite exerting significant antiarrhythmic activity. Approximately 25% of dose converted to NAPA, up to 40% conversion occurs in patients who are rapid acetylators.

Excretion: The $t_{\frac{1}{2}}$ is 3 to 4 hr (normal renal function, procainamide) and approximately 6 hr (NAPA). Urinary excretion (6% to 52% NAPA, 30% to 60% as unchanged procainamide); a trace amount is excreted in urine as free and conjugated p-aminobenzoic acid.

Peak: 60 to 90 min (oral), 15 to 60 min (IM), and immediate (IV).

Special Populations:
Renal Function Impairment – Elimination $t_{\frac{1}{2}}$ is prolonged.
Elderly – Elimination $t_{\frac{1}{2}}$ is prolonged.
Children – In infants, $t_{\frac{1}{2}}$ and renal clearance are reduced.

Indications Treatment of documented ventricular arrhythmias that are life threatening.

Contraindications Complete heart block; idiosyncratic hypersensitivity; lupus erythematosus; torsades de pointes.

Route/Dosage
ADULTS: PO 50 mg/kg/day in divided doses (q 3 hr for regular release; q 6 to 12 hr for sustained release, depending on the formulation).
IV 20 mg/min for 25 to 30 min as loading dose, then 2 to 6 mg/min for maintenance.
IM 50 mg/kg/day in divided doses q 3 to 6 hr until oral therapy is possible.

CHILDREN: Safety not established. Following doses have been used:
PO 15 to 50 mg/kg/day in divided doses q 3 to 6 hr, max of 4 g/day;
IM 20 to 30 mg/kg/day in divided doses q 4 to 6 hr, max 4 g/day;
IV 3 to 6 mg/kg/dose over 5 min for loading dose, then 20 to 80 mcg/kg/min continuous infusion (max, 100 mg/dose or 2 g/day).

Interactions
Amiodarone, cimetidine, trimethoprim: May increase procainamide and NAPA concentrations.
Cisapride, quinolone antibiotics (eg, gatifloxacin), thioridazine, ziprasidone: May increase the risk of life-threatening cardiac arrhythmias, including torsades de pointes.
Group 1a antiarrhythmic agents (eg, quinidine): Coadministration with procainamide is contraindicated.

Lab Test Interferences
None well documented.

Adverse Reactions
CV: Proarrhythmic effects; hypotension.
CNS: Dizziness; weakness; depression; psychosis with hallucinations.
DERM: Angioneurotic edema; urticaria; pruritus; flushing; rash.
EENT: Bitter taste.
GI: Nausea; vomiting; anorexia; abdominal pain.
HEMA: Neutropenia; thrombocytopenia; hemolytic anemia; agranulocytosis.
OTHER: Lupus erythematosus-like syndrome.

> **WARNING:**
> *Cardiovascular effects:* Procainamide has proarrhythmic effects. May cause or aggravate CHF or produce severe hypotension, especially in patients with CHF, acute ischemic heart disease, or cardiomyopathy.
> *Hematological:* Agranulocytosis, bone marrow depression, neutropenia, hypoplastic anemia, and thrombocytopenia have been reported and may occur, usually within first 12 wk of therapy at recommended doses. Use caution in patients with pre-existing marrow failure or cytopenia.
> *Positive ANA titer:* Chronic administration may result in positive titers with or without symptoms of lupus erythematosus-like syndrome.
> Approximately 50% of patients will develop ANA within 2 to 18 mo of starting therapy.

Precautions
Pregnancy: Category C.
Lactation: Excreted in breast milk.
Children: Safety and efficacy not established.
Hypersensitivity: Consider the possibility of cross-sensitivity to procainamide in patients sensitive to procaine or other ester-type local anesthetics.
Renal function impairment: Individual dose adjustment may be necessary.
Special risk patients: Elderly patients and patients with renal, hepatic or cardiac insufficiency will require smaller or less frequent doses. Individual dosage adjustment will be necessary.
Tartrazine sensitivity: Some tablet forms contain tartrazine.
Sulfite sensitivity: Parenteral forms contain sulfites.
Asymptomatic PVCs: Avoid use of product in treatment of patients with this condition.
Blood dyscrasias: Agranulocytosis, bone marrow depression, neutropenia, hypoplastic anemia, and thrombocytopenia have been reported; monitor carefully.
Complete heart block: Do not administer to patients with complete heart block because of effects in suppressing nodal or ventricular pacemakers and hazard of asystole.
Concurrent antiarrhythmic agents: May see enhanced prolongation of conduction or depression of contractility and hypotension.
Digitalis intoxication: Use with caution treating arrhythmias associated with digitalis intoxication.
First-degree heart block: Use with caution if first-degree heart block develops during procainamide therapy.
Myasthenia gravis: Patients may experience increase of muscle weakness. Observe closely.
Predigitalization for atrial flutter or fibrillation: Cardiovert or digitalize patient prior to procainamide therapy to avoid enhancement of AV conduction.

Overdosage: Signs and Symptoms
Hypotension, widening of QRS complex, prolonged QT and PR intervals, ventricular tachyarrhythmias.

PATIENT CARE CONSIDERATIONS
Administration/Storage
- Give sustained-release forms whole. Do not crush or allow patient to bite or chew them.
- Digitalize or cardiovert patients with atrial flutter or fibrillation as prescribed prior to administration.
- Prepare IV infusion solution using D5W. Use controlled infusion device.
- IV solutions may turn slightly yellow or light amber on standing, but potency is not affected.
- For direct IV injection, do not exceed maximal IV rate of 50 mg/min and do not give more than 100 mg in any 5-min period.
- Wait 3 to 4 hr after last IV dose before first oral dose.
- IV solutions may be stored at room temperature (59° to 86°F) for 24 hr or for 7 days if refrigerated. Discard IV infusion solutions that are darker than light amber.
- Store oral dosage forms at room temperature in tightly closed container.

Assessment/Interventions
- Obtain patient history, including drug history and any known allergies.
- Repeat ECG as ordered.
- Be aware that patients with decreased renal function and elderly patients will metabolize drug more slowly.
- Monitor ECG and BP regularly during parenteral administration.
- Monitor muscle weakness in patients with myasthenia gravis.
- Monitor results of CBC (including WBC differential and platelet count) weekly during first 3 mo of therapy and periodically thereafter, as well as at any time patient develops signs of infection, bruising, or bleeding.
- Monitor procainamide and NAPA levels as ordered.
- Report diarrhea, vomiting, anorexia, abdominal pain, dizziness, or altered mental status to health care provider.
- In prolonged therapy, observe for lupus erythematosus-like syndrome with arthralgia, pleural or abdominal pain and possible fever, chills, myalgia, pericarditis, pleural effusion, arthritis, or skin lesions and report to health care provider.

Patient/Family Education
- Tell patient to take medication with full glass of water.
- Caution patient not to crush or chew sustained-release capsules.
- Explain that this medication should be taken throughout 24-hr period.
- Explain importance of informing other health care providers or dentists about therapy before surgical or dental procedures.
- Emphasize importance of drug compliance. Caution patient not to make up for missed doses.
- Instruct patient to report the following symptoms to health care provider immediately: difficulty breathing, pounding or irregular heartbeat, joint pain, fever, chills, skin rash, continued dizziness.
- Explain that diarrhea, nausea, dizziness, or loss of appetite may occur and to contact health care provider if symptoms are bothersome.
- Advise patient that drug may cause dizziness and to use caution when driving or performing other tasks requiring mental alertness.

Procarbazine
(pro-CAR-buh-ZEEN)
Class Alkylating agent

How Supplied
Matulane Capsules 50 mg

Action
PHARMACOLOGY: The mode of cytotoxic action is not clear; procarbazine may inhibit protein, RNA, and DNA synthesis.

PHARMACOKINETICS/DYNAMICS:
Absorption: Rapidly and completely absorbed from the GI tract. T_{max} is 60 min (oral).

Distribution: Quickly equilibrates between plasma and CSF.

Metabolism: Metabolized in the liver and kidneys to cytotoxic products.

Excretion: Urine (mostly as N-isopropylterephthalamic acid, less than 5% as unchanged). Plasma $t_{1/2}$ approximately 10 min (IV).

Indications
Adult and Pediatric: Advanced Hodgkin disease (stage III and IV) as part of the MOPP (nitrogen mustard, vincristine, procarbazine, prednisone) regimen. **Unlabeled use(s):** Non-Hodgkin lymphoma, brain tumors, small cell lung cancer (adult use).

Contraindications Hypersensitivity to procarbazine. Inadequate marrow reserve demonstrated by bone marrow aspiration.

Route/Dosage
Base dosages on patient's actual weight. The following doses are for administration of procarbazine as a single agent. When used in com-

bination with other anticancer drugs, appropriately reduce procarbazine dosage. In the MOPP regimen, the dose is 100 mg/m² daily for 14 days.

Hodgkin Disease
ADULTS: **PO** To minimize nausea and vomiting, give single or divided doses of 2 to 4 mg/kg/day for the first wk. Maintain daily dosage at 4 to 6 mg/kg/day until the WBC falls below 4000/mm³ or the platelets fall below 100,000/mm³, or until max response is obtained. Upon evidence of hematologic toxicity, discontinue the drug until there has been satisfactory recovery. Resume treatment at 1 to 2 mg/kg/day. When max response is obtained, maintain the dose at 1 to 2 mg/kg/day.

PEDIATRIC: **PO** Individualize dosage. The dosage schedule is a guideline only: 50 mg/m²/day for the first week. Maintain daily dosage at 100 mg/m² until leukopenia or thrombocytopenia occurs or max response is obtained. When max response is attained, maintain the dose at 50 mg/m²/day. Upon evidence of hematologic or other toxicity, discontinue drug until there has been satisfactory recovery.

Interactions
Alcohol: Alcohol consumption may cause a disulfiram-like reaction in patients on procarbazine.

CNS depressants (eg, narcotics, analgesics, alcohol, antiemetics, benzodiazepines, sedatives, and tranquilizers): Concurrent use may potentiate CNS effects.

Digitalis glycosides: May result in a decrease in digoxin plasma levels, even several days after stopping chemotherapy.

High-tyramine foods (eg, wine, yogurt, ripe cheese, bananas), OTC antihistamines, and sympathomimetics: Avoid known high-tyramine foods, OTC antihistamines, and sympathomimetics. Procarbazine is a weak MAO inhibitor.

Levodopa: Flushing and a significant rise in BP may result within 1 hr of levodopa administration.

Methotrexate: May increase methotrexate-induced nephrotoxicity.

Radiation or other chemotherapy: May depress bone marrow activity.

Sympathomimetics (indirect-acting): May cause an abrupt increase in BP, resulting in a potentially fatal hypertensive crisis.

Tricyclic antidepressants: Severe toxic and fatal reactions including excitability, fluctuations in BP, convulsions, and coma may occur.

Lab Test Interferences
None well documented.

Adverse Reactions
CV: Hypotension; tachycardia; syncope.

CNS: Coma; neuropathy; nystagmus; diminished reflexes; falling; foot drop; headache; unsteadiness; paresthesias; dizziness; depression; insomnia; hallucinations; ataxia; seizures; apprehension; nervousness; confusion; nightmares.

DERM: Dermatitis; pruritus; urticaria; alopecia; flushing; herpes; hyperpigmentation; rash; flushing.

GI: Hepatic dysfunction; jaundice; stomatitis; hematemesis; melena; nausea; vomiting; anorexia; dry mouth; dysphagia; abdominal pain; diarrhea; constipation.

GU: Amenorrhea; azoospermia; hematuria; urinary frequency; nocturia.

HEMA: Leukopenia; anemia; thrombopenia; pancytopenia; eosinophilia; hemolytic anemia; petechiae; purpura; epistaxis; hemoptysis; bone marrow suppression; nadir at approximately 4 wk.

OPHTH: Retinal hemorrhage; photophobia; diplopia; papilledema; inability to focus.

RESP: Pneumonitis; pleural effusion; cough.

OTHER: Acute myelocytic leukemia; malignant myelosclerosis; lung cancer; fever; generalized allergic reactions; gynecomastia in prepubertal and early pubertal boys; intercurrent infections; hearing loss; pyrexia; diaphoresis; lethargy; weakness; fatigue; edema; chills; slurred speech; hoarseness; drowsiness.

> **WARNING:**
> Recommend procarbazine be given only by or under the supervision of a physician experienced in the use of potent antineoplastic drugs. Adequate clinical and laboratory facilities should be made available to patients for proper monitoring of treatment.

Precautions
Pregnancy: Category D.

Lactation: Undetermined. Not recommended.

Children: Close clinical monitoring is mandatory. Toxicity, evidenced by tremors, convulsions, and coma, has occurred.

Renal function impairment: Undue toxicity may occur.

Hepatic function impairment: Undue toxicity may occur.

Carcinogenesis: Tobacco use during procarbazine therapy increases risk of developing secondary lung cancer. Advise patients not to use tobacco.

Fertility impairment: Azoospermia and antifertility effects associated with procarbazine coadministered with other antineoplastics for treating Hodgkin disease have been reported.

Bone-marrow suppression: If radiation or a chemotherapeutic agent known to have marrow-depressant activity has been used, wait at least 1 mo before starting procarbazine.

Toxicity: Toxicity includes hemolysis and the appearance of Heinz-Ehrlich inclusion bodies in erythrocytes.

Discontinue: Discontinue if any of the following occurs: CNS signs or symptoms; leukopenia (WBC less than 4000/mm^3); thrombocytopenia (platelets less than 100,000/mm^3); hypersensitivity reaction; stomatitis (the first small ulceration or persistent spot soreness); diarrhea; hemorrhage or bleeding tendencies Resume therapy after side effects clear; adjust to a lower dosage schedule.

Overdosage: Signs and Symptoms

Nausea, vomiting, enteritis, diarrhea, hypotension, tremors, convulsions, coma.

PATIENT CARE CONSIDERATIONS

Administration/Storage

- Administer in combination with other chemotherapy medications.
- Administer prescribed dose without regard to meals. Administer with food if GI upset occurs.
- Follow procedures for proper handling and disposal of anticancer drugs.
- Store capsules at controlled room temperature (59° to 86°F).

Assessment/Interventions

- Obtain patient history, including drug history and any known allergies. Note renal or hepatic impairment, inadequate bone marrow reserve, previous treatment with radiation or chemotherapeutic agent known to suppress bone marrow function.
- Ensure that patient's diet contains no food with high-tyramine content.
- Ensure that dose is calculated based on patient's actual weight. Use estimated lean body mass (dry weight) if patient is obese or if there has been a spurious weight gain caused by fluid accumulation (eg, edema, ascites).
- Ensure that reticulocyte count and CBC with differential and platelet count are obtained before starting and q 3 to 4 days during treatment.
- Ensure that urinalysis, BUN, creatinine, transaminases, and alkaline phosphatase are obtained before starting and q wk during treatment.
- Discontinue treatment if any of the following occur: WBC count less than 4000/mm^3; platelet count less than 100,000/mm^3; hemorrhage; paresthesia; neuropathy; confusion; allergic reaction.
- Ensure women of childbearing potential are using effective contraception before initiating therapy and for duration of treatment.
- Monitor patient for CNS, GI, GU, respiratory, DERM, and general body side effects. Report to health care provider if noted and significant.

Patient/Family Education

- Explain name, action, and potential side effects of drug.
- Advise patient or caregiver that medication may usually be used in combination with other chemotherapy agents to achieve max benefit possible.
- Review dosing schedule with patient or caregiver.
- Advise patient to take prescribed dose without regard to meals but to take with food if GI upset occurs.
- Advise patient or caregiver that if a dose is missed not to take the missed dose and not to double the next dose. Take the next dose at the regularly scheduled time.
- Instruct patient to avoid foods with high tyramine content. Review common foods known to have high tyramine content (eg, aged cheeses, soy sauce, fermented or air-dried meats, sauerkraut, tap beers, red wines).
- Advise patient to discontinue therapy and immediately notify health care provider if any of the following occur: diarrhea; fever, chills or other signs of infection; bleeding; abnormal skin sensations; confusion; allergic reaction; pain, burning, or numbness of feet, legs, or hands.
- Advise patient that medication may cause muscle or joint pain, nausea, vomiting, tiredness, weakness, constipation, headache, difficulty swallowing, loss of appetite, loss of hair, and mental depression and to notify health care provider if any develop and are intolerable.
- Caution patient to avoid alcohol, other CNS depressants (eg, antihistamines), and decongestants (eg, pseudoephedrine) while taking procarbazine.
- Advise patient who smokes that a second malignancy, including lung cancer, can develop following treatment and that tobacco use increases the risk. Advise patient who smokes to discontinue smoking to reduce the risk of developing a secondary lung cancer.
- Caution patient that medication may cause drowsiness and dizziness and to use caution while driving or performing hazardous tasks until tolerance is determined.
- Caution women of childbearing potential to avoid becoming pregnant while being treated.

- Advise women to notify health care provider if pregnant, planning to become pregnant, or breastfeeding.
- Instruct patient not to take any prescription or OTC medications or dietary supplements unless advised by health care provider.
- Advise patient that frequent follow-up visits and laboratory tests will be required to monitor therapy and to keep appointments.

Prochlorperazine
(pro-klor-PURR-uh-zeen)
Class Antipsychotic/Phenothiazine/Antiemetic
How Supplied
Compazine Tablets 5 mg (as maleate), Tablets 10 mg (as maleate), Spansules (sustained-release capsules as maleate) 10 mg, Spansules (sustained-release capsules as maleate) 15 mg, Suppositories 2.5 mg, Suppositories 5 mg, Suppositories 25 mg, Syrup (as edisylate) 5 mg/5 mL, Injection (as edisylate) 5 mg/mL ♦ *Compro* Suppositories 25 mg
🍁 *Apo-Prochlorazine* ♦ *Nu-Prochlor* ♦ *Stemetil*

Action
PHARMACOLOGY: Effects apparently related to dopamine receptor blocking in CNS. Antiemetic activity may be caused by direct inhibition on medullary chemoreceptor trigger zone.

PHARMACOKINETICS/DYNAMICS:
Absorption: May be erratic. C_{max} shows large interindividual differences. Food slows the absorption and decreases C_{max} 23% and AUC 13%.

Distribution: Large volume of distribution; crosses the placenta and is distributed into breast milk. Protein binding is at least 90%.

Metabolism: Hepatic to active and inactive metabolites.

Excretion: Renal and biliary, with some enterohepatic recycling.

Onset: 10 to 20 min (IM).

Peak: 4 to 7 days (antipsychotic effect).

Duration: 3 to 4 hr (IM).

Indications
Treatment of schizophrenia; short-term treatment of generalized nonpsychotic anxiety; control of severe nausea and vomiting. **Unlabeled use(s):** Treatment of migraines (IV).

Contraindications
Coma or severely depressed states; allergy to any phenothiazine; presence of large amounts of other CNS depressants; pediatric patients under 2 yr of age or less than 20 lb; surgery in pediatric patients.

Route/Dosage
Individualize dosage. SC administration is not advised because of local irritation.

Nonpsychotic Anxiety
ADULTS: **PO** 5 mg tid to qid; 15 mg (sustained-release formulation) in morning or 10 mg (sustained-release formation) q 12 hr. Do not exceed 20 mg/day or give for more than 12 wk.

Schizophrenia
ADULTS: **IM** Start with 10 to 20 mg for immediate control of schizophrenic patients with severe symptomatology; if necessary, repeat initial dose q 2 to 4 hr to gain control of patient. More than 3 or 4 doses are seldom necessary. If IM therapy is needed for a prolonged period, give 10 to 20 mg q 4 to 6 hr.

Mild conditions: **PO** 5 to 10 mg tid or qid. Moderate to severe conditions: **PO** 10 mg tid qid, increasing dosage gradually (q 2 or 3 days) until symptoms are controlled or side effects become bothersome. Some patients respond satisfactorily on 50 to 75 mg/day; in more severe disturbances, the optimum dosage is usually 100 to 150 mg/day.

CHILDREN 2 TO 12 YR: **PO/PR** 2.5 mg bid or tid. Do not exceed 10 mg the first day.

CHILDREN 2 TO 5 YR: **PO/PR** Do not exceed 20 mg/day.

CHILDREN 6 TO 12 YR: **PO/PR** Do not exceed 25 mg/day. **IM** For children under 12 yr, calculate each dose on the basis of 0.03 mg/kg given by deep IM injection.

Nausea and Vomiting
ADULTS: **PO** 5 or 10 mg tablet tid to qid; 15 mg (sustained-release formulation) on arising or 10 mg q 12 hr. **PR** 25 mg bid. **IM** 5 to 10 mg. May repeat q 3 to 4 hr. Do not exceed 40 mg/day. **IV** 2.5 to 10 mg by slow IV or infusion at a rate not to exceed 5 mg/min (single dose not to exceed 10 mg; max, 40 mg/day).

CHILDREN: Adjust according to patient response and severity of symptoms.

CHILDREN 18 TO 38.5 KG: **PO/PR** 2.5 mg tid or 5 mg bid; do not exceed 15 mg/day. **IM** 0.03 mg/kg given by deep IM injection.

CHILDREN 13.6 TO 17.6 KG: **PO/PR** 2.5 mg given bid to tid; do not exceed 10 mg/day. **IM** 0.03 mg/kg given by deep IM injection.

CHILDREN 9 TO 13 KG: **PO/PR** 2.5 mg given qd or bid; do not exceed 7.5 mg/day. **IM** 0.03 mg/kg given by deep IM injection.

Nausea and Vomiting (Surgery)
ADULTS: **IM** 5 to 10 mg 1 to 2 hr prior to induction of anesthesia (may repeat once in 30 min) or to control acute symptoms during and after surgery (may repeat once).

ADULTS: **IV injection** or **infusion** 5 to 10 mg 15 to 30 min before induction of anesthesia or to control acute symptoms during or after surgery. Repeat once if necessary. Rate of administration should not exceed 5 mg/min and a single dose should not exceed 10 mg.

Interactions

Alcohol or other CNS depressants: May result in increased CNS depression and may precipitate dystonic reactions.

Anticholinergics: May reduce therapeutic effects of prochlorperazine and worsen anticholinergic effects.

Barbiturate anesthetics: Frequency and severity of neuromuscular excitation and hypotension may be increased.

Beta-blockers: May result in increased plasma levels of beta-blocker and prochlorperazine.

Cisapride, sparfloxacin: The risk of life-threatening cardiac arrhythmias, including torsades de pointes, may be increased.

Guanethidine: Hypotensive action of guanethidine may be inhibited.

Metrizamide: Possibility of seizure may be increased when subarachnoid metrizamide injection is used.

Paroxetine: Plasma levels of prochlorperazine may be elevated, increasing the risk of side effects.

INCOMPATIBILITIES: Do not mix prochlorperazine injection with other agents in syringe. Do not dilute with any diluent containing parabens as preservative.

Lab Test Interferences May discolor urine pink to red-brown. False-positive pregnancy tests may occur but are less likely to occur with serum test. Increases in protein-bound iodine reported.

Adverse Reactions

CV: Orthostatic hypotension; hypertension; tachycardia; bradycardia; syncope; cardiac arrest; circulatory collapse; ECG changes.

CNS: Lightheadedness; faintness; dizziness; pseudoparkinsonism; dystonia; dyskinesia; motor restlessness; oculogyric crises; opisthotonos; hyperreflexia; tardive dyskinesia; drowsiness; headache; weakness; tremor; fatigue; slurring of speech; insomnia; vertigo; abnormalities of CSF proteins; paradoxical excitement or exacerbation of psychotic symptoms; catatonic-like states; paranoid reactions; lethargy; seizures; hyperactivity; nocturnal confusion; bizarre dreams.

DERM: Photosensitivity; skin pigmentation; dry skin; pruritus; exfoliative dermatitis; urticarial rash; maculopapular hypersensitivity reaction; seborrhea; eczema.

EENT: Pigmentary retinopathy; glaucoma; photophobia; blurred vision; mydriasis; glaucoma; dry mouth or throat; nasal congestion.

GI: Nausea; vomiting; dyspepsia, adynamic ileus (which may result in death); constipation.

GU: Urinary hesitancy or retention; impotence, sexual dysfunction; menstrual irregularities; priapism; breast enlargement; galactorrhea.

HEPA: Jaundice.

HEMA: Agranulocytosis; eosinophilia; leukopenia; hemolytic anemia; thrombocytopenic purpura; pancytopenia; aplastic anemia.

METAB: Hyperglycemia; hypoglycemia; increased cholesterol levels.

RESP: Laryngospasm; bronchospasm; dyspnea.

OTHER: Increases in appetite and weight; polydipsia; increased prolactin levels; heat stroke.

Precautions

Pregnancy: Undetermined.
Lactation: Undetermined.

Children: Do not give to children under 9 kg or 2 yr. Do not use in pediatric surgery. Extrapyramidal side effects may develop even at moderate doses. Use lowest effective dose. Some children respond with restlessness and excitement; do not give additional doses. Use with caution in children with acute illnesses or dehydration.

Elderly: More susceptible to effects; consider lower dose.

Special risk patients: Use caution in patients with CV disease or mitral insufficiency, history of glaucoma, EEG abnormalities or seizure disorders, prior brain damage, hepatic or renal impairment, or those who will be exposed to extreme heat.

Sulfite sensitivity: Some parenteral products may contain sulfites.

Aspiration: As result of suppression of cough reflex, aspiration of vomitus possible.

Bone marrow suppression: Patients with bone marrow depression or who have previously demonstrated a hypersensitivity reaction with a phenothiazine should not receive prochlorperazine unless, in the judgment of the health care provider, the potential benefits outweigh the possible risks.

CNS effects: May impair mental or physical abilities, especially during first few days of therapy.

Hepatic effects: Jaundice usually occurs between wk 2 and 4 of treatment; considered hypersensitivity reaction. Usually reversible.

Neuroleptic malignant syndrome (NMS): NMS has occurred with agents in this class; is potentially fatal. Signs and symptoms are hyperpyrexia, muscle rigidity, altered mental status, irregular pulse, fluctuating BP, tachycardia, and diaphoresis.

Pulmonary: Cases of bronchopneumonia (some fatal) occurred.

Sudden death: Sudden death reported; predisposing factors may be seizures or previous brain damage. Flare-ups of psychotic behavior may precede death.

Tardive dyskinesia: Syndrome of potentially irreversible involuntary body and facial movements may develop. Prevalence highest in elderly, especially women. Use smallest effective doses for shortest possible time.

Overdosage: Signs and Symptoms

CNS depression (somnolence to coma), fever, agitation, restlessness, hypotension, extrapyramidal effects, circulatory collapse, seizures, arrhythmias.

PATIENT CARE CONSIDERATIONS

Administration/Storage

- Dose and frequency of administration are variable, depending on condition being treated.
- Administer tablets as prescribed, without regard to meals. Administer with food if GI upset occurs.
- Administer sustained-release capsules 1 hr before or 2 hr after meals. Administer with food if GI upset occurs.
- Administer sustained-release capsules whole; do not crush; do not allow patient to bite or chew capsule.
- Measure prescribed dose of syrup using calibrated dropper or dosing syringe.
- Double check pediatric dosage for suppositories (2.5 mg) to avoid confusion with adult dose (25 mg).
- Administer IM dose by slow, deep injection into outer quadrant of buttock.
- Administer IV dose by slow IV injection or infusion at rate not exceeding 5 mg/mL. Injection may be administered undiluted or diluted in isotonic solution (eg, normal saline, D5W). Do not administer as bolus.
- Injection is not for intradermal or SC administration.
- Do not administer injection if particulate matter or marked discoloration are noted. A slight yellowish discoloration is normal and will not alter potency.
- Do not mix injection with other drugs in syringe.
- If injection is spilled on skin or clothing, rinse area immediately with water to prevent contact dermatitis.
- Store injection below 86°F. Do not freeze. Store tablets, syrup, and suppositories at controlled room temperature (59° to 86°F); protect from light.

Assessment/Interventions

- Obtain patient history, including drug history and any known allergies. Note allergy to prochlorperazine or other phenothiazines, previous episode of jaundice with phenothiazine therapy, renal impairment, hepatic impairment, ischemic heart disease, heart failure, arrhythmias, cerebrovascular disease, asthma, emphysema, narrow angle glaucoma, epilepsy, mitral insufficiency, pheochromocytoma, prostatic hypertrophy, condition predisposing to hypotension (eg, dehydration, hypovolemia), concomitant use of antihypertensive drugs, or previous episodes of NMS.
- Ensure that medication is discontinued at least 48 hr before myelography and not resumed until at least 24 hr after procedure to reduce chance of seizures occurring.
- Frequently assess patient for response to treatment. Notify health care provider if condition is not improving or is worsening.
- Ensure therapy is periodically reviewed to determine if it needs to be continued without change or if a dose change (eg, increase, decrease, discontinuation) is indicated.
- Avoid sudden discontinuation of therapy if possible. Attempt to gradually reduce dose if decision to discontinue medication is made.
- Inform health care provider immediately if hyperpyrexia, muscle rigidity, altered mental status, irregular pulse and BP, tachycardia, or diaphoresis develop.
- Notify health care provider immediately if palpitations or syncope occur.
- Assess neurologic status before and during treatment. Observe for involuntary body and facial movements, excessive drowsiness, agitation, tremor, or anxiety. Inform health care provider if noted.
- Administer IM dose to patient who is bedfast. Keep patient lying down for at least 30 min after injection to minimize hypotensive effects.
- Monitor patient for CNS, CV, GI, GU, psychiatric, musculoskeletal, and general body side effects. Inform health care provider if noted and significant.
- Assess medication compliance.

Patient/Family Education

- Explain name, dose, action, and potential side effects of drug.
- Advise patient, family, or caregiver that dose will be adjusted periodically until max benefit has been obtained.
- Advise patient, family, or caregiver not to change the dose or stop taking unless advised by health care provider.
- Instruct patient, family, or caregiver to measure prescribed dose of syrup using calibrated

dropper or dosing syringe.
- Instruct patient, family, or caregiver to immediately report fainting or loss of consciousness, palpitations, dizziness, high fever, muscle rigidity, altered mental status, irregular pulse, sore throat, unusual bruising, yellowing of the skin or eyes.
- Advise patient, family, or caregiver to notify health care provider of the following: excessive drowsiness, increased agitation or anxiety, involuntary body or facial movements.
- Advise patient to avoid strenuous activity during periods of high temperature or humidity.
- Instruct patient to avoid alcoholic beverages and other depressants while taking this medication.
- Instruct patient to get up slowly from lying or sitting position and to avoid sudden position changes to prevent postural hypotension. Advise patient to report dizziness with position changes to health care provider. Caution patient that hot tubs and hot showers or baths may make dizziness worse.
- Advise patient to take sips of water, suck on ice chips or sugarless hard candy, or chew sugarless gum if dry mouth occurs.
- Advise patient drug may cause drowsiness and impaired judgment or thinking skills and to use caution while driving or performing other tasks requiring mental alertness until tolerance is determined.
- Caution patient that medication may cause sensitivity to sunlight and to avoid unnecessary exposure to UV light (eg, sunlight, tanning booths) and to use sunscreen and wear protective clothing when exposed to UV light until tolerance is determined.
- Advise women to notify health care provider if pregnant, planning to pregnant, or breastfeeding.
- Instruct patient not to take any prescription or OTC medications or dietary supplements unless advised by health care provider.
- Advise patient that follow-up visits may be required to monitor therapy and to keep appointments.

Procyclidine

(pro-SIGH-klih-deen)
Class Antiparkinson/Anticholinergic
How Supplied
Kemadrin Tablets 5 mg
✤ *Procyclid*

Action
PHARMACOLOGY: Has atropine-like action and exerts antispasmodic effect on smooth muscle. Is potent mydriatic and inhibits salivation; normally has no sympathetic ganglion-blocking activity.
PHARMACOKINETICS/DYNAMICS:
Absorption: Procyclidine hydrochloride is well-absorbed from the GI tract. T_{max} is 1.1 to 2 hr. C_{max} is 80 mcg/L. Bioavailability is 52% to 97% (oral).
Excretion: The t½ is 11.5 to 12.6 hr.
Duration: 4 hr (oral).

Indications Treatment of parkinsonism, including postencephalitic, arteriosclerotic and idiopathic types. Usually more efficacious in relief of rigidity than of tremor and can be used alone in mild to moderate cases. Also can be given to treat drug-induced extrapyramidal symptoms of phenothiazine or rauwolfia therapy and to control sialorrhea associated with neuroleptic medication.

Contraindications Angleclosure glaucoma; pyloric and duodenal obstruction; stenosing peptic ulcers; prostatic hypertrophy; bladder neck obstruction; achalasia; myasthenia gravis; megacolon.

Route/Dosage
Parkinsonism (No Prior Therapy)
ADULTS: PO 2.5 mg tid after meals initially. If well tolerated, dose may be gradually increased to 5 mg tid. Bedtime dose can be added if necessary.

Transferring from Prior Therapy
Substitute 2.5 mg tid for all or part of original agent. Increase prn while other drug is lowered or omitted. Individualize (max dose, 60 mg/day).

Drug-Induced Extrapyramidal Symptoms
ADULTS: Begin with 2.5 mg tid; increase by 2.5 mg increments until symptoms are relieved. Usually 10 to 20 mg/day is adequate.

Interactions
Haloperidol: Schizophrenic symptoms may worsen, haloperidol levels may decrease and tardive dyskinesia may develop.
Phenothiazines: Actions of phenothiazines may be decreased. Anticholinergic side effects may increase.

Lab Test Interferences None well documented.

Adverse Reactions
CV: Tachycardia; palpitations; orthostatic hypotension.
CNS: Disorientation; confusion; memory loss; hallucinations; agitation; nervousness; depression; drowsiness; giddiness; lightheadedness.
DERM: Rash; urticaria; decreased sweating.
EENT: Mydriasis; blurred vision.

GI: Dry mouth; nausea; vomiting; epigastric distress; constipation; paralytic ileus.
GU: Urinary retention; urinary hesitancy.
OTHER: Muscle weakness; acute suppurative parotitis; hyperthermia; heat stroke.

Precautions
Pregnancy: Category C.
Lactation: Undetermined.
Children: Safety and efficacy not established.
Elderly: More susceptible to adverse effects. Occasionally may exhibit confusion, disorientation, agitation, hallucinations, and psychotic-like symptoms.
Special risk patients: Use caution in concurrent illness in which anticholinergic effects may be undesirable (ie, tachycardia, urinary retention, marked prostatic hypertrophy). Closely observe hypotensive patients.
Anticholinergic effects: Administration of other drugs with anticholinergic effects will increase incidence and severity of these effects.
CNS: Psychotic episode may be precipitated in treating drug-induced extrapyramidal side effects of phenothiazines or rauwolfia derivatives.
Heat illness: Give with caution during hot weather.
Ophthalmic: Incipient narrow-angle glaucoma may be precipitated.

Overdosage: Signs and Symptoms
Circulatory collapse, respiratory depression or arrest, CNS depression preceded or followed by stimulation, psychosis, stupor, coma, seizures, fever, hot/dry/flushed skin, dry mucous membranes, paralytic ileus.

PATIENT CARE CONSIDERATIONS
Administration/Storage
- Give with food if GI upset is experienced.
- Give before meals if excessive drying of mouth occurs.
- Offer water or ice chips to aid patient comfort.
- Give with caution during hot weather (anhidrosis and hyperthermia may occur).
- Store at room temperature in tightly closed containers.

Assessment/Interventions
- Obtain patient history, including drug history and any known allergies.
- Observe hypotensive patients closely.
- Inform health care provider of dizziness, orthostatic hypotension, tachycardia or mild bradycardia, dry mouth, constipation, blurred vision, disorientation, confusion, urinary retention or hesitancy, or other side effects.
- Observe elderly patients for signs of mental confusion and disorientation.

Patient/Family Education
- Advise patient to use caution in hot weather as drug increases susceptibility to heat stroke.
- Instruct patient to report the following symptoms to health care provider immediately: pounding heartbeat, eye pain, confusion or skin rash. Also tell patient to report bothersome side effects including blurred vision, urinary retention or hesitancy, nausea, vomiting, constipation, dizziness, drowsiness or dry mouth, nose, or throat.
- Tell patient to take sips of water frequently, suck on ice chips or sugarless hard candy or chew sugarless gum if dry mouth occurs.
- Instruct patient to avoid intake of alcoholic beverages or other CNS depressants.
- Advise patient that drug may cause drowsiness or dizziness and to use caution while driving or performing tasks requiring mental alertness.
- Instruct patient not to take any OTC medications without consulting health care provider.

Progesterone
(pro-JESS-ter-ohn)
Class Progestin

How Supplied
Crinone Vaginal gel 4% (45 mg), Vaginal gel 8% (90 mg) ♦ *Prochieve* Vaginal gel 4% (45 mg), Vaginal gel 8% (90 mg) ♦ *Prometrium* Capsules 100 mg (micronized progesterone), Capsules 200 mg (micronized progesterone) ♦ *Progesterone in Oil* Injection 50 mg/mL

Action
PHARMACOLOGY: Inhibits secretion of pituitary gonadotropins, thereby preventing follicular maturation and ovulation (contraceptive effect); inhibits spontaneous uterine contraction; transforms proliferative endometrium into secretory endometrium.

PHARMACOKINETICS/DYNAMICS:
Absorption: Rapidly absorbed from the GI tract (oral); rapidly absorbed (IM). T_{max} is 1 to 2 hr (oral); 6.8 hr (8% gel); and 9.2 hr (90 mg IM). C_{max} is 17.3 to 72.5 ng/mL (100 to 300 mg/day for oral).

Distribution: Protein binding is 96% to 99%, primarily to serum albumin (50% to 54%) and transcortin (43% to 48%). Undergoes enterohepatic recycling and distributes into breast milk.

Metabolism: Metabolized in the liver to pregnanediols and pregnenolones metabolites, which are conjugated to glucuronide and sulfate metabolites.

Excretion: Excreted in the kidney (50% to 60% metabolites), bile/feces (approximately 10% metabolites), and small amount as unchanged in the bile. The t½ is approximately 2 to 3 hr (after first 6-hr oral ingestion) and approximately 8 to 9 hr thereafter (oral). Absorption t½ is a few minutes (IM) and 25 to 50 hr (gel). Elimination t½ is approximately 10 wk (IM) and 5 to 20 min (gel).

Duration: 3 to 6 mo (IM, long-acting).

Special Populations:
Renal Function Impairment – Use with caution and only with careful monitoring because metabolites are eliminated this way.
Severe liver insufficiency – Contraindicated.

Indications
Injection: Amenorrhea and abnormal uterine bleeding caused by hormonal imbalance in the absence of organic pathology (eg, uterine cancer).
Gel: Progesterone supplementation or replacement as part of an assisted reproductive technology (ART) treatment for infertile women with progesterone deficiency.
Capsule: Prevention of endometrial hyperplasia in nonhysterectomized postmenopausal women receiving conjugated estrogen tablets.
Capsules and gel: Use in secondary amenorrhea.

Contraindications Hypersensitivity to progestins; thrombophlebitis, thromboembolic disorders, cerebral hemorrhage (or history of these disorders); impaired liver function; breast or genital organ cancer; undiagnosed vaginal bleeding; missed abortion; diagnostic test for pregnancy; pregnancy or suspected pregnancy.

Route/Dosage
Amenorrhea
ADULTS: **IM** 5 to 10 mg/day for 6 to 8 consecutive days.

ART
ADULTS (8% GEL): **Intravaginal** 90 mg once daily for women requiring progesterone supplementation. In women with partial or complete ovarian failure, who require progesterone replacement, 90 mg bid.

Functional Uterine Bleeding
ADULTS: **IM** 5 to 10 mg/day for 6 days.

Prevention of Endometrial Hyperplasia
ADULTS: **PO** 200 mg in the evening for 12 days, sequentially per 28-day cycle.

Secondary Amenorrhea
ADULTS: **PO** Single 400 mg dose in the evening for 10 days. **Intravaginal** 45 mg of 4% gel every other day for up to 6 doses. Women who fail to respond, 90 mg of 8% gel every other day for up to 6 doses.

Interactions
CYP3A4 inhibitors (eg, ketoconazole): May inhibit progesterone metabolism, increasing plasma levels and the risk of side effects.

Lab Test Interferences Altered metyrapone test; increased sulfobromophthalein retention and other hepatic function tests; increase in prothrombin factors VII, VIII, IX, and X; altered pregnanediol determination; increase in protein bound iodine and butanol extractable protein bound iodine; decrease in T3 uptake.

Adverse Reactions
CV: Hypertension, palpitation, angina pectoris (less than 5%); syncope with and without hypotension.
CNS: Headache, depression, dizziness, worry, fatigue, emotional lability, irritability (at least 5%); confusion, somnolence, speech disorder, anxiety, impaired concentration, insomnia, personality disorder (less than 5%); asthenia, anorexia, increased appetite, nervousness (clinical trials); migraine, decreased libido.
DERM: Acne, verruca, wound debridement (less than 5%); pain at injection site, melasma, chloasma, photosensitivity.
EENT: Earache, nasal congestion, pharyngitis, abnormal vision (less than 5%).
GI: Abdominal bloating and pain, nausea, vomiting, diarrhea (at least 5%); constipation (at least 2%); dry mouth, dyspepsia, gastroenteritis, hemorrhagic rectum, hiatus hernia (less than 5%); tooth disorder (clinical trials).
GU: Breast tenderness, urinary problems, vaginal discharge, breast pain, vaginal dryness (at least 5%); breast carcinoma (at least 2%); leucorrhea, uterine fibroid, vaginal dryness, fungal vaginitis, vaginitis, UTI (less than 5%); breast enlargement (clinical trials); breakthrough bleeding, spotting, change in menstrual flow, amenorrhea, changes in cervical squamocolumnar junction and cervical secretions, vaginal candidiasis, pruritus vulvae, endometriosis, spontaneous abortion, pelvic infection.
HEPA: Cholecystectomy (at least 2%); hepatitis, elevated transaminases (postmarketing); cholestatic jaundice.
HEMA/LYMPH: Lymphadenopathy (less than 5%).
M/N: Edema, peripheral edema (less than 5%); increase or decrease in weight.
MUSC: Joint or musculoskeletal pain, back pain (at least 5%); arthritis, leg cramps, hypertonia, muscle disorder, myalgia (less than 5%).
RESP: Upper respiratory tract infection, coughing (at least 5%); bronchitis, pneumonitis, sinusitis (less than 5%).

OTHER: Hot flashes, chest pain, night sweats, swelling of hands and feet, viral infection (at least 5%); accidental injury, chest pain, fever (less than 5%); abscess, herpes simplex (less than 5%); increased sweating (clinical trials); anaphylaxis and anaphylactoid reactions, pyrexia, masculinization of female fetus.

Precautions

Pregnancy: Category X; Category B (*Prometrium* capsule).
Lactation: Excreted in breast milk.
Children: Safety and efficacy not established.
Depression: Carefully observe patients with history of depression.
Fluid retention: Use cautiously when conditions that might be affected by this factor are present (eg, asthma, cardiac or renal dysfunction, epilepsy).
Ophthalmic effects: Discontinue medication if there are any sudden changes in vision or other serious ophthalmic effects.
Peanut oil: Capsule contains peanut oil and should not be used in patients allergic to peanuts.
Thrombotic disorder: Discontinue if these conditions occur or are suspected.
Vaginal bleeding: With irregular vaginal bleeding, including breakthrough bleeding, nonfunctional causes should be considered and adequate diagnostic measures undertaken.

PATIENT CARE CONSIDERATIONS

Administration/Storage

- Store capsules, vaginal gel, and injection at controlled room temperature (59° to 86°F). Protect capsules from excessive moisture.

Capsules:

- Because medication can cause drowsiness, administer prescribed dose in the evening.
- To prevent endometrial hyperplasia, administer prescribed dose once daily for 12 days per 28-day cycle.
- For secondary amenorrhea, administer prescribed dose once daily for 10 days.
- Administer without regard to meals, but administer with food if GI upset occurs.

Gel:

- For intravaginal administration only. Not for dermal, ophthalmic, or oral administration.
- Administer gel using prefilled disposable applicator.
- Discard applicator after delivering dose. Do not save for future use.
- For treating secondary amenorrhea, administer prescribed dose every other day.
- If using vaginal gel for ART, administer once or twice daily as prescribed.
- Do not use concurrently with other intravaginal therapy. If other intravaginal therapy is used, administer at least 6 hr before or after progesterone vaginal gel.

Injection:

- For IM injection only. Not for intradermal, subcutaneous, or intra-arterial administration.
- Do not administer if particulate matter, cloudiness, or discoloration is noted.
- Rotate injection sites.

Assessment/Interventions

- Obtain patient history, including drug history and any known allergies. Note renal or hepatic impairment, depression or history of depression, epilepsy, migraine headaches, asthma, or cardiac dysfunction.
- Review patient's health history for any condition that would contraindicate use of progesterone: previous allergic reaction to progesterone; known or suspected pregnancy; known or suspected cancer of the breast or genital organs; undiagnosed vaginal bleeding; active or past history of thromboembolic disorders or stroke; severe liver dysfunction or disease; missed abortion; allergy to peanuts (capsules and injection containing peanut oil only), or allergy to sesame seed oil or seeds (injection containing sesame oil only).
- Ensure breast, abdominal, and pelvic examination and Pap smear have been completed and documented before starting therapy.
- Monitor blood sugar in diabetic patient when therapy with estrogen and progesterone therapy is started. Report significant changes to health care provider.
- Assess BP at beginning of therapy with estrogen and progesterone and periodically during treatment.
- Assess patient for GI, CNS, PSYCH, GU, and general body side effects. Inform health care provider if noted and significant.
- Inform health care provider immediately if any of the following are noted: pain in groin or calves; sharp chest pain, coughing blood, or sudden shortness of breath; crushing chest pain or heaviness in chest; abnormal vaginal bleeding; breast lumps; sudden severe headache; dizziness or fainting; tremors or seizures; vision or speech problems; weakness or numbness of arms or legs; abdominal swelling or severe pain; jaundice; symptoms of depression.

Injection:

- Document site of each injection.

- Assess injection sites for reaction. Inform health care provider if noted and significant.

Patient/Family Education
- Explain name, dose, action, and potential side effects of drug.
- Advise patient to read *Patient Information* leaflet before using the first time and with each refill.
- Instruct diabetic patient taking estrogen and progesterone to monitor blood glucose more frequently when therapy is started and to inform health care provider of significant changes in readings.
- Teach patient proper method of breast self-examination, and remind patient to perform monthly.
- Instruct patient to immediately report any of the following symptoms to health care provider: pain in groin or calves; sharp chest pain, coughing blood, or sudden shortness of breath; crushing chest pain or heaviness in chest; abnormal vaginal bleeding; breast lumps; sudden severe headache; dizziness or fainting; tremors or seizure; vision or speech problems; weakness or numbness of arms or legs; severe abdominal pain; depression; yellowing of the skin or eyes; or persistent pain, pus, or bleeding at injection site.
- Advise patient that drug may cause dizziness and/or drowsiness and to use caution while driving or performing other tasks requiring mental alertness, coordination, or physical dexterity until tolerance is determined.
- Advise women to notify health care provider if pregnant, planning to become pregnant, or breastfeeding.
- Advise patient that follow-up visits and examinations, including Pap smear, at least once a year, will be required to monitor therapy and to keep appointments.

Capsules:
- Advise patient to take prescribed dose in the evening to minimize problems with medication-induced drowsiness or dizziness.
- Remind patient using progesterone for prevention of endometrial hyperplasia to take prescribed dose once daily for 12 days per 28-day cycle.
- Remind patient using progesterone for treating secondary amenorrhea that prescribed dose is taken once daily for 10 days.
- Advise patient to take each dose without regard to meals but to take with food if stomach upset occurs.

Vaginal Gel:
- Review instructions for preparing the applicator and administering the gel.
- If gel will be used at altitudes above 762 m, review special instructions for preparing the applicator to prevent partial release of gel before vaginal insertion.
- Instruct patient to discard applicator after use and not to save for future use.
- Advise patient that gel should not be used at the same time as other intravaginal products. If other intravaginal therapy is being used, instruct patient to administer at least 6 hr before or after the progesterone vaginal gel.
- Advise patient that small, white globules may appear as a discharge, even several days after using gel, but that this is normal and of no concern.
- Advise patient to discontinue use and notify health care provider if vaginal irritation develops while using the medication.

Injection:
- Advise patient that injection will be prepared and administered by a health care provider in a medical setting.

Promethazine Hydrochloride

(pro-METH-uh-zeen HIGH-droe-KLOR-ide)
Class Antihistamine/Antiemetic/Antivertigo

How Supplied
Phenergan Tablets 25 mg, Tablets 50 mg, Suppositories 12.5 mg, Suppositories 25 mg, Suppositories 50 mg, Injection 25 mg/mL, Injection 50 mg/mL (IM use only)

Action
PHARMACOLOGY: Competitively antagonizes histamine at H_1 receptor sites. Produces sedative and antiemetic effects.

PHARMACOKINETICS/DYNAMICS:
Absorption: Well absorbed from the GI tract.
Distribution: Protein binding is 65% to 95%. Small amounts may distribute into breast milk.
Metabolism: Metabolized in the liver; sulfoxides and n-demethylpromethazine are the predominant metabolites.
Excretion: Urine (metabolites appear here). $T_{1/2}$ is 7 to 14 hr.
Onset: 15 to 60 min (oral); 20 min (IM); 3 to 5 min (IV); 20 min (rectal).
Duration: Duration of action is 4 to 6 hr; may persist up to 12 hr (oral).

Indications
Oral/Rectal: Temporary relief of runny nose and sneezing caused by common cold; symptomatic relief of perennial and seasonal allergic rhinitis,

vasomotor rhinitis, allergic conjunctivitis, allergic and nonallergic pruritic symptoms, mild, uncomplicated skin manifestations of urticaria, and angioedema; amelioration of allergic reactions to blood or plasma; treatment of dermographism; adjunctive therapy in anaphylactic reactions; preoperative, postoperative or obstetric sedation; prevention and control of nausea and vomiting associated with certain types of anesthesia and surgery; adjunctive therapy to analgesics for postoperative pain; sedation and relief of apprehension; induction of light sleep; active and prophylactic treatment of motion sickness; antiemetic therapy in postoperative patients.
Parenteral: Treatment of motion sickness; prevention and control of nausea and vomiting associated with anesthesia and surgery; allergic reactions.

IV: Adjunct to anesthesia and analgesia with reduced amounts of meperidine or other narcotic analgesics in special surgical situations (eg, repeated bronchoscopy, ophthalmic surgery, poor-risk patients).

Contraindications Hypersensitivity to antihistamines; narrow-angle glaucoma; stenosing peptic ulcer; symptomatic prostatic hypertrophy; asthmatic attack; bladder neck obstruction; pyloroduodenal obstruction; comatose patients; CNS depression from barbiturates, general anesthetics, tranquilizers, alcohol, narcotics, or narcotic analgesics; previous phenothiazine idiosyncrasy, jaundice or bone marrow depression; acutely ill or dehydrated children; intra-arterial injection; nursing mothers; MAOI use.

Route/Dosage
Allergy
ADULTS AND CHILDREN (OVER 2 YR): **PO/PR** 25 mg at bedtime; 12.5 mg before meals and at bedtime may be given if necessary. Single 25 mg doses at bedtime or 6.25 to 12.5 mg tid will usually suffice.
ADULTS: **IM/IV** 25 mg; may repeat dose within 2 hr if needed.
CHILDREN (AT LEAST 2 YR): **IM/IV** Do not exceed 50% the adult dose.

Motion Sickness
ADULTS: **PO** 25 mg bid with initial dose taken 30 min to 1 hr before travel and repeated in 8 to 12 hr if needed. Thereafter 25 mg on rising and before evening meal.
CHILDREN (OVER 2 YR): **PO/PR** 12.5 to 25 mg bid.

Nausea and Vomiting
ADULTS: **PO/PR** 25 mg. Repeat doses of 12.5 to 25 mg prn q 4 to 6 hr.
ADULTS: **IM/IV** 12.5 to 25 mg not more than q 4 hr.

CHILDREN (OVER 2 YR): **PO/PR** 1 mg/kg q 4 to 6 hr prn.

Prophylaxis of Nausea and Vomiting
ADULTS: **PO/PR** 25 mg q 4 to 6 hr prn.
CHILDREN (OVER 2 YR): **PO/PR** 1 mg/kg q 4 to 6 hr prn.

Nighttime Sedation
ADULTS: **PO/PR/IM/IV** 25 to 50 mg.
CHILDREN (OVER 2 YR): **PO/PR/IM/IV** 12.5 to 25 mg.

Preoperative Sedation
ADULTS: **PO/PR/IM/IV** 25 to 50 mg night before surgery.
CHILDREN (OVER 2 YR): **PO/PR** 1 mg/kg.
CHILDREN (2 TO 12 YR): **IM/IV** 1 mg/kg.

Postoperative Sedation and Adjunctive Use with Analgesics
ADULTS: **PO/PR/IM/IV** 25 to 50 mg.
CHILDREN (OVER 2 YR): **PO/PR/IM/IV** 12.5 to 25 mg.

Sedation During Labor
ADULTS: **IM/IV** 50 mg in early stages of labor. When labor is established, 25 to 75 mg with reduced dose of narcotic (max total dose, 100 mg/24 hr).

Interactions
Anticholinergics: May decrease action of promethazine.
Barbiturate anesthetics: Risk of neuromuscular excitation and hypotension may increase.
CNS depressants (eg, alcohol, narcotics): May have additive CNS depressant effects.
MAO inhibitors: May prolong and intensify anticholinergic effects; may cause hypotension and extrapyramidal effects.
Metrizamide: May increase risk of seizure.

Lab Test Interferences Diagnostic pregnancy tests based on immunologic reactions between hCG and anti-hCG may result in false-negative or false-positive interpretations. Following interferences also have occurred: increased serum cholesterol, blood glucose, spinal fluid protein, and urinary urobilinogen concentrations; decreased protein-bound iodine; false positive urine bilirubin tests; interference with urinary ketone and steroid determinations; false-positive phenylketonuria test results.

Adverse Reactions
CV: Orthostatic hypotension; palpitations; bradycardia; tachycardia; reflex tachycardia; extrasystoles.
CNS: Drowsiness; sedation; dizziness; faintness; disturbed coordination; extrapyramidal effects (usually dose related and include three forms: pseudoparkinsonism, akathisia, dystonias); tardive dyskinesia; adverse behavioral effects.

EENT: Blurred vision; nasal stuffiness; dry nose; dry or sore throat.
GI: Epigastric distress; dry mouth; nausea; vomiting; diarrhea; constipation.
GU: Urinary retention/frequency.
HEMA: Hemolytic anemia; thrombocytopenia; agranulocytosis.
METAB: Increased appetite, weight gain.
RESP: Thickening of bronchial secretions; chest tightness; wheezing; respiratory depression.
OTHER: Hypersensitivity reactions; photosensitivity; elevated prolactin levels; neuroleptic malignant syndrome.

Precautions
Pregnancy: Category C. Do not use during third trimester.
Lactation: Undetermined. Contraindicated in nursing mothers.
Children: Contraindicated in children who are acutely ill or dehydrated. Tablets and suppositories are not recommended in children less than 2 yr. Antihistamines may diminish mental alertness and may produce paradoxical excitation. Administer IV form with caution. Not recommended for treatment of uncomplicated vomiting in children; use only when vomiting is prolonged and of unknown cause. Extrapyramidal symptoms that can occur secondary to IV use may be confused with CNS signs of undiagnosed primary disease (eg, encephalopathy, Reye syndrome). Avoid use in children with history of sleep apnea, family history of Sudden Infant Death Syndrome (SIDS) or hepatic diseases, and in children with Reye syndrome.
Elderly: Greater likelihood of dizziness, excessive sedation, syncope, toxic confusional states, and hypotension in patients over 60 yr. Dosage reduction may be required.
Hypersensitivity: Hypersensitivity may occur. Have 1:1000 epinephrine immediately available.
Special risk patients: Use drug with caution in patients with predisposition to urinary retention, history of bronchial asthma, IOP, hyperthyroidism, sleep apnea, cardiovascular disease or hypertension, bone marrow depression, liver dysfunction, ulcer disease, or respiratory impairment.
Lower seizure threshold: Drug may lower seizure threshold; use drug with caution in people with known seizure disorders or when giving in combination with narcotics or local anesthetics that may alter seizure control.
Respiratory disease: Drug is generally not recommended to treat lower respiratory tract symptoms including asthma.
Skin test procedures: May prevent or diminish positive reactions to dermal reactivity indicators. If possible, discontinue 4 days prior to skin test.

Overdosage: Signs and Symptoms
CNS depression (sedation to coma), apnea, diminished mental alertness, cardiovascular collapse, insomnia, hallucinations, tremors, convulsions, profound hypotension. respiratory depression, dizziness, ataxia, tinnitus, blurred vision, fixed dilated pupils, flushing, dry mouth, fever, oral and facial dystonic reactions.

PATIENT CARE CONSIDERATIONS
Administration/Storage
- Give oral form with food if GI upset occurs.
- When administering drug parenterally, preferred route is IM injection.
- If drug must be administered IV, use caution; do not inject directly into vein and inject through appropriate site in IV tubing. Promethazine may be mixed with meperidine in same syringe.
- Do not exceed IV concentration of 25 mg/mL and do not exceed IV rate of 25 mg/min.
- Do not administer SC or intra-arterially.
- Dose of barbiturates must be reduced by ½ and of narcotics by ¼ to ½ when using this drug concomitantly.
- Avoid use of this drug in cases of vomiting of unknown origin.
- Discontinue drug 4 days before skin testing procedures.
- Store suppositories in refrigerator and use while cold and firm.
- Store oral dosage form at room temperature in tightly closed, light-resistant container.
- Store parenteral form at room temperature, protected from light. Do not freeze.

Assessment/Interventions
- Obtain patient history, including drug history and any known allergies. Note presence of glaucoma, ulcer disease, urinary retention, hypertension, seizure disorder, bone marrow depression, history of bronchial asthma, hyperthyroidism, cardiovascular disease, or liver dysfunction.
- Monitor for possible increased blood glucose.
- In children, check for history of sleep apnea, Reye syndrome, hepatic disease, or family history of SIDS.
- Observe for sedation, fatigue, insomnia, dry mouth, sore throat, thickening of mucus, unusual bleeding, or nervousness, and report to health care provider.

Patient/Family Education
- Instruct patient using drug for motion sickness to take drug 30 min to 1 hr before travel.
- Teach patient to store suppositories in refrigerator and to use while cold and firm.
- Advise patient to notify all health care professionals of this drug therapy.

- Inform patient that drug may cause dryness of mouth, nose, or throat and to notify health care provider if this dryness continues for more than 2 wk.
- Instruct patient to report the following symptoms to health care provider: sore throat, thickening of mucus, fever, unusual bleeding, drowsiness, unusual weakness.
- Advise patient to take sips of water frequently or to suck on ice chips or sugarless candy, or chew sugarless gum if dry mouth occurs.
- Caution patient to avoid sudden position changes to prevent orthostatic hypotension.
- Instruct patient to avoid intake of alcoholic beverages and other CNS depressants.
- Advise patient that drug may cause drowsiness and to use caution while driving or performing other tasks requiring mental alertness.
- Caution patient to avoid exposure to sunlight and to use sunscreen or wear protective clothing to avoid photosensitivity reaction.

Promethazine Hydrochloride/Codeine Phosphate

(Pro-METH-uh-zeen HIGH-droe-KLOR-ide/ KOE-deen FOSS-fate)

Class Antihistamine/Antitussive/Narcotic Analgesic

How Supplied
Prometh with Codeine Syrup 10 mg codeine phosphate and 6.25 mg promethazine hydrochloride

Action
PHARMACOLOGY:
Promethazine: Competitively antagonizes histamine at H_1-receptor sites and produces sedative as well as antiemetic effects.
Codeine: Stimulates opiate receptors in the CNS in addition to causing respiratory depression, peripheral vasodilation, inhibition of intestinal peristalsis, stimulation of the chemoreceptors that cause vomiting, increased bladder tone, and suppression of cough.

Indications Temporary relief of coughs and upper respiratory tract symptoms associated with allergy or the common cold.

Contraindications Treatment of lower respiratory tract symptoms, including asthma; known hypersensitivity or idiosyncratic reaction to promethazine or other phenothiazines; hypersensitivity to any component of the product.

Route/Dosage
ADULTS AND CHILDREN 12 YR AND OLDER: PO 1 tsp (5 mL) q 4 to 6 hr (max, 30 mL/24 hr).
CHILDREN 6 YR TO UNDER 12 YR: PO ½ to 1 tsp (2.5 to 5 mL) q 4 to 6 hr (max, 30 mL/24 hr).
CHILDREN UNDER 6 YR (WEIGHT 18 KG OR 40 LBS): PO ¼ to ½ tsp (1.25 to 2.5 mL) q 4 to 6 hr (max, 9 mL/24 hr).
CHILDREN UNDER 6 YR (WEIGHT 16 KG OR 35 LBS): PO ¼ to ½ tsp (1.25 to 2.5 mL) q 4 to 6 hr (max, 8 mL/24 hr).
CHILDREN UNDER 6 YR (WEIGHT 14 KG OR 30 LBS): PO ¼ to ½ tsp (1.25 to 2.5 mL) q 4 to 6 hr (max, 7 mL/24 hr).
CHILDREN UNDER 6 YR (WEIGHT 12 KG OR 25 LBS): PO ¼ to ½ tsp (1.25 to 2.5 mL) q 4 to 6 hr (max, 6 mL/24 hr).

Interactions
Codeine:
CNS depressants (eg, tranquilizers, sedatives, alcohol) – Additive CNS depression.
MAO inhibitors (eg, isocarboxazid) – Excessive narcotic or MAO inhibitor interaction may occur.
Quinidine – May decrease the analgesic effect of codeine by interference with metabolism of codeine to morphine.
Promethazine:
Alcohol, barbiturates, narcotic analgesics, sedative-hypnotics, tricyclic antidepressants, tranquilizers or other CNS depressants – Sedative effects of promethazine is additive with these agents.

Lab Test Interferences
Codeine: Increased plasma levels of amylase or lipase, making determination of these enzyme levels unreliable for 24 hr after taking codeine.
Promethazine: False-negative or false-positive interpretations of diagnostic pregnancy tests based on immunological reactions between HCG and anti-HCG; increased blood glucose tests.

Adverse Reactions
CV:
Codeine – Circulatory depression; tachycardia; bradycardia; palpitation; faintness; syncope; orthostatic hypotension.
Promethazine – Increased or decreased BP.
CNS:
Codeine – Lightheadedness; dizziness; sedation; euphoria; dysphoria; headache; transient hallucination; disorientation; convulsions.
Promethazine – Sedation; sleepiness; dizziness; confusion; disorientation; extrapyramidal symptoms (including oculogyric crisis); torticollis; tongue depression.

DERM:
Promethazine – Rash; photosensitivity.
EENT:
Codeine – Visual disturbances.
Promethazine – Blurred vision.
GI:
Codeine – Nausea; vomiting; constipation; biliary tract spasms increased colonic motility (in patients with chronic ulcerative colitis).
Promethazine – Dry mouth; nausea; vomiting.
GU:
Codeine – Oliguria; urinary retention; antidiuretic effect.
HEMA:
Promethazine – Leukopenia; thrombocytopenia; agranulocytosis.
RESP:
Codeine – Respiratory depression.
OTHER:
Codeine – Allergy (including pruritus, giant urticaria, angioneurotic edema, laryngeal edema); flushing; sweating; weakness.

Precautions
Pregnancy: Category C.
Lactation:
Codeine – Excreted in breast milk.
Promethazine – Undetermined.
Children: Safety and efficacy not established in children under 2 yr.
Special risk patients: Use with caution in the very young, elderly, or debilitated patient. Use with caution in patients with acute abdominal conditions, convulsive disorders, significant hepatic or renal impairment, fever, hypothyroidism, Addison disease, ulcerative colitis, prostatic hypertrophy, cardiovascular disease, recent GI or urinary tract surgery, head injury or increased intracranial pressure, and in atopic children (because of possible histamine release), narrowangle glaucoma, stenosing peptic ulcer, pyloroduodenal obstruction, narrowing of the bladder neck.
Cholestatic jaundice: May occur.
Dependency: Codeine has abuse potential. Psychological and physical dependence as well as tolerance may occur.
Seizure threshold: Seizure threshold may be lowered; use with caution in patients with known seizure disorders or when given in combination with narcotics or local anesthetics that may also affect seizure threshold.

Overdosage: Signs and Symptoms
Codeine: Respiratory depression, extreme somnolence progressing to stupor or coma, skeletal muscle flaccidity, cold clammy skin, bradycardia, hypotension, apnea, circulatory collapse, cardiac arrest, death; promethazine is additive to depressant effects of codeine.
Promethazine: Range from mild depression of the CNS and cardiovascular system to profound hypotension, respiratory depression and unconsciousness, stimulation (especially in children and geriatric patients), paradoxical hyperexcitability and nightmares in children, convulsions, dry mouth, fixed dilated pupils, flushing, GI symptoms.

PATIENT CARE CONSIDERATIONS
Administration/Storage
- Give prescribed dose of syrup q 4 to 6 hr as needed.
- Give with food or milk if GI upset occurs.
- Use dosing spoon or syringe for pediatric doses.
- Store syrup at controlled room temperature (59° to 86°F). Keep tightly capped and protect from light.

Assessment/Interventions
- Obtain patient history, including drug history and any known allergies. Note history of liver disease, kidney disease, cardiovascular disease, acute abdominal conditions, peptic ulcer disease, seizures, hypothyroidism, Addison disease, ulcerative colitis, enlarged prostate, asthma, narrow angle glaucoma, urinary retention, head injury, increased intracranial pressure, or recent GI or urinary tract surgery.
- Assess for allergy or cold symptoms (eg, cough, rhinitis, sneezing, itching, watery eyes) before and periodically throughout therapy.
- Monitor patient for GI, CNS, CV, and general body side effects. Inform health care provider if noted and significant.

Patient/Family Education
- Explain name, dose, action, and potential side effects of drug.
- Advise patient to take prescribed dose q 4 to 6 hr as needed.
- Advise caregiver to use dosing spoon or syringe when giving suspension to children.
- Advise patient to take with food or milk if GI upset occurs.
- Advise patient that if a dose is missed to take as soon as remembered unless it is nearing time for the next dose. Caution patient to not double the dose to catch up.
- Advise patient that if cough, allergy, or cold symptoms are not controlled, not to increase the dose of medication but to inform health care provider.
- Caution patient that drug may cause drowsiness and to use caution while driving or performing other tasks requiring mental alertness until tolerance is determined.

- Advise patient to avoid alcohol and other CNS depressants because of risk of excessive sedation.
- Caution patient not to take any OTC antihistamines or decongestants while taking this medication unless advised by health care provider.
- If patient is to have allergy skin testing, advise to not take the medication for at least 6 days before the skin testing.
- Advise women to notify health care provider if pregnant, planing to become pregnant, or breastfeeding.
- Instruct patient to stop taking drug and immediately report any of these symptoms to health care provider: abnormal muscle movements, unusual sensitivity to sunlight, dizziness, excessive drowsiness.
- Caution patient not to take any prescription or OTC medications or dietary supplements unless advised by health care provider.

Promethazine Hydrochloride/ Phenylephrine Hydrochloride

(Pro-METH-uh-zeen HIGH-droe-KLOR-ide/ fen-ill-EFF-rin HIGH-droe-KLOR-ide)

Class Antihistamine/Decongestant

How Supplied
Prometh VC Plain Syrup 5 mg phenylephrine hydrochloride and 6.25 promethazine hydrochloride

Action
PHARMACOLOGY:
Promethazine: Competitively antagonizes histamine at H_1-receptor sites and produces sedative as well as antiemetic effects.
Phenylephrine: Stimulates postsynaptic alpha-receptors, resulting in rise in arterial peripheral vasoconstriction.

Indications Temporary relief of upper respiratory tract symptoms, including nasal congestion, associated with allergy or the common cold.

Contraindications Treatment of lower respiratory tract symptoms, including asthma; patients with hypertension or peripheral vascular insufficiency; patients receiving MAO inhibitors; known hypersensitivity or an idiosyncratic reaction to promethazine or other phenothiazines; allergy to any component of the product.

Route/Dosage
ADULTS AND CHILDREN 12 YR AND OVER: **PO** 1 tsp (5 mL) q 4 to 6 hr (max, 6 tsp [30 mL] in 24 hr).
CHILDREN 6 TO UNDER 12 YR: **PO** ½ to 1 tsp (2.5 to 5 mL) q 4 to 6 hr (max, 6 tsp [30 mL] in 24 hr).
CHILDREN 2 TO UNDER 6 YR: **PO** ¼ to ½ tsp (1.25 to 2.5 mL) q 4 to 6 hr.

Interactions
Promethazine:
Alcohol, barbiturates, narcotic analgesics, sedative-hypnotics, tricyclic antidepressants, tranquilizers, or other CNS depressants – Sedative effects of promethazine is additive with these agents.
Phenylephrine:
Alpha-adrenergic blockers (eg, Phentolamine) – Decreased pressor response.
Anorexiants (eg, amphetamines, phenylpropanolamine) – Synergistic adrenergic response.
Atropine – Reflex bradycardia may be blocked or pressor response enhanced.
Beta-adrenergic blockers (eg, propranolol) – Cardiostimulating effects may be blocked.
Bronchodilators, sympathomimetic agents – Tachycardia or other arrhythmias may occur.
Ergot derivatives – Excessive increase in BP may occur.
MAO inhibitors (eg, isocarboxazid) – Because acute hypertensive crisis may occur, coadministration of these agents is contraindicated.
Tricyclic antidepressants – Pressor effects of phenylephrine may be increased.

Lab Test Interferences False-negative or false-positive interpretations of diagnostic pregnancy tests based on immunological reactions between HCG and anti-HCG; increased blood glucose tests.

Adverse Reactions
CV:
Promethazine – Hypertension; hypotension.
Phenylephrine – Hypertension.
CNS:
Promethazine – Sedation; sleepiness; dizziness; confusion; disorientation; extrapyramidal symptoms (including oculogyric crisis, torticollis, tongue protrusion).
Phenylephrine – Restlessness; anxiety; nervousness; dizziness; tremor; weakness.

DERM:
Promethazine – Rash; photosensitivity.
EENT:
Promethazine – Blurred vision.
GI:
Promethazine – Nausea; vomiting; dryness of mouth.
HEMA:
Promethazine – Leukopenia; thrombocytopenia; agranulocytosis.
RESP:
Phenylephrine – Respiratory distress.
OTHER:
Phenylephrine – Precordial pain.

Precautions
Pregnancy: Category C.
Lactation: Undermined.
Children: Safety and efficacy not established in children under 2 yr.
Special risk patients: Use with caution in patients with narrow-angle glaucoma, stenosing peptic ulcer, pyloroduodenal obstruction, urinary bladder obstruction due to symptomatic prostatic hypertrophy or narrowing of the bladder neck, thyroid disease, diabetes mellitus, cardiovascular disease, hepatic function impairment.
Cholestatic jaundice: May occur.
Seizure threshold: Seizure threshold may be lowered; use with caution in persons with known seizure disorders or when given in combination with narcotics or local anesthetics that may also affect seizure threshold.
Sleep apnea: Avoid use in patients with history of sleep apnea.

Overdosage: Signs and Symptoms
Range from mild depression of the CNS and cardiovascular system to profound hypotension, respiratory depression, and unconsciousness, stimulation (especially in children and geriatric patients), paradoxical hyperexcitability and nightmares in children, convulsions, dry mouth, fixed dilated pupils, flushing, GI symptoms, hypertension, headache, cerebral hemorrhage, vomiting, ventricular tachycardia.

PATIENT CARE CONSIDERATIONS

Administration/Storage
- Give prescribed dose of syrup q 4 to 6 hr as needed.
- Give with food or milk if GI upset occurs.
- Use dosing spoon or syringe for pediatric doses.
- Store syrup at controlled room temperature (59° to 86°F). Keep tightly capped and protect from light.

Assessment/Interventions
- Obtain patient history, including drug history and any known allergies. Note history of liver disease, peptic ulcer disease, diabetes, peripheral vascular disease, hypertension, seizures, hyperthyroidism, enlarged prostate, asthma, narrow angle glaucoma, urinary retention, coronary artery disease, concurrent use of tricyclic antidepressants, or concurrent use of or within 2 wk of stopping MAO-inhibitor therapy.
- Assess for allergy or cold symptoms (eg, rhinitis, nasal congestion, sneezing, itching, watery eyes) before and periodically throughout therapy.
- Monitor pulse and BP periodically during therapy.
- Monitor patient for GI, CNS, CV, and general body side effects. Inform health care provider if noted and significant.

Patient/Family Education
- Explain name, dose, action, and potential side effects of drug.
- Advise patient to take prescribed dose q 4 to 6 hr as needed.
- Advise caregiver to use dosing spoon or syringe when giving suspension to children.
- Advise patient to take with food or milk if GI upset occurs.
- Advise patient that if a dose is missed to take as soon as remembered unless it is nearing time for the next dose. Caution patient to not double the dose to catch up.
- Advise patient that if allergy symptoms are not controlled not to increase the dose of medication but to inform health care provider.
- Caution patient that drug may cause drowsiness and to use caution while driving or performing other tasks requiring mental alertness until tolerance is determined.
- Advise patient to avoid alcohol and other CNS depressants because of risk of excessive sedation.
- Caution patient not to take any OTC antihistamines or decongestants while taking this medication unless advised by health care provider.
- If patient is to have allergy skin testing, advise to not take the medication for at least 6 days before the skin testing.
- Advise women to notify health care provider if pregnant, planning to become pregnant, or breastfeeding.
- Instruct patient to stop taking drug and immediately report any of these symptoms to health care provider: abnormal muscle movements, unusual sensitivity to sunlight nervousness, dizziness, excessive drowsiness.
- Caution patient not to take any prescription or OTC medications or dietary supplements unless advised by health care provider.

Promethazine Hydrochloride/ Phenylephrine Hydrochloride/Codeine Phosphate

(Pro-METH-uh-zeen HIGH-droe-KLOR-ide/ fen-ill-EFF-rin HIGH-droe-KLOR-ide/KOE-deen FOSS-fate)

Class Antihistamine/Decongestant/Antitussive/ Narcotic Analgesic

How Supplied
Prometh VC w/Codeine Syrup 6.25 mg promethazine hydrochloride/5 mg phenylephrine hydrochloride/10 mg codeine phosphate/5 mL

Action
PHARMACOLOGY:
Promethazine: Competitively antagonizes histamine at H_1-receptor sites and produces sedative as well as antiemetic effects.
Phenylephrine: Stimulates postsynaptic alpha-receptors, resulting in rise in arterial peripheral vasoconstriction.
Codeine: Stimulates opiate receptors in the CNS in addition to causing respiratory depression, peripheral vasodilation, inhibition of intestinal peristalsis, stimulation of the chemoreceptors that cause vomiting, increased bladder tone, and suppression of cough.

Indications Temporary relief of coughs and upper respiratory tract symptoms, including nasal congestion, associated with allergy or the common cold.

Contraindications Patients with hypertension; peripheral vascular insufficiency; known hypersensitivity to any component of the product; hypersensitivity or idiosyncratic reaction to promethazine or other phenothiazines; patients receiving MAO inhibitors; treatment of lower respiratory tract symptoms, including asthma.

Route/Dosage
ADULTS: **PO** 1 tsp (5 mL) q 4 to 6 hr (max, 30 mL/24 hr).
CHILDREN 6 YR THROUGH 11 YR: **PO** ½ to 1 tsp (2.5 to 5 mL) q 4 to 6 hr (max, 30 mL/24 hr).
CHILDREN UNDER 6 YR (WEIGHT 18 KG OR 40 LBS): **PO** ¼ to ½ tsp (1.25 to 2.5 mL) q 4 to 6 hr (max, 9 mL/24 hr).
CHILDREN UNDER 6 YR (WEIGHT 16 KG OR 35 LBS): **PO** ¼ to ½ tsp (1.25 to 2.5 mL) q 4 to 6 hr (max, 8 mL/24 hr).
CHILDREN UNDER 6 YR (WEIGHT 14 KG OR 30 LBS): **PO** ¼ to ½ tsp (1.25 to 2.5 mL) q 4 to 6 hr (max, 7 mL/24 hr).
CHILDREN UNDER 6 YR (WEIGHT 12 KG OR 25 LBS): **PO** ¼ to ½ tsp (1.25 to 2.5 mL) q 4 to 6 hr (max, 6 mL/24 hr).

Interactions
Codeine:
CNS depressants (eg, tranquilizers, sedatives, alcohol) – Causes additive CNS depression.
MAO inhibitors (eg, isocarboxazid) – Excessive narcotic or MAO inhibitor interaction may occur.
Quinidine – May decrease the analgesic effect of codeine by interference with metabolism of codeine to morphine.
Promethazine:
Alcohol, barbiturates, narcotic analgesics, sedative-hypnotics, tricyclic antidepressants, tranquilizers, or other CNS depressants – Sedative effects of promethazine is additive with these agents.
Phenylephrine:
Alpha-adrenergic blockers (eg, phentolamine) – Decreased pressor response.
Anorexiants (eg, amphetamines, phenylpropanolamine) – Synergistic adrenergic response.
Atropine – Reflex bradycardia may be blocked or pressor response enhanced.
Beta-adrenergic blockers (eg, propranolol) – Cardiostimulating effects may be blocked.
Bronchodilators, sympathomimetic agents – Tachycardia or other arrhythmias may occur.
Ergot derivatives – Excessive increase in BP may occur.
MAO inhibitors (eg, isocarboxazid) – Because acute hypertensive crisis may occur, coadministration of these agents is contraindicated.
Tricyclic antidepressants – Pressor effects of phenylephrine may be increased.

Lab Test Interferences
Codeine: Increased plasma levels of amylase or lipase, making determination of these enzyme levels unreliable for 24 hr after taking codeine.
Promethazine: False-negative or false-positive interpretations of diagnostic pregnancy tests based on immunological reactions between HCG and anti-HCG; increased blood glucose tests.

Adverse Reactions
CV:
Codeine – Circulatory depression; tachycardia; bradycardia; palpitation; faintness; syncope; orthostatic hypotension.
Phenylephrine – Hypertension.
Promethazine – Increased or decreased BP.
CNS:
Codeine – Lightheadedness; dizziness; sedation; euphoria; dysphoria; headache; transient hallucination; disorientation; convulsions.

Phenylephrine – Restlessness; anxiety; nervousness; dizziness; tremor; weakness.
Promethazine – Sedation; sleepiness; dizziness; confusion; disorientation; extrapyramidal symptoms (including oculogyric crisis); torticollis; tongue depression.
DERM:
Promethazine – Rash; photosensitivity.
EENT: Visual disturbances
Promethazine – Blurred vision.
GI:
Codeine – Nausea; vomiting; constipation; biliary tract spasm increased colonic motility (in patients with chronic ulcerative colitis).
Promethazine – Dry mouth; nausea; vomiting.
GU:
Codeine – Oliguria; urinary retention; antidiuretic effect.
HEMA:
Promethazine – Leukopenia; thrombocytopenia; agranulocytosis.
RESP:
Codeine – Respiratory depression.
Phenylephrine – Respiratory distress.
OTHER:
Codeine – Allergy (including pruritus, giant urticaria, angioneurotic edema, laryngeal edema); flushing; sweating; weakness.
Phenylephrine – Precordial pain.

Precautions

Pregnancy: Category C.
Lactation:
Codeine – Excreted in breast milk.
Promethazine and phenylephrine – Undetermined.
Children: Safety and efficacy not established in children under 2 yr.
Special risk patients: Use with caution in patients with narrow-angle glaucoma, stenosing peptic ulcer, acute abdominal conditions, convulsive disorders, significant hepatic or renal impairment, fever, thyroid disease, diabetes mellitus, Addison disease, ulcerative colitis, prostatic hypertrophy, pyloroduodenal obstruction caused by symptomatic prostatic hypertrophy or narrowing of the bladder, CV disease, recent GI or urinary tract surgery, head injury or increased intracranial pressure, and in atopic children (because of possible histamine release), in the very young or elderly or debilitated patient; patients receiving tricyclic antidepressants or diet preparations (eg, amphetamines).
Dependency: Codeine has abuse potential. Psychological and physical dependence as well as tolerance may occur.
Seizure threshold: Seizure threshold may be lowered; use with caution in persons with known seizure disorders or when given in combination with narcotics or local anesthetics that may also affect seizure threshold.
Sleep apnea: Avoid use in patients with history of sleep apnea.

Overdosage: Signs and Symptoms

Codeine: Respiratory depression, extreme somnolence progressing to stupor or coma, skeletal muscle flaccidity, cold clammy skin, bradycardia, hypotension, apnea, circulatory collapse, cardiac arrest, death, promethazine is additive to depressant effects of codeine.
Phenylephrine: Hypertension, headache, convulsions, cerebral hemorrhage, vomiting, ventricular premature beats, short paroxysms of ventricular tachycardia, bradycardia.
Promethazine: Range from mild depression of the CNS and CV system to profound hypotension, respiratory depression, and unconsciousness; stimulation (especially in children and geriatric patients); paradoxical hyperexcitability and nightmares in children; convulsions; dry mouth; fixed dilated pupils; flushing; GI symptoms.

PATIENT CARE CONSIDERATIONS

Administration/Storage

- Give prescribed dose of syrup q 4 to 6 hr prn.
- Give with food or milk if GI upset occurs.
- Use dosing spoon or syringe for pediatric doses.
- Store syrup at controlled room temperature (59° to 77°F). Keep tightly capped and protect from light.

Assessment/Interventions

- Obtain patient history, including drug history and any known allergies. Note history of liver disease, kidney disease, acute abdominal conditions, peptic ulcer disease, diabetes, peripheral vascular disease, hypertension, seizures, hyperthyroidism, enlarged prostate, asthma, narrow angle glaucoma, urinary retention, coronary artery disease, head injury, increased intracranial pressure, concurrent use of tricyclic antidepressants, or concurrent use of or within 2 wk of stopping MAO inhibitor therapy.
- Assess for allergy or cold symptoms (eg, cough, rhinitis, nasal congestion, sneezing, itching, watery eyes) before and periodically throughout therapy.
- Monitor pulse and BP periodically during therapy.
- Monitor patient for GI, CNS, CV, and general body side effects. Inform health care provider if noted and significant.

Patient/Family Education
- Explain name, dose, action, and potential side effects of drug.
- Advise patient to take prescribed dose q 4 to 6 hr prn.
- Advise caregiver to use dosing spoon or syringe when giving suspension to children.
- Advise patient to take with food or milk if GI upset occurs.
- Advise patient that if a dose is missed to take as soon as remembered unless it is nearing time for the next dose. Caution patient not to double the dose to catch up.
- Advise patient that if allergy symptoms are not controlled, to not increase the dose of medication but to inform the health care provider.
- Caution patient that drug may cause drowsiness and to use caution while driving or performing other tasks requiring mental alertness until tolerance is determined.
- Advise patient to avoid alcohol and other CNS depressants because of risk of excessive sedation.
- Caution patient not to take any OTC antihistamines or decongestants while taking this medication unless advised by health care provider.
- If patient is to have allergy skin testing, advise against taking the medication for at least 6 days before the skin testing.
- Advise women to notify health care provider if pregnant, planning to become pregnant, or breastfeeding.
- Instruct patient to stop taking drug and immediately report any of the following symptoms to health care provider: abnormal muscle movements, unusual sensitivity to sunlight, nervousness, dizziness, excessive drowsiness.
- Caution patient not to take any prescription or OTC medications or dietary supplements unless advised by health care provider.

Propafenone

(proe-pa-FEEN-one)

Class Antiarrhythmic

How Supplied
Rythmol Tablets, immediate release 150 mg, Tablets, immediate release 225 mg, Tablets, immediate release 300 mg, Capsule, extended release 225 mg, Capsule, extended release 325 mg, Capsule, extended release 425 mg

Action
PHARMACOLOGY: Reduces fast inward current carried by sodium ion in the Purkinje fibers, and to a lesser extent myocardial fibers.

PHARMACOKINETICS/DYNAMICS:

Absorption: Nearly completely absorbed. T_{max} is approximately 3.5 hr for immediate release (IR) and approximately 3 to 8 hours for extended release (ER). Bioavailability is dose- and dosage-form dependent and is 3.4% (150 mg), 10.6% (300 mg), and 21.4% (300 mg solution). Steady state is 4 to 5 days. Food increased peak blood levels and bioavailability in single dose study; however, multiple doses did not change bioavailability significantly.

Distribution: Protein binding is greater than 95%. Propafenone and 5-hydroxypropafenone are distributed into breast milk. Total Vd is about 252 L.

Metabolism: Exhibits extensive first-pass metabolism in the liver producing 2 main active metabolites: 5-hydroxypropafenone and n-depropylpropafenone, which have antiarrhythmic activity comparable with propafenone, but present in concentrations less than 20%. Two genetically metabolism groups exist: fast and slow metabolizers; 90% are fast and 10% are slow metabolizers.

Excretion: Renal (38% as metabolites, less than 1% as unchanged); fecal (53% as metabolites). The t½ is 2 to 10 hr (rapid metabolizers); 10 to 32 hr (slower metabolizers).

Special Populations:
Hepatic Function Impairment – Cl is reduced and elimination t½ is increased.

Indications
IR: Prolong time to recurrence of paroxysmal atrial fibrillation/flutter or paroxysmal supraventricular tachycardia associated with disabling symptoms in patients without structural heart disease; treatment of ventricular arrhythmias (eg, sustained ventricular tachycardia [VT]) that are life-threatening.

ER: Prolong the time to recurrence of symptomatic atrial fibrillation in patients with structural heart disease.

Contraindications
Uncontrolled CHF; cardiogenic shock; sinoatrial, AV and intraventricular disorders of impulse generation and/or conduction (eg, sick sinus node syndrome, AV block) in the absence of an artificial pacemaker; bradycardia; marked hypotension; bronchospastic disorders; manifest electrolyte imbalance; known hypersensitivity to the drug.

Route/Dosage
Individually titrate dose based on response and tolerance.

ADULTS: **PO (IR)** 150 mg q 8 hr initially, increasing at a minimum of 3- to 4-day intervals to 225 mg q 8 hr and, if necessary, to 300 mg q 8 hr.

ADULTS: **PO (ER)** 225 mg q 12 hr initially, increasing at a minimum of 5-day intervals to 325 mg q 12 hr (max, 425 mg q 12 hr).

Interactions

Cimetidine, certain serotonin reuptake inhibitors (eg, fluoxetine, paroxetine, sertraline), quinidine, ritonavir: May increase propafenone plasma concentrations, potentially increasing pharmacologic and adverse effects.

Cyclosporine, desipramine, digoxin, metoprolol, propranolol, theophylline, venlafaxine, warfarin: Propafenone may increase plasma concentrations of these agents, increasing the risk of side effects and toxicity.

Drugs that prolong the QT interval (eg, cisapride, bepridil, tricyclic antidepressants), antiarrhythmic agents (class Ia and III antiarrhythmic agents [eg, amiodarone, quinidine]): Coadministration with propafenone is not recommended because of the increased risk of life-threatening cardiac arrhythmias.

Local anesthetics: May increase the risk of CNS side effects.

Mexiletine: Mexiletine metabolism may be inhibited, elevating plasma levels in extensive metabolizers and increasing the risk of side effects.

Rifamycins (eg, rifabutin, rifapentine): May decrease propafenone plasma concentrations, decreasing the therapeutic effect.

Lab Test Interferences None well documented.

Adverse Reactions

CV: Angina, proarrhythmia (5%); CHF (4%); first-degree AV block, palpitation, VT (3%); PVCs, increased QRS duration, syncope, bradycardia, chest pain, weakness (2%); bundle branch block, atrial fibrillation, hypotension, intraventricular conduction delay (1%); atrial flutter, AV dissociation, cardiac arrest, sick sinus syndrome, sinus pause or arrest, supraventricular tachycardia, prolongation of PR and QRS intervals (less than 1%).
CNS: Dizziness (13%); fatigue (6%); headache (5%); insomnia, anorexia, anxiety, ataxia (2%); drowsiness, tremor (1%).
DERM: Rash (3%).

PATIENT CARE CONSIDERATIONS
Administration/Storage

- May be used alone or in combination with other antiarrhythmic medications.
- Store IR tablets and ER capsules at controlled room temperature (59° to 86°F).

IR tablet:
- Administer IR tablets q 8 hr as prescribed.

EENT: Blurred vision (4%).
GI: Nausea and vomiting (11%); unusual taste (9%); constipation (7%); diarrhea, dyspepsia (3%); dry mouth, abdominal pain, cramps (2%); flatulence (1%).
HEMA/LYMPH: Agranulocytosis, anemia, bruising, granulocytopenia, leukopenia, thrombocytopenia.
MUSC: Joint pain (1%).
OTHER: Dyspnea (5%); edema, diaphoresis (1%).

> **WARNING:**
> Mortality risks noted for flecainide and/or encainide (type 1C antiarrhythmics). Reserved for use in patients with life-threatening ventricular arrhythmias.

Precautions

Pregnancy: Category C.
Lactation: Excreted in breast milk.
Children: Safety and efficacy not established.
Elderly: Because of the increased risk of impaired renal and hepatic function, use with caution.
Renal function impairment: Use with caution.
Hepatic function impairment: Use with caution.
Antinuclear antibody (ANA) titers: Positive ANA titers may occur.
CV effects: Has proarrhythmic effect; evaluate patients electrocardiographically and clinically prior to and during therapy to determine if response supports continued use.
CHF: Because propafenone exerts beta-blockade and a negative inotropic effect, fully compensate patients before giving propafenone.
Conduction disturbances: Dose-related first degree AV block, average PR interval prolongation, and increases in QRS duration may occur.
Nonallergic bronchospasm: Avoid propafenone administration.
Pacemaker threshold: Pacing and sensing thresholds of artificial pacemakers may be altered.

Overdosage: Signs and Symptoms

Hypotension, somnolence, bradycardia, intra-atrial and intraventricular conduction disturbances, convulsions, high-grade ventricular arrhythmias.

- Administer without regard to meals but administer with food if GI upset occurs.
- Do not increase dose more often than q 3 days during dosage titration as optimal effect may not be achieved during the first 3 days following initiation of therapy or dose change.

ER capsule:
- Administer ER capsules q 12 hr as prescribed. Caution patient to swallow capsule whole and not chew, crush, or open the capsule.
- Administer without regard to meals but administer with food if GI upset occurs.
- Do not increase dose more often than q 5 days during dosage titration as optimal effect may not be achieved during the first 5 days following initiation of therapy or dose change.

Assessment/Interventions
- Obtain patient history, including drug history and any known allergies. Note renal or hepatic impairment, myasthenia gravis, heart failure or myocardial dysfunction, sick sinus syndrome, concurrent therapy with drugs known to prolong QT interval, concurrent therapy with class Ia or class III antiarrhythmic agent, or concurrent therapy with drugs known to inhibit CYP2D6, CYP1A2, or CYP3A4.
- Review patient's health history and current situation for any of the following conditions that would contraindicate propafenone therapy: hypersensitivity to propafenone; uncontrolled CHF; bradycardia; marked hypotension; bronchospastic disorder; electrolyte imbalance; cardiogenic shock; sinoatrial, AV or intraventricular disorder of impulse generation or conduction (eg, sick sinus syndrome, AV block) unless pacemaker is present.
- Ensure class Ia or III antiarrhythmic has been withheld for at least 5 half-lives before initiating therapy with propafenone.
- Ensure renal function (BUN, Scr) and liver enzymes are evaluated before initiating therapy and periodically thereafter during long-term treatment.
- Ensure CBC with differential is evaluated before starting therapy and periodically thereafter during prolonged treatment. Notify health care provider if decrease in granulocytes and/or platelets is noted.
- Review baseline ECG. Monitor cardiac rhythm while initiating therapy or when adjusting dose. Notify health care provider immediately of increase in ventricular rate, new or worsening premature ventricular contractions, VT, or ventricular fibrillation. Be prepared to treat appropriately.
- Measure PR, QRS, and QT intervals before initiating therapy and closely thereafter while adjusting dose. Notify health care provider immediately of significant prolongation. Be prepared to reduce dose if significant widening of QRS complex or second- or third-degree AV block develops.
- Ensure preexisting electrolyte disorders have been corrected before initiating therapy.
- Ensure pacing threshold is determined before starting therapy, and periodically thereafter, in patient with pacemaker.
- Ensure reduced initial dose and slower dose titration are used in elderly patient or patient with hepatic impairment.
- Monitor and record BP and pulse frequently during treatment. Notify health care provider of any significant changes.
- Monitor patient with heart failure or myocardial dysfunction for evidence of worsening heart failure (eg, new or worsening shortness of breath, peripheral edema, rapid weight gain). Inform health care provider if noted or suspected.
- Monitor patient for CV, GI, CNS, and general body side effects. Inform health care provider if noted and significant. Immediately report bleeding, unusual bruising, fever, chills, sore throat, or any other sign or symptom of possible infection.
- Monitor patient for signs or symptoms of propafenone toxicity (eg, hypotension, drowsiness, bradycardia). Immediately report to health care provider if noted or suspected.

Patient/Family Education
- Explain name, dose, action, and potential side effects of drug.
- Advise patient that dose of medication will be changed periodically to obtain max benefit.
- Caution patient taking ER capsules to take prescribed dose q 12 hr exactly as ordered.
- Caution patient taking IR tablets to take prescribed dose q 8 hr exactly as ordered.
- Caution patient that serious heart disturbances can result from missing doses.
- Advise patient to take each dose without regard to meals but to take with food if stomach upset occurs.
- Caution patient not to change the dose or stop taking unless advised by health care provider. Advise patient that serious side effects can result from increasing or decreasing the dose without medical supervision.
- Advise patient that if a dose is missed to skip that dose and take the next dose at the regularly scheduled time. Caution patient not to double the dose to catch up.
- Inform patient that drug controls, but does not cure, abnormal heart rhythm and to continue taking as prescribed once the heart rhythm has been controlled.

- Instruct patient to continue taking other heart medications as prescribed by health care provider.
- Instruct patient in BP and pulse measurement skills.
- Advise patient to monitor and record BP and pulse at home and to inform health care provider if abnormal measurements are noted. Also advise patient to take record of BP and pulse to each follow-up visit.
- Advise patient with heart failure or those taking other medications with negative inotropic effect to monitor and record weight on a daily basis and to inform health care provider if unexplained or rapid weight gain is noted.
- Instruct patient to lie or sit down if they experience dizziness or lightheadedness when standing.
- Advise patient to notify health care provider if any of the following occur: frequent episodes of dizziness or lightheadedness, persistent fatigue, persistent headache, constipation, vision changes, any other unusual or unexplained symptom or sign.
- Instruct patient to immediately report the following to health care provider: fainting, pounding in chest, new or worsening shortness of breath, change in pulse or heart rhythm, swelling in feet or ankles, any symptom affecting electrolyte balance (eg, excessive or prolonged diarrhea, excessive sweating, vomiting), any sign or symptom of infection (eg, fever, sore throat, chills), bleeding, or unusual bruising.
- Caution patient that drug may cause dizziness or drowsiness and to use caution while driving or performing other tasks requiring mental alertness or coordination until tolerance is determined.
- Advise patient to carry medical identification (eg, *Medi-Alert*) describing cardiac condition and medication regimen.
- Advise women to notify health care provider if pregnant, planning to become pregnant, or breastfeeding.
- Caution patient not to take any prescription, herbal preparations, or OTC medications or dietary supplements unless advised by health care provider.
- Offer family instruction in basic life support.
- Advise patient that follow-up visits and lab tests will be required to monitor therapy and to keep appointments.

Propranolol Hydrochloride/Hydrochlorothiazide (HCTZ)

(pro-PRAN-oh-lahl HIGH-droe-KLOR-ide/high-droe-klor-THIGH-uh-zide)

Class Antihypertensive combination

How Supplied
Inderide Tablets 40 mg propranolol/25 mg HCTZ, Tablets 80 mg propranolol/25 mg HCTZ

Action
PHARMACOLOGY:

Propranolol: Blocks beta receptors, primarily affecting the cardiovascular system (decreases heart rate, cardiac contractility, and BP) and lungs (promotes bronchospasm).

HCTZ: Increases chloride, sodium, and water excretion by interfering with transport of sodium ions across renal tubular epithelium.

Indications Management of hypertension.

Contraindications Cardiogenic shock; sinus bradycardia and greater than first-degree block; bronchial asthma; CHF (unless failure is secondary to a tachy-arrhythmia treatable with propranolol); anuria; hypersensitivity to sulfonamide-derived drugs or any component of this product.

Route/Dosage
The fixed combination is not indicated for initial therapy. The combination may be substituted for the titrated components.

ADULTS: PO HCTZ can be given at 12.5 to 50 mg/day when used alone. The initial propranolol dose is 80 mg/day and may be increased gradually until optimal BP control is achieved. The usual effective dose when used alone is 160 to 480 mg/day. One *Inderide* tablet bid can be used to administer up to 160 mg propranolol and 50 mg HCTZ. For propranolol doses greater than 160 mg, the combination products are inappropriate because their use would lead to excessive doses of HCTZ.

Interactions
Propranolol:

Aluminum hydroxide – May decrease intestinal absorption of propranolol.

Antipyrine, lidocaine – May reduce the clearance of propranolol.

Calcium-channel blocking agent (eg, verapamil) – May have additive of synergistic effects with propranolol, depressing myocardial contractility or atrioventricular conduction.

Catecholamine-depleting drugs (eg, reserpine) – May produce excessive reduction of resting sym-

pathetic nervous activity, which may result in hypotension, marked bradycardia, vertigo, syncopal attacks, or orthostatic hypotension.
Chlorpromazine – Increased plasma concentrations of both chlorpromazine and propranolol.
Cimetidine – May decrease the metabolism of propranolol, delaying elimination and increasing the blood level.
Ethanol – May slow the rate of propranolol absorption.
Haloperidol – Hypotension and cardiac arrest have been reported with concurrent use of propranolol.
Phenobarbital, phenytoin, rifampin – May increase the rate of propranolol elimination.
Theophylline – Plasma levels may be increased by propranolol; in addition, propranolol may antagonize the effect of theophylline.
Thyroxine – May result in lower T_3 concentrations when used concomitantly with propranolol.
HCTZ:
Alcohol, barbiturates, narcotics – Increased risk of orthostatic hypotension.
Antidiabetic agents (oral agents and insulin) – Dosage adjustment of antidiabetic agent may be necessary.
Antihypertensive agent – Additive or potentiation of effects.
Cholestyramine, colestipol resins – Impaired absorption of HCTZ.
Corticosteroids, ACTH – Increased electrolyte depletion, increasing the risk of hypokalemia.
Lithium – Renal clearance of lithium may be reduced, increasing the risk of lithium toxicity.
Nondepolarizing skeletal muscle relaxants (eg, tubocurarine) – Increased effect of the muscle relaxant.
Nonsteroidal anti-inflammatory agents – The diuretic, natriuretic, and antihypertensive effects of loop, potassium-sparing, and thiazide diuretics may be reduced.
Pressor amines (eg, norepinephrine) – Decreased responsiveness to the pressor amine.

Lab Test Interferences May decrease serum protein-bound iodine levels without signs of thyroid disturbances. May cause diagnostic interference of serum electrolyte levels, blood and urine glucose levels, serum bilirubin levels, and serum uric acid levels.

Adverse Reactions
CV:
HCTZ – Orthostatic hypotension.
Propranolol – CHF, hypotension, intensification of AV block, bradycardia, thrombocytopenia purpura, arterial insufficiency (usually of the Raynaud type), paresthesia of hands.
CNS:
HCTZ – Dizziness, vertigo, headache, xanthopsia, paresthesias, weakness, restlessness.
Propranolol – Mental depression (progressing to catatonia); mental depression (manifested by insomnia, lassitude, weakness, fatigue); acute syndrome characterized by disorientation for time and place, short-term memory loss, emotional lability, slightly clouded sensorium, decreased performance on neuropsychometrics; hallucinations; vivid dreams; lightheadedness; fatigue; lethargy.
DERM:
Propranolol – Alopecia, psoriaform rashes, oculomucocutaneous reactions (involving the skin, serous membranes, and conjunctivae).
EENT:
HCTZ – Blurred vision.
Propranolol – Visual disturbances, dry eyes.
GI:
HCTZ – Pancreatitis, sialadenitis, anorexia, nausea, vomiting, gastric irritation, cramping, diarrhea, constipation.
Propranolol – Mesenteric arterial thrombosis; ischemic colitis; nausea; vomiting; epigastric distress; abdominal cramping; diarrhea; constipation.
GU:
Propranolol – Impotence.
HEMA:
HCTZ – Aplastic anemia, agranulocytosis, leukopenia, thrombocytopenia.
Propranolol – Agranulocytosis, nonthrombocytopenic purpura, thrombocytopenic purpura.
HEPA:
HCTZ – Jaundice (intrahepatic cholestatic).
METAB:
HCTZ – Hypokalemia, hyperuricemia, hyponatremia, hyperglycemia, glucosuria.
RESP:
Propranolol – Bronchospasm.
OTHER:
HCTZ – Hypersensitivity (including anaphylactic reactions, necrotizing angiitis, respiratory distress, fever, urticaria, rash, purpura, photosensitivity); muscle spasm.
Propranolol – Allergic reaction (including laryngospasm, respiratory distress, pharyngitis, agranulocytosis, fever, aching and sore throat, erythematous rash); systemic lupus erythematosus; Peyronie disease.

Precautions
Pregnancy: Category C.
Lactation: Propranolol and HCTZ secreted in breast milk.
Children: Safety and efficacy not established.

Elderly: Select dose with caution, reflecting greater frequency of decreased hepatic, renal, or cardiac function and comorbidity.

Renal function impairment: Use with caution; minor alterations of fluid and electrolyte balance may precipitate hepatic coma (HCTZ).

Hepatic function impairment: Use with caution; minor alterations of fluid and electrolyte balance may precipitate hepatic coma (HCTZ).

Anesthesia and major surgery: Withdrawing beta blockers prior to major surgery is controversial; beta blockade impairs the heart's ability to respond to beta-adrenergically mediated reflex stimuli.

Angina pectoris: Exacerbation of angina and MI may occur following abrupt discontinuation of propranolol; therefore, discontinue propranolol by gradually reducing the dosage and carefully monitoring the patient.

Cardiac failure: Increased risk of further depressing myocardial contractility and precipitating cardiac failure. In patients receiving digitalis, propranolol may reduce the positive inotropic action of digitalis.

Diabetes and hypoglycemia: Propranolol may prevent the appearance of certain premonitory signs and symptoms (eg, pulse rate and BP changes) of acute hypoglycemia.

Electrolyte imbalance: Do not use in patients with hyponatremia, hypochloremic alkalosis, hypokalemia, or hypomagnesemia prior to correction of imbalance.

Hyperucemia: May occur or frank gout may be precipitated by thiazide therapy.

Nonallergic bronchospasm (eg, chronic bronchitis, emphysema): Use beta blockers with caution because it may block bronchodialation produced by endogenous and exogenous catecholamine stimulation of beta receptors.

Systemic lupus erythematosus (HCTZ): Exacerbation or activation may occur.

Thyrotoxicosis: Propranolol may mask certain clinical signs of hyperthyroidism (eg, tachycardia).

Wolff-Parkinson-White syndrome: In several reported cases, tachycardia was replaced by severe bradycardia requiring a demand pacemaker.

Overdosage: Signs and Symptoms

Bradycardia, cardiac failure, hypotension, bronchospasm, diuresis, lethargy, coma, depression of respiration and cardiac function, CNS depression, GI irritation and hypermotility, temporary elevated BUN.

PATIENT CARE CONSIDERATIONS

Administration/Storage

- Administer prescribed dose bid with or without food.
- Administer last dose late in the afternoon to reduce nighttime urination.
- Administer alone or in combination with other antihypertensives.
- Store tablets at controlled room temperature (less than 77°F).
- Keep container tightly closed. Protect from moisture, freezing, and excessive heat.

Assessment/Interventions

- Obtain patient history, including drug history and any known allergies. Note history of CHF, coronary artery disease, COPD, asthma, diabetes, hyperthyroidism, Wolff-Parkinson-White Syndrome, anuria, lupus erythematosus, kidney or liver disease, gout, or allergy to any sulfonamide-derived medications.
- Ensure that serum electrolytes and renal function are monitored periodically.
- Monitor and record BP and pulse. If bradycardia or hypotension occur, hold medication and notify health care provider.
- Take safety precautions if orthostatic hypotension occurs.
- Monitor blood sugar in diabetic patient when drug is started or dose is changed. Report significant changes to health care provider.

Patient/Family Education

- Explain name, dose, action, and potential side effects of drug.
- Advise patient to take prescribed dose bid, without regard to meals, but to take with food if GI upset occurs.
- Advise patient to take last dose late in the afternoon to reduce chances of nighttime urination.
- Advise patient to try to take each dose at about the same time each day.
- Inform patient that drug controls, but does not cure, hypertension and to continue taking drug as prescribed even when BP is not elevated.
- Caution patient not to change the dose or stop taking unless advised by health care provider.
- Advise patient that if medication needs to be discontinued that the dose will be slowly reduced and then stopped.
- Instruct patient to continue taking other BP medications as prescribed by health care provider.

- Instruct patient in BP and pulse measurement skills.
- Advise patient to monitor and record BP and pulse at home and to inform health care provider if abnormal measurements are noted. Also, advise patient to take record of BP and pulse to each follow-up visit.
- Instruct patient to lie or sit down if experiencing dizziness or lightheadedness when standing.
- Caution patient that inadequate fluid intake, excessive perspiration, diarrhea, or vomiting can lead to excessive fall in BP resulting in lightheadedness or fainting.
- Instruct patient to notify health provider immediately if any of the following occur: dryness of mouth, thirst, weakness, lethargy, unexplained drowsiness or restlessness, persistent muscle pain or cramps, persistent nausea or vomiting, decreased urine production, rapid or slow heartbeat, depressed feeling.
- Instruct diabetic patient to monitor blood glucose more frequently when drug is started or dose is changed and to inform health care provider of significant changes in readings.
- Caution patient to avoid unnecessary exposure to UV light (sunlight, tanning booths) and to use sunscreen and wear protective clothing when exposed to UV light to avoid photosensitivity reaction.
- Emphasize to hypertensive patient importance of other modalities on BP: weight control, regular exercise, smoking cessation, and moderate intake of alcohol and salt.
- Advise women to notify health care provider if pregnant, planning to become pregnant, or breastfeeding.
- Caution patient not to take any prescription or OTC medications or dietary supplements unless advised by health care provider.
- Advise patient that follow-up visits and lab tests may be required to monitor therapy and to keep appointments.
- Instruct patient that beta blockers can cause reduction of IOP and may interfere with glaucoma screening test.

Propantheline Bromide

(pro-PAN-thuh-leen BROE-mide)
Class Anticholinergic/Antispasmodic
How Supplied
Pro-Banthine Tablets 7.5 mg, Tablets 15 mg
✤ *Propanthel*

Action
PHARMACOLOGY: Exerts anticholinergic effects, resulting in GI smooth muscle relaxation and diminished volume and acidity of GI secretions.

PHARMACOKINETICS/DYNAMICS:
Absorption: Poor GI absorption, only 10% to 25% of oral dose is absorbed. T_{max} is approximately 1 hr.
Distribution: Not fully determined.
Metabolism: Extensively metabolized by hydrolysis to inactive metabolites.
Excretion: Renal (70%, mostly as metabolites and 3% as propantheline). Half-life is 1.6 hr.
Duration: 6 hr.

Indications Adjunctive therapy in treatment of peptic ulcer. **Unlabeled use(s):** Treatment of secretory and spastic disorders of GI tract, biliary tract, urinary tract, and bladder.

Contraindications Hypersensitivity to anticholinergic drugs; narrow-angle glaucoma; adhesions between iris and lens; obstructive uropathy; obstructive disease of GI tract; paralytic ileus; intestinal atony of elderly or debilitated patient; severe ulcerative colitis; toxic megacolon complicating ulcerative colitis; hepatic or renal disease; tachycardia; myocardial ischemia; unstable cardiovascular status in acute hemorrhage; myasthenia gravis.

Route/Dosage
Peptic Ulcer
ADULTS: PO 15 mg 30 min before meals and 30 mg at bedtime.

PATIENTS WITH MILD MANIFESTATIONS, ELDERLY PATIENTS OR THOSE OF SMALL STATURE: PO 7.5 mg tid.

Secretory Disorders
ADULTS: PO 1.5 mg/kg/day in 3 to 4 divided doses.

Spastic Disorders
ADULTS: PO 2 to 3 mg/kg/day in divided doses q 4 to 6 hr and at bedtime.

Interactions
Antacids: Decrease absorption of propantheline if given together.
Drugs with anticholinergic effects (eg, antihistamines, antiparkinson drugs, tricyclic antidepressants): Additive peripheral anticholinergic side effects.
Haloperidol: May cause decreased serum haloperidol levels, worsened schizophrenic symptoms and tardive dyskinesia.
Phenothiazines: May decrease antipsychotic effectiveness of phenothiazines; may produce additive anticholinergic effects.

Lab Test Interferences None well documented.

Adverse Reactions

CV: Palpitations; tachycardia.
CNS: Headache; flushing; nervousness; drowsiness; weakness; dizziness; confusion; insomnia; fever; mental confusion or excitement; restlessness; tremor.
DERM: Severe allergic reactions including anaphylaxis, urticaria and dermal manifestations.
EENT: Blurred vision; mydriasis; photophobia; cycloplegia; increased intraocular pressure; dilated pupils; nasal congestion; altered taste perception.
GI: Dry mouth; nausea; vomiting; dysphagia; heartburn; constipation; bloated feeling; paralytic ileus.
GU: Urinary hesitancy and retention; impotence.
OTHER: Suppression of lactation; decreased sweating.

Precautions

Pregnancy: Category C.
Lactation: Undetermined.
Children: Safety and efficacy not established.
Elderly: For elderly or debilitated patients, drug may cause excitement, agitation, drowsiness, and other untoward manifestations, even in small doses.

Special risk patients: Use drug with caution in patients with glaucoma, autonomic neuropathy, hepatic or renal disease, ulcerative colitis, hyperthyroidism, coronary artery disease, CHF, cardiac tachyarrhythmias, tachycardia, hypertension, prostatic hypertrophy and hiatal hernia associated with reflux esophagitis.
Diarrhea: May be symptom of incomplete intestinal obstruction, especially in patients with ileostomy or colostomy. Treatment of diarrhea with drug is inappropriate and possibly harmful.
Gastric ulcer: May delay gastric emptying rate and complicate therapy.
Heat prostration: Can occur in presence of high environmental temperature.

Overdosage: Signs and Symptoms

Dry mouth, thirst, vomiting, nausea, abdominal distention, paralytic ileus, difficulty swallowing, muscular weakness, paralysis, CNS stimulation (restlessness, anxiety), delirium (disorientation, hallucinations), drowsiness, stupor, fever, dizziness, headache, seizures, ataxia, coma, circulatory failure, rapid pulse and respiration, vasodilation, tachycardia with weak pulse, hypertension, hypotension, respiratory depression, palpitations, urinary urgency with difficulty in micturition, blurred vision, photophobia, dilated pupils, leukocytosis, flushed hot dry skin, rash.

PATIENT CARE CONSIDERATIONS

Administration/Storage

- Do not crush or allow patient to chew tablets.
- Administer antacids 1 hr before or after propantheline.
- Administer 30 min before meals and at bedtime (at least 2 hr after last meal) unless otherwise directed.
- Store at room temperature in tight container.

Assessment/Interventions

- Obtain patient history, including drug history and any known allergies.
- Check patient's vital signs.
- Monitor I&O.
- Observe for drowsiness, dizziness, urinary hesitancy or retention, blurred vision, diarrhea or constipation and other anticholinergic side effects and report to health care provider.

Patient/Family Education

- Advise patient to take drug 30 min before meals and at bedtime unless directed otherwise by health care provider.
- Instruct patient not to chew or crush tablets.
- Warn patient that drug increases risk of heat prostration and caution patient to avoid becoming overheated by exercise or high environmental temperatures.
- Instruct patient to report the following symptoms to health care provider: drowsiness, dizziness, urinary hesitancy and retention, blurred vision, diarrhea or constipation, skin rash, flushing, or eye pain.
- Tell patient to take sips of water frequently, suck on ice chips or sugarless hard candy or chew sugarless gum if dry mouth occurs.
- Advise patient that drug may cause drowsiness and to use caution while driving or performing other tasks requiring mental alertness.

Propofol

(PRO-puh-FOLE)
Class General anesthetic
How Supplied
Diprivan Injection 10 mg/mL
Action
PHARMACOLOGY: Produces sedation/hypnosis rapidly (within 40 sec) and smoothly with minimal excitation; decreases intraocular pressure and systemic vascular resistance; rarely is associated with malignant hyperthermia and histamine release; suppresses cardiac output and respiratory drive.

PHARMACOKINETICS/DYNAMICS:
Absorption: Rapidly and extensively distributed. Vd is approximately 60 L/kg (10-day infusion), highly lipophilic. Crosses blood brain barrier and placenta; distributes into breast milk. Protein binding is 95% to 99%.

Metabolism: Liver conjugation to inactive metabolites.

Excretion: 50% of dose is excreted in the kidney (metabolites). Clearance is 23 to 50 mL/kg/min. Terminal $t_{1/2}$ is 1 to 3 days (10-day infusion). $T_{1/2}$ of rapid distribution is 2 to 4 min. $T_{1/2}$ of slower distribution is 30 to 64 min.

Onset: Rapid onset, usually within 40 sec from start of injection.

Duration: 3 to 5 min (single bolus).

Special Populations:
Elderly – With increasing age, the dose requirement decreases because of occurrence of higher peak plasma concentrations.

Indications Induction and maintenance of anesthesia in adults; induction anesthesia in children at least 3 yr; maintenance anesthesia in pediatric patients at least 2 mo; initiation and maintenance of monitored anesthesia care sedation in adults; sedation in intubated or respiratory-controlled adult ICU patients.

Contraindications Situations in which general anesthesia or sedation are contraindicated.

Route/Dosage
Anesthesia
ADULTS UNDER 55 YR: **IV Induction** 40 mg q 10 sec until onset. Usual dose is 2 to 2.5 mg/kg total. For maintenance infusion, titrate to 100 to 200 mcg/kg/min (6 to 12 mg/kg/hr). For maintenance intermittent bolus, use 25 to 50 mg increments, as needed.
ELDERLY, DEBILITATED, OR ASA III/IV: (American Society of Anesthesiologists classification of heart disease, cardiac function, angina, and physical status used to assign risk for anesthesia.) **IV** 20 mg q 10 sec until onset. Usual dose is 1 to 1.5 mg/kg. For maintenance infusion, titrate to 50 to 100 mcg/kg/min (3 to 6 mg/kg/hr).
NEUROSURGICAL PATIENTS: **IV Induction** 20 mg q 10 sec until onset. Usual dose is 1 to 2 mg/kg. For maintenance infusion, use 100 to 200 mcg/kg/min (6 to 12 mg/kg/hr).
CHILDREN AT LEAST 3 YR: **IV Induction** 2.5 to 3.5 mg/kg over 20 to 30 sec. For maintenance infusion (at least 2 mo), use 200 to 300 mcg/kg/min immediately following the induction dose, then, after the first 30 min of maintenance, use infusion rates of 125 to 150 mcg/kg/min titrated to achieve the desired clinical effect, are typically needed.

Sedation
ADULTS UNDER 55 YR: **IV Initiation** 100 to 150 mcg/kg/min (6 to 9 mg/kg/hr) for 3 to 5 min (preferred method) or slow injection of 0.5 mg/kg over 3 to 5 min; follow by maintenance infusion. For maintenance, use 25 to 75 mcg/kg/min (1.5 to 4.5 mg/kg/hr) (preferred method) or incremental bolus doses of 10 to 20 mg.
ELDERLY, DEBILITATED, OR ASA III/IV: **IV Initiation** Same as adults; not as rapid bolus. For maintenance, use 20% reduction of adult dose; avoid rapid bolus doses.

ICU Sedation
ADULTS: **IV Initiation** 5 mcg/kg/min (0.3 mg/kg/hr) for at least 5 min; increments of 5 to 10 mcg/kg/min (0.2 to 0.6 mg/kg/hr) over 5 to 10 min may be used until desired level of sedation is achieved. For maintenance, use 5 to 50 mcg/kg/min (0.3 to 3 mg/kg/hr) or higher may be required; use minimum dose required for sedation.

Interactions
CNS depressants (eg, barbiturates, benzodiazepines, narcotics): Increased CNS depression.
INCOMPATIBILITIES: For IV, do not mix with other therapeutic agents prior to administration. Avoid mixing blood or plasma in same IV catheter.

Lab Test Interferences None well documented.

Adverse Reactions
CV: Myocardial ischemia; hypotension; bradycardia; decreased cardiac output; hypertension (especially in children).
CNS: Amorous behavior; movement hypotonia; hallucinations; neuropathy; opisthotonos.
DERM: Rash.

EENT: Conjunctival hyperemia; nystagmus.
METAB: Hyperlipidemia.
RESP: Apnea; cough; respiratory acidosis during weaning.
OTHER: Asthenia; burning, stinging, or pain at injection site; fever.

Precautions
Pregnancy: Category B.
Lactation: Excreted in breast milk.
Children: Safety and efficacy not established for induction anesthesia in children under 3 yr or maintenance anesthesia in children under 2 mo.
Labor and delivery: Not recommended for obstetrical anesthesia (neonatal depression).
Special risk patients: Use lower induction and maintenance doses in elderly debilitated, and ASA III/IV patients, and monitor continuously for sign of hypotension or bradycardia. Use with caution in patients with lipid metabolism disorders, because propofol is an emulsion. Epileptics may be at risk of convulsions during recovery phase. Avoid significant decreases in mean arterial pressure (and cerebral perfusion) in patients with increased intracranial pressure or impaired cerebral circulation.
Anaphylaxis: Has occurred rarely; relationship to drug has not been established.

Overdosage: Signs and Symptoms
Cardiorespiratory and cardiovascular depression.

PATIENT CARE CONSIDERATIONS

Administration/Storage
- Should be administered only by personnel who are trained in administration of general anesthesia and familiar with drug.
- Administer only in settings in which resuscitation equipment is immediately available.
- Shake well before use. Do not use if there is evidence of separation of phases of emulsion.
- Maintain strict aseptic technique in handling; rapid growth of organisms may occur if contaminated.
- Dilute with 5% Dextrose Injection, but do not dilute to concentration less than 2 mg/mL. Drug is compatible with 5% Dextrose; Lactated Ringer's Injection; Lactated Ringer's and 5% Dextrose Injection; 5% Dextrose and 0.45% Sodium Chloride Injection; 5% Dextrose and 0.2% Sodium Chloride Injection.
- Minimize pain associated with administration by infusing into larger veins.
- Discard any unused portions of drug or solution at end of anesthetic procedure; do not keep for more than 6 hr.
- In ICU sedation discard after 12 hr if administered directly from vial or after 6 hr if transferred to syringe or other container.
- Store at room temperature. Do not refrigerate. Protect from light.

Assessment/Interventions
- Obtain patient history, including drug history and any known allergies. Note epilepsy, cardiac and respiratory status, and lipid disorders.
- Monitor patient carefully; be especially alert for apnea, hypotension, or cardiovascular depression (bradycardia). Notify health care provider if these symptoms occur.
- Be prepared for possible alterations in mental status including confusion, combativeness and hallucinations and for possible neurological changes, including increases in movement, hypertonia, clonic/myoclonic movement, and bucking, jerking, or thrashing.
- Monitor for increases in serum triglycerides or serum turbidity in patients at risk of hyperlipidemia and notify health care provider.
- Observe for possible respiratory acidosis during weaning after prolonged administration.

Patient/Family Education
- Advise patient that mental alertness, coordination, and physical dexterity may be impaired for some time after administration.

Propoxyphene

(pro-POX-ee-feen)

Class Narcotic analgesic

How Supplied
Propoxyphene Hydrochloride
Darvon-N Tablets 100 mg (as napsylate) ♦
Darvon Pulvules Capsules 65 mg (as hydrochloride)

 642

Action
PHARMACOLOGY: Relieves pain by stimulating opiate receptors in CNS; also causes respiratory depression, peripheral vasodilation, inhibition of intestinal peristalsis, sphincter of Oddi spasm, stimulation of chemoreceptor that cause vomiting and increased bladder tone.

PHARMACOKINETICS/DYNAMICS:
Absorption: T_{max} is 2 to 2.5 hr. C_{max} is 0.05 to 0.1 mcg/mL.

Distribution: Distributes into breast milk.

Metabolism: Propoxyphene metabolizes in the liver to norpropoxyphene metabolite.

Excretion: Renal (less than 10% unchanged) and biliary. The $t_{1/2}$ is 6 to 12 hr (parent drug) and 30 to 36 hr (metabolite).

Onset: 30 to 60 min.
Peak: 120 min.
Duration: 4 to 6 hr.
Special Populations:
Elderly – Half-life may be increased because of decreased clearance rate.

Indications Relief of mild to moderate pain.

Contraindications Upper airway obstruction; acute asthma; diarrhea caused by poisoning or toxins.

Route/Dosage

PROPOXYPHENE HYDROCHLORIDE
ADULTS: PO 65 mg q 4 hr prn; not to exceed 390 mg/day.

PROPOXYPHENE NAPSYLATE
ADULTS: PO 100 mg q 4 hr prn; not to exceed 600 mg/day.

Interactions
Carbamazepine: Increased carbamazepine serum concentrations.
Charcoal: Charcoal decreases the GI absorption of propoxyphene.
Cigarette smoking: Decreased propoxyphene effect caused by liver enzyme induction.
CNS depressants (eg, alcohol, barbiturate anesthetics, sedatives, tranquilizers): Additive CNS depression.
Protease inhibitors: Avoid combination with propoxyphene.
Warfarin: Potentiation of hypoprothrombinemic effect.

Lab Test Interferences Increased amylase and lipase for up to 24 hr after administration.

Adverse Reactions
CV: Hypotension.
CNS: Lightheadedness; dizziness; sedation; disorientation; incoordination; paradoxical excitement; hallucinations; euphoria; dysphoria; insomnia.
DERM: Sweating; pruritus; urticaria.
GI: Nausea; vomiting; constipation; abdominal pain.
GU: Urinary retention or hesitancy.
HEPA: Jaundice; abnormal LFTs.
RESP: Depression of cough reflex.
OTHER: Tolerance; psychological and physical dependence with chronic use; weakness.

> **WARNING:**
> Not for use in patients who are suicidal or addiction prone. Do not exceed recommended dose. Propoxyphene products in excessive doses or in drug interactions with CNS depressants (including alcohol) are major causes of drug-related deaths.

Precautions
Pregnancy: Category C. Category D if used for long periods.
Lactation: Excreted in breast milk.
Children: Not recommended for children.
Elderly: The rate of propoxyphene metabolism may be reduced in some patients. Consider increased dosing interval.
Renal function impairment: Duration of action may be prolonged; may need to reduce dose.
Hepatic function impairment: Duration of action may be prolonged; may need to reduce dose.
Special risk patients: Use with caution in patients with myxedema, acute alcoholism, acute abdominal conditions, ulcerative colitis, decreased respiratory reserve, head injury or increased intracranial pressure, hypoxia, supraventricular tachycardia, depleted blood volume or circulatory shock.
Drug dependence: Has abuse potential.

Overdosage: Signs and Symptoms
CNS depression (stupor to coma), respiratory depression, hypotension, seizures, pulmonary edema, cardiac arrhythmias, respiratory-metabolic acidosis.

PATIENT CARE CONSIDERATIONS

Administration/Storage
- Administer with food if GI upset occurs.
- Be aware that 65 mg of hydrochloride form is equivalent to 100 mg of napsylate form in delivering same amount of propoxyphene.
- Store in light-resistant container at room temperature.

Assessment/Interventions
- Obtain patient history, including drug history and any known allergies. Note potential for suicide or drug dependence.
- Assess pain prior to and 30 to 60 min after administration.
- Provide safety measures (eg, accessible call bell, side rails, night light) and assist with ambulation.
- Monitor for prolonged duration of action in cases of hepatic or renal impairment and report to health care provider; dose may need to be reduced.
- Observe for respiratory depression, dizziness, sedation, nausea, vomiting, or constipation; notify health care provider if these symptoms occur.

Patient/Family Education
- Advise patient to take drug with food if GI upset occurs.
- Explain that increasing fluid and fiber intake may help decrease constipation. Use of stool softeners and laxatives may also be suggested.
- Advise patient not to wait until pain level is high to self-medicate because drug will not be as effective.
- For long-term therapy, explain that dosage will be tapered gradually to prevent withdrawal symptoms.
- Tell patient to notify health care provider if drug does not provide pain relief.
- Instruct patient to report the following symptoms to health care provider: shortness of breath or difficulty breathing, nausea, vomiting, constipation or other effects of drug.
- Caution patient to avoid sudden position changes to prevent orthostatic hypotension.
- Instruct patient to avoid intake of alcoholic beverages or other CNS depressants.
- Advise patient that drug may cause drowsiness or dizziness and to use caution while driving or performing other tasks requiring mental alertness.

Propoxyphene/Acetaminophen

(pro-POX-ee-feen/ass-cet-ah-MEE-noe-fen)

Class Narcotic analgesic combination

How Supplied

Propoxyphene Hydrochloride/Acetaminophen
Wygesic Tablets 65 mg propoxyphene hydrochloride/650 mg acetaminophen

Propoxyphene Napsylate/Acetaminophen
Darvocet-N 50 Tablets 50 mg propoxyphene napsylate/325 mg acetaminophen ◆ Darvocet A500 Tablets 100 mg propoxyphene napsylate/500 mg acetaminophen ◆ Darvocet-N 100 Tablets 100 mg propoxyphene napsylate/650 mg acetaminophen

Action

PHARMACOLOGY: Propoxyphene relieves pain by stimulating opiate receptors in CNS; causes respiratory depression; peripheral vasodilation, inhibition of intestinal peristalsis, sphincter of hepatopancreatic ampulla spasm, stimulation of receptors that cause vomiting, increased bladder tone. Acetaminophen inhibits synthesis of prostaglandins; does not have significant anti-inflammatory effects or antiplatelet effects; produces antipyresis by direct action on the hypothalamic heat-regulating center.

Indications Relief of mild to moderate pain; as analgesic-antipyretic in presence of aspirin allergy, hemostatic disturbances, bleeding diatheses, upper GI disease, and gouty arthritis.

Contraindications Standard considerations.

Route/Dosage

PROPOXYPHENE NAPSYLATE
ADULTS: PO 100 mg (with 500 or 650 mg acetaminophen) q 4 hr prn; max, 600 mg/day.

PROPOXYPHENE HYDROCHLORIDE
ADULTS: PO 65 mg (with 650 mg acetaminophen) q 4 hr; max, 390 mg/day.
ELDERLY: The rate of propoxyphene metabolism may be reduced; consider increasing dosing interval.

Interactions

Carbamazepine: Increased carbamazepine serum levels; increased risk of acetaminophen hepatotoxicity.
Charcoal: Decreased propoxyphene absorption.
Cigarette smoking: Decreased propoxyphene effect because of liver enzyme induction.
CNS depressants (alcohol, antidepressants, barbiturates, muscle relaxants, sedatives, tranquilizers): Increased CNS and respiratory depression.
Hydantoins: Increased risk of acetaminophen hepatotoxicity.
Sulfinpyrazone: Increased risk of acetaminophen hepatotoxicity.
Warfarin: Acetaminophen may potentiate the hypoprothrombinemic effect.

Lab Test Interferences Increased amylase and lipase for up to 24 hr after administration.

Adverse Reactions

CV: Hypotension.
CNS: Lightheadedness; weakness; fatigue; sedation; dizziness; disorientation; incoordination; paradoxical excitement; euphoria; dysphoria; insomnia; headache; hallucinations.
HEPA: Abnormal LFTs; reversible jaundice (including cholestatic jaundice).
GI: Nausea; vomiting; constipation; anorexia; abdominal pain; biliary spasm.
GU: Urinary retention or hesitancy.
RESP: Dyspnea; depression of cough reflex.
SPEC SENSE: Minor visual disturbances.
OTHER: Tolerance; psychological and physical dependence with long-term use; histamine release; skin rashes.

> **Warning:**
> Do not prescribe propoxyphene for patients who are suicidal or addiction-prone. Prescribe with caution for patients taking tranquilizers or antidepressant drugs and patients who use alcohol in excess.

Precautions
Pregnancy: Category C (Category D if used for prolonged periods).
Lactation: Excreted in breast milk.
Children: Safety and efficacy not established.
Renal function impairment: Use drug with caution; reduce total daily dosage; advise chronic alcoholics to limit acetaminophen intake to less than 2 g/day.
Hepatic function impairment: Use drug with caution; reduce total daily dosage; advise chronic alcoholics to limit acetaminophen intake to less than 2 g/day.
Special risk patients: Use with caution in patients with myxedema, acute alcoholism, acute abdominal conditions, ulcerative colitis, decreased respiratory reserve, head injury or increased cranial pressure, hypoxia, supraventricular tachycardia, depleted blood volume or circulatory shock.
Drug dependence: Has abuse potential.
Fatalities: Excessive doses, either alone or in combination with other CNS depressants (including alcohol), are major cause of drug-induced death.

Overdosage: Signs and Symptoms
CNS depression (stupor to coma), respiratory depression, hypotension, seizures, pulmonary edema, cardiac arrhythmias, respiratory-metabolic acidosis, Cheyne-Stokes respiration, apnea, circulatory collapse, death.

PATIENT CARE CONSIDERATIONS
Administration/Storage
- Administer prescribed dose without regard to meals but administer with food if GI upset occurs.
- Do not exceed manufacturer's recommended max daily doses.
- Store at controlled room temperature (68° to 77°F).

Assessment/Interventions
- Obtain patient history, including drug history and any known allergies. Note hepatic or renal impairment, emotional disorder, suicidal ideation, hypothyroidism, head injury, increased intracranial pressure, acute abdominal conditions, concurrent use of CNS depressant medications, concurrent use of acetaminophen or other medications containing acetaminophen, or history of excessive alcohol use, substance abuse, or addiction.
- Assess pain before starting therapy and periodically during treatment. Notify health care provider if pain control is not achieved.
- Monitor patient for CNS, GI, and general body side effects. Report to health care provider if noted and significant.

Patient/Family Education
- Explain name, dose, action, and potential side effects of drug.
- Advise patient to review patient information leaflet before using the first time and with each refill.
- Advise patient to take prescribed dose without regard to meals but to take with food if GI upset occurs.
- Advise patient using medication as needed to control pain not to wait until pain level is high to medicate because the medication may not be as effective.
- Advise patient not to change the dose or stop taking unless advised by health care provider.
- Caution patient not to exceed prescribed dose and to inform health care provider if prescribed dose does not adequately control pain.
- Instruct patient to avoid alcoholic beverages and other depressants while taking this medication.
- Advise patient that drug may impair judgment, thinking, or motor skills or cause drowsiness and to use caution while driving or performing other tasks requiring mental alertness until tolerance is determined.
- Advise women to notify health care provider if pregnant, planning to become pregnant, or breastfeeding.
- Warn patient not to take any prescription or OTC drugs or dietary supplements without consulting health care provider. Caution patient that taking acetaminophen or other medications containing acetaminophen can be dangerous.
- Advise patient that follow-up visits may be necessary to monitor therapy and to keep appointments.

Propoxyphene Hydrochloride/Aspirin/Caffeine

(pro-POX-ih-feen HIGH-droe-KLOR-ide/ ASS-pihr-in/kaff-EEN)

Class Narcotic Analgesic

How Supplied
Darvon Compound-65 Pulvules 65 mg propoxyphene hydrochloride, 389 mg aspirin, 32.4 mg caffeine

Action
PHARMACOLOGY:
Propoxyphene: Relieves pain by stimulating opiate receptors in CNS.
Aspirin: Inhibits prostaglandin synthesis, resulting in analgesia, anti-inflammatory activity and inhibition of platelet aggregation.
Caffeine: Is thought to produce constriction of cerebral blood vessels.

Indications
Relief of mild to moderate pain.

Contraindications
Patients who are suicidal or addiction-prone; hypersensitivity to any component of this product.

Route/Dosage
ADULTS: PO 65 mg propoxyphene hydrochloride, 389 mg aspirin and 32.4 mg caffeine q 4 hr as needed for pain (maximum 390 mg/day of propoxyphene hydrochloride)

Interactions
Alcohol, CNS depressants: Additive CNS-depressant effects.
Uricosuric agents (Probenecid): Effects may be inhibited by aspirin.
Warfarin: Anticoagulant effect of warfarin may be increased by aspirin.

Lab Test Interferences
None well documented.

Adverse Reactions
CNS: Dizziness; sedation; lightheadedness; headache; weakness; euphoria; dysphoria; hallucinations.
DERM: Skin rashes.
EENT: Minor visual disturbances.
GI: Nausea; vomiting; constipation; abdominal pain.
HEPA: Jaundice (including cholestatic).

Precautions
Pregnancy: Undetermined.
Lactation: Propoxyphene and aspirin secreted in breast milk.
Children: Safety and efficacy not established. Reye syndrome has been associated with aspirin administration to children (including teenagers) with acute febrile illness.
Elderly: Rate of propoxyphene metabolism may be reduced; consider increasing the dosing interval.
Special risk patients: Use with caution in patients with peptic ulcer, coagulation abnormalities, hepatic or renal impairment.
Dependence: Propoxyphene has abuse potential; may be habit forming.
Fatalities: Prescribe with caution to patients taking tranquilizers or antidepressants or who use alcohol. Excessive doses of propoxyphene, alone or in combination with other CNS depressants (including alcohol), are a major cause of drug-related deaths

Overdosage: Signs and Symptoms
Propoxyphene: Somnolence, stupor, coma, convulsions, respiratory depression, decreased respiratory rate and tidal volume, cyanosis, hypoxia, pinpoint pupils becoming dilated as hypoxia increases, Cheyne-Stokes respiration; apnea, decreased BP, decreased cardiac function, pulmonary edema, circulatory collapse, cardiac arrhythmias, conduction delay, respiratory-metabolic acidosis, lactic acid formed, death.
Aspirin: Nausea, vomiting, tinnitus, deafness, vertigo, headaches, mental dullness, confusion, diaphoresis, rapid pulse, increase respiration, respiratory alkalosis.

PATIENT CARE CONSIDERATIONS

Administration/Storage
- Be aware that the 65 mg of hydrochloride form is equivalent to 100 mg of napsylate form in delivering same amount of propoxyphene.
- Administer 1 to 2 capsules as prescribed q 4 hr if needed for pain.
- Administer without regard to meals but administer with food if GI upset occurs.
- Do not exceed 6 capsules in 24 hr.
- Store at controlled room temperature (59° to 86°F).

Assessment/Interventions
- Obtain patient history, including drug history and any known allergies. Note history of addiction, suicidal behavior, alcohol abuse, bleeding or coagulation disorders, hepatic or renal impairment, peptic ulcer or other serious GI lesions, syndrome of nasal polyps, rhinitis and bronchospastic reactivity to aspirin or other NSAIDs, or concurrent use of tranquilizers or antidepressants.
- Assess pain before starting therapy and periodically during treatment.

- Monitor patient for RESP, CNS, GI, and general body side effects. Report to health care provider if noted and significant.
- Provide safety measures (eg, accessible call bell, side rails, night light) and assist with ambulation if patient experiences dizziness or excessive sedation.
- Discontinue therapy and notify health care provider immediately if any of the following occur: allergic reaction, unusual bleeding or bruising, shortness of breath, black or tarry stools, vomiting of blood or coffee ground-like material.

Patient/Family Education
- Explain name, dose, action, and potential side effects of drug.
- Advise patient to take 1 to 2 capsules as prescribed q 4 hr if needed for pain but to not take more than 6 capsules in 24 hr.
- Advise patient to take without regard to meals but to take with food if GI upset occurs.
- Advise patient not to wait until pain level is high to self-medicate because drug may not be as effective.
- Instruct patient that if a dose is missed to take as soon as remembered unless it is nearing time for the next dose, which should be taken as scheduled. Caution patient to not double the dose to catch up.
- Instruct patient to avoid alcoholic beverages and other depressants while taking this medication.
- Advise patient that drug may impair judgment, thinking, or motor skills or cause drowsiness and to use caution while driving or performing other tasks requiring mental alertness until tolerance is determined
- Advise patient to stop taking the drug and notify their health care provider if any of the following occur: allergic reaction, unusual bleeding or bruising, shortness of breath, black or tarry stools, vomiting of blood or coffee ground-like material, excessive sedation, persistent nausea or vomiting, or bothersome constipation.
- Advise women to notify health care provider if pregnant, planning to become pregnant, or breastfeeding.
- Warn patient not to take any prescription or OTC drugs or dietary supplements without consulting their health care provider.
- Advise patient that follow-up visits may be necessary to monitor therapy and to keep appointments.

Propranolol Hydrochloride

(pro-PRAN-oh-lahl HIGH-droe-KLOR-ide)

Class Beta-adrenergic blocker

How Supplied
Inderal Tablets 10 mg, Tablets 20 mg, Tablets 40 mg, Tablets 60 mg, Tablets 80 mg, Injection 1 mg/mL ◆ *Inderal LA* Capsules, sustained-release 60 mg, Capsules, sustained-release 80 mg, Capsules, sustained-release 120 mg, Capsules, sustained-release 160 mg ◆ *InnoPran XL* Capsules, extended-release 80 mg ◆ *Propranolol Intensol* Solution, concentrated oral 80 mg/mL
🍁 *APO-Propranolol* ◆ *Detensol* ◆ *Nu-Propranolol*

Action

PHARMACOLOGY: Blocks beta receptors, primarily affecting the CV system (decreased heart rate, decreased cardiac contractility, decreased BP) and lungs (promotes bronchospasm).

PHARMACOKINETICS/DYNAMICS:

Absorption: Well-absorbed from the GI tract. Extent of absorption is less than 90%. Bioavailability is 30% (immediate release) and 9% to 18% (long acting). Food enhances bioavailability. T_{max} is 1 to 1.5 hr (immediate release) and 6 hr (long acting).

Distribution: Protein binding is 90%. Readily enters the CNS. Crosses the placenta.

Metabolism: Significant first-pass hepatic metabolism.

Excretion: Urine is less than 1% excreted unchanged. Plasma t½ is 3 to 5 hr (immediate release) and 8 to 11 hr (long acting).

Indications Angina pectoris (except *InnoPran XL*); cardiac arrhythmias (except sustained release); essential tremor (except sustained release); hypertension; hypertrophic subaortic stenosis (except *InnoPran XL*); migraine prophylaxis (except *InnoPran XL*); MI (except sustained release); pheochromocytoma (except sustained release).

Contraindications Hypersensitivity to beta-blockers; greater than first-degree heart block; CHF unless secondary to tachyarrhythmia or untreated hypertension treatable with beta-blockers; overt cardiac failure; sinus bradycardia; cardiogenic shock; untreated bronchial asthma or bronchospasm, including severe COPD.

Route/Dosage

Angina
ADULTS: PO 80 to 320 mg/day in 2 to 4 divided doses or 80 mg/day of sustained-release medication (max, 320 mg/day).

Arrhythmias
ADULTS: PO 10 to 30 mg tid to qid before meals and at bedtime.

Arrhythmias (Life-Threatening)
ADULTS: **IV** 1 to 3 mg at rate of 1 mg/min; may repeat after 2 min; give subsequent doses q 4 hr.

Essential Tremor
ADULTS: **PO** 40 mg bid initially; titrate to response. The maintenance dose is 120 to 320 mg/day in 2 to 3 divided doses (max, 320 mg/day).

Hypertension
ADULTS: **PO** The initial dose is 40 mg bid initially or 80 mg sustained-release medication/day; titrate to response. The usual maintenance dose is 120 to 240 mg/day in 2 to 3 divided doses or 120 to 160 mg/day sustained-release medication, except for *InnoPran XL* (do not exceed 120 mg/day). Do not exceed 640 mg/day.
CHILDREN: **PO** 0.5 mg/kg bid; titrate q 3 to 5 days to max dose of 16 mg/kg/day.

Hypertrophic Aortic Stenosis
ADULTS: **PO** 20 to 40 mg tid to qid before meals and at bedtime or 80 to 160 mg sustained-release medication once daily.

Migraine
ADULTS: **PO** 80 mg in divided doses daily or once daily (sustained release); titrate to response (max dose, 240 mg/day); discontinue after 6 wk if no response.

MI
ADULTS: **PO** 180 to 240 mg/day in 3 to 4 divided doses up to 240 mg/day.

Pheochromocytoma
ADULTS: **PO** 60 mg/day for 3 days prior to surgery, given with alpha-blocker.

Interactions

ACE inhibitors (eg, captopril): Increased risk of hypotension, especially in patients with acute MI; bronchial hyper-reactivity may be increased.
Aluminum hydroxide gel: Greatly reduces GI absorption of propranolol.
Amiodarone: Has additive antiarrhythmic and negative chronotropic properties with propranolol.
Anesthetic agents (eg, methoxyflurane, trichloroethylene): Depression in myocardial contractility may occur.
Barbiturates: Decreased bioavailability of propranolol.
Cimetidine: Increased propranolol levels.
Clonidine: Attenuation or reversal of antihypertensive effect; potentially life-threatening increases in BP, especially on withdrawal.
Disopyramide: Has been associated with severe bradycardia, asystole, and heart failure, when given with propranolol.
Dobutamine, isoproterenol: May reverse effects of propranolol.
Epinephrine: Initial hypertensive episode followed by bradycardia.
Ergot derivatives: Peripheral ischemia, manifested by cold extremities and possible gangrene.
Ethanol: Slows rate of propranolol absorption.
Hydantoins, rifabutin, rifampin: Decreased effects of propranolol.
Hydralazine: Increased serum levels of both drugs.
Insulin: Prolonged hypoglycemia with masking of symptoms.
Lidocaine: Increased lidocaine levels, leading to toxicity.
Methimazole, propafenone, propylthiouracil, quinidine: Increased effects of propranolol.
NSAIDs: Some agents may impair antihypertensive effect.
Phenothiazines: Increased effects of either drug.
Prazosin: Increased orthostatic hypotension.
Reserpine: Hypotension, marked bradycardia, vertigo, syncopal attacks, and orthostatic hypotension may result from excessive reduction of resting sympathetic nervous activity caused by reserpine-induced catecholamine-depletion.
Theophylline: Reduces elimination of theophylline; pharmacologic antagonism.
Thyroxin: May result in decreased T3 concentration when coadministered with propranolol.
Verapamil: Increased effects of both drugs.

Lab Test Interferences May interfere with glaucoma screening tests; may increase BUN, serum transaminases, alkaline phosphatase, or LDH.

Adverse Reactions

CV: AV block; bradycardia; CHF; edema; hypotension; peripheral ischemia; torsades de pointes; worsening angina.
CNS: Bizarre dreams; decreased performance on neuropsychometric tests; depression; dizziness; emotional lability; fatigue; hallucinations; insomnia; lethargy; short-term memory loss; sleep disturbances; slightly clouded sensorium; tiredness; weakness.
DERM: Erythema multiforme; exfoliative dermatitis; pruritus; rash; Stevens-Johnson syndrome; toxic epidermal necrolysis; urticaria.
EENT: Dry eyes; visual disturbances.
GI: Dyspepsia; nausea; vomiting; diarrhea; dry mouth; epigastric distress; abdominal cramping; constipation; mesenteric arterial thrombosis; ischemic colitis.
GU: Impotence; urinary retention; difficulty with urination.
HEMA: Agranulocytosis; nonthrombocytopenic and thrombocytopenic purpura.
HEPA: Elevated liver enzymes.
METAB: Hyperglycemia; hypoglycemia.
RESP: Wheezing; dyspnea; bronchospasm; difficulty breathing.
OTHER: Decreased exercise tolerance; hypersensitivity, including anaphylactic/anaphylactoid

reactions; increased sensitivity to cold (Raynaud phenomenon); oculomucocutaneous reactions; pharyngitis, agranulocytosis, erythematous rash, fever, laryngospasm, and respiratory distress; psoriasis-like eruptions; skin necrosis; systemic lupus erythematosus.

> **WARNING:**
>
> *Abrupt withdrawal:* In patients with angina pectoris or coronary artery disease (CAD), abrupt withdrawal may cause exacerbation of angina, occurrence of MI, and ventricular arrhythmias. Monitor patients closely. Because CAD is common and unrecognized, it may be prudent not to discontinue beta-blocker therapy abruptly in patients treated only for hypertension.

Precautions

Pregnancy: Category C.
Lactation: Excreted in breast milk.
Children: Safety and efficacy not established. IV use not recommended, but oral propranolol has been used.
Elderly: Use with caution because of the greater frequency of decreased hepatic, renal, or cardiac function, and concomitant diseases or other drug therapy.
Renal function impairment: Reduce dose.
Hepatic function impairment: Reduce dose.

Abrupt withdrawal: A beta-blocker withdrawal syndrome (eg, hypertension, tachycardia, anxiety, angina, MI) may occur 1 to 2 wk after sudden discontinuation of systemic beta-blockers. If possible, gradually withdraw therapy over 1 to 2 wk.
Anaphylaxis: Deaths have occurred; aggressive therapy may be required.
CHF: Avoid in patients with overt CHF; administer cautiously in patients whose CHF is controlled by digitalis and diuretics.
Diabetes mellitus: May mask symptoms of hypoglycemia (eg, tachycardia, BP changes). May potentiate insulin-induced hypoglycemia.
Nonallergic bronchospastic diseases: Give drug with caution in patients with bronchospastic diseases.
Peripheral vascular disease: May precipitate or aggravate symptoms of arterial insufficiency.
Thyrotoxicosis: May mask clinical signs (eg, tachycardia) of developing or continuing hyperthyroidism. Abrupt withdrawal may exacerbate symptoms of hyperthyroidism, including thyroid storm.
Wolff-Parkinson-White syndrome: In several cases, tachycardia was replaced by severe bradycardia requiring a demand pacemaker.

Overdosage: Signs and Symptoms

Bradycardia, hypotension, CHF, AV block, intraventricular conduction defects, asystole, bronchospasm, coma.

PATIENT CARE CONSIDERATIONS

Administration/Storage

- May be used alone or in combination with other CV medications for the treatment of hypertension, angina, or cardiac arrhythmias, and in combination with other medications for the treatment or prevention of migraine headaches.
- Immediate-release and extended-release dose forms may not be interchangeable on a mg to mg basis. Be prepared to retitrate dose to maintain desired therapeutic effect.
- Store extended-release capsules at controlled room temperature (59° to 86°F). Store immediate-release tablets, oral solution, concentrated oral solution, and injection at controlled room temperature (68° to 77°F). Protect from light, freezing, or excessive heat. Protect tablets and capsules from moisture.

Immediate-release tablets:

- Administer prescribed dose bid to qid as ordered.
- Administer without regard to meals but administer with food if GI upset occurs.

Extended-release capsules:

- Administer prescribed dose once daily (*InnoPran XL* should be administered at bedtime).
- Administer without regard to meals but administer with food if GI upset occurs. Administer consistently either with or without food.
- Have patient swallow capsules whole and not crush, chew, break, or open capsule.

Oral solution:

- Measure and administer prescribed dose using dosing syringe, spoon, or cup.
- Administer without regard to meals but administer with food if GI upset occurs.

Concentrated oral solution:

- Use supplied dropper to measure prescribed dose. Squeeze dropper contents into a liquid (eg, water, juice, soda, soda-like beverage) or semisolid food (eg, applesauce, pudding) and mix by gently stirring the mixture. Entire amount of mixture should be consumed immediately.

- Do not prepare mixtures ahead of time and store for future use.

Injection:
- For IV administration only. Not for intradermal, subcutaneous, IM, or intra-arterial administration.
- For treatment of life-threatening cardiac arrhythmias only.
- Do not administer if solution is discolored or cloudy, or if particulate matter is noted.
- Administer IV bolus dose at rate not exceeding 1 mg (1 mL) per minute. A second dose may be administered 2 min later if response to first dose is inadequate. Additional drug should not be given in less than 4 hr.
- Discard any unused solution. Do not save for future use.

Assessment/Interventions
- Obtain patient history, including drug history and any known allergies. Note hepatic or renal impairment, sinus bradycardia, and greater than first-degree AV block, asthma, heart failure, cardiogenic shock, coronary artery disease, COPD, asthma, diabetes, hyperthyroidism, Wolff-Parkinson-White Syndrome, or concurrent treatment with catecholamine-depleting drugs or calcium channel blocker.
- Assess response to therapy. Notify health care provider if condition is not improving or appears to be worsening.
- Ensure that therapy is periodically reviewed to determine if therapy needs to be continued without change or if a dose change (eg, increase, decrease, discontinuation) is indicated.
- Monitor and record BP and pulse. If bradycardia or hypotension occur, hold medication and notify health care provider.
- Take safety precautions if orthostatic hypotension occurs.
- If treatment is to be discontinued in patient with angina pectoris, or in patient at risk of having occult atherosclerotic heart disease, gradually taper the dose over several weeks to prevent exacerbation of angina or precipitation of MI.
- Monitor patient for CV, CNS, GI, RESP, DERM, and general body side effects. Inform health care provider if noted and significant.

Patient/Family Education
- Explain name, dose, action, and potential side effects of drug.
- Advise patient to read *Patient Information* leaflet before using the first time and to reread each time the medication is renewed.
- Advise patient or caregiver that IV propranolol will be prepared and administered by health care professionals in a medical setting and that conversion to oral therapy will be made as soon as possible.
- Advise patient using oral dose forms to take prescribed dose without regard to meals but to take with food if stomach upset occurs. Advise patient to take propranolol consistently either with or without food.
- Caution patient not to change the dose or stop taking unless advised by health care provider.
- Advise patient taking immediate-release tablets to take bid to qid as prescribed.
- Advise patient taking extended-release products to take once daily as prescribed. Caution patient to swallow extended-release products whole and not to crush, chew, break, or open the capsule.
- Advise patient or caregiver using oral solution to measure and administer prescribed dose using dosing syringe, spoon, or cup.
- Advise patient or caregiver using concentrated oral solution to use supplied dropper to measure prescribed dose then squeeze dropper contents into a liquid (eg, water, juice, soda, soda-like beverage) or semisolid food (eg, applesauce, pudding) and mix by gently stirring the mixture. Advise patient or caregiver that entire amount of mixture should be consumed immediately. Caution patient or caregiver not to prepare mixtures ahead of time and store for future use.
- Advise patient that if a dose is missed to take it as soon as remembered. However, if the next regular dose is less than 4 hr away (8 hr for extended-release capsule) to skip the missed dose and take the next dose at the regularly scheduled time. Caution patient never to double the dose to catch up.
- Inform patient or caregiver that drug controls, but not does cure, condition being treated and to continue taking as prescribed even when condition or symptoms are controlled.
- Caution patients to never stop taking propranolol on their own because sudden discontinuation could cause worsening angina pectoris or a heart attack. Advise patient that if treatment is to be discontinued it will usually be done gradually over a period of several weeks.
- Instruct patient to continue taking other medications for the condition as prescribed by health care provider.
- Instruct patient in BP and pulse measurement skills.
- Advise patient to monitor and record BP and pulse at home and to inform health care provider if abnormal measurements are noted.

Also advise patient to take record of BP and pulse to each follow-up visit.
- Caution patient with insulin-dependent diabetes that propranolol may reduce or minimize warning signs and symptoms (eg, pulse rate and BP changes) associated with a hypoglycemic reaction.
- Instruct patient to lie or sit down if experiencing dizziness or lightheadedness when standing.
- Instruct patient to notify health provider immediately if any of the following occur: weakness, lethargy, unexplained drowsiness, slow or irregular heartbeat, depressed feeling, new or worsening chest pain, swelling of feet or ankles, unexplained shortness of breath or difficulty breathing, skin rash or itching.
- Emphasize to hypertensive patient importance of other modalities on BP control: Weight control, regular exercise, smoking cessation, moderate intake of alcohol and salt.
- Advise women to notify health care provider if pregnant, planning to become pregnant, or breastfeeding.
- Caution patient not to take any prescription or OTC medications, herbal preparations, or dietary supplements unless advised by health care provider.
- Advise patient that follow-up visits and lab tests may be required to monitor therapy and to keep appointments.

Propylthiouracil (PTU)

(pro-puhl-thigh-oh-YOU-rah-sill)
Class Antithyroid

How Supplied
Available as generic only
✤ *Propyl-Thyracil*

Action
PHARMACOLOGY: Inhibits synthesis of thyroid hormones.

PHARMACOKINETICS/DYNAMICS:
Absorption: Readily absorbed from the GI tract. Bioavailability is 80% to 95%. T_{max} is 1.99 hr; C_{max} is 7.12 mcg/mL.

Distribution: Protein binding is 75% to 80%, primarily to albumin. Vd is approximately 0.4 L/kg.

Metabolism: Actively concentrated by the thyroid. Metabolized rapidly in the liver; undergoes glucuronidation.

Excretion: Urine (35%); less than 1% as unchanged. $T_{1/2}$ is 1 to 2 hr. Total body clearance is approximately 7 L/hr.

Peak: Approximately 17 wk to normalize serum T_3 and T_4 concentrations.

Indications Long-term therapy of hyperthyroidism; amelioration of hyperthyroidism in preparation for subtotal thyroidectomy or radioactive iodine therapy; when thyroidectomy is contraindicated or not advisable. **Unlabeled use(s):** Management of alcoholic liver disease.

Contraindications Hypersensitivity to antithyroid drugs; lactating women.

Route/Dosage
ADULTS: **PO** The initial dose is 300 mg/day in 3 equal doses q 8 hr. In patients with severe hyperthyroidism or very large goiters, initial dose is usually 400 mg/day, occasionally up to 600 or 900 mg/day. The maintenance dose is 100 to 150 mg/day in divided doses q 8 hr.

CHILDREN OVER 10 YR: **PO** The initial dose is 150 to 300 mg/day in divided doses q 8 hr. The maintenance dose is determined by response.

CHILDREN 6 TO 10 YR: **PO** The initial dose is 50 to 150 mg/day in divided doses q 8 hr.

ALTERNATE DOSING FOR CHILDREN: **PO** The initial dose is 5 to 7 mg/kg/day in divided doses q 8 hr. The maintenance dose is ⅓ to ⅔ initial dose, beginning when patient is euthyroid.

Interactions
Anticoagulants: Altered anticoagulant action.
Beta blockers: Increased effects of beta blockers.
Digitalis glycosides: Increased digitalis levels, resulting in toxicity.
Theophylline: Altered theophylline clearance in hyperthyroid or hypothyroid patients.

Lab Test Interferences None well documented.

Adverse Reactions
CNS: Paresthesias; neuritis; headache; vertigo; drowsiness; neuropathies; CNS stimulation; depression.
DERM: Rash; urticaria; pruritus; erythema nodosum; skin pigmentation; exfoliative dermatitis; lupus-like syndrome (splenomegaly, hepatitis, periarteritis; hypoprothrombinemia; bleeding).
EENT: Loss of taste; sialadenopathy.

GI: Nausea; vomiting; epigastric distress.
GU: Nephritis.
HEPA: Jaundice; hepatitis.
HEMA: Inhibition of myelopoiesis (eg, agranulocytosis, leukopenia, granulocytopenia, thrombocytopenia); aplastic anemia; hypoprothrombinemia; periarteritis.
OTHER: Abnormal hair loss; arthralgia; myalgia; edema; lymphadenopathy; drug fever; interstitial pneumonitis; insulin autoimmune syndrome (hypoglycemia).

Precautions
Pregnancy: Category D.
Lactation: Avoid nursing. However, if antithyroid drug is essential, PTU is preferred antithyroid agent while nursing.
Children: Hepatotoxicity has occurred in pediatric patients. Discontinue drug immediately if signs and symptoms of hepatic dysfunction develop.
Agranulocytosis: Potentially most serious side effect. Discontinue drug if agranulocytosis, aplastic anemia, hepatitis, fever, or exfoliative dermatitis occur.
Hemorrhagic effects: May cause hypoprothrombinemia and bleeding.

Overdosage: Signs and Symptoms
Nausea, vomiting, epigastric distress, headache, fever, arthralgia, pruritus, edema, pancytopenia; most serious effect: agranulocytosis.

PATIENT CARE CONSIDERATIONS
Administration/Storage
- Give with meals to minimize GI irritation.
- Administer q 8 hr to maintain serum drug levels.
- Encourage fluid intake of 3 to 4 L/day, unless contraindicated.
- Store in tight, light-resistant container at room temperature.

Assessment/Interventions
- Obtain patient history, including drug history and any known allergies.
- Obtain baseline weight, BP, body temperature and pulse rate and monitor periodically during therapy.
- Ensure that baseline thyroid function has been evaluated prior to therapy and reassess q 2 to 3 mo during therapy.
- Determine baseline WBC count and differential before administration and monitor for agranulocytosis during first 3 mo of therapy.
- Monitor I&O and check for edema.
- Before discharge, obtain dietary consult for patient regarding iodine intake; shellfish and iodine-containing foods may be restricted.
- Assess for signs of hypoprothrombinemia; monitor prothrombin time during therapy, especially during surgical procedures.
- Assess patient for development and tolerance of symptoms of hyperthyroidism or hypothyroidism.
- If symptoms of hypersensitivity occur (eg, swollen lymph nodes, skin eruption or itching), notify health care provider. Drug may be discontinued.

Patient/Family Education
- Instruct patient to take resting pulse daily and encourage patient to keep recorded chart.
- Advise patient to monitor weight at least 2 to 3 times/wk or per health care provider instruction, obtaining weight at same time, using same scale. Encourage patient to keep recorded chart.
- Emphasize importance of following dietary restrictions regarding shellfish, iodized salt and other foods high in iodine.
- Explain that desired response may take several months if the thyroid is greatly enlarged.
- Advise patient to carry *Medi-Alert* identification at all times describing medications.
- Instruct patient to notify dentist or health care provider of drug regimen before surgical or dental procedures.
- Emphasize importance of follow-up visits to monitor effectiveness of drug therapy.
- Caution patient not to stop taking medication abruptly to avoid thyroid crisis.
- Instruct patient to report the following symptoms to health care provider: Sore throat, fever, rash, mouth sores; cold intolerance, mental depression; tachycardia, irritability; persistent nausea, steatorrhea or vomiting, drowsiness, yellowing of skin or whites of eyes; unusual bleeding or bruising.
- Advise patient that drug may cause drowsiness and to use caution while driving or performing other activities requiring mental alertness.
- Instruct patient not to take *otc* medications without consulting health care provider.

Protamine Sulfate

(PRO-tuh-meen SULL-fate)

Class Heparin antagonist

How Supplied *Available as generic only*

Action

PHARMACOLOGY: Neutralizes heparin by forming heparin-protamine complex.

PHARMACOKINETICS/DYNAMICS:

Metabolism: May be partially metabolized or may be cleaved by fibrinolysin, thus freeing heparin.

Onset: Rapid, neutralization occurs within 5 min.

Duration: Duration is 2 hr, dependent on body temperature.

Indications Treatment of heparin overdose.

Contraindications Standard considerations.

Route/Dosage

ADULTS: IV 1 mg for each 90 USP units of heparin derived from lung tissue or 115 USP units of heparin derived from intestinal mucosa. Because heparin disappears rapidly from circulation, the dose of protamine required decreases rapidly with time following IV injection of heparin. For example, if protamine is administered 30 min after heparin, ½ the usual dose may be sufficient. The dose of protamine should be determined by blood coagulation studies.

Interactions None well documented.

INCOMPATIBILITIES: Protamine should not be mixed with other drugs without knowledge of their compatibility.

Lab Test Interferences None well documented.

Adverse Reactions

CV: Hypotension; bradycardia; circulatory collapse.

CNS: Lassitude.

GI: Nausea; vomiting.

RESP: Shortness of breath; pulmonary edema; acute pulmonary hypertension.

OTHER: Anaphylaxis (severe respiratory distress, circulatory collapse, capillary leak, noncardiogenic pulmonary edema); transient flushing and feeling of warmth; back pain.

Precautions

Pregnancy: Category C.

Lactation: Undetermined.

Children: Safety and efficacy not established.

Hypersensitivity: Fatal anaphylaxis may occur.

Circulatory collapse: Can occur along with myocardial failure and reduced cardiac output.

Heparin rebound: When used to neutralize large doses of heparin, protamine can be inactivated by blood; treatment consists of giving additional protamine.

Pulmonary edema: High-protein noncardiogenic pulmonary edema has occurred with use of protamine in patients on cardiopulmonary bypass undergoing cardiovascular surgery.

Too rapid administration: Can result in severe hypotension and anaphylactoid reactions.

Overdosage: Signs and Symptoms

Bleeding.

PATIENT CARE CONSIDERATIONS

Administration/Storage

- Discontinue IV heparin infusion and maintain IV route access.
- Flush IV line completely to clear previously administered medications.
- When given via direct IV injection, use 10 mg/mL concentration and administer slowly over 1 to 3 min. No more than 50 mg should be given in any 10-min period.
- Protamine sulfate injection is not intended to be further diluted. If further dilution is desired, dilute with D5W or normal saline.
- Store protamine sulfate injection in refrigerator. Do not freeze.

Assessment/Interventions

- Obtain patient history, including drug history and any known allergies, particularly hypersensitivity to drug, fish (salmon) or previous reaction to or use of isophane or protamine insulins. Note if male patient has had vasectomy or history of infertility (either can increase risk of hypersensitivity reaction).
- Assess for hypovolemia before initiating therapy, because peripheral vasodilation of protamine sulfate can result in cardiovascular collapse if hypovolemia is uncorrected.
- Have resuscitation equipment available.
- Monitor patient for urticaria, edema, rash, wheezing and coughing (hypersensitivity symptoms).
- Monitor activated clotting time, activated partial thromboplastin time, and thrombin time 5 to 15 min after therapy is begun and prn.
- Monitor vital signs frequently.
- Assess for bleeding during and after therapy (heparin rebound can precipitate hemorrhage 8 to 9 hr after therapy; after cardiopulmonary bypass, rebound can occur as late as 18 hr after therapy). Monitor for severe headache, gingival erythema or bleeding, complaint of abdominal or back pain, petechiae or bruises and excessive bleeding from cuts or venipuncture sites. Check urine and stool for visible

and occult blood. Ask female patient about increased amount of menstrual discharge.
- To prevent bleeding, avoid injections and rectal temperatures and provide gentle mouth care.

Patient/Family Education
- Instruct patient to notify health care provider immediately if any bleeding occurs.
- Tell patient to report the following symptoms to health care provider: Shortness of breath, dizziness, or swelling.
- Advise patient to avoid activities that could damage blood vessels or precipitate bleeding (eg, shaving, vigorous brushing of teeth, ambulation) until risk of hemorrhage has passed.

Protriptyline Hydrochloride
(pro-TRIP-tih-leen HIGH-droe-KLOR-ide)
Class Tricyclic antidepressant
How Supplied
Vivactil Tablets 5 mg, Tablets 10 mg
Action
PHARMACOLOGY: Inhibits reuptake of norepinephrine and serotonin in CNS.
PHARMACOKINETICS/DYNAMICS:
Absorption: Well absorbed from GI tract and rapidly sequestered into tissues. T_{max} is 8 to 12 hr. Steady state is 14 to 19 days.
Distribution: Widely distributed into tissues, including CNS. Penetrates into the brain rapidly. Small amounts are found in breast milk. Protein binding is 90%, in plasma and tissues. Vd is 22 L/kg.
Metabolism: Metabolized in the liver by demethylation of secondary amine moiety.
Excretion: In the urine (small amounts unchanged). $T_{1/2}$ is 67 to 89 hr.
Onset: 2 to 3 wk (antidepressant effect.)
Indications Relief of symptoms of mental depression in patients who are under close medical supervision. **Unlabeled use(s):** Treatment of obstructive sleep apnea and panic disorder.
Contraindications Hypersensitivity to tricyclic antidepressants. Generally not to be given in combination with or within 14 days of treatment with MAO inhibitors, nor during acute recovery phases of MI.
Route/Dosage
ADULTS: PO 15 to 60 mg/day in divided doses. The maintenance dose may be given as a single dose.
ELDERLY AND ADOLESCENTS: PO The initial dose is 5 mg tid. Increase slowly if needed.
Interactions
Cimetidine, fluoxetine: Increased protriptyline blood levels and effects.
CNS depressants: Additive depressant effects.
Clonidine: Hypertensive crisis.
Dicumarol: Increased anticoagulant actions.
Guanethidine: Inhibition of hypotensive action by guanethidine.
MAO inhibitors: Hyperexcitability, hyperthermia, convulsions, and death may occur.
Sympathomimetics, direct-acting (eg, norepinephrine, phenylephrine): Increased pressor response.
Sympathomimetics, indirect-acting (eg, dopamine, ephedrine): Decreased pressor response.
Lab Test Interferences None well documented.
Adverse Reactions
CV: Orthostatic hypotension; hypertension; tachycardia; palpitations; arrhythmias; ECG changes; heart block; CHF.
CNS: Confusion; hallucinations; disorientation; delusions; nervousness; restlessness; anxiety; agitation; panic; insomnia; nightmares; mania; exacerbation of psychosis; drowsiness; dizziness; weakness; fatigue; emotional lability; seizures; tremors.
DERM: Rash; pruritus; photosensitivity reaction; dry skin; acne; itching.
EENT: Mydriasis; blurred vision; increased intraocular pressure; tinnitus; peculiar taste.
GI: Nausea; vomiting; anorexia; GI distress; diarrhea; flatulence; dry mouth; constipation.
GU: Impotence; sexual dysfunction; nocturia; dysmenorrhea; amenorrhea; urinary retention and hesitancy.
HEMA: Bone marrow depression, including agranulocytosis; eosinophilia; purpura; thrombocytopenia; leukopenia.
METAB: Elevation or depression of blood glucose.
RESP: Pharyngitis, rhinitis; sinusitis; laryngitis; cough.
OTHER: Numbness; breast enlargement; extrapyramidal symptoms (eg, pseudoparkinsonism, movement disorders, akathisia).
Precautions
Pregnancy: Pregnancy category undetermined.
Lactation: Excreted in breast milk.
Children: Not recommended for use in children.
Special risk patients: Use drug with caution in patients with history of seizures, urinary retention, urethral or ureteral spasm, angle-closure

glaucoma or increased intraocular pressure, cardiovascular disorders, hyperthyroid patients or those receiving thyroid medication, hepatic or renal impairment, schizophrenic or paranoid patients.

Anticholinergic effects: Additive with other medications with anticholinergic effects.

Tachycardia/Postural hypotension: Tachycardia and postural hypotension may occur more frequently with protriptyline.

Overdosage: Signs and Symptoms
CNS stimulation (agitation, irritability, delirium) followed by depression (drowsiness to coma), hypertension followed by hypotension, hyperpyrexia followed by hypothermia, cardiac arrhythmias, seizures.

PATIENT CARE CONSIDERATIONS

Administration/Storage
- Give with food or milk to minimize GI irritation.
- Maintenance doses may be given as a single daily dose, in the morning and not at night, because of the mild stimulant effect of the drug.
- Store at room temperature in tightly-closed, light-resistant container.

Assessment/Interventions
- Obtain patient history, including drug history and any known allergies. Note recent MI, seizure disorder or prostatic hypertrophy.
- Ensure that baseline CBC with differential, ECG and hepatic studies have been obtained before beginning therapy and monitor regularly.
- Obtain baseline weight, BP (standing and lying), and pulse.
- Supervise patient closely during initiation of therapy. Assess appearance, behavior, speech pattern, level of interest, and mood.
- Monitor for weight gain (appetite may increase), dysrhythmias, and drop in BP. Withhold drug and notify health care provider if systolic pressure drops 20 mm Hg.
- Closely monitor cardiovascular response of elderly patients receiving more than 20 mg/day.
- Assist with ambulation at start of therapy and provide safety measures (eg, side rails up), especially for elderly patients.
- Monitor for headache, nausea, vertigo, malaise, and nightmares (symptoms of withdrawal when drug is abruptly discontinued or dose reduced).
- Monitor pattern of daily bowel activity, stool consistency, and urinary output. Modify fluid and bulk in diet to offset constipation.

Patient/Family Education
- Explain that therapeutic effect of drug may be seen within 2 to 5 days, but full effectiveness of drug may not occur for 2 to 3 wk.
- Tell patient that dosage will be tapered slowly before stopping to prevent withdrawal symptoms.
- Warn patient to monitor food intake; weight gain can occur because of increased appetite.
- Emphasize importance of follow-up visits to monitor effectiveness of therapy.
- Instruct patient to report the following symptoms to health care provider: Visual disturbances, mental status changes (especially increase in depression or panic), urinary retention and extrapyramidal symptoms (frequently noted in elderly) such as rigidity or fine hand tremors.
- Advise patient to take sips of water frequently or to suck on ice chips, sugarless hard candy or chew sugarless gum to relieve dry mouth.
- Caution patient to avoid sudden position changes to avoid dizziness.
- Instruct patient to avoid intake of alcoholic beverages or other CNS depressants.
- Advise patient that drug may cause drowsiness and to use caution while driving or performing other activities requiring mental alertness while dose is being stabilized.
- Caution patient to avoid exposure to sunlight and use sunscreen or wear protective clothing to avoid photosensitivity reaction.
- Instruct patient to avoid taking OTC medications without consulting health care provider.

Pseudoephedrine (d-Isoephedrine)

(SUE-doe-eh-FED-rin)

Class Nasal decongestant

How Supplied
Allermed Capsules 60 mg ♦ Cenafed Tablets 60 mg, Liquid 30 mg/5 mL ♦ Children's Congestion Relief Liquid 30 mg/5 mL ♦ Congestion Relief Tablets 30 mg ♦ Children's Silfedrine Liquid 30 mg/5 mL ♦ Decofed Syrup Liquid 30 mg/5 mL ♦ Defed-60 Tablets 60 mg ♦ Dorcol Children's Decongestant Liquid 15 mg/5 mL ♦ Dynafed Pseudo Tablets 60 mg ♦ Genaphed Tablets 30 mg ♦ Halofed Tablets 30 mg, Tablets 60 mg ♦ Mini Thin Pseudo Tablets 60 mg ♦ PediaCare Infant's Decongestant Drops 7.5 mg/0.8 mL ♦ PediaCare Nasal Decongestant Drops 7.5 mg/0.8 mL ♦ Pseudo Liquid 30 mg/5 mL ♦ Pseudo-Gest Tablets 30 mg, Tablets 60 mg ♦ Seudotabs Tablets 30 mg ♦ Sinustop Pro Capsules 60 mg ♦ Sudafed Tablets 30 mg, Tablets 60 mg ♦ Sudafed 12 Hour Caplets Tablets, extended-release 120 mg ♦ Sudex Tablets 30 mg ♦ Triaminic Infant Oral Decongestant Drops Liquid 7.5 mg/0.8 mL ♦ Triaminic AM Decongestant Formula Liquid 15 mg/5 mL
✽ Balminil Decongestant Syrup ♦ Benylin Decongestant ♦ Contac Cold 12 Hour Nondrowsy ♦ Eltor 120 ♦ Pseudofrin ♦ Sudafed Decongestant 12 Hour ♦ Sudafed Decongestant Children's ♦ Sudafed Decongestant Extra Strength ♦ Triaminic Pediatric

Action
PHARMACOLOGY: Causes vasoconstriction and subsequent shrinkage of nasal mucous membranes by alpha-adrenergic stimulation, promoting nasal drainage.

PHARMACOKINETICS/DYNAMICS:
Distribution: Distributes into breast milk.
Metabolism: Partially metabolized in the liver.
Excretion: Renal (55% to 75% as unchanged); acidic urine accelerates rate of excretion.
Onset: 15 to 30 min.
Peak: 30 to 60 min.
Duration: 3 to 4 hr; 8 to 12 hr (extended-release).

Indications Relief of nasal or eustachian tube congestion.

Contraindications Hypersensitivity to sympathomimetic amines; severe hypertension; coronary artery disease; MAO inhibitor therapy; breast-feeding mothers.

Route/Dosage
PSEUDOEPHEDRINE SULFATE
ADULTS AND CHILDREN OLDER THAN 12 YR: PO 120 mg sustained-release q 12 hr.

PSEUDOEPHEDRINE HYDROCHLORIDE
ADULTS: PO 60 mg q 4 to 6 hr or 120 mg sustained-release q 12 hr. Not to exceed 240 mg/day.
CHILDREN 6 TO 12 YR: PO 30 mg q 4 to 6 hr. Not to exceed 120 mg/day.
CHILDREN 2 TO 5 YR: PO 15 mg q 4 to 6 hr. Not to exceed 60 mg/day.
CHILDREN 1 TO 2 YR: PO 7 drops (0.2 mL)/kg q 4 to 6 hr. Not to exceed 4 doses/day.
CHILDREN 3 TO 12 MO: PO 3 drops/kg q 4 to 6 hr. Not to exceed 4 doses/day.

Interactions
Furazolidone, guanethidine, methyldopa: Increased BP.
MAO inhibitors: Severe headache, hypertension and hyperpyrexia; can cause hypertensive crisis.
Urinary acidifiers (eg, ammonium chloride): Increased elimination of pseudoephedrine.
Urinary alkalinizers (eg, sodium bicarbonate): Decreased elimination of pseudoephedrine.

Lab Test Interferences None well documented.

Adverse Reactions
CV: Arrhythmias; cardiovascular collapse with hypotension; tachycardia; bradycardia; transient hypertension.
CNS: Nervousness; excitability; dizziness; tremor; insomnia; restlessness; depression.
DERM: Pallor.
GI: Anorexia; nausea; vomiting; dry mouth.
GU: Difficulty urinating.

Precautions
Pregnancy: Category C.
Lactation: Do not give to breastfeeding mothers.
Children: Use drug only under health care provider's advice in children under 3 mo.
Elderly: Ensure that short-acting product is tolerated before giving sustained-release product.
Special risk patients: Use drug with caution in patients with hyperthyroidism, diabetes, cardiovascular disease, increased intraocular pressure or prostatic hypertrophy. Patients with hypertension should use only under medical advice.
Excessive use: Systemic effects (eg, nervousness, dizziness, sleeplessness) are more common in elderly and infants.

Overdosage: Signs and Symptoms
Somnolence; sedation, which may be accompanied by profuse sweating, hypotension or shock; coma. Symptoms in elderly include hallucinations, seizures, CNS depression, and death.

PATIENT CARE CONSIDERATIONS

Administration/Storage
- Tell patient to swallow sustained-release preparations whole, and not to break, crush or chew.
- Contents of capsule may be mixed with food (eg, jelly, applesauce) if patient has difficulty swallowing.
- Administer at least 2 hr before bedtime to diminish insomnia.
- Store at room temperature.

Assessment/Interventions
- Obtain patient history, including drug history, special risk factors (eg, hypertension) and any known allergies. Note hypersensitivity to pseudoephedrine or other sympathomimetic amines.
- Assess congestion (eg, nasal, sinus, eustachian tubes), vital signs, lung sounds and characteristics of respiratory secretions prior to and during therapy.
- Provide sufficient fluid intake to liquefy secretions and maintain hydration.

Patient/Family Education
- Advise patient not to exceed recommended dose.
- Instruct patient not to chew or crush sustained-release form.
- Teach patient to use calibrated measuring device to administer liquid and calibrated dropper to administer drops.
- Instruct patient to report the following symptoms to health care provider: Breathing difficulties, hallucinations, seizures (symptoms of overdose); lack of improvement within 7 days; high fever.
- Instruct patient to take sips of water frequently or suck on ice chips, sugarless hard candy or chew sugarless gum if dry mouth occurs.
- Advise patient to avoid taking other OTC medications containing sympathomimetic amines.

Pseudoephedrine Hydrochloride/Guaifenesin/ Dextromethorphan HBr

(SUE-doe-eh-FED-rin HIGH-droe-KLOR-ide /GWHY-fen-ah-sin/ DEX-troe-meth-OR-fan HIGH-droe-BROE-mide)

Class Decongestant/Expectorant/Antitussive

How Supplied
PanMist-DM Syrup 15 mg dextromethorphan HBr, 100 mg guaifenesin, 40 mg pseudoephedrine hydrochloride per 5 mL, Tablets 32 mg dextromethorphan HBr, 595 mg guaifenesin, 48 mg pseudoephedrine hydrochloride

Action
PHARMACOLOGY:
Pseudoephedrine: Causes vasoconstriction and subsequent shrinkage of nasal mucous membranes by alpha-adrenergic stimulation, which promotes nasal drainage.
Guaifenesin: May enhance output of respiratory tract fluid by reducing adhesiveness and surface tension, enhancing removal of viscous mucus and making nonproductive coughs more productive and less frequent.
Dextromethorphan: Suppresses cough by central action on cough center in medulla.

Indications Temporary relief of nasal congestion and cough associated with respiratory tract infections and related conditions, such as sinusitis, pharyngitis, bronchitis, and asthma, when these conditions are complicated by tenacious mucus or mucus plugs and congestion.

Contraindications Hypertension; severe coronary artery disease; MAO inhibitor therapy; pregnancy; nursing; hypersensitivity to any component of product or idiosyncrasy to sympathomimetic amines, which may manifest as insomnia, dizziness, weakness, tremor, or arrhythmias.

Route/Dosage
ADULTS AND CHILDREN OVER 12 YR: **PO** 1 or 2 tablets q 12 hr (max, 4 tablets in 24 hr) or up to 2 tsp of syrup 3 to 4 times daily.
CHILDREN 6 TO 12 YR: **PO** 1 tablet q 12 hr (max, 2 tablets in 24 hr) or up to 1 tsp 3 to 4 times daily, not to exceed 4 mg per kilogram of body weight of pseudoephedrine in 24 hr.

Interactions
Digitalis: Ectopic pacemaker activity may be increased by pseudoephedrine.
Guanethidine, mecamylamine, methyldopa, reserpine, veratrum alkaloids: Antihypertensive effects may be reduced by pseudoephedrine.
Kaolin: May increase pseudoephedrine absorption.
MAO Inhibitors (eg, isocarboxazid): May increase the effects of pseudoephedrine. Dextromethorphan is contraindicated with MAO inhibitors.

Lab Test Interferences Guaifenesin may interfere with the interpretation of the test for urinary 5-hydroxyindoleacetic acid for the diagnosis of carcinoid syndrome.

Adverse Reactions
CV: Tachycardia; palpitations; arrhythmias; cardiovascular collapse with hypotension.

CNS: Headache; dizziness; fear; anxiety; nervousness; restlessness; tremor; weakness; insomnia; hallucinations; convulsions; CNS depression.
GI: Nausea.
GU: Dysuria.
RESP: Respiratory difficulty.
OTHER: Pallor.

Precautions

Pregnancy: Category C.
Lactation: Contraindicated in nursing women.
Children: Safety and efficacy in children under 6 yr not established for tablets and in children under 2 yr of age for syrup.
Elderly: Geriatric patients are more likely to exhibit adverse effects, such as confusion or CNS depression.
Special risk patients: Use with caution in patients with hypertension, heart disease, asthma, hyperthyroidism, increased intraocular pressure, diabetes mellitus, prostatic hypertrophy.
Cough: To determine that appropriate therapy for the primary disease is instituted, ascertain underlying cause of cough prior to use of cough suppressants.
Drug abuse: Has abuse potential.

Overdosage: Signs and Symptoms

Pseudoephedrine: Excessive CNS stimulation (eg, excitement, tremor, restlessness, insomnia), tachycardia, hypertension, pallor, mydriasis, hyperglycemia, urinary retention, tachypnea, hyperpnea, hallucinations, convulsions, delirium, arrhythmias, hypotension, circulatory collapse, hypokalemia.
Dextromethorphan: Drowsiness, ataxia, nystagmus, opisthotonos, convulsive disorders.

PATIENT CARE CONSIDERATIONS

Administration/Storage
- Give prescribed dose every 12 hr as needed.
- Give with food if GI upset occurs.
- Tablets may be broken in half for ease of administration. Do not crush or chew tablets or half-tablets.
- Store tablets at controlled room temperature (59° to 86°F).

Assessment/Interventions
- Obtain patient history, including drug history and any known allergies. Note history of diabetes, hypertension, hyperthyroidism, enlarged prostate, narrow-angle glaucoma, urinary retention, severe coronary artery disease, pregnancy, or concurrent use of or within 2 wk of stopping MAO inhibitor therapy.
- Assess symptoms (eg, cough, sputum viscosity, color and volume, sinus congestion) before and periodically throughout therapy.
- Monitor patient for nervousness, dizziness, tachycardia, and palpitations. If noted, hold therapy and notify health care provider.

Patient/Family Education
- Explain name, dose, action, and potential side effects of drug.
- Advise patient to take prescribed dose every 12 hr as needed.
- Advise patient to take with food if GI upset occurs.
- Advise patient that if a dose is missed to take as soon as remembered unless it is nearing time for the next dose. Caution patient not to double the dose to catch up.
- Instruct patient to discontinue use and report any of these symptoms to health care provider: nervousness, dizziness, sleeplessness.
- Advise patient that if symptoms are not controlled, not to increase the dose of medication but to inform health care provider.
- Advise women to notify health care provider if pregnant, planning to become pregnant, or breastfeeding.
- Caution patient to not take any prescription or OTC medications or dietary supplements unless advised by health care provider.

Pyrazinamide

(peer-uh-ZIN-uh-mide)

Class Anti-infective/Antitubercular

How Supplied
Pyrazinamide Tablets 500 mg
♣ Tebrazid

Action
PHARMACOLOGY: Pyrazine analog of nicotinamide may be bacteriostatic or bactericidal against *Mycobacterium tuberculosis*.

PHARMACOKINETICS/DYNAMICS:
Absorption: Rapid and almost complete from GI tract. T_{max} is 1 to 2 hr (pyrazinamide) and 4 to 5 hr (pyrazinoic acid). C_{max} is 19 to 39 mcg/mL (pyrazinamide) and 3 to 4.5 mcg/mL (pyrazinoic acid).

Distribution: Widely distributed to most fluids and tissues, including the liver, lungs, kidney, and bile. Excellent penetration into CSF (87% to 105%). Vd is 0.57 to 0.74 L/kg. Protein binding is 10% to 20% (pyrazinamide) and 31% (pyrazinoic acid). Distributes into breast milk.

Metabolism: Hepatic; hydrolyzed by microsomal deamidase to active metabolites pyrazinoic acid, then hydroxylated by xanthine oxidase to 5-hydroxypyrazinoic acid.

Excretion: Renal (3% as unchanged pyrazinamide, 33% pyrazinoic acid). The t½ distribution is approximately 1.6 hr. Elimination t½ is approximately 9.5 hr (pyrazinamide, normal renal function), approximately 26 hr (pyrazinamide, chronic renal failure), approximately 12 hr (pyrazinoic acid, normal renal function), and approximately 22 hr (pyrazinoic acid, chronic renal failure).

Special Populations:
Renal Function Impairment – The t½ of pyrazinamide and metabolite is increased.

Indications Initial treatment of active tuberculosis in adults and selected children when combined with other antituberculosis agents.

Contraindications Severe hepatic damage; acute gout.

Route/Dosage
ADULTS: PO 15 to 30 mg/kg qd (max, 2 g/day) or 50 to 70 mg/kg 2 times/week (max, 4 g/dose) or 50 to 70 mg/kg 3 times/wk (max, 3 g).
CHILDREN: PO 15 to 30 mg/kg qd (max, 2 g/day) or 50 to 70 mg/kg 2 times/wk (max, 4 g) or 50 to 70 mg/kg 3 times/wk (max, 3 g).

Interactions None well documented.

Lab Test Interferences May interfere with *Acetest* and *Ketostix* urine tests, producing pink-brown color.

Adverse Reactions
DERM: Rash; acne; photosensitivity.
GI: Nausea; vomiting; anorexia.
HEPA: Hepatotoxicity.
METAB: Gout; porphyria.
OTHER: Arthralgia and myalgia; hypersensitivity reactions (eg, urticaria, pruritus); fever.

Precautions
Pregnancy: Category C.
Lactation: Excreted in breast milk.
Children: Safety and efficacy not established. Use only if therapy is essential.
Hepatic function impairment: Closely follow patients with pre-existing liver disease or patients at increased risk (eg, alcohol abusers). It may be necessary to discontinue drug; do not resume therapy if signs of hepatocellular damage appear.
Diabetes mellitus: Management of diabetes mellitus may be more difficult.
Hyperuricemia: May inhibit renal excretion of urates, resulting in hyperuricemia.

Overdosage: Signs and Symptoms
Abnormal LFTs.

PATIENT CARE CONSIDERATIONS

Administration/Storage
- Drug should always be part of multi-drug therapy to decrease chance of resistant organisms. Question doses more than 35 mg/kg/day.
- Administer with food to decrease GI irritation.
- Store at room temperature in tightly closed, light-resistant container.

Assessment/Interventions
- Obtain patient history, including drug history and any known allergies.
- Assess for signs of anemia (eg, hematocrit, hemoglobin, evidence of fatigue).
- Ensure that serum AST, ALT, and uric acid concentration have been determined before beginning therapy and repeated q 2 to 4 wk.
- Obtain culture and sensitivity monthly to detect resistance and ensure sensitivity to medication.
- Monitor patient for signs of liver disease or gout.

Patient/Family Education
- Emphasize need to be compliant with regimen and not to miss any doses.
- Explain that long-term therapy (6 mo to 2 yr) will be necessary.
- Inform diabetic patients that drug may interfere with urine ketone values.
- Emphasize importance of follow-up examinations to monitor effectiveness of therapy and identify side effects.
- Instruct patient to report the following symptoms to health care provider: fever; loss of appetite; malaise; nausea and vomiting; darkened urine, yellowish skin or eye discoloration; pain or swelling joints.
- Advise patient to avoid intake of alcoholic beverages and alcohol-containing products.

Pyridostigmine Bromide

(pihr-id-oh-STIG-meen BROE-mide)

Class Cholinergic muscle stimulant/Anticholinesterase

How Supplied
Mestinon Tablets 60 mg, Tablets, extended-release 180 mg, Syrup 60 mg/5 mL, Injection 5 mg/mL

Action
PHARMACOLOGY: Facilitates myoneural junction impulse transmission by inhibiting acetylcholine destruction by cholinesterase.

PHARMACOKINETICS/DYNAMICS:
Excretion: Primarily excreted unchanged by the kidney.

Indications Treatment of myasthenia gravis; reversal agent or antagonist to nondepolarizing muscle relaxants such as curariform drugs and gallamine triethiodide (IV only).

Contraindications Mechanical intestinal or urinary obstruction; hypersensitivity to anticholinesterase agents.

Route/Dosage
ADULTS: **PO** Individualize dosage to meet the needs of the patients.
Syrup/Conventional tablet: Average dose is ten 5 mL tsp (60 mg/5 mL) daily or ten 60 mg tablets spaced to provide max relief when max strength is needed (range is usually 1 to 25 tablets or tsp/day).
Extended-release tablets: One to three 180 mg tablets, qd or bid with at least 6 hr between doses.
IV To supplement oral dosage preoperatively and postoperatively during labor and postpartum, during myasthenic crisis, or when oral therapy is impractical, give approximately 1/30 the oral dose, either IM or very slow IV.
NEONATES: **IV** Neonates of myasthenic mothers may have transient difficulty in swallowing, sucking, and breathing. Injectable pyridostigmine may be indicated (by symptoms and use of the edrophonium test) until syrup can be taken. Dosage requirements range from 0.05 to 0.15 mg/kg IM.

Reversal of Nondepolarizing Muscle Relaxants
Injection – Give atropine sulfate (0.6 to 1.2 mg) IV immediately prior to pyridostigmine to minimize side effects. Pyridostigmine 10 or 20 mg IV is usually sufficient. Full recovery usually occurs in no more than 15 min but at least 30 min may be required.

Interactions
Atropine: May mask signs of overdosage, leading to inadvertent induction of cholinergic crisis.
Corticosteroids: The therapeutic effects of pyridostigmine may be antagonized.
Succinylcholine: Neuromuscular blockade produced by succinylcholine may be prolonged or antagonized.

Lab Test Interferences None well documented.

Adverse Reactions
DERM: Skin rash.
EENT: Miosis.
GI: Nausea; vomiting; diarrhea; abdominal cramps; increased peristalsis; increased salivation.
MUSC: Muscle cramps and fasciculation; weakness.
RESP: Increased bronchial secretions.
OTHER: Increased sweating.

Precautions
Pregnancy: Category C.
Lactation: Excreted in breast milk.
Renal function impairment: Lower doses may be required in patients with renal disease.
Bronchial asthma: Use with caution.
Cardiac dysrhythmias (IV only): Use with caution. Transient bradycardia may occur and be relieved by atropine sulfate.
Cholinergic crisis: Observe patients closely for cholinergic reactions, particularly if the IV route is used. May be difficult to distinguish from myasthenic crisis. Differentiation is important because increasing the dose of pyridostigmine or other drugs of this class may have grave consequences in patients in cholinergic crisis.

Overdosage: Signs and Symptoms
Cholinergic crisis, characterized by increasing muscle weakness (including respiratory paralysis and death).

PATIENT CARE CONSIDERATIONS
Administration/Storage
- Administer as prescribed. Size of dose (eg, number of tablets or tsp of syrup) and frequency of administration will be adjusted to provide max relief of myasthenia gravis symptoms.
- Administer without regard to meals. Administer with food if GI upset occurs.
- Do not chew or crush extended-release tablet. Instruct patient to swallow tablet(s) whole.
- Store tablets and syrup at controlled room temperature (59° to 86°F).

Assessment/Interventions
- Obtain patient history, including drug history and any known allergies. Note kidney disease, asthma, mechanical intestinal, or urinary obstruction.

- Assess pulse, BP, and respiratory rate before starting therapy and periodically during treatment. Notify health care provider immediately of any significant changes.
- Ensure that emergency airway and resuscitation equipment are available.
- Ensure that parenteral atropine is available for emergency treatment of cholinergic crisis.
- Frequently assess muscle strength and function. Notify health care provider immediately of increasing muscle weakness and/or respiratory distress.
- Assess patient for GI, respiratory, musculoskeletal, and general body side effects. Inform health care provider if noted and significant.

Patient/Family Education
- Explain name, dose, action, and potential side effects of drug.
- Advise patient that dose and frequency of administration may be adjusted to achieve max benefit.
- Advise patient to take exactly as prescribed and not to change the dose or stop taking unless advised by health care provider.
- Advise patient to take prescribed dose without regard to meals but to take with food if upset stomach occurs.
- Instruct patient to contact health care provider immediately if any of the following occur: worsening muscle weakness, difficulty breathing, slow heart rate, dizziness, fainting.
- Advise women to notify health care provider if pregnant, planning to become pregnant, or breastfeeding.
- Instruct patient not to take any prescription or OTC medications or dietary supplements unless advised by health care provider.
- Advise patient that follow-up visits will be required to monitor therapy and to keep appointments.

Pyridoxine Hydrochloride (B_6)

(peer-ih-DOX-een HIGH-droe-KLOR-ide)

Class Vitamin

How Supplied
Aminoxin Tablets, enteric-coated 20 mg (as pyridoxal-5'-phosphate) ◆ *Nestrex* Tablets 25 mg
✤ *Hexa-Betalin*

Action
PHARMACOLOGY: Vitamin B_6 functions as coenzyme in amino acid, carbohydrate and lipid metabolism.

PHARMACOKINETICS/DYNAMICS:

Absorption: Absorbed by passive diffusion in the jejunum and to a lesser extent in the ileum.

Distribution: Primarily stored in the liver, lesser amount in the muscle and brain. Not protein bound.

Metabolism: Metabolized in the liver and converted to 4-pyridoxic acid metabolite.

Excretion: Excreted mostly as 4-pyridoxic acid in the urine. $T_{1/2}$ is 15 to 20 days.

Indications Pyridoxine deficiency, including inadequate diet, drug-induced causes (eg, isoniazid, hydralazine, oral contraceptives) or inborn errors of metabolism. Parenteral use is indicated when oral therapy is not feasible.

Unlabeled use(s): Treatment of hydrazine poisoning, PMS, hyperoxaluria type I, nausea and vomiting in pregnancy, sideroblastic anemia associated with high serum iron, carpal tunnel syndrome, tardive dyskinesia.

Contraindications Standard considerations.

Route/Dosage
Dietary Deficiency
ADULTS: **PO/IM/IV** 10 to 20 mg/day for 3 wk.

Drug-Induced Deficiency Anemia or Neuritis
ADULTS: **PO/IM/IV** 100 to 200 mg/day for 3 wk; follow with 25 to 100 mg/day.

Neuropathy
ADULTS: **PO/IM/IV** 50 to 200 mg/day.

Vitamin B_6 Dependency Syndrome
ADULTS: **PO/IM/IV** 600 mg, followed by 30 mg/day for life. Dependency has been noted in adults administered 200 mg/day.
PYRIDOXINE-DEPENDENT INFANTS: **IM/IV** 10 to 100 mg, followed by 2 to 100 mg/day.

Metabolic Disorders
ADULTS: **PO/IM/IV** 100 to 500 mg/day.

Isoniazid (INH) Poisoning
ADULTS AND CHILDREN: **IV** 4 g IV followed by 1 g IM q 30 min until pyridoxine dose equal to INH dose has been given.

Interactions
Cycloserine, INH, hydralazine, oral contraceptives, penicillamine: Increased need for pyridoxine.

Levodopa: Decreased effect of levodopa. (Interaction does not occur with levodopa/carbidopa in combination with pyridoxine.)

Phenytoin: Phenytoin serum levels may be decreased.

INCOMPATIBILITIES: Incompatible with alkaline solutions, iron salts and oxidizing agents (parenteral).

Lab Test Interferences May result in false-positive urobilinogen in the spot test using Ehrlich's reagent.

Adverse Reactions
CNS: Neuropathy; unstable gait; drowsiness; somnolence.
EENT: Perioral numbness.
OTHER: Numbness of feet; decreased sensation to touch, temperature or vibration; paresthesia; low serum folic acid levels; burning/stinging at IM injection site; photoallergic reaction; ataxia.

PATIENT CARE CONSIDERATIONS
Administration/Storage
- Instruct patient to swallow sustained-release preparation whole and not to break, crush or chew.
- When giving via IM route, rotate sites.
- IV preparation may be given undiluted or added to standard compatible IV solutions.
- Store all forms of drug at room temperature in tightly-closed, light-resistant containers. Avoid freezing injection.

Assessment/Interventions
- Obtain patient history, including drug history and any known allergies.
- Assess for signs of vitamin B_6 deficiency (eg, irritability, seizures, anemia, dermatitis, nausea, vomiting) prior to and during therapy.

Precautions
Pregnancy: Category A. (Category C in doses that exceed the RDA.)
Lactation: Excreted in breast milk; may inhibit lactation.
Children: Safety and efficacy not established in doses exceeding nutritional requirements.

Overdosage: Signs and Symptoms
Ataxia, sensory neuropathy.

- Institute seizure precautions in pyridoxine-dependent infants.
- Obtain dietary consultation to review importance of well-balanced meals and sources of B_6 prior to discharge home.

Patient/Family Education
- Emphasize importance of complying with prescribed dietary recommendations.
- Teach patient about foods high in B_6 (whole grain cereals, meat [eg, liver], potatoes, green vegetables, legumes [eg, lima beans], yeast and bananas).
- If patient is self-medicating with vitamin supplements, caution that megadosing may cause side effects such as unsteady gait, impaired hand coordination and numbness of feet.

Pyrimethamine
(pihr-ih-METH-ah-meen)
Class Anti-infective/Antimalarial
How Supplied
Daraprim Tablets 25 mg
Action
PHARMACOLOGY: Pyrimethamine is a folic acid antagonist, and the therapeutic action is based on differential requirements between host and parasite for nucleic acid precursors involved in growth.

PHARMACOKINETICS/DYNAMICS:
Absorption: Well absorbed, reaching C_{max} in 2 to 6 hr.
Distribution: Plasma protein binding is 87%.
Excretion: Plasma t½ is approximately 96 hr.

Indications Treatment of toxoplasmosis (in conjunction with a sulfonamide); treatment of acute malaria (in conjunction with a schizonticide [eg, chloroquine, quinine] but a sulfonamide [eg, sulfadoxine] will initiate transmission control and suppression of susceptible strains of plasmodia); chemoprophylaxis of malaria.

Contraindications Patients with documented megaloblastic anemia caused by folate deficiency; hypersensitivity to any component of the product.

Route/Dosage
Acute Malaria
ADULTS AND CHILDREN OLDER THAN 10 YR: PO 50 mg/day for 2 days.
CHILDREN 4 TO 10 YR: PO 25 mg/day for 2 days. Follow with the once weekly chemoprophylaxis regimen described below. Regimens that include suppression should be extended through any characteristic periods of early recrudescence and late relapse (for at least 10 wk).

Chemoprophylaxis of Malaria
ADULTS AND CHILDREN OLDER THAN 10 YR: PO 25 mg once/wk.
CHILDREN 4 THROUGH 10 YR: PO 12.5 mg once/wk.
INFANTS AND CHILDREN YOUNGER THAN 4 YR: PO 6.25 mg once/wk.

Toxoplasmosis
ADULTS: PO Start with 50 to 75 mg/day, together with 1 to 4 g of a sulfapyrimidine type sulfonamide (eg, sulfadoxine). Continue for 1 to 3 wk, depending on response and tolerance. Dosage may then be reduced to about one-half that previously given for each drug and continued for an additional 4 to 5 wk.
CHILDREN: PO 1 mg/kg/day in 2 equally divided doses; after 2 to 4 days, reduce dose to one-half and continue for about 1 mo. Coadminister the

usual pediatric sulfonamide dosage with pyrimethamine.

Interactions

Antifolate drugs or agents associated with myelosuppression (eg, cytostatic agents [eg, methotrexate], sulfonamides, trimethoprim-sulfamethoxazole, proguanil, zidovudine): May increase risk of bone marrow suppression.
Lorazepam: Mild hepatotoxicity has been reported.

Lab Test Interferences None well documented.

Adverse Reactions

CV: Rhythm disorders.
GI: Anorexia; vomiting (with large doses); atrophic glossitis.
HEMA: Megaloblastic anemia; leukopenia; thrombocytopenia; pancytopenia; hematuria.
OTHER: Hypersensitivity (may include Stevens-Johnson syndrome, toxic epidermal necrolysis, erythema multiforme, anaphylaxis); pulmonary eosinophilia (rare).

Precautions

Pregnancy: Category C.
Lactation: Excretion in breast milk.
Children: See Route/Dosage section.
Elderly: Use with caution, usually starting at the low end of the dosing range because of the greater frequency of decreased hepatic, renal, or cardiac function, and concomitant diseases or other drug therapy.
Renal function impairment: Use with caution.
Hepatic function impairment: Use with caution.
Accidental ingestion: Keep out of the reach of infants and children as they are extremely susceptible to adverse effects from an overdose; death may occur.
Folic acid deficiency: The dose of pyrimethamine required to treat toxoplasmosis approaches the toxic level. Use with caution in possible folate deficiency.
Hemolytic anemia: Large doses may precipitate hemolytic anemia in patients with glucose-6-phosphate dehydrogenase deficiency.
Resistance: Resistance to pyrimethamine is prevalent worldwide; it is not considered suitable as a prophylactic agent for travelers to most areas.

Overdosage: Signs and Symptoms

Convulsions, abdominal pain, nausea, severe and repeated vomiting (including hematemesis), CNS toxicity (manifested as excitability), generalized and prolonged convulsions, respiratory depression, circulatory collapse, death.

PATIENT CARE CONSIDERATIONS

Administration/Storage

- May be used alone or in combination with other antimalarial medications or sulfonamide antibiotics.
- Administer prescribed dose with food to minimize anorexia and vomiting.
- Store tablets at controlled room temperature (59° to 77°F). Protect from light and moisture.

Assessment/Interventions

- Obtain patient history, including drug history and any known allergies. Note renal or hepatic impairment, malabsorption syndrome, chronic alcoholism, pregnancy, breastfeeding, megaloblastic anemia caused by folate deficiency, seizure disorder, or concurrent use of medications know to reduce folate levels (eg, phenytoin).
- Ensure that a sulfonamide antibiotic is used concurrently with pyrimethamine when treating patient with acute malaria or toxoplasmosis.
- Ensure that CBC, including platelet count, is performed before starting therapy and semiweekly thereafter in patient being treated for toxoplasmosis. If signs of folate deficiency develop (eg, megaloblastic changes, glossitis), discontinue pyrimethamine and administer folinic acid (leucovorin) until normal hematopoiesis is restored.
- Ensure that patient being treated for toxoplasmosis is evaluated for need for concurrent folinic acid (leucovorin) therapy.
- Monitor patient for GI, DERM, and general body side effects. Report to health care provider if noted and significant. If patient develops skin rash, notify health care provider immediately and be prepared to discontinue the medication if lesions progress.

Patient/Family Education

- Explain name, dose, action, and potential side effects of drug.
- Advise patient to continue to take any concurrently prescribed therapy (eg, folinic acid, sulfonamide) in order to achieve maximum benefit and reduce risk of side effects.
- Advise patient to take each dose with food to reduce chances of appetite loss and vomiting.
- Advise patient that protective clothing, insect repellants, and bednets are important components of malaria prophylaxis.
- Advise patient to stop using and contact health care provider immediately if skin rash, sore throat, paleness, red or inflamed tongue or mouth, or small purple spots under skin develop.

- Advise women of childbearing potential to use effective contraception while taking pyrimethamine.
- Advise women to notify health care provider if pregnant, planning to become pregnant, or breastfeeding.
- Instruct patient not to take any prescription or OTC medications or dietary supplements unless advised by health care provider.
- Advise patient that if a febrile illness develops during or after return from a malaria-endemic area, to seek health care and inform health care provider of possible malaria exposure.
- Advise patient that follow-up examinations and lab tests may be required to monitor therapy and to keep appointments.

Quazepam
(KWAY-zuh-pam)
Class Sedative/Hypnotic/Benzodiazepine

How Supplied
Doral Tablets 7.5 mg, Tablets 15 mg

Action
PHARMACOLOGY: Potentiates action of GABA, an inhibitory neurotransmitter, resulting in increased neuronal inhibition and CNS depression, especially in limbic system and reticular formation.

PHARMACOKINETICS/DYNAMICS:
Absorption: Well absorbed from GI tract. The $t_{1/2}$ is 30 min; C_{max} is about 20 ng/mL; T_{max} is about 2 hr.

Distribution: Protein binding is 95%. Quazepam is present in breast milk (less than 0.1% of dose).

Metabolism: It is extensively metabolized in the liver to 2 active metabolites, 2-oxoquazepam and N-desalkyl-2-oxoquazepam.

Excretion: Eliminated in the urine (31%) and feces (23%) as trace amounts of unchanged drug. The $t_{1/2}$ for parent and 2-oxoquazepam is 39 hr and 73 hr for N-desalkyl-2-oxoquazepam.

Special Populations:
Hepatic Function Impairment – The potential for excessive sedation or impaired coordination exists.
Elderly – Elimination $t_{1/2}$ of N-desalkyl-2-oxoquazepam is increased 2-fold that of young adults.
Alcoholism – The potential for excessive sedation or impaired coordination exists.

Indications Short-term management of insomnia.

Contraindications Hypersensitivity to benzodiazepines; pregnancy; sleep apnea.

Route/Dosage
ADULTS: **PO** 15 mg at bedtime initially; may reduce to 7.5 mg once individual response is determined.

ELDERLY OR DEBILITATED PATIENTS: Attempt dosage reduction after 1 to 2 nights.

Interactions
Alcohol, CNS depressants: May cause additive CNS depressant effects.
Cimetidine, disulfiram, omeprazole: May increase quazepam effects.
Digoxin: May increase serum digoxin concentrations.
Theophylline: May antagonize sedative effects.

Lab Test Interferences None well documented.

Adverse Reactions
CV: Palpitations, tachycardia.
CNS: Daytime drowsiness; dizziness; lethargy; confusion; memory impairment; euphoria; relaxed feeling; falling; ataxia; hallucinations; paradoxical reactions (eg, anger, hostility, mania); headache.
DERM: Rash.
EENT: Blurred vision; difficulty focusing.
GI: Anorexia; diarrhea; abdominal cramping; constipation; nausea and vomiting.
HEMA: Leukopenia; agranulocytopenia.
HEPA: Hepatic dysfunction.
OTHER: Tolerance; physical and psychological dependence; weakness; slurred speech.

Precautions
Pregnancy: Category X.
Lactation: Excreted in breast milk.
Children: Contraindicated in children less than 18 yr.
Special risk patients: Use drug with caution in patients with renal or hepatic impairment, depression or suicidal tendencies, drug abuse and dependence, chronic pulmonary insufficiency, seizure disorders.
Dependence/Withdrawal: Prolonged use can lead to psychologic or physical dependence. Withdrawal syndrome may occur; dose must be tapered gradually.

Overdosage: Signs and Symptoms
Somnolence, confusion with reduced or absent reflexes, respiratory depression, apnea, hypotension, impaired coordination, slurred speech, seizures, coma.

PATIENT CARE CONSIDERATIONS

Administration/Storage
- Administer 30 min to 1 hr before bedtime with full glass of water. If GI upset occurs, administer with snack.
- Check to see that medication is swallowed.
- After long-term use, drug must be discontinued gradually. When drug is discontinued, expect nighttime sleep to be disturbed briefly (a few days).
- Store in tight container in cool area.

Assessment/Interventions
- Obtain patient history, including drug history and any known allergies. Note potential for suicide or drug dependence.
- Assess type of sleep difficulty (eg, falling asleep, remaining asleep).

- Assess sleep pattern prior to and during therapy.
- Assess mental status (eg, sensorium, affect, mood, and long-term and short-term memory).
- Provide safety measures (eg, removal of cigarettes, side rails up, night light, easily accessible call bell) and assistance with ambulation.

Patient/Family Education
- Caution patient that this medication must not be taken during pregnancy or when pregnancy is possible. Advise patient to use reliable form of birth control while taking this drug.
- Discuss with patient ways to facilitate sleep (eg, quiet, darkened room; avoidance of caffeine and nicotine; warm bath; warm milk; deep breathing; relaxation; self-hypnosis).
- Instruct patient not to increase dose.
- Emphasize importance of follow-up evaluation with health care provider to monitor progress of therapy. Instruct patient to inform health care provider if drug does not seem to be working.
- Instruct patient not to discontinue medication abruptly after prolonged therapy (eg, more than 2 wk).
- Advise patient that disturbed nocturnal sleep may be experienced for 1 to 2 nights after discontinuing drug.
- Instruct patient to report the following symptoms to health care provider: sudden onset of vision changes, irregular heart beat, fever, sore throat, bruising, rash, jaundice, unusual bleeding (eg, epistaxis), or if pregnancy is detected.
- Advise patient to avoid intake of alcoholic beverages or other CNS depressants.
- Advise patient that drug may cause drowsiness and to use caution while driving or performing other tasks requiring mental alertness.

Quetiapine Fumarate

(cue-TIE-ah-peen)
Class Antipsychotic

How Supplied
Seroquel Tablets 25 mg, Tablets 100 mg, Tablets 200 mg, Tablets 300 mg

Action
PHARMACOLOGY: Has antipsychotic effects, apparently caused by dopamine and serotonin receptor blockade in the CNS.

PHARMACOKINETICS/DYNAMICS:
Absorption: Rapid absorption. T_{max} is 1.5 hr. Bioavailability is 100%. Food increases C_{max} 25% and AUC 15%.

Distribution: Widely distributed throughout. Vd is about 10 L/kg. It is 83% bound to plasma proteins.

Metabolism: Highly metabolized by the liver via 3A4 isoenzyme. Major metabolic pathways are sulfoxidation to the sulfoxide metabolite and oxidation to parent acid metabolite, both inactive.

Excretion: Mainly via hepatic metabolism, less than 1% excreted as unchanged drug. About 73% of dose recovered in urine and 20% in feces. The mean terminal t½ is 6 hr.

Special Populations:
Renal Function Impairment – Ccr 10 to 30 mL/min had 25% lower Cl; dosage adjustment not needed.
Hepatic Function Impairment – 30% lower Cl; AUC and C_{max} 3-fold higher; dosage adjustment may be needed.
Elderly – Oral Cl is reduced 40%. Dosage adjustments may be needed.

Indications Treatment of schizophrenia; short-term treatment of acute manic episodes associated with bipolar I disorder.

Contraindications Standard considerations.

Route/Dosage
Acute Bipolar Mania
ADULTS: PO Start with 100 mg/day in bid divided doses on day 1; increase to 400 mg/day on day 4 in increments of up to 100 mg/day in bid divided doses. Further dosage adjustments up to 800 mg/day by day 6 should be in increments no greater than 200 mg/day. Safety of doses greater than 800 mg/day has not been evaluated.

Schizophrenia
ADULTS: PO 25 mg bid initially; may increase 25 to 50 mg bid to tid on the second and third day to target range of 300 to 400 mg/day by the fourth day. Therapeutic dose range is 150 to 750 mg/day.

Hepatic Impairment
ADULTS: PO Start with 25 mg/day; increase in daily increments of 25 to 50 mg/day to an effective dose.

Interactions
Alcohol, CNS-acting drugs: Possible additive CNS depressant effects; use with caution.
Antihypertensive agents: Hypotensive effects may be enhanced.
Dopamine agonists (eg, ropinirole, pramipexole), levodopa: Quetiapine may antagonize therapeutic effects of dopamine agonists and levodopa.
Hepatic enzyme inducers (eg, carbamazepine, barbiturates, phenytoin, rifampin, glucocorticoids): May

decrease the effects of quetiapine; increased doses of quetiapine may be necessary to maintain control of psychotic symptoms.

Inhibitors of CYP3A (eg, ketoconazole, itraconazole, fluconazole, erythromycin): May increase the effects of quetiapine; use with caution.

Lorazepam: Quetiapine increases the effects of lorazepam.

Thioridazine: May decrease the effects of quetiapine.

Lab Test Interferences None well documented.

Adverse Reactions

CV: Postural hypotension (7%); tachycardia (6%); palpitation (at least 1%).

CNS: Somnolence (34%); headache (21%); agitation (20%); dizziness (11%); tremor (8%); anxiety (4%); hypertonia, dysarthria (at least 1%).

DERM: Rash (4%); sweating (at least 1%); Stevens-Johnson syndrome (postmarketing).

EENT: Pharyngitis (6%); rhinitis (3%); amblyopia (2%).

GI: Dry mouth (19%); constipation (10%); abdominal pain (7%); vomiting (6%); dyspepsia (5%); gastroenteritis (2%); anorexia (at least 1%).

HEMA: Leukopenia (at least 1%); agranulocytosis (postmarketing).

HEPA: Increased ALT (5%); increased AST (3%).

M/N: Weight gain (6%); peripheral edema (at least 1%); hyponatremia, SIADH (postmarketing).

MUSC: Rhabdomyolysis (postmarketing).

RESP: Increased cough, dyspnea (at least 1%).

OTHER: Asthenia (10%); pain (7%); back pain (5%); fever (2%); flu-like syndrome (at least 1%); anaphylaxis (postmarketing).

Precautions

Pregnancy: Category C.

Lactation: Undetermined.

Children: Safety and efficacy not established.

Elderly: Elderly and debilitated patients may be more susceptible to effects. Consider lower starting dose, slower titration, and careful monitoring. At increased risk of tardive dyskinesia, especially elderly women.

Hepatic function impairment: Dosage adjustment may be needed.

Aspiration pneumonia: Antipsychotics have been associated with esophageal dysmotility and aspiration. Use with caution in patients at risk for aspiration pneumonia.

Body temperature regulation: Antipsychotics can disrupt the body's ability to reduce core temperature.

Cataracts: Lens changes have been observed in patients during long-term treatment.

Cognitive and motor performance: Because of initial sedation, mental and/or physical abilities may be impaired, especially during the first few days of therapy.

Hyperglycemia and diabetes mellitus: Hyperglycemia, in some cases extreme and associated with ketoacidosis or hyperosmolar coma or death, may occur. Monitor patients with established diagnosis of diabetes mellitus regularly for worsening of glucose control.

Long-term use (more than 6 wk): Long-term use not evaluated. Periodically reevaluate usefulness.

Neuroleptic malignant syndrome (NMS): NMS has occurred with antipsychotics and is potentially fatal. Signs and symptoms are hyperpyrexia, muscle rigidity, altered mental status, irregular pulse, irregular BP, tachycardia, and diaphoresis.

Orthostatic hypotension: May occur during the initial dose-titration period. Follow dosing guidelines carefully to reduce risk. Use with caution in patients with known CV disease, cerebral vascular disease, or conditions that predispose to hypotension (eg, dehydration).

Seizures: Seizures have occurred. Use with caution in patients with a history of seizures or with conditions that potentially lower the seizure threshold (eg, Alzheimer dementia).

Suicide: Closely supervise high-risk patients; do not give access to excessive quantities.

Tardive dyskinesia: A potentially irreversible syndrome of involuntary body and facial movements may occur.

Overdosage: Signs and Symptoms

Drowsiness, sedation, tachycardia, hypotension.

PATIENT CARE CONSIDERATIONS

Administration/Storage

- Administer dose bid or tid as prescribed without regard to meals.
- Administer with food if GI upset occurs.
- Store at controlled room temperature (59° to 86°F).

Assessment/Interventions

- Obtain patient history, including drug history and any known allergies. Note kidney or liver disease, CV disease, cerebrovascular disease, cardiac arrhythmias, previous episodes of NMS, seizures or conditions that predispose to seizures (eg, Alzheimer disease), conditions that would predispose to hypotension (eg, dehydration, hypovolemia, treatment with antihypertensive medications), and concur-

rent use of medications that induce CYP3A4 (eg, phenytoin) or inhibit CYP3A4 (eg, ketoconazole).
- Ensure that patient has eye examination and is evaluated for cataract formation before starting therapy and q 6 mo during treatment.
- Monitor patient during titration of drug for hypotension; notify health care provider if noted and be prepared to return to previous dose.
- Take safety precautions if orthostatic hypotension occurs.
- Monitor blood sugar in diabetic patient when drug is started or dose is changed. Report significant changes to health care provider.
- Ensure that fasting blood glucose is evaluated before starting therapy and periodically thereafter during therapy in patient with risk factors for diabetes mellitus (eg, obesity, family history of diabetes).
- Inform health care provider immediately if hyperpyrexia, muscle rigidity, altered mental status, irregular pulse and BP, tachycardia, or diaphoresis develop.
- Notify health care provider if any of the following develops: hypotension, tachycardia, excessive drowsiness, constipation, persistent indigestion, symptoms of hyperglycemia (polyuria, polydipsia, polyphagia).
- Assess baseline neurologic status and during treatment observe for involuntary body and facial movements, drowsiness, agitation, anxiety, aggressive reaction, or seizure activity.
- Frequently assess patient for response to treatment. Notify health care provider if condition does not appear to be improving or is worsening.
- Ensure that therapy is periodically reviewed to determine if it needs to be continued without change or if a dose change (eg, increase, decrease, discontinuation) is indicated.
- Monitor patient for suicidal tendencies often associated with schizophrenia and bipolar disorder.
- Assess medication compliance.

Patient/Family Education
- Explain name, dose, action, and potential side effects of drug.
- Instruct patient to take dose bid or tid as prescribed, without regard to meals. Advise patient to take with food if GI upset occurs.
- Advise patient that if a dose is missed to take it as soon as possible and then return to the normal schedule. Instruct patient that if a dose is skipped not to double the dose to catch up.
- Advise patient that dose will be started low and then increased until max benefit is obtained.
- Instruct patient not to change the dose or stop taking unless advised by health care provider.
- Instruct patient not to stop taking quetiapine when feeling better.
- Caution patient that if medication is stopped for more than 1 wk and then restarted that the initial dose and titration schedule should be followed.
- Instruct diabetic patient to monitor blood glucose more frequently when drug is started or dose is changed and to inform health care provider of significant changes in readings.
- Tell patient to immediately report high fever, muscle rigidity, altered mental status, irregular pulse, sweating, seizures, or rash to health care provider.
- Advise patient to notify health care provider of the following: excessive drowsiness, weight gain, involuntary body or facial movements, rapid pulse, excessive urination and thirst.
- Advise patient to take frequent sips of water, suck on ice chips or sugarless hard candy, or chew sugarless gum if dry mouth occurs.
- Advise patient to avoid strenuous activity during periods of high temperature or humidity.
- Instruct patient to avoid alcoholic beverages and sedatives (eg, diazepam) while taking quetiapine.
- Instruct patient to get up slowly from lying or sitting position and to avoid sudden position changes to prevent postural hypotension. Advise patient to report dizziness with position changes to health care provider. Caution patient that hot tubs and hot showers or baths may make dizziness worse.
- Advise patient taking antihypertensives to monitor BP at regular intervals.
- Advise patient that drug may impair judgment, thinking, or motor skills or cause drowsiness and to use caution while driving or performing other tasks requiring mental alertness until tolerance is determined.
- Advise women to notify health care provider if pregnant, planning to become pregnant, or breastfeeding.
- Instruct patient not to take any prescription or OTC medications, herbal preparations, or dietary supplements unless advised by health care provider.
- Advise patient that follow-up visits will be required to monitor therapy and to keep appointments.

Quinapril Hydrochloride

(KWIN-uh-PRILL HIGH-droe-KLOR-ide)

Class Antihypertensive/Angiotensin-converting enzyme (ACE) inhibitor

How Supplied

Accupril Tablets 5 mg, Tablets 10 mg, Tablets 20 mg, Tablets 40 mg

Action

PHARMACOLOGY: Competitively inhibits angiotensin I-converting enzyme, resulting in prevention of angiotensin I conversion to angiotensin II, a potent vasoconstrictor that also stimulates aldosterone release. Clinical consequences are decrease in BP, reduced sodium resorption, and potassium retention.

PHARMACOKINETICS/DYNAMICS:

Absorption: T_{max} is 1 hr for the parent drug, quinapril. T_{max} is 2 hr for the metabolite, quinaprilat. Food decreases rate 25% and extent of absorption 30% when administered with a high-fat meal.

Distribution: Protein binding is about 97%.

Metabolism: De-esterified to major active metabolite quinaprilat (about 38% of dose).

Excretion: Renal (96% of quinaprilat) IV dose. The t½ accumulation is about 3 hr for quinaprilat; t½ elimination is about 2 hr for quinaprilat; and t½ prolonged terminal phase is about 25 hr for quinaprilat.

Onset: Within 1 hr.

Peak: 2 to 4 hr.

Duration: 24 hr.

Special Populations:

Renal Function Impairment – When Ccr decreases, the elimination t½ increases for quinaprilat.

Elderly – Elimination of quinaprilat is decreased.

Heart failure – Elimination of quinaprilat is decreased.

Alcoholic cirrhosis – Quinaprilat concentrations are decreased because of impaired de-esterification of quinapril.

Indications Treatment of hypertension; adjunctive therapy of CHF.

Contraindications Hypersensitivity to ACE inhibitors; history of angioedema related to previous treatment with an ACE inhibitor.

Route/Dosage

CHF

ADULTS: **PO** 5 mg bid initially; may increase dose weekly for clinical control, usually 20 to 40 mg in 2 equally divided doses.

RENAL FUNCTION IMPAIRMENT: Initial dose is 5 mg with Ccr more than 30 mL/min or 2.5 mg with Ccr 10 to 30 mL/min. If well tolerated, it may be given the following day as a bid regimen. In the absence of excessive hypotension or significant deterioration of renal function, the dose may be increased at weekly intervals based on clinical and hemodynamic response.

Hypertension

ADULTS: **PO** 10 or 20 mg qd initially; adjust dosage at intervals of at least 2 wk.

ADULTS (MAINTENANCE): **PO** 20, 40, or 80 mg/day as single dose or 2 equally divided doses.

ELDERLY: **PO** 10 mg qd followed by titration to the optimal response.

RENAL FUNCTION IMPAIRMENT: Initial dose varies based on Ccr: more than 60 mL/min is 10 mg; 30 to 60 mL/min is 5 mg; 10 to 30 mL/min is 2.5 mg.

Interactions

Antacids: Quinapril bioavailability may be decreased. Separate administration times by 1 to 2 hr.

Capsaicin: Cough may be exacerbated.

Digoxin: May cause increased or decreased digoxin levels.

Diuretics: Increased risk of hypotension.

Food: Food (especially fat) reduces bioavailability of quinapril.

Indomethacin, salicylates (eg, aspirin): May reduce hypotensive effects, especially in low renin or volume-dependent hypertensive patients.

Lithium: May cause increased lithium levels and symptoms of lithium toxicity.

Loop diuretics: Effects of loop diuretics may be decreased.

Phenothiazines: Enhanced hypotensive effect.

Potassium supplements and potassium-sparing diuretics: Hyperkalemia.

Tetracycline: Decreased tetracycline absorption.

Lab Test Interferences False elevation of liver enzymes, serum bilirubin, uric acid, and blood glucose may occur.

Adverse Reactions

CV: Hypotension (3%).

CNS: Dizziness (8%); headache (6%); fatigue (3%).

DERM: Rash (1%).

GI: Nausea, vomiting, diarrhea (2%).

HEMA: Neutropenia; agranulocytosis.

LABTESTABS: BUN (11%); serum creatinine (8%).

METAB: Hyperkalemia (2%).

RESP: Cough (4%).

OTHER: Chest pain (2%); abdominal pain, back pain (1%); angioedema (0.1%); anaphylactoid reactions.

> **WARNING:**
> *Pregnancy:* Use in second and third trimesters may cause injury and death to fetus.

Precautions
Pregnancy: Category D (second, third trimester); category C (first trimester). Avoid use in pregnant patients and discontinue drug as soon as pregnancy is detected; closely observe infants with histories of in utero exposure.
Lactation: Undetermined.
Children: Safety and efficacy not established.
Elderly: May show higher peak blood levels of metabolite.
Renal function impairment: May further decrease renal function with elevations in BUN and serum creatinine because of decreased renal perfusion. Furthermore, dosage should be reduced to compensate for reduced drug elimination.
Hepatic function impairment: Use drug with caution; dosage reduction may be necessary because of impaired metabolism.

PATIENT CARE CONSIDERATIONS
Administration/Storage
- Administer alone or in combination with other antihypertensives.
- Do not administer to pregnant women during second and third trimesters as fetal and neonatal morbidity and death can occur.
- Give prescribed dose without regard to meals. Administer with food if GI upset occurs.
- Store tablets at controlled room temperature (59° to 89°F). Protect from light.

Assessment/Interventions
- Obtain patient history, including drug history and any known allergies. Note renal or hepatic impairment, conditions predisposing to volume depletion (eg, prolonged diuretic therapy), diabetes, heart failure, anuria, hereditary or idiopathic angioedema, lupus erythematosus, left ventricular outflow obstruction, allergy to any other ACE inhibitor, and concurrent use of potassium-containing salt substitutes, potassium supplements, or potassium-sparing diuretics.
- Ensure that small initial dose and gradual escalation of dose are used in patient with heart failure or moderate to severe renal impairment (Ccr less than 60 mL/min) or following vigorous diuresis.
- Ensure that patient at risk of excessive hypotension or complications from hypotension (eg, ischemic heart or cerebrovascular disease) is closely monitored for the first 2 wk after starting therapy and following dosing escalation.

Angioedema: May occur and is potentially fatal if laryngeal edema occurs. Intestinal angioedema has occurred. Use drug with extreme caution in patients with hereditary angioedema.
Cough: Chronic cough may occur during treatment; more common in women.
Hepatic failure: Rarely, ACE inhibitors have been associated with a syndrome that starts with cholestatic jaundice and progresses to fulminant hepatic necrosis and sometimes death.
Hypotension/first-dose effect: Significant decreases in BP may occur after first dose, especially in severely salt- or volume-depleted patients (eg, patients on aggressive diuretic therapy) or in those with heart failure.
Neutropenia and agranulocytosis: Have occurred rarely; risk appears greater with renal dysfunction, heart failure, or immunosuppression.
Proteinuria: Has occurred with similar agents, especially with high doses or prior renal disease.

Overdosage: Signs and Symptoms
Hypotension.

- Ensure that volume and/or salt depletion have been corrected before initiating therapy.
- Ensure that serum electrolytes and renal function are monitored periodically.
- Ensure that CBC with differential are evaluated prior to starting therapy, at 2 wk intervals for 3 mo, and then periodically thereafter in patient with renal impairment.
- Monitor and record BP and pulse. Should symptomatic hypotension occur, hold medication and notify health care provider.
- Take safety precautions if orthostatic hypotension occurs.
- Assess heart failure patient for evidence of worsening failure (eg, daily weights, evaluation of peripheral edema, shortness of breath). Inform health care provider if rapid weight gain (eg, 2 pounds in 1 day or 5 pounds in 1 wk) is noted or if patient is experiencing worsening edema or other symptoms of heart failure (eg, worsening shortness of breath).
- Monitor for signs of hypersensitivity including angioedema involving swelling of the face, lips, eyelids, and tongue. Discontinue medication and notify health care provider immediately if noted. Be prepared to treat appropriately.
- Assess patient for GI, CNS, and general body side effects. Inform health care provider if noted and significant.

Patient/Family Education
- Explain name, dose, action, and potential side effects of drug.
- Advise patient to take prescribed dose without regard to meals but to take with food if stomach upset occurs.
- Advise patient to try to take each dose at about the same time each day
- Inform hypertensive patient that drug controls, but does not cure, hypertension and to continue taking drug as prescribed even when BP is not elevated.
- Caution patient not to change the dose or stop taking unless advised by health care provider.
- Instruct patient to continue taking other medications for condition as prescribed by health care provider.
- Instruct patient in BP and pulse measurement skills.
- Advise patient to monitor and record BP and pulse at home and to inform health care provider should abnormal measurements be noted. Also advise patient to take record of BP and pulse to each follow-up visit.
- Caution patient to avoid sudden position changes to prevent orthostatic hypotension.
- Instruct patient to lie or sit down if experiencing dizziness or lightheadedness when standing.
- Emphasize to hypertensive patient the importance of the following other modalities on BP control: weight control, regular exercise, smoking cessation, and moderate intake of alcohol and salt.
- Emphasize to heart failure patient the importance of the following other modalities that can help control heart failure symptoms: weight control, progressive exercise program, smoking cessation, and moderate intake of alcohol and salt.
- Advise heart failure patient to weigh daily, keep a record of daily weights, and notify health care provider if rapid weight gain (eg, 5 pounds in 1 wk) is noted or if edema or shortness of breath worsen.
- Caution patient that inadequate fluid intake, excessive perspiration, diarrhea, or vomiting can lead to excessive fall in BP resulting in lightheadedness or fainting.
- Advise patient that medication may cause dizziness or lightheadedness and to use caution while driving or performing other tasks requiring mental alertness until tolerance is determined.
- Caution patient to avoid unnecessary exposure to UV light (sunlight, tanning booths) and to use sunscreen and wear protective clothing when exposed to UV light to avoid photosensitivity reaction.
- Advise women to notify health care provider if pregnant, planning to become pregnant, or breastfeeding.
- Instruct patient to stop taking drug and immediately report any of the following symptoms to health care provider: sore throat, fever, swelling of the hands or feet, irregular heartbeat, chest pains, fainting, swelling of the face, lips, eyelids, or tongue, difficulty breathing
- Instruct patient to inform health care provider if a persistent cough develops while taking this medication.
- Caution patient not to take any prescription or OTC medications, potassium-containing salt substitutes, potassium supplements, or dietary supplements unless advised by health care provider.
- Advise patient that follow-up visits and lab tests will be required to monitor therapy and to keep appointments.

Quinapril Hydrochloride/ Hydrochlorothiazide (HCTZ)

(KWIN-uh-PRILL HIGH-droe-KLOR-ide/ high-droe-klor-THIGH-uh-zide)

Class Antihypertensive combination

How Supplied
Accuretic Tablets 10 mg quinapril/12.5 mg HCTZ, Tablets 20 mg quinapril/12.5 mg HCTZ, Tablets 20 mg quinapril/25 mg HCTZ

Action

PHARMACOLOGY:

Quinapril: Competitively inhibits angiotensin I-converting enzyme, resulting in the prevention of angiotensin I conversion to angiotensin II, a potent vasoconstrictor that stimulates aldosterone secretion. This action results in a decrease in sodium and fluid retention, an increase in diuresis, and a decrease in BP.

Hydrochlorothiazide (HCTZ): Increases chloride, sodium, and water excretion by interfering with transport of sodium ions across renal tubular epithelium.

Indications Treatment of hypertension.

Contraindications Patients with a history of angioedema related to previous treatment with an ACE inhibitor; patients with anuria; hypersensitivity to sulfonamide-derived drugs or any component of the product.

Route/Dosage

The fixed combination is not indicated for initial therapy. The combination may be substituted for the titrated components.

ADULTS: **PO** Quinapril monotherapy is an effective treatment of hypertension over a dose range of 10 to 80 mg/day administered qd. HCTZ is effective in doses of 12.5 to 50 mg qd. Patients whose BP is not adequately controlled with quinapril monotherapy may be given quinapril/HCTZ (10/12.5 or 20/12.5). Further increases in dose of either or both components depend on the clinical response. Generally, the dose of HCTZ should not be increased until 2 to 3 wk have elapsed.

Renal Function Impairment

ADULTS: No adjustment required as long as Ccr is greater than 30 mL/min; in severe renal impairment, loop diuretics are preferred to thiazides.

Interactions

ACTH, corticosteroids: Electrolyte depletion may be intensified, especially hypokalemia.
Alcohol, barbiturates (eg, phenobarbital), narcotics: Orthostatic hypotension may be potentiated.
Anticoagulants (eg, warfarin): Anticoagulant effect may be decreased.
Antidiabetic agents (eg, insulin, sulfonylureas), antigout agents (eg, probenecid): Dosage adjustment may be necessary because of possible HCTZ-induced elevation in blood glucose levels.
Cardiac glycosides (eg, digoxin): Possible digitalis toxicity associated with hypokalemia.
Cholestyramine, colestipol: May impair the absorption of HCTZ.
Insulin: In diabetic patients, requirements of insulin may be increased, decreased, or unchanged.
Lithium: Plasma levels of lithium may be elevated, increasing the risk of toxicity.
NSAIDs: May reduce the natriuretic and antihypertensive effect of HCTZ.
Potassium supplements, potassium-sparing diuretics (eg, spironolactone): Increased risk of hyperkalemia.
Nondepolarizing muscle relaxants (eg, tubocurarine): Effects may be increased.
Pressor amines (eg, norepinephrine): Response to pressor amines may be decreased.
Tetracycline and other drugs that interact with magnesium: Because of the magnesium content in quinapril, absorption of tetracycline may be reduced, decreasing the therapeutic effect.

Lab Test Interferences

HCTZ: May decrease serum protein-bound iodine levels without signs of thyroid disturbances.

Adverse Reactions

CV: Bradycardia; cor pulmonale; vasculitis; deep thrombosis; vasodilatation; chest pain.
Quinapril – Syncope.
HCTZ – Orthostatic hypotension.
CNS: Dizziness; somnolence; paralysis; hemiplegia; speech disorder; abnormal gait; meningism; amnesia; headache; fatigue; insomnia; vertigo; asthenia.
Quinapril – Depression.
HCTZ – Lightheadedness; paresthesia; weakness; restlessness.
DERM: Urticaria; macropapular rash; petechiases.
EENT: Esophagitis; abnormal vision; rhinitis.
Quinapril – Amblyopia.
HCTZ – Transient blurred vision; xanthopsia.
GI: GI carcinoma; vomiting diarrhea; nausea; abdominal pain; constipation; dyspepsia.
HCTZ – Pancreatitis; sialadenitis; diarrhea; cramping; gastric irritation; anorexia.
GU: Abnormal kidney function; albuminuria; pyuria; hematuria; nephrosis.
HCTZ – Renal failure; renal dysfunction; interstitial nephritis.
HEMA: Anemia.
HCTZ – Aplastic anemia; agranulocytosis; leukopenia; thrombocytopenia; hemolytic anemia.
HEPA: Cholestatic jaundice; hepatitis.
HCTZ – Jaundice (intrahepatic cholestatic).
METAB: Weight loss.
HCTZ – Hyperglycemia; glucosuria; hyperuricemia; hypokalemia; hyponatremia; hypochloremic alkalosis.
RESP: Coughing; pneumonia; asthma; respiratory infiltration; lung disorder; upper respiratory tract infection; bronchitis.
OTHER: Shock; accidental injury; neoplasm; cellulitis; ascites; generalized edema; hernia; myopathy; myositis; arthritis; myalgia; viral infection; angioedema.
Quinapril – Back pain; anaphylactoid reactions.
HCTZ – Muscle spasm; hypersensitivity (including necrotizing angiitis, Stevens-Johnson syndrome, respiratory distress [including pneumonia and pulmonary edema], purpura, urticaria, rash, and photosensitivity).

Precautions

Pregnancy: Category D (second and third trimester); Category C (first trimester). ACE inhibitors (eg, quinapril) can cause injury or death to fetus if used during second or third trimester. When pregnancy is detected, discontinue as soon as possible.
Lactation: Excreted in breast milk.
Children: Safety and efficacy not established.
Elderly: Select dose with caution, reflecting greater frequency of decreased hepatic, renal, or cardiac function and comorbidity.

Renal function impairment: Use with caution.
Hepatic function impairment: Use with caution.
Anaphylactoid reactions: Reported in patients with a history of angioedema, undergoing desensitizing treatment with Hymenoptera venom, and in patients dialyzed with high-flux membranes.
Angioedema: Use with extreme caution in patients with a history of angioedema. Angioedema associated with laryngeal edema may be fatal. Angioedema may occur more frequently in black patients receiving an ACE inhibitor compared with non-black patients.
Cough: Chronic cough may occur during treatment.
Electrolyte imbalance: Treatment with thiazide diuretics has been associated with hypokalemia, hyponatremia, hypochloremic alkalosis, hypercalcemia, and hypomagnesemia. Do not initiate therapy prior to correction of imbalance.
Hepatic failure: Rarely, ACE inhibitors have been associated with a syndrome that starts with cholestatic jaundice and progresses to fulminant hepatic necrosis and death.
Hypotension: Decreases in BP may occur, especially in salt- or volume-depleted patients as a result of dialysis, prolonged diuretic therapy, dietary salt restriction, diarrhea, or vomiting. Volume and salt depletion should be corrected before initiating therapy with quinapril/HCTZ.
Metabolic disturbances: Thiazide diuretics tend to reduce glucose tolerance, raise cholesterol, triglycerides, and uric acid levels.
Neutropenia/Agranulocytosis: Has occurred with other ACE inhibitors.
Surgery/Anesthesia: In patients undergoing surgery or during anesthesia with agents that produce hypotension, angiotensin II formation, secondary to compensatory renal release, may be blocked.
Systemic Lupus Erythematosus (SLE): HCTZ may exacerbate or activate SLE.

Overdosage: Signs and Symptoms
Dehydration, electrolyte imbalance (hypokalemia [which may accentuate cardiac arrhythmias in patients receiving digitalis], hypochloremia, hyponatremia), hypotension.

PATIENT CARE CONSIDERATIONS
Administration/Storage
- Give qd in the morning with or without food.
- Administer with food if GI upset occurs.
- Administer alone or in combination with other antihypertensives.
- Do not administer to pregnant women as fetal and neonatal morbidity and death can occur.
- Store tablets at controlled room temperature (68° to 77°F). Keep container tightly closed.

Assessment/Interventions
- Obtain patient history, including drug history and any known allergies. Note history of diabetes, anuria, angioedema, lupus erythematosus, kidney or liver disease, or allergy to any other ACE inhibitor or sulfonamide-derived medications. Note concurrent use of potassium-containing salt substitutes, potassium supplements, or potassium-sparing diuretics.
- Ensure that serum electrolytes and renal function are monitored periodically.
- Ensure that volume and/or salt depletion have been corrected before initiating therapy.
- Monitor and record BP and pulse. If hypotension results, hold medication and notify health care provider.
- Take safety precautions if orthostatic hypotension occurs.
- Monitor blood sugar in diabetic patient when drug is started or dose is changed. Report significant changes to health care provider.
- Monitor for signs of hypersensitivity, including angioedema involving swelling of the face, lips, eyelids, and tongue. Discontinue medication and notify health care provider immediately if noted. Be prepared to treat appropriately.

Patient/Family Education
- Explain name, dose, action, and potential side effects of drug.
- Advise patient to take prescribed dose qd without regard to meals.
- Advise patient to try to take each dose at about the same time qd.
- Inform patient that drug controls, but does not cure, hypertension and to continue taking drug as prescribed even when BP is not elevated.
- Caution patient not to change the dose or stop taking unless advised by health care provider.
- Instruct patient to continue taking other BP medications as prescribed by health care provider.
- Instruct patient in BP and pulse measurement skills.
- Advise patient to monitor and record BP and pulse at home and to inform health care provider if abnormal measurements are noted. Also, advise patient to take record of BP and pulse to each follow-up visit.
- Caution patient to avoid sudden position changes to prevent orthostatic hypotension.
- Instruct patient to lie or sit down if experiencing dizziness or lightheadedness when standing.

- Caution patient that inadequate fluid intake, excessive perspiration, diarrhea, or vomiting can lead to excessive fall in BP resulting in lightheadedness or fainting.
- Instruct diabetic patient to monitor blood glucose more frequently when drug is started or dose is changed and to inform health care provider of significant changes in readings.
- Caution patient to avoid unnecessary exposure to UV light (sunlight, tanning booths) and to use sunscreen and wear protective clothing when exposed to UV light to avoid photosensitivity reaction.
- Emphasize to hypertensive patient importance of other modalities on BP: weight control, regular exercise, smoking cessation, and moderate intake of alcohol and salt.
- Advise women to notify health care provider if pregnant, planning to become pregnant, or breastfeeding.
- Instruct patient to stop taking drug and immediately report any of the following symptoms to health care provider: fainting, swelling of the face, lips, eyelids or tongue, difficulty breathing.
- Instruct patient to inform health care provider if a persistent cough develops while taking this medication.
- Caution patient not to take any prescription or OTC medications, potassium-containing salt substitutes, potassium supplements, or dietary supplements unless advised by health care provider.
- Advise patient that follow-up visits and lab tests may be required to monitor therapy and to keep appointments.

Quinidine

(KWIN-ih-deen)

Class Antiarrhythmic

How Supplied

Quinidine Sulfate
Quinora Tablets 300 mg
✽ Apo-Quinidine ◆ Biquin Durules

Quinidine Gluconate
Quinaglute Dura-Tabs Tablets, sustained-release 324 mg ◆ Quinalan Tablets, sustained-release 324 mg

Quinidine Polygalacturonate
Cardioquin Tablets 275 mg (equiv. to 200 mg sulfate)

Action

PHARMACOLOGY: Depresses myocardial excitability, conduction velocity and contractility; prolongs effective refractory period and increases conduction time; indirect anticholinergic effects; may decrease vagal tone at low doses paradoxically increasing conduction through the AV node.

PHARMACOKINETICS/DYNAMICS:

Absorption:
Quinidine gluconate – Rapidly absorbed from GI tract. Bioavailability is 70% to 80% (extended-release). T_{max} is 3 to 5 hr. With food, absorption is increased in both rate (27%) and extent (17%).
Quinidine sulfate – Bioavailability is about 70%, varies widely (45% to 100%) between patients. T_{max} is about 2 hr. The rate of absorption is somewhat slower when taken with food.

Distribution: Vd is 2 to 3 L/kg (healthy adults), decreased to 0.5 L/kg (CHF), increased to 3 to 5 L/kg (liver cirrhosis). Protein binding occurs in adults 80% to 88%, decreased protein binding in pregnant women, infants, and neonates (about 50% to 70%). Protein binding is increased in chronic renal failure.

Metabolism: Occurs in the liver (60% to 80%) to some active metabolites, mainly to the active 3-hydroxy-quinidine (3HQ).

Excretion: T½ is 6 to 8 hr (adult), 3 to 5 hr (children), and 12 hr (3HQ). Cl is 3 to 5 mL/min/kg (adult), may be 2 to 3 times as rapid in children. Elimination occurs in the urine (20% unchanged). Urine acidification increases excretion, alkalinization decreases excretion.

Special Populations:
Renal Function Impairment – Vd and renal Cl may be reduced.
Elderly – Elimination t½ may be increased.
CHF – Total Cl and Vd are decreased.
Hepatic cirrhosis – Elimination t½ may be prolonged and increase Vd.

Indications Treatment of premature atrial, atrioventricular junctional, and ventricular contractions; treatment of paroxysmal supraventricular tachycardia, paroxysmal atrioventricular junctional rhythm, atrial flutter, paroxysmal and chronic atrial fibrillation, and paroxysmal ventricular tachycardia not associated with complete heart block; maintenance therapy after electrical conversion of atrial fibrillation or flutter.
Quinidine gluconate (IV administration): Treatment of life-threatening Plasmodium falciparum malaria.

Contraindications Myasthenia gravis; history of thrombocytopenic purpura associated with quinidine administration; digitalis intoxication; complete heart block; left bundle branch block; complete atrioventricular (AV) block with AV nodal or idioventricular pacemaker; aberrant ectopic impulses and abnormal rhythms because of escape mechanisms; history of drug-induced torsade de pointes; history of long QT syndrome.

Route/Dosage

The following oral doses are expressed as quinidine sulfate salt:

Premature Atrial and Ventricular Contractions
ADULTS: PO 200 to 300 mg tid/qid.
CHILDREN: PO 30 mg/kg/day or 900 mg/m^2/day in 5 divided doses.

Paroxysmal Supraventricular Tachycardia
ADULTS: PO 400 to 600 mg q 2 to 3 hr until event is abated.

Atrial Flutter
Administer after digitalization and individualize dose.

Conversion of Atrial Fibrillation
ADULTS: PO 200 mg q 2 to 3 hr for 5 to 8 doses, then maintain with 200 to 300 mg tid to qid (immediate-release tablets) or 300 to 600 mg bid to tid (sustained-release tablets); do not exceed 3 to 4 g/day.

QUINIDINE GLUCONATE
ADULTS: PO 324 to 648 mg (1 to 2 tablets) q 8 to 12 hr.

QUINIDINE POLYGALACTURONATE
ADULTS: PO Maintenance dose: 275 mg q 8 to 12 hr.

PARENTERAL QUINIDINE GLUCONATE
Acute Tachycardia
Adults: IM 600 mg initially, then 400 mg prn up to q 2 hr.
Children: IV 2 to 10 mg/kg/dose q 3 to 6 hr prn.

P. falciparum Malaria
ADULTS: IV 15 mg/kg infused over 4 hr initially, then 7.5 mg/kg over 4 hr q 8 hr for 7 days or until oral therapy can be instituted or 10 mg/kg over 1 to 2 hr initially, then 0.02 mg/kg/min for up to 72 hr or until oral therapy can be instituted.

Interactions

Amiodarone, antacids, cimetidine, verapamil: May increase quinidine levels.
Anticoagulants: May increase effect of anticoagulant; may cause hemorrhage.
Barbiturates, nifedipine, primidone, sucralfate: May decrease quinidine levels.
Beta-blockers: May increase effect of beta-blocker.
Dextromethorphan: May increase plasma dextromethorphan concentrations.
Digitoxin, digoxin: May increase digoxin plasma levels.
Hydantoins: May reduce therapeutic effect of quinidine.
Nondepolarizing neuromuscular blocking agents, succinylcholine: May increase neuromuscular blockade effect.
Propafenone: Increased propafenone levels.
Rifampin: May increase quinidine metabolism.

Lab Test Interferences Triamterene will interfere with the fluorescent measurement of quinidine levels.

Adverse Reactions

CV: Widening of QRS complex; cardiac asystole; ventricular ectopy; hypotension; paradoxical tachycardia.
CNS: Headache; fever; vertigo; excitement; confusion; delirium; syncope.
DERM: Rash; urticaria; pruritus; flushing; photosensitivity.
EENT: Mydriasis; blurred vision; photophobia, diplopia, night blindness; tinnitus.
GI: Nausea; vomiting; anorexia; abdominal pain; diarrhea.
GU: Lupus nephritis.
HEMA: Acute hemolytic anemia; agranulocytosis; thrombocytopenic purpura.
HEPA: Hepatitis.
OTHER: Lupus erythematosus-like syndrome; cinchonism (headache, tinnitus, nausea, disturbed vision, deafness, dizziness, vertigo, lightheadedness); hypersensitivity reactions; arthralgia; myalgia.

> **WARNING:**
> Mortality rates increased when used to treat non-life-threatening arrhythmias.

Precautions

Pregnancy: Category C.
Lactation: Excreted in breast milk.
Children: Safety and efficacy not established.
Hypersensitivity: May occur; administer single 200 mg tablet of quinidine sulfate or 200 mg IM injection of quinidine gluconate before starting therapy to determine if patient has idiosyncrasy to quinidine.
Renal function impairment: Use drug with caution because of potential for toxicity.
Hepatic function impairment: Use drug with caution because of potential for toxicity.
Atrial flutter or fibrillation: Pretreat these patients with digitalis preparation.
Bioequivalence: Different salts have different amounts of quinidine base. Do not interchange without taking this into consideration.
Cardiotoxicity: May occur; immediately discontinue drug.
Hepatotoxicity (including granulomatous hepatitis): Has occurred. Consider possibility if unexplained fever or elevated hepatic enzymes develop.
Malaria: Dose schedules may result in hypotension, ECG changes, and cinchonism.
Parenteral therapy: Use only when oral therapy is not possible or when rapid therapeutic effect is required.

Potassium balance: Effect of quinidine is enhanced by potassium and reduced if hypokalemia is present.
Cardiac impairment: Use drug with caution because of potential for toxicity.
Syncope: Occasionally occurs in patients on long-term therapy; may be fatal. Often caused by torsades de pointes.
Vagolytic effects: May antagonize vagal maneuvers or administration of cholinergic drugs used to terminate paroxysmal supraventricular tachycardia.

Overdosage: Signs and Symptoms
Cardiorespiratory depression, lethargy, confusion, coma, seizures, headache, paresthesia, vertigo, vomiting, abdominal pain, diarrhea, nausea, tachyarrhythmias, depressed automaticity and conduction, hypotension, syncope, heart failure, cinchonism, hypokalemia, visual/auditory disturbances, tinnitus, acidosis.

PATIENT CARE CONSIDERATIONS
Administration/Storage
- Use IV route only when rapid response is needed or oral route is not feasible.
- Give test dose of 200 mg as ordered to evaluate intolerance/sensitivity.
- Position patient supine during IV administration to minimize hypotension.
- For direct IV push, administer slowly at 1 mL/min.
- For intermittent IV infusion, dilute 800 mg/50 mL or more with D5W; give at a rate of 16 mg/min or less. Use infusion device for accuracy/safety.
- Administer IM injection in deltoid muscle.
- Give oral preparation with full glass of water on empty stomach (1 hr before or 2 hr after other medication) to enhance absorption; if GI distress develops, administer with or just after meal.
- Do not break or crush or allow patient to chew sustained-release preparations. Instruct patient to swallow whole.
- Store vial at room temperature. Parenteral solution must be clear and colorless. Solution is stable for 24 hr.
- Store tablets in tight, light-resistant container.

Assessment/Interventions
- Obtain patient history, including drug history and any known allergies.
- Determine if patient has myasthenia gravis.
- When drug is used as antiarrhythmic agent, assess ECG prior to and continuously throughout therapy. Therapy is discontinued if severe heart block occurs (50% widening of QRS complex, PR, or QT interval are prolonged) or tachycardia or frequent ventricular ectopic beats develops.
- Obtain baseline BP and pulse and assess continuously during therapy.
- Monitor CBC and hepatic and renal function tests during long-term therapy.
- When drug is used as antimalarial agent, monitor BP, ECG, and plasma quinidine levels closely during therapy, especially if drug is being administered parenterally.
- If patient had been receiving digoxin, measure digoxin concentration to ensure it does not increase to toxic levels.
- Observe for hypotension, tachycardia, and arrhythmias.

Patient/Family Education
- Instruct patient/family to administer medication around clock as directed and to continue taking medication even if symptoms improve.
- Advise patient to take with food if GI upset occurs.
- Tell patient that sustained-release tablet should not be crushed or chewed.
- Instruct patient/family how to take pulse. Advise them to check pulse prior to each dose and to contact health care provider if rate or rhythm changes.
- Advise patient to carry identification (eg, Medi-Alert) indicating disease and drug therapy at all times.
- Advise patient to notify other health care providers/dentist prior to other therapy/surgery.
- Emphasize importance of regular medical follow-up, even in absence of side effects or problems related to this drug therapy.
- Caution patient to wear dark glasses as needed to decrease light sensitivity and inform patient that dark glasses may be needed both indoors and outside.
- Instruct patient to report the following symptoms to health care provider immediately: visual disturbances (eg, blurring), tinnitus, bleeding, bruising, fever, headache, dizziness, severe diarrhea, or skin rash/eruption.
- Advise patient that drug causes dizziness and blurred vision and to use caution while driving or performing other tasks requiring mental alertness.
- Caution patient to avoid exposure to sunlight and to use sunscreen or wear protective clothing to avoid photosensitivity reaction.
- Instruct patient not to take OTC medications without consulting health care provider.

Quinine Sulfate

(KWIE-nine SULL-fate)

Class Anti-infective/Antimalarial

How Supplied
Quinine sulfate Capsules 200 mg, Capsules 260 mg, Capsules 325 mg, Tablets 260 mg
✤ Quinine-Odan

Action
PHARMACOLOGY: Causes pH elevation in intracellular organelles of parasites; also has skeletal muscle relaxant effects and cardiovascular effects similar to those of quinidine.

PHARMACOKINETICS/DYNAMICS:
Absorption: Complete and readily absorbed PO, mainly from upper small intestines. T_{max} is 1 to 3 hr (single dose). Bioavailability is about 80%.
Distribution: Protein binding is 70% to 85%, increases up to more than 90% in patients with cerebral malaria, pregnant women, and children. Crosses placenta and into fetal tissues and CSF. Vd is about 1.2 L/kg (cerebral malaria in adult patients), 1.7 L/kg (adult uncomplicated malaria), and 0.8 L/kg (children with uncomplicated malaria).
Metabolism: Metabolized in the liver. Metabolites have less activity than the parent drug.
Excretion: Occurs in the urine (less than 5% as unchanged), metabolites excreted in urine mainly as hydroxy derivatives, small amounts appear in feces, gastric juice, and bile. Urine excretion of drug is twice as fast as when urine is acidic.

Indications Treatment of chloroquine-resistant falciparum malaria; alternative treatment for chloroquine-sensitive strains of *P. falciparum*, *P. malariae*, *P. ovale*, and *P. vivax*.

Unlabeled use(s): Prevention and treatment of nocturnal recumbency leg cramps.

Contraindications G-6-PD deficiency; optic neuritis; tinnitus; history of blackwater fever and thrombocytopenic purpura associated with previous quinine ingestion; pregnancy.

Route/Dosage
Chloroquine-resistant P. falciparum Malaria
ADULTS: PO 650 mg q 8 hr for 5 to 7 days.
CHILDREN: PO 25 mg/kg/day in divided doses q 8 hr for 5 to 7 days.
Chloroquine-Sensitive Malaria
ADULTS: PO 600 mg q 8 hr for 5 to 7 days.
CHILDREN: PO 10 mg/kg q 8 hr for 5 to 7 days.
Nocturnal Leg Cramps
ADULTS: PO 260 to 300 mg at bedtime.

Interactions
Aluminum-containing antacids: Causes delayed or decreased quinine absorption.
Anticoagulants, oral: May cause depression of hepatic enzyme system that synthesizes vitamin K-dependent clotting factors and may enhance action of oral anticoagulants.
Cimetidine: May reduce quinine's clearance and prolong its half-life in body.
Digoxin: May cause increased digoxin serum concentration.
Mefloquine: May cause ECG abnormalities or cardiac arrest and may increase risk of convulsions. Do not use concurrently. Delay administration 12 hr after last dose of quinine.
Neuromuscular blocking agents: May potentiate neuromuscular blockade and may result in respiratory difficulties.
Urinary alkalinizers: May increase quinine serum concentrations and potentiate toxicity.

Lab Test Interferences Urinary 17-ketogenic steroids may have elevated values with Zimmerman method.

Adverse Reactions
CV: Anginal symptoms.
CNS: Vertigo; dizziness; headache; fever; apprehension; restlessness; confusion; syncope; excitement; delirium; hypothermia; seizures.
EENT: Visual disturbances (eg, photophobia, blurred vision with scotomata, night blindness, amblyopia, diplopia, diminished visual fields, mydriasis, optic atrophy) tinnitus; deafness.
GI: Nausea; vomiting; diarrhea; epigastric pain.
GU: Renal tubular damage; anuria.
HEMA: Acute hemolysis; hemolytic anemia; thrombocytopenic purpura; agranulocytosis; hypoprothrombinemia.
HEPA: Hepatitis.
OTHER: Cinchonism (headache, tinnitus, nausea, diarrhea, disturbed vision, skin, CV and CNS symptoms at very high doses); hypersensitivity (rash, pruritus, flushing, sweating, facial edema, asthmatic symptoms).

Precautions
Pregnancy: Category X.
Lactation: Excreted in breast milk.
Cardiac disease: Patients with cardiac arrhythmias may have exacerbation of symptoms with quinine, which acts similarly to quinidine. May cause cardiotoxicity. In patients with atrial fibrillation, quinine requires same precautions as for quinidine.
Hemolysis: Has been associated with G-6-PD deficiency. Discontinue immediately if hemolysis appears.

Overdosage: Signs and Symptoms
Tinnitus, dizziness, skin rash, GI disturbance, diarrhea, arrhythmias, convulsions, blurred vision, headache, nausea/vomiting, fever, confusion.

PATIENT CARE CONSIDERATIONS
Administration/Storage
- Give with food or after meals to minimize GI irritation; give bedtime dose with milk or snack.
- Administer around clock (q 8 hr) to maintain serum drug levels if being used to treat malaria.
- Administer at bedtime if being used to treat or prevent nocturnal leg cramps.
- Do not crush tablets; have patient swallow tablets whole.
- Store in tight, light-resistant container.

Assessment/Interventions
- Obtain patient history, including drug history and any known allergies.
- Determine whether patient has any contraindications to quinine (eg, G-6PD deficiency, pregnancy).
- Obtain baseline ECG, hepatic studies, and CBC prior to therapy.
- Assess pulse and ECG during therapy to detect arrhythmias.
- Assess for evidence of hematological abnormalities (eg, sore throat, fever, bleeding/bruising, fatigue, weakness).
- Assess for the following signs of cinchonism: blurred vision, headache, tinnitus, vertigo, lightheadedness, nausea. Report these adverse effects immediately to the health care provider.

Patient/Family Education
- Caution patient that this medication must not be taken during pregnancy or when pregnancy is possible. Advise patient to use reliable form of birth control while taking this drug.
- If medication is being used to treat malaria, advise patient to take medication around clock and to take full course of treatment even if feeling better.
- Emphasize importance of medical follow-up when this course of therapy has been completed to ensure that therapy has been successful.
- If medication is being used to treat nocturnal leg cramps, advise patient to take drug before bedtime.
- Instruct patient to consult health care provider before combining any new medications with this drug.
- Advise patient to take medication with or after meals or snack to minimize GI distress.
- Instruct patient to report the following symptoms to the health care provider: flushing, itching, rash, fever, difficulty breathing, vision problems, ringing in ears, diarrhea, nausea/vomiting, vertigo.
- Advise patient that drug may cause dizziness and vision problems, and to use caution while driving or performing other tasks requiring mental alertness.
- Instruct patient not to take OTC medications (especially cold preparations) without consulting health care provider.

Quinupristin/Dalfopristin

(kwih-NEW-priss-tin/dal-FOE-priss-tin)

Class Anti-infective/Streptogramin

How Supplied
Synercid Injection, lyophilized 500 mg (150 mg quinupristin; 350 mg dalfopristin)/10 mL

Action
PHARMACOLOGY: Quinupristin inhibits the late phase of protein synthesis; dalfopristin inhibits the early phase of protein synthesis.

Indications Treatment of serious or life-threatening infections associated with VREF; treatment of complicated skin and skin structure infections caused by *Staphylococcus aureus* (methicillin-susceptible) or *Streptococcus pyogenes*.

Contraindications Hypersensitivity to any component of product or prior hypersensitivity to other streptogramins.

Route/Dosage
VREF
ADULTS AND CHILDREN (16 YR AND OLDER):
IV 7.5 mg/kg, infused over a 60-min period, q 8 hr. Duration of therapy based on site and severity of infection.

Complicated Skin and Skin Structure Infection
ADULTS AND CHILDREN (16 YR AND OLDER):
IV 7.5 mg/kg, infused over a 60-min period, q 12 hr for at least 7 days.

Interactions
Drugs metabolized by cytochrome P450 3A4 (CYP3A4) enzyme system (eg, carbamazepine, cisapride, cyclosporine, delavirdine, diazepam, diltiazem, disopyramide, HMG-CoA reductase inhibitors [eg, simvastatin], docetaxel, indinavir, lidocaine, methylprednisolone, midazolam, nevirapine, nifedipine, paclitaxel, quinidine, ritonavir, tacrolimus, verapamil, vinca alkaloids [eg, vinblastine]): Plasma concentrations of these agents may be elevated, increasing or prolonging

their therapeutic or adverse effects. Avoid drugs metabolized by CYP3A4 and that prolong the QTc interval.

INCOMPATIBILITIES: Saline solutions.

Lab Test Interferences None well documented.

Adverse Reactions

CV: Thrombophlebitis; palpitations; phlebitis; vasodilation.
CNS: Headache.
DERM: Pain, edema and inflammation at infusion site; rash; pruritus.
GI: Nausea; diarrhea; vomiting.
GU: Hematuria.
OTHER: Pain; abdominal pain; leg cramps; allergic reactions; chest pain.

> **WARNING:**
> One of quinupristin/dalfopristin's approved indications is for the treatment of patients with serious of life-threatening infections associated with VREF bacteremia. Quinupristin/dalfopristin has been approved for this indication under the FDA's accelerated approval regulations.

Precautions

Pregnancy: Category B.
Lactation: Undetermined.
Children: Safety and efficacy in children less than 16 yr not established.
Superinfection: May result in bacterial or fungal overgrowth of nonsusceptible microorganisms.
Pseudomembranous colitis: Consider in patients who develop diarrhea.

PATIENT CARE CONSIDERATIONS

Administration/Storage

- For IV administration only. Not for intradermal, SC, or IM administration.
- Follow manufacturer's instructions for reconstituting the Powder for Injection and subsequent further dilution.
- Dilute reconstituted solution within 30 min of reconstitution.
- Do not administer if particulate matter, cloudiness, or discoloration noted.
- Administer IV infusion over 60 min.
- After completing IV infusion, flush vein with 5% Dextrose in Water to minimize vein irritation.
- If other drugs are being administered through same IV line, flush IV line before and after infusion of quinupristin/dalfopristin with 5% Dextrose in Water solution.
- Store vials in refrigerator (36° to 46°F). Store diluted solution for up to 5 hr at room temperature or 54 hr under refrigeration (36° to 46°F).

Assessment/Interventions

- Obtain patient history, including drug history and any known allergies. Note history of hypersensitivity to quinupristin/dalfopristin or other streptogramins.
- Review results of culture and sensitivity testing as available.
- Assess venous access site for irritation. If moderate to severe irritation noted, change infusion site or infuse by peripherally inserted central catheter (PICC) or central venous catheter.
- Monitor for signs of infection and for positive response to antibiotic therapy.
- Monitor patient for signs and symptoms of anaphylactic or serious allergic reaction. Immediately discontinue infusion, notify health care provider, and be prepared to treat appropriately.
- Monitor patient for GI, CNS, and general body side effects. Report to health care provider if noted and significant.

Patient/Family Education

- Explain name, dose, action, and potential side effects of drug.
- Advise patient, family, or caregiver that medication will be prepared and administered by a health care provider in a health care setting.
- Review dosing schedule and prescribed length of therapy with patient, family, or caregiver. Advise patient that dose and duration of therapy are dependent on site and cause of infection.
- Advise patient that infusion site reaction, muscle pain, and joint pain are the most common side effects, and to inform health care provider if they occur and are intolerable.
- Advise patient to report the following signs of superinfection to health care provider: black "furry" tongue, white patches in mouth, foul-smelling stools, vaginal itching, or discharge.
- Warn patient, family, or caregiver that diarrhea containing blood or pus may be a sign of a serious disorder and to inform health care provider if noted.

Rabeprazole Sodium

(ra-BE-pray-zole)

Class Gastrointestinal/Proton Pump Inhibitor

How Supplied
Aciphex Tablets, delayed-release 20 mg
✤ *Pariet*

Action
PHARMACOLOGY: Suppresses gastric acid secretion by blocking "acid (proton) pump" within gastric parietal cells.

PHARMACOKINETICS/DYNAMICS:
Absorption: T_{max} is 2 to 5 hr. Oral bioavailability is about 52%.

Distribution: Protein binding is 96.3%.

Metabolism: Extensively metabolized in liver by CYP3A to sulfone metabolite and CYP2C19 to desmethyl rabeprazole. Thioether metabolite is formed by reduction of rabeprazole. These metabolites do not have significant antisecretory activity. Poor metabolizers of rabeprazole, CYP2C19 exhibits genetic polymorphism due to its deficiency (white 3% to 5%; Asians 17% to 20%).

Excretion: Plasma $t_{1/2}$ is 1 to 2 hr. Eliminated in urine (90% as thioether carboxylic acid, glucuronide and mercapturic acid); its remainder recovered in feces. No unchanged drug recovered.

Special Populations:
Hepatic Function Impairment – For chronic mild to moderate, AUC approximately doubled, elimination $t_{1/2}$ was 2 to 3 fold higher, total clearance decreased to less than half. For mild to moderate, C_{max} increased about 20% (not significant).
Elderly – AUC values doubled, C_{max} decreased 60%.

Indications
Short-term treatment in healing and symptomatic relief of duodenal ulcers and erosive or ulcerative gastroesophageal reflux disease (GERD); maintaining healing and reducing relapse rates of heartburn symptoms in patients with GERD; treatment of daytime and nighttime heartburn and other symptoms associated with GERD; long-term treatment of pathological hypersecretory conditions, including Zollinger-Ellison syndrome in combination with amoxicillin and clarithromycin to eradicate *H. pylori*.

Contraindications
Known hypersensitivity to substituted benzimidazoles.

Route/Dosage
Treatment of Erosive or Ulcerative GERD
ADULTS: **PO** 20 mg/day for 4 to 8 wk, an additional 8 wk may be considered for patients who do not heal.

Maintenance of Erosive or Ulcerative GERD
ADULTS: **PO** 20 mg/day.

Healing of Duodenal Ulcers
ADULTS: **PO** 20 mg/day after the morning meal for 4 wk, additional therapy may be required for some patients.

Treatment of Pathological Hypersecretory Conditions
ADULTS: **PO** 60 mg/day. Doses up to 100 mg qd or 60 mg bid have been administered.

H. Pylori Eradication to Reduce Risk of Duodenal Ulcer Recurrence
ADULTS: **PO** 20 mg rabeprazole plus amoxicillin 1000 mg plus clarithromycin 500 mg bid for 7 days with morning and evening meals.

Interactions
Drugs dependent on gastric pH for absorption (eg, digoxin, ketoconazole): Plasma levels of digoxin may be increased, while ketoconazole concentrations may be decreased.

Lab Test Interferences None well documented.

Adverse Reactions
CV: Hypertension; MI; ECG abnormalities; migraine; syncope; angina pectoris; bundle branch block; palpitation; sinus bradycardia; tachycardia.
CNS: Headache; insomnia; anxiety; dizziness; depression; nervousness; somnolence; hypertonia; neuralgia; vertigo; convulsion; extrapyramidal syndrome; hyperkinesias.
DERM: Rash; pruritus; sweating; urticaria; alopecia.
EENT: Cataract; amblyopia; glaucoma; dry eyes; abnormal vision; tinnitus; otitis media.
GI: Diarrhea; nausea; abdominal pain; vomiting; dyspepsia; flatulence; constipation; dry mouth; eructation; gastroenteritis; rectal hemorrhage; melena; anorexia; mouth ulceration; stomatitis; dysphagia; gingivitis; increased appetite; abnormal stools; proctitis; colitis; esophagitis; glossitis; pancreatitis; cholelithiasis; cholecystitis.
GU: Cystitis; urinary frequency; dysmenorrhea; dysuria; kidney calculus; metrorrhagia; polyuria.
HEMA: Anemia; ecchymosis; lymphadenopathy; hypochromic anemia.
METAB: Hyperthyroidism; hypothyroidism; peripheral edema; edema; weight gain/loss; gout; dehydration.
RESP: Dyspnea; asthma; epistaxis; laryngitis; hiccough; hyperventilation.
OTHER: Asthenia; fever; allergic reaction; chills; malaise; substernal chest pain; neck rigidity; photosensitivity reaction; myalgia; arthritis; leg cramps; bone pain; arthrosis; bursitis.

Precautions
Pregnancy: Category B.

Lactation: Undetermined.
Children: Safety and efficacy not established.
Gastric malignancy: Symptomatic response to rabeprazole does not preclude gastric malignancy.

PATIENT CARE CONSIDERATIONS
Administration/Storage
- Give prescribed dose once daily, at least 1 hr before eating.
- Do not chew, crush, or split. Instruct patient to swallow tablet whole.
- Store tablets at controlled room temperature. Protect from moisture.

Assessment/Interventions
- Obtain patient history, including drug history and any known allergies. Note history of liver disease.
- Assess for bloody or coffee ground emesis and black tarry stools.
- Assess for symptoms of esophageal reflux (eg, heart burn, acid regurgitation) or peptic ulcer activity (eg, indigestion, abdominal pain, nausea).
- Monitor patient for CNS, GI, musculoskeletal, and general body side effects. Report to health care provider if noted and significant.

Patient/Family Education
- Explain name, dose, action, and potential side effects of drug.
- Advise patient to not chew, crush, or split medication; swallow the tablet whole.
- Remind patient to take each dose at least 1 hr before eating.
- Inform patients that antacids may be taken concurrently with rabeprazole.
- Remind patient that rabeprazole is to be taken every day and not "as needed" nor only when symptoms are present.
- Instruct women to notify health care provider if pregnant, planing to become pregnant, or breastfeeding.
- Advise patient to report any of the following events: bloody or coffee ground emesis, black tarry stools, recurrent heart burn, recurrent indigestion or abdominal pain, increasing need for antacid use.

Rabies Immune Globulin, Human (RIG)

(RAY-beez ih-MYOON GLAB-byoolin)

Class Immune serum

How Supplied
Hyperab Injection 150 IU/mL ♦ Imogam Injection 150 IU/mL

Action
PHARMACOLOGY: Directly neutralizes rabies virus.

PHARMACOKINETICS/DYNAMICS:
Absorption: Absorbed slowly (IM). T_{max} is 2 to 13 days.
Distribution: Distribution into milk and across placenta likely due to passage of other immunoglobulins.
Excretion: $T_{1/2}$ serum is about 24 days.

Indications
Passive, transient postexposure prevention of rabies infection in susceptible individuals.

Contraindications
Repeated doses once vaccine treatment has been initiated. RIG may theoretically be contraindicated in people who have had life-threatening reactions to human IgG antibody products or any RIG components. Previous complete immunization with rabies vaccine and presence of adequate antibody titer.

Route/Dosage
ADULTS AND CHILDREN: **IM** 20 IU/kg (0.133 mL/kg) as soon as possible after exposure, preferably with first dose of vaccine.

Interactions
Measles, mumps, polio, or rubella live vaccines: Other antibodies in RIG preparation may interfere with response to these live vaccines.

Lab Test Interferences
None well documented.

Adverse Reactions
DERM: Urticaria; skin rash.
GU: Nephrotic syndrome.
OTHER: Local tenderness, soreness, or stiffness at injection site; low-grade fever; angioedema; sensitization to repeated injections; anaphylactic shock.

Precautions
Pregnancy: Category C.
Lactation: Unknown.
Hypersensitivity to thimerosal or human immunoglobulins: Give drug with caution.
Live vaccines: To avoid inactivating live vaccines, do not give live vaccines within 4 mo after RIG.
Bloodborne viral transmission: Because RIG is made from human plasma, there is a risk of transmitting infectious agents (eg, viruses).

PATIENT CARE CONSIDERATIONS

Administration/Storage
- Use up to ½ dose to infiltrate wound site if nature and location of wound site permits. Administer balance of dose IM at different site and in different extremity from rabies vaccine, preferably in gluteal muscle (upper, outer quadrant only) or deltoid muscle.
- Administer as soon as possible after exposure up to 8 days after first vaccine dose.
- RIG is used in conjunction with rabies vaccine. Administer human diploid cell culture (HDCV) rabies vaccine as soon as possible after rabies exposure.
- Do not give more than 5 mL in 1 injection site.
- Store under refrigeration; do not freeze.

Assessment/Interventions
- Obtain complete history, including drug history, and any known allergies. Verify that prior vaccine treatment has not been initiated and that hypersensitivity to human immune globulins and thimerosal (chemical found in contact lens solutions) does not exist.
- Assess for signs of immediate (within 15 min) and delayed allergic reaction: shortness of breath, rash, pruritus, and fever. Report symptoms to health care provider immediately.
- Note date of last tetanus immunization. Vaccinate if needed.

Patient/Family Education
- Advise patient that pain, itching, and swelling may temporarily occur at injection site.
- Advise patient to take acetaminophen to alleviate headache, fever, and pain.
- Teach patient wound care and signs of infection (eg, fever, wound drainage, increased pain at wound site) if applicable prior to discharge.
- Encourage patient to return for medical follow-up within 7 to 10 days after discharge.
- Advise female patients to contact health care provider if pregnant, planning on becoming pregnant, or breastfeeding.

Rabies Vaccine

(RAY-beez vaccine)

Class Vaccine, inactivated virus

How Supplied
Imovax Rabies Vaccine (Human Diploid Cell) Powder for injection Freeze-dried suspension of Wistar rabies virus strain PM-1503-3M grown in human diploid cell cultures (inactivated whole virus). Contains 2.5 IU or more rabies antigen/mL. ♦ *Imovax Rabies I.D. Vaccine (Human Diploid Cell)* Powder for injection Freeze-dried suspension of Wistar rabies virus strain PM-1503-3M grown in human diploid cell cultures. Contains 0.25 IU rabies antigen/0.1 mL intradermal use. (For pre-exposure use only via intradermal route) ♦ *RabAvert* Powder for injection Freeze-Dried fixed-virus strain Flury LEP grown in cultures of chicken fibroblasts. Contains 2.5 IU or more rabies antigen/mL IM dose. ♦ *Rabies Vaccine (Adsorbed)* Injection Challenge Virus Standard (CVS) Kissling/MDPH strain

Action
PHARMACOLOGY: Induces neutralizing antibodies and cellular immunity.

Indications Induction of active immunity against rabies virus either before or after viral exposure.

Contraindications May theoretically be contraindicated in people who have had life-threatening allergic reactions to rabies vaccine or any of its components. Pre-exposure treatment: developing febrile illness.

Route/Dosage
Preexposure Prophylaxis
ADULTS & CHILDREN: **IM** 1 mL or **Intradermal** 0.1 mL (*Imovax ID* only) on days 0, 7, and 21 or 28.

Postexposure Prophylaxis
ADULTS & CHILDREN: Following RIG administration, **IM** 1 mL on days 0, 3, 7, 14, and 28. Patients who previously received preexposure prophylaxis: **IM** 1 mL on only days 0 and 3. Do not give RIG.

Interactions
Chloroquine: Long-term therapy with chloroquine may suppress immune response to intradermal rabies vaccine. Complete pre-exposure rabies vaccination 1 to 2 mo before starting chloroquine administration.

Immunosuppressant drugs (including high-dose corticosteroids): May result in insufficient response to immunization. If possible, do not give immunosuppressive agents during postexposure therapy.

Lab Test Interferences None well documented.

Adverse Reactions
CNS: Headache; dizziness.
GI: Nausea; abdominal pain.
LOCAL: Swelling; erythema; pruritus; local pain; discomfort.

OTHER: Muscle aches; slight fever; fatigue; serum-sickness-like reactions with intradermal booster doses.

Precautions

Pregnancy: Category C. Vaccinate if risk of disease outweighs risk to patients.

Lactation: Unknown.

Hypersensitivity: In people who experience immune-complex-like (or serum-sickness-like) hypersensitivity reactions during pre-exposure prophylaxis, do not give further doses of rabies vaccine unless they are exposed to rabies or they are likely to be unapparently or unavoidably exposed to rabies virus and have unsatisfactory antibody titers.

Intradermal route: Indicated only for preexposure immunization.

Pre-exposure immunization: Those at high risk of exposure to the rabies virus require preexposure immunization: veterinarians, certain laboratory workers, animal handlers, forest rangers, spelunkers, and people staying longer than 1 mo in other countries where rabies is constant threat (eg, India).

Postexposure prophylaxis: If bite from animal is unprovoked, animal is not apprehended and rabies is present in that species in area, administer RIG and rabies vaccine. Consider vaccine recipients adequately immunized if they previously completed preexposure or postexposure prophylaxis with either current rabies vaccine (but not *Wyvac* brand from Wyeth) or have documented adequate antibody response.

Radiation therapy: People undergoing radiation therapy may experience insufficient response to immunization and remain susceptible.

Travelers: Travelers to endemic areas may receive vaccine by intradermal route if 3-dose series can be completed 30 days or more before departure; otherwise give vaccine IM.

PATIENT CARE CONSIDERATIONS

Administration/Storage

- Reconstitute vaccine with 1 mL of diluent using a needle longer than the intradermal needle used for administration. Stir contents until dissolved and withdraw amount needed. Remove reconstitution needle and replace with smaller needle for administration.
- For postexposure vaccination, do not administer intradermally; administer IM in deltoid area in older children and adults and in vastis lateralis in young children. Never administer rabies vaccine in gluteal area; this may result in inadequate immune response.
- May administer pre-exposure prophylaxis vaccine intradermally. Intradermal injections in lateral aspect of upper arm are less likely to cause adverse reactions than intradermal injections in forearm.
- Follow careful recordkeeping when administering vaccine: note manufacturer, lot number, expiration date of vaccine, date of administration, and signature of person administering vaccine.
- Report severe reaction to FDA through local/state health departments; note reaction on patient chart.
- Store under refrigeration; do not freeze.

Assessment/Interventions

- Obtain patient history, including drug history and any known allergies. Note previous life-threatening allergic reaction to rabies vaccine or any of its components.
- Determine if patient is receiving immunosuppressive therapy.
- Assess for allergic reaction (eg, urticaria, breathing difficulty, nausea and vomiting, fever) within 15 min of administration and document patient tolerance of vaccine.
- Have epinephrine and antihistamines (eg, diphenhydramine) readily available.

Pre-exposure prophylaxis:

- Assess temperature; withhold pre-exposure dose if patient has febrile illness.

Postexposure prophylaxis:

- Immediately and thoroughly scrub wounds/scratches with antibacterial soap and water. Dress wound as necessary.
- Give tetanus prophylaxis and control bacterial infection (wound management, antibiotics) as ordered.

Patient/Family Education

- Advise patient at risk for ongoing rabies exposure to receive rabies booster every 2 yr or more often (per serology q 6 mo) if very high risk (eg, veterinarians).
- Advise patient to seek immediate medical attention should future rabies exposure occur. Emphasize danger of wound infection and need to evaluate rabies antibody response.
- Teach patient/family wound care and signs of infection (eg, fever, wound drainage, increased pain at wound) prior to discharge.
- Advise patient that aspirin/antihistamines can be taken to treat mild local or systemic reactions.
- Encourage medical follow-up within 7 to 10 days after discharge for wound evaluation.
- Advise female patients to contact health care provider if pregnant, planning on becoming pregnant, or breastfeeding.

Raloxifene Hydrochloride

(ral-OX-ih-FEEN)

Class Selective estrogen receptor modulator

How Supplied
Evista Tablets 60 mg

Action

PHARMACOLOGY: The biological actions of raloxifene are mediated largely through binding to estrogen receptors, which results in activation of certain estrogenic pathways and blockade of others. Raloxifene decreases resorption of bone and reduced biochemical markers of bone turnover to the premenopausal range. Effects on bone are manifested as reductions in the serum and urine levels of bone turnover markers, decreases in bone resorption based on radiocalcium kinetics studies, increases in bone mineral density, and decreases in incidence of fractures. Raloxifene also effects lipid metabolism, decreasing total and LDL cholesterol levels but does not increase triglyceride levels or change total HDL cholesterol levels.

PHARMACOKINETICS/DYNAMICS:

Absorption: Absorbed rapidly after oral administration. Bioavailability is 2%.

Distribution: Vd is 2348 L/kg. Protein binding is 95%. Binds albumin and alpha-1-acid glycoprotein.

Metabolism: Extensive first pass metabolism to glucuronide conjugates.

Excretion: Primarily excreted in feces. Less than 0.2% is excreted unchanged in urine. Cl (oral) is 44.1 L/kg/hr and t½ is 27.7 to 32.5 hr. Chronic dosing Cl is 40 to 60 L/kg/hr.

Special Populations:
Cirrhosis – Plasma concentrations increase 2.5 times. Safety and efficacy have not been evaluated any further.

Indications For the prevention and treatment of osteoporosis in postmenopausal women.

Contraindications Women who are or may become pregnant; women with active or history of venous thromboembolic events, including deep venous thrombosis, pulmonary embolism, and retinal vein thrombosis; allergy to raloxifene or other constituents of the tablet; coadministration of cholestyramine.

Route/Dosage
ADULT WOMEN: PO 60 mg qd.

Interactions
Cholestyramine: Major reduction in absorption and enterohepatic cycling of raloxifene; avoid concurrent use.
Highly protein-bound drugs (eg, clofibrate, indomethacin, naproxen, ibuprofen, diazepam, diazoxide): May displace raloxifene from protein-binding sites, increasing the effects of raloxifene.
Warfarin: Raloxifene may decrease anticoagulant effect.

Lab Test Interferences None well documented.

Adverse Reactions
CV: Hot flashes.
CNS: Migraine; depression; insomnia.
DERM: Rash; sweating.
EENT: Sinusitis; pharyngitis; laryngitis.
GI: Nausea; dyspepsia; vomiting; flatulence; gastroenteritis; abdominal pain.
GU: Vaginitis; UTI; cystitis; leukorrhea; endometrial disorder.
RESP: Cough; pneumonia.
OTHER: Infection; flu-syndrome; leg cramps; chest pain; fever; weight gain; edema; arthralgia; myalgia; arthritis.

Precautions
Pregnancy: Category X.
Lactation: Undetermined.
Children: Safety and efficacy not established.
Hepatic function impairment: Safety and efficacy not evaluated in patients with severe hepatic insufficiency.
Breast abnormality: Investigate any unexplained breast abnormality during therapy.
Concurrent estrogen therapy: Concurrent use with systemic estrogens is not recommended.
Endometrium: Because raloxifene does not affect endometrial proliferation unexplained uterine bleeding should be investigated as clinically indicated.
History of breast cancer: Raloxifene has not been adequately studied in women with history of breast cancer.
Lipid metabolism: Raloxifene lowers serum total and LDL cholesterol but does not affect total HDL or triglycerides.
Premenopausal use: Safety and efficacy not established. Use is not recommended.
Use in men: Safety and efficacy not established.
Venous thromboembolic events: Increased risk of thromboembolic events.

PATIENT CARE CONSIDERATIONS

Administration/Storage
- Administer once daily.
- Can be administered any time of the day without regard to meals.
- Store at controlled room temperature.

Assessment/Interventions
- Obtain patient history, including drug history

and any known allergies. Note previous history of thromboembolic disease or breast cancer.
- Ensure that patient has adequate calcium intake via diet or supplement.
- Ensure that medication is discontinued 72 hr or more prior to and during any event associated with prolonged immobilization.
- Monitor patient for signs of thromboembolic event and notify health care provider.
- Assess patient for side effects.

Patient/Family Education
- Advise patient to read package insert before starting therapy and each time the prescription is refilled.
- Teach name, expected action, and potential side effects to patient.
- Advise patient that drug is taken once a day without regard to meals.
- Advise patient that if a dose is missed, to start taking the drug on the normal schedule as soon as possible. Do not make up for the missed dose.
- Advise patient that this drug is for postmenopausal women only. It should not be given to men or premenopausal women to prevent osteoporosis.
- Advise patient that estrogen therapy comes as a pill, patch, or injection and should not be used in conjunction with this drug.
- Advise patient that drug does not reduce hot flashes and may actually cause hot flashes in women who are closer to menopause.
- Instruct patient to take supplemental calcium (1500 mg) and vitamin D (400 IU) daily if dietary intake is not adequate.
- Encourage patient to perform weight-bearing exercises and avoid behaviors that promote osteoporosis (eg, alcohol consumption, cigarette smoking).
- Advise patient to avoid prolonged restrictions of movement during travel.
- Advise patient that medication will need to be discontinued 72 hr or more prior to any event that would cause prolonged immobilization (eg, postsurgical recovery) and can only be restarted once patient is fully mobile.
- Instruct patient to report the following symptoms to health care provider: pain in groin or calves; leg swelling; sudden chest pain; shortness of breath or coughing blood; abnormal vaginal bleeding; breast lumps; sudden vision problems.
- Advise women to contact health care provider if pregnant, planning to become pregnant, or breastfeeding.

Ramipril

(ruh-MIH-prill)

Class Antihypertensive/Angiotensin converting enzyme (ACE inhibitor)

How Supplied
Altace Capsules 1.25 mg, Capsules 2.5 mg, Capsules 5 mg, Capsules 10 mg

Action
PHARMACOLOGY: Competitively inhibits angiotensin I-converting enzyme, resulting in prevention of angiotensin I conversion to angiotensin II, a potent vasoconstrictor. Clinical consequences include decrease in BP and indirect (by inhibiting aldosterone) decrease in sodium and fluid retention and increase in diuresis.

PHARMACOKINETICS/DYNAMICS:

Absorption: Extent of absorption in GI tract is at least 50% to 60%. T_{max} is 1 hr (parent compound) or 2 to 4 hr (metabolite, ramiprilat). Bioavailability is 28% (ramipril) or 44% (ramiprilat).

Distribution: Protein binding is about 73% (parent) or about 56% (metabolite). Plasma concentrations of ramiprilat decline in a triphasic manner: initial rapid decline (representing distribution into peripheral compartment), apparent elimination phase, and terminal elimination phase.

Metabolism: In liver to active metabolite ramiprilat, which had 6 times the ACE inhibitory activity.

Excretion: Eliminated in urine (60% of parent and metabolites) and feces (40%). Less than 2% of drug recovered in urine is unchanged. The $t_{½}$ is less than 50 hr (ramiprilat).

Special Populations:
Renal Function Impairment – In patients with Ccr less than 40 mL/min, peak levels of metabolite approximately doubled. AUC was 3 to 4 times larger. Urinary excretion of metabolite is reduced. Higher peak and trough ramiprilat levels.

Hepatic Function Impairment – Slowed metabolism of ramiprilat. Ramipril plasma levels increase about 3-fold.

Indications Treatment of hypertension; for stable patients who have demonstrated clinical signs of CHF within the first few days after sustaining acute MI; reduce risk of MI, stroke, or death from CV causes in patients at high risk.

Contraindications Hypersensitivity to ACE inhibitors (particularly history of angioedema).

Route/Dosage
Heart Failure Post-MI
ADULTS: PO 2.5 mg bid. Switch to 1.25 mg bid if hypotension occurs. Titrate to target dose of 5 mg bid.

Hypertension
ADULTS: PO Initial dose is 2.5 mg qd initially. Maintenance dose is 2.5 to 20 mg/day as single dose or in 2 equally divided doses.

Patients with Renal Impairment
PO 1.25 mg qd in patients with Ccr below 40 mL/min (serum creatinine higher than 2.5 mg/dL; max, 5 mg/day).

Reduction in Risk of MI, Stroke, and Death from CV Causes
ADULTS: PO Initial dose is 2.5 mg qd for 1 wk, 5 mg qd for 3 wk, then increase the dose as tolerated to maintenance dose. Maintenance dose is 10 mg qd or in divided doses if patient is hypertensive or recently post-MI.

Interactions
Antacids: Ramipril bioavailability may be decreased. Separate administration times by 1 to 2 hr.
Capsaicin: May exacerbate cough.
Digoxin: Increased or decreased digoxin levels.
Diuretics: Increased risk of hypotension.
Indomethacin, salicylates (eg, aspirin): May reduce hypotensive effects, especially in low-renin or volume-dependent hypertensive patients.
Lithium: May cause increased lithium levels and symptoms of lithium toxicity.
Loop diuretics: Effects of loop diuretics may be decreased.
Phenothiazines: Enhanced hypotensive effects.
Potassium supplements, potassium-sparing diuretics: May cause increased potassium serum levels.

Lab Test Interferences
False elevation of liver enzymes, serum bilirubin, uric acid, and blood glucose may occur.

Adverse Reactions
CV: Hypotension (11%); angina pectoris (3%); postural hypotension, syncope (2%).
CNS: Dizziness (4%).
EENT: Vertigo (2%).
GI: Nausea, vomiting (2%); diarrhea (1%).
GU: Abnormal renal function (1%).
HEMA: Neutropenia, agranulocytosis.
METAB: Hyperkalemia (1%).
RESP: Cough (8%).

OTHER: Angioedema (0.3%); anaphylactoid reactions.

> **WARNING:**
> *Pregnancy:* Use in second and third trimesters may cause injury and death to fetus.

Precautions
Pregnancy: Category D (second, third trimester); category C (first trimester). Discontinue use in pregnant patients; fetal/neonatal injury and death have occurred. Closely observe infants with histories of in utero exposure.
Lactation: Undetermined.
Children: Safety and efficacy not established.
Elderly: May show higher blood levels of active metabolite.
Renal function impairment: Dosage reduction is required in patients with renal impairment. May further decrease renal function with elevations in BUN and serum creatinine caused by decreased renal perfusion.
Hepatic function impairment: Use drug with caution. Dosage reduction may be required because of impaired metabolism.
Angioedema: Angioedema may occur. Use drug with extreme caution in patients with hereditary angioedema.
Cough: Chronic cough may occur during treatment; it is more common in women.
Hepatic failure: Rarely, ACE inhibitors have been associated with a syndrome that starts with cholestatic jaundice and progresses to fulminant hepatic necrosis and sometimes death.
Hypotension/first-dose effect: Significant decreases in BP may occur following first dose, especially in severely salt- or volume-depleted patients (such as those receiving diuretics) or those with heart failure.
Neutropenia and agranulocytosis: Neutropenia and agranulocytosis have occurred with similar agents; risk appears greater in presence of renal dysfunction, heart failure, or immunosuppression.
Proteinuria: Proteinuria has occurred with agents in this class, especially with high doses or prior renal disease.

Overdosage: Signs and Symptoms
Hypotension.

PATIENT CARE CONSIDERATIONS
Administration/Storage
- Administer alone or in combination with other antihypertensives.
- Do not administer to pregnant women during second and third trimesters as fetal and neonatal morbidity and death can occur.
- Give prescribed dose without regard to meals. Administer with food if GI upset occurs.
- Store tablets at controlled room temperature (59° to 89°F). Protect from moisture.

Assessment/Interventions

- Obtain patient history, including drug history and any known allergies. Note renal or hepatic impairment, conditions predisposing to volume depletion (eg, prolonged diuretic therapy), diabetes, heart failure, anuria, hereditary or idiopathic angioedema, lupus erythematosus, left ventricular outflow obstruction, allergy to any other ACE inhibitor, and concurrent use of potassium-containing salt substitutes, potassium supplements, or potassium-sparing diuretics.
- Ensure that small initial dose and gradual escalation of dose are used in patient with heart failure and moderate to severe renal impairment (Ccr less than 50 mL/min) or following vigorous diuresis.
- Ensure that volume and/or salt depletion have been corrected before initiating therapy.
- Ensure that serum electrolytes and renal function are monitored periodically.
- Ensure that CBC with differential are evaluated prior to starting therapy, at 2 wk intervals for 3 mo, and periodically thereafter in patient with renal impairment
- Monitor and record BP and pulse. Should symptomatic hypotension occur, hold medication and notify health care provider.
- Take safety precautions if orthostatic hypotension occurs.
- Assess heart failure patient for evidence of worsening failure (eg, daily weights, evaluation of peripheral edema, shortness of breath). Inform health care provider if rapid weight gain (eg, 2 pounds in 1 day or 5 pounds in 1 wk) is noted or if patient is experiencing worsening edema or other symptoms of heart failure (eg, worsening shortness of breath).
- Monitor for signs of hypersensitivity including angioedema involving swelling of the face, lips, eyelids, and tongue. Discontinue medication and notify health care provider immediately if noted. Be prepared to treat appropriately.
- Assess patient for GI, CNS, and general body side effects. Inform health care provider if noted and significant.

Patient/Family Education

- Explain name, dose, action, and potential side effects of drug.
- Advise patient to take prescribed dose without regard to meals but to take with food if stomach upset occurs.
- Advise patient to try to take each dose at about the same time each day.
- Inform hypertensive patient that drug controls, but does not cure, hypertension and to continue taking drug as prescribed even when BP is not elevated.
- Caution patient not to change the dose or stop taking unless advised by health care provider.
- Instruct patient to continue taking other medications for condition as prescribed by health care provider.
- Instruct patient in BP and pulse measurement skills.
- Advise patient to monitor and record BP and pulse at home and to inform health care provider should abnormal measurements be noted. Also advise patient to take record of BP and pulse to each follow-up visit.
- Caution patient to avoid sudden position changes to prevent orthostatic hypotension.
- Instruct patient to lie or sit down if experiencing dizziness or lightheadedness when standing.
- Emphasize to hypertensive patient the importance of the following other modalities on BP control: weight control, regular exercise, smoking cessation, and moderate intake of alcohol and salt.
- Emphasize to heart failure patient the importance of the following other modalities that can help control heart failure symptoms: weight control, progressive exercise program, smoking cessation, and moderate intake of alcohol and salt.
- Advise heart failure patient to weigh daily, keep a record of daily weights, and notify health care provider if rapid weight gain (eg, 5 pounds in 1 wk) is noted or if edema or shortness of breath are getting worse.
- Caution patient that inadequate fluid intake, excessive perspiration, diarrhea, or vomiting can lead to excessive fall in BP resulting in lightheadedness or fainting.
- Advise patient that medication may cause dizziness or lightheadedness and to use caution while driving or performing other tasks requiring mental alertness until tolerance is determined.
- Caution patient to avoid unnecessary exposure to UV light (sunlight, tanning booths) and to use sunscreen and wear protective clothing when exposed to UV light to avoid photosensitivity reaction.
- Advise women to notify health care provider if pregnant, planning to become pregnant, or breastfeeding.
- Instruct patient to stop taking drug and immediately report any of the following symptoms to health care provider: sore throat, fever, swelling of the hands or feet, irregular heartbeat, chest pains, fainting, swelling of the face, lips, eyelids, or tongue, difficulty breathing.

- Instruct patient to inform health care provider if a persistent cough develops while taking this medication.
- Caution patient not to take any prescription or OTC medications, potassium-containing salt substitutes, potassium supplements, or dietary supplements unless advised by health care provider.
- Advise patient that follow-up visits and lab tests will be required to monitor therapy and to keep appointments.

Ranitidine

(ran-EYE-tih-DEEN)

Class Histamine H_2 antagonist

How Supplied

Zantac Injection 0.5 mg (as hydrochloride)/mL, Injection 25 mg (as hydrochloride)/mL, Syrup 15 mg (as hydrochloride)/mL, Tablets 150 mg (as hydrochloride), Tablets 300 mg (as hydrochloride) ◆ *Zantac 75* Tablets 75 mg ◆ *Zantac EFFERdose* Tablets, effervescent 150 mg, Granules, effervescent 150 mg

❋ *Alti-Ranitidine Hydrochloride* ◆ *Apo-Ranitidine* ◆ *Nu-Ranit* ◆ *Novo-Ranitidine* ◆ *PMS-Ranitidine* ◆ *ratio-Ranitidine* ◆ *Rhoxal-ranitidine*

Action

PHARMACOLOGY: Reversibly and competitively blocks histamine at H_2 receptors, particularly those in gastric parietal cells, leading to inhibition of gastric acid secretion.

PHARMACOKINETICS/DYNAMICS:

Absorption: Absorbed rapidly (IV and IM), 50% absorbed orally. C_{max} is 576 ng/mL (IM) or 440 to 545 ng/mL (oral). T_{max} is 15 min (IM) or 2 to 3 hr (oral). Bioavailability is 90% to 100% (IV) or 50% (oral).

Distribution: Protein binding is 15%. Vd is 1.4 L/kg.

Metabolism: Hepatic to N-oxide (main metabolite), s-oxide and desmethyl ranitidine.

Excretion: Excreted in urine (70% unchanged when given IV, 30% unchanged when given orally), main metabolite is N-oxide (less than 4%), also S-oxide (1%), desmethyl ranitidine (1%), remainder found in feces. Renal clearance is 530 mL/min (IM), 410 mL/min (oral). Total clearance is 760 mL/min. $T_{1/2}$ elimination is 2 to 2.5 hr (IM) or 2.5 to 3 hr (oral).

Special Populations:
Renal Function Impairment – Plasma half-life, clearance, volume of distribution are all altered in proportion to creatinine clearance.
Hepatic Function Impairment – Alterations in half-life, distribution, clearance, and bioavailability are minor but clinically insignificant.
Elderly – Plasma half-life is prolonged and total clearance is lowered.

Indications Treatment and maintenance of duodenal ulcer; management of gastroesophageal reflux disease (GERD; including erosive or ulcerative disease); short-term treatment of benign gastric ulcer; treatment of pathologic hypersecretory conditions (Zollinger-Ellison).

Unlabeled use(s): Prevention of upper GI bleeding; treatment of aspiration pneumonia; stress ulcer; and gastric NSAID damage. Used as a part of a multi-drug regimen to eradicate *Helicobacter pylori* in the treatment of peptic ulcer; protection against aspiration of acid during anesthesia; prevention of gastro duodenal mucosal damage that may be associated with long-term NSAIDS; to control acute upper GI bleeding; prevention of stress ulcers.

Contraindications Hypersensitivity to ranitidine or other H_2 antagonists.

Route/Dosage

Duodenal Ulcer (Active)
ADULTS: PO 150 mg bid or 300 mg at bedtime. Maintenance dose is 150 mg at bedtime. **IM/IV/Intermittent IV** 50 mg q 6 to 8 hr.

Acute Benign Gastric Ulcer and GERD
ADULTS: PO 150 mg bid. **IM/IV/Intermittent IV** 50 mg q 6 to 8 hr.

Pathologic Hypersecretory Conditions
ADULTS: PO 150 mg bid. Individualize.

Erosive Esophagitis
ADULTS: PO 75 to 150 mg cid. **IM/IV/Intermittent IV** 50 mg q 6 to 8 hr. **Continuous IV** 6.25 mg/hr. For patients with Zollinger-Ellison, start infusion at rate of 1 mg/kg/hr and adjust upward in 0.5 mg/kg/hr increments according to gastric acid output (max, 2.5 mg/kg/hr; infusion rate 220 mg/hr).

Renal Insufficiency (Ccr less than 50 mL/min)
ADULTS: PO 150 mg q 24 hr. **IM/IV** 50 mg q 18 to 24 hr.

Interactions

Diazepam: Pharmacologic effects may be decreased due to decreased GI absorption by ranitidine. Staggering administration times may avoid this reaction.
Ethanol: May increase plasma ethanol levels.
Glipizide: Possible increased hypoglycemia effect.
Ketoconazole: May decrease effects of ketoconazole.
Lidocaine: May cause increased lidocaine levels.
Warfarin: Ranitidine may interfere with warfarin clearance. Hypoprothrombinemic effects may increase; may need adjustment.

Lab Test Interferences False-positive test results for urine protein with *Multistix* may occur during ranitidine therapy; testing with sulfosalicylic acid is recommended.

Adverse Reactions
CV: Cardiac arrhythmias; bradycardia.
CNS: Headache; somnolence; fatigue; dizziness; hallucinations; depression; insomnia.
DERM: Alopecia; rash; erythema multiforme.
GI: Nausea; vomiting; abdominal discomfort; diarrhea; constipation; pancreatitis.
HEMA: Agranulocytosis; autoimmune hemolytic or aplastic anemia; thrombocytopenia, granulocytopenia.
HEPA: Cholestatic or hepatocellular effects.
OTHER: Hypersensitivity reactions.

Precautions
Pregnancy: Category B.
Lactation: Excreted in breast milk.
Children: Safety and efficacy not established.
Elderly: May have reduced renal function; therefore, decreased drug clearance may be more common.
Hypersensitivity: Rare cases of anaphylaxis have occurred as well as rare episodes of hypersensitivity.
Renal function impairment: Decreased clearance may occur; dosage reduction may be needed. Hemodialysis reduces level of ranitidine-dosage timing must be adjusted so that scheduled dose coincides with end of hemodialysis.
Hepatic function impairment: Use drug with caution; decreased clearance may occur.
Hepatocellular injury: May occur, manifested as reversible hepatitis, hepatocellular or hepatocanalicular or mixed, with or without jaundice.
Rapid IV administration: May rarely result in bradycardia, tachycardia, or premature ventricular beats, usually in patients predisposed to cardiac rhythm disturbances.

Overdosage: Signs and Symptoms
Rapid respiration, respiratory failure, tachycardia, muscle tremors, vomiting, restlessness, pallor of mucous membranes, redness of mouth and ears, hypotension, collapse, lacrimation, salivation, diarrhea, miosis.

PATIENT CARE CONSIDERATIONS
Administration/Storage
- For IV use, medication is stable in 5% or 10% Dextrose Injection, 0.9% Sodium Chloride or Lactated Ringer's Solution.
- Administer without regard to meals.
- When administering via IV push, dilute to volume of 20 mL with Saline for Injection and inject over at least 5 min.
- For intermittent infusion, dilute 50 mg in 50 to 100 mL D5W and infuse over 15 to 20 min.
- Do not mix with other IV medications.
- Administer continuous infusion at rate of 6.25 mg/hr except for patients with Zollinger-Ellison syndrome.
- Store diluted IV solutions at room temperature. Discard after 48 hr.
- Do not give oral drug at same time as other antacids. Separate administration by at least 1 hr.
- Store syrup form in refrigerator.
- Dissolve *EFFERdose* tablets in 6 to 8 oz of water.

Assessment/Interventions
- Obtain patient history, including drug history and any known allergies.
- Obtain baseline CBC, renal, and LFT results and monitor at regular intervals.
- Assess mental status before starting drug and monitor for changes.
- Notify health care provider if patient develops right upper quadrant abdominal pain, nausea, vomiting, change in color or consistency of stools, and jaundice.
- Slow rate of IV administration if bradycardia, tachycardia, or premature ventricular contractions develop. If these conditions persist, stop infusion and notify health care provider.
- Notify health care provider if patient has arrhythmias, headache, fatigue, dizziness, hallucinations, depression, insomnia, alopecia, rash or erythema multiforme, or severe or persistent diarrhea.

Patient/Family Education
- Instruct patient not to take antacids at same time as drug. Separate administration by at least 1 hr.
- Advise patient to report these symptoms to health care provider: abdominal pain, nausea, vomiting, change in color or consistency of stools, black stools or coffee ground emesis, jaundice, headache, excessive fatigue, dizziness, unusual bruising or bleeding, petechiae, rash, or shortness of breath.
- Discuss necessary dietary changes or restrictions appropriate for patient. Refer patient to dietitian if indicated.
- Advise patient with ulcers to avoid alcohol and smoking.
- Discuss stress reduction with patient if indicated.
- Instruct patient to dissolve effervescent formulation in 6 to 8 oz of water before drinking.
- Advise patient that drug may cause dizziness

and to use caution while driving or performing other tasks requiring mental alertness.

Ranitidine Bismuth Citrate

(ran-EYE-tih-DEEN BISS-muth)
Class Histamine H_2 antagonist/H. Pylori Agent

How Supplied
Tritec Tablets 400 mg

Action
PHARMACOLOGY: Suppresses gastric acid secretion and bismuth, which may aid in *Helicobacter pylori* eradication. Used in combination with clarithromycin, a macrolide antibiotic.

PHARMACOKINETICS/DYNAMICS:
Absorption: Variable oral absorption. C_{max} is 455 ng/mL (400 mg oral dose) (ranitidine); 3.3 ng/mL (400 mg dose) (bismuth). T_{max} is 0.5 to 5 hr (ranitidine); 15 to 60 min (bismuth). Rate of absorption decreased 50% and extent of absorption decreased 25% when taken 30 min after a meal.

Distribution: Vd is 1.7 L/kg (ranitidine). Protein binding is 15% (ranitidine); 98% (bismuth) (primarily albumin).

Metabolism: Ranitidine metabolized to N-oxide, S-oxide, and N-desmethyl metabolites. Not known whether bismuth undergoes any biotransformation.

Excretion: Eliminated in urine (30%; less than 1% of bismuth excreted in urine) and feces (28% bismuth). $T_{1/2}$ is 2.8 to 3.1 hr (ranitidine); 11 to 28 days (bismuth). Renal clearance is 530 mL/min (ranitidine); 30 to 60 mL/min (bismuth). Total clearance is 760 mL/min (ranitidine).

Special Populations:
Renal Function Impairment – Ranitidine and bismuth concentrations may be elevated, not recommended when Ccr is below 25 mL/min.

PATIENT CARE CONSIDERATIONS
Administration/Storage
- Can be taken with or without food.
- Administer in combination with antibiotic agent (eg, clarithromycin) for first 14 days of therapy for the treatment of active duodenal ulcer.
- Refrigerate or store at room temperature. Protect from light in tightly closed container. Protect from moisture.

Assessment/Interventions
- Obtain patient history including drug history and any known allergies. Note renal impairment and history of acute porphyria.

- Advise female patients to contact health care provider if pregnant, planning on becoming pregnant, or breastfeeding.

Indications Treatment of active duodenal ulcers associated with *H. pylori* infection when used in combination with clarithromycin. Eradication of this bacterium reduces the risk of ulcer recurrence.

Contraindications Standard considerations.

Route/Dosage
ADULTS: **PO** 400 mg bid for 28 days in conjunction with clarithromycin (*Biaxin*) 500 mg tid for the first 14 days.

Interactions
Antacids: High doses lower ranitidine and possibly bismuth levels.
Clarithromycin: Increased ranitidine and bismuth levels. However, the combination is indicated to eradicate *H. pylori* and is not likely to be clinically relevant.

Lab Test Interferences False positive urine protein with the *Multistix* may occur while on ranitidine. Alternate testing with sulfosalicylic acid is recommended.

Adverse Reactions
CNS: Headache.
GI: Diarrhea; constipation; benign dark or black coloration of the tongue or feces.

Precautions
Pregnancy: Category C.
Lactation: Undetermined.
Children: Safety and efficacy not established
Renal function impairment: Not recommended for use in patients with Ccr 25 mL/min or less.
Porphyria: Do not use in patients with history of porphyria.
Treatment failure: Patients who fail to respond to therapy should not be retreated with a regimen containing clarithromycin.

Overdosage: Signs and Symptoms
Bismuth: Neurotoxicity, nephrotoxicity.

- Monitor CBC, renal, and LFT results.
- Ensure that clarithromycin is used concurrently during first 14 days of therapy.
- Monitor the adverse effects and report significant findings to health care provider.

Patient/Family Education
- Instruct the patient to take ranitidine bismuth citrate twice daily as prescribed.
- Inform patient that in order for therapy to work, clarithromycin must be taken tid for first 14 days of therapy.
- Instruct patient not to take OTC medications without consulting health care provider.

- Instruct the patient not to take an antacid at the same time as this combination therapy. This action may result in a decrease in plasma concentration of bismuth and ranitidine.
- Advise patient to complete full course of therapy even if symptoms have resolved.
- Inform patient of potential adverse effects and precautions associated with separate drugs in this combination therapy
- Advise patient that bismuth may cause a temporary darkening of the tongue and stool.
- Instruct patient not to confuse the stool darkening with blood in the stool (melena). Occult blood testing may be necessary.
- Instruct patient to report any signs of bleeding to primary care provider.
- Instruct patient to notify primary care provider of any adverse reactions.
- Advise female patients to contact health care provider if pregnant, planning on becoming pregnant, or breastfeeding.
- Advise patients not to breastfeed while taking this medication.

Rasburicase

(raz-BYOOR-ih-kays)

Class Antimetabolite

How Supplied
Elitek Powder for injection, lyophilized 1.5 mg/vial

Action
PHARMACOLOGY: Catalyzes enzymatic oxidation of uric acid into an inactive and soluble metabolite (allantoin).

PHARMACOKINETICS/DYNAMICS:
Distribution: Vd is 110 to 127 mL/kg (pediatrics).
Excretion: $T_{1/2}$ is about 18 hr.

Indications Initial management of plasma uric acid levels in pediatric patients with leukemia, lymphoma, and solid tumor malignancies who are receiving anticancer therapy expected to result in tumor lysis and subsequent elevation of plasma uric acid.

Contraindications Individuals with G-6-PD deficiency; known history of anaphylaxis or hypersensitivity; hemolytic or methemoglobinemia reactions to product or any of its excipients.

Route/Dosage
PEDIATRICS: **IV** 0.15 or 0.2 mg/kg, infused over 30 min, as a single dose for 5 days.

Interactions None well documented.
INCOMPATIBILITIES: Reconstitute with diluent provided and infuse through a different line than that used for the infusion of other concomitant medications. If separated line is not possible, flush line with at least 15 mL of saline solution prior to and after infusion.

Lab Test Interferences At room temperature, causes enzymatic degradation of uric acid in blood/plasma/serum samples, potentially resulting in spuriously low plasma uric acid assay readings.

Adverse Reactions
CV: Arrhythmia; cardiac failure; cardiac arrest; cerebrovascular disorder; MI.
CNS: Convulsions; headache.
DERM: Rash.
EENT: Retinal hemorrhage.
GI: Diarrhea; ileus; intestinal obstruction; vomiting; nausea; abdominal pain; constipation.
GU: Acute renal failure.
HEMA: Hemolysis; methemoglobinemia; neutropenia with and without fever; hemorrhage; pancytopenia; thrombosis.
METAB: Dehydration.
RESP: Respiratory distress; pneumonia; pulmonary edema; pulmonary hypertension.
OTHER: Allergic reactions including anaphylaxis; sepsis; mucositis; cellulitis; chest pain; cyanosis; hot flashes; infection; paresthesia; rigors; thrombophlebitis; fever.

Precautions
Pregnancy: Category C.
Lactation: Undetermined.
Children: Safety and efficacy was studied in pediatric patients ranging from 1 mo to 17 yr. Children under 2 yr had higher mean uric acid AUC than those 2 to 17 yr. In addition, children under 2 yr had a lower rate of success at achieving maintenance uric acid levels by 48 hr. Children under 2 yr experienced more toxicity (eg, vomiting, diarrhea, fever, rash).
Anaphylaxis: Hypersensitivity reactions, including anaphylaxis may occur.
Hemolysis: Can cause severe hemolysis in patients with G-6-PD deficiency. Prior to use, screen patients at high risk of G-6-PD deficiency (eg, patients of African or Mediterranean ancestry).
Methemoglobinemia: May occur.

Overdosage: Signs and Symptoms
Low or undetectable plasma uric acid levels.

PATIENT CARE CONSIDERATIONS
Administration/Storage
- For IV infusion only. Not for intradermal, SC, IM, or IV bolus administration.
- Follow manufacturer's instructions for reconstituting the Powder for Injection and subsequent further dilution.
- Do not administer if particulate matter, cloudiness, or discoloration are noted.
- Infuse diluted solution over 30 min 4 to 24 hr before chemotherapy is started.
- Do not use an in-line IV filter.
- Store vials in refrigerator (36° to 46°F). Do not freeze. Protect from light. Store reconstituted solution in refrigerator for up to 24 hr. Discard unused product after 24 hr.

Assessment/Interventions
- Obtain patient history, including drug history and any known allergies. Note history of G-6-PD deficiency, previous anaphylactic or hypersensitivity reactions, hemolytic reactions, or methemoglobinemia reactions to rasburicase.
- Ensure that patient at high risk of G-6-PD deficiency (eg, African or Mediterranean ancestry) is screened for G-6-PD deficiency prior to starting therapy.
- Monitor patient for signs and symptoms of hemolysis (eg, dark urine, jaundice) and methemoglobinemia (eg, dizziness, nausea, headache, dyspnea, confusion, seizures). Immediately discontinue infusion and inform health care provider if noted.
- When collecting blood for uric acid measurements, carefully follow the procedure recommended by the manufacturer.
- Monitor patient for signs and symptoms of anaphylactic or serious allergic reactions. Immediately discontinue infusion, notify health care provider and be prepared to treat appropriately.
- Monitor patient for CNS, GI, and general body side effects. Report to health care provider if noted and significant.

Patient/Family Education
- Explain name, dose, action, and potential side effects of drug.
- Advise patient, family, or caregiver that medication will be prepared and administered by a health care professional in a medical facility.
- Advise patient or caregiver to report the following: dark urine, yellowing of skin or eyes, dizziness, nausea, headache, difficulty breathing, intolerable injection site reactions, any unusual symptoms to health care provider.
- Advise female patients to contact health care provider if pregnant, planning on becoming pregnant, or breastfeeding

Remifentanil Hydrochloride
(reh-mih-FEN-tah-nill HIGH-droe-KLOR-ide)

Class Narcotic Agonist Analgesic

How Supplied
Ultiva Powder for injection, lyophilized 1 mg/mL after reconstitution

Action
PHARMACOLOGY: Opioid agonist.

PHARMACOKINETICS/DYNAMICS:

Absorption: Plasma concentrations are proportional to the administered dose.

Distribution: Initial V_d is approximately 100 mL/kg and distributes into peripheral tissue with a V_{dss} of approximately 350 mL/kg. Plasma protein binding is approximately 70%.

Metabolism: Metabolized by nonspecific esterases in blood and tissue.

Excretion: Elimination t½ is approximately 3 to 10 minutes.

Special Populations:
Elderly – The clearance is reduced approximately 25%.
Children – In pediatric patients, 5 days to 17 yr, the clearance and Vd are increased.

Indications Analgesic for use during the induction and maintenance of general anesthesia for inpatient and outpatient procedures and for continuation as an analgesic into the immediate postoperative period under supervision of an anesthesia practitioner; as an analgesic component of monitored anesthesia care.

Contraindications Epidural or intrathecal administration; hypersensitivity to fentanyl analogs; any component of the product.

Route/Dosage
General Anesthesia
Not recommended as the sole agent in general anesthesia.

ADULTS: Induction of anesthesia through intubation: **IV** 0.5 to 1 mcg/kg/min by continuous infusion. If endotracheal intubation is to occur less than 8 min after the start of infusion, then an initial dose of 1 mcg/kg may be given over 30 to 60 sec.

Maintenance Of Anesthesia With Nitrous Oxide (66%)
ADULTS: **IV** 0.4 mcg/kg/min by continuous infusion (range, 0.1 to 2 mcg/kg/min), supplemental bolus dose of 1 mcg/kg.

Maintenance of Anesthesia with Isoflurane (0.4 to 1.5 MAC) or Propofol (100 to 200 mcg/kg/min)
ADULTS: **IV** 0.25 mcg/kg/min (range, 0.05 to 2 mcg/kg/min), supplemental bolus of 1 mcg/kg.

Continuation As An Analgesic Into Immediate Postoperative Period
ADULTS: **IV** 0.1 mcg/kg/min (range, 0.025 to 0.2 mcg/kg/min), supplemental bolus not recommended.

Analgesic Component Of Monitored Anesthesia Care
Supplemental oxygen should be supplied.
ADULTS: Single dose: **IV** 0.5 to 1 mcg/kg administered over 30 to 60 sec given 90 sec before placement of the local or regional anesthetic block.
ADULTS: Continuous infusion: **IV** 0.1 mcg/kg/min beginning 5 min before placement of local or regional anesthetic block.

Individualization of Dosage
ELDERLY (OVER 65 YR OF AGE): **IV** Decrease the starting dose by 50% and cautiously titrate to effect.
CHILDREN (2 YR AND OVER): **IV** Same doses per kg as adults.
OBESITY: **IV** Base starting dose on ideal body weight in patients more than 30% over ideal body weight.

Interactions
Agonist/Antagonist analgesics: Withdrawal may be precipitated.
Barbiturate anesthetics: May cause increased CNS and respiratory depression.

Lab Test Interferences None well documented.

Adverse Reactions
CV: Bradycardia; hypotension; tachycardia; hypertension; premature ventricular beats; MI; atrial fibrillation; atrial flutter; decreased cardiac output; arrhythmia; ventricular fibrillation; third degree heart block.
CNS: Dizziness; agitation; headache; somnolence; anxiety; hallucinations; decreased mental acuity.
DERM: Pruritus.
EENT: Visual disturbance; pharyngitis.
GI: Nausea; vomiting; constipation.
GU: Oliguria.
HEMA: Coagulation disorder; hemorrhage; anemia; thrombocytopenia.
RESP: Respiratory depression; apnea; pleural effusion; pneumonia; cough; dyspnea.
OTHER: Skeletal muscle rigidity; shivering; chills; fever; postoperative pain; hypoxia; sweating; flushing; warm sensation; pain at IV site; postoperative and perioperative complications; involuntary movements; edema; heartburn.

Precautions
Pregnancy: Category C.
Lactation: Undetermined.
Children: Safety and efficacy not established in children under 2 yr.
Elderly: Reduce dose in patients over 65 yr.
Drug dependence: Has abuse potential of the morphine type.

PATIENT CARE CONSIDERATIONS

Administration/Storage
- For IV administration only. Do not administer via epidural, intrathecal, intradermal, IM, or SC routes.
- Follow manufacturer's instructions for reconstitution of powder and dilution of reconstituted solution.
- Refer to manufacturer's insert for compatibility with IV fluids and other medications.
- Inspect solution visually before administration. Do not administer if solution is cloudy, discolored, or contains particulate matter.
- IV infusion must be administered by an infusion device.
- IV bolus administration should be used only during maintenance of general anesthesia.
- Bolus injections or infusion should be made into IV tubing at or close to the venous cannula.
- Following IV bolus dose or discontinuation of IV infusion flush tubing to clear residual medication to prevent inadvertent administration at a later time.
- Do not administer in same IV tubing with blood.
- Store powder for injection in refrigerator (36° to 46°F) or at room temperature (less than 78°F). Reconstituted and diluted solutions are stable for up to 24 hr at room temperature.

Assessment/Interventions
- Obtain patient history, including drug history and any known allergies.
- Ensure that resuscitative and tracheal intubation equipment, oxygen, and an opioid antagonist are available at all times.
- Ensure that vital signs and oxygenation are continuously monitored by an appropriate health care professional who is not involved in the conduct of the surgical or diagnostic intervention.
- Do not administer IV bolus doses simultaneously with a continuous infusion to a spontaneously breathing patient or to treat pain in the postoperative period
- Administer reduced doses to patient 65 yr or older.

- Use ideal body weight to determine dose in obese patient.
- Assess pain type and intensity during postoperative recovery and effectiveness of infusion.
- Assess respiratory rate, heart rate, and BP frequently during postoperative recovery. Report significant changes to health care provider.

Overdosage: Signs and Symptoms
Extension of the pharmacologic effects including, apnea, chest-wall rigidity, seizures, hypoxemia, hypotension, bradycardia

Patient/Family Education
- Explain name, action, and potential side effects of drug.
- Advise patient, family, or caregiver that medication will be prepared and administered by a health care provider in a health care setting.
- Reassure patient, family, or caregiver that breathing will be closely monitored and supported while medication is being administered and that breathing and function will quickly return to normal after medication has been discontinued.
- Advise patient, family, or caregiver that nausea, vomiting, itching, or headache may occur during recovery period and to inform health care provider if noted and bothersome.

Repaglinide

(reh-PAG-lih-nide)
Class Antidiabetic/Meglitinide

How Supplied
Prandin Tablets 0.5 mg, Tablets 1 mg, Tablets 2 mg
✤ GlucoNorm

Action
PHARMACOLOGY: Decreases blood glucose by stimulating insulin release from the pancreas.

PHARMACOKINETICS/DYNAMICS:
Absorption: Rapidly and completely absorbed from GI tract. T_{max} is 1 hr (single and multiple doses). Absolute bioavailability is 56%. Mean C_{max} is decreased 20%; AUC is decreased 12.4% by food.
Distribution: Vd is 31 L (IV). Protein binding is less than 98%, albumin.
Metabolism: Completely metabolized by oxidative biotransformation and direct conjugation with glucuronic acid. CYP450 enzymes, mainly CYP3A4, are involved in N-dealkylation to oxidized dicarboxylic acid (M2), then to the aromatic amine (M1), and acyl glucuronide (M7) (inactive metabolites).
Excretion: Eliminated in feces (90% recovered) and urine (8%). Total body Cl is 38 L/hr (IV). The t½ is about 1 hr.
Special Populations:
Renal Function Impairment – AUC and C_{max} increased in severe renal impairment. Dosage adjustment does not appear to be necessary, but make subsequent increases carefully.
Hepatic Function Impairment – Higher and more prolonged serum concentrations.

Indications Adjunct to diet and exercise to lower blood glucose in patients with non-insulin-dependent diabetes mellitus (type 2) whose hyperglycemia cannot be controlled by diet and exercise alone. Can be used with metformin or thiazolidinediones (eg, rosiglitazone) when hyperglycemia cannot be controlled by exercise, diet, and monotherapy with metformin, sulfonylureas, repaglinide, or thiazolidinediones.

Contraindications Insulin-dependent (type 1) diabetes; diabetic ketoacidosis with or without coma; hypersensitivity to repaglinide or its ingredients.

Route/Dosage
No fixed dosage regimen; periodically monitor blood glucose to determine minimum effective dose. Double preprandial dose up to 4 mg with each meal until satisfactory response is achieved (max dose, 16 mg/day). Allow 1 wk to elapse after each dose adjustment to assess response.
Patients Not Previously Treated or Whose HbA_{1c} is Less Than 8%
ADULTS: PO Initial dose is 0.5 mg with each meal.
Patients Previously Treated or Whose HbA_{1c} is More Than or Equal to 8%
ADULTS: PO Initial dose 1 to 2 mg with each meal.

COMBINATION THERAPY
ADULTS: PO The starting dose and dosage adjustments for combination therapy are the same as repaglinide monotherapy.

Interactions
Drugs that induce CYP3A4 (eg, barbiturates, carbamazepine, rifampin, troglitazone): May increase repaglinide metabolism.
Drugs that inhibit CYP3A4 (eg, erythromycin, ketoconazole, miconazole): May inhibit repaglinide metabolism.
Drug that produce hyperglycemia (eg, calcium channel blockers, corticosteroids, diuretics, estrogens and oral contraceptives, isoniazid, nicotinic acid, phenothiazines, phenytoin, sympathomimetics, thyroid products): May lead to loss of

glycemic control. Monitor patient and adjust therapy when these agents are started or stopped.

Gemfibrozil: May result in enhanced and prolonged blood glucose-lowering effects of repaglinide. Patients receiving repaglinide should not start gemfibrozil; patients receiving gemfibrozil should not start taking repaglinide.

Gemfibrozil plus itraconazole: Itraconazole and gemfibrozil have a synergistic inhibitory effect on repaglinide metabolism. Patients taking gemfibrozil and repaglinide should not receive itraconazole.

Levonorgestrel and ethinyl estradiol: Plasma levels of these agents as well as those of repaglinide may be elevated.

Protein bound drugs (eg, NSAIDs, salicylates, sulfonamides, probenecid, MAO inhibitors, beta-adrenergic blocking agents): May potentiate hypoglycemic effect of repaglinide.

Simvastatin: Repaglinide plasma levels may be increased.

Lab Test Interferences None well documented.

Adverse Reactions
CV: Serious CV events (4%); cardiac ischemic events (2%); deaths caused by CV events (0.5%).
CNS: Headache (11%).
DERM: Alopecia, Stevens-Johnson syndrome (postmarketing).
EENT: Rhinitis (7%).
GI: Diarrhea, nausea (5%); dyspepsia (4%); constipation, vomiting (3%); tooth disorder (2%); pancreatitis (postmarketing).
GU: UTI (3%).
HEMA/LYMPH: Thrombocytopenia, leukopenia (less than 1%); hemolytic anemia, severe hepatic dysfunction (postmarketing).
M/N: Hypoglycemia (31%).
MUSC: Arthralgia, back pain (6%).
RESP: Upper respiratory tract infection (16%); sinusitis, bronchitis (6%).
OTHER: Chest pain, paresthesia (3%); allergy (2%).

Precautions
Pregnancy: Category C. Insulin is recommended to maintain blood glucose levels during pregnancy.
Lactation: Undetermined.
Children: Safety and efficacy not established.
Elderly: Elderly, malnourished, or debilitated patients are particularly susceptible to the hypoglycemic action of repaglinide. Hypoglycemia may be difficult to recognize in the elderly. Administer with meals to lessen risk of hypoglycemia.
Renal function impairment: Use caution when titrating repaglinide.
Hepatic function impairment: Use with caution. Allow longer intervals between dosage adjustments.
Secondary failure: Patients stabilized on any diabetic regimen may experience loss of glycemic control when exposed to stress, including trauma, fever, infection, or surgery. At such times, it may be necessary to discontinue repaglinide and administer insulin.

Overdosage: Signs and Symptoms
Hypoglycemia, seizure, neurologic impairment, coma.

PATIENT CARE CONSIDERATIONS

Administration/Storage
- May be used alone or in combination with metformin or a thiazolidinedione. Do not use for the treatment of type 1 diabetes.
- Administer prescribed dose immediately before or up to 30 min before each meal.
- If a meal is skipped, the dose should be skipped to reduce the risk of hypoglycemia.
- Store tablets at controlled room temperature (below 77°F). Keep tightly closed and protect from moisture.

Assessment/Interventions
- Obtain patient history, including drug history and any known allergies. Note renal impairment, liver disease, nature of the patient's diabetes (type 1 vs type 2), and concurrent use of gemfibrozil or itraconazole.
- Check blood sugars frequently and observe for signs of hypoglycemia and hyperglycemia. Inform health care provider if blood sugar readings are outside target range or if hypoglycemic events are noted. Be prepared to treat hypoglycemic reactions.
- Ensure therapy is periodically reviewed to determine if it needs to be continued without change or if a dose change (eg, increase, decrease, discontinuation) is indicated.

Patient/Family Education
- Explain name, dose, action, and potential side effects of drug.
- Advise patient or caregiver to read *Patient Information* leaflet before using the first time and with each refill.
- Instruct patient to take prescribed dose immediately before or up to 30 min before each meal. Advise patient to add a dose before an extra meal.
- Instruct patient that if meal is missed, to skip the dose for that meal to reduce risk of hypoglycemia.
- Educate patient or caregiver regarding diabetes and its management, including target

ranges for blood sugar control. Instruct patient or caregiver that this medication is not a substitute for diet and exercise and to continue to follow prescribed regimens.
- Educate patient or caregiver regarding potential long-term complications of diabetes and need for regular general physical and eye examinations.
- Ensure patient or caregiver understands how to use home glucose monitor and has a plan for monitoring and recording blood sugar measurements (eg, log). Advise patient to take log to each visit with health care provider.
- Educate patient regarding value of periodic A_{1c} testing to confirm level of glucose control.
- Review symptoms of hypoglycemia (eg, low blood sugar) and hyperglycemia (eg, high blood sugar) and action plans to undertake in the event either occur.
- Advise patient to discuss with health care provider a plan for managing each of the following situations: medication dosing during intercurrent conditions (eg, vomiting, infection, trauma, stress, sick days); accidental ingestion of too little or too much medication; missed dose of medication; inadequate food intake or a skipped meal; travel across time zones; change in physical activity.
- Instruct patient to notify health care provider if experiencing severe, continuous, or frequent hypoglycemic episodes; hypoglycemic episodes with few or no warning symptoms; or continuous or severe hyperglycemia.
- Advise patient to carry medical identification of diabetes (eg, Medi-Alert).
- Advise women to notify health care provider if pregnant, planning to become pregnant, or breastfeeding.
- Instruct patient not to take prescription or OTC drugs, dietary supplements, or herbal preparations without consulting health care provider.
- Advise patient that follow-up visits and lab tests will be required to monitor therapy and to keep appointments.

Reserpine/Hydralazine Hydrochloride/ Hydrochlorothiazide

(reh-SER-peen/high-DRAL-uh-zeen HIGH-droe-KLOR-ide/high-droe-klor-oh-THIGH uh-zide)

Class Antihypertensive/Vasodilator/Thiazide diuretic

How Supplied
Hydrap-ES Tablets 15 mg hydrochlorothiazide, 0.1 mg reserpine, and 25 mg hydralazine hydrochloride ♦ Ser-Ap-Es Tablets 15 mg hydrochlorothiazide, 0.1 mg reserpine, and 25 mg hydralazine hydrochloride

Action
PHARMACOLOGY:
Reserpine: Depletes stores of catecholamines and 5-hydroxytryptamine, resulting in decreased heart rate and lowering of arterial BP.
Hydralazine: Directly relaxes vascular smooth muscle to cause peripheral vasodilation, decreasing arterial BP, and peripheral vascular resistance.
Hydrochlorothiazide: Increases chloride, sodium, and water excretion by interfering with transport of sodium ions across renal tubular epithelium.

Indications Treatment of hypertension.

Contraindications Hypersensitivity to any components of product; hypersensitivity to sulfonamide-derived drugs; mental depression or history of mental depression; active peptic ulcer; ulcerative colitis; patients receiving electroconvulsive therapy; coronary artery disease; mitral valvular rheumatic heart disease; anuria.

Route/Dosage
ADULTS: PO Dosage should be determined by individual titration (max, 0.25 mg reserpine/day).

Interactions
Reserpine:
Digoxin, quinidine – Risk of cardiac arrhythmias may be increased.
Direct- (eg, epinephrine) and indirect- (eg, amphetamines) acting amines – The effects of direct-acting amines may be prolonged while the effects of indirect-acting amines may be inhibited.
MAO inhibitors – Avoid concurrent use or use with extreme caution.
Tricyclic antidepressants – Antihypertensive effects of reserpine may be decreased.
Hydralazine:
MAO inhibitors – Use with caution.
Potent parenteral antihypertensive agents (eg, diazoxide) – Profound hypotensive episodes may occur.
Hydrochlorothiazide:
Insulin – Insulin requirements may be increased, decreased, or unchanged.
Lithium – Renal clearance of lithium may be decreased, increasing the risk of toxicity.
Methyldopa – The risk of hemolytic anemia may be increased.
Norepinephrine – Arterial responsiveness may be decreased by hydrochlorothiazide.

NSAIDs (eg, indomethacin) – The diuretic, natriuretic, and antihypertensive effect of hydrochlorothiazide may be reduced.

Tubocurarine – Responsiveness to tubocurarine may be decreased.

Lab Test Interferences

Hydrochlorothiazide: May decrease serum protein-bound iodine levels without signs of thyroid disturbances. May cause diagnostic interference of serum electrolyte levels, blood and urine glucose levels, serum bilirubin levels, and serum uric acid levels.

Adverse Reactions

CV: Arrhythmias; syncope; angina-like symptoms; bradycardia; edema; angina pectoris; hypotension; paradoxical pressor response; tachycardia; palpitations; orthostatic hypotension.

CNS: Parkinsonian syndrome and other extrapyramidal tract symptoms; dizziness; headache; paradoxical anxiety; depression; nervousness; nightmares; dull sensorium; drowsiness; disorientation; peripheral neuritis including paresthesia; numbness and tingling; tremors; vertigo; xanthopsia; weakness; restlessness.

EENT: Nasal congestion; deafness; optic atrophy; glaucoma; uveitis; conjunctival injection; conjunctivitis; lacrimation; transient blurred vision.

GI: Vomiting; diarrhea; nausea; anorexia; dry mouth; hypersecretion; paralytic ileus; constipation; pancreatitis.

GU: Pseudolactation; impotence; dysuria; gynecomastia; decreased libido; breast engorgement; difficulty in urination.

HEMA: Blood dyscrasias including reduction in hemoglobin and RBCs; leukopenia; agranulocytosis; lymphadenopathy; splenomegaly; eosinophilia; aplastic anemia; thrombocytopenia.

HEPA: Hepatitis; jaundice (intrahepatic cholestatic); sialadenitis; vomiting; diarrhea; cramping; nausea; gastric irritation; constipation; anorexia.

METAB: Hyperglycemia ;glycosuria; hyperuricemia.

RESP: Dyspnea; epistaxis; pneumonitis; pulmonary edema.

OTHER: Muscular aches; flushing; muscle cramps; arthralgia; muscle spasm; hypersensitivity (including necrotizing angiitis, Stevens-Johnson syndrome, purpura, urticaria, rash, pruritus); photosensitivity.

Precautions

Pregnancy: Category C.

Lactation: Reserpine and hydrochlorothiazide are excreted in breast milk.

Children: Safety and efficacy not established.

Special risk patients: Use with caution in patients with severe renal disease, impaired hepatic function, peptic ulcer, ulcerative colitis, or gallstones.

Postsympathectomy patients: Drug may enhance antihypertensive effects.

Systemic lupus erythematosus (SLE): Hydralazine may produce an SLE-like reaction while hydrochlorothiazide may exacerbate or activate SLE.

Overdosage: Signs and Symptoms

Impaired consciousness including drowsiness, coma, flushing, conjunctival injection, papillary constriction, hypotension, hypothermia, central respiratory depression, bradycardia, increased salivary and gastric secretions, diarrhea, tachycardia, headache, generalized skin flushing, myocardial ischemia, MI, cardiac arrhythmia, profound shock, loss of fluid and electrolytes, shock, weakness, confusion, dizziness, cramps of calf muscles, paresthesia, fatigue, vomiting, nausea, thirst, polyuria, oliguria, anuria, hypokalemia, hyponatremia, hypochloremia, alkalosis, increased BUN.

PATIENT CARE CONSIDERATIONS

Administration/Storage

- Administer prescribed dose daily without regard to meals. Administer with food if GI upset occurs.
- Administer alone or in combination with other antihypertensives.
- Store tablets at controlled room temperature (59° to 86°F).

Assessment/Interventions

- Obtain patient history, including drug history and any known allergies. Note history of depression, diabetes, lupus erythematosus, hyperkalemia, anuria, kidney disease, liver disease, peptic ulcer disease, ulcerative colitis, gallstones, electroconvulsive therapy, coronary artery disease, mitral valvular rheumatic heart disease, or allergy to sulfonamides.
- Ensure that serum electrolytes, BUN, creatinine, complete blood counts, and antinuclear antibody titers are monitored before and periodically during therapy.
- Monitor and record BP and pulse. Should hypotension result, hold medication and notify health care provider.
- Take safety precautions if orthostatic hypotension occurs.
- Monitor blood sugar in diabetic patient when drug is started or dose is changed. Report significant changes to health care provider.
- Monitor patient for GI, CV, and general body side effects. Inform health care provider if muscle cramps, depression, weakness, fatigue, or other significant effects are noted.

Patient/Family Education
- Explain name, dose, action, and potential side effects of drug.
- Advise patient to take prescribed dose daily, without regard to meals but to take with food if GI upset occurs.
- Inform patient that drug controls, but does not cure, hypertension and to continue taking medication as prescribed even when BP is not elevated.
- Caution patient not to change the dose or stop taking unless advised to do so by health care provider.
- Instruct patient to continue taking other BP medications as prescribed by health care provider.
- Instruct patient in BP and pulse measurement skills.
- Advise patient to monitor and record BP and pulse at home and to inform health care provider should abnormal measurements be noted. Also advise patient to take record of BP and pulse to each follow-up visit.
- Instruct patient to lie or sit down if experiencing dizziness or lightheadedness when standing.
- Caution patient that inadequate fluid intake, excessive perspiration, diarrhea, or vomiting can lead to excessive fall in BP resulting in lightheadedness or fainting.
- Instruct diabetic patient to monitor blood glucose more frequently when drug is started or dose is changed and to inform health care provider of significant changes in readings.
- Caution patient to avoid unnecessary exposure to UV light (sunlight, tanning booths) and to use sunscreen and wear protective clothing when exposed to UV light to avoid photosensitivity reaction.
- Emphasize to hypertensive patient importance of other modalities on BP: weight control, regular exercise, smoking cessation, and moderate intake of alcohol and salt.
- Advise women to notify health care provider if pregnant, planning to become pregnant, or breastfeeding.
- Instruct patient to immediately report any of these symptoms to health care provider: depression, drowsiness, weakness, decreased urination, or rapid heart rate.
- Advise patient that follow-up visits and lab tests may be required to monitor therapy and to keep appointments.

Reteplase, Recombinant

(REH-tuh-place)
Class Tissue plasminogen activator

How Supplied
Retavase Powder for injection, lyophilized 10.4 U (18.1 mg)

Action
PHARMACOLOGY: Aids in dissolution of blood clots.

PHARMACOKINETICS/DYNAMICS:
Excretion: Cleared primarily by liver and kidneys. Plasma Cl is 250 to 450 mL/min. The $t_{1/2}$ is 13 to 16 min.

Indications Management of acute MI, to reduce incidence of CHF and mortality associated with an acute MI.

Contraindications Active internal bleeding; history of cerebrovascular accident; recent intracranial or intraspinal surgery or trauma; intracranial neoplasm, arteriovenous malformation or aneurysm; bleeding diathesis or severe uncontrolled hypertension because thrombolytic therapy increases the risk of bleeding.

Route/Dosage
ADULTS: **IV** 10 + 10 U double-bolus injection, each bolus given over 2 min. The second bolus given 30 min after initiation of the first.

Interactions
Abciximab, aspirin, dipyridamole, heparin, vitamin K antagonists: May increase the risk of bleeding.
INCOMPATIBILITIES:
Heparin: Do not add other medications to the same IV.

Lab Test Interferences Results of coagulation tests may be unreliable if precautions are not taken to prevent in vitro artifacts.

Adverse Reactions
HEMA: Bleeding, both superficial (eg, venous cutdowns, arterial punctures, sites of surgical intervention) and internal (eg, GI tract, GU tract, intracranial, pericardial, retroperitoneal sites).

Precautions
Pregnancy: Category C.
Lactation: Undetermined.
Children: Safety and efficacy not established.
Antithrombotic use: Heparin and aspirin have been administered concomitantly with reteplase.
Arrhythmias: Antiarrhythmic therapy should be available because coronary reperfusion may result in arrhythmias.
Bleeding: Most frequent and serious side effect.
Cholesterol embolism: May occur rarely in patients treated with thrombolytic agents.
Readministration: There is no experience with readministration of reteplase.

Overdosage: Signs and Symptoms
Bleeding.

PATIENT CARE CONSIDERATIONS

Administration/Storage

- Administer only by IV bolus injection. Not for intradermal, SC, IM, or intra-arterial administration.
- Reconstitute lyophilized powder following manufacturer's recommendations using supplied diluent (sterile water for injection) and dispensing pin. Do not reconstitute with bacteriostatic water for injection.
- Mix by gentle swirling. Avoid excessive agitation during reconstitution.
- Use reconstituted solution immediately or within 4 hr if stored properly.
- Do not administer if particulate matter or discoloration noted.
- Administer reconstituted solution as IV bolus injection over 2 min via IV line in which no other medication, including heparin, is being administered. If administration through an IV line containing heparin is necessary, flush line with normal saline or 5% dextrose in water prior to and following reteplase administration.
- Administer second bolus injection 30 min after initiation of first bolus.
- Discard any unused solution.
- Store unopened vials in refrigerator (36° to 46°F) or at controlled room temperature (less than 77°F). Protect from exposure to light. Reconstituted solution may be stored for up to 4 hr in refrigerator (36° to 46°F) or at controlled room temperature (less than 86°F).

Assessment/Interventions

- Obtain patient history, including drug history and any known allergies. Note renal or hepatic impairment.
- Review patient's health history for any of the following conditions that would contraindicate reteplase use: active internal bleeding; history of cerebrovascular accident, including cardiopulmonary resuscitation; recent intracranial or intraspinal surgery or trauma; intracranial neoplasm, arteriovenous malformation, or aneurysm; severe uncontrolled hypertension; known bleeding diatheses; hypersensitivity to alteplase.
- Review patient's health history for any of the following conditions that could increase the risk of bleeding complications: recent trauma, major surgery, GI bleeding, obstetrical delivery, organ biopsy, previous puncture of noncompressible vessel, or recent GI or GU bleeding; hypertension; likelihood of left heart thrombus; subacute bacterial endocarditis; acute pericarditis; hemostatic defects including those caused by liver or kidney disease; pregnancy; diabetic hemorrhagic retinopathy or other hemorrhagic ophthalmic conditions; septic thrombophlebitis or occluded AV cannula at seriously infected site; cerebrovascular disease; age greater than 75 yr; concurrent use of oral anticoagulants.
- Review patient's medication record for use of drugs that present special risks when used in conjunction with reteplase (other thrombolytic agents, anticoagulants, or antiplatelet agents).
- Monitor patient for signs of internal and superficial bleeding throughout therapy, paying particular attention to recent puncture and cutdown sites. If bleeding develops (eg, epistaxis, hematuria, hematemesis, bloody or black, tarry stools), notify health care provider immediately. Should uncontrollable bleeding occur, discontinue reteplase therapy and concurrent heparin. Be prepared to administer protamine to reverse heparin effects.
- Ensure that second bolus of reteplase is not administered if serious bleeding occurs following the first dose.
- Monitor BP during administration. If hypertension or hypotension develops, notify health care provider immediately. Be prepared to treat appropriately.
- Monitor patient for signs of anaphylaxis or severe allergic reaction. Discontinue therapy and immediately notify health care provider if noted. Be prepared to treat appropriately.
- Avoid IM injections, noncompressible arterial punctures, internal jugular and subclavian venous punctures, and nonessential handling of patient during treatment. Perform venipunctures carefully and as infrequently as possible during therapy.
- If arterial puncture is necessary, ensure that upper extremity vessel is used. Following puncture, apply pressure for at least 30 min. Apply pressure dressing and check puncture site frequently.

Patient/Family Education

- Explain name, action, and potential side effects of drug.
- Advise patient, family, or caregiver that medication will be prepared and administered by a health care professional in a medical setting.
- Instruct patient, family, or caregiver to report any unusual symptoms or feelings, signs of bleeding, or allergic reaction immediately.
- Caution patient to avoid getting out of bed without assistance during treatment.

Rh₀(D) Immune Globulin (RhIG)

(ih-MYOON GLAB-byoo-lin)

Class Immune serum

How Supplied
Gamulin Rh Package Vial of Rho(D) Immune Globulin dissolved in 0.3 M glycine with 0.01% thimersol. ◆ *HypRho-D* Package Syringe of Rho(D) Immune Globulin dissolved in 0.21 to 0.32 M glycine with 80 to 120 mcg thimersol. ◆ *HypRho-D Mini-Dose* Package Syringe of Rho(D) Immune Globulin microdose dissolved in 0.21 to 0.32 M glycine with 80 to 120 mcg thimerosal. ◆ *MICRhoGAM* Package Syringe of Rho(D) Immune Globulin dissolved in glycine 15 mg/mL with 0.003% thimersol. ◆ *RhoGAM* Package Vial of Rho(D) Immune Globulin microdose dissolved in glycine 15 mg/mL with 0.003% thimersol, 2.9 mg sodium chloride, and 0.01% polysorbate 80.

Action
PHARMACOLOGY: By binding Rh₀(D) antigen on red blood cells (RBCs), RhIG prevents production of anti-Rh₀(D) antibodies in Rh₀(D) antigen-negative people. Prevention of Rh sensitization, in turn, prevents hemolytic disease of fetus and newborn in subsequent Rh₀(D) antigen-positive children.

PHARMACOKINETICS/DYNAMICS:
Absorption: T_{max} is 2 hr (IV) or 5 to 10 days (IM). C_{max} is 36 to 48 ng/mL (IV) or 18 to 19 ng/mL (IM).

Excretion: $T_{1/2}$ is about 24 days (IV) or about 30 days (IM).

Indications
Passive, transient protection against development of endogenous anti-Rh antibodies (isoimmunization) in nonsensitized Rh antigen-negative people who receive Rh antigen-positive blood. Such exposure may result from fetomaternal hemorrhage occurring during delivery, spontaneous or induced abortion, abdominal trauma, ectopic pregnancy, chorionic villus sampling (CVS), percutaneous umbilical cord blood sampling (PUBS), amniocentesis, fetal surgery or manipulation, or as result of transfusion accident. RhIG prevents hemolytic disease of fetus and newborn (including erythroblastosis fetalis and hydrops fetalis) in subsequent Rh antigen-positive children. If Rh typing of fetus is not possible, assume fetus is Rh antigen-positive and give mother RhIG. Do not perform Rh cross-match prior to administration.
Term delivery: To warrant RhIG administration, (1) mother must be Rh antigen-negative, (2) mother should not have been previously sensitized to Rh factor (and thus produce her own anti-Rh antibodies), and (3) infant must be Rh antigen-positive and direct antiglobulin negative. (4) If father can be determined to be Rh antigen-negative, RhIG need not be given.

Other obstetric conditions: Administer RhIG to all nonsensitized Rh antigen-negative women after spontaneous or induced abortions, after ruptured ectopic pregnancies, amniocentesis, other abdominal trauma, CVS, PUBS, fetal surgery or manipulation, or any transplacental hemorrhage, unless blood type of fetus has been determined to be Rh antigen-negative. Sensitization occurs more frequently in women undergoing induced abortions than in those aborting spontaneously.

Transfusion accidents: RhIG can be used to prevent Rh sensitization in Rh antigen-negative patients who accidentally receive transfusions with RBCs or blood components containing RBCs, platelets, or granulocytes prepared from Rh antigen-positive blood. Administer within 72 hr following Rh-incompatible transfusion.

Contraindications
Hypersensitivity to thimerosal, any immune globulin, or any of the product's components.
MICRhoGAM: Any indication with continuation of pregnancy or beyond 12 wk gestation.

Route/Dosage
For IM administration only. Contents of total dose may be injected as divided dose at different injection sites at same time, or total dosage may be divided and injected at intervals, provided total dosage to be given is injected within 72 hr.

Postpartum Prophylaxis, Miscarriage, Abortion, or Ectopic Pregnancy
1 full-dose vial or syringe of RhIG prevents maternal sensitization if RBC volume that entered mother's circulation is less than 15 mL. When fetomaternal hemorrhage exceeds 15 mL of RBCs, administer 1 or more containers of RhIG. One minidose container of RhIG will prevent formation of anti-Rh antibodies resulting from spontaneous or induced abortion up to 12 wk gestation. After 12 wk gestation, give full-dose container.

Antepartum Prophylaxis
1 full-dose container of RhIG at 28 wk gestation and again within 72 hr after Rh-incompatible delivery is highly effective in preventing Rh isoimmunization during pregnancy.

Threatened Abortion
Following threatened abortion at any stage of gestation with continuation of pregnancy, give 1 full-dose container of RhIG, unless larger dose is needed.

Amniocentesis or Abdominal Trauma
Following amniocentesis at either 15 to 18 wk gestation or during third trimester, or following abdominal trauma in second or third trimester, give 1 full-dose container of RhIG, unless larger dose is needed.

Transfusion Accidents
Dose of RhIG is dependent on volume of red cells or whole blood transfused. To determine amount of RhIG needed, multiply volume (measured in mL) of Rh antigen-positive whole blood administered by Hct of donor unit. This value equals volume of RBCs transfused. Divide volume of RBCs by 15 to obtain dose of RhIG needed. If dose calculation results in fraction, administer next higher whole number of full-dose vials or syringes of RhIG. Rh antigen-negative patients who receive Rh antigen-positive blood have received as many as 15 to 33 vials of RhIG without adverse reaction. If any event requires administration of RhIG at 13 to 18 wk gestation, give another full dose at 26 to 28 wk gestation. Give additional full dose of RhIG within 72 hr after delivery if infant is Rh antigen-positive. If delivery occurs within 3 wk after last dose, postpartum dose may be withheld, unless there is fetomaternal hemorrhage of more than 15 mL RBCs.

Interactions Antibodies in RhIG may interfere with response to live vaccines. Do not give live vaccines within 14 to 30 days before or 3 mo after RhIG administration. Nonetheless, RhIG does not usually impair response to rubella vaccine. Rubella-susceptible postpartum women who received blood products or RhIG may receive rubella vaccine prior to discharge, provided that rubella antibody titer is drawn 6 to 8 wk after vaccination to ensure seroconversion.

Lab Test Interferences Infants born of women given RhIG antepartum may have weakly positive antiglobulin (*Coombs*) test result at birth. Anti-Rh antibodies may be detected in maternal serum within several wk of administration of RhIG. Such finding does not preclude further RhIG doses. Presence of RhIG antibodies in maternal blood sample can affect interpretation of tests to identify patient as candidate for RhIG. In case of doubt as to patient's Rh group or immune status, give RhIG. Significant fetomaternal hemorrhage late in pregnancy or following delivery may cause weak, mixed-field positive D^u test result. If there is any doubt about mother's Rh type, give RhIG. Screening test for fetal RBCs may help in such cases.

Adverse Reactions
OTHER: As with most IgG products, adverse reactions are infrequent, usually mild in nature and generally confined to site of injection. Occasional patient may react more strongly with localized tenderness, erythema, or low-grade fever. Fever, splenomegaly, myalgia, lethargy, and elevated bilirubin levels occur in some individuals receiving multiple doses of RhIG following mismatched transfusions. This latter reaction may be due to relatively rapid rate of foreign red cell destruction, not to RhIG. Hypersensitivity and systemic reactions and induced sensitization with repeated injections occur rarely.

Precautions
Pregnancy: Category C.
Lactation: Undetermined.
Children: For suppression of Rh isoimmunization in the mother. Do not administer to infants.
IM administration: As with other drugs administered by IM injection, give RhIG with caution to patients on anticoagulant therapy.

PATIENT CARE CONSIDERATIONS

Administration/Storage
- Administer IM only.
- If desirable, divide total dose and give at different injection sites or inject at intervals.
- Give total dosage within 72 hr.
- Store in refrigerator.
- Confirm mother is $Rh_o(D)$ negative prior to administration.
- Obtain blood type and direct antiglobulin test on infant immediately postpartum, prior to administration.

Assessment/Interventions
- Obtain patient history, including drug history and any known allergies.
- Observe injection site for tenderness or erythema.
- Administer with caution if patient is receiving anticoagulants.
- Notify health care provider if fever, splenomegaly, myalgia, or lethargy develop.
- Assess bilirubin levels prior to and following treatment.

Patient/Family Education
- Tell patient to report fever, myalgia, lethargy, abdominal pain, or jaundice to health care provider.
- Instruct patient not to receive any live vaccines within 30 days before or 3 mo after administration of drug.
- Explain how future Rh_o-positive infants will be protected.
- Advise female patients to contact health care provider if pregnant, planning on becoming pregnant, or breastfeeding.

$Rh_o(D)$ Immune Globulin IV (Human) [RhIVIG]

(ih-MYOON GLAB-byoo-lin)

Class Immune globulin

How Supplied
WinRho SDF Powder for Injection, lyophilized 600 IU (120 mcg) (2.5 mL 0.9% Sodium Chloride Injection diluent), Powder for Injection, lyophilized 1500 IU (300 mcg) (2.5 mL 0.9% Sodium Chloride Injection diluent), Powder for Injection, lyophilized 5000 IU (1000 mcg) (8.5 mL 0.9% Sodium Chloride Injection diluent)

Action
PHARMACOLOGY: By binding $Rh_o(D)$ antigen and red blood cells, RhIGIV prevents production of anti-$Rh_o(D)$ antibodies in $Rh_o(D)$ antigen-negative people, which prevents hemolytic disease of the fetus and newborn in subsequent $Rh_o(DP)$ antigen-positive children. Increases platelets in immune thrombocytopenia purpura (ITP) patients.

PHARMACOKINETICS/DYNAMICS:
Absorption: C_{max} is 36 to 48 ng/mL (IV), 18 to 19 ng/mL (IM). T_{max} is 2 hr (IV). 5 to 10 days (IM).

Excretion: $T_{1/2}$ is about 24 days (IV); about 30 days (IM).

Duration: Duration of protective effect is about 30 days.

Indications
Treatment of ITP: Treatment of nonsplenectomized $Rh_o(D)$-positive children with chronic or acute ITP, adults with chronic ITP, or children and adults with ITP secondary to HIV infection.

Suppression of Rh isoimmunization:
Pregnancy and other obstetric conditions – Suppression of Rh isoimmunization in nonsensitized, $Rh_o(D)$-negative women after spontaneous or induced abortions, amniocentesis, chorionic villus sampling, ruptured tubal pregnancy, abdominal trauma, or transplacental hemorrhage, or in the normal course of pregnancy unless the blood type of fetus or father is known to be $Rh_o(D)$-negative. To warrant RhIGIV administration for an Rh-incompatible pregnancy, mother must be $Rh_o(D)$-negative, mother is carrying a child whose father is $Rh_o(D)$-positive or $Rh_o(D)$ unknown, baby is $Rh_o(D)$-positive or $Rh_o(D)$ unknown, and mother must not be previously sensitized to $Rh_o(D)$ factor.

Transfusion – Suppression of Rh isoimmunization in $Rh_o(D)$-negative female children and female adults in their childbearing years transfused with $Rh_o(D)$-positive RBCs or blood components containing $Rh_o(D)$-positive RBCs.

Contraindications Individuals known to have had an anaphylactic or severe systemic reaction to human globulin.

Route/Dosage
ITP
IV Initial dose of 50 mcg/kg (250 IU/kg) as a single dose or in 2 divided doses given on separate days; if patient has hemoglobin less than 10 g/dL, reduce dose to 25 to 40 mcg/kg (125 to 200 IU/kg). If subsequent therapy is required to elevate platelet count, a dose of 25 to 60 mcg/kg (125 to 300 IU/kg) is recommended.

Pregnancy
IM/IV 300 mcg (1500 IU) given at 28 wk gestation. If administered early in pregnancy, administration at 12-wk intervals is recommended. Administer 120 mcg (600 IU) as soon as possible after delivery of a confirmed $Rh_o(D)$ baby, normally no later than 72 hr after delivery. If Rh status of baby is not known at 72 hr, administer RhIGIV to mother 72 hr after delivery. If more than 72 hr have elapsed, administer RhIGIV as soon as possible, up to 28 days after delivery.

Other Obstetric Conditions
IM/IV Administer 120 mcg (600 IU) immediately after abortion, amniocentesis (after 34-wk gestation), or any other manipulation late in pregnancy (after 34-wk gestation) associated with increased risk of Rh isoimmunization. Give RhIGIV within 72 hr after the event.

IM/IV Administer 300 mcg (1500 IU) immediately after amniocentesis, before 34 wk gestation, or after chorionic villus sampling; repeat dose q 12 wk while woman is pregnant. In threatened abortion, give RhIGIV as soon as possible.

Transfusion
Administer within 72 hr after exposure for treatment of incompatible blood transfusions or massive fetal hemorrhage.

IV When patient is exposed to $Rh_o(D)$-positive whole blood, administer 600 mcg (3000 IU) q 8 hr, until 9 mcg (45 IU)/mL of blood is given. When patient is exposed to $Rh_o(D)$-positive red blood cells, administer 600 mcg (3000 IU) q 8 hr, until 18 mcg (90 IU)/mL of cells is given. **IM** When patient is exposed to $Rh_o(D)$-positive whole blood, administer 1200 mcg (6000 IU) q 12 hr, until 12 mcg (60 IU)/mL of blood is given. When patient is exposed to $Rh_o(D)$-positive red blood cells, administer 1200 mcg (6000 IU) q 12 hr, until 24 mcg (120 IU)/mL of cells is given.

Interactions
Live virus vaccines (eg, measles, mumps, polio, rubella): RhIGIV may interfere with the response to live virus vaccines.

INCOMPATIBILITIES: Do not administer RhIGIV concurrently with other products.

Lab Test Interferences

Treatment of ITP: RhIGIV contains trace amounts of anti-A, anti-B, anti-C, and anti-E antibodies which may be detectable in direct and indirect antiglobulin (eg, *Coombs*) tests obtained following RhIGIV administration.
Suppression of Rh isoimmunization: Presence of passively administered anti-Rh_o(D) in maternal or fetal blood can lead to a positive direct antiglobulin (eg, *Coombs*) test.

Adverse Reactions

OTHER:
Treatment of ITP – Headache, fever, chills. When RhIGIV is administered to Rh_o(D)-positive patients with ITP, side effects related to the destruction of Rh_o(D)-positive red blood cells (eg, decreased hemoglobin) can be expected. In most cases, RBC destruction is believed to occur in the spleen; however, signs and symptoms consistent with intravascular hemolysis (IVH), including back pain, shaking, chills, and hemoglobinuria may occur. Complications associated with IVH include death, acute onset or exacerbation of anemia, and acute onset or exacerbation of renal insufficiency.
Suppression of Rh isoimmunization – Adverse reactions to RhIGIV are infrequent in Rh_o(D)-negative patients. Discomfort and slight swelling at site of injection and slight elevation in temperature have been reported.
General – Asthenia; abdominal or back pain; hypotension; pallor; diarrhea; increased LDH; arthralgia; myalgia; dizziness; hyperkinesias; somnolence; vasodilatation; pruritus; rash; sweating; anaphylaxis.

Precautions

Pregnancy: Category C.
Lactation: Undetermined.
Children: Do not administer to infants.
Infection: Because RhIGIV is made from human plasma, there is a risk of transmitting infectious agents (eg, viruses) and theoretically, Creutzfeldt-Jakob disease.
Monitoring: When administering RhIGIV to Rh_o(D)-positive ITP patients, monitor for signs and symptoms of IVH, clinically compromising anemia, and renal insufficiency.

PATIENT CARE CONSIDERATIONS

Administration/Storage

- Administer IV for treatment of ITP RhIGIV (human).
- Use product within 12 hr of reconstitution; discard unused portion.
- Infuse IV-administered dose into a suitable vein over 3 to 5 min, separately from other drugs.
- Administer IM into deltoid muscle of upper arm or anterolateral aspects of upper thigh.
- Administer total dose to patient within 72 hr.
- Store in refrigerator; do not freeze.
- If reconstituted product is not used immediately, store at room temperature for no longer than 12 hr; do not freeze reconstituted product; discard if not administered within 12 hr.
- Confirm mother is Rh_o(D)-negative prior to administration.
- Obtain blood type and direct antiglobulin test on infant immediately postpartum, prior to administration.

Assessment/Interventions

- Obtain patient history, including drug history and any known allergies.
- Observe injection site for tenderness or erythema.
- Notify health care provider if fever, splenomegaly, myalgia, or lethargy develop.

Patient/Family Education

- Tell patient to report fever, myalgia, lethargy, or abdominal pain to health care provider.
- Instruct patient not to receive any live vaccines within 30 days before or 3 mo after administration of drug.
- Explain how future Rh_o-positive infants will be protected.
- Advise female patients to contact health care provider if pregnant, planning on becoming pregnant, or breastfeeding.

Ribavirin

(rye-buh-VIE-rin)

Class Anti-infective/Antiviral

How Supplied

Copegus Tablets 200 mg ♦ *Rebetol* Capsules 200 mg ♦ *Virazole* Lyophilized powder for aerosol reconstitution 6 g ribavirin/100 mL vial. Contains 20 mg/mL when reconstituted with 300 mL sterile water.

Action

PHARMACOLOGY: Has antiviral inhibitory activity against respiratory syncytial virus (RSV), influenza virus, and herpes simplex virus. Exact mechanism is unknown.

PHARMACOKINETICS/DYNAMICS:
Absorption: Absorbed systemically following nasal and oral inhalation. Bioavailability is

unknown and depends on the method of drug delivery.

Distribution: Highest concentrations found in respiratory tract and erythrocytes.

Metabolism: Metabolized to deribosylated ribavirin in the liver.

Excretion: Mostly excreted in urine as unchanged drug and metabolites. The $t_{1/2}$ is 40 days (of erythrocytes). Plasma $t_{1/2}$ is 9.5 hr (children).

Indications
Aerosol: Treatment of carefully selected hospitalized infants and young children with severe lower respiratory tract infections caused by RSV.
Capsule: In combination with recombinant interferon alfa-2b injection for the treatment of chronic hepatitis C in patients with compensated liver disease previously untreated with alpha interferon or who have relapsed following alpha interferon therapy.
Tablet: In combination with peginterferon alfa-2a for the treatment of adults with chronic hepatitis C virus infection who have compensated liver disease and have not been previously treated with interferon alpha.

Contraindications
Women who are pregnant or in men whose female partners are pregnant; patients with a history of hypersensitivity to ribavirin or any component of the product; patients with hemoglobinopathies (eg, thalassemia major or sickle cell anemia); ribavirin tablet/peginterferon alfa-2a combination is contraindicated in patients with autoimmune hepatitis and hepatic decompensation (Child-Pugh class B and C) before or during treatment; ribavirin capsules/interferon alfa-2b is contraindicated in patients with autoimmune hepatitis.

Route/Dosage
RSV

INFANTS AND CHILDREN: **Inhalation** 6 g reconstituted with 300 mL Sterile Water aerosolized and administered over 12 to 18 hr/day for 3 to 7 days.

CAPSULES
ADULTS:
For patients 75 kg or less: **PO** Two 200 mg capsules in the morning and three 200 mg capsules in the evening.

For patients more than 75 kg: **PO** Three 200 mg capsules in the morning and evening. In patients whose hemoglobin levels fall below 10 g/dL, reduce the ribavirin dose to 600 mg/day (one 200 mg capsule in the morning and two 200 mg capsules in the evening). Permanently discontinue ribavirin in patients whose hemoglobin levels fall below 8.5 g/dL. In patients with a history of stable cardiovascular disease, a permanent dose reduction of ribavirin to 600 mg/day is required if the hemoglobin decreased by 2 g/dL or more during any 4-wk treatment period. Permanently discontinue ribavirin therapy in patients with cardiac history if the hemoglobin remains less than 12 g/dL after 4 wk on a reduced ribavirin dose.

TABLETS
ADULTS: **PO** 800 to 1200 mg/day in 2 divided doses with food. Individualize dose depending on baseline disease characteristics (eg, genotype), response to therapy and tolerability of the regimen. Duration of treatment, for patients previously untreated with ribavirin and interferon, is 24 to 48 wk. If severe adverse reactions or laboratory abnormalities develop during combined treatment with ribavirin tablets and peginterferon alfa-2a, modify or discontinue the dose, if appropriate, until adverse reactions subside. If intolerance persists after dosage adjustment, discontinue therapy with these agents. Once ribavirin tablets have been withheld because of clinical manifestation or laboratory abnormality, an attempt may be made to restart ribavirin at 600 mg/day with a further increase in the dose to 800 mg/day. Increasing the dose to the original assigned dose of 1000 to 1200 mg is not recommended.

Interactions
None well documented.

Lab Test Interferences
None well documented.

Adverse Reactions
CV: Cardiac arrest, hypotension, digitalis toxicity (aerosol).
CNS: Headache, dizziness, insomnia, irritability, depression, emotional lability, impaired concentration, nervousness, fatigue (capsules).
DERM: Rash; alopecia, pruritus, injection site inflammation and reaction (capsules).
EENT: Conjunctivitis (aerosol); sinusitis, taste perversion, hearing disorders, vertigo (capsules).
GI: Nausea, anorexia, dyspepsia, vomiting (capsules).
HEMA: Anemia (aerosol); hemolytic anemia, changes in hemoglobin, WBC, neutrophil, and platelet values (capsules).
RESP: Worsening of respiratory status, bacterial pneumonia, pneumothorax, apnea, ventilator dependence (aerosol); dyspnea (capsules).
OTHER: Myalgia, arthralgia, musculoskeletal pain, rigors, fever, flu-like symptoms, asthenia, chest pain (capsules).

WARNING:

Oral: Ribavirin monotherapy is not effective for the treatment of chronic hepatitis C virus infection and should not be used alone for this indication. Primary toxicity is hemolytic anemia, which may result in worsening of cardiac disease that has led to fatal and nonfatal MIs. Do not treat patients with a history of significant or unstable cardiac disease with ribavirin. Contraindicated in women who are pregnant and in the male partners of women who are pregnant. Avoid pregnancy during therapy and for 6 mo after completion of treatment.

Aerosol: Sudden deterioration of respiratory function has been associated with initiation of aerosolized ribavirin use in infants. Carefully monitor respiratory function. If treatment appears to produce sudden deterioration of respiratory function, stop treatment and reinstitute only with extreme caution, continuous monitoring, and consideration of coadministration of bronchodilators. Ribavirin has been shown to produce testicular lesions in rodents.

Precautions
Pregnancy: Category X.
Lactation: Undetermined.
Children: Safety and efficacy of ribavirin capsules not established.
Elderly: Administer ribavirin capsules with caution, reflecting greater frequency of decreased hepatic, renal, or cardiac function and comorbidity.
Renal function impairment: Do not use in patients with Ccr below 50 mL/min.

PATIENT CARE CONSIDERATIONS

Administration/Storage
- Administer by aerosol using only Small Particle Aerosol Generator (SPAG-2). Refer to manufacturer instructions for use of device.
- Reconstitute with 100 mL of preservative-free Sterile Water for Injection, then transfer solution to reservoir.
- Dilute to final volume of 300 mL with Sterile Water for Injection. Concentration should be 20 mg/mL.
- Do not administer with other aerosol medications.
- Discard solutions placed in SPAG-2 unit q 24 hr or longer and when liquid level is low before adding newly reconstituted solution.
- Store reconstituted solution at room temperature and discard after 24 hr.
- Store powder form of drug at room temperature.
- Minimize environmental exposure to ribavirin by use of an aerosol delivery hood or other shielding techniques. Do not allow pregnant women near patient when aerosol is being delivered.

Assessment/Interventions
- Obtain patient history, including drug history and any known allergies.
- Obtain baseline reticulocyte count and monitor daily.
- Monitor I&O.
- Obtain baseline vital signs and monitor at regular intervals during administration.
- Assess respiratory status prior to starting drug and monitor closely during treatment.
- If respiratory status deteriorates rapidly, discontinue treatment and notify health care provider.
- Obtain baseline digoxin levels on patients who are concomitantly receiving digoxin and monitor for digoxin toxicity.
- Assess skin prior to starting drug and observe for changes.

Patient/Family Education
- Caution patient that this medication must not be taken during pregnancy or when pregnancy is possible.
- Advise women to contact health care provider if pregnant, planning to become pregnant, or breastfeeding.
- Tell family to notify health care provider if change in respiratory status or rash occurs.

Riboflavin (Vitamin B₂)

(RYE-boh-FLAY-vin)
Class Vitamin
How Supplied
Riboflavin Tablets 50 mg, Tablets 100 mg
Action
PHARMACOLOGY: Is converted in body to coenzyme necessary in oxidation reduction. Also necessary in maintaining integrity of RBCs.

PHARMACOKINETICS/DYNAMICS:
Absorption: Absorbed from duodenum.
Distribution: Riboflavin and metabolites distributed into all body tissues and breast milk. Small amount stored in liver, spleen, kidneys, and heart. Protein binding is 60% (metabolites FAD and FMN).
Metabolism: Hepatic.
Excretion: Eliminated in urine (excreted mostly as metabolites), small amount in bile, feces, and sweat. $T_{1/2}$ is 66 to 84 min (oral or IM).
Indications Prevention and treatment of riboflavin deficiency.
Contraindications None well documented.

Route/Dosage
Supplement
ADULTS: PO 1.4 to 1.8 mg (men), 1.2 to 1.3 mg (women), 1.6 to 1.8 mg (pregnant or lactating women).
CHILDREN: PO 0.8 to 1.2 mg/day.

Treatment of Deficiency
ADULTS: PO 5 to 10 mg/day.
CHILDREN: PO 2 to 10 mg/day.

Interactions None well documented.
Lab Test Interferences Large doses produce bright-yellow urine, which may contain fluorescent substances and interfere with urinalysis based on spectrometry or color reactions.
Adverse Reactions
GU: Yellow-orange discoloration of urine.
Precautions
Pregnancy: Category A (Category C in doses that exceed the RDA).
Lactation: Excreted in breast milk.
Deficiency: Riboflavin deficiency rarely occurs alone; often associated with deficiency of other B vitamins and protein.

PATIENT CARE CONSIDERATIONS

Administration/Storage
- May be given IM or IV as component of multivitamin.
- Administer with food for optimal absorption.
- Store in cool place in light-resistant container.

Assessment/Interventions
- Obtain patient history, including drug history and any known allergies.
- Assess for deficiency of other B vitamins and protein.
- Evaluate diet history.
- Perform nutritional assessment if indicated.

Patient/Family Education
- Instruct patient to take medication with meals to increase drug absorption.
- Inform patient that urine may turn yellow-orange color.
- Advise patient to take only recommended dose.
- Teach patient about nutritious diet and refer to dietitian if necessary.
- Review diet of foods high in riboflavin (B_2): eggs, organ meats, whole grain cereals and breads, green vegetables, mushrooms, avocados, kidney beans, cashews, chestnuts, cheeses.
- Advise female patients to contact health care provider if pregnant, planning on becoming pregnant, or breastfeeding.

Rifabutin

(RIFF-uh-BYOO-tin)
Class Anti-infective/Antitubercular
How Supplied
Mycobutin Capsules 150 mg
Action
PHARMACOLOGY: Inhibits DNA-dependent RNA polymerase in susceptible strains of bacteria.

PHARMACOKINETICS/DYNAMICS:
Absorption: Readily absorbed from GI tract (53%). C_{max} is 375 ng/mL. T_{max} is 3.3 hr. Bioavailability is 20% (HIV-positive patients) or 85% (healthy patients). High fat meals slow the rate without influencing extent of absorption. Steady state is 9.3 L/kg.

Distribution: High lipophilicity demonstrates a high propensity for distribution and intracellular uptake. Protein binding is about 85%. Vd is 9.3 L/kg.

Metabolism: In the liver, there are 5 metabolites identified, 25-0-desacetyl and 31-hydroxy are the most predominant.

Excretion: Eliminated in the urine (53% excreted primarily as metabolites, 5% unchanged) and feces (30%; 5% unchanged). Systemic cl is 0.69 L/hr/kg. Terminal $t_{1/2}$ is 45 hr.

Special Populations:
Renal Function Impairment – Ccr is less than 30 mL/min. AUC is increased 71%. Reduction in dosage is recommended.

Indications Prevention of disseminated *Mycobacterium avium* complex (MAC) disease in patients with advanced HIV infection.

Contraindications Hypersensitivity to rifabutin or other rifamycins; active tuberculosis.

Route/Dosage
ADULTS: **PO** 300 to 450 mg once daily.
INFANTS AND CHILDREN: **PO** Up to 5 mg/kg/day.

Interactions
Azole antifungal agents, benzodiazepines, beta blockers, buspirone, chloramphenicol, clarithromycin, clozapine, oral contraceptives, corticosteroids, cyclosporine, delavirdine, digitoxin, disopyramide, doxycycline, erythromycin, estrogens, haloperidol, hydantoins, indinavir, losartan, methadone, mexiletine, morphine, nelfinavir, ondansetron, oral anticoagulants, quinidine, quinine, ritonavir, sulfonylureas, tacrolimus, tamoxifen, theophyllines, tocainide, toremifene, tricyclic antidepressants, troleandomycin, verapamil, zolpidem: Therapeutic efficacy may be decreased because of liver enzyme-inducing properties of rifabutin.
Indinavir, itraconazole, ritonavir: May elevate rifabutin plasma levels, increasing the risk of side effects.
Ketoconazole: May reduce rifabutin plasma levels, decreasing the therapeutic effects.
Zidovudine: May decrease plasma levels of zidovudine.

Lab Test Interferences None well documented.

Adverse Reactions
CV: Chest pain.
CNS: Asthenia; headache; insomnia.
DERM: Rash.
EENT: Taste perversion.
GI: Anorexia; diarrhea; dyspepsia; abdominal pain; eructation; flatulence; nausea; vomiting.
GU: Discolored urine.
HEMA: Anemia; eosinophilia; leukopenia; neutropenia; thrombocytopenia.
METAB: Increased alkaline phosphatase, AST, and ALT.
OTHER: Myalgia; fever; discolored saliva, sputum, tears, or skin.

Precautions
Pregnancy: Category B.
Lactation: Unknown. Discontinue nursing or discontinue drug.
Children: Safety and efficacy not established. Based on the limited data available, there is no evidence that doses higher than 5 mg/kg daily are useful.

PATIENT CARE CONSIDERATIONS

Administration/Storage
- Administer on empty stomach. If nausea and vomiting develop, give in divided doses mixed with food such as applesauce.
- Store at room temperature, in tightly closed container.

Assessment/Interventions
- Obtain patient history, including drug history and any known allergies.
- Obtain baseline CBC and monitor at regular intervals during drug therapy. Report decreased neutrophil count.
- Inform health care provider if signs or symptoms of MAC or tuberculosis develops.
- Obtain baseline LFT results and monitor during treatment.

Patient/Family Education
- Inform patient that body fluids (eg, urine, feces, saliva, sputum, perspiration, tears) may be brown-orange in color and that soft contact lenses may be permanently stained. Suggest use of glasses during drug therapy.
- Instruct patient to use nonhormonal methods of birth control while taking drug.
- Instruct patient to notify health care provider of rash, nausea, vomiting, anorexia, diarrhea, abdominal pain, change in color or consistency of stools, jaundice, arthralgias, myositis, chest pressure or pain with shortness of breath, seizure activity, parathesia, aphasia, confusion, insomnia, excessive fatigue, fever, or infection.
- Instruct patient to report photophobia, excessive tearing, or eye pain immediately.
- Advise women to contact health care provider if pregnant, planning to become pregnant, or breastfeeding.

Rifaximin

(riff-AX-ih-min)

Class Antidiarrheal/Anti-infective

How Supplied
Xifaxan Tablets 200 mg

Action

PHARMACOLOGY: Inhibits bacterial RNA synthesis.

PHARMACOKINETICS/DYNAMICS:

Absorption: Systemic absorption is low. Mean C_{max} 4.3 ng/mL; median T_{max} is 1.25 hr; mean AUC 19.5 ng•hr/mL.

Metabolism: Induces CYP3A4 in in vitro studies; however, because of low systemic absorption, clinically important interactions are unlikely.

Excretion: The t½ is 5.9 hr. Excreted primarily in feces (97% of administered dose) and 0.32% unchanged in the urine.

Indications Treatment of travelers' diarrhea by noninvasive strains of *Escherichia coli*.

Contraindications Hypersensitivity to any rifamycins or any component of product.

Route/Dosage

ADULTS AND CHILDREN 12 YR OF AGE AND OLDER: PO 200 mg tid for 3 days.

Interactions None well documented.

Lab Test Interferences None well documented.

Adverse Reactions

CNS: Headache (10%); abnormal dreams, dizziness, migraine, syncope, loss of taste, insomnia fatigue (less than 2%).

DERM: Sunburn, clamminess, rash, increased sweating (less than 2%).

EENT: Ear pain, motion sickness, tinnitus, nasal passage irritation, nasopharyngitis, pharyngitis, pharyngolaryngeal pain, rhinitis, rhinorrhea (less than 2%).

GI: Constipation (4%); vomiting (2%); abdominal distension, diarrhea, dry throat, fecal abnormality, gingival disorder, inguinal hernia, dry lips, stomach discomfort, dysentery, blood in stool, anorexia (less than 2%).

GU: Blood in urine, cholura, dysuria, hematuria, polyuria, proteinuria, urinary frequency (less than 2%).

HEMA/LYMPH: Lymphocytosis, monocytosis, neutropenia (less than 2%).

HYPERSEN: Allergic dermatitis, rash, angioneurotic edema, urticaria, pruritus (postmarketing).

LABTESTABS: Increased aspartate aminotransferase (less than 2%).

M/N: Weight loss, dehydration (less than 2%).

MUSC: Arthralgia, muscle spasms, myalgia, neck pain (less than 2%).

RESP: Respiratory tract infection, upper respiratory tract infection, dyspnea (less than 2%).

OTHER: Chest pain, malaise, pain, weakness, hot flashes (less than 2%).

Precautions

Pregnancy: Category C.

Lactation: Undetermined.

Children: Safety and efficacy not established in children less than 12 yr of age.

Clostridia overgrowth: Treatment with rifaximin may permit overgrowth of *Clostridia*.

Efficacy: Not found to be effective in treating travelers' diarrhea caused by pathogens other than *E. coli*.

Pseudomembranous colitis: Should be considered in patients in whom diarrhea develops subsequent to treatment.

Superinfection: Use may result in bacterial or fungal overgrowth.

PATIENT CARE CONSIDERATIONS

Administration/Storage

- Dose, dosing frequency, and duration of therapy are dependent on condition being treated.
- Administer prescribed dose without regard to meals. Administer with food if GI upset occurs.
- Store tablets at controlled room temperature (59° to 86°F).

Assessment/Interventions

- Obtain patient history, including drug history and any known allergies. Note hypersensitivity to rifamycin antimicrobial agents.
- Ensure medication is not used to treat patient with fever, blood in the stool, or diarrhea caused by pathogens other than *E. coli*.
- Monitor response to therapy. Notify health care provider if diarrhea symptoms worsen or persist more than 48 hr. Be prepared to discontinue therapy and institute alternative antibiotic therapy.
- Monitor patient for GI, CNS, general body side effects, and signs of superinfection. Report to health care provider if noted and significant. Immediately report severe diarrhea, diarrhea containing blood or pus, or severe abdominal cramping.

Patient/Family Education

- Explain name, dose, action, and potential side effects of drug.
- Advise patient to read *Patient Information Leaflet* before starting therapy.

- Review the following decision-making skills that reduce the chances of getting travelers' diarrhea: eat only thoroughly cooked foods; drink bottled water, boiled water, or beverages made with boiled water; drink carbonated beverages in bottles or cans; avoid tap water, fountain drinks, and beverages containing ice.
- Review dosing schedule and prescribed length of therapy with patient.
- Caution patient that medication is to be taken only if they get diarrhea while traveling, but not to take in an effort to prevent diarrhea.
- Instruct patient not to take rifaximin if they have diarrhea and a fever, or have blood in their stools. Instruct patient to seek medical care if either of these occurs.
- Advise patient to take prescribed dose without regard to meals but to take with food if stomach upset occurs.
- Instruct patient to complete entire course of therapy, even if symptoms of travelers' diarrhea have disappeared.
- Advise patient that diarrhea should resolve within 24 to 48 hr after starting therapy. Instruct patient to notify health care provider if diarrhea symptoms worsen or persist more than 48 hr.
- Caution patient that although this medication is an antibiotic, it does not get into the bloodstream and will not work to treat other infections such as chest, sinus, or lung infections caused by bacteria.
- Advise patient to report the following signs of superinfection to health care provider: black "furry" tongue, white patches in mouth, foul-smelling stools, vaginal itching or discharge.
- Warn patient that diarrhea containing blood or pus may be a sign of a serious disorder and to seek medical care if noted and not treat at home.
- Advise patient that drug may cause dizziness and to use caution while driving or performing other tasks requiring mental alertness until tolerance is determined.
- Advise women to notify health care provider if pregnant, planning to become pregnant, or breastfeeding.
- Caution patient not to take any prescription or OTC medications, herbal preparations, or dietary supplements unless advised by health care provider.
- Advise patient that follow-up examinations and lab tests may be required to monitor therapy and to keep appointments.

Rifampin

(RIFF-am-pin)

Class Anti-infective/Antitubercular

How Supplied
Rifadin Capsules 150 mg, Capsules 300 mg, Powder for injection 600 mg ◆ *Rimactane* Capsules 300 mg
✣ *Rofact*

Action

PHARMACOLOGY: Inhibits DNA-dependent RNA polymerase in susceptible strains of bacteria.

PHARMACOKINETICS/DYNAMICS:

Absorption: Almost completely absorbed (oral). T_{max} is 1 to 4 hr (oral). C_{max} is 7 mcg/mL (oral average), may vary 4 to 32 mcg/mL (oral adults); 3.5 to 15 mcg/mL (oral, children); 9 to 17 mcg/mL (IV). Absorption decreased 30% when taken with food.

Distribution: Vd is about 0.64 L/kg (600 mg IV); 0.66 L/kg (300 mg IV). Diffuses well into most body tissues and fluids, including CSF. Crosses placenta and distributes into breast milk. Protein binding is 89%.

Metabolism: Metabolized in liver by deacetylation to active metabolite 25-0-desacetylrifampin. Undergoes enterohepatic circulation.

Excretion: Primarily through bile/fecal (60% to 65% in feces); renal (6% to 15% excreted as unchanged, 15% excreted as active metabolites, 7% as inactive metabolites).

Indications Adjunctive treatment of tuberculosis; short-term management to eliminate meningococci from nasopharynx in *Neisseria meningitidis* carriers. **Unlabeled use(s):** Treatment of infections caused by *Staphylococcus aureus* and *Staphylococcus epidermidis*; treatment of gram-negative bacteremia in infancy; treatment of *Legionella*; management of leprosy; prophylaxis of *Haemophilus influenzae* meningitis.

Contraindications Hypersensitivity to any rifamycin.

Route/Dosage

Tuberculosis

IV dosage form is for initial treatment or retreatment when drug cannot be taken by mouth.

ADULTS: **PO/IV** 10 mg/kg/day (max, 600 mg/day) or 10 mg/kg 2 or 3 times/wk (max, 600 mg).

CHILDREN: **PO/IV** 10 to 20 mg/kg/day (max, 600 mg/day) or 10 to 20 mg/kg 2 or 3 times/wk (max, 600 mg).

Meningococcal Carriers
ADULTS: **PO/IV** 600 mg qd for 4 consecutive days.
CHILDREN 1 MO OR OLDER: **PO/IV** 10 mg/kg q 12 hr for 2 consecutive days.
CHILDREN YOUNGER THAN 1 MO: 5 mg/kg q 12 hr for 2 consecutive days.

Interactions
Azole antifungal agents, benzodiazepines, beta-blockers, buspirone, chloramphenicol, clarithromycin, clozapine, oral contraceptives, corticosteroids, cyclosporine, delavirdine, digitoxin, disopyramide, doxycycline, erythromycin, estrogens, haloperidol, hydantoins, indinavir, losartan, methadone, mexiletine, morphine, nelfinavir, ondansetron, oral anticoagulants, quinidine, quinine, ritonavir, sulfonylureas, tacrolimus, tamoxifen, theophyllines, tocainide, toremifene, tricyclic antidepressants, troleandomycin, verapamil, zolpidem: Therapeutic efficacy may be decreased because of liver enzyme-inducing properties of rifampin.
Digoxin: May decrease digoxin serum concentrations.
Enalapril: May significantly increase BP.
Halothane: Hepatotoxicity and hepatic encephalopathy have been reported with coadministration.
Isoniazid: May result in higher rate of hepatotoxicity.
Ketoconazole: May cause treatment failure of either ketoconazole or rifampin.
Probenecid: Elevates rifampin levels.

Lab Test Interferences
May inhibit standard microbiological assays for serum folate and vitamin B_{12}. Thus, use alternate assay methods. Transient abnormalities in LFTs (eg, elevation in serum bilirubin, abnormal bromsulfophthalein excretion, alkaline phosphatase, serum transaminases) and reduced biliary excretion of contrast media used for visualization of gallbladder may occur. Therefore, perform these tests before the morning dose of rifampin.

Adverse Reactions
CV: Hypotension; shock.
CNS: Headache; drowsiness; fatigue; dizziness; inability to concentrate; mental confusion; generalized numbness; behavioral changes; myopathy.
DERM: Rash; pruritus; urticaria; pemphigoid reaction; flushing.
EENT: Visual disturbances; exudative conjunctivitis.
GI: Heartburn; epigastric distress; anorexia; nausea; vomiting; gas; cramps; diarrhea; sore mouth and tongue; pseudomembranous colitis; pancreatitis.
GU: Hemoglobinuria; hematuria; renal insufficiency; acute renal failure.
HEMA: Eosinophilia; transient leukopenia; hemolytic anemia; decreased hemoglobin; hemolysis; thrombocytopenia.
HEPA: Asymptomatic elevations of liver enzymes and hepatitis.
RESP: Shortness of breath; wheezing.
OTHER: Ataxia; muscular weakness; pain in extremities; osteomalacia; myopathy; menstrual disturbances; fever; elevations in BUN; elevated serum uric acid; possible immunosuppression; abnormal growth of lung tumors; reduced 25-hydroxycholecalciferol levels; edema of face and extremities; discoloration of body fluids.

Precautions
Pregnancy: Category C.
Lactation: Excreted in breast milk. Discontinue nursing or drug.
Hepatic function impairment: Dosage adjustment is necessary.
Body fluids: Medication may cause harmless red-orange discoloration of urine, feces, saliva, sputum, sweat, and tears. Soft contact lenses may be permanently stained.

Overdosage: Signs and Symptoms
Nausea, vomiting, increasing lethargy, unconsciousness, liver enlargement, jaundice, increased direct and total bilirubin levels, altered hepatic enzyme levels.

PATIENT CARE CONSIDERATIONS
Administration/Storage
- Administer oral form 1 hr before or 2 hr after meals.
- Observe IV site closely for extravasation.
- For IV infusion, reconstitute powder in 10 mL of Sterile Water for Injection and swirl gently. Reconstituted solution is stable at room temperature for 24 hr. Withdraw appropriate dose of drug, mix with 500 mL of D5W, and infuse over 3 hr. If ordered, drug may be added to 100 mL and infused over 30 min. A less concentrated solution infused over a longer period is preferred.
- If D5W is contraindicated, use sterile saline. Do not mix with other solutions.
- Initial dilutions of drug in vial are stable for 24 hr at room temperature.
- Use final dilution (500 or 100 mL volumes) within 24 hr because precipitation may occur after this time period.

- Administer solution for injection by IV route only. Do not administer IM or SC.

Assessment/Interventions
- Obtain patient history, including drug history, history of medication noncompliance, and any known allergies.
- Obtain baseline CBC and liver and renal function test results, and monitor at regular intervals.
- Assess skin prior to starting drug and during treatment for rash, pruritus, flushing, urticaria, and jaundice.
- Assess baseline neurologic status and observe for changes.
- Monitor I&O and assess for development of edema.

Patient/Family Education
- Instruct patient to take drug on empty stomach, 1 hr before or 2 hr after meals.
- Inform patient that body fluids may turn red-orange in color and that soft contact lenses may become permanently stained. Advise patient to wear glasses during course of therapy.
- Instruct patient to notify health care provider of persistent anorexia, nausea, vomiting, diarrhea, jaundice, fever, change in color or consistency of stools, malaise or right upper quadrant abdominal pain, unusual bleeding or bruising, petechiae, hematuria, bleeding gums, or pallor.
- Tell patient to notify health care provider of drowsiness, fatigue, dizziness, inability to concentrate, confusion, or visual or behavioral changes.
- Advise patient who uses oral contraceptives to use nonhormonal form of contraception during therapy.
- Advise women to contact health care provider if pregnant, planning to become pregnant, or breastfeeding.
- Advise patient that drug may cause drowsiness and to use caution while driving or performing other tasks requiring mental alertness.
- Advise patient of importance of medication compliance in treatment of tuberculosis. Medication noncompliance reduces efficacy and promotes resistance.
- Caution patient to avoid alcohol.

Rifapentine

(Riff-ah-pen-teen)

Class Anti-infective/Antitubercular

How Supplied
Priftin Tablets 150 mg

Action
PHARMACOLOGY: Inhibits DNA-dependent RNA polymerase in susceptible strains of *Mycobacterium tuberculosis*. Bactericidal for intracellular and extracellular *M. tuberculosis* organisms.

PHARMACOKINETICS/DYNAMICS:

Absorption: Rapid and well absorbed. Absolute bioavailability is not determined. Relative bioavailability is 70% (oral solution). T_{max} is 5 to 6 hr (rifapentine); 11.25 hr (metabolite). C_{max} is 15.05 mcg/mL (rifapentine); 6.26 mcg/mL (25-desacetyl rifapentine metabolite). Food increased AUC and C_{max}. Steady state is 10 days.

Distribution: Vd is 70 L. Protein binding is 97.7% (rifapentine); 93.2% (25-desacetyl rifapentine metabolite). Both bound mainly to albumin.

Metabolism: Hepatic; rifapentine undergoes enzymatic transformation to active 25-desacetyl rifapentine.

Excretion: Eliminated in urine (17%) and feces (70%).

Indications
Treatment of pulmonary tuberculosis in conjunction with 1 or more other antituberculosis drug to which the isolate is susceptible.

Contraindications
Hypersensitivity to any of the rifamycins (rifabutin, rifampin).

Route/Dosage
ADULTS AND CHILDREN (12 YR OR OLDER): **PO** Intensive phase: 600 mg twice weekly (with an interval of 3 days or more) for 2 mo. Continuation phase: 600 mg once weekly for 4 mo.

Interactions
Amitriptyline, azole antifungal agents, barbiturates, buspirone, chloramphenicol, clarithromycin, clofibrate, clozapine, oral contraceptives, corticosteroids, cyclosporine, dapsone, delavirdine, diazepam, digitalis glycosides, disopyramide, doxycycline, erythromycin, fluconazole, fluoroquinolones, haloperidol, indinavir, itraconazole, ketoconazole, levothyroxine, losartan, methadone, mexiletine, morphine, nelfinavir, nifedipine, nortriptyline, ondansetron, phenytoin, progestins, quinidine, quinine, ritonavir, saquinavir, sildenafil, sulfonylureas, tacrolimus, tamoxifen, theophylline, tocainide, toremifene, tricyclic antidepressants, troleandomycin, verapamil, warfarin, zidovudine, zolpidem: Has same interaction potential as rifampin. Potent inducer of hepatic drug metabolizing enzymes. Reduced levels and efficacy of target drugs may occur.
Ketoconazole: May reduce rifapentine plasma levels, decreasing the therapeutic effects.

Lab Test Interferences May alter microbiological assays for folate and vitamin B_{12}.

Adverse Reactions
CV: Hypertension.
CNS: Headache; dizziness.
DERM: Rash; acne; pruritus.
GI: Nausea; vomiting; dyspepsia; diarrhea; hemoptysis.
GU: Pyuria; proteinuria; hematuria; urinary casts.
HEMA: Neutropenia; lymphopenia; anemia; leukopenia; thrombocytosis.
HEPA: Increased AST and ALT; hepatitis.
OTHER: Anorexia; arthralgia; pain; hyperuricemia.

Precautions
Pregnancy: Category C.

PATIENT CARE CONSIDERATIONS
Administration/Storage
- Administer pyridoxine (vitamin B_6) concomitantly in patients who are malnourished, adolescent, and predisposed to neuropathy.
- If GI upset occurs or is anticipated, give drug with food.
- Store at room temperature. Protect from heat and humidity.

Assessment/Interventions
- Obtain patient history, including drug history, history of noncompliance, and any known allergies.
- Assess for diarrhea with blood or pus, which may be a symptom of pseudomembranous colitis. Symptoms may occur after antiinfective treatment is completed.
- Avoid administration to pregnant or nursing women.
- Obtain baseline CBC, hepatic enzyme, and platelet counts.

Lactation: Undetermined.
Children: Safety and efficacy in children younger than 12 yr not established.
Monitoring: Conduct baseline measurements of hepatic enzymes, bilirubin, CBC, and platelet counts. Question patients monthly concerning symptoms of adverse reactions. Follow up on abnormalities, including laboratory tests.
Body fluids: May produce a reddish-orange discoloration of the feces, urine saliva, sweat, sputum, tears, and other body fluids. Contact lenses may become permanently discolored.
Pseudomembranous colitis: Should be considered in patients in whom diarrhea develops.

Overdosage: Signs and Symptoms
Headache, urinary frequency, heartburn, transient elevations of hepatic enzymes.

Patient/Family Education
- Provide patient information pamphlet.
- Instruct patient to take drug only as prescribed and for the full course of therapy.
- Inform patient that body fluids may turn reddish color, including urine sweat, sputum, and tears, and that contact lenses may be permanently stained.
- Advise patient to take with food if prone to nausea, vomiting, or GI upset.
- Instruct patient to notify health care provider if any of the following symptoms are noted: fever; anorexia; malaise; nausea; vomiting; dark urine; yellowed skin or eyes; pain or swelling of joints.
- Advise patients who are using oral contraceptives to use a nonhormonal form of contraception during therapy.
- Advise women to contact health care provider if pregnant, planning to become pregnant, or breastfeeding.

Riluzole

(RILL-you-zole)
Class Neuroprotective
How Supplied
Rilutek Tablets 50 mg

Action
PHARMACOLOGY: Unknown; however, the following properties may be related to effects: inhibits glutamate release; inactivates voltage-dependent sodium channels; interferes with intra-cellular events following transmitter binding at excitatory amino acid receptors. These effects may protect neural tissues against degenerative changes.

PHARMACOKINETICS/DYNAMICS:
Absorption: Well absorbed (about 90%). Oral bioavailability is about 50%. High fat meals decrease absorption, decrease AUC about 20% and peak blood levels by about 45%. Steady state is less than 5 days.

Distribution: Protein binding is 96%, mainly to albumin and lipoproteins. Penetrates brain readily.

Metabolism: Extensively metabolized to 6 major and a number of minor metabolites via CYP450 dependent hydroxylation and glucuronidation. CYP450 1A2 is the main isoenzyme involved in N-hydroxylation.

Excretion: Eliminated in urine (more than 85% glucuronide metabolites; 2% unchanged) and small amount in feces. $T_{1/2}$ is 12 hr (after multiple dosing).

Special Populations:
Renal Function Impairment – Reduced clearance of riluzole and its metabolites leading to higher plasma levels.
Hepatic Function Impairment – Reduced clearance of riluzole and its metabolites, leading to higher plasma levels.
Elderly – Age-related decreased renal function will give higher plasma levels of riluzole and metabolites.
Gender – CYP1A2 activity has been reported to be lower in women and may result in higher blood concentrations and metabolites.
Race – Clearance of drug in Japanese subjects was found to be 50% lower; may possess a lower capacity (oxadative or conjugative) for metabolizing riluzole.
Smoking – Induces CYP1A2 and will eliminate riluzole faster; no information on need to adjust dose in these patients.

Indications Treatment of patients with amyotrophic lateral sclerosis (ALS; Lou Gehrig disease).

Contraindications Standard considerations.

Route/Dosage
ADULTS: PO 50 mg q 12 hr.

Interactions
Caffeine, theophylline, amitriptyline, quinolones: May reduce riluzole elimination.
Cigarette smoke, rifampin, omeprazole: May enhance riluzole elimination.

Lab Test Interferences None well documented.

Adverse Reactions
CV: Hypertension; tachycardia; palpitations; peripheral edema.
CNS: Headache; hypertonia; depression; dizziness; insomnia; somnolence; vertigo; circumoral paresthesia; aggravation reaction; agitation; tremor.
DERM: Pruritus; eczema; alopecia; exfoliative dermatitis.
EENT: Rhinitis; sinusitis.
HEPA: Abnormal LFTs.
GI: Nausea; vomiting; dyspepsia; anorexia; diarrhea; constipation; flatulence; abdominal pain; stomatitis; dry mouth; oral moniliasis.
GU: Urinary tract infection; dysuria.
METAB: Weight loss.
RESP: Decreased lung function; cough.
OTHER: Asthenia; arthralgia; back pain; malaise.

Precautions
Pregnancy: Category C.
Lactation: Undetermined.
Children: Safety and efficacy not established.
Elderly: Age-related compromised renal and hepatic function may cause a decrease in clearance of riluzole.
Renal function impairment: Use with caution in patients with renal impairment.
Hepatic function impairment: Use with caution in patients with current evidence or history of abnormal liver function indicated by significant elevations of liver enzymes. Baseline elevations of several LFTs (especially elevated bilirubin) should preclude use of riluzole.
Monitoring: Measure serum aminotransferases before and during therapy. Evaluate serum SGPT levels every month during the first 3 mo of treatment, every 3 mo during the remainder of the first yr and periodically thereafter.
Special risk patients: Females and Japanese patients may possess a lower metabolic capacity to eliminate riluzole as compared to males and Caucasian subjects, respectively.

PATIENT CARE CONSIDERATIONS

Administration/Storage
- Medication is most effective on an empty stomach. Take at least 1 hr before or 2 hr after a meal for best effect.
- Store at room temperature; protect from bright light.

Assessment/Interventions
- Obtain patient history.
- Obtain baseline laboratory tests, including BUN, SGPT, Hgb, and Hct. Perform and evaluate these tests periodically during treatment, (eg, SGPT levels monthly for 3 mo, every 3 mo during the remainder of the yr and periodically thereafter).
- Monitor for effectiveness and reduction in symptom progression of the disease.
- Assess patient for development of asthenia, nausea, dizziness, diarrhea, decreased level of consciousness, and respiratory distress.

Patient/Family Education
- Instruct patient to take medication 30 min before or 2 hr after a meal.
- Take with a full glass of water.
- Instruct patient to take medicine at same time each day. If a dose is missed, take the next dose as originally planned.
- Instruct patient not to change dose or discontinue medication without consulting health care provider. Larger than prescribed doses do not increase effectiveness, but do increase the side effects.

- Instruct patient to check with health care provider before taking any OTC or prescription medications and vaccinations.
- Have patient report any serious side effects to health care provider, including: asthenia, nausea, dizziness, diarrhea, decreased level of consciousness, respiratory distress.
- Inform patient of need for frequent laboratory tests while taking medication. Be sure to keep appointments.
- Instruct patient to report any fevers to health care provider.
- Instruct patient to avoid drinking alcohol in excess while taking this medication.
- Advise patient that drug may cause dizziness, vertigo, or somnolence and not to drive or operate machinery until patient has gained enough experience to gauge whether or not it affects mental or motor performance adversely.
- Advise female patients to contact health care provider if pregnant, planning on becoming pregnant, or breastfeeding.

Rimantadine Hydrochloride

(rih-MAN-tuh-deen HIGH-droe-KLOR-ide)

Class Anti-infective/Antiviral

How Supplied
Flumadine Syrup 50 mg/5 mL, Tablets 100 mg

Action
PHARMACOLOGY: Inhibits viral replication cycle in various strains of influenza A virus.

PHARMACOKINETICS/DYNAMICS:
Absorption: Well absorbed. C_{max} is 74 ng/mL (single dose). T_{max} is 6 hr (single dose).

Distribution: Protein binding is 40%, mainly albumin.

Metabolism: Extensively metabolized in the liver to 3 hydroxylated metabolites.

Excretion: Eliminated in the urine (less than 25% as unchanged drug). $T_{1/2}$ is 25.4 hr (single dose) and 32 hr (elderly older than 70 yr).

Special Populations:
Renal Function Impairment – Apparent clearance for Ccr 31 to 50 mL/min was 37% lower; apparent clearance for Ccr 11 to 30 mL/min was 16% lower and plasma metabolite concentrations were higher; apparent clearance for Ccr 0 to 10 mL/min was 40% lower with a 1.6-fold increase in elimination half-life.

Elderly – In patients older than 70 years of age, the average AUC, peak concentrations, and elimination half-life at steady state were 20% to 30% higher.

Severe hepatic insufficiency – AUC was about 3-fold larger, elimination half-life was about 2-fold longer, and the apparent clearance was 50% lower.

Indications
Adults: Prophylaxis and treatment of infection caused by various strains of influenza A virus.
Children: Prophylaxis against influenza A virus.

Contraindications Hypersensitivity to drugs of adamantine class including rimantadine and amantadine.

Route/Dosage
Prophylaxis and Treatment
ADULTS: PO 100 mg bid.
ELDERLY NURSING HOME PATIENTS, HEPATIC AND RENAL IMPAIRMENT (CCR LESS THAN 10 ML/MIN): Reduce to 100 mg/day.

Prophylaxis
CHILDREN 10 YR OR OLDER: PO 100 mg bid.
CHILDREN YOUNGER THAN 10 YR: PO 5 mg/kg/day (max, 150 mg/dose).

Interactions
Acetaminophen, aspirin: Decreased peak serum concentration of rimantadine.
Cimetidine: Increased serum concentration caused by decreased clearance.

Lab Test Interferences None well documented.

Adverse Reactions
CNS: Insomnia; dizziness; headache; nervousness; asthenia; impaired concentration.
EENT: Eye pain.
GI: Nausea; vomiting; anorexia; dry mouth; abdominal pain.

Precautions
Pregnancy: Category C.
Lactation: Undetermined. Do not administer to nursing mothers.
Children: Safety and efficacy for prophylaxis not established in children younger than 1 yr.
Elderly: CNS symptoms may occur more frequently.
Seizures: Increased incidence of seizures in patients with seizure history and who receive amantadine.

Overdosage: Signs and Symptoms
Agitation, cardiac arrhythmias, hallucinations, death.

PATIENT CARE CONSIDERATIONS
Administration/Storage
- Administer orally only.
- Store at room temperature.

Assessment/Interventions
- Obtain patient history, including drug history and any known allergies.
- Assess baseline renal and LFT results.
- Notify health care provider if patient has seizure activity, severe or persistent diarrhea, dizziness, impaired concentration, asthenia, or dyspnea.

Patient/Family Education
- Tell patient with history of seizures to discontinue drug and notify health care provider if seizure activity develops.
- Instruct patient to report insomnia, dizziness, headache, nervousness, asthenia, impaired concentration, nausea, vomiting, anorexia, persistent diarrhea, dry mouth, abdominal pain, dyspnea, cough, palpitations, or syncope.
- Caution patient to avoid driving or operating hazardous equipment if dizziness or confusion develops.
- Advise patient to take drug several hours before going to bed if insomnia develops.
- Advise female patients to contact health care provider if pregnant, planning on becoming pregnant, or breastfeeding.

Risedronate Sodium

(riss-ED-row-nate)

Class Hormone/Bisphosphonate

How Supplied
Actonel Tablets 30 mg

Action
PHARMACOLOGY: Inhibits normal and abnormal bone resorption.

PHARMACOKINETICS/DYNAMICS:
Absorption: Relatively rapid and occurs in upper GI tract (oral). T_{max} is about 1 hr. Steady state is about 57 days. Bioavailability is 0.63%.

Distribution: 60% of dose is distributed to bone. Vd is 6.3 L/kg. Protein binding is about 24%.

Excretion: Eliminated in urine (about 40%), unabsorbed drug is eliminated in feces. Mean renal clearance is 105 mL/min. Mean total clearance is 122 mL/min. Initial $T_{1/2}$ is about 1.5 hr. Terminal exponential $t_{1/2}$ is about 480 hr.

Special Populations:
Renal Function Impairment – Ccr is 30 mL/min, clearance decreased by about 70%. Not recommended for use in patients with severe renal impairment.

Indications
Treatment of osteoporosis in postmenopausal women; prevention of osteoporosis in postmenopausal women at risk of developing osteoporosis; prevention and treatment of glucocorticoid-induced osteoporosis in men and women; treatment of Paget disease of the bone.

PATIENT CARE CONSIDERATIONS
Administration/Storage
- Store at room temperature in tightly closed container.
- Administer 30 min before the first meal of the day.
- Administer in upright position with a full glass of water.
- Ensure adequate intake of calcium and vitamin D in patients with Paget disease.

Contraindications
Hypocalcemia.

Route/Dosage
Paget Disease
ADULTS: PO 30 mg once daily for 2 mo.

Treatment and Prevention of Postmenopausal Osteoporosis; Glucocorticoid-Induced Osteoporosis
ADULTS: PO 5 mg/day.

Interactions
Antacids, calcium supplements, oral medicines containing divalent cations: Decrease risedronate absorption, which may decrease activity.

Lab Test Interferences
Interferes with bone-imaging agents.

Adverse Reactions
CNS: Headache; dizziness.
DERM: Rash.
EENT: Amblyopia; tinnitus; dry eye; sinusitis.
GI: Diarrhea; abdominal pain; nausea; constipation; belching; colitis; dysphagia; esophagitis; esophageal ulcers; gastric ulcer.
RESP: Bronchitis.
OTHER: Flu syndrome; chest pain; asthenia; neoplasm; arthralgia; bone pain; leg cramps; myasthenia; peripheral edema.

Precautions
Pregnancy: Category C.
Lactation: Undetermined.
Children: Safety and efficacy not established.
Renal function impairment: Not recommended in patients with Ccr less than 30 mL/min.

Overdosage: Signs and Symptoms
Hypocalcemia.

- Administer with caution to patients with a history of upper GI disorders.
- Exercise caution when administering concomitantly with aspirin or any other NSAID medications.

Assessment/Interventions
- Obtain a complete history of prescription and nonprescription drugs and any history of hypersensitivities.
- Assess for possible drug interactions and potential adverse reactions.
- Ensure that hypocalcemia or other disturbance of the bone and mineral metabolism are effectively treated before administration of risedronate.
- Monitor for signs and symptoms of upper GI disorders such as dysphagia, epigastric pain, esophagitis, esophageal ulcer, and gastric ulcer.

Patient/Family Education
- Instruct patient to take the medication exactly as directed, as clinical benefits may be negatively affected by failure to take the drug according to instructions.
- Instruct patient to take in an upright position with a full 8 oz glass of water 30 min or more before the first food or liquid of the day.
- Remind patient to avoid lying down for 30 min after taking this medication.
- Instruct patient to take any supplement containing calcium or antacids containing magnesium or aluminum 1 hr or more prior or 2 hr after taking risedronate tablets to prevent interference with absorption.
- Warn nursing mothers that a decision to use the drug or continue nursing should be made in collaboration with their primary health care provider.
- Advise female patients to contact health care provider if pregnant, planning on becoming pregnant, or breastfeeding.

Risperidone

(RISS-PURR-ih-dohn)

Class Antipsychotic/Benzisoxazole

How Supplied
Risperdal Tablets 0.25 mg, Tablets 0.5 mg, Tablets 1 mg, Tablets 2 mg, Tablets 3 mg, Tablets 4 mg, Oral solution 1 mg/mL ♦ *Risperdal Consta* Powder for Injection 25 mg, Powder for Injection 37.5 mg, Powder for Injection 50 mg ♦ *Risperdal M-TAB* Tablets, orally disintegrating 0.5 mg, Tablets, orally disintegrating 1 mg, Tablets, orally disintegrating 2 mg

Action
PHARMACOLOGY: Has antipsychotic effect, apparently caused by dopamine and serotonin receptor blocking in CNS.

PHARMACOKINETICS/DYNAMICS:
Absorption: Well absorbed. Bioavailability is 94% (oral). T_{max} is 3 hr (9-hydroxyrisperidone extensive metabolizers) or 20 hr (9-hydroxyrisperidone poor metabolizers). Steady state is about 1 day (extensive metabolizers), about 5 days (poor metabolizers), or about 5 to 6 days (9-hydroxyrisperidone extensive metabolizers). **IM** The main release of the drug starts from 3 wk after injection, is maintained from 4 to 6 wk, and subsides by 7 wk.

Distribution: Vd is 1 to 2 L/kg. Protein binding is about 90% (parent compound) or about 77% (9-hydroxyrisperidone). Once absorbed, the IM form is rapidly distributed.

Metabolism: Extensively metabolized in the liver by CYP450 2D6 to major active metabolite 9-hydroxyrisperidone. CYP450 2D6 is subject to genetic polymorphism (about 6% to 8% white patients, low percentage of Asian patients), has little or no activity, and is considered a poor metabolizer. Extensive metabolizers have low risperidone and high 9-hydroxyrisperidone concentrations; the opposite is true for poor metabolizers.

Excretion: Eliminated in urine (70%) and feces (14%). The t½ is about 21 hr (9-hydroxyrisperidone extensive metabolizers), about 30 hr (9-hydroxyrisperidone poor metabolizers), or about 20 hr (risperidone and active metabolite).

Special Populations:
Renal Function Impairment – (Moderate to severe) Cl of parent drug and active metabolite decreased 60%. Dosage reduction recommended.
Hepatic Function Impairment – Mean free fraction of risperidone in plasma increased about 35%. Dosage reduction is recommended.
Elderly – Renal Cl of both parent drug and active metabolite was decreased. Elimination t½ was prolonged. Modify dose accordingly.

Indications Treatment of schizophrenia; bipolar mania (oral only).

Contraindications Standard considerations.

Route/Dosage
Bipolar Mania
ADULTS: **PO** 2 to 3 mg per day on a once daily schedule. Adjust dose at intervals of no less than 24 hr in increments of 1 mg daily (max, 6 mg daily). No data to support acute treatment beyond 3 wk.

Schizophrenia
ADULTS: **PO** 1 mg bid on first day, 2 mg bid on second day, and 3 mg bid on third day. Dosage adjustment thereafter should occur at intervals

of at least 1 wk in increments of 1 mg bid. Max effect generally occurs in a range of 4 to 8 mg/day (max, 16 mg/day). **IM** 25 mg q 2 wk (max, 50 mg q 2 wk). Oral risperidone should be given with the first injection and continued for 3 wk to ensure adequate plasma concentrations. Do not make upward dosage adjustments more frequently than q 4 wk.

Special Populations

ELDERLY AND PATIENTS WITH RENAL OR HEPATIC IMPAIRMENT WHO CAN TOLERATE AT LEAST 2 MG OF ORAL RISPERIDONE: **IM** 25 mg q 2 wk. ELDERLY OR DEBILITATED PATIENTS WITH SEVERE RENAL OR HEPATIC IMPAIRMENT AND PATIENTS PREDISPOSED TO HYPOTENSION OR FOR WHOM HYPOTENSION WOULD POSE A RISK: **PO** 0.5 mg bid initially; increase in 0.5 mg increments bid thereafter. Increases above 1.5 mg bid should generally occur at intervals of at least 1 wk.

Interactions

Alcohol, CNS depressants: May cause additive CNS depressant effects.

Antihypertensives: Risperidone may enhance hypotensive effects of some antihypertensives.

Carbamazepine: May decrease risperidone plasma levels.

Clozapine, fluoxetine, paroxetine: May increase risperidone plasma levels.

Levodopa and other dopamine agonists: The effects of levodopa and other dopamine agonists may be antagonized.

Lab Test Interferences None well documented.

Adverse Reactions

CV:

Long-acting injection – Hypertension (3%).
Oral – Tachycardia (5%); orthostatic dizziness, palpitations (dose related); atrial fibrillation, cerebrovascular disorder (postmarketing).
CNS:

Long-acting injection – Insomnia (16%); akathisia (9%); hallucinations (7%); somnolence (6%); suicide attempts (4%); abnormal thinking, tremor (3%); abnormal dreaming, hypoesthesia (2%); psychosis, depression, paranoid reaction, delusion, apathy, hypertonia, dystonia (at least 1%).

Oral – Extrapyramidal symptoms (up to 34%); insomnia, agitation (26%); headache (22%); anxiety (20%); dizziness (11%); somnolence (8%); aggressive reaction (3%); increased dream activity, diminished sexual desire, nervousness, increased sleep duration (at least 1%); sleepiness, increased duration of sleep, parkinsonism, extrapyramidal symptoms, asthenia, lassitude, increased fatigability (dose related); mania, Parkinson disease aggravation (postmarketing).

DERM:

Oral – Rash (5%); dry skin (4%); seborrhea (1%); photosensitivity (at least 1%); increased pigmentation (dose related).
EENT:

Long-acting injection – Ear disorder (3%).
Oral – Rhinitis (14%); increased saliva (6%); tooth ache, abnormal vision (3%); accommodation disturbances (dose related).
GI:

Long-acting injection – Diarrhea (5%).
Oral – Constipation (13%); dyspepsia (10%); vomiting (7%); nausea (6%); abdominal pain (4%); increased salivation, toothache (2%); anorexia, reduced salivation (at least 1%); intestinal obstruction (postmarketing).
GU:

Long-acting injection – Amenorrhea (at least 1%).

Oral – Polyuria, polydipsia, menorrhagia, dry vagina, erectile dysfunction (at least 1%); ejaculatory and orgastic dysfunction (dose related).
HEMA:

Long-acting injection – Anemia (at least 1%).
HEPA:

Long-acting injection – Increased hepatic enzymes (at least 1%).

Oral – Jaundice (postmarketing).
METAB:

Long-acting injection – Decreased weight (4%).
Oral – Weight gain (dose related); aggravated diabetes mellitus (including diabetic ketoacidosis), hyperglycemia (postmarketing).
RESP: Coughing (5%); pharyngitis, upper respiratory tract infection, sinusitis (3%); dyspnea (1%); apnea, pulmonary embolism (postmarketing).
OTHER:

Long-acting injection – Pain (10%); leg pain, myalgia (4%); peripheral edema (3%); syncope (2%); arthralgia, skeletal pain, injection site pain (at least 1%).

Oral – Chest pain, fever, arthralgia (3%); back pain (2%); increased prolactin levels; anaphylactic reaction, angioedema, pancreatitis, sudden unexpected death (postmarketing).

Precautions

Pregnancy: Category C.
Lactation: Undetermined; do not breastfeed.
Children: Safety and efficacy not established.
Elderly: Elderly and debilitated patients may have reduced ability to eliminate risperidone. At increased risk of tardive dyskinesia, especially in elderly women, cerebrovascular adverse events and fatalities may occur.

Renal function impairment: Patients with renal impairment may experience enhanced effect of risperidone because of reduced ability to eliminate risperidone. Dose adjustment may be required.

Hepatic function impairment: Patients with hepatic impairment may experience enhanced effect of risperidone because of reduced ability to eliminate risperidone. Dose adjustment may be required.

Aspiration pneumonia: Antipsychotics have been associated with esophageal dysmotility and aspiration. Use with caution in patients at risk for aspiration pneumonia.

Body temperature regulation: Antipsychotics can disrupt the body's ability to reduce core temperature.

Cardiac effects: Appears to have proarrhythmic effects. Orthostatic hypotension may also occur.

Cerebrovascular adverse events (CVAE): CVAE (eg, stroke, transient ischemic attack), including fatalities may occur.

Change in drug therapy: When patient is switched from another antipsychotic to risperidone, it is recommended that the other antipsychotic be discontinued before starting risperidone therapy or to minimize period of overlap.

Cognitive and motor impairment: Caution patients about operating potentially hazardous machinery (eg, driving) until they know whether the drug impairs their ability. Avoid use of alcohol.

Hyperglycemia: Hyperglycemia, in some cases extreme and associated with ketoacidosis, hyperosmolar coma, or death, may occur.

Hyperprolactinemia: May elevate prolactin levels.

Long-term use (more than 8 wk): Long-term use not well evaluated. Periodically reevaluate usefulness.

Neuroleptic malignant syndrome (NMS): NMS has occurred with antipsychotics and is potentially fatal. Signs and symptoms are hyperpyrexia, muscle rigidity, altered mental status, irregular pulse, irregular BP, tachycardia, and diaphoresis.

Priapism: Although reported rarely and a causal relationship has not been established, other drugs with alpha-adrenergic blocking effects have been implicated. Severe priapism may require surgical intervention.

Seizures: Seizures may occur. Use with caution in patients with a history of seizures.

Suicide: Possible suicide attempts are inherent in schizophrenia and bipolar disorder. Closely supervise high-risk patients. Write prescriptions for the smallest quantity consistent with good patient management.

Tardive dyskinesia: A potentially irreversible syndrome of involuntary body and facial movements may occur.

Overdosage: Signs and Symptoms

Drowsiness, tachycardia, hypotension, extrapyramidal symptoms, hyponatremia, hypokalemia, prolonged QT and widened QRS intervals, seizures.

PATIENT CARE CONSIDERATIONS

Administration/Storage

- Oral tablets and disintegrating tablets are bioequivalent and can be interchanged on a mg to mg basis.
- Administer prescribed dose daily or bid as prescribed without regard to meals. Administer with food if GI upset occurs.
- Store tablets, orally disintegrating tablets, and oral solution at controlled room temperature (59° to 77°F). Protect tablets from light and moisture. Protect oral solution from light and freezing. Store injection dose pack in refrigerator (36° to 46°F). If refrigeration is unavailable, store at temperatures not exceeding 77°F for no more than 7 days prior to reconstitution. Once in suspension, avoid exposure to temperatures exceeding 77°F. Discard suspension if not administered within 6 hr of reconstitution.

Oral solution:

- Use calibrated pipette supplied with oral solution to measure prescribed dose. Oral solution can be mixed with 3 to 4 oz of water, coffee, orange juice, or low-fat milk (but not with cola or tea) prior to administration.

Orally disintegrating tablet:

- Contains phenylalanine. Do not administer orally disintegrating tablet to patient with phenylketonuria without first discussing with health care provider.
- Do not open pouch until ready to administer medication.
- Administer disintegrating tablet by peeling back foil on blister pack (do not push tablet through foil) and, using dry hands, remove tablet from foil and place on patient's tongue in patient's mouth; tablet will disintegrate with or without liquid. Advise patient not to chew tablet.

Powder for injection:

- For IM administration only. Not for intradermal, subcutaneous, IV, or intra-arterial administration.
- Administer prescribed dose by deep IM gluteal injection q 2 wk. Alternate injections between the 2 buttocks.
- Allow dose pack from refrigerator to reach room temperature before reconstituting powder for injection.

- Reconstitute powder for injection following manufacturer's guidelines and supplied diluent.
- Administer suspension immediately after reconstitution. If not administered immediately after reconstitution, the suspension must be administered within 6 hr. Resuspend injection following manufacturer's guidelines if injection is not administered immediately after reconstitution.
- Administer oral risperidone, or other antipsychotic medication, as ordered, with the first risperidone injection and for 3 wk, then discontinue.

Assessment/Interventions

- Obtain patient history, including drug history and any known allergies. Note renal or hepatic impairment, dementia-related psychosis, diabetes, CV disease, cerebrovascular disease, cardiac arrhythmias, previous episodes of NMS, seizures, conditions that predispose to seizures (eg, Alzheimer disease), or conditions that would predispose to hypotension (eg, dehydration, hypovolemia, treatment with antihypertensive medications).
- Ensure that lower dose and slower dose escalation is used in elderly or debilitated patient, patient with severe renal or hepatic impairment, or patient who is predisposed to hypotension or in whom hypotension would pose a risk.
- Monitor cardiac patients initiating therapy and following dose increases for orthostatic hypotension; implement safety precautions if orthostatic hypotension occurs and notify health care provider.
- Monitor blood sugar in diabetic patient when drug is started or dose is changed. Report significant changes to health care provider.
- Ensure that fasting blood glucose is evaluated before starting therapy and periodically thereafter during therapy in patient with risk factors for diabetes mellitus (eg, obesity, family history of diabetes).
- Monitor patient for symptoms of hyperglycemia (eg, polydipsia, polyuria, polyphagia, weakness). Inform health care provider if noted.
- Inform health care provider immediately if hyperpyrexia, muscle rigidity, altered mental status, irregular pulse and BP, tachycardia, and diaphoresis develop.
- Assess baseline neurologic status and during treatment observe for involuntary body and facial movements, drowsiness, agitation, anxiety, aggressive reaction, or seizure activity.
- Monitor patient for suicidal tendencies often associated with schizophrenia.
- Ensure that therapy is periodically reviewed to determine if therapy needs to be continued without change or if a dose change (eg, increase, decrease, discontinuation) is indicated.
- Monitor patient for CNS, PSYCH, GI, CV, and general body side effects. Inform health care provider if noted and significant.
- Assess medication compliance.

Patient/Family Education

- Explain name, dose, action, and potential side effects of drug.
- Advise patient to read *Patient Information* leaflet before starting therapy and with each refill.
- Instruct patient to take prescribed dose once daily or bid as prescribed, without regard to meals. Advise patient to take with food if GI upset occurs.
- Advise patient receiving risperidone by injection that medication will be prepared and administered by a health care professional in a medical setting.
- Instruct patient using oral solution to use calibrated pipette to measure each dose. Advise patient that solution may be mixed with 3 to 4 oz of water, coffee, orange juice, or low-fat milk (but not with cola or tea) prior to administration.
- Caution patient using disintegrating tablet not to open the blister until ready to take the dose.
- Advise patient that if a dose is missed to take it as soon as possible and then return to the normal schedule. However, if it is almost time for the next dose, to skip the missed dose and take the next dose at the regularly scheduled time. Instruct patient not to double the dose to catch up.
- Advise patient that dose will be started low and then increased until max benefit is obtained.
- Instruct patient not to change the dose or stop taking the medicine unless advised by health care provider.
- Instruct patient not to stop taking risperidone when feeling better.
- Tell patient to immediately report high fever, muscle rigidity, altered mental status, irregular pulse, sweating, seizures, or rash to health care provider.
- Instruct patient to contact health care provider if symptoms do not appear to be getting better or are getting worse.
- Advise patient to notify health care provider of the following: excessive drowsiness, weight gain, involuntary body or facial movements,

change in personality or mood, frequent urination, excessive thirst.
- Advise patient to avoid strenuous activity during periods of high temperature or humidity.
- Instruct diabetic patient to monitor blood glucose more frequently when drug is started or dose is changed and to inform health care provider of significant changes in readings.
- Instruct patient to avoid alcoholic beverages and sedatives (eg, diazepam) while taking risperidone.
- Instruct patient to get up slowly from lying or sitting position and to avoid sudden position changes to prevent postural hypotension. Advise patient to report dizziness with position changes to health care provider. Caution patient that hot tubs and hot showers or baths may make dizziness worse.
- Advise patient taking antihypertensives to monitor BP at regular intervals.
- Advise patient that drug may impair judgment, thinking, or motor skills or cause drowsiness and to use caution while driving or performing other tasks requiring mental alertness until tolerance is determined.
- Advise patient that medication may cause photosensitivity and to use sunscreen or wear protective clothing until tolerance to the sun or UV light is determined.
- Advise women to notify health care provider if pregnant, planning to become pregnant, or breastfeeding.
- Instruct patient not to take any prescription or OTC medications, dietary supplements, or herbal preparations unless advised by health care provider.
- Advise patient that follow-up visits will be required to monitor therapy and to keep appointments.

Ritodrine Hydrochloride

(RIH-toe-dreen HIGH-droe-KLOR-ide)

Class Uterine relaxant

How Supplied
Ritodrine Hydrochloride in 5% Dextrose Injection 0.3 mg/mL • *Yutopar* Injection 10 mg/mL, Injection 15 mg/mL

Action
PHARMACOLOGY: Inhibits contractility of uterine smooth muscle through beta-adrenergic receptor stimulation.

PHARMACOKINETICS/DYNAMICS:
Absorption: Bioavailability is 100% (60 min IV infusion). C_{max} is 32 to 52 ng/mL.
Distribution: Protein binding is 32%, mainly albumin. Crosses placenta.
Metabolism: Hepatic, metabolized to conjugates.
Excretion: Eliminated in urine (90% as metabolites). Distribution phase $t_{1/2}$ is 6 to 9 min (IV). Second phase $t_{1/2}$ is 1.7 to 2.6 hr (IV). Elimination $t_{1/2}$ is 15 to 17 hr (IV).
Onset: 5 min (IV).

Indications Management of preterm labor in suitable patients.

Contraindications Before 20th wk of pregnancy and when continuation of pregnancy is hazardous to mother or fetus; hypersensitivity; pre-existing maternal conditions that would be seriously affected by pharmacologic properties of beta-mimetic agent.

Route/Dosage
ADULTS: **IV** 0.05 mg/min initially, increasing by 0.05 mg/min q 10 min until desired result is obtained. The usual effective dose is between 0.15 to 0.35 mg/min, continued for at least 12 hr after uterine contractions cease.

Interactions
Atropine: Systemic hypertension may be exaggerated.
Beta-adrenergic blockers: Effects are antagonistic; avoid coadministration.
Corticosteroids: Concomitant use may lead to pulmonary edema.
Magnesium sulfate; diazoxide; meperidine; general anesthetics: Cardiovascular effects of ritodrine may be potentiated.
Sympathomimetics: Effects may be additive or potentiated.

Lab Test Interferences None well documented.

Adverse Reactions
CV: Palpitations; chest pain or tightness; heart murmur; angina pectoris; myocardial ischemia; alterations in BP; pulmonary edema; sinus bradycardia upon drug withdrawal; arrhythmias; drowsiness; weakness; mild tachycardia.
CNS: Tremor, headache (including migraines); nervousness; jitteriness; restlessness; emotional upset; anxiety; malaise; hyperventilation.
DERM: Erythema; rash
GI: Nausea; constipation; diarrhea; vomiting; epigastric distress; ileus; bloating.
HEMA: Leukopenia; agranulocytosis.
HEPA: Hemolytic icterus; impaired liver function.
METAB: Lactic acidosis; glycosuria.
RESP: Dyspnea.
OTHER: Sweating; chills; hypokalemia; hyperglycemia.

Precautions
Pregnancy: Contraindicated before 20th wk of pregnancy; otherwise, Category B.
Lactation: Undetermined.
Sulfite sensitivity: May cause allergic-type reaction in susceptible patients.
Cardiovascular responses: Are common and more pronounced with IV administration.
Maternal pulmonary edema: Has been reported. Closely monitor and avoid fluid overload.
Mild-to-moderate preeclampsia, hypertension, or diabetes: Do not use in these patients unless benefits clearly outweigh risks.
Advanced labor: Safety and efficacy in advanced labor (cervical dilation greater than 4 cm or effacement greater than 80%) are not established.

Overdosage: Signs and Symptoms
Symptoms relate to excessive beta-adrenergic stimulation and include tachycardia, palpitations, cardiac arrhythmias, hypotension, dyspnea, nervousness, tremor, nausea, vomiting.

PATIENT CARE CONSIDERATIONS
Administration/Storage
- 150 mg in 500 mL fluid yields a final concentration of 0.3 mg/mL. When fluid restriction is desirable, may prepare a more concentrated solution. Dilute with 5% Dextrose. Because of increased probability of pulmonary edema, reserve saline diluents for cases where D5W is undesirable.
- Do not use if solution is discolored or contains any precipitate.
- Administer IV infusion with patient in left lateral position to minimize risk of hypotension.
- Use controlled infusion device to deliver medication.
- Use diluted drug within 48 hr. Store at room temperature and avoid excessive heat.
- Store at room temperature, protected from excessive heat.

Assessment/Interventions
- Obtain patient history, including drug history and any known allergies.
- Monitor maternal HR, BP, lung sounds, and fetal HR frequently during IV administration.
- Evaluate strength and frequency of contractions at regular intervals.
- Notify health care provider if patient develops persistent tachycardia or tachypnea or increased systolic BP with widening pulse pressure.
- Discontinue drug, notify health care provider and obtain ECG if chest pain or tightness develops.
- Assess baseline serum glucose (in patients with diabetes) and electrolytes and monitor at regular intervals with IV administration.
- Assess baseline ECG prior to starting drug.
- Notify health care provider if palpitations, tremor, nausea, vomiting, headache, erythema, nervousness, restlessness, anxiety, or malaise develops.
- Monitor I&O for possible fluid overload.
- Assess newborn for ileus and hypotension.
- Monitor glucose and electrolytes of newborn.

Patient/Family Education
- Tell patient to report palpitations, chest pain or tightness, tremor, headache, nervousness, emotional upset, anxiety, malaise, hyperventilation, nausea, vomiting, epigastric distress, bloating, chills, or sweating.
- Advise female patients to contact health care provider if pregnant, planning on becoming pregnant, or breastfeeding.

Ritonavir
(rih-TON-a-veer)

Class Antiretroviral/Protease inhibitor

How Supplied
Norvir Capsules 100 mg, Oral solution 80 mg/mL

Action
PHARMACOLOGY: Inhibits human immunodeficiency virus (HIV) protease, the enzyme required to form functional proteins in HIV-infected cells.

PHARMACOKINETICS/DYNAMICS:
Absorption: Well absorbed. T_{max} is 2 hr (fasting) or 4 hr (non-fasting). Under non-fasting conditions, the oral solution's peak concentration is decreased 23% and the extent of absorption is decreased 7%. The C_{max} is 11.2 mcg/mL.

Distribution: Vd is 0.41 L/kg. Protein binding is 98% to 99%, mainly albumin and alpha-1 acid glycoprotein.

Metabolism: Liver via CYP3A is the major isoform involved in metabolism; CYP2D6 also contributes. Five metabolites have been identified. The major metabolite is isopropylthiazole oxidation metabolite (M-2), which has antiviral activity similar to that of the parent drug.

Excretion: Eliminated in the urine (3.5% excreted as unchanged drug) and feces (33.8% as unchanged drug). $T_{1/2}$ is 3 to 5 hr. Systemic

Cl is 8.8 L/hr (multiple dose), 4.6 L/hr (single dose). Renal Cl is less than 0.1 L/hr.

Special Populations:
Children – Steady state oral clearance for pediatric patients was about 1.5 times faster.

Indications Treatment of HIV infections in combination with other antiretroviral agents.

Contraindications Hypersensitivity to product; concomitant therapy with amiodarone, bepridil, cisapride, flecainide, pimozide, propafenone, quinidine, ergot derivatives, midazolam, triazolam.

Route/Dosage

ADULTS: **PO** 600 mg bid. If adverse reactions occur, relief may be provided by dose titration: 300 mg bid and increased at 2- to 3-day intervals by 100 mg bid.

CHILDREN 2 YR OR OLDER: **PO** Start at 250 mg/m² bid and increase dose at 2- to 3-day intervals by 50 mg/m² bid (max, 600 mg bid).

Interactions

Alprazolam, clorazepate, diazepam, estazolam, fentanyl, flurazepam, midazolam, triazolam, zolpidem: Ritonavir may increase blood levels of these drugs, which may produce extreme sedation and respiratory depression. Do not coadminister.

Amiodarone, bepridil, bupropion, cisapride, clarithromycin, clozapine, encainide, fentanyl, flecainide, lovastatin, meperidine, pimozide, piroxicam, propafenone, propoxyphene, quinidine, rifabutin, sildenafil, simvastatin, tramadol: Ritonavir may elevate blood levels of these drugs, which may increase the risk of arrhythmias, hematologic abnormalities, seizures, or other potential serious adverse effects.

Azole antifungal agents (eg, ketoconazole), clarithromycin, interleukins: May elevate ritonavir plasma levels, increasing the risk of side effects.

Carbamazepine, dexamethasone, phenobarbital, phenytoin, rifabutin, rifampin, St. John's wort: May decrease plasma concentrations of ritonavir.

Desipramine: Desipramine levels may be increased.

Didanosine, methadone, theophylline: Levels may be decreased by ritonavir.

Disulfiram, metronidazole: Ritonavir contains alcohol and may produce a disulfiram-like reaction with these drugs.

Ergot derivatives (eg, ergotamine): Because the risk of ergot toxicity may be increased, coadministration with ritonavir is contraindicated.

Indinavir, saquinavir: Ritonavir may inhibit indinavir and saquinavir metabolism and increase their levels.

Oral contraceptives: Concentrations of ethinyl estradiol, a component of oral contraceptives, may be reduced.

Ritonavir: Consult product labeling for complete list of potential drug interactions.

Warfarin: The anticoagulant effect may be decreased.

Lab Test Interferences None well documented.

Adverse Reactions

CV: Vasodilation; hypotension; palpitations, postural hypotension; tachycardia; syncope.
CNS: Headache; malaise; circumoral paresthesia; paresthesia; dizziness; insomnia; somnolence; abnormal thinking; depression; anxiety.
DERM: Rash; sweating.
EENT: Pharyngitis; sore throat; abnormal taste.
GI: Anorexia; constipation; diarrhea; dyspepsia; flatulence; nausea; vomiting; abdominal pain.
GU: Impotence; dysuria; kidney failure.
HEPA: Hepatitis; hepatomegaly; abnormal LFTs.
METAB: Increased CPK; hyperlipidemia; diabetes mellitus.
OTHER: Asthenia; fever; myalgia.

> **WARNING:**
> Drug interactions with certain drugs may result in serious/life-threatening adverse events.

Precautions

Pregnancy: Category B.
Lactation: Undetermined. HIV-infected mothers should not breastfeed their infants.
Children: Not recommended for children less than 2 yr.
Hepatic function impairment: Use caution; decreased ritonavir clearance may occur.
Diabetes: Monitor glucose closely.
Fat redistribution: Redistribution/accumulation of body fat observed in patients receiving antiretroviral therapy.
Hemophilia: There have been reports of increased bleeding, including skin hematomas and hemarthrosis in patients with hemophilia type A and B.
Pancreatitis: Major toxicity; may be fatal. Consider if patient develops abdominal pain, nausea, vomiting, or lab test abnormalities.

Overdosage: Signs and Symptoms

Paresthesia.

PATIENT CARE CONSIDERATIONS
Administration/Storage
- The medication should be taken with food.
- The oral solution may be mixed with chocolate milk, Ensure, or Advera within 1 hr of dosing to improve the taste.
- Shake the solution well before use.
- Store capsules in the refrigerator in a light-resistant container. Refrigeration is not required if used within 30 days and stored below 77°F.
- Store oral solution at room temperature (59° to 86°F); do not refrigerate. Keep in original container with cap tightly closed.
- Do not switch between oral solution and capsules, as the absorption rates are different.

Assessment/Interventions
- Obtain patient history.
- Assess for history of impaired hepatic function. This medication is metabolized in, and toxic to, the liver.
- Obtain baseline triglycerides, ALT, AST, GGT, CPK, and uric acid. Monitor periodically during treatment.
- Monitor WBC and differential. Note any significant changes.
- Monitor Hct and Hgb frequently (severe anemia may require blood transfusions).

Patient/Family Education
- Advise patient to take ritonavir with food.
- Advise patient to take medication exactly as prescribed.
- Warn patient not to alter the dose or discontinue the medication without consulting health care provider.
- If patient misses a dose, take the next dose as soon as possible. If a dose is skipped, do not double the next dose.
- Instruct patient not to take any other medications, including OTC medications, without checking with health care provider first. This medication interacts with a wide range of all types of medications.
- Explain that the patient will be required to have frequent follow-up blood and urine tests during the course of the treatment and to keep appointments.
- Inform patient that this medication is not a cure for HIV infection and they may continue to acquire secondary illnesses associated with the disease.
- Emphasize to patient, family, and significant others that this medication does not reduce the risk of transmitting HIV to others through sexual contact or blood contamination.
- Inform patient to report symptoms associated with paresthesia (eg, sensations of burning, prickling, formication) to health care provider for a possible reduction in dosage.
- Inform patient to report any other serious side effects to health care provider.
- Explain that the long-term effects of this medication are not known at this time.
- Advise women to contact health care provider if pregnant, planning to become pregnant, or breastfeeding.

Rituximab

(rih-TUCK-sih-mab)

Class Monoclonal antibody

How Supplied
Rituxan Solution for injection 10 mg/mL

Action
PHARMACOLOGY: Rituximab is a monoclonal antibody directed against the CD20 antigen found on the surface of normal and malignant B lymphocytes. The CD20 antigen is also expressed on more than 90% of B-cell non-Hodgkin lymphomas (NHL).

PHARMACOKINETICS/DYNAMICS:
Absorption: Intravenous absorption is immediate and results in a rapid and sustained depletion of circulating and tissue based cells.

Distribution: Binds to lymphoid cells in thymus, white pulp of spleen, and a majority of B lymphocytes in peripheral blood and lymph nodes.

Excretion: Mean serum $t_{1/2}$ is 59.8 hr after first infusion and 174 hr after fourth infusion. Wide range of half-lives reflect the variable tumor burden and changes in CD-20 positive, B-cell populations.

Duration: Detectable in serum 3 to 6 months after completion of treatment. B-cell recovery began at about 6 months following completion of treatment. Median B-cell levels returned to normal by 12 months following completion of treatment.

Indications Relapsed or refractory low-grade or follicular, CD-20 positive, B-cell non-Hodgkin lymphoma.

Contraindications IgE-mediated hypersensitivity or anaphylactic reactions to murine proteins or to any component of this product.

Route/Dosage

Non-Hodgkin Lymphoma
ADULTS: **IV infusion** Initial therapy: 375 mg/m^2 given once weekly for 4 or 8 doses.
RETREATMENT: Patients who subsequently develop progressive disease may be safely retreated with rituximab 375 mg/m^2 once weekly for 4 doses. Currently, there are limited data concerning more than 2 courses.

Pretreatment Regimens
ADULTS: Give acetaminophen 650 mg (**PO** or **rectal**) and diphenhydramine 25 to 50 mg (**PO** or **IV**) 30 to 60 min before administering rituximab.

Interactions No specific drug interactions have been reported. Coadministration of drugs with similar pharmacologic effects may cause additive side effects, including toxicity.

Lab Test Interferences None well documented.

Adverse Reactions
CV: Hypotension, arrhythmias, angina.
CNS: Headache, dizziness, asthenia.
DERM: Pruritus, rash, urticaria.
GI: Nausea and vomiting, abdominal pain.
HEMA: Mild thrombocytopenia, neutropenia, anemia.
RESP: Rhinitis, bronchospasm, dyspnea.
OTHER: Fever, chills, rigor, angioedema, flushing.

> **WARNING:**
> *Fatal infusion reaction:* Deaths within 24 hr of infusion reported. Reaction complex consists of hypoxia, pulmonary infiltrates, acute respiratory distress syndrome, MI, ventricular fibrillation or cardiogenic shock. Approximately 80% of fatal infusion reactions occur with first infusion. Interrupt the rituximab infusion for severe reactions and institute supportive care measures as medically indicated (eg, IV fluids, vasopressors, oxygen, bronchodilators, diphenhydramine, acetaminophen).
>
> *Mucocutaneous reactions (severe):*
> Reported with fatal outcomes.
>
> *Tumor lysis syndrome:* Rapid reduction in tumor volume followed by acute renal failure, hyperkalemia, hypocalcemia, hyperuricemia, or hyperphosphatasemia reported within 12 to 24 hr after the first rituximab infusion.

Precautions
Pregnancy: Category C.
Lactation: Because human IgG is excreted in breast milk and the potential for absorption and immunosuppression in the infant is unknown, advise women to discontinue nursing until circulating drug levels are no longer detectable.
Children: Safety and efficacy have not been established.
Hypersensitivity: Rituximab is associated with hypersensitivity reactions (non-IgE-mediated reactions), which may respond to adjustments in the infusion rate and in medical management.
Cardiac arrhythmias: Discontinue infusions in the event of serious or life-threatening cardiac arrhythmias.
Severe mucocutaneous reactions: Mucocutaneous reactions, some with fatal outcome, have been reported in patients treated with rituximab.

PATIENT CARE CONSIDERATIONS

Administration/Storage

- Do not mix or dilute rituximab with other drugs.
- Rituximab vials are stable at 2° to 8°C (36° to 46°F). Do not use beyond expiration date stamped on carton. Protect vials from direct sunlight. Refer to Preparation for information on the stability and storage of solutions of rituximab diluted for infusion. Rituximab solutions for infusion may be stored at 2° to 8°C (36° to 46°F) for 24 hr and are stable at room temperature for an additional 24 hr. However, since rituximab solutions do not contain a preservative, store diluted solutions refrigerated at 2° to 8°C (36° to 46°F).
- Withdraw appropriate dose from vial and dilute with 0.9% Sodium Chloride or 5% Dextrose to a final concentration of 1 to 4 mg/mL. Gently invert the bag to mix the solution. Discard unused portion in vial.
- Administer IV. Do not give as an IV push or bolus.

- Infusion rate: Start the initial infusion at 50 mg/hr. If no infusion reaction occurs, increase the infusion rate in increments of 50 mg/hr q 30 min up to 400 mg/hr. Subsequent infusions may be started at 100 mg/hr and increased in increments of 100 mg/hr q 30 min up to 400 mg/hr. If an infusion reaction occurred with the first dose, start subsequent infusions at 50 mg/hr.
- Infusion reactions: Slow or stop the infusion if the patient experiences a reaction. When symptoms improve, restart the infusion at 50% of the prior rate and administer the remainder of the dose.

Assessment/Interventions
- Obtain CBC and platelet counts at regular intervals during therapy and more frequently in patients who develop cytopenias. The duration of cytopenias caused by rituximab can extend well beyond the treatment period.
- To avoid excessive infusion-related hypotension, consider avoiding antihypertensive medications for 12 hr prior to the rituximab infusion.
- Women of childbearing age should use effective contraception methods during treatment and for up to 12 mo following rituximab therapy.

Patient/Family Education
- Explain name, action, and potential side effects of drug.
- Advise patient, family, or caregiver that medication will be prepared and administered by health care provider in a health care setting.
- Review dosing schedule with patient, family, or caregiver.
- Advise patient, family, or caregiver to immediately report any of the following to health care provider: rash; itching; hives; shortness of breath or difficulty breathing; decreased urine output; chest pain; fever, chills, or other signs of infection; sores in mouth; unusual bleeding or bruising.
- Advise patient, family, or caregiver to report any of the following to health care provider: persistent nausea, vomiting, diarrhea, or appetite loss; persistent or worsening general body weakness.
- Instruct patient to not take any prescription or OTC medications or dietary supplements unless advised to do so by health care provider.
- Advise female patients to contact health care provider if pregnant, planning on becoming pregnant, or breastfeeding.
- Advise patient that frequent follow-up visits and laboratory tests will be required to monitor therapy and to keep appointments.

Rivastigmine Tartrate

(riv-vah-STIGG-meen TAR-trate)

Class Cholinesterase inhibitor

How Supplied
Exelon Capsules 1.5 mg (as base), Capsules 3 mg (as base), Capsules 4.5 mg (as base), Capsules 6 mg (as base), Solution 2 mg/mL (as base)

Action
PHARMACOLOGY: Unknown; however, may increase acetylcholine by inhibiting acetylcholinesterase, thereby increasing cholinergic function.

PHARMACOKINETICS/DYNAMICS:
Absorption: Rapidly and completely absorbed. T_{max} is about 1 hr. Bioavailability is 36% to 40%. Food delays absorption T_{max} by 90 min, lowers C_{max} by 30%, increases AUC 30%.

Distribution: Widely distributed throughout the body, penetrates blood brain barrier, and distributes equally between blood and plasma. Vd is 1.8 to 2.7 L/kg. Protein binding is 40%.

Metabolism: Rapidly and extensively metabolized, primarily via cholinesterase-mediated hydrolysis to the decarbamylated metabolite. CYP-450 is minimally involved. Shows linear pharmakokinetics up to 3 mg twice daily, but is nonlinear at higher doses.

Excretion: Eliminated in urine (97%, no parent drug detected) and feces (0.4%).

Special Populations:
Renal Function Impairment – Moderate to mean oral clearance is 64% lower. Severe to mean oral clearance is 43% higher for unexplained reasons. Dosage adjustment may be necessary, since dose is individually titrated.
Hepatic Function Impairment – Mean oral clearance is 60% lower. Dosage adjustment is not necessary.
Elderly – Mean oral clearance was 30% lower.
Nicotine users – Increased oral clearance 23%.

Indications Treatment of mild to moderate dementia of the Alzheimer type.

Contraindications Hypersensitivity to rivastigmine or carbamate derivatives.

Route/Dosage
ADULTS: **PO** 1.5 mg twice daily initially, then the dose may be increased by increments of 1.5 mg twice daily at intervals of 2 wk or more (max, 6 mg twice daily).

Interactions

Anticholinergic drugs: Possible reduction in anticholinergic effects.

Cholinesterase inhibitors, cholinomimetics: Synergistic effects may occur.

Lab Test Interferences None well documented.

Adverse Reactions

CV: Hypertension; syncope; chest pain; peripheral edema; hypotension; postural hypotension; cardiac failure; atrial fibrillation; bradycardia; palpitation; angina pectoris; MI; AV block; bundle branch block; sick sinus syndrome; cardiac arrest; supraventricular tachycardia; peripheral ischemia; pulmonary embolism; thrombosis; deep thrombophlebitis; aneurysm; intracranial hemorrhage; extrasystoles; tachycardia.

CNS: Dizziness; headache; insomnia; confusion; depression; anxiety; somnolence; hallucination; tremor; aggression; vertigo; agitation; nervousness; delusion; paranoid reaction; abnormal gait; ataxia; paresthesia; convulsions.

DERM: Increased sweating; rash (eg, maculopapular, eczema, bullous, exfoliative, psoriaform, erythematous).

EENT: Rhinitis; coughing; pharyngitis; bronchitis; tinnitus; cataract.

GI: Nausea; vomiting; anorexia; diarrhea; dyspepsia; abdominal pain; constipation; hemorrhoids; flatulence; eructation; fecal incontinence; gastritis.

GU: Urinary tract infection; urinary incontinence; hematuria.

HEMA: Anemia; epistaxis; hypochromic anemia; thrombocytopenia; lymphadenopathy; leukocytosis.

HEPA: Abnormal hepatic function; cholecystitis.

METAB: Weight decrease; dehydration; hypokalemia.

RESP: Upper respiratory tract infection; bronchoconstriction.

OTHER: Asthenia; accidental trauma; fatigue; malaise; flu-like syndrome; back pain; arthralgia; pain; bone fracture; infection; arthritis; leg cramps; myalgia; fever; edema; allergy; hot flashes.

Precautions

Pregnancy: Category B.

Lactation: Undetermined.

Children: Safety and efficacy not established.

Concomitant medical conditions: Increases cholinergic activity and, therefore, can affect other organ systems, possibly leading to bradycardia, bladder outflow obstruction, increased gastric acid secretion, or bronchoconstriction.

Overdosage: Signs and Symptoms

Cholinergic crisis (eg, severe nausea, vomiting, salivation, sweating, bradycardia, hypotension, respiratory depression, muscle weakness, collapse, convulsions), death.

PATIENT CARE CONSIDERATIONS

Administration/Storage

- Administer twice daily, preferably with morning and evening meal.
- Dose is gradually increased at 2-wk intervals.
- Administer oral solution using the dosing syringe provided with each bottle of medication.
- Dose of oral solution may be swallowed directly from syringe or first mixed with a small glass of water, cold fruit juice, or soda. If mixed with water, juice, or soda, stir completely and have patient drink entire mixture.
- Oral solution and capsules can be interchanged at equal doses.
- Store capsules and oral solution below 77°F (25°C). Store solution upright and protect from freezing.

Assessment/Interventions

- Obtain patient history, including drug history and any known allergies.
- Evaluate patient's mental status and function prior to initiation of therapy.
- Monitor patient for signs of improvement after therapy is started.
- Assess patient for GI, CNS, CV, psychiatric, and general body side effects. Report to health care provider if noted and significant.

Patient/Family Education

- Explain name, dose, action, and potential side effects of drug.
- Advise patient or caregiver that medication is started at a low dose and gradually increased (no more often than every 2 wk) as tolerated to reduce the risk of severe nausea and vomiting occurring.
- Advise patient or caregiver that medication is taken 2 times a day, preferably with the morning and evening meal.
- Ensure that patient or caregiver understands the correct procedure for administering the oral solution. Urge patient or caregiver to review Instruction Sheet included in each package of oral solution.
- Advise patient or caregiver that oral solution may be swallowed directly from syringe or first mixed with a small glass of water, cold fruit juice, or soda. If mixing with water, juice, or soda, stir the mixture well and drink entire mixture.

- Advise patient or caregiver if nausea, vomiting, abdominal pain, or anorexia occur during treatment to discontinue medication for several doses and then restart at the same or next lower dose level.
- Caution patient or caregiver that if medication has been stopped for several days or longer to restart at the lowest dose and gradually increase to the current dose.
- Advise patient or caregiver that nausea and vomiting are the most common side effects and that taking the medication with food may reduce these side effects. If nausea and vomiting become a problem the patient or caregiver should inform the health care provider.
- Advise patient, family, and caregiver not to discontinue the drug or change the dose unless advised to do so by the health care provider.
- Advise patient, family, and caregiver that this drug does not alter the Alzheimer's process and that the effectiveness of the medication may lessen over time.
- Advise patient or caregiver that follow-up visits may be required to monitor therapy and to be sure and keep appointments.

Rizatriptan

(rye-zah-TRIP-tan)

Class Analgesic/Migraine

How Supplied
Maxalt Tablets 5 mg, Tablets 10 mg ◆ Maxalt-MLT Tablets, orally disintegrating 5 mg, Tablets, orally disintegrating 10 mg
✤ Maxalt RPD

Action
PHARMACOLOGY: Binds to serotonin 1_B and 1_D receptors in intracranial arteries leading to vasoconstriction and subsequent relief of migraine headache.

PHARMACOKINETICS/DYNAMICS:
Absorption: Completely absorbed orally. Bioavailability is about 45%. T_{max} is about 1 to 1.5 hr. C_{max} is about 19.8 mg/L.

Distribution: Vd is 140 L in men and 110 L in women. Protein binding is 14%.

Metabolism: Extensive first pass metabolism via oxidative deamination by monoamine oxidase-A (MAO-A) to the indole acetic acid metabolite (inactive) and N-monodesmethyl-rizatriptan (active metabolite).

Excretion: Eliminated in urine (82%; 14% excreted as unchanged, 51% excreted as indole acetic acid metabolite) and feces (12%). Plasma t½ is 2 to 3 hr.

Special Populations:
Gender – AUC is about 30% higher and C_{max} is 11% higher in women than in men.
Hemodialysis patients – Ccr is less than 2 mL/min per $1.73 m^2$; AUC was 44% greater.

Indications Treatment of acute migraine attacks with or without aura.

Contraindications Patients with ischemic heart disease (eg, angina, MI history, silent ischemia, coronary artery vasospastic disease, uncontrolled hypertension, basal or hemiplegic migraine). Rizatriptan is contraindicated within 24 hr of use with other serotonin agonists, ergotamine compounds, or methysergide, or concurrent treatment with MAO inhibitors or within 14 days following discontinuation of an MAO inhibitor.

Route/Dosage
ADULTS: **PO** 5 or 10 mg tablet with the onset of migraine headache. Individualize dose based on response and side effects. Doses may be repeated after a minimum of 2 hr as needed with a max dose of 30 mg in a 24-hr period. Patients taking propanolol should receive the 5 mg dose with a max of 3 doses (15 mg) in a 24-hr period. The MLT formulation is a rapidly disintegrating tablet that may be taken without water. It is placed on the tongue where it rapidly breaks apart and can then be swallowed with normal saliva production.

Interactions
5-HT₁ agonists (eg, sumatriptan): Increased risk of vasospastic reactions; therefore, coadministration of two 5-HT₁ agonists within 24 hr of each other is contraindicated.
Ergot-containing drugs: Additive and prolonged vasospasm.
MAO inhibitors: Use of rizatriptan with MAO inhibitors or within 14 days following discontinuation of an MAO inhibitor is contraindicated.
Propanolol: Increased rizatriptan plasma concentrations.
Selective serotonin reuptake inhibitors (eg, citalopram, fluoxetine, fluvoxamine, sertraline): Weakness, hyperreflexia, and incoordination have been rarely reported.
Sibutramine: Serotonin syndrome, including CNS irritability, motor weakness, shivering, myoclonus, and altered consciousness may occur.

Lab Test Interferences None well documented.

Adverse Reactions
CV: Palpitation (at least 1%); coronary artery vasospasm, transient myocardial ischemia, ventricular tachycardia, ventricular fibrillation

(rare); MI, myocardial ischemia, stroke (postmarketing).
CNS: Dizziness (9%); somnolence (8%); paresthesia (4%); headache (2%); hypesthesia, decreased mental acuity, euphoria, tremor (at least 1%).
DERM: Flushing (at least 1%).
GI: Nausea (6%); dry mouth (3%); diarrhea, vomiting (at least 1%); dysgeusia (postmarketing).
GU: Hot flashes (at least 1%).
RESP: Dyspnea (at least 1%).
OTHER: Asthenia, fatigue (7%); atypical sensations (5%); pain, tightness, pressure, or heaviness of chest, localized pain (3%); tightness, pain, or pressure of neck, throat, or jaw, regional tightness, pressure, or heaviness (2%); warm or cold sensations (at least 1%); hypersensitivity (including angioedema), wheezing, or toxic epidermal necrolysis (postmarketing).

Precautions
Pregnancy: Category C.

PATIENT CARE CONSIDERATIONS
Administration/Storage
- Do not administer with or within 14 days of MAO inhibitor.
- Administer prescribed dose at onset of migraine symptoms.
- Administer without regard to meals.
- Do not administer within 24 hr of treatment with another 5-HT$_1$ agonist or ergot-containing drug.
- If headache recurs after initial relief, a second tablet may be administered, provided there is an interval of at least 2 hr between doses.
- If first dose is ineffective, do not administer a second dose unless prescribed by health care provider.
- Do not administer more than 30 mg per 24-hr period.
- Store tablets and orally disintegrating tablets at ambient room temperature (59° to 86°F).

Orally Disintegrating Tablet:
- Contains phenylalanine. Do not administer orally disintegrating tablet to patient with phenylketonuria without first discussing with health care provider.
- Do not remove orally disintegrating tablets from the outer aluminum pouch until ready to consume.
- Peel open blister pack with dry hands and place orally disintegrating tablet on patient's tongue. Advise patient to allow tablet to dissolve and then swallow with saliva. Advise patient not to chew tablet.

RIZATRIPTAN 1597

Lactation: Undetermined.
Children: Safety and efficacy not established.
Renal function impairment: Cl is decreased; use with caution.
Hepatic function impairment: Cl is decreased; use with caution.
Cardiac: May cause coronary vasospasm in patients with CAD. Administer first dose in health care provider's office or similarly staffed and equipped facility to patients at possible risk of unrecognized coronary disease.
Cerebrovascular events: Cerebral hemorrhage, subarachnoid hemorrhage, stroke, and other cerebrovascular events have been reported with 5-HT$_1$ agonists.
Hypertensive crisis: Elevation in BP, including hypertensive crisis, have been reported with administration of 5-HT$_1$ agonists.
Phenylketonurics: The MLT formulation contains phenylalanine.

Overdosage: Signs and Symptoms
Hypertension.

Assessment/Interventions
- Obtain patient history, including drug history and any known allergies. Note renal or hepatic impairment, ischemic or vasospastic CAD, uncontrolled hypertension, peripheral vascular disease, ischemic bowel disease, stroke, transient ischemic attacks, hemiplegic or basilar migraine, concurrent use of propranolol, or concurrent or recent (within 14 days) use of MAO inhibitor.
- Note recent (within 24 hr) use of other 5-HT$_1$ agonists or ergotamine-containing or ergot-type drugs.
- Ensure that patient receiving propranolol is given the 5 mg dose only and does not take more than 15 mg in any 24-hr period.
- Assess pain location, intensity, duration, and associated symptoms of migraine attack and response to treatment.
- Provide quiet, calm environment. Decrease stimuli, noise, and light.
- Ensure that patients with potential for CAD, including postmenopausal women, men over 40 yr of age, patients with risk factors for CAD (eg, hypertension, hypercholesterolemia, obesity, diabetes, smokers, family history), undergo a CV evaluation before initiating therapy.
- Administer first dose in physician's office or other adequately staffed medical facility to patient with potential for CAD whose CV evaluation provided clinical evidence that

patient is reasonably free of coronary artery and ischemic myocardial disease or other significant underlying CV disease. Consider obtaining an ECG during the interval immediately following administration of the first dose of medication to patient with potential for CAD.
- Monitor patient for signs of allergic reaction. Discontinue therapy and immediately notify health care provider if noted. Be prepared to treat appropriately.
- Ensure that patient who is a long-term user of triptans, such as rizatriptan, undergoes periodic CV evaluation.
- Monitor patient for CNS, CV, GI, and general body side effects. Report to health care provider if noted and significant.

Patient/Family Education
- Explain name, dose, action, and potential side effects of drug.
- Advise patient to read the *Patient Information* leaflet before starting therapy and again with each refill.
- Caution patient using disintegrating tablet not to open the blister until ready to take the dose.
- Explain that drug is to be used only during migraine and does not prevent or reduce the number of attacks. Emphasize that drug is used only to treat actual migraine attack and should not be used to prevent migraine headaches or treat headaches caused by other conditions.
- Advise patient that drug is to be taken as soon as symptoms of migraine appear. A second dose may be taken if symptoms return, but no sooner than 2 hr following the first dose. For a given attack, if there is no response to the first tablet, do not take a second tablet without first consulting with health care provider. Do not take more than 30 mg in any 24-hr period.
- Advise patient that safety of treating more than 4 headaches in a 30-day period has not been established and to inform health care provider if headaches are occurring more frequently.
- Advise patient to immediately notify health care provider if any of the following occur after taking a dose of rizatriptan: severe chest pain or chest pain that does not go away; sudden and/or severe stomach pain; shortness of breath; wheezing; swelling of eyelids, face, or lips.
- Advise patient that if tightness, pain, pressure, or heaviness in chest, throat, neck, or jaw occurs when using sumatriptan, to discuss these symptoms with health care provider before using again.
- Advise patient to notify health care provider if feelings of tingling, heat, flushing, tiredness, dizziness, heaviness, or pressure occur after treatment.
- Advise patient that drug may cause fatigue or dizziness and to use caution while driving or performing other activities requiring mental alertness.
- Advise patient to avoid unnecessary exposure to sunlight or tanning lamps and to use sunscreen and wear protective clothing to avoid photosensitivity reactions.
- Instruct patient to continue taking prescribed migraine prophylactic medications daily as directed.
- Advise patient not currently taking a migraine prophylactic drug to discuss the use of such drugs with health care provider.
- Advise women to notify health care provider if pregnant, planning to become pregnant, or breastfeeding.
- Warn patient not to take any prescription or OTC drugs, dietary supplements, or herbal preparations without consulting health care provider.
- Advise patient that follow-up visits may be necessary to monitor therapy and to keep appointments.

Rocuronium Bromide

(row-kuhr-OH-nee-uhm BROE-mide)

Class Nondepolarizing neuromuscular blocking agent

How Supplied
Zemuron Injection 10 mg/mL

Action
PHARMACOLOGY: Binds competitively to cholinergic receptors on motor end-plate to antagonize action of acetylcholine, resulting in block of neuromuscular transmission.

PHARMACOKINETICS/DYNAMICS:
Distribution: Rapid distribution t½ is 1 to 2 min and the slower distribution t½ is 14 to 18 min. Plasma protein binding is approximately 30%.

Indications As an adjunct to general anesthesia for inpatients and outpatients to facilitate both rapid sequence and routine tracheal intubation and to provide skeletal muscle relaxation during surgery or mechanical ventilation.

Contraindications Standard considerations.

Route/Dosage

Use of a peripheral nerve stimulator is recommended to monitor drug response and determine the need for additional relaxant and adequacy of spontaneous recovery or antagonism.

Continuous Infusion

ADULTS: **IV** 0.01 to 0.012 mg/kg per min initiated only after early evidence of spontaneous recovery from the intubating dose.

Individualization of Dosage

CHILDREN: **IV** 0.6 mg/kg as an initial dose in children under halothane anesthesia produces excellent to good intubating conditions within 1 min.

Maintenance dose: 0.075 to 0.125 mg/kg administered at 25% recovery of control T_1 provides relaxation for 7 to 10 min.

ELDERLY (65 YR OF AGE AND OLDER): **IV** exhibited slightly prolonged median clinical duration under opioid/nitrous oxide/oxygen anesthesia following doses of 0.6, 0.9, and 1.2 mg/kg, respectively.

Maintenance dose: 0.1 to 0.15 mg/kg administered at 25% recovery of T_1.

Maintenance

ADULTS: **IV** 0.1, 0.15, and 0.2 mg/kg administered at 25% recovery of control T_1 (defined as 3 twitches of train-of-four).

Rapid Sequence Intubation

ADULTS: **IV** 0.6 to 1.2 mg/kg provides excellent to good intubating conditions in most patients in less than 2 min.

Tracheal Intubation

ADULTS: **IV** 0.6 mg/kg as a recommended initial dose. Good intubation conditions usually occur within 2 min.

Interactions

Antibiotics (eg, aminoglycoside antibiotics [eg, kanamycin], bacitracin, clindamycin, lincomycin, polymyxins, sodium colistimethate, tetracyclines), lithium, local anesthetics, magnesium salts, procainamide, quinidine: May enhance the neuromuscular blocking action of rocuronium.

Carbamazepine, phenytoin: Resistance to neuromuscular blocking action of rocuronium may occur.

Nitrous oxide/oxygen with either enflurane or isoflurane: May prolong the clinically effective duration of action of initial and maintenance doses of rocuronium and decrease the required infusion rate.

PATIENT CARE CONSIDERATIONS

Administration/Storage

- For IV administration only. Do not administer intradermally, IM, or subcutaneously.
- Follow manufacturer's instructions for prepara-

Succinylcholine: Time of onset of max block following rocuronium may be faster with prior administration of succinylcholine.

INCOMPATIBILITIES: Should not be mixed with alkaline solutions (eg, barbiturates) in the same syringe or administered simultaneously during IV infusion through the same needle.

Lab Test Interferences None well documented.

Adverse Reactions

CV: Arrhythmia, abnormal ECG, tachycardia, transient hypotension and hypertension (less than 1%).

DERM: Rash, injection site edema, pruritus (less than 1%).

GI: Nausea, vomiting (less than 1%).

RESP: Asthma (bronchospasm, wheezing, rhonchi), hiccup (at least 1%).

Precautions

Pregnancy: Category C.

Lactation: Undetermined.

Children: Safety and efficacy has not been established in children less than 3 mo of age. Use in pediatric patients less than 3 mo or greater than 14 yr of age have not been studied.

Hypersensitivity: Rare, severe, or life-threatening anaphylactic reactions have been reported.

Hepatic function impairment: Use with caution.

Special risk patients: May have profound effect in patients with neuromuscular disease (eg, myasthenia gravis). Patients with burns, hemiparesis, or paraparesis may have resistance to rocuronium.

Administration: Under the supervision of experienced clinicians who are familiar with rocuronium action and complications. Personnel and facilities for resuscitation and life support and an antagonist of rocuronium should be immediately available.

Malignant hyperthermia: May occur.

Onset time: May be delayed in patients with slower circulation time (eg, CV disease).

Pulmonary hypertension: Because rocuronium may be associated with increased pulmonary vascular resistance, use with caution in patients with pulmonary hypertension or valvular heart disease.

Tolerance: Tolerance may develop during chronic administration in the intensive care unit.

Overdosage: Signs and Symptoms

Prolonged neuromuscular block.

tion and storage of solutions for continuous IV infusion.

- Inspect solution visually before administration. Solution may have a slightly yellow or greenish-yellow color.

- Do not administer if solution is cloudy, discolored, or contains particulate matter.
- Store vials in refrigerator (36° to 46°F). Do not freeze. May be removed from refrigerator and stored at controlled room temperature (less than 77°F), but injection must be used within 60 days. Once vial has been opened, use within 30 days.

Assessment/Interventions
- Obtain patient history, including drug history and any known allergies. Note liver or kidney disease, myasthenia gravis or myasthenic syndrome, pulmonary hypertension, valvular heart disease, coadministration of antibiotics or magnesium salts, or acid-base abnormality.
- Ensure that resuscitative and tracheal intubation equipment, oxygen, and an antagonist (eg, neostigmine) are available at all times.
- Ensure that peripheral nerve stimulator is used to monitor neuromuscular function during administration in order to monitor effectiveness of dosing, need for additional doses, and confirm recovery from neuromuscular blockade.
- Ensure that patient has adequate anesthesia or sedation before administering rocuronium.
- Administer reduced dose to patient with neuromuscular disease (eg, myasthenia gravis).
- To avoid inaccurate dosing in patient with hemiparesis or paraparesis, monitor neuromuscular function on a nonparetic limb.
- Provide total care for immobilized patient.
- Check mechanical ventilator settings frequently.
- Assess respiratory status frequently. Inform health care provider immediately if deterioration in respiratory status or blood gases are noted.
- Monitor vital signs frequently. Inform health care provider immediately if CV instability is noted.
- Assess infusion site frequently. If extravasation occurs, discontinue infusion or injection immediately and restart in another vein.

Patient/Family Education
- Explain name, action, and potential side effects of drug.
- Advise patient, family, or caregiver that medication will be prepared and administered by a health care provider in a health care setting.
- Reassure patient, family, or caregiver that breathing will be closely monitored and supported while medication is being administered and that breathing and muscle function will return to normal after medication has been discontinued.

Rofecoxib†

(roe-feh-cox-ib)

Class Analgesic/NSAID

How Supplied
Vioxx Tablets 12.5 mg, Tablets 25 mg, Tablets 50 mg

Action
PHARMACOLOGY: Decreases inflammation, pain, and fever, probably by inhibition of prostaglandin, by way of inhibition of cyclooxygenase-2.

PHARMACOKINETICS/DYNAMICS:
Absorption: Bioavailability is about 93%. T_{max} is about 2 to 3 hours. Steady state is reached in 4 days after multiple dosing.

Distribution: Protein binding is about 87% (human plasma). Vd is 86 to 91 L.

Metabolism: Hepatic, primarily mediated through reduction by cytosolic enzymes. Main metabolic products are cis-dihydro and trans-dihydro derivatives of rofecoxib. CYPA50 plays a minor role in metabolism.

Excretion: Eliminated in urine (less than 1% unchanged, 72% excreted as metabolites) and feces (14% unchanged). Plasma clearance is 120 to 141 mL/min. $T_{1/2}$ is about 17 hours.

Special Populations:
Hepatic Function Impairment – (Moderate): AUC increased 55%, C_{max} increased 53%.
Elderly – AUC increased 34%; dosage adjustment not necessary. Initiate lowest recommended dose.
Race – AUC increased 10 to 15% in black and Hispanic patients; no dosage adjustment necessary.
End stage renal disease – Peak plasma levels decreased 18%, AUC decreased 9%; use is not recommended.

Indications Relief of signs and symptoms of osteoarthritis and rheumatoid arthritis; treatment of primary dysmenorrhea; management of acute pain in adults.

Contraindications History of asthma, urticaria, or allergic-type reactions to aspirin or other NSAIDs.

Route/Dosage
Osteoarthritis
ADULTS: **PO** 12.5 to 25 mg once daily.

Rheumatoid Arthritis
ADULTS: **PO** 25 mg once daily (max, 25 mg/day).

† Withdrawn from the market

Primary Dysmenorrhea and Management of Acute Pain
ADULTS: PO 50 mg once daily.

Interactions
ACE inhibitors: Antihypertensive effects may be decreased.
Aspirin: Risk of GI complications (eg, ulceration) may be increased.
Lithium, methotrexate: Rofecoxib may increase plasma levels of these drugs, which may increase activity and adverse effects.
Loop diuretics, thiazide diuretics: Diuretic effects may be decreased.
Rifampin: May decrease rofecoxib plasma levels, which may cause a decrease in activity.
Warfarin: The risk of bleeding may be increased.

Lab Test Interferences
None well documented.

Adverse Reactions
CV: Hypertension; angina pectoris; irregular heartbeat; bradycardia; premature ventricular contraction; tachycardia; palpitations.
CNS: Asthenia; fatigue; dizziness; headache; syncope; hypesthesia; insomnia; migraine; muscular spasm; parethesia; sciatica; somnolence; vertigo; anxiety; depression; decreased mental acuity.
DERM: Alopecia; atopic dermatitis; basal cell carcinoma; blister; cellulitis; contact dermatitis; nail disorder; perspiration; rash; pruritus; erythema; urticaria; xerosis.
EENT: Sinusitis; dry mouth; esophagitis; blurred vision; cerumen impaction; conjunctivitis; dry throat; epistaxis; laryngitis; nasal congestion; nasal secretion; ophthalmic injection; otic pain; otitis; otitis media; pharyngitis; tinnitus; tonsillitis.
GI: Abdominal pain, tenderness, and distension; GI bleeding; diarrhea; dyspepsia; epigastric discomfort; heartburn; duodenal ulcers; nausea; aphthous stomatitis; constipation; gas symptoms; dysgeusia; flatulence; gastritis; gastroenteritis; bloody stools; hemorrhoids; vomiting.
GU: UTI; breast mass; cystitis; dysuria; menopausal symptoms; menstrual disorder; nocturia; urinary retention; vaginitis.
METAB: Hypercholesterolemia.
RESP: Upper respiratory tract infection; bronchitis; asthma; cough; dyspnea; pneumonia; pulmonary congestion.
OTHER: Flu-like condition; pain; back pain; chest pain; pelvic pain; flushing; peripheral edema; upper extremity edema; allergy; muscle pain, cramp, stiffness, and weakness; myalgia.

Precautions
Pregnancy: Category C. Avoid in late pregnancy because rofecoxib may cause premature closure of ductus arteriosus.
Lactation: Undetermined.
Children: Safety and efficacy not established.
Elderly: Initiate therapy with lowest recommended dose.
Renal function impairment: Use with caution.
Hepatic function impairment: Not recommended in patients with moderate or severe hepatic insufficiency.
Asthma: Use with caution in patients with pre-existing asthma.
GI effects: Serious GI toxicity (eg, bleeding, ulceration, performation) can occur at any time, with or without warning symptoms.

PATIENT CARE CONSIDERATIONS
Administration/Storage
- Store tablet and suspension at 25°C (77°F); excursions permitted to (59° to 86°F).
- Shake suspension before use.
- Administer orally using the lowest effective dose as prescribed for each patient.

Assessment/Interventions
- Assess for signs and symptoms of hypersensitivity.
- Obtain a complete history of prescription and nonprescription drug use and any history of hypersensitivity.
- Assess for possible drug interactions and potential adverse reactions.
- Monitor for signs and symptoms of decreased renal function: serum creatinine, BUN, unexpected weight gain, edema.

Patient/Family Education
- Instruct patient to take the medication as prescribed.
- Advise patient to inform primary care provider if taking or planning to take any OTC medications.
- Stress the importance of promptly reporting signs or symptoms of GI ulceration or bleeding, skin rash, unexplained weight gain, or edema to primary caregiver.
- Inform patients of the warning signs and symptoms of hepatotoxicity (eg, nausea, fatigue, lethargy, pruritus, jaundice, right upper quadrant tenderness, flu-like symptoms) and to stop therapy and contact primary care provider should any of these occur.
- Instruct patient to seek immediate emergency help in event of an anaphylactoid reaction.
- Caution patient on prolonged corticosteroid therapy not to stop treatment abruptly but to taper the dosage slowly as directed by health care provider or primary caregiver if the decision has been to discontinue the medication.

- Advise female patients to contact health care provider if pregnant, planning on becoming pregnant, or breastfeeding.
- Warn nursing mothers that a decision to discontinue the drug or nursing should be made in collaboration with their primary health care provider.
- Instruct patient to report any unusual reaction or concern to primary care provider.

Ropinirole Hydrochloride

(row-PIN-ih-role)

Class Antiparkinson/Non-ergot dopamine receptor agonist

How Supplied
Requip Tablets 0.25 mg, Tablets 0.5 mg, Tablets 1 mg, Tablets 2 mg, Tablets 5 mg

Action

PHARMACOLOGY: Stimulates dopamine receptors in the corpus striatum, relieving parkinsonian symptoms.

PHARMACOKINETICS/DYNAMICS:

Absorption: T_{max} is 1 to 2 hr. T_{max} is increased by 2.5 hr when taken with food. Steady state is 2 days. Bioavailability is 55%.

Distribution: Widely distributed throughout the body. Bound to plasma proteins up to 40%. Vd is 7.5 L/kg.

Metabolism: Extensively metabolized by liver to inactive metabolites; major enzyme in metabolism is CYP1A2.

Excretion: Eliminated in the urine (less than 10% as unchanged, 40% N-despropylropinirole, 10% carboxylic acid, 10% hydroxy metabolite). Clearance is 47 L/hr. $T_{1/2}$ elimination is about 6 hr.

Special Populations:
Elderly – In patients older than 65 years of age, oral clearance is reduced by 30%; dosage adjustment is not necessary.

Cigarette smoking – Effect of clearance with smoking has not been evaluated, however, smoking is expected to increase clearance since the CYP1A2 is known to be induced by smoking.

Indications Treatment of the signs and symptoms of idiopathic Parkinson disease. May be used in conjunction with L-dopa.

Contraindications Standard considerations.

Route/Dosage

Individualize by careful titration.

ADULTS: **PO** 0.25 mg tid initially. Then dosage may be increased weekly by 0.75 mg/day until taking 3 mg/day, then by 1.5 mg/day until taking 9 mg/day, then by 3 mg/day to total dose of 24 mg/day.

Interactions

Estrogen: May reduce clearance of ropinirole. Ropinirole dosage adjustments may be needed if estrogen therapy is started or stopped during treatment with ropinirole.

CYP1A2 inducers (eg, smoking, omeprazole): May increase metabolic clearance of ropinirole.

CYP1A2 inhibitors (eg, cimetidine, ciprofloxacin, diltiazem, enoxacin, erythromycin, fluvoxamine, mexiletine, norfloxacin, tacrine): May decrease metabolic clearance of ropinirole. Ropinirole dosage adjustment may be needed if CYP1A2 inhibitor is started or stopped during treatment with ropinirole.

Dopamine antagonists (eg, butyrophenones, metoclopramide, phenothiazines, thioxanthenes): May reduce effectiveness of ropinirole.

Lab Test Interferences None well documented.

Adverse Reactions

CV: Syncope; orthostatic hypotension; hypotension; hypertension; tachycardia; palpitations; arrhythmias; peripheral ischemia.

CNS: Dizziness; somnolence; headache; confusion; hallucinations; abnormal dreams; tremor; anxiety; insomnia; aggravated Parkinson's disease; hyperkinesia; hypokinesia; dyskinesia; paresthesia; vertigo; amnesia; impaired concentration.

DERM: Sweating; flushing.

EENT: Abnormal vision; xerophthalmia; rhinitis; pharyngitis.

GI: Nausea; vomiting; dyspepsia; constipation; abdominal pain; dry mouth; anorexia; diarrhea; flatulence; dysphagia; increased salivation.

GU: Urinary tract infection; urinary frequency; urinary incontinence; impotence.

HEMA: Anemia.

RESP: Bronchitis; dyspnea; pneumonia.

OTHER: Fatigue; viral infection; pain; asthenia; edema; chest pain; malaise; yawning; arthralgia; falls; injury.

Precautions

Pregnancy: Category C.

Lactation: Inhibits prolactin secretion. Do not give to nursing mothers.

Children: Safety and efficacy not established.

Elderly: Incidence of hallucinations appears to be increased with age.

Renal function impairment: Use with caution in presence of severe renal function impairment.

Hepatic function impairment: Use with caution in presence of severe hepatic function impairment.

Hypotension: Postural hypotension may occur, especially during dose escalation.

Syncope: Syncope, sometimes associated with bradycardia, may occur. Most events occur more than 4 wk after starting therapy and are usually associated with a recent increase in dose.
Hallucinations: Can occur during ropinirole therapy. Frequency is greater when used in conjunction with L-dopa.
Dyskinesia: Ropinirole may potentiate dopaminergic effects of L-dopa and may cause or exacerbate pre-existing dyskinesias.
Abrupt withdrawal: Rapid withdrawal or dose reduction of antiparkinsonism drugs may produce symptoms resembling the neuroleptic malignant syndrome.
Retinal pathology: Pathological changes were observed in the retinas of albino rats receiving dopaminergic receptor agonists. The importance of this effect in humans has not been established but cannot be disregarded.
CNS effects: Use concomitant CNS depressants with caution because of additive sedative effects.
Concurrent L-dopa use: When ropinirole is administered as adjunct therapy to levodopa, the dose of levodopa may be decreased as tolerated.

Overdosage: Signs and Symptoms
Nausea, vomiting, agitation, dyskinesia, grogginess, sedation, orthostatic hypotension, chest pain, confusion.

PATIENT CARE CONSIDERATIONS

Administration/Storage
- Administer tid without regard to meals or food.
- If nausea occurs administer each dose with food.
- Store at controlled room temperature protected from light.

Assessment/Interventions
- Obtain patient history, including drug history and any known allergies.
- Note hepatic or renal function impairment.
- Complete baseline assessment of parkinsonian symptoms before instituting therapy.
- Assess for therapeutic effects, adverse reactions and drug interactions throughout course of therapy.
- Assess for orthostatic hypotension, dizziness and mental status changes during initial phase of therapy or following dose escalation.
- Assist patient with position changes and ambulation during initial therapy to prevent falling.
- Monitor BP and pulse routinely during therapy.
- Do not administer if significant changes in BP, pulse, or mental status occur; notify health care provider.

Patient/Family Education
- Instruct patient to take exactly as prescribed. Advise patient that dose may be taken without regard to meals but to take with food if nausea occurs.
- Inform patient that drug may cause drowsiness and to use caution while driving or performing other tasks requiring mental alertness.
- Instruct patient to avoid sudden position changes to prevent orthostatic hypotension.
- Instruct patient to report these symptoms to health care provider: uncontrollable movements, dizziness, mood or mental changes, irregular heartbeat, severe or persistent nausea or vomiting, headache.
- Inform patient that hallucinations can occur and that elderly are more susceptible.
- Advise patient to use caution when taking other drugs with CNS depressant effects (eg, alcohol, sedatives).
- Advise patient not to take any other medications (including OTC) without consulting health care provider.
- Advise female patients to contact health care provider if pregnant, planning on becoming pregnant, or breastfeeding.

Rosiglitazone Maleate
(roe-sih-GLIH-tah-sone MAL-ee-ate)
Class Antidiabetic/Thiazolidinedione

How Supplied
Avandia Tablets 2 mg, Tablets 4 mg, Tablets 8 mg

Action
PHARMACOLOGY: Increases insulin sensitivity; improves sensitivity to insulin in muscles, adipose tissue, and inhibits hepatic gluconeogenisis.

PHARMACOKINETICS/DYNAMICS:
Absorption: Bioavailability is 99%. T_{max} is 1 hr. When administered with food, C_{max} is lowered 28% with a delay in T_{max} by 1.75 hr.

Distribution: Vd is about 17.6 L. Protein binding is 99.8%, primarily albumin.

Metabolism: Extensively metabolized by isoenzyme 2C8 with CYP2C9 as minor pathway. Metabolites are less potent than parent with no contribution to insulin-sensitizing activity.

Excretion: Eliminated in urine (64%) and feces (23%). Plasma t½ is 103 to 158 hr. Elimination t½ is 3 to 4 hr.

Special Populations:
Hepatic Function Impairment – (Moderate to severe) Unbound oral Cl was significantly lower, C_{max} and AUC was increased 2- to 3-fold, and elimination t½ was about 2 hr longer. Do not initiate therapy if patient has active liver disease.

Gender – Mean oral Cl in women was about 6% lower; no dosage adjustment is necessary.

Indications Improves glycemic control of type 2 diabetes mellitus as monotherapy and as an adjunct to diet and exercise; in combination with metformin, insulin, or a sulfonylurea when diet, exercise, and a single agent does not result in adequate glycemic control in patients with type 2 diabetes mellitus.

Contraindications Standard considerations.

Route/Dosage
Monotherapy
ADULTS: **PO** Initiate therapy at 4 mg/day, administered as a single dose or 2 divided doses. For patients not responding adequately, the dose may be increased to 8 mg/day after 8 to 12 wk of therapy.

METFORMIN
Combination Therapy
ADULTS: **PO** In combination with metformin, initiate therapy with 4 mg rosiglitazone as a single dose or 2 divided doses.

SULFONYLUREAS
Combination Therapy
ADULTS: **PO** In combination with sulfonylureas, the recommended dose of rosiglitazone is 4 mg as a single dose or 2 divided doses. If patient reports hypoglycemia, decrease the sulfonylurea dose.

INSULIN
Combination Therapy
ADULTS: **PO** In combination with insulin, the recommended dose of rosiglitazone is 4 mg/day. If the patient reports hypoglycemia or if fasting blood glucose concentrations decrease to less than 100 mg/dL, it is recommended that the insulin dose be decreased 10% to 25%. Individualize further adjustment based on glucose-lowering response.

Interactions None well documented.

Lab Test Interferences Mean hemoglobin and hematocrit may decrease, WBC also may decrease; may be related to increased plasma volume.

Adverse Reactions
CNS: Headache (6%); fatigue (4%).
EENT: Sinusitis (3%).
GI: Diarrhea (2%).
HEMA: Dose-related decreases in hemoglobin (up to 1 g/dL) and hematocrit (up to 3%); anemia (2%).
METAB: Hyperglycemia (4%); hypoglycemia (0.6%).
RESP: Upper respiratory tract infection (10%).
OTHER: Injury (8%); edema (5%); back pain (4%).
Postmarketing – Adverse reactions potentially related to volume expansion (eg, CHF, pulmonary edema, pleura effusions).

Precautions
Pregnancy: Category C.
Lactation: Undetermined.
Children: Safety and efficacy not established.
Hepatic function impairment: Use with caution. Do not initiate therapy with rosiglitazone if patient exhibits clinical evidence of active liver disease or increased serum transaminase levels (ALT more than 2.5 times the upper limit of normal) at start of therapy.
Cardiac failure: Fluid retention may occur, which may exacerbate or lead to heart failure.
Edema: Use with caution; can cause fluid retention.
Ovulation: May result in resumption of ovulation in premenopausal, anovulatory women with insulin resistance.
Weight gain: Dose-related weight gain has been seen alone and in combination with other hypoglycemic agents.

PATIENT CARE CONSIDERATIONS

Administration/Storage
* Do not administer to patients with clinical evidence of active liver disease or elevated liver enzymes (ALT greater than 2.5 times upper limit of normal) or to patients with type 1 diabetes mellitus.
* Administer dose qd or bid as prescribed without regard to meals.
* Administer with food if GI upset occurs.
* Store at controlled room temperature (59° to 86°F). Protect from moisture and humidity.

Assessment/Interventions
* Obtain patient history, including drug history and any known allergies. Note history of liver disease or CHF.
* Ensure that liver enzymes are determined before starting therapy and periodically during therapy (eg, q 2 mo for first yr then periodically thereafter).
* Monitor patients with heart failure for fluid retention (eg, rapid weight gain, edema) and symptoms of heart failure. Notify health care provider if noted.
* Check blood sugars frequently and observe for signs of hypoglycemia and hyperglycemia and report to health care provider.

Patient/Family Education
- Explain name, dose, action, and potential side effects of drug.
- Advise patient to take qd or bid as prescribed.
- Advise patient that medication can be taken without regard to meals but to take with food if GI upset occurs.
- Educate patient, family, and/or caregiver regarding type 2 diabetes and its management.
- Instruct patient that this drug is not a substitute for diet and exercise and that patient should continue to follow prescribed regimens.
- Emphasize the importance of regular daily blood glucose monitoring and periodic glycosylated hemoglobin (A_{1c}) tests.
- Advise patient to carry medical identification of diabetes (eg, Medi-Alert).
- Advise patient to report any of the following to health care provider immediately: nausea, vomiting, abdominal pain, fatigue, anorexia, dark urine, or yellowing of skin or eyes.
- Review symptoms of hypoglycemia and hyperglycemia and action plans to undertake in the event either occur.
- Instruct patient to notify health care provider if experiencing hypoglycemic or hyperglycemic episodes.
- Advise patient that blood will be drawn to check liver function prior to starting therapy and about q 2 mo for the first yr and periodically thereafter and to keep appointments.
- Caution women that drug can cause resumption of ovulation in premenopausal, anovulatory women with insulin resistance. Adequate contraceptive measures for these women should be addressed.
- Advise women to notify health care provider if pregnant, planning to become pregnant, or breastfeeding.
- Instruct patient not to take prescription or OTC drugs or dietary supplements without consulting health care provider.

Rosiglitazone Maleate/Metformin Hydrochloride

(roe-sih-GLIH-tah-sone MAL-ee-ate/ met-FORE-min HIGH-droe-KLOR-ide)

Class Antidiabetic combination/Thiazolinedione/Biguanide

How Supplied
Avandamet Tablets 1 mg/500 mg, Tablets 2 mg/500 mg, Tablets 2 mg/1000 mg, Tablets 4 mg/500 mg, Tablets 4 mg/1000 mg

Action
PHARMACOLOGY:
Rosiglitazone: Increases insulin sensitivity.
Metformin: Decreases blood glucose by reducing hepatic glucose production, increases peripheral glucose uptake and utilization, and may decrease intestinal absorption of glucose.

Indications As an adjunct to diet and exercise to improve glycemic control in patients with type 2 diabetes mellitus who are already treated with combination rosiglitazone and metformin or who are not adequately controlled on metformin alone.

Contraindications Patients with renal disease or renal dysfunction that may also result from conditions such as CV collapse, acute MI, and septicemia; CHF requiring pharmacologic treatment; acute or chronic metabolic acidosis, with or without coma; known hypersensitivity to any component of the product.

Route/Dosage
Base dosage selection of rosiglitazone and metformin on the patient's current doses of rosiglitazone or metformin (max, 8 mg rosiglitazone/2000 mg metformin/day).

Patients Inadequately Controlled on Metformin Monotherapy
ADULTS: PO Start with 4 mg rosiglitazone qd plus the metformin dose already being taken. If prior therapy consists of 1000 mg/day of metformin, start with 2 mg/500 mg and administer 1 tablet bid. If prior therapy consists of 2000 mg/day metformin, start with 2 mg/1000 mg and administer 1 tablet bid.

Patients Inadequately Controlled on Rosiglitazone Monotherapy
ADULTS: PO Start with 1000 mg metformin qd plus the rosiglitazone dose already being taken. If prior therapy consists of 4 mg/day of rosiglitazone, start with 2 mg/500 mg and administer 1 tablet bid. If prior therapy consists of 8 mg/day of rosiglitazone, start with 4 mg/500 mg and administer 1 tablet bid.

Switching From Separate Doses of Rosiglitazone and Metformin To Combination Therapy
ADULTS: PO Start with the doses of rosiglitazone and metformin already being taken. Increase the dose in increments of 4 mg rosiglitazone and/or 500 mg metformin up to the max recommended total daily dose of 8 mg/2000 mg.

Interactions
Alcohol: The effects of metformin on lactate metabolism may be potentiated.
Calcium channel blocking agents, corticosteroids, estrogens, isoniazid, nicotinic acid, oral contraceptives, phenothiazines, phenytoin, sympatho-

mimetics, thiazides and other diuretics, thyroid products: These agents tend to produce hyperglycemia and may lead to loss of blood glucose control.

Cationic drugs (eg, amiloride, digoxin, morphine, procainamide, ranitidine, trimethoprim): Use with caution; may interact with metformin by competing for common renal tubular transport systems.

Cimetidine: Increased metformin plasma levels.

Furosemide: Metformin plasma levels may be elevated while furosemide levels may be decreased.

Nifedipine: Metformin plasma levels may be increased.

Lab Test Interferences None well documented.

Adverse Reactions
CV: Cardiac failure (3%).
CNS: Headache, fatigue (at least 5%).
EENT: Sinusitis (at least 5%).
GI: Diarrhea (at least 5%).
HEMA: Anemia (at least 5%).
RESP: Upper respiratory tract infection, pulmonary edema, pleural effusions (at least 5%).
OTHER: Injury, back pain, viral infection, arthralgia, edema (at least 5%).

> **WARNING:**
> Lactic acidosis is a rare, but serious metabolic complication that can occur because of metformin accumulation during treatment with rosiglitazone/metformin. It is fatal in approximately 50% of cases.

Precautions
Pregnancy: Category C.
Lactation: Undetermined.
Children: Safety and efficacy not established.
Elderly: In general, elderly patients are not titrated to the max dose because of age-related decreases in renal function.
Renal function impairment: Decreased renal function results in decreased renal Cl and prolongation of the metformin t½. Concomitant medications that affect renal function may result in hemodynamic changes or interfere with disposition of metformin (eg, cationic drugs) and should be used with caution. Avoid metformin in patients whose serum creatinine levels exceed the upper limit of normal for their age.

Hepatic function impairment: Avoid metformin in patients with clinical or laboratory evidence of hepatic disease.

Special risk patients: Use with caution in patients with edema; avoid use in patients with type 1 diabetes.

Cardiac failure: Fluid retention, which may exacerbate or lead to heart failure, may occur.

Iodinated contrast materials: Metformin therapy should be withheld at the time of or prior to parenteral contrast studies with iodinate materials. Reinstitute therapy 48 hr after the study and after renal function has been determined to be normal.

Lactic acidosis: Can occur as a result of metformin accumulation (eg, renal impairment) or in pathophysiologic conditions associated with tissue hypoperfusion and hypoxia. The risk of lactic acidosis increases with the degree of renal dysfunction and the age of the patient.

Ovulation: Rosiglitazone therapy may result in ovulation in some premenopausal anovulatory women, increasing the risk of pregnancy.

Surgical procedures: Treatment should be temporarily suspended for any surgical procedure, except minor procedures not associated with restricted intake of food and fluids, and should not be restarted until oral intake has resumed and renal function has been evaluated as normal.

Vitamin B_{12} levels: Metformin may decrease vitamin B_{12} levels.

Weight gain: Dose-related weight gain was seen with rosiglitazone.

Overdosage: Signs and Symptoms
Lactic acidosis.

PATIENT CARE CONSIDERATIONS

Administration/Storage
- Do not administer to patients with renal impairment, clinical evidence of active liver disease, elevated liver enzymes (ALT greater than 2.5 × upper limit of normal), or type 1 diabetes mellitus.
- Refer to manufacturer's dosing chart when converting patients from rosiglitazone or metformin monotherapy to combination therapy.
- Administer dose bid as prescribed.
- Administer each dose with food to prevent GI distress.
- Store at controlled room temperature (59° to 86°F).

Assessment/Interventions
- Obtain patient history, including drug history and any known allergies. Note renal disease, liver disease, CHF, edema, dehydration, chronic metabolic acidosis, acute metabolic acidosis (eg, diabetic ketoacidosis), previous episode of jaundice while taking troglitazone.
- Ensure that renal function, hemoglobin, hematocrit, and RBC indices have been assessed prior to starting therapy and at least annually during therapy.

- Ensure that Ccr has been determined in patients older than 80 yr before initiating therapy.
- Ensure that liver enzymes are determined before starting therapy, q 2 mo during therapy for the first year, and then periodically thereafter.
- Ensure that medication is discontinued in patients who develop symptoms of hepatic dysfunction or whose liver enzymes increase to 3 × upper limit of normal.
- Check blood sugars frequently and observe for signs of hypoglycemia. Inform health care provider if blood sugar readings are outside target range or if hypoglycemic events are noted. Be prepared to treat hypoglycemic reactions.
- Monitor patient for signs or symptoms of metabolic acidosis (eg, malaise, myalgia, respiratory distress, unexplained drowsiness, nausea, vomiting, abdominal pain) and hepatitis (eg, right upper quadrant pain, dark urine, jaundice). Inform health care provider immediately if noted and be prepared to discontinue therapy.
- Monitor patient for fluid retention (eg, edema, rapid weight gain) or other symptoms or signs of heart failure. Inform health care provider if noted.
- Assess patient for GI, CNS, and general body side effects. Inform health care provider if noted and significant.
- Ensure that medication is withheld before, and for 48 hr after, undergoing a radiologic study with intravascular administration of iodinated contrast material and is not restarted until renal function has been documented to be normal.
- Hold therapy in patient undergoing surgical procedure until oral intake has resumed and renal function has been documented to be normal.
- Ensure that premenopausal anovulatory patient is on an effective contraception regimen.

Patient/Family Education

- Explain name, dose, action, and potential side effects of drug.
- Educate patient regarding diabetes and its management, including target ranges for blood sugar control. Instruct patient that medication is not a substitute for diet and exercise and to continue to follow prescribed regimens.
- Educate patient or caregiver regarding potential long-term complications of diabetes and the need for regular physical and eye examinations.
- Advise patient to read *Patient Information* leaflet before starting therapy and with each refill.
- Advise patient to take prescribed dose bid and to take with food to decrease GI distress.
- Advise patient that dose may be gradually increased q 2 wk until max benefit is obtained but that it can take up to 2 to 3 mo for full benefit to be noted.
- Advise patient not to stop taking or change the dose unless advised by health care provider.
- Ensure that patient understands how to use home glucose monitor and has a plan for monitoring and recording blood sugar measurements (eg, log). Advise patient to take log to each visit with health care provider.
- Educate patient regarding value of periodic HbA1c testing to confirm level of glucose control.
- Advise patient to discuss with health care provider a plan for managing each of the following situations: medication dosing during intercurrent conditions (eg, vomiting, infection, trauma, stress, sick days); accidental administration of too little or too much medication; missed dose; inadequate food intake or a skipped meal; travel across time zones; change in physical activity.
- Advise patient to carry medical identification of diabetes (eg, *Medi-Alert*).
- Caution patient to avoid excessive alcohol intake to reduce risk of metabolic acidosis.
- Instruct patient to report any of the following to health care provider immediately: general body discomfort, muscle aches, unexplained rapid breathing or shortness of breath, unexplained drowsiness, nausea, vomiting, abdominal pain, fatigue, anorexia, dark urine, yellowing of the skin or eyes, rapid weight gain.
- Review symptoms of hypoglycemia and hyperglycemia and action plans to undertake in the event either occur.
- Instruct patient to notify health care provider if experiencing hypoglycemic episodes or if measured blood sugars are outside target range.
- Caution premenopausal women that drug can cause resumption of ovulation in premenopausal anovulatory women with insulin resistance. Address adequate contraceptive measures for these women.
- Advise women to notify health care provider if pregnant, planning to become pregnant, or breastfeeding.
- Instruct patient not to take prescription or OTC drugs or dietary supplements without consulting health care provider.
- Advise patient that follow-up visits and lab tests will be necessary to monitor therapy and to keep appointments.

Rosuvastatin Calcium

(row-SEU-vah-stat-in KAL-see-uhm)

Class Antihyperlipidemic/HMG-CoA reductase inhibitor

How Supplied
Crestor Tablets 5 mg, Tablets 10 mg, Tablets 20 mg, Tablets 40 mg

Action
PHARMACOLOGY: Inhibits HMG-CoA reductase, the rate-limiting enzyme that converts 3-hydroxy-3-methyl-glutaryl coenzyme A to mevalonate, a precursor of cholesterol.

PHARMACOKINETICS/DYNAMICS:
Absorption: Absolute bioavailability is about 20%. C_{max} is reached in 3 to 5 hr.
Distribution: The mean Vd_{ss} is about 134 L. Rosuvastatin is 88% protein bound, mainly to albumin.
Metabolism: Not extensively metabolized; about 10% recoverable as a metabolite.
Excretion: Primarily excreted in the feces (90%). The elimination t½ is about 19 hr.

Special Populations:
Hepatic Function Impairment – C_{max} and AUC are increased.
Renal insufficiency – Plasma concentrations increase about 3-fold in patient with severe renal impairment (Ccr less than 30 mL/min). Mild to moderate renal impairment did not affect plasma levels.

Indications As an adjunct to diet to reduce elevated total cholesterol (C), LDL-C, nonHDL-C, ApoB, and TG levels and to increase HDL-C in patients with primary hypercholesterolemia and mixed dyslipidemia; as an adjunct to diet for the treatment of patients with elevated serum TG levels; to reduce LDL-C, total-C, and ApoB in patients with homozygous familial hypercholesterolemia as an adjunct to other lipid-lowering treatments or if such treatments are not available.

Contraindications Pregnancy; breastfeeding; patients with active liver disease or with unexplained persistent elevations of serum transaminases; hypersensitivity to any component of the product.

Route/Dosage
Hypercholesterolemia and Mixed Dyslipidemia
ADULTS: PO 5 to 40 mg once daily, based on goal of therapy and response.

Homozygous, Familial Hypercholesterolemia
ADULTS: PO Start with 20 mg once daily (max, 40 mg/day).

Concurrent Cyclosporine Therapy
ADULTS: PO Limit dose of rosuvastatin to 5 mg/day.

Concurrent Lipid-Lowering Therapy
ADULTS: PO Effect of rosuvastatin may be enhanced with bile acid-binding resin. Limit dose of rosuvastatin to 10 mg/day in patients receiving gemfibrozil.

Renal Insufficiency
ADULTS: PO In patients with severe renal impairment (Ccr less than 30 mL/min/1.73 m^2) not on hemodialysis, start with 5 mg once daily (max, 10 mg once daily).

Interactions
Cyclosporine, gemfibrozil: Plasma concentrations of rosuvastatin may be elevated, increasing the risk of side effects.
Warfarin: Anticoagulant effect of warfarin may be enhanced, increasing the risk of bleeding.

Lab Test Interferences None well documented.

Adverse Reactions
CV: Hypertension (at least 2%); angina pectoris, vasodilatation, palpitation (at least 1%).
CNS: Headache (6%); dizziness, insomnia, hypertonia, paresthesia, depression (at least 2%); anxiety, vertigo, neuralgia (at least 1%).
DERM: Rash (at least 2%); pruritus (at least 1%).
EENT: Pharyngitis (9%); rhinitis, sinusitis (2%).
GI: Diarrhea, dyspepsia, nausea (3%); constipation, gastroenteritis (at least 2%); vomiting, flatulence, periodontal abscess, gastritis (at least 1%).
ENDO: Diabetes mellitus (at least 1%).
GU: UTI (2%).
HEMA: Anemia, ecchymosis (at least 1%).
LABTESTABS: Elevated creatinine phosphokinase, transaminases, hyperglycemia, glutamyl transpeptidase, alkaline phosphatase, bilirubin, thyroid function abnormalities, proteinuria, microscopic hematuria (at least 1%).
METAB: Peripheral edema (at least 2%).
MUSC: Myalgia, asthenia (3%); arthritis, arthralgia (at least 2%); pathological fracture (at least 1%).
RESP: Bronchitis, increased cough (at least 2%); dyspnea, pneumonia, asthma (at least 1%).

OTHER: Back pain (3%); flu syndrome (2%); abdominal pain, accidental injury, chest pain, infection, pain (at least 2%); pelvic pain, neck pain (at least 1%).

Precautions

Pregnancy: Category X.
Lactation: Contraindicated.
Children: Safety and efficacy not established.
Lab test abnormalities: It is recommended that LFTs be performed before and at 12 wk following both the initiation of therapy and any elevation in dose and periodically (eg, semiannually) thereafter.
Endocrine effects: Use caution when administering with drugs that affect steroid levels or activity.
Skeletal muscle effects: Rhabdomyolysis with renal dysfunction secondary to myoglobinuria has been reported with rosuvastatin. Temporarily withhold therapy in any patient experiencing an acute or serious condition predisposing to the development of renal failure secondary to rhabdomyolysis (eg, sepsis, hypotension). The risk of myopathy with other drugs in this class was found to be increased if therapy with cyclosporine, gemfibrozil, or niacin is coadministered. Consider myopathy in any patient with diffuse myalgia, muscle tenderness or weakness, or marked elevation of CPK.

PATIENT CARE CONSIDERATIONS

Administration/Storage

- Give prescribed dose once daily with or without food. Administer with food if GI upset occurs.
- Administer alone or in combination with other lipid-lowering therapy.
- Administer aluminum and magnesium hydroxide combination antacid at least 2 hr after rosuvastatin administration.
- Store tablets at controlled room temperature (68° to 77°F). Protect from moisture.

Assessment/Interventions

- Obtain patient history, including drug history and any known allergies. Note presence of active liver disease, hepatic insufficiency, unexplained elevations of serum transaminases, renal impairment, alcohol consumption, and concurrent therapy with medications known to increase the risk of myopathy (eg, cyclosporine, gemfibrozil).
- Ensure that secondary causes of hypercholesterolemia (eg, poorly controlled diabetes, hypothyroidism) are excluded before starting therapy.
- Ensure that patient is on a cholesterol-lowering diet before starting therapy and that diet is continued during treatment.
- Ensure that reduced doses are administered to patient with severe renal impairment (eg, Ccr less than 30 mL/min) or receiving cyclosporine or gemfibrozil.
- Ensure that therapy is temporarily withheld in patient with an acute, serious condition suggestive of myopathy or predisposing to the development of renal failure secondary to rhabdomyolysis (eg, sepsis, hypotension).
- Ensure that serum cholesterol and triglycerides are measured before therapy is started and within 2 to 4 wk of starting therapy or changing the rosuvastatin dose and periodically thereafter.
- Ensure that LFTs (transaminases) are determined before and 12 wk following initiation of therapy, or after increase in dose, and periodically thereafter (eg, q 6 mo).
- If elevated serum transaminase levels develop during treatment, repeat levels more frequently. If transaminase levels rise to 3 times upper limit of normal and persist, notify health care provider. Be prepared to reduce dose or discontinue therapy if ordered.
- If muscle tenderness and/or weakness develop during therapy, determine CPK levels. Notify health care provider if CPK levels are markedly increased or if muscle symptoms continue or worsen.
- Assess patient for GI, CNS, musculoskeletal, and general body side effects. If noted and significant, inform health care provider.

Patient/Family Education

- Explain name, dose, action, and potential side effects of drug.
- Advise patient to take once daily as prescribed, without regard to meals but to take with food if stomach upset occurs.
- Advise patient to try to take each dose at about the same time each day.
- Inform patient that drug helps control, but does not cure, cholesterol abnormality and to continue taking drug as prescribed if cholesterol levels are lowered.
- Caution patient not to change the dose or stop taking unless advised by health care provider.
- Advise patient that if a dose is missed to take as soon as remembered but to never take more than 1 dose of medicine a day.
- Instruct patient to continue taking other cholesterol-lowering medications as prescribed by health care provider.
- Emphasize to patient importance of other modalities on cholesterol control: dietary changes (reduced saturated fat intake,

increase soluble fiber intake), weight control, regular exercise, and smoking cessation.
- Advise women of childbearing potential to use effective contraception during treatment with rosuvastatin.
- Advise women to notify health care provider if pregnant, planning to become pregnant, or breastfeeding.
- Advise patient who is also using an aluminum and magnesium hydroxide combination antacid to take the antacid at least 2 hr after taking rosuvastatin.
- Caution patient not to take any prescription or OTC medications or dietary supplements unless advised by health care provider.
- Instruct patient to notify health care provider if experiencing any unexplained muscle pain, tenderness, and/or weakness, or any other unusual feelings.
- Advise patient that follow-up visits and lab tests will be required to monitor therapy and to keep appointments.

Salicylate Combination

(suh-LIS-ih-late)

Class Analgesic/Salicylate combination

How Supplied
Choline Magnesium Trisalicylate Liquid 500 mg salicylate (as 294 mg choline salicylate, 362 mg magnesium salicylate), Tablets 500 mg salicylate (as 293 mg choline salicylate, 362 mg magnesium salicylate), Tablets 750 mg salicylate (as 440 mg choline salicylate, 544 mg magnesium salicylate), Tablets 1000 mg salicylate (as 587 mg choline salicylate, 725 mg magnesium salicylate)
♦ *Tricosal* Tablets 500 mg salicylate (as 293 mg choline salicylate, 362 mg magnesium salicylate), Tablets 750 mg salicylate (as 440 mg choline salicylate, 544 mg magnesium salicylate)

Action
PHARMACOLOGY: Relieves pain by inhibiting prostaglandin synthesis and release; reduces fever by vasodilation of peripheral vessels. Unlike aspirin, does not inhibit platelet aggregation.

PHARMACOKINETICS/DYNAMICS:
Absorption: Salicylate is absorbed rapidly and reaches C_{max} in approximately 1 to 2 hr after a single dose of a tablet or liquid doseform.

Metabolism: The primary salicylate metabolites are glycine and glucuronide conjugates.

Excretion: The primary route of excretion of salicylate is renal. Serum salicylate concentrations are increased by conditions that decrease glomerular filtration rate or proximal tubular secretion. Salicylate t½ is approximately 9 to 17 hr.

Indications Relief of mild-to-moderate pain; treatment of rheumatic fever and rheumatoid arthritis including juvenile arthritis and osteoarthritis; management of fever.

Contraindications Hypersensitivity to nonacetylated salicylates, NSAIDs or aspirin; advanced chronic renal insufficiency; bleeding disorders; GI bleeding.

Route/Dosage
Inflammatory Conditions
ADULTS: PO 1500 mg bid or 3000 mg qd.
ELDERLY PATIENTS: PO 750 mg tid.

Fever, Mild-to-Moderate Pain
ADULTS: PO 1000 to 1500 mg bid.
CHILDREN UNDER 37 KG: PO 50 mg/kg/day in 2 divided doses.
CHILDREN OVER 37 KG: PO 2250 mg/day in 2 divided doses. Doses are adjusted based on patient's response, tolerance and serum salicylate concentration.

Interactions
Carbonic anhydrase inhibitors (eg, acetazolamide): Accumulation of carbonic anhydrase inhibitor and toxicity.
Corticosteroids: Decreased plasma salicylate concentration.
Methotrexate: Could cause methotrexate toxicity.
Oral hypoglycemics or insulin: Could cause hypoglycemia.
Urinary acidifiers: Increased salicylate serum concentration.
Urinary alkalinizers (eg, chronic antacids): Decreased salicylate serum concentration.
Warfarin: Enhanced anticoagulant activity of oral anticoagulants. Creates potential for increased prothrombin time due to protein-binding displacement.

Lab Test Interferences
Phenolsulfonphthalein: Salicylates decrease renal excretion.
Thyroid function tests: Drug causes increased free T_4 and decreased total T_4; thyroid function is not affected.
Urine glucose: Drug causes false-negative results by glucose oxidase method and false-positive results by copper reduction method with moderate to high doses of salicylates.
Urine 5-HIAA: Salicylates interfere with fluorescent method.
Urine ketones: Drug causes interference with ferric chloride (Gerhardt) method by turning urine a reddish color.
Urine vanillylmandelic acid: Salicylates can interfere with determination.

Adverse Reactions
DERM: Hives; rash; angioedema.
EENT: Tinnitus.
GI: Nausea; dyspepsia; gastric ulceration.
HEMA: Prolonged bleeding time.
HEPA: Hepatotoxicity.
METAB: Uric acid levels elevated by salicylate concentrations less than 10 mg/dL and decreased by levels greater than 10 mg/dL.
RESP: Bronchospasm.
OTHER: Anaphylaxis; salicylism may occur with large doses or chronic therapy (symptoms include dizziness, tinnitus, vomiting, diarrhea, confusion, CNS depression, headache, sweating, hyperventilation, and lassitude); fever.

Precautions
Pregnancy: Category C. Do not use during third trimester; could prematurely close ductus arteriosus in the fetus.
Lactation: Excreted in breast milk.
Children: May increase risk of Reye's syndrome;

do not use in individuals under 18 yr if chickenpox or flu symptoms are suspected.
Special risk patients: Use drug with caution in patients with renal or hepatic dysfunction, peptic ulcer disease, or gastritis.
Aspirin or NSAID hypersensitivity: Nonacetylated salicylates have been tolerated in aspirin-sensitive asthmatic patients; however, cases of cross-sensitivity including bronchospasm have been reported.

PATIENT CARE CONSIDERATIONS
Administration/Storage
- May cause GI upset; take with food or after meals. Take with a full glass of water.
- Store in tight, light-resistant container.

Assessment/Interventions
- Obtain patient history, including drug history and any known allergies.
- Assess quality of pain (location, onset, type, and duration) or temperature prior to therapy.
- Monitor pain relief and temperature after medication administration.
- Inspect affected joints. Assess mobility, swelling/deformities, and skin condition.
- Monitor improvement during therapy (fever reduction, relief from joint tenderness and pain; increased movement).
- Assess areas of bruising prior to and during therapy. Report increased bruising immediately to health care provider.
- If tinnitus, flushing, tachycardia, hyperventilation, sweating, or thirst occurs, withhold medication and immediately notify health care provider.
- Obtain baseline hepatic and renal studies and CBC, PT, and PTT. Monitor periodically if patient is undergoing long-term therapy.
- Monitor salicylate serum levels as ordered by health care provider.

Patient/Family Education
- Advise patient to take medication with food or after meals with full glass of water.
- Emphasize need to avoid alcohol ingestion and use of NSAIDs during therapy (which increase risk of GI irritation/GI bleeding), especially if patient is undergoing long-term therapy.
- Instruct patients with diabetes to monitor blood levels closely during treatment.
- Instruct patient to call health care provider immediately if ringing in ears or persistent GI pain occurs while taking this medication.

Overdosage: Signs and Symptoms
Respiratory alkalosis, hyperpnea, tachypnea, nausea, vomiting, hypokalemia, tinnitus, neurologic abnormalities (disorientation, irritability, lethargy, stupor), dehydration, hyperthermia, seizures, coma.

Salmeterol
(sal-MEET-ah-rahl)

Class Bronchodilator/Sympathomimetic

How Supplied
Serevent Diskus Inhalation powder 50 mcg salmeterol (as salmeterol xinafoate salt)

Action
PHARMACOLOGY: Produces bronchodilation by relaxing bronchial smooth muscle through beta-2 receptor stimulation.

PHARMACOKINETICS/DYNAMICS:
Absorption: Salmeterol acts locally in the lung. Plasma levels do not predict therapeutic effect. Depending on dose, T_{max} is 5 to 45 min and mean C_{max} is 167 pg/mL.
Distribution: Salmeterol is highly protein bound (greater than 99%).
Metabolism: Salmeterol is extensively metabolized by hydroxylation.
Excretion: Salmeterol is eliminated predominantly in feces and t½ is 11 days.

Special Populations:
Hepatic Function Impairment – Liver function impairment may lead to accumulation of salmeterol in plasma.

Indications Maintenance treatment of asthma and prevention of bronchospasm with reversible obstructive airway disease; prevention of exercise-induced bronchospasm; maintenance treatment of bronchospasm associated with COPD (including emphysema and chronic bronchitis).

Contraindications Standard considerations.

Route/Dosage
Asthma/Bronchospasm
ADULTS AND CHILDREN 4 YR AND OLDER FOR INHALATION POWDER: **Inhalation** 1 inhalation (50 mcg) bid, approximately 12 hr apart.

Exercise-Induced Bronchospasm
ADULTS AND CHILDREN 4 YR AND OLDER FOR INHALATION POWDER: **Inhalation** 1 inhalation at least 30 min before exercise; additional doses should not be used for up to 12 hr.

COPD
ADULTS: **Inhalation** 1 inhalation (50 mcg) bid, approximately 12 hr apart.

Interactions
Diuretics: ECG changes and hypokalemia associated with diuretics may worsen with coadministration.

MAO inhibitors, tricyclic antidepressants: May increase CV effects of salmeterol.

Lab Test Interferences
None well documented.

Adverse Reactions
CV: Arrhythmias (including atrial fibrillation, supraventricular tachycardia, extrasystoles), hypertension (4%); tachycardia, palpitations (1% to 3%).

CNS: Headache (28%); tremor (4%); dizziness/giddiness, nervousness, malaise/fatigue (3%); anxiety, insomnia, migraine, paresthesia, sleep disturbance (1% to 3%).

DERM: Rash (4%); contact dermatitis, eczema, urticaria, skin eruption (1% to 3%).

EENT: Nasopharyngitis (14%); nasal sinus congestion, pallor (9%); sore throat (8%); disease of nasal cavity/sinus, pharyngitis (6%); rhinitis (5%); sinus headache (4%); allergic rhinitis, rhinorrhea (3%); laryngitis, cold symptoms, earache, epistaxis, nasal congestion, sneezing, keratitis, conjunctivitis (1% to 3%).

GI: Diarrhea (5%); stomachache (4%); nausea, viral gastroenteritis, vomiting, abdominal pain, dental pain, dyspepsia, gastric pain, gastric upset, constipation, heartburn, oral candidiasis, xerostomia, surgical removal of tooth, hyposalivation (1% to 3%).

GU: Dysmenorrhea, UTI (1% to 3%).

MUSC: Back pain (4%); pain in joints, muscle cramp/contraction, myalgia/myositis, muscular soreness, leg cramps, neck pain, pain in arm, shoulder pain, neck muscle injury, arthralgia, articular rheumatism, muscle stiffness, tightness, and rigidity, inflammation (1% to 3%).

RESP: Upper respiratory tract infection (14%); bronchitis, cough, tracheitis (7%); lower respiratory infection, chest congestion (4%); asthma, common cold, influenza (3%); acute bronchitis, dyspnea, pneumonia, wheezing (1% to 3%); serious exacerbations of asthma (some fatal), laryngeal spasm, irritation or swelling (including stridor or choking), oropharyngeal irritation (postmarketing).

OTHER: Influenza (5%); fever, body pain, chest discomfort, pain, edema, hyperglycemia, swelling (1% to 3%).

> **WARNING:**
> When added to usual asthma therapy, there may be a small increase in asthma-related deaths in patients receiving salmeterol compared with placebo. The risk may be greater in black patients compared with white patients.

Precautions
Pregnancy: Category C.

Lactation: Undetermined.

Children: Not recommended for children younger than 4 yr.

Hypersensitivity: Allergic reactions can occur after administration.

Acute asthma attacks: Do not use to treat acute symptoms.

CV disease: Use with caution in patients with CV disease; toxic symptoms may occur.

Excessive use: Paradoxical bronchospasm and cardiac arrest have been associated with excessive inhalant use.

Hypokalemia: Decreases in potassium levels may occur.

Overdosage: Signs and Symptoms
Tremor, palpitations, tachycardia, headache, hypokalemia, hyperglycemia, cardiac arrest.

PATIENT CARE CONSIDERATIONS
Administration/Storage
- For oral inhalation only.
- Not to be used for the acute treatment of bronchospasm or asthma symptoms.
- May be used alone or in combination with inhaled or systemic corticosteroid therapy.
- If patient is also receiving short-acting bronchodilator by inhalation, administer short-acting bronchodilator 5 min before salmeterol to enhance penetration of latter drug into bronchial tree.
- Administer 1 inhalation bid, morning and evening, as prescribed.
- Activate and use the inhalation device in a level, horizontal position. Do not shake inhalation device before or during inhalation.
- Prepare dose by activating inhalation device immediately prior to administration. Have patient exhale fully, then place inhaler mouthpiece between lips. Teeth should not be closed. Instruct patient to take slow, deep breath and hold breath for 5 to 10 sec and then breathe out slowly. Have patient rinse mouth after inhalations are complete.
- Do not use with a spacer device (eg, *Aerochamber*). Do not exhale into the inhalation device, wash, or attempt to take the inhalation device apart.
- Store powder for oral inhalation at controlled room temperature (68° to 77°F) in a dry place. Protect from direct heat or sunlight. Discard 6 wk after removal from moisture-

protective foil pouch or when the dose indicator reads "0."

Assessment/Interventions

- Obtain patient history, including drug history and any known allergies. Note hepatic impairment, coronary artery disease, arrhythmias, hypertension, hyperthyroidism, seizures, or concurrent use of MAO inhibitors, tricyclic antidepressants, other products containing salmeterol, or another long-acting bronchodilator.
- Ensure that therapy is not initiated in patient who is experiencing rapidly deteriorating or potentially life-threatening episode of asthma.
- Ensure that patient is not receiving another inhaled, long-acting bronchodilator simultaneously.
- Ensure that baseline pulmonary function tests have been completed.
- Note frequency and severity of asthma attacks. Notify health care provider if patient needs increasing doses of short-acting bronchodilator or if effectiveness of short-acting bronchodilator appears to be decreasing.
- Assess patient for respiratory, CNS, GI, and general body side effects. Inform health care provider if noted and significant.

Patient/Family Education

- Explain name, dose, action, and potential side effects of drug.
- Instruct patient on the proper storage, handling, and use of the dry powder inhaler, referring to the *Patient's Instructions for Use* instruction sheet included with the medication.
- Advise patient that medication should never be administered with a spacer device.
- Caution patient not to exceed prescribed dose. Inform patient that medication is still inhaled even if not tasted or felt when delivered.
- Instruct patient not to stop the medication once symptoms have been controlled. Continued daily use is necessary to continue to control symptoms.
- Advise patient not to change the dose or stop using unless advised by health care provider.
- Caution patient not to use other salmeterol-containing products or other long-acting bronchodilators while using salmeterol.
- Warn patient that salmeterol is a maintenance medication and is not to be used to treat an acute asthma attack. "Rescue medication" (short-acting bronchodilator) must be used to obtain rapid relief of asthma symptoms.
- Advise patient using salmeterol for prevention of exercise-induced bronchospasm to take medication at least 30 to 60 min before exercise and to wait 12 hr before using again.
- Advise patient that medication does not replace inhaled or oral corticosteroids and to continue to use as prescribed by health care provider.
- Advise patient not to increase dose and to inform health care provider if symptoms do not improve or worsen or if more short-acting bronchodilator than usual is needed or if short-acting bronchodilator appears to become less effective.
- Advise patient to carry *Medi-Alert* card if experiencing acute severe asthma attacks requiring rapid systemic treatment.
- Advise patient to report these symptoms to health care provider: worsening asthma symptoms, sore throat or mouth, persistent cough, palpitations, chest pain, rapid heart rate, tremor, nervousness.
- Advise women to notify health care provider if pregnant, planning to become pregnant, or breastfeeding.
- Caution patient not to take any prescription or OTC medications or dietary supplements unless advised by health care provider.
- Advise patient that follow-up visits may be required to monitor therapy and to keep appointments.

Samarium SM 153 Lexidronam

(sah-MARE-ee-uhm SM 153 lex-IH-drah-nam)

Class Radiopharmaceuticals

How Supplied
Quadramet Injection 1850 MBq/mL

Action

PHARMACOLOGY: Consisting of radioactive samarium and a tetraphosphonate chelator, EDTMP. The mechanism of action of samarium in relieving the pain of bone metastases is not known.

Indications Relief of pain in patients with osteoblastic metastatic bone lesions that enhance on radionuclide bone scan. **Unlabeled use(s):** Ankylosing spondylitis; Paget's disease; rheumatoid arthritis.

Contraindications Hypersensitivity to EDTMP or similar phosphonate compounds.

Route/Dosage
Bone Lesions
ADULTS: IV 1 mCi/kg, administered over a period of 1 min through a secure indwelling catheter and followed with a saline flush. Exercise caution when determining the dose in very thin or very obese patients.

Interactions
Chemotherapy: Do not give samarium concurrently with chemotherapy or external beam radiation therapy unless the benefit outweighs the risks. Do not give samarium after either of these treatments until there has been time for adequate marrow recovery.

Lab Test Interferences None well documented.

Adverse Reactions
CV: Arrhythmias; chest pain; hypertension; hypotension; sinus bradycardia; vasodilation.
CNS: Dizziness; paresthesia; spinal cord compression; cerebrovascular accident/stroke.
DERM: Purpura; rash.
GI: Abdominal pain; diarrhea; nausea; vomiting.
HEMA:
Bleeding manifestations – Ecchymosis; epistaxis; hematuria; bone marrow suppression; coagulation disorder; hemoglobin decreased; leukopenia; lymphadenopathy; thrombocytopenia; bone marrow toxicity.
RESP: Bronchitis; cough increased; pneumonia.
OTHER: Fever; chills; unspecified infection; oral moniliasis; myasthenia; pathologic fracture.

PATIENT CARE CONSIDERATIONS
Administration/Storage
- Have the patient ingest (or receive by IV administration) a minimum of 500 mL (2 cups) of fluids prior to injection and void as often as possible after injection to minimize radiation exposure to the bladder.
- Samarium contains calcium and may be incompatible with solutions that contain molecules that can complex with and form calcium precipitates.
- Do not dilute or mix with other solutions.
- Thaw at room temperature before administration and use within 8 hr. Store frozen at -20° to -10°C (-4° to 14°F) in a lead shielded container.
- Women of childbearing age should have a negative pregnancy test before administration of samarium.

Assessment/Interventions
- Measure the dose by a suitable radioactivity calibration system, such as a radioisotope dose

Precautions
Pregnancy: Category C.
Lactation: Discontinue breastfeeding or discontinue the drug.
Children: Safety and efficacy in pediatric patients less than 16 yr have not been established.
Pain flare reactions: Some patients have reported a transient increase in bone pain shortly after injection (flare reaction). This is usually mild and self-limiting and occurs within 72 hr of injection.
Bone marrow suppression: Samarium causes bone marrow suppression. Use with caution in patients with compromised bone marrow reserves.
Radioactivity: Verify dose.
ECG changes: Use caution and appropriate monitoring.
Skeletal effects: Spinal cord compression frequently occurs in patients with known metastases to the cervical, thoracic, or lumbar spine. Administration for pain relief of metastatic bone cancer does not prevent the development of spinal cord compression.
Incontinence: Take special precautions with bladder catherization in incontinent patients to minimize the risk of radioactive contamination.
Hypocalcemia: Exercise caution when administering to patients at risk for developing hypocalcemia.
Flare reactions: A transient increase in bone pain shortly after injection (flare reaction) may occur.

Overdosage: Signs and Symptoms
Bone marrow suppression.

calibrator, immediately before administration.
- Before administering samarium, give consideration to the patient's current clinical and hematologic status and bone marrow response history to treatment with myelotoxic agents. Exercise caution in treating cancer patients whose platelet counts are falling or who have other clinical or laboratory findings suggesting DIC. Monitor blood counts weekly for at least 8 wk or until recovery of adequate bone marrow function.
- Do not give concurrently with chemotherapy or external beam radiation therapy unless clinical benefits outweigh the risks.
- Verify the dose of radioactivity to be administered to the patient before administering samarium. Do not release patient until radioactivity levels and exposure rates comply with federal and local regulations.
- Take special precautions with bladder catheterization in incontinent patients to mini-

mize the risk of radioactive contamination of clothing, bed linen, and the patient's environment. Urinary excretion of radioactivity occurs within approximately 12 hr.

Patient/Family Education
- Advise patients that for several hours following administration, radioactivity will be present in excreted urine. To help protect themselves and others in their environment, precautions need to be taken for 12 hr following administration. Whenever possible, use a toilet rather than a urinal and flush the toilet several times after each use. Clean up spilled urine completely and wash hands thoroughly. If blood or urine gets onto clothing, wash the clothing separately or store for 1 to 2 wk to allow for decay of the samarium.
- Women of childbearing age should have a negative pregnancy test before administration of samarium. If this drug is used during pregnancy, or if a patient becomes pregnant after taking this drug, apprise her of the potential hazard to the fetus. Advise women of childbearing potential to avoid becoming pregnant soon after receiving samarium. Advise male and female patients to use an effective method of contraception after samarium administration.

Saquinavir Mesylate

(sack-KWIN-uh-vihr MEH-sih-LATE)

Class Antiretroviral/Protease inhibitor

How Supplied
Fortovase Capsules 200 mg ♦ *Invirase* Capsules 200 mg (as mesylate)
✤ *Fortovase Roche*

Action
PHARMACOLOGY: Inhibits human immunodeficiency virus (HIV) protease, the enzyme required to form functional proteins in HIV-infected cells.

PHARMACOKINETICS/DYNAMICS:

Absorption: Absorption is poor, but is increased with a high fat meal. The effect of food has been shown to persist for up to 2 hr. Bioavailability averaged 4% (*Invirase*).

Distribution: Saquinavir is approximately 98% protein bound and Vd is 700 L.

Metabolism: Saquinavir undergoes extensive first-pass metabolism. Metabolism is cytochrome P450–mediated with the specific isoenzyme CYP3A4 responsible for more than 90% of the hepatic metabolism.

Excretion: Systemic clearance is rapid (1.14 L/hr/kg after IV doses of 6, 36, and 72 mg).

Special Populations:
Renal Function Impairment – Approximately 1% is excreted via urine. Impact of renal impairment on elimination should be minimal.

Indications Treatment of advanced HIV infection. Saquinavir is given in combination with nucleoside analogs (eg, zidovudine).

Contraindications Coadministration with cisapride, ergot derivatives, midazolam, triazolam.

Route/Dosage
ADULTS AND CHILDREN AT LEAST 16 YR: **PO** Three 200 mg capsules (600 mg) tid within 2 hr after a full meal.

Interactions
Aldesleukin, cyclosporine, grapefruit juice: May increase saquinavir serum levels.
Carbamazepine, dexamethasone, nevirapine, phenobarbital, phenytoin, rifabutin, rifampin, rifapentine, St. John's wort, other cytochrome P450 3A4 inducers: May increase metabolism of saquinavir and decrease serum levels.
Cisapride, cyclosporine, ergot derivatives, fentanyl, midazolam, triazolam, other drugs metabolized by cytochrome P450 3A4: Serum levels of these drugs may be elevated, increasing the risk of toxicity.
Clarithromycin, delavirdine, indinavir, ketoconazole, nelfinavir, ritonavir: May decrease metabolism of saquinavir and increase serum levels.
Clarithromycin, nelfinavir, sildenafil: Saquinavir may increase levels of these drugs.
Warfarin: The anticoagulant effect may be decreased.

Lab Test Interferences None well documented.

Adverse Reactions
CNS: Paresthesia; numbness; confusion; seizures; headache; depression; insomnia; anxiety; libido disorder.
DERM: Rash; photosensitivity; eczema; verruca; Stevens-Johnson syndrome; bullous skin eruption.
EENT: Taste alteration.
GI: Diarrhea; abdominal pain and discomfort; nausea; dyspepsia; flatulence; vomiting; constipation; intestinal obstruction.
GU: Nephrolithiasis; acute renal insufficiency.
HEMA: Acute myeloblastic leukemia; hemolytic anemia; thrombocytopenia.
HEPA: Elevated LFTs; jaundice; portal hypertension.
OTHER: Ataxia; fatigue; pain weakness; ascites; pancreatitis; drug fever; intracranial hemorrhage.

> **WARNING:**
> *Invirase* (capsules) and *Fortovase* (soft gelatin capsules) are not bioequivalent and are not interchangeable. When using saquinavir as part of an antiviral regimen, *Fortovase* is the recommended formulation. In rare circumstances, *Invirase* may be considered if combined with antiretrovirals that significantly inhibit saquinavir's metabolism.

Precautions
Pregnancy: Category B.
Lactation: Undetermined. HIV-infected mothers should not breastfeed their infants.
Children: Not recommended for children less than 16 yr.

PATIENT CARE CONSIDERATIONS
Administration/Storage
- The medication should be taken within 2 hr after a full meal.
- Doses less than 600 mg tid are not effective.
- Store capsules at room temperature in a tightly closed bottle.
- Store *Invirase* capsules at room temperature in a tightly closed bottle.
- Store *Fortovase* capsules in the refrigerator 2° to 8°C (36° to 46°F).

Assessment/Interventions
- Obtain patient history.
- Assess for history of impaired hepatic function.
- Obtain baseline triglycerides, ALT, AST, GGT, CPK, and uric acid. Monitor periodically during treatment.
- Monitor WBC and differential. Note any significant changes.
- Monitor Hct and Hgb frequently (severe anemia may require blood transfusions).

Patient/Family Education
- Advise patient to take the medication exactly as prescribed.
- Advise patient regarding importance of taking after a meal.
- Warn patient not to alter the dose or discontinue the medication without consulting the health care provider.
- Instruct patient not to take any other medications, including OTC medications, without consulting a health care provider.

Hepatic function impairment: Exercise caution when administering to patients with hepatic insufficiency (LFTs greater than 5 times upper limit of normal).
Photosensitivity: May occur; take protective measures against exposure to ultraviolet light or sunlight until tolerance is determined.
Clinical chemistry: Perform clinical chemistry tests prior to and at appropriate intervals during therapy.
Dosage adjustment: Do not reduce dose; lower doses do not exhibit antiviral activity.
Nucleoside analog therapy: Saquinavir must be used in combination with nucleoside analog (eg, AZT [zidovudine], ddC [zalcitabine]) therapy.

Overdosage: Signs and Symptoms
No acute toxicities or sequelae have been reported.

- Explain that a patient will be required to have frequent follow-up blood and urine tests during the course of the treatment and to keep appointments.
- Inform patient that this medication is NOT a cure for HIV infection and secondary illnesses associated with the disease may continue to be acquired.
- Emphasize to patient, family, and significant others that this medication does NOT reduce the risk of transmitting HIV to others through sexual contact or blood contamination.
- Inform patient to report any serious side effects to a health care provider.
- Explain that the long-term effects of this medication are not known, and the initial results have not demonstrated a reduction in symptoms or prolongation of life.
- Caution patient regarding possibility of photosensitivity and to use protective measures until tolerance is determined.
- Advise patient that saquinavir is recommended for use in combination with active antiretroviral therapy and adherence to the prescribed regimen is strongly recommended.
- Advise patient to store *Fortovase* capsules in the refrigerator 2° to 8°C (36° to 46°F) until the expiration date; once brought to room temperature, use capsules within 3 mo.
- Inform patient that redistribution or accumulation of body fat may occur and that long-term health effects are not known.

Sargramostim

(sar-GRUH-moe-STIM)

Class Colony-stimulating factor

How Supplied
Leukine Powder for injection, lyophilized 250 mcg, Powder for injection, lyophilized 500 mcg, Liquid 500 mcg/mL

Action
PHARMACOLOGY: Supports survival, proliferation, and differentiation of hematopoietic progenitor cells; induces partially committed progenitor cells to divide and differentiate in granulocyte-macrophage pathways; activates mature granulocytes and macrophages; promotes proliferation of megakaryocytic and erythroid progenitors.

PHARMACOKINETICS/DYNAMICS:
Absorption: C_{max} is 5 to 5.4 ng/mL, AUC is 640 to 680 ng/mL•min, and T_{max} is 1 to 3 hr postinjection.

Excretion: Mean clearance rate is 420 to 430 mL/min/m^2 and t½ is 60 minutes.

Indications
Myeloid reconstitution after autologous bone marrow transplantation and after bone marrow transplantation failure or graft failure; promotion of early engraftment or engraftment delay; treatment of neutropenia associated bone marrow transplant; induction chemotherapy in acute myelogenous leukemia (AML); mobilization and following transplantation of autologous PBPC; and myeloid reconstitution after allogeneic BMT. **Unlabeled use(s):** Increase WBC counts in patients with myelodysplastic syndromes and in AIDS patients receiving zidovudine; decrease nadir of leukopenia secondary to myelosuppressive chemotherapy; decrease myelosuppression in preleukemic patients; correct neutropenia in aplastic anemia patients; decrease transplantation-associated organ system damage.

Contraindications
Excessive leukemic myeloid blasts in bone marrow or peripheral blood; hypersensitivity to granulocyte-macrophage colony-stimulating factor, yeast-derived products, or any component of product; simultaneous administration with cytotoxic chemotherapy or radiotherapy, or administration 24 hrs preceding or following chemotherapy or radiotherapy.

Route/Dosage
Bone Marrow Transplant Failure or Engraftment Delay
ADULTS: IV 250 mcg/m^2/day for 14 days.

Myeloid Reconstitution After Bone Marrow Transplantation
ADULTS: IV 250 mcg/m^2/day for 21 days (first dose given 2 to 4 hr after transplant).

Neutrophil Recovery Following Chemotherapy in AML
ADULTS: IV 250 mcg/m^2/day over a 4-hr period starting around day 11 or 4 days following the completion of induction chemotherapy, if the day 10 bone marrow is hypoplastic with less than 5% blasts.

Mobilization of PBPC
ADULTS: IV 250 mcg/m^2/day over 24 hr or SC once daily. Continue at the same dose through the period of PBPC collection.

Postperipheral Blood Progenitor Cell Transplantation
ADULTS: IV 250 mcg/m^2/day over 24 hr or SC once daily beginning immediately following infusion of progenitor cells and continuing until an ANC of more than 1500 for 3 consecutive days is attained.

Interactions
Antineoplastics: Do not use concomitantly.
Corticosteroids or lithium: May potentiate myeloproliferative effects of sargramostim.

Lab Test Interferences
None well documented.

Adverse Reactions
CV: Tachycardia.
CNS: Anxiety.
DERM: Pruritus.
EENT: Eye hemorrhage.
GI: Abdominal pain; hematemesis; dysphagia.
HEMA: Bilirubinemia.
METAB: Metabolic disorder; weight gain.
RESP: Pharyngitis.
OTHER: Bone pain; arthralgia; malaise; chest pain.

Precautions
Pregnancy: Category C.
Lactation: Undetermined.
Children: Safety and efficacy not established. However, available data indicate that sargramostim does not exhibit any greater toxicity in children than in adults.
Hypersensitivity: Reactions are infrequent and have ranged from serious allergic or anaphylactic reactions to transient rashes and local injection site reactions.
Renal function impairment: Monitor patients closely and use with caution.
Hepatic function impairment: Monitor patients closely and use with caution.

Benzyl alcohol: Benzyl alcohol as a preservative has been associated with fatal "gasping syndrome" in premature infants.
Concomitant chemotherapy and radiotherapy: Since rapidly dividing cells are particularly sensitive to cytotoxic chemotherapy and radiotherapy, sargramostim should not be given within 24 hr of chemotherapy or within 12 hr of radiotherapy.
Growth factor potential: Administer with caution in patients with myeloid malignancies.

PATIENT CARE CONSIDERATIONS
Administration/Storage
- Reconstitute with 1 mL Sterile Water for Injection (without preservative); do not re-enter vial. Discard any unused portion.
- During reconstitution, direct sterile water at side of vial and gently swirl contents to prevent foaming during dissolution. Avoid excessive or vigorous agitation; do not shake.
- Dilute in 0.9% Sodium Chloride Injection to prepare IV infusion. If final concentration is less than 10 mcg/mL, add human albumin to make final concentration of 0.1% to saline before adding sargramostim to prevent absorption to drug delivery system. For final concentration of 0.1% albumin, add 1 mg human albumin/1 mL 0.9% saline injection. Give within 6 hr after reconstitution. Discard any unused portion after 6 hr.
- Administer each dose over 2 hr as IV infusion.
- Do not use in-line membrane filter for IV infusion.
- Do not add other medications to IV solution.
- Administer 2 to 4 hr after autologous bone marrow infusion, not less than 24 hr after last dose of antineoplastics, and 12 hr after last dose of radiotherapy, bone marrow transplantation failure or engraftment delay.
- Refrigerate sterile powder, reconstituted solution, and diluted solution for injection. Do not freeze or shake.

Assessment/Interventions
- Obtain patient history, including drug history and any known allergies.
- Monitor CBC and differential biweekly during therapy. If ANC is more than 20,000/mm^3 or platelet count is more than 500,000 cells/mm^3, discontinue or reduce dose by one half. Leukocytosis may occur.
- Monitor renal and hepatic studies before treatment, including BUN, creatinine, urinalysis, AST, ALT, alkaline phosphatase, and monitor biweekly during therapy if renal or hepatic disease is present.
- Observe for hypersensitivity reactions, including rashes and local injection site reactions, which are usually transient.
- Monitor I&O, hydration status and weight. Observe for fluid retention or edema; pleural and pericardial effusions have occurred.
- Monitor vital signs during therapy; supraventricular arrhythmias have occurred in patients with cardiac disease. Hypotension with flushing and syncope has rarely occurred with first dose.
- Monitor for respiratory symptoms during and immediately following infusion, especially in patients with history of pulmonary disease. If dyspnea occurs during infusion, reduce rate by one half. If symptoms worsen, notify health care provider and discontinue infusion.

Patient/Family Education
- Reassure patient that hypotension with flushing and syncope has rarely occurred with first dose.
- Stress importance of follow-up for laboratory tests.
- Instruct patient to inform health care provider if any of the following symptoms occur: dyspnea, malaise, nausea, fever, rash, rapid heart rate, headache, chills.

Cardiac patients: Monitor patients closely and use with caution.
Respiratory symptoms: It may be necessary to decrease rate of infusion by 50% if dyspnea occurs during administration.

Overdosage: Signs and Symptoms
Dyspnea, malaise, nausea, fever, rash, sinus tachycardia, headache and chills, increases in WBC no more than 200,000 cells/mm^3.

Scopolamine HBr (Hyoscine HBr)
(skoe-PAHL-uh-meen HIGH-droe-BRO-mide)
Class Antiemetic/Antivertigo/Anticholinergic

How Supplied
Isopto Hyoscine Solution 0.25% ♦ *Scopace* Tablets, soluble 0.4 mg
🍁 *Transderm-V*

Action
PHARMACOLOGY: Competitively inhibits

action of acetylcholine at muscarinic receptors. Principal effects are on iris and ciliary body (pupil dilations and blurred vision), secretory glands (dry mouth), drowsiness, euphoria, fatigue, decreased nausea, and vomiting.

PHARMACOKINETICS/DYNAMICS:

Absorption: Scopolamine is well absorbed percutaneously. T_{max} is reached within 24 hr; C_{max} is 87 pg/mL (free scopolamine) and 354 pg/mL (total scopolamine).

Distribution: Scopolamine crosses the placenta and the blood-brain barrier. It may be reversibly bound to plasma proteins.

Metabolism: Scopolamine is extensively metabolized and conjugated with less than 5% of the total dose appearing unchanged in urine.

Excretion: Less than 10% of the total dose is excreted in urine as parent and metabolites over 108 hr; t½ is 9.5 hr.

Indications Accomplishment of cycloplegia and mydriasis for diagnostic procedures and for preoperative and postoperative states in treatment of iridocyclitis (ophthalmic use); prevention of nausea and vomiting associated with motion sickness (transdermal); preanesthetic sedation and obstetric amnesia in conjunction with analgesics and to calm delirium (parenteral).

Contraindications Hypersensitivity to any product component, glaucoma; adhesions between iris and lens; children with previous severe reaction to atropine.

Route/Dosage

Ophthalmic

ADULTS: 1 to 2 gtt of 1% solution into eye 1 hr prior to refraction; or 1 to 2 gtt up to qid for uveitis.

CHILDREN: 1 to 2 gtt of 0.5% solution into eye 1 hr prior to refraction; or 1 to 2 gtt of 0.5% solution up to tid for uveitis.

Parenteral

ADULTS: **IM/SQ/IV** 0.32 to 0.65 mg.

CHILDREN: 0.006 mg/kg (max, 0.3 mg).

Transdermal

ADULTS: One transdermal patch placed behind ear at least 4 hr prior to event. Wear only 1 patch at a time. Approximately 1 mg will be delivered over 3 days.

Interactions

Haloperidol: Worsened schizophrenia, decreased haloperidol levels, and tardive dyskinesia may occur.

IV incompatibilities: Solutions are incompatible with alkalies.

Phenothiazines: Actions of phenothiazines may be decreased.

Lab Test Interferences None well documented.

Adverse Reactions

CV: Increased heart rate.
CNS: Drowsiness; disorientation; delirium.
DERM: Contact dermatitis; erythema.
EENT: Blurred vision; stinging; increased IOP; photophobia; conjunctivitis.
GI: Dry mouth.
RESP: Decreased respiratory rate.

Precautions

Pregnancy: Category C.
Lactation: Undetermined.
Children: Safety and efficacy not established for transdermal use. Use with caution in children and infants.
Elderly: Use with caution in geriatric patients.
Hypersensitivity: Contact dermatitis for transdermal system has been reported. Potentially alarming idiosyncratic reactions may occur with therapeutic doses.
Diabetes: Use with caution in those with diabetes.
Thyroid abnormalities: Use with caution in thyroid abnormalities.
Glaucoma: Use with caution in those with glaucoma.
Other: Dizziness, nausea, vomiting, headache, and disturbances with equilibrium have been reported upon discontinuation after several days of use.

Overdosage: Signs and Symptoms

Somnolence, dry mouth, dilated pupils, delirium, disorientation, memory disturbances, dizziness, restlessness, hallucinations.

PATIENT CARE CONSIDERATIONS

Administration/Storage

Direct IV:

- Dilute with Sterile Water for Injection and give slowly; position patient recumbent and keep in bed for 1 hr after administration to prevent orthostatic hypotension.

Transdermal route:

- Apply patch 4 hr prior to expected motion. Apply to clean, hairless, dry area behind ear. Do not touch exposed adhesive area of patch; wash hands thoroughly before and after application. Rotate application sites; place only 1 patch at a time; change patch every 72 hr.

- Store transdermal patches in packages until ready for use; note expiration date; store ophthalmic and parenteral solutions at room temperature and protect from light.

Ophthalmic route:

- Wash hands before and after instillation. Position patient supine or with head tilted back in "star-gazing" position (looking at ceiling) to administer drops. Pull down lower lid to form pocket and instill solution as ordered. Avoid contact between dispenser and eye. Close eye gently and apply pressure to inner canthus for 1 to 2 min to prevent systemic absorption and drainage into nose/throat. Blot excessive solution from around eye with tissue. Wait 5 min before instilling additional ophthalmic solutions.

Assessment/Interventions
- Obtain patient history, including drug history and any known allergies.
- Assess vital signs (heart rate, BP), presence of pain and intake/output ratio (watch for urinary retention) prior to and during therapy.
- Provide pain medication concomitantly as needed; remember medication alone can precipitate behavior changes such as excitation and delirium.
- Assess mouth for dryness; provide mouth care, hard candy, or frequent sips of water as needed.
- Assess for blurred vision, drowsiness, and dizziness; implement safety precautions (call bell, side rails) and assist with ambulation.

Patient/Family Education
Oral/Parenteral/Transdermal:
- Tell patient if dose is missed to take as soon as remembered, but caution against doubling doses.
- Advise patient to avoid use of alcohol or other CNS depressants (eg, sedatives, antihistamines) while taking this medication.
- Advise patient that drug may cause drowsiness or dizziness and to use caution while driving or performing other tasks requiring mental alertness.
- Explain that rinsing mouth, good oral hygiene, and sugarless gum or candy will help to counteract mouth dryness.
- Encourage medical follow-up to monitor effects of therapy.
- Instruct patient and family in correct technique for application of patches; explain that patch is waterproof and not affected by showering or bathing.
- Remind patient to wash hands before and after applying patch.
- Explain to patient that if patch is dislodged, to replace it with a new unit at a different site.

Ophthalmic Preparation:
- Instruct patient to wash hands before and after instillation.
- Instruct patient and family in correct technique for instillation of drops for ophthalmic use.
- Explain that blurring of vision will decrease with repeated use of drug and to avoid hazardous activities until vision clears.
- Explain that eyes may become sensitive to light and advise patient to use dark glasses indoors and outdoors.
- Emphasize need to contact health care provider immediately if patient notices change in vision, eye pain, loss of sight, inability to breath, or flushing.
- Tell patient to notify health care provider if light sensitivity persists 1 wk or more after medication has been discontinued.

Secobarbital Sodium

(see-koe-BAR-bih-tahl SO-dee-uhm)

Class Sedative and hypnotic/Barbiturate

How Supplied
Seconal Sodium Pulvules Capsules 100 mg

Action
PHARMACOLOGY: Depresses sensory cortex, decreases motor activity, alters cerebellar function, and produces drowsiness, sedation, and hypnosis.

PHARMACOKINETICS/DYNAMICS:

Absorption: Secobarbital absorption is rapid; the rate is increased if the sodium salt is ingested as a dilute solution or taken on an empty stomach.

Distribution: Secobarbital has very high lipid solubility and high protein binding. The drug is distributed to all tissues and fluids, with high concentrations in the brain, liver, and kidneys.

Metabolism: Metabolism of secobarbital is primarily by the hepatic microsomal enzyme system.

Excretion: Secobarbital is eliminated renally. The inactive metabolites are excreted as conjugates of glucuronic acid. T½ is 15 to 40 hr (mean, 28 hr).

Onset: Secobarbital's onset of action is 10 to 15 min (PO).

Duration: Secobarbital's duration of action is 3 to 4 hr (PO).

Indications Short-term (up to 2 wk) treatment of insomnia; induction of basal hypnosis before anesthesia (parenteral form); sedation (parenteral form). **Unlabeled use(s):** Control of status epilepticus or acute seizure episodes.

Contraindications Hypersensitivity to barbiturates; history of addiction to sedative/hypnotic drugs; history of porphyria; severe liver impairment; respiratory disease with dyspnea; nephritic patients.

Route/Dosage

Insomnia
ADULTS: **PO** At bedtime 100 mg.

Hypnotic
ADULTS: **IM** 100 to 200 mg; **IV** 50 to 250 mg.

Sedation
ADULTS: **PO** 30 to 50 mg tid or qid.
CHILDREN: **PO/PR** 2 to 6 mg/kg. For rectal administration, dilute 1% to 1.5% solution.

Preoperative Sedation
ADULTS: **PO** 200 to 300 mg 1 to 2 hr before surgery.
CHILDREN: **PO** 2 to 6 mg/kg (max, 100 mg) 1 to 2 hr before surgery.

Sedation/Preanesthesia
ADULTS: **IM** (light sedation) 1 mg/kg 15 min before procedure.
CHILDREN: **IM** 4 to 5 mg/kg.

Convulsions
ADULTS: **IM/IV** 1.1 to 2.2 mg/kg. Maximum IV rate 50 mg/15 sec. Maximum adult IM dose 500 mg or 5 mL volume regardless of concentration.

Interactions

Alcohol, CNS depressants: May produce additive CNS depressant effects.
Anticoagulants (eg, warfarin), beta blockers (eg, metoprolol, propranolol), verapamil, quinidine, theophyllines: May reduce activity of these drugs.
Anticonvulsants: May reduce serum concentrations of carbamazepine, valproic acid, and succinimides. Valproic acid may increase barbiturate serum levels.
Corticosteroids: May reduce effectiveness of corticosteroids.
Estrogens, estrogen-containing oral contraceptives: May reduce contraceptive effect and estrogen effect.

Lab Test Interferences
May increase bromsulphalein retention; may cause decreased serum bilirubin concentrations; false-positive phentolamine test results; decreased response to metyrapone; impaired absorption of radioactive cyanocobalamin.

Adverse Reactions
CV: Bradycardia; hypotension; syncope.
CNS: Drowsiness; agitation; confusion; headache; hyperkinesia; ataxia; CNS depression; paradoxical excitement; nightmares; psychiatric disturbances; hallucinations; insomnia; dizziness.
GI: Nausea; vomiting; constipation.
HEMA: Blood dyscrasias (eg, agranulocytosis, thrombocytopenia).
RESP: Hypoventilation; apnea; laryngospasm; bronchospasm.
OTHER: Hypersensitivity reactions (eg, angioedema, rashes, exfoliative dermatitis); fever; liver damage; injection site reactions (eg, local pain, thrombophlebitis).

Precautions
Pregnancy: Category D.
Lactation: Excreted in breast milk.
Children: May respond with excitement rather than depression.
Elderly: More sensitive to drug effects; dosage reduction is required.
Renal function impairment: Use drug with caution; dosage reduction may be required.
Hepatic function impairment: Use drug with caution; dosage reduction may be required.
Dependence: Tolerance or psychological and physical dependence may occur with continued use.
IV administration: Do not exceed maximum IV rate 50 mg/15 sec; respiratory depression, apnea, and hypotension may result. Parenteral solutions are highly alkaline; extravasation may cause tissue damage and necrosis. Inadvertent intra-arterial injection may lead to arterial spasm, thrombosis and gangrene.
Seizure disorders: Status epilepticus may result from abrupt discontinuation.

Overdosage: Signs and Symptoms
CNS and respiratory depression, Cheyne-Stokes respiration, areflexia, oliguria, tachycardia, hypotension, lowered body temperature, coma, pulmonary edema, death.

PATIENT CARE CONSIDERATIONS

Administration/Storage
- Administer on empty stomach with full glass of water to enhance absorption. Tablet may be crushed and mixed with food or swallowed whole.
- For insomnia, give ½ to 1 hr before bedtime.
- Check to see that medication is swallowed.
- For IM administration: inject deep into large muscle using Z-track technique to diminish tissue irritation and potential sloughing. Do not inject SC. Do not exceed 5 mL at any 1 site. Rotate injection sites.
- For direct IV administration, may give undiluted or diluted with Sterile Water for Injection, normal saline (0.9% Sodium Chloride) or Ringer's solution. Do not use lactated Ringer's solution.
- Administer IV no faster than 50 mg/15 sec; too rapid administration can cause respiratory depression and hypotension. Have resuscitative equipment readily available.
- Use diluted solution within 30 min of mixing. Rotate; do not shake vial.

- For rectal administration in children preoperatively, after cleansing enema, give diluted parenteral solution (1% to 1.5%) as ordered.
- Store oral preparation at room temperature. Refrigerate parenteral form. Use only clear solution; discard if precipitate forms or solution becomes cloudy.

Assessment/Interventions
- Obtain patient history, including drug history and any known allergies. Note history of respiratory disease with dyspnea or hypersensitivity to barbiturates or sedative/hypnotic drug addiction.
- Assess type of sleep difficulty: falling asleep, remaining asleep.
- Assess sleep pattern prior to and during therapy.
- Assess vital signs q 15 to 30 min after parenteral administration for 2 hr and then prn.
- Assess mental status: sensorium, affect, mood, and long- and short-term memory.
- Obtain baseline Hct, Hgb, RBC, and LFT results (transaminase levels and bilirubin). Periodically evaluate those results if patient is on long-term therapy.
- Provide safety measures (removal of cigarettes, side rails up, night light, easily accessible callbell) and assistance with ambulation.

Patient/Family Education
- Explain that this medication may cause psychological and physical dependence. Emphasize that it is important not to increase dose without consulting health care provider.
- Discuss ways to facilitate sleep (quiet, darkened room; avoidance of caffeine and nicotine; warm bath, warm milk; deep breathing; relaxation; self-hypnosis).
- Inform patient that it may take a few doses to achieve noticeable sleep benefit.
- Instruct patient to notify health care provider immediately of sudden onset of fever, sore throat, bruising, rash, jaundice, or unusual bleeding (eg, epistaxis).
- Instruct patient to avoid intake of alcoholic beverages or other CNS depressants (eg, pain relievers, antihistamines, sedatives) to prevent serious CNS depression.
- Emphasize importance of follow-up evaluation with health care provider to monitor progress of therapy.
- Inform patient that after discontinuation of drug, nighttime sleeping might be disturbed for a few days and increased dreaming may occur.
- Advise patient that drug may cause daytime drowsiness and to use caution while driving or performing other tasks requiring mental alertness.
- Instruct patient not to discontinue medication abruptly without consulting health care provider.

Secretin

(SEH-kreh-tin)

Class Diagnostic aid/Gastrointestinal function test

How Supplied
SecreFlo Powder for injection, lyophilized 16 mcg of purified secretin

Action
PHARMACOLOGY: Increase the volume and bicarbonate content of secreted pancreatic juices.

PHARMACOKINETICS/DYNAMICS:
Distribution: Vd approximately 2 L.

Excretion: After IV bolus administration of 0.4 mcg/kg, plasma concentration rapidly declines to baseline secretin levels within 90 min. Elimination t½ 27 min.

Indications Stimulation of pancreatic secretions, including bicarbonate, to aid in diagnosis of pancreatic exocrine dysfunction; stimulation of gastrin secretion to aid in diagnosis of gastrinoma; stimulation of pancreatic secretions to facilitate the identification of ampulla of Vater and accessory papilla during endoscopic retrograde cholangiopancreatography.

Contraindications Acute pancreatitis.

Route/Dosage
Stimulation of Gastrin Secretion
ADULTS: IV 0.4 mcg/kg over 1 min.

Stimulate Pancreatic Secretions; Facilitation of Identification of Ampulla of Vater
ADULTS: IV 0.2 mcg/kg over 1 min.

Interactions
Anticholinergics: May make patient hyporesponsive, producing false positive results.

Lab Test Interferences None well documented.

Adverse Reactions
CV: Decreased BP (6%); mild bradycardia (2%); thready pulse (1%).
CNS: Lightheadedness (3%); headache, numbness/tingling in extremities (2%); fatigue, seizure (1%).
DERM: Diaphoresis, flushing (6%); pallor, abdominal rash, urticaria secondary to contrast media (1%).
GI: Nausea (8%); abdominal discomfort (7%);

burning in stomach (3%); abdominal cramps (2%); diarrhea, hunger pangs, vomiting (1%).
OTHER: Sphincterectomy bleeding (6%); upper GI bleeding secondary to endoscopic abrasion, endoscopic perforation of pancreatic duct, transient respiratory distress (2%); bloating, fever, hot sensation, leukocytoclastic vasculitis, transient low oxygen saturation (1%).

PATIENT CARE CONSIDERATIONS
Administration/Storage
- For IV administration only. Not for intradermal, SC, IM, or intra-arterial administration.
- Reconstitute powder using 8 mL sodium chloride injection following manufacturer's instructions. Shake vigorously to dissolve. Each mL of reconstituted solution contains 2 mcg of secretin.
- Use immediately after reconstitution. Discard any unused portion.
- Do not administer if particulate matter, cloudiness, or discoloration noted.
- Withdraw prescribed dose into syringe for injection. Do not filter reconstituted solution.
- Do not add other medications to secretin nor reconstitute with other diluents.
- Administer 0.1 mL test dose. If no allergic reaction is noted after 1 min, recommended dose for specific indication may be injected slowly over 1 min.
- Store vials in freezer (-4°F).

Precautions
Pregnancy: Category C.
Lactation: Undetermined.
Children: Safety and efficacy not established.
Allergy: Because of potential allergic reaction, patients should receive an IV test dose of 0.2 mcg (0.1 mL).

Assessment/Interventions
- Obtain patient history, including drug history and any known allergies. Note acute pancreatitis, liver disease, inflammatory bowel disease, history of vagotomy, or concurrent use of drugs with anticholinergic activity.
- Do not administer to patient with acute pancreatitis until the episode has resolved.
- Monitor patient for signs and symptoms of anaphylactic or serious allergic reactions. Be prepared to treat appropriately.
- Monitor patient for CV, GI, CNS, general body side effects, and injection site reactions. Report to health care provider if noted and significant.

Patient/Family Education
- Explain name, action, potential side effects of drug, and how drug will be used during the specific procedure that is going to be performed.
- Advise patient that medication will be prepared and administered by a health care provider in a medical setting.

Selegiline Hydrochloride (L-Deprenyl)

(seh-LEH-jih-leen HIGH-droe-KLOR-ide)
Class Antiparkinson
How Supplied
Carbex Tablets 5 mg ♦ *Eldepryl* Capsules 5 mg
❋ *Apo-Selegiline* ♦ *Gen-Selegiline* ♦ *Novo-Selegiline* ♦ *Nu-Selegiline*

Action
PHARMACOLOGY: Selective type B monoamine oxidase (MAO) inhibitor thought to increase dopaminergic activity. MAO enzyme breaks down catecholamines and serotonin. Selegiline may also interfere with dopamine reuptake at synapse.

PHARMACOKINETICS/DYNAMICS:
Absorption: C_{max} of metabolites following a single oral dose of 10 mg are from 4 to almost 20 times greater than that of maximum plasma concentration of selegiline (1 ng/mL). Bioavailability is increased 3- to 4-fold when taken with food.

Metabolism: Selegiline undergoes extensive metabolism. Major metabolites are N-desmethylselegiline, L-amphetamine, and L-methamphetamine. Only N-desmethylselegiline has MAO-B inhibiting activity.

Excretion: Following a single oral dose, the mean $t_½$ is 2 hr. The $t_½$ increases to 10 hr under steady-state conditions.

Special Populations:
Elderly – Systemic exposure is about twice as great in elderly as compared to a younger population given a single 10 mg oral dose.

Indications
Adjunct to levodopa/carbidopa in idiopathic Parkinson's disease, postencephalitic parkinsonism/symptomatic parkinsonism.

Contraindications
Standard considerations.

Route/Dosage
ADULTS: PO 10 mg/day as divided dose of 5 mg each taken at breakfast and lunch. Do not exceed 10 mg/day. After 2 to 3 days of treatment, try reducing levodopa/carbidopa dose by 10% to 30%. Further reductions may be possible during continued selegiline therapy.

Interactions
Fluoxetine: May produce a "serotonin" syndrome (CNS irritability, increased muscle tone, altered consciousness).
Meperidine: Could result in agitation, seizures, diaphoresis, and fever, which may progress to coma, apnea, and death. Reactions may occur several weeks following withdrawal of selegiline.

Lab Test Interferences None well documented.

Adverse Reactions
CV: Palpitations; orthostatic hypotension; arrhythmia; hypertension; new or increased angina; syncope.
CNS: Dizziness; lightheadedness; fainting; confusion; hallucinations; vivid dreams; headache; anxiety; tension; insomnia; lethargy; depression; loss of balance; delusions; dyskinesias; increased akinetic involuntary movements; bradykinesia; chorea.
DERM: Sweating; rash; photosensitivity.
EENT: Diplopia; blurred vision.
GI: Nausea; abdominal pain; dry mouth; diarrhea.
GU: Sexual dysfunction; urinary retention, frequency, hesitancy.
OTHER: Generalized ache; leg pain; low back pain; weight loss.

Precautions
Pregnancy: Category C.
Lactation: Undetermined.
Children: Effects have not been evaluated.
Maximum: Do not exceed recommended daily dose of 10 mg/day because of risks associated with nonselective inhibition of MAO (potentially serious food or drug interactions may occur at higher doses).
Hypertensive crisis risk: Selegiline can be given with active amine-containing medications and tyramine foods as long as recommended dose is not exceeded. However, report any possible symptoms suggestive of hypertensive crisis.

Overdosage: Signs and Symptoms
Hypotension, psychomotor agitation.

PATIENT CARE CONSIDERATIONS
Administration/Storage
- Administer 5 mg with breakfast and with lunch.
- Do not exceed 10 mg/day.

Assessment/Interventions
- Obtain patient history, including drug history and any known allergies.
- Monitor vital signs, especially BP and respirations.
- Assess patient for decrease in akathisia and mood.
- Assess patient's mental status: affect, mood, behavioral changes, depression.
- Dosage of levodopa/carbidopa may be reduced after 2 to 3 days of treatment.
- Assess for side effects, particularly nausea, dizziness, lightheadedness, abdominal pain, confusion, hallucination.
- Assist patient with ambulation at beginning of therapy.
- Assess diet for tyramine-containing foods.
- Implement safety measures to prevent falls, especially during initial treatment.

Patient/Family Education
- Encourage patient to change position slowly to prevent orthostatic hypotension.
- Instruct patient to avoid driving or other potentially hazardous activities until effect of medication is determined.
- Explain that dosage of levodopa/carbidopa may be reduced after initiation of adjunctive therapy.
- Identify tyramine-containing foods; explain rationale for exclusion from diet.
- Instruct patient to report these side effects: twitching, eye spasms.
- Caution patient to use drug exactly as prescribed. Explain that if drug is discontinued, parkinsonian crisis may occur.
- Advise patient not to exceed 10 mg/day dose.
- Inform patient and family of symptoms of hypertensive crisis and when to call health care provider. Instruct them to report severe headache or other unusual symptoms.

Selenium (as selenious acid)
(seh-LEE-nee-uhm)

Class Trace Metal

How Supplied
Sele-Pak Injection 40 mcg/mL (as 65.4 mcg selenious acid) ◆ *Selepen* Injection 40 mcg/mL (as 65.4 mcg selenious acid)

Action
PHARMACOLOGY: Part of glutathione peroxidase, which protects cell components from oxidative damage caused by peroxidases produced in cellular metabolism.

PHARMACOKINETICS/DYNAMICS:
Excretion: Primarily by the kidney but endogenous losses occur through the feces.

Indications Use as a supplement to IV total parenteral nutrition (TPN) solutions to prevent depletion of endogenous stores and subsequent deficiency symptoms.

Contraindications Do not give undiluted by direct IV injection.

Route/Dosage
ADULTS: **TPN Additive** Metabolically stable patients: 20 to 40 mcg/day. In selenium deficiency states resulting from long-term TPN support: 100 mcg/day for 24 to 31 days.
CHILDREN: **TPN Additive** 3 mcg/kg/day.

Interactions None well documented.

Lab Test Interferences None well documented.

Adverse Reactions Unlikely to occur at recommended dosage level.

Precautions
Pregnancy: Category C.

PATIENT CARE CONSIDERATIONS
Administration/Storage
- For admixture in TPN solution only. Not for intradermal, SC, IM, or direct IV administration.
- Add prescribed additive dose to TPN solution using aseptic technique, preferably under a laminar flow hood.
- Do not administer if particulate matter, cloudiness, or discoloration are noted.
- Discard any unused solution in single-dose vial. Do not save for future use.
- Store vials at controlled room temperature (59° to 86°F).

Assessment/Interventions
- Obtain patient history, including drug history and any known allergies. Note renal impairment, GI dysfunction, or recent blood transfusion(s).

Renal function impairment: Supplement dosage may be adjusted, reduced, or omitted.
Benzyl alcohol: Contains benzyl alcohol in multidoses preparation.
GI malfunction: Dose may be adjusted, reduced, or omitted.

Overdosage: Signs and Symptoms
Acute: Death (preceded by coma) with histopathological changes, including fulminating peripheral vascular collapse, internal vascular congestion, edematous lungs, brick-red color gastric mucosa
Chronic: Hair loss, weakened nails, dermatitis, dental defects, GI disorders, nervousness, mental depression, metallic taste, vomiting, garlic odor of breath and sweat

- Ensure plasma selenium levels are frequently measured during TPN support.
- Ensure that renal function is evaluated before starting therapy and periodically during treatment.
- Frequently assess vascular access site for signs of inflammation or infection. Inform health care provider if noted.

Patient/Family Education
- Explain name, action, and potential side effects of drug.
- Advise patient, family, or caregiver that medication will be added to TPN solution.
- Advise patient to report pain, redness, warmth, or swelling of TPN access site.
- Advise patient that follow-up visits and lab tests will be required to monitor therapy and to keep appointments.

Senna
(SEN-ah)

Class Laxative

How Supplied
Agoral Liquid 25 mg ♦ *Black-Draught* Granules 20 mg/5 mL, Tablets 6 mg ♦ *ex•lax* Tablets 15 mg ♦ *ex•lax chocolate* Tablets 15 mg ♦ *Fletcher Castoria* Liquid 33.3 mg/mL ♦ *Senexon* Tablets 8.5 mg ♦ *Senna-Gen* Tablets 8.6 mg ♦ *Senokot* Granules 15 mg/5 mL, Syrup 8.8 mg/5 mL, Tablets 8.6 mg ♦ *SenokotXTRA* Tablets 17 mg
✤ *Glysennid*

Action
PHARMACOLOGY: Directly acts on intestinal mucosa by altering water and electrolyte secretion, inducing peristalsis and defecation.

Indications Short-term treatment of constipation; preoperative and preradiographic bowel evacuation for procedures involving GI tract.

Contraindications Nausea, vomiting, or other symptoms of appendicitis; acute surgical abdomen; fecal impaction; intestinal obstruction; undiagnosed abdominal pain.

Route/Dosage
ADULTS: **PO** 2 tablets, 1 tsp of granules or 10 to 15 mL of syrup, usually at bedtime.
PR 1 suppository at bedtime; may repeat in 2 hr.
CHILDREN: Generally, for children 6 to 12 yr or more than 60 lb, give (at bedtime) 1 tablet or ½ tsp granules **PO** or ½ suppository **PR**. Liquid dose ranges from 1.25 to 15 mL depending on age and product formulation.

Interactions None well documented.

Lab Test Interferences None well documented.

Adverse Reactions
CV: Palpitations.
CNS: Dizziness; fainting.

GI: Excessive bowel activity (eg, griping, diarrhea, nausea, vomiting); perianal irritation; bloating; flatulence; abdominal cramping.
OTHER: Sweating; weakness.

Precautions
Pregnancy: Category C.
Lactation: Undetermined.
Abuse/dependency: Long-term use may lead to laxative dependency, which may result in fluid and electrolyte imbalances, steatorrhea, osteomalacia and vitamin and mineral deficiencies. Cathartic colon, a poorly functioning colon, results from long-term abuse. Pathologic presentation may resemble ulcerative colitis.
Discoloration of acidic urine: May result in yellow-brown urine.
Discoloration of alkaline urine: May result in pink to red urine.
Fluid and electrolyte imbalance: Excessive laxative use may lead to significant fluid and electrolyte imbalance.
Melanosis Coli: Darkened pigmentation of colonic mucosa may occur after long-term use, usually resolving within 5 to 11 mo of discontinuation.
Rectal bleeding or failure to respond: May indicate serious condition requiring further attention.

Overdosage: Signs and Symptoms
Gripping pain, diarrhea.

PATIENT CARE CONSIDERATIONS

Administration/Storage
- Administer at bedtime on empty stomach.
- Shake liquid solution before administering.
- Dissolve granules before administering.
- For preoperative or prediagnostic bowel preparation, give between 2 to 4 PM on day before procedure.
- Limit patient's diet to clear liquids until after procedure.
- Give oral dosages with full glass of water or juice.
- Administer suppository with patient lying on left side.

Assessment/Interventions
- Obtain patient history, including drug history and any known allergies.
- Assess bowel function, including normal frequency, type, last bowel movement, bowel sounds, abdominal distention.
- Assess for presence of abdominal pain, nausea, vomiting.
- Assess for fluid and electrolyte imbalance associated with long-term laxative use.
- Identify factors potentially contributing to constipation (ie, opioid analgesics), inactivity.
- Monitor effectiveness of therapy.
- Implement measures to prevent constipation (eg, fluids, activity, dietary bulk).

Patient/Family Education
- Explain potential hazards (eg, dependence) associated with long-term laxative use.
- Advise that senna may result in discolored yellow-brown or reddish urine.
- Explain that bowel patterns are very individual.
- Identify measures to improve bowel function, ie, fluids, activity, dietary bulk.
- Caution against taking laxatives in presence of acute abdominal pain or in presence of nausea or vomiting.

Sertaconazole Nitrate

(SIR-tah-KAHN-uh-zole NYE-trate)
Class Anti-infective/Antifungal

How Supplied
Ertaczo Cream 2%

Action
PHARMACOLOGY: Alters permeability of fungal cell membrane, leading to cell death.

Indications
Topical treatment of interdigital tinea pedis caused by *Trichophyton rubrum*, *Trichophyton mentagrophytes*, and *Epidermophyton floccosum* in immunocompetent patients.

Contraindications
Sensitivity to imidazoles or any component of the product.

Route/Dosage
ADULTS AND CHILDREN 12 YR AND OLDER:
Topical Apply bid for 4 wk, applying a sufficient amount to cover affected areas between the toes and immediately surrounding skin. Review the diagnosis if no improvement is noted 2 wk after starting treatment.

Interactions
None well documented.

Lab Test Interferences
None well documented.

Adverse Reactions
DERM: Contact dermatitis, dry skin, burning skin, application site reaction, skin tenderness (2%).

Precautions
Pregnancy: Category C.
Lactation: Undetermined.
Children: Safety and efficacy not established in children under 12 yr.
Diagnosis: Should be confirmed by direct microscopic examination of infected superficial epidermal tissue or by culture on appropriate medium.

PATIENT CARE CONSIDERATIONS
Administration/Storage
- For topical use only. Not for ophthalmic, oral, or intravaginal use.
- Thoroughly dry affected areas of skin before application of cream.
- Apply cream in sufficient quantity to cover affected areas between toes and the immediately surrounding healthy skin bid.
- Avoid contact with the eyes, nose, mouth, and other mucus membranes.
- Do not apply occlusive dressings unless ordered by health care provider.
- Store cream at controlled room temperature (59° to 86°F). Keep tube tightly capped.

Assessment/Interventions
- Obtain patient history, including drug history and any known allergies. Note pregnancy, breastfeeding, or sensitivity to other imidazoles antifungal agents (eg, econazole).
- Assess and document skin condition before initial application and periodically throughout treatment. Inform health care provider if condition does not improve, worsens, or if application site reactions are bothersome.

Patient/Family Education
- Explain name, action, and potential side effects of drug.
- Advise patient to try to keep affected areas as dry as possible because moist skin favors growth of fungi.
- Advise patient to carefully dry between the toes after showering or bathing, apply drying and dusting powders as necessary, and change socks frequently.
- Teach patient or caregiver proper technique for applying cream: wash hands; apply sufficient cream to cover affected areas between the toes and the immediately surrounding healthy skin and gently massage into skin. Wash hands after applying cream. Caution patient not to cover with occlusive dressing unless advised by health care provider.
- Advise patient to apply cream to affected areas bid as directed by health care provider.
- Caution patient to avoid contact with eyes, nose, mouth, and other mucus membranes. Advise patient that if cream does come into contact with the eyes, to wash eyes with large amounts of cool water and contact health care provider if eye irritation occurs.
- Advise patient that symptoms should begin to improve fairly soon after starting treatment but to continue applying cream as directed for full treatment period to prevent recurrence of infection.
- Advise patient to notify health care provider if condition does not improve, worsens, or if application site reactions (eg, irritation, burning, stinging, redness, itching, blistering, swelling, oozing) develop and are bothersome.
- Advise women to notify health care provider if pregnant, planning to become pregnant, or breastfeeding.
- Warn patient not to take any prescription or OTC drugs or dietary supplements without consulting health care provider.
- Advise patient that follow-up visits to monitor response to treatment may be required and to keep appointments.

Sertraline Hydrochloride

(SIR-truh-leen HIGH-droe-KLOR-ide)

Class Antidepressant

How Supplied
Zoloft Tablets 25 mg, Tablets 50 mg, Tablets 100 mg, Oral concentrate 20 mg/mL
✤ *Apo-Sertraline* ♦ *Novo-Sertraline* ♦ *ratio-Sertraline*

Action
PHARMACOLOGY: Selectively blocks reuptake of serotonin, enhancing serotonergic function.

PHARMACOKINETICS/DYNAMICS:
Absorption: T_{max} is 4 to 9 hr postdose. Steady state should be achieved after approximately 1 wk of qd dosing.
Tablet bioavailability – AUC was slightly increased when the drug was given with food and C_{max} was 25% greater while T_{max} decreased from 8 hr postdosing to 5.5 hr.
Oral concentrate bioavailability – T_{max} was prolonged from 5.9 to 7 hr with food.

Distribution: Sertraline is 98% protein bound.

Metabolism: Sertraline undergoes extensive first-pass metabolism. The principal initial metabolic pathway is N-demethylation. The liver is the primary site of metabolism.

Excretion: Sertraline t½ is 26 hr.

Special Populations:
Hepatic Function Impairment – Liver impairment can affect the elimination of sertraline. Give a lower, less frequent dose.
Children – Pediatric patients metabolize sertraline with slightly greater efficacy than adults.

Indications Treatment of major depression; treatment of obsessions and compulsions in patients with obsessive-compulsive disorder (OCD), as defined in the DSM-III-R; treatment of panic disorder with or without agoraphobia, as defined in DSM-IV; posttraumatic stress disorder (PTSD); treatment of premenstrual dysphoric disorder; treatment of social anxiety disorder (social phobia).

Contraindications Hypersensitivity to any components; concomitant use in patients taking monoamine oxidase inhibitors (MAOIs), pimozide, disulfiram (due to alcohol content in oral concentrate).

Route/Dosage
Major Depressive Disorders
ADULTS: **PO** 50 mg qd (max, 200 mg/day). Dose changes should not occur at intervals of less than 1 wk.

OCD
ADULTS AND CHILDREN 13 TO 17 YR: **PO** 50 mg qd (max, 200 mg/day). Dose changes should not occur at intervals of less than 1 wk.
CHILDREN 6 TO 12 YR: **PO** 25 mg qd (max, 200 mg/day). Dose changes should not occur at intervals of less than 1 wk.

Panic Disorder, Social Anxiety Disorder, and PTSD
ADULTS: **PO** 25 mg qd; the dose may be increased to 50 mg qd after 1 wk (max, 200 mg/day). Dose changes should not occur at intervals of less than 1 wk.

Premenstrual Dysphoric Disorder
ADULTS: **PO** 50 mg/day, either daily throughout the menstrual cycle or limited to the luteal phase of the menstrual cycle, depending on physician assessment. Patients not responding to 50 mg/day may benefit from increases (at 50 mg increments/menstrual cycle) up to 150 mg/day when dosing throughout the menstrual cycle, or 100 mg/day when dosing during the luteal phase of the menstrual cycle. If a 100 mg/day dose has been established with luteal dosing, use a 50 mg/day titration step for 3 days at the beginning of each luteal phase dosing period.

Switching patients to or from MAOIs
At least 14 days should elapse between discontinuation of an MAOI and initiation of therapy with sertraline.

Interactions
5-HT$_1$ agonists (eg, naratriptan, rizatriptan, sumatriptan, zolmitriptan): Weakness, hyperreflexia, and incoordination reported rarely.
Alcohol, CNS depressants: May enhance CNS depressant effects.
Cimetidine: Increased sertraline AUC (50%), C$_{max}$ (24%), and t½ (26%). Clinical significance is unknown.
Clozapine: Elevated serum clozapine levels occurred. Closely monitor patients on coadministration.
Hydantoins (eg, phenytoin): Plasma levels may be increased by sertraline, increasing the pharmacologic and adverse effects.
MAO inhibitors: May cause serious, even fatal reactions. Discontinue MAO inhibitors at least 14 days before starting sertraline.
Pimozide: Increase in pimozide AUC and C$_{max}$ of about 40%; concomitant administration is contraindicated.
St. John's wort: Sedative-hypnotic effects of sertraline may be increased.
Sympathomimetics (eg, amphetamine, fenfluramine): Increased sensitivity to sympathomimetics; increased risk of "serotonin syndrome."
Tolbutamide: Sertraline significantly decreased the Cl of tolbutamide (16%). Clinical significance is unknown.
Tricyclic antidepressants (eg, amitriptyline): Pharmacologic and toxic effects may be increased by sertraline; "serotonin syndrome" has been reported.
Type 1C antiarrhythmics (eg, propafenone, flecainide): Plasma levels may be increased. Monitor cardiac function.
Zolpidem: Onset of action of zolpidem may be shortened and the effect increased.

Lab Test Interferences None well documented.

Adverse Reactions
CV: Palpitations; hot flushes; hypotension (postural); hypertension; syncope; tachycardia; chest pain.
CNS: Agitation; anxiety; nervousness; headache; insomnia; dizziness; tremor; fatigue; tingling; diminished sensation; twitching; hypertonia; decreased concentration; confusion; somnolence; depression; decreased libido; agitation; emotional lability; vertigo; hypesthesia; apathy; hypokinesia/hyperkinesia; abnormal dreams; manic reaction.
DERM: Sweating, rash; pruritus; acne.
EENT: Abnormal vision; ringing in the ears; rhinitis; pharyngitis; change in taste perception.
GI: Nausea; diarrhea; dry mouth; anorexia; vomiting; flatulence; constipation; abdominal pain; increased appetite; dyspepsia; gastroenteritis; tooth disorder/caries; dysphagia; melena.
GU: Sexual dysfunction; urinary frequency; urinary disorder; menstrual disorder; pain; abnormal ejaculation; impotence.
HEMA: Lymphadenopathy; purpura.
LABTESTABS: Increase in total cholesterol, decrease in serum uric acid.
METAB: Dehydration; hypoglycemia.
RESP: Upper respiratory tract infection; pharyngitis; sinusitis; increased cough; dyspnea; bronchitis; rhinitis; epistaxis.
OTHER: Muscle pain; weight loss or gain; myalgia; arthralgia; asthenia; fever; allergy/

allergic reaction; chills; back pain; malaise; edema; yawning.

Precautions

Pregnancy: Category C.
Lactation: Undetermined.
Children: Safety and efficacy not established.
Elderly: Dosage reduction may be required.
Renal function impairment: Use drug with caution. Lower or less frequent dosing schedule may be required.
Hepatic function impairment: Use drug with caution. Lower or less frequent dosing schedule may be required.
Activation of mania/hypomania: Activation of mania/hypomania occurs infrequently in patients taking selective serotonin reuptake inhibitors.

Hyponatremia: Several cases of sertraline-induced hyponatremia have occurred.
MAO inhibitors: Cases of serious sometimes fatal reactions have been reported when an MAO inhibitors is used in combination with sertraline.
Seizures: Use drug with caution in patients with history of seizures.
Suicide: Supervise depressed patients at risk during initial therapy.

Overdosage: Signs and Symptoms

Somnolence, nausea, vomiting, tachycardia, ECG changes, anxiety, dilated pupils, serotonin syndrome, agitation, tremor, ejaculation disorder, convulsions, hypertension.

PATIENT CARE CONSIDERATIONS

Administration/Storage

- Administer qd in morning or evening.
- Do not change dosage at intervals of less than 1 wk.
- Do not administer to patients who have used MAO inhibitors in the past 14 days.
- Store at room temperature (59° to 86°F).
- Oral concentrate must be diluted before use. May mix with 4 oz of water, ginger ale, lemon/lime soda, lemonade, or orange juice only.
- Oral concentrate dose should be taken immediately after mixing.

Assessment/Interventions

- Obtain patient history, including drug history and any known allergies. Determine whether any MAO inhibitors have been used in the past 14 days. Note history of seizure disorders and renal and hepatic impairment.
- Observe for common side effects (eg, agitation, insomnia, somnolence, dizziness, headache, tremor, anorexia, diarrhea/loose stools, nausea, fatigue) and notify health care provider.
- Take appropriate safety measures because possibility of suicide may persist until significant remission occurs.

Patient/Family Education

- Discuss with family members precautionary measures to be taken to prevent suicide attempt.
- Inform patient that improvement may not be evident for 2 to 4 wk after treatment has started.
- Advise women to notify health care provider if pregnant, planning to become pregnant, or breastfeeding.
- Inform men of possible sexual dysfunction (primarily ejaculatory delay), and advise them to notify health care provider if it occurs.
- Explain that anorexia, nausea, diarrhea, and weight loss may occur. Advise patient to notify health care provider if these symptoms persist.
- Instruct patient to report these symptoms to health care provider: agitation, insomnia, somnolence, dizziness, headache, tremor, anorexia, diarrhea/loose stools, nausea, fatigue, other physical complaints.
- Tell patient to avoid intake of alcoholic beverages or other CNS depressants.
- Advise patient that drug may cause drowsiness and dizziness and to use caution while driving or performing other tasks requiring mental alertness.
- Advise patient to notify health care provider if rash, hives, or a related allergic phenomenon develops.
- While patient may notice improvement in 1 to 4 wk, advise continuation of therapy as directed.

Sevelamer Hydrochloride

(seh-VELL-ah-meer)
Class Polymeric phosphate binder
How Supplied
Renagel Tablets 400 mg, Tablets 800 mg

Action

PHARMACOLOGY: Decreases intestinal phosphate absorption by binding to phosphate in the GI tract.

PHARMACOKINETICS/DYNAMICS:
Absorption: Studies indicate that sevelamer is not systemically absorbed.

Indications Reduction of serum phosphorus in patient with chronic kidney disease who are on hemodialysis.

Contraindications Hypophosphatemia, bowel obstruction, or hypersensitivity to any component of the product.

Route/Dosage

Patients Not Taking Phosphate Binders
ADULTS: **PO** Serum phosphate greater than 5.5 and less than 7.5 mg/dL, start with 800 mg tid with meals. Serum phosphate 7.5 or greater and less than 9 mg/dL, start with 1,200 or 1,600 mg tid with meals. Serum phosphate 9 mg/dL or greater, start with 1,600 mg tid with meals.

Patients Switching from Calcium Acetate
ADULTS: **PO** Start with 800 mg sevelamer with meals in patients receiving 667 mg calcium acetate. Start with 1,200 mg or 1,600 mg sevelamer with meals in patients receiving 1,334 mg of calcium acetate. Start with 2,000 mg or 2,400 mg sevelamer with meals in patients receiving 2,001 mg of calcium acetate.

Dose Titration
ADULTS: **PO** Adjust dosage based on the serum phosphorus concentration with a goal of lowering serum phosphorus to 5.5 mg/dL or less. If serum phosphorus is greater than 5.5 mg/dL, increase sevelamer by 1 tablet per meal at 2-wk intervals. If serum phosphorus is 3.5 to 5.5 mg/dL, maintain current dose. If serum phosphorus is less than 3.5 mg/dL, decrease sevelamer by 1 tablet per meal.

Interactions None well documented.

Lab Test Interferences None well documented.

Adverse Reactions
CV: Hypertension (10%).
CNS: Headache (9%).
DERM: Pruritus (13%); rash (postmarketing).
EENT: Nasopharyngitis (14%).
GI: Vomiting (22%); nausea (20%); diarrhea (19%); dyspepsia (16%); constipation (8%); abdominal pain (postmarketing).
MUSC: Limb pain (13%); arthralgia (12%); back pain (4%).
RESP: Bronchitis (11%); dyspnea (10%); cough (7%); upper respiratory tract infection (5%).
OTHER: Mechanical complication of implant (6%); pyrexia (5%).

Precautions
Pregnancy: Category C.
Lactation: Not absorbed systemically.
Children: Safety and efficacy not established.
GI disorders: Use with caution in patients with dysphagia, swallowing disorders, severe GI motility disorders, or major GI tract surgery.

PATIENT CARE CONSIDERATIONS

Administration/Storage
- Dose is individualized depending on serum phosphorous.
- Administer prescribed dose with meals.
- Because sevelamer may bind concomitantly with administered medications and reduce their bioavailability, administer sevelamer 1 hr after or 3 hr before other medications.
- Because sevelamer expands in water, have patient swallow tablets whole and do not chew, crush, or break tablets.
- Store tablets at ambient room temperature (59° to 86°F). Protect from moisture.

Assessment/Interventions
- Obtain patient history, including drug history and any known allergies. Note hypophosphatemia, bowel obstruction, dysphagia, swallowing disorder, GI motility disorder, or major GI tract surgery.
- Ensure that serum calcium, phosphorous, bicarbonate, and chloride levels are determined before starting therapy and periodically during treatment.
- Ensure that sevelamer dose is adjusted as necessary in order to lower serum phosphorous to 5.5 mg/dL or less.
- Assess patient for GI, CV, and general body side effects. Inform health care provider if noted and significant.

Patient/Family Education
- Explain name, dose, action, and potential side effects of drug.
- Advise patient that medication does not replace diet changes and to continue to adhere to the prescribed diet.
- Advise patient that dose may be adjusted periodically in order to achieve max benefit.
- Advise patient to take each dose with food. Caution patient that medication swells when exposed to water and not to chew, break, or crush tablets.
- Advise women to notify health care provider if pregnant, planning to become pregnant, or breastfeeding.
- Instruct patient not to take any prescription or OTC medications, dietary supplements, or herbal preparations unless advised by health care provider.
- Advise patient that follow-up examinations and lab tests will be required to monitor therapy and to keep appointments.

Sibutramine Hydrochloride

(sih-BYOO-trah-meen)

Class CNS stimulant/Anorexiant

How Supplied
Meridia Capsules 5 mg, Capsules 10 mg, Capsules 15 mg

Action
PHARMACOLOGY: Inhibits reuptake of norepinephrine, serotonin, and dopamine. May stimulate satiety center in brain, causing appetite suppression.

PHARMACOKINETICS/DYNAMICS:
Absorption: Sibutramine T_{max} is 1.2 hr; food delays T_{max} by approximately 3 hr. Approximately 77% of a single oral dose is absorbed. Steady state is reached within 4 days.

Distribution: Sibutramine is extensively bound and is rapidly and extensively distributed into tissues. Highest concentrations are in liver and kidneys.

Metabolism: Sibutramine undergoes extensive first-pass metabolism and is metabolized primarily by the cytochrome P4503A4 isoenzyme. The pharmacologically active metabolites are mono- and di-desmethyl M_1 and M_2.

Excretion: Sibutramine t½ is 1.1 hr. Oral clearance is 1750 L/hr, and approximately 85% is excreted in urine.

Special Populations:
Renal Function Impairment – Do not use in severe renal impairment.
Hepatic Function Impairment – Do not use in severe hepatic impairment.
Elderly – Dose selection should be cautious, reflecting the greater frequency of decreased hepatic, renal, or cardiac function, and of concomitant disease or other drug therapy.

Indications
As an adjunct to a reduced calorie diet for the management of obesity, including weight loss and maintenance of weight loss. Recommended for patients with an initial body mass index greater than 30 kg/m^2 or greater than 27 kg/m^2 in the presence of other risk factors (eg, hypertension, diabetes, dyslipidemia).

Contraindications
Concurrent use of, or within 2 wk of discontinuing, an MAO inhibitor; anorexia nervosa; concurrent use of other centrally acting appetite suppressants; allergy to sibutramine or any product component; uncontrolled or poorly controlled hypertension.

Route/Dosage
ADULTS AND CHILDREN GREATER THAN 16 YR: PO 10 mg once daily. May titrate to 15 mg/day after 4 wk if necessary.

Interactions
5-HT receptor agonists (eg, sumatriptan), bupropion, dextromethorphan, ergots (eg, dihydroergotamine), fentanyl, lithium, meperidine, pentazocine, selective serotonin reuptake inhibitors (eg, fluoxetine), tetracyclic antidepressants (eg, trazodone), tricyclic antidepressants (eg, amitriptyline), tryptophan: May precipitate "serotonin syndrome" if used concurrently with sibutramine. Avoid concurrent use.

Centrally acting appetite suppressants (eg, prescription, otc, and herbal products): Concurrent use is contraindicated.

Ephedrine, phenylpropanolamine, pseudoephedrine: Use with caution. Potential additive effects on BP and pulse.

MAO inhibitors: Do not use concomitantly with sibutramine. Separate therapy with either agent by at least 2 wk.

Lab Test Interferences None well documented.

Adverse Reactions
CV: Tachycardia; vasodilation; hypertension; palpitations.
CNS: Headache; migraine; dizziness; nervousness; anxiety; depression; paresthesia; somnolence; CNS stimulation; emotional lability; agitation; hypertonia; abnormal thinking; insomnia.
DERM: Rash; sweating; herpes simplex; acne; pruritus.
EENT: Amblyopia; ear disorder; ear pain; rhinitis; sinusitis; laryngitis; pharyngitis.
GI: Abdominal pain; anorexia; constipation; increased appetite; nausea; dyspepsia; gastritis; vomiting; rectal disorder; dry mouth; taste perversion; diarrhea; flatulence; gastroenteritis; tooth disorder; thirst.
GU: Dysmenorrhea; urinary tract infection; vaginitis; metrorrhagia; menstrual disorder.
RESP: Cough; bronchitis; dyspnea.
OTHER: Back, chest, or neck pain; flu syndrome; accidental injury; asthenia; allergic reactions; edema; arthralgia; myalgia; tenosynovitis; fever; leg cramps.

Precautions
Pregnancy: Category C.
Lactation: Undetermined.
Children: Safety and efficacy in children less than 16 yr not established.
Elderly: Use with caution in patients greater than 65 yr.
Renal function impairment: Do not use in patients with severe renal impairment.
Hepatic function impairment: Do not use in patients with severe hepatic impairment.
Blood pressure/Pulse: Sibutramine can cause

tachycardia and hypertension. Use with caution in patients with a history of hypertension. Do not administer to patients with uncontrolled or poorly controlled hypertension.
Concomitant cardiovascular disease: Do not use in patients with a history of coronary artery disease, CHF, arrhythmias, or stroke.
Glaucoma: Use with caution in patients with narrow angle glaucoma.
Seizures: Use with caution in patients with a history of seizures. Discontinue use in any patient who develops seizures.

PATIENT CARE CONSIDERATIONS
Administration/Storage
- Administer as a single daily dose without regard to meals.
- Consider administering in the morning.
- Store at room temperature in a tightly closed container. Protect from heat and moisture.

Assessment/Interventions
- Obtain patient history, including drug history and any known allergies. Note cardiovascular disease, hepatic or renal impairment, history of seizures, or glaucoma.
- Obtain baseline BP and pulse and then regularly thereafter. Notify health care provider if patient develops hypertension or tachycardia.
- Monitor patient weight.
- Implement protective measures and supervise and assist with ambulation if dizziness or drowsiness are problems.
- Monitor patient for side effects. Report significant findings to health care provider.

Patient/Family Education
- Advise patient to take drug daily as prescribed. Remind patient that it can be taken without regard to food.
- Instruct patient not to change the dose or discontinue therapy unless advised to do so by their health care provider.
- Encourage patient to follow medically supervised weight reduction program. Emphasize that this medication will only work in conjunction with a diet and exercise program.
- Advise patient to avoid alcohol and other CNS depressants.
- Emphasize importance of follow-up visits for monitoring BP and pulse as well as weight loss.
- Advise patient to contact their health care provider if they note any of the following: unexplained shortness of breath, swelling of ankles, decreased exercise tolerance, skin rash, hives, or other signs of an allergic reaction.
- Advise patient that drug may cause drowsiness or dizziness and to use caution while driving or performing other tasks requiring mental alertness.
- Advise women of childbearing potential to use an effective birth control method while on this drug.
- Instruct patient to notify health care provider if they become pregnant, plan on becoming pregnant, or are breastfeeding.
- Instruct patient not to take any other medications (including otc and herbal products) unless advised to do so by their health care provider. Many drugs can interact with sibutramine and cause potentially life-threatening reactions.
- Advise patient that safety of long term (longer than 1 yr) use has not been determined.

Gallstones: Weight loss can precipitate or exacerbate gallstone formation.
Drug abuse: Carefully evaluate patients for a history of drug abuse. Follow such patients closely, observing for signs of misuse or abuse.
Primary pulmonary hypertension/Cardiac valve dysfunction: Although not reported with sibutramine, these have occurred in patients receiving certain other centrally acting appetite suppressants.

Overdosage: Signs and Symptoms
Tachycardia, hypertension.

Sildenafil Citrate

(sill-DEN-ah-fil)

Class Agent for impotence

How Supplied
Viagra Tablets 25 mg, Tablets 50 mg, Tablets 100 mg

Action
PHARMACOLOGY: Enhances the effect of nitric oxide by inhibiting phosphodiesterase type 5 in the corpus cavernosum of the penis. This results in vasodilation, increased inflow of blood into the corpora cavernosa, and ensuing penile erection upon sexual stimulation.

PHARMACOKINETICS/DYNAMICS:
Absorption: Sildenafil bioavailability is 40%; T_{max} is 30 to 120 min (mean, 60 min). The drug is rapidly absorbed; when taken with a high-fat meal, the absorption rate is reduced with a mean delay in T_{max} of 60 min and a mean reduction of C_{max} of 29%.

Distribution: Vd of sildenafil is 105 L and it is 96% bound to plasma proteins.

Metabolism: Sildenafil undergoes hepatic

metabolism (mainly cytochrome P450 3A4). The major circulating metabolite results from N-desmethylation.

Excretion: Sildenafil t½ is 4 hr. The drug is cleared primarily by the CYP3A4 (major route) and CYP2C9 (minor route) hepatic microsomal isoenzymes, and is excreted primarily in feces (approximately 80%) and to a lesser extent in urine (approximately 13%).

Duration: Duration of action is up to 4 hr.

Special Populations:
Renal Function Impairment – Severe renal impairment is associated with increased plasma levels. Consider a starting dose of 25 mg in these patients.

Hepatic Function Impairment – Hepatic impairment is associated with increased plasma levels. Consider a starting dose of 25 mg in these patients.

Elderly – Age greater than 65 yr is associated with increased plasma levels. Consider a starting dose of 25 mg in these patients.

Indications Treatment of impotence related to erectile dysfunction of the penis.

Contraindications
Patients using any type of organic nitrates (eg, nitroglycerin, isosorbide mono, dinitrate): Enhanced effects leading to prolonged hypotension.

Route/Dosage
ADULTS: PO 50 mg once 0.5 to 4 hr prior to sexual activity. Titration to a 25- or a 100-mg dose may be used based on tolerability or efficacy. The max recommended use is once daily.

Dosage Adjustments
ADULTS: PO Consider a starting dose of 25 mg in patients older than 65 yr or in patients with hepatic impairment, severe renal impairment, or concurrent use of potent cytochrome P450 3A4 inhibitors (eg, erythromycin, ketoconazole, itraconazole, saquinavir).

PROTEASE INHIBITORS: Do not exceed a max single dose of 25 mg sildenafil in a 48-hr period.
ALPHA-BLOCKERS: Do not take 50 or 100 mg doses of sildenafil within 4 hr of alpha-blocker administration; however, a 25 mg dose of sildenafil may be taken at any time.

Interactions
Amlodipine, alpha-blockers (eg, doxazosin): Administration may result in an additional decrease in BP.
Cimetidine, erythromycin, ketoconazole, itraconazole, tacrolimus: Increased sildenafil levels potentially leading to increased adverse effects.
Nitrates: Hypotension (see Contraindications).
Protease inhibitors (eg, ritonavir, saquinavir): Sildenafil plasma concentration may be increased, requiring a modification in sildenafil dosage.
Inducers of CYP3A4 (eg, rifampin): May decrease sildenafil levels.

Lab Test Interferences None well documented.

Adverse Reactions
CV: Angina pectoris, AV block, syncope, tachycardia, palpitation, hypotension, postural hypotension, myocardial ischemia, cerebral thrombosis, cardiac arrest, heart failure, abnormal ECG, cardiomyopathy (less than 2%); sudden cardiac death, MI, ventricular arrhythmia, cerebrovascular hemorrhage, transient ischemic attack, hypertension, subarachnoid and intracerebral hemorrhages, pulmonary hemorrhage (postmarketing).
CNS: Headache (16%); dizziness (2%); ataxia, hypertonia, neuralgia, paresthesia, tremor, vertigo, depression, insomnia, somnolence, migraine, neuropathy, abnormal dreams, decreased reflexes, hypesthesia (less than 2%); seizure, anxiety (postmarketing).
DERM: Flushing (10%); rash (2%); urticaria, herpes simplex, pruritus, sweating, skin ulcer, contact dermatitis, exfoliative dermatitis (less than 2%).
EENT: Nasal congestion (4%); abnormal vision (mild and transient, predominantly color tinge vision, increased sensitivity to light or blurred vision [3%]); mydriasis, conjunctivitis, photophobia, tinnitus, eye pain, deafness, ear pain, eye hemorrhage, cataract, dry eyes (less than 2%); diplopia, temporary vision loss/decreased vision, ocular redness, bloodshot appearance, ocular burning, ocular swelling/pressure, increased IOP, retinal vascular disease or bleeding, vitreous detachment/traction, paramacular edema, epistaxis (postmarketing).
GI: Dyspepsia (7%); diarrhea (3%); vomiting, glossitis, colitis, dysphagia, gastritis, gastroenteritis, esophagitis, stomatitis, dry mouth, rectal hemorrhage, gingivitis (less than 2%).
GU: UTI (3%); cystitis, nocturia, urinary frequency, breast enlargement, urinary incontinence, abnormal ejaculation, genital edema, anorgasmia (less than 2%); prolonged erection, priapism, hematuria (postmarketing).
HEMA: Anemia, leukopenia (less than 2%).
HEPA: Abnormal LFTs (less than 2%).
METAB: Thirst, edema, gout, unstable diabetes, hyperglycemia, peripheral edema, hyperuricemia, hypoglycemic reaction, hypernatremia.
MUSC: Arthritis, arthrosis, myalgia, tendon rupture, tenosynovitis, bone pain, myasthenia, synovitis.
RESP: Asthma, dyspnea, laryngitis, pharyngitis, sinusitis, bronchitis, increased sputum, increased

cough (less than 2%).
OTHER: Face edema, photosensitivity, shock, asthenia, pain, chills, accidental falls, abdominal pain, allergic reaction, chest pain, accidental injury (less than 2%).

Precautions
Pregnancy: Category B.
Lactation: Undetermined.
Children: Not indicated for use in children.
Renal function impairment: Consider an initial dose of 25 mg.
Hepatic function impairment: Consider an initial dose of 25 mg.
Anatomical deformation: Use with caution in patients with anatomical deformation of the penis (eg, Peyronie disease) or patients prone to priapism (eg, patients with sickle cell disease).
Cardiac risk: Exertion from renewed sexual activity may pose a risk of cardiac events such as MI, sudden cardiac death, ventricular arrhythmia, cerebrovascular hemorrhage, transient ischemic attack, and hypertension.

PATIENT CARE CONSIDERATIONS

Administration/Storage
- Administer prescribed dose approximately 60 min before sexual activity.
- Administer dose greater than 25 mg 4 hr before or after an alpha-blocker (eg, doxazosin).
- Administer without regard to meals. Administer with food if GI upset occurs.
- Max dosing frequency is once daily.
- Store tablets at controlled room temperature (59° to 86°F).

Assessment/Interventions
- Obtain patient history, including drug history and any known allergies. Note liver disease, kidney disease, left ventricular outflow obstruction, unstable angina, hypotension, uncontrolled hypertension, anatomical deformation of penis (eg, Peyronie disease), conditions predisposing to priapism (eg, sickle cell anemia, multiple myeloma, leukemia), congenital degenerative retinal disorder, heart failure, recent (eg, within 6 mo) history of stroke, life-threatening arrhythmia or MI, and concurrent use of other treatments for erectile dysfunction, nitrates (eg, nitroglycerin), strong CYP3A4 inhibitors (eg, ritonavir, indinavir, ketoconazole, itraconazole, erythromycin), or alpha-blockers (eg, doxazosin).
- Ensure that CV status of patient has been assessed before therapy is started.
- Ensure that a lower starting dose is used in patient over 65 or with hepatic or severe renal impairment (CrCl less than 30 mL/min), or who is concurrently taking a strong CYP3A4 inhibitor.
- Assess patient for CV, CNS, GI, and general body side effects. Inform health care provider if noted and significant.

Patient/Family Education
- Explain name, dose, action, and potential side effects of drug.
- Instruct patient to read the *Patient Information* leaflet before starting therapy and with each refill.
- Advise patient that medication may be most effective if taken approximately 60 min before anticipated sexual activity, but that medication can be taken anywhere from 30 min to 4 hr before sexual activity.
- Advise patient not to take more than 1 dose in a 24-hr period.
- Caution patient who is taking 50 or 100 mg dose of sildenafil and an alpha-blocker to take sildenafil at least 4 hr before or after the alpha-blocker.
- Advise patient to take prescribed dose without regard to meals but to take with food if stomach upset occurs.
- Advise patient that sexual stimulation will be required for medication to work and an erection to occur.
- Instruct patient not to change the dose unless advised by health care provider.
- Advise patient to contact health care provider if not satisfied with sexual performance after taking medication or if bothersome side effects occur.
- Instruct patient to stop using and contact health care provider immediately if any of the following occur: dizziness, fainting, chest pain, vision changes, erection persisting longer than 4 hr, painful erection.
- Caution patient to avoid using "poppers" (eg, amyl nitrate, butyl nitrate) while taking this medication.
- Caution patient that medication is not a male form of birth control nor does it provide protection against sexually transmitted diseases and to use protective measures as indicated.
- Instruct patient not to take any prescription or OTC medications or dietary supplements unless advised by health care provider.
- Advise patient that follow-up visits may be required to monitor therapy and to keep appointments.

Simethicone

(sih-METH-ih-kone)

Class Antiflatulent

How Supplied
Degas Tablets, chewable 80 mg ♦ *Extra Strength Gas-X* Capsules, softgel 125 mg, Tablets, chewable 125 mg ♦ *Flatulex* Drops 40 mg/0.6 mL ♦ *Genasyme* Tablets, chewable 80 mg ♦ *Genasyme Drops* Drops 40 mg/0.6 mL ♦ *Gas-X* Tablets, chewable 80 mg ♦ *Maalox Anti-Gas* Tablets, chewable 80 mg ♦ *Mylanta Gas* Tablets, chewable 40 mg, Tablets, chewable 80 mg ♦ *Maximum Strength Mylanta Gas* Tablets, chewable 125 mg ♦ *Mylicon* Drops 40 mg/0.6 mL ♦ *Phazyme* Drops 40 mg/0.6 mL, Tablets 60 mg ♦ *Phazyme 95* Tablets, chewable 95 mg ♦ *Phazyme 125* Tablets, chewable 125 mg

✤ *Ovol* ♦ *Ovol Drops*

Action
PHARMACOLOGY: Relieves flatulence by dispersing and preventing formation of mucus-surrounded gas pockets in GI tract.

Indications Relief of painful symptoms and pressure of excess gas in digestive tract. Adjunct in treatment of many conditions in which gas retention may be problem, such as postoperative gaseous distention and pain, endoscopic examination, air swallowing, functional dyspepsia, peptic ulcer, spastic or irritable colon, diverticulosis. **Unlabeled use(s):** Treatment of infant colic.

Contraindications Standard considerations.

Route/Dosage

CAPSULES

ADULTS: PO 125 mg qid after meals and at bedtime.

TABLETS

ADULTS: PO 40 to 125 mg qid after meals and at bedtime.

LIQUID (DROPS)

ADULTS: PO 40 to 80 mg qid (up to 500 mg/day).
CHILDREN 2 TO 12 YR: PO 40 mg qid.
CHILDREN LESS THAN 2 YR: PO 20 mg qid (up to 240 mg/day).

Interactions None well documented.

Lab Test Interferences None well documented.

Adverse Reactions None well documented.

Precautions None well documented.

PATIENT CARE CONSIDERATIONS

Administration/Storage
- Tablets: Be certain patient chews tablet thoroughly or allows tablet to dissolve in mouth.
- Liquid: Shake well before using.
- Store tablets/capsules at room temperature in well closed container.
- Store suspension at room temperature in tight, light-resistant container. Do not freeze.

Assessment/Interventions
- Obtain patient history, including drug history and any known allergies.
- Assess baseline bowel sounds and GI status prior to therapy, and continue to monitor bowel sounds throughout therapy.
- Assess for belching and flatus as evidence of drug action.
- Monitor effectiveness of therapy, documenting decreased abdominal distention and discomfort.

Patient/Family Education
- Advise patient to report any worsening of GI symptoms to health care provider.

Simvastatin

(SIM-vuh-STAT-in)

Class Antihyperlipidemic/HMG-CoA reductase inhibitor

How Supplied
Zocor Tablets 5 mg, Tablets 10 mg, Tablets 20 mg, Tablets 40 mg, Tablets 80 mg

Action
PHARMACOLOGY: Increases rate at which body removes cholesterol from blood and reduces production of cholesterol by inhibiting enzyme that catalyzes early rate-limiting step in cholesterol synthesis.

PHARMACOKINETICS/DYNAMICS:
Absorption: Simvastatin T_{max} is 4 hr and 85% of an oral dose is absorbed. Higher drug concentrations appear in the liver than in nontarget tissues.

Distribution: Simvastatin is approximately 95% bound to plasma proteins.

Metabolism: Simvastatin undergoes extensive first-pass metabolism in the liver (approximately 60%), its primary site of action. Higher concentrations are achieved in the liver than in nontarget tissues.

Excretion: Thirteen percent of the drug is excreted in urine; 60% in feces.

Indications Adjunct to diet for reducing elevated total cholesterol and LDL cholesterol levels in patients with primary hypercholesterolemia (types IIa and IIb) when response to diet and other nonpharmacologic measures alone are inadequate; to reduce the risk of stroke or transient ischemic attack. **Unlabeled use(s):** Lower elevated cholesterol levels in patients with heterozygous familial hypercholesterolemia, familial combined hyperlipidemia, diabetic dyslipidemia in noninsulin-dependent diabetic patients, hyperlipidemia secondary to nephrotic syndrome, and homozygous familial hypercholesterolemia in patients who have defective, rather than absent, LDL receptors.

Contraindications Active liver disease or unexplained persistent elevations of liver function values; pregnancy; lactation.

Route/Dosage
ADULTS: PO 5 to 40 mg/day in evening.

Interactions
Azole antifungal agents (eg, ketoconazole), cyclosporine, macrolide antibiotics (eg, erythromycin), gemfibrozil, grapefruit juice, niacin, protease inhibitors (eg, ritonavir), verapamil: Severe myopathy or rhabdomyolysis may occur.
Rifamycins (eg, rifampin): May reduce simvastatin plasma levels, decreasing the pharmacologic effect.

Lab Test Interferences None well documented.

Adverse Reactions
CNS: Headache; asthenia; paresthesia; peripheral neuropathy.
EENT: Dysfunction of certain cranial nerves (including alteration of taste, impairment of extraocular movement, facial paresis); progression of cataracts.
GI: Nausea; vomiting; diarrhea; abdominal pain; constipation; flatulence; dyspepsia; pancreatitis.
HEPA: Hepatitis; jaundice; fatty change in liver; cirrhosis; fulminant hepatic necrosis; hepatoma; increased serum transaminases.
RESP: Upper respiratory tract infection.
OTHER: Myopathy; rhabdomyolysis; fatigue. Apparent hypersensitivity syndrome has been reported rarely that has included 1 or more of the following features: anaphylaxis; angioedema; lupus erythematous-like syndrome; polymyalgia rheumatica; vasculitis; purpura; thrombocytopenia; leukopenia; hemolytic anemia; positive antinuclear antibody; erythrocyte sedimentation rate increase; arthritis; arthralgia; urticaria; asthenia; photosensitivity; fever; chills; flushing; malaise; dyspnea; toxic epidermal necrolysis; erythema multiforme, including Stevens-Johnson syndrome.

Precautions
Pregnancy: Category X. Use a reliable form of birth control.
Lactation: Undetermined.
Children: Use in children not recommended.
Renal function impairment: High doses may result in severe renal insufficiency.
Liver dysfunction: Use drug with caution in patients who consume substantial quantities of alcohol or who have history of liver disease. Marked, persistent increases in serum transaminases have occurred.
Skeletal muscle effects: Rhabdomyolysis with renal dysfunction secondary to myoglobinuria has occurred in this class of drugs. Consider myopathy in any patient with diffuse myalgias, muscle tenderness, or weakness, or marked CPK elevation.

PATIENT CARE CONSIDERATIONS
Administration/Storage
- Adjust dosage as indicated, usually at 4-wk intervals.
- Administer at bedtime for best results. Hepatic cholesterol production is highest during night.
- Store at room temperature.

Assessment/Interventions
- Obtain patient history, including drug history and any known allergies.
- Maintain patient on standard cholesterol diet for at least 3 to 6 mo.
- Determine baseline serum cholesterol and triglyceride levels and monitor at 4- to 6-wk intervals and again at 3 mo.
- Determine baseline LFT values and monitor q 6 wk for first 3 mo, q 8 wk for remainder of first year, then q 6 mo thereafter.
- In patients with renal impairment, monitor for possible severe renal insufficiency.
- Periodic CPK determinations may be necessary.
- Notify the health care provider if cholesterol levels are unchanged or if there is a significant rise in triglyceride levels.

Patient/Family Education
- Caution patient that this medication must not be taken during pregnancy or when pregnancy is possible. Advise patient to use reliable form of birth control while taking this drug.
- Advise patient to control weight and to adhere to prescribed dietary regimen.
- Tell patient to notify health care provider or pharmacist if taking, will be taking, or stopping any prescription or OTC medication.

- Advise patient that exercise and diet that reduces intake of cholesterol and saturated fats are helpful.
- Instruct patient to report the following symptoms to health care provider: any unexplained muscle pain, tenderness, or weakness, especially if accompanied by fever or malaise; yellowing of skin or eyes.
- Tell patient to avoid alcoholic beverages.

Sirolimus

(SER-oh-lih-muss)

Class Immunosuppressive

How Supplied
Rapamune Solution, oral 1 mg/mL, Tablets 2 mg

Action
PHARMACOLOGY: Inhibits T-lymphocyte activation and proliferation that occurs in response to antigenic and cytokine stimulation; inhibits antibody production.

PHARMACOKINETICS/DYNAMICS:

Absorption: Sirolimus t_{max} is 1 hr; absorption is rapid. Bioavailability is 14% (oral solution) and 41% (tablet). To minimize variability, both oral solution and tablets should be taken consistently with or without food.

Distribution: Sirolimus is 97% protein bound (albumin) and Vd is 7.52 L/kg.

Excretion: 91% is recovered from feces; 2.2% is excreted in urine.

Special Populations:
Renal Function Impairment – There is minimal (2.2%) renal excretion of the drug and its metabolites. No dosage adjustments are necessary in renal insufficiency.
Hepatic Function Impairment – Dosage adjustment is recommended for patients with mild to moderate hepatic impairment.

Indications
Prophylaxis of organ rejection in patients receiving renal transplants. **Unlabeled use(s):** Treatment of psoriasis.

Contraindications
Standard considerations.

Route/Dosage
Only physicians experienced in immunosuppressive therapy and management of renal transplant patients should use sirolimus.

ADULTS: **PO** Recommended loading dose of 6 mg with a daily maintenance dose of 2 mg (loading dose 3 times the maintenance dose) in a regimen with cyclosporine and corticosteroids.

ADULTS AND CHILDREN AT LEAST 13 YR WHO WEIGH LESS THAN 40 KG: **PO** Adjust dose to 1 mg/m^2/day based on body surface area. The loading dose should be 3 mg/m^2.

Hepatic Impairment – **PO** Reduce maintenance dose by approximately 33%; do not modify loading dose.

Interactions
Cyclosporine: Sirolimus plasma concentrations may be increased; administer sirolimus 4 hr after cyclosporine.
Cytochrome P450 3A4 inhibitors (eg, erythromycin, protease inhibitors [eg, ritonavir], verapamil): Sirolimus plasma levels may be elevated, increasing the pharmacologic and adverse effects.
Cytochrome P450 3A4 inducers (eg, carbamazepine, phenytoin, St. John's wort): Sirolimus plasma levels may be reduced, decreasing the pharmacologic effects.
Diltiazem, ketoconazole, voriconazole: Sirolimus plasma concentrations may be increased.
Rifampin: Sirolimus plasma concentrations may be decreased.
Vaccination: Response to vaccination may be less effective.

Lab Test Interferences None well documented.

Adverse Reactions
CV: Hypertension (at least 20%); hypotension, atrial fibrillation, CHF, hemorrhage, hypervolemia, palpitation, peripheral vascular disorder, postural hypotension, syncope, tachycardia, thrombophlebitis, thrombosis, vasodilation (less than 20%).
CNS: Headache, insomnia, tremor (at least 20%); insomnia, anxiety, confusion, depression, dizziness, emotional lability, hypertonia, hypesthesia, hypotonia, insomnia, neuropathy, paresthesia, somnolence, tremor (less than 20%).
DERM: Acne, rash (at least 20%); skin ulcer, fungal dermatitis, hirsutism, pruritus, skin hypertrophy, skin ulcer, sweating (less than 20%).
EENT: Pharyngitis (at least 20%); rhinitis, abnormal vision, cataract, conjunctivitis, deafness, ear pain, otitis media, tinnitus (less than 20%).
GI: Constipation, abdominal pain, diarrhea, dyspepsia, nausea, vomiting (at least 20%); anorexia, dysphagia, eructation, esophagitis, flatulence, gastritis, gastroenteritis, gingivitis, gum hyperplasia, ileus, mouth, ulceration, oral moniliasis, stomatitis (less than 20%).

GU: UTI (at least 20%); pyelonephritis, albuminuria, bladder pain, dysuria, hematuria, hydronephrosis, impotence, kidney pain, kidney tubular necrosis, nocturia, oliguria, pyelonephritis, pyuria, scrotal edema, testis disorder, toxic nephropathy, urinary frequency, urinary incontinence, urinary retention, menorrhagia, metrorrhagia (less than 20%).
HEMA: Anemia, leukopenia, thrombocytopenia (at least 20%); thrombotic thrombocytopenic purpura (hemolytic-uremic syndrome), ecchymosis, leukocytosis, lymphadenopathy, polycythemia (less than 20%).
HEPA: Hepatotoxicity (including fatal hepatic necrosis), abnormal LFTs, increased ALT and AST (less than 20%).
LABTESTABS: Increased creatinine, hypercholesterolemia, hyperkalemia, hyperlipidemia, hypokalemia, hypophosphatemia, peripheral edema, weight gain (at least 20%); increased LDH, alkaline phosphatase, BUN and creatine phosphokinase, dehydration, abnormal healing, Cushing syndrome, diabetes mellitus, glycosuria, acidosis, increased alkaline phosphatase, hypercalcemia, hyperglycemia, hyperphosphatemia, hypocalcemia, hypoglycemia, hypomagnesemia, hyponatremia, weight loss (less than 20%).
RESP: Dyspnea, upper respiratory tract infection (at least 20%); bronchitis, pneumonia, asthma, atelectasis, bronchitis, increased cough, epistaxis, hypoxia, lung edema, pleural effusion, pneumonia, sinusitis, interstitial lung disease (less than 20%).
OTHER: Asthenia, back pain, chest pain, fever, pain, arthralgia (at least 20%); herpes simplex, epistaxis, lymphocele, facial edema, arthrosis, bone necrosis, leg cramps, myalgia, osteoporosis, tetany, enlarged abdomen, abscess, ascites, cellulitis, chills, flu syndrome, generalized edema, hernia, herpes zoster infection, pelvic pain, peritonitis, sepsis, malaise, abnormal healing following transplant surgery (less than 20%).

WARNING:
Immunosuppression: Increased susceptibility to infection and possible development of lymphoma may result from immunosuppression.

Liver transplantation-excess mortality, graft loss, and hepatic artery thrombosis (HAT): The use of sirolimus in combination with cyclosporine or tacrolimus was associated with an increase in HAT; most cases of HAT occurred within 30 days post-transplantation and most led to graft loss or death.

Lung transplantation-bronchial anastomotic dehiscence: Cases of bronchial anastomotic dehiscence, most fatal, have been reported in de novo lung transplant patients when sirolimus has been used as part of an immunosuppressive regimen. The safety and efficacy of sirolimus as immunosuppressive therapy have not been established in liver or lung transplant patients, and therefore, such use is not recommended.

Precautions
Pregnancy: Category C.
Lactation: Undetermined.
Children: Safety and efficacy not established in children younger than 13 yr.
Renal function impairment: Decreased renal function may occur; monitor closely.
Antimicrobial prophylaxis: Pneumocystis carinii pneumonia has occurred in patients not receiving antimicrobial prophylaxis. Administration of antimicrobial prophylaxis for 1 yr following transplantation is recommended. Cytomegalovirus prophylaxis for 3 mo after transplantation is recommended.

Interstitial lung disease: Interstitial lung diseases (including pneumonitis, and infrequently bronchiolitis fibrosa obliterans organizing pneumonia and pulmonary fibrosis), some fatal, have occurred in patients receiving immunosuppressive regimens including sirolimus. In some cases, interstitial lung disease resolved upon discontinuation of sirolimus. The risk may be increased as the sirolimus trough level increases.
Lipids: Increased serum cholesterol and triglycerides, requiring treatment, may occur.
Liver transplantation: Sirolimus, in combination with tacrolimus, has been associated with excess mortality and graft loss in de novo liver transplant recipients. Many patients have had evidence of infection at or near the time of death. Sirolimus, in combination with cyclosporine or tacrolimus, has been associated with an increase in hepatic artery thrombosis in de novo liver transplant recipients; most cases occurred within 30 days posttransplantation and often led to graft loss or death.
Lung transplantation: Bronchial anastomotic dehiscence, mostly fatal, has occurred in de novo lung transplant patients when sirolimus was used as part of an immunosuppressive regimen.
Lymphocele: Lymphocele, a surgical complication of renal transplantation, has occurred more often in a dose-related fashion in sirolimus-treated patients.

Overdosage: Signs and Symptoms
Atrial fibrillation.

PATIENT CARE CONSIDERATIONS
Administration/Storage
- Administer prescribed dose qd.
- Administer consistently either with or without food to minimize variability in blood levels and effectiveness.
- Administer 4 hr after cyclosporine solution (modified) or cyclosporine capsules (modified).
- 2 mg tablet is interchangeable with 2 mL oral solution. It is not known if higher doses of solution and tablets are interchangeable.

Oral solution - bottle:
- Check bottle for haze before withdrawing dose. If haze is noted, allow bottle to stand at room temperature (47° to 77°F) and shake gently until haze disappears.
- Use amber oral dosage syringe to withdraw prescribed amount of sirolimus and empty into a glass or plastic container with at least 2 oz of water or orange juice (no other liquids, including grapefruit juice, should be used for dilution). Stir vigorously and instruct patient to drink at once. Refill container with 4 oz of water or orange juice, stir vigorously, and instruct patient to drink at once.
- Amber dosage syringe may be capped and stored at controlled room temperature for up to 24 hr.
- Discard dosage syringe after 1 use.
- Store bottle in refrigerator (36° to 46°F). Protect from light. Once opened the contents should be used within 1 mo. If necessary the bottle can be stored at room temperature for up to 15 days.

Oral solution - pouch:
- Squeeze entire contents of pouch into a glass or plastic container with at least 2 oz of water or orange juice (no other liquids, including grapefruit juice, should be used for dilution). Stir vigorously and have patient drink at once. Refill container with 4 oz of water or orange juice, stir vigorously, and have patient drink at once.
- Store pouches in refrigerator. Protect from light. If necessary pouch can be kept at controlled room temperature for up to 24 hr.

Tablets:
- Store tablets at controlled room temperature (68° to 77°F). Protect from light.

Assessment/Interventions
- Obtain patient history, including drug history and any known allergies. Note history of: concurrent use of medications known to impair renal function (eg, amphotericin B); or concurrent use of medications known to induce (eg, carbamazepine, St. John's wort) or inhibit (eg, fluconazole) CYP3A4.
- Ensure that initial use of sirolimus is in a regimen with cyclosporine and corticosteroids.
- Ensure that whole blood sirolimus trough concentrations are monitored in patients: over 13 yr who weigh less than 40 kg; with hepatic impairment; receiving concentration-controlled sirolimus; receiving potent CYP3A4 inducer or inhibitor or whose cyclosporine is discontinued or the dose is markedly changed.
- Ensure that patient receives antimicrobial prophylaxis for *Pneumocystis carinii* for 1 yr and Cytomegalovirus (CMV) prophylaxis for 3 mo following transplantation.
- Ensure that renal function is periodically assessed in patient receiving sirolimus in combination with cyclosporine. Be prepared to adjust the immunosuppression regimen if elevated or increasing serum creatinine levels are noted.
- Ensure that patient at low to moderate immunologic risk is evaluated for possible gradual reduction of cyclosporine dose. If cyclosporine

is withdrawn, be prepared to increase sirolimus dose to maintain recommended blood concentrations.
- Ensure that reduced dose is administered to patient with mild to moderate hepatic impairment.
- Ensure that patient is monitored for development of hyperlipidemia. Be prepared to treat appropriately if lipid abnormalities are noted.
- Ensure that women of childbearing potential use effective contraception before initiating therapy, during, and for 12 wk following discontinuation of sirolimus.
- Monitor patient for signs and symptoms of infection and immediately report to health care provider if noted.
- Monitor patient for signs and symptoms of anaphylactic or serious allergic reactions. Be prepared to discontinue therapy and treat appropriately.
- Monitor patient for CNS, GI, respiratory, and general body side effects. Report to health care provider if noted and significant.
- Do not administer live virus vaccines while patient is on sirolimus therapy.

Patient/Family Education
- Explain name, dose, action, and potential side effects of drug.
- Advise patient receiving oral solution to review "Patient Instructions" for oral solution administration before using and with each refill.
- Instruct patient to take each dose consistently with or without food to minimize variability in blood levels and effectiveness.
- Advise patient taking cyclosporine solution (modified) or capsules (modified), to take sirolimus 4 hr after taking the cyclosporine.
- Caution patient to avoid ingesting grapefruit and grapefruit juice while taking this medication.
- Instruct patient to continue taking other immunosuppressive and prophylactic medications prescribed by health care provider. Caution patient to not change the dose or stop taking any of their medications unless advised by health care provider.
- Instruct female patient of childbearing potential to use effective contraception before starting therapy, during therapy, and for 12 wk following discontinuation of sirolimus.
- Advise women to notify health care provider if pregnant, planning to become pregnant, or breastfeeding.
- Warn patient to avoid exposure to sun and sun lamps while using this medication because of increased risk of skin cancer. Advise patient to use sunscreens with high protective factor and wear protective clothing when exposure cannot be avoided.
- Advise patient to immediately report any of the following to health care provider: signs or symptoms of transplant rejection (fever, pain over transplant site, rapid weight gain), fever or other signs of infection, sore throat, bothersome side effects.
- Instruct patient not to take any prescription or OTC medications or dietary supplements unless advised by health care provider.
- Remind patient that office visits and laboratory tests will be required to monitor therapy and to keep appointments.

Smallpox Vaccine

(SMAHL-pocks vak-SEEN)

Class Viral vaccine

How Supplied
Dryvax Powder for injection Dried, calf lymph type live-virus preparation of vaccinia virus (polymyxin B sufate, dihydrostreptomycin sulfate, chlortetracycline hydrochloride, and neomycin sulfate are added in trace amounts). The reconstituted vaccine contains approximately 100 million infectious vaccinia viruses/mL.

Action
PHARMACOLOGY: Introduction of infectious vaccinia virus into superficial layers of the skin results in viral multiplication, immunity and cellular hypersensitivity.

Indications Immunization against smallpox disease.

Contraindications Infants younger than 12 mo (nonemergency use in children younger than 18 yr); individuals with eczema or history of eczema or whose household contacts have eczema, other acute, chronic, or exfoliative skin conditions (eg, atopic dermatitis) and siblings or other household contacts of such individuals; individuals and household contacts of individuals receiving systemic corticosteroid therapy at certain doses (eg, at least 2 mg/kg body weight or at least 20 mg/day of prednisone for 2 wk or longer), immunosuppressive drugs (eg, alkylating agents), or radiation; individuals and household contacts of individuals with congenital or acquired deficiencies of immune system, including individuals infected with HIV; individuals with immunosuppression (eg, leukemia) or household contacts of such individuals; during pregnancy, suspected pregnancy, or household contacts of such individuals; hypersensitivity to any component of the product, including polymyxin B sulfate, dihydrostreptomycin sulfate, chlortetracycline hydrochloride, and neomycin sulfate.

Route/Dosage

ADULTS: **SCARIFICATION** Using bifurcated end of needle, deposit drop of vaccine onto clean, dry site previously prepared for vaccination. With same end of needle, and using multiple-puncture technique, vaccinate through drop of vaccine. Holding needle perpendicular to the skin, rapidly make punctures with strokes vigorous enough to allow a trace of blood to appear after 15 to 20 sec. Two or 3 punctures are recommended for primary vaccinations; 15 punctures for revaccinations. Wipe off any remaining vaccine with dry sterile gauze and dispose of gauze in a biohazard waste container.

Interactions None well documented.

Lab Test Interferences None well documented.

Adverse Reactions

CNS: Postvaccinial encephalitis; encephalomyelitis; encephalopathy; progressive vaccinia; eczema vaccinatum; permanent neurological sequelae.
DERM: Generalize rashes; secondary pyogenic infections at the site of vaccination; bullous erythema multiforme (Stevens-Johnson syndrome); inadvertent inoculation at other sites (eg, face, eyelids, genitalia).
EENT: Blindness (from inadvertent infection [autoinoculation] of the eye).
OTHER: Fever; death (from complications [eg, encephalitis]).

Precautions

Pregnancy: Category C.
Lactation: Undetermined.
Children: Not recommended for use in nonemergency situations and contraindicated in children less than 12 mo in nonemergency situations.
Elderly: Not recommended in nonemergency situations.
Latex sensitivity: Vial stopper is dry, natural rubber that may produce hypersensitivity when handled or administered by individuals with latex sensitivity.
Prevention of transmission: Vaccinia virus may be cultured from the site of primary vaccination beginning at the time of development of a papule (2 to 5 days after vaccination) until the scab separates from the skin (14 to 21 days after vaccination). During this time, care must be taken to prevent spread of the virus to another area of the body or to another individual.
Vaccine complications: The CDC can assist physicians diagnose and manage patients with suspected complications of smallpox vaccination.

PATIENT CARE CONSIDERATIONS

Administration/Storage

- For conventional smallpox vaccination (scarification) only. Not for IM, IV, SC, or intradermal administration.
- Follow manufacturer's instructions for reconstituting the powder for injection. Record date of reconstitution.
- Prepare appropriate vaccination site (skin over insertion of deltoid muscle or posterior aspect of arm over triceps) before withdrawing vaccine. If alcohol is used to prepare the site, the skin must be allowed to dry thoroughly to prevent inactivation of the vaccine.
- Carefully remove rubber stopper from reconstituted vial and aseptically retain stopper in inverted position for subsequent use.
- Obtain 1 confirmed drop of vaccine on bifurcated needle and deposit on prepared skin site. Using same needle and using multiple puncture technique, perform 2 to 3 punctures for primary immunization or 15 punctures for revaccination. Remove any remaining vaccine with dry sterile gauze.
- Do not redip the needle into vaccine if needle has touched skin.
- Vaccine site may be left uncovered or can be covered with a porous bandage (eg, gauze).

- If vaccine is to be stored for subsequent use, carefully restop the vial with rubber stopper and place unused vaccine in refrigerator.
- For reuse, gently swirl suspension to ensure resuspension and then carefully remove rubber stopper.
- Always record manufacturer's name and vaccine lot number in patient's permanent medical record file along with date of administration, name, and title of person administering vaccine.
- Dispose of any used equipment (eg, gauze, venting needle, immunization needle) in biohazard waste container. The contents of the biohazard waste container must be burned, boiled, or autoclaved before disposal.
- Store unreconstituted and reconstituted vaccine in refrigerator (36° to 46° F). Do not freeze. Reconstituted vaccine may be used for no more than 15 days after reconstitution. Do not use vaccine after expiration date regardless of whether it is in the dry or reconstituted form.

Assessment/Interventions

- Obtain patient history, including drug history and any known allergies. Note presence of or history of the following: latex sensitivity;

eczema or any acute, chronic, or exfoliative skin lesion in patient or household contacts of patient; immunosuppressant therapy (eg, corticosteroids, immunosuppressive drugs, radiation therapy) or conditions involving immunosuppression (eg, leukemia, organ transplant, bone marrow transplant, immunity disorders) in patient or household contact of patient; immune deficiency (eg, HIV) in patient or household contact of patient; suspected or confirmed pregnancy in patient or household contact of patient.
- Ensure that a plan for handling vaccine complications is in place before initiating vaccination program.
- Wash hands thoroughly after any contact with the vaccine site (eg, changing dressings).
- Apply and change dressings as appropriate. Discard dressing material in biohazard waste container.
- Vaccine site is infectious from the time the papule develops (2 to 5 days after vaccination) until the scab separates from the skin lesion (14 to 21 days after vaccination) during which time care must be taken to prevent spread of the virus to another area of the body or another person.
- Ensure that vaccination site is inspected 6 to 8 days after vaccination to determine whether patient experienced a major reaction (eg, vesicular or pustular lesion or area of definite palpable induration or congestion) or equivocal reaction (any response other than major reaction).
- Repeat vaccination using vaccine from another vial or lot (if possible) in patient who develops equivocal reaction. If this fails to generate a major reaction consult the CDC or state or local health department before giving another vaccination.
- Monitor patient for evidence of autoinoculation of virus from vaccine site to other sites (eg, face, eyelid, nose, mouth, genitalia, rectum), generalized vaccinia (vesicular rash), or evidence of encephalopathy. Inform health care provider immediately if noted.
- Monitor febrile patient's temperature. Acetaminophen or NSAIDs may be administered as ordered to reduce fever. Notify health care provider if temperature exceeds 104°F or if antipyretic measures are ineffective.
- Monitor patient for signs of anaphylaxis or severe allergic reaction. Discontinue therapy and immediately notify health care provider if noted. Be prepared to treat appropriately.
- No information exists regarding safety or efficacy of simultaneous administration of other live-virus vaccines with small pox vaccine.

Defer immunization with other live-virus vaccines if possible.

Patient/Family Education
- Explain name, action, and potential side effects of vaccine.
- Educate patient regarding expected progressive response to initial vaccination: a small, solid elevation (papule) should form 2 to 5 days after vaccination; this should become a blister (vesicle) by day 5 or 6; this progresses and the blister fills with pus, becomes harder and redder between days 3 to 12 during which fever, general body discomfort, and swollen glands may be noted; the pus and redness then go away and a scab (crust) forms over the vaccination site which then come off between days 14 and 21.
- Advise patient that OTC acetaminophen or NSAIDs may be used for fever or general body discomfort but to notify health care provider if symptoms persist or worsen.
- Caution patient that the vaccine site is infectious from the time the papule develops (2 to 5 days after vaccination) until the scab separates from the skin lesion (14 to 21 days after vaccination) during which time care must be taken to prevent spread of the virus to another area of the body or another person.
- Instruct patient to thoroughly wash hands after changing bandages or any other contact with the vaccination site.
- Instruct patient to not apply any salves or ointments to the vaccination site.
- Advise patient that vaccine site may be left uncovered or can be covered with a porous bandage (eg, gauze) until the scab has separated and the underlying skin has healed. Caution patient to not use an occlusive bandage unless it is changed q 1 to 2 days to prevent maceration of the vaccine site.
- Instruct patient to place any contaminated bandages or wraps in a sealed plastic bag before disposal in trash.
- Advise patient that clothing or other cloth materials than have had contact with the vaccine site while it is infectious can be decontaminated with routine laundering in hot water and bleach.
- Advise patient that normal bathing can continue but to keep vaccination site dry at other times.
- Instruct patient to notify health care provider if the following occur: papules are noted on any part of the body other than the vaccination site (autoinoculation); vesicular (blisters) rash develops; or if headache, changes in behavior or alertness, stiff neck, or other unexplained feelings or symptoms occur.

- If patient is a health care worker, avoid contact with patients, particularly those with immunodeficiencies, until the scab has separated from the skin at the vaccination site. If this is not possible, then the vaccination site must be well covered (semipermeable polyurethane dressing over gauze pad) and good hand-washing technique must be maintained.
- Provide patient with immunization history record.

Sodium Bicarbonate

(SO-dee-uhm by-CAR-boe-nate)

Class Urinary tract product/Alkalinizer/Electrolyte/Antacid

How Supplied
Bell/ans Tablets 520 mg ♦ *Neut* Neutralizing additive solution 4% (0.48 mEq/mL) ♦ *Sodium Bicarbonate* Injection 4.2% (0.5 mEq/mL), Injection 5% (0.6 mEq/mL), Injection 7.5% (0.9 mEq/mL), Injection 8.4% (1 mEq/mL), Neutralizing additive solution 4.2% (0.5 mEq/mL), Powder 120 g, Tablets 325 mg, Tablets 650 mg

Action
PHARMACOLOGY: Increases plasma bicarbonate; buffers excess hydrogen ion concentrations; raises blood pH; reverses metabolic acidosis.

Indications
Treatment of metabolic acidosis; promotion of gastric, systemic, and urinary alkalinization; replacement therapy in severe diarrhea; used to reduce incidence of chemical phlebitis (used as neutralizing additive solution).

Contraindications
Loss of chloride from vomiting or continuous GI suction when patient is receiving diuretics known to produce hypochloremic alkalosis; metabolic and respiratory alkalosis; hypocalcemia in which alkalosis may produce tetany, hypertension, convulsions, or CHF; when administration of sodium could be clinically detrimental.

Route/Dosage
ADULTS AND CHILDREN GREATER THAN 2 YR: IV Administration performed in concentrations ranging from 1.5% (isotonic) to 8.4% depending on clinical condition and requirements of patient.
SC After dilution to isotonicity (1.5%). The dose depends on the clinical condition and requirements of the patient (including age and weight).
PO 325 mg to 2 g 1 to 4 times daily (patients less than 60 yr, max dose 16 g/day; patients greater than 60 yr max dose 8 g/day).

INFANTS UP TO 2 YR: IV 4.2% solution at rate up to 8 mEq/kg/day.

Interactions
Amphetamine, dextroamphetamine, ephedrine, flecainide, mecamylamine, methamphetamine, pseudoephedrine, quinidine: Sodium bicarbonate can decrease elimination of these drugs, thus increasing their therapeutic effects.
Chlorpropamide, lithium, methotrexate, salicylates, tetracyclines: Sodium bicarbonate can increase elimination of these drugs, thus decreasing their therapeutic effect.
Ketoconazole: PO sodium bicarbonate may decrease the dissolution of ketoconazole in the GI tract, reducing the effectiveness.
INCOMPATIBILITIES: Do not mix with IV solutions containing catecholamines, such as dobutamine, dopamine, and norepinephrine.

Lab Test Interferences
None well documented.

Adverse Reactions
CV: Exacerbation of CHF.
GI: Rebound hyperacidity; milk-alkali syndrome.
LAB TESTS ABS: Hypernatremia; alkalosis.
OTHER: Extravasation with cellulitis, tissue necrosis, ulceration, and sloughing; local pain; venous irritation; tetany; edema.

Precautions
Pregnancy: Category C.
Lactation: Undetermined.
Children:
Newborns and children younger than 2 yr – Administration of at least 10 mL/min of hypertonic sodium bicarbonate may produce hypernatremia, decreased CSF pressure, and possible intracranial hemorrhage.
Special risk patients: Use drug with caution in edematous sodium-retaining states, CHF, liver cirrhosis, toxemia of pregnancy, or renal impairment.
Sodium content: May be significant, especially in patients with hypertension or CHF or in patients on low-sodium diets.

Overdosage: Signs and Symptoms
Alkalosis, hyperirritability, tetany, nausea, vomiting.

PATIENT CARE CONSIDERATIONS
Administration/Storage
- For IV solution preparation, use Sterile Water for Injection, Sodium Chloride Injection, 5% Dextrose, or other standard electrolyte solutions as diluent.
- With chewable tablets, instruct patient to

chew thoroughly before swallowing and then to drink a glass of water.
- Do not administer other oral drugs within 1 to 2 hr of oral sodium bicarbonate (antacid) administration.

Assessment/Interventions
- Obtain patient history, including drug history and any known allergies.
- Evaluate pH and electrolytes with preadministration values. If there is evidence of alkalosis, notify health care provider.
- Assess baseline BP and respiratory rate and rhythm.
- Assess serum pH, PaO_2, $PaCO_2$, and serum electrolytes frequently during therapy. Inform health care provider of results.
- Test urine to determine pH.
- If patient has edematous tendency, notify health care provider.
- If patient exhibits shortness of breath and hyperpnea, notify health care provider.
- If patient is vomiting, withhold medication and notify health care provider.
- Notify health care provider if relief is not obtained or if patient demonstrates any symptoms that suggest bleeding such as black tarry stools or coffee ground emesis.

Patient/Family Education
- Instruct patient not to take medication with milk because renal calculi can develop.
- Explain need to avoid OTC medications containing sodium bicarbonate, such as *Alka-Seltzer*. Excessive use of sodium bicarbonate can result in increase acid secretion or systemic alkalosis.
- Instruct patient not to use maximum dose of antacids for more than 2 wk except under supervision of health care provider.
- Advise patient not to take sodium bicarbonate on routine or long-term basis. Tell patient to notify health care provider if symptoms of gastric distress continue.
- Caution patient to report these symptoms to health care provider immediately: nausea, vomiting, anorexia.

Sodium Citrate/Citric Acid

(SO-dee-uhm SIH-trate/SIH-trik ASS-id)
Class Systemic alkalinizer/Urinary alkalinizer

How Supplied
Bicitra Solution 500 mg sodium citrate/334 mg citric acid per 5 mL (1 mEq sodium equiv. to 1 mEq bicarbonate/mL) • *Oracit* Solution 490 mg sodium citrate/640 mg citric acid per 5 mL (1 mEq sodium equiv. to 1 mEq bicarbonate/mL)

Action
PHARMACOLOGY: Sodium citrate is metabolized to sodium bicarbonate, thus acting as a systemic alkalizer.

Indications Long-term maintenance of an alkaline urine; alleviation of chronic metabolic acidosis; buffering and neutralizing gastric hydrochloric acid.

Contraindications Patients on sodium-restricted diets; impaired renal function with oliguria, azotemia, or anuria; untreated Addison disease; adynamia episodica hereditaria; acute dehydration; heat cramps; severe myocardial damage; hyperkalemia.

Route/Dosage
Systemic Alkalization
ADULTS: **PO** 2 to 6 tsp (10 to 30 mL), diluted in 1 to 3 oz of water, after meals and at bedtime, or as directed by health care provider.
CHILDREN 2 YR AND OLDER: **PO** 1 to 3 tsp (5 to 15 mL), diluted in 1 to 3 oz of water, after meals and at bedtime, or as directed by health care provider.
Neutralizing Buffer
ADULTS: **PO** 3 tsp (15 mL), diluted in 15 mL of water, taken as a single dose, or as directed by health care provider.

Interactions
Sodium citrate:
Anorexiants, flecainide, mecamylamine, quinidine, sympathomimetics – Urinary alkalinizers may decrease the excretion and increase the serum levels of these agents, possibly increasing their pharmacologic effects.
Chlorpropamide, lithium, methenamine, methotrexate, salicylates, tetracyclines – Urinary alkalinizers may increase the excretion and decrease the serum levels of these agents, possibly decreasing their pharmacologic effects.

Lab Test Interferences None well documented.

Adverse Reactions Generally well tolerated when taken in recommended doses by patients with normal renal function and urinary output.
METAB: Hypernatremia; metabolic alkalosis.
GI: Diarrhea; loose bowel movements.

Precautions
Pregnancy: Category C.
Lactation: Undetermined.
Renal function impairment: Because alkalosis can occur, especially in the presence of hypocalcemia, use with caution.
Special risk patients: Sodium salts should be used with caution in patients with cardiac failure, hypertension, impaired renal function, periph-

eral and pulmonary edema, and toxemia of pregnancy.

GI effects: Dilute with water to minimize GI disturbance. Take after meals to avoid saline laxative effect.

Urolithiasis: Citrate mobilizes calcium from bones and increases its renal excretion; this, along with the elevated urine pH, may predispose to urolithiasis.

Overdosage: Signs and Symptoms
Diarrhea, nausea, vomiting, hypernoia (excessive mental activity), convulsions.

PATIENT CARE CONSIDERATIONS

Administration/Storage
- Refrigerate solution prior to administration to enhance palatability.
- Dilute each dose with 1 to 3 oz of water and administer after meals to reduce saline laxative effect.
- Additional water may be given after the dose if desired by the patient.
- Store syrup at controlled room temperature (59° to 86°F). Keep tightly capped and protect from freezing or excessive heat.

Assessment/Interventions
- Obtain patient history, including drug history and any known allergies. Note history of sodium-restricted diet, renal impairment, low urine output, heart failure, hypertension, edema states, toxemia of pregnancy, or coadministration of aluminum-based antacids.
- Ensure that serum electrolytes and acid-base states are determined before and periodically throughout therapy.
- Notify health care provider if any of the following occur: edema, decreased urine output, persistent diarrhea.

Patient/Family Education
- Explain name, dose, action, and potential side effects of drug.
- Advise patient to take as prescribed and not to change the dose or stop taking unless advised by health care provider.
- Advise patient to dilute each dose with 1 to 3 oz of cold water and take after meals if possible to prevent laxative effect. Additional water may follow the dose if desired.
- Advise patient that if a dose is missed, to take as soon as remembered unless it is nearing time for the next dose. Caution patient against doubling the dose to catch up.
- Advise patient to inform health care provider if any of the following occur: edema, nausea, stomach pain, vomiting, decreased urine production, persistent diarrhea, or any other bothersome side effects.
- Advise women to notify health care provider if pregnant, planning to become pregnant, or breastfeeding.
- Caution patient not to take any prescription or OTC medications or dietary supplements unless advised by health care provider.
- Advise patient that follow-up visits and lab tests will be required to monitor therapy and to keep appointments.
- Advise patient to avoid salty foods and use of extra table salt.

Sodium Ferric Gluconate

(SO-dee-uhm FER-ick GLUE-koe-nate)

Class Trace elements

How Supplied
Ferrlecit Injection 62.5 mg/5 mL (12.5 mg/mL) of elemental iron

Action
PHARMACOLOGY: Provides iron to replenish hemoglobin and depleted iron stores.

Indications Treatment of iron deficiency anemia in patients undergoing chronic hemodialysis and supplemental erythropoietin.

Contraindications All anemias not associated with iron deficiency; evidence of iron overload; hypersensitivity to any component of the product.

Route/Dosage
Dosage is expressed as mg of elemental iron.

ADULTS: **IV Iron Replacement Dose** 10 mL (125 mg iron) diluted in 100 mL of 0.9% sodium chloride. Infuse over 1 hr. Most patients require a minimum cumulative dose of 1 g over 8 sessions at sequential dialysis treatments.

Interactions None well documented.
INCOMPATIBILITIES: Do not mix with other medications or add to parenteral nutrition solutions.

Lab Test Interferences None well documented.

Adverse Reactions
CV: Hypotension (29%); hypertension (13%); syncope (6%); tachycardia (5%); bradycardia; vasodilatation; angina pectoris; MI; pulmonary edema.
CNS: Dizziness (13%); fatigue, paresthesia (6%); agitation; somnolence; malaise; nervousness (postmarketing).
DERM: Pruritus (6%); rash; increased sweating.

EENT: Conjunctivitis; abnormal vision; ear disorder.
GI: Nausea, vomiting, diarrhea (35%); anorexia; dyspepsia; eructation; flatulence; GI disorder; melena; rectal disorder; dry mouth (postmarketing).
GU: UTI.
HEMA: Abnormal erythrocytes (11%); sepsis; anemia; leukocytosis; lymphadenopathy; hemorrhage (postmarketing).
LOCAL: Injection site reactions (33%).
M/N: Hyperkalemia (6%); generalized edema (5%); leg edema; peripheral edema; hypoglycemia; edema; hypervolemia; hypokalemia.
MUSC: Leg cramps (10%); myalgia; arthralgia.
OTHER: Cramps (25%); chest pain, pain (10%); fever (5%); infection; abscess; back pain; chills; rigors; arm pain; flu-like syndrome; hypersensitivity; hypertonia (postmarketing).

Precautions
Pregnancy: Category B.

Lactation: Undetermined.
Children: Safety and efficacy are not established.
Elderly: Dose cautiously, starting at low end of range.
Hypersensitivity: Rare cases of serious hypersensitivity reported.
Flushing and hypotension reactions: Associated with too rapid administration. Do not exceed 125 mg/hr (2.1 mg/min).
Hypotension: Hypotension associated with lightheadedness, malaise, fatigue, weakness or severe chest, back, flank, or groin pain reported. This reaction has not been associated with hypersensitivity and usually resolves within 1 to 2 hr.

Overdosage: Signs and Symptoms
Accumulation of iron in iron storage sites, abdominal pain, diarrhea, vomiting, pallor, cyanosis, lassitude, drowsiness, hyperventilation (caused by acidosis), CV collapse.

PATIENT CARE CONSIDERATIONS
Administration/Storage
- Discontinue oral iron preparations before administering parenteral iron products.
- For IV administration only. Not for intradermal, SC, or IM.
- Administer prescribed dose directly into dialysis line or peripheral IV access either by slow injection or by infusion.
- For slow IV injection, administer undiluted solution at rate no greater than 1 mL/min (max, 10 mL [2 vials]).
- For IV infusion, dilute contents of 2 vials in 100 mL 0.9% NaCl immediately prior to infusion and infuse over 1 hr. Discard any unused diluted solution.
- Do not mix with other IV medications or add to parenteral nutrition solutions
- Do not administer if particulate matter or discoloration noted.
- Store vials at controlled room temperature (59° to 86°F). Protect from freezing.

Assessment/Interventions
- Obtain patient history, including drug history and any known allergies.
- Review patient's health history for any condition that could contraindicate sodium ferric gluconate such as evidence of iron overload or anemia not caused by iron deficiency.
- Ensure that patient is also receiving erythropoietin therapy.

- Ensure that hemoglobin, hematocrit, serum ferritin, and transferrin saturation are determined before and periodically during treatment.
- Monitor BP during infusion. If hypotension occurs, slow infusion rate. If hypotension continues, discontinue infusion and be prepared to treat appropriately.
- Monitor patient for signs and symptoms of anaphylactic or serious allergic reactions during and shortly after infusion. Be prepared to discontinue therapy and treat appropriately.
- Monitor patient for CNS, CV, respiratory, GI, and general body side effects, and injection site reactions. Report to health care provider if noted and significant.

Patient/Family Education
- Explain name, dose, action, and potential side effects of drug.
- Advise patient that medication will be prepared and administered by health care provider during dialysis sessions and that medication will not be administered at home.
- Instruct patient to inform health care provider if any of the following occur during the administration of drug: anxiety, sweating, rapid heart beat, shortness of breath or difficulty breathing, swelling of the throat, rash, itching.
- Advise patient that follow-up visits and laboratory tests will be required to monitor therapy and to keep appointments.

Sodium Iodide I 131

(So-dee-uhm EYE-uh-dide I 131)

Class Radiopharmaceuticals

How Supplied
Iodotope Capsules 1 to 50 mCi, Oral Solution 7.05 mCi ♦ *Sodium Iodide I 131* Capsules 0.75 to 100 mCi, Oral Solution 3.5 to 150 mCi

Action
PHARMACOLOGY: After rapid GI absorption, iodine 131 is primarily distributed within extracellular fluid. It is trapped and rapidly converted to protein-bound iodine by the thyroid; it is concentrated, but not protein bound, by the stomach and salivary glands. It is promptly excreted by kidneys. About 90% of the local irradiation is caused by beta radiation and 10% is caused by gamma radiation. Iodine 131 has a physical half-life of 8.04 days.

Indications Thyroid carcinoma, hyperthyroidism.

Contraindications Preexisting vomiting and diarrhea; women who are or may become pregnant.

Route/Dosage
Thyroid Carcinoma, Hyperthyroidism
ADULTS: PO Individualize dosage. *Usual dose for ablation of normal thyroid tissue:* 50 mCi, with subsequent therapeutic doses usually 100 to 150 mCi.

Interactions
Iodine, thyroid, and antithyroid agents: Uptake of iodine 131 will be affected by recent intake of stable iodine in any form, or by use of thyroid, antithyroid, and certain other drugs.

Lab Test Interferences None well documented.

Adverse Reactions
ENDO: Acute thyroid crises.
HEMA: Depression of hematopoietic system with large doses; bone marrow depression; acute leukemia; anemia; blood dyscrasia; leukopenia; thrombocytopenia; death.
OTHER: Radiation sickness; severe sialoadenitis; increased clinical symptoms; chest pain; tachycardia; rash; hives; chromosomal abnormalities; tenderness and swelling of neck; pain on swallowing; sore throat and cough may occur around third day after treatment; temporary hair thinning (may occur 2 to 3 mo after treatment).

Precautions
Pregnancy: Category X.
Lactation: Discontinue nursing during therapy. Do not resume nursing until all radiation is absent from breast milk (approximately 14 days).
Children: Safety and efficacy have not been established.
Sulfite sensitivity: Contains sulfites that may cause allergic-type reactions, including anaphylactic symptoms.
Radiation exposure: Ensure minimum radiation exposure to patients and occupational workers consistent with proper patient management.

Overdosage: Signs and Symptoms
Hypothyroidism.

PATIENT CARE CONSIDERATIONS

Administration/Storage
- Dose will be prepared by a person authorized by the Nuclear Regulatory Commission and will be delivered ready to administer.
- Store in transport container until time of administration.
- Administer prescribed dose via equipment supplied (eg, glass straw) and then return equipment to transport container for disposal.

Assessment/Interventions
- Obtain patient history, including drug history and any known allergies. Note history of thyroid medications, antithyroid medications, or recent procedures involving radiographic contrast material.
- Ensure that patient is not vomiting or has diarrhea before administering dose.
- Ensure that women of childbearing potential are not pregnant at time of administration.

Patient/Family Education
- Explain name, action, and potential side effects of drug.
- Advise patient that medication will be prepared and administered by health care provider in a health care setting.
- Advise patient, family, or caregiver that medication is usually administered 1 time only.
- Advise patient, family, or caregiver to report any of the following to the health care provider: persistent or worsening tenderness or swelling of the neck; pain on swallowing; sore throat; cough; persistent nausea or vomiting; worsening symptoms of hyperthyroidism; any other unexplained sensation.
- Instruct patient not to take any prescription or OTC medications or dietary supplements unless advised to do so by health care provider.
- Instruct women of childbearing potential to notify health care provider if pregnant, planning to become pregnant, or breastfeeding.
- Advise patient that frequent follow-up visits and laboratory tests will be required to monitor therapy and to keep appointments.

Sodium Phosphate P 32

(SO-dee-uhm FOSS-fate P 32)

Class Radiopharmaceuticals

How Supplied
Sodium Phosphate P 32 Injection 0.67 mCi/mL

Action
PHARMACOLOGY: Phosphorus is necessary to the metabolic and proliferative activity of cells. Radioactive phosphorus concentrates to a very high degree in rapidly proliferating tissue. Sodium phosphate P 32 decays by beta emission with a physical half-life of 14.3 days. The mean energy of the sodium phosphate P 32 beta particle is 695 keV.

Indications Treatment of polycythemia vera, chronic myelocytic leukemia, and chronic lymphocytic leukemia; skeletal metastases.

Contraindications Do not use as part of sequential treatment with a chemotherapeutic agent. Do not administer when the leukocyte count is less than 5000/mm^3 or platelet count is less than 150,000/mm^3. Do not administer when the leukocyte count is less than 20,000/mm^3. Usually not administered when the leukocyte count is less than 5000/mm^3 and the platelet count is less than 100,000/mm^3.

Route/Dosage
Administer IV. Do not administer as an intracavity injection. Oral administration of high-specific-activity sodium phosphate P 32 in the fasting state may equal IV administration.

Polycythemia Vera
ADULTS: **IV** 1 to 8 mCi. Individualize. Repeat doses depending upon stage of disease and size of patient.

Chronic Leukemia
ADULTS: **IV** 6 to 15 mCi usually with concomitant hormone manipulation.

Interactions None well documented.

Lab Test Interferences None well documented.

Adverse Reactions None well documented.

Precautions
Pregnancy: Category C.
Lactation: Discontinue nursing during therapy.
Children: Safety and efficacy have not been established.
Retinoblastomas: Sodium phosphate P 32 does not usually localize in retinoblastomas.
Radiation exposure: Ensure minimum radiation exposure to patients and occupational workers consistent with proper patient management.

Overdosage: Signs and Symptoms
May produce serious effects on the hematopoietic system.

PATIENT CARE CONSIDERATIONS

Administration/Storage
- Dose will be prepared by a person authorized by the Nuclear Regulatory Commission and will be delivered ready to administer.
- Store in transport container until time of administration.
- Following administration return all equipment to transport container for disposal.

Assessment/Interventions
- Obtain patient history, including drug history and any known allergies.
- Ensure that CBC and differential are determined at baseline, prior to each course, and as indicated during therapy.
- Withhold dose in polycythemia vera patient if leukocyte count is less than 5000/mm^3 or if platelet count is less than 150,000/mm^3.
- Withhold dose in chronic myelocytic leukemia patient if leukocyte count is less than 20,000/mm^3.
- Withhold dose in patient with bone metastases if leukocyte count is less than 5000/mm^3 or if platelet count is less than 100,000/mm^3.
- Implement infection control measures if WBC drops; implement bleeding precautions if platelet count drops.

Patient/Family Education
- Explain name, action, and potential side effects of drug.
- Advise patient, family, or caregiver that medication will be prepared and administered by health care provider in a health care setting.
- Advise patient, family, or caregiver that medication may be repeated depending on response to therapy and size of the patient. It is usually administered 1 time only.
- Advise patient to immediately report any of the following to the health care provider: fever, chills, or other signs of infection; unusual bruising or bleeding.
- Instruct patient not to take any prescription or OTC medications or dietary supplements unless advised to do so by the health care provider.
- Instruct women of childbearing potential to notify health care provider if pregnant, planning to become pregnant, or breastfeeding.
- Advise patient that frequent follow-up visits and laboratory tests will be required to monitor therapy and to keep appointments.

Sodium Polystyrene Sulfonate

(SO-dee-uhm pah-lee-STYE-reen SULL-fuh-nate)

Class Potassium-removing resin

How Supplied
Kayexalate Powder Finely powdered sodium polystyrene sulfonate. Sodium content approximately 100 mg (4.1 mEq)/g ♦ *SPS* Suspension 15 g/60 mL. Sodium content 1.5 g (65 mEq) ♣ *Sodium Polystyrene Sulfonate*

Action
PHARMACOLOGY: Resin that exchanges sodium ions for potassium in large intestine.

PHARMACOKINETICS/DYNAMICS:
Absorption: Sodium polystyrene sulfonate is not absorbed from the GI tract.
Onset: Onset of action is hours to days.

Indications
Treatment of hyperkalemia.

Contraindications
Hypokalemia.

Route/Dosage
ADULTS: **PO** or via **NG tube** 15 g 1 to 4 times/day. **PR** 30 to 50 g q 6 hr has been given as daily enema.
CHILDREN: **PO** Calculate children's dose by exchange ratio of 1 mEq potassium per gram of resin. (1 g/kg q 6 hr has been recommended.)

Interactions
Digitalis: If hypokalemia occurs, likelihood of toxic effects of digoxin may be increased.
Nonabsorbable cation donating antacids and laxatives (eg, aluminum carbonate, magnesium hydroxide): Systemic alkalosis has occurred. Potassium exchange capability of sodium polystyrene sulfonate may be reduced. Intestinal obstruction due to concretions of aluminum hydroxide when used in combination has occurred.

Lab Test Interferences
None well documented.

Adverse Reactions
GI: Gastric irritation; anorexia; nausea; vomiting; constipation; fecal impaction.
METAB: Hypokalemia; hypocalcemia; sodium retention.

Precautions
Pregnancy: Category C.
Lactation: Undetermined.
Electrolyte abnormalities: Serious potassium deficiency can occur. Sodium polystyrene sulfonate is not totally selective for potassium and small amounts of magnesium and calcium can be lost. Use with caution in patients who cannot tolerate even small increase in sodium load (ie, severe CHF, severe hypertension, marked edema).
Severe hyperkalemia: Treatment with this drug alone may be insufficient to rapidly correct severe hyperkalemia associated with states of rapid tissue breakdown (eg, burns, renal failure) or hyperkalemia so marked as to constitute medical emergency.

Overdosage: Signs and Symptoms
Nausea, vomiting, constipation (fecal impaction), hypokalemia, hypocalcemia, sodium retention.

PATIENT CARE CONSIDERATIONS

Administration/Storage
Oral powder:
- Shake bottle well before administration. Give each dose as suspension in water or, for greater palatability, in syrup. Use sorbitol to combat constipation. Oral suspensions contain sorbitol and sodium. Resin may be introduced into stomach through plastic tube; if desired, mixed with appropriate diet. Never mix with orange juice because of high potassium content.

Retention enema:
- After initial cleansing enema, insert soft, large (28°F) rubber tube into the rectum about 20 cm, with tip well into sigmoid colon, and tape in place. Elevate hips to prevent leakage. After administration, flush suspension with 50 to 100 mL of fluid, clamp tube, and leave in place. Keep suspension in sigmoid colon for several hours. Then irrigate colon with approximately 2 L of non-sodium-containing solution. Drain return through Y-tube connection.

- Store at room temperature. Store repackaged product in refrigerator and use within 14 days. Do not store freshly prepared suspensions longer than 24 hr. Do not heat, because this may alter exchange of properties of resin.

Assessment/Interventions
- Obtain patient history, including drug history and any known allergies.
- Assess GI function. Use caution in elderly because of predisposition to fecal impaction.
- Assess electrolyte levels including sodium, potassium, calcium, and magnesium.
- Use caution with patients who have tendencies toward hypernatremia or hypertension or who are receiving digitalis preparations.
- Assess vital signs each shift.
- Monitor serum potassium and sodium daily and observe for signs and symptoms of hypo-

kalemia, including irritability, confusion, cardiac arrhythmias, ECG changes, and muscle weakness.
- Observe for signs of sodium overload, such as edema.
- Closely monitor patients on sodium restriction.
- Monitor serum calcium levels. If deficient, patient may require supplements.
- Observe for changes in bowel function. Report to health care provider if patient becomes constipated.

Sodium Sulfacetamide/Sulfur

(SO-dee-uhm sul-fah-SEE-tah-mide/SULL-fer)

Class Antibacterial/Sulfonamide/Keratolytic agent

How Supplied
Avar Cleanser 10% sodium sulfacetamide and 5% sulfur, Gel 10% sodium sulfacetamide and 5% sulfur ◆ *Clenia* Cream 10% sodium sulfacetamide and 5% sulfur, Foam 10% sodium sulfacetamide and 5% sulfur ◆ *Rosula* Gel 10% sodium sulfacetamide and 5% sulfur ◆ *Sulfacet-R* Lotion 10% sodium sulfacetamide and 5% sulfur ◆ *Zetacet* Topical suspension 10% sodium sulfacetamide and 5% sulfur

Action
PHARMACOLOGY:
Sulfacetamide: Competitively antagonizes PABA, an essential component of folic acid synthesis.
Sulfur: Inhibits the growth of *Propionibacterium acnes* and the formation of free fatty acids.

Indications Topical control of acne vulgaris, acne rosacea, and seborrheic dermatitis.

Contraindications Kidney disease; known hypersensitivity to sulfonamides, sulfur, or any component of the product.

PATIENT CARE CONSIDERATIONS
Administration/Storage
- For topical use only. Not for ophthalmic or otic use.
- Shake well before use.
- Apply a thin film to affected area(s) qd to tid as ordered. Use gloves or applicator as applicable.
- Do not apply near the eyes.
- Store at controlled room temperature (59° to 86°F). Keep bottle tightly closed.

Assessment/Interventions
- Obtain patient history, including drug history and any known allergies. Note history of kidney disease or sulfite-sensitivity.
- Monitor patient's response to therapy. Notify health care provider if skin inflammation, irritation, or sensitization are noted or if symptoms do not improve or worsen.

Patient/Family Education
- Explain name, action, and potential side effects of medication.
- Review prescribed dosing schedule with patient or caregiver.
- Remind patient or caregiver that product is not to be used in the eye or ear.
- Teach patient or caregiver proper technique

Patient/Family Education
- Tell patient not to mix medication with fruit juice.
- Instruct patient to shake bottle well before taking medication.
- Advise patient to report any water retention or edema.
- Instruct patient to report these symptoms to health care provider: anorexia, nausea, vomiting, any changes in bowel function.
- Tell patient not to take OTC medications without consulting health care provider.

Route/Dosage
ADULTS AND CHILDREN 12 YR AND OLDER:
Topical Apply a thin film to affected areas qd to tid with light massaging to blend in each application.

Interactions None well documented.
Lab Test Interferences None well documented.

Adverse Reactions
DERM: Local irritation; dryness; erythema; itching.
OTHER: Allergic hypersensitivity.

Precautions
Pregnancy: Category C.
Lactation: Undetermined; however, small amounts of orally administered sulfonamides are secreted in breast milk.
Children: Safety and efficacy not determined in children under 12 yr.
Irritation: If irritation develops, discontinue use and institute appropriate therapy.
Sensitivity: May occur; use caution and careful supervision when prescribing this drug for patients who may be prone to hypersensitivity to topical sulfonamides.
Sodium metabisulfite: May contain sodium metabisulfite, which can cause allergic-type reactions, including anaphylactic symptoms and life-threatening or less severe asthmatic episodes in susceptible individuals.

for applying product: wash hands; shake lotion and suspension well, then apply thin film to affected area(s) using fingers. Wash hands after applying product.
- Advise patient or caregiver to contact health care provider if local redness or swelling develops or if skin lesions do not improve or worsen.

Somatrem

(so-muh-TREM)

Class Growth hormone

How Supplied
Protropin Powder for injection, lyophilized 5 mg (approximately 13 IU)/vial, Powder for injection, lyophilized 10 mg (approximately 26 IU)/vial

Action
PHARMACOLOGY: Mimics actions of naturally occurring growth hormone to stimulate linear and skeletal growth; increases number and size of muscle cells; increases RBC mass and internal organ size; increases cellular protein synthesis; reduces body fat stores and lipid mobilization; increases plasma fatty acids.

PHARMACOKINETICS/DYNAMICS:

Absorption: Somatrem's extent of absorption is approximately 590 ng•hr/mL.

Indications Long-term treatment of children with growth failure caused by lack of adequate endogenous growth hormone secretion.

Contraindications Benzyl alcohol sensitivity; closed epiphyses; evidence of tumor activity; intracranial lesions must be inactive and antitumor therapy complete prior to instituting therapy.

PATIENT CARE CONSIDERATIONS

Administration/Storage
- Reconstitute with Bacteriostatic Water for Injection, USP (benzyl alcohol preserved) only. Roll or swirl gently; do not shake.
- Use syringe small enough to permit accurate measurement of drug. Needle should be at least 1 inch to ensure ability to reach muscle layer.
- Reconstitute with Water for Injection when administering to newborns. Use only 1 dose per vial. Discard unused portion.
- Rotate injection sites.
- Do not use if solution is cloudy.
- Store before and after reconstitution in the refrigerator. Store reconstituted drug in refrigerator for up to 14 days. Avoid freezing.

- Advise women to notify health care provider if pregnant, planning to become pregnant, or breastfeeding.
- Remind patient or caregiver that follow-up examinations may be necessary while using this medication and to keep appointments.

Route/Dosage
CHILDREN: **SC/IM** Up to 0.1 mg/kg 3 times/wk.

Interactions
Glucocorticoids: May inhibit growth-promoting effects of somatrem.

Lab Test Interferences None well documented.

Adverse Reactions
OTHER: Persistent antibodies to growth hormone.

Precautions
Pregnancy: Category C.
Lactation: Undetermined.
Hypothyroidism: May develop during therapy.
Insulin resistance: May be induced with therapy.
Intracranial hypertension: Intracranial hypertension with papilledema, visual changes, headache, nausea, or vomiting has been reported in a few patients.
Intracranial lesion: Frequently examine patient with history of intracranial lesion for progression or recurrence of lesion.
Slipped capital epiphysis: Slipped capital epiphysis may occur more frequently in patients treated with growth hormone.

Overdosage: Signs and Symptoms
Hypoglycemia, hyperglycemia, acromegaly.

Assessment/Interventions
- Obtain patient history, including drug history and any known allergies. Determine if epiphyses are closed and if intracranial lesions and tumor activity are present.
- Examine patients with intracranial lesions frequently to make sure that the lesions are not active.
- Check thyroid function periodically to detect possible hypothyroidism.
- Monitor for signs of acromegaly and report to health care provider.
- Monitor for glucose intolerance; insulin resistance may develop.
- Monitor patient's growth.

- Observe for common side effects of headache, weakness, localized muscle pain, or mild transient edema and report to health care provider.
- Notify health care provider of any limp or complaints of hip or knee pain in children; these symptoms indicate slipped capital femoral epiphyses.

Patient/Family Education
- Instruct diabetic patient to monitor blood sugars closely and to report variations to health care provider.
- Teach children and parents to report any limp or complaints of hip or knee pain to health care provider as soon as possible.
- Instruct patient to report the following symptoms to health care provider: headache, weakness, localized muscle pain, or mild transient edema.

Somatropin

(SO-muh-TROE-pin)
Class Growth hormone

How Supplied
Genotropin Powder for injection, lyophilized 1.5 mg (approximately 4.5 IU)/vial, Powder for injection, lyophilized 5.8 mg (approximately 17.4 IU)/vial, Powder for injection, lyophilized 13.8 mg (approximately 41.4 IU)/vial ♦ *Genotropin Miniquick* Powder for injection, lyophilized 0.2 mg/vial, Powder for injection, lyophilized 0.4 mg/vial, Powder for injection, lyophilized 0.6 mg/vial, Powder for injection, lyophilized 0.8 mg/vial, Powder for injection, lyophilized 1 mg/vial, Powder for injection, lyophilized 1.2 mg/vial, Powder for injection, lyophilized 1.4 mg/vial, Powder for injection, lyophilized 1.6 mg/vial, Powder for injection, lyophilized 1.8 mg/vial, Powder for injection, lyophilized 2 mg/vial ♦ *Humatrope* Powder for injection, lyophilized 5 mg (approximately 15 IU)/vial, Powder for injection, lyophilized 6 mg (18 IU)/cartridge, Powder for injection, lyophilized 12 mg (36 IU)/cartridge, Powder for injection, lyophilized 24 mg (72 IU)/cartridge ♦ *Norditropin* Powder for injection, lyophilized 4 mg (approximately 12 IU)/vial, Powder for injection, lyophilized 8 mg (approximately 24 IU)/vial, Injection 5 mg/1.5 mL, Injection 10 mg/1.5 mL, Injection 15 mg/1.5 mL ♦ *Nutropin* Powder for injection, lyophilized 5 mg (approximately 15 IU)/vial, Powder for injection, lyophilized 10 mg (approximately 26 IU)/vial ♦ *Nutropin AQ* Injection 10 mg (approximately 30 IU)/vial ♦ *Nutropin Depot* Powder for injection 13.5 mg, Powder for injection 18 mg, Powder for injection 22.5 mg ♦ *Saizen* Powder for injection, lyophilized 5 mg (approximately 15 IU)/vial ♦ *Serostim* Powder for injection, lyophilized 4 mg (approximately 12 IU)/vial, Powder for injection, lyophilized 5 mg (approximately 15 IU)/vial, Powder for injection, lyophilized 6 mg (approximately 18 IU)/vial

Action
PHARMACOLOGY: Mimics actions of naturally occurring growth hormone to stimulate linear and skeletal growth; increases number and size of skeletal muscle cells; increases RBC mass and internal organ size; increases cellular protein synthesis; reduces body fat stores and lipid mobilization, and increases plasma fatty acids.

PHARMACOKINETICS/DYNAMICS:
Absorption: Somatropin C_{max} with concentrations of 5.3 mg/mL is approximately 23 ng/mL. C_{max} with concentrations of 1.3 mg/mL is approximately 17.4 ng/mL. Following a 0.03 mg/kg SC injection of 1.3 mg/mL, about 80% was systemically available as compared with that available following IV dosing.

Distribution: Vd is approximately 1.3 L/kg.

Metabolism: Somatropin undergoes classical protein catabolism in both liver and kidneys.

Excretion: Somatropin's $t_{½}$ is approximately 0.4 hr (IV) and approximately 3 hr (SC). Mean clearance of SC administration is about 0.3 L/hr/kg.

Indications Long-term treatment of children with growth failure caused by lack of adequate endogenous growth hormone secretion (except *Serostim*); (*Genotropin* only) long-term treatment of children with growth failure caused by Prader-Willi syndrome (PWS); (*Genotropin, Nutropin, Nutropin AQ,* and *Humatrope* only) long-term replacement therapy in adults with growth hormone deficiency of either childhood- or adult-onset etiology; (*Nutropin* and *Nutropin AQ* only) treatment of growth failure associated with chronic renal insufficiency up to time of renal transplantation; (*Nutropin, Nutropin AQ,* and *Humatrope* only) long-term treatment of short stature associated with Turner syndrome; (*Serostim* only) treatment of AIDS wasting or cachexia.

Contraindications Closed epiphyses; evidence of tumor activity or active neoplasm; intracranial lesion must be inactive and antitumor therapy complete prior to instituting therapy; sensitivity to benzyl alcohol (*Nutropin* diluent) glycerin or M-cresol (*Humatrope* diluent).

Route/Dosage

Growth Failure
CHILDREN: (*Genotropin*) **SC** 0.16 to 0.24 mg/kg/wk (divided into 6 or 7 injections) (*Humatrope*). **IM/SC** 0.18 mg/kg/wk (divided into equal doses given on 3 alternate days, 6 times/wk, or daily) to a max of 0.3 mg/kg of body weight; (*Norditropin*) **SC** 0.024 to 0.034 mg/kg 6 to 7 times/wk, (*Nutropin/Nutropin AQ*) **SC** 0.3 mg/kg/wk (divided into daily injections); (*Saizen*) **IM/SC** 0.06 mg/kg 3 times/wk.

Growth Failure PWS
CHILDREN: (*Genotropin*) **SC** 0.24 mg/kg/wk.

Growth Hormone Deficiency
ADULTS: (*Genotropin*) **SC** Start with up to 0.04 mg/kg/wk (divided into 6 or 7 injections), increasing the dose at 4- to 8-wk intervals according to patient requirements (max, 0.08 mg/kg/wk); (*Humatrope*) **SC** start with up to 0.006 mg/kg/day, increasing the dose according to patient requirements (maximum 0.0125 mg/kg/day); (*Nutropin/Nutropin AQ*) **SC** start with up to 0.006 mg/kg/day, increasing the dose according to patient requirements to a maximum of 0.025 mg/kg/day in patients less than 35 yr and maximum of 0.0125 mg/kg daily in patients greater than 35 yr.

Growth Failure Associated with Chronic Renal Insufficiency
ADULTS: (*Nutropin/Nutropin AQ*) **SC** Up to 0.35 mg/kg weekly (divided into daily injections) continued up to time of renal transplantation.

Short Stature Associated with Turner Syndrome
CHILDREN: (*Humatrope*) **SC** Up to 0.375 mg/kg/wk (divided into equal doses given either daily or on 3 alternate days); (*Nutropin/Nutropin AQ*) **SC** up to 0.375 mg/kg/wk (divided into equal doses 3 to 7 times/wk).

AIDS Wasting or Cachexia
ADULTS: (*Serostim*) **SC** (at bedtime) greater than 55 kg body weight 6 mg daily; 45 to 55 kg body weight 5 mg daily; 35 to 45 kg body weight 4 mg daily; less than 35 kg body weight 0.1 mg/kg.

Interactions
Glucocorticoids: May inhibit growth-promoting effects of somatropin.

Lab Test Interferences
None well documented.

Adverse Reactions
CNS: Headache; weakness; recurrent growth of intracranial tumor.
DERM: Rash; urticaria; pain; inflammation at injection site.
GU: Glucosuria; hypercalciuria.
METAB: Hypothyroidism; hyperglycemia.
OTHER: Localized muscle pain; mild, transient edema; antibodies to growth hormone.

Precautions
Pregnancy: Category C.
Lactation: Undetermined.
Concomitant glucocorticoid therapy: May inhibit growth-promoting effects.
Hypothyroidism: May develop during therapy; monitor thyroid function.
Insulin resistance: May be induced with therapy; monitor for glucose intolerance.
Intracranial hypertension: Intracranial hypertension, with papilledema, visual changes, headache, nausea, or vomiting has been reported in few patients.
Intracranial lesion: Frequently examine patients with history of lesion.
Slipped capital epiphysis: May be seen in children with advanced renal osteodystrophy; may be affected by growth hormone. Be alert to development of limp or complaints of hip or knee pain.

Overdosage: Signs and Symptoms
Hypoglycemia followed by hyperglycemia; acromegaly (chronic overdosage).

PATIENT CARE CONSIDERATIONS

Administration/Storage
- Reconstitute each 5 mg vial with 1 to 5 mL or each 10 mg vial with 1 to 10 mL of Bacteriostatic Water for Injection, USP (benzyl alcohol preserved) only.
- Store before and after administration in refrigerator. Use reconstituted drug within 14 days; refrigerate until used; avoid freezing.
- In patients with sensitivity to M-cresol, glycerin, or benzyl alcohol reconstitute with Sterile Water for Injection; use reconstituted dose within 24 hr; refrigerate until used; do not freeze; use only 1 dose per vial; discard unused portion.

Assessment/Interventions
- Obtain patient history, including drug history and any known allergies.
- Be aware that use of product with glucocorticoid therapy may inhibit growth-promoting effects.
- Frequently examine patients with history of intracranial lesion for evidence of recurrence or progression.
- Monitor thyroid function test results.
- Be aware that insulin resistance may develop and monitor for signs of glucose intolerance.

- Be alert for signs of acromegaly and report to health care provider.
- Assess for common side effects: headache, weakness, localized muscle pain, or transient edema and report to health care provider.
- Report any limp or complaints of hip or knee pain in children to health care provider; this may indicate slipped epiphyses.

Patient/Family Education
- Instruct diabetic patients to monitor blood sugar closely and to report variations to health care provider.
- Tell children and parents to report limp or complaints of hip or knee pain to health care provider as soon as possible.
- Instruct patient to report these symptoms to health care provider: headache, weakness, localized muscle pain, or mild, transient edema.

Sotalol Hydrochloride

(SOTT-uh-lahl HIGH-droe-KLOR-ide)
Class Beta-adrenergic blocker

How Supplied
Betapace Tablets 80 mg, Tablets 120 mg, Tablets 160 mg, Tablets 240 mg ◆ *Betapace AF* Tablets 80 mg, Tablets 120 mg, Tablets 160 mg
✤ *Apo-Sotalol* ◆ *Gen-Sotalol* ◆ *Novo-Sotalol* ◆ *Nu-Sotalol* ◆ *PMS-Sotalol* ◆ *ratio-Sotalol* ◆ *Rhoxal-sotalol* ◆ *Sotacor*

Action
PHARMACOLOGY: Blocks beta receptors, which primarily affect heart (slows rate), vascular musculature (decreases blood pressure), and lungs (reduces function).

PHARMACOKINETICS/DYNAMICS:

Absorption: Oral bioavailability of sotalol is 90% to 100% and T_{max} is 2.5 to 4 hr. Absorption was reduced approximately 20% compared to fasting when administered with a standard meal. Steady state is reached after 1 to 2 days.

Distribution: Sotalol does not bind to plasma proteins.

Metabolism: Sotalol is not metabolized.

Excretion: Sotalol t½ is 12 hr and it is excreted predominantly via the kidney in unchanged form.

Special Populations:
Renal Function Impairment – Lower doses are necessary in renal impairment.
Hepatic Function Impairment – Patients with hepatic impairment show no alteration in sotalol clearance.

Indications
Betapace: Management or prevention of life-threatening ventricular arrhythmias.
Betapace AF: Maintenance of normal sinus rhythm in patients with highly symptomatic atrial fibrillation/atrial flutter (AFIB/AFL) (*Betapace AF*).

Contraindications
Betapace: Hypersensitivity to beta-blockers; greater than first-degree heart block; CHF unless secondary to tachyarrhythmia treatable with beta-blockers; overt cardiac failure; sinus bradycardia; cardiogenic shock; bronchial asthma or bronchospasm, including severe COPD; congenital or acquired long QT syndromes.
Betapace AF: Sinus bradycardia (less than 50 bpm during waking hours); sick sinus syndrome or second and third degree AV block (unless a functioning pacemaker is present); congenital or acquired QT syndromes; baseline QT interval greater than 450 msec; cardiogenic shock; uncontrolled heart failure; hypokalemia (less than 4 mEq/L); Ccr less than 40 mL/min; bronchial asthma; previous evidence of hypersensitivity to sotalol.

Route/Dosage
Do not substitute *Betapace* for *Betapace AF* because of significant differences in labeling (eg, patient package insert, dosing administration, safety information).

Ventricular Arrhythmias

BETAPACE

ADULTS: **PO** 80 mg twice daily; may increase up to 320 mg/day in 2 or 3 divided doses. Patients with a history of symptomatic AFIB/AFL currently receiving *Betapace* should be transferred to *Betapace AF* because of the significant differences in labeling.

BETAPACE AF

Therapy with *Betapace AF* must be initiated and, if necessary, titrated in a setting that provides continuous ECG monitoring and in the presence of personnel trained in the management of serious ventricular arrhythmias. Monitor patients in this way for a minimum of 3 days on the maintenance dose and do not discharge within 12 hr of electrical or pharmacological conversion to normal sinus rhythm.

ADULTS: **PO** Initiate therapy at 80 mg bid if Ccr is greater than 60 mL/min, and 80 mg once daily if the Ccr is 40 to 60 mL/min. Begin continuous ECG monitoring with QT interval measurements 2 to 4 hr after each dose. If the 80 mg dose level is tolerated and QT interval remains less than 500 msec after at least 3 days, the patient may be discharged. Alternatively, during hospitalization, if 80 mg level does not reduce the frequency of relapse of AFIB/AFL and is tolerated without excessive QT interval prolongation (ie, greater than 520 msec), after following the patient for 3 days, the dose level may be increased to 120 mg (once or twice daily depending on Ccr). The max recommended dose in patients with Ccr greater than 60 mL/min is 160 mg bid.

Interactions
Amiodarone, disopyramide, procainamide, quinidine: May prolong cardiac refractoriness.
Calcium channel blockers: Increased risk of hypotension; possible increased effect on atrioventricular conduction or ventricular function.
Clonidine: May enhance or reverse antihypertensive effects; may enhance clonidine rebound hypertension.
Gatifloxacin, moxifloxacin, sparfloxacin: Do not use in patients receiving sotalol because of increased risk of life-threatening cardiac arrhythmias.
Guanethidine, reserpine: Increased hypotension or bradycardia.
Insulin, oral sulfonylurea hypoglycemic agents: Hyperglycemia; symptoms of hypoglycemia may be masked.
NSAIDs: Some agents may impair antihypertensive effect.

Lab Test Interferences May interfere with glucose or insulin tolerance tests, may result in falsely elevated urinary levels of metanephrine.

Adverse Reactions
CV: Arrhythmias; sustained ventricular tachycardia or fibrillation; torsades de pointes.
CNS: Depression; dizziness; headache; lethargy; paresthesias; vivid dreams.
DERM: Rash.
GI: Anorexia; constipation; diarrhea; dry mouth; dyspepsia; flatulence; nausea; vomiting.
GU: Decreased libido; dysuria; impotence; nocturia; urinary retention or frequency; urinary tract infection.
HEMA: May increase or decrease blood glucose.
HEPA: Elevated liver enzymes.
RESP: Bronchospasm; difficulty breathing; wheezing.

> **WARNING:**
> *Equipped facility:* To minimize risk of induced arrhythmia, initiate or re-initiate therapy for at least 3 days in facility that can provide cardiac resuscitation and EKG monitoring.
> Do not substitute *Betapace* for *Betapace AF*. *Betapace* does not have an atrial fibrillation indication or package insert information for patient.

Precautions
Pregnancy: Category B.
Lactation: Excreted in breast milk.
Children: Safety and efficacy not established.
Renal function impairment: Alteration of dosage interval and reduced daily dose are advised.
Hepatic function impairment: Alteration of dosage interval and reduced daily dose are advised.
Abrupt withdrawal: Has been associated with adverse effects; gradually decrease dose over 1 to 2 wk.
Anaphylaxis: Deaths have occurred; aggressive therapy may be required.
CHF: Administer cautiously in patients with CHF controlled by digitalis and diuretics.
Diabetic patients: Drug may mask signs and symptoms of hypoglycemia (eg, tachycardia, BP changes). Drug may potentiate insulin-induced hypoglycemia.
Nonallergic bronchospasm: Give drug with caution in patients with bronchospastic disease.
Peripheral vascular disease: May precipitate or aggravate symptoms of arterial insufficiency.
Proarrhythmia: May provoke new or worsened arrhythmias. Correct hypokalemia or hypomagnesemia before administering sotalol. Anticipate proarrhythmic events with initial dose and with every dose adjustment.
Thyrotoxicosis: May mask clinical signs (eg, tachycardia) of developing or continuing hyperthyroidism. Abrupt withdrawal may exacerbate symptoms of hyperthyroidism, including thyroid storm.

Overdosage: Signs and Symptoms
Bradycardia, CHF, hypotension, bronchospasm, prolongation of QT interval, torsades de pointes, ventricular tachycardia, premature ventricular complexes, hypoglycemia.

PATIENT CARE CONSIDERATIONS
Administration/Storage
- Adjust dosage gradually to attain steady-state plasma concentrations.
- Before initiating therapy, carefully monitor response to withdrawal of previous antiarrhythmic therapy.
- Give on empty stomach.
- Store at room temperature.

Assessment/Interventions
- Obtain patient history, including drug history and any known allergies.
- Obtain complete cardiac assessment prior to initiation of therapy.
- Closely monitor patient during initiation of therapy and with each dosage change.

- Monitor pulse and BP, ECG, and heart rate and rhythm routinely.
- Monitor potassium, magnesium, and glucose levels routinely.
- Assess apical pulse and BP prior to each dose.
- If extremes in pulse rates are detected, withhold medication and call health care provider immediately.
- Notify health care provider immediately of any signs of CHF or of any unexplained respiratory symptoms.

Patient/Family Education
- Explain importance of not discontinuing drug suddenly, and advise that dosage will be decreased over 1 to 2 wk.
- Explain that drug may mask signs and symptoms of hypoglycemia.
- Teach patient to take pulse daily and to notify health care provider if pulse is less than 60.
- Tell patient to call health care provider if adverse reaction occurs.
- Instruct patient not to take OTC medications without consulting health care provider.

Sparfloxacin

(spar-FLOX-ah-sin)

Class Antibiotic/Fluoroquinolone

How Supplied
Zagam Tablets 200 mg

Action
PHARMACOLOGY: Interferes with microbial DNA synthesis.

PHARMACOKINETICS/DYNAMICS:

Absorption: Oral bioavailability of sparfloxacin is 92%; antacids containing aluminum hydroxide or magnesium hydroxide reduce bioavailability by as much as 50%. C_{max} is approximately 1.3 mcg/mL; AUC is approximately 34 mcg•hr/mL; T_{max} is between 3 and 6 hr. Oral absorption is unaffected by milk, food, or high fat meals.

Distribution: Sparfloxacin distributes well into the body. Vd is approximately 3.9 L/kg. Sparfloxacin has low protein binding (approximately 45%).

Metabolism: Sparfloxacin is metabolized by the liver and does not interfere with cytochrome P450.

Excretion: Total Cl is approximately 11.4 L/hr; renal Cl is approximately 1.5 L/hr. Ten percent of an orally administered dose is excreted in urine. Sparfloxacin t½ is about 20 hr.

Special Populations:
Renal Function Impairment – In Ccr below 50 mL/min, t½ is lengthened. Single or multiple doses in patients with varying degrees of renal impairment typically produce plasma concentrations that are twice those observed in healthy subjects.
Hepatic Function Impairment – The kinetics of sparfloxacin are not altered in patients with mild to moderate hepatic impairment without cholestasis.

Indications Treatment of community acquired pneumonia or bacterial exacerbation of chronic bronchitis caused by susceptible organisms.

Contraindications History of hypersensitivity or photosensitivity reactions; drugs known to prolong the electrocardiogram QT_c interval such as disopyramide and amiodarone or patients with underlying QT_c prolongation (torsades de pointes has been reported in such patients); patients whose lifestyle or occupation prevents avoidance of sun, bright natural light, or ultraviolet rays while taking this drug and for 5 days after treatment is stopped; tendonitis or tendon rupture associated with quinolone use.

Route/Dosage
ADULTS: PO 400 mg on day 1 (loading dose) followed by 200 mg qd for a total 10 days of therapy.

Renal Function Impairment (Ccr less than 50 mL)
ADULTS: PO 400 mg on day 1 (loading dose) followed by 200 mg q 48 hr for a total of 9 days of therapy.

Tuberculosis
ADULTS: PO 200 mg/day (max, 200 mg/day).

Interactions
Aluminum-magnesium antacids, sucralfate, zinc, iron salts: Reduced absorption leading to lower bioavailability and efficacy.
Bepridil, cisapride, erythromycin, pentamidine, phenothiazines and related antipsychotics, tricyclic antidepressants, any other drug known to prolong the QT_c interval: Increased risk of torsades de pointes or other malignant ventricular arrhythmias.

Lab Test Interferences False-negative results for *Mycobacterium tuberculosis* cultures.

Adverse Reactions
CV: QT_c prolongation (possibly leading to serious ventricular arrhythmias); vasodilation.
CNS: Headache; dizziness; insomnia; somnolence.
DERM: Photosensitivity; pruritus; rash.
EENT: Taste perversion.

GI: Diarrhea; nausea; dyspepsia; abdominal pain; dry mouth; vomiting; flatulence.
GU: Vaginal moniliasis.
OTHER: Asthenia.

Precautions

Pregnancy: Category C.
Lactation: Excreted in breast milk.
Children: Safety and efficacy not established.
Hypersensitivity: Acute anaphylactic reactions and serious dermatologic hypersensitivity reactions have been reported. Stop sparfloxacin if a rash or any other sign of photosensitivity develops.
Renal function impairment: Dose adjustment necessary if Ccr is less than 50 mL/min.
Superinfection: Use of antibiotics may result in bacterial or fungal overgrowth.
Phototoxicity: Moderate to severe phototoxic reactions have been reported. Patients must avoid exposure to direct or indirect sunlight or other sources of UV light while taking this medication and for 5 days thereafter. Patients must discontinue therapy at first sign or symptom of a phototoxic reaction (eg, sensation of skin burning, redness, swelling, blistering, rash, itching, dermatitis).
Convulsions and toxic psychosis: CNS stimulation, lowering of the seizure threshold, and psychotic reactions have been reported. Use with caution in patients with seizures or other CNS disorders.
Pseudomembranous colitis: Consider possibility in patients with diarrhea.
Tendonitis: Inflammation and rupture of tendons has been associated with the use of fluoroquinolone antibiotics.
QT interval: May be prolonged in some patients.

Overdosage: Signs and Symptoms

Possible QT_c prolongation.

PATIENT CARE CONSIDERATIONS

Administration/Storage

- Administer without regard to meals but with a full glass of water.
- Administer antacids, sucralfate, zinc, and iron salts at least 4 hr after sparfloxacin administration.
- Store at room temperature in tightly closed container.

Assessment/Interventions

- Obtain patient history, including drug history and any known allergies.
- Obtain specimens as ordered for culture and sensitivity before beginning treatment.
- Monitor signs and symptoms of infection throughout course of therapy.
- Obtain baseline CBC, renal, LFTs, and electrolytes.
- Monitor I&O.
- Monitor for symptoms of superinfections such as vaginitis, stomatitis, and diarrhea. Notify health care provider if present.
- Notify health care provider if symptoms of pseudomembranous colitis occur (loose or foul-smelling stools).
- Discontinue immediately and notify health care provider at the first appearance of a rash or any other signs of hypersensitivity and institute support measures.
- Discontinue immediately if signs of increased intracranial pressure, or CNS reactions such as restlessness, agitation, tremors, confusion, hallucinations, or other signs of psychoses should appear.

Patient/Family Education

- Instruct patient to take medication as directed with a full glass of water without regard to meals.
- Instruct patient that sparfloxacin may be taken with food or milk. However, mineral supplements, vitamins with iron, zinc calcium, and magnesium- and aluminum-containing antacids, and sucralfate should be taken 4 hr after antibiotic administration.
- Instruct patients to drink fluids liberally while taking medication.
- Advise patient to avoid exposure to direct or indirect sunlight (including through glass, while using sunscreen or sunblocks, reflected sunlight, and cloudy weather) and exposure to artificial UV light during treatment with sparfloxacin and for at least 5 days after therapy. If exposure to sun cannot be avoided, patient should cover as much of the skin as possible with clothing.
- Caution patient to discontinue sparfloxacin therapy at first sign or symptom of phototoxicity (eg, sensation of skin burning, redness, swelling, blisters, rash, itching, dermatitis) and to contact the primary care provider at once.
- Advise patient who has experienced a phototoxic reaction to the medicine to avoid further exposure to sunlight or artificial UV light until completely recovered from the reaction or for 5 days following discontinuation of treatment, whichever is longer. In rare cases, reactions have recurred up to several weeks following discontinuation.

- Advise patient not to drive, operate machinery, or engage in other activities that require mental alertness and coordination until reaction to sparfloxacin is known (eg, dizziness, light-headedness).
- Instruct patient to discontinue medication and inform primary caregiver if pain or inflammation of a tendon is experienced and to rest and not exercise until tendonitis or tendon rupture has been ruled out.
- Instruct patient to report these symptoms to health care provider: diarrhea, foul-smelling stools, stomatitis, vaginitis, black, furry appearance of tongue.
- Instruct patient to discontinue the drug and to contact health care provider at the first sign of a rash or other allergic reaction.
- Instruct patient to complete full course of therapy, even if symptoms of infection have resolved.
- Advise patient to consult with health care provider before taking any other medications, including OTC products.

Spectinomycin

(speck-TIN-oh-MY-sin)

Class Anti-infective

How Supplied
Trobicin Powder for injection 400 mg (as hydrochloride) per mL when reconstituted

Action
PHARMACOLOGY: Inhibits protein synthesis in bacterial cells (30S ribosomal subunit).

PHARMACOKINETICS/DYNAMICS:
Absorption: Rapid after IM injection. Following a 2 g dose, C_{max} is about 100 mcg/mL at approximately 1 hr; and 160 mcg/mL 2 hr after a 4 g dose. Eight hours after a 2 or 4 g dose, average serum levels are 15 and 31 mcg/mL, respectively.

Indications
Treatment of acute gonorrheal urethritis and proctitis in men and acute gonorrheal cervicitis and proctitis in women.

Contraindications
Standard considerations.

Route/Dosage
ADULTS: IM 2 g deep into upper outer quadrant of the gluteal muscle. In geographic locations where antibiotic resistance is known to be prevalent, treat with 4 g divided between 2 gluteal injection sites.

PATIENT CARE CONSIDERATIONS

Administration/Storage
- For IM administration only. Not for intradermal, subcutaneous, IV, or intra-arterial administration.
- Reconstitute powder for injection using 3.2 mL of supplied diluent. Shake vial vigorously immediately after adding diluent.
- Do not administer if particulate matter, cloudiness, or discoloration noted.
- To minimize injection site reactions, administer prescribed dose by deep IM injection into upper outer quadrant of gluteal muscle.
- Discard any unused solution. Do not save unused solution for later administration.
- Store unopened vials at controlled room temperature (68° to 77°F). Store reconstituted suspension at controlled room temperature and use within 24 hr.

Assessment/Interventions
- Obtain patient history, including drug history and any known allergies.
- Review results of culture and sensitivity testing as available.
- Ensure a serologic test for syphilis is performed at time of diagnosis and again 3 mo after treatment for gonorrhea.
- Ensure cultures are re-evaluated 3 to 5 days after treatment for pharyngeal infection to verify eradication.

Interactions None well documented.

Lab Test Interferences None well documented.

Adverse Reactions
CNS: Dizziness; insomnia.
DERM: Soreness at injection site; urticaria.
GI: Nausea.
GU: Decreased urine output.
HYPERSEN: Anaphylaxis or anaphylactoid reactions.
LABTESTABS: Decreased hemoglobin, hematocrit, and Ccr; elevated alkaline phosphatase, BUN, and ALT.
OTHER: Chills; fever.

Precautions
Pregnancy: Category B.
Lactation: Undetermined.
Children: Safety and efficacy not established.
Benzyl alcohol: Contains benzyl alcohol, which has been associated with fatal gasping syndrome in premature infants and increased incidence of neurologic and other complications.
Efficacy: Monitor to detect evidence of *Neisseria gonorrhoeae* resistance.
Syphilis: Spectinomycin is not effective in treating syphilis, and high doses for short periods of time to treat gonorrhea may mask or delay symptoms of incubating syphilis.

- Monitor patient for signs of allergic reaction. Discontinue therapy and immediately notify health care provider if noted. Be prepared to treat appropriately.

Patient/Family Education
- Explain name, action, and potential side effects of drug.
- Advise patient or caregiver that medication will be prepared and administered by a health care provider in a health care setting.
- Advise patient to report injection site pain or redness.

Spironolactone

(SPEER-oh-no-LAK-tone)

Class Potassium-sparing diuretic

How Supplied
Aldactone Tablets 25 mg, Tablets 50 mg, Tablets 100 mg ♦ *Spironolactone* Tablets 25 mg
✤ *Novo-Spiroton* ♦ *Novo-Spirozine*

Action
PHARMACOLOGY: Competitively inhibits aldosterone in distal tubules, resulting in increased excretion of sodium and water and decreased excretion of potassium.

PHARMACOKINETICS/DYNAMICS:

Absorption: Spironolactone is rapidly and extensively metabolized. Food increases bioavailability by almost 100%.

Distribution: Spironolactone is greater than 90% bound to plasma proteins.

Metabolism: Sulfur-containing products are predominant metabolites and are thought to be primarily responsible together with spironolactone for the therapeutic effect of the drug.

Excretion: Metabolites are excreted primarily in the urine and secondarily in bile.

Indications Short-term preoperative treatment of primary hyperaldosteronism; long-term maintenance therapy for idiopathic hyperaldosteronism; management of edematous conditions in CHF, cirrhosis of liver and nephrotic syndrome; management of essential hypertension; treatment of hypokalemia. **Unlabeled use(s):** Treatment of hirsutism; relief of PMS symptoms; short-term treatment of familial male precocious puberty; and short-term treatment of acne vulgaris.

Contraindications Anuria; acute renal insufficiency; impaired renal excretory function; hyperkalemia.

Route/Dosage

Diagnosis of Primary Hyperaldosteronism
ADULTS: PO 400 mg/day for 4 days (short test) or 3 to 4 wk (long test).

Maintenance Therapy for Hyperaldosteronism
ADULTS: PO 100 to 400 mg daily in single or divided doses.

Edema
ADULTS: PO 25 to 200 mg/day in single or divided doses.
CHILDREN: PO 3.3 mg/kg/day in single or divided doses.

Essential Hypertension
ADULTS: PO 50 to 100 mg/day in single or divided doses.
CHILDREN: PO 1 to 2 mg/kg bid.

Diuretic-Induced Hypokalemia
ADULTS: PO 25 to 100 mg/day when oral potassium or other potassium-sparing regimens are inappropriate.

Interactions
ACE inhibitors: May result in severely elevated serum potassium levels.
Digitalis glycosides: May decrease digoxin clearance, resulting in increased serum digoxin levels and toxicity; may attenuate inotropic action of digoxin.
Mitotane: May decrease therapeutic response to mitotane.
Potassium preparations: May severely increase serum potassium levels, possibly resulting in cardiac arrhythmias or cardiac arrest. Do not take with potassium preparations.
Salicylates: May result in decreased diuretic effect.

Lab Test Interferences Drug may cause falsely elevated serum digoxin values with radioimmunoassay (assay specific) for measuring digoxin.

Adverse Reactions
CNS: Drowsiness; lethargy; headache; mental confusion; ataxia.
DERM: Maculopapular or erythematous cutaneous eruptions; urticaria.
GI: Cramping; diarrhea; gastric bleeding; gastric ulceration; gastritis; vomiting.
GU: Inability to achieve or maintain erection.
HEMA: Agranulocytosis.
HEPA: Hyperchloremic metabolic acidosis in decompensated hepatic cirrhosis.
OTHER: Gynecomastia; irregular menses or amenorrhea; postmenopausal bleeding; hirsutism; deepening of voice; drug fever; carcinoma of breast.

Precautions
Pregnancy: Category D.
Lactation: Excreted in breast milk.

Electrolyte imbalances and BUN increase: Hyperkalemia (serum potassium greater than 5.5 mEq/L), hyponatremia, hypochloremia and increases in BUN may occur.

Overdosage: Signs and Symptoms
Electrolyte imbalance.

PATIENT CARE CONSIDERATIONS
Administration/Storage
- If single dose is prescribed, administer in morning.
- Take medication with food.
- May crush tablets and administer as suspension.
- Suspension is stable for 30 days under refrigeration. Protect from light.
- Store tablets at room temperature.

Assessment/Interventions
- Obtain patient history, including drug history and any known allergies.
- Assess fluid and electrolyte status prior to therapy.
- Monitor potassium levels. If level is greater than 5.5 mEq/L, withhold medication and notify health care provider.
- Monitor serum electrolytes, I&O, weight, and BP daily.
- Monitor ABGs, liver, and renal function studies.
- If deep rapid respirations or headaches develop, notify health care provider.
- Assess urinary status. If patient develops urinary frequency, dysuria, edema, or reduced urinary output, notify health care provider.
- Assess for any changes in hepatic status. If patient appears jaundiced and mentally confused, notify health care provider.
- If nausea, vomiting, distention, diarrhea, or anorexia occur, notify health care provider.
- Note any changes in neurologic status. If drowsiness, ataxia, lethargy, confusion, or headache occurs, notify health care provider.

Patient/Family Education
- Explain that medication's full diuretic effect may not be achieved for 1 to 2 wk.
- Instruct patient to avoid large quantities of potassium-rich foods or potassium salt substitutes.
- For patient being treated for hypertension, explain that patient may feel tired for several weeks because body needs to adjust to lowered BP.
- Instruct patient to take drug with food to minimize GI irritation.
- Tell patient to weigh self twice weekly and to notify health care provider of any increase.
- Instruct patient to notify health care provider if new symptoms develop.
- Tell patient to report these symptoms to health care provider: GI cramping, diarrhea, lethargy, thirst, headache, skin rash, menstrual abnormalities, deepening of voice, and breast enlargement in men.
- Advise patient that drug may cause drowsiness and to use caution while driving or performing other tasks requiring mental alertness.
- Instruct patient not to take prescription or otc medications without consulting health care provider.

Spironolactone/ Hydrochlorothiazide

(SPEER-oh-no-LAK-tone/high-droe-klor-THIGH-uh-zide)

Class Diuretic combination

How Supplied
Aldactazide Tablets 25 mg spironolactone and 25 mg hydrochlorothiazide, Tablets 50 mg spironolactone and 50 mg hydrochlorothiazide

Action
PHARMACOLOGY:
Spironolactone: Competitively inhibits aldosterone in distal tubules, resulting in increased excretion of sodium and water and decreased excretion of potassium.
Hydrochlorothiazide: Increases chloride, sodium, and water excretion by interfering with transport of sodium ions across renal tubular epithelium.

Indications Edematous conditions for patients with CHF, cirrhosis of the liver accompanied edema or ascites, nephrotic syndrome, or essential hypertension.

Contraindications Patients with anuria; acute renal insufficiency, significant impairment of renal excretory function; severe hepatic failure; hyperkalemia; hypersensitivity to any component of product or sulfonamide-derived drugs.

Route/Dosage
Edema (CHF, hepatic cirrhosis, nephrotic syndrome)
ADULTS: PO Usual maintenance dose is 100 mg each of spironolactone and hydrochlorothiazide daily, administered in a single dose or divided doses, ranging from 25 to 200 mg of each component daily, depending on the response to the initial titration.

Essential Hypertension
ADULTS: PO Varies depending on titration of

individual ingredients; however, many patients have an optimal response to 50 to 100 mg each of spironolactone and hydrochlorothiazide daily, given in a single dose or divided doses.

Interactions

ACE inhibitors (eg, captopril): Severe hyperkalemia may occur.
Alcohol, barbiturates, narcotics: Orthostatic hypotension may be potentiated.
Antidiabetic agents (oral and insulin): May require dosage adjustment of antidiabetic agent.
Corticosteroids, ACTH: Electrolyte depletion, particularly hypokalemia, may occur.
Digoxin: The t½ of digoxin may be prolonged and serum levels may be elevated, increasing the risk of toxicity.
Lithium: Renal clearance of lithium may be decreased, increasing the risk of toxicity.
Nondepolarizing skeletal muscle relaxants (eg, tubocurarine): Unresponsiveness to muscle relaxant may occur.
NSAIDs (eg, indomethacin): The diuretic, natriuretic, and antihypertensive effect of hydrochlorothiazide may be reduced.
Pressor amines (eg, norepinephrine): The vascular response to norepinephrine may be reduced.

Lab Test Interferences

Hydrochlorothiazide: May decrease serum protein-bound iodine levels without signs of thyroid disturbances. May cause diagnostic interference of serum electrolyte levels, blood and urine glucose levels, serum bilirubin levels, and serum uric acid levels.

Adverse Reactions

CV: Hypotension (including orthostatic).
CNS: Mental confusion; ataxia; headache; drowsiness; lethargy; vertigo; paresthesia; dizziness; restlessness.
DERM: Urticaria; rash; purpura; erythema multiforme; pruritus.
EENT: Transient blurred vision; xanthopsia.
GI: Gastric bleeding; ulceration; gastritis; diarrhea and cramping; nausea; vomiting; sialadenitis; constipation; gastric irritation; anorexia; pancreatitis.
GU: Gynecomastia; inability to achieve and maintain erection; irregular menses; amenorrhea; postmenopausal bleeding; renal dysfunction; renal failure; interstitial nephritis.
HEMA: Agranulocytosis; aplastic anemia; leukopenia; hemolytic anemia; thrombocytopenia.
HEPA: Mixed cholestatic/hepatocellular toxicity; jaundice (intrahepatic cholestatic jaundice).
METAB: Electrolyte imbalance; hyperglycemia; glycosuria; hyperuricemia.
RESP: Respiratory distress (including pneumonitis and pulmonary edema.)
OTHER: Hypersensitivity (fever, urticaria, maculopapular or erythematous cutaneous eruptions); vasculitis; weakness; anaphylactic reactions; necrotizing angiitis; photosensitivity; fever; muscle spasm.

Precautions

Pregnancy: Category C.
Lactation: Canrenone, a major and active metabolite of spironolactone, is excreted in breast milk.
Children: Safety and efficacy not established.
Special risk patients: Use with caution in patients with severe renal disease or impaired hepatic function.
Combination Therapy: Fixed-dose combination therapy is not indicated for initial therapy of edema or hypertension. Therapy should be titrated to the individual. If the fixed combination represents the dosage so determined, its use may be more convenient in patient management.
Electrolyte imbalance and BUN increase: Hyperkalemia (serum potassium greater than 5.5 mEq/L) hyponatremia, hypochloremia, and increases in BUN may occur.
Systemic lupus erythematosus (SLE): Hydrochlorothiazide may exacerbate or activate SLE.

Overdosage: Signs and Symptoms

Drowsiness, mental confusion, maculopapular or erythematous rash, nausea, vomiting, dizziness, diarrhea, hyperkalemia, electrolyte imbalance, hypokalemia and/or hyponatremia, thirst, restlessness, depression, lethargy, fatigue.

PATIENT CARE CONSIDERATIONS

Administration/Storage

- Administer qd or bid as prescribed without regard to meals. Administer with food if GI upset occurs.
- Administer alone or in combination with other antihypertensives.
- Store tablets at controlled room temperature (59° to 86°F).

Assessment/Interventions

- Obtain patient history, including drug history and any known allergies. Note history of diabetes, lupus erythematosus, hyperkalemia, anuria, kidney disease, liver disease, concurrent use of potassium-conserving medications or potassium-containing salt substitute, or allergy to sulfonamides.
- Ensure that serum electrolytes, BUN, and creatinine are monitored periodically.
- Monitor and record BP and pulse. Should hypotension result, hold medication and notify health care provider.
- Take safety precautions if orthostatic hypotension occurs.

- Monitor blood sugar in diabetic patient when drug is started or dose is changed. Report significant changes to health care provider.
- Monitor patient for GI, CV, and general body side effects. Inform health care provider if muscle cramps, paresthesia, weakness, fatigue, tachycardia or bradycardia, or other significant effects are noted.

Patient/Family Education
- Explain name, dose, action, and potential side effects of drug.
- Advise patient to take qd or bid as prescribed, without regard to meals but to take with food if GI upset occurs.
- Inform patient that drug controls, but does not cure, hypertension and to continue taking medication as prescribed even when BP is not elevated.
- Caution patient not to change the dose or stop taking unless advised to do so by health care provider.
- Instruct patient to continue taking other BP medications as prescribed by health care provider.
- Instruct patient in BP and pulse measurement skills.
- Advise patient to monitor and record BP and pulse at home and to inform health care provider should abnormal measurements be noted. Also advise patient to take record of BP and pulse to each follow-up visit.
- Instruct patient to lie or sit down if experiencing dizziness or lightheadedness when standing.
- Caution patient that inadequate fluid intake, excessive perspiration, diarrhea, or vomiting can lead to excessive fall in BP resulting in lightheadedness or fainting.
- Instruct diabetic patient to monitor blood glucose more frequently when drug is started or dose is changed and to inform health care provider of significant changes in readings.
- Caution patient to avoid unnecessary exposure to UV light (sunlight, tanning booths) and to use sunscreen and wear protective clothing when exposed to UV light to avoid photosensitivity reaction.
- Emphasize to hypertensive patient importance of other modalities on BP: weight control, regular exercise, smoking cessation, and moderate intake of alcohol and salt.
- Advise women to notify health care provider if pregnant, planning to become pregnant, or breastfeeding.
- Instruct patient to stop taking drug and immediately report any of these symptoms to health care provider: abnormal skin sensations, muscle weakness, or slow pulse.
- Caution patient not to take any prescription or OTC medications, salt substitutes, or dietary supplements unless advised by health care provider.
- Advise patient that follow-up visits and lab tests may be required to monitor therapy and to keep appointments.

Stavudine

(STAV-yoo-deen)

Class Antiretroviral/Nucleoside reverse transcriptase inhibitor

How Supplied
Zerit Capsules 15 mg, Capsules 20 mg, Capsules 30 mg, Capsules 40 mg, Powder for oral solution 1 mg/mL solution after reconstitution (200 mL bottle) ◆ *Zerit XR* Capsules, extended-release 37.5 mg, Capsules, extended-release 50 mg, Capsules, extended-release 75 mg, Capsules, extended-release 100 mg

Action
PHARMACOLOGY: Inhibits replication of HIV.

PHARMACOKINETICS/DYNAMICS:

Absorption: Stavudine is rapidly absorbed. C_{max} and AUC range from 0.03 to 4 mg/kg. T_{max} occurs 1 hr after dosing.

Distribution: Stavudine distributes equally between RBCs and plasma. Protein binding ranges from 0.01 to 11.4 mcg/mL.

Excretion: Renal elimination accounts for approximately 40% of overall clearance regardless of the route of administration. Stavudine undergoes active tubular secretion as well as glomerular filtration.

Special Populations:
Renal Function Impairment – Oral Cl and Ccr decreases in patients with renal insufficiency. Adjust dosage in patients with reduced Ccr and patients receiving maintenance hemodialysis.

Indications For the treatment of HIV-1 infection in combination with other antiretroviral agents.

Contraindications Standard considerations.

Route/Dosage
ADULTS:
Immediate-release: **PO** 40 mg q 12 hr for patients weighing at least 60 kg; 30 mg q 12 hr for patients weighing under 60 kg. May be taken without regard to food.
Extended-release: **PO** 100 mg qd for patients weighing at least 60 kg; 75 mg qd for patients weighing under 60 kg.

CHILDREN: PO 1 mg/kg/dose q 12 hr for patients weighing under 30 kg; give those weighing at least 30 kg the adult dosage.

Renal Function Impairment
Use drug cautiously in patients with renal impairment. Dosage adjustment based on renal function may be required (see table).

Renal Function Impairment Dosage		
Ccr (mL/min)	≥ 60 kg	< 60 kg
> 50	40 mg q 12 hr	30 mg q 12 hr
26 to 50	20 mg q 12 hr	15 mg q 12 hr
10 to 25	20 mg q 24 hr	15 mg q 24 hr

Interactions
Didanosine: Pancreatitis has occurred when in combination with stavudine (with or without hydroxyurea).
Zidovudine: May competitively inhibit the phosphorylation of stavudine; this combination is not recommended.

Lab Test Interferences
None well documented.

Adverse Reactions
CNS: Peripheral neuropathy; headache; insomnia.
DERM: Rash.
GI: Pancreatitis (may be fatal); diarrhea; nausea and vomiting; abdominal pain; anorexia.
HEMA: Anemia; leukopenia; thrombocytopenia.
HEPA: Lactic acidosis; hepatomegaly with hepatic steatosis.
METAB: AST greater than 5 times the ULN; ALT greater than 5 times ULN; amylase at least 1.4 times the ULN.
OTHER: Allergic reaction; chills/fever; myalgia.

> **WARNING:**
> *Pancreatitis:* Fatal and nonfatal cases have occurred in combination with didanosine with or without hydroxyurea.
> *Lactic acidosis and hepatomegaly:* Reported with steatosis (including fatal cases) with the use of nucleoside analogues alone or in combination.
> Reported in pregnant women who have received didanosine and stavudine with other antiretroviral agents. Use the combination with caution in pregnant women.

Precautions
Pregnancy: Category C.
Lactation: Undetermined; do not breastfeed.
Children: Safety and efficacy of extended-release dosage form not established.
Fat redistribution: Accumulation/redistribution of body fat including central obesity, dorsocervical fat enlargement (buffalo hump), peripheral wasting, facial wasting, breast enlargement, and "cushingoid appearance" have occurred in patients receiving antiretroviral therapy. A causal relationship has not been established.
Hemodialysis: 20 mg q 24 hr (patients at least 60 kg) or 15 mg q 24 hr (patients less than 60 kg) administered after the completion of hemodialysis and at the same time of the day on nondialysis days.
Peripheral neuropathy: Symptoms may worsen temporarily following therapy discontinuation. If symptoms of peripheral neuropathy develop, then interrupt therapy. Symptoms may resolve if therapy is withdrawn promptly. If symptoms resolve completely, then resume therapy at 50% of the recommended dose. If neuropathy recurs after resumption of stavudine, consider permanent discontinuation. Manage clinically significant elevations of hepatic transaminases in the same way.

PATIENT CARE CONSIDERATIONS

Administration/Storage
- Administer bid q 12 hr without regard to meals.
- Shake solution vigorously before measuring each dose. Use measuring cup provided.
- Administer reduced dose to patient with renal impairment.
- Store tablets at controlled room temperature (59° to 86°F) in a tightly closed container protected from moisture. Store solution in refrigerator. Keep bottle tightly closed. Discard any unused solution after 30 days.

Assessment/Interventions
- Obtain patient history, including drug history and any known allergies. Note renal or liver impairment, history of pancreatitis, and prior response to stavudine.
- Ensure that liver and renal function tests are obtained before beginning therapy and repeated periodically during therapy.
- Monitor patient for development of pancreatitis. If patient develops abdominal pain, nausea, or vomiting, or has elevated amylase

or LFT results, withhold medication and contact health care provider.
- Monitor patient for signs of lactic acidosis. If patient develops profound weakness or tiredness, unexpected stomach discomfort, coldness, dizziness, lightheadedness, or slow or irregular heartbeat, withhold drug and contact health care provider.
- Assess for evidence of peripheral neuropathy (eg, numbness, tingling, burning, or pain in hands or feet) or evidence of opportunistic infections. Notify health care provider if these occur.

Patient/Family Education
- Explain name, dose, action, and potential side effects of drug.
- Warn patient that this drug is not to be used by itself but is combined with other antiviral agents.
- Advise patient to take drug bid q 12 hr without regard to meals.
- Remind patient using solution to use measuring cup provided with drug and to shake bottle vigorously before measuring each dose.
- Instruct patient to report the following symptoms immediately to the health care provider: abdominal pain; nausea; vomiting; numbness, tingling, burning, or pain in hands or feet; profound weakness or tiredness; unexpected stomach discomfort; feeling cold, dizzy, or lightheaded; slow or irregular heartbeat.
- Inform patient that drug does not completely eliminate HIV virus and therefore does not reduce risk of transmitting HIV. Appropriate precautions must be followed.
- Advise patient that drug is not a cure for HIV infection and that the patient may continue to acquire illnesses associated with HIV infection, including opportunistic infections and to remain under a health care provider's care.
- Instruct patient to not take any prescription or OTC medications or dietary supplements unless advised by health care provider.
- Advise women to notify health care provider if pregnant, planning to become pregnant, or breastfeeding.
- Advise patient that follow-up visits and lab tests may be required to monitor therapy and to keep appointments.

Streptokinase

(STREP-toe-KIN-ace)
Class Thrombolytic enzyme
How Supplied
Streptase Powder for Injection 250,000 IU, Powder for Injection 750,000 IU, Powder for Injection 1,500,000 IU

Action
PHARMACOLOGY: Converts plasminogen to the enzyme plasmin, which aids in dissolution of blood clots.

PHARMACOKINETICS/DYNAMICS:
Metabolism: No metabolites identified.
Excretion: Streptokinase is cleared by the liver. The t½ is approximately 23 min (for activator complex).

Indications Acute MI, lysis of intracoronary thrombi, improvement of ventricular function, and reduction of mortality associated with acute MI (IV or intracoronary route); reduction of infarct size and CHF associated with acute MI (IV); lysis of objectively diagnosed (eg, angiography) pulmonary emboli (involving obstruction of blood flow to a lobe or multiple segments, with or without unstable hemodynamics); lysis of objectively diagnosed (eg, ascending venography), acute, extensive thrombi of the deep veins (eg, those involving the popliteal vessels); lysis of acute arterial thrombi and emboli; alternative to surgical revision for clearing totally or partially occluded arteriovenous cannulae when acceptable flow cannot be achieved.

Contraindications Active internal bleeding; recent cerebrovascular accident (within 2 mo); intracranial or intraspinal surgery; intracranial neoplasm; severe uncontrolled hypertension.

Route/Dosage
Acute Evolving Transmural MI
ADULTS: **IV infusion** Administer as soon as possible after symptom onset (greatest benefit when administered within 4 hr, but benefit has been reported up to 24 hr). Infuse a total dose of 1,500,000 IU within 60 min. **Intracoronary infusion** Administer 20,000 IU by bolus followed by 2000 IU/min for 60 min (total dose, 140,000 IU).

Pulmonary Embolism, Deep Vein Thrombosis (DVT), Arterial Thrombosis, or Embolism
ADULTS: **IV infusion** Administer as soon as possible after onset of thrombolic event, preferably within 7 days. A loading dose of 250,000 IU infused into a peripheral vein over 30 minutes has been found appropriate in over 90% of patients. If thrombin time or any parameter of lysis after 4 hr of therapy is not significantly different from the normal control level, discontinue streptokinase because excessive resistance is present. Dose and duration of therapy (following the loading dose of 250,000 IU/30 min): pulmonary embolism 100,000 IU/hr for 24 hr (72 hr if concurrent

DVT is suspected); DVT 100,000 IU/hr for 72 hr; arterial thrombosis or embolism 100,000 IU/hr for 24 to 72 hr.

Arteriovenous Cannulae Occlusion
Slowly instill 250,000 in 2 mL of solution into each occluded limb of the cannula. Clamp off cannula limb(s) for 2 hr. Closely observe patient for adverse effects. After treatment, aspirate contents of infused cannula limb(s) and flush with saline before reconnecting cannula.

Interactions
Anticoagulants, agents that alter platelet function (eg, aspirin, other NSAIDs, dipyridamole), other thrombolytic agents, agents that alter coagulation: May increase the risk of bleeding.
INCOMPATIBILITIES: Do not add other medication to the streptokinase container.

Lab Test Interferences
Will cause marked decreases in plasminogen and fibrinogen levels and increases in thrombin time, activated partial thromboplastin time, and prothrombin time, which usually normalize within 12 to 24 hr.

Adverse Reactions
CV: Hypotension (sometimes severe).
HEMA: Bleeding (major and minor).
RESP: Respiratory depression.
OTHER: Allergic reactions (eg, fever and shivering, urticaria, itching, flushing, nausea, headache, musculoskeletal pain); anaphylactic and anaphylactoid reactions (ranging from minor breathing difficulty to bronchospasm, periorbital swelling or angioneurotic edema); transient elevations of serum transaminases; back pain.

Precautions
Pregnancy: Category C.
Children: Safety and efficacy not established.

Special risk patients: Use with caution in patients with recent (within 10 days) major surgery, obstetrical delivery, organ biopsy, previous puncture of noncompressible vessels; recent (within 10 days) serious GI bleeding, recent (within 10 days) trauma including cardiopulmonary resuscitation, hypertension (systolic BP greater than 180 mm Hg or diastolic BP greater then 110 mm Hg), high likelihood of left heart thrombus (eg, mitral stenosis with atrial fibrillation), subacute bacterial endocarditis, hemostatic defects including those secondary to severe hepatic or renal disease, cerebrovascular disease, diabetic hemorrhagic retinopathy, septic thrombophlebitis, occluded AV cannula at seriously infected site, or any condition in which bleeding constitutes a significant hazard or would be particularly difficult to manage because of location; use with caution in patients who are pregnant or over age 75 yr.
Arrhythmia: Rapid lysis of coronary thrombi has been shown to cause reperfusion arterial or ventricular dysrhythmias, requiring immediate treatment.
Bleeding: Major and minor bleeding may occur. Severe, sometimes fatal, internal bleeding involving GI, hepatic, GU, or intracerebral sites has occurred.
Cholesterol embolism: Serious and fatal cholesterol embolism may occur.
Repeat administration: Because of increased likelihood of resistance caused by antistreptokinase antibodies, streptokinase may not be effective if administered within 5 days to 12 mo of prior streptokinase or anistreplase administration, or streptococcal infections (eg, streptococcal pharyngitis).

PATIENT CARE CONSIDERATIONS

Administration/Storage
- Administer only by IV infusion, intracororary artery infusion, or into arteriovenous cannulae. Not for SC or IM administration.
- Reconstitute lyophilized powder following manufacturer's recommendations.
- Avoid shaking or agitating vial during reconstitution process.
- Use reconstituted solution immediately or within 8 hr if stored at 36° to 46°F.
- Do not add any other medications to reconstituted solution.
- Do not administer if particulate matter or discoloration noted. A slight yellowish color is normal and is of no concern.
- Discard any unused solution.
- Store unopened vials at controlled room temperature (59° to 86°F).

Assessment/Interventions
- Obtain patient history, including drug history and any known allergies.
- Review patient's health history for any of the following conditions that would contraindicate streptokinase use: active internal bleeding; recent (within 2 mo) cerebrovascular accident; intracranial or intraspinal surgery; intracranial neoplasm; severe uncontrolled hypertension; hypersensitivity to streptokinase.
- Review patient's health history for any of the following conditions that could increase the risk of complications: recent (within 10 days) major surgery; GI bleeding; cardiopulmonary resuscitation; obstetrical delivery; organ biopsy; previous puncture of noncompressible vessel; hypertension; likelihood of left heart thrombus; subacute bacterial endocarditis; hemostatic defects including those caused by liver or kidney disease; pregnancy; age greater than 75 yr; diabetic hemorrhagic retinopathy; cerebrovascular disease.

- Note prior use of streptokinase administration or history of streptococcal infection.
- Review patient's medication record for use of drugs that present special risks when used in conjunction with streptokinase (anticoagulants or antiplatelet agents).
- Ensure that patient has been evaluated for bleeding disorders before administration of streptokinase.
- Monitor patient for signs of bleeding throughout therapy. If bleeding develops (eg, epistaxis, hematuria, hematemesis, bloody or black, tarry stools) notify health care provider immediately. Should uncontrollable bleeding occur, discontinue streptokinase therapy.
- Monitor patient with acute MI for arrhythmias during and immediately following administration. Be prepared to treat appropriately.
- Monitor BP during administration. If hypotension develops notify health care provider immediately. Be prepared to treat appropriately.
- Monitor patient for signs of anaphylaxis or severe allergic reaction. Discontinue therapy and immediately notify health care provider if noted. Be prepared to treat appropriately.
- Ensure that TT, aPTT, PT, or fibrinogen levels are determined prior to therapy and periodically, as indicated, throughout therapy.
- Ensure that hematocrit, platelet count and TT, aPTT, PT, or fibrinogen levels are determined before beginning therapy. Monitor hematocrit periodically, as indicated, throughout therapy.
- Discontinue heparin before therapy and ensure that TT or aPTT is less than twice the normal value before beginning streptokinase.
- If heparin is to be (re)instituted following streptokinase administration, ensure that TT or aPTT is less than twice the normal value before starting heparin.
- Avoid IM injections during and for 24 hr following administration.
- Perform venipunctures carefully and as infrequently as possible during therapy.
- If arterial puncture is necessary, ensure that upper extremity vessel is used. Following puncture, apply pressure for at least 30 min. Apply pressure dressing and check puncture site frequently.

Patient/Family Education
- Explain name, dose, action, and potential side effects of drug.
- Advise patient, family, or caregiver that medication will be prepared and administered by a health care professional in a medical setting.
- Instruct patient, family member, or caregiver to report any signs of bleeding or allergic reaction immediately.

Streptomycin Sulfate

(strep-toe-MY-sin Sull-fate)
Class Anti-infective/Antitubercular

How Supplied
Streptomycin Sulfate Injection 400 mg/mL, Lyophilized cake/Powder for injection 200 mg/mL

Action
PHARMACOLOGY: Interferes with protein synthesis.

PHARMACOKINETICS/DYNAMICS:

Absorption: Peak serum levels are reached within 1 hr following IM injection.

Distribution: Appreciable concentrations are found in all organ tissue except the brain.

Excretion: Following a single 600 mg dose, 29% to 89% is excreted in the urine within 24 hr.

Indications
Treatment of moderate to severe infections caused by susceptible strains of *Mycobacterium tuberculosis* and nontuberculosis infections.

Contraindications
Hypersensitivity to aminoglycosides or any component of the product.

Route/Dosage
Tuberculosis
ADULTS: **IM** 15 mg/kg/day (max, 1 g) or 25 to 30 mg/kg 2 or 3 times weekly (max, 1.5 g).
CHILDREN: **IM** 20 to 40 mg/kg/day (max, 1 g) or 25 to 30 mg/kg 2 or 3 times weekly (max, 1.5 g).

Tularemia
IM 1 to 2 g/day in divided doses for 7 to 14 days until patient is afebrile for 5 to 7 days.

Plague
IM 2 g/day in 2 divided doses for minimum of 10 days.

Bacterial Endocarditis
Streptococcal – **IM** 1 g bid for 1 wk then 0.5 g bid for the second week in combination with penicillin. In patients over 60 yr, give 0.5 g bid for the entire 2 wk period.
Enterococcal – **IM** 1 g bid for 2 wk and 0.5 g bid for 4 wk in combination with penicillin.

Concomitant Use with Other Agents
ADULTS: **IM** 1 to 2 g in divided doses q 6 to

12 hr for moderate to severe infections (max, 2 g/day).
CHILDREN: **IM** 20 to 40 mg/kg/day in divided doses q 6 to 12 hr, avoiding excessive doses.

Interactions
Ethacrynic acid, furosemide, mannitol, possibly other diuretics: May potentiate the ototoxic effects of streptomycin.
Neurotoxic or nephrotoxic agents (eg, colistin, cyclosporine, gentamicin, kanamycin, neomycin, paromomycin, polymyxin B, tobramycin): May increase the risk of neuro- or nephrotoxicity and should be avoided.

Lab Test Interferences
None well documented.

Adverse Reactions
DERM: Rash; urticaria; exfoliative dermatitis.
EENT: Vestibular ototoxicity (eg, nausea, vomiting, vertigo); cochlear ototoxicity (deafness); amblyopia.
GU: Azotemia; nephrotoxicity.
HEMA: Eosinophilia; leukopenia; thrombocytopenia; pancytopenia; hemolytic anemia.
OTHER: Paresthesia of face; fever; angioneurotic edema; anaphylaxis; muscular weakness.

> **WARNING:**
> *Neurotoxicity:* Risk of severe neurotoxic reactions (including cochlear and vestibular dysfunction, optic nerve dysfunction, peripheral neuritis, arachnoiditis, and encephalopathy) increase in patients with impaired renal function or pre-renal azotemia.
> *Nephrotoxicity:* Avoid concurrent use of nephrotoxic/neurotoxic drugs.
> Monitor renal function carefully. Patients with reduced function should have reduced doses. Peak serum concentrations in patients with renal dysfunction should be 20 to 25 mcg/mL or less.

Precautions
Pregnancy: Category D. Crosses the placenta and may cause fetal harm.
Lactation: Excreted in breast milk.
Children: See Route/Dosage section.
Elderly: Because of increased risk of side effects, reduce the dose in patients over 60 yr.
Superinfection: May result in bacterial or fungal overgrowth of nonsusceptible microorganisms.
Ototoxicity: May occur.
Nitrogen retention: Reduced doses are necessary.

PATIENT CARE CONSIDERATIONS

Administration/Storage
- For IM administration only. Do not administer SC, intradermal, or IV.
- Reconstitute following manufacturer's instructions.
- Inspect reconstituted solution visually before administration. Do not administer if solution is cloudy, discolored, or contains particulate matter.
- Administer prescribed dose by deep IM injection into large muscle mass taking precautions to avoid injection near peripheral nerves.
- Store injection in refrigerator (36° to 46°F).
- Store cake/powder for injection at controlled room temperature (59° to 86°F). Reconstituted solution may be stored for up to 1 wk at controlled room temperature (59° to 86°F). Protect reconstituted solution from light.

Assessment/Interventions
- Obtain patient history, including drug history and any known allergies. Note history of previous reaction to aminoglycosides, auditory impairment, renal impairment, or coadministration of medications with neurotoxic or nephrotoxic potential.
- Ensure that culture and susceptibility test results indicate sensitivity to streptomycin.
- Ensure that caloric and audiometric measurements are performed prior to starting therapy and periodically during therapy.
- Ensure that renal function is evaluated prior to starting therapy and periodically during therapy.
- Assess patient for auditory and vestibular dysfunction. Notify health care provider immediately if noted.

Patient/Family Education
- Explain name, dose, action, and potential side effects of drug.
- Advise patient that medication will be prepared and administered by a health care provider in a health care setting.
- Review dosing schedule and prescribed length of therapy with patient.
- Instruct patient to immediately report the following to health care provider: headache, nausea, vomiting, ringing in the ears, vertigo (feeling of whirling motion), dizziness, roaring noises, sense of fullness in ears, hearing loss, itching, rash.
- Advise women to contact health care provider if pregnant, planning to become pregnant, or breastfeeding.
- Caution patient to not take any prescription or OTC medications or dietary supplements unless advised to do so by health care provider.
- Advise patient that follow-up visits and lab tests will be required to monitor therapy and to keep appointments.

Streptozocin

(STREP-toe-ZOE-sin)

Class Alkylating agent/Nitrosoureas

How Supplied
Zanosar Powder for injection 1 g

Action
PHARMACOLOGY: Streptozocin is a naturally occurring nitrosourea that contains a glucose moiety not present in the other compounds. The glucose moiety is believed to contribute to reduced myelotoxicity. Streptozocin inhibits DNA synthesis without significantly affecting RNA or protein synthesis in bacterial and mammalian cells. The biochemical mechanism leading to mammalian cell death has not been established but is at least partially caused by DNA alkylation causing intrastrand crosslinks. After rapid IV injection, unchanged drug is rapidly cleared from the plasma (half-life, 35 min).

PHARMACOKINETICS/DYNAMICS:

Absorption: Streptozocin disappears from blood very quickly.

Distribution: Streptozocin concentrates in liver and kidneys

Metabolism: As much as 20% of the drug (or metabolites containing an N-nitrosourea group) is metabolized and/or excreted by the kidney.

Excretion: As much as 20% of the drug (or metabolites containing an N-nitrosourea group) is metabolized and/or excreted by the kidney.

Indications
Adult/Pediatric: Symptomatic or progressive metastatic islet cell carcinoma of the pancreas.

Contraindications
Standard considerations.

Route/Dosage
Pancreatic Islet Cell Carcinoma
ADULT: **IV** 500 mg/m^2/day for 5 days q 4 to 6 wk; or 1000 mg/m^2 once a week for the first 2 wk, increased to a max of 1500 mg/m^2 if necessary. Do not give more than 1500 mg/m^2 in a single dose because of dose-related nephrotoxicity. Median total dose to maximal response is 4000 mg/m^2.
PEDIATRIC: **IV** No pediatric dosing information is available.

Adjustment in Renal Insufficiency
ADULT: **IV** If Ccr is more than 50 mL/min, administer 100% of usual dose. If Ccr is 10 to 50 mL/min, administer 75% of usual dose. If Ccr is less than 10 mL/min, administer 50% of usual dose.

Interactions
Nephrotoxic agents: Because streptozocin is nephrotoxic, do not use in combination with other nephrotoxic agents.

Lab Test Interferences
None well documented.

Adverse Reactions
CNS: Confusion, lethargy, depression (observed with 5 day continuous infusion).
GI: Very high potential for nausea and vomiting, diarrhea, jaundice, transient elevation of LFTs, hypoalbuminemia.
HEMA: Bone marrow suppression, nadir at 7 to 14 days.
METAB: Hypoglycemia, usually within 24 hr of the dose.
RENAL: Dose-related and cumulative renal tubular damage in 25% to 75% of patients, renal failure, reversible if streptozocin stopped early.

> **WARNING:**
> GI: Nausea and vomiting usually begin 1 to 4 hr after administration and last for 24 hr; occasionally requiring discontinuation of drug therapy.
> *Liver dysfunction, hematological changes:* Have been observed.
> *Renal toxicity:* Renal toxicity occurs in up to 2/3 of all patients treated with streptozocin, as evidenced by azotemia, anuria, hypophosphatemia, glycosuria, and renal tubular acidosis. Such toxicity is dose-related and cumulative and may be severe or fatal.

Precautions
Pregnancy: Category C.
Lactation: Undetermined.
Extravasation risk: Local irritation or phlebitis may occur. Refer to your institution specific protocol.
Hypoglycemia: Mild to moderate abnormalities of glucose tolerance have generally been reversible, but insulin shock with hypoglycemia has occurred.
Hydration: Because of renal toxicity, keep the patient well hydrated.
Topical exposure: May pose a carcinogenic hazard following topical exposure if not properly handled.

PATIENT CARE CONSIDERATIONS
Administration/Storage
- Refrigerate. Protect from light.
- Add 9.5 mL of 5% Dextrose Injection or 0.9% Sodium Chloride to the vial producing a clear, pale gold solution (concentration is 100 mg/mL). Dilute further for IV infusion with 5% Dextrose or 0.9% Sodium Chloride.
- Reconstituted solutions are stable for up to 48 hr at room temperature and for up to 96 hr under refrigeration. Use streptozocin solutions within 24 hr because they are preservative-free. The manufacturer recommends disposal within 12 hr of reconstitution. A color change from pale gold to dark brown indicates decomposition.
- Diluted 2 mg/mL solutions prepared with 5% Dextrose or 0.9% Sodium Chloride are stable for up to 48 hr at room temperature and for up to 96 hr under refrigeration.
- Rapid IV injection, or IV infusion over 15 min to 6 hr. Bolus administration may cause intense venous pain.

Assessment/Interventions
- Monitor renal function before and after each course of therapy. Obtain serial urinalysis, BUN, plasma creatinine, serum electrolytes, and Ccr prior to, at least weekly during, and for 4 wk after drug administration. Serial urinalysis is particularly important for the early detection of proteinuria; quantitate with a 24-hr collection when proteinuria is detected. Mild proteinuria is one of the first signs of renal toxicity. Reduce the dose or discontinue treatment in the presence of significant renal toxicity. In patients with preexisting renal disease, judge potential benefit of streptozocin against known risk of serious renal damage. Do not use in combination or concomitantly with other potential nephrotoxins.
- Have 50% Dextrose Injection on hand, especially when the first dose is administered, because of the risk of hypoglycemia.
- Assess renal function prior to, weekly during, and for 4 wk after streptozocin therapy.
- Ample fluid intake and subsequent increase in urine output may aid excretion and reduce renal toxicity.
- Closely monitor for evidence of renal, hepatic, and hematopoietic toxicity. Perform CBCs and LFTs at least weekly. Dosage adjustments or discontinuance of the drug may be indicated, depending upon the degree of toxicity.

Patient/Family Education
- Explain name, action, and potential side effects of drug.
- Advise patient, family, or caregiver that medication will be prepared and administered by health care provider in a health care setting.
- Review dosing schedule (daily or weekly dose) with patient, family, or caregiver.
- Advise patient, family, or caregiver to immediately report any of the following to the health care provider: decreased urination; fever, chills, or other signs of infection; unusual bleeding or bruising; pain, redness, or swelling at injection site.
- Advise patient, family, or caregiver to report any of the following to the health care provider: persistent nausea, vomiting, diarrhea, or appetite loss; persistent or worsening general body weakness.
- Caution patient that medication may cause confusion, drowsiness, and depression and to use caution when driving or performing other tasks that require mental alertness or coordination.
- Instruct patient not to take any prescription or OTC medications or dietary supplements unless advised to do so by health care provider.
- Caution women of childbearing potential to avoid becoming pregnant during therapy.
- Instruct women of childbearing potential to notify health care provider if pregnant, planning to become pregnant, or breastfeeding.
- Advise patient, family, or caregiver that frequent follow-up visits and laboratory tests will be required to monitor therapy and to keep appointments.

Strontium-89 Chloride
(STRAHN-shee-uhm 89 KLOR-ide)
Class Radiopharmaceuticals
How Supplied
Metastron Injection 148 MBq, 4 mCi
Action
PHARMACOLOGY: Following IV injection, soluble strontium compounds behave like their calcium analogs, clearing rapidly from blood and selectively localizing in bone mineral. Uptake of strontium by bone occurs preferentially in sites of active osteogenesis. Selectively irradiates sites of primary metastatic bone involvement with minimal effect on soft tissues distant from bone lesions.

Indications Painful skeletal metastases.
Contraindications None well documented.

Route/Dosage
Painful Skeletal Metastases
ADULTS: **IV** 148 MBq, 4 mCi given by slow IV injection (1 to 2 min). Alternatively, a dose of 1.5 to 2.2 MBq/kg, 40 to 60 mcCi/kg may be used. Repeat doses are generally not recommended at intervals of less than 90 days.

Interactions
None well documented.

Lab Test Interferences
None well documented.

Adverse Reactions
OTHER: Fatal septicemia following neutropenia; transient increase in bone pain at 36 to 72 hr after injection; chills and fever 12 hr after injection without long-term sequelae.

Precautions
Pregnancy: Category D.
Lactation: It is recommended that nursing be discontinued by mothers.
Children: Safety and efficacy in children less than 18 yr have not been established.
Carcinogenesis: It is a potential carcinogen.
Bone metastases: Not indicated for use in patients with cancer not involving bone. Confirm presence of bone metastases prior to therapy.
Radiopharmaceuticals: Only health care providers who are qualified by training and experience in the safe use and handling of radionuclides and whose experience and training have been approved by the appropriate government agency authorized to license the use of radionuclides should use radiopharmaceuticals.
Flushing sensation: A calcium-like flushing sensation has been observed following a rapid (less than 30 sec injection) administration.

PATIENT CARE CONSIDERATIONS
Administration/Storage
- The vial is shipped in a transportation shield with an approximately 3 mm lead wall thickness. Store the vial and its contents inside its transportation container at room temperature (15° to 25°C; 59° to 77°F).

Assessment/Interventions
- Measure dose by suitable radioactivity calibration system immediately prior to use.
- Bone marrow toxicity is to be expected following administration, particularly WBCs and platelets. It is recommended that the patient's peripheral blood cell counts be monitored at least once every other wk.
- Recovery occurs slowly, typically reaching pre-administration levels 6 mo after treatment unless the patient's disease or additional therapy intervenes.
- In considering repeat administration, carefully evaluate hematologic response to initial dose, current platelet level, and other evidence of marrow depletion.
- Verification of dose and patient identification is necessary prior to use because strontium-89 delivers a relatively high dose of radioactivity.
- In patients with renal dysfunction, weigh the possible risks of administering strontium-89 against the possible benefits.
- Restrict treatment to patients with well-documented metastatic bone disease.
- Use with caution in patients with platelet counts less than 60,000 and white cell counts less than 2400.
- Like other radioactive drugs, handle with care and take safety measures to minimize radiation to clinical personnel.
- Administration to patients with very short life expectancy is not recommended.
- Take special precautions, such as urinary catheterization, following administration to patients who are incontinent to minimize the risk of radioactive contamination of clothing, bed linen, and the patient's environment.

Patient/Family Education
- The patient may feel a slight increase in pain for 2 or 3 days beginning 2 or 3 days after injection. The health care provider may suggest a temporary increase in the dose of pain medication until the pain is under control. After about 1 to 2 wk, the pain should begin to diminish.
- The patient can eat and drink normally and there is no need to avoid alcohol or caffeine unless already advised to do so. The health care provider may want to carry out periodic, routine blood tests.
- Advise patients to tell any health practitioner who is giving them medical treatment that they have received strontium-89.
- During the first week after injection, strontium-89 will be present in the blood and urine. It is therefore important to consider the following precautions for 1 wk: 1) Where a normal toilet is available, use in preference to a urinal. Flush the toilet twice; 2) Wipe up any spilled urine with a tissue and flush it away; 3) Always wash hands after using the toilet; 4) Immediately wash any linen or clothes that become stained with urine or blood. Wash them separately from other clothes, and rinse thoroughly; 5) If any urine collection device is used, follow instructions on its use; 6) Wash away any spilled blood if a cut occurs.
- In many people who receive strontium-89, the effect lasts for several months. If pain returns, consult the health care provider.

Succimer

(SUX-ih-mer)
Class Detoxification/Chelating agent
How Supplied
Chemet Capsules 100 mg
Action
PHARMACOLOGY: Forms water soluble chelate with lead, increasing the urinary excretion.

PHARMACOKINETICS/DYNAMICS:
Absorption: Rapid but variable absorption with peak levels in 1 to 2 hr.

Excretion: Approximately 49% of the dose excreted (39% feces, 9% urine, 1% as carbon dioxide via the lungs). Elimination $t_½$ about 2 days.

Indications Treatment of lead poisoning in children with blood levels above 45 mcg/dL.
Unlabeled use(s): Treatment of heavy metal poisonings (mercury, arsenic); however, further study is needed.

Contraindications Standard considerations.
Route/Dosage
CHILDREN 12 MO AND OLDER: **PO** Start with 10 mg/kg or 350 mg/m^2 q 8 hr for 5 days. Reduce frequency of administration to 10 mg/kg or 350 mg/m^2 q 12 hr for an additional 14 days. A course of treatment lasts 19 days. Repeated courses may be necessary if indicated by weekly monitoring of lead blood concentration. A minimum of 14 days between courses is recommended unless lead blood levels indicate the need for more prompt treatment. In young children unable to swallow capsules, the contents of the capsule can be sprinkled on a small amount of soft food or placed on a spoon and followed with fruit drink.

Interactions
Chelating therapy: Coadministration with other chelation therapy is not recommended.

Lab Test Interferences May interfere with serum and urinary laboratory tests (in vitro, succimer caused false-positive results with ketones in urine using nitroprusside reagents [eg, Ketostix] and falsely decreased serum uric acid and CPK measurements).

Adverse Reactions Incidence of adverse reactions stated for children (unless adult is stated), most reactions occur more frequently in adults.
CV: Arrhythmia (1.8% adults).
CNS: Head pain, heavy head/tired, head cold, headache (5.2% children, 15.7% adults); drowsiness, dizziness, sensorimotor neuropathy, sleepiness, paresthesia (1% children, 12.7% adults).
DERM: Papular rash, herpetic rash, rash, mucocutaneous eruptions, pruritus (2.6% children, 11.2% adults).
GI: Nausea, vomiting, diarrhea, appetite loss, hemorrhoidal symptoms, loose stools, metallic taste in mouth (12% children, 20.9% adults); abdominal cramps, stomach pains (5.2% children, 15.7% adults).
GU: Moniliasis (5.2% children, 15.7% adults); decreased urination, voiding difficulty, proteinuria increased (3.7% adults).
HEMA: Mild to moderate neutropenia, increased platelet count, intermittent eosinophilia (0.5% children, 1.5% adults).
METAB: Elevated AST, ALT, alkaline phosphatase, elevated serum cholesterol (4.2% children, 10.4% adults).
MUSC: Back pain, rib pain (5.2% children, 15.7% adults); kneecap pain, leg pains (3% adults).
RESP: Throat sore, rhinorrhea, nasal congestion, cough (3.7% children, 0.7% adults).
SPEC SENSE: Cloudy film in eye, ears plugged, otitis media, eyes watery (1% children, 12.7% adults).
OTHER: Chills, flank pain, fever, flu-like symptoms (5.2% children, 15.7% adults)

Precautions
Pregnancy: Category C.
Lactation: Undetermined.
Children: Safety and efficacy not established in children under 12 mo.
Hypersensitivity: Consider the possibility upon readministration and during the initial courses.
Renal function impairment: Adequately hydrate patients undergoing treatment. Use with caution in patients with compromised renal function. While succimer appears to be dialyzable, lead chelates are not.
Hepatic function impairment: Transient mild elevations of serum transaminases have been reported. Monitor serum transaminases before the start of therapy and at least weekly during therapy. Closely monitor patients with a history of liver disease.
Infection: If an infection is suspected, a CBC with WBC differential and direct platelet count should be obtained.
Lead poisoning: Not a substitute for effective abatement of lead exposure.
Neutropenia: Mild to moderate neutropenia has been reported; however, a causal relationship has not been established.
Rebound lead blood levels: Due to redistribution of lead from bone stores to soft tissue and blood, elevated lead blood levels and associated symptoms may return rapidly after discontinuation of succimer. Therefore, monitor for rebound lead blood levels at least weekly.

PATIENT CARE CONSIDERATIONS
Administration/Storage
- For treatment of lead poisoning only. Not to be used for prophylaxis of lead poisoning in a lead-containing environment.
- Administer prescribed dose once q 8 hr for 5 days then q 12 hr for 2 wk.
- Swallow capsules whole. Do not crush, cut, or chew.
- If patient has difficulty swallowing whole capsules, the capsules may be opened and the medicated beads sprinkled on a small amount of soft food or placed in a spoon and followed with a fruit drink.
- Store at controlled room temperature (59° to 77°F).

Assessment/Interventions
- Obtain patient history, including drug history and any known allergies. Note history of renal impairment, liver disease, or concurrent or recent (eg, within 4 wk) therapy with other chelation therapy.
- Ensure that at least 4 wk separate treatment with succimer from previous treatment with other chelation therapy.
- Ensure that patient is adequately hydrated during therapy.
- Ensure that transaminases and CBC with WBC differential and direct platelet counts are obtained prior to and weekly during therapy with succimer.
- Discontinue or withhold therapy if absolute neutrophil count is less than 1200/µL. Monitor patient closely to document recovery of absolute neutrophil count to above 1500/µL or to patient's baseline neutrophil count. Restart succimer only if benefit of therapy clearly outweighs potential risk of another episode of neutropenia.
- Assess patient for any sign of infection. Inform health care provider immediately if infection is suspected. Be prepared to obtain CBC with WBC differential.
- Assess patient for side effects. Inform health care provider if noted and significant.
- Ensure that blood lead levels are determined at least once/wk until stable following discontinuation of therapy.
- Ensure that efforts are undertaken to identify and remove the source of lead exposure.

Patient/Family Education
- Explain name, dose, action, and potential side effects of drug.
- Advise patient or caregiver that prescribed dose is to be taken q 8 hr for 5 days and then q 12 hr for 2 wk. Advise patient or caregiver that regimen may need to be repeated if blood lead levels are still elevated.
- Advise patient or caregiver that good hydration will be important during therapy.
- Instruct patient or caregiver to immediately report rash or any signs of infection to health care provider.
- Advise women to notify health care provider if pregnant, planning to become pregnant, or breastfeeding.
- Instruct patient not to take any prescription or OTC medications or dietary supplements unless advised by health care provider.
- Advise patient or caregiver that the source of lead exposure must be identified and removed to prevent further exposure to lead.
- Advise patient that follow-up visits and lab tests will be required to monitor therapy and to keep appointments.

Sucralfate

(sue-KRAL-fate)

Class Gastrointestinal

How Supplied
Carafate Tablets 1 g, Suspension 1 g/10 mL
✣ Novo-Sucralfate ♦ Nu-Sucralfate ♦ PMS-Sucralfate

Action
PHARMACOLOGY: Adheres to ulcer in acidic gastric juice, forming protective layer that serves as barrier against acid, bile salts, and enzymes present in stomach and duodenum.

PHARMACOKINETICS/DYNAMICS:
Absorption: Sucralfate is minimally absorbed from the GI tract. Binding to the ulcer site has been shown for up to 6 hr; approximately 30% of a dose is retained within the GI tract for at least 3 hr.

Distribution: Approximately 95% of a dose remains in the GI tract, with only minute amounts being distributed into liver, kidneys, skeletal muscle, adipose tissue, and skin.

Excretion: Sucralfate is eliminated primarily in urine. Following reaction of sucralfate with hydrochloric acid, nonmetabolized sucrose sulfate is formed in the GI tract.

Duration: Duration of action of sucralfate depends on the time that the drug is in contact with the site because sucralfate exerts its effects directly at the site of the ulcer.

Indications Short-term treatment of duodenal ulcer; maintenance therapy of duodenal ulcer (tablets only). **Unlabeled use(s):** Treatment of gastric ulcers; reflux and peptic esophagitis; treatment of NSAID- or aspirin-induced GI symptoms and mucosal damage; prevention of stress ulcers and GI bleeding in critically ill patients; treatment of oral and esophageal ulcers caused by radiation, chemotherapy, and sclerotherapy; treatment of oral ulcerations and dysphagia in patients with epidermolysis bullosa.

Contraindications Standard considerations.

Route/Dosage
Active Duodenal Ulcer
ADULTS: **PO** 1 g qid on empty stomach (1 hr before meals and at bedtime) for 4 to 8 wk. Maintenance (tablets only): 1 g bid.

Interactions
Aluminum-containing antacids: May increase total body burden of aluminum.
Cimetidine, ciprofloxacin (and other quinolone antibiotics), diclofenac, digoxin, hydantoins (eg, phenytoin), ketoconazole, levothyroxine, penicillamine, quinidine, ranitidine, tetracycline, theophylline: Oral absorption and pharmacologic action of these agents may be reduced if given with sucralfate. Administer 2 hr apart from sucralfate.

Lab Test Interferences None well documented.

Adverse Reactions
CNS: Dizziness; insomnia; vertigo; headache.
DERM: Rash; pruritus.
GI: Constipation (2%); diarrhea; nausea; vomiting; dry mouth; indigestion; flatulence.
OTHER: Back pain.

Precautions
Pregnancy: Category B.
Lactation: Undetermined.
Children: Safety and efficacy not established.
Chronic renal failure/dialysis: Small amounts of aluminum may be absorbed from sucralfate, and concomitant use of other aluminum-containing products may increase total body burden of aluminum. Aluminum is not removed by dialysis and excretion through kidneys is impaired in patients with chronic renal failure. Aluminum accumulation and toxicity (eg, aluminum osteodystrophy, osteomalacia, encephalopathy) have occurred.

Overdosage: Signs and Symptoms
Dyspepsia, abdominal pain, nausea, vomiting.

PATIENT CARE CONSIDERATIONS

Administration/Storage
- Administer with full glass of water, on empty stomach, at least 1 hr before meals and at bedtime.
- Shake suspension well before measuring dose. Use dosing cup or spoon to measure prescribed dose.
- Administer antacids, if needed for pain relief, ½ hr before or after sucralfate.
- Administer other medications either 2 hr before or after sucralfate to minimize effects on absorption.
- Store tablets and suspension at controlled room temperature (68° to 77°F).

Assessment/Interventions
- Obtain patient history, including drug history and any known allergies. Note renal impairment.
- Ensure that other products containing aluminum (eg, some antacids) are not used concurrently in patients with chronic renal failure.
- Assess symptoms before starting therapy and periodically during treatment. Inform health care provider if symptoms do not improve or appear to be getting worse.
- Ensure that progress of the peptic ulcer under treatment is being followed appropriately (eg, contrast radiology, endoscopy) and that tests for occult blood in the stool, hemoglobin, and hematocrit are being periodically evaluated to rule out bleeding from the ulcer.
- Monitor patient for GI, CNS, and general body side effects. Inform health care provider if noted and significant.

Patient/Family Education
- Explain name, dose, action, and potential side effects of drug.
- Advise patient to take prescribed dose with a full glass of water, on empty stomach, at least 1 hr before meals and at bedtime.
- Advise patient that initial treatment of ulcer requires taking prescribed dose qid, but that maintenance treatment is usually just 2 doses/day. Advise patient taking 2 doses/day to take first dose before breakfast and the second dose before bedtime.
- Advise patient using suspension to shake suspension well before measuring dose and to use a dosing cup or spoon to measure prescribed dose.
- Advise patient to continue to take as prescribed, even after ulcer symptoms have gone away, to ensure max healing of the ulcer.
- Advise patient that antacids can be used as needed for pain relief, but to take at least 30 min before or after the sucralfate.
- Advise patient to take other medications either 2 hr before or after sucralfate to minimize effects on absorption.

- Advise patient that constipation is the most common side effect and that increasing fluid and fiber intake may prevent this problem from developing.
- Advise patient to notify health care provider if symptoms do not improve or appear to be getting worse, or if intolerable side effects (eg, constipation) develop.
- Advise women to notify health care provider if pregnant, planning to become pregnant, or breastfeeding.
- Advise patient not to take any prescription or OTC drugs or dietary supplements without consulting health care provider.
- Advise patient that follow-up visits may be necessary to monitor therapy and to keep appointments.

Sufentanil Citrate

(sue-FEN-tuh-nill SIH-trate)

Class Narcotic analgesic

How Supplied
Sufenta Injection 50 mcg (as citrate)/mL

Action

PHARMACOLOGY: Relieves pain by stimulating opiate receptors in CNS; causes respiratory depression, peripheral vasodilation, inhibition of intestinal peristalsis, sphincter of Oddi spasm, stimulation of chemoreceptors that cause vomiting and increased bladder tone.

PHARMACOKINETICS/DYNAMICS:

Absorption: Sufentanil T_{max} is 1.4 min. After epidural administration totalling 5 to 40 mcg during labor and delivery, maternal and neonatal plasma concentrations were at or near the 0.05 to 0.1 ng/mL limit of detection and were slightly higher in mothers than infants.

Distribution: Sufentanil is 93% protein bound in males, 91% bound in mothers, and 79% bound in neonates.

Metabolism: Sufentanil is metabolized in liver and small intestines.

Excretion: Sufentanil t½ is 164 min. Approximately 80% is excreted within 24 hr and only 2% of the dose is eliminated as unchanged drug.

Onset: Onset of action is immediate.

Indications Adjunct for surgical analgesia; induction of primary anesthesia for major surgical procedures requiring favorable myocardial or cerebral oxygen balance or when extended postoperative ventilation is anticipated; epidural analgesia with bupivacaine during labor and vaginal delivery.

Contraindications Upper airway obstruction; acute asthma; diarrhea caused by poisoning or toxins.

Route/Dosage

General Surgery (with Nitrous Oxide/Oxygen)
ADULTS: **IV** 1 to 2 mcg/kg initially; 10 to 25 mcg prn for maintenance.

Major Surgical Procedures (with Nitrous Oxide/Oxygen)
ADULTS: **IV** 2 to 8 mcg/kg initially; 10 to 50 mcg prn for maintenance.

Major Cardiovascular Surgery/Neurosurgery (with 100% Oxygen)
ADULTS: **IV** 8 to 30 mcg/kg initially; 25 to 50 mcg prn for maintenance.
CHILDREN LESS THAN 12 YR: **IV** 10 to 25 mcg/kg initially; 25 to 50 mcg prn for maintenance.

Labor and Delivery
ADULTS: **Epidural** 10 to 15 mcg sufentanil mixed with 10 mL bupivacaine 0.125% with or without epinephrine. Can give total of 3 doses at least 1 hr intervals until delivery.

Interactions

Barbiturate anesthetics: May cause increased CNS and respiratory depression.

Beta blockers: The incidence and degree of bradycardia and hypotension during induction of sufentanil may be greater in patients on chronic beta blocker therapy.

Calcium channel blockers: The incidence and degree of bradycardia and hypotension during induction of sufentanil may be greater in patients on chronic calcium channel blocker therapy.

Nitrous oxide: Nitrous oxide may cause cardiovascular depression with high-dose sufentanil.

Lab Test Interferences Increased amylase and lipase for up to 24 hr after dose may occur.

Adverse Reactions

CV: Hypotension; orthostatic hypotension; hypertension; bradycardia; tachycardia; arrhythmias.
CNS: Sedation.
DERM: Pruritus.
GI: Nausea; vomiting.
RESP: Bronchospasm; depression of cough reflex; respiratory depression; postoperative respiratory depression; chest wall rigidity.
OTHER: Chills; intraoperative muscle movement; tolerance.

Precautions

Pregnancy: Category C.
Lactation: Undetermined.
Children: Safety and efficacy have been demonstrated in limited number of children less than 2 yr undergoing cardiovascular surgery.
Elderly: May require dosage reduction.

Renal function impairment: Duration of action may be prolonged; dosage reduction may be required.
Hepatic function impairment: Duration of action may be prolonged; dosage reduction may be required.
Special risk patients: Use drug with caution in patients with decreased respiratory reserve, head injury, increased intracranial pressure, or hypoxia.
Drug dependence: Has abuse potential.
Hypoventilation: Naloxone and intubation equipment must be available in case hypoventilation occurs.
Obese patients: If patient is greater than 20% above ideal weight, dose must be adjusted based on ideal body weight.
Skeletal muscle rigidity: May cause skeletal muscle rigidity, particularly of the truncal muscles. The incidence and severity of muscle rigidity is usually dose-related.

Overdosage: Signs and Symptoms
Miosis, respiratory and CNS depression, circulatory collapse, seizures, cardiopulmonary arrest, death.

PATIENT CARE CONSIDERATIONS

Administration/Storage
- For direct IV administration, administer slowly over 1 to 2 min.
- Store at room temperature. Protect from light.
- Limit epidural or intrathecal administration of preservative free sufentanil to the lumbar area.

Assessment/Interventions
- Obtain patient history, including drug history and any known allergies.
- Assess patient for head injury, pulmonary disease, or decreased respiratory reserve.
- Maintain narcotic antagonist and resuscitative equipment at bedside.
- Monitor respiratory rate and BP closely during administration.
- Observe for evidence of effective induction of anesthesia.
- Monitor vital signs at frequent intervals postoperatively.

Patient/Family Education
- Inform patient that nausea, vomiting or constipation may occur and advise patient to notify health care provider should these symptoms become prominent.
- Advise patient to ask for assistance with ambulation.
- Instruct patient to report these symptoms to health care provider: shortness of breath or difficulty breathing.
- Caution patient to avoid sudden position changes to prevent orthostatic hypotension.

Sulfadiazine

(SULL-fah-DIE-ah-zeen)

Class Anti-infective/Sulfonamide

How Supplied
Sulfadiazine Tablets 500 mg

Action
PHARMACOLOGY: Exerts bacteriostatic action by competing with PABA, an essential component in folic acid synthesis, therefore preventing synthesis of folic acid needed by bacteria for growth.

PHARMACOKINETICS/DYNAMICS:

Absorption: Absorbed rapidly from the GI tract. A peak level of 6.04 mg per 100 mL is reached 4 hr after a single 2 g oral dose (4.65 mg per 100 mL is free or active drug).

Distribution: Protein binding is 38% to 48%. Diffuses into CSF, reaching concentrations of 32% to 65% of blood levels.

Metabolism: At least 1 acetylated form.

Excretion: Excreted primarily in the urine, reaching concentrations that are 10 to 25 times higher then serum levels. About 10% of a single oral dose is excreted in the first 6 hr, 50% within 24 hr, and 60% to 85% in 48 to 72 hr. 15% to 40% is excreted in the acetyl form.

Indications Treatment of chancroid, trachoma, inclusion conjunctivitis, nocardiosis, UTI, toxoplasmosis encephalitis, malaria, meningococcal meningitis, acute otitis media; prophylaxis against meningococcal meningitis and recurrences of rheumatic fevers; with streptomycin as adjunctive therapy for *Haemophilus influenza* meningitis.

Contraindications Hypersensitivity to sulfonamides; infants less than 2 mo of age (except as adjunctive therapy with pyrimethamine in treating congenital toxoplasmosis); pregnancy at term; nursing period.

Route/Dosage

ADULTS: **PO** 2 to 4 g, divided into 3 to 6 doses, q 24 hr.

CHILDREN OLDER THAN 2 MO OF AGE: **PO** Initially, one-half the 24-hr dose.

Maintenance
150 mg/kg or 4 g/m^2, divided into 4 to 6 doses, q 24 hr.

Rheumatic Fever Prophylaxis
Under 30 kg give 500 mg q 24 hr; over 30 kg give 1 g q 24 hr.

Interactions
Anticoagulants, hydantoins (eg, phenytoin), methotrexate, sulfonylureas, thiazide diuretics, uricosuric agents: Effects of these agents may be enhanced by sulfadiazine.
Indomethacin, probenecid, salicylates: May increase free sulfadiazine plasma levels, increasing the pharmacologic and adverse effects.

Lab Test Interferences
None well documented.

Adverse Reactions
CNS: Headache; peripheral neuritis; mental depression; convulsions; ataxia; hallucinations; vertigo; insomnia.
EENT: Tinnitus.
GI: Nausea; emesis; abdominal pain; diarrhea; anorexia; pancreatitis; stomatitis.
GU: Crystalluria; stone formation; toxic nephrosis with oliguria and anuria; periarteritis nodosa; lupus erythematosus phenomenon.
HEMA: Agranulocytosis; aplastic anemia; thrombocytopenia; leukopenia; hemolytic anemia; purpura; hypoprothrombinemia; methemoglobinemia.
HEPA: Hepatitis.
OTHER: Allergic reactions including erythema multiforme (Stevens-Johnson syndrome), generalized skin eruptions, toxic epidermal necrolysis, urticaria, serum sickness, pruritus, exfoliative dermatitis, anaphylactoid reactions, periorbital edema, conjunctival and scleral injection, photosensitization, arthralgia, allergic myocarditis, drug fever, and chills.

Precautions
Pregnancy: Category C.
Lactation: Excreted in breast milk; use is contraindicated.
Children: Contraindicated in children under 2 mo of age (except as adjunctive therapy with pyrimethamine in treating toxoplasmosis).
Special risk patients: Use with caution in patients with impaired renal or hepatic function and those with severe allergy, or bronchial asthma.
Crystalluria: May occur if adequate fluid intake is not maintained.
Group A beta-hemolytic streptococcal infections: Do not use drug for this infection.
Hemolytic anemia: May occur in G-6-PD-deficient individuals.
Severe reactions: Severe reactions, including deaths, have been associated with hypersensitivity reactions, agranulocytosis, aplastic anemia, other blood dyscrasias, and renal and hepatic damage.
Sulfonamides: Has chemical similarities to some goitrogens, diuretics (eg, acetazolamide, thiazides), and oral hypoglycemic agents. Goiter production, diuresis, and hypoglycemia have occurred rarely in patients receiving sulfonamides; cross-sensitivity may exist.

PATIENT CARE CONSIDERATIONS

Administration/Storage
- Administer prescribed dose with a full glass of water.
- Administer without regard to meals but administer with food if GI upset occurs.
- Store tablets at ambient room temperature (59° to 86°F).

Assessment/Interventions
- Obtain patient history, including drug history and any known allergies. Note renal or hepatic impairment, glucose-6-phosphate dehydrogenase deficiency, asthma, allergic history, pregnancy at term, breastfeeding, or allergy to sulfonamide antibiotics or chemically related drugs (eg, sulfonylureas, thiazide and loop diuretics, carbonic anhydrase inhibitors).
- Review results of culture and sensitivity testing as available.
- Ensure that CBC and urinalysis are performed frequently during prolonged or high-dose therapy.
- Monitor for signs of infection, especially fever, and for positive response to antibiotic therapy.
- Ensure that patient is well-hydrated to prevent sulfonamide crystalluria and stone formation.
- Monitor patient for signs of allergic reaction. Discontinue therapy and immediately notify health care provider if noted. Be prepared to treat appropriately.
- Monitor patient for GI, CNS, and general body side effects. Report to health care provider if noted and significant.
- Withhold drug and notify health care provider immediately if any of the following symptoms occur: sore throat, fever, pallor, purpura, hematuria, jaundice

Patient/Family Education
- Explain name, dose, action, and potential side effects of drug.
- Review dosing schedule and prescribed length of therapy with patient.
- Advise patient to take each dose with a full (8 oz) glass of water without regard to meals.

- Advise patient to take with food if stomach upset occurs.
- Remind patient to complete entire course of therapy, even if symptoms of infection have disappeared.
- Advise patient to contact health care provider if infection does not seem to be improving or is worsening.
- Advise patient to drink fluids liberally (eg, eight 8-oz glasses of water daily) while taking this medication.
- Advise patient to discontinue therapy and contact health care provider immediately if any of the following symptoms occur: rash, hives, itching, sore throat, unexplained fever, pallor, purple spots under the skin, blood in urine, yellowing of the skin or eyes.
- Warn patient that diarrhea containing blood or pus may be a sign of a serious disorder and to seek medical care if noted and not treat at home.
- Advise patient to avoid unnecessary exposure to sunlight or tanning lamps and to use sunscreen and wear protective clothing to avoid photosensitivity reactions.
- Advise women to notify health care provider if pregnant, planning to become pregnant, or breastfeeding.
- Instruct patient not to take any prescription or OTC medications, dietary supplements, or herbal preparations unless advised by health care provider.
- Advise patient that follow-up examinations and lab tests may be required to monitor therapy and to keep appointments.

Sulfadoxine/Pyrimethamine

(SULL-fah-DOX-een/pihr-ih-METH-ah-meen)

Class Antimalarial

How Supplied
Fansidar Tablets 500 mg sulfadoxine and 25 mg pyrimethamine

Action
PHARMACOLOGY: The 2 components sequentially block 2 enzymes involved in the biosynthesis of folinic acid within the parasites.

Indications Treatment of *Plasmodium falciparum* malaria for those patients in whom chloroquine resistance is suspected; prophylaxis of malaria for travelers to areas where chloroquine-resistant *P. falciparum* malaria is endemic.

Contraindications Patients with severe renal insufficiency; marked liver parenchymal damage; blood dyscrasias; documented megaloblastic anemia caused by folate deficiency; infants less than 2 mo; pregnancy at term; during the nursing period; hypersensitivity to pyrimethamine, sulfonamides, or any component of the product.

Route/Dosage
Acute Attack of Malaria
ADULTS: **PO** Single dose of 2 to 3 tablets.
CHILDREN 9 TO 14 YR: **PO** Single dose of 2 tablets.
CHILDREN 4 TO 8 YR: **PO** Single dose of 1 tablet.
CHILDREN UNDER 4 YR: **PO** Single dose of ½ tablet.

Malaria Prophylaxis
Take first dose 1 or 2 days before departure to an endemic area; continue administration during the stay and for 4 to 6 wk after returning.

ADULTS: **PO** 1 tablet once/wk or 2 tablets once q 2 wk.
CHILDREN 9 TO 14 YR: **PO** ¾ tablet once/wk or 1½ tablets once q 2 wk.
CHILDREN 4 TO 8 YR: **PO** ½ tablet once/wk or 1 tablet once q 2 wk.
CHILDREN UNDER 4 YR: **PO** ¼ tablet once/wk or ½ tablet once q 2 wk.

Interactions
Antifolic drugs (eg, sulfonamides, trimethoprim-sulfamethoxazole): Should not be taken by patients receiving sulfadoxine/pyrimethamine.
Chloroquine: Incidence and severity of adverse reactions may be increased compared with taking sulfadoxine/pyrimethamine alone.

Lab Test Interferences None well documented.

Adverse Reactions
CNS: Headache; peripheral neuritis; mental depression; convulsions; ataxia; hallucinations; insomnia; apathy; fatigue; muscle weakness; nervousness; vertigo.
EENT: Tinnitus.
GI: Glossitis; stomatitis; nausea; emesis; abdominal pain; diarrhea; pancreatitis.
GU: Toxic nephrosis with oliguria and anuria.
HEMA: Agranulocytosis; aplastic anemia; megaloblastic anemia; thrombopenia; leukopenia; hemolytic anemia; purpura; hypoprothrombinemia; methemoglobinemia; eosinophilia.
HEPA: Hepatitis; hepatocellular necrosis.
RESP: Pulmonary infiltrates.
OTHER: Allergic reactions including erythema multiforme, Stevens-Johnson syndrome, generalized skin eruptions, toxic epidermal necrolysis, urticaria, serum sickness, pruritus, exfoliative dermatitis, anaphylactoid reactions, periorbital edema, conjunctival and scleral injection, photosensitization, arthralgia and allergic myocardi-

tis; drug fever; chills; periarteritis nodosa; lupus erythematosus.

> **WARNING:**
> Fatalities have occurred because of severe reactions, including Stevens-Johnson syndrome and toxic epidermal necrolysis. Discontinue sulfadoxine and pyrimethamine prophylaxis at the first appearance of skin rash, if a significant reduction in the count of any formed blood elements is noted, or upon the occurrence of active bacterial or fungal infections.

Precautions
Pregnancy: Category C. Contraindicated in pregnancy at term (may cross placenta, causing kernicterus).
Lactation: Secreted in breast milk (may cause kernicterus).
Children: Should not be given to infants under 2 mo because of inadequate development of glucuronide-forming enzyme system.
Elderly: Use with caution because of the greater frequency of decreased hepatic, renal, or cardiac function, and concomitant diseases or other drug therapy.
Special risk patients: Use with caution in patients with impaired renal or hepatic function, possible folate deficiency, severe allergy or bronchial asthma, or glucose-6-phosphate dehydrogenase deficiency.
Severe reaction: Fatalities have occurred because of fulminant hepatic necrosis, agranulocytosis, aplastic anemia, and other blood dyscrasias.

Overdosage: Signs and Symptoms
Anorexia, vomiting, CNS stimulation (including convulsions), megaloblastic anemia, leukopenia, thrombocytopenia, glossitis, crystalluria.

PATIENT CARE CONSIDERATIONS
Administration/Storage
Malaria Treatment:
- May be used alone or combined with quinine.
- Administer prescribed dose 1 time only with or without food.

Malaria Prophylaxis:
- Prescribed dose is taken 1 or 2 days before departure, once/wk or q 2 wk during stay in malaria-infected area, and for 4 to 6 wk following return.
- Store tablets at controlled room temperature (59° to 77°F).

Assessment/Interventions
- Obtain patient history, including drug history and any known allergies. Note presence of severe renal insufficiency, liver damage, blood dyscrasia, megaloblastic anemia caused by folate deficiency, folate deficiency, severe allergies, asthma, glucose-6-phosphate deficiency, pregnancy at term, breastfeeding, or history of allergy to pyrimethamine or sulfonamides.
- Ensure that microscopic urinalysis and renal function tests are performed periodically during therapy in patients with renal impairment.
- Ensure that CBCs are obtained periodically during prolonged therapy.
- Ensure that adequate fluid intake is maintained during therapy.
- Monitor patient for GI, CNS, DERM, and MUSC side effects. Inform health care provider if noted and significant.
- Discontinue medication and notify health care provider immediately if any of the following are noted: significant reduction in the count of any formed blood element (eg, RBCs, platelets, granulocytes), skin rash, fever or other signs of infection (eg, sore throat), joint pain, unexplained cough or shortness of breath, paleness, skin discoloration, yellowing of skin or eyes, tongue inflammation.

Patient/Family Education
- Explain name, dose, action, and potential side effects of drug.
- Advise patient to maintain adequate fluid intake (eg, 8 glasses of water/day) while taking medication.
- Instruct patient taking medication for prophylaxis that first dose should be taken 1 to 2 days prior to arrival in malaria-infected area and that subsequent doses should be taken on the same day of the week (or every other week if ordered) while in the malaria-infected area and for 4 to 6 wk after leaving the malaria-infected area.
- Advise patient that protective clothing, insect repellents, and bednets are important components of malaria prophylaxis
- Advise patient to discontinue therapy and notify health care provider immediately if any of the following occur: skin rash; fever or other signs of infection (eg, sore throat); joint pain; unexplained cough or shortness of breath; paleness; skin discoloration; yellowing of skin or eyes; tongue inflammation.
- Advise patient to notify health care provider if severe or persistent vomiting or diarrhea develop, other bothersome side effects occur, or if therapy is prematurely discontinued for any reason.
- Advise women of childbearing potential to use effective contraception while taking medi-

cation for malaria prophylaxis.
- Advise women to notify health care provider if pregnant, planning to become pregnant, or breastfeeding.
- Instruct patient not to take any prescription or OTC medications or dietary supplements unless advised by health care provider.
- Advise patient if a febrile illness develops during or after return from a malaria-endemic area to seek health care and inform health care provider of possible exposure to malaria.

Sulfasalazine

(SULL-fuh-SAL-uh-zeen)

Class Anti-infective/Sulfonamide

How Supplied
Azulfidine Tablets 500 mg ♦ *Azulfidine EN-tabs* Tablets, delayed-release 500 mg
✥ *ratio-Sulfasalazine* ♦ *Salazopyrin* ♦ *Salazopyrin Desensitizing Kit* ♦ *Salazopyrin EN-tabs*

Action
PHARMACOLOGY: Competitively antagonizes PABA, an essential component in folic acid synthesis.

PHARMACOKINETICS/DYNAMICS:

Absorption: Bioavailability of sulfasalazine is less than 15%; T_{max} is 6 hr (range, 3 to 12 hr) post-ingestion; C_{max} is 6 mcg/mL. Sulfasalazine is partially absorbed. Approximately 1/3 of a dose of sulfasalazine is absorbed from the small intestine. The remaining 2/3 passes to the colon where the compound is split into 5-aminosalicylic acid (5-ASA) and sulfinpyridine. Detectable serum concentrations are found within 90 min after ingestion of a 2 g dose.

Distribution: Sulfasalazine is highly bound to albumin (more than 99.3%); Vd is approximately 7.5 L.

Metabolism: Sulfasalazine is extensively metabolized.

Excretion: Sulfasalazine t½ (IV) is approximately 7.6 hr. Clearance following IV administration is approximately 1 L/hr.

Special Populations:
Elderly – Elderly patients with rheumatoid arthritis showed a prolonged plasma t½ for sulfasalazine, sulfinpyridine, and their metabolites. The clinical impact of this is unknown.

Indications Treatment of ulcerative colitis; rheumatoid arthritis and juvenile rheumatoid arthritis (enteric-coated tablets). **Unlabeled use(s):** Treatment of ankylosing spondylitis, collagenous colitis, Crohn disease, psoriasis, psoriatic arthritis.

Contraindications Hypersensitivity to sulfonamides or chemically related drugs (eg, sulfonylureas, thiazide and loop diuretics, carbonic anhydrase inhibitors, sunscreens containing PABA, local anesthetics); pregnancy at term; lactation; infants less than 2 mo; porphyria; hypersensitivity to salicylates; intestinal or urinary obstruction.

Route/Dosage
Ulcerative Colitis
ADULTS: **PO** 3 to 4 g/day in evenly divided doses. More than 4 g/day is associated with higher incidence of side effects. May begin with 1 to 2 g/day to lessen GI effects.
Maintenance: 2 g/day in 4 divided doses.
CHILDREN AT LEAST 2 YR: **PO** 40 to 60 mg/kg/24 hr initially in 3 to 6 divided doses.
Maintenance: 20 to 30 mg/kg/day in 4 divided doses. Max, 2 g/day.

Rheumatoid Arthritis
ADULTS: **PO** *Enteric-coated:* 2 g/day in 2 evenly divided doses. May initiate therapy with a lower dosage (eg, 0.5 to 1 g/day) to reduce possible GI intolerance.
CHILDREN AT LEAST 6 YR: **PO** *Enteric-coated:* 30 to 50 mg/kg/day in 2 evenly divided doses. Initiate therapy with 25% to 33% of the planned maintenance dose to lessen GI effects; increase weekly until reaching maintenance dose at 1 mo. Max, 2 g/day.

Interactions
Folic acid: Signs of folate deficiency have occurred, but specific symptoms related to deficiency have not been reported.
Methotrexate: Risk of methotrexate-induced bone marrow suppression may be enhanced.
Sulfonylureas: Increased sulfonylurea half-lives and hypoglycemia have occurred.

Lab Test Interferences May produce false-positive urinary glucose tests when performed by *Benedict* method.

Adverse Reactions
CNS: Headache; insomnia; peripheral neuropathy; depression; convulsions.
DERM: Orange-yellow discoloration of skin.
GI: Nausea; vomiting; abdominal pain; diarrhea; anorexia; pancreatitis; impaired folic acid absorption; pseudomembranous enterocolitis.
GU: Orange-yellow urine; crystalluria; hematuria; proteinuria; elevated creatinine; nephrotic syndrome; toxic nephrosis with oliguria and anuria.
HEMA: Agranulocytosis; aplastic anemia; thrombocytopenia; leukopenia; hemolytic anemia; purpura; hypoprothrombinemia; methemoglobinemia; megaloblastic (macrocytic) anemia; Heinz body anemia.

HEPA: Hepatitis; hepatocellular necrosis.
HYPERSEN: May present as erythema multiforme of Stevens-Johnson type; generalized skin eruptions; allergic myocarditis; epidermal necrolysis, with or without corneal damage; urticaria; serum sickness; pruritus; exfoliative dermatitis; anaphylactoid reactions; periorbital edema; photosensitization; arthralgia; transient pulmonary changes with eosinophilia and decreased pulmonary function.
RESP: Pulmonary infiltrates.
OTHER: Drug fever; chills; pyrexia; arthralgia; myalgia; periarteritis nodosum; lupus erythematosus phenomenon.

Precautions
Pregnancy: Category B.
Lactation: Excreted in breast milk.
Children: Do not use in infants less than 2 mo.
Renal function impairment: Use drug with caution in patients with impaired renal function.
Hepatic function impairment: Use drug with caution in patients with impaired hepatic function.

Allergy or asthma: Use drug with caution in patients with severe allergy or bronchial asthma. Hemolytic anemia may occur in G-6-PD deficient individuals.
Contact lenses: May permanently stain soft contact lenses yellow.
Porphyria: May precipitate acute attack of porphyria.
Severe reactions: Reactions, including deaths, have been associated with hypersensitivity reactions, agranulocytosis, aplastic anemia, other blood dyscrasias, and renal and hepatic damage. Irreversible neuromuscular and CNS changes and fibrosing alveolitis may occur.
Sulfonamides: Bear chemical similarities to some goitrogens, diuretics (acetazolamide and thiazides), and oral hypoglycemic agents. Goiter production, diuresis, and hypoglycemia have occurred rarely in patients receiving sulfonamides. Cross-sensitivity may exist.

Overdosage: Signs and Symptoms
Anuria, nausea, vomiting, gastric distress, drowsiness, seizures.

PATIENT CARE CONSIDERATIONS
Administration/Storage
- Have resuscitative equipment readily available during administration.
- Give after meals or with food (to minimize GI irritation and prolong intestinal passage). Administer around clock (q 6 to 8 hr) in evenly spaced doses.
- Give each dose with full glass of water; encourage fluids between meals up to 2000 mL/day (to maintain hydration and decrease crystallization in kidneys).
- Do not allow patient to chew or crush enteric-coated tablet.
- Shake oral suspension well prior to administration; measure dose accurately with calibrated device.
- Store tables in tight, light-resistant container at room temperature; refrigerate suspension after opening and discard unused portion after 14 days.

Assessment/Interventions
- Obtain patient history, including drug history and any known allergies.
- Assess results of CBC, hepatic function, and renal function studies (BUN, creatinine, urinalysis) prior to and during therapy if on long-term regimen.
- Assess stool pattern (eg, frequency, consistency [dose increased if diarrhea recurs/continues], quantity) and document abdominal pain prior to and during therapy; sigmoidoscopy and proctoscopy may be used to verify response or adjust dosage.
- Monitor I&O; note urine color, pH, and character (high urine acidity may require alkalinization).
- Assess skin for rash, bleeding, bruising, jaundice; note fever, sore throat, mouth sores, or joint pain. Report any of these symptoms to health care provider (may require discontinuation of medication).
- Enteric-coated tablets: Careful monitoring is recommended for doses greater than 2 g/day.

Patient/Family Education
- Advise patient to take with or after meals if GI intolerance occurs.
- Instruct patient and family to adhere to around the clock schedule as directed. Explain that if dose is missed patient should take it as soon as remembered. Emphasize that patient should not double up doses.
- Tell patient to notify other health care providers/dentist of therapy prior to other treatments/surgery.
- Explain that medication may cause urine and skin to have yellow-orange discoloration (expected effect) and that it may permanently stain soft contact lenses yellow.
- Encourage medical follow-up to ensure success of therapy and to evaluate continuing symptoms.
- Advise patient to take each oral dose with full glass of water to prevent crystalluria.
- Instruct patient to report the following symptoms to health care provider immediately: difficulty breathing, skin rash, fever, chills, mouth sores, sore throat, ringing in ears, or unusual bleeding/bruising.

- Advise patient that drug may cause dizziness and to use caution while driving or performing other activities requiring mental alertness.
- Caution patient to avoid exposure to sunlight and to wear protective clothing or use sunscreen to avoid photosensitivity reaction.
- Instruct patient not to take OTC medications (even vitamins) without consulting health care provider.

Sulfisoxazole

(sull-fih-SOX-uh-zole)

Class Anti-infective/Sulfonamide

How Supplied
Gantrisin Pediatric Suspension 500 mg per 5 mL

Action
PHARMACOLOGY: Exerts bacteriostatic action by competing with PABA, an essential component in folic acid synthesis, thus preventing synthesis of folic acid, needed by bacteria for growth.

PHARMACOKINETICS/DYNAMICS:

Absorption: Sulfisoxazole is rapidly and completely absorbed. The major site of absorption is the small intestine, but some drug is absorbed from the stomach. Steady-state plasma concentrations are about 49 to 89 mcg/mL. C_{max} is approximately 169 mcg/mL.

Distribution: Sulfisoxazole is approximately 85% bound to plasma proteins and is only distributed in extracellular body fluids. The drug readily crosses the placental barrier and enters into fetal circulation. Sulfisoxazole crosses the blood-brain barrier.

Metabolism: N_1-acetyl sulfisoxazole is metabolized to sulfisoxazole and is absorbed as sulfisoxazole.

Excretion: Sulfisoxazole is excreted primarily by the kidneys through glomerular filtration. Drug concentrations are higher in urine than in blood. Sulfisoxazole t½ is 4.6 to 7.8 hr after oral administration.

Special Populations:
Elderly – Elimination has been shown to be slower in the elderly (63 to 75 years of age) with diminished renal function (Ccr 37 to 68 mL/min).

Indications
Oral: Treatment of UTI, chancroid, inclusion conjunctivitis, malaria, meningitis caused by *Haemophilus influenzae* or meningococci, nocardiosis, acute otitis media, toxoplasmosis, and trachoma.
Ophthalmic: Treatment of conjunctivitis, corneal ulcer, and superficial ocular infections, adjunct to systemic sulfonamide therapy of trachoma.

Unlabeled use(s):
Oral – Treatment of recurrent otitis media.

Contraindications Hypersensitivity to sulfonamides or chemically related drugs (eg, sulfonylureas, thiazide and loop diuretics, carbonic anhydrase inhibitors, sunscreens containing PABA, local anesthetics); hypersensitivity to salicylates; porphyria; children younger than 2 mo of age; pregnancy at term.

Route/Dosage
ADULTS: **PO** 2 to 4 g initially, then 4 to 8 g/day in 4 to 6 divided doses. **Ophthalmic** Instill 1 to 2 drops into lower conjunctival sac q 1 to 3 hr daily.

CHILDREN AND INFANTS OLDER THAN 2 MO OF AGE: **PO** 75 mg/kg initially, then 120 to 150 mg/kg/day in 4 to 6 divided doses (max, 6 g/day).

Interactions
Anticoagulants, oral: May enhance anticoagulant action.
Cyclosporine: Reduced concentration of cyclosporine and reduced efficacy; may have additive nephrotoxicity.
Hydantoins: May increase hydantoin serum levels.
Methotrexate: May enhance risk of methotrexate-induced bone marrow suppression.
Sulfonylureas: May increase sulfonylurea half-life and produce hypoglycemia.

Lab Test Interferences May produce false-positive urinary glucose test results when performed by *Benedict's* method; may interfere with *Urobilistix* test; may produce false-positive results with sulfosalicylic acid tests for urinary protein.

Adverse Reactions
CNS: Headache; peripheral neuropathy; depression; convulsions; dizziness; ataxia.
GI: Nausea; vomiting; abdominal pain; diarrhea; anorexia; pancreatitis; impaired folic acid absorption; pseudomembranous enterocolitis.
GU: Crystalluria; hematuria; proteinuria; elevated creatinine; nephrotic syndrome; toxic nephrosis with oliguria and anuria.
HEMA: Agranulocytosis; aplastic anemia; thrombocytopenia; leukopenia; hemolytic anemia; purpura; hypoprothrombinemia; anemia; methemoglobinemia; megaloblastic (macrocytic) anemia.
HEPA: Hepatitis; hepatocellular necrosis.
OPHTH: Browache; local irritation; transient epithelial keratitis; reactive hyperemia; conjunctival edema; burning; stinging; sensitivity to bright light.
RESP: Pulmonary infiltrates.
OTHER: Drug fever; chills; pyrexia; arthralgia; myalgia; periarteritis nodosum; lupus

erythematosus phenomenon. Hypersensitivity reactions may present as erythema multiforme of Stevens-Johnson type, generalized skin eruptions, allergic myocarditis, epidermal necrolysis with or without corneal damage, urticaria, serum sickness; pruritus, exfoliative dermatitis, anaphylactoid reactions, periorbital edema, photosensitization, arthralgia, and transient pulmonary changes with eosinophilia and decreased pulmonary function.

Precautions
Pregnancy: Category C. Sulfonamides cross placenta and can produce jaundice, hemolytic anemia, and kernicterus in newborn; therefore, they are contraindicated at term.
Lactation: Excreted in breast milk in low concentrations. Do not nurse premature infants or those with hyperbilirubinemia or G-6-PD deficiency.
Children: Contraindicated in infants younger than 2 mo of age.
Renal function impairment: Use drug with caution.
Hepatic function impairment: Use drug with caution.
Photosensitivity: Photosensitization may occur.

Allergy or asthma: Use drug with caution in patients with severe allergy or bronchial asthma.
Dry eye (ophthalmic): Use with caution in patients with severe dry eye.
Group A beta-hemolytic streptococcal infections: Do not use drug for these infections.
Hemolytic anemia: May occur in G-6-PD-deficient individuals.
Porphyria: Drug may precipitate acute attack of porphyria.
Severe reactions: Reactions, including deaths, have been associated with hypersensitivity reactions, agranulocytosis, aplastic anemia, other blood dyscrasias, and renal and hepatic damage. Irreversible neuromuscular and CNS changes and fibrosing alveolitis may occur.
Sulfonamides: Have chemical similarities to some goitrogens, diuretics (acetazolamide and the thiazides), and oral hypoglycemic agents. Goiter production, diuresis, and hypoglycemia have occurred rarely in patients receiving sulfonamides. Cross-sensitivity may exist.

Overdosage: Signs and Symptoms
Anorexia, nausea, vomiting, abdominal cramping, dizziness, headache, drowsiness, coma.

PATIENT CARE CONSIDERATIONS

Administration/Storage
Oral Administration:
- Give on empty stomach with full glass of water 1 hr before meal or 2 hr after meal for best absorption.
- Administer around the clock at equal intervals.
- May crush tablet and mix with liquid for ease of swallowing. May allow patient to chew tablet.
- Shake oral suspension well prior to administration. Measure dose accurately with calibrated device.
- Store oral suspension in refrigerator.

Ophthalmic Solution:
- Do not use solution if it is discolored or contains precipitate.
- Wash hands thoroughly before and after instillation.
- Position patient supine or have patient tilt head back in "star-gazing" position (looking at ceiling). Pull down lower lid to form pocket and instill drops as ordered. Avoid contact between dispensing container and eye. Close eye gently and apply pressure to inner canthus for 1 to 2 min to prevent systemic absorption and draining into nose/throat.
- Store at room temperature and protect from light.

Assessment/Interventions
- Obtain patient history, including drug history and any known allergies. Note hypersensitivity to salicylates, sulfonamides, or chemically related drugs (eg, thiazides, acetazolamide, probenecid); severe hepatic/renal dysfunction; G-6-PD deficiency; porphyria.
- Assess patient for infection (vital signs; appearance of wound, sputum, urine, and stool).
- Obtain CBC, culture, and sensitivity. First dose may be given before results are available.
- Culture and sensitivity may be repeated when full course of therapy is completed.
- Encourage fluids between meals (up to 2,000 mL/day) to maintain hydration and decrease crystallization in kidneys.
- Assess diabetic patients taking oral hypoglycemic agents frequently for hypoglycemia prior to and during therapy.
- Monitor I&O. Note urine color, pH, and character.
- Assess skin for rash, bleeding, bruising, and jaundice. Note fever, chills, sore throat, mouth sores or joint pain. Report any of these symptoms immediately to health care provider.

Patient/Family Education
Oral:
- Advise patient to administer medication around the clock.
- Advise patient to notify other health care providers/dentists of this drug therapy prior to

other treatments or surgery.
- Instruct patient to report these symptoms to health care provider immediately: difficulty breathing, skin rash, fever, chills, mouth sores, sore throat, ringing in ears or unusual bleeding/bruising.
- Caution patient to avoid exposure to sunlight and to use sunscreen or wear protective clothing to avoid photosensitivity reaction. Inform patient that photosensitivity may persist for several months after therapy is completed.
- Advise patient not to take OTC medications without consulting health care provider.

Ophthalmic:
- Instruct patient/family in correct instillation of drops. Inform patient that stinging, burning, and blurred vision may occur after instillation of ophthalmic preparations. Advise patient to avoid hazardous activities until vision clears. Emphasize need for patient to contact health care provider immediately if patient notices a change in vision, eye pain, increased redness, itching, swelling, loss of sight, inability to breath, or flushing after ophthalmic application of this medication.
- Advise patient to note color change or precipitate in container and to discard if these are present.
- Tell patient to notify health care provider if improvement is not noted within 7 days.

Sulfinpyrazone

(sull-fin-PEER-uh-zone)

Class Uricosuric/Gout

How Supplied
Anturane Capsules 200 mg, Tablets 100 mg
✤ *Apo-Sulfinpyrazone* ◆ *Nu-Sulfinpyrazone*

Action
PHARMACOLOGY: Potent uricosuric agent that inhibits renal tubular reabsorption of uric acid and reduces renal tubular secretion of other organic anions; possesses antithrombotic and platelet-inhibiting effects.

PHARMACOKINETICS/DYNAMICS:
Absorption: Sulfinpyrazone is well absorbed after oral administration.

Distribution: 98% to 99% of sulfinpyrazone is bound to plasma proteins.

Excretion: Around 50% of an orally administered dose appears in urine after 24 hr, 90% as unchanged drug and 10% as its active metabolite, N^1-p-hydroxyphenol.

Indications Treatment of chronic and intermittent gouty arthritis. Not intended for relief of acute attack of gout. **Unlabeled use(s):** Post MI treatment (within 1 to 6 mo of acute MI) to decrease incidence of sudden cardiac death. May also be used to reduce frequency of systemic embolism in rheumatic mitral stenosis.

Contraindications Active peptic ulcer or symptoms of GI inflammation or ulceration; hypersensitivity to phenylbutazone or other pyrazoles; blood dyscrasias.

Route/Dosage
ADULTS: **PO** *Initial:* 200 to 400 mg daily in 2 divided doses with meals or milk, gradually increasing to full maintenance dosage in 1 wk.
Maintenance: 200 to 800 mg daily, given in 2 divided doses; may increase or decrease after serum urate level is controlled. In case of acute exacerbations, administer concomitant treatment with indomethacin (or another NSAID) or colchicine.

Interactions
Acetaminophen: Increased hepatotoxicity and reduced efficacy of acetaminophen may occur.
Anticoagulants, sulfonylureas (eg, tolbutamide): Blood levels and toxicity of these agents may increase.
Salicylates: Uricosuric action of sulfinpyrazone may be reduced.
Verapamil: Reduced efficacy of verapamil may occur.

Lab Test Interferences None well documented.

Adverse Reactions
DERM: Rash.
GI: Nausea; vomiting; epigastric distress.
HEMA: Blood dyscrasias, including anemia; leukopenia; agranulocytosis; thrombocytopenia; aplastic anemia.
RESP: Bronchoconstriction (in aspirin-sensitive patients).

Precautions
Pregnancy: Use only when clearly needed.
Lactation: Undetermined.
Children: Safety and efficacy not established.
Renal function impairment: Periodically assess renal function.
Alkalinization of urine: Sulfinpyrazone use may precipitate acute gouty arthritis, urolithiasis and renal colic. Adequate fluid intake (10 to 12 eight oz glasses of fluid) and alkalinization of urine are recommended to reduce potential for renal complications.
Healed peptic ulcer: Administer with care to these patients.

Overdosage: Signs and Symptoms
Nausea, vomiting, diarrhea, epigastric pain, ataxia, labored respiration, convulsions, coma.

PATIENT CARE CONSIDERATIONS

Administration/Storage
- Administer with food or milk; add antacid if needed.

Assessment/Interventions
- Obtain patient history, including drug history and any known allergies.
- Maintain adequate fluid intake and alkalinization of urine. Monitor I&O.
- Monitor blood uric acid levels to evaluate efficacy of treatment.
- Monitor complete blood cell counts for evidence of blood dyscrasias.
- In patients with impaired renal function, monitor renal function test values.
- Observe for upper GI disturbances, rash, or bronchoconstriction and report to health care provider.

Patient/Family Education
- Tell patient that medication is taken on daily basis to provide long-term protection from attacks of gout.
- Point out that gout attacks may worsen during initial treatment but continue the drug.
- Explain that other medications may be needed to control attacks of gout.
- Explain that drug may cause GI distress and to take with food or milk and antacid if needed.
- Instruct patient to report these symptoms to health care provider: rash, difficulty breathing, unusual bleeding or bruising, sore throat, fatigue, or fever.
- Explain importance of adequate hydration and instruct patient to drink 10 to 12 full glasses of fluid each day.
- Advise patient to consult health care provider before using aspirin or other salicylates, acetaminophen, or drinking alcohol.
- Tell patient to notify health care provider if GI distress continues.

Sulfuric Acid/Sulfonated Phenolics

(SULL-fyoor-ick acid/SULL-fun-ated FEE-nahl-icks)

Class Topical astringent/Tissue denaturant

How Supplied
Debacterol Liquid 30% sulfuric acid and 22% sulfonated phenolics

Action
PHARMACOLOGY:
Sulfuric acid: Tissue denaturant and sterilizing agent.
Sulfonated phenolics: Antiseptic agents with topical analgesic properties.

Indications Topical treatment of ulcerating lesions of the oral cavity (eg, recurrent aphthous stomatitis [canker sores]); relief of pain and discomfort of oral mucosal ulcers; decrease risk of infection of ulcerated tissue.

Contraindications Standard considerations.

Route/Dosage
ADULTS AND CHILDREN 12 YR AND OLDER:
TOPICAL Before applying, dry the ulcerated area of oral mucosa using a sterile cotton-tipped applicator or similar method. Apply coated applicator directly to the dried ulcer bed, holding the applicator in contact with the ulcer for at least 5 sec, but not more than 10 sec, while using a rolling motion to thoroughly coat the entire ulcer bed, the ulcer rim, and surrounding halo of normal mucosa. Then, thoroughly rinse mouth with water and spit out the water. The stinging sensation and ulcer pain should subside almost immediately after rinsing. If the ulcer pain returns shortly after rinsing with water, some part of the ulcer may not have been covered during the application. A second application should be applied to the ulcer immediately during the same treatment session until it remains pain-free after rinsing. More than 1 treatment session is not recommended on an individual mucosal ulcer.

Interactions None well documented.

Lab Test Interferences None well documented.

Adverse Reactions Stinging and local irritation upon application.

Precautions
Pregnancy: Category C.
Children: Safety and efficacy not established in children under 12 yr.
Application: For external use only. Avoid prolonged use on normal tissue. Apply carefully because all tissue to which product is applied in sufficient volume will eventually necrotize and slough.
Ophthalmic exposure: Immediately remove any contact lenses and irrigate eyes for at least 15 min with lukewarm water and contact a health care provider.

PATIENT CARE CONSIDERATIONS
Administration/Storage
- For external use in oral cavity only. Avoid contact with eyes and other tissues outside the oral cavity.
- Dry ulcerated area of oral cavity with sterile cotton-tipped applicator immediately before application. Hold applicator swab with colored ring up; bend colored ring tip gently to side until it snaps and releases liquid inside. Liquid flows down into the white tip of applicator. Apply coated applicator directly to the dried ulcer bed. A brief stinging sensation should be felt immediately.
- Hold cotton-tipped applicator in contact with ulcer for at least 5 sec, but no longer than 10 sec. Gently roll applicator tip to thoroughly coat the entire ulcer bed, ulcer rim, and surrounding halo of normal mucosa.
- Thoroughly rinse mouth with water and spit out rinse water. The stinging sensation and ulcer pain will subside almost immediately.
- If ulcer pain returns shortly after rinsing, a second application should be performed immediately during the same treatment session until the ulcer remains pain-free after rinsing.
- Return used swabs to pouch for disposal.
- Store applicator at controlled room temperature (59° to 86°F).

Assessment/Interventions
- Obtain patient history, including drug history and any known allergies.
- Ensure that ulcer to be treated is not a vascular lesion (eg, cold sore, fever blister).
- Assess patient for resolution of pain and stinging and evidence of tissue irritation from treatment. If excess irritation is noted, instruct patient to rinse with sodium bicarbonate solution (½ tsp baking soda in 120 mL water).
- Do not reapply medication to same lesion after achieving pain-free status.

Patient/Family Education
- Explain name, action, and potential side effects of drug.
- Advise patient that medication will be applied by a health care provider in a medical setting.
- Advise patient to inform health care provider if pain, burning, or stinging are felt after rinsing mouth.

Sulindac
(sull-IN-dak)
Class Analgesic/NSAID

How Supplied
Clinoril Tablets 150 mg, Tablets 200 mg
✤ *APO-Sulin* ♦ *Novo-Sundac* ♦ *Nu-Sulindac*

Action
PHARMACOLOGY: Decreases inflammation, pain, and fever, probably through inhibition of cyclooxygenase activity and prostaglandin synthesis.

PHARMACOKINETICS/DYNAMICS:

Absorption: Sulindac T_{max} is 2 hr (when fasting) and 3 to 4 hr (when given with food). Approximately 90% of the drug is absorbed after oral administration. Bioavailability is unchanged by concomitant magnesium or aluminum antacid administration.

Metabolism: Recirculation of sulindac and its sulfone metabolite is more active and extensive than that of the active sulfide metabolite.

Excretion: Sulindac t½ is 7.8 hr. The main route of excretion is via the urine. Approximately 25% is found in feces, primarily as the sulfone and sulfide metabolites.

Special Populations:
Renal Function Impairment – Because sulindac is excreted in urine, it may possibly affect renal function to a lesser extent than other NSAIDs.

Indications Treatment of acute and chronic rheumatoid and osteoarthritis, ankylosing spondylitis, acute gouty arthritis, acute painful shoulder, tendonitis, bursitis. **Unlabeled use(s):** Treatment of juvenile rheumatoid arthritis and sunburn.

Contraindications Hypersensitivity to aspirin, iodides, or any NSAID.

Route/Dosage
Osteoarthritis, Rheumatoid Arthritis, Ankylosing Spondylitis
ADULTS: PO 150 mg bid.

Acute Painful Shoulder, Acute Gouty Arthritis
ADULTS: PO 200 mg bid for 7 to 14 days. Max, 400 mg/day.

Interactions
Anticoagulants: May increase effect of anticoagulants because of decreased plasma protein binding. May increase risk of gastric erosion and bleeding.
Cimetidine: Sulindac has increased cimetidine bioavailability.
Dimethyl sulfoxide: DMSO may decrease formation of active metabolite of sulindac, possibly resulting in decreased therapeutic effect. Also, topical DMSO with sulindac has resulted in severe peripheral neuropathy.
Lithium: May decrease lithium clearance.

Loop diuretics: Decreased diuresis may result.
Methotrexate: May increase methotrexate levels.
Ranitidine: Sulindac has increased ranitidine bioavailability.

Lab Test Interferences May prolong bleeding time.

Adverse Reactions
CV: Edema; weight gain; CHF; alterations in blood pressure; vasodilation; palpitations; tachycardia; arrhythmia.
CNS: Dizziness; headaches; nervousness; anxiety; vertigo; lightheadedness; drowsiness; somnolence; tiredness; insomnia; depression; psychic disturbances; seizures; syncope; aseptic meningitis.
DERM: Rash; pruritus; ecchymosis; sweating; photosensitivity; alopecia; erythema multiforme; toxic epidermal necrolysis; exfoliative dermatitis.
EENT: Tinnitus; blurred vision; visual disturbances; decreased hearing.
GI: Peptic ulceration; GI bleeding; GI pain; dyspepsia; nausea; vomiting; diarrhea; constipation; pancreatitis; flatulence; anorexia; GI cramps; abdominal distress; stomatitis.
GU: Discoloration of urine; dysuria; proteinuria; hematuria; interstitial nephritis; nephrotic syndrome; acute renal insufficiency; hyperkalemia; hyponatremia; renal papillary necrosis.
HEMA: Increased bleeding time; thrombocytopenia; purpura; leukopenia; agranulocytosis; neutropenia; bone marrow depression.
HEPA: Increased LFTs; hepatitis; hepatic failure; cholestasis; jaundice.
RESP: Bronchospasm; laryngeal edema; rhinitis, dyspnea, pharyngitis; hemoptysis; shortness of breath.
OTHER: Dry mucous membranes.

Precautions
Pregnancy: Pregnancy category undetermined.
Lactation: Undetermined.
Children: Safety and efficacy not established.
Elderly: Increased risk of adverse reactions.
Hypersensitivity: May occur; use caution in aspirin-sensitive individuals because of possible cross-sensitivity. Potentially fatal reaction.
Renal function impairment: Assess function before and during therapy, because NSAID metabolites are eliminated renally.
Hepatic function impairment: Use with caution.
GI effects: Serious GI toxicity (eg, bleeding, ulceration, perforation) can occur at any time, with or without warning symptoms. Do not give to patients with active GI lesions or history of recurrent lesions, except in special circumstances and with close monitoring.
Renal lithiasis: Use with caution in patients with a history of renal lithiasis.

Overdosage: Signs and Symptoms
Drowsiness, dizziness, confusion, disorientation, lethargy, vomiting, abdominal pain, headache, tinnitus, sweating, seizures, stupor, coma.

PATIENT CARE CONSIDERATIONS

Administration/Storage
- Give with food, milk, or antacids if needed to minimize GI irritation.
- Crush tablet and mix with food for patient with swallowing difficulty.
- Keep patient well hydrated while receiving drug.
- Store in tight, light-resistant container at room temperature.

Assessment/Interventions
- Obtain patient history, including drug history and any known allergies, noting chronic alcohol use, fluid retention, nasal polyps, bronchospastic disease, or hypersensitivity to aspirin or NSAIDs.
- Assess hearing and vision (audiometry, ophthalmic exam) prior to and during therapy if long-term.
- Assess areas of bruising prior to and during therapy; report increased bruising immediately to health care provider.
- Assist with ambulation if drowsiness or dizziness is present; provide for safety at all times (call bell, side rails).
- Assess quality of pain (location, onset, type, and duration) and body temperature prior to therapy; monitor pain relief and body temperature after medication administration.
- Assess affected joints (mobility, swelling/deformities, skin condition); monitor improvement during therapy (relief from joint tenderness and pain; increased movement and improved strength of upper extremities).
- Monitor for fever, chills, and joint pain (symptoms of acute hypersensitivity reaction); withhold medication and report symptoms immediately to health care provider.
- Monitor CBC, renal, and LFT results periodically if on long-term therapy.

Patient/Family Education
- Advise patient/family to take medication with food or after meals.
- Tell patient to take medication with full glass of water to prevent medication from lodging in esophagus.
- Emphasize importance of regular medical followup, even in absence of side effects or problems related to drug therapy.
- Instruct patient to report these symptoms of toxicity to health care provider immediately: ringing in ears, blurred vision, change in urine (pattern, blood in urine).

- Tell patient to avoid intake of alcoholic beverages or other NSAIDs/ASA during therapy (increases risk of GI irritation/GI bleeding), especially during long-term therapy.
- Advise patient that drowsiness or dizziness may occur and to use caution while driving or performing other activities requiring mental alertness.
- Caution patient to avoid exposure to sunlight and to use sunscreen or wear protective clothing to prevent photosensitivity reaction.

Sumatriptan

(SUE-muh-TRIP-tan)

Class Analgesic/Migraine

How Supplied

Imitrex Injection 6 mg per 0.5 mL (as succinate), Nasal, spray 5 mg, Nasal, spray 20 mg, Tablets 25 mg (as succinate), Tablets 50 mg (as succinate), Tablets 100 mg (as succinate)

Action

PHARMACOLOGY: Selective agonist for vascular serotonin (5-HT) receptor subtype, causing vasoconstriction of cranial arteries.

PHARMACOKINETICS/DYNAMICS:

Absorption: Sumatriptan T_{max} for subcutaneous, oral, and intranasal administration is 0.17, 1.5, and 1.5 hr, respectively. C_{max} for subcutaneous, oral, and intranasal administration is 72, 54, and 13 mg/L, respectively. AUC for subcutaneous, oral, and intranasal administration is 90, 158, and 48 mcg/L•hr, respectively. Bioavailability for subcutaneous, oral, and intranasal administration is 96%, 14%, and 15.8%, respectively.

Distribution: Sumatriptan protein binding is 14% to 21%.

Excretion: Sumatriptan t½ for subcutaneous, oral, and intranasal administration is 2, 2, and 1.8 hr, respectively.

Special Populations:
Hepatic Function Impairment – The max single dose should be 50 mg or less. Bioavailability following oral administration may be markedly increased in patients with liver disease.

Indications Acute treatment of migraine attacks with/without aura; treatment of acute cluster headaches (injection only).

Contraindications IV use (causes coronary vasospasm); patients with history, signs or symptoms of ischemic heart disease (eg, angina, including Prinzmetal variant, MI, silent myocardial ischemia), cerebrovascular or peripheral vascular syndromes; uncontrolled hypertension; concurrent use or within 24 hr of ergotamine-containing preparations; management of hemiplegic or basilar migraine; concurrent MAO inhibitor therapy or within 2 wk of discontinuing an MAO inhibitor; severe hepatic impairment; hypersensitivity to any component of the product.

Route/Dosage

ADULTS: **PO** Recommended dose is up to 100 mg taken with fluids. Doses of 100 mg have not been proven to provide a greater effect than 50 mg. If headache returns, a single additional dose may be taken after 2 hr up to a max of 200 mg per day. If headache returns following an initial dose with the injection, additional doses of single tablets (up to 100 mg per day) may be given with an interval of at least 2 hr between tablet doses. **Subcutaneous** Administer as soon as symptoms appear. Max single adult dose is 6 mg. Max dose per 24 hr is two 6 mg injections separated by at least 1 hr. Available in auto-injection prefilled syringe devices that deliver 6 mg for easy use; however, lower doses should be used in patients who have side effects at usual dose.

Intranasal Administer a single dose of 5, 10, or 20 mg in 1 nostril. A 10 mg dose can be achieved by the administration of a single 5 mg dose in each nostril. If headache returns, the dose may be repeated once after 2 hr. Do not exceed a total daily dose of 40 mg.

Hepatic Function Impairment
Maximum single dose is up to 50 mg.

Interactions

5-HT₁ agonists (eg, naratriptan): Increased risk of vasospastic reactions; therefore, coadministration of two $5-HT_1$ agonists within 24 hr of each other is contraindicated.
Ergot-containing drugs: May cause additive prolonged vasospastic reactions. Avoid use within 24 hr of each other.
MAO inhibitors: Use of sumatriptan with MAO inhibitors or within 14 days following discontinuation of an MAO inhibitor is contraindicated.
Selective serotonin reuptake inhibitors (eg, citalopram, fluoxetine, fluvoxamine, paroxetine, sertraline): Weakness, hyperreflexia, and incoordination have been reported rarely.
Sibutramine: Serotonin syndrome, including CNS irritability, motor weakness, shivering, myoclonus, and altered consciousness may occur.

Lab Test Interferences None well documented.

Adverse Reactions

CV: Flushing (7%); palpitation, syncope, decreased or increased BP (at least 1%); atrial fibrillation, cardiomyopathy, colonic ischemia,

Prinzmetal variant angina, pulmonary embolism, shock, thrombophlebitis (postmarketing).
CNS: Dizziness/vertigo (12%); paresthesia (5%); drowsiness/sedation, malaise or fatigue (3%); headache (2%); anxiety (1%); phonophobia, photophobia (at least 1%); vasculitis, cerebrovascular accident, dysphasia, subarachnoid hemorrhage, panic disorder (postmarketing).
DERM: Sweating (2%); exacerbation of sunburn (postmarketing).
EENT: Unusual taste (25% [intranasal]); discomfort in nasal cavity or sinuses (4%); throat discomfort (3%); visual alterations (1%); sinusitis, tinnitus, allergic rhinitis, upper respiratory inflammation, ear, nose, and throat hemorrhage, external otitis, hearing loss, nasal inflammation, sensitivity to noise (at least 1%); deafness, ischemic optic neuropathy, retinal artery occlusion, retinal vein thrombosis, loss of vision (postmarketing).
GI: Mouth or tongue discomfort (5%); nausea, vomiting (4% [14% intranasal]); jaw discomfort (2%); abdominal discomfort, dysphagia (1%); diarrhea, gastric symptoms (at least 1%); ischemic colitis with rectal bleeding, xerostomia (postmarketing).
GU: Acute renal failure (postmarketing).
HEMA: Hemolytic anemia, pancytopenia, thrombocytopenia (postmarketing).
HEPA: Elevated LFTs (postmarketing).
HYPERSEN: Allergic vasculitis, erythema, pruritus, rash, shortness of breath, urticaria, anaphylaxis/anaphylactoid reactions (postmarketing).
LOCAL: Injection site reaction (59%); pain, redness, stinging, induration, swelling, contusion, subcutaneous bleeding, lipoatrophy, lipohypertrophy (subcutaneous administration [postmarketing]).
MUSC: Weakness, neck pain or stiffness (5%); myalgia (2%); muscle cramps (1%).

PATIENT CARE CONSIDERATIONS
Administration/Storage
- Do not administer with or within 14 days of MAO inhibitor.
- Do not administer within 24 hr of treatment with another 5-HT$_1$ agonist or ergot-containing drug.
- Store tablets, nasal spray, and injection at ambient room temperature (47° to 86°F) or in refrigerator (36° to 46°F). Protect nasal spray and injection from light.

Tablets:
- Administer prescribed dose at onset of migraine symptoms.
- Administer without regard to meals.

RESP: Bronchospasm (1%); dyspnea (at least 1%).
OTHER: Tingling (14%); warm/hot sensation (11%); burning sensation (8%); feeling of heaviness or pressure (7%); feeling of tightness, numbness (5%); tightness in chest, cold sensation (3%); pressure in chest, feeling strange, head tightness, pain (2%).

Precautions
Pregnancy: Category C.
Lactation: Excreted in breast milk.
Children: Safety and efficacy not established.
Elderly: Safety and efficacy in patients greater than 65 yr of age not thoroughly evaluated.
Hypersensitivity: Hypersensitivity reactions (including anaphylaxis and anaphylactoid reactions) may occur.
Renal function impairment: Use caution.
Hepatic function impairment: Use caution.
Cardiac events/Vasoconstriction: Serious coronary events, though extremely rare, can occur after sumatriptan use. Administer first dose in health care provider's office to patients at possible risk of unrecognized coronary disease. If symptoms consistent with angina occur, conduct ECG evaluation for ischemic changes. May cause coronary vasospasm in patients with history of coronary heart disease (CAD). Rare reports of MI, major arrhythmias, angina symptoms, and death.
Cerebrovascular events: Cerebral hemorrhage, subarachnoid hemorrhage, stroke, and other cerebrovascular events have been reported.
Hypertensive crisis: Elevation in BP, including hypertensive crisis, have been reported.

Overdosage: Signs and Symptoms
Convulsions, tremor, inactivity, erythema of extremities, reduced respiratory rate, cyanosis, ataxia, mydriasis, injection site reactions (eg, desquamation, hair loss, scab formation), paralysis.

- If headache recurs after initial relief, a second dose may be administered, providing there is an interval of at least 2 hr between doses.
- If first dose is ineffective, do not administer a second dose unless prescribed by health care provider.
- Do not administer greater than 200 mg per 24 hr-period.

Nasal Spray:
- For intranasal use only. Avoid spraying into the eyes or mouth.
- If headache recurs after initial relief, a second dose may be administered, providing there is an interval of at least 2 hr between doses.

- If first dose is ineffective, do not administer a second dose unless prescribed by health care provider.
- Do not administer more than 40 mg per 24-hr period.

Injection:
- For subcutaneous administration only. Not for intradermal, IM, IV, or intra-arterial administration.
- Do not administer if particulate matter, cloudiness, or discoloration noted.
- Administer prescribed dose at onset of migraine or cluster headache symptoms.
- If headache recurs after initial relief, a second dose may be administered, provided there is an interval of at least 1 hr between doses.
- If first dose is ineffective, do not administer a second dose unless prescribed by health care provider.
- Do not administer greater than 12 mg per 24-hr period.

Assessment/Interventions
- Obtain patient history, including drug history and any known allergies. Note renal or hepatic impairment, ischemic or vasospastic CAD, uncontrolled hypertension, peripheral vascular disease, ischemic bowel disease, seizures, stroke, transient ischemic attacks, hemiplegic or basilar migraine, or current or recent (within 14 days) use of MAO inhibitor.
- Note recent (within 24 hr) use of other 5-HT$_1$ agonists or ergotamine-containing or ergot-type drugs.
- Assess pain location, intensity, duration, and associated symptoms of migraine attack and response to treatment.
- Provide quiet, calm environment. Decrease stimuli, noise, and light.
- Ensure that patients with potential for CAD, including postmenopausal women, men over 40 yr of age, patients with risk factors for CAD (eg, hypertension, hypercholesterolemia, obesity, diabetes, smokers, family history), undergo a CV evaluation before initiating therapy.
- Administer first dose in physician's office or other adequately staffed medical facility to patient with potential for CAD whose CV evaluation provided clinical evidence that patient is reasonably free of coronary artery and ischemic myocardial disease or other significant underlying CV disease. Consider obtaining an ECG during the interval immediately following administration of the first dose of medication to patient with potential for CAD.
- Monitor patient for signs of allergic reaction. Discontinue therapy and immediately notify health care provider if noted. Be prepared to treat appropriately.
- Ensure that patient who is a long-term user of triptans, such as sumatriptan, undergoes periodic CV evaluation.
- Monitor patient for CNS, CV, GI, and general body side effects. Report to health care provider if noted and significant.

Patient/Family Education
- Explain name, dose, action, and potential side effects of drug.
- Advise patient to read the *Patient Information* leaflet before starting therapy and again with each refill.
- Explain that drug is to be used only during migraine (or cluster headache if using injection) and does not prevent or reduce the number of attacks. Emphasize that drug is used only to treat actual migraine attack (or cluster headache if using injection) and should not be used to prevent headaches or treat headaches caused by other conditions.
- Advise patient that drug is to be taken as soon as symptoms of migraine appear. A second dose may be taken if symptoms return, but no sooner than 2 hr (1 hr for injection) following the first dose. For a given attack, if there is no response to the first tablet, do not take a second dose without first consulting with health care provider.
- Advise patient not to take more than 200 mg per day if using tablets, 40 mg per day if using nasal spray, or 12 mg per day if using injection.
- Advise patient that safety of treating more than 4 headaches in a 30-day period has not been established and to inform health care provider if headaches are occurring more frequently.
- Advise patient to immediately notify health care provider if any of the following occur after taking a dose of sumatriptan: severe chest pain or chest pain that does not go away; sudden and/or severe stomach pain; shortness of breath; wheezing; swelling of eyelids, face, or lips.
- Advise patient that if tightness, pain, pressure or heaviness in chest, throat, neck, or jaw occurs when using sumatriptan, to discuss these symptoms with their health care provider before using again.
- Advise patient to notify health care provider if feelings of tingling, heat, flushing, tiredness, dizziness, heaviness, or pressure occur after treatment.

- Advise patient that drug may cause fatigue or dizziness and to use caution while driving or performing other activities requiring mental alertness.
- Advise patient to avoid unnecessary exposure to sunlight or tanning lamps and to use sunscreen and wear protective clothing to avoid photosensitivity reactions.
- Instruct patients to continue taking prescribed migraine prophylactic medications daily as directed.
- Advise patients not currently taking a migraine prophylactic drug to discuss the use of such drugs with health care provider.
- Advise women to notify health care provider if pregnant, planning to become pregnant, or breastfeeding.
- Warn patient not to take any prescription or OTC drugs, dietary supplements, or herbal preparations without consulting health care provider.
- Advise patient that follow-up visits may be necessary to monitor therapy and to keep appointments.

Injection:
- Ensure that the patient or caregiver understands how to store, prepare, and administer the dose and dispose of used equipment and supplies.

Tacrine Hydrochloride (Tetrahydroaminoacridine; THA)

(TAK-reen HIGH-droe-KLOR-ide)

Class Reversible cholinesterase inhibitor

How Supplied
Cognex Capsules 10 mg, Capsules 20 mg, Capsules 30 mg, Capsules 40 mg

Action
PHARMACOLOGY: Believed to inhibit (reversibly) cholinesterase in CNS, leading to increased concentrations of acetylcholine.

PHARMACOKINETICS/DYNAMICS:

Absorption: Tacrine is rapidly absorbed after oral administration. T_{max} is 1 to 2 hr. Tacrine bioavailability is approximately 17%; food reduces bioavailability about 30% to 40%; however, there is no food effect if given at least 1 hr before meals. Steady state is achieved within 24 to 36 hr.

Distribution: Vd is about 349 L and it is approximately 55% bound to plasma proteins.

Metabolism: Extensively metabolized by the cytochrome P450 system. Cytochrome P450 1A2 is the principal isozyme involved in metabolism. The extent of first-pass metabolism depends on the dose administered.

Excretion: The t½ is approximately 2 to 4 hr.

Special Populations:
Hepatic Function Impairment – Hepatic impairment may reduce Cl.
Gender – Plasma concentrations are about 50% higher in women than men.
Smoking – Mean plasma concentrations in people who currently smoke are approximately one third the concentrations in nonsmokers.

Indications Treatment of mild to moderate dementia of Alzheimer type.

Contraindications Hypersensitivity to acridine derivatives; previous treatment with tacrine that resulted in jaundice (confirmed by elevated total bilirubin greater than 3 mg/dL); signs or symptoms of hypersensitivity (eg, rash, fever) in association with ALT elevations.

Route/Dosage
ADULTS:
Initial dose: PO 40 mg/day (10 mg qid). Maintain this dose for at least 4 wk with every-other-week monitoring of transaminase levels beginning at week 4 of therapy.

Titration: PO Increase the dose to 80 mg/day (20 mg qid), providing there are no significant transaminase elevations and the patient is tolerating treatment. Titrate patients to higher doses (120 and 160 mg/day in divided doses on a qid schedule) at 4-wk intervals on the basis of tolerance.

Dose adjustment: If transaminase levels are greater than 2 to 3 × ULN or less, continue treatment according to recommended titration. Monitor transaminase levels weekly until levels return to normal limits. If transaminase levels are greater than 3 to 5 × ULN or less, reduce the daily dose by 40 mg/day. Monitor ALT levels weekly. Resume dose titration and every other wk monitoring when transaminase levels return to within normal limits. If transaminase levels are greater than 5 × ULN, stop treatment. Monitor the patient closely for signs and symptoms associated with hepatitis and follow transaminase levels until within normal limits. Rechallenge: Initial dose of 40 mg/day (10 mg qid) and monitor transaminase levels weekly. If after 6 wk on 40 mg/day the patient is tolerating the dosage with no unacceptable elevations in transaminases, recommended dose titration and transaminase monitoring may be resumed.

Interactions
Cimetidine, fluvoxamine: Increased tacrine concentrations.
Levodopa: The antiparkinsonism effects of levodopa may be inhibited.
Theophylline: Increased theophylline concentrations.

Lab Test Interferences None well documented.

Adverse Reactions
CV: Hypotension, hypertension (at least 1%).
CNS: Dizziness (12%); headache (11%); agitation, confusion (7%); ataxia, insomnia (6%); depression, fatigue, somnolence (4%); abnormal thinking, anxiety (3%); tremor, hallucinations, hostility (2%); convulsions, vertigo, syncope, hyperkinesias, paresthesia, nervousness (at least 1%).
DERM: Rash (7%); facial/skin flushing (3%); increased sweating (at least 1%).
EENT: Rhinitis (8%); conjunctivitis, pharyngitis, sinusitis (at least 1%).
GI: Nausea/vomiting (28%); diarrhea (16%); dyspepsia, anorexia (9%); abdominal pain (8%); flatulence, constipation (4%).
GU: Urinary incontinence, urinary frequency, UTI (3%).
M/N: Weight decrease (3%).
MUSC: Myalgia (9%); fracture, arthralgia, arthritis, hypertonia (at least 1%).
RESP: Coughing, upper respiratory tract infection (3%); bronchitis, pneumonia, dyspnea (at least 1%).

OTHER: Elevated transaminases (29%); chest pain (4%); back pain, asthenia, purpura (2%); chills, fever, malaise, peripheral edema (at least 1%).

Precautions
Pregnancy: Category C.
Lactation: Undetermined.
Children: Safety and efficacy not established in any dementing illness.
Hepatic function impairment: Use drug with caution in patients with history of abnormal liver function.
Carcinogenesis: May be carcinogenic.
Anesthesia: Use of muscle relaxants (eg, succinylcholine) during anesthesia, while receiving tacrine, may lead to exaggerated effects.
Concomitant medical conditions: Increases cholinergic activity and therefore can affect other organ systems, possibly leading to bradycardia, bladder outflow obstruction, increased gastric acid secretion, or bronchoconstriction. Use drug with caution in patients susceptible to these effects.
Hematology: An absolute neutrophil count (ANC) less than 500/mcL occurred in 4 patients who received tacrine during the course of clinical trials.
Neurologic conditions: Drug may contribute to seizures. Cognitive function may worsen after discontinuation or large dose reductions.

Overdosage: Signs and Symptoms
Cholinergic crisis, severe nausea, vomiting, salivation, sweating, bradycardia, hypotension, collapse, convulsions.

PATIENT CARE CONSIDERATIONS

Administration/Storage
- Administer prescribed dose between meals whenever possible. Administer with food if GI upset occurs; however, food reduces absorption. Administer consistently either with or without food.
- Dose is gradually increased no more often than q 4 wk as tolerated by patient.
- May be administered alone or in combination with other medications for dementia or behavior.
- Store capsules at controlled room temperature (59° to 86°F). Protect from moisture.

Assessment/Interventions
- Obtain patient history, including drug history and any known allergies. Note bradycardia, sick sinus syndrome, conduction abnormalities, peptic ulcer disease or history of peptic ulcer disease, concurrent use of NSAIDs, current evidence of or history of abnormal liver function, asthma, prostatic hypertrophy, seizure disorder or condition predisposing to seizures, history of jaundice, elevated bilirubin, or hypersensitivity (eg, skin rash or fever) in association with elevated liver enzymes during previous treatment with tacrine.
- Ensure that patient who has previously experienced tacrine-induced jaundice or hypersensitivity reaction (eg, fever, rash) in association with elevated liver enzymes does not receive tacrine again.
- Ensure that liver enzymes are evaluated every wk from wk 4 through 16 of treatment and then q 3 mo thereafter. If patient discontinues tacrine and then restarts 4 or more wk later, ensure that this monitoring program is reinstituted.
- Ensure that dose and frequency of liver enzyme monitoring are adjusted, following manufacturer's guidelines, in patient whose liver enzymes are greater than 2 times ULN.
- Evaluate patient's mental status and function prior to initiation of therapy and frequently during treatment. Report decline in mental function or behavior to health care provider.
- Assess patient for CNS, GI, GU, psychiatric, respiratory, and general body side effects, especially after any increase in dose. Report to health care provider if noted and significant.
- Notify health care provider immediately if sensitivity reaction (eg, fever, rash) and elevated liver enzymes are noted or if jaundice or bilirubin greater than 3 mg/dL are noted.

Patient/Family Education
- Explain name, dose, action, and potential side effects of drug.
- Advise patient or caregiver that this drug does not alter the Alzheimer process and that effectiveness of the medication may lessen over time.
- Instruct patient or caregiver to continue using other medications for dementia or behavior as prescribed by health care provider.
- Advise patient or caregiver that medication is started at a low dose and gradually increased (no more often than q 4 wk) as tolerated until max benefit is obtained.
- Advise patient or caregiver to take prescribed doses at regular intervals between meals but to take with food if GI upset occurs. Encourage consistency in dosage schedule (eg, either always between meals or always with food) to prevent fluctuations in effectiveness and side effects.
- Caution patient or caregiver not to discontinue the drug or change the dose unless

- advised by health care provider.
- Caution patient or caregiver that if medication is discontinued for more than 1 wk to notify health care provider before restarting the medication.
- Advise patient or caregiver that nausea, vomiting, and diarrhea are common side effects and to notify health care provider if they occur and are intolerable.
- Advise patient that drug may cause drowsiness or dizziness and to use caution while driving or performing other tasks requiring mental alertness until tolerance is determined.
- Advise patient or caregiver to notify health care provider immediately if any of the following are noted: rash, fever, persistent nausea or vomiting, yellowing of skin or eyes.
- Advise patient or caregiver to report changes in thinking or behavior, bothersome side effects, or unexplained feelings or symptoms.
- Advise women to notify health care provider if pregnant, planning to become pregnant, or breastfeeding.
- Instruct patient or caregiver not to use any prescription or OTC medications or dietary supplements unless advised by health care provider.
- Advise patient or caregiver that follow-up visits and laboratory tests will be required to monitor therapy and to keep appointments.

Tacrolimus

(tack-CROW-lih-muss)

Class Immunosuppressive

How Supplied
Prograf Capsules 0.5 mg, Capsules 1 mg, Capsules 5 mg, Injection 5 mg/mL ◆ *Protopic* Ointment 0.03%, Ointment 0.1%

Action
PHARMACOLOGY: Suppresses cell-mediated immune reactions and some humoral immunity, but exact mechanism is not known.

PHARMACOKINETICS/DYNAMICS:

Absorption: In healthy volunteers, as well as kidney and liver transplant patients, tacrolimus C_{max} ranged from approximately 19.2 to 68.5 ng/mL, T_{max} ranged from 1.5 to 3 hr, AUC ranged from 203 to 3300 ng•hr/mL, t½ was from 11.7 to 34.8 hr, and bioavailability ranged from approximately 17% to 22%.

Food effects – The rate and extent of absorption were greatest under fasted conditions. The presence and composition of food decrease the rate and extent of absorption. The effect was most pronounced with a high-fat meal. Mean AUC and C_{max} were decreased 37% and 77%, respectively. T_{max} was lengthened 5-fold. A high carbohydrate meal decreased mean AUC and mean C_{max} 28% and 65%, respectively.

Distribution: Tacrolimus Vd is about 0.85 to 1.94 L/kg. Protein binding is about 99%, mainly to albumin and alpha-1 glycoprotein.

Metabolism: Tacrolimus is extensively metabolized by the mixed function oxidation system, primarily the cytochrome P450 system (CYP3A). The major metabolite identified is 13-demethyl tacrolimus.

Excretion: Clearance is about 0.04 to 0.83 L/hr/kg. Less than 1% of an administered dose is excreted unchanged in the urine. The t½ is approximately 31.9 to 48.1 hr (PO and IV).

Special Populations:
Hepatic Function Impairment – The mean clearance was substantially lower and t½ prolonged in patients with severe hepatic dysfunction.
Children – Children under 12 yr need higher doses than adults to achieve similar trough concentrations.

Indications
PO and IV: Prophylaxis of organ rejection in patients receiving allogenic liver or kidney transplants. Used in conjunction with adrenal corticosteroids.
Topical: Atopic dermatitis. **Unlabeled use(s):** Prophylaxis of rejection for patients receiving kidney, bone marrow, cardiac, pancreas, pancreatic island cell, and small bowel transplantation.

Contraindications Hypersensitivity to polyoxyl 60 hydrogenated castor oil, which is present in the injection, or any component of the product.

Route/Dosage
Prophylaxis of Organ Rejection Liver Transplants
ADULTS: **PO** 0.1 to 0.15 mg/kg/day in 2 divided daily doses q 12 hr no sooner than 6 hr after transplantation. **IV** 0.03 to 0.05 mg/kg/day as continuous infusion.

CHILDREN: **PO** 0.15 to 0.2 mg/kg/day in 2 divided daily doses q 12 hr. **IV** 0.03 to 0.05 mg/kg/day as continuous infusion.

Prophylaxis of Organ Rejection Kidney Transplants
ADULTS: **PO** 0.2 mg/kg/day in 2 divided daily doses q 12 hr, starting within 24 hr of transplantation but delayed until renal function is recovered (eg, serum creatinine of 4 mg/dL or less). Black patients may require higher doses to achieve comparable blood concentration.

Topical Dermatitis
ADULTS: **Topical** Apply thin layer of 0.03% or 0.1% to affected skin areas bid and rub in gently and completely; continue for 1 wk after clearing

of atopic dermatitis.
CHILDREN (AT LEAST 2 YR): **Topical** Apply thin layer of 0.03% to affected skin areas bid and rub in gently and completely; continue for 1 wk after clearing of atopic dermatitis.

Interactions

Azole antifungal agents (eg, fluconazole, ketoconazole), calcium channel blockers (eg, diltiazem, nifedipine), clotrimazole, macrolide antibiotics (eg, erythromycin): Tacrolimus plasma levels may be elevated, increasing the risk of toxicity.
Cyclosporine: Additive nephrotoxicity.
Hydantoins (eg, phenytoin): Tacrolimus plasma levels may be reduced, while hydantoin concentrations may be increased.
Mycophenolate mofetil: Plasma levels of mycophenolate mofetil may be elevated.
Rifamycins (eg, rifampin, St. John's wort): Tacrolimus plasma levels may be reduced, increasing the risk of rejection.

Lab Test Interferences
None well documented.

Adverse Reactions

CV: Hypertension; edema; peripheral edema, angina pectoris, arrhythmia, cerebrovascular accident, palpitations, peripheral vascular disorder, vasodilation (topical).
CNS: Headache; insomnia; anxiety; paresthesia; tremor, weakness, abnormal dreams, agitation, confusion (oral and IV); depression, dizziness, migraine, neuritis (topical).
DERM: Rash; pruritus; burning sensation, erythema, infection, herpes simplex, eczema herpeticum, pustular rash, folliculitis, urticaria, maculopapular rash, fungal dermatitis, acne, sunburn, skin disorder, vesiculobullous rash, skin tingling, dry skin, benign skin neoplasm, contact dermatitis, eczema, exfoliative dermatitis, alopecia, cellulitis, ecchymosis, skin discoloration, sweating, furunculosis (topical).
EENT: Abnormal vision, tinnitus (oral and IV); pharyngitis, rhinitis, sinusitis, otitis media, conjunctivitis, laryngitis, ear pain, eye disorder, eye pain, taste perversion (topical).
GI: Diarrhea; nausea; constipation; anorexia; vomiting; abdominal pain; dyspepsia, gastroenteritis, gastritis (topical).
GU: Renal dysfunction, UTI, oliguria (oral and IV); dysmenorrhea, increased creatinine, unintended pregnancy, vaginal moniliasis (topical).
HEMA: Leukocytosis; anemia; thrombocytopenia (oral and IV); leukopenia (topical).
HEPA: Abnormal LFTs; bilirubinemia (topical).

PATIENT CARE CONSIDERATIONS
Administration/Storage
Capsules and Injection:
- Dilute IV form of the medication prior to use with 0.9% normal saline or 5% dextrose

METAB: Hyperglycemia; hyperkalemia, hypomagnesemia, hyperuricemia (oral and IV); hypoglycemia (topical).
RESP: Dyspnea; pleural effusion, atelectasis (oral and IV); Increased cough, asthma, bronchitis, pneumonia, hypoxia, lung disorder (topical).
OTHER: Fever; pain; back pain; ascites (oral and IV); flu-like symptoms, allergic reaction, infection, accidental injury, lack of drug effect, lymphadenopathy, face edema, hyperesthesia, varicella zoster/herpes zoster asthenia, periodontal abscess, myalgia, cyst, arthralgia, arthritis, anaphylactoid reaction, angioedema, breast pain, cheilitis, chills, dehydration, epistaxis, exacerbation of untreated area, hernia, malaise, neck pain, photosensitivity (topical).

> **WARNING:**
> Increased risk of lymphoma and increased susceptibility to infection may be related to immunosuppression.
> Should be administered under the supervision of an experienced physician/equipped facility.

Precautions
Pregnancy: Category C.
Lactation: Excreted in breast milk. Avoid nursing.
Children: Children generally require higher doses to maintain trough tacrolimus levels similar to adults (oral and IV). Safety and efficacy not established in children at least 2 yr (topical).
Renal function impairment: May require reduced doses; monitor closely.
Hepatic function impairment: Patients with hepatic disease may require reduced doses.
Anaphylactic reactions: May occur with IV injection.
Hyperglycemia: Frequently occurs with tacrolimus; may require treatment.
Lymphadenopathy: Investigate the etiology of lymphadenopathy occurring in patients receiving the topical ointment.
Viral infections: The topical ointment may be associated with increased risk of varicella zoster virus infection (chicken pox or shingles), herpes simplex virus infection, or eczema herpeticum.

Overdosage: Signs and Symptoms
No acute toxicities have been reported.

injection to a concentration between 0.004 and 0.02 mg/mL.
- Diluted solution must be stored in glass or polyethylene containers for up to 24 hr after

mixing. Storage in PVC containers reduces stability.
- Do not use solutions that contain particulate matter or are discolored.
- The initial IV or oral dose of this medication should be no sooner than 6 hr after transplantation.
- Switch patients to the oral form of the medication as soon as possible.
- When converting from IV to oral dosage form, the first oral dose should be no sooner than 8 to 12 hr after discontinuation of IV administration.
- Oral medication is most effective on an empty stomach.
- Do not use this medication simultaneously with cyclosporine. Discontinue cyclosporine at least 24 hr before administering this drug.
- Diluted IV solution may be stored at controlled room temperature (59° to 86°F).
- Store capsules at room temperature.

Ointment:
- For topical use only. Not for ophthalmic, oral, or intravaginal use.
- Avoid contact with eyes and areas of active cutaneous viral or bacterial infections.
- Ointment is usually applied to affected areas bid.
- Apply a thin film of ointment to cover the affected area(s).
- Store ointment at controlled room temperature (59° to 86°F). Keep tube tightly capped.

Assessment/Interventions
Capsules and Injection:
- Obtain patient history. Note hypersensitivity to other antirejection drugs such as cyclosporine and polyoxyethylated castor oil.
- Obtain baseline laboratory tests, including BUN, creatinine, lipid levels, potassium, WBC with differential, and CBC. Perform and evaluate these tests periodically during treatment.
- Assess for pre-existing hypertension, particularly in children.
- Assess for any signs of infection, bleeding, or bruising.
- Remain with patient for the first 30 min of the initial IV administration of this medication and assess for symptoms of anaphylactic reaction. Assess frequently during all IV administrations.
- Maintain medical asepsis and eliminate any potential sources of environmental contamination.
- Monitor patient and lab tests for evidence of organ rejection.

Ointment:
- Obtain patient history, including drug history and any known allergies. Note Netherton syndrome, current viral or bacterial infection of affected skin, concurrent light therapy (eg, phototherapy), and concurrent use of other skin products.
- Ensure that clinical infections at treatment sites have been treated before starting therapy.
- Assess the skin and identify areas where medication is to be applied and areas that should be avoided (eg, infected site).
- Do not apply other topical products unless advised by health care provider.
- Assess and document skin condition before initial application and periodically throughout treatment. Inform health care provider if condition does not improve, worsens, or if application site reactions are bothersome.
- Monitor patient for development of lymphadenopathy. If noted inform health care provider.
- Assess patient for respiratory, CNS, GI, general body side effects, and application site reactions. Inform health care provider if noted and significant.

Patient/Family Education
Capsules and Injection:
- Warn patient not to alter the dose or discontinue the medication without consulting the health care provider.
- Instruct patient to check with health care provider before taking any OTC or prescription medications, or receiving any vaccinations.
- Patient should report any serious side effects to the health care provider.
- Inform patient of the need for frequent laboratory tests to assess the effectiveness of the treatment regimen and the need to keep appointments.
- Direct patient to avoid contact with others who may have any type of infection.
- Direct patient to take the medication 30 min before or 2 hr after meals. If the medication causes GI upset, take with a full glass of water. May be taken with food but is less effective.
- Advise patient to minimize or avoid exposure to natural or artificial sunlight while using tacrolimus ointment.
- Instruct patient to be sure skin is completely dry before applying tacrolimus ointment after a shower or bath.
- Instruct patient not to use tacrolimus with occlusive dressings.

Ointment:
- Explain name, dose, action, and potential side effects of drug.
- Advise patient or caregiver to carefully read the "Patient Package Insert" before using the first time and with each refill.
- Advise patient or caregiver that ointment is applied topically to skin lesions bid.
- Teach patient or caregiver proper technique for applying ointment: Wash hands. Apply a thin film of ointment to cover involved areas. Wash hands after applying ointment unless hands are also being treated.
- Advise patient or caregiver that before applying ointment after a bath or shower to be sure that skin is completely dry.
- Advise patient to continue therapy for 1 wk after signs and symptoms of dermatitis have resolved and then to stop using the ointment. If symptoms return, start applying the ointment again.
- Caution patient not to cover treated areas with bandages, dressings, or wraps.
- Warn patient to avoid contact with the eyes.
- Advise patient that if ointment comes in contact with the eyes to wash eyes with large amounts of cool water and to contact health care provider if eye irritation persists.

- Advise patient that burning sensations, stinging, soreness, or itching at the application site are the most common side effects and to notify health care provider if symptoms become severe or persist for more than several days.
- Advise patient that if condition does not improve after 2 wk of treatment or if condition worsens, to contact health care provider.
- Advise patient to talk to health care provider before using any other topical agents (eg, medicated soaps, astringents, cosmetics) on treated skin.
- Warn patient to avoid unnecessary exposure to sun and sunlamps while using this medication. Advise patient to use sunscreens, with minimum SPF of 15, and protective clothing over treated areas when exposure cannot be avoided.
- Advise women to notify health care provider if pregnant, planning to become pregnant, or breastfeeding.
- Warn patient not to take any prescription or OTC drugs or dietary supplements without consulting health care provider.
- Advise patient that follow-up visits to examine the skin lesions may be necessary and to keep appointments.

Tadalafil

(tah-DAH-lah-fil)

Class Agent for impotence

How Supplied
Cialis Tablets 5 mg, Tablets 10 mg, Tablets 20 mg

Action

PHARMACOLOGY: Enhances the effect of nitric oxide at the nerve ending and endothelial cells in the corpus cavernosum by inhibiting phosphodiesterase type 5 in the corpus cavernosum of the penis. This results in vasodilation, increased inflow of blood into the corporus cavernosum, and ensuing penile erection upon sexual stimulation.

PHARMACOKINETICS/DYNAMICS:

Absorption: Bioavailability undetermined; T_{max} is 30 min to 6 hr (median 2 hr).

Distribution: Vd of tadalafil is approximately 63 L, and it is 94% protein bound.

Metabolism: Predominantly metabolized by CYP3A4 to a catechol metabolite, which undergoes further metabolism to the major circulating metabolite, a methylcatechol glucuronide.

Excretion: Mean oral Cl is 2.5 L/hr and the mean t½ is 17.5 hr. Tadalafil is excreted predominantly as metabolites, mainly in the feces (approximately 61%) and to a lesser degree in the urine (about 36%).

Special Populations:
Elderly – Subjects over 65 yr have a 25% higher exposure compared with subjects 19 to 45 yr; however, no dosage adjustment is warranted based on age alone.

Indications Treatment of erectile dysfunction.

Contraindications Administration with nitrates and nitric oxide donors, alpha-blockers (except 0.4 mg/day tamsulosin); hypersensitivity to any component of the product.

Route/Dosage

ADULTS: **PO** 10 mg prior to anticipated sexual activity. The dose may be titrated to 5 or 20 mg based on efficacy and tolerability. The max recommended frequency is qd for most patients.

Renal Insufficiency
ADULTS: **PO** Mild renal insufficiency: No dosage adjustment is required. Moderate renal insufficiency (Ccr 31 to 50 mL/min): Start with 5 mg not more than qd (max, 10 mg q 48 hr). Severe renal insufficiency (Ccr less than 30 mL/min) on hemodialysis: Max recommended dose is 5 mg.

Hepatic Impairment
ADULTS: **PO** Mild to moderate hepatic impairment: Dose should not exceed 10 mg qd. Severe

hepatic impairment: Use is not recommended.

Interactions
Alpha-blockers (eg, terazosin), nitrates: Coadministration of these agents with tadalafil is contraindicated (except 0.4 mg/day tamsulosin).

CYP3A4 inducers (eg, carbamazepine, phenytoin, rifampin): Plasma levels may be decreased, reducing tadalafil exposure; however, no dosage adjustment is warranted.

CYP3A4 inhibitors (eg, ketoconazole, ritonavir): Plasma levels of tadalafil may be elevated, increasing the risk of side effects and necessitating dosage adjustment. Do not exceed 10 mg once every 72 hr.

Lab Test Interferences None well documented.

Adverse Reactions
CV: Angina pectoris, chest pain, hypotension, MI, postural hypotension, palpitation, syncope, tachycardia (less than 2%).
CNS: Headache (15%); fatigue, dizziness, hypesthesia, insomnia, paresthesia, somnolence, vertigo (less than 2%).
DERM: Pruritus, rash, sweating (less than 2%).
EENT: Nasal congestion (3%); blurred vision, changes in color vision, conjunctivitis (including hyperemia), eye pain, increased lacrimation, swelling of eyelids (less than 2%).
GI: Dyspepsia (10%); diarrhea, dry mouth, dysphagia, esophagitis (less than 2%).
GU: Increased erection, spontaneous penile erection (less than 2%).
HEPA: Abnormal LFTs (less than 2%).
MUSC: Myalgia (4%); arthralgia, neck pain (less than 2%).
RESP: Epistaxis, pharyngitis (less than 2%).
OTHER: Back pain (6%); limb pain, flushing (3%); asthenia, face edema, pain (less than 2%).

Precautions
Pregnancy: Category B.
Lactation: Undetermined.
Children: Safety and efficacy not established.
Renal function impairment: Dosage adjustment may be needed.
Hepatic function impairment: Dosage adjustment may be needed.
Special risk patients: Because there are no clinical data on safety and efficacy, use is not recommended in patients with unstable angina or angina occurring during sexual intercourse, MI within last 90 days, New York Heart Association Class II or greater heart failure in last 6 mo, uncontrolled arrhythmias, hypotension, uncontrolled hypertension, stroke within last 6 mo, hereditary degenerative retinal disorder (eg, retinitis pigmentosa).
CV risk: CV status and left ventricular outflow obstruction (eg, aortic stenosis) should be evaluated before treatment.
Priapism: Prolonged erections, exceeding 4 hr, may occur and require immediate medical attention.

PATIENT CARE CONSIDERATIONS

Administration/Storage
- Administer prescribed dose at least 30 min before sexual activity.
- Administer without regard to meals. Administer with food if GI upset occurs.
- Max dosing frequency is qd.
- Store tablets at controlled room temperature (59° to 86°F).

Assessment/Interventions
- Obtain patient history, including drug history and any known allergies. Note hepatic impairment, renal impairment, left ventricular outflow obstruction, unstable angina or angina occurring during sexual intercourse, hypotension, uncontrolled hypertension, anatomical deformation of penis (eg, Peyronie disease), conditions predisposing to priapism (eg, sickle cell anemia, multiple myeloma, leukemia), congenital degenerative retinal disorder, recent history of stroke (within 6 mo), heart failure (within 6 mo) or MI (within 90 days), uncontrolled arrhythmia. Note also concurrent use of antihypertensive medications, other treatments for erectile dysfunction, nitrates (eg, nitroglycerin), strong CYP3A4 inhibitors (eg, ritonavir, indinavir, ketoconazole, intraconazole, erythromycin), or alpha-blockers (eg, doxazosin).
- Ensure that CV status of patient has been assessed before therapy is started.
- Ensure that manufacturer's recommendations regarding use of lower doses and/or prolonged dosing intervals are followed for patient with moderate hepatic impairment, moderate or severe renal impairment, or who is concurrently taking a strong CYP3A4 inhibitor.
- Assess patient for CV, CNS, GI, musculoskeletal, and general body side effects. Inform health care provider if noted and significant.

Patient/Family Education
- Explain name, dose, action, and potential side effects of drug.
- Instruct patient to read the *Information for the Patient* leaflet before starting therapy and with each refill.
- Advise patient that medication may be most effective if taken approximately 60 min before anticipated sexual activity, but that medication can be taken anywhere from 30 min to 4 hr before sexual activity.

- Advise patient to take prescribed dose at least 30 min before anticipated sexual activity.
- Advise patient to take each dose without regard to meals but to take with food if stomach upset occurs.
- Advise patient that sexual stimulation will be required for medication to work and an erection to occur.
- Caution patient not to increase the dose or frequency of use unless advised by health care provider.
- Advise patient to contact health care provider if unsatisfied with sexual performance after taking medication or if bothersome side effects occur.
- Instruct patient to stop using and contact health care provider immediately if any of the following occur: dizziness, fainting, chest pain, vision changes, erection persisting longer than 4 hr, painful erection.
- Caution patient to limit alcohol intake while using tadalafil.
- Caution patient regarding concurrent use of nitrates and alpha-blockers (except 0.4 mg qd tamsulosin).
- Caution patient to avoid using "poppers" (eg, amyl nitrate, butyl nitrate) while taking this medication.
- Caution patient that medication is not a male form of birth control nor does it provide protection against sexually transmitted diseases and to use protective measures as indicated.
- Instruct patient not to take any prescription or OTC medications or dietary supplements unless advised by health care provider.
- Advise patient that follow-up visits may be required to monitor therapy and to keep appointments.

Talc, Sterile Powder

(TALK)

Class Sclerosing agent

How Supplied
Sclerosol Aerosol 4 g talc ♦ *Sterile Talc Powder* Powder 5 g talc

Action
PHARMACOLOGY: Induces an inflammatory reaction, which promotes adherence of the visceral and parietal pleura, obliterating the pleural space and preventing reaccumulation of pleural fluid.

Indications Decrease or prevent recurrence of malignant pleural effusions.

Contraindications Standard considerations.

Route/Dosage
ADULTS: **Powder** 5 g dissolved in 50 to 100 mL sodium chloride injection is recommended. **Aerosol** Single 4 to 8 g dose delivered from spray canister (1 to 2 cans), which delivers talc at a rate of 0.4 g/sec.

Interactions None well documented.

PATIENT CARE CONSIDERATIONS
Administration/Storage
Aerosol:
- Shake canister well immediately before use.
- Remove protective cap and securely attach actuator button with delivery tube (either 15 or 25 cm) to the valve stem of canister.
- Insert delivery tube through pleural trocar, taking care not to place distal end of delivery tube adjacent to the lung parenchyma or directly against chest wall. Hold delivery tube and pleural trocar together in 1 hand and

Lab Test Interferences None well documented.

Adverse Reactions
CV: Tachycardia; MI; hypotension; hypovolemia; asystolic arrest.
RESP: Hypoxemia; dyspnea; unilateral pulmonary edema; pneumonia; acute respiratory distress syndrome; bronchopleural fistula; hemoptysis; pulmonary emboli.
OTHER: Fever; empyema; pain; infection at site of thoracostomy or thoracoscopy; localized bleeding; subcutaneous emphysema.

Precautions
Pregnancy: Category B.
Children: Safety and efficacy not established.
Curable diseases: Because talc has no antineoplastic activity, it should not be used alone for potentially curable malignancies where systemic therapy is appropriate.
Future procedures: Sclerosis of the pleural space may preclude subsequent diagnostic procedures of the pleura on the treated side.
Pulmonary complications: Acute pneumonitis and acute respiratory distress syndrome may occur.

gently apply pressure to actuator button on the canister. Aerosol is not delivered by metered dose but depends on the extent and duration of manual compression of the actuator button on the canister. Point the distal end of the delivery tube in several different directions while administering short bursts in order to distribute talc powder equally and extensively on all visceral and parietal pleural surfaces. Discard canister and delivery tube after application is complete.

- Keep canister in upright position during talc instillation to ensure optimal distribution of talc powder.
- Store aerosol at controlled room temperature (59° to 86°F). Avoid freezing. Protect against sunlight. Do not expose to temperature greater than 120°F or canister may rupture. Contents under pressure. Do not puncture or incinerate canister.

Powder:

- Prepare talc slurry by adding 50 mL sodium chloride injection to talc bottle following manufacturer's instructions. Divide the content of the talc bottle into two 60 mL irrigation syringes by withdrawing 25 mL of the slurry into each syringe while swirling the bottle to prevent the talc from settling. Add sufficient quantity of sodium chloride injection to each syringe so that total volume is 50 mL. Draw air into each syringe to the 60 mL mark to provide a headspace for mixing prior to administration.
- Use slurry within 12 hr or discard and prepare a fresh slurry.
- Label syringes appropriately, noting the expiration date and time, and statements "For pleurodesis only - Not for IV administration," and "Shake well before use."
- Prior to administration, completely and continuously agitate the syringes to redisperse the talc and avoid settlement. Immediately prior to administration, vent the 10 mL air headspace and attach adapter and syringe tip. Maintain continuous agitation of the syringes. Shake well before instillation.
- Administer talc slurry through chest tube, then flush chest tube with 10 to 25 mL sodium chloride solution to ensure the complete talc dose is delivered. Clamp chest tube and follow manufacturer's guidelines regarding patient movement and distribution of talc within chest cavity.
- Store powder at controlled room temperature (64° to 77°F). Protect against sunlight.

Assessment/Interventions

- Obtain patient history, including drug history and any known allergies. Note potentially curable malignancy.
- Ensure that pleural fluid has been adequately drained and the lung fully re-expanded before instilling talc powder.
- Ensure that future diagnostic and therapeutic procedures involving the hemithorax have been considered before administering talc powder.
- Monitor patient for CV, RESP, and general body side effects. Report to health care provider if noted and significant.

Patient/Family Education

- Explain name, action, and potential side effects of drug, and how drug will be delivered into pleural space.
- Advise patient that medication will be prepared and administered by a health care provider in a medical setting.

Tamoxifen Citrate

(ta-MOX-ih-fen)

Class Antiestrogen hormone

How Supplied
Nolvadex Tablets 10 mg, Tablets 20 mg
✤ Apo-Tamox ♦ Gen-Tamoxifen ♦ Nolvadex-D ♦ Novo-Tamoxifen ♦ PMS-Tamoxifen ♦ Tamofen

Action
PHARMACOLOGY: A nonsteroidal agent with antiestrogenic properties.

PHARMACOKINETICS/DYNAMICS:

Absorption: Tamoxifen C_{max} is 40 ng/mL (range, 35 to 45 ng/mL), T_{max} is approximately 5 hr after dosing, and steady state is achieved in about 4 wk.

Metabolism: Tamoxifen is extensively metabolized. The major metabolite is N-desmethyl tamoxifen. It is a substrate of cytochrome P450 3A, 2C9, 2D6, and an inhibitor of P-glycoprotein.

Excretion: Tamoxifen t½ is 5 to 7 days; 65% of a dose is excreted over a period of 2 wk, with fecal excretion as the primary route of elimination.

Indications Breast carcinoma in women; metastatic breast carcinoma in men and women; reduction in risk of breast cancer in high-risk women; lower risk of invasive breast cancer in women with ductal carcinoma in situ (DCIS). **Unlabeled use(s):** Mastalgia; decreasing the size and pain of gynecomastia; McCune-Albright syndrome in female pediatric patients (in combination with other agents).

Contraindications Hypersensitivity to drug; women who require concomitant coumarin-type anticoagulant therapy; women with a history of deep vein thrombosis or pulmonary embolus (reduction in breast cancer incidence and DCIS indications).

Route/Dosage
Tamoxifen Alone as Adjunct to Surgery
ADULTS: **PO** 20 mg/day in 1 to 2 divided doses.

Duration of therapy of more than 2 yr is most effective.

Combination Chemotherapy as Adjunct to Surgery
ADULTS: PO 10 mg bid in postmenopausal women or women greater than 50 yr with positive axillary nodes for 5 yr.

Advanced Breast Carcinoma in Postmenopausal Women
ADULTS: PO 10 to 20 mg bid. Response to therapy should occur within 4 to 10 wk.

Prevention of Breast Cancer in High-Risk Women
ADULTS: PO 20 mg/day in 1 to 2 divided doses. Continue for 5 yr.

Interactions
Aminoglutethimide, phenobarbital: Tamoxifen concentrations may be reduced.
Bromocriptine: Tamoxifen concentrations may be increased.
Rifamycins (eg, rifampin): Tamoxifen plasma levels may be reduced, decreasing the antiestrogenic effect.
Tacrolimus, other drugs metabolized by cytochrome P450 3A4 (eg, amitriptyline, carbamazepine, cyclosporine, lovastatin, sertraline, verapamil): Coadministration may result in reduced clearance and increased serum concentrations of these agents.
Warfarin: Increased hypoprothrombinemic effect.

Lab Test Interferences
T_4 elevations; increased AST; increased bilirubin; increased creatinine. Variations in the karyopyknotic index on vaginal smears and various degrees of estrogen effect on Pap smears. In oligospermic males treated with tamoxifen, LH, FSH, testosterone, and estrogen levels were elevated.

Adverse Reactions
CV: Peripheral edema.
CNS: Headache; dizziness; depression.
DERM: Rash.
ENDO: Hot flashes.
GI: Moderate to low potential for nausea and vomiting; food distaste.
GU: Vaginal discharge; pruritus vulvae.
METAB: Hypercalcemia.
MUSC: Bone and tumor pain at initiation of therapy; soft tissue lesions can increase in size.
SPEC SENSE: Retinopathy; superficial corneal opacity.
OTHER: At doses of 40 mg/day, tamoxifen has increased the risk of endometrial cancer.

> **WARNING:**
> Uterine malignancies, stroke, and pulmonary embolism reported with use in risk reduction setting (women with ductal carcinoma in situ and women at high risk for breast cancer); some were fatal. Patient counseling in above patient groups may be necessary. Benefits outweigh risk in women with diagnosed breast cancer.

Precautions
Pregnancy: Category D.
Lactation: It is not known whether this drug is excreted in breast milk.
Children: Safety and efficacy in pediatric patients have not been established. Safety and efficacy for girls 2 to 10 yr with McCune-Albright syndrome and precocious puberty have not been studied beyond 1 yr of treatment. Long-term effects of therapy for girls have not been established.
Disease of bone: Increased bone pain, tumor pain, and local disease flare are sometimes associated with a good tumor response shortly after starting tamoxifen, and generally subside rapidly.
Hepatic effects: Changes in liver enzyme levels.
Hypercalcemia: If occurs, institute appropriate measures and, if severe, discontinue use.
Thromboembolic effects: Including deep vein thrombosis and pulmonary embolism.
Visual disturbances: Visual disturbances, including corneal changes, cataracts, the need for cataract surgery, decrement in color vision perception, retinal vein thrombosis, and retinopathy have occurred with use.

Overdosage: Signs and Symptoms
Respiratory difficulties, convulsions.

PATIENT CARE CONSIDERATIONS

Administration/Storage
- Store at room temperature (59° to 86°F). Protect from light.
- Administer PO.

Assessment/Interventions
- Monitor periodic CBC.
- Monitor periodic serum calcium levels during initial therapy in women with metastatic disease.
- Tamoxifen related tumor flare may be managed with supportive care, temporarily stopping tamoxifen with reintroduction at 5 to 10 mg/day, and concomitant prednisone for 1 to 2 wk.
- Perform periodic LFTs.
- Perform a breast examination, a mammogram, and a gynecologic examination prior to the initiation of therapy for women taking tamoxifen to reduce the incidence of breast cancer.

- Repeat CBC, LFTs, and gynecologic examinations at regular intervals while on therapy.
- Periodic monitoring of plasma triglycerides and cholesterol may be indicated in patients with preexisting hyperlipidemias.

Patient/Family Education

- Tamoxifen can induce ovulation.
- Tamoxifen reduces the incidence of breast cancer, but may not eliminate risk.
- Women should have regular gynecologic examinations and promptly inform their health care provider of menstrual irregularities, abnormal vaginal bleeding, change in vaginal discharge, or pelvic pain or pressure.
- Women should not become pregnant during therapy.
- Notify health care provider of pain/swelling/tenderness of legs or calves, unexplained shortness of breath, changes in vision, new breast lumps, vaginal bleeding, gynecologic symptoms (eg, menstrual irregularities, changes in vaginal discharge, pelvic pain or pressure), sudden chest pain, or coughing up blood.

Tamsulosin Hydrochloride

(tam-SOO-loe-sin HIGH-droe-KLOR-ide)

Class Antiadrenergic, peripherally acting

How Supplied

Flomax Capsules 0.4 mg

Action

PHARMACOLOGY: Selectively blocks alpha$_1$-adrenergic receptors causing relaxation of prostate smooth muscle resulting in an increase in urinary flow rate and a reduction in symptoms of BPH.

PHARMACOKINETICS/DYNAMICS:

Absorption: Tamsulosin absorption is greater than 90% (fasting), and T_{max} is 4 to 5 hr (fasting) and 6 to 7 hr (with food). Taking tamsulosin under fasted conditions results in a 30% increase in bioavailability (AUC) and 40% to 70% increase in peak concentrations.

Distribution: Steady state is achieved by the fifth day of qd dosing. Vd is about 16 L. Tamsulosin is widely distributed to most tissues, including kidney, prostate, liver, gall bladder, heart, aorta, and brown fat. There is minimal distribution to brain, spinal cord, and testes. The drug is 94% to 99% protein bound.

Metabolism: Tamsulosin is extensively metabolized by cytochrome P450 in the liver.

Excretion: Tamsulosin t½ is 5 to 7 hr. Approximately 10% is excreted unchanged in urine.

Special Populations:

Elderly – AUC is 40% higher in subjects 55 to 75 yr compared with subjects 20 to 32 yr.

Indications Treatment of signs and symptoms of benign prostatic hyperplasia.

PATIENT CARE CONSIDERATIONS

Administration/Storage

- Do not chew, crush, or open capsule. Instruct patient to swallow capsule whole.
- Give once daily about 30 min after the same meal each day.

Contraindications Standard considerations.

Route/Dosage

ADULTS: PO 0.4 mg/day, administered approximately 30 min following the same meal each day. If the patient fails to respond after 2 to 4 wk, the dose may be increased to 0.8 mg/day.

Interactions

Cimetidine: Concomitant use may decrease tamsulosin clearance and increase the AUC. Use with caution.

Lab Test Interferences None well documented.

Adverse Reactions

CNS: Headache (21%); dizziness (17%); somnolence (4%); decreased libido (2%); insomnia (1%).
EENT: Rhinitis (18%); pharyngitis (5%); amblyopia (2%).
GI: Diarrhea (6%); nausea (4%); tooth disorder (2%).
GU: Abnormal ejaculation (18%).
RESP: Increased cough (5%); sinusitis (4%).
OTHER: Infection (11%); asthenia (9%); back pain (8%); chest pain (4%).

Precautions

Pregnancy: Category B.
Lactation: Not indicated for use in women.
Children: Safety and efficacy not established.
Hypertension: Tamsulosin is currently not indicated for the treatment of hypertension.
Priapism: Association is rare; can lead to permanent impotence if not properly treated.
Prostate cancer: Rule out before starting therapy.

Overdosage: Signs and Symptoms

Hypotension, severe headache.

- Store at controlled room temperature (59° to 86°F). Protect from excessive moisture.
- Not indicated for use in women.

Assessment/Interventions
- Obtain patient history, including drug history and any known allergies. Note current use of antihypertensives.
- Assess BP and pulse after administration.
- Monitor changes in urination (eg, frequency, volume, dribbling).
- Monitor patient for GI, CNS, CV, and general body side effects. Report to health care provider if noted and significant.
- Monitor patient for orthostatic hypotension. Notify health care provider if symptomatic orthostatic hypotension is noted.
- Implement safety precautions for patients who experience dizziness.

Patient/Family Education
- Explain name, dose, action, and potential side effects of drug.
- Advise about the possibility of priapism, which requires immediate medical attention.
- Advise patient to take prescribed dose qd, about 30 min after the same meal each day.
- Advise patient not to crush, chew, or open capsule and to swallow the capsule whole with a full glass of water.
- Advise patient that dose may be increased after 2 to 4 wk to increase beneficial effects on the prostate gland. Caution patient that if a larger dose is being used and is interrupted for several days to restart therapy with the lower dose.
- Caution patient to avoid sudden position changes to prevent orthostatic hypotension. If orthostatic hypotension does occur, instruct patient to sit or lie down
- Caution patient that drug may cause dizziness or drowsiness and to use caution while driving or performing other tasks requiring mental alertness until tolerance is determined.
- Instruct patient to report the following symptoms to the health care provider: dizziness, fainting, excessive drowsiness, sexual dysfunction.
- Advise patient to contact health care provider if urinary symptoms do not improve or if they worsen while taking this medication.
- Advise patient to read Patient Information insert before starting therapy and with each refill.
- Caution patient not to take any prescription or OTC drugs or dietary supplements unless advised by health care provider.
- Advise patient that follow-up visits may be necessary to monitor therapy and to keep appointments.

Tazarotene

(tazz-AHR-oh-teen)

Class Retinoid

How Supplied
Avage Cream 0.1% ♦ Tazorac Cream 0.05%, Cream 0.1%, Gel 0.05%, Gel 0.1%

Action
PHARMACOLOGY: Undefined; however, inhibits cornified envelope formation, which is an element of psoriatic scales.

Indications
Treatment of acne (*Tazorac* cream and gel), psoriasis (*Tazorac* gel); as an adjunctive agent in mitigation of facial fine wrinkling, facial mottled hyper- and hypopigmentation, and benign facial lentigines in patients who use comprehensive skin care and sunlight avoidance programs (*Avage*).

Contraindications
Pregnancy; hypersensitivity to any component of the product.

Route/Dosage
Acne
ADULTS AND CHILDREN (12 YR AND OLDER): Topical After gently cleansing and drying the face, apply a thin film (2 mg/cm^2) once daily in the evening where acne lesions appear.

Psoriasis
ADULTS (18 YR AND OLDER): Topical Apply once a day in the evening to psoriatic lesions, using enough (2 mg/cm^2) to cover only the lesion with a thin film.

Wrinkling, Hyper- and Hypopigmentation, Lentigines
ADULTS (18 YR AND OLDER): Topical Apply pea-sized amount once daily at bedtime to lightly cover the entire face including the eyelids if desired.

Interactions
None well documented.

Lab Test Interferences
None well documented.

Adverse Reactions
DERM: Skin pain (*Tazorac*); skin inflammation, worsening of psoriasis, rash (*Tazorac* for psoriasis); desquamation; stinging; dry skin; erythema; pruritus; skin irritation; burning sensation; fissuring localized edema, skin discoloration (*Tazorac* gel for acne); irritant contact dermatitis; fissuring; bleeding (*Tazorac* gel for psoriasis); contact dermatitis; dermatitis; eczema; peripheral edema (*Tazorac* cream for psoriasis); irritant contact dermatitis; acne; rash; cheilitis (*Avage*).
METAB: Hypertriglyceridemia (*Tazorac* cream for psoriasis)

Precautions
Pregnancy: Category X.
Lactation: Undetermined.
Children: Safety and efficacy not established in patients with psoriasis under 18 yr or under 12 yr with acne (cream). Safety and efficacy not established in children under 12 yr (gel). Safety and efficacy not established in patients under 17 yr with facial fine wrinkling, facial mottled hypo- and hyperpigmentation and benign facial lentigines (*Avage*).

Special risk patients: Avoid use on eczematous skin and avoid concurrent use of medications and cosmetics that have a strong drying effect; assess facial pigmented lesions before use.
Photosensitivity: Use with caution if patient is known to be taking a photosensitizing drug because of increased risk of photosensitivity.

Overdosage: Signs and Symptoms
Marked redness, peeling, discomfort.

PATIENT CARE CONSIDERATIONS

Administration/Storage
- For topical use only. Not for ophthalmic, oral, or intravaginal use.
- Avoid contact with eyes, eyelids, lips, and mucus membranes.
- Cream or gel is usually applied to affected areas once daily at nighttime.
- For treatment of acne, cleanse area with a mild or soapless cleanser before applying cream or gel. Skin should be dry before application.
- For treatment of wrinkling, hyper- or hypopigmentation, or lentigines, cleanse area with a mild soap before applying cream. Skin should be dry before application.
- Apply a thin film of cream or gel to cover the affected area(s). Avoid application to unaffected areas of the skin.
- Store gel at controlled room temperature (59° to 86°F). Cream may be stored in refrigerator or at room temperature (23° to 86°F). Keep tube tightly capped.

Assessment/Interventions
- Obtain patient history, including drug history and any known allergies. Note sensitivity to sunlight, concurrent use of medications which increase sensitivity to sunlight, or concurrent use of vitamin A supplements.
- Ensure that women of childbearing potential are not pregnant before starting therapy and that effective birth control measures are being used.
- Initiate therapy in women of childbearing potential during a normal menstrual period.
- Assess the skin and identify areas where medication is to be applied and areas that should be avoided (eg, eczema, sunburned skin).
- Assess and document skin condition before initial application and periodically throughout treatment.
- Monitor for side effects, including redness, scaling, dryness, or persistent itching or burning. Inform health care provider if noted and significant.

Patient/Family Education
- Advise patient to carefully read the "Information For Patients" leaflet before using the first time and with each refill.
- Explain name, dose, action, and potential side effects of drug.
- Advise patient that medication is applied topically to skin lesions once daily at nighttime.
- Teach patient with psoriasis proper technique for applying medication: ensure that skin is dry if shower or bath were taken; wash hands; apply a thin film of cream or gel to cover skin areas with psoriasis plaques or scales; wash medication off unaffected areas that may have had medication applied. Wash hands after applying medication unless medication is being used to treat psoriasis on hands.
- Teach patient with acne proper technique for applying medication: wash hands; cleanse area with mild or soapless cleanser first then apply a thin film of cream or gel to cover skin areas with acne lesions. Wash hands after applying medication.
- Teach patient with winkling, hypo- or hyperpigmentation or lentigines proper technique for applying medication: wash hands; cleanse area with mild soap first, allow to dry and then apply a "pea-sized" amount of cream and lightly spread to cover the entire face, including the eyelids if desired. Wash hands after applying medication. Remind patient that facial moisturizers may be used as frequently as desired and to always apply a moisturizing sunscreen, SPF 15 or greater, each morning.
- Advise patient using creams or lotions to soften or lubricate skin to apply medication only after ensuring that the cream or lotion has been absorbed and the skin is dry.
- Caution patient not to cover treated areas with bandages or dressings.
- Inform patient that a mild sensation of warmth or slight stinging or burning may be

felt shortly after application and that this is expected and should be of no concern.
- Warn patient that applying medication more often than prescribed or in excessive quantities will not produce more rapid improvement or better results but will result in greater side effects such as redness, scaling, and discomfort.
- Advise patient that if they miss an application to not try to make it up but to return to normal application schedule as soon as possible.
- Warn patient to avoid contact with the eyes, eyelids, lips, and mucous membranes.
- Advise patient that if cream or gel comes in contact with the eyes to wash eyes with large amounts of cool water and to contact health care provider if eye irritation persists.
- Advise patient to not apply to skin areas with eczema or that are sunburned.
- Advise patient with psoriasis that plaques and scales will begin to improve in 1 to 4 wk but that the redness may take longer to improve and to continue using the medication.
- Advise patient with acne that improvement may not be seen for at least 4 wk and to continue using the medication.
- Advise patient that local redness, drying, scaling, burning, or itching are the most common side effects and to notify health care provider if becoming bothersome.
- Advise patient that if severe dermal reactions occur to stop using the medication and contact health care provider.
- Advise patient to talk to health care provider before using any other topical agents (eg, medicated soaps, astringents, cosmetics, other acne products) on treated skin.
- Warn patient to avoid unnecessary exposure to sun and sun lamps while using this medication. Advise patient to use sunscreens, with minimum SPF of 15, and protective clothing over treated areas when exposure cannot be avoided.
- Caution patient that while using the medication, exposure to extreme weather conditions (eg, wind, cold air) may be irritating to the treated areas.
- Advise women to inform health care provider if pregnant, planning to become pregnant, or breastfeeding.
- Warn patient not to take any prescription or OTC drugs or dietary supplements without consulting health care provider.
- Advise patient that follow-up visits to examine the skin lesions may be necessary and to keep appointments.

Tegaserod Maleate

(teg-ah-SER-odd MAL-ee-ate)
Class 5-HT$_4$ receptor agonist
How Supplied
Zelnorm Tablets 2 mg, Tablets 6 mg
Action
PHARMACOLOGY: Binds with high affinity to human 5-HT$_4$ receptors, acting as an agonist at neuronal 5-HT$_4$ receptors to trigger the release of neurotransmitters.

PHARMACOKINETICS/DYNAMICS:
Absorption: Tegaserod T$_{max}$ is 1 hr. Bioavailability is approximately 10% when given to fasting subjects. When given with food, tegaserod bioavailability is decreased 40% to 65%, and C$_{max}$ is decreased approximately 20% to 40%.
Distribution: Tegaserod is approximately 98% protein bound (predominantly to alpha-1-acid glycoprotein) and exhibits pronounced distribution into tissues following IV dosing. Vd is approximately 368 L.
Metabolism: Tegaserod is metabolized 1) by presystemic acid catalyzed hydrolysis in stomach followed by oxidation and conjugation, and 2) by direct glucuronidation. The main metabolite is a 5-methoxyindole-3-carboxylic acid glucuronide and has negligible affinity.
Excretion: Plasma Cl of tegaserod is approximately 77 L/hr. Elimination t½ is approximately 11 hr following IV dosing. About ⅔ of the orally administered dose is excreted unchanged in the feces; ⅓ is excreted in the urine primarily as the main metabolite.

Special Populations:
Renal Function Impairment – Tegaserod is not recommended in severe renal impairment because AUC is increased 10-fold.
Hepatic Function Impairment – Mean AUC is approximately 31% higher, but no dosage adjustment is required in mild hepatic impairment; however, caution is recommended when using tegaserod in this population.

Indications Short-term treatment of women with irritable bowel syndrome (IBS) whose primary symptom is constipation.

Contraindications Severe renal impairment; moderate to severe hepatic impairment; history of bowel obstruction; symptomatic gall bladder disease; suspected sphincter of Oddi dysfunction; abdominal adhesions; known hypersensitivity to the drug or any of its excipients.

Route/Dosage
ADULTS (WOMEN): **PO** 6 mg bid before meals for 4 to 6 wk.

Interactions
Digoxin, oral contraceptives: Plasma concentrations of these drugs may be reduced; however, adjustments in therapy are unlikely to be necessary.

Lab Test Interferences None well documented.

Adverse Reactions
CV: Hypotension; angina pectoris; syncope; arrhythmia; bundle branch block; supraventricular tachycardia; syncope (postmarketing).
CNS: Headache (15%); dizziness (4%); migraine (2%); vertigo; attempted suicide; impaired concentration; emotional lability; increased appetite; sleep disorder; depression.
DERM: Flushing; pruritus; increased sweating.
GI: Abdominal pain (12%); diarrhea (9%); nausea (8%); flatulence (6%); irritable colon; fecal incontinence; tenesmus; increased appetite; eructation; appendicitis; subileus; ischemic colitis, mesenteric ischemia, gangrenous bowel, rectal bleeding, suspected sphincter of Oddi spasm, bile duct stone (postmarketing).
GU: Ovarian cyst; miscarriage; menorrhagia; breast carcinoma; albuminuria; frequent micturition: polyuria; renal pain.
HEPA: Increased AST and ALT; bilirubinemia; cholecystitis.
METAB: Increased creatine phosphokinase.
MUSC: Back pain (5%); arthropathy (2%); cramps.
RESP: Asthma.
OTHER: Accidental trauma (3%); leg pain (1%); pain, facial edema.

Precautions
Pregnancy: Category B.
Lactation: Undetermined.
Children: Safety and efficacy in children younger than 18 yr of age not established.
Abdominal pain: Discontinue immediately in patients with new or sudden worsening of abdominal pain.
Diarrhea: Do not initiate therapy in patients who are experiencing or frequently experience diarrhea.
Ischemic colitis: May occur. Discontinue immediately in patients who develop symptoms of ischemic colitis, such as rectal bleeding, bloody diarrhea, or new or worsening abdominal pain.

Overdosage: Signs and Symptoms
Diarrhea, headache, intermittent abdominal pain, flatulence, nausea, vomiting.

PATIENT CARE CONSIDERATIONS
Administration/Storage
- For use in women only. Do not administer to men.
- Administer prescribed dose bid at least 30 min before meals.
- Store tablets at controlled room temperature (59° to 86°F). Protect from moisture.

Assessment/Interventions
- Obtain patient history, including drug history and any known allergies. Note severe renal impairment, moderate or severe hepatic impairment, symptomatic gallbladder disease, suspected sphincter of Oddi dysfunction, abdominal adhesions, history of bowel obstruction, or history of ischemic colitis while taking tegaserod previously.
- Do not administer to patient who is experiencing diarrhea or frequently experiences diarrhea.
- Assess and document effect of medication on IBS symptoms.
- Monitor patient for CNS, GI, and general body side effects. Report to health care provider if noted and significant.
- Discontinue use and notify health care provider immediately if patient experiences new or sudden worsening of abdominal pain, rectal bleeding, bloody diarrhea, hypotension, or syncope.

Patient/Family Education
- Explain name, dose, action, and potential side effects of drug.
- Advise patient to read *Patient Information* provided with medication.
- Instruct patient to take prescribed dose bid at least 30 min before a meal.
- Instruct patient that if a dose is missed to skip that dose and take the next dose at the regularly scheduled time. Warn patient not to double the dose to make up the missed dose.
- Warn patient not to start medication if currently or frequently experiencing diarrhea.
- Advise patient that medication does not cure IBS, should be taken as prescribed, and not to stop taking or change the dose unless advised by health care provider. Advise patient that IBS symptoms may return within 1 to 2 wk of discontinuing therapy.
- Advise patient that medication is usually taken for 4 to 6 wk and if improvement is noted, health care provider may recommend an additional 4 to 6 wk of therapy.
- Instruct patient to discontinue use and immediately notify health care provider if any of

the following occur: new or worsening abdominal pain; severe diarrhea or diarrhea accompanied by severe cramping, stomach pain, or dizziness; rectal bleeding or bloody diarrhea; fainting.
- Advise women to notify health care provider if pregnant, planning to become pregnant, or breastfeeding.
- Warn patient not to take any prescription or OTC drugs, dietary supplements, or herbal preparations without consulting health care provider.
- Advise patient that follow-up visits may be necessary to monitor therapy and to keep appointments.

Telithromycin

(tel-ITH-roe-MY-sin)

Class Antibiotic

How Supplied
Ketek Tablets 400 mg

Action
PHARMACOLOGY: Interferes with microbial protein synthesis.

PHARMACOKINETICS/DYNAMICS:
Absorption: Bioavailability 57%. C_{max} approximately 2 mcg/mL after an 800 mg oral dose, and peak level is reached in about 1 hr. Steady-state plasma level reached in 2 to 3 days.
Distribution: Protein binding is 60% to 70%. Vd is 2.9 L/kg.
Metabolism: Approximately 70% of dose is metabolized. About 50% of metabolism is mediated by CYP3A4.
Excretion: Terminal elimination t½ is about 10 hr. Elimination consists of 7% unchanged in feces, 13% unchanged in the urine, and 37% metabolized by the liver.

Indications Treatment of acute bacterial exacerbation of chronic bronchitis, acute bacterial sinusitis, and community-acquired pneumonia caused by strains of susceptible organisms.

Contraindications Coadministration of cisapride or pimozide; history of hypersensitivity to any macrolide antibiotic or any component of this product.

Route/Dosage
Acute Bacterial Exacerbation of Chronic Bronchitis; Acute Bacterial Sinusitis
ADULTS: PO 800 mg daily for 5 days.

Community-Acquired Pneumonia
ADULTS: PO 800 mg daily for 7 to 10 days.

Interactions
Atorvastatin, lovastatin, simvastatin: Telithromycin may elevate plasma levels of these agents increasing the risk of side effects (eg, myopathy).
Carbamazepine, cyclosporine, hexobarbital, metoprolol, midazolam, phenytoin, sirolimus, tacrolimus: Telithromycin may elevate plasma levels of these agents, increasing the pharmacologic and adverse effects.
Carbamazepine, phenobarbital, phenytoin, rifampin: May decrease telithromycin plasma concentrations, resulting in subtherapeutic levels and loss of efficacy.
Cisapride, pimozide: Concurrent use of these agents with telithromycin is contraindicated.
Ergot alkaloid derivatives (eg ergotamine, dihydroergotamine): Acute ergot toxicity characterized by severe peripheral vasospasm and dyesthesia may occur.
Itraconazole, ketoconazole: May increase telithromycin plasma concentrations.
Sotalol: Plasma levels may be decreased by telithromycin.

Lab Test Interferences None well documented.

Adverse Reactions
CV: Atrial arrhythmias (postmarketing).
CNS: Headache (6%); dizziness (4%); dry mouth, somnolence, insomnia, vertigo, increased sweating, fatigue (less than 2%).
DERM: Rash (less than 2%).
EENT: Visual adverse effects (including blurred vision, diplopia, difficulty focusing [less than 2%]).
GI: Diarrhea (11%); nausea (8%); vomiting (3%); loose stools, dysgeusia (2%); abdominal distension, dyspepsia, GI upset, flatulence, constipation, gastroenteritis, gastritis, anorexia, oral candidiasis, glossitis, stomatitis, watery stools, abdominal pain, upper abdominal pain (less than 2%).
GU: Vaginal candidiasis, vaginitis, vaginal fungal infection (less than 2%).
HEMA: Increased platelet count (less than 2%).
HEPA: Abnormal LFTs, increased transaminases, increased liver enzymes (eg, ALT, AST) (less than 2%); hepatic dysfunction, including hepatocellular and/or cholestatic hepatitis, with or without jaundice (postmarketing).
MUSC: Muscle cramps, exacerbation of myasthenia gravis (postmarketing).
OTHER: Allergy, including face edema, angioedema, anaphylaxis (postmarketing).

Precautions
Pregnancy: Category C.
Lactation: Undetermined.
Children: Safety and efficacy not established.

Superinfection: Prolonged use of antibiotics may result in bacterial or fungal overgrowth of nonsusceptible microorganisms.
Hepatitis/Jaundice: Use with caution in patients with history of hepatitis or jaundice associated with telithromycin use.
Myasthenia gravis: Exacerbation of myasthenia gravis have been reported, in some cases within hours after the first dose of telithromycin. Life-threatening acute respiratory failure with rapid onset in patients with myasthenia gravis treated for respiratory tract infections with telithromycin has been reported.
Pseudomembranous colitis: Consider possibility in patients in whom diarrhea develops.
QT interval: May be prolonged in some patients.
Visual disturbances: Ability to accommodate and ability to release accommodation may be slowed.

Overdosage: Signs and Symptoms
Carefully monitor ECG and electrolytes.

PATIENT CARE CONSIDERATIONS
Administration/Storage
- Duration of therapy depends on site of infection.
- Administer daily without regard to meals. Administer with food if GI upset occurs.
- Store tablets at controlled room temperature (59° to 86°F).

Assessment/Interventions
- Obtain patient history, including drug history and any known allergies. Note renal or hepatic impairment, myasthenia gravis, congenital QT prolongation, hypokalemia, hypomagnesemia, bradycardia, hepatitis, or jaundice associated with previous use of telithromycin, concurrent use of class IA (eg, quinidine) or class III (eg, dofetilide) antiarrhythmic agents, concurrent use of simvastatin, lovastatin, or atorvastatin, or hypersensitivity to any other macrolide antibiotic.
- Review results of culture and sensitivity testing as available.
- Monitor for signs of infection, especially fever, and for positive response to antibiotic therapy.
- Monitor patient for GI, CNS, general body side effects, and signs of superinfection. Report to health care provider if noted and significant. Immediately report severe diarrhea, diarrhea containing blood or pus, or severe abdominal cramping.

Patient/Family Education
- Explain name, dose, action, and potential side effects of drug.
- Instruct patient to take exactly as prescribed and not to change the dose or discontinue therapy unless advised by health care provider.
- Instruct patient to take prescribed dose at the same time once daily. Advise patient that medication can be taken without regard to meals, but to take with food if stomach upset occurs.
- Instruct patient to complete entire course of therapy, even if symptoms of infection have disappeared.
- Instruct patient to notify health care provider if infection does not appear to be improving or appears to be getting worse.
- Advise patient to discontinue therapy and contact health care provider immediately if skin rash, hives, itching, shortness of breath, palpitations, or fainting occur.
- Advise patient to report signs of superinfection to health care provider: black "furry" tongue, white patches in mouth, foul-smelling stools, vaginal itching or discharge.
- Warn patient that diarrhea containing blood or pus may be a sign of a serious disorder and to seek medical care if noted and not treat at home. Caution patient that this may occur even weeks after completing therapy.
- Caution patient that drug may cause visual disturbances (eg, blurred vision, difficulty focusing, double vision) and to use caution while driving or performing other potentially hazardous activities until tolerance is determined. Advise patient that if visual problems develop that avoiding quick changes in viewing objects in the distance and nearby may help decrease the effects. Advise patient to contact health care provider if visual difficulties interfere with daily activities.
- Advise patient to report any other bothersome side effect to health care provider.
- Advise women to notify physician if pregnant, planning to become pregnant, or breastfeeding.
- Instruct patient not to take any prescription or OTC medications, dietary supplements, or herbal preparations unless advised by health care provider.
- Advise patient that follow-up examinations and lab tests may be required to monitor therapy and to keep appointments.

Telmisartan

(tell-mih-SAHR-tan)

Class Antihypertensive/Angiotensin II antagonist

How Supplied
Micardis Tablets 20 mg, Tablets 40 mg, Tablets 80 mg

Action
PHARMACOLOGY: Antagonizes the effect of angiotensin II (vasoconstriction and aldosterone secretion) by blocking the angiotensin II (AT_1) receptor) in vascular smooth muscle and the adrenal gland, producing decreased BP.

PHARMACOKINETICS/DYNAMICS:

Absorption: Telmisartan T_{max} is 0.5 to 1 hr after dosing. Food slightly reduces bioavailability of telmisartan, with an AUC reduction of about 6% with a 40 mg tablet and 20% with a 160 mg dose. At 40 and 160 mg, the bioavailability was 42% and 58%. Trough plasma concentrations with qd dosing are about 10% to 25% of peak plasma concentrations.

Distribution: Telmisartan is greater than 99.5% protein bound. Vd is about 500 L.

Metabolism: Telmisartan is metabolized by conjugation to form a pharmacologically inactive acylglucuronide. The glucuronide of the parent compound is the only metabolite that has been identified in human plasma and urine.

Excretion: Telmisartan t½ is approximately 24 hr and total plasma Cl is greater than 800 mL/min. After IV or oral administration, more than 97% is eliminated unchanged in feces via biliary excretion.

Special Populations:
Hepatic Function Impairment – Plasma concentrations are increased and absolute bioavailability approaches 100%.
Gender – Plasma concentrations are generally 2 to 3 times higher in women than in men.

Indications Treatment of hypertension.

Contraindications Standard considerations.

Route/Dosage
ADULTS: **PO** 20 to 80 mg/day; usual starting dose, 40 mg/day.

PATIENT CARE CONSIDERATIONS

Administration/Storage
* Store at room temperature (59° to 86°F).
* Do not remove tablets from blisters or containers until immediately before administration.

Interactions
Digoxin: May increase plasma levels of digoxin, that may increase toxicity.
Lithium: Plasma concentrations may be increased by telmisartan, resulting in an increase in the pharmacologic and adverse effects of lithium.

Lab Test Interferences None well documented.

Adverse Reactions
EENT: Sinusitis (3%); pharyngitis (1%).
GI: Diarrhea (3%).
RESP: Upper respiratory tract infection (7%).
OTHER: Back pain (3%).

> WARNING:
>
> *Pregnancy:* Use in second and third trimesters may cause injury and death to fetus.

Precautions
Pregnancy: Category C (first trimester); Category D (second and third trimester).
Lactation: Undetermined.
Children: Safety and efficacy not established.
Renal function impairment: Use with caution in patients whose renal function may depend on the activity of the renin-angiotensin-aldosterone system (eg, patients with severe CHF); use may be associated with oliguria, progressive azotemia, acute renal failure, and death.
Hepatic function impairment: Use with caution.
Black patients: Telmisartan may not be as effective in black patients.
Dialysis: Patients on dialysis may develop orthostatic hypotension.
Hypotension/Volume-depleted patients: Symptomatic hypotension may occur after telmisartan initiation in intravascularly volume-depleted patients (eg, those treated with diuretics). Correct these conditions prior to administration or use lower starting dose.

Overdosage: Signs and Symptoms
Hypotension, dizziness, tachycardia, bradycardia.

* Anticipate combination with a diuretic if target BP values are not reached.
* Administer without regard to food.
* Do not administer to patients with intravascular volume depletion until the condition has been corrected.

- Administer with caution and under close medical supervision to patients with biliary obstructive disorders or hepatic insufficiency.
- Do not administer to pregnant women.

Assessment/Interventions
- Obtain patient history and drug history including allergies.
- Monitor patient for potential adverse effects and drug interactions.
- Monitor BP and pulse. Should hypotension, tachycardia, or bradycardia occur, withhold the medication and notify health care provider.
- Closely monitor patients on dialysis for orthostatic hypotension.
- Monitor BP, especially patients on dialysis.
- Monitor patient for signs of hypersensitivity including angioedema involving swelling of the face, lips, and tongue, or difficulty breathing.

Patient/Family Education
- Instruct patient to take the medication as prescribed at the same time each day.
- Inform patient that telmisartan controls but does not cure hypertension.
- Caution patient to take the dose exactly as prescribed and not to stop taking the medication even if feeling better. Instruct patient not to increase or decrease the dosage.
- Instruct family and patient in BP and pulse measurement skills. Caution patient to call primary health care provider should abnormal measurements occur.
- Instruct patient in methods of fall prevention including rising slowly and sitting on the side of the bed before standing, especially early in therapy.
- Inform patient of the importance of adjunct therapies such as dietary planning, regular exercise program, weight reduction, low sodium diet, alcohol reduction, smoking cessation, and stress management.
- Instruct patient to report symptoms of weakness, fatigue, dizziness, or lightheadedness to health care provider.
- Caution patient to notify health care provider or dentist of use of this product prior to surgery or treatment.
- Advise women to contact health care provider if pregnant, planning to become pregnant, or breastfeeding. Inform the patient of potential harm to the fetus.

Telmisartan/Hydrochlorothiazide

(tell-mih-SAHR-tan/high-droe-klor-THIGH-uh-zide)

Class Antihypertensive combination

How Supplied
Micardis HCT Tablets 40 mg telmisartan and 12.5 mg hydrochorothiazide, Tablets 80 mg telmisartan and 12.5 mg hydrochorothiazide

Action
PHARMACOLOGY:
Telmisartan: Antagonizes the effect of angiotensin II (vasoconstriction and aldosterone secretion) by blocking the angiotensin II (AT_1 receptor) in vascular smooth muscle and the adrenal gland, producing decreased BP.
Hydrochlorothiazide (HCTZ): Increases chloride, sodium, and water excretion by interfering with transport of sodium ions across renal tubular epithelium.

Indications Treatment of hypertension.

Contraindications Patients with anuria; hypersensitivity to sulfonamide-derived drugs or any component of this product.

Route/Dosage
The fixed combination is not indicated for initial therapy. The combination may be substituted for the titrated components.

ADULTS: PO Telmisartan may be used over a dose range of 20 to 80 mg/day, administered qd. HCTZ is effective in doses of 12.5 to 50 mg qd. The dose may be titrated up to 160 mg telmisartan plus 25 mg of HCTZ, if necessary.

Interactions
Telmisartan:
Digoxin – Peak and trough plasma levels may be elevated by telmisartan.
HCTZ:
Alcohol, barbiturates, narcotics – Increased risk of orthostatic hypotension.
Antidiabetic agents (oral agents and insulin) – Dosage adjustment of antidiabetic agent may be necessary.
Antihypertensive agent – Additive or potentiation of effects.
Cholestyramine, colestipol resins – Impaired absorption of hydrochlorothiazide.
Corticosteroids, ACTH – Increased electrolyte depletion, increasing the risk of hypokalemia.
Lithium – Renal Cl of lithium may be reduced, increasing the risk of lithium toxicity.
Nondepolarizing skeletal muscle relaxants (eg, tubocurarine) – Increased effect of the muscle relaxant.
Nonsteroidal anti-inflammatory agents – The diuretic, natriuretic, and antihypertensive effects of loop, potassium-sparing, and thiazide diuretics may be reduced.

Potassium supplements – Salt substitutes containing potassium or potassium supplements should not be used without consulting the prescribing physician.

Pressor amines (eg, norepinephrine) – Decreased responsiveness to the pressor amine.

Lab Test Interferences

HCTZ: May decrease serum protein-bound iodine levels without signs of thyroid disturbances. May cause diagnostic interference of serum electrolyte levels, blood and urine glucose levels, serum bilirubin levels, and serum uric acid levels.

Adverse Reactions

CV: Tachycardia; postural hypotension.
Telmisartan – Palpitations; dependent edema; angina pectoris; leg edema; abnormal ECG; hypertension; peripheral edema; cerebral vascular disorder.
CNS: Fatigue; dizziness.
Telmisartan – Insomnia; somnolence; migraine; vertigo; paresthesia; involuntary muscle contraction; anxiety; depression; nervousness; hypoaesthesia.
HCTZ – Restlessness.
DERM: Rash.
Telmisartan – Increased sweating; flushing; dermatitis; eczema; pruritus.
HCTZ – Erythema multiforme (including Stevens-Johnson syndrome); exfoliative dermatitis (including toxic epidermal necrolysis).
EENT: Sinusitis; pharyngitis.
Telmisartan – Otitis media; rhinitis; abnormal vision; conjunctivitis; tinnitus; earache.
HCTZ – Blurred vision; xanthopsia.
GI: Diarrhea; nausea; dyspepsia; vomiting; abdominal pain.
Telmisartan – Flatulence; constipation; gastritis; dry mouth; hemorrhoids; gastroenteritis; enteritis; gastroesophageal reflux; toothache; nonspecific GI disorders.
HCTZ – Pancreatitis; sialadenitis; cramping; gastric irritation.
GU:
Telmisartan – Impotence; micturition frequency; cystitis.
HCTZ – Renal failure; renal dysfunction; interstitial nephritis.
HEMA:
HCTZ – Agranulocytosis; aplastic anemia; leukopenia; hemolytic anemia; thrombocytopenia.
HEPA:
HCTZ – Jaundice (intrahepatic cholestatic).
METAB:
Telmisartan – Gout; hypercholesterolemia; diabetes mellitus.
HCTZ – Hyperglycemia; glycosuria; hyperuricemia.
RESP: Upper respiratory tract infection; bronchitis.
Telmisartan – Asthma; dyspnea; epistaxis.
OTHER: Flu-like symptoms; back pain.
Telmisartan – Allergy; fever; leg pain and cramps; malaise; chest pain; arthritis; arthralgia; myalgia; infection (including fungal); abscess.
HCTZ – Hypersensitivity (including purpura, photosensitivity, urticaria, necrotizing angiitis [vasculitis, cutaneous vasculitis], fever, respiratory distress [including pneumonitis, pulmonary edema], anaphylactic reactions); muscle spasm.

Precautions

Pregnancy: Category D (second and third trimester); Category C (first trimester), drugs that act directly on the renin-angiotensin system can cause injury and even death to the developing fetus.
Lactation:
Telmisartan – Undetermined.
Hydrochlorothiazide – Excreted in breast milk.
Children: Safety and efficacy not established.
Hypersensitivity: May occur in patients with or without history of allergy or bronchial asthma; cross-sensitivity with sulfonamides also may occur.
Renal function impairment: Decreases in renal function may occur in patients whose renal function is dependent on the renin-angiotensin system; patients with renal artery stenosis may experience acute renal failure. Use caution in treating patients whose renal function may depend on the activity of renin-angiotensin-aldosterone system (eg, severe CHF). In addition, HCTZ may precipitate azotemia and cumulative effects of the drug may develop in patients with impaired renal function.
Hepatic function impairment: Use with caution. Minor alterations of fluid and electrolyte balance may precipitate hepatic coma.
Diabetics: May require adjustments of insulin or oral hypoglycemic agents. Hyperglycemia may occur with thiazide diuretics.
Hyperuricemia: May occur or frank gout may be precipitated in certain patients receiving thiazide therapy.
Hypotension/Volume-depleted patients: Symptomatic hypotension may occur after initiation of telmisartan therapy in patients who are intravascularly volume depleted (eg, those treated with diuretics). Correct these conditions prior to administration of telmisartan or start treatment under close medical supervision.

Lightheadedness can occur, especially during the first days of therapy.
Systemic lupus erythematosus: Exacerbation or activation may occur.

Overdosage: Signs and Symptoms
Hypotension, dizziness, tachycardia, bradycardia, electrolyte depletion (eg, hypokalemia, hypochloremia, hyponatremia), dehydration.

PATIENT CARE CONSIDERATIONS
Administration/Storage
- Do not remove tablet from blister until immediately before administration.
- Administer prescribed dose qd in the morning, with or without food.
- Administer with food if GI upset occurs.
- Administer alone or in combination with other antihypertensives.
- Do not administer to pregnant women as fetal and neonatal morbidity and death can occur.
- Administer with caution and reduce dosage in patients with possible depletion of intravascular volume.
- Store tablets at controlled room temperature (59° to 86°F).

Assessment/Interventions
- Obtain patient history, including drug history and any known allergies. Note history of diabetes, anuria, lupus erythematosus, kidney or liver disease, or allergy to sulfonamide-derived drugs.
- Ensure that serum electrolytes are monitored periodically.
- Monitor and record BP and pulse. If hypotension results, hold medication and notify health care provider.
- Take safety precautions if orthostatic hypotension occurs.
- Monitor blood sugar in diabetic patient when drug is started or dose is changed. Report significant changes to health care provider.
- Monitor for signs of hypersensitivity including angioedema involving swelling of the face, lips, eyelids, and tongue. Discontinue medication and notify health care provider immediately if noted.

Patient/Family Education
- Explain name, dose, action, and potential side effects of drug.
- Instruct patient not to remove tablet from blister until immediately before taking the dose.
- Advise patient to take qd as prescribed without regard to meals but to take with food if GI upset occurs.
- Advise patient to try to take each dose at about the same time each day.
- Inform patient that drug controls, but does not cure, hypertension and to continue taking drug as prescribed even when BP is not elevated.
- Caution patient not to change the dose or stop taking unless advised by health care provider.
- Instruct patient to continue taking other BP medications as prescribed by health care provider.
- Instruct patient in BP and pulse measurement skills.
- Advise patient to monitor and record BP and pulse at home and to inform health care provider if abnormal measurements are noted. Also advise patient to take record of BP and pulse to each follow-up visit.
- Caution patient to avoid sudden position changes to prevent orthostatic hypotension.
- Instruct patient to lie or sit down if experiencing dizziness or lightheadedness when standing.
- Caution patient that inadequate fluid intake, excessive perspiration, diarrhea, or vomiting can lead to excessive fall in BP resulting in lightheadedness or fainting.
- Instruct diabetic patient to monitor blood glucose more frequently when drug is started or dose is changed and to inform health care provider of significant changes in readings.
- Emphasize to hypertensive patient the importance of other modalities on BP: weight control, regular exercise, smoking cessation, moderate intake of alcohol and salt.
- Advise women to notify health care provider if pregnant, planning to become pregnant, or breastfeeding.
- Instruct patient to stop taking drug and immediately report any of the following symptoms to health care provider: fainting, swelling of the face, lips, eyelids, or tongue.
- Caution patient not to take any prescription or OTC medications, salt substitutes, or dietary supplements unless advised by health care provider.
- Advise patient that follow-up visits and lab tests may be required to monitor therapy and to keep appointments.

Temazepam

(tem-AZE-uh-pam)

Class Sedative/Hypnotic/Benzodiazepine

How Supplied
Restoril Capsules 7.5 mg, Capsules 15 mg, Capsules 30 mg

✤ Apo-Temazepam ♦ Gen-Temazepam ♦ Novo-Temazepam ♦ Nu-Temazepam ♦ PMS-Temazepam

Action

PHARMACOLOGY: Potentiates action of GABA (gamma-aminobutyric acid), an inhibitory neurotransmitter, resulting in increased neuronal inhibition and CNS depression, especially in limbic system and reticular formation.

PHARMACOKINETICS/DYNAMICS:

Absorption: Temazepam is completely absorbed. T_{max} is 2 to 3 hr.

Distribution: Steady state is reached on the third day after a once-daily regimen.

Metabolism: Temazepam undergoes minimal (about 8%) first-pass metabolism and is 96% bound to plasma proteins.

Excretion: Temazepam t½ is approximately 10 hr and 80% to 90% is excreted in urine.

Onset: Onset of action is 20 to 40 min.

Indications Short-term management of insomnia.

Contraindications Hypersensitivity to benzodiazepines; pregnancy.

Route/Dosage

ADULTS: **PO** 7.5 to 30 mg at bedtime; individualize.

ELDERLY OR DEBILITATED PATIENTS: **PO** 15 mg until individual response is determined.

Interactions

Alcohol, other CNS depressants: Additive CNS depressant effects.

Digoxin: Serum digoxin concentrations may increase.

Theophylline: May antagonize sedative effects.

Lab Test Interferences None well documented.

Adverse Reactions

CV: Palpitations; tachycardia.
CNS: Drowsiness; dizziness; lethargy; confusion; euphoria; weakness; falling; ataxia; hallucinations; paradoxical reactions (eg, excitement, agitation); headache; memory impairment.
EENT: Blurred vision; difficulty focusing.
GI: Anorexia; diarrhea; abdominal cramping; constipation; nausea; vomiting.
HEMA: Leukopenia; agranulocytopenia.
OTHER: Tolerance; physical and psychological dependence; slurred speech; elevated AST, ALT, bilirubin.

Precautions

Pregnancy: Category X.
Lactation: Similar drugs excreted in breast milk.
Children: Not for use in children less than 18 yr.
Elderly: Increased side effects start with lowest dose.
Renal function impairment: Observe caution. Abnormal blood dyscrasias have occurred.
Hepatic function impairment: Observe caution. Abnormal LFT results and blood dyscrasias have occurred.
Anterograde amnesia: Has occurred with similar drugs. Alcohol may increase risk.
Dependence/withdrawal: Prolonged use can lead to psychological or physical dependence. Withdrawal syndrome may occur; dose must be tapered gradually.

Overdosage: Signs and Symptoms

Symptoms of decreased CNS function: somnolence, confusion, respiratory depression, decreased BP, seizures, coma, impaired coordination, slurred speech.

PATIENT CARE CONSIDERATIONS

Administration/Storage

- Administer ½ hr before bedtime with full glass of water.
- If GI upset occurs, administer with food.
- Store in tightly closed container at cool temperature.

Assessment/Interventions

- Obtain patient history, including drug history and any known allergies. Note drug dependence and potential for suicide.
- Assess type of sleep difficulty (eg, falling asleep, remaining asleep).
- Provide safety measures (eg, side rails up, night light, call bell accessible) and assist with ambulation.

- Carefully document response to initial dose; dose may be increased to 30 mg.
- Assess results of baseline liver and kidney function test and complete blood count with differential. Periodically reevaluate these values throughout long-term therapy.
- Assess and document mental and psychological parameters such as hallucinations, dreaming and nightmares, depression, euphoria, apprehension affect, mood, and memory. Report potential problems to health care provider.
- Notify health care provider if any of these symptoms occur: palpitations, increased heart rate, visual disturbances along with nausea

and vomiting or headache, excitation, dermatitis, sweating, flushing, pruritus, body or joint pain, tinnitus, and nasal congestion.

Patient/Family Education

- Caution patient that this medication must not be taken during pregnancy or when pregnancy is possible. Advise patient to use reliable form of birth control while taking this drug.
- Discuss with patient ways to facilitate sleep: quiet, avoidance of caffeine and nicotine, warm baths, deep breathing, relaxation techniques.
- Explain that disturbed nocturnal sleep may occur for first or second night after discontinuing use.
- Tell patient not to discontinue medication abruptly after prolonged therapy (longer than 2 wk).
- Explain safety precautions with regard to falls, especially for elderly and debilitated patients.
- Instruct patient to report these symptoms to health care provider: visual disturbances, abdominal pain or palpitations, fever, sore throat, bruising, rash, jaundice, unusual bleeding.
- Advise patient to avoid intake of alcoholic beverages or other CNS depressants.
- Caution patient that drug may cause drowsiness and to use caution while driving or performing other tasks requiring mental alertness.

Temozolomide

(te-moe-ZOE-loe-mide)

Class Alkylating agent

How Supplied

Temodar Gelatin capsules for oral use 5, 20, 100, and 250 mg

Action

PHARMACOLOGY: Temozolomide is a pro-drug that undergoes rapid nonenzymatic conversion. Cytotoxicity and antiproliferative activity against tumor cells are thought to be primarily caused by methylation of specific guanine-rich areas of DNA that initiates transcription. Temozolomide is rapidly and completely absorbed after oral administration, demonstrating a 98% oral bioavailability. Peak plasma concentrations occur in 1 hr and has a mean elimination half-life of 1.8 hr.

PHARMACOKINETICS/DYNAMICS:

Absorption: Temozolomide is rapidly and completely absorbed after oral administration; T_{max} is 1 hr. Food reduces the rate and extent of absorption.

Distribution: Temozolomide is weakly bound to plasma proteins (about 15%); Vd is 0.4 L/kg.

Metabolism: Cytochrome P450 plays only a minor role in the metabolism of temozolomide's active metabolites.

Excretion: Temozolomide's t½ is 1.8 hr. Overall clearance is approximately 5.5 L/hr/m².

Special Populations:
Renal Function Impairment – Exercise caution.
Hepatic Function Impairment – Exercise caution.
Gender – Women have approximately 5% lower clearance than men.

Indications Refractory anaplastic astrocytoma. **Unlabeled use(s):** Metastatic melanoma.

Contraindications Hypersensitivity to any component of the product; hypersensitivity to dacarbazine; pregnancy.

Route/Dosage

Anaplastic Astrocytoma, Single Agent Therapy

ADULTS: PO 150 mg/m²/day for 5 days; may repeat at 28-day intervals. Based on hematologic response, titrate up to target maintenance dose of 200 mg/m²/day for 5 days of each cycle. Continue therapy until disease progression occurs.

DOSAGE ADJUSTMENT BASED ON LOWEST POST-TREATMENT BLOOD COUNTS: If platelets are greater than 100,000/mm³ and neutrophils are greater than 1500/mm³ then increase dose 50 mg/m²/day for next cycle. Do not increase above max dose of 200 mg/m²/day. If platelets are 50,000 to 100,000/mm³ and neutrophils are 1000 to 1500/mm³ then no dosage adjustment is necessary. Delay next course until neutrophils are greater than 1500/mm³ and platelets greater than 100,000/mm³. If platelets are less than 50,000/mm³ and neutrophils are less than 1000/mm³ then reduce dose 50 mg/m²/day for next cycle. Do not reduce below minimum dose of 100 mg/m²/day. Discontinue therapy if patient cannot tolerate 100 mg/m²/day.

Interactions

Food: Food reduces the rate and extent of temozolomide absorption.
Valproic acid: Valproic acid decreases temozolomide clearance about 5%.

Lab Test Interferences None well documented.

Adverse Reactions

CV: Peripheral edema.
CNS: Headache; fatigue; seizures; hemiparesis; weakness; dizziness; abnormal coordination; amnesia; insomnia; paresthesias.

Temazepam

(tem-AZE-uh-pam)

Class Sedative/Hypnotic/Benzodiazepine

How Supplied
Restoril Capsules 7.5 mg, Capsules 15 mg, Capsules 30 mg

✤ Apo-Temazepam ♦ Gen-Temazepam ♦ Novo-Temazepam ♦ Nu-Temazepam ♦ PMS-Temazepam

Action

PHARMACOLOGY: Potentiates action of GABA (gamma-aminobutyric acid), an inhibitory neurotransmitter, resulting in increased neuronal inhibition and CNS depression, especially in limbic system and reticular formation.

PHARMACOKINETICS/DYNAMICS:

Absorption: Temazepam is completely absorbed. T_{max} is 2 to 3 hr.

Distribution: Steady state is reached on the third day after a once-daily regimen.

Metabolism: Temazepam undergoes minimal (about 8%) first-pass metabolism and is 96% bound to plasma proteins.

Excretion: Temazepam t½ is approximately 10 hr and 80% to 90% is excreted in urine.

Onset: Onset of action is 20 to 40 min.

Indications Short-term management of insomnia.

Contraindications Hypersensitivity to benzodiazepines; pregnancy.

Route/Dosage

ADULTS: **PO** 7.5 to 30 mg at bedtime; individualize.

ELDERLY OR DEBILITATED PATIENTS: **PO** 15 mg until individual response is determined.

Interactions
Alcohol, other CNS depressants: Additive CNS depressant effects.
Digoxin: Serum digoxin concentrations may increase.
Theophylline: May antagonize sedative effects.

Lab Test Interferences None well documented.

Adverse Reactions
CV: Palpitations; tachycardia.
CNS: Drowsiness; dizziness; lethargy; confusion; euphoria; weakness; falling; ataxia; hallucinations; paradoxical reactions (eg, excitement, agitation); headache; memory impairment.
EENT: Blurred vision; difficulty focusing.
GI: Anorexia; diarrhea; abdominal cramping; constipation; nausea; vomiting.
HEMA: Leukopenia; agranulocytopenia.
OTHER: Tolerance; physical and psychological dependence; slurred speech; elevated AST, ALT, bilirubin.

Precautions
Pregnancy: Category X.
Lactation: Similar drugs excreted in breast milk.
Children: Not for use in children less than 18 yr.
Elderly: Increased side effects; start with lowest dose.
Renal function impairment: Observe caution. Abnormal blood dyscrasias have occurred.
Hepatic function impairment: Observe caution. Abnormal LFT results and blood dyscrasias have occurred.
Anterograde amnesia: Has occurred with similar drugs. Alcohol may increase risk.
Dependence/withdrawal: Prolonged use can lead to psychological or physical dependence. Withdrawal syndrome may occur; dose must be tapered gradually.

Overdosage: Signs and Symptoms
Symptoms of decreased CNS function: somnolence, confusion, respiratory depression, decreased BP, seizures, coma, impaired coordination, slurred speech.

PATIENT CARE CONSIDERATIONS

Administration/Storage
- Administer ½ hr before bedtime with full glass of water.
- If GI upset occurs, administer with food.
- Store in tightly closed container at cool temperature.

Assessment/Interventions
- Obtain patient history, including drug history and any known allergies. Note drug dependence and potential for suicide.
- Assess type of sleep difficulty (eg, falling asleep, remaining asleep).
- Provide safety measures (eg, side rails up, night light, call bell accessible) and assist with ambulation.
- Carefully document response to initial dose; dose may be increased to 30 mg.
- Assess results of baseline liver and kidney function test and complete blood count with differential. Periodically reevaluate these values throughout long-term therapy.
- Assess and document mental and psychological parameters such as hallucinations, dreaming and nightmares, depression, euphoria, apprehension affect, mood, and memory. Report potential problems to health care provider.
- Notify health care provider if any of these symptoms occur: palpitations, increased heart rate, visual disturbances along with nausea

and vomiting or headache, excitation, dermatitis, sweating, flushing, pruritus, body or joint pain, tinnitus, and nasal congestion.

Patient/Family Education
- Caution patient that this medication must not be taken during pregnancy or when pregnancy is possible. Advise patient to use reliable form of birth control while taking this drug.
- Discuss with patient ways to facilitate sleep: quiet, avoidance of caffeine and nicotine, warm baths, deep breathing, relaxation techniques.
- Explain that disturbed nocturnal sleep may occur for first or second night after discontinuing use.
- Tell patient not to discontinue medication abruptly after prolonged therapy (longer than 2 wk).
- Explain safety precautions with regard to falls, especially for elderly and debilitated patients.
- Instruct patient to report these symptoms to health care provider: visual disturbances, abdominal pain or palpitations, fever, sore throat, bruising, rash, jaundice, unusual bleeding.
- Advise patient to avoid intake of alcoholic beverages or other CNS depressants.
- Caution patient that drug may cause drowsiness and to use caution while driving or performing other tasks requiring mental alertness.

Temozolomide

(te-moe-ZOE-loe-mide)

Class Alkylating agent

How Supplied
Temodar Gelatin capsules for oral use 5, 20, 100, and 250 mg

Action
PHARMACOLOGY: Temozolomide is a pro-drug that undergoes rapid nonenzymatic conversion. Cytotoxicity and antiproliferative activity against tumor cells are thought to be primarily caused by methylation of specific guanine-rich areas of DNA that initiates transcription. Temozolomide is rapidly and completely absorbed after oral administration, demonstrating a 98% oral bioavailability. Peak plasma concentrations occur in 1 hr and has a mean elimination half-life of 1.8 hr.

PHARMACOKINETICS/DYNAMICS:

Absorption: Temozolomide is rapidly and completely absorbed after oral administration; T_{max} is 1 hr. Food reduces the rate and extent of absorption.

Distribution: Temozolomide is weakly bound to plasma proteins (about 15%); Vd is 0.4 L/kg.

Metabolism: Cytochrome P450 plays only a minor role in the metabolism of temozolomide's active metabolites.

Excretion: Temozolomide's t½ is 1.8 hr. Overall clearance is approximately 5.5 L/hr/m².

Special Populations:
Renal Function Impairment – Exercise caution.
Hepatic Function Impairment – Exercise caution.
Gender – Women have approximately 5% lower clearance than men.

Indications Refractory anaplastic astrocytoma. **Unlabeled use(s):** Metastatic melanoma.

Contraindications Hypersensitivity to any component of the product; hypersensitivity to dacarbazine; pregnancy.

Route/Dosage
Anaplastic Astrocytoma, Single Agent Therapy
ADULTS: **PO** 150 mg/m²/day for 5 days; may repeat at 28-day intervals. Based on hematologic response, titrate up to target maintenance dose of 200 mg/m²/day for 5 days of each cycle. Continue therapy until disease progression occurs.
DOSAGE ADJUSTMENT BASED ON LOWEST POST-TREATMENT BLOOD COUNTS: If platelets are greater than 100,000/mm³ and neutrophils are greater than 1500/mm³ then increase dose 50 mg/m²/day for next cycle. Do not increase above max dose of 200 mg/m²/day. If platelets are 50,000 to 100,000/mm³ and neutrophils are 1000 to 1500/mm³ then no dosage adjustment is necessary. Delay next course until neutrophils are greater than 1500/mm³ and platelets greater than 100,000/mm³. If platelets are less than 50,000/mm³ and neutrophils are less than 1000/mm³ then reduce dose 50 mg/m²/day for next cycle. Do not reduce below minimum dose of 100 mg/m²/day. Discontinue therapy if patient cannot tolerate 100 mg/m²/day.

Interactions
Food: Food reduces the rate and extent of temozolomide absorption.
Valproic acid: Valproic acid decreases temozolomide clearance about 5%.

Lab Test Interferences None well documented.

Adverse Reactions
CV: Peripheral edema.
CNS: Headache; fatigue; seizures; hemiparesis; weakness; dizziness; abnormal coordination; amnesia; insomnia; paresthesias.

DERM: Rash; pruritus.
GI: Moderate potential for nausea and vomiting; constipation; diarrhea; abdominal pain; anorexia.
GU: Fetal malformations in rabbits.
HEMA: Dose-limiting bone marrow suppression; neutrophil and platelet nadirs at 26 to 28 days with recovery by day 40 to 42; elderly patients (at least 70 yr) may experience more severe myelosuppression.
MUSC: Back pain.
OTHER: Fever.

Precautions

Pregnancy: Category D.
Lactation: Undetermined; discontinue nursing.
Children: Safety and efficacy have not been established.
Elderly: Elderly patients at least 70 yr had a higher incidence of Grade 4 neutropenia and Grade 4 thrombocytopenia in the first cycle of therapy; exercise caution when treating.
Renal function impairment: Dosage reduction may be necessary in severely impaired renal function (eg, Ccr less than 36 mL/min or Child's-Pugh Class worse than grade I to II). Specific recommendations are not available. Exercise caution when administering to patients with severe renal impairment.
Hepatic function impairment: Dosage reduction may be necessary in severely impaired hepatic function (eg, Ccr less than 36 mL/min or Child's-Pugh Class worse than grade I to II). Specific recommendations are not available. Exercise caution when administering to patients with severe hepatic impairment.
Carcinogenesis: In rats treated with 200 mg/m^2 (equivalent to the max recommended daily human dose) on 5 consecutive days, mammary carcinomas were found in males and females.
Mutagenesis: Temozolomide was mutagenic in vitro in bacteria and clastogenic in mammalian cells.
Fertility impairment: Multicycle toxicology studies in rats and dogs have demonstrated testicular toxicity.
Special risk patients: Pharmacokinetic analysis indicates that women have an approximately 5% lower clearance (adjusted for body surface area) for temozolomide than men. Women have higher incidences than men of Grade 4 neutropenia and thrombocytopenia in the first cycle of therapy.
Myelosuppression: Prior to dosing, patients must have an absolute neutrophil count (ANC) at least 1.5×10^9/L and a platelet count at least 100×10^9/L. Myelosuppression generally occurred late in the treatment.

Overdosage: Signs and Symptoms

Hematologic: Neutropenia and thrombocytopenia.

PATIENT CARE CONSIDERATIONS

Administration/Storage

- Store capsules at room temperature.
- Do not open or split capsules. Round the dose to the nearest 5 mg. If capsules are accidentally opened or damaged, take rigorous precautions with the capsule contents to avoid inhalation or contact with the skin or mucous membranes.
- Administer PO.
- To achieve dependable plasma levels, patients should be consistent about the timing of temozolomide with regard to meals. Administration on an empty stomach or at bedtime may reduce the risk of nausea and vomiting.
- Follow procedures for proper handling and disposal of anticancer drugs. Wear gloves and avoid skin exposure and inhalation of fumes.
- Do not crush or chew capsules; swallow whole.
- Administer at bedtime. Antiemetic therapy may be administered prior to or following temozolomide administration.

Assessment/Interventions

- Monitor CBC at baseline, between days 20 and 24 of each cycle, and weekly until the neutrophil count is greater than 1500/mm^3 and platelets are greater than 100,000/mm^3.

Patient/Family Education

- Inform patients that the most frequently occurring adverse effects are nausea and vomiting. These were usually self-limiting or readily controlled with standard antiemetic therapy.
- There are no dietary restrictions with temozolomide. To reduce nausea and vomiting, take on an empty stomach.
- Do not open capsules. If capsules are accidentally opened or damaged, take rigorous precautions with the capsule contents to avoid inhalation or contact with the skin or mucous membranes.
- Keep the medication away from children and pets.
- If this drug is used during pregnancy or if patient becomes pregnant while on this drug, inform patient of potential hazard to the fetus.

Teniposide
(TEN-ih-POE-side)

Class Podophyllotoxin derivative

How Supplied
Vumon Injection concentrate 50 mg/5 mL

Action
PHARMACOLOGY: Teniposide is a phase-specific cytotoxic drug, acting in the late S or early G_2 phase of the cell cycle, thus preventing cells from entering mitosis. Teniposide causes single- and double-stranded breaks in DNA and DNA:protein cross-links. The mechanism of action appears to be related to the inhibition of type II topoisomerase activity. The terminal half-life is 5 hr. The volume of distribution is 3 to 11 L in children and 8 to 44 L in adults. Renal elimination is 44%, fecal elimination is up to 10%, and 4% to 12% is excreted unchanged in the urine.

PHARMACOKINETICS/DYNAMICS:

Distribution: Teniposide is highly protein bound (greater than 99%).

Excretion: Teniposide $t_½$ is about 5 hr. Total body clearance is approximately 25%; 44% is recovered in urine within 120 hr after dosing, and 0% to 10% is recovered in feces after 72 hr.

Special Populations:

Hepatic Function Impairment – Exercise caution in patients with hepatic dysfunction.

Indications
Adult: Refractory childhood acute lymphoblastic leukemia.
Pediatric: Refractory acute lymphoblastic leukemia. **Unlabeled use(s):** Adult acute lymphocytic leukemia, non-Hodgkin's lymphoma.

Contraindications
Hypersensitivity to teniposide or *Cremophor EL* (polyoxyethylated castor oil).

Route/Dosage
Acute Lymphoblastic Leukemia
ADULTS: **IV** 165 mg/m² on days 1, 4, 8, and 11 during consolidation on the "Linker" regimen. *Dosage adjustment:* Reduce dose 50% during the first treatment course in patients with Down's syndrome and leukemia. Higher doses may be administered during subsequent courses, depending on the degree of myelosuppression.

Acute Lymphoblastic Leukemia, Combination Therapy
PEDIATRIC: **IV** 165 mg/m²/dose twice weekly for 8 to 9 doses; or 250 mg/m²/dose once a week for 4 to 8 wk in combination with other chemotherapeutic drugs. *Dosage adjustment:* Reduce dose 50% for the initial course of therapy. Depending on the degree of myelosuppression and mucositis which occur, higher doses may be given during subsequent courses.

Interactions
Methotrexate: Plasma clearance of methotrexate may be slightly increased.
Phenytoin: May increase clearance of teniposide, resulting in decreased therapeutic effects.
Tolbutamide, sodium salicylate, and sulfamethizole: May displace protein bound teniposide.

Lab Test Interferences
None well documented.

Adverse Reactions
CV: Hypotension (with rapid IV administration or large doses).
DERM: Alopecia, rash.
GI: Moderate to low potential for nausea and vomiting, mucositis, diarrhea. Mucositis may be more severe in patients with Down's syndrome and leukemia.
HEMA: Bone marrow suppression, nadir at 3 to 14 days (usually occurs in 7 days), infection, bleeding.
HYPERSEN: Acute anaphylactoid reaction (5% frequency), incidence may be higher in brain tumor or neuroblastoma patients.
OTHER: The risk of secondary acute non-lymphocytic leukemia was 12 times higher in children treated once or twice weekly for acute lymphoblastic leukemia than with regimens using less frequent administration schedules; fever.

> **WARNING:**
> *Myelosuppression:* Severe cases resulting in infection or bleeding may occur. Dose-limiting bone marrow suppression is the most significant toxicity.
> *Hypersensitivity reactions:* May occur at initial dose or repeat doses.

Precautions
Pregnancy: Category D.
Lactation: Undetermined.
Hypersensitivity: Note hypersensitivity reactions to polyoxyethylated castor oil.
Renal function impairment: Dosage reduction is advised in patients with impaired renal function. Specific recommendations are currently unavailable.
Hepatic function impairment: Exercise caution in patients with hepatic dysfunction. Dosage reduction is advised in patients with impaired hepatic function. Specific recommendations are currently unavailable.
Anaphylaxis: Anaphylaxis manifested by chills, fever, tachycardia, bronchospasm, dyspnea, facial flushing, hypertension, or hypotension may occur.

Extravasation risk: Local irritation or phlebitis may occur. Refer to your institution specific protocol.

Hypotension: Administer by slow IV infusion since hypotension may occur with rapid IV injection.

PATIENT CARE CONSIDERATIONS
Administration/Storage
- Refrigerate unopened ampules in original package to protect from light.
- Dilute with 5% Dextrose or 0.9% Sodium Chloride for a final concentration of 0.1, 0.2, 0.4, or 1 mg/mL.
- Diluted solutions may leach DEHP from PVC infusion sets or bags. Use glass, polypropylene, or polyolefin containers.
- Solutions with a final concentration up to 0.4 mg/mL are stable at room temperature for up to 24 hr. Administer solutions with a final concentration of 1 mg/mL within 4 hr of preparation to prevent precipitation. Excessive shaking can cause precipitation. Refrigeration of diluted teniposide is not recommended.
- Administer IV.
- Infuse over at least 30 to 60 min to decrease risk of hypotension.
- During 24-hr continuous infusion, teniposide can precipitate and obstruct a central venous catheter.
- The use of a non-PVC IV administration set is recommended.
- Heparin can cause precipitation of teniposide. Flush well with heparin-free solutions before and after administration.

Assessment/Interventions
- Observe patients during and after the infusion for signs of hypersensitivity.
- Perform at the start of therapy and prior to each subsequent dose: platelet count, hemoglobin, WBC, and differential. A platelet count less than 50,000/mm^3 or an absolute neutrophil count less than 500/mm^3 is an indication to withhold further therapy until the blood counts have sufficiently recovered.
- Carefully monitor renal and hepatic function tests prior to and during therapy.

Patient/Family Education
- Contraceptive measures are recommended during treatment.
- Notify health care provider of the following: Fever; chills; rapid heartbeat; difficult breathing.

Overdosage: Signs and Symptoms
Bone marrow suppression.

Tenofovir Disoproxil Fumarate

(teh-NOE-fo-veer DIE-so-prox-ill FYU-mah-rate)

Class Antiretroviral/Nucleotide analog reverse transcriptase inhibitor

How Supplied
Viread Tablets 300 mg (equivalent to 245 mg tenofovir disoproxil)

Action
PHARMACOLOGY: Tenofovir disoproxil fumarate is a prodrug of tenofovir, which inhibits the activity of HIV reverse transcriptase by competing with deoxyadenosine 5'-triphosphate and by DNA chain termination after incorporation into DNA.

PHARMACOKINETICS/DYNAMICS:

Absorption: Tenofovir C_{max} is approximately 296 ng/mL and approximately 326 ng/mL in fasting and fed states, respectively. AUC is approximately 2,287 ng•hr/mL and approximately 3,324 ng•hr/mL in fasting and fed states, respectively. T_{max} is about 1.5 hr and bioavailability is approximately 25%. Administration following a high-fat meal increases the oral bioavailability, with an increase in AUC of about 40% and C_{max} increase of about 14%. Tenofovir should be taken with a meal to enhance bioavailability.

Distribution: Vd of tenofovir is approximately 1.3 L/kg.

Metabolism: Tenofovir is not a P450 substrate.

Excretion: Elimination of tenofovir is by glomerular filtration and tubular secretion. Approximately 70% to 80% is recovered in urine as unchanged drug.

Special Populations:
Renal Function Impairment – In patients with Ccr less than 50 mL/min or with end-stage renal disease requiring dialysis, C_{max} and AUC of tenofovir were increased to approximately 372 to 601 ng/mL and 6,008 to 15,984 ng•hr/mL, respectively. It is recommended that the dosing interval be modified in these patients. Tenofovir is efficiently removed by hemodialysis with an extraction coefficient of approximately 54%. Following a single 300 mg dose, a 4-hr hemodi-

alysis session removed approximately 10% of the administered tenofovir dose.

Indications Treatment of HIV-1 infection in combination with other antiretroviral agents.

Contraindications Standard considerations.

Route/Dosage

ADULTS: **PO** 300 mg/day without regard to food.

Renal Impairment
ADULTS: **PO** Ccr at least 50 mL/min, give 300 mg q 24 hr; Ccr 30 to 49 mL/min, give 300 mg q 48 hr; 10 to 29 mL/min, give 300 mg twice weekly.
Hemodialysis: Give 300 mg q 7 days or after a total of about 12 hr of dialysis.

Interactions

Didanosine: Plasma concentrations of didanosine may be increased, increasing the risk of side effects.
Drugs that reduce renal function or compete for active tubular secretion (eg, acyclovir, adefovir, dipivoxil, ganciclovir): May increase serum levels of tenofovir.
Indinavir, lopinavir/ritonavir: May increase tenofovir plasma levels. Indinavir plasma concentrations may be decreased by tenofovir.

Lab Test Interferences None well documented.

Adverse Reactions

CNS: Asthenia (11%); headache, depression (8%); peripheral neuropathy (5%); insomnia (4%); dizziness (3%).
DERM: Rash (including pruritus, maculopapular rash, urticaria, vesiculobullous rash, pustular rash) (7%); sweating (3%).
GI: Diarrhea (16%); nausea (11%); abdominal pain, vomiting (7%); anorexia, dyspepsia, flatulence (4%); pancreatitis (postmarketing).
GU: Renal insufficiency, renal failure, acute renal failure, Fanconi syndrome, proximal tubulopathy, proteinuria, acute tubular necrosis (postmarketing).
LABTESTABS: Increased creatinine (postmarketing).
M/N: Weight loss (4%); hypophosphatemia, lactic acidosis (postmarketing).
MUSC: Myalgia, back pain (4%).
RESP: Pneumonia (3%), dyspnea (postmarketing).
OTHER: Pain (12%); fever (4%); chest pain (3%).

> **WARNING:**
> Lactic acidosis and hepatomegaly with steatosis (including fatal cases) was reported with the use of nucleoside analogues alone or in combination with other antiretrovirals.

Precautions

Pregnancy: Category B.
Lactation: Undetermined. HIV-infected mothers should not breastfeed infants.
Children: Safety and efficacy not established.
Elderly: Select dose with caution, reflecting greater frequency of decreased hepatic, renal, or cardiac function and comorbidity.
Renal function impairment: See Route/Dosage section for recommended adjustments.
Fat redistribution: Accumulation and redistribution of body fat including central obesity, dorsocervical fat enlargement (buffalo hump), peripheral wasting, facial wasting, breast enlargement, and cushingoid appearance may occur.
Hepatitis B: Test HIV patients for hepatitis B virus (HBV) before starting antiretroviral therapy.
Hepatomegaly: Severe hepatomegaly with steatosis, including fatal cases, may occur.

PATIENT CARE CONSIDERATIONS

Administration/Storage

- Administer once daily without regard to meals. Administer with food if GI upset occurs.
- If coadministering with didanosine enteric-coated tablets, administer with a light meal or under fasted conditions. If coadministering with didanosine buffered tablet, administer under fasted conditions.
- Store tablets at controlled room temperature (59° to 86°F).

Assessment/Interventions

- Obtain patient history, including drug history and any known allergies. Note renal or hepatic impairment, osteopenia or osteoporosis, or concurrent use of nephrotoxic agents.
- Ensure tenofovir is used in combination with other antiretroviral agents.
- Ensure renal function is evaluated before starting therapy and repeated periodically during prolonged treatment.
- Ensure dosing interval is adjusted, following manufacturer's guidelines, in patient with Ccr less than 50 mL/min.
- Ensure liver enzymes are evaluated before starting therapy and periodically thereafter during prolonged treatment.

- Ensure patient has been tested for HBV before starting therapy. In patient coinfected with HBV and HIV, closely monitor with clinical and laboratory follow-up for at least several months after discontinuation of tenofovir because of risk of potential exacerbation of HBV.
- Ensure bone density monitoring is performed in HIV-infected patient with history of pathologic bone fracture or at substantial risk for osteopenia.
- Ensure supplementation with calcium and vitamin D has been considered in patient with HIV-associated osteopenia or osteoporosis.
- Monitor patient for GI, CNS, and general body side effects. Notify health care provider if noted and significant.
- Monitor patient for signs of lactic acidosis. If patient develops profound weakness or tiredness, unexpected stomach discomfort, fatty diarrhea, feeling cold, dizzy, or lightheaded, or slow or irregular heartbeat, withhold drug and notify health care provider immediately.

Patient/Family Education
- Explain name, dose, action, and potential side effects of drug.
- Advise patient or caregiver to review the *Patient Information Leaflet* before starting therapy and with each refill.
- Advise patient to take tenofovir once daily without regard to meals, but to take with food if stomach upset occurs.
- Instruct patient that if a dose is missed, to take it as soon as possible and then take the next dose at the regularly scheduled time. If it is almost time for the next dose, advise patient not to take the missed dose and wait and take the next dose as scheduled. Caution patient not to double the dose to catch up.
- Warn patient that this drug is not to be used by itself but is combined with other antiviral agents.
- Instruct patient to report the following symptoms immediately to health care provider: abdominal swelling or enlargement, fatty diarrhea, profound weakness or tiredness, unexpected stomach discomfort, feeling cold, dizzy or lightheaded, slow or irregular heartbeat.
- Inform patient that drug does not completely eliminate HIV virus and therefore does not reduce risk of transmitting HIV to others. Appropriate precautions must still be followed.
- Advise patient that drug is not a cure for HIV infection, and illnesses associated with HIV infection, including opportunistic infections, may continue to occur. Patient should remain under a physician's care.
- Advise patient with HIV-associated osteopenia or osteoporosis to discuss need for supplementation with calcium and vitamin D with health care provider.
- Advise women to notify health care provider if pregnant, planning to become pregnant, or breastfeeding. Advise HIV-infected mothers not to breastfeed to prevent infecting infants with HIV.
- Instruct patient not to take any prescription or OTC medications, dietary supplements, or herbal preparations unless advised by health care provider.
- Remind patient that follow-up visits and laboratory tests will be required to monitor therapy and to keep appointments.

Terazosin

(ter-AZE-oh-sin)

Class Antihypertensive/Antiadrenergic, peripherally acting

How Supplied
Hytrin Capsules 1 mg, Capsules 2 mg, Capsules 5 mg, Capsules 10 mg
🍁 Apo-Terazosin ♦ Novo-Terazosin ♦ Nu-Terazosin ♦ PMS-Terazosin ♦ ratio-Terazosin

Action
PHARMACOLOGY: Selectively blocks postsynaptic alpha$_1$-adrenergic receptors, resulting in dilation of arterials and veins.

PHARMACOKINETICS/DYNAMICS:
Absorption: Oral terazosin is completely absorbed. Food delayed the time to peak concentration by 1 hr. T_{max} occurs 1 hr after dosing.

Distribution: Terazosin is 90% to 94% bound to plasma proteins.

Metabolism: Terazosin undergoes minimal first-pass metabolism.

Excretion: Terazosin t½ is approximately 12 hr. Approximately 40% of an orally administered dose is excreted in urine and approximately 60% is excreted in feces.

Special Populations:
Elderly – After oral administration, plasma clearance was decreased 31.7% in patients over 70 yr vs patients 20 to 39 yr.

Indications Management of hypertension and symptomatic benign prostatic hyperplasia.

Contraindications Hypersensitivity to doxazosin or prazosin.

Route/Dosage
Hypertension
ADULTS: **PO** *Initial:* 1 mg at bedtime. (Do not exceed this as initial dose to avoid severe hypotensive effects; reinstitute at this dose if drug is discontinued for several days). *Maintenance:* 1 to 5 mg q day; may consider bid dosing (max, 20 mg/day).

Benign Prostatic Hyperplasia
ADULTS: **PO**.
Initial: 1 mg at bedtime. (Do not exceed this as initial dose); increase dose in step-wise fashion. Usual maintenance: 10 mg q day for minimum of 4 to 6 wk (max, 20 mg/day).

Interactions
None well documented.

Lab Test Interferences
None well documented.

Adverse Reactions
CV: Palpitations; orthostatic hypotension; hypotension; tachycardia; arrhythmias; vasodilation.
CNS: Dizziness; nervousness; paresthesia; somnolence; anxiety; headache; insomnia; weakness; drowsiness.
DERM: Pruritus; rash; sweating.
EENT: Blurred or abnormal vision; conjunctivitis; tinnitus; nasal congestion; sinusitis; epistaxis; pharyngitis.
GI: Nausea; vomiting; dry mouth; diarrhea; constipation; abdominal discomfort or pain; flatulence.
GU: Impotence; urinary frequency; urinary tract infection.
RESP: Dyspnea; bronchitis; bronchospasm; flu symptoms; increased cough.
OTHER: Shoulder, neck, back, or extremity pain; arthralgia; edema; fever; weight gain.

Precautions
Pregnancy: Category C.
Lactation: Undetermined.
Children: Safety and efficacy not established.
BPH complications: Long-term effects on incidence of surgery, acute urinary obstruction, or other complications of BPH have not been determined.
First-dose effect: May cause marked hypotension (especially orthostatic) and syncope at 15 to 90 min after first few doses, after reintroduction, with rapid increase in dosing, or after addition of another antihypertensive; to avoid, initiate dosing with low dose and gradually increase after 2 wk; monitor patients carefully.
Hemodilution: Small decreases in hematocrit, hemoglobin, WBCs, total protein, and albumin may occur, possibly because of hemodilution.

Overdosage: Signs and Symptoms
Severe hypotension.

PATIENT CARE CONSIDERATIONS
Administration/Storage
- Give PO. Maximum dosage should not exceed 20 mg.
- For benign prostatic hypertrophy, increase dose in step-wise fashion, as prescribed.
- Store in tight container in cool location.

Assessment/Interventions
- Obtain patient history, including drug history and any known allergies
- Assess BP response and pulse after administration to aid dosage adjustment.
- Check weight daily.
- Monitor I&O.
- Implement safety precautions for patients who experience dizziness. Fainting occasionally occurs after the first dose.
- Observe for symptoms of decreased BP, such as dizziness.
- Assess for potential respiratory side effects, including dyspnea, bronchospasm, or cough.

Patient/Family Education
- Explain to patient that first few doses may cause hypotension and syncope. Therefore, initially, terazosin should be taken at bedtime and patient should be warned to stay prone after taking dose. After first few doses, orthostatic hypotension with syncope is rare.
- Advise patient to avoid OTC cough, cold, and allergy medicines containing sympathomimetics, and identify common examples.
- Instruct patient to avoid driving or other activities that require alertness for first 24 hr after initial dose.
- Advise patient to follow up with health care provider to monitor BP.
- Caution patient to rise slowly from lying or sitting position to minimize dizziness.
- Instruct patient to report these symptoms to health care provider: dizziness, visual changes, palpitations.
- Alert male patients that impotence may be side effect.
- Explain potential adverse reactions: arthralgia, weight gain, tinnitus, pruritus, epistaxis, blurred vision. Be certain patient understands that health care provider should be made aware of any significant adverse reactions.
- Caution patient to avoid sudden position changes to prevent orthostatic hypotension.

Terbinafine

(TER-bin-a-feen)

Class Anti-infective/Antifungal

How Supplied
Lamisil Tablets 250 mg ♦ Lamisil AT Cream 1% ♣ Apo-Terbinafine ♦ Gen-Terbinafine ♦ Novo-Terbinafine ♦ PMS-Terbinafine

Action
PHARMACOLOGY: Inhibits squalene epoxidase, resulting in ergosterol deficiency and a corresponding accumulation of squalene within the fungal cell leading to fungal cell death.

PHARMACOKINETICS/DYNAMICS:

Absorption: Absorption from oral terbinafine is greater than 70%; bioavailability is about 40%. Terbinafine C_{max} is 1 mcg/mL, T_{max} occurs 2 hr after a 250 mg dose. AUC is 4.56 mcg•hr/mL and is increased less than 20% with food. At steady state in comparison to single dose, C_{max} is 25% higher and AUC is increased 2.5 times.

Distribution: Terbinafine is more than 99% protein bound and there are no specific binding sites. It is distributed to the sebum and skin.

Metabolism: Prior to excretion, terbinafine is extensively metabolized. There are no major metabolites that have antifungal activity similar to terbinafine.

Excretion: Terbinafine t½ is 200 to 400 hr and the drug is about 70% eliminated in the urine.

Special Populations:
Renal Function Impairment – In renal impairment (Ccr approximately 50 mL/min), terbinafine clearance is decreased 50%.
Hepatic Function Impairment – In hepatic cirrhosis, terbinafine clearance is decreased 50%.

Indications Treatment of onychomycosis of the toenail or fingernail caused by dermatophytes.
Topical: Interdigital tinea pedis, tinea cruris, or tinea corporis caused by *E. floccosum*, *T. mentagrophytes*, or *T. rubrum*. **Unlabeled use(s):** Cutaneous candidiasis, pityriasis (tinea) versicolor (topical).

Contraindications Preexisting liver disease or renal impairment (Ccr up to 50 mL/min).

Route/Dosage
ADULTS: PO 250 mg/day for 6 wk for fingernail onychomycosis; 250 mg/day for 12 wk for toenail onychomycosis.
Topical Apply to affected areas and surrounding skin once or twice daily.

Interactions
Caffeine: Terbinafine decreases the clearance of IV caffeine 19%.
Cimetidine: Terbinafine clearance is decreased 33% by cimetidine.
Cyclosporine: Terbinafine increases the clearance of cyclosporine 15%.
Dextromethorphan: Plasma dextromethorphan concentrations may be elevated, increasing the pharmacologic and adverse effects. Terbinafine inhibits dextromethorphan metabolism via the cytochrome P450 2D6 enzyme.
Rifampin: Terbinafine clearance is increased 100% by rifampin.

Lab Test Interferences None well documented.

Adverse Reactions
DERM: Pruritus; rash; urticaria.
GI: Abdominal pain; diarrhea; dyspepsia; flatulence; nausea.
OTHER: Headache; liver enzyme abnormalities; taste disturbance; visual disturbance.

Precautions
Pregnancy: Category B.
Lactation: Excreted in breast milk.
Children: Safety and efficacy not established.
Renal function impairment: Do not use in patients with renal impairment (Ccr up to 50 mL/min).
Hepatic function impairment: LFTs are recommended if used more than 6 wk and in the presence of possible signs of liver dysfunction. Insufficient information on risks in presence of preexisting liver or renal disease. Transient decreases in absolute lymphocyte counts have occurred. Risk to immune deficient patients is unknown. Severe neutropenia has been reported.
Ophthalmic: Changes in the ocular lens and retina have been reported.

PATIENT CARE CONSIDERATIONS

Administration/Storage
- Administer 1 tablet daily without regard to meals.
- Store tablets below 77°F (25°C). Keep tightly closed and protect from light.

Assessment/Interventions
- Obtain patient history, including drug history and any known allergies. Note history of renal or liver impairment.
- Ensure that nail specimens have been obtained for laboratory testing to confirm diagnosis of onychomycosis prior to starting therapy.
- Ensure that liver enzymes are determined before starting therapy and if clinical evidence of liver injury develops during therapy.

- Monitor CBC in patient with known or suspected immunodeficiency receiving drug for more than 6 wk.
- Monitor patient for signs and symptoms of liver dysfunction (eg, persistent nausea, anorexia, vomiting, right upper abdominal pain, fatigue, dark urine, yellowing of the skin or eyes). Notify health care provider immediately if noted.
- Monitor patient for headache and dermatologic and GI side effects. Report to health care provider if noted and significant.

Patient/Family Education
- Explain name, dose, action, and potential side effects of drug.
- Review dosing schedule and prescribed length of therapy with patient. 1 tablet daily for 6 wk (fingernail onychomycosis) or 12 wk (toenail onychomycosis).
- Instruct patient to take 1 tablet daily without regard to meals.
- Advise patient that if a dose is missed, take it as soon as possible, but if close to the next dose, do not double up and take the next dose as scheduled.
- Emphasize importance of completing full course of therapy, even if signs and symptoms of infection have disappeared.
- Warn patient to report any of the following to their health care provider immediately: skin rash, persistent nausea, vomiting, right upper abdominal pain, fatigue, anorexia, dark urine, yellowing of the skin or eyes.
- Advise female patient to inform health care provider if they become pregnant, plan on becoming pregnant, or are breastfeeding.
- Instruct patient to not take any prescription or OTC medications or dietary supplements unless advised to do so by their health care provider.
- Advise patient that follow-up examinations and lab tests may be required to monitor therapy and to be sure and keep appointments.

Terbutaline Sulfate

(ter-BYOO-tuh-leen SULL-fate)
Class Bronchodilator/Sympathomimetic
How Supplied
Brethaire Aerosol 0.2 mg/actuation ♦ *Brethine* Tablets 2.5 mg, Tablets 5 mg, Injection 1 mg/mL ♦ *Bricanyl* Tablets 2.5 mg, Tablets 5 mg, Injection 1 mg/mL
🍁 *Bricanyl Turbuhaler*

Action
PHARMACOLOGY: Produces bronchodilation by relaxing bronchial smooth muscle through $beta_2$-receptor stimulation.

PHARMACOKINETICS/DYNAMICS:
Absorption: Terbutaline C_{max} is approximately 8.5 ng/mL; T_{max} is about 1 to 3 hr, and AUC is approximately 54 hr•ng/mL. Terbutaline bioavailability is 103%.

Metabolism: The sulfate conjugate is the major metabolite.

Excretion: Terbutaline $t_{1/2}$ is about 3.4 hr. Approximately 90% is excreted in urine at 96 hr after SC administration, with about 60% being unchanged drug. Urinary excretion is the primary route of elimination.

Onset: Onset of action is 30 min.

Peak: Time to peak effect of terbutaline is 120 to 180 min.

Duration: Duration of action is 4 hr or longer.

Indications Treatment of reversible bronchospasm associated with asthma, bronchitis, and emphysema.

Contraindications Cardiac arrhythmias associated with tachycardia.

Route/Dosage
ADULTS AND CHILDREN OVER 15 YR: **PO** 2.5 to 5 mg at 6 hr intervals, tid during waking hours. Do not exceed 15 mg in 24 hr.
CHILDREN 12 TO 15 YR: **PO** 2.5 mg tid. Do not exceed 7.5 mg in 24 hr. **SC** 0.25 mg given in lateral deltoid area. May repeat in 15 to 30 min. Do not exceed 0.5 mg in 4 hr.

Interactions
Beta-blockers: Block bronchodilator effect of terbutaline.
MAOIs: Hypertension may occur.
Tricyclic antidepressants: Cardiovascular effects of terbutaline may be enhanced.

Lab Test Interferences None well documented.

Adverse Reactions
CV: Palpitations; tachycardia; chest discomfort or pain; arrhythmias; BP changes/hypertension.
CNS: Stimulation; tremor; dizziness; nervousness; drowsiness; headache; weakness.
GI: Nausea; vomiting; GI distress.
HEPA: Elevated liver enzymes.
METAB: Hypokalemia (with high doses).
RESP: Dyspnea.
OTHER: Flushing; sweating; muscle cramps; hypersensitivity vasculitis; ECG changes (eg, sinus pause, atrial premature beats, AV block, ventricular premature beats, ST-T-wave depression, T-wave inversion, sinus bradycardia, atrial escape beat with aberrant conduction); increased heart rate; muscle cramps; central stimulations;

pain at injection site; elevations in liver enzymes; seizures; hypersensitivity vasculitis.

Precautions

Pregnancy: Category B.
Lactation: Excreted in breast milk.
Children: Safety and efficacy in children younger than 12 yr not established.
Elderly: Lower doses may be required.
Labor and delivery: May inhibit uterine contractions and delay preterm labor.
Hypersensitivity: Hypersensitivity (allergic) reactions can occur after administration.
Carcinogenesis: A significant increase in the incidence of leiomyomas of the mesovarium and ovarian cysts has been demonstrated.
Cardiovascular effects: Toxic symptoms in patients with cardiovascular disorders may occur.

CNS effects: CNS stimulation may occur; use cautiously in patients with history of seizures or hyperthyroidism.
Diabetes: Dosage adjustment of insulin or oral hypoglycemic agent may be required.
Excessive use: Paradoxical bronchospasm and cardiac arrest have been associated with excessive inhalant use.
Hypokalemia: Decreases in potassium levels have occurred.
Tolerance: If previously effective dose fails to provide relief, therapy may need to be reassessed.

Overdosage: Signs and Symptoms

Tremor, palpitations, increased heart rate, decreased BP, seizures, hypokalemia, muscle cramps, headache, hyperglycemia.

PATIENT CARE CONSIDERATIONS

Administration/Storage

- For IV administration, obtain baseline potassium level prior to administration and place patient on cardiac monitor to assess for tachycardia or arrhythmias. Toxic symptoms have been documented in patients with cardiovascular disorders.
- Do not allow patient to use inhaler form of medication more than 6 times/day.
- Limit SC doses to up to 0.5 mg in 4 hr.
- For patients who are also using steroid inhaler, make sure that terbutaline is used first and 5 min elapse before steroid inhaler is used.
- Do not use medication if discolored.
- Store at room temperature. Protect from light.

Assessment/Interventions

- Obtain patient history, including drug history and any known allergies.

- Be alert for drug tolerance, which may occur with long-term use.

Patient/Family Education

- Instruct patient on proper technique for use of inhalers and evaluate return demonstration.
- Demonstrate use of spacer or peak flow meter if prescribed.
- Caution patient not to use inhaler form of medication more than 6 times/day.
- Advise patient to take tablets with food to avoid GI upset.
- Inform patient that the drug can stop working over time. If this is noted or if the inhalation makes breathing worse, notify the health care provider at once.
- Instruct patient to report these symptoms to health care provider: chest pain, dizziness or headache, persisting symptoms of asthma.

Terconazole

(ter-CONE-uh-zole)

Class Topical/Antifungal

How Supplied

Terazole 3 Vaginal cream 0.8%, Vaginal suppositories 80 mg ◆ *Terazole 7* Vaginal cream 0.4%
 Terazol

Action

PHARMACOLOGY: May alter permeability of fungus cell membrane, allowing leakage of essential intracellular components.

PHARMACOKINETICS/DYNAMICS:

Absorption: Terconazole C_{max} is approximately 5.9 ng/mL or 0.006 mcg/mL and T_{max} is about 6.6 hr.

Distribution: Terconazole is 94.9% protein bound. The degree of binding is independent of the drug concentration.

Metabolism: Terconazole is extensively metabolized.

Excretion: Terconazole t½ is 6.9 hr (range, 4 to 11.3 hr). Excretion of radioactivity is by both renal (32% to 56%) and fecal (47% to 52%) routes.

Special Populations:

Gender – Following terconazole administration, absorption varies in hysterectomized subjects (5% to 8% absorption) vs nonhysterectomized subjects (12% to 16% absorption). Other than this, overall absorption is similar in all women.

Indications Local treatment of vulvovaginal candidiasis.

Contraindications Standard considerations.

Route/Dosage
ADULTS: **Intravaginal** 1 suppository at bedtime for 3 days or 1 applicatorful of 0.4% cream at bedtime for 7 days or 1 applicatorful of 0.8% cream for 3 days.

Interactions None well documented.

Lab Test Interferences None well documented.

Adverse Reactions
CNS: Headache.
GI: Abdominal pain.
GU: Dysmenorrhea; genitalia pain; vulvovaginal burning; itching; irritation; burning.
OTHER: Body pain; fever; chills.

Precautions
Pregnancy: Category C. Avoid during first trimester because of absorption possibility.
Lactation: Undetermined.
Children: Safety and efficacy not established.
Recurrent infections: May indicate underlying medical cause, including diabetes or HIV infection.

PATIENT CARE CONSIDERATIONS

Administration/Storage
- Insert applicator high in vagina.
- Store at room temperature.

Assessment/Interventions
- Obtain patient history, including drug history and any known allergies.
- Ask patient about local reactions. If reactions are severe or symptoms of infection persist or worsen, notify health care provider.

Patient/Family Education
- Instruct patient to complete full course of therapy. This medication must be used continuously even through menses.
- Alert patient to potential side effects of vulvovaginal itching or burning, head or body aches. Advise patient to discontinue medication and notify health care provider if irritation occurs.
- Instruct patient to insert applicator high into vagina.
- Wash hands before and after application.
- Also, maintain external clean genitalia but avoid use of douches or other vaginal *otc* products while using the medication.
- Advise patient to wash applicator with mild soap and rinse thoroughly.
- Caution patient to refrain from sexual intercourse during course of therapy in order to help to prevent reinfection.
- Advise patient that sanitary napkin or minipad may be used to prevent stains on clothing.
- Instruct patient to consult with health care provider if infection recurs. Diabetes, AIDS, and chronic antibiotic or steroid therapy place patient at increased risk for recurrent infection.
- Explain that ingredients in product may interact with latex and weaken latex condoms and diaphragms. Advise patient to avoid use of these forms of birth control for 72 hr after application of medication.

Teriparatide

(TEH-rih-PAR-ah-TIDE)

Class Parathyroid hormone

How Supplied
Forteo Injection 250 mcg/mL

Action
PHARMACOLOGY: Regulates bone metabolism, renal tubular reabsorption of calcium and phosphate, and intestinal calcium reabsorption.

PHARMACOKINETICS/DYNAMICS:
Absorption: Bioavailability is approximately 95% and T_{max} is approximately 30 min.

Distribution: Vd is approximately 0.12 L/kg (IV dose).

Metabolism: Metabolized by nonspecific enzymatic mechanisms in the liver.

Excretion: Cl is approximately 62 L/hr (women) and 94 L/hr (men). $T_{1/2}$ is 5 min (IV) and 1 hr (SC). Excreted via the kidneys.

Onset: 2 hr (serum calcium concentrations begin to increase).

Peak: 4 to 6 hr (peak serum calcium concentrations).

Duration: 16 to 24 hr (serum calcium concentrations return to baseline).

Special Populations:
Renal Function Impairment – In patients with severe renal insufficiency (Ccr less than 30 mL/min), the AUC and $t_{1/2}$ increased 73% and 77%, respectively.
Gender – Systemic exposure is approximately 20% to 30% lower in men; no dosage adjustment needed.

Indications Treatment of postmenopausal women with osteoporosis who are at high risk for fracture (eg, history of osteoporotic fracture); increase bone mass in men with primary or hypogonadal osteoporosis who are at high risk of fracture (eg, history of osteoporotic fracture).

Contraindications Standard considerations.

Route/Dosage
ADULTS: **SC** 20 mcg once daily into thigh or abdominal wall.

Interactions
Digoxin: Because teriparatide may increase serum calcium, which may predispose patients to digitalis toxicity, use with caution in patients receiving digoxin.

Lab Test Interferences Transient increases in serum calcium, with the maximal effect observed at approximately 4 to 6 hr postdose.

Adverse Reactions
CV: Hypertension; syncope; angina pectoris.
CNS: Dizziness; headache; insomnia; depression; vertigo.
DERM: Rash; sweating.
GI: Nausea; constipation; dyspepsia; diarrhea; vomiting; GI disorder; tooth disorder.
RESP: Rhinitis; increased cough; pharyngitis; pneumonia; dyspnea.
OTHER: Arthralgia; leg cramp; pain; asthenia; neck pain.

> WARNING:
>
> *Osteosarcoma:* Increased incidence in rats. Dose and duration dependent. Should not be prescribed in patients who are at increased baseline risk for osteosarcoma (eg, Paget disease, unexplained elevations of alkaline phosphatase, open epiphyses, prior radiation therapy involving skeleton).

Precautions
Pregnancy: Category C.
Lactation: Not established; however, since it is indicated for osteoporosis in postmenopausal women, it should not be administered to women who are nursing their children.
Children: Safety and efficacy not established.
Special risk patients: Do not administer to patients at increased risk of osteosarcoma (ie, patients with Paget disease of the bone, pediatric population, patients with a history of radiation therapy involving the skeleton); do not use in patients with bone metastases or history of skeletal malignancies, metabolic bone diseases other than osteoporosis or preexisting hypercalcemia or underlying hypercalcemia disorder (eg, primary hyperparathyroidism).
Orthostatic hypotension: Symptomatic orthostatic hypotension may occur.
Urolithiasis: Use with caution.

Overdosage: Signs and Symptoms
Delayed hypercalcemic effect orthostatic hypotension, nausea, vomiting, dizziness, headache.

PATIENT CARE CONSIDERATIONS

Administration/Storage
- For SC administration only. Not for intradermal, IM, or IV administration.
- Inject prescribed dose once daily into the thigh or abdominal wall.
- Rotate injection sites (thigh, abdominal wall). Give new injections at least 1 inch from old site and never into areas where the skin is tender, bruised, red, or hard.
- Do not administer if particulate matter or discoloration noted.
- Store pen in refrigerator (36° to 46°F) at all times. During the use period, minimize time out of the refrigerator; the dose can be administered immediately following removal from the refrigerator. Recap pen when not in use. Pen can be used for up to 28 days after first injection; discard pen after 28-day use period even if it still contains unused solution. Do not freeze. Discard if pen has been frozen.

Assessment/Interventions
- Obtain patient history, including drug history and any known allergies. Note hypercalcemia and history of Paget disease of the bone, prior radiation therapy to skeleton, bone metastases, skeletal malignancies, urolithiasis, hypercalcemic disorders, and metabolic bone disease other than osteoporosis.
- Monitor patient for signs/symptoms of orthostatic hypotension following dose administration. Be prepared to treat appropriately. If orthostatic hypotension occurs administer subsequent doses with patient in lying or sitting position.
- Assess patient for CV, GI CNS, and general body side effects. Report to health care provider if noted and significant.

Patient/Family Education
- Explain name, dose, action, and potential side effects of drug.

- Instruct patient to read "Medication Guide" and pen "User Manual" before starting therapy and each time the prescription is renewed.
- Ensure that the patient understands how to store, prepare, and administer the dose, and dispose of used equipment and supplies. The first injection should be performed under the supervision of a qualified health professional.
- Advise patient to inject prescribed dose at about the same time every day.
- Advise patient that if a dose is missed, take it as soon as remembered but to never administer more than 1 injection in the same day.
- Advise patient to administer the first few doses in an area where they can sit or lie down quickly if they get dizzy.
- Advise patient that if they feel lightheaded or have palpitations after the injection to sit or lie down until symptoms resolve. Advise patient to notify health care provider if these symptoms persist or worsen.
- Advise patient regarding other ways they can help their osteoporosis: supplemental calcium and vitamin D, weight-bearing exercises, reduction of cigarette smoking and alcohol consumption.
- Instruct patient to report the following symptoms to health care provider: persistent nausea, vomiting, constipation, tingling, lethargy, muscle weakness.
- Advise women to inform health care provider if pregnant, planning to become pregnant, or breastfeeding.
- Instruct patient to not take any prescription or OTC medications or dietary supplements unless advised by their health care provider.
- Advise patient that follow-up visits and laboratory tests will be required to monitor therapy and to keep appointments.

Testosterone

(teh-STAHS-tuh-RONE)

Class Androgen

How Supplied

Testosterone

Androderm Transdermal system 5 mg/24 hr, 44 cm^2 surface area, 24.3 mg total testosterone, Transdermal system 2.5 mg/24 hr, 37 cm^2 surface area, 12.2 mg total testosterone ◆ *Testoderm* Transdermal system 4 mg/24 hr, 40 cm^2 surface area, 10 mg total testosterone, Transdermal system 6 mg/24 hr, 60 cm^2 surface area, 15 mg total testosterone ◆ *Testopel* Implant Pellets 75 mg ◆ *Testoderm with Adhesive* Transdermal system 6 mg/24 hr, 60 cm^2 surface area, 15 mg total testosterone

Testosterone Cypionate

Depo-Testosterone Injection 100 mg/mL, Injection 200 mg/mL

Testosterone Enanthate

Delatestryl Injection 200 mg/mL

Testosterone Gel

AndroGel Gel 1%

Testosterone Buccal System

Striant Mucoadhesive 30 mg

Action

PHARMACOLOGY: Promotes growth and development of male reproductive organs, maintains secondary sex characteristics, increases protein anabolism and decreases protein catabolism.

PHARMACOKINETICS/DYNAMICS:

Absorption: Testosterone transdermal T_{max} is 2 to 4 hr. Slowly released following buccal application, reaching the C_{max} within 10 to 12 hr.

Distribution: After transdermal administration, steady-state testosterone levels occur in 3 to 4 wk; 98% is bound to proteins.

Metabolism: Transdermal testosterone is metabolized in the liver.

Excretion: Transdermal testosterone t½ is 10 to 100 min. Approximately 90% is excreted in urine, and approximately 6% is excreted in feces.

Indications

Men: Replacement therapy in primary hypogonadism and hypogonadotropic hypogonadism; stimulation of puberty in delayed puberty (testosterone enanthate and pellets).
Women: Ablation of ovaries in metastatic breast cancer (testosterone enanthate). **Unlabeled use(s):** Reversible contraception in men.

Contraindications Hypersensitivity to product; serious cardiac, hepatic, or renal disease; men with carcinoma of breast or prostate; women who are or may become pregnant; testosterone gel and buccal system are contraindicated in women.

Route/Dosage

Androgen Replacement Therapy

ADULTS: **IM** 50 to 400 mg q 2 to 4 wk (testosterone enanthate, testosterone cypionate). **SC** 150 to 450 mg q 3 to 6 mo (testosterone pellets). **Transdermal** 6 mg/day system applied daily or 4 mg/day system applied qd if scrotal area is small (*Testoderm*); 5 mg applied qd (*Androderm*). **Topical** Start by applying entire packet of testosterone gel 5 g (delivering 50 mg testosterone systemically) to clean, dry skin of shoulders and upper arms or abdomen. Based on measurements of serum testosterone levels and clinical response 14 days after initiation of therapy, dose may be increased from 5 to 7.5 g and from 7.5 to 10 g. **Buccal** 30 mg applied to the gum region bid, morning and evening (about 12 hr apart). Place in a comfortable position just above 1 of the incisor teeth.

Delayed Puberty
ADOLESCENTS: **IM** 50 to 200 mg q 2 to 4 wk for limited duration (testosterone enanthate, testosterone cypionate) or **IM** 40 to 50 mg/m^2/dose monthly until growth rate falls to prepubertal levels (testosterone, testosterone propionate). **SC** 150 to 450 mg q 4 to 6 mo (testosterone pellets).

Breast Cancer
ADULTS: **IM** 200 to 400 mg q 2 to 4 wk (testosterone enanthate).

Interactions
Anticoagulants: May potentiate anticoagulant effects.
Insulin, oral hypoglycemics: May decrease glucose levels and antidiabetic drug requirements.
Oxyphenbutazone: Coadministration may result in elevated serum levels of oxyphenbutazone.

Lab Test Interferences
Thyroid function tests: Testosterone may cause decreased levels of thyroid hormones.
Clotting factors II, V, VII, X: Testosterone may suppress expression.

Adverse Reactions
CV: Edema.
CNS: Depression; headache; increased or decreased libido; anxiety.
DERM: Acne; hirsutism; male pattern baldness; seborrhea; rash.
GI: Gum or mouth irritation (9%); bitter taste (4%); gum pain and tenderness (3%); gum edema and taste perversion (2%, buccal system); nausea.
GU: Gynecomastia, penile erections, decreased ejaculatory volume (men); amenorrhea, virilization (deepening of voice and clitoral enlargement [women]).
HEPA: Cholestatic jaundice (elevated LFT results).
METAB: Increased cholesterol; decreased serum glucose.

OTHER: Inflammation at injection site; fluid and electrolyte retention; hypersensitivity; application site reactions (topical).

Precautions
Pregnancy: Category X.
Lactation: Undetermined. Testosterone gel, cypionate, buccal, and transdermal are not indicated for women.
Children: Use drug with great caution; may effect bone maturation.
Testosterone gel and buccal system – Safety and efficacy not established.
Elderly: Elderly men may be at increased risk of developing prostatic hypertrophy or carcinoma.
Acute intermittent porphyria: Acute intermittent porphyria has been reported. Use drug with caution in patients known to have this condition.
Athletic performance: Abuse of these agents to enhance athletic performance has potential risk of serious side effects.
Breast cancer and immobilized patients: May develop hypercalcemia.
Edema: Use drug with caution in patients with conditions that might be affected by fluid retention (eg, asthma, cardiac or renal dysfunction, epilepsy).
Gynecomastia: Frequently occurs and may persist. Use drug with caution in patients with pre-existing gynecomastia.
Hepatic effects: Prolonged use of high doses of androgens may result in potentially life-threatening peliosis, cholestatic jaundice, hepatitis, hepatic neoplasms, or hepatocellular carcinoma.
Oligospermia and reduced ejaculatory volume: May occur after prolonged use.
Product interchange: Do not interchange products because of their differences in duration of action.
Serum cholesterol: Levels may increase with androgen use; use drug with caution in patients with history of MI or coronary artery disease.

Overdosage: Signs and Symptoms
Chronic overdose: virilization, MI, thrombosis, movement disorders, hepatitis, nausea, vomiting, acne, seborrheic dermatitis.

PATIENT CARE CONSIDERATIONS
Administration/Storage
- Administer IM injections deep in gluteal muscle. Rotate sites.
- Shake vial well before withdrawing solution. Warming and shaking vial dissolves crystals that may have formed.
- Using wet needle or syringe may cause solution to become cloudy; however, this does not affect potency of drug.
- The number of pellets to be implanted depends upon the minimum daily requirement of testosterone propionate required weekly. Usual ratio is as follows: implant 2 pellets for each 25 mg testosterone propionate required weekly. When a patient requires injections of 75 mg/wk, it is usually necessary to implant 450 mg (6 pellets). With injection of 50 mg/wk, implantation of 300 mg (4 pel-

lets) may suffice for approximately 3 mo. With lower requirements by injection, correspondingly lower amounts may be implanted.
- Ascertain whether health care provider desires aqueous suspension or oil-based testosterone. Do not interchange products. Different salt forms have different duration of action.
- Wear gloves while handling transdermal patches. Apply *Testoderm* patches to clean, dry, and shaved scrotal skin. Patch should be worn 22 to 24 hr/day. Apply *Androderm* to a clean, dry area of the skin on the back, abdomen, upper arms, or thighs. Do not apply to the scrotum. Rotate application sites. Fold used patches with adhesive edges together. Discard patches so that they cannot be handled.
- Store IM preparation at room temperature (59° to 86°F).
- Store pellets in a cool place.

Buccal System:
- Have patient place buccal system in a comfortable position on the gum just above the incisor tooth on either side of the mouth.
- Have patient place rounded side of buccal system against the gum and hold firmly in place with finger over the lip and against the product for 30 sec.
- Have patient remove old system (gently slide system downward from gum toward tooth) and replace with a new system on other side of mouth bid (about q 12 hr).
- Discard used buccal system in trash in a manner that prevents accidental exposure to children or pets.
- Store blister packs at controlled room temperature (68° to 77°F). Protect from heat and moisture. Do not remove buccal system from blister pack until ready to apply.

Assessment/Interventions
- Obtain patient history, including drug history and any known allergies.
- Determine if patient has serious cardiac, hepatic, or renal disease; carcinoma of breast or prostate; clotting problems; epilepsy; or migraine headaches.
- Monitor and record I&O. Notify health care provider of fluid retention.
- Report jaundice or inflamed injection site to health care provider.
- Monitor serum cholesterol and report to health care provider if total cholesterol has increased and is greater than 200 mg/dL.
- In male adolescents being treated for delayed puberty, monitor bone maturation by assessing bone age of the wrist and hand q 6 mo by x-ray evaluation.
- Perform periodic LFTs.
- Observe for hypercalcemia, especially in breast cancer patients and immobilized patients.
- Monitor for signs of virilization in women.
- Report frequent, persistent erections, nausea, vomiting, changes in skin color, or ankle swelling.

Buccal System:
- Inspect application site frequently. Report tenderness or irritation to health care provider.

Patient/Family Education
- Caution patient that this medication must not be taken during pregnancy or when pregnancy is possible. Advise patient to use reliable form of birth control while taking this drug.
- Advise patient to consult with health care provider before taking OTC or prescription drugs.
- Instruct patient to remain as active as possible. Hypercalcemia may result if patient is inactive, and therapy will have to be discontinued.
- Advise patient to report the following symptoms to health care provider: depression, headache, nausea, yellow skin or yellowing of whites of eyes, swelling of ankles, painful or difficult urination, severe acne, painful or prolonged penile erections.
- Inform patient of the following potential side effects: increased facial or body hair and loss of scalp hair (in both men and women); breast enlargement and decreased ejaculatory volume (in men); deep voice, enlarged clitoris, and cessation of menses (in women).
- Warn patients being treated for hypogonadism that gynecomastia caused by testosterone therapy may persist.
- Caution patient not to take this drug without prescription and not to increase prescribed dosage in an effort to increase athletic performance. Side effects can be very serious.
- Instruct patient not to accept brands, types, or forms of drug different from the one originally prescribed.
- Advise patient using *Testoderm* transdermal patches to wear briefs instead of boxer shorts underwear to keep the patch from falling off.
- Instruct patient using the transdermal scrotal patch to shave scrotum with dry disposable razor about once/wk. Apply patch to dry scrotum. Patch should be temporarily removed while bathing or swimming. Patch is adhesive-free and clings to skin by an electrostatic effect.

- Male adolescent patients should have bone development checked q 6 mo if receiving treatment for delayed puberty.

Buccal System:
- Advise patient to read Patient Information leaflet before starting therapy and with each refill.
- Review application and removal process with patient.
- Instruct patient to apply buccal system bid, morning and evening (about 12 hr apart).
- Caution patient not to chew or swallow the buccal system.
- Advise patient to avoid dislodging the buccal system and check to see if the system is in place following toothbrushing, use of mouthwash, and eating or drinking.
- Advise patient that if the buccal system fails to properly adhere to the gum or falls off during the 12-dosing interval, the old system should be discarded and a new one applied. If the buccal system falls out of position within 4 hr of the next dose, a new system should be applied and may remain in place until the time of the next regularly scheduled dose.
- Advise patient to regularly inspect gum region where buccal system is applied and to report any abnormality (including gum tenderness or irritation) to health care professional.

Testosterone Cypionate/Estradiol Cypionate

(tess-TAHS-ter-ohn SIP-ee-oh-nate/ESS-truh-DIE-ole SIP-ee-oh-nate)

Class Androgen/Estrogen combination

How Supplied
Depo-Testadiol Injection 2 mg/mL estradiol, 50 mg/mL testosterone

Action
PHARMACOLOGY:
Testosterone: Promotes growth and development of male reproductive organs, increases protein anabolism, and decreases protein catabolism.
Estradiol: Promotes growth and development of female reproductive system and secondary sex characteristics; affects release of pituitary gonadotropins; inhibits ovulation and prevents postpartum breast engorgement; conserves calcium and phosphorus and encourages bone formation; overrides stimulatory effects of testosterone.

Indications Treatment of moderate to severe vasomotor symptoms associated with menopause.

Contraindications Known or suspected pregnancy; undiagnosed abnormal genital bleeding; known or suspected cancer of the breast except in appropriately selected patients being treated for metastatic disease; known or suspected estrogen-dependent neoplasm; active thrombophlebitis or thromboembolic disorder.

Route/Dosage
ADULTS: **IM** Use the lowest dose and regimen that will control symptoms and discontinue medication as promptly as possible. Usual dose is 1 mL (2 mg estradiol and 50 mg testosterone) at 4-wk intervals. Attempt to discontinue or taper medication at 3- to 6-mo intervals.

Interactions
Acetaminophen, ascorbic acid: Estrogen plasma levels may be elevated, increasing the risk of side effects.
Anticoagulants: Anticoagulant effects may be increased, requiring a dosage reduction.
Insulin: Insulin requirements may be reduced by the anabolic effects of testosterone.

Lab Test Interferences Endocrine and LFT results may be affected; possible decreased PT and increased platelet aggregability; increased thyroid binding globulin and total T_4; impaired glucose tolerance; decreased serum triglyceride and phospholipid concentrations; increased corticosteroid binding globulin and sex-hormone binding globulin; increased plasma HDL concentration; reduced LDL cholesterol concentrations; increased triglyceride levels; reduced response to metyrapone test; reduced folate concentration. The estrogenic effect on these values may be altered by the coadministration of testosterone.

Adverse Reactions
CNS: Headache; migraine; dizziness; mental depression; chorea; changes in libido.
DERM: Chloasma; melasma; erythema multiforme; erythema nodosum; hemorrhagic eruption; loss of scalp hair; hirsutism; acne.
EENT: Steepening of corneal curvature; intolerance to contact lenses.
GI: Nausea; vomiting; abdominal cramps; bloating; increased incidence of gallbladder disease.
GU: Vaginal bleeding; abnormal withdrawal bleeding or flow; breakthrough bleeding; increase in size of uterine leiomyomata; vaginal candidiasis; breast tenderness and enlargement; virilization.
HEPA: Cholestatic jaundice.
METAB: Increased or decreased weight; reduced carbohydrate tolerance; edema; hypercalcemia.

OTHER: Aggravation of porphyria; hypersensitivity (including anaphylactoid reactions); local irritation.

Precautions

Pregnancy: Category X.
Lactation: Estrogens are excreted in breast milk and may decrease the quantity and quality of milk.
Hepatic function impairment: Use with caution.
Carcinogenesis: Estrogens may increase the risk of endometrial carcinoma and other carcinomas in postmenopausal women.
Calcium/Phosphorus metabolism: Use with caution in patients with metabolic bone diseases.
Edema: Edema with or without CHF may occur.
Familial hyperlipoproteinemia: Estrogen use may be associated with massive elevations of plasma triglycerides.
Fluid retention: Because estrogens may cause fluid retention, use with caution when conditions that might affect fluid retention are present (eg, asthma, cardiac or renal dysfunction, epilepsy).
Gallbladder disease: Risk of gallbladder disease may increase in women receiving postmenopausal estrogens.
Hypercalcemia: Estrogens may cause severe hypercalcemia in patients with breast cancer and bone metastases.
Hypercoagulability: May occur because of decreased antithrombin activity.
Liver disease: Androgen therapy has been associated with peliosis hepatitis, cholestatic hepatitis, jaundice, and hepatocellular carcinoma.
Uterine bleeding: Undesirable manifestations of estrogenic stimulation (eg, abnormal uterine bleeding, mastodynia) may occur.
Virilization: Women receiving androgens may develop masculine characteristics.

Overdosage: Signs and Symptoms

Nausea, vomiting, withdrawal bleeding in women, estrogenic and androgenic effects.

PATIENT CARE CONSIDERATIONS

Administration/Storage

- For IM administration only. Not for intradermal, SC, or IV administration.
- Usual dose is 1 mL administered q 4 wk.
- Do not administer if particulate matter, cloudiness, or discoloration noted.
- Crystals may form if vial is stored at temperatures below those recommended. Should this occur, warming and gently shaking the vial should redissolve the crystals.
- Store at controlled room temperature (59° to 86°F).

Assessment/Interventions

- Obtain patient history, including drug history and any known allergies. Note history of the following: hypertension; diabetes; breast cancer with bone metastases; metabolic bone disease other than osteoporosis; liver disease; renal disease; cardiac disease; epilepsy; or asthma.
- Review patient's health history for any conditions that could contraindicate testosterone/estradiol (eg, previous allergic reaction to either drug, known or suspected pregnancy, known or suspected cancer of the breast, known or suspected estrogen-dependent cancer, undiagnosed abnormal uterine bleeding, active or past history of thromboembolic disorders or stroke, liver dysfunction or disease).
- Ensure that breast, abdominal, and pelvic examination and Pap smear have been completed and documented before starting therapy.
- Ensure that a progestin is used to prevent endometrial hyperplasia in women with an intact uterus.
- Monitor blood sugar in patients with diabetes when drug is started or dose is changed. Report significant changes to health care provider.
- Assess BP at beginning of therapy and periodically during treatment.
- Monitor patient for GI, GU, and general body side effects. Inform health care provider if noted and significant.
- Notify health care provider of pain, swelling, redness, or warmth in calves; sudden severe headache; visual disturbances; weakness or numbness of arms or legs; signs of liver dysfunction (eg, dark urine, jaundice); or signs of depression.
- Ensure that attempts are made to discontinue or taper the medication at 3- to 6-mo intervals.

Patient/Family Education

- Explain name, dose, action, and potential side effects of drug.
- Advise patient that medication will be prepared and administered by a health care professional in a medical setting.
- Instruct patients with diabetes to monitor blood glucose more frequently when drug is started or dose is changed and to inform health care provider of significant changes in readings.

- Review nonhormonal modalities that help prevent osteoporosis: 1500 mg/day of calcium; vitamin D supplementation; and exercise.
- Instruct patient to report the following symptoms to health care provider: pain in groin or calves; sharp chest pain or sudden shortness of breath; abnormal vaginal bleeding; breast lumps; sudden severe headache; dizziness or fainting; vision or speech problems; weakness or numbness of arms or legs; severe abdominal pain; yellowing of skin or eyes; or severe depression.
- Advise women to contact health care provider if pregnant, planning to become pregnant, or breastfeeding.
- Teach patient proper method of breast self-examination.
- Advise patient that follow-up visits and examinations, including Pap smear, at least once a year will be required to monitor therapy and to keep appointments.

Tetanus Immune Globulin (TIG)

(TET-ah-nus ih-MYOON GLAH-byoo-lin)

Class Immune serum

How Supplied
Baytet Solution 250 units/syringe

Action
PHARMACOLOGY: Directly neutralizes toxin excreted by *Clostridium tetani*, cause of tetanus.

PHARMACOKINETICS/DYNAMICS:
Absorption: Tetanus immune globulin T_{max} is approximately 2 days after IM injection.
Excretion: Tetanus immune globulin $T_{½}$ is 23 days.

Indications Passive, transient protection against tetanus in any person that may be contaminated with tetanus spores when: (1) patient's personal history of immunization with tetanus toxoid is unknown or uncertain, (2) person received less than 2 prior doses of tetanus toxoid, or (3) person received 2 prior doses of tetanus toxoid, but delay of more than 24 hr occurred between time of injury and initiation of tetanus prophylaxis. **Unlabeled use(s):** Treatment of clinical tetanus.

Contraindications Hypersensitivity to human antibody product, thimerosal, or other components; circulating anti-IgA antibodies.

Route/Dosage
ADULTS:
Prophylactic dose: **IM** 250 U. Give 500 U if wounds are severe or treatment is delayed. Dosage may be increased to 1000 to 2000 U. For therapy of tetanus, give 500 to 3000 or 6000 U. Give deep IM, preferably in upper outer quadrant of gluteal muscle.
CHILDREN: **IM** Dose is calculated on basis of body weight (4 U/kg); however, it may be advisable to administer 250 U regardless of the size of the child. The same amount of toxin is produced by the bacteria in adults and children.

Interactions There is no significant interaction between TIG and tetanus toxoid if given at different injection sites. To avoid inactivating vaccines containing live viruses or bacteria, give live vaccines 2 to 4 wk before or 12 wk after TIG.

Lab Test Interferences None well documented.

Adverse Reactions Local and systemic reactions following TIG are infrequent and usually mild. Expect some pain, tenderness, and muscle stiffness at injection site, persisting for several hours. Hives, angioedema, nephrotic syndrome, and local inflammation occur occasionally. Anaphylactic reactions are very infrequent.

Precautions
Pregnancy: Category C.
Lactation: Undetermined. Use TIG as soon as possible after tetanus-prone injuries. Do not inject IV.

PATIENT CARE CONSIDERATIONS

Administration/Storage
- Administer by IM injection only; do not give IV.
- Refer to appropriate immunization schedule or CDC wound management guideline for correct dosing.
- Use different syringe and injection site for the tetanus toxoid.
- Remember that history of tetanus "shots" is not reliable unless it can be confirmed that these shots were tetanus toxoid. However, U.S. Armed Forces personnel since 1940 have received at least 1 dose and probably complete immunizing series. If tetanus toxoid is needed, give in a separate site.
- Store in the refrigerator.

Assessment/Interventions
- Obtain patient history, including drug history and any known allergies.
- Observe patient for possible anaphylactic reaction after administration.

Patient/Family Education
- Alert patient that pain, soreness, inflammation, or stiffness at site of injection may be experienced.
- Advise patient who is also receiving tetanus toxoid series to complete pending immunizations since TIG protection is only temporary.

Tetanus and Diphtheria Toxoids (Adult Strength, Td)

(TET-ah-nus and diff-THEER-ee-uh toxoids)

Class Vaccine/Inactivated bacteria

How Supplied
Available as generic only

Action
PHARMACOLOGY: Induces antibodies against toxins made by *Corynebacterium diphtheriae* and *Clostridium tetani*.

Indications Achievement of active immunity against diphtheria and tetanus. Tetanus and diphtheria toxoids (Td) for adult use is preferred agent for immunizing most adults and children after 7 yr.

Contraindications Immediate hypersensitivity to product, thimerosal or any product components; during immunosuppression, acute respiratory tract infection (except for emergency booster recall doses).

Route/Dosage
Primary Immunizing Series
ADULTS AND CHILDREN 7 YR AND OLDER: **IM** A total of 3 doses (0.5 mL each): 1 dose now followed by 1 dose 4 to 8 wk later and then 1 dose 6 to 12 mo after first dose.

Booster Doses
ADULTS: **IM** 0.5 mL at 10-yr intervals throughout life to maintain immunity.

Interactions None well documented.

Lab Test Interferences None well documented.

PATIENT CARE CONSIDERATIONS

Administration/Storage
- Shake vial before withdrawing dose.
- Give IM only; do not administer IV or SC.
- Inject into deltoid muscle. Take care to avoid major peripheral nerve trunks.
- Several routine vaccines may safely and effectively be administered simultaneously at separate injection sites (eg, measles-mumps-rubella, oral polio vaccine, inactivated poliomyelitis vaccine, *Haemophilus influenzae* Type b, hepatitis B, influenza). Authorities recommend simultaneous immunization at separate sites as indicated by age or health risk.

Adverse Reactions
LOCAL: Small amount of erythema, induration, pain, tenderness, heat, and edema surrounding injection site, persisting for a few days, is not unusual. Nodule may be palpable at injection site for a few weeks. Allow such nodules to recede spontaneously. Sterile abscess and SC atrophy occur rarely. Adverse reactions often associated with multiple prior booster doses may be manifested 2 to more than 12 hr after administration by erythema, boggy edema, pruritus, lymphadenopathy, and induration surrounding point of injection. Pain and tenderness, if present, are usually not primary complaints.
SYST: Transient low-grade fever (temperatures over 38°C [100°F]) following Td administration are unusual; chills, malaise, generalized aches and pains, headaches, flushing, generalized urticaria or pruritus, tachycardia, anaphylaxis, hypotension, neurologic complications. People developing significant adverse reactions should not be given Td, even emergency doses, more frequently than every 10 yr.

Precautions
Pregnancy: Category C.
Lactation: Undetermined.
Anticoagulant therapy: As with all IM injections, give drug with caution to people receiving anticoagulant therapy.
Susceptibility: Like all inactivated vaccines, administration of Td to people receiving immunosuppressant drugs, including high-dose corticosteroids or radiation therapy, may result in insufficient response to immunization. They may remain susceptible despite immunization.

- Document in patient's medical record the manufacturer name and lot number, date of administration, and name, address, and title of person administering vaccine.
- Report adverse events to Vaccine Adverse Event Reporting System (VAERS), 1-800-822-7967.
- Store under refrigeration.

Assessment/Interventions
- Obtain patient history, including drug history and any known allergies.
- Use caution when administering to patient on anticoagulant therapy.

- Observe patient after injection for symptoms of anaphylaxis. Have 1:1000 epinephrine on hand.
- Monitor for significant side effects, including tachycardia, hypotension, neurologic complications, fever, chills, generalized arthralgias, headache, and flushing.

Patient/Family Education
- Explain that pain, edema, or pruritus may be experienced at site of injection.
- Stress to family that patient must receive all 3 doses for immunization to be effective.
- Explain need for booster at 10-yr intervals.

Tetracycline Hydrochloride

(teh-truh-SIGH-kleen HIGH-droe-KLOR-ide)

Class Antibiotic/Tetracycline

How Supplied
Sumycin 250 Tablets 250 mg ♦ Sumycin 500 Tablets 500 mg ♦ Sumycin Syrup Oral Suspension 125 mg per 5 mL
🍁 Apo-Tetra ♦ Novo-Tetra ♦ Nu-Tetra

Action
PHARMACOLOGY: Inhibits bacterial protein synthesis.

PHARMACOKINETICS/DYNAMICS:

Absorption: Tetracycline is adequately, but incompletely, absorbed from the GI tract.

Distribution: Tetracycline is about 65% bound to plasma proteins (short-acting). The protein binding for intermediate and long-acting analogs is usually greater. Penetration into most body fluids and tissues is excellent. Tetracycline is distributed in varying degrees in liver, bile, lung, kidney, prostate, urine, CSF, synovial fluid, mucosa of the maxillary sinus, brain, sputum, and bone. Tetracycline crosses the placenta and enters fetal circulation and amniotic fluid.

Metabolism: Tetracycline is concentrated by the liver in the bile.

Excretion: Tetracycline is excreted in both urine and feces at high concentrations in a biologically active form.

Special Populations:
Renal Function Impairment – Because renal Cl is by glomerular filtration, excretion is significantly affected by the state of renal function.

Indications Treatment of infections caused by susceptible strains of gram-positive and gram-negative bacteria; treatment of *Rickettsia, Mycoplasma pneumoniae*; chlamydial infections including treatment of trachoma; adjunctive treatment in severe acne; treatment of susceptible infections when penicillins are contraindicated; adjunctive treatment of acute intestinal amebiasis; treatment of nongonococcal urethritis caused by *Ureaplasma urealyticum*; treatment of relapsing fever due to *Borrelia recurrentis*.

Contraindications Hypersensitivity to tetracyclines or any component.

Route/Dosage
ADULTS: **PO** Usual dose: 1 to 2 g/day in 2 or 4 equal doses.
Mild to Moderate Infections: 500 mg bid or 250 mg qid.
Severe Infections: 500 mg qid.
CHILDREN OLDER THAN 8 YR OF AGE: **PO** 25 to 50 mg/kg/day in 4 equally divided doses.

Brucellosis
ADULTS: **PO** 500 mg qid for 3 wk, accompanied by 1 g streptomycin IM bid the first week and daily the second week.

Severe Acne
ADULTS: **PO** Start with 1 g/day in divided doses; for maintenance, 125 to 500 mg/day (alternate-day or intermittent therapy may be adequate in some patients).

Streptococcal Infections
Treat streptococcal infections for at least 10 days.

Syphilis
ADULTS: **PO** Sumycin only: Total dose of 30 to 40 g in equally divided doses over 10 to 15 days. All except Sumycin: Early (less than 1 yr duration) - 500 mg qid for 15 days. More than 1 yr duration - 500 mg qid for 30 days. CDC-recommended treatment for penicillin-allergic patients: Early (less than 1 yr duration) - 500 mg qid for 14 days. More than 1 yr duration - 500 mg qid for 28 days.

Uncomplicated Gonorrhea
ADULTS: **PO** 500 mg q 6 hr for 7 days.

Uncomplicated Urethral, Endocervical, or Rectal Infections Caused by Chlamydia trachomatis
ADULTS: **PO** 500 mg qid for at least 7 days.

Interactions
Antacids (containing aluminum, calcium, and magnesium), dairy products, food, iron salts: May decrease oral absorption of tetracycline.
Anticoagulants: The action of oral anticoagulants may be increased.
Methoxyflurane: Increased potential for nephrotoxicity exists; do not use together.

Oral contraceptives: May reduce effect of oral contraceptives.
Penicillins: May interfere with bactericidal action of penicillins.

Lab Test Interferences None well documented.

Adverse Reactions
CV: Pericarditis (as component of hypersensitivity reaction).
CNS: Dizziness; headache.
DERM: Rash; photosensitivity.
GI: Diarrhea; nausea; vomiting; abdominal pain or discomfort; bulky, loose stools; sore throat; glossitis; anorexia; stomatitis; black hairy tongue; dysphagia; hoarseness; enterocolitis; inflammatory lesions; epigastric distress.
GU: Increased BUN.
HEMA: Hemolytic anemia; thrombocytopenia; neutropenia; anemia; thrombocytopenic purpura; eosinophilia.
OTHER: Hypersensitivity, including anaphylaxis.

Precautions
Pregnancy: Category D. Avoid during pregnancy.
Lactation: Excreted in breast milk.
Children: Avoid in children younger than 8 yr of age because abnormal bone formation and discoloration of teeth may occur.
Renal function impairment: Excessive accumulation may occur in patients with renal impairment, resulting in possible liver toxicity; dosage reduction may be required.
Superinfection: Prolonged use may result in bacterial or fungal overgrowth.
Ophthalmic use: May retard corneal epithelial healing.
Outdated product: Do not use because degradation products are highly nephrotoxic.
Pseudomembranous colitis: Consider in patients in whom diarrhea develops.
Pseudotumor cerebri (benign intracranial hypertension): Reported in adults. Usual manifestations are headache and blurred vision.
Sensitivity reactions: Because sensitivity reactions are more likely to occur in persons with a history of allergy, hay fever, or urticaria, the preparation should be used with caution in such individuals. Cross-sensitization among the various tetracyclines is extremely common.

Overdosage: Signs and Symptoms
Nausea, vomiting, headache, increased intracranial pressure, skin pigmentation.

PATIENT CARE CONSIDERATIONS
Administration/Storage
- Dose, dosing frequency, and duration of therapy are dependent on condition treated.
- Administer prescribed dose at least 2 hr before or after meals.
- Administer tablets and capsules with a full glass of water to reduce risk of esophageal irritation and ulceration.
- Shake suspension well before measuring dose.
- Administer prescribed dose of suspension using dosing syringe, dosing spoon, or medicine cup.
- Administer tetracycline 2 hr before or after antacids containing aluminum, calcium, or magnesium, preparations containing iron or zinc, milk, or other dairy products.
- Store capsules, tablets, and oral suspension at controlled room temperature (59° to 86°F). Protect from light and excessive heat.

Assessment/Interventions
- Obtain patient history, including drug history and any known allergies. Note renal or hepatic impairment, history of allergy or intolerance to other tetracycline antibiotics, or sulfite sensitivity (suspension only).
- Ensure that expiration date has not been exceeded.
- Review results of culture and sensitivity testing as appropriate.
- Ensure that women are not pregnant or breastfeeding.
- Ensure that CBC, liver enzymes, and renal function are periodically evaluated during prolonged therapy.
- Monitor patient's response to therapy. Notify health care provider if infection does not appear to be improving or is worsening.
- Monitor patient for signs of allergic reaction. Discontinue therapy and immediately notify health care provider if noted. Be prepared to treat appropriately.
- Monitor patient for GI, CNS, DERM, general body side effects, and signs of superinfection. Report to health care provider if noted and significant. Immediately report severe diarrhea, diarrhea containing blood or pus, or severe abdominal cramping.

Patient/Family Education
- Explain name, dose, action, and potential side effects of drug.
- Review dosing schedule and prescribed length of therapy with patient. Advise patient that dose, dosing frequency, and duration of therapy are dependent on site and cause of infection.

- Instruct patient using capsules or tablets to take prescribed dose with a full glass of water to reduce risk of esophageal irritation or ulceration.
- Instruct patient or caregiver using oral suspension to measure and administer prescribed dose using dosing spoon, dosing syringe, or medicine cup.
- Advise patient to take prescribed dose at least 2 hr before or after meals.
- Advise patient to take 2 hr before or after antacids containing aluminum, calcium, or magnesium, preparations containing iron or zinc, milk, or other dairy products.
- Instruct patient to complete entire course of therapy, even if symptoms of infection disappear.
- Advise patient to discontinue therapy and contact health care provider immediately if skin rash, hives, itching, shortness of breath, or headache and blurred vision occur.
- Advise patient that medication may cause photosensitivity (sensitivity to sunlight) and to avoid unnecessary exposure to sunlight or tanning lamps, use sunscreens, and wear protective clothing to avoid photosensitivity reactions.
- Caution women taking oral contraceptives that tetracycline may make birth control pills less effective and to use nonhormonal forms of contraception during treatment.
- Advise women to notify health care provider if pregnant, planning to become pregnant, or breastfeeding.
- Caution patient that drug may cause dizziness, lightheadedness, or feeling of a whirling motion and to use caution while driving or performing other hazardous tasks until tolerance is determined.
- Advise patient to report following signs of superinfection to health care provider: black furry tongue, white patches in mouth, foul-smelling stools, vaginal itching or discharge.
- Warn patient that diarrhea containing blood or pus may be a sign of a serious disorder and to seek medical care if noted and not treat at home.
- Caution patient to not take any prescription or OTC medications, dietary supplements, or herbal preparations unless advised by health care provider.
- Advise patient to discard any unused tetracycline by the expiration date noted on the label.
- Advise patient that follow-up examinations and lab tests may be required to monitor therapy and to keep appointments.

Thalidomide

(the-LID-oh-mide)

Class Leprostatic

How Supplied
Thalomid Capsules 50 mg, Capsules 100 mg, Capsules 200 mg

Action
PHARMACOLOGY: Immunomodulatory agent, mechanism of action not fully understood.

PHARMACOKINETICS/DYNAMICS:
Absorption: Thalidomide T_{max} is 2.9 to 5.7 hr. Coadministration with a high-fat meal causes minor (less than 10%) changes in AUC and C_{max}; however, it causes an increase in T_{max} to approximately 6 hr.

Metabolism: Thalidomide is not hepatically metabolized to any large extent, but appears to undergo nonenzymatic hydrolysis in plasma to multiple metabolites.

Excretion: Thalidomide $t_{½}$ is 5 to 7 hr. Renal Cl 1.15 mL per min with less than 0.7% of the dose excreted in urine as unchanged drug.

Duration: Urinary levels were undetectable 48 hr after dosing.

Indications Acute treatment of cutaneous manifestations of moderate to severe erythema nodosum leprosum (ENL); maintenance therapy for prevention and suppression of cutaneous manifestations of ENL recurrence.

Contraindications Pregnancy.

Route/Dosage
ADULTS: PO Initial dose 100 to 300 mg daily, preferably 1 hr after the evening meal. Give 400 mg daily at bedtime or in divided doses at least 1 hr after meals to patients with severe cutaneous ENL reaction or to those who have previously required higher doses to control reaction.

Tapering Schedule
Dosing should continue until signs and symptoms have subsided, usually for at least 2 wk. Taper in 50 mg decrements q 2 to 4 wk. Patients requiring prolonged maintenance treatment to prevent recurrence or who flare during tapering, decrease medication q 3 to 6 mo in decrements of 50 mg q 2 to 4 wk.

Interactions
Barbiturates, chlorpromazine, ethanol, reserpine: The sedative effect of these drugs may be enhanced.

Lab Test Interferences None well documented.

Adverse Reactions

CV: Bradycardia; hypertension; hypotension; vasodilation; orthostatic hypotension; peripheral vascular disorder; tachycardia; angina pectoris; arrhythmia; atrial fibrillation; cerebral ischemia; cerebrovascular accident; CHF; deep thrombophlebitis; heart arrest; heart failure; murmur; MI; palpitation; pericarditis; thrombophlebitis; thrombosis; sick sinus syndrome, EKG abnormalities (postmarketing).

CNS: Drowsiness; somnolence; peripheral neuropathy; dizziness; agitation; insomnia; nervousness; paresthesia; tremor; vertigo; headache; malaise; abnormal thinking; agitation; amnesia; anxiety; causalgia; circumoral paresthesia; confusion; depression; euphoria; hyperesthesia; neuralgia; neuropathy; psychosis; abnormal gait; ataxia; decreased libido; decreased reflexes; dementia; dysesthesia; dyskinesia; emotional lability; hostility; hypalgesia; hyperkinesias; incoordination; meningitis; neurologic disorder; neuritis; peripheral neuritis; mental status or mood changes (including depression and suicide attempts), disturbances in consciousness (including lethargy), syncope, loss of consciousness or stupor, seizures (including grand mal convulsions and status epilepticus), migraine, hangover effect (postmarketing).

DERM: Rash; acne; fungal dermatitis; nail disorder; pruritus; maculopapular rash; sweating; alopecia; dry skin; eczematous rash; exfoliative dermatitis; ichthyosis; perifollicular thickening; skin necrosis; seborrhea; urticaria; vesiculobullous rash; angioedema; benign skin neoplasm; eczema; herpes simplex; incomplete Stevens-Johnson syndrome; psoriasis; skin discoloration; skin disorder; erythema multiforme, erythema nodosum, petechiae, purpura (postmarketing).

EENT: Amblyopia; deafness; dry eyes; eye pain; sinusitis; tinnitus; conjunctivitis; lacrimation disorder; retinitis; taste perversion; diplopia, nystagmus (postmarketing).

GI: Anorexia; constipation; diarrhea; dry mouth; flatulence; nausea; oral moniliasis; tooth pain; abdominal pain; cholangitis; cholestatic jaundice; colitis; dyspepsia; dysphagia; esophagitis; gastroenteritis; GI disorder; GI hemorrhage; increased appetite; gum disorder; pancreatitis; parotid gland enlargement; periodontitis; stomatitis; tongue discoloration; tooth disorder; enlarged abdomen; aphthous stomatitis, stomach ulcer (postmarketing).

GU: Albuminuria; hematuria; impotence; decreased Ccr; orchitis; proteinuria; pyuria; urinary frequency; acute renal failure; amenorrhea, enuresis; gynecomastia, galactorrhea, metrorrhagia, oliguria (postmarketing).

HEMA: Neutropenia; leukopenia; decreased erythrocyte sedimentation rate; eosinophilia; granulocytopenia; hypochromic anemia; leukemia; leukocytosis; elevated mean cell volume; abnormal RBC; palpable spleen; thrombocytopenia; erythroleukemia; myelogenous leukemia, aplastic anemia; macrocytic anemia; megaloblastic anemia; microcytic anemia; WBC decrease (including neutropenia and febrile neutropenia), PT changes, chronic myelogenous leukemia, erythroleukemia, pancytopenia (postmarketing).

HEPA: Abnormal LFTs; increased AST; enlarged liver; hepatitis; bile duct obstruction (postmarketing).

METAB: Hyperlipidemia; inappropriate antidiuretic hormone; amyloidosis; bilirubinemia; increased BUN; cyanosis; diabetes; abnormal electrolytes; hyperkalemia; hyperuricemia; hypocalcemia; hypoproteinemia; increased LDH; decreased phosphate; avitaminosis; dehydration; hypercholesteremia; hyperglycemia; hypoglycemia; increased alkaline phosphatase; increased lipase; increased serum creatinine; peripheral edema; hypomagnesemia; edema; peripheral edema; facial edema; hyponatremia, hypothyroidism, myxedema (postmarketing).

MUSC: Arthritis; bone tenderness; hypertonia; joint disorder; leg cramps; myalgia; myasthenia; periosteal disorder.

RESP: Pharyngitis; rhinitis; cough; emphysema; epistaxis; pulmonary embolus; rales; upper respiratory tract infection; voice alteration; apnea; bronchitis; lung disorder; lung edema; pneumonia (including *Pneumocystis carinii* pneumonia); rhinitis; pleural effusion, dyspnea (postmarketing).

OTHER: Teratogenicity; hypersensitivity; HIV viral load increase; lymphadenopathy; accidental injury; asthenia; back pain; chills; fever; infection; neck pain; neck rigidity; pain; photosensitivity; upper extremity pain; ascites; AIDS; allergic reactions; cellulitis; chest pain; cyst; decreased CD4 count; flu syndrome; hernia; altered thyroid hormone level; moniliasis; sarcoma; sepsis; viral infection; carpal tunnel, dysesthesia, foot drop, lymphadenopathy, lymphopenia, nodular sclerosing Hodgkin disease (postmarketing).

> **WARNING:**
> If thalidomide is taken during pregnancy, it can cause severe birth defects or death to an unborn baby. Thalidomide should never be used by women who are pregnant or who could become pregnant while taking the drug. It is approved for marketing only under a special restricted distribution program approved by the FDA. This program is called the System for Thalidomide Education and Prescribing Safety (S.T.E.P.S.). Only prescribers and pharmacists registered with the program are allowed to prescribe and dispense the product. Patients must be advised of, agree to, and comply with the requirements of the S.T.E.P.S. program in order to receive the product.

Precautions

Pregnancy: Category X.
Lactation: Undetermined.
Children: Safety and efficacy in children younger than 12 yr of age not established.
Hypersensitivity: Has been reported, including fever, tachycardia, and hypotension.
Photosensitivity: May occur; avoid exposure to sunlight or UV light.
Females: Contraindicated in women of childbearing potential unless alternative therapies are inappropriate and patient meets the following conditions (ie, unable to become pregnant while on thalidomide): understands and can carry out instructions; is capable of complying with mandatory contraceptive measures, pregnancy testing, patient registration, and patient survey described in System for Thalidomide Education in Prescribing Safety (S.T.E.P.S.) program; received both oral and written warning of hazards of taking thalidomide during pregnancy and of exposing fetus to drug; received oral and written warnings or risk of possible contraception failure and need to use 2 reliable forms of contraception simultaneously, unless continuous abstinence from reproductive heterosexual intercourse is chosen (sexually mature women who have not undergone hysterectomy or who have not been postmenopausal for at least 24 consecutive mo [who have had menses at some time in the preceding 24 consecutive mo] are considered to be of childbearing potential); acknowledges in writing understanding of these warnings and of need for using 2 reliable methods of contraception for 1 mo prior to starting thalidomide therapy, during therapy, and for 1 mo after stopping thalidomide; has had negative pregnancy test with sensitivity of 50 mIU/mL or greater within 24 hr of starting therapy; parent or legal guardian reads this material and agrees to ensure compliance with above for patients between 12 and 18 yr of age.
Males: Contraindicated in sexually mature males unless the following: understands and can carry out instructions; is capable of complying with mandatory contraceptive measures appropriate for men; patient registration and patient survey as described in S.T.E.P.S. program; received both oral and written warnings of risk of possible contraception failure and of need for barrier contraception in women of childbearing potential (latex condom [even if has undergone vasectomy]); acknowledges in writing understanding of these warnings and the need for barrier contraception; parent or legal guardian reads this material and agrees to ensure compliance with above for patients between 12 and 18 yr of age.
Dermatology: Serious and life-threatening dermatologic reactions, including Stevens-Johnson syndrome and toxic epidermal necrolysis, may occur.
Drug abuse and dependence: Physical and psychological dependence not reported in patients taking thalidomide.
HIV patients: Plasma HIV RNA levels were found to increase.
Neutropenia: Decreased WBC, including neutropenia, have been reported. Treatment should not be initiated with an absolute neutrophil count (ANC) of less than 750/mm^3. Monitor WBC and differential on an ongoing basis.
Peripheral neuritis: May cause permanent nerve damage. Not indicated as monotherapy for ENL treatment in presence of moderate-to-severe neuritis.
Prescribers/Dispensers: May only be prescribed and dispensed by individuals in the S.T.E.P.S. program.
Thrombotic events: Thrombotic events have been reported. Patients with neoplastic and various inflammatory conditions may have an increased incidence of pulmonary embolism, thrombophlebitis, deep vein thrombophlebitis, or thrombosis with thalidomide therapy.

PATIENT CARE CONSIDERATIONS

Administration/Storage

- Thalidomide can only be prescribed by physicians registered in the S.T.E.P.S. program.
- Administer single daily dose with a full glass of water, preferably at bedtime, and at least 1 hr after the evening meal.
- Administer divided doses with a full glass of water at least 1 hr after meals.

- Remove capsule from blister pack immediately before administration. Avoid extensive handling of the capsule. Do not open the capsule. If there is accidental contact with a non-intact thalidomide capsule or the powder contents, wash the exposed area with soap and water.
- Store capsules at controlled room temperature (59° to 86°F). Protect from light.

Assessment/Interventions
- Obtain patient history, including drug history and any known allergies. Note pregnancy, seizure disorder, or concurrent therapy with medications known to interfere with hormonal contraception (eg, carbamazepine).
- Ensure that patient has received both oral and written warnings of the hazards of taking thalidomide during pregnancy and of exposing a fetus to the drug and has signed the authorization form before starting therapy.
- Ensure that a negative pregnancy test has been obtained within 24 hr of starting therapy.
- Ensure that a pregnancy test is obtained weekly during the first mo of therapy and then monthly thereafter in woman with regular menstrual cycle. For woman with irregular menstrual cycles, pregnancy testing should be done q 2 wk.
- Ensure that a woman of childbearing potential who has not had a hysterectomy or has not been postmenopausal for at least 24 mo, has been using 2 reliable forms of contraception for at least 1 mo before starting therapy and that contraception is continued during therapy and for 1 mo following discontinuation of therapy.
- Ensure that men, even with a vasectomy, use a latex condom during any sexual contact with women of childbearing potential.
- Ensure that patient is examined monthly for the first 3 mo of therapy and periodically thereafter for early signs of neuropathy (numbness, tingling, pain) in the hands or feet. Discontinue thalidomide immediately if symptoms of drug-induced neuropathy are noted.
- Ensure that CBC with differential is evaluated before starting therapy and periodically during treatment. Do not initiate treatment if absolute neutrophil count (ANC) is less than 750/mm^3. If ANC decreases to less than 750/mm^3 reevaluate therapy and consider withholding thalidomide.
- Ensure that viral loads are measured in HIV-seropositive patient after the first and third mo of therapy and q 3 mo thereafter for duration of therapy.
- Monitor patient for development of orthostatic hypotension; if noted, implement safety precautions and have patient sit upright for a few min before standing up from a recumbent position. Notify health care provider if orthostatic hypotension persists and is bothersome.
- Frequently assess patient for response to treatment. Notify health care provider if cutaneous manifestations of erythema nodosum leprosum do not improve or appear to worsen.
- Ensure that therapy is periodically reviewed to determine if therapy needs to be continued without change or if a dose change (eg, increase, decrease, discontinuation) is indicated.
- Monitor patient for GI, CNS, DERM, and general body side effects. Report to health care provider if noted and significant. Immediately discontinue thalidomide and notify health care provider if symptoms of peripheral neuropathy are detected.
- Discontinue thalidomide if skin rash occurs and only resume following appropriate clinical evaluation.
- If caregiver is going to be exposed to body fluids of patient receiving thalidomide, utilize appropriate precautions (eg, wearing gloves) to prevent potential cutaneous exposure to thalidomide. If accidental, unprotected contact with body fluids does occur, wash the exposed area with soap and water.

Patient/Family Education
- Explain name, dose, action, and potential side effects of drug.
- Carefully instruct patient about the potential teratogenicity of thalidomide and the precautions (eg, pregnancy tests, use of effective contraception in women, condom use in men) that must be taken to prevent fetal exposure according to the S.T.E.P.S. program and boxed Warnings.
- Caution patient that under no circumstances should this drug be shared with anyone and that even a single dose taken by a pregnant woman could cause severe birth defects.
- Advise patient not to donate blood while taking thalidomide. Advise men not to donate sperm while taking thalidomide.
- Instruct patient to take exactly as prescribed and not to change the dose or stop taking unless advised by health care provider.
- Instruct patient not to extensively handle or open thalidomide capsules and to maintain storage of capsules in blister packs until time to take dose. Advise patient that if there is accidental contact with a non-intact thalidomide capsule or the powder contents, to wash the exposed area with soap and water.

- Advise patient to take each dose with a full glass of water at least 1 hr after meals. Advise patient taking single daily dose to try to take at bedtime, at least 1 hr after the evening meal.
- Advise patient that if medication needs to be discontinued it will be slowly withdrawn over a period of several wk unless safety concerns (eg, rash) require a more rapid withdrawal.
- Caution patient that drug may cause drowsiness and to use caution while driving or performing other tasks requiring mental alertness until tolerance is determined.
- Advise patient that medication can cause dizziness and orthostatic hypotension and to sit upright for a few min before standing from a lying position.
- Instruct patient to stop using and immediately notify health care provider if numbness, tingling, or pain in the hands or feet occur.
- Advise women to notify health care provider if they suspect that they may be pregnant (eg, change in menstrual pattern, missed period, contraceptive failure).
- Advise patient that medication may cause photosensitivity (sensitivity to sunlight) and to avoid unnecessary exposure to sunlight or tanning lamps and to use sunscreens and wear protective clothing to avoid photosensitivity reactions.
- Caution patient to avoid alcohol and other central nervous system depressants while taking this medication.
- Caution patient not to take any prescription or OTC medications, dietary supplements, or herbal preparations unless advised by health care provider.
- Advise patient that follow-up visits will be required to monitor therapy and to keep appointments.

Theophylline

(thee-AHF-ih-lin)

Class Bronchodilator/Xanthine derivative

How Supplied
Accurbron Syrup 150 mg/15 mL (50 mg/5 mL) ◆ *Asmalix* Elixir 80 mg/15 mL (26.7 mg/5 mL) ◆ *Bronkodyl* Capsules 100 mg, Capsules 200 mg ◆ *Elixomin* Elixir 80 mg/15 mL (26.7 mg/5 mL) ◆ *Elixophyllin* Capsules 100 mg, Capsules 200 mg, Elixir 80 mg/15 mL (26.7 mg/5 mL) ◆ *Lanophyllin* Elixir 80 mg/15 mL (26.7 mg/5 mL) ◆ *Quibron-T Dividose* Tablets 300 mg ◆ *Quibron-T/SR Dividose* Tablets, timed-release (8 to 12 hours) 300 mg ◆ *Slo-bid Gyrocaps* Capsules, timed-release (8 to 12 hours) 100 mg, Capsules, timed-release (8 to 12 hours) 125 mg, Capsules, timed-release (8 to 12 hours) 200 mg, Capsules, timed-release (8 to 12 hours) 300 mg ◆ *Slo-Phyllin* Tablets 100 mg, Tablets 200 mg, Syrup 80 mg/15 mL (26.7 mg/5 mL) ◆ *T-Phyl* Tablets, timed-release (8 to 12 hours) 200 mg ◆ *Theo-24* Capsules, timed-release (24 hours) 100 mg, Capsules, timed-release (24 hours) 200 mg, Capsules, timed-release (24 hours) 300 mg ◆ *Theo-Dur* Tablets, timed-release (8 to 24 hours) 100 mg, Tablets, timed-release (8 to 24 hours) 200 mg, Tablets, timed-release (8 to 24 hours) 300 mg, Tablets, timed-release (8 to 24 hours) 450 mg ◆ *Theochron* Tablets, extended-release 100 mg, Tablets, extended-release 200 mg, Tablets, extended-release 300 mg ◆ *Theolair* Tablets 125 mg, Tablets 250 mg ◆ *Uni-Dur* Tablets, extended-release (24 hours) 400 mg, Tablets, extended-release (24 hours) 600 mg ◆ *Uniphyl* Tablets, timed-release (24 hours) 400 mg, Tablets, timed-release (24 hours) 600 mg

🍁 *Apo-Theo LA* ◆ *Novo-Theophyl SR*

Action

PHARMACOLOGY: Relaxes bronchial smooth muscle and stimulates central respiratory drive.

PHARMACOKINETICS/DYNAMICS:

Absorption: Theophylline is rapidly and completely absorbed in solution or immediate-release. Theophylline C_{max} is 10 mcg/mL (range, 5 to 15 mcg/mL) and T_{max} is 1 to 2 hr. Food and antacids do no cause any clinically significant changes. The therapeutic range is 10 to 20 mcg/mL.

Distribution: Theophylline is approximately 40% protein bound (primarily to albumin). Unbound theophylline distributes throughout body water, but distributes poorly into body fat. Vd is approximately 0.45 L/kg (range, 0.3 to 0.7 L/kg) based on idea body weight. Theophylline freely passes across the placenta, into breast milk, and into CSF.

Metabolism: Theophylline does not undergo any measurable first-pass elimination. In adults and children over 1 yr of age, about 90% of the dose is metabolized in the liver. Caffeine and 3-methylxanthine are the only theophylline metabolites with pharmacologic activity.

Excretion: Excretion is via the kidneys. In neonates, approximately 50% of a theophylline dose is excreted unchanged in urine. Beyond 0 to 3 mo, 10% of a theophylline dose is excreted unchanged in urine.

Special Populations:
Renal Function Impairment – No dosage adjustment is required for renal insufficiency in adults and children over 3 mo. In neonates with reduced renal function, dose reduction and frequent monitoring of serum concentrations is required.

Hepatic Function Impairment – A prolonged t½ may occur in liver dysfunction. Pharmacokinetics vary widely among similar patients and cannot be predicted by age, sex, body weight, or other demographic characteristics. A prolonged t½ may occur in CHF, alcoholism, and respiratory infections.

Indications Prevention or treatment of reversible bronchospasm associated with asthma or chronic obstructive pulmonary disease.
Unlabeled use(s): Treatment of apnea and bradycardia of prematurity; reduction of essential tremor.

Contraindications Hypersensitivity to xanthines; seizure disorders not adequately controlled with medication.

Route/Dosage
Dosage based on lean body weight.
Acute Therapy in Patients Not Currently Receiving Theophylline
Loading dose:
ADULTS AND CHILDREN: **PO** 5 mg/kg.
MAINTENANCE:
Children 9 to 16 yr and Young Adult Smokers: **PO** 3 mg/kg q 6 hr.
Children 1 to 9 yr: **PO** 4 mg/kg q 6 hr.
Elderly and Cor Pulmonale Patients: **PO** 2 mg/kg q 8 hr.
Patients With CHF: **PO** 1 to 2 mg/kg q 12 hr.
Nonsmoking Adults: **PO** 3 mg/kg q 8 hr.

Acute Therapy in Patients Receiving Theophylline
Each 0.5 mg/kg theophylline administered as a loading dose will increase serum theophylline concentration approximately 1 mcg/mL. If a serum theophylline concentration can be obtained rapidly, defer the loading dose. If this is not possible, clinical judgment must be exercised, using close monitoring. Maintenance doses as per above.

Chronic Therapy
Slow clinical titration preferred.
Initial dose – 16 mg/kg/24 hr or 400 mg/24 hr, whichever is less.
Increasing dose – Increase the above dosage 25% increments at 3-day intervals as long as the drug is tolerated or until the following maximum dose is reached (not to exceed 900 mg, whichever is less).
MAXIMUM DOSE (WHERE SERUM CONCENTRATION IS NOT MEASURED): Do not attempt to maintain any dose that is not tolerated.
ADULTS AND CHILDREN OVER 16 YR: 13 mg/kg/day.
CHILDREN 12 TO 16 YR: 18 mg/kg/day.
CHILDREN 9 TO 12 YR: 24 mg/kg/day.
CHILDREN 1 TO 9 YR: 24 mg/kg/day.

Adjustments Based on Serum Theophylline Concentrations (Recommended for Final Adjustments in Dosage)
If serum theophylline concentration is within the desired range (10 to 20 mcg/mL), maintain dosage if tolerated. If too high (20 to 25 mcg/mL) decrease doses by approximately 10% and recheck in 3 days; (25 to 30 mcg/mL) skip the next dose, decrease subsequent doses by about 25% and recheck after 3 days; (over 30 mcg/mL) skip the next 2 doses, decrease subsequent doses by approximately 50% and recheck in 3 days. If too low (less than 10 mcg/mL) increase dosage 25% at 3-day intervals until either the desired clinical response or serum concentration is achieved.

Infant Guidelines
INFANTS 26 TO 52 WK: Dosing interval is q 6 hr.
INFANTS 26 WK OR YOUNGER: Dosing interval is q 8 hr.
INFANTS 6 TO 52 WK: **PO** 24 hr dose in mg [(0.2 × age in wk) + 5] × weight in kg.
PREMATURE INFANTS OVER 24 DAYS: **PO** 1.5 mg/kg q 12 hr.
PREMATURE INFANTS 24 DAYS AND YOUNGER: **PO** 1 mg/kg q 12 hr. Final dosage guided by serum concentration after steady state is achieved.

Interactions
Allopurinol, nonselective beta-blockers, calcium channel blockers, cimetidine, oral contraceptives, corticosteroids, disulfiram, ephedrine, influenza virus vaccine, interferon, macrolide antibiotics (eg, erythromycin), mexiletine, quinolone antibiotics (eg, ciprofloxacin), thyroid hormones: Increase theophylline levels.
Aminoglutethimide, barbiturates, hydantoins, ketoconazole, rifampin, smoking (cigarettes and marijuana), sulfinpyrazone, sympathomimetics: Decrease theophylline levels.
Benzodiazepines and propofol: Theophylline may antagonize sedative effects.
Beta-agonists: Cardiovascular adverse effects may be additive. However, may be used together for additive beneficial effects.
Carbamazepine, isoniazid, and loop diuretics: May increase or decrease theophylline levels.
Halothane: Coadministration has caused catecholamine-induced arrhythmias.
Ketamine: Coadministration may result in seizures.
Lithium: Theophylline may reduce lithium levels.
Nondepolarizing muscle relaxants: Theophylline may antagonize neuromuscular blockade.

INCOMPATIBILITIES: Do not mix following solutions with theophylline in IV fluids: ascorbic acid; chlorpromazine; corticotropin; dimenhydrinate; epinephrine hydrochloride; erythromycin gluceptate; hydralazine; hydroxyzine hydrochloride; insulin; levorphanol tartrate; meperidine; methadone; methicillin sodium; morphine sulfate; norepinephrine bitartrate; oxytetracycline; papaverine; penicillin G potassium; phenobarbital sodium; phenytoin sodium; procaine; prochlorperazine maleate; promazine; promethazine; tetracycline; vancomycin; vitamin B complex with C.

Lab Test Interferences None well documented.

Adverse Reactions
CV: Palpitations; tachycardia; hypotension; arrhythmias.
CNS: Irritability; headache; insomnia; muscle twitching; seizures.
GI: Nausea; vomiting; gastroesophageal reflux; epigastric pain.

PATIENT CARE CONSIDERATIONS
Administration/Storage
- Some sustained-release preparations should be given on empty stomach to avoid rapid drug release.
- Do not crush or allow patient to chew sustained release preparations.
- If GI irritation occurs, give with food or full glass of water.
- When administering parenterally, use a pump or controller to maintain a constant infusion rate.

Assessment/Interventions
- Obtain patient history, including drug history and any known allergies.
- Carefully monitor patients with history of arrhythmias, seizures, peptic ulcer, or gastroesophageal reflux.
- Monitor theophylline levels. The usual therapeutic range is 7 to 20 mcg/mL but some toxicity may be noted at the upper end of this range.
- Assess baseline LFT results.
- Implement cardiac monitoring as ordered for patients receiving IV form of theophylline.
- Monitor vital signs and I&O.

Thiabendazole
(THIGH-uh-BEND-uh-zole)
Class Anti-infective/Anthelmintic
How Supplied
Mintezol Tablets, chewable 500 mg, Oral suspension 500 mg/5 mL

GU: Proteinuria; diuresis.
RESP: Tachypnea; respiratory arrest.
OTHER: Fever; flushing; hyperglycemia; inappropriate antidiuretic hormone secretion; sensitivity reactions (exfoliative dermatitis and urticaria).

Precautions
Pregnancy: Category C.
Lactation: Excreted in breast milk.
Cardiac effects: Theophylline may cause or worsen preexisting arrhythmias.
GI effects: Theophylline may cause or worsen preexisting ulcers or gastroesophageal reflux.
Toxicity: Patients with liver impairment, cardiac failure, or over 55 yr are at greatest risk; monitor theophylline levels to prevent toxicity.

Overdosage: Signs and Symptoms
Anorexia, nausea and vomiting, nervousness, insomnia, agitation, irritability, headache, tachycardia, extrasystoles, tachypnea, fasciculations, seizures, ventricular arrhythmias, hyperamylasemia.

Patient/Family Education
- Emphasize importance of follow-up with health care provider to monitor drug levels.
- Explain to patient that the medication is used to prevent asthma attacks and should be used continuously.
- Explain that some sustained-release forms should be taken on empty stomach. Sustained-release products should not be crushed or chewed.
- Explain that low-protein, high-carbohydrate diets may increase theophylline levels while high-protein, low-carbohydrate diets and charcoal-broiled foods may decrease theophylline levels.
- Alert patients to common adverse reactions including stomach upset, nausea, insomnia, tremors, palpitations, exfoliative dermatitis, and urticaria.
- Tell patient to avoid food products containing caffeine.
- Instruct patient not to take extra doses of theophylline for acute asthma attack.
- Advise patient to consult with health care provider before taking any OTC preparations.

Action
PHARMACOLOGY: Inhibits helminth-specific enzyme fumarate reductase; suppresses egg or larval production and may inhibit subsequent development of eggs or larvae that are passed in the stool.

PHARMACOKINETICS/DYNAMICS:

Absorption: Thiabendazole is rapidly absorbed. T_{max} is within 1 to 2 hr.

Metabolism: Thiabendazole is almost completely metabolized to the 5-hydroxy form, which appears in the urine as glucuronide or sulfate conjugates.

Excretion: In 48 hr, about 5% of a thiabendazole dose is recovered from feces and 90% from urine.

Indications Treatment of strongyloidiasis (threadworm infection), cutaneous larva migrans (creeping eruption), and visceral larva migrans alone or in conjunction with enterobiasis (pinworm). Secondary therapy for uncinariasis (hookworm: *Necator americanus* and *Ancylostoma duodenale*), trichuriasis (whipworm), and ascariasis (large roundworm); alleviation of symptoms of trichinosis during invasive phase.

Contraindications Standard considerations.

Route/Dosage

ADULTS AT LEAST 150 LB (68 KG): **PO** 1.5 g/dose bid (max, 3 g/day).

ADULTS AND CHILDREN 30 TO 150 LB (13.6 TO 68 KG): **PO** 10 mg/lb/dose (22 mg/kg/dose) (max, 3 g/day).

Strongyloidiasis, Ascariasis, Uncinariasis, Trichuriasis, Cutaneous larva migrans – Two doses daily for 2 successive days (may repeat for some indications).

Trichinosis – Two doses daily for 2 to 4 successive days.

Visceral larva migrans – Two doses daily for 7 successive days.

Interactions

Xanthines: Thiabendazole may increase serum concentrations of theophylline to potentially toxic levels.

Lab Test Interferences None well documented.

Adverse Reactions

CV: Hypotension.
CNS: Dizziness; fatigue; drowsiness; giddiness; headache; numbness; hyperirritability; seizures; collapse.
EENT: Tinnitus; abnormal sensation in eyes; xanthopsia; blurring of vision; drying of mucous membranes; appearance of live ascaris in mouth and nose.
GI: Anorexia; nausea; vomiting; diarrhea; epigastric distress.
GU: Hematuria; enuresis; malodor of urine; crystalluria.
HEMA: Transient leukopenia.
HEPA: Jaundice; cholestasis; parenchymal liver damage, transient rise in cephalin flocculation and AST.
OTHER: Hypersensitivity reaction (pruritus, fever, facial flush, chills, conjunctival injection (red eye), angioedema, anaphylaxis, skin rashes, erythema multiforme, lymphadenopathy).

Precautions

Pregnancy: Category C.
Lactation: Unknown.
Children: Safety and efficacy in children weighing less than 13.6 kg (30 lb) not established.
Mixed infections with Ascaris lumbricoides: Thiabendazole may cause these worms to migrate. Drug should not be used prophylactically.
Supportive therapy: Anemic, dehydrated, or malnourished patients may need concomitant therapy to reverse these conditions.

Overdosage: Signs and Symptoms

Transient visual disturbances, psychic alterations.

PATIENT CARE CONSIDERATIONS

Administration/Storage

- Shake suspension before administering.
- Administer with food to reduce stomach upset.
- Instruct patient to chew tablets thoroughly before swallowing.
- Store at room temperature.

Assessment/Interventions

- Obtain patient history, including drug history and any known allergies. Monitor patient closely for signs of hypersensitivity reactions: Stevens-Johnson syndrome and erythema multiforme.
- If anemic, dehydrated, or malnourished, provide supportive measures.
- If patient is taking theophylline or aminophylline, monitor theophylline serum levels; dosage adjustment may be necessary.
- Assess patient for possible hypotension after administration.
- Obtain baseline LFTs.

Patient/Family Education

- Instruct patient to take medicine with food. No special diets are needed.
- Advise patient that all family members should be treated and that treatment may need to be repeated in 7 days to prevent reinfection.
- Instruct patient to bathe daily and to launder bedlinens, clothes, and towels daily. Instruct patient on proper technique for hygiene and hand-washing.

- Advise patient to avoid consuming excessive amounts of caffeine-containing beverages, such as coffee.
- Instruct patient to inform health care provider immediately of any symptoms of hypersensitivity or overdosage.
- Advise patient that drug can cause drowsiness and dizziness and to use caution while driving or performing other tasks requiring mental alertness.

Thiamin Hydrochloride (B_1)

(THIGH-uh-min HIGH-droe-KLOR-ide)

Class Vitamin

How Supplied
Thiamilate Tablets, enteric coated 20 mg
 Betaxin

Action
PHARMACOLOGY: Thiamin, after conversion to thiamin pyrophosphate, functions with adenosine triphosphate (ATP) in carbohydrate metabolism. Deficiencies result in beriberi, characterized by GI manifestations, peripheral neuropathy, and cerebral deficits.

PHARMACOKINETICS/DYNAMICS:
Absorption: Thiamin is a water-soluble vitamin. It is absorbed by both diffusion and active transport mechanisms. Absorption following IM administration is rapid and complete.

Distribution: Thiamin is widely distributed in all tissues, with highest concentrations in liver, brain, kidney, and heart. When thiamin intake exceeds needs, tissue stores increase more than 2 to 3 times. If intake is insufficient, tissues become depleted of their vitamin content.

Metabolism: Thiamin undergoes rapid metabolism. Thiamine + ATP → thiamine pyrophosphate (cocarboxylase) coenzyme.

Excretion: Excess thiamin is excreted in urine. Depletion of vitamin B_1 occurs about 3 wk with absence of thiamin in diet.

Indications Prophylaxis or treatment of thiamin deficiency (beriberi). Parenteral use indicated when oral therapy not feasible or advisable. **Unlabeled use(s):** Mosquito repellant; treatment of ulcerative colitis, chronic diarrhea, cerebellar syndrome, polyneuritis; appetite stimulant; prevention of Wernicke-Korsakoff syndrome.

Contraindications Standard considerations.

Route/Dosage
ADULTS: **PO** 0.5 mg/1000 kcal intake. RDA is 1.2 to 1.5 mg (adult males), 1 to 1.1 mg (adult females).
(CHILDREN 6 TO 10 YR): 0.8 to 1 mg.
(CHILDREN LESS THAN 6 YR): 0.3 to 0.5 mg (infants).

Wet Beriberi with Myocardial Failure
ADULTS: **IV** 10 to 30 mg tid. Treat as emergency cardiac condition.

Beriberi
ADULTS: **IM** 10 to 20 mg tid for 2 wk, then **PO** 5 to 10 mg (as part of multivitamin) for 1 mo.
CHILDREN: **IV** 10 mg initially followed by **IM** 10 mg bid for 3 days, then 10 mg daily for 6 wk.

Thiamin Deficiency Secondary to Alcoholism (Wernicke's Encephalopathy)
ADULTS: **IV** 50 to 100 mg; then **IM/IV** 50 to 100 mg/day until consuming normal diet; then **PO** 40 mg/day.

Metabolic Disorders
ADULTS: **PO** 10 to 20 mg daily; maximum doses of 4 g daily have been used.

Interactions
IV incompatibilities: Unstable in neutral or alkaline solutions. Incompatible with sulfite containing solutions. Incompatible with barbiturates, erythromycin, lactobionate, citrates.

Lab Test Interferences None well documented.

Adverse Reactions
CV: Cardiovascular collapse; hypotension; death.
CNS: Weakness; restlessness
DERM: Pruritus; urticaria.
EENT: Tightness of throat.
GI: Nausea; hemorrhage into GI tract.
RESP: Pulmonary edema; cyanosis.
OTHER: Feeling of warmth; sweating; anaphylaxis; angioneurotic edema; local tenderness and induration (after IM use).

Precautions
Pregnancy: Category A. (Category C if used in doses greater than the RDA.)
Lactation: Undetermined.
Hypersensitivity: Can occur. Deaths have resulted from IV administration. Intradermal test dose is recommended if sensitivity is suspected.
Deficiency: Single vitamin B_1 deficiency is rare; suspect multiple vitamin deficiencies.
Wernicke's encephalopathy: May occur or worsen suddenly in thiamin-deficient patients given glucose. If deficiency is suspected, give thiamin before or with dextrose-containing fluids.

PATIENT CARE CONSIDERATIONS
Administration/Storage
- As a nutritional supplement, calculate dosage based on standard dose of 0.5 mg/1000 kcal daily intake.
- For IV infusion, give at rate of up to 100 mg/at least 5 min.
- For IM injection, rotate injection sites if pain and inflammation occur. Administer via Z-track method to minimize pain. Application of cold may decrease pain.
- Store in light-resistant container.

Assessment/Interventions
- Obtain patient history including drug history and any known allergies.
- Give intradermal test dose first if hypersensitivity is suspected.
- Assess the patient for other nutritional deficiencies, since single vitamin deficiencies are rare.
- Administer thiamin before giving IV solutions containing glucose as glucose administration may cause sudden worsening of Wernicke's encephalopathy.
- Monitor for adverse reactions and notify health care provider of signs of weakness, restlessness, cardiovascular collapse, pulmonary edema, throat tightness, nausea, GI hemorrhage, pruritus, urticaria, feeling of warmth, diaphoresis, cyanosis, angioneurotic edema.

Patient/Family Education
- Alert patient to potential lab test abnormalities.
- Inform patient of all potential adverse reactions and of importance of reporting problems to health care provider.
- Teach patient about proper nutritional balance needed in diet. Thiamin-rich foods are yeast, beef, liver, legumes, beans, and whole grains.

Thioguanine

(THIGH-oh-GWAHN-een)

Class Purine antimetabolite

How Supplied
Tabloid Tablets 40 mg

Action
PHARMACOLOGY: Thioguanine, an analog of the nucleic acid constituent guanine, is closely related structurally and functionally to 6-mercaptopurine. Thioguanine nucleotides are incorporated into RNA and DNA by phosphodiester linkages and incorporation of such fraudulent bases may contribute to the cytotoxicity of thioguanine.

PHARMACOKINETICS/DYNAMICS:

Absorption: Thioguanine absorption is incomplete and variable, averaging about 30%. T_{max} is 8 hr and C_{max} is seldom over 1 to 2 mcg/mL.

Distribution: Thioguanine has very low distribution.

Metabolism: Thioguanine undergoes rapid metabolism to active intracellular derivatives.

Excretion: Trace quantities of thioguanine are found in urine; some metabolites are found in urine after about 22 hr.

Indications
Adults/Children: For remission induction, remission consolidation, and maintenance therapy of acute nonlymphocytic leukemia; busulfan is the preferred drug for treating the chronic phase of chronic myelogenous leukemia, however, thioguanine has activity in treating this condition.
Unlabeled use(s): Crohn disease.

Contraindications Prior resistance to this drug. There is usually complete cross-resistance between mercaptopurine and thioguanine.

Route/Dosage
ADULTS AND CHILDREN: PO 2 mg/kg/day; if there is no clinical improvement and no leukocyte or platelet depression after 4 wk on this dosage, the dosage may be cautiously increased to 3 mg/kg/day given as a single dose.

Interactions
Busulfan: Concomitant therapy may increase risk of hepatotoxicity, esophageal varices, and portal hypertension.

Lab Test Interferences None well documented.

Adverse Reactions
GI: Anorexia; intestinal necrosis and perforation (with multiple-drug regimens); nausea; stomatitis; vomiting.
GU: Hyperuricemia.
HEMA/LYMPH: Myelosuppression; pancytopenia (with multiple-drug regimens).
HEPA: Abnormal liver enzymes; hepatomegaly; jaundice; esophageal varices (in combination with busulfan); veno-occlusive liver disease (with multiple-drug regimens).

Precautions
Pregnancy: Category D.
Lactation: Undetermined.
Elderly: Use with caution because of the greater frequency of decreased hepatic, renal, or cardiac function, and concomitant diseases or other drug therapy.
Renal function impairment: Dosage reduction is advised in adult patients with impaired renal

function. Specific recommendations are currently unavailable.
Hepatic function impairment: Dosage reduction is advised in adult patients with impaired hepatic function. Specific recommendations are currently unavailable.
Bone marrow suppression: May be manifested by anemia, leukopenia, or thrombocytopenia.
Enzyme deficiency: There are patients with inherent deficiency of the enzyme thiopurine methyltransferase who may be unusually sensitive to the myelosuppressive effects of thioguanine and prone to developing rapid bone marrow suppression.
Hepatotoxicity: Jaundice has occurred. Withhold thioguanine if there is evidence of toxic hepatitis, biliary stasis, clinical jaundice, hepatomegaly, or anorexia with tenderness in the right hypochondrium.
Myelosuppression: May occur during induction phase of adult acute nonlymphocytic leukemias.

Overdosage: Signs and Symptoms
Nausea, vomiting, malaise, hypotension, diaphoresis, myelosuppression, azotemia.

PATIENT CARE CONSIDERATIONS
Administration/Storage
- Follow institutional and NIH procedures for handling, administration, and disposal of anticancer drugs.
- Administer as single daily dose.
- Store tablets at controlled room temperature (59° to 77°F). Protect from moisture.

Assessment/Interventions
- Obtain patient history, including drug history and any known allergies. Note prior resistance to thioguanine or mercaptopurine, liver disease, bone marrow impairment, or concurrent treatment with medications that inhibit thiopurine-S-methyltransferase (eg, olsalazine, mesalazine).
- Advise women of childbearing potential to avoid becoming pregnant during therapy and to use effective contraception during treatment.
- Ensure that risk of developing hyperuricemia is evaluated before starting therapy and that hypouricemic therapy, including adequate fluid intake, and monitoring of uric acid, is initiated before starting treatment in patient determined to be at risk for developing hyperuricemia and urate precipitation.
- Ensure that CBC with differential and quantitative platelet count is evaluated before starting therapy and then frequently during therapy.
- Implement infection control measures if WBC drops; implement bleeding precautions if platelet count drops. Be prepared to administer platelet transfusions for bleeding, and antibiotics and granulocyte transfusions for sepsis.
- Ensure that thioguanine is temporarily withdrawn at the first sign of an unexpected abnormally large fall in any of the formed elements of the blood, if not attributable to another drug or disease process.
- Ensure that thiopurine-S-methyltransferase (TPMT) testing is considered for patient who exhibits clinical or laboratory evidence of severe toxicity, particularly myelosuppression.
- Ensure that serum transaminase levels, alkaline phosphatase, and bilirubin levels are monitored weekly when therapy is initiated and then monthly thereafter during prolonged treatment. Consider more frequent monitoring in patient with preexisting liver disease or concurrently taking potentially hepatotoxic drugs. Inform health care provider if abnormalities are noted or if symptoms of hepatic injury (eg, jaundice, hepatomegaly, anorexia with tenderness in right upper quadrant) are documented. Be prepared to discontinue therapy.
- Monitor patient for signs of anaphylactic or serious allergic reactions. Discontinue therapy and immediately notify health care provider if noted. Be prepared to treat appropriately.
- Monitor patient for HEMA, GI, DERM, and general body side effects. Report to health care provider if noted and significant.
- Monitor patient for signs and symptoms of bacterial, viral, or fungal infection. Report to health care provider immediately if noted.

Patient/Family Education
- Explain name, action, and potential side effects of the treatment regimen. Review the treatment regimen including dosing schedule, duration of treatment, and monitoring that will be required.
- Advise patient, family, or caregiver that medication may be used in combination with other agents to achieve maximum benefit possible.
- Advise patient to take as a single daily dose.
- Advise patient, family, or caregiver to immediately report any of the following to health care provider: rash; hives; difficulty breathing; fever, chills, or other signs of infection; bleeding or unusual bruising; sores in mouth; dark urine; yellowing of skin or eyes.
- Advise patient, family, or caregiver to report any of the following to health care provider:

persistent nausea, vomiting, diarrhea, or appetite loss; persistent or worsening general body weakness.
- Instruct patient not to take any prescription or OTC medications, herbal preparations, or dietary supplements unless advised by health care provider.
- Advise women of childbearing potential to avoid becoming pregnant during therapy.
- Advise women to notify health care provider if pregnant, planning to become pregnant, or breastfeeding.
- Advise patient, family, or caregiver that frequent follow-up visits and laboratory tests will be required to monitor therapy and to keep appointments.

Thiopental Sodium

(thigh-oh-PEN-tahl SC-dee-uhm)
Class General anesthetic/Barbiturate

How Supplied
Pentothal Powder for Injection 2% (20 mg/mL), Powder for Injection 2.5% (25 mg/mL)

Action
PHARMACOLOGY: Depresses CNS to produce hypnosis and anesthesia without analgesia.
PHARMACOKINETICS/DYNAMICS:
Distribution: Thiopental is 80% bound to plasma proteins. The partition coefficient is 580.
Metabolism: Thiopental is degraded in liver and to a smaller extent, kidney and brain. The concentrations in spinal fluid is slightly less than in plasma.
Excretion: Thiopental is eliminated in urine and t½ is 3 to 8 hr.

Indications Induction of anesthesia; supplementation of other anesthetic agents; IV anesthesia for short surgical procedures with minimal painful stimuli; induction of hypnotic state; control of convulsions and increased intracranial pressure (IV administration); induction of preanesthetic sedation or basal narcosis (PR administration).

Contraindications Hypersensitivity to barbiturates; variegate or acute intermittent porphyria; absence of suitable veins for IV administration; status asthmaticus
Rectal administration: Patients undergoing rectal surgery; lesions of bowel.

Route/Dosage
Test Dose
ADULTS: **IV** 25 to 75 mg; observe for 60 sec.
Anesthesia
ADULTS: **IV** 50 to 75 mg slowly q 20 to 40 sec until anesthesia is established then 25 to 50 mg prn or continuous infusion of 0.2% or 0.4%.
CHILDREN: **IV** 5 to 6 mg/kg then 1 mg/kg prn.
INFANTS: **IV** 5 to 8 mg/kg then 1 mg/kg prn.
NEWBORNS: **IV** 3 to 4 mg/kg then 1 mg/kg prn.
Convulsive States
ADULTS: **IV** 75 to 125 mg; may need 125 to 250 mg over 10 min.
CHILDREN: **IV** 2 to 3 mg/kg/dose; repeat prn.
Increased Intracranial Pressure
ADULTS: **IV** 1.5 to 3.5 mg/kg.
CHILDREN: **IV** 1.5 to 5 mg/kg/dose; repeat prn.
Psychiatric Disorders
ADULTS: **IV** 100 mg/min slowly with patient counting backwards or as infusion of 50 mL/min of 0.2% solution.
Preanesthetic Sedation
ADULTS: **PR** 1 g/34 kg (30 mg/kg).
Basal Narcosis
ADULTS: **PR** 1 g/22.5 kg (44 mg/kg) (max, 3 to 4 g for adults weighing over 90 kg).
CHILDREN OVER 3 MO: **PR** 25 mg/kg/dose; if not sedated within 15 to 20 min, may repeat with single dose of 15 mg/kg/dose (max, 1.15 g for children over 34 kg).
CHILDREN UNDER 3 MO: **PR** 15 mg/kg/dose; if not sedated within 15 to 20 min, may repeat with single dose of less than 7.5 mg/kg/dose.

Interactions
Narcotics: May cause additive barbiturate effects and increase risk of apnea.
Phenothiazines: May increase frequency and severity of neuromuscular excitation and hypotension.
Probenecid: May extend barbiturate effects or effects may be achieved at lower doses.
Sulfisoxazole: May enhance barbiturate effects.
INCOMPATIBILITIES: Tubocurarine, succinylcholine, or other acid pH solutions.

Lab Test Interferences
LFTs: Drug may falsely elevate results.
Serum potassium: Drug may falsely elevate results.

Adverse Reactions
CV: Myocardial depression; arrhythmias.
CNS: Delirium, headache; amnesia; seizures.
DERM: Rash.
GI: Abdominal pain; rectal irritation; diarrhea; cramping; rectal bleeding (rectal suspension).
RESP: Apnea; laryngospasm; bronchospasm; hiccoughs; sneezing; coughing.
OTHER: Thrombophlebitis; pain at injection site; salivation; shivering.

Precautions
Pregnancy: Category C; readily crosses placental barrier.
Lactation: Excreted in breast milk.

Elderly: At increased risk of prolonged or potentiated hypnotic effects. Dosage reduction is required when administered rectally.
Renal function impairment: Use drug with caution in patients with renal disease. Dosage reduction is required (75% of normal dose if Ccr is less than 10 mL/min).
Hepatic function impairment: Use drug with caution in patients with hepatic disease.
Special risk patients: Use drug with caution in patients with severe cardiovascular, respiratory, renal, hepatic, or endocrine disease, hypotension or shock, conditions in which hypnotic effects may be prolonged or potentiated, potential rectal surgery (rectal suspension), or presence of inflammatory, ulcerative, bleeding, or neoplastic lesions of lower bowel (rectal suspension).
Repeated doses: May result in prolonged drug effect because of accumulation.

Overdosage: Signs and Symptoms
Respiratory depression, hypotension, shock, apnea, occasional laryngospasm, coughing, respiratory difficulties.

PATIENT CARE CONSIDERATIONS
Administration/Storage
- Use Sterile Water for Injection, Sodium Chloride Injection, or 5% Dextrose Injection as diluent.
- Avoid extravascular or intra-arterial injection since ulceration, necrosis, and gangrene may result.
- Patients with renal dysfunction require dosage reduction.
- Use freshly prepared solutions promptly. Discard unused portions after 24 hr.
- When preparing rectal suspension, observe caution when filling applicator. Cleansing enema is not required.
- Dosage reduction of thiopental may be required if thiopental is administered concomitantly with narcotic analgesics.
- Store at room temperature, protected from light.

Assessment/Interventions
- Obtain patient history, including drug history and any known allergies.
- Give test dose to assess reaction.
- Monitor vital signs before, during, and after administration.
- Monitor ventilation carefully when drug is being administered to neurosurgical patients with increased intracranial pressure who are not receiving mechanical ventilation.
- Maintain airway patency at all times and have oxygen and resuscitation equipment nearby.
- Monitor respiration rate carefully.
- If patient is receiving drug IV, monitor cardiac function on cardiac monitor to assess for arrhythmias.
- Observe for thrombophlebitis, which may occur with IV administration.
- Observe for symptoms of anaphylaxis including pruritus, urticaria, and erythema.

Patient/Family Education
- Instruct patient to notify health care provider of any signs of hypersensitivity to barbiturates.
- Inform patient to avoid alcohol or other CNS depressants for 24 hr.
- Advise patient that drug can continue to impair abilities for 24 hr following administration and caution patient to avoid driving or performing other tasks requiring mental alertness.

Thioridazine Hydrochloride
(THIGH-oh-RID-uh-zeen HIGH-droe-KLOR-ide)
Class Antipsychotic/Phenothiazine

How Supplied
Thioridazine Hydrochloride Tablets 10 mg, Tablets 15 mg, Tablets 25 mg, Tablets 50 mg, Tablets 100 mg, Tablets 150 mg, Tablets 200 mg, Oral Concentrate 30 mg/mL, Oral Concentrate 100 mg/mL
✤ *Apo-Thioridazine*

Action
PHARMACOLOGY: Effects apparently caused by dopamine receptor blocking in CNS.

Indications Management of schizophrenia.

Contraindications Congenital QT interval prolongation; concurrent drugs that prolong the QT interval; history of cardiac arrhythmias; comatose or severely depressed states; allergy to this or any phenothiazine; presence of large amounts of other CNS depressants; severe hypotension or hypertension.

Route/Dosage
ADULTS: **PO** Start with 50 to 100 mg tid, increasing the dose gradually in increments (max, 800 mg/day). Total daily dose ranges from 200 to 800 mg divided into 2 to 4 doses.
CHILDREN: **PO** Start with 0.5 mg/kg/day in divided doses, increasing the dose gradually until

optimal therapeutic effect is obtained (max, 3 mg/kg/day).

Interactions
Alcohol and other CNS depressants: May result in increased CNS depression and may precipitate extrapyramidal reaction.
Anticholinergics: May reduce therapeutic effects of thioridazine and worsen anticholinergic effects of thioridazine. May lead to tardive dyskinesia.
Barbiturate anesthetics: Frequency and severity of neuromuscular excitation and hypotension may increase.
Beta-blockers: May result in increased plasma levels of beta-blocker and thioridazine.
Drugs that prolong the QT interval (eg, cisapride), drugs that inhibit CYP2D6 (eg, fluoxetine, paroxetine): May increase the risk of life-threatening cardiac arrhythmias, including torsades de pointes. Coadministration of these agents is contraindicated.
Drugs that reduce the clearance of thioridazine by other mechanisms (eg, fluvoxamine, propranolol, pindolol): May elevate plasma levels of thioridazine, increasing the risk of side effects including life-threatening cardiac arrhythmias. Avoid coadministration of these agents.
Epinephrine: May antagonize effects of epinephrine.
Lithium: May cause disorientation, unconsciousness, and extrapyramidal effects.

Lab Test Interferences
May discolor urine pink to red-brown. False-positive pregnancy test results may occur, but are less likely to occur with serum test. Increases in protein bound iodine have been reported.

Adverse Reactions
CV: Orthostatic hypotension; hypertension; tachycardia; bradycardia; syncope; cardiac arrest; circulatory collapse; lightheadedness; faintness; dizziness; EKG changes, including dose-related prolongation of the QTc interval.
CNS: Pseudoparkinsonism; dystonias; motor restlessness; headache; weakness; tremor; fatigue; slurring; insomnia; vertigo; seizures; tardive dyskinesia; drowsiness; paradoxical excitement; headache; confusion.
DERM: Photosensitivity skin pigmentation; dry skin; exfoliative dermatitis; urticarial rash; maculopapular hypersensitivity reaction; seborrhea; eczema.
EENT: Pigmentary retinopathy; glaucoma; photophobia; blurred vision; mydriasis; increased IOP; dry throat; nasal congestion.
GI: Dyspepsia; constipation; dry mouth; adynamic ileus; nausea; vomiting; diarrhea.
GU: Urinary hesitancy or retention; impotence; sexual dysfunction; dysmenorrhea; menstrual irregularities; uremia; breast enlargement; galactorrhea.
HEMA: Agranulocytosis; eosinophilia; leukopenia; hemolytic anemia; thrombocytopenic purpura.
HEPA: Jaundice; biliary stasis.
METAB: Decreased cholesterol.
RESP: Laryngospasm; respiratory depression; bronchospasm; dyspnea.
OTHER: Increase in appetite and weight; polydipsia; neuroleptic malignant syndrome (NMS); allergy (including fever, laryngeal edema, angioneurotic edema, asthma); elevated prolactin levels.

> **WARNING:**
> QTc prolongation is dose related. Torsades de pointes-type arrhythmias and sudden death.
>
> Reserved for use only in refractory schizophrenia that failed to show an acceptable response to adequate course of other antipsychotics.

Precautions
Pregnancy: Safety not established.
Lactation: Safety not established.
Children: See Route/Dosage.
Elderly: More susceptible to effects; consider lower dose.
Special risk patients: Use caution in patients with CV disease or mitral insufficiency, history of glaucoma, EEG abnormalities, or seizure disorders, prior brain damage, hepatic or renal impairment, or in those exposed to extreme heat.
CNS effects: May impair mental or physical abilities, especially during first few days of therapy.
Hepatic effects: Jaundice usually occurs between second and fourth wk of treatment; considered hypersensitivity reaction. Usually reversible.
NMS: Has occurred with agents of this class; is potentially fatal. Signs and symptoms are hyperpyrexia, muscle rigidity, altered mental status, irregular pulse, irregular BP, tachycardia, and diaphoresis.
Pulmonary: Cases of bronchopneumonia (some fatal) occurred.
Sudden death: Sudden death reported; predisposing factors may be seizures or previous brain damage. Flare-ups of psychotic behavior may precede death.
Tardive dyskinesia: Syndrome of potentially irreversible involuntary body and facial movements may develop. Prevalence highest in the elderly, especially women. Use smallest effective doses for shortest possible time.

THIORIDAZINE HYDROCHLORIDE 1749

Overdosage: Signs and Symptoms
Decreased consciousness, arrhythmias, extrapyramidal effects, confusion, agitation, respiratory depression, anticholinergic effects.

PATIENT CARE CONSIDERATIONS
Administration/Storage
- Dose and frequency of administration are variable, depending on condition being treated.
- Administer tablets as prescribed, without regard to meals. Administer with food if GI upset occurs.
- Measure prescribed dose of oral concentrate using calibrated dropper supplied with medication.
- Oral concentrate may be diluted with 1 to 2 oz of distilled water, acidified tap water, or tomato or fruit juice just prior to administration. Do not prepare dilutions ahead of time and store.
- If oral concentrate is spilled on skin or clothing, rinse area immediately with water to prevent contact dermatitis.
- Store tablets and oral concentrate at controlled room temperature (59° to 86°F).

Assessment/Interventions
- Obtain patient history, including drug history and any known allergies. Note allergy to thioridazine or other phenothiazines, previous episode of jaundice with phenothiazine therapy, renal impairment, hepatic impairment, ischemic heart disease, heart failure, arrhythmias, cerebrovascular disease, asthma, emphysema, narrow angle glaucoma, epilepsy, mitral insufficiency, pheochromocytoma, prostatic hypertrophy, condition predisposing to hypotension (eg, dehydration, hypovolemia), concomitant use of antihypertensive drugs, or previous episodes of NMS.
- Review patient's health history for any condition that could contraindicate therapy with thioridazine: current use of drugs known to prolong the QTc interval (eg, cisapride, erythromycin); current use of medications that inhibit CYP4502D6 (eg, fluoxetine, paroxetine); history of cardiac arrhythmia; congenital long QTc interval.
- Ensure that baseline ECG is performed and serum potassium level is determined before starting therapy and periodically during treatment.
- Do not administer to patient with QTc interval greater than 450 msec at baseline. Discontinue therapy if QTc interval prolongs to greater than 500 msec during therapy.
- Ensure that medication is discontinued at least 48 hr before myelography and not resumed until at least 24 hr after procedure to reduce chance of seizures occurring.
- Frequently assess patient for response to treatment. Notify health care provider if condition being treated is not improving or is worsening.
- Ensure that therapy is periodically reviewed to determine if therapy needs to be continued without change or if a dose change (eg, increase, decrease, discontinuation) is indicated.
- Avoid sudden discontinuation of therapy if possible. Attempt to gradually reduce dose if decision to discontinue medication is made.
- Inform health care provider immediately if hyperpyrexia, muscle rigidity, altered mental status, irregular pulse and BP, tachycardia, or diaphoresis develop.
- Notify health care provider immediately if palpitations or syncope occur.
- Assess neurologic status before and during treatment. Observe for involuntary body and facial movements, excessive drowsiness, agitation, tremor, or anxiety. Inform health care provider if noted.
- Monitor patient for CNS, CV, GI, GU, psychiatric, musculoskeletal, and general body side effects. Inform health care provider if noted and significant.
- Assess medication compliance.

Patient/Family Education
- Explain name, dose, action, and potential side effects of drug.
- Advise patient, family, or caregiver that dose will be adjusted periodically until max benefit has been obtained.
- Advise patient, family, or caregiver not to change the dose or stop taking unless advised by health care provider.
- Instruct patient, family, or caregiver to measure prescribed dose of oral concentrate using calibrated dropper supplied with medication.
- Advise patient, family, or caregiver that oral concentrate may be diluted with 1 to 2 oz of distilled water, acidified tap water, or tomato or fruit juice just prior to administration. Caution patient, family, or caregiver to not prepare dilutions ahead of time and store.
- Instruct patient not to stop taking thioridazine when feeling better.
- Instruct patient, family, or caregiver to immediately report fainting or loss of consciousness, palpitations, dizziness, high fever, muscle rigidity, altered mental status, irregular pulse, sore throat, unusual bruising, or yellowing of the skin or eyes.
- Advise patient, family, or caregiver to notify health care provider of the following: exces-

sive drowsiness, increased agitation or anxiety, involuntary body or facial movements, vision problems (eg, fuzzy vision, brownish coloring, impairment of night vision).
- Advise patient to avoid strenuous activity during periods of high temperature or humidity.
- Instruct patient to avoid alcoholic beverages and other depressants while taking this medication.
- Instruct patient to get up slowly from lying or sitting position and to avoid sudden position changes to prevent postural hypotension. Advise patient to report dizziness with position changes to health care provider. Caution patient that hot tubs and hot showers or baths may make dizziness worse.
- Advise patient to take sips of water, suck on ice chips or sugarless hard candy, or chew sugarless gum if dry mouth occurs.
- Advise patient that drug may cause drowsiness or impaired judgment or thinking skills and to use caution while driving or performing other tasks requiring mental alertness until tolerance is determined.
- Caution patient that medication may cause sensitivity to sunlight and to avoid unnecessary exposure to UV light (eg, sunlight, tanning booths) and to use sunscreen and wear protective clothing when exposed to UV light until tolerance is determined.
- Advise women to notify health care provider if pregnant, planning to become pregnant, or breastfeeding.
- Instruct patient not to take any prescription or OTC medications or dietary supplements unless advised by health care provider.
- Advise patient that follow-up visits may be required to monitor therapy and to keep appointments.

Thiotepa

(thigh-oh-TEP-uh)
Class Alkylating agent/Ethylenimines/Methylmelamines

How Supplied
Thioplex Powder for Injection 15 mg

Action
PHARMACOLOGY: Thiotepa is a cell cycle nonspecific alkylating agent related to nitrogen mustard. Its radiomimetic action is believed to occur through the release of ethylenimine radicals, which disrupt the bonds of DNA. TEPA possesses cytotoxic activity.

PHARMACOKINETICS/DYNAMICS:
Absorption: Following a 30-mg dose, thiotepa C_{max} is approximately 131 ng/mL and AUC is approximately 2832 ng/hr.mL.

Excretion: Following a 60-mg dose, thiotepa $t_{½}$ is approximately 2.4 hr and total clearance is approximately 446 mL/min.

Indications Bladder cancer, palliative therapy of breast and ovarian carcinoma. **Unlabeled use(s):** Prevention of pterygium recurrence after postoperative β-irradiation, autologous bone marrow transplantation.

Contraindications History of hypersensitivity reaction, hepatic disease, renal disease, or bone marrow toxicity. Administer reduced doses if therapy is necessary in these patients.

Route/Dosage
Breast and Ovarian Carcinoma
ADULTS: IV 0.3 to 0.4 mg/kg every 1 to 4 wk. Alternative regimens, 0.2 mg/kg/day for 4 to 5 days every 2 to 4 wk; or 5 mg/m²/day for 4 to 5 days every 2 to 4 wk.

Bladder Tumors
ADULTS: **Intravesically** 30 to 60 mg instilled (in 60 mL of sterile water) once weekly for 4 wk. Retain fluid in bladder for 2 hr. If patient cannot retain for 2 hr, dilute successive doses in 30 mL of sterile water instead of 60 mL. It may be necessary to repeat course of therapy or give maintenance therapy with 30 to 60 mg intravesically once monthly for up to 1 yr. After local resection or fulguration of bladder tumors, prophylaxis with thiotepa 30 to 60 mg has been used.

Interactions
Pancuronium: Prolonged apnea and paralysis because of pancuronium occurred in a patient who received thiotepa.
Succinylcholine: Prolonged apnea because of succinylcholine occurred in a patient who had received thiotepa and other antineoplastics.

Lab Test Interferences None well documented.

Adverse Reactions
CNS: Confusion and somnolence at high doses used for bone marrow transplantation. With intrathecal use lower extremity weakness or pain, spinal cord demyelination, transient paresthesias.
DERM: Rash, hives, bronze hyperpigmentation after bone marrow transplantation.
GI: Low potential for nausea and vomiting, anorexia, mucositis, intestinal ulceration, lower abdominal pain with intravesical use.
GU: Chemical and hemorrhagic cystitis, hematuria with intravesical use, amenorrhea, interference with spermatogenesis.
HEMA: Bone marrow suppression, leukocyte nadir at 10 to 30 days, bone marrow suppression

from systemically absorbed thiotepa can occur after bladder instillation.
SPEC SENSE: Eye irritation and delayed periorbital skin depigmentation with ophthalmic use.
OTHER: Acute leukemia and myelodysplastic syndrome with long-term intravesical use.

Precautions
Pregnancy: Category D.
Lactation: Undetermined.
Children: Safety and efficacy have not been established.
Renal function impairment: If the benefits outweigh the potential risks, use in low doses and monitor renal function.
Hepatic function impairment: If the benefits outweigh the potential risks, use in low doses and monitor hepatic function.
Mutagenesis: In vitro, it causes chromatid-type chromosomal aberations.
Fertility impairment: Thiotepa impaired fertility in male mice and inhibited implantation in female rats.
Hematopoietic toxicity: This drug is highly toxic to the hematopoietic system. Perform weekly blood and platelet counts during therapy and for 3 wk or more after therapy discontinuation. The most serious complication of excessive therapy is bone marrow depression, causing leukopenia, thrombocytopenia, and anemia. If WBC count falls to 3000/mm^3 or less, discontinue use. If the platelet count falls to 150,000/mm^3, discontinue therapy.

Overdosage: Signs and Symptoms
Hematopoietic toxicity, decrease in WBC count, decrease in platelets, bleeding manifestations may develop, increased infection vulnerability.

PATIENT CARE CONSIDERATIONS
Administration/Storage
- Refrigerate powder for injection and protect from light.
- Reconstitute powder for injection by adding 1.5 mL sterile water for injection to each 15 mg vial to yield 10 mg/mL solution.
- Reconstituted solution is hypotonic and should be further diluted with 0.9% Sodium Chloride before administration. Do not use solutions which are opaque or contain precipitate.
- Reconstituted 10 mg/mL solution is stable for 24 hr or longer under refrigeration; however, thiotepa contains no preservative and the manufacturer recommends using the product within 8 hr.
- Diluted 5 mg/mL solutions prepared with 0.9% Sodium Chloride are stable for up to 24 hr at room temperature or under refrigeration. Diluted 0.5 mg/mL solutions must be used within 8 hr.
- IV, intravesical, or ophthalmic instillation.
- Prior to intravesical instillation, patients should not drink for 8 to 12 hr. While thiotepa is instilled, patient may be repositioned q 15 min to maximize area of contact.

Assessment/Interventions
- Monitor CBC with differential at baseline, at least once weekly during therapy, and for 3 wk or more after discontinuing therapy. Discontinue therapy for WBC less than 3000/mm^3 or platelet count less than 150,000/mm^3.

Patient/Family Education
- Notify the health care provider in the case of any sign of bleeding (eg, epistaxis, easy bruising, change in color of urine, black stool) or infection (eg, fever, chills).
- Notify the health care provider if patient or partner may be pregnant. Use effective contraception during therapy.

Thiothixene

(THIGH-oh-THIX-een)

Class Antipsychotic/Thioxanthene

How Supplied
Navane Capsules 1 mg, Capsules 2 mg, Capsules 5 mg, Capsules 10 mg, Capsules 20 mg

Action
PHARMACOLOGY: Produces antipsychotic effects apparently because of dopamine receptor blocking in CNS.
PHARMACOKINETICS/DYNAMICS:
Absorption: Thiothixene absorption is erratic and varies. T_{max} occurs 2 to 4 hr after oral use.
Distribution: Thiothixene is highly lipophilic, is widely distributed in tissues, and is 91% to 99% protein bound.
Metabolism: Thiothixene is extensively metabolized in the liver.
Excretion: About 50% of excretion occurs via the kidneys; the other 50% occurs through enterohepatic circulation. Thiothixene t½ is 20 to 40 hr. Less than 1% is excreted as unchanged drug.

Indications Management of schizophrenia.
Contraindications Comatose or severely

depressed states; circulatory collapse; CNS depression from any cause; bone marrow depression; blood dyscrasias.

Route/Dosage
Mild Conditions
ADULTS AND CHILDREN 12 YR AND OLDER: PO Start with 2 mg tid, an increase to 15 mg/day is often effective if needed.

Severe Conditions
ADULTS AND CHILDREN 12 YR AND OLDER: PO Start with 5 mg bid. The usual optimal dose is 20 to 30 mg/day. If indicated, an increase to 60 mg/day may be effective. Doses above 60 mg/day rarely increase the beneficial response.

Interactions
Alcohol, other CNS depressants: May cause additive CNS depressant effects.
Anticholinergics: May reduce therapeutic effects and increase anticholinergic effects of thiothixene; may lead to tardive dyskinesia.
Guanethidine: May inhibit hypotensive effect of guanethidine.

Lab Test Interferences
False-positive pregnancy test results may occur but are less likely to occur with serum test. Increases in protein-bound iodine have been reported.

Adverse Reactions
CV: Orthostatic hypotension; tachycardia; syncope; lightheadedness; ECG changes.
CNS: Tardive dyskinesia; extrapyramidal symptoms (eg, pseudoparkinsorism, akathisia, dystonias); drowsiness; insomnia; restlessness; agitation; seizures; paradoxical exacerbation of psychotic symptoms.
DERM: Rash; pruritus; urticaria; photosensitivity.
EENT: Pigmentary retinopathy; lenticular pigmentation; blurred vision; nasal congestion.
GI: Dry mouth; anorexia; diarrhea; nausea; vomiting; constipation.
GU: Impotence, sexual dysfunction; amenorrhea; breast enlargement; lactation; gynecomastia.
HEMA: Leukopenia; leukocytosis.
METAB: Elevations of serum transaminase and alkaline phosphatase.
RESP: Laryngospasm; bronchospasm; increased depth of respiration.
OTHER: Hypoglycemia; hyperglycemia; glycosuria; polydipsia; increase in appetite and weight; peripheral edema; elevated prolactin levels; increased sweating or salivation.

Precautions
Pregnancy: Pregnancy category undetermined.
Lactation: Undetermined.
Children: Not recommended in children less than 12 yr.
Elderly: More susceptible to adverse effects.
Special risk patients: Use drug with caution in patients with CV disease or mitral insufficiency, history of glaucoma, EEG abnormalities, seizure disorders, prior brain damage, hepatic or renal impairment, or those exposed to extreme heat.
CNS effects: Drug may impair mental or physical abilities, especially during first few days of therapy.
Hepatic effects: Jaundice (usually reversible) may occur, usually between second and fourth week of treatment, and is considered a hypersensitivity reaction.
Neuroleptic malignant syndrome (NMS): NMS has occurred with similar agents and is potentially fatal. Signs and symptoms are hyperpyrexia, muscle rigidity, altered mental status, irregular pulse, irregular BP, tachycardia, and diaphoresis.
Pulmonary effects: Cases of bronchopneumonia, some fatal, have occurred.
Sudden death: Has been reported; predisposing factors may be seizures or previous brain damage. Flare-ups of psychotic behavior may precede death.
Tardive dyskinesia: Potentially irreversible involuntary body and facial movements may occur. Prevalence highest in elderly, especially women.

Overdosage: Signs and Symptoms
Twitching muscles, drowsiness, dizziness, CNS depression, rigidity, weakness, torticollis, tremor, salivation, dysphagia, hypotension, disturbed gait, coma.

PATIENT CARE CONSIDERATIONS
Administration/Storage
- Dose and frequency of administration are variable, depending on condition being treated.
- Administer tablets as prescribed, without regard to meals. Administer with food if GI upset occurs.
- Store tablets at controlled room temperature (59° to 86°F).

Assessment/Interventions
- Obtain patient history, including drug history and any known allergies. Note allergy to phenothiazines, blood dyscrasia, renal impairment, hepatic impairment, ischemic heart disease, heart failure, cerebrovascular disease, epilepsy, or previous episodes of NMS.
- Frequently assess patient for response to treatment. Notify health care provider if condition being treated is not improving or is worsening.
- Ensure therapy is periodically reviewed to determine if it needs to be continued without change or if a dose change (eg, increase,

decrease, discontinuation) is indicated.
- Avoid sudden discontinuation of therapy if possible. Attempt to gradually reduce dose if decision to discontinue medication is made.
- Inform health care provider immediately if hyperpyrexia, muscle rigidity, altered mental status, irregular pulse and BP, tachycardia, and diaphoresis develop.
- Notify health care provider immediately if palpitations or syncope occur.
- Assess neurologic status before and during treatment. Observe for involuntary body and facial movements, excessive drowsiness, agitation, tremor, or anxiety. Inform health care provider if noted.
- Monitor patient for CNS, CV, GI, GU, psychiatric, musculoskeletal, and general body side effects. Inform health care provider if noted and significant.
- Assess medication compliance.

Patient/Family Education
- Explain name, dose, action, and potential side effects of drug.
- Advise patient, family, or caregiver that dose will be adjusted periodically until max benefit has been obtained.
- Advise patient, family, or caregiver not to change the dose or stop taking unless advised by health care provider.
- Instruct patient not to stop taking thiothixene when feeling better.
- Instruct patient, family, or caregiver to immediately report fainting, dizziness, high fever, muscle rigidity, altered mental status, and irregular pulse.
- Advise patient, family, or caregiver to notify health care provider of the following: excessive drowsiness, increased agitation or anxiety, involuntary body or facial movements.
- Advise patient to avoid strenuous activity during periods of high temperature or humidity.
- Instruct patient to avoid alcoholic beverages and other depressants while taking this medication.
- Instruct patient to get up slowly from lying or sitting position and to avoid sudden position changes to prevent postural hypotension. Advise patient to report dizziness with position changes to health care provider. Caution patient that hot tubs and hot showers or baths may worsen dizziness.
- Advise patient to take sips of water, suck on ice chips or sugarless hard candy, or chew sugarless gum if dry mouth occurs.
- Advise patient that drug may cause drowsiness or impaired judgment or thinking skills and to use caution while driving or performing other tasks requiring mental alertness until tolerance is determined.
- Caution patient that medication may cause sensitivity to sunlight and to avoid unnecessary exposure to UV light (sunlight, tanning booths) and to use sunscreen and wear protective clothing when exposed to UV light until tolerance is determined.
- Advise women to notify health care provider if pregnant, planning to become pregnant, or breastfeeding.
- Instruct patient not to take any prescription or OTC medications or dietary supplements unless advised by health care provider.
- Advise patient that follow-up visits may be required to monitor therapy and to keep appointments.

Thyroid, Desiccated (Thyroid USP)

(THIGH-royd, DESS-ih-KATE-uhd)

Class Thyroid

How Supplied
Armour Thyroid Tablets 15 mg (¼ grain), Tablets 30 mg (½ grain), Tablets 60 mg (1 grain), Tablets 90 mg (1½ grain), Tablets 120 mg (2 grain), Tablets 180 mg (3 grain), Tablets 240 mg (4 grain), Tablets 300 mg (5 grain) ◆ *S-P-T* Capsules 60 mg (1 grain) (Pork thyroid suspended in soybean oil), Capsules 120 mg (2 grain) (Pork thyroid suspended in soybean oil), Capsules 180 mg (3 grain) (Pork thyroid suspended in soybean oil), Capsules 300 mg (5 grain) (Pork thyroid suspended in soybean oil) ◆ *Thyrar* Tablets 30 mg (½ grain) (Bovine thyroid), Tablets 60 mg (1 grain) (Bovine thyroid), Tablets 120 mg (2 grain) (Bovine thyroid) ◆ *Thyroid Strong* Tablets 30 mg (½ grain) (50% stronger than thyroid USP. Each grain is eq. to 1½ grain of thyroid USP.), Tablets 60 mg (1 grain) (50% stronger than thyroid USP. Each grain is eq. to 1½ grain of thyroid USP.), Tablets 120 mg (2 grain) (50% stronger than thyroid USP. Each grain is eq. to 1½ grain of thyroid USP.), Tablets 180 mg (3 grain) (50% stronger than thyroid USP. Each grain is eq. to 1½ grain of thyroid USP.)

Action

PHARMACOLOGY: Increases metabolic rate of body tissues.

PHARMACOKINETICS/DYNAMICS:
Absorption: Levothyroxine (T_4) is only partially absorbed from the GI tract. Absorption

varies from 48% to 79%. Fasting increases absorption. Liothyronine (T_3) is almost totally absorbed (95%) in 4 hr.

Distribution: More than 99% is bound to serum proteins.

Metabolism: Deiodination of levothyroxine (T_4) occurs at a number of sites, including liver, kidney, and other tissues.

Indications Replacement or supplemental therapy in hypothyroidism; TSH suppression (in thyroid cancer, nodules, goiters, and enlargement in chronic thyroiditis); diagnostic agent to differentiate suspected hyperthyroidism from euthyroidism.

Contraindications Hypersensitivity to any ingredient; acute MI and thyrotoxicosis uncomplicated by hypothyroidism. Also contraindicated when hypothyroidism and hypoadrenalism (Addison disease) coexist, unless treatment of hypoadrenalism with adrenocortical steroids precedes initiation of thyroid therapy.

Route/Dosage

Optimal dosage determined by clinical response and laboratory findings.

Hypothyroidism

ADULTS: PO 30 mg/day initially, increasing by 15 mg increments q 2 to 3 wk. In patients with long-standing myxedema, 15 mg/day, particularly if cardiovascular impairment is suspected. Reduce dosage if angina occurs.
Maintenance: 60 to 120 mg/day.
CHILDREN: PO See table for recommended dose in congenital hypothyroidism.

CONGENITAL HYPOTHYROIDISM DOSE

Age	Dose per day (mg)	Daily dose per kg (mg)
> 12 yr	> 90	1.2 to 1.8
6 to 12 yr	60 to 90	2.4 to 3
1 to 5 yr	45 to 60	3 to 3.6
6 to 12 mo	30 to 45	3.6 to 4.8
0 to 6 mo	7.5 to 30	2.4 to 6

Thyroid Cancer
Larger doses required.

Interactions

Anticoagulants: Anticoagulant effects may be increased.
Cholestyramine: May decrease thyroid efficacy.
Digitalis glycosides: Digitalis levels may increase, resulting in toxicity.
Theophyllines: Theophylline clearance may be altered in hyperthyroid or hypothyroid patients.

Lab Test Interferences Consider changes in thyroid-binding globulin concentration when interpreting T_4 and T_3 values. Medicinal or dietary iodine interferes with all in vivo tests of radioiodine uptake, producing low uptakes that may not reflect true decrease in hormone synthesis.

Adverse Reactions

CV: Palpitations; tachycardia; cardiac arrhythmias; angina pectoris; cardiac arrest.
CNS: Tremors; headache; nervousness; insomnia.
GI: Diarrhea; vomiting.
GU: Menstrual irregularities.
OTHER: Hypersensitivity; weight loss; sweating; heat intolerance; fever. Adverse reactions generally indicate hyperthyroidism caused by therapeutic overdosage.

Precautions

Pregnancy: Category A.
Lactation: Excreted in breast milk.
Children:
Congenital hypothyroidism – Routine determinations of serum T_4 or TSH are strongly advised in newborns. Initiate treatment immediately on diagnosis and continue for life, unless transient hypothyroidism is suspected. In infants, excessive doses of thyroid hormone preparations may produce craniosynostosis. Children may experience transient partial hair loss in first few months of thyroid therapy.
Cardiovascular disease: Use caution when integrity of CV system, particularly coronary arteries is suspect (eg, angina, elderly). Development of chest pain or worsening CV disease requires decrease in dosage. Observe patients with coronary artery disease during surgery, since possibility of cardiac arrhythmias may be greater in those treated with thyroid hormones.
Endocrine disorders: Therapy in patients with concomitant diabetes mellitus or insipidus or adrenal insufficiency (Addison disease) exacerbates intensity of symptoms. Therapy of myxedema coma requires simultaneous administration of glucocorticoids. In patients whose hypothyroidism is secondary to hypopituitarism, adrenal insufficiency, if present, should be corrected with corticosteroids before administering thyroid hormones.
Hyperthyroid effects: May rarely precipitate hyperthyroid state or may aggravate existing hyperthyroidism.
Morphologic hypogonadism and nephrosis: Rule out before therapy.
Myxedema: Patients are particularly sensitive to thyroid preparations. Begin with small doses.
Obesity: Should not be used for weight reduction; may produce serious or even life-threatening toxicity in larger doses, particularly when given with anorexiants.

Overdosage: Signs and Symptoms
Tachycardia, arrhythmias, hypertension, angina, fever, tremor, vomiting, diarrhea, insomnia, headache, seizures, coma.

PATIENT CARE CONSIDERATIONS
Administration/Storage
- Assess baseline T_4 or TSH as ordered by health care provider.
- When administered as single dose, give in morning to avoid sleeplessness.
- Adjust dose to administer lowest dose possible to relieve symptoms.
- Do not interchange different thyroid products. Absorption may vary.
- Store at room temperature in tightly closed container.

Assessment/Interventions
- Obtain patient history, including drug history and any known allergies.
- Before each dose assess BP and pulse.
- Monitor vital signs and weight.
- In children, monitor height and weight to document normal growth rate.
- Notify health care provider of any changes from baseline status in physical assessment or laboratory testing.

Patient/Family Education
- Explain that children may have short-term temporary hair loss at start of therapy.
- Tell patient to report fever, weight loss, menstrual irregularity, palpitations, chest pain, headache, faint feeling, sweatiness, diarrhea, vomiting, inability to sleep, excitability, irritability, anxiety, nervousness, or any changes to health care provider.
- Teach patient to avoid OTC preparations and food with iodine: iodinated salt, soy beans, tofu, turnips, some seafood, some types of bread.
- Instruct patient not to switch drug brands unless health care provider approves.
- Caution patients not to take thyroid for weight control.

Tiagabine Hydrochloride
(TIE-egg-un-bine)
Class Anticonvulsant

How Supplied
Gabitril Filmtabs Tablets 4 mg, Tablets 12 mg, Tablets 16 mg, Tablets 20 mg

Action
PHARMACOLOGY: Mechanism unknown; may block GABA uptake into presynaptic neurons, allowing more GABA to be available for binding with the GABA receptor of post-synaptic cells.

PHARMACOKINETICS/DYNAMICS:
Absorption: Tiagabine is rapidly and well absorbed, with food slowing absorption rate, but not altering the extent of absorption. T_{max} is 45 min following oral dosing in the fasting state. Bioavailability is 90%. Steady state is achieved within 2 days following multiple dosing.

Distribution: Tiagabine is 96% bound to plasma proteins.

Metabolism: At least 2 metabolic pathways have been identified in humans: 1) thiophene ring oxidation leading to the formation of 5-oxo-tiagabine, and 2) glucuronidation. Tiagabine is metabolized primarily by the 3A isoform subfamily of hepatic cytochrome P450 (CYP3A4), although contributions to the metabolism from CYP1A2, 2D6, or 2C19 have not been excluded.

Excretion: Tiagabine t½ is 7 to 9 hr in healthy people, and 4 to 7 hr in patients receiving hepatic enzyme-inducing drugs (carbamazepine, phenytoin, primidone, phenobarbital).

Peak: Mean steady-state values were 40% lower in the evening that in the morning. Steady-state AUC values were also found to be 15% lower following the evening dose compared with AUC following the morning dose.

Special Populations:
Hepatic Function Impairment: – Moderate hepatic impairment caused a 60% decrease in the clearance of unbound tiagabine. Patients with impaired liver function may require reduced initial and maintenance doses or longer dosing intervals.

Indications
Adjunctive treatment in treatment of partial seizures.

Contraindications
Standard considerations.

Route/Dosage
ADULTS: **PO** Initial dose 4 mg qd. Increase by 4 to 8 mg at weekly intervals until response achieved or total of 56 mg/day.

ADOLESCENTS 12 TO 18 YR: **PO** Initial dose 4 mg qd. Increase dose by 4 mg after 1 wk and thereafter by 4 to 8 mg at weekly intervals until response achieved or total of 32 mg/day.

Interactions
Enzyme-inducing antiepileptic drugs (eg, carbamazepine, phenytoin, primidone, phenobarbital): Increased tiagabine clearance.

Lab Test Interferences
None well documented.

Adverse Reactions
CNS: Dizziness; lightheadedness; somnolence; nervousness; irritability; agitation; hostility; lan-

guage problem; tremor; abnormal gait; ataxia; abnormal thinking; concentration/attention difficulty; depression; confusion; insomnia; speech disorder; difficulty with memory; paresthesia; emotional lability.
DERM: Rash; pruritus; ecchymosis.
EENT: Nystagmus; amblyopia; pharyngitis.
GI: Nausea; abdominal pain; diarrhea; vomiting; increased appetite; mouth ulceration; gingivitis.
OTHER: Asthenia; lack of energy; pain; cough; myasthenia; accidental injury; infection; flu syndrome; myalgia; urinary tract infection; vasodilation.

Precautions
Pregnancy: Category C.
Lactation: Undetermined.
Children: Safety and efficacy in children under 12 yr not established.
Hepatic function impairment: Dosage reduction or longer dosing interval may be necessary.

PATIENT CARE CONSIDERATIONS
Administration/Storage
- Administer medication with food.
- Titrate dose at weekly intervals to effective or maximum dose.
- Administer initial dose as single daily dose. The total daily dose should be given as equally divided doses bid to qid.
- Discontinue medication gradually over minimum of 1 wk.
- Store at room temperature, protected from light and moisture.

Assessment/Interventions
- Obtain patient history, including drug history and any known allergies. Note hepatic function impairment and seizure pattern.
- Assess baseline vital signs.
- Assess for development of side effects. Notify health care provider if noted.
- Withdraw medication gradually to avoid the possibility of increasing seizure frequency.

Patient/Family Education
- Advise patient that medication should be

Serious adverse effects: During clinical trials some patients experienced status epilepticus, and 10 sudden unexplained deaths occurred. The association of these events with tiagabine use is unclear.
Withdrawal: Do not discontinue antiepileptic drugs abruptly because of possible increased seizure frequency on drug withdrawal.
EEG: Patients with a history of spike and wave discharges on EEG may have exacerbations of EEG abnormalities associated with cognitive/neuropsychiatric events, which may be a manifestation of underlying seizure activity. Dosage reduction of tiagabine may be necessary.

Overdosage: Signs and Symptoms
Somnolence, impaired consciousness, agitation, confusion, speech difficulty, hostility, depression, weakness, myoclonus, ataxia, lethargy, drowsiness.

taken with food.
- Explain that missed dose should be taken as soon as possible but that 2 doses should not be taken together. Instruct patient to call health care provider if 2 or more doses are missed.
- Instruct patient to report these symptoms to health care provider: somnolence, excessive fatigue or weakness, dizziness, concentration or attention difficulty, difficulty with memory, speech disorder, ataxia.
- Advise patient that drug may cause drowsiness and to use caution while driving or performing other tasks requiring mental alertness.
- Advise patient to use caution when taking these other drugs with CNS depressant effects (eg, alcohol, sedatives).
- Advise patient to notify their health care provider if they become pregnant, plan on becoming pregnant, or are breastfeeding while taking this medication.

Ticarcillin (Ticarcillin Disodium)
(TIE-car-sill-in)
Class Antibiotic/Penicillin

How Supplied
Ticar Powder for Injection 3 g

Action
PHARMACOLOGY: Inhibits bacterial cell wall mucopeptide synthesis.

PHARMACOKINETICS/DYNAMICS:
Absorption: Ticarcillin is not absorbed orally. It must be given IM or IV. T_{max} is ½ to 1 hr.
Distribution: Ticarcillin is not highly bound to serum protein (approximately 45%). The drug can be detected in tissues and interstitial fluid following IV administration. Penetration into CSF, bile, and pleural fluid has been documented.
Excretion: Ticarcillin is eliminated by glomerular filtration and tubular secretion. It is excreted unchanged in high concentrations in the urine. Ticarcillin t½ is about 70 min.

Special Populations:
Renal Function Impairment – The dosage of

ticarcillin need only be adjusted in severe renal impairment. The drug may be removed from patients undergoing dialysis; the actual amount removed depends on the duration and type of dialysis.

Indications Treatment of bacterial septicemia, skin and soft tissue infections, acute and chronic respiratory tract infections, GU tract infections and infections caused by susceptible strains of anaerobic bacteria, *Pseudomonas aeruginosa*, *Proteus* species, and *Escherichia coli*.

Contraindications Hypersensitivity to penicillins.

Route/Dosage

Bacterial Septicemia, Respiratory Tract Infections, Skin and Soft Tissue Infections, Intra-Abdominal Infections, and Infections of the Female Pelvis and Genital Tract
ADULTS AND CHILDREN: **IV** 200 to 300 mg/kg/day in divided doses q 4 to 6 hr. In adults, the usual dose is IV 3 to 4 g q 4 to 6 hr.

Complicated UTIs
ADULTS AND CHILDREN: **IV** 150 to 200 mg/kg/day in divided doses q 4 to 6 hr (usual dose for 70 kg adult is 3 g qid).

Uncomplicated UTIs
ADULTS: **IM/IV** 1 g q 6 hr.
CHILDREN WEIGHING LESS THAN 40 KG: **IM/IV** 50 to 100 mg/kg/day in divided doses q 6 to 8 hr.

Severe infections (sepsis) caused by susceptible strains of Pseudomonas *sp.,* Proteus *sp., and* E. coli
NEONATES: **IM/IV** For children weighing less than 2 kg and less than 7 days of age, give 75 mg/kg q 12 hr. For children weighing less than 2 kg and more than 7 days of age, give 75 mg/kg q 8 hr. For children weighing 2 kg or more and less than 7 days of age, give 75 mg/kg q 8 hr. For children weighing 2 kg or more and more than 7 days of age, give 100 mg/kg q 8 hr.

Interactions

Anticoagulants: May increase bleeding risks of anticoagulant by prolonging bleeding time.
Chloramphenicol: Synergism or antagonism may develop.
Contraceptives, oral: May reduce efficacy of oral contraceptives. Use additional form of contraception during ticarcillin therapy.
Erythromycin: Synergism or antagonism may develop.
Heparin: May increase bleeding risks of heparin by prolonging bleeding time.
Probenecid: May increase ticarcillin concentration.
Tetracyclines: May impair bactericidal effects of ticarcillin.
INCOMPATIBILITIES:
Aminoglycosides, parenteral: Parenteral aminoglycosides may inactivate aminoglycosides in vitro; do not mix in same IV solution. May be used in combination for synergy.

Lab Test Interferences May cause false-positive urine glucose test results with *Benedict's* solution, *Fehling's* solution, or *Clinitest* tablets but not with enzyme-based tests (eg, *Clinistix*, *Tes-tape*); false-positive direct *Coombs'* test result in certain patient groups; false-positive protein reactions with sulfosalicylic acid and boiling test, acetic acid test, biuret reaction, and nitric acid test but not with bromphenol blue test (*Multi-Stix*).

Adverse Reactions

CV: Phlebitis; vein irritation; deep vein thrombosis.
CNS: Neurotoxicity (eg, lethargy, neuromuscular irritability, hallucinations, convulsions, seizures).
DERM: Rash; pruritus; urticaria.
EENT: Itchy eyes.
GI: Nausea; vomiting; diarrhea or bloody diarrhea; pseudomembranous colitis.
GU: Elevated creatinine or BUN; vaginitis.
HEMA: Anemia; hemolytic anemia; thrombocytopenia; thrombocytopenic purpura; eosinophilia; leukopenia; granulocytopenia; neutropenia; bone marrow depression; prolongation of bleeding and prothrombin time; increase in platelets.
HEPA: Transient hepatitis (elevated AST).
METAB: Elevated serum alkaline phosphatase; hypernatremia; reduced serum potassium.
OTHER: Hypersensitivity reactions; hyperthermia; pain at site of injection; hematomas.

Precautions

Pregnancy: Category B.
Lactation: Excreted in breast milk.
Hypersensitivity: Reactions range from mild to life-threatening. Administer drug with caution to cephalosporin-sensitive patients because of possible crossreactivity.
Renal function impairment: Dosage and interval adjustments are necessary.
Superinfection: May result in bacterial or fungal overgrowth of nonsusceptible organisms.
Bleeding abnormalities: Hemorrhagic manifestations associated with abnormalities of coagulation tests (eg, bleeding time, prothrombin time, platelet aggregation) may occur. Abnormalities should revert to normal once drug is discontinued.
Pseudomembranous colitis: May occur because of overgrowth of clostridia.
Sodium content: Contains 4.7 to 5 mEq sodium/g.

Overdosage: Signs and Symptoms

May result in neuromuscular hyperexcitability or seizures.

PATIENT CARE CONSIDERATIONS
Administration/Storage
IM:
- Reconstitute with sterile water, sodium chloride or 1% lidocaine hydrochloride solution (without epinephrine) to obtain 1 g ticarcillin/2.6 mL solution.
- Use promptly after reconstitution.
- Inject into relatively large muscle.
- Do not exceed 1 g/injection.

IV:
- Do not mix gentamicin, amikacin, or tobramycin in same IV solution.
- Administer slowly over 30 min to 2 hr to avoid vein irritation.
- To reconstitute, add 4 mL of sodium chloride injection, dextrose injection 5%, or lactated ringer's injection to each gram of ticarcillin powder to obtain 200 mg/mL. When dissolved, dilute further to desired volume.
- Reconstitute 3 g piggyback bottles with minimum of 30 mL of desired IV solution. A dilution of no more than 50 mg/mL will reduce incidence of vein irritation.
- After reconstitution, ticarcillin may be stored frozen for up to 30 days.
- Store IV solutions mixed in sodium chloride or dextrose no longer than 72 hr at room temperature or 14 days under refrigeration.
- Store IV solutions mixed in Ringer's solution no longer than 48 hr at room temperature or 14 days under refrigeration.

Assessment/Interventions
- Obtain patient history, including drug history and any known allergies.
- Obtain urine and culture and sensitivity specimens and send to lab. Therapy may be initiated before results are received, but collect cultures prior to drug therapy.
- Request WBC and differential counts prior to initiation of therapy and at least weekly during therapy.
- Request AST, ALT, H&H, BUN, and creatinine studies at appropriate intervals during therapy.
- Perform periodic hemoccult tests on stool.
- Monitor and record skin integrity; report ecchymosis, bleeding, and rashes.
- Assess neurologic status and report lethargy and irritability.
- Assess GI status and report changes in appetite or bowel habits.
- Assess GU status and report hematuria, oliguria, and proteinuria.
- Monitor lab results and report abnormal H&H, potassium, WBC and differential counts, blood coagulation tests, and LFTs.
- Monitor results of culture and sensitivity to ensure bacteria is sensitive to ticarcillin.
- Monitor IV site and report signs of vein irritation.
- Monitor I&O and report imbalances. Ensure adequate fluid intake, especially if patient has diarrhea episodes.
- Apply ice pack if pain and induration occur at injection site.
- Monitor for signs of superinfection.

Patient/Family Education
- Advise patient to report rash, hives, fever, itching, severe diarrhea, shortness of breath, wheezing, black tongue, sore throat, nausea, vomiting, swollen joints, unusual bleeding, or bruising.
- Tell diabetic patients to use *Clinistix* or *Testape* for urine monitoring. Solutions used for urine glucose testing may indicate false-positive results if taking penicillin therapy over period of time.

Ticarcillin/Clavulanate (Ticarcillin Disodium and Clavulanate Potassium)
(TIE-car-sill-in/CLAV-you-luh-nate)

Class Antibiotic/Penicillin

How Supplied
Timentin Powder for Injection 3 g ticarcillin (as disodium) and 0.1 g clavularic acid (as potassium) (contains 4.75 mEq sodium and 0.15 mEq potassium/g), Injection, solution 3 g ticarcillin (as disodium) and 0.1 g clavulanic acid (as potassium)/100 mL (contains 18.7 mEq sodium and 0.5 mEq potassium/100 mL)

Action
PHARMACOLOGY: Ticarcillin inhibits bacterial cell wall mucopeptide synthesis. Clavulanate lactamase enzymes commonly found in microorganisms resistant to ticarcillin.

PHARMACOKINETICS/DYNAMICS:
Absorption: T_{max} is achieved immediately after completion of the infusion. C_{max} is 330 mcg/mL (ticarcillin) and 8 to 16 mcg/mL (clavulanic acid). AUC is about 485 mcg•hr/mL and about

8.2 mcg•hr/mL for ticarcillin and clavulanic acid, respectively.

Distribution: The drugs are not highly protein bound (approximately 45% and 9% for ticarcillin and clavulanic acid, respectively). Ticarcillin/Clavulanate is detected in tissues and interstitial fluid following IV administration. Penetration into bile and pleural fluid has been demonstrated.

Excretion: Serum t½ is about 1.1 hr. Approximately 60% to 70% of ticarcillin and approximately 35% to 45% of clavulanic acid are excreted unchanged in urine during the first 6 hr after a single dose.

Special Populations:
Renal Function Impairment – The dosage of ticarcillin need only be adjusted in severe renal impairment. The drugs may be removed from patients undergoing dialysis; the actual amount removed depends on the duration and type of dialysis.

Indications Treatment of bacterial septicemia, skin and skin structure infections, lower respiratory tract infections, bone and joint infections, GU and gynecologic infections, and intra-abdominal infections caused by susceptible strains of bacteria.

Contraindications Hypersensitivity to penicillin.

Route/Dosage
Systemic and Urinary Tract Infections
ADULTS AND CHILDREN 60 KG AND OVER: **IV** 3.1 g q 4 to 6 hr.
ADULTS AND CHILDREN LESS THAN 60 KG: **IV** 200 to 300 mg/kg/day in divided doses q 4 to 6 hr.

Gynecologic Infections
ADULTS: **IV** 200 to 300 mg/kg/day in divided doses q 4 to 6 hr.

Interactions
Anticoagulants: May increase bleeding risks of anticoagulant by prolonging bleeding time.
Chloramphenicol: Synergism or antagonism may develop.
Contraceptives, oral: May reduce efficacy of oral contraceptives. Use additional form of contraception during ticarcillin/clavulanate therapy.
Erythromycin: Synergism or antagonism may develop.
Heparin: May increase bleeding risks of heparin by prolonging bleeding time.
Probenecid: May increase ticarcillin levels.
Sodium bicarbonate: Ticarcillin/clavulanate is incompatible with sodium bicarbonate; not recommended as diluent.
Tetracyclines: May impair bactericidal effects of ticarcillin/clavulanate.
INCOMPATIBILITIES: Aminoglycosides, parenteral: May inactivate aminoglycosides in vitro; do not mix in same IV solution. May be used in combination for synergy.

Lab Test Interferences May cause false-positive urine glucose test results with *Benedict's* Solution, *Fehling's* Solution, or *Clinitest* tablets but not with enzyme-based tests (eg, *Clinistix, Tes-tape*); false-positive direct Coombs' test in certain patient groups; positive direct antiglobulin tests (DAT); false-positive protein reactions with sulfosalicylic acid and boiling test, acetic acid test, biuret reaction, and nitric acid test but not with bromphenol blue test (*Multi-Stix*).

Adverse Reactions
CV: Deep vein thrombosis; vein irritation; phlebitis.
CNS: Neurotoxicity (lethargy, neuromuscular irritability, and seizures).
DERM: Rash; pruritus; urticaria; ecchymosis.
GI: Nausea; vomiting; abdominal pain or cramp; diarrhea; pseudomembranous colitis.
GU: Elevated creatinine or BUN; vaginitis.
HEMA: Anemia; hemolytic anemia; thrombocytopenia; eosinophilia; leukopenia; granulocytopenia; neutropenia; prolongation of bleeding and prothrombin time.
HEPA: Transient hepatitis; cholestatic jaundice.
METAB: Elevated serum alkaline phosphatase; hypernatremia; reduced serum potassium.
OTHER: Hypersensitivity reactions; pain at site of injection; hematomas; hyperthermia.

Precautions
Pregnancy: Category B.
Lactation: Excreted in breast milk.
Hypersensitivity: Reactions range from mild to life-threatening. Administer cautiously to cephalosporin-sensitive patients due to possible cross-reactivity.
Renal function impairment: Dosage and interval adjustments necessary in renal insufficiency.
Superinfection: May result in bacterial or fungal overgrowth of non-susceptible organisms.
Bleeding abnormalities: Hemorrhagic manifestations associated with abnormalities of coagulation tests (bleeding time, prothrombin time, platelet aggregation) may occur. Abnormalities should revert to normal once drug is discontinued.
Hypokalemia: Ticarcillin has rarely decreased potassium levels.
Pseudomembranous colitis: May occur due to overgrowth of clostridia.
Sodium content: Powder for injection contains 4.75 mEq Na/g of ticarcillin.

Overdosage: Signs and Symptoms
Neuromuscular hyperexcitability, seizures.

PATIENT CARE CONSIDERATIONS
Administration/Storage
- To reconstitute: Add approximately 13 mL of Sterile Water for Injection or Sodium Chloride Injection. Then dilute further to concentrations of 10 to 100 mg/mL with NaCl, 5% Dextrose or Lactated Ringer's.
- Administer IV over 30 min by direct infusion or by piggyback.
- Discontinue other solutions while this drug is being infused via piggy-back.
- Do not mix sodium bicarbonate, gentamicin, amikacin, or tobramycin in same IV solution.
- Store concentrated stock solution (200 mg/mL) no longer than 6 hr at room temperature or 72 hr under refrigeration.
- Store concentrations of 10 to 100 mg/mL in Sodium Chloride for Injection or Lactated Ringer's no longer than 24 hr at room temperature; 7 days under refrigeration or 30 days frozen. Store solutions made with 5% Dextrose no longer than 24 hr at room temperature, 3 days under refrigeration, or 7 days frozen.
- Thaw premixed, frozen solutions at room temperature or in refrigerator.
- Do not immerse in water baths or microwave to thaw.
- After thawing, store refrigerated no longer than 7 days or 24 hr at room temperature.
- Do not refreeze.

Assessment/Interventions
- Obtain patient history, including drug history and any known allergies.
- Assess results of AST, ALT, H&H, BUN, and creatinine studies at appropriate intervals during therapy.
- Send urine and culture and sensitivity specimens to lab. Therapy may be initiated before results are received, but cultures should be collected prior to drug therapy.
- Request WBC and differential counts prior to initiation of therapy and at least weekly during therapy.
- Perform periodic hemoccult tests on stool.
- Monitor and record skin integrity. Report ecchymosis, bleeding, and rashes.
- Assess neurologic status and report lethargy and irritability.
- Assess GI status and report changes in appetite or bowel habits. If patient has diarrhea, consider possibility of pseudomembranous colitis.
- Assess GU status and report hematuria, oliguria, and proteinuria.
- Monitor data throughout therapy and report abnormalities to health care provider.
- Monitor I&O and report imbalances to health care provider. Ensure adequate fluid intake, especially if client has diarrhea episodes.
- Assess IV site regularly and report signs of vein irritation to health care provider.
- If pain and induration occur at injection site, apply ice pack.
- Monitor for signs of superinfection.

Patient/Family Education
- Advise patient to report rash, hives, fever, itching, severe diarrhea, shortness of breath, wheezing, black tongue, sore throat, nausea, vomiting, fever, swollen joints, unusual bleeding or bruising.
- Explain that intermittent urinalysis may be required several months after treatment.
- Tell diabetic patients to use *Clinistix* or *Testape* for urine monitoring. Solutions used for urine glucose testing may indicate false-positive results if taking penicillin therapy over period of time.

Ticlopidine Hydrochloride
(tie-KLOE-pih-DEEN HIGH-droe-KLOR-ide)

Class Antiplatelet

How Supplied
Ticlid Tablets 250 mg
✹ *Apo-Ticlopidine* ◆ *Gen-Ticlopidine* ◆ *Nu-Ticlopidine* ◆ *PMS-Ticlopdine* ◆ *Rhoxal-ticlopidine*

Action
PHARMACOLOGY: Produces time- and dose-dependent inhibition of both platelet aggregation and release of platelet granule constituents as well as prolongation of bleeding time; interferes with platelet membrane function by inhibiting platelet-fibrinogen binding and subsequent platelet-platelet interactions.

PHARMACOKINETICS/DYNAMICS:
Absorption: Ticlopidine is rapidly absorbed with peak levels (T_{max}) occurring about 2 hr after dose. The drug is greater than 80% absorbed. Administration after meals results in a 20% increase in the AUC. Ticlopidine is 98% bound to plasma proteins.

Metabolism: Ticlopidine is metabolized extensively by the liver; only trace amounts are detected in urine.

Excretion: Ticlopidine t½ is 4 to 5 days.

Special Populations:
Hepatic Function Impairment – Average plasma concentration is slightly higher in cirrhosis.

Indications Reduction of risk of thrombotic stroke in patients who have experienced stroke precursors and in patients who have had completed thrombotic stroke. Reserved for patients intolerant to aspirin because of greater risk of adverse reactions. **Unlabeled use(s):** Improved walking distance in intermittent claudication; vascular improvement in chronic arterial occlusion; reduced incidence of neurologic deficit in subarachnoid hemorrhage; reduced incidence of vascular occlusion in uremic patients with arteriovenous shunts or fistulas; control of platelet count in open heart surgery; decreased graft occlusion in coronary artery bypass grafts; reduced degree of proteinuria and hematuria in primary glomerulonephritis; reduced incidence, duration, and severity of infarctive crises in sickle cell disease.

Contraindications Presence of hematopoietic disorders (eg, neutropenia, thrombocytopenia); history of thrombotic thrombocytopenic purpura (TTP); presence of hemostatic disorder or active pathologic bleeding (eg, bleeding, peptic ulcer, intracranial bleeding, hemophilia, other coagulation defects); severe liver impairment.

Route/Dosage
ADULTS: PO 250 mg bid with food.

Interactions
Antacids: May reduce ticlopidine absorption.
Aspirin: Increased effect of aspirin on collagen-induced platelet aggregation.
Cimetidine: Elevated ticlopidine levels with possible increase in therapeutic and toxic effects.
Theophylline: Elevated serum theophylline concentrations, increasing risk of toxicity.
Phenytoin: Elevated phenytoin plasma levels with associated somnolence and lethargy have been reported. Exercise caution when administering with ticlopidine.

Lab Test Interferences None well documented.

Adverse Reactions
CV: Vasculitis.
CNS: Headache; peripheral neuropathy; dizziness.
DERM: Maculopapular or urticarial rash; rash; pruritus.
EENT: Tinnitus.
GI: Diarrhea; nausea; fullness; dyspepsia; GI pain; purpura; vomiting; flatulence; anorexia.
GU: Nephrotic syndrome.
HEMA: Prolonged bleeding time; bleeding complications (ecchymosis, epistaxis, hematuria, conjunctival hemorrhage, GI bleeding, perioperative bleeding); neutropenia; pancytopenia; hemolytic anemia; serum sickness; immune thrombocytopenia; abnormal LFTs; TTP; agranulocytosis; eosinophilia; bone marrow depression.
HEPA: Hepatitis; cholestatic jaundice; increased alkaline phosphatase, serum transaminases, and bilirubin.
METAB: Increased cholesterol and triglycerides.
OTHER: Weakness; pain; allergic pneumonitis; systemic lupus erythematosus; arthropathy; myositis; hyponatremia; aplastic anemia; hepatic necrosis; peptic ulcer; renal failure; sepsis; angioedema; hepatocellular jaundice.

> **WARNING:**
> *Hematological:* Life-threatening events including neutropenia, agranulocytosis, thrombotic thrombocytopenic purpura (TTP), and aplastic anemia. Severe hematological problems may occur within a few days after the start of therapy. Thus, monitor hematologically and clinically. Immediately discontinue therapy at any evidence of neutropenia or TTP. TTP incidence peaks at 3 to 4 wk posttherapy initiation. Neutropenia risk peaks at 4 to 6 wk posttherapy initiation. Aplastic anemia risk peaks at 4 to 8 wk posttherapy initiation. Perform CBC with ANC, platelet count, and appearance of the peripheral smear at baseline and q 2 wk during therapy for the first 3 mo.

Precautions
Pregnancy: Category B.
Lactation: Undetermined.
Children: Safety and efficacy in children under 18 yr not established.
Elderly: Require dosage reduction.
Hypersensitivity: Reactions range from minor to life-threatening.
Renal function impairment: Dosage reduction or discontinuation of therapy may be required if hemorrhagic or hematopoietic complications occur.
Hepatic function impairment: Use not recommended because patient may have preexisting bleeding diathesis.
Cholesterol elevation: May cause increased serum cholesterol and triglycerides.
GI bleeding: Use with caution in patients who have lesions with a propensity to bleed.
Hematologic effects: Fatal reactions (eg, pancytopenia) have occurred.
Increased bleeding risk: Use with caution in

patients who may be at risk of increased bleeding from trauma, surgery, or pathological conditions.

PATIENT CARE CONSIDERATIONS
Administration/Storage
- Administer medication with food.
- Anticoagulant or fibrinolytic drugs must be discontinued before initiation of ticlopidine administration.
- Ticlopidine must be discontinued 10 to 14 days before surgery.
- Store at room temperature.

Assessment/Interventions
- Obtain patient history, including drug history and any known allergies. Note ulcers and bleeding problems.
- Monitor patients for evidence of neutropenia or TTP. Immediately discontinue ticlopidine if there is any evidence of neutropenia or TTP.
- Ensure that patient does not have preexisting bleeding tendency by monitoring PT/PTT. Measure periodically during therapy.
- Check results of CBC with platelets and ANC (absolute neutrophil count); check platelet count and the appearance of the peripheral smear.
- Take vital signs including orthostatic BP and pulse.
- Assess for signs of infection.
- Obtain CBC with platelets and ANC as baseline and then every 2 wk during first 3 mo of therapy. Assess more frequently if ANC decreases constantly or is 30% less than baseline. After 3 mo, if CBC, platelet, and ANC are stable, assess these values only if there are signs of infection or bleeding.
- When drug is discontinued, perform CBC with platelet and ANC 1 to 3 wk after last dose.

Overdosage: Signs and Symptoms
Increased bleeding time, increased ALT.

- Monitor LFTs periodically during therapy.
- Monitor for nausea, vomiting, or diarrhea.
- Monitor for signs of bleeding, including petechiae or unusual bruising.

Patient/Family Education
- Instruct patient to take with food.
- Inform patient of increased risk of bleeding and caution patient to take precautionary measures (eg, not to use manual razor, use soft toothbrush, handle knives carefully, always wear shoes when walking).
- Instruct patient to report signs of infection (eg, fever, white overgrowth in mouth, vaginal yeast, nonhealing wounds or wounds that appear red with drainage) to health care provider.
- Advise patient to notify health care provider of signs of blood or changes in stool or urine, unusual bruising, decreased appetite, dark urine, light-colored stools, or yellow skin color.
- Instruct patient to inform health care providers/dentists of drug regimen before undergoing any treatments or surgery or receiving new drugs.
- Suggest that patient carry identification (eg, Medi-Alert) indicating drug regimen and condition.
- Advise patient to separate administration of ticlopidine and antacids by at least 2 hr.
- Advise patients to immediately report symptoms and signs of TTP (eg, fever, weakness, difficulty speaking, seizures, yellowing of skin or eyes, dark or bloody urine, pallor, or pinpoint hemorrhagic spots on the skin).

Tiludronate Disodium
(tie-LOO-droe-nate)

Class Hormone/Biphosphonate

How Supplied
Skelid Tablets 240 mg (eq. to 200 mg tiludronic acid)

Action
PHARMACOLOGY: Inhibits normal and abnormal bone resorption.

PHARMACOKINETICS/DYNAMICS:
Absorption: Tiludronate bioavailability is 6%. In clinical studies, efficacy was seen when dosed at least 2 hr before or after meals. Tiludronate C_{max} is 3 mg/L; T_{max} occurs with 2 hr of dose.

Distribution: Tiludronate is widely distributed in bones and soft tissue and is about 90% bound to proteins.

Excretion: The primary route of elimination is in urine. Approximately 60% of a dose is excreted in urine. Tiludronate $t_½$ is 150 hr.

Special Populations:
Renal Function Impairment – Tiludronate is not recommended for patients with severe renal failure (Ccr less than 30 mL/min) because of lack of clinical experience.

Indications Treatment of Paget disease of bone.

Contraindications Standard considerations.
Route/Dosage
ADULTS: PO 400 mg qd for 3 mo.
Interactions
Aspirin, calcium, aluminum- or magnesium-containing antacids: Decrease tiludronate bioavailability.
Indomethacin: Increases tiludronate bioavailability.
Lab Test Interferences None well documented.
Adverse Reactions
CV: Hypertension; syncope.
CNS: Paresthesia; vertigo; somnolence; anxiety; nervousness; insomnia; involuntary muscle contractions.
DERM: Rash; pruritus; sweating.
EENT: Cataract; conjunctivitis; glaucoma; rhinitis; sinusitis; pharyngitis.
GI: Diarrhea; nausea; constipation; vomiting; flatulence; abdominal pain; anorexia; dry mouth; gastritis.
METAB: Hyperparathyroidism.
OTHER: Fatigue; asthenia; chest pain; edema; arthrosis; flushing.
Precautions
Pregnancy: Category C.
Lactation: Undetermined.
Children: Safety and efficacy not established.
Renal function impairment: Not recommended in patients with Ccr less than 30 mL/min.
Overdosage: Signs and Symptoms
Hypocalcemia.

PATIENT CARE CONSIDERATIONS
Administration/Storage
- Have patient take drug on empty stomach 2 hr before or after meals.
- Swallow tablet with 6 to 8 oz of plain water. Do not use beverages other than plain water (eg, mineral water).
- Calcium or mineral supplements should be taken at least 2 hr before or after tiludronate.
- Aluminum or magnesium-containing antacids, if needed, should be taken at least 2 hr after taking tiludronate.
- Administer aspirin or indomethacin, if ordered, either 2 hr before or after tiludronate.
- The 3 mo course of treatment may be repeated in some patients following a 3 mo tiludronate-free interval.
- Store at controlled room temperature. Do not remove from foil strip until ready for administration.

Assessment/Interventions
- Obtain patient history, including drug history and any known allergies. Note any hypersensitivity to biphosphonates and evidence of renal function impairment.
- Record dates of any previous treatment with tiludronate.
- Monitor patient for side effects.

Patient/Family Education
- Instruct patient to take drug with 6 to 8 oz of plain water. Advise patient to not use any other beverage (eg, mineral water).
- Instruct patient to avoid eating 2 hr before and 2 hr after taking medication since absorption of drug is reduced by food.
- Instruct patient to maintain adequate intake of vitamin D and calcium.
- Advise patient to take calcium or mineral supplements 2 hr before or 2 hr after tiludronate.
- Advise patient to take aluminum- or magnesium-containing antacids at least 2 hr after tiludronate.
- Advise patients taking aspirin or indomethacin to take these 2 hr before or after tiludronate.
- Advise patient to not remove medication from foil strip until just before administration.

Timolol Maleate
(TI-moe-lahl MAL-ee-ate)
Class Beta-adrenergic blocker
How Supplied
Betimol Solution 0.25%, Solution 0.5% ♦ Blocadren Tablets 5 mg, Tablets 10 mg, Tablets 20 mg ♦ Istalol Solution 0.5% ♦ Timoptic Solution 0.25%, Solution 0.5% ♦ Timoptic Ocudose Solution 0.25%, Solution 0.5% ♦ Timoptic-XE Solution, gel-forming 0.25%, Solution, gel-forming 0.5%

✤ Apo-Timol ♦ Apo-Timop ♦ Gen-Timolol ♦ Novo-Timol Tablets ♦ Nu-Timolol ♦ PMS-Timolol ♦ ratio-Timolol ♦ Rhoxal-timolol

Action
PHARMACOLOGY: Blocks beta-receptors, which primarily affect heart (slows rate), vascular musculature (decreases BP), and lungs (reduces function). Reduces elevated and normal IOP via decreasing production of aqueous humor or increasing flow.

PHARMACOKINETICS/DYNAMICS:
Absorption: Timolol is rapidly and about 90% absorbed following oral administration. T_{max} is approximately 1 to 2 hr.

Distribution: Timolol is not extensively bound to plasma proteins.
Metabolism: Timolol undergoes approximately 50% first-pass metabolism.
Excretion: Timolol t½ is approximately 4 hr.

Indications Treatment of hypertension, alone or in combination with other agents; reduction of risk of reinfarction post-MI; migraine prophylaxis; treatment of elevated IOP in chronic open-angle glaucoma, ocular hypertension, aphakic glaucoma patients, patients with secondary glaucoma, and in patients with elevated IOP who need ocular pressure lowering.

Contraindications Hypersensitivity to beta-blockers; greater than first-degree heart block; CHF unless secondary to tachyarrhythmia treatable with beta-blockers; overt cardiac failure; sinus bradycardia; cardiogenic shock; bronchial asthma or bronchospasm, including severe COPD.

Route/Dosage
Hypertension
ADULTS: **PO** 10 mg bid, titrate to response q 7 days (max, 60 mg/day).

MI Prophylaxis
ADULTS: **PO** 10 mg bid.

Migraine Prophylaxis
ADULTS: **PO** 10 mg bid (max, 30 mg/day); if no response in 6 wk then discontinue.

Glaucoma
ADULTS: **Ophthalmic** 1 drop 0.25% to 0.5% solution in affected eye(s) bid.

Interactions
Clonidine: May enhance or reverse antihypertensive effect; potentially life-threatening situations may occur, especially on withdrawal.
Epinephrine: Initial hypertensive episode followed by bradycardia may occur.
Ergot derivatives: Peripheral ischemia, manifested by cold extremities and possible gangrene, may occur.
Insulin: Prolonged hypoglycemia with masking of symptoms may occur.
NSAIDs: Some agents may impair antihypertensive effect.
Prazosin: Orthostatic hypotension may be increased.
Theophyllines: Elimination of theophylline may be reduced. Effects of both drugs may be reduced.
Verapamil: Effects of both drugs may be increased.

Lab Test Interferences None well documented.

Adverse Reactions
CV: Hypotension; heart palpitations; bradycardia; heart failure, edema.
CNS: Dizziness; depression; lethargy; headache; insomnia; anxiety; tremor; paresthesia.
DERM: Increased sensitivity to cold; rash; pruritus; alopecia; sweating.
EENT: Transient irritation, burning, tearing, and conjunctival edema, blurred vision, light sensitivity (topical use).
GI: Abdominal pain; diarrhea; nausea.
GU: Impotence; sexual dysfunction; decreased libido; dysuria; urinary retention or frequency; nocturia; increased BUN.
HEMA: Decreased Hgb, Hct.
METAB: Alteration of glucose metabolism; masking of hypoglycemia; increased triglycerides, uric acid, potassium.
RESP: Wheezing; cough; breathing difficulties, especially in asthmatics or patients with COPD.
OTHER: Joint pain; muscle cramps.

> **WARNING:**
> *Abrupt withdrawal:* In patients with angina pectoris or CAD, may cause exacerbation of angina, occurrence of MI, and ventricular arrhythmias. Monitor patients closely. Because CAD is common and unrecognized it may be prudent not to discontinue beta-blocker therapy abruptly in patients treated only for hypertension.

Precautions
Pregnancy: Category C.
Lactation: Excreted in breast milk.
Children: Safety and efficacy not established.
Renal function impairment: Dosage reduction may be required.
Hepatic function impairment: Dosage reduction may be required.
Abrupt withdrawal: Has been associated with increased angina and MI; gradually decrease dose over 1 to 2 wk.
Anaphylaxis: Deaths have occurred; aggressive therapy may be required.
Bronchospasm: Oral and ophthalmic forms may precipitate bronchospasm in susceptible patients.
CHF: Administer drug with caution to patients with CHF controlled by digitalis and diuretics. Notify health care provider at first sign or symptom of CHF or of unexplained respiratory symptoms in any patient.
Diabetic patients: Drug may mask signs and symptoms of hypoglycemia (eg, tachycardia, BP changes). Drug may potentiate insulin-induced hypoglycemia.
Peripheral vascular disease: Drug may precipitate or aggravate symptoms of arterial insufficiency.
Thyrotoxicosis: Drug may mask clinical signs (eg, tachycardia) of developing or continuing hyperthyroidism. Abrupt withdrawal may exac-

erbate symptoms of hyperthyroidism, including thyroid storm.

PATIENT CARE CONSIDERATIONS
Administration/Storage
- Administer tablets orally with meals and at bedtime. Administer ophthalmic solutions via dropper provided.
- Tablets may be crushed or swallowed whole.
- Store tablets at room temperature, away from moisture and sunlight.
- Store ophthalmic solution at room temperature away from sunlight. Do not freeze.
- Discard ophthalmic solution if brown, cloudy, or if it contains particles.

Assessment/Interventions
- Obtain patient history, including drug history and any known allergies.
- Monitor and record BP, especially that of renal dialysis patients (report hypotension); pulse (report tachycardia); blood glucose of diabetic patients on regular basis (report hypoglycemia).
- Assess apical/radial pulse before administration. Notify health care provider of any changes.
- Assess and document muscle strength of myasthenia gravis patients and report increased weakness.
- Contact health care provider immediately if patient shows signs of cardiac failure.
- Have available isoproterenol, dopamine, dobutamine, or norepinephrine to reverse effects in emergency.
- Use ophthalmic solution cautiously if patient is taking oral beta-blockers, because solution may be absorbed systemically and create an additive effect.
- If drug is for migraine prevention, monitor effectiveness and consult health care provider if satisfactory response is not obtained after 6 to 8 wk of maximum daily dose.
- Monitor I&O and weight daily. Monitor hydration status.
- Assess for edema in feet and legs daily.

Patient/Family Education
- Explain that eye drops commonly produce transient stinging or discomfort and to notify health care provider if symptoms are severe.
- Teach patient how to instill eye drops: shake once before using. Wash hands; do not allow dropper to touch eye. Tilt head back, look up; pull lower eyelid down; instill prescribed number of drops. Close eye for 1 to 2 min and apply gentle pressure over bridge of nose. Do not rub eye.
- Explain that if using eye drops, health care provider may need to monitor eye pressure at regular intervals and at different times of day.
- Tell patient to consult health care provider before using OTC cough, cold, or allergy medications, including nasal decongestants.
- Encourage diabetic patient to use glucometer regularly. This drug may increase chances of hypoglycemic reactions to insulin or may mask signs and symptoms of hypoglycemia.
- Inform patient to notify health care provider immediately of shortness of breath (especially if lying down), feet swelling, night cough, and slow pulse rate.
- Tell patient to notify health care provider of skin rash, fever, lightheadedness, confusion, depression, sore throat, unusual bleeding or bruising, jaundice, and changes in urination.
- Explain ways to avoid sudden changes in posture, and caution against hot baths or showers, especially if dizziness is experienced.
- Tell patient to contact health care provider quickly if nausea, vomiting, or diarrhea develop. Dehydration may occur and may lower BP severely. Health care provider may decrease dose during episode.
- Explain need to be cautious when driving or participating in activities needing coordination. This drug may produce drowsiness, dizziness, lightheadedness, or blurred vision, especially during first days of therapy or when dose is increased.
- Tell patient that before any surgery, health care provider should be informed that this drug is being used (even as eye drops). Health care provider may wish to discontinue drugs temporarily.
- Explain to patient that abrupt withdrawal of the drug is dangerous and dose is generally tapered according to health care provider's instructions.
- Encourage patient to wear support hose.
- Instruct patient to avoid alcohol, smoking, and sodium intake.
- Teach patient to take pulse at home and when to notify health care provider.

Overdosage: Signs and Symptoms
Severe bradycardia, severe hypotension, bronchospasm, acute cardiac failure.

Tinidazole

(tie-NIH-dah-zole)

Class Anti-infective/Antiprotozoal

How Supplied
Tindamax Tablets 250 mg; Tablets 500 mg

Action

PHARMACOLOGY: Unknown; however, may be related to action of free nitro radical generated as a result of reduction by cell extracts of *Trichomonas*.

PHARMACOKINETICS/DYNAMICS:

Absorption: Rapid and complete after oral administration. C_{max} is 47.7 mcg/mL; T_{max} is 1.6 hr; AUC is 901.6 mcg•hr/mL at 72 hr. Steady-state conditions reached in 2.5 to 3 days.

Distribution: Distributed to virtually all tissues and body fluid and crosses the blood-brain barrier. Vd is about 50 L. Protein binding is 12%.

Metabolism: Partly metabolized by oxidation, hydroxylation, and conjugation. Metabolized by CYP3A4.

Excretion: Plasma t½ is 12 to 14 hr. Elimination t½ is 13.2 hr. About 20% to 25% excreted unchanged in urine and 12% in feces.

Indications Treatment of trichomoniasis caused by *T. vaginalis*, giardiasis caused by *G. duodenalis*, and amebiasis caused by *E. histolytica*.

Contraindications First trimester of pregnancy; hypersensitivity to nitroimidazole derivatives (eg, metronidazole); any component of product.

Route/Dosage

Amebiasis, Intestinal
ADULTS: PO 2 g dose daily for 3 days with food.
CHILDREN OVER 3 YR OF AGE: PO 50 mg/kg daily (max, 2 g/day) for 3 days with food.

Amebic Liver Abscess
ADULTS: PO 2 g dose daily for 3 to 5 days with food.
CHILDREN OLDER THAN 3 YR OF AGE: PO 50 mg/kg daily (max, 2 g/day) for 3 to 5 days with food.

Giardiasis
ADULTS: PO Single 2 g dose with food.
CHILDREN OVER 3 YR OF AGE: PO Single 50 mg/kg (max, 2 g) dose with food.

Trichomoniasis
ADULTS: PO Single 2 g dose with food. Treat sexual partners at same time.

Interactions The following interactions were reported with metronidazole, which is chemically-related to tinidazole.

Alcohol, disulfiram: Avoid during tinidazole use and for 3 days afterward because cramps, nausea, vomiting, headaches, and flushing may occur.

Anticoagulants, oral (eg, warfarin): Anticoagulant effects may be increased. Anticoagulant dose may need to be adjusted during coadministration and for up to 8 days after discontinuation.

Cholestyramine: Bioavailability of tinidazole may be decreased.

Cyclosporine, lithium, tacrolimus: Levels may be elevated by tinidazole, increasing the risk of toxicity.

Drugs that induce CYP3A4 (eg, fosphenytoin, phenobarbital, phenytoin, rifampin): May increase metabolism of tinidazole, decreasing plasma levels and therapeutic effect.

Drugs that inhibit CYP3A4 (eg, cimetidine, ketoconazole): May prolong t½ and decrease tinidazole Cl, increasing plasma levels and risk of side effects.

Fluorouracil: Cl may be decreased by tinidazole, increasing the risk of side effects.

Oxytetracycline: Therapeutic effect of tinidazole may be decreased.

Phenytoin, fosphenytoin: The t½ may be prolonged and Cl reduced by tinidazole, increasing the risk of side effects.

Lab Test Interferences May interfere with chemical analysis for AST, ALT, LDH, triglycerides, and hexokinase glucose; zero values may occur.

Adverse Reactions

CV: Palpitation.
CNS: Weakness/fatigue/malaise (2%); dizziness, headache (1%); convulsions; transient peripheral neuropathy (including numbness and paresthesia); vertigo; ataxia; giddiness; insomnia; drowsiness.
GI: Metallic/bitter taste (6%); nausea (5%); anorexia (3%); dyspepsia/cramps/epigastric discomfort, vomiting (2%); constipation (1%); tongue discoloration, stomatitis, diarrhea, oral candidiasis.
GU: Dark urine; increased vaginal discharge.
HEMA: Transient neutropenia; transient leukopenia.
HEPA: Hepatic abnormalities (including elevated transaminase levels).
HYPERSEN: Urticaria; pruritus; rash; flushing; sweating; dryness of mouth; fever; burning sensation; thirst; salivation; angioedema.
MUSC: Arthralgia; myalgia; arthritis.
OTHER: *Candida* overgrowth.

> **WARNING:**
> Carcinogenicity has been seen in mice and rats treated chronically with another nitroimidazole (metronidazole).

Precautions
Pregnancy: Category C. Contraindicated in the first trimester.
Lactation: Excreted in breast milk.
Children: Other than use in giardiasis and amebiasis in pediatric patients older than 3 yr of age, safety and efficacy not established.
Elderly: Use with caution because of the greater frequency of decreased hepatic, renal, or cardiac function, and concomitant diseases or other drug therapy.
Hepatic function impairment: Use with caution.
Blood dyscrasias: Use with caution in patients with history of blood dyscrasias.
Neurologic effects: Convulsive seizures and peripheral neuropathy have occurred. Use with caution.

PATIENT CARE CONSIDERATIONS
Administration/Storage
- Duration of therapy varies, depending on condition being treated.
- Administer prescribed dose with food to minimize GI side effects.
- Oral suspension can be prepared by grinding four 500 mg tablets to a fine powder with a mortar and pestle. Add 10 mL cherry syrup and mix until smooth. Transfer the suspension to an amber bottle and, using several small rinses of cherry syrup, transfer any remaining drug in mortar to the final suspension for a final volume of 30 mL and a final concentration of 66.6 mg/mL.
- Shake suspension well before measuring dose. Administer suspension using dosing cup, dosing spoon, or dosing syringe.
- Store tablets and extemporaneous suspension at controlled room temperature (59° to 86°F). Protect from light. Discard any unused suspension after 7 days.

Assessment/Interventions
- Obtain patient history, including drug history and any known allergies. Note renal impairment, severe hepatic impairment, CNS disease, blood dyscrasia or history of blood dyscrasia, pregnancy, current or recent (within 2 wk) use of disulfiram, current or recent use of alcohol, or hypersensitivity to metronidazole.
- Ensure medication is not administered to pregnant patient during first trimester of pregnancy.
- Ensure breastfeeding is interrupted during tinidazole therapy and for 3 days following the last dose.
- Ensure partner of patient being treated for trichomoniasis is simultaneously treated to prevent reinfection.
- Ensure total and differential leukocyte count is evaluated if retreatment is necessary.
- Monitor patient for GI, CNS, and general body side effects. Report to health care provider if noted and significant. Immediately report any abnormal neurologic signs or symptoms (eg, seizures, extremity numbness, abnormal skin sensations).

Patient/Family Education
- Explain name, dose, action, and potential side effects of drug.
- Instruct patient to take exactly as prescribed and not to change the dose or discontinue therapy unless advised by health care provider.
- Advise patient to take prescribed dose with food to minimize GI side effects.
- Caution patient to avoid alcoholic beverages while taking tinidazole and for at least 3 days following completion of therapy.
- Advise patient that metallic taste is a common side effect of therapy but that this will resolve when therapy has been completed.
- Advise patient to report any other bothersome side effects to health care provider and to immediately report any abnormal neurologic signs or symptoms (eg, seizures, extremity numbness, abnormal skin sensations).
- Advise women to notify health care provider if pregnant, planning to become pregnant, or breastfeeding.
- Instruct patient to not take any prescription or OTC medications, dietary supplements, or herbal preparations unless advised by health care provider.
- Advise patient that follow-up visits may be required to monitor therapy and to keep appointments.

Tinzaparin Sodium
(tin-ZA-pa-rin SO-dee-uhm)
Class Anticoagulants
How Supplied
Innohep Injection 20,000 IU/mL

Action
PHARMACOLOGY: Inhibits reactions that lead to the clotting of blood, including the formation of fibrin clots.

PHARMACOKINETICS/DYNAMICS:
Absorption: Tinzaparin T_{max} is about 4 to 5 hr

and C_{max} is approximately 0.25 to 0.87 IU/mL. Bioavailability is 86.7%.

Distribution: Tinzaparin Vd is 3.1 to 5 L.

Excretion: Tinzaparin t½ is approximately 3 to 4 hr. Clearance is approximately 1.7 L/hr and the primary route of elimination is renal.

Special Populations:
Renal Function Impairment – Patients with severe renal impairment should be dosed with caution.

Indications Treatment of acute symptomatic deep vein thrombosis with or without pulmonary embolism when administered with warfarin.

Contraindications Active major bleeding, heparin-induced thrombocytopenia, hypersensitivity to heparin, sulfites, benzyl alcohol, or pork products.

Route/Dosage
ADULTS: SC 175 anti-Xa IU/kg once daily for more than 6 days and until patient is adequately anticoagulated with warfarin.

Interactions
Anticoagulants, platelet inhibitors (eg, dipyridamole, NSAIDs, salicylates): Use with caution because of increased risk of bleeding.

Lab Test Interferences Asymptomatic reversible increases in AST and ALT concentrations.

Adverse Reactions
CV: Cardiac arrhythmia, hypertension; hypotension; pulmonary embolism tachycardia; thrombophlebitis.
CNS: Confusion; dizziness; headache; insomnia.
DERM: Bullous eruption; epidermal necrolysis; rash; skin disorder; skin necrosis.
EENT: Epistaxis; hearing impairment; ocular hemorrhage.
GI: Abdominal pain; constipation; dyspepsia; flatulence; nausea; vomiting.
GU: Dysuria; hematuria; priapism; urinary retention; urinary tract infection.
HEMA: Anemia; bleeding ecchymosis; hematoma; hemorrhage; thrombocytopenia.
HEPA: Elevated ALT and AST.
RESP: Dyspnea; pneumonia; respiratory disorder.

OTHER: Anaphylactoid reactions; back pain; chest pain; fever; hypersensitivity; local irritation; pain; pruritus; rectal bleeding.

> **WARNING:**
>
> *Spinal/Epidural hematomas:* Risk of spinal/epidural hematomas increased in patients receiving neuraxial anesthesia or spinal puncture and are anticoagulated with low molecular weight heparins or heparinoids. Other risk factors include indwelling epidural catheters, repeated/traumatic epidural/spinal puncture, or other drugs affecting hemostasis (eg, NSAIDs, platelet inhibitors, anticoagulants). Risk of long-term or permanent paralysis. Frequent monitoring for signs/symptoms of neurological impairment.

Precautions
Pregnancy: Category B.
Lactation: Undetermined.
Children: Safety and efficacy not established.
Hypersensitivity: Allergic-type reactions may occur caused by sodium metabisulfite present in tinzaparin.
Renal function impairment: Effect of tinzaparin may be prolonged.
Special risk patients: Use drug with caution in patients with diabetic retinopathy, bleeding diathesis, uncontrolled arterial hypertension, or history of recent GI ulceration and hemorrhage.
Fatal gasping syndrome: Fatal gasping syndrome in premature infants has been associated with benzyl alcohol preservative present in tinzaparin.
Hemorrhage: Use with caution in conditions with increased risk of hemorrhage (eg, bacterial endocarditis, severe uncontrolled hypertension, active ulcerative GI disease).
Interchangeability with heparin: Cannot be used interchangeably (unit for unit) with heparin or other low molecular weight heparins.
Priapism: Has been reported as a rare occurrence.

Overdosage: Signs and Symptoms
Bleeding complications, nosebleeds, blood in urine, tarry stools, bruising, petechial hemorrhage, frank bleeding.

PATIENT CARE CONSIDERATIONS

Administration/Storage

- Store at room temperature (77°F; 25°C) range allowed (59° to 86°F; 15° to 30°C).
- Inspect the clear, colorless to slightly yellow solution, and do not administer if particulate matter or discoloration is present.
- Assess all patients for bleeding disorders before administration of tinzaparin.
- Administer weight-adjusted dose by deep SC injection only.
- Place the patient in the supine or sitting position before administration.
- Alternate injection sites between the left and right anterolateral and left and right posterolateral abdominal wall.
- Hold skinfold between the thumb and forefinger until the injection is completed.

- Introduce the full length of the needle into the skinfold and inject without aspiration.
- To minimize bruising, do not massage the injection site.
- Do not administer IM or IV or mix with other injections or infusions.
- Do not administer to patients with active major bleeding, a history of heparin-induced thrombocytopenia, or hypersensitivity to heparin, sulfites, benzyl alcohol, or pork products.
- Administer with extreme caution and under close medical supervision to patients with increased risk of hemorrhage, uncontrolled arterial hypertension, history of GI ulceration, and diabetic retinopathy.
- Administer with caution to patients with impaired liver function, renal failure, and those at risk for decreased renal function such as the elderly.
- Administer to pregnant women with caution and only if clearly needed as benzyl alcohol may cross the placenta causing fatalities in premature infants.
- Administer with caution to nursing mothers as tinzaparin is found in low concentrations in breast milk.
- Do not interchange unit for unit with heparin or any other low-molecular weight anticoagulant.

Assessment/Interventions

- Obtain a complete drug history and assess for allergies and potential drug interactions (eg, oral anticoagulants, platelet inhibitors, salicylates, dipyridamole, sulfinpyrazone, dextran and NSAIDs, thrombolytics).
- If coadministration with these medications is necessary, close laboratory and clinical monitoring is needed.
- Assess periodic hematocrit, hemoglobin, and platelet counts.
- Neither aPTT or PT can be used for therapeutic monitoring of tinzaparin sodium.
- Assess patient for signs and symptoms that might indicate bleeding or other adverse occurrences. These could include hypertension or hypotension, dizziness, irritability, insomnia, confusion, dyspepsia or other symptoms of ulcers, occult blood in stool, tachycardia, angina, thrombocytopenia, priapism, anemia, impaired healing, infection, dysuria, calf tenderness or pain, purpura, hematoma, or other skin indications of problems.
- Closely monitor patients following spinal or epidural anesthesia as they are at risk for developing an epidural or spinal hematoma which can result in long-term or permanent paralysis.
- The risk is increased if an indwelling epidural catheter is used; repeated or traumatic epidural or spinal procedures are employed; or concomitant use of anticoagulant drugs including NSAIDs and platelet inhibitors are utilized.
- Most bleeding complications can be controlled by discontinuing tinzaparin and applying pressure to the site.
- Tinzaparin has a $t_{1/2}$ of approximately 3 to 4 hr.
- If needed, blood elements and volume can be replaced.
- In case of serious bleeding or large overdose, protamine sulfate can be given by slow IV infusion.
- Only give protamine sulfate when resuscitation facilities are readily available, as fatal reactions have occurred.

Patient/Family Education

- Instruct patient to take safety precautions to avoid cuts and bruises (eg, soft toothbrush, electric razor, handrails).
- Caution patient to avoid aspirin or other *otc* anticoagulants.
- Instruct patients to report any current or future prescription, *otc*, or herbal medication use to primary care provider.
- Advise patient to report bruises, bleeding, nosebleeds, bleeding gums, coffee-ground emesis, red-flecked sputum, or tarry, black, or red stools.
- Explain the rationale for follow-up examinations and laboratory studies to ensure effectiveness of medication and prevention of complications or side effects.

Tiotropium Bromide

(tye-oh-TROE-pee-uhm BROE-mide)
Class Bronchodilator/Anticholinergic
How Supplied
Spiriva Powder for inhalation 18 mcg (as base)
Action
PHARMACOLOGY: Inhibits smooth muscle receptors, leading to bronchodilation.

PHARMACOKINETICS/DYNAMICS:
Absorption: Bioavailability is about 19.5%.
Distribution: Vd is 32 L/kg. Protein binding is 72%. At steady-state, peak and trough plasma levels are 17 to 19 picograms/mL and 3 to 4 picograms/mL, respectively.
Excretion: Approximately 14% is eliminated unchanged in the urine; the remainder is not absorbed in the gut and is eliminated in the feces. Terminal elimination $t_{1/2}$ is 5 to 6 days.

Special Populations:
Elderly – Advanced age is associated with a decrease in tiotropium renal Cl, which is explained by decreased renal function.
Renal impairment: Reduced Cl and increased plasma concentrations may occur.

Indications Long-term maintenance treatment of bronchospasm associated with COPD, including chronic bronchitis and emphysema.

Contraindications Hypersensitivity to atropine or its derivatives, including ipratropium, or any component of this product.

Route/Dosage
ADULTS: **Inhalation** Contents of 1 capsule daily, using the *HandiHaler* inhalation device.

Interactions None well documented.

Lab Test Interferences None well documented.

Adverse Reactions
CV: Angina pectoris (including aggravated angina pectoris, [1% to 3%]).
CNS: Dysphonia, paresthesia, depression (1% to 3%).
DERM: Rash (4%).
EENT: Pharyngitis (9%); cataract (1% to 3%).
GI: Dry mouth (16%); dyspepsia (6%); abdominal pain (5%); constipation, vomiting (4%); stomatitis (including ulcerative stomatitis), gastroesophageal reflux (1% to 3%).
GU: UTI (7%).
M/N: Hypercholesterolemia, hyperglycemia (1% to 3%).
MUSC: Myalgia (4%); skeletal pain (1% to 3%).
RESP: Upper respiratory tract infection (41%); sinusitis (11%); rhinitis (6%); epistaxis (4%); coughing (at least 3%); laryngitis (1% to 3%).
OTHER: Accidents (13%); non-specific chest pain (7%); dependent edema (5%); infection, moniliasis (4%); arthritis, flu-like symptoms (at least 3%); allergic reaction, leg pain, herpes zoster infection (1% to 3%).

Precautions
Pregnancy: Category C.
Lactation: Undetermined.
Children: Safety and efficacy not established.
Hypersensitivity: Immediate hypersensitivity reactions, including angioedema, may occur.
Renal function impairment: Monitor therapy closely in patients with moderate to severe renal impairment.
Special risk patients: Use with caution in patients with narrow-angle glaucoma, prostatic hyperplasia, or bladder-neck obstruction.
Acute bronchospasm: Not indicated for initial treatment of acute episodes of bronchospasm.
Bronchospasm: Paradoxical bronchospasm may occur.

Overdosage: Signs and Symptoms
Anticholinergic signs and symptoms.

PATIENT CARE CONSIDERATIONS

Administration/Storage
- For oral inhalation only. Not to be taken by mouth.
- Not to be used for the acute treatment of bronchospasm.
- May be used alone or in combination with short- and long-acting bronchodilators, and inhaled or systemic corticosteroid therapy.
- If patient is also receiving short-acting bronchodilator by inhalation administer short-acting bronchodilator 5 min before tiotropium to enhance penetration of latter drug into bronchial tree.
- Administer contents of 1 capsule daily as prescribed.
- Administer using supplied inhalation device (*HandiHaler*) only. Place capsule in center chamber of inhalation device and pierce by pressing and releasing button on side of inhalation device.
- Prepare dose by activating inhalation device immediately prior to administration. Have patient exhale fully then place inhaler mouthpiece between lips. Do not close teeth. Instruct patient to take slow, deep breath, and to hold breath for 5 to 10 sec and then breathe out slowly. Have patient repeat this process 1 more time to ensure receiving full dose.
- Do not use with a spacer device (eg, *Aerochamber*). Do not exhale into the inhalation device.
- Store capsules for oral inhalation in sealed blisters at ambient room temperature (59° to 86°F). Protect from extreme temperature and moisture. Do not remove capsule from sealed blister until immediately before use. Discard any capsule that is inadvertently removed from the sealed blister and not used immediately. Do not store capsules in inhalation device.

Assessment/Interventions
- Obtain patient history, including drug history and any known allergies. Note renal impairment, narrow-angle glaucoma, prostatic hyperplasia, bladder neck obstruction, or hypersensitivity to atropine or its derivatives (eg, ipratropium).
- Note frequency and severity of bronchospastic attacks. Notify health care provider if patient needs increasing doses of short-acting bronchodilator or if effectiveness of short-acting bronchodilator appears to be decreasing.

- Monitor patient's respiratory status during each treatment. If bronchospasm worsens during or shortly after a treatment, discontinue the treatment and notify health care provider immediately.
- Monitor patient for signs and symptoms of anaphylactic or serious allergic reactions. If noted, discontinue therapy and be prepared to treat appropriately.
- Monitor patient for signs and symptoms of acute narrow-angle glaucoma (eg, eye pain, blurred vision, visual halos, conjunctival congestion). If noted, discontinue therapy and inform health care provider immediately.
- Assess patient for RESP, GI, GU, and general body side effects. Inform health care provider if noted and significant.

Patient/Family Education

- Explain name, dose, action, and potential side effects of drug.
- Advise patient to continue taking other medications for same condition as prescribed by health care provider.
- Instruct patient on the proper storage, handling, and use of the capsules and inhalation device, referring to the *Patient's Instructions for Use* instruction sheet included with the medication. Ensure that patient understands how to clean the inhalation device.
- Advise patient that medication should never be administered with a spacer device or with any other inhalation device than that provided. Caution patient not to administer other inhaled medications with the inhalation device.
- Caution patient not to exceed prescribed dose. Inform patient that medication is being inhaled even if the dose being delivered is not tasted or felt.
- Instruct patient not to stop the medication once symptoms have improved. Continued daily use is necessary to control symptoms.
- Advise patient not to change the dose or stop using unless advised by health care provider.
- Warn patient that tiotropium is a maintenance medication and is not to be used for immediate relief of breathing problems. Advise patient to use rescue medication (short-acting bronchodilator) to obtain rapid relief of breathing problems.
- Advise patient that medication does not replace inhaled or oral corticosteroids and to continue to use those drugs as prescribed by health care provider.
- Advise patient to inform health care provider if symptoms do not improve or worsen, if more short-acting bronchodilator than usual is needed, or if the short-acting bronchodilator appears to become less effective.
- Instruct patient to discontinue use and immediately notify health care provider if eye pain or discomfort, blurred vision, vision halos, or colored images develop in association with red eyes. Advise patient that these symptoms may be associated with a serious problem that will require immediate medical care.
- Advise patient to carry Medi-Alert card indicating that they have COPD.
- Advise women to notify health care provider if pregnant, planning to become pregnant, or breastfeeding.
- Caution patient not to take any prescription or OTC medications, dietary supplements, or herbal preparations unless advised by health care provider.
- Advise patient that follow-up visits will be required to monitor therapy and to keep appointments.

Tizanidine Hydrochloride

(tye-ZAN-i-deen)

Class Skeletal muscle relaxant/Centrally acting

How Supplied
Zanaflex Tablets 2 mg, Tablets 4 mg

Action
PHARMACOLOGY: Unknown; may increase presynaptic inhibition of motor neurons.

PHARMACOKINETICS/DYNAMICS:
Absorption: Tizanidine is completely absorbed. T_{max} is approximately 1.5 hr. Food increases C_{max} by about 1/3 and shortens time to peak by about 40 min, but extent of absorption is not affected. Bioavailability is about 40%.

Distribution: Tizanidine is widely distributed. Vd is about 2.4 L/kg. About 30% is bound to plasma proteins and about 95% of a dose is metabolized.

Excretion: Tizanidine t½ is about 2.5 hr.

Special Populations:
Renal Function Impairment – Clearance is reduced more than 50% in elderly patients with renal insufficiency (Ccr less than 25 mL/min) compared with healthy subjects; this would be expected to lead to a longer duration of clinical effect. Use caution in renally impaired patients.
Elderly – Younger subjects cleared the drug 4 times faster than elderly subjects.

Indications Acute and intermittent management of increased muscle tone associated with spasticity.

Contraindications Standard considerations.

Route/Dosage
ADULTS: **PO** Initiate therapy with a 4 mg dose, increasing the dose gradually in 2 to 4 mg increments to optimum effect. The dose can be repeated at 6- to 8-hr intervals as needed (max, 3 doses in 24 hr not to exceed 36 mg/day).

Interactions
Alcohol: Plasma levels of tizanidine may be elevated, increasing the side effects.
Antihypertensive agents: Use with caution; do not administer with other alpha$_2$-adrenergic agonists (eg, clonidine).
Oral contraceptives: Clearance of tizanidine may be reduced; decrease the dosage requirement.

Lab Test Interferences
None well documented.

Adverse Reactions
CV: Vasodilation; postural hypotension; syncope; arrhythmia; migraine.
CNS: Somnolence; dizziness; dyskinesia; nervousness; depression; anxiety; paresthesia.
DERM: Rash; sweating; skin ulcer.
EENT: Pharyngitis; amblyopia; rhinitis; ear pain; tinnitus; deafness; glaucoma; conjunctivitis; eye pain; optic neuritis; otitis media; retinal hemorrhage; visual field defect.
GI: Dry mouth; constipation; vomiting; abdominal pain; diarrhea; dyspepsia.
GU: Urinary frequency; urinary tract infection; urinary urgency; cystitis; menorrhagia; pyelonephritis; urinary retention; kidney calculus; enlarged uterine fibroids; vaginal moniliasis; vaginitis.
HEMA: Ecchymosis; hypercholesterolemia; anemia; hyperlipemia; leukopenia; leukocytosis; sepsis.
HEPA: Increased ALT and liver function tests.
RESP: Sinusitis; pneumonia; bronchitis.
OTHER: Asthenia; increased spasm or tone; flu-like syndrome; infection; speech disorder; myasthenia; back pain; fever; allergic reaction; malaise; abscess; neck pain; cellulitis.

Precautions
Pregnancy: Category C.
Lactation: Undetermined.
Children: Safety and efficacy not established.
Elderly: Use with caution because clearance may be decreased 4-fold.
Renal function impairment: Use with caution.
Hepatic function impairment: Use with caution.
Hypotension: Hypotension may occur; patients are at increased risk for orthostatic effects.
Hepatotoxicity: Hepatocellular liver injury may occur.
Psychotic-like symptoms: Hallucinations or delusions may occur.
Sedation: Sedation severe enough to interfere with every day activities may occur.

Overdosage: Signs and Symptoms
Coma, respiratory depression with Cheyne-Stokes respiration.

PATIENT CARE CONSIDERATIONS

Administration/Storage
- Administer prescribed dose at 6- to 8-hr intervals as needed for spasticity, to maximum of 3 doses in 24-hr period.
- Administer without regard to meals. Administer with food if GI upset occurs.
- Store at controlled room temperature (59° to 86°F).

Assessment/Interventions
- Obtain patient history, including drug history and any known allergies. Note history of liver disease, renal disease, and concurrent use of antihypertensive drugs.
- Ensure that LFTs are determined before starting therapy and periodically during treatment.
- Assess effect of medication on spasticity.
- Monitor BP when starting therapy or changing dose. Inform health care provider if hypotension occurs.
- Initiate safety precautions if orthostatic hypotension occurs.
- Monitor patient for CV, CNS, GI, and general body side effects.
- Inform health care provider if any of the following are noted: bradycardia, orthostatic hypotension; lightheadedness; dizziness; excessive sedation; fainting; jaundice; dark urine; right upper quadrant abdominal pain.

Patient/Family Education
- Explain name, dose, action, and potential side effects of drug.
- Instruct patient to take prescribed dose at 6- to 8-hr intervals as needed for spasticity, to a max of 3 doses in 24-hr period.
- Advise patient that medication can be taken without regard to meals but to take with food if GI upset occurs.
- Advise patient that medication is started at a low dose and gradually increased as tolerated until maximum benefit is achieved.
- Instruct patient to avoid alcohol and other CNS depressant medications.
- Instruct patient to get up slowly from lying or sitting position and to avoid sudden position changes to prevent postural hypotension. Advise patient to report dizziness with position changes to health care provider. Caution patient that hot tubs and hot showers or baths may make dizziness worse.
- Instruct patient to lie or sit down if experi-

encing dizziness or lightheadedness when standing.
• Advise patient to take sips of water, suck on ice chips or sugarless hard candy, or chew sugarless gum if dry mouth occurs.
• Advise patient that drug may cause drowsiness and to use caution while driving or performing other tasks requiring mental alertness.
• Instruct women to notify health care provider if they become pregnant, plan on becoming pregnant, or are breastfeeding.
• Advise patient to notify health care provider of the following: excessive drowsiness, yellowing of skin or eyes, dark urine, right upper abdominal pain.
• Instruct patient not to take any prescription or *otc* medications or dietary supplements unless advised to do so by health care provider.
• Advise patient that follow-up visits and lab tests will be required to monitor therapy and to be sure and keep appointments.

Tobramycin

(TOE-bruh-MY-sin)
Class Antibiotic/Aminoglycoside
How Supplied
AKTob Solution 0.3% ♦ *Defy* Solution 0.3% ♦ Nebcin Injection 10 mg/mL, Injection 40 mg/mL, Powder for Injection 1.2 g ♦ *Nebcin Pediatric* Injection 10 mg/mL ♦ *TOBI* Nebulizer solution 300 mg/5 mL ♦ *Tobrex* Solution 0.3%, Ointment 3 mg/g
♣ PMS-*Tobramycin* ♦ *Scheinpharm Tobramycin*
Action
Pharmacology: Inhibits bacterial protein synthesis, causing cell death.
Pharmacokinetics/Dynamics:
Absorption:
Injection (IM) – IM tobramycin is rapidly absorbed. C_{max} is 4 mcg/mL (IM dose 1 mg/kg). T_{max} is 30 to 90 min. Levels persist approximately 8 hr. Therapeutic serum levels are about 4 to 6 mcg/mL. The injectable dose form is poorly absorbed in the GI tract.
Inhalation – Bioavailability varies because of individual differences in nebulizer performance and airway pathology. C_{max} is 35 to 7414 mcg/g in sputum.
Distribution:
Injection (IM) – Tobramycin can be detected in tissues and body fluids. The drug appears in low concentrations in CSF and concentrations are dose-dependent, dependent on rate of penetration, and degree of meningeal inflammation. Concentrations in the renal cortex are several times higher than usual serum levels.
Inhalation – Tobramycin is concentrated primarily in airways.
Metabolism:
Injection (IM) – Little, if any, metabolic transformation occurs.
Excretion:
Injection (IM) – Tobramycin is eliminated almost exclusively by glomerular filtration. In healthy renal function, up to 84% of a dose is recoverable from urine in 8 hr and up to 93% in 24 hr. Tobramycin t½ is 2 hr.
Onset:
Inhalation – Onset of action is 10 min.
Duration:
Injection (IM) – Duration of action is up to 8 hr following an IM dose.
Special Populations:
Renal Function Impairment –
Injection (IM): Serum concentrations are usually higher and can be measured for longer periods of time than in healthy adults. Dosage adjustment is recommended. Excretion is slow and accumulation of the drug may cause toxic blood levels.
Dialysis patients: 25% to 70% of the administered dose may be removed depending on duration and type of dialysis.
Neonates – Serum concentrations are usually higher and can be measured for longer periods of time than in healthy adults. Dosage adjustment is recommended.

Indications Treatment of serious infections caused by susceptible strains of gram-negative bacteria; treatment of serious susceptible staphylococcal infections when other, less toxic drugs are contraindicated. *Ophthalmic use:* Treatment of superficial ocular infections. Management of cystic fibrosis patients with *Pseudomonas aeruginosa*.

Contraindications Previous reactions to aminoglycosides. *Ophthalmic use:* Epithelial herpes simplex keratitis; vaccinia; varicella; mycobacterial infections of eye; fungal infections.

Route/Dosage
ADULTS: **IM/IV** 3 to 5 mg/kg/day in 3 to 4 equal doses. **Ophthalmic** 1.25 cm ribbon of ointment bid to tid (q 3 to 4 hr for severe infections) or 1 to 2 gtt 4 to 6 times/day (for severe infections, q hr until improvement; then frequency of administration is reduced).
CHILDREN: **IM/IV** 6 to 7.5 mg/kg/day in 3 to 4 equally divided doses. **Ophthalmic** 1.25 cm ribbon of ointment bid to tid (q 3 to 4 hr for severe infections) or 1 to 2 gtt 4 to 6 times/day (for severe infections, q hr until improvement;

then frequency of administration is reduced).
PREMATURE OR FULL-TERM NEWBORNS 1 WK OLD OR YOUNGER: **IM/IV** Up to 4 mg/kg/day in 2 divided doses.

Interactions
Depolarizing and nondepolarizing muscle relaxants: May enhance neuromuscular blocking effects. Protracted respiratory depression may occur.
Loop diuretics: May increase auditory toxicity.
Nephrotoxic drugs (eg, amphotericin B, cephalosporins, enflurane, methoxyflurane, vancomycin): May increase risk of nephrotoxicity.
Penicillins: Penicillins, particularly carbenicillin and ticarcillin, can inactivate tobramycin in admixture, assay procedures, or patients with renal failure.
Polypeptide antibiotics: May increase risk of respiratory paralysis and renal dysfunction.
INCOMPATIBILITIES: Do not mix with other drugs.

Lab Test Interferences
None well documented.

Adverse Reactions
CNS: Headache; fever; confusion; lethargy; disorientation; delirium.
DERM: Rash; urticaria; itching; pain and irritation at injection site.
EENT: Tinnitus; vertigo; dizziness; hearing loss. With ophthalmic preparation: localized ocular toxicity and hypersensitivity; lid itching; lid swelling; conjunctival erythema.
GI: Nausea; vomiting; diarrhea.
GU: Oliguria; proteinuria; increased serum creatinine and BUN.
HEMA: Anemia; leukopenia; leukocytosis; eosinophilia.
METAB: Decreased serum calcium, sodium, potassium, or magnesium; increased LFT results.
RESP: Apnea.

> **WARNING:**
> Renal and eight nerve function closely monitored in patients with suspected renal dysfunction. Monitor peak and trough concentration.
> Dosage adjustments required in renal impairment.
> *Nephrotoxicity:* Usually reversible.
> *Neurotoxicity:* Manifests as both auditory and vestibular ototoxicity, and primarily occurs in patients with preexisting renal damage or with prolonged therapy. Partial or total irreversible deafness may continue to develop after drug is stopped. Other features of neurotoxicity include paresthesias, twitching, and seizures.
> *Teratogenic:* In pregnancy.

Precautions
Pregnancy: Category D (parenteral); Category B (ophthalmic).
Lactation: Undetermined.
Children: Use parenteral form cautiously in premature infants and newborns due to renal immaturity.
Burn patients: Pharmacokinetics may be altered; serum levels are important for determining appropriate dosing.
Hypomagnesemia: Occurs often, especially in those with restricted diets or who eat poorly.
Long-term therapy: Generally not indicated; greatly increases risk of toxic reactions.
Neuromuscular blockade: Potential curare-like effects may aggravate muscle weakness or cause neurotoxicity. Use drug with caution in patients with neuromuscular disorders, hypomagnesemia, hypocalcemia, or hypokalemia; with anesthesia or muscle relaxants, and in newborns whose mothers received magnesium sulfate.
Ophthalmic ointment: May retard corneal healing.

Overdosage: Signs and Symptoms
Nephrotoxicity, neuromuscular blockade, respiratory paralysis, ototoxicity. With ophthalmic preparation (topical overdose): punctate keratitis, erythema, increased lacrimation, edema, lid itching.

PATIENT CARE CONSIDERATIONS
Administration/Storage
- Administer separately. Do not mix with other drugs.
- For IV administration dilute in 50 to 100 mL of 0.9% Sodium Chloride Injection or 5% Dextrose Injection. Use less diluent for children. Administer at least 20 min to 60 min.
- Administer IM injection deep into large muscle.
- For ophthalmic preparations, wash hands before and after instillation. Have patient tilt head back; place medication in conjunctival sac and have patient close eyes. Apply light finger pressure on lacrimal duct for 1 min following instillation. Do not touch tip of container to any surface.
- Store ophthalmic preparations at room temperature away from sunlight. Do not freeze.

- Discard if solution is brown or cloudy or contains particles.

Nebulizer solution:
- Do not adjust dosage by age or weight.
- Administer as close to 12 hr apart as possible. Do not administer less than 6 hr apart.
- Administer by inhalation over 10 to 15 min period.
- Do not dilute or mix with dornase alfa in the nebulizer.

Assessment/Interventions
- Obtain culture and susceptibility before initiating drug therapy. Treatment can be initiated before results are obtained.
- Obtain patient history, including drug history and any known allergies. Determine if patient has renal impairment, hearing loss, neuromuscular disorders, muscle weakness, Parkinson's disease, myasthenia gravis, mycobacterial infections, or fungal infections.
- If patient may be intubated or ventilated, inform anesthetist that patient is taking this drug. Neuromuscular effects may be enhanced with succinylcholine or other neuromuscular blocking agent.
- Do not administer to newborns if mother received magnesium sulfate.
- Monitor and record respiratory status.
- Schedule hearing test prior to administration. Periodically test hearing throughout treatment and 1 mo after treatment is discontinued. Deafness may occur after drug has been discontinued, especially if treated more than 10 days.
- Monitor renal function (especially in elderly patients), Ccr rate, and BUN. Report any changes from baseline to health care provider.
- Request periodic urine studies.
- Monitor peak and trough drug levels, especially in elderly patients, and use to guide dosing. Obtain these values within 48 hr of start of therapy and every 3 to 4 days.
- Monitor for signs of superinfection.
- Monitor I&O and report imbalances to health care provider.
- Monitor magnesium, sodium, calcium, and potassium blood levels. Report low levels to health care provider.
- Monitor neurologic status and function of cranial nerve VIII. Report tinnitus, vertigo, numbness, tingling, muscle twitching or weakness, and convulsions to health care provider.
- Keep patient well hydrated.
- If toxicity is detected, immediately notify health care provider. Discontinuation of drug or adjustment of dose or dosing interval may be required.

Patient/Family Education
- Instruct patient how to administer ophthalmic preparation, including need for careful handwashing.
- Encourage patient to drink plenty of fluids while taking drug.
- Instruct patient to notify health care provider of headache, fever, confusion, nausea, vomiting, diarrhea, rashes, itching, pain at injection site, ringing or roaring in ears, dizziness, or hearing loss.
- Advise patient to consult with health care provider before taking any other OTC or prescription medications.
- Inform patient that health care provider will want follow-up blood studies and audiograms.
- Inform patient that ophthalmic preparations may cause temporary blurring of vision or stinging and instruct patient to report excessive stinging, burning, persistent or increased pain, tearing, lid itching, swelling or redness of eyes to health care provider.
- Instruct patient not to wear contact lenses during treatment.
- For patient using ophthalmic solution, stress need for compliance with complete course of therapy.

Nebulizer solution:
- Instruct patient to take as close to 12 hr apart as possible. Do not take less than 6 hr apart.
- Should be taken over a 10- to 15-min period using a hand-held *PARI LC PLUS* reusable nebulizer with a *DeVilbiss Pulmo-Aide* compressor.
- If patient is on multiple therapies, other therapies should be taken first followed by tobramycin.
- Inhale while sitting or standing upright and breathing normally through the mouthpiece of the nebulizer. Nose clips may help the patient breathe through the mouth.

Tolazamide

(tole-AZE-uh-mid)
Class Antidiabetic/Sulfonylurea

How Supplied
Tolinase Tablets 100 mg, Tablets 250 mg, Tablets 500 mg

Action
PHARMACOLOGY: Decreases blood glucose by stimulating release of insulin from pancreas.

PHARMACOKINETICS/DYNAMICS:
Absorption: Tolazamide T_{max} is 3 to 4 hr. The drug is well absorbed from the GI tract.

Metabolism: There are 5 major metabolites ranging in hypoglycemic activity from 0% to 70%.

Excretion: Tolazamide $t_½$ is 7 hr. Tolazamide is excreted principally in the urine (85%), and 7% in feces over a 5-day period.

Onset: Onset of action of tolazamide is 4 to 6 hr.

Peak: Time to peak effect of tolazamide is 4 to 6 hr.

Duration: Duration of action is 10 hr.

Indications Adjunct to diet to lower blood glucose in patients with non-insulin-dependent diabetes mellitus (type 2) whose hyperglycemia cannot be controlled by diet alone. **Unlabeled use(s):** Temporary adjunct to insulin therapy in selected patients with non-insulin-dependent diabetes mellitus to improve diabetic control.

Contraindications Hypersensitivity to sulfonylureas; diabetes complicated by ketoacidosis, with or without coma; sole therapy of insulin-dependent (type 1) diabetes mellitus; gestational diabetes.

Route/Dosage
ADULTS: PO 100 to 250 mg/day with breakfast or first main meal. If fasting blood sugar (FBS) is less than 200 mg/dL, initial dose is 100 mg/day or if FBS is greater than 200 mg/dL, initial dose is 250 mg/day. In malnourished, underweight, elderly patients use 100 mg/day. May adjust dose by 100 to 250 mg/wk as needed to a maximum of 1000 mg/day. If more than 500 mg/day is required, give in divided doses bid. Doses greater than 1 g/day are not likely to improve control.
MAINTENANCE DOSE: PO Usual dose is 100 to 1000 mg/day with the average 250 to 500 mg/day. Following initiation of therapy, dosage adjustment is made in increments of 100 to 250 mg at weekly intervals based on patient's blood glucose response.

Interactions
Androgens, anticoagulants, azole antifungals, chloramphenicol, clofibrate, fenfluramine, fluconazole, gemfibrozil, histamine H_2 antagonists, magnesium salts, methyldopa, MAO inhibitors, phenylbutazone, probenecid, salicylates, sulfinpyrazone, sulfonamides, tricyclic antidepressants, urinary acidifiers: Increased hypoglycemic effect.
Beta-blockers, calcium channel blockers, cholestyramine, corticosteroids, diazoxide, estrogens, hydantoins, isoniazid, nicotinic acid, oral contraceptives, phenothiazines, rifampin, sympathomimetics, thiazide diuretics, thyroid agents, urinary alkalinizers: Decreased hypoglycemic effect.
Charcoal: Charcoal can reduce the absorption; depending on clinical situation, this will reduce sulfonylureas efficacy or toxicity.
Digitalis glycosides: Coadministration may result in increased digitalis serum levels.

Lab Test Interferences None well documented.

Adverse Reactions
CV: Increased risk of cardiovascular mortality.
CNS: Dizziness; vertigo.
DERM: Allergic skin reactions; eczema; pruritus; erythema; urticaria; morbilliform or maculopapular eruptions; lichenoid reactions.
GI: Nausea; epigastric fullness; heartburn; cholestatic jaundice.
GU: Mild diuresis.
HEMA: Leukopenia; thrombocytopenia; aplastic anemia; agranulocytosis; hemolytic anemia; pancytopenia; hepatic porphyria.
METAB: Hypoglycemia.
OTHER: Disulfiram-like reaction; weakness; paresthesia; fatigue; malaise.

Precautions
Pregnancy: Category C.
Lactation: Undetermined.
Children: Safety and efficacy in children not established.
Elderly: Elderly and debilitated patients are particularly susceptible to hypoglycemic action of sulfonylureas.
Renal function impairment: Use drug with caution and monitor renal function frequently.
Hepatic function impairment: Use drug with caution and monitor liver function frequently.
Hypoglycemia: Tolazamide may produce severe hypoglycemia, which may be more difficult to recognize in elderly or in patients receiving beta-blockers.
Disulfiram-like syndrome: Administration with alcohol may include facial flushing reaction and occasional breathlessness. This reaction has been reported more commonly with other sulfonylureas.

Hyperglycemia: Hyperglycemia is major risk factor in development of diabetic complications. Measurement of glycosylated hemoglobin and self-monitoring of blood glucose are useful.
Loss of blood glucose control: Stress (including fever, trauma, infection, or surgery) or secondary failure (wherein drug's effectiveness in lowering blood glucose diminishes over time) may precipitate loss of blood glucose control.

Overdosage: Signs and Symptoms
Hypoglycemia including symptoms of the following: tingling of lips and tongue, nausea, lethargy, confusion, agitation, nervousness, tachycardia, sweating, tremor, hunger, convulsions, stupor, coma.

PATIENT CARE CONSIDERATIONS
Administration/Storage
- Give with breakfast or with first meal of day.
- Crush tablet if patient unable to swallow tablet whole.

Assessment/Interventions
- Obtain patient history, including drug history and any known allergies.
- Closely monitor glucose control in elderly patients and promptly adjust dose if hypoglycemia is noted.
- Initially monitor blood glucose and urine ketones tid. Once glucose control is established monitor less often in type 2 diabetic patients.

Patient/Family Education
- Teach signs and symptoms of hypoglycemia (eg, profuse sweating, excessive hunger, weakness, dizziness, tremor, tachycardia, anxiety, numbness of extremities) and of hyperglycemia (eg, excessive thirst or urination, urinary glucose or ketones, fever, sore throat, unusual bleeding or rash). Remind patient to keep source of quick-acting sugar available at all times.
- When adjusting the dose, tell patient to check urine for ketones and blood for glucose 3 times a day; 1 to 2 times a day after stable control is established. Tell patient to notify health care provider if planning surgery or experiencing vomiting, injury, infection, or fever.
- Demonstrate correct technique for performing blood glucose and urine glucose and ketone tests, and ensure correct return demonstrations.
- Tell patient to report repeated abnormal glucose or ketone results to health care provider.
- Emphasize importance of continuing diet restrictions and exercise regimen.
- Caution about disulfiram-like syndrome (eg, facial flushing, abdominal cramping, nausea) when consuming alcohol. Advise patient to avoid alcohol.
- Inform patient that therapy will not cure disease.

Tolbutamide

(tole-BYOO-tuh-mide)

Class Antidiabetic/Sulfonylurea

How Supplied
Orinase Tablets 500 mg ◆ *Orinase Diagnostic* Powder for injection 1 g (as sodium)/vial
✥ *Apo-Tolbutamide* ◆ *Novo-Butamide*

Action
PHARMACOLOGY: Decreases blood glucose by stimulating release of insulin from pancreas.

PHARMACOKINETICS/DYNAMICS:
Absorption: Orally administered tolbutamide is readily absorbed from the GI tract.
Metabolism: Tolbutamide has no p-amino group, cannot be acetylated; however, presence of p-methyl group makes it susceptible to oxidation. A major metabolite is 1-butyl-3-p-carboxyphenylsulfonylurea (inactive).
Excretion: Tolbutamide t½ is 4.5 to 6.5 hr.
Onset: Onset of action is 20 min.
Peak: Time to peak effect is 3 to 4 hr.
Duration: Tolbutamide duration of action is 24 hr.

Indications
Oral form: Adjunct to diet to lower blood glucose in patients with non-insulin-dependent diabetes mellitus (type 2) whose hyperglycemia cannot be controlled by diet alone.
IV form (tolbutamide sodium): Aid in diagnosis of pancreatic islet cell adenoma.

Contraindications
Hypersensitivity to sulfonylureas; diabetes complicated by ketoacidosis with or without coma; sole therapy of insulin-dependent (type 1) diabetes mellitus; diabetes occurring during pregnancy.

Route/Dosage
ADULTS: **PO** Usually 1 to 2 g/day (range, 0.25 to 3 g) in 1 to 2 divided doses.

For Diagnostic Purposes
ADULTS: **IV** 1 g over 2 to 3 min.

Interactions
Androgens, anticoagulants, azole antifungals, chloramphenicol, clofibrate, dicumarol, fenfluramine, fluconazole, gemfibrozil, histamine H_2 antagonists, magnesium salts, methyldopa, MAO

inhibitors, phenylbutazone, probenecid, salicylates, sulfinpyrazone, sulfonamides, tricyclic antidepressants, urinary acidifiers:* May increase hypoglycemic effect.
Beta-blockers, calcium channel blockers, cholestyramine, corticosteroids, diazoxide, estrogens, hydantoins, isoniazid, nicotinic acid, oral contraceptives, phenothiazines, rifampin, sympathomimetics, thiazide diuretics, thyroid agents, urinary alkalinizers: May decrease hypoglycemic effect.
Charcoal: Charcoal can reduce the absorption of sulfonylureas; depending on the clinical situation, this will reduce their efficacy or toxicity.
Digitalis glycosides: Coadministration may result in increased digitalis serum levels.
Digoxin: May cause increased digoxin serum concentrations.
Ethanol: May cause disulfiram-like reaction.

Lab Test Interferences Drug may cause false-positive reaction for albumin with acidification-after-boiling test; no interference occurs with sulfosalicyclic acid test. Elevated LFTs and elevations in BUN and creatinine may occur.

Adverse Reactions

CV: Increased risk of cardiovascular mortality.
CNS: Dizziness; vertigo.
DERM: Allergic skin reactions; eczema; pruritus; erythema; urticaria; morbilliform or maculopapular eruptions; lichenoid reactions; porphyria; photosensitivity.
EENT: Tinnitus.
GI: Nausea; epigastric fullness; heartburn.
HEMA: Leukopenia; thrombocytopenia; aplastic anemia; agranulocytosis; hemolytic anemia; pancytopenia.

PATIENT CARE CONSIDERATIONS

Administration/Storage

- Administer 30 min prior to meal. May administer with food if GI upset occurs.
- May administer total dose in morning or give in divided doses to decrease GI upset or to decrease blood glucose fluctuation.
- Inject at constant rate over 2 to 3 min.
- Refer to manufacturer's product information for specific test methodology and interpretation of test results.
- Use within 1 hr of reconstitution but only if solution is complete and clear.

Assessment/Interventions

- Obtain patient history, including drug history and any known allergies. Note diabetes complicated by ketoacidosis, decreased renal or hepatic function, or sensitivity to sulfa drugs.
- If renal or hepatic function is diminished, use cautiously and monitor function.

HEPA: Cholestatic jaundice.
METAB: Hypoglycemia; SIADH with water retention and dilutional hyponatremia, especially in patients with CHF or hepatic cirrhosis.
OTHER: Disulfiram-like reaction; weakness; paresthesia; fatigue; malaise; slight burning sensation along course of vein during IV injection; thrombophlebitis with thrombosis of injected vein.

Precautions

Pregnancy: Category C. Insulin is recommended to control elevated blood glucose levels during pregnancy.
Lactation: Excreted into breast milk.
Children: Safety and efficacy have not been established.
Elderly: Particularly susceptible to hypoglycemic action. Hypoglycemia may be difficult to recognize in elderly.
Renal function impairment: Use drug with caution.
Hepatic function impairment: Use drug with caution.
Disulfiram-like syndrome: Administration of drug with alcohol may induce facial flushing and breathlessness.
Cardiovascular risk: Patients treated for 5 to 8 yr with diet plus tolbutamide (1.5 g/day) had a rate of cardiovascular mortality approximately 2.5 times that of patients treated with diet alone.

Overdosage: Signs and Symptoms

Hypoglycemia including symptoms of the following: tingling of lips and tongue, nausea, lethargy, confusion, agitation, nervousness, tachycardia, sweating, tremor, hunger, convulsions, stupor, coma.

- Monitor elderly closely for hypoglycemic effects.
- Monitor vital signs, blood sugar, weight, and I&O daily.
- If jaundice occurs, discontinue drug and notify health care provider.

Patient/Family Education

- Instruct patient to follow the diet and exercise regimen prescribed by health care provider.
- Inform patient of symptoms of and treatment for low blood sugar and advise patient to carry source of sugar at all times.
- Instruct patient to avoid alcohol. Inform patient that alcohol may react with tolbutamide and cause *Antabuse*-like reaction (eg, flushing, headache, dizziness, high BP).

- Instruct patient to monitor weight and to inform health care provider if steady weight gain occurs.
- Inform patient that surgery, illness, or trauma may require temporary use of insulin.
- Instruct patient to alert health care provider to following problems: nausea, vomiting, GI distress, diarrhea, fever, sore throat, rash, itching, weakness, unusual bruising or bleeding, spilling of glucose or ketones in urine.
- Caution patient to avoid exposure to sunlight and to use sunscreen or wear protective clothing to avoid photosensitivity reaction.
- Recommended that patient carry identification card (eg, *Medi-Alert*) indicating condition and drug therapy.

Tolcapone

(TOLE-kah-pone)

Class Antiparkinson

How Supplied
Tasmar Tablets 100 mg, Tablets 200 mg

Action

PHARMACOLOGY: The exact mechanism of action is unknown. Inhibits catechol-O-methyl transferase (COMT) thus blocking the degradation of catechols including dopamine and levodopa. This may lead to more sustained levels of dopamine and consequently a more prolonged antiparkinson's effect.

PHARMACOKINETICS/DYNAMICS:

Absorption: Tolcapone T_{max} is about 2 hr. Bioavailability is 65%. Food given within 1 hr before and 2 hr after dosing decreases the bioavailability 10% to 20%.

Distribution: Tolcapone Vd is 9 L and it does not distribute widely into tissues. Protein binding is about 99%.

Metabolism: Tolcapone's main metabolic pathway is glucuronidation. The drug is almost completely metabolized prior to excretion, with only a very small amount (0.5% of a dose) found unchanged in urine.

Excretion: Tolcapone's t½ is 2 to 3 hr. Systemic clearance is about 7 L/hr.

Special Populations:
Hepatic Function Impairment – In patients with moderate cirrhotic liver disease, clearance and Vd is reduced about 50%. Do not initiate therapy if the patient exhibits clinical evidence of active liver disease or 2 ALT or AST values greater than the ULN.

Indications As an adjunct to levodopa/carbidopa for the management of signs and symptoms of Parkinson's disease.

Contraindications Hypersensitivity to the drug or its ingredients; patients with liver disease; patients who were withdrawn from tolcapone because of evidence of tolcapone-induced hepatocellular injury; patients with a history of non-traumatic rhabdomyolysis or hyperpyrexia and confusion possibly related to medication.

Route/Dosage

ADULTS: **PO** 100 or 200 mg tid. The maximum recommended dose is 600 mg/day.

Interactions None well documented.

Lab Test Interferences None well documented.

Adverse Reactions

CV: Orthostatic complaints; syncope; chest pain; hypotension; chest discomfort.
CNS: Sleep disorder; excessive dreaming; somnolence; confusion; dizziness; headache; hallucination; dyskinesia; dystonia; fatigue; balance loss; hyperkinesia; paresthesia; hypokinesia; agitation; irritability; mental deficiency; hyperactivity; panic reaction; euphoria; hypertonia.
DERM: Dermal bleeding; skin tumor; alopecia.
EENT: Xerostomia; cataract; eye inflammation.
GI: Nausea; diarrhea; vomiting; constipation; abdominal pain; dyspepsia; flatulence.
GU: Urinary tract infection; urine discoloration; micturition disorder; uterine tumor.
HEPA: Severe hepatocellular injury, including fulminant liver failure resulting in death.
RESP: Upper respiratory tract infection; dyspnea; sinus congestion.
OTHER: Muscle cramps; anorexia; falling; increased sweating; rhabdomyolysis; stiffness; arthritis; neck pain; influenza; burning; malaise; fever.

> WARNING:
> Hepatotoxicity may be fatal, thus reserve for use in Parkinson patients on levodopa/carbidopa with symptom fluctuations and not satisfactorily responding. If no benefit observed after 3 wk of therapy, discontinue drug. Do not initiate therapy if patient exhibits clinical evidence of liver disease or 2 AST or ALT values greater than upper limit of normal. Monitor baseline AST and ALT and q 2 wk for first yr, q 4 wk for next 6 mo, and q 8 wk thereafter. Withdraw therapy if patient exhibits clinical evidence of liver disease. Use with caution in patients with severe dystonia/dyskinesias.

Precautions

Pregnancy: Category C.
Lactation: Undetermined.
Children: Safety and efficacy not established.
Diarrhea: Diarrhea is the most common reason for stopping therapy. Follow up all cases with appropriate work-up, including occult blood.
Dosage reduction: Decrease levodopa dosage appropriately when used concurrently.
Dyskinesia: Tolcapone may potentiate the dopaminergic side effects of levodopa and may cause or exacerbate preexisting dyskinesia.
Fibrotic complications: Cases of retroperitoneal fibrosis, pulmonary infiltrates, pleural effusion, and pleural thickening have been reported in some patients treated with ergot-derived dopaminergic agents.
Hallucinations: Patients treated with placebo, 100, and 200 mg tolcapone tid developed hallucinations at an incidence of approximately 5%, 8%, and 10%, respectively. Hallucinations present shortly after the initiation of therapy with tolcapone (typically within the first 2 wk).
Hepatic enzyme abnormalities: Elevations usually occurred within 6 wk to 6 mo of starting treatment. In about half the cases, enzyme levels returned to baseline within 1 to 3 mo and when treatment was discontinued, enzymes generally declined within 2 to 3 wk, but in some cases it took as long as 1 to 2 mo to return to normal.
Hypertension/Syncope: Dopaminergic therapy in Parkinson disease patients has been associated with orthostatic hypotension.
Monoamine oxidase (MAO) inhibitors: Avoid concurrent use of MAO inhibitors. Administration of MAO inhibitors may result in inhibition of the majority of pathways for catecholamine metabolism.
Rhabdomyolysis: Cases of severe rhabdomyolysis, with 1 case of multiorgan failure rapidly progressing to death, have been reported.
Withdrawal-emergent hyperpyrexia and confusion: Cases resembling the neuroleptic malignant syndrome (characterized by elevated temperature, muscular rigidity, and altered consciousness), similar to that reported in association with the rapid dose reduction or withdrawal of other dopaminergic drugs, have been reported.

Overdosage: Signs and Symptoms
Nausea, vomiting, dizziness.

PATIENT CARE CONSIDERATIONS

Administration/Storage
- May be given without regard to meals.
- Store at room temperature.

Assessment/Interventions
- Obtain patient history including drug history and any known allergies.
- Do not use tolcapone until there has been a complete discussion of the risks and the patients has provided written informed consent.
- Perform complete baseline assessment of parkinsonian signs and symptoms before instituting therapy.
- Monitor liver enzymes
- Check for occult blood in stool if diarrhea occurs.
- Assist with ambulation during initial phase of therapy because of dizziness due to hypotension.
- Offer support to patient and family because relief of parkinsonian symptoms may take several weeks to months after therapy is initiated.
- Conduct appropriate tests to exclude the presence of liver disease before starting treatment with tolcapone. Determine baseline levels of ALT and AST and every 2 wk for the first year of therapy, every 4 wk for the next 6 mo, and every 8 wk thereafter.

Patient/Family Education
- Provide patient information pamphlet.
- Instruct patient to take drug only as prescribed.
- Inform patient that postural hypotension with or without symptoms (eg, dizziness, syncope) may occur and caution patients against rising rapidly after sitting or lying down.
- Inform patient that nausea may occur.
- Advise patient of the possibility of an increase in dyskinesia and dystonia.
- Instruct patient to notify their health care provider if they become pregnant or intend to become pregnant during therapy.
- Advise patient to notify their health care provider if they intend to breastfeed an infant.
- Advise patients about the need for self-monitoring for classical signs of liver disease (eg, clay-colored stools, jaundice) and nonspecific ones (eg, fatigue, appetite loss, lethargy).
- Inform patient of the clinical signs and symptoms that suggest the onset of hepatic injury (eg, persistent nausea, fatigue, lethargy, anorexia, jaundice, dark urine, pruritus, right upper quadrant tenderness).

Tolmetin Sodium

(TOLE-mee-tin SO-dee-uhm)
Class Analgesic/NSAID

How Supplied
Tolectin 200 Tablets 200 mg (as sodium) ◆
Tolectin 600 Tablets 600 mg (as sodium)

Action
PHARMACOLOGY: Decreases inflammation, pain, and fever, probably through inhibition of cyclooxygenase activity and prostaglandin synthesis.

PHARMACOKINETICS/DYNAMICS:
Absorption: Tolmetin is rapidly and completely absorbed. T_{max} is about 30 to 60 min and C_{max} is about 40 mcg/mL.

Metabolism: Tolmetin is recovered in urine partially as an inactive oxidative metabolite.

Excretion: Almost all of the tolmetin dose is recovered in urine in 24 hr.

Indications Treatment of chronic and acute rheumatoid arthritis and osteoarthritis and juvenile rheumatoid arthritis.

Contraindications Hypersensitivity to aspirin, iodides, or any NSAID.

Route/Dosage
Osteoarthritis/Rheumatoid Arthritis
ADULTS: **PO** 400 mg tid initially; titrate to 600 to 1600 mg/day for osteoarthritic patients or 600 to 1800 mg/day in divided doses for rheumatoid arthritis patients. Daily doses exceeding 1800 mg/day are not recommended.

Juvenile Rheumatoid Arthritis
CHILDREN 2 YR OR OLDER: **PO** 20 mg/kg/day in 3 to 4 divided doses initially; titrate to 15 to 30 mg/kg/day (max, 30 mg/kg/day).

Interactions
Anticoagulants: May increase effect of anticoagulants due to decreased plasma protein binding. May increase risk of gastric erosion and bleeding.
Cyclosporine: May potentiate nephrotoxicity of both agents.
Methotrexate: May increase methotrexate levels.

Lab Test Interferences May prolong bleeding time. May produce false-positive test result for proteinuria using sulfosalicylic acid. Increases in serum uric acid, LFTs, serum creatinine, BUN.

Adverse Reactions
CV: Edema; sodium retention; hypertension; CHF.
CNS: Dizziness; drowsiness; lightheadedness; confusion; increased sweating; vertigo; headache; nervousness; migraine; anxiety; aggravated Parkinson's disease or epilepsy; paresthesia; peripheral neuropathy; myalgia; fatigue; asthenia; depression.
DERM: Rash; pruritus; urticaria; purpura; erythema multiforme; skin irritation; sweating.
EENT: Blurred vision; tinnitus; visual disturbances.
GI: Nausea; dyspepsia; abdominal pain or discomfort; flatulence; diarrhea; constipation; vomiting; gastritis; anorexia; glossitis; stomatitis; mouth ulcers; peptic ulcer; GI distress.
GU: Hematuria; proteinuria; dysuria; elevations in BUN; acute renal insufficiency; interstitial nephritis; hyperkalemia; hyponatremia; renal papillary necrosis; UTIs.
HEMA: Increased bleeding time; anemia; decreases in Hgb or Hct; leukopenia; thrombocytopenia; hemolytic anemia.
HEPA: Hepatitis; increased LFT results; elevated liver enzymes.
METAB: Weight decrease or increase.
RESP: Bronchospasm; laryngeal edema; rhinitis; dyspnea; pharyngitis; hemoptysis; shortness of breath.

Precautions
Pregnancy: Category C.
Lactation: Excreted in breast milk.
Children: Safety and efficacy not established in children under 2 yr.
Elderly: Increased risk of adverse reactions.
Renal function impairment: Use drug with caution in patients with compromised cardiac function, hypertension, or other conditions predisposing to fluid retention.
GI effects: Serious GI toxicity (eg, bleeding, ulceration, perforation) can occur at any time with or without warning symptoms.
Anaphylactoid reactions: Have occurred in patients with aspirin hypersensitivity and in patients who discontinued tolmetin, then restarted it.

Overdosage: Signs and Symptoms
Drowsiness, dizziness, mental confusion, paresthesia, vomiting, abdominal pain, intense headache, tinnitus, sweating, convulsions, visual disturbances, elevated serum creatinine and BUN levels, hypotension.

PATIENT CARE CONSIDERATIONS
Administration/Storage
- Administer capsules or tablets PO tid with schedule including morning dose and evening dose.
- Do not administer with food, milk, or sodium bicarbonate.
- If GI distress occurs, give with antacids that do not contain sodium bicarbonate.
- Store at room temperature. Do not expose to sunlight or moisture.

Assessment/Interventions
- Obtain patient history, including drug history and any known allergies.
- Assess renal function before and during therapy, especially in patients with renal impairment.
- Monitor serum uric acid, serum creatinine, and BUN and report if increased.
- Monitor periodic urine tests for blood and protein and report positive results to health care provider. Be aware when testing for proteinuria that using sulfosalicylic acid may cause false-positive results. Use dye-impregnated reagent strips.
- Monitor results of LFTs and report dyscrasias to health care provider.
- Monitor serum potassium (report hyperkalemia) and sodium (report hyponatremia).
- Monitor Hgb and Hct and notify health care provider of decrease.
- Obtain periodic occult blood test in stool if patient is receiving long-term therapy.
- Monitor BP and I&O throughout therapy.
- Notify health care provider of any shortness of breath or other signs of edema.
- Assess visual acuity and hearing with periodic exams for patients on prolonged therapy, especially if patient experiences blurred vision or changes in color vision.

Patient/Family Education
- Explain that product should not be taken with aspirin or other NSAIDs without consulting health care provider.
- Explain that full antirheumatic action may not occur for up to 7 days and may not reach maximum effect for up to 1 mo after starting therapy.
- Tell patient to avoid taking with food or milk or immediately after meal. If medication causes stomach upset tell patient to take with antacids that do not contain sodium bicarbonate. Instruct patient to call health care provider if pain continues.
- Tell patient to avoid smoking or drinking alcohol while taking this drug.
- Explain that dizziness or black stools should be reported to health care provider immediately.
- Explain that if drowsiness, dizziness, or blurred vision occur, patient should observe caution while driving or performing other tasks requiring alertness.
- Explain that photosensitivity may occur and to use sunscreens and protective clothing when exposed to ultraviolet or sunlight until tolerance is determined.
- Identify potential clinically important adverse reactions: drowsiness, blurred vision, edema, headache, lightheadedness, confusion, fatigue, swelling feet, ringing of ears, nausea, vomiting, mouth ulcers, unusual bleeding or bruising, rash, itching, skin irritation. Tell patient to notify health care provider if persistent or severe.
- Tell patient not to store drug in bathroom but in cool, dry place.

Tolnaftate

(tahl-NAFF-tate)

Class Topical/Antifungal

How Supplied
Absorbine Athlete's Foot Cream Cream 1% ♦ *Absorbine Footcare* Spray liquid 1% ♦ *Aftate for Athlete's Foot* Gel 1%, Spray powder 1%, Spray liquid 1% ♦ *Aftate for Jock Itch* Gel 1%, Spray powder 1% ♦ *Blis-To-Sol Liquid* Liquid 1% ♦ *Genaspor* Cream 1% ♦ *NP-27* Liquid 1% ♦ *Quinsana Plus Foot Powder* Powder 1% ♦ *Tinactin* Cream 1%, Solution 1%, Powder 1%, Spray powder 1%, Spray liquid 1% ♦ *Tinactin for Jock Itch* Cream 1%, Spray powder 1% ♦ *Ting* Cream 1%

❧ *Pitrex* ♦ *Tinactin Plus*

Action
PHARMACOLOGY: Distorts hyphae and inhibits mycelial growth in susceptible fungi.

Indications
Treatment and prophylaxis of tinea pedia (athlete's foot); treatment of tinea cruris (jock itch) or tinea corporis (ringworm) caused by specific fungi; treatment of onchomycosis, chronic scalp infections, palm and sole infections with kerion formation; treatment of tinea versicolor.

Contraindications
Standard considerations.

Route/Dosage
ADULTS AND CHILDREN: **Topical** Apply small amount of ointment, cream, or powder or 1 to 3 gtt of solution to affected area bid for 2 to 3 wk (6 wk if skin is thickened); continue treatment to maintain remission. Reserve powder for mild infections.

Interactions None well documented.

Lab Test Interferences None well documented.

PATIENT CARE CONSIDERATIONS

Administration/Storage
- Cleanse skin with soap and water and dry thoroughly before applying.
- Apply small quantities of ointment, cream, solution, spray liquid, or gel as primary therapy.
- Use powder or powder aerosol as adjunctive therapy or prophylaxis for athlete's foot. Use as primary therapy only in very mild conditions.
- Consult health care provider if no improvement after 10 days.
- To prevent recurrence, continue treatment for 2 wk beyond disappearance of symptoms.
- Store at room temperature. Avoid moisture and sunlight. Keep powders from getting wet or damp.

Assessment/Interventions
- Obtain patient history, including drug history and any known allergies.
- Monitor for sensitization, irritation, pruritus, rash, or stinging.

Patient/Family Education
- Tell patient to cleanse skin with soap and water and dry thoroughly before applying.

Adverse Reactions
DERM: Sensitization; mild irritation; pruritus; contact dermatitis; stinging.

Precautions
Pregnancy: Undetermined.
Lactation: Undetermined.
External use only: Avoid contact with eyes.
Nail and scalp infections: Do not use drug except as adjunct to systemic treatment.
Sensitization or irritation: Discontinue treatment if sensitization or irritation occurs.

- Emphasize to use only externally in small amounts massaged well into affected area and surrounding skin.
- Instruct patient to wash hands before and after applying medication.
- Tell patient to avoid contact with eyes.
- Advise patient to wear well-fitting, ventilated shoes and to change shoes and socks at least daily.
- Tell patient not to cover treated site with bandages unless ordered specifically by health care provider.
- Instruct patient to notify health care provider if there has been no apparent improvement after 10 days of treatment.
- Emphasize that product should not be used on nail and scalp infections unless using in addition to internal medication prescribed by health care provider.
- Tell patient to store at room temperature and not in bathroom (especially powders).
- Instruct patient to report these symptoms to health care provider: persistent or severe irritation, itching, rash, stinging.

Tolterodine Tartrate

(tole-THE-roe-deen)

Class Urinary tract product/Muscarinic antagonist

How Supplied
Detrol Tablets 1 mg, Tablets 2 mg ◆ *Detrol LA* Capsule, extended-release 2 mg, Capsule, extended-release 4 mg
🍁 *Unidet*

Action
PHARMACOLOGY: Antagonizes muscarinic receptor, which mediates urinary bladder contraction and salivation.

PHARMACOKINETICS/DYNAMICS:
Absorption: Tolterodine is rapidly absorbed. After dosing, T_{max} is within 1 to 2 hr (immediate-release) and 2 to 6 hr (extended-release). Food increases bioavailability (about 53%) of immediate-release, but has no effect on extended-release formulation.

Distribution: Tolterodine is highly protein bound. Vd is about 113 L.

Metabolism: Tolterodine is extensively metabolized by the liver following oral dosing. The primary metabolic route involves oxidation of the 5-methyl group and is mediated by the cytochrome P-450 2D6 isoenzyme and leads to a pharmacologically active 5-hydroxymethyl metabolite.

Excretion: 77% is recovered in urine and 17% is recovered in feces within 7 days. Tolterodine's t½ is approximately 2 to 4 hr

Special Populations:
Renal Function Impairment – Patients with reduced renal function should receive no more

than 2 mg tolterodine/day. Use caution.
Hepatic Function Impairment – Patients with significantly reduced hepatic function should not receive doses more than 1 mg bid.

Indications Treatment of overactive bladder with symptoms of urinary frequency, urgency, or urge incontinence.

Contraindications Urinary retention; gastric retention; uncontrolled narrow-angle glaucoma.

Route/Dosage
IMMEDIATE-RELEASE
ADULTS: PO 1 to 2 mg daily.

EXTENDED-RELEASE
PO 2 to 4 mg daily.

Interactions
Clarithromycin, erythromycin, itraconazole, ketoconazole, miconazole (and other cytochrome P450 3A4 inhibitors): May increase tolterodine plasma levels, which may increase activity and side effects.
Fluoxetine: Plasma levels of tolterodine may be decreased while the AUC of the active 5-hydroxymethyl metabolite may be increased; requires no dosage adjustment.

Lab Test Interferences None well documented.

Adverse Reactions
CV: Hypertension.
CNS: Headache; somnolence; paresthesia, nervousness (immediate-release); dizziness, anxiety (extended-release).
DERM: Pruritus; dry skin.
EENT: Abnormal vision (accommodation abnormalities); xerophthalmia; sinusitis (extended-release).
GI: Dry mouth; constipation; abdominal pain; dyspepsia; flatulence, vomiting, nausea (immediate-release).
GU: Dysuria (extended-release).
METAB: Weight gain.
RESP: Bronchitis; coughing.
OTHER: Chest pain; infection; fungal infection; falling (immediate-release); fatigue (extended-release).

Precautions
Pregnancy: Category C.
Lactation: Undetermined.
Children: Safety and efficacy not established.
Renal function impairment: Use with caution.
Hepatic function impairment: Use with caution.
Controlled narrow-angle glaucoma: Use with caution.
Urinary/Gastric retention: Use with caution.

Overdosage: Signs and Symptoms
Dry mouth, thirst, cardiac slowing followed by acceleration, palpitations, hypertension, hypotension, inhibition of sweating, flushing, hot skin, photophobia, dilated pupils, blurred vision, speech disturbances, CNS stimulation, delirium, restlessness, drowsiness, stupor, headache, decreased intestinal peristalsis, abdominal distension, ataxia, hallucinations, seizures, coma.

PATIENT CARE CONSIDERATIONS
Administration/Storage
- Store at room temperature in tightly closed container.
- Do not administer to nursing mothers and pregnant women unless the potential benefit for the mother justifies the potential risk for the fetus.
- Do not administer more than 1 mg dose bid to patients receiving cytochrome P450 3A4 inhibitors (ie, macrolide antibiotic and antifungal agents) or to patients with reduced hepatic function.

Assessment/Interventions
- Obtain a complete history of prescription and OTC drug use and history of hypersensitivities.
- Assess for possible drug interactions and potential adverse reactions.

Patient/Family Education
- Instruct patient to take the medication as prescribed at the same time each day.
- Advise patient that antimuscarinic agents such as tolterodine may produce side effects including blurred vision and to notify primary health care giver if side effects occur or if there are any other concerns.
- Caution female patients to notify the health care provider immediately should they become or plan to become pregnant.

Topiramate

(Toe-PEER-ah-mate)
Class Anticonvulsant

How Supplied
Topamax Tablets 25 mg, Tablets 50 mg, Tablets 100 mg, Tablets 200 mg, Capsules, sprinkle 15 mg, Capsules, sprinkle 25 mg

Action
PHARMACOLOGY: Precise mechanism is unknown but topiramate may block repetitively elicited action potentials, affect ability of chloride ion to move into neurons, and antagonize an excitatory amino acid receptor.

PHARMACOKINETICS/DYNAMICS:
Absorption: Topiramate absorption is rapid. T_{max} is 2 hr. Bioavailability is about 80% and is not affected by food.

Distribution: Topiramate is 13% to 17% bound to plasma proteins.

Metabolism: Topiramate is not extensively metabolized.

Excretion: Topiramate is primarily eliminated unchanged in urine (about 70% of a dose). Plasma Cl is about 20 to 30 mL per min following oral administration. Topiramate t½ is 21 hr.

Special Populations:
Renal Function Impairment – Cl is reduced 42% in moderately impaired and 54% in severely impaired patients.
Hepatic Function Impairment – Cl may be decreased in this population.
Children – Pediatric patients have a 50% higher Cl and shorter t½ than adults. Consequently, plasma concentrations for the same mg/kg dose may be lower in pediatric patients than adults.

Indications Adjunctive therapy for partial onset seizures; primary generalized tonic-clonic seizures; seizures associated with Lennox-Gastaut syndrome.

Contraindications Standard considerations.

Route/Dosage
ADULTS 17 YR OF AGE AND OLDER: **PO** 200 to 400 mg daily in 2 divided doses in adults with partial seizures and 400 mg daily in 2 divided doses in adults with primary, generalized, tonic-clonic seizures. Initiate therapy at 25 to 50 mg daily and titrate to an effective dose in increments of 25 to 50 mg weekly. Doses over 400 mg have not been shown to improve response.
CHILDREN 2 TO 16 YR OF AGE: **PO** 5 to 9 mg/kg per day in 2 divided doses. Initiate therapy at 25 mg or less (based on range of 1 to 3 mg/kg per day) nightly for first wk and titrate to an effective dose at 1- to 2-wk intervals by increments of 1 to 3 mg/kg per day in 2 divided doses.
Renal Function Impairment (Ccr 70 mL per min or less) – Dosage adjustment of 50% of the usual adult dose is recommended.

Interactions
Alcohol, CNS depressants: CNS depression and side effects may be increased.
Carbamazepine: Effects of topiramate may be decreased.
Carbonic anhydrase inhibitors (eg, acetazolamide): Increased risk of renal stone formation.
Oral contraceptives: Efficacy of oral contraceptives may be decreased and possible increased breakthrough bleeding.
Phenytoin: Effects of phenytoin may be increased while those of topiramate may decrease.
Valproic acid: Effects of valproic acid and topiramate may both be decreased.

Lab Test Interferences None well documented.

Adverse Reactions
CV: Hypertension (2%).
CNS: Dizziness (32%); fatigue (30%); somnolence (29%); psychomotor slowing (21%); nervousness, paresthesia (19%); ataxia (16%); difficulty with memory, confusion, difficulty with concentration (14%); speech disorders/related speech problems, depression (13%); nystagmus (11%); language problems (10%); tremor, mood problems (9%); abnormal coordination (4%); agitation, aggressive reaction, apathy, emotional lability, abnormal gait (3%); hypesthesia, depersonalization, decreased libido, involuntary muscle contractions, stupor, vertigo (2%); hypertonia, hallucination, euphoria, psychosis, headache, anxiety, convulsions, insomnia, suicide attempt (1% or more).
DERM: Skin disorder (2%); acne, urticaria (1% or more); erythematous rash, increased sweating (1%); bullous skin reactions (including erythema multiforme, Stevens-Johnson syndrome, toxic epidermal necrolysis, pemphigus) (postmarketing).
EENT: Abnormal vision (13%); diplopia (10%); pharyngitis (6%); taste perversion (4%); decreased hearing (2%); tinnitus, conjunctivitis, eye pain (1% or more).
GI: Nausea, anorexia (12%); dyspepsia, abdominal pain (7%); constipation, dry mouth (4%); gastroenteritis (2%); gingivitis, GI disorder (1%); diarrhea, vomiting (1% or more).
GU: Breast pain (4%); UTI (3%); amenorrhea, menorrhagia, menstrual disorder, hematuria, micturition frequency, urinary incontinence, prostatic disorder (2%); abnormal urine (1%); dysuria, impotence, renal calculus, dysmenorrhea (1% or more).
HEMA: Leukopenia (2%); anemia (1% or more).
HEPA: Hepatitis, hepatic failure (postmarketing).
METAB: Weight decrease (13%); dehydration (1% or more).
MUSC: Myalgia (2%); arthralgia, muscle weakness (1% or more)
RENAL: Renal tubular acidosis (postmarketing).
RESP: Rhinitis (7%); sinusitis (6%); dyspnea (2%); coughing, upper respiratory tract infection (1% or more).
OTHER: Asthenia (6%); back pain (5%); chest pain, flu-like symptoms, leg pain (4%); myalgia, epistaxis, hot flashes, infection, viral

infection, allergy (2%); fever, pain (1% or more); edema; body odor, moniliasis, rigors, skeletal pain (1%); pancreatitis (postmarketing).

Precautions

Pregnancy: Category C.
Lactation: Undetermined.
Children: Safety and efficacy in children under 2 yr of age not established.
Elderly: No age-related differences in safety and efficacy have been seen, but consider age-related changes in renal function.
Renal function impairment: Reduce dose 50% if Ccr less than 70 mL per min.
Hepatic function impairment: Administer with caution.
Acute myopia: Acute myopia secondary to angle-closure glaucoma has been reported.
Hemodialysis: Supplemental dose may be necessary before prolonged dialysis.
Kidney stones: Risk of developing kidney stones may be increased.
Metabolic acidosis: Hyperchloremic, non-anion gap, metabolic acidosis has been associated with topiramate treatment.
Oligohidrosis and hyperthermia: Have been reported with the majority in children.
Withdrawal: Gradually withdraw therapy to minimize potential of increased seizure frequency.

Overdosage: Signs and Symptoms

Convulsions, drowsiness, speech disturbance, blurred vision, diplopia, mentation impaired, lethargy, abnormal coordination, stupor, hypotension, abdominal pain, agitation, dizziness, depression, deaths, severe metabolic acidosis.

PATIENT CARE CONSIDERATIONS

Administration/Storage

- Use in combination with other antiepileptic drugs (AEDs).
- Tablets and sprinkle capsules are interchangeable on mg for mg basis.
- Administer prescribed dose without regard to meals. Administer with food if GI upset occurs.
- Administer tablets whole. Chewing, breaking, or crushing tablet may leave a bitter taste.
- Sprinkle capsules may be swallowed whole or the capsule can be opened and the entire contents sprinkled on a small amount (eg, teaspoon) of soft food (eg, applesauce) that should be swallowed immediately without chewing and then washed down with a fluid (eg, water, juice).
- Store tablets at controlled room temperature (59° to 86°F). Store capsules at temperature less than 77°F. Keep tightly capped and protect from moisture.

Assessment/Interventions

- Obtain patient history, including drug history and any known allergies. Note renal or hepatic impairment, condition or therapy predisposing to metabolic acidosis (eg, severe respiratory disorder, diarrhea, ketogenic diet, surgery), and concurrent use of phenytoin and/or carbamazepine or medications that predispose to heat-related disorders (eg, anticholinergics).
- Ensure that reduced dose is administered to patient with renal impairment (Ccr less than 70 mL per min).
- Ensure that patient is well hydrated during therapy to reduce kidney stone formation.
- Ensure serum bicarbonate is evaluated before starting therapy and periodically thereafter. Consider reducing the dose or discontinuing topiramate if metabolic acidosis develops and persists. Consider adding alkali therapy if decision is made to continue topiramate in the face of persistent acidosis.
- Frequently assess patient for response to treatment. Notify health care provider if seizures do not improve or appear to worsen.
- Ensure that therapy is periodically reviewed to determine if it needs to be continued without change or if a dose change (eg, increase, decrease, discontinuation) is indicated.
- Avoid sudden discontinuation of therapy if possible. Attempt to gradually reduce dose over a period of 2 wk or more if decision to discontinue medication is made.
- Monitor patient for GI, CNS, GU, DERM, and general body side effects. Inform health care provider if noted and significant.
- Implement safety precautions for patients who experience dizziness or ataxia.

Patient/Family Education

- Explain name, dose, action, and potential side effects of drug.
- Advise patient, family, or caregiver to read the *Patient Information* leaflet before starting therapy and with each refill.
- Instruct patient, family, or caregiver to continue other medications for seizures unless advised to do otherwise by health care provider.
- Advise patient, family, or caregiver that medication will be started at a low dose and then gradually increased as tolerated until max benefit has been obtained.
- Instruct patient, family, or caregiver to take (give) exactly as prescribed and not to change the dose or discontinue therapy unless advised by health care provider.

- Advise patient to swallow tablet whole. Chewing the tablet may leave a bitter taste.
- Advise patient, family, or caregiver that sprinkle capsules may be swallowed whole or opened and the entire contents sprinkled onto a small amount (eg, teaspoon) of soft food (eg, applesauce) and then consumed immediately without chewing. Advise patient, family, or caregiver that fluid (eg, water) should be given to help wash the sprinkle/food mixture down. Caution patient, family, or caregiver to not prepare ahead of time and store for future use.
- Advise patient, family, or caregiver that each dose may be taken without regard to meals but to take with food if stomach upset occurs.
- Instruct patient, family, or caregiver that if a dose is missed to skip that dose and not to double the next dose.
- Advise patient, family, or caregiver to maintain adequate fluid intake to reduce chance of kidney stones developing.
- Instruct patient, family, or caregiver to discontinue therapy and immediately notify health care provider of any of the following: sudden change in vision, eye pain or pain around the eye, decreased sweating, elevated body temperature.
- Advise patient, family, or caregiver that if medication needs to be discontinued it will be slowly withdrawn over a period of 2 wk or more unless safety concerns (eg, rash) require a more rapid withdrawal.
- Advise patient to avoid alcoholic beverages and other depressants while taking this medication.
- Caution patient that drug may cause dizziness, drowsiness, confusion, or difficulty concentrating and to use caution while driving or performing other tasks requiring mental alertness or coordination until tolerance is determined.
- Advise women using oral contraceptives that topiramate may reduce their effectiveness and to consider using an alternate method of contraception.
- Advise women to notify health care provider if pregnant, planning to become pregnant, or breastfeeding.
- Advise patient that medication may cause photosensitivity (sensitivity to sunlight) and to avoid unnecessary exposure to UV light (sunlight, tanning booths), use sunscreen, and wear protective clothing when exposed to UV light until tolerance is determined.
- Instruct patient, family, or caregiver to contact health care provider if seizures get worse or if new types of seizures occur.
- Advise patient, family, or caregiver to contact health care provider if bothersome side effects occur.
- Advise patient to carry identification (eg, Medic Alert) indicating medication usage and epilepsy.
- Advise patient, family, or caregiver not to take (give) any prescription or OTC medications, dietary supplements, or herbal preparations unless advised by health care provider.
- Advise patient, family, or caregiver that laboratory tests and follow-up visits will be required to monitor therapy and to keep appointments.

Topotecan Hydrochloride

(toe-poe-TEE-kan)

Class Topoisomerase I inhibitor

How Supplied
Hycamtin Powder for Injection 4 mg

Action
PHARMACOLOGY: Topotecan hydrochloride is an antitumor drug with topoisomerase I-inhibitory activity.

PHARMACOKINETICS/DYNAMICS:
Absorption: Topotecan AUC is approximately dose-proportional.

Distribution: Topotecan is approximately 35% protein bound. The mean Vd_{ss} is between 17 to 22 L/m^2 for topotecan and 26 to 563 L/m^2 for its active lactone form.

Metabolism: Topotecan undergoes a reversible, pH-dependent hydrolysis of its lactone moiety. The lactone form is pharmacologically active.

Excretion: Topotecan $t_{1/2}$ is 2 to 3 hr. 30% is excreted in urine. Renal Cl is an important determinant of elimination.

Special Populations:
Renal Function Impairment – With Ccr approximately 40 to 60 mL/min, plasma Cl decreased to about 67%. With Ccr approximately 20 to 39 mL/min, plasma Cl decreased to about 34%. Dosage adjustment is recommended in these patients.
Hepatic Function Impairment – Plasma Cl is decreased to approximately 67% in hepatic impaired patients with bilirubin 1.7 to 15 mg/dL. No dosage adjustment is necessary.
Elderly – Decreased renal Cl is common in the elderly, an important determinant of topotecan Cl.
Gender – Overall plasma Cl is about 24% higher in men than women.

Indications Metastatic carcinoma of the ovary after failure of initial or subsequent chemotherapy; small cell lung cancer sensitive disease after failure of first-line chemotherapy.

Contraindications Hypersensitivity to topotecan or to any of its ingredients; pregnancy or breastfeeding; severe bone marrow depression.

Route/Dosage

Dosage Adjustment

ADULTS: **IV** If neutropenia develops (defined as absolute neutrophil count less than 1500/mm^3), reduce the dose by 0.25 mg/m^2 for subsequent doses. Alternately, a course of filgrastim may be started on day 6 of each subsequent cycle; give the first filgrastim dose 24 hr after the final topotecan dose.

Ovarian or Small-Cell Lung Cancer

ADULTS: **IV** Topotecan 1.5 mg/m^2/day over 30 min daily for 5 consecutive days starting on day 1 of a 21-day cycle. Tumor response may be delayed; administer at least 4 cycles provided the tumor is not progressing. Before giving each dose, the patient should have a neutrophil count greater than 1500/mm^3 and a platelet count greater than 100,000/mm^3.

Renal Function Impairment

ADULTS: **IV** Dosage adjustment is recommended in patients with moderate renal impairment (Ccr of 20 to 39 mL/min); give 50% of usual dose. For Ccr less than 20 mL/min, reduce dose; specific recommendations not available.

Interactions

Cisplatin: Myelosuppression is more severe when topotecan is given in combination with cisplatin.

Filgrastim: Coadministration can prolong the duration of neutropenia. If filgrastim is used, do not initiate until day 6 of the course of therapy, 24 hr after completion of treatment with topotecan.

Lab Test Interferences None well documented.

Adverse Reactions

CNS: Headache (18%); paresthesia (7%).
DERM: Alopecia (49%); rash (16%); severe dermatitis, severe pruritus (postmarketing).
GI: Nausea (64%); vomiting (45%); diarrhea (32%); constipation (29%) abdominal pain (22%); anorexia (19%); stomatitis (18%); intestinal obstruction (5%).
HEMA: Neutropenia (less than 1500 cells/mm^3 [97%], less than 500 cells/mm^3 [78%]); leukopenia (less than 3000 cells/mm^3 [97%], less than 1000 cells/mm^3 [32%]); thrombocytopenia (less than 75,000/mm^3 [69%], less than 25,000/mm^3 [27%]); anemia (less than 10 g/dL [89%], less than 8 g/dL [37%]), sepsis (23%); RBC transfusions (52%); platelet transfusions (15%); rare severe bleeding (postmarketing).
HEPA: Elevated hepatic enzymes (8%).
HYPERSEN: Allergic manifestations, anaphylactic reactions, angioedema (postmarketing).
MUSC: Arthralgia (1%).
RESP: Dyspnea (22%); coughing (15%); pneumonia (8%).
OTHER: Fatigue (29%); fever (28%); asthenia (25%); pain (23%); malaise, chest pain (2%).

> **WARNING:**
> *Bone marrow suppression (primarily neutropenia):* Bone marrow suppression is the dose-limiting toxicity of topotecan. Administer only to patients with adequate bone marrow reserves, including baseline neutrophil counts of at least 1500 cells/mm^3 and platelet counts of at least 100,000/mm^3.

Precautions

Pregnancy: Category D.
Lactation: Undetermined. Discontinue breastfeeding.
Children: Safety and efficacy have not been established.
Anemia: Severe anemia (grade 3/4, Hgb less than 8 g/dL) occurred.
Extravasation: Topotecan is an irritant; inadvertent extravasation may produce mild local reactions such as erythema and bruising.
Neutropenia: Grade 4 (less than 500 cells/mm^3) neutropenia was most common during course 1 of treatment.
Thrombocytopenia: Grade 4 thrombocytopenia (less than 25,000 cells/mm^3) occurred.

Overdosage: Signs and Symptoms

Bone marrow suppression.

PATIENT CARE CONSIDERATIONS

Administration/Storage

- For IV infusion only. Not for IV bolus, intradermal, SC, IM, or intra-arterial administration.
- Follow institutional procedures for handling, administration, and disposal of anticancer drugs.
- Reconstitute powder for injection with 4 mL sterile water for injection then dilute appropriate volume of reconstituted solution with either 0.9% sodium chloride IV infusion or 5% dextrose IV infusion following manufacturer's guidelines.
- If topotecan solution contacts the skin, wash the skin immediately and thoroughly with soap and water.
- If topotecan contacts mucous membranes, flush thoroughly with water.

- Discard unused portions of vial. Do not save any unused portions for future use.
- Do not mix with any other medications.
- Do not administer if particulate matter or cloudiness is noted.
- Administer prescribed dose by IV infusion over 30 min.
- Store unopened vials at controlled room temperature (68° to 77°F) in original container, protected from light. Reconstituted solution should be used immediately or used within 24 hr if stored at 68° to 77°F and in ambient lighting conditions. Discard solution if not used within 24 hr.

Assessment/Interventions
- Obtain patient history, including drug history and any known allergies. Note renal impairment, bone marrow suppression, pregnancy, or breast feeding.
- Ensure that CBC with differential and platelet count is evaluated before starting therapy and frequently during treatment.
- Do not administer if baseline absolute neutrophil count is less than 1500/mm^3 or if platelet count is less than 100,000/mm^3. Do not administer subsequent courses of topotecan until neutrophils recover to greater than 1000/mm^3, platelets recover to greater than 100,000/mm^3, and hemoglobin levels recover to 9 g/dL (with transfusion if necessary).
- Ensure that reduced dose is administered to patient with moderate renal impairment (Ccr 20 to 39 mL/min) following manufacturer's guidelines.
- Ensure that women of childbearing potential are not pregnant or attempting to become pregnant.
- Monitor patient for signs or symptoms of infection or bleeding. Inform health care provider immediately if noted and be prepared to treat appropriately.
- Assess patient for GI, CNS, RESP, DERM, HEMA, and general body side effects. Report to health care provider if noted and significant.

Patient/Family Education
- Explain name, action, and potential side effects of drug.
- Advise patient, family, or caregiver that medication will be prepared and administered by health care provider in a health care setting.
- Review dosing schedule with patient, family, or caregiver.
- Advise patient, family, or caregiver that medication may cause hair loss but that this is reversible when therapy is stopped.
- Advise patient, family, or caregiver to immediately report any of the following to health care provider: fever, chills, or other signs of infection; unusual bleeding or bruising; pain, redness, or swelling at injection site.
- Advise patient, family, or caregiver to report any of the following to health care provider: persistent nausea, vomiting, diarrhea or appetite loss; persistent or worsening general body weakness.
- Caution patient that medication may cause weakness or fatigue and to use caution when driving or performing other tasks that require mental alertness or coordination.
- Caution women of childbearing potential to avoid becoming pregnant during therapy.
- Advise women of childbearing potential to notify health care provider if pregnant, planning to become pregnant, or breastfeeding.
- Instruct patient not to take any prescription or OTC medications or dietary supplements unless advised by health care provider.
- Advise patient, family, or caregiver that frequent follow-up visits and laboratory tests will be required to monitor therapy and to keep appointments.

Toremifene Citrate

(TORE-EM-ih-feen)

Class Antiestrogen hormone

How Supplied
Fareston Oral tablets 60 mg

Action
PHARMACOLOGY: A nonsteroidal antiestrogen that blocks the growth-stimulating effects of estrogen in the tumor.

PHARMACOKINETICS/DYNAMICS:
Absorption: Toremifene is well absorbed and is not influenced by food. T_{max} is 3 hr. Steady state is reached in about 4 to 6 wk.

Distribution: Vd of toremifene is 580 L. Approximately 99.5% of the drug is bound to plasma proteins, mainly albumin. Mean distribution t½ is approximately 4 hr.

Metabolism: Toremifene is extensively metabolized, principally by CYP3A4 to N-demethyltoremifene.

Excretion: Mean total clearance is about 5 L/hr. Elimination is primarily in feces (as metabolites) with about 10% excreted in urine during a 1-wk period. Elimination is slow. Toremifene t½ is about 5 days.

Special Populations:
Hepatic Function Impairment – The mean elimination t½ was increased by less than 2-fold in patients with cirrhosis or fibrosis.
Elderly – Increases of elimination t½ and Vd were observed in elderly women.

Indications Metastatic breast cancer in postmenopausal women.

Contraindications Standard considerations.

Route/Dosage
Breast Cancer
ADULTS: PO 60 mg once daily with or without food.

Interactions
Anticonvulsants: May increase toremifene clearance by 2-fold.
CYP3A4: Toremifene may be altered by drugs that inhibit (eg, ketoconazole, itraconazole, macrolides) or induce (eg, phenobarbital, phenytoin, carbamazepine) this enzyme.
Thiazide diuretics: May cause hypercalcemia with agents that reduce renal excretion of calcium.
Warfarin: May increase the hypoprothrombinemic effect of warfarin.

Lab Test Interferences None well documented.

Adverse Reactions
CV: Edema; pulmonary embolism; thrombophlebitis; thrombosis; cerebrovascular accident; transient ischemic attack; cardiac failure; MI.
CNS: Dizziness.
ENDO: Hot flashes; sweating.
GI: Nausea and vomiting; elevated LFTs.
GU: Vaginal discharge; vaginal bleeding; endometrial thickening.
METAB: Hypercalcemia.
MUSC: Bone and tumor pain at initiation of therapy; soft tissue lesions can temporarily increase in size.
SPEC SENSE: Cataracts; dry eyes; abnormal visual fields; corneal keratopathy; glaucoma; abnormal vision; diplopia.

Precautions
Pregnancy: Category D.
Lactation: Undetermined.
Children: Safety and efficacy not established.
Hepatic function impairment: Metabolized in the liver; dose reduction may be necessary in patients with liver disease.
Hypercalcemia and tumor flare: Drugs that decrease renal calcium excretion (eg, thiazide diuretics) may increase the risk of hypercalcemia in patients receiving toremifene.
Preexisting endometrial hyperplasia: Avoid long-term use.
Thromboembolic disease: Caution in patients with thromboembolic diseases.

Overdosage: Signs and Symptoms
Vertigo, headache, dizziness, nausea, vomiting, reversible hallucinations, ataxia.

PATIENT CARE CONSIDERATIONS
Administration/Storage
* Store at room temperature. Protect from heat and light.
* Administer PO without regards to food.

Assessment/Interventions
* Tumor flare and hypercalcemia may occur during the first few weeks of treatment. Monitor serum calcium concentrations periodically.
* Monitor CBC and LFTs periodically during therapy.
* Monitor leukocyte and platelet counts.

Patient/Family Education
* Instruct patient to contact the health care provider if vaginal bleeding occurs.
* Inform patient with bone metastases of typical signs/symptoms of hypercalcemia. Contact the health care provider if such signs or symptoms occur.

Torsemide

(TORE-suh-MIDE)
Class Loop diuretic

How Supplied
Demadex Tablets 5 mg, Tablets 10 mg, Tablets 20 mg, Tablets 100 mg, Injection 10 mg/mL

Action
PHARMACOLOGY: Inhibits sodium/potassium/chloride carrier system in ascending loop of Henle, resulting in increased urinary excretion of sodium, chloride, and water. Does not significantly alter glomerular filtration rate, renal plasma flow, or acid-base balance.

PHARMACOKINETICS/DYNAMICS:
Absorption: Bioavailability of oral torsemide is approximately 80%, T_{max} is 1 hr, and AUC is 2.5 to 200 mg; food delays the time by approximately 30 min, but there is no effect on bioavailability.

Distribution: Torsemide is more than 99% protein bound. Vd is 12 to 15 L in healthy adults or mild to moderate renal function impairment or CHF; Vd is doubled in hepatic cirrhosis.

Metabolism: The major metabolite is a carboxylic acid derivative and is biologically inactive.

Excretion: Torsemide is cleared by hepatic metabolism (about 80%) and about 20% is excreted into urine. Torsemide t½ is 3.5 hr in healthy adults.

Special Populations:
Renal Function Impairment – Renal clearance is decreased, but total plasma clearance is not significantly altered. A diuretic response in renal failure may still be achieved if patients are given higher doses.
Hepatic Function Impairment – In patients with hepatic cirrhosis, the Vd, plasma t½, and renal clearance are all increased, but total clearance is not changed.
Elderly – There may be a decrease in renal clearance related to the decline in renal function that commonly occurs with aging.
Decompensated CHF – With oral torsemide, in decompensated CHF, hepatic and renal clearances are decreased.

Indications Management of edema associated with CHF, hepatic cirrhosis, and renal disease; treatment of hypertension.

Contraindications Hypersensitivity to sulfonylureas; anuria; severe electrolyte depletion.

Route/Dosage

ADULTS: PO/IV 5 to 20 mg once daily. Titrate dose upward until desired response is obtained. Single doses greater than 200 mg have not been studied.

Interactions

Aminoglycosides: May increase ototoxicity.
Anticoagulants: May enhance anticoagulant activity.
Cisplatin: May cause additive ototoxicity.
Digitalis glycosides: Electrolyte disturbances may predispose to digitalis-induced arrhythmias.
Lithium: May increase plasma lithium levels and toxicity.
Nondepolarizing muscle relaxants: May antagonize or potentiate response to muscle relaxants.
NSAIDs: May decrease effects of torsemide.
Probenecid: May reduce action of torsemide.
Salicylates: May impair diuretic response in patients with cirrhosis and ascites.
Sulfonylureas: May decrease glucose tolerance, resulting in need for increased sulfonylurea dose.
Thiazide diuretics: May cause synergistic effects that may result in profound diuresis and serious electrolyte abnormalities.

Lab Test Interferences None well documented.

Adverse Reactions

CV: ECG abnormality; chest pain; atrial fibrillation; orthostatic hypotension; ventricular tachycardia; shunt thrombosis.
CNS: Headache; dizziness; asthenia; insomnia; nervousness; syncope.
DERM: Rash; pruritus.
EENT: Hearing loss; sore throat.
GI: Diarrhea; constipation; nausea; dyspepsia; GI hemorrhage; rectal bleeding.
GU: Excessive urination.
METAB: Hyperglycemia; hyperuricemia; hypomagnesemia; hypokalemia; hypocalcemia; hyponatremia; hypochloremia; hypovolemia.
RESP: Rhinitis; cough increase.
OTHER: Arthralgia; myalgia.

Precautions

Pregnancy: Category B.
Lactation: Unknown.
Children: Safety and efficacy not established.
Hypersensitivity: Patients with known sulfonamide sensitivity may show allergic reactions to torsemide.
Photosensitivity: Photosensitization may occur.
Hepatic cirrhosis and ascites: Sudden alterations of electrolyte balance may precipitate hepatic encephalopathy and coma.
Hyperuricemia: Asymptomatic hyperuricemia or gout may occur.
Lipids: Increases in LDL, total cholesterol, and triglycerides with decreases in HDL cholesterol may occur.
Ototoxicity: Associated with rapid injection or very large doses.

Overdosage: Signs and Symptoms

Dehydration, arrhythmias, decreased renal function, blood volume and electrolyte depletion, weakness, dizziness, mental confusion, anorexia, lethargy, vomiting, cramps, circulatory collapse, vascular thrombosis and embolism.

PATIENT CARE CONSIDERATIONS

Administration/Storage

- Administer oral form with or without food.
- Administer IV form once daily via slow (over 2 min) infusion.
- Store in dry area away from sunlight.

Assessment/Interventions

- Obtain patient history, including drug history and any known allergies. Note whether patient has lupus erythematosus, kidney dysfunction, or cirrhosis.
- Assess gross hearing acuity before administration and periodically during drug therapy, especially if drug is being given at high doses or concurrently with another ototoxic drug.
- Monitor lying and standing BP before drug administration. Consult with health care provider if patient is hypotensive.
- Monitor I&O and body weight.

- Monitor electrolytes. Notify health care provider of electrolyte imbalances, especially hypokalemia.
- Monitor hepatic and renal function.

Patient/Family Education
- Instruct patient to inform health care provider of all *otc* or prescription drugs being taken, especially NSAIDs, digitalis, or lithium.
- Advise hypertensive patient to avoid foods or medications that may increase BP, including *otc* drugs for appetite suppression or cold symptoms, *otc* drugs to help keep awake, and excessive consumption of coffee or other substances containing caffeine.
- Instruct patient to eat potassium-rich foods daily. These foods include banana, cantaloupe, and potatoes.
- Advise patient not to store drug in bathroom, but in a cool, dry place.
- Inform patient that drug may raise blood sugar levels. Instruct diabetic patients to monitor blood glucose regularly and report patterns of hyperglycemia.
- Advise patient that this drug increases urination. Advise patient to take medication early in morning to avoid disrupted sleep.
- Caution patient to notify health care provider immediately if vomiting and diarrhea occur or if signs of excessive potassium loss (eg, cramps, muscle weakness, nausea, dizziness) are noted.
- Instruct patient to report these symptoms to health care provider: chest pain, dizziness, rapid heart beat, headache, nausea, increased swelling of feet, black stools, rectal bleeding, rash, face rash, fatigue, or hearing loss.
- Caution patient to avoid sudden position changes to prevent dizziness or fainting.
- Advise patient that drug may cause dizziness and to use caution while driving or performing other tasks requiring mental alertness.
- Caution patient to avoid exposure to sunlight and to use sunscreen or wear protective clothing to avoid photosensitivity reaction.

Tositumomab and Iodine ^{131}I-Tositumomab

(TOE-sih-too-MOE-mab EYE-uh-dine)
Class Murine monoclonal antibody

How Supplied
Bexxar Injection kits

Action
PHARMACOLOGY: Blocks (complement-dependent cytotoxicity) CD20 antigen, which is found on the surface of normal and malignant B lymphocytes. Cell death is associated with ionizing radiation from the radioisotope.

Indications Treatment of patients with CD20 positive, follicular, non-Hodgkin lymphoma, with and without transformation, whose disease is refractory to rituximab and has relapsed following chemotherapy.

Contraindications Hypersensitivity to murine proteins or any component of the therapeutic regimen.

Route/Dosage
ADULTS: **IV** The therapeutic regimen consists of 4 components administered in 2 discrete steps: the dosimetric step followed in 7 to 14 days by the therapeutic step.
Dosimetric step: **IV** Tositumomab 450 mg over 60 min. Reduce the rate 50% for mild to moderate infusional toxicity; interrupt infusion for severe infusional toxicity. After resolution of severe infusional toxicity, resume infusion at a 50% reduction in infusion rate. IV ^{131}I-tositumomab, which contains 5 mCi ^{131}I and 35 mg tositumomab, in 30 mL of 0.9% sodium chloride infused over 20 min. Reduce the rate 50% for mild to moderate infusional toxicity; interrupt infusion for severe infusional toxicity. After resolution of severe infusional toxicity, resume infusion at a 50% reduction in infusion rate.
Therapeutic step (7 to 14 days after dosimetric step; do not administer if biodistribution is altered): **IV** Tositumomab 450 mg over 60 min. Reduce the rate by 50% for mild to moderate infusional toxicity; interrupt infusion for severe infusional toxicity. After resolution of severe infusional toxicity, resume infusion at a 50% reduction in infusion rate. IV ^{131}I-tositumomab, reduce the rate 50% for mild to moderate infusional toxicity; interrupt infusion for severe infusional toxicity. After resolution of severe infusional toxicity, resume infusion at a 50% reduction in rate.

Premedication
ADULTS: **PO** Thyroid protective agents: Saturated solution of potassium iodide (SSKI) 4 drops tid; Lugol's solution 20 drops tid; or potassium iodide tablets 130 mg qd. Start thyroid protective agents at least 24 hr prior to administration of ^{131}I-tositumomab dosimetric dose and continue until 2 wk after administration of the ^{131}I-tositumomab therapeutic dose. Ameliorate/prevent infusion reaction: Acetaminophen 650 mg and diphenhydramine 50 mg, 30 min prior to administration of tositumomab in the dosimetric and therapeutic steps.

Interactions None well documented.

Lab Test Interferences None well documented.

Adverse Reactions
CV: Hypotension (7%); vasodilation (5%).
CNS: Headache (16%); dizziness, somnolence (5%).
DERM: Rash (17%); pruritus (10%); sweating (8%).
EENT: Pharyngitis (12%); rhinitis (10%).
GI: Nausea (36%); abdominal pain, vomiting (15%); anorexia (14%); diarrhea (12%); constipation, dyspepsia (6%).
HEMA: Hematologic toxicities (most frequently observed adverse event); hemorrhage in thrombocytopenic patients; secondary leukemia; myelodysplasia.
METAB: Peripheral edema (9%); weight loss (6%); dehydration.
MUSC: Myalgia (13%); arthralgia (10%).
RESP: Increased cough (21%); dyspnea (11%); pneumonia (6%)
OTHER: Asthenia (46%); infection (eg, sepsis [45%]); fever (37%); pain (19%); chills (18%); hypothyroidism (14%); back pain (8%); chest pain (7%); neck pain, hypersensitivity (6%); severe and prolonged cytopenias; allergic reactions; infusional toxicity (including fever, rigors/chills, sweating); pleural effusion.

> **WARNING:**
> *Hypersensitivity reactions:* Medications for treatment of severe hypersensitivity, including anaphylaxis, should be available.
> *Cytopenias:* Prolonged and severe thrombocytopenia and neutropenia may occur.
> *Pregnancy:* Fetal harm can occur.
> *Special requirements:* Only physicians and other health care professionals qualified by training in the safe use and handling of therapeutic radionuclides should administer ^{131}I-tositumomab.

Precautions
Pregnancy: Category X.
Lactation: Excreted in breast milk.
Children: Safety and efficacy not established.
Elderly: Rate and duration of response were decreased in patients 65 yr and older.
Hypersensitivity: Hypersensitivity reactions, including anaphylaxis, may occur.
Renal function impairment: Impaired renal function may decrease rate of excretion of radiolabeled iodine, increasing exposure to the radioactive component.
Carcinogenesis: Radiation is a potential carcinogen.
Malignancies: Myelodysplastic syndrome and/or acute leukemia may occur.
Hypothyroidism: May occur. All patients must receive thyroid blocking agents.

Overdosage: Signs and Symptoms
Hematologic toxicity.

PATIENT CARE CONSIDERATIONS
Administration/Storage
- Do not administer to patient with greater than 25% lymphoma marrow involvement and/or impaired bone marrow reserve, platelet count less than 100,000 cells/mm^3, neutrophil count less than 1500 cells/mm^3, pregnant women, or to patient who has not received adequate doses of thyroid protective agents.
- For IV administration only. Not for intradermal, SC, or IM administration.
- Administer premedication (acetaminophen and diphenhydramine) 30 min before infusion.
- Carefully follow manufacturer's instructions for dosimetric and therapeutic steps, including dilution, administration set-up, and administration times. Iodine ^{131}I-tositumomab should be prepared, assayed, and administered by personnel who are licensed to handle and/or administer radionuclides.
- Appropriate radiation shielding should be used during preparation and administration of Iodine ^{131}I-tositumomab.

- Therapeutic step is administered 7 to 14 days following dosimetric step.
- Administer dosimetric and therapeutic dose through the same IV tubing set with in-line 0.22 micro filter. Changing IV tubing and filter between doses can result in loss of drug.
- Do not administer if particulate matter, cloudiness or discoloration noted.
- Discard any unused solution.
- Store tositumomab in refrigerator (36° to 46°F) prior to dilution. Protect from strong light. Do not shake and do not freeze. Diluted solutions can be stored for up to 24 hr in refrigerator (34° to 46°F) or for up to 8 hr at room temperature (59° to 86°F). Discard any unused portions in the vial.
- Store iodine ^{131}I-tositumomab in original lead pot in freezer (-4°F or below) prior to dilution. Diluted solution can be stored for up to 8 hr in refrigerator (36° to 46°F) or at room temperature.

Assessment/Interventions

- Obtain patient history, including drug history and any known allergies. Note renal impairment, and concurrent use of anticoagulants or agents that inhibit platelet function (eg, NSAIDs). Note history of allergy to murine proteins (eg, mouse) or previous treatment with products containing murine proteins.
- Ensure that the institution's radiation safety practices are followed while handling and administering Iodine ^{131}I-tositumomab.
- Ensure that CBC with differential and platelet count is obtained and evaluated before starting therapy and then at least weekly for at least 10 to 12 wk.
- Ensure that TSH is obtained and evaluated before starting therapy and then annually thereafter.
- Ensure that serum creatinine is obtained and evaluated immediately prior to administration of therapeutic regimen.
- Ensure that patient who has previously received therapy with murine proteins has been screened for human antimouse antibodies.
- Ensure that thyroid-blocking medications (eg, SSKI) are initiated at least 24 hr before receiving the dosimetric dose and continued until 14 days after the therapeutic dose.
- Ensure that women of childbearing potential use effective contraception before starting treatment, during therapy, and for 12 mo after therapy has been completed.
- Ensure that sexually active men use effective contraception during therapy and for 12 mo after therapy has been completed.
- Ensure that patient receives premedication (acetaminophen and diphenhydramine) 30 min prior to both dosimetric and therapeutic doses to ameliorate or prevent infusion reactions.
- Ensure that whole body dosimetry and biodistribution are determined and evaluated before administration of therapeutic dose.
- Monitor patient for infusion-related toxicity (eg, fever, rigors, chills, sweating, dyspnea, nausea), which can occur during and for up to 14 days following infusion. If reaction occurs during infusion, notify health care provider and be prepared to slow rate of infusion or temporarily discontinue infusion according to manufacturer's guidelines.
- Monitor patient for bleeding or signs of infection. Report immediately to health care provider if noted.
- Monitor patient for signs and symptoms of anaphylactic or serious allergic reactions. Be prepared to treat appropriately.
- Assess patient for CV, CNS, GI, respiratory, and general body side effects. Report to health care provider if noted and significant.
- Do not administer live virus vaccines while patient is undergoing therapy.

Patient/Family Education

- Explain name, dose, action, and potential side effects of drug.
- Advise patient, family, or caregiver that medication will be prepared and administered in a health care setting by a health care provider.
- Reinforce need for compliance with thyroid blocking agents and life-long monitoring of thyroid function.
- Advise patient of the risks associated with cytopenias and the need for frequent monitoring of blood counts for up to 12 wk after treatment and possibly longer.
- Advise patient that radioactive material will be in the body for several days following each dose. Provide and review with patient, family, or caregiver written instructions for minimizing radiation exposure of family members, friends, and the general public.
- Advise patient to immediately report any of the following to health care provider: fever or other signs of infection, sore throat, bleeding, unusual bruising or small purple spots under the skin, signs of an allergic reaction (eg, shortness of breath, rash, hives).
- Instruct women of childbearing potential to use effective contraception before starting treatment, during therapy, and for 12 mo after therapy has been completed.
- Advise women to notify physician if preg-

nant, planning to become pregnant, or breastfeeding.
- Instruct sexually active men to use effective contraception during therapy and for 12 mo after therapy has been completed.
- Instruct patient not to take any prescription or OTC medications or dietary supplements unless advised by health care provider.
- Remind patient that office visits and laboratory tests will be required to monitor therapy and to keep appointments.

Tramadol Hydrochloride

(TRAM-uh-dole HIGH-droe-KLOR-ide)

Class Analgesic

How Supplied
Ultram Tablets 50 mg

Action

PHARMACOLOGY: Binds to certain opioid receptors and inhibits reuptake of norepinephrine and serotonin; exact mechanism of action unknown.

PHARMACOKINETICS/DYNAMICS:
Absorption: Mean absolute bioavailability of tramadol is 75%. Food has no effect. T_{max} is 2 to 3 hr. Steady state plasma concentration of both tramadol and the metabolite are achieved within 2 days.

Distribution: Tramadol is 20% protein bound and is independent of concentrations up to 10 mcg/mL. Vd is approximately 2.7 L/kg. Tramadol follows linear kinetics.

Metabolism: There is no evidence of self-induction. Production of M1 (metabolite) is dependent on cytochrome P450 CYP2D6. The O-demethylated metabolite is M1. Tramadol is extensively metabolized after administration. The major metabolic pathway is N- and O-demethylation and glucuronidation or sulfation in liver.

Excretion: 30% of a dose is excreted in urine unchanged; 60% is excreted as metabolites. The t½ is 6.3 hr for tramadol and 7.4 hr for the metabolite.

Onset: The onset of action is 1 hr.

Peak: Time to peak effect is 2 to 3 hr.

Special Populations:
Renal Function Impairment – In patients with renal impairment, there is a decreased rate and extent of excretion of tramadol and M1. In patients with Ccr less than 30 mL/min, dose adjustment is recommended.

Hepatic Function Impairment – Metabolism of tramadol and M1 is reduced in patients with advanced cirrhosis. In cirrhotic patients, dose adjustment is recommended.

Elderly – In patients over 75 yr, dose adjustment is recommended.

Indications Relief of moderate to moderately severe pain.

Contraindications Acute intoxication with alcohol, hypnotics, centrally acting analgesics, opioids, or psychotropic agents.

Route/Dosage
ADULTS AND CHILDREN 16 YR AND OLDER: **PO** Start with 25 mg/day in the morning and titrate in 25 mg increments as separate doses q 3 days to reach 100 mg/day (25 mg qid). Thereafter, increase the dose by 50 mg as tolerated q 3 days to reach 200 mg/day (50 mg qid). After titration, administer 50 to 100 mg q 4 to 6 hr as needed for pain relief (max, 400 mg/day).
ELDERLY (OVER 65 YR): **PO** Start with low end of dosing (max, 300 mg/day in patients 75 yr and older).
RENAL IMPAIRMENT (CCR LESS THAN 30 ML/MIN): **PO** Increase the dosing interval to 12 hr (max, 200 mg/day).
HEPATIC IMPAIRMENT: **PO** 50 mg q 12 hr.

Interactions
Carbamazepine: May reduce serum tramadol levels, leading to decreased effectiveness.
Digoxin: Digoxin toxicity has been reported.
MAO inhibitors: Risk of seizures may be increased.
SSRIs (eg, fluoxetine): Increased risk of serotonin syndrome.
Warfarin: Anticoagulant effect of warfarin may be increased.

Lab Test Interferences None well documented.

Adverse Reactions
CV: Vasodilation.
CNS: Dizziness/vertigo; headache; somnolence; stimulation; anxiety; confusion; coordination disturbances; euphoria; nervousness; sleep disorder; seizures.
DERM: Pruritus; sweating; rash.
EENT: Visual disturbances; dry mouth.
GI: Nausea; diarrhea; constipation; vomiting; dyspepsia; abdominal pain; anorexia; flatulence.
GU: Urinary retention/frequency; menopausal symptoms; increased creatinine; proteinuria.
HEMA: Decreased hemoglobin.
HEPA: Elevated liver enzymes.
OTHER: Asthenia; hypertonia.

Precautions
Pregnancy: Category C.
Lactation: Excreted in breast milk.
Children: Not recommended for children under 16 yr.
Elderly: In elderly patients over 75 yr, concentrations may be slightly elevated; may have less ability to tolerate adverse effects; use reduced dosage.
Hypersensitivity: Serious and, rarely, fatal anaphylactoid reactions may occur.
Renal function impairment: Dosage adjustments may be required.
Hepatic function impairment: Dosage adjustments may be required in patients with cirrhosis.
Acute abdominal conditions: Tramadol may complicate the assessment of acute abdominal conditions.
CNS depressants: Use with caution and in reduced dosage when administering to patients receiving CNS depressants or SSRIs.
Drug abuse: May induce psychic and physical dependence of the morphine type. Do not use in opioid-dependent patients.
Head trauma: Use with caution in patients with increased intracranial pressure or head trauma.
MAO inhibitors (eg, isocarboxazid): Use with great caution in patients taking MAO inhibitors.
Opioid dependence: Not recommended for patients who are opioid-dependent; use caution when administering to patients who have recently received substantial amounts of opioids.
Respiratory depression: Use with caution.
Seizures: Seizures may occur within the recommended dosage range.
Withdrawal: If tramadol is discontinued abruptly, withdrawal symptoms may occur.

Overdosage: Signs and Symptoms
Respiratory depression, seizures, vomiting.

PATIENT CARE CONSIDERATIONS

Administration/Storage
- Can be taken without regard to meals.
- Administer medication before pain becomes severe.
- Store at room temperature (59° to 86°F), in a tightly closed container.

Assessment/Interventions
- Obtain patient history.
- Assess degree, location, and characteristics of pain before administering.
- Assess vital signs before administering medication. If patient is hypotensive or dyspneic, notify health care provider before administering.
- Monitor I&O and check for urinary retention.
- Assess the effectiveness of the medication in relieving pain.

Patient/Family Education
- Instruct patient to take the prescribed dose at the recommended intervals.
- Inform patient to check with health care provider first before taking any OTC or prescription medications, including analgesics.
- Have patient report any serious side effects to health care provider.
- Advise patient not to wait until pain level is high to self-medicate, because drug will not be as effective.
- Advise patient to avoid using alcohol or other CNS depressants (eg, sleeping pills).
- Advise the patient that this medication may cause drowsiness and to use caution while driving or using heavy equipment or performing other tasks requiring mental alertness.
- Advise patient to notify health care provider if the pain is not relieved by the medication at the prescribed dosage.

Tramadol Hydrochloride/Acetaminophen

(TRAM-uh-dole HIGH-droe-KLOR-ide/ass-cet-ah-MEE-noe-fen)

Class Nonnarcotic Analgesic Combination

How Supplied
Ultracet Tablets 325 mg acetaminophen/37.5 mg tramadol hydrochloride

Action
PHARMACOLOGY:
Tramadol: Exact mechanism is unknown; however, it binds to certain opioid receptors and inhibits reuptake of norepinephrine and serotonin.
Acetaminophen: Inhibits prostaglandin in CNS and reduces fever through direct action on hypothalamic heat-regulating center.

PHARMACOKINETICS/DYNAMICS:
Absorption: The absolute bioavailability of tramadol after administration of a single 100 mg dose is approximately 75%. The mean peak plasma concentration of racemic tramadol occurs at approximately 2 hr. Oral absorption of acetaminophen occurs primarily in the small intestine. Peak concentrations of acetaminophen occur within 1 hr.

Distribution: The Vd of tramadol is 2.6 and 2.9 L/kg in men and women, respectively, following IV administration of 100 mg. Tramadol is approximately 20% protein bound. Acetaminophen is widely distributed throughout the body tissue except fat. The Vd is approximately 0.9 L/kg. Less than 20% is bound to plasma protein.

Metabolism: Tramadol is extensively metabolized in the liver by a number of pathways, including CYP2D6 and 3A4, as well as by conjugation. The O-desmethyltramadol metabolite is pharmacologically active. Plasma levels of tramadol are approximately 20% higher in poor metabolizers (CYP2D6) compared with extensive metabolizers. Acetaminophen is primarily metabolized in the liver. In adults, the majority of acetaminophen is conjugated with glucuronic acid, and is not active. In premature infants, newborns and young infants, the predominant metabolite is the sulfate conjugate.

Excretion: Approximately 30% of the tramadol dose is excreted unchanged in the urine and 60% is excreted as metabolites. The plasma elimination t½ of tramadol and the active metabolite are approximately 5 to 6 hr and 7 hr, respectively. The apparent t½ of racemic tramadol increases to 7 to 9 hr with multiple dosing. The t½ of acetaminophen is approximately 2 to 3 hr in adults and somewhat shorter in children, while being somewhat longer in neonates and patients with cirrhotic disease. Acetaminophen is eliminated in the urine, primarily as metabolites (less than 9% excreted unchanged).

Special Populations: Use in patients with hepatic impairment is not recommended. Clearance of tramadol is 20% higher in women compared with men.

Indications Short-term (5 days or less) management of acute pain.

Contraindications Any situation in which opioids are contraindicated, including acute intoxication with any of the following: alcohol, hypnotics, narcotics, centrally acting analgesics, opioids, or psychotropic drugs; hypersensitivity to any component of the product or opioids.

Route/Dosage

ADULTS: PO 2 tablets (37.5 mg tramadol/325 mg acetaminophen/tablet) q 4 to 6 hr as needed for pain relief (max, 8 tablets/day). In patients with Ccr less than 30 mL/min, it is recommended that the dosing interval be increased not to exceed 2 tablets q 12 hr.

Interactions

Alcohol: Do not use.
Carbamazepine: Concurrent use with tramadol is not recommended because carbamazepine increases tramadol metabolism and tramadol increases the risk of seizures.
CNS depressants (eg, anesthetic agents, narcotics, opioids, phenothiazines, sedative-hypnotics, tranquilizers): Use with caution and in reduced doses.
MAO inhibitors (eg, isocarboxazid), serotonin reuptake inhibitors (eg, fluoxetine): Use with caution because of increased risk of side effects, including seizures and serotonin syndrome.
Quinidine, inhibitors of CYP2D6 (eg, fluoxetine, amitriptyline): Plasma concentrations of tramadol may be increased; the clinical importance of these interactions is not known.
Warfarin: Anticoagulant effect of warfarin may be altered (eg, elevation in PT).

Lab Test Interferences Acetaminophen may cause more than a 20% decrease in mean glucose as measured with *Chemstrip bG* home blood glucose system.

Adverse Reactions

CV: Hypertension; hypotension; arrhythmia; palpitation; tachycardia.
CNS: Somnolence; anorexia; insomnia; dizziness; headache; tremor; anxiety; confusion; euphoria; nervousness; amnesia; hallucination.
DERM: Increased sweating; pruritus; rash.
GI: Constipation; diarrhea; nausea; dry mouth; abdominal pain; dyspepsia; flatulence; vomiting.
GU: Prostatic disorder; urinary retention.
HEMA: Anemia.
HEPA: Abnormal hepatic function.
RESP: Dyspnea.
OTHER: Asthenia; fatigue; hot flushes; allergic reactions.

Precautions

Pregnancy: Category C.
Lactation: Undetermined.
Children: Safety and efficacy not established.
Elderly: Use with caution, reflecting the greater frequency of decreased hepatic, renal, or cardiac function, and concomitant disease and multiple drug therapy.
Abdominal conditions: Assessment of patients with acute abdominal conditions may be more difficult.
Acetaminophen-containing products: Do not use concurrently with other acetaminophen-containing products because of increased risk of hepatotoxicity.
Anaphylactoid reactions: Serious and rarely fatal anaphylactoid reactions may occur.
Head injury: Use with caution in patients with increased intracranial pressure or head injury.
Dependence: Psychic and physical dependence of the morphine-type may occur with tramadol.
Hepatic disease: Use is not recommended in patients with hepatic impairment.
Respiratory depression: Use with caution in patients at risk of respiratory depression.

Seizures: May occur.
Withdrawal: Symptoms (eg, anxiety, sweating, insomnia, rigors, pain, tremors) may occur if tramadol is discontinued abruptly.

Overdosage: Signs and Symptoms
Tramadol: Respiratory depression, seizures, lethargy, coma, cardiac arrest, death
Acetaminophen: Anorexia, nausea, vomiting, malaise, pallor, diaphoresis, hepatic centrilobular necrosis (leading to hepatic failure and death), renal tubular necrosis, hypoglycemia, coagulation defects

PATIENT CARE CONSIDERATIONS

Administration/Storage
- Administer 2 tablets q 4 to 6 hr as prescribed if needed for pain.
- Do not exceed 8 tablets in 24 hr.
- Administer without regard to meals but administer with food if GI upset occurs.
- Store at controlled room temperature (59° to 86°F).

Assessment/Interventions
- Obtain patient history, including drug history and any known allergies. Note history of addiction, hepatic or renal impairment, seizures, drug or alcohol withdrawal, COPD, head injury, increased intracranial pressure, acute abdominal conditions, or concurrent use of MAO inhibitors tricyclic antidepressants, SSRIs, neuroleptics, or other opioids.
- Administer reduced dose to patient with renal impairment.
- Assess type, location, and intensity of pain before starting therapy and frequently during treatment.
- Monitor patient for GI, PSYCH, CNS, RESP, and general body side effects. Report to health care provider if noted and significant.
- Discontinue therapy and notify health care provider immediately if any of the following occur: allergic reaction, respiratory depression, seizures.

Patient/Family Education
- Explain name, dose, action, and potential side effects of drug.
- Advise patient to take 2 tablets q 4 to 6 hr if needed for pain but to not take more than 8 tablets in 24 hr.
- Advise patient to take without regard to meals but to take with food if GI upset occurs.
- Caution patient to not take more tablets than prescribed or more frequently than prescribed. Serious toxicity may develop if prescribed dose is exceeded or doses are taken too close together.
- Advise patient that medication is for short-term use (5 days or less) only and if symptoms persist to contact health care provider regarding other therapies for pain control.
- Instruct patient to avoid taking acetaminophen or other acetaminophen-containing products, tramadol, or other tramadol-containing products.
- Instruct patient to avoid alcoholic beverages and other depressants while taking this medication.
- Advise patient that drug may impair judgment, thinking, or motor skills or cause dizziness and to use caution while driving or performing other tasks requiring mental alertness until tolerance is determined.
- Advise women to inform the health care provider if pregnant, planning to become pregnant, or breastfeeding.
- Warn patient not to take any prescription or OTC drugs or dietary supplements without consulting the health care provider.
- Advise patient that follow-up visits may be necessary to monitor therapy and to keep appointments.

Trandolapril

(tran-DOE-lah-prill)

Class Antihypertensive/Angiotensin converting enzyme (ACE) inhibitor

How Supplied
Mavik Tablets 1 mg, Tablets 2 mg, Tablets 4 mg

Action
PHARMACOLOGY: Reduces the formation of the vasopressor hormone angiotensin II by inhibiting ACE. Results in decreased BP and reduced sodium reabsorption and potassium retention.

PHARMACOKINETICS/DYNAMICS:
Absorption: Food slows absorption, but does not affect AUC. Plasma concentration and AUC are dose-proportional. Bioavailability is 10% as trandolapril and 70% as trandolaprilat (metabolite). T_{max} is 1 hr for trandolapril and 4 to 10 hr for trandolaprilat.

Distribution: Trandolapril is 80% protein bound and is independent of concentration. Binding of trandolaprilat is concentration-dependent (from 65% to 94%). Vd is 18 L.

Metabolism: Trandolaprilat is the major metabolite and is 8 times more active than trandolapril. Other metabolites are glucuronides or de-esterification products.

Excretion: 33% of parent drug and metabolites are recovered in urine and 66% in feces. Trandolapril t½ is 6 hr. The t½ of trandolaprilat is 10 hr.

Peak: Time to peak effect is 4 hr.

Duration: Duration of action is 24 hr.

Special Populations:
Renal Function Impairment – Plasma trandolapril and trandolaprilat are approximately 2-fold greater and renal Cl is decreased approximately 85% in patients with Ccr less than 30 mL/min and in hemodialysis patients.
Hepatic Function Impairment – In patients with mild to moderate alcoholic cirrhosis, plasma concentration of trandolapril and trandolaprilat were 9- and 2-fold greater, respectively, but inhibition of ACE activity was not affected. Consider lower doses in hepatic insufficiency.
Elderly – In patients 65 yr and older, plasma concentrations of trandolapril are increased in hypertension.

Indications
Heart Failure Post-MI/Left-Ventricular Dysfunction Post-MI: For stable patients who have evidence of left-ventricular systolic dysfunction (identified by wall motion abnormalities) or who are symptomatic from CHF within the first few days after sustaining acute MI.
Hypertension: Treatment of hypertension either alone or in combination with other antihypertensive drugs.

Contraindications Hypersensitivity or history of angioedema with any ACE inhibitor.

Route/Dosage
Heart Failure Post-MI/Left-Ventricular Dysfunction Post-MI
ADULTS: PO 1 mg/day. Following initial dose, titrate patients (as tolerated) toward a target dosage of 4 mg/day.
RENAL/HEPATIC FUNCTION IMPAIRMENT: PO For patients with a Ccr less than 30 mL/min or with hepatic cirrhosis, starting dosage is 0.5 mg/day.

Hypertension
ADULTS: PO 1 to 2 mg qd initially with usual maintenance doses of 2 to 4 mg qd.

Interactions
Capsaicin: Cough may be exacerbated.
Digoxin: May cause increased or decreased digoxin levels.
Diuretics: Possible hypotensive effect. Use lower starting doses.
Indomethacin, salicylates (eg, aspirin): May reduce hypotensive effects, especially in low renin or volume-dependent hypertensive patients.
Lithium salts: Increased serum lithium levels and increased risk of lithium toxicity.
Loop diuretics: Effects of loop diuretics may be decreased.
Phenothiazines: Enhanced hypotensive effect.
Potassium supplements or potassium-sparing drugs: May increase serum potassium levels.

Lab Test Interferences None well documented.

Adverse Reactions
CV: Hypotension (11%); syncope (6%); bradycardia (5%); cardiogenic shock, intermittent claudication (4%); stroke (3%).
CNS: Dizziness (23%).
GI: Dyspepsia (6%); gastritis (4%); diarrhea (1%).
LABTESTABS: Elevated serum uric acid (15%); elevated BUN (9%); elevated creatinine (5%).
METAB: Hyperkalemia, hypocalcemia (5%).
MUSC: Myalgia (5%).
RESP: Cough (35%).
OTHER: Asthenia (3%); angioedema (0.13%); anaphylactoid reactions.

> **WARNING:**
> *Pregnancy:* Use in second and third trimesters may cause injury and death to fetus.

Precautions
Pregnancy: Category D (second and third trimester); category C (first trimester).
Lactation: Undetermined. Avoid use in nursing women, if possible.
Children: Safety and efficacy not established.
Elderly: Reduce doses if needed.
Renal function impairment: Reduce dosage. Decreases in renal function may occur if renal function is dependent on the renin-angiotensin system; patients with renal artery stenosis may experience acute renal failure.
Anaphylactoid reactions: Angioedema and anaphylactoid reactions are rarely reported but are potentially life-threatening.
Angioedema: Use with extreme caution in patients with hereditary angioedema.
Cough: Chronic nonproductive cough may occur.
Hepatic failure: May occur. Discontinue drug if patient develops jaundice.
Hypotension/first-dose effect Hypotension may occur during initiation of therapy, especially in patients with severe salt or volume depletion or those with CHF.
Neutropenia or agranulocytosis: Has occurred with other ACE inhibitors; risk appears greater in patients with renal dysfunction, heart failure,

PATIENT CARE CONSIDERATIONS
Administration/Storage
- Administer alone or in combination with other antihypertensives.
- Do not administer to pregnant women during second and third trimesters as fetal and neonatal morbidity and death can occur.
- Give prescribed dose without regard to meals. Administer with food if GI upset occurs.
- Store tablets at controlled room temperature (68° to 77°F).

Assessment/Interventions
- Obtain patient history, including drug history and any known allergies. Note renal or hepatic impairment, conditions predisposing to volume depletion (eg, prolonged diuretic therapy), diabetes, heart failure, anuria, hereditary or idiopathic angioedema, lupus erythematosus, left ventricular outflow obstruction, allergy to any other ACE inhibitor, and concurrent use of potassium-containing salt substitutes, potassium supplements, or potassium-sparing diuretics.
- Ensure that small initial dose and gradual escalation of dose are used in patient with moderate to severe renal impairment (Ccr less than 30 mL/min), hepatic cirrhosis, or in patient on concurrent diuretic therapy.
- Ensure that volume and/or salt depletion have been corrected before initiating therapy.
- Ensure that serum electrolytes and renal function are monitored periodically.
- Ensure that CBC with differential are evaluated prior to starting therapy, at 2 wk intervals for 3 mo, and periodically thereafter in patient with renal impairment.
- Monitor and record BP and pulse. Should symptomatic hypotension occur, hold medication and notify health care provider.
- Take safety precautions if orthostatic hypotension occurs.
- Assess heart failure patient for evidence of worsening failure (eg, daily weights, evaluation of peripheral edema, shortness of breath). Inform health care provider if rapid weight gain (eg, 2 pounds in 1 day or 5 pounds in 1 wk) is noted or if patient is experiencing worsening edema or other symptoms of heart failure (eg, worsening shortness of breath).
- Monitor for signs of hypersensitivity including angioedema involving swelling of the face, lips, eyelids, and tongue. Discontinue medication and notify health care provider immediately if noted. Be prepared to treat appropriately.
- Assess patient for GI, CNS, and general body side effects. Inform health care provider if noted and significant.

Patient/Family Education
- Explain name, dose, action, and potential side effects of drug.
- Advise patient to take prescribed dose without regard to meals but to take with food if stomach upset occurs.
- Advise patient to try to take each dose at about the same time each day.
- Inform hypertensive patient that drug controls, but does not cure, hypertension and to continue taking drug as prescribed even when BP is not elevated.
- Caution patient not to change the dose or stop taking unless advised by health care provider.
- Instruct patient to continue taking other medications for condition as prescribed by health care provider.
- Instruct patient in BP and pulse measurement skills.
- Advise patient to monitor and record BP and pulse at home and to inform health care provider should abnormal measurements be noted. Also advise patient to take record of BP and pulse to each follow-up visit.
- Caution patient to avoid sudden position changes to prevent orthostatic hypotension.
- Instruct patient to lie or sit down if experiencing dizziness or lightheadedness when standing.
- Emphasize to hypertensive patient the importance of the following other modalities on BP control: weight control, regular exercise, smoking cessation, and moderate intake of alcohol and salt.
- Emphasize to heart failure patient the importance of the following other modalities that can help control heart failure symptoms: weight control, progressive exercise program, smoking cessation, and moderate intake of alcohol and salt.
- Advise heart failure patient to weigh daily, keep a record of daily weights, and notify health care provider if rapid weight gain (eg, 5 pounds in 1 wk) is noted or if edema or shortness of breath are getting worse.
- Caution patient that inadequate fluid intake, excessive perspiration, diarrhea, or vomiting can lead to excessive fall in BP resulting in lightheadedness or fainting.

Overdosage: Signs and Symptoms
Hypotension.

- Advise patient that medication may cause dizziness or lightheadedness and to use caution while driving or performing other tasks requiring mental alertness until tolerance is determined.
- Advise women to notify health care provider if pregnant, planning to become pregnant, or breastfeeding.
- Instruct patient to stop taking drug and immediately report any of the following symptoms to health care provider: sore throat, fever, swelling of the hands or feet, irregular heartbeat, chest pains, fainting, swelling of the face, lips, eyelids, or tongue, difficulty breathing.
- Instruct patient to inform health care provider if a persistent cough develops while taking this medication.
- Caution patient not to take any prescription or OTC medications, potassium-containing salt substitutes, potassium supplements, or dietary supplements unless advised by health care provider.
- Advise patient that follow-up visits and lab tests will be required to monitor therapy and to keep appointments.

Trandolapril/Verapamil Hydrochloride

(tran-DOE-lah-prill/veh-RAP-uh-mill HIGH-droe-KLOR-ide)

Class Antihypertensive combination/ACE inhibitor/Calcium channel blocker

How Supplied
Tarka Tablets 1 mg trandolapril and 240 mg verapamil, Tablets 2 mg trandolapril and 180 mg verapamil, Tablets 2 mg trandolapril and 240 mg verapamil, Tablets 4 mg trandolapril and 240 mg verapamil

Action
Pharmacology:
Trandolapril: Reduces formation of the vasopressor hormone angiotensin II by inhibiting angiotensin-converting enzyme (ACE), resulting in decreased BP and reduced sodium reabsorption and potassium retention.
Verapamil: Inhibits movement of calcium ions across cell membrane, resulting in depression of mechanical contraction of myocardial and vascular smooth muscle and depression of both impulse formation (automaticity) and conduction velocity.

Indications Treatment of hypertension.

Contraindications Patients with severe left ventricular dysfunction; hypotension (systolic pressure less than 90 mm Hg) or cardiogenic shock; sick sinus syndrome (except in patients with a functioning artificial ventricular pacemaker); atrial flutter or atrial fibrillation and an accessory bypass tract (eg, Wolff-Parkinson-White syndrome); history of angioedema related to previous treatment with an ACE inhibitor; hypersensitivity to any component of the product; second- or third-degree AV block (except in patients with a functioning artificial ventricular pacemaker).

Route/Dosage
The fixed combination is not indicated for initial therapy. The combination may be substituted for the titrated components.

ADULTS: PO The recommended dose range of trandolapril for hypertension is 1 to 4 mg/day in a single dose or 2 divided doses. The recommended dose range of sustained-release verapamil is 120 to 480 mg/day in a single dose or 2 divided doses. For convenience, patients receiving trandolapril (up to 8 mg) and verapamil (up to 240 mg) in separate tablets administered qd may instead substitute *Tarka* containing the same component doses.

Interactions
Trandolapril:
Agents increasing serum potassium (eg, potassium-sparing diuretics [amiloride, spironolactone, triamterene]; potassium supplements, potassium-containing salt substitutes) – Risk of hyperkalemia may be increased.
Diuretics – Increased risk of excessive reduction in BP.
Thiazide diuretics (eg, hydrochlorothiazide) – Potassium loss caused by thiazides may be attenuated.
Verapamil:
Beta-blockers (eg, propranolol) – Additive negative effects on heart rate, AV conduction, and/or cardiac contractility.
Carbamazepine, cyclosporine, digitalis, theophylline – Serum levels may be elevated by verapamil, resulting in toxicity of these agents.
Disopyramide – Do not administer within 48 hr before or 24 hr after verapamil.
Flecainide – Additive effects on myocardial contractility, AV conduction, repolarization, negative inotropic effect, and prolongation of AV conduction.
Lithium – Increased sensitivity to the effects of lithium and increased lithium serum levels, resulting in toxicity.
Neuromuscular blocking agents (curare-like and depolarizing) – Activity may be potentiated.

Phenobarbital – May increase verapamil Cl.
Quinidine – Increased risk of hypotension in patients with hypertrophic cardiomyopathy. Verapamil may counteract the effects of quinidine on AV conduction.
Rifampin – Bioavailability of verapamil may be reduced, decreasing the therapeutic effect.

Lab Test Interferences None well documented.

Adverse Reactions

CV: First degree AV block; bradycardia; chest pain; angina; second degree AV block; bundle branch block; edema; hypotension; MI; palpitation; premature ventricular contractions; nonspecific ST-T changes; near syncope; tachycardia; hypotension.
Verapamil – CHF/pulmonary edema; third degree AV block; syncope.

CNS: Dizziness; drowsiness; hypesthesia; insomnia; loss of balance; paresthesia; vertigo; anxiety; abnormal mentation; malaise; weakness; headaches; fatigue.
Trandolapril – Decreased libido.
Verapamil – Cerebrovascular accident; confusion; psychotic symptoms; shakiness; somnolence.

DERM: Pruritus; rash.
Verapamil – Ecchymosis; bruising; exanthema; hair loss; hyperkeratosis; maculae; sweating; urticaria; Stevens-Johnson syndrome; erythema multiforme.

EENT: Epistaxis; tinnitus; blurred vision.
GI: Constipation; diarrhea; nausea; dyspepsia; dry mouth.
Trandolapril – Pancreatitis.
Verapamil – Gingival hyperplasia; reversible, nonobstructive paralytic ileus.

GU: Endometriosis; impotence; hematuria; nocturia; polyuria; proteinuria
Verapamil – Gynecomastia; galactorrhea/hyperprolactinemia; increased urination; spotty menstruation.

HEMA: Decreased leukocytes; decreased neutrophils; decreased platelets; decreased WBC.
HEPA: Increased liver enzymes (ALT, AST, alkaline phosphatase).
METAB: Gout (increased uric acid).
RESP: Bronchitis; cough; dyspnea; upper respiratory tract infection.
OTHER: Flushing; arthralgias/myalgias; angioedema; back and joint pain.

Precautions

Pregnancy: Category D (second and third trimester). Category C (first trimester). ACE inhibitors (eg, trandolapril) can cause injury or death to fetus if used during second or third trimester. When pregnancy is detected, discontinue as soon as possible.
Lactation:
Trandolapril – Not established.
Verapamil – Excreted in breast milk.
Children: Safety and efficacy not established.
Elderly: Greater sensitivity compared with younger patients should be considered.
Hepatic effects:
Trandolapril – ACE inhibitors rarely have been associated with a syndrome of cholestatic jaundice, fulminant hepatic necrosis, and death.
Verapamil – Elevations of transaminases with and without concomitant elevations in alkaline phosphatase and bilirubin have been reported.
Hepatic/Renal impairment: Use with caution.
Angioedema: ACE inhibitors including trandolapril may cause angioedema of the face, extremities, lips, tongue, glottis, and larynx.
Cardiac conduction: Verapamil may be associated with a variety of cardiac conduction abnormalities including first-, second-, or third-degree AV block; bradycardia; asystole; severe hypotension; nodal escape rhythms, PR prolongation and ventricular tachycardia in patients with atrial flutter/fibrillation and Wolff-Parkinson-White syndrome caused by antigrade conduction.
Heart failure: Verapamil should be avoided in patients with severe left ventricular dysfunction or any degree of ventricular dysfunction if receiving a beta-adrenergic blocker.
Hypertrophic cardiomyopathy: Serious adverse effects where seen in patients with hypertrophic cardiomyopathy who received verapamil.
Hypotension:
Trandolapril – May cause excessive hypotension in patients with CHF or salt or volume depletion.
Verapamil – Hypotension may occur during initial therapy or with dosage increases and is more likely in patients taking beta-blockers.
Neutropenia/Agranulocytosis: May occur with trandolapril; risk appears greatest in patients with renal dysfunction, heart failure, or immunosuppression.
Neuromuscular transmission: It may be necessary to reduce the dose of verapamil in patients with attenuated neuromuscular transmission.

Overdosage: Signs and Symptoms

Trandolapril: Severe hypotension
Verapamil: Pronounced hypotension, bradycardia and conduction system abnormalities, symptoms secondary to hypoperfusion (eg, metabolic acidosis, hyperglycemia, hyperkalemia, renal dysfunction, convulsions)

PATIENT CARE CONSIDERATIONS
Administration/Storage
- Administer qd or bid as prescribed.
- Administer each dose with food.
- Administer alone or in combination with other antihypertensives.
- Do not administer to pregnant women as fetal and neonatal morbidity and death can occur.
- Administer with caution and reduced dosage in patients with possible depletion of intravascular volume.
- Store tablets at controlled room temperature (59° to 77°F). Keep container tightly closed.

Assessment/Interventions
- Obtain patient history, including drug history and any known allergies. Note history of kidney or liver disease, heart failure, hypotension, sick sinus syndrome without pacemaker, second- or third-degree block without pacemaker, atrial flutter or fibrillation and accessory bypass tract, diabetes, hypertrophic cardiomyopathy, lupus erythematosus, or allergy to any other ACE inhibitor or sulfonamide-derived medications. Note concurrent use of potassium-containing salt substitutes, potassium supplements, or potassium-sparing diuretics.
- Perform periodic monitoring of liver function tests.
- Ensure that serum electrolytes and renal function are monitored periodically.
- Ensure that volume and/or salt depletion have been corrected before initiating therapy.
- Monitor and record BP and pulse. If hypotension results, hold medication and notify health care provider.
- Take safety precautions if orthostatic hypotension occurs.
- Monitor for signs of hypersensitivity, including angioedema involving swelling of the face, lips, eyelids, and tongue. Discontinue medication and notify health care provider immediately if noted. Be prepared to treat appropriately.

Patient/Family Education
- Explain name, dose, action, and potential side effects of drug.
- Advise patient to take qd or bid as prescribed and to take each dose with food.
- Advise patient to try to take each dose at about the same time each day.
- Inform patient that drug controls but does not cure hypertension and to continue taking drug as prescribed even when BP is not elevated.
- Caution patient not to change the dose or stop taking unless advised by health care provider.
- Instruct patient to continue taking other BP medications as prescribed by health care provider.
- Instruct patient in BP and pulse measurement skills.
- Advise patient to monitor and record BP and pulse at home and to inform health care provider if abnormal measurements are noted. Also, advise patient to take record of BP and pulse to each follow-up visit.
- Caution patient to avoid sudden position changes to prevent orthostatic hypotension.
- Instruct patient to lie or sit down if experiencing dizziness or lightheadedness when standing.
- Caution patient that inadequate fluid intake, excessive perspiration, diarrhea, or vomiting can lead to excessive fall in BP, resulting in lightheadedness or fainting.
- Emphasize to hypertensive patient importance of other modalities on BP: weight control, regular exercise, smoking cessation, and moderate intake of alcohol and salt.
- Advise women to notify health care provider if pregnant, planning to become pregnant, or breastfeeding.
- Instruct patient to stop taking the drug and immediately report any of the following symptoms to health care provider: fainting; swelling of the face, lips, eyelids, or tongue; difficulty breathing; yellowing of the skin or eyes.
- Instruct patient to inform health care provider if a persistent cough or bothersome constipation develop while taking this medication.
- Caution patient not to take any prescription or OTC medications, potassium-containing salt substitutes, potassium supplements, or dietary supplements unless advised by health care provider.
- Advise patient that follow-up visits and lab tests may be required to monitor therapy and to keep appointments.

Tranylcypromine Sulfate

(tran-ill-SIP-row-meen SULL-fate)

Class Antidepressant/MAO inhibitor

How Supplied
Parnate Tablets 10 mg

Action
PHARMACOLOGY: Tranylcypromine blocks activity of enzyme MAO thereby increasing monoamine (eg, epinephrine, norepinephrine, serotonin) concentrations in CNS.

PHARMACOKINETICS/DYNAMICS:

Absorption: Tranylcypromine appears to be well absorbed following oral administration of 30 mg/day. T_{max} is 3 hr; however, maximum inhibition of MAO occurs within 5 to 7 days. There is a rapid onset of activity.

Metabolism: Tranylcypromine is metabolized with the release of the active metabolite. In activation is primarily by acetylation.

Excretion: The drug is excreted in 24 hr.

Onset: Onset of action is from 48 hr to 3 wk.

Special Populations:
Slow acetylators – Slow acetylators may yield exaggerated effects after standard dosing.

Indications Treatment of reactive depression.
Unlabeled use(s): Bulimia; treatment of panic disorders with associated agoraphobia.

Contraindications Hypersensitivity to MAO inhibitors; pheochromocytoma; CHF; abnormal liver function; history of liver disease; severe renal impairment; cerebrovascular defect; concurrent use of another MAO inhibitor, tricyclic or SSRI antidepressants, dextromethorphan, or CNS depressants (eg, alcohol), meperidine, sympathomimetic drugs (eg, amphetamines, dopamine, pseudoephedrine), or related drugs (eg, methyldopa, levodopa), buspirone, cheese or food with high tyramine content; cardiovascular disease; hypertension; history of headache; patients older than 60 yr (possibility of cerebral sclerosis).

Route/Dosage
ADULTS: **PO** 10 mg tid initially; if no improvement after 2 wk, titrate up to 60 mg/day in 10 mg/day increments at intervals of 1 to 3 wk.

Interactions
Amine-containing foods: May cause severe hypertension or hemorrhagic strokes.
Anorexiants: May cause exaggerated pharmacologic effects (eg, severe headaches, hypertension, hyperpyrexia) of anorexiants (eg, amphetamines, related compounds).
CNS depressants: May enhance CNS effects.
Dextromethorphan: Concurrent use has been associated with severe reactions (eg, hyperpyrexia, hypotension, death).
Fluoxetine, fluvoxamine, nefazodone, paroxetine, sertraline, trazodone, venlafaxine: Although data are limited, interactions comparable to those of tricyclic antidepressants and tranylcypromine may occur.
Guanethidine: MAO inhibitors may antagonize antihypertensive effect. Insulin and sulfonylureas may enhance hypoglycemic action.
Levodopa: May cause hypertensive reactions.
Meperidine: May lead to severe reactions, including agitation, convulsions, diaphoresis, fever, respiratory depression, and vascular collapse.
Sympathomimetics: May cause severe headache, hypertensive crisis, and hyperpyrexia.
Tricyclic antidepressants, buspirone, carbamazepine, CNS stimulants, cyclobenzaprine, maprotiline, tyramine: May lead to potentially fatal reactions, including seizures and hypertensive crisis, mental status changes, hyperthermia.

Lab Test Interferences None well documented.

Adverse Reactions
CV: Orthostatic hypotension; edema; hypertensive crisis; palpitations; tachycardia.
CNS: Dizziness; headache; sleep disturbances; tremors; hyperreflexion; manic symptoms; muscle twitching; convulsions; vertigo; confusion; memory impairment; toxic delirium; hypomania; coma.
DERM: Rash; sweating; photosensitivity.
EENT: Blurred vision; glaucoma; dry mouth.
GI: Constipation; nausea; diarrhea; anorexia; abdominal pain.
GU: Sexual dysfunction; urinary retention; incontinence.
HEMA: Anemia; leukopenia; agranulocytosis; thrombocytopenia.
HEPA: Fatal progressive necrotizing hepatocellular damage; elevated serum transaminases; hepatitis.
METAB: Weight gain; hypermetabolic syndrome (eg, fever, tachycardia, rapid breathing, rigidity, metabolism, acidosis, coma); hypernatremia.

Precautions
Pregnancy: Category undetermined.
Lactation: Excreted in breast milk.
Children: Not recommended for patients under 16 yr.
Elderly: Use with caution; older patients may suffer more morbidity than younger patients.
Diabetes: May alter glucose control.
Epilepsy: May lower seizure threshold.
Depression: May aggravate coexisting symptoms such as anxiety and agitation.
Hyperthyroidism: Use with caution because of increased sensitivity to pressor amines.

Suicidal patients: Strict supervision may be necessary in patients at risk.

Overdosage: Signs and Symptoms
Excitement, hypotension, dizziness, movement disorders, irritability, insomnia, weakness, severe headache, anxiety, restlessness, drowsiness, coma, convulsions, flushing, hypertension, sweating, tachypnea, acidosis, hyperpyrexia, tachycardia, cardiorespiratory arrest, incoherence, agitation, mental confusion, shock.

PATIENT CARE CONSIDERATIONS
Administration/Storage
- Tablets may be crushed before administration and taken with food or fluids if patient has difficulty swallowing pills.
- Avoid administering medication in the evening due to the possibility of insomnia.
- Do not administer unless the patient has been on a tyramine-free diet for at least 2 to 3 days. Continue this diet for 2 wk after discontinuing medication.
- Do not administer other antidepressants and MAO inhibitors for at least 2 wk after discontinuing.
- Store tablets at room temperature in a tightly closed container.

Assessment/Interventions
- Obtain complete patient history. Note history of liver and cardiac disease, cerebrovascular disorders, hypertension, renal disorders, pheochromocytoma, or severe headaches.
- Monitor BP both lying and standing before initiating therapy. Monitor BP frequently during initial therapy and periodically thereafter. Tranylcypromine produces hypertensive reactions more frequently than other MAO inhibitors.
- Obtain baseline liver function, CBC, and renal function tests prior to initiating therapy. Monitor periodically during treatment with this medication.
- Observe for onset of desired effects (eg, improved mood, improved sleep patterns, better socialization, improved personal hygiene, lower suicidal potential). These should occur with 7 to 14 days with maximal response in 6 wk.
- Monitor for signs of hypertensive crisis (eg, severe headache, chest pain, palpitations, diaphoresis, nausea, vomiting, dilated pupils, photophobia, elevated BP).

Patient/Family Education
- Advise patient that antidepressants restore depressed people to normal moods.
- Inform patient and family that it may be 3 to 4 wk before a noticeable improvement in mood is noted.
- Instruct patient to take the medication at the same time every day.
- Advise patient not to take any other medications, including *otc* or prescription medications without checking with their health care provider first. This medication interacts with a large number of other medications.
- Teach patient to avoid sudden position changes to prevent orthostatic hypotension.
- Instruct patient and family on how to take BP. If the BP is markedly higher than normal, they should notify the health care provider.
- Warn patient that eating foods that contain tyramine or tryptophan while taking this medication can produce hypertensive crisis which is potentially fatal. These foods include, but are not limited to, protein foods that are aged or fermented such as cheeses, pickled herring, liver, hard sausage, pods of broad beans, beer, red wine, yeast extract, yogurt, ginseng, soy sauce, bananas, raisins, and avocados. Arrange for a consultation with a dietitian.
- Instruct patient to ingest caffeine and chocolate only in small amounts.
- Inform patient to avoid the use of alcohol and other recreational drugs.
- Advise patient to use caution while driving or performing other tasks requiring mental alertness until effect is determined.
- Instruct patient to stop taking the medication and notify the health care provider immediately if any of the following occurs: severe headache, chest pain, rapid heart beat, eye pain or photophobia, severe sweating, stiff neck, nausea, or vomiting.

Trastuzumab

(tras-TOO-ze-mab)

Class Humanized monoclonal anti-HER2 antibody

How Supplied
Herceptin Sterile Powder for Injection, Lyophilized 440 mg

Action
PHARMACOLOGY: Recombinant DNA-derived humanized monoclonal antibody that selectively binds with high affinity to the extracellular domain of the HER2. It inhibits the proliferation of human tumor cells that overexpress HER2 and mediates antibody-dependent cellular cytotoxicity (ADCC).

PHARMACOKINETICS/DYNAMICS:

Absorption: At a dose of 500 mg, trastuzumab C_{max} is 377 mcg/mL. Between weeks 16 and 32, serum concentrations reached a steady state with C_{min} 79 mcg/mL and C_{max} 123 mcg/mL.

Distribution: Vd is 44 mL/kg.

Excretion: Trastuzumab kinetics are dose-dependent. Mean t½ increases and clearance decreases with increasing dose level. Mean t½ is 5.8 days (range, 1 to 32 days).

Indications Breast cancer.

Contraindications None well documented.

Route/Dosage
Breast Cancer
ADULTS: **IV** The recommended initial loading dose is 4 mg/kg infused over 90 min. The recommended weekly maintenance dose is 2 mg/kg and can be infused over 30 min if the initial loading dose was tolerated. Trastuzumab may be administered in an outpatient setting. Do not administer as an IV push or bolus.

Interactions There have been no formal drug interaction studies performed with trastuzumab in humans. Administration of paclitaxel in combination with trastuzumab resulted in a 2-fold decrease in trastuzumab clearance in a nonhuman primate study and in a 1.5-fold increase in trastuzumab serum levels in clinical studies. The incidence and severity of cardiac dysfunction increases in patients who receive trastuzumab in combination with anthracyclines and cyclophosphamide.

Lab Test Interferences None well documented.

Adverse Reactions
CV: CHF; peripheral edema; tachycardia; ventricular dysfunction.
CNS: Headache; depression; dizziness; insomnia; neuropathy; paresthesia; peripheral neuritis; asthenia.
DERM: Acne (rare); herpes simplex; rash.
GI: Moderate to low potential for nausea and vomiting; diarrhea (25%); anorexia; abdominal pain.
GU: Urinary tract infection.
HEMA: Mild anemia; leukopenia.
HYPERSEN: Allergic reactions rarely, including anaphylactoid reactions, asthma, hives, rash.
METAB: Peripheral edema.
MUSC: Arthralgia; bone pain; back pain.
RESP: Cough; dyspnea; pharyngitis; rhinitis; sinusitis.
OTHER: Chills; pain; fever; flu syndrome (eg, fever, chills, malaise); infection. Chills and fever reported in approximately 40% within 1 to 2 hr of the initial infusion. Rigors, dyspnea, and hypotension also may occur. Reactions are usually mild to moderate in severity and do not require discontinuation of therapy. The incidence decreases approximately 20% with subsequent doses.

> **WARNING:**
> *Cardiomyopathy:* Ventricular dysfunction and CHF. Increased risk with concurrent anthracycline and cyclophosphamide.
>
> *Hypersensitivity (anaphylaxis, infusion reactions, pulmonary events):* Most cases occur during or within 24 hr of infusion. Rarely fatal.

Precautions
Pregnancy: Category B.
Lactation: Advise women to discontinue nursing during trastuzumab therapy and for 6 mo after the last dose because human IgG is excreted in breast milk, and the potential for absorption and harm to the infant is unknown.
Children: Safety and efficacy have not been established.
Elderly: The risk of cardiac dysfunction may be increased. The reported clinical experience is not adequate to determine whether older patients respond differently than younger patients.

Overdosage: Signs and Symptoms
There is no experience with overdosage in human clinical trials. Single doses greater than 500 mg have not been tested.

PATIENT CARE CONSIDERATIONS

Administration/Storage
- Refrigerate.
- Reconstitute vial aseptically with 20 mL of Bacteriostatic Water for Injection (supplied) or Sterile Water for Injection (not supplied). The final concentration will be 21 mg/mL.
- Withdraw appropriate dose from vial and dilute in 250 mL 0.9% Sodium Chloride.
- Do not reconstitute or dilute with 5% Dextrose since aggregation may occur.
- Trastuzumab is stable for 28 days refrigerated.
- Trastuzumab solutions reconstituted with sterile water are preservative-free; use within 24 hr. The possibility of microbial contamination must be considered.
- Refrigerate diluted solutions and use within 24 hr when stored in PVC or polyethylene bags.

Assessment/Interventions
- Frequently monitor patients for deteriorating cardiac function. Assess baseline cardiac function including history and physical exam and

at least 1 of the following: ECG, echocardiogram, and MUGA scan. Monitoring may not identify all patients who will develop cardiac dysfunction.
- Use with caution in patients with known hypersensitivity to trastuzumab, Chinese Hamster ovary cell proteins, or any component of this product.
- For patients with a known hypersensitivity to benzyl alcohol (the preservative in Bacteriostatic Water for Injection), reconstitute trastuzumab with Sterile Water for Injection, and discard following a single use.

Immunogenicity:
- Human anti-human antibody to trastuzumab was detected in 1 patient.

Patient/Family Education
- Explain name, action, and potential side effects of drug.
- Advise patient, family, or caregiver that medication will be prepared and administered by health care provider in a health care setting.
- Advise patient, family, or caregiver that medication will be used in combination with other agents to achieve maximum benefit possible.
- Review dosing schedule with patient, family, or caregiver.
- Advise patient, family, or caregiver to immediately report any of the following to health care provider: rash; itching; hives; shortness of breath or difficulty breathing; unexplained cough; swelling in arms or legs; fever, chills, or other signs of infection.
- Advise patient, family, or caregiver to report any of the following to health care provider: persistent nausea, vomiting, diarrhea, or appetite loss; persistent or worsening general body weakness.
- Instruct patient not to take any prescription or OTC medications or dietary supplements unless advised to do so by health care provider.
- Instruct women of childbearing potential to notify health care provider if pregnant, planning to become pregnant, or breastfeeding.
- Advise patient that frequent follow-up visits, ECG, heart function tests, and laboratory tests will be required to monitor therapy and to keep appointments.

Travoprost

(tra-voe-prost)

Class Ophthalmic prostaglandin agonist

How Supplied
Travatan Solution 0.004%

Action
PHARMACOLOGY: May reduce intraocular pressure (IOP) by increasing uveoscleral outflow.

Indications
Reduction of IOP in patients with open-angle glaucoma or ocular hypertension who are intolerant of other IOP-lowering agents or insufficiently responsive to other IOP-lowering medications.

Contraindications
Standard considerations; pregnancy.

Route/Dosage
ADULTS: **Ophthalmic** Instill 1 drop in affected eye(s) in evening.

Interactions
None well documented.

Lab Test Interferences
None well documented.

Adverse Reactions
CV: Angina pectoris; bradycardia; chest pain; hypertension; hypotension.
CNS: Anxiety; depression; headache.
EENT: Ocular and conjunctival hyperemia; decreased visual acuity; eye discomfort and disorder; foreign body sensation; pain; pruritus; abnormal vision; blepharitis; blurred vision; cataract; conjunctivitis; dry eye; flare; iris discoloration; keratitis; lid margin crusting; photophobia; subconjunctival hemorrhage; tearing; sinusitis.
GI: Dyspepsia; GI disorder.
GU: Prostate disorder; urinary incontinence; UTI.
METAB: Hypercholesterolemia.
RESP: Bronchitis.
OTHER: Arthritis; back pain; cold symptoms; infection; pain.

Precautions
Pregnancy: Category C.
Lactation: Undetermined.
Children: Safety and efficacy not established.
Active intraocular inflammation: Use with caution in patients with iritis/uveitis.
Bacterial keratitis: Bacterial keratitis has been reported with multiple-dose containers as a result of patient contamination.
Contact lenses: Remove contact lenses prior to and 15 min following administration.
Macular edema: Use with caution in aphakic patients, pseudophakic patients with a risk of torn posterior lens capsule, or in patients with risk factors for macular edema.
Pigmentation changes: Permanent changes to pigmented tissue may occur most frequently involving pigmentation of the iris and eyelid and increased pigmentation and growth of eyelashes. Gradual change in eye color (ie, increased amount of brown pigmentation in the iris) may occur.

PATIENT CARE CONSIDERATIONS

Administration/Storage
- If instilling other ophthalmic eye drops, separate each medication by at least 5 min.
- Store at controlled room temperature. Keep container tightly closed.

Assessment/Interventions
- Obtain patient history, including drug history and any known allergies.
- Ensure that IOP has been measured and documented in the patient's record.
- Ensure that women of childbearing potential are not pregnant or attempting to become pregnant.

Patient/Family Education
- Explain name, dose, action, and potential side effects of drug.
- Warn patient to not instill more often than once a day in the evening. More frequent use may decrease effectiveness of the medication.
- Teach patient proper technique for instilling eye drops. Wash hands; do not allow dropper to touch eye. Tilt head back, look up; pull lower eyelid down; instill drop. Close eye for 1 to 2 min and apply gentle pressure to bridge of nose. Do not rub eye.
- Advise patients who wear contact lenses to remove lenses before instilling this medicine and to wait at least 15 min after instilling eye drop before inserting lenses.
- Advise patient that if more than 1 topical ophthalmic drug is being used, administer the drugs at least 5 min apart.
- Inform patient that this medication may cause a gradual increase in brown pigment in the pupil, which may slowly change eye color.
- Inform patient that this medication may also cause eyelid skin darkening and increases in length, thickness, color, and number of eyelashes.
- Advise patient to contact eye doctor if eye or eyelid inflammation is noted, if eye is injured, or if having surgery on the eye.
- Remind patient that eye examinations and measurement of IOP are necessary while using this medication; advise patient to keep appointments.

Trazodone Hydrochloride
(TRAY-zoe-dohn HIGH-droe-KLOR-ide)

Class Antidepressant

How Supplied
Desyrel Tablets 50 mg, Tablets 100 mg ◆ *Desyrel Dividose* Tablets 150 mg, Tablets 300 mg ◆ *Alti-Trazodone* ◆ *Alti-Trazodone Dividose* ◆ *Apo-Trazodone* ◆ *Apo-Trazodone D* ◆ *Gen-Trazodone* ◆ *Novo-Trazodone* ◆ *Nu-Trazodone* ◆ *Nu-Trazodone-D* ◆ *PMS-Trazodone* ◆ *ratio-Trazodone*

Action
PHARMACOLOGY: Undetermined; may affect serotonin uptake at presynaptic neuronal membrane.

PHARMACOKINETICS/DYNAMICS:

Absorption: Trazodone is well absorbed after administration. T_{max} is 1 hr on an empty stomach and 2 hr with food.

Excretion: Trazodone undergoes biphasic elimination with an initial phase ($t_½$ 3 to 6 hr) followed by a slower phase ($t_½$ 5 to 9 hr).

Peak: Time to peak effect is 1 hr.

Indications Treatment of depression.
Unlabeled use(s): Treatment of neurogenic pain, aggression, panic disorder, cocaine withdrawal.

Contraindications Hypersensitivity to trazodone; initial recovery phase of MI.

Route/Dosage
ADULTS: PO 150 mg/day in divided doses initially; increase in 50 mg increments up to maximum of 400 mg/day (outpatients) or 600 mg/day (inpatients).

ELDERLY PATIENTS: PO Start with 75 mg/day in divided doses.

Interactions
Alcohol, barbiturates, CNS depressants: CNS depressant effects may be additive.
Carbamazepine: Plasma concentrations of trazodone and its active metabolite may be decreased, producing a decrease in therapeutic effect.
Fluoxetine: May increase trazodone serum levels.
Hypotensive agents: May cause additive hypotensive effects.
MAO inhibitors: It is unknown whether interactions may take place. Initiate trazodone therapy cautiously if patient is currently taking or has recently stopped taking MAO inhibitors.
Phenothiazines: Elevated trazodone serum concentrations have occurred, increasing the pharmacologic and toxic effects.
SSRIs: A serotonin syndrome, including irritability, increased muscle tone, shivering, myoclonus, and altered consciousness may occur.

Lab Test Interferences None well documented.

Adverse Reactions
CV: Hypertension; orthostatic hypotension;

shortness of breath; syncope; tachycardia; palpitations; chest pain; MI; arrhythmias; sinus bradycardia; conduction block; cardiac arrest; CHF; conduction block.
CNS: Anger; hostility; nightmares/vivid dreams; confusion; disorientation; decreased concentration; dizziness; drowsiness; excitement; fatigue; headache; insomnia; impaired memory; nervousness; tingling; tremors; convulsions; incoordination; paresthesia; agitation; anxiety; grand mal seizures; hallucinations/delusions.
EENT: Blurred vision; red eyes; ringing in ears; nasal or sinus congestion; tinnitus.
GI: Abdominal/gastric disorders; unpleasant taste; dry mouth; nausea; vomiting; diarrhea; constipation; flatulence.
GU: Altered libido; impotence; priapism; urinary retention; breast enlargement or engorgement; delayed urine flow; early menses.
HEMA: Anemia; hemolytic anemia; decreased WBC.
HEPA: Jaundice; increased LFTs.
OTHER: Hypersensitivity reaction (eg, skin conditions, edema, rash, itching, purpura); muscle aches and pains; decreased appetite; sweating; changes in weight; malaise; allergic skin condition/edema; nasal/sinus congestion; akathisia; allergic reaction; alopecia; anemia; aphasia; apnea; ataxia; cardiac arrest; cardiospasm; cerebrovascular accident; chills; cholestasis; clitorism; diplopia; extrapyramidal symptoms; hematuria; hemolytic anemia; hirsutism; hyperbilirubinemia.

Precautions
Pregnancy: Category C.
Lactation: Excreted in breast milk.
Children: Safety and efficacy in children under 18 yr not established.
Cardiac disease: Not recommended for patients in acute recovery from MI. Trazodone may also cause arrhythmias; patients with preexisting cardiac disease should be closely monitored.
Lab tests: Patients who develop fever, sore throat, or other signs of infection during therapy should have WBC and differential taken, because trazodone may lower WBC and neutrophil counts.
Priapism: Priapism (prolonged, painful inappropriate penile erection) has been reported. Condition may require surgical intervention. Any patient experiencing inappropriate or prolonged erection should stop taking trazodone immediately and notify health care provider.
Suicide: Patients at risk should be closely monitored and not be given access to excessive quantities.

Overdosage: Signs and Symptoms
Priapism, respiratory arrest, seizures, ECG changes, death, drowsiness, vomiting.

PATIENT CARE CONSIDERATIONS
Administration/Storage
- Administer with meals or with light snack.
- Increase dosage gradually; drowsiness may require administration of bedtime dosage or reduced dosage.
- Assess for initial improvement in 1 wk, with optimal effect evident within 2 to 4 wk of therapy.
- Store in tight, light-resistant container at room temperature.

Assessment/Interventions
- Obtain patient history, including drug history and any known allergies.
- Obtain blood studies (CBC, differential) and hepatic studies in patients undergoing long-term therapy.
- Assess mood and mental status before and during therapy.
- Check to be sure oral medication is taken.
- Implement oral hygiene measures in presence of dry mouth or unpleasant taste.
- Implement safety precautions to prevent injury, especially during initial therapy until effect is known. Assist with ambulation.
- Monitor patient for urinary retention.
- Monitor BP and pulse throughout therapy.
- Monitor ECG in patients with cardiac disorders.
- Monitor weight weekly.
- Monitor for side effects, particularly drowsiness, dizziness, lightheadedness, changes in BP or pulse, dry mouth, GI disturbances, altered libido.
- Assess for hypotension, particularly when used concurrently with antihypertensives and nitrates.

Patient/Family Education
- Tell patient that maximal effect may not be evident for up to 4 wk.
- Instruct family to monitor mood during therapy. Observe for suicidal tendencies.
- Advise patient to check weight weekly because appetite may increase with drug.
- Tell patient taking antihypertensives or nitrates about potential for additive hypotensive effect.
- Instruct patient to report these symptoms to health care provider: shortness of breath, chest pain, confusion, convulsions, impotence.
- Advise patient to take sips of water frequently, suck on ice chips or sugarless hard

candy, or chew sugarless gum to prevent dry mouth or unpleasant tastes.
- Instruct patient to avoid intake of alcoholic beverages, sedatives/hypnotics, or other CNS depressants.
- Advise patient to use caution while driving or performing other tasks requiring mental alertness until effect is determined.

Tretinoin (trans-Retinoic Acid, Vitamin A Acid)

(TREH-tih-NO-in)

Class Retinoids

How Supplied

Avita Cream 0.025% ♦ *Renova* Cream 0.02%, Cream 0.05% ♦ *Retin-A* Cream 0.025%, Cream 0.05%, Cream 0.1%, Gel 0.025%, Gel 0.01%, Liquid 0.05% ♦ *Retin-A Micro* Gel 0.04%, Gel 0.1% ♦ *Vesanoid* Capsules 10 mg
❀ *Retisol-A* ♦ *Stieva-A*

Action

PHARMACOLOGY:

Topical: Decreases cohesiveness and stimulates mitotic activity and turnover of follicular epithelial cells, resulting in decreased formation and increased extrusion of comedones.

PO: Induces maturation of acute promyelocytic leukemia cells. When given PO, time to reach peak concentration was between 1 and 2 hr. Tretinoin is more than 95% bound in plasma, predominantly to albumin. CYP450 enzymes have been implicated in the oxidative metabolism of tretinoin.

PHARMACOKINETICS/DYNAMICS:

Absorption: C_{max} is approximately 347 ng/mL. T_{max} is 1 or 2 hr. Orally, tretinoin is well absorbed into systemic circulation.

Distribution: Vd is not yet determined. Tretinoin is more than 95% protein bound (primarily to albumin). Binding remains constant over the concentration range of 10 to 500 ng/mL.

Metabolism: Cytochrome P450 (CYP3A4, 2C8, and 2E) enzymes have been implicated in the oxidative metabolism of tretinoin. Metabolites are 13-cis retinoic acid, 4-oxo trans retinoic acid, 4-oxo cis retinoic acid, 4-oxo trans retinoic acid glucuronide. Metabolites have been identified in plasma and urine. Tretinoin's activity is primarily caused by the parent drug. There is evidence that tretinoin induces its own metabolism.

Excretion: Tretinoin's t½ is 0.5 to 2 hr. 63% is excreted in urine and 31% in feces.

Peak: 1 to 2 hr.

Indications Topical treatment of acne vulgaris; as an adjunctive agent for use in the mitigation of fine wrinkles, mottled hyperpigmentation, and tactile roughness of facial skin. PO treatment for acute promyelocytic leukemia. **Unlabeled use(s):** Treatment of skin cancer; various dermatologic conditions including lamellar ichthyosis, warts, and Darier disease.

Contraindications Do not use if sunburned or have eczema, highly sensitive to the sun, or with skin irritation (*Renova* only).

Route/Dosage

Treatment of Acne

ADULTS AND PEDIATRIC: **Topical** Apply lightly to affected area qd before bedtime.

Treatment of Fine Wrinkles, Hyperpigmentation, and Tactile Roughness of Facial Skin

ADULT: **Topical** Apply lightly to affected area. Use smallest amount possible.

Acute Myelocytic Leukemia

ADULT AND PEDIATRIC (MORE THAN 1 YR): **PO** 45 mg/m²/day in 2 divided doses. Continue therapy for a max duration of 90 days or for 30 days after achieving complete remission, whichever is shorter.

Interactions

Benzoyl peroxide, cosmetics with drying effects, resorcinol, salicylic acid, soaps, or sulfur: May result in significant skin irritation.
CYP450: Elimination may be altered by agents that inhibit or induce CYP450 enzymes.
Photosensitizers (eg, fluoroquinolones, phenothiazines, tetracyclines, thiazide diuretics, sulfonamides): May augment photosensitivity.

Lab Test Interferences None well documented.

Adverse Reactions

CV: Fluid retention; chest discomfort; arrhythmias; flushing; hypotension; hypertension; phlebitis.
CNS: Fatigue; weakness; headache; fever; malaise; dizziness; anxiety; paresthesia; insomnia; depression; confusion; agitation; hallucination; severe headache may be more common in children; cerebral hemorrhage; intracranial hypertension; pseudotumor cerebri.
DERM: Dry skin and mucous membranes; rash; pruritus; increased sweating; alopecia.
ENDO: Hypercholesterolemia; hypertriglyceridemia; weight gain/loss.
GI: Nausea and vomiting; elevated LFTs; GI hemorrhage; abdominal pain; mucositis; diarrhea; anorexia; constipation; dyspepsia.
GU: Renal insufficiency; flank pain; dysuria; spontaneous abortion; fetal malformations.

HEMA: Hemorrhage; DIC.
MUSC: Bone pain; shivering; myalgia.
RESP: Upper and lower respiratory tract disorders; dyspnea; pleural effusion.
SPEC SENSE: Visual or ocular disturbances; ear fullness; earache.
OTHER: Retinoic acid-acute promyelocytic leukemia syndrome, characterized by fever, dyspnea, weight gain, radiographic pulmonary infiltrates, and pleural or pericardial effusions; infections.

> **WARNING:**
>
> *Retinoic acid-APL syndrome:* Occurs in about 25% of APL patients treated with tretinoin, typically occurring within 1 mo of therapy. It is characterized by fever, dyspnea, weight gain, radiographic pulmonary infiltrates, and pleural or pericardial effusions. It is occasionally accompanied by impaired myocardial contractility and episodic hypotension.
>
> *Leukocytosis:* It has been reported in about 40% of patients during therapy. High WBC (greater than 5×10^9/L) at diagnosis indicates increased risk. If signs and symptoms of the RA-APL syndrome are present together with leukocytosis, initiate treatment with high-dose steroids immediately.
>
> *Teratogenicity: Pregnancy:* Category D. There is a high risk that a severely deformed infant will result if tretinoin is administered during pregnancy. The patient must receive full information and warnings of the risk to the fetus. Instruct in the need to use 2 reliable forms of contraception simultaneously during therapy and for 1 mo following discontinuation of therapy.
>
> Within 1 wk prior to institution of tretinoin therapy, the patient should have blood or urine collected for a serum or urine pregnancy test. Repeat pregnancy testing and contraception counseling monthly throughout the period of treatment.

Precautions
Pregnancy: Category C (topical); Category D (PO).
Lactation: Undetermined.
Children: Safety and efficacy in patients younger than 18 yr of age not established (*Renova* only).
Photosensitivity: Tumorigenic potential of ultraviolet radiation may be accelerated. Photosensitization may occur.
External use only: Keep away from eyes, mouth, angles of nose, mucous membranes, and open wounds.
Irritation: May cause severe local irritation. May need to use less often or discontinue temporarily or completely.
Lipids: Up to 60% of patients experienced hypercholesterolemia or hypertriglyceridemia, which were reversible upon completion of treatment.
Pseudotumor cerebri: Retinoids, including tretinoin, have been associated with pseudotumor cerebri (benign intracranial hypertension), especially in children.

Overdosage: Signs and Symptoms
Redness, pain, blistering, cracking of the skin (topical); headache, facial flushing, cheilosis, abdominal pain, dizziness, ataxia (PO).

PATIENT CARE CONSIDERATIONS
Administration/Storage
Cream/Gel:
- Apply at bedtime.
- Wash hands and cleanse affected area thoroughly and dry completely before topical application.
- Apply lightly to affected area using gauze pad, cotton swab, or fingertip. Wash hands immediately after application.
- Avoid applying around eyes, mouth, angles of nose, mucus membranes, and open wounds.
- Do not apply other topical acne products at same time as tretinoin. In some cases other topical acne products may be applied at other times of the day.

Oral capsules:
- Administer bid in evenly divided doses with food.
- Store capsules at controlled room temperature. Protect from light.

Assessment/Interventions
Cream/Gel:
- Assess and document skin condition before initial application and throughout treatment.
- Monitor for side effects including red, irritated, blistered, or crusted skin.
- Assess for photosensitivity reactions.

Oral capsules:
- Obtain patient history, including drug history and any known allergies. Note history of allergy to parabens.

- Ensure that CBC and differential are determined before and periodically during therapy.
- Ensure that liver enzymes are determined before and periodically during therapy. Be prepared to temporarily withhold therapy if liver enzymes elevate to greater than 5 times ULN values.
- Ensure that sexually active women have negative pregnancy tests before starting therapy.
- Ensure that sexually active women, including those with history of infertility or menopause, are using 2 reliable forms of contraception during and for 1 mo following therapy unless a hysterectomy has been performed.
- Monitor patient for signs and symptoms of RA-APL syndrome (eg, fever, dyspnea, weight gain). Inform health care provider if noted.
- Monitor patient for signs and symptoms of pseudotumor cerebri (eg, headache, nausea, vomiting, visual changes). Inform health care provider if noted.
- Monitor patient for GI, CV, CNS, RESP, and general body side effects. Inform health care provider if noted and significant.

Patient/Family Education
Cream/Gel:

- Advise patient that this is a serious medicine and use only as part of a comprehensive program that includes the use of sunscreens, non-oil-based moisturizers, and avoidance of exposure to direct sunlight and the use of sunlamps.
- Inform patient that topical therapeutic response should be seen after 2 to 3 wk, but may not be optimal for 6 wk.
- Advise patient that acne symptoms may worsen initially, but do not discontinue therapy at this time.
- Instruct patient to thoroughly cleanse area before topical application; to avoid application around eyes, mouth, angle of nose, mucus membranes, and open wounds and to thoroughly wash hands immediately after application.
- Advise patient that normal use of cosmetics is allowed but instruct patient to avoid oil-based cosmetics.
- Advise patient not to apply other acne products at the same time as tretinoin, and not to apply tretinoin more than once daily.
- Advise patient that medicated soaps and cosmetics that have a strong drying effect and products with high concentrations of alcohol, astringents, spices, or lime (eg, shaving lotion) may worsen dry skin.
- Explain that temporary hypopigmentation or hyperpigmentation may occur at application site.
- Instruct patient to discontinue use and consult health care provider if sensitivity or increased irritation occurs.

Oral capsules:

- Explain name, dose, action, and potential side effects of drug.
- Explain that medication is used for induction of remission of leukemia and that maintenance therapy will be needed following successful induction.
- Advise patient to take prescribed dose bid with meals.
- Advise patient that if a dose is missed, take it as soon as possible, but if close to the next dose, do not double the dose to catch up, and take the next dose as scheduled.
- Advise patient, family, or caregiver to immediately report any of the following to the health care provider: difficulty breathing; rapid weight gain; visual changes; fever, chills, or other signs of infection; sore throat; unusual bruising or bleeding.
- Advise patient, family, or caregiver to inform health care provider of any of the following: persistent severe headache; persistent nausea, vomiting; severe skin or mucus membrane dryness.
- Advise patient that drug may cause dizziness or confusion and to use caution while driving or performing other tasks requiring mental alertness.
- Instruct sexually active women, unless they have had a hysterectomy, to use 2 reliable forms of contraception during and for 1 mo following completion of therapy.
- Instruct women of child bearing potential to notify health care provider if pregnant, planning to become pregnant, or breastfeeding.
- Instruct patient not to take any prescription or OTC medications or dietary supplements unless advised to do so by the health care provider.
- Advise patient that follow-up examinations and lab tests will be required to monitor therapy and to keep appointments.

Triamcinolone

(TRY-am-SIN-oh-lone)
Class Corticosteroid
How Supplied
Triamcinolone
Aristocort Tablets 4 mg

Triamcinolone Acetonide
Aristocort Ointment 0.1%, Cream 0.025%, Cream 0.1%, Cream 0.5% ♦ *Aristocort A* Ointment 0.1%, Cream 0.025%, Cream 0.1%, Cream 0.5% ♦ *Azmacort* Aerosol 100 mcg/actuation (Inhaler contains 60 mg) ♦ *Kenalog* Ointment 0.025%, Ointment 0.1%, Cream 0.025%, Cream 0.5%, Aerosol 2 sec. Spray ♦ *Kenalog-10* Injection 10 mg/mL suspension ♦ *Kenalog-40* Injection 40 mg/mL suspension ♦ *Kenalog-H* Cream 0.1% ♦ *Kenalog in Orabase* Paste 0.1% ♦ *Nasacort AQ* Spray 55 mcg/actuation ♦ *Tac-3* Injection 3 mg/mL suspension ♦ *Triacet* Cream 0.1% ♦ *Triderm* Cream 0.1% ❋ Aristospan ♦ Oracort

Triamcinolone Diacetate
Amcort Injection 40 mg/mL suspension ♦ Aristocort Intralesional Injection 25 mg/mL suspension ♦ Cinacort Injection 40 mg/mL suspension ♦ Triam Forte Injection 40 mg/mL suspension ♦ Trilone Injection 40 mg/mL suspension ♦ Tristoject Injection 40 mg/mL suspension ❋ Aristocort Parenteral ♦ Aristocort Syrup

Triamcinolone Hexacetonide
Aristospan Intra-articular Injection 20 mg/mL suspension ♦ Aristospan Intralesional Injection 5 mg/mL suspension

Action
PHARMACOLOGY: Anti-inflammatory effect by depressing formation, release, and activity of endogenous mediators of inflammation including prostaglandins, kinins, histamine, liposomal enzymes, and complement system. Also modifies body's immune response.

Indications
PO/IM/IV administration: Replacement therapy in endocrine disorders; adjunctive therapy for short-term administration in rheumatic disorders; maintenance therapy or control of exacerbation of collagen diseases; treatment of dermatologic diseases; control of allergic states; management of allergic and inflammatory ophthalmic processes; treatment of respiratory diseases, including pulmonary emphysema and diffuse interstitial pulmonary fibrosis; treatment of selected hematologic disorders; palliative management of selective neoplastic diseases; induction of diuresis in edematous states caused by nephrotic syndrome or refractory CHF, and in ascites caused by cirrhosis of liver; control of exacerbation in selected GI diseases (eg, inflammatory bowel disease); control of exacerbation of multiple sclerosis; adjunctive treatment of tuberculous meningitis; treatment of trichinosis with neurologic or myocardial involvement; management of postoperative dental inflammatory reactions.
Intra-articular or soft tissue administration: Short-term adjunctive therapy in synovitis of osteoarthritis, rheumatoid arthritis, bursitis, acute gouty arthritis, epicondylitis, acute nonspecific tenosynovitis, posttraumatic osteoarthritis.
Intralesional administration: Management of keloids; treatment of localized hypertrophic, infiltrated, inflammatory lesions of lichen planus, psoriatic plaques, granuloma annulare, lichen simplex chronicus; treatment of discoid lupus erythematosus, necrobiosis lipoidica diabeticorum, alopecia areata, cystic tumors of aponeurosis or tendon.
Topical application: Relief of inflammatory and pruritic manifestations of corticosteroid-responsive dermatoses.
Oral inhalation: Maintenance treatment of asthma as prophylactic therapy; use in asthma patients requiring systemic corticosteroid administration.
Intranasal administration: Relief of seasonal and perennial allergic rhinitis symptoms.

Contraindications Systemic fungal infections; IM use in idiopathic thrombocytopenic purpura; administration of live virus vaccines; topical monotherapy in primary bacterial infections; topical use on face, groin, or axilla; oral inhalation as primary treatment for status asthmaticus or other acute episodes of asthma; intranasal administration in untreated localized infections involving nasal mucosa.

Route/Dosage
TRIAMCINOLONE
ADULTS: **PO** 4 to 100 mg/day.
CHILDREN: **PO** 0.117 to 1.66 mg/kg/day.

TRIAMCINOLONE ACETONIDE
ADULTS AND CHILDREN: **Topical** Apply sparingly bid to qid.
ADULTS AND CHILDREN OLDER THAN 12 YR OF AGE: **IM** 2.5 to 60 mg/day. **Intra-articular/intrasynovial/soft tissue** 2.5 to 40 mg prn. **Intradermal** 1 mg/intradermal injection site. **Inhalation** 2 inhalations bid to qid or 4 inhalations bid (max, 16 inhalations/day).
Nasacort: **Intranasal** Start with 220 mcg/day as 2 sprays (55 mcg/spray) in each nostril daily. The dose may be increased to 440 mcg/day either as once-a-day dosage or divided up to qid (ie, bid [2 sprays/nostril] or qid [1 spray/nostril]). Some

patients may be maintained with 1 spray/nostril daily.

Nasacort AQ: **Intranasal** Recommended starting and max dose is 220 mcg/day as 2 sprays in each nostril daily. When the max benefit is achieved and symptoms controlled at 220 mcg/day, decreasing the dose to 110 mcg/day (1 spray in each nostril/day) may be effective in maintaining control of allergic rhinitis symptoms.

CHILDREN 6 TO 12 YR OF AGE: **IM** 0.03 to 0.2 mg/kg q 1 to 7 days. **Inhalation** 1 to 2 inhalations tid to qid or 2 to 4 inhalations bid (max, 12 inhalations/day).

CHILDREN 6 TO 11 YR OF AGE:

Nasacort: **Intranasal** Recommended starting dose is 220 mcg/day as 2 sprays in each nostril daily. Once the max effect has been achieved, titrate to minimum effective dose.

Nasacort AQ: **Intranasal** Recommended starting dose is 110 mcg/day as 1 spray in each nostril daily. Maximum recommended dose is 220 mcg/day as 2 sprays per nostril daily. Once symptoms are controlled, pediatric patients may be maintained on 110 mcg/day (1 spray in each nostril/day).

TRIAMCINOLONE DIACETATE

ADULTS: **IM** 40 mg/wk. **Intra-articular/intrasynovial/soft tissue** 2 to 40 mg prn. **Intradermal** 5 to 48 mg (no more than 12.5 mg per injection site) prn.

TRIAMCINOLONE HEXACETAMIDE

ADULTS: **Intra-articular** 2 to 20 mg prn. **Intradermal** No more than 0.5 mg/square inch of affected area.

Interactions

Anticholinesterases: May antagonize anticholinesterase effects in myasthenia gravis.
Barbiturates: May decrease pharmacologic effect of systemically administered triamcinolone.
Hydantoins, rifampin: May increase Cl and decrease efficacy of systemically administered triamcinolone.
Salicylates: Systemic administration may reduce serum levels and efficacy of salicylates.
Somatrem: May inhibit growth-promoting effects of somatrem.
Troleandomycin: May increase triamcinolone effects.

Lab Test Interferences

Uptake of thyroid I^{131} may be decreased; false-negative results with nitroblue-tetrazolium test may occur; skin test reactions may be suppressed.

Adverse Reactions

CV: Edema; thromboembolism or fat embolism; thrombophlebitis; necrotizing angiitis; cardiac arrhythmias or ECG changes; syncopal episodes; hypertension; myocardial rupture; CHF.
CNS: Convulsions; pseudotumor cerebri; vertigo; headache; neuritis; paresthesias; psychosis.
DERM: Impaired wound healing; thin fragile skin; petechiae and ecchymoses; erythema; lupus erythematosus-like lesions; subcutaneous fat atrophy; striae; hirsutism; acneiform eruptions; allergic dermatitis; urticaria; angioneurotic edema; perineal irritation; hyperpigmentation or hypopigmentation (injection); burning, itching, irritation, erythema, dryness, folliculitis, hypertrichosis, perioral dermatitis, allergic contact dermatitis, stinging, cracking, and tightening of skin, secondary infections, miliaria, telangiectasia (topical).
EENT: Posterior subcapsular cataracts; increased IOP; glaucoma; exophthalmos; throat irritation, hoarseness, dysphonia, coughing, thrush, dry mouth (oral); nasal irritation, burning, stinging, dryness, epistaxis or bloody mucus, congestion, occasional sneezing attacks, rhinorrhea, anosmia, loss of sense of taste, throat discomfort (intranasal); sinusitis, pharyngitis (oral inhalation/intranasal).
GI: Pancreatitis; nausea; vomiting; increased appetite and weight gain; peptic ulcer; bowel perforation.
HEMA: Leukocytosis.
METAB: Sodium and fluid retention; hypokalemia; hypokalemic metabolic alkalosis; hypocalcemia.
RESP: Wheezing (oral).
OTHER: Musculoskeletal effects (eg, weakness, myopathy, muscle mass loss, osteoporosis, spontaneous fractures); endocrine abnormalities (eg, menstrual irregularities, cushingoid state, growth suppression in children, sweating, decreased carbohydrate tolerance or hyperglycemia, glycosuria, increased insulin or sulfonylurea requirements in diabetic patients, hirsutism); anaphylactoid or hypersensitivity reactions; aggravation or masking of infections; osteonecrosis, tendon rupture, infection, skin atrophy, postinjection flare, hypersensitivity, facial flushing (intra-articular); may cause adverse effects similar to systemic use because of absorption (topical).

Precautions

Pregnancy: Undetermined. Category C (oral inhalation/nasal/topical).
Lactation: Undetermined.
Children: Children may be more susceptible to adverse effects from topical use. Monitor growth and development of infants and children on prolonged therapy. Intranasal/oral inhalation form not recommended in children younger than 6 yr of age.

Elderly: The elderly may require lower doses.
Hypersensitivity: Reactions including anaphylaxis may occur.
Renal function impairment: Use drug with caution.
Special risk patients: Use inhaled corticosteroids with caution in patients with active or quiescent tuberculosis infection, untreated systemic fungal, bacterial, parasitic or viral infections, or ocular herpes simplex.
Tartrazine sensitivity: Some oral dosage forms of these products contain tartrazine, which may cause allergic-type reactions in susceptible individuals.
Acute asthma: Oral inhalation is not indicated for rapid relief of bronchospasm.
Adrenal suppression: Prolonged therapy may lead to hypothalamic-pituitary-adrenal (HPA) suppression.
Allergy: Transfer of patients from systemic steroids therapy to inhalation therapy may unmask allergic conditions previously suppressed by systemic steroid therapy (eg, rhinitis).
Bronchospasm: Bronchospasm may occur with an immediate increase in wheezing following dosing, requiring immediate treatment with a fast-acting inhaled bronchodilator.
CV effects: Use drug with caution after recent MI.
Hepatitis: Drug may be harmful in chronic active hepatitis positive for hepatitis B surface antigen.
Immunosuppression: Do not administer live virus vaccines while patient is on therapy.

PATIENT CARE CONSIDERATIONS
Administration/Storage
PO:
- Administer with meals or snacks.
- If drug is to be taken only once daily, administer early in morning.
- Administer multiple doses at evenly spaced intervals throughout day.
- When large doses are given, consider administering antacids between meals to help prevent peptic ulcers.
- Store at controlled room temperature (59° to 86°F).
- Avoid freezing of oral solution and suspension.
- Protect from light.

IM:
- Shake vial well before withdrawing drug from vial.
- Inject deeply into well-developed muscle.
- Rotate injection sites.
- Avoid injection into deltoid muscle.
- Store at controlled room temperature (59° to 86°F).

Infections: Drug may mask signs of infection and may decrease host-defense mechanisms to prevent dissemination of infection.
Inhalant only: Transfer from oral corticosteroids to inhaled corticosteroids has resulted in death caused by adrenal insufficiency related to a lower systemic availability. A number of months are required for recovery of HPA axis suppression. Patients maintained in at least 20 mg prednisone/day may be at higher risk. During periods of stress or severe asthma attack, patients who have been withdrawn from systemic corticosteroids should be instructed to resume oral steroids immediately.
Ocular effects: Use drug with caution in ocular herpes simplex because of possible corneal perforation.
Peptic ulcer: Drug may contribute to peptic ulceration, especially in large doses.
Repository injections: Do not inject subcutaneously. Avoid injection into deltoid muscle and repeated IM injection into same site.
Stress: Increased dosage of rapidly acting corticosteroid may be needed before, during, and after stressful situations.
Withdrawal: Abrupt discontinuation may result in adrenal insufficiency.

Overdosage: Signs and Symptoms
Moonface, central obesity, striae, hirsutism, acne, ecchymoses, hypertens.on, osteoporosis, myopathy, sexual dysfunction, hyperglycemia, hyperlipidemia, peptic ulcer, electrolyte and fluid imbalance (excessive or long-term use).

Oral Inhalation:
- May be administered alone or in combination with systemic corticosteroids.
- For oral inhalation only. Avoid spraying into the nose or eyes.
- If patient is also receiving bronchodilators by inhalation, administer bronchodilator 5 min before triamcinolone to enhance penetration of latter drug into bronchial tree.
- Open inhaler so that medication canister is vertical and locked into position on built-in spacer.
- Thoroughly shake inhaler. Have patient take drink of water to moisten throat. Place adapter mouthpiece in mouth. Have patient tilt head back slightly, activate inhaler into spacer, and take slow, deep breath for 3 to 5 sec while inhaler is activated. Have patient hold breath for 10 sec and breathe out slowly. Allow at least 1 min between inhalations. Have patient rinse mouth with water or mouthwash after each use.

- Store inhalation aerosol at controlled room temperature (68° to 77°F), away from heat or open flame. Do not puncture or discard pressurized canister in incinerator.

Nasal Inhalation:

- For intranasal use only. Avoid spraying into the nose or mouth.
- Shake gently before each use.
- Actuate the pump 5 times to prime before first use. If pump has not been used for more than 14 days, reprime the pump with 1 spray.
- Clear nasal passages of secretions prior to use. If patient is congested, use topical, short-acting decongestant just before administration to ensure adequate penetration of spray. Saline nasal lavage may help remove secretions.
- Shake canister, place nasal adapter into 1 nostril, and gently close other nostril with finger. While inhaling from nostril, activate canister. Repeat process on other side.
- Do not blow nose immediately after administration.
- If 2 sprays per dose are ordered, administer 1 spray in each nostril, wait a few seconds, and administer second spray into each nostril.
- Store nasal spray at controlled room temperature (68° to 77°F). Discard bottle when labeled number of sprays have been used, even if bottle is not completely empty.

Topical:

- To increase drug penetration, wash or soak area before application.
- May use occlusive dressing such as plastic wrap to increase skin penetration. However, do not use occlusive dressings for more than 12 hr/day.
- Apply cream, ointment, or lotion sparingly in light film; rub in gently.
- Do not place bandages, dressings, cosmetics, or other skin products over treated area unless directed by health care provider.
- Avoid contact with eyes.

Dental Paste:

- For oral use only. Not for use in the eye or on the skin.
- If medication is to be applied once daily, apply at bedtime. If medication is to be applied bid or tid, apply at bedtime and after meals during the day.
- Press a small dab (about 1/4 inch) on the lesion until a thin film develops. Do not rub in.
- Store tube at controlled room temperature (59° to 77°F). Keep tube tightly capped.

Assessment/Interventions

- Obtain patient history, including drug history and any known allergies. Note untreated fungal, bacterial, or systemic viral infection, active or quiescent tuberculosis, ocular herpes simplex, recent nasal surgery, trauma, or septal ulcers (intranasal only).

Oral/IM:

- Document baseline disease state activity. Reassess periodically to document response to therapy.
- Ensure that electrolytes are periodically evaluated during prolonged treatment with systemic product.
- Plot growth pattern in children on prolonged therapy with systemic product. Inform health care provider if abnormalities noted.
- Ensure that therapy is periodically reviewed to determine if therapy needs to be continued without change or if a dose change (eg, increase, decrease, discontinuation) is indicated.
- Monitor blood sugar in diabetic patient when drug is started or dose is changed. Report significant changes to health care provider.
- Ensure that fasting blood glucose is evaluated before starting therapy and periodically thereafter during therapy in patient with risk factors for diabetes mellitus (eg, obesity, family history of diabetes).
- Monitor patient for symptoms of hyperglycemia (eg, polydipsia, polyuria, polyphagia, weakness). Inform health care provider if noted.
- If treatment is to be discontinued after long-term use, ensure that dose is gradually tapered to prevent adrenal insufficiency from occurring. If symptoms of adrenal insufficiency occur, reinstitute previous dosing schedule and attempt a less rapid tapering regimen after patient has stabilized.
- Monitor patient for GI, CNS, CV, DERM, and general body side effects. Notify health care provider if noted and significant.

Oral Inhalation/Intranasal:

- If change is made from systemic (oral) corticosteroids to inhaled or intranasal corticosteroids, observe patient carefully for signs of adrenal insufficiency (eg, nausea, fatigue, dizziness, hypotension, depression, or abdominal, joint, or muscle pain). Notify health care provider if these signs occur. Deaths caused by adrenal insufficiency have occurred during and after converting to aerosol corticosteroids.
- Assess patient's symptoms before initiating therapy and periodically during treatment. Notify health care provider if symptoms do not improve or worsen.
- Notify health care provider if oral, nasal, or pharyngeal irritation occurs or if symptoms worsen.

Patient/Family Education
- Explain name, dose, action, and potential side effects of drug.
- Advise patient to read the *Patient Information* leaflet before starting therapy and again with each refill.
- Advise patient to continue taking other medications for same condition as prescribed by health care provider.
- Advise patient that dose may be changed periodically, depending on how well symptoms are controlled.
- Explain that effects of drug are not immediate. Benefit requires daily use as instructed and usually begins to occur within 1 or 2 days, but full benefit may take 1 to 2 wk, depending on the condition being treated and the dose and route of administration of medication being used.
- Caution patient not to decrease the dose or stop taking unless advised by health care provider.
- Caution patient not to increase dose but to inform health care provider if symptoms do not seem to be improving or are worsening.
- Instruct diabetic patient to monitor blood glucose more frequently when drug is started or dose is changed and to inform health care provider of significant changes in readings.
- Advise patient to immediately notify health care provider if any of the following occur: swelling of feet or ankles, muscle weakness, black tarry stools, vomiting of blood, fever, sore throat, or other signs of infection.
- Advise patient to avoid exposure to chickenpox and measles and to seek medical advice immediately if exposed.
- Advise women to notify health care provider if pregnant, planning to become pregnant, or breastfeeding.
- Caution patient not to take any prescription or OTC medications, dietary supplements, or herbal preparations unless advised by health care provider.
- Advise patient that follow-up visits may be required to monitor therapy and to keep appointments.

Oral Inhalation:
- Review proper administration technique. Have patient demonstrate technique to ensure effective use of the MDI and attached spacer.
- Warn patient that drug is an asthma controller and is not to be used to treat an acute asthma attack. Rescue medication (bronchodilator) must be used to obtain rapid relief of asthma symptoms.
- Instruct patient not to stop the medication once symptoms have been controlled. Continued daily use is necessary to control symptoms.
- Advise patient to discard the aerosol canister when the labeled number of doses has been used.
- Instruct patient to carry Medi-Alert card if experiencing acute severe asthma attacks requiring rapid systemic treatment.
- Advise patient to report the following symptoms to health care provider: sore throat or mouth, cough, dry mouth, rash, facial swelling, worsening asthma symptoms (increasing need for bronchodilator).

Nasal Inhalation:
- Review proper administration technique. Have patient demonstrate technique to ensure effective use of the nasal spray.
- Instruct patient not to stop the medication once symptoms have been controlled. Continued daily use is necessary to control symptoms.
- Instruct patient to use with caution if sores develop or injuries occur in nasal passages. Drug may prevent or slow proper healing.
- Advise patient to report the following symptoms to health care provider: sneezing, nasal irritation, nosebleed.
- Advise patient to discard bottle when labeled number of sprays have been used even if bottle is not completely empty.

Oral/IM:
- Advise patient to carry Medi-Alert card indicating use of corticosteroids, the condition(s) being treated, and possible need of supplemental systemic corticosteroids during periods of stress.
- Caution patient not to suddenly stop taking this medication after more than 1 mo of use. Advise patient that if medication needs to be discontinued after prolonged therapy (eg, greater than 1 mo), it will be slowly withdrawn to prevent adrenal insufficiency.
- Review signs and symptoms of adrenal insufficiency (eg, nausea, fatigue, dizziness, hypotension, depression, abdominal, joint, or muscle pain). Instruct patient to immediately seek medical care if symptoms suggestive of adrenal insufficiency develop.
- If patient is being converted from oral to inhaled or intranasal corticosteroids, review signs and symptoms of adrenal insufficiency, which may occur days or weeks after conversion is complete. Advise patient to carry Medi-Alert card indicating possible need of supplemental systemic corticosteroids during periods of stress or a severe asthma attack.

Dental Paste:
- Teach patient proper technique for applying the paste: press a small dab (about ¼ inch) on the lesion until a thin film develops. Caution patient not to rub the paste into the lesion.
- Advise patient to apply at bedtime if being used once a day and after meals if being used more than once a day.
- Advise patient to stop using and inform health care provider if any of the following local reactions occur: burning, itching, new blistering or peeling, irritation, new sores.

Triamterene

(try-AM-tur-een)

Class Potassium-sparing diuretic

How Supplied
Dyrenium Capsules 50 mg, Capsules 100 mg

Action
PHARMACOLOGY: Interferes with sodium reabsorption at distal renal tubule, resulting in increased excretion of sodium and water and decreased excretion of potassium.

PHARMACOKINETICS/DYNAMICS:

Absorption: C_{max} is 30 ng/mL and T_{max} is 3 hr. Triamterene is rapidly absorbed; maximum effect is seen in several days.

Distribution: Triamterene crosses the placental barrier.

Metabolism: Triamterene is primarily metabolized to sulfate conjugate of hydroxytriamterene.

Excretion: Less than 50% of triamterene is excreted in urine.

Onset: Onset of action is 2 to 4 hr after ingestion.

Peak: Time to peak effect is 3 hr.

Duration: Duration of diuresis depends on several factors, especially renal function, but generally it tapers off 7 to 9 hr after administration.

Indications Treatment of edema associated with CHF, hepatic cirrhosis and nephrotic syndrome; treatment of steroid-induced edema, idiopathic edema, and edema caused by secondary hyperaldosteronism; management of hypertension in patient with diuretic-induced hypokalemia or at risk of hypokalemia.

Contraindications Treatment with spironolactone or amiloride; anuria severe hepatic disease; hyperkalemia; severe or progressive kidney disease or dysfunction, with exception of nephrosis.

Route/Dosage
ADULTS: PO 100 mg bid after meals (max, 300 mg/day).
CHILDREN: PO 2 to 4 mg/kg/day given in 1 dose or 2 divided doses (max, 300 mg/day).

Interactions
ACE inhibitors: May result in severely elevated serum potassium levels.
Indomethacin: May cause rapid progression into acute renal failure.
Potassium preparations and salt substitutes: May severely increase serum potassium levels, possibly resulting in cardiac arrhythmias or cardiac arrest. Do not take with potassium preparations.

Lab Test Interferences May interfere with fluorometry such as quinidine serum levels and LDH determination.

Adverse Reactions
CV: Hypotension.
CNS: Weakness; fatigue; dizziness; headache.
DERM: Photosensitivity; rash.
GI: Diarrhea; nausea; vomiting; dry mouth.
GU: Azotemia; elevated BUN and creatinine; renal stones; bluish discoloration to urine; interstitial nephritis.
HEMA: Thrombocytopenia; megaloblastic anemia.
HEPA: Jaundice; liver enzyme abnormalities.
METAB: Hyponatremia; hyperchloremic metabolic acidosis; hyperkalemia.
OTHER: Anaphylaxis; muscle cramps.

Precautions
Pregnancy: Category B.
Lactation: Undetermined.
Renal function impairment: Use drug with caution; monitor renal function.
Adult-onset diabetes mellitus: Blood glucose levels may be increased; dosage adjustments of hypoglycemic agents may be needed.
Concurrent diuretic therapy: Dosage reduction may be necessary.
Electrolyte imbalances and BUN increase: Hyperkalemia (serum potassium greater than 5.5 mEq/L), hyponatremia, hyperchloremia, and increases in BUN may occur. Monitor serum electrolytes and BUN levels.
Hematologic effects: Triamterene is weak folic acid antagonist and may contribute to appearance of megaloblastosis.
Metabolic acidosis: May decrease alkali reserve with possibility of metabolic acidosis.
Renal stones: Triamterene has been found in renal stones. Use drug with caution in patients with history of stone formation.

Overdosage: Signs and Symptoms
Hypotension, hyperkalemia, metabolic acidosis, nausea, vomiting, weakness, acute renal failure.

PATIENT CARE CONSIDERATIONS

Administration/Storage
- Administer after meals.
- Administer once daily dose in morning to avoid disturbing sleep.
- Open capsules and mix with food or fluids if appropriate for patient needs.
- Store at room temperature in tight, light resistant container.

Assessment/Interventions
- Obtain patient history, including drug history and any known allergies.
- Assess renal status, BUN, creatinine levels, and fluid and electrolyte status.
- Assess I&O, body weight, and hydration status.
- Assess lung sounds and peripheral edema.
- Assess vital signs, especially BP.
- Institute safety precautions to prevent falls, particularly with initial doses.
- Monitor for signs and symptoms of hyperkalemia, especially with diabetic patients.
- Monitor for signs and symptoms of side effects, (eg, hyperkalemia, GI disturbances, weakness, dizziness, unusual bleeding or bruising).
- Monitor patient for signs of metabolic acidosis; hyperventilation, drowsiness, restlessness.

Patient/Family Education
- Tell patient to avoid salt substitutes and limit potassium-rich foods.
- Inform patients taking antihypertensives that additive effects are possible; identify signs and symptoms of hypotension and precautions to be taken.
- Advise patient that medication may cause urine to become blue tinged.
- Explain potential GI side effects and to take medication after meals.
- Tell patient that drug may cause weakness, headache, nausea, vomiting, or dry mouth and to notify health care provider if they become severe or persistent.
- Instruct patient to report these symptoms to health care provider: fever, sore throat, mouth sores, unusual bleeding or bruising.
- Caution patient to avoid intake of alcoholic beverages or other CNS depressants.
- Advise patient to use caution while driving or performing other tasks requiring mental alertness.
- Caution patient to avoid exposure to sunlight or ultraviolet light and to use sunscreen or wear protective clothing to prevent photosensitivity reaction.

Triazolam

(try-AZE-oh-lam)

Class Sedative and hypnotic/Benzodiazepine

How Supplied
Halcion Tablets 0.125 mg, Tablets 0.25 mg
✤ *Alti-Triazolam* ◆ *APO-Triazo* ◆ *Gen-Triazolam*

Action
PHARMACOLOGY: Potentiates action of GABA (gamma-aminobutyric acid), an inhibitory neurotransmitter, resulting in increased neuronal inhibition and CNS depression, especially in limbic system and reticular formation.

PHARMACOKINETICS/DYNAMICS:
Absorption: Triazolam's T_{max} is 2 hr; C_{max} is 1 to 6 ng/mL. Plasma levels achieved are proportional to the dose given.

Metabolism: Metabolites are mainly conjugated glucuronides presumably inactive.

Excretion: Triazolam plasma t½ is 1.5 to 5.5 hr. Metabolites are primarily excreted in urine (79.9%). Urinary excretion is biphasic in its time course.

Indications
Treatment of insomnia.

Contraindications
Hypersensitivity to benzodiazepines; pregnancy.

Route/Dosage
ADULTS: PO 0.125 to 0.5 mg at bedtime.
ELDERLY OR DEBILITATED PATIENTS: Initiate with 0.125 mg until individual response is determined.

Interactions
Alcohol, CNS depressants (eg, narcotic sedatives): May cause additive CNS depressant effects.
Cimetidine, disulfiram, omeprazole, oral contraceptives: Triazolam effects may increase.
Digoxin: Serum digoxin concentrations may be increased.
Theophylline: May antagonize sedative effects.

Lab Test Interferences
None well documented.

Adverse Reactions
CNS: Anterograde amnesia; headache; nervousness; drowsiness; confusion; talkativeness; apprehension; irritability; euphoria; weakness; tremor; incoordination; memory impairment; depression; ataxia; dizziness; dreaming/nightmares; hallucinations; paradoxical reactions (eg, anger, hostility, mania, muscle spasms).
DERM: Rash; photosensitivity.
EENT: Visual or auditory disturbances; depressed hearing; taste disturbances.

GI: Heartburn; nausea; vomiting; diarrhea; constipation; dry mouth; anorexia.
HEMA: Blood dyscrasias including agranulocytosis; anemia; thrombocytopenia; leukopenia; neutropenia.
HEPA: Hepatic dysfunction including hepatitis and jaundice.
OTHER: Dependence/withdrawal syndrome (eg, confusion, abnormal perception of movement, depersonalization, muscle twitching, psychosis, paranoid delusions, seizures). Rebound sleep disorder (recurrence of insomnia worse than before treatment) may occur during first 3 nights after abrupt discontinuation.

Precautions
Pregnancy: Category X.
Lactation: Undetermined.
Children: Not for use in children under 18 yr.
Special risk patients: Use drug with caution in elderly patients and patients with renal or hepatic impairment, depression or suicidal tendencies, drug abuse and dependence, chronic pulmonary insufficiency or apnea, seizure disorder.
Dependence: Prolonged use (more than 1 to 2 wk) can lead to dependence. Withdrawal syndrome may occur; taper dose gradually.

Overdosage: Signs and Symptoms
Somnolence, confusion, delirium, lack of coordination, ataxia, slurred speech, respiratory depression, coma, seizures.

PATIENT CARE CONSIDERATIONS

Administration/Storage
- Administer at bedtime with full glass of water.
- Administer with food if GI upset occurs.
- Administer lowest dosage until response is determined.
- If patient exhibits possible suicidal tendencies, ensure that patient swallows drug and that patient does not have access to large quantities.
- Store at room temperature in a tight, light-resistant container.

Assessment/Interventions
- Obtain patient history, including drug history and any known allergies. Identify potential for abuse and underlying depression.
- Assess usual sleep patterns and define type of sleep alteration, (eg, insomnia). Assess for modifiable causes of sleep disturbance, such as environmental noise, daytime sleeping, and caffeine use.
- Assess therapeutic response to therapy throughout usage.
- Implement safety precautions to prevent injury (eg, assist with ambulation), particularly during initial treatment until individual response is determined.
- Utilize general comfort measures to encourage sleep.
- Implement environmental control measures when appropriate to enhance sleep.
- Monitor for side effects, such as dizziness, drowsiness, headache, change in mood or mental status, GI disturbance, paradoxical excitation.
- Monitor for daytime drowsiness or lethargy.
- Assess for signs of dependence.

Patient/Family Education
- Caution patient that this medication must not be taken during pregnancy or when pregnancy is possible. Advise patient to use reliable form of birth control while taking this drug.
- Remind patient that medication should not be abruptly discontinued.
- Review with patient and family other general sleep promotion measures, as well as what to avoid, such as caffeine and excessive exercise at bedtime.
- Explain that medication may cause morning drowsiness or tiredness.
- Caution patient regarding dependence potential.
- Explain potential side effects and what to report to health care provider (eg, confusion, paradoxical excitement, headache, bleeding, recurrent sleep disorder).
- Instruct patient to avoid intake of alcoholic beverages or other CNS depressants.
- Advise patient to use caution while driving or performing other tasks requiring mental alertness.
- Instruct patient not to take OTC medications without consulting health care provider.

Trientine Hydrochloride

(TRY-eh-TEEN HIGH-droe-KLOR-ide)

Class Detoxification/Chelating agent

How Supplied
Syprine Capsules 250 mg

Action
PHARMACOLOGY: Forms chelate with copper, facilitating removal from the body.

Indications Treatment of Wilson disease in patients intolerant of penicillamine.

Contraindications Standard considerations.

Route/Dosage
ADULTS: PO Initially, 750 to 1250 mg/day in divided doses bid, tid, or qid (max, 2000 mg/day).
CHILDREN 12 YR AND UNDER: PO Initially, 500 to 750 mg/day in divided doses bid, tid, or qid (max, 1500 mg/day).

Interactions
Mineral supplements: In general, do not give mineral supplements because they may block the absorption of trientine. Because iron deficiency may develop, iron may be given in short courses if necessary, separating the administration times of iron and trientine by 2 hr.
Food, other drugs: To permit maximum absorption, administer trientine on an empty stomach at least 1 hr before or 2 hr after meals and at least 1 hr apart from any other drug, food, or milk.

Lab Test Interferences None well documented.

Adverse Reactions
CNS: Malaise; weakness.
DERM: Thickening, fissuring, and flaking of the skin.
GI: Heartburn; epigastric pain and tenderness; acute gastritis; abdominal pain; anorexia; cramps.
HEMA: Hypochromic microcytic anemia.
METAB: Iron deficiency.
RESP: Asthma; bronchitis.
OTHER: System lupus erythematosus; dystonia; muscular spasm; myasthenia gravis; aphthoid ulcers; melena; muscle pain; rhabdomyolysis.

Precautions
Pregnancy: Category C.
Lactation: Undetermined.
Children: Safety and efficacy not established; however, trientine has been used clinically in children as young as 6 yr without reported adverse effects.
Elderly: Use with caution because of the greater frequency of decreased hepatic, renal, or cardiac function and concomitant diseases or other drug therapy.
Hypersensitivity: Although not reported, observe patients for signs of possible hypersensitivity.

PATIENT CARE CONSIDERATIONS

Administration/Storage
- Total daily dose is divided and administered as either bid, tid, or qid.
- Administer each dose on an empty stomach, 1 hr before or 2 hr after meals and at least 1 hr apart from any other drug, food, or milk. Separate trientine and iron administration by at least 2 hr.
- Swallow capsules whole with a full glass of water. Do not crush, cut, or chew.
- If skin contact with capsule contents occurs, thoroughly wash exposed skin with water promptly after exposure.
- Store capsules in refrigerator (36° to 46°F). Keep container tightly closed.

Assessment/Interventions
- Obtain patient history, including drug history and any known allergies.
- Ensure that patient is on a low copper diet.
- Measure and record temperature nightly during the first month of treatment. Report fever to health care provider.
- Assess patient for skin eruptions and report immediately to health care provider if noted.
- Ensure that therapy is monitored with periodic (eg, q 6 to 12 mo) serum-free copper levels and 24 hr urinary copper analysis.
- With the exception of iron, avoid concurrent use of mineral supplements or mineral-containing products.

Patient/Family Education
- Explain name, dose, action, and potential side effects of drug.
- Remind patient or caregiver that following a low-copper diet is an important part of therapy and that medication therapy will be continued for months to years.
- Advise patient or caregiver that each dose should be taken with a full glass of water on an empty stomach, 1 hr before or 2 hr after meals and at least 1 hr apart from any other drug, food, or milk. Advise patient who is also taking iron supplements to separate trientine and iron administration by at least 2 hr.
- Advise patient or caregiver that capsules should be swallowed whole. Do not crush, chew, cut, or open capsules.
- Advise patient or caregiver that if accidental skin contact occurs with contents of capsule

to immediately flush exposed skin with water to remove medication.
- Instruct patient or caregiver to take and record temperature each night for the first month of therapy and to report any fever or elevated temperature to health care provider.
- Instruct patient or caregiver to immediately report skin rash or eruption to health care provider.
- Advise women to notify health care provider if pregnant, planning to become pregnant, or breastfeeding.
- Instruct patient not to take any prescription or OTC medications or dietary supplements, including mineral supplements, unless advised by health care provider.
- Advise patient that follow-up visits and lab tests will be required to monitor therapy and to keep appointments.

Trifluoperazine Hydrochloride

(try-flew-oh-PURR-uh-zeen HIGH-droe-KLOR-ide)

Class Antipsychotic/Phenothiazine

How Supplied
Trifluoperazine Hydrochloride Tablet 1 mg, Tablet 2 mg, Tablet 5 mg, Tablet 10 mg
✤ *Apo-Trifluoperazine*

Action
PHARMACOLOGY: Effects apparently related to dopamine receptor blocking in CNS.

PHARMACOKINETICS/DYNAMICS:
Absorption: Absorption is erratic and variable. T_{max} occurs 2 to 4 hr after oral use.

Distribution: Trifluoperazine is widely distributed in tissues. CNS concentrations exceed those in plasma. Approximately 91% to 99% of the drug is protein bound. Because trifluoperazine is highly lipophilic, parent drug and metabolites accumulate in brain, lungs, and other tissues with high blood supply. The drug may be found in urine for up to 6 mo after the last dose.

Metabolism: Extensive biotransformation occurs in the liver. Numerous active metabolites, which persist for prolonged periods, have important side effects and contribute to the biological activity of the parent drug.

Excretion: 50% of excretion occurs via kidneys; the other 50% is through enterohepatic circulation. The t½ is approximately 20 to 40 hr. Less than 1% is excreted as unchanged drug.

Special Populations:
Elderly – The elderly have diminished capacity to metabolize and eliminate trifluoperazine.
Children – Fetuses and infants have diminished capacity to metabolize and eliminate trifluoperazine; children tend to metabolize more rapidly than adults.

Indications Management of schizophrenia; short-term treatment (less than 12 wk) of nonpsychotic anxiety.

Contraindications Sensitivity to phenothiazines; comatose or severely depressed states; presence of large amounts of other CNS depressants; bone marrow depression or blood dyscrasias; liver disease.

Route/Dosage
Individualize dose.
Schizophrenia
ADULTS: **PO** 2 to 5 mg bid initially. *Maintenance:* 15 to 20 mg/day in single or divided doses. Few patients may require 40 mg/day or more.
CHILDREN: Individualize dosage based on weight of child and severity of symptoms.
CHILDREN 6 TO 12 YR: **PO** 1 mg qd or bid initially. *Maintenance:* Rarely over 15 mg/day in single or divided doses.

Nonpsychotic Anxiety
ADULTS: **PO** 1 to 2 mg bid (max, 6 mg/day).

Interactions
Alcohol and other CNS depressants (eg, narcotics, sedatives): May result in increased CNS depression and may precipitate dystonic reactions.
Anticholinergics: May reduce therapeutic effects of trifluoperazine and worsen anticholinergic effects of trifluoperazine. May lead to tardive dyskinesia.
Barbiturate anesthetics: May increase frequency and severity of neuromuscular excitation and hypotension.
Beta-blockers: May result in increased plasma levels of beta-blocker and trifluoperazine.
Cisapride, sparfloxacin: The risk of life-threatening cardiac arrhythmias, including torsades de pointes, may be increased.
Guanethidine: May inhibit hypotensive action of guanethidine.
Metrizamide: Possibility of seizure may be increased when subarachnoid metrizamide injection is used.
Paroxetine: Plasma levels of trifluoperazine may be elevated, increasing the risk of side effects.

Lab Test Interferences Drug may discolor urine pink to red-brown. False-positive pregnancy tests may occur but are less likely to occur with serum test. Increases in protein-bound iodine reported. False-positive test for phenylketonuria may occur.

Adverse Reactions
CV: Orthostatic hypotension; tachycardia; syncope; cardiac arrest; circulatory collapse; ECG changes.
CNS: Lightheadedness; faintness; headache; weakness; tremor; fatigue; slurring of speech; insomnia; sedation; vertigo; seizures; twitching; ataxia; tardive dyskinesia; drowsiness; lethargy; paradoxical excitement; pseudoparkinsonism; motor restlessness; oculogyric crises; opisthotonos; hyperreflexia; tardive dyskinesia; dizziness; dystonia.
DERM: Photosensitivity; skin pigmentation; dry skin; exfoliative dermatitis; urticarial rash; maculopapular hypersensitivity reaction; seborrhea; contact dermatitis.
EENT: Pigmentary retinopathy; glaucoma; photophobia; blurred vision; miosis; mydriasis; increased IOP; dry mouth or throat; nasal congestion.
GI: Dyspepsia; constipation; adynamic ileus (may result in death); nausea; anorexia.
GU: Urinary hesitancy or retention; impotence; sexual dysfunction; menstrual irregularities; priapism; breast enlargement; galactorrhea.
HEMA: Agranulocytosis; eosinophilia; leukopenia; hemolytic anemia; thrombocytopenic purpura; pancytopenia.
HEPA: Cholestatic jaundice.
METAB: Decreased cholesterol.
RESP: Laryngospasm; bronchospasm; shortness of breath.
OTHER: Increases in appetite and weight; polydipsia; heat-illness; neuroleptic malignant syndrome (NMS); elevated prolactin levels.

Precautions
Pregnancy: Undetermined.
Lactation: Excreted in breast milk.
Children: In general, not recommended for children less than 12 yr. When drug is used in children with acute illnesses (eg, chickenpox, measles, gastroenteritis, dehydration), they are more susceptible to neuromuscular reactions than adults. Avoid use of drug in children and adolescents with signs and symptoms suggestive of Reye syndrome.
Renal function impairment: Use with caution. Lower dose may be necessary.
Hepatic function impairment: Use with caution.
Special risk patients: Use with caution in patients with CV disease or mitral insufficiency, history of glaucoma, EEG abnormalities, seizure disorders, prior brain damage, or in those exposed to extreme heat.
CNS effects: Drug may impair mental or physical abilities, especially during first few days of therapy.
Elderly, debilitated, or emaciated patients: More susceptible to hypotensive and neuromuscular effects. Require lower initial dosage and more gradual increase in dosage.
Hepatic effects: Jaundice usually occurs between second and fourth weeks of treatment and is considered a hypersensitivity reaction; usually reversible.
NMS: NMS occurred with agents in this class and is potentially fatal. Signs and symptoms are hyperpyrexia, muscle rigidity, altered mental status, irregular pulse, irregular BP, tachycardia, and diaphoresis.
Pulmonary effects: Cases of bronchopneumonia, some fatal, have occurred.
Sudden death: Sudden death reported. Predisposing factors may be seizures or previous brain damage. Flare-ups of psychotic behavior may precede death.
Tardive dyskinesia: Syndrome of potentially irreversible involuntary body and facial movements may develop. Prevalence highest in elderly, especially women. Use smallest effective doses for shortest possible time.

Overdosage: Signs and Symptoms
CNS depression (somnolence to coma), hypotension, extrapyramidal symptoms, agitation, restlessness, seizures, fever, hypothermia, hyperthermia, autonomic reactions, ECG changes, cardiac arrhythmias.

PATIENT CARE CONSIDERATIONS
Administration/Storage
- Dose and frequency of administration are variable, depending on condition being treated.
- Administer tablets as prescribed, without regard to meals. Administer with food if GI upset occurs.
- Store tablets at controlled room temperature (59° to 86°F).

Assessment/Interventions
- Obtain patient history, including drug history and any known allergies. Note allergy to trifluoperazine or other phenothiazines, previous episode of jaundice with phenothiazine therapy, renal impairment, hepatic impairment, ischemic heart disease, heart failure, arrhythmias, cerebrovascular disease, asthma, emphysema, narrow angle glaucoma, epilepsy, mitral insufficiency, pheochromocytoma, prostatic hypertrophy, condition predisposing to hypotension (eg, dehydration, hypovolemia), concomitant use of antihypertensive drugs, or

previous episodes of NMS.
- Ensure that medication is discontinued at least 48 hr before myelography and not resumed until at least 24 hr after procedure to reduce chance of seizures occurring.
- Frequently assess patient for response to treatment. Notify health care provider if condition being treated is not improving or is worsening.
- Ensure that therapy is periodically reviewed to determine if therapy needs to be continued without change or if a dose change (eg, increase, decrease, discontinuation) is indicated.
- Avoid sudden discontinuation of therapy if possible. Attempt to gradually reduce dose if decision to discontinue medication is made.
- Inform health care provider immediately if hyperpyrexia, muscle rigidity, altered mental status, irregular pulse or BP, tachycardia, or diaphoresis develop.
- Notify health care provider immediately if palpitations or syncope occur.
- Assess neurologic status before and during treatment. Observe for involuntary body and facial movements, excessive drowsiness, agitation, tremor, or anxiety. Inform health care provider if noted.
- Monitor patient for CNS, CV, GI, GU, PSYCH, musculoskeletal, and general body side effects. Inform health care provider if noted and significant.
- Assess medication compliance.

Patient/Family Education
- Explain name, dose, action, and potential side effects of drug.
- Advise patient, family, or caregiver that dose will be adjusted periodically until max benefit has been obtained.
- Advise patient, family, or caregiver not to change the dose or stop taking unless advised by health care provider.
- Instruct patient not to stop taking trifluoperazine when feeling better.
- Instruct patient, family, or caregiver to immediately report fainting or loss of consciousness, palpitations, dizziness, high fever, muscle rigidity, altered mental status, irregular pulse, unusual bruising, yellowing of the skin or eyes, sore throat, or other signs of infection.
- Advise patient, family, or caregiver to notify health care provider of excessive drowsiness, increased agitation or anxiety, or involuntary body or facial movements.
- Advise patient to avoid strenuous activity during periods of high temperature or humidity.
- Instruct patient to avoid alcoholic beverages and other depressants while taking this medication.
- Instruct patient to get up slowly from lying or sitting position and to avoid sudden position changes to prevent postural hypotension. Advise patient to report dizziness with position changes to health care provider. Caution patient that hot tubs and hot showers or baths may worsen dizziness.
- Advise patient to take sips of water, suck on ice chips or sugarless hard candy, or chew sugarless gum if dry mouth occurs.
- Advise patient that drug may cause drowsiness or impaired judgment or thinking skills and to use caution while driving or performing other tasks requiring mental alertness until tolerance is determined.
- Caution patient that medication may cause sensitivity to sunlight and to avoid unnecessary exposure to UV light (sunlight, tanning booths) and use sunscreen and wear protective clothing when exposed to UV light until tolerance is determined.
- Advise women to notify health care provider if pregnant, planning to become pregnant, or breastfeeding.
- Instruct patient to not take any prescription or OTC medications or dietary supplements unless advised by health care provider.
- Advise patient that follow-up visits may be required to monitor therapy and to keep appointments.

Trihexyphenidyl Hydrochloride

(try-hex-ee-FEN-in-dill HIGH-droe-KLOR-ide)

Class Antiparkinson/Anticholinergic

How Supplied
Artane Tablets 2 mg, Tablets 5 mg, Elixir 2 mg/5 mL ◆ *Artane Sequels* Capsules, sustained-release 5 mg ◆ *Trihexy-2* Tablets 2 mg ◆ *Trihexy-5* Tablets 5 mg

🍁 *Apo-Trihex* ◆ *Trihexyphen*

Action
PHARMACOLOGY: Exerts direct inhibitory effect on parasympathetic nervous system by inhibiting actions of acetylcholine; has relaxing effect on smooth musculature.

PHARMACOKINETICS/DYNAMICS:
Absorption: T_{max} is 1 to 1.3 hr, C_{max} is 87.2 mcg/L, and oral bioavailability is approximately 100%. Trihexyphenidyl is tolerated best in divided doses and taken at mealtimes.

Excretion: Trihexyphenidyl t½ is 5.6 to 10.2 hr.

Indications Adjunct in treatment of all forms of parkinsonism (postencephalitic, arteriosclerotic, and idiopathic); adjuvant therapy with levodopa for control of drug-induced extrapyramidal disorders.

Sustained-release: Maintenance therapy after patients have been stabilized on tablets or elixir.

Contraindications Standard considerations.

Route/Dosage
Parkinsonism
ADULTS: **PO** 1 or 2 mg first day; increase by 3 mg increments at intervals of 3 to 5 days, until 6 to 10 mg given daily in divided doses. Some postencephalitic patients may require total daily dose of 12 to 15 mg. Usually given tid at mealtimes. High doses may be taken qid, at mealtimes and at bedtime.

Concomitant use with other anticholinergics – Gradually initiate trihexyphenidyl with progressive reduction of other anticholinergic.

Drug-Induced Extrapyramidal Disorders
Amount and frequency is individualized. Start with single 1 mg dose. If symptoms are not controlled in few hr, progressively increase until controlled. Daily dosage usually ranges 5 to 15 mg in divided doses.

Sustained-Release
Not for initial therapy. Once patient is stabilized, may switch on equipotent daily basis. Give as single dose after breakfast or in bid doses 12 hr apart.

Interactions
Haloperidol: Schizophrenic symptoms may worsen; haloperidol levels may decrease and tardive dyskinesia may develop.

Phenothiazines: Actions of phenothiazines may be decreased.

PATIENT CARE CONSIDERATIONS
Administration/Storage
- Do not crush sustained-release product or allow patient to chew.
- Store at room temperature in light-resistant container. Avoid freezing the elixir.

Assessment/Interventions
- Obtain patient history, including drug history and any known allergies.
- Assess Parkinson's symptoms prior to and throughout therapy.
- Implement safety precautions to prevent injury, particularly during initial therapy until individual response is determined.
- Encourage frequent oral hygiene.
- Implement measures to prevent constipation, (eg, fluids, activity, dietary bulk).

Lab Test Interferences None well documented.

Adverse Reactions
CV: Tachycardia; palpitations; hypotension.
CNS: Dizziness; nervousness; psychiatric manifestations such as delusions or hallucinations; mental confusion; agitation; disturbed behavior.
DERM: Rash.
EENT: Blurred vision; angle-closure glaucoma; difficulty swallowing.
GI: Dry mouth; nausea; vomiting; constipation; suppurative parotitis; dilation of colon; paralytic ileus.
GU: Urinary retention; urinary hesitancy; impotence.
OTHER: Fever; flushing; decreased sweating; heat illness.

Precautions
Pregnancy: Category C.
Lactation: Undetermined.
Children: Safety and efficacy not established.
Elderly: More susceptible to adverse effects.
Special risk patients: Use drug with caution in patients with tachycardia, arrhythmias, hypertension, hypotension, prostatic hypertrophy, liver or kidney disorders, obstructive disease of GI tract.
Anticholinergic effect: Concomitant use of other drugs with anticholinergic effects will have additive effects.
Heat illness: Give with caution during hot weather. Severe anhidrosis and fatal hyperthermia may occur.
Ophthalmic: Incipient narrow-angle glaucoma may be precipitated by drug use; therefore, closely monitor patient for symptoms and evaluate IOP at regular, periodic intervals.

- Monitor the following for side effects: dry mouth, nausea, dizziness, nervousness, blurred vision. If dry mouth occurs, provide patient with ice chips, sugarless hard candy, or sugarless gum.
- Monitor for other anticholinergic side effects: constipation, difficulty voiding. If these effects are noted, increase patient's fluid intake and notify health care provider if problematic.
- Monitor vital signs per routine and more frequently when increasing dose.
- Monitor frequency of bowel movements, I&O.
- If patient complains of sudden onset of eye pain and blurred vision, discontinue drug and notify health care provider.
- Assess for behavioral changes, particularly in individuals with history of mental disorder.

Trimethobenzamide Hydrochloride

(try-meth-oh-BEN-zuh-mide HIGH-droe-KLOR-ide)

Class Antiemetic/Antivertigo/Anticholinergic

How Supplied
Pediatric Tiban Pediatric suppositories 100 mg ♦ *T-Gen* Pediatric suppositories 100 mg, Adult suppositories 200 mg ♦ *Tebamide* Pediatric suppositories 100 mg, Adult suppositories 200 mg ♦ *Ticon* Injection 100 mg/mL ♦ *Tigan* Capsules 100 mg, Capsules 250 mg, Pediatric suppositories 100 mg, Adult suppositories 200 mg, Injection 100 mg/mL ♦ *Triban* Adult suppositories 200 mg ♦ *Trimazide* Pediatric suppositories 100 mg, Adult suppositories 200 mg

Action
PHARMACOLOGY: Believed to directly affect medullary chemoreceptor trigger zone to inhibit nausea.

PHARMACOKINETICS/DYNAMICS:
Absorption: Following IM administration, T_{max} is 30 min. After PO administration T_{max} is 45 min. 300 mg oral capsules are equivalent to 200 mg IM. The bioavailability of the capsule formulation compared with the solution is 100%.
Excretion: Trimethobenzamide t½ is 7 to 9 hr.

Indications Prevention and treatment of nausea and vomiting.

PATIENT CARE CONSIDERATIONS

Administration/Storage
- Do not use oral route with vomiting.
- If necessary, open capsule and mix with food or liquids for administration.
- Use Z-track technique for IM administration.
- Avoid exposure to light; store at room temperature.
- Avoid freezing injectable.

Assessment/Interventions
- Obtain patient history, including drug history and any known allergies.
- Assess bowel sounds and severity of nausea and vomiting.
- Implement safety precautions, particularly during initial therapy until individual response is determined.
- Implement general comfort measures.
- Monitor response to therapy.

Overdosage: Signs and Symptoms
CNS depression, dry skin, dry mucous membranes, fever, dilated, sluggish pupils, respiratory depression, circulatory collapse, coma.

Contraindications Hypersensitivity to benzocaine or other local anesthetics. Suppositories contraindicated in newborns or premature infants; parenteral use contraindicated in children.

Route/Dosage
ADULTS: PO 250 mg tid to qid. PR 200 mg tid to qid. IM 200 mg tid to qid.
CHILDREN 14 TO 41 KG: PO 100 to 200 mg tid to qid. PR 100 to 200 mg tid to qid.
CHILDREN UNDER 14 KG: PR 100 mg tid to qid.

Interactions None well documented.

Lab Test Interferences None well documented.

Adverse Reactions
CV: Hypotension (after injection).
CNS: Mood depression; disorientation; headache; drowsiness; opisthotonos; dizziness; seizures; coma; Parkinson-like symptoms.
EENT: Blurred vision.
GI: Diarrhea.
HEMA: Blood dyscrasias.
HEPA: Jaundice.
OTHER: Local pain, burning, stinging, redness and swelling (after injection); hypersensitivity reactions; muscle cramps.

Precautions
Pregnancy: Safety not established.
Lactation: Undetermined.
Hypersensitivity: Has been reported; discontinue use of drug at first signs of sensitivity.

- Monitor I&O.
- Monitor vital signs, particularly BP.
- Monitor for potential side effects, particularly drowsiness and hypotension.

Patient/Family Education
- Instruct patient that when used for motion sickness, medication should be taken 30 min before exposure to motion.
- Advise patient to report these symptoms to health care provider: dizziness, yellowing of skin or eyes, muscle cramps, abnormal movements.
- Instruct patient to avoid intake of alcoholic beverages or other CNS depressants.
- Advise patient that drug may cause drowsiness or dizziness and to use caution while driving or performing tasks requiring mental alertness.

Trimethoprim Sulfate/Polymyxin B Sulfate

(try-METH-oh-prim SULL-fate/pahl-ee-MIX-in BEE SULL-fate)

Class Ophthalmic antibiotic combination

How Supplied
Polytrim Ophthalmic Solution 1 mg/mL trimethoprim sulfate and 10,000 units/g polymyxin B sulfate

Action
PHARMACOLOGY:
Trimethoprim: Blocks production of tetrahydrofolic acid by inhibiting the enzyme dihydrofolate reductase.
Polymyxin B: Interacts with phospholipid components of bacterial cell membranes, increasing cell wall permeability.

Indications Treatment of surface ocular bacterial infections, including acute bacterial conjunctivitis and blepharoconjunctivitis caused by susceptible organisms.

Contraindications Standard considerations.

PATIENT CARE CONSIDERATIONS

Administration/Storage
- For ophthalmic use only. Not for use in the ears or on the skin.
- Instill 1 gtt into affected eye(s) q 3 hr to max of 6 doses/day.
- Do not allow tip of dropper bottle to touch eye, eyelid, fingers, or any other surface.
- If using other topical ophthalmic medications, instill gtt first, wait at least 5 min, and instill ointment last.
- Store at controlled room temperature (59° to 77°F). Keep bottle tightly capped and protect from light.

Assessment/Interventions
- Obtain patient history, including drug history and any known allergies.
- Monitor patient's response to therapy. Notify health care provider if eye or eyelid inflammation is noted or if symptoms do not improve or worsen.

Patient/Family Education
- Explain name, dose, action, and potential side effects of drug.
- Review prescribed dosing schedule with patient, family, or caregiver.
- Remind patient, family, or caregiver that solution is for use in the eye only.

Route/Dosage
ADULTS AND CHILDREN 2 MO AND OLDER:
Topical Instill 1 gtt in the affected eye(s) q 3 hr (max, 6 doses/day) for 7 to 10 days.

Interactions None well documented.

Lab Test Interferences None well documented.

Adverse Reactions
EENT: Local irritation (including increased redness, burning, stinging, and itching); hypersensitivity (including lid edema, itching, increased redness, tearing, and circumocular rash).
OTHER: Photosensitivity (has occurred with oral trimethoprim).

Precautions
Pregnancy: Category C.
Lactation: Undetermined.
Children: Safety and efficacy not established in children younger than 2 mo.
Superinfection: Prolonged use may result in bacterial or fungal overgrowth of nonsusceptible microorganisms.

- Teach patient, family, or caregiver proper technique for instilling solution: wash hands; do not allow tip of dropper bottle to touch eye, eyelid, fingers, or any other surface. Tilt head back, look up; pull lower eyelid down to form pocket; place prescribed number of gtt in the pocket. Look downward before closing eye. Do not rub eye.
- Advise patient, family, or caregiver that if more than 1 topical ophthalmic drug is being used, instill eye gtt first, wait at least 5 min, and instill ointment last.
- Inform patient that temporary blurred vision and stinging of the eye are the most common side effects and to contact health care provider if they occur and are bothersome.
- Advise patient to contact eye doctor if eye or eyelid inflammation is noted or if eye symptoms do not improve or worsen.
- Advise patient that the entire course of therapy must be completed to ensure max benefit and to complete full course of therapy even if symptoms have resolved.
- Instruct patient not to wear contact lenses during treatment.
- Remind patient, family, or caregiver that follow-up eye examinations may be necessary while using this medication and to keep appointments.

Trimethoprim/ Sulfamethoxazole (Co-trimoxazole; TMP-SMZ)

(try-METH-oh-prim/suhl-fuh-meth-OX-uh-zole)

Class Anti-infective

How Supplied
Bactrim Tablets 80 mg trimethoprim and 400 mg sulfamethoxazole ♦ *Bactrim D.S.* Tablets, double-strength 160 mg trimethoprim and 800 mg sulfamethoxazole ♦ *Bactrim IV* Injection 80 mg trimethoprim and 400 mg sulfamethoxazole/5 mL ♦ *Bactrim Pediatric* Oral suspension 40 mg trimethoprim and 200 mg sulfamethoxazole/5 mL ♦ *Cotrim* Tablets 80 mg trimethoprim and 400 mg sulfamethoxazole ♦ *Cotrim D.S.* Tablets, double-strength 160 mg trimethoprim and 800 mg sulfamethoxazole ♦ *Cotrim Pediatric* Oral suspension 40 mg trimethoprim and 200 mg sulfamethoxazole/5 mL ♦ *Septra* Tablets 80 mg trimethoprim and 400 mg sulfamethoxazole, Oral suspension 40 mg trimethoprim and 200 mg sulfamethoxazole/5 mL ♦ *Septra DS* Tablets, double-strength 160 mg trimethoprim and 800 mg sulfamethoxazole ♦ *Septra IV* Injection 80 mg trimethoprim and 400 mg sulfamethoxazole/5 mL ♦ *Sulfatrim* Oral suspension 40 mg trimethoprim and 200 mg sulfamethoxazole/5 mL ♦ *Uroplus DS* Tablets 160 mg trimethoprim and 800 mg sulfamethoxazole ♦ *Uroplus SS* Tablets 80 mg trimethoprim and 400 mg sulfamethoxazole

❧ *Apo-Sulfatrim* ♦ *Bactrim Roche* ♦ *Novo-Trimel* ♦ *Novo-Trimel D.S.* ♦ *Nu-Cotrimox* ♦ *Septra Injection*

Action
PHARMACOLOGY: Sulfamethoxazole (SMZ) inhibits bacterial synthesis of dihydrofolic acid by competing with PABA. Trimethoprim (TMP) blocks production of tetrahydrofolic acid by inhibiting the enzyme dihydrofolate reductase. This combination blocks 2 consecutive steps in bacterial biosynthesis of essential nucleic acids and proteins and is usually bactericidal.

PHARMACOKINETICS/DYNAMICS:

Absorption: TMP/SMZ is rapidly absorbed following PO administration. T_{max} is 1 to 4 hr. Steady state is achieved after 3 days.

Distribution: 70% of sulfamethoxazole and 44% of trimethoprim is protein bound. TMP/SMZ is distributed to sputum, vaginal fluid, and middle ear fluid. TMP/SMZ passes the placental barrier and is excreted in human milk.

Metabolism: Metabolism of SMZ is primarily by N_4-acetylation. The principal metabolites of trimethoprim are the 1- and 3-oxides and the 3- and 4-hydroxy derivatives. The free forms are considered therapeutically active.

Excretion: Serum t½ of SMZ and TMP is 10 hr and 8 to 10 hr, respectively. TMP/SMZ is primarily eliminated by kidneys through glomerular filtration and tubular secretion. Urine concentrations are higher than blood concentrations.

Onset: Onset of action is 24 hr after administration.

Special Populations:
Renal Function Impairment – Patients with severely impaired renal function exhibit an increase in the half lives of both components, requiring dosage adjustments.

Indications
PO/Parenteral: Treatment of UTIs caused by susceptible strains of bacteria, shigellosis enteritis, and *Pneumocystis carinii* pneumonitis.
PO: Treatment of acute otitis media and acute exacerbations of chronic bronchitis; treatment of traveler's diarrhea. **Unlabeled use(s):** Treatment of cholera, salmonella-type infections and nocardiosis; prevention of recurrent UTIs in women; prophylaxis of bacterial infections in susceptible patients; treatment of prostatitis; prophylaxis of *Pneumocystis carinii* pneumonitis.

Contraindications
Hypersensitivity to sulfonamides; megaloblastic anemia caused by folate deficiency; pregnancy at term; lactation; infants less than 2 mo.

Route/Dosage
UTIs, Shigellosis, Acute Otitis Media
ADULTS: PO 160 mg TMP/800 mg SMZ q 12 hr for 10 to 14 days and 5 days for shigellosis. IV 8 to 10 mg/kg/day (based on TMP) in 2 to 4 divided doses q 6 to 12 hr for up to 14 days for severe UTIs and 5 days for shigellosis.
CHILDREN OVER 2 MO: PO 8 mg/kg TMP/ 40 mg/kg SMZ daily in 2 divided doses q 12 hr for 10 days and 5 days for shigellosis.

Pneumocystis carinii Pneumonitis
ADULTS: PO 20 mg/kg TMP/100 mg/kg SMZ daily in divided doses q 6 hr for 14 days. IV 15 to 20 mg/kg/day (based on TMP) in 3 to 4 divided doses for up to 14 days.

Traveler's Diarrhea
ADULTS: PO 160 mg TMP/800 mg SMZ q 12 hr for 5 days.

Exacerbation of Chronic Bronchitis
ADULTS: PO 160 mg TMP/800 mg SMZ q 12 hr for 14 days.

Interactions
Cyclosporine: May cause decrease in therapeutic effect of cyclosporine and increased risk of nephrotoxicity.
Methotrexate: May displace methotrexate from

protein-binding sites, thus increasing free methotrexate levels.
Phenytoin: Trimethoprim may inhibit metabolism of phenytoin or other hydantoins.
Procainamide: Trimethoprim may inhibit renal elimination of procainamide and its metabolites.
Sulfonylureas: May increase hypoglycemic response to sulfonylureas because of displacement from protein-binding sites or inhibition of hepatic metabolism.
Warfarin: May cause prolonged PT.
INCOMPATIBILITIES: Do not mix with other drugs or solutions other than D5W.

Lab Test Interferences Can interfere with serum methotrexate assay as determined by competitive binding protein technique when bacterial dihydrofolate reductase is used as binding protein. May interfere with Jaffe alkaline picrate reaction assay for creatinine, resulting in overestimations.

Precautions

Pregnancy: Category C. Do not use at term because of risk of neonatal kernicterus.
Lactation: Undetermined. Not recommended during nursing because sulfonamides are excreted in breast milk and may cause kernicterus. Premature infants and infants with hyperbilirubinemia or G-6-PD deficiency are also at risk for adverse effects.
Children: Not recommended for infants less than 2 mo.
Elderly: Are at increased risk of severe adverse reactions.
Renal function impairment: Use drug with caution. Dosage adjustment may be required.
Hepatic function impairment: Use drug with caution. Dosage adjustment may be required.

Special risk patients: Use drug with caution in patients with possible folate deficiency (eg, elderly patients, chronic alcoholics, patients undergoing anticonvulsant therapy, patients with malabsorption syndromes or malnutrition), patients with severe allergy or bronchial asthma, patients who have sulfite sensitivity and G-6-PD-deficient individuals.
Ulceration: Take tablets with water or food to prevent lodging in esophagus and subsequent ulceration.
Hematologic effects: Sulfonamide-associated deaths, although rare, have occurred from hypersensitivity of respiratory tract, Stevens-Johnson syndrome, toxic epidermal necrolysis, fulminant hepatic necrosis, agranulocytosis, aplastic anemia, and other blood dyscrasias. Both components can interfere with hematopoiesis. IV use at high doses for extended periods of time may cause bone marrow depression.
Patients with AIDS: Incidence of side effects, especially rash, fever, and leukopenia, is greatly increased.
Streptococcal pharyngitis: Do not use for streptococcal pharyngitis.
Sulfonamides: Are chemically similar to some goitrogens, diuretics (acetazolamide and the thiazides), and oral hypoglycemic agents. Goiter production, diuresis, and hypoglycemia occur rarely in patients receiving sulfonamides. Cross-sensitivity may occur.

Overdosage: Signs and Symptoms

Anorexia, colic, nausea, vomiting, dizziness, headache, drowsiness, depression, confusion, altered mental status, fever, hematuria, crystalluria, blood dyscrasias, jaundice, bone marrow depression.

PATIENT CARE CONSIDERATIONS

Administration/Storage

- Administer with full glass of water.
- May administer with food if GI upset occurs.
- For IV infusion, must dilute in 75 or 125 mL of D5W only. Administer each dose over 60 to 90 min. Flush IV line after infusion. Do not use IV solution if cloudy or precipitates are noted.
- If local irritation or inflammation because of extravascular infiltration occurs, discontinue infusion and restart at another site.
- Avoid rapid or direct IV injection. Do not inject IM.
- Shake oral suspension well before use.
- Store IV solution at room temperature. Do not refrigerate. Discard prepared IV solution if not used within 2 hr (75 mL) or 6 hr (125 mL).
- Store tablets or suspension at room temperature in a tight, light-resistant container.

Assessment/Interventions

- Obtain patient history, including drug history and any known allergies. Note decreased renal or hepatic function and sensitivity to sulfonamides (including sulfonylureas or thiazide diuretics) and trimethoprim.
- Obtain culture and sensitivity before beginning drug therapy.
- Monitor I&O.
- Encourage fluid intake.
- Monitor renal function during prolonged treatment.
- Notify health care provider of GI upset, fever, chills, headache, rash, decreased urine output, wheezing, shortness of breath, dizziness, sore throat, unusual bleeding or bruising, arthralgia.

Patient/Family Education

- Advise patient to complete full course of therapy.

- Encourage patient to maintain adequate fluid intake.
- Advise patient to take tablet with full glass of water.
- Educate patient and family to report any signs of superinfection such as fever, vaginitis, oral candidiasis, and fatigue.
- Instruct patient to report these symptoms to health care provider: skin rash, sore throat, fever, unusual bruising or bleeding.
- Caution patient to avoid exposure to sunlight and to use sunscreen or wear protective clothing to avoid photosensitivity reaction.

Trimetrexate Glucuronate

(TRY-meh-TREK-sate glue-CURE-uh-nate)

Class Folic acid antimetabolite/Anti-infective/Antiprotozoal

How Supplied

Neutrexin Powder for injection, lyophilized 25 mg

Action

PHARMACOLOGY: Inhibits dihydrofolate reductase necessary for DNA, RNA, and protein synthesis, leading to cell death. Following a single-dose of 10 to 130 mg/m^2 the alpha phase t½ was about 57 min followed by a terminal phase with a t½ of approximately 16 hr. Clearance has been reported as about 53 mL/min and about 32 mL/min following single-dose administration.

PHARMACOKINETICS/DYNAMICS:

Distribution: There are inconsistencies in reporting of protein binding; in vitro, trimetrexate is 95% protein bound (over concentration of 18.75 to 100 ng/mL). Others report greater than 98% bound at concentrations 0.1 to 10 mcg/mL. Vd in AIDS patients is approximately 20 L/m^2.

Metabolism: Metabolism has not been characterized. Preclinical trial suggest major metabolic pathway is oxidative O-demethylation followed by conjugation to either glucuronide or the sulfate.

Excretion: Terminal t½ in HIV is approximately 11 hr and terminal t½ in cancer is approximately 16 hr. Clearance is approximately 38 mL/min/m^2.

Indications As alternative therapy, with concurrent leucovorin administration, for treatment of moderate-to-severe *Pneumocystis carinii* pneumonia in immunocompromised patients in whom trimethoprim-sulfamethoxazole cannot be used. **Unlabeled use(s):** Treatment of non-small cell lung, prostate, and colorectal cancer.

Contraindications Clinically significant sensitivity to trimetrexate, leucovorin, or methotrexate.

Route/Dosage

ADULTS: **IV** 45 mg/m^2 q/day by **IV** infusion over 60 to 90 min for 21 days. Leucovorin may be administered **IV** at dose of 20 mg/m^2 over 5 to 10 min q 6 hr for total daily dose of 80 mg/m^2 or **PO** at dose of 20 mg/m^2 q 6 hr for 24 days. Adjust dose of trimetrexate and leucovorin according to hematologic toxicity. Interruption of therapy may be necessary for hematologic, hepatic, renal, or mucosal toxicity or for uncontrolled fever. See manufacturer's recommendations.

Interactions

Hepatic enzyme inducers (eg, phenobarbital, phenytoin, carbamazepine, rifampin, rifabutin): Decreased trimetrexate concentrations and reduced efficacy are possible.

Hepatic enzyme inhibitors (eg, ketoconazole, itraconazole, macrolides, cimetidine): Increased trimetrexate concentrations and increased toxicity are possible.

Hepatotoxic drugs (eg, NSAIDs, etretinate, ethanol, methotrexate, asparaginase): Increased risk of hepatotoxicity may occur.

Nephrotoxic drugs (eg, aminoglycosides, amphotericin B, cisplatin, co-trimoxazole, cyclosporine, ganciclovir, melphalan, NSAIDs): Increased risk of nephrotoxicity may occur.

Pneumococcal vaccine: Reduced vaccine efficacy may occur.

Pyrimethamine, trimethoprim: Increased antifolate effects and increased toxicity may occur.

Yellow fever vaccine, other live vaccines: Increased risk of infection (ie, vaccine toxicity).

Zidovudine: Zidovudine should be discontinued during trimetrexate therapy to allow for full therapeutic doses of trimetrexate.

INCOMPATIBILITIES: Do not mix with solutions containing either chloride ion (eg, sodium chloride) or leucovorin, because precipitation occurs instantly.

Lab Test Interferences None well documented.

Adverse Reactions

CNS: Confusion; fatigue.
DERM: Rash; pruritus.
GI: Nausea; vomiting; increased serum transaminases; increased alkaline phosphatase; increased bilirubin; mucositis; hepatotoxicity.
GU: Increased serum creatinine.
HEMA: Neutropenia; thrombocytopenia; anemia; myelosuppression.
METAB: Hyponatremia; hypocalcemia.
OTHER: Fever.

> **WARNING:**
> Concurrent leucovorin must be used to avoid potentially serious or life-threatening toxicities including bone marrow suppression, oral and GI mucosal ulceration, and renal and hepatic dysfunction.

Precautions
Pregnancy: Category D.
Lactation: Undetermined.
Children: Safety and efficacy not established.
Hypersensitivity: Has rarely occurred.
Renal function impairment: Use drug with caution in patients with impaired renal function.
Hepatic function impairment: Use drug with caution in patients with impaired hepatic function.
Special risk patients: Use drug with caution in patients with impaired hematologic function and in patients who require concomitant therapy with nephrotoxic, myelosuppressive, or hepatotoxic drugs.
Hepatic toxicity: Transient elevations of transaminases and alkaline phosphatase have occurred. Interrupt therapy if levels increase to more than 5 times upper limit of normal.
Seizures: Have rarely occurred.

Overdosage: Signs and Symptoms
Severe neutropenia, severe thrombocytopenia, severe anemia, nausea, vomiting.

PATIENT CARE CONSIDERATIONS
Administration/Storage
- Administer IV trimetrexate and leucovorin solutions separately. Leucovorin solution may be administered prior to or after trimetrexate. In either case flush IV line thoroughly with at least 10 mL of 5% Dextrose Injection between infusions.
- Avoid contact with skin or mucosa. If trimetrexate contacts skin or mucosa, immediately and thoroughly wash with soap and water.
- Reconstitute with 2 mL of 5% Dextrose for Injection or Sterile Water to yield concentration of 12.5 mg/mL. Do not reconstitute with solutions containing either chloride ion or leucovorin, because precipitation will occur instantly.
- Filter solution (0.22 mcm) prior to dilution.
- Further dilute reconstituted solution with 5% Dextrose Injection to yield final concentration of 0.25 to 2 mg/mL.
- Administer diluted solution by IV infusion over 60 to 90 min.
- Flush IV line with at least 10 mL of 5% Dextrose Injection before and after administering trimetrexate.
- Store vials at controlled room temperature and protect from exposure to light.
- After reconstitution, retain solution at room temperature or under refrigeration for up to 24 hr. Do not freeze reconstituted solution.
- Use cytotoxic drug precautions for proper disposal.

Assessment/Interventions
- Obtain patient history, including drug history and any known allergies.
- Assess for signs and symptoms of oral and GI mucosal ulceration, changes in mental status, fatigue, and signs and symptoms of infection.
- Monitor CBC, differential and platelet counts, and hepatic and renal function tests at baseline and at least twice weekly during therapy.
- Consider termination of treatment if fever (oral temperature 105°F or greater; 40.5°C) cannot be controlled by antipyretics.
- Consider discontinuation of therapy if serum creatinine is greater than 2.5 mg/dL or if transaminase or alkaline phosphatase levels become more than 5 times normal.

Patient/Family Education
- Explain that continued, frequent monitoring by health care provider is necessary.
- Inform patient that blood test must be performed at least twice weekly.
- Explain that leucovorin therapy must be continued for 72 hr or more after last dose of trimetrexate.
- Describe potential side effects, and what should be reported to health care provider (eg, fever, mucosal toxicity).

Trimipramine Maleate
(TRY-MIH-prah-meen MAL-ee-ate)
Class Tricyclic antidepressant
How Supplied
Surmontil Capsules 25 mg, Capsules 50 mg, Capsules 100 mg

Action
PHARMACOLOGY: Mechanism of action is not known.

Indications Relief of symptoms of depression.

Contraindications Hypersensitivity to any tricyclic antidepressant; not to be given with or within 14 days of treatment with an MAO inhibitor; during acute recovery phase following an MI; cross-sensitivity may occur among the dibenzazepines.

Route/Dosage
ADOLESCENTS AND ELDERLY: **PO** Initially, 50 mg/day, with gradual incremental increases up to 100 mg/day, depending on response and tolerance.

Hospitalized Patients
ADULTS: **PO** Initially, 100 mg/day. This may be gradually increased in a few days to 200 mg/day, depending on response and tolerance. If improvement does not occur in 2 to 3 wk, the dose may be increased to a max of 250 to 300 mg/day.

Outpatients and Office Patients
ADULTS: **PO** Initially, 75 mg/day in divided doses, increased to 150 mg/day. Dosages over 200 mg/day are not recommended. Maintenance therapy ranges from 50 to 150 mg/day.

Interactions
Alcohol, CNS depressants: Depressant effects may be additive.
Catecholamines/anticholinergics: Effects of the catecholamine may be potentiated.
Cimetidine: May cause increased trimipramine blood levels.
Drugs inhibiting CYP2D6 (amiodarone, fluoxetine, quinidine): Trimipramine blood levels may be elevated, increasing the pharmacologic and adverse effects.
MAO inhibitors: May cause hyperpyretic crisis, severe convulsions, and death when given with trimipramine.

Lab Test Interferences
None well documented.

Adverse Reactions
CV: Hypotension; hypertension; tachycardia; palpitation; MI; arrhythmias; heart block; stroke.
CNS: Confusional states (especially in the elderly); hallucinations; disorientation; delusions; anxiety; restlessness; agitation; insomnia; nightmares; hypomania; exacerbation of psychosis; numbness; tingling; paresthesias of extremities; incoordination; ataxia; tremors; peripheral neuropathy; extrapyramidal symptoms; seizures; alterations in EEG patterns; manic and hypomanic episodes; drowsiness; dizziness; weakness; fatigue; headache.
DERM: Perspiration; alopecia.
EENT: Tinnitus; blurred vision; disturbances of accommodation; mydriasis.
ENDO: Gynecomastia (males); breast enlargement and galactorrhea (females); increased and decreased libido; impotence; testicular swelling; increased and decreased blood glucose.
GI: Dry mouth; constipation; paralytic ileus; nausea; vomiting; anorexia; epigastric distress; diarrhea; peculiar taste; stomatitis; abdominal cramps; black tongue.
GU: Urinary retention; delayed micturation; dilation of urinary tract; urinary frequency.
HEMA: Bone marrow suppression (including agranulocytosis, eosinophilia, purpura, thrombocytopenia).
HEPA: Jaundice; altered liver function.
METAB: SIADH; weight gain or loss.
OTHER: Allergy (including skin rash, petechiae, urticaria, itching, photosensitivity, edema of face and hands); flushing; parotid swelling.

Precautions
Pregnancy: Category C.
Children: Safety and efficacy not established.
Hepatic function impairment: Use with caution.
Schizophrenia: Activation of psychosis may occur.
Suicide: Supervise depressed patients at risk during initial therapy. Prescribe the smallest quantity consistent with good patient management in order to reduce the risk of overdose.
Withdrawal: Though not indicative of addiction, abrupt cessation of treatment after prolonged use may produce nausea, headache, and malaise.

Overdosage: Signs and Symptoms
Cardiac arrhythmias, severe hypotension, convulsions, confusion, disturbed concentration, transient visual hallucinations, dilated pupils, agitation, hyperactive reflexes, stupor, drowsiness, muscle rigidity, vomiting, hypothermia, hyperpyrexia, CNS depression including coma.

PATIENT CARE CONSIDERATIONS

Administration/Storage
- Do not administer with or within 14 days of MAO inhibitor administration.
- Can be administered as a single dose at bedtime or in divided doses.
- Administer prescribed dose without regard to meals. Administer with food if GI upset occurs.
- Store tablets at controlled room temperature (68° to 77°F).

Assessment/Interventions
- Obtain patient history, including drug history and any known allergies. Determine whether any MAO inhibitors have been used in the past 14 days. Note liver disease, glaucoma, prostatic hypertrophy, hyperthyroidism, CV disease, arrhythmias, heart failure, recent MI, seizure disorder, or current use of selective serotonin reuptake inhibitors.

- Continue suicide monitoring of high-risk patients.
- Observe for signs of mood change and report to health care provider.
- Assess patient for CNS, GI, CV, PSYCH, GU, and general body side effects. Report to health care provider if noted and significant.
- If treatment needs to be discontinued, attempt to gradually taper the dose over at least a 2-wk interval in patient who has been on prolonged therapy.

Patient/Family Education

- Explain name, dose, action, and potential side effects of drug.
- Advise patient that medication will be started at a low dose and then increased as tolerated until max benefit is obtained.
- Advise patient to take prescribed dose without regard to meals but to take with food if stomach upset occurs.
- Advise patient that if a dose is missed to skip that dose and take the next dose at the regularly scheduled time. Caution patient to never take 2 doses at the same time.
- Advise patient not to change the dose or stop taking unless advised by health care provider.
- Inform patient that it may take 1 to 4 wk to note improvement in symptoms and to continue with the prescribed therapy once improvement has been noted.
- Advise patient to take frequent sips of water, suck on ice chips or sugarless hard candy, or chew sugarless gum if dry mouth occurs.
- Advise patient to avoid alcoholic beverages.
- Advise patient that drug may impair judgment, thinking, or reflexes and to use caution while driving or performing other tasks requiring mental alertness until tolerance is determined.
- Advise patient to contact health care provider if rash, hives, or other symptoms of an allergic reaction occur, or if experiencing bothersome side effects such as unusual sweating, headache, drowsiness, nausea, tremors, or changes in sexual function.
- Caution patient to avoid unnecessary exposure to UV light (sunlight, tanning booths) and to use sunscreen and wear protective clothing when exposed to UV light until tolerance is determined.
- Instruct patient not to take prescription or OTC drugs or dietary supplements unless advised by health care provider.
- Advise women to notify health care provider if pregnant, planning to become pregnant, or breastfeeding.
- Advise patient that follow-up visits will be necessary to monitor therapy and to keep appointments.

Triprolidine Hydrochloride

(try-PRO-lih-deen HIGH-droe-KLOR-ide)

Class Antihistamine/Alkylamine

How Supplied
Zymine Liquid 1.25 mg/5 mL

Action
PHARMACOLOGY: Competitively blocks histamine at H_2 receptor sites.

PHARMACOKINETICS/DYNAMICS:
Absorption: C_{max} is about 5.5 to 6 ng/mL. T_{max} is about 2 and 1.5 hr for tablets and syrup, respectively.

Excretion: Plasma t½ is about 3.2 hr. Only about 1% of an administered dose is eliminated unchanged over a 24 hr period.

Indications Symptomatic relief of perennial and seasonal allergic rhinitis, vasomotor rhinitis, allergic conjunctivitis; management of allergic and non-allergic pruritic symptoms, mild uncomplicated urticaria and angioedema.

Contraindications Hypersensitivity to antihistamines; newborn or premature infants; nursing mothers; narrow-angle glaucoma; stenosing peptic ulcer; symptomatic prostatic hypertrophy; asthmatic attack; bladder neck obstruction; pyloroduodenal obstruction; MAO therapy.

Route/Dosage
ADULTS AND CHILDREN (AT LEAST 12 YR): PO 2.5 mg q 4 to 6 hr (max, 10 mg/24 hr).
CHILDREN (6 TO 12 YR): PO 1.25 mg q 4 to 6 hr (max, 5 mg/24 hr).
CHILDREN (4 TO 6 YR): PO 0.94 mg q 4 to 6 hr (max, 3.75 mg/24 hr).
CHILDREN (2 TO 4 YR): PO 0.625 mg q 4 to 6 hr (max, 2.5 mg/24 hr).
CHILDREN (4 MO TO 2 YR): PO 0.31 mg q 4 to 6 hr (max, 1.25 mg/24 hr).

Interactions
Alcohol, CNS depressants (eg, narcotics, sedatives): Additive CNS depression possible.
MAO inhibitors: Anticholinergic effects may increase.

Lab Test Interferences In skin testing procedures, may prevent or diminish otherwise positive reaction to dermal reactivity indicators.

Adverse Reactions
CV: Orthostatic hypotension; palpitations; tachycardia; faintness.
CNS: Drowsiness (often transient); sedation;

dizziness; faintness; disturbed coordination; excitation.
EENT: Blurred vision; nasal stuffiness; dry mouth, nose, and throat sore throat.
GI: Epigastric distress; nausea; vomiting; diarrhea; constipation; change in bowel habits.
METAB: Increased appetite, weight gain.
RESP: Thickening of bronchial secretions.
OTHER: Hypersensitivity reactions; photosensitivity.

Precautions
Pregnancy: Category C.
Lactation: Undetermined.
Children: Overdosage may cause hallucinations, convulsions, and death. Antihistamines may diminish mental alertness. In young children, triprolidine may produce paradoxical excitation.
Elderly: Greater likelihood of dizziness, excessive sedation, syncope, toxic confusional states, and hypotension in patients over 60 yr. Dosage reduction may be required.
Special risk patients: Use drug with caution in patients with predisposition to urinary retention, history of bronchial asthma, increased intraocular pressure, hyperthyroidism, sleep apnea, cardiovascular disease, or hypertension.
Respiratory disease: Generally not recommended to treat lower respiratory tract symptoms including asthma.

Overdosage: Signs and Symptoms
CNS depression, CNS stimulation, hypotension, respiratory depression, coma, seizures.

PATIENT CARE CONSIDERATIONS

Administration/Storage
- Give with food.
- Store tablets and oral solution at room temperature in a tight, light-resistant container. Do not freeze oral solution.

Assessment/Interventions
- Obtain patient history, including drug history and any known allergies.
- Monitor for potential neurologic side effects especially in elderly and young.
- Obtain CBC if signs of blood dyscrasias are noted.
- Assess LFT results and BUN and serum creatinine as indicated.

Patient/Family Education
- Explain potential side effects and adverse reactions, and identify problems that should be reported to health care provider.
- Tell patient not to take within 4 days before skin testing procedures.
- Advise patient to take sips of water frequently, suck on ice chips or sugarless hard candy, or chew sugarless chewing gum if dry mouth occurs.
- Instruct patient to avoid alcohol and other CNS depressants.
- Advise patient that drug may cause drowsiness or dizziness and to use caution while driving or performing other tasks requiring mental alertness.

Triptorelin Pamoate
(trip-toe-REL-in PAM-on-ate)

Class Gonadotropin-releasing hormone

How Supplied
Trelstar Depot Microgranules for injection, lyophilized Equivalent to 3.75 mg triptorelin peptide base ♦ *Trelstar LA* Microgranules for injection, lyophilized Equivalent to 11.25 mg triptorelin peptide base

Action
PHARMACOLOGY: Synthetic analog of gonadotropin-releasing hormone (GnRH) that acts as potent inhibitor of gonadotropin secretion.

PHARMACOKINETICS/DYNAMICS:
Absorption: Triptorelin is not active when given orally. It is given IM only. C_{max} is approximately 28.43 ng/mL. T_{max} is 1 hr (range, 1 to 3 hr). AUC is approximately 224 hr•ng/mL.

Distribution: Vd is 30 to 33 L (from a dose of 0.5 mg). There is no evidence of protein binding.

Metabolism: No metabolites are found. Metabolism in humans is unknown, but unlikely to involve hepatic microsomal enzyme P450.

Excretion: Triptorelin is eliminated by both the liver and kidneys. 41.7% of a dose is excreted in urine.

Peak: Time-to-peak effect occurs on day 4.

Duration: Duration of action is up to 4 wk.

Special Populations:
Renal Function Impairment – There is a decrease in total Cl proportional to decrease in Ccr and increased Vd and $t_{½}$.
Hepatic Function Impairment – The decrease in triptorelin Cl is more pronounced. Triptorelin $t_{½}$ increase is similar to renal impairment.
Young healthy men 20 to 22 yr – Increased Ccr caused triptorelin to be eliminated twice as fast.

Indications
Palliative treatment of advanced prostate cancer and as an alternative treatment for prostate cancer when orchiectomy or estrogen administration are not indicated or are unacceptable to the patient.

Contraindications Hypersensitivity to triptorelin or any component of product; other gonadotropin-releasing hormone agonists; pregnancy.

Route/Dosage
ADULTS: **IM** 3.75 mg in a depot formulation administered as a single monthly injection (*Trelstar Depot*); 11.25 mg in a long-acting formulation q 84 days as a single injection in either buttock (*Trelstar LA*).

Interactions
Hyperprolactinemic drugs: Do not administer concurrently with triptorelin.

Lab Test Interferences Because chronic or continuous administration of triptorelin suppresses pituitary-gonadal axis, diagnostic tests of pituitary-gonadal function performed during triptorelin treatment or after cessation of therapy may be misleading.

Adverse Reactions
CV: Hypertension (4%); chest pain (2%).
CNS: Headache (7%); dizziness (3%); fatigue, insomnia (2%); emotional lability, asthenia (1%).
DERM: Rash (2%); pruritus (1%).
EENT: Conjunctivitis, eye pain (1%).
GI: Nausea (3%); vomiting, anorexia, constipation, dyspepsia (2%); diarrhea, abdominal pain (1%).
GU: Impotence (7%); dysuria (4%); breast pain, decreased libido, gynecomastia (2%); UTI, urinary retention (1%).
HEMA: Anemia (1%).
HEPA: Abnormal hepatic function (1%).
MUSC: Skeletal pain (13%); arthralgia, leg cramps (2%); myalgia (1%).
RESP: Coughing (2%); dyspnea, pharyngitis (1%).
OTHER: Hot flushes (73%); leg edema (6%); leg pain (5%); injection site pain (4%); back pain, pain (3%); dependent edema, increased alkaline phosphatase (2%); peripheral edema (1%).

Precautions
Pregnancy: Category X.
Lactation: Undetermined.
Children: Safety and efficacy not established.
Hypersensitivity: Anaphylactic reactions reported.
Special risk patients: Spinal cord compression or renal impairment reported.
Worsening of signs and symptoms: Drug initially causes transient increase in testosterone, which may lead to worsening of signs and symptoms of prostate cancer (eg, bone pain) during first few weeks of treatment.

PATIENT CARE CONSIDERATIONS

Administration/Storage
- For IM administration only. Not for intradermal, SC, or IV administration.
- Administer prescribed dose of *Trelstar Depot* dose form q 28 days into either buttock.
- Administer prescribed dose of *Trelstar LA* dose form q 84 days into either buttock.
- Rotate injection sites.
- Reconstitute powder for injection following manufacturer's guidelines using sterile water for injection. Shake well to thoroughly disperse particles to obtain a uniform suspension.
- Administer suspension immediately after reconstitution. Discard any suspension that is not used immediately after reconstitution.
- Store microgranules for injection at controlled room temperature (59° to 86°F). Do not freeze long-acting triptorelin.

Assessment/Interventions
- Obtain patient history, including drug history and any known allergies. Note hepatic or renal impairment or history of hypersensitivity to other luteinizing hormone-releasing hormone (LHRH) agonists (eg, goserelin) or LHRHs.
- Ensure that serum testosterone and prostate-specific antigen levels are measured to monitor response to therapy. Serum testosterone levels should be measured immediately prior to or immediately after dosing.
- Closely monitor patient with metastatic vertebral lesions and/or lower urinary tract obstruction for signs or symptoms indicating possible spinal cord compression (eg, weakness or paralysis of lower extremities) or complete obstruction of the urinary tract (eg, inability to urinate). Inform health care provider immediately if noted and be prepared to treat appropriately.
- Monitor patient for signs and symptoms of anaphylactic or serious allergic reaction. Notify health care provider immediately and be prepared to treat appropriately.
- Monitor patient for CNS, GI, GU, and general body side effects, and injection site reactions. Report to health care provider if noted and significant.

Patient/Family Education
- Explain name, dose, action, and potential side effects of drug.

- Advise patient, family, or caregiver that medication will be prepared and administered by a health care professional in a health care setting.
- Educate patient, family, or caregiver of importance of returning as scheduled for additional injections in order to achieve maximal benefits from the medication.
- Advise patient, family, or caregiver that medication may temporarily worsen signs and symptoms of the disease (eg, bone pain, blood in urine, difficult or painful urination) but that these should improve after 2 or 3 wk.
- Advise patient, family, or caregiver to immediately report any of the following to the health care provider: rash; itching or hives; swelling of the face, lips, eyes, or tongue; wheezing; shortness of breath; difficulty breathing; weakness or paralysis of legs; inability to urinate.
- Instruct patient, family, or caregiver not to use any prescription or OTC medications or dietary supplements unless advised by health care provider.
- Advise patient, family, or caregiver that follow-up office visits will be required to administer medication, and lab tests will be required to monitor response to therapy.

Trospium Chloride

(TROSE-pee-um KLOR-ide)

Class Anticholinergic/Antispasmodic

How Supplied
Sanctura Tablets 20 mg

Action
PHARMACOLOGY: Antagonizes effect of acetylcholine on muscarinic receptors in cholinergically innervated organs. Its parasympatholytic action reduces tonus of smooth muscle in the bladder.

PHARMACOKINETICS/DYNAMICS:

Absorption: Less than 10% absorbed after oral dose (bioavailability 9.6%). C_{max} occurs 5 to 6 hr postdose. Dose increases from 20 to 40 mg or 60 mg result in an increase in C_{max} of 3- or 4-fold, respectively. There is a diurnal variability with a decrease in C_{max} and AUC of up to 59% and 33%, respectively, for evening compared with morning doses. Because high-fat meals reduce absorption, it is recommended that trospium be taken at least 1 hr before meals or on an empty stomach.

Distribution: Vd is 395 L after a 20 mg dose. Protein binding is 50% to 85%.

Metabolism: Of 10% absorbed, metabolites account for about 40% of excreted dose. Hypothesized metabolic pathway is ester hydrolysis with subsequent conjugation of benzylic acid.

Excretion: Plasma t½ is approximately 20 hr. Majority of dose (85.2%) recovered in feces and 5.8% in urine.

Indications
Treatment of overactive bladder with symptoms of urinary incontinence, urgency, and urinary frequency.

Contraindications
Patients with or at risk of urinary retention; gastric retention; uncontrolled narrow-angle glaucoma; hypersensitivity to any component of product.

Route/Dosage
ADULTS: PO 20 mg bid on an empty stomach or at least 1 hr before meals.

Severe Renal Impairment (Ccr less than 30 mL/min)
ADULTS: PO 20 mg once daily at bedtime.
ELDERLY (75 YR OF AGE AND OLDER): PO Titrate dose down to 20 mg once daily based on tolerability.

Interactions
Anticholinergics: Additive effects, leading to increased dry mouth, constipation, and other anticholinergic effects.

Drugs eliminated by active tubular secretion (eg, digoxin, metformin, morphine, pancuronium, procainamide, tenofovir, vancomycin): Serum concentrations of these agents as well as trospium may be increased.

Lab Test Interferences None well documented.

Adverse Reactions
CV: Tachycardia; palpitations, supraventricular tachycardia, chest pain, syncope, hypertensive crisis (postmarketing).
CNS: Headache (4%); fatigue (2%); hallucinations, delirium (postmarketing).
DERM: Stevens-Johnson syndrome (postmarketing).
EENT: Dry eyes (1%); abnormal vision (postmarketing).
GI: Dry mouth (20%); constipation (10%); upper abdominal pain (2%); aggravated constipation, dyspepsia, flatulence (1%); gastritis (postmarketing).
HYPERSEN: Anaphylactic reactions (postmarketing).
MUSC: Rhabdomyolysis (postmarketing).
RENAL: Urinary retention (1%).

Precautions
Pregnancy: Category C.
Lactation: Undetermined.
Children: Safety and efficacy not established.

Elderly: May have increased sensitivity to effects of anticholinergic agents.

Renal function impairment: In patients with severe renal insufficiency, there is a 4.5- and 2-fold increase in mean AUC and C_{max}, respectively, and prolonged elimination t½. Dose modification is recommended with Ccr less than 30 mL/min.

Special risk patients: Use with caution in patients with GI obstruction (risk of gastric retention), hepatic impairment, or clinically important bladder overflow obstruction (risk of urinary retention).

Controlled narrow-angle glaucoma: Use only if benefits outweigh risks.

Overdosage: Signs and Symptoms
Severe anticholinergic effects.

PATIENT CARE CONSIDERATIONS

Administration/Storage
- Administer prescribed dose on an empty stomach 1 hr before or 2 hr after meals.
- Store tablets at controlled room temperature (59° to 86°F).

Assessment/Interventions
- Obtain patient history, including drug history and any known allergies. Note renal or hepatic impairment, urinary retention, gastric retention, narrow angle glaucoma, GI obstructive disorder, ulcerative colitis, intestinal atony, myasthenia gravis, or concurrent therapy with other anticholinergics agents or drugs eliminated by tubular secretion (eg, digoxin).
- Ensure reduced dose is administered to patient older than 75 yr of age or to patient with severe renal insufficiency (Ccr less than 30 mL/min).
- Assess changes in urinary symptoms (eg, urinary frequency, urgency, urge incontinence). Notify health care provider if symptoms are not improving or are worsening.
- Monitor patient for GI, CNS, and general body side effects. Inform health care provider if noted and significant.

Patient/Family Education
- Explain name, dose, action, and potential side effects of drug.
- Advise patient to take prescribed dose on an empty stomach at least 1 hr before or 2 hr after a meal.
- Advise patient if a dose is missed to skip that dose and take the next dose at least 1 hr before the next meal.
- Advise patient to contact health care provider if urinary symptoms do not improve or worsen while taking this medication.
- Advise patient to take sips of water, chew sugarless gum, or suck on sugarless candy to relieve symptoms of dry mouth.
- Advise patient to avoid strenuous activity during periods of high temperature or humidity.
- Advise patient to avoid alcoholic beverages and sedatives (eg, diazepam) while taking trospium.
- Advise patient that drug may cause dizziness or blurred vision and to use caution while driving or performing other tasks requiring coordination and mental alertness until tolerance is determined.
- Advise women to notify health care provider if pregnant, planning to become pregnant, or breastfeeding.
- Caution patient not to take any prescription or OTC drugs, herbal preparations, or dietary supplements unless advised by health care provider.
- Advise patient that follow-up visits may be necessary to monitor therapy and to keep appointments.

Trovafloxacin Mesylate/ Alatrofloxacin Mesylate

(TROE-vah-FLOX-ah-sin MEH-sih-LATE/al-at-row-FLOX-ah-sin)

Class Antibiotic/Fluoroquinolone

How Supplied
Trovan Tablets 100 mg (as trovafloxacin mesylate), Tablets 200 mg (as trovafloxacin mesylate), Solution for injection 5 mg/mL alatrofloxacin mesylate

Action
PHARMACOLOGY: The IV form is rapidly converted to trovafloxacin, which interferes with microbial DNA synthesis.

PHARMACOKINETICS/DYNAMICS:

Absorption: Absorption is not altered by food. Trovafloxacin is well absorbed from the GI tract. Trovafloxacin bioavailability is approximately 88%. No dosage adjustment is necessary when switching from parenteral to oral administration. Steady state concentrations are achieved by the third daily oral or IV dose.

Distribution: Trovafloxacin is approximately 76% protein bound and is concentration-dependent. The drug is widely distributed throughout the body.

Metabolism: Trovafloxacin is metabolized by conjugation (the role of cytochrome P450 oxidative metabolism of trovafloxacin is minimal). The metabolites are ester glucuronide and N-acetyl.

Excretion: Trovafloxacin is about 50% excreted unchanged: 43% in feces and 6% in urine.

Special Populations:
Hepatic Function Impairment – In mild to moderate cirrhosis, dosage adjustment is recommended because clearance was reduced and t½ is prolonged.

Gender – After a 200 mg dose, C_{max} and AUC were 60% and 32% higher, respectively, in females compared to males.

Indications Treatment of nosocomial pneumonia, community-acquired pneumonia, complicated intra-abdominal infections, complicated skin and skin structure infections, gynecologic, and pelvic infections caused by susceptible organisms.

Contraindications Hypersensitivity to fluoroquinolones, quinolone antibiotics, or any product component; tendonitis or tendon rupture associated with quinolone use.

Route/Dosage
Nosocomial Pneumonia
ADULTS: **IV** 300 mg followed by **PO** 200 mg q 24 hr for 10 to 14 days.

Community Acquired Pneumonia
ADULTS: **PO/IV** 200 mg followed by **PO** 200 mg q 24 hr for 7 to 14 days.

Complicated Intra-Abdominal; Gynecologic; Pelvic Infections
ADULTS: **IV** 300 mg followed by **PO** 200 mg q 24 hr for 7 to 14 days.

Complicated Skin and Skin Structure Infections
ADULTS: **PO/IV** 200 mg followed by **PO** 200 mg q 24 hr for 10 to 14 days.

Interactions
Magnesium-aluminum-containing antacids, antacids containing citric acid buffered with sodium citrate, iron salts, vitamins, minerals containing iron, sucralfate: May decrease oral absorption of trovafloxacin. Stagger administration times by at least 2 hr.

IV morphine sulfate: May decrease oral absorption of trovafloxacin. Administer IV morphine 2 hr after administration of trovafloxacin in fasted state or 4 hr after administration with food.

Lab Test Interferences None well documented.

Adverse Reactions
CNS: Headache; dizziness; lightheadedness.
DERM: Pruritus; rash (IV use).
GI: Nausea; diarrhea; vomiting; abdominal pain.
GU: Vaginitis (PO use).
OTHER: Application/injection/insertion site reaction (IV use).

> **WARNING:**
> Severe hepatotoxicity leading to transplantation and death has occurred with trovafloxacin. Risk increased with more than 2 wk duration. Use only in life-threatening infections and in an inpatient facility. Do not use when safer alternatives are available.

Precautions
Pregnancy: Category C.
Lactation: Excreted in breast milk.
Children: Safety and efficacy in children less than 18 yr not established.
Hypersensitivity: Serious and potentially fatal reactions have occurred.
Hepatic function impairment: Dosage reduction is recommended for patients with mild or moderate cirrhosis. Refer to manufacturer's package insert for dose calculations. There is no information regarding use in patients with severe cirrhosis.
Superinfection: Use of antibiotics may result in bacterial or fungal overgrowth.
Photosensitivity: Moderate to severe reactions may occur.
Convulsions: CNS stimulation can occur; use drug with caution in patients with known or suspected CNS disorder.
LFTs (PO Use): Elevation of LFTs have occurred during or soon after prolonged therapy (over 21 days).
Long-term safety: Safety and efficacy of therapy given for more than 4 wk have not been studied.
Pseudomembranous colitis: Consider possibility in patients who develop diarrhea.

PATIENT CARE CONSIDERATIONS
Administration/Storage
PO use:
- Do not administer for over 2 wk.
- Administer without regard to food with full glass of water.
- Administer 2 hr before or after antacids containing magnesium or aluminum; antacids containing citric acid buffered with sodium citrate, sucralfate; vitamins or minerals with iron, iron salts.
- Administer IV morphine sulfate 2 hr after trovafloxacin is administered without food or 4 hr after administration with food.

- Store at room temperature in tightly closed container.

IV use:
- Do not administer for over 2 wk.
- For IV administration only. Do not administer via IM, intrathecal, intraperitoneal, or SC route.
- Must be diluted with appropriate solution before administration. Refer to the manufacturer's package insert for compatible fluids and dilution guidelines.
- Infuse over 60 min. Avoid rapid or bolus injection.
- Do not use if particulate matter or discoloration is noted.
- Other medications or additives should not be combined with alatrofloxacin nor infused simultaneously through the same IV line.
- If same IV line is used for sequential infusion of several different drugs, the line should be flushed before and after each medication with a mutually compatible solution.
- Discard any unused solution.
- Patients started on alatrofloxacin may be switched to trovafloxacin tablets using comparable dosages (ie, no adjustment necessary), when clinically indicated at the discretion of the health care provider.
- Store undiluted vials at room temperature protected from light. Do not freeze.
- Diluted solution is stable for 3 days at room temperature or 7 days when refrigerated.

Assessment/Interventions
- Limit the use of trovafloxacin/alatrofloxacin to patients who receive initial treatment in a hospital or long-term nursing facility.
- Obtain patient history, including drug history and any known allergies. Note hepatic impairment.
- Monitor for signs of infection throughout course of therapy.
- Monitor I&O.
- Monitor for signs of anaphylaxis (eg, pharyngeal or facial edema, dyspnea, urticaria and itching, hypotension).
- Monitor for symptoms of pseudomembranous colitis (eg, loose or foul-smelling stools) or symptoms of CNS stimulation (eg, tremor, restlessness, confusion).

Patient/Family Education
PO use:
- Inform patient that tablets may be taken orally without regard to meals.
- Inform patient to take tablets 2 hr before or after antacids containing magnesium or aluminum, citric acid buffered with sodium citrate, sucralfate, vitamins and minerals containing iron and iron salts.
- Caution patient to avoid exposure to sunlight, and to use sunscreen or protective clothing until tolerance is determined.
- Instruct patient to report any signs of bacterial or fungal overgrowth (eg, black, furry appearance of tongue, vaginal itching or discharge, loose or foul-smelling stools).
- Caution patient that drug may cause dizziness or lightheadedness and to use caution while driving or performing other tasks requiring mental alertness.
- Emphasize importance of completing entire dose regimen.
- Instruct patient to discontinue treatment and inform health care provider if experiencing any of the following: pain, inflammation, or rupture of a tendon; skin rash or hives; difficulty swallowing or breathing; swelling of lips, tongue, or face; tightness of throat.
- Instruct patient to notify health care provider if experiencing persistent diarrhea or diarrhea containing mucous.

IV use:
- Inform patient that IV form is administered until health care provider decides it is appropriate to convert to oral therapy with trovafloxacin.

Trypsin/Balsam Peru/Castor Oil

(TRIP-sin/BOLL-sam peh-RUH/KASS-ter oil)

Class Topical Enzyme

How Supplied
Granulex Aerosol 0.12 mg trypsin/87 mg balsam peru/788 mg castor oil per g

Action
PHARMACOLOGY: Physiologically debrides tissue; improves epithelization by reducing premature epithelial desiccation and cornification.

Indications In acute and chronic conditions such as varicose ulcers, decubital ulcers, eschar, dehiscent wounds and sunburn, relieves pain and promotes healing; debrides eschar and necrotic tissue; stimulates vascular bed; improves epithelization; reduces odor from necrotic wounds.

Contraindications Standard considerations.

Route/Dosage
Topical:
Aerosol Shake well and hold upright approximately 12 inches from the area to be treated.

Apply bid or as often as necessary. To remove, wash gently with water.

Interactions None well documented.

Lab Test Interferences None well documented.

Adverse Reactions
DERM: Stinging or burning sensation; irritation.

PATIENT CARE CONSIDERATIONS
Administration/Storage
- For topical use only. Not for ophthalmic or otic use.
- Shake well before each use.
- Hold can upright and approximately 12 inches from area to be treated. Press valve and coat wound rapidly. Area may be covered with a wet bandage or left uncovered.
- Avoid spraying in the eyes.
- Apply bid or as often as necessary. Wash gently with water to remove before next application.
- Contents are flammable and under pressure. Do not expose spray to fire or open flame, and do not puncture or incinerate can.
- Store at controlled room temperature (less than 86°F). Do not expose can to temperatures above 120°F.

Assessment/Interventions
- Obtain patient history, including drug history and any known allergies. Note presence of

Precautions
Arterial clots: Do not spray on fresh arterial clots.
External use only: Avoid spraying in eyes.
Flammable: Do not expose to fire or open flame.

Overdosage: Signs and Symptoms
Concentrating and inhaling the contents can be harmful or fatal.

fresh arterial clots.
- Monitor patient's response to therapy.

Patient/Family Education
- Explain name, action, and potential side effects of medication.
- Advise patient, family, or caregiver that medication will usually be prepared and applied by a health care provider in a medical setting but may also be used in a home environment.
- Review prescribed dosing schedule and application process with patient, parent, or caregiver.
- Advise patient, parent, or caregiver that spray may produce a temporary stinging sensation when applied to sensitive skin, but that this should be tolerable. If it persists or is intolerable, notify health care provider.
- Remind patient, parent, or caregiver that follow-up examinations may be necessary while using this medication and to keep appointments.

Tuberculin, Purified Protein Derivative (PPD)

(too-BURR-kyoo-lin)

Class Diagnostic skin test

How Supplied
Tuberculin PPD Multiple Puncture Device
Aplitest Injection 5 TU activity/test ♦ *Tine Test PPD* Injection 5 TU activity/test

Tuberculin Purified Protein Derivative
Aplisol Injection 5 TU/0.1 mL ♦ *Tubersol* Injection 1 TU/0.1 mL, Injection 5 TU/0.1 mL, Injection 250 TU/0.1 mL

Action
PHARMACOLOGY: Contains soluble products from mycobacterium, which react with lymphocytes to release mediators of cellular hypersensitivity. Some of these mediators induce inflammatory response. Positive reaction is consistent with previous or current tuberculosis infection or previous BCG vaccination.

Indications Detection of delayed hypersensitivity to *Mycobacterium tuberculosis*; aid in diagnosis of infection with *M. tuberculosis*; routine testing for tuberculosis; testing individuals suspected of having contact with active tuberculosis; follow-up verification testing in individuals who have had reactions to tuberculin multipuncture devices used as screening test.

Contraindications People known to be tuberculin-positive reactors.

Route/Dosage
ADULTS AND CHILDREN: **Intradermal** 0.1 mL of 5 TU/0.1 mL concentration (Mantoux test) or multiple puncture device.

HIGHLY SENSITIZED PEOPLE: **Intradermal** 0.1 mL of 1 TU/0.1 mL concentration.

INDIVIDUALS WHO FAIL TO REACT TO PREVIOUS INJECTION OF 5 TU: **Intradermal** 0.1 mL of 250 TU/0.1 mL concentration.

Routine Tuberculin Screening
CHILDREN: Perform at 12 mo, 4 to 6 yr, and 14 to 16 yr.

Interactions
BCG vaccine, previous: May result in positive PPD test (see Precautions).

Corticosteroids or other immunosuppressive drugs: May suppress reactivity to any tuberculin test.
Recent immunization with live virus vaccines (including influenza, measles, mumps, rubella, polio virus, smallpox, yellow fever): May suppress reactivity to any tuberculin test. If tuberculin skin testing is indicated, perform it either before or simultaneous with immunization or 4 to 6 wk after immunization.

Lab Test Interferences None well documented.

Adverse Reactions

DERM: Immediate erythematous reactions, vesiculation, pain, ulceration, necrosis, or scarring at administration site; bleeding at puncture site (tine test).

Precautions

Pregnancy: Category C. Use if needed. Unrecognized tuberculosis places infant in grave danger of tuberculosis and tuberculous meningitis. No adverse effects on fetus from tuberculin have been reported.
Lactation: Undetermined.
Children: A child who has been exposed to tuberculosis must not be judged free of infection until there is negative tuberculin reaction at least 10 wk after ending contact with tuberculous person.
Elderly: Skin-test responsiveness may be delayed or reduced in magnitude among older people. Two-step testing is especially important in people 35 yr or older. Reactions may peak after 72 hr.
BCG vaccine: People previously immunized with BCG vaccine may test positive to tuberculin skin test. Tuberculin reactions caused by BCG cannot reliably be distinguished from reactions caused by natural mycobacterial infections. Tuberculin reactivity in BCG vaccinees does not reliably predict protection against M. tuberculosis.

Bioequivalency: The various PPD solutions are generically equivalent but differ from PPD multipuncture devices and from old tuberculin (OT) products.
Immunodeficiency: Skin-test responsiveness may be suppressed during or for as much as 6 wk after viral infection, live viral vaccination, miliary or pulmonary tuberculosis infection, bacterial infection, severe febrile illness, malnutrition, sarcoidosis, malignancy or immunosuppression (eg, corticosteroids or other immunosuppressive pharmacotherapy). In most patients who are very sick with tuberculosis, a previously negative tuberculin test becomes positive after a few weeks of chemotherapy.
Interpretation of test results: Positive PPD reaction indicates hypersensitivity to tuberculin and implies past or present infection with M. tuberculosis. Positive reactions do not necessarily signify active disease. Further diagnostic procedures (eg, chest radiograph, microbiological examination of sputum) must be conducted before a diagnosis of tuberculosis can be made.
Multipuncture devices: Multipuncture devices are screening tools that aid in determining tuberculin hypersensitivity. They may contain either PPD or OT. These devices are comparable to 5 TU of PPD but may yield false-positive reactions because quantity of tuberculin deposited into skin cannot be precisely controlled. Positive reactions to multipuncture devices must be confirmed with intradermal injection of PPD solution. OT cross-reacts with other mycobacteria (eg, *Mycobacterium avium*). Multipuncture devices are useful in people who object to use of needle and syringe (eg, children).
Repeated testing of uninfected individuals: Does not sensitize to tuberculin.

Overdosage: Signs and Symptoms
Vesiculation, ulceration, necrosis.

PATIENT CARE CONSIDERATIONS
Administration/Storage
- Cleanse site with 70% isopropyl alcohol, acetone, ether, or soap and water and allow to dry before test injection.
- Avoid areas with rash, hair, scars, pimples, moles, and other marks.
- Use fresh solution for injection.
- For intradermal injection, use 26- or 27-gauge ½-inch needle to administer intradermal injection into flexor or dorsal surface of forearm, creating white bleb 6 to 10 mm in diameter. No dressing is required.
- For multiple puncture device, apply unit firmly and without twisting to volar surface of upper ⅓ of forearm for 1 sec. Make sure all 4 tines penetrate skin.
- If performing retest, perform on opposite forearm.
- Do not use 250 TU/0.1 mL concentration for initial testing.
- PPD multi-puncture devices should be stored at room temperature.
- PPD solution should be stored in refrigerator.

Assessment/Interventions
- Obtain patient history, including prior PPD test results, BCG vaccination, drug history, and any known allergies. Individuals who may have received BCG vaccination will likely exhibit false-positive reactions.
- Assess appropriate timing of testing; viral febrile illnesses, liver virus vaccination, mal-

nutrition, or immunosuppression may suppress results. Tuberculin skin testing cannot be performed until 4 to 6 wk after immunization with live virus vaccines.
- Obtain history of exposure to tuberculous people prior to skin testing.
- Assess for hypersensitivity, especially in patients with high risk of disease. Have epinephrine readily available.
- Assess ability of patient to accurately read test results.
- Interpret results 48 to 72 hr after administration. Delayed hypersensitivity reactions begin within 5 to 6 hr and peak after 48 to 72 hr. Reactions in elderly people and those never before tested may peak sometime after 72 hr.
- Measure induration along transverse diameter at right angle to long axis of forearm.
- Detect induration by gently palpating double skinfold between thumb and forefinger, starting in normal area around test site and moving toward test site until thickened area is felt. Consider only induration in interpreting test. If erythema is greater than 10 mm in diameter occurs without induration, injection may have been made too deeply; retest patient.

Interpretation:

- Induration less than 5 mm in diameter are classified as negative. This indicates lack of hypersensitivity to tuberculin and implies that tuberculous infection is highly unlikely.
- Reactions to PPD with induration at least 5 mm diameter are classified as positive in (1) people with HIV infection or risk factors for HIV infection (including IV drug use) whose HIV status is unknown, (2) people with close recent contact with infectious tuberculosis cases, and (3) people with chest radiographs consistent with old healed tuberculosis.
- Induration at least 10 mm diameter are classified as positive in (1) foreign-born people from high-prevalence countries in Asia, Africa, or Latin America; (2) HIV-negative IV drug users; (3) medically underserved low-income populations (eg, high-risk racial or ethnic minority populations); (4) residents of long-term care facilities (eg, correctional institutions, nursing homes, institutions for disabled people); (5) people with conditions that increase risk of tuberculosis (eg, silicosis, gastrectomy, jejunoileal bypass, body weight at least 10% below ideal weight, chronic renal failure, diabetes mellitus, immunosuppressive therapy, leukemias, lymphomas, or other malignancies); (6) other high-risk populations defined locally.
- Induration at least 15 mm diameter are classified as positive in all other people not listed above, especially in people greater than 35 yr.
- Reactions to either OT or PPD multipuncture devices with induration at least 2 mm in diameter or presence of any vesiculation at application site are classified as positive. Positive response indicates hypersensitivity to tuberculin and implies past or present infection with M. *tuberculosis*. Retesting with PPD solution is necessary in patients who exhibit positive responses (any size induration) to multipuncture devices.
- If patient is BCG positive, use alternative measurement for accuracy of results.
- Apply cold packs or topical corticosteroid preparations to administration site for symptomatic relief of associated pain, pruritus, and discomfort.
- If patient is considered at risk for immunodeficiency, PPD should be applied with other skin tests (eg, mumps, candida) to evaluate cell-mediated immunity. Skin tests should be at least 5 to 10 cm apart.

Patient/Family Education

- Inform patient to return in 48 to 72 hr for test interpretation or explain how to interpret skin results. Provide card for interpretation.
- Advise patient of significance of test results and stress importance of reporting results.
- If test results are positive, provide information on where patient can obtain further evaluation.

Unoprostone Isopropyl

(YOU-no-PROSTE-ohn eye-so-PRO-pill)
Class Ophthalmic prostaglandin agonists

How Supplied
Rescula Solution 0.15%

Action
PHARMACOLOGY: May reduce IOP by increasing the outflow of aqueous humor.

PHARMACOKINETICS/DYNAMICS:
Absorption: Absorbed through cornea and conjunctival epithelium where it is hydrolyzed by esterases to unoprostone-free acid. The C_{max} is less than 1.5 ng/mL.
Excretion: The t½ is 14 min. Metabolites are excreted primarily in urine.

Indications Reduction of IOP in patients with open-angle glaucoma or ocular hypertension who are intolerant of other IOP-lowering agents or insufficiently responsive to other IOP-lowering medications.

Contraindications Standard considerations.

Route/Dosage
ADULTS: **Ophthalmic** Instill 1 drop in affected eye(s) bid.

Interactions None well documented.

Lab Test Interferences None well documented.

Adverse Reactions
CV: Hypertension.
CNS: Dizziness; headache; insomnia.
EENT: Burning/stinging eyes upon instillation; dry eyes; itchy eyes; increased eyelash length; decreased eyelash length; abnormal vision; eyelid disorders; foreign body sensations; lacrimation disorder; blepharitis; cataract; conjunctivitis; corneal lesions; eye discharge; eye hemorrhage; eye pain; keratitis; irritation; photophobia; vitreous disorder; pharyngitis; rhinitis; sinusitis.
METAB: Diabetes mellitus.
RESP: Bronchitis; increased cough.
OTHER: Flu symptoms; accidental injury; allergy; back pain; pain.

Precautions
Pregnancy: Category C.
Lactation: Undetermined.
Children: Safety and efficacy not established.
Active intraocular inflammation: Use with caution in patients with iritis/uveitis.
Bacterial keratitis: Bacterial keratitis has been reported with multiple-dose containers as a result of patient contamination.
Contact lenses: Remove contact lenses prior to administration and for 15 min following administration.
Macular edema: Use with caution in aphakic patients, pseudophakic patients with a risk of torn posterior lens capsule, or in patients with risk factors for macular edema.
Pigmentation changes: Permanent changes to pigmented tissue may occur, most frequently involving pigmentation of the iris and eyelid and increased pigmentation and growth of eyelashes. Gradual change in eye color (ie, increased amount of brown pigmentation in the iris) may occur.

PATIENT CARE CONSIDERATIONS

Administration/Storage
- If using other topical ophthalmic drugs, separate each medication by at least 5 min.
- Store at controlled room temperature. Keep container tightly closed.

Assessment/Interventions
- Obtain patient history, including drug history and any known allergies.
- Ensure that IOP has been measured and documented in the patient's record.

Patient/Family Education
- Explain name, dose, action, and potential side effects of drug.
- Teach patient proper technique for instilling eye drops. Wash hands; do not allow dropper to touch eye. Tilt head back, look up; pull lower eyelid down; instill drop. Close eye for 1 to 2 min and apply gentle pressure to bridge of nose. Do not rub eye.
- Advise patients who wear contact lenses to remove lenses before instilling medicine and to wait at least 15 min after instilling eye drops before inserting lenses.
- Advise patient that if more than 1 topical ophthalmic drug is being used, administer the drugs at least 5 min apart.
- Inform patient that medication may cause a gradual increase in brown pigment in the pupil, which may slowly change eye color.
- Advise patient to contact eye doctor if eye or eyelid inflammation is noted, if eye is injured, or if having surgery on eye.
- Remind patient that eye examinations and measurement of IOP is necessary while using this medication. Advise patient to keep appointments.

Urea/Hydrocortisone Acetate

(you-REE-ah/HIGH-droe-core-tih-sone ASS-uh-TATE)

Class Corticosteroid

How Supplied
Carmol HC Cream 1% hydrocortisone acetate and 10% urea

Action
PHARMACOLOGY:
Hydrocortisone: Depresses formation, release, and activity of endogenous mediators of inflammation as well as modifying body's immune response.
Urea: Hydrating and keratolytic properties.

Indications Relief of inflammatory and pruritic manifestations of corticosteroid-responsive dermatoses.

Contraindications Standard considerations.

Route/Dosage
ADULTS AND CHILDREN: **TOPICAL** Apply thin film to affected area bid to qid, depending on the seriousness of the condition. Administration of topical corticosteroids to children should be limited to the least amount compatible with an effective therapeutic regimen.

PATIENT CARE CONSIDERATIONS

Administration/Storage
- For topical use only. Not for ophthalmic or otic use.
- Apply a thin film to affected area(s) bid to qid, as ordered. Use gloves or applicator as applicable.
- Do not apply an occlusive dressing unless ordered by health care provider.
- Store at controlled room temperature (59° to 86°F). Keep tube tightly closed and protect from freezing.

Assessment/Interventions
- Obtain patient history, including drug history and any known allergies. Note history of sulfite sensitivity or bacterial, viral, fungal, or mycobacterial skin infections.
- Monitor patient's response to therapy. Notify health care provider if skin inflammation, irritation, or sensitization are noted or if symptoms do not improve or worsen.

Interactions None well documented.

Lab Test Interferences None well documented.

Adverse Reactions
DERM: Burning; itching; irritation; dryness; folliculitis; hypertrichosis; acneiform eruptions; hypopigmentation; perioral dermatitis; allergic contact dermatitis; maceration of the skin; secondary infection; skin atrophy; striae; miliaria.

Precautions
Pregnancy: Category C.
Lactation: Undetermined; however, systemic hydrocortisone is excreted in breast milk.
Children: Pediatric patients may demonstrate greater susceptibility to topical corticosteroid-induced hypothalamic-pituitary-adrenal (HPA) axis suppression and Cushing syndrome than mature patients because of a larger skin surface area to body weight ratio.
Topical absorption: Systemic absorption of topical corticosteroids can produce reversible HPA axis suppression, manifestations of Cushing syndrome, hyperglycemia, and glucosuria.

Overdosage: Signs and Symptoms
HPA axis suppression; manifestations of Cushing syndrome; hyperglycemia and glucosuria, especially when large surface areas, prolonged use, or occlusive dressings are involved.

Patient/Family Education
- Explain name, action, and potential side effects of medication.
- Review prescribed dosing schedule with patient or caregiver.
- Remind patient or caregiver that cream is not to be used in the eye or ear.
- Teach patient or caregiver proper technique for applying cream: wash hands; apply thin film to affected area(s) using fingers or applicator. Wash hands after applying cream.
- Caution patient or caregiver not to cover area with an occlusive dressing unless advised by health care provider.
- Advise patient or caregiver to contact health care provider if local redness or swelling develops or if skin lesions do not improve or worsen.
- Remind patient or caregiver that follow-up examinations may be necessary while using this medication and to keep appointments.

Urofollitropin

(YOUR-oh-fole-lih-TROE-pin)
Class Sex hormone/Ovulation stimulant

How Supplied
Bravelle Powder for injection, lyophilized 75 units follicle stimulating hormone (FSH) activity

Action
PHARMACOLOGY: Stimulates ovarian follicular growth in women who do not have primary ovarian failure.

PHARMACOKINETICS/DYNAMICS:
Absorption: Subcutaneous administration T_{max} occurs in about 20 hr; 17 hr in IM administration.

Excretion: Mean elimination t½ for subcutaneous and IM single dosing are approximately 32 and 37 hr, respectively.

Indications
To be administered in conjunction with human chorionic gonadotropin (hCG) for ovulation induction in patients who have previously received pituitary suppression; in conjunction with hCG for multiple follicular development (controlled ovarian stimulation) during assisted reproductive technologies (ART) cycles in patients who have previously received pituitary suppression.

Contraindications
Women who have high FSH levels, indicating primary ovarian failure; uncontrolled thyroid and adrenal dysfunction; organic intracranial lesion (eg, pituitary tumor); presence of any cause of infertility other than anovulation; abnormal bleeding of undetermined origin; ovarian cysts or enlargement not caused by polycystic ovary syndrome; pregnancy; prior hypersensitivity to urofollitropin.

Route/Dosage
Infertility
ADULTS: **Subcutaneous/IM** In patients who have received gonadotropin-releasing hormone (GnRH) agonist or antagonist pituitary suppression, start with 150 units/day for 5 days, then based on patient response, adjust dose. Do not make adjustments more frequently than once q 2 days and do not exceed 75 to 150 units per adjustment (max, 450 units/day). In most cases, do not dose beyond 12 days. If response is appropriate, give hCG 5,000 to 10,000 units 1 day following the last dose of urofollitropin. Withhold hCG if serum estradiol is greater than 2,000 pg/mL.

ART
ADULTS: **Subcutaneous** 225 units/day for the first 5 days for patients undergoing in vitro fertilization and donor egg patients who have received GnRH agonist or antagonist pituitary suppression. Adjust subsequent dosing according to individual patient response based on clinical monitoring (including serum estradiol levels and vaginal ultrasound results). Dosage adjustments should not be more frequent than once q 2 days and should not exceed 75 to 150 units/adjustment (max, 450 units/day). In most cases, dosing beyond 12 days is not recommended. Once adequate follicular development is evident, administer 5,000 to 10,000 units of hCG to induce final follicular maturation in preparation for oocyte retrieval. To reduce the chance of developing ovarian hyperstimulation syndrome (OHSS), withhold hCG administration in cases where ovaries are abnormally enlarged on the last day of therapy.

Interactions None well documented.

Lab Test Interferences None well documented.

Adverse Reactions
CV: Hypertension (3%).
CNS: Headache (13%); emotional lability, depression (3%).
DERM: Rash, acne, exfoliative dermatitis (3%).
GI: Abdominal cramps (14%); nausea (9%); abdominal fullness/enlargement (7%); abdominal pain (5%); constipation (3%).
GU: OHSS (11%); vaginal hemorrhage (9%); postretrieval pain (8%); pelvic pain (7%); hot flashes (6%); uterine spasms, vaginal bleeding, vaginal discharge, UTI, cervix disorder (3%); ovarian disorder, breast tenderness, fungal infections (2%).
METAB: Weight gain, dehydration (3%).
RESP: Respiratory disorder (6%); accidental injury (2%).
OTHER: Pain (6%); injection site reaction (4%); neck pain, fever, accidental injury (3%); anaphylactic reactions.

Precautions
Pregnancy: Category X.
Lactation: Undetermined.
Children: Safety and efficacy not established.
Elderly: Safety and efficacy not established.
Multiple births: Multiple pregnancies have occurred.
Health care provider use: Urofollitropin should only be used by health care providers thoroughly familiar with infertility problems and their management.
Ovarian enlargement: Mild to moderate uncomplicated ovarian enlargement may occur in approximately 20% of women treated with follitropin and hCG and generally regresses without treatment within 2 to 3 wk.
OHSS: Warning signs include difficulty breathing, severe pelvic pain, nausea, vomiting, rapid weight gain, stomach pain or bloating, diarrhea,

or infrequent urination. May progress within 24 hr to several days to become a serious medical event. Treatment must be stopped and patient hospitalized.

Pulmonary and vascular complications: Intravascular thrombosis and embolism can reduce blood flow to critical organs (may result in pulmonary infarct) or extremities (may cause loss of limbs).

Overdosage: Signs and Symptoms
OHSS, multiple gestations.

PATIENT CARE CONSIDERATIONS
Administration/Storage
- Urofollitropin stimulates ovarian follicular growth and must be used in conjunction with hCG, which induces ovulation.
- Dose and duration of therapy are variable, depending on indication for use and patient response. Max daily dose should not exceed 450 units. Dosing beyond 12 days is not recommended.
- For subcutaneous or IM administration only when used for ovulation induction. Not for intradermal, IV, or intra-arterial administration.
- For subcutaneous administration only when used for multifollicular development during ART. Not for intradermal, IM, IV, or intra-arterial administration.
- Reconstitute powder for injection by adding 1 mL sterile 0.9% sodium chloride injection and swirl gently until solution is clear. Do not shake vial during reconstitution.
- For patient requiring a single injection from multiple vials of urofollitropin, up to 6 vials can be reconstituted with 1 mL of sterile 0.9% sodium chloride injection. Reconstitute the first vial as described above, then draw the entire contents of the first vial into a syringe and inject the contents into the second vial of lyophilized urofollitropin. Gently swirl the second vial until solution is clear. Repeat this process with 4 additional vials for a total of up to 6 vials of lyophilized urofollitropin into 1 mL of diluent.
- Do not administer if solution is discolored or cloudy, or if particulate matter is noted.
- Immediately administer reconstituted solution either as subcutaneous or IM injection as ordered.
- Administer subcutaneous doses in either side of lower abdomen in alternating fashion. Vary the actual injection site with each injection. Do not administer subcutaneously into thigh unless the lower abdomen is not usable because of scarring, surgical deformity, or other medical conditions.
- For subcutaneous injection, insert needle at a 90° angle to the skin surface.
- Administer IM doses into the upper outer quadrant of the buttock muscle near the hip. Stretching the skin helps the needle go in more easily and pushes the tissue beneath the skin out of the way. This helps the solution disperse correctly.
- For IM administration, insert needle at a 90° angle to the skin surface. Pushing in with a quick thrust causes the least discomfort.
- Gently massage injection site to help disperse solution and relieve any discomfort.
- Discard any unused solution. Do not save unused solution for later administration.
- Store lyophilized powder in refrigerator or at room temperature (37° to 77°F). Protect from light.

Assessment/Interventions
- Obtain patient history, including drug history and any known allergies. Note uterine or tubal pathology.
- Review patient's health history for any condition that could contraindicate urofollitropin therapy: previous allergic reaction to urofollitropin; high levels of FSH; uncontrolled thyroid or adrenal dysfunction; intracranial lesion; abnormal uterine bleeding of undetermined origin; ovarian cyst or enlargement not caused by polycystic ovary syndrome; any cause of infertility other than anovulation; pregnancy.
- Ensure that patient and her partner have been advised of the potential risk of multiple births before treatment is started.
- Ensure that patient has had a thorough gynecological and endocrinologic evaluation before starting therapy.
- To reduce risk of overstimulation of the ovary in women, ensure that ovarian response to therapy is closely monitored (eg, serum estradiol levels, ultrasonography). Do not administer hCG to patient if serum estradiol level is greater than 2,000 pg/mL. If the ovaries are abnormally enlarged or abdominal pain occurs, discontinue urofollitropin therapy, do not administer hCG, and caution patient to avoid intercourse.
- Monitor patient for signs and symptoms of overstimulation of the ovary (eg, dyspnea, severe pelvic pain, nausea, vomiting, diarrhea, rapid weight gain, abdominal pain or distension, oliguria) during therapy and for 2 wk after hCG has been discontinued. Report to health care provider immediately if noted or suspected.

- Monitor patient for signs and symptoms of thromboembolic events (eg, venous thrombophlebitis, pulmonary embolism, pulmonary infarction, stroke, arterial occlusion). Report to health care provider immediately if noted or suspected.
- Assess patient for GU, GI, and general body side effects and injection site reactions. Inform health care provider if noted and significant.

Patient/Family Education
- Explain names, actions, and potential side effects of the treatment regimen, including risk of multiple births. Review the treatment regimen, including duration of treatment and monitoring that will be required.
- If patient will be self-administering at home, ensure the patient understands how to store, prepare, and administer the dose, and dispose of used equipment and supplies.
- Caution patient not to change the dose or stop taking the medicine unless advised by health care provider.
- Caution patient that if a dose is missed not to double the dose to catch up. Advise patient to contact health care provider for further instructions.
- Remind patient that drug is administered to promote follicular growth and egg production, and that hCG will need to be administered to induce ovulation.
- Encourage patient receiving drug for infertility to have intercourse daily, beginning on the day prior to administration of hCG until ovulation has become apparent.
- Warn patient that close monitoring for overstimulation of the ovary is required and to report any of the following immediately to health care provider: difficulty breathing, severe pelvic pain, nausea, vomiting, diarrhea, rapid weight gain, stomach pain or bloating, infrequent urination.
- Advise patient to inform health care provider of any side effects, symptoms, physical changes, or bothersome injection site reactions.
- Caution patient not to take any prescription or OTC medications, herbal preparations, or dietary supplements unless advised by health care provider.
- Advise patient that follow-up visits and frequent lab tests will be required to monitor therapy and to keep appointments.

Urokinase

(YOUR-oh-KIN-ace)

Class Thrombolytic enzyme

How Supplied
Abbokinase Injection 250,000 IU

Action
PHARMACOLOGY: Converts plasminogen to the enzyme plasmin, which aids in dissolution of blood clots.

PHARMACOKINETICS/DYNAMICS:
Distribution: Vd is 11.5 L.

Excretion: Small amounts of urokinase are excreted in the bile and urine. The t½ is 12.6 min (for biologic activity).

Special Populations:
Hepatic Function Impairment – Clearance may be reduced.

Indications Lysis of acute massive pulmonary emboli (defined as obstruction of blood flow to a lobe or multiple segments); lysis of pulmonary emboli accompanied by unstable hemodynamics (ie, failure to maintain BP without supportive measures).

Contraindications Active internal bleeding; recent cerebrovascular accidents (eg, within 2 mo); recent intracranial or intraspinal surgery (eg, within 2 mo); recent trauma including cardiopulmonary resuscitation; intracranial neoplasm, arteriovenous malformation, or aneurysm; known bleeding diatheses; severe uncontrolled arterial hypertension; known hypersensitivity to any component of the product.

Route/Dosage
ADULTS: IV Loading dose of 2000 IU/lb (4400 IU/kg) admixture (0.9% sodium chloride injection, or 5% dextrose injection) instituted soon after onset of pulmonary embolism and infused at a rate of 90 mL/hr over 10-min period, followed by continuous infusion of 2000 IU/lb/hr (4400 IU/kg/hr) at a rate of 15 mL/hr for 12 hr. Flush tubing with solution (0.9% sodium chloride injection, or 5% dextrose injection) approximately equal to the volume of the tubing in the infusion set. The pump should be set to administer the flush solution at the rate of 15 mL/hr.

Interactions
Anticoagulants, agents that alter platelet function (eg, aspirin, other NSAIDs, dipyridamole), other thrombolytic agents, agents that alter coagulation: May increase the risk of serious bleeding.
INCOMPATIBILITIES: Do not use bacteriostatic water for injection; do not add any other medication to urokinase solution.

Lab Test Interferences None well documented.

Adverse Reactions

CV: MI; cardiac arrest; vascular embolism (including cholesterol embolism); cerebral vascular accidents; hyperfusion ventricular arrhythmias.
CNS: Stroke.
HEMA: Bleeding (including fatal hemorrhage, bronchospasm, orolingual edema, urticaria, rash, and pruritus); decreased hematocrit; thrombocytopenia.
RESP: Pulmonary embolism; pulmonary edema.
OTHER: Hemiplegia; hypersensitivity (including fatal anaphylaxis); substernal pain; diaphoresis; chest pain.

Precautions

Pregnancy: Category B.
Lactation: Undetermined.
Children: Safety and efficacy not established.
Elderly: Use with caution.
Hypersensitivity: Anaphylaxis, bronchospasm, orolingual edema, and urticaria may occur.

PATIENT CARE CONSIDERATIONS

Administration/Storage

- Administer only by IV infusion. Not for SC or IM administration.
- Reconstitute lyophilized powder following manufacturer's recommendations.
- Avoid shaking the vial during reconstitution.
- Use reconstituted solution immediately.
- Do not add any other medications to reconstituted solution.
- Do not administer if particulate matter or discoloration noted. A slight yellowish color is normal and is of no concern.
- Discard any unused solution.
- Store unopened vials in refrigerator (36° to 46°F).

Assessment/Interventions

- Obtain patient history, including drug history and any known allergies.
- Review patient's health history for any of the following conditions that would contraindicate urokinase use: active internal bleeding; recent (within 2 mo) cerebrovascular accident; trauma; including cardiopulmonary resuscitation; intracranial or intraspinal surgery; intracranial neoplasm, arteriovenous malformation, or aneurysm; severe uncontrolled hypertension; known bleeding diatheses; hypersensitivity to urokinase.
- Review patient's health history for any of the following conditions that could increase the risk of complications: recent (within 10 days) major surgery, GI bleeding, obstetrical delivery, organ biopsy, previous puncture of noncompressible vessel; hypertension; likelihood of left heart thrombus; subacute bacterial endocarditis; hemostatic defects including those caused by liver or kidney disease; pregnancy; diabetic hemorrhagic retinopathy; cerebrovascular disease.

Special risk patients: The risk of bleeding may be increased in patients with the following conditions: recent major surgery (within 10 days), obstetrical delivery, organ biopsy, previous puncture of noncompressible vessels; recent serious GI bleeding (within 10 days); high likelihood of a left heart thrombus (eg, mitral stenosis with arterial fibrillation); subacute bacterial endocarditis; hemostatic defects including those secondary to severe hepatic or renal disease; pregnancy; cerebrovascular accident; diabetic hemorrhagic retinopathy; any condition in which bleeding might constitute a hazard or be particularly difficult to manage because of location.

Bleeding: Risk of serious bleeding (eg, intracranial hemorrhage) is increased. Careful attention should be paid to all potential bleeding sites (eg, catheter insertion sites, cutdown sites, needle puncture sites).

Cholesterol embolism: Serious and fatal cholesterol embolism may occur.

- Review patient's medication record for use of drugs that present special risks when used in conjunction with urokinase (other thrombolytic agents, anticoagulants, or antiplatelet agents).
- Ensure that patient has been evaluated for bleeding disorders before administration of urokinase.
- Monitor patient for signs of bleeding throughout therapy. If bleeding develops (eg, epistaxis, hematuria, hematemesis, bloody or black, tarry stools) notify health care provider immediately. Should uncontrollable bleeding occur discontinue urokinase therapy.
- Monitor BP during administration. If hypotension develops notify health care provider immediately. Be prepared to treat appropriately.
- Monitor patient for signs of anaphylaxis or severe allergic reaction. Discontinue therapy and immediately notify health care provider if noted. Be prepared to treat appropriately.
- Ensure that TT, aPTT, PT, or fibrinogen levels are determined prior to therapy and periodically, as indicated, throughout therapy.
- Ensure that hematocrit, platelet count and TT, aPTT, PT, or fibrinogen levels are determined before beginning therapy and periodically, as indicated, throughout therapy.
- Discontinue heparin before therapy and ensure that TT or aPTT is less than twice the normal value before beginning urokinase.

- If heparin is to be (re)instituted following urokinase administration, ensure that TT or aPTT is less than twice the normal value before starting heparin.
- Avoid IM injections during and for 24 hr following administration.
- Perform venipunctures carefully and as infrequently as possible during therapy.
- If arterial puncture is necessary, ensure that upper extremity vessel is used. Following puncture apply pressure for at least 30 min. Apply pressure dressing and check puncture site frequently.

Patient/Family Education
- Explain name, dose, action, and potential side effects of drug.
- Advise patient, family, or caregiver that medication will be prepared and administered by a health care professional in a medical setting.
- Instruct patient, family member, or caregiver to report any signs of bleeding or allergic reaction immediately.

Valacyclovir Hydrochloride

(val-lay-SIGH-kloe-vihr HIGH-droe-KLOR-ide)

Class Anti-infective/Antiviral

How Supplied
Valtrex Tablets 500 mg, Tablets 1 g

Action
PHARMACOLOGY: Converted to acyclovir, which then inhibits viral DNA replication by interfering with viral DNA polymerase.

PHARMACOKINETICS/DYNAMICS:
Absorption: Rapidly absorbed from the GI tract. Bioavailability is about 55%. C_{max} is less than 0.5 mcg/mL.

Metabolism: Converted to acyclovir and L-valine by first-pass intestinal or hepatic metabolism.

Excretion: About 46% is recovered in urine. About 47% is recovered in feces.

Special Populations:
Renal Function Impairment – Dose reduction is recommended.
Elderly – Dose modification may be necessary in geriatric patients with reduced renal function.

Indications Treatment of herpes zoster (shingles); treatment or suppression of genital herpes; treatment of herpes labialis (cold sores).

Contraindications Hypersensitivity or intolerance to valacyclovir, acyclovir, or any component of the formulation.

Route/Dosage
Herpes Zoster
ADULTS: **PO** 1 g tid for 7 days (initiate therapy within 48 hr of onset of rash).

Genital Herpes
ADULTS:
Initial Episodes: **PO** 1 g bid for 10 days (initiate therapy within 48 to 72 hr of onset of signs and symptoms).
Recurrent Episodes: **PO** 500 mg bid for 3 days (initiate therapy within 24 hr of onset of signs or symptoms).
Suppressive Therapy: **PO** 1 g once daily. If history of recurrence up to 9 recurrences/yr, 500 mg/day may be administered.

HIV-Infected Patients
ADULTS: **PO** 500 mg bid for HIV-infected patients with CD4 cell count of at least 100 cells/mm^3 (efficacy beyond 6 mo of therapy has not been established).

Herpes Labialis
ADULTS: **PO** 2 g bid for 1 day approximately 12 hr apart, initiated at earliest symptoms of cold sore (eg, tingling, burning, itching).

Interactions
Cimetidine, probenecid: Increased acyclovir serum concentrations.

Lab Test Interferences None well documented.

Adverse Reactions
CV: Hypertension, tachycardia (postmarketing).
CNS: Headache (38%); depression (7%); dizziness (4%); aggressive behavior, agitation, ataxia, coma, confusion, decreased consciousness, dysarthria, encephalopathy, mania, psychosis (including audio and visual hallucinations), seizures (postmarketing).
DERM: Erythema multiforme, rashes (including photosensitivity), alopecia (postmarketing).
EENT: Visual abnormalities (postmarketing).
GI: Nausea (15%); abdominal pain (11%); vomiting (6%); diarrhea (postmarketing).
GU: Dysmenorrhea (8%); renal failure (postmarketing).
HEPA: Hepatitis (postmarketing).
LABTESTABS: Increased AST (4%); increased serum creatinine, leukopenia, thrombocytopenia, decreased hemoglobin (1%); abnormal liver enzymes, elevated creatinine, aplastic anemia (postmarketing).
OTHER: Arthralgia (6%); acute hypersensitivity reactions (including anaphylaxis, angioedema, dyspnea, pruritus, rash, and urticaria), facial edema, leukocytoclastic vasculitis (postmarketing).

Precautions
Pregnancy: Category B.
Lactation: Undetermined (acyclovir is excreted in breast milk).
Children: Safety and efficacy not established.
Elderly: Dosage reduction may be necessary, depending on underlying renal status.
Renal function impairment: Dosage reduction is recommended; exercise caution when giving valacyclovir to patients with renal impairment or those receiving potentially nephrotoxic drugs.
Immunocompromised: Valacyclovir is not indicated for use in immunocompromised patients.
Thrombotic thrombocytopenic purpura/hemolytic uremic syndrome: May occur and has resulted in death in patients with advanced HIV disease and also in allergenic bone marrow and renal transplant recipients receiving 8 g/day of valacyclovir.

Overdosage: Signs and Symptoms
Acute renal failure, anuria.

PATIENT CARE CONSIDERATIONS
Administration/Storage
- Administer prescribed dose without regard to meals. Administer with food if GI upset occurs.
- Dose and duration of therapy is dependent on condition being treated.
- Store at controlled room temperature (59° to 77°F).

Assessment/Interventions
- Obtain patient history, including drug history and any known allergies. Note impaired renal function or HIV infection.
- Ensure that reduced dose is administered to patient with renal impairment.
- For herpes zoster (shingles) assess for history of present illness and time of rash onset. Treatment should be started no later than 72 hr after onset of rash.
- For genital herpes assess for history of present illness and time of onset of symptoms.
- Treatment should be started no later than 72 hr after onset of symptoms for first episode or 24 hr for recurrent episode.
- For recurrent genital herpes assess history of frequency of recurrence.
- Monitor for effectiveness of treatment.
- Monitor patient for CNS, GI, and general body side effects. Report to health care provider if noted and significant.

Patient/Family Education
- Explain name, dose, action, and potential side effects of drug.
- Review dose and appropriate dosing schedule depending on condition being treated (shingles, cold sores, or genital herpes). Instruct patient to take medication exactly as prescribed and not to stop taking or change the dose unless advised by health care provider.
- Advise patient that medication can be taken without regard to meals but to take with food if stomach upset occurs.
- Remind patient using medication for cold sores that it is not a cure and to initiate therapy at the first symptom of a cold sore (eg, tingling, itching, burning). Remind patient that treatment should not exceed 2 doses taken about 12 hr apart.
- Remind patient using medication for recurrent episodes of genital herpes to initiate therapy at the first sign or symptom or recurrence and that medication may not be effective if started more than 24 hr after onset of signs or symptoms of recurrence.
- Advise patient with genital herpes that this drug is not a cure for genital herpes and does not prevent transmission of virus. Instruct patient to avoid sexual intercourse when lesions and/or symptoms are present to avoid infecting partner.
- Advise patient to contact health care provider if medication does not seem to be controlling lesions and/or symptoms or if intolerable side effects develop.
- Caution patient to avoid unnecessary exposure to UV light (sunlight, tanning booths) and to use sunscreen and wear protective clothing until tolerance is determined.
- Advise women to contact health care provider if pregnant, planning to become pregnant, or breastfeeding.
- Instruct patient not to take any prescription or OTC medications or dietary supplements unless advised by health care provider.
- Advise patient that follow-up visits may be necessary to monitor therapy and to keep appointments.

Valdecoxib

(Val-deh-cox-ib)
Class Analgesic/NSAID

How Supplied
Bextra Tablets 10 mg, Tablets 20 mg

Action
PHARMACOLOGY: Inhibits inflammation, pain and fever, probably by inhibition of cyclooxygenase-2 (COX-2).

PHARMACOKINETICS/DYNAMICS:
Absorption: T_{max} is about 3 hr. Bioavailability is 83%. Steady state is achieved by 4 days. AUC is about 1480 hr•ng/mL. C_{max} is about 160 ng/mL. C_{min} is about 22 ng/mL.

Distribution: Protein binding is 98%. Vd is 86 L.

Metabolism: Extensive hepatic metabolism involving both P450 isoenzymes (3A4 and 2C9) and non-P450 dependent pathways (ie, glucoronidation).

Excretion: $T_{½}$ is 8 to 11 hr. Eliminated primarily via hepatic metabolism with about 5% of the dose excreted unchanged in the urine and feces. Clearance is about 6 L/hr.

Special Populations:
Hepatic Function Impairment – Plasma concentrations increased about 130% in patients with moderate hepatic impairment. Initiate valdecoxib treatment with caution. Do not use in severe hepatic impairment.

Indications Relief of signs and symptoms of osteoarthritis and adult rheumatoid arthritis; treatment of primary dysmenorrhea.

Contraindications Asthma; urticaria; allergic-type reactions after taking aspirin or NSAIDs; sensitivity to valdecoxib.

Route/Dosage
Osteoarthritis, Rheumatoid Arthritis
ADULTS: PO 10 mg once daily.

Primary Dysmenorrhea
ADULTS: PO 20 mg bid as needed.

Interactions
ACE inhibitors: Antihypertensive effect may be decreased.
Aspirin: Risk of GI complications (eg, ulceration) may be increased.
Dextromethorphan: Plasma levels may be reduced by valdecoxib, decreasing the pharmacologic effect.
Fluconazole, ketoconazole, lithium: Plasma levels may be elevated by valdecoxib, increasing the pharmacologic and adverse effects.
Loop diuretics (eg, furosemide): Diuretic effect may be decreased.
Warfarin: Risk of bleeding may be increased.

Lab Test Interferences None well documented.

Adverse Reactions
CV: Hypertension; aneurysm; angina pectoris; arrhythmia; cardiomyopathy; CHF; coronary artery disorder; heart murmur; hypotension; generalized edema; bradycardia; palpitation; tachycardia; intermittent claudication; acquired hemagioma; varicose veins.
CNS: Dizziness; headache; cerebrovascular disorder; hypertonia; hypoesthesia; migraine; neuralgia; neuropathy; paresthesia; tremor; twitching; vertigo; fatigue; anorexia; anxiety; increased appetite; confusion; depression; aggravated depression; insomnia; nervousness; morbid dreaming; somnolence.
DERM: Rash; cellulitis; contact dermatitis; acne; alopecia; dermatitis; fungal dermatitis; eczema; photosensitivity allergic reaction; pruritus; erythematous rash; maculopapular rash; psoriaform rash; dry skin; skin hypertrophy; skin ulceration; increased sweating; urticaria.
EENT: Sinusitis; ear abnormality; earache; tinnitus; otitis media; blurred vision; cataract; conjunctivitis; eye pain; keratitis; abnormal vision.
GI: Abdominal fullness; abdominal pain; diarrhea; dyspepsia; flatulence; nausea; abnormal stools; constipation; diverticulosis; dry mouth; duodenal ulcer; duodenitis; eructation; esophagitis; fecal incontinence; gastric ulcer; gastritis; gastroenteritis; gastroesophageal reflux; hematemesis; hematochezia; hemorrhoids; bleeding hemorrhoids; hiatal hernia; melena; stomatitis; increased stool frequency tenesmus; tooth disorder; vomiting; taste perversion.
GU: Amenorrhea; dysmenorrhea; leukorrhea; mastitis; menstrual disorder; menorrhagia; menstrual bloating; vaginal hemorrhage; impotence; prostatic disorder; genital moniliasis; albuminuria; cystitis; dysuria; hematuria; increased micturition frequency; pyuria; urinary incontinence; urinary tract infection.
HEMA: Anemia; ecchymosis; epistaxis; hematoma NOS; thrombocytopenia; eosinophilia; leukopenia; leukocytosis; lymphadenopathy; lymphangitis; lymphopenia.
HEPA: Abnormal hepatic function; hepatitis; increased ALT and AST.
METAB: Increased alkaline phosphatase, BUN, CPK, creatinine, and LDH; diabetes mellitus; glycosuria; gout; hypercholesterolemia; hyperglycemia; hyperkalemia; hyperlipemia; hyperuricemia; hypocalcemia; hypokalemia; increased thirst; decreased and increased weight; xerophthalmia.
RESP: Upper respiratory tract infection; abnormal breath sounds; bronchitis; bronchospasm; coughing; dyspnea; emphysema; laryngitis; pneumonia; pharyngitis; pleurisy; rhinitis.
OTHER: Back pain; peripheral edema; flu-like symptoms; accidental injury; myalgia; goiter; allergic reaction; aggravated allergy; asthenia; chest pain; chills; cyst; face edema; fever; hot flushes; malaise; pain; periorbital swelling; peripheral pain; halitosis; arthralgia; accidental fracture; neck stiffness; osteoporosis; synovitis; tendonitis; breast neoplasm; lipoma; malignant ovarian cyst; herpes simplex; herpes zoster; fungal infection; soft tissue infection; viral infection; moniliasis.

Precautions
Pregnancy: Category C.
Lactation: Undetermined.
Children: Safety and efficacy not established.
Renal function impairment: Use with caution.
Hepatic function impairment: Use with caution in patients with mild to moderate hepatic impairment; avoid use in severe hepatic impairment.
GI effects: Serious GI toxicity (eg, ulceration, bleeding, perforation) can occur at any time, with or without warning symptoms.
Anaphylaxis: Anaphylaxis may occur in patients without known exposure to valdecoxib; do not administer to patients with aspirin triad.
Dehydration: Use with caution and rehydrate patient before use.

Overdosage: Signs and Symptoms
Lethargy, drowsiness, nausea, vomiting, epigastric pain, GI bleeding, hypertension, acute renal failure, respiratory depression, coma, anaphylaxis.

PATIENT CARE CONSIDERATIONS

Administration/Storage
- May administer each dose without regard to meals or antacids.
- Store tablets at controlled room temperature.

Assessment/Interventions
- Obtain patient history, including drug history and any known allergies. Note history of GI bleeding or ulcers, "aspirin triad" (eg, asthma, rhinitis with or without nasal polyps), allergic reactions to aspirin or other NSAIDs, hypertension, CHF, edema, renal or hepatic impairment.
- Obtain baseline assessments of pain and ability to perform activities of daily living in patient with arthritis. Monitor periodically during therapy.
- Ensure that renal function has been assessed prior to initiating therapy and periodically during therapy in patient with renal impairment.
- Notify health care provider if indigestion, epigastric pain, unusual bleeding or bruising, or dark tarry stools occur.
- Monitor patient for GI, CNS, and general body side effects. Report to health care provider if noted and significant.

Patient/Family Education
- Explain name, dose, action, and potential side effects of drug.
- Instruct patient to take exactly as prescribed.
- Advise patient that each dose may be taken without regard to food.
- Advise patient that dose is individualized based upon severity of symptoms and response to therapy.
- Advise patient to continue other arthritis medications as recommended by their health care provider.
- Caution patient to avoid smoking, alcohol, and aspirin-containing medications while taking this drug.
- Advise patient that if a dose is missed, take it as soon as possible, but if close to the next dose, do not double up and take the next dose as scheduled.
- Instruct patient to discontinue drug and notify health care provider if any of the following occur: persistent GI upset, skin rash, itching, black stools, weight gain, edema, changes in urine patterns, persistent nausea, "flu-like" symptoms, right upper abdominal pain, yellowing of skin or eyes, unexplained fatigue or lethargy.
- Advise patient to inform the health care provider if becoming pregnant, planning on becoming pregnant, or are breastfeeding.
- Instruct patient not to take any prescription or *otc* medications or dietary supplements unless advised to do so by their health care provider.
- Advise patient that follow-up examinations and lab tests may be required to monitor therapy and to be sure and keep appointments.

Valganciclovir

(val-gan-sye-kloh-veer)

Class Antiviral agent

How Supplied
Valcyte Tablets 450 mg

Action
PHARMACOLOGY: Valganciclovir is a prodrug of ganciclovir, which inhibits cytomegalovirus (CMV) replication by inhibition of viral DNA synthesis.

PHARMACOKINETICS/DYNAMICS:

Absorption: Well absorbed from the GI tract. Bioavailability is about 60%. T_{max} is about 1 to 3 hr. When administered with high-fat meal, AUC increased 30%, and C_{max} increased 14%. It should be administered with food.

Distribution: Valganciclovir is metabolized to ganciclovir. Protein binding of ganciclovir is about 1% to 2%. Vd of ganciclovir is about 0.703 L/kg.

Metabolism: Rapidly metabolized in the intestinal wall and liver to ganciclovir.

Excretion: Major route of elimination is by renal excretion. The t½ is about 4.08 hr (tablets) and about 3.81 hr (IV).

Special Populations:
Renal Function Impairment – Dosage reductions according to Ccr are required for valganciclovir.

Indications Treatment of CMV retinitis in patients with AIDS; prevention of CMV disease in kidney, heart, and kidney-pancreas transplant patients at high risk (donor CMV seropositive/recipient CMV seronegative [D+/R-]).

Contraindications Hypersensitivity to ganciclovir or valganciclovir.

Route/Dosage
CMV Retinitis
ADULTS: **PO** 900 mg bid with food for 21 days. Following this induction phase, or in patients with inactive CMV retinitis, give 900 mg qd with food.

Decreased Renal Function
INDUCTION (ADULTS): **PO** 900 mg bid (Ccr 60 mL/min or more); 450 mg bid (Ccr 40 to 59 mL/min); 450 mg qd (Ccr 25 to 39 mL/min); 450 mg q 2 days (Ccr 10 to 24 mL/min).
MAINTENANCE (ADULTS): **PO** 900 mg/day (Ccr 60 mL/min or more); 450 mg qd (Ccr 40 to 59 mL/min); 450 mg q 2 days (Ccr 25 to 39 mL/min); 450 mg twice/wk (Ccr 10 to 24 mL/min).

Prevention of CMV Disease in Heart, Kidney, and Kidney-Pancreas Transplantation
ADULTS: **PO** 900 mg qd with food, starting within 10 days of transplantation until 100 days posttransplantation.

Interactions Interaction studies have not been conducted; however, because valganciclovir is converted to ganciclovir, interactions associated with ganciclovir are expected to occur for valganciclovir.
Amphotericin B, cyclosporine, nephrotoxic drugs: May increase serum creatinine.
Cytotoxic drugs: May increase the risk of toxicity.
Didanosine: Plasma levels of didanosine may be increased, while didanosine may decrease levels of ganciclovir.
Imipenem-cilastatin: May cause generalized seizures.
Probenecid: May reduce renal Cl and increase serum levels of ganciclovir.
Zidovudine: Both ganciclovir and zidovudine can cause granulocytopenia.

Lab Test Interferences None well documented.

Adverse Reactions
CV: Hypertension (18%); hypotension (at least 5% or serious adverse events).
CNS: Headache (22%); insomnia (20%); peripheral neuropathy (9%); paresthesia (8%); dizziness, convulsions, depression, psychosis, hallucinations, confusion, agitation (at least 5% or serious adverse events).
DERM: Dermatitis, pruritus, acne (at least 5% or serious adverse events).
EENT: Retinal detachment (15%); pharyngitis/nasopharyngitis, rhinorrhea (at least 5% or serious adverse events).
GI: Diarrhea (41%); nausea (30%); vomiting (21%); abdominal pain (15%); constipation, dyspepsia, abdominal distention, ascites (at least 5% or serious adverse events).
GU: UTI, renal impairment, dysuria, decreased Ccr (at least 5% or serious adverse events).
HEMA: Neutropenia (27%); anemia (26%); leukopenia (14%); thrombocytopenia (including life-threatening bleeding) (6%); pancytopenia, bone marrow depression, aplastic anemia (at least 5% or serious adverse events).
HEPA: Abnormal hepatic function (at least 5% or serious adverse events).
M/N: Hyperkalemia, hypokalemia, hypomagnesemia, hyperglycemia, decreased appetite, dehydration, hypophosphatemia, hypocalcemia (at least 5% or serious adverse events).
MUSC: Back pain, arthralgia, muscle cramps, limb pain (at least 5% or serious adverse events).
RESP: Upper respiratory tract infection, cough, dyspnea, pleural effusion (at least 5% or serious adverse events).
OTHER: Pyrexia (31%); tremors (28%); graft rejection (24%); catheter-related infections (3%); hypersensitivity, fatigue, pain, edema, peripheral edema, weakness, local and systemic infections and sepsis, postoperative pain, wound infection and complications, increased wound drainage, wound dehiscence (at least 5% or serious adverse events).

> **WARNING:**
> Toxicity includes granulocytopenia, anemia, and thrombocytopenia. In animal studies, ganciclovir was carcinogenic, teratogenic, and caused aspermatogenesis.

Precautions
Pregnancy: Category C.
Lactation: Undetermined; however, the CDC recommends that HIV-infected mothers not breastfeed infants to avoid risk of HIV transmission.
Children: Safety and efficacy not established.
Renal function impairment: Use with caution and adjust dosage.
Cytopenia: Severe leukopenia, neutropenia, bone marrow depression, and aplastic anemia have been reported; therefore, use with caution in patients with preexisting cytopenias, or those who have received or are receiving myelosuppressive drugs or irradiation.

Overdosage: Signs and Symptoms
Pancytopenia, bone marrow depression, medullary aplasia, leukopenia, neutropenia, granulocytopenia, hepatitis, liver function disorder, worsening of hematuria, acute renal failure, elevated creatinine, abdominal pain, diarrhea, vomiting, generalized tremor, convulsion.

PATIENT CARE CONSIDERATIONS
Administration/Storage
- Valganciclovir tablets cannot be substituted for ganciclovir capsules on a one-to-one basis.
- Administer with food to maximize absorption.
- Have patient swallow tablet whole. Do not crush, break, split, or chew tablets.

- If broken or crushed tablet comes in contact with skin or mucus membranes, wash thoroughly with soap and water and rinse eyes thoroughly with plain water.
- Store at controlled room temperature (59° to 86°F).

Assessment/Interventions
- Obtain patient history, including drug history and any known allergies. Note renal impairment, cytopenia, sensitivity to ganciclovir, or concurrent treatment with myelosuppressive drugs or radiation.
- Ensure that reduced dose is administered to patient with renal impairment (Ccr less than 60 mL/min) following manufacturer's recommendations.
- Ensure that baseline CBC, platelet count, and serum creatinine are determined before starting therapy and frequently during therapy.
- Do not administer to patient if absolute neutrophil count is less than 500/mm^3, platelet count is less than 25,000/mm^3, or hemoglobin is less than 8 g/dL.
- Monitor patient for GI, CNS, DERM, and general body side effects. Report to health care provider if noted and significant.

Patient/Family Education
- Explain name, dose, action, and potential side effects of drug.
- Advise patient to read *Patient Information* leaflet before beginning therapy and with each refill.
- Warn patient that valganciclovir tablets cannot be substituted for ganciclovir capsules on a one-to-one basis.
- Review dosing schedule with patient.
- Instruct patient to take each dose with food to maximize absorption into the body.
- Advise patient not to chew, crush, break, or split tablets. If direct contact with broken or crushed tablets occurs, advise patient to wash thoroughly with soap and water and rinse eyes thoroughly with plain water.
- Advise patient that if a dose is missed to take as soon as remembered and to take the next dose at the usual time. However, if it is nearing the time for the next dose, to skip the dose and take the next dose at the regularly scheduled time.
- Advise patient that this drug is not a cure for CMV retinitis and that retinitis may continue to progress during or following treatment.
- Advise patient that valganciclovir is converted to ganciclovir in the body and that it may cause infertility and birth defects. Advise men to use barrier contraception during and for at least 90 days following treatment and women to use effective contraception during treatment.
- Advise men that drug may cause temporary or permanent infertility.
- Advise patient that drug may cause sedation, dizziness and/or confusion and to use caution while performing tasks requiring alertness, including driving and operating machinery.
- Advise patient to immediately report any of the following to health care provider: fever or other signs of infection, sore throat, unusual bruising or bleeding.
- Advise patient that diarrhea, nausea, vomiting, and headache are common side effects and to inform health care provider if they occur and are intolerable.
- Advise women to notify health care provider if pregnant, planning to become pregnant, or breastfeeding. Advise HIV-infected mothers not to breastfeed infants to avoid risk of HIV transmission to the infant.
- Instruct patient not to take any prescription or OTC medications or dietary supplements unless advised by health care provider.
- Remind patient that office visits, ophthalmic examinations, and laboratory tests will be required to monitor therapy and to keep appointments.

Valproic Acid and Derivatives (Sodium Valproate, Divalproex Sodium)

(VAL-pro-ik acid)
Class Anticonvulsant

How Supplied

Sodium Valproate
Depakene Capsules 250 mg (as valproic acid), Syrup 250 mg per 5 mL ♦ *Depacon* Injection 100 mg/mL

🍁 *Alti-Valproic* ♦ *Apo-Divalproex* ♦ *Apo-Valproic* ♦ *Epiject* ♦ *Gen-Valproic* ♦ *Novo-Divalproex* ♦ *Novo-Valproic* ♦ *Nu-Divalproex* ♦ *Nu-Valproic* ♦ *PMS-Valproic Acid* ♦ *ratio-Valproic* ♦ *Rhoxal-valproic* ♦ *Rhoxal-valproic EC*

Divalproex Sodium
Depakote Tablets, delayed-release 125 mg, Tablets, delayed-release 250 mg, Tablets, delayed-release 500 mg, Capsules, sprinkle 125 mg ♦ *Depakote ER* Tablets, extended-release 250 mg, Tablets, extended-release 500 mg

Action
PHARMACOLOGY: Believed to work by increas-

ing brain levels of gamma-aminobutyric acid (GABA). It may also inhibit catabolism of GABA, potentiate postsynaptic GABA responses, and affect potassium channels or directly stabilize membranes.

PHARMACOKINETICS/DYNAMICS:

Absorption: Valproic acid is rapidly absorbed in the GI tract. Divalproex dissociates into valproic acid in the GI tract. T_{max} is 4 to 17 hr (extended-release tablets).

Distribution: Vd of total or free valproic acid is 11 and 92 L per 1.73 m^2, respectively. 80% to 90% protein bound (concentration-dependent).

Metabolism: Metabolized primarily in the liver.

Excretion: 30% to 50% excreted as glucuronide conjugate in the urine. The $t_{½}$ is 9 to 16 hr for valproate.

Special Populations:
Renal Function Impairment – Protein binding in renal failure patients is substantially reduced.
Hepatic Function Impairment – Cl may be decreased and unbound fraction of valproate may be increased.
Elderly – Intrinsic Cl is reduced 39%; the free fraction is increased 44%.

Indications Sole and adjunctive therapy in simple (petit mal) and complex absence seizures; adjunctive therapy in multiple seizure types, including absence seizures; monotherapy and adjunctive therapy in complex partial seizures that occur in isolation or with other seizure types; manic episodes associated with bipolar disorder (divalproex sodium delayed-release tablets); prophylaxis of migraine headaches (divalproex sodium delayed-release and extended-release [ER] tablets). **Unlabeled use(s):** Treatment of atypical absence, myoclonic, and tonic-clonic (grand mal) seizures and atonic, elementary partial, and infantile spasm seizures; prevention of recurrent pediatric febrile seizures; intractable status epilepticus in patients who have not responded to other therapies; treatment of minor incontinence after ileoanal anastomosis (subchronic administration); management of anxiety disorders and panic attacks.

Contraindications Hepatic disease dysfunction; known urea cycle disorders; hypersensitivity to the drug.

Route/Dosage

Therapeutic serum levels for most patients with seizures range from 50 to 100 mcg/mL; however, a good correlation has not been established between daily dose, serum level, and therapeutic effect.

Complex Partial Seizures
ADULTS AND CHILDREN 10 YR OF AGE AND OLDER:

Monotherapy: **PO/IV** Start at 10 to 15 mg/kg daily and increase by 5 to 10 mg/kg per wk to achieve optimal clinical response, which usually occurs below 60 mg/kg daily.

Conversion to monotherapy: **PO/IV** Start at 10 to 15 mg/kg daily and increase by 5 to 10 mg/kg per wk to achieve optimal clinical response, which usually occurs below 60 mg/kg daily. Concomitant antiepilepsy drug dosage can usually be reduced approximately 25% q 2 wk. The reduction may be started at initiation of therapy or delayed by 1 to 2 wk if there is a concern that reductions may result in seizures. If the total daily dose exceeds 250 mg, administer in divided doses.

Adjunctive therapy: **PO/IV** Divalproex sodium or valproic acid may be added to the patient's regimen at a dosage of 10 to 15 mg/kg daily. The dosage may be increased by 5 to 10 mg/kg per wk to achieve optimal response, which usually occurs below 60 mg/kg daily. If the total daily dose exceeds 250 mg, administer in divided doses.

Conversion from Depakote to Depakote ER
ADULTS AND CHILDREN 10 YR OF AGE AND OLDER: Patients with epilepsy previously receiving *Depakote* should be administered *Depakote ER* daily using a dose that is 8% to 20% higher than the daily dose of *Depakote*. For patients whose *Depakote* total daily dose cannot be directly converted to *Depakote ER*, consideration may be given, at the clinician's discretion, to an increase in the patient's *Depakote* total daily dose to the next higher dosage before converting to the appropriate total daily dose of *Depakote ER*.

Mania (Divalproex Sodium Delayed-Release Tablets)
ADULTS: **PO** 750 mg daily in divided doses. Increase dose as rapidly as possible to achieve the lowest therapeutic dose that produces the desired clinical effect (max, 60 mg/kg daily).

Migraine (Divalproex Sodium)
Divalproex sodium delayed-release tablets – **PO** Start with 250 mg bid (max, 1,000 mg daily).
Divalproex sodium ER tablets – **PO** Start with 500 mg daily for 1 wk, thereafter increasing to 1,000 mg daily.

Simple and Complex Absence Seizures
PO/IV Start at 15 mg/kg daily, increasing at 1-wk intervals by 5 to 10 mg/kg daily until seizures are controlled or side effects preclude further increases (max, 60 mg/kg daily). If the total daily dose exceeds 250 mg, administer in divided doses.

Interactions
Alcohol, CNS depressants: Enhanced CNS depression.

Amitriptyline/Nortriptyline, barbiturates, diazepam, ethosuximide: May increase levels and actions of these drugs.
Carbamazepine, hydantoins: May result in increased levels of these drugs and reduced efficacy of valproic acid.
Charcoal, cholestyramine: May reduce absorption of valproic acid.
Chlorpromazine, cimetidine, erythromycin, rifampin, salicylates: May increase valproic acid levels.
Clonazepam: May increase risk of absence status in patients with history of absence-type seizures.
Felbamate: Increased valproic acid levels.
Lamotrigine: Decreased valproic acid levels; increased lamotrigine levels.
Meropenem: May decrease valproic acid levels.
Zidovudine: Increased AUC of zidovudine.

Lab Test Interferences Valproic acid may yield false-positive results on urine ketone tests; altered thyroid function tests.

Adverse Reactions

CV: Hypertension, hypotension, postural hypotension, palpitation, tachycardia, bradycardia (more than 1% and less than 5%).
CNS: Tremor (57%); somnolence (30%); asthenia (21%); dizziness (18%); insomnia (15%); nervousness (11%); amnesia (7%); headache (5% or more); depression (5%); ataxia, emotional lability, abnormal thinking, paresthesia (1% to 5%); anxiety, confusion, abnormal gait, hypertonia, incoordination, abnormal dreams, personality disorder, agitation, catatonic reaction, dysarthria, hallucinations, hypokinesia, increased reflexes, tardive dyskinesia, speech disorder, vertigo (more than 1% and less than 5%).
DERM: Alopecia (7%); rash (6%); dry skin, pruritus, petechiae, discoid lupus erythematosus, furunculosis, maculopapular rash, seborrhea (more than 1% and less than 5%); erythema multiforme, photosensitivity, Stevens-Johnson syndrome, toxic epidermal necrolysis (rare).
EENT: Pharyngitis, amblyopia, blurred vision (8%); nystagmus, tinnitus (7%); diplopia, taste perversion (1% to 5%); abnormal vision, deafness, otitis media, conjunctivitis, dry eyes, ear pain/disorder, eye pain (more than 1% and less than 5%).
GI: Nausea (34%); diarrhea, vomiting (23%); dyspepsia (13%); abdominal pain (12%); anorexia (11%); increased appetite (6%); constipation (1% to 5%); flatulence, hematemesis, eructation, periodontal abscess, fecal incontinence, gastroenteritis, glossitis, periodontal abscess, dry mouth, GI disorder, stomatitis, tooth disorder (more than 1% and less than 5%).
GU: Amenorrhea, dysmenorrhea, urinary frequency, urinary incontinence, vaginitis, cystitis, metrorrhagia, vaginal hemorrhage (more than 1% and less than 5%).
HEMA/LYMPH: Thrombocytopenia (24% [high dose]); ecchymosis (5%); frank hemorrhage; relative lymphocytosis; macrocytosis; leucopenia; eosinophilia; anemia; bone marrow suppression; pancytopenia; aplastic anemia; acute intermittent porphyria.
HEPA: Hepatotoxicity.
LABTESTABS: Increase ALT, AST, LDH, bilirubin.
METAB: Weight gain (9%); edema (more than 1% and less than 5%); hyperammonemia; Fanconi syndrome (primarily in children); hyperglycemia.
MUSC: Arthralgia, leg cramps, myalgia, myasthenia, twitching arthrosis (more than 1% and less than 5%).
RESP: Infection (20%); flu-like syndrome (12%); rhinitis; dyspnea (1% to 5%); epistaxis, pneumonia, sinusitis, increased cough (more than 1% and less than 5%).
OTHER: Infection (15%); back pain (8%); injection site pain (3%); injection site reaction (2%); fever, chest pain, vasodilation, peripheral edema, accidental injury, chills, face edema, viral infection (1% to 5%); malaise (more than 1% and less than 5%); lupus erythematosus; anaphylaxis.

> **WARNING:**
>
> *Hepatotoxicity:* Increased risk in children younger than 2 yr of age, especially those on multiple anticonvulsants or those with congenital metabolic disorders, severe seizure disorders, mental retardation, or organic brain syndrome. Onset is typically during the first 6 mo.
>
> *Pancreatitis, some cases life-threatening:* Occurs in children and adults after initial or long-term therapy.
>
> *Teratogenicity:* Can produce teratogenic effects such as neural tube defects (eg, spina bifida).

Precautions

Pregnancy: Category D.
Lactation: Excreted in breast milk.
Children: Use with extreme caution in children younger than 2 yr of age (see Warning box). Safety and efficacy of divalproex sodium for treatment of acute mania have not been established in patients younger than 18 yr of age. Safety and efficacy of divalproex sodium for the prophylaxis of migraines have not been established in patients younger than 16 yr of age. Safety and efficacy of divalproex sodium ER

tablets for the prophylaxis of migraine headaches in pediatric patients have not been established. Safety and efficacy of divalproex ER for the treatment of complex partial seizures, simple and complex absence seizures, and multiple seizure types that include absence seizures have not been established in pediatric patients younger than 10 yr of age. Safety and efficacy of valproate sodium injection have not been established in children younger than 2 yr of age.
Elderly: Reduce starting dose and base therapeutic dose on clinical response.
Acute head injuries: Because IV valproic acid has been associated with a higher incidence of death than IV phenytoin, do not use in the prevention of posttraumatic seizures in patients with acute head injuries.
Discontinuation: Abrupt discontinuation may precipitate status epilepticus with attendant life-threatening hypoxia in patients receiving valproic acid to prevent major seizures.
Hematologic effects: Thrombocytopenia, inhibition of secondary phase of platelet aggregation and abnormal coagulation parameters (eg, low fibrinogen) may occur. Risk of bleeding may be increased.
Hepatotoxicity: Reactions usually occur within first 6 mo of therapy and are preceded by symptoms such as lost seizure control, malaise, weakness, lethargy, facial edema, anorexia, jaundice, and vomiting. Use drug with caution in patients with prior history of liver disease. Monitor results of LFTs frequently.
Hyperammonemia: May occur with or without lethargy and coma and contribute to hepatotoxicity.
Mania: Clinical data from long-term studies (more than 3 wk) are not available.
Pancreatitis: Life-threatening pancreatitis has been reported.
Suicide: Suicidal ideation may be a manifestation of certain psychiatric disorders and may persist until significant remission of symptoms occurs.

Overdosage: Signs and Symptoms
Motor restlessness, somnolence, heart block, visual hallucinations, asterixis, deep coma, death.

PATIENT CARE CONSIDERATIONS
Administration/Storage
- Injection and oral dose forms are interchangeable on a mg for mg basis.
- Double check oral dose form being ordered. Multiple dose forms with different dosing guidelines are available.
- Follow manufacturer's dosing guidelines when converting from Depakote to Depakote ER.
- Administer prescribed oral dose without regard to meals. Administer with food if GI upset occurs.
- Store syrup, tablets, and unopened injection vials at controlled room temperature (59° to 86°F). Store capsules and sprinkle capsules at temperature less than 77°F. Diluted injection may be stored at controlled room temperature for up to 24 hr.

Tablets, delayed-release tablets, and extended-release tablets:
- Have patient swallow whole. Do not crush, chew, or divide.
- Extended-release tablets can be administered daily at bedtime to reduce daytime sedation.

Capsules:
- Have patient swallow whole. Do not open, crush, or chew to avoid irritation of mouth and throat.

Sprinkle capsules:
- Sprinkle capsules may be swallowed whole or the capsule can be opened and the entire contents sprinkled on a small amount (eg, teaspoon) of soft food (eg applesauce) that should be swallowed immediately without chewing and then washed down with a fluid (eg, water, juice).

Syrup:
- Measure prescribed dose using dosing spoon or dosing syringe.

Injection:
- Administer by IV route only. Not for intradermal, subcutaneous, or IM administration.
- Dilute prescribed dose in at least 50 mL of 5% dextrose injection, 0.9% sodium chloride injection, or lactated Ringer's solution.
- Do not administer if particulate matter, cloudiness, or discoloration noted.
- Administer prescribed dose as a 60-min infusion or at a rate not to exceed 20 mg per min.
- Discard any unused portion of vial. Do not save for future use.

Assessment/Interventions
- Obtain patient history, including drug history and any known allergies. Note renal impairment, hepatic impairment, urea cycle disorder, or acute head trauma.
- Attempt to switch patient from IV medication to oral dose form as soon as possible.
- Ensure that lower starting dose and slower dose titration are used in elderly patient.
- Ensure that liver enzymes are determined before starting therapy and at frequent intervals thereafter, especially during the first 6 mo of therapy.

- Ensure that platelet counts and clotting parameters are evaluated before starting therapy, periodically thereafter, and before any surgical procedure.
- Ensure that plasma valproate levels are determined periodically to monitor therapy and during concurrent use of other medications capable of enzyme induction.
- Frequently assess patient for response to treatment. Notify health care provider if condition does not appear to be improving or is worsening.
- Ensure that therapy is periodically reviewed to determine if therapy needs to be continued without change or if a dose change (eg, increase, decrease, discontinuation) is indicated.
- Avoid sudden discontinuation of therapy in epileptic patient if possible. Attempt to gradually reduce dose over a period of 2 wk or more if decision to discontinue medication is made.
- Assess patient with bipolar disorder for suicide potential. Closely supervise high-risk patient during initial drug therapy.
- Monitor patient for GI, CNS, GU, MUSC, and general body side effects. Inform health care provider if noted and significant.
- Immediately notify health care provider of any of the following: loss of seizure control in epileptic patient, malaise, weakness, lethargy, facial edema, anorexia, persistent nausea or vomiting, sudden onset of abdominal pain, mental status changes. Be prepared to discontinue therapy.
- Implement safety precautions for patients who experience dizziness or ataxia.

Patient/Family Education

- Explain name, dose, action, and potential side effects of drug.
- Advise patient, family, or caregiver to read the *Patient Information* leaflet before starting therapy and with each refill.
- Instruct patient, family, or caregiver to continue to take other medications unless advised otherwise by health care provider.
- Advise patient, family, or caregiver that medication will be started at a low dose and gradually increased as tolerated until max benefit has been obtained.
- Instruct patient, family, or caregiver to take (give) exactly as prescribed and not change the dose or discontinue therapy unless advised by health care provider.
- Advise patient, family, or caregiver that each dose may be taken without regard to meals but to take with food if stomach upset occurs.
- Instruct patient, family, or caregiver that if a dose is missed to skip that dose and not to double up on the next dose.
- Instruct patient, family, or caregiver to immediately contact health care provider if any of the following occur: loss of seizure control in epileptic patient, general body discomfort, weakness, lethargy, facial swelling, appetite loss, persistent nausea or vomiting, sudden onset of stomach pain, mental status changes.
- Advise patient, family, or caregiver that if medication needs to be discontinued it will usually be slowly withdrawn over a period of 2 wk or more unless safety concerns (eg, rash) require a more rapid withdrawal.
- Caution patient that drug may cause dizziness or drowsiness and to use caution while driving or performing other tasks requiring mental alertness or coordination until tolerance is determined.
- Caution women of childbearing potential that medication may be harmful if taken while pregnant and to use effective contraception to avoid becoming pregnant.
- Advise women to notify health care provider if pregnant, planning to become pregnant, or breastfeeding.
- Instruct patient, family, or caregiver to contact health care provider if seizures get worse, new types of seizures occur, bipolar symptoms do not improve or worsen, or migraine headaches do not improve or worsen.
- Advise patient, family, or caregiver to contact health care provider if bothersome side effects (eg, drowsiness, indigestion) occur.
- Advise diabetic patient that medication may interfere with urine ketone tests.
- Advise patient, family, or caregiver not to take (give) any prescription or OTC medications or dietary supplements unless advised by health care provider.
- Advise patient, family, or caregiver that laboratory tests and follow-up visits will be required to monitor therapy and to keep appointments.

Syrup:
- Advise patient, family, or caregiver to measure prescribed dose using dosing spoon or dosing syringe.

Tablets, delayed-release tablets, and extended-release tablets:
- Advise patient to swallow whole and not to crush, chew, or divide.
- Advise patient, family, or caregiver that extended-release tablets given daily can be taken at night to reduce daytime sedation.

Capsules:
* Advise patient to swallow whole and not to open, crush, or chew to avoid local irritation of mouth and throat.

Sprinkle capsules:
* Advise patient, family, or caregiver that sprinkle capsules may be swallowed whole or the capsule can be opened and the entire contents of the capsule sprinkled on a small amount (eg, teaspoon) of soft food (eg, applesauce) that should be swallowed immediately without chewing and then washed down with a fluid (eg, water, juice). Caution patient, family, or caregiver not to prepare ahead of time and store for future use.

Injection:
* Advise patient, family, or caregiver that medication will be prepared and administered by a health care professional in a health care setting.
* Advise patient, family, or caregiver that injection will only be used to control seizures if it is not possible or not feasible to take medications by mouth.

Valrubicin

(val-ROO-bih-sin)

Class Antineoplastic antibiotic/Anthracycline

How Supplied

Valstar Preservative-free solution for intravesical use 40 mg/mL (with 50% Dehydrated Alcohol and 50% *Cremophor EL*), in 5 mL vials.
🍁 *Valtaxin*

Action

PHARMACOLOGY: Valrubicin, a semisynthetic analog of the anthracycline doxorubicin, readily penetrates into cells, causes extensive chromosomal damage, and arrests the G_2 phase of the cell cycle.

PHARMACOKINETICS/DYNAMICS:

Absorption: Significant penetration into the bladder wall.

Distribution: Distribution is dependent on the condition of the bladder wall.

Metabolism: Major metabolites are N-trifluoroacetyladriamycin and N-trifluoroacetyladriamycinol.

Excretion: Almost completely excreted by voiding (urine).

Indications Intravesical use for the treatment of BCG-refractory carcinoma in-situ of the urinary bladder when immediate cystectomy is contraindicated.

Contraindications Concurrent urinary tract infection, perforated bladder, compromised integrity of the bladder wall, bladder capacity less than 75 mL, or hypersensitive to anthracyclines or *Cremophor EL*. Use with caution in patients with severe irritable bladder symptoms.

Route/Dosage

ADULTS: **Urethral catheter** 300 mg (contents of 4 vials) instilled in the bladder once weekly for 6 wk starting at least 14 days after fulguration or transurethral resection. Do not use IV or IM. Insert a urethral catheter into the patient's bladder under aseptic conditions, drain the bladder, and instill the diluted 75 mL solution slowly via gravity flow for several minutes. Withdraw the catheter. The patient should retain the drug for 2 hr before voiding. At the end of 2 hr, all patients should void.

Interactions No specific drug interactions have been reported.

Lab Test Interferences None well documented.

Adverse Reactions

CNS: Weakness; dizziness.
GI: Abdominal pain; very low potential for nausea and vomiting.
GU: Urinary frequency and urgency; painful urination; bladder spasm; hematuria; bladder pain; urinary incontinence; urinary tract infection; nocturia; urinary retention; local reactions occur shortly after instillation and resolve within 1 to 7 days.
HEMA: Dose-limiting leukopenia and neutropenia in patients with increased systemic exposure. Nadir seen by week 2 and recovery by week 3.

Precautions

Pregnancy: Category C.
Lactation: Discontinue nursing before the initiation of valrubicin therapy.
Children: Safety and efficacy have not been established.
Extravasation risk: Local irritation or phlebitis may occur. Refer to your institution specific protocol.
Cystectomy: Inform patients that valrubicin induces complete response in about 20% with BCG-refractory CIS and that delaying cystectomy could lead to development of metastatic bladder cancer, which is lethal.
Bladder integrity: Do not administer to patients with a perforated bladder or to those in whom the integrity of the bladder mucosa has been compromised.
Irritable bladder symptoms: Use with caution in patients with severe irritable bladder symptoms. Bladder spasm and spontaneous discharge of the intravesical instillate may occur; clamping of the urinary catheter is not advised; if performed,

execute under medical supervision and with caution.

PATIENT CARE CONSIDERATIONS
Administration/Storage
- Refrigerate intravesical solution. Do not freeze. Do not heat vials.
- Allow solution to warm slowly to room temperature. Do not heat or microwave.
- Dilute with 0.9% Sodium Chloride providing 75 mL of a diluted solution.
- Valrubicin may be prepared in glass containers using a non-PVC-containing administration set.
- Solutions diluted with 0.9% Sodium Chloride are chemically stable for 12 hr at room temperature.
- Solutions should be clear and red in color.
- Visually inspect the product for particulate matter prior to administration. *Cremophor EL* may form a waxy precipitate at temperatures less than 4°C (39°F); warm the vial by hand to dissolve the precipitate. If particles remain after warming, discard the dose.
- Do not mix with other drugs.
- Intravesical administration.
- Instill into bladder slowly by gravity via a urethral catheter. During the first hour following installation, the patient should lie for 15 min each in the prone and supine position and also on each side. The patient is then allowed to be up, but retains the suspension for another 60 min (total of 2 hr). All patients should void in the seated position for safety reasons.
- Aseptic techniques must be used during administration of intravesical valrubicin to avoid introducing contaminants into the urinary tract or unduly traumatizing the urinary mucosa.
- Follow Safe Handling procedures.
- Urine voided for 6 hr after instillation should be collected and disposed of as chemotherapy waste.

Overdosage: Signs and Symptoms
Irritable bladder symptoms; myelosuppression.

Assessment/Interventions
- Valrubicin contains *Cremophor EL* (polyoxyethylated castor oil), which may cause hypersensitivity reactions. Patients with hypersensitivity reactions to valrubicin who require further therapy should be pretreated with a corticosteroid and an antihistamine.
- Assess bladder status at baseline and prior to instilling each dose. Delay therapy if bladder integrity is compromised.
- Monitor for refractory CIS closely for disease recurrence or progression. Recommended evaluations include cystoscopy, biopsy, and urine cytology every 3 mo.
- Assess patient response after 3 mo or if disease recurs. In the absence of a complete response, reconsider cystectomy.

Patient/Family Education
- Patients should not drink fluids for 4 hr before administration. They should void before instillation of valrubicin into the bladder.
- Instruct patients to maintain adequate hydration after treatment.
- Inform patients that the major acute toxicities from valrubicin are related to irritable bladder symptoms that may occur during instillation and retention of valrubicin and for a limited period following voiding.
- Valrubicin may cause red discoloration of urine for up to 24 hr after administration.
- Patients should report prolonged irritable bladder symptoms or prolonged passage of red-colored urine immediately to their health care provider.
- Advise women of childbearing potential not to become pregnant during treatment. Advise men to refrain from engaging in procreative activities while receiving therapy. Advise all patients of reproductive age to use an effective contraception method during the treatment period.

Valsartan

(VAL-sahr-tan)

Class Antihypertensive/Angiotensin II antagonist

How Supplied
Diovan Capsules 80 mg, Capsules 160 mg

Action
PHARMACOLOGY: Antagonizes the effect of angiotensin II (vasoconstriction and aldosterone secretion) by blocking the angiotensin II receptor (AT_1 receptor) in vascular smooth muscle and the adrenal gland, producing decreased BP.

PHARMACOKINETICS/DYNAMICS:
Absorption: T_{max} is 2 to 4 hr after dosing. Bioavailability is about 10% to 35%. Food decreases the AUC by about 40% and decreases C_{max} by about 50%. Valsartan does not accumulate appreciably in plasma following repeated administration.

Distribution: Vd is about 17 L. Valsartan does not distribute into tissues extensively. It is highly bound to albumin (about 95%).

Metabolism: The major metabolite, valeryl

4-hydroxy valsartan, accounts for about 9% of the dose.

Excretion: T½ is about 5 hr. Valsartan is primarily recovered in the feces (about 83%) and urine (about 13% of the dose). Recovery is mainly unchanged drug, with only about 20% of the dose recovered as metabolite. The plasma clearance is about 2 L/hr.

Onset: Renal clearance is about 0.62 L/hr (about 30% total clearance).

Special Populations:
Renal Function Impairment – In severe renal disease, exercise care with dosing valsartan.
Hepatic Function Impairment – Patients with mild-to-moderate chronic liver disease have about twice the AUC value. No dosage adjustments are necessary. Exercise care in patients with liver disease.
Elderly – AUC is about 70% higher and t½ is about 35% longer in elderly. No dosage adjustment is necessary.

Indications Treatment of hypertension either alone or in combination with other antihypertensive drugs; heart failure.

Contraindications Standard considerations.

Route/Dosage
Hypertension
ADULTS:
Initial dose: **PO** 80 mg qd.
Maintenance: **PO** 80 to 320 mg qd.

Heart Failure
ADULTS:
Initial dose: **PO** 40 mg bid; titration to 80 and 160 mg bid should be done to the highest dose, as tolerated by the patient.

Interactions
Lithium: Plasma concentrations may be increased by valsartan, resulting in an increase in the pharmacologic and adverse effects of lithium.

Lab Test Interferences None well documented.

Adverse Reactions
CNS: Headache; dizziness; fatigue.
EENT: Sinusitis; pharyngitis; rhinitis.
GI: Abdominal pain; diarrhea; nausea.
HEMA: Neutropenia.
METAB: Hyperkalemia.
RESP: Cough.
OTHER: Fatigue; viral infection; edema; arthralgia.

> **WARNING:**
> *Pregnancy:* Use in second and third trimesters may cause injury and death to fetus.

Precautions
Pregnancy: Category D (second and third trimester); Category C (first trimester).
Lactation: Undetermined.
Children: Safety and efficacy not established.
Renal function impairment: Decreases in renal function may occur in patients whose renal function is dependent on the renin-angiotensin system; patients with renal artery stenosis may experience acute renal failure. Use caution in treating patients whose renal function may depend on the activity of renin-angiotensin-aldosterone system (eg, severe CHF).
Hypotension/Volume-depleted patients: Symptomatic hypotension may occur after initiation of valsartan therapy in patients who are intravascularly volume depleted (eg, those treated with diuretics). Correct these conditions prior to administration of valsartan or start treatment under close medical supervision.
Liver disease: Use with caution. Valsartan is excreted hepatically and higher levels are possible in patients with decreased hepatic function.

Overdosage: Signs and Symptoms
Hypotension, tachycardia.

PATIENT CARE CONSIDERATIONS
Administration/Storage
- Administer once daily without regard to food.
- Store at room temperature in tightly closed container. Protect from moisture.
- Can be administered alone or in combination with other antihypertensives.
- Administer with caution and reduced dosage to patients with possible depletion of intravascular volume or a history of hepatic impairment.

Assessment/Interventions
- Obtain patient history, including drug history and any known allergies.
- Monitor BP and pulse. Should hypotension, tachycardia, or bradycardia result, withhold the medication and notify health care provider.
- Monitor for signs of hypersensitivity including angioedema involving swelling of face, lips, and tongue.
- Ensure that baseline blood and renal function studies have been obtained before administration and monitor during therapy.
- Obtain base BP and pulse and monitor closely for at least 2 hr after initial dose and during first 2 wk of therapy. If systolic BP is less than 90 or if patient has symptoms of hypotension, withhold medication and notify health care provider.

- Monitor for hyperkalemia in patients with impaired renal function or diabetes mellitus and in patients receiving potassium supplements or potassium-sparing diuretics.
- Assist patient with position changes and ambulation during initial phase of therapy. Orthostatic hypotension is common.
- Keep side rails raised if hypotension or dizziness occur.

Patient/Family Education
- Instruct patient to take medication as prescribed at same time each day.
- Inform patients that valsartan controls but does not cure hypertension.
- Caution patients to take dose exactly as prescribed and not to stop taking medication even if they feel better. Instruct patient not to decrease or increase their dosage.
- Instruct patient not to take OTC medications without consulting health care provider.
- Instruct the patient in BP and pulse measuring skills. Advise patient to call health care provider should abnormal readings occur.
- Instruct patients in methods of fall prevention including arising slowly and sitting on side of bed before standing especially early in therapy.
- Inform patients of importance of adjunct therapies such as dietary planning, a regular exercise program, weight reduction, a low sodium diet, smoking cessation program, alcohol reduction, and stress management.
- Instruct patient to report the following symptoms to health care provider: changes in urinary output, discomfort during urination, weakness, fatigue, dizziness, lightheadedness, jaundice.
- Advise women to contact health care provider if pregnant, planning to become pregnant, or breastfeeding.
- Emphasize importance of follow-up visits and frequent assessment of BP while taking drug.

Valsartan/Hydrochlorothiazide

(VAL-sahr-tan/ high-droe-klor-oh-THIGH-uh-zide)

Class Antihypertensive combination

How Supplied
Diovan HCT Tablets 12.5 mg hydrochlorothiazide and 80 mg valsartan, Tablets 12.5 mg hydrochlorothiazide and 160 mg valsartan, Tablets 25 mg hydrochlorothiazide and 160 mg valsartan

Action
PHARMACOLOGY:
Valsartan: Antagonizes the effect of angiotensin II (vasoconstriction and aldosterone secretion) by blocking the angiotensin II receptor (AT_1 receptor) in vascular smooth muscle and the adrenal gland, producing decreased BP.
Hydrochlorothiazide (HCTZ): Increases chloride, sodium, and water excretion by interfering with transport of sodium ions across renal tubular epithelium.

Indications Treatment of hypertension.

Contraindications Hypersensitivity to any component of this product; anuria; hypersensitivity to sulfonamide-derived drugs (HCTZ).

Route/Dosage
Dosage must be individualized. The fixed combination is not indicated for initial therapy. The combination may be substituted for the titrated components.
ADULTS: **PO** Valsartan may be used over a dose range of 80 to 320 mg/day, administered qd. HCTZ is effective in doses of 12.5 to 50 mg qd. There are no studies evaluating doses of valsartan greater than 160 mg in combination with HCTZ 25 mg.

Renal Impairment (Ccr greater than 30 mL/min)
Loop diuretics are preferred to thiazides.

Interactions
Valsartan:
Lithium – Plasma concentrations may be elevated by valsartan, increasing the pharmacologic and toxic effects of lithium.
HCTZ:
Alcohol, barbiturates, narcotics – Increased risk of orthostatic hypotension.
Anticholinergic agents (eg, atropine, biperiden) – May increase bioavailability of thiazide-type diuretics.
Antidiabetic agents (oral agents and insulin) – Dosage adjustment of antidiabetic agent may be necessary.
Antihypertensive agent – Additive or potentiation of effects.
Cholestyramine, colestipol resins – Impaired absorption of HCTZ.
Corticosteroids, ACTH – Increased electrolyte depletion, increasing the risk of hypokalemia.
Cyclosporin – Concomitant use may increase risk of hyperuricemia and gout-type complications.
Digoxin – Thiazide-induced electrolyte disturbances may predispose to digitalis-induced arrhythmias.
Lithium – Renal Cl of lithium may be reduced, increasing the risk of lithium toxicity.
Methyldopa – Reports of hemolytic anemia occurring with concomitant use.
Nondepolarizing skeletal muscle relaxants (eg, tubocurarine) – Increased effect of the muscle

relaxant.

Nonsteroidal anti-inflammatory agents – The diuretic, natriuretic, and antihypertensive effects of loop, potassium-sparing, and thiazide diuretics may be reduced.

Potassium supplements – Do not use salt substitutes containing potassium or potassium supplements without consulting the prescribing physician.

Pressor amines (eg, norepinephrine) – Decreased responsiveness to the pressor amine.

Vitamin D/Calcium salts – May potentiate rise in serum calcium.

Lab Test Interferences

Valsartan: None well documented.

HCTZ: May decrease serum protein-bound iodine levels without signs of thyroid disturbances. May cause diagnostic interference of serum electrolyte levels, blood and urine glucose levels, serum bilirubin levels, and serum uric acid levels.

Adverse Reactions

CV: Palpitations; syncope; tachycardia; hypotension.

CNS: Headache; fatigue; dizziness; increased appetite; anxiety; insomnia decreased libido; paresthesia; somnolence; asthenia.

DERM: Flushing; rash; increased sweating.

HCTZ – Erythema multiforme (including Stevens-Johnson syndrome); exfoliative dermatitis (including toxic epidermal necrolysis).

EENT: Pharyngitis; sinusitis; tinnitus; vertigo; abnormal vision; rhinitis; epistaxis.

HCTZ – Transient blurred vision; xanthopsia.

GI: Diarrhea; constipation; dyspepsia; flatulence; dry mouth; nausea; abdominal pain; vomiting.

HCTZ – Pancreatitis; sialadenitis; cramping; gastric irritation.

GU: Dysuria; impotence; micturition frequency; UTI.

HCTZ – Renal failure; renal dysfunction; interstitial nephritis.

HEMA:

HCTZ – Aplastic anemia; leukopenia; thrombocytopenia; microcytic anemia; neutropenia.

HEPA: Elevated liver enzymes; jaundice (intrahepatic cholestatic); hepatitis.

METAB: Dehydration; gout; edema.

HCTZ – Hyperglycemia; glycosuria; hyperuricemia.

RESP: Cough; upper respiratory tract infection; dyspnea; epistaxis; bronchitis.

OTHER: Viral infection; back pain; chest pain; allergic reaction; anaphylaxis; asthenia; dependent edema; arthralgia; muscle cramps; muscle weakness; arm pain; leg pain; angioedema.

HCTZ – Hypersensitivity (including purpura, photosensitivity, urticaria, necrotizing angiitis, fever, respiratory distress, anaphylactic reactions).

Precautions

Pregnancy: Category D (second and third trimester); Category C (first trimester). Drugs that act directly on the renin-angiotensin system can cause injury and death to the developing fetus.

Lactation:

Valsartan – Undetermined.

HCTZ – Excreted in breast milk.

Children: Safety and efficacy not established.

Hypersensitivity: May occur in patients with or without history of allergy or bronchial asthma; cross-sensitivity with sulfonamides may also occur.

Renal function impairment: Decreases in renal function may occur in patients whose renal function is dependent on the renin-angiotensin system; patients with renal artery stenosis may experience acute renal failure. Use caution in treating patients whose renal function may depend on the activity of renin-angiotensin-aldosterone system (eg, severe CHF). In addition, HCTZ may precipitate azotemia and cumulative effects of the drug may develop in patients with impaired renal function.

Hepatic disease: Use with caution. Minor alterations of fluid and electrolyte balance may precipitate hepatic coma.

Hyperuricemia: May occur, or acute gout may be precipitated in thiazide therapy.

Hypotension/Volume-depleted patients: Symptomatic hypotension may occur after initiation of valsartan therapy in patients who are intravascularly volume depleted (eg, those treated with diuretics). Correct these conditions prior to administration of valsartan or start treatment under close medical supervision.

Lightheadedness can occur, especially during the first days of therapy.

Systemic lupus erythematosus: Exacerbation or activation may occur.

Valvular stenosis: May increase the risk of decreased coronary perfusion when treated with vasodilators.

Overdosage: Signs and Symptoms

Hypotension, tachycardia, bradycardia, electrolyte depletion (eg, hypokalemia, hypochloremia, hyponatremia), dehydration.

PATIENT CARE CONSIDERATIONS

Administration/Storage

- Administer prescribed dose qd in the morning, with or without food.
- Administer with food if GI upset occurs.
- Administer alone or in combination with other antihypertensives.

- Do not administer to pregnant women as fetal and neonatal morbidity and death can occur.
- Administer with caution and reduce dosage in patients with possible depletion of intravascular volume.
- Store tablets at controlled room temperature (59° to 86°F). Protect from moisture.

Assessment/Interventions

- Obtain patient history, including drug history and any known allergies. Note history of diabetes, anuria, lupus erythematosus, kidney or liver disease, gout, or allergy to sulfonamide-derived drugs.
- Ensure that serum electrolytes are monitored periodically.
- Ensure that volume and/or salt depletion have been corrected before initiating therapy.
- Monitor and record BP and pulse. If hypotension results, hold medication and notify health care provider.
- Take safety precautions if orthostatic hypotension occurs.
- Monitor blood sugar in diabetic patients when drug is started or dose is changed. Report significant changes to health care provider.
- Monitor for signs of hypersensitivity, including angioedema with swelling of the face, lips, eyelids, and tongue. Discontinue medication and notify health care provider immediately if noted.

Patient/Family Education

- Explain name, dose, action, and potential side effects of drug.
- Advise patient to take qd as prescribed, without regard to meals but to take with food if GI upset occurs.
- Advise patient to try to take each dose at about the same time each day.
- Inform patient that drug controls but does not cure hypertension and to continue taking drug as prescribed even when BP is not elevated.
- Caution patient not to change the dose or stop taking unless advised by health care provider.
- Instruct patient to continue taking other BP medications as prescribed by health care provider.
- Instruct patient in BP and pulse measurement skills.
- Advise patient to monitor and record BP and pulse at home and to inform health care provider if abnormal measurements are noted. Advise patient to take record of BP and pulse to each follow-up visit.
- Caution patient to avoid sudden position changes to prevent orthostatic hypotension.
- Instruct patient to lie or sit down if experiencing dizziness or lightheadedness when standing.
- Caution patient that inadequate fluid intake, excessive perspiration, diarrhea, or vomiting can lead to excessive fall in BP, resulting in lightheadedness or fainting.
- Instruct diabetic patient to monitor blood glucose more frequently when drug is started or dose is changed and to inform health care provider of significant changes in readings.
- Caution patient to avoid unnecessary exposure to UV light (sunlight, tanning booths) and to use sunscreen and wear protective clothing when exposed to UV light to avoid photosensitivity reaction.
- Emphasize to hypertensive patient importance of the following modalities on BP: weight control, regular exercise, smoking cessation, moderate intake of alcohol and salt.
- Advise women to notify health care provider if pregnant, planning to become pregnant, or breastfeeding.
- Instruct patient to stop taking drug and immediately report any of the following symptoms to health care provider: fainting, swelling of the face, lips, eyelids, or tongue.
- Caution patient not to take any prescription or OTC medications, salt substitutes, or dietary supplements unless advised by health care provider.
- Advise patient that follow-up visits and lab tests may be required to monitor therapy and to keep appointments.

Vancomycin

(van-koe-MY-sin)

Class Anti-infective/Antibiotic

How Supplied

Lyphocin Powder for Injection, lyophilized 500 mg, Powder for Injection, lyophilized 1 g, Powder for Injection, lyophilized 5 g, Powder for Injection, lyophilized 10 g ◆ *Vancocin* Pulvules 125 mg, Pulvules 250 mg, Powder for Oral Solution 1 g, Powder for Oral Solution 10 g, Powder for Injection 500 mg, Powder for Injection 1 g, Powder for Injection 10 g ◆ *Vancoled* Powder for Injection 500 mg, Powder for Injection 1 g, Powder for Injection 5 g

Action

PHARMACOLOGY: Inhibits bacterial cell wall synthesis and alters cell-membrane permeability and RNA synthesis.

PHARMACOKINETICS/DYNAMICS:
Absorption: Poorly absorbed (orally). C_{max} is 63 mcg/mL. T_{max} is 1 hr.

Distribution: 55% protein bound. Vd is 0.3 to 0.43 L/kg. Distributes to pleural, pericardial, ascitic, and synovial fluids; in urine; in peritoneal dialysis fluid; and atrial appendage tissue.

Metabolism: No apparent metabolism of the drug.

Excretion: Mean t½ is 4 to 6 hr. 75% is excreted in urine by glomerular filtration (in the first 24 hr). Mean plasma clearance is 0.058 L/kg/hr. Renal clearance is 0.048 L/kg/hr.

Special Populations:
Renal Function Impairment – Renal dysfunction slows excretion of vancomycin in anephric patients, t½ is 7.5 days.
Elderly – Total systemic and renal clearance may be reduced.

Indications
Parenteral: Treatment of serious or severe infections due to susceptible bacteria not treatable with other antimicrobials (eg, staphylococcus).
Oral: Treatment of pseudomembranous colitis caused by *Clostridium difficile*; treatment of staphylococcal enterocolitis. **Unlabeled use(s):** IV prophylaxis against bacterial endocarditis in penicillin-allergic patients

Contraindications
Standard considerations.

Route/Dosage
ADULTS: **PO** 500 mg to 2 g/day in 3 or 4 divided doses for 7 to 10 days.
CHILDREN: **PO** 40 mg/kg/day (up to 2 g/day) in 3 or 4 divided doses for 7 to 10 days.
NEWBORNS: **PO** 10 mg/kg/day in divided doses.
ADULTS: **IV** 500 mg by IV infusion q 6 hr or 1 g q 12 hr.
CHILDREN: **IV** 10 mg/kg/dose q 6 hr.
INFANTS & NEWBORNS: **IV** 15 mg/kg initially, followed by 10 mg/kg q 12 hr for newborns in first week of life, and q 8 hr for ages up to 1 mo.

Interactions
Aminoglycosides: May increase risk of nephrotoxicity.
Neurotoxic and nephrotoxic agents: May give additive toxicity.
Nondepolarizing muscle relaxants: Neuromuscular blockade may be enhanced.

INCOMPATIBILITIES: IV solution is incompatible with alkaline injections.

Lab Test Interferences None well documented.

Adverse Reactions
CV: Hypotension.
DERM: Rash; urticaria; pruritus; inflammation at site of injection.
EENT: Hearing loss.
GI: Nausea.
GU: Increased serum creatinine and BUN; renal failure.
HEMA: Neutropenia; eosinophilia.
RESP: Wheezing; dyspnea.
OTHER: Anaphylaxis; drug fever; chills; Red Man Syndrome (hypotension with or without rash over face, neck, upper chest, and extremities).

Precautions
Pregnancy: Category C.
Lactation: Excreted in breast milk.
Children: Confirming serum levels may be appropriate in newborns. Use of vancomycin with anesthetics may cause erythema and flushing.
Special risk patients: Use with caution in patients with preexisting hearing loss, patients receiving ototoxic or nephrotoxic drugs, patients receiving drugs that cause neutropenia; patients with renal impairment; elderly; newborns.
Hypotension: Too rapid IV infusion or bolus administration may be associated with exaggerated hypotension, including shock and cardiac arrest, with or without maculopapular rash over face, neck, upper chest, and extremities (Red Man or Redneck syndrome). Reaction has been rarely associated with slow infusion or oral or intraperitoneal administration.
Reversible neutropenia: May occur after total dose of 25 g.
Tissue irritation, thrombophlebitis: Give by secure IV route. May minimize thrombophlebitis by giving slowly as dilute infusion.

Overdosage: Signs and Symptoms
Increase serum creatinine, increase BUN, hearing loss, ringing in ears, vertigo.

PATIENT CARE CONSIDERATIONS

Administration/Storage
- Prepare oral solution by adding 115 mL of water to 10 g vial or 20 mL of water to 1 g vial. Further dilute prepared oral solution dose with 30 mL of water or flavoring syrups may be used with oral solution.
- May give oral solution via nasogastric tube as indicated or ordered.
- Reconstitute parenteral form with Sterile Water for Injection.
- Further dilute parenteral medication with compatible solution (eg, 5% Dextrose Injection, 0.9% Sodium Chloride, Lactated Ringer's)
- Parenteral form may be administered by oral route.
- Reconstituted oral solution may be stored in refrigerator for 2 wk after bottle is opened.
- Dilute to minimum dilution of 2.5 mL and infuse parenteral solution over at least 60 min. Intermittent infusion preferred.

- Pretreat with antihistamine if patient has previously experienced Red Man Syndrome.
- Dosage or dosage interval may be changed based upon vancomycin serum levels.
- Reconstituted powder for injection is stable at room temperature for 2 wk.
- Dilute solutions (sodium chloride or D5W) are stable at room temperature for 24 hr.

Assessment/Interventions
- Obtain patient history, including drug history and any known allergies.
- Assess results of culture and sensitivity to determine sensitivity.
- Assess hearing acuity before and after therapy. Anticipate ototoxicity.
- Monitor for signs of superinfection.
- Monitor skin for Red Man Syndrome with each dose infused.
- Notify health care provider of elevated BUN and creatinine, which indicate nephrotoxicity.
- Document hematuria and notify health care provider.
- Monitor I&O, BP for hypotension, and respirations for wheezing or dyspnea.
- Maintain adequate fluid intake.
- Obtain blood levels, new order, or protocol. Keep blood levels between 10 to 20 mcg/mL.
- Ensure that resuscitation equipment is available.

Patient/Family Education
- Explain that IV medication is given at regular intervals to maintain blood levels.
- Tell patient to report hearing loss, ringing in ears, or vertigo to health care provider.
- Explain signs of superinfection (eg, vaginitis).
- Identify symptoms of potential adverse reactions.
- Tell patient to maintain adequate fluid intake.

Vardenafil Hydrochloride

(var-DEN-ah-fil HIGH-droe-KLOR-ide)

Class Agent for impotence

How Supplied
Levitra Tablets 2.5 mg, Tablets 5 mg, Tablets 10 mg, Tablets 20 mg

Action
PHARMACOLOGY: Enhances the effect of nitric oxide at the nerve ending and endothelial cells in the corpus cavernosum by inhibiting phosphodiesterase type 5 in the corpus cavernosum of the penis. This results in vasodilation, increased inflow of blood into the corpora cavernosa, and ensuing penile erection upon sexual stimulation.

PHARMACOKINETICS/DYNAMICS:
Absorption: Rapidly absorbed with bioavailability of about 15%. C_{max} reached between 30 min and 2 hr after an oral dose.

Distribution: Vd_{ss} is 208 L. Protein binding is about 95%.

Metabolism: Metabolized predominantly by CYP3A4 and to a lesser degree by CYP3A5 and CYP2C isoforms. The M1 metabolite accounts for 7% of the total activity.

Excretion: Excretion as metabolites (91% to 95% in feces; 2% to 6% in urine). Total body Cl is 56 L/hr, t½ is approximately 4 to 5 hr.

Special Populations:
Renal Function Impairment – The AUC was 20% to 30% higher in moderate or severe renal impairment.

Hepatic Function Impairment – Hepatic impairment is associated with increased plasma levels. A starting dose of 5 mg is recommended in patients with moderate hepatic impairment and the max dose should not exceed 10 mg.
Elderly – In men 65 yr and older, the C_{max} and AUC are increased 34% and 52%, respectively, compared with men 18 to 45 yr.

Indications Treatment of erectile dysfunction.

Contraindications Administration with nitrates, nitric oxide donors, or alpha blockers; hypersensitivity to any component of the product.

Route/Dosage
ADULTS: PO Recommended starting dose is 10 mg approximately 60 min prior to sexual activity. Depending on efficacy and side effects, the dose may be decreased to 5 mg or increased to 20 mg.
GERIATRIC (65 YR AND OLDER): PO A 5 mg starting dose is recommended.

Hepatic Impairment
ADULTS: PO A 5 mg starting dose is recommended in patients with moderate hepatic impairment (max, 10 mg). Do not use in severe hepatic impairment.

Concomitant Therapy
ADULTS: PO In patients receiving ritonavir, do not exceed a single 2.5 mg dose in a 72-hr period. In patients receiving indinavir, itraconazole (400 mg/day), or ketoconazole (400 mg/day), do not exceed a single 2.5 mg dose in a 24-hr period. In patients receiving erythromycin, itraconazole (200 mg/day), or ketoconazole (200 mg/day), do not exceed a single 5 mg dose in a 24-hr period.

Interactions
Alpha blockers (eg, terazosin), nitrates: Coadministration of these agents with vardenafil is contraindicated.

Class IA (eg, quinidine, procainamide), class III (eg, amiodarone, sotalol) antiarrhythmic agents: Patients with congenital QT prolongation and those receiving these agents should avoid use of vardenafil.

Cytochrome P450 3A4/5 and CYP2C9 (eg, erythromycin, indinavir, itraconazole, ketoconazole, ritonavir): Plasma levels of vardenafil may be elevated, increasing the risk of side effects and necessitating dosage adjustment.

Lab Test Interferences
None well documented.

Adverse Reactions
CV: Angina pectoris, chest pain, hypertension, hypotension, MI, myocardial ischemia, palpitation, postural hypotension, syncope, tachycardia (less than 2%).
CNS: Headache (15%); dizziness (2%); hypertonia, hypesthesia, insomnia, paresthesia, somnolence, vertigo (less than 2%).
DERM: Photosensitivity reaction, pruritus, rash, sweating (less than 2%).
EENT: Rhinitis (9%); sinusitis (3%); tinnitus, pharyngitis, abnormal vision, blurred vision, chromatopsia, color vision changes, conjunctivitis, dim vision, eye pain, glaucoma, photophobia, watery eyes (less than 2%).
GI: Dyspepsia (4%); nausea (2%); abdominal pain, diarrhea, dry mouth, dysphagia, esophagitis, gastritis, gastroesophageal reflux, vomiting, gamma-glutamyl-transpeptidase increase (less than 2%).
GU: Abnormal ejaculation, priapism (less than 2%).
HEPA: Abnormal LFTs (less than 2%).
LABTESTABS: Increased creatine kinase (2%).
MUSC: Arthralgia, back pain, myalgia, neck pain (less than 2%).
RESP: Dyspnea, epistaxis (less than 2%).
OTHER: Flushing (11%); accidental injury, flu syndrome (3%); anaphylactic reactions, asthenia, face edema, pain (less than 2%).

Precautions
Pregnancy: Category B.
Lactation: Undetermined.
Children: Not indicated for use in children.
Elderly: Because men 65 yr and older may have higher plasma levels, a lower starting dose is recommended.
Hepatic function impairment: Reduce starting dose in patients with moderate hepatic impairment.
Cardiac risk: Evaluate CV status, left ventricular outflow obstruction (eg, aortic stenosis), and BP before treatment.
Priapism: Prolonged erections (exceeding 4 hr) may occur and require immediate medical assistance.
Special populations: Because there are no clinical data on safety and efficacy, use is not recommended in patients with unstable angina, hypotension, uncontrolled hypertension, recent history of stroke, life-threatening arrhythmia, MI, severe cardiac failure, severe hepatic impairment, or end stage renal disease or known hereditary degenerative retinal disorder, including retinitis pigmentosa.

Overdosage: Signs and Symptoms
Back pain/myalgia, abnormal vision.

PATIENT CARE CONSIDERATIONS
Administration/Storage
- Administer prescribed dose approximately 60 min before sexual activity.
- Administer without regard to meals. Administer with food if GI upset occurs.
- Max dosing frequency is once daily.
- Store tablets at controlled room temperature (59° to 86°F).

Assessment/Interventions
- Obtain patient history, including drug history and any known allergies. Note liver disease, kidney disease, left ventricular outflow obstruction, unstable angina, hypotension, uncontrolled hypertension, anatomical deformation of penis (eg, Peyronie disease), conditions predisposing to priapism (eg, sickle cell anemia, multiple myeloma, leukemia), congenital degenerative retinal disorder, severe heart failure, congenital or acquired QT prolongation, recent history (eg, within 6 mo) of stroke, life-threatening arrhythmia or MI, and concurrent use of other treatments for erectile dysfunction, strong CYP3A4 inhibitors (eg, ritonavir, indinavir, ketoconazole, itraconazole, erythromycin), Class 1A antiarrhythmics (eg, procainamide), or Class III antiarrhythmics (eg, amiodarone, sotalol).
- Review patient's health history for any condition that could contraindicate therapy with vardenafil: current use of nitrates (eg, nitroglycerin) or alpha blockers (eg, terazosin, tamsulosin).
- Ensure that CV status of patient has been assessed before therapy is started.
- Ensure that a lower starting dose is used in patients over 65 yr or in patient with moderate hepatic impairment.
- Ensure that reduced dose is used in patient concurrently taking strong CYP3A4 inhibitors.

- Assess patient for CV, CNS, GI, and general body side effects. Inform health care provider if noted and significant.

Patient/Family Education
- Explain name, dose, action, and potential side effects of drug.
- Instruct patient to read the patient information leaflet before starting therapy and with each refill.
- Advise patient to take prescribed dose 60 min before anticipated sexual activity and not to take more than 1 dose in a 24 hr period.
- Advise patient to take prescribed dose without regard to meals but to take with food if stomach upset occurs.
- Advise patient that sexual stimulation will be required for medication to work and an erection to occur.
- Instruct patient not to change the dose unless advised by health care provider.
- Advise patient to contact health care provider if they are not satisfied with their sexual performance after taking medication or if bothersome side effects occur.
- Instruct patient to stop using and contact health care provider immediately if any of the following occur: dizziness, fainting, chest pain, vision changes, erection persisting longer than 4 hr, painful erection.
- Caution patient to avoid using poppers (eg, amyl nitrate, butyl nitrate) while taking this medication.
- Caution patient that the medication is not a male form of birth control, nor does it provide protection against sexually transmitted diseases and to use protective measures as indicated.
- Instruct patient not to take any prescription or OTC medications or dietary supplements unless advised by health care provider.
- Advise patient that follow-up visits may be required to monitor therapy and to keep appointments.

Vasopressin (8-Arginine-Vasopressin)

(VAY-so-PRESS-in)

Class Posterior pituitary hormone

How Supplied
Pitressin Injection 20 pressor units/mL
♣ *Pressyn*

Action
PHARMACOLOGY: Promotes resorption of water through kidney. At high doses, stimulates contraction of smooth muscle causing vasoconstriction, increased peristaltic activity, and gallbladder contractions.

PHARMACOKINETICS/DYNAMICS:
Absorption: T_{max} is about 2 to 8 hr.
Metabolism: Majority of dose is metabolized and rapidly destroyed in the liver and kidneys.
Excretion: $T_{1/2}$ is about 10 to 20 min. About 5% of the dose is excreted unchanged in the urine after 4 hr.

Indications Treatment of neurogenic diabetes insipidus; prevention and treatment of postoperative abdominal distention; facilitation of abdominal roentgenography. **Unlabeled use(s):** Treatment of bleeding esophageal varices.

Contraindications Standard considerations.

Route/Dosage
Diabetes Insipidus
ADULTS: **IM/SC** 5 to 10 U 2 or 3 times daily as needed. Intranasal injection solution may be given as an individualized dosage intranasally on cotton pledgets, by nasal spray, or dropper.
CHILDREN: Reduce dosage proportionally.

Abdominal Distention
ADULTS: **IM** 5 U initially; subsequent injections q 3 to 4 hr prn. May increase the dose to 10 U if necessary.

Abdominal Roentgenography
ADULTS: **IM/SC** 2 injections of 10 U each administered 2 hr and 30 min before films are exposed.

Bleeding Esophageal Varices
ADULTS: **IV** Infuse initially at 0.2 to 0.4 U/min and increase to 0.9 U/min if necessary.

Interactions
Alcohol, demeclocycline, heparin, lithium, norepinephrine: May decrease the antidiuretic effect of vasopressin.
Carbamazepine, chlorpropamide, clofibrate, fludrocortisone, tricyclic antidepressants, urea: May potentiate antidiuretic effect of vasopressin.
Ganglionic blocking agents: May markedly increase sensitivity to vasopressin pressor effects.

Lab Test Interferences None well documented.

Adverse Reactions
CV: Angina.
GI: Abdominal cramps; nausea; vomiting; gas.
OTHER: Gangrene; ischemic colitis; tissue necrosis (with extravasation); allergic reaction (cardiac arrest, tremor, vertigo, sweating).

Precautions
Pregnancy: Category C.
Lactation: Undetermined.
Hypersensitivity: Local or systemic reactions,

including anaphylaxis, may occur.
Special risk patients: Use drug with caution in patients with epilepsy, migraine, asthma, heart failure, or any condition where a rapid rise in extracellular water may result in further compromise.

Chronic nephritis with nitrogen retention: Contraindicates use until reasonable nitrogen blood levels have been attained.

Extravasation: Severe vasoconstriction and local tissue necrosis may result if drug extravasates during IV infusion.

Vascular disease: Use extreme caution in patients with vascular disease.

Water intoxication: Water intoxication may occur. Early signs include confusion, drowsiness, listlessness, and headache.

Overdosage: Signs and Symptoms
Confusion, lethargy, drowsiness, listlessness, headache.

PATIENT CARE CONSIDERATIONS

Administration/Storage
* Store at room temperature. Do not freeze.
* Give 1 to 2 glasses of water with dose to prevent skin blanching, abdominal cramps, and nausea.
* If administering via IV infusion, dilute with 0.9% Normal Saline or D5W to a concentration of 0.1 to 1 U/mL. Ensure patency of venous access and use infusion control device.

Assessment/Interventions
* Obtain patient history, including drug history and any known allergies.
* Monitor for allergic reactions, including tremors, sweating, vertigo, circumoral pallor, "pounding in head," abdominal cramps, flatus, nausea, vomiting, urticaria, or bronchial constriction.
* Monitor I&O and weight daily.
* Monitor urine specific gravity and osmolarity.
* Monitor vital signs.
* Monitor ECG and fluid and electrolyte status at frequent intervals during prolonged therapy.
* Monitor patient for evidence of water intoxication (eg, confusion, drowsiness, listlessness, headache). Report to health care provider immediately if noted.
* Monitor the following for therapeutic responses: decreased urine output; decreased thirst.
* Assess reduction of thirst.
* In abdominal distention, assess bowel sounds and presence or absence of flatus.

Patient/Family Education
* Tell patient to take with 1 to 2 glasses of water to prevent skin blanching, nausea, or abdominal cramping.
* Caution patient to withhold medication and to notify health care provider of chest pain.
* Tell patient to report drowsiness, listlessness, and headache to health care provider, and to restrict water intake.
* Explain that urine output should decrease after use.
* Tell patient to monitor weight daily.
* Instruct patient to avoid alcohol intake during therapy.
* Remind patients with diabetes insipidus to carry appropriate medical identification.

Vecuronium Bromide

(veh-CUE-row-nee-uhm BROE-mide)

Class Nondepolarizing neuromuscular blocker/Muscle relaxant/Anesthetic adjunct

How Supplied
Norcuron Powder for Injection 10 mg, Powder for Injection 20 mg

Action
PHARMACOLOGY: Causes paralysis of skeletal muscles by binding competitively to cholinergic receptors on motor end-plate to antagonize action of acetylcholine, resulting in block of neuromuscular transmission.

PHARMACOKINETICS/DYNAMICS:
Distribution: About 60% to 80% bound to plasma proteins. Distribution t½ is about 4 min. Vd is 300 to 400 mL/kg.

Metabolism: One metabolite, 3-desacetyl vecuronium, has been recovered in urine of some patients in quantities that account for up to 10% of an injected dose. 3-desacetyl vecuronium also has been recovered by T-tube in some patients accounting for up to 25% of the injected dose.

Excretion: The t½ is 65 to 75 min. In late pregnancy, the t½ is about 35 to 40 min. Systemic rate of clearance is about 3 to 4.5 mL/min/kg. Urine recovery varies from 3% to 35% within 42 hr.

Indications Adjunct to general anesthesia to facilitate endotracheal intubation and provide skeletal muscle relaxation during surgery or mechanical ventilation.

Contraindications Hypersensitivity to vecuronium or bromides.

Route/Dosage

ADULTS & CHILDREN YOUNGER THAN 10 YR OF AGE: **IV** *Initial dose:* for inhalation 0.08 to 0.1 mg/kg. Reduce initial dose by 15% (0.06 to 0.85 mg/kg) if inhalation agents are already in use. If intubation is performed using succinylcholine, reduce initial dose to 0.04 to 0.06 mg/kg with inhalation anesthesia and 0.05 to 0.06 mg/kg with balanced anesthesia. *Maintenance:* IV bolus 0.01 to 0.015 mg/kg within 25 to 40 min of initial dose, then q 12 to 15 min. *IV infusion:* 1 mcg/kg/min initially beginning 20 to 40 min after IV bolus. Titrate to desired clinical response.

CHILDREN 1 TO 10 YR OF AGE: **IV** Slightly higher initial doses and more frequent supplementation.

INFANTS 7 WK TO 1 YR OF AGE: **IV** Slightly lower doses and 1.5 times less frequent.

Interactions

Aminoglycosides, verapamil, inhalation anesthetics (eg, enflurane, isoflurane), lincosamides (eg, clindamycin, lincomycin), magnesium salts, polypeptide antibiotics (eg, bacitracin, polymyxin B): May enhance action of vecuronium (eg, respiratory depression).

Hydantoins, carbamazepine: May cause vecuronium to have shorter duration or decreased effectiveness.

Quinidine, quinine: Recurrent paralysis may occur with injection of quinidine during recovery from use of other muscle relaxants.

Theophyllines: Dose-dependent reversal of neuromuscular blockade is possible.

Thiopurines (eg, mercaptopurine): May decrease or reverse vecuronium action.

Trimethaphan: May cause prolonged apnea.

Lab Test Interferences
None well documented.

Adverse Reactions
RESP: Respiratory insufficiency; apnea.

OTHER: Skeletal muscle weakness; profound and prolonged skeletal muscle paralysis.

> **WARNING:**
> Must be administered via trained personnel in an equipped facility to monitor, assist, and control respiration.

Precautions

Pregnancy: Category C.
Lactation: Undetermined.
Children: Infants are moderately more sensitive and take longer to recover. Not recommended in newborns; diluent contains benzyl alcohol (fatal-gasping syndrome).
Elderly: May experience delayed onset of action.
Circulatory disease (eg, cardiovascular disease, elderly, edematous states): May cause delayed onset of action, do not increase dosage.
Consciousness: Vecuronium has no known effect on consciousness, pain threshold, or cerebration. Accompany administration of this drug by adequate anesthesia.
Electrolyte imbalance: Neuromuscular blockade may be altered depending on nature of imbalance.
Hepatic/Renal/Biliary disease: Prolonged neuromuscular blockade may occur due to reduced elimination. Higher doses may be needed due to increased volume of distribution.
Malignant hyperthermia: Monitor patient closely.
Myasthenia gravis: Small doses may have profound effects; administer test dose in monitoring response to muscle relaxants.
Severe obesity or neuromuscular disease: May pose airway or ventilation problems requiring special care before, during, or after vecuronium.

Overdosage: Signs and Symptoms
Skeletal muscle weakness, neuromuscular block beyond time needed, hypotension, decreased respiratory reserve, low tidal volume, apnea.

PATIENT CARE CONSIDERATIONS

Administration/Storage
- Administer IV only. Not for IM administration.
- Administer only if intubation, artificial respiration, oxygen, and reversal agents are immediately available.
- Reconstitute with 0.9% sodium chloride, 5% dextrose, 5% dextrose in saline, Lactated Ringer's solution, or sterile water for injection.
- May reconstitute with bacteriostatic water for injection. However, when this diluent is used, solution contains benzyl alcohol and is contraindicated in newborns.
- Store unopened vial at room temperature. Protect from light.
- Following reconstitution, refrigerate. Use within 8 hr.
- Intended for single use only. Discard unused portions.

Assessment/Interventions
- Obtain patient history, including drug history and any known allergies.
- In patients with myasthenia gravis, perform test dose.
- Observe for histamine-release symptoms, bronchospasm, flushing, redness, hypotension, and tachycardia.
- Monitor respirations and be prepared to assist or control respiration.

- Monitor BP and pulse.
- Assess skeletal muscle tone.
- Monitor I&O.
- Check for urinary retention.
- Monitor carefully for signs of increased or decreased efficacy and pharmacologic activity (eg, muscle twitch response to peripheral nerve stimulation).

Patient/Family Education
- Explain to patient and family that patient will recover from anesthesia in 25 to 40 min.
- Inform patient and family that patient may have difficulty speaking when recovering postoperatively but that speech will improve as effects of medication wear off.
- Inform patient that postoperative urinary retention is possible.

Venlafaxine

(VEN-luh-fax-EEN)

Class Antidepressant

How Supplied
Effexor Tablets 25 mg, Tablets 37.5 mg, Tablets 50 mg, Tablets 75 mg, Tablets 100 mg ♦ *Effexor* XR Capsules, extended-release 37.5 mg, Capsules, extended-release 75 mg, Capsules, extended-release 150 mg

Action
PHARMACOLOGY: Potentiates norepinephrine, serotonin, and dopamine neurotransmitter activity in CNS.

PHARMACOKINETICS/DYNAMICS:

Absorption: Absolute bioavailability (oral) is 45% and well absorbed (at least 92%). Steady-state concentrations of venlafaxine and O-desmethylvenlafaxine (ODV) in plasma are attained within 3 days of oral dose. Exhibits linear kinetics over dose range 75 to 450 mg/day. Time of administration AM vs PM has no affect. Food has no significant effect on absorption.

Distribution: Vd is 1.8 L/kg; 27% venlafaxine and 30% ODV is protein bound.

Metabolism: Extensively metabolized in the liver. The major metabolite is ODV.

Excretion: Renal elimination of venlafaxine and its metabolite is the primary route of excretion. Within 48 hr, 87% is recovered in urine.

Special Populations:
Renal Function Impairment – Dosage adjustment is necessary with Ccr 10 to 70 mL/min. Venlafaxine t½ was prolonged about 50%, Cl was reduced about 24%; ODV t½ was prolonged 40% although Cl was unchanged.
Hepatic Function Impairment – In patients with hepatic cirrhosis, dosage adjustment is necessary. Venlafaxine t½ was prolonged to about 30%, Cl decreased 50%; ODV t½ was prolonged about 60%, Cl decreased 30%.
Dialysis – Dose adjustment is necessary. Venlafaxine t½ was prolonged about 180% and Cl was reduced about 57%. ODV t½ was prolonged about 142% and Cl was reduced 56%.
Poor/Extensive Metabolizer – Plasma concentrations of venlafaxine were higher in CYP2D6 poor metabolizers than in extensive metabolizers. However, AUC of both venlafaxine and ODV were similar in both groups, so there is no need for dose adjustment.

Indications Treatment of depression; generalized anxiety disorder (*Effexor ER*).

Contraindications Concomitant use with MAO inhibitors.

Route/Dosage
Depression
ADULTS (IMMEDIATE RELEASE): **PO** 75 mg/day in 2 or 3 divided doses; titrate to clinical effect, adding up to 75 mg/day at intervals of at least 4 days (max, 375 mg/day).

ADULTS (EXTENDED RELEASE): **PO** 75 mg/day administered in single dose either in morning or evening at approximately same time qd. Some patients may need to start at 37.5 mg/day for 4 to 7 days before increasing to 75 mg/day. Make dose increases in increments of up to 75 mg/day prn and at intervals of at least 4 days.

Generalized Anxiety Disorder
ADULTS (EXTENDED RELEASE): **PO** The usual dosage is 75 to 225 mg/day. Some patients may need to start with 37.5 mg/day to avoid overstimulation.

Interactions
Desipramine, haloperidol: Plasma levels of these drugs may be elevated by venlafaxine, increasing the risk of adverse effects.
MAO inhibitors: MAO inhibitors have produced serious, even fatal, reactions when given concomitantly with venlafaxine. Do not use venlafaxine together with MAO inhibitors or within 14 days of MAO inhibitor use. Wait at least 7 days after stopping venlafaxine before using MAO inhibitors.
St. John's wort: Increased sedative-hypnotic effects may occur.
Sibutramine, sumatriptan, trazodone: Serotonin syndrome, including irritability, increased muscle tone, shivering, myoclonus, and altered consciousness may occur.

Lab Test Interferences None well documented.

Adverse Reactions
CV: Vasodilation (6%); hypertension (5%); palpitation (3%); tachycardia (2%); postural hypotension (1%); deep vein thrombophlebitis, EKG abnormalities (eg, QT prolongation), cardiac arrhythmias (including atrial fibrillation, torsades de pointes [postmarketing]).
CNS: Headache (34%); nervousness (32%); somnolence (26%); dizziness (24%); insomnia (23%); asthenia (17%); anxiety (11%); tremor (10%); decreased libido (9%); abnormal dreams (7%); agitation (4%); depression, hypertonia, paresthesia (3%); twitching, abnormal thinking, confusion (2%); depersonalization (1%); migraine, trismus, vertigo, emotional lability, amnesia, hypesthesia (at least 1%); catatonia, delirium, extrapyramidal symptoms, neuroleptic malignant syndrome-like events, involuntary movements, serotonin syndrome, shock-like electrical sensations, panic (postmarketing).
DERM: Sweating (19%); rash (3%); pruritus (1%); epidermal necrolysis/Stevens-Johnson syndrome, erythema multiforme (postmarketing).
EENT: Abnormality of accommodation (9%); pharyngitis (7%); abnormal vision (6%); mydriasis, taste perversion, tinnitus, sinusitis (2%).
GI: Nausea (58%); dry mouth (22%); anorexia (20%); constipation (15%); diarrhea, vomiting, abdominal pain (8%); dyspepsia (7%); flatulence (3%).
GU: Abnormal ejaculation (16%); impotence (10%); anorgasmia (female [8%]), urinary frequency (3%); eructation, impaired urination, orgasm disturbance (2%); decreased libido, urinary retention (1%); metrorrhagia, prostatitis, vaginitis (at least 1%).
HEMA: Ecchymosis (at least 1%); agranulocytosis, aplastic anemia, neutropenia, pancytopenia (postmarketing).
HEPA: Hepatic events (including elevated GGT, unspecified LFT abnormalities, liver damage necrosis, failure and fatty liver [postmarketing]).
LABTESTABS: Increased CFK and LDH (postmarketing).
M/N: Weight loss (4%); weight gain, edema (at least 1%).
RESP: Dyspnea (at least 1%).
OTHER: Yawn (8%); chills (7%); infection, flu-like syndrome (6%); accidental injury (5%); chest pain, trauma (2%); arthralgia (at least 1%); congenital anomalies, night sweats, pancreatitis, hemorrhage, anaphylaxis, renal failure, rhabdomyolysis, pulmonary eosinophilia, increased prolactin (postmarketing).

Precautions
Pregnancy: Category C.
Lactation: Excreted in breast milk.
Children: Safety and efficacy not established.
Elderly: Take extra care when increasing dose in elderly patients.
Renal function impairment: Reduction of dose may be necessary. Use drug with caution.
Hepatic function impairment: Reduction of dose may be necessary. Use drug with caution.
Special risk patients: Use drug with caution in patients whose underlying condition might be compromised by increases in heart rate (eg, hyperthyroidism, heart failure) and in patients with history of seizure, mania, suicidal tendencies, drug abuse or dependence.
Discontinuation: After 1 wk of therapy, dosage requires tapering if discontinuing; after 6 wk of treatment, taper over 2-wk period.
Hypertension: Regular monitoring of BP is recommended. Venlafaxine is associated with sustained but small increases in BP (usually associated with doses less than 300 mg/day).
Hyponatremia: Hyponatremia and/or syndrome of inappropriate antidiuretic hormone secretion may occur.

Overdosage: Signs and Symptoms
Somnolence, sinus tachycardia.

PATIENT CARE CONSIDERATIONS
Administration/Storage
- Do not administer with or within 14 days of MAO inhibitor administration.
- Patient on immediate-release tablet may be switched to extended-release capsule at nearest equivalent mg/day dose.

Immediate-release tablets:
- Administer bid or tid with food as prescribed.

Extended-release capsules:
- Administer prescribed dose qd with food in the morning or evening.
- Have patient swallow capsule whole with fluid. Do not cut, chew, or place capsule in water.
- For patients having difficulty swallowing capsule, it can be opened and the contents sprinkled on a spoonful of applesauce. Have patient swallow mixture immediately without chewing and follow with full glass of water to ensure complete swallowing.
- Store tablets and capsules at controlled room temperature (68° to 77°F).

Assessment/Interventions
- Obtain patient history, including drug history and any known allergies. Determine whether any MAO inhibitors have been used in the past 14 days. Note kidney or liver disease, glaucoma, hyperthyroidism, heart failure,

recent MI, seizure disorder, or current use of triptans, SSRIs, or lithium.
- Ensure that initial dose does not exceed 75 mg/day and that dosage increases are made no more than q 4 days
- Ensure that dose is reduced in patient with renal and/or hepatic impairment.
- Continue suicide monitoring of high-risk patients.
- Observe for signs of mood change and report to physician.
- Monitor and record BP and pulse periodically during treatment. If hypertension develops, notify health care provider. Be prepared to reduce dose or discontinue therapy if hypertension persists.
- Assess patient for CNS, GI, psychiatric, musculoskeletal, GU, and general body side effects. Report to health care provider if noted and significant.
- If treatment needs to be discontinued, attempt to gradually taper the dose over at least a 2-wk interval in patient who has been on therapy for longer than 1 wk.

Patient/Family Education
- Explain name, dose, action, and potential side effects of drug.
- Advise patient that medication will be started at a low dose and then increased as tolerated until max benefit is obtained.
- Advise patient taking immediate-release tablets to take bid or tid with food as prescribed.
- Advise patient taking extended-release capsules to take prescribed dose qd with food, in the morning or evening. Caution patient not to crush or chew capsule. If patient can't swallow the capsule, it can be opened and the contents sprinkled on a spoonful of applesauce. Have patient swallow mixture immediately without chewing and follow with full glass of water to ensure complete swallowing.
- Advise patient that if a dose is missed to skip that dose and take the next dose at the regularly scheduled time. Caution patient to never take 2 doses at the same time.
- Advise patient not to change the dose or stop taking unless advised by health care provider.
- Inform patient that it may take 1 to 4 wk to note improvement in symptoms and to continue with the prescribed therapy once improvement has been noted.
- Advise patient to take frequent sips of water, suck on ice chips or sugarless hard candy, or chew sugarless gum if dry mouth occurs.
- Advise patient to avoid alcoholic beverages.
- Advise patient that drug may impair judgment, thinking, or reflexes and to use caution while driving or performing other tasks requiring mental alertness until tolerance is determined.
- Advise patient to contact health care provider if rash, hives, or other symptoms of an allergic reaction develop, if experiencing painful or prolonged erection, or if experiencing bothersome side effects such as unusual sweating, headache, drowsiness, insomnia, nausea, tremors, or changes in sexual function.
- Instruct patient not to take prescription or OTC drugs or dietary supplements unless advised by health care provider.
- Advise women to notify health care provider if pregnant, planning to become pregnant, or breastfeeding.
- Advise patient that follow-up visits will be necessary to monitor therapy and to keep appointments.

Verapamil Hydrochloride

(veh-RAP-uh-mill HIGH-droe-KLOR-ide)
Class Calcium channel blocker

How Supplied
Calan Tablets 40 mg, Tablets 80 mg, Tablets 120 mg ◆ *Calan SR* Tablets, sustained release 120 mg, Tablets, sustained release 180 mg, Tablets, sustained release 240 mg ◆ *Covera-HS* Tablets, extended release 180 mg, Tablets, extended release 240 mg ◆ *Isoptin* Tablets 40 mg, Tablets 80 mg, Tablets 120 mg ◆ *Isoptin SR* Tablets, sustained release 120 mg, Tablets, sustained release 180 mg, Tablets, sustained release 240 mg ◆ *Verelan* Capsules, sustained release 120 mg, Capsules, sustained release 180 mg, Capsules, sustained release 240 mg, Capsules, sustained release 360 mg ◆ *Verelan PM* Capsules, sustained release 100 mg, Capsules, sustained release 200 mg, Capsules, sustained release 300 mg ◆ *Verapamil* Injection 2.5 mg/mL
🍁 *Alti-Verapamil* ◆ *APO-Verap* ◆ *Chronovera* ◆ *Gen-Verapamil* ◆ *Gen-Verapamil SR* ◆ *Isoptin I.V.* ◆ *Novo-Veramil* ◆ *Novo-Veramil SR* ◆ *Nu-Verap*

Action
PHARMACOLOGY: Inhibits movement of calcium ions across cell membrane resulting in depression of mechanical contraction of myocardial and vascular smooth muscle and depression of impulse formation (automaticity) and conduction velocity.

PHARMACOKINETICS/DYNAMICS:
Distribution: Rapid early distribution phase ($t_{½}$ about 4 min).

Metabolism: Rapidly metabolized. Extensive metabolism in the liver with 12 metabolites having been identified, most only in trace amounts. Major metabolites are N- and O-dealkylated products of verapamil.

Excretion: Terminal elimination t½ is about 2 to 5 hr. About 70% of dose is excreted in the urine and 16% more in feces within 5 days. About 3% to 4% is excreted as unchanged drug.

Special Populations:
Elderly – Elimination t½ may be prolonged.

Indications

Oral: Treatment of vasospastic (Prinzmetal variant), chronic stable (classic effort-associated), and unstable (crescendo, preinfarction) angina; adjunctive treatment with digitalis to control ventricular rate at rest and during stress in atrial flutter or fibrillation; prophylaxis of repetitive paroxysmal supraventricular tachycardia (PSVT); management of essential hypertension.
Sustained-release – Management of essential hypertension.
Parenteral: Rapid conversion of PSVTs to sinus rhythm; temporary control of rapid ventricular rate in atrial flutter or fibrillation. **Unlabeled use(s):** Treatment of migraine and cluster headaches; treatment of hypertrophic cardiomyopathy.

Contraindications

Hypersensitivity to verapamil; sick sinus syndrome or second- or third-degree atrioventricular (AV) block except with functioning pacemaker; hypotension (less than 90 mm Hg systolic); severe left ventricular dysfunction; cardiogenic shock and severe CHF, unless secondary to supraventricular tachycardia amenable to verapamil; patients with atrial flutter or fibrillation and accessory bypass tract. IV verapamil should not be used concomitantly (within few hours) of IV beta-adrenergic blocking agents or in ventricular tachycardia.

Route/Dosage

ADULTS: **PO** 40 to 160 mg tid. Do not exceed 480 mg/day.
Sustained release: **PO** 120 to 480 mg/day. Lower doses are given once daily; larger doses divided into 2 doses.
ADULTS: **IV** 5 to 10 mg bolus over 2 min. May repeat with 10 mg, 30 min after first dose. Give slower (over at least 3 min) in older patients.
CHILDREN 1 TO 15 YR OF AGE: **IV** 0.1 to 0.3 mg/kg (not to exceed 5 mg) over at least 2 min. May repeat in 30 min.
CHILDREN LESS THAN 1 YR OF AGE: **IV** 0.1 to 0.2 mg/kg (usual range, 0.75 to 2 mg) bolus over 2 min with continuous ECG monitoring.

Interactions

Other antihypertensive agents: Additive hypotension.
Beta-blockers: May result in increased hypotension and adverse effects because of additive depressant effects on myocardial contractility or AV conduction.
Buspirone: Pharmacologic and adverse effects may be increased by verapamil.
Calcium salts: Clinical effects and toxicities of verapamil may be reversed.
Carbamazepine: Increased carbamazepine serum levels.
Cyclosporine: Increased cyclosporine levels may result.
Dofetilide: Risk of life-threatening ventricular arrhythmias, including torsades de pointes, may be increased. Coadministration with verapamil is contraindicated.
Digitalis glycosides: Increased serum digoxin or digitoxin levels may occur.
Disopyramide: Do not use 48 hr before or 24 hr after verapamil.
Flecainide: May prolong AV conduction.
Nondepolarizing muscle relaxants: Enhanced muscle relaxant effects and prolonged respiratory depression may occur.
Prazosin: Increased prazosin serum levels may result.
Quinidine: Hypotension, bradycardia, ventricular tachycardia, AV block, and pulmonary edema may occur.
Rifampin: Loss of effectiveness of oral verapamil may occur.
Simvastatin: Plasma levels may be elevated by verapamil, increasing the risk of toxicity (eg, rhabdomyolysis).
INCOMPATIBILITIES: Do not mix with sodium lactate in polyvinyl chloride bags, albumin, amphotericin B, hydralazine, aminophylline, sodium bicarbonate, nafcillin, or trimethoprim-sulfamethoxazole. Do not mix in solution with pH greater than 6.

Lab Test Interferences

None well documented.

Adverse Reactions

CV: Peripheral edema; hypotension; AV block; bradycardia; CHF; pulmonary edema; cerebrovascular accident.
CNS: Dizziness; lightheadedness; headache; asthenia.
DERM: Dermatitis; rash; sweating; gingival hyperplasia.
GI: Nausea; constipation.
HEPA: Increased transaminases; hepatitis.
RESP: Shortness of breath; dyspnea; wheezing.

Precautions

Pregnancy: Category C.
Lactation: Excreted in breast milk.
Children: Children younger than 6 mo of age may not respond to IV use. Rare severe hemodynamic side effects have occurred in newborns and infants after IV use.
Elderly: May have greater hypotensive effects in elderly. Elderly may respond to lower doses.
Renal function impairment: Use caution.

Hepatic function impairment: Hepatic cirrhosis can significantly alter pharmacokinetics of verapamil.
Antiplatelet effects: Calcium channel blockers may inhibit platelet function.
Cardiac conduction: May be associated with variety of cardiac conduction abnormalities including first-, second-, or third-degree AV block; bradycardia; asystole; severe hypotension; nodal escape rhythms; PR prolongation; and ventricular tachycardia in patients with atrial flutter/fibrillation and W-P-W syndrome caused by antegrade conduction.
CHF: Use verapamil with caution in patients with CHF.
Duchenne muscular dystrophy: May decrease neuromuscular transmission in patients with Duchenne muscular dystrophy and prolong recovery from neuromuscular blocking agent vecuronium.
Hypertrophic cardiomyopathy: Serious adverse effects were seen in patients with hypertrophic cardiomyopathy who received oral verapamil.
Hypotension: Hypotension may occur during initial therapy or with dosage increases and is more likely in patients taking beta blockers.
Increased intracranial pressure: IV verapamil has increased intracranial pressure in patients with supratentorial tumors at time of anesthesia induction.
Premature ventricular contractions (PVCs): May occur after IV use; consider possibility with oral use.

Overdosage: Signs and Symptoms
Hypotension, bradycardia, AV block, asystole.

PATIENT CARE CONSIDERATIONS
Administration/Storage
- Administer with milk or meals if GI upset or intolerance occurs.
- Give IV slowly over 2 min.
- Implement cardiac monitor when administering drug IV and monitor BP.
- Do not give concomitantly with IV beta-adrenergic blockers (within few hours).
- Administer Covera-HS once daily at bedtime. Swallow tablet whole; do not crush or chew.
- Store injection at room temperature, protected from light. Avoid freezing.
- Store oral form at room temperature in tight, light-resistant container.

Assessment/Interventions
- Obtain patient history, including drug history and any known allergies.
- Report any cardiovascular changes to health care provider.
- Report any chest pain to health care provider.
- If drug is to be discontinued, aid in gradual reduction of dosage.

Patient/Family Education
- Tell patient if dose is missed to take as soon as possible. If several hours have passed or if it is nearing time for next dose, tell patient not to double dose to catch up unless advised by health care provider.
- If more than one dose is missed, tell patient to contact health care provider.
- Caution patient not to change dose unless directed by health care provider.
- Advise patient not to suddenly stop taking medication.
- Remind patient to brush and floss teeth and see dentist regularly.
- Instruct patient to report any irregular heart beat, shortness of breath, swelling of hands and feet, pronounced dizziness, constipation, nausea, or hypotension.
- Advise patient to avoid use of alcohol and OTC medications without consulting health care provider.
- Instruct patient to limit caffeine consumption.
- Advise patient that drug may cause dizziness and to use caution while driving or performing other tasks requiring mental alertness until effects of drug have stabilized.
- Stress to patient the importance of compliance in all areas of treatment regimen: diet, exercise, stress reduction, drug therapy.

Vinblastine Sulfate

(vin-BLAST-een)
Class Vinca alkaloid

How Supplied
Vinblastine Sulfate Injection 10 mg

Action
PHARMACOLOGY: Vinblastine interferes with metabolic pathways of amino acids leading from glutamic acid to the citric acid cycle and urea. Vinblastine has an effect on cell energy production required for mitosis and interferes with nucleic acid synthesis.

PHARMACOKINETICS/DYNAMICS:
Absorption: Rapidly absorbed 15 to 30 min following IV triphasic serum decay pattern.

Distribution: Undergoes rapid distribution (from blood to tissue) and extensive tissue binding.

Metabolism: Metabolized by the hepatic P450 3A cytochromes. The metabolite, deacetyl vinblastine, is more active than parent drug.

Excretion: Major route of excretion is the biliary system (liver). Terminal t½ is 24.8 hr.

Special Populations:
Hepatic Function Impairment – Toxicity may be enhanced. A dose reduction is recommended. In patients with a direct serum bilirubin value more than 3 mg/dL, a 50% dose reduction is recommended.

Pregnancy – Category D. Information is very limited.

Indications
Adult: Hodgkin's disease, non-Hodgkin's lymphoma, mycosis fungoides, advanced testicular carcinoma, Kaposi's sarcoma, choriocarcinoma, breast cancer.

Pediatric: Hodgkin's disease, non-Hodgkin's lymphoma, mycosis fungoides, Letterer-Siwe disease, choriocarcinoma. **Unlabeled use(s):** Non-small cell lung carcinoma, bladder cancer, cervical cancer, refractory idiopathic thrombocytopenic purpura, autoimmune hemolytic anemia.

Contraindications
Leukopenia; presence of bacterial infection (infections must be under control prior to initiating therapy); significant granulocytopenia unless it is a result of the disease being treated.

Route/Dosage
Initial
ADULTS: **IV** Initially 3.7 mg/m² as a single dose/wk. Then increase at weekly intervals in 1.8 mg/m² increments until the leukocyte count decreases to about 3000/mm³. The maximum weekly dose is 18.5 mg/m².

PEDIATRIC: **IV** Initially 2.5 mg/m² as a single dose/wk. Then increase at weekly intervals in 1.25 mg/m² increments until the leukocyte count decreases to about 3000/mm³. The maximum weekly dose is 12.5 mg/m².

Maintenance
ADULTS: **IV** The maintenance dose is 1.8 mg/m² less than the dose required to produce a leukocyte count of 3000/mm³ every 7 to 14 days. The optimum weekly dose is normally 5.5 to 7.4 mg/m². Maintenance doses should not be given until the WBC reaches 4000/mm³. For an adequate trial, vinblastine must be continued for at least 4 to 6 wk.

PEDIATRIC: **IV** The maintenance dose is 1.25 mg/m² less than the dose required to produce a leukocyte count of 3000/mm³ every 7 to 14 days. Maintenance doses should not be given until the WBC reaches 4000/mm³. For an adequate trial, vinblastine must be continued for at least 4 to 6 wk.

Adjustment in Hepatic Insufficiency
ADULTS: **IV** Reduce the dose 50% in patients with a direct serum bilirubin exceeding 3 mg/dL.

Interactions
CYP450 inhibitors: Vinblastine elimination may be reduced by cytochrome P450 enzyme inhibitors.

Erythromycin: Erythromycin may decrease metabolism of vinblastine causing increased toxicity.

Mitomycin: Acute shortness of breath and severe bronchospasm have occurred following concomitant or previous use of mitomycin.

Phenytoin: May reduce phenytoin plasma concentration.

Lab Test Interferences
None well documented.

Adverse Reactions
CV: Hypertension.
CNS: Malaise; weakness; dizziness; numbness of digits or paresthesia; loss of deep tendon reflexes; peripheral neuritis; mental depression; headache; convulsions.
DERM: Alopecia; photosensitivity.
ENDO: Syndrome of inappropriate antidiuretic hormone secretion.
GI: Pharyngitis; vesiculation of the mouth; mucositis; ileus; diarrhea; constipation; anorexia; abdominal pain; rectal bleeding; hemorrhagic enterocolitis; bleeding from an old peptic ulcer.
GU: Amenorrhea; loss of sperm or semen.
HEMA: Bone marrow suppression, usually selective for leukocytes, nadir at 5 to 10 days.
MUSC: Bone or jaw pain acutely.
RESP: Acute bronchospasm, especially in combination with mitomycin.

> **WARNING:**
>
> *IV use only:* Intrathecal use of other vinca alkaloids has been fatal. Label syringe "Warning - For IV Use Only; fatal if given intrathecally."
>
> *Granulocytopenia:* May be severe and predispose to infection. Do not administer to patients with granulocyte counts less than 1000 cells/mm³.
>
> *Avoid extravasation:* Proper placement of needle/catheter prior to administration. Extravasation can cause severe local necrosis. Local irritation or phlebitis may occur. Refer to your institution specific protocol.

Precautions
Pregnancy: Category D.
Lactation: Undetermined.
Hepatic function impairment: Toxicity may be enhanced in the presence of hepatic insufficiency. A dose reduction is recommended.
Dosage adjustment guidelines (pediatric): Follow dosage adjustment guidelines recommended for adults.

Hematologic effects: Leukopenia is expected. If leukopenia (less than 2000 WBC/mm³) occurs following a dose of this drug, carefully watch the patient for evidence of infection until a safe WBC count has returned
Pulmonary reactions: Acute shortness of breath and severe bronchospasm have occurred. These reactions occur most frequently when used with mitomycin.

Overdosage: Signs and Symptoms
Side effects are dose-related. Expect exaggerated effects.

PATIENT CARE CONSIDERATIONS
Administration/Storage
- Refrigerate. Protect from light. Unopened vials are stable at room temperature for 2 wk, but this is not recommended for storage. Solutions reconstituted with bacteriostatic 0.9% Sodium Chloride are stable for 30 days in the refrigerator. Solutions reconstituted with preservative-free 0.9% Sodium Chloride should be used within 24 hr.
- Reconstitute sterile powder with 10 mL of bacteriostatic 0.9% Sodium Chloride containing phenol or benzyl alcohol (final concentration 1 mg/mL). Powder also may be reconstituted with 10 mL of preservative-free 0.9% Sodium Chloride.
- Give IV push injection or IV side arm into a running infusion.

Assessment/Interventions
- Monitor CBC closely.
- Carefully watch the patient for evidence of infection until a safe WBC count has returned.
- Hyperuricemia may occur because of rapid cell lysis; monitor serum uric acid. Minimize effects of hyperuricemia with hydration, urinary alkalinization, and allopurinol.

Patient/Family Education
- Immediately report sore throat, fever, chills, or sore mouth to the health care provider.
- The following may occur: alopecia, jaw pain, pain in the organs containing tumor tissue, nausea, and vomiting. Scalp hair will regrow to its pretreatment extent, even with continued treatment. Report any other serious medical event to the health care provider.
- Avoid constipation.

Vincristine Sulfate
(vin-KRISS-teen)
Class Vinca alkaloid
How Supplied
Oncovin Solution for Injection 1 mg/mL

Action
PHARMACOLOGY: Mode of action is unknown. In vitro, vincristine arrests mitotic division at metaphase. It reversibly binds to microtubule and spindle proteins in the S phase.

PHARMACOKINETICS/DYNAMICS:
Absorption: Very rapidly absorbed via IV (15 to 30 min).
Distribution: More than 90% of drug is distributed from blood to tissue, where it remains tightly but not irreversibly. Penetration across the blood brain barrier is poor.
Metabolism: Triphasic serum decay following rapid IV injection.
Excretion: Terminal t½ is 85 hr (19 to 155 hr). Liver is the major excretory organ. 80% of the dose appears in the feces, 10% to 20% in the urine.
Onset: 15 to 30 min.
Special Populations:
Hepatic Function Impairment – A 50% reduction in dose is recommended for patients having a direct serum bilirubin more than 3 mg/dL.

Indications
Adult/Pediatric: Acute lymphocytic leukemia, lymphomas, rhabdomyosarcoma, neuroblastoma, Wilms tumor. **Unlabeled use(s):** Small-cell lung carcinoma, brain tumors, multiple myeloma, Kaposi sarcoma, chronic lymphocytic and myelocytic leukemias, autoimmune hemolytic anemia, idiopathic thrombocytopenic purpura.

Contraindications
Patients with demyelinating form of Charcot-Marie-Tooth syndrome.

Route/Dosage
Acute Lymphocytic Leukemia, Lymphomas, Rhabdomyosarcoma, Neuroblastoma, Wilms Tumor
ADULT: IV 1.4 mg/m² weekly (typical dose, 2 mg).
CHILDREN WEIGHING MORE THAN 10 KG (OR BODY SURFACE AREA AT LEAST 1 M²): IV 1.4 to 2 mg/m² weekly for 3 to 8 wk. Do not exceed a max of 2 mg/dose.
CHILDREN WEIGHING UP TO 10 KG (OR BODY SURFACE AREA LESS THAN 1 M²): IV 0.05 mg/kg weekly initially. Titrate dose as tolerated, up to a max of 2 mg/dose. Continue therapy for 3 to 8 wk.

Adjustment in Hepatic Insufficiency
ADULT: **IV** A 50% reduction in dose is recommended for patients having a direct serum bilirubin value more than 3 mg/dL.

Neuroblastoma, Combination Therapy
CHILDREN WEIGHING MORE THAN 10 KG (OR BODY SURFACE AREA AT LEAST 1 M^2): **IV** Vincristine 1 mg/m^2/day by continuous infusion over 24 hr for 3 days (total dose of 3 mg/m^2 over a 3-day period).

Interactions
CYP450 inhibitors: Vincristine elimination may be reduced by cytochrome P450 enzyme inhibitors.
Digoxin: May decrease digoxin plasma concentration.
Itraconazole: Vincristine neurotoxicity has occurred during coadministration.
L-asparaginase: Vincristine clearance may decrease when L-asparaginase is given prior to vincristine. Give vincristine 12 to 24 hr prior to L-asparaginase.
Mitomycin: Acute shortness of breath and severe bronchospasm have occurred following concomitant or previous use of mitomycin.
Phenytoin: May reduce phenytoin plasma concentration.
Quinolone antibiotics: Vincristine may decrease oral absorption of quinolone antibiotics.

Lab Test Interferences None well documented.

Adverse Reactions
CV: Hypertension; hypotension; MI.
CNS: Autonomic and peripheral neuropathy; headache.
DERM: Alopecia; rash
GI: Mucositis; abdominal cramps; diarrhea; anorexia; intestinal necrosis or perforation; constipation that can lead to upper colon impaction; paralytic ileus; weight loss.
GU: Amenorrhea; polyuria; dysuria; urinary retention because of bladder atony; azoospermia.
HEMA: Bone marrow suppression; nadir less than 7 days.
MUSC: Acute bone or jaw pain.
RESP: Acute shortness of breath; severe bronchospasm.
SPEC SENSE: Optic atrophy with blindness; transient cortical blindness; ptosis; diplopia; photophobia.
OTHER: Fever.

> **WARNING:**
>
> *IV use only:* Intrathecal use of other vinca alkaloids has been fatal. Label syringe "Warning - For IV Use Only; fatal if given intrathecally."
>
> *Granulocytopenia:* May be severe and predispose to infection. Do not administer to patients with granulocyte counts less than 1000 cells/mm^3.
>
> *Avoid extravasation:* Proper placement of needle/catheter prior to administration. Local irritation or phlebitis may occur. Refer to your institution specific protocol.

Precautions
Pregnancy: Category D. Can cause fetal harm when administered to pregnant women.
Lactation: Undetermined.
Hypersensitivity: Hypersensitivity temporally related to vincristine therapy has occurred.
Dosage adjustment (pediatric): Follow dosage adjustment guidelines recommended for adults.
CNS leukemia: CNS leukemia has occurred. Additional agents may be required.
Pulmonary reactions: Acute shortness of breath and severe bronchospasm have occurred, most frequently when the drug was used with mitomycin-C.

Overdosage: Signs and Symptoms
Side effects are dose-related. Expect exaggerated side effects.

PATIENT CARE CONSIDERATIONS
Administration/Storage
- Refrigerate. Protect from light.
- Do not dilute vincristine for routine IV use. For continuous IV infusion, vincristine may be diluted with 0.9% Sodium Chloride or 5% Dextrose.
- Administer by IV injection or continuous IV infusion.
- Do not filter.
- Give over a 1-min period by IV push injection or IV side arm into a running infusion.
- Continuous infusions can only be administered through a central venous catheter resting in the vena cava. A peripherally-inserted central catheter, or PICC line, may also be appropriate.

Assessment/Interventions
- Consider routine prophylaxis for constipation.
- Hyperuricemia may occur because of rapid cell lysis; monitor serum uric acid. Minimize effects of hyperuricemia with hydration, urinary alkalinization, and allopurinol.
- Perform CBC before each dose.

Patient/Family Education
- Explain name, action, and potential side effects of drug.

- Advise patient, family, or caregiver that medication will be prepared and administered by health care provider in a health care setting.
- Advise patient, family, or caregiver that medication may be used in combination with other agents to achieve max benefit possible.
- Review dosing schedule with patient, family, or caregiver.
- Advise patient, family, or caregiver that medication may cause hair loss but that it is reversible when therapy is stopped.
- Advise patient, family, or caregiver to immediately report any of the following to health care provider: rash; shortness of breath or difficulty breathing; abnormal skin sensations; stumbling; muscle wasting; fever, chills, or other signs of infection, redness or swelling at injection site.
- Advise patient, family, or caregiver to report any of the following to health care provider: persistent nausea, vomiting, constipation, diarrhea, or appetite loss; persistent or worsening general body weakness.
- Instruct patient not to take any prescription or OTC medications or dietary supplements unless advised to do so by health care provider.
- Caution women of childbearing potential to avoid becoming pregnant during therapy.
- Instruct women of childbearing potential to notify health care provider if pregnant, planning to become pregnant, or breastfeeding.
- Advise patient, family, or caregiver that following discharge, frequent follow-up visits and laboratory tests will be required to monitor therapy and to keep appointments.

Vinorelbine Tartrate

(vih-NORE-ell-bean)

Class Vinca alkaloid

How Supplied
Navelbine Solution for Injection 10 mg/mL

Action
PHARMACOLOGY: Vinorelbine interferes with microtubule assembly primarily by inhibiting mitosis at metaphase through its interaction with tubulin.

PHARMACOKINETICS/DYNAMICS:
Distribution: Vd is 25 to 40.1 L/kg.

Metabolism: One metabolite, deacetylvinorelbine, has been shown to possess antitumor activity.

Excretion: T½ is 28 to 44 hr. Mean plasma clearance is about 1 to 1.25 L/hr/kg. Substantial hepatic elimination in humans, with large amounts recovered in feces after IV administration.

Special Populations:
Hepatic Function Impairment – Based on experience with other anticancer vinca alkaloids, dosage adjustments are recommended for patients with impaired hepatic function taking vinorelbine.

Indications Unresectable, advanced non-small cell lung cancer. **Unlabeled use(s):** Breast cancer, cisplatin-resistant ovarian cancer, Hodgkin lymphoma.

Contraindications Pretreatment granulocyte counts less than 1000 cells/mm^3.

Route/Dosage
Unresectable, Advanced Non-Small Cell Lung Cancer
ADULTS: **IV** 30 mg/m^2 once weekly until either disease progression or dose-limiting toxicity occur.

Dosage Adjustment for Hematologic Toxicity
Granulocyte counts should be at least 1000 cells/mm^3 prior to the administration of vinorelbine. Base dosage adjustments on granulocyte counts. See manufacturer's recommendations.

Dosage Adjustment in Hepatic Dysfunction
ADULTS: **IV** Reduce dose 50% if total bilirubin is 2.1 to 3 mg/dL. Reduce dose 25% if total bilirubin is more than 3 mg/dL.

Interactions
Cisplatin: Incidence of granulocytopenia increases when vinorelbine is used in combination with cisplatin.
Cytochrome P450 3A enzyme inhibitors (eg ketoconazole, itraconazole, macrolides): May increase vinorelbine serum levels and toxicity.
Mitomycin: Acute pulmonary reactions were noted when vinca alkaloids were given with mitomycin.
Paclitaxel: Monitor for signs and symptoms of neuropathy with concomitant use of vinorelbine and paclitaxel.
Radiation: Radiation recall reactions may occur.

Lab Test Interferences None well documented.

Adverse Reactions
CV: Chest pain.
CNS: Fatigue; mild to moderate peripheral neuropathy.
DERM: Mild alopecia; rash and injection site reactions; pain at injection site.
GI: Transient elevations in LFTs; constipation; paralytic ileus; mild stomatitis; anorexia; diarrhea.
HEMA: Dose-limiting granulocytopenia occurs with a nadir of 7 to 10 days.

HYPERSEN: Anaphylaxis; angioedema; pruritus.
MUSC: Jaw pain; myalgia; arthralgia.
RESP: Dyspnea.

> **WARNING:**
>
> *IV use only:* Intrathecal use of other vinca alkaloids has been fatal. Label syringe "Warning - For IV Use Only; fatal if given intrathecally."
>
> *Granulocytopenia:* May be severe and predispose to infection. Do not administer to patients with granulocyte counts less than 1000 cells/mm^3.
>
> *Avoid extravasation:* Proper placement of needle/catheter prior to administration. Extravasation can cause severe local necrosis.

Precautions
Pregnancy: Category D.
Lactation: Undetermined.
Children: Safety and efficacy in children have not been established.
Hepatic function impairment: Administer with caution to patients with hepatic insufficiency.
GI: May cause severe constipation, paralytic ileus, intestinal obstruction, necrosis, and perforation.
Interstitial pulmonary changes: Cases of interstitial pulmonary changes and ARDS, most of which were fatal, occurred in patients.

Overdosage: Signs and Symptoms
Paralytic ileus, stomatitis, esophagitis, bone marrow aplasia, sepsis, paresis.

PATIENT CARE CONSIDERATIONS
Administration/Storage
- Refrigerate but do not freeze. Protect from light. Unopened vials may be stored at room temperature up to 25°C (77°F) for up to 72 hr. Diluted solutions may be stored at room temperature or under refrigeration for up to 24 hr in polypropylene syringes or PVC bags. Solutions are preservative-free and should be discarded within 24 hr of preparation.
- Vinorelbine must be further diluted prior to administration.
- Administer by IV infusion
- Infuse IV over 6 to 10 min into the side port of a freely flowing IV line closest to the IV bag. Follow injection with at least 75 to 125 mL 5% Dextrose or 0.9% Sodium Chloride.

Assessment/Interventions
- Monitor CBC with differential and serum bilirubin concentrations at baseline and prior to each dose.
- Use with caution in patients receiving other bone marrow suppressants, with prior radiation therapy, or with a history of neuropathy or pulmonary dysfunction.
- Patients who develop bronchospasm during infusions may be treated with supplemental oxygen, bronchodilators, or corticosteroids.
- Monitor patients developing severe granulocytopenia for evidence of infection or fever.
- Monitor patients with a history of or with preexisting neuropathy, for new or worsening signs and symptoms of neuropathy.
- Promptly evaluate patients with alterations in their baseline pulmonary symptoms or with new onset of dyspnea, cough, hypoxia, or other symptoms.

Patient/Family Education
- Advise patients to report fever or chills immediately.
- Advise women of childbearing potential to avoid pregnancy during treatment.
- Advise patients to contact the health care provider if experiencing increased shortness of breath, cough, or other new pulmonary symptoms, or if experiencing symptoms of abdominal pain or constipation.

Voriconazole

(vore-ih-KOE-nuh-zole)
Class Anti-infective/Antifungal

How Supplied
Vfend Tablets 50 mg, Tablets 200 mg, Powder for injection, lyophilized 200 mg, Powder for oral suspension 45 g (40 mg/mL after reconstitution)

Action
PHARMACOLOGY: Inhibition of fungal cytochrome P450-mediated 14 alpha-lanosterol demethylation, an essential step in fungal ergosterol biosynthesis.

PHARMACOKINETICS/DYNAMICS:
Absorption: Oral bioavailability is 96%. T_{max} is 1 to 2 hr. AUC decreases with high-fat meals 24% (tablet) and 37% (oral suspension). The C_{max} decreases 34% (tablet) and 58% (oral suspension).

Distribution: Vd is 4.6 L/kg, suggesting extensive distribution into tissues. It is 58% protein bound.

Metabolism: Nonlinear. Metabolized by hepatic cytochrome P450-enzymes, CYP2C19, CYP2C9, and CYP3A4, with CYP2C19 significantly involved; this enzyme also exhibits genetic polymorphism. The major metabolite, N-oxide, accounts for 72% of the circulating radiolabeled metabolites in the plasma. It has minimal antifungal activity.

Excretion: Eliminated via hepatic metabolism with less than 2% of the dose excreted unchanged in the urine. Terminal t½ is dose-dependent and is not useful in predicting the accumulation/elimination.

Special Populations:
Renal Function Impairment – IV voriconazole should be avoided in patients with moderate to severe (Ccr less than 50 mL/min) accumulation of IV vehicle SBECD (sulfobutyl ether beta-cyclodextrin sodium) may occur.
Hepatic Function Impairment – It is recommended that the standard loading-dose regimens be used but that the maintenance dose be halved in patients with mild to moderate hepatic cirrhosis.

Indications Treatment of invasive aspergillosis; treatment of *Scedosporium apiospermum* and *Fusarium* spp., including *Fusarium solani*, in patients intolerant of or refractory to other therapy; treatment of esophageal candidiasis.

Contraindications Hypersensitivity to voriconazole or any of it excipients, coadministration of carbamazepine, cisapride, efavirenz, ergot derivatives (eg, ergotamine, dihydroergotamine), long-acting barbiturates, pimozide, quinidine, rifabutin, rifampin, ritonavir, sirolimus.

Route/Dosage
ADULTS AND CHILDREN 12 YR OF AGE AND OLDER: **IV** Loading dose of 6 mg/kg q 12 hr for 2 doses, followed by a maintenance dose of 4 mg/kg q 12 hr. If patients are unable to tolerate treatment, reduce the IV maintenance dose to 3 mg/kg q 12 hr.
ADULTS AND CHILDREN 12 YR OF AGE AND OLDER: **PO** Once an oral dose can be tolerated, patients weighing more than 40 kg should receive 200 mg q 12 hr. If response is inadequate, the oral dose may be increased to 300 mg q 12 hr. If patients are unable to tolerate oral treatment, reduce the oral dose by 50 mg increments to a minimum of 200 mg q 12 hr. Patients weighing less than 40 kg should receive 100 mg q 12 hr. If the response is inadequate, the oral dose may be increased to 150 mg q 12 hr. If patients weighing less than 40 kg are unable to tolerate oral treatment, reduce the oral dose by 50 mg increments to a minimum of 100 mg q 12 hr.

Esophageal Candidiasis
PO In patients weighing 40 kg or more, the recommended dosing regimen is 200 mg q 12 hr. In patients weighing less than 40 kg, the recommended dose is 100 mg q 12 hr. Treat for a minimum of 14 days and for at least 7 days after resolution of symptoms.

Hepatic Insufficiency
ADULTS AND CHILDREN 12 YR OF AGE AND OLDER: **IV or PO** It is recommended that the standard loading-dose regimens be used but that the maintenance dose be halved in patients with mild to moderate hepatic cirrhosis.

Phenytoin Coadministration
Increase the IV maintenance dose of voriconazole to 5 mg/kg q 12 hr, or the oral maintenance dose to 400 mg q 12 hr. In patients weighing less than 40 kg, use 100 mg q 12 hr.

Renal Insufficiency
In patients with Ccr less than 50 mL/min, accumulation of the IV vehicle SBECD occurs. Use only if benefit/risk to patient justifies the use.

Interactions
Benzodiazepines (eg, alprazolam), cyclosporine, dihydropyridine calcium channel blockers (eg, felodipine), HMG-CoA reductase inhibitors (eg, lovastatin), NNRT (eg, efavirenz), omeprazole, phenytoin, protease inhibitors (eg, ritonavir), sulfonylurea hypoglycemic agents (eg, glipizide), tacrolimus, vinca alkaloids (eg, vinblastine), warfarin: Plasma exposure to these agents may be increased by voriconazole, increasing the pharmacologic and adverse effects.
Carbamazepine, cisapride, efavirenz, ergot derivatives (eg, dihydroergotamine, ergotamine), long-acting barbiturates, pimozide, quinidine, rifabutin, rifampin, ritonavir, sirolimus: Coadministration of these agents with voriconazole is contraindicated.
Nonnucleoside reverse transcriptase (NNRT) inhibitors (eg, efavirenz), phenytoin: May decrease voriconazole plasma levels, reducing the pharmacologic effect.
NNRT inhibitors (eg, efavirenz), protease inhibitors (eg, ritonavir): May elevate voriconazole plasma levels, increasing the pharmacologic and adverse effect.
INCOMPATIBILITIES:
Aminofusin 10%: Do not infuse voriconazole into the same line or cannula with other drug infusions, including parenteral nutrition; do not infuse with blood products or electrolyte supplementations; do not dilute with 4.2% sodium bicarbonate infusion.

Adverse Reactions
CV: Tachycardia (3%); hypertension, hypotension, vasodilatation (2%).
CNS: Hallucinations (5%); headache (4%); dizziness (3%).

DERM: Rash (6%); pruritus, maculopapular rash (1%).
EENT: Abnormal vision (28%); photophobia (4%); chromatopsia (1%).
GI: Nausea (7%); vomiting (6%); diarrhea, dry mouth (2%).
GU: Abnormal kidney function (2%).
HEMA: Thrombocytopenia (1%); pancytopenia.
HEPA: Abnormal LFTs (5%); increased hepatic enzymes, peripheral edema (4%); hypokalemia, cholestatic jaundice (2%); hypomagnesemia (1%).
LABTESTABS: Increased creatinine (21%); increased AST (20%); elevated total bilirubin, increased ALT (19%); decreased potassium (17%); increased alkaline phosphatase (16%).
M/N: Increased alkaline phosphatase (4%).
OTHER: Fever (6%); chills (4%); abdominal pain (3%); chest pain (2%).

PATIENT CARE CONSIDERATIONS
Administration/Storage
Tablets and Oral Suspension:
- Administer prescribed dose q 12 hr, at least 1 hr before or 1 hr following a meal.
- Follow manufacturer's guidelines for reconstituting powder for oral suspension.
- Shake reconstituted oral suspension for approximately 10 sec before measuring dose. Administer only using the supplied oral dispenser.
- Do not mix reconstituted oral suspension with any other medication or flavoring agent or further dilute with water or other vehicles.
- Store powder for oral suspension in refrigerator (37° to 46°F) before reconstitution. Store tablets and reconstituted oral suspension at controlled room temperature (59° to 86°F). Do not refrigerate or freeze reconstituted oral suspension. Discard any remaining reconstituted oral suspension 14 days after reconstitution.

Injection:
- For IV infusion only. Not for intradermal, subcutaneous, IM, IV bolus, or intra-arterial administration.
- Carefully follow manufacturer's instructions for reconstitution, dilution, and administration.
- Inspect solution visually before administration. Do not administer if solution is cloudy, discolored, or contains particulate matter.
- Administer loading doses and maintenance doses at max rate of 3 mg/kg/hr over 1 to 2 hr.
- Do not administer concomitantly with other drug infusions, blood products, or electrolyte replacements
- Store powder for injection at controlled room temperature (59° to 86°F). Reconstituted injection should be used immediately or stored in refrigerator (37° to 46°F) for up to 24 hr. Discard any unused solution or solution stored for more than 24 hr.

Precautions
Pregnancy: Category D.
Lactation: Undetermined.
Children: Safety and efficacy not established in children younger than 12 yr of age.
Hepatic function impairment: Serious hepatic reactions including hepatitis, cholestasis, and fulminant hepatic failure have been reported.
Special risk patients: Administer with caution to patients with proarryhthmic conditions.
Dermatological reaction: Rarely serious cutaneous reactions such as Stevens-Johnson syndrome have occurred.
Galactose intolerance: The tablets contain galactose and should not be given to patients with hereditary galactose intolerance, Lapp lactose deficiency, or glucose-galactose malabsorption.

Overdosage: Signs and Symptoms
Photophobia.

Assessment/Interventions
- Obtain patient history, including drug history and any known allergies. Note history of sensitivity to azole antifungals, liver disease, kidney disease, concurrent use of rifampin, rifabutin, carbamazepine, long-acting barbiturates, sirolimus, ritonavir, efavirenz, cisapride, pimozide, quinidine, or ergot alkaloids, galactose intolerance (tablets only), fructose intolerance, sucrase-isomaltase deficiency, or glucose-galactose malabsorption (oral suspension only).
- Do not administer to pregnant patient.
- Ensure that women of child-bearing potential use effective contraception during therapy.
- Ensure that fungal culture, as appropriate, has been obtained before beginning therapy.
- Monitor patient's response to therapy. Notify health care provider if infection does not appear to be improving or is worsening.
- Ensure that electrolyte abnormalities have been corrected before initiating therapy.
- Administer reduced maintenance dose to patient with mild to moderate hepatic cirrhosis (Child-Pugh Class A and B).
- Administer reduced maintenance dose, following manufacturer's guidelines, to patient who cannot tolerate treatment with standard dose.
- Ensure that LFTs are evaluated prior to initiating therapy and periodically during therapy. Closely monitor patient who develops abnor-

mal LFTs during therapy for development of more severe hepatic injury. Withhold therapy and notify health care provider if signs and symptoms consistent with liver disease are noted.
* Ensure that visual acuity, visual field, and color perception are monitored if treatment duration exceeds 28 days.
* Ensure that renal function is evaluated prior to initiating therapy and periodically during therapy.
* Monitor renal function closely if injectable dose form is administered to patient with renal impairment (Ccr less than 50 mL/min). Consider changing to oral voriconazole if increase in serum creatinine is noted.
* Monitor patient during IV infusion for anaphylactoid-type reaction and discontinue infusion if noted.
* Monitor IV infusion site for signs of reaction or phlebitis.
* Assess patient for visual CNS, GI, CV, MUSC, DERM, and general body side effects. Report to health care provider if noted and significant. Be prepared to discontinue therapy if patient develops a rash.
* Convert from IV dose form to tablets or oral suspension when patient can tolerate medication given by mouth.

Patient/Family Education
* Explain name, dose, action, and potential side effects of drug.
* Advise patient that injectable form of drug will be prepared and administered by a health care professional in a medical facility.
* Explain need for prolonged therapy and for close monitoring during course of therapy.
* Advise patient to take tablets or oral suspension at least 1 hr before or 1 hr after a meal.
* Advise patient or caregiver using oral suspension to shake suspension for approximately 10 sec before measuring dose and to only use the oral dispenser supplied with the medication.
* Advise patient to report any of the following to health care provider: injection site reaction, visual disturbances, fever, chills, rash, persistent vomiting, nausea or diarrhea, headache, swelling of the feet, ankles, or calves.
* Advise patient that medication may cause photosensitivity (sensitivity to sunlight) and to avoid unnecessary exposure to sunlight or tanning lamps, to use sunscreens, and wear protective clothing to avoid photosensitivity reactions.
* Caution patient not to drive at night while taking this medication because it may cause changes in vision including blurring and sensitivity to bright light. Advise patient to avoid driving or operating machinery if any change in vision is noted.
* Instruct women of child-bearing potential to use effective contraception while taking voriconazole.
* Advise women to notify health care provider if pregnant, planning to become pregnant, or breastfeeding.
* Instruct patient not to take any prescription or OTC medications, dietary supplements, or herbal preparations unless advised by health care provider.
* Advise patient that follow-up visits and lab tests will be required to monitor therapy and to keep appointments.

Warfarin

(WORE-fuh-rin)
Class Anticoagulants

How Supplied
Coumadin Tablets 1 mg, Tablets 2 mg, Tablets 2.5 mg, Tablets 3 mg, Tablets 4 mg, Tablets 5 mg, Tablets 6 mg, Tablets 7.5 mg, Tablets 10 mg, Powder for Injection, lyophilized 2 mg
✤ *Apo-Warfarin* ◆ *Gen-Warfarin* ◆ *Taro-Warfarin*

Action
PHARMACOLOGY: Interferes with hepatic synthesis of vitamin K-dependent clotting factors, resulting in in-vivo depletion of clotting factors II, VII, IX, and X.

PHARMACOKINETICS/DYNAMICS:
Absorption: It is completely absorbed. The T_{max} is 4 hr.
Distribution: Vd is about 0.14 L/kg. It is about 99% bound to plasma protein.
Metabolism: The elimination of warfarin is almost entirely by metabolism. It is metabolized by cytochrome P450 to inactive hydroxylated metabolites (predominant route) and by reductases to reduced metabolites (warfarin alcohols).
Excretion: Metabolites are principally excreted into urine and to a lesser extent into the bile. The t½ after a single dose is about 1 wk; however, the effective t½ ranges from 20 to 60 hr. The clearance of R-warfarin is 50% that of S-warfarin. The t½ of R-warfarin is about 37 to 89 hr and it is about 21 to 43 hr in S-warfarin. About 92% of orally administered doses are recovered in urine.

Special Populations:
Hepatic Function Impairment – Hepatic dysfunction can potentiate the response to warfarin through impaired synthesis of clotting factors and decrease metabolism of warfarin.
Elderly – Patients at least 60 yr appear to exhibit greater than expected prothrombin time (PT)/international normalized ratio (INR) response to warfarin. As a patient's age increases, a lower dose is usually required to produce a therapeutic level of anticoagulation.

Indications Prophylaxis and treatment of venous thrombosis and its extension; prophylaxis and treatment of atrial fibrillation with embolization; prophylaxis and treatment of pulmonary embolism; adjunct in prophylaxis of systemic embolism after MI. **Unlabeled use(s):** Prevention of recurrent transient ischemic attacks and reduction of risk of recurrent MI; adjunctive treatment of small cell carcinoma of lung.

Contraindications Pregnancy; hemorrhagic tendencies; hemophilia; thrombocytopenic purpura; leukemia; recent or contemplated surgery of eye or CNS, major regional lumbar block anesthesia, or surgery resulting in large, open surfaces; patients bleeding from GI, respiratory, or GU tract; threatened abortion; aneurysm; ascorbic acid deficiency; history of bleeding diathesis; prostatectomy; continuous tube drainage of small intestine; polyarthritis; diverticulitis; emaciation; malnutrition; cerebrovascular hemorrhage; eclampsia and preeclampsia; blood dyscrasias; severe uncontrolled or malignant hypertension; severe renal or hepatic disease; pericarditis and pericardial effusion; subacute bacterial endocarditis; visceral carcinoma; following spinal puncture and other diagnostic or therapeutic procedures (eg, IUD insertion) with potential for uncontrollable bleeding; history of warfarin-induced necrosis.

Route/Dosage
ADULTS: PO 2 to 5 mg/day initially for 2 to 4 days; adjust daily dose according to PT or INR determinations. Usual maintenance dose is PO 2 to 10 mg/day.
ELDERLY: Lower dosages are recommended.
ADULTS: IV Provides an alternative administration route for patients who cannot receive oral drugs. The IV dosages would be the same as those that would be used orally. Administer as a slow bolus injection over 1 to 2 min in a peripheral vein.

Interactions
Aminoglutethimide, azathioprine, barbiturates, carbamazepine, cholestyramine, ethchlorvynol, ginseng, glutethimide, griseofulvin, mercaptopurine, rifabutin, rifampin, St. John's wort, trazodone, ubiquinone, and vitamin K: Decreased anticoagulant effect of warfarin.
Androgens, amiodarone, cefamandole, cefazolin, cefoperazone, cefotetan, cefoxitin, ceftriaxone, chloramphenicol, cimetidine clofibrate, danshen, dextrothyroxine, disulfiram, dong quai, erythromycin, fluconazole, glucagon, methimazole, metronidazole, miconazole, moxalactam, nalidixic acid, NSAIDs, phenylbutazone, propylthiouracil, quinidine, quinine, salicylates, sulfinpyrazone, sulfonamides, thyroid hormones, tricyclic antidepressants, and vitamin E: Increased anticoagulant effect of warfarin.
Hydantoins: Serum hydantoin concentration may be elevated, increasing risk of toxicity.

Lab Test Interferences Oral anticoagulants may cause red-orange discoloration of alkaline urine, interfering with some laboratory tests.

Adverse Reactions
DERM: Skin necrosis; gangrene; exfoliative dermatitis; urticaria; alopecia.

EENT: Mouth ulcers.
GI: Nausea; vomiting; diarrhea; paralytic ileus; intestinal obstruction; anorexia; abdominal cramps.
GU: Red-orange urine.
HEMA: Hemorrhage; leukopenia.
HEPA: Hepatotoxicity; cholestatic jaundice.
OTHER: Fever; cholesterol microembolization (purple toe syndrome); hypersensitivity.

Precautions

Pregnancy: Category X.
Lactation: Excreted in breast milk.
Children: Safety and efficacy not established in children under 18 yr.
Elderly: May be more sensitive to effects.
Hypersensitivity: Reactions range from mild to life-threatening. Symptoms may be dermatologic (eg, erythema, eczematous rash, exfoliative dermatitis, exudative erythema multiforme, alopecia), hematologic (eg, eosinophilia, leukopenia, thrombocytopenia), renal, (eg, nephropathy, nephritis, oliguria), GI (eg enanthema, severe stomatitis), or hepatic (eg, mixed hepatocellular damage, cholestasis, jaundice). If signs or symptoms occur, discontinue therapy and notify health care provider.
Hepatic function impairment: Use cautiously.
Special risk patients: There is increased risk associated with using warfarin in patients with trauma, infection, renal insufficiency, dietary insufficiency, uncontrolled hypertension, polycythemia vera, vasculitis, indwelling catheters. Evaluate benefits of therapy vs risks.
Adrenal hemorrhage: Discontinue therapy if patient develops signs and symptoms of adrenal insufficiency.
Hemorrhage/Necrosis: Most serious risks of therapy; may result in death.
Monitoring/PT: Individualize treatment based on PT or INR.
Protein C deficiency: Hereditary, familial, or clinical protein C deficiency has been associated with necrosis following warfarin therapy. If warfarin is suspected cause of necrosis, discontinue administration.
Purple toe syndrome: Systemic cholesterol microembolization from release of atheromatous plaque emboli. Discontinue therapy.
Surgical/Dental procedures: Adjust dose to maintain PT or INR at low end of therapeutic range for patients who must be anticoagulated during dental or surgical procedures.

Overdosage: Signs and Symptoms

Hematuria, excessive menstrual bleeding, melena, petechiae, oozing from superficial injuries.

PATIENT CARE CONSIDERATIONS

Administration/Storage

- Do not give large loading dose.
- Do not switch brands.
- Administer at same time each day.
- Store at room temperature in tight, light-resistant container.
- For IV use, give a slow bolus injection over 1 to 2 min in a peripheral vein.
- Reconstitute IV vial with 2.7 mL of Sterile Water for Injection.
- After reconstitution, solution is stable for 4 hr at room temperature.
- Check solution for particle matter or discoloration immediately before use. If either is present, do not use.
- Discard unused solution.

Assessment/Interventions

- Obtain patient history, including drug history and any known allergies.
- Use care in determining cooperation of patient to ensure compliance.
- Monitor PT or INR.
- Test urine, stool, and drainage for occult blood.
- Observe for low back pain and GI symptoms.
- Avoid IM injection and venipuncture if possible.
- If purple toe syndrome, tissue necrosis, or signs of adrenal insufficiency (eg, fever, myalgia, arthralgia, anorexia, nausea, diarrhea) are observed, stop drug and report to health care provider immediately.
- If bleeding occurs, report to health care provider immediately.

Patient/Family Education

- Caution patient that this medication must not be taken during pregnancy or when pregnancy is possible. Advise patient to use reliable form of birth control while taking this drug.
- Advise patient not to change dose unless advised by health care provider.
- Advise patient not to drastically change diet or consume alcohol.
- Advise patient not to change brands of medicine.
- Advise patient to limit intake of vitamin K-rich foods, including avocados, bananas, broccoli, dried fruits, grapefruit, lima beans, nuts, oranges, peaches, potatoes, sunflower seeds, spinach, and tomatoes.
- Instruct patient to report any GI upset, pink or red discoloration of urine, red or tar-black stools or diarrhea, rash, yellowish tint of skin

or eyes, unusual bleeding (eg, heavier than normal menstrual flow), or bruising.
- Caution patient not to take aspirin or other salicylates without consulting health care provider.
- Instruct patient in safety practices: Use of soft toothbrush, electric razor, night lights, and avoidance of activities that could result in bruising or bleeding.
- Tell patient not to take any OTC or prescription medications without consulting health care provider.
- Remind patient to wear Medi-Alert identification bracelet.

Zafirlukast

(zah-fur-LOO-cast)

Class Leukotriene receptor antagonist

How Supplied
Accolate Tablets 10 mg, Tablets 20 mg

Action
PHARMACOLOGY: Inhibits 3 leukotriene receptor types. Leukotrienes have been associated with the longer, inflammatory component of asthma.

PHARMACOKINETICS/DYNAMICS:
Absorption: Rapidly absorbed. T_{max} is 3 hr. Bioavailability is unknown. Administration with food reduced the mean bioavailability about 40%.

Distribution: At least 99% bound to proteins (predominantly albumin). V/d is 70 L. Minimal distribution across blood-brain barrier.

Metabolism: Extensively metabolized. Most common metabolic products are hydroxylated metabolites, which are excreted in feces. These metabolites are formed through the cytochrome P450 2C9 pathway. Inhibits CYP3A4 and CYP2C9 isoenzymes.

Excretion: Oral Cl is about 20 L/hr. Biliary route is primary route of excretion. Urinary excretion accounts for about 10% of the dose, while the rest is excreted in feces. The terminal $t_{1/2}$ is about 10 hr. The plasma $t_{1/2}$ is about 8 to 16 hr.

Special Populations:
Hepatic Function Impairment – Approximately 50% to 60% greater C_{max} and AUC compared with healthy subjects.

Elderly – Oral Cl decreases with age. In patients older than 65 yr of age, there are about 2- to 3-fold greater C_{max} and AUC compared with young adults.

Indications
Prophylaxis and chronic treatment of asthma in adults and children 5 yr of age and older.

Contraindications
Standard considerations.

Route/Dosage
ADULTS AND CHILDREN 12 YR OF AGE OR OLDER: PO 20 mg bid.
CHILDREN 5 TO 11 YR OF AGE: PO 10 mg bid.

Interactions
Aspirin: Increased zafirlukast plasma levels.
Erythromycin, theophylline: Lowered zafirlukast plasma concentrations.
Warfarin: Zafirlukast potentiates the hypoprothrombinemic effect of warfarin. Significant increase in the PT may result.

Lab Test Interferences
None well documented.

Adverse Reactions
CNS: Headache (13%); dizziness (2%).
GI: Nausea, diarrhea (3%); vomiting (2%); dyspepsia (1%).
HEMA: Agranulocytosis.
HEPA: ALT elevations (2%).
HYPERSEN: Hypersensitivity (including urticaria, angioedema, rashes).
MUSC: Myalgia (2%).
OTHER: Infection (4%); pain, asthenia, abdominal pain, accidental injury, fever, back pain (2%).

Precautions
Pregnancy: Category B.
Lactation: Excreted in breast milk.
Children: Safety and efficacy in children younger than 5 yr of age not established.
Elderly: Drug Cl decreases with age.
Acute asthma: Zafirlukast is not effective in treating acute asthmatic symptoms, but it can be continued during these times.
Infections: Elderly patients experienced an increased frequency of infections (primarily respiratory) compared with placebo-treated patients. These appeared to be associated with coadministration of inhaled corticosteroids.

Overdosage: Signs and Symptoms
Rash, upset stomach.

PATIENT CARE CONSIDERATIONS

Administration/Storage
- Not to be used for the acute treatment of bronchospasm or asthma symptoms.
- May be used alone or in combination with bronchodilators and inhaled or systemic corticosteroids.
- Administer prescribed dose 1 hr before or 2 hr after meals.
- Store tablets at controlled room temperature (68° to 77°F). Protect from light and moisture.

Assessment/Interventions
- Obtain patient history, including drug history and any known allergies. Note hepatic impairment or history of hepatitis with previous use of zafirlukast.
- Ensure that medication is not administered to patient who is breastfeeding.
- Ensure that baseline pulmonary function tests have been completed.
- Document baseline disease state activity (eg, frequency and severity of asthma episodes).

Reassess periodically to document response to therapy.
- Monitor patient for GI, CNS, and general body side effects. Notify health care provider if noted and significant.

Patient/Family Education
- Explain name, dose, action, and potential side effects of drug.
- Advise patient to take each dose on an empty stomach, either 1 hr before or 2 hr after meals.
- Advise patient to continue taking other medications for asthma as prescribed by health care provider.
- Warn patient that drug is an asthma controller and is not to be used to treat an acute asthma attack. Advise patient to continue to take zafirlukast during an acute attack but use rescue medication (bronchodilator) to obtain rapid relief of asthma symptoms.
- Instruct patient not to stop the medication once symptoms have been controlled. Continued daily use is necessary to control symptoms.
- Advise patient not to change the dose or stop using unless advised by health care provider.
- Instruct patient not to exceed prescribed dose. Advise patient to contact health care provider if this medication no longer seems to control asthma symptoms.
- Advise patient to discontinue therapy and contact health care provider immediately if any of the following occur: persistent nausea; unexplained fatigue; excessive sleepiness or drowsiness; stomach pain; flu-like symptoms; itching; yellowing of skin or eyes; appetite loss.
- Advise patient to carry Medi-Alert card indicating asthma.
- Advise women to notify health care provider if pregnant, planning to become pregnant, or breastfeeding.
- Caution patient not to take any prescription or OTC medications, dietary supplements, or herbal preparations unless advised by health care provider.
- Advise patient that follow-up visits will be required to monitor therapy and to keep appointments.

Zalcitabine (Dideoxycytidine; ddC)

(zal-SITE-uh-BEAN)

Class Antiretroviral/Nucleoside reverse transcriptase inhibitor

How Supplied
Hivid Tablets 0.375 mg, Tablets 0.75 mg

Action
PHARMACOLOGY: Inhibits replication of DNA in HIV.

PHARMACOKINETICS/DYNAMICS:
Absorption: Oral bioavailability is about 80%. Absorption rate of a 1.5 mg oral dose was reduced with food. C_{max} is 25.2 ng/mL. T_{max} is 0.8 hr. AUC is 72 ng•hr/mL.

Distribution: Vd is 0.534 L/kg. Less than 4% protein bound. Drug interaction involved in binding site is unlikely.

Metabolism: Major metabolite is dideoxyuridine.

Excretion: Renal elimination is the primary route of elimination. The t½ is about 2 hr.

Special Populations:
Renal Function Impairment – Prolonged elimination may be expected.
Children – Mean bioavailability is 54%.

Indications
Combination therapy: For the treatment of selected patients with advanced HIV infection.

Contraindications Standard considerations.

Route/Dosage
Combination therapy
ADULTS AND ADOLESCENTS MORE THAN 13 YR: PO 0.75 mg (coadministered with other antiviral agents) q 8 hr (total daily dose 2.25 mg zalcitabine).

Interactions
Aminoglycosides, amphotericin, foscarnet: May increase risk of peripheral neuropathy and other zalcitabine toxicities caused by decreased clearance of zalcitabine.

Chloramphenicol, cisplatin, dapsone, disulfiram, ethionamide, glutethimide, gold, hydralazine, iodoquinol, isoniazid, metronidazole, nitrofurantoin, phenytoin, ribavirin, vincristine: May increase risk of peripheral neuropathy.

Drugs associated with pancreatitis (eg, pentamidine): Fatal pancreatitis has occurred, possibly related to zalcitabine and IV pentamidine given concurrently.

Lab Test Interferences None well documented.

Adverse Reactions
CV: Chest pain; cardiomyopathy; CHF.
CNS: Headache; dizziness; confusion; impaired concentration; peripheral neuropathy.
DERM: Rash; pruritus; dermatitis.
EENT: Pharyngitis.
GI: Pancreatitis; oral ulcers; nausea; dysphagia; anorexia; abdominal pain; vomiting; diarrhea; dry mouth; esophageal ulcers; dyspepsia; glossitis.

METAB: Weight decrease; weight gain; increased amylase; hyperglycemia; hyponatremia; hypoglycemia; loss of appetite.
RESP: Nasal discharge; cough; respiratory distress.
OTHER: Myalgia; arthralgia; foot pain; fatigue; anaphylactoid reaction; abnormal GGT.

> **WARNING:**
>
> *Hepatitis B:* Hepatic failure and death, possibly related to underlying hepatitis B and zalcitabine, have been reported.
>
> *Lactic acidosis and hepatomegaly:* Have been reported with steatosis (including fatal cases) reported with the use of nucleoside analogues alone or in combination with other antiretrovirals.
>
> *Neuropathy:* Severe peripheral neuropathy, use with extreme caution in patients with preexisting neuropathy.
>
> *Pancreatitis:* Rarely occurs; monitor.

Precautions

Pregnancy: Category C.
Lactation: Undetermined. It is recommended that HIV-positive women do not breastfeed.

PATIENT CARE CONSIDERATIONS

Administration/Storage

- Administer on empty stomach 1 hr before or 2 hr after meals for maximum absorption.
- Administer q 8 hr around clock.
- If Ccr is decreased, reduced dose (0.75 mg) may be given q 12 hr (Ccr 10 to 40 mL/min) or q 24 hr (Ccr less than 10 mL/min).
- Store at room temperature in tight containers.

Assessment/Interventions

- Obtain patient history, including drug history, and any known allergies. Note cardiac, hepatic and renal dysfunction. peripheral neuropathy; and pancreatitis.
- Perform clinical chemistry tests before and periodically during therapy. Monitor CBC, renal function studies (eg, BUN, serum uric acid, urine creatinine clearance), liver function tests (bilirubin, AST ALT, alkaline phosphatase), and baseline serum amylase and triglyceride levels in patients with prior history of pancreatitis, increased amylase or ethanol abuse, and those on parenteral nutrition.
- Prior to therapy and throughout treatment, assess for signs of peripheral neuropathy: Tingling, burning, or pain in distal extremities. In patients with moderate symptoms of peripheral neuropathy, discontinue drug then reintroduce at 50% of initial dose only if neuropathy symptoms have improved to mild. Use of drug may be discontinued permanently if severe discomfort due to neuropathy or moderate discomfort progresses at least 1 wk.
- Assess the following for pancreatitis: abdominal pain, nausea, vomiting, elevated liver enzymes. Withhold zalcitabine and zidovudine and notify health care provider of these symptoms immediately.
- Observe for signs of infection; monitor temperature q 4 hr. Antibiotics may be ordered prophylactically.
- Frequently monitor hematologic indices to detect serious anemia or granulocytopenia. Development of anemia (hemoglobin less than 7.5/dL or reduction more than 25% of baseline) or granulocytopenia (granulocyte count less than 750/min^3 or reduction more than 50% of baseline) may require interruption of treatment with both zalcitabine and zidovudine until marrow recovers. Transfusion may be needed.
- In patients developing hematologic toxicity, decreases in hemoglobin may occur as early as 2 to 4 wk after therapy begins and granulocytopenia may occur after 6 to 8 wk of therapy.
- Reduction of dose is not required for patients weighing at least 30 kg.

Children: Safety and efficacy in children less than 13 yr not established.
Renal function impairment: Patients with renal impairment (Ccr less than 55 mL/min) may be at greater risk of toxicity because of decreased drug clearance. Dosage reduction may be needed.
Hepatic function impairment: In patients with history of liver disease or alcoholism, zalcitabine may exacerbate hepatic dysfunction. Dosage reduction or interruption of therapy may be needed.
Anaphylactoid reaction: Anaphylactoid reaction has occurred. Urticaria has occurred without other signs of anaphylaxis.
Cardiomyopathy/CHF: Cardiomyopathy/CHF may develop. Use drug with caution in patients with history of cardiomyopathy or CHF.
Esophageal ulcers: Esophageal ulcers have occurred.
HIV infection complications: Patients receiving zalcitabine or any other antiretroviral therapy may continue to develop opportunistic infections and other complications of HIV infection.

Overdosage: Signs and Symptoms

Rash, fever, peripheral neuropathy.

Patient/Family Education

- Advise patient to take around the clock as prescribed and not to increase the dose.

- Advise patient not to share the drug with others.
- Inform patient and family that patient may continue to develop opportunistic infections and other complications of HIV infection and should remain under close medical supervision.
- Explain that zalcitabine is not a cure but may offer symptomatic improvement.
- Reinforce fact that zalcitabine does not decrease risk of transmission of HIV through sexual contact or blood contamination.
- Instruct patient to notify health care provider immediately of signs of peripheral neuropathy (numbness and burning feeling in arms and legs) or pancreatitis (abdominal pain, nausea, vomiting).
- Encourage patient to report all changes in conditions to health care provider.
- Inform patient that long-term effects of this drug alone and in combination with zidovudine are unknown.

Zaleplon

(ZAL-eh-plahn)
Class Sedative and hypnotic
How Supplied
Sonata Capsules 5 mg, Capsules 10 mg
✤ *Sotacor*

Action
PHARMACOLOGY: Interacts with the gamma-aminobutyric acid receptor complex.

PHARMACOKINETICS/DYNAMICS:
Absorption: Rapid absorption. T_{max} is about 1 hr. Absolute bioavailability is about 30% because it undergoes significant presystemic metabolism. High fat meals prolonged the absorption, delaying T_{max} about 2 hr and reducing C_{max} about 35%.

Distribution: Vd is about 1.4 L/kg. Protein binding is about 60%.

Metabolism: Extensively metabolized with about 1% of dose excreted unchanged in the urine. Primarily metabolized by aldehyde oxidase to form 5-oxo-zaleplon. Metabolized to a lesser extent by cytochrome P450 3A4. Metabolites converted to glucuronides and eliminated in the urine.

Excretion: $T_½$ is about 1 hr. It is rapidly eliminated. Oral dose plasma Cl is about 3 L/hr/kg. IV dose plasma Cl is about 1 L/hr/kg. 70% of dose recovered in urine within 48 hr.

Special Populations:
Renal Function Impairment – No dose adjustment in mild to moderate renal insufficiency. It has not been studied in severe renal insufficiency.
Hepatic Function Impairment – Primarily metabolized by the liver and undergoes presystemic metabolism. Oral Cl was reduced 70% and 87% in compensated and decompensated patients, respectively. Reduce dose in mild to moderate hepatic impairment. Do not use in severe hepatic insufficiency.
Race – C_{max} and AUC were increased 37% and 64%, respectively in Asian populations.

Indications Short-term treatment of insomnia.

Contraindications Standard considerations.

Route/Dosage
ADULTS: PO 5 to 20 mg at bedtime.
ELDERLY/DEBILITATED PATIENTS: PO 5 to 10 mg at bedtime.
HEPATIC IMPAIRMENT (MILD TO MODERATE): PO 5 mg at bedtime.

Interactions
Alcohol, other CNS depressants: Additive or potentiation of CNS depressant effects.
Cimetidine: May elevate zaleplon plasma levels, increasing the therapeutic and adverse effects.
Rifampin: May reduce zaleplon plasma levels, reducing the effectiveness.

Lab Test Interferences None well documented.

Adverse Reactions
CV: Migraine.
CNS: Depression; hypertonia; nervousness; abnormal thinking; headache; anxiety; amnesia; dizziness; depersonalization; hallucinations; hypesthesia; paresthesia; somnolence; tremor; vertigo.
DERM: Pruritus; rash; photosensitivity.
EENT: Conjunctivitis; abnormal vision; ear pain; eye pain; hyperacusis; parosmia.
GI: Constipation; dry mouth; anorexia; colitis; dyspepsia; nausea.
GU: Dysmenorrhea.
RESP: Bronchitis; epistaxis.
OTHER: Back pain; chest pain; arthritis; abdominal pain; asthenia; fever; malaise; peripheral edema.

Precautions
Pregnancy: Category C.
Lactation: Excreted in breast milk.
Children: Safety and efficacy not established.
Elderly: Impaired motor or cognitive function with repeated exposure or unusual sensitivity is a concern.
Hepatic function impairment: Use with caution and in reduced dosage.
Amnesia: May occur.
Depression: Administer with caution to depressed patients or those with suicidal tenden-

cies. Signs and symptoms of depression may be intensified.

Withdrawal: Rebound insomnia on the first night following withdrawal occurs in some patients.

PATIENT CARE CONSIDERATIONS

Administration/Storage
- Store at room temperature in tightly closed, light-resistant container out of the reach of children.
- Do not administer with or immediately after a high fat or heavy meal.
- Anticipate administering the lowest dose possible, especially to patients at risk (ie, elderly and patients with decreased hepatic function).

Assessment/Interventions
- Obtain patient history, including drug history, and any known allergies.
- Ensure that side rails are raised after administration.
- Assist patient with ambulation after administration.
- Assess depressed patient for suicidal thoughts. If present, institute protective measures.
- Monitor for problems of tolerance, dependence, changes in behavior and thinking, memory problems, and withdrawal symptoms if medication is abruptly stopped.

Patient/Family Education
- Instruct patient to take the medication exactly as directed. Do not increase or decrease the dose or use longer than as directed by health care provider.
- Instruct patient to take zaleplon immediately before going to bed or after going to bed if patient has difficulty falling asleep. Avoid taking medication after a high-fat or heavy meal.

Overdosage: Signs and Symptoms
Drowsiness, mental confusion, lethargy, ataxia, hypotonia, hypotension, respiratory depression, coma, death.

- Instruct patient not to take zaleplon if able to get at least 4 hours of sleep before active again and only for a short period of time (1 or 2 days and generally less than 1 or 2 weeks) to avoid the problems of prolonged use.
- Discuss with primary caregiver and patient the benefits and risks of prolonged use including: memory problems, tolerance, dependence, changes in behavior and thinking, and withdrawal symptoms.
- Instruct patient to inform primary caregiver if taking or planning to take any OTC or prescription medications.
- Warn patient of the dangers of drinking alcohol and taking zaleplon or any other sleeping pill or CNS depressant.
- Caution patient that zaleplon may have some residual sedation at first and to not drive an automobile, operate dangerous machinery, or engage in activities that require mental alertness and coordination until knowing how the patient will react to this drug.
- Instruct patient to inform health care provider if experiencing any unusual or disturbing thoughts or if signs of depression occur.
- Inform patient of potential sleeping problems the first few nights after stopping the medication.
- Caution patient to inform the health care provider if pregnant, planning to become pregnant, or breastfeeding.

Zanamivir

(za-NA-mi-veer)

Class Antiviral agent

How Supplied
Relenza Blisters of powder for oral inhalation 5 mg

Action
PHARMACOLOGY: Inhibition of influenza virus neuraminidase, with the possibility of alteration of virus particle aggregation and release.

PHARMACOKINETICS/DYNAMICS:
Absorption: About 4% to 17% of orally inhaled dose is systemically absorbed. C_{max} is 17 to 142 ng/mL, and T_{max} is 1 to 2 hr following a 10 mg dose. The AUC is 111 to 1,364 ng•hr/mL.

Distribution: Less than 10% protein bound.
Metabolism: No metabolites detected in humans.
Excretion: Renally excreted as unchanged drug in urine. Serum t½ is 2.5 to 5.1 hr. Total Cl is 2.5 to 10.9 L/hr. Unabsorbed drug is excreted in feces.

Special Populations:
Renal Function Impairment – After IV administration, significant decrease in renal Cl and increase in t½ (range, 3.1 to 18.5 hr). Safety and efficacy have not been documented in severe renal impairment.

Indications Uncomplicated acute illness caused by influenza A and B virus in adults and pediatric patients at least 7 yr of age who have been symptomatic for no longer than 2 days.

Contraindications Standard considerations.

Route/Dosage

ADULTS/CHILDREN AT LEAST 7 YR OF AGE:
Oral inhalation 2 inhalations (one 5 mg blister per inhalation). Give bid (approximately 12 hr apart) for 5 days.

Interactions None well documented.

Lab Test Interferences None well documented.

Adverse Reactions

CV: Arrhythmias, syncope (postmarketing).
CNS: Headache, dizziness (2%); seizures (postmarketing).
DERM: Urticaria (less than 1.5%); facial edema, rash, serious cutaneous reactions (postmarketing).
EENT: Ear, nose, and throat infections, nasal signs and symptoms (2%).
GI: Diarrhea, nausea (3%); vomiting (1%); abdominal pain (less than 1.5%).
MUSC: Myalgia, arthralgia (less than 1.5%).
RESP: Sinusitis (3%); bronchitis, cough (2%); bronchospasm, dyspnea (postmarketing).
OTHER: Malaise, fatigue, fever (less than 1.5%); allergic or allergic-like reactions including oropharyngeal edema (postmarketing).

Precautions

Pregnancy: Category C.
Lactation: Undetermined.
Children: Safety and efficacy not established in patients younger than 7 yr of age.
Bronchospasm: Bronchospasm and decline in lung function have been reported. Discontinue use if this occurs.
High-risk patients: Safety and efficacy not demonstrated in patients with high-risk underlying medical conditions.
Prevention of influenza: Not established for prophylactic use to prevent influenza.
Underlying respiratory disease: Safety and efficacy not demonstrated in patients with underlying chronic pulmonary disease (severe COPD or asthma); its use is not recommended.

PATIENT CARE CONSIDERATIONS

Administration/Storage

- For oral inhalation only. Not for intranasal inhalation.
- Initiate therapy within 48 hr of onset of influenza symptoms.
- Follow manufacturer's instructions for loading medicine disks into *Diskhaler*, puncturing the blisters, and inhaling the medication.
- Have patient inhale contents from 2 blisters bid for 5 days. Two doses should be taken on the first day, provided there is at least 2 hr between doses. On subsequent days, doses should be approximately 12 hr apart at approximately the same time each day.
- If patient is scheduled to use an inhaled bronchodilator at the same time as zanamivir, have patient use the inhaled bronchodilator before inhaling zanamivir.
- Store *Diskhaler* and blister packs at controlled room temperature (59° to 86°F). Do not puncture any blister until just before inhaling a dose.

Assessment/Interventions

- Obtain patient history, including drug history and any known allergies. Note asthma or COPD.
- If decision is made to use zanamivir in patient with chronic pulmonary disease (eg, asthma, COPD), ensure patient is under close observation, respiratory function is carefully monitored, and a fast-acting bronchodilator is available for use, if needed.
- Monitor patient's response to therapy. Inform health care provider if influenza symptoms are not improving, are worsening, or if new symptoms develop during treatment.
- Monitor patient for signs of allergic reaction. Discontinue therapy and immediately notify health care provider if noted. Be prepared to treat appropriately.
- Monitor patient closely for evidence of bronchospasm or decline in respiratory function. Discontinue therapy and immediately inform health care provider if noted. Be prepared to treat appropriately.
- Monitor patient for RESP, GI, CNS, and general body side effects. Report to health care provider if noted and significant.

Patient/Family Education

- Explain name, dose, action, and potential side effects of drug.
- Advise patient to read and carefully follow *Patient's Instructions for Use* leaflet before starting therapy.
- Review and demonstrate proper use of the delivery system.
- Caution parent or caregiver of child receiving zanamivir that medication should be used only under adult supervision and instruction. Review, and demonstrate if possible, proper use of the delivery system with supervising adult.
- Review dosing schedule and prescribed length of therapy with patient. Advise patient to inhale contents from 2 blisters bid for 5 days. Inform patient that 2 doses should be taken on the first day, provided there is at least 2 hr between doses. On subsequent days, doses should be approximately 12 hr apart at approximately the same time. Caution patient

- that medication must be started within 48 hr of onset of influenza symptoms in order to be effective.
- Advise patient using an inhaled bronchodilator at the same time as zanamivir to use the inhaled bronchodilator before inhaling zanamivir.
- Advise patient that if a dose is missed to take as soon as remembered; however, if it is within 2 hr of the time for the next dose, to skip the dose and take the next dose at the regularly scheduled time.
- Review other modalities for alleviating influenza symptoms (eg, rest, hydration, OTC antipyretics and analgesics).
- Remind patient to complete entire course of therapy, even if feeling better.
- Advise patient that medication does not prevent the flu nor does it reduce risk of transmission of flu virus to others and to continue to take appropriate precautions to prevent spreading the infection.
- Advise patient that zanamivir is not a substitute for flu vaccination, and to continue to obtain an annual flu vaccination.
- Advise patient to inform health care provider if flu symptoms do not appear to be improving, are worsening, or if new symptoms develop during or after treatment.
- Instruct patient to discontinue therapy and contact health care provider immediately if experiencing increased respiratory symptoms (eg, worsening wheezing, shortness of breath) or signs or symptoms of an allergic reaction (eg, rash, hives, swelling of throat).
- Advise women to notify health care provider if pregnant, planning to become pregnant, or breastfeeding.
- Instruct patient not to take any prescription or OTC medications, herbal preparations, or dietary supplements unless advised by health care provider.
- Advise patient that follow-up examinations and lab tests may be required to monitor therapy and to keep appointments.

Zidovudine (Azidothymidine; AZT; Compound S)

(zid-OH-vue-deen)

Class Antiretroviral/Nucleoside reverse transcriptase inhibitor

How Supplied
Retrovir Tablets 300 mg, Capsules 100 mg, Syrup 50 mg/5 mL, Injection 10 mg/mL
✤ *APO-Zidovudine* ◆ *Novo-AZT*

Action

PHARMACOLOGY: Inhibits replication of retroviruses including HIV.

PHARMACOKINETICS/DYNAMICS:

Absorption: Rapidly absorbed, not affected by food. T_{max} is 0.5 to 1.5 hr. Oral bioavailability is 64%. AUC is equivalent whether it is tablets or capsules.

Distribution: It is extensively distributed. Binding to plasma protein is low, less than 38%. Apparent Vd is about 1.6 L/kg.

Metabolism: Hepatic metabolism. Major metabolites are D-glucopyranuronosylthymidine (GZDV) and 3′-amino-3′-deoxythymidine. GZDV AUC is about 3-fold greater than zidovudine.

Excretion: Primarily eliminated by hepatic metabolism. $T_{½}$ is 0.5 to 3 hr GZDV (74%) and zidovudine (14%) are recovered in the urine.

Special Populations:
Renal Function Impairment – Ccr is at least 15 mL/min. Dose adjustment is not necessary; however, Cl decreases resulting in an increased t½ of drug and metabolite and increased AUC. A dose adjustment is necessary for patients undergoing hemodialysis or peritoneal dialysis.
Hepatic Function Impairment – Limited information; however, it is expected Cl would decrease and plasma concentration would increase.
Children – Children older than 3 mo are similar to those in adults.
HIV-infected mothers – Mothers should not breastfeed their infants to avoid risking postnatal transmission of HIV.

Indications In combination with other antiretroviral agents for the treatment of HIV infections; prevention of maternal-fetal HIV transmission.

Contraindications Life-threatening hypersensitivity to any component.

Route/Dosage
HIV Infection
ADULTS: PO 600 mg/day in divided doses in combination with other antiretroviral agents.

Maternal-Fetal HIV Transmission
MATERNAL DOSING: PO Greater than 14 wk of pregnancy-100 mg orally 5 times/day until the start of labor. During labor and delivery, administer IV zidovudine at 2 mg/kg over 1 hr followed by a continuous IV infusion of 1 mg/kg/hr until clamping of the umbilical cord.

INFANT DOSING: **PO** 2 mg/kg orally q 6 hr starting within 12 hr after birth and continuing through 6 wk of age. Infants unable to receive oral dosing may be given zidovudine IV at 1.5 mg/kg, infused over 30 min, q 6 hr.

Interactions
Acetaminophen, nelfinavir, ribavirin, rifamycin, ritonavir, stavudine: May decrease zidovudine serum concentrations, reducing the therapeutic effect.
Acyclovir: Possible increased risk of neurotoxicity (lethargy or seizure).
Adriamycin, amphotericin B, dapsone, flucytosine, interferon, pentamidine, vinblastine, vincristine: May increase risk of toxicity, including nephrotoxicity, cytotoxicity, or hematologic toxicity.
Aspirin, atovaquone, fluconazole, indomethacin, methadone, probenecid, trimethoprim, valproic acid: May increase serum concentration and potential toxicity of zidovudine.
Doxorubicin: May antagonize the effect of zidovudine.
Experimental nucleoside analogs: May affect RBC/WBC counts or function and may increase potential for hematologic toxicity.
Ganciclovir: Life-threatening hematologic toxicity may occur.

Lab Test Interferences
None well documented.

Adverse Reactions
CV: ECG abnormality; vasodilation; syncope; cardiomyopathy; CHF.
CNS: Headache; dizziness; insomnia; paresthesia; malaise; asthenia; decreased reflexes; nervousness or irritability.
DERM: Rash; acne.
EENT: Taste perversion; hearing loss.
GI: Anorexia; constipation; dyspepsia; nausea; vomiting; dysphagia; flatulence; bleeding of the gums; rectal hemorrhage; mouth ulcers; edema of the tongue; eructation; abdominal pain.
HEMA: Anemia; granulocytopenia; pancytopenia.
RESP: Dyspnea; cough; epistaxis; pharyngitis; rhinitis; sinusitis; hoarseness.
OTHER: Fever, diaphoresis; myalgia; arthralgia; muscle spasm; body odor; chills; edema of the lip; flu syndrome; hyperalgesia; abdominal/back/chest pain; hypersensitivity reaction; anemia, neutropenia (infants).

> **WARNING:**
> Neutropenia and severe anemia, particularly in patients with advanced HIV disease have been reported. Myopathy has been associated with prolonged use. Lactic acidosis and hepatomegaly with steatosis (including fatal cases) have been reported with the use of nucleoside analogues alone or in combination with other antiretrovirals.

Precautions
Pregnancy: Category C.
Lactation: Undetermined. HIV-infected mothers should not breastfeed.
Children: Dosing regimen not established in children less than 3 mo.
Hypersensitivity: Sensitization reactions, including anaphylaxis, have occurred.
Renal function impairment: May have greater risk of toxicity.
Hepatic function impairment: May have greater risk of toxicity.
Hematologic effects: Use with extreme caution in patients with bone marrow compromise (Hgb less than 9.5 g/dL or granulocyte count less than $1000/mm^3$).

Overdosage: Signs and Symptoms
Nausea, vomiting, fatigue, headache, hematologic changes.

PATIENT CARE CONSIDERATIONS
Administration/Storage
- Use syrup, tablet, or capsule form for oral administration according to patient needs. Do *not* interchange between syrup and capsules. Syrup form absorbs faster than capsule form.
- Dilute IV preparation prior to administration. Remove calculated dose from vial; add to 5% dextrose to achieve concentration of up to 4 mg/mL.
- Do *not* mix with biologic or colloidal fluids (eg, blood products, protein solutions).
- Infuse over 1 hr at constant rate. Avoid rapid infusion or bolus.
- Awake patient to administer around clock unless otherwise instructed by health care provider.
- Do not administer with probenecid, acetaminophen, aspirin, or indomethacin (may inhibit metabolism or decrease clearance of zidovudine; serum concentrations may increase to potentially toxic levels).
- Store capsules at room temperature in a tight, light-resistant container Protect from heat and moisture.
- Store syrup at room temperature. Protect from light.
- After dilution, the solution is physically and chemically stable for 24 hr at room temperature and 48 hr if refrigerated. As an additional precaution, administer the diluted solution within 8 hr if stored at room temperature or 24 hr if refrigerated to minimize the potential

administration of a microbially contaminated solution. Store undiluted vials at room temperature and protect from light.

Assessment/Interventions
- Obtain patient history, including drug history, and any known allergies.
- Assess periodic ECGs.
- Monitor and record WBC and differential q 2 wk. Report decreased WBC, especially granulocytes immediately.
- Assess skin for signs of sensitization reactions (eg, report rash).
- Assess Hct and Hgb q 2 wk; severe anemia may require immediate blood transfusion.
- Monitor respiratory and cardiac status (eg, report dyspnea, edema, other signs of CHF).
- Monitor results of liver and renal function studies.

Patient/Family Education
- Advise patient to take exactly as prescribed.
- Advise patient not to share medication and not to exceed the recommended dose.
- Inform patient that fever, sore throat, shortness of breath, and dizziness require immediate attention by health care provider. These may be signs of severe anemia or decreased WBCs and may indicate need for blood transfusion.
- Explain that health care provider will request follow-up blood or urine studies; do not skip appointments.
- Tell patient to notify health care provider of headache, insomnia, nausea, muscle aches, dyspnea, numbness or tingling, nervousness, loss of appetite, diarrhea, GI pain, vomiting, rash, excessive sweating, swelling of feet and legs, and taste perversions.
- Explain that drug does not prevent transmission of disease.
- Caution patient not to take any other drugs without consulting health care provider. This especially includes acetaminophen (eg, *Tylenol*), aspirin, indomethacin, and acyclovir.
- Instruct patient to increase fluid intake to 2 to 3 L/day.
- Advise patient to record weight daily.
- Tell patient to protect medication from light during storage.
- Advise patient that drug may cause drowsiness and to use caution while driving or performing other tasks requiring mental alertness.
- Explain that long-term effects of drug are not known at this time.
- Advise patient that zidovudine therapy has not been shown to reduce the risk of transmission of HIV to others through sexual contact or blood contamination.
- Advise pregnant women considering use of the drug to prevent maternal-fetal transmission of HIV that transmission may still occur in some cases despite therapy. Long-term consequences of in utero and infant exposure are unknown.

Zileuton

(zill-LOO-tuhn)
Class Leukotriene receptor antagonist
How Supplied
Zyflo Tablets 600 mg
Action
PHARMACOLOGY: Attenuates bronchoconstriction by inhibiting leukotriene-dependent smooth muscle contractions.

PHARMACOKINETICS/DYNAMICS:
Absorption: Rapidly absorbed. T_{max} is about 1.7 hr. C_{max} is about 4.98 mcg/mL. AUC is about 19.2 mcg•hr/mL. Food caused a 27% increase in C_{max}; administer with or without food.

Distribution: Vd is about 1.2 L/kg. It is about 93% bound to plasma proteins, primarily albumin.

Metabolism: Two diastereomeric O-glucuronide conjugates (major metabolites) and an N-dehydroxylated metabolite have been identified. The N-dehydroxylated metabolite can be oxidatively metabolized by cytochrome P450 isoenzyme 1A2, 2C9, and 3A4.

Excretion: Predominantly via metabolism with a mean $t_½$ of about 2.5 hr. Oral Cl is about 7 mL/min/kg. It is 94.5% recovered in urine with 2.2% recovered in feces.

Special Populations:
Renal Function Impairment – Dosage adjustments in patients with renal dysfunction or undergoing hemodialysis are not necessary.
Hepatic Function Impairment – Contraindicated in patients with active liver disease. Because treatment with zileuton may result in increased hepatic transaminases, use zileuton with caution in patients who consume substantial quantities of alcohol or have a history of liver disease.

Indications Prophylaxis and chronic treatment of asthma.

Contraindications Active liver disease; elevations in transaminases at least 3 times the ULN.

Route/Dosage
ADULTS AND CHILDREN AT LEAST 12 YR: **PO** 600 mg qid.

Interactions
Propranolol, theophylline, warfarin: Effects of these agents may be increased.

Lab Test Interferences None well documented.

Adverse Reactions
CNS: Pain; dizziness; insomnia; somnolence; malaise; nervousness; hypertonia.
EENT: Conjunctivitis.
GI: Abdominal pain; dyspepsia; nausea; vomiting; constipation; flatulence.
GU: Urinary tract infection; vaginitis.
HEPA: Elevated LFTs.
OTHER: Asthenia; myalgia; arthralgia; chest pain; fever; lymphadenopathy; muscle rigidity; pruritus.

PATIENT CARE CONSIDERATIONS

Administration/Storage
- Available only in PO form.
- Store tablets at room temperature (20° to 25°C; 68° to 77°F).
- Keep in tightly sealed container, protected from light.
- May be taken with meals and at bed time

Assessment/Interventions
- Obtain patient history, including drug history, and any known allergies. Note history of liver disease or alcohol consumption.
- Assess patient's respiratory status prior to and during therapy.
- Ensure that liver function tests are monitored during therapy.
- Monitor patient medication for effectiveness and side effects, including signs and symptoms of liver dysfunction.

Patient/Family Education
- Inform the patient that this medication is for long-term treatment of asthma.
- Instruct patient to take the medication exactly as prescribed even when symptom free.

Precautions
Pregnancy: Category C.
Lactation: Undetermined.
Children: Safety and efficacy in pediatric patients less than 12 yr not established.
Acute asthma attacks: Not indicated for treatment of acute asthma attacks. Continue therapy during acute exacerbations of asthma.
Hematologic: Transient decreases in WBCs may occur.
Hepatotoxicity: Elevations in LFTs may occur. Use with caution in patients who consume substantial quantities of alcohol or who have history of liver disease. Monitor hepatic transaminases at initiation of, and during therapy.

- Advise patient to take medication 4 times/day with each meal and at bedtime.
- Warn the patient that this is not a bronchodilator and should not be used for the treatment of acute asthma attacks. However, advise the patient to continue during acute asthma attacks.
- Instruct the patient to continue to take other asthma medications as prescribed.
- Instruct the patient to avoid taking other medication, including OTC, without discussing it with his/her health care provider.
- Advise patient that elevation of liver enzyme is most serious side effect and that he/she must have liver function tests periodically. Instruct the patient to notify his/her health care provider if experiencing any signs or symptoms of liver disease: Flu-like symptoms; nausea; right upper quadrant pain; fatigue; lethargy; pruritus; jaundice.
- Instruct patient to notify health care provider if the use of short-acting bronchodilators increases or if more than the maximal number of inhalations of short-acting bronchodilators are needed.

Zinc Sulfate

(zink SULL-fate)
Class Mineral

How Supplied
Eye-Sed Solution 0.25% ♦ *Orazinc* Tablets 110 mg (25 mg zinc), Capsules 220 mg (50 mg zinc) ♦ *Verazinc* Capsules 220 mg (50 mg zinc) ♦ *Zinc 15* Tablets 66 mg (15 mg zinc) ♦ *Zinc-220* Capsules 220 mg (50 mg zinc) ♦ *Zinca-Pak* Injection 1 mg/ml (as sulfate [as 4.39 mg heptahydrate or 2.46 mg anhydrous]), Injection 5 mg/ml (as 21.95 mg sulfate) ♦ *Zincate* Capsules 220 mg (50 mg zinc)
✤ *Neosporin Ointment*

Action
PHARMACOLOGY: Acts as integral part of several enzymes important to protein and carbohydrate metabolism, wound healing, maintenance of normal growth and skin hydration, and senses of taste and smell.

PHARMACOKINETICS/DYNAMICS:
Absorption: Some studies indicate that ingestion with certain foods may inhibit zinc absorption. It is poorly absorbed from the GI tract (only 20% to 30%).

Distribution: Major stores of zinc are in the skeletal muscle and bone.

Excretion: About 90% is excreted through the intestines; about 2% in the urine.

Indications Dietary supplementation; supplement to IV solutions given for TPN; treatment or prevention of zinc deficiencies. Ophthalmic solution used as mild astringent for relief of eye irritation. **Unlabeled use(s):** Treatment of acrodermatitis enteropathica and delayed wound healing associated with zinc deficiency; treatment of acne, rheumatoid arthritis, Wilson's disease.

Contraindications Direct injection of undiluted solution into peripheral vein.

Route/Dosage
Dietary Supplement
ADULTS: **PO** 25 to 50 mg/day.

Supplement to IV Solutions
METABOLICALLY STABLE ADULTS: **IV** 2.5 to 4 mg/day. Add 2 mg/day for acute catabolic state.
STABLE ADULTS WITH FLUID LOSS FROM SMALL BOWEL: **IV** Increase dose by 12.2 mg/L TPN or 17.1 mg/kg loose stool or ileostomy output.
FULL-TERM INFANTS AND CHILDREN UNDER 5 YR: **IV** 100 mcg/kg/day.
PREMATURE INFANTS UNDER 3 KG: **IV** 300 mcg/kg/day.

Astringent
ADULTS: **Ophthalmic** 1 to 2 gtt into eye(s) up to qid.

Interactions
Fluoroquinolones; tetracyclines: Absorption of these agents may be decreased.

Lab Test Interferences None well documented.

Adverse Reactions
GI: Nausea; vomiting (especially in large oral doses).

Precautions
Pregnancy: Category C. Routine supplementation during pregnancy is not recommended.
Lactation: Excreted in breast milk.
Renal function impairment: Dosage reduction may be required in patients with renal dysfunction.
Excessive intake: In healthy people may be harmful.
Benzyl alcohol: Some of these products contain benzyl alcohol, which has been associated with a fatal "gasping" syndrome in premature infants.
IV products: Some contain benzyl alcohol, which is associated with fatal "gasping syndrome" in infants.

Overdosage: Signs and Symptoms
Nausea, vomiting, dehydration, restlessness, sideroblastic anemia, profuse sweating, hyperamylasemia.

PATIENT CARE CONSIDERATIONS
Administration/Storage
- If GI upset occurs, administer oral form with food but not with dairy products, bran, or foods containing caffeine.
- Dilute IV solutions prior to administration.
- To prevent contamination of ophthalmic solution, avoid contacting tip of container with any other surface and tightly close container after use.
- Do not use ophthalmic solution if becomes discolored or cloudy.

Assessment/Interventions
- Obtain patient history, including drug history, and any known allergies.
- If eye irritation persists or increases or pain or vision change occurs, consult health care provider.

Patient/Family Education
- Tell patient to contact health care provider if nausea, severe vomiting, dehydration, or restlessness occurs.
- Identify food sources of zinc (eg, seafood, organ meats, wheat germ).
- Inform patient that sense of taste and smell, skin hydration, and wound healing should improve.
- Instruct patient to follow RDA guidelines and limitations in terms of vitamin and mineral supplementation.
- Tell patient to take with food if GI upset occurs but to avoid foods high in calcium, phosphorus, and phytate. Inform patient that bran, caffeine, and dairy products may decrease absorption.
- Tell patient to notify health care provider if change in vision occurs or if eye irritation or pain persists or increases while using ophthalmic form.
- Teach patient proper administration technique for eye drops.

Ziprasidone

(zi-PRAY-si-done)

Class Antipsychotic/Benzisoxazole

How Supplied
Geodon Capsules 20 mg (as hydrochloride), Capsules 40 mg (as hydrochloride), Capsules 60 mg (as hydrochloride), Capsules 80 mg (as hydrochloride), Injection 20 mg/mL (as mesylate)

Action
PHARMACOLOGY: Antipsychotic activity, apparently because of dopamine and serotonin receptor antagonism.
PHARMACOKINETICS/DYNAMICS:
Absorption: Well absorbed after oral administration. T_{max} is about 6 to 8 hr. Bioavailability is about 60%. Absorption increased 2-fold in the presence of food.
Distribution: Vd is 1.5 L/kg. About 99% bound to plasma proteins, primarily albumin and $alpha_1$-acid glycoprotein.
Metabolism: Unlikely to interfere with metabolism of drugs metabolized by cytochrome P450. It is extensively metabolized. CYP3A4 is the major CYP contributing to the oxidative metabolism of ziprasidone.
Excretion: The t½ is about 7 hr. Cl is about 7.5 mL/min/kg. About 20% of the dose is excreted in urine and 66% eliminated in feces. Unchanged ziprasidone represents about 44% of total-drug related material in serum.
Special Populations:
Hepatic Function Impairment – Hepatic impairment would increase the AUC of ziprasidone.

Indications Treatment of schizophrenia; treatment of acute agitation in schizophrenic patients (injection only).

Contraindications Drugs known to prolong the QT interval (eg, quinidine, pimozide, sotalol); patients with a history of QT prolongation; recent acute MI; uncompensated heart failure; known hypersensitivity to the product.

Route/Dosage
ADULTS: **PO** 20 to 80 mg bid.
ADULTS: **IM** 10 to 20 mg/day (max, 40 mg/day).

Interactions
Alcohol, CNS-acting drugs: May cause additive CNS effects.
Amiodarone, dofetilide, dolasetron, droperidol, levomethadyl, moxifloxacin, pimozide, quinidine, sotalol, sparfloxacin, tacrolimus, thioridazine, any other drug known to prolong the QT interval: Contraindicated because of increased risk of torsades de pointes or other malignant ventricular arrhythmias.
Antihypertensive agents: Hypotensive effects may be enhanced.
Carbamazepine: May reduce ziprasidone levels, decreasing the effectiveness.
Ketoconazole, other inhibitors of cytochrome P450 3A4 metabolism: May elevate ziprasidone levels, increasing the risk of toxicity.
Dopamine agonists, levodopa: Effects may be antagonized.

Lab Test Interferences None well documented.

Adverse Reactions
CV: Tachycardia (2%); postural hypotension (1%); hypertension (at least 1%); hypertension, bradycardia, vasodilation (IM).
CNS: Somnolence (14%); akathisia, dizziness (8%); extrapyramidal syndrome (5%); dystonia (4%); hypertonia (3%); agitation, tremor, dyskinesia, hostility, paresthesia, confusion, vertigo, hypokinesia, hyperkinesias, abnormal gait, hypesthesia, ataxia, amnesia, cogwheel rigidity, delirium, hypotonia, akinesia, dysarthria, withdrawal syndrome, buccoglossal syndrome, choreoathetosis, incoordination, neuropathy (at least 1%); anxiety, tremor (dose related); headache, insomnia, personality disorder, psychosis, speech disorder (IM).
DERM: Rash (4%); fungal dermatitis (2%); sweating (1%).
EENT: Rhinitis (4%); abnormal vision (3%); oculogyric crisis, diplopia (at least 1%).
GI: Nausea (10%); constipation (9%); dyspepsia (8%); diarrhea (5%); dry mouth (4%); anorexia (2%); vomiting (at least 1%); increased salivation (dose related); tooth disorder (IM).
GU: Dysmenorrhea, priapism (IM).
METAB: Weight gain (10%).
RESP: Respiratory disorder (eg, cold symptoms, upper respiratory tract infection [8%]); increased cough (3%); dyspnea (at least 1%).
OTHER: Asthenia (5%); accidental injury (4%); myalgia (1%); abdominal pain, flu-like syndrome, fever, accidental fall, face edema, chills, photosensitivity reaction, flank pain, hypothermia, motor vehicle accident (at least 1%); arthralgia (dose related); injection site pain, back pain (IM).

Precautions
Pregnancy: Category C.
Lactation: Undetermined.
Children: Safety and efficacy not established.
Elderly: Use with caution
Body temperature regulation: Antipsychotic agents disrupt the ability to reduce core body temperature. Use with caution in patients who will experience conditions that may contribute

to an elevation in core body temperature (eg, strenuous exercise, exposure to extreme heat, concomitant anticholinergic therapy, subject to dehydration).

CV effects: QT prolongation with increased risk of life-threatening CV events may occur. Certain circumstances may increase the risk of the occurrence of torsades de pointes and/or sudden death in association with the use of drugs that prolong the QTc interval including bradycardia; hypokalemia or hypomagnesemia; concomitant use of other drugs that prolong the QTc interval; and the presence of congenital prolongation of the QT interval.

Cognitive and motor performance: Because of initial sedation, mental and/or physical abilities may be impaired, especially during the first few days or weeks of therapy.

Dysphagia: Use with caution in patients at risk of aspiration pneumonia.

Neuroleptic malignant syndrome (NMS): This potentially fatal condition has been reported in association with antipsychotic agents. Signs and symptoms include hyperpyrexia, muscle rigidity, altered mental status, irregular pulse or BP, tachycardia, diaphoresis, and cardiac arrhythmias.

Orthostatic hypotension: Orthostatic hypotension may occur.

Seizures: May occur; use with caution in patients with a history of seizures.

Suicide: Inherent in psychotic illness; use with caution and dispense in small quantities.

Tardive dyskinesia: A potentially irreversible syndrome of involuntary body and facial movements may occur.

Overdosage: Signs and Symptoms
Sedation, slurred speech, transient hypertension.

PATIENT CARE CONSIDERATIONS
Administration/Storage
Capsules:
- Administer prescribed dose bid with food.
- Have patient swallow capsules whole. Do not crush, chew, or open capsules.
- Store capsules at controlled room temperature (59° to 86°F).

Injection:
- For IM administration only. Not for intradermal, SC, or IV administration.
- Reconstitute powder for injection with 1.2 mL sterile water for injection. Each mL of reconstituted solution contains 20 mg ziprasidone.
- Do not mix with other medications or use other diluents.
- Do not administer if particulate matter, cloudiness, or discoloration noted.
- Discard any unused solution. Do not save unused solution for later administration.
- Store powder for injection at controlled room temperature (59° to 86°F). Protect from light. Following reconstitution, the injection can be stored for up to 24 hr at controlled room temperature or up to 7 days if refrigerated (36° to 46°F).

Assessment/Interventions
- Obtain patient history, including drug history and any known allergies. Note history of renal disease, liver disease, QT prolongation, congenital long QT syndrome, recent MI, uncompensated heart failure, CV disease, cerebrovascular disease, cardiac arrhythmias, previous episodes of NMS, seizures or conditions that predispose to seizures (eg, Alzheimer disease), conditions that would predispose to hypotension (eg, dehydration, hypovolemia, treatment with antihypertensive medications), or coadministration of medications known to prolong the QT interval (eg, pimozide), induce CYP3A4 (eg, carbamazepine), or inhibit CYP3A4 (eg, ketoconazole).
- Ensure that electrolytes are determined before starting and periodically during therapy in patients at risk of hypokalemia and/or hypomagnesemia (eg, concurrent diuretic therapy, diarrhea).
- Ensure that hypokalemia and/or hypomagnesemia are corrected before initiating therapy and normal potassium and magnesium levels are maintained during therapy.
- Ensure that ECG is performed before initiating therapy and periodically thereafter, especially during periods of dose adjustment. Discontinue therapy if QTc interval is consistently greater than 500 msec.
- Ensure that lower dose and slower dose escalation is used in elderly or debilitated patient, or patient who is predisposed to hypotension or in whom hypotension would pose a risk.
- Monitor cardiac patient during initiation of drug for orthostatic hypotension; notify health care provider if noted.
- Take safety precautions if orthostatic hypotension occurs.
- Inform health care provider immediately if hyperpyrexia, muscle rigidity, altered mental status, irregular pulse and BP, tachycardia, or diaphoresis develop.
- Notify health care provider immediately if rash, dizziness, palpitations, or syncope occur.

- Assess baseline neurologic status and during treatment observe for involuntary body and facial movements, drowsiness, agitation, anxiety, aggressive reaction, or seizure activity.
- Monitor patient for suicidal tendencies often associated with schizophrenia.
- Monitor patient for CNS, PSYCH, GI, CV, RESP, and general body side effects. Inform health care provider if noted and significant.
- Assess medication compliance.

Patient/Family Education
- Explain name, dose, action, and potential side effects of drug.
- Advise patient receiving injectable ziprasidone that medication will be prepared and administered by a health care provider in a medical setting because oral therapy is not feasible.
- Advise patient to review *Patient Package Insert* before starting therapy and with each refill.
- Instruct patient to take prescribed dose bid.
- Advise patient to take each dose with food to increase absorption and effectiveness.
- Advise patient to swallow capsules whole.
- Advise patient that if a dose is missed to take it as soon as possible and then return to the normal schedule. Instruct patient not to double the dose to catch up.
- Advise patient that dose will be started low and then increased until maximum benefit is obtained.
- Instruct patient to not change the dose or stop taking unless advised by health care provider.
- Instruct patient to not stop taking ziprasidone when feeling better.
- Tell patient to immediately report dizziness, palpitations, fainting, high fever, muscle rigidity, altered mental status, irregular pulse, sweating, seizures, or rash to health care provider.
- Advise patient to notify health care provider of the following: excessive drowsiness, weight gain, involuntary body or facial movements, rapid pulse, change in personality or mood.
- Advise patient to avoid strenuous activity during periods of high temperature or humidity.
- Instruct patient to avoid alcoholic beverages and sedatives (eg, diazepam) while taking ziprasidone.
- Instruct patient to get up slowly from lying or sitting position and to avoid sudden position changes to prevent postural hypotension. Advise patient to report dizziness with position changes to health care provider. Caution patient that hot tubs and hot showers or baths may make dizziness worse.
- Advise patient taking antihypertensives to monitor BP at regular intervals.
- Advise patient that drug may impair judgment, thinking, or motor skills or cause drowsiness and to use caution while driving or performing other tasks requiring mental alertness until tolerance is determined.
- Advise women to notify health care provider if pregnant, planning to become pregnant, or breastfeeding.
- Instruct patient not to take any prescription or OTC medications or dietary supplements unless advised by health care provider.
- Advise patient that follow-up visits will be required to monitor therapy and to keep appointments.

Zoledronic Acid

(zoe-leh-DROE-nik acid)
Class Bisphosphonate
How Supplied
Zometa Reconstituted Solution 4 mg per vial
Action
PHARMACOLOGY: Inhibition of bone resorption.

PHARMACOKINETICS/DYNAMICS:
Absorption: AUC is about 2 to 16 mg.
Distribution: Protein binding is about 22%.
Metabolism: It does not inhibit CYP450 in vitro.
Excretion: The $t_{1/2}$ is about 146 hr. The 0- to 24-hr renal Cl was about 3.7 L/hr.
Special Populations:
Renal Function Impairment – Mild renal impairment averaged increases in AUC of 15%. Moderate renal impairment averaged increases in AUC of 43%. The risk of renal deterioration appears to increase with AUC, which doubled at a Ccr of 10 mL/min.

Indications Treatment of hypercalcemia of malignancy; treatment of patients with multiple myeloma and bone metastases from solid tumors in conjunction with standard antineoplastic therapy.

Contraindications Zoledronic acid or other bisphosphonates, or any excipients in the formulation.

Route/Dosage
Hypercalcemia of Malignancy
ADULTS: **IV** 4 mg max dose given as single infusion over more than 15 min. Retreatment with 4 mg may be considered if serum calcium does not return to normal or remain normal

after initial treatment. To allow a full response, it is recommended that a min of 7 days should elapse before retreatment.

Multiple Myeloma and Metastatic Bone Lesions from Solid Tumors
ADULTS: **IV** 4 mg infused over 15 min q 3 or 4 wk.

Interactions
Aminoglycosides, loop diuretics (eg, furosemide): Increased risk of hypocalcemia.
Thalidomide: Increased risk of renal dysfunction.

Lab Test Interferences
None well documented.

Adverse Reactions
CV: Hypotension.
CNS: Insomnia; anxiety; confusion; agitation; fatigue; weakness; anorexia; decreased appetite; headache; dizziness; insomnia; paresthesia; hypoesthesia; depression.
DERM: Redness and swelling at injection site; rash; pruritus; alopecia; dermatitis.
EENT: Conjunctivitis.
GI: Nausea; vomiting; constipation; diarrhea; abdominal pain; anorexia; dysphagia.
GU: UTI.
HEMA: Anemia; granulocytopenia; thrombocytopenia; pancytopenia; neutropenia.
METAB: Hypomagnesemia; hypokalemia; hypophosphatemia; weight decrease; dehydration.
RESP: Dyspnea; coughing; upper respiratory tract infection.
OTHER: Flu-like symptoms; chest pain; fever; moniliasis; skeletal pain; asthenia; mucositis; metastases; non-specific infection; pyrexia; lower limb edema; rigors; bone pain; myalgia; arthralgia; back pain; aggravated malignant neoplasm.

Precautions
Pregnancy: Category D.
Lactation: Undetermined.
Children: Safety and efficacy not established.
Elderly: Because renal function may be decreased more often in this age group, special care should be taken to monitor renal function.
Renal function impairment: Use not recommended in patients with severe renal impairment.
Asthma: Use with caution in patients with aspirin-sensitive asthma.
Hepatic insufficiency: Insufficient data available; use with caution.

Overdosage: Signs and Symptoms
Hypocalcemia, hypophosphatemia, hypomagnesemia.

PATIENT CARE CONSIDERATIONS

Administration/Storage
- Administer by IV route only. Not for IM or SQ administration.
- To reduce risk of renal failure, maximum recommended dose is 4 mg and minimum duration of infusion is at least 15 min.
- Reconstitute lyophilized powder (4 mg) with 5 mL Sterile Water for Injection. Completely dissolve drug before withdrawing for further dilution.
- Further dilute reconstituted solution in 100 mL 0.9% Sodium Chloride or 5% Dextrose Injection.
- Infuse over more than 15 min via separate IV line.
- Do not mix with calcium-containing IV solutions (eg, Lactated Ringer's solution) or other IV medications.
- Do not administer if particulate matter or discoloration noted.
- Store unopened vials at controlled room temperature. Reconstituted solution may be stored in refrigerator (36° to 46°F). The total time between reconstitution, dilution, storage in refrigerator, and end of administration must not exceed 24 hr.

Hypercalcemia of malignancy:
- Do not retreat for at least 7 days.

Multiple myeloma and bone metastases of solid tumors:
- May repeat dose every 3 to 4 wk.

Assessment/Interventions
- Obtain patient history, including drug history and any known allergies. Note hypersensitivity to bisphosphonates. Note presence of renal impairment or dehydration.
- Record dates and response to any previous treatment with zoledronic acid.
- Ensure that serum creatinine is assessed prior to each treatment. Notify health care provider if serum creatinine is increasing.
- Ensure that serum calcium, phosphate, magnesium, electrolytes, and hemoglobin/hematocrit are monitored and recorded before and periodically following initiation of therapy. Notify health care provider if abnormalities are noted and be prepared to treat appropriately.
- Withhold therapy in patient with hypercalcemia of malignancy whose renal function deteriorates until renal function returns to baseline.
- Ensure that vigorous saline hydration is utilized in patients being treated for hypercalcemia of malignancy.

- Monitor patient for signs of fluid overload during saline hydration. Notify health care provider if noted and be prepared to administer diuretics if ordered.
- Monitor and record temperature before and during treatment.
- Assess patient for infusion site reaction, GI, CNS, RESP, and general body side effects. Report to health care provider if noted and significant.

Patient/Family Education
- Explain name, dose, action, and potential side effects of drug.
- Advise patient that medication will be prepared and administered by a qualified health care provider in a health care setting and that medication will not be administered at home.
- Advise patient that infusion-site reactions (eg, redness, swelling, hardness, pain) can be treated with local measures (eg, warm or cold packs) and oral otc analgesics (eg, acetaminophen, ibuprofen). Advise patient to report infusion-site reactions that do not respond to symptomatic treatment to health care provider.
- Instruct patient to report the following symptoms to health care provider: tingling, numbness, muscle spasms, stomach pain, fever, fatigue, swelling, nausea, appetite loss, constipation, diarrhea, vomiting, difficulty breathing, muscle, joint or bone pain.
- Advise women to inform their health care provider if they become pregnant, plan on becoming pregnant, or are breastfeeding.
- Instruct patient to not take any prescription or OTC medications or dietary supplements unless advised to do so by their health care provider.
- Advise patient that follow-up visits and laboratory tests will be required to monitor therapy and to be sure to keep appointments.

Zolmitriptan

(ZOLE-mih-TRIP-tan)
Class Analgesic/Migraine
How Supplied
Zomig Tablets 2.5 mg, Tablets 5 mg ♦ Zomig Spray, nasal 5 mg ♦ Zomig ZMT Tablets, orally disintegrating 2.5 mg
♣ Zomig Rapimelt

Action
PHARMACOLOGY: Selective agonist for the vascular serotonin (5-HT) receptor subtype, causing vasoconstriction of cranial arteries and inhibition of pro-inflammatory neuropeptide release.

PHARMACOKINETICS/DYNAMICS:
Absorption: Vd is about 7 L/kg. It is well absorbed after oral administration of both conventional tablets and the orally disintegrating tablets. T_{max} for oral disintegrating tablets is 3 hr and for conventional tablets is 1.5 hr. Bioavailability is about 40%.

Distribution: Plasma protein binding is about 25%.

Metabolism: Converted to an active N-desmethyl metabolite such that the metabolite concentrations are about ⅔ that of zolmitriptan.

Excretion: The t½ is 3 hr. About 8% of the dose is recovered in urine as unchanged drug. Mean total plasma Cl is about 31.5 mL/min/kg and 25.9 mL/min/kg for nasal spray. Cl is renal tubular secretion.

Special Populations:
Renal Function Impairment – Cl was reduced 25% in patients with severe renal impairment. No change in Cl was found in moderately renally impaired patients.
Hepatic Function Impairment – In severely hepatically impaired patients, the C_{max}, T_{max}, and AUC were increased 1.5-, 2-, and 3-fold, respectively. When dosed orally, the effect of hepatic disease on zolmitriptan nasal spray has not been evaluated. Administer with caution in subjects with liver disease, generally using doses less than 2.5 mg.
Gender – Mean plasma concentrations were up to 1.5-fold higher in women than men.

Indications Short-term treatment of migraine attacks with/without aura.

Contraindications Ischemic heart disease or in patients with Prinzmetal angina; symptoms consistent with possible ischemic heart disease; uncontrolled hypertension; symptomatic Wolff-Parkinson-White syndrome; use within 24 hr of treatment with another 5-HT agonist or an ergotamine-containing or ergot-like medication; coadministration of, or within 2 wk of discontinuation of, an MAO inhibitor, management of hemiplegic or basilar migraines.

Route/Dosage
ADULTS: **PO** Initial recommended dose is up to 2.5 mg (eg, ½ tablet) with fluids; max recommended single dose is 5 mg. If headache returns, the dose may be repeated after 2 hr, not to exceed 10 mg within a 24-hr period. The effectiveness of a second dose, if the initial dose is ineffective, has not been determined.
ADULTS: **Intranasal** One dose of 5 mg for acute migraine. If headache returns, dose may be repeated after 2 hr (max, 10 mg per 24 hr).

Response is individual. Doses lower than 5 mg can only be achieved through the use of an oral formulation. Make the choice of dose and route of administration on an individual basis.

Interactions

5-HT₁ agonists (eg, sumatriptan): Avoid use within 24 hr of each other.

Cimetidine: Zolmitriptan levels and t½ may be increased.

Ergot-containing or ergot-type drugs (eg, methysergide): May cause additive prolonged vasospastic reactions. Avoid use within 24 hr of each other.

MAO inhibitors (eg, phenelzine): Do not use zolmitriptan concurrently or within 2 wk of discontinuation of a MAO inhibitor.

Selective serotonin reuptake inhibitors (eg, fluoxetine): Combined use may cause weakness, hyperreflexia, and incoordination.

Sibutramine: Serotonin syndrome, including CNS irritability, motor weakness, shivering, myoclonus, and altered consciousness, may occur.

Lab Test Interferences None well documented.

Adverse Reactions

CV: Palpitations; coronary artery vasospasm, transient myocardial ischemia, angina pectoris, MI (postmarketing).

CNS: Paresthesia, dizziness, somnolence, vertigo, hyperesthesia (at least 2%); headache (postmarketing).

EENT: Nasal cavity discomfort (at least 2%).
GI: Unusual taste (21% intranasal); dry mouth, dyspepsia, dysphagia, nausea (at least 2%); ischemic colitis, GI infarction or necrosis (postmarketing).

HYPERSEN: Anaphylaxis or anaphylactoid reactions, angioedema (postmarketing).

MUSC: Myalgia.

OTHER: Asthenia, pain, chest/throat/neck pain, tightness, or heaviness, warm or cold sensations, sweating (at least 2%).

Precautions

Pregnancy: Category C.
Lactation: Undetermined.
Children: Safety and efficacy not established.
Elderly: Safety and efficacy in patients older than 65 yr of age not established.
Hepatic function impairment: Use with caution; use doses less than 2.5 mg.
Cardiac events/Vasoconstriction: Serious coronary events, though extremely rare, can occur after administration of 5-HT₁ agonists. Administer first dose in health care provider's office to patients at possible risk of unrecognized coronary disease. If symptoms consistent with angina occur, conduct ECG evaluation for ischemic changes. May cause coronary vasospasm in patients with history of coronary artery disease (CAD).
Cerebrovascular events: Cerebral hemorrhage, subarachnoid hemorrhage, stroke, and other cerebrovascular events have been reported with 5-HT₁ agonists.
Hypertensive crisis: Elevation in BP, including hypertensive crisis, have been reported.

Overdosage: Signs and Symptoms
Sedation.

PATIENT CARE CONSIDERATIONS

Administration/Storage

- Do not administer with or within 14 days of MAO inhibitor.
- Do not administer within 24 hr of treatment with another 5-HT₁ agonist or ergot-containing drug.
- Administer prescribed dose at onset of migraine symptoms.
- If headache recurs after initial relief, a second dose may be administered, provided there is an interval of at least 2 hr between doses.
- If first dose is ineffective, do not administer a second dose unless prescribed by health care provider.
- Do not administer greater than 10 mg per 24-hr period.
- Store tablets, orally-disintegrating tablets, and nasal spray at controlled room temperature (68° to 77°F). Protect from light and moisture.

Tablets:

- Administer without regard to meals.

Orally Disintegrating Tablet:

- Contains phenylalanine. Do not administer orally disintegrating tablet to patient with phenylketonuria without first discussing with health care provider.
- Remove tablet from blister pack just prior to administering dose.
- Peel open blister pack with dry hands and place orally disintegrating tablet on patient's tongue. Advise patient to allow tablet to dissolve and then swallow with saliva. Advise patient not to break or chew tablet.

Nasal Spray:

- For intranasal use only. Avoid spraying into the eyes or mouth.
- Remove gray protection cap immediately before administering.
- Discard spray unit after administering.

Assessment/Interventions

- Obtain patient history, including drug history and any known allergies. Note renal or hepatic impairment, ischemic or vasospastic CAD, uncontrolled hypertension, peripheral vascular disease, ischemic bowel disease, seizures, stroke, transient ischemic attacks, hemiplegic or basilar migraine, Wolff-Parkinson-White syndrome, or other arrhythmias associated with other cardiac accessory conduction pathway disorders, or current or recent (ie, within 14 days) use of MAO inhibitor.
- Note recent (within 24 hr) use of other 5-HT$_1$ agonists or ergotamine-containing or ergot-type drugs.
- Assess pain location, intensity, duration, and associated symptoms of migraine attack and response to treatment.
- Provide quiet, calm environment. Decrease stimuli, noise, and light.
- Ensure that patients with potential for CAD, including postmenopausal women, men over 40 yr of age, patients with risk factors for CAD (eg, hypertension, hypercholesterolemia, obesity, diabetes, smokers, family history), undergo a CV evaluation before initiating therapy.
- Administer first dose in physician's office or other adequately staffed medical facility to patient with potential for CAD whose CV evaluation provided clinical evidence that patient is reasonably free of coronary artery and ischemic myocardial disease or other significant underlying CV disease. Consider obtaining an ECG during the interval immediately following administration of the first dose of medication to patient with potential for CAD.
- Monitor patient for signs of allergic reaction. Discontinue therapy and immediately notify health care provider if noted. Be prepared to treat appropriately.
- Ensure that patient who is a long-term user of triptans, such as zolmitriptan, undergoes periodic CV evaluation.
- Monitor patient for CNS, CV, GI, and general body side effects. Report to health care provider if noted and significant.

Patient/Family Education

- Explain name, dose, action, and potential side effects of drug.
- Advise patient to read the *Patient Information* leaflet before starting therapy and again with each refill.
- Explain that drug is to be used only during migraine and does not prevent or reduce the number of attacks. Emphasize that the drug is used only to treat actual migraine attack and should not be used to prevent headaches or treat headaches caused by other conditions.
- Advise patient that drug is to be taken as soon as symptoms of migraine appear. A second dose may be taken if symptoms return, but no sooner than 2 hr following the first dose. For a given attack, if there is no response to the first tablet, do not take a second dose without first consulting with health care provider.
- Advise patient not to take more than 10 mg per day.
- Advise patient that safety of treating more than 4 headaches in a 30-day period with nasal spray (or 3 headaches in a 30-day period with tablets) has not been established and to inform health care provider if headaches are occurring more frequently.
- Advise patient to immediately notify health care provider if any of the following occur after taking a dose of sumatriptan: severe chest pain or chest pain that does not go away; sudden and/or severe stomach pain; shortness of breath; wheezing; swelling of eyelids, face, or lips.
- Advise patient that if tightness, pain, pressure, or heaviness in chest, throat, neck, or jaw occurs when using sumatriptan, to discuss these symptoms with health care provider before using again.
- Advise patient to notify health care provider if feelings of tingling, heat, flushing, tiredness, dizziness, heaviness, or pressure occur after treatment.
- Advise patient that drug may cause fatigue or dizziness and to use caution while driving or performing other activities requiring mental alertness.
- Advise patient to avoid unnecessary exposure to sunlight or tanning lamps and to use sunscreen and wear protective clothing to avoid photosensitivity reactions.
- Instruct patient to continue taking prescribed migraine prophylactic medications daily as directed.
- Advise patient not currently taking a migraine prophylactic drug to discuss the use of such drugs with health care provider.
- Advise women to notify health care provider if pregnant, planning to become pregnant, or breastfeeding.
- Warn patient not to take any prescription or OTC drugs, dietary supplements, or herbal preparations without consulting health care provider.
- Advise patient that follow-up visits may be necessary to monitor therapy and to keep appointments.

Zolpidem Tartrate

(ZOLE-pih-dem)

Class Sedative and hypnotic

How Supplied
Ambien Tablets 5 mg, Tablets 10 mg

Action
PHARMACOLOGY: Mechanism is unknown but may involve subunit modulation of the aminobutyrate activase (GABA) receptor chloride channel macromolecular complex.

PHARMACOKINETICS/DYNAMICS:
Absorption: Rapid absorption from the GI tract. Do not administer with or immediately after a meal. The T_{max} is 1.6 hr. The C_{max} (5 mg tablet) is about 29 to 113 ng/mL; the C_{max} (10 mg tablet) is about 58 to 272 ng/mL.

Distribution: Protein binding is about 92.5%.

Excretion: The t½ (5 mg tablet) is 2.6 hr; the t½ (10 mg tablet) is 2.5 hr.

Special Populations:
Hepatic Function Impairment – C_{max} and AUC were found to be 2 times and 5 times higher, respectively, in hepatically compromised patients. Modify dosing accordingly in patients with hepatic insufficiency.
Elderly – The dose should be 5 mg, based on several studies in which the mean C_{max} and AUC were significantly increased when compared with results in young adults.

Indications
Short-term treatment of insomnia.

Contraindications
Standard considerations.

Route/Dosage
ADULTS: PO 10 mg immediately before bedtime.
ELDERLY, DEBILITATED, OR HEPATIC INSUFFICIENT PATIENTS: An initial 5 mg dose is recommended. Max dose, no more than 10 mg.

PATIENT CARE CONSIDERATIONS

Administration/Storage
- Available only in PO tablet form.
- Administer immediately before bedtime on an empty stomach.
- Store at room temperature (19° to 30°C; 66° to 86°F).
- Keep in tightly sealed, child-proof container.

Assessment/Interventions
- Obtain patient history, including drug history, and any known allergies. Note hepatic impairment, debilitated status, and respiratory status.
- Ensure that side rails are raised after administration.

Interactions
Food: Reduces absorption of zolpidem.
Ritonavir: Possible severe sedation and respiratory depression.

Lab Test Interferences
None well documented.

Adverse Reactions
CV: Palpitations.
CNS: Amnesia; daytime drowsiness; dizziness; headache; lethargy; "drugged feelings," lightheadedness; depression; abnormal dreams; ataxia; confusion; euphoria; insomnia; vertigo.
EENT: Sinusitis; pharyngitis; diplopia, abnormal vision.
GI: Diarrhea; constipation; dry mouth.
OTHER: Allergy; back pain; flu-like symptoms; chest pain.

Precautions
Pregnancy: Category B.
Lactation: Excreted in breast milk.
Children: Safety and efficacy not established.
Elderly: Closely monitor elderly/debilitated patients. Recommended dosage is 5 mg.
Hepatic function impairment: Dosage modification may be necessary.
Duration of therapy: Generally limit to 7 to 10 days, reevaluate patient if to be taken for more than 2 to 3 wk.
Abrupt discontinuation: Abrupt discontinuation associated with withdrawal symptoms similar to those associated with other CNS depressant drugs.
Abuse/Dependence: Use with caution in patients with history of drug or alcohol abuse, depression, or suicidal tendencies.
Respiratory depression: Use with caution in patients with compromised respiratory function.

Overdosage: Signs and Symptoms
Somnolence, light coma, cardiovascular, respiratory compromise.

- Assist patient with ambulation after administration of drug.
- Assess sleep patterns prior to and during therapy.
- Assess for the development of abnormal thinking or behavior changes during therapy.

Patient/Family Education
- Advise patient to take immediately before going to bed. Advise patient to take on an empty stomach.
- Warn patient to never stop taking medication suddenly; withdrawal symptoms may develop.
- Instruct patient to avoid alcohol and other CNS depressants while taking drug.

- Caution patients to avoid driving or other tasks requiring alertness, coordination, or physical dexterity due to drowsiness that may occur.
- Instruct patient to take medication exactly as directed; do not increase dosage without health care provider approval.
- Emphasize the importance of follow-up appointments to monitor progress of therapy.

Zonisamide

(zoe-NIS-ah-MIDE)
Class Anticonvulsant/Sulfonamide
How Supplied
Zonegran Capsules 25 mg, Capsules 50 mg, Capsules 100 mg
Action
PHARMACOLOGY: Unknown; however, may produce anticonvulsant effects through action at sodium and calcium channels.
PHARMACOKINETICS/DYNAMICS:
Absorption: The C_{max} is 2 to 5 mcg/mL and T_{max} is 2 to 6 hr. In the presence of food, T_{max} is delayed to 4 to 6 hr, but has no effect on bioavailability.
Distribution: Vd is about 1.45 L/kg. It is about 40% bound to plasma proteins and extensively binds to erythrocytes, resulting in an 8-fold higher concentration in RBCs than plasma.
Metabolism: It undergoes acetylation to form N-acetyl zonisamide and reduction to form the open ring metabolite, 2-sulfamoylacetyl phenol (SMAP).
Excretion: Renal Cl is about 3.5 mL/min. Elimination t½ is about 63 hr. It is excreted primarily in urine as parent drug and as glucuronide metabolite. About 62% is recovered in urine and about 3% in feces by day 10. Plasma Cl is about 0.3 to 0.35 mL/min/kg in patients not receiving enzyme-inducing antiepilepsy drugs.
Special Populations:
Renal Function Impairment – Renal Cl decreases with decreased renal function. Marked renal impairment was associated with an increase in zonisamide AUC of 35%.
Indications Adjunctive therapy in the treatment of partial seizures in adult epileptic patients.
Contraindications Hypersensitivity to sulfonamides or zonisamide.
Route/Dosage
ADULTS (OVER 16 YR): **PO** 100 mg/day initially, then the dose may be increased by 100 mg/day at intervals of at least 2 wk (max, 600 mg/day).
Interactions
Drugs that induce liver enzymes (eg, carbamazepine, phenobarbital, phenytoin): May increase the metabolism and Cl and decrease the t½ of zonisamide.
Lab Test Interferences None well documented.
Adverse Reactions Because zonisamide is used as adjunctive therapy, figures obtained when zonisamide is added to concomitant antiepileptic drug therapy cannot be used to predict the frequency of adverse events in the course of usual medical practice. Except for potentially serious adverse effects (eg, blood dyscrasias, CV events), which have been reported to occur in less than 1% of the patients, the following adverse reactions have been reported in at least 1% of zonisamide-treated patients:
CV: Vascular insufficiency; atrial fibrillation; heart failure; ventricular extrasystoles.
CNS: Somnolence; dizziness; headache; agitation; irritability; fatigue; tiredness; difficulty concentrating; memory difficulty mental slowing; ataxia; paresthesia; confusion; depression; insomnia; anxiety; nervousness; schizophrenic/schizophreniform behavior; speech abnormalities; difficult verbal expression; tremor; convulsion; abnormal gait; hyperesthesia; incoordination.
DERM: Rash; pruritus.
EENT: Nystagmus; diplopia; taste perversion; amblyopia; tinnitus.
GI: Nausea; anorexia; vomiting; abdominal pain; diarrhea; dyspepsia; constipation; dry mouth.
HEMA: Ecchymosis; leukopenia; anemia; lymphadenopathy; thrombocytopenia; microcytic anemia.
HEPA: Increased ALT and AST.
METAB: Weight loss.
RESP: Rhinitis; pulmonary embolus; pharyngitis; increased cough.
OTHER: Flu-like syndrome; asthenia; accidental injury.
Precautions
Pregnancy: Category C.
Lactation: Undetermined.
Children: Safety and efficacy in children younger than 16 yr not established.
Elderly: Select dose with caution, reflecting the greater frequency of decreased hepatic, renal, or cardiac function and comorbidity.

Hypersensitivity: May present as fatal or severe reactions such as Stevens-Johnson syndrome, toxic epidermal necrolysis, fulminant hepatic necrosis, agranulocytosis, aplastic anemia, and other blood dyscrasias.
Renal function impairment: Do not use if glomerular filtration rate is less than 50 mL/min.
Cognitive adverse events: Frequent CNS adverse events, including depression, psychosis, psychomotor slowing, somnolence, fatigue, and difficulty with concentration, speech, or language problems have occurred.
Kidney stones: May occur.
Oligohydrosis and hyperthermia in pediatric patients: Oligohydrosis, sometimes resulting in heat stroke and hospitalization, has been reported in pediatric patients.
Serious skin reactions: Consider discontinuing drug.
Sudden death: Sudden unexplained death has occurred.
Withdrawal seizures: Abrupt withdrawal may precipitate increased seizure frequency or status epilepticus; gradually discontinue or decrease dose.

Overdosage: Signs and Symptoms
CNS symptoms, bradycardia, hypotension, respiratory depression, coma.

PATIENT CARE CONSIDERATIONS

Administration/Storage
- Administer qd or bid as prescribed.
- May be administered without regard to meals. Administer with food if GI upset occurs.
- Administer capsules whole. Do not chew or break capsules.
- Increase dose no more often than q 2 wk.
- Do not administer to patient with Ccr less than 50 mL/min.
- Store capsules at controlled room temperature (59° to 86°F). Protect from moisture and light.

Assessment/Interventions
- Obtain patient history, including drug history, and any known allergies. Note history of sulfonamide allergy.
- Ensure that patient has reviewed the *Patient Information* leaflet before starting therapy.
- Ensure that renal function studies are performed before starting therapy and periodically during therapy.
- Have patient increase fluid intake (6 to 8 glasses of water/day) to reduce risk of kidney stones.
- Frequently assess patient for response to treatment. Notify health care provider if seizures do not improve or appear to worsen.
- Ensure that therapy is periodically reviewed to determine if it needs to be continued without change or if a dose change (eg, increase, decrease, discontinuation) is indicated.
- Avoid sudden discontinuation of therapy if possible. Attempt to gradually reduce dose over a period of several weeks if decision to discontinue medication is made.
- Monitor patient for skin rash, fever, hives, sores in the mouth, unusual bruising, or lack of sweating. Notify health care provider immediately if noted.
- Monitor patient for GI, CNS, PSYCH, and general body side effects. Report to health care provider if noted and significant.
- Implement safety precautions for patients who experience dizziness or ataxia.

Patient/Family Education
- Explain name, dose, action, and potential side effects of drug.
- Advise patient to read the *Patient Information* leaflet before starting therapy and with each refill.
- Instruct patient to take exactly as prescribed and not to change the dose or discontinue unless advised by health care provider.
- Advise patient that dose is gradually increased no more often than q 2 wk until max benefit has been obtained.
- Advise patient to swallow capsule whole. Do not chew, crush, or break capsule.
- Advise patient that each dose may be taken without regard to meals but to take with food if stomach upset occurs.
- Warn patient that if a dose is missed not to double up on the next dose.
- Advise patient to increase fluid intake (6 to 8 glasses of water/day) while taking this medication to reduce the risk of kidney stones from forming.
- Advise patient that if medication needs to be discontinued it will be slowly withdrawn over a period of weeks unless safety concerns (eg, rash) require a more rapid withdrawal.
- Caution patient that drug may cause drowsiness and to use caution while driving or performing other tasks requiring mental alertness until tolerance is determined.
- Advise women of childbearing potential to use effective contraception during treatment with zonisamide.

- Advise women to notify health care provider if pregnant, planning to become pregnant, or breastfeeding.
- Instruct patient to contact health care provider immediately if developing a skin rash, sudden back pain, abdominal pain, blood in urine, fever, sore throat, oral ulcers, easy bruising, depression, unusual thoughts, speech or language problems, decreased sweating, or rise in body temperature.
- Instruct parent or caregiver to contact health care provider immediately if a child taking zonisamide is not sweating as usual with or without a fever.
- Instruct patient to inform health care provider if seizures become worse or if new types of seizures occur.
- Advise patient to inform health care provider if experiencing symptoms of depression.
- Advise patient not to take any prescription or OTC medications or dietary supplements unless advised by health care provider.
- Advise patient that laboratory tests and follow-up visits will be required to monitor therapy and to keep appointments.

Appendix

Antihyperlipidemic Combinations

Components of these combination products may include:

Lovastatin:

Lovastatin is an antihyperlipidemic agent and HMG-CoA reductase inhibitor used to reduce elevated cholesterol and LDL cholesterol levels in patients with primary hypercholesterolemia (types IIa and IIb); slow progression of coronary atherosclerosis in patients with coronary heart disease; reduce risk of MI, unstable angina, and coronary revascularization procedures.

Niacin:

Niacin is a vitamin and antihyperlipidemic agent used for the treatment of hyperlipidemia (types IV and V); adjunct to diet for reduction of elevated total and LDL cholesterol levels in patients with primary hypercholesterolemia.

Antihyperlipidemic Combinations		
Trade name	Strength/Ingredient	Dosage
Advicor	500 mg niacin (extended-release); 20 mg lovastatin	Niacin extended-release/lovastatin tablets may be substituted for equivalent doses of niacin extended-release tablets but should not be substituted for other modified- or immediate-release niacin preparations
	750 mg niacin (extended-release); 20 mg lovastatin	
	1000 mg niacin (extended-release); 20 mg lovastatin	

Gastrointestinal Anticholinergic Combinations

GI anticholinergic agents are used primarily to decrease motility (smooth muscle tone) in the GI, biliary, and urinary tracts and for their antisecretory effects.

Combination anticholinergic preparations may include the following components:

Barbiturates, prochlorperazine, hydroxyzine, meprobamate, chlordiazepoxide: These components are used as sedatives and antianxiety agents.

Ergotamine tartrate: Ergotamine tartrate provides inhibition of the sympathetic nervous system.

Antihistamines: Antihistamines are used for antihistaminic effects, sedative, or anticholinergic side effects.

Kaolin: Kaolin is used for its adsorbent properties.

Anticholinergic Combinations		
Trade Name	Strength/Ingredient	Average Dose
Butibel Tablets	15 mg belladonna extract, 15 mg butabarbital sodium	4 to 8 tablets daily
Librax Capsules	2.5 mg clidinium, 5 mg chlordiazepoxide HCl	3 to 8 capsules daily
Butibel Elixir	15 mg belladonna extract, 15 mg butabarbital sodium per 5 mL, 7% alcohol, saccharin	20 to 40 mL/day

Migraine Combinations

Components of these combinations include:

Ergotamine tartrate: Ergotamine tartrate is used for its specific action against migraine.

Caffeine: Caffeine, a cranial vasoconstrictor, is added to ergotamine to enhance vasoconstrictive effects. It may enhance the absorption of ergotamine.

Barbiturates: Barbiturates are used for sedation.

Belladonna alkaloids: Belladonna alkaloids are used for their anticholinergic and antiemetic effects in individuals experiencing excessive nausea and vomiting during attacks.

Migraine Combinations		
Trade Name	Strength/Ingredient	Average Dose
Wigraine Tablets	1 mg ergotamine tartrate, 100 mg caffeine	2 tablets at first sign of attack; follow with 1 tablet q 30 min, if needed Max dose: 6 tablets per attack (do not exceed 10 tablets per wk)
Cafergot Suppository	2 mg ergotamine tartrate, 100 mg caffeine	Max dose: 2 suppositories per attack

Narcotic Analgesic Combinations

Components of these combinations include:

Narcotic analgesics: Codeine, hydrocodone bitartrate, dihydrocodeine bitartrate, opium, oxycodone HCl, oxycodone terephthalate, meperidine HCl, propoxyphene HCl, propoxyphene napsylate.

Nonnarcotic analgesics: Acetaminophen, salicylates, salicylamide. Caffeine, a traditional component of many analgesic formulations, may be beneficial to certain vascular headaches.

Magnesium-aluminum hydroxides and calcium carbonate: Magnesium-aluminum hydroxides and calcium carbonate are used as buffers.

Barbiturates, acetylcarbromal, carbromal, and bromisovalum: Barbiturates, acetylcarbromal, carbromal, and bromisovalum are used for their sedative effects.

Promethazine HCl: Promethazine HCl (a phenothiazine derivative with antihistamine properties) is used for its sedative effect.

Belladonna alkaloids: Belladonna alkaloids are used as an antispasmodic.

Narcotic Analgesic Combinations		
Trade Name	Strength/Ingredient	Average Dose
Alor 5-500 Tablets, *Lortab ASA* Tablets	5 mg hydrocodone bitartrate, 500 mg aspirin	1 or 2 tablets q 4 to 6 hr up to 8 tablets daily
Lortab Elixir	2.5 hydrocodone bitartrate, 167 mg acetaminophen per 5 mL. 7% alcohol, saccharin, sorbitol, sucrose, parabens	15 mL q 4 to 6 hr
Synalgos-DC Capsules	16 mg dihydrocodeine bitartrate, 356.4 mg aspirin, 30 mg caffeine	2 capsules q 4 hr
Percodan-Demi Tablets	2.25 mg oxycodone HCl and 0.19 mg oxycodone terephthalate, 325 mg aspirin	1 or 2 tablets q 6 hr
Percodan Tablets, *Roxiprin* Tablets	4.5 mg oxycodone HCl and 0.38 mg oxycodone terephthalate, 325 mg aspirin	1 tablets q 6 hr

Narcotic Analgesic Combinations

Trade Name	Strength/Ingredient	Average Dose
Darvon Compound-32 Pulvules	32 mg propoxyphene, 389 mg aspirin, 32.4 caffeine	1 tablet q 4 hr
Darvon Compound-65 Pulvules	65 mg propoxyphene, 389 mg aspirin, 32.4 mg caffeine	1 tablet q 4 hr
B & O Supprettes No. 15A Suppositories	30 mg powdered opium, 16.2 mg powdered belladonna extract, polyethylene glycol base	1 or 2 suppositories daily
B & O Supprettes No. 16A Suppositories	60 mg powdered opium, 16.2 mg powdered belladonna extract, polyethylene glycol base	1 or 2 suppositories daily

Nonnarcotic Analgesic Combinations

Components of these combinations include:

Nonnarcotic analgesics: Acetaminophen, salicylates, salsalate, salicylamide.

Barbiturates, meprobamate, and antihistamines: Barbiturates, meprobamate, and antihistamines are used for their sedative effects.

Antacids: Antacids are used to minimize gastric upset from salicylates.

Caffeine: Caffeine, a traditional component of many analgesic formulations, may be beneficial in treating certain vascular headaches.

Belladonna: Belladonna alkaloids are used as antispasmodics.

Pamabrom: Pamabrom is used as a diuretic.

Cinnamedrine: Cinnamedrine, a sympathomimetic amine claimed to have a relaxant effect in the uterus, is used in products for premenstrual syndrome. Its real value has not been established.

Aminobenzoate: Aminobenzoate retards the conjugation of salicylic acid and prolongs the action of salicylates.

Other components listed but not contributing to the analgesic properties of these products include: Calcium gluconate, ipecac, and camphor.

Nonnarcotic Analgesic Combinations

Trade Name	Strength/Ingredient	Average Dose
Micrainin Tablets	325 mg aspirin, 200 mg meprobamate	1 or 2 tablets q 2 to 6 hr
Magsal Tablets	600 mg magnesium salicylate, 25 mg phenyltoloxamine citrate	1 or 2 tablets q 2 to 6 hr
Phrenilin Tablets	325 mg acetaminophen, 50 mg butalbital	1 or 2 tablets or capsules q 2 to 6 hr
Bupap, Phrenilin Forte Capsules, Repan CF, Sedapap Tablets, Tencon	650 mg acetaminophen, 50 mg butalbital	1 or 2 tablets or capsules q 2 to 6 hr

Respiratory Combination Products

These combination products are presented in groups based on the components of their formulations.

Antiasthmatic Combinations:

Antiasthmatic combinations contain xanthine derivatives and sympathomimetics for bronchodilation. Many products also contain expectorants to facilitate mobilization of mucus.

Upper Respiratory Combinations:

Upper respiratory combinations are used primarily for relief of symptoms associated with colds, upper respiratory infections, and allergic conditions (eg, acute rhinitis, sinusitis).

Ingredients:

Antihistamines: Antihistamines are used for symptomatic relief from allergic rhinitis (hay fever) including runny nose, sneezing, itching of the nose or throat, and itchy and watery eyes. The anticholinergic effects of antihistamines may cause a thickening of bronchial secretions; therefore, these agents may be counterproductive in respiratory conditions characterized by congestion. Antihistamines may cause drowsiness.

Xanthines: Xanthines, primarily theophylline, relieve bronchial spasm by direct action on the bronchial smooth muscle in bronchospastic conditions such as asthma and chronic bronchitis. Some xanthine-containing combination products are available OTC, but asthmatic patients should use them only under physician supervision.

Sympathomimetics: Sympathomimetics are used for their vasoconstrictor/decongestant or bronchodilator effects.

Decongestants: Decongestants are used for temporary relief of nasal congestion caused by colds or allergy. Given orally, they are less effective than topical nasal decongestants and have a potential for systemic side effects. Frequent or prolonged topical use may lead to local irritation and rebound congestion.

Bronchodilators: Ephedrine is common in these combinations; however, it stimulates cardiac (β_1) receptors. Bronchodilation is weaker than with the catecholamines: α-adrenergic effects may decrease congestion of mucous membranes. Other β-active agents are effective bronchodilators, but pseudoephedrine is not.

Analgesics: Analgesics (eg, acetaminophen, aspirin, ibuprofen, sodium salicylate) are frequently included for symptoms of headache, fever, muscle aches, and pain.

Anticholinergics: Anticholinergics are included for their drying effects on mucous secretions. This action may be beneficial in acute rhinorrhea; however, drying of respiratory secretions may lead to obstruction. Traditionally, anticholinergics have been avoided in patients with asthma or chronic obstructive pulmonary disease (COPD); however, some patients respond well to these agents. Caution is still advised in this group.

An anticholinergic for oral inhalation is available as a bronchodilator for maintenance of bronchospasm associated with COPD, including chronic bronchitis and emphysema.

Papaverine HCl: Papaverine HCl relaxes the smooth muscle of the bronchial tree.

Barbiturates: Barbiturates are included for their sedative effects as "correctives" in combination with xanthines or sympathomimetics, which may cause CNS stimulation. The sedative efficacy of low doses (eg, 8 mg phenobarbital) is questionable.

Caffeine: Caffeine is included in some combinations for CNS stimulation to counteract antihistamine depression and to enhance concomitant analgesics.

Combination Drugs

Antiasthmatic Combinations		
Trade Name	**Strength/Ingredient**	**Average Dose**
Dyflex-G Tablets	200 mg dyphylline, 200 mg guaifenesin	1 or 2 qid
Dyline G.G. Tablets	200 mg dyphylline, 200 mg guaifenesin	1 tid or qid
Lufyllin-GG Tablets	200 mg dyphylline, 200 mg guaifenesin	1 qid
Theolate Liquid	150 mg theophylline, 90 mg guaifenesin per 15 mL	15 mL q 6 to 8 h
Elixophyllin GG Liquid[1]	100 mg theophylline, 100 mg guaifenesin per 15 mL	3 mg/kg q 8 h
Elixophyllin-KI Elixir[2,3]	80 mg theophylline, 130 mg potassium iodide, per 15 mL, 10% alcohol, sodium bisulfite, anise oil	3 mg/kg q 8 h
Dilor-G Liquid,[1-3] Dyline-GG Liquid[1-3]	300 mg dyphylline, 300 mg guaifenesin per 15 mL	5 or 10 mL tid or qid
Brondelate Elixir	192 mg theophylline (300 mg oxtriphylline), 150 mg guaifenesin per 15 mL, alcohol	10 mL qid

[1] Contains sorbitol.
[2] Contains sucrose.
[3] Contains saccharin.

Upper Respiratory Combinations		
Trade Name	**Strength/Ingredient**	**Average Adult Dose**
Colfed-A Capsules, Deconamine SR Capsules, Deconomed SR Capsules, Kronofed-A Capsules, Time-Hist Capsules	120 mg pseudoephedrine HCl, 8 mg chlorpheniramine maleate	1 q 12 h
Dallergy Jr Capsules[1]	20 mg phenylephrine HCl, 4 mg chlorpheniramine maleate	Children (6 to 12 yr): 1 q 12 h Adults (over 12 yr): 2 q 12 h up to 4/day
Ed A-Hist Tablets	20 mg phenylephrine HCl, 8 mg chlorpheniramine maleate	1 q 12 h
Bromfed Capsules, ULTRAbrom Capsules	120 mg pseudoephedrine HCl, 12 mg brompheniramine maleate	1 q 12 h
Rondec-TR Tablets	120 mg pseudoephedrine HCl, 8 mg carbinoxamine maleate	1 bid
Trinalin Repetabs	120 mg pseudoephedrine sulfate, 1 mg azatadine maleate	1 bid
Bromfenex PD,[1] Lodrane LD Capsules, Respahist Capsules	60 mg pseudoephedrine HCl, 6 mg brompheniramine maleate	1 or 2 q 12 h
Deconamine Tablets, Klerist-D Tablets	60 mg pseudoephedrine HCl, 4 mg chlorpheniramine maleate	1 tid or qid
Semprex-D Capsules	60 mg pseudoephedrine HCl, 8 mg acrivastine	1 q 4 to 6 h up to 4/day
Bromfenex[1]	120 mg pseudoephedrine HCl, 12 mg brompheniramine maleate	1 q 12 h
Drixomed	120 mg pseudoephedrine sulfate, 6 mg dexbrompheniramine maleate	1 q 12 h up to 2/day
Kronofed-A Jr. Capsules, Rescon JR Capsules	60 mg pseudoephedrine HCl, 4 mg chlorpheniramine maleate	Children (6 to 11 yr): 1 q 12 h
Bromfed-PD Capsules, ULTRAbrom PD Capsules	60 mg pseudoephedrine HCl, 6 mg brompheniramine maleate	Children (6 to 12 yr): 1 q 12 h
Rondec-TR[2,3]	8 mg carbinoxamine maleate, 120 mg pseudoephedrine HCl	1 bid
ED-TLC Liquid,[4] Endagen-HD,[4] Vanex HD[4]	5 mg phenylephrine HCl, 2 mg chlorpheniramine maleate, 1.67 mg hydrocodone bitartrate per 5 mL	10 mL tid or qid

Upper Respiratory Combinations

Trade Name	Strength/Ingredient	Average Adult Dose
Brofed Liquid	30 mg pseudoephedrine HCl, 4 mg brompheniramine maleate per 5 mL	10 mL tid
Ed A-Hist Liquid	10 mg phenylephrine HCl, 4 mg chlorpheniramine maleate per 5 mL, 5% alcohol	5 mL tid or qid
AH-chew	10 mg phenylephrine HCl, 2 mg chlorpheniramine maleate, 1.25 mg methscopolamine nitrate	1 or 2 q 4 h
Extendryl Chewable Tablets		2 q 4 h up to 12/day
Extendryl Syrup		10 mL q 4 h up to 40 mL/day
Cardec-S Liquid	60 mg pseudoephedrine HCl, 4 mg carbinoxamine per 5 mL	5 mL qid
Deconamine Syrup	30 mg pseudoephedrine HCl, 2 mg chlorpheniramine maleate per 5 mL	5 to 10 mL tid or qid
Rondec Oral Drops	15 mg pseudoephedrine HCl, 1 mg carbinoxamine maleate per mL	Infants: 0.25 to 1 mL qid
Extendryl S.R. Capsules, OMNIhist L.A. Tablets	20 mg phenylephrine HCl, 8 mg chlorpheniramine, 2.5 mg methscopolamine nitrate	1 q 12 h
Stahist Tablets	25 mg phenylephrine HCl, 40 mg pseudoephedrine, 8 mg chlorpheniramine maleate, 0.19 mg hyoscyamine sulfate, 0.04 mg atropine sulfate, 0.01 mg scopolamine HBr	1 q 12 h
Mescolor Tablets	120 mg pseudoephedrine HCl, 8 mg chlorpheniramine maleate, 2.5 mg methscopolamine nitrate	1 q 12 h up to 2/day
Deconsal II, Defen-LA, Guaifenex PSE 60, Respa-1st	600 mg guaifenesin, 60 mg pseudoephedrine HCl	1 or 2 q 12 h
Duratuss, Entex PSE,[3] Guaifenex PSE 120, Guaimax-D	600 mg guaifenesin, 120 mg pseudoephedrine HCl	1 q 12 h
Nasatab LA	500 mg guaifenesin, 120 mg pseudoephedrine HCl	1 bid
Mytussin DAC Liquid,[1,4-6] Novagest Expectorant w/Codeine Liquid,[4,6]	100 mg guaifenesin, 30 mg pseudoephedrine HCl, 10 mg codeine phosphate per 5 mL	10 mL q 4 h up to 40 mL/day
Dallergy Tablets	10 mg phenylephrine HCl, 4 mg chlorpheniramine maleate, 1.25 mg methscopolamine nitrate	1 q 4 to 6 h up to 4/day
AH-chew Tablets, Extendryl Chewable Tablets	10 mg phenylephrine HCl, 2 mg chlorpheniramine maleate, 1.25 mg methscopolamine nitrate	1 or 2 q 4 h
Extendryl Syrup	10 mg phenylephrine HCl, 2 mg chlorpheniramine maleate, 1.25 mg methscopolamine nitrate	10 mL q 4 h up to 40 mL/day
Dallergy Syrup	10 mg phenylephrine HCl, 2 mg chlorpheniramine maleate, 0.625 mg methscopolamine nitrate	10 mL q 4 to 6 h up to 40 mL/day
Extendryl JR Capsules	10 mg phenylephrine HCl, 4 mg chlorpheniramine maleate, 1.25 mg methscopolamine maleate	Children (6 to 12 yr): 1 q 12 h
Poly-Histine	4 mg phenyltoloxamine, 4 mg pyrilamine, 4 mb pheniramine per 5 mL	Adults and children (at least 12 yr): 10 mL q 4 hr Children (6 to 12 yr): 5 mL q 4 hr Children (2 to 6 yr): 2.5 mL q 4 hr

[1] Contains sucrose.
[2] Contains lactose.
[3] Contains sugar.
[4] Controlled substance.
[5] Contains saccharin.
[6] Contains alcohol.

Orphan Drugs

The Orphan Drug Act defines an orphan drug as a drug or biological product for the diagnosis, treatment, or prevention of a rare disease or condition. A rare disease is one that affects less than 200,000 people in the United States or one that affects greater than 200,000 people but for which there is no reasonable expectation that the cost of developing the drug and making it available will be recovered from sales of that drug in the United States.

The FDA Office of Orphan Products Development (OOPD) provides an information package that includes an overview of the FDA's orphan drug program, a brief description of the orphan products grant program, and a current list of designated orphan products. OOPD's information package also contains a directory sheet listing sources of information about the treatment of rare diseases, patient organizations, and availability of orphan drugs. Requests for the Rare Disease Information Directory or the entire orphan drugs information package may be made by contacting OOPD:

>Office of Orphan Products Development (HF-35)
>Food and Drug Administration
>5600 Fishers Lane
>Rockville, MD 20857
>(301) 827-3666 or (800) 300-7469; fax: (301) 443-4915
>Internet: http://www.fda.gov/orphan/

Those agents that have been approved for marketing or whose specific indication has been approved for marketing are denoted with the footnote a.

Orphan Drugs		
Drug (Trade name)	**Proposed use**	**Sponsor**
(+/-)-7-[3-(4-acetyl-3-methoxy-2-propylphenoxy)-propoxy]-3,4-dihydro-8-propyl-2H-1-benzopyran-2-2 carboxylic acid	To prevent serious adverse events associated with vascular leak syndrome caused by interleukin-2 therapy	BioMedicines
(1S)-1-(9-deazahypoxanthin-9-yl)-1,4-dideoxy-1,4-imino-D-ribitol-hydrochloride	T-cell non-Hodgkin lymphoma	BioCryst Pharm
(4S)-4-ethyl-4-hydroxy-3,14-dioxo-3,4,12,14-tetra-hydro-1-H-pyrano[3?,4?:6,7]-indolizino-]-quinoline-11-carbaldehyde O-(tert-butyl)-(E)-oxime (*Gimatecan*)	Malignant glioma	Sigma-Tau Res
[5,10,15,20-tetrakis(1,3-diethylimidazolium-2-yl)-porphyrinato] manganese(III)pentachloride	Amyotrophic lateral sclerosis	Aeolus Pharm
1,1'-[1,4-phenylenebis-(methylane]-bis-1,4,8,11-tetraazacyclotetradecan	With filgrastim to improve the yield of progentor cells in the apheresis product for subsequent stem cell transplantation following myelosuppressive or myeloablative chemotherapy	AnorMED
1,5-(Butylimino)-1,5 dideoxy,D-glucitol	Fabry disease	Oxford GlycoSciences
1-(11-dodecylamino-10-hydroxyundecyl)-3-7-dimethylxanthine hydrogen methanesulfonate	Hormone refractory prostate carcinoma	Cell Therapeutics
[111]Indium pentetreotide (*SomatoTher*)	Somatostatin receptor-positive neuroendocrine tumors	Louisiana State Univ Medical Center Foundation
166Ho-DOTMP	Multiple myeloma	NeoRx
2'-3'-dideoxyadenosine	AIDS	National Cancer Inst
2',3',5'-tri-o-acetyluridine	Mitochondrial disease	Repigen
2'-deoxycytidine	Host-protective agent in acute myelogenous leukemia	Steven Grant, MD

Orphan Drugs

Drug (Trade name)	Proposed use	Sponsor
2-0-Butyryl-1-0-octyl-myo-inositol 3,4,5,6-tetrakisphosphate	Cystic fibrosis	Inologic
2-0-desulfated heparin (Aeropin)	Cystic fibrosis	Kennedy and Hoidal, MDs
2-(3-diethylaminopropyl)-3,8-dipropyl-2-azaspiro[4,5]-decan dimaleate (Atiprimod)	Multiple myeloma and associated bone resorption	Callisto Pharm
24,25 dihydroxycholecalciferol	Uremic osteodystrophy	Lemmon
2-chloroethyl-3-sarcosinamide-1-nitrosourea (Sarmustine)	Malignant glioma	Pangene
		Lawrence Panasci, MD
2-methoxyestradiol (Panzem)	Multiple myeloma	EntreMed
3-(3,5-dimethyl-1H-2ylmethylene)-1,3-dihydro-indol-2-one	Kaposi sarcoma; von Hippel-Lindau disease	Sugen
3,4-diaminopyridine	Lambert-Eaton myasthenic syndrome	Jacobus Pharm
3-(4′aminoisoindoline-1′-one)-1-piperidine-2,6-dione (CC-5013) (Revimid)	Multiple myeloma; myelodysplastic syndromes	Celgene
3,5,3′-triiodothyroacetate	Well-differentiated papillary, follicular, or combined papillary/follicular carcinomas of the thyroid gland	Elliot Danforth Jr., MD
3′-azido-2′,3′dideoxyuridine (AZDU)	AIDS	Berlex Labs
4,5-dibromorhodamine 123 (Theralux Irradiation Device)	Chronic myelogenous leukemia	Celmed BioSciences
4-aminosalicylic acid	Mild to moderate ulcerative colitis in patients intolerant to sulfasalazine	Warren Beeken, MD
(Pamisyl)		Parke-Davis
(Rezipas)		Squibb
40SD02	Chronic iron overload resulting from conventional transfusional treatment of beta-thalassemia major and sickle cell anemia	Biomedical Frontiers
5,5′,5′′-[Phosphinothioyli-dyne tris(imino-2,1-ethanediyl)]tris[5-methyl-chelidoninium]trihydroide hexahydrochloride	Pancreatic cancer	Now Pharm AG
5,6-dihydro-5-azacytidine	Malignant mesothelioma	ILEX Oncology
506U78	Chronic lymphocytic leukemia	GlaxoSmithKline
5a8, monoclonal antibody to CD4	Postexposure prophylaxis for occupational exposure to human immunodeficiency virus (HIV)	Biogen
5-aza-2′-deoxycytidine	Acute leukemia	SuperGen
6-hydroxymethylacylfulvene	Histologically confirmed advanced or metastatic pancreatic cancer	MGI Pharma
8-cyclopentyl 1,3-dipropylxanthine	Cystic fibrosis	SciClone Pharm
8-methoxsalen (Uvadex)	In conjunction with the UVAR photopheresis system to treat diffuse systemic sclerosis; to prevent acute rejection of cardiac allografts	Therakos
9-cis retinoic acid (Panretin)	To prevent retinal detachment caused by proliferative vitreoretinopathy	Allergan
	Acute promyelocytic leukemia	Ligand Pharm
9-nitro-20-(S)-camptothecin (Camvirex)	Pancreatic cancer	SuperGen
	Pediatric HIV infection/AIDS	NovoMed Pharm

Orphan Drugs

Drug (Trade name)	Proposed use	Sponsor
90Y-hPAMA4 (PAN-Cide)	Pancreatic cancer	Immunomedics
a-(3-aminophthalimido) glutaramide (Actimid[a])	Multiple myeloma	Celgene
Abetimus	Lupus nephritis	La Jolla Pharm
ACA125	Epithelial ovarian cancer	CellControl Biomedical Labs
Acetylcysteine (Acetadote)[a]	IV treatment for moderate to severe acetaminophen overdose	Ligand
(Mucomyst/Mucomyst 10 IV)		Bristol-Myers Squibb
Acid sphingomyelinase	Niemann-Pick disease type B	Genzyme
Aconiazide	Tuberculosis	Lincoln Diagnostics
Adeno-associated viral-based vector cystic fibrosis gene therapy	Cystic fibrosis	Targeted Genetics
Adeno-associated viral vector containing the gene for human coagulation Factor IX (Coagulin-B)	Intrahepatic and IM treatment of moderate to severe hemophilia	Avigen
Adenosine	With BCNU (carmustine) in the treatment of brain tumors	Medco Res
Adenovirus-based vector Factor VIII complementary DNA to somatic cells (MiniAdFVIII)	Hemophilia A	GenStar Therapeutics
Adenovirus-mediated herpes simplex virus-thymidine kinase gene	With gancyclovir in the treatment of malignant glioma	Ark Therapeutics Ltd
Aerosolized pooled immune globulin	Respiratory syncytial virus lower respiratory tract disease	Pediatric Pharm
α-Galactosidase A (Plant-Produced Human α-Galactosidase)	Fabry disease	Large Scale Biology
AI-RSA	Autoimmune uveitis	Autoimmune
Albendazole (Albenza)	Hydatid disease (cystic echinococcosis caused by *Echinococcus granulosus* larvae or alveolar echinococcosis caused by *E. multilocularis* larvae);[a] neurocysticercosis caused by *Taenia solium* as: 1) Chemotherapy of parenchymal, subarachnoidal, and racemose (cysts in spinal fluid) neurocysticercosis in symptomatic cases and 2) prophylaxis of epilepsy and other sequelae in asymptomatic neurocysticercosis[a]	SmithKline Beecham
Albuterol	To prevent paralysis caused by spinal cord injury	MotoGen
Aldesleukin (Proleukin)	Metastatic renal cell carcinoma[a]; metastatic melanoma[a]; primary immunodeficiency disease associated with T-cell defects; acute myelogenous leukemia; non-Hodgkin lymphoma	Chiron
Alemtuzumab (Campath)	Chronic lymphocytic leukemia[a]	Millennium and ILEX Partners, LP
Alendronate (Fosamax)	Osteogenesis imperfecta in pediatric patients 4 years of age and older	Merck
Alendronate disodium (Fosamax)	Bone manifestations of Gaucher disease	Richard J. Wenstrup, MD
Alglucerase injection (Ceredase)	Replacement therapy in Gaucher disease type I,[a] II, and III	Genzyme
Alitretinoin (Panretin)	Topical treatment of cutaneous lesions in AIDS-related Kaposi sarcoma[a]	Ligand Pharm
Allantoin (Alwextin)	Skin blistering and erosions associated with inherited epidermolysis bullosa	Alwyn Co.

Orphan Drugs

Drug (Trade name)	Proposed use	Sponsor
Allogeneic human retinal pigment epithelial cells on gelatin microcarriers (Spheramine)	Hoehn and Yahr stage 3 and 4 Parkinson disease	Titan Pharm
Allogeneic peripheral blood mononuclear cells (sensitized against patient alloantigens by mixed lymphocyte culture) (CYTOIMPLANT)	Pancreatic cancer	Applied Immunothera-
Allogenic thymic tissue for transplantation, cultured, partially T-cell depleted	Therapy for primary immune deficiency resulting from athymia associated with complete DiGeorge syndrome	Duke University Medical Center
Allopurinol riboside	Chagas disease; cutaneous and visceral leishmaniasis	Burroughs Wellcome
Allopurinol sodium (Aloprim for Injection)	Ex-vivo preservation of cadaveric kidneys for transplantation	Burroughs Wellcome
	Management of patients with leukemia, lymphoma, and solid tumor malignancies who are receiving cancer therapy that causes elevations of serum and urinary uric acid levels and who cannot tolerate oral therapy[a]	Catalytica Pharm
Alpha-1-antitrypsin (recombinant DNA origin)	Supplementation therapy for alpha-1-antitrypsin deficiency in the ZZ phenotype population	Chiron
Alpha$_1$-proteinase inhibitor (human) (Prolastin)	To slow the progression of emphysema in alpha$_1$-antitrypsin deficient patients	Aventis Behring LLC
	Replacement therapy in the alpha$_1$-proteinase inhibitor congenital deficiency state[a]	Bayer
Alpha-galactosidase A (CC-Galactosidase)	Alpha-galactosidase A deficiency (Fabry disease)	Orphan Medical
(Fabrase)	Fabry disease	Robert J. Desnick, MD
(Replagal)	Long-term enzyme replacement therapy for treatment of Fabry disease	Transkaryotic Therapies
Alpha-melanocyte stimulating hormone	To prevent and treat intrinsic acute renal failure caused by ischemia	National Institute of Diabetes, and Digestive and Kidney Diseases
Alprostadil	For severe peripheral arterial occlusive disease (critical limb ischemia) when other procedures, grafts, or angioplasty are not indicated	Schwarz Pharma
Alteplase (Activase)	Intraventricular hemorrhage associated with intracerebral hemorrhage	Daniel F. Hanley, MD
Altretamine (Hexalen)	Advanced ovarian adenocarcinoma[a]	Medimmune Oncology
AMG 531	Immune thrombocytopenic purpura	Amgen
Amifostine (Ethyol)	To reduce the incidence of moderate to severe xerostomia in postoperative radiation treatment for head and neck cancer[a]; to reduce the incidence and severity of toxicities associated with cisplatin administration; myelodysplastic syndromes; chemoprotective agent for the following: Cisplatin in metastatic melanoma, cisplatin in advanced ovarian carcinoma,[a] cyclophosphamide in advanced ovarian carcinoma	MedImmune Oncology
Amiloride HCl solution for inhalation	Cystic fibrosis	GlaxoWellcome R&D
Aminocaproic acid (Caprogel)	Topical treatment of traumatic hyphema of the eye	Eastern Virginia Medical
Aminosalicylate sodium	Crohn disease	Syncom Pharm
Aminosalicylic acid (Paser Granules)	Tuberculosis infections[a]	Jacobus Pharm

Orphan Drugs

Drug (Trade name)	Proposed use	Sponsor
Aminosidine (*Gabbromicina*)	Tuberculosis; *Mycobacterium avium* complex	Thomas P. Kanyok,
(*Paromomycin*)	Visceral leishmaniasis (kala-azar)	
Amiodarone (*Amio-Aqueous*)	Incessant ventricular tachycardia	Academic Pharm
Amiodarone HCl (*Cordarone*)	Acute treatment and prophylaxis of life-threatening ventricular tachycardia or ventricular fibrillation[a]	Wyeth-Ayerst Labs
Ammonium tetrathiomolybdate	Wilson disease	George J. Brewer, MD
Amphotericin B lipid complex (*Abelcet*)	Invasive prototheocosis, sporotrichosis, coccidioidomycosis, zygomycosis, and candidiasis; invasive fungal infections[a]	Liposome
Amsacrine (*Amsidyl*)	Acute adult leukemia	Warner-Lambert
Anagrelide (*Agrylin*)	Polycythemia vera; essential thrombocythemia[a]; thrombocytosis in chronic myelogenous leukemia	Roberts Pharm
Ananain, comosain (*Vianain*)	Enzymatic debridement of severe burns	Genzyme
Anaritide acetate (*Auriculin*)	Acute renal failure; improvement of early renal allograft function following renal transplantation	Scios
Ancestim (*Stemgen*)	With filgrastim to decrease the number of phereses required to collect peripheral blood progenitor cells capable of providing rapid multilineage hematopoietic reconstitution following myelosuppressive or myeloablative therapy	Amgen
Ancrod (*Viprinex*)	To establish and maintain anticoagulation in heparin-intolerant patients undergoing cardiopulmonary bypass	Knoll Pharm
Angiotensin 1-7 (*MARstem*)	Neutropenia associated with autologous bone marrow transplantation; myelodysplastic syndrome	Maret Pharm
Anti pan T lymphocyte monoclonal antibody (*Anti-t Lymphocyte Immunotoxin Xmmly-h65-rta*)	In-vivo treatment of bone marrow recipients to prevent graft rejection and graft vs host disease; ex-vivo treatment to eliminate mature T-cells from potential bone marrow grafts	Xoma
Antiangiogenic components extracted from marine cartilage (*Neovastat [AE-941]*)	Renal cell carcinoma	AEterna Labs
Anti-CD23 IgG1, kappa monoclonal antibody	Chronic lymphocytic leukemia	IDEC Pharm
Anti-CD45 monoclonal antibodies	To prevent acute graft rejection of human organ transplants	Baxter Healthcare
Anti-CEA Sheep-human chimeric monoclonal antibody labeled w/iodine-131 (*KAb201*)	Pancreatic cancer	KS Biomedix Ltd
Anti-cytomegalovirus monoclonal antibodies	To prevent/treat human cytomegalovirus infection in bone marrow and organ transplantation and in AIDS	Biomedical Res Inst
Antiepilepsirine	Drug-resistant generalized tonic-clonic epilepsy in children and adults	Children's Hospital, Columbus, OH
Antihemophilic factor (human) (*Alphanate*)	von Willebrand disease	Alpha Therapeutic
Antihemophilic factor (recombinant) (*Kogenate*)	Prophylaxis/Treatment of bleeding in hemophilia A[a] or for prophylaxis when surgery is required in these patients[a]	Bayer

Orphan Drugs

Drug (Trade name)	Proposed use	Sponsor
(ReFacto)	To control/prevent hemorrhagic episodes; for surgical prophylaxis in patients with hemophilia A (congenital factor VIII deficiency or classic hemophilia)	Genetics Institute
Antihemophilic factor/von Willebrand factor complex (human), dried, pasteurized (Humate-P)	To treat/prevent bleeding in hemophilia A (classical hemophilia) in adult patients; treat spontaneous and trauma-induced bleeding episodes in severe von Willebrand disease, and in mild to moderate von Willebrand disease where use of desmopressin is known or suspected to be inadequate in adult and pediatric patients[a]	Aventis Behring LLC
Anti-interferon-gamma Fab from goats	Immunologic corneal allograft rejection	Advanced Biotherapy
Antimelanoma antibody XMMME-001-DTPA 111 Indium (Antimelanoma Antibody XMMME-001-DTPA 111 Indium)	Diagnostic use in imaging systemic and nodal melanoma metastasis	Xoma
Antimelanoma antibody XMMME-001-RTA (Antimelanoma Antibody XMMME-001-RTA)	Stage III melanoma not amenable to surgical resection	Xoma
Antipyrine test	For use as an index of hepatic drug metabolizing capacity	Upsher-Smith Labs
Antisense 20-mer phosphorothioate oligonucleotide [complementary to the coding region of R2 component of the human ribonucleotide reductase mRNA] (GTI-2040)	Renal cell carcinoma	Lorus Therapeutics
Anti-tap-72 immunotoxin (Xomazyme-791)	Metastatic colorectal adenocarcinoma	Xoma
Antithrombin III (human) (Antithrombin III human)	To prevent/arrest episodes of thrombosis in congenital AT-III deficiency and/or to prevent the occurrence of thrombosis in AT-III deficiency who have undergone trauma or who are about to undergo surgery or parturition	American National Red Cross
(ATnativ)	Hereditary antithrombin III deficiency in connection with surgical or obstetrical procedures or thromboembolism[a]	Pharmacia & Upjohn AB
(Thrombate III)	Replacement therapy in congenital deficiency of AT-III to prevent and treat thrombosis and pulmonary emboli[a]	Bayer
Antithrombin III (human) concentrate IV (Kybernin P)	Prophylaxis/Treatment of thromboembolic episodes in genetic AT-III deficiency	Aventis Behring LLC
Anti-thymocyte globulin (Rabbit) (Thymoglobulin)	Myelodysplastic syndrome (MDS)	SangStat Medical
Anti-thymocyte serum (Nashville Rabbit Antithymocyte Serum)	Allograft rejection, including solid organ (kidney, liver, heart, lung, pancreas) and bone marrow transplantation	Applied Medical Res
Antivenin crotaline (pit-viper) equine immune F(ab)2 (Antivipmyn)	Envenomation by Crotaline snakes	Rare Disease Therapeutics
Antivenin crotalidae polyvalent immune Fab (ovine) (CroFab)	Envenomations inflicted by North American crotalid snakes[a]	Protherics
Antivenom (crotalidae) purified (avian)	Envenomation by poisonous snakes belonging to the Crotalidae family	Ophidian Pharm
AP1903	Acute graft vs host disease in patients undergoing bone marrow transplantation	Ariad Gene Therapeutics

Orphan Drugs

Drug (Trade name)	Proposed use	Sponsor
APL 400-020 V-Beta DNA vaccine	Cutaneous T-cell lymphoma	Wyeth-Lederle Vaccines & Pediatrics
Apomorphine	Treatment of the on-off fluctuations associated with late-stage Parkinson disease	Pentech Pharm
	Rescue treatment for early morning motor dysfunction in late-stage Parkinson disease	Scherer DDS
Apomorphine HCl (*Apokyn*)	Treatment of the on-off fluctuations associated with late-stage Parkinson disease	Mylan
Aprotinin (*Trasylol*)	Prophylaxis to reduce perioperative blood loss and the homologous blood transfusion requirement in patients undergoing cardiopulmonary bypass surgery in the course of repeat coronary artery bypass graft (CABG) surgery, and in selected cases of primary CABG surgery when the risk of bleeding is especially high (impaired hemostasis), or where transfusion is unavailable or unacceptable[a]	Bayer
Arcitumomab (*99m Tc-labeled CEA-Scan*)	Diagnosis and localization of primary, residual, recurrent, and metastatic medullary thyroid carcinoma	Immunomedics
Arginine butyrate	Beta-hemoglobinopathies and beta-thalassemia	Susan P. Perrine, MD
	Sickle cell disease and beta-thalassemia	Vertex Pharm
Arsenic trioxide (*Trisenox*)	Acute promyelocytic leukemia[a]; chronic myeloid leukemia; multiple myeloma; myelodysplastic syndrome; acute myelocytic leukemia subtypes M0, M1, M2, M4, M5, M6, and M7; chronic lymphocytic leukemia; liver cancer	Cell Therapeutics
Artesunate	Malaria	World Health Organization
As-101	AIDS	NPDC-AS101
AT1001	Fabry disease	Amicus Therapeutics
Atomoxetine HCl (*Strattera*)	Tourette syndrome	Eli Lilly
Atovaquone (*Mepron*)	AIDS-associated *Pneumocystis carinii* pneumonia (PCP)[a]; to prevent PCP in high-risk, HIV-infected patients (defined by ≥ 1 episode of PCP and/or a peripheral CD4+ lymphocyte count ≤ 200/mm^3)[a]; treatment and suppression of *Toxoplasma gondii* encephalitis; primary prophylaxis of HIV-infected people at high risk for developing *T. gondii* encephalitis	GlaxoWellcome GlaxoWellcome R & D
Augmerosen (*Genasense*)	Multiple myeloma; acute myelocytic leukemia; chronic lymphocytic leukemia	Genta
Autologous antigen presenting cells pulsed with autologous tumor Ig idiotype (*Mylovenge*)	Multiple myeloma	Dendreon
Autologous dendritic cells pulsed with autologous glioblastoma multiforme acid-eluted tumor antigens (*DCVax-Brain*)	Glioblastoma multiforme	Northwest Biotherapeutics
Autologous DNP-conjugated tumor vaccine (*M-Vax*)	Adjuvant therapy in melanoma patients with surgically resectable lymph node metastasis (stage III and limited stage IV disease)	Avax Technologies
Autologous tumor-derived gp96 heat shock protein-peptide complex (*Oncophage*)	Renal cell carcinoma; metastatic melanoma	Antigenics
Autolymphocyte therapy	Renal cell carcinoma	Cytogen
Azacitadine	Myelodysplastic syndromes	Pharmion
Azathioprine (*Imuran*)	Oral manifestations of graft vs host disease	Oral Solutions

Orphan Drugs

Drug (Trade name)	Proposed use	Sponsor
Aztreonam	Inhalation therapy for control of gram-negative bacteria in the respiratory tract with cystic fibrosis	Corus Pharma
B lymphocyte stimulator (BLyS)	Common variable immunodeficiency	Human Genome Sciences
Bacitracin (Altracin)	Antibiotic-associated pseudomembranous enterocolitis caused by toxins A and B elaborated by Clostridium difficile	AL Labs
Baclofen (Lioresal Intrathecal)	Intractable spasticity caused by multiple sclerosis or spinal cord injury	Infusaid
	Intractable spasticity caused by spinal cord injury, multiple sclerosis, and other spinal diseases (eg, spinal ischemia, spinal tumor, transverse myelitis, cervical spondylosis, degenerative myelopathy)[a]; spasticity associated with cerebral palsy	Medtronic
	Dystonia	Medronic Neurological
Basiliximab (Simulect)	Prophylaxis of solid organ rejection[a]	Novartis
Beclomethasone 17,21-dipropionate	To prevent GI graft vs host disease	Enteron Pharm
Beclomethasone dipropicnate	Oral administration for intestinal graft vs host disease	George B. McDonald, MD
Benzoate and phenylacetate (Ucephan)	Adjunctive therapy to prevent/treat hyperammonemia in patients with urea cycle enzymopathy caused by carbamylphosphate synthetase, ornithine, transcarbamylase, or argininosuccinate synthetase deficiency[a]	Immunex
Benzoate/Phenylacetate (Ammonul)	Acute hyperammonemia and associated encephalopathy in patients with deficiencies in enzymes of the urea cycle	Medicis Pharm
Benzophenone-3, octylmethoxycinnamate, avobenzone, titanium dioxide, zinc oxide (Total Block VL SPF 75)	To prevent visible light-induced skin photosensitivity as a result of porfimer sodium photodynamic therapy	Fallien Cosmeceuticals Ltd
Benzydamine HCl (Tantum)	Prophylactic treatment of oral mucositis resulting from radiation therapy for head and neck cancer	Angelini Pharm
Benzylpenicillin, benzylpenicilloic, benzylpenilloic acid (Pre-Pen/MDM)	To assess risk of penicillin administration when it is the preferred drug of choice in adult patients who have previously received penicillin and in adults who have a history of clinical penicillin sensitivity	Hollister-Stier Labs LLC
Beractant (Survanta Intratracheal Suspension)	To prevent/treat neonatal respiratory distress syndrome (RDS)[a]; for full-term newborns with respiratory failure caused by meconium aspiration syndrome, persistent pulmonary hypertension of the newborn, or pneumonia and sepsis	Ross
Beraprost	Pulmonary arterial hypertension associated with any New York Heart Association classification (class I, II, III, or IV)	United Therapeutics
Beta alethine (Betathine)	Multiple myeloma; metastatic melanoma	Dovetail Tech
Betaine (Cystadane)	Homocystinuria[a]	Orphan Medical
Bethandidine sulfate	To prevent recurrence of primary ventricular fibrillation; treat primary ventricular fibrillation	Medco Res
Bexarotene (Targretin)	Cutaneous manifestations of cutaneous T-cell lymphoma in patients who are refractory to ≥ 1 prior systemic therapy[a]	Ligand Pharm
Bifidobacterium longum infantis 35624	Pediatric Crohn disease	Alimentary Health Ltd
Bindarit	Lupus nephritis	Angelini Pharm

Orphan Drugs

Drug (Trade name)	Proposed use	Sponsor
Bioartificial liver system utilizing xenogenic hepatocytes in a hollow fiber bioreactor cartridge (BAL)	In acute liver failure presenting with encephalopathy deteriorating beyond Parson grade 2	Excorp Medical
Bis(4-fluorophenyl)phenylacetamide	Sickle cell disease	ICAgen
Bleomycin (Blenoxane)	Pancreatic cancer	Genetronics
Bleomycin sulfate (Blenoxane)	Malignant pleural effusion[a]	Bristol-Myers Squibb Pharm Res Inst
BMY-45622	Ovarian cancer	Bristol-Myers Squibb
Bortezomib (Velcade)	Multiple myeloma[a]	Millennium Pharm
Bosentan (Tracleer)	Pulmonary arterial hypertension[a]	Actelion Life Sciences
Botulinum toxin type A	Synkinetic closure of the eyelid associated with VII cranial nerve aberrant regeneration	Botulinim Toxin Res
(Botox)	Blepharospasm and strabismus associated with dystonia in adults ≥ 12 years of age[a]; cervical dystonia[a]; dynamic muscle contracture in pediatric cerebral palsy	Allergan
(Dysport)	Spasmodic torticollis (cervical dystonia); dynamic muscle contractures in pediatric cerebral palsy; essential blepharospasm	Ipsen Limited
Botulinum toxin type B (NeuroBloc)	Cervical dystonia[a]	Elan Pharm
Botulinum toxin type F	Spasmodic torticollis (cervical dystonia); essential blepharospasm	Ipsen Limited
Botulism immune globulin (BabyBIG)	Infant botulism[a]	CA Dept Health Services
Bovine colostrum	AIDS-related diarrhea	Donald Hastings, DVM
Bovine immunoglobulin concentrate, Cryptosporidium parvum (Sporidin-G)	Treatment and symptomatic relief of Cryptosporidium parvum infection of the GI tract in immunocompromised patients	GalaGen
Bovine whey protein concentrate (Immuno-C)	Cryptosporidiosis caused by Cryptosporidium parvum in the GI tract of patients who are immunodeficient/immunocompromised or immunocompetent	Biomune Systems
Branched chain amino acids	Amyotrophic lateral sclerosis	Mount Sinai Medical Center
Brimonidine (Alphagan)	Anterior ischemic optic neuropathy	Allergan
Bromhexine (Bisolvon)	Mild to moderate keratoconjunctivitis sicca in Sjogren syndrome	Boehringer Ingelheim
Broxuridine (Broxine/Neomark)	Radiation sensitizer in the treatment of primary brain tumors	NeoPharm
Bryostatin-1	With paclitaxel in the treatment of esophageal cancer	GPC Biotech
Buffered intrathecal electrolyte/dextrose injection (Elliotts B Solution)	Diluent in intrathecal administration of methotrexate and cytarabine for prevention or treatment of meningeal leukemia or lymphocytic lymphoma[a]	Orphan Medical
Buprenorphine HCl (Subutex)	Opiate addictions in opiate users[a]	Reckitt Benckiser Pharm
Buprenorphine in combination with naloxone (Suboxone)	Opiate addiction in opiate users[a]	Reckitt Benckiser Pharm
Busulfan (Busulfex)	Preparative therapy in the treatment of malignancies with bone marrow transplantation[a]	Orphan Medical
(Partaject)	Preparative therapy for pediatric patients undergoing bone marrow transplantation	SuperGen

Orphan Drugs

Drug (Trade name)	Proposed use	Sponsor
(Spartaject)	Preparative therapy for malignancies treated with bone marrow transplantation	Sparta Pharm
	Primary brain malignancies	SuperGen
(Spartaject-Busulfan)	Intrathecal therapy for neoplastic meningitis	SuperGen
Butyrylcholinesterase	Reduction and clearance of toxic blood levels of cocaine encountered during a drug overdose; postsurgical apnea	Shire Labs
BW 12C	Sickle cell disease	Burroughs Wellcome
C1 esterase inhibitor (human)	To prevent and treat angioedema caused by C1-esterase inhibitor deficiency	Alpha Therapeutic
C1-esterase inhibitor, human, pasteurized (Berinert P)	To prevent and/or treat acute attacks of hereditary angioedema	Aventis Behring LLC
C1-inhibitor (C1-Inhibitor [human] Vapor Heated, Immuno)	To treat acute attacks of angioedema; to prevent acute attacks of angioedema, including short-term prophylaxis for patients requiring dental or other surgical procedures	Baxter Healthcare
Caffeine (Cafcit)	Apnea of prematurity[a]	OPR Development, LP
Calcitonin-human for injection (Cibacalcin)	Symptomatic Paget disease (osteitis deformans)[a]	Novartis
Calcitonin-salmon nasal spray (Miacalcin Nasal Spray)	Symptomatic Paget disease (osteitis deformans)	Sandoz Pharm
Calcium acetate (Phos-Lo)	Hyperphosphatemia in end-stage renal disease	Pharmedic
	Hyperphosphatemia in end-stage renal failure[a]	Braintree Labs
Calcium carbonate (R & D Calcium Carbonate/600)	Hyperphosphatemia in end-stage renal disease	R & D Labs
Calcium gluconate (Calgonate)	A wash for hydrofluoric acid spills on human skin	Calgonate
Calcium gluconate gel (H-F Gel)	Emergency topical treatment of hydrogen fluoride (hydrofluoric acid) burns	LTR Pharm
Calcium gluconate gel 2.5%	Emergency topical treatment of hydrogen fluoride (hydrofluoric acid) burns	Paddock Labs
Calfactant (Infasurf)	Acute respiratory distress syndrome	ONY
Capsaicin	Painful HIV-associated neuropathy; erythromelalgia	NeurogesX
Carbamic acid,[[4-[[3-[[4-[1 (4-hydroxyphenyl)-1-methylethyl]phenoxy]methyl]phenyl]methoxy]-phenyl]-iminomethyl]-,ethyl ester	Management of cystic fibrosis	Boeringer Ingelheim
Carbamylglutamic acid	N-acetylglutamate synthetase deficiency	Orphan Europe
Carbovir	AIDS and symptomatic HIV infection with CD4 count less than 200/mm^3	GlaxoWellcome
Carboxypeptidase G2	To treat patients at risk of methotrexate toxicity	Protherics
Carmustine	Intracranial malignancies	Direct Therapeutics
Cascara sagrada fluid extract	For oral drug overdosage to speed lower bowel evacuation	Intramed
CD4 human truncated 369 AA polypeptide (Soluble T4)	AIDS	SmithKline Beecham
CD5-T lymphocyte immunotoxin (Xomazyme-H65)	Graft vs host disease and/or rejection in bone marrow transplant recipients	Xoma
CDP571	Crohn disease	Celltech Chiroscience Ltd

Orphan Drugs

Drug (Trade name)	Proposed use	Sponsor
Cells produced using the AastromReplicelle System and SC-I Therapy Kit	For patients receiving high-dose chemotherapy who are unable to generate an acceptable dose of peripheral blood stem cells and have a sufficient bone marrow aspirate without morphological evidence of tumor	Aastrom Biosciences
Centruroides immune F(ab)2 (Alacramyn)	Scorpion envenomations requiring medical attention	Silanes Labs SA de CV
Ceramide trihexosidase/ alpha-galactosidase A (Fabrazyme)	Fabry disease[a]	Genzyme
Cetiedil citrate injection	Sickle cell disease crisis	Baker Cummins Pharm
Cetuximab	Squamous cell cancer of the head and neck in patients who express epidermal growth factor receptor	ImClone Systems
Chenodeoxycholic acid (Chenofalk)	Cerebrotendinous xanthomatosis	Dr. Falk Pharma GmbH
Chenodiol (Chenix)	Radiolucent stones in well-opacifying gallbladders where elective surgery would be undertaken except for presence of increased surgical risk caused by systemic disease or age[a]	Solvay
Chimeric (human-murine) G250 IgG monoclonal antibody	Renal cell carcinoma	Wilex Biotechnology GmbH
Chimeric, humanized monoclonal antibody to Staphylococcus	Prophylaxis of *Staphylococcus epidermidis* sepsis in low birth weight (≤ 1500 g) infants	Biosynexus
Chimeric M-T412 (human-murine) IgG monoclonal anti-CD4	Multiple sclerosis	Centocor
Chlorhexidine gluconate mouth rinse (Peridex)	Amelioration of oral mucositis associated with cytoreductive therapy used in conditioning patients for bone marrow transplantation therapy	Procter & Gamble
Cholic acid (3 alpha, 7 alpha, 12 alpha trihydroxy 5-beta cholanolic acid) (Falkochol)	Inborn errors of cholesterol and bile acid synthesis and metabolism	Dr. Falk Pharma GmbH
Choline chloride (Intrachol)	Choline deficiency (specifically the choline deficiency, hepatic steatosis, and cholestasis associated with long-term parenteral nutrition)	Orphan Medical
Chondrocyte-alginate gel suspension	To correct vesicoureteral reflux in the pediatric population	Curis
Chondroitinase	Patients undergoing vitrectomy	Bausch & Lomb
Ciliary neurotrophic factor	Amyotrophic lateral sclerosis	Regeneron Pharm
Ciliary neurotrophic factor, recombinant human	Motor neuron disease (including amyotrophic lateral sclerosis, progressive muscular atrophy, progressive bulbar palsy, and primary lateral sclerosis); spinal muscular atrophies	Syntex-Synergen Neuroscience
Cinacalcet	Hypercalcemia in patients with parathyroid carcinoma	Amgen
Cisplatin/Epinephrine (IntraDose)	Metastatic malignant melanoma; squamous cell carcinoma of the head and neck	Matrix Pharm
Citric acid, glucono-delta-lactone, and magnesium carbonate (Renacidin Irrigation)	Renal and bladder calculi of the apatite or struvite variety[a]	United-Guardian
Civamide (Zucapsaicin)	Postherpetic neuralgia of the trigeminal nerve	Winston Labs
Cladribine (Leustatin Injection)	Hairy-cell leukemia[a]; chronic lymphocytic leukemia; non-Hodgkin lymphoma; acute myeloid leukemia	RW Johnson Pharm Res Inst
(Mylinax)	Chronic progressive multiple sclerosis	
Clindamycin (Cleocin)	To treat and prevent *Pneumocystis carinii* pneumonia associated with AIDS	Pharmacia & Upjohn Pfizer

Orphan Drugs

Drug (Trade name)	Proposed use	Sponsor
Clofarabine (Clofarex)	Acute lymphoblastic and myelogenous leukemia	Ilex Products
Clofazimine (Lamprene)	Lepromatous leprosy, including dapsone-resistant lepromatous leprosy and lepromatous leprosy complicated by erythema nodosum leprosum[a]	Novartis
Clonazepam (Klonopin)	Hyperekplexia (startle disease)	Hoffmann-La Roche
Clonidine (Duraclon)	For continuous epidural administration as adjunctive therapy with intraspinal opiates for pain in cancer patients tolerant or unresponsive to intraspinal opiates[a]	Roxane Labs
Clostridial collagenase	Advanced (involutional or residual stage) Dupuytren disease	L. Hurst, MD and
Clotrimazole	Sickle cell disease	Carlo Brugnara, MD
Coagulation factor VIIa (recombinant) (NovoSeven)	Bleeding episodes in hemophilia A or B patients with inhibitors to Factor VIII or Factor IX[a]	Novo Nordisk
Coagulation factor IX (Mononine)	Replacement treatment and prophylaxis of hemorrhagic complications of hemophilia B[a]	Armour Pharm
Coagulation factor IX (human) (AlphaNine)	Replacement therapy in hemophilia B for prevention and control of bleeding episodes and during surgery to correct defective hemostasis[a]	Alpha Therapeutic
Coagulation factor IX (recombinant) (BeneFix)	Hemophilia B[a]	Genetics Inst
Coenzyme Q10	Huntington disease	Vitaline
Colchicine	Arrest the progression of neurologic disability caused by chronic progressive multiple sclerosis	Pharmacontrol
Colfosceril palmitate, cetyl alcohol, tyloxapol (Exosurf)	Adult respiratory distress syndrome	GlaxoSmithKline
(Exosurf Neonatal for Intratracheal Suspension)	To prevent hyaline membrane disease (respiratory distress syndrome) in infants born at ≤ 32 weeks gestation[a]; to treat established hyaline membrane disease at all gestational ages[a]	GlaxoWellcome
Collagenase (lyophilized) for injection (Plaquase)	Peyronie disease	Advance Biofactures
Combretastatin A4 phosphate	Anaplastic thyroid cancer, medullary thyroid cancer, and stage VI papillary or follicular thyroid cancer	OXiGENE
Conjugate of human transferrin and a mutant diphtheria toxin (CRM 107) (TransMID)	Malignant tumors of the CNS	INTELLigene Expressions
Conjugated bile acids (COBARTin)	Steatorrhea in short bowel syndrome	Jarrow Formulas
Corticorelin ovine triflutate (Acthrel)	To differentiate between pituitary and ectopic production of adrenocorticotropic hormone (ACTH) in ACTH-dependent Cushing syndrome[a]	Ferring Labs
Corticotropin-releasing factor, human (Xerecept)	Peritumoral brain edema	Neurobiological Technologies
Coumarin (Onkolox)	Renal cell carcinoma	Drossapharm Ltd
Creatine (Creapure)	Amyotrophic lateral sclerosis	Avicena Group
Cromolyn sodium (Gastrocrom)	Mastocytosis[a]	Fisons

Orphan Drugs		
Drug (Trade name)	*Proposed use*	*Sponsor*
Cromolyn sodium 4% ophthalmic solution (*Opticrom 4% Ophthalmic Solution*)	Vernal keratoconjunctivitis[a]	Fisons
***Cryptosporidium* hyperimmune bovine colostrum IgG concentrate**	Diarrhea in AIDS patients caused by infection with *Cryptosporidium parvum*	ImmuCell
CT-2584 mesylate	Adult soft tissue sarcoma; malignant mesothelioma	Cell Therapeutics
CY-1503 (*Cylexin*)	Postischemic pulmonary reperfusion edema following surgical treatment for chronic thromboembolic pulmonary hypertension; for neonates and infants undergoing cardiopulmonary bypass during surgical repair of congenital heart lesions	Cytel
CY-1899	Chronic active hepatitis B infection in HLA-A2 positive patients	Cytel
Cyclosporin	Prophylaxis of acute rejection in patients requiring allogenic lung transplant	Chiron
Cyclosporine	Refractory acute rejection in patients requiring allogenic lung transplants	Chiron
Cyclosporine 2% ophthalmic ointment	Treatment of patients at high risk of graft rejection following penetrating keratoplasty; corneal melting syndromes of known or presumed immunologic etiopathogenesis, including Mooren ulcer	Allergan
Cyclosporine in combination with omega-3 polyunsaturated fatty acids	To prevent solid organ graft rejection	RTP Pharma
Cyclosporine ophthalmic (*Optimmune*)	Severe keratoconjunctivitis sicca associated with Sjogren syndrome	University of Georgia
Cyproterone acetate (*Androcur*)	Severe hirsutism	Berlex Labs
Cysteamine (*Cystagon*)	Nephropathic cystinosis	Jess G. Thoene, MD
	Nephropathic cystinosis[a]	Mylan
Cysteamine HCl	Corneal cystine crystal accumulation in cystinosis patients	Sigma-Tau Pharm
Cystic fibrosis gene therapy	Cystic fibrosis	Genzyme
Cystic fibrosis Tr gene therapy (recombinant adenovirus) (*AdGVCFTR.10*)	Cystic fibrosis	GenVec
Cystic fibrosis transmembrane conductance regulator	Cystic fibrosis transmembrane conductance regulator protein replacement therapy in cystic fibrosis	Genzyme
Cystic fibrosis transmembrane conductance regulator gene	Cystic fibrosis	Genetic Therapy
Cytarabine liposomal (*DepoCyt*)	Neoplastic meningitis[a]	DepoTech
Cytomegalovirus immune globulin IV (human) (*CytoGam*)	With ganciclovir sodium for the treatment of cytomegalovirus pneumonia in bone marrow transplant patients	Bayer
	Prevention or attenuation of primary cytomegalovirus disease in immunosuppressed recipients of organ transplants[a]	MA Public Health Bio Labs
Daclizumab (*Zenapax*)	To prevent acute renal allograft rejection[a]	Hoffmann-LaRoche
Dantrolene sodium (*Dantrium*)	Neuroleptic malignant syndrome	Norwich Eaton Pharm
Dapsone	Prophylaxis of toxoplasmosis in severely immunocompromised patients with CD4 counts < 100	Jacobus Pharm

Orphan Drugs

Drug (Trade name)	Proposed use	Sponsor
Dapsone, USP (Dapsone)	Prophylaxis of Pneumocystis carinii pneumonia (PCP); with trimethoprim for treatment of PCP	Jacobus Pharm
Daunorubicin citrate liposome injection (DaunoXome)	Advanced HIV-associated Kaposi sarcoma[a]	NeXstar
Debrase (Debridase)	Debridement of acute, deep dermal burns in hospitalized patients	MediWound Ltd
Decitabine	Myelodysplastic syndromes; chronic myelogenous leukemia; sickle cell anemia	SuperGen
Deferasirox	Chronic iron overload in patients with transfusion-dependent anemias	Novartis
Deferiprone (Ferriprox)	Iron overload in patients with hematologic disorders requiring chronic transfusion therapy	Apotex Res
Defibrotide	Thrombotic thrombocytopenic purpura	Crinos
	Hepatic veno-occlusive disease	Gentium SpA
Dehydroepiandrosterone (DHEA) (Fidelin)	Systemic lupus erythematosus (SLE) and reduction of steroid use in steroid-dependent SLE patients	Genelabs Tech
	Replacement therapy in patients with adrenal insufficiency	Paladin Labs
Dehydroepiandrosterone sulfate sodium	To treat serious burns requiring hospitalization; to accelerate re-epithelialization of donor sites in those hospitalized burn patients who must undergo autologous skin grafting	Pharmadigm
Denileukin diftitox (Ontak)	Persistent or recurrent cutaneous T-cell lymphoma whose malignant cells express the CD25 component of the IL-2 receptor[a]	Ligand Pharm
Deoxyribose, phosphorothioate	Advanced malignant melanoma (stages II, III, and IV)	Genta
Desmopressin acetate	Mild hemophilia A and von Willebrand disease[a]	Aventis Behring LLC
Dexamethasone	Used in posterior segment drug delivery system in idiopathic intermediate uveitis	Oculex Pharm
Dexrazoxane (Zinecard)	T prevent cardiomyopathy associated with doxorubicin administration[a]	Pharmacia & Upjohn
Dextran 1	Cystic fibrosis	BCY LifeSciences
Dextran 70 (Dehydrex)	Recurrent corneal erosion unresponsive to conventional therapy	Holles Labs
Dextran and deferoxamine (Bio-Rescue)	Acute iron poisoning	Biomedical Frontiers
Dextran sulfate (inhaled, aerosolized) (Uendex)	As an adjunct to the treatment of cystic fibrosis	Kennedy and Hoidal, MDs
Dextran sulfate sodium	AIDS	Ueno Fine Chemicals
DHA-paclitaxel (Taxoprexin)	Pancreatic cancer; metastatic malignant melanoma; adenocarcinoma of the stomach or lower esophagus	Protarga
Dianeal peritoneal dialysis solution with 1.1% amino acids (Nutrineal [Peritoneal Dialysis Solution with 1.1% Amino Acid])	Nutritional supplement for malnourishment in patients undergoing continuous ambulatory peritoneal dialysis	Baxter Healthcare
Diazepam viscous solution for rectal administration	For the management of selected, refractory patients with epilepsy on stable regimens of antiepileptic drugs who require intermittent use of diazepam to control bouts of increased seizure activity[a]	Xcel
Diaziquone	Primary brain malignancies (grade III and IV astrocytomas)	Warner-Lambert
Dideoxyinosine	AIDS	Bristol-Myers Squibb

Orphan Drugs		
Drug (Trade name)	*Proposed use*	*Sponsor*
Diethyldithiocarbamate (*Imuthiol*)	AIDS	Connaught Labs
Diferuloylmethane	Cystic fibrosis	Seer Pharm
Digitoxin	Soft tissue sarcomas; ovarian cancer	PrimeCyte
Digoxin immune FAB (ovine) (*Digibind*)	To treat potentially life-threatening digitalis intoxication in patients refractory to management by conventional therapy[a]	GlaxoWellcome
(*Digidote*)	Life-threatening acute cardiac glycoside intoxication manifested by conduction disorders, ectopic ventricular activity, and, in some cases, hyperkalemia	Boehringer Mannheim
Dihydrotestosterone (*Androgel-DHT*)	Weight loss in AIDS with HIV-associated wasting	Unimed
Dimethyl sulfoxide	Topical treatment for the prevention of soft tissue injury following extravasation of cytotoxic drugs; palmar-plantar-erythrodysesthesia syndrome	Cancer Technologies
	Increased intracranial pressure in patients with severe, closed-head injury (traumatic brain coma) for whom no other effective treatment is available	Pharma 21
	Cutaneous manifestations of scleroderma	Research Industries
Dipalmitoylphosphatidyl-choline/Phosphatidylglycerol (*ALEC*)	To prevent/treat neonatal respiratory distress syndrome	Forum Products
Diphenylcyclopenone	Chronic severe forms of alopecia areata (alopecia totalis/alopecia universalis)	Lloyd E. King, Jr.
Disaccharide tripeptide glycerol dipalmitoyl (*Immther*)	Pulmonary and hepatic metastases in colorectal adenocarcinoma	ImmunoTherapeutics
Disodium clodronate	Hypercalcemia of malignancy	Discovery Experimental & Development
Disodium clodronate tetrahydrate (*Bonefos*)	Increased bone resorption caused by malignancy	Anthra Pharm
Disodium silibinin dihemisuccinate (*Legalon*)	Hepatic intoxication by *Amanita phalloides* (mushroom poisoning)	Pharmaquest
DMP 777	Therapeutic management of lung disease attributable to cystic fibrosis	DuPont
DNA-lipid complex (DMRIE/DOPE)/plasmid vector (VCL-1102, Vical) expressing human interleukin-2 (*Leuvectin*)	Renal cell carcinoma	Vical
DNP-modified autologous tumor vaccine (*O-Vax*)	Adjuvant therapy for the treatment of ovarian cancer	AVAX Technologies
Docosahexanoic acid-paclitaxel (*Taxoprexin*)	Hormone-refractory prostate cancer	Protarga
Dornase alfa (*Pulmozyme*)	Reduces mucous viscosity and enables the clearance of airway secretions in cystic fibrosis[a]	Genentech
Doxorubicin liposome (*Doxil*)	Ovarian cancer[a]	Alza
D-peptide of the sequence AKRHHGYKRKFH-NH2 (*PulmaDex*)	Cystic fibrosis	Demegen
Dronabinol (*Marinol*)	Stimulation of appetite and prevention of weight loss in patients with a confirmed diagnosis of AIDS[a]	Unimed
Duramycin	Cystic fibrosis	Mol Chem Medicines

Orphan Drugs

Drug (Trade name)	Proposed use	Sponsor
Dynamine	Lambert-Eaton myasthenic syndrome; hereditary motor and sensory neuropathy type I (Charcot-Marie-Tooth disease)	Mayo Foundation
Eculizumab	Idiopathic membranous glomerular nephropathy; paroxysmal nocturnal hemoglobinuria	Alexion Pharm
Eflornithine HCl (*Ornidyl*)	*Trypanosoma brucei* gambiense infection (sleeping sickness)[a]	Hoechst Marion Roussel
	Pneumocystis carinii pneumonia in AIDS	Marion Merrell Dow
Elcatonin	Intrathecal treatment of intractable pain	Innapharma
Enadoline HCl	Severe head injury	Warner-Lambert
Encapsulated porcine islet preparation (*BetaRx*)	For patients with type I diabetes already on immunosuppression	VivoRx
Enisoprost	In organ transplantation to diminish the nephrotoxicity induced by cyclosporine; with cyclosporine in organ transplantation to reduce acute transplant rejection	G.D. Searle
Epidermal growth factor (human)	Acceleration of corneal epithelial regeneration and healing of stromal tissue in nonhealing corneal defects	Chiron Vision
	To promote cutaneous wound healing in extreme burn treatment protocols	Ethicon
Epirubicin (*Ellence*)	Breast cancer[a]	Pharmacia & Upjohn
Epoetin alfa	Myelodysplastic syndrome	Johnson & Johnson Pharm R & D
(*Epogen*)	Anemia associated with end-stage renal disease[a] or HIV infection or treatment[a]	Amgen
(*Procrit*)	Anemia associated with end-stage renal disease; anemia of prematurity in preterm infants; HIV-associated anemia related to HIV infection or treatment	RW Johnson Pharm Res Inst
Epoetin beta (*Marogen*)	Anemia associated with end-stage renal disease	Chugai-USA
Epoprostenol (*Cycloprostin*)	Replacement of heparin in patients requiring hemodialysis and who are at increased risk of hemorrhage	Upjohn
(*Flolan*)	Primary pulmonary hypertension[a]; secondary pulmonary hypertension caused by intrinsic precapillary pulmonary vascular disease[a]; replacement of heparin in patients requiring hemodialysis and who are at increased risk of hemorrhage	GlaxoSmithKline
Epratuzumab (*LymphoCIDE*)	Non-Hodgkin lymphoma	Amgen
Erlotinib HCl (*Tarceva*)	Malignant gliomas	Genentech
Erwinia L-asparaginase	Alternative to *Escherichia coli* asparaginase in those situations where repeat courses of asparaginase therapy for acute lymphoblastic leukemia are required or when allergic reactions force the discontinuance of the *E. coli* preparation	Lyphomed
(*Erwinase*)	Acute lymphocytic leukemia	Porton International
Erythropoietin (recombinant human)	Anemia associated with end-stage renal disease	McDonnell Douglas
		Organon Teknika
Etanercept (*Enbrel*)	Reduction in signs and symptoms of moderately to severely active polyarticular-course juvenile rheumatoid arthritis where there has been inadequate response to ≥ 1 disease-modifying anti-rheumatic drug[a]; Wegener granulomatosis	Immunex
Ethanolamine oleate (*Ethamolin*)	To prevent rebleeding of esophageal varices that have recently bled[a]	Block Drug

Orphan Drugs

Drug (Trade name)	Proposed use	Sponsor
Ethinyl estradiol, USP	Turner syndrome	Bio-Technology General
Ethiofos	A chemoprotective agent for cisplatin and cyclophosphamide in ovarian cancer	US Bioscience
Ethyl eicosapentaenoate	Huntington disease	Laxdale Ltd
Etidronate disodium (Didronel)	Hypercalcemia of malignancy inadequately managed by dietary modification and/or oral hydration[a]	MGI Pharma
(Didronel IV Infusion)	To prevent/treat degenerative metabolic bone disease in patients who require long-term ($\geq$ 6 months) total parenteral nutrition	
Etiocholanedione	Aplastic anemia; Prader-Willi syndrome	SuperGen
Exemestane (Aromasin)	Advanced breast cancer in postmenopausal women whose disease has progressed following tamoxifen therapy[a]	Pharmacia & Upjohn
Exisulind	Suppression and control of colonic adenomatous polyps in the inherited disease adenomatous polyposis coli	Cell Pathways
Factor XIII [A2] homodimer, recombinant DNA orgin	Congenital FXIII deficiency; prophylaxis of bleeding associated with congenital FXIII deficiency	ZymoGenetics
Factor XIII concentrate (human) pasteurized (Fibrogammin P)	Congenital Factor XIII deficiency	Aventis Behring LLC
Factor XIII, recombinant	Congenital Factor XIII deficiency	Zymogenetics
Fampridine (Neurelan)	For the relief of symptoms of multiple sclerosis; chronic, incomplete spinal cord injury	Acorda Therapeutics
Felbamate (Felbatol)	Lennox-Gastaut syndrome[a]	Wallace Labs
Ferric hexacyanoferrate (II) "Prussian Blue"	Known or suspected internal contamination with radioactive or nonradioactive cesium or thallium	Degussa AG
FIAU	Adjunctive treatment of chronic active hepatitis B	Oclassen Pharm
Fibrinogen (human)	Control of bleeding and prophylactic treatment of patients deficient in fibrinogen	Alpha Therapeutics
Fibronectin (human plasma-derived)	For nonhealing corneal ulcers or epithelial defects unresponsive to conventional therapy and the underlying cause has been eliminated	Melville Biologics
Fibronectin (plasma-derived)	For nonhealing corneal ulcers or epithelial defects unresponsive to conventional therapy and for which any infectious cause of the defect has been eliminated	Chiron Vision
Filgrastim (Neupogen)	Severe chronic neutropenia (absolute neutrophil count < 500/mm^3)[a]; neutropenia associated with bone marrow transplants[a]; AIDS patients with cytomegalovirus retinitis being treated with ganciclovir; mobilization of peripheral blood progenitor cells for collection in patients who will receive myeloablative or myelosuppressive chemotherapy[a]; to reduce duration of neutropenia, fever, antibiotic use, and hospitalization following induction and consolidation treatment for acute myeloid leukemia[a]; myelodysplastic syndrome	Amgen
Flucinolone	Uveitis involving the posterior segment of the eye	Bausch & Lomb
Fludarabine phosphate (Fludara)	Treatment and management of non-Hodgkin lymphoma; chronic lymphocytic leukemia (CLL) including refractory CLL[a]	Berlex Labs
Flumecinol (Zixoryn)	Hyperbilirubinemia in newborn infants unresponsive to phototherapy	Farmacon
Flunarizine (Sibelium)	Alternating hemiplegia	Janssen Res

Orphan Drugs

Drug (Trade name)	Proposed use	Sponsor
Fluorouracil	With interferon alpha-2a, recombinant, for advanced colorectal and esophageal carcinomas	Hoffmann-La Roche
	Glioblastoma multiforme	Ethypharm SA
(Adrucil)	With leucovorin for metastatic adenocarcinoma of the colon and rectum	Lederle Labs
Fluoxetine (Prozac)	Autism	Eric Hollander, MD
Follitropin alfa, recombinant (Gonal-F)	Induction of spermatogenesis in men with primary and secondary hypogonadotropic hypogonadism in whom the cause of infertility is not caused by primary testicular failure[a]	Serono Labs
Fomepizole (Antizol)	Methanol or ethylene glycol poisoning[a]	Orphan Medical
Fosphenytoin (Cerebyx)	Acute treatment of patients with status epilepticus of the grand mal type[a]	Warner-Lambert
Fructose-1,6-diphosphate (Cordox)	For painful vaso-occlusive episodes associated with sickle cell disease	Questcor Pharm
G17DT immunogen	Adenocarcinoma of the pancreas; gastric cancer	Aphton
Gabapentin (Neurontin)	Amyotrophic lateral sclerosis	Warner-Lambert
Gallium nitrate injection (Ganite)	Hypercalcemia of malignancy[a]	Solopak Pharm
Gamma hydroxybutyrate	Narcolepsy and auxiliary symptoms of cataplexy, sleep paralysis, hypnagogic hallucinations, and automatic behavior	Biocraft Labs
Gamma hydroxybutyric acid	Narcolepsy and auxiliary symptoms of cataplexy, sleep paralysis, hypnagogic hallucinations, and automatic behavior	Sigma Chemical
Gammalinolenic acid	Juvenile rheumatoid arthritis	Robert B. Zurier, MD
Ganaxolone	Infantile spasms	Purdue Pharma LP
Ganciclovir intravitreal implant (Vitrasert Implant)	Cytomegalovirus retinitis[a]	Bausch & Lomb Surgical, Chiron Vision Products
Ganciclovir sodium (Cytovene)	Cytomegalovirus retinitis in immunocompromised patients with AIDS[a]	Syntex (USA)
Gancyclovir	Severe human cytomegalovirus infections in specific immunosuppressed patient populations	Burroughs Wellcome
Gangliosides as sodium salts (Cronassial)	Retinitis pigmentosa	Fidia Pharm
Gavilimomab	Acute graft vs host disease	Abgenix
Gemtuzumab ozogamicin (Mylotarg)	CD33-positive acute myeloid leukemia[a]	Wyeth-Ayerst Labs
Gene plasmid hVEGF165 driven by human cytomegalovirus, and [2,3-bis(oleoyl)propyl]trimethyl ammonium and dioleoyl phosphatidyl ethanolamine (Trinam)	To prevent complications caused by neointimal hyperplasia disease in certain vascular anastomoses	Ark Therapeutics
Gentamicin impregnated PMMA beads on surgical wire (Septopal)	Chronic osteomyelitis of posttraumatic, postoperative, or hematogenous origin	Lipha Pharm
Gentamicin liposome injection (Maitec)	Disseminated Mycobacterium avium-intracellulare infection	Liposome
Glatiramer acetate (Copaxone)	Multiple sclerosis[a]	Teva

Orphan Drugs

Drug (Trade name)	Proposed use	Sponsor
Glatiramer acetate for injection (Copaxone)	Primary-progressive multiple sclerosis	Teva
Glutamine	With human growth hormone in the treatment of short bowel syndrome (nutrient malabsorption from the GI tract resulting from an inadequate absorptive surface)	Nutritional Restart Pharm
Glyceol	To decrease intracranial hypertension and/or alleviate cerebral edema in patients who may benefit from osmotherapy	Chugai Pharm
Glyceryl trioleate and glyceryl trierucate	Adrenoleukodystrophy	Hugo W. Moser, MD
Gonadorelin acetate (Lutrepulse)	Ovulation induction in women with hypothalamic amenorrhea caused by a deficiency or absence in quantity or pulse pattern of endogenous GnRH secretion[a]	Ferring Labs
Gossypol	Cancer of the adrenal cortex	Marcus M. Reidenberg, MD
Gp100 adenoviral gene therapy	Metastatic melanoma	Genzyme
Granulocyte macrophage-colony stimulating factor (Leucomax)	Neutropenia caused by hairy cell leukemia; neutropenia associated with bone marrow transplants; severe thermal injuries in patients with > 40% full or partial thickness burns; myelodysplastic syndrome; chronic lymphocytic leukemia to increase granulocyte count	Schering
Group B streptococcus immune globulin	Disseminated group B streptococcal infection in neonates	North American Biologicals
Growth hormone releasing factor	Long-term treatment of children who have growth failure caused by a lack of adequate endogenous growth hormone secretion	Valeant Pharm
Guanethidine monosulfate (Ismelin)	Moderate to severe sympathetic reflex dystrophy and causalgia	Novaris
Guanfacine (Tenex)	Fragile X syndrome	Watson Labs
Gusperimus (Spanidin)	Acute renal graft rejection episodes	Bristol-Myers Squibb Pharm Res Inst
h5G1.1-mAb	Dermatomyositis	Alexion Pharm
Halofantrine (Halfan)	Mild to moderate acute malaria caused by susceptible strains of Plasmodium falciparum and P. vivax[a]	SmithKline Beecham
Halofuginone (Stenorol)	Systemic sclerosis	Collgard Biopharmaceuticals Ltd
Heme arginate (Normosang)	Symptomatic stage of acute porphyria; myelodysplastic syndromes	Berlex Labs
Hemin (Panhematin)	Amelioration of recurrent attacks of acute intermittent porphyria (AIP) temporarily related to the menstrual cycle in susceptible women and similar symptoms that occur in other patients with AIP, porphyria variegata, and hereditary coproporphyria[a]	Abbott Labs
Hemin and zinc mesoporphyrin (Hemex)	Acute porphyric syndromes	Herbert L. Bonkovsky, MD
Heparin, oral unfractionated	Sickle cell disease	TRF Technologies
Hepatitis B immune globulin IV (human) (Nabi-HB)	Prophylaxis against hepatitis B virus reinfection in liver transplant patients	NABI
Hepatitis C virus immune globulin (human)	Prophylaxis of hepatitis C infection in liver transplant recipients	NABI
HepeX-B	To prevent hepatitis B virus reinfection in liver transplant patients	XTL Biopharmaceuticals
Herpes simplex virus gene	Primary and metastatic brain tumors	Genetic Therapy

Orphan Drugs

Drug (Trade name)	Proposed use	Sponsor
Herpes simplex virus, genetically engineered (G207)	Malignant glioma	MediGene
Histamine (Maxamine)	Adjunctive to cytokine therapy in treatment of acute myeloid leukemia and malignant melanoma	Maxim Pharm
Histrelin	Treatment of acute intermittent porphyria, hereditary coproporphyria, and variegate porphyria	Karl E. Anderson, MD
Histrelin acetate (Supprelin Injection)	Central precocious puberty[a]	Roberts Pharm
HIV neutralizing antibodies (Immupath)	AIDS	Hemacare
HLA-B7/Beta2M DNA Lipid (DMRIE/DOPE) Complex (Allovectin-7)	Invasive and metastatic melanoma (stages II, III, IV)	Vical Incorporated
Homoharringtonine	Chronic myelogenous leukemia	American BioScience
HPA-23	AIDS	Rhone-Poulenc Rorer
Hsp E7	Recurrent respiratory papillomatosis	StressGen Biotechnologies
Hu1D10, humanized, monoclonal antibody (Remitogen)	1D10+ B cell non-Hodgkin lymphoma	Protein Design Labs
Human acid precursor alpha-glucosidase, recombinant	Glycogen storage disease type II	Pharming/Genzyme LLC
Human anti-transforming growth factor beta 1 monoclonal antibody	Systemic sclerosis	Genzyme
Human anti-tumor necrosis factor alpha monoclonal antibody	Uveitis of the posterior segment of noninfectious etiology, and uveitis of the anterior segment of noninfectious etiology and refractory to conventional therapy	Centocor
Human gammaglobulin	Juvenile rheumatoid arthritis; GI disturbances (eg, constipation, diarrhea, abdominal pain) associated with regression-onset autism in pediatric patients; idiopathic inflammatory myopathies	Protein Therapeutics
Human IgM monoclonal antibody (C-58) to cytomegalovirus (Centovir)	Cytomegalovirus infections in allogenic bone marrow transplant patients; prophylaxis of cytomegalovirus infections in bone marrow transplant patients	Centocor
Human immunodeficiency virus immune globulin (Hivig)	AIDS; HIV-infected pregnant women and pediatric patients; infants of HIV-infected mothers	NABI
Human T-lymphotropic virus type III Gp 160 antigens (Vaxsyn HIV-1)	AIDS	MicroGeneSys
Humanized anti-CD2 monoclonal antibody	Graft vs host disease	MedImmune
Humanized anti-human CD2 MAb (MEDI-507)	Induction of donor-specific immunologic unresponsiveness resulting in prophylaxis of organ rejection without the need for chronic immunosuppressive therapy in allogeneic renal transplants	Biotransplant
Humanized anti-tac (Zenapax)	To treat acute graft vs host disease following bone marrow transplantation	Hoffmann-La Roche
Humanized MAb (IDEC-131) to CD40L	Systemic lupus erythematosus	Idec Pharm
Humanized monoclonal antibody against Shiga-like toxin II	To prevent the development of or to decrease the incidence and severity of hemolytic uremic syndrome and associated sequelae of Shiga-like toxin-producing Escherichia coli	Teijin America
Hyaluronic acid	Emphysema caused by alpha-1 antitrypsin deficiency	Exhale Therapeutics

Orphan Drugs

Drug (Trade name)	Proposed use	Sponsor
Hydroxocobalamin (*Cyanokit*)	Acute cyanide poisoning	Orphan Medical
		EMD Pharm
Hydroxycobalamin/Sodium thiosulfate	Severe acute cyanide poisoning	Alan H. Hall, MD
Hydroxyurea (*Droxia*)	Sickle cell anemia as shown by the presence of hemoglobin S[a]	Bristol-Myers Squibb Pharm Res Inst
Hypericin	Glioblastoma multiforme; cutaneous T-cell lymphoma	Nexell Therapeutics
I(131)-TM-601 (chlorotoxin)	Malignant glioma	TransMolecular
Ibritumomab tiuxetan (*Zevalin*)	B-cell non-Hodgkin lymphoma[a]	IDEC Pharm
Ibuprofen IV solution (*Salprofen*)	To prevent/treat patent ductus arteriosus	Farmacon-IL LLC
Icatbant	Angioedema	Jerini AG
Icodextrin 7.5% with electrolytes peritoneal dialysis solution (*Extraneal [with 7.5% Icodextrin] Peritoneal Dialysis Solution*)	End-stage renal disease requiring peritoneal dialysis treatment[a]	Baxter Healthcare
Idarubicin (*Idamycin*)	Myelodysplastic syndromes; chronic myelogenous leukemia	Pharmacia & Upjohn
Idarubicin HCl for injection (*Idamycin*)	Acute lymphoblastic leukemia in pediatric patients	Pharmacia & Upjohn
	Acute myelogenous leukemia (acute nonlymphocytic leukemia)[a]	Adria Labs
IDN 6556	Patients undergoing solid organ transplantation	Idun Pharm
Idoxuridine	Nonparenchymatous sarcomas	NeoPharm
Iduronate-2-sulfatase	Long-term enzyme replacement therapy for mucopolysaccharidosis II (Hunter syndrome)	Transkaryotic Therapies
Ifosfamide (*Ifex*)	Testicular cancer[a]; bone sarcomas; soft tissue sarcomas	Bristol-Myers Squibb Pharm Res Inst
IL-4 pseudomonas toxin fusion protein (IL-4(38-37)-PE38KDEL)	Astrocytic glioma	Neurocrine Biosciences
IL-13-PE38QQR	Malignant glioma	NeoPharm
Iloprost solution for infusion	Heparin-associated thrombocytopenia; Raynaud phenomenon secondary to systemic sclerosis	Berlex Labs
Imatinib mesylate (*Gleevec*)	Chronic myelogenous leukemia[a]; GI stromal tumors[a]	Novartis
Imciromab pentetate (*Myoscint*)	To detect early necrosis as an indication of rejection of orthotopic cardiac transplants	Centocor
Imexon	Multiple myeloma; metastatic malignant melanoma; pancreatic adenocarcinoma	AmpliMed
Imiglucerase (*Cerezyme*)	Replacement therapy in patients with types I, II, and III Gaucher disease[a]	Genzyme
Immune globulin IV (human) (*Gamimune N*)	Infection prophylaxis in pediatric patients with HIV[a]	Bayer
(*Immuno, Iveegam*)	Acute myocarditis; polymyositis/dermatomyositis; juvenile rheumatoid arthritis	Immuno Clin Res
Imported fire ant venom, allergenic extract	Skin testing for victims of fire ant stings to confirm fire ant sensitivity and, if positive, as immunotherapy for prevention of IgE-mediated anaphylactic reactions	ALK Labs
Indium In-111 altumomab pentetate (*Hybri-ceaker*)	To detect suspected and previously unidentified tumor foci of recurrent colorectal carcinoma	Hybritech

Orphan Drugs

Drug (Trade name)	Proposed use	Sponsor
Indium In 111 murine monoclonal antibody FAB to myosin (*Myoscint*)	To aid in diagnosis of myocarditis	Centocor
Infliximab (*Remicade*)	Moderately to severely active Crohn disease for the reduction of the signs and symptoms in patients who have an inadequate response to conventional therapy; fistulizing Crohn disease for the reduction in the number of draining enterocutaneous fistula(s)[a]; chronic sarcoidosis; giant cell arteritis; juvenile rheumatoid arthritis; Crohn disease and ulcerative colitis in pediatric (0 to 16 years of age) patients	Centocor
INGN 201 (*Advexin*)	Head and neck cancer	Introgen Therapeutics
INH-A00021 (*Veronate*)	To reduce (prevent) nosocomial bacteremia caused by staphylococci in very low birth weight infants	Inhibitex
Inolimomab (*Leukotac*)	Graft vs host disease	Opi
Inosine pranobex (*Isoprinosine*)	Subacute sclerosing panencephalitis	Newport Pharm
Interferon alfa-1b	Multiple myeloma	Ernest C. Borden
Interferon alfa-2a (recombinant) (*Roferon-A*)	AIDS-related Kaposi sarcoma[a]; renal-cell carcinoma; with fluorouracil for esophageal carcinoma or advanced colorectal cancer; with teceleukin for metastatic renal cell carcinoma or metastatic malignant melanoma; chronic myelogenous leukemia[a]	Hoffmann-La Roche
Interferon alfa-2b (recombinant) (*Intron A*)	AIDS-related Kaposi sarcoma[a]; metastatic renal cell carcinoma; chronic myelogenous leukemia; laryngeal (respiratory) papillomatosis; acute hepatitis B; primary malignant brain tumors; invasive carcinoma of the cervix; carcinoma in situ of the urinary bladder; chronic delta hepatitis; ovarian carcinoma	Schering
Interferon alfa-n1 (*Wellferon*)	AIDS-related Kaposi sarcoma	Burroughs Wellcome
	Human papillomavirus in severe resistant/recurrent respiratory (laryngeal) papillomatosis	Glaxo Wellcome
Interferon beta-1a (recombinant human) (*Avonex*)	Acute non-A, non-B hepatitis; primary brain tumors; juvenile rheumatoid arthritis; multiple sclerosis[a]; pulmonary fibrosis	Biogen
(*Betaseron*)	Multiple sclerosis[a]	Berlex Labs and Chiron
	AIDS	Berlex Labs
(*r-HuIFN-beta*)	Systemic treatment of cutaneous T-cell lymphoma and cutaneous malignant melanoma; intralesional and/or systemic treatment of AIDS-related Kaposi sarcoma	Biogen
(*R-IFN-beta*)	Systemic treatment of metastatic renal cell carcinoma	Biogen
(*Rebif*)	Symptomatic patients with AIDS (including CD4 T-cell counts < 200 cells/mm^3); secondary progressive multiple sclerosis	Serono Labs
Interferon gamma-1b (*Actimmune*)	Renal cell carcinoma	Genentech
	Chronic granulomatous disease[a]; delaying time to disease progression in patients with severe, malignant osteopetrosis[a]; idiopathic pulmonary fibrosis	InterMune
Interleukin-1 alpha, human recombinant	Hematopoietic potentiation in aplastic anemia; promotion of early engraftment in bone marrow transplantation	Immunex
Interleukin-1 receptor antagonist (human recombinant) (*Antril*)	Juvenile rheumatoid arthritis; to prevent/treat graft vs host disease in transplant recipients	Amgen

Orphan Drugs

Drug (Trade name)	Proposed use	Sponsor
Interleukin-2 (*Teceleukin*)	Alone or with interferon alfa-2a for metastatic renal-cell carcinoma; alone or with interferon alfa-2a for metastatic malignant melanoma	Hoffmann-La Roche
Interleukin-3 human (recombinant)	Promotion of erythropoiesis in Diamond-Blackfan anemia (congenital pure red cell aplasia)	Immunex
	Sequential administration with sargramostim to accelerate neutrophil and platelet recovery in patients undergoing autologous bone marrow transplantation for Hodgkin disease or non-Hodgkin lymphoma	Sandoz Pharm
Intraoral fluoride releasing system (IFRS)	To prevent dental caries caused by radiation-induced xerostomia in head and neck cancer	Digestive Care
Iobenguane sulfate I 131	Diagnostic adjunct in patients with pheochromocytoma[a]	University of Michigan
Iodine I 123 murine monoclonal antibody to alpha-fetoprotein	Detection of hepatocellular carcinoma and hepatoblastoma and alpha-fetoprotein-producing germ-cell tumors	Immunomedics
Iodine I 123 murine monoclonal antibody to hCG	Detection of hCG-producing tumors (eg, germ-cell, trophoblastic-cell tumors)	Immunomedics
Iodine I 131 6B-iodomethyl-19-norcholesterol	Adrenal cortical imaging	David E. Kuhl, MD
Iodine I 131 bis(indium-diethylenetriaminepentaacetic acid)tyrosyllysine/hMN-14x m734 F(ab')2 bispecific monoclonal antibody (*Pentacea*)	Small-cell lung cancer	IBC Pharm
Iodine I 131 Lym-1 monoclonal antibody	B-cell lymphoma	Lederle Labs
Iodine I 131 murine monoclonal antibody IgG2a to B cell (*Immurait, LI-2-I-131*)	B-cell leukemia and B-cell lymphoma	Immunomedics
Iodine I 131 murine monoclonal antibody to alpha-fetoprotein	Hepatocellular carcinoma and hepatoblastoma; alpha-fetoprotein-producing germ-cell tumors	Immunomedics
Iodine I 131 murine monoclonal antibody to hCG	hCG-producing tumors (eg, germ-cell, trophoblastic-cell tumors)	Immunomedics
Iodine I 131 radiolabeled chimeric MAb tumor necrosis treatment (TNT-1B) (*131IchTNT-1*)	Glioblastoma multiforme and anaplastic astrocytoma	Peregrine Pharm
Irofulven	Renal cell carcinoma; ovarian cancer	MGI Pharma
Iron(III)-hexacyanoferrate(II) (*Radiogardase*)	Known or suspected internal contamination with radioactive or nonradioactive cesium or thallium[a]	Hey Chemisch-
Isobutyramide	Sickle cell disease and beta-thalassemia	Alpha Therapeutics
(*Isobutyramide Oral Solution*)	Beta-hemoglobinopathies and beta-thalassemia syndromes	Susan P. Perrine, MD
Japanese encephalitis vaccine (live, attenuated)	To prevent Japanese encephalitis	Boran Pharm
Ketoconazole (*Nizoral*)	With cyclosporine A to diminish the nephrotoxicity induced by cyclosporine in organ transplantation	Pharmedic
L-2-oxothiazolidine-4-carboxylic acid (*Procysteine*)	Adult respiratory distress syndrome; amyotrophic lateral sclerosis	Transcend Therapeutics
L-5-hydroxytryptophan	Tetrahydrobiopterin deficiency	Watson Labs
L-baclofen	Trigeminal neuralgia	Gerhard Fromm, MD

Orphan Drugs

Drug (Trade name)	Proposed use	Sponsor
(Neuralgon)	Trigeminal neuralgia; intractable spasticity from spinal cord injury or multiple sclerosis; intractable spasticity in children with cerebral palsy	Pharmascience
L-cycloserine	Gaucher disease	Meir Lev, MD
L-cysteine	To prevent and lessen photosensitivity in erythropoietic protoporphyria	Orphan Pharm USA
L-glutamine	Sickle cell disease	Orphan Drugs International LLC
L-glutamyl-L-tryptophan	AIDS-related Kaposi sarcoma	Cytran
L-leucovorin (Isovorin)	With high-dose methotrexate in the treatment of osteosarcoma; in combination chemotherapy with the approved agent 5-fluorouracil in the palliative treatment of metastatic adenocarcinoma of the colon and rectum	Lederle Labs
L-threonine	Spasticity associated with familial spastic paraparesis	Interneuron Pharm
(Threostat)	Amyotrophic lateral sclerosis	Tyson & Assoc
Lactic acid (Aphthaid)	Severe aphthous stomatitis in severely, terminally immunocompromised patients	Frontier Pharm
Lactic acid bacteria (Lactobacilli, Bifidobacteria, and Streptococcus sp.)	Chronic active pouchitis; to prevent disease relapse in patients with chronic pouchitis	VSL Pharm
Lactobin (Lactobin)	AIDS-associated diarrhea unresponsive to initial antidiarrheal therapy	Roxane Labs
Lactoferrin alpha	To prevent and treat graft vs host disease	Agennix
Lamotrigine (Lamictal)	Lennox-Gastaut syndrome[a]	GlaxoWellcome R & D
Lanreotide, Somatostatin (Ipstyl)	Acromegaly	IPSEN
Laronidase (Aldurazyme)	Patients with mucopolysaccharidosis-I[a]	BioMarin Pharm
Latrodectus immune F(ab)2 (Aracmyn)	Black widow spider envenomations	Rare Disease Therapeutics
Leflunomide	To prevent acute and chronic rejection in patients with solid organ transplants	James W. Williams, MD
Lepirudin (Refludan)	Heparin-associated thrombocytopenia type II[a]	Hoechst Marion Roussel
Leucovorin (Leucovorin calcium)	With 5-fluorouracil for metastatic colorectal cancer[a]; rescue use after high-dose methotrexate therapy in the treatment of osteosarcoma[a]	Immunex
Leucovorin calcium (Wellcovorin)	With 5-fluorouracil for the treatment of metastatic colorectal cancer	GlaxoWellcome R & D
Leupeptin	As an adjunct to microsurgical peripheral nerve repair	Neuromuscular Adjuncts
Leuprolide acetate (Lupron Injection)	Central precocious puberty[a]	Tap Pharm
Levocabastine HCl ophthalmic suspension 0.05%	Vernal keratoconjunctivitis	Iolab Pharm
Levocarnitine (Carnitor)	Genetic carnitine deficiency[a]; primary and secondary carnitine deficiency of genetic origin[a]; to prevent/treat secondary carnitine deficiency in valproic acid toxicity; pediatric cardiomyopathy; to treat zidovudine-induced mitochondrial myopathy; manifestations of carnitine deficiency in patients with end-stage renal disease who require dialysis[a]	Sigma-Tau Pharm
Levodopa and carbidopa (Duodopa)	Late-stage Parkinson disease	Nouvel Pharma
Levomethadyl acetate HCl (ORLAAM)	Heroin addiction suitable for maintenance on opiate agonists[a]	Biodevelopment

Orphan Drugs

Drug (Trade name)	Proposed use	Sponsor
Lidocaine patch 5% (Lidoderm Patch)	To relieve allodynia (painful hypersensitivity) and chronic pain in postherpetic neuralgia[d]	Teikoku Pharma USA
Lintuzumab (Zamyl)	Acute myelogenous leukemia	Protein Design Labs
Liothyronine sodium injection (Triostat)	Myxedema coma/precoma[a]	SmithKline Beecham
Lipase, amylase, and protease (TheraCLEC-Total)	Pancreatic insufficiency	Altus Biologics
Lipid/DNA human cystic fibrosis gene	Cystic fibrosis	Genzyme
Liposomal amphotericin B (AmBisome)	Cryptococcal meningitis[a]; visceral leishmaniasis[a]; histoplasmosis	Fujisawa USA
Liposomal-cis-bis-neodecanoato-trans-R,R-1,2-diaminocyclohexane-Pt (II)	Malignant mesothelioma	Antigenics
Liposomal cyclosporin A (Cyclospire)	For aerosolized administration to prevent/treat lung allograft rejection and pulmonary rejection events associated with bone marrow transplantation	Vernon Knight, MD
Liposomal N-Acetylglucosminyl-N-Acetylmuramyl-L-Ala-D-isoGln-L-Ala-glycerolidpalmitoyl (ImmTher)	Osteosarcoma; Ewing sarcoma	Endorex
Liposomal nystatin (Nyotran)	Invasive fungal infections	Antigenics
Liposomal p-ethoxy growth receptor bound protein-2 antisense product	Chronic myelogenous leukemia	Interpath Pharm
Liposomal prostaglandin E1 injection	Acute respiratory distress syndrome	Liposome
Liposome encapsulated recombinant interleukin-2	Brain and CNS tumors; kidney and renal pelvis cancers	Biomira USA
Lisofylline	To treat patients undergoing induction therapy for acute myeloid leukemia	Cell Therapeutics
Lodoxamide tromethamine (Alomide Ophthalmic Solution)	Vernal keratoconjunctivitis[a]	Alcon Labs
Loxoribine	Common variable immunodeficiency	RW Johnson Pharm
Lucinactant (Surfaxin)	Meconium aspiration syndrome in newborn infants; respiratory distress syndrome in premature infants; acute adult respiratory distress syndrome	Discovery Labs
Lysine acetylsalicylate injectable	Pain and fever secondary to sickle cell disease crisis	GD Searle
Mafenide acetate solution (Sulfamylon solution)	Adjunctive topical antimicrobial agent to control bacterial infection when used under moist dressings over meshed autografts on excised burn wounds[a]	Mylan
Mafosfamide	Neoplastic meningitis	Baxter Oncology GmbH
Marijuana	HIV-associated wasting syndrome	Multidisciplinary Assoc for Psychedelic Studies
MART-1 adenoviral gene therapy for malignant melanoma	Metastatic melanoma	Genzyme
Matrix metalloproteinase inhibitor (Galardin)	Corneal ulcers	Glycomed
MaxAdFVIII	Hemophilia A	GenStar Therapeutics
Mazindol (Sanorex)	Duchenne muscular dystrophy	Platon J. Collipp, MD

Orphan Drugs

Drug (Trade name)	Proposed use	Sponsor
Mecamylamine (*Inversine*)	Tourette syndrome	Targacept
Mecasermin	Growth hormone insufficiency syndrome	Genentech
(*Myotrophin*)	Amyotrophic lateral sclerosis	Cephalon
Medroxyprogesterone acetate (*Hematrol*)	Immune thrombocytopenic purpura	InKine Pharm
Mefloquine HCl (*Lariam*)	Acute malaria caused by *Plasmodium falciparum* and *P. vivax*[a]; prophylaxis of *P. falciparum* malaria resistant to other available drugs[a]	Hoffman-La Roche
(*Mephaquin*)	To prevent/treat chloroquine-resistant *Falciparum* malaria	Mepha AG
Megestrol acetate (*Megace*)	Anorexia, cachexia, or significant weight loss (≥ 10% of baseline body weight) with confirmed diagnosis of AIDS[a]	Bristol-Myers Squibb Pharm Res Inst
Melanoma cell vaccine	Invasive melanoma	CancerVax
Melanoma vaccine (*Melacine*)	Stage III-IV melanoma	Ribi ImmunoChem Res
Melatonin	Circadian rhythm sleep disorders in blind people with no light perception	Robert Sack, MD
Meloxicam (*Mobic*)	Juvenile rheumatoid arthritis	Boehringer Ingelheim
Melphalan (*Alkeran for Injection*)	Hyperthermic regional limb perfusion to treat metastatic melanoma of the extremity; multiple myeloma for whom oral therapy is inappropriate[a]	GlaxoWellcome
Meropenem (*Merrem IV*)	Manage acute pulmonary exacerbations in cystic fibrosis patients caused by respiratory tract infections with susceptible organisms	Zeneca
Mesna	Inhibition of the urotoxic effects induced by oxazaphosphorine compounds (eg, cyclophosphamide)	Asta Medica
(*Mesnex*)	As a prophylactic to reduce the incidence of ifosfamide-induced hemorrhagic cystitis[a]	Degussa
Methionine/L-methionine	AIDS myelopathy	Alessandro Di Rocco,
Methotrexate (*Rheumatrex*)	Juvenile rheumatoid arthritis	Wyeth-Ayerst Labs
Methotrexate sodium (*Methotrexate*)	Osteogenic sarcoma[a]	Lederle Labs
Methotrexate with laurocapram (*Methotrexate/Azone*)	Topical treatment of *Mycosis fungoides*	Durham Pharm
Methoxsalen (*Uvadex*)	Used in conjunction with the UVAR photopheresis system to treat graft vs host disease	Therakos
Methylbicyclone	Cystic fibrosis	Sucampo Pharm
Methylnaltrexone	Chronic opioid-induced constipation unresponsive to conventional therapy	University of Chicago
Metreleptin	Metabolic disorders secondary to lipodystrophy; leptin deficiency secondary to generalized lipodystrophy and partial familial lipodystrophy	Amgen
Metronidazole (*Metrogel*)	Perioral dermatitis	Galderma Labs
Metronidazole (topical) (*Flagyl*)	Grade III and IV anaerobically infected, decubitus ulcers	Searle
(*Metrogel*)	Acne rosacea[a]	Galderma Labs
Microbubble contrast agent (*Filmix Neurosonographic Contrast Agent*)	Intraoperative aid in the identification and localization of intracranial tumors	Cav-Con

Orphan Drugs

Drug (Trade name)	Proposed use	Sponsor
Midodrine HCl (*Amatine*)	Symptomatic orthostatic hypotension[a]	Schier Ridgewood FKA
Miglustat (*Zavesca*)	Gaucher disease[a]	Actelion Pharm
Minocycline HCl (*Minocin Intravenous*)	Chronic malignant pleural effusion	Lederle Labs
Mitoguazone (*apep*)	Diffuse non-Hodgkin lymphoma, including AIDS-related diffuse non-Hodgkin lymphoma	ILEX Oncology
Mitolactol	Adjuvant therapy in the treatment of primary brain tumors; recurrent invasive or metastatic squamous carcinoma of the cervix	Biopharmaceutics
Mitomycin-C	Refractory glaucoma as an adjunct to ab externo glaucoma surgery	IOP
Mitoxantrone (*Novantrone*)	Progressive-relapsing multiple sclerosis[a]; secondary-progressive multiple sclerosis[a]	Immunex
	Hormone-refractory prostate cancer[a]	Serono Labs
Mitoxantrone HCl (*Novantrone*)	Acute myelogenous leukemia (acute nonlymphocytic leukemia)[a]	Lederle Labs
MN14 monoclonal antibody to carcinoembryonic antigen (*Cea-Cide*)	Small-cell lung cancer; pancreatic cancer	Immunomedics
Modafinil (*Provigil*)	Excessive daytime sleepiness in narcolepsy[a]	Cephalon
Molgramostim (*Leucomax*)	Aplastic anemia; AIDS patients with neutropenia caused by the disease, AZT, or ganciclovir	Schering
Monarsen	Myasthenia gravis	Medica Venture Partners
Monoclonal Ab(murine) anti-idiotype melanoma-associated antigen (*Melimmune*)	Invasive cutaneous melanoma	IDEC Pharm
Monoclonal antibodies (murine or human) to B-cell lymphoma	B-cell lymphoma	IDEC Pharm
Monoclonal antibody 17-1a (*Panorex*)	Pancreatic cancer	Centocor
Monoclonal antibody-B43.13 (*Ovarex MAb-B43.13*)	Epithelial ovarian cancer	AltaRex US
Monoclonal antibody for immunization against lupus nephritis	Lupus nephritis	VivoRx Autoimmune
Monoclonal antibody to cytomegalovirus (human)	Treatment of cytomegalovirus retinitis in AIDS; prophylaxis of cytomegalovirus disease in solid organ transplantation	Protein Design Labs
Monoclonal antibody to hepatitis B virus (human)	Prophylaxis of hepatitis B reinfection in liver transplantation secondary to end-stage chronic hepatitis B infection	Protein Design Labs
Monoclonal antiendotoxin antibody XMMEn-0e5	Gram-negative sepsis that has progressed to shock	Pfizer
Monoctanoin (*Moctanin*)	Dissolution of cholesterol gallstones retained in the common bile duct[a]	Ethitek Pharm
Monolaurin (*Glylorin*)	Congenital primary ichthyosis	GlaxoWellcome
Morphine sulfate concentrate (preservative free) (*Infumorph*)	In microinfusion devices for intraspinal administration for intractable chronic pain[a]	Elkins-Sinn
Motexafin gadolinium (*Xcytrin*)	With whole brain radiation for the treatment of brain metastases arising from solid tumors	Pharmacyclics
MTC-DOX for injection	Hepatocellular carcinoma	FeRx
Mucoid exopolysaccharide *Pseudomonas* hyperimmune globulin (*MEP IGIV*)	To prevent and treat pulmonary infections caused by *Pseudomonas aeruginosa* in cystic fibrosis	North American Biologicals

Orphan Drugs		
Drug (Trade name)	Proposed use	Sponsor
Multi-vitamin infusion (neonatal formula)	To establish and maintain total parenteral nutrition in very low birth weight infants	Astra Pharm
Muramyltripeptide, phosphatidyl-ethanolamine encased in multi-lamellar liposomes	Children and adolescent osteosarcoma	Immuno-Designed Molecules
Murine MAb (Lym-1) and Iodine 131-I radiolabeled murine MAb (Lym-1) to human B-cell lymphoma (Oncolym)	B-cell non-Hodgkin lymphoma	Peregrine Pharm
Murine MAb to polymorphic epithelial mucin, human milk fat globule 1 (Theragyn)	Adjunctive treatment for ovarian cancer	Antisoma plc
Mx-dnG1 or Rexin-G retroviral vector (Rexin-G)	Pancreatic cancer	Epeius Biotechnologies
Mycobacterium avium sensitin RS-10	In the diagnosis of invasive Mycobacterium avium disease in immunocompetent individuals	Statens Seruminstitut
Mycobacterium with immunomodulator, heat killed (CADI Mw)	Adjunctive to multi-drug therapy in the management of multibacillary leprosy	CPL, Inc.
Myelin	Multiple sclerosis	Autoimmune
Myristoylated recombinant SCR1-3 of human complement reseptor type I (APT070)	To prevent delayed graft function in solid organ transplant	Adprotech
N-5-yl)phenyl]-N'-methyl)phenyl]urea	Sickle cell disease	NeuroSearch A/S
N-acetylcysteinate lysine (Nacystelyn Dry Powder Inhaler)	Management of cystic fibrosis	Galephar Pharm Res
N-acetylcysteine	Acute liver failure	William M. Lee, MD, FACP
N-acetylprocainamide	To prevent life-threatening ventricular arrhythmias in documented procainamide-induced lupus	NAPA of the Bahamas
(Napa)	Lower the defibrillation energy requirement sufficiently to allow automatic implantable cardioverter defibrillator therapy in patients who could otherwise not use the device	Medco Res
N-acetylgalactosamine-4-sulfatase, recombinant human	Mucopolysaccharidosis type VI (Maroteaux-Lamy syndrome)	BioMarin Pharm
N-acetyl-sarcosyl-glycyl-L-valyl-D-alloisoleucyl-L-threonyl-L-norvaly-L-isoleucyl-L-arginyl-L-prolylethylaminde acetate	Soft tissue sarcoma	Abbott
Nafarelin acetate (Synarel Nasal Solution)	Central precocious puberty[a]	Syntex (USA)
Naltrexone HCl (Trexan)	Blockade of the pharmacological effects of exogenous opioids as an adjunct to maintain opioid-free state in detoxified, formerly opioid-dependent individuals[a]	DuPont Pharm
Natural human lymphoblastoid interferon-alpha	Polycythemia vera	Amarillo Biosciences
	Papillomavirus warts in the oral cavity of HIV-positive patients; Behcet disease	Atrix Labs
NDROGE	Postanoxic intention myoclonus	Watson Labs
Nebacumab (Centoxin)	Gram-negative bacteremia that has progressed to endotoxin shock	Centocor

Orphan Drugs

Drug (Trade name)	Proposed use	Sponsor
Neurotrophin-1	Motor neuron disease/amyotrophic lateral sclerosis	Arthur Dale Ericsson, MD
NG-29 (*Somatrel*)	Diagnostic measure of the capacity of the pituitary gland to release growth hormone	Ferring Labs
Nifedipine	Interstitial cystitis	Jonathan Fleischmann,
Niprisan (*Hemoxin*)	Sickle cell disease	Xechem
Nitazoxanide (*Alinia*)	Intestinal giardiasis[a]; cryptosporidiosis[a]	Romark Labs
(*Cryptaz*)	Intestinal amebiasis	
Nitisinone (*Orfadin*)	Tyrosinemia type 1[a]; alkaptonuria	Swedish Orphan AB
Nitric oxide (*INOmax*)	Persistent pulmonary hypertension in the newborn[a]; acute adult respiratory distress syndrome	INO Therapeutics
Nitroprusside	To prevent and treat cerebral vasospasm following subarachnoid hemorrhage	Jeffrey Evan Thomas, MD
Nolatrexed (*THYMITAQ*)	Hepatocellular carcinoma	Zarix
Novel acting thrombolytic (NAT)	Peripheral arterial occlusion	Amgen
NZ-1002	Enzyme replacement therapy in patients with all subtypes of mucopolysaccharidosis I	Novazyme Pharm
Octavalent *Pseudomonas aeruginosa* O-polysaccharide-toxin A conjugate (*Aerugen*)	To prevent *Pseudomonas aeruginosa* infections in cystic fibrosis	Orphan Europe
Octreotide (*Sandostatin LAR*)	Acromegaly[a]; severe diarrhea and flushing associated with malignant carcinoid tumors[a]; diarrhea associated with vasoactive intestinal peptide tumors (VIPoma)[a]	Novartis
Ofloxacin (*Ocuflox Ophthalmic Solution*)	Bacterial corneal ulcers[a]	Allergan
Oglufanide disodium	Ovarian cancer	Cytran
OM 401 (*Drepanol*)	Prophylactic treatment of sickle cell disease	Omex International
Omega-3 (n-3) polyunsaturated fatty acid (with all double bonds in the cis configuration)	To prevent organ graft rejection	Research Triangle Pharm
Omega-3 (n-3) polyunsaturated fatty acids (*Omacor*)	IgA nephropathy	Pronova Biocare, AS
Oncorad Ov103	Ovarian cancer	Cytogen
Oprelvekin (*Neumega*)	To prevent severe chemotherapy-induced thrombocytopenia[a]	Genetics Institute
Orgotein for injection	Familial amyotrophic lateral sclerosis associated with a mutation of the gene (on chromosome 21q) for copper, zinc superoxide dismutase	Oxis International
Oxaliplatin	Ovarian cancer	Debio Pharm SA
Oxandrolone	Constitutional delay of growth and puberty	Bio-Technology General
(*Hepandrin*)	For moderate/severe acute alcoholic hepatitis in the presence of moderate protein calorie malnutrition	
(*Oxandrin*)	Duchenne and Becker muscular dystrophy; adjunctive therapy for AIDS patients with HIV-wasting syndrome; short stature associated with Turner syndrome	
Oxybate (*Xyrem*)	Narcolepsy[a]	Orphan Medical

Orphan Drugs

Drug (Trade name)	Proposed use	Sponsor
Oxymorphone (Numorphan H.P.)	To relieve severe intractable pain in narcotic-tolerant patients	DuPont Merck
Oxypurinol	Hyperuricemia in patients intolerant to allopurinol	Cardiome Pharma
P1, P4-Di(uridine 5'-tetraphosphate), tetrasodium salt	Cystic fibrosis	Inspire Pharm
p1-(uridine 5'-)-p4-(2'-deoxycytidine 5'-) tetraphosphate, tetrasodium salt	Cystic fibrosis	Inspire Pharm
PA mAb (Abthrax)	Treat anthrax	Human Genome Sciences
Paclitaxel (Paxene)	AIDS-related Kaposi sarcoma	Baker Norton Pharm
(Taxol)[a]		Bristol-Myers Squibb
Papain, trypsin, and chymotrypsin (Wobe-Mugos)	Multiple myeloma	Marlyn Nutraceuticals
Papaverine topical gel	Sexual dysfunction in spinal cord injury	Pharmedic
Parvovirus B19 (recombinant VP1 and VP2; *Spodoptera frugiperda* cells) vaccine (MEDI-491)	To prevent transient aplastic crisis in patients with sickle cell anemia	MedImmune
Patul-end	Patulous eustachian tube	Ear Foundation
Pegademase bovine (Adagen)	Enzyme replacement for adenosine deaminase deficiency in patients with severe combined immunodeficiency[a]	Enzon
Pegaspargase (Oncaspar)	Acute lymphocytic leukemia[a]	Enzon
PEG-glucocerebrosidase (Lysodase)	Chronic enzyme replacement therapy in Gaucher disease patients deficient in glucocerebrosidase	National Institute of Mental Health, NIH
Peginterferon alfa-2a (PEGASYS)	Renal cell carcinoma; chronic myelogenous leukemia	Hoffmann-La Roche
PEG-interleukin-2	Primary immunodeficiencies associated with T-cell defects	Chiron
Pegvisomant (Somavert)	Acromegaly[a]	Sensus
Pegylated arginine deiminase (Hepacid)	Hepatocellular carcinoma	Phoenix Pharmacologics
(Melanocid)	Invasive malignant melanoma	
Pegylated recombinant human megakaryocyte growth and development factor (MEGAGEN)	To reduce the period of thrombocytopenia in patients undergoing hematopoietic stem cell transplantation	Amgen
Peldesine	Cutaneous T-cell lymphoma	BioCryst Pharm
Pemetrexed disodium (Alimta)	Malignant pleural mesothelioma	Eli Lilly
Pentamidine isethionate	*Pneumocystis carinii* pneumonia	Aventis Behring
(Nebupent)	*Pneumocystis carinii* pneumonia prevention in high-risk patients[a]	Fujisawa USA
(Pentam 300)	*Pneumocystis carinii* pneumonia[a]	Fujisawa USA
Pentamidine isethionate (inhalation) (Pneumopent)	To prevent *Pneumocystis carinii* pneumonia in high-risk patients	Fisons
Pentastarch (Pentaspan)	Adjunctive in leukapheresis to improve the harvesting and increase the yield of leukocytes by centrifugal means[a]	DuPont Pharm

Orphan Drugs

Drug (Trade name)	Proposed use	Sponsor
Pentosan polysulphate sodium (Elmiron)	Interstitial cystitis[a]	Alza
Pentostatin (Nipent)	Chronic lymphocytic leukemia; cutaneous T-cell lymphoma; peripheral T-cell lymphomas	SuperGen
Pentostatin for injection (Nipent)	Hairy-cell leukemia[a]	SuperGen
Perflubron (LiquiVent)	Acute adult respiratory distress syndrome	Alliance Pharm
Perfosfamide (Pergamid)	Ex-vivo treatment of autologous bone marrow and subsequent reinfusion in acute myelogenous leukemia, also referred to as acute nonlymphocytic leukemia	Scios Nova
Pergolide (Permax)	Tourette syndrome	Floyd R. Sallee, MD, PhD
Phenylacetate	Adjunctive to surgery, radiation therapy, and chemotherapy for the treatment of patients with primary or recurrent malignant glioma	Elan Drug Delivery
Phenylalanine ammonia-lyase (Phenylase)	Hyperphenylalaninemia	Ibex Technologies
Phenylbutyrate	Acute promyelocytic leukemia	Elan Drug Delivery
Phenylephrine	Ileal pouch anal anastomosis related fecal incontinence	SLA Pharma
Phosphocysteamine	Cystinosis	Medea Res Labs
Pilocarpine HCl (Salagen)	Xerostomia induced by radiation therapy for head and neck cancer[a]; xerostomia and keratoconjunctivitis sicca in Sjogren syndrome[a]	MGI Pharma
Piracetam (Nootropil)	Myoclonus	UCE Pharma
Pirfenidone	Idiopathic pulmonary fibrosis	InterMune
Piritrexim isethionate	Infections caused by Pneumocystis carinii, Toxoplasma gondii, and Mycobacterium avium-intracellulare	Burroughs Wellcome
Polifeprosan 20 with carmustine (Gliadel)	Malignant glioma[a]	Guilford Pharm
Poloxamer 188 (Flocor)	Vasospasm in subarachnoid hemorrhage patients following surgical repair of a ruptured cerebral aneurysm; sickle cell crisis; severe burns requiring hospitalization	CytRx
Poloxamer 331 (Protox)	Initial therapy for toxoplasmosis in AIDS patients	CytRx
Poly I: poly C12U (Ampligen)	AIDS; renal cell carcinoma; chronic fatigue syndrome; invasive metastatic melanoma (stage IIB, III, IV)	Hemispherx Biopharma
Poly-ICLC	Primary brain tumors	Oncovir
Polyethylene glycol (PEG)-uricase	To control the clinical consequences of hyperuricemia in patients with severe gout in whom conventional therapy is contraindicated or has been ineffective	Bio-Technology General
Polyethylene glycol-modified uricase (Zurase)	Tumor lysis syndrome in cancer patients undergoing chemotherapy; prophylaxis of hyperuricemia in cancer patients prone to develop tumor lysis syndrome during chemotherapy	Phoenix Pharmacologics
Polyinosinic-polycytidilic acid (Poly-ICLC)	Adjuvant to smallpox vaccination; flavivirus infections including those caused by West Nile, Japanese encephalitis, dengue, St. Louis encephalitis, yellow fever, Murray valley, and Banzai viruses	Oncovir

Orphan Drugs		
Drug (Trade name)	*Proposed use*	*Sponsor*
Polyinosinic-polycytidilic acid (Poly-ICLC) (Hiltonol)	Orthopox virus infections	Oncovir
Polymeric oxygen	Sickle cell anemia	Capmed USA
Porcine fetal neural dopaminergic cells and/or precursors aseptically prepared and coated with anti-MHC-1 Ab for intracerebral implantation (NeuroCell-PD)	Hoehn and Yahr stage 4 and 5 Parkinson disease	Diacrin/Genzyme LLC
Porcine fetal neural dopaminergic cells and/or precursors aseptically prepared for intracerebral implantation (NeuroCell-PD)	Hoehn and Yahr stage 4 and 5 Parkinson disease	Diacrin/Genzyme LLC
Porcine fetal neural gabaergic cells and/or precursors aseptically prepared and coated with anti-MHC-1 Ab for intracerebral implantation (NeuroCell-HD)	Huntington disease	Diacrin/Genzyme LLC
Porcine fetal neural gabaergic cells and/or precursors aseptically prepared for intracerebral implantation for Huntington disease (NeuroCell-HD)	Huntington disease	Diacrin/Genzyme LLC
Porcine Sertoli cells aseptically prepared for intracerebral co-implantation with fetal neural tissue (N-Graft)	Hoehn and Yahr stage 4 and 5 Parkinson disease	Titan Pharm
Porfimer (Photofrin)	Ablation of high-grade dysplasia in Barrett esophagus in patients who are not considered to be candidates for esophagectomy[a]	Axcan Scandipharm
Porfimer sodium (Photofrin)	Photodynamic therapy of patients with primary or recurrent obstructing (partially or completely) esophageal carcinoma[a]; photodynamic therapy of patients with transitional cell carcinoma in situ of the urinary bladder	QLT Phototherapeutics
Porfiromycin (Promycin)	Head, neck, and cervical cancer	Boehringer Ingelheim
Potassium citrate (Urocit-K)	To prevent uric acid nephrolithiasis[a]; to prevent calcium renal stones in patients with hypocitraturia[a]; to avoid the complication of calcium stone formation in uric lithiasis[a]	University of Texas Health Sciences Center at Dallas
Potassium citrate and citric acid	Dissolution and control of uric acid and cysteine calculi in the urinary tract	Willen Drug
Pr-122 (redox-phenytoin)	Emergency rescue treatment of status epilepticus, grand mal type	Pharmos
PR-225 (redox-acyclovir)	Herpes simplex encephalitis in AIDS	Pharmos
PR-239 (redox penicillin G)	AIDS-associated neurosyphilis	Pharmos
Pr-320 (molecusol-carbamazepine)	Emergency rescue treatment of status epilepticus, grand mal type	Pharmos
Pramiracetam sulfate	Management of cognitive dysfunction and enhancement of antidepressant activity with electroconvulsive therapy	Cambridge Neuroscience
Praziquantel	Neurocysticercosis	EM Pharm
Prednimustine (Sterecyt)	Malignant non-Hodgkin lymphomas	Pharmacia
Primaquine phosphate	With clindamycin HCl in AIDS-associated *Pneumocystis carinii* pneumonia	Sanofi Winthrop

Orphan Drugs		
Drug (Trade name)	Proposed use	Sponsor
Progesterone	Establish and maintain pregnancy in women undergoing in vitro fertilization or embryo transfer procedures	Watson Labs
Propamidine isethionate 0.1% ophthalmic solution (Brolene)	Acanthamoeba keratitis	Bausch & Lomb
Prostaglandin E1 enol ester (AS-013)	Fontaine stage IV chronic, critical limb ischemia	Mitsubishi Pharma
Prostaglandin E1 in lipid emulsion (Lipo-PGE1)	Ischemic ulceration of the lower limbs caused by peripheral arterial disease	Alpha Therapeutic
Protaxel	Ovarian cancer	Biophysica
Protein C concentrate (Protein C Concentrate [human] Vapor Heated, Immuno)	Replacement therapy in patients with congenital or acquired protein C deficiency to prevent/treat warfarin-induced skin necrosis during oral anticoagulation; to prevent and treat purpura fulminans in meningococcemia	Immuno Clin Res
	Replacement therapy in congenital protein C deficiency to prevent and treat thrombosis, pulmonary emboli, and purpura fulminans	Baxter Healthcare
Protirelin	To prevent infant respiratory distress syndrome associated with prematurity	UCB Pharma
Protirelin injection	Amyotrophic lateral sclerosis	Abbott Labs
Pulmonary surfactant replacement	To prevent and treat infant respiratory distress syndrome	Scios Nova
Pulmonary surfactant replacement, porcine (Curosurf)	To prevent and treat respiratory distress syndrome in premature infants	Dey Labs
Purified extract of Pseudomonas aeruginosa (ImmuDyn)	Immune thrombocytopenic purpura where it is required to increase platelet counts	DynaGen
Purified type II collagen (Colloral)	Juvenile rheumatoid arthritis	AutoImmune
pVGI.1(VEGF2)	Thromboangiitis obliterans	Vascular Genetics
Pyruvate	Interstitial lung disease	Cellular Sciences
Quinacrine HCl	To prevent recurrence of pneumothorax in high-risk patients	Lyphomed
R-etodolac	Chronic lymphocytic leukemia	Salmedix
(R)-N-[2-(6-chloro-5-methoxy-1H-indol-3-yl)-propyl]acetamide	Circadian rhythm sleep disorders in blind people with no light perception; neuroleptic-induced tardive dyskinesia in patients with schizophrenia	Phase 2 Discovery
Rasburicase (Elitek)	Malignancy-associated or chemotherapy-induced hyperuricemia[a]	Sanofi-Synthelabo
Recombinant adeno-associated virus alpha 1-antitrypsin vector (rAAV-AAT)	Alpha1-antitrypsin deficiency	Applied Genetic Technologies
Recombinant bactericidal/permeability-increasing protein (Neuprex)	Severe meningococcal disease	Xoma
Recombinant glycine2-human glucagon-like peptide-2	Short bowel syndrome	NPS Allelix
Recombinant human acid alpha-glucosidase	Glycogen storage disease type II	Genzyme

Orphan Drugs

Drug (Trade name)	Proposed use	Sponsor
Recombinant human alpha-1 antitrypsin (rAAT)	Cystic fibrosis	Arriva Pharm
		PPL Therapeutics (Scotland) Ltd
	To delay progression of chronic obstructive pulmonary disease resulting from AAT deficiency-mediated emphysema and bronchiectasis	Baxter Healthcare
Recombinant human alpha-fetoprotein (rhAFP)	Myasthenia gravis	Merrimack Pharm
Recombinant human antithrombin III	Antithrombin III-dependent heparin resistance requiring anticoagulation	AT III LLC
Recombinant human C1-esterase inhibitor	Prophylactic treatment of angioedema caused by hereditary or acquired C1-esterase inhibitor deficiency; treatment of acute attacks of angioedema caused by hereditary or acquired C1-esterase inhibitor deficiency	Pharming NV
Recombinant human CD4 immunoglobulin G	AIDS resulting from HIV-1 infection	Genentech
Recombinant human Clara Cell 10kDa protein	To prevent neonatal bronchopulmonary dysplasia in premature neonates with respiratory distress syndrome	Claragen
Recombinant human endostatin protein	Neuroendocrine tumors; metastatic melanoma	EntreMed
Recombinant human fibroblast growth factor-20	Radiation-induced oral mucositis	CuraGen
Recombinant human gelsolin	Respiratory symptoms of cystic fibrosis; acute and chronic respiratory symptoms of bronchiectasis	Biogen
Recombinant human highly phosphorylated acid alpha-glucosidase	For enzyme replacement therapy in patients with all subtypes of glycogen storage disease type II (GSDII, Pompe disease)	Novazyme Pharm
Recombinant human insulin-like growth factor-I	Postpoliomyelitis syndrome	Cephalon
(IGF-1)	Growth hormone receptor deficiency; antibody-mediated growth hormone resistance with isolated growth hormone deficiency Ia	Pharmacia & Upjohn
(PV802)	Short-bowel syndrome as a result of resection of the small bowel or congenital dysfunction of the intestines	GroPep Pty Ltd
Recombinant human insulin-like growth factor-I/insulin-like growth factor binding protein-3	Major burns that require hospitalization	Celtrix Pharm
(SomatoKine)	Growth hormone insensitivity syndrome	
Recombinant human interleukin-12	Renal cell carcinoma	Genetics Institute
Recombinant human keratinocyte growth factor	To reduce the incidence and severity of radiation-induced xerostomia	Amgen
Recombinant human luteinizing hormone (LHadi)	With recombinant human follicle stimulating hormone for women with chronic anovulation caused by hypogonadotropic hypogonadism	Serono Labs
Recombinant human monoclonal antibody to hsp90 (Mycograb)	Invasive candidiasis	NeuTec Pharma plc
Recombinant human nerve growth factor	HIV-associated sensory neuropathy	Genentech
Recombinant human neutrophil inhibitor (hNE)	Cystic fibrosis	Dyax
Recombinant human porphobilinogen deaminase (Porphozyme)	Acute intermittent porphyria attacks	HemeBiotech A/S

Orphan Drugs

Drug (Trade name)	Proposed use	Sponsor
Recombinant human porphobilinogen deaminase, erythropoetic form	To prevent acute intermittent porphyria attacks	HemeBiotech A/S
Recombinant human relaxin	Progressive systemic sclerosis	Connetics
Recombinant human thrombopoietin	To accelerate platelet recovery in patients undergoing hematopoietic stem-cell transplantation	Genentech
Recombinant humanized MAb 5c8	To prevent and treat Factor VIII/Factor IX inhibitors in hemophilia A or B; to prevent rejection of solid organ transplants; to prevent rejection of pancreatic islet cell transplants; immune thrombocytopenic purpura; systemic lupus erythematosus	Biogen
Recombinant inhibitor of human plasma kallikrein	Angioedema	Dyax
Recombinant methionyl brain-derived neurotrophic factor	Amyotrophic lateral sclerosis	Amgen
Recombinant methionyl human stem cell factor	Primary bone marrow failure	Amgen
Recombinant retroviral vector - glucocerebrosidase	Enzyme replacement therapy for types I, II, or III Gaucher disease	Genetic Therapy
Recombinant secretory leucocyte protease inhibitor	Congenital alpha-1 antitrypsin deficiency; cystic fibrosis	Amgen
Recombinant soluble human CD4 (rCD4)	AIDS	Genentech
(Receptin)		Biogen
Recombinant T-cell receptor ligand	Patients with multiple sclerosis who are HLA-DR2 positive and autoreactive to myelin oligo-dendrocyte glycoprotein residues 35-55	Virogenomics
Recombinant urate oxidase	Prophylaxis of chemotherapy-induced hyperuricemia	Sanofi-Synthelabo
Recombinant vaccinia (human papillomavirus) (TA-HPV)	Cervical cancer	Xenova Res Ltd
Reduced L-glutathione (Cachexon)	AIDS-associated cachexia	Telluride Pharm
Remacemide (Ecovia)	Huntington disease	AstraZeneca LP
Repertaxin	To prevent delayed graft function in solid organ transplant	Dompe s.p.a.
Repository corticotropin or adrenocorticotropic hormone (H.P. Acthar Gel)	Infantile spasms	Questcor
Resiniferatoxin	Intractable pain at end-stage disease	Andrew J. Mannes, MD
Respiratory syncytial virus (RSV) immune globulin (human) (Hypermune RSV)	To treat respiratory syncytial virus lower respiratory tract infections in hospitalized infants and young children	MedImmune
(Respigam)	Prophylaxis of respiratory syncytial virus (RSV) lower respiratory tract infections in infants and young children at high risk of RSV disease[a]	MedImmune and MA
Retroviral gamma-c cDNA containing vector	X-linked severe combined immune deficiency disease	AVAX Tech
Retroviral vector, R-GC and GC gene 1750	Gaucher disease	Genzyme
Reviparin sodium (Clivarine)	Deep vein thrombosis that may lead to pulmonary embolism in pediatric patients; long-term treatment of acute deep vein thrombosis with or without pulmonary embolism in pregnant patients	Knoll AG
RGG0853, E1A lipid complex	Ovarian cancer	Targeted Genetics

Orphan Drugs

Drug (Trade name)	Proposed use	Sponsor
rhIGF-I/rhIGFBP-3 (SomatoKine)	Extreme insulin-resistance syndromes (type A, Rabson-Mendenhall syndrome, Leprechaunism, type B syndrome)	Insmed
Rho (D) immune globulin IV (human) (WinRho SD)	Immune thrombocytopenic purpura[a]	Rh Pharm
rhuMAb VEGF (bevacizumab) (Avastin)	Renal cell carcinoma	Genentech
Ribavirin (Rebetol)	Chronic hepatitis C in pediatric patients[a]	Schering
(Virazole)	Hemorrhagic fever with renal syndrome	Valeant
Ricin (blocked) conjugated murine MCA (anti-B4)	B-cell leukemia and B-cell lymphoma; ex vivo purging of leukemic cells from the bone marrow of non-T-cell acute lymphocytic leukemia patients who are in complete remission	ImmunoGen
Ricin (blocked) conjugated murine MCA (anti-my9)	Myeloid leukemia, including acute myelogenous leukemia, and blast crisis of chronic myeloid leukemia; ex vivo treatment of autologous bone marrow and subsequent reinfusion in acute myelogenous leukemia	ImmunoGen
Ricin (blocked) conjugated murine MCA (n901)	Small-cell lung cancer	ImmunoGen
Ricin (blocked) conjugated murine monoclonal antibody (CD6)	Cutaneous T-cell lymphomas, acute T-cell leukemia-lymphoma, and related mature T-cell malignancies	ImmunoGen
Rifabutin	To treat disseminated *Mycobacterium avium* complex disease	Pfizer
(Mycobutin)	To prevent disseminated *Mycobacterium avium* complex disease in advanced HIV infection[a]	Adria Labs
Rifalazil	Pulmonary tuberculosis	PathoGenesis
Rifampin (Rifadin IV)	Antituberculosis treatment when oral doseform is not feasible[a]	Hoechst Marion Roussel
Rifampin, isoniazid, pyrazinamide (Rifater)	Short-course treatment of tuberculosis[a]	Hoechst Marion Roussel
Rifapentine (Priftin)	Pulmonary tuberculosis[a]; *Mycobacterium avium* complex (MAC) in patients with AIDS; prophylaxis of MAC in patients with AIDS and a CD4+ count ≤ 75/mm^3	Hoechst Marion Roussel
Rifaximin (Normix)	Hepatic encephalopathy	Salix Pharm
RII Retinamide	Myelodysplastic syndromes	Sparta Pharm
Riluzole (Rilutek)	Amyotrophic lateral sclerosis[a]; Huntington disease	Rhone-Poulenc Rorer
Rituximab (Rituxan)	Non-Hodgkin B-cell lymphoma[a]; chronic lymphocytic leukemia	IDEC Pharm
	Immune thrombocytopenic purpura	Genentech
Roquinimex (Linomide)	To prolong time to relapse in leukemia patients who have undergone autologous bone marrow transplantation	Pharmacia & Upjohn
rSP-C lung surfactant (Venticute)	Adult respiratory distress syndrome	Byk Gulden Pharm
Rubitecan	HIV- and AIDS-infected pediatric patients	SuperGen
S(-)-3-]-glutaramide	Multiple myeloma	EntreMed
Sacrosidase (Sucraid)	Congenital sucrase-isomaltase deficiency[a]	Orphan Medical
S-adenosylmethionine	AIDS-myelopathy	Alessandro Di Rocco, MD

Orphan Drugs

Drug (Trade name)	Proposed use	Sponsor
Sargramostim (*Leukine*)	Neutropenia associated with bone marrow transplant, graft failure, and delay of engraftment[a] and for promotion of early engraftment[a]; to reduce neutropenia and leukopenia and decrease the incidence of death caused by infection in patients with acute myelogenous leukemia[a]	Immunex
Satumomab pendetide (*OncoScint CR/OV*)	Detect ovarian carcinoma[a]	Cytogen
SB-408075	Pancreatic cancer	SmithKline Beecham
SC-1 monoclonal antibody	CD55 (sc-1) positive gastric tumors	H3 Pharma
SCH 58500	Primary ovarian cancer	Schering
Secalciferol (*Osteo-D*)	Familial hypophosphatemic rickets	Teva Pharm USA
Secretory leukocyte protease inhibitor	Bronchopulmonary dysplasia	Synergen
Selegiline HCl (*Eldepryl*)	Adjuvant to levodopa and carbidopa in idiopathic Parkinson disease (paralysis agitans), postencephalitic Parkinsonism, and symptomatic Parkinsonism[a]	Somerset Pharm
Sermorelin acetate (*Geref*)	Idiopathic or organic growth hormone deficiency in children with growth failure[a]; adjunctive to gonadotropin in ovulation induction in anovulatory or oligo-ovulatory infertility after failure of clomiphene citrate or gonadotropin alone; AIDS-associated catabolism/weight loss	Serono Labs
Serratia marcescens extract (polyribosomes) (*Imuvert*)	Primary brain malignancies	Cell Technology
SGN-30 (anti-CD30 mAb)	Hodgkin disease	Seattle Genetics
Short chain fatty acid enema (*Colomed*)	Chronic radiation proctitis	Richard I. Breuer, MD
Short chain fatty acid solution (*Colomed*)	Active phase of ulcerative colitis with involvement restricted to the left side of the colon	Richard I. Breuer, MD
Silver sulfadiazine and cerium nitrate (*Flammacerium*)	To prevent mortality in severely burned patients	Synthes (USA)
Siplizumab	T-cell lymphomas	Medimmune Oncology
SK&F 110679	Long-term treatment of children who have growth failure caused by a lack of adequate endogenous growth hormone secretion	SmithKline Beecham
Sodium 1,3-propanedisulfonate	Secondary amyloidosis	Neurochem
Sodium dichloroacetate	Congenital lactic acidosis	Peter W. Stacpoole, Questcor Pharm
	Lactic acidosis in severe malaria; homozygous familial hypercholesterolemia	Peter W. Stacpoole, PhD, MD
	Antidote in managing systemic monochloroacetic acid poisoning	EBD Group
(*Ceresine*)	Severe head injury	Questcor Pharm
Sodium monomercaptoundecahydro-closo-dodecaborate	In conjunction with a thermal or epithermal neutron beam in boron nuclear capture therapy of glioblastoma multiforme	Theragenics
(*Borocell*)	In boron neutron capture therapy in glioblastoma multiforme	Neutron Technology & Neutron R & D Partner
Sodium phenylbutyrate	Adjunctive to surgery, radiation therapy, and chemotherapy for primary or recurrent malignant glioma	Elan Drug Delivery

Orphan Drugs

Drug (Trade name)	Proposed use	Sponsor
(Buphenyl)	The following urea cycle disorders: Carbamylphosphate synthetase deficiency; ornithine transcarbamylase deficiency[a]; arginiosuccinic acid synthetase deficiency; sickling disorders including S-S, S-C, and S-thalassemia hemoglobinopathy	Medicis Pharm
Sodium pyruvate	Cystic fibrosis	Cellular Sciences
Sodium tetradecyl sulfate (Sotradecol)	Bleeding esophageal varices	Elkins-Sinn
Sodium thiosulfate	To prevent platinum-induced ototoxicity in pediatric patients	Adherex Technologies
Soluble complement receptor type 1	To prevent postcardiopulmonary bypass syndrome in children undergoing cardiopulmonary bypass	Avant Immunotherapeutics
Soluble recombinant human complement receptor type 1	To prevent and reduce adult respiratory distress syndrome	T Cell Sciences
Somatostatin	Bleeding esophageal varices	UCB Pharm
(Zecnil)	Adjunctive to nonoperative management of secreting cutaneous fistulas of the stomach, duodenum, small intestine (jejunum and ileum), or pancreas	Ferring Labs
Somatrem for injection (Protropin)	Long-term treatment of children with growth failure caused by lack of adequate endogenous growth hormone secretion[a]; short stature associated with Turner syndrome	Genentech
Somatropin (Biotropin)	Cachexia associated with AIDS	Bio-Technology General
(Genotropin)	Adults with growth hormone deficiency[a]	Pharmacia & Upjohn
(Humatrope)	Short stature associated with Turner syndrome[a]	Eli Lilly
(Norditropin)	Adjunctive in ovulation induction in women with infertility caused by hypogonadotropic hypogonadism or bilateral tubal occlusion or unexplained infertility who are undergoing in vivo or in vitro fertilization procedures; short stature associated with Turner syndrome	Novo Nordisk Pharm
(Nutropin)	Long-term treatment of children with growth failure caused by lack of adequate endogenous growth hormone secretion[a]	Genentech
Somatropin for injection (Nutropin)	Growth retardation associated with chronic renal failure[a]; short stature associated with Turner syndrome[a]; replacement therapy for growth hormone deficiency in adults after epiphyseal closure[a]	Genentech
(Humatrope)	Long-term treatment of children who have growth failure caused by inadequate secretion of normal endogenous growth hormone[a]	Eli Lilly
(Serostim)	AIDS-associated catabolism/weight loss[a]	Serono Labs
Somatropin (rDNA) (Genotropin)	Growth failure in children who were born small for gestational age[a]; short stature in patients with Prader-Willi syndrome[a]	Pharmacia & Upjohn
(Nutropin Depot)	Long-term treatment of children who have growth failure caused by a lack of adequate endogenous growth hormone secretion	Genentech
(Saizen)	Enhancement of nitrogen retention in hospitalized patients suffering from severe burns; idiopathic or organic growth hormone deficiency in children with growth failure	Serono Labs
(Serostim)	Alone or with glutamine in short bowel syndrome	Serono Labs
Somatropin (rDNA) for injection (Serostim)	Children with AIDS-associated failure-to-thrive, including AIDS-associated wasting	Serono Labs

Orphan Drugs

Drug (Trade name)	Proposed use	Sponsor
Somatropin (rDNA origin) injection (*Norditropin*)	Growth failure in children caused by inadequate growth hormone secretion	Novo Nordisk
Sorivudine (*BRAVAVIR*)	Herpes zoster (shingles) in immunocompromised patients	Bristol-Myers Squibb
Sotalol HCl (*Betapace*)	To prevent and treat[a] life-threatening ventricular tachyarrhythmias	Berlex Labs
Spiramycin (*Rovamycine*)	Symptomatic relief and parasitic cure of chronic cryptosporidiosis in immunodeficiency	Rhone-Poulenc Rorer
Squalamine lactate	Ovarian cancer refractory or resistant to standard chemotherapy	Genaera
SS1(dsFv)-PE38	Malignant mesothelioma; epithelial ovarian cancer	NeoPharm
***Staphylococcus aureus* immune globulin (human)** (*Altastaph*)	Prophylaxis against *Staphylococcus aureus* infections in low birth weight neonates	NABI
ST1-RTA immunotoxin (SR 44163)	To prevent acute graft vs host disease in allogenic bone marrow transplantation; treat B-chronic lymphocytic leukemia	Sanofi Winthrop
SU101	Malignant glioma; ovarian cancer	Sugen
Suberoylanilide hydroxamic acid	Multiple myeloma	Aton Pharma
Succimer (*Chemet*)	To prevent cystine kidney stones in patients with homozygous cystinuria who are prone to stone development; mercury intoxication	Sanofi Winthrop
(*Chemet capsules*)	Lead poisoning in children[a]	Bock Pharmacal
Sucralfate	Oral mucositis and stomatitis following radiation therapy for head and neck cancer	Fuisz Tech
Sucralfate suspension	Oral complications of chemotherapy in bone marrow transplants; oral ulcerations and dysphagia in epidermolysis bullosa	Darby Pharm
Sulfadiazine	With pyrimethamine for *Toxoplasma gondii* encephalitis in patients with and without AIDS[a]	Eon Labs
Sulfapyridine	Dermatitis herpetiformis	Jacobus Pharm
Superoxide dismutase (human)	To protect donor organ tissue from damage or injury mediated by oxygen-derived free radicals that are generated during the necessary periods of ischemia (hypoxia, anoxia) and especially reperfusion associated with the operative procedure	Pharmacia-Chiron Partnership
Superoxide dismutase (recombinant human) (*Oxsodrol*)	To prevent reperfusion injury to donor organ tissue	Bio-Technology General
Suramin (*Metaret*)	Hormone-refractory prostate cancer	Warner-Lambert
Surface active extract of saline lavage of bovine lungs (*Infasurf*)	To prevent and treat respiratory failure caused by pulmonary surfactant deficiency in preterm infants	ONY
Surfactant (human) (amniotic fluid derived) (*Human Surf*)	To prevent and treat neonatal respiratory distress syndrome	T Allen Merritt, MD
Synsorb Pk	Verocytotoxigenic *Escherichia coli* infections	Synsorb Biotech
Synthetic human parathyroid hormone 1-34	Hypoparathyroidism	Orphan Pharm US
Synthetic human secretin	To evaluate exocrine pancreas function; obtaining desquamated pancreatic cells for cytopathologic examination in pancreatic carcinoma; diagnosing gastrinoma associated with Zollinger-Ellison syndrome; with diagnostic procedures for pancreatic disorders to increase pancreatic fluid secretion	ChiRhoClin

Orphan Drugs

Drug (Trade name)	Proposed use	Sponsor
Synthetic porcine secretin	To evaluate exocrine pancreas function[a]; obtaining desquamated pancreatic cells for cytopathologic examination in pancreatic carcinoma; diagnosing gastrinoma associated with Zollinger-Ellison syndrome[a]; with diagnostic procedures for pancreatic disorders to increase pancreatic fluid secretion[a]	ChiRhoClin
T4 endonuclease V, liposome encapsulated	To prevent cutaneous neoplasms and other skin abnormalities in xeroderma pigmentosum	AGI Dermatics
Tacrolimus (Prograf)	Prophylaxis of graft vs host disease	Fujisawa USA
TAK-603	Crohn disease	Tap Holdings
Talc, sterile (Steritalc)	Malignant pleural effusion; pneumothorax	Novatech SA
Talc powder, sterile (Sclerosol Intrapleural Aercsol)	Malignant pleural effusion[a]	Bryan
T-cell depleted stem cell enriched cellular product from peripheral blood stem cells	Chronic granulomatous disease	Nexell Therapeutics
Technetium Tc99m anti-melanoma murine monoclonal antibody (Oncotrac Melanoma Imaging Kit)	To detect, by imaging, metastases of malignant melanoma	NeoRx
Technetium Tc99m murine monoclonal antibody (IgG2a) to B cell (LymphoScan)	Diagnostic imaging in evaluating the extent of disease in patients with histologically confirmed diagnosis of non-Hodgkin B-cell lymphoma, acute B-cell lymphoblastic leukemia (in children and adults), and chronic B-cell lymphocytic leukemia	Immunomedics
Technetium Tc99m murine monoclonal antibody to hCG (Immuraid, hCG-Tc-99m)	To detect human chorionic gonadotropin-producing tumors such as germ-cell and trophoblastic cell tumors	Immunomedics
Technetium Tc99m murine monoclonal antibody to human AFP (AFP-Scan)	To detect alpha-fetoprotein producing germ-cell tumors; detect hepatocellular carcinoma and hepatoblastoma	Immunomedics
(Immuraid)	To detect hepatocellular carcinoma and hepatoblastoma	
Technetium Tc99m pterotetramide	Identification of ovarian carcinomas	Endocyte
Technetium Tc99m rh-Annexin V (Apomate)	Diagnosis or assessment of rejection status in heart, heart-lung, single lung, or bilateral lung transplants	Theseus Imaging
Temoporfin (Foscan)	Palliative treatment of recurrent, refractory, or second primary squamous cell carcinomas of the head and neck considered to be incurable with surgery or radiotherapy	Scotia Pharm
Temozolomide (Temodal)	Advanced metastatic melanoma	Schering-Plough Res Inst
(Temodar)	Recurrent malignant glioma[a]	
Teniposide (Vumon for Injection)	Refractory childhood acute lymphocytic leukemia[a]	Bristol-Myers Squibb Pharm Res Inst
Teriparatide (Parathar)	Diagnostic agent for patients with clinical and laboratory evidence of hypocalcemia caused by hypoparathyroidism or pseudohypoparathyroidism	Rhone-Poulenc Rorer
	Idiopathic osteoporosis	Henri Beaufour InstituteUSA
Terlipressin (Glypressin)	Bleeding esophageal varices	Ferring Labs
Testosterone (Androgel)	Weight loss in AIDS patients with HIV-associated wasting	Unimed

Orphan Drugs

Drug (Trade name)	Proposed use	Sponsor
(TheraDerm Testosterone Transdermal System)	Physiologic testosterone replacement in androgen-deficient, HIV-positive patients with an associated weight loss	Watson Labs
Testosterone propionate ointment 2%	Vulvar dystrophies	Star Pharm
Testosterone sublingual	Constitutional delay of growth and puberty in boys	Bio-Technology General
Tetrabenazine	Moderate/Severe tardive dyskinesia; Huntington disease	Prestwick Pharm
Tetrahydrobiopterin	Hyperphenylalaninemia	Biomarin Pharm
Tetraiodothyroacetic acid	Suppression of thyroid stimulating hormone in patients with well-differentiated cancer of the thyroid gland	Elliot Danforth Jr., MD
Tezacitabine	Adenocarcinoma of the esophagus and stomach	Chiron
TGF(beta)2-specific phosphorothioate antisense oligodeoxynucleotide (Oncomun)	Malignant glioma	Antisense Pharma GmbH
Thalidomide	To treat and prevent recurrent aphthous ulcers in severely, terminally immunocompromised patients; to treat/prevent graft vs host disease	Andrulis Res
	Clinical manifestations of mycobacterial infection caused by *Mycobacterium tuberculosis* and nontuberculous mycobacteria; primary brain malignancies; severe recurrent aphthous stomatitis in severely, terminally immunocompromised patients; Kaposi sarcoma	Celgene
	To treat and prevent graft vs host disease in bone marrow transplantation; to treat and maintain reactional lepromatous leprosy	Pediatric Pharm
(Synovir)	HIV-associated wasting syndrome	Celgene
(Thalomid)	Erythema nodosum leprosum[a]; multiple myeloma; Crohn disease	Celgene
Thymalfasin (Zadaxin)	Chronic active hepatitis B; DiGeorge anomaly with immune defects; hepatocellular carcinoma	SciClone Pharm
Thymoxamine HCl	To reverse phenylephrine-induced mydriasis in patients who have narrow anterior angles and are at risk of developing an acute attack of angle-closure glaucoma following mydriasis	Iolab Pharm
Thyrotropin alfa (Thyrogen)	Well-differentiated papillary, follicular, or combined papillary/follicular carcinomas of the thyroid; adjunct in the diagnosis of thyroid cancer[a]	Genzyme
Tiapride	Tourette syndrome	Sanofi-Synthelabo
Tiazofurin (2-Beta-D-ribofuranosyl-4-thiazolecarboxamide)	Chronic myelogenous leukemia	Ribapharm
Tin ethyl etiopurpurin	To prevent access graft disease in hemodialysis patients	Miravant Medical Technologies
Tinidazole	Giardiasis; amebiasis	Presutti Labs
Tiopronin (Thiola)	To prevent cystine nephrolithiasis in patients with homozygous cystinuria[a]	Charles Y. C. Pak, MD
Tirapazamine	Head and neck cancer	Sanofi-Synthelabo
Tiratricol (Triacana)	With levothyroxine to suppress thyroid stimulating hormone in patients with well-differentiated thyroid cancer who are intolerant to adequate doses of levothyroxine alone	Laphal Labs
Tizanidine HCl (Zanaflex)	Spasticity associated with multiple sclerosis and spinal cord injury	Athena Neurosciences

Orphan Drugs

Drug (Trade name)	Proposed use	Sponsor
Tobramycin (Tobi)	Bronchiectasis patients infected with Pseudomonas aeruginosa	Chiron
Tobramycin for inhalation (TOBI)	Bronchopulmonary infections of P. aeruginosa in cystic fibrosis patients[a]	Pathogenesis
Tocophersolan oral solution (vitamin E-tpgs)	Vitamin E deficiency resulting from malabsorption caused by prolonged cholestatic hepatobililary disease	Sterling Winthrop
Topiramate (Topamax)	Lennox-Gastaut syndrome[a]	RW Johnson Pharm Res Inst
Toralizumab	Immune thrombocytopenic purpura	IDEC Pharm
Toremifene (Fareston)	Hormonal therapy of metastatic breast carcinoma[a]; desmoid tumors	Orion
Tositumomab and iodine I 131 tositumomab (Bexxar)	Non-Hodgkin B-cell lymphoma[a]	Corixa
Tranexamic acid (Cyklokapron)	Patients with congenital coagulopathies who are undergoing surgical procedures (eg, dental extractions)[a]; undergoing prostatectomy where there is hemorrhage or risk of hemorrhage as a result of increased fibrinolysis or fibrinogenolysis; hereditary angioneurotic edema	Pharmacia
Tranilast (Rizaben)	Malignant glioma	Angiogen Pharm
Transforming growth factor-beta 2	Full-thickness macular holes	Celtrix Pharm
Transgenic human alpha 1 antitrypsin	Emphysema secondary to alpha 1 antitrypsin deficiency	PPL Therapeutics (Scotland) Ltd
Trastuzumab (Herceptin)	Pancreatic cancer that overexpresses p185HER2	Genentech
Treosulfan (Ovastat)	Ovarian cancer	Medac GmbH
Treprostinil (Remodulin)	Treatment of pulmonary arterial hypertension[a]	United Therapeutics
Tretinoin	Squamous metaplasia of the ocular surface epithelia (conjunctiva and/or cornea) with mucous deficiency and keratinization	Hannan Ophthalmic Marketing Service
(ATRA-IV)	Acute and chronic leukemia; T-cell non-Hodgkin lymphoma	Antigenics
(Vesanoid)	Acute promyelocytic leukemia[a]	Hoffmann-La Roche
Tri-antennary glycotripeptide derivative of 5-fluorodeoxyuridine monophosphate	Hepatocellular carcinoma	Cell Works
Trientine HCl (Syprine)	Wilson disease intolerant or inadequately responsive to penicillamine[a]	Merck Sharp & Dohme Res
Trimetrexate glucuronate (Neutrexin)	Metastatic carcinoma of head and neck (buccal cavity, pharynx, larynx); metastatic colorectal adenocarcinoma; pancreatic adenocarcinoma; Pneumocystis carinii pneumonia in AIDS patients[a]; advanced non-small-cell carcinoma of the lung; metastatic osteogenic sarcoma	Medimmune Oncology
Triptorelin pamoate (Decapeptyl Injection)	In palliative treatment of advanced ovarian carcinoma of epithelial origin	Debio R.A.

Orphan Drugs		
Drug (Trade name)	*Proposed use*	*Sponsor*
Trisaccharides A and B (*Biosynject*)	Moderate to very severe clinical forms of transfusion reactions arising from ABO incompatible transfusions of blood, blood products, and blood derivatives; moderate to severe clinical forms of hemolytic disease in newborns arising from placental transfer of antibodies against blood groups A and B; ABO-incompatible solid organ transplantation including kidney, heart, liver, and pancreas; to prevent ABO hemolytic reactions arising from ABO-incompatible bone marrow transplantation	Chembiomed Ltd
Trisodium citrate concentration (*Hemocitrate*)	Used in leukapheresis procedures	Hemotec Medical
Tumor necrosis factor-binding protein I	Symptomatic AIDS patients including all patients with CD4 T-cell counts < 200 cells/mm^3	Serono Labs
Tumor necrosis factor-binding protein II	Symptomatic AIDS patients including all patients with CD4 T-cell counts < 200 cells/mm^3	Serono Labs
Tyloxapol (*Supervent*)	Cystic fibrosis	Kennedy and Hoidal, MDs
Ubiquinone (*Ubi-Q-Gel*)	Mitochondrial cytopathies	Gel-Tec, Division of Tishcon
Unconjugated chimeric (human-murine) G250 IgG monoclonal antibody	Renal cell carcinoma	Wilex Biotechnolog GmbH
Uridine 5'-triphosphate	Cystic fibrosis; facilitate removal of lung secretions in primary ciliary dyskinesia	Inspire Pharm
Urofollitropin (*Fertinex*)	For the initiation and reinitiation of spermatogenesis in adult males with reproductive failure caused by hypothalamic or pituitary dysfunction, hypogonadotropic hypogonadism	Serono Labs
(*Metrodin*)	Ovulation induction in patients with polycystic ovarian disease who have an elevated luteinizing hormone/follicle-stimulating hormone ratio and who have failed to respond to adequate clomiphene citrate therapy[a]	
Urogastrone	To accelerate corneal epithelial regeneration and healing of stromal incisions from corneal transplant surgery	Chiron Vision
Ursodiol (*Actigall*)	Management of clinical signs and symptoms associated with primary biliary cirrhosis	Novartis
(*URSO*)	Primary biliary cirrhosis[a]	Axcan Pharma
Valine, isoleucine, and leucine (*VIL*)	Hyperphenylalaninemia	Leas Res Products
Valrubicin (*Valstar*)	Carcinoma in situ of the urinary bladder[a]	Anthra Pharm
Vapreotide (*Octastatin*)	GI and pancreatic fistulas; to prevent early postoperative complications following pancreatic resection; esophageal variceal hemorrhage patients with portal hypertension	Debiopharm S.A.
Vapreotide pamoate (*Sanvar*)	Acromegaly	H3 Pharma
Vasoactive intestinal peptide	Acute respiratory distress syndrome	Sami I. Said, MD
Vasoactive intestinal polypeptide	Acute esophageal food impaction	Research Triangle Pharm
Vigabatrin (*Sabril*)	Infantile spasms	Aventis
Viloxazine HCl (*Catatrol*)	Narcolepsy; cataplexy	Stuart Pharm
Virulizin (*Virulizin*)	Pancreatic cancer	Lorus Therapeutics

Orphan Drugs		
Drug (Trade name)	Proposed use	Sponsor
Xenogeneic hepatocytes (HepatAssist Liver Assist System)	Severe liver failure	Circe Biomedical
XL119	Bile duct tumors	Exelixis
Yttrium-90 radiolabeled humanized monoclonal anti-carcinoembryonic antigen IgG antibody (Cea-Cide)	Ovarian carcinoma	Immunomedics
Zalcitabine	AIDS	National Cancer Inst, DCT
(Hivid)	AIDS[a]	Hoffman-La Roche
Zidovudine (Retrovir)	AIDS[a]; AIDS-related complex[a]	GlaxoWellcome
Zinc acetate (Galzin)	Wilson disease[a]	Lemmon
Zoledronate (Zometa, Zabel)	Tumor-induced hypercalcemia[a]	Novartis

[a] Approved for marketing.

AIDS Drugs in Development

Drug	Drug type	FDA status	Treatment sponsor
AIDS Drugs in Development			
Adipose redistribution syndrome			
Serostim[2] (somatropin [rDNA origin])	growth hormone	Phase II/III	Serono
AIDS			
ACT (activated cellular therapy)	other	Phase II	Neoprobe
BMS-234475	nd[1]	Phase I	Bristol-Myers Squibb
Cytolin	nontoxic AIDS monoclonal antibody	Phase I/II	CytoDyn Inc.
MDX-240	virus-specific bispecific antibody	Phase I/II	Medarex Inc.
SPD 754	nd[1]	Phase I	Shire Pharmaceutical
SPD 756	nd[1]	Phase I	Shire Pharmaceutical
Tipranavir	protease inhibitor	Phase II	Boehringer-Ingelheim Pharmaceuticals
Aphthous ulcers			
Thalomid (thalidomide)[2]	nd[1]	Phase III	Celgene
Cachexia			
Testosterone[2]	anabolic steroid	Phase II	TheraTech
CMV infection			
Benzimidavir (1263W94)	CMV-DNA inhibitor	Phase II	GlaxoSmithKline
T902611 (T611)	nd[1]	Phase I	Tularik
CMV retinitis			
GW275175	CMV-DNA maturation inhibitor	Phase I	GlaxoSmithKline
Dementia			
Memantine[2]	NMDA receptor antagonist/ neuroprotective agent	Phase II	Neurobiological Technologies
Diarrhea			
DiffGAM	nd[1]	Phase II	Immucell
Letrazurile	nd[1]	Phase II	Janssen Pharmaceutica
Synsorb CD (due to *Clostridium difficile*)	GI	Phase II	Synsorb Biotech
Fungal infections			
FK463[1]	nd[1]	Phase III	Fujisawa
Oramed[1]	nd[1]	Phase I	Biosyn
Posaconazole[1] (oral triazole)	nd[1]	Phase III	Schering-Plough
Hepatitis B co-infection			
Entecavir (BMS 200475)	nd[1]	Phase II	Bristol-Myers Squibb
Herpes co-infection			
Forvade (cidofovir gel)	antiviral	Phase I/II completed	Gilead Sciences
ME-609 cream	nd[1]	Phase II completed	Medivir
HIV infection			
AIDS vaccine	vaccine	Phase I	United Biomedical
Alferon N (interferon alfa-n3)[2] injection	nd[1]	Phase III	Interferon Sciences

AIDS Drugs in Development

Drug	Drug type	FDA status	Treatment sponsor
ALVAC-E120TMG (vCP1521)	nd[1]	Phase II	Aventis Pasteur
ALVAC-MN120TMG (vCP205)	nd[1]	Phase I/II	Aventis Pasteur
Amdoxovir	nucleoside analog	Phase II	Gilead
Ampligen	nucleic acid	Phase II	HemispheRx Biopharma
Ancer 20 injection	nd[1]	Phase I	Zeria USA
Anticort[2] (procaine HCl)	nd[1]	Phase II completed	Samaritan
Aztec (zidovudine) controlled-release	antiviral	Phase III completed	Verex Pharmaceuticals
BAY 50-4798	nd[1]	Phase I	Bayer
Beta-L-Fd4C	nd[1]	Phase II	Achillion Pharmaceuticals
BMS-234475	second generation protease inhibitor	Phase II	Bristol-Myers Squibb
BMS 561390	NNRTI[3]	Phase II	Bristol-Myers Squibb
Calanolide A	NNRTI[3]	Phase I/II	Sarawak MediChem
CCR5	receptor antagonist	Phase I	Schering-Plough
Crixivan in NanoCrystal formulation (indinavir)	protease inhibitor	Phase II	NanoSystems LLC/Merck and Co. Inc.
CS-92	NRTI[4]	Phase I/II	Triangle Pharmaceuticals
Cytolin	nd[1]	Phase I/II	Amerimmune Pharmaceuticals
Epivir/lamivudine (once-daily dosing)	nd[1]	application submitted	GlaxoSmithKline
Epivir and Ziagen combination tablet	nd[1]	Phase III	GlaxoSmithKline
GEM 92	nd[1]	Phase I	Hybridon
HGP-30 and sargramostim[2]	nd[1]	Phase I	Cel-Sci Corp./Immunex Corp.
HGTV43	gene therapy	Phase I	Enzo Biochem
HIV Therapeutic	nd[1]	Phase I	United Biomedical
HIV-IT	nd[1]	Phase II	Chiron Viagene
IL-2	nd[1]	Phase I/II	Bayer
ISIS 5320	nd[1]	Phase I	Isis Pharmaceuticals, Inc.
L-708,906	integrase inhibitor	nd[1]	nd[1]
MIV-150	NNRTI[3]	Phase I	Chiron
MIV-310[2]	nd[1]	Phase II	Medivir
Multikine	immunotherapeutic agent	Phase I	Cel-Sci Corp.
PA-457	budding inhibitor	preclinical	Panacos Pharmaceuticals
Pro 542	recombinant fusion inhibitor	Phase II	Progenics/Genzyme Transgenics
Pro 2000 gel	antiviral agent/microbicide	Phase II	Interneuron
Proleukin[2] (aldesleukin) interleukin-2 (IL-2)	interleukin	Phase III	Chiron
Rev 123	nd[1]	Phase I/II	Novartis
S-1360 (GW810781)	integrase inhibitor	Phase II	GlaxoSmithKline
Savvy	vaginal gel microbicide and spermicide	Phase I/II	Biosyn
T-1249	fusion inhibitor	Phase I/II	Trimeris
TAT antagonist	antiviral	Phase I/II	Hoffman-LaRoche

AIDS Drugs in Development

Drug	Drug type	FDA status	Treatment sponsor
Timunox (thymopentin)	immunomodulator	Phase III	Immunobiology Research Institute
Tipranavir	nonpeptidic protease inhibitor	Phase III	Boehringer-Ingelheim Pharmaceuticals
TM 114	protease inhibitor	Phase II	Tibotec
TMC125	NNRTI[3]	Phase II	Tibotec
TNX-355	anti-CD4 monoclonal antibody	Phase I	Tanox
Tucaresol (immunopotentiator)	immunomodulator/ immunopotentiator	Phase II	GlaxoWellcome
Tumor necrosis factor (TNF)	antiviral	Phase I	Immunex
UK-427,857	entry inhibitor	Phase I	nd[1]
Ushercell	nd[1]	Phase I	Polydex
VX-175 (GW433908)	protease inhibitor	Phase III	Vertex Pharmaceuticals
VX-385	nd[1]	Phase I	Vertex Pharmaceuticals
WF10 OXO[2]	nd[1]	Phase III	Chemie
Zerit (stavudine) extended-release	nd[1]	application submitted	Bristol-Myers Squibb
HIV infection and AIDS			
Abavca/Perthon	plant derivative	Phase I/II	Advanced Plant Pharmaceuticals
Ampligen	nd[1]	Phase II/III	HemispheRx Biopharma
Capravirine	NNRTI[3]	Phase II	Agouron Pharmaceuticals
Emtriva and *Viread*	nd[1]	Research stage	Gilead
GS 4338	nd[1]	Research stage	Gilead
GS 7340	nd[1]	Phase I	Gilead
HE 2000	cellular energy regulators	Phase II	Hollis-Eden Pharmaceuticals
T-1249	peptide fusion inhibitor	Phase I/II	Trimeris
Tipranavir	protease inhibitor	Phase III	Boehringer-Ingelheim Pharmaceuticals
Zadaxin	nd[1]	Phase II	SciClone
HIV wasting			
Androderm[2]	testosterone replacement	Phase III	SmithKline Beecham
Androgel DHT (dihydrotestosterone gel)	steroid	Phase II	Unimed
Thalomid[2] (thalidomide)	TNF-alpha selective inhibitor	Phase III	Celgene
HPV co-infection			
Low-dose oral interferon alpha	nd[1]	Phase I	Atrix Laboratories
Multikine (leukocyte interleukin injection)	interleukin	Phase I	Cel-Sci Corp.
Veldona Lozenge (interferon alpha)	natural human interferon alpha	Phase III	Amarillo Biosciences
Kaposi sarcoma			
A-007	nd[1]	Phase I	Dekk-Tec
Panretin (alitretinoin) oral	retinoic acid	Phase II	Ligand Pharmaceuticals
BMS 275291	nd[1]	Phase I/II	National Cancer Institute
Cidofovir[2]	antiviral	Phase II completed	Gilead Sciences
Interleukin-12	interleukin	Phase III	National Cancer Institute

AIDS Drugs in Development

Drug	Drug type	FDA status	Treatment sponsor
Metastat (4-dedimethysancycline)	matrix metallo proteinase inhibitor	Phase II	CollaGenex Pharmaceuticals
Panretin and interferon	nd[1]	Phase I/II	Ligand Pharmaceuticals
Paxene (paclitaxel), Taxol[2]	nd[1]	Phase III/Phase II/III	IVAX/National Cancer Institute
SU5416	angiogenesis inhibitor	Phase II completed	SUGEN
Thalidomide[2]	cytokine-selective inhibitor	Phase II completed	National Cancer Institute
Virulizin	macrophage activator	Phase III	Imutec Pharma
Lymphomas			
Bryostatin	nd[1]	Phase I	National Cancer Institute
Proleukin[2] (aldesleukin, interleukin-2 [IL-2])	nd[1]	Phase II	National Cancer Institute
Rituxan (rituximab)	nd[1]	Phase II	National Cancer Institute/ IDEC Pharmaceuticals
Virulizin	macrophage activator	Phase III	Imutec Pharma
Mycobacterial infection			
MiKasome (amikasin)	nd[1]	Phase II	NeXstar Pharmaceuticals
Mycobacterial avium complex			
Rifalazil (PA-1648)	rifampin derivative	Phase II	PathoGenesis
Non-Hodgkin lymphoma			
ATRA-IV (tretinoin)	liposomal all-transretinoic acid	Phase II	Aronex Pharmaceuticals
G3139	antisense compound	Phase I/II	Genta
LymphoCide	nd[1]	Phase III	Immunomedics
Proleukin[2] (aldesleukin, interleukin-2 [IL-2])	nd[1]	Phase II	National Cancer Institute
Rituxan (rituximab)	nd[1]	Phase II	National Cancer Institute/ IDEC Pharmaceuticals
Pain			
DPI3290	nd[1]	Phase II	Ardent
Morphelan ROER (morphine sulfate rapid-onset extended-release)	nd[1]	application submitted	Elan Pharmaceuticals/ Ligand Pharmaceuticals
Ziconotide	nd[1]	application submitted	Elan Pharmaceuticals
PCP infection			
Dapsone[2]	nd[1]	Phase III	Jacobus
Dapsone/pyrimethamine/ folinic acid[2]	nd[1]	Phase III	Jacobus
Dapsone/trimethoprim[2]	nd[1]	Phase III	Jacobus
DB 289	nd[1]	Phase I	Immtech
Pediatric HIV			
Combivir[2] (zidovudine/ lamivudine)	nucleoside analog reverse transcriptase inhibitor combination	nd[1]	GlaxoSmithKline
Crixivan[2] (indinavir)	protease inhibitor	nd[1]	Merck
Fortovase[2] (saquinavir)	protease inhibitor	nd[1]	Roche
HIV-1 immunogen	nd[1]	Phase I completed	Agouron Pharmaceuticals
Hivid[2] (zalcitabine, ddC)	NRTI[4]	nd[1]	Roche
Invirase[2] (saquinavir)	protease inhibitor	nd[1]	Roche
MKC-442	nd[1]	Phase II	Triangle Pharmaceuticals
Rescriptor[2] (delavirdine)	NNRTI[3]	Phase II	Pfizer

Drug	Drug type	FDA status	Treatment sponsor
	**AIDS Drugs in Development**		
Viread (tenofovir disoproxil fumarate)	nucleoside analog reverse transcriptase inhibitor	Phase I	Gilead Sciences
	***Progressive multifocal leukoencephalopathy (PML)***		
Topotecan (hycamtin)[1,2]	semi-synthetic derivative of camptothecin, toposiomerase I-inhibitor	Phase II completed	GlaxoSmithKline
	***Vaccines***		
AIDS vaccine	multi-envelope HIV vaccine component	Phase I	St. Jude Children's Research Hospital
Aidsvax	vaccine	Phase III	VaxGen
ALVAC (vCP1452)	vaccine	Phase II	Aventis Pasteur
ALVAC (vCP1521)	vaccine	Phase II	Aventis Pasteur
Genevax-HIV/APL-400-003 (end/rev) facilitated DNA-based vaccine	vaccine	Phase I	Wyeth
Genevax-HIV/APL-400-047 (gag/pol) facilitated DNA-based vaccine	vaccine	Phase I	Wyeth
HIV vaccine	vaccine	Phase I	GlaxoSmithKline
HIV-1 peptide vaccine	vaccine	Phase I	National Cancer Institute
Remune	vaccine	Phase III	Immune Response
TBC-3B	vaccine, recombinant	Phase I	Therion Biologics

[1] nd = no data.
[2] Approved for other indications; refer to individual monographs.
[3] NNRTI = Non-nucleoside reverse transcriptase inhibitor.
[4] NRTI = Nucleoside reverse transcriptase inhibitor.

Summary Acquired Immunodeficiency Syndrome (AIDS) is an immunodeficiency state caused by an infection with the human immunodeficiency virus, HIV. There are several drugs being studied for HIV, AIDS, and AIDS-related illnesses. Listed above are some antiviral, cytokine, immunomodulating drugs, and vaccines currently undergoing clinical trials.

FDA Pregnancy Categories

The rational use of any medication requires a risk vs benefit assessment. Among the myriad of risk factors which complicate this assessment, pregnancy is one of the most perplexing.

The FDA has established 5 categories to indicate the potential of a systemically absorbed drug for causing birth defects. The key differentiation among the categories rests upon the degree (reliability) of documentation and the risk vs benefit ratio. Pregnancy Category X is particularly notable in that if any data exists that may implicate a drug as a teratogen and the risk vs benefit ratio does not support use of the drug, the drug is contraindicated during pregnancy. These categories are summarized below:

FDA Pregnancy Categories	
Pregnancy Category	**Definition**
A	Controlled studies show no risk. Adequate, well-controlled studies in pregnant women have failed to demonstrate risk to the fetus.
B	No evidence of risk in humans. Either animal findings show risk, but human findings do not; or if no adequate human studies have been done, animal findings are negative.
C	Risk cannot be ruled out. Human studies are lacking, and animal studies are either positive for fetal risk or lacking. However, potential benefits may justify the potential risks.
D	Positive evidence of risk. Investigational or postmarketing data show risk to the fetus. Nevertheless, potential benefits may outweigh the potential risks. If needed in a life-threatening situation or a serious disease, the drug may be acceptable if safer drugs cannot be used or are ineffective.
X	Contraindicated in pregnancy. Studies in animals or human, or investigational or post-marketing reports have shown fetal risk which clearly outweighs any possible benefit to the patients.

Regardless of the designated pregnancy category or presumed safety, no drug should be administered during pregnancy unless it is clearly needed and potential benefits outweigh potential hazards to the fetus.

General Management of Acute Overdosage

Rapid intervention is essential to minimize morbidity and mortality in an acute toxic ingestion. Institute measures to prevent absorption and hasten elimination as soon as possible; however, symptomatic and supportive care takes precedence over other therapy. It is assumed that basic life support measures, (eg, cardiopulmonary resuscitation [CPR]) have been instituted. Specific antidotes are discussed in the overdosage section of individual or group monographs. The discussion below outlines procedures used in the management of acute overdosage of orally ingested systemic drugs.

ADVANCED LIFE SUPPORT MEASURES:

Adequate airway: Adequate airway must be established and maintained, generally via oropharyngeal or endotracheal airways, cricothyrotomy, or tracheostomy.

Ventilation: Ventilation may then be performed via mouth-to-mouth insufflation, hand-operated bag (ambu bag), or by mechanical ventilator.

Circulation: Circulation must be maintained.
- *Hypotension:* If hypotension/hypoperfusion occurs, place the patient in shock position (head lowered, feet elevated); specific therapy may include:
    Establish IV access and initiate IV fluids (eg, 0.9% or 0.45% Saline, Lactate Ringer's, Dextrose). A maintenance flow rate is generally 100 to 200 mL/hour; individualize as necessary.
    Plasma, plasma protein fractions, whole blood, or plasma expanders may be required.
    Severe hypotension may required judicious use of cardiovascular active agents. The most commonly recommended agents are dopamine, dobutamine, and norepinephrine.
- *Arrhythmia:* Treatment is dictated by the offending drug.
- *Hypertension:* Sometimes severe, hypertension may occur. (See Nitroprusside and Diazoxide, Parenteral in the Agents for Hypertensive Emergencies section.)
- *Seizures:* Simple isolated seizures may require only observation and supportive care. Repetitive seizures or status epilepticus require therapy. Give IV diazepam or lorazepam followed by fosphenytoin and/or phenobarbital. Pancuronium may also be considered.

REDUCTION OF DRUG ABSORPTION:

Gastric emptying: Gastric emptying is generally recommended as soon as possible; hwoever, this is generally not very effective unless employed within the first 1 to 2 hours after ingestion. Syrup of ipecac and gastric lavage are the 2 most commonly employed methods for gastric emptying.
- *Syrup of ipecac:* This is the preferred method of choice outside the hospital. Do not induce vomiting if the medication is caustic or a petroleum or if the patient is in a coma or having seizures. Syrup of ipecac takes 20 to 30 minutes to work. Consider gastric lavage if response is needed immediately. The following dosage is recommended for syrup of ipecac and may be followed by a glass of water. A second dose may be given if results do not occur within 20 to 30 minutes.
    6 months to 1 year – 10 mL
    1 year to 12 years – 15 mL
    more than 12 years – 30 mL
- *Gastric lavage:* This is indicated in the comatose patient or for those in whom syrup of ipecac failes to produce emesis. Gastric lavage is immediate and does not have a delay reaction, and is preferred over forced emesis. Airway protection via endotracheal intubation is appropriate for the patient without a gag reflex or comatose patients. Position the patient on left side, face down and use a large bore tube. Instill warm water or saline 300 to 360 mL for adults. Avoid water for infants and children; use warm saline or 5% to 6% polyethylene glycol solution. Give until lavage solution becomes clear. Add charcoal before removing the tube.

Adsorption: Adsorption, using activated charcoal alone or after completion of emesis or lavage, is indicated for virtually all significant toxic ingestions. It adsorbs a wide variety of toxins and there are no contraindications. However, it adsorbs many orally administered antidotes as well, so space dosage properly. Give an adult 50 to 100 g of activated charcoal mixed in 240 mL of water; the pediatric dose is 1 g/kg, or 25 to 50 g in 120 mL of water.

Cathartics: Cathartics increases the elimination of charcoal-poison complex. Generally using a saline or osmotic cathartic (eg, magnesium sulfate or citrate or sorbital) with 3 mL/kg of a 35% to 75% solution of sorbitol has the most rapid effect.

Whole bowel irrigation (WBI): Whole bowel irrigation utilizes rapid administration of large volumes of lavage solutions, such as PEG. The dose is 4 to 6 L over 1 to 2 hours for adults and 0.5 L/hr for children. It may be most useful to remove iron tables, sustained-release capsules or cocaine-containing condoms or balloons.

ELIMINATION OF ABSORBED DRUG:

Interruption of enterohepatic circulation: Interruption of enterohepatic circulation by "gastric dialysis" uses scheduled doses of activated charcoal for 1 to 2 days. Gastric dialysis not only interrupts the enterohepatic cycle of some drugs, but also creates an osmotic gradient, drawing drug from the plasma back into the GI lumen where it is bound by the charcoal and excreted in the feces.

Diuresis: Diuresis may be effective as identified in the individual drug monographs.
- *Forced diuresis:* Occasionally useful, forced diuresis may cause volume overload or electrolyte disturbances. Forced diuresis is useful for phenobarbital, bromides, lithium, salicylate, or amphetamines overdosages. Do not use for tricyclic antidepressants, sedative-hypnotics, or highly protein-bound medications. The most common agents employed are furosemide and osmotic diuretics with mannitol.
- *Alkaline diuresis:* Alkaline diuresis promotes elimination of weak acids (eg, barbiturates, salicylates) and is accomplished by the administration of IV sodium bicarbonate.
- *Acid diuresis:* Acid diuresis may be indicated in overdoses with weak bases (eg, amphetamines, fenfluramine, quinine) but use with caution in patients with renal or liver disease. It is usually accomplished with oral or IV ascorbic acid or ammonium chloride.

Dialysis: Dialysis is indicated in a minority of severe overdosage cases. Drug factors that alter dialysis effectiveness include volume of distribution, drug compartmentalization, protein binding, and lipid/water solubility.
- *Hemodialysis:* Hemodialysis may be used after an overdosage and when the patient is having complications (eg, severe metabolic acidosis, electrolyte imbalances, renal failure).
- *Peritoneal dialysis:* Peritoneal dialysis is even less effective than hemodialysis.
- *Charcoal hemoperfusion:* Charcoal hemoperfusion is useful when a drug can be adsorbed by charcoal (eg, theophylline, barbiturates).

Poison Control Center: Consultation with a regional poison control center is highly recommended.

Management of Acute Hypersensitivity Reactions

Type I hypersensitivity reactions (immediate hypersensitivity or anaphylaxis) are immunologic responses to a foreign antigen to which a patient has been previously sensitized. Anaphylactoid reactions are not immunologically mediated; however, symptoms and treatment are similar.

Signs and symptoms: Acute hypersensitivity reactions typically begin within 1 to 30 minutes of exposure to the offending antigen. Tingling sensations and a generalized flush may proceed to a fullness in the throat, chest tightness, or a "feeling of impending doom." Generalized urticaria and sweating are common. *Severe* reactions include life-threatening involvement of the airway and cardiovascular system.

Treatment: Appropriate and immediate treatment is imperative. The following general measures are commonly employed:

Epinephrine: 1:1000, 0.2 to 0.5 mg (0.2 to 0.5 mL) SC is primary treatment. In children, administer 0.01 mg/kg or 0.1 mg. Doses may be repeated every 5 to 15 minutes if needed. A succession of small doses is more effective and less dangerous than a single large dose. Additionally, 0.1 mg may be introduced into an injection site where the offending drug was administered. If appropriate, the use of a tourniquet above the site of injection of the causative agent may slow its absorption and distribution. However, remove or loosen the tourniquet every 10 to 15 minutes to maintain circulation.

Epinephrine IV (generally indicated in the presence of hypotension) is often recommended in a 1:10,000 dilution, 0.3 to 0.5 mg over 5 minutes; repeat every 15 minutes, if necessary. In children, inject 0.1 to 0.2 mg or 0.01 mg/kg/dose over 5 minutes; repeat every 30 minutes.

A conservative IV epinephrine protocol includes 0.1 mg of a 1:100,000 dilution (0.1 mg of a 1:1000 dilution mixed in 10 mL normal saline) given over 5 to 10 minutes. If an IV infusion is necessary, administer at a rate of 1 to 4 mcg/min. In children, infuse 0.1 to 1.5 (maximum) mcg/kg/min.

Dilute epinephrine 1:10,000 may be administered through an endotracheal tube, if no other parenteral access is available, directly into the bronchial tree. It is rapidly absorbed there from the capillary bed of the lung.

Airway: Ensure a patent airway via endotracheal intubation or cricothyrotomy (ie, inferior laryngotomy, used prior to tracheotomy) and administer oxygen. Severe respiratory difficulty may respond to IV aminophylline or to other bronchodilators.

Hypotension: The patient should be recumbent with feet elevated. Depending upon the severity, consider the following measures:
- Establish a patent IV catheter in a suitable vein.
- Administer IV fluids (eg, Normal Saline, Lactated Ringer's).
- Administer plasma expanders.
- Administer cardioactive agents (see group and individual monographs). Commonly recommended agents include dopamine, dobutamine, norepinephrine, and phenylephrine.

Adjunctive therapy: Adjunctive therapy does not alter acute reactions, but may modify an ongoing or slow-onset process and shorten the course of the reaction.
- *Antihistamines: Diphenhydramine* – 50 to 100 mg IM or IV, continued orally at 5 mg/kg/day or 50 mg every 6 hours for 1 to 2 days. For children, give 5 mg/kg/day, maximum 300 mg/day.
  Chlorpheniramine – Adults, 10 to 20 mg; children, 5 to 10 mg IM or slowly IV.
  Hydroxyzine – 10 to 25 mg orally or 25 to 50 mg IM 3 to 4 times daily.
- *Corticosteroids:* Eg, hydrocortisone IV 100 to 1000 mg or equivalent, followed by 7 mg/kg/day IV or oral for 1 to 2 days. The role of corticosteroids is controversial.
- H_2 *antagonists: Cimetidine* – Children, 25 to 30 mg/kg/day IV in 6 divided doses; Adults, 300 mg every 6 hours.
  Ranitidine – 50 mg IV over 3 to 5 minutes. May be of value in addition to H_1 antihistamines, although this opinion is not universally shared.

Calculations

To calculate milliequivalent weight: $mEq = \dfrac{\text{gram molecular weight/valence}}{1000}$

$mEq = \dfrac{mg}{eq\ wt}$ equivalent weight or $eq\ wt = \dfrac{\text{gram molecular weight}}{\text{valence}}$

Commonly Used mEq Weights			
Chloride	35.5 mg = 1 mEq	Magnesium	12 mg = 1 mEq
Sodium	23 mg = 1 mEq	Potassium	39 mg = 1 mEq
Calcium	20 mg = 1 mEq		

To convert temperature °C ↔ °F: $\dfrac{°C}{°F - 32} = 5/9$ or °C = 5/9 (°F - 32)

°F = 32 + 9/5 °C

To calculate creatinine clearance (Ccr) from serum creatinine:

Males: $\dfrac{\text{Weight (kg)} \times (140 - \text{age})}{72 \times \text{serum creatinine (mg/dL)}} = Ccr$

Females   0.85 × above value

To calculate ideal body weight (kg):

Male = 50 kg + 2.3 kg (each inch > 5 ft)

Female = 45.5 kg + 2.3 kg (each inch > 5 ft)

Body Surface Area: To calculate body surface area (BSA) in adults and children:

1) Dubois method:

SA (cm^2) = wt (kg)$^{0.425}$ × ht (cm)$^{0.725}$ × 71.84

SA (m^2) = K × $\sqrt[3]{wt^2\ (kg)}$ (common K value 0.1 for toddlers, 0.103 for neonates)

2) Simplified method

BSA (m^2) = $\sqrt{\dfrac{\text{ht (cm)} \times \text{wt (kg)}}{3600}}$

To approximate surface area (m^2) of children from weight (kg):

Weight range (kg)	≈ Surface area (m^2)
1 to 5	(0.05 × kg) + 0.05
6 to 10	(0.04 × kg) + 0.10
11 to 20	(0.03 × kg) + 0.20
21 to 40	(0.02 × kg) + 0.40

Suggested Weights for Adults	
Height[1]	*Weight in pounds[2]*
4'10"	91-119
4'11"	94-124
5'0"	97-128
5'1"	101-132
5'2"	104-137
5'3"	107-141
5'4"	111-146
5'5"	114-150
5'6"	118-155
5'7"	121-160
5'8"	125-164
5'9"	129-169
5'10"	132-174
5'11"	136-179
6'0"	140-184
6'1"	144-189
6'2"	148-195
6'3"	152-200
6'4"	156-205
6'5"	160-211
6'6"	164-216

[1] Without shoes.
[2] Without clothes.

The higher weights in the ranges generally apply to people with more muscle and bone. Source: Nutrition and Your Health: Dietary Guidelines for Americans, 4th ed, 1995. US Department of Agriculture, US Department of Health and Human Services. At press time, these new guidelines had not been officially released. It is possible some changes to this chart will occur.

International System of Units

The *Système international d'unités* (International System of Units) or *SI* is a modernized version of the metric system. The primary goal of the conversion to SI units is to revise the present confused measurement system and to improve test-result communications.

The SI has 7 basic units from which other units are derived:

Base Units of SI		
Physical quantity	Base unit	SI symbol
length	meter	m
mass	kilogram	kg
time	second	s
amount of substance	mole	mol
thermodynamic temperature	kelvin	K
electric current	ampere	A
luminous intensity	candela	cd

Combinations of these base units can express any property, although, for simplicity, special names are given to some of these derived units.

Representative Derived Units		
Derived unit	Name and symbol	Derivation from base units
area	square meter	m^2
volume	cubic meter	m^3
force	newton (N)	$kg \cdot m \cdot s^{-2}$
pressure	pascal (Pa)	$kg \cdot m^{-1} \cdot s^{-2} (N/m^2)$
work, energy	joule (J)	$kg \cdot m^2 \cdot s^{-2} (N \cdot m)$
mass density	kilogram per cubic meter	kg/m^3
frequency	hertz (Hz)	$1 \text{ cycles}/s^{-1}$
temperature degree	Celsius (°C)	°C = °K −273.15
concentration		
mass	kilogram/liter	kg/L
substance	mole/liter	mol/L
molality	mole/kilogram	mol/kg
density	kilogram/liter	kg/L

Prefixes to the base unit are used in this system to form decimal multiples and submultiples. The preferred multiples and submultiples listed below change the quantity by increments of 10^3 or 10^{-3}. The exceptions to these recommended factors are within the middle rectangle.

Prefixes and Symbols for Decimal Multiples and Submultiples		
Factor	Prefix	Symbol
10^{18}	exa	E
10^{15}	peta	P
10^{12}	tera	T
10^{9}	giga	G
10^{6}	mega	M
10^{3}	kilo	k
10^{2}	hecto	h
10^{1}	deka	da

Prefixes and Symbols for Decimal Multiples and Submultiples		
Factor	Prefix	Symbol
10^{-1}	deci	d
10^{-2}	centi	c
10^{-3}	milli	m
10^{-6}	micro	µ
10^{-9}	nano	n
10^{-12}	pico	p
10^{-15}	femto	f
10^{-18}	atto	a

To convert drug concentrations to or from SI units:

- Conversion factor (CF) = $\dfrac{1000}{\text{mol wt}}$
- Conversion *to* SI units: µmol/L
- Conversion *from* SI units: µmol/L ÷ CF = µg/mL

Normal Laboratory Values

In the following tables, normal reference values for commonly requested laboratory tests are listed in traditional units and in SI units. The tables are a guideline only. Values are method dependent and "normal values" may vary between laboratories.

Blood, Plasma or Serum		
	Reference Value	
Determination	Conventional units	SI units
Alpha-fetoprotein	Adult: < 15 ng/mL Pregnant (16-18 weeks): 38-45 ng/mL	Adult: < 15 mcg/L Pregnant (16-18 weeks): 38-45 mcg/L
Ammonia (NH_3) - diffusion	20-120 mcg/dL	12-70 mcmol/L
Ammonia nitrogen	15-45 µg/dL	11-32 µmol/L
Amylase	20-100 units/dL	37-185 U/L
Anion gap ($Na^+ - [Cl^- + HCO_3^-]$) (P)	7-16 mEq/L	7-16 mmol/L
Antinuclear antibodies	negative at 1:10 dilution of serum	negative at 1:10 dilution of serum
Antithrombin III (AT III)	80-120 U/dL	800-1200 U/L
Bicarbonate: Arterial Venous	21-28 mEq/L 22-29 mEq/L	21-28 mmol/L 22-29 mmol/L
Bilirubin: Conjugated (direct) Total	≤ 0.2 mg/dL 0.1-1 mg/dL	≤ 4 mcmol/L 2-18 mcmol/L
Calcitonin: Female Male	≤ 20 pg/mL ≤ 40 pg/mL	≤ 20 ng/L ≤ 40 ng/L
Calcium: Total Ionized	8.6-10.3 mg/dL 4.4-5.1 mg/dL	2.2-2.74 mmol/L 1-1.3 mmol/L
Carbon dioxide content (plasma)	21-32 mmol/L	21-32 mmol/L
Carcinoembryonic antigen	< 3 ng/mL	< 3 mcg/L
Chloride	95-110 mEq/L	95-110 mmol/L
Coagulation screen: Bleeding time Prothrombin time Partial thromboplastin time (activated) Protein C Protein S	3-9.5 min 10-13 sec 22-37 sec 0.7-1.4 µ/mL 0.7-1.4 µ/mL	180-570 sec 10-13 sec 22-37 sec 700-1400 U/mL 700-1400 U/mL
Copper, total	70-160 mcg/dL	11-25 mcmol/L
Corticotropin (ACTH [adrenocorticotropic hormone]) - 0800 hr	< 60 pg/mL	< 13.2 pmol/L
Cortisol: 0800 hr 1800 hr 2000 hr	5-30 mcg/dL 2-15 mcg/dL ≤ 50% of 0800 hr	138-810 nmol/L 50-410 nmol/L ≤ 50% of 0800 hr
Creatine kinase: Female Male	20-170 IU/L 30-220 IU/L	0.33-2.83 mckat/L 0.5-3.67 mckat/L
Creatinine kinase isoenzymes, MB fraction	0-12 IU/L	0-0.2 mckat/L
Creatinine	0.5-1.7 mg/dL	44-150 mcmol/L
Fibrinogen (coagulation factor I)	150-360 mg/dL	1.5-3.6 g/L
Follicle-stimulating hormone (FSH): Female Midcycle Male	2-13 mIU/mL 5-22 mIU/mL 1-8 mIU/mL	2-13 IU/L 5-22 IU/L 1-8 IU/L
Glucose, fasting	65-115 mg/dL	3.6-6.3 mmol/L
Glucose Tolerance Test (Oral) Fasting 60 min 90 min 120 min	mg/dL Normal / Diabetic 70-105 / > 140 120-170 / ≥ 200 100-140 / ≥ 200 70-120 / ≥ 140	mmol/L Normal / Diabetic 3.9-5.8 / > 7.8 6.7-9.4 / ≥ 11.1 5.6-7.8 / ≥ 11.1 3.9-6.7 / ≥ 7.8
(γ) - Glutamyltransferase (GGT): Male Female	9-50 units/L 8-40 units/L	9-50 units/L 8-40 units/L
Haptoglobin	44-303 mg/dL	0.44-3.03 g/L

Blood, Plasma or Serum		
	Reference Value	
Determination	Conventional units	SI units
Hematologic tests:		
Fibrinogen	200-400 mg/dL	2-4 g/L
Hematocrit (Hct), female	36%-44.6%	0.36-0.446 fraction of 1
male	40.7%-50.3%	0.4-0.503 fraction of 1
Hemoglobin A_{1C}	4%-6%	0.053-0.075
Hemoglobin (Hb), female	12-16 g/dL	7.49-9.9 mmol/L
male	14-18 g/dL	8.7-11.2 mmol/L
Leukocyte count (WBC)	3800-9800/mcL	$3.8-9.8 \times 10^9$/L
Erythrocyte count (RBC), female	$3.5-5 \times 10^6$/mcL	$3.5-5 \times 10^{12}$/L
male	$4.3-5.9 \times 10^6$/mcL	$4.3-5.9 \times 10^{12}$/L
Mean corpuscular volume (MCV)	80-97.6 mcm^3	80-97.6 fl
Mean corpuscular hemoglobin (MCH)	27-33 pg/cell	1.66-2.09 fmol/cell
Mean corpuscular hemoglobin concentration (MCHC)	33-36 g/dL	20.3-22 mmol/L
Erythrocyte sedimentation rate (sedrate, ESR)	≤ 30 mm/hr	≤ 30 mm/hr
Erythrocyte enzymes:		
Glucose-6-phosphate dehydrognase (G-6-PD)	250-5000 units/10^6 cells	250-5000 mcunits/cell
Ferritin	10-300 ng/mL	10-300 pmol/L
Folic acid: normal	> 3.1-12.4 ng/mL	7-28.1 nmol/L
Platelet count	150-450 x 10^3/mcL	150-450 x 10^9/L
Reticulocytes	0.5%-1.5% of erythrocytes	0.005-0.015
Vitamin B_{12}	223-1132 pg/mL	165-835 pmol/L
Iron: Female	30-160 mcg/dL	5.4-31.3 mcmol/L
Male	45-160 mcg/dL	8.1-31.3 mcmol/L
Iron binding capacity	220-420 mcg/dL	39.4-75.2 mcmol/L
Isocitrate dehydrogenase	1.2-7 units/L	1.2-7 units/L
Isoenzymes		
Fraction 1	14%-26% of total	0.14-0.26 fraction of total
Fraction 2	29%-39% of total	0.29-0.39 fraction of total
Fraction 3	20%-26% of total	0.20-0.26 fraction of total
Fraction 4	8%-16% of total	0.08-0.16 fraction of total
Fraction 5	6%-16% of total	0.06-0.16 fraction of total
Lactate dehydrogenase	100-250 IU/L	1.67-4.17 mckat/L
Lactic acid (lactate)	6-19 mg/dL	0.7-2.1 mmol/L
Lead	≤ 20 mcg/dL	≤ 2.41 mcmol/L
Lipase	10-150 IU/L	10-150 IU/L
Lipids:		
Total Cholesterol		
Desirable	< 200 mg/dL	< 5.2 mmol/L
Borderline-high	200-239 mg/dL	< 5.2-6.2 mmol/L
High	> 239 mg/dL	> 6.2 mmol/L
LDL		
Desirable	< 130 mg/dL	< 3.36 mmol/L
Borderline-high	130-159 mg/dL	3.36-4.11 mmol/L
High	> 159 mg/dL	> 4.11 mmol/L
HDL		
Low	< 40 mg/dL	
High	≥ 60 mg/dL	
Triglycerides		
Desirable	< 150 mg/dL	
Borderline-high	150-199 mg/dL	
High	200-499 mg/dL	
Very high	> 500 mg/dL	
Magnesium	1.3-2.2 mEq/L	0.65-1.1 mmol/L
Osmolality	280-300 mOsm/kg	280-300 mmol/kg
Oxygen saturation (arterial)	94%-100%	0.94-1 fraction of 1
PCO_2, arterial	35-45 mm Hg	4.7-6 kPa
pH, arterial	7.35-7.45	7.35-7.45
PO_2, arterial: Breathing room air[1]	80-105 mm Hg	10.6-14 kPa
On 100% O_2	> 500 mm Hg	
Phosphatase (acid), total at 37°C	0.13-0.63 IU/L	2.2-10.5 IU/L or 2.2-10.5 mckat/L
Phosphatase alkaline[2]	20-130 IU/L	20-130 IU/L or 0.33-2.17 mckat/L
Phosphorus, inorganic,[3] (phosphate)	2.5-5 mg/dL	0.8-1.6 mmol/L
Potassium	3.5-5 mEq/L	3.5-5 mmol/L

Normal Laboratory Values

Blood, Plasma or Serum		
	Reference Value	
Determination	Conventional units	SI units

Progesterone
Female
  Follicular phase
  Luteal phase
Male
	
	0.1-1.5 ng/mL
	2.5-28 ng/mL
	< 0.5 ng/mL
		
		0.32-4.8 nmol/L
		8-89 nmol/L
		< 1.6 nmol/L

Prolactin	1.4-24.2 ng/mL	1.4-24.2 mcg/L
Prostate specific antigen	0-4 ng/mL	0-4 ng/mL

Protein: Total
  Albumin
  Globulin
	6-8 g/dL
	3.6-5 g/dL
	2.3-3.5 g/dL
		60-80 g/L
		36-50 g/L
		23-35 g/L

Rheumatoid factor	< 60 IU/mL	< 60 kIU/L
Sodium	135-147 mEq/L	135-147 mmol/L
Testosterone: Female Male	6-86 ng/dL 270-1070 ng/dL	0.21-3 nmol/L 9.3-37 nmol/L
Thyroid Hormone Function Tests: Thyroid-stimulating hormone (TSH) Thyroxine-binding globulin capacity Total triiodothyronine (T_3) Total thyroxine by RIA (T_4) T_3 resin uptake	 0.35-6.2 mcU/mL 10-26 mcg/dL 75-220 ng/dL 4-11 mcg/dL 25%-38%	 0.35-6.2 mU/L 100-260 mcg/L 1.2-3.4 nmol/L 51-142 nmol/L 0.25-0.38 fraction of 1
Transaminase, AST (aspartate aminotransferase, SGOT)	11-47 IU/L	0.18-0.78 mckat/L
Transaminase, ALT (alanine aminotransferase, SGPT)	7-53 IU/L	0.12-0.88 mckat/L
Transferrin	220-400 mg/dL	2.20-4.00 g/L
Urea nitrogen (BUN)	8-25 mg/dL	2.9-8.9 mmol/L
Uric acid	3-8 mg/dL	179-476 mcmol/L
Vitamin A (retinol)	15-60 mcg/dL	0.52-2.09 mcmol/L
Zinc	50-150 mcg/dL	7.7-23 mcmol/L

[1] Age dependent
[2] Infants and adolescents up to 104 U/L
[3] Infants in the first year up to 6 mg/dL

Urine		
	Reference value	
Determination	Conventional units	SI units
Calcium[1]	50-250 mcg/day	1.25-6.25 mmol/day
Catecholamines: Epinephrine Norepinephrine	 < 20 mcg/day < 100 mcg/day	 < 109 nmol/day < 590 nmol/day
Catecholamines, 24-hr	< 110 µg	< 650 nmol
Copper[1]	15-60 mcg/day	0.24-0.95 mcmol/day
Creatinine: Child Adolescent Female Male	8-22 mg/kg 8-30 mg/kg 0.6-1.5 g/day 0.8-1.8 g/day	71-195 µmol/kg 71-265 µmol/kg 5.3-13.3 mmol/day 7.1-15.9 mmol/day
pH	4.5-8	4.5-8
Phosphate[1]	0.9-1.3 g/day	29-42 mmol/day
Potassium[1]	25-100 mEq/day	25-100 mmol/day
Protein Total At rest	 1-14 mg/dL 50-80 mg/day	 10-140 mg/L 50-80 mg/day
Protein, quantitative	< 150 mg/day	< 0.15 g/day
Sodium[1]	100-250 mEq/day	100-250 mmol/day
Specific gravity, random	1.002-1.030	1.002-1.030
Uric acid, 24-hr	250-750 mg	1.48-4.43 mmol

[1] Diet Dependent

Drug Levels*			
		Reference value	
	Drug determination	Conventional units	SI units
Aminoglycosides	Amikacin (trough) (peak)	1-8 mcg/mL 20-30 mcg/mL	1.7-13.7 mcmol/L 34-51 mcmol/L
	Gentamicin (trough) (peak)	0.5-2 mcg/mL 6-10 mcg/mL	1-4.2 mcmol/L 12.5-20.9 mcmol/L
	Kanamycin (trough) (peak)	5-10 mcg/mL 20-25 mcg/mL	nd[1] nd
	Netilimicin (trough) (peak)	0.5-2 mcg/mL 6-10 mcg/mL	nd nd
	Streptomycin (trough) (peak)	< 5 mcg/mL 20-30 mcg/mL	nd nd
	Tobramycin (trough) (peak)	0.5-2 mcg/mL 6-10 mcg/mL	1.1-4.3 mcmol/L 12.8-21.8 mcmol/L
Antiarrhythmics	Amiodarone	0.5-2.5 mcg/mL	1.5-4 mcmol/L
	Bretylium	0.5-1.5 mcg/mL	nd
	Digitoxin	9-25 mcg/L	11.8-32.8 nmol/L
	Digoxin	0.8-2 ng/mL	0.9-2.5 nmol/L
	Disopyramide	2-8 mcg/mL	6-18 mcmol/L
	Flecainide	0.2-1 mcg/mL	nd
	Lidocaine	1.5-6 mcg/mL	4.5-21.5 mcmol/L
	Mexiletine	0.5-2 mcg/mL	nd
	Procainamide	4-8 mcg/mL	17-34 mcmol/mL
	Propranolol	50-100 ng/mL	190-390 nmol/L
	Quinidine	2-6 mcg/mL	4.6-9.2 mcmol/L
	Tocainide	5-12 mcg/mL	22-52 mcmol/L
	Verapamil	50-200 ng/mL	100-420 nmol/L
Anticonvulsants	Carbamazepine	4-12 mcg/mL	17-51 mcmol/L
	Phenobarbital	10-40 mcg/mL	43-172 mcmol/L
	Phenytoin	10-20 mcg/mL	40-80 mcmol/L
	Primidone	5-15 mg/mL	23-69 mcmol/L
	Valproic Acid	50-100 mcg/L	346-693 mcmol/L
Antidepressants	Amitriptyline	110-250 ng/mL[2]	500-900 nmol/L
	Amoxapine	200-500 ng/mL	637-1594 nmol/L
	Bupropion	50-100 ng/mL	nd
	Clomipramine	80-100 ng/mL	nd
	Desipramine	115-300 ng/mL	281-1125 nmol/L
	Doxepin	30-250 ng/mL	107-537 nmol/L
	Imipramine	100-300 ng/mL	nd
	Maprotiline	200-300 ng/mL	nd
	Nortriptyline	50-150 ng/mL	190-665 nmol/L
	Protriptyline	70-250 ng/mL	266-950 nmol/L
	Trazodone	800-1600 ng/mL	nd

Drug Levels[*]			
		Reference value	
	Drug determination	Conventional units	SI units
Antipsychotics	Chlorpromazine	50-300 ng/mL	157-942 nmol/L
	Fluphenazine	5-20 ng/mL	nd
	Haloperidol	5-20 ng/mL	10-30 nmol/L
	Perphenazine	2-6 ng/mL	nd
	Thiothixene	2-57 ng/mL	nd
Miscellaneous	Amantadine	300 ng/mL	nd
	Amrinone	3.7 mcg/mL	nd
	Chloramphenicol	10-20 mcg/mL	31-62 mcmol/L
	Cyclosporine[3]	250-800 ng/mL (whole blood, RIA) 50-300 ng/mL (plasma, RIA)	nd nd
	Ethanol[4]	0 mg/dL	0 mmol/L
	Hydralazine	100 ng/mL	nd
	Lithium	0.6-1.2 mEq/L	0.6-1.2 mmol/L
	Salicylate	100-300 mg/L	724-2172 mcmol/L
	Sulfonamide	5-15 mg/dL	nd
	Theophylline	10-20 mcg/mL	55-110 mcmol/L
	Vancomycin (trough) (peak)	5-15 ng/mL 20-40 mcg/mL	nd nd

[*] The values given are generally accepted as desirable for treatment without toxicity for most patients. However, exceptions are not uncommon.
[1] nd = No data available.
[2] Parent drug plus N-desmethyl metabolite.
[3] 24-hour trough values.
[4] Toxic: 50-100 mg/dL (10.9–21.7 mmol/L).

The following table is adopted from the Seventh Report of the Joint National Committee on Prevention, Detection, Evaluation, and Treatment of High Blood Pressure, National Institutes of Health.

Classification of Blood Pressure[1]			
	Reference value		
Category	Systolic (mm Hg)		Diastolic (mm Hg)
Normal	< 120	and	< 80
Prehypertension	120-139	or	80-89
Hypertension – Stage 1	140-159	or	90-99
Hypertension – Stage 2	≥ 160	or	≥ 100

[1] For adults age 18 and older who are not taking antihypertensive drugs and not acutely ill. Based on the average of two or more readings taken at each of two or more visits after an initial screening. When systolic and diastolic blood pressures fall into different categories, the higher category should be selected to classify the individual's blood pressure status. In addition to classifying stages of hypertension on the basis of average blood pressure levels, clinicians should specify presence or absence of target organ disease and additional risk factors.

Drug Names That Look and Sound Alike

This list has been prepared to sensitize health professionals and their support personnel for the need to properly communicate when writing, speaking, reading, and hearing drug names.

No drug name is without problems. Any name can be written or spoken poorly enough so that it can be mistaken for another.

Listed in the accompanying table are drug names that can look and/or sound alike. Some are dangerously close, whereas others require incomplete prescribing information, poor communications skills, poor listening, and/or lack of knowledge about the drugs for an error to result.

To reduce errors, practitioners must share the common goal of drug name safety with pharmaceutical manufacturers, the Food and Drug Administration (FDA), the World Health Organization (WHO), the United States Adopted Name Council (USANC), and the United States Pharmacopeia (USP).

The potential errors can be reduced by:
- Pretesting proposed names for error potential
- Careful selection of brand names and generic names by manufacturers, FDA, WHO, and USANC
- Legible handwriting
- Clear oral communications
- Writing complete drug orders
- Specifying the dosage form (eg, tablet)
- Specifying the drug strength (eg, 100 mg)
- Specifying directions (eg, take one daily with breakfast)
- Specifying the purpose/indication (eg, take one daily with breakfast to control blood pressure)
- Printing orders for new or rarely prescribed drugs
- Using computer-generated orders
- For those involved in drug dispensing and administration, being aware of the drugs that are available and paying careful attention to the work at hand
- Knowing the patient's condition/problems, to ascertain if the drug name which has been read or heard is indicated
- Double-checking completed prescriptions in the pharmacy
- Educating patients about their drug regimens (this serves as another final check that the prescription was properly read and dispensed)

Proprietary names are capitalized; other names are in lower case letters.

A

Accolate	Accupril
Accolate	Aclovate
Accupril	Accolate
Accupril	Accutane
Accupril	Aciphex
Accurbron	Accutane
Accutane	Accupril
Accutane	Accurbron
acetazolamide	acetohexamide
acetohexamide	acetazolamide
acetylcholine	acetylcysteine
acetylcysteine	acetylcholine
Aciphex	Accupril
Aciphex	Aricept
Aclovate	Accolate
Acthar	Acthrel
Acthar	Acular
Acthrel	Acthar
Acular	Acthar
adapalene	Adapin
Adapin	adapalene
Adderall	Inderal
Adeflor M	Aldoclor
Adriamycin	Idamycin
Afrin	aspirin
Aggrastat	Aggrenox
Aggrenox	Aggrastat
Albutein	albuterol
albuterol	Albutein
albuterol	atenolol
Alcaine	Alcare
Alcare	Alcaine
Aldactazide	Aldactone
Aldactone	Aldactazide

Aldoclor	Adeflor M	Antabuse	Anturane
Aldoclor	Aldoril	Anturane	Antabuse
Aldomet	Aldoril	Anturane	Artane
Aldomet	Anzemet	Anusol	Aplisol
Aldoril	Aldoclor	Anusol	Aquasol
Aldoril	Aldomet	Anzemet	Aldomet
Alesse	Aleve	Aplisol	Anusol
Aleve	Alesse	Aplisol	Aplitest
Alfenta	Sufenta	Aplisol	Atropisol
alfentanil	Anafranil	Aplitest	Aplisol
alfentanil	fentanyl	Apresazide	Apresoline
alfentanil	sufentanil	Apresoline	Apresazide
Alkeran	Leukeran	Aquasol	Anusol
Alor 5/500	Alora	Aricept	Aciphex
Alora	Alor 5/500	Aricept	Ascriptin
alprazolam	lorazepam	Artane	Altace
alprazolam	alprostadil	Artane	Anturane
alprostadil	alprazolam	Asacol	Os-Cal
Altace	alteplase	Ascriptin	Aricept
Altace	Artane	Asendin	aspirin
alteplase	Altace	aspirin	Afrin
alteplase	anistreplase	aspirin	Asendin
Alupent	Atrovent	Atarax	Ativan
Amaryl	Amerge	Atarax	Marax
Ambenyl	Aventyl	atenolol	albuterol
Ambien	Amen	atenolol	timolol
Amen	Ambien	Atgam	Ativan
Amerge	Amaryl	Ativan	Atarax
Amicar	amikacin	Ativan	Atgam
Amicar	Amikin	Ativan	Avitene
amikacin	Amicar	Atropisol	Aplisol
Amikin	Amicar	Atrovent	Alupent
amiloride	amiodarone	Avelox	Avonex
amiloride	amlodipine	Aventyl	Ambenyl
aminophylline	amitriptyline	Aventyl	Bentyl
aminophylline	ampicillin	Avitene	Ativan
amiodarone	amiloride	Avonex	Avelox
amitriptyline	aminophylline	azatadine	azathioprine
amitriptyline	nortriptyline	azathioprine	azatadine
amlodipine	amiloride	azathioprine	azidothymidine
amoxapine	amoxicillin	azathioprine	Azulfidine
amoxicillin	amoxapine	azidothymidine	azathioprine
ampicillin	aminophylline	azithromycin	erythromycin
Anafranil	alfentanil	Azulfidine	azathioprine
Anafranil	enalapril		
Anafranil	nafarelin	**B**	
Anaprox	Anaspaz	bacitracin	Bactrim
Anaspaz	Anaprox	bacitracin	Bactroban
Ancobon	Cncovin	baclofen	Bactroban
anisindione	anisotropine	baclofen	Becolvent
anisotropine	anisindione	Bactrim	bacitracin
anistreplase	alteplase	Bactroban	bacitracin

DRUG NAMES THAT LOOK AND SOUND ALIKE

Bactroban .... baclofen
Banthine .... Brethine
Becolvent .... baclofen
Beminal .... Benemid
Benadryl .... benazepril
Benadryl .... Bentyl
Benadryl .... Benylin
benazepril .... Benadryl
Benemid .... Beminal
Benoxyl .... Brevoxyl
Benoxyl .... Peroxyl
Bentyl .... Aventyl
Bentyl .... Benadryl
Benylin .... Benadryl
Benylin .... Ventolin
benztropine .... bromocriptine
bepridil .... Prepidil
Betadine .... betaine
Betagan .... Betagen
Betagen .... Betagan
betaine .... Betadine
betaxolol .... bethanechol
bethanechol .... betaxolol
Betoptic .... Betoptic S
Betoptic S .... Betoptic
Bicillin .... Wycillin
Brethaire .... Brethine
Brethine .... Banthine
Brethine .... Brethaire
Brevoxyl .... Benoxyl
bromocriptine .... benztropine
Bronkodyl .... Bronkosol
Bronkosol .... Bronkodyl
bupivacaine .... mepivacaine
bupropion .... buspirone
buspirone .... bupropion
butabarbital .... Butalbital
Butalbital .... butabarbital

C

Cafergot .... Carafate
Caladryl .... calamine
calamine .... Caladryl
calcifediol .... calcitriol
calciferol .... calcitriol
calcitonin .... calcitriol
calcitriol .... calcifediol
calcitriol .... calcitonin
calcium glubionate .... calcium gluconate
calcium gluconate .... calcium glubionate
Capastat .... Cepastat
Capitrol .... Captopril

Captopril .... Capitrol
Carafate .... Cafergot
Carbatrol .... Cartrol
Carbex .... Surbex
Carboplatin .... Cisplatin
Cardene .... Cardura
Cardene .... codeine
Cardene SR .... Cardizem SR
Cardizem SR .... Cardene SR
Cardura .... Cardene
Cardura .... Cordarone
Cardura .... Coumadin
Cardura .... K-Dur
carteolol .... carvedilol
Cartrol .... Carbatrol
carvedilol .... carteolol
Catapres .... Cetapred
Catapres .... Combipres
cefamandole .... cefmetazole
cefazolin .... cefprozil
cefmetazole .... cefamandole
Cefobid .... cefonicid
cefonicid .... Cefobid
Cefotan .... Ceftin
cefotaxime .... cefoxitin
cefotaxime .... ceftizoxime
cefotaxime .... cefuroxime
cefotetan .... cefoxitin
cefoxitin .... cefotaxime
cefoxitin .... cefotetan
cefoxitin .... Cytoxan
cefprozil .... cefazolin
ceftazidime .... ceftizoxime
Ceftin .... Cefotan
Ceftin .... Cefzil
ceftizoxime .... cefotaxime
ceftizoxime .... ceftazidime
cefuroxime .... cefotaxime
cefuroxime .... deferoxamine
Cefzil .... Ceftin
Cefzil .... Kefzol
Celebrex .... Cerebyx
Cepastat .... Capastat
cephapirin .... cephradine
cephradine .... cephapirin
Cerebyx .... Celebrex
Cerebyx .... Cerezyme
Ceredase .... Cerezyme
Cerezyme .... Cerebyx
Cerezyme .... Ceredase
Cetaphil .... Cetapred
Cetapred .... Catapres

1984 Drug Names That Look and Sound Alike

Cetapred	Cetaphil	Coumadin	Cardura
Chenix	Cystex	Coumadin	Kemadrin
chlorambucil	Chloromycetin	Cozaar	Zocor
Chloromycetin	chlorambucil	cyclobenzaprine	cycloserine
chlorpromazine	chlorpropamide	cyclobenzaprine	cyproheptadine
chlorpromazine	clomipramine	cyclophosphamide	cyclosporine
chlorpromazine	prochlorperazine	cycloserine	cyclobenzaprine
chlorpropamide	chlorpromazine	cycloserine	cyclosporine
Chorex	Chymex	cyclosporine	cyclophosphamide
Chymex	Chorex	cyclosporine	cycloserine
Cidex	Lidex	cyclosporine	Cyklokapron
Ciloxan	cinoxacin	Cyklokapron	cyclosporine
Ciloxan	Cytoxan	cyproheptadine	cyclobenzaprine
cimetidine	simethicone	Cystex	Chenix
cinoxacin	Ciloxan	Cytadren	cytarabine
Cisplatin	Carboplatin	cytarabine	Cytadren
Citracal	Citrucel	cytarabine	vidarabine
Citrucel	Citracal	CytoGam	Cytoxan
Clinoril	Clozaril	Cytosar U	Cytovene
clofazimine	clozapine	Cytosar U	Cytoxan
clofibrate	clorazepate	Cytotec	Cytoxan
clomiphene	clomipramine	Cytovene	Cytosar U
clomiphene	clonidine	Cytoxan	cefoxitin
clomipramine	chlorpromazine	Cytoxan	Ciloxan
clomipramine	clomiphene	Cytoxan	CytoGam
clonazepam	lorazepam	Cytoxan	Cytosar U
clonidine	clomiphene	Cytoxan	Cytotec
clonidine	quinidine		
clorazepate	clofibrate	**D**	
clotrimazole	co-trimoxazole	dacarbazine	Dicarbosil
Cloxapen	clozapine	dacarbazine	procarbazine
clozapine	clofazimine	Dacriose	Danocrine
clozapine	Cloxapen	dactinomycin	daunorubicin
Clozaril	Clinoril	dactinomycin	doxorubicin
Clozaril	Colazal	Dalmane	Demulen
co-trimoxazole	clotrimazole	Dalmane	Dialume
codeine	Cardene	Danocrine	Dacriose
codeine	Lodine	Dantrium	Daraprim
Colazal	Clozaril	dapsone	Diprosone
Combipres	Catapres	Daranide	Daraprim
Combivent	Combivir	Daraprim	Dantrium
Combivir	Combivent	Daraprim	Daranide
Compazine	Copaxone	Darvocet-N	Darvon-N
Comvax	Recombivax	Darvon-N	Darvocet-N
Copaxone	Compazine	daunorubicin	dactinomycin
Cordarone	Cordran	daunorubicin	doxorubicin
Cordarone	Cardura	deferoxamine	cefuroxime
Cordran	Cordarone	Delsym	Desyrel
Cort-Dome	Cortone	Demerol	Demulen
Cortone	Cort-Dome	Demerol	Dymelor
Cortrosyn	Cotazym	Demulen	Dalmane
Cotazym	Cortrosyn	Demulen	Demerol

Depen	Endep	Donnatal	Donnagel
Depo-Estradiol	Depo-Testadiol	dopamine	dobutamine
Depo-Medrol	Solu-Medrol	dopamine	Dopram
Depo-Testadiol	Depo-Estradiol	Dopar	Dopram
Dermatop	Dimetapp	Dopram	dopamine
Desferal	Disophrol	Dopram	Dopar
desipramine	disopyramide	doxacurium	doxapram
desipramine	imipramine	doxacurium	doxorubicin
desoximetasone	dexamethasone	doxapram	doxacurium
Desoxyn	digoxin	doxapram	doxazosin
Desyrel	Delsym	doxapram	doxepin
Desyrel	Zestril	doxapram	Doxinate
dexamethasone	desoximetasone	doxapram	doxorubicin
Dexedrine	Dextran	doxazosin	doxapram
Dexedrine	Excedrin	doxazosin	doxepin
Dextran	Dexedrine	doxazosin	doxorubicin
DiaBeta	Zebeta	doxepin	digoxin
Dialume	Dalmane	doxepin	doxapram
Diamox	Trimox	doxepin	doxazosin
diazepam	diazoxide	doxepin	Doxidan
diazepam	Ditropan	Doxidan	doxepin
diazoxide	diazepam	Doxil	Doxy
diazoxide	Dyazide	Doxil	Paxil
Dicarbosil	dacarbazine	Doxinate	doxapram
dichloroacetic acid	trichloracetic acid	doxorubicin	dactinomycin
diclofenac	Diflucan	doxorubicin	daunorubicin
diclofenac	Duphalac	doxorubicin	doxacurium
dicyclomine	doxycycline	doxorubicin	doxapram
dicyclomine	dyclonine	doxorubicin	doxazosin
Diflucan	diclofenac	doxorubicin	idarubicin
Diflucan	disulfiram	Doxy	Doxil
digoxin	Desoxyn	doxycycline	dicyclomine
digoxin	doxepin	doxycycline	doxylamine
Dilantin	Dilaudid	doxylamine	doxycycline
Dilaudid	Dilantin	dronabinol	droperidol
dimenhydrinate	diphenhydramine	droperidol	dronabinol
Dimetane	Dimetapp	Duphalac	diclofenac
Dimetapp	Dermatop	Dyazide	diazoxide
Dimetapp	Dimetane	dyclonine	dicyclomine
diphenhydramine	dimenhydrinate	Dymelor	Demerol
Diprosone	dapsone	Dynabac	Dynacin
dipyridamole	disopyramide	Dynabac	DynaCirc
Disophrol	Desferal	Dynacin	Dynabac
disopyramide	desipramine	Dynacin	DynaCirc
disopyramide	dipyridamole	DynaCirc	Dynabac
disulfiram	Diflucan	DynaCirc	Dynacin

E

dithranol	Ditropan
Ditropan	diazepam
Ditropan	dithranol
dobutamine	dopamine
...bid	Slo-bid
...agel	Donnatal

Ecotrin	Edecrin
Edecrin	Ecotrin
Efidac	Efudex
Efudex	Efidac

Elavil	Equanil
Elavil	Mellaril
Eldepryl	enalapril
Eldopaque Forte	Eldoquin Forte
Eldoquin Forte	Eldopaque Forte
Elmiron	Imuran
Emcyt	Eryc
enalapril	Anafranil
enalapril	Eldepryl
Endep	Depen
Enduronyl Forte	Inderal 40 mg
enflurane	isoflurane
Entex	Tenex
ephedrine	epinephrine
epinephrine	ephedrine
Epogen	Neupogen
Equagesic	EquiGesic (veterinary)
Equanil	Elavil
EquiGesic (veterinary)	Equagesic
Eryc	Emcyt
Erythrocin	Ethmozine
erythromycin	azithromcyin
erythromycin	Ethmozine
Esimil	Estinyl
Esimil	Ismelin
Estinyl	Esimil
Estraderm	Testoderm
Ethamolin	ethanol
ethanol	Ethamolin
ethanol	Ethyol
Ethmozine	Erythrocin
Ethmozine	erythromycin
ethosuximide	methsuximide
Ethyol	ethanol
etidocaine	etidronate
etidronate	etidocaine
etidronate	etomidate
etomidate	etidronate
Eurax	Evoxac
Eurax	Serax
Eurax	Urex
Evoxac	Eurax
Excedrin	Dexedrine

F

Factrel	Sectral
fentanyl	alfentanil
Feosol	Fer-in-Sol
Fer-in-Sol	Feosol
Feridex	Fertinex
Fertinex	Feridex
Fioricet	Fiorinal
Fiorinal	Fioricet
Fiorinal	Florinef
flecainide	fluconazole
Flexeril	Floxin
Flexon	Floxin
Flomax	Fosamax
Flomax	Volmax
Florinef	Fiorinal
Florvite	Flovite
Floxin	Flexeril
Floxin	Flexon
fluconazole	flecainide
Fludara	FUDR
Flumadine	flunisolide
Flumadine	flutamide
flunisolide	Flumadine
flunisolide	fluocinonide
fluocinolone	fluocinonide
fluocinonide	flunisolide
fluocinonide	fluocinolone
fluoxetine	fluvastatin
flutamide	Flumadine
fluvastatin	fluoxetine
folic acid	folinic acid
folinic acid	folic acid
Folvite	Florvite
Fosamax	Flomax
fosinopril	lisinopril
FUDR	Fludara
Fulvicin	Furacin
Furacin	Fulvicin
furosemide	Torsemide

G

Gantanol	Gantrisin
Gantrisin	Gantanol
Genpril	Genprin
Genprin	Genpril
Glaucon	glucagon
glimepiride	glipizide
glipizide	glimepiride
glipizide	glyburide
glucagon	Glaucon
Glucotrol	glyburide
glutethimide	guanethidine
glyburide	glipizide
glyburide	Glucotrol
GoLYTELY	NuLytely
gonadorelin	gonadotropin
gonadorelin	guanadrel
gonadotropin	gonadorelin
guaifenesin	guanfacine

guanabenz	guanadrel
guanabenz	guanfacine
guanadrel	gonadorelin
guanadrel	guanabenz
guanethidine	glutethimide
guanethidine	guanidine
guanfacine	guaifenesin
guanfacine	guanabenz
guanfacine	guanidine
guanidine	guanethidine
guanidine	guanfacine

H

halcinonide	Halcion
Halcion	halcinonide
Halcion	Haldol
Halcion	Healon
Haldol	Halcion
Haldol	Halog
Halog	Haldol
Halotestin	Halotex
Halotestin	halothane
Halotex	Halotestin
halothane	Halotestin
Healon	Halcion
heparin	Hespan
Hespan	heparin
Humalog	Humulin
Humulin	Humalog
Hycodan	Hycomine
Hycodan	Vicodin
Hycomine	Hycodan
hydralazine	hydroxyzine
hydrochlorothiazide	hydroflumethiazide
hydrocortisone	hydroxychloroquine
hydroflumethiazide	hydrochlorothiazide
hydromorphone	morphine
hydroxychloroquine	hydrocortisone
hydroxyprogesterone	medroxyprogesterone
hydroxyurea	hydroxyzine
hydroxyzine	hydralazine
hydroxyzine	hydroxyurea
Hygroton	Regroton
Hyperstat	Nitrostat
Hytone	Vytone

I

Idamycin	Adriamycin
idarubicin	doxorubicin
Iletin	Lente
imipenem	Omnipen
imipramine	desipramine
Imodium	Indocin

Imodium	Ionamin
Imuran	Elmiron
Imuran	Inderal
indapamide	iodamide
indapamide	iopamidol
indapamide	Iopidine
Inderal	Adderall
Inderal	Imuran
Inderal	Inderide
Inderal	Isordil
Inderal 40 mg	Enduronyl Forte
Inderide	Inderal
Indocin	Imodium
Indocin	Vicodin
interferon 2	interleukin 2
interferon alfa-2a	interferon alfa-2b
interferon alfa-2b	interferon alfa-2a
interleukin 2	interferon 2
interleukin 2	interleukin 11
interleukin 11	interleukin 2
Intropin	Isoptin
iodamide	indapamide
iodamide	Iopidine
iodine	Iopidine
iodine	Lodine
Ionamin	Imodium
iopamidol	indapamide
Iopidine	indapamide
Iopidine	iodamide
Iopidine	iodine
Iopidine	Lodine
Ismelin	Estimil
Ismelin	Isuprel
isoflurane	enflurane
Isoptin	Intropin
Isopto Carbachol	Isopto Carpine
Isopto Carpine	Isopto Carbachol
Isordil	Inderal
Isordil	Isuprel
Isuprel	Ismelin
Isuprel	Isordil

K

K-Dur	Cardura
K-Lor	Kaochlor
K-Phos Neutral	Neutra-Phos-K
Kaochlor	K-Lor
Kefzol	Cefzil
Kemadrin	Coumadin
Klaron	Klor-Con
Klor-Con	Klaron

L

lactose	lactulose
lactulose	lactose
Lamictal	Lamisil
Lamictal	Lomotil
Lamisil	Lamictal
lamivudine	lamotrigine
lamotrigine	lamivudine
Lanoxin	Levsinex
Lanoxin	Lonox
Lantus	Lente
Lasix	Lidex
Lasix	Luvox
Lasix	Luxiq
Lente	Iletin
Lente	Lantus
Leukeran	Alkeran
Leukeran	Leukine
Leukine	Leukeran
Leustatin	lovastatin
Levatol	Lipitor
Levbid	Lithobid
levothyroxine	liothyronine
Levsinex	Lanoxin
Librax	Librium
Librium	Librax
Lidex	Cidex
Lidex	Lasix
Lioresal	lisinopril
liothyronine	levothyroxine
Lipitor	Levatol
lisinopril	fosinopril
lisinopril	Lioresal
Lithobid	Levbid
Lithobid	Lithostat
Lithobid	Lithotabs
Lithonate	Lithostat
Lithostat	Lithobid
Lithostat	Lithonate
Lithostat	Lithotabs
Lithotabs	Lithobid
Lithotabs	Lithostat
Livostin	lovastatin
Lodine	codeine
Lodine	iodine
Lodine	Iopidine
Lomotil	Lamictal
Loniten	Lotensin
Lonox	Lanoxin
Lonox	Loprox
Lopressor	Lopurin
Loprox	Lonox
Lopurin	Lopressor
Lopurin	Lupron
Lorabid	Lortab
lorazepam	alprazolam
lorazepam	clonazepam
Lortab	Lorabid
Lotensin	Loniten
Lotensin	lovastatin
Lotronex	Lovenox
Lotronex	Protonix
lovastatin	Leustatin
lovastatin	Livostin
lovastatin	Lotensin
Lovenox	Lotronex
Luminal	Tuinal
Lupron	Lopurin
Lupron	Nuprin
Luvox	Lasix
Luxiq	Lasix

M

Maalox	Maolate
Maalox	Marax
magnesium sulfate	manganese sulfate
manganese sulfate	magnesium sulfate
Maolate	Maalox
Maranox	Marax
Marax	Atarax
Marax	Maalox
Marax	Maranox
Maxidex	Maxzide
Maxzide	Maxidex
Mebaral	Medrol
Mebaral	Mellaril
mecamylamine	mesalamine
Medrol	Mebaral
medroxyprogesterone	hydroxyprogesterone
medroxyprogesterone	methylprednisolone
medroxyprogesterone	methyltestosterone
Mellaril	Elavil
Mellaril	Mebaral
melphalan	Mephyton
mephenytoin	Mephyton
mephenytoin	phenytoin
mephobarbital	methocarbamol
Mephyton	melphalan
Mephyton	mephenytoin
mepivacaine	bupivacaine
mesalamine	mecamylamine
Mesantoin	Mestinon
Mestinon	Mesantoin
Mestinon	Metatensin

metaproterenol	metipranolol	Mycitracin	Myciguent
metaproterenol	metoprolol	Mydfrin	Midrin
Metatensin	Mestinon	Mylanta	Milontin
methazolamide	metolazone	Mylanta	Mynatal
methenamine	methionine	Myleran	Mylicon
methicillin	mezlocillin	Mylicon	Myleran
methionine	methenamine	Mynatal	Mylanta
methocarbamol	mephobarbital	Myoflex	Mycelex
methsuximide	ethosuximide		
methylprednisolone	medroxyprogesterone	**N**	
methyltestosterone	medroxyprogesterone	nafarelin	Anafranil
metipranolol	metaproterenol	Naldecon	Nalfon
metolazone	methiazolamine	Nalfon	Naldecon
metolazone	metoprolol	naloxone	naltrexone
metoprolol	metaproterenol	naltrexone	naloxone
metoprolol	metolazone	Narcan	Norcuron
metyrapone	metyrosine	Nasarel	Nizoral
metryrosine	metyrapone	Navane	Norvasc
Mevacor	Mivacron	Navane	Nubain
mezlocillin	methicillin	Nembutal	Myambutol
miconazole	Micronase	Nephro-Calci	Nephrocaps
miconazole	Micronor	Nephrocaps	Nephro-Calci
Micro-K	Micronase	Neumega	Neupogen
Micronase	miconazole	Neupogen	Epogen
Micronase	Micro-K	Neupogen	Neumega
Micronase	Micronor	Neupogen	Nutramigen
Micronor	miconazole	Neurontin	Noroxin
Micronor	Micronase	Neutra-Phos-K	K-Phos Neutral
Midrin	Mydfrin	niacin	Minocin
Mifeprex	Mirapex	nicardipine	nifedipine
Milontin	Miltown	Nicobid	Nitro-Bid
Milontin	Mylanta	Nicoderm	Nitroderm
Miltown	Milontin	Nicorette	Nordette
Minocin	Mithracin	nifedipine	nicardipine
Minocin	niacin	nifedipine	nimodipine
MiraLax	Mirapex	Nilstat	Nitrostat
Mirapex	Mifeprex	Nilstat	Nystatin
Mirapex	MiraLax	nimodipine	nifedipine
Mithracin	Minocin	Nitro-Bid	Nicobid
mithramycin	mitomycin	Nitroderm	Nicoderm
mitomycin	mithramycin	nitroglycerin	nitroprusside
Mivacron	Mevacor	Nitrol	Nizoral
Moban	Mobidin	nitroprusside	nitroglycerin
Mobidin	Moban	Nitrostat	Hyperstat
Modane	Mudrane	Nitrostat	Nilstat
Monopril	Monurol	Nitrostat	Nystatin
Monurol	Monopril	Nizoral	Nasarel
morphine	hydromorphone	Nizoral	Nitrol
Mudrane	Modane	Norcuron	Narcan
Myambutol	Nembutal	Nordette	Nicorette
Mycelex	Myoflex	Norgesic #40	Norgesic Forte
Myciguent	Mycitracin	Norgesic Forte	Norgesic #40

Noroxin	Neurontin
nortriptyline	amitriptyline
Norvasc	Navane
Norvasc	Vascor
Nubain	Navane
NuLytely	GoLYTELY
Nuprin	Lupron
Nutramigen	Neupogen
Nystatin	Nilstat
Nystatin	Nitrostat

O

OctreoScan	octreotide
OctreoScan	OncoScint
octreotide	OctreoScan
Ocufen	Ocuflox
Ocuflox	Ocufen
olanzapine	olsalazine
olsalazine	olanzapine
Omnipen	imipenem
Omnipen	Unipen
OncoScint	OctreoScan
Oncovin	Ancobon
Ophthaine	Ophthetic
Ophthetic	Ophthaine
Optiray	Optival
Optivar	Optiray
Oretic	Oreton
Oreton	Oretic
Orinase	Ornade
Orinase	Ornex
Ornade	Orinase
Os-Cal	Asacol
oxaprozin	oxazepam
oxazepam	oxaprozin
oxybutynin	OxyContin
OxyContin	oxybutynin
oxymetazoline	oxymetholone
oxymetholone	oxymetazoline
oxymetholone	oxymorphone
oxymorphone	oxymetholone

P

paclitaxel	paroxetine
paclitaxel	Paxil
Panadol	pindolol
pancuronium	pipecuronium
Paraplatin	Platinol
paregoric	Percogesic
Parlodel	pindolol
paroxetine	paclitaxel
paroxetine	pyridoxine
Patanol	Platinol
Pathilon	Pathocil
Pathocil	Pathilon
Pathocil	Placidyl
Paxil	Doxil
Paxil	paclitaxel
Paxil	Plavix
Paxil	Taxol
Pediapred	Pediazole
Pediazole	Pediapred
Penetrex	Pentrax
penicillamine	penicillin
penicillin	penicillamine
penicillin G potassium	penicillin G procaine
penicillin G procaine	penicillin G potassium
pentobarbital	phenobarbital
pentosan	pentostatin
pentostatin	pentosan
Pentrax	Penetrex
Pentrax	Permax
Perative	Periactin
Percocet	Percodan
Percodan	Percocet
Percodan	Percogesic
Percodan	Periactin
Percogesic	paregoric
Percogesic	Percodan
Periactin	Perative
Periactin	Percodan
Periactin	Persantine
Peridex	Precedex
Permax	Pentrax
Permax	Pernox
Pernox	Permax
Peroxyl	Benoxyl
Persantine	Periactin
phenobarbital	pentobarbital
phentermine	phentolamine
phentolamine	phentermine
phenytoin	mephenytoin
pHisoDerm	pHisoHex
pHisoHex	pHisoDerm
pHisoHex	Phos-Ex
Phos-Ex	pHisoHex
Phos-Flur	PhosLo
PhosChol	PhosLo
PhosChol	Phosphocol P32
PhosLo	Phos-Flur
PhosLo	PhosChol
Phosphocol P32	PhosChol
physostigmine	Prostigmin
physostigmine	pyridostigmine
pindolol	Panadol

pindolol	Parlodel	Prokine	procaine
pindolol	Plendil	Proloprim	Protropin
pipecuronium	pancuronium	promazine	promethazine
Pitocin	Pitressin	promethazine	promazine
Pitressin	Pitocin	Pronestyl	Ponstel
Placidyl	Pathocil	propranolol	Pravachol
Platinol	Paraplatin	Proscar	Posicor
Platinol	Patanol	Proscar	ProSom
Plavix	Paxil	Proscar	Prozac
Plendil	pindolol	Proscar	Psorcon
Plendil	Pletal	ProSom	Proscar
Pletal	Plendil	ProSom	Prozac
Polocaine	prilocaine	ProSom	Psorcon
Ponstel	Pronestyl	Prostigmin	physostigmine
Posicor	Proscar	protamine	ProAmatine
Posicor	Psorcon	protamine	Protopam
pralidoxime	Pramoxine	protamine	Protropin
pralidoxime	pyridoxine	Protonix	Lotronex
Pramoxine	pralidoxime	Protopam	protamine
Pravachol	Prevacid	Protopam	Protropin
Pravachol	propranolol	Protropin	Proloprim
PreCare	Precose	Protropin	protamine
Precedex	Peridex	Protropin	Protopam
Precose	PreCare	Proventil	Prinivil
prednisolone	prednisone	Prozac	Prilosec
prednisone	prednisolone	Prozac	Proscar
prednisone	primidone	Prozac	ProSom
Premarin	Primaxin	Psorcon	Posicor
Premarin	Remeron	Psorcon	Proscar
Premphase	Prempro	Psorcon	ProSom
Prempro	Premphase	Pyridium	pyridoxine
Prepidil	bepridil	pyridostigmine	physostigmine
Prevacid	Pravachol	pyridoxine	paroxetine
Prevacid	Prevpac	pyridoxine	pralidoxime
Preven	Prevnar	pyridoxine	Pyridium
Prevnar	Preven		
Prevpac	Prevacid		
prilocaine	Polocaine		

Q

Quarzan	quazepam
Quarzan	Questran
quazepam	Quarzan
Questran	Quarzan
quinidine	clonidine
quinidine	quinine
quinidine	Quinora
quinine	quinidine
Quinora	quinidine

prilocaine	Prilosec		
Prilosec	prilocaine		
Prilosec	Prinivil		
Prilosec	Prozac		
Primaxin	Premarin		
primidone	prednisone		
Prinivil	Prilosec		
Prinivil	Proventil		
ProAmatine	protamine		
probenecid	Procanbid		
procaine	Prokine		
Procanbid	probenecid		
procarbazine	dacarbazine		
prochlorperazine	chlorpromazine		

R

ranitidine	rimantadine
ranitidine	ritodrine
Recombivax	Comvax
Reglan	Regonol
Reglan	Renagel

Regonol	Reglan	Serax	Eurax
Regonol	Regroton	Serax	Xerac
Regonol	Renagel	Serentil	Serevent
Regranex	Repronex	Serentil	sertraline
Regroton	Hygroton	Serevent	Serentil
Regroton	Regonol	Serophene	Sarafem
Remeron	Premarin	sertraline	Serentil
Remicade	Renacidin	simethicone	cimetidine
Renacidin	Remicade	Sinequan	saquinavir
Renagel	Reglan	Slo-bid	Dolobid
Renagel	Regonol	Slow FE	Slow-K
Repronex	Regranex	Slow-K	Slow FE
reserpine	risperidone	Solu-Medrol	Depo-Medrol
Restasis	Retavase	somatrem	somatropin
Restoril	Vistaril	somatropin	somatrem
Restoril	Zestril	somatropin	sumatriptan
Retavase	Restasis	sotalol	Stadol
Retrovir	ritonavir	Sporanox	Suprax
Revex	ReVia	Stadol	sotalol
ReVia	Revex	Stelazine	selegiline
Ribavirin	riboflavin	Sufenta	Alfenta
riboflavin	Ribavirin	Sufenta	Survanta
rifabutin	rifampin	sufentanil	alfentanil
Rifadin	Ritalin	sulfadiazine	sulfasalazine
Rifamate	rifampin	sulfamethizole	sulfamethoxazole
rifampin	rifabutin	sulfamethoxazole	sulfamethizole
rifampin	Rifamate	sulfasalazine	sulfadiazine
rifampin	rifapentine	sulfasalazine	sulfisoxazole
rifapentine	rifampin	sulfisoxazole	sulfasalazine
rimanatadine	ranitidine	sumatriptan	somatropin
risperidone	reserpine	Suprax	Sporanox
Ritalin	Rifadin	Surbex	Carbex
ritodrine	ranitidine	Surbex	Surfak
ritonavir	Retrovir	Surfak	Surbex
Roxanol	Roxicet	Survanta	Sufenta
Roxicet	Roxanol	Synagis	Synalgos-DC
		Synalgos-DC	Synagis

S

Sandimmune	Sandoglobulin
Sandimmune	Sandostatin
Sandoglobulin	Sandimmune
Sandoglobulin	Sandostatin
Sandostatin	Sandimmune
Sandostatin	Sandoglobulin
saquinavir	Sinequan
Sarafem	Serophene
Sectral	Factrel
Sectral	Septra
selegiline	Stelazine
Septa	Septra
Septra	Sectral
Septra	Septa

T

Taxol	Paxil
Taxol	Taxotere
Taxotere	Taxol
Tazicef	Tazidime
Tazidime	Tazicef
Tegretol	Toradol
Tegretol	Trental
Ten-K	Tenex
Tenex	Entex
Tenex	Ten-K
Tenex	Xanax
terbinafine	terbutaline
terbutaline	terbinafine

terbutaline	tolbutamide	triflupromazine	trifluoperazine
terconazole	tioconazole	TriHemic	Triaminic
Testoderm	Estraderm	trimeprazine	trimipramine
testolactone	testosterone	trimipramine	triamterene
testosterone	testolactone	trimipramine	trimeprazine
Theolair	Thyrolar	Trimox	Diamox
Thera-Flur	TheraFlu	Trimox	Tylox
TheraFlu	Thera-Flur	Trobicin	tobramycin
thiamine	Thorazine	Tronolane	Tronothane
thioridazine	thiothixene	Tronothane	Tronolane
thioridazine	Thorazine	Tuinal	Luminal
thiothixene	thioridazine	Tuinal	Tylenol
Thorazine	thiamine	Tylenol	Tuinal
Thorazine	thioridazine	Tylenol	Tylox
Thyrogen	Thyrolar	Tylox	Trimox
Thyrolar	Theolair	Tylox	Tylenol
Thyrolar	Thyrogen		
timolol	atenolol	**U**	
Timoptic	Viroptic	Ultane	Ultram
tioconazole	terconazole	Ultram	Ultane
TobraDex	Tobrex	Unicap	Unipen
tobramycin	Trobicin	Unipen	Omnipen
Tobrex	TobraDex	Unipen	Unicap
tolazamide	tolbutamide	Urex	Eurax
tolbutamide	terbutaline	Urised	Urispas
tolbutamide	tolazamide	Urispas	Urised
tolnafate	Tornalate		
Toradol	Tegretol	**V**	
Toradol	Torecan	Valcyte	Valium
Toradol	tramadol	Valium	Valcyte
Torecan	Toradol	valsartan	Valstar
Tornalate	tolnaftate	Valstar	valsartan
Torsemide	furosemide	Vancenase	Vanceril
tramadol	Toradol	Vanceril	Vancenase
tramadol	Trandate	Vanceril	Vansil
Trandate	tramadol	Vaniqa	Viagra
Trandate	Trental	Vansil	Vanceril
Travatan	Xalatan	Vantin	Ventolin
Trental	Tegretol	Vascor	Norvasc
Trental	Trandate	Vasocidin	Vasodilan
tretinoin	trientine	Vasodilan	Vasocidin
triamcinolone	Triaminicin	Vasosulf	Velosef
triamcinolone	Triaminicol	Velosef	Vasosulf
Triaminic	Triaminicin	Ventolin	Benylin
Triaminic	TriHemic	Ventolin	Vantin
Triaminicin	triamcinolone	VePesid	Versed
Triaminicin	Triaminic	Verelan	Virilon
Triaminicol	triamcinolone	Verelan	Vivarin
triamterene	trimipramine	Verelan	Voltaren
trichloracetic acid	dichlotoacetic acid	Versed	VePesid
trientine	tretinoin	Vexol	VoSol
trifluoperazine	triflupromazine	Viagra	Vaniqa
		Vicodin	Hycodan

Vicodin	Indocin	Xanax	Zantac
vidarabine	cytarabine	Xerac	Serax
vinblastine	vincristine	Xopenex	Xanax
vinblastine	vinorelbine		

Z

vincristine	vinblastine	Zagam	Zyban
vinorelbine	vinblastine	Zantac	Xanax
Vioxx	Zyvox	Zantac	Zofran
Virilon	Verelan	Zarontin	Zaroxolyn
Viroptic	Timoptic	Zaroxolyn	Zarontin
Visine	Visken	Zebeta	DiaBeta
Visken	Visine	Zestril	Desyrel
Vistaril	Restoril	Zestril	Restoril
Vivarin	Verelan	Zestril	Zostrix
Volmax	Flomax	Zocor	Cozaar
Voltaren	Verelan	Zofran	Zantac
VoSol	Vexol	Zofran	Zosyn
Vytone	Hytone	ZORprin	Zyloprim
		Zostrix	Zestril

W

Wellbutrin	Wellcovorin	Zostrix	Zovirax
Wellbutrin	Wellferon	Zosyn	Zofran
Wellcovorin	Wellbutrin	Zosyn	Zyvox
Wellcovorin	Wellferon	Zovirax	Zostrix
Wellferon	Wellbutrin	Zyban	Zagam
Wellferon	Wellcovorin	Zyloprim	ZORprin
Wycillin	Bicillin	Zyprexa	Zyrtec
		Zytrec	Zyprexa

X

Xalatan	Travatan	Zyvox	Vioxx
Xanax	Tenex	Zyvox	Zosyn
Xanax	Xopenex		

This list was compiled by Neil M. Davis MS, PharmD, FASHP, President, Safe Medication Practices Consulting, Inc., 1143 Wright Drive, Huntingdon Valley, PA, 19006.

Oral Dosage Forms That Should Not Be Crushed or Chewed

The purpose of this feature is to alert health care professionals about medications that should not be crushed or chewed because of their special pharmaceutical formulations or characteristics. Oral dosage forms that are sustained release (slow release) comprise the vast majority of this designation. Crushing or chewing such products may substantially alter their intended pharmacokinetics. Additional reasons for not chewing or crushing drugs include poor taste, irritant properties, or carcinogenic potential. Alternative liquid forms of these products are listed if available. Refer to the end of the table for a complete explanation of references.

It is important to understand that the inability to crush or chew drugs with slow-release properties does not always mean the dosage form cannot be divided or halved. Some newer slow-release dosage forms (eg, *Toprol XL*) are commercially available as scored tablets. This reference addresses those drugs that cannot be crushed or chewed.

Anyone who visits any acute- or long-term care facility can observe personnel meticulously grinding tablets or the contents of capsules in a mortar and pestle. Their rationale is well-intentioned: they have an order to administer medication to a patient with an nasogastric tube or who cannot swallow solids and have to incorporate the drug into a liquid vehicle. However, they do so at the risk of changing the pharmacokinetics of the solid dosage formulation. Examples of special formulations include sublingual or buccal, enteric-coated, and extended-release tablets or capsules. Products containing extended-release dosage forms frequently have an abbreviation affixed to their brand name that serves as a clue that crushing may affect the formulation (Table 1). In addition, some medications are inherently corrosive to the oral mucosa and/or upper gastrointestinal tract, remarkably bitter to the taste, or capable of staining the oral mucosa and teeth.

Finally, several medications are potentially carcinogenic and require limited handling by medical personnel. Crushing or breaking of products that have carcinogenic/teratogenic potential (ie, antineoplastics) may not alter the dosage form or delivery mechanisms but may cause aerosolization of particles, exposing health care workers who handle these products. The reader is encouraged to review the American Society of Health-System Pharmacists' (previously the American Society of Hospital Pharmacists) bulletin on handling cytotoxic and hazardous drugs.

A more detailed description of the dosage forms mentioned above has been published in previous versions of this article and is summarized in Table 2.

Alternatives to Crushing: For patients who cannot swallow whole tablets or capsules, the most logical approach is to use liquid suspension forms of the same medication. Table 3 identifies examples of medications that have a liquid form commercially available. In some cases, there must be a dosage adjustment when the liquid is substituted. This is especially true if the tablet or capsule is an extended-release medication. If a liquid or suspension is not commercially available, the pharmacist should be consulted to determine if a liquid formulation could be extemporaneously prepared.

Occasionally, it is possible to substitute the injectable form of the medication by placing the appropriate amount of injection in some suitable fluid, such as juice. This should be done, however, only after consultation with a pharmacist to ensure that there are no problems regarding compatibility, stability, or changes in absorption of the drug. Another alternative is to use a chemically different but clinically similar medication that is available in a liquid form. Some medications that cannot be crushed may be administered in other ways, such as administering the contents of a capsule in soft food. This type of information is provided in Table 3 and indexed in the footnote.

Updates to List: Inherent with a listing of this type is the difficulty in keeping such lists current. The author encourages manufacturers, pharmacist, nurses, and other health professionals to notify us of any changes or updates.

References:
1. American Society of Hospital Pharmacists. ASHP technical assistance bulletin on handling cytotoxic and hazardous drugs. *Am J Hosp Pharm*. 1990;47:1033-1049.
2. Mitchell JF. Oral dosage forms that should not be crushed: 200 update. *Hosp Pharm*. 2000;35:553-567.

Table 1: Common Abbreviations for Extended-Release Products

CD	controlled dose
CR	controlled release
CRT	controlled release tablet
LA	long acting
SR	sustained release
TR	time release
TD	time delay
SA	sustained action
XL	extended release
XR	extended release

Table 2: Summary of Drug Formulations that Preclude Crushing

Type	Reason(s) for the formulation
Enteric coated	Designed to pass through the stomach intact with drug being released in the intestines to: (1) prevent destruction of drug by stomach acids (2) prevent stomach irritation (3) delay onset of action
Extended release	Designed to release drug over an extended period of time. Such products include: (1) multiple-layered tablets releasing drug as each layer is dissolved (2) mixed release pellets that dissolve at different time intervals (3) special matrixes that are themselves inert, but slowly release drug from the matrix
Sublingual	Designed to dissolve quickly in oral fluids for rapid absorption by the abundant blood supply of the mouth.
Miscellaneous	Drugs that: (1) produce oral mucosa irritation (2) are extremely bitter (3) contain dyes or inherently could stain teeth and mucosal tissue (4) drugs that, if handled without adequate protection, are potentially carcinogenic

Table 3: Medications That Should Not Be Crushed or Chewed

Drug Product	Dosage Form	Reason/Comments
Aciphex	Tablet	Slow release
Accuhist	Tablet	Slow release[6]
Accutane	Capsule	Mucous membrane irritant
Adalat CC	Tablet	Slow release
Aggrenox	Capsule	Slow release Note: Capsule may be opened. Contents include an aspirin tablet that may be chewed and dipyridamole pellets that may be sprinkled.
Adderall XR	Capsule	Slow release[2]
Advicor	Tablet	Slow release
AeroHist Plus	Tablet	Slow release[6]
Afeditab CR	Tablet	Slow release
Alavert Allergy Sinus 12 Hour	Tablet	Slow release
Allegra D	Tablet	Slow release
Altocor	Tablet	Slow release
Arthritis Bayer Time Release	Capsule	Slow release
Arthrotec	Tablet	Enteric coated
ASA Enseals	Tablet	Enteric coated
Asacol	Tablet	Slow release
Ascriptin A/D	Tablet	Enteric coated
Ascriptin Extra Strength	Tablet	Enteric coated
Augmentin XR	Tablet	Slow release[1,6]
Avinza	Capsule	Slow release[2] (not padding)
Avodart	Capsule	Teratogenic potential[7]
Azulfidine EN-tabs	Tablet	Enteric coated
Bayer Enteric-Coated	Caplet	Enteric coated
Bayer Low Adult 81 mg	Tablet	Enteric coated
Bayer Regular Strength 325 mg	Caplet	Enteric coated
Bellahist-D LA	Tablet	Slow release
Biaxin-XL	Tablet	Slow release
Biltricide	Tablet	Taste[6]
Biohist LA	Tablet	Slow release[6]
Bisacodyl	Tablet	Enteric coated[5]
Bontril-SR	Capsule	Slow release
Bromafed PD	Capsule	Slow release
Bromafed SR	Capsule	Slow release
Budeprion SR	Tablet	Slow release
Calan SR	Tablet	Slow release[6]
Carbatrol	Capsule	Slow release[2]
Cardene SR	Capsule	Slow release
Cardizem	Tablet	Slow release
Cardizem CD	Capsule	Slow release[2]
Cardizem LA	Tablet	Slow release
Cardizem SR	Capsule	Slow release[2]
Carter's Little Pills	Tablet	Enteric coated
CartiaXT	Capsule	Slow release
Ceclor CD	Tablet	Slow release
Ceftin	Tablet	Taste[1] Note: Use suspension for children

Table 3: Medications That Should Not Be Crushed or Chewed

Drug Product	Dosage Form	Reason/Comments
CellCept	Capsule, Tablet	Teratogenic potential[7]
Charcoal Plus	Tablet	Enteric coated
Chloral Hydrate	Capsule	Note: Product is in liquid form within a special capsule[1]
Chlor-Trimeton 12-Hour	Tablet	Slow release[1]
Cipro	Tablet	Taste[4]
Cipro XR	Tablet	Slow release
Claritin-D 12 Hour	Tablet	Slow release
Claritin-D 24 Hour	Tablet	Slow release
Colace	Capsule	Taste[4]
Colestid	Tablet	Slow release
Comhist LA	Capsule	Slow release[2]
Compazine Spansule	Capsule	Slow release[1]
Concerta	Tablet	Slow release
Commit	Lozenge	Note: Integrity compromised by chewing or crushing
Contac 12-Hour	Capsule	Slow release[1,2]
Cotazym-S	Capsule	Enteric coated[2]
Covera-HS	Tablet	Slow release
Creon 5, 10, 20	Capsule	Enteric coated[2]
Crixivan	Capsule	Taste Note: Capsule may be opened and mixed with fruit puree (eg, banana).
Cytovene	Capsule	Skin irritant
Cytoxan	Tablet	Note: Drug may be crushed, but manufacturer recommends injection
Dallergy	Capsule	Slow release
Dallergy-JR	Capsule	Slow release
Deconamine SR	Capsule	Slow release[1]
Defen-LA	Tablet	Slow release[6]
Depakene	Capsule	Slow release, mucous membrane irritant[1]
Depakote	Capsule	Enteric coated
Depakote ER	Tablet	Slow release
Desoxyn	Tablet	Slow release
Desyrel	Tablet	Taste[4]
Detrol LA	Capsule	Slow release
Dexedrine Spansule	Capsule	Slow release
Diamox Sequels	Capsule	Slow release
Dilacor XR	Capsule	Slow release
Dilatrate-SR	Capsule	Slow release
Diltia XT	Capsule	Slow release
Ditropan XL	Tablet	Slow release
Dolobid	Tablet	Irritant
Donnatal Extentab	Tablet	Slow release[1]
Drisdol	Capsule	Liquid filled[8]
DriHist SR	Tablet	Slow release[6]
Drixoral	Tablet	Slow release[1]
Drixoral Plus	Tablet	Slow release
Drixoral Sinus	Tablet	Slow release
Dulcolax	Tablet	Enteric coated[5]
Dulcolax	Capsule	Liquid filled

Table 3: Medications That Should Not Be Crushed or Chewed

Drug Product	Dosage Form	Reason/Comments
DuraHist	Tablet	Slow release[6]
Duratuss G, GP	Tablet	Slow release[6]
Dynabac	Tablet	Enteric coated
DynaCirc CR	Tablet	Slow release
Easprin	Tablet	Enteric coated
EC-Naprosyn	Tablet	Enteric coated
Ecotrin Adult Low Strength	Tablet	Enteric coated
Ecotrin Maximum Strength	Tablet	Enteric coated
Ecotrin Regular Strength	Tablet	Enteric coated
E.E.S. 400	Tablet	Enteric coated[1]
Effexor XR	Capsule	Slow release
Efidac/24	Tablet	Slow release
Efidac/24 Pseudoephedrine	Tablet	Slow release
E-Mycin	Tablet	Enteric coated
Entex LA	Tablet	Slow release[1]
Entex PSE	Tablet	Slow release
Entocort EC	Capsule	Enteric coated[2]
Ergomar	Tablet	Sublingual form[9]
Eryc	Capsule	Enteric coated[2]
Ery-Tab	Tablet	Enteric coated
Erythrocin Stearate	Tablet	Enteric coated
Erythromycin Base	Tablet	Enteric coated
Eskalith CR	Tablet	Slow release
Evista	Tablet	Taste; teratogenic potential[7]
Extendryl JR	Capsule	Slow release
Extendryl SRC	Capsule	Slow release[1]
Feldene	Capsule	Mucous membrane irritant
Feosol	Tablet	Enteric coated[1]
Feratab	Tablet	Enteric coated[1]
Fergon	Capsule	Slow release[2]
Fero-Grad 500 mg	Tablet	Slow release
Ferro-Sequels	Tablet	Slow release
Flagyl ER	Tablet	Slow release
Flomax	Capsule	Slow release
Fosamax	Tablet	Mucous membrane irritant
Fumatinic	Capsule	Slow release
Geocillin	Tablet	Taste
GFN/PSE/DM	Tablet	Slow release
Gleevec	Tablet	Taste[6] Note: May be dissolved in mineral oil or apple juice.
Glucophage XR	Tablet	Slow release
Glucotrol XL	Tablet	Slow release
Gris-PEG	Tablet	Note: Crushing may result in precipitation as larger particles
Guiafed	Capsule	Slow release
Guiafed-PD	Capsule	Slow release
Guaifenex DM	Tablet	Slow release[6]
Guaifenex LA	Tablet	Slow release[6]
Guaifenex PSE	Tablet	Slow release[6]

Table 3 Medications That Should Not Be Crushed or Chewed

Drug Product	Dosage Form	Reason/Comments
Guaifenex-Rx DM	Tablet	Slow release
Guaimax-D	Tablet	Slow release
Hista-Vent DA	Tablet	Slow release[6]
Humibid DM	Tablet	Slow release
Humibid LA	Tablet	Slow release
Iberet Filmtab	Tablet	Slow release[1]
Iberet 500	Tablet	Slow release[1]
Iberet-Folic	Tablet	Slow release
ICaps Time Release	Tablet	Slow release
Imdur	Tablet	Slow release[6]
Inderal LA	Capsule	Slow release
Inderide LA	Capsule	Slow release
Indocin SR	Capsule	Slow release[1,2]
Innopran XL	Capsule	Slow release
Ionamin	Capsule	Slow release
Isoptin SR	Tablet	Slow release
Isordil Sublingual	Tablet	Sublingual form[9]
Isosorbide Dinitrate Sublingual	Tablet	Sublingual form[9]
Isosorbide SR	Tablet	Slow release
K + 8	Tablet	Slow release[1]
K + 10	Tablet	Slow release[1]
Kadian	Capsule	Slow release[2]
Kaon Cl	Tablet	Slow release[1]
K-Dur	Tablet	Slow release
Klor-Con	Tablet	Slow release[1]
Klor-Con M	Tablet	Slow release[1]
Klotrix	Tablet	Slow release[1]
K-Lyte	Tablet	Effervescent tablet[3]
K-Lyte CL	Tablet	Effervescent tablet[3]
K-Lyte DS	Tablet	Effervescent tablet[3]
K-Tab	Tablet	Slow release[1]
Lescol XL	Tablet	Slow release
Levbid	Tablet	Slow release[6]
Levsinex Timecaps	Capsule	Slow release
Lexxel	Tablet	Slow release
Lipram 4500	Capsule	Enteric coated[2]
Lipram CR, PN, UL	Capsule	Enteric coated[2]
Lipram (all)	Capsule	Slow release[2]
Liquibid-D 1200	Tablet	Slow release[6]
Liquibid-PD	Tablet	Slow release[6]
Lithobid	Tablet	Slow release
Lodine XL	Tablet	Slow release
Lodrane LD	Capsule	Slow release[2]
Mag-Tab SR	Tablet	Slow release
Maxifed	Tablet	Slow release
Maxifed DM	Tablet	Slow release
Maxifed G	Tablet	Slow release
Medent-DM	Tablet	Slow release
Medent LD	Tablet	Slow release

Table 3: Medications That Should Not Be Crushed or Chewed

Drug Product	Dosage Form	Reason/Comments
Mestinon Timespan	Tablet	Slow release[1]
Metadate CD	Capsule	Slow release[2]
Metadate ER	Tablet	Slow release
Methylin ER	Tablet	Slow release
Micro K	Capsule	Slow release[1,2]
Motrin	Tablet	Taste[4]
MS Contrin	Tablet	Slow release[1]
Mucinex	Tablet	Slow release
Muco-Fen-DM	Tablet	Slow release[6]
Myfortic	Tablet	Slow release
Naprelan	Tablet	Slow release
Nasatab LA	Tablet	Slow release[6]
Nexium	Capsule	Slow release[2]
Niaspan	Tablet	Slow release
Nicotinic Acid	Capsule, Tablet	Slow release
Nifediac CC	Tablet	Slow release
Nitrostat	Tablet	Sublingual form[9]
Norflex	Tablet	Slow release
Norpace CR	Capsule	Slow release form within a special capsule
Ondrox	Tablet	Slow release
Optilets 500	Tablet	Enteric coated
Optilets-M 500	Tablet	Enteric coated
Oramorph SR	Tablet	Slow release[1]
Oruvail	Capsule	Slow release
OxyContin	Tablet	Slow release
Palgic-D Extended Release	Tablet	Slow release[6]
Pancrease	Capsule	Enteric coated[2]
Pancrease MT	Capsule	Enteric coated[2]
Pancrecarb MS	Capsule	Enteric coated[2]
PanMist Jr, LA	Tablet	Slow release[6]
PanMist DM	Tablet	Slow release[6]
Pannaz	Tablet	Slow release[6]
Papaverine Sustained Action	Capsule	Slow release
Paxil CR	Tablet	Slow release
Pentasa	Tablet	Slow release
Perdiem	Granules	Wax coated
Phena Vent D	Tablet	Slow release
Pre-Hist-D	Tablet	Slow release[6]
Plendil	Tablet	Slow release
Prelu-2	Capsule	Slow release
Prevacid	Capsule	Slow release
Prevacid Suspension	Suspension	Slow release Note: Contains enteric coated granules.
Prilosec	Capsule	Slow release
Procainamide HCl SR	Tablet	Slow release
Procanbid	Tablet	Slow release
Procardia	Capsule	Delays absorption[1,2]
Procardia XL	Tablet	Slow release Note: AUC is unaffected
Profen II	Tablet	Slow release[6]

Table 3: Medications That Should Not Be Crushed or Chewed

Drug Product	Dosage Form	Reason/Comments
Profen II DM	Tablet	Slow release[6]
Profen Forte DM	Tablet	Slow release
Pronestyl SR	Tablet	Slow release
Propecia	Tablet	Note: Women who are or may become pregnant should not handle crushed or broken tablets
Proscar	Tablet	Note: Women who are or may become pregnant should not handle crushed or broken tablets
Protonix	Tablet	Slow release
Protuss DM	Tablet	Slow release
Pytest	Capsule	Note: Radiopharmaceutical
QDALL	Capsule	Slow release
Quibron-T SR	Tablet	Slow release[1]
Quinidex Extentabs	Tablet	Slow release
Rescon JR	Tablet	Slow release
Rescon MX	Tablet	Slow release
Respa-1st	Tablet	Slow release[6]
Respa-DM	Tablet	Slow release[6]
Respahist	Capsule	Slow release[2]
Respaire 120 SR	Capsule	Slow release
Ritalin SR	Tablet	Slow release
Rondec TR	Tablet	Slow release[1]
R-Tanna	Tablet	Slow release
Rythmol SR	Capsule	Slow release
Sinemet CR	Tablet	Slow release
Singlet for Adults	Tablet	Slow release
SINUtuss DM CR	Tablet	Slow release[6]
SINUvent PE	Tablet	Slow release[6]
Slo-Niacin	Tablet	Slow release[6]
Slow-K	Tablet	Slow release[1]
Slow-Mag	Tablet	Slow release
Somnote	Capsule	Liquid filled
Sudafed 12 hour	Capsule	Slow release[1]
Sudal 60/500	Tablet	Slow release
Sular	Tablet	Slow release
Symax SR	Tablet	Slow release
Taztia XT	Capsule	Slow release
Tegretol-XR	Tablet	Slow release
Temodar	Capsule	Note: If capsules are accidentally opened or damaged, rigorous precautions should be taken to avoid inhalation or contact of contents with the skin or mucous membranes.[7]
Tessalon Perles	Capsule	Slow release
Theo-24	Tablet	Slow release[1]
Theochron	Tablet	Slow release
Theo-Time SR	Tablet	Slow release
Tiazac	Capsule	Slow release
Topamax	Tablet	Taste
Topamax	Capsule	Taste[2]

Table 3: Medications That Should Not Be Crushed or Chewed

Drug Product	Dosage Form	Reason/Comments
Touro CC	Tablet	Slow release
Touro EX	Tablet	Slow release
Touro LA	Tablet	Slow release
Trental	Tablet	Slow release
Triptone	Tablet	Slow release
Tussafed LA	Tablet	Slow release
Tylenol Arthritis	Tablet	Slow release
Tylenol 8 Hour	Tablet	Slow release
Ultrace	Capsule	Enteric coated[2]
Ultrace MT	Capsule	Enteric coated[2]
Uniphyl	Tablet	Slow release
Urocit-K	Tablet	Wax coated
Verelan	Capsule	Slow release[2]
Videx EC	Capsule	Slow release
Voltaren XR	Tablet	Slow release
VoSpire ER	Tablet	Slow release
Wellbutrin SR, XL	Tablet	Slow release
Xanax XR	Tablet	Slow release
Z-Cof LA	Tablet	Slow release[6]
Zephrex LA	Tablet	Slow release
ZORprin	Tablet	Slow release
Zyban	Tablet	Slow release

[1] Liquid dosage forms of the product are available; however, dose, frequency of administration, and manufacturers may differ from that of the solid dosage form.

[2] Capsule may be opened and the contents taken without crushing or chewing; soft food such as applesauce or pudding may facilitate administration; contents may generally be administered via nasogastric tube using an appropriate fluid, provided entire contents are washed down the tube.

[3] Effervescent tablets must be dissolved in the amount of diluent recommended by the manufacturer.

[4] The taste of this product in a liquid form would likely be unacceptable to the patient; administration via nasogastric tube should be acceptable.

[5] Antacids and/or milk may prematurely dissolve the coating of the tablet.

[6] Tablet is scored and may be broken in half without affecting release characteristics.

[7] Skin contact may enhance tumor production; avoid direct contact.

[8] Capsule may be opened and the liquid contents removed for administration.

[9] Tablets are made to disintegrate under the tongue.

Revised by John F. Mitchell, PharmD, FASHP and Michelle A. Leady, PharmD, from an article that originally appeared in *Hosp Pharm.* 1996.;1:27–37.

Childhood Immunization Schedule

Recommended Childhood and Adolescent Immunization Schedule – United States, 2005[1]

Vaccine	Birth	1 Mo.	2 Mos.	4 Mos.	6 Mos.	12 Mos.	15 Mos.	18 Mos.	24 Mos.	4-6 Yrs.	11-12 Yrs.	13-18 Yrs.
Hepatitis B[2]	Hep B #1	only if mother HBsAg (-)										
			Hep B #2			Hep B #3					Hep B series	
Diphtheria, Tetanus, Pertussis[3]			DTaP	DTaP	DTaP		DTaP			DTaP	Td	Td
Haemophilus influenzae Type b[4]			Hib	Hib	Hib	Hib						
Inactivated Polio			IPV	IPV		IPV				IPV		
Measles, Mumps, Rubella[5]						MMR #1				MMR #2	MMR #2	
Varicella[6]						Varicella					Varicella	
Pneumococcal[7]			PCV	PCV	PCV	PCV			PCV	PPV		
Influenza[8]					Influenza (yearly)					Influenza (Yearly)		
Vaccines below this line are for selected populations												
Hepatitis A[9]										Hep A series		

▢ Range of recommended ages

■ Catch-up vaccination – Indicates age groups that warrant special effort to administer those vaccines not previously given.

▨ Preadolescent assessment

[1] This schedule indicates the recommended ages for routine administration of currently licensed childhood vaccines, as of December 1, 2004, for children through 18 years of age. Any dose not given at the recommended age should be given at any subsequent visit when indicated and feasible.
Indicates age groups that warrant special effort to administer those vaccines not previously given. Additional vaccines may be licensed and recommended during the year. Licensed combination vaccines may be used whenever any components of the combination are indicated and the vaccine's other components are not contraindicated. Providers should consult the manufacturers' package inserts for detailed recommendations. Clinically significant adverse events that follow immunization should be reported to the Vaccine Adverse Event Reporting System (VAERS). Guidance about how to obtain and complete a VAERS form can be found on the Internet: http://www.vaers.org/ or by calling 1-800-822-7967.

[2] **Hepatitis B vaccine (HepB).** All infants should receive the first dose of hepatitis B vaccine soon after birth and before hospital discharge; the first dose may also be given by 2 months of age if the infant's mother is hepatitis B surface antigen (HBsAg) negative. Only monovalent HepB can be used for the birth dose. Monovalent or combination vaccine containing HepB may be used to complete the series. Four doses of vaccine may be administered when a birth dose is given. The second dose should be given at least 4 weeks after the first dose, except for combination vaccines which cannot be administered before 6 weeks of age. The third dose should be given at least 16 weeks after the first dose and at least 8 weeks after the second dose. The last dose in the vaccination series (third or fourth dose) should not be administered before 24 weeks of age.

Infants born to HBsAg-positive mothers should receive HepB and 0.5 mL hepatitis B immune globulin (HBIG) within 12 hours of birth at separate sites. The second dose is recommended at 1 to 2 months of age. The last dose in the vaccination series should not be administered before 24 weeks of age. These infants should be tested for HBsAg and antibody to HBsAg (anti-HBs) at 9 to 15 months of age.

Infants born to mothers whose HBsAg status is unknown should receive the first dose of the HepB series within 12 hours of birth. Maternal blood should be drawn as soon as possible to determine the mother's HBsAg status; if the HBsAg test is positive, the infant should receive HBIG as soon as possible (no later than 1 week of age). The second dose is recommended at 1 to 2 months of age. The last dose in the vaccination series should not be administered before 24 weeks of age.

[3] **Diphtheria and tetanus toxoids and acellular pertussis vaccine (DTaP).** The fourth dose of DTaP may be administered as early as 12 months of age, provided 6 months have elapsed since the third dose and the child is unlikely to return at 15 to 18 months of age. The final dose in the series should be given at 4 years of age or older. **Tetanus and diphtheria toxoids (Td)** is recommended at 11 to 12 years of age if at least 5 years have elapsed since the last dose of tetanus and diphtheria toxoid-containing vaccine. Subsequent routine Td boosters are recommended every 10 years.

[4] *Haemophilus influenza* **type b (Hib) conjugate vaccine.** Three Hib conjugate vaccines are licensed for infant use. If PRP-OMP (*PedvaxHIB* or *ComVax* [Merck]) is administered at 2 and 4 months of age, a dose at 6 months of age is not required. DTaP/Hib combination products should not be used for primary immunization in infants at 2, 4, or 6 months of age, but can be used as boosters following any Hib vaccine. The final dose in the series should be given at 12 months of age or older.

[5] **Measles, mumps, and rubella vaccine (MMR).** The second dose of the MMR is recommended routinely at 4 to 6 years of age but may be administered during any visit, provided at least 4 weeks have elapsed since the first dose and that both doses are administered beginning at or after 12 months of age. Those who have not previously received the second dose should complete the schedule by the 11– to 12–year-old visit.

[6] **Varicella vaccine.** Varicella vaccine is recommended at any visit at or after 12 months of age for susceptible children (ie, those who lack a reliable history of chickenpox). Susceptible people 13 years of age or older should receive 2 doses, given at least 4 weeks apart.

[7] **Pneumococcal vaccine.** The heptavalent **pneumococcal conjugate vaccine (PCV)** is recommended for all children 2 to 23 months of age. It is also recommended for certain children 24 to 59 months of age. The final dose in the series should be given at age 12 months or older. **Pneumococcal polysaccharide vaccine (PPV)** is recommended in addition to PCV for certain high-risk groups. See *MMWR*. 2000;49(RR-9);1–35.

[8] **Influenza vaccine.** Influenza vaccine is recommended annually for children 6 months of age or older with certain risk factors (including but not limited to asthma, cardiac disease, sickle cell disease, HIV, diabetes, health care workers, and household members of persons in high-risk groups [see *MMWR*. 2004;53(RR-6);1-40]), and can be administered to all others wishing to obtain immunity. In addition, healthy children 6 to 23 months of age and close contacts of healthy children 0 to 23 months of age are encouraged to receive influenza vaccine if feasible because children in this age group are at substantially increased risk for influenza-related hospitalizations. For healthy persons 5 to 49 years of age, the intranasally administered live-attenuated influenza vaccine (LAIV) is an acceptable alternative to the intramuscular trivalent inactivated influenza vaccine (TIV). See *MMWR*. 2004;53(RR-6):1-40. Children receiving TIV should be administered a dosage appropriate for their age (0.25 mL if 6 to 35 months of age or 0.5 mL if 3 years of age or older). Children 8 years of age or less who are receiving influenza vaccine for the first time should receive 2 doses (separated by at least 4 weeks for TIV and at least 6 weeks for LAIV).

[9] **Hepatitis A vaccine.** Hepatitis A vaccine is recommended for children and adolescents in selected states and regions, and for certain high-risk groups; consult your local public health authority. All children and adolescents in these states, regions, and high-risk groups who have not been immunized against hepatitis A can begin the hepatitis A vaccination series during any visit. The two doses in the series should be administered at least 6 months apart. See *MMWR*. 1999;48(RR–12);1-37.

Source: Advisory Committee on Immunization Practices (ACIP), http://www.cdc.gov/nip/acip; the American Academy of Pediatrics (AAP), http://www.aap.org; and the American Academy of Family Physicians (AAFP), http://www.aafp.org.

Reference: CDC. Recommended childhood & immunization schedule – United States, 2005.

Index

INDEX

.44 Magnum, 269
½ Halfprin, 139
1-Deamino-8-D-Arginine Vasopressin, 507
(1S)-1-(9-Deazahypoxanthin-9-yl)-1,4-dideoxy-1,4-imino-D-ribitol-hydrochloride, 1919
1,5-(Butylimino)-1,5 dideoxy,D-glucitol, 1919
2-O-Burtyryl-1-O-octyl-myo-inositol 3,4,5,6-tetrakisphosphate, 1920
2-Chloroethyl-3-sarcosinamide-1-nitrosourea, 1920
3′-Azido-2′,3′dideoxyuridine, 1920
(4S)-4-ethyl-4-hydroxy-3, 14-dioxo-3,4,12,14-tetrahydro-1-H-pyrano[3?,4?:6,7]-indolizino-[1,2-b]-quinoline-11-carbaldehyde O-(tert-butyl)-(E)-oxime, 1919
5-ASA, 1125
5-Aza-2′-deoxycytidine, 1920
8-Cyclopentyl 1,3-dipropylxanthine, 1920
8-MOP, 1151
9-nitro-20-(S)-Camptothecin, 1920
20-20, 269
40 Winks, 556
357 HR Magnum, 269
642, [C], 1511

A

A-007, 1965
A-Hydrocort, 889
A-Methapred, 1166
A-Spas S/L, 901
A/T/S, 659
Abacavir Sulfate, 1
Abacavir Sulfate/Lamivudine/Zidovudine, 2
Abarelix, 4
Abavca/Perthon, 1965
Abbokinase, 1847
Abciximab, 6
Abelcet, 108, 1923
Abenol, [C], 12
Abetimus, 1921
Abilify, 17
Absorbine Antifungal Foot Powder, 1186
Absorbine Athlete's Foot Cream, 1782
Absorbine Footcare, 1782
Abthrax, 1948
ACA125, 1921
Acamprosate Calcium, 7
Acarbose, 7
Accolate, 1888
Accupril, 1538
Accurbron, 1739
Accuretic, 1540

Accutane, 975
Accutane Roche, [C], 975
Acebutolol Hydrochloride, 10
Acellular Pertussis Vaccine (DTaP), 561
Aceon, 1402
Acephen, 12
Aceta, 12
Aceta w/Codeine, 13
Acetadote, 19, 1921
Acetaminophen, 12, 1915
Acetaminophen/Caffeine/Butalbital, 259
Acetaminophen/Caffeine/Codeine Phosphate/Butalbital, 261
Acetaminophen/Hydrocodone Bitartrate, 880
Acetaminophen/Isometheptene Mucate/Dichloralphenazone, 969
Acetaminophen/Oxycodone, 1340
Acetaminophen/Propoxyphene, 1513
Acetaminophen/Tramadol Hydrochloride, 1796
Acetaminophen Uniserts, 12
Acetaminophen with Codeine Phosphate, 13
Acetazolamide, 15
Acetohexamide, 17
Acetoxyl 2.5% and 5%, [C], 190
Acetoxyl 10%, [C], 190
N-Acetyl-p-Aminophenol, 12
(+/-)-7-[3-(4-Acetyl-3-methoxy-2-propylphenoxy)-propoxy]-3,4-dihydro-8-propyl-2H-1-benzopyran-2-2carboxylic Acid, 1919
N-Acetyl-sacrosyl-glycyl-L-valyl-D-alloisoleucyl-L-threonyl-L-norvaly-L-isoleucyl-L-arginyl-L-prolylethylaminde Acetate, 1946
Acetylcarbromal, 1914
Acetylcysteine, 19, 1921
N-Acetylcysteinate Lysine, 1946
N-Acetylgalactosamine-4-sulfatase, Recombinant Human, 1946
N-Acetylprocainamide, 1946
Acetylsalicylic Acid, 139
Achtrel, 1930
Aciphex, 1549
Acitretin, 22
Aclovate, 40
Aconiazide, 1921
Acrivastine/Pseudoephedrine Hydrochloride, 25
ACT (Activated Cellular Therapy), 1963
ACTH, 453

ACTH, Synthetic, 457
Acthar, 453
ActHIB, 853
Acticin, 1404
Actidose-Aqua, 360
Actidose with Sorbitol, 360
Actigall, 1961
Actimid, 1921
Actimmune, 953, 1940
Actinex, 1088
Actiq, 724
Activase, 68, 1922
Activase rt-PA, [C], 68
Activated Cellular Therapy, 1963
Actonel, 1584
Actos, 1439
Acular, 990
Acular LS, 990
Acyclovir, 26
Adagen, 1948
Adalat, 1283
Adalat CC, 1283
Adalat XL, [C], 1283
Adalimumab, 30
Adapalene, 32
Adderall, 106, 520
Adderall XR, 520
Adefovir Dipivoxil, 33
Adeno-Associated Viral-Based Vector Cystic Fibrosis Gene Therapy, 1921
Adeno-Associated Viral Vector Containing the Gene for Human Coagulation Factor IX, 1921
Adenocard, 35
Adenoscan, 35
Adenosine, 35, 1921
S-Adenosylmethionine, 1954
Adenovirus-based Vector Factor VIII Complementary DNA to Somatic Cells, 1921
Adenovirus-mediated Herpes Simplex Virus-Thyimidine Kinase Gene, 1921
Adipex-P, 1418
Adoxa, 597
Adrenalin, [C], 637
Adrenalin Chloride, 637
Adrenocorticotropic Hormone, 453
Adrenocorticotropic Hormone, Repository Corticotropin or Adrenocorticotropic Hormone, 1953
Adriamycin PFS, 591
Adriamycin RDF, 591
Adrucil, 755, 1936
Adsorbocarpine, 1432
Advair Diskus, 773
Advexin, 1940
Advicor, 1276, 1913
Advil, 903
Advil, Children's, 903

(Trade names appear in italics. Canadian products are indicated with a [C], withdrawn products with a [D].)

Advil Drops, Pediatric, 903
Advil, Junior Strength, 903
Advil Liqui-Gels, 903
Advil Migraine, 903
Aerius, [C], 506
AeroBid, 750
AeroBid-M, 750
Aeropin, 1920
Aeroseb-Dex, 511
Aerosolized Pooled Immune Globulin, 1921
Aerugen, 1947
Afeditab CR, 1283
Aftate for Athlete's Foot, 1782
Aftate for Jock Itch, 1782
Agalsidase Beta, 36
Agenerase, 116
Aggrenox, 567
Agoral, 1626
Agrylin, 119, 1923
AH-chew, 377, 1918
AH-chew D, 1421
AI-RSA, 1921
AIDS Drugs in Development, 1963
AIDS Vaccine, 1963, 1967
Aidsvax, 1967
Airet, 39
Airomir, [C], 39
AK-Beta, 1021
AK-Dex, 511
AK-Dilate, 1421
AK-Poly-Bac, 172
AK-Pred, 1467
AK-Trol, 1266
Akarpine, 1432
Akineton, 209
Akne-mycin, 659
AKTob, 1773
Ala-Cort, 889
Ala-Scalp, 889
Alacramyn, 1929
Alatrofloxacin Mesylate/Trovafloxacin Mesylate, 837
Alavert, 1064
Albendazole, 1921
Albenza, 1921
Albumin Human (Normal Serum Albumin), 37
Albuminar-5, 37
Albuminar-25, 37
Albunex, 37
Albutein 5%, 37
Albutein 25%, 37
Albuterol, 39, 1921
Albuterol Sulfate/Ipratropium Bromide, 958
Alclometasone Dipropionate, 40
Alconefrin, 1421
Alconefrin 12, 1421
Alconefrin 25, 1421
Aldactazide, 1661
Aldactone, 1660
Aldara, 917
Aldesleukin, 42, 1921, 1964, 1966
Aldomet, 1159
Aldurazyme, 1008, 1942
ALEC, 1933
Alefacept, 46

Alemtuzumab, 47, 1921
Alendronate, 1921
Alendronate Disodium, 1921
Alendronate Sodium, 50
Alertec, [C], 1214
Alesse, 450
Aleve, 1251
Alfenta, 51
Alfentanil Hydrochloride, 51
Alferon N, 947
Alferon N Injection, 1963
Alfuzosin Hydrochloride, 52
Alglucerase Injection, 1921
Alimta, 1377, 1948
Alinia, 1947
Alitretinoin, 54, 1921
Alka-Seltzer Flavoured, [C], 139
Alka-Seltzer Plus Cold & Cough, 526
Alkeran, 1109
Alkeran for Injection, 1944
Allegra, 729
Allegra 12 Hour, [C], 729
Allegra 24 Hour, [C], 729
Allegra-D, 731
Allentoin, 1921
Aller-Chlor, 375
Allerdryl, [C], 556
Allergy, 375
Allergy Medication, 556
AllerMax, 556
AllerMax Allergy and Cough Formula, 556
Allermed, 1525
Allernix, [C], 556
Allfen Jr, 848
Allogeneic Human Retinal Pigment Epithelial Cells on Gelatin Microcarriers, 1922
Allogeneic Peripheral Blood Mononuclear Cells (Sensitized Against Patient Alloantigens by Mixed Lymphocyte Culture), 1922
Allogeneic Thymic Tissue for Transplantation, Cultured, Partially T-cell Depleted, 1922
Allopurinol, 55
Allopurinol Riboside, 1922
Allopurinol Sodium, 1922
Allovectin-7, 1938
Almotriptan Malate, 57
Alocril, 1257
Alomide Ophthalmic Solution, 1943
Aloprim, 55
Aloprim for Injection, 1922
Alor 5-500 Tablets, 1914
Alora, 672
Alosetron, 59
Aloxi, 1352
Alpha-galactosidase A, 1922
Alpha-Melanocyte Stimulating Hormone, 1922
Alpha$_1$-Proteinase Inhibitor (Human), 61, 1922
Alphagan, 1927
Alphagan P, 232
Alphanate, 1923

AlphaNine, 1930
AlphaNine SD, 714
Alprazolam, 62
Alprazolam Intensol, 62
Alprostadil, 65, 1922
Altace, 1554
Altastaph, 1957
Alteplase, 1922
Alteplase, Recombinant, 68
Altertamine, 1922
Alti-Pindolol, [C], 1438
Alti-Piroxicam, [C], 1445
Alti-Prazosi, [C], 1466
Alti-Prednisone, [C], 1473
Alti-Ranitidine Hydrochloride, [C], 1557
Alti-Salbutamol Sulfate, [C], 39
Alti-Trazodone, [C], 1808
Alti-Trazodone Dividose, [C], 1808
Alti-Triazolam, [C], 1819
Alti-Valproic, [C], 1855
Alti-Verapamil, [C], 1874
Altoprev, 1074
Altoprev, [C], 1074
Altracin, 1926
Altretamine, 71
Alupent, 1130
ALVAC (vCP205), 1964
ALVAC (vCP1452), 1967
ALVAC (vCP1521), 1964, 1967
ALVAC-E120TMG, 1964
ALVAC-MN120TMG, 1964
Aluextin, 1921
Amantadine Hydrochloride, 72
Amaryl, 825
Amascrine, 1923
Amatine, 1945
Ambien, 1906
AmBisome, 108, 1943
Amcort, 1813
Amdoxovir, 1964
Amen, 1098
Amerge, 1253
Amerituss AD, 526
Amevive, 46
AMG 531, 1922
Amicar, 81
Amifostine, 74, 1922
Amikacin Sulfate, 76
Amikin, 76
Amiloride Hydrochloride, 77
Amiloride Hydrochloride/Hydrochlorothiazide, 79
Amiloride Hydrochloride Solution for Inhalation, 1922
Aminobenzoate, 1915
Aminocaproic Acid, 81, 1922
Aminoglutethimide, 82
3-(4'Aminoisoindoline-1'-one)-1-piperidine-2,6-dione(CC-5013), 1920
a-(3-Aminophthalimido) Glutaramide, 1921
Aminophylline, 83
Aminosalicylate Sodium, 85, 1922
Aminosalicylic Acid, 1922

(*Trade names appear in italics. Canadian products are indicated with a [C], withdrawn products with a [D].*)

4-Aminosalicylic Acid, 1920
5-Aminosalicylic Acid, 1125
Aminosidine, 1923
Aminoxin, 1530
Amio-Aqueous, 1923
Amiodarone, 86, 1923
Amiodarone Hydrochloride, 1923
Amitriptyline/ Chlordiazepoxide, 368
Amitriptyline Hydrochloride, 89
Amitriptyline/Perphenazine, 1408
Amlodipine, 91
Amlodipine/Benazepril Hydrochloride, 95
Amlodipine Besylate/ Atorvastatin Calcium, 92
Ammonium Tetrathiomolybdate, 1923
Ammonul, 1926
Amobarbital/Secobarbital, 98
Amobarbital Sodium, 97
Amoxapine, 99
Amoxicillin, 101
Amoxicillin/Clavulanate Potassium, 103
Amoxicillin/Lansoprazole/ Clarithromycin, 105
Amoxil, 101
Amoxil Pediatric Drops, 101
Amphetamine, 106
Amphetamine Aspartate Monohydrate, 520
Amphetamine Sulfate, 520
Amphetamine Sulfate, Racemic, 106
Amphotec, 108, 111
Amphotericin B, 108
Amphotericin B Cholesteryl, 108
Amphotericin B Cholesteryl Sulfate Complex, 111
Amphotericin B Desoxycholate, 108
Amphotericin B Lipid-Based, 108
Amphotericin B Lipid Complex, 1923
Ampicillin, 112
Ampicillin Sodium, 112
Ampicillin Sodium/Sulbactam Sodium, 114
Ampligen, 1949, 1964, 1965
Amprenavir, 116
Amsidyl, 1923
Amyl Nitrite, 118
Amyl Nitrite Aspirols, 118
Amyl Nitrite Vaporole, 118
Amytal, [C], 97
Amytal Sodium, 97
Anafranil, 423
Anagrelide, 119, 1923
Anakinra, 121
Analpram HC, 892
Ananain, Comosain, 1923
Anandron, [C], 1285
Anaprox, 1251
Anaprox DS, 1251
Anaritide Acetate, 1923

Anaspaz, 901
Anastrozole, 122
Ancef, 321
Ancer 20 Injection, 1964
Ancestim, 1923
Ancobon, 743
Ancrod, 1923
Androcur, 1931
Androderm, 1726
Androgel, 1726, 1958
Androgel-DHT, 1933, 1965
Android, 1169
Anestacon, 1035
Anexate, [C], 748
Anexsia 5/500, 880
Anexsia 7.5/650, 880
Anexsia 10/660, 880
Angiomax, 217
Angiotensin 1-7, 1923
Anistreplase, 123
Ansaid, 767
Antabuse, 571
Anti-CD4 Monoclonal Antibody, 1965
Anti-CD23 lgG1, Kappa Monclonal Antibody, 1923
Anti-CD45 Monoclonal Antibodies, 1923
Anti-CEA Sheep-Human Chimeric Monoclonal Antibody Labeled w/Iodine-131 (KAb201), 1923
Anti-Cytomegalovirus Monoclonal Antibodies, 1923
Anti-Interferon-Gamma Fab from Goats, 1924
Anti Pan T Lymphocyte Monoclonal Antibody, 1923
Anti-T Lymphocyte immunotoxin Xmmly-h65-rta, 1923
Anti-Tap-72-Immunotoxin, 1924
Anti-Thymocyte Globulin (Rabbit), 125, 1924
Anti-Thymocyte Serum, 1924
Anti-Tuss, 848
Antiangiogenic Components Extracted From Marine Cartilege, 1923
Anticort, 1964
Antiepilepsirine, 1923
Antihemophilic Factor (Human), 1923
Antihemophilic Factor (Recombinant), 1923
Antihemophilic Factor/von Willebrand Factor Complex (Human), Dried, Pasteurized, 1924
Antihyperlipidemic Combinations, 1913
Antimelanoma Antibody XMMME-001-DTPA 111 Indium, 1924
Antimelanoma Antibody XMMME-001-RTA, 1924
Antiphlogistine Rub A-535 Capsaicin, [C], 284
Antipyrine/Benzocaine/ Glycerin Dehydrated, 126

Antipyrine Test, 1924
Antisense 20-mer Phosphorothioate Oligonucleotide [Complementary to the Coding Region of R2 Component of the Human Ribonucleotide Reductase mRNA], 1924
Antispas, 540
Antithrombin III (Human), 1924
Antithrombin III (Human) Concentrate IV, 1924
Alpha-1-Antitrypsin (Recombinant DNA Origin), 1922
Antivenin Crotalidae Polyvalent Immune Fab (Ovine), 1924
Antivenin Crotaline (Pit-Viper) Ecuine Immune F(ab)2, 1924
Antivenom (Crotalidae) Purified (Avian), 1924
Antivert, 1095
Antivipmyn 1924
Antizol, 1956
Antrizine, 1095
Anturane, 1684
Anucort-HC, 889
Anumed HC, 889
Anusol-HC, 889
Anusol HC-1 Hydrocortisone Anti-Itch, 889
Anzemet, 579
AP1903, 1924
Apacet, 12
APAP, 12
Aphthaid, 1942
Apidra, 935
APL 400-C20 V-Beta DNA Vaccine, 1925
Aplisol, 1840
Aplitest, 1840
Apo-Acebutolol, [C], 10
Apo-Acetaminophen, [C], 12
APO-Acetazolamide, [C], 15
Apo-Acyclovir, [C], 26
Apo-Allopurinol, [C], 55
Apo-Alpraz, [C], 62
Apo-Alpraz TS, [C], 62
Apo-Amilzide, [C], 79
APO-Amitriptyline, [C], 89
APO-Amoxi, [C], 101
Apo-Amoxi-Clav, [C], 103, 1459
APO-Ampi, [C], 112
APO-Atenol, [C], 144
Apo-Azathioprine, [C], 161
APO-Baclofen, [C], 173
Apo-Beclomethasone, [C], 179
Apo-Benztropine, [C], 193
APO-Bisacodyl, [C], 210
Apo-Bromocriptine, [C], 234
Apo-Buspirone, [C], 254
Apo-Butorphanol, [C], 267
APO-Capo, [C], 285
APO-Carbamazepine, [C], 290
Apo-Cefaclor, [C], 316

(*Trade* names appear in italics. Canadian products are indicated with a [C], withdrawn products with a [D].)

Apo-Cefadroxil, [C], 318
Apo-Cefuroxime, [C], 347
APO-Cephalex, [C], 352
Apo-Cetirizine, [C], 354
Apo-Chlordiazepoxide, [C], 366
Apo-Chlorhexidine, [C], 370
APO-Chlorpropamide, [C], 384
Apo-Chlorthalidone, [C], 385
Apo-Cimetidine, [C], 398
Apo-Clomipramine, [C], 423
Apo-Clonazepam, [C], 425
APO-Clonidine, [C], 427
Apo-Clorazepate, [C], 434
Apo-Cromolyn Nasal Spray, [C], 458
Apo-Cromolyn Sterules, [C], 458
Apo-Cyclobenzaprine, [C], 463
Apo-Desipramine, [C], 502
Apo-Desmopressin, [C], 507
Apo-Diazepam, [C], 527
Apo-Diclo, [C], 533
Apo-Diclo Rapide, [C], 533
Apo-Diclo SR, [C], 533
Apo-Diflunisal, [C], 545
Apo-Diltiaz, [C], 550
Apo-Diltiaz CD, [C], 550
Apo-Diltiaz Injectable, [C], 550
Apo-Diltiaz SR, [C], 550
Apo-Dimenhydrinate, [C], 553
Apo-Divalproex, [C], 1855
Apo-Doxazosin, [C], 588
Apo-Doxepin, [C], 589
Apo-Doxy, [C], 597
Apo-Doxy-Tabs, [C], 597
Apo-Erythro Base, [C], 659
Apo-Erythro E-C, [C], 659
Apo-Erythro-ES, [C], 659
Apo-Erythro-S, [C], 659
Apo-Etodolac, [C], 705
Apo-Famotidine, [C], 716
Apo-Feno-Micro, [C], 721
Apo-Fenofibrate, [C], 721
Apo-Ferrous Sulfate, [C], 723
Apo-Fluconazole, [C], 740
Apo-Fluconazole-150, [C], 740
Apo-Flunisolide, [C], 750
Apo-Fluoxetine, [C], 759
Apo-Fluphenazine, [C], 763
Apo-Fluphenazine Decanoate Injection, [C], 763
Apo-Flurazepam, [C], 765
Apo-Flurbiprofen, [C], 767
Apo-Flutamide, [C], 768
Apo-Fluvoxamine, [C], 778
Apo-Folic, [C], 780
Apo-Furosemide, [C], 802
Apo-Gabapentin, [C], 805
APO-Gain Topical Solution, [C], 1201
Apo-Gemfibrozil, [C], 815
Apo-Glyburide, [C], 832
Apo-Haloperidol, [C], 859

Apo-Haloperidol Decanoate Injection, [C], 860
Apo-Hydralazine, [C], 874
Apo-Hydro, [C], 875
Apo-Hydroxyzine, [C], 899
Apo-Ibuprofen, [C], 903
Apo-Imipramine, [C], 915
Apo-Indapamide, [C], 921
Apo-Indomethacin, [C], 924
Apo-Ipravent, [C], 957
APO-ISDN, [C], 973
APO-K, [C], 1459
APO-Keto, [C], 989
APO-Keto-E, [C], 989
APO-Keto SR, [C], 989
Apo-Ketoconazole, [C], 987
Apo-Ketorolac, [C], 990
Apo-Ketorolac Injection, [C], 990
Apo-Labetalol, [C], 995
Apo-Lactulose, [C], 996
Apo-Levobunolol, [C], 1021
Apo-Levocarb, [C], 1024
Apo-Lisinopril, [C], 1048
Apo-Loperamide, [C], 1059
Apo-Loratadine, [C], 1064
Apo-Lorazepam, [C], 1068
Apo-Lovastatin, [C], 1074
Apo-Loxapine, [C], 1076
Apo-Mefenamic, [C], 1102
Apo-Megestrol, [C], 1105
Apo-Meprobamate, [C], 1120
Apo-Metformin, [C], 1135
Apo-Methyldopa, [C], 1159
APO-Metoclop, [C], 1174
Apo-Metoprolol, [C], 1177
Apo-Metoprolol (Type L), [C], 1177
Apo-Metronidazole, [C], 1179
Apo-Midazolam, [C], 1188
Apo-Minocycline, [C], 1198
Apo-Misoprostol, [C], 1205
Apo-Nabumetone, [C], 1239
Apo-Nadol, [C], 1240
Apo-Napro-Na, [C], 1251
Apo-Napro-Na DS, [C], 1251
Apo-Naproxen, [C], 1251
Apo-Naproxen SR, [C], 1251
Apo-Nefazodone, [C], 1258
Apo-Nifed, [C], 1283
Apo-Nifed PA, [C], 1283
Apo-Nitrofurantoin, [C], 1289
Apo-Nizatidine, [C], 1294
Apo-Norflox, [C], 1298
Apo-Nortriptyline, [C], 1300
Apo-Oflox, [C], 1305
Apo-Oxaprozin, [C], 1330
Apo-Oxazepam, [C], 1332
Apo-Oxybutynin, 1336
APO-Pen VK, [C], 1388
Apo-Perphenazine, [C], 1405
APO-Pindol, [C], 1438
Apo-Piroxicam, [C], 1445
Apo-Pravastatin, [C], 1463

APO-Prazo, [C], 1466
Apo-Prednisone, [C], 1473
Apo-Primidone, [C], 1476
Apo-Procainamide, [C], 1481
Apo-Prochlorazine, [C], 1486
APO-Propranolol, [C], 1516
Apo-Quinidine, [C], 1543
Apo-Ranitidine, [C], 1557
Apo-Salvent, [C], 39
Apo-Selegiline, [C], 1624
Apo-Sertraline, [C], 1628
Apo-Sotalol, [C], 1655
Apo-Sulfatrim, [C], 1828
Apo-Sulfinpyrazone, [C], 1684
APO-Sulin, [C], 1686
Apo-Tamox, [C], 1700
Apo-Temazepam, [C], 1713
Apo-Terazosin, [C], 1719
Apo-Terbinafine, [C], 1721
Apo-Tetra, [C], 1733
Apo-Theo LA, [C], 1739
Apo-Thioridazine, [C], 1747
Apo-Ticlopidine, [C], 1760
Apo-Timol, [C], 1763
Apo-Timop, [C], 1763
Apo-Tolbutamide, [C], 1777
Apo-Trazodone, [C], 1808
Apo-Trazodone D, [C], 1808
Apo-Triazide, [C], 878
APO-Triazo, [C], 1819
Apo-Trifluoperazine, [C], 1822
Apo-Trihex, [C], 1824
Apo-Valproic, [C], 1855
APO-Verap, [C], 1874
Apo-Warfarin, [C], 1885
APO-Zidovudine, [C], 1894
Apokyn, 1924, 1925
Apomate, 1958
Apomorphine, 1925
Apomorphine Hydrochloride, 1924, 1925
Apraclonidine, 127
Aprepitant, 127
Apresoline, 874
Apri, 450
Aprotinin, 1924, 1925
APT070, 1946
Aquachloral Supprettes, 361
Aquacort, [C], 889
AquaMEPHYTON, 1430, 1930
Aracmyn, 1942
Aralast, 61
Aralen, [C], 371
Aralen Hydrochloride, 371
Aralen Phosphate, 371
Aramine, 1132
Aranesp, 490
Arava, 1010
Arcitumomab, 1924, 1925
Aredia, 1353
Arestin, 1198
Argatroban, 129
Argatroban, 129
Arginine Butyrate, 1925
8-Arginine-Vasopressin, 1869
Aricept, 581

Arimidex, 122
Aripiprazole, 131
Aristocort, 1813
Aristocort A, 1813
Aristocort Intralesional, 1813
Aristocort Parenteral, [C], 1813
Aristocort Syrup, [C], 1813
Aristospan, [C], 1813
Aristospan Intra-articular, 1813
Aristospan Intralesional, 1813
Arixtra, 786
Armour Thyroid, 1753
Aromasin, 708, 1935
Arsenic Trioxide, 134, 1925
Artane, 1824
Artane Sequels, 1824
Artesunate, 1925
Arthritis Foundation Pain Reliever, 139
Arthrotec, 537
As-101, 1925
ASA, 139
Asacol, 1125
Asaphen, [C], 139
Asaphen E. C., [C], 139
Ascorbic Acid, 136
Asendin, 99
Asmalix, 1739
Asparaginase, 137
Aspergum, 139
Aspirin, 139, 567
Aspirin/Caffeine/Butalbital, 262
Aspirin/Caffeine/Codeine Phosphate/Butalbital, 263
Aspirin/Caffeine/Orphenadrine Citrate, 1326
Aspirin/Codeine Phosphate/Carisoprodol, 306
Aspirin/Methocarbamol, 1145
Aspirin/Oxycodone Hydrochloride, 1342
Aspirin/Propoxyphene Hydrochloride/Caffeine, 1515
Aspirin Free Anacin Maximum Strength, 12
Aspirin Free Pain Relief, 12
Astelin, 165
Astramorph PF, 1226
AT 1001, 1925
A/T/S, 659
Atacand, 276
Atacand HCT, 278
Atacand Plus, [C], 278
Atarax, 899
Atasol, [C], 12
Atazanavir Sulfate, 141
Atenolol, 144
Atenolol/Chlorthalidone, 146
Atgam, 1077
Atiprimrod, 1920
Ativan, 1068
ATnativ, 1924
Atomoxetine, 147
Atomoxetine Hydrochloride, 1925
Atorvastatin Calcium, 149
Atorvastatin Calcium/Amlodipine Besylate, 92
Atovaquone, 151, 1925

Atovaquone/Proguanil Hydrochloride, 152
ATRA-IV, 1960, 1966
Atridox, 597
Atropine, 154
Atropine, [C], 154
Atropine-1, 154
Atropine Care, 154
Atropine Injection, [C], 154
Atropine Sulfate, 558
Atropine Ointment, [C], 154
Atropine Sulfate/Scopolamine Hydrobromide/Hyoscyamine Sulfate/Phenobarbital, 156
Atrovent, 957
Augmented Betamethasone Dipropionate, 197
Augmentin, 103
Augmentin ES-600, 103
Augmentin XR, 103
Augmerosen, 1925
Auralgan, 126
Auranofin, 157
Auriculin, 1923
Aurolate, 839
Autologous Antigen Presenting Cells Pulsed with Autologous Tumor Ig Idiotype, 1925
Autologous Dendritic Cells Pulsed with Autologous Glioblatoma Multiforme Acid-Eluted Tumor Antigens, 1925
Autologous DNP-Conjugated Tumor Vaccine, 1925
Autologous Tumor-Derived gp96 Heat Shock Protein-Peptide Complex, 1925
Autolymphocyte Therapy, 1925
Avage, 1703
Avandamet, 1605
Avandia, 1603
Avapro, 960
Avar, 1651
Avastin, 203, 1954
Avaxim, [C], 865
Avaxim Pediatric, [C], 865
Avelox, 1229
Avelox IV, 1229
Aventyl Hydrochloride, 1300
Aventyl Hydrochloride Pulvules, 1300
Aviane, 450
Avita, 1810
Avodart, 607
Avonex, 948, 1940
Axert, 57
Axid AR, 1294
Axid Pulvules, 1294
Aygestin, 1297
Azacitadine, 158, 1925
Azactam, 169
Azasan, 161
Azathioprine, 161, 1925
AZDU, 1920
Azelaic Acid, 163
Azelastine Hydrochloride, 165
Azelex, 163
Azidothymidine, 1894
Azithromycin, 167

Azmacort, 1813
Azo-Standard, 1410
Azopt, 233
AZT, 1894
Aztec, 1964
Aztreonam, 169, 1926
Azulfidine, 1680
Azulfidine EN-tabs, 1680

B

B_1, 1743
B_6, 1530
B & O Supprettes No. 15A, 181, 1915
B & O Supprettes No. 16A, 181, 1915
B Lymphocyte Stimulator, 1926
BabyBIG, 229, 1927
Bacitracin, 1926
Bacitracin Zinc/Neomycin/Polymyxin B Sulfates, 1264
Bacitracin Zinc/Neomycin/Polymyxin B Sulfates/Hydrocortisone, 171
Bacitracin Zinc/Polymyxin B Sulfate, 172
Baclofen, 173, 1926
L-Baclofen, 1941
Bactoshield, 370
Bactoshield 2, 370
Bactrim, 1828
Bactrim D.S., 1828
Bactrim IV, 1828
Bactrim Pediatric, 1828
Bactrim Roche, [C], 1828
Bactroban, 1232
Bactroban Nasal, 1232
Balminil Decongestant Syrup, [C], 1525
Balminil DM, [C], 524
Balminil DM Children, [C], 524
Balminil Expectorant, [C], 848
Balsalazide Disodium, 175
Balsam Peru/Castor Oil/Trypsin, 1839
Bancap-HC, 880
Banflex, 1325
Banophen, 556
Barbidonna, 156
Barbidonna No. 2, 156
Baridium, 1410
Basiliximab, 176, 1926
BAY 50-4798, 1964
Bayer 8-Hour, Extended Release, 139
Bayer Children's Aspirin, 139
Bayer Enteric 500 Aspirin, Extra Strength, 139
Bayer Enteric Coated Caplets, Regular Strength, 139
Bayer Low Adult Strength, 139
Bayer, Maximum, 139
BayGam, 918
BayHep B, 867
Baytet, 1731
BCG Live, 177
Beclomethasone 17,21-dipropionate, 1926

(Trade names appear in italics. Canadian products are indicated with a [C], withdrawn products with a [D].)

Beclomethasone Dipropionate, 179, 1926
Beepen-VK, 1388
Bell/ans, 1644
Belladonna (levorotatory alkaloids)/Phenobarbital/ Ergotamine Tartrate, 182
Belladonna/Opium, 181
Bellamine, 182
Bellatol, 1415
Bemote, 540
Benadryl, 556
Benadryl Allergy, 556
Benadryl Allergy Ultratabs, 556
Benadryl Dye Free, 556
Benadryl Dye Free Allergy Liqui Gels, 556
Benazepril Hydrochloride, 184
Benazepril Hydrochloride/ Amlodipine, 95
Benazepril Hydrochloride/ Hydrochlorothiazide, 186
Bendroflumethiazide, 188
BeneFix, 714, 1930
Benicar, 1314
Bentyl, 540
Bentylol, [C], 540
Benuryl, [C], 1478
Benylin Adult, 524
Benylin Decongestant, [C], 1525
Benylin DM, 524
Benylin DM, [C], 524
Benylin DM 12 Hour, [C], 524
Benylin DM for Children, [C], 524
Benylin DM for Children 12 Hour, [C], 524
Benylin E Extra Strength, [C], 848
Benylin Pediatric, 524
Benzac, 190
Benzagel, 190
Benzamycin, 661
Benzimidavir, 1963
Benzoate/Phenylacetate, 1926
Benzocaine, 525
Benzonatate, 190
Benzophenone-3, Octylmethyoxycinnamate, Avobenzone, Titanium Dioxide, Zinc Oxide, 1926
Benzoyl Peroxide, 190, 661
Benzphetamine Hydrochloride, 192
Benztropine Mesylate, 193
Benztropine Omega, [C], 193
Benzydamine Hydrochloride, 1926
Benzylpenicillin, Benzylpenicilloic, Benzylpenilloic Acid, 1926
Bepridil, 194
Beractant, 196, 1926
Beraprost, 1926
Berinert P, 1928
Beta Alethrine, 1926
Beta-L-Fd4C, 1964
Beta-Val, 197
Betacort, [C], 197
Betagan, [C], 1021

Betagan Liquifilm, 1021, 1953
Betaine, 1926
Betaloc, [C], 1177
Betaloc Durules, [C], 1177
Betamethasone, 197
Betamethasone/Clotrimazole, 199
Betamethasone Dipropionate, 197
Betamethasone Dipropionate, Augmented, 197
Betamethasone Sodium Phosphate, 197
Betamethasone Sodium Phosphate/Betamethasone Acetate, 197
Betamethasone Valerate, 197
Betapace, 1655, 1957
Betapace AF, 1655
Betaprolene, [C], 197
BetaRx, 1934
Betasept, 370
Betaseron, 951, 1940
Betathine, 1926
Betaxin, [C], 1743
Betaxolol Hydrochloride, 200
Bethandidine Sulfate, 1926
Bethanechol Chloride, 202
Betimol, 1763, 1954
Betnesol, [C], 197
Betoptic, 200
Betoptic S, 200
Bevacizumab, 203
Bexarotene, 205, 1926
Bextra, 1851
Bexxar, 1792, 1960
Biaxin, 414
Biaxin BID, [C], 414
Biaxin XL, 414
Bicalutamide, 207
Bicillin C-R, 1387
Bicillin C-R 900/300, 1387
Bicillin L-A, 1384
Bicitra, 1645
BiCNU, 308
Bifidobacterium Longum Infantis 35624, 1926
BIG-IV, 229
Big Shot B-12, 461
Bilotropin, 1956
Biltricide, 1465
Bimatoprost, 208
Bindarit, 1926
Bioartificial Liver System Utilizing Xenogenic Hepatocytes in a Hollow Fiber Bioreactor Cartridge (BAL), 1927
Biocef, 352
Biosynject, 1961
Biperiden, 209
Biquin Durules, [C], 1543
Bisac-Evac, 210
Bis(4-fluorophenyl)phenylacetamide, 1927
Bisacodyl, 210
Bisacodyl Uniserts, 210
Bismatrol, 212
Bismatrol Extra Strentgh, 212
Bismuth Subsalicylate, 212

Bismuth Subsalicylate/ Metronidazole/Tetracycline, 213
Bisolvon, 1927
Bisoprolol Fumarate/ Hydrochlorothiazide, 214
Bitolterol Mesylate, 216
Bivalirudin, 217
Black-Draught, 1626
Blenoxane, 219, 1927
Bleomycin, 1927
Bleomycin Sulfate, 219, 1927
Blis-To-Sol Liquid, 1782
Blocadren, 1763
BLyS, 1926
BMS 200475, 1963
BMS-234475, 1963, 1964
BMS 275291, 1965
BMS 561390, 1964
BMY-45622, 1927
Bonamine, [C], 1095
Bonefos, 1933
Bontril PDM, 1411
Bontril Slow-Release, 1411
Borocell, 1955
Bortezomib, 222, 1927
Bosentan, 224, 1927
Botox, 226, 1927
Botox Cosmetic, 226
Botulinum Toxin Type A, 226, 1927
Botulinum Toxin Type B, 228, 1927
Botulinum Toxin Type F, 1927
Botulism Immune Globulin, 1927
Botulism Immune Globulin Intravenous, 229
Bovine Colostrum, 1927
Bovine Immunoglobulin Concentrate, 1927
Bovine Whey Protein Concentrate, 1927
Branched Chain Amino Acids, 1927
BRAVAVIR, 1957
Bravelle, 1845
Breezee Mist Antifungal, 1186
Breonesin, 848
Brethaire, 1722
Brethine, 1722
Bretylium Tosylate, 231
Bretylium Tosylate in 5% Dextrose, 231
Brevibloc, 666
Brevicon, 450
Brevoxyl, 190
Bricanyl, 1722
Bricanyl Turbuhaler, [C], 1722
Brimonidine, 1927
Brimonidine Tartrate, 232
Brinzolamide, 233
Brofed Liquid, 1918
Brolene, 1951
Bromfed Capsules, 1917
Bromfed-PD Capsules, 1917
Bromfenex, 1917
Bromfenex PD, 1917
Bromhexine, 1927
Bromisovalum, 1914
Bromocriptine Mesylate, 234

(Trade names appear in italics. Canadian products are indicated with a [C], withdrawn products with a [D].)

Brompheniramine Maleate/ Pseudoephedrine Hydrochloride, 236
Brompheniramine Maleate/ Pseudoephedrine Hydrochloride/ Dextromethorphan Hydrobromide, 237
Brompheniramine Tannate, 239
Brondelate Elixir, 1917
Bronkodyl, 1739
Brovex, 239
Broxine, 1927
Broxuridine, 1927
Bryostatin, 1966
Bryostatin-1, 1927
Budesonide, 241
Buffered Intrathecal Electrolyte/Dextrose Injection, 1927
Bumetanide, 245
Bumex, 245
Buminate 5%, 37
Buminate 25%, 37
Bupap, 1915
Buphenyl, 1956
Buprenex, 247
Buprenorphine Hydrochloride, 247, 1927
Buprenorphine Hydrochloride/ Naloxone Hydrochloride, 249, 1927
Bupropion Hydrochloride, 250
Burinex, [C], 245
Burn-o-Jel, 1035
BuSpar, 254
Buspirone Hydrochloride, 254
Busulfan, 256, 1927
Busulfex, 1927
Butabarbital Sodium, 258
Butalbital/Acetaminophen/ Caffeine, 259
Butalbital/Acetaminophen/ Caffeine/Codeine Phosphate, 261
Butalbital/Aspirin/Caffeine, 262
Butalbital/Aspirin/Caffeine/ Codeine Phosphate, 263
Butalbital Compound, 262
Butenafine Hydrochloride, 265
Butibel, 1913
Butisol Sodium, 258
Butoconazole Nitrate, 266
Butorphanol Tartrate, 267
Butyrylcholinestrase, 1928
BW 12C, 1928
Byclomine, 540
Bydramine Cough, 556

C

C1-Esterase Inhibitor (Human), 1928
C1-Esterase Inhibitor (Human), Pasteurized, 1928
C1-inhibitor, 1928
Cachexon, 1953
CADI Mw, 1946
Caduet, 92
Caelyx, [C], 592
Cafcit, 269, 1928

Cafergot Suppository, 1914
Caffedrine, 269
Caffeine, 269, 1914, 1915, 1916, 1928
Caffeine/Butalbital/ Acetaminophen, 259
Caffeine/Butalbital/Aspirin, 262
Caffeine/Codeine Phosphate/ Butalbital/Acetaminophen, 261
Caffeine/Codeine Phosphate/ Butalbital/Aspirin, 263
Caffeine/Propoxyphene Hydrochloride/Aspirin, 1515
Caffeine/Orphenadrine Citrate/ Aspirin, 1326
Calan, 1874
Calan SR, 1874
Calanolide A, 1964
Calcijex, 273
Calcimar, 271
Calcipotriene, 270
Calcitonin-Human for Injection, 1928
Calcitonin-Salmon, 271
Calcitonin-Salmon, Nasal Spray, 1928
Calcitriol, 273
Calcitriol Injection, 273
Calcium Acetate, 1928
Calcium Carbonate, 1914, 1928
Calcium Disodium Versenate, 610
Calcium EDTA, 610
Calcium Gluconate, 1928
Calcium Gluconate Gel, 1928
Calcium Gluconate Gel 2.5%, 1928
Calculations, 1972
Caldecort Hydrocortisone Anti-Itch, 889
Calfactant, 275, 1928
Calgonate, 1928
Calm-X, 553
Caltine, [C], 271
Camitor, 1942
Campath, 47, 1921
Campral, 7
Camptosar, 962
Camvirex, 1920
Cancidas, 315
Candesartan Cilexetil, 276
Candesartan Cilexetil/ Hydrochlorothiazide, 278
Candistatin, [C], 1301
Canesten, [C], 436
Cantil, 1114
Capastat Sulfate, 283
Capecitabine, 281
Capital w/Codeine, 13
Capoten, 285
Capozide 25/15, 287
Capozide 25/25, 287
Capozide 50/15, 287
Capozide 50/25, 287
Capravirine, 1965
Capreomycin, 283
Caprogel, 1922
Capsaicin, 284, 1928
Capsaicin HP, [C], 284

Capsin, 284
Captopril, 285
Captopril/Hydrochlorothiazide, 287
Capzasin • P, 284
Carac, 755
Carafate, 1573
Carbamazepine, 290
Carbamic Acid,[[4-[[3-[[4-[1(4-hydroxyphenyl)-1-methylethyl]phenoxy]methyl]phenyl]methoxy]-phenyl]iminomethyl]-,ethyl ester, 1928
Carbamylglutamic Acid, 1928
Carbatrol, 290
Carbenicillin Indanyl Sodium, 294
Carbex, 1624
Carbidopa, 295
Carbidopa/Levodopa/ Entacapone, 296
Carbinoxamine Maleate, 299
Carbinoxamine Maleate/ Pseudoephedrine Hydrochloride/ Dextromethorphan Hydrobromide, 301
Carbolith, [C], 1053
Carboplatin, 302
Carbovir, 1928
Carboxypeptidase G2, 1928
Carbromcl, 1914
Cardec DM, 301
Cardec-S Liquid, 1918
Cardene, 1279
Cardene I.V., 1279
Cardene SR, 1279
Cardioquin, 1543
Cardizem, 550
Cardizem CD, 550
Cardizem LA, 550
Cardura, 588
Cardura-1, [C], 588
Cardura-2, [C], 588
Cardura-4, [C], 588
Carisoprodol, 305
Carisoprodol/Aspirin/Codeine Phosphate, 306
Carmol HC, 1844
Carmustine, 308, 1928
Caroid, 210
Carteolol Hydrochloride, 310
Cartia XT, 550
Cartrol, 310
Carved lol, 312
Cascara Sagrada Fluid Extract, 1928
Casodex, 207
Caspofungin Acetate, 315
Castor Oil/Trypsin/Balsam Peru, 1839
Cataflam, 533
Catapres, 427
Catapres-TTS-1, 427
Catapres-TTS-2, 427
Catapres-TTS-3, 427
Catatrol, 1961
Cathflo Activase, 68
Caverject, 65

(*Trade* names appear in italics. Canadian products are indicated with a [C], withdrawn products with a [D].)

CCR5

5, 1964
4 Human Truncated 369 AA Polypeptide, 1928
CD5-T Lymphocyte Immunotoxin, 1928
CDP571, 1928
Cea-Cide, 1945, 1962
Ceclor, 316
Ceclor Pulvules, 316
Cecon, 136
Cedax, 343
CeeNu, 1057
Cefaclor, 316
Cefadroxil, 318
Cefamandole Nafate, 319
Cefazolin Sodium, 321
Cefdinir, 323
Cefditoren Pivoxil, 324
Cefepime, 326
Cefixime, 328
Cefizox, 344
Cefmetazole Sodium, 329
Cefobid, 331
Cefoperazone Sodium, 331
Cefotan, 334
Cefotaxime Sodium, 333
Cefotetan Disodium, 334
Cefoxitin Sodium, 336
Cefpodoxime Proxetil, 338
Cefprozil, 339
Ceftazidime, 341
Ceftibuten, 343
Ceftin, 347
Ceftizoxime Sodium, 344
Ceftriaxone Sodium, 346
Cefuroxime, 347
Cefzil, 339
Celebrex, 350
Celecoxib, 350
Celestoderm-V, [C], 197
Celestoderm-V/2, [C], 197
Celestone, 197
Celestone Phosphate, 197
Celestone Soluspan, 197
Celexa, 411
CellCept, 1236
CellCept I.V., [C], 1236
Cells Produced Using the AnastromReplicelle System and SC-I Therapy Kit, 1929
Celontin, 1156
Cena-K, 1458
Cenafed, 1525
Cenestin, 686
Centovir, 1938
Centoxin, 1946
Centuroides immune F(ab)2, 1929
Cephalexin, 352
Cephradine, 353
Cephulac, 996
Ceptaz, 341
Ceramide Trihexosidase/Alpha Galactosidase A, 1929
Cerebyx, 797, 1936
Ceredase, 1921
Ceresine, 1955
Cerezyme, 1939
Cerubidine, 495
Cervidil, 555
C.E.S., [C], 684

Ceta-Plus, 880
Cetacort, 889
Cetiedil Citrate Injection, 1929
Cetirizine, 354
Cetuximab, 356, 1929
Cevi-Bid, 136
Cevimeline Hydrochloride, 358
CharcoAid, 360
CharcoAid 2000, 360
Charcoal, Activated, 360
Charcodote, [C], 360
Charcodote Aqueous, [C], 360
Charcodote TFS, [C], 360
Chemet, 1672, 1957
Chenix, 1929
Chenodeoxycholic Acid, 1929
Chenodiol, 1929
Chenofalk, 1929
Chewable Vitamin C, 136
Chibroxin, 1298
Childhood Immunization Schedule, 2004
Children's Advil, 903
Children's Congestion Relief, 1525
Children's Dramamine, 553
Children's Dynafed Jr., 12
Children's Feverall, 12
Children's Genapap, 12
Children's Halenol, 12
Children's Mapap, 12
Children's Motrin, 903
Children's Nostril, 1421
Children's Panadol, 12
Children's Silapap, 12
Children's Silfedrine, 1525
Children's Tylenol, 12
Children's Tylenol Soft Chews, 12
Chimeric, Humanized Monoclonal Antibody to Staphylococcus, 1929
Chimeric (Human-Murine) G250 IgG Monoclonal Antibody, 1929
Chimeric M-T412 (Human-Marine) IgG Monoclonal Anti-CD4, 1929
Chlo-Amine, 375
Chlor-Trimeton Allergy 8 Hour, 375
Chlor-Trimeton Allergy 12 Hour, 375
Chlor-Tripolon, [C], 375
Chlor-Tripolon N.D., [C], 1066
Chloral Hydrate, 361
Chlorambucil, 362
Chloramphenicol, 364
Chlordiazepoxide, 366, 1913
Chlordiazepoxide/ Amitriptyline, 368
Chlorhexidine Gluconate, 370
Chlorhexidine Gluconate Mouth Rinse, 1929
(R)-N-[2-(6-Chloro-5-methoxy-1H-indol-3-yl)-propyl]acetamide, 1951
Chloromycetin Sodium Succinate, 364
Chloroquine, 371

Chloroquine Hydrochloride, 371
Chloroquine Phosphate, 371
Chlorothiazide, 372
Chlorpheniramine Maleate, 375, 526
Chlorpheniramine Maleate/ Hydrocodone Bitartrate, 881
Chlorpheniramine Maleate/ Phenylephrine Hydrochloride/ Methscopolamine Nitrate, 377
Chlorpheniramine Maleate/ Pseudoephedrine Hydrochloride/Codeine Phosphate, 379
Chlorpheniramine Polistirex/ Codeine Polistirex, 443
Chlorpheniramine Tannate/ Phenylephrine Tannate, 1423
Chlorpheniramine Tannate/ Pyrilamine Tannate/ Phenylephrine Tannate, 1425
Chlorpromazine Hydrochloride, 380
Chlorpropamide, 384
Chlorthalidone, 385
Chlorthalidone/Atenolol, 146
Chlorthalidone/Clonidine Hydrochloride, 430
Chlorzoxazone, 387
Cholac, 996
Cholestyramine, 388
Cholic Acid (3 alpha, 7 alpha, 12 alpha trihydroxy 5-beta cholanolic acid), 1929
Choline Chloride, 1929
Choline Magnesium Trisalicylate, 1611
Chondrocyte-Alginate Gel Suspension, 1929
Chondroitinase, 1929
Chorex-10, 389
Chorionic Gonadotropin, 389
Chorionic Gonadotropin, 389
Chroma-Pak, 391
Chromic Chloride, 391
Chromic Phosphate P 32, 390
Chromium, 391
Chromium Chloride, 391
Chronovera, [C], 1874
Chronulac, 996
Cialis, 1697
Cibacalcin, 1928
Ciclopirox, 392
Cidofovir, 394, 1965
Cidofovir Gel, 1963
Ciliary Neurotrophic Factor, 1929
Ciliary Neurotrophic Factor, Recombinant Human, 1929
Cilostazol, 396
Ciloxan, 401
Cimetidine, 398
Cinacalcet, 1929
Cinacalcet Hydrochloride, 400
Cinacort, 1813
Cinnamedrine, 1915
Cipro, 401, 1418
Cipro HC Otic, 405

(Trade names appear in italics. Canadian products are indicated with a [C], withdrawn products with a [D].)

Cipro IV, 401
Cipro XR, 401
Ciprofloxacin, 401
Ciprofloxacin Hydrochloride/ Hydrocortisone, 405
Cisatracurium Besylate, 406
Cisplatin, 408
Cisplatin/Epinephrine, 1929
Citalopram, 411
Citrate of Magnesia, 1082
Citric Acid, Glucono-Delta-Lactone, and Magnesium Carbonate, 1929
Citric Acid/Sodium Citrate, 1645
Citric Acid/Potassium Citrate/ Sodium Citrate, 1461
Citro-Mag, [C], 1082
Citro-Nesia, 1082
Citrovorum Factor, 1015
Civamide, 1929
Cladribine, 413, 1929
Claforan, 333
Claravis, 975
Clarinex, 506
Clarinex RediTabs, 506
Clarithromycin, 414
Clarithromycin/Amoxicillin/ Lansoprazole, 105
Claritin, 1064
Claritin-D 12 Hour, 1066
Claritin-D 24 Hour, 1066
Claritin Extra, [C], 1066
Claritin Kids, [C], 1064
Claritin Liberator, [C], 1066
Claritin RediTabs, 1064
Claritin Skin Itch Relief, [C], 889
Clavulanate Potassium/ Amoxicillin, 103
Clavulanate/Ticarcillin, 1758
Clavulin, [C], 103
Clearasil, 190
Clemastine Fumarate, 416
Clenia, 1651
Cleocin, 417, 1929
Cleocin Pediatric, 417
Cleocin Phosphate, 417
Cleocin T, 417
Climara, 672
Clinac, 190
Clindagel, 417
ClindaMax, 417
ClindaMax Lotion, 417
Clindamycin, 417, 1929
Clindamycin Hydrochloride, 417
Clindamycin Palmitate Hydrochloride, 417
Clindamycin Phosphate, 417
Clindets, 417
Clinoril, 1686
Clivarine, 1953
Clobetasol Propionate, 421
Clobex, 421
Clofarabine, 1930
Clofarex, 1930
Clofazimine, 1930
Clomid, 422
Clomiphene Citrate, 422

Clomipramine Hydrochloride, 423
Clonazepam, 425, 1930
Clonidine, 1930
Clonidine Hydrochloride, 427
Clonidine Hydrochloride/ Chlorthalidone, 430
Clopidogrel, 432
Clorazepate Dipotassium, 434
Clorpres, 430
Clostridial Collagenase, 1930
Clotrimazole, 436, 1930
Clotrimazole/Betamethasone, 199
Clozapine, 438
Clozaril, 438
CO Fluoxetine, [C], 759
Co-Gesic, 880
Co-Trimoxazole, 1828
Coagulin-B, 1921
Coagulation Factor VIIa (Recombinant), 1930
Coagulation Factor IX, 1930
Coagulation Factor IX (Human), 1930
Coagulation Factor IX (Recombinant), 1930
COBARTin, 1930
Cobalamin, 781
Codeine, 442
Codeine Contin, [C], 442
Codeine Phosphate, 849
Codeine Phosphate/Butalbital/ Acetaminophen/Caffeine, 261
Codeine Phosphate/Butalbital/ Aspirin/Caffeine, 263
Codeine Phosphate/ Carisoprodol/Aspirin, 306
Codeine Phosphate/ Chlorpheniramine Maleate/ Pseudoephedrine Hydrochloride, 379
Codeine Phosphate/ Promethazine Hydrochloride, 1496
Codeine Phosphate/ Promethazine Hydrochloride/ Phenylephrine Hydrochloride, 1500
Codeine Polistirex/ Chlorpheniramine Polistirex, 443
Codeprex, 443
Codiclear DH, 882
Coenzyme Q10, 1930
Cogentin, 193
Cognex, 1692
Colace, 576, 836
Colazal, 175
Colchicine, 445, 1930
Colchicine/Probenecid, 1480
Colesevelam Hydrochloride, 446
Colestid, 447
Colestipol Hydrochloride, 447
Colfed-A Capsules, 1917
Colfosceril Palmitate, Cetyl Alcohol, Tyloxapol, 1930

Colistin Sulfate/Neomycin Sulfate/Thonzonium Br/Hydrocortisone Acetate, 448
Collagenase (Lyphoilized) for Injection, 1930
Colloral, 1951
Colomed, 1955
Coly-Mycin S Otic, 448
CoLyte, 1455
CombiPatch, 680
Combivent, 958
Combivent Inhalation Solution, [C], 957
Combivir, 1000, 1966
Combretastasin A4 Phosphate, 1930
Commit, 1280
Compazine, 1486
Complement Receptor Type 1, Soluble, 1956
Complement Receptor Type 1, Soluble Recombinant Human, 1956
Compound S, 1894
Compoz Gel Caps, 556
Compoz Nighttime Sleep Aid, 556
Compro, 1486
Comtan, 633
Comvax, 858
Concerta, 1163
Congest, [C], 684
Congestion Relief, 1525
Conjugate of Human Transferrin and a Mutant Diphtheria Toxin (CRM 107), 1930
Conjugated Bile Acids, 1930
Conjugated Estrogens, 684
Conjugated Estrogens, Synthetic A or B, 686
Constilac, 996
Constulose, 996
Contac Cold 12 Hour Nondrowsy, [C], 1525
Contraceptives, Oral (Combination Products), 450
Contraceptives, Oral (Progestin-Only Products), 452
Copaxone, 823, 1936, 1937
Copegus, 1572
Cordarone, 86, 1923
Cordox, 1936
Coreg, 312
Corgard, 1240
Correctol, 210
Cort-Dome, 889
CortaGel, Extra Strength, 889
Cortaid, Maximum Strength, 889
Cortaid Topical Spray, 889
Cortaid with Aloe, 889
Cortef, 889
Cortenema, 889
Corticorelin Ovine Triflutate, 1930
Corticotropin, 453
Corticotropin-Releasing Factor, Human, 1930

...opin, Repository ...otropin or Adrenocor-...opic Hormone, 1953
...cotropin, Synthetic, 457
...tisol, 889
...ortisone, 455
Cortisone Acetate, 455
Cortisporin, 171
Cortisporin-TC Otic, 448
Cortizone-5, 889
Cortizone-10, 889
Cortizone-10 Plus Maximum Strength, 889
Cortizone 10 Quickshot Spray, 889
Cortizone for Kids, 889
Cortoderm, [C], 889
Cortone Acetate, 455
Cortrosyn, 457
Corvert, 904
Cosmegen, 480
Cosopt, 585, 1967
Cosyntropin, 457
Cotrim, 1828
Cotrim D.S., 1828
Cotrim Pediatric, 1828
Cough-X, 525
Coumadin, 1885
Coumarin, 1930
Covera-HS, 1874
Coversyl, [C], 1402
Cozaar, 1070
Creapure, 1930
Creatine, 1930
Creo-Terpin, 524
Creon 5, 1355
Creon 5, [C], 1356
Creon 10, 1355
Creon 10, [C], 1356
Creon 20, 1355
Creon 20, [C], 1356
Crestor, 1608
Crinone, 1490
Crixivan, 923, 1966
Crixivan in NanoCrystal Formulation, 1964
CroFab, 1924
Crolom, 458
Cromolyn Sodium, 458, 1930
Cromolyn Sodium 4% Ophthalmic Solution, 1931
Cronassial, 1936
Crotamiton, 460
Cruex, 436
Cryptaz, 1947
Cryptosporidium Hyperimmune Bovine Colostrum IgG Concentrate, 1931
Cryselle, 450
Crystamine, 461
Crystapen, [C], 1384
CS-92, 1964
CT-2584 Mesylate, 1931
Cubicin, 489
Cuprimine, 1383
Curosurf, 1951
Curretab, 1098
CY-1503, 1931
CY-1899, 1931
Cyanocobalamin, 461

Cyanoject, 461
Cyclessa, 450
Cyclobenzaprine Hydrochloride, 463
Cyclomen, [C], 484
Cyclomydril, 464
Cyclopentolate Hydrochloride/Phenylephrine Hydrochloride, 464
Cyclophosphamide, 465
Cycloprostin, 1934
Cycloserine, 467
L-Cycloserine, 1942
Cyclospire, 1943
Cyclosporin, 1931
Cyclosporin A, 469
Cyclosporine, 469, 1931
Cyclosporine Ophthalmic, 1931
Cycrin, 1098
Cyklokapron, 1960
Cylert, 1379
Cylexin, 1931
Cymbalta, 604
Cyomin, 461
Cyproheptadine Hydrochloride, 471
Cyproterone Acetate, 1931
Cystadane, 1926
Cystagon, 1931
Cysteamine, 1931
Cysteamine Hydrochloride, 1931
L-Cysteine, 1942
Cystic Fibrosis Gene Therapy, 1931
Cystic Fibrosis Tr Gene Therapy (Recombinant Adenovirus), 1931
Cystic Fibrosis Transmembrane Conductance Regulator, 1931
Cystic Fibrosis Transmembrane Conductance Regulator Gene, 1931
Cystospaz, 901
Cytadren, 82
Cytarabine, 472
Cytarabine, Liposomal, 475, 1931
CytoGam, 1931
CYTOIMPLANT, 1922
Cytolin, 1963
Cytomegalovirus Immune Globulin IV (Human), 1931
Cytomel, 1044
Cytosar, [C], 472
Cytosar-U, 472
Cytotec, 1205
Cytovene, 809, 1936
Cytoxan, 465

D

D-peptide of the Sequence AKRHHGYKRKFH-NH2, 1933
D-S-S, 576
D.A. Chewable, 377
Dacarbazine, 477
Daclizumab, 478, 1931
Dactinomycin, 480

Dalacin C, [C], 417
Dalacin C Phosphate, [C], 417
Dalacin T Topical, [C], 417
Dalalone, 511
Dalalone DP, 511
Dalalone LA, 511
Dalfopristin/Quinupristin, 1547
Dallergy, 377
Dallergy Jr Capsules, 1917
Dallergy Syrup, 1918
Dallergy Tablets, 1918
Dalmane, 765
Dalteparin Sodium, 483
Danazol, 484
Danocrine, 484
Dantrium, 485, 1931
Dantrium Intravenous, 485
Dantrolene Sodium, 485, 1931
Dapacin, 12
Dapsone, 487, 1932, 1966
Dapsone/Pyrimethamine/Folinic Acid, 1966
Dapsone/Trimethoprim, 1966
Daptacel, 561
Daptomycin, 489
Daraprim, 1531
Darbepoetin Alfa, 490
Darvocet A500, 1513
Darvocet-N 50, 1513
Darvocet-N 100, 1513
Darvon Compound-65, 1515, 1915
Darvon Compound-32 Pulvules, 1915
Darvon-N, 1511
Darvon Pulvules, 1511
Daunorubicin Citrate Liposomal, 492
Daunorubicin Citrate Liposome Injection, 1932
Daunorubicin Hydrochloride, 495
DaunoXome, 492, 1932
Dayhist-1, 416
Daypro, 1330
DB 289, 1966
DC Softgels, 576
DCVax-Brain, 1925
DDAVP, 507
DDAVP Rhinyle Nasal Solution, [C], 507
ddC, 1889
ddI, 541
Debacterol, 1685
Debrase, 1932
Debridase, 1932
Decadron, 511
Decadron-LA, 511
Decadron Phosphate, 511
Decaject, 511
Decaject-L.A., 511
Decapeptyl Injection, 1960
Decaspray, 511
Decitabine, 1932
Declomycin, 499
Decofed Syrup, 1525
Decohistine DH, 379
Deconamine SR Capsules, 1917
Deconamine Syrup, 1918
Deconamine Tablets, 1917

Deconomed SR Capsules, 1917
Deconsal II, 1918
4-Dedimethysancycline, 1966
Defed-60, 1525
Defen-LA, 1918
Deferasirox, 1932
Deferiprone, 1932
Defibrotide, 1932
Defy, 1773
Degas, 1636
Dehistine, 377
Dehydrex, 1932
Dehydroepiandrosterone (DHEA), 1932
Dehydroepiandrosterone Sulfate Sodium, 1932
Del-Mycin, 659
Delatestryl, 1726
Delavirdine, 1966
Delavirdine Mesylate, 497
Delestrogen, 673
Delsym, 524
Delta-Cortef, 1467
Deltasone, 1473
Demadex, 1790
Demeclocycline, 499
Demerol Hydrochloride, 1116
Demulen 1/35, 450
Demulen 1/50, 450
Denavir, 1382
Denileukin Diftitox, 501, 1932
Dentipatch, 1035
2′-Deoxycytidine, 1919
Deoxyribonuclease, Recombinant Human, 583
Deoxyribose, Phosphorothioate, 1932
Depacon, 1855
Depakene, 1855
Depakote, 1855
Depakote ER, 1855
Depen, 1383
depMedalone 40, 1166
depMedalone 80, 1166
Depo-Estradiol, 673
Depo-Medrol, 1166
Depo-Medrol, [C], 1166
Depo-Provera, 1098
Depo-Testadiol, 1729
Depo-Testosterone, 1726
DepoCyt, 475, 1931
Deponit, 1290
Depopred-40, 1166
Depopred-80, 1166
L-Deprenyl, 1624
Dermacort, 889
DermaFlex, 1035
Dermol HC, 889
Dermovate, [C], 421
Dermtex HC Maximum Strength Spray, 889
Desenex, 436
Desenex Antifungal, Maximum Strength, 1186
Deserpidine/Methyclothiazide, 1157
Desipramine Hydrochloride, 502
Desirudin, 504
Desloratadine, 506

Desmopressin Acetate, 507, 1932
Desocort, [C], 509
Desogen, 450
Desonide, 509
DesOwen, 509
Desoxi, [C], 510
Desoximetasone, 510
Desoxyephedrine Hydrochloride, 1138
Desoxyn, 1138
Desquam, 190
2-0-Desulfated heparin, 1920
Desyrel, 1808
Desyrel Dividose, 1808
Detensol, [C], 1516
Detrol, 1783
Detrol LA, 1783
Detussin, 887
Dexacine, 1266
Dexair, [C], 511
Dexameth, 511
Dexamethasone, 511, 1932
Dexamethasone Acetate, 511
Dexamethasone/Neomycin Sulfate/Polymyxin B Sulfate, 1266
Dexamethasone Sodium Phosphate, 511
Dexamethasone/Tobramycin, 514
Dexasone, 511
Dexasone-L.A., 511
Dexchlorpheniramine Maleate, 515
Dexchlorpheniramine Maleate, 515
Dexedrine, 522
Dexedrine Spansules, 522
DexFerrum, 728, 964
Dexiron, [C], 964
Dexmethylphenidate Hydrochloride, 517
Dexone, 511
Dexone LA, 511
Dexrazoxane, 518, 1932
Dextran 1, 1932
Dextran 70, 1932
Dextran Sulfate (Inhaled, Aerosolized), 1932
Dextran Sulfate Sodium, 1932
Dextroamphetamine Saccharate/Amphetamine Aspartate Monohydrate/ Dextroamphetamine Sulfate/ Amphetamine Sulfate, 520
Dextroamphetamine Sulfate, 520, 522
Dextromethorphan HBr/ Brompheniramine Maleate/ Pseudoephedrine Hydrochloride, 237
Dextromethorphan HBr/ Carbinoxamine Maleate/ Pseudoephedrine Hydrochloride, 301
Dextromethorphan Hydrobromide, 524

Dextromethorphan Hydrobromide/Benzocaine, 525
Dextromethorphan Hydrobromide/Phenylephrine Hydrochloride/ Chlorpheniramine Maleate, 526
Dextromethorphan Hydrobromide/ Pseudoephedrine Hydrochloride/Guaifenesin, 1526
Dextrostat, 522
DHA-paclitaxel, 1932
D.H.E. 45, 548
DHPG, 809
Di-Spaz, 540
DiaBeta, 832
Diabetes CF, 524
Diabetic Tussin EX, 848
Diabinese, 384
DiaβBeta, [C], 832
Dialose, 576
3,4-Diaminopyridine, 1920
Diamox Sequels, 15
Dianeal Peritoneal Dialysis Solution with 1.1% Amino Acids, 1932
Diar-aid, 1059
Diastat, 527
Diazemuls, [C], 527
Diazepam, 527
Diazepam Intensol, 527
Diazepam Viscous Solution for Rectal Administration, 1932
Diaziquone, 1932
Diazoxide, Oral, 531
Diazoxide, Parenteral, 532
Dibent, 540
Dibenzyline, 1417
4,5-Dibromorhodamine 123, 1920
Dichloralphenazone/ Acetaminophen/ Isometheptene Mucate, 969
Diclofenac, 533
Diclofenac Sodium/ Misoprostol, 537
Dicloxacillin Sodium, 538
Dicyclomine Hydrochloride, 540
Didanosine, 541
2′-3′-Dideoxyadenosine, 1919
Dideoxycytidine, 1889
Dideoxyinosine, 541, 1932
Didrex, 192
Didronel 704, 1935
Didronel IV, 704
Didronel IV Infusion, 1935
2-(3-Diethylaminopropyl)-9,8-dipropyl-2-azaspiro[4,5]-decan dimaleate, 1920
Diethyldithiocarbamate, 1933
Diethylpropion Hydrochloride, 543
Diferulcylmethane, 1933
Differin, 32
DiffGAM, 1963
Diflorasone Diacetate, 544
Diflucan, 740

(*Trade* names appear in italics. Canadian products are indicated with a [C], withdrawn products with a [D].)

50, [C], 740
., 545
., 1933
.te, 1933
.ek, 546
.gitoxin, 1933
Digoxin, 546
Digoxin immune FAB (ovine), 1933
Dihistine DH, 379
5,6-Dihydro-5-azacytidine, 1920
Dihydroergotamine Mesylate, 548
Dihydroergotoxine, 653
Dihydrogenated Ergot Alkaloids, 653
Dihydrotestosterone, 1933
Dihydrotestosterone Gel, 1965
24,25- Dihydroxycholecalciferol, 1920
Dilacor XR, 550
Dilantin, 1428
Dilantin-30 Pediatric, [C], 1428
Dilantin-125, 1428
Dilantin Infatab, 1428
Dilantin Kapseals, 1428
Dilatrate-SR, 973
Dilaudid, 893
Dilaudid-HP, 893
Dilaudid-HP Plus, [C], 893
Dilaudid Sterile Powder, [C], 893
Dilaudid-XP, [C], 893
Dilocaine, 1035
Dilomine, 540
Dilor, 608
Dilor-G Liquid, 1917
Diltia XT, 550
Diltiazem Hydrochloride, 550
Diltiazem Hydrochloride Extended Release, 550
Dimenhydrinate, 553
Dimetabs, 553
3-(3,5-Dimethyl-1H-2ylmethylene)-1,3-dihydroindol-2-one, 1920
Dimethyl Sulfoxide, 1933
Dinate, 553
Dinoprostone, 555
Diocto, 576
Diocto-K, 576
Dioctyl Calcium Sulfosuccinate, 576
Dioctyl Potassium Sulfosuccinate, 576
Dioctyl Sodium Sulfosuccinate, 576
Diovan, 1861
Diovan HCT, 1863
Dipalmitoylphosphatidylcholine/Phospatidylglycerol, 1933
Dipentum, 1316
Diphen AF, 556
Diphen Cough, 556
Diphenhist, 556
Diphenhist Captabs, 556
Diphenhydramine Hydrochloride, 556
Diphenoxylate Hydrochloride/Atropine Sulfate, 558

Diphenylcyclopenone, 1933
Diphtheria and Tetanus Toxoids and Acellular Pertussis Vaccine, Adsorbed, Hepatitis B (Recombinant) and Inactivated Poliovirus Vaccine Combined, 559
Diphtheria/Tetanus Toxoids/Acellular Pertussis Vaccine, 561
Dipivefrin Hydrochloride, 564
Diprivan, 1510
Diprolene, 197
Diprolene AF, 197
Diprolene Glycol, [C], 197
Diprosone, 197
Dipyridamole, 565
Dipyridamole/Aspirin, 567
Dirithromycin, 568
Disaccharide Tripeptide Glycerol Dipalmitoyl, 1933
Disodium Clodronate, 1933
Disodium Clodronate Tetrahydrate, 1933
Disodium Cromoglycate, 458
Disodium Silibinin Dihemisuccinate, 1933
Disopyramide, 569
Disulfiram, 571
Ditropan, 1336
Ditropan XL, 1336
Diurigen, 372
Diuril, 372
Divalproex Sodium, 1855
Dixarit, [C], 427
DMP 777, 1933
DNA-liquid Complex (DMRIE/DOPE)/plasmid Vector (VCL-1102, Vical) Expressing Human Interleukin-2, 1933
DNase, 583
DNP-modified Autologous Tumor Vaccine, 1933
Dobutamine, 573
Dobutrex, 573
Docetaxel, 574
Docosahexanoic Acid-paclitaxel, 1933
Docu, 576
Docusate, 576
Docusate Calcium, 576
Docusate Potassium, 576
Docusate Sodium, 576
1-(11-Dodecylamino-10-hydroxyundecyl)-3-7-dimethylxanthine hydrogen methanesulfonate, 1919
Dofetilide, 578
Dolacet, 880
Dolasetron Mesylate, 579
Dolobid, 545
Dolophine Hydrochloride, 1137
Dolorac, 284
Donepezil, 581
Donnamar, 901
Donnatal, 156
Dopamine Hydrochloride, 582
Dopamine Hydrochloride in 5% Dextrose, 582
Dopar, 1022

Dopram, 586
Doral, 1534
Dorcol Children's Decongestant, 1525
Dormin, 556
Dornase Alfa, 583, 1933
Doryx, 597
Dorzolamide, 584
Dorzolamide Hydrochloride/Timolol Maleate, 585
D.O.S., 576
Dovonex, 270
Doxapram Hydrochloride, 586
Doxazosin Mesylate, 588
Doxepin Hydrochloride, 589
Doxil, 594, 1933
Doxorubicin, Conventional, 591
Doxorubicin, Liposomal, 594, 1933
Doxy 100, 597
Doxy 200, 597
Doxycin, [C], 597
Doxycycline, 597
DPI3290, 1966
Dramamine, 553
Dramamine, Children's, 553
Dramamine Less Drowsy, 1095
Dramanate, 553
Drepanol, 1947
DriHist, 377
Drixomed, 1917
Drixoral Cough Liquid Caps, 524
Dronabinol, 600, 1933
Droperidol, 602
Drotrecogin Alfa (Activated), 603
Droxia, 897, 1939
Drug Names that Look and Sound Alike, 1981
Dryvax, 1641
DSS, 576
DTaP, 561
DTIC-Dome, 477
Dulcolax, 210
Dull-C, 136
Duloxetine Hydrochloride, 604
Duo-Trach kit, 1035
Duocet, 880
Duodopa, 1942
DuoNeb, 958
Duphalac, 996
Duraclon, 427, 1930
Duradryl, 377
Duradyne DHC, 880
Duragesic, [C], 726
Duragesic-25, 726
Duragesic-50, 726
Duragesic-75, 726
Duragesic-100, 726
Duralith, [C], 1053
Duralone-40, 1166
Duralone-80, 1166
Duramorph, 1226
Duramycin, 1933
Duratuss, 1918
Duricef, 318
Dutasteride, 607
Duvoid, 202
Dyazide, 878
Dyflex-G Tablets, 1917

(*Trade* names appear in italics. Canadian products are indicated with a [C], withdrawn products with a [D].)

Dyline G.G. Tablets, 1917
Dyline GG Liquid, 1917
Dymelor, 17
Dymenate, 553
Dyna-Hex 2 Skin Cleanser, 370
Dyna-Hex Skin Cleanser, 370
Dynabac, 568
Dynacin, 1198
DynaCirc, 979
DynaCirc CR, 979
Dynafed E.X., Extra Strength, 12
Dynafed Jr., Children's, 12
Dynafed Pseudo, 1525
Dynamine, 1934
Dyphylline, 608
Dyrenium, 1818
Dysport, 1927

E

E-Base, 659
E-Mycin, 659
Easprin, 139
EC Naprosyn, 1251
Econazole Nitrate, 609
Econopred, 1467
Econopred Plus, 1467
Ecostatin, [C], 609
Ecotrin, 139
Ecotrin Adult Low Strength, 139
Ecotrin Maximum Strength, 139
Ecovia, 1953
Eculizumab, 1934
Ed A-Hist Liquid, 1918
Ed A-Hist Tablets, 1917
ED-IN-SOL, 728
ED-SPAZ, 901
ED-TLC Liquid, 1917
Edecrin, 695
Edecrin Sodium, 695
Edetate Calcium Disodium, 610
Edetate Disodium, 611
Edex, 65
Edrophonium Chloride, 612
EDTA, 611
E.E.S. 200, 659
E.E.S. 400, 659
E.E.S. Granules, 659
EES 600, [C], 659
Efalizumab, 613
Efavirenz, 615
Effer-K, 1458
Effexor, 1872
Effexor XR, 1872
Efidac 24, 375
Eflornithine Hydrochloride, 1934
Efudex, 755
ELA-Max, 1035
Elavil, 89
Elcatonin, 1934
Eldepryl, 1624, 1955
Elestat, 636
Eletriptan Hydrobromide, 617
Elidel, 1434
Elimite, 1404
Elitek, 1560, 1951
Elixomin, 1739
Elixophyllin, 1739

Elixophyllin GG Liquid, 1917
Elixophyllin-KI Elixir, 1917
Ellence, 640, 1934
Elliotts B Solution, 1927
Elmiron, 1395, 1949
Elocom, [C], 1221
Elocon, 1221
Elspar, 137
Eltor 120, [C], 1525
Embeline, 421
Embeline E, 421
Emcyt, 682
Emend, 127
Emgel, 659
Eminase, 123
EMLA, 1038
EMLA Patch, 1038
EMLA Patch, [C], 1038
Emo-Cort, [C], 889
Empirin, 139
Emtricitabine, 619
Emtricitabine/Tenofovir Disoproxil Fumarate, 621
Emtriva, 619
Emtriva and Viread, 1965
Enadoline Hydrochloride, 1934
Enalapril Maleate, 623
Enalapril Maleate/Felodipine, 626
Enalapril Maleate/Hydrochlorothiazide, 628
Enbrel, 693, 1934
Encapsulated Porcine Islet Preparation, 1934
Endagen-HD, 1917
Endal Nasal Decongestant, 1426
Endantadine, [C], 72
Endocodone, 1339
Endrate, 611
Enduronyl, 1157
Enerjets, 269
Enfuvirtide, 630
Engerix-B, 868
Enisoprost, 1934
Enjuvia, 686
Enlon, 612
Enoxaparin Sodium, 631
Enpresse, 450
Entacapone, 633
Entacapone/Carbidopa/Levodopa, 296
Entecavir, 1963
Entex, 1426
Entex ER, 1426
Entex LA, 1426
Entex PSE, 1918
Entocort Capsules, [C], 241
Entocort EC, 241
Entocort Enema, [C], 241
Entrophen, [C], 139
Enulose, 996
Enzone, 892
Epaxal Berna, [C], 865
Ephedrine, 635
Epidermal Growth Factor (Human), 1934
Epiject, [C], 1855
Epinastine Hydrochloride, 636
Epinephrine, 637

Epinephrine/Lidocaine Hydrochloride, 1037
EpiPen, 637
EpiPen Jr., 637
Epirubicin, 1934
Epirubicin Hydrochloride, 640
Epitol, 290
Epivir, 998
Epivir-HBV, 998
Epivir/Lamivudine, 1964
Epivir/Ziagen Combination Tablet, 1964
Eplerenone, 644
EPO, 646
Epoetin Alfa, 646, 1934
Epoetin Beta, 1934
Epogen, 646, 1934
Epoprostenol, 1934
Epoprostenol Sodium, 648
Epratuzumab, 1934
Eprex, [C], 646
Eprosartan Mesylate, 650
Epsom Salt, 1083
Eptifibatide, 651
Equanil, 1120
Erbitux, 356
Ergoloid Mesylates, 653
Ergomar, 655
Ergonovine Maleate, 654
Ergotamine Tartrate, 655, 1913, 1914
Ergotamine Tartrate/Belladonna (levorotary alkaloids)/Phenobarbital, 182
Ergotrate, 554
Erlotinib Hydrochloride, 1934
Ertaczo, 1627
Ertapenem, 657
Erwinase, 1934
Erwinia L-Asparaginase, 1934
Ery-Tab, 659
Erybid, [C], 659
Eryc, 659
Erycette, 659
Eryderm, 659
Erymax, 659
EryPed, 659
EryPed 200, 659
EryPed 400, 659
EryPed Drops, 659
Erythra-Derm, 659
Erythrocin Stearate, 659
Erythromycin, 659
Erythromycin/Benzoyl Peroxide, 661
Erythromycin Ethylsuccinate/Sulfisoxazole, 662
Erythropoietin, 646
Erythropoietin, Recombinant Human, 1934
Eryzole, 662
Escitalopram Oxalate, 663
Esclim, 672
Esgic, 259
Esgic-Plus, 259
Esidrix, 875
Eskalith, 1053
Eskalith CR, 1053
Esmolol Hydrochloride, 666
Esomeprazole Magnesium, 667
Estazolam, 668

(Trade names appear in italics. Canadian products are indicated with a [C], withdrawn products with a [D].)

Estrogens, 684
Estrogens/
 yltestosterone, 670
 e, 672
aderm, 672
straderm 25, [C], 673
Estradiol, 672
Estradiol Cypionate, 673
Estradiol Cypionate/
 Medroxyprogesterone Acetate, [D], 678, 1100
Estradiol Cypionate/
 Testosterone Cypionate, 1729
Estradiol/Norethindrone Acetate, 680
Estradiol Valerate, 673
Estradot, [C], 673
Estramustine Phosphate Sodium, 682
Estrasorb, 673
Estratest, 670
Estratest HS, 670
Estring, 673
Estrogens, Conjugated, 684
Estrogens, Conjugated/
 Medroxyprogesterone Acetate, 689
Estrogens, Esterified, 684
Estrogens, Synthetic Conjugated, A or B, 686
Estropipate, 691
Estrostep 21, 450
Estrostep Fe, 450
Etanercept, 693, 1934
Ethacrynate, 695
Ethacrynic Acid, 695
Ethambutol Hydrochloride, 597
Ethanolamine Oleate, 1934
Ethchlorvynol, 698
Ethinyl Estradiol/
 Levonorgestrel, 699
Ethinyl Estradiol, USP, 1935
Ethiofos, 1935
Ethionamide, 700
Ethmozine, 1224
Ethosuximide, 701
Ethotoin, 702
(4S)-4-Ethyl-4-hydroxy-3,14 dioxo-3,4,12,14-tetra-hydro-1-H-pyrano[3?,4?:6,7]-indolizino-]-quinoline-11-carbaldehyde O-(tert-butyl)-(E)-oxime, 1919
Ethyl Eicosapentaneonate, 1935
Ethyol, 74, 1922
Etidronate Disodium, 704, 1935
Etiocholanedione, 1935
Etodolac, 705
Etopophos, 707
Etoposide, 707
Etrafon, 1408
Etrafon 2-10, 1408
Etrafon-A, 1408
Etrafon-Forte, 1408
Euflex, [C], 768
Euglycon, [C], 832
Eulexin, 768
Eurax, 460

Evista, 1553
Evoxac, 358
Ex-Histine, 377
Exelon, 1594
Exemestane, 708, 1935
Exidine-2 Scrub, 370
Exidine-4 Scrub Care, 370
Exidine Skin Cleanser, 370
Exisulind, 1935
ex•lax, 1626
ex•lax chocolate, 1626
ex-lax Stool Softener, 576
Exosurf, 1930
Exosurf Neonatal for Intratracheal Suspension, 1930
Extended Release Bayer 8-Hour, 139
Extendryl, 377
Extendryl Chewable Tablets, 1918
Extendryl JR Capsules, 1918
Extendryl S.R. Capsules, 1918
Extendryl Syrup, 1918
Extra Strength Bayer Enteric 500 Aspirin, 139
Extra Strength Dynafed E.X., 12
Extra Strength Gas-X, 1636
Extraneal (with 7.5% Icodextrin) Peritoneal Dialysis Solution, 1939
Eye-Sed, 1897
Ezetimibe, 709
Ezetimibe/Simvastatin, 711
Ezide, 875

F

Fabrase, 1922
Fabrazyme, 36, 1929
Factive, 816
Factor IX Concentrates, 714
Factor XIII, Recombinant, 1935
Factor XIII [A2] Homodimer, Recombinant DNA Origin, 1935
Factor XIII Concentrate (Human) Pasteurized, 1935
Falkochol, 1929
Famciclovir, 715
Famotidine, 716
Fampridine, 1935
Famvir, 715
Fansidar, 1678
Fareston, 1789, 1960
Faslodex, 801
Fastlene, 269
Father John's Medicine Plus, 526
FDA Pregnancy Categories, 1968
Feen-a-mint, 210
Felbamate, 718, 1935
Felbatol, 718, 1935
Feldene, 1445
Felodipine, 626, 720
Femara, 1014
Femiron, 728
Femizol-M, 1186
Femstat 3, 266
Fenesin, 848
Fenofibrate, 721

Fenoprofen Calcium, 723
Fentanyl Citrate, 724
Fentanyl Oralet, 724
Fentanyl Transdermal System, 726
FeoSol, 728
Feostat, 728
Fer-gen-sol, 728
Fer-Iron, 728
Feratab, 728
Fergon, 728
Ferodan, [C], 728
Ferrex, 728
Ferric Hexacyanoferrate (II) "Prussian Blue," 1935
Ferriprox, 1932
Ferrlecit, 1646
Ferro-Sequels, 728
Ferrous Fumarate, 728
Ferrous Gluconate, 728
Ferrous Salts, 728
Ferrous Sulfate, 728
Ferrous Sulfate Exsiccated, 728
Fertinex, 1961
Feverall, Children's, 12
Feverall, Infants, 12
Feverall, Junior Strength, 12
Fexofenadine Hydrochloride, 729
Fexofenadine Hydrochloride/
 Pseudoephedrine Hydrochloride, 731
FIAU, 1935
Fibrinogen (Human), 1935
Fibrogrammin P, 1935
Fibronectin (Human Plasma-derived), 1935
Fibronectin (Plasma-derived), 1935
Fidelin, 1932
Filgrastim, 732, 1935
Filmix Neurosonographic Contrast Agent, 1944
Finacea, 163
Finasteride, 733
Fioricet, 259
Fioricet with Codeine, 261
Fiorinal, 262
Fiorinal with Codeine, 263
Fiortal, 262
FK463, 1963
Flagyl, 1179, 1944
Flagyl 375, 1179
Flagyl ER, 1179
Flagyl I.V., 1179
Flagyl I.V. RTU, 1179
Flatulex, 1636
Flavocoxid, 735
Flavoxate, 736
Flecainide Acetate, 736
Fleet Babylax, 836
Fleet Laxative, 210
Fletcher Castoria, 1626
Flexeril, 463
Flexoject, 1325
Flocor, 1949
Flolan, 648, 1934
Flomax, 1702
Flonase, 769
Florazole ER, [C], 1179
Florinef, [C], 769

(*Trade* names appear in italics. Canadian products are indicated with a [C], withdrawn products with a [D].)

Florinef Acetate, 746
Floven HFA, [C], 769
Flovene, 769
Flovent Diskus, 769
Flovent Rotadisk, 769
Floxin, 1305
Floxuridine, 739
Flucinolone, 1935
Fluconazole, 740
Flucytosine, 743
Fludara, 744, 1935
Fludarabine Phosphate, 744, 1935
Fludrocortisone Acetate, 746
Flumadine, 1583
Flumarizine, 1935
Flumazenil, 748
Flumecinol, 1935
FluMist, 928
Flunisolide, 750
Fluocinolone Acetonide, 752
Fluocinonide, 753
Fluoderm, [C], 752
Fluoracaine, 758
Fluorescein Sodium/ Proparacaine Hydrochloride, 758
Fluorometholone/ Sulfacetamide, 753
Fluoroplex, 755
Fluorouracil, 755, 1936
Fluoxetine, 1936
Fluoxetine Hydrochloride, 759
Fluoxetine Hydrochloride/ Olanzapine, 1311
Fluoxymesterone, 761
Fluoxymesterone, 761
Fluphenazine, 763
Fluphenazine Decanoate, 763
Fluphenazine Hydrochloride, 763
Fluphenazine Hydrochloride, 763
Fluphenazine Omega, [C], 763
Flurazepam Hydrochloride, 765
Flurbiprofen, 767
Flurbiprofen Sodium, 767
Flutamide, 768
Fluticasone Propionate, 769
Fluticasone Propionate/ Salmeterol, 773
Fluvastatin, 776
Fluviral S/F, [C], 928
Fluvirin, 928
Fluvoxamine Maleate, 778
Fluzone, 928
FML-s, 753
Focalin, 517
Folic Acid, 780
Folic Acid/Cobalamin/ Pyridoxine Hydrochloride, 781
Folinic Acid, 1015
Folinic Acid/Dapsone/ Pyrimethamine, 1966
Follistim, 784
Follitropin Alfa, 781
Follitropin Alfa, Recombinant, 1936
Follitropin Beta, 784

Foltx, 781
Folvite, [C], 780
Fomepizole, 1936
Fondaparinux Sodium, 786
Foradil Aerosolizer, 788
Formoterol Fumarate, 788
Fortaz, 341
Forteo, 1724
Fortovase, 1616
Fortovase Roche, [C], 1616
Forvade, 1963
Fosamax, 50, 1921
Fosamprenavir Calcium, 789
Foscan, 1958
Foscarnet Sodium, 792
Foscavir, 792
Fosfomycin Tromethamine, 794
Fosinopril Sodium, 795
Fosphenytoin, 797, 1936
Fragmin, 483
Froben, [C], 767
Froben SR, [C], 767
Frova, 799
Frovatriptan Succinate, 799
Fructose-1,6-diphosphate, 1936
Fruit C 100, 136
Fruit C 200, 136
Fruit C 500, 136
FUDR, 739
Fulvestrant, 801
Fulvicin P/G, 847
Fungizone, 108
Fungoid Cream, 1186
Fungoid Tincture, 1186
Furadantin, 1289
Furosemide, 802
Furosemide Special, [C], 802
Fuzeon, 630

G

G3139, 1966
G-CSF, 732
G-myticin, 821
Gabapentin, 805, 1936
Gabbromicina, 1923
Gabitril Filmtabs, 1755
CC-Galactosidase, 1922
α-Galactosidase A, 1921
Galantamine Hydrobromide, 806
Galardin, 1943
Gallium Nitrate, 807
Gallium Nitrate Injection, 1936
Galzin, 1962
Gamimune N, 919, 1939
Gamma Globulin, 918
Gamma Hydroxybutyrate, 1936
Gamma Hydroxybutyric Acid, 1936
Gammagard S/D, 919
Gammalinolenic Acid, 1936
Gammar-P.I.V., 919
Gamulin Rh, 1569
Ganaxolone, 1936
Ganciclovir, 809, 1936
Ganciclovir Intravitreal Implant, 1936
Ganciclovir Sodium, 1936

Gangliosides as Sodium Salts, 1936
Ganite, 807, 1936
Gantrisin PediaTRIC, 1682
Garamycin, 321
Gas-X, 1636
Gas-X, Extra Strength, 1636
Gastrocrom, 458, 1930
Gastrointestinal Anticholinergic Combinations, 1913
Gastrosed, 901
Gatifloxacin, 811
Gavilimomab, 1936
G17DT Immunogen, 1936
Gee-Gee, 848
GEM 92, 1964
Gemcitabine Hydrochloride, 814
Gemfibrozil, 815
Gemifloxacin Mesylate, 816
Gemtuzumab Ozogamicin, 818, 1936
Gemzar, 814
Gen-Acebutolol, [C], 10
Gen-Acebutolol Type S, [C], 10
Gen-Acyclovir, [C], 26
Gen-Alprazolam, [C], 62
Gen-Amantadine, [C], 72
Gen-Amiodarone, [C], 86
Gen-Amoxicillin, [C], 101
Gen-Atenolol, [C], 144
Gen-Azathioprine, [C], 161
Gen-Baclofen, [C], 173
Gen-Beclo Aq., 179
Gen-Budesonide AQ, [C], 241
Gen-Buspirone, [C], 254
Gen-Captopril, [C], 285
Gen-Carbamazepine CR, [C], 290
Gen-Cimetidine, [C], 398
Gen-Clobetasol Cream/Ointment, [C], 421
Gen-Clobetasol Scalp Application, [C], 421
Gen-Clomipramine, [C], 423
Gen-Clonazepam, [C], 425
Gen-Cyclobenzaprine, [C], 463
Gen-Diltiazem, [C], 550
Gen-Doxazosin, [C], 588
Gen-Famotidine, [C], 716
Gen-Fenofibrate Micro, [C], 721
Gen-Fluoxetine, [C], 759
Gen-Gemfibrozil, [C], 815
Gen-Glybe, [C], 832
Gen-Hydroxyurea, [C], 897
Gen-Indapamide, [C], 921
Gen-Ipratropium, [C], 957
Gen-K, 1458
Gen-Lovastatin, [C], 1074
Gen-Medroxy, [C], 1098
Gen-Metformin, [C], 1135
Gen-Metoprolol, [C], 1177
Gen-Minocycline, [C], 1198
Gen-Nabumetone, [C], 1239
Gen-Naproxen EC, [C], 1251
Gen-Nitro, [C], 1290

(*Trade* names appear in italics. Canadian products are indicated with a [C], withdrawn products with a [D].)

rtyline, [C], 1300
.utynin, 1336
.dolol, [C], 1438
iroxicam, [C], 1445
.-Salbutamol Respirator Solution, 39
Gen-Salbutamol Sterinebs P.F., 39
Gen-Selegiline, [C], 1624
Gen-Sotalol, [C], 1655
Gen-Tamoxifen, [C], 1700
Gen-Temazepam, [C], 1713
Gen-Terbinafine, [C], 1721
Gen-Ticlopidine, [C], 1760
Gen-Timolol, [C], 1763
Gen-Trazodone, [C], 1808
Gen-Triazolam, [C], 1819
Gen-Valproic, [C], 1855
Gen-Verapamil, [C], 1874
Gen-Verapamil SR, [C], 1874
Gen-Warfarin, [C], 1885
Genahist, 556
Genapap, 12
Genapap, Children's, 12
Genapap Extra Strength, 12
Genapap, Infants' Drops, 12
Genaphed, 1525
Genasense, 1925
Genasoft, 576
Genaspor, 1782
Genasyme, 1636
Genasyme Drops, 1636
Genatuss, 848
Gene Plasmid hVEGF165 Driven by Human Cytomegalovirus, and [2,3-bis(oleoyl)propyl]trimethyl ammonium and dioleoyl phosphatidyl ethanlamine, 1936
Genebs, 12
General Management of Acute Overdosage, 1969
Genebs Extra Strength, 12
Genevax-HIV/APL-400-003 (end/rev) Facilitated DNA-Based Vaccine, 1967
Genevax-HIV/APL-400-047 (gag/pol) Facilitated DNA-Based Vaccine, 1967
Genoptic, 821
Genoptic S.O.P., 821
Genotropin, 1653, 1956
Genotropin Miniquick, 1653
Genpril, 903
Genprin, 139
Gent-AK, [C], 821
Gentacidin, 821
Gentak, 821
Gentamicin, 821
Gentamicin Impregnated PMMA Beads on Surgical Wire, 1936
Gentamicin Liposome Injection, 1936
Gentamicin Sulfate/Prednisolone Acetate, 1470
Genuine Bayer, 139
Geocillin, 294

Geodon, 1899
Geref, 1955
Geridium, 1410
Gerimal, 653
GFN 600/Phenylephrine 20, 1426
GG-Cen, 848
Gimatecan, 1919
Glatiramer Acetate, 823, 1936
Glatiramer Acetate for Injection, 1937
Gleevec, 910, 1939
Gliadel, 308, 1949
Glimepiride, 825
Glipizide, 826
Glipizide/Metformin Hydrochloride, 828
Glucagen, 830
Glucagon, 830
Glucagon Diagnostic Kit, 830
Glucagon Emergency Kit, 830
GlucoNorm, [C], 1563
Glucophage, 1135
Glucophage XR, 1135
Glucotrol, 826
Glucotrol XL, 826
Glucovance, 834
Glutamine, 1937
L-Glutamine, 1942
L-Glutamyl-L-Tryptophan, 1942
S(-)-3-]-Glutaramide, 1954
Glyate, 848
Glyburide, 832
Glyburide/Metformin Hydrochloride, 834
Glyceol, 1937
Glycerin, 836
Glycerol, 836
Glyceryl Guaiacolate, 848
Glycopyrrolate, 837
Glycotuss, 848
Glylorin, 1945
Glynase PresTab, 832
Glypressin, 1958
Glysennid, [C], 1626
Glyset, 1194
Glytuss, 848
Gold Sodium Thiomalate, 839
GoLYTELY, 1455
Gonadorelin Acetate, 841, 1937
Gonal-f, 781, 1936
Gonal-f RFF Pen, 781
Goserelin Acetate, 842
Gossypol, 1937
Gp100 Adenoviral Gene Therapy, 1937
Gramicidin/Neomycin Sulfate/Polymyxin B Sulfate, 1267
Granisetron Hydrochloride, 845
Granulex, 1839
Granulocyte Macrophage Colony Stimulating Factor, 1937
Gravol, [C], 553
Grifulvin V, 847
Gris-PEG, 847
Grisactin 250, 847
Grisactin 500, 847

Grisactin Ultra, 847
Griseofulvin, 847
Griseofulvin, Microsize, 847
Griseofulvin, Ultrasize, 847
Group B Streptococcus Immune Globulin, 1937
Growth Hormone Releasing Factor, 1937
GS 4338, 1965
GS 7340, 1965
GTI-2040, 1924
Guaifed, 1426
Guaifed-PD, 1426
Guaifenesin, 848
Guaifenesin/Codeine Phosphate, 849
Guaifenesin/Pseudoephedrine Hydrochloride/Dextromethorphan Hydrobromide, 1526
Guaifenesin/Phenylephrine Hydrochloride, 1426
Guaifenesin/Hydrocodone Bitartrate, 882
Guaifenex PSE 60, 1918
Guaifenex PSE 120, 1918
Guaimax-D, 1918
Guaitussin AC, 849
Guanabenz Acetate, 851
Guanadrel, 852
Guanethidine Monosulfate, 853
Guanfacine, 1937
Guanfacine Hydrochloride, 855
Guanidine, 856
Guanidine Hydrochloride, 856
GuiaCough CF, 848
GuiaCough PE, 848
Guiafenex LA, 848
Guiatuss, 848
Gusperimus, 1937
GW275175, 1963
GW433908, 1965
GW810781, 1964
Gyceryl Trioleate and Glyceryl Trierucate, 1937
Gyne-Lotrimin 3, 436
Gyne-Lotrimin 3 Combination Pack, 436
Gyne-Lotrimin 7, 436
Gynecort 10, Extra Strength, 889
Gynodiol, 673

H

Haemophilus b Conjugate Vaccine, 858
Halcinonide, 859
Halcion, 1819
Haldol, 859
Haldol Decanoate 50, 859
Haldol Decanoate 100, 859
Halenol, Children's, 12
Halfprin 81, 139
Halobetasol Propionate, 859
Halofed, 1525
Halofuginone, 1937
Halog, 859
Halog-E, 859
Haloperidol, 859
Haloperidol Decanoate, 859

(Trade names appear in italics. Canadian products are indicated with a [C], withdrawn products with a [D].)

Haloperidol-LA Omega, [C], 859
Haltran, 903
Havrix, 865
HBIG, 867
HCTZ/Triamterene, 878
HE 2000, 1965
Heartline, 139
Helidac, 213
Hematrol, 1944
Heme Arginate, 1937
Hemex, 1937
Hemin and Zinc Mesoporphyrin, 1937
Hemocitrate, 1961
Hemocyte, 728
Hemonyne, 714
Hemorrhoidal HC, 889
Hemoxin, 1947
Hemril-HC Uniserts, 889
Hep-Lock, 862
Hep-Lock U/P, 862
Hepacid, 1948
Hepalean, [C], 862
Hepalean-Lok, [C], 862
Hepandrink, 1947
Heparin, 862
Heparin, Oral Unfractionated, 1937
Heparin Leo, [C], 862
Heparin Lock Flush, [C], 862
Heparin Sodium, 862
HepatAssist Liver Assist System, 1962
Hepatitis A, Inactivated & Hepatitis B (Recombinant) Vaccine, 866
Hepatitis A Vaccine, Inactivated, 865
Hepatitis B Immune Globulin, 867
Hepatitis B Immune Globulin IV (Human), 1937
Hepatitis B Vaccine, 868
Hepatitis C Virus Immune Gobulin (Human), 1937
HepeX-B, 1937
Hepsera, 33
Heptovir, [C], 998
Herceptin, 1805, 1960
Hermin, 1937
Herpes Simplex Virus, Genetically Engineered (G207), 1938
Herpes Simplex Virus Gene, 1937
Herplex, 908
Herplex-D, [C], 908
HES, 870
Hespan, 870
Hetastarch, 870
Hexa-Betalin, [C], 1530
Hexadrol, 511
Hexadrol Phosphate, 511
Hexalen, 71, 1922
Hexit, [C], 1040
h5g1.1-mAb, 1937
HGP-30 and Sargromostim, 1964
HGTV43, 1964
Hi-Cor 1.0, 889

Hi-Cor 2.5, 889
Hibiclens, 370
Hibiclens Antiseptic/Antimicrobial Skin Cleanser, 370
Hibistat Germicidal Hand Rinse, 370
Hibistat Towelettes, 370
HibTITER, 858
Hiltonol, 1950
Hiprex, 1140
Hista-Vent DA, 377
Histamine, 1938
Histex CT, 299
Histex Pd, 299
Histrelin, 1938
Histrelin Acetate, 1938
Histussin D, 887
HIV-1 Immunogen, 1966
HIV-1 Peptide Vaccine, 1967
HIV-IT, 1964
HIV Neutralizing Antibodies, 1938
HIV Therapeutic, 1964
HIV Vaccine, 1967
Hivid, 1889, 1962
Hivig, 1938
HLA-B7/Beta2M DNA Lipid (DMRIE/DOPE) Complex, 1938
166Ho-DOTMP, 1919
Hold DM, 524
Homatropine Methylbromide/ Hydrocodone Bitartrate, 884
Homoharringtonine, 1938
H.P. Acthar Gel, 1953
Hp-PAC, [C], 105
HPA-23, 1938
Hsp E7, 1938
Hu1D10, Humanized, Monoclonal Antibody, 1938
Humalog, 933
Humalog Mix 75/25, 933
Human Acid Precursor Alpha-Glucosidase, Recombinant, 1938
Human Albumin Grifols, 37
Human Anti-Transforming Growth Factor Beta 1 Monoclonal Antibody, 1938
Human Anti-Tumor Necrosis Factor Alpha Monoclonal Antibody, 1938
Human Gammaglobulin, 1938
Human Immunodeficiency Virus Immune Globulin, 1938
Human IgM Monoclonal Antibody (C-58) to Cytomegalovirus, 1938
Human Surf, 1957
Human T-Lymphotropic Virus Type III Gp 160 Antigens, 1938
Humanized Anti-CD2 Monoclonal Antibody, 1938
Humanized Anti-Human CD2 MAb, 1938
Humanized Anti-Tac, 1938
Humanized MAb (IDEC-131) to CD40L, 1938

Humanized Monoclonal Antibody Against Shiga-Like Toxin II, 1938
Humate-P, 1924
Humatin, 1363
Humatrope, 1653, 1956
Humibid LA, 848
Humibid Sprinkle, 848
Humira, 30
Humulin 7C/30, 931
Humulin L, 931
Humulin N, 931
Humulin R, 931
Hy-Phen, 880
Hyalgan, 871
Hyaluronic Acid, 1938
Hyaluronic Acid Derivatives, 871
Hybri-Ceaker, 1939
Hycamtin, 1787, 1967
Hycodan, 834
Hycosin Expectorant, 882
Hycotuss Expectorant, 882
Hydeltrasol, 1468
Hydergine, 653
Hyderm, [C], 889
Hydralazine Hydrochloride, 874
Hydralazine Hydrochloride/ Hydrochlorothiazide/ Reserpine, 1565
Hydrap-ES, 1565
Hydrate, 553
Hydrea, 897
Hydro-DIURIL, 875
Hydro-Par, 875
Hydrocet, 880
Hydrochlorothiazide, 628, 875
Hydrochlorothiazide/Amiloride Hydrochloride, 79
Hydrochlorothiazide/Benazepril Hydrochloride, 186
Hydrochlorothiazide/Bisoprolol Fumarate, 214
Hydrochlorothiazide/ Candesartan Cilexetil, 278
Hydrochlorothiazide/Captopril, 287
Hydrochlorothiazide/Lisinopril, 877, 1051
Hydrochlorothiazide/Losartan Potassium, 1072
Hydrochlorothiazide/Quinapril Hydrochloride, 1540
Hydrochlorothiazide/Reserpine/ Hydralazine Hydrochloride, 1565
Hydrochlorothiazide/ Spironolactone, 1661
Hydrochlorothiazide/ Telmisartan, 1710
Hydrochlorothiazide/ Triamterene, 878
Hydrochlorothiazide/Valsartan, 1863
Hydrocodone Bitartrate/ Acetaminophen, 880
Hydrocodone Bitartrate/ Chlorpheniramine Maleate, 881
Hydrocodone Bitartrate/ Guaifenesin, 882

(*Trade* names appear in italics. Canadian products are indicated with a [C], withdrawn products with a [D].)

Hydrocodone Bitartrate/
  Homatropine
  Methylbromide, 884
Hydrocodone Bitartrate/
  Ibuprofen, 885
Hydrocodone Bitartrate/
  Pseudoephedrine Hydrochloride, 887
Hydrocodone GF, 882
Hydrocortisone, 889
Hydrocortisone/Bacitracin
  Zinc/Neomycin/Polymyxin B
  Sulfates, 171
Hydrocortisone/Ciprofloxacin
  Hydrochloride, 405
Hydrocortisone Acetate, 889
Hydrocortisone Acetate/
  Pramoxine Hydrochloride, 892
Hydrocortisone Acetate/
  Colistin Sulfate/Neomycin
  Sulfate/Thonzonium Br, 448
Hydrocortisone Acetate/Urea, 1844
Hydrocortisone Buteprate, 889
Hydrocortisone Butyrate, 889
Hydrocortisone Cypionate, 889
Hydrocortisone Phosphate, 889
Hydrocortisone Valerate, 889
Hydrogesic, 880
Hydromorph Contin, [C], 893
Hydromorphone HP 10, [C], 893
Hydromorphone HP 20, [C], 893
Hydromorphone HP 50, [C], 893
Hydromorphone HP Forte, [C], 893
Hydromorphone Hydrochloride, 893
HydroVal, [C], 889
Hydroxocobalamin, 1939
Hydroxychloroquine Sulfate, 894
Hydroxycobalamin/Sodium
  Thiosulfate, 1939
Hydroxyethyl Starch, 870
Hydroxymagnesium Aluminate, 1081
6-Hydroxymethylacylfulvene, 1920
L-5-Hydroxytryptophan, 1941
Hydroxyurea, 897, 1939
Hydroxyzine, 899, 1913
Hydroxyzine Hydrochloride, 899
Hygroton, 385
Hylorel, 852
Hyoscine Hydrobromide, 1619
Hyoscyamine Sulfate, 901
Hyosyamine Sulfate/
  Phenobarbital/Atropine
  Sulfate/Scopolamine
  Hydrobromide, 156
Hyosophen, 156
Hyperab, 1550
Hypericin, 1939
Hypermune RSV, 1953
Hyperstat IV, 532
HypoRho-D, 1569
HypoRho-D Mini-Dose, 1569
Hyrexin-50, 556
Hytinic, 728
Hytone, 889
Hytrin, 1719
Hytuss, 848
Hytuss 2x, 848
Hyzaar, 1072

I

I(131)-TM-601 (Chlorotoxin), 1939
Ibritumomab Tiuxetan, 1939
Ibuprofen, 903
Ibuprofen/Hydrocodone Bitartrate, 885
Ibuprofen IV Solution, 1939
Ibutilide Fumarate, 904
Icar, 728
Icatibant, 1939
131IchTNT-1, 1941
Icodextrin 7.5% with Electrolytes Peritoneal Dialysis Solution, 1939
Idamycin, 1939
Idamycin PFS, 906
Idarubicin, 906, 1939
IDN 6556, 1939
Idoxuridine, 908, 1939
Idrarubicin Hydrochloride for Injection, 1939
Iduronate-2-Sulfatase, 1939
Ifex, 909, 1939
Ifosfamide, 909, 1939
IG, 918
IGF-1, 1952
IGIM, 918
IGIV, 919
IL-2, 1964, 1966
IL-4 *Pseudomonas* Toxin Fusion Protein (IL-4(38-37)-PE38KDEL), 1939
IL-13-PE38QQR, 1939
Iletin II, Regular, 931
Iloprost Solution for Infusion, 1939
Ilosone, 659
Ilotycin, 659
Ilotycin Gluceptate, 659
Imatinib, 910
Imatinib Mesylate, 1939
Imciromab Pentetate, 1939
Imdur, 974
Imexon, 1939
Imiglucerase, 1939
Imipenem-Cilastatin, 913
Imipramine Hydrochloride, 915
Imipramine Pamoate, 915
Imiquimod, 917
Imitrex, 1688
ImmTher, 1933, 1943
ImmuDyn, 1951
Immune Globulin Intramuscular, 918
Immune Globulin IV, 919
Immune Globulin IV (human), 1939
Immunine VH, [C], 714
Immuno, 1939
Immuno-C, 1927
Immupath, 1938
Immuraid, 1958
Immurait, 1941
Imodium, 1059
Imodium A-D, 1059
Imogam, 1550
Imovax Rabies I. D. Vaccine (Human Diploid Cell), 1551
Imovax Rabies Vaccine (Human Diploid Cell), 1551
Imported Fire Ant Venom, Allergenic Extract, 1939
Impril, [C], 915
Imuran, 161, 1925
Imuthiol, 1933
Imuvert, 1955
Inamrinone, 920
Inapsine, 602
Indapamide, 921
Inderal, 1516
Inderal LA, 1516
Inderide, 1505
Indinavir, 1964, 1966
Indinavir Sulfate, 923
Indium-111 Altumomab Pentetate, 1939
Indium-111 Murine Monoclonal Antibody FAB to Myosin, 1940
Indium-111 Pentetreotide, 1919
Indocid, [C], 924
Indocid P.D.A., [C], 924
Indocin, 924
Indocin IV, 924
Indocin SR, 924
Indomethacin, 924
Indomethacin Sodium Trihydrate, 924
Infanrix, 561
Infant's Motrin, 903
Infants' Pain Reliever, 12
Infants' Silapap, 12
Infasurf, 275, 1928, 1957
InFeD, 964
Infergen, 937
Inflamase Forte, 1468
Inflamase Mild, 1468
Infliximab, 926, 1940
Influenza Virus Vaccine, 928
Infufer, [C], 964
Infumorph, 1226, 1945
INGN 201, 1940
INH, 970
INH-A00021, 1940
Innohep, 1767
InnoPran XL, 1516
Inocor, 920
Inolimomab, 1940
INOMax, 1947
Inosine Pranobex, 1940
Inspra, 644
Insulin, 931
Insulin Analogs, 933
Insulin Aspart, 933
Insulin Glargine, 933
Insulin Glulisine, 933
Insulin Injection, Regular, 931
Insulin Lispro, 933
Insulin Zinc Suspension, 931
Intal, 458
Integrilin, 651
Interferon Alfa-2a, 940

Interferon Alfa-2a (Recombinant), 1940
Interferon Alfa-1b, 1940
Interferon Alfa-2b, 941
Interferon Alfa-2b, Recombinant, 1940
Interferon Alfa-2b, Recombinant/Ribavirin, 945
Interferon Alfa-n1, 1940
Interferon Alfa-n3, 947
Interferon Alfa-n3 Injection, 1963
Interferon Alfacon-I, 937
Interferon Alpha, Low-Dose Oral, 1965
Interferon Alpha (Natural Human), 1965
Interferon Beta-1a, 948
Interferon Beta-1a (Recombinant Human), 1940
Interferon Beta-1b, 951
Interferon Gamma-1b, 953, 1940
Interleukin-2, 1941, 1964, 1966
Interleukin-12, 1965
Interleukin-1 Alpha, Human Recombinant, 1940
Interleukin-3 Human (Recombinant), 1941
Interleukin-1 Receptor Antagonist (Human Recombinant), 1940
International System of Units, 1974
Intrachol, 1929
IntraDose, 1929
Intraoral Fluoride Releasing System (IFRS), 1941
Intron A, 941, 1940
Invanz, 657
Inversine, 1091, 1944
Invirase, 1616
Iobenguane Sulfate I 131, 1941
Iodine, 954
Iodine-123 Murine Monoclonal Antibody to Alpha-Fetoprotein, 1941
Iodine-123 Murine Monoclonal Antibody to hCG, 1941
Iodine-131 6B-iodomethyl-19-norcholestorol, 1941
Iodine-131 bis (indium-diethylenetriaminepentaacetic Acid)tyrosyllysine/hMN-14xm734 F(ab')2 Bispecific Monoclonal Antibody, 1941
Iodine-131 Lym-1 Monoclonal Antibody, 1941
Iodine-131 Murine Monoclonal Antibody IgG2a to BCell, 1941
Iodine-131 Murine Monoclonal Antibody to Alpha-Fetoprotein, 1941
Iodine-131 Murine Monoclonal Antibody to hCG, 1941
Iodine-131 Radiolabeled Chimeric MAb Tumor Necrosis Treatment (TNT-1B), 1941
Iodine-131 Tositumomab, 1792
Iodine Tincture, 954

Iodopen, 954
Iodotope, 1648
Ionamin, 1418
Iopidine, 127
Iopidine 0.5%, [C], 127
Iopidine 1%, [C], 127
Iosopan, 1081
Ipecac Syrup, 955
IPOL, 1451
Ipratropium Bromide, 957
Ipratropium Bromide/Albuterol Sulfate, 958
Iprivask, 504
Ipstyl, 1942
IPV, 1451
Irbesartan, 960
Ircon, 728
Irinotecan, 962
Irofulven, 1941
Iron Dextran, 964
Iron(III)-Hexyacyanoferrate(II), 1941
Iron Sucrose, 965
ISG, 918
ISIS 5320, 1964
Ismelin, 853
ISMO, 974
Isobutyramide, 1941
Isobutyramide Oral Solution, 1941
Isocarboxazid, 967
Isocom, 969
d-Isoephedrine, 1525
Isometheptene Mucate/Dichloralphenazone/Acetaminophen, 969
Isoniazid, 970
Isonicotinic Acid Hydrazide, 970
Isopap, 969
Isoprinosine, 1940
Isoproterenol, 971
Isoproterenol Hydrochloride, 971
Isoproterenol Sulfate, 971
Isoptin, 1874
Isoptin I.V., [C], 1874
Isoptin SR, 1874
Isopto Atropine, 154
Isopto-Carpine, 1432
Isopto Hyoscine, 1619
Isordil, 973
Isordil Titradose, 973
Isosorbide Dinitrate, 973
Isosorbide Mononitrate, 974
Isotamine, [C], 970
Isotretinoin, 975
Isotrex, [C], 975
Isovorin, 1942
Isoxsuprine Hydrochloride, 978
Isradipine, 979
Istalol, 1763
Isuprel, 971
Itraconazole, 980
Iveegam, 919, 1939
Iveegam Immuno, [C], 919

J

Jaa Prednisone, [C], 1473

Japanese Encephalitis Vaccine (Live, Attenuated), 1941
Jenest-28, 450
Junior Strength Advil, 903
Junior Strength Motrin, 903

K

K + 8, 1458
K + 10, 1458
K + Care, 1458
K + Care ET, 1458
K-10 Solution, [C], 1459
K-Dur 10, 1458
K-Dur 20, 1458
K-G Elixir, 1458
K-Lor, 1459
K-Lor, [C], 1459
K-Tab, 1459
K-vescent Potassium Chloride, 1459
Kadian, 1226
Kaletra, 1060
Kanamycin Sulfate, 984
Kantrex, 984
Kao-Spen, 985
Kaoch, [C], 1459
Kaochlor-20 Concentrate, [C], 1459
Kaolin, 1913
Kaolin/Pectin, 985
Kaon, 1459
Kaon Cl, 1459
Kaon Cl-10, 1459
Kaon-Cl 20%, 1459
Kaopectate II Caplets, 1059
Kapectolin, 985
Kariva, 450
Kasof, 576
Kay Ciel, 1459
Kayexalate, 1650
Kaylixir, 1459
Keep Alert, 269
Keep Going, 269
Keflex, 352
Keftab, 352
Kemadrin, 1489
Kenalog, 1813
Kenalog-10, 1813
Kenalog-40, 1813
Kenalog-H, 1813
Kenalog in Orabase, 1813
Keppra, 1019
KeriCort-10, 889
Kerlone, 200
Ketalar, 986
Ketamine Hydrochloride, 986
Ketek, 1707
Ketoconazole, 987, 1941
Ketoprofen, 989
Ketorolac Tromethamine, 990
Ketotifen Fumarate, 993
Key-Pred 25, 1467
Key-Pred 50, 1467
Key-Pred-SP, 1468
Kidrolase, [C], 137
Kineret, 121
Klerist-D Tablets, 1917
Klonopin, 425, 1930
Klor-Con, 1459

(*Trade* names appear in italics. Canadian products are indicated with a [C], withdrawn products with a [D].)

Klor-Con 8, 1459
Klor-Con 10, 1459
Klor-Con/25, 1459
Klor-Con/EF, 1459
Klor-Con M10, 1459
Klor-Con M15, 1459
Klor-Con M20, 1459
Klorvess, 1459
Klotrix, 1459
K•Lyte, 1459
K•Lyte/Cl, 1459
K•Lyte/Cl 50, 1459
K•Lyte DS, 1459
Koffex DM, [C], 524
Kogenate, 1923
Kolyum, 1459
Konyne 80, 714
Kronofed-A Capsules, 1917
Kronofed-A Jr. Capsules, 1917
Ku-Zyme, 1355
Ku-Zyme HP, 1355
Kutrase, 1355
Kwelcof, 882
Kybernin P, 1924
Kytril, 845

L

L-708,906, 1964
L1-2-I-131, 1941
Labetalol Hydrochloride, 955
Lactic Acid, 1942
Lactic Acid Bacteria (*Lactobacilli, Bifidobacteria,* and *Streptococcus* species), 1942
LactiCare-HC, 889
Lactobin, 1942
Lactoferrin Alpha, 1942
Lactulose, 996
Lamictal, 1001, 1942
Lamictal Chewable Dispersible, 1001
Lamisil, 1721
Lamisil AT, 1721
Lamivudine, 998
Lamivudine/Zidovudine, 1000, 1966
Lamivudine/Zidovudine/ Abacavir Sulfate, 2
Lamotrigine, 1001, 1942
Lamoxicaps, 546
Lamprene, 1930
Lanacort 5, 889
Lanacort 10, 889
Lanacort Maximum Strength Cool Creme, 889
Lanophyllin, 1739
Lanoxin, 546
Lanreotide, Somatostatin, 1942
Lansoprazole, 1005
Lansoprazole/Clarithromycin/ Amoxicillin, 105
Lantus, 933
Largactil, [C], 380
Lariam, 1104, 1944
Laronidase, 1008, 1942
Lasix, 802
Lasix Special, [C], 802
Latanoprost, 1009

Latrodectus Immune F(ab)2, 1942
Laxilose, [C], 996
Lederle Leucovorin Calcium, [C], 1015
Leflunomide, 1010, 1942
Legalon, 1933
Lente Iletin II, 931
Lepirudin, 1012
Lescol, 776
Lescol XL, 776
Lessina, 450
Letrazurile, 1963
Letrozole, 1014
Leucomax, 1937, 1945
Leucovorin, 1942
L-Leucovorin, 1942
Leucovorin Calcium, 1015, 1942
Leukeran, 362
Leukine, 1618, 1955
Leukotac, 1940
Leupeptin, 1942
Leuprolide Acetate, 1016, 1942
Leustatin, 413
Leustatin Injection, 1929
Leuvectin, 1933
Levalbuterol Hydrochloride, 1017
Levaquin, 1026
Levarterenol, 1296
Levatol, 1380
Levbid, 901
Levetiracetam, 1019
Levitra, 1867
Levlen, 450
Levlite, 450
Levo-Dromoran, 1031
Levobunolol, 1021
Levocabastine Hydrochloride Ophthalmic Solution 0.05%, 1942
Levocarnitine, 1942
Levodopa, 1022
Levodopa/Carbidopa, 1024, 1942
Levodopa/Entacapone/ Carbidopa, 296
Levofloxacin, 1026
Levomethadyl Acetate Hydrochloride, 1942
Levonorgestrel, 699, 1029
Levophed, 1296
Levora 0.15/30, 450
Levorphanol Tartrate, 1031
Levothroid, 1032
Levothyroxine Sodium, 1032
Levoxyl, 1032
Levsin, 901
Levsin Drops, 901
Levsin/SL, 901
Levsinex Timecaps, 901
Lexapro, 663
Lexiva, 789
Lexxel, 626
LHadi, 1952
Librax, 1913
Librium, 366
Lidex, 753
Lidex-E, 753
Lidocaine Hydrochloride, 1035

Lidocaine Hydrochloride/ Epinephrine, 1037
Lidocaine Hydrochloride for Cardiac Arrhythmias, 1035
Lidocaine Hydrochloride in 5% Dextrose, 1035
Lidocaine Hydrochloride/ Prilocaine, 1038
Lidocaine Path 5%, 1943
Lidodan Endotracheal, [C], 1035
Lidodan Ointment, [C], 1035
Lidodan Viscous, [C], 1035
Lidoderm Patch, 1943
Lidoject-1, 1035
Lidoject-2, 1035
Lidopen Auto-Injector, 1035
Limbitrol DS 10-25, 368
Limbrel, 735
Lin-Amox, [C], 101
Lin-Buspirone, [C], 254
Lin-Nefazodone, [C], 1258
Lindane, [D], 1040
Linezolid, 1042
Linmegestrol, [C], 1105
Linomide, 1954
Lintuzumab, 1943
Lioresal, 173
Lioresal Intrathecal, 1926
Liothyronine Sodium, 1044
Liothyronine Sodium Injection, 1943
Liotrix, 1046
Lipase, Amylase, and Protease, 1943
Lipid/DNA Human Cystic Fibrosis Gene, 1943
Lipidil Micro, [C], 721
Lipidil Supra, [C], 721
Lipitor, 149
Lipo-PGE1, 1951
Liposomal all-transretinoic Acid, 1966
Liposomal Amphotericin B, 1943
Liposomal-cis-bis- neodeconoato-trans-R,R-1,2- diaminocyclohexane-Pt (II), 1943
Liposomal Cyclosporin A, 1943
Liposomal N-Acetylglucosaminyl-N- Acetylmuramyl-L-Ala-D- isoGln-L-Ala- glycerolidpalmitoyl, 1943
Liposomal Nystatin, 1943
Liposomal p-ethoxy Growth Receptor Bound Protein-2 Antisense Product, 1943
Liposomal Prostaglandin E1 Injection, 1943
Liposome Encapsulated Recombinant Interleukin-2, 1943
Lipram 4500, 1355
Lipram-CR5, 1355
Lipram-CR10, 1355
Lipram-CR20, 1355
Lipram-PN10, 1355
Lipram-PN16, 1355
Lipram-PN20, 1355

(*Trade* names appear in italics. Canadian products are indicated with a [C], withdrawn products with a [D].)

Lipram-UL12, 1355
Lipram-UL18, 1355
Lipram-UL20, 1355
Liqui-Char, 360
Liquibid, 848
Liquibid-D, 1426
Liquibid-D 1200, 1426
Liquibid-PD, 1426
Liquid Pred, 1473
Liquiprin Drops for Children, 12
LiquiVent, 1949
Lisinopril, 1048
Lisinopril/Hydrochlorothiazide, 877, 1051
Lisofylline, 1943
Lithane, [C], 1053
Lithium, 1053
Lithobid, 1053
Lithonate, 1053
Lithotabs, 1053
Lo/Ovral, 450
LoCHOLEST, 388
LoCHOLEST Light, 388
Locoid, 889
Lodine, 705
Lodine XL, 705
Lodosyn, 295
Lodoxamide Tromethamine, 1943
Lodrane, 236
Lodrane 12 D, 236
Lodrane LD, 236
Lodrane LD Capsules, 1917
Loestrin 21 1/20, 450
Loestrin 21 1.5/30, 450
Loestrin Fe 1.5/30, 450
Loestrin Fe 1/20, 450
Lofibra, 721
Logen, 558
Lomanate, 558
Lomefloxacin Hydrochloride, 1055
Lomine, [C], 540
Lomotil, 558
Lomustine, 1057
Loniten, 1201
Lonox, 558
Loperamide Hydrochloride, 1059
Lopid, 815
Lopinavir/Ritonavir, 1060
Lopressor, 1177
Loprox, 392
Lorabid, 1062
Loracarbef, 1062
Loratadine/Pseudoephedrine Sulfate, 1066
Lorazepam, 1068
Lorazepam Intensol, 1068
Lorcet 10/650, 880
Lorcet-HD, 880
Lorcet Plus, 880
Lortab 5/500, 880
Lortab 7.5/500, 880
Lortab 10/500, 880
Lortab ASA Tablets, 1914
Lortab Elixir, 1914
Losartan Potassium, 1070
Losartan Potassium/Hydrochlorothiazide, 1072
Losec, [C], 1319

Lotensin, 184
Lotensin HCT, 186
Lotrel, 95
Lotrimin AF, 436, 1186
Lotrimin Ultra, 265
Lotrisone, 199
Lotronex, 59
Lovastatin, 1074, 1913
Lovastatin/Niacin, 1276
Lovenox, 631
Lovenox HP, [C], 631
Low-Ogestrel, 450
Loxapac, [C], 1076
Loxapine, 1076
Loxitane, 1076
Loxoribine, 1943
Lozide, [C], 921
Lozol, 921
Lucinactant, 1943
Ludiomil, 1087
Lufyllin, 608
Lufyllin-GG Tablets, 1917
Lugol's Solution, 954
Lumigan, 208
Luminal Sodium, 1415
Lunelle, [D], 678, 1100
rSP-C Lung surfactant, 1954
Lupron Depot, 1016
Lupron Depot 3.75 mg/11.25 mg, [C], 1016
Lupron Depot-3 Month, 1016
Lupron Depot-4 Month, 1016
Lupron Depot-Ped, 1016
Lupron for Pediatric Use, 1016
Lupron Injection, 1942
Lupron/Lupron Depot 3.75 mg/7.5 mg, [C], 1016
Lupron/Lupron Depot 7.5 mg/22.5 mg/30 mg, [C], 1016
Lutrepulse, 841, 1937
Luvox, 778
Luxiq, [C], 197
LymphoCide, 1934, 1966
Lymphocyte Immune Globulin, 1077
LymphoScan, 1958
Lyphocin, 1865
Lysine Acetylsalicylate Injectable, 1943
Lysodase, 1948
Lysodren, 1208

M

M-M-R II, 1089
M-oxy, 1339
M-Vax, 1925
M-Zole 3 Combination Pack, 1186
M-Zole 7 Dual Pack, 1186
Maalox Anti-Gas, 1636
Macrobid, 1289
Macrodantin, 1289
Mafosfamide, 1943
Mag-Ox 400, 1083
Magaldrate, 1081
Magnesium-Aluminum Hydroxides, 1914
Magnesium Citrate, 1082
Magnesium Oxide, 1083

Magnesium Sulfate, 1083
Magsal, 1915
Maitec, 1936
Malarone, 152
Malarone Pediatric, 152
Malathion 1086
Management of Acute Hypersensitivity Reactions, 1971
Mandameth, 1140
Mandelamine, 1140
Mandol, 319
Manfenide Acetate Solution, 1943
Maox 420, 1083
Mapap, Children's, 12
Mapap Extra Strength, 12
Mapap Infant Drops, 12
Mapap Regular Strength, 12
Maprotiline Hydrochloride, 1087
Maranox, 12
Margesic, 259
Margesic H, 880
Marijuana, 1943
Marinol, 630, 1933
Marogen, 1934
Marplan, 967
MARstem, 1923
MART-1 Adenoviral Gene Therapy for Malignant Melanoma, 1943
Masoprocol, 1088
Matrix Metalloproteinase Inhibitor, 1943
Matulane, 1483
Mavik, 1798
MaxAdFVIII, 1943
Maxair Autohaler, 1444
Maxalt, 1596
Maxalt-MLT, 1596
Maxalt RFD, [C], 1596
Maxamine, 1938
Maxaquin, 1055
Maxeran, [C], 1174
Maxidex, 511
Maximum Bayer, 139
Maximum Strength Desenex Antifungal, 1186
Maximum Strength Mylanta Gas, 1636
Maximum Strength NoDoz, 269
Maximum Strength Nytol, 556
Maximum Strength Sleepinal Capsules and Soft Gels, 556
Maximum Strength Unisom SleepGels, 556
Maxipime, 326
Maxitrol, 1266
Maxivate, 197
Maxolon, 1174
Maxzide, 378
Maxzide-25MG, 878
Mazindol 1943
MDX-240, 1963
ME-609 Cream, 1963
Measles, Mumps and Rubella Vaccine, Live, 1089
Mebaral, 1118
Mebendazole, 1090
Mecamylamine, 1944

(Trade names appear in italics. Canadian products are indicated with a [C], withdrawn products with a [D].)

Mecamylamine Hydrochloride, 1091
Mechlorethamine Hydrochloride, 1093
Meclizine, 1095
Meclofenamate Sodium, 1096
Med-Atenolol, [C], 144
Med-Baclofen, [C], 173
Meda Cap, 12
Meda Tab, 12
MEDI-491, 1948
MEDI-507, 1938
Medigesic, 259
Medihaler-ISO, 971
Medralone 40, 1166
Medralone 80, 1166
Medrol, 1166
Medroxyprogesterone Acetate, 678, 689, 1098, 1944
Medroxyprogesterone Acetate/ Estradiol Cypionate, [D], 1100
Mefenamic Acid, 1102
Mefloquine Hydrochloride, 1104
Mefloquine Hydrochloride, 1104, 1944
Mefoxin, 336
Megace, 1105, 1944
Megace OS, [C], 1105
MEGAGEN, 1948
Megestrol Acetate, 1105, 1944
Melacine, 1944
Melanocid, 1948
Melanoma Cell Vaccine, 1944
Melanoma Vaccine, 1944
Melatonin, 1944
Melfiat-105 Unicelles, 1411
Melimmune, 1945
Meloxicam, 1107, 1944
Melphalan, 1109, 1944
Memantine, 1963
Memantine Hydrochloride, 1111
Menadol, 903
Menest, 684
Meni-D, 1095
Menotropins, 1112
Mentax, 265
Mepenzolate Bromide, 1114
Meperidine Hydrochloride, 1116
Mephaquin, 1944
Mephentermine Sulfate, 1117
Mephobarbital, 1118
Mephyton, 1430
Meprobamate, 1120, 1913, 1915
Mepron, 151, 1925
Mercaptopurine, 1122
Meridia, 1632
Meropenem, 1124, 1944
Merrem, 1124
Merrem IV, 1944
Mesacal, [C], 1125
Mesalamine, 1125
Mescasermin, 1944
Mescolor Tablets, 1918
Mesna, 1126, 1944
Mesnex, 1126, 1944
Mesoridazine, 1128

Mestinon, 1529
Metadate CD, 1163
Metadate ER, 1163
Metadol, [C], 1137
Metaglip, 828
Metaproterenol Sulfate, 1130
Metaraminol, 1132
Metaret, 1957
Metastat, 1966
Metastron, 1670
Metaxalone, 1133
Metformin Hydrochloride, 828, 834, 1135
Metformin Hydrochloride/ Rosiglitazone Maleate, 1605
Methadone Hydrochloride, 1137
Methadose, 1137
Methamphetamine Hydrochloride, 1138
Methazolamide, 1140
Methenamine, 1140
Methenamine Hippurate, 1140
Methenamine Mandelate, 1140
Methenamine Salts, 1140
Methergine, 1162
Methimazole, 1142
Methionine/L-Methionine, 1944
Methitest, 1169
Methocarbamol, 1143
Methocarbamol/Aspirin, 1145
Methotrexate, 1146, 1944
Methotrexate/Azone, 1944
Methotrexate LPF Sodium, 1146
Methotrexate Sodium, 1146, 1944
Methotrexate with Laurocapram, 1944
Methoxsalen, 1151, 1944
8-Methoxsalen, 1920
2-Methoxyestradiol, 1920
Methscopolamine Bromide, 1154
Methscopolamine Nitrate/ Chlorpheniramine Maleate/ Phenylephrine Hydrochloride, 377
Methsuximide, 1156
Methyclothiazide/Deserpidine, 1157
Methylbicyclone, 1944
Methyldopa, 1159
Methyldopate Hydrochloride, 1159
Methylergonovine Maleate, 1162
Methylin, 1163
Methylin ER, 1163
Methylnaltrexone, 1944
Methylphenidate Hydrochloride, 1163
Methylphytyl Naphthoquinone, 1430
Methylprednisolone, 1166
Methylprednisolone Acetate, 1166
Methylprednisolone Sodium Succinate, 1166
Methyltestosterone, 670, 1169
Methysergide Maleate, 1171

Meticorten, 1473
Metipranolol, 1172
Metoclopramide, 1174
Metoclopramide Omega, [C], 1174
Metolazone, 1176
Metoprolol, 1177
Metreleptin, 1944
Metric 21, 1179
MetroCream, 1179
Metrodin, 1961
MetroGel, 1179, 1944
MetroGel-Vaginal, 1179
MetroLotion, 1179
Metronidazole, 1179, 1944
Metronidazole/Tetracycline/ Bismuth Subsalicylate, 213
Metronidazole (Topical), 1944
Mevacor, [C], 1074
Mexiletine Hydrochloride, 1183
Mexitil, 1183
Mezlin, 1185
Mezlocillin Sodium, 1185
Miacalcin, 271
Miacalcin Nasal Spray, 1928
Miacalcin NS, [C], 271
Micardis, 1709
Micardis HCT, 1710
Micatin, 1186
Miconazole, 1186
MICRhoGAM, 1569
Micro-K Extencaps, 1459
Micro-K LS, 1459
Microbubble Contrast Agent, 1944
Microgestin Fe 1/20, 450
Microgestin Fe 1.5/30, 450
Micronase, 832
microNefrin, 637
Micronor, 452
Microzide, 875
Midamor, 77
Midazolam Hydrochloride, 1188
Midchlor, 969
Midodrine Hydrochloride, 1191, 1945
Midol Maximum Strength Cramp Formula, 903
Midol PM, 556
Midrin, 969
Mifeprex, 1193
Mifepristone, 1193
Miglitol, 1194
Miglustat, 1195, 1945
Migranal, 548
Migratine, 969
MiKasome, 1966
Miles Nervine, 556
Milophene, 422
Milrinone Lactate, 1197
Miltown, 1120
Mini-Thin Pseudo, 1525
MiniAdFVIII, 1921
Minims Atropine, [C], 154
Minims Gentamicin, [C], 821
Minims Phenylephrine, [C], 1421
Minims-Pilocarpine, [C], 1432
Minims Prednisolone, 1467

(*Trade* names appear in italics Canadian products are indicated with a [C], withdrawn products with a [D].)

Minipress, 1466
Minirin, [C], 507
Minitran, 1290
Minocin, 1198
Minocin Intravenous, 1945
Minocycline, 1198
Minocycline Hydrochloride, 1945
Minoxidil, 1201
Minoxidil for Men, 1201
Mintezol, 1741
MiraLax, 1454
Mirapex, 1462
Mircette, 450
Mirena, 1029
Mirtazapine, 1203
Misoprostol, 537, 1205
Mitomycin, 1206
Mitomycin-C, 1945
Mitotane, 1208
Mitoxantrone, 1210, 1945
Mitoxantrone Hydrochloride, 1945
MIV-150, 1964
MIV-310, 1964
Mivacron, 1212
Mivacurium Chloride, 1212
MKC-442, 1966
MN14 Monoclonal Antibody for Immunization Against Lupus Nephritis, 1945
Moban, 1218
Mobic, 1107, 1944
Mobicox, [C], 1107
Moctanin, 1222, 1945
Modafinil, 1214, 1945
Modane, 210
Modecate, [C], 763
Modecate Concentrate, [C], 763
Modicon, 450
Moditen Hydrochloride, [C], 763
Moduret, [C], 79
Moduretic, 79
Moexipril Hydrochloride, 1216
Molgramostim, 1945
Molie, 269
Molindone Hydrochloride, 1218
Mometasone, 1219
Mometasone Furoate, 1221
Monafed, 848
Monarsen, 1945
Monistat 3, 1186
Monistat 7, 1186
Monistat 7 Combination Pack, 1186
Monistat Derm, 1186
Monitan, [C], 10
Monoclonal Ab(murine) Anti-idiotype melanoma-associated Antigen, 1945
Monoclonal Antibodies (Murine or Human) to B-Cell Lymphoma, 1945
Monoclonal Antibody-17-1a, 1945
Monoclonal Antibody-B43.13, 1945

Monoclonal Antibody for Immunization Against Lupus Nephritis, 1945
5a8, Monoclonal Antibody to CD4, 1920
Monoclonal Antibody to Cytomegalovirus (Human), 1945
Monoclonal Antibody to Hepatitis B Virus (Human), 1945
Monoclonal Antiendotoxin Antibody XMMEn-0e5, 1945
Monoctanoin, 1222, 1945
Monodox, 597
Monoket, 974
Monolaurin, 1945
Mononessa, 450
Mononine, 714
Monopril, 795
Monoxidil, 1201
Montelukast Sodium, 1223
Monurol, 794
Moricizine Hydrochloride, 1224
Morphelan ROER, 1966
Morphine Sulfate, 1226
Morphine Sulfate, Rapid-Onset Extended-Release, 1966
Morphine Sulfate Concentrate (Preservative Free), 1945
Motexafin Gadolinium, 1945
Motrin, 903
Motrin, Children's, 903
Motrin IB, 903
Motrin IB Extra Strength, [C], 903
Motrin IB Super Strength, [C], 903
Motrin, Infants, 903
Motrin, Junior Strength, 903
Motrin Migraine Pain, 903
Moxifloxacin Hydrochloride, 1229
MS Contin, 1226
MSD Enteric Coated ASA, [C], 139
MSIR, 1226
MTC-DOX for Injection, 1945
MTX, 1146
Mucinex, 848
Muco-Fen-LA, 848
Mucoid Exopolysaccharide, 1945
Mucomyst, 19
Mucomyst/Mucomyst 10 IV, 1921
Mucrainin, 1915
Multi-vitamin Infusion (Neonatal Formula), 1946
Multikine, 1964, 1965
Mumps, Measles, and Rubella Vaccine, Live, 1089
Mupirocin, 1232
Muramyltripeptide, Phosphatidyl-ethanolamine Encased in Multi-lamellar Liposomes, 1946

Murine MAb (Lym-1) and Iodine 131-I Radiolabeled Murine MAb (Lym-1) to Human B-Cell Lymphoma, 1946
Muromonab-CD3, 1233
Muse, 65
Mustargen 1093
Mutamycin, 1206
Mx-dnG1 or Rexin-G Retroviral Vector, 1946
Myambutol, 697
Mycelex, 436
Mycelex-7, 436
Mycelex-7 Combination Pack, 436
Mycobacterium with Immunomodulator, Heat Killed, 1946
Mycobutin, 1575, 1954
Mycogen II, 1302
Mycograb, 1952
Mycolog II, 1302
Mycophenolate Mofetil, 1236
Mycostatin, 1301
Mycostatin Pastilles, 1301
Mydfrin 2.5%, 1421
Myelin, 1946
Mykrox, 1176
Mylanta Gas, 1636
Mylanta Gas, Maximum Strength, 1636
Myleran, 256
Mylicon, 1636
Mylinax, 1929
Mylocel, 897
Mylotarg, 818, 1936
Mylovenge, 1925
Myobloc, 228
Myocet, [C], 592
Myoscint, 1939
Myotonachol, 202
Myristoylated Recombinant SCR1-3 of Human Complement Reseptor Type I, 1946
Myscint, 1940
Mysoline, 1476
Mytotrophin, 1944
Mytrex, 1302
Mytussin, 848
Mytussin AC, 849
Mytussin DAC Liquid, 1918

N

N-[4-bromo-2-(1H-1,2,3,4-tetrazol-5-yl) phenyl]-N'-[3,5-bis(trifluoromethyl)phenyl]urea, 1946
N-Graft, 1950
Nabi-HB, 867, 1937
Nabumetone, 1239
Nacystelyn Dry Powder Inhaler, 1946
Nadolol, 1240
Nadopen-V, [C], 1388
Nafarelin Acetate, 1242, 1946
Nafcillin Sodium, 1243
Nalbuphine Hydrochloride, 1245
Nalcrom, [C], 458

(Trade names appear in italics. Canadian products are indicated with a [C], withdrawn products with a [D].)

Naldecon Senior EX, 848
Nalfon Pulvules, 723
Nalidixic Acid, 1246
Naloxone Hydrochloride, 1247
Naloxone Hydrochloride/Buprenorphine Hydrochloride, 249
Naltrexone Hydrochloride, 1249, 1946
Namenda, 1111
Napa, 1946
Naprelan, 1251
Naprosyn, 1251
Naproxen, 1251
Naproxen Sodium, 1251
Naratriptan, 1253
Narcan, 1247
Nardil, 1412
Nasacort AQ, 1813
Nasalcrom, 458
Nasarel, 750
Nasatab LA, 1918
Nascobal, 461
Nashville Rabbit Anti-thymocyte Serum, 1924
Nasonex, 1219
Natacyn, 1255
Natamycin, 1255
Nateglinide, 1256
Natrecor, 1270
Natural Human Lymphoblastoid Interferon-Alpha, 1946
Naturetin, 188
Navane, 1751
Navelbine, 1880
Naxen, [C], 1251
NDROGE, 1946
Nebacumab, 1946
Nebcin, 1773
Nebcin Pediatric, 1773
NebuPent, 1390, 1948
Necon 0.5/35, 450
Necon 1/35, 450
Necon 1/50, 450
Necon 10/11, 450
Nedocromil Sodium, 1257
Nefazodone Hydrochloride, 1258
NegGram, 1246
Nelfinavir Mesylate, 1261
Nembutol Sodium, 1393
Neo-Diaral, 1059
Neo-fradin, 1263
Neo-Synephrine, 1421
Neomark, 1927
Neomycin/Polymyxin B Sulfates/Bacitracin Zinc, 1264
Neomycin/Polymyxin B Sulfates/Bacitracin Zinc/Hydrocortisone, 171
Neomycin Sulfate, 1263
Neomycin Sulfate/Polymyxin B Sulfate/Dexamethasone, 1266
Neomycin Sulfate/Polymyxin B Sulfate/Gramicidin, 1267
Neomycin Sulfate/Thonzonium Br/Hydrocortisone Acetate/Colistin Sulfate, 448

Neomycin Sulfate/Polymyxin B Sulfate/Prednisolone Acetate, 1472
Neopap, 12
Neoral, 469
Neosar, 465
Neosporin, 1264, 1267
Neosporin Eye and Ear Solution, [C], 1267
Neosporin Ointment, [C], 1264, 1897
Neostigmine, 1268
Neovastat [AE-941], 1923
Nephro-Fer, 728
Nervocaine, 1035
Nesiritide, 1270
Nestrex, 1530
Neumega, 1322, 1947
Neupogen, 732, 1935
Neuprex, 1951
Neuralgon, 1942
Neurelan, 1935
NeuroBloc, 1927
NeuroCell-HD, 1950
NeuroCell-PD, 1950
Neurontin, 805, 1936
Neurotrophin-1, 1947
Neutrexin, 1830, 1960
Neutrogena, 190
Nevirapine, 1272
Nexium, 667
NG-29, 1947
Niacin, 1274, 1913
Niacin/Lovastatin, 1276
Niaspan, 1274
Nicardipine Hydrochloride, 1279
N'ice Vitamin C Drops, 136
Nicoderm, 1280
Nicorette, 1280
Nicorette DS, 1280
Nicorette Plus, [C], 1280
Nicotine, 1280
Nicotinic Acid, 1274
Nicotrol, 1280
Nicotrol Inhaler, 1280
Nicotrol NS, 1280
Nida Gel, [C], 1179
Nifedical XL, 1283
Nifedipine, 1283, 1947
Niferex, 728
Niferex-150, 728
Nighttime Sleep Aid, 556
Nilandron, 1285
Nilstat, 1301
Nilutamide, 1285
Nimbex, 406
Nimodipine, 1286
Nimotop, 1286
Nipent, 1396, 1949
Nipirisan, 1947
Nisoldipine, 1287
Nitazoxanide, 1947
Nitisinone, 1947
Nitrek, 1290
Nitric Oxide, 1947
Nitro-Bid, 1290
Nitro-Bid IV, 1290
Nitro-Dur, 1290

Nitro-Time, 1290
Nitrodisc, 1290
Nitrofurantoin, 1289
Nitrogard, 1290
Nitroglycerin, 1290
Nitrol, 1290
Nitrolingual, 1290
Nitrolingual Pumpspray, [C], 1290
Nitropress, 1293
Nitroprusside, 1947
Nitroprusside Sodium, 1293
NitroQuick, 1290
Nitrostat, 1290
Nix Cream Rinse, 1404
Nix Creme Rinse, [C], 1404
Nix Dermal Cream, [C], 1404
Nizatidine, 1294
Nizoral, 987, 1941
No Pain-HP, 284
NoDoz, Maximum Strength, 269
Nolahist, 1414
Nolatrexed, 1947
Nolvadex, 1700
Nolvadex-D, [C], 1700
Non-Habit Forming Stool Softener, 576
Nonnarcotic Analgesic Combinations, 1915
Nootropil, 1949
Nor-Q.D., 452
Norco, 880
Norcuron, 1870
Nordette, 450
Norditropin, 1653, 1956, 1957
Norel DM, 526
Norepinephrine, 1296
Norethindrone Acetate, 680, 1297
Norflex, 1325
Norfloxacin, 1298
Norgesic, 1326
Norgesic Forte, 1326
Norinyl 1+35, 450
Norinyl 1+50, 450
Noritate, 1179
Norlutate, [C], 1297
Normal Laboratory Values, 1976
Normix, 1954
Normodyne, 995
Normosang, 1937
Noroxin, 1298
Norpace, 569
Norpace CR, 569
Norplant System, 1029
Norpramin, 502
Nortrel 0.5/35, 450
Nortrel 1/35, 450
Nortriptyline Hydrochloride, 1300
Norvasc, 91
Norvir, 1590
Norwich Extra-Strength, 139
Nostril, 1421
Nostril, Children's, 1421
Novagest Expectorant w/Codeine Liquid, 1918
Novahistine Decongestant, [C], 1421

(Trade names appear in italics. Canadian products are indicated with a [C], withdrawn products with a [D].)

Novamilor, [C], 79
Novamoxin, [C], 101
Novantrone, 1210, 1945
Novarel, 389
Novasen, [C], 139
Novel Acting Thrombolytic (NAT), 1947
Novo-5 ASA, [C], 1125
Novo-Acebutolol, [C], 10
Novo-Alprazol, [C], 62
Novo-Amiodarone, [C], 86
Novo Ampicillin, 112
Novo-Atenol, [C], 144
Novo-AZT, [C], 1894
Novo-Buspirone, [C], 254
Novo-Butamide, [C], 1777
Novo-Captoril, [C], 285
Novo-Carbamaz, [C], 290
Novo-Cefaclor, [C], 316
Novo-Cefadroxil, [C], 318
Novo-Cholamine, [C], 388
Novo-Cholamine Light, [C], 388
Novo-Cimetine, [C], 398
Novo-Clobetasol, [C], 421
Novo-Clonazepam, [C], 425
Novo-Clonidine, [C], 427
Novo-Clopamine, [C], 423
Novo-Clopate, [C], 434
Novo-Cycloprine, [C], 463
Novo-Desipramine, [C], 502
Novo-Difenac, [C], 533
Novo-Difenac K, [C], 533
Novo-Difenac SR, [C], 533
Novo-Diflunisal, [C], 545
Novo-Diltiazem, [C], 550
Novo-Diltiazem SR, [C], 550
Novo-Divalproex, [C], 1855
Novo-Doxasozin, [C], 588
Novo-Doxepin, [C], 589
Novo-Doxylin, [C], 597
Novo-Famotidine, [C], 716
Novo-Fluoxetine, [C], 759
Novo-Flupam, [C], 765
Novo-Flurbiprofen, [C], 767
Novo-Flurprofen, [C], 767
Novo-Flutamide, [C], 768
Novo-Fluvoxamine, [C], 778
Novo-Furantoin, [C], 1289
Novo-Gabapentin, [C], 805
Novo-Gemfibrozil, [C], 815
Novo-Glyburide, [C], 832
Novo-Hydroxyzin, [C], 899
Novo-Hylazin, [C], 874
Novo-Indapamide, [C], 921
Novo-Ipramide, [C], 957
Novo-Keto, [C], 989
Novo-Keto-EC, [C], 989
Novo-Ketoconazole, [C], 987
Novo-Ketorolac, [C], 990
Novo-Levobunolol, [C], 1021
Novo-Levocarbidopa, [C], 1024
Novo-Lexin, [C], 352
Novo-Lorazem, [C], 1068

Novo-Maprotiline, [C], 1087
Novo-Medrone, [C], 1098
Novo-Metformin, [C], 1135
Novo-Methacin, [C], 924
Novo-Metoprol, [C], 1177
Novo-Mexiletine, [C], 1183
Novo-Minocycline, [C], 1198
Novo-Misoprostol, [C], 1205
Novo-Nadolol, [C], 1240
Novo-Naprox, [C], 1251
Novo-Naprox EC, [C], 1251
Novo-Naprox Sodium, [C], 1251
Novo-Naprox Sodium DS, [C], 1251
Novo-Naprox SR, [C], 1251
Novo-Nidazol, [C], 1179
Novo-Nifedin, [C], 1283
Novo-Nizatidine, [C], 1294
Novo-Norfloxacin, [C], 1298
Novo-Nortriptyline, [C], 1300
Novo-Oxybutynin, 1336
Novo-Pen-VK, [C], 1388
Novo-Peridol, [C], 859
Novo-Pindol, [C], 1438
Novo-Piroxicam, [C], 1445
Novo-Prazin, [C], 1466
Novo-Prednisolone, 1467
Novo-Profen, [C], 903
Novo-Purol, [C], 55
Novo-Ranitidine, [C], 1557
Novo-Salmol, [C], 39
Novo-Selegiline, [C], 1624
Novo-Sertraline, [C], 1628
Novo-Sotalol, [C], 1655
Novo-Spiroton, [C], 1660
Novo-Spirozine, [C], 1660
Novo-Sucralfate, [C], 1673
Novo-Sundac, [C], 1686
Novo-Tamoxifen, [C], 1700
Novo-Temazepam, [C], 1713
Novo-Terazosin, [C], 1719
Novo-Terbinafine, [C], 1721
Novo-Tetra, [C], 1733
Novo-Theophyl SR, [C], 1739
Novo-Timol Tablets, [C], 1763
Novo-Trazodone, [C], 1808
Novo-Triamzide, [C], 878
Novo-Trimel, [C], 1828
Novo-Trimel D.S., [C], 1828
Novo-Valproic, [C], 1855
Novo-Veramil, [C], 1874
Novo-Veramil SR, [C], 1874
Novolin 70/30, 931
Novolin ge 30/70, [C], 931
Novolin ge 40/60, [C], 931
Novolin ge 50/50, [C], 931
Novolin ge Lente, [C], 931
Novolin ge NPH, [C], 931
Novolin ge Toronto, [C], 931
Novolin ge Ultralente, [C], 931
Novolin L, 931
Novolin N, 931
Novolin R, 931

NovoLog, 933
NovoLog Mix 70/30, 933
Novorythro Encap, [C], 659
NovoSeven, 1930
NP-27, 1782
70% NPH, Human Insulin Isophane Suspension and 30% Regular, Human Insulin Injection ([rDNA Origin)], 931
NPH, Isophane Insulin Suspension, 931
NPH Iletin II, 931
Nu-Acebutolol, [C], 10
Nu-Acyclovir, [C], 26
Nu-Alpraz, [C], 62
Nu-Amilzide, [C], 79
Nu-Amoxi, [C], 101
Nu-Ampi, 112
Nu-Atenol, [C], 144
Nu-Baclo, [C], 173
Nu-Beclomethasone, [C], 179
Nu-Buspirone, [C], 254
Nu-Captc, [C], 285
Nu-Carbcmazepine, [C], 290
Nu-Cefaclor, [C], 316
Nu-Cephalex, [C], 352
Nu-Cimet, [C], 398
Nu-Clonazepam, [C], 425
Nu-Clonidine, [C], 427
Nu-Cotrimox, [C], 1828
Nu-Cromolyn, [C], 458
Nu-Cyclobenzaprine, [C], 463
Nu-Desipramine, [C], 502
Nu-Diclo, [C], 533
Nu-Diclo-SR, [C], 533
Nu-Diflunisal, [C], 545
Nu-Diltiaz, [C], 550
Nu-Diltiaz-CD, [C], 550
Nu-Divalproex, [C], 1855
Nu-Doxycycline, [C], 597
Nu-Erythromycin-S, [C], 659
Nu-Famotidine, [C], 716
Nu-Fenofibrate, [C], 721
Nu-Fluoxetine, [C], 759
Nu-Flurbiprofen, [C], 767
Nu-Fluvoxamine, [C], 778
Nu-Gemfibrozil, [C], 815
Nu-Glyburide, [C], 832
Nu-Hydral, [C], 874
Nu-Hydroxyzine, [C], 899
Nu-Ibuprofen, [C], 903
Nu-Indapamide, [C], 921
Nu-Indo, [C], 924
Nu-Ipratropium, [C], 957
Nu-Iron, 728
Nu-Iron 150, 728
Nu-Ketoprofen, [C], 989
Nu-Ketoprofen-SR, [C], 989
Nu-Levocarb, [C], 1024
Nu-Loraz, [C], 1068
Nu-Loxapine, [C], 1076
Nu-Medopa, [C], 1159
Nu-Mefenamic, [C], 1102

(Trade names appear in italics. Canadian products are indicated with a [C], withdrawn products with a [D].)

Nu-Megestrol, [C], 1105
Nu-Metformin, [C], 1135
Nu-Metoclopramide, [C], 1174
Nu-Metop, [C], 1177
Nu-Naprox, [C], 1251
Nu-Nifed, [C], 1283
Nu-Nifedipine, [C], 1283
Nu-Nortriptyline, [C], 1300
Nu-Oxybutynin, 1336
Nu-Pen-VK, [C], 1388
Nu-Pentoxifylline, [C], 1399
Nu-Pindol, [C], 1438
Nu-Pirox, [C], 1445
Nu-Pravastatin, [C], 1463
Nu-Prazo, [C], 1466
Nu-Prochlor, [C], 1486
Nu-Propranolol, [C], 1516
Nu-Ranit, [C], 1557
Nu-Salbutamol Solution, 39
Nu-Selegiline, [C], 1624
Nu-Sotalol, [C], 1655
Nu-Sucralfate, [C], 1673
Nu-Sulfinpyrazone, [C], 1684
Nu-Sulindac, [C], 1686
Nu-Temazepam, [C], 1713
Nu-Terazosin, [C], 1719
Nu-Tetra, [C], 1733
Nu-Ticlopidine, [C], 1760
Nu-Timolol, [C], 1763
Nu-Trazodone, [C], 1808
Nu-Trazodone-D, [C], 1808
Nu-Triazide, [C], 878
Nu-Valproic, [C], 1855
Nu-Verap, [C], 1874
Nubain, 1245
Nubain, [C], 1245
Nuhist, 1423
NuLev, 901
NuLYTELY, 1455
Numby Stuff, 1035
Numorphan, 1343
Numorphan H.P., 1948
Nuprin, 903
Nutrineal (Peritoneal Dialysis Solution with 1.1% Amino Acid), 1932
Nutracort, 889
Nutropin, 1653, 1956
Nutropin AQ, 1653
Nutropin Depot, 1653, 1956
Nyaderm, [C], 1301
Nydrazid, 970
Nyotran, 1943
Nystatin, 1301
Nystatin/Triamcinolone Acetonide, 1302
Nytol, 556
Nytol Extra Strength, [C], 555
Nytol, Maximum Strength, 556
NZ-1002, 1947

O

O-Vax, 1933
Obe-Nix, 1418
OCL, 1455
Octamide, 1174
Octamide PFS, 1174
Octastatin, 1961
Octavalent Pseudomonas Aeruginosa O-polysaccharide-toxin A conjugate, 1947
Octocaine, 1035
Octostim, [C], 507
Octostim Spray, [C], 507
Octreocide, 1947
Octreotide Acetate, 1304
Ocufen, 767
Ocuflox, 1305
Ocuflox Ophthalmic Solution, 1947
Ocupress, 310, 1953
Ocusert Pilo-20, 1432, 1957
Ocusert Pilo-40, 1432
Ofloxacin, 1305, 1947
Ogen, 691
Ogestrel 0.5/50, 450
Oglufanide Disodium, 1947
Olanzapine, 1307
Olanzapine/Fluoxetine Hydrochloride, 1311
Olmesartan Medoxomil, 1314
Olopatadine Hydrochloride, 1315
Olsalazine Sodium, 1316
Olux, 421
OM 401, 1947
Omacor, 1947
Omalizumab, 1317
Omega-3 (N-3) Polyunsaturated Fatty Acids, 1947
Omega-3 (N-3) Polyunsaturated Fatty Acids, with all double bonds in the cis configuration, 1947
Omeprazole, 1319
Omnicef, 323
OMNIhist L.A., 377, 1918
OMS Concentrate, 1226
Oncaspar, 1367, 1948
Oncolym, 1946
Oncomun, 1959
Oncophage, 1925
Oncovin, 1878
Ondansetron Hydrochloride, 1320
Onkolox, 1930
Onocrad Ov103, 1947
Onoctrac Melanoma Imaging Kit, 1958
OnoScint CR/OV, 1955
Ontak, 501, 1932
Ophthalgan, 836
Opium/Belladonna, 181
Oprelvekin, 1322, 1947
Opticrom 4% Ophthalmic Solution, 1931
Optimyxin Ointment, [C], 172
Optimyxin Plus Solution, [C], 1267
OptiPranolol, 1172
Optivar, 165
OPV, 1449
Or-Tyl, 540
Oracit, 1645

Oracort, [C], 1813
Oral Contraceptives, Combination Products, 450
Oral Contraceptives, Progestin-Only, 452
Oral Dosage Forms that Should Not be Crushed or Chewed, 1995
Oramed, 1963
Oramorph SR, 1226
Orap, 1435
Oraphen-PD, 12
Orasone, 1473
Orazinc, 1897
Oretic, 875
Orfadin, 1947
Orfenace, [C], 1325
Organidin NR, 848
Orgotein for Injection, 1947
Orimune, 1449
Orinase, 1777
Orinase Diagnostic, 1777
ORLAAM, 1942
Orlistat, 1323
Ornidyl, 1934
Orphan Drugs, 1919
Orphenadrine Citrate, 1325
Orphenadrine Citrate/Aspirin/Caffeine, 1326
Ortho-Cept, 450
Ortho-Cyclen, 450
Ortho-Novum 1/35, 450
Ortho-Novum 1/50, 450
Ortho-Novum 10/11, 450
Ortho-Novum 7/7/7, 450
Ortho Tri-Cyclen, 450
Ortho Tri-Cyclen Lo, 450
Orthoclone OKT3, 1233
Orthoest, 691
Orudis, 989
Orudis SR, [C], 989
Oruvail, 989
Oseltamivir Phosphate, 1327
Osmoglyn, 836
Osteo-D, 1955
Osteocalcin, 271
Ovarex MAb-B43.13, 1945
Ovastat, 1960
Ovcon-35, 450
Ovcon-50, 450
Overtime, 269
Ovide, 1086
Ovol, [C], 1636
Ovol Drops, [C], 1636
Ovral-28, 450
Ovrette, 452
Oxacillin Sodium, 1329
Oxaliplatin, 1947
Oxandrin, 1947
Oxandrolone, 1947
Oxaprozin, 1330
Oxazepam, 1332
Oxcarbazepine, 1333
Oxeze Turbuhaler, [C], 788
L-2-Oxothiazolidine-4-Carboxylic Acid, 1941
Oxsodrol, 1957
Oxsoralen, 1151
Oxsoralen-Ultra, 1151
Oxy, 190

Oxybate, 1947
Oxybutynin Chloride, 1336
Oxycodone/Acetaminophen, 1340
Oxycodone Hydrochloride, 1339
Oxycodone Hydrochloride/Aspirin, 1342
OxyContin, 1339
Oxyderm 5%, [C], 190
Oxyderm 10%, [C], 190
Oxyderm 20%, [C], 190
Oxydose, 1339
OxyFAST, 1339
OxyIR, 1339
Oxymorphone, 1948
Oxymorphone Hydrochloride, 1343
Oxypurinol, 1948
Oxytetracycline Hydrochloride/Polymyxin B Sulfate, 1347
Oxytocin, 1345
Oxytrol, 1336

P

P1, P4-Di(uridine 5'-tetraphosphate), Tetrasodium Salt, 1948
P-V-Tussin, 887
PA-457, 1964
PA-1648, 1966
PA mAb, 1948
Pacerone, 86
Paclitaxel, 1349, 1948, 1966
Pain Doctor, 284
Pain-X, 284
Palafer, [C], 728
Palivizumab, 1351
Palonosetron, 1352
Pamabrom, 1915
Pamelor, 1300
Pamidronate Disodium, 1353
Pamine, 1154
Pamine Forte, 1154
Pamisyl, 1920
PAN-Cide, 1921
Panacet 5/500, 880
Panadol, 12
Panadol, Children's, 12
Panadol, Infants' Drops, 12
Panasol-S, 1473
Pancrease, 1355
Pancrease MT, [C], 1356
Pancrease MT 4, 1355
Pancrease MT 10, 1355
Pancrease MT 16, 1356
Pancrease MT 20, 1356
Pancrecarb MS-4, 1356
Pancrecarb MS-8, 1356
Pancrelipase, 1355, 1356
Pancuronium Bromide, 1358
Pandel, 889
Panhematin, 1937
PanMist-DM, 1526
Panokase, 1356
Panorex, 1945
PanOxyl, 190
Panoxyl 5% Wash, [C], 190
Panoxyl 10%, [C], 190

Panoxyl 15%, [C], 190
Panoxyl 20%, [C], 190
Panoxyl Aquagel 2.5% and 5%, [C], 190
Panoxyl Aquagel 10% and 20%, [C], 190
Panretin, 54, 1920, 1921, 1965
Panretin and Interferon, 1966
Panto IV, [C], 1359
Pantoloc, [C], 1359
Pantoprazole Sodium, 1359
Panzem, 1920
Papain, Trypsin, and Chymotrypsin, 1948
Papaverine Hydrochloride, 1361
Papaverine Topical Gel, 1948
Para-Aminosalicylate Sodium, 85
Paraflex, 387
Parafon Forte DSC, 387
Paraplatin, 302
Paraplatin-AQ, [C], 302
Parathar, 1958
Parathyroid Hormone 1-34, Synthetic Human, 1957
Pariet, [C], 1549
Parlodel, 234
Parlodel, [C], 234
Parnate, 1804
Paromomycin, 1923
Paromomycin Sulfate, 1363
Paroxetine, 1364
Paroxetine Hydrochloride, 1364
Paroxetine Mesylate, 1364
Partaject, 1927
Parvolex, [C], 19
Parvovirus B19 (Recombinant VP1 and VP2; *S. frugiperda* Cells) Vaccine, 1948
PAS, 85
Paser, 85
Paser Granules, 1922
Patanol, 1315
Patul-end, 1948
Pavabid Plateau Caps, 1361
Pavagen, 1361
Paxene, 1948, 1966
Paxil, 1364
Paxil CR, 1364
PCE Dispertab, 659
Pectin/Kaolin, 985
Pedi-Dri, 1301
PediaCare Fever, 903
PediaCare Infant's Decongestant, 1525
PediaCare Nasal Decongestant, 1525
Pediapred, 1468
Pediarix, 559
Pediatex, 299
Pediatric Advil Drops, 903
Pediatric Tiban, 1826
Pediatric Vicks 44d Dry Hacking Cough and Head Congestion, 524
Pediatrix, [C], 12
Pediazole, 662

PedvaxHIB, Liquid, 858
PEG, 1454
PEG-ES, 1455
PEG-glucocerebrosidase, 1948
PEG-interleukin-2, 1948
PEG-Intron, 1373
Pegademase Bovine, 1948
Peganone, 702
Pegaspargase, 1367, 1948
PEGASYS, 1370, 1948
Pegfilgrastim, 1369
Peginterferon Alfa-2a, 1370, 1948
Peginterferon Alfa-2b, 1373
Pegvisomant, 1375, 1948
Pegylated Arginine Deiminase, 1948
Pegylated Recombinant Human Megakaryocyte Growth and Development Factor, 1948
Peldesine, 1948
Pemetrexed, 1377
Pemetrexed Disodium, 1948
Pemoline, 1379
Pen-Vee, [C], 1388
Pen-Vee K, 1388
Penbutolol Sulfate, 1380
Penciclovir, 1382
Penecort, 889
Penicillamine, 1383
Penicillin G, 1384
Penicillin G Benzathine, 1384
Penicillin G Benzathine/Penicillin G Procaine, 1387
Penicillin G Potassium, 1384
Penicillin G Procaine, 1384
Penicillin G Procaine/Penicillin G Benzathine, 1387
Penicillin G Sodium, 1384
Penicillin G Sodium, 1384
Penicillin V, 1388
Penicillin V Potassium, 1388
Penicillin VK, 1388
Penlac Nail Lacquer, 392
Pentacarinat, 1390
Pentacea, 1941
Pentam 300, 1390, 1660, 1948
Pentamidine Isethionate, 1390
Pentamidine Isethionate (Inhalation), 1948
Pentamycetin, [C], 364
Pentasa, 1125
Pentaspan, 1948
Pentastarch, 1948
Pentazocine, 1392
Pentobarbital Sodium, 1393
Pentosan Polysulfate Sodium, 1395, 1949
Pentostatin, 1396, 1949
Pentostatin for Injection, 1949
Pentothal, 1746
Pentoxifylline, [C], 1399
Pentoxifylline, 1399
Pepcid, 716
Pepcid AC, 716
Pepcid IV, [C], 716
Pepcid RPD, 716
Pepto-Bismol, 212

(Trade names appear in italics. Canadian products are indicated with a [C], withdrawn products with a [D].)

Pepto-Bismol Maximum Strength, 212
Pepto Diarrhea Control, 1059
Percocet, 1340
Percocet-Demi, [C], 1340
Percodan, 1342, 1914
Percodan-Demi Tablets, 1914
Percolone, 1339
Perestan, 576
Perflubron, 1949
Perfosfamide, 1949
Pergamid, 1949
Pergolide, 1949
Pergolide Mesylate, 1400
Pergonal, 1112
Periactin, 471
Peridex, 370
Perindopril Erbumine, 1402
PerioChip, 370
PerioGard, 370
Periostat, 597
Permapen, 1384
Permax, 1400, 1949
Permethrin, 1404
Perphenazine, 1405
Perphenazine/Amitriptyline, 1408
Persantine, 565
Pertussin CS, 524
Pertussin ES, 524
Pexeva, 1364
Pfizerpen, 1384
PGE_1, 65
PGE_2, 555
Pharmorubicin PFS, [C], 640
Phazyme, 1636
Phazyme 95, 1636
Phazyme 125, 1636
Phenaphen w/Codeine No. 3, 13
Phenaphen w/Codeine No. 4, 13
Phenazo, [C], 1410
Phenazopyridine Hydrochloride, 1410
Phendimetrazine Tartrate, 1411
Phenelzine Sulfate, 1412
Phenergan, 1493
Phenindamine Tartrate, 1414
Phenobarbital, 1415
Phenobarbital/Atropine Sulfate/Scopolamine Hydrobromide/Hyosyamine Sulfate, 156
Phenobarbital/Ergotamine Tartrate/Belladonna (levorotary alkaloids), 182
Phenobarbital Sodium, 1415
Phenoptic, 1421
Phenoxybenzamine Hydrochloride, 1417
Phenoxymethyl Penicillin, 1388
Phentermine Hydrochloride, 1418
Phentermine Resin, 1418
Phentolamine, 1420
Phentolamine Mesylate, 1420
Phenylacetate, 1949
Phenylacetate/Benzoate, 1926
Phenylalanine Ammonia-Lyase, 1949
Phenylase, 1949
Phenylbutyrate, 1949
1,1'-[1,4-Phenylenebis-methylane]-bis-1,4,8,11-tetraazacyclotradecan, 1919
Phenylephrine, 1949
Phenylephrine Hydrochloride, 526, 1421
Phenylephrine Hydrochloride/Codeine Phosphate/Promethazine Hydrochloride, 1500
Phenylephrine Hydrochloride/Cyclopentolate Hydrochloride, 464
Phenylephrine Hydrochloride/Guaifenesin, 1426
Phenylephrine Hydrochloride/Methscopolamine Nitrate/Chlorpheniramine Maleate, 377
Phenylephrine Hydrochloride/Promethazine Hydrochloride, 1498
Phenylephrine Tannate/Chlorpheniramine Tannate, 1423
Phenylephrine Tannate/Chlorpheniramine Tannate/Pyrilamine Tannate, 1425
Phenytoin, 1428
Phenytoin Sodium, 1428
Phillips' Liqui-Gels, 576
Phos-Lo, 1928
5,5',5''-[Phosphinothioylidyne tris(imino-2,1-ethanediyl)]tris[5-methylchelidoninium]trihydroide hexahydrochloride, 1920
Phosphocol P 32, 390
Phosphocysteamine, 1949
Phosphonoformic Acid, 792
Photofrin, 1456, 1950
Phrenilin, 1915
Phrenilin Forte, 1915
Phrenilin Forte Capsules, 1915
Phrenilin Tablets, 1915
Phyllocontin, 83
Phyllocontin, [C], 83
Phyllocontin-350, [C], 83
Phylloquinone, 1430
Phytonadione, 1430
α_1-*PI*, 61
Pilocar, 1432, 1956
Pilocarpine, 1432
Pilocarpine Hydrochloride, 1949
Pilopine HS, 1432, 1956
Piloptic-1, 1432
Piloptic-2, 1432
Piloptic-3, 1432
Piloptic-4, 1432
Piloptic-6, 1432
Piloptic-1/2, 1432
Pilostat, 1432
Pimecrolimus, 1434
Pimozide, 1435
Pindolol, 1438
Pink Bismuth, 212
Pink Bismuth, [C], 212
Pioglitazone, 1439

Piperacillin Sodium, 1441
Piperacillin Sodium/Tazobactam Sodium, 1443
Piperazine Estrone Sulfate, 691
Pipracil, 1441
Piracetam, 1949
Pirbuterol Acetate, 1444
Pirfenidone, 1949
Piritrexim Isethionate, 1949
Piroxicam, 1445
Pitocin, 1345
Pitressin, 1869
Pitrex, [C], 1782
Placidyl, 698
Plant-Produced Human α-Galactosidase, 1921
Plaquase, 1930
Plaquenil Sulfate, 894
Plaretase 8000, 1356
Plasbumin-5, 37
Plasbumin-25, 37
Platinol AQ, 408
Plavix, 432
Plenaxis, 4
Plendil, 720
Pletal, 396
PMS-Atenolol, [C], 144
PMS-Baclofen, [C], 173
PMS-Bethanechol, [C], 202
PMS-Bromocriptine, [C], 234
PMS-Buspirone, [C], 254
PMS-Captopril, [C], 285
PMS-Carbamazepine CR, [C], 290
PMS-Cefaclor, [C], 316
PMS-Chloral Hydrate, [C], 361
PMS-Clonazepam, [C], 425
PMS-Desipramine, [C], 502
PMS-Dexamethasone, [C], 511
PMS-Diclofenac, [C], 533
PMS-Diclofenac SR, [C], 533
PMS-Diphenhydramine, [C], 556
PMS-Erythromycin, [C], 659
PMS-Fenofibrate Micro, [C], 721
PMS-Fluoxetine, [C], 759
PMS-Fluphenazine Decanoate, [C], 763
PMS-Flutamide, [C], 768
PMS-Fluvoxamine, [C], 778
PMS-Gabapentin, [C], 805
PMS-Gemfibrozil, [C], 815
PMS-Glyburide, [C], 832
PMS-Haloperidol LA, [C], 859
PMS-Hydromorphone, [C], 893
PMS-Hydroxyzine, [C], 899
PMS-Indapamide, [C], 921
PMS-Ipratropium, [C], 957
PMS-Isoniazid, [C], 970
PMS-Lactulose, [C], 996
PMS-Levobunolol, [C], 1021
PMS-Lindane, [C], 1040
PMS-Lithium Carbonate, [C], 1053
PMS-Lithium Citrate, [C], 1053
PMS-Loperamide Hydrochloride, [C], 1059

(*Trade* names appear in italics Canadian products are indicated with a [C], withdrawn products with a [D].)

PMS-Loxapine, [C], 1076
PMS-Mefenamic Acid, [C], 1102
PMS-Metformin, [C], 1135
PMS-Methylphenidate, [C], 1163
PMS-Metoprolol-B, [C], 1177
PMS-Metoprolol-L, [C], 1177
PMS-Minocycline, [C], 1198
PMS-Nizatidine, [C], 1294
PMS-Nortriptyline, [C], 1300
PMS-Nystatin, [C], 1301
PMS-Oxybutynin, 1336
PMS-Pindolol, [C], 1438
PMS-Ranitidine, [C], 1557
PMS-Salbutamol Respirator Solution, [C], 39
PMS-Sotalol, [C], 1655
PMS-Sucralfate, [C], 1673
PMS-Tamoxifen, [C], 1700
PMS-Temazepam, [C], 1713
PMS-Terazosin, [C], 1719
PMS-Terbinafine, [C], 1721
PMS-Ticlopidine, [C], 1760
PMS-Timolol, [C], 1763
PMS-Tobramycin, [C], 1773
PMS-Trazodone, [C], 1808
PMS-Valproic Acid, [C], 1855
Pneumococcal 7-Valent Conjugate Vaccine, 1448
Pneumococcal Vaccine, Polyvalent, 1447
Pneumomist, 848
Pneumopent, 1948
Pneumotussin, 882
Pneumotussin 2.5, 882
Pneumovax 23, 1447
Pnu-Imune 23, 1447
Polifeprosan 20 with Carmustine, 1949
Poliovirus Vaccine, Inactivated, 1451
Poliovirus Vaccine, Live, Oral Trivalent, 1449
Poloxamer 188, 1949
Poloxamer 331, 1949
Poly-L-Lactic Acid, 1452
Poly-Histine, 1918
Poly I: Poly C12U, 1949
Poly-ICLC, 1949, 1950
Poly-Pred Liquifilm, 1472
Polycitra, 1461
Polycitra-LC, 1461
Polyethylene Glycol, 1454
Polyethylene Glycol (PEG)-uricase, 1949
Polyethylene Glycol-Electrolyte Solution, 1455
Polygam, 919
Polygam S/D, 919
Polyinosinic-polucytidillic Acid, 1949, 1950
Polymeric Oxygen, 1950
Polymyxin B Sulfate/Bacitracin Zinc, 172
Polymyxin B Sulfate/Dexamethasone/Neomycin Sulfate, 1266

Polymyxin B Sulfate/Gramicidin/Neomycin Sulfate, 1267
Polymyxin B Sulfate/Oxytetracycline Hydrochloride, 1347
Polymyxin B Sulfate/Prednisolone Acetate/Neomycin Sulfate, 1472
Polymyxin B Sulfate/Trimethoprim Sulfate, 1827
Polymyxin B Sulfates/Bacitracin Zinc/Neomycin, 1264
Polymyxin B Sulfates/Hydrocortisone/Bacitracin Zinc/Neomycin, 171
Polysporin, 172
Polytrim, 1827
Ponstan, [C], 1102
Ponstel, 1102
Porcine Fetal Neural Dopaminergic Cells or Precursors Aseptically Prepared and Coated with Anti-MHC-1 Ab for Intracerebral Implantation, 1950
Porcine Fetal Neural Dopaminergic Cells or Precursors Aseptically Prepared for Intracerebral Implantation for Huntington Disease, 1950
Porcine Fetal Neural Gabaergic Cells or Precursors Aseptically Prepared and Coated with Anti-MHC-1 Ab for Intracerebral Implantation, 1950
Porcine Sertoli Cells (Aseptically Prepared for Intracerebral Co-Implantation with Fetal Neural Tissue), 1950
Porfimer, 1950
Porfimer Sodium, 1456, 1950
Porfiromycin, 1950
Porphozyme, 1952
Portia, 450
Posaconazole, 1963
Potasalan, 1459
Potassium Acetate, 1458
Potassium Bicarbonate, 1458
Potassium Chloride, 1458
Potassium Citrate, 1458, 1950
Potassium Citrate/Citric Acid, 1950
Potassium Citrate/Sodium Citrate/Citric Acid, 1461
Potassium Gluconate, 1458
Potassium Products, 1458
Potassium-Sparing Diuretics, 79
PPD, 1840
Pr-122 (Redox-phenytoin), 1950
PR-225 (Redox-acyclovir), 1950
PR-239 (Redox Penicillin G), 1950
Pr-320 (Molescusol-carbamazepine), 1950

Pramipexole Dihydrochloride, 1462
Pramiracetam Sulfate, 1950
Pramosone, 892
Pramox HC, [C], 892
Pramoxine Hydrochloride/Hydrocortisone Acetate, 892
Prandin, 1563
Pravachol, 1463
Pravastatin Sodium, 1463
Praziquantel, 1465, 1950
Prazosin, 1466
Pre-Hist-D, 377
Pre-Pen/MDM, 1926
Precose, 8
Pred Forte, 1467
Pred-G, 1470
Pred-G S.O.P., 1470
Pred Mild, 1467
Predalone 50, 1467
Predcor-50, 1467
Prednimustine, 1950
Prednisol TBA, 1468
Prednisolone, 1467
Prednisolone Acetate/Gentamicin Sulfate, 1470
Prednisolone Acetate/Neomycin Sulfate/Polymyxin B Sulfate, 1472
Prednisolone Sodium Phosphate, 1467
Prednisolone Tebutate, 1468
Prednisone, 1473
Prednisone Intensol Concentrate, 1473
Prefrin Liquifilm, 1421
Pregnyl, 389
Prelone, 1467
Prelu-2, 1411
Premarin, 684
Premarin IV, 684
Premphase, 689
Prempro, 689
Prepidil, 555
Pressyn, [C], 1869
Pretz-D, 635
Prevacid, 1005
Prevacid I.V., 1005
Prevalite, 388
Preven, 699
Prevex B, [C], 197
Prevex HC, [C], 889
Prevnar, 1448
Prevpac, 105
Priftin, 1580, 1954
Prilosec, 1319
Primacor, 1197
Primaquine Phosphate, 1475, 1950
Primatene Mist, 637
Primaxin IM, 913
Primaxin IV, 913
Primidone, 1476
Principen, 112
Prinivil, 1048
Prinzide, 877
Prinzide 10/12.5 mg, 1051
Prinzide 20/12.5 mg, 1051
Prinzide 20/25 mg, 1051
Priorix, [C], 1089

(*Trade* names appear in italics. Canadian products are indicated with a [C], withdrawn products with a [D].)

Pro 542, 1964
Pro 2000 Gel, 1964
Pro-Banthine, 1508
ProAmatine, 1191
Probenecid, 1478
Probenecid/Colchicine, 1480
Procainamide Hydrochloride, 1481
Procan SR, [C], 1481
Procanbid, 1481
Procarbazine, 1483
Procardia, 1283
Prochieve, 1490
Prochlorperazine, 1913
Prochlorperazine, 1486
Procrit, 646, 1934
Proctocort, 889
ProctoCream-HC, 889, 892
ProctoFoam-HC, 892
Procyclid, [C], 1489
Procyclidine, 1489
Procysteine, 1941
Procytox, [C], 465
Prodium, 1410
Profilnine SD, 714
Proflavanol, [C], 136
Progesterone, 1490, 1951
Progesterone in Oil, 1490
Proglycem, 531
Prograf, 1694, 1958
Proguanil Hydrochloride/
 Atovaquone, 152
Prolastin, 61, 1922
Proleukin, 42, 1921, 1964, 1966
Prolixin Decanoate, 763
Promoth VC Plain, 1498
Prometh VC w/Codeine, 1500
Prometh with Codeine, 1496
Promethazine Hydrochloride, 1493
Promethazine Hydrochloride/
 Codeine Phosphate, 1496
Promethazine Hydrochloride/
 Phenylephrine Hydrochloride, 1498
Promethazine Hydrochloride/
 Phenylephrine
 Hydrochloride/Codeine Phosphate, 1500
Prometrium, 1490
Promycin, 1950
Pronestyl, 1481
Pronestyl-SR, 1481
Propafenone, 1502
Propamidine Isethionate 0.1%
 Ophthalmic Solution, 1951
Propanthel, [C], 1508
Propantheline Bromide, 1508
Proparacaine Hydrochlorie, 758
Propecia, 733
Prophasi, 389
Propine, 564, 1948
Proplex T, 714
Propofol, 1510
Propoxyphene, 1511
Propoxyphene/Acetaminophen, 1513
Propoxyphene Hydrochloride, 1511

Propoxyphene Hydrochloride/
 Acetaminophen, 1513
Propoxyphene Hydrochloride/
 Aspirin/Caffeine, 1515
Propoxyphene Napsylate/
 Acetaminophen, 1513
Propranolol Hydrochloride, 1516
Propranolol Hydrochloride/
 Hydrochlorothiazide, 1505
Propranolol Intensol, 1516
Propyl-Thyracil, [C], 1520
Propylthiouracil, 1520
Proscar, 733
ProSom, 668
Prostaglandin E$_1$, 65
Prostaglandin E1 Enol Ester
 (AS-013), 1951
Prostaglandin E1 in Lipid
 Emulsion, 1951
Prostaglandin E$_2$, 555
ProStep, 1280
Prostigmin, 1268
Prostin E2, 555
Prostin VR Pediatric, 65
Protamine Sulfate, 1522
Protaxel, 1951
Protein C Concentrate, 1951
Protirelin, 1951
Protirelin Injection, 1951
Protonix, 1359
Protonix IV, 1359
Protopic, 1694
Protostat, 1179
Protox, 1949
Protriptyline Hydrochloride, 1523
Protropin, 1652, 1956
Proventil, 39
Proventil HFA, 39
Provera, 1098
Provigil, 1214, 1945
Prozac, 759, 1936
Prozac Weekly, 759
Pseudo, 1525
Pseudo-Gest, 1525
Pseudoephedrine, 1525
Pseudoephedrine Hydrochloride, 731
Pseudoephedrine
 Hydrochloride/Acrivastine, 25
Pseudoephedrine
 Hydrochloride/
 Brompheniramine Maleate, 236
Pseudoephedrine
 Hydrochloride/
 Brompheniramine Maleate/
 Dextromethorphan HBr, 237
Pseudoephedrine
 Hydrochloride/Codeine
 Phosphate/Chlorpheniramine
 Maleate, 379
Pseudoephedrine
 Hydrochloride/
 Dextromethorphan HBr/
 Carbinoxamine Maleate, 301

Pseudoephedrine
 Hydrochloride/Guaifenesin/
 Dextromethorphan
 Hydrobromide, 1526
Pseudoephedrine
 Hydrochloride/Hydrocodone
 Bitartrate, 887
Pseudoephedrine Sulfate/
 Loratadine, 1066
Pseudofrin, [C], 1525
*Pseudomonas Hyperimmune
 Globulin*, 1945
Psorcon E, 544
PTU, 1520
PulmaDex, 1933
Pulmicort Nebuamp, [C], 241
Pulmicort Respules, 241
Pulmicort Turbuhaler, 241
Pulmonary Surfactant Replacement, 1951
Pulmonary Surfactant Replacement, Porcine, 1951
Pulmozyme, 583, 1933
Puregon, [C], 784
Purified Extract of *Pseudomonas
 aeruginosa*, 1951
Purified Type II Collagen, 1951
Purinethol, 1122
PV802, 1952
PVF K, [C], 1388
pVGI.1(VEGF2), 1951
Pyrazinamide, 1527
Pyridiate, 1410
Pyridium, 1410
Pyridium Plus, 1410
Pyridostigmine Bromide, 1529
Pyridoxine Hydrochloride, 781, 1530
Pyrilamine Tannate/
 Phenylephrine Tannate/
 Chlorpheniramine Tannate, 1425
Pyrimethamine, 1531
Pyrimethamine/Folinic Acid/
 Dapsone, 1966
Pyrimethamine/Sulfadoxine, 1678
Pyruvate, 1951

Q

Quadramet, 1614
Quazepam, 1534
Questran, 388
Questran Light, 388
Quetiapine Fumarate, 1535
Quibron-T Dividose, 1739
Quibron-T/SR, 1739
Quinacrine Hydrochloride, 1951
Quinaglute Dura-Tabs, 1543
Quinalan, 1543
Quinapril Hydrochloride, 1538
Quinapril Hydrochloride/
 Hydrochlorothiazide, 1540
Quinidine, 1543
Quinidine Gluconate, 1543
Quinidine Polygalacturonate, 1543
Quinidine Sulfate, 1543

(*Trade* names appear in italics. Canadian products are indicated with a [C], withdrawn products with a [D].)

Quinine-Odan, [C], 1546
Quinine Sulfate, 1546
Quinora, 1543
Quinsana Plus Foot Powder, 1782
Quinupristin/Dalfopristin, 1547
Quixin, 1026
QVAR, 179

R

R & D Calcium Carbonate/600, 1928
R-etodolac, 1951
R-Gel, 284
r-HuIFN-Beta, 1940
R-IFN-Beta, 1940
R-Tanna S, 1423
RabAvert, 1551
Rabeprazole Sodium, 1549
Rabies Immune Globulin, Human, 1550
Rabies Vaccine, 1551
Rabies Vaccine (Adsorbed), 1551
Racemice Amphetamine Sulfate, 106
Radiogardase, 1941
Raloxifene Hydrochloride, 1553
Ramipril, 1554
Ranitidine, 1557
Ranitidine Bismuth Citrate, 1559
Rapamune, 1638
Raptiva, 613
Rasburicase, 1560, 1951
Raspertaxin, 1953
ratio-Alprazolam, [C], 62
ratio-Amiodarone, [C], 86
ratio-Amoxi Clav, [C], 103
ratio-Atenolol, [C], 144
ratio-Azathioprine, [C], 161
ratio-Baclofen, [C], 173
ratio-Bisacodyl, [C], 210
ratio-Brimonidine, [C], 232
ratio-Buspirone, [C], 254
ratio-Captopril, [C], 285
ratio-Clindamycin, [C], 417
ratio-Clonazepam, [C], 425
ratio-Codeine, [C], 442
ratio-Colchicine, [C], 445
ratio-Cyclobenzaprine, [C], 463
ratio-Desipramine, [C], 502
ratio-Dexamethasone, [C], 511
ratio-Diltiazem CD, [C], 550
ratio-Docusate Calcium, [C], 576
ratio-Docusate Sodium, [C], 576
ratio-Doxasozin, [C], 588
ratio-Doxycycline, [C], 597
ratio-Famotidine, [C], 716
ratio-Flunisolide, [C], 750
ratio-Fluoxetine, [C], 759
ratio-Flurbiprofen, [C], 767
ratio-Fluvoxamine, [C], 778
ratio-Gentamicin, [C], 821
ratio-Glyburide, [C], 832
ratio-Haloperidol, [C], 859
ratio-Indomethacin, [C], 924
ratio-Ipratropium, [C], 957
ratio-Ipratropium UDV, [C], 957
ratio-Lactulose, [C], 996
ratio-Levobunolol, [C], 1021
ratio-Lovastatin, [C], 1074
ratio-Metformin, [C], 1135
ratio-Methotrexate, [C], 1146
ratio-Methylphenidate, [C], 1163
ratio-Minocycline, [C], 1198
ratio-MPA, [C], 1098
ratio-Nadolol, [C], 1240
ratio-Naproxen, [C], 1251
ratio-Nortriptyline, [C], 1300
ratio-Nystatin, [C], 1301
ratio-Oxycocet, [C], 1340
ratio-Oxycodan, [C], 1342
ratio-Oxycodone, [C], 1342
ratio-Ranitidine, [C], 1557
ratio-Salbutamol, [C], 39
ratio-Sertraline, [C], 1628
ratio-Sotalol, [C], 1655
ratio-Sulfasalazine, [C], 1680
ratio-Terazosin, [C], 1719
ratio-Timolol, [C], 1763
ratio-Topilene, [C], 197
ratio-Topisone, [C], 197
ratio-Trazodone, [C], 1808
ratio-Valproic, [C], 1855
Reactine, [C], 354
Rebetol, 1572, 1954
Rebetron, 945
Rebif, 948, 1940
Receptin, 1953
Recombinant Bactericidal/Permeability-Increasing Protein, 1951
Recombinant Glycine2-Human Glucagon-Like Peptide-2, 1951
Recombinant Human Acid Alpha-Glucosidase, 1951
Recombinant Human Alpha-1 Antitrypsin (rAAT), 1952
Recombinant Human Alpha-Fetoprotein (rhAFP), 1952
Recombinant Human Antithrombin III, 1952
Recombinant Human C1-Esterase Inhibitor, 1952
Recombinant Human CD4 Immunoglobulin G, 1952
Recombinant Human Clara Cell 10kDa Protein, 1952
Recombinant Human Deoxyribonuclease, 583
Recombinant Human Endostatin Protein, 1952
Recombinant Human Fibroblast Growth Factor-20, 1952
Recombinant Human Gelsolin, 1952
Recombinant Human Highly Phosphorylated Acid Alpha-Glucosidase, 1952
Recombinant Human Insulin-Like Growth Factor-I, 1952
Recombinant Human Insulin-Like Growth Factor-I/Insulin-Like Growth Factor Binding Protein-3, 1952
Recombinant Human Interleukin-12, 1952
Recombinant Human Keratinocyte Growth Factor, 1952
Recombinant Human Luteinizing Hormone, 1952
Recombinant Human Monoclonal Antibody to hsp90, 1952
Recombinant Human Nerve Growth Factor, 1952
Recombinant Human Neutrophil Inhibitor (hNE), 1952
Recombinant Human Porphobilinogen Deaminase, 1952
Recombinant Human Porphobilinogen Deaminase, Erythopoetic Form, 1953
Recombinant Human Relaxin, 1953
Recombinant Human Thrombopoietin, 1953
Recombinant Humanized MAb 5c8, 1953
Recombinant Inhibitor of Human Plasma Kallikrein, 1953
Recombinant Methionyl Brain-Derived Neurotrophic Factor, 1953
Recombinant Reteplase, 1567
Recombinant Retroviral Vector - Glucocerebrosidase, 1953
Recombinant Secretory Leucocyte Protease Inhibitor, 1953
Recombinant Soluble Human CD4 (rCD4), 1953
Recombinant T-Cell Receptor Ligand, 1953
Recombinant Urate Oxidase, 1953
Recombinant Vaccinia (Human Papillomavirus), 1953
Recombivax HB, 868
Reduced L-glutothione, 1953
Redutemp, 12
ReFacto, 1924
Refludan, 1012, 1942
Reglan, 1174
Regular, Insulin Injection, 931
Regular Iletin II, 931
Regular Strength Bayer Enteric Coated Caplets, 139
Regulax SS, 576
Relafen, 1239
Relenza, 1892
Reliable Gentle Laxative, 210
Relief, 1421
Relpax, 617
Remacemide, 1953
Remeron, 1203
Remicade, 926, 1940
Remifentanil Hydrochloride, 1561

(*Trade* names appear in italics. Canadian products are indicated with a [C], withdrawn products with a [D].)

Reminyl, 806
Remitogen, 1938
Remodulin, 1960
Remular-S, 387
Remune, 1967
Renacidin Irrigation, 1929
Renagel, 1630
Renedil, [C], 720
Renova, 1810
Respiratory Combination Products, 1916
ReoPro, 6
Repaglinide, 1563
Repain CF, 1915
Repan, 259
Replagal, 1922
Repository Corticotropin o-Adrenocorticotropic Hormone, 1953
Repronex, 1112
Requip, 1602
Rescon-CG, 1426
Rescon JR Capsules, 1917
Rescriptor, 497
Rescula, 1843, 1965
Reserpine/Hydralazine Hydrochloride/Hydrochlorothiazide, 1565
Resiniferatoxin, 1953
Respa-1st, 1918
Respahist Capsules, 1917
Respigam, 1953
Respiratory Syncytial Virus (RSV) Immune Globulin (Human), 1953
Restoril, 1713
Restylane, 871
Retavase, 1567
Reteplase, Recombinant, 1567
Retin-A, 1810
Retin-A Micro, 1810
9-cis Retinoic Acid, 1920
13-cis-Retinoic Acid, 975
trans-Retinoic Acid, 1810
Retisol-A, [C], 1810
Retrovir, 1894, 1962
Retroviral Gamma-c cDNA Containing Vector, 1953
Retroviral vector, R-GC and GC Gene 1750, 1953
Rev 123, 1964
Reversol, 612
ReVia, 1249
Revimid, 1920
Reviparin Sodium, 1953
Revitalose-C-1000, [C], 136
Rexin-G, 1946
Reyataz, 141
Rezipas, 1920
RGG0853, E1A Lipid Complex, 1953
Rheumatex, 1944
Rheumatrex Dose Pack, 1146
RhIG, 1569
Rhinall, 1421
Rhinatate-NF, 1423
Rhinocort Aqua, 241
Rhinocort Turbuhaler, [C], 241
RhIVIG, 1571
rhIGF-I/rhIGFBP-3, 1954

Rh$_o$ (D) Immune Globulin, 1569
Rh$_o$ (D) Immune Globulin IV (Human), 1954
Rh$_o$ (D) Immune Globulin IV (Human), 1571
Rho-Salbutamol, [C], 39
Rhodacine, [C], 924
Rhodis, [C], 989
Rhodis-EC, [C], 989
Rhodis SR, [C], 989
RhoGAM, 1569
Rhotral, [C], 10
Rhovail, [C], 989
Rhoxal-amiodarone, [C], 86
Rhoxal-atenolol, [C], 144
Rhoxal-clonazepam, [C], 425
Rhoxal-clozapine, [C], 438
Rhoxal-cyclosporine, [C], 469
Rhoxal-diltiazem CD, [C], 550
Rhoxal-famotidine, [C], 716
Rhoxal-fluoxetine, [C], 759
Rhoxal-loperamide, [C], 1059
Rhoxal-metformin, [C], 1135
Rhoxal-metformin FC, [C], 1135
Rhoxal-minocycline, [C], 1198
Rhoxal-nabumetone, [C], 1239
Rhoxal-orphenadrine, [C], 1325
Rhoxal-oxaprozin, [C], 1330
Rhoxal-ranitidine, [C], 1557
Rhoxal-salbutamol, [C], 39
Rhoxal-sotalol, [C], 1655
Rhoxal-ticlopidine, [C], 1760
Rhoxal-timolol, [C], 1763
Rhoxal-valproic, [C], 1855
Rhoxal-valproic EC, [C], 1855
rhuMAb VEGF, 1954
Rhythmodon, [C], 569
Rhythmodon-LA, [C], 569
Ribavirin, 1572, 1954
Riboflavin, 1575
Ricin (Blocked) Conjugated Murine MCA (Anti-B4), 1954
Ricin (Blocked) Conjugated Murine MCA (Anti-my9), 1954
Ricin (Blocked) Conjugated Murine MCA (m901), 1954
Ricin (Blocked) Conjugated Murine Monoclonal Antibody (CD6), 1954
Ridaura, 157
Ridenol, 12
Rifabutin, 1575, 1954
Rifadin, 1578
Rifadin IV, 1954
Rifalazil, 1954, 1966
Rifampin, 1578, 1954
Rifampin, Isoniazid, Pyrazinamide, 1954
Rifapentine, 1580, 1954
Rifater, 1954
Rifaximin, 1577, 1954
RIG, 1550
RII Retinamide, 1954
Rilutek, 1581, 1954

Riluzole, 1581, 1954
Rimactane, 1578
Rimantadine Hydrochloride, 1583
Riopan, 1081
Risedronate Sodium, 1584
Risperdal, 1585
Risperdal Consta, 1585
Risperdal M-TAB, 1585
Risperidone, 1585
Ritalin, 1163
Ritalin LA, 1163
Ritalin-SR, 1163
Ritodrine Hydrochloride, 1589
Ritodrine Hydrochloride in 5% Dextrose, 1589
Ritonavir, 1590
Rituxan, 1592, 1954, 1966
Rituximab, 1592, 1954, 1966
Rivanase AQ, 179
Rivastigmine Tartrate, 1594
Rivotril, [C], 425
Rizaben, 1960
Rizatriptan, 1596
Robaxin, 1143
Robaxin-750, 1143
Robaxisal, 1145
Robinul, 837
Robinul Forte, 837
Robitussin, 848
Robitussin Children's, [C], 524
Robitussin Cough Calmers, 524
Robitussin Extra Strength, [C], 848
Robitussin Honey Cough DM, [C], 524
Robitussin Pediatric, 524
Rocaltrol, 273
Rocephin, 346
Rocuronium Bromide, 1598
Rofact, [C], 1578
Rofecoxib, [D], 1600
Roferon-A, 940, 1940
Rogaine, 1201
Rogitine, [C], 1420
Romazicon, 748
Romilar AC, 849
Rondec-DM, 237
Rondec Oral Drops, 1918
Rondec-TR, 1917
Rondec-TR Tablets, 1917
Ropinirole Hydrochloride, 1602
Roquinimex, 1954
Rosiglitazone Maleate, 1603
Rosiglitazone Maleate/Metformin Hydrochloride, 1605
Rosula, 1651
Rosuvastatin Calcium, 1608
Rovamycine, 1957
Rowasa, 1125
Roxanal, 1226
Roxanal 100, 1226
Roxanal T, 1226
Roxanol Rescudose, 1226
Roxanol UD, 1226
Roxicet, 1340
Roxicet 5/500, 1340
Roxicodone, 1339
Roxicodone Intensol, 1339

Roxilox, 1340
Roxiprin, 1914
Rubella Vaccine, Live, Measles, and Mumps, 1089
Rubesol-1000, 461
Rubex, 591
Rubitecan, 1954
Rum-K, 1459
Ryna-C, 379
Rynatan, 1423
Rythmodan, 569
Rythmodan LA, 569
Rythmol, 1502

S

S(-)-3-[3-amino-phthalimido]-glutaramide, 1954
S2, 637
S-1360, 1964
S-P-T, 1753
S-T Cort, 889
S-T Forte 2, 881
Sabril, 1961
Sacrosidase, 1954
Sagramostim, 1955
St. Joseph Adult Chewable Aspirin, 139
St. Joseph Cough Suppressant, 524
Saizen, 1653, 1956
Sal-Tropine, 154
Salagen, 1432, 1949
Salazopyrin, [C], 1680
Salazopyrin Desensitizing Kit, [C], 1680
Salazopyrin EN-tabs, [C], 1680
Salicylamide, 1915
Salicylate Combination, 1611
Salmeterol, 773, 1612
Salmonine, 271
Salofalk, [C], 1125
Salprofen, 1939
Salsalate, 1915
Sama HC, [C], 889
Samarium SM 153 Lexidronam, 1614
Sanctura, 1836
Sandimmune, 469
Sandimmune, [C], 469
Sandostatin, 1304
Sandostatin LAR, 1304, 1947
SangCya, 469
Sani-Supp, 836
Sanorex, 1943
Sansert, 1171
Sanvar, 1961
Saquinavir Mesylate, 1616
Sarafem, 759
Sargramostim, 1618
Sarmustine, 1920
Satumomab Pendetide, 1955
Savvy, 1964
SB-408075, 1955
SC-1 Monoclonal Antibody, 1955
Scalpicin, 889
SCH 58500, 1955
Scheinpharm Tobramycin, [C], 1773

Sclerosol, 1699
Sclerosol Intrapleural Aerosol, 1958
Scopace, 1619
Scopolamine Hydrobromide, 1619
Scopolamine Hydrobromide/Hyoscyamine Sulfate/Phenobarbital/Atropine Sulfate, 156
Scot-Tussin Allergy DM, 556
Scot-Tussin DM Cough Chasers, 524
Scot-tussin Expectorant, 848
Sculptra, 1452
40SD02, 1920
Seasonale, 450
Secalciferol, 1955
Secobarbital/Amobarbital, 98
Secobarbital Sodium, 1621
Seconal Sodium Pulvules, 1621
SecreFlo, 1623
Secretin, 1623
Secretin, Synthetic Human, 1957
Secretin, Synthetic Porcine, 1958
Secretory Leukocyte Protease Inhibitor, 1955
Sectral, 10
Sedapap, 1915
Sedapap Tablets, 1915
Selax, [C], 576
Sele-Pak, 1625
Selegiline Hydrochloride, 1624, 1955
Selenium, 1625
Selepen, 1625
Semprex-D, 25
Semprex-D Capsules, 1917
Senexon, 1626
Senna, 1626
Senna-Gen, 1626
Senokot, 1626
SenokotXTRA, 1626
Sensipar, 400
Septopal, 1936
Septra, 1828
Septra DS, 1828
Septra Injection, [C], 1828
Septra IV, 1828
Ser-Ap-Es, 1565
Serax, 1332
Serentil, 1128
Serevent, 1612
Sermorelin Acetate, 1955
Seromycin Pulvules, 467
Serophene, 422
Seroquel, 1535
Serostim, 1653, 1956
Serratia Marcescens Extract, 1955
Sertaconazole Nitrate, 1627
Sertan, [C], 1476
Sertraline Hydrochloride, 1628
Serzone, 1258
Serzone-5HT2, [C], 1258
Seudotabs, 1525
Sevelamer Hydrochloride, 1630

Short Chain Fatty Acid Enema, 1955
Sibelium, 1935
Sibutramine Hydrochloride, 1632
Silace, 576
Siladryl, 556
Silapap, Infants', 12
Sildenafil Citrate, 1633
Silfedrine Children's, 1525
Silphen DM, 524, 1658
Siltussin SA, 848
Silver Sulfadizine and Cerium Nitrate, 1955
Simethicone, 1636
Simply Sleep, [C], 556
Simulect, 176, 1926
Simvastatin, 711, 1636
Sinemet 10/100, 1024
Sinemet 25/100, 1024
Sinemet 25/250, 1024
Sinemet CR, 1024
Sinequan, 589
Sinex, 1421
Singulair, 1223
Sinumist-SR Capsulets, 848
Sinustop Pro, 1525
SINUvent PE, 1426
Sipilizumab, 1955
Sirolimus, 1638
Skelaxin, 1133
Skelid, 1762
SK&F 110679, 1955
Sleep-Eze 3, 556
Sleepinall Capsules and Soft Gels, Maximum Strength, 556
Sleepwell 2-nite, 556
Slo-bid Gyrocaps, 1739
Slo-Niacin, 1274
Slo-Phyllin, 1739
Slow-FE, 728
Smallpox Vaccine, 1641
Snoozefast, 556
Sodium 1,3-propanedisulfonate, 1955
Sodium Bicarbonate, 1644
Sodium Citrate/Citric Acid, 1645
Sodium Citrate/Citric Acid/Potassium Citrate, 1461
Sodium Dichloroacetate, 1955
Sodium Ferric Gluconate, 1646
Sodium Iodide I 131, 1648
Sodium monomercaptoundecahydrocloso-dodecaborate, 1955
Sodium Phenylbutyrate, 1955
Sodium Phosphate P 32, 1649
Sodium Polystyrene Sulfonate, [C], 1650
Sodium Polystyrene Sulfonate, 1650
Sodium Pyruvate, 1956
Sodium Sulfacetamide/Sulfur, 1651
Sodium Tetradecyl Sulfate, 1956
Sodium Thiosulfate, 1956
Sodium Valproate, 1855
Soflax, [C], 576
Solaraze, 533

(*Trade* names appear in italics. Canadian products are indicated with a [C], withdrawn products with a [D].)

Solarcaine Aloe Extra Burn Relief, 1035
Solatol Hydrochloride, 1957
Solfoton, 1215
Solu-Cortef, 889
Solu-Medrol, 1166
Soluble Complement Receptor Type 1, 1956
Soluble Recombinant Human Complement Receptor Type 1, 1956
Soluble T4, 1928
Solugel 4, [C], 190
Solugel 8, [C], 190
Solurex, 511
Solurex LA, 511
Soma, 305
Soma Compound with Codeine, 306
SomatoKine, 1952, 1954
Somatostatin, 1956
SomatoTher, 1919
Somatrel, 1947
Somatrem, 1652
Somatrem for Injection, 1956
Somatropin, 1653, 1956
Somatropin (rDNA), 1956, 1963
Somatropin for Injection, 1956
Somatropin (rDNA) for Injection, 1956
Somatropin (rDNA Origin) Injection, 1957
Somavert, 1375, 1948
Sominex, 556
Sonata, 1891
Sorbitrate, 973
Soriatane, 22
Sorivudine, 1957
Sotacor, [C], 1655, 1891
Sotalol Hydrochloride, 1655
Sotradecol, 1956
Spanidin, 1937
Sparfloxacin, 1657
Spartaject, 1928
Spartaject-Busulfan, 1928
Spasmolin, 156
SPD 754, 1963
SPD 756, 1963
Spectazole, 609
Spectinomycin, 1659
Spectracef, 324
Spheramine, 1922
Spiramycin, 1957
Spiriva, 1769
Spironolactone, 1660
Spironolactone/Hydrochlorothiazide, 1661
Sporanox, 980
Sporidin-G, 1927
Sprintec, 450
SPS, 1650
Squalamine Lactate, 1957
SS1(dsFv)-PE38, 1957
ST1-RTA Immunotoxin (SE 44163), 1957
Stadol, 267
Stagesic, 880
Stahist Tablets, 1918
Stalevo 50, 296
Stalevo 100, 296

Stalevo 150, 296
Staphylococcus aureus Immune Globulin (Human), 1957
Starlix, 1256
Stavudine, 1663
Stay Awake, 269
STCC-Fluoxetine, [C], 759
Stemetil, [C], 1486
Stemgen, 1923
Stenorol, 1937
Sterapred, 1473
Sterapred DS, 1473
Sterecyt, 1950
Sterile Talc Powder, 1699
Steritalc, 1958
Stieva-A, [C], 1810
Stimate, 507
Stool Softener, 576
Stool Softener DC, 576
Strattera, 147, 1925
Streptase, 1665
Streptokinase, 1665
Streptomycin Sulfate, 1667
Streptozocin, 1669
Striant, 1726
Strong Iodine, 954
Strong Iodine Tincture, 954
Strontium-89 Chloride, 1670
SU101, 1957
SU5416, 1966
Suberoylanilide Hydroxamic Acid, 1957
Sublimaze, 724
Suboxone, 249, 1927
Subutex, 247, 1927
Succimer, 1672, 1957
Sucraid, 1954
Sucralfate, 1673, 1957
Sucrets 4-hr Cough, 524
Sucrets Cough Control, 524
Sudafed, 1525
Sudafed 12 Hour Caplets, 1525
Sudafed Decongestant 12 Hour, [C], 1525
Sudafed Decongestant Children's, [C], 1525
Sudafed Decongestant Extra Strength, [C], 1525
Sudex, 1525
Sufenta, 1675
Sufentanil Citrate, 1675
Sular, 1287
Sulbactam Sodium/Ampicillin Sodium, 114
Sulfacet-R, 1651
Sulfacetamide, 753
Sulfadiazine, 1676
Sulfadiazine, 1676, 1957
Sulfadoxine/Pyrimethamine, 1678
Sulfamethoxazole/Trimethoprim, 1828
Sulfamylon Solution, 1943
Sulfapyridine, 1957
Sulfasalazine, 1680
Sulfatrim, 1828
Sulfinpyrazone, 1684
Sulfisoxazole, 662, 1682
Sulfonated Phenolics/Sulfuric Acid, 1685

Sulfur/Sodium Sulfacetamide, 1651
Sulfuric Acid/Sulfonated Phenolics, 1685
Sulindac, 1686
Sumatriptan, 1688
Sumycin 250, 1733
Sumycin 500, 1733
Sumycin Syrup, 1733
Sunkist Vitamin C, 136
Supartz, 871
Superoxide Dismutase (Human), 1957
Superoxide Dismutase (Recombinant Human), 1957
Supervent, 1961
Supeudol, [C], 1339
Supprelin Injection, 1938
Suppress, 524
Suprax, 328
Suramin, 1957
Surface Active Extract of Saline Lavage of Bovine Lungs, 1957
Surfactant (Human) (Amniotic Fluid Derived), 1957
Surfak Liquigels, 576
Surfaxin, 1943
Surmontil, 1831
Survanta, 196
Survanta Intratracheal Suspension, 1926
Sustiva, 615
Sylphen Cough, 556
Symbyax, 1311
Symmetrel, 72
Symmetrel, [C], 72
Sympathomimetics, 1916
Synagis, 1351
Synalar, 752
Synalgos-DC Capsules, 1914
Synarel, 1242
Synarel Nasal Solution, 1946
Synercid, 1547
Synovir, 1959
Synsorb CD, 1963
Synsorb Pl, 1957
Synthetic ACTH, 457
Synthetic Corticotropin, 457
Synthetic Human Parathyroid Hormone 1-34, 1957
Synthetic Human Secretin, 1957
Synthetic Porcine Secretin, 1958
Synthroid, 1032
Synvisc, 871
Syprine, 1821, 1960
Syrup Ipecac, USP, 955

T

T_3, 1044
T_4, 1032
T-1249, 1964
T902611 (T611), 1963
T-Cell Depleted Stem Cell Enriched Cellular Product From Peripheral Blood Stem Cells, 1958

(Trade names appear in italics. Canadian products are indicated with a [C], withdrawn products with a [D].)

T4 Endonuclease V, Liposome Encapsulated, 1958
T-Gen, 1826
T-Gesic, 880
T-Phyl, 1739
T/Scalp, 889
TA-HPV, 1953
Tabloid, 1744
Tac-3, 1813
Tacrine Hydrochloride, 1692
Tacrolimus, 1694, 1958
Tadalafil, 1697
Tagamet, 398
Tagamet HB, 398
TAK-603, 1958
Talacen, 1392
Talc, Sterile Powder, 1699, 1958
Talwin, 1392
Talwin Compound, 1392
Talwin NX, 1392
Tambocor, 736
Tamiflu, 1327
Tamofen, [C], 1700
Tamoxifen Citrate, 1700
Tamsulosin Hydrochloride, 1702
Tantum, 1926
Tapanol Extra Strength, 12
Tapanol Regular Strength, 12
Tapazole, 1142
Targretin, 205, 1926
Tarka, 1801
Taro-Carbamazepine, [C], 290
Taro-Sone, [C], 197
Taro-Warfarin, [C], 1885
Tasmar, 1779
TAT Antagonist, 1964
Tavist Allergy, 416
Tavist ND, 1064
Taxol, 1349, 1948, 1966
Taxoprexin, 1932, 1933
Taxotere, 574
Tazarotene, 1703
Tazicef, 341
Tazidime, 341
Tazobactam Sodium/ Piperacillin Sodium, 1443
Tazorac, 1703
Taztia XT, 550
TBC-3B, 1967
Tebamide, 1826
Tebrazid, [C], 1527
Teceleukin, 1941
Technetium-99m Antimelanoma Murine Monoclonal Antibody, 1958
Technetium-99m Antimelanoma Murine Monoclonal Antibody (IgG2a) to B Cell, 1958
Technetium-99m Antimelanoma Murine Monoclonal Antibody to hCG, 1958
Technetium-99m-labeled CEA-Scan, 1925
Technetium-99m Pteroteramide, 1958

Technetium-99m rh-Annexin V, 1958
Tegaserod Maleate, 1705
Tegretol, 290
Tegretol XR, 290
Teladar, 197
Telithromycin, 1707
Telmisartan, 1709
Telmisartan/ Hydrochlorothiazide, 1710
Temazepam, 1713
Temodal, 1958
Temodar, 1714, 1958
Temoporfin, 1958
Temovate, 421
Temovate Emollient, 421
Temozolomide, 1714, 1958
Tempra, 12
Tempra 1, 12
Tempra 3, 12
Tempra 2 Syrup, 12
Ten-K, 1459
Tencon, 1915
Tenex, 855, 1937
Teniposide, 1716, 1958
Tenofovir Disoproxil Fumarate, 621, 1717
Tenoretic-50, 146
Tenoretic-100, 146
Tenormin, 144
Tensilon, 612
Tenuate, 543
Tenuate Dospan, 543
Tequin, 811
Terak with Polymyxin B Sulfate, 1347
Terazol, [C], 1723
Terazole 3, 1723
Terazole 7, 1723
Terazosin, 1719
Terbinafine, 1721
Terbutaline Sulfate, 1722
Terconazole, 1723
Teriparatide, 1724, 1958
Terlipressin, 1958
Terramycin with Polymyxin B Sulfate, 1347
Tessalon, 190
Testoderm, 1726
Testoderm with Adhesive, 1726
Testopel, 1726
Testosterone, 1726, 1958, 1963, 1965
Testosterone Buccal System, 1726
Testosterone Cypionate, 1726
Testosterone Cypionate/ Estradiol Cypionate, 1729
Testosterone Enanthate, 1726
Testosterone Gel, 1726
Testosterone Propionate Ointment 2%, 1959
Testosterone Sublingual, 1959
Testred, 1169
Tetanus and Diphtheria Toxoids (Adult Strength, Td), 1732
Tetanus Immune Globulin, 1731
Tetanus Toxoids, 561
Tetra-Formula, 525

Tetrabenazine, 1959
Tetracycline/Bismuth Subsalicylate/Metronidazole, 213
Tetracycline Hydrochloride, 1733
Tetrahydroaminoacridine, 1692
Tetrahydrobiopterin, 1959
Tetraiodothyroacetic Acid, 1959
[5,10,15,20-Tetrakis(1,3-diethylimidazolium-2-yl)-porphyrinato] manganese(III)pentachloride, 1919
Teveten, 650
Texacort unc, 889
Tezacitabine, 1959
TGF(Beta)2-specific Phosphorothioate Antisense Oligodeoxynucleotide, 1959
THA, 1692
Thalidomide, 1735, 1959, 1963, 1965, 1966
Thalitone, 385
Thalomid, 1735, 1959, 1963, 1965
Theo-24, 1739
Theo-Dur, 1739
Theochron, 1739
Theolair, 1739
Theolate Liquid, 1917
Theophylline, 1739
Theophylline Ethylenediamine, 83
TheraCLEC-Total, 1943
TheraCys, 177
TheraDerm Testosterone Transdermal System, 1959
Theragyn, 1946
Theralux Irradiation Device, 1920
Theramycin Z, 659
Thiabendazole, 1741
Thiamilate, 1743
Thiamin Hydrochloride, 1743
Thioguanine, 1744
Thiola, 1959
Thiopental Sodium, 1746
Thioplex, 1750
Thioridazine Hydrochloride, 1747
Thiotepa, 1750
Thonzonium Br/Hydrocortisone Acetate/Colistin Sulfate/ Neomycin Sulfate, 448
Thiothixene, 1751
Thorazine, 380
L-Threonine, 1942
Threostat 1942
Thrombase III, 1924
Thymalfasin, 1959
THYMITAQ, 1947
Thymoglobulin, 125, 1924
Thymopentin, 1965
Thymoxamine Hydrochloride, 1959
Thyrar, 1753
Thyrogen, 1959
Thyroid, Desiccated, 1753
Thyroid Strong, 1753

(Trade names appear in italics. Canadian products are indicated with a [C], withdrawn products with a [D].)

Thyroid USP, 1753
Thyrolar 1/4, 1046
Thyrolar 1/2, 1046
Thyrolar 1, 1046
Thyrolar 2, 1046
Thyrolar 3, 1046
Thyrotropin Alfa, 1959
L-Thyroxine, 1032
Tiagabine Hydrochloride, 1755
Tiamol, [C], 753
Tiapride, 1959
Tiazac, 550
Tiazofurin (2-Beta-D-ribofuranosyl-4-thiazolecarboxamide), 1959
Tiban, Pediatric, 1826
Ticar, 1756
Ticarcillin, 1756
Ticarcillin/Clavulanate, 1758
Ticarcillin Disodium, 1756
Ticarcillin Disodium/Clavulanate Potassium, 1758
TICE BCG, 177
Ticlid, 1760
Ticlopidine Hydrochloride, 1760
Ticon, 1826
TIG, 1731
Tigan, 1826
Tikosyn, 578
Tilade, 1257
Tiludronate Disodium, 1762
Time-Hist Capsules, 1917
Timedose Vitamin C, [C], 136
Timentin, 1758
Timolol Maleate, 585, 1763
Timoptic, 1763, 1954
Timoptic Ocudose, 1763
Timoptic-XE, 1763, 1954
Timunox, 1965
Tin ethyl etiopurpurin, 1959
Tinactin, 1782
Tinactin for Jock Itch, 1782
Tinactin Plus, [C], 1782
Tindamax, 1766
Tine Test PPD, 1840
Ting, 1782
Tinidazole, 1766, 1959
Tinzaparin Sodium, 1767
Tiopronin, 1959
Tiotropium Bromide, 1769
Tipranavir, 1963, 1965
Tirapazamine, 1959
Tiratricol, 1959
Tizanidine Hydrochloride, 1771, 1959
TM 114, 1965
TMC125, 1965
TMP-SMZ, 1828
TNX-355, 1965
TOBI, 1773, 1960
Tobi, 1960
TobraDex, 514
Tobramycin, 514, 1773, 1960
Tobramycin for Inhalation, 1960
Tobrex, 1773
Tocophersolan Oral-Solution (Vitamin E-tpgs), 1960
Tofranil, 915
Tofranil-PM, 915

Tolazamide, 1776
Tolbutamide, 1777
Tolcapone, 1779
Tolectin 200, 1781
Tolectin 600, 1781
Tolinase, 1776
Tolmetin Sodium, 1781
Tolnaftate, 1782
Tolterodine Tartrate, 1783
Topamax, 1784, 1960
Topicort, 510
Topicort LP, 510
Topilene, [C], 197
Topiramate, 1784, 1960
Toposar, 707
Topotecan Hydrochloride, 1787, 1967
Toprol XL, 1177
Topsyn, [C], 753
Toradol, 990
Toradol IM, [C], 990
Torazlizumab, 1960
Toremifene, 1960
Toremifene Citrate, 1789
Tornalate, 216
Torsemide, 1790
Tositumomab and Iodine-131 I-Tositumomab, 1792, 1960
Total Block VL SPF 75, 1926
Tracleer, 224, 1927
Tramadol Hydrochloride, 1795
Tramadol Hydrochloride/Acetaminophen, 1796
Trandate, 995
Trandolapril, 1798
Trandolapril/Verapamil Hydrochloride, 1801
Tranexamic Acid, 1960
Tranilast, 1960
Transderm-Nitro, 1290
Transderm-V, [C], 1619
Transforming Growth Factor-Beta 2, 1960
Transgenic Human Alpha 1 Antitrypsin, 1960
TransMD, 1930
Tranxene-SD, 434
Tranxene-SD Half Strength, 434
Tranxene T-tab, 434
Tranylcypromine Sulfate, 1804
Trastuzumab, 1805, 1960
Trasylol, 1924, 1925
Travatan, 1807, 1963
Travoprost, 1807
Trazodone Hydrochloride, 1808
Trecator-SC, 700
Trelstar Depot, 1834
Trelstar LA, 1834
Trental, 1399
Treosulfan, 1960
Treprostinil, 1960
Tretinoin, 1810, 1960, 1966
Trexall, 1146
Trexan, 1946
Tri-antennary Glycotripeptide Derivative of 5-fluorodeoxyuridine Monophosphate, 1960
Tri-K, 1459
Tri-Levlen, 450

Tri-Norinyl, 451
2′,3′,5′-Tri-o-acetyluridine, 1919
Triacana, 1959
Triacet, 1813
Triad, 259
Triam Forte, 1813
Triamcinolone, 1813
Triamcinolone Acetonide, 1813
Triamcinolone Acetonide/Nystatin, 1302
Triamcinolone Diacetate, 1813
Triamcinolone Hexacetonide, 1813
Triaminic AM Decongestant Formula, 1525
Triaminic Infant Oral Decongestant Drops, 1525
Triaminic Pediatric, [C], 1525
Triamterene, 1818
Triamterene/Hydrochlorothiazide, 878
Triatec-30, [C], 13
Triaz, 190
Triaz Cleanser, 190
Triazine, 477
Triazolam, 1819
Triban, 1826
Tricor, 721
Tricosal, 1611
Triderm, 1813
Tridesilon, 509
Trientine Hydrochloride, 1821, 1960
Trifluoperazine Hydrochloride, 1822
Trihexy-2, 1824
Trihexy-5, 1824
Trihexyphen, [C], 1824
Trihexyphenidyl Hydrochloride, 1824
3,5,3′-Triiodothyroacetate, 1920
Triiodothyronine, 1044
Trileptal, 1333
Trilone, 1813
Trimazide, 1826
Trimethobenzamide Hydrochloride, 1826
Trimethoprim/Dapsone, 1966
Trimethoprim/Sulfamethoxazole, 1828
Trimethoprim Sulfate/Polymyxin B Sulfate, 1827
Trimetrexate Glucuronate, 1830, 1960
Trimipramine Maleate, 1831
Trimox, 101
Trinalin Repetabs, 1917
Trinam, 1936
Triostat, 1044, 1943
Triotann Pediatric, 1425
Triotann-S Pediatric, 1425
Tripedia, 561
Triphasil, 451
Triprolidine Hydrochloride, 1833
Triptone, 553
Triptorelin Pamoate, 1834, 1960
Trisaccharides A and B, 1961